PDR®

58

EDITION

2004

PHYSICIANS' DESK REFERENCE®

Supplement A

For important errata, turn the page.

IMPORTANT NOTICE

Supplements to PHYSICIANS' DESK REFERENCE are published twice yearly to provide readers with significant revisions of existing product listings as well as comprehensive information on new drugs and other products not included in the current annual edition. Before prescribing or administering any product described in PHYSICIANS' DESK REFERENCE, be sure to consult this supplement to determine whether revisions have occurred since the 2004 edition of PDR went to press.

This supplement is a compilation of information submitted by the products' manufacturers. Each entry has been prepared, edited, and approved by the manufacturer's medical department, medical director, and/or medical consultant. The publisher does not warrant or guarantee any of the products described herein nor is the publisher responsible for misuse of a product due to typographical error. The publisher does not perform any independent analysis in connection with the product information contained herein.

ERRATA

PDR 2004

1. The header at the top of the first column on page 1904 should read “Loprox Gel” rather than “Loprox Lotion.”
2. On page 6 in the Manufacturers' Index, there is a cross-reference to “Faulding Pharmaceutical Company.” The cross-reference should be to “Faulding Laboratories.”

NEW PRODUCT LISTINGS INDEX

Listed below are new *PDR* listings first appearing in 2004 *PDR Supplement A.* These listings include comprehensive descriptions of new pharmaceutical products introduced since publication of the 2004 *PDR*, new dosage forms of products already described, and existing pharmaceutical products not described in the 2004 *PDR*.

REVISED PRODUCT INFORMATION INDEX

As new research data and clinical findings become available, the product information in *PDR* is revised accordingly. Revisions submitted since the 2004 edition went to press can be found below. To remind yourself of a revision, write "See Supplement A" next to the product's heading in the book.

Brand or Generic Name (Manufacturer, PDR Page No.) — Supplement Page

NEW PRODUCT LISTINGS

This section contains comprehensive descriptions of new pharmaceutical products introduced since publication of the 2004 *PDR*, new dosage forms of products already described, and existing pharmaceutical products not described in the 2004 *PDR*.

Andrx Laboratories, Inc.
411 HACKENSACK AVENUE, 3RD FLOOR
HACKENSACK, NJ 07601

Direct Inquiries to:
phone (800) 595-1883

FORTAMET™ ℞
[fōr-tă mĕt]
(metformin hydrochloride) Extended-Release Tablets
℞ only

DESCRIPTION
FORTAMET™ (metformin hydrochloride) Extended-Release Tablets contain an oral antihyperglycemic drug used in the management of type 2 diabetes. Metformin hydrochloride (N, N-dimethylimidodicarbonimidic diamide hydrochloride) is a member of the biguanide class of oral antihyperglycemics and is not chemically or pharmacologically related to any other class of oral antihyperglycemic agents. The empirical formula of metformin hydrochloride is $C_4H_{11}N_5 \cdot HCl$ and its molecular weight is 165.63. Its structural formula is:

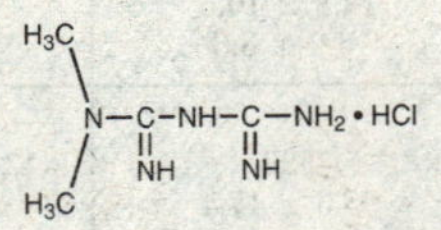

Metformin hydrochloride is a white to off-white crystalline powder that is freely soluble in water and is practically insoluble in acetone, ether, and chloroform. The pKa of metformin is 12.4. The pH of a 1% aqueous solution of metformin hydrochloride is 6.68.

FORTAMET™ Extended-Release Tablets are designed for once-a-day oral administration and deliver 500 mg or 1000 mg of metformin hydrochloride. In addition to the active ingredient metformin hydrochloride, each tablet contains the following inactive ingredients: candellila wax, cellulose acetate, hypromellose, magnesium stearate, polyethylene glycols (PEG 400, PEG 8000), polysorbate 80, povidone, sodium lauryl sulfate, synthetic black iron oxides, titanium dioxide, and triacetin.

SYSTEM COMPONENTS AND PERFORMANCE

FORTAMET™ was developed as an extended-release formulation of metformin hydrochloride and designed for once-a-day oral administration using the patented single-composition osmotic technology (SCOT™). The tablet is similar in appearance to other film-coated oral administered tablets but it consists of an osmotically active core formulation that is surrounded by a semipermeable membrane. Two laser drilled exit ports exist in the membrane, one on either side of the tablet. The core formulation is composed primarily of drug with small concentrations of excipients. The semipermeable membrane is permeable to water but not to higher molecular weight components of biological fluids. Upon ingestion, water is taken up through the membrane, which in turn dissolves the drug and excipients in the core formulation. The dissolved drug and excipients exit through the laser drilled ports in the membrane. The rate of drug delivery is constant and dependent upon the maintenance of a constant osmotic gradient across the membrane. This situation exists so long as there is undissolved drug present in the core tablet. Following the dissolution of the core materials, the rate of drug delivery slowly decreases until the osmotic gradient across the membrane falls to zero at which time delivery ceases. The membrane coating remains intact during the transit of the dosage form through the gastrointestinal tract and is excreted in the feces.

CLINICAL PHARMACOLOGY
Mechanism of Action

Metformin is an antihyperglycemic agent which improves glucose tolerance in patients with type 2 diabetes, lowering both basal and postprandial plasma glucose. Its pharmacologic mechanisms of action are different from other classes of oral antihyperglycemic agents. Metformin decreases hepatic glucose production, decreases intestinal absorption of glucose, and improves insulin sensitivity by increasing peripheral glucose uptake and utilization. Unlike sulfonylureas, metformin does not produce hypoglycemia in either patients with type 2 diabetes or normal subjects (except in special circumstances, see **PRECAUTIONS**) and does not cause hyperinsulinemia. With metformin therapy, insulin secretion remains unchanged while fasting plasma insulin levels and day-long plasma insulin response may actually decrease.

PHARMACOKINETICS AND DRUG METABOLISM

Absorption and Bioavailability

The appearance of metformin in plasma from a FORTAMET™ Extended-Release Tablet is slower and more prolonged compared to immediate-release metformin.

In a multiple-dose crossover study, 23 patients with type 2 diabetes mellitus were administered either FORTAMET™ 2000 mg once a day (after dinner) or immediate-release (IR) metformin hydrochloride 1000 mg twice a day (after breakfast and after dinner). After 4 weeks of treatment, steady-state pharmacokinetic parameters, area under the concentration-time curve (AUC), time to peak plasma concentration (Tmax), and maximum concentration (Cmax) were evaluated. Results are presented in Table 1.

Table 1
FORTAMET™ vs. Immediate-Release Metformin Steady-State Pharmacokinetic Parameters at 4 Weeks

Pharmacokinetic Parameters (mean ± SD)	FORTAMET™ 2000 mg (administered q.d. after dinner)	Immediate-Release Metformin 2000 mg (1000 mg b.i.d.)
$AUC_{0\text{-}24\,hr}$ (ng•hr/mL)	26,811 ± 7055	27,371 ± 5,781
T_{max} (hr)	6 (3-10)	3 (1-8)
C_{max} (ng/mL)	2849 ± 797	1820 ± 370

In four single-dose studies and one multiple-dose study, the bioavailability of FORTAMET™ 2000 mg given once daily, in the evening, under fed conditions [as measured by the area under the plasma concentration versus time curve (AUC)] was similar to the same total daily dose administered as immediate-release metformin 1000 mg given twice daily. The geometric mean ratios (FORTAMET™/immediate-release metformin) of $AUC_{0\text{-}24hr}$, $AUC_{0\text{-}72hr}$, and $AUC_{0\text{-}inf}$ for these five studies ranged from 0.96 to 1.08.

In a single-dose, four-period replicate crossover design study, comparing two 500 mg FORTAMET™ tablets to one 1000 mg FORTAMET™ tablet administered in the evening with food to 29 healthy male subjects, two 500 mg FORTAMET™ tablets were found to be equivalent to one 1000 mg FORTAMET™ tablet.

In a study carried out with FORTAMET™, there was a dose-associated increase in metformin exposure over 24 hours following oral administration of 1000, 1500, 2000, and 2500 mg.

In three studies with FORTAMET™ using different treatment regimens (2000 mg after dinner; 1000 mg after breakfast and after dinner; and 2500 mg after dinner), the pharmacokinetics of metformin as measured by AUC appeared linear following multiple-dose administration.

The extent of metformin absorption (as measured by AUC) from FORTAMET™ increased by approximately 60% when given with food. When FORTAMET™ was administered with food, Cmax was increased by approximately 30% and Tmax was more prolonged compared with the fasting state (6.1 versus 4.0 hours).

Distribution

Distribution studies with FORTAMET™ have not been conducted. However, the apparent volume of distribution (V/F) of metformin following single oral doses of immediate-release metformin 850 mg averaged 654 ± 358 L. Metformin is negligibly bound to plasma proteins, in contrast to sulfonylureas, which are more than 90% protein bound. Metformin partitions into erythrocytes, most likely as a function of time. At usual clinical doses and dosing schedules of immediate-release metformin, steady state plasma concentrations of metformin are reached within 24-48 hours and are generally <1 μg/mL. During controlled clinical trials of immediate-release metformin, maximum metformin plasma levels did not exceed 5 μg/mL, even at maximum doses.

Metabolism and Excretion

Metabolism studies with FORTAMET™ have not been conducted.

Intravenous single-dose studies in normal subjects demonstrate that metformin is excreted unchanged in the urine and does not undergo hepatic metabolism (no metabolites have been identified in humans) nor biliary excretion.

In healthy nondiabetic adults (N=18) receiving 2500 mg q.d. FORTAMET™, the percent of the metformin dose excreted in urine over 24 hours was 40.9% and the renal clearance was 542 ± 310 mL/min. After repeated administration of FORTAMET™, there is little or no accumulation of metformin in plasma, with most of the drug being eliminated via renal excretion over a 24-hour dosing interval. The $t_{1/2}$ was 5.4 hours for FORTAMET™.

Renal clearance of metformin (Table 2) is approximately 3.5 times greater than creatinine clearance, which indicates that tubular secretion is the major route of metformin elimination. Following oral administration, approximately 90% of the absorbed drug is eliminated via the renal route within the first 24 hours, with a plasma elimination half-life of approximately 6.2 hours. In blood, the elimination half-life is approximately 17.6 hours, suggesting that the erythrocyte mass may be a compartment of distribution.

Special Populations

Geriatrics

Limited data from controlled pharmacokinetic studies of immediate-release metformin in healthy elderly subjects suggest that total plasma clearance of metformin is decreased, the half-life is prolonged, and C_{max} is increased, compared to healthy young subjects. From these data, it appears that the change in metformin pharmacokinetics with aging is primarily accounted for by a change in renal function (Table 2). FORTAMET™ treatment should not be initiated in patients 80 years of age unless measurement of creatinine clearance demonstrates that renal function is not reduced. (See **WARNINGS**, **PRECAUTIONS** and **DOSAGE AND ADMINISTRATION**.)

Pediatrics

No pharmacokinetic data from studies of pediatric patients are currently available. (See **PRECAUTIONS**.)

Gender

Five studies indicated that with FORTAMET™ treatment, the pharmacokinetic results for males and females were comparable.

[See table 2 at top of next page]

Renal Insufficiency

In patients with decreased renal function (based on measured creatinine clearance), the plasma and blood half-life

Continued on next page

Fortamet—Cont.

of metformin is prolonged and the renal clearance is decreased in proportion to the decrease in creatinine clearance (Table 2; also see **WARNINGS**).

Hepatic Insufficiency

No pharmacokinetic studies of metformin have been conducted in patients with hepatic insufficiency.

Race

No studies of metformin pharmacokinetic parameters according to race have been performed. In controlled clinical studies of immediate-release metformin in patients with type 2 diabetes, the antihyperglycemic effect was comparable in whites (n=249), blacks (n=51), and Hispanics (n=24).

Clinical Studies

In a double-blind, randomized, active-controlled, multicenter U.S. clinical study, which compared FORTAMET™ q.d. to immediate-release metformin b.i.d., 680 patients with type 2 diabetes who had been taking metformin-containing medication at study entry were randomly assigned in equal numbers to double-blind treatment with either FORTAMET™ or immediate-release metformin. Doses were adjusted during the first six weeks of treatment with study medication based on patients' FPG levels and were then held constant over a period of 20 weeks. The primary efficacy endpoint was the change in HbA_{1c} from baseline to endpoint. The primary objective was to demonstrate the clinical non-inferiority of FORTAMET™ compared to immediate-release metformin on the primary endpoint.

FORTAMET™ and metformin patients had mean HbA_{1c} changes from baseline to endpoint equal to +0.40 and +0.14, respectively (Table 3). The least-square (LS) mean treatment difference was 0.25 (95% CI = 0.14, 0.37) demonstrating that FORTAMET™ was clinically similar to metformin according to the pre-defined criterion to establish efficacy.

[See table 3 at right]

Footnote: Patients were taking metformin-containing medications at baseline that were prescribed by their personal physician.

The mean changes for FPG (Table 3) and plasma insulin (Table 3) were small for both FORTAMET™ and immediate-release metformin, and were not clinically meaningful. Seventy-six (22%) and 49 (14%) of the FORTAMET™ and immediate-release patients, respectively, discontinued prematurely from the trial. Eighteen (5%) patients on FORTAMET™ withdrew because of a stated lack of efficacy, as compared with 8 patients (2%) on immediate-release metformin (p=0.047).

Results from this study also indicated that neither FORTAMET™ nor immediate-release metformin were associated with weight gain or increases in body mass index.

A 24-week, double blind, placebo-controlled study of immediate-release metformin plus insulin, versus insulin plus placebo, was conducted in patients with type 2 diabetes who failed to achieve adequate glycemic control on insulin alone (Table 4). Patients randomized to receive immediate-release metformin plus insulin achieved a reduction in HbA_{1c} of 2.10%, compared to a 1.56% reduction in HbA_{1c} achieved by insulin plus placebo. The improvement in glycemic control was achieved at the final study visit with 16% less insulin, 93.0 U/day versus 110.6 U/day, immediate-release metformin plus insulin versus insulin plus placebo, respectively, p=0.04.

Table 4
Combined Immediate-Release Metformin/Insulin vs. Placebo/Insulin: Summary of Mean Changes from Baseline in HbA_{1c} and Daily Insulin Dose

	Immediate-Release Metformin/ Insulin (n = 26)	Placebo/ Insulin (n = 28)	Treatment difference Mean ± SE
HbA_{1c} (%)			
Baseline	8.95	9.32	
Change at FINAL VISIT	-2.10	-1.56	-0.54 ± 0.43[a]
Insulin Dose (U/day)			
Baseline	93.12	94.64	
Change at FINAL VISIT	-0.15	15.93	-16.08 ± 7.77[b]

[a] Statistically significant using analysis of covariance with baseline as covariate (p=0.04)
Not significant using analysis of variance (values shown in table)
[b] Statistically significant for insulin (p=0.04)

A second double-blind, placebo-controlled study (n=51), with 16 weeks of randomized treatment, demonstrated that in patients with type 2 diabetes controlled on insulin for 8 weeks with an average HbA_{1c} of 7.46 ± 0.97%, the addition of immediate-release metformin maintained similar glycemic control (HbA_{1c} 7.15 ± 0.61 versus 6.97 ± 0.62 for immediate-release metformin plus insulin and placebo plus insulin, respectively) with 19% less insulin versus baseline (reduction of 23.68 ± 30.22 versus an increase of 0.43 ± 25.20 units for immediate-release metformin plus insulin and placebo plus insulin, p<0.01). In addition, this study demonstrated that the combination of immediate-release metformin plus insulin resulted in reduction in body weight of 3.11 ± 4.30 lbs, compared to an increase of 1.30 ± 6.08 lbs for placebo plus insulin, p=0.01.

Table 2
Select Mean (±SD) Metformin Pharmacokinetic Parameters Following Single or Multiple Oral Doses of Immediate-Release Metformin

Subject Groups: Immediate-Release Metformin dose[a] (number of subjects)	C_{max}[b] (μg/mL)	T_{max}[c] (hrs)	Renal Clearance (mL/min)
Healthy, nondiabetic adults:			
500 mg single dose (24)	1.03 (±0.33)	2.75 (±0.81)	600 (±132)
850 mg single dose (74)[d]	1.60 (±0.38)	2.64 (±0.82)	552 (±139)
850 mg three times daily for 19 doses[e] (9)	2.01 (±0.42)	1.79 (±0.94)	642 (±173)
Adults with type 2 diabetes:			
850 mg single dose (23)	1.48 (±0.5)	3.32 (±1.08)	491 (±138)
850 mg three times daily for 19 doses[e] (9)	1.90 (±0.62)	2.01 (±1.22)	550 (±160)
Elderly[f], healthy nondiabetic adults:			
850 mg single dose (12)	2.45 (±0.70)	2.71 (±1.05)	412 (±98)
Renal-impaired adults:			
850 mg single dose			
Mild (CL_{cr}[g] 61-90 mL/min) (5)	1.86 (±0.52)	3.20 (±0.45)	384 (±122)
Moderate (CL_{cr} 31-60 mL/min) (4)	4.12 (±1.83)	3.75 (±0.50)	108 (±57)
Severe (CL_{cr} 10-30 mL/min) (6)	3.93 (±0.92)	4.01 (±1.10)	130 (±90)

[a] All doses given fasting except the first 18 doses of the multiple dose studies
[b] Peak plasma concentration
[c] Time to peak plasma concentration
[d] Combined results (average means) of five studies: mean age 32 years (range 23-59 years)
[e] Kinetic study done following dose 19, given fasting
[f] Elderly subjects, mean age 71 years (range 65-81 years)
[g] CL_{cr} = creatinine clearance normalized to body surface area of 1.73 m^2

Table 3
FORTAMET™ vs. Immediate-Release Metformin
Switch Study: Summary of Mean Changes in HbA_{1c}, Fasting Plasma Glucose, Body Weight, Body Mass Index, and Plasma Insulin

	FORTAMET™	Immediate-Release Metformin	Treatment difference for change from baseline (FORTAMET™ minus Immediate-Release Metformin) LS mean (2-sided 95% CI[a])
HbA_{1c} (%)			
N	327	332	0.25
Baseline (mean ± SD)	7.04 ± 0.88	7.07 ± 0.76	(0.14, 0.37)[b]
Change from baseline (mean ±SD)	0.40 ± 0.75	0.14 ± 0.75	
Fasting Plasma Glucose (mg/dL)			
N	329	333	6.43
Baseline (mean ± SD)	146.8 ± 32.1	145.6 ± 29.5	(0.57, 12.29)
Change from baseline (mean ±SD)	10.0 ± 40.8	4.2 ± 35.9	
Plasma Insulin (μu/mL)			
N	304	316	0.02
Baseline (mean ± SD)	17.9 ± 15.1	17.3 ± 10.5	(-1.47, 1.50)
Change from baseline (mean ±SD)	-3.6 ± 13.8	-3.2 ± 8.6	
Body Weight (kg)			
N	313	320	0.30
Baseline (mean ± SD)	94.1 ± 17.8	93.3 ± 17.4	(-0.22, 0.81)
Change from baseline (mean ±SD)	0.3 ± 2.9	0.0 ± 3.7	
Body Mass Index (kg/m^2)			
N	313	320	0.08
Baseline (mean ± SD)	31.1 ± 4.7	31.4 ± 4.5	(-0.11, 0.26)
Change from baseline (mean ±SD)	0.1 ± 1.1	0.0 ± 1.3	

[a] CI = Confidence Interval
[b] FORTAMET was clinically similar to immediate-release metformin based on the pre-defined criterion to establish efficacy. While demonstrating clinical similarity, the response to FORTAMET compared to immediate-release metformin was also shown to be statistically smaller as seen by the 95% CI for the treatment difference which did not include zero.

Pediatric Clinical Studies

No pediatric clinical studies have been conducted with FORTAMET™. In a double-blind, placebo-controlled study in pediatric patients aged 10 to 16 years with type 2 diabetes (mean FPG 182.2 mg/dL), treatment with immediate-release metformin (up to 2000 mg/day) for up to 16 weeks (mean duration of treatment 11 weeks) resulted in a significant mean net reduction in FPG of 64.3 mg/dL compared with placebo (Table 5).

Table 5
Immediate-Release Metformin vs. Placebo (Pediatrics[a]): Summary of Mean Changes from Baseline* in Plasma Glucose and Body Weight at Final Visit

	Immediate-Release Metformin	Placebo	p-Value
FPG (mg/dL)	**(n = 37)**	**(n = 36)**	
Baseline	162.4	192.3	
Change at FINAL VISIT	-42.9	21.4	<0.001
Body Weight (lbs)	**(n = 39)**	**(n = 38)**	
Baseline	205.3	189.0	
Change at FINAL VISIT	-3.3	-2.0	NS**

[a] Pediatric patients mean age 13.8 years (range 10-16 years)
* All patients on diet therapy at Baseline
** Not statistically significant

INDICATIONS AND USAGE

FORTAMET™ (metformin hydrochloride) Extended-Release Tablets, used as a once per day monotherapy, are indicated as an adjunct to diet and exercise to lower blood glucose. FORTAMET™ can be used concomitantly with a sulfonylurea or insulin to improve glycemic control in adults. FORTAMET™ is indicated in patients 17 years of age and older as either monotherapy or in combination therapy.

CONTRAINDICATIONS

FORTAMET™ is contraindicated in patients with:

1. Renal disease or renal dysfunction (e.g., as suggested by serum creatinine levels ≥1.5 mg/dL [males], ≥1.4 mg/dL [females] or abnormal creatinine clearance) which may also result from conditions such as cardiovascular collapse (shock), acute myocardial infarction, and septicemia (see **WARNINGS** and **PRECAUTIONS**).
2. Congestive heart failure requiring pharmacologic treatment.
3. Known hypersensitivity to metformin.
4. Acute or chronic metabolic acidosis, including diabetic ketoacidosis, with or without coma. Diabetic ketoacidosis should be treated with insulin.

FORTAMET™ should be temporarily discontinued in patients undergoing radiologic studies involving intravascular administration of iodinated contrast materials, because use of such products may result in acute alteration of renal function. (See also **PRECAUTIONS**.)

WARNINGS

Lactic Acidosis:

Lactic acidosis is a rare, but serious, metabolic complication that can occur due to metformin accumulation during treatment with FORTAMET™ (metformin hydrochloride) Extended-Release Tablets; when it occurs, it is fatal in approximately 50% of cases. Lactic acidosis may also occur in association with a number of pathophysiologic conditions, including diabetes mellitus, and whenever there is significant tissue hypoperfusion and hypoxemia. Lactic acidosis is characterized by elevated blood lactate levels (>5 mmol/L), decreased blood pH, electrolyte disturbances with an increased anion gap, and an increased lactate/pyruvate ratio. When metformin is implicated as the cause of lactic acidosis, metformin plasma levels >5 μg/mL are generally found.

The reported incidence of lactic acidosis in patients receiving metformin hydrochloride is very low (approximately 0.03 cases/1000 patient-years, with approximately 0.015 fatal cases/1000 patient-years). Reported cases have occurred primarily in diabetic patients with significant renal insufficiency, including both intrinsic renal disease and renal hypoperfusion, often in the setting of multiple concomitant medical/surgical problems and multiple concomitant medications. Patients with congestive heart failure requiring pharmacologic management, in particular those with unstable or acute congestive heart failure who are at risk of hypoperfusion and hypoxemia, are at increased risk of lactic acidosis. The risk of lactic acidosis increases with the degree of renal dysfunction and the patient's age. The risk of lactic acidosis may, therefore, be significantly decreased by regular monitoring of renal function in patients taking FORTAMET™ (metformin hydrochloride) Extended-Release Tablets and by use of the minimum effective dose of FORTAMET™. In particular, treatment of the elderly should be accompanied by careful monitoring of renal function. FORTAMET™ treatment should not be initiated in patients ≥80 years of age unless measurement of creatinine clearance demonstrates that renal function is not reduced, as these patients are more susceptible to developing lactic acidosis. In addition, FORTAMET™ should be promptly withheld in the presence of any condition associated with hypoxemia, dehydration, or sepsis. Because impaired hepatic function may significantly limit the ability to clear lactate, FORTAMET™ should generally be avoided in patients with clinical or laboratory evidence of hepatic disease. Patients should be cautioned against excessive alcohol intake, either acute or chronic, when taking FORTAMET™, since alcohol potentiates the effects of metformin hydrochloride on lactate metabolism. In addition, FORTAMET™ should be temporarily discontinued prior to any intravascular radiocontrast study and for any surgical procedure (see also PRECAUTIONS).

The onset of lactic acidosis often is subtle, and accompanied only by nonspecific symptoms such as malaise, myalgias, respiratory distress, increasing somnolence, and nonspecific abdominal distress. There may be associated hypothermia, hypotension, and resistant bradyarrhythmias with more marked acidosis. The patient and the patient's physician must be aware of the possible importance of such symptoms and the patient should be instructed to notify the physician immediately if they occur (see also PRECAUTIONS). FORTAMET™ should be withdrawn until the situation is clarified. Serum electrolytes, ketones, blood glucose and, if indicated, blood pH, lactate levels, and even blood metformin levels may be useful. Once a patient is stabilized on any dose level of FORTAMET™, gastrointestinal symptoms, which are common during initiation of therapy, are unlikely to be drug related. Later occurrence of gastrointestinal symptoms could be due to lactic acidosis or other serious disease. Levels of fasting venous plasma lactate above the upper limit of normal but less than 5 mmol/L in patients taking FORTAMET™ do not necessarily indicate impending lactic acidosis and may be explainable by other mechanisms, such as poorly controlled diabetes or obesity, vigorous physical activity, or technical problems in sample handling. (See also PRECAUTIONS.)

Lactic acidosis should be suspected in any diabetic patient with metabolic acidosis lacking evidence of ketoacidosis (ketonuria and ketonemia).

Lactic acidosis is a medical emergency that must be treated in a hospital setting. In a patient with lactic acidosis who is taking FORTAMET™, the drug should be discontinued immediately and general supportive measures promptly instituted. Because metformin hydrochloride is dialyzable (with a clearance of up to 170 mL/min under good hemodynamic conditions), prompt hemodialysis is recommended to correct the acidosis and remove the accumulated metformin. Such management often results in prompt reversal of symptoms and recovery. (See also CONTRAINDICATIONS and PRECAUTIONS.)

PRECAUTIONS

General

Monitoring of renal function – Metformin is known to be substantially excreted by the kidney, and the risk of metformin accumulation and lactic acidosis increases with the degree of impairment of renal function. Thus, patients with serum creatinine levels above the upper limit of normal for their age should not receive FORTAMET™. In patients with advanced age, FORTAMET™ should be carefully titrated to establish the minimum dose for adequate glycemic effect, because aging is associated with reduced renal function. In elderly patients, particularly those ≥80 years of age, renal function should be monitored regularly and, generally, FORTAMET™ should not be titrated to the maximum dose (see **WARNINGS** and **DOSAGE AND ADMINISTRATION**).

Before initiation of FORTAMET™ therapy and at least annually thereafter, renal function should be assessed and verified as normal. In patients in whom development of renal dysfunction is anticipated, renal function should be assessed more frequently and FORTAMET™ discontinued if evidence of renal impairment is present.

Use of concomitant medications that may affect renal function or metformin disposition – Concomitant medication(s) that may affect renal function or result in significant hemodynamic change or may interfere with the disposition of metformin, such as cationic drugs that are eliminated by renal tubular secretion (see **PRECAUTIONS: Drug Interactions**), should be used with caution.

Radiologic studies involving the use of intravascular iodinated contrast materials (for example, intravenous urogram, intravenous cholangiography, angiography, and computed tomography (CT) scans with intravascular contrast materials) – Intravascular contrast studies with iodinated materials can lead to acute alteration of renal function and have been associated with lactic acidosis in patients receiving metformin (see **CONTRAINDICATIONS**). Therefore, in patients in whom any such study is planned, FORTAMET™ should be temporarily discontinued at the time of or prior to the procedure, and withheld for 48 hours subsequent to the procedure and reinstituted only after renal function has been re-evaluated and found to be normal.

Hypoxic states – Cardiovascular collapse (shock) from whatever cause, acute congestive heart failure, acute myocardial infarction and other conditions characterized by hypoxemia have been associated with lactic acidosis and may also cause prerenal azotemia. When such events occur in patients on FORTAMET™ therapy, the drug should be promptly discontinued.

Surgical procedures – FORTAMET™ therapy should be temporarily suspended for any surgical procedure (except minor procedures not associated with restricted intake of food and fluids) and should not be restarted until the patient's oral intake has resumed and renal function has been evaluated as normal.

Alcohol intake – Alcohol is known to potentiate the effect of metformin on lactate metabolism. Patients, therefore, should be warned against excessive alcohol intake, acute or chronic, while receiving FORTAMET™.

Impaired hepatic function – Since impaired hepatic function has been associated with some cases of lactic acidosis, FORTAMET™ should generally be avoided in patients with clinical or laboratory evidence of hepatic disease.

Vitamin B_{12} levels – In controlled clinical trials of immediate-release metformin of 29 weeks duration, a decrease to subnormal levels of previously normal serum Vitamin B_{12} levels, without clinical manifestations, was observed in approximately 7% of patients. Such decrease, possibly due to interference with B_{12} absorption from the B_{12}-intrinsic factor complex, is, however, very rarely associated with anemia and appears to be rapidly reversible with discontinuation of immediate-release metformin or Vitamin B_{12} supplementation. Measurement of hematologic parameters on an annual basis is advised in patients on FORTAMET™ and any apparent abnormalities should be appropriately investigated and managed (see **PRECAUTIONS: Laboratory Tests**).

Certain individuals (those with inadequate Vitamin B_{12} or calcium intake or absorption) appear to be predisposed to developing subnormal Vitamin B_{12} levels. In these patients, routine serum Vitamin B_{12} measurements at two- to three-year intervals may be useful.

Change in clinical status of patients with previously controlled type 2 diabetes – A patient with type 2 diabetes previously well controlled on FORTAMET™ who develops laboratory abnormalities or clinical illness (especially vague and poorly defined illness) should be evaluated promptly for evidence of ketoacidosis or lactic acidosis. Evaluation should include serum electrolytes and ketones, blood glucose and, if indicated, blood pH, lactate, pyruvate, and metformin levels. If acidosis of either form occurs, FORTAMET™ must be stopped immediately and other appropriate corrective measures initiated (see also **WARNINGS**).

Hypoglycemia – Hypoglycemia does not occur in patients receiving FORTAMET™ alone under usual circumstances of use, but could occur when caloric intake is deficient, when strenuous exercise is not compensated by caloric supplementation, or during concomitant use with other glucose-lowering agents (such as sulfonylureas and insulin) or ethanol. Elderly, debilitated, or malnourished patients, and those with adrenal or pituitary insufficiency or alcohol intoxication are particularly susceptible to hypoglycemic effects. Hypoglycemia may be difficult to recognize in the elderly, and in people who are taking beta-adrenergic blocking drugs.

Loss of control of blood glucose – When a patient stabilized on any diabetic regimen is exposed to stress such as fever, trauma, infection , or surgery, a temporary loss of glycemic control may occur. At such times, it may be necessary to withhold FORTAMET™ and temporarily administer insulin. FORTAMET™ may be reinstituted after the acute episode is resolved.

The effectiveness of oral antidiabetic drugs in lowering blood glucose to a targeted level decreases in many patients over a period of time. This phenomenon, which may be due to progression of the underlying disease or to diminished responsiveness to the drug, is known as secondary failure, to distinguish it from primary failure in which the drug is ineffective during initial therapy. Should secondary failure occur with FORTAMET™ or sulfonylurea monotherapy, combined therapy with FORTAMET™ and sulfonylurea may result in a response. Should secondary failure occur with combined FORTAMET™/sulfonylurea therapy, it may be necessary to consider therapeutic alternatives including initiation of insulin therapy.

Information for Patients

Patients should be informed of the potential risks and benefits of FORTAMET™ and of alternative modes of therapy. They should also be informed about the importance of adherence to dietary instructions, of a regular exercise program, and of regular testing of blood glucose, glycosylated hemoglobin, renal function, and hematologic parameters.

The risks of lactic acidosis, its symptoms, and conditions that predispose to its development, as noted in the **WARNINGS** and **PRECAUTIONS** sections, should be explained to patients. Patients should be advised to discontinue FORTAMET™ immediately and to promptly notify their health practitioner if unexplained hyperventilation, myalgia, malaise, unusual somnolence, or other nonspecific symptoms occur. Once a patient is stabilized on any dose level of FORTAMET™, gastrointestinal symptoms, which are common during initiation of metformin therapy, are unlikely to be drug related. Later occurrence of gastrointestinal symptoms could be due to lactic acidosis or other serious disease.

Patients should be counseled against excessive alcohol intake, either acute or chronic, while receiving FORTAMET™.

FORTAMET™ alone does not usually cause hypoglycemia, although it may occur when FORTAMET™ is used in conjunction with oral sulfonylureas and insulin. When initiating combination therapy, the risks of hypoglycemia, its symptoms and treatment, and conditions that predispose to its development should be explained to patients and responsible family members. (See **Patient Information** Printed Below.)

Patients should be informed that FORTAMET™ must be swallowed whole and not chewed, cut, or crushed, and that the inactive ingredients may occasionally be eliminated in the feces as a soft mass that may resemble the original tablet. (See **Patient Information**.)

Laboratory Tests

Response to all diabetic therapies should be monitored by periodic measurements of fasting blood glucose and glycosylated hemoglobin levels, with a goal of decreasing these levels toward the normal range. During initial dose titration, fasting glucose can be used to determine the therapeutic response. Thereafter, both glucose and glycosylated hemoglobin should be monitored. Measurements of glycosylated hemoglobin may be especially useful for evaluating long-term control (see also **DOSAGE AND ADMINISTRATION**).

Initial and periodic monitoring of hematologic parameters (e.g., hemoglobin/hematocrit and red blood cell indices) and renal function (serum creatinine) should be performed, at least on an annual basis. While megaloblastic anemia has rarely been seen with immediate-release metformin therapy, if this is suspected, Vitamin B_{12} deficiency should be excluded.

Drug Interactions (Clinical Evaluation of Drug Interactions Conducted with Immediate-Release Metformin)

Glyburide – In a single-dose interaction study in type 2 diabetes patients, co-administration of metformin and glyburide did not result in any changes in either metformin pharmacokinetics or pharmacodynamics. Decreases in glyburide AUC and C_{max} were observed, but were highly variable. The single-dose nature of this study and the lack of correlation between glyburide blood levels and pharmacodynamic effects, makes the clinical significance of this interaction uncertain. (See **DOSAGE AND ADMINISTRATION: Concomitant FORTAMET™ and Oral Sulfonylurea Therapy in Adult Patients**.)

Furosemide – A single-dose, metformin-furosemide drug interaction study in healthy subjects demonstrated that phar-

Continued on next page

Fortamet—Cont.

macokinetic parameters of both compounds were affected by co-administration. Furosemide increased the metformin plasma and blood C_{max} by 22% and blood AUC by 15%, without any significant change in metformin renal clearance. When administered with metformin, the C_{max} and AUC of furosemide were 31% and 12% smaller, respectively, than when administered alone, and the terminal half-life was decreased by 32%, without any significant change in furosemide renal clearance. No information is available about the interaction of metformin and furosemide when co-administered chronically.

Nifedipine – A single-dose, metformin-nifedipine drug interaction study in normal healthy volunteers demonstrated that co-administration of nifedipine increased plasma metformin C_{max} and AUC by 20% and 9%, respectively, and increased the amount excreted in the urine. T_{max} and half-life were unaffected. Nifedipine appears to enhance the absorption of metformin. Metformin had minimal effects on nifedipine.

Cationic drugs – Cationic drugs (e.g., amiloride, digoxin, morphine, procainamide, quinidine, quinine, ranitidine, triamterene, trimethoprim, or vancomycin) that are eliminated by renal tubular secretion theoretically have the potential for interaction with metformin by competing for common renal tubular transport systems. Such interaction between metformin and oral cimetidine has been observed in normal healthy volunteers in both single- and multiple-dose, metformin-cimetidine drug interaction studies, with a 60% increase in peak metformin plasma and whole blood concentrations and a 40% increase in plasma and whole blood metformin AUC. There was no change in elimination half-life in the single-dose study. Metformin had no effect on cimetidine pharmacokinetics. Although such interactions remain theoretical (except for cimetidine), careful patient monitoring and dose adjustment of FORTAMET™ and/or the interfering drug is recommended in patients who are taking cationic medications that are excreted via the proximal renal tubular secretory system.

Other – Certain drugs tend to produce hyperglycemia and may lead to loss of glycemic control. These drugs include the thiazides and other diuretics, corticosteroids, phenothiazines, thyroid products, estrogens, oral contraceptives, phenytoin, nicotinic acid, sympathomimetics, calcium channel blocking drugs, and isoniazid. When such drugs are administered to a patient receiving FORTAMET™, the patient should be closely observed for loss of blood glucose control. When such drugs are withdrawn from a patient receiving FORTAMET™, the patient should be observed closely for hypoglycemia.

In healthy volunteers, the pharmacokinetics of metformin and propranolol, and metformin and ibuprofen were not affected when co-administered in single-dose interaction studies.

Metformin is negligibly bound to plasma proteins and is, therefore, less likely to interact with highly protein-bound drugs such as salicylates, sulfonamides, chloramphenicol, and probenecid, as compared to the sulfonylureas, which are extensively bound to serum proteins.

Carcinogenesis, Mutagenesis, Impairment of Fertility

Long-term carcinogenicity studies with metformin have been performed in rats (dosing duration of 104 weeks) and mice (dosing duration of 91 weeks) at doses up to and including 900 mg/kg/day and 1500 mg/kg/day, respectively. These doses are both approximately four times the maximum recommended human daily dose of 2000 mg based on body surface area comparisons. No evidence of carcinogenicity with metformin was found in either male or female mice. Similarly, there was no tumorigenic potential observed with metformin in male rats. There was, however, an increased incidence of benign stromal uterine polyps in female rats treated with 900 mg/kg/day.

There was no evidence of mutagenic potential of metformin in the following *in vitro* tests: Ames test (*S. typhimurium*), gene mutation test (mouse lymphoma cells), or chromosomal aberrations test (human lymphocytes). Results in the *in vivo* mouse micronucleus test were also negative.

Fertility of male or female rats was unaffected by metformin when administered at doses as high as 600 mg/kg/day, which is approximately three times the maximum recommended human daily dose based on body surface area comparisons.

Pregnancy

Teratogenic Effects: Pregnancy Category B

Recent information strongly suggests that abnormal blood glucose levels during pregnancy are associated with a higher incidence of congenital abnormalities. Most experts recommend that insulin be used during pregnancy to maintain blood glucose levels as close to normal as possible. Because animal reproduction studies are not always predictive of human response, FORTAMET™ should not be used during pregnancy unless clearly needed.

There are no adequate and well-controlled studies in pregnant women with immediate-release metformin or FORTAMET™. Metformin was not teratogenic in rats and rabbits at doses up to 600 mg/kg/day. This represents an exposure of about two and six times the maximum recommended human daily dose of 2000 mg based on body surface area comparisons for rats and rabbits, respectively. Determination of fetal concentrations demonstrated a partial placental barrier to metformin.

Nursing Mothers

Studies in lactating rats show that metformin is excreted into milk and reaches levels comparable to those in plasma. Similar studies have not been conducted in nursing mothers. Because the potential for hypoglycemia in nursing infants may exist, a decision should be made whether to discontinue nursing or to discontinue the drug, taking into account the importance of the drug to the mother. If FORTAMET™ is discontinued, and if diet alone is inadequate for controlling blood glucose, insulin therapy should be considered.

Pediatric Use

No pediatric clinical studies have been conducted with FORTAMET™. The safety and effectiveness of immediate-release metformin for the treatment of type 2 diabetes have been established in pediatric patients ages 10 to 16 years (studies have not been conducted in pediatric patients below the age of 10 years). Use of immediate-release metformin in this age group is supported by evidence from adequate and well-controlled studies of immediate-release metformin in adults with additional data from a controlled clinical study in pediatric patients ages 10-16 years with type 2 diabetes, which demonstrated a similar response in glycemic control to that seen in adults. (See **CLINICAL PHARMACOLOGY: Pediatric Clinical Studies.**) In this study, adverse effects were similar to those described in adults. (See **ADVERSE REACTIONS: Pediatric Patients.**) A maximum daily dose of 2000 mg of immediate-release metformin is recommended.

FORTAMET™

The safety and efficacy of FORTAMET™ has not been evaluated in pediatric patients.

Geriatric Use

Of the 389 patients who received FORTAMET™ in controlled Phase III clinical studies, 26.5% [103/389] were 65 years and older. No overall differences in effectiveness or safety were observed between these patients and younger patients.

Controlled clinical studies of immediate-release metformin did not include sufficient numbers of elderly patients to determine whether they respond differently from younger patients, although other reported clinical experience has not identified differences in responses between the elderly and younger patients. Metformin is known to be substantially excreted by the kidney and because of the risk of serious adverse reactions to the drug is greater in patients with impaired renal function, immediate-release metformin should only be used in patients with normal renal function (see **CONTRAINDICATIONS**, **WARNINGS**, and **CLINICAL PHARMACOLOGY: Pharmacokinetics**). Because aging is associated with reduced renal function, immediate-release metformin should be used with caution as age increases. Care should be taken in dose selection and should be based on careful and regular monitoring of renal function. Generally, elderly patients should not be titrated to the maximum dose of immediate-release metformin (see also **WARNINGS** and **DOSAGE AND ADMINISTRATION**).

ADVERSE REACTIONS

FORTAMET™ Clinical Studies

In the controlled clinical studies of FORTAMET™ in patients with type 2 diabetes, a total of 424 patients received FORTAMET™ therapy (up to 2500 mg/day) and 430 patients received immediate-release metformin. Adverse reactions reported in ≥5% of the FORTAMET™ or immediate-release metformin patients are listed in Table 6. These pooled results show that the most frequently reported adverse reactions in the FORTAMET™ group were infection, diarrhea, and nausea. Similar incidences of these adverse reactions were seen in the immediate-release metformin group.

Table 6
Number and Percentage of Patients With the Most Common (Incidence ≥5%) Treatment-Emergent Signs or Symptoms by Body System and Preferred Term – Pooled Phase II and III Studies

	FORTAMET™ (N=424)		Immediate-Release Metformin (N=430)	
Body System Preferred Term	**n**	**(%)**	**n**	**(%)**
Body as a Whole				
Accidental Injury	31	(7.3)	24	(5.6)
Headache	20	(4.7)	22	(5.1)
Infection	87	(20.5)	90	(20.9)
Digestive System				
Diarrhea	71	(16.7)	51	(11.9)
Dyspepsia	18	(4.2)	22	(5.1)
Nausea	36	(8.5)	32	(7.4)
Respiratory System				
Rhinitis	18	(4.2)	24	(5.6)

The most frequent adverse events thought to be related to FORTAMET™ were diarrhea, nausea, dyspepsia, flatulence, and abdominal pain. The frequency of dyspepsia was 4.2% in the FORTAMET™ group compared to 5.1% in the immediate-release group, the frequency of flatulence was 3.5% in the FORTAMET™ group compared to 3.7% in the immediate-release group, and the frequency of abdominal pain was 3.3% in the FORTAMET™ group compared to 4.4% in the immediate-release group.

In the controlled studies, 4.7% of patients treated with FORTAMET™ and 4.9% of patients treated with immediate-release metformin were discontinued due to adverse events.

Immediate-Release Metformin

Immediate-Release Metformin Phase III Clinical Studies

In a U.S. double-blind clinical study of immediate-release metformin in patients with type 2 diabetes, a total of 141 patients received immediate-release metformin therapy (up to 2550 mg per day) and 145 patients received placebo. Adverse reactions reported in greater than 5% of the immediate-release metformin patients, and that were more common in immediate-release metformin- than placebo-treated patients, are listed in Table 7.

Table 7
Most Common Adverse Reactions (>5.0%) in a Placebo-Controlled Clinical Study of Immediate-Release Metformin Monotherapy*

	Immediate-Release Metformin Monotherapy (n = 141)	Placebo (n = 145)
Adverse Reaction	**% of Patients**	
Diarrhea	53.2	11.7
Nausea/Vomiting	25.5	8.3
Flatulence	12.1	5.5
Asthenia	9.2	5.5
Indigestion	7.1	4.1
Abdominal Discomfort	6.4	4.8
Headache	5.7	4.8

* Reactions that were more common in immediate-release metformin than placebo-treated patients

Diarrhea led to discontinuation of study medication in 6% of patients treated with immediate-release metformin. Additionally, the following adverse reactions were reported in ≥1.0 - ≤5.0% of immediate-release metformin patients and were more commonly reported with immediate-release metformin than placebo: abnormal stools, hypoglycemia, myalgia, lightheaded, dyspnea, nail disorder, rash, sweating increased, taste disorder, chest discomfort, chills, flu syndrome, flushing, palpitation.

Pediatric Patients

No pediatric clinical studies have been conducted with FORTAMET™. In clinical trials with immediate-release metformin in pediatric patients with type 2 diabetes, the profile of adverse reactions was similar to that observed in adults.

OVERDOSAGE

Hypoglycemia has not been seen even with ingestion of up to 85 grams of immediate-release metformin, although lactic acidosis has occurred in such circumstances (see **WARNINGS**). Metformin is dialyzable with a clearance of up to 170 mL/min under good hemodynamic conditions. Therefore, hemodialysis may be useful for removal of accumulated drug from patients in whom metformin overdosage is suspected.

DOSAGE AND ADMINISTRATION

There is no fixed dosage regimen for the management of hyperglycemia in patients with type 2 diabetes with FORTAMET™ or any other pharmacologic agent. Dosage of FORTAMET™ must be individualized on the basis of both effectiveness and tolerance, while not exceeding the maximum recommended daily dose. The maximum recommended daily dose of FORTAMET™ Extended-Release Tablets in adults is 2500 mg.

FORTAMET™ should generally be given once daily with the evening meal. FORTAMET™ should be started at a low dose, with gradual dose escalation, both to reduce gastrointestinal side effects and to permit identification of the minimum dose required for adequate glycemic control of the patient.

During treatment initiation and dose titration (see **Recommended Dosing Schedule**), fasting plasma glucose should be used to determine the therapeutic response to FORTAMET™ and identify the minimum effective dose for the patient. Thereafter, glycosylated hemoglobin should be measured at intervals of approximately three months. The therapeutic goal should be to decrease both fasting plasma glucose and glycosylated hemoglobin levels to normal or near normal by using the lowest effective dose of FORTAMET™, either when used as monotherapy or in combination with sulfonylurea or insulin.

Monitoring of blood glucose and glycosylated hemoglobin will also permit detection of primary failure, i.e., inadequate lowering of blood glucose at the maximum recommended dose of medication, and secondary failure, i.e., loss of an adequate blood glucose lowering response after an initial period of effectiveness.

Short-term administration of FORTAMET™ may be sufficient during periods of transient loss of control in patients usually well-controlled on diet alone.

Recommended Dosing Schedule

The usual starting dose of FORTAMET™ (metformin hydrochloride) Extended-Release Tablets is 1000 mg once daily with the evening meal, although 500 mg may be utilized when clinically appropriate. Dosage increases should be made in increments of 500 mg weekly, up to a maximum of 2500 mg once daily with the evening meal. (See **CLINICAL PHARMACOLOGY, Clinical Studies.**)

In randomized trials, patients currently treated with immediate-release metformin were switched to FORTAMET™. Results of this trial suggest that patients receiving immediate-release metformin treatment may be safely switched to FORTAMET™ once daily at the same total daily dose, up to 2500 mg once daily. Following a switch from immediate-release metformin to FORTAMET™, glycemic control should be closely monitored and dosage adjustments made accordingly (see **CLINICAL PHARMACOLOGY, Clinical Studies.**)

Pediatrics – There is no pediatric information available for FORTAMET™.

Transfer From Other Antidiabetic Therapy

When transferring patients from standard oral hypoglycemic agents other than chlorpropamide to FORTAMET™, no transition period generally is necessary. When transferring patients from chlorpropamide, care should be exercised during the first two weeks because of the prolonged retention of chlorpropamide in the body, leading to overlapping drug effects and possible hypoglycemia.

Concomitant FORTAMET™ and Oral Sulfonylurea Therapy in Adult Patients

If patients have not responded to four weeks of the maximum dose of FORTAMET™ monotherapy, consideration should be given to gradual addition of an oral sulfonylurea while continuing FORTAMET™ at the maximum dose, even if prior primary or secondary failure to a sulfonylurea has occurred. Clinical and pharmacokinetic drug-drug interaction data are currently available only for metformin plus glyburide (also known as glibenclamide). With concomitant FORTAMET and sulfonylurea therapy, the desired control of blood glucose may be obtained by adjusting the dose of each drug. However, attempts should be made to identify the minimum effective dose of each drug to achieve this goal. With concomitant FORTAMET™ and sulfonylurea therapy, the risk of hypoglycemia associated with sulfonylurea therapy continues and may be increased. Appropriate precautions should be taken. (See Package Insert of the respective sulfonylurea.)

If patients have not satisfactorily responded to one to three months of concomitant therapy with the maximum dose of FORTAMET™ and the maximum dose of an oral sulfonylurea, consider therapeutic alternatives including switching to insulin with or without FORTAMET™.

Concomitant FORTAMET™ and Insulin Therapy in Adult Patients

The current insulin dose should be continued upon initiation of FORTAMET™ therapy. FORTAMET™ therapy should be initiated at 500 mg once daily in patients on insulin therapy. For patients not responding adequately, the dose of FORTAMET™ should be increased by 500 mg after approximately 1 week and by 500 mg every week thereafter until adequate glycemic control is achieved. The maximum recommended daily dose for FORTAMET™ Extended-Release Tablets is 2500 mg. It is recommended that the insulin dose be decreased by 10% to 25% when fasting plasma glucose concentrations decrease to less than 120 mg/dL in patients receiving concomitant insulin and FORTAMET™. Further adjustment should be individualized based on glucose-lowering response.

Specific Patient Populations

FORTAMET™ is not recommended for use in pregnancy, and is not recommended in patients below the age of 17 years.

The initial and maintenance dosing of FORTAMET™ should be conservative in patients with advanced age, due to the potential for decreased renal function in this population. Any dosage adjustment should be based on a careful assessment of renal function. Generally, elderly, debilitated, and malnourished patients should not be titrated to the maximum dose of FORTAMET™.

Monitoring of renal function is necessary to aid in prevention of lactic acidosis, particularly in the elderly. (See **WARNINGS.**)

HOW SUPPLIED

FORTAMET™ (metformin hydrochloride) Extended-Release Tablets are supplied as biconvex-shaped, film-coated extended-release tablets containing 500 mg or 1000 mg of metformin hydrochloride.

NDC 62022 574 60: 500 mg extended-release white-colored tablets imprinted with Andrx logo and 574 on one side, bottles of 60.

NDC 62022 575 60: 1000 mg extended-release white-colored tablets imprinted Andrx logo and 575 on one side, bottles of 60.

STORAGE

Store at 25°C (77°F); excursions permitted to 15°-30°C (59°-86°F) [see USP Controlled Room Temperature]. Keep tightly closed (protect from moisture). Protect from light. Avoid excessive heat and humidity.

Distributed by:
Andrx Laboratories, Inc.
Weston, Florida 33331

Manufactured by:
Andrx Pharmaceuticals, Inc.
Ft. Lauderdale, Florida 33314
Copyright© ANDRX LABS, INC., 2003
7420
Rev. 04/04

PATIENT INFORMATION ABOUT FORTAMET™

(metformin hydrochloride) extended-release tablets

Q1. Why do I need to take FORTAMET™?

Your doctor has prescribed FORTAMET™ to treat your type 2 diabetes, a condition in which blood sugar (blood glucose) is elevated. There are two types of diabetes. FORTAMET™ is indicated for the most common type, known as type 2 diabetes.

Q2. Why is it important to control type 2 diabetes?

Type 2 diabetes has multiple possible complications, including blindness, kidney failure, and circulatory and heart problems. Lowering your blood sugar to a normal level may prevent or delay these complications.

Q3. How is type 2 diabetes usually controlled?

High blood sugar can be lowered by diet and exercise, by a number of oral medications and by insulin injections. Your doctor may recommend that you try lifestyle modifications such as improved diet and exercise before initiating drug treatment for type 2 diabetes. Each patient will be treated individually by his or her physician, and should follow all treatment recommendations.

Q4. Does FORTAMET™ work differently from other glucose-control medications?

Yes. FORTAMET™, as well as other formulations of metformin, lowers the amount of sugar in your blood by controlling how much sugar is released by the liver. FORTAMET™ (metformin hydrochloride) does not cause your body to produce more insulin. FORTAMET™ rarely causes hypoglycemia (low blood sugar) and it does not usually cause weight gain when taken alone. However, if you do not eat enough, if you take other medications to lower blood sugar, or if you drink alcohol, you can develop hypoglycemia. Specifically, when FORTAMET™ is taken together with a sulfonylurea or with insulin, hypoglycemia and weight gain are more likely to occur.

Q5. What happens if my blood sugar is still too high?

If your blood sugar is high, consult your physician. When blood sugar cannot be lowered enough by either FORTAMET™ (metformin hydrochloride) Extended-Release Tablets or a sulfonylurea, the two medications can be effective when taken together. Other alternatives involve switching to other oral antidiabetic drugs (e.g., alpha glucoside inhibitors or glitazones). FORTAMET™ may be stopped and replaced with other drugs and/or insulin. If you are unable to maintain your blood sugar with diet, exercise and glucose-control medications taken orally, then your doctor may prescribe injectable insulin to control your diabetes.

Q6. Why should I take FORTAMET in addition to insulin if I am already on insulin alone?

Adding FORTAMET™ to insulin can help you better control your blood sugar while reducing the insulin dose and possibly reducing your weight.

Q7. Can FORTAMET™ cause side effects?

FORTAMET™, like all blood sugar-lowering medications, can cause side effects in some patients. Most of these side effects are minor and will go away after you've taken FORTAMET™ for a while. However, there are also serious but rare side effects related to FORTAMET™ (see below).

Q8. What kind of side effects can FORTAMET™ cause?

If side effects occur, they usually occur during the first few weeks of therapy. They are normally minor ones such as diarrhea, nausea, abdominal pain and upset stomach. FORTAMET™ is generally taken with meals, which reduce these side effects.

Although these side effects are likely to go away, call your doctor if you have severe discomfort or if these effects last for more than a few weeks. Some patients may need to have their doses lowered or stop taking FORTAMET™, either temporarily or permanently. You should tell your doctor if the problems come back or start later on during the therapy.

WARNING: A rare number of people who have taken metformin have developed a serious condition called lactic acidosis. Properly functioning kidneys are needed to help prevent lactic acidosis. You should not take FORTAMET™ if you have impaired kidney function, as measured by a blood test (see Q9-13).

Q9. Are there any serious side effects that FORTAMET™ can cause?

FORTAMET™ rarely causes serious side effects. The most serious side effect that FORTAMET™ can cause is called lactic acidosis.

Q10. What is lactic acidosis and can it happen to me?

Lactic acidosis is caused by a build-up of lactic acid in the blood. Lactic acidosis associated with metformin is rare and has occurred mostly in people whose kidneys were not working normally. Lactic acidosis has been reported in about one in 33,000 patients taking metformin over the course of a year. Although rare, if lactic acidosis does occur, it can be fatal in up to half the cases.

It is also important for your liver to be working normally when you take FORTAMET™. Your liver helps to remove lactic acid from your bloodstream. Your doctor will monitor your diabetes and may perform blood tests on you from time to time to make sure your kidneys and your liver are functioning normally. There is no evidence that FORTAMET™ causes harm to the kidneys or liver.

Q11. Are there other risk factors for lactic acidosis?

Your risk of developing lactic acidosis from taking FORTAMET™ is very low as long as your kidneys and liver are healthy. However, some factors can increase your risk because they can affect kidney and liver function. You should discuss your risk with your physician. You should not take FORTAMET™ if:

- You have some forms of kidney or liver problems
- You have congestive heart failure which is treated with medications, e.g., digoxin (Lanoxin®) or furosemide (Lasix®)
- You drink alcohol excessively (all the time or short-term "binge" drinking)
- You are seriously dehydrated (have lost a large amount of body fluids)
- You are going to have, within a few days, certain x-ray tests with injectable contrast agents
- You are going to have surgery
- You develop a serious condition such as a heart attack, severe infection, or a stroke
- You are 80 years of age or older and have NOT had your kidney function tested

Q12. What are the symptoms of lactic acidosis?

Some of the symptoms include feeling very weak, tired or uncomfortable, unusual muscle pain, trouble breathing, unusual or unexpected stomach discomfort, feeling cold, feeling dizzy or lightheaded, or suddenly developing a slow or irregular heartbeat. If you notice these symptoms, or if your medical condition has suddenly changed, stop taking FORTAMET™ and call your doctor right away. Lactic acidosis is a medical emergency that must be treated in a hospital.

Q13. What does my doctor need to know to decrease my risk of lactic acidosis?

Tell your doctor if you have an illness that results in severe vomiting, diarrhea and/or fever, or if your intake of fluids is generally reduced. These situations can lead to severe dehydration, and it may be necessary to stop taking FORTAMET™ temporarily. You should let your doctor know if you are going to have any surgery or specialized x-ray procedures that require injection of contrast agents. FORTAMET™ therapy will need to be stopped temporarily in such instances.

Q14. Can I take FORTAMET™ with other medications?

Remind your doctor and/or pharmacist that you are taking FORTAMET™ when any new drug is prescribed or a change is made in how you take a drug already prescribed. FORTAMET™ may interfere with the way some drugs work and some drugs may interfere with the action of FORTAMET™.

Q15. What if I become pregnant while taking FORTAMET™?

Tell your doctor if you plan to become pregnant or have become pregnant. As with other oral glucose-control medications, you should not take FORTAMET™ during pregnancy. Usually your doctor will prescribe insulin while you are pregnant.

Q16. How do I take FORTAMET™?

FORTAMET™ tablets should be swallowed whole. FORTAMET™ should not be cut, crushed, or chewed. FORTAMET™ should be taken once a day with food. You will be started on a low dose of FORTAMET™ and your dosage will be increased gradually until your blood sugar is controlled.

Q17. Where can I get more information about FORTAMET™?

This leaflet is a summary of the most important information about FORTAMET™. If you have any questions or problems, you should talk to your doctor or other healthcare provider about type 2 diabetes as well as FORTAMET™ and its side effects.

Distributed by:
Andrx Laboratories, Inc.
Weston, Florida 33331

Manufactured by:
Andrx Pharmaceuticals, Inc.
Ft. Lauderdale, Florida 33314
www.Fortamet.com
Copyright© ANDRX LABS, INC., 2003
7446
Rev. 02/04

To keep your **PDR** up to date throughout the year, note these revisions on the corresponding pages of the annual volume. Simply write **"See Supplement A"** next to the product heading.

AstraZeneca Pharmaceuticals LP
1800 CONCORD PIKE
WILMINGTON, DE 19850-5437 USA

For Product and Business Information, and Adverse Drug Experiences:
Information Center
1-800-236-9933

For Product Ordering:
Trade Customer Service
1-800-842-9920

Internet: www.astrazeneca-us.com

CRESTOR® ℞
[krĕs-tōr]
(rosuvastatin calcium)

DESCRIPTION

CRESTOR® (rosuvastatin calcium) is a synthetic lipid-lowering agent. Rosuvastatin is an inhibitor of 3-hydroxy-3-methylglutaryl-coenzyme A (HMG-CoA) reductase. This enzyme catalyzes the conversion of HMG-CoA to mevalonate, an early and rate-limiting step in cholesterol biosynthesis. Rosuvastatin calcium is bis[(E)-7-[4-(4-fluorophenyl)-6-isopropyl-2-[methyl(methylsulfonyl)amino] pyrimidin-5-yl](3R,5S)-3,5-dihydroxyhept-6-enoic acid] calcium salt. The empirical formula for rosuvastatin calcium is $(C_{22}H_{27}FN_3O_6S)_2Ca$. Its molecular weight is 1001.14. Its structural formula is:

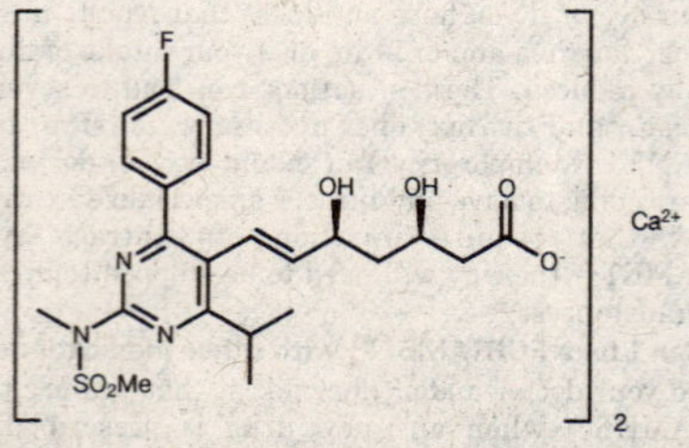

Rosuvastatin calcium is a white amorphous powder that is sparingly soluble in water and methanol, and slightly soluble in ethanol. Rosuvastatin is a hydrophilic compound with a partition coefficient (octanol/water) of 0.13 at pH of 7.0.

CRESTOR Tablets for oral administration contain 5, 10, 20, or 40 mg of rosuvastatin and the following inactive ingredients: microcrystalline cellulose NF, lactose monohydrate NF, tribasic calcium phosphate NF, crospovidone NF, magnesium stearate NF, hypromellose NF, triacetin NF, titanium dioxide USP, yellow ferric oxide, and red ferric oxide NF.

CLINICAL PHARMACOLOGY

General: In the bloodstream, cholesterol and triglycerides (TG) circulate as part of lipoprotein complexes. With ultracentrifugation, these complexes separate into very-low-density lipoprotein (VLDL), intermediate-density lipoprotein (IDL), and low-density lipoprotein (LDL) fractions that contain apolipoprotein B-100 (ApoB-100) and high-density lipoprotein (HDL) fractions.

Cholesterol and TG synthesized in the liver are incorporated into VLDL and secreted into the circulation for delivery to peripheral tissues. TG are removed by the action of lipases, and in a series of steps, the modified VLDL is transformed first into IDL and then into cholesterol-rich LDL. IDL and LDL are removed from the circulation mainly by high affinity ApoB/E receptors, which are expressed to the greatest extent on liver cells. HDL is hypothesized to participate in the reverse transport of cholesterol from tissues back to the liver.

Epidemiologic, experimental, and clinical studies have established that high LDL cholesterol (LDL-C), low HDL cholesterol (HDL-C), and high plasma TG promote human atherosclerosis and are risk factors for developing cardiovascular disease. In contrast, higher levels of HDL-C are associated with decreased cardiovascular risk.

Like LDL, cholesterol-enriched triglyceride-rich lipoproteins, including VLDL, IDL, and remnants, can also promote atherosclerosis. Elevated plasma triglycerides are frequently found with low HDL-C levels and small LDL particles, as well as in association with non-lipid metabolic risk factors for coronary heart disease (CHD). As such, total plasma TG has not consistently been shown to be an independent risk factor for CHD. Furthermore, the independent effect of raising HDL or lowering TG on the risk of coronary and cardiovascular morbidity and mortality has not been determined.

Mechanism of Action: Rosuvastatin is a selective and competitive inhibitor of HMG-CoA reductase, the rate-limiting enzyme that converts 3-hydroxy-3-methylglutaryl coenzyme A to mevalonate, a precursor of cholesterol. *In vivo* studies in animals, and *in vitro* studies in cultured animal and human cells have shown rosuvastatin to have a high uptake into, and selectivity for, action in the liver, the target organ for cholesterol lowering. In *in vivo* and *in vitro* studies, rosuvastatin produces its lipid-modifying effects in two ways. First, it increases the number of hepatic LDL receptors on the cell-surface to enhance uptake and catabolism of LDL. Second, rosuvastatin inhibits hepatic synthesis of VLDL, which reduces the total number of VLDL and LDL particles.

Rosuvastatin reduces total cholesterol (total-C), LDL-C, ApoB, and nonHDL-C (total cholesterol minus HDL-C) in patients with homozygous and heterozygous familial hypercholesterolemia (FH), nonfamilial forms of hypercholesterolemia, and mixed dyslipidemia. Rosuvastatin also reduces TG and produces increases in HDL-C. Rosuvastatin reduces total-C, LDL-C, VLDL-cholesterol (VLDL-C), ApoB, nonHDL-C, and TG, and increases HDL-C in patients with isolated hypertriglyceridemia. The effect of rosuvastatin on cardiovascular morbidity and mortality has not been determined.

Pharmacokinetics and Drug Metabolism

Absorption: In clinical pharmacology studies in man, peak plasma concentrations of rosuvastatin were reached 3 to 5 hours following oral dosing. Both peak concentration (C_{max}) and area under the plasma concentration-time curve (AUC) increased in approximate proportion to rosuvastatin dose. The absolute bioavailability of rosuvastatin is approximately 20%.

Administration of rosuvastatin with food decreased the rate of drug absorption by 20% as assessed by C_{max}, but there was no effect on the extent of absorption as assessed by AUC.

Plasma concentrations of rosuvastatin do not differ following evening or morning drug administration.

Significant LDL-C reductions are seen when rosuvastatin is given with or without food, and regardless of the time of day of drug administration.

Distribution: Mean volume of distribution at steady-state of rosuvastatin is approximately 134 liters. Rosuvastatin is 88% bound to plasma proteins, mostly albumin. This binding is reversible and independent of plasma concentrations.

Metabolism: Rosuvastatin is not extensively metabolized; approximately 10% of a radiolabeled dose is recovered as metabolite. The major metabolite is N-desmethyl rosuvastatin, which is formed principally by cytochrome P450 2C9, and *in vitro* studies have demonstrated that N-desmethyl rosuvastatin has approximately one-sixth to one-half the HMG-CoA reductase inhibitory activity of rosuvastatin. Overall, greater than 90% of active plasma HMG-CoA reductase inhibitory activity is accounted for by rosuvastatin.

Excretion: Following oral administration, rosuvastatin and its metabolites are primarily excreted in the feces (90%). The elimination half-life ($t_{1/2}$) of rosuvastatin is approximately 19 hours.

After an intravenous dose, approximately 28% of total body clearance was via the renal route, and 72% by the hepatic route.

Special Populations

Race: A population pharmacokinetic analysis revealed no clinically relevant differences in pharmacokinetics among Caucasian, Hispanic, and Black or Afro-Caribbean groups. However, pharmacokinetic studies show an approximate 2-fold elevation in median exposure (AUC) in Japanese subjects residing in Japan and in Chinese subjects residing in Singapore when compared with Caucasians residing in North America and Europe. No studies directly examining Asian ethnic populations residing in the U.S. are available, so the contribution of environmental and genetic factors to the observed increases in rosuvastatin drug levels have not been determined. (See WARNINGS, Myopathy/Rhabdomyolysis, and PRECAUTIONS, General.)

Gender: There were no differences in plasma concentrations of rosuvastatin between men and women.

Geriatric: There were no differences in plasma concentrations of rosuvastatin between the nonelderly and elderly populations (age ≥65 years).

Pediatric: In a pharmacokinetic study, 18 patients (9 boys and 9 girls) 10 to 17 years of age with heterozygous FH received single and multiple oral doses of rosuvastatin. Both C_{max} and AUC of rosuvastatin were similar to values observed in adult subjects administered the same doses.

Renal Insufficiency: Mild to moderate renal impairment (creatinine clearance ≥30 mL/min/1.73m^2) had no influence on plasma concentrations of rosuvastatin when oral doses of 20 mg rosuvastatin were administered for 14 days. However, plasma concentrations of rosuvastatin increased to a clinically significant extent (about 3-fold) in patients with severe renal impairment (CL_{cr} < 30 mL/min/1.73m^2) compared with healthy subjects (CL_{cr} > 80 mL/min/1.73m^2) (see PRECAUTIONS, General).

Hemodialysis: Steady-state plasma concentrations of rosuvastatin in patients on chronic hemodialysis were approximately 50% greater compared with healthy volunteer subjects with normal renal function.

Hepatic Insufficiency: In patients with chronic alcohol liver disease, plasma concentrations of rosuvastatin were modestly increased. In patients with Child-Pugh A disease, C_{max} and AUC were increased by 60% and 5%, respectively, as compared with patients with normal liver function. In patients with Child-Pugh B disease, C_{max} and AUC were increased 100% and 21%, respectively, compared with patients with normal liver function (see CONTRAINDICATIONS and WARNINGS, Liver Enzymes).

Drug-Drug Interactions

Cytochrome P450 3A4: *In vitro* and *in vivo* data indicate that rosuvastatin clearance is not dependent on metabolism by cytochrome P450 3A4 to a clinically significant extent. This has been confirmed in studies with known cytochrome P450 3A4 inhibitors (ketoconazole, erythromycin, itraconazole).

Ketoconazole: Coadministration of ketoconazole (200 mg twice daily for 7 days) with rosuvastatin (80 mg) resulted in no change in plasma concentrations of rosuvastatin.

Erythromycin: Coadministration of erythromycin (500 mg four times daily for 7 days) with rosuvastatin (80 mg) decreased AUC and C_{max} of rosuvastatin by 20% and 31%, respectively. These reductions are not considered clinically significant.

Itraconazole: Itraconazole (200 mg once daily for 5 days) resulted in a 39% and 28% increase in AUC of rosuvastatin after 10 mg and 80 mg dosing, respectively. These increases are not considered clinically significant.

Fluconazole: Coadministration of fluconazole (200 mg once daily for 11 days) with rosuvastatin (80 mg) resulted in a 14% increase in AUC of rosuvastatin. This increase is not considered clinically significant.

Cyclosporine: Coadministration of cyclosporine with rosuvastatin resulted in no significant changes in cyclosporine plasma concentrations. However, C_{max} and AUC of rosuvastatin increased 11- and 7-fold, respectively, compared with historical data in healthy subjects. These increases are considered to be clinically significant (see PRECAUTIONS, Drug Interactions, WARNINGS, Myopathy/Rhabdomyolysis, and DOSAGE AND ADMINISTRATION).

Warfarin: Coadministration of warfarin (20 mg) with rosuvastatin (40 mg) did not change warfarin plasma concentrations but increased the International Normalized Ratio (INR) (see PRECAUTIONS, Drug Interactions).

Digoxin: Coadministration of digoxin (0.5 mg) with rosuvastatin (40 mg) resulted in no change to digoxin plasma concentrations.

Fenofibrate: Coadministration of fenofibrate (67 mg three times daily) with rosuvastatin (10 mg) resulted in no significant changes in plasma concentrations of rosuvastatin or fenofibrate (see PRECAUTIONS, Drug Interactions and WARNINGS, Myopathy/Rhabdomyolysis).

Gemfibrozil: Coadministration of gemfibrozil (600 mg twice daily for 7 days) with rosuvastatin (80 mg) resulted in a 90% and 120% increase for AUC and C_{max} of rosuvastatin, respectively. This increase is considered to be clinically significant (see PRECAUTIONS, Drug Interactions, WARNINGS, Myopathy/Rhabdomyolysis, DOSAGE AND ADMINISTRATION).

Antacid: Coadministration of an antacid (aluminum and magnesium hydroxide combination) with rosuvastatin (40 mg) resulted in a decrease in plasma concentrations of rosuvastatin by 54%. However, when the antacid was given 2 hours after rosuvastatin, there were no clinically significant changes in plasma concentrations of rosuvastatin (see PRECAUTIONS, Information for Patients).

Oral contraceptives: Coadministration of oral contraceptives (ethinyl estradiol and norgestrel) with rosuvastatin resulted in an increase in plasma concentrations of ethinyl estradiol and norgestrel by 26% and 34%, respectively.

Clinical Studies

Hypercholesterolemia (Heterozygous Familial and Nonfamilial) and Mixed Dyslipidemia (Fredrickson Type IIa and IIb)

CRESTOR reduces total-C, LDL-C, ApoB, nonHDL-C, and TG, and increases HDL-C, in patients with hypercholesterolemia and mixed dyslipidemia. Therapeutic response is seen within 1 week, and maximum response is usually achieved within 4 weeks and maintained during long-term therapy.

CRESTOR is effective in a wide variety of adult patient populations with hypercholesterolemia, with and without hypertriglyceridemia, regardless of race, gender, or age and in special populations such as diabetics or patients with heterozygous FH. Experience in pediatric patients has been limited to patients with homozygous FH.

Dose-Ranging Study: In a multicenter, double-blind, placebo-controlled, dose-ranging study in patients with hypercholesterolemia, CRESTOR given as a single daily dose for 6 weeks significantly reduced total-C, LDL-C, nonHDL-C, and ApoB, across the dose range (Table 1).

Table 1.
Dose-Response in Patients With Primary Hypercholesterolemia (Adjusted Mean % Change From Baseline at Week 6)

Dose	N	Total-C	LDL-C	Non HDL-C	ApoB	TG	HDL-C
Placebo	13	-5	-7	-7	-3	-3	3
5	17	-33	-45	-44	-38	-35	13
10	17	-36	-52	-48	-42	-10	14
20	17	-40	-55	-51	-46	-23	8
40	18	-46	-63	-60	-54	-28	10

Active-Controlled Study: CRESTOR was compared with the HMG-CoA reductase inhibitors atorvastatin, simvastatin, and pravastatin in a multicenter, open-label, dose-ranging study of 2,240 patients with Type IIa and IIb hypercholesterolemia. After randomization, patients were treated for 6 weeks with a single daily dose of either CRESTOR, atorvastatin, simvastatin, or pravastatin (Figure 1 and Table 2).

Figure 1.
Percent LDL-C Change by Dose of CRESTOR, Atorvastatin, Simvastatin, and Pravastatin at Week 6 in Patients With Type IIa/IIb Dyslipidemia

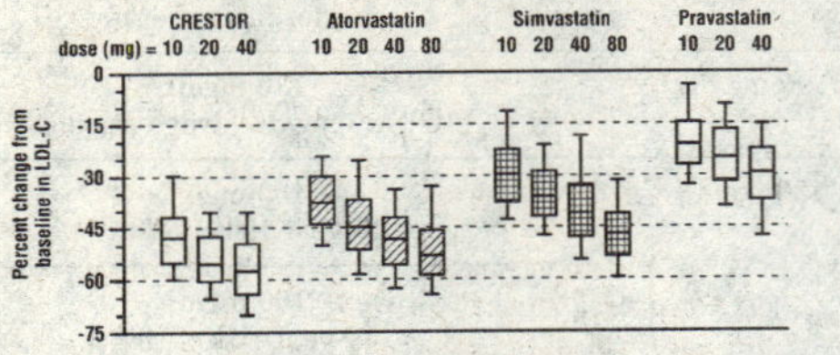

Box plots are a representation of the 25th, 50th, and 75th percentile values, with whiskers representing the 10th and 90th percentile values. Mean baseline LDL-C: 189 mg/dL.

Table 2.
Percent Change in LDL-C From Baseline to Week 6 (LS means§) by Treatment Group (sample sizes ranging from 156-157 patients per group)

Treatment	Treatment Daily Dose 10 mg	20 mg	40 mg	80 mg
CRESTOR	-46*	-52†	-55‡	—
Atorvastatin	-37	-43	-48	-51
Pravastatin	-20	-24	-30	—
Simvastatin	-28	-35	-39	-46

*CRESTOR 10 mg reduced LDL-C significantly more than atorvastatin 10 mg; pravastatin 10 mg, 20 mg, and 40 mg; simvastatin 10 mg, 20 mg, and 40 mg. ($p<0.002$)
† CRESTOR 20 mg reduced LDL-C significantly more than atorvastatin 20 mg and 40 mg; pravastatin 20 mg, and 40 mg; simvastatin 20 mg, 40 mg, and 80 mg. ($p<0.002$)
‡ CRESTOR 40 mg reduced LDL-C significantly more than atorvastatin 40 mg; pravastatin 40 mg; simvastatin 40 mg and 80 mg. ($p<0.002$)
§ Corresponding standard errors are approximately 1.00

Heterozygous Familial Hypercholesterolemia

In a study of patients with heterozygous FH (baseline mean LDL of 291), patients were randomized to CRESTOR 20 mg or atorvastatin 20 mg. The dose was increased by 6-week intervals. Significant LDL-C reductions from baseline were seen at each dose in both treatment groups (Table 3).

Table 3.
Mean LDL-C Percentage Change from Baseline

		CRESTOR (n=435) LS Mean* (95% CI)	Atorvastatin (n=187) LS Mean (95% CI)
Week 6	20 mg	-47% (-49%, -46%)	-38% (-40%, -36%)
Week 12	40 mg	-55% (-57%, -54%)	-47% (-49%, -45%)
Week 18	80 mg	NA	-52% (-54%, -50%)

*LS Means are least square means adjusted for baseline LDL.

Hypertriglyceridemia
(Fredrickson Type IIb & IV)

In a double-blind, placebo-controlled dose-response study in patients with baseline TG levels from 273 to 817 mg/dL, CRESTOR given as a single daily dose (5 to 40 mg) over 6 weeks significantly reduced serum TG levels (Table 4).
[See table 4 above]

Homozygous Familial Hypercholesterolemia

In an open-label, forced-titration study, homozygous FH patients (n=40, 8-63 years) were evaluated for their response to CRESTOR 20 to 40 mg titrated at a 6-week interval. In the overall population, the mean LDL-C reduction from baseline was 22%. About one-third of the patients benefited from increasing their dose from 20 mg to 40 mg with further LDL lowering of greater than 6%. In the 27 patients with at least a 15% reduction in LDL-C, the mean LDL-C reduction was 30% (median 28% reduction). Among 13 patients with an LDL-C reduction of <15%, 3 had no change or an increase in LDL-C. Reductions in LDL-C of 15% or greater were observed in 3 of 5 patients with known receptor negative status.

INDICATIONS AND USAGE

CRESTOR is indicated:

1. as an adjunct to diet to reduce elevated total-C, LDL-C, ApoB, nonHDL-C, and TG levels and to increase HDL-C in patients with primary hypercholesterolemia (heterozygous familial and nonfamilial) and mixed dyslipidemia (Fredrickson Type IIa and IIb);
2. as an adjunct to diet for the treatment of patients with elevated serum TG levels (Fredrickson Type IV);
3. to reduce LDL-C, total-C, and ApoB in patients with homozygous familial hypercholesterolemia as an adjunct to other lipid-lowering treatments (e.g., LDL apheresis) or if such treatments are unavailable.

According to NCEP-ATPIII guidelines, therapy with lipid-altering agents should be a component of multiple-risk-factor intervention in individuals at increased risk for coronary heart disease due to hypercholesterolemia. The two major modalities of LDL-lowering therapy are therapeutic lifestyle changes (TLC) and drug therapy. The TLC Diet stresses reductions in saturated fat and cholesterol intake. Table 5 defines LDL-C goals and cutpoints for initiation of TLC and for drug consideration.

Table 4.
Dose-Response in Patients With Primary Hypertriglyceridemia Over 6 Weeks Dosing Median (Min, Max) Percent Change From Baseline

Dose	Placebo N=26	CRESTOR 5 mg N=25	CRESTOR 10 mg N=23	CRESTOR 20 mg N=27	CRESTOR 40 mg N=25
Triglycerides	1 (-40, 72)	-21 (-58, 38)	-37 (-65, 5)	-37 (-72, 11)	-43 (-80, -7)
NonHDL-C	2 (-13, 19)	-29 (-43, -8)	-49 (-59, -20)	-43 (-74, 12)	-51 (-62, -6)
VLDL-C	2 (-36, 53)	-25 (-62, 49)	-48 (-72, 14)	-49 (-83, 20)	-56 (-83, 10)
Total-C	1 (-13, 17)	-24 (-40, -4)	-40 (-51, -14)	-34 (-61, -11)	-40 (-51, -4)
LDL-C	5 (-30, 52)	-28 (-71, 2)	-45 (-59, 7)	-31 (-66, 34)	-43 (-61, -3)
HDL-C	-3 (-25, 18)	3 (-38, 33)	8 (-8, 24)	22 (-5, 50)	17 (-14, 63)

[See table 5 at top of next page]

After the LDL-C goal has been achieved, if the TG is still ≥ 200 mg/dL, nonHDL-C (total-C minus HDL-C) becomes a secondary target of therapy. NonHDL-C goals are set 30 mg/dL higher than LDL-C goals for each risk category.
At the time of hospitalization for a coronary event, consideration can be given to initiating drug therapy at discharge if the LDL-C is ≥ 130 mg/dL (see NCEP Treatment Guidelines, above).
Patients >20 years of age should be screened for elevated cholesterol levels every 5 years.
Prior to initiating therapy with CRESTOR, secondary causes for hypercholesterolemia (e.g., poorly-controlled diabetes mellitus, hypothyroidism, nephrotic syndrome, dysproteinemias, obstructive liver disease, other drug therapy, and alcoholism) should be excluded, and a lipid profile performed to measure total-C, LDL-C, HDL-C, and TG. For patients with TG <400 mg/dL (<4.5 mmol/L), LDL-C can be estimated using the following equation: LDL-C = total-C - (0.20 × [TG] + HDL-C). For TG levels >400 mg/dL (>4.5 mmol/L), this equation is less accurate and LDL-C concentrations should be determined by ultracentrifugation.
CRESTOR has not been studied in Fredrickson Type I, III, and V dyslipidemias.

CONTRAINDICATIONS

CRESTOR is contraindicated in patients with a known hypersensitivity to any component of this product.
Rosuvastatin is contraindicated in patients with active liver disease or with unexplained persistent elevations of serum transaminases (see WARNINGS, Liver Enzymes).

Pregnancy and Lactation

Atherosclerosis is a chronic process and discontinuation of lipid-lowering drugs during pregnancy should have little impact on the outcome of long-term therapy of primary hypercholesterolemia. Cholesterol and other products of cholesterol biosynthesis are essential components for fetal development (including synthesis of steroids and cell membranes). Since HMG-CoA reductase inhibitors decrease cholesterol synthesis and possibly the synthesis of other biologically active substances derived from cholesterol, they may cause fetal harm when administered to pregnant women. Therefore, HMG-CoA reductase inhibitors are contraindicated during pregnancy and in nursing mothers. ROSUVASTATIN SHOULD BE ADMINISTERED TO WOMEN OF CHILDBEARING AGE ONLY WHEN SUCH PATIENTS ARE HIGHLY UNLIKELY TO CONCEIVE AND HAVE BEEN INFORMED OF THE POTENTIAL HAZARDS. If the patient becomes pregnant while taking this drug, therapy should be discontinued immediately and the patient apprised of the potential hazard to the fetus.

WARNINGS

Liver Enzymes

HMG-CoA reductase inhibitors, like some other lipid-lowering therapies, have been associated with biochemical abnormalities of liver function. The incidence of persistent elevations (>3 times the upper limit of normal [ULN] occurring on 2 or more consecutive occasions) in serum transaminases in fixed dose studies was 0.4, 0, 0, and 0.1% in patients who received rosuvastatin 5, 10, 20, and 40 mg, respectively. In most cases, the elevations were transient and resolved or improved on continued therapy or after a brief interruption in therapy. There were two cases of jaundice, for which a relationship to rosuvastatin therapy could not be determined, which resolved after discontinuation of therapy. There were no cases of liver failure or irreversible liver disease in these trials.
It is recommended that liver function tests be performed before and at 12 weeks following both the initiation of therapy and any elevation of dose, and periodically (e.g., semiannually) thereafter. Liver enzyme changes generally occur in the first 3 months of treatment with rosuvastatin. Patients who develop increased transaminase levels should be monitored until the abnormalities have resolved. Should an increase in ALT or AST of >3 times ULN persist, reduction of dose or withdrawal of rosuvastatin is recommended.
Rosuvastatin should be used with caution in patients who consume substantial quantities of alcohol and/or have a history of liver disease (see CLINICAL PHARMACOLOGY, Special Populations, Hepatic Insufficiency). Active liver disease or unexplained persistent transaminase elevations are contraindications to the use of rosuvastatin (see CONTRAINDICATIONS).

Myopathy/Rhabdomyolysis

Rare cases of rhabdomyolysis with acute renal failure secondary to myoglobinuria have been reported with rosuvastatin and with other drugs in this class.
Uncomplicated myalgia has been reported in rosuvastatin-treated patients (see ADVERSE REACTIONS). Creatine kinase (CK) elevations (>10 times upper limit of normal) occurred in 0.2% to 0.4% of patients taking rosuvastatin at doses up to 40 mg in clinical studies. Treatment-related myopathy, defined as muscle aches or muscle weakness in conjunction with increases in CK values >10 times upper limit of normal, was reported in up to 0.1% of patients taking rosuvastatin doses of up to 40 mg in clinical studies. Rare cases of rhabdomyolysis were seen with higher than recommended doses (80 mg) of rosuvastatin in clinical trials. Factors that may predispose patients to myopathy with HMG-CoA reductase inhibitors include advanced age (≥65 years), hypothyroidism, and renal insufficiency. The incidence of myopathy increased at doses of rosuvastatin above the recommended dosage range.
Consequently:

1. Rosuvastatin should be prescribed with caution in patients with predisposing factors for myopathy, such as, renal impairment (see DOSAGE AND ADMINISTRATION), advanced age, and hypothyroidism.
2. Patients should be advised to promptly report unexplained muscle pain, tenderness, or weakness, particularly if accompanied by malaise or fever. Rosuvastatin therapy should be discontinued if markedly elevated CK levels occur or myopathy is diagnosed or suspected.
3. The risk of myopathy during treatment with rosuvastatin may be increased with concurrent administration of other lipid-lowering therapies or cyclosporine, (see CLINICAL PHARMACOLOGY, Drug Interactions, PRECAUTIONS, Drug Interactions, and DOSAGE AND ADMINISTRATION). **The benefit of further alterations in lipid levels by the combined use of rosuvastatin with fibrates or niacin should be carefully weighed against the potential risks of this combination. Combination therapy with rosuvastatin and gemfibrozil should generally be avoided. (See DOSAGE AND ADMINISTRATION and PRECAUTIONS, Drug Interactions).**
4. **The risk of myopathy during treatment with rosuvastatin may be increased in circumstances which increase rosuvastatin drug levels (see CLINICAL PHARMACOLOGY, Special Populations, Race and Renal Insufficiency, and PRECAUTIONS, General).**
5. **Rosuvastatin therapy should also be temporarily withheld in any patient with an acute, serious condition suggestive of myopathy or predisposing to the development of renal failure secondary to rhabdomyolysis (e.g., sepsis, hypotension, major surgery, trauma, severe metabolic, endocrine, and electrolyte disorders, or uncontrolled seizures).**

PRECAUTIONS

General

Before instituting therapy with rosuvastatin, an attempt should be made to control hypercholesterolemia with appropriate diet and exercise, weight reduction in obese patients, and treatment of underlying medical problems (see INDICATIONS AND USAGE).
Administration of rosuvastatin 20 mg to patients with severe renal impairment (CL_{cr} <30 mL/min/1.73 m^2) resulted in a 3-fold increase in plasma concentrations of rosuvastatin compared with healthy volunteers (see WARNINGS, Myopathy/Rhabdomyolysis and DOSAGE AND ADMINISTRATION).
Pharmacokinetic studies show an approximate 2-fold elevation in median exposure in Japanese subjects residing in Japan and in Chinese subjects residing in Singapore compared with Caucasians residing in North America and Europe. The contribution of environmental and genetic factors to the difference observed has not been determined. However, these increases should be considered when making rosuvastatin dosing decisions for patients of Japanese and Chinese ancestry. (See WARNINGS Myopathy/Rhabdomyolysis; CLINICAL PHARMACOLOGY, Special Populations, Race.)

Information for Patients

Patients should be advised to report promptly unexplained muscle pain, tenderness, or weakness, particularly if accompanied by malaise or fever.
When taking rosuvastatin with an aluminum and magnesium hydroxide combination antacid, the antacid should be taken at least 2 hours after rosuvastatin administration (see CLINICAL PHARMACOLOGY, Drug Interactions).

Laboratory Tests

In the rosuvastatin clinical trial program, dipstick-positive proteinuria and microscopic hematuria were observed among rosuvastatin treated patients, predominantly in patients dosed above the recommended dose range (i.e., 80 mg). However, this finding was more frequent in patients taking rosuvastatin 40 mg, when compared to lower doses of rosuvastatin or comparator statins, though it was generally transient and was not associated with worsening renal function. Although the clinical significance of this finding is unknown, a dose reduction should be considered for patients on rosuvastatin 40 mg therapy with unexplained persistent proteinuria during routine urinalysis testing.

Continued on next page

Crestor—Cont.

Drug Interactions

Cyclosporine: When rosuvastatin 10 mg was coadministered with cyclosporine in cardiac transplant patients, rosuvastatin mean C_{max} and mean AUC were increased 11-fold and 7-fold, respectively, compared with healthy volunteers. These increases are considered to be clinically significant and require special consideration in the dosing of rosuvastatin to patients taking concomitant cyclosporine (see WARNINGS, Myopathy/Rhabdomyolysis, and DOSAGE AND ADMINISTRATION).

Warfarin: Coadministration of rosuvastatin to patients on stable warfarin therapy resulted in clinically significant rises in INR (>4, baseline 2-3). In patients taking coumarin anticoagulants and rosuvastatin concomitantly, INR should be determined before starting rosuvastatin and frequently enough during early therapy to ensure that no significant alteration of INR occurs. Once a stable INR time has been documented, INR can be monitored at the intervals usually recommended for patients on coumarin anticoagulants. If the dose of rosuvastatin is changed, the same procedure should be repeated. Rosuvastatin therapy has not been associated with bleeding or with changes in INR in patients not taking anticoagulants.

Gemfibrozil: Coadministration of a single rosuvastatin dose to healthy volunteers on gemfibrozil (600 mg twice daily) resulted in 2.2- and 1.9-fold, respectively, increase in mean C_{max} and mean AUC of rosuvastatin (see DOSAGE AND ADMINISTRATION).

Endocrine Function

Although clinical studies have shown that rosuvastatin alone does not reduce basal plasma cortisol concentration or impair adrenal reserve, caution should be exercised if any HMG-CoA reductase inhibitor or other agent used to lower cholesterol levels is administered concomitantly with drugs that may decrease the levels or activity of endogenous steroid hormones such as ketoconazole, spironolactone, and cimetidine.

CNS Toxicity

CNS vascular lesions, characterized by perivascular hemorrhages, edema, and mononuclear cell infiltration of perivascular spaces, have been observed in dogs treated with several other members of this drug class. A chemically similar drug in this class produced dose-dependent optic nerve degeneration (Wallerian degeneration of retinogeniculate fibers) in dogs, at a dose that produced plasma drug levels about 30 times higher than the mean drug level in humans taking the highest recommended dose. Edema, hemorrhage, and partial necrosis in the interstitium of the choroid plexus was observed in a female dog sacrificed moribund at day 24 at 90 mg/kg/day by oral gavage (systemic exposures 100 times the human exposure at 40 mg/day based on AUC comparisons). Corneal opacity was seen in dogs treated for 52 weeks at 6 mg/kg/day by oral gavage (systemic exposures 20 times the human exposure at 40 mg/day based on AUC comparisons). Cataracts were seen in dogs treated for 12 weeks by oral gavage at 30 mg/kg/day (systemic exposures 60 times the human exposure at 40 mg/day based on AUC comparisons). Retinal dysplasia and retinal loss were seen in dogs treated for 4 weeks by oral gavage at 90 mg/kg/day (systemic exposures 100 times the human exposure at 40 mg/day based on AUC). Doses ≤30 mg/kg/day (systemic exposures ≤60 times the human exposure at 40 mg/day based on AUC comparisons) following treatment up to one year, did not reveal retinal findings.

Carcinogenesis, Mutagenesis, Impairment of Fertility

In a 104-week carcinogenicity study in rats at dose levels of 2, 20, 60, or 80 mg/kg/day by oral gavage, the incidence of uterine stromal polyps was significantly increased in females at 80 mg/kg/day at systemic exposure 20 times the human exposure at 40 mg/day based on AUC. Increased incidence of polyps was not seen at lower doses.

In a 107-week carcinogenicity study in mice given 10, 60, 200 mg/kg/day by oral gavage, an increased incidence of hepatocellular adenoma/carcinoma was observed at 200 mg/kg/day at systemic exposures 20 times human exposure at 40 mg/day based on AUC. An increased incidence of hepatocellular tumors was not seen at lower doses.

Rosuvastatin was not mutagenic or clastogenic with or without metabolic activation in the Ames test with *Salmonella typhimurium* and *Escherichia coli*, the mouse lymphoma assay, and the chromosomal aberration assay in Chinese hamster lung cells. Rosuvastatin was negative in the *in vivo* mouse micronucleus test.

In rat fertility studies with oral gavage doses of 5, 15, 50 mg/kg/day, males were treated for 9 weeks prior to and throughout mating and females were treated 2 weeks prior to mating and throughout mating until gestation day 7. No adverse effect on fertility was observed at 50 mg/kg/day (systemic exposures up to 10 times human exposure at 40 mg/day based on AUC comparisons). In testicles of dogs treated with rosuvastatin at 30 mg/kg/day for one month, spermatidic giant cells were seen. Spermatidic giant cells were observed in monkeys after 6-month treatment at 30 mg/kg/day in addition to vacuolation of seminiferous tubular epithelium. Exposures in the dog were 20 times and in the monkey 10 times human exposure at 40 mg/day based on body surface area comparisons. Similar findings have been seen with other drugs in this class.

Pregnancy

Pregnancy Category X

See CONTRAINDICATIONS.

Table 5.
NCEP Treatment Guidelines: LDL-C Goals and Cutpoints for Therapeutic Lifestyle Changes and Drug Therapy in Different Risk Categories

Risk Category	LDL Goal	LDL level at which to initiate TLC	LDL level at which to consider drug therapy
CHD[a] or CHD Risk Equivalent (10-year risk > 20%)	<100 mg/dL	≥100 mg/dL	≥130 mg/dL (100-129 mg/dL: drug optional)[c]
2+ Risk Factors (10-year risk ≤ 20%)	<130 mg/dL	≥ 130 mg/dL	≥130 mg/dL 10-year risk 10-20%
			≥160 mg/dL 10-year risk <10%
0-1 Risk Factor[b]	<160 mg/dL	≥160 mg/dL	≥190 mg/dL (160-189 mg/dL (LDL-lowering drug optional)

[a] CHD = coronary heart disease.
[b] Some authorities recommend use of LDL-lowering drugs in this category if an LDL-C <100 mg/dL cannot be achieved by TLC. Others prefer use of drugs that primarily modify triglycerides and HDL-C, e.g., nicotinic acid or fibrate. Clinical judgment also may call for deferring drug therapy in this subcategory.
[c] Almost all people with 0-1 risk factor have 10-year risk <10%; thus, 10-year risk assessment in people with 0-1 risk factor is not necessary.

Rosuvastatin may cause fetal harm when administered to a pregnant woman. Rosuvastatin is contraindicated in women who are or may become pregnant. Safety in pregnant women has not been established. There are no adequate and well-controlled studies of rosuvastatin in pregnant women. Rosuvastatin crosses the placenta and is found in fetal tissue and amniotic fluid at 3% and 20%, respectively, of the maternal plasma concentration following a single 25 mg/kg oral gavage dose on gestation day 16 in rats. A higher fetal tissue distribution (25% maternal plasma concentration) was observed in rabbits after a single oral gavage dose of 1 mg/kg on gestation day 18. If this drug is administered to a woman with reproductive potential, the patient should be apprised of the potential hazard to a fetus.

In female rats given oral gavage doses of 5, 15, 50 mg/kg/day rosuvastatin before mating and continuing through day 7 postcoitus results in decreased fetal body weight (female pups) and delayed ossification at the high dose (systemic exposures 10 times human exposure at 40 mg/day based on AUC comparisons).

In pregnant rats given oral gavage doses of 2, 20, 50 mg/kg/day from gestation day 7 through lactation day 21 (weaning), decreased pup survival occurred in groups given 50 mg/kg/day, systemic exposures ≥12 times human exposure at 40 mg/day based on body surface area comparisons.

In pregnant rabbits given oral gavage doses of 0.3, 1, 3 mg/kg/day from gestation day 6 to lactation day 18 (weaning), exposures equivalent to human exposure at 40 mg/day based on body surface area comparisons, decreased fetal viability and maternal mortality was observed.

Rosuvastatin was not teratogenic in rats at ≤25 mg/kg/day or in rabbits ≤3 mg/kg/day (systemic exposures equivalent to human exposure at 40 mg/day based on AUC or body surface comparison, respectively).

Nursing Mothers

It is not known whether rosuvastatin is excreted in human milk. Studies in lactating rats have demonstrated that rosuvastatin is secreted into breast milk at levels 3 times higher than that obtained in the plasma following oral gavage dosing. Because many drugs are excreted in human milk and because of the potential for serious adverse reactions in nursing infants from rosuvastatin, a decision should be made whether to discontinue nursing or administration of rosuvastatin taking into account the importance of the drug to the lactating woman.

Pediatric Use

The safety and effectiveness in pediatric patients have not been established. Treatment experience with rosuvastatin in a pediatric population is limited to 8 patients with homozygous FH. None of these patients was below 8 years of age.

Geriatric Use

Of the 10,275 patients in clinical studies with rosuvastatin, 3,159 (31%) were 65 years and older, and 698 (6.8%) were 75 years and older. The overall frequency of adverse events and types of adverse events were similar in patients above and below 65 years of age. (See WARNINGS, Myopathy/Rhabdomyolysis.)

The efficacy of rosuvastatin in the geriatric population (≥65 years of age) was comparable to the efficacy observed in the non-elderly.

ADVERSE REACTIONS

Rosuvastatin is generally well tolerated. Adverse reactions have usually been mild and transient. In clinical studies of 10,275 patients, 3.7% were discontinued due to adverse experiences attributable to rosuvastatin.

The most frequent adverse events thought to be related to rosuvastatin were myalgia, constipation, asthenia, abdominal pain, and nausea.

Clinical Adverse Experiences

Adverse experiences, regardless of causality assessment, reported in ≥2% of patients in placebo-controlled clinical studies of rosuvastatin are shown in Table 6; discontinuations due to adverse events in these studies of up to 12 weeks duration occurred in 3% of patients on rosuvastatin and 5% on placebo.

Table 6. Adverse Events in Placebo-Controlled Studies

Adverse Event	Rosuvastatin N=744	Placebo N=382
Pharyngitis	9.0	7.6
Headache	5.5	5.0
Diarrhea	3.4	2.9
Dyspepsia	3.4	3.1
Nausea	3.4	3.1
Myalgia	2.8	1.3
Asthenia	2.7	2.6
Back Pain	2.6	2.4
Flu syndrome	2.3	1.8
Urinary tract infection	2.3	1.6
Rhinitis	2.2	2.1
Sinusitis	2.0	1.8

In addition, the following adverse events were reported, regardless of causality assessment, in ≥1% of 10,275 patients treated with rosuvastatin in clinical studies. The events in *italics* occurred in ≥2% of these patients.

Body as a Whole: *Abdominal pain, accidental injury, chest pain, infection, pain*, pelvic pain, and neck pain.

Cardiovascular System: *Hypertension*, angina pectoris, vasodilatation, and palpitation.

Digestive System: *Constipation, gastroenteritis*, vomiting, flatulence, periodontal abscess, and gastritis.

Endocrine: Diabetes mellitus.

Hemic and Lymphatic System: Anemia and ecchymosis.

Metabolic and Nutritional Disorders: *Peripheral edema*.

Musculoskeletal System: *Arthritis, arthralgia*, and pathological fracture.

Nervous System: *Dizziness, insomnia, hypertonia, paresthesia, depression*, anxiety, vertigo and neuralgia.

Respiratory System: *Bronchitis, cough increased*, dyspnea, pneumonia, and asthma.

Skin and Appendages: *Rash* and pruritus.

Laboratory Abnormalities: In the rosuvastatin clinical trial program, dipstick-positive proteinuria and microscopic hematuria were observed among rosuvastatin-treated patients, predominantly in patients dosed above the recommended dose range (i.e., 80 mg). However, this finding was more frequent in patients taking rosuvastatin 40 mg, when compared to lower doses of rosuvastatin or comparator statins, though it was generally transient and was not associated with worsening renal function. (See PRECAUTIONS, Laboratory Tests.)

Other abnormal laboratory values reported were elevated creatinine phosphokinase, transaminases, hyperglycemia, glutamyl transpeptidase, alkaline phosphatase, bilirubin, and thyroid function abnormalities.

Other adverse events reported less frequently than 1% in the rosuvastatin clinical study program, regardless of causality assessment, included arrhythmia, hepatitis, hypersensitivity reactions (i.e., face edema, thrombocytopenia, leukopenia, vesiculobullous rash, urticaria, and angioedema), kidney failure, syncope, myasthenia, myositis, pancreatitis, photosensitivity reaction, myopathy, and rhabdomyolysis.

OVERDOSAGE

There is no specific treatment in the event of overdose. In the event of overdose, the patient should be treated symptomatically and supportive measures instituted as required. Hemodialysis does not significantly enhance clearance of rosuvastatin.

DOSAGE AND ADMINISTRATION

The patient should be placed on a standard cholesterol-lowering diet before receiving CRESTOR and should continue on this diet during treatment. CRESTOR can be administered as a single dose at any time of day, with or without food.

Hypercholesterolemia (Heterozygous Familial and Nonfamilial) and Mixed Dyslipidemia (Fredrickson Type IIa and IIb)

The dose range for CRESTOR is 5 to 40 mg once daily. Therapy with CRESTOR should be individualized according to goal of therapy and response. The usual recommended starting dose of CRESTOR is 10 mg once daily. Initiation of therapy with 5 mg once daily may be considered for patients requiring less aggressive LDL-C reductions or who have predisposing factors for myopathy (see WARNINGS, Myopathy/Rhabdomyolysis). For patients with marked hypercholesterolemia (LDL-C > 190 mg/dL) and aggressive lipid targets, a 20-mg starting dose may be considered. The 40-mg dose of CRESTOR should be reserved for those patients who have not achieved goal LDL-C at 20 mg (see WARNINGS, Myopathy/Rhabdomyolysis). After initiation and/or upon titration of CRESTOR, lipid levels should be analyzed within 2 to 4 weeks and dosage adjusted accordingly.

Homozygous Familial Hypercholesterolemia

The recommended starting dose of CRESTOR is 20 mg once daily in patients with homozygous FH. The maximum recommended daily dose is 40 mg. CRESTOR should be used in these patients as an adjunct to other lipid-lowering treatments (e.g., LDL apheresis) or if such treatments are unavailable. Response to therapy should be estimated from pre-apheresis LDL-C levels.

Dosage in Patients Taking Cyclosporine

In patients taking cyclosporine, therapy should be limited to CRESTOR 5 mg once daily (see WARNINGS, Myopathy/Rhabdomyolysis, and PRECAUTIONS, Drug Interactions).

Concomitant Lipid-Lowering Therapy

The effect of CRESTOR on LDL-C and total-C may be enhanced when used in combination with a bile acid binding resin. If CRESTOR is used in combination with gemfibrozil, the dose of CRESTOR should be limited to 10 mg once daily (see WARNINGS, Myopathy/Rhabdomyolysis, and PRECAUTIONS, Drug Interactions).

Dosage in Patients With Renal Insufficiency

No modification of dosage is necessary for patients with mild to moderate renal insufficiency. For patients with severe renal impairment (CL_{cr} <30 mL/min/1.73 m^2) not on hemodialysis, dosing of CRESTOR should be started at 5 mg once daily and not to exceed 10 mg once daily (see PRECAUTIONS, General, and CLINICAL PHARMACOLOGY, Special Populations, Renal Insufficiency).

HOW SUPPLIED

CRESTOR® (rosuvastatin calcium) Tablets are supplied as:

5 mg tablets: Yellow, round, biconvex, coated tablets identified as "ZD4522" and "5" debossed on one side and plain on the other side of the tablet.

(NDC 0310-0755-90) bottles of 90

10 mg tablets: Pink, round, biconvex, coated tablets identified as "ZD4522" and "10" debossed on one side and plain on the other side of the tablet.

(NDC 0310-0751-90) bottles of 90
(NDC 0310-0751-39) unit dose packages of 100

20 mg tablets: Pink, round, biconvex, coated tablets identified as "ZD4522" and "20" debossed on one side and plain on the other side of the tablet.

(NDC 0310-0752-90) bottles of 90
(NDC 0310-0752-39) unit dose packages of 100

40 mg tablets: Pink, oval, biconvex, coated tablets identified as "ZD4522" debossed on one side and "40" debossed on the other side of the tablet.

(NDC 0310-0754-30) bottles of 30
(NDC 0310-0754-39) unit dose packages of 100

Storage

Store at controlled room temperature, 20-25°C (68-77°F) [see USP]. Protect from moisture.

Rx only

CRESTOR is a trademark of the AstraZeneca group of companies.

Licensed from SHIONOGI & CO., LTD., Osaka, Japan
Manufactured for:
AstraZeneca Pharmaceuticals LP
Wilmington, DE 19850
By: IPR Pharmaceuticals, Inc.
Carolina, PR 00984
IPR (trade) 630100
IPR (sample) 630200
API (sample) 23073-00
Rev. 08/03
AstraZeneca

In the PDR annual,
the **Brand and Generic Name Index**
(PINK section)
alphabetizes drugs under both
brand and generic names.

Aventis Pharmaceuticals Inc.

**300 SOMERSET CORPORATE BOULEVARD
BRIDGEWATER, NJ 08807-2854**

Direct Inquiries to:
Customer Service
300 Somerset Corporate Boulevard
Bridgewater, NJ 08807-2854
(800) 207-8049

For Medical Information Contact:
Generally:
Medical Information Services
300 Somerset Corporate Boulevard
Bridgewater, NJ 08807-2854
(800) 633-1610
For Oncology Medical Information
call (866) 662-6411

KETEK™ ℞

[*kē-tĕk*]
(telithromycin) Tablets

To reduce the development of drug-resistant bacteria and maintain the effectiveness of KETEK and other antibacterial drugs, KETEK should be used only to treat infections that are proven or strongly suspected to be caused by bacteria.

DESCRIPTION

KETEK™ tablets contain telithromycin, a semisynthetic antibacterial in the ketolide class for oral administration. Chemically, telithromycin is designated as Erythromycin, 3-de[(2,6-dideoxy-3-C-methyl-3-O-methyl-α-L-ribo-hexopyranosyl)oxy]-11,12-dideoxy-6-O-methyl-3-oxo-12,11-[oxycarbonyl[[4-[4-(3-pyridinyl)-1H-imidazol-1-yl]butyl]imino]]-.

Telithromycin, a ketolide, differs chemically from the macrolide group of antibacterials by the lack of α-L-cladinose at position 3 of the erythronolide A ring, resulting in a 3-keto function. It is further characterized by a C11-12 carbamate substituted by an imidazolyl and pyridyl ring through a butyl chain. Its empirical formula is $C_{43}H_{65}N_5O_{10}$ and its molecular weight is 812.03.

Telithromycin is a white to off-white crystalline powder. The following represents the chemical structure of telithromycin.

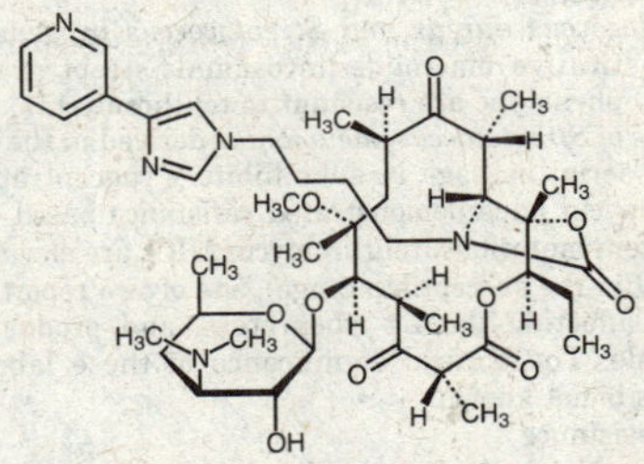

KETEK tablets are light-orange, oval, film-coated tablets, each containing 400 mg telithromycin, plus the following inactive ingredients: cornstarch, croscarmellose sodium, hypromellose, lactose monohydrate, magnesium stearate, microcrystalline cellulose, polyethylene glycol, povidone, red ferric oxide, talc, titanium dioxide, and yellow ferric oxide.

CLINICAL PHARMACOLOGY

Pharmacokinetics

Absorption:

Following oral administration, telithromycin reached maximal concentration at about 1 hour (0.5 - 4 hours). It has an absolute bioavailability of 57% in both young and elderly subjects.

The rate and extent of absorption are unaffected by food intake, thus KETEK tablets can be given without regard to food.

In healthy adult subjects, peak plasma telithromycin concentrations of approximately 2 µg/mL are attained at a median of 1 hour after an 800-mg oral dose.

Steady-state plasma concentrations are reached within 2 to 3 days of once daily dosing with telithromycin 800 mg. Following oral dosing, the mean terminal elimination half-life of telithromycin is 10 hours.

The pharmacokinetics of telithromycin after administration of single and multiple (7 days) once daily 800-mg doses to healthy adult subjects are shown in Table 1.

Table 1

	Mean (SD)	
Parameter	**Single dose (n=18)**	**Multiple dose (n=18)**
C_{max}(µg/mL)	1.9 (0.80)	2.27 (0.71)
T_{max}(h)*	1.0 (0.5-4.0)	1.0 (0.5-3.0)
$AUC_{(0-24)}$ (µg.h/mL)	8.25 (2.6)	12.5 (5.4)
Terminal $t_{1/2}$ (h)	7.16 (1.3)	9.81 (1.9)
C_{24h}(µg/mL)	0.03 (0.013)	0.07 (0.051)

* Median (min-max) values
SD=Standard deviation
C_{max}=Maximum plasma concentration
T_{max}=Time to C_{max}
AUC=Area under concentration vs. time curve
$t_{1/2}$=Terminal plasma half-life
C_{24h} =Plasma concentration at 24 hours post-dose

In a patient population, mean peak and trough plasma concentrations were 2.9 µg/mL (±1.55), (n=219) and 0.2 µg/mL (±0.22), (n=204), respectively, after 3 to 5 days of KETEK 800 mg once daily.

Distribution: Total *in vitro* protein binding is approximately 60% to 70% and is primarily due to human serum albumin.

Protein binding is not modified in elderly subjects and in patients with hepatic impairment.

The volume of distribution of telithromycin after intravenous infusion is 2.9 L/kg.

Telithromycin concentrations in bronchial mucosa, epithelial lining fluid, and alveolar macrophages after 800 mg once daily dosing for 5 days in patients are displayed in Table 2.

[See table 2 at bottom of next page]

Telithromycin concentration in white blood cells exceeds the concentration in plasma and is eliminated more slowly from white blood cells than from plasma. Mean white blood cell concentrations of telithromycin peaked at 72.1 µg/mL at 6 hours, and remained at 14.1 µg/mL 24 hours after 5 days of repeated dosing of 600 mg once daily. After 10 days, repeated dosing of 600 mg once daily, white blood cell concentrations remained at 8.9 µg/mL 48 hours after the last dose.

Metabolism: In total, metabolism accounts for approximately 70% of the dose. In plasma, the main circulating compound after administration of an 800-mg radiolabeled dose was parent compound, representing 56.7% of the total radioactivity. The main metabolite represented 12.6% of the AUC of telithromycin. Three other plasma metabolites were quantified, each representing 3% or less of the AUC of telithromycin.

It is estimated that approximately 50% of its metabolism is mediated by CYP 450 3A4 and the remaining 50% is CYP 450-independent.

Elimination: The systemically available telithromycin is eliminated by multiple pathways as follows: 7% of the dose is excreted unchanged in feces by biliary and/or intestinal secretion; 13% of the dose is excreted unchanged in urine by renal excretion; and 37% of the dose is metabolized by the liver.

Special populations

Gender: There was no significant difference between males and females in mean AUC, C_{max}, and elimination half-life in two studies; one in 18 healthy young volunteers (18 to 40 years of age) and the other in 14 healthy elderly volunteers (65 to 92 years of age), given single and multiple once daily doses of 800 mg of KETEK.

Hepatic insufficiency: In a single-dose study (800 mg) in 12 patients and a multiple-dose study (800 mg) in 13 patients with mild to severe hepatic insufficiency (Child Pugh Class A, B and C), the C_{max}, AUC and $t_{1/2}$ of telithromycin were similar to those obtained in age- and sex-matched healthy subjects. In both studies, an increase in renal elimination was observed in hepatically impaired patients indicating that this pathway may compensate for some of the decrease in metabolic clearance. No dosage adjustment is recommended due to hepatic impairment. (See **PRECAUTIONS, General** and **DOSAGE AND ADMINISTRATION.**)

Renal insufficiency: In a multiple-dose study, 36 subjects with varying degrees of renal impairment received 400 mg, 600 mg, or 800 mg KETEK once daily for 5 days. There was a 1.4-fold increase in $C_{max,ss}$, and a 1.9-fold increase in AUC $(0\text{-}24)_{ss}$ at 800 mg multiple doses in the severely renally impaired group (CL_{CR} < 30 mL/min) compared to healthy volunteers. Renal excretion may serve as a compensatory elimination pathway for telithromycin in situations where metabolic clearance is impaired. Patients with severe renal impairment are prone to conditions that may impair their metabolic clearance.

In a single-dose study in patients with end-stage renal failure on hemodialysis (n=10), the mean C_{max} and AUC values were similar to normal healthy subjects when KETEK was administered 2 hours post-dialysis. However, the effect of dialysis on removing telithromycin from the body has not been studied.

At present, no dose has been established in severely renal-impaired patients including those who need dialysis. (See **DOSAGE AND ADMINISTRATION.**)

Multiple insufficiency: The effects of co-administration of ketoconazole in 12 subjects (age ≥ 60 years), with impaired renal function were studied (CL_{CR}=24 to 80 mL/min). In this study, when severe renal insufficiency (CL_{CR} < 30 mL/min, n=2) and concomitant impairment of CYP 3A4 metabolism pathway were present, telithromycin exposure (AUC (0-24) was increased by approximately 4- to 5-fold compared with the exposure in healthy subjects with normal renal function receiving telithromycin alone. In the presence of severe renal impairment (CL_{CR} < 30 mL/min), no dose has been established.

Geriatric: Pharmacokinetic data show that there is an increase of 1.4-fold in exposure (AUC) in 20 patients ≥ 65 years of age with community acquired pneumonia in a Phase III study, and a 2.0-fold increase in exposure (AUC)

Continued on next page

Ketek—Cont.

in 14 subjects ≥ 65 years of age as compared with subjects less than 65 years of age in a Phase I study. No dosage adjustment is required based on age alone.

Drug-drug interactions

Studies were performed to evaluate the effect of CYP 3A4 inhibitors on telithromycin and the effect of telithromycin on drugs that are substrates of CYP 3A4 and CYP 2D6. In addition, drug interaction studies were conducted with several other concomitantly prescribed drugs.

CYP 3A4 inhibitors:

Itraconazole: A multiple-dose interaction study with itraconazole showed that C_{max} of telithromycin was increased by 22% and AUC by 54%.

Ketoconazole: A multiple-dose interaction study with ketoconazole showed that C_{max} of telithromycin was increased by 51% and AUC by 95%.

Grapefruit juice: When telithromycin was given with 240 mL of grapefruit juice after an overnight fast to healthy subjects, the pharmacokinetics of telithromycin were not affected.

CYP 3A4 substrates:

Cisapride: Steady-state peak plasma concentrations of cisapride (an agent with the potential to increase QT interval) were increased by 95% when co-administered with repeated doses of telithromycin, resulting in significant increases in QTc. (See **CONTRAINDICATIONS**.)

Simvastatin: When simvastatin was co-administered with telithromycin, there was a 5.3-fold increase in simvastatin C_{max}, an 8.9-fold increase in simvastatin AUC, a 15-fold increase in the simvastatin active metabolite C_{max}, and a 12-fold increase in the simvastatin active metabolite AUC. (See **PRECAUTIONS**.)

In another study, when simvastatin and telithromycin were administered 12 hours apart, there was a 3.4-fold increase in simvastatin C_{max}, a 4.0-fold increase in simvastatin AUC, a 3.2-fold increase in the active metabolite C_{max}, and a 4.3-fold increase in the active metabolite AUC. (See **PRECAUTIONS**.)

Midazolam: Concomitant administration of telithromycin with intravenous or oral midazolam resulted in 2- and 6-fold increases, respectively, in the AUC of midazolam due to inhibition of CYP 3A4-dependent metabolism of midazolam. (See **PRECAUTIONS**.)

CYP 2D6 substrates:

Paroxetine: There was no pharmacokinetic effect on paroxetine when telithromycin was co-administered.

Metoprolol: When metoprolol was co-administered with telithromycin, there was an increase of approximately 38% on the C_{max} and AUC of metoprolol, however, there was no effect on the elimination half-life of metoprolol. Telithromycin exposure is not modified with concomitant single-dose administration of metoprolol. (See **PRECAUTIONS, Drug interactions**.)

Other drug interactions:

Digoxin: The plasma peak and trough levels of digoxin were increased by 73% and 21%, respectively, in healthy volunteers when co-administered with telithromycin. However, trough plasma concentrations of digoxin (when equilibrium between plasma and tissue concentrations has been achieved) ranged from 0.74 to 2.17 ng/mL. There were no significant changes in ECG parameters and no signs of digoxin toxicity. (See **PRECAUTIONS**.)

Theophylline: When theophylline was co-administered with repeated doses of telithromycin, there was an increase of approximately 16% and 17% on the steady-state C_{max} and AUC of theophylline. Co-administration of theophylline may worsen gastrointestinal side effects such as nausea and vomiting, especially in female patients. It is recommended that telithromycin should be taken with theophylline 1 hour apart to decrease the likelihood of gastrointestinal side effects.

Sotalol: Telithromycin has been shown to decrease the C_{max} and AUC of sotalol by 34% and 20%, respectively, due to decreased absorption.

Warfarin: When co-administered with telithromycin, there were no pharmacodynamic or pharmacokinetic effects on racemic warfarin in healthy subjects.

Oral contraceptives: When oral contraceptives containing ethinyl estradiol and levonorgestrel were co-administered with telithromycin, the steady-state AUC of ethinyl estradiol did not change and the steady-state AUC of levonorgestrel was increased by 50%. The pharmacokinetic/pharmacodynamic study showed that telithromycin did not interfere with the antiovulatory effect of oral contraceptives containing ethinyl estradiol and levonorgestrel.

Ranitidine, antacid: There was no clinically relevant pharmacokinetic interaction of ranitidine or antacids containing aluminum and magnesium hydroxide on telithromycin.

Rifampin: During concomitant administration of rifampin and KETEK in repeated doses, C_{max} and AUC of telithromycin were decreased by 79%, and 86%, respectively. (See **PRECAUTIONS, Drug Interactions**.)

Microbiology

Telithromycin belongs to the ketolide class of antibacterials and is structurally related to the macrolide family of antibiotics. Telithromycin concentrates in phagocytes where it exhibits activity against intracellular respiratory pathogens. *In vitro,* telithromycin has been shown to demonstrate concentration-dependent bactericidal activity against isolates of *Streptococcus pneumoniae* (including multi-drug resistant isolates [MDRSP*]).

*MDRSP=Multi-drug resistant *Streptococcus pneumoniae* includes isolates known as PRSP (penicillin-resistant *Streptococcus pneumoniae*), and are isolates resistant to two or more of the following antimicrobials: penicillin, 2nd generation cephalosporins (e.g., cefuroxime), macrolides, tetracyclines, and trimethoprim/sulfamethoxazole.

Mechanism of action

Telithromycin blocks protein synthesis by binding to domains II and V of 23S rRNA of the 50S ribosomal subunit. By binding at domain II, telithromycin retains activity against gram-positive cocci (e.g., *Streptococcus pneumoniae*) in the presence of resistance mediated by methylases (*erm* genes) that alter the domain V binding site of telithromycin. Telithromycin may also inhibit the assembly of nascent ribosomal units.

Mechanism of resistance

Staphylococcus aureus and *Streptococcus pyogenes* with the constitutive macrolide-lincosamide-streptogramin B ($cMLS_B$) phenotype are resistant to telithromycin.

Mutants of *Streptococcus pneumoniae* derived in the laboratory by serial passage in subinhibitory concentrations of telithromycin have demonstrated resistance based on L22 riboprotein mutations (telithromycin MICs are elevated but still within the susceptible range), one of two reported mutations affecting the L4 riboprotein, and production of K-peptide. The clinical significance of these laboratory mutants is not known.

Cross resistance

Telithromycin does not induce resistance through methylase gene expression in erythromycin-inducibly resistant bacteria, a function of its 3-keto moiety. Telithromycin has not been shown to induce resistance to itself.

List of Microorganisms

Telithromycin has been shown to be active against most strains of the following microorganisms, both *in vitro* and in clinical settings as described in the **INDICATIONS AND USAGE** section.

Aerobic gram-positive microorganisms

Staphylococcus aureus (methicillin and erythromycin susceptible isolates only)

Streptococcus pneumoniae (including multi-drug resistant isolates [MDRSP*])

*MDRSP=Multi-drug resistant *Streptococcus pneumoniae* includes isolates known as PRSP (penicillin-resistant *S. pneumoniae*), and are isolates resistant to two or more of the following antimicrobials: penicillin, 2nd generation cephalosporins (e.g., cefuroxime), macrolides, tetracyclines, and trimethoprim/sulfamethoxazole.

Aerobic gram-negative microorganisms

Haemophilus influenzae

Moraxella catarrhalis

Other microorganisms

Chlamydophila (Chlamydia) pneumoniae

Mycoplasma pneumoniae

The following *in vitro* data are available, **but their clinical significance is unknown.**

At least 90% of the following microorganisms exhibit *in vitro* minimum inhibitory concentrations (MICs) less than or equal to the susceptible breakpoint for telithromycin. However, the safety and efficacy of telithromycin in treating clinical infections due to these microorganisms have not been established in adequate and well-controlled clinical trials.

Aerobic gram-positive microorganisms

Streptococcus pyogenes (erythromycin susceptible isolates only)

Streptococci (Lancefield groups C and G)

Viridans group streptococci

Anaerobic bacteria

Prevotella bivia

Prevotella intermedia

Peptostreptococcus spp.

Other microorganisms

Legionella pneumophila

Susceptibility Test Methods

When available, the clinical microbiology laboratory should provide cumulative results of *in vitro* susceptibility test results for antimicrobial drugs used in local hospitals and practice areas to the physician as periodic reports that describe the susceptibility profile of nosocomial and community-acquired pathogens. These reports should aid the physician in selecting the most effective antimicrobial.

Dilution techniques:

Quantitative methods are used to determine antimicrobial minimum inhibitory concentrations (MICs). These MICs provide estimates of the susceptibility of bacteria to antibacterial compounds. The MICs should be determined using a standardized procedure. Standardized procedures are based on dilution methods (broth or agar dilution)[1,3] or equivalent with standardized inoculum and concentrations of telithromycin powder. The MIC values should be interpreted according to criteria provided in Table 3.

Diffusion techniques:

Quantitative methods that require measurement of zone diameters also provide reproducible estimates of the susceptibility of bacteria to antibiotics. One such standardized procedure[2,3] requires the use of standardized inoculum concentrations. This procedure uses paper disks impregnated with 15 µg telithromycin to test the susceptibility of microorganisms to telithromycin. Disc diffusion zone sizes should be interpreted according to criteria in Table 3.

[See table 3 at left]

A report of "Susceptible" indicates that the antimicrobial is likely to inhibit growth of the pathogen if the antibacterial compound in the blood reaches the concentrations usually achievable. A report of "Intermediate" indicates that the result should be considered equivocal, and, if the microorganism is not fully susceptible to alternative, clinically feasible drugs, the test should be repeated. This category implies possible clinical applicability in body sites where the drug is physiologically concentrated or in situations where high dosage of drug can be used. This category also provides a buffer zone that prevents small uncontrolled technical factors from causing major discrepancies in interpretation. A report of "Resistant" indicates that the antimicrobial is not likely to inhibit growth of the pathogen if the antimicrobial compound in the blood reaches the concentrations usually achievable; other therapy should be selected.

Quality control:

Standardized susceptibility test procedures require the use of quality control microorganisms to determine the performance of the test procedures[1,2,3]. Standard telithromycin powder should provide the MIC ranges for the quality control organisms in Table 4. For the disk diffusion technique, the 15-µg telithromycin disk should provide the zone diameter ranges for the quality control organisms in Table 4.

Table 2

	Hours post-dose	Mean concentration (µg/mL) Tissue or fluid	Plasma	Tissue/Plasma Ratio
Bronchial mucosa	2	3.88*	1.86	2.11
	12	1.41*	0.23	6.33
	24	0.78*	0.08	12.11
Epithelial lining fluid	2	14.89	1.86	8.57
	12	3.27	0.23	13.8
	24	0.84	0.08	14.41
Alveolar macrophages	2	65	1.07	55
	8	100	0.605	180
	24	41	0.073	540

*Units in mg/kg

Table 3. Susceptibility Test Result Interpretive Criteria for Telithromycin

Pathogen	Minimal Inhibitory Concentrations (µg/mL) S	I	R[a]	Disk Diffusion (zone diameters in mm) S	I	R[a]
Staphylococcus aureus	≤ 0.25			≥ 22		
Streptococcus pneumoniae	≤ 1	2	≥ 4	≥ 19	16–18	≤ 15
Haemophilus influenzae	≤ 4	8	≥ 16	≥ 15	12–14	≤ 11

[a] The current absence of data on resistant isolates precludes defining any category other than "Susceptible". If strains yield MIC results other than susceptible, they should be submitted to a reference laboratory for further testing.

Table 4. Acceptable Quality Control Ranges for Telithromycin

QC Strain	Minimal Inhibitory Concentrations (µg/mL)	Disk Diffusion (Zone diameters in mm)
Staphylococcus aureus ATCC® 29213	0.06-0.25	Not Applicable
Staphylococcus aureus ATCC 25923	Not Applicable	24-30
Streptococcus pneumoniae		

ATCC 49619	0.004-0.03	27-33
Haemophilus influenzae		
ATCC 49247	1.0-4.0	17-23

ATCC = American Type Culture Collection

INDICATIONS AND USAGE

KETEK tablets are indicated for the treatment of infections caused by susceptible strains of the designated microorganisms in the conditions listed below for patients 18 years old and above.

Acute bacterial exacerbation of chronic bronchitis due to *Streptococcus pneumoniae, Haemophilus influenzae*, or *Moraxella catarrhalis.*

Acute bacterial sinusitis due to *Streptococcus pneumoniae, Haemophilus influenzae, Moraxella catarrhalis*, or *Staphylococcus aureus.*

Community-acquired pneumonia (of mild to moderate severity) due to *Streptococcus pneumoniae*, (including multi-drug resistant isolates [MDRSP*]), *Haemophilus influenzae, Moraxella catarrhalis, Chlamydophila pneumoniae*, or *Mycoplasma pneumoniae.*

*MDRSP, Multi-drug resistant *Streptococcus pneumoniae* includes isolates known as PRSP (penicillin-resistant *Streptococcus pneumoniae*), and are isolates resistant to two or more of the following antibiotics: penicillin, 2nd generation cephalosporins, e.g., cefuroxime, macrolides, tetracyclines and trimethoprim/sulfamethoxazole.

To reduce the development of drug-resistant bacteria and maintain the effectiveness of KETEK and other antibacterial drugs, KETEK should be used only to treat infections that are proven or strongly suspected to be caused by susceptible bacteria. When culture and susceptibility information are available, they should be considered in selecting or modifying antibacterial therapy. In the absence of such data, local epidemiology and susceptibility patterns may contribute to the empiric selection of therapy.

CONTRAINDICATIONS

KETEK is contraindicated in patients with a history of hypersensitivity to telithromycin and/or any components of KETEK tablets, or any macrolide antibiotic.

Concomitant administration of KETEK with cisapride or pimozide is contraindicated. (See **CLINICAL PHARMACOLOGY, Drug-drug Interactions** and **PRECAUTIONS.**)

WARNINGS

Pseudomembranous colitis has been reported with nearly all antibacterial agents, including telithromycin, and may range in severity from mild to life-threatening. Therefore, it is important to consider this diagnosis in patients who present with diarrhea subsequent to the administration of any antibacterial agents.

Treatment with antibacterial agents alters the flora of the colon and may permit overgrowth of clostridia. Studies indicate that toxin-producing strains of *Clostridium difficile* are the primary cause of "antibiotic-associated colitis".

After the diagnosis of pseudomembranous colitis has been established, therapeutic measures should be initiated. Mild cases of pseudomembranous colitis usually respond to drug discontinuation alone. In moderate to severe cases, consideration should be given to management with fluids and electrolytes, protein supplementation, and treatment with an antibacterial drug clinically effective against *C. difficile* colitis. (See **ADVERSE REACTIONS.**)

Telithromycin has the potential to prolong the QTc interval of the electrocardiogram in some patients. QTc prolongation may lead to an increased risk for ventricular arrhythmias, including torsades de pointes. Thus, telithromycin should be avoided in patients with congenital prolongation of the QTc interval, and in patients with ongoing proarrhythmic conditions such as uncorrected hypokalemia or hypomagnesemia, clinically significant bradycardia, and in patients receiving Class IA (e.g., quinidine and procainamide) or Class III (e.g., dofetilide) antiarrhythmic agents.

No cardiovascular morbidity or mortality attributable to QTc prolongation occurred with telithromycin treatment in 4780 patients in clinical efficacy trials, including 204 patients having a prolonged QTc at baseline.

Exacerbations of myasthenia gravis have been reported in patients with myasthenia gravis treated with telithromycin. This has sometimes occurred within a few hours after intake of the first dose of telithromycin. Reports have included life-threatening acute respiratory failure with a rapid onset in patients with myasthenia gravis treated for respiratory tract infections with telithromycin. Telithromycin is not recommended in patients with myasthenia gravis unless no other therapeutic alternatives are available. If other therapeutic alternatives are not available, patients with myasthenia gravis taking telithromycin must be closely monitored. Patients must be advised that if they experience exacerbation of their symptoms, they should discontinue treatment of KETEK and immediately seek medical attention. Supportive measures should be instituted as medically necessary.

PRECAUTIONS

General

Prescribing KETEK in the absence of a proven or strongly suspected bacterial infection or a prophylactic indication is unlikely to provide benefit to the patient and increases the risk of the development of drug-resistant bacteria.

Table 5

All and Possibly Related Treatment-Emergent Adverse Events Reported in Controlled Phase III Clinical Studies (Percent Incidence)

Adverse Event*	All TEAEs		Possibly-Related TEAEs	
	KETEK	Comparator†	KETEK	Comparator†
	n= 2702	n= 2139	n= 2702	n= 2139
Diarrhea	10.8%	8.6%	10.0%	8.0%
Nausea	7.9%	4.6%	7.0%	4.1%
Headache	5.5%	5.8%	2.0%	2.5%
Dizziness (excl. vertigo)	3.7%	2.7%	2.8%	1.5%
Vomiting	2.9%	2.2%	2.4%	1.4%
Loose Stools	2.3%	1.5%	2.1%	1.4%
Dysgeusia	1.6%	3.6%	1.5%	3.6%

*Based on a frequency of all and possibly related treatment-emergent adverse events of ≥ 2% in KETEK or comparator groups.
†Includes comparators from all controlled Phase III studies.

Table 6

Infection	Daily dose and route of administration	Frequency of administration	Duration of treatment
Acute bacterial exacerbation of chronic bronchitis	800 mg oral (2 tablets of 400 mg)	once daily	5 days
Acute bacterial sinusitis	800 mg oral (2 tablets of 400 mg)	once daily	5 days
Community-acquired pneumonia	800 mg oral (2 tablets of 400 mg)	once daily	7-10 days

Table 7. CAP: Clinical cure rate at post-therapy follow-up (17–24 days)

Controlled Studies	Patients (n)		Clinical cure rate	
	KETEK	Comparator	KETEK	Comparator
KETEK vs. clarithromycin 500 mg BID for 10 days	162	156	88.3%	88.5%
KETEK vs. trovafloxacin* 200 mg QD for 7 to 10 days	80	86	90.0%	94.2%
KETEK vs. amoxicillin 1000 mg TID for 10 days	149	152	94.6%	90.1%
KETEK for 7 days vs. clarithromycin 500 mg BID for 10 days	161	146	88.8%	91.8%

*This study was stopped prematurely after trovafloxacin was restricted for use in hospitalized patients with severe infection.

Table 10. Acute Sinusitis: Clinical cure rate at post-therapy follow-up (17–24 days)

Controlled Studies	Patients (n)		Clinical cure rate	
	KETEK (5 day treatment)	Comparator (10 day treatment)	KETEK (5 day treatment)	Comparator (10 day treatment)
KETEK vs. amoxicillin/clavulanic acid 500/125 mg TID	146	137	75.3%	74.5%
KETEK vs. cefuroxime axetil 250 mg BID	189	89	85.2%	82.0%

Table 12. AECB: Clinical cure rate at post-therapy follow-up (17–24 days)

Controlled Studies	Patients (n)		Clinical cure rate	
	KETEK	Comparator	KETEK	Comparator
KETEK (5 day therapy) vs. cefuroxime axetil 500mg BID (10 day therapy)	140	142	86.4%	83.1%
KETEK (5 day therapy) vs. amoxicillin/clavulanic acid 500/125 mg TID (10 day therapy)	115	112	86.1%	82.1%
KETEK (5 day therapy) vs. clarithromycin 500mg BID (10 day therapy)	225	231	85.8%	89.2%

KETEK may cause visual disturbances particularly in slowing the ability to accommodate and the ability to release accommodation. Visual disturbances included blurred vision, difficulty focusing, and diplopia. Most events were mild to moderate; however, severe cases have been reported. Patients should be cautioned about the potential effects of these visual disturbances on driving a vehicle, operating machinery or engaging in other potentially hazardous

Continued on next page

Ketek—Cont.

activities. (See **ADVERSE REACTIONS, CLINICAL STUDIES.**)

Hepatic dysfunction, including increased liver enzymes and hepatitis, with or without jaundice, has been reported with the use of KETEK. These events were generally reversible. Caution should be used in patients with a previous history of hepatitis/jaundice associated with the use of KETEK. (See **ADVERSE REACTIONS, Liver and biliary system.**)

Telithromycin is principally excreted via the liver and kidney. Telithromycin may be administered without dosage adjustment in the presence of hepatic impairment. In the presence of severe renal impairment (CL_{CR} < 30 mL/min), the dose of KETEK has not been established. (See **DOSAGE AND ADMINISTRATION.**)

Information for patients

The following information and instructions should be communicated to the patient.

KETEK may cause problems with vision particularly when looking quickly between objects close by and objects far away. These events include blurred vision, difficulty focusing, and objects looking doubled. Most events were mild to moderate; however, severe cases have been reported. Problems with vision were reported as having occurred after any dose during treatment, but most occurred following the first or second dose. These problems lasted several hours and in some patients came back with the next dose. (See **PRECAUTIONS, General** and **ADVERSE REACTIONS.**)

If visual difficulties occur:

- patients should avoid driving a motor vehicle, operating heavy machinery, or engaging in otherwise hazardous activities.
- avoiding quick changes in viewing between objects in the distance and objects nearby may help to decrease the effects of these visual difficulties.
- patients should contact their physician if these visual difficulties interfere with their daily activities.

Patients should also be advised:

- that antibacterial drugs including KETEK should only be used to treat bacterial infections. They do not treat viral infections (e.g., the common cold). When KETEK is prescribed to treat a bacterial infection, patients should be told that although it is common to feel better early in the course of therapy, the medication should be taken exactly as directed. Skipping doses or not completing the full course of therapy may (1) decrease the effectiveness of the immediate treatment and (2) increase the likelihood that bacteria will develop resistance and will not be treatable by KETEK or other antibacterial drugs in the future.
- that KETEK has the potential to produce changes in the electrocardiogram (QTc interval prolongation) and that they should report any fainting occurring during drug treatment.
- that KETEK should be avoided in patients receiving Class 1A (e.g., quinidine, procainamide) or Class III (e.g., dofetilide) antiarrhythmic agents.
- to inform their physician of any personal or family history of QTc prolongation or proarrhythmic conditions such as uncorrected hypokalemia, or clinically significant bradycardia.
- that telithromycin is not recommended in patients with myasthenia gravis. Patients should inform their physician if they have myasthenia gravis.
- that simvastatin, lovastatin, or atorvastatin should be avoided in patients receiving KETEK. If KETEK is prescribed, therapy with simvastatin, lovastatin, or atorvastatin should be stopped during the course of treatment.
- that KETEK tablets can be taken with or without food.
- to inform their physician of any other medications taken concurrently with KETEK, including over-the-counter medications and dietary supplements.

Drug interactions

Telithromycin is a strong inhibitor of the cytochrome P450 3A4 system. Co-administration of KETEK tablets and a drug primarily metabolized by the cytochrome P450 3A4 enzyme system may result in increased plasma concentration of the drug co-administered with telithromycin that could increase or prolong both the therapeutic and adverse effects. Therefore, appropriate dosage adjustments may be necessary for the drug co-administered with telithromycin.

The use of KETEK is contraindicated with cisapride. (See **CONTRAINDICATIONS** and **CLINICAL PHARMACOLOGY, Drug-drug interactions.**)

The use of KETEK is contraindicated with pimozide. Although there are no studies looking at the interaction between KETEK and pimozide, there is a potential risk of increased pimozide plasma levels by inhibition of CYP 3A4 pathways by KETEK as with macrolides. (See **CONTRAINDICATIONS.**)

In a pharmacokinetic study, simvastatin levels were increased due to CYP 3A4 inhibition by telithromycin. (See **CLINICAL PHARMACOLOGY, Other drug interactions.**) Similarly, an interaction may occur with lovastatin or atorvastatin, but not with pravastatin or fluvastatin. High levels of HMG-CoA reductase inhibitors increase the risk of myopathy. Use of simvastatin, lovastatin, or atorvastatin concomitantly with KETEK should be avoided. If KETEK is prescribed, therapy with simvastatin, lovastatin, or atorvastatin should be suspended during the course of treatment. Monitoring of digoxin side effects or serum levels should be considered during concomitant administration of digoxin and KETEK. (See **CLINICAL PHARMACOLOGY, Drug-drug interactions.**)

Patients should be monitored with concomitant administration of midazolam and dosage adjustment of midazolam should be considered if necessary. Precaution should be used with other benzodiazepines, which are metabolized by CYP 3A4 and undergo a high first-pass effect (e.g., triazolam). (See **CLINICAL PHARMACOLOGY, Drug-drug interactions.**)

Concomitant treatment of KETEK with rifampin, a CYP 3A4 inducer, should be avoided. Concomitant administration of other CYP 3A4 inducers such as phenytoin, carbamazepine, or phenobarbital is likely to result in subtherapeutic levels of telithromycin and loss of effect. (See **CLINICAL PHARMACOLOGY, Other drug interactions.**)

In patients treated with metoprolol for heart failure, the increased exposure to metoprolol, a CYP 2D6 substrate, may be of clinical importance. Therefore, co-administration of KETEK and metoprolol in patients with heart failure should be considered with caution. (See **CLINICAL PHARMACOLOGY, Drug-drug interactions.**)

No specific drug interaction studies have been performed to evaluate the following potential drug-drug interactions with KETEK. However, these drug interactions have been observed with macrolide products.

Drugs metabolized by the cytochrome P450 system such as carbamazepine, cyclosporine, tacrolimus, sirolimus, hexobarbital, and phenytoin: elevation of serum levels of these drugs may be observed when co-administered with telithromycin. As a result, increases or prolongation of the therapeutic and/or adverse effects of the concomitant drug may be observed.

Ergot alkaloid derivatives (such as ergotamine or dihydroergotamine): acute ergot toxicity characterized by severe peripheral vasospasm and dysesthesia has been reported when macrolide antibiotics were co-administered. Without further data, the co-administration of KETEK and these drugs is not recommended.

Laboratory test interactions

There are no reported laboratory test interactions.

Carcinogenesis, mutagenesis, impairment of fertility

Long-term studies in animals to determine the carcinogenic potential of KETEK have not been conducted.

Telithromycin showed no evidence of genotoxicity in four tests: gene mutation in bacterial cells, gene mutation in mammalian cells, chromosome aberration in human lymphocytes, and the micronucleus test in the mouse.

No evidence of impaired fertility in the rat was observed at doses estimated to be 0.61 times the human daily dose on a mg/m^2 basis. At doses of 1.8-3.6 times the human daily dose, at which signs of parental toxicity were observed, moderate reductions in fertility indices were noted in male and female animals treated with telithromycin.

Pregnancy

Teratogenic effects: Pregnancy Category C. Telithromycin was not teratogenic in the rat or rabbit. Reproduction studies have been performed in rats and rabbits, with effect on pre-post natal development studied in the rat. At doses estimated to be 1.8 times (900 mg/m^2) and 0.49 times (240 mg/m^2) the daily human dose of 800 mg (492 mg/m^2) in the rat and rabbit, respectively, no evidence of fetal terata was found. At doses higher than the 900 mg/m^2 and 240 mg/m^2 in rats and rabbits, respectively, maternal toxicity may have resulted in delayed fetal maturation. No adverse effects on prenatal and postnatal development of rat pups were observed at 1.5 times (750 mg/m^2/d) the daily human dose.

There are no adequate and well-controlled studies in pregnant women. Telithromycin should be used during pregnancy only if the potential benefit justifies the potential risk to the fetus.

Nursing mothers

Telithromycin is excreted in breast milk of rats. Telithromycin may also be excreted in human milk. Because many drugs are excreted in human milk, caution should be exercised when KETEK is administered to a nursing mother.

Pediatric use

The safety and effectiveness of KETEK in pediatric patients has not been established.

Geriatric use

In all Phase III clinical trials (n=4,780), KETEK was administered to 694 patients who were 65 years and older, including 231 patients who were 75 years and older. Efficacy and safety in elderly patients ≥ 65 years were generally similar to that observed in younger patients; however, greater sensitivity of some older individuals cannot be ruled out. No dosage adjustment is required based on age alone. (See **CLINICAL PHARMACOLOGY, Special populations, Geriatric** and **DOSAGE AND ADMINISTRATION.**)

ADVERSE REACTIONS

In Phase III clinical trials, 4,780 patients (n=2702 in controlled trials) received daily oral doses of KETEK 800 mg once daily for 5 days or 7 to 10 days. Most adverse events were mild to moderate in severity. In the combined Phase III studies, discontinuation due to treatment-emergent adverse events occurred in 4.4% of KETEK-treated patients and 4.3% of combined comparator-treated patients. Most discontinuations in the KETEK group were due to treatment-emergent adverse events in the gastrointestinal body system, primarily diarrhea (0.9% for KETEK vs. 0.7% for comparators), nausea (0.7% for KETEK vs. 0.5% for comparators).

All and possibly related treatment-emergent adverse events (TEAEs) occurring in controlled clinical studies in ≥ 2.0% of all patients are included below:

[See table 5 at top of previous page]

The following events judged by investigators to be at least possibly drug related were observed infrequently (≥ 0.2% and < 2%), in KETEK-treated patients in the controlled Phase III studies.

Gastrointestinal system: abdominal distension, dyspepsia, gastrointestinal upset, flatulence, constipation, gastroenteritis, gastritis, anorexia, oral candidiasis, glossitis, stomatitis, watery stools.

Liver and biliary system: abnormal liver function tests: increased transaminases, increased liver enzymes (e.g., ALT, AST) were usually asymptomatic and reversible. ALT elevations above 3 times the upper limit of normal were observed in 1.6%, and 1.7% of patients treated with KETEK and comparators, respectively. Hepatitis, with or without jaundice, occurred in 0.07% of patients treated with KETEK, and was reversible. (See **PRECAUTIONS, General.**)

Nervous system: dry mouth, somnolence, insomnia, vertigo, increased sweating

Body as a whole: abdominal pain, upper abdominal pain, fatigue

Special senses: Visual adverse events most often included blurred vision, diplopia, or difficulty focusing. Most events were mild to moderate; however, severe cases have been reported. Some patients discontinued therapy due to these adverse events. Visual adverse events were reported as having occurred after any dose during treatment, but most visual adverse events (65%) occurred following the first or second dose. Visual events lasted several hours and recurred upon subsequent dosing in some patients. For patients who continued treatment, some resolved on therapy while others continued to have symptoms until they completed the full course of treatment. (See **PRECAUTIONS, General** and **PRECAUTIONS, Information for patients.**)

Females and patients under 40 years old experienced a higher incidence of telithromycin-associated visual adverse events. (See **CLINICAL STUDIES.**)

Urogenital system: vaginal candidiasis, vaginitis, vaginosis fungal

Skin: rash

Hematologic: increased platelet count

Other possibly related clinically-relevant events occurring in <0.2% of patients treated with KETEK from the controlled Phase III studies included: anxiety, bradycardia, eczema, elevated blood bilirubin, erythema multiforme, flushing, hypotension, increased blood alkaline phosphatase, increased eosinophil count, paresthesia, pruritus, urticaria.

Post-Marketing Adverse Event Reports:

In addition to adverse events reported from clinical trials, the following events have been reported from worldwide post-marketing experience with KETEK.

Allergic: face edema, rare reports of severe allergic reactions, including angioedema and anaphylaxis.

Cardiovascular: atrial arrhythmias

Liver and biliary system: Hepatic dysfunction, including increased liver enzymes, and hepatocellular and/or cholestatic hepatitis, with or without jaundice, has been infrequently reported with telithromycin. This hepatic dysfunction may be severe and is usually reversible.

Musculoskeletal: muscle cramps, rare reports of exacerbation of myasthenia gravis. (See **WARNINGS.**)

OVERDOSAGE

In the event of acute overdosage, the stomach should be emptied by gastric lavage. The patient should be carefully monitored (e.g., ECG, electrolytes) and given symptomatic and supportive treatment. Adequate hydration should be maintained. The effectiveness of hemodialysis in an overdose situation with KETEK is unknown.

DOSAGE AND ADMINISTRATION

The dose of KETEK tablets is 800 mg taken orally once every 24 hours. The duration of therapy depends on the infection type and is described below. KETEK tablets can be administered with or without food.

[See table 6 at top of previous page]

KETEK may be administered without dosage adjustment in the presence of hepatic impairment.

In the presence of severe renal impairment (CL_{CR} < 30 mL/min), including patients who need dialysis, the dose of KETEK has not been established.

HOW SUPPLIED

KETEK™ 400 mg tablets are supplied as light-orange, oval, film-coated tablets, imprinted "H3647" on one side and "400" on the other side. These are packaged in bottles and blister cards (Ketek Pak™ and unit dose) as follows:

Bottles of 60	(NDC 0088-2225-41)
Ketek Pak™, 10-tablet cards (2 tablets per blister cavity)	(NDC 0088-2225-07)
Unit dose package of 100 (blister pack)	(NDC 0088-2225-49)

Store at 25°C (77°F); excursions permitted to 15-30°C (59-86°F) [see USP Controlled Room Temperature].

CLINICAL STUDIES

Community-acquired pneumonia (CAP)

KETEK was studied in four randomized, double-blind, controlled studies and four open-label studies for the treatment of community-acquired pneumonia. Patients with mild to moderate CAP who were considered appropriate for oral outpatient treatment were enrolled in these trials. Patients with severe pneumonia were excluded based on any one of the following: ICU admission, need for parenteral antibiotics, respiratory rate > 30/minute, hypotension, altered mental status, < 90% oxygen saturation by pulse oximetry, or white blood cell count < 4000/mm^3. Total number of clinically evaluable patients in the telithromycin group included 2016 patients.

[See table 7 at top of page 11]

Clinical cure rates by pathogen from the four CAP controlled clinical trials in microbiologically evaluable patients given KETEK for 7-10 days or a comparator are displayed in Table 8.

Table 8. CAP: Clinical cure rate by pathogen at post-therapy follow-up (17-24 days)

Pathogen	KETEK	Comparator
Streptococcus pneumoniae	73/78 (93.6%)	63/70 (90.0%)
Haemophilus influenzae	39/47 (83.0%)	42/44 (95.5%)
Moraxella catarrhalis	12/14 (85.7%)	7/9 (77.8%)
Chlamydophila (Chlamydia) pneumoniae	23/25 (92.0%)	18/19 (94.7%)
Mycoplasma pneumoniae	22/23 (95.7%)	20/22 (90.9%)

Clinical cure rates for patients with CAP due to *Streptococcus pneumoniae* were determined from patients in controlled and uncontrolled trials. Of 333 evaluable patients with CAP due to *Streptococcus pneumoniae*, 312 (93.7%) achieved clinical success. Only patients considered appropriate for oral outpatient therapy were included in these trials. More severely ill patients were not enrolled. Blood cultures were obtained in all patients participating in the clinical trials of mild to moderate community-acquired pneumonia. In a limited number of outpatients with incidental pneumococcal bacteremia treated with KETEK, a clinical cure rate of 88% (67/76) has been observed. KETEK is not indicated for the treatment of severe community-acquired pneumonia or suspected pneumococcal bacteremia.

Clinical cure rates for patients with CAP due to multi-drug resistant *Streptococcus pneumoniae* (MDRSP*) were determined from patients in controlled and uncontrolled trials. Of 36 evaluable patients with CAP due to MDRSP, 33 (91.7%) achieved clinical success.

*MDRSP: Multi-drug resistant *Streptococcus pneumoniae* includes isolates known as PRSP (penicillin-resistant *Streptococcus pneumoniae*), and are isolates resistant to two or more of the following antibiotics: penicillin, 2nd generation cephalosporins, e.g., cefuroxime, macrolides, tetracyclines and trimethoprim/sulfamethoxazole.

Table 9. Clinical cure rate for 36 evaluable patients with MDRSP treated with KETEK in studies of community-acquired pneumonia

Screening Susceptibility	Clinical Success in Evaluable MDRSP Patients	
	n/N[a]	%
Penicillin-resistant	20/23	86.9
2nd generation cephalosporin-resistant	20/22	90.9
Macrolide-resistant	25/28	89.3
Trimethoprim/ sulfamethoxazole-resistant	24/27	88.9
Tetracycline-resistant[b]	11/13	84.6

[a] n = the number of patients successfully treated; N = the number with resistance to the listed drug of the 36 evaluable patients with CAP due to MDRSP.

[b] Includes isolates tested for resistance to either tetracycline or doxycycline.

Acute bacterial sinusitis

KETEK was studied in two randomized, double-blind, comparative studies for the treatment of acute sinusitis. Clinical cure rates with KETEK given for 5 days and comparator drug are shown in Table 10.

[See table 10 on page 11]

A third study compared 5 days with 10 days of KETEK for the treatment of acute bacterial sinusitis, clinical cure rates for the two treatments were similar (91.1% vs. 91.0% respectively).

Clinical cure rates in microbiologically evaluable patients for KETEK against the most common pathogens from the two acute sinusitis controlled clinical trials are displayed in Table 11.

Table 11. Acute Sinusitis: Clinical cure rate by pathogen

Pathogen	KETEK 5 days	Comparator 10-days
Streptococcus pneumoniae	27/31 (87.1%)	14/16 (87.5%)
Haemophilus influenzae	28/34 (82.4%)	13/15 (86.7%)
Moraxella catarrhalis	7/7 (100%)	7/7 (100%)
Staphylococcus aureus	8/8 (100%)	2/3 (66.7%)

Acute bacterial exacerbation of chronic bronchitis (AECB)

KETEK was studied in three randomized, double-blind, controlled studies for the treatment of acute exacerbation of chronic bronchitis. Clinical cure rates are displayed in Table 12.

[See table 12 at bottom of page 11]

Clinical cure rates in microbiologically evaluable patients treated with KETEK against the most common pathogens from the three acute exacerbation of chronic bronchitis clinical trials are displayed in Table 13.

Table 13. AECB: Clinical cure rate by pathogen at post-therapy follow-up (17–24 days)

Pathogen	KETEK	Comparator
Streptococcus pneumoniae	22/27 (81.5%)	15/19 (78.9%)
Haemophilus influenzae	44/60 (73.3%)	45/53 (84.9%)
Moraxella catarrhalis	27/29 (93.1%)	29/34 (85.3%)

Visual Adverse Events

Table 14 provides the incidence of all treatment-emergent visual adverse events in controlled Phase III studies by age and gender. The group with the highest incidence was females under the age of 40, while males over the age of 40 had rates of visual adverse events similar to comparator-treated patients.

Table 14. Incidence of All Treatment-Emergent Visual Adverse Events in Controlled Phase III Studies

Gender/Age	Telithromycin	Comparators*
Female ≤ 40	2.1% (14/682)	0.0% (0/534)
Female > 40	1.0% (7/703)	0.35% (2/574)
Male ≤ 40	1.2% (7/563)	0.48% (2/417)
Male > 40	0.27% (2/754)	0.33% (2/614)
Total	1.1% (30/2702)	0.28% (6/2139)

* Includes all comparators combined

ANIMAL PHARMACOLOGY

Repeated dose toxicity studies of 1, 3, and 6 months' duration with telithromycin conducted in rat, dog and monkey showed that the liver was the principal target for toxicity with elevations of liver enzymes and histological evidence of damage. There was evidence of reversibility after cessation of treatment. Plasma exposures based on free fraction of drug at the no observed adverse effect levels ranged from 1 to 10 times the expected clinical exposure.

Phospholipidosis (intracellular phospholipid accumulation) affecting a number of organs and tissues (e.g., liver, kidney, lung, thymus, spleen, gall bladder, mesenteric lymph nodes, GI-tract) has been observed with the administration of telithromycin in rats at repeated doses of 900 mg/m^2/day (1.8× the human dose) or more for 1 month, and 300 mg/m^2/day (0.61× the human dose) or more for 3–6 months. Similarly, phospholipidosis has been observed in dogs with telithromycin at repeated doses of 3000 mg/m2/day (6.1× the human dose) or more for 1 month and 1000 mg/ m^2/day (2.0× the human dose) or more for 3 months. The significance of these findings for humans is unknown.

Pharmacology/toxicology studies showed an effect both in prolonging QTc interval in dogs *in vivo* and *in vitro* action potential duration (APD) in rabbit Purkinje fibers. These effects were observed at concentrations of free drug at least 8.8 (in dogs) times those circulating in clinical use. *In vitro* electrophysiological studies (hERG assays) suggested an inhibition of the rapid activating component of the delayed rectifier potassium current (I_{Kr}) as an underlying mechanism.

Rev. March 2004

Aventis Pharmaceuticals Inc.
Kansas City, MO 64137

US Patent Nos.: 5,527,780; 5,969,161; and 6,022,965

Rx only

www.aventispharma-us.com

References

1. National Committee for Clinical Laboratory Standards. Methods for Dilution Antimicrobial Susceptibility Tests for Bacteria That Grow Aerobically – Sixth Edition; Approved Standard, NCCLS Document M7-A6, Vol. 23, No. 2, NCCLS, Wayne, PA, January, 2003.
2. National Committee for Clinical Laboratory Standards. Performance Standards for Antimicrobial Disk Susceptibility Tests - Eighth Edition; Approved Standard, NCCLS Document M2-A8, Vol. 23, No. 1, NCCLS, Wayne, PA, January, 2003.
3. National Committee for Clinical Laboratory Standards. Performance Standards for Antimicrobial Susceptibility Testing: Twelfth Informational Supplement; Approved Standard, NCCLS Document M2-A8 and M7-A6, Vol. 23, No. 1, NCCLS, Wayne, PA, January, 2004.

Rx only

Patient Information About:
KETEK™
(telithromycin) Tablets
400mg Tablets

Before beginning your treatment, please read this section to learn important information about KETEK™ (telithromycin). Although the information presented here will be useful during your therapy, not all the benefits and risks of treatment with KETEK are discussed in this document. This section is not intended to take the place of conversations with your doctor or healthcare provider about your treatment or medical condition. The medicine described here can only be prescribed by a licensed healthcare provider. With this in mind, be sure to talk to your healthcare provider if you have any questions. It's important to note that only a doctor or healthcare provider can determine if KETEK is right for you.

What is KETEK?

KETEK (*KEE tek*) is an antibiotic used to treat adults 18 years of age and older with certain respiratory (lung and sinus) infections caused by certain germs called bacteria. KETEK kills many of the types of bacteria that can infect the lungs and sinuses, and has been found to treat these infections safely and effectively in clinical trials.

Not all respiratory infections are caused by bacteria. For example, common colds are caused by viruses. KETEK, like other antibiotics, does not kill viruses.

KETEK Tablets are light orange, oval, film-coated tablets, imprinted with "H3647" on one side and "400" on the other side, and each containing 400 mg of active drug.

How and when should I take KETEK?

The usual dose is two KETEK Tablets taken at the same time once daily for 5 to 10 days.

KETEK tablets should be swallowed whole and may be taken with or without food. Try to take your tablets at the same time every day, unless your healthcare provider tells you otherwise.

Follow the dosing instructions carefully, and do not take more than the prescribed amount. If you miss a dose, take it as soon as you remember. Do not take more than one dose (e.g., two tablets) of KETEK in a 24-hour period. If you have any questions, talk to your healthcare provider.

To make sure that all bacteria are killed, take all of the medicine that was prescribed for you even if you begin to feel better, unless instructed otherwise. You should contact your healthcare provider if your condition is not improving while taking KETEK.

Who should not take KETEK?

You must not take KETEK if:

- You have ever had a severe allergic reaction to KETEK or to any of the group of antibiotics known as "macrolides" such as erythromycin, azithromycin (Zithromax®), clarithromycin (Biaxin®) or dirithromycin (Dynabac®).
- You are currently taking cisapride (Propulsid®) or pimozide (Orap®).

You should be sure to talk to your healthcare provider before taking KETEK if any of the following are true, so he/she can determine if KETEK is right for you:

- If you have, or if a relative has, a rare heart condition known as congenital prolongation of the QT interval.
- If you are being treated for heart rhythm disturbances with certain medicines known as antiarrhythmics (such as quinidine, procainamide, or dofetilide) or if you have low blood potassium (hypokalemia), or low blood magnesium (hypomagnesemia).
- If you have a disease known as myasthenia gravis.
- If you are pregnant, planning to become pregnant, or are nursing.
- If you have ever experienced jaundice (yellow color of the skin and/or eyes) while taking KETEK.
- If you have any other serious medical conditions, including heart, liver, or kidney disease.

What about other medications I am taking?

It is important to let your healthcare provider know about all of the medicines you are taking, including those obtained without a prescription. Also see section **"Who should not take KETEK?"**

It is important to tell your healthcare provider if you are taking:

- Simvastatin, lovastatin, or atorvastatin (used for lowering cholesterol). You should stop treatment with these medications while you are taking KETEK.
- Medicines that correct heart rhythm called "antiarrhythmics" (such as quinidine, procainamide, or dofetilide).
- Any of the following medicines: itraconazole, ketoconazole, midazolam, digoxin, ergot alkaloid derivatives, cyclosporine, carbamazepine, hexobarbital, phenytoin, tacrolimus, sirolimus, metoprolol, theophylline or rifampin.
- Medicines called diuretics (also sometimes called water pills) such as furosemide or hydrochlorothiazide.

What are the possible side effects of KETEK?

KETEK is generally well tolerated. Most side effects are mild to moderate.

Continued on next page

Ketek—Cont.

The most common side effects are nausea, headache, dizziness, vomiting, and diarrhea. If diarrhea persists call your healthcare provider.

KETEK may cause problems with vision, particularly when looking quickly between objects close by and objects far away. These events include blurred vision, difficulty focusing, and objects looking doubled. Most events were mild to moderate; however, severe cases have been reported. Problems with vision were reported as having occurred after any dose during treatment, but most occurred following the first or second dose. These problems lasted several hours and sometimes came back with the next dose.

If visual difficulties occur:

- You should avoid driving a motor vehicle, operating heavy machinery, or engaging in otherwise hazardous activities.
- Avoiding quickly looking between objects in the distance and objects nearby may help you to decrease these visual difficulties.
- You should contact your physician if these visual difficulties interfere with your daily activities.

There have been reports of side effects on the liver. If you develop jaundice (yellow color of the skin and/or eyes), stop your medication and contact your healthcare provider.

KETEK has the potential to affect the heart, as seen on an electrocardiogram (EKG) test. In very rare cases, this condition may result in a serious abnormal heartbeat. Contact your healthcare provider if you have a fainting spell.

There have been reports of worsening of myasthenia gravis symptoms in patients with myasthenia gravis. If you have myasthenia gravis and experience any worsening of your symptoms (such as muscle weakness, difficulty breathing) during treatment with KETEK, you should stop taking KETEK and seek immediate medical attention.

If you have other side effects not mentioned in this section or have concerns about side effects, be sure to talk to your healthcare provider.

How can I find out more about KETEK?

This is a summary of selected key points about KETEK. If you'd like more information or if you have concerns, talk to your healthcare provider. You can also visit the KETEK website at www.KETEK.com. But remember, neither this Patient Information nor the website can replace discussions with your doctor or healthcare provider.

Other key points to remember:

- Take your prescribed dose of KETEK once a day at the same time each day.
- Complete the course of medication (take all the tablets prescribed), even if you start to feel better, unless instructed otherwise.
- As with all other medications, do not use KETEK for other conditions or give tablets to others.
- Store KETEK tablets at room temperature.
- Keep this medication out of the reach of children.
- Do not take your tablets after the expiration date noted.
- Talk to your healthcare provider if you have questions or concerns.

Patient Information as of March 2004

BIAXIN® (clarithromycin) is a registered trademark of Abbott Laboratories.

ZITHROMAX® (azithromycin) is a registered trademark of Pfizer Inc.

DYNABAC® (dirithromycin) is a registered trademark of Eli Lilly and Company.

PROPULSID® (cisapride) is a registered trademark of Johnson & Johnson.

ORAP® (pimozide) is a registered trademark of Teva Pharmaceuticals USA, Inc.

Aventis Pharmaceuticals Inc.
Kansas City, MO 64137
US Patent Nos.: 5,527,780; 5,969,161; and 6,022,965
Rx only

KET-PI-15249-1

To keep your **PDR** up to date throughout the year, note these revisions on the corresponding pages of the annual volume. Simply write **"See Supplement A"** next to the product heading.

Barr Laboratories, Inc.

2 QUAKER RD. P.O. BOX 2900
POMONA, NY 10970

Direct Inquiries to:
1-800-BARRLAB (227-7522)

PLAN B® ℞

[*plăn b*]
(Levonorgestrel)
Tablets, 0.75 mg

Plan B® is intended to prevent pregnancy after known or suspected contraceptive failure or unprotected intercourse. Emergency contraceptive pills (like all oral contraceptives) do not protect against infection with HIV (the virus that causes AIDS) and other sexually transmitted diseases.

DESCRIPTION

Emergency contraceptive tablet. Each Plan B® tablet contains 0.75 mg of a single active steroid ingredient, levonorgestrel [18,19-Dinorpregn-4-en-20-yn-3-one-13-ethyl-17-hydroxy-, (17α)-(-)-], a totally synthetic progestogen. The inactive ingredients present are colloidal silicon dioxide, potato starch, gelatin, magnesium stearate, talc, corn starch, and lactose monohydrate. Levonorgestrel has a molecular weight of 312.45, and the following structural and molecular formulas:

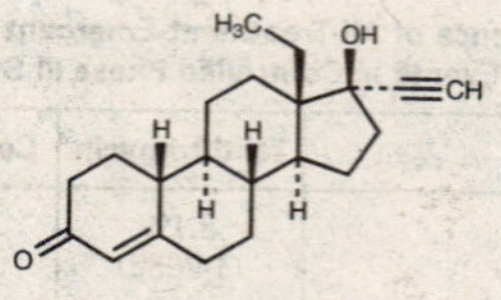

$C_{21}H_{28}O_2$

CLINICAL PHARMACOLOGY

Emergency contraceptives are not effective if the woman is already pregnant. Plan B® is believed to act as an emergency contraceptive principally by preventing ovulation or fertilization (by altering tubal transport of sperm and/or ova). In addition, it may inhibit implantation (by altering the endometrium). It is not effective once the process of implantation has begun.

Pharmacokinetics

Absorption

No specific investigation of the absolute bioavailability of Plan B® in humans has been conducted. However, literature indicates that levonorgestrel is rapidly and completely absorbed after oral administration (bioavailability about 100%) and is not subject to first pass metabolism.

After a single dose of Plan B® (0.75 mg) administered to 16 women under fasting conditions, maximum serum concentrations of levonorgestrel are 14.1 ± 7.7 ng/mL (mean ± SD) at an average of 1.6 ± 0.7 hours. No formal study of the effect of food on the absorption of levonorgestrel has been undertaken.

Table 1 Pharmacokinetic Parameter Values Following Single Dose Administration of Plan B® (Levonorgestrel) Tablets, 0.75 mg to Healthy Female Volunteers

N	Mean (± S.D.)					
	C_{max} (ng/mL)	T_{max} (h)	CL (L/h)	V_d (L)	$T_{1/2}$ (h)	$AUC_{0-\infty}$ (ng/mL/h)
16	14.1± 7.7	1.6 ± 0.7	7.7 ± 2.7	260.0	24.4 ± 5.3	123.1 ± 50.1

Distribution

Levonorgestrel in serum is primarily protein bound. Approximately 50% is bound to albumin and 47.5% is bound to sex hormone binding globulin (SHBG).

Metabolism

Following a single oral dosage, levonorgestrel does not appear to be extensively metabolized by the liver. The primary metabolites are 3α,5β- and 3α,5α-tetrahydrolevonorgestrel with 16β-hydroxynorgestrel also identified. Together, these account for less than 10% of parent plasma levels. Urinary metabolites hydroxylated at the 2α and 16β positions have also been identified. Small amounts of the metabolites are present in plasma as sulfate and glucuronide conjugates.

Excretion

The elimination half-life of levonorgestrel following single dose administration as Plan B® (0.75 mg) is 24.4 ± 5.3 hours. Excretion following single dose administration as emergency contraception is unknown, but based on chronic, low-dose contraceptive use, levonorgestrel and its metabolites are primarily excreted in the urine, with smaller amounts recovered in the feces.

Special Populations

Geriatric

This product is not intended for use in geriatric (age 65 years or older) populations and pharmacokinetic data are not available for this population.

Pediatric

This product is not intended for use in pediatric (premenarcheal) populations, and pharmacokinetic data are not available for this population.

Race

No formal studies have evaluated the effect of race. However, clinical trials demonstrated a higher pregnancy rate in the Chinese population with both Plan B® and the Yuzpe regimen (another form of emergency contraception consisting of two doses of ethinyl estradiol 0.1 mg + levonorgestrel 0.5 mg). The reason for this apparent increase in the pregnancy rate of emergency contraceptives in Chinese women is unknown.

Hepatic Insufficiency and Renal Insufficiency

No formal studies have evaluated the effect of hepatic insufficiency or renal insufficiency on the disposition of emergency contraceptive tablets.

Drug-Drug Interactions

No formal studies of drug-drug interactions were conducted.

INDICATIONS & USAGE

Indication

Plan B® is an emergency contraceptive that can be used to prevent pregnancy following unprotected intercourse or a known or suspected contraceptive failure. To obtain optimal efficacy, the first tablet should be taken as soon as possible within 72 hours of intercourse. The second tablet must be taken 12 hours later.

Clinical Studies

A double-blind, controlled clinical trial in 1,955 evaluable women compared the efficacy and safety of Plan B® (one 0.75 mg tablet of levonorgestrel taken within 72 hours of intercourse, and one tablet taken 12 hours later) to the Yuzpe regimen (two tablets of 0.25 mg levonorgestrel and 0.05 mg ethinyl estradiol, taken within 72 hours of intercourse, and two tablets taken 12 hours later). Plan B® was at least as effective as the Yuzpe regimen in preventing pregnancy. After a single act of intercourse, the expected pregnancy rate of 8% (with no contraception) was reduced to approximately 1% with Plan B®. Thus, Plan B® reduced the expected number of pregnancies by 89%.

Emergency contraceptives are not as effective as routine contraception since their failure rate, while low based on a single use, would accumulate over time with repeated use (see Warnings). See Table 2 below.

Table 2 Percentage of Women Experiencing an Unintended Pregnancy During the First Year of Typical Use and the First Year of Perfect Use of Contraception, and the Percentage Continuing Use at the End of the first Year – United States

	% of Women Experiencing an Unintended Pregnancy within the First Year of Use		% of Women Continuing Use at One Year
Method (1)	Typical Use[1] (2)	Perfect Use[2] (3)	(4)[3]
Chance[4]	85	85	
Spermicide[5]	26	6	40
Periodic Abstinence	25		63
Calendar		9	
Ovulation Method		3	
Symptom-thermal[6]		2	
Post-ovulation		1	
Withdrawal	19	4	
Cap[7]			
Parous Women	40	26	42
Nulliparous Women	20	9	56
Sponge			
Parous Women	40	20	42
Nulliparous Women	20	9	56
Diaphragm[7]	20	6	56
Condom[8]			
Female (Reality)	21	5	56
Male	14	3	56
Oral Contraceptives	5		71
Progestin Only		0.5	
Combined		0.1	
IUD			
Progestin T	2.0	1.5	81
Copper T 380A	0.8	0.6	78
LNG	0.1	0.1	81
Depo-Provera	0.3	0.3	
Norplant and Norplant-2	0.05	0.05	88

Female Sterilization	0.5	0.5	100
Male Sterilization	0.15	0.10	100

Emergency Contraceptive Pills: Treatment initiated within 72 hours after unprotected intercourse reduces the risk of pregnancy by at least 75%.
Lactational Amenorrhea Method: LAM is a highly effective temporary method of contraception.[9]

1. Among typical couples who initiate use of a method (not necessarily for the first time) who experience an accidental pregnancy during the first year if they do not stop use for any other reason.
2. Among couples who initiate use of a method (not necessarily for the first time) and who use it perfectly (both consistently and correctly) the percentage who experience an accidental pregnancy during the first year if they do not stop use for any other reason.
3. Among couples attempting to avoid pregnancy, the percentage (column 4) who continue to use a method for 1 year.
4. The percent becoming pregnant in columns (2) and (3) are based on data from populations where contraception is not used and from women who cease using contraception in order to become pregnant. Among such populations, about 89% become pregnant within 1 year among women now relying on reversible methods of contraception if they abandoned contraception altogether.
5. Foams, creams, gels, vaginal suppositories, and vaginal film.
6. Cervical mucus (ovulation) method supplemented by calendar in the pre-ovulatory and basal body temperature in the post-ovulatory phase.
7. With spermicidal cream or jelly.
8. Without spermicides.
9. However, to maintain an effective protection against pregnancy, another method of contraception must be used as soon as menstruation resumes, the frequency or duration of breast feeds is reduced, bottle feeds are introduced, or the baby reaches 6 months of age.

Source: Trussell J. Contraceptive efficacy. In Hatcher RA, Trussell J, Stewart F, Cates W, Stewart GK, Guest F, Kowal D. Contraceptive Technology; Seventeenth Revised Edition. New York, NY: Irvington Publishers, 1998.

CONTRAINDICATIONS

Progestin-only contraceptive pills (POPs) are used as a routine method of birth control over longer periods of time, and are contraindicated in some conditions. It is not known whether these same conditions apply to the Plan B® regimen consisting of the emergency use of two progestin pills. POPs however, are not recommended for use in the following conditions:

- Known or suspected pregnancy
- Hypersensitivity to any component of the product
- Undiagnosed abnormal genital bleeding

WARNINGS

Plan B® is not recommended for routine use as a contraceptive.
Plan B® is not effective in terminating an existing pregnancy.

Effects on Menses
Menstrual bleeding patterns are often irregular among women using progestin-only oral contraceptives and in clinical studies of levonorgestrel for postcoital and emergency contraceptive use. Some women may experience spotting a few days after taking Plan B®. At the time of expected menses, approximately 75% of women using Plan B® had vaginal bleeding similar to their normal menses, 12–13% bled more than usual, and 12% bled less than usual. The majority of women (87%) had their next menstrual period at the expected time or within ± 7 days, while 13% had a delay of more than 7 days beyond the anticipated onset of menses. If there is a delay in the onset of menses beyond 1 week, the possibility of pregnancy should be considered.

Ectopic Pregnancy
Ectopic pregnancies account for approximately 2% of reported pregnancies (19.7 per 1,000 reported pregnancies). Up to 10% of pregnancies reported in clinical studies of routine use of progestin-only contraceptives are ectopic. A history of ectopic pregnancy need not be considered a contraindication to use of this emergency contraceptive method. Health providers, however, should be alert to the possibility of an ectopic pregnancy in women who become pregnant or complain of lower abdominal pain after taking Plan B®.

PRECAUTIONS

Pregnancy
Many studies have found no effects on fetal development associated with long-term use of contraceptive doses of oral progestins (POPs). The few studies of infant growth and development that have been conducted with POPs have not demonstrated significant adverse effects.

STD/HIV
Plan B®, like progestin-only contraceptives, does not protect against HIV infection (AIDS) and other sexually transmitted diseases.

Physical Examination and Follow-up
A physical examination is not required prior to prescribing Plan B®. A follow-up physical or pelvic examination, however, is recommended if there is any doubt concerning the general health or pregnancy status of any woman after taking Plan B®.

Carbohydrate Metabolism
The effects of Plan B® on carbohydrate metabolism are unknown. Some users of progestin-only oral contraceptives (POPs) may experience slight deterioration in glucose tolerance, with increases in plasma insulin; however, women with diabetes mellitus who use POPs do not generally experience changes in their insulin requirements. Nonetheless, diabetic women should be monitored while taking Plan B®.

Drug Interactions
Theoretically, the effectiveness of low-dose progestin-only pills is reduced by hepatic enzyme-inducing drugs such as the anticonvulsants phenytoin, carbamazepine, and barbiturates, and the antituberculosis drug rifampin. No significant interaction has been found with broad-spectrum antibiotics. It is not known whether the efficacy of Plan B® would be affected by these or any other medications.

Nursing Mothers
Small amounts of progestin pass into the breast milk in women taking progestin-only pills for long-term contraception resulting in steroid levels in infant plasma of 1–6% of the levels of maternal plasma. However, no adverse effects due to progestin-only pills have been found on breastfeeding performance, either in the quality or quantity of the milk, or on the health, growth or development of the infant.

Pediatric Use
Safety and efficacy of progestin-only pills have been established in women of reproductive age for long-term contraception. Safety and efficacy are expected to be the same for postpubertal adolescents under the age of 16 and for users 16 years and older. Use of Plan B® emergency contraception before menarche is not indicated.

Fertility Following Discontinuation
The limited available data indicate a rapid return of normal ovulation and fertility following discontinuation of progestin-only pills for emergency contraception and long-term contraception.

ADVERSE REACTIONS

The most common adverse events in the clinical trial for women receiving Plan B® included nausea (23%), abdominal pain (18%), fatigue (17%), headache (17%), and menstrual changes. The table below shows those adverse events that occurred in ≥5% of Plan B® users.

Table 3 Adverse Events in ≥5% of Women, by % Frequency

Most Common Adverse Events	Plan B® Levonorgestrel N=977 (%)
Nausea	23.1
Abdominal Pain	17.6
Fatigue	16.9
Headache	16.8
Heavier Menstrual Bleeding	13.8
Lighter Menstrual Bleeding	12.5
Dizziness	11.2
Breast Tenderness	10.7
Other complaints	9.7
Vomiting	5.6
Diarrhea	5.0

Plan B® demonstrated a superior safety profile over the Yuzpe regimen for the following adverse events:

- Nausea: Occurred in 23% of women taking Plan B® (compared to 50% with Yuzpe)
- Vomiting: Occurred in 6% of women taking Plan B® (compared to 19% with Yuzpe)

DRUG ABUSE AND DEPENDENCE

There is no information about dependence associated with the use of Plan B®.

OVERDOSAGE

There are no data on overdosage of Plan B®, although the common adverse event of nausea and its associated vomiting may be anticipated.

DOSAGE AND ADMINISTRATION

One tablet of Plan B® should be taken orally within 72 hours after unprotected intercourse. The second tablet should be taken 12 hours after the first dose. Efficacy is better if Plan B® is taken as directed as soon as possible after unprotected intercourse. Plan B® can be used at any time during the menstrual cycle.
The user should be instructed that if she vomits within one hour of taking either dose of medication she should contact her health care professional to discuss whether to repeat that dose.

HOW SUPPLIED

Plan B® (Levonorgestrel) Tablets, 0.75 mg are available for a single course of treatment in PVC/aluminum foil blister packages of two tablets each. The tablet is white, round and marked: INOR.

Available as:
Unit-of-use NDC 51285-038-93
Store Plan B® tablets at controlled room temperature, 20° to 25°C (68° to 77°F); excursions permitted between 15° to 30°C (59° to 86°F) [See USP].
Mfg. by Gedeon Richter, Ltd., Budapest, Hungary
for Duramed Pharmaceuticals, Inc.
Subsidiary of Barr Pharmaceuticals, Inc.
Pomona, New York 10970
Phone: 1-800-330-1271 Website: www.go2planb.com
Revised FEBRUARY 2004
BR- 038 / 21000382503

SEASONALE® ℞

[*sē-sōn-āl*]
(levonorgestrel/ethinyl estradiol tablets)
0.15 mg/0.03 mg

Patients should be counseled that this product does not protect against HIV-infection (AIDS) and other sexually transmitted diseases.

DESCRIPTION

Seasonale® (levonorgestrel/ethinyl estradiol tablets) is an extended-cycle oral contraceptive consisting of 84 pink active tablets each containing 0.15 mg of levonorgestrel, a synthetic progestogen and 0.03 mg of ethinyl estradiol, and 7 white inert tablets (without hormones). The chemical formula of levonorgestrel USP is 18,19-Dinorpregn-4-en-20-yn-3-one, 13-ethyl-17-hydroxy-, (17α)-, (-)-, and the chemical formula of ethinyl estradiol USP is 19-Norpregna-1,3,5(10)-trien-20-yne-3,17-diol, (17α)-. The structural formulas are as follows:

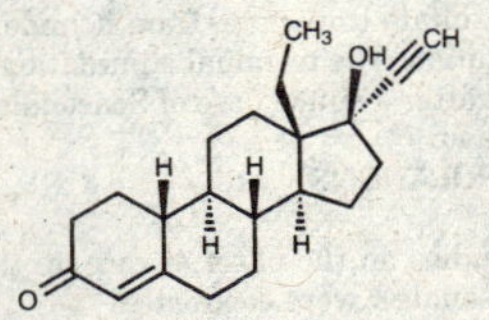

Levonorgestrel
$C_{21}H_{28}O_2$ MW: 312.4

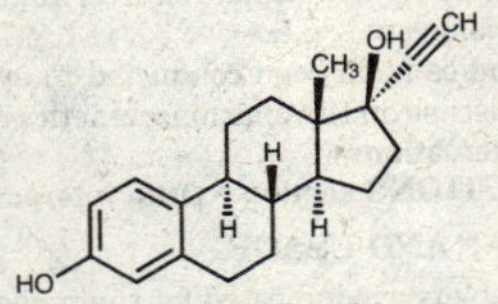

Ethinyl Estradiol
$C_{20}H_{24}O_2$ MW: 296.4

Each pink active tablet contains the following inactive ingredients: anhydrous lactose NF, FD&C blue no. 1, FD&C red no. 40, hydroxypropyl methylcellulose USP, microcrystalline cellulose NF, polyethylene glycol NF, magnesium stearate NF, polysorbate 80 NF, and titanium dioxide USP.
Each white inert tablet contains the following inactive ingredients: anhydrous lactose NF, hydroxypropyl methylcellulose USP, microcrystalline cellulose NF, and magnesium stearate NF.

CLINICAL PHARMACOLOGY

Mode of Action
Combination oral contraceptives act by suppression of gonadotropins. Although the primary mechanism of this action is inhibition of ovulation, other alterations include changes in the cervical mucus (which increase the difficulty of sperm entry into the uterus) and changes in the endometrium (which reduce the likelihood of implantation).

Pharmacokinetics
Absorption
No specific investigation of the absolute bioavailability of Seasonale® in humans has been conducted. However, literature indicates that levonorgestrel is rapidly and completely absorbed after oral administration (bioavailability nearly 100%) and is not subject to first-pass metabolism. Ethinyl estradiol is rapidly and almost completely absorbed from the gastrointestinal tract but, due to first-pass metabolism in gut mucosa and liver, the bioavailability of ethinyl estradiol is approximately 43%.
[See table 1 at bottom of next page]
The effect of food on the rate and the extent of levonorgestrel and ethinyl estradiol absorption following oral administration of Seasonale® has not been evaluated.
Distribution
The apparent volume of distribution of levonorgestrel and ethinyl estradiol are reported to be approximately 1.8 L/kg and 4.3 L/kg, respectively. Levonorgestrel is about 97.5-99% protein-bound, principally to sex hormone binding globulin (SHBG) and, to a lesser extent, serum albumin. Ethinyl estradiol is about 95–97% bound to serum albumin. Ethinyl estradiol does not bind to SHBG, but induces SHBG synthesis, which leads to decreased levonorgestrel clearance. Following repeated daily dosing of combination levonorgestrel/ethinyl estradiol oral contraceptives, levonorgestrel plasma concentrations accumulate more than predicted based on

Continued on next page

Seasonale—Cont.

single-dose kinetics, due in part, to increased SHBG levels that are induced by ethinyl estradiol, and a possible reduction in hepatic metabolic capacity.

Metabolism

Following absorption, levonorgestrel is conjugated at the 17β-OH position to form sulfate and to a lesser extent, glucuronide conjugates in plasma. Significant amounts of conjugated and unconjugated 3α,5β-tetrahydrolevonorgestrel are also present in plasma, along with much smaller amounts of 3α,5α-tetrahydrolevonorgestrel and 16β-hydroxylevonorgestrel. Levonorgestrel and its phase I metabolites are excreted primarily as glucuronide conjugates. Metabolic clearance rates may differ among individuals by several-fold, and this may account in part for the wide variation observed in levonorgestrel concentrations among users.

First-pass metabolism of ethinyl estradiol involves formation of ethinyl estradiol-3-sulfate in the gut wall, followed by 2-hydroxylation of a portion of the remaining untransformed ethinyl estradiol by hepatic cytochrome P-450 3A4 (CYP3A4). Levels of CYP3A4 vary widely among individuals and can explain the variation in rates of ethinyl estradiol hydroxylation. Hydroxylation at the 4-, 6-, and 16- positions may also occur, although to a much lesser extent than 2-hydroxylation. The various hydroxylated metabolites are subject to further methylation and/or conjugation.

Excretion

About 45% of levonorgestrel and its metabolites are excreted in the urine and about 32% are excreted in feces, mostly as glucuronide conjugates. The terminal elimination half-life for levonorgestrel after a single dose of Seasonale® was about 30 hours.

Ethinyl estradiol is excreted in the urine and feces as glucuronide and sulfate conjugates, and it undergoes enterohepatic recirculation. The terminal elimination half-life of ethinyl estradiol after a single dose of Seasonale® was found to be about 15 hours.

SPECIAL POPULATIONS

Race

No formal studies on the effect of race on the pharmacokinetics of Seasonale® were conducted.

Hepatic Insufficiency

No formal studies have been conducted to evaluate the effect of hepatic disease on the pharmacokinetics of Seasonale®. However, steroid hormones may be poorly metabolized in patients with impaired liver function.

Renal Insufficiency

No formal studies have been conducted to evaluate the effect of renal disease on the pharmacokinetics of Seasonale®.

Drug-Drug Interactions

See PRECAUTIONS section – Drug Interactions.

INDICATIONS AND USAGE

Seasonale® tablets are indicated for the prevention of pregnancy in women who elect to use oral contraceptives as a method of contraception.

In a 1-year controlled clinical trial, 4 pregnancies occurred in women 18-35 years of age during 809 completed 91-day cycles of Seasonale® during which no backup contraception was utilized. This represents an overall use-efficacy (typical user efficacy) pregnancy rate of 1.98 per 100 women-years of use.

Oral contraceptives are highly effective for pregnancy prevention. Table 2 lists the typical unintended pregnancy rates for users of combination oral contraceptives and other methods of contraception. The efficacy of these contraceptive methods, except sterilization, and Norplant® Implant System, depends upon the reliability with which they are used. Correct and consistent use of methods can result in lower failure rates.

TABLE 2

Percentage of women experiencing an unintended pregnancy during the first year of typical use and the first year of perfect use of contraception and the percentage continuing use at the end of the first year: United States.

	% of Women Experiencing an Unintended Pregnancy within the First Year of Use		% of Women Continuing Use at One Year[3]
Method (1)	Typical Use[1] (2)	Perfect Use[2] (3)	(4)
Chance[4]	85	85	
Spermicides[5]	26	6	40
Periodic abstinence	25		63
Calendar		9	
Ovulation method		3	
Sympto-thermal[6]		2	
Post-ovulation		1	
Withdrawal	19	4	
Cap[7]			
Parous women	40	26	42
Nulliparous women	20	9	56
Sponge			
Parous women	40	20	42
Nulliparous women	20	9	56
Diaphragm[7]	20	6	56
Condom[8]			
Female (Reality)	21	5	56
Male	14	3	61
Pill	5		71
Progestin only		0.5	
Combined		0.1	
IUD:			
Progesterone T	2.0	1.5	81
Copper T 380A	0.8	0.6	78
LNg 20	0.1	0.1	81
Depo Provera	0.3	0.3	70
Norplant and Norplant-2	0.05	0.05	88
Female sterilization	0.5	0.5	100
Male sterilization	0.15	0.10	100

Emergency Contraceptive Pills: Treatment initiated within 72 hours after unprotected intercourse reduces the risk of pregnancy by at least 75%.[9]

Lactational Amenorrhea Method: LAM is a highly effective, *temporary* method of contraception.[10]

Source: Trussell J, Contraceptive efficacy. In Hatcher RA, Trussell J, Stewart F, Cates W, Stewart GK, Kowal D, Guest F, Contraceptive Technology: Seventeenth Revised Edition. New York NY: Irvington Publishers, 1998.

[1] Among *typical* couples who initiate use of a method (not necessarily for the first time), the percentage who experience an unintended pregnancy during the first year if they do not stop use for any other reason.

[2] Among couples who initiate use of a method (not necessarily for the first time) and who use it *perfectly* (both consistently and correctly), the percentage who experience an unintended pregnancy during the first year if they do not stop use for any other reason.

[3] Among couples attempting to avoid pregnancy, the percentage who continue to use a method for one year.

[4] The percentages of women becoming pregnant in columns (2) and (3) are based on data from populations where contraception is not used and from women who cease using contraception in order to become pregnant. Among such populations, about 89% become pregnant within one year. This estimate was lowered slightly (to 85%) to represent the percentage who would become pregnant within one year among women now relying on reversible methods of contraception if they abandoned contraception altogether.

[5] Foams, creams, gels, vaginal suppositories and vaginal film.

[6] Cervical mucus (ovulation) method supplemented by calendar in the pre-ovulatory and basal body temperature in the post-ovulatory phases.

[7] With spermicidal cream or jelly.

[8] Without spermicides.

[9] The treatment schedule is one dose within 72 hours after unprotected intercourse and a second dose 12 hours after the first dose. The Food and Drug Administration has declared the following brands of oral contraceptives to be safe and effective for emergency contraception: Ovral (1 dose is 2 white pills), Alesse (1 dose is 5 pink pills), Nordette or Levlen (1 dose is 2 light-orange pills), Lo/Ovral (1 dose is 4 white pills), Triphasil or Tri-Levlen (1 dose is 4 yellow pills).

[10] However, to maintain effective protection against pregnancy, another method of contraception must be used as soon as menstruation resumes, the frequency or duration of breastfeeds is reduced, bottle feeds are introduced or the baby reaches six months of age.

Table 1: Mean ± SD Pharmacokinetic Parameters Following A Single Dose Administration of Two Tablets of Seasonale® in Healthy Female Subjects Under Fasting Conditions

Analyte	AUC_t (mean ± SD)	C_{max} (mean ± SD)	T_{max} (mean ± SD)	$T_{1/2}$ (mean ± SD)
Levonorgestrel	60.8 ± 25.6 ng*hr/mL	5.6 ± 1.5 ng/mL	1.4 ± 0.3 hours	29.8 ± 8.3 hours
Ethinyl estradiol	1307 ± 361 pg*hr/mL	145 ± 45 pg/mL	1.6 ± 0.5 hours	15.4 ± 3.2 hours

CONTRAINDICATIONS

Oral contraceptives should not be used in women who currently have the following conditions:

- Thrombophlebitis or thromboembolic disorders
- A past history of deep vein thrombophlebitis or thromboembolic disorders
- Cerebrovascular or coronary artery disease (current or history)
- Valvular heart disease with thrombogenic complications
- Uncontrolled hypertension
- Diabetes with vascular involvement
- Headaches with focal neurological symptoms
- Major surgery with prolonged immobilization
- Known or suspected carcinoma of the breast or personal history of breast cancer
- Carcinoma of the endometrium or other known or suspected estrogen-dependent neoplasia
- Undiagnosed abnormal genital bleeding
- Cholestatic jaundice of pregnancy or jaundice with prior pill use
- Hepatic adenomas or carcinomas, or active liver disease
- Known or suspected pregnancy
- Hypersensitivity to any component of this product

WARNINGS

Cigarette smoking increases the risk of serious cardiovascular side effects from oral contraceptive use. This risk increases with age and with heavy smoking (15 or more cigarettes per day) and is quite marked in women over 35 years of age. Women who use oral contraceptives should be strongly advised not to smoke.

The use of oral contraceptives is associated with increased risk of several serious conditions including venous and arterial thrombotic and thromboembolic events (such as myocardial infarction, thromboembolism, and stroke), hepatic neoplasia, gallbladder disease, and hypertension. The risk of serious morbidity or mortality is very small in healthy women without underlying risk factors. The risk of morbidity and mortality increases significantly in the presence of other underlying risk factors such as certain inherited thrombophilias, hypertension, hyperlipidemias, obesity and diabetes.

Practitioners prescribing oral contraceptives should be familiar with the following information relating to these risks. The information contained in this package insert is principally based on studies carried out in patients who used oral contraceptives with higher formulations of estrogens and progestogens than those in common use today. The effect of long-term use of the oral contraceptives with lower doses of both estrogens and progestogens remains to be determined.

Throughout this labeling, epidemiological studies reported are of two types: retrospective or case control studies and prospective or cohort studies. Case control studies provide a measure of the relative risk of a disease, namely, a ratio of the incidence of a disease among oral contraceptive users to that among nonusers. The relative risk does not provide information on the actual clinical occurrence of a disease. Cohort studies provide a measure of attributable risk, which is the difference in the incidence of disease between oral contraceptive users and nonusers. The attributable risk does provide information about the actual occurrence of a disease in the population. For further information, the reader is referred to a text on epidemiological methods.

1. Thromboembolic Disorders and Other Vascular Problems

Use of Seasonale® provides women with more hormonal exposure on a yearly basis than conventional monthly oral contraceptives containing similar strength synthetic estrogens and progestins (an additional 9 weeks per year). While this added exposure may pose an additional risk of thrombotic and thromboembolic disease, studies to date with Seasonale have not suggested an increased risk of these disorders.

a. *Myocardial Infarction:* An increased risk of myocardial infarction has been attributed to oral contraceptive use. This risk is primarily in smokers or women with other underlying risk factors for coronary artery disease such as hypertension, hypercholesterolemia, morbid obesity, and diabetes. The relative risk of heart attack for current oral contraceptive users has been estimated to be two to six. The risk is very low under the age of 30. Smoking in combination with oral contraceptive use has been shown to contribute substantially to the incidence of myocardial infarction in women in their mid-thirties or older with smoking accounting for the majority of excess cases. Mortality rates associated with circulatory disease have been shown to increase substantially in smokers over the age of 35 and nonsmokers over the age of 40 (Figure 1) among women who use oral contraceptives.

Figure 1

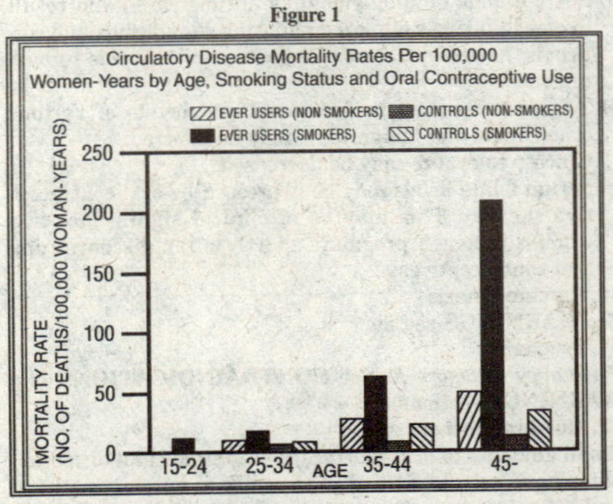

Adapted from P.M. Layde and V. Beral, Lancet, *1*:541–546, 1981

Oral contraceptives may compound the effects of well-known risk factors, such as hypertension, diabetes, hyperlipidemias, age and obesity. In particular, some progestogens are known to decrease HDL cholesterol and cause glucose intolerance, while estrogens may create a state of hyperinsulinism. Oral contraceptives have been shown to increase blood pressure among users (see section 9 in **WARNINGS**). The severity and number of risk factors increase heart disease risk. Oral contraceptives must be used with caution in women with cardiovascular disease risk factors.

b. *Thromboembolism:* An increased risk of thromboembolic and thrombotic disease associated with the use of oral contraceptives is well established. Case control studies have found the relative risk of users compared to non-users to be 3 for the first episode of superficial venous thrombosis, 4 to 11 for deep vein thrombosis or pulmonary embolism, and 1.5 to 6 for women with predisposing conditions for venous thromboembolic disease. Cohort studies have shown the relative risk to be somewhat lower, about 3 for new cases and about 4.5 for new cases requiring hospitalization. The approximate incidence of deep vein thrombosis and pulmonary embolism in users of low dose (<50 µg ethinyl estradiol) combination oral contraceptives is up to 4 per 10,000 woman-years compared to 0.5-3 per 10,000 woman-years for non-users. However, the incidence is less than that associated with pregnancy (6 per 10,000 woman-years). The risk of thromboembolic disease due to oral contraceptives is not related to length of use and disappears after pill use is stopped.

A two- to four-fold increase in relative risk of postoperative thromboembolic complications has been reported with the use of oral contraceptives. The relative risk of venous thrombosis in women who have predisposing conditions is twice that of women without such medical conditions. If feasible, oral contraceptives should be discontinued at least four weeks prior to and for two weeks after elective surgery of a type associated with an increase in risk of thromboembolism and during and following prolonged immobilization. Since the immediate postpartum period is also associated with an increased risk of thromboembolism, oral contraceptives should be started no earlier than four weeks after delivery in women who elect not to breast-feed.

c. *Cerebrovascular Diseases:* Oral contraceptives have been shown to increase both the relative and attributable risks of cerebrovascular events (thrombotic and hemorrhagic strokes), although, in general, the risk is greatest among older (>35 years), hypertensive women who also smoke. Hypertension was found to be a risk factor for both users and nonusers, for both types of strokes, while smoking interacted to increase the risk for hemorrhagic strokes. In a large study, the relative risk of thrombotic strokes has been shown to range from 3 for normotensive users to 14 for users with severe hypertension. The relative risk of hemorrhagic stroke is reported to be 1.2 for non-smokers who used oral contraceptives, 2.6 for smokers who did not use oral contraceptives, 7.6 for smokers who used oral contraceptives, 1.8 for normotensive users and 25.7 for users with severe hypertension. The attributable risk is also greater in older women. Oral contraceptives also increase the risk for stroke in women with other underlying risk factors such as certain inherited or acquired thrombophilias, hyperlipidemias, and obesity. Women with migraine (particularly migraine with aura) who take combination oral contraceptives may be at an increased risk of stroke.

d. *Dose-Related Risk of Vascular Disease from Oral Contraceptives:* A positive association has been observed between the amount of estrogen and progestogen in oral contraceptives and the risk of vascular disease. A decline in serum high-density lipoproteins (HDL) has been reported with many progestational agents. A decline in serum high-density lipoproteins has been associated with an increased incidence of ischemic heart disease. Because estrogens increase HDL cholesterol, the net effect of an oral contraceptive depends on a balance achieved between doses of estrogen and progestogen and the nature and absolute amount of progestogen used in the contraceptive. The amount of both hormones should be considered in the choice of an oral contraceptive.

Minimizing exposure to estrogen and progestogen is in keeping with good principles of therapeutics. For any particular estrogen/progestogen combination, the dosage regimen prescribed should be one which contains the least amount of estrogen and progestogen that is compatible with a low failure rate and the needs of the individual patient. New acceptors of oral contraceptive agents should be started on preparations containing the lowest estrogen content which is judged appropriate for the individual patient.

e. *Persistence of Risk of Vascular Disease:* There are two studies which have shown persistence of risk of vascular disease for ever-users of oral contraceptives. In a study in the United States, the risk of developing myocardial infarction after discontinuing oral contraceptives persists for at least 9 years for women 40 to 49 years old who had used oral contraceptives for five or more years, but this increased risk was not demonstrated in other age groups. In another study in Great Britain, the risk of developing cerebrovascular disease persisted for at least 6 years after discontinuation of oral contraceptives, although excess risk was very small. However, both studies were performed with oral contraceptive formulations containing 50 micrograms or higher of estrogens.

2. Estimates of Mortality from Contraceptive Use

One study gathered data from a variety of sources which have estimated the mortality rate associated with different methods of contraception at different ages (Table 3). These estimates include the combined risk of death associated with contraceptive methods plus the risk attributable to pregnancy in the event of method failure. Each method of contraception has its specific benefits and risks. The study concluded that with the exception of oral contraceptive users 35 and older who smoke and 40 and older who do not smoke, mortality associated with all methods of birth control is less than that associated with childbirth. The observation of a possible increase in risk of mortality with age for oral contraceptive users is based on data gathered in the 1970's--but not reported until 1983. However, current clinical practice involves the use of lower estrogen dose formulations combined with careful restriction of oral contraceptive use to women who do not have the various risk factors listed in this labeling. Because of these changes in practice and, also, because of some limited new data which suggest that the risk of cardiovascular disease with the use of oral contraceptives may now be less than previously observed, the Fertility and Maternal Health Drugs Advisory Committee was asked to review the topic in 1989. The Committee concluded that although cardiovascular disease risks may be increased with oral contraceptive use after age 40 in healthy nonsmoking women (even with the newer low-dose formulations), there are greater potential health risks associated with pregnancy in older women and with the alternative surgical and medical procedures which may be necessary if such women do not have access to effective and acceptable means of contraception.

Therefore, the Committee recommended that the benefits of oral contraceptive use by healthy nonsmoking women over 40 may outweigh the possible risks. Of course, older women, as all women who take oral contraceptives, should take the lowest possible dose formulation that is effective.

TABLE 3: ANNUAL NUMBER OF BIRTH-RELATED OR METHOD-RELATED DEATHS ASSOCIATED WITH CONTROL OF FERTILITY PER 100,000 NONSTERILE WOMEN, BY FERTILITY-CONTROL METHOD AND ACCORDING TO AGE

Method of control and outcome	AGE 15-19	20-24	25-29	30-34	35-39	40-44
No fertility - control methods*	7.0	7.4	9.1	14.8	25.7	28.2
Oral contraceptives non-smoker**	0.3	0.5	0.9	1.9	13.8	31.6
Oral contraceptives smoker**	2.2	3.4	6.6	13.5	51.1	117.2
IUD**	0.8	0.8	1.0	1.0	1.4	1.4
Condom*	1.1	1.6	0.7	0.2	0.3	0.4
Diaphragm/ spermicide*	1.9	1.2	1.2	1.3	2.2	2.8
Periodic abstinence*	2.5	1.6	1.6	1.7	2.9	3.6

* Deaths are birth related
** Deaths are method related

Adapted from H.W. Ory, Family Planning Perspectives, *15*: 57-63, 1983.

3. Carcinoma of the Reproductive Organs and Breasts

Numerous epidemiological studies have been performed on the incidence of breast, endometrial, ovarian and cervical cancer in women using oral contraceptives. Although the risk of having breast cancer diagnosed may be slightly increased among current and recent users of combined oral contraceptives (RR=1.24), this excess risk decreases over time after combination oral contraceptive discontinuation and by 10 years after cessation the increased risk disappears. The risk does not increase with duration of use and no consistent relationships have been found with dose or type of steroid. The patterns of risk are also similar regardless of a woman's reproductive history or her family breast cancer history. The subgroup for whom risk has been found to be significantly elevated is women who first used oral contraceptives before age 20, but because breast cancer is so rare at these young ages, the number of cases attributable to this early oral contraceptive use is extremely small. Breast cancers diagnosed in current or previous oral contraceptive users tend to be less clinically advanced than in never-users. Women who currently have or have had breast cancer should not use oral contraceptives because breast cancer is a hormone sensitive tumor.

Some studies suggest that oral contraceptive use has been associated with an increase in the risk of cervical intraepithelial neoplasia or invasive cervical cancer in some populations of women. However, there continues to be controversy about the extent to which such findings may be due to differences in sexual behavior and other factors. In spite of many studies of the relationship between oral contraceptive use and breast cancer and cervical cancers, a cause-and-effect relationship has not been established.

4. Hepatic Neoplasia

Benign hepatic adenomas are associated with oral contraceptive use, although their occurrence is rare in the United States. Indirect calculations have estimated the attributable risk to be in the range of 3.3 cases/100,000 for users, a risk that increases after four or more years of use. Rupture of hepatic adenomas may cause death through intra-abdominal hemorrhage.

Studies from Britain have shown an increased risk of developing hepatocellular carcinoma in long-term (>8 years) oral contraceptive users. However, these cancers are extremely rare in the U.S., and the attributable risk (the excess incidence) of liver cancers in oral contraceptive users approaches less than one per million users.

5. Ocular Lesions

There have been clinical case reports of retinal thrombosis associated with the use of oral contraceptives that may lead to partial or complete loss of vision. Oral contraceptives should be discontinued if there is unexplained partial or complete loss of vision; onset of proptosis or diplopia; papilledema; or retinal vascular lesions. Appropriate diagnostic and therapeutic measures should be undertaken immediately.

6. Oral contraceptive Use Before or During Early Pregnancy

Because women using Seasonale® will likely have withdrawal bleeding only 4 times per year, pregnancy should be ruled out at the time of any missed menstrual period (see **DOSAGE AND ADMINISTRATION** section). Oral contraceptive use should be discontinued if pregnancy is confirmed.

Extensive epidemiological studies have revealed no increased risk of birth defects in women who have used oral contraceptives prior to pregnancy. Studies also do not suggest a teratogenic effect, particularly in so far as cardiac anomalies and limb-reduction defects are concerned, when taken inadvertently during early pregnancy (see **CONTRAINDICATIONS** section).

The administration of oral contraceptives to induce withdrawal bleeding should not be used as a test for pregnancy. Oral contraceptives should not be used during pregnancy to treat threatened or habitual abortion.

7. Gallbladder Disease

Earlier studies have reported an increased lifetime relative risk of gallbladder surgery in users of oral contraceptives and estrogens. More recent studies, however, have shown that the relative risk of developing gallbladder disease among oral contraceptive users may be minimal. The recent findings of minimal risk may be related to the use of oral contraceptive formulations containing lower hormonal doses of estrogens and progestogens.

8. Carbohydrate and Lipid Metabolic Effects

Oral contraceptives have been shown to cause glucose intolerance in a significant percentage of users. Oral contraceptives containing greater than 75 micrograms of estrogens cause hyperinsulinism, while lower doses of estrogen cause less glucose intolerance. Progestogens increase insulin secretion and create insulin resistance,

Continued on next page

Seasonale—Cont.

this effect varying with different progestational agents. However, in the nondiabetic woman, oral contraceptives appear to have no effect on fasting blood glucose. Because of these demonstrated effects, prediabetic and diabetic women should be carefully observed while taking oral contraceptives.

A small proportion of women will have persistent hypertriglyceridemia while on the pill. As discussed earlier (see **WARNINGS** 1a. and 1d.), changes in serum triglycerides and lipoprotein levels have been reported in oral contraceptive users.

9. Elevated Blood Pressure

Women with significant hypertension should not be started on hormonal contraceptive. An increase in blood pressure has been reported in women taking oral contraceptives and this increase is more likely in older oral contraceptive users and with continued use. Data from the Royal College of General Practitioners and subsequent randomized trials have shown that the incidence of hypertension increases with increasing concentrations of progestogens.

Women with a history of hypertension or hypertension-related diseases, or renal disease should be encouraged to use another method of contraception. If women with hypertension elect to use oral contraceptives, they should be monitored closely, and if significant elevation of blood pressure occurs, oral contraceptives should be discontinued (see **CONTRAINDICATIONS** section). For most women, elevated blood pressure will return to normal after stopping oral contraceptives, and there is no difference in the occurrence of hypertension among ever- and never-users.

10. Headache

The onset or exacerbation of migraine or development of headache with a new pattern that is recurrent, persistent, or severe requires discontinuation of oral contraceptives and evaluation of the cause. (See **WARNINGS**, 1c.)

11. Bleeding Irregularities

When prescribing Seasonale®, the convenience of fewer planned menses (4 per year instead of 13 per year) should be weighed against the inconvenience of increased intermenstrual bleeding and/or spotting.

The clinical trial (SEA 301) that compared the efficacy of Seasonale® (91-day cycles) to an equivalent dosage 28-day cycle regimen also assessed intermenstrual bleeding. The participants in the study were composed primarily of women who had used oral contraceptives previously as opposed to new users. Women with a history of breakthrough bleeding/spotting ≥ 10 consecutive days on oral contraceptives were excluded from the study. More Seasonale® subjects, compared to subjects on the 28-day cycle regimen, discontinued prematurely for unacceptable bleeding (7.7% [Seasonale®] vs. 1.8% [28-day cycle regimen]).

Table 4 shows the percentages of women with ≥ 7 days and ≥ 20 days of intermenstrual spotting and/or bleeding in the Seasonale® and the 28-day cycle treatment groups.

Table 4. Percentage of Subjects with Intermenstrual Bleeding and/or Spotting

Days of intermenstrual bleeding and/or spotting	Percentage of Subjects*	
Seasonale®	Cycle 1 (N=385)	Cycle 4 (N=261)
≥ 7 days	65%	42%
≥ 20 days	35%	15%
28-day regimen	Cycles 1-4 (N=194)	Cycles 10-13 (N=158)
≥ 7 days	38%	39%
≥ 20 days	6%	4%

* Based on spotting and/or bleeding on days 1-84 of a 91 day cycle in the Seasonale subjects and days 1-21 of a 28 day cycle over 4 cycles in the 28-day dosing regimen.

Total days of bleeding and/or spotting (withdrawal plus intermenstrual) were similar over one year of treatment for Seasonale® subjects and subjects on the 28-day cycle regimen.

As in any case of bleeding irregularities, nonhormonal causes should always be considered and adequate diagnostic measures taken to rule out malignancy or pregnancy.

In the event of amenorrhea, pregnancy should be ruled out. Some women may encounter post-pill amenorrhea or oligomenorrhea (possibly with anovulation), especially when such a condition was preexistent.

PRECAUTIONS

1. Sexually Transmitted Diseases

Patients should be counseled that this product does not protect against HIV infection (AIDS) and other sexually transmitted diseases.

2. Physical Examination and Follow-up

A periodic history and physical examination are appropriate for all women, including women using oral contraceptives. The physical examination, however, may be deferred until after initiation of oral contraceptives if requested by the woman and judged appropriate by the clinician. The physical examination should include special reference to blood pressure, breasts, abdomen and pelvic organs, including cervical cytology, and relevant laboratory tests. In case of undiagnosed, persistent or recurrent abnormal vaginal bleeding, appropriate diagnostic measures should be conducted to rule out malignancy. Women with a strong family history of breast cancer or who have breast nodules should be monitored with particular care.

3. Lipid Disorders

Women who are being treated for hyperlipidemias should be followed closely if they elect to use oral contraceptives. Some progestogens may elevate LDL levels and may render the control of hyperlipidemias more difficult. (See **WARNINGS** 1d.)

In patients with familial defects of lipoprotein metabolism receiving estrogen-containing preparations, there have been case reports of significant elevations of plasma triglycerides leading to pancreatitis.

4. Liver Function

If jaundice develops in any woman receiving such drugs, the medication should be discontinued. Steroid hormones may be poorly metabolized in patients with impaired liver function.

5. Fluid Retention

Oral contraceptives may cause some degree of fluid retention. They should be prescribed with caution, and only with careful monitoring, in patients with conditions, which might be aggravated by fluid retention.

6. Emotional Disorders

Women with a history of depression should be carefully observed and the drug discontinued if depression recurs to a serious degree. Patients becoming significantly depressed while taking oral contraceptives should stop the medication and use an alternate method of contraception in an attempt to determine whether the symptom is drug related.

7. Contact Lenses

Contact-lens wearers who develop visual changes or changes in lens tolerance should be assessed by an ophthalmologist.

8. Drug Interactions

Changes in contraceptive effectiveness associated with co-administration of other products

a. Anti-infective agents and anticonvulsants

Contraceptive effectiveness may be reduced when hormonal contraceptives are co-administered with antibiotics, anticonvulsants, and other drugs that increase the metabolism of contraceptive steroids. This could result in unintended pregnancy or breakthrough bleeding. Examples include rifampin, barbiturates, phenylbutazone, phenytoin, carbamazepine, felbamate, oxcarbazepine, topiramate, and griseofulvin. Several cases of contraceptive failure and breakthrough bleeding have been reported in the literature with concomitant administration of antibiotics such as ampicillin and tetracyclines. However, clinical pharmacology studies investigating drug interaction between combined oral contraceptives and these antibiotics have reported inconsistent results.

b. Anti-HIV protease inhibitors

Several of the anti-HIV protease inhibitors have been studied with co-administration of oral combination hormonal contraceptives; significant changes (increase and decrease) in the plasma levels of the estrogen and progestin have been noted in some cases. The safety and efficacy of combination oral contraceptive products may be affected with co-administration of anti-HIV protease inhibitors. Healthcare providers should refer to the label of the individual anti-HIV protease inhibitors for further drug-drug interaction information.

c. Herbal products

Herbal products containing St. John's Wort (hypericum perforatum) may induce hepatic enzymes (cytochrome P450) and p-glycoprotein transporter and may reduce the effectiveness of contraceptive steroids. This may also result in breakthrough bleeding.

Increase in plasma levels of estradiol associated with co-administered drugs

Co-administration of atorvastatin and certain combination oral contraceptives containing ethinyl estradiol increase AUC values for ethinyl estradiol by approximately 20%. Ascorbic acid and acetaminophen may increase plasma ethinyl estradiol levels, possibly by inhibition of conjugation. CYP 3A4 inhibitors such as itraconazole or ketoconazole may increase plasma hormone levels.

Changes in plasma levels of co-administered drugs

Combination hormonal contraceptives containing some synthetic estrogens (e.g., ethinyl estradiol) may inhibit the metabolism of other compounds. Increased plasma concentrations of cyclosporin, prednisolone, and theophylline have been reported with concomitant administration of combination oral contraceptives. Decreased plasma concentrations of acetaminophen and increased clearance of temazepam, salicylic acid, morphine and clofibric acid, due to induction of conjugation have been noted when these drugs were administered with combination oral contraceptives.

9. Interactions with Laboratory Tests

Certain endocrine and liver function tests and blood components may be affected by oral contraceptives:

a) Increased prothrombin and factors VII, VIII, IX, and X; decreased antithrombin 3; increased norepinephrine-induced platelet aggregability.

b) Increased thyroid-binding globulin (TBG) leading to increased circulating total thyroid hormone, as measured by protein-bound iodine (PBI), T4 by column or by radioimmunoassay. Free T3 resin uptake is decreased, reflecting the elevated TBG, free T4 concentration is unaltered.

c) Other binding proteins may be elevated in serum.

d) Sex hormone binding globulins are increased and result in elevated levels of total circulating sex steroids and corticoids; however, free or biologically active levels remain unchanged.

e) Triglycerides may be increased and levels of various other lipids and lipoproteins may be affected.

f) Glucose tolerance may be decreased.

g) Serum folate levels may be depressed by oral contraceptive therapy. This may be of clinical significance if a woman becomes pregnant shortly after discontinuing oral contraceptives.

10. Carcinogenesis

See **WARNINGS** section.

11. Pregnancy

Pregnancy Category X. See **CONTRAINDICATIONS** and **WARNINGS** sections.

12. Nursing Mothers

Small amounts of oral contraceptive steroids and/or metabolites have been identified in the milk of nursing mothers, and a few adverse effects on the child have been reported, including jaundice and breast enlargement. In addition, oral contraceptives given in the postpartum period may interfere with lactation by decreasing the quantity and quality of breast milk. If possible, the nursing mother should be advised not to use oral contraceptives but to use other forms of contraception until she has completely weaned her child.

13. Pediatric Use:

Safety and efficacy of Seasonale® tablets have been established in women of reproductive age. Safety and efficacy are expected to be the same in postpubertal adolescents under the age of 16 and users 16 and older. Use of Seasonale® before menarche is not indicated.

14. Geriatric Use:

Seasonale® tablets have not been studied in women who have reached menopause.

INFORMATION FOR THE PATIENT

See Patient Labeling Printed Below.

ADVERSE REACTIONS

An increased risk of the following serious adverse reactions has been associated with the use of oral contraceptives (see **WARNINGS** section):

- Thrombophlebitis
- Arterial thromboembolism
- Pulmonary embolism
- Myocardial infarction
- Cerebral hemorrhage
- Cerebral thrombosis
- Hypertension
- Gallbladder disease
- Hepatic adenomas or benign liver tumors

There is evidence of an association between the following conditions and the use of oral contraceptives:

- Mesenteric thrombosis
- Retinal thrombosis

The following adverse reactions have been reported in patients receiving oral contraceptives and are believed to be drug related:

- Nausea
- Vomiting
- Gastrointestinal symptoms (such as abdominal cramps and bloating)
- Breakthrough bleeding
- Spotting
- Change in menstrual flow
- Amenorrhea
- Temporary infertility after discontinuation of treatment
- Edema/fluid retention
- Melasma/chloasma which may persist
- Breast changes: tenderness, enlargement, and secretion
- Change in weight or appetite (increase or decrease)
- Change in cervical ectropion and secretion
- Possible diminution in lactation when given immediately postpartum
- Cholestatic jaundice
- Migraine headache
- Rash (allergic)
- Mood changes, including depression
- Vaginitis, including candidiasis
- Change in corneal curvature (steepening)
- Intolerance to contact lenses
- Decrease in serum folate levels
- Exacerbation of systemic lupus erythematosus
- Exacerbation of porphyria
- Exacerbation of chorea
- Aggravation of varicose veins
- Anaphylactic/anaphylactoid reactions, including urticaria, angioedema, and severe reactions with respiratory and circulatory symptoms

The following adverse reactions have been reported in users of oral contraceptives and the association has been neither confirmed nor refuted:

- Premenstrual syndrome
- Cataracts
- Optic neuritis which may lead to partial or complete loss of vision

- Cystitis-like syndrome
- Headache
- Nervousness
- Dizziness
- Hirsutism
- Loss of scalp hair
- Erythema multiforme
- Erythema nodosum
- Hemorrhagic eruption
- Impaired renal function
- Hemolytic uremic syndrome
- Budd-Chiari syndrome
- Acne
- Changes in libido
- Colitis
- Pancreatitis
- Dysmenorrhea

OVERDOSAGE

Serious ill effects have not been reported following acute ingestion of large doses of oral contraceptives by young children. Overdosage may cause nausea, and withdrawal bleeding may occur in females.

NONCONTRACEPTIVE HEALTH BENEFITS

The following noncontraceptive health benefits related to the use of oral contraceptives are supported by epidemiological studies which largely utilized oral contraceptive formulations containing doses exceeding 0.035 mg of ethinyl estradiol or 0.05 mg of mestranol.

Effects on menses:
- May decrease blood loss and may decrease incidence of iron-deficiency anemia
- May decrease incidence of dysmenorrhea

Effects related to inhibition of ovulation:
- May decrease incidence of functional ovarian cysts
- May decrease incidence of ectopic pregnancies

Effects from long-term use:
- May decrease incidence of fibroadenomas and fibrocystic disease of the breast
- May decrease incidence of acute pelvic inflammatory disease
- May decrease incidence of endometrial cancer
- May decrease incidence of ovarian cancer

DOSAGE AND ADMINISTRATION

Although the occurrence of pregnancy is unlikely if Seasonale® is taken according to directions, if withdrawal bleeding does not occur while taking white (inactive) tablets, the possibility of pregnancy must be considered. Appropriate diagnostic measures to rule out pregnancy should be taken at the time of any missed menstrual period. Seasonale should be discontinued if pregnancy is confirmed.

The dosage of Seasonale® is one pink (active) tablet daily for 84 consecutive days, followed by 7 days of white (inert) tablets. To achieve maximum contraceptive effectiveness, Seasonale® must be taken exactly as directed and at intervals not exceeding 24 hours. Ideally, the tablets should be taken at the same time of the day on each day of active treatment. The tablets should not be removed from the protective blister packaging and outer plastic dispenser to avoid damage to the product. The plastic dispenser should be kept in the foil pouch until dispensed to the patient.

During the first cycle of medication, the patient is instructed to begin taking Seasonale® on the first Sunday after the onset of menstruation. If menstruation begins on a Sunday, the first tablet (pink) is taken that day. One pink tablet should be taken daily for 84 consecutive days, followed by 7 days on which a white (inert) tablet is taken. Withdrawal bleeding should occur during the 7 days following discontinuation of pink active tablets. During the first cycle, contraceptive reliance should not be placed on Seasonale® until a pink (active) tablet has been taken daily for 7 consecutive days and a non-hormonal back-up method of birth control (such as condoms or spermicide) should be used during those 7 days. The possibility of ovulation and conception prior to initiation of medication should be considered.

The patient begins her next and all subsequent 91-day courses of tablets without interruption on the same day of the week (Sunday) on which she began her first course, following the same schedule: 84 days on which pink tablets are taken followed by 7 days on which white tablets are taken. If in any cycle the patient starts tablets later than the proper day, she should protect herself against pregnancy by using a non-hormonal back-up method of birth control until she has taken a pink tablet daily for 7 consecutive days.

If spotting or breakthrough bleeding occurs, the patient is instructed to continue on the same regimen. This type of bleeding may be transient and without significance; however, if the bleeding is persistent or prolonged, the patient is advised to consult her healthcare provider.

For patient instructions regarding missed pills, see the **"WHAT TO DO IF YOU MISS PILLS"** section in the **DETAILED PATIENT LABELING.** Any time the patient misses two or more pink tablets, she should also use another method of non-hormonal back-up contraception until she has taken a pink tablet daily for seven consecutive days. If the patient misses one or more white tablets, she is still protected against pregnancy provided she begins taking pink tablets again on the proper day. The possibility of ovulation increases with each successive day that scheduled pink tablets are missed. The risk of pregnancy increases with each active (pink) tablet missed.

In the nonlactating mother, Seasonale® may be initiated no earlier than day 28 postpartum, for contraception due to the increased risk for thromboembolism. When the tablets are administered in the postpartum period, the increased risk of thromboembolic disease associated with the postpartum period must be considered (See **CONTRAINDICATIONS, WARNINGS** and **PRECAUTIONS** concerning thromboembolic disease). The patient should be advised to use a nonhormonal back-up method for the first 7 days of tablet-taking. However, if intercourse has already occurred, the possibility of ovulation and conception prior to initiation of medication should be considered. Seasonale® may be initiated immediately after a first-trimester abortion; if the patient starts Seasonale® immediately, additional contraceptive measures are not needed.

HOW SUPPLIED

Seasonale® tablets (levonorgestrel/ethinyl estradiol tablets) 0.15 mg/0.03 mg are available in Extended-Cycle Tablet Dispensers (**NDC 51285-058-66**), each containing a 13-week supply of tablets: 84 pink tablets, each containing 0.15 mg of levonorgestrel and 0.03 mg ethinyl estradiol, and 7 white inert tablets. The active pink tablets are round, film-coated, biconvex, unscored tablets with a debossed ***S*** on one side and **62** on the other side. The inert tablets are white, round, biconvex, unscored tablet debossed with ***S*** on one side and **197** on the other side. Store at controlled room temperature 20°–25° C (68°–77° F) [See USP].

References available upon request.

Brief Summary Patient Package Insert

This product (like all oral contraceptives) is intended to prevent pregnancy. It does not protect against HIV infection (AIDS) and other sexually transmitted diseases such as chlamydia, genital herpes, genital warts, gonorrhea, hepatitis B, and syphilis.

Oral contraceptives, also known as "birth control pills" or "the pill", are taken to prevent pregnancy, and when taken correctly, have a failure rate of approximately 1.0% per year (1 pregnancy per 100 women per year of use). The typical failure rate of pill users is approximately 5% per year when women who miss pills are included.

For the majority of women, oral contraceptives can be taken safely. But for some women oral contraceptive use is associated with certain serious diseases that can be life-threatening or may cause temporary or permanent disability or death. The risks associated with taking oral contraceptives increase significantly if you:
- smoke
- have high blood pressure, diabetes, high cholesterol or are obese
- have or have had clotting disorders, heart attack, stroke, angina pectoris, cancer of the breast or sex organs, jaundice, or malignant or benign liver tumors

You should not take the pill if you are pregnant.

Although cardiovascular disease risks may be increased with oral contraceptive use after age 40 in healthy, non-smoking women (even with the newer low-dose formulations), there are also greater potential health risks associated with pregnancy in older women.

Cigarette smoking increases the risk of serious cardiovascular side effects from oral contraceptive use. This risk increases with age and with the amount of smoking (15 or more cigarettes per day has been associated with a significantly increased risk) and is quite marked in women over 35 years of age. Women who use oral contraceptives should not smoke.

Most side effects of the pill are not serious. The most common are nausea, vomiting, bleeding or spotting between menstrual periods, weight gain, breast tenderness, and difficulty wearing contact lenses. Some of these side effects, especially nausea and vomiting, may subside within the first 3 months of use.

The serious side effects of the pill occur very infrequently, especially if you are in good health and do not smoke. However, you should know that the following medical conditions have been associated with or made worse by the pill:

1. Blood clots in the legs (thrombophlebitis), lungs (pulmonary embolism), stoppage or rupture of a blood vessel in the brain (stroke), blockage of blood vessels in the heart (heart attack or angina pectoris) or other organs of the body. As mentioned above, smoking increases the risk of heart attacks and strokes and subsequent serious medical consequences. Women with migraine also may be at increased risk of stroke when taking the pill.
2. Liver tumors, which may rupture and cause severe bleeding. A possible but not definite association has been found with the pill and liver cancer. However, liver cancers are extremely rare. The chance of developing liver cancer from using the pill is thus even rarer.
3. High blood pressure, although blood pressure usually returns to normal when the pill is stopped.

The symptoms associated with these serious side effects are discussed in the detailed patient information leaflet. Notify your healthcare provider if you notice any unusual physical disturbances while taking the pill. In addition, drugs such as rifampin, as well as some anticonvulsants and some antibiotics, and herbal preparations containing St. John's Wort (hypericum perforatum) may decrease oral contraceptive effectiveness.

Breast cancer has been diagnosed slightly more often in women who use the pill than in women of the same age who do not use the pill. This very small increase in the number of breast cancer diagnoses gradually disappears during the 10 years after stopping use of the pill. It is not known whether the difference is caused by the pill. It may be that women taking the pill were examined more often, so that breast cancer was more likely to be detected. You should have regular breast examinations by a healthcare provider and examine your own breasts monthly. Tell your healthcare provider if you have a family history of breast cancer or if you have had breast nodules or an abnormal mammogram. Women who currently have or have had breast cancer should not use hormonal contraceptives because breast cancer is usually a hormone-sensitive tumor.

Some studies have found an increase in the incidence of cancer or precancerous lesions of the cervix in women who use the pill. However, this finding may be related to factors other than the use of the pill.

Be sure to discuss any medical condition you may have with your healthcare provider. Your healthcare provider will take a medical and family history before prescribing oral contraceptives and will examine you. The physical examination may be delayed to another time if you request it and the healthcare provider believes that it is appropriate to postpone it. You should be reexamined at least once a year while taking oral contraceptives. The detailed patient information leaflet gives you further information, which you should read and discuss with your healthcare provider.

What You Should Know About Your Menstrual Cycle When Taking Seasonale®

When you take Seasonale®, which has a 91-day treatment cycle, you should expect to have 4 menstrual periods per year (bleeding when you are taking the 7 white pills). However, you also should expect to have more bleeding or spotting between your menstrual periods than if you were taking an oral contraceptive with a 28-day treatment cycle. During the first Seasonale® treatment cycle, about 1 in 3 women may have 20 or more days of unplanned bleeding or spotting (bleeding when you are taking pink pills). This bleeding or spotting tends to decrease during later cycles. Do not stop Seasonale® because of the bleeding. If the spotting continues for more than 7 consecutive days or if the bleeding is heavy, call your healthcare provider.

If You Miss Your Menstrual Period When Taking Seasonale

You should consider the possibility that you are pregnant if you miss your menstrual period (no bleeding on the days that you are taking white tablets). Since scheduled menstrual periods are less frequent when you are taking Seasonale®, notify your healthcare provider that you have missed your period and are taking Seasonale®. Also notify your healthcare provider if you have symptoms of pregnancy such as morning sickness or unusual breast tenderness. It is important that your healthcare provider evaluates you to determine if you are pregnant. Stop taking Seasonale® if it is determined that you are pregnant.

HOW TO TAKE SEASONALE®

IMPORTANT POINTS TO REMEMBER *BEFORE* YOU START TAKING SEASONALE®

1. BE SURE TO READ THESE DIRECTIONS:
   - Before you start taking your pills.
   - Anytime you are not sure what to do.
2. THE RIGHT WAY TO TAKE SEASONALE® IS TO TAKE ONE PILL EVERY DAY AT THE SAME TIME. If you miss pills you could get pregnant. This includes starting the pack late. The more pills you miss, the more likely you are to get pregnant.
3. MANY WOMEN MAY FEEL SICK TO THEIR STOMACH DURING THE FIRST FEW WEEKS OF TAKING PILLS. If you feel sick to your stomach, do not stop taking the pill. The problem will usually go away. If it doesn't go away, check with your healthcare provider.
4. MANY WOMEN HAVE SPOTTING OR LIGHT BLEEDING DURING THE FIRST FEW MONTHS OF TAKING SEASONALE®. **Do not stop taking your pills even if you are having irregular bleeding.** If the bleeding lasts for more than 7 consecutive days, talk to your healthcare provider.
5. MISSING PILLS CAN ALSO CAUSE SPOTTING OR LIGHT BLEEDING, even when you make up these missed pills. On the days you take 2 pills to make up for missed pills, you could also feel a little sick to your stomach.
6. IF YOU HAVE VOMITING OR DIARRHEA, or IF YOU TAKE SOME MEDICINES, including some antibiotics and the herbal supplement St. John's Wort, Seasonale may not work as well. Use a back-up method (such as condoms or spermicides) until you check with your healthcare provider.
7. IF YOU HAVE TROUBLE REMEMBERING TO TAKE SEASONALE®, talk to your healthcare provider about how to make pill-taking easier or about using another method of birth control.
8. IF YOU HAVE ANY QUESTIONS OR ARE UNSURE ABOUT THE INFORMATION IN THIS LEAFLET, call your healthcare provider.

***BEFORE* YOU START TAKING SEASONALE®**

1. DECIDE WHAT TIME OF DAY YOU WANT TO TAKE YOUR PILL. It is important to take it at about the same time every day.
2. LOOK AT YOUR EXTENDED-CYCLE TABLET DISPENSER. Your Tablet Dispenser consists of 3 trays with cards that hold 91 individually sealed pills (a 13-week or 91-day cycle). The 91 pills consist of 84 pink pills (active

Continued on next page

Seasonale—Cont.

pills with hormones) and 7 white pills (inactive pills without hormone). Trays 1 and 2 each contain 28 pink pills (4 rows of 7 pills). Tray 3 contains 35 pills consisting of 28 pink pills (4 rows of 7 pills) and 7 white pills (1 row of 7 pills).

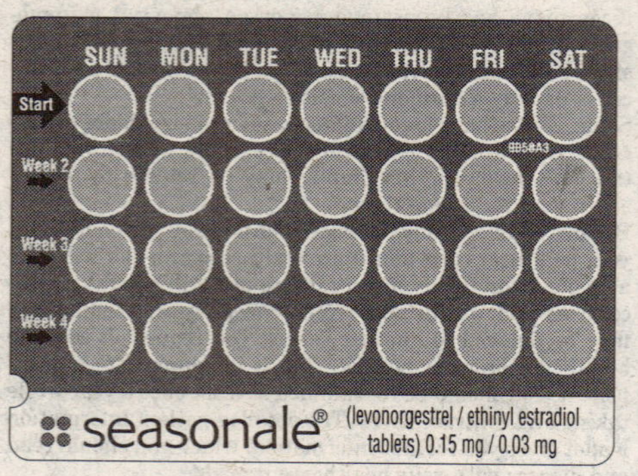

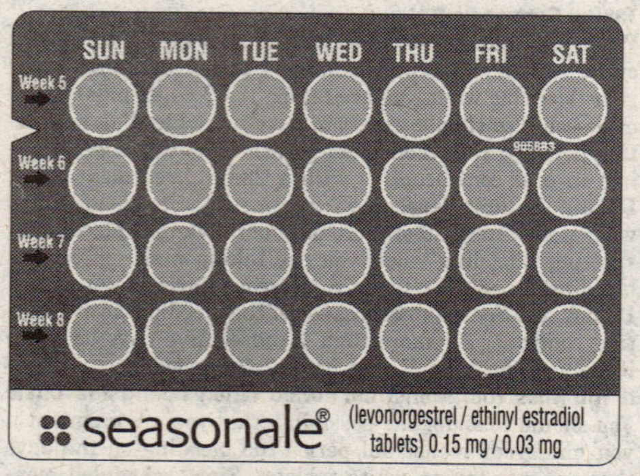

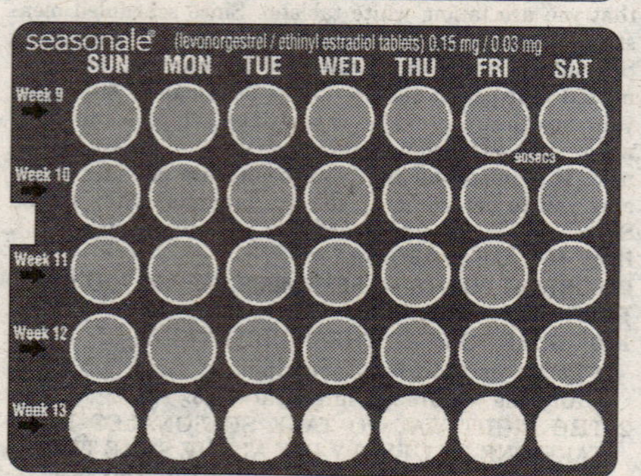

3. ALSO FIND:
   - Where on the first tray in the pack to start taking pills (upper left corner at the start arrow) and
   - In what order to take the pills (follow the weeks and arrow).
4. BE SURE YOU HAVE READY AT ALL TIMES ANOTHER KIND OF BIRTH CONTROL (such as condoms or spermicides), to use as a back-up in case you miss pills.

WHEN TO START SEASONALE®

1. Take the first "active" pink pill on the *Sunday after your period starts*, even if you are still bleeding. If your period begins on Sunday, start the first pink pill that same day.
2. *Use another method of birth control (such as condom or spermicide)* as a back-up method if you have sex anytime from the Sunday you start your first pink pill until the next Sunday (first 7 days).

HOW TO TAKE SEASONALE®

1. **Take one pill at the same time every day until you have taken the last pill in the tablet dispenser.**
   Do not skip pills even if you are spotting or bleeding or feel sick to your stomach (nausea).
   Do not skip pills even if you do not have sex very often.
2. **WHEN YOU FINISH A TABLET DISPENSER.**
   After taking the last white pill, start taking the first pink pill from a new Extended-Cycle Tablet Dispenser **the very next day** regardless of when your period started. This should be on a Sunday.
3. **If you miss your period when you are taking the white pills, call your healthcare provider because you may be pregnant.**

WHAT TO DO IF YOU MISS PILLS

If you **MISS 1** pink "active" pill:
1. Take it as soon as you remember. Take the next pill at your regular time. This means you may take 2 pills in 1 day.
2. You do not need to use a back-up birth control method if you have sex.

If you **MISS 2** pink "active" pills in a row:
1. Take 2 pills on the day you remember, and 2 pills the next day.
2. Then take 1 pill a day until you finish the pack.
3. You COULD BECOME PREGNANT if you have sex in the *7 days after* you restart your pills. You MUST use another birth control method (such as condoms or spermicide) as a back-up on the 7 days after you restart your pills.

If you **MISS 3 OR MORE** pink "active" pills in a row:
1. Do not remove the missed pills from the pack as they will not be taken. Keep taking 1 pill every day as indicated on the pack until you have completed all of the remaining pills in the pack. For example: If you resume taking the pill on Thursday, take the pill under "Thursday" and do not take the missed pills. You may experience bleeding during the week following the missed pills.
2. You COULD BECOME PREGNANT if you have sex during the days of missed pills or during the first 7 days after restarting your pills.
3. You **must** use a non-hormonal birth control method (such as condoms or spermicide) as a back-up when you miss pills and for the first 7 days after you restart your pills. **If you miss your period when you are taking the white pills, call your healthcare provider because you may be pregnant.**

If you **MISS ANY** of the 7 white inactive pills.
1. Throw away the missed pills.
2. Keep taking the scheduled pills until the pack is finished.
3. You do not need a back-up method of birth control.

FINALLY, IF YOU ARE STILL NOT SURE WHAT TO DO ABOUT THE PILLS YOU HAVE MISSED
1. Use a BACK-UP METHOD anytime you have sex.
2. KEEP TAKING ONE PILL EACH DAY until you contact your healthcare provider.

DETAILED PATIENT LABELING

This product (like all oral contraceptives) is intended to prevent pregnancy. Oral contraceptives do not protect against transmission of HIV (AIDS) and other sexually transmitted diseases such as chlamydia, genital herpes, genital warts, gonorrhea, hepatitis B, and syphilis.

INTRODUCTION

Any woman who considers using oral contraceptives ("the birth control pill" or "the pill") should understand the benefits and risks of using this form of birth control. Although oral contraceptives have important advantages over other methods of contraception, they have certain risks that no other method has, and some of these risks may continue after you have stopped using the oral contraceptive. This leaflet will give you much of the information you will need to make this decision and will also help you determine if you are at risk of developing any of the serious side effects of the pill. It will tell you how to use Seasonale® properly so that it will be as effective as possible. However, this leaflet is not a replacement for a careful discussion between you and your healthcare provider. You should discuss the information provided in this leaflet with your healthcare provider, both when you first start taking Seasonale® and during your revisits. You should also follow your healthcare provider's advice with regard to regular check-ups while you are on Seasonale®.

EFFECTIVENESS OF ORAL CONTRACEPTIVES

Oral contraceptives or "the birth control pill" or "the pill" are used to prevent pregnancy and are more effective than most other nonsurgical methods of birth control. The chance of becoming pregnant is approximately 1.0% per year (1 pregnancy per 100 women per year of use) when the pills are used correctly, and no pills are missed. Typical failure rates are approximately 5.0% per year when women who miss pills are included. The chance of becoming pregnant increases with each missed pill during the menstrual cycle. In comparison, typical failure rates for other methods of birth control during the first year of use are as follows:

No methods: 85%
Vaginal sponge: 20 to 40%
Cervical cap: 20 to 40%
Spermicides alone: 26%
Periodic abstinence: 25%
Condom (female): 21%
Diaphragm with spermicides: 20%
Withdrawal: 19%
Condom (male): 14%
Female sterilization: 0.5%
IUD: 0.1 to 2.0%
Injectable progestogen: 0.3%
Male sterilization: 0.15%
Norplant system: 0.05%

WHO SHOULD NOT TAKE ORAL CONTRACEPTIVES

> **Cigarette smoking increases the risk of serious cardiovascular side effects from oral contraceptive use. This risk increases with age and with the amount of smoking (15 or more cigarettes per day has been associated with a significantly increased risk) and is quite marked in women over 35 years of age. Women who use oral contraceptives should not smoke.**

Some women should not use the pill. You should not use the pill if you have any of the following conditions:
- A history of heart attack or stroke
- A history of blood clots in the legs (thrombophlebitis), lungs (pulmonary embolism), or eyes
- A history of blood clots in the deep veins of your legs
- Chest pain (angina pectoris)
- Known or suspected breast cancer or cancer of the lining of the uterus, cervix, vagina, or certain hormonally-sensitive cancers
- Unexplained vaginal bleeding (until a diagnosis is reached by your healthcare provider)
- Yellowing of the whites of the eyes or of the skin (jaundice) during pregnancy or during previous use of the pill
- Liver tumor (benign or cancerous)
- Known or suspected pregnancy
- Heart valve or heart rhythm disorders that may be associated with formation of blood clots
- Diabetes affecting your circulation
- Uncontrolled high blood pressure
- Active liver disease with abnormal liver function tests
- Allergy or hypersensitivity to any of the components of Seasonale®
- A need for surgery with prolonged bedrest

Tell your healthcare provider if you have any of the above conditions. Your healthcare provider can recommend a safer method of birth control.

OTHER CONSIDERATIONS BEFORE TAKING ORAL CONTRACEPTIVES

Tell your healthcare provider if you or any family member has ever had:
- Breast nodules, fibrocystic disease of the breast, an abnormal breast X-ray or mammogram
- Diabetes
- Elevated cholesterol or triglycerides
- High blood pressure
- Migraine or other headaches or epilepsy
- Depression
- Gallbladder, liver, heart or kidney disease
- History of scanty or irregular menstrual periods

Women with any of these conditions should be checked often by their healthcare provider if they choose to use oral contraceptives. Also, be sure to inform your healthcare provider if you smoke or are on any medications.

RISKS OF TAKING ORAL CONTRACEPTIVES

If you use Seasonale® you will receive more exposure to hormones on a yearly basis than if you used a conventional 28-day cycle oral contraceptives containing a similar amount of estrogen and progestin (an additional 9 weeks exposure per year). While this added exposure may pose an additional risk of thrombotic and thromboembolic disease, studies to date with Seasonale have not suggested an increased risk of these disorders.

1. **Risk of Developing Blood Clots**
   Blood clots and blockage of blood vessels are the most serious side effects of taking oral contraceptives and can cause death or serious disability. In particular, a clot in the legs can cause thrombophlebitis and a clot that travels to the lungs can cause a sudden blocking of the vessel carrying blood to the lungs. Rarely, clots occur in the blood vessels of the eye and may cause blindness, double vision, or impaired vision. If you take oral contraceptives and need elective surgery, need to stay in bed for a prolonged illness, or have recently delivered a baby, you may be at risk of developing blood clots. You should consult your healthcare provider about stopping oral contraceptives three to four weeks before surgery and not taking oral contraceptives for two weeks after surgery or during bed rest. You should also not take oral contraceptives soon after delivery of a baby. It is advisable to wait for at least four weeks after delivery if you are not breastfeeding. If you are breastfeeding, you should wait until you have weaned your child before using the pill (See also the section on **Breastfeeding** in **"GENERAL PRECAUTIONS"**.)
   The risk of circulatory disease in oral contraceptive users may be higher in users of high-dose pills (containing 50 micrograms or higher of ethinyl estradiol) and may be greater with longer duration of oral contraceptive use. In addition, some of these increased risks may continue for a number of years after stopping oral contraceptives. The risk of abnormal blood clotting increases with age in both users and nonusers of oral contraceptives, but the increased risk from the oral contraceptive appears to be present at all ages. For women aged 20 to 44, it is estimated that about 1 in 2,000 using oral contraceptives will be hospitalized each year because of abnormal clotting. Among nonusers in the same age group, about 1 in 20,000 would be hospitalized each year. For oral contraceptive users in general, it has been estimated that in women between the ages of 15 and 34 the risk of death due to a circulatory disorder is about 1 in 12,000 per year, whereas for nonusers the rate is about 1 in 50,000 per year. In the age group 35 to 44, the risk is estimated to be about 1 in 2,500 per year for oral contraceptive users and about 1 in 10,000 per year for nonusers.
2. **Heart Attacks and Strokes**
   Oral contraceptives may increase the tendency to develop strokes (stoppage or rupture of blood vessels in the brain) and angina pectoris and heart attacks (blockage of blood vessels in the heart). Any of these conditions can cause death or serious disability. Smoking greatly increases the possibility of suffering heart attacks and strokes. Furthermore, smoking and the use of oral contraceptives greatly increase the chances of developing and dying of heart disease.
   Women with migraine (especially migraine with aura) who take oral contraceptives also may be at higher risk of stroke.
3. **Gallbladder Disease**
   Oral contraceptive users probably have a greater risk

than nonusers of having gallbladder disease, although this risk may be related to pills containing high doses of estrogens.

4. **Liver Tumors**
In rare cases, oral contraceptives can cause benign but dangerous liver tumors. These benign liver tumors can rupture and cause fatal internal bleeding. In addition, a possible but not definite association has been found with the pill and liver cancers in two studies in which a few women who developed these very rare cancers were found to have used oral contraceptives for long periods. However, liver cancers in general are extremely rare and the chance of developing liver cancer from using the pill is thus even rarer.

5. **Cancer of the Breast and Reproductive Organs**
Breast cancer has been diagnosed slightly more often in women who use the pill than in women of the same age who do not use the pill. This small increase in the number of breast cancer diagnoses gradually disappears during the 10 years after stopping use of the pill. It is not known whether the difference is caused by the pill. It may be that women taking the pill are examined more often, so that breast cancer is more likely to be detected. You should have regular breast examinations by a healthcare provider and examine your own breasts monthly. Tell your healthcare provider if you have a family history of breast cancer or if you have had breast nodules or an abnormal mammogram.
Women who currently have or have had breast cancer should not use oral contraceptives because breast cancer is usually a hormone-sensitive tumor.
Some studies have found an increase in the incidence of cancer or precancerous lesions of the cervix in women who use oral contraceptives. However, this finding may be related to factors other than the use of oral contraceptives. There is insufficient evidence to rule out the possibility that the pill may cause such cancers.

6. **Lipid Metabolism and Inflammation of the Pancreas**
In patients with inherited defects of the lipid metabolism, there have been reports of significant elevations of plasma triglycerides during estrogen therapy. This has led to pancreatitis in some cases.

ESTIMATED RISK OF DEATH FROM A BIRTH CONTROL METHOD OR PREGNANCY

All methods of birth control and pregnancy are associated with a risk of developing certain diseases, which may lead to disability or death. An estimate of the number of deaths associated with different methods of birth control and pregnancy has been calculated and is shown in the following table.

ANNUAL NUMBER OF BIRTH-RELATED OR METHOD-RELATED DEATHS ASSOCIATED WITH CONTROL OF FERTILITY PER 100,000 NONSTERILE WOMEN, BY FERTILITY-CONTROL METHOD AND ACCORDING TO AGE

Method of control and outcome	AGE 15-19	20-24	25-29	30-34	35-39	40-44
No fertility - control methods*	7.0	7.4	9.1	14.8	25.7	28.2
Oral contraceptives non-smoker**	0.3	0.5	0.9	1.9	13.8	31.6
Oral contraceptives smoker**	2.2	3.4	6.6	13.5	51.1	117.2
IUD**	0.8	0.8	1.0	1.0	1.4	1.4
Condom*	1.1	1.6	0.7	0.2	0.3	0.4
Diaphragm/ spermicide*	1.9	1.2	1.2	1.3	2.2	2.8
Periodic abstinence*	2.5	1.6	1.6	1.7	2.9	3.6

* Deaths are birth related
** Deaths are method related

In the above table, the risk of death from any birth control method is less than the risk of childbirth, except for oral contraceptive users over the age of 35 who smoke and pill users over the age of 40 even if they do not smoke. It can be seen in the table that for women aged 15 to 39, the risk of death was highest with pregnancy (7 to 26 deaths per 100,000 women, depending on age). Among pill users who do not smoke, the risk of death was always lower than that associated with pregnancy for any age group, although over the age of 40, the risk increases to 32 deaths per 100,000 women, compared to 28 associated with pregnancy at that age. However, for pill users who smoke and are over the age of 35, the estimated number of deaths exceeds those for other methods of birth control. If a woman is over the age of 40 and smokes, her estimated risk of death is four times higher (117/100,000 women) than the estimated risk associated with pregnancy (28/100,000 women) in that age group. The suggestion that women over 40 who don't smoke should not take oral contraceptives is based on information from older high-dose pills. An Advisory Committee of the FDA discussed this issue in 1989 and recommended that the benefits of oral contraceptive use by healthy, nonsmoking women over 40 years of age may outweigh the possible risks. Older women, as all women who take oral contraceptives, should take an oral contraceptive that contains the least amount of estrogen and progestin that is compatible with the individual patient needs.

WARNING SIGNALS

If any of these adverse effects occur while you are taking oral contraceptives, call your healthcare provider immediately:

- Sharp chest pain, coughing of blood, or sudden shortness of breath (indicating a possible clot in the lung).
- Pain in the calf (indicating a possible clot in the leg).
- Crushing chest pain or heaviness in the chest (indicating a possible heart attack).
- Sudden severe headache or vomiting, dizziness or fainting, disturbances of vision or speech, weakness, or numbness in an arm or leg (indicating a possible stroke).
- Sudden partial or complete loss of vision (indicating a possible clot in the eye).
- Breast lumps (indicating possible breast cancer or fibrocystic disease of the breast; ask your doctor or healthcare provider to show you how to examine your breasts).
- Severe pain or tenderness in the stomach area (indicating a possibly ruptured liver tumor).
- Difficulty in sleeping, weakness, lack of energy, fatigue, or change in mood (possibly indicating severe depression).
- Jaundice or a yellowing of the skin or eyeballs, accompanied frequently by fever, fatigue, loss of appetite, dark-colored urine, or light-colored bowel movements (indicating possible liver problems).

SIDE EFFECTS OF ORAL CONTRACEPTIVES

In addition to the risks and more serious side effects discussed above (see **RISKS OF TAKING ORAL CONTRACEPTIVES, ESTIMATED RISK OF DEATH FROM A BIRTH CONTROL METHOD OR PREGNANCY** and **WARNING SIGNALS** sections), the following may also occur:

1. **Irregular vaginal bleeding**
Irregular vaginal bleeding or spotting (bleeding or spotting between your expected period) is likely to occur while you are taking Seasonale®. Irregular bleeding may vary from slight staining between menstrual periods to breakthrough bleeding which is a flow much like a regular period. Irregular bleeding occurs most often during the first few 91-day cycles of Seasonale® use, tends to decrease during later cycles, but may also occur after you have been taking Seasonale® for some time. Such bleeding usually does not indicate any serious problems. **It is important to continue taking your pills on schedule even if you are having irregular bleeding.** If the bleeding lasts for more than 7 consecutive days, talk to your healthcare provider.
When you take Seasonale®, you need to consider the convenience of fewer expected menstrual periods (4 per year instead of 13) and the inconvenience of more irregular vaginal bleeding or spotting. In a clinical trial comparing Seasonale® (91-day cycles) to a conventional equivalent dosage 28-day cycle oral contraceptive, more women using Seasonale® discontinued treatment because of bleeding problems (7.7% of the Seasonale® users compared to 1.8% of the 28-day cycle users).
The following Table shows the percentages of women with 7 or more and 20 or more days of intermenstrual bleeding and/or spotting in the Seasonale® and the 28-day cycle treatment groups.

Percentages (%) of Women with Intermenstrual Bleeding and/or Spotting

Number of days of intermenstrual bleeding and/or spotting	Percentage of subjects with intermenstrual bleeding or spotting*	
Seasonale®	Cycle 1	Cycle 4
7 or more days	65%	42%
20 or more days	35%	15%
28-day cycle pill	Cycles 1-4	Cycles 10-13
7 or more	38%	39%
20 or more days	6%	4%

* Based on spotting and/or bleeding on days 1-84 of a 91 day cycle in the Seasonale® subjects and days 1-21 of a 28 day cycle over 4 cycles in the 28-day dosing regimen.

Total days of bleeding and/or spotting (withdrawal plus intermenstrual) were similar over one year of treatment for Seasonale® subjects and subjects on the 28-day cycle regimen.

2. **Contact lenses**
If you wear contact lenses and notice a change in vision or an inability to wear your lenses, contact your healthcare provider.

3. **Fluid retention**
Oral contraceptives may cause edema (fluid retention) with swelling of the fingers or ankles and may raise your blood pressure. If you experience fluid retention, contact your healthcare provider.

4. **Melasma**
A spotty darkening of the skin is possible, particularly of the face.

5. **Other side effects**
Other side effects may include nausea and vomiting, change in appetite, breast tenderness, headache, nervousness, depression, dizziness, loss of scalp hair, rash, vaginal infections, and allergic reactions.
If any of these side effects bother you, call your healthcare provider.

GENERAL PRECAUTIONS

1. **Missed Periods and Use of Oral Contraceptives Before or During Early Pregnancy**
If you miss any periods (no bleeding on the days that you take white pills), you must consider the possibility that you may be pregnant. Notify your healthcare provider that you are taking Seasonale® and have missed your period. Also notify your healthcare provider if you have symptoms of pregnancy such as morning sickness or unusual breast tenderness. Because you are taking Seasonale®, it is very important that your healthcare provider evaluates you to determine if you are pregnant. Stop taking Seasonale® if you are pregnant.
There is no conclusive evidence that oral contraceptive use is associated with an increase in birth defects, when taken inadvertently during early pregnancy. Previously, a few studies had reported that oral contraceptives might be associated with birth defects, but these studies have not been confirmed. Nevertheless, oral contraceptives should not be used during pregnancy. You should check with your healthcare provider about risks to your unborn child of any medication taken during pregnancy.

2. **While Breastfeeding**
If you are breastfeeding, consult your healthcare provider before starting oral contraceptives. Some of the drug will be passed on to the child in the milk. A few adverse effects on the child have been reported, including yellowing of the skin (jaundice) and breast enlargement. In addition, oral contraceptives may decrease the amount and quality of your milk. If possible, do not use oral contraceptives while breastfeeding. You should use another method of contraception since breastfeeding provides only partial protection from becoming pregnant and this partial protection decreases significantly as you breast-feed for longer periods of time. You should consider starting oral contraceptives only after you have weaned your child completely.

3. **Laboratory Tests**
If you are scheduled for any laboratory tests, tell your healthcare provider you are taking birth control pills. Certain blood tests may be affected by birth control pills.

4. **Drug Interactions**
Certain drugs may interact with birth control pills to make them less effective in preventing pregnancy or cause an increase in breakthrough bleeding. Such drugs include rifampin, drugs used for epilepsy such as barbiturates (for example, phenobarbital), carbamazepine (Tegretol is one brand of this drug), and phenytoin (Dilantin® is one brand of this drug), primidone (Mysoline®), topiramate (Topamax®), phenylbutazone (Butazolidin® is one brand), some drugs used for HIV such as ritonavir (Norvir®), modafinil (Provigil®) and possibly certain antibiotics (such as ampicillin and other penicillins, and tetracyclines). Pregnancies and breakthrough bleeding have been reported by users of combined hormonal contraceptives who also used some form of the herbal supplement St. John's Wort. You may need to use a non-hormonal method of contraception during any cycle in which you take drugs that can make oral contraceptives less effective. Be sure to tell your healthcare provider if you are taking or start taking any other medications, including nonprescription products or herbal products while taking birth control pills.
You may be at higher risk of a specific type of liver dysfunction if you take troleandomycin and oral contraceptives at the same time.

5. **Sexually transmitted diseases**
This product (like all oral contraceptives) is intended to prevent pregnancy. It does not protect against transmission of HIV (AIDS) and other sexually transmitted diseases such as chlamydia, genital herpes, genital warts, gonorrhea, hepatitis B, and syphilis.

What You Should Know About Your Menstrual Cycle When Taking Seasonale®

When you take Seasonale®, which has a 91-day treatment cycle, you should expect to have 4 menstrual periods per year (bleeding when you are taking the 7 white pills). However, you should expect to have more bleeding or spotting between your menstrual periods than if you were taking an oral contraceptive with a 28-day treatment cycle. During the first Seasonale® treatment cycle, about 1 in 3 women may have 20 or more days of unplanned bleeding or spotting (bleeding when you are taking pink pills). This bleeding or spotting tends to decrease during later cycles. Do not stop Seasonale® because of the bleeding. If the spotting continues for more than 7 consecutive days or if the bleeding is heavy, call your healthcare provider.

HOW TO TAKE SEASONALE®

IMPORTANT POINTS TO REMEMBER *BEFORE* YOU START TAKING SEASONALE®

1. BE SURE TO READ THESE DIRECTIONS:
   - Before you start taking your pills.
   - Anytime you are not sure what to do.
2. THE RIGHT WAY TO TAKE SEASONALE® IS TO TAKE ONE PILL EVERY DAY AT THE SAME TIME.

Continued on next page

Seasonale—Cont.

If you miss pills you could get pregnant. This includes starting the pack late. The more pills you miss, the more likely you are to get pregnant.

3. MANY WOMEN MAY FEEL SICK TO THEIR STOMACH DURING THE FIRST FEW WEEKS OF TAKING PILLS.
   If you feel sick to your stomach, do not stop taking the pill. The problem will usually go away. If it doesn't go away, check with your healthcare provider.
4. MANY WOMEN HAVE SPOTTING OR LIGHT BLEEDING DURING THE FIRST FEW MONTHS OF TAKING SEASONALE®. **Do not stop taking your pills even if you are having irregular bleeding.** If the bleeding lasts for more than a few days, talk to your healthcare provider.
5. MISSING PILLS CAN ALSO CAUSE SPOTTING OR LIGHT BLEEDING, even when you make up these missed pills. On the days you take 2 pills to make up for missed pills, you could also feel a little sick to your stomach.
6. IF YOU HAVE VOMITING OR DIARRHEA, or IF YOU TAKE SOME MEDICINES, including some antibiotics and the herbal supplement St. John's Wort, Seasonale may not work as well. Use a back-up method (such as condoms or spermicides) until you check with your healthcare provider.
7. IF YOU HAVE TROUBLE REMEMBERING TO TAKE SEASONALE®, talk to your healthcare provider about how to make pill-taking easier or about using another method of birth control.
8. IF YOU HAVE ANY QUESTIONS OR ARE UNSURE ABOUT THE INFORMATION IN THIS LEAFLET, call your healthcare provider.

***BEFORE* YOU START TAKING SEASONALE®**

1. DECIDE WHAT TIME OF DAY YOU WANT TO TAKE YOUR PILL. It is important to take it at about the same time every day.
2. LOOK AT YOUR EXTENDED-CYCLE TABLET DISPENSER. Your Tablet Dispenser consists of 3 trays with cards that hold 91 individually sealed pills (a 13-week or 91-day cycle). The 91 pills consist of 84 pink pills (active pills with hormones) and 7 white pills (inactive pills without hormone). Trays 1 and 2 each contain 28 pink pills (4 rows of 7 pills). Tray 3 contains 35 pills consisting of 28 pink pills (4 rows of 7 pills) and 7 white pills (1 row of 7 pills).

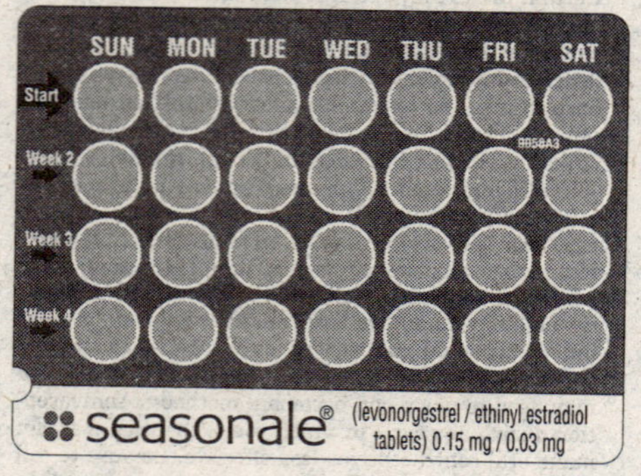

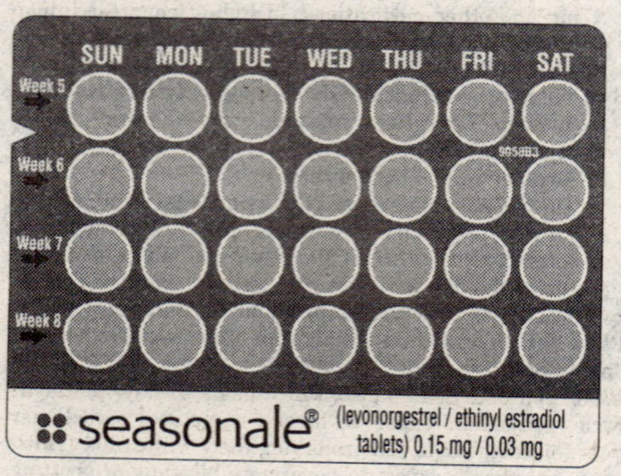

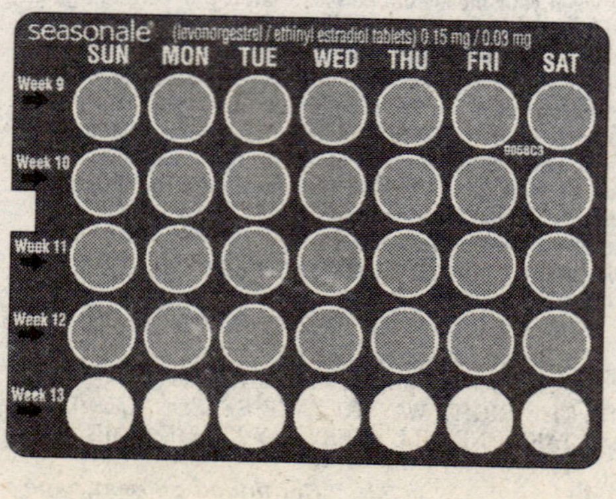

3. ALSO FIND:
   - Where on the first tray in the pack to start taking pills (upper left corner at the start arrow) and
   - In what order to take the pills (follow the weeks and arrow).
4. BE SURE YOU HAVE READY AT ALL TIMES ANOTHER KIND OF BIRTH CONTROL (such as condoms or spermicides), to use as a back-up in case you miss pills.

WHEN TO START SEASONALE®

1. Take the first "active" pink pill on the *Sunday after your period starts*, even if you are still bleeding. If your period begins on Sunday, start the first pink pill that same day.
2. *Use another method of birth control (such as condom or spermicide)* as a back-up method if you have sex anytime from the Sunday you start your first pink pill until the next Sunday (first 7 days).

HOW TO TAKE SEASONALE®

1. **Take one pill at the same time every day until you have taken the last pill in the tablet dispenser. Do not skip pills even if you are spotting or bleeding** or feel sick to your stomach (nausea).
   Do not skip pills even if you do not have sex very often.
2. **WHEN YOU FINISH A TABLET DISPENSER.**
   After taking the last white pill, start taking the first pink pill from a new Extended-Cycle Tablet Dispenser **the very next day** regardless of when your period started. This should be on a Sunday.
3. **If you miss your period when you are taking the white pills, call your healthcare provider because you may be pregnant.**

WHAT TO DO IF YOU MISS PILLS

If you **MISS 1** pink "active" pill:

1. Take it as soon as you remember. Take the next pill at your regular time. This means you may take 2 pills in 1 day.
2. You do not need to use a back-up birth control method if you have sex.

If you **MISS 2** pink "active" pills in a row:

1. Take 2 pills on the day you remember, and 2 pills the next day.
2. Then take 1 pill a day until you finish the pack.
3. You COULD BECOME PREGNANT if you have sex in the *7 days* after you restart your pills. You MUST use another birth control method (such as condoms or spermicide) as a back-up on the 7 days after you restart your pills.

If you **MISS 3 OR MORE** pink "active" pills in a row:

1. Do not remove the missed pills from the pack as they will not be taken. Keep taking 1 pill every day as indicated on the pack until you have completed all of the remaining pills in the pack. For example: If you resume taking the pill on Thursday, take the pill under "Thursday" and do not take the missed pills. You may experience bleeding during the week following the missed pills.
2. You COULD BECOME PREGNANT if you have sex during the days of missed pills or during the first 7 days after restarting your pills.
3. You **must** use a non-hormonal birth control method (such as condoms or spermicide) as a back-up when you miss pills and for the first 7 days after you restart your pills. **If you miss your period when you are taking the white pills, call your healthcare provider because you may be pregnant.**

If you **MISS ANY** of the 7 white inactive pills.

1. Throw away the missed pills.
2. Keep taking the scheduled pills until the pack is finished.
3. You do not need a back-up method of birth control.

FINALLY, IF YOU ARE STILL NOT SURE WHAT TO DO ABOUT THE PILLS YOU HAVE MISSED

1. Use a BACK-UP METHOD anytime you have sex.
2. KEEP TAKING ONE PILL EACH DAY until you contact your healthcare provider.

PREGNANCY DUE TO PILL FAILURE

If taken every day as directed, the incidence of pill failure resulting in pregnancy is approximately 1 % (ie, one pregnancy per 100 women per year), but more typical failure rates are about 5%. If failure does occur, the risk to the fetus is minimal.

PREGNANCY AFTER STOPPING THE PILL

There may be some delay in becoming pregnant after you stop using oral contraceptives, especially if you had irregular menstrual cycles before you used oral contraceptives. It may be advisable to postpone conception until you begin menstruating regularly once you have stopped taking the pill and desire pregnancy.

There does not appear to be any increase in birth defects in newborn babies when pregnancy occurs soon after stopping the pill.

OVERDOSAGE

Serious ill effects have not been reported following ingestion of large doses of oral contraceptives by young children. Overdosage may cause nausea and withdrawal bleeding in females. In case of overdosage, contact your healthcare provider or pharmacist.

OTHER INFORMATION

Your healthcare provider will take a medical and family history before prescribing oral contraceptives and will examine you. The physical examination may be delayed to another time if you request it and the healthcare provider believes that it is appropriate to postpone it. You should be reexamined at least once a year. Be sure to inform your healthcare provider if there is a family history of any of the conditions listed previously in this leaflet. Be sure to keep all appointments with your healthcare provider, because this is a time to determine if there are early signs of side effects of oral contraceptive use.

Do not use the drug for any condition other than the one for which it was prescribed. This drug has been prescribed specifically for you; do not give it to others who may want birth control pills.

NONCONTRACEPTIVE HEALTH BENEFITS

The following noncontraceptive health benefits related to the use of oral contraceptives are supported by epidemiological studies which largely utilized oral contraceptive formulations containing doses exceeding 0.035 mg of ethinyl estradiol or 0.05 mg of mestranol.

Effects on menses:

- May decrease blood loss and may decrease incidence of iron-deficiency anemia
- May decrease incidence of dysmenorrhea

Effects related to inhibition of ovulation:

- May decrease incidence of functional ovarian cysts
- May decrease incidence of ectopic pregnancies

Effects from long-term use:

- May decrease incidence of fibroadenomas and fibrocystic disease of the breast
- May decrease incidence of acute pelvic inflammatory disease
- May decrease incidence of endometrial cancer
- May decrease incidence of ovarian cancer

If you want more information about birth control pills, ask your doctor or pharmacist. They have a more technical leaflet called the Professional Labeling which you may wish to read.

MANUFACTURED BY:
DURAMED PHARMACEUTICALS, INC.
A subsidiary of Barr Laboratories, Inc.
Pomona, NY 10970-0519
Revised September 2003
310905825001
BR 9058

Bayer Pharmaceuticals Corporation

400 MORGAN LANE
WEST HAVEN, CT 06516

For Medical Information Contact:
Director, Medical Services
(800) 468-0894
(203) 812-2000

LEVITRA® ℞
[lĕ-vē-trā]
(vardenafil HCl)
TABLETS

DESCRIPTION

LEVITRA® is an oral therapy for the treatment of erectile dysfunction. This monohydrochloride salt of vardenafil is a selective inhibitor of cyclic guanosine monophosphate (cGMP)-specific phosphodiesterase type 5 (PDE5).

Vardenafil HCl is designated chemically as piperazine, 1-[[3-(1,4-dihydro-5-methyl-4-oxo-7-propylimidazo[5,1-*f*][1,2,4]triazin-2-yl)-4-ethoxyphenyl]sulfonyl]-4-ethyl-, monohydrochloride and has the following structural formula:

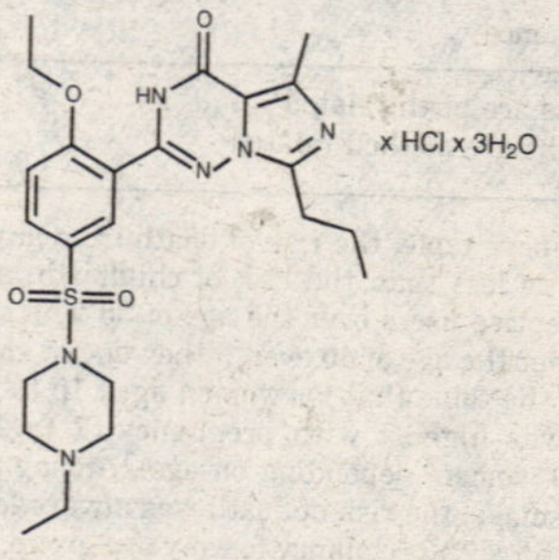

Vardenafil HCl is a nearly colorless, solid substance with a molecular weight of 579.1 g/mol and a solubility of 0.11 mg/mL in water. LEVITRA is formulated as orange, round, film-coated tablets with "BAYER" cross debossed on one side and "2.5", "5", "10", and "20" on the other side corresponding to 2.5 mg, 5 mg, 10 mg, and 20 mg of vardenafil, respectively. In addition to the active ingredient, vardenafil HCl, each tablet contains microcrystalline cellulose, crospovidone, colloidal silicon dioxide, magnesium stearate, hypromellose, polyethylene glycol, titanium dioxide, yellow ferric oxide, and red ferric oxide.

CLINICAL PHARMACOLOGY

Mechanism of Action

Penile erection is a hemodynamic process initiated by the relaxation of smooth muscle in the corpus cavernosum and its associated arterioles. During sexual stimulation, nitric oxide is released from nerve endings and endothelial cells in the corpus cavernosum. Nitric oxide activates the enzyme guanylate cyclase resulting in increased synthesis of cyclic guanosine monophosphate (cGMP) in the smooth muscle cells of the corpus cavernosum. The cGMP in turn triggers smooth muscle relaxation, allowing increased blood flow into the penis, resulting in erection. The tissue concentration of cGMP is regulated by both the rates of synthesis and degradation via phosphodiesterases (PDEs). The most abundant PDE in the human corpus cavernosum is the cGMP-specific phosphodiesterase type 5 (PDE5); therefore, the inhibition of PDE5 enhances erectile function by increasing the amount of cGMP. Because sexual stimulation is required to initiate the local release of nitric oxide, the inhibition of PDE5 has no effect in the absence of sexual stimulation.

In vitro studies have shown that vardenafil is a selective inhibitor of PDE5. The inhibitory effect of vardenafil is more selective on PDE5 than for other known phosphodiesterases (>15-fold relative to PDE6, >130-fold relative to PDE1, >300-fold relative to PDE11, and >1,000-fold relative to PDE2, 3, 4, 7, 8, 9, and 10).

Pharmacokinetics

The pharmacokinetics of vardenafil are approximately dose proportional over the recommended dose range. Vardenafil is eliminated predominantly by hepatic metabolism, mainly by CYP3A4 and to a minor extent, CYP2C isoforms. Concomitant use with strong CYP3A4 inhibitors such as ritonavir, indinavir, ketoconazole, itraconazole as well as moderate CYP3A inhibitors such as erythromycin results in significant increases of plasma levels of vardenafil (see **PRECAUTIONS, WARNINGS** and **DOSAGE AND ADMINISTRATION**). Mean vardenafil plasma concentrations measured after the administration of a single oral dose of 20 mg to healthy male volunteers are depicted in Figure 1.

Figure 1: Plasma Vardenafil Concentration (Mean ± SD) Curve for a Single 20 mg LEVITRA Dose

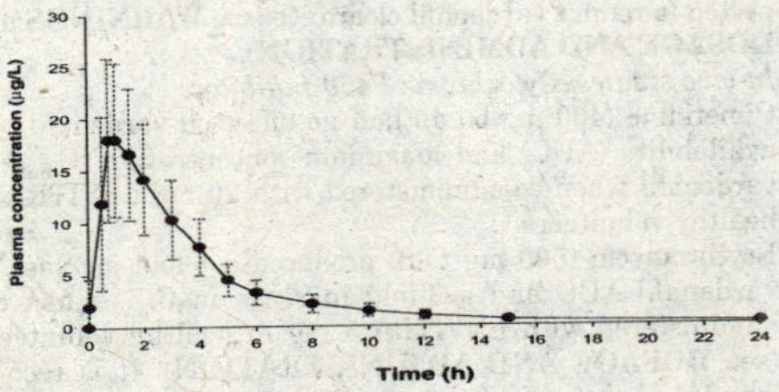

Absorption: Vardenafil is rapidly absorbed with absolute bioavailability of approximately 15%. Maximum observed plasma concentrations after a single 20 mg dose in healthy volunteers are usually reached between 30 minutes and 2 hours (median 60 minutes) after oral dosing in the fasted state. Two food-effect studies were conducted which showed that high-fat meals caused a reduction in C_{max} by 18%-50%.

Distribution: The mean steady-state volume of distribution (Vss) for vardenafil is 208 L, indicating extensive tissue distribution. Vardenafil and its major circulating metabolite, M1, are highly bound to plasma proteins (about 95% for parent drug and M1). This protein binding is reversible and independent of total drug concentrations.

Following a single oral dose of 20 mg vardenafil in healthy volunteers, a mean of 0.00018% of the administered dose was obtained in semen 1.5 hours after dosing.

Metabolism: Vardenafil is metabolized predominantly by the hepatic enzyme CYP3A4, with contribution from the CYP3A5 and CYP2C isoforms. The major circulating metabolite, M1, results from desethylation at the piperazine moiety of vardenafil. M1 is subject to further metabolism. The plasma concentration of M1 is approximately 26% that of the parent compound. This metabolite shows a phosphodiesterase selectivity profile similar to that of vardenafil and an *in vitro* inhibitory potency for PDE5 28% of that of vardenafil. Therefore, M1 accounts for approximately 7% of total pharmacologic activity.

Excretion: The total body clearance of vardenafil is 56 L/h, and the terminal half-life of vardenafil and its primary metabolite (M1) is approximately 4-5 hours. After oral administration, vardenafil is excreted as metabolites predominantly in the feces (approximately 91-95% of administered oral dose) and to a lesser extent in the urine (approximately 2–6% of administered oral dose).

Pharmacokinetics in Special Populations

Pediatrics: Vardenafil trials were not conducted in the pediatric population.

Geriatrics: In a healthy volunteer study of elderly males (≥ 65 years) and younger males (18–45 years), mean C_{max} and AUC were 34% and 52% higher, respectively, in the elderly males (see **PRECAUTIONS, Geriatric Use** and **DOSAGE AND ADMINISTRATION**). Consequently, a lower starting dose of LEVITRA (5 mg) in patients ≥ 65 years of age should be considered.

Renal Insufficiency: In volunteers with mild renal impairment (CL_{cr} = 50–80 ml/min), the pharmacokinetics of vardenafil were similar to those observed in a control group with normal renal function. In the moderate (CL_{cr} = 30–50 ml/min) or severe (CL_{cr} <30 ml/min) renal impairment groups, the AUC of vardenafil was 20–30% higher compared to that observed in a control group with normal renal function (CL_{cr} >80 ml/min). Vardenafil pharmacokinetics have not been evaluated in patients requiring renal dialysis (see **PRECAUTIONS, Renal Insufficiency,** and **DOSAGE AND ADMINISTRATION**).

Table 1. Mean QT and QT_c changes in msec (90% CI) from baseline relative to placebo at 1 hour post-dose with different methodologies to correct for the effect of heart rate.

Drug/Dose	QT Uncorrected (msec)	Fridericia QT Correction (msec)	Individual QT Correction (msec)
Vardenafil 10 mg	-2 (-4, 0)	8 (6, 9)	4 (3, 6)
Vardenafil 80 mg	-2 (-4, 0)	10 (8, 11)	6 (4, 7)
Moxifloxacin* 400 mg	3 (1, 5)	8 (6, 9)	7 (5, 8)

* Active control (drug known to prolong QT)

Hepatic Insufficiency: In volunteers with mild hepatic impairment (Child-Pugh A), the C_{max} and AUC following a 10 mg vardenafil dose were increased by 22% and 17%, respectively, compared to healthy control subjects. In volunteers with moderate hepatic impairment (Child-Pugh B), the C_{max} and AUC following a 10 mg vardenafil dose were increased by 130% and 160%, respectively, compared to healthy control subjects. Consequently, a starting dose of 5 mg is recommended for patients with moderate hepatic impairment, and the maximum dose should not exceed 10 mg (see **PRECAUTIONS** and **DOSAGE AND ADMINISTRATION**). Vardenafil has not been evaluated in patients with severe (Child-Pugh C) hepatic impairment.

Pharmacodynamics

Effects on Blood Pressure: In a clinical pharmacology study of patients with erectile dysfunction, single doses of vardenafil 20 mg caused a mean maximum decrease in supine blood pressure of 7 mm Hg systolic and 8 mm Hg diastolic (compared to placebo), accompanied by a mean maximum increase of heart rate of 4 beats per minute. The maximum decrease in blood pressure occurred between 1 and 4 hours after dosing. Following multiple dosing for 31 days, similar blood pressure responses were observed on Day 31 as on Day 1. Vardenafil may add to the blood pressure lowering effects of antihypertensive agents (see **CONTRAINDICATIONS, PRECAUTIONS, Drug Interactions**).

Effects on Blood Pressure and Heart Rate when LEVITRA is Combined with Nitrates: A study was conducted in which the blood pressure and heart rate response to 0.4 mg nitroglycerin (NTG) sublingually was evaluated in 18 healthy subjects following pretreatment with LEVITRA 20 mg at various times before NTG administration. LEVITRA 20 mg caused an additional time-related reduction in blood pressure and increase in heart rate in association with NTG administration. The blood pressure effects were observed when LEVITRA 20 mg was dosed 1 or 4 hours before NTG and the heart rate effects were observed when 20 mg was dosed 1, 4, or 8 hours before NTG. Additional blood pressure and heart rate changes were not detected when LEVITRA 20 mg was dosed 24 hours before NTG. (See Figure 2.)

Figure 2: Placebo-subtracted point estimates (with 90% CI) of mean maximal blood pressure and heart rate effects of pre-dosing with LEVITRA 20 mg at 24, 8, 4, and 1 hour before 0.4 mg NTG sublingually.

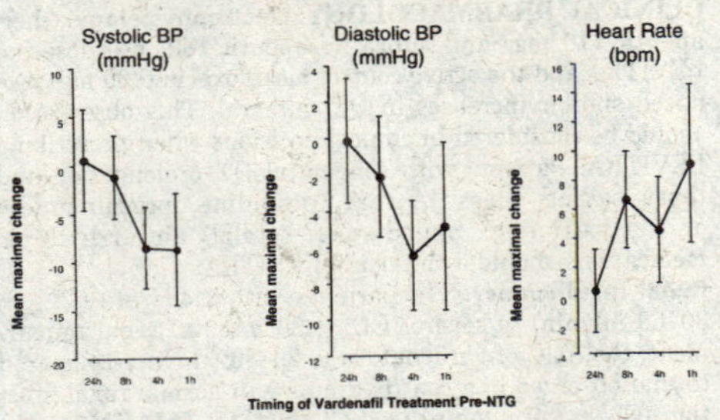

Because the disease state of patients requiring nitrate therapy is anticipated to increase the likelihood of hypotension, the use of vardenafil by patients on nitrate therapy or on nitric oxide donors is contraindicated (see **CONTRAINDICATIONS**).

Electrophysiology: The effect of 10 mg and 80 mg vardenafil on QT interval was evaluated in a single-dose, double-blind, randomized, placebo- and active-controlled (moxifloxacin 400 mg) crossover study in 59 healthy males (81% White, 12% Black, 7% Hispanic) aged 45-60 years. The QT interval was measured at one hour post dose because this time point approximates the average time of peak vardenafil concentration. The 80 mg dose of LEVITRA (four times the highest recommended dose) was chosen because this dose yields plasma concentrations covering those observed upon co-administration of a low-dose of LEVITRA (5 mg) and 600 mg BID of ritonavir. Of the CYP3A4 inhibitors that have been studied, ritonavir causes the most significant drug-drug interaction with vardenafil. Table 1 summarizes the effect on mean uncorrected QT and mean corrected QT interval (QT_c) with different methods of correction (Fridericia and a linear individual correction method) at one hour post-dose. No single correction method is known to be more valid than the other. In this study, the mean increase in heart rate associated with a 10 mg dose of LEVITRA compared to placebo was 5 beats/minute and with an 80 mg dose of LEVITRA the mean increase was 6 beats/minute. [See table 1 above]

Therapeutic and supratherapeutic doses of vardenafil and the active control moxifloxacin produced similar increases in QT_c interval. This study, however, was not designed to make direct statistical comparisons between the drug or the dose levels. The clinical impact of these QT_c changes is unknown (see **PRECAUTIONS**).

Effects on Exercise Treadmill Test in Patients with Coronary Artery Disease (CAD): In two independent trials that assessed 10 mg (n=41) and 20 mg (n=39) vardenafil, respectively, vardenafil did not alter the total treadmill exercise time compared to placebo. The patient population included men aged 40–80 years with stable exercise-induced angina documented by at least one of the following: 1) prior history of MI, CABG, PTCA, or stenting (not within 6 months); 2) positive coronary angiogram showing at least 60% narrowing of the diameter of at least one major coronary artery; or 3) a positive stress echocardiogram or stress nuclear perfusion study.

Results of these studies showed that LEVITRA did not alter the total treadmill exercise time compared to placebo (10 mg LEVITRA vs. placebo: 433±109 and 426±105 seconds, respectively; 20 mg LEVITRA vs. placebo: 414±114 and 411±124 seconds, respectively). The total time to angina was not altered by LEVITRA when compared to placebo (10 mg LEVITRA vs. placebo: 291±123 and 292±110 seconds; 20 mg LEVITRA vs. placebo: 354±137 and 347±143 seconds, respectively). The total time to 1 mm or greater ST-segment depression was similar to placebo in both the 10 mg and the 20 mg LEVITRA groups (10 mg LEVITRA vs. placebo: 380±108 and 334±108 seconds; 20 mg LEVITRA vs. placebo: 364±101 and 366±105 seconds, respectively).

Effects on Vision: Single oral doses of phosphodiesterase inhibitors have demonstrated transient dose-related impairment of color discrimination (blue/green) using the Farnsworth-Munsell 100-hue test and reductions in electroretinogram (ERG) b-wave amplitudes, with peak effects near the time of peak plasma levels. These findings are consistent with the inhibition of PDE6 in rods and cones, which is involved in phototransduction in the retina. The findings were most evident one hour after administration, diminishing but still present 6 hours after administration. In a single dose study in 25 normal males, LEVITRA 40 mg, twice the maximum daily recommended dose, did not alter visual acuity, intraocular pressure, fundoscopic and slit lamp findings.

CLINICAL STUDIES

LEVITRA was evaluated in four major double-blind, randomized, placebo-controlled, fixed-dose, parallel design, multicenter trials in 2431 men aged 20–83 (mean age 57 years; 78% White, 7% Black, 2% Asian, 3% Hispanic and 10% Other/Unknown). The doses of LEVITRA in these studies were 5 mg, 10 mg, and 20 mg. Two of these trials were conducted in the general ED population and two in special ED populations (one in patients with diabetes mellitus and one in post-prostatectomy patients). LEVITRA was dosed without regard to meals on an as needed basis in men with erectile dysfunction (ED), many of whom had multiple other medical conditions. The primary endpoints were assessed at 3 months.

Primary efficacy assessment in all four major trials was by means of the Erectile Function (EF) Domain score of the validated International Index of Erectile Function (IIEF) Questionnaire and two questions from the Sexual Encounter Profile (SEP) dealing with the ability to achieve vaginal penetration (SEP2), and the ability to maintain an erection long enough for successful intercourse (SEP3).

In all four fixed-dose efficacy trials, LEVITRA showed clinically meaningful and statistically significant improvement in the EF Domain, SEP2, and SEP3 scores compared to placebo. The mean baseline EF Domain score in these trials was 11.8 (scores range from 0–30 where lower scores represent more severe disease). LEVITRA (5 mg, 10 mg, and 20 mg) was effective in all age categories (<45, 45 to <65, and ≥65 years) and was also effective regardless of race (White, Black, Other).

Trials in a General Erectile Dysfunction Population: In the major North American fixed-dose trial, 762 patients (mean age 57, range 20–83 years; 79% White, 13% Black, 4% Hispanic, 2% Asian and 2% Other) were evaluated. The mean baseline EF Domain scores were 13, 13, 13, 14 for the LEVITRA 5 mg, 10 mg, 20 mg and placebo groups, respectively. There was significant improvement (p<0.0001) at 3 months with LEVITRA (EF Domain scores of 18, 21, 21, for the 5 mg, 10 mg, and 20 mg dose groups, respectively) compared to the placebo group (EF Domain score of 15). The

Continued on next page

Levitra—Cont.

European trial (total N=803) confirmed these results. The improvement in mean score was maintained at all doses at 6 months in the North American trial.

In the North American trial, LEVITRA significantly improved the rates of achieving an erection sufficient for penetration (SEP2) at doses of 5 mg, 10 mg, and 20 mg compared to placebo (65%, 75%, and 80%, respectively, compared to a 52% response in the placebo group at 3 months; p< 0.0001). The European trial confirmed these results.

LEVITRA demonstrated a clinically meaningful and statistically significant increase in the overall per-patient rate of maintenance of erection to successful intercourse (SEP3) (51% on 5 mg, 64% on 10 mg, and 65% on 20 mg, respectively, compared to 32% on placebo; p< 0.0001) at 3 months in the North American trial. The European trial showed comparable efficacy. This improvement in mean score was maintained at all doses at 6 months in the North American trial.

Trial in Patients with ED and Diabetes Mellitus: LEVITRA demonstrated clinically meaningful and statistically significant improvement in erectile function in a prospective, fixed-dose (10 and 20 mg LEVITRA), double-blind, placebo-controlled trial of patients with diabetes mellitus (n=439; mean age 57 years, range 33–81; 80% White, 9% Black, 8% Hispanic, and 3% Other).

Significant improvements in the EF Domain were shown in this study (EF Domain scores of 17 on 10 mg LEVITRA and 19 on 20 mg LEVITRA compared to 13 on placebo; p< 0.0001).

LEVITRA significantly improved the overall per-patient rate of achieving an erection sufficient for penetration (SEP2) (61% on 10 mg and 64% on 20 mg LEVITRA compared to 36% on placebo; p< 0.0001).

LEVITRA demonstrated a clinically meaningful and statistically significant increase in the overall per-patient rate of maintenance of erection to successful intercourse (SEP3) (49% on 10 mg, 54% on 20 mg LEVITRA compared to 23% on placebo; p< 0.0001).

Trial in Patients with ED after Radical Prostatectomy: LEVITRA demonstrated clinically meaningful and statistically significant improvement in erectile function in a prospective, fixed-dose (10 and 20 mg LEVITRA), double-blind, placebo-controlled trial in post-prostatectomy patients (n=427, mean age 60, range 44-77 years; 93% White, 5% Black, 2% Other).

Significant improvements in the EF Domain were shown in this study (EF Domain scores of 15 on 10 mg LEVITRA and 15 on 20 mg LEVITRA compared to 9 on placebo; p< 0.0001).

LEVITRA significantly improved the overall per-patient rate of achieving an erection sufficient for penetration (SEP2) (47% on 10 mg and 48% on 20 mg LEVITRA compared to 22% on placebo; p<0.0001).

LEVITRA demonstrated a clinically meaningful and statistically significant increase in the overall per-patient rate of maintenance of erection to successful intercourse (SEP3) (37% on 10 mg, 34% on 20 mg LEVITRA compared to 10% on placebo; p< 0.0001).

INDICATIONS AND USAGE

LEVITRA is indicated for the treatment of erectile dysfunction.

CONTRAINDICATIONS

Nitrates: Administration of LEVITRA with nitrates (either regularly and/or intermittently) and nitric oxide donors is contraindicated (see **CLINICAL PHARMACOLOGY, Pharmacodynamics, Effects on Blood Pressure and Heart Rate when LEVITRA is Combined with Nitrates**). Consistent with the effects of PDE5 inhibition on the nitric oxide/cyclic guanosine monophosphate pathway, PDE5 inhibitors may potentiate the hypotensive effects of nitrates. A suitable time interval following LEVITRA dosing for the safe administration of nitrates or nitric oxide donors has not been determined.

Alpha-Blockers: Because the co-administration of alpha-blockers and LEVITRA can produce hypotension, LEVITRA is contraindicated in patients taking alpha-blockers (see **PRECAUTIONS, Drug Interactions**).

Hypersensitivity: LEVITRA is contraindicated for patients with a known hypersensitivity to any component of the tablet.

WARNINGS

Cardiovascular effects

General: Physicians should consider the cardiovascular status of their patients, since there is a degree of cardiac risk associated with sexual activity. In men for whom sexual activity is not recommended because of their underlying cardiovascular status, any treatment for erectile dysfunction, including LEVITRA, generally should not be used.

Left Ventricular Outflow Obstruction: Patients with left ventricular outflow obstruction, e.g., aortic stenosis and idiopathic hypertrophic subaortic stenosis, can be sensitive to the action of vasodilators including Type 5 phosphodiesterase inhibitors.

Blood Pressure Effects: LEVITRA has systemic vasodilatory properties that resulted in transient decreases in supine blood pressure in healthy volunteers (mean maximum decrease of 7 mmHg systolic and 8 mmHg diastolic) (see **CLINICAL PHARMACOLOGY, Pharmacodynamics**). While this normally would be expected to be of little consequence in most patients, prior to prescribing LEVITRA, physicians should carefully consider whether their patients with underlying cardiovascular disease could be affected adversely by such vasodilatory effects.

Effect of Co-administration of Strong CYP3A4 Inhibitors

Long-term safety information is not available on the concomitant administration of vardenafil with HIV protease inhibitors. Concomitant administration with ritonavir or indinavir substantially increases plasma concentrations of vardenafil. To decrease the chance of adverse events in patients concomitantly taking ritonavir or indinavir, which are strong inhibitors of CYP3A4 metabolism, a maximum single dose of 2.5 mg LEVITRA should not be exceeded. Because ritonavir prolongs LEVITRA elimination half-life (5-6-fold), no more than a single 2.5 mg dose of LEVITRA should be taken in a 72-hour period by patients also taking ritonavir. Patients taking indinavir, ketoconazole 400 mg daily, or itraconazole 400 mg daily should not exceed LEVITRA 2.5 mg once daily. For patients taking ketoconazole or itraconazole 200 mg daily, a single dose of 5 mg LEVITRA should not be exceeded in a 24-hour period (see **PRECAUTIONS, Drug Interactions** and **DOSAGE AND ADMINISTRATION**).

Other Effects

There have been rare reports of prolonged erections greater than 4 hours and priapism (painful erections greater than 6 hours in duration) for this class of compounds, including vardenafil. In the event that an erection persists longer than 4 hours, the patient should seek immediate medical assistance. If priapism is not treated immediately, penile tissue damage and permanent loss of potency may result.

Patient Subgroups Not Studied in Clinical Trials

There is no controlled clinical data on the safety or efficacy of LEVITRA in the following patients; and therefore its use is not recommended until further information is available.

- unstable angina; hypotension (resting systolic blood pressure of <90 mm Hg); uncontrolled hypertension (>170/110 mm Hg); recent history of stroke, life-threatening arrhythmia, or myocardial infarction (within the last 6 months); severe cardiac failure
- severe hepatic impairment (Child-Pugh C)
- end stage renal disease requiring dialysis
- known hereditary degenerative retinal disorders, including retinitis pigmentosa

PRECAUTIONS

The evaluation of erectile dysfunction should include a determination of potential underlying causes, a medical assessment, and the identification of appropriate treatment. Before prescribing LEVITRA, it is important to note the following:

Hepatic Insufficiency: In volunteers with moderate impairment (Child-Pugh B), the C_{max} and AUC following a 10 mg vardenafil dose were increased 130% and 160%, respectively, compared to healthy control subjects. Consequently, a starting dose of 5 mg is recommended for patients with moderate hepatic impairment and the maximum dose should not exceed 10 mg (see **CLINICAL PHARMACOLOGY, Pharmacokinetics in Special Populations,** and **DOSAGE AND ADMINISTRATION**). Vardenafil has not been evaluated in patients with severe hepatic impairment (Child-Pugh C).

Congenital or Acquired QT Prolongation: In a study of the effect of LEVITRA on QT interval in 59 healthy males (see **CLINICAL PHARMACOLOGY, Electrophysiology**), therapeutic (10 mg) and supratherapeutic (80 mg) doses of LEVITRA and the active control moxifloxacin (400 mg) produced similar increases in QT_c interval. This observation should be considered in clinical decisions when prescribing LEVITRA. Patients with congenital QT prolongation and those taking Class IA (e.g., quinidine, procainamide) or Class III (e.g., amiodarone, sotalol) antiarrhythmic medications should avoid using LEVITRA.

Renal Insufficiency: In patients with moderate (CL_{cr} = 30–50 ml/min) to severe (CL_{cr} <30 ml/min) renal impairment, the AUC of vardenafil was 20–30% higher compared to that observed in a control group with normal renal function (CL_{cr} >80 ml/min) (see **CLINICAL PHARMACOLOGY, Pharmacokinetics in Special Populations**). Vardenafil pharmacokinetics have not been evaluated in patients requiring renal dialysis.

General: In humans, vardenafil alone in doses up to 20 mg does not prolong the bleeding time. There is no clinical evidence of any additive prolongation of the bleeding time when vardenafil is administered with aspirin. Vardenafil has not been administered to patients with bleeding disorders or significant active peptic ulceration. Therefore LEVITRA should be administered to these patients after careful benefit-risk assessment.

Treatment for erectile dysfunction should generally be used with caution by patients with anatomical deformation of the penis (such as angulation, cavernosal fibrosis, or Peyronie's disease), or by patients who have conditions that may predispose them to priapism (such as sickle cell anemia, multiple myeloma, or leukemia).

The safety and efficacy of LEVITRA used in combination with other treatments for erectile dysfunction have not been studied. Therefore, the use of such combinations is not recommended.

Information for Patients

Physicians should discuss with patients the contraindication of LEVITRA with regular and/or intermittent use of organic nitrates. Patients should be counseled that concomitant use of LEVITRA with nitrates could cause blood pressure to suddenly drop to an unsafe level, resulting in dizziness, syncope, or even heart attack or stroke.

Physicians should inform their patients that concomitant use of LEVITRA with alpha-blockers is contraindicated because co-administration can produce hypotension.

Physicians should discuss with patients the appropriate use of LEVITRA and its anticipated benefits. It should be explained that sexual stimulation is required for an erection to occur after taking LEVITRA. LEVITRA should be taken approximately 60 minutes before sexual activity. Patients should be counseled regarding the dosing of LEVITRA. Patients should be advised to contact their healthcare provider for dose modification if they are not satisfied with the quality of their sexual performance with LEVITRA or in the case of an unwanted effect. Patients should be advised to contact the prescribing physician if new medications that may interact with LEVITRA are prescribed by another healthcare provider.

Physicians should discuss with patients the potential cardiac risk of sexual activity for patients with preexisting cardiovascular risk factors.

The use of LEVITRA offers no protection against sexually transmitted diseases. Counseling of patients about protective measures necessary to guard against sexually transmitted diseases, including the Human Immunodeficiency Virus (HIV), should be considered.

Physicians should inform patients that there have been rare reports of prolonged erections greater than 4 hours and priapism (painful erections greater than 6 hours in duration) for LEVITRA and this class of compounds. In the event that an erection persists longer than 4 hours, the patient should seek immediate medical assistance. If priapism is not treated immediately, penile tissue damage and permanent loss of potency may result.

Drug Interactions

Effect of other drugs on LEVITRA

In vitro studies: Studies in human liver microsomes showed that vardenafil is metabolized primarily by cytochrome P450 (CYP) isoforms 3A4/5, and to a lesser degree by CYP2C9. Therefore, inhibitors of these enzymes are expected to reduce vardenafil clearance (see **WARNINGS** and **DOSAGE AND ADMINISTRATION**).

In vivo studies: Cytochrome P450 Inhibitors

Cimetidine (400 mg b.i.d.) had no effect on vardenafil bioavailability (AUC) and maximum concentration (C_{max}) of vardenafil when co-administered with 20 mg LEVITRA in healthy volunteers.

Erythromycin (500 mg t.i.d) produced a 4-fold increase in vardenafil AUC and a 3-fold increase in C_{max} when co-administered with LEVITRA 5 mg in healthy volunteers (see **DOSAGE AND ADMINISTRATION**). It is recommended not to exceed a single 5 mg dose of LEVITRA in a 24-hour period when used in combination with erythromycin.

Ketoconazole (200 mg once daily) produced a 10-fold increase in vardenafil AUC and a 4-fold increase in C_{max} when co-administered with LEVITRA (5 mg) in healthy volunteers. A 5-mg LEVITRA dose should not be exceeded when used in combination with 200 mg once daily ketoconazole. Since higher doses of ketoconazole (400 mg daily) may result in higher increases in C_{max} and AUC, a single 2.5 mg dose of LEVITRA should not be exceeded in a 24-hour period when used in combination with ketoconazole 400 mg daily (see **WARNINGS** and **DOSAGE AND ADMINISTRATION**).

HIV Protease Inhibitors:

Indinavir (800 mg t.i.d.) co-administered with LEVITRA 10 mg resulted in a 16-fold increase in vardenafil AUC, a 7-fold increase in vardenafil C_{max} and a 2-fold increase in vardenafil half-life. It is recommended not to exceed a single 2.5 mg LEVITRA dose in a 24-hour period when used in combination with indinavir (see **WARNINGS** and **DOSAGE AND ADMINISTRATION**).

Ritonavir (600 mg b.i.d.) co-administered with LEVITRA 5 mg resulted in a 49-fold increase in vardenafil AUC and a 13-fold increase in vardenafil C_{max}. The interaction is a consequence of blocking hepatic metabolism of vardenafil by ritonavir, a highly potent CYP3A4 inhibitor, which also inhibits CYP2C9. Ritonavir significantly prolonged the half-life of vardenafil to 26 hours. Consequently, it is recommended not to exceed a single 2.5 mg LEVITRA dose in a 72-hour period when used in combination with ritonavir (see **WARNINGS** and **DOSAGE AND ADMINISTRATION**).

Other Drug Interactions: No pharmacokinetic interactions were observed between vardenafil and the following drugs: glyburide, warfarin, digoxin, Maalox, and ranitidine. In the warfarin study, vardenafil had no effect on the prothrombin time or other pharmacodynamic parameters.

Effects of LEVITRA on other drugs

In vitro studies:

Vardenafil and its metabolites had no effect on CYP1A2, 2A6, and 2E1 (Ki > 100µM). Weak inhibitory effects toward other isoforms (CYP2C8, 2C9, 2C19, 2D6, 3A4) were found, but Ki values were in excess of plasma concentrations achieved following dosing. The most potent inhibitory activity was observed for vardenafil metabolite M1, which had a Ki of 1.4 µM toward CYP3A4, which is about 20 times higher than the M1 C_{max} values after an 80 mg LEVITRA dose.

In vivo studies:

Nitrates: The blood pressure lowering effects of sublingual nitrates (0.4 mg) taken 1 and 4 hours after vardenafil and increases in heart rate when taken at 1, 4 and 8 hours were potentiated by a 20 mg dose of LEVITRA in 2 healthy middle-aged subjects. These effects were not observed when LEVITRA 20 mg was taken 24 hours before the NTG. Potentiation of the hypotensive effects of nitrates for patients with ischemic heart disease has not been evaluated, and concomitant use of LEVITRA and nitrates is contraindicated (see **CLINICAL PHARMACOLOGY, Pharmacodynamics, Effects on Blood Pressure and Heart Rate when LEVITRA is Combined with Nitrates; CONTRAINDICATIONS**).

Nifedipine: Vardenafil 20 mg, when co-administered with slow-release nifedipine 30 mg or 60 mg once daily, did not affect the relative bioavailability (AUC) or maximum concentration (C_{max}) of nifedipine, a drug that is metabolized via CYP3A4. Nifedipine did not alter the plasma levels of LEVITRA when taken in combination. In these patients whose hypertension was controlled with nifedipine, LEVITRA 20 mg produced mean additional supine systolic/diastolic blood pressure reductions of 6/5 mm Hg compared to placebo.

Alpha-blockers: When LEVITRA 10 or 20 mg was given to healthy volunteers either simultaneously or 6 hours after a 10 mg dose of terazosin, significant hypotension developed in a substantial number of subjects. With simultaneous dosing of LEVITRA 10 mg and terazosin 10 mg, 6 of 8 subjects experienced a standing systolic blood pressure of less than 85 mm Hg. With simultaneous dosing of LEVITRA 20 mg and terazosin 10 mg, 2 of 9 subjects experienced a standing systolic blood pressure of less than 85 mm Hg. When LEVITRA dosing was separated from terazosin 10 mg by 6 hours, 7 of 28 subjects who received 20 mg of LEVITRA experienced a decrease in standing systolic blood pressure below 85 mm Hg. In a similar study with tamsulosin in healthy volunteers, 1 of 24 subjects dosed with LEVITRA 20 mg and tamsulosin 0.4 mg separated by 6 hours experienced a standing systolic blood pressure below 85 mm Hg. Two of 16 subjects dosed simultaneously with LEVITRA 10 mg and tamsulosin 0.4 mg experienced a standing systolic blood pressure below 85 mm Hg. The administration of lower doses of LEVITRA with alpha-blockers has not been completely evaluated to determine if they can be safely administered together. Based on these data, LEVITRA should not be used in patients on alpha-blocker therapy (see **CONTRAINDICATIONS**).

Ritonavir and indinavir: Upon concomitant administration of 5 mg of LEVITRA with 600 mg BID ritonavir, the C_{max} and AUC of ritonavir were reduced by approximately 20%. Upon administration of 10 mg of LEVITRA with 800 mg TID indinavir, the C_{max} and AUC of indinavir were reduced by 40% and 30%, respectively.

Alcohol: Alcohol (0.5 g/kg body weight: approximately 40 mL of absolute alcohol in a 70 kg person) and vardenafil plasma levels were not altered when dosed simultaneously. LEVITRA (20 mg) did not potentiate the hypotensive effects of alcohol during the 4-hour observation period in healthy volunteers when administered with alcohol (0.5 g/kg body weight).

Aspirin: LEVITRA (10 mg and 20 mg) did not potentiate the increase in bleeding time caused by aspirin (two 81 mg tablets).

Other interactions: LEVITRA had no effect on the pharmacodynamics of glyburide (glucose and insulin concentrations) and warfarin (prothrombin time or other pharmacodynamic parameters).

Carcinogenesis, Mutagenesis, Impairment of Fertility

Vardenafil was not carcinogenic in rats and mice when administered daily for 24 months. In these studies systemic drug exposures (AUCs) for unbound (free) vardenafil and its major metabolite were approximately 400- and 170-fold for male and female rats, respectively, and 21- and 37-fold for male and female mice, respectively, the exposures observed in human males given the Maximum Recommended Human Dose (MRHD) of 20 mg. Vardenafil was not mutagenic as assessed in either the *in vitro* bacterial Ames assay or the forward mutation assay in Chinese hamster V79 cells. Vardenafil was not clastogenic as assessed in either the *in vitro* chromosomal aberration test or the *in vivo* mouse micronucleus test. Vardenafil did not impair fertility in male and female rats administered doses up to 100 mg/kg/day for 28 days prior to mating in male, and for 14 days prior to mating and through day 7 of gestation in females. In a corresponding 1-month rat toxicity study, this dose produced an AUC value for unbound vardenafil 200 fold greater than AUC in humans at the MRHD of 20 mg.

There was no effect on sperm motility or morphology after single 20 mg oral doses of vardenafil in healthy volunteers.

Pregnancy, Nursing Mothers and Pediatric Use

LEVITRA is not indicated for use in women, newborns, or children. Vardenafil was secreted into the milk of lactating rats at concentrations approximately 10-fold greater than found in the plasma. Following a single oral dose of 3 mg/kg, 3.3% of the administered dose was excreted into the milk within 24 hours. It is not known if vardenafil is excreted in human breast milk.

Pregnancy Category B: No evidence of specific potential for teratogenicity, embryotoxicity or fetotoxicity was observed in rats and rabbits that received vardenafil at up to 18 mg/kg/day during organogenesis. This dose is approximately 100 fold (rat) and 29 fold (rabbit) greater than the AUC values for unbound vardenafil and its major metabolite in humans given the MRHD of 20 mg. In the rat pre-and postnatal development study, the NOAEL (no observed adverse effect level) for maternal toxicity was 8 mg/kg/day. Retarded physical development of pups in the absence of maternal effects was observed following maternal exposure to 1 and 8 mg/kg possibly due to vasodilatation and/or secretion of the drug into milk. The number of living pups born to rats exposed pre- and postnatally was reduced at 60 mg/kg/day. Based on the results of the pre- and postnatal study, the developmental NOAEL is less than 1 mg/kg/day. Based on plasma exposures in the rat developmental toxicity study, 1mg/kg/day in the pregnant rat is estimated to produce total AUC values for unbound vardenafil and its major metabolite comparable to the human AUC at the MRHD of 20 mg. There are no adequate and well-controlled trials of vardenafil in pregnant women.

Geriatric Use

Elderly males age 65 years and older have higher vardenafil plasma concentrations than younger males (18 – 45 years), mean C_{max} and AUC were 34% and 52% higher, respectively (see **CLINICAL PHARMACOLOGY, Pharmacokinetics in Special Populations,** and **DOSAGE AND ADMINISTRATION**). Phase 3 clinical trials included more than 834 elderly patients, and no differences in safety or effectiveness of LEVITRA 5, 10, or 20 mg were noted when these elderly patients were compared to younger patients. However, due to increased vardenafil concentrations in the elderly, a starting dose of 5 mg LEVITRA should be considered in patients ≥ 65 years of age.

ADVERSE REACTIONS

LEVITRA was administered to over 4430 men (mean age 56, range 18-89 years; 81% White, 6% Black, 2% Asian, 2% Hispanic and 9% Other) during controlled and uncontrolled clinical trials worldwide. Over 2200 patients were treated for 6 months or longer, and 880 patients were treated for at least 1 year.

In placebo-controlled clinical trials, the discontinuation rate due to adverse events was 3.4% for LEVITRA compared to 1.1% for placebo.

When LEVITRA was taken as recommended in placebo-controlled clinical trials, the following adverse events were reported (see Table 2).

Table 2: Adverse Events Reported By ≥ 2% of Patients Treated with LEVITRA and More Frequent on Drug than Placebo in Fixed and Flexible[γ] Dose Randomized, Controlled Trials of 5 mg, 10 mg, or 20 mg Vardenafil

Adverse Event	Percentage of Patients Reporting Event	
	Placebo N = 1199	LEVITRA N = 2203
Headache	4%	15%
Flushing	1%	11%
Rhinitis	3%	9%
Dyspepsia	1%	4%
Accidental Injury*	2%	3%
Sinusitis	1%	3%
Flu Syndrome	2%	3%
Dizziness	1%	2%
Increased Creatinine Kinase	1%	2%
Nausea	1%	2%

* All the events listed in the above table were deemed to be adverse drug reactions with the exception of accidental injury.

γ Flexible dose studies started all patients at LEVITRA 10 mg and allowed decrease in dose to 5 mg or increase in dose to 20 mg based on side effects and efficacy.

Back pain was reported in 2.0% of patients treated with LEVITRA and 1.7% of patients on placebo.

Placebo-controlled trials suggested a dose effect in the incidence of some adverse events (headache, flushing, dyspepsia, nausea, rhinitis) over the 5 mg, 10 mg, and 20 mg doses of LEVITRA. The following section identifies additional, less frequent events (<2%) reported during the clinical development of LEVITRA. Excluded from this list are those events that are infrequent and minor, those events that may be commonly observed in the absence of drug therapy, and those events that are not reasonably associated with the drug.

BODY AS A WHOLE: anaphylactic reaction (including laryngeal edema), asthenia, face edema, pain

AUDITORY: tinnitus

CARDIOVASCULAR: angina pectoris, chest pain, hypertension, hypotension, myocardial ischemia, myocardial infarction, palpitation, postural hypotension, syncope, tachycardia

DIGESTIVE: abdominal pain, abnormal liver function tests, diarrhea, dry mouth, dysphagia, esophagitis, gastritis, gastroesophageal reflux, GGTP increased, vomiting

MUSCULOSKELETAL: arthralgia, back pain, myalgia, neck pain

NERVOUS: hypertonia, hypesthesia, insomnia, paresthesia, somnolence, vertigo

RESPIRATORY: dyspnea, epistaxis, pharyngitis

SKIN AND APPENDAGES: photosensitivity reaction, pruritus, rash, sweating

OPHTHALMOLOGIC: abnormal vision, blurred vision, chromatopsia, changes in color vision, conjunctivitis (increased redness of the eye), dim vision, eye pain, glaucoma, photophobia, watery eyes

UROGENITAL: abnormal ejaculation, priapism (including prolonged or painful erections)

OVERDOSAGE

The maximum dose of LEVITRA for which human data are available is a single 120 mg dose administered to eight healthy male volunteers. The majority of these subjects experienced reversible back pain/myalgia and/or "abnormal vision."

In cases of overdose, standard supportive measures should be taken as required. Renal dialysis is not expected to accelerate clearance because vardenafil is highly bound to plasma proteins and is not significantly eliminated in the urine.

DOSAGE AND ADMINISTRATION

For most patients, the recommended starting dose of LEVITRA is 10 mg, taken orally approximately 60 minutes before sexual activity. The dose may be increased to a maximum recommended dose of 20 mg or decreased to 5 mg based on efficacy and side effects. The maximum recommended dosing frequency is once per day. LEVITRA can be taken with or without food. Sexual stimulation is required for a response to treatment.

Geriatrics: A starting dose of 5 mg LEVITRA should be considered in patients ≥ 65 years of age (see **CLINICAL PHARMACOLOGY, Pharmacokinetics in Special Populations** and **PRECAUTIONS**).

Hepatic Impairment: For patients with mild hepatic impairment (Child-Pugh A), no dose adjustment of LEVITRA is required. Vardenafil clearance is reduced in patients with moderate hepatic impairment (Child-Pugh B), and a starting dose of 5 mg LEVITRA is recommended. The maximum dose in patients with moderate hepatic impairment should not exceed 10 mg. LEVITRA has not been evaluated in patients with severe hepatic impairment (Child-Pugh C) (see **CLINICAL PHARMACOLOGY, Metabolism and Excretion, WARNINGS** and **PRECAUTIONS**).

Renal Impairment: For patients with mild (CL_{cr} = 50-80 ml/min); moderate (CL_{cr} = 30-50 ml/min), or severe (CL_{cr} <30 ml/min) renal impairment, no dose adjustment is required. LEVITRA has not been evaluated in patients on renal dialysis (see **CLINICAL PHARMACOLOGY, Metabolism and Excretion,** and **PRECAUTIONS**).

Concomitant Medications: The dosage of LEVITRA may require adjustment in patients receiving certain CYP3A4 inhibitors (e.g., ketoconazole, itraconazole, ritonavir, indinavir, and erythromycin) (see **WARNINGS, PRECAUTIONS, Drug Interactions**). For ritonavir, a single dose of 2.5 mg LEVITRA should not be exceeded in a 72-hour period. For indinavir, ketoconazole 400 mg daily, and itraconazole 400 mg daily, a single dose of 2.5 mg LEVITRA should not be exceeded in a 24-hour period. For ketoconazole 200 mg daily, itraconazole 200 mg daily, and erythromycin, a single dose of 5 mg LEVITRA should not be exceeded in a 24-hour period.

HOW SUPPLIED

LEVITRA (vardenafil HCl) is formulated as orange, film-coated round tablets with debossed "BAYER" cross on one side and "2.5", "5", "10", and "20" on the other side equivalent to 2.5 mg, 5 mg, 10 mg, and 20 mg of vardenafil, respectively.

Package	Strength	NDC Code
Bottles of 30	2.5 mg	0026-8710-69
	5 mg	0026-8720-69
	10 mg	0026-8730-69
	20 mg	0026-8740-69
Packages of 6	10 mg	0026-8730-05
	20 mg	0026-8740-05

Recommended Storage: Store at 25°C (77°F); excursions permitted to 15-30°C (59-86°F) [see USP Controlled Room Temperature].

Bayer HealthCare
Bayer Pharmaceuticals Corporation
400 Morgan Lane
West Haven, CT 06516
Made in Germany
℞ Only
08669034, R.1 1/04

Patient Information

LEVITRA® (Luh-VEE-Trah)
(vardenafil HCl) Tablets

Read the Patient Information about LEVITRA before you start taking it and again each time you get a refill. There may be new information. You may also find it helpful to share this information with your partner. This leaflet does not take the place of talking with your doctor. You and your doctor should talk about LEVITRA when you start taking it and at regular checkups. If you do not understand the information, or have questions, talk with your doctor or pharmacist.

WHAT IMPORTANT INFORMATION SHOULD YOU KNOW ABOUT LEVITRA?

LEVITRA can cause your blood pressure to drop suddenly to an unsafe level if it is taken with certain other medicines. With a sudden drop in blood pressure, you could get dizzy, faint, or have a heart attack or stroke.

Do not take LEVITRA if you:

- **take any medicines called "nitrates."**
- **use recreational drugs called "poppers" like amyl nitrate and butyl nitrate.**
- **take medicines called alpha-blockers.**

(See "Who Should Not Take LEVITRA?")

Continued on next page

Levitra—Cont.

Tell all your healthcare providers that you take LEVITRA. If you need emergency medical care for a heart problem, it will be important for your healthcare provider to know when you last took LEVITRA.

WHAT IS LEVITRA?

LEVITRA is a prescription medicine taken by mouth for the treatment of erectile dysfunction (ED) in men.

ED is a condition where the penis does not harden and expand when a man is sexually excited, or when he cannot keep an erection. A man who has trouble getting or keeping an erection should see his doctor for help if the condition bothers him. LEVITRA may help a man with ED get and keep an erection when he is sexually excited.

LEVITRA does not:
- cure ED
- increase a man's sexual desire
- protect a man or his partner from sexually transmitted diseases, including HIV. Speak to your doctor about ways to guard against sexually transmitted diseases.
- serve as a male form of birth control

LEVITRA is only for men with ED. LEVITRA is not for women or children. LEVITRA must be used only under a doctor's care.

HOW DOES LEVITRA WORK?

When a man is sexually stimulated, his body's normal physical response is to increase blood flow to his penis. This results in an erection. LEVITRA helps increase blood flow to the penis and may help men with ED get and keep an erection satisfactory for sexual activity. Once a man has completed sexual activity, blood flow to his penis decreases, and his erection goes away.

WHO CAN TAKE LEVITRA?

Talk to your doctor to decide if LEVITRA is right for you. LEVITRA has been shown to be effective in men over the age of 18 years who have erectile dysfunction, including men with diabetes or who have undergone prostatectomy.

WHO SHOULD NOT TAKE LEVITRA?

Do not take LEVITRA if you:
- **take any medicines called "nitrates"** (See "What important information should you know about LEVITRA?"). Nitrates are commonly used to treat angina. Angina is a symptom of heart disease and can cause pain in your chest, jaw, or down your arm.
  Medicines called nitrates include nitroglycerin that is found in tablets, sprays, ointments, pastes, or patches. Nitrates can also be found in other medicines such as isosorbide dinitrate or isosorbide mononitrate. Some recreational drugs called "poppers" also contain nitrates, such as amyl nitrate and butyl nitrate. Do not use LEVITRA if you are using these drugs. Ask your doctor or pharmacist if you are not sure if any of your medicines are nitrates.
- **take medicines called "alpha-blockers."** Alpha-blockers are sometimes prescribed for prostate problems or high blood pressure. If LEVITRA is taken with alpha-blockers, your blood pressure could suddenly drop to an unsafe level. You could get dizzy and faint.
- **you have been told by your healthcare provider to not have sexual activity because of health problems.** Sexual activity can put an extra strain on your heart, especially if your heart is already weak from a heart attack or heart disease.
- **are allergic to LEVITRA or any of its ingredients.** The active ingredient in LEVITRA is called vardenafil. See the end of this leaflet for a complete list of ingredients.

WHAT SHOULD YOU DISCUSS WITH YOUR DOCTOR BEFORE TAKING LEVITRA?

Before taking LEVITRA, tell your doctor about all your medical problems, including if you:
- **have heart problems** such as angina, heart failure, irregular heartbeats, or have had a heart attack. Ask your doctor if it is safe for you to have sexual activity.
- **have low blood pressure** or have high blood pressure that is not controlled
- **have had a stroke**
- **or any family members have a rare heart condition known as prolongation of the QT interval (long QT syndrome)**
- **have liver problems**
- **have kidney problems and require dialysis**
- **have retinitis pigmentosa**, a rare genetic (runs in families) eye disease
- **have stomach ulcers**
- **have a bleeding problem**
- **have a deformed penis shape** or Peyronie's disease
- **have had an erection that lasted more than 4 hours**
- **have blood cell problems** such as sickle cell anemia, multiple myeloma, or leukemia

CAN OTHER MEDICATIONS AFFECT LEVITRA?

Tell your doctor about all the medicines you take including prescription and non-prescription medicines, vitamins, and herbal supplements. LEVITRA and other medicines may affect each other. Always check with your doctor before starting or stopping any medicines. Especially tell your doctor if you take any of the following:
- medicines called nitrates (See "What important information should you know about LEVITRA?")
- medicines called alpha-blockers. These include Hytrin® (terazosin HCl), Flomax® (tamsulosin HCl), Cardura® (doxazosin mesylate), Minipress® (prazosin HCl) or Uroxatral® (alfuzosin HCl).
- medicines that treat abnormal heartbeat. These include quinidine, procainamide, amiodarone and sotalol.
- ritonavir (Norvir®) or indinavir sulfate (Crixivan®)
- ketoconazole or itraconazole (such as Nizoral® or Sporanox®)
- erythromycin
- other medicines or treatments for ED

HOW SHOULD YOU TAKE LEVITRA?

Take LEVITRA exactly as your doctor prescribes. LEVITRA comes in different doses (2.5 mg, 5 mg, 10 mg, and 20 mg). For most men, the recommended starting dose is 10 mg. **Take LEVITRA no more than once a day.** Doses should be taken at least 24 hours apart. Some men can only take a low dose of LEVITRA because of medical conditions or medicines they take. Your doctor will prescribe the dose that is right for you.
- If you are older than 65 or have liver problems, your doctor may start you on a lower dose of LEVITRA.
- If you are taking certain other medicines your doctor may prescribe a lower starting dose and limit you to one dose of LEVITRA in a 72-hour (3 days) period.

Take 1 LEVITRA tablet about 1 hour (60 minutes) before sexual activity. Some form of sexual stimulation is needed for an erection to happen with LEVITRA. LEVITRA may be taken with or without meals.

Do not change your dose of LEVITRA without talking to your doctor. Your doctor may lower your dose or raise your dose, depending on how your body reacts to LEVITRA.

If you take too much LEVITRA, call your doctor or emergency room right away.

WHAT ARE THE POSSIBLE SIDE EFFECTS OF LEVITRA?

The most common side effects with LEVITRA are headache, flushing, stuffy or runny nose, indigestion, upset stomach, or dizziness. These side effects usually go away after a few hours. Call your doctor if you get a side effect that bothers you or one that will not go away.

LEVITRA may uncommonly cause:
- **an erection that won't go away (priapism).** If you get an erection that lasts more than 4 hours, get medical help right away. Priapism must be treated as soon as possible or lasting damage can happen to your penis including the inability to have erections.
- **vision changes,** such as seeing a blue tinge to objects or having difficulty telling the difference between the colors blue and green.

These are not all the side effects of LEVITRA. For more information, ask your doctor or pharmacist.

HOW SHOULD LEVITRA BE STORED?
- Store LEVITRA at room temperature between 59° and 86° F (15° to 30° C).
- **Keep LEVITRA and all medicines out of the reach of children.**

GENERAL INFORMATION ABOUT LEVITRA.

Medicines are sometimes prescribed for conditions other than those described in patient information leaflets. Do not use LEVITRA for a condition for which it was not prescribed. Do not give LEVITRA to other people, even if they have the same symptoms that you have. It may harm them. This leaflet summarizes the most important information about LEVITRA. If you would like more information, talk with your healthcare provider. You can ask your doctor or pharmacist for information about LEVITRA that is written for health professionals.

For more information you can also visit www.LEVITRA.com, or call 1-866-LEVITRA.

WHAT ARE THE INGREDIENTS OF LEVITRA?

Active Ingredient: vardenafil hydrochloride

Inactive Ingredients: microcrystalline cellulose, crospovidone, colloidal silicon dioxide, magnesium stearate, hypromellose, polyethylene glycol, titanium dioxide, yellow ferric oxide, and red ferric oxide.

Norvir (ritonavir) is a trademark of Abbott Laboratories

Crixivan (indinavir sulfate) is a trademark of Merck & Co., Inc.

Nizoral (ketoconazole) is a trademark of Johnson & Johnson

Sporanox (itraconazole) is a trademark of Johnson & Johnson

Hytrin (terazosin HCl) is a trademark of Abbott Laboratories

Flomax (tamsulosin HCl) is a trademark of Yamanouchi Pharmaceutical Co., Ltd.

Cardura (doxazosin mesylate) is a trademark of Pfizer Inc.

Minipress (prazosin HCl) is a trademark of Pfizer Inc.

Uroxatral (alfuzosin HCl) is a trademark of Sanofi-Synthelabo

Bayer HealthCare
Bayer Pharmaceuticals Corporation
400 Morgan Lane
West Haven, CT 06516
Made in Germany

℞ Only

08669034IP, R.1 1/04

To keep your **PDR** up to date throughout the year, note these revisions on the corresponding pages of the annual volume. Simply write **"See Supplement A"** next to the product heading.

Boehringer Ingelheim Pharmaceuticals, Inc.

A subsidiary of Boehringer Ingelheim Corporation
900 RIDGEBURY ROAD
POST OFFICE BOX 368
RIDGEFIELD, CT 06877-0368

For Medical Information Contact:
1–800–542–6257
or email:
druginfo@rdg.boehringer-ingelheim.com

MIRAPEX® ℞
[*mĭ-ră-pĕks*]
(pramipexole dihydrochloride)
0.125 mg, 0.25 mg, 0.5 mg, 1 mg, and 1.5 mg Tablets

DESCRIPTION

MIRAPEX® (pramipexole dihydrochloride) Tablets contain pramipexole, a dopamine agonist indicated for the treatment of the signs and symptoms of idiopathic Parkinson's disease. The chemical name of pramipexole dihydrochloride is (S)-2-amino-4,5,6,7-tetrahydro-6-(propylamino)benzothiazole dihydrochloride monohydrate. Its empirical formula is $C_{10}H_{17}N_3S \bullet 2\ HCl \bullet H_2O$, and its molecular weight is 302.27. The structural formula is:

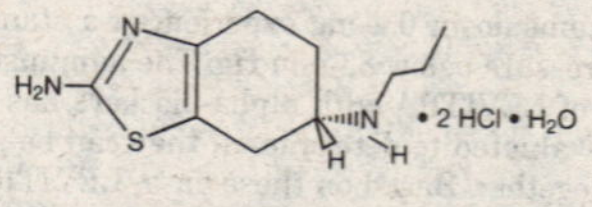

Pramipexole dihydrochloride is a white to off-white powder substance. Melting occurs in the range of 296°C to 301°C, with decomposition. Pramipexole dihydrochloride is more than 20% soluble in water, about 8% in methanol, about 0.5% in ethanol, and practically insoluble in dichloromethane.

MIRAPEX (pramipexole dihydrochloride) Tablets, for oral administration, contain 0.125 mg, 0.25 mg, 0.5 mg, 1.0 mg, or 1.5 mg of pramipexole dihydrochloride monohydrate. Inactive ingredients consist of mannitol, corn starch, colloidal silicon dioxide, povidone, and magnesium stearate.

CLINICAL PHARMACOLOGY

Pramipexole is a nonergot dopamine agonist with high relative in vitro specificity and full intrinsic activity at the D_2 subfamily of dopamine receptors, binding with higher affinity to D_3 than to D_2 or D_4 receptor subtypes. The relevance of D_3 receptor binding in Parkinson's disease is unknown.

The precise mechanism of action of pramipexole as a treatment for Parkinson's disease is unknown, although it is believed to be related to its ability to stimulate dopamine receptors in the striatum. This conclusion is supported by electrophysiologic studies in animals that have demonstrated that pramipexole influences striatal neuronal firing rates via activation of dopamine receptors in the striatum and the substantia nigra, the site of neurons that send projections to the striatum.

Pharmacokinetics

Pramipexole is rapidly absorbed, reaching peak concentrations in approximately 2 hours. The absolute bioavailability of pramipexole is greater than 90%, indicating that it is well absorbed and undergoes little presystemic metabolism. Food does not affect the extent of pramipexole absorption, although the time of maximum plasma concentration (T_{max}) is increased by about 1 hour when the drug is taken with a meal.

Pramipexole is extensively distributed, having a volume of distribution of about 500 L (coefficient of variation [CV]=20%). It is about 15% bound to plasma proteins. Pramipexole distributes into red blood cells as indicated by an erythrocyte-to-plasma ratio of approximately 2.

Pramipexole displays linear pharmacokinetics over the clinical dosage range. Its terminal half-life is about 8 hours in young healthy volunteers and about 12 hours in elderly volunteers (see CLINICAL PHARMACOLOGY, Pharmacokinetics in Special Populations). Steady-state concentrations are achieved within 2 days of dosing.

Metabolism and elimination: Urinary excretion is the major route of pramipexole elimination, with 90% of a pramipexole dose recovered in urine, almost all as unchanged drug. Nonrenal routes may contribute to a small extent to pramipexole elimination, although no metabolites have been identified in plasma or urine. The renal clearance of pramipexole is approximately 400 mL/min (CV=25%), approximately three times higher than the glomerular filtration rate. Thus, pramipexole is secreted by the renal tubules, probably by the organic cation transport system.

Pharmacokinetics in Special Populations

Because therapy with pramipexole is initiated at a subtherapeutic dosage and gradually titrated upward according to clinical tolerability to obtain the optimum therapeutic effect, adjustment of the initial dose based on gender, weight, or age is not necessary. However, renal insufficiency, which can cause a large decrease in the ability to eliminate pramipexole, may necessitate dosage adjustment (see CLINICAL PHARMACOLOGY, Renal Insufficiency).

Gender: Pramipexole clearance is about 30% lower in women than in men, but most of this difference can be accounted for by differences in body weight. There is no difference in half-life between males and females.

Age: Pramipexole clearance decreases with age as the half-life and clearance are about 40% longer and 30% lower, respectively, in elderly (aged 65 years or older) compared with young healthy volunteers (aged less than 40 years). This difference is most likely due to the well-known reduction in renal function with age, since pramipexole clearance is correlated with renal function, as measured by creatinine clearance (see CLINICAL PHARMACOLOGY, Renal Insufficiency).

Parkinson's disease patients: A cross-study comparison of data suggests that the clearance of pramipexole may be reduced by about 30% in Parkinson's disease patients compared with healthy elderly volunteers. The reason for this difference appears to be reduced renal function in Parkinson's disease patients, which may be related to their poorer general health. The pharmacokinetics of pramipexole were comparable between early and advanced Parkinson's disease patients.

Pediatric: The pharmacokinetics of pramipexole in the pediatric population have not been evaluated.

Hepatic insufficiency: The influence of hepatic insufficiency on pramipexole pharmacokinetics has not been evaluated. Because approximately 90% of the recovered dose is excreted in the urine as unchanged drug, hepatic impairment would not be expected to have a significant effect on pramipexole elimination.

Renal insufficiency: The clearance of pramipexole was about 75% lower in patients with severe renal impairment (creatinine clearance approximately 20 mL/min) and about 60% lower in patients with moderate impairment (creatinine clearance approximately 40 mL/min) compared with healthy volunteers. A lower starting and maintenance dose is recommended in these patients (see PRECAUTIONS and DOSAGE AND ADMINISTRATION). In patients with varying degrees of renal impairment, pramipexole clearance correlates well with creatinine clearance. Therefore, creatinine clearance can be used as a predictor of the extent of decrease in pramipexole clearance. Pramipexole clearance is extremely low in dialysis patients, as a negligible amount of pramipexole is removed by dialysis. Caution should be exercised when administering pramipexole to patients with renal disease.

CLINICAL STUDIES

The effectiveness of MIRAPEX (pramipexole dihydrochloride) Tablets in the treatment of Parkinson's disease was evaluated in a multinational drug development program consisting of seven randomized, controlled trials. Three were conducted in patients with early Parkinson's disease who were not receiving concomitant levodopa, and four were conducted in patients with advanced Parkinson's disease who were receiving concomitant levodopa. Among these seven studies, three studies provide the most persuasive evidence of pramipexole's effectiveness in the management of patients with Parkinson's disease who were and were not receiving concomitant levodopa. Two of these three trials enrolled patients with early Parkinson's disease (not receiving levodopa), and one enrolled patients with advanced Parkinson's disease who were receiving maximally tolerated doses of levodopa. In all studies, the Unified Parkinson's Disease Rating Scale (UPDRS), or one or more of its subparts, served as the primary outcome assessment measure. The UPDRS is a four-part multi-item rating scale intended to evaluate mentation (part I), activities of daily living (part II), motor performance (part III), and complications of therapy (part IV).

Part II of the UPDRS contains 13 questions relating to activities of daily living (ADL), which are scored from 0 (normal) to 4 (maximal severity) for a maximum (worst) score of 52. Part III of the UPDRS contains 27 questions (for 14 items) and is scored as described for part II. It is designed to assess the severity of the cardinal motor findings in patients with Parkinson's disease (eg, tremor, rigidity, bradykinesia, postural instability, etc), scored for different body regions, and has a maximum (worst) score of 108.

Studies In Patients With Early Parkinson's Disease

Patients (N=599) in the two studies of early Parkinson's disease had a mean disease duration of 2 years, limited or no prior exposure to levodopa (generally none in the preceding 6 months), and were not experiencing the "on-off" phenomenon and dyskinesia characteristic of later stages of the disease.

One of the two early Parkinson's disease studies (N=335) was a double-blind, placebo-controlled, parallel trial consisting of a 7-week dose-escalation period and a 6-month maintenance period. Patients could be on selegiline, anticholinergics, or both, but could not be on levodopa products or amantadine. Patients were randomized to MIRAPEX (pramipexole dihydrochloride) or placebo. Patients treated with MIRAPEX (pramipexole dihydrochloride) had a starting daily dose of 0.375 mg and were titrated to a maximally tolerated dose, but no higher than 4.5 mg/day in three divided doses. At the end of the 6-month maintenance period, the mean improvement from baseline on the UPDRS part II (ADL) total score was 1.9 in the group receiving MIRAPEX (pramipexole dihydrochloride) and –0.4 in the placebo group, a difference that was statistically significant. The mean improvement from baseline on the UPDRS part III total score was 5.0 in the group receiving MIRAPEX (pramipexole dihydrochloride) and –0.8 in the placebo group, a difference that was also statistically significant. A statistically significant difference between groups in favor of MIRAPEX (pramipexole dihydrochloride) was seen beginning at week 2 of the UPDRS part II (maximum dose 0.75 mg/day) and at week 3 of the UPDRS part III (maximum dose 1.5 mg/day).

The second early Parkinson's disease study (N=264) was a double-blind, placebo-controlled, parallel trial consisting of a 6-week dose-escalation period and a 4-week maintenance period. Patients could be on selegiline, anticholinergics, amantadine, or any combination of these, but could not be on levodopa products. Patients were randomized to 1 of 4 fixed doses of MIRAPEX (pramipexole dihydrochloride) (1.5 mg, 3.0 mg, 4.5 mg, or 6.0 mg per day) or placebo. At the end of the 4-week maintenance period, the mean improvement from baseline on the UPDRS part II total score was 1.8 in the patients treated with MIRAPEX (pramipexole dihydrochloride), regardless of assigned dose group, and 0.3 in placebo-treated patients. The mean improvement from baseline on the UPDRS part III total score was 4.2 in patients treated with MIRAPEX (pramipexole dihydrochloride) and 0.6 in placebo-treated patients. No dose-response relationship was demonstrated. The between-treatment differences on both parts of the UPDRS were statistically significant in favor of MIRAPEX (pramipexole dihydrochloride) for all doses.

No differences in effectiveness based on age or gender were detected. There were too few non-Caucasian patients to evaluate the effect of race. Patients receiving selegiline or anticholinergics had responses similar to patients not receiving these drugs.

Studies In Patients With Advanced Parkinson's Disease

In the advanced Parkinson's disease study, the primary assessments were the UPDRS and daily diaries that quantified amounts of "on" and "off" time.

Patients in the advanced Parkinson's disease study (N=360) had a mean disease duration of 9 years, had been exposed to levodopa for long periods of time (mean 8 years), used concomitant levodopa during the trial, and had "on-off" periods.

The advanced Parkinson's disease study was a double-blind, placebo-controlled, parallel trial consisting of a 7-week dose-escalation period and a 6-month maintenance period. Patients were all treated with concomitant levodopa products and could additionally be on concomitant selegiline, anticholinergics, amantadine, or any combination. Patients treated with MIRAPEX (pramipexole dihydrochloride) had a starting dose of 0.375 mg/day and were titrated to a maximally tolerated dose, but no higher than 4.5 mg/day in three divided doses. At selected times during the 6-month maintenance period, patients were asked to record the amount of "off," "on," or "on with dyskinesia" time per day for several sequential days. At the end of the 6-month maintenance period, the mean improvement from baseline on the UPDRS part II total score was 2.7 in the group treated with MIRAPEX (pramipexole dihydrochloride) and 0.5 in the placebo group, a difference that was statistically significant. The mean improvement from baseline on the UPDRS part III total score was 5.6 in the group treated with MIRAPEX (pramipexole dihydrochloride) and 2.8 in the placebo group, a difference that was statistically significant. A statistically significant difference between groups in favor of MIRAPEX (pramipexole dihydrochloride) was seen at week 3 of the UPDRS part II (maximum dose 1.5 mg/day) and at week 2 of the UPDRS part III (maximum dose 0.75 mg/day). Dosage reduction of levodopa was allowed during this study if dyskinesia (or hallucinations) developed; levodopa dosage reduction occurred in 76% of patients treated with MIRAPEX (pramipexole dihydrochloride) versus 54% of placebo patients. On average, the levodopa dose was reduced 27%.

The mean number of "off" hours per day during baseline was 6 hours for both treatment groups. Throughout the trial, patients treated with MIRAPEX (pramipexole dihydrochloride) had a mean of 4 "off" hours per day, while placebo-treated patients continued to experience 6 "off" hours per day.

No differences in effectiveness based on age or gender were detected. There were too few non-Caucasian patients to evaluate the effect of race.

INDICATIONS AND USAGE

MIRAPEX (pramipexole dihydrochloride) Tablets are indicated for the treatment of the signs and symptoms of idiopathic Parkinson's disease.

The effectiveness of MIRAPEX (pramipexole dihydrochloride) was demonstrated in randomized, controlled trials in patients with early Parkinson's disease who were not receiving concomitant levodopa therapy as well as in patients with advanced disease on concomitant levodopa (see CLINICAL STUDIES).

CONTRAINDICATIONS

MIRAPEX (pramipexole dihydrochloride) Tablets are contraindicated in patients who have demonstrated hypersensitivity to the drug or its ingredients.

WARNINGS

Falling Asleep During Activities of Daily Living:

Patients treated with MIRAPEX (pramipexole dihydrochloride) have reported falling asleep while engaged in activities of daily living, including the operation of motor vehicles which sometimes resulted in accidents. Although many of these patients reported somnolence while on MIRAPEX (pramipexole dihydrochloride), some perceived that they had no warning signs such as excessive drowsiness, and believed that they were alert immediately prior to the event. Some of these events have been reported as late as one year after the initiation of treatment.

Somnolence is a common occurrence in patients receiving MIRAPEX (pramipexole dihydrochloride) at doses above 1.5 mg/day. Many clinical experts believe that falling asleep while engaged in activities of daily living always occurs in a setting of pre-existing somnolence, although patients may not give such a history. For this reason, prescribers should continually reassess patients for drowsiness or sleepiness, especially since some of the events occur well after the start of treatment. Prescribers should also be aware that patients may not acknowledge drowsiness or sleepiness until directly questioned about drowsiness or sleepiness during specific activities.

Before initiating treatment with MIRAPEX (pramipexole dihydrochloride), patients should be advised of the potential to develop drowsiness and specifically asked about factors that may increase the risk with MIRAPEX (pramipexole dihydrochloride) such as concomitant sedating medications, the presence of sleep disorders, and concomitant medications that increase pramipexole plasma levels (e.g., cimetidine — see PRECAUTIONS, Drug Interactions). If a patient develops significant daytime sleepiness or episodes of falling asleep during activities that require active participation (e.g., conversations, eating, etc.), MIRAPEX (pramipexole dihydrochloride) should ordinarily be discontinued. If a decision is made to continue MIRAPEX (pramipexole dihydrochloride), patients should be advised to not drive and to avoid other potentially dangerous activities. While dose reduction clearly reduces the degree of somnolence, there is insufficient information to establish that dose reduction will eliminate episodes of falling asleep while engaged in activities of daily living.

Symptomatic Hypotension: Dopamine agonists, in clinical studies and clinical experience, appear to impair the systemic regulation of blood pressure, with resulting orthostatic hypotension, especially during dose escalation. Parkinson's disease patients, in addition, appear to have an impaired capacity to respond to an orthostatic challenge. For these reasons, Parkinson's disease patients being treated with dopaminergic agonists ordinarily require careful monitoring for signs and symptoms of orthostatic hypotension, especially during dose escalation, and should be informed of this risk (see PRECAUTIONS, Information for Patients).

In clinical trials of pramipexole, however, and despite clear orthostatic effects in normal volunteers, the reported incidence of clinically significant orthostatic hypotension was not greater among those assigned to MIRAPEX (pramipexole dihydrochloride) Tablets than among those assigned to placebo. This result is clearly unexpected in light of the previous experience with the risks of dopamine agonist therapy.

While this finding could reflect a unique property of pramipexole, it might also be explained by the conditions of the study and the nature of the population enrolled in the clinical trials. Patients were very carefully titrated, and patients with active cardiovascular disease or significant orthostatic hypotension at baseline were excluded.

Hallucinations: In the three double-blind, placebo-controlled trials in early Parkinson's disease, hallucinations were observed in 9% (35 of 388) of patients receiving MIRAPEX (pramipexole dihydrochloride), compared with 2.6% (6 of 235) of patients receiving placebo. In the four double-blind, placebo-controlled trials in advanced Parkinson's disease, where patients received MIRAPEX (pramipexole dihydrochloride) and concomitant levodopa, hallucinations were observed in 16.5% (43 of 260) of patients receiving MIRAPEX (pramipexole dihydrochloride) compared with 3.8% (10 of 264) of patients receiving placebo. Hallucinations were of sufficient severity to cause discontinuation of treatment in 3.1% of the early Parkinson's disease patients and 2.7% of the advanced Parkinson's disease patients compared with about 0.4% of placebo patients in both populations.

Age appears to increase the risk of hallucinations attributable to pramipexole. In the early Parkinson's disease patients, the risk of hallucinations was 1.9 times greater than placebo in patients younger than 65 years and 6.8 times greater than placebo in patients older than 65 years. In the advanced Parkinson's disease patients, the risk of hallucinations was 3.5 times greater than placebo in patients younger than 65 years and 5.2 times greater than placebo in patients older than 65 years.

PRECAUTIONS

Rhabdomyolysis: A single case of rhabdomyolysis occurred in a 49-year-old male with advanced Parkinson's disease treated with MIRAPEX (pramipexole dihydrochloride) Tablets. The patient was hospitalized with an elevated CPK (10,631 IU/L). The symptoms resolved with discontinuation of the medication.

Renal: Since pramipexole is eliminated through the kidneys, caution should be exercised when prescribing MIRAPEX (pramipexole dihydrochloride) to patients with renal insufficiency (see DOSAGE AND ADMINISTRATION).

Dyskinesia: MIRAPEX (pramipexole dihydrochloride) may potentiate the dopaminergic side effects of levodopa and may cause or exacerbate preexisting dyskinesia. Decreasing the dose of levodopa may ameliorate this side effect.

Retinal pathology in albino rats: Pathologic changes (degeneration and loss of photoreceptor cells) were observed in the retina of albino rats in the 2-year carcinogenicity study. While retinal degeneration was not diagnosed in pigmented

Continued on next page

Mirapex—Cont.

rats treated for 2 years, a thinning in the outer nuclear layer of the retina was slightly greater in rats given drug compared with controls. Evaluation of the retinas of albino mice, monkeys, and minipigs did not reveal similar changes. The potential significance of this effect in humans has not been established, but cannot be disregarded because disruption of a mechanism that is universally present in vertebrates (ie, disk shedding) may be involved (see ANIMAL TOXICOLOGY).

Events Reported With Dopaminergic Therapy

Although the events enumerated below have not been reported in association with the use of pramipexole in its development program, they are associated with the use of other dopaminergic drugs. The expected incidence of these events, however, is so low that even if pramipexole caused these events at rates similar to those attributable to other dopaminergic therapies, it would be unlikely that even a single case would have occurred in a cohort of the size exposed to pramipexole in studies to date.

Withdrawal-emergent hyperpyrexia and confusion: Although not reported with pramipexole in the clinical development program, a symptom complex resembling the neuroleptic malignant syndrome (characterized by elevated temperature, muscular rigidity, altered consciousness, and autonomic instability), with no other obvious etiology, has been reported in association with rapid dose reduction, withdrawal of, or changes in antiparkinsonian therapy.

Fibrotic complications: Although not reported with pramipexole in the clinical development program, cases of retroperitoneal fibrosis, pulmonary infiltrates, pleural effusion, and pleural thickening have been reported in some patients treated with ergot-derived dopaminergic agents. While these complications may resolve when the drug is discontinued, complete resolution does not always occur.

Although these adverse events are believed to be related to the ergoline structure of these compounds, whether other, nonergot derived dopamine agonists can cause them is unknown.

Information for Patients: Patients should be instructed to take MIRAPEX (pramipexole dihydrochloride) only as prescribed.

Patients should be alerted to the potential sedating effects associated with MIRAPEX (pramipexole dihydrochloride), including somnolence and the possibility of falling asleep while engaged in activities of daily living. Since somnolence is a frequent adverse event with potentially serious consequences, patients should neither drive a car nor engage in other potentially dangerous activities until they have gained sufficient experience with MIRAPEX (pramipexole dihydrochloride) to gauge whether or not it affects their mental and/or motor performance adversely. Patients should be advised that if increased somnolence or new episodes of falling asleep during activities of daily living (e.g., watching television, passenger in a car, etc.) are experienced at any time during treatment, they should not drive or participate in potentially dangerous activities until they have contacted their physician. Because of possible additive effects, caution should be advised when patients are taking other sedating medications or alcohol in combination with MIRAPEX (pramipexole dihydrochloride) and when taking concomitant medications that increase plasma levels of pramipexole (e.g., cimetidine).

Patients should be informed that hallucinations can occur and that the elderly are at a higher risk than younger patients with Parkinson's disease.

Patients may develop postural (orthostatic) hypotension, with or without symptoms such as dizziness, nausea, fainting or blackouts, and sometimes, sweating. Hypotension may occur more frequently during initial therapy. Accordingly, patients should be cautioned against rising rapidly after sitting or lying down, especially if they have been doing so for prolonged periods and especially at the initiation of treatment with MIRAPEX (pramipexole dihydrochloride).

Because the teratogenic potential of pramipexole has not been completely established in laboratory animals, and because experience in humans is limited, patients should be advised to notify their physicians if they become pregnant or intend to become pregnant during therapy (see PRECAUTIONS, Pregnancy).

Because of the possibility that pramipexole may be excreted in breast milk, patients should be advised to notify their physicians if they intend to breast-feed or are breast-feeding an infant.

If patients develop nausea, they should be advised that taking MIRAPEX (pramipexole dihydrochloride) with food may reduce the occurrence of nausea.

Laboratory Tests: During the development of MIRAPEX (pramipexole dihydrochloride), no systematic abnormalities on routine laboratory testing were noted. Therefore, no specific guidance is offered regarding routine monitoring; the practitioner retains responsibility for determining how best to monitor the patient in his or her care.

Drug Interactions

Carbidopa/levodopa: Carbidopa/levodopa did not influence the pharmacokinetics of pramipexole in healthy volunteers (N=10). Pramipexole did not alter the extent of absorption (AUC) or the elimination of carbidopa/levodopa, although it caused an increase in levodopa C_{max} by about 40% and a decrease in T_{max} from 2.5 to 0.5 hours.

Selegiline: In healthy volunteers (N=11), selegiline did not influence the pharmacokinetics of pramipexole.

Amantadine: Population pharmacokinetic analysis suggests that amantadine is unlikely to alter the oral clearance of pramipexole (N=54).

Cimetidine: Cimetidine, a known inhibitor of renal tubular secretion of organic bases via the cationic transport system, caused a 50% increase in pramipexole AUC and a 40% increase in half-life (N=12).

Probenecid: Probenecid, a known inhibitor of renal tubular secretion of organic acids via the anionic transporter, did not noticeably influence pramipexole pharmacokinetics (N=12).

Other drugs eliminated via renal secretion: Population pharmacokinetic analysis suggests that coadministration of drugs that are secreted by the cationic transport system (eg, cimetidine, ranitidine, diltiazem, triamterene, verapamil, quinidine, and quinine) decreases the oral clearance of pramipexole by about 20%, while those secreted by the anionic transport system (eg, cephalosporins, penicillins, indomethacin, hydrochlorothiazide, and chlorpropamide) are likely to have little effect on the oral clearance of pramipexole.

CYP interactions: Inhibitors of cytochrome P450 enzymes would not be expected to affect pramipexole elimination because pramipexole is not appreciably metabolized by these enzymes in vivo or in vitro. Pramipexole does not inhibit CYP enzymes CYP1A2, CYP2C9, CYP2C19, CYP2E1, and CYP3A4. Inhibition of CYP2D6 was observed with an apparent Ki of 30 µM, indicating that pramipexole will not inhibit CYP enzymes at plasma concentrations observed following the highest recommended clinical dose (1.5 mg tid).

Dopamine antagonists: Since pramipexole is a dopamine agonist, it is possible that dopamine antagonists, such as the neuroleptics (phenothiazines, butyrophenones, thioxanthenes) or metoclo- pramide, may diminish the effectiveness of MIRAPEX (pramipexole dihydrochloride).

Drug/Laboratory Test Interactions: There are no known interactions between MIRAPEX (pramipexole dihydrochloride) and laboratory tests.

Carcinogenesis, Mutagenesis, Impairment of Fertility: Two-year carcinogenicity studies with pramipexole have been conducted in mice and rats. Pramipexole was administered in the diet to Chbb:NMRI mice at doses of 0.3, 2, and 10 mg/kg/day (0.3, 2.2, and 11 times the highest recommended clinical dose [1.5 mg tid] on a mg/m^2 basis). Pramipexole was administered in the diet to Wistar rats at 0.3, 2, and 8 mg/kg/day (plasma AUCs equal to 0.3, 2.5, and 12.5 times the AUC in humans receiving 1.5 mg tid). No significant increases in tumors occurred in either species.

Pramipexole was not mutagenic or clastogenic in a battery of assays, including the in vitro Ames assay, V79 gene mutation assay for HGPRT mutants, chromosomal aberration assay in Chinese hamster ovary cells, and in vivo mouse micronucleus assay.

In rat fertility studies, pramipexole at a dose of 2.5 mg/kg/day (5.4 times the highest clinical dose on a mg/m^2 basis), prolonged estrus cycles and inhibited implantation. These effects were associated with reductions in serum levels of prolactin, a hormone necessary for implantation and maintenance of early pregnancy in rats.

Pregnancy: Pregnancy Category C. When pramipexole was given to female rats throughout pregnancy, implantation was inhibited at a dose of 2.5 mg/kg/day (5.4 times the highest clinical dose on a mg/m^2 basis). Administration of 1.5 mg/kg/day of pramipexole to pregnant rats during the period of organogenesis (gestation days 7 through 16) resulted in a high incidence of total resorption of embryos. The plasma AUC in rats dosed at this level was 4.3 times the AUC in humans receiving 1.5 mg tid. These findings are thought to be due to the prolactin-lowering effect of pramipexole, since prolactin is necessary for implantation and maintenance of early pregnancy in rats (but not rabbits or humans). Because of pregnancy disruption and early embryonic loss in these studies, the teratogenic potential of pramipexole could not be adequately evaluated. There was no evidence of adverse effects on embryo-fetal development following administration of up to 10 mg/kg/day to pregnant rabbits during organogenesis (plasma AUC was 71 times that in humans receiving 1.5 mg tid). Postnatal growth was inhibited in the offspring of rats treated with 0.5 mg/kg/day (approximately equivalent to the highest clinical dose on a mg/m^2 basis) or greater during the latter part of pregnancy and throughout lactation.

There are no studies of pramipexole in human pregnancy. Because animal reproduction studies are not always predictive of human response, pramipexole should be used during pregnancy only if the potential benefit outweighs the potential risk to the fetus.

Nursing Mothers: A single-dose, radio-labeled study showed that drug-related materials were excreted into the breast milk of lactating rats. Concentrations of radioactivity in milk were three to six times higher than concentrations in plasma at equivalent time points.

Other studies have shown that pramipexole treatment resulted in an inhibition of prolactin secretion in humans and rats.

It is not known whether this drug is excreted in human milk. Because many drugs are excreted in human milk and because of the potential for serious adverse reactions in nursing infants from pramipexole, a decision should be made as to whether to discontinue nursing or to discontinue the drug, taking into account the importance of the drug to the mother.

Pediatric Use: The safety and efficacy of MIRAPEX® (pramipexole dihydrochloride) in pediatric patients has not been established.

Geriatric Use: Pramipexole total oral clearance was approximately 30% lower in subjects older than 65 years compared with younger subjects, because of a decline in pramipexole renal clearance due to an age-related reduction in renal function. This resulted in an increase in elimination half-life from approximately 8.5 hours to 12 hours. In clinical studies, 38.7% of patients were older than 65 years. There were no apparent differences in efficacy or safety between older and younger patients, except that the relative risk of hallucination associated with the use of MIRAPEX (pramipexole dihydrochloride) was increased in the elderly.

ADVERSE EVENTS

During the premarketing development of pramipexole, patients with either early or advanced Parkinson's disease were enrolled in clinical trials. Apart from the severity and duration of their disease, the two populations differed in their use of concomitant levodopa therapy. Patients with early disease did not receive concomitant levodopa therapy during treatment with pramipexole; those with advanced Parkinson's disease all received concomitant levodopa treatment. Because these two populations may have differential risks for various adverse events, this section will, in general, present adverse-event data for these two populations separately.

Because the controlled trials performed during premarketing development all used a titration design, with a resultant confounding of time and dose, it was impossible to adequately evaluate the effects of dose on the incidence of adverse events.

Early Parkinson's Disease

In the three double-blind, placebo-controlled trials of patients with early Parkinson's disease, the most commonly observed adverse events (>5%) that were numerically more frequent in the group treated with MIRAPEX (pramipexole dihydrochloride) Tablets were nausea, dizziness, somnolence, insomnia, constipation, asthenia, and hallucinations.

Approximately 12% of 388 patients with early Parkinson's disease and treated with MIRAPEX (pramipexole dihydrochloride) who participated in the double-blind, placebo-controlled trials discontinued treatment due to adverse events compared with 11% of 235 patients who received placebo. The adverse events most commonly causing discontinuation of treatment were related to the nervous system (hallucinations [3.1% on MIRAPEX (pramipexole dihydrochloride) vs 0.4% on placebo]; dizziness [2.1% on MIRAPEX (pramipexole dihydrochloride) vs 1% on placebo]; somnolence [1.6% on MIRAPEX (pramipexole dihydrochloride) vs 0% on placebo]; extrapyramidal syndrome [1.6% on MIRAPEX (pramipexole dihydrochloride) vs 6.4% on placebo]; headache and confusion [1.3% and 1.0%, respectively, on MIRAPEX (pramipexole dihydrochloride) vs 0% on placebo]); and gastrointestinal system (nausea [2.1% on MIRAPEX (pramipexole dihydrochloride) vs 0.4% on placebo]).

Adverse-event incidence in controlled clinical studies in early Parkinson's disease: Table 1 lists treatment-emergent adverse events that occurred in the double-blind, placebo-controlled studies in early Parkinson's disease that were reported by ≥1% of patients treated with MIRAPEX (pramipexole dihydrochloride) and were numerically more frequent than in the placebo group. In these studies, patients did not receive concomitant levodopa. Adverse events were usually mild or moderate in intensity.

The prescriber should be aware that these figures cannot be used to predict the incidence of adverse events in the course of usual medical practice where patient characteristics and other factors differ from those that prevailed in the clinical studies. Similarly, the cited frequencies cannot be compared with figures obtained from other clinical investigations involving different treatments, uses, and investigators. However, the cited figures do provide the prescribing physician with some basis for estimating the relative contribution of drug and nondrug factors to the adverse-event incidence rate in the population studied.

Table 1: Treatment-Emergent Adverse-Event* Incidence in Double-Blind, Placebo-Controlled Trials in Early Parkinson's Disease (Events ≥ 1% of Patients Treated With MIRAPEX (pramipexole dihydrochloride) and Numerically More Frequent Than in the Placebo Group)

Body System/ Adverse Event	MIRAPEX (pramipexole (dihydrochloride) N=388	Placebo N=235
Body as a Whole		
Asthenia	14	12
General edema	5	3
Malaise	2	1
Reaction unevaluable	2	1
Fever	1	0
Digestive System		
Nausea	28	18
Constipation	14	6

Anorexia	4	2
Dysphagia	2	0
Metabolic & Nutritional System		
Peripheral edema	5	4
Decreased weight	2	0
Nervous System		
Dizziness	25	24
Somnolence	22	9
Insomnia	17	12
Hallucinations	9	3
Confusion	4	1
Amnesia	4	2
Hypesthesia	3	1
Dystonia	2	1
Akathisia	2	0
Thinking abnormalities	2	0
Decreased libido	1	0
Myoclonus	1	0
Special Senses		
Vision abnormalities	3	0
Urogenital System		
Impotence	2	1

* Patients may have reported multiple adverse experiences during the study or at discontinuation; thus, patients may be included in more than one category.

Other events reported by 1% or more of patients with early Parkinson's disease and treated with MIRAPEX (pramipexole dihydrochloride) but reported equally or more frequently in the placebo group were infection, accidental injury, headache, pain, tremor, back pain, syncope, postural hypotension, hypertonia, depression, abdominal pain, anxiety, dyspepsia, flatulence, diarrhea, rash, ataxia, dry mouth, extrapyramidal syndrome, leg cramps, twitching, pharyngitis, sinusitis, sweating, rhinitis, urinary tract infection, vasodilation, flu syndrome, increased saliva, tooth disease, dyspnea, increased cough, gait abnormalities, urinary frequency, vomiting, allergic reaction, hypertension, pruritis, hypokinesia, increased creatine PK, nervousness, dream abnormalities, chest pain, neck pain, paresthesia, tachycardia, vertigo, voice alteration, conjunctivitis, paralysis, accommodation abnormalities, tinnitus, diplopia, and taste perversions.

In a fixed-dose study in early Parkinson's disease, occurrence of the following events increased in frequency as the dose increased over the range from 1.5 mg/day to 6 mg/day: postural hypotension, nausea, constipation, somnolence, and amnesia. The frequency of these events was generally 2-fold greater than placebo for pramipexole doses greater than 3 mg/day. The incidence of somnolence with pramipexole at a dose of 1.5 mg/day was comparable to that reported for placebo.

Advanced Parkinson's Disease

In the four double-blind, placebo-controlled trials of patients with advanced Parkinson's disease, the most commonly observed adverse events (>5%) that were numerically more frequent in the group treated with MIRAPEX (pramipexole dihydrochloride) and concomitant levodopa were postural (orthostatic) hypotension, dyskinesia, extrapyramidal syndrome, insomnia, dizziness, hallucinations, accidental injury, dream abnormalities, confusion, constipation, asthenia, somnolence, dystonia, gait abnormality, hypertonia, dry mouth, amnesia, and urinary frequency.

Approximately 12% of 260 patients with advanced Parkinson's disease who received MIRAPEX (pramipexole dihydrochloride) and concomitant levodopa in the double-blind, placebo-controlled trials discontinued treatment due to adverse events compared with 16% of 264 patients who received placebo and concomitant levodopa. The events most commonly causing discontinuation of treatment were related to the nervous system (hallucinations [2.7% on MIRAPEX (pramipexole dihydrochloride) vs 0.4% on placebo]; dyskinesia [1.9% on MIRAPEX (pramipexole dihydrochloride) vs 0.8% on placebo]; extrapyramidal syndrome [1.5% on MIRAPEX (pramipexole dihydrochloride) vs 4.9% on placebo]; dizziness [1.2% on MIRAPEX (pramipexole dihydrochloride) vs 1.5% on placebo]; confusion [1.2% on MIRAPEX (pramipexole dihydrochloride) vs 2.3% on placebo]); and cardiovascular system (postural [orthostatic] hypotension [2.3% on MIRAPEX (pramipexole dihydrochloride) vs 1.1% on placebo]).

Adverse-event incidence in controlled clinical studies in advanced Parkinson's disease: Table 2 lists treatment-emergent adverse events that occurred in the double-blind, placebo-controlled studies in advanced Parkinson's disease that were reported by ≥1% of patients treated with MIRAPEX (pramipexole dihydrochloride) and were numerically more frequent than in the placebo group. In these studies, MIRAPEX (pramipexole dihydrochloride) or placebo was administered to patients who were also receiving concomitant levodopa. Adverse events were usually mild or moderate in intensity.

The prescriber should be aware that these figures cannot be used to predict the incidence of adverse events in the course of usual medical practice where patient characteristics and other factors differ from those that prevailed in the clinical studies. Similarly, the cited frequencies cannot be compared with figures obtained from other clinical investigations involving different treatments, uses, and investigators. However, the cited figures do provide the prescribing physician with some basis for estimating the relative contribution of drug and nondrug factors to the adverse-events incidence rate in the population studied.

Table 2: Treatment-Emergent Adverse-Event* Incidence in Double-Blind, Placebo-Controlled Trials in Advanced Parkinson's Disease (Events ≥ 1% of Patients Treated With MIRAPEX (pramipexole dihydrochloride) and Numerically More Frequent Than in the Placebo Group)

Body System/ Adverse Event	MIRAPEX† (pramipexole (dihydrochloride) N=260	Placebo† N=264
Body as a Whole		
Accidental injury	17	15
Asthenia	10	8
General edema	4	3
Chest pain	3	2
Malaise	3	2
Cardiovascular System		
Postural hypotension	53	48
Digestive System		
Constipation	10	9
Dry mouth	7	3
Metabolic & Nutritional System		
Peripheral edema	2	1
Increased creatine PK	1	0
Musculoskeletal System		
Arthritis	3	1
Twitching	2	0
Bursitis	2	0
Myasthenia	1	0
Nervous System		
Dyskinesia	47	31
Extrapyramidal syndrome	28	26
Insomnia	27	22
Dizziness	26	25
Hallucinations	17	4
Nervous System		
Dream abnormalities	11	10
Confusion	10	7
Somnolence	9	6
Dystonia	8	7
Gait abnormalities	7	5
Hypertonia	7	6
Amnesia	6	4
Akathisia	3	2
Thinking abnormalities	3	2
Paranoid reaction	2	0
Delusions	1	0
Sleep disorders	1	0
Respiratory System		
Dyspnea	4	3
Rhinitis	3	1
Pneumonia	2	0
Skin & Appendages		
Skin disorders	2	1
Special Senses		
Accommodation abnormalities	4	2
Vision abnormalities	3	1
Diplopia	1	0
Urogenital System		
Urinary frequency	6	3
Urinary tract infection	4	3
Urinary incontinence	2	1

* Patients may have reported multiple adverse experiences during the study or at discontinuation; thus, patients may be included in more than one category.
† Patients received concomitant levodopa.

Other events reported by 1% or more of patients with advanced Parkinson's disease and treated with MIRAPEX (pramipexole dihydrochloride) but reported equally or more frequently in the placebo group were nausea, pain, infection, headache, depression, tremor, hypokinesia, anorexia, back pain, dyspepsia, flatulence, ataxia, flu syndrome, sinusitis, diarrhea, myalgia, abdominal pain, anxiety, rash, paresthesia, hypertension, increased saliva, tooth disorder, apathy, hypotension, sweating, vasodilation, vomiting, increased cough, nervousness, pruritus, hypesthesia, neck pain, syncope, arthralgia, dysphagia, palpitations, pharyngitis, vertigo, leg cramps, conjunctivitis, and lacrimation disorders.

Adverse Events; Relationship to Age, Gender, and Race: Among the treatment-emergent adverse events in patients treated with MIRAPEX (pramipexole dihydrochloride), hallucination appeared to exhibit a positive relationship to age. No gender-related differences were observed. Only a small percentage (4%) of patients enrolled were non-Caucasian, therefore, an evaluation of adverse events related to race is not possible.

Other Adverse Events Observed During All Phase 2 and 3 Clinical Trials: MIRAPEX (pramipexole dihydrochloride) has been administered to 1,408 individuals during all clinical trials (Parkinson's disease and other patient populations), 648 of whom were in seven double-blind, placebo-controlled Parkinson's disease trials. During these trials, all adverse events were recorded by the clinical investigators using terminology of their own choosing. To provide a meaningful estimate of the proportion of individuals having adverse events, similar types of events were grouped into a smaller number of standardized categories using modified COSTART dictionary terminology. These categories are used in the listing below. The events listed below occurred in less than 1% of the 1,408 individuals exposed to MIRAPEX (pramipexole dihydrochloride) and occurred on at least two occasions (on one occasion if the event was serious). All reported events, except those already listed above, are included, without regard to determination of a causal relationship to MIRAPEX (pramipexole dihydrochloride).

Events are listed within body-system categories in order of decreasing frequency.

Body as a whole: enlarged abdomen, death, fever, suicide attempt.

Cardiovascular system: peripheral vascular disease, myocardial infarction, angina pectoris, atrial fibrillation, heart failure, arrhythmia, atrial arrhythmia, pulmonary embolism.

Digestive system: thirst.

Musculoskeletal system: joint disorder, myasthenia.

Nervous system: agitation, CNS stimulation, hyperkinesia, psychosis, convulsions.

Respiratory system: pneumonia.

Special senses: cataract, eye disorder, glaucoma.

Urogenital system: dysuria, abnormal ejaculation, prostate cancer, hematuria, prostate disorder.

Falling Asleep During Activities of Daily Living: Patients treated with MIRAPEX (pramipexole dihydrochloride) have reported falling asleep while engaged in activities of daily living, including operation of a motor vehicle which sometimes resulted in accidents (see bolded WARNING).

DRUG ABUSE AND DEPENDENCE

Pramipexole is not a controlled substance. Pramipexole has not been systematically studied in animals or humans for

Continued on next page

Mirapex—Cont.

its potential for abuse, tolerance, or physical dependence. However, in a rat model on cocaine self-administration, pramipexole had little or no effect.

OVERDOSAGE

There is no clinical experience with massive overdosage. One patient, with a 10-year history of schizophrenia, took 11 mg/day of pramipexole for 2 days; this is two to three times the protocol recommended daily dose. No adverse events were reported related to the increased dose. Blood pressure remained stable although pulse rate increased to between 100 and 120 beats/minute. The patient withdrew from the study at the end of week 2 due to lack of efficacy. There is no known antidote for overdosage of a dopamine agonist. If signs of central nervous system stimulation are present, a phenothiazine or other butyrophenone neuroleptic agent may be indicated; the efficacy of such drugs in reversing the effects of overdosage has not been assessed. Management of overdose may require general supportive measures along with gastric lavage, intravenous fluids, and electrocardiogram monitoring.

DOSAGE AND ADMINISTRATION

In all clinical studies, dosage was initiated at a subtherapeutic level to avoid intolerable adverse effects and orthostatic hypotension. MIRAPEX (pramipexole dihydrochloride) should be titrated gradually in all patients. The dosage should be increased to achieve a maximum therapeutic effect, balanced against the principal side effects of dyskinesia, hallucinations, somnolence, and dry mouth.

Dosing in Patients With Normal Renal Function

Initial Treatment: Dosages should be increased gradually from a starting dose of 0.375 mg/day given in three divided doses and should not be increased more frequently than every 5 to 7 days. A suggested ascending dosage schedule that was used in clinical studies is shown in the following table:

Table 3: Ascending Dosage Schedule of MIRAPEX (pramipexole dihydrochloride)

Week	Dosage (mg)	Total Daily Dose (mg)
1	0.125 tid	0.375
2	0.25 tid	0.75
3	0.5 tid	1.50
4	0.75 tid	2.25
5	1.0 tid	3.0
6	1.25 tid	3.75
7	1.5 tid	4.50

Maintenance Treatment: MIRAPEX (pramipexole dihydrochloride) Tablets were effective and well tolerated over a dosage range of 1.5 to 4.5 mg/day administered in equally divided doses three times per day with or without concomitant levodopa (approximately 800 mg/day).

In a fixed-dose study in early Parkinson's disease patients, doses of 3 mg, 4.5 mg, and 6 mg per day of MIRAPEX (pramipexole dihydrochloride) were not shown to provide any significant benefit beyond that achieved at a daily dose of 1.5 mg/day. However, in the same fixed-dose study, the following adverse events were dose related: postural hypotension, nausea, constipation, somnolence, and amnesia. The frequency of these events was generally 2-fold greater than placebo for pramipexole doses greater than 3 mg/day. The incidence of somnolence reported with pramipexole at a dose of 1.5 mg/day was comparable to placebo.

When MIRAPEX (pramipexole dihydrochloride) is used in combination with levodopa, a reduction of the levodopa dosage should be considered. In a controlled study in advanced Parkinson's disease, the dosage of levodopa was reduced by an average of 27% from baseline.

Table 4: Patients with Renal Impairment

Pramipexole Dosage in the Renally Impaired

Renal Status	Starting Dose (mg)	Maximum Dose (mg)
Normal to mild impairment (creatinine Cl > 60 mL/min)	0.125 tid	1.5 tid
Moderate impairment (creatinine Cl = 35 to 59 mL/min)	0.125 bid	1.5 bid
Severe impairment (creatinine Cl = 15 to 34 mL/min)	0.125 qd	1.5 qd
Very severe impairment (creatinine Cl < 15 mL/min and hemodialysis patients)	The use of MIRAPEX (pramipexole dihydrochloride) has not been adequately studied in this group of patients.	

Discontinuation of Treatment: It is recommended that MIRAPEX (pramipexole dihydrochloride) be discontinued over a period of 1 week; in some studies, however, abrupt discontinuation was uneventful.

HOW SUPPLIED

MIRAPEX (pramipexole dihydrochloride) Tablets are available as follows:

0.125 mg: white, round tablet with "U" on one side and "2" on the reverse side.
Bottles of 63 NDC 0597-0083-53

0.25 mg: white, oval, scored tablet with "U" twice on one side and "4" twice on the reverse side.
Bottles of 90 NDC 0597-0084-90
Unit dose packages of 100 NDC 0597-0084-61

0.5 mg: white, oval, scored tablet with "U" twice on one side and "8" twice on the reverse side.
Bottles of 90 NDC 0597-0085-90
Unit dose packages of 100 NDC 0597-0085-61

1 mg: white, round, scored tablet with "U" twice on one side and "6" twice on the reverse side.
Bottles of 90 NDC 0597-0090-90
Unit dose packages of 100 NDC 0597-0090-61

1.5 mg: white, round, scored tablet with "U" twice on one side and "37" twice on the reverse side.
Bottles of 90 NDC 0597-0091-90
Unit dose packages of 100 NDC 0597-0091-61

Store at 25°C (77°F); excursions permitted to 15°–30°C (59°–86°F) [see USP Controlled Room Temperature]. Protect from light.

℞ **only**

ANIMAL TOXICOLOGY

Retinal Pathology in Albino Rats

Pathologic changes (degeneration and loss of photoreceptor cells) were observed in the retina of albino rats in the 2-year carcinogenicity study with pramipexole. These findings were first observed during week 76 and were dose dependent in animals receiving 2 or 8 mg/kg/day (plasma AUCs equal to 2.5 and 12.5 times the AUC in humans that received 1.5 mg tid). In a similar study of pigmented rats with 2 years exposure to pramipexole at 2 or 8 mg/kg/day, retinal degeneration was not diagnosed. Animals given drug had thinning in the outer nuclear layer of the retina that was only slightly greater than that seen in control rats utilizing morphometry.

Investigative studies demonstrated that pramipexole reduced the rate of disk shedding from the photoreceptor rod cells of the retina in albino rats, which was associated with enhanced sensitivity to the damaging effects of light. In a comparative study, degeneration and loss of photoreceptor cells occurred in albino rats after 13 weeks of treatment with 25 mg/kg/day of pramipexole (54 times the highest clinical dose on a mg/m^2 basis) and constant light (100 lux) but not in pigmented rats exposed to the same dose and higher light intensities (500 lux). Thus, the retina of albino rats is considered to be uniquely sensitive to the damaging effects of pramipexole and light. Similar changes in the retina did not occur in a 2-year carcinogenicity study in albino mice treated with 0.3, 2, or 10 mg/kg/day (0.3, 2.2 and 11 times the highest clinical dose on a mg/m^2 basis). Evaluation of the retinas of monkeys given 0.1, 0.5, or 2.0 mg/kg/day of pramipexole (0.4, 2.2, and 8.6 times the highest clinical dose on a mg/m^2 basis) for 12 months and minipigs given 0.3, 1, or 5 mg/kg/day of pramipexole for 13 weeks also detected no changes.

The potential significance of this effect in humans has not been established, but cannot be disregarded because disruption of a mechanism that is universally present in vertebrates (ie, disk shedding) may be involved.

Fibro-osseous Proliferative Lesions in Mice

An increased incidence of fibro-osseous proliferative lesions occurred in the femurs of female mice treated for 2 years with 0.3, 2.0, or 10 mg/kg/day (0.3, 2.2, and 11 times the highest clinical dose on a mg/m^2 basis). Lesions occurred at a lower rate in control animals. Similar lesions were not observed in male mice or rats and monkeys of either sex that were treated chronically with pramipexole. The significance of this lesion to humans is not known.

Distributed by: Boehringer Ingelheim Pharmaceuticals, Inc.
Ridgefield, CT 06877 USA

Co-marketed by: Boehringer Ingelheim Pharmaceuticals, Inc.
and
Pfizer Inc, New York, NY 10017

Licensed from: Boehringer Ingelheim International GmbH

Trademark under license from:
Boehringer Ingelheim International GmbH
U.S. Patent Nos. 4,886,812 and 4,843,086

Revised October 2003 819898001/US/1

SPIRIVA® HANDIHALER® ℞

[*spĭ-rī-vă*]

(tiotropium bromide inhalation powder)

For Oral Inhalation Only

Prescribing Information

DESCRIPTION

SPIRIVA® HandiHaler® (tiotropium bromide inhalation powder) consists of a capsule dosage form containing a dry powder formulation of SPIRIVA (tiotropium bromide) intended for oral inhalation only with the HandiHaler inhalation device.

Each light green, hard gelatin capsule contains 18 mcg tiotropium (equivalent to 22.5 mcg tiotropium bromide monohydrate) blended with lactose monohydrate as the carrier.

The dry powder formulation within the capsule is intended for oral inhalation only.

The active component of SPIRIVA is tiotropium. The drug substance, tiotropium bromide monohydrate, is an anticholinergic with specificity for muscarinic receptors. It is chemically described as (1α, 2β, 4β, 5α, 7β)-7-[(Hydroxydi-2-thienylacetyl)oxy]-9,9-dimethyl-3-oxa-9-azoniatricyclo [3.3.1.0^{2,4}]nonane bromide monohydrate. It is a synthetic, non-chiral, quaternary ammonium compound. Tiotropium bromide is a white or yellowish white powder. It is sparingly soluble in water and soluble in methanol.

The structural formula is:

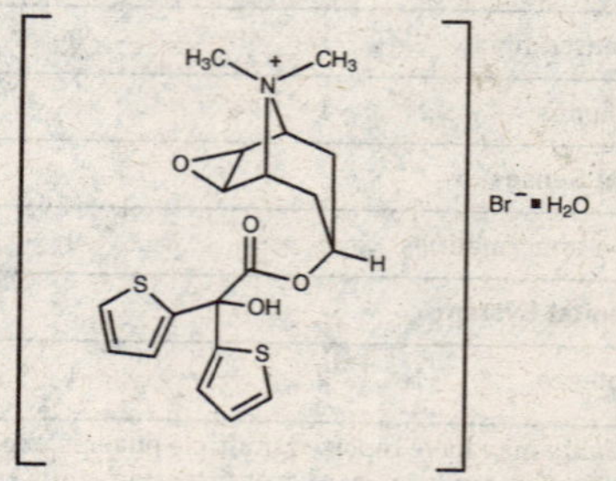

Tiotropium bromide (monohydrate) has a molecular mass of 490.4 and a molecular formula of $C_{19}H_{22}NO_4S_2Br \cdot H_2O$.

The HandiHaler is an inhalation device used to inhale the dry powder contained in the SPIRIVA capsule. The dry powder is delivered from the HandiHaler device at flow rates as low as 20 L/min. Under standardized *in vitro* testing, the HandiHaler device delivers a mean of 10.4 mcg tiotropium when tested at a flow rate of 39 L/min for 3.1 seconds (2L total). In a study of 26 adult patients with chronic obstructive pulmonary disease (COPD) and severely compromised lung function [mean FEV_1 1.02 L (range 0.45 to 2.24 L); 37.6% of predicted (range 16%–65%)], the median peak inspiratory flow (PIF) through the HandiHaler device was 30.0 L/min (range 20.4 to 45.6 L/min). The amount of drug delivered to the lungs will vary depending on patient factors such as inspiratory flow and peak inspiratory flow through the HandiHaler device, which may vary from patient to patient, and may vary with the exposure time of the capsule outside the blister pack.

For administration of SPIRIVA, a capsule is placed into the center chamber of the HandiHaler device. The capsule is pierced by pressing and releasing the button on the side of the inhalation device. The tiotropium formulation is dispersed into the air stream when the patient inhales through the mouthpiece. (see **Patient's Instructions For Use**)

CLINICAL PHARMACOLOGY

Mechanism of Action

Tiotropium is a long-acting, antimuscarinic agent, which is often referred to as an anticholinergic. It has similar affinity to the subtypes of muscarinic receptors, M_1 to M_5. In the airways, it exhibits pharmacological effects through inhibition of M_3-receptors at the smooth muscle leading to bronchodilation. The competitive and reversible nature of antagonism was shown with human and animal origin receptors and isolated organ preparations. In preclinical *in vitro* as well as *in vivo* studies prevention of methacholine-induced bronchoconstriction effects were dose-dependent and lasted longer than 24 hours. The bronchodilation following inhalation of tiotropium is predominantly a site-specific effect.

Pharmacokinetics

Tiotropium is administered by dry powder inhalation. In common with other inhaled drugs, the majority of the delivered dose is deposited in the gastrointestinal tract and, to a lesser extent, in the lung, the intended organ. Many of the pharmacokinetic data described below were obtained with higher doses than recommended for therapy.

Absorption:

Following dry powder inhalation by young healthy volunteers, the absolute bioavailability of 19.5% suggests that the fraction reaching the lung is highly bioavailable. It is expected from the chemical structure of the compound (quaternary ammonium compound) that tiotropium is poorly absorbed from the gastrointestinal tract. Food is not expected to influence the absorption of tiotropium for the same reason. Oral solutions of tiotropium have an absolute bioavailability of 2–3%. Maximum tiotropium plasma concentrations were observed five minutes after inhalation.

Distribution:
Tiotropium shows a volume of distribution of 32 L/kg indicating that the drug binds extensively to tissues. The drug is bound by 72% to plasma proteins. At steady state, peak tiotropium plasma levels in COPD patients were 17–19 pg/mL when measured 5 minutes after dry powder inhalation of an 18 mcg dose and decreased rapidly in a multi-compartmental manner. Steady state trough plasma concentrations were 3–4 pg/mL. Local concentrations in the lung are not known, but the mode of administration suggests substantially higher concentrations in the lung. Studies in rats have shown that tiotropium does not readily penetrate the blood-brain barrier.

Biotransformation:
The extent of biotransformation appears to be small. This is evident from a urinary excretion of 74% of unchanged substance after an intravenous dose to young healthy volunteers. Tiotropium, an ester, is nonenzymatically cleaved to the alcohol *N*-methylscopine and dithienylglycolic acid, neither of which bind to muscarinic receptors.

In vitro experiments with human liver microsomes and human hepatocytes suggest that a fraction of the administered dose (74% of an intravenous dose is excreted unchanged in the urine, leaving 25% for metabolism) is metabolized by cytochrome P450-dependent oxidation and subsequent glutathione conjugation to a variety of Phase II metabolites. This enzymatic pathway can be inhibited by CYP450 2D6 and 3A4 inhibitors, such as quinidine, ketoconazole, and gestodene. Thus, CYP450 2D6 and 3A4 are involved in the metabolic pathway that is responsible for the elimination of a small part of the administered dose. *In vitro* studies using human liver microsomes showed that tiotropium in supra-therapeutic concentrations does not inhibit CYP450 1A1, 1A2, 2B6, 2C9, 2C19, 2D6, 2E1, or 3A4.

Elimination:
The terminal elimination half-life of tiotropium is between 5 and 6 days following inhalation. Total clearance was 880 mL/min after an intravenous dose in young healthy volunteers with an inter-individual variability of 22%. Intravenously administered tiotropium is mainly excreted unchanged in urine (74%). After dry powder inhalation, urinary excretion is 14% of the dose, the remainder being mainly non-absorbed drug in the gut which is eliminated via the feces. The renal clearance of tiotropium exceeds the creatinine clearance, indicating active secretion into the urine. After chronic once-daily inhalation by COPD patients, pharmacokinetic steady state was reached after 2–3 weeks with no accumulation thereafter.

Drug Interactions:
An interaction study with tiotropium (14.4 mcg intravenous infusion over 15 minutes) and cimetidine 400 mg three times daily or ranitidine 300 mg once daily was conducted. Concomitant administration of cimetidine with tiotropium resulted in a 20% increase in the AUC_{0-4h}, a 28% decrease in the renal clearance of tiotropium and no significant change in the C_{max} and amount excreted in urine over 96 hours. Co-administration of tiotropium with ranitidine did not affect the pharmacokinetics of tiotropium. Therefore, no clinically significant interaction occurred between tiotropium and cimetidine or ranitidine.

Electrophysiology:
In a multicenter, randomized, double-blind trial that enrolled 198 patients with COPD, the number of subjects with changes from baseline-corrected QT interval of 30–60 msec was higher in the SPIRIVA group as compared with placebo. This difference was apparent using both the Bazett (QTcB) [20 (20%) patient vs. 12 (12%) patients] and Fredericia (QTcF) [16 (16%) patients vs. 1 (1%) patient] corrections of QT for heart rate. No patients in either group had either QTcB or QTcF of >500 msec. Other clinical studies with SPIRIVA did not detect an effect of the drug on QTc intervals.

Special Populations:
Elderly Patients:
As expected for drugs predominantly excreted renally, advanced age was associated with a decrease of tiotropium renal clearance (326 mL/min in COPD patients <58 years to 163 mL/min in COPD patients >70 years), which may be explained by decreased renal function. Tiotropium excretion in urine after inhalation decreased from 14% (young healthy volunteers) to about 7% (COPD patients). Plasma concentrations were numerically increased with advancing age within COPD patients (43% increase in AUC_{0-4} after dry powder inhalation), which was not significant when considered in relation to inter- and intra-individual variability. (See **DOSAGE AND ADMINISTRATION SECTION**)

Hepatically-impaired Patients:
The effects of hepatic impairment on the pharmacokinetics of tiotropium were not studied. However, hepatic insufficiency is not expected to have relevant influence on tiotropium pharmacokinetics. Tiotropium is predominantly cleared by renal elimination (74% in young healthy volunteers) and by simple non-enzymatic ester cleavage to products that do not bind to muscarinic receptors. (See **DOSAGE AND ADMINISTRATION SECTION**)

Renally-impaired Patients:
Since tiotropium is predominantly renally excreted, renal impairment was associated with increased plasma drug concentrations and reduced drug clearance after both intravenous infusion and dry powder inhalation. Mild renal impairment (CrCl 50–80 mL/min), which is often seen in elderly patients, increased tiotropium plasma concentrations (39% increase in AUC_{0-4} after intravenous infusion). In COPD patients with moderate to severe renal impairment (CrCl <50 mL/min), the intravenous administration of tiotropium resulted in doubling of the plasma concentrations (82% increase in AUC_{0-4}), which was confirmed by plasma concentrations after dry powder inhalation. (See **DOSAGE AND ADMINISTRATION** and **PRECAUTIONS Sections**)

Figure 1: Mean FEV_1 Over Time (prior to and after administration of study drug) on Days 1 and 169 for Trial A (a Six-Month Placebo-Controlled Study)*

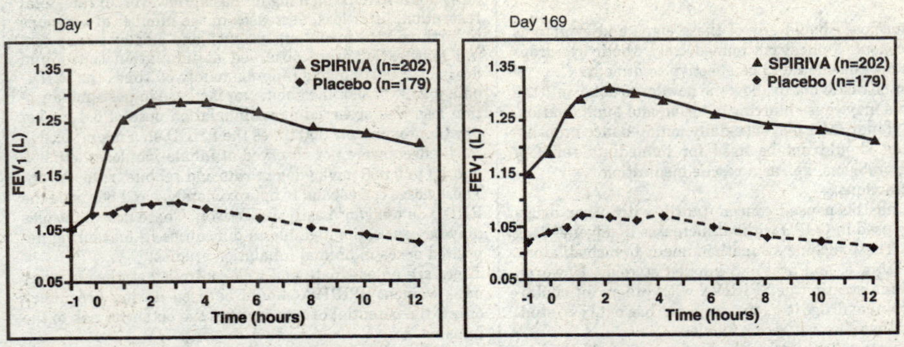

*Means adjusted for center, treatment, and baseline effect. On Day 169, a total of 183 and 149 patients in the SPIRIVA and placebo groups, respectively, completed the trial. The data for the remaining patients were imputed using last observation or least favorable observation carried forward.

Figure 2: Mean FEV_1 Over Time (0 to 6 hours postdose) on Days 1 and 92, respectively for one of the two Ipratropium-Controlled Studies*

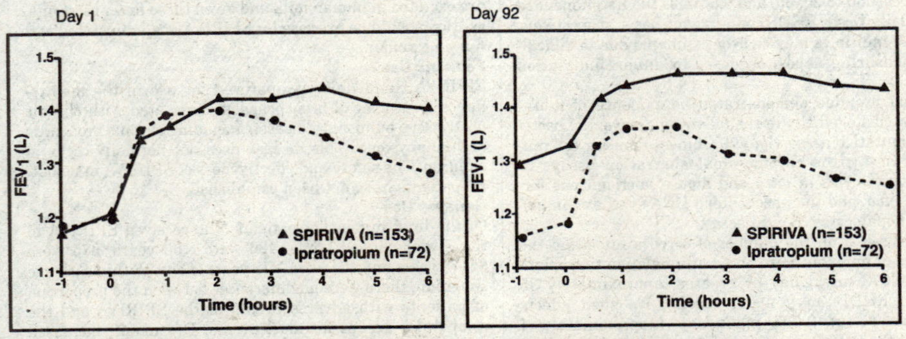

*Means adjusted for center, treatment, and baseline effect. On Day 92 (primary endpoint), a total of 151 and 69 patients in the SPIRIVA and ipratropium groups, respectively, completed through three months of observation.The data for the remaining patients were imputed using last observation or least favorable observation carried forward.

CLINICAL STUDIES

The SPIRIVA HandiHaler clinical development program consisted of six phase 3 studies in 2,663 patients with COPD (1,308 receiving SPIRIVA): two 1-year, placebo-controlled studies, two 6-month, placebo-controlled studies and two 1-year, ipratropium-controlled studies. These studies enrolled patients who had a clinical diagnosis of COPD, were 40 years of age or older, had a history of smoking greater than 10 pack-years, had an FEV_1 less than or equal to 60 or 65% of predicted, and a ratio of FEV_1/FVC of less than or equal to 0.7.

In these studies, SPIRIVA, administered once-daily in the morning, provided improvement in lung function (forced expiratory volume in one second, FEV_1), with peak effect occurring within 3 hours following the first dose.

In the 1-year, placebo controlled trials, the mean improvement in FEV_1 at 30 minutes was 0.13 liters (13%) with a peak improvement of 0.24 liters (24%) relative to baseline after the first dose (day 1). Further improvements in FEV_1 and FVC were observed with pharmacodynamic steady state reached by day 8 with once-daily treatment. The mean peak improvement in FEV_1, relative to baseline, was 0.28 to 0.31 liters (28% to 31%), after 1 week (day 8) of once-daily treatment. Improvement of lung function was maintained for 24 hours after a single dose and consistently maintained over the 1-year treatment period with no evidence of tolerance.

In the two 6-month, placebo-controlled trials, serial spirometric evaluations were performed throughout daytime hours in Trial A (12 hours) and limited to 3 hours in Trial B. The serial FEV_1 values over 12 hours (Trial A) are displayed in Figure 1. These trials further support the improvement in pulmonary function (FEV_1) with SPIRIVA, which persisted over the spirometric observational period. Effectiveness was maintained for 24 hours after administration over the 6-month treatment period.

[See figure 1 above]

Results of each of the one-year ipratropium-controlled trials were similar to the results of the one-year placebo-controlled trials. The results of one of these trials are shown in Figure 2.

[See figure 2 above]

A randomized, placebo-controlled clinical study in 105 patients with COPD demonstrated that bronchodilation was maintained throughout the 24-hour dosing interval in comparison to placebo, regardless of whether SPIRIVA was administered in the morning or in the evening.

Throughout each week of the one-year treatment period in the two placebo-controlled trials, patients taking SPIRIVA had a reduced requirement for the use of rescue short-acting $beta_2$-agonists. Reduction in the use of rescue short-acting $beta_2$-agonists, as compared to placebo, was demonstrated in one of the two 6-month studies.

INDICATIONS AND USAGE

SPIRIVA HandiHaler is indicated for the long-term, once-daily, maintenance treatment of bronchospasm associated with chronic obstructive pulmonary disease (COPD), including chronic bronchitis and emphysema.

CONTRAINDICATIONS

SPIRIVA HandiHaler is contraindicated in patients with a history of hypersensitivity to atropine or its derivatives, including ipratropium, or to any component of this product.

WARNINGS

SPIRIVA HandiHaler is intended as a once-daily maintenance treatment for COPD and is not indicated for the initial treatment of acute episodes of bronchospasm, i.e., rescue therapy.

Immediate hypersensitivity reactions, including angioedema, may occur after administration of SPIRIVA. If such a reaction occurs, therapy with SPIRIVA should be stopped at once and alternative treatments should be considered.

Inhaled medicines, including SPIRIVA, may cause paradoxical bronchospasm. If this occurs, treatment with SPIRIVA should be stopped and other treatments considered.

PRECAUTIONS

General
As an anticholinergic drug, SPIRIVA may potentially worsen symptoms and signs associated with narrow-angle glaucoma, prostatic hyperplasia or bladder-neck obstruction and should be used with caution in patients with any of these conditions.

As a predominantly renally excreted drug, patients with moderate to severe renal impairment (creatinine clearance of ≤50 mL/min) treated with SPIRIVA should be monitored closely. (See **CLINICAL PHARMACOLOGY, Pharmacokinetics**, Special Populations: *Renally-impaired Patients*)

Information for Patients
It is important for patients to understand how to correctly administer SPIRIVA capsules using the HandiHaler inhalation device. (See **Patient's Instructions for Use**) SPIRIVA capsules should only be administered via the HandiHaler device and the HandiHaler device should not be used for administering other medications.

Capsules should always be stored in sealed blisters and only removed immediately before use. The blister strip should be carefully opened to expose only one capsule at a time. Open the blister foil as far as the *STOP* line to remove only one capsule at a time. The drug should be used immediately after the packaging over an individual capsule is opened, or else its effectiveness may be reduced. Capsules that are inadvertently exposed to air (i.e., not intended for immediate use) should be discarded.

Eye pain or discomfort, blurred vision, visual halos or colored images in association with red eyes from conjunctival congestion and corneal edema may be signs of acute narrow-

Continued on next page

Spiriva—Cont.

angle glaucoma. Should any of these signs and symptoms develop, consult a physician immediately. Miotic eye drops alone are not considered to be effective treatment.
Care must be taken not to allow the powder to enter into the eyes as this may cause blurring of vision and pupil dilation.
SPIRIVA HandiHaler is a once-daily maintenance bronchodilator and should not be used for immediate relief of breathing problems, i.e., as a rescue medication.

Drug Interactions

SPIRIVA has been used concomitantly with other drugs commonly used in COPD without increases in adverse drug reactions. These include sympathomimetic bronchodilators, methylxanthines, and oral and inhaled steroids. However, the co-administration of SPIRIVA with other anticholinergic-containing drugs (e.g., ipratropium) has not been studied and is therefore not recommended.

Drug/Laboratory Test Interactions

None known.

Carcinogenesis, Mutagenesis, Impairment of Fertility

No evidence of tumorigenicity was observed in a 104-week inhalation study in rats at tiotropium doses up to 0.059 mg/kg/day, in an 83-week inhalation study in female mice at doses up to 0.145 mg/kg/day, and in a 101-week inhalation study in male mice at doses up to 0.002 mg/kg/day. These doses correspond to 25, 35, and 0.5 times the Recommended Human Daily Dose (RHDD) on a mg/m^2 basis, respectively. These dose multiples may be over-estimated due to difficulties in measuring deposited doses in animal inhalation studies.
Tiotropium bromide demonstrated no evidence of mutagenicity or clastogenicity in the following assays: the bacterial gene mutation assay, the V79 Chinese hamster cell mutagenesis assay, the chromosomal aberration assays in human lymphocytes *in vitro* and mouse micronucleus formation *in vivo*, and the unscheduled DNA synthesis in primary rat hepatocytes *in vitro* assay.
In rats, decreases in the number of corpora lutea and the percentage of implants were noted at inhalation tiotropium doses of 0.078 mg/kg/day or greater (approximately 35 times the RHDD on a mg/m^2 basis). No such effects were observed at 0.009 mg/kg/day (approximately 4 times than the RHDD on a mg/m^2 basis). The fertility index, however, was not affected at inhalation doses up to 1.689 mg/kg/day (approximately 760 times the RHDD on a mg/m^2 basis). These dose multiples may be over-estimated due to difficulties in measuring deposited doses in animal inhalation studies.

Pregnancy

Pregnancy Category C

No evidence of structural alterations was observed in rats and rabbits at inhalation tiotropium doses of up to 1.471 and 0.007 mg/kg/day, respectively. These doses correspond to approximately 660 and 6 times the recommended human daily dose (RHDD) on a mg/m^2 basis. However, in rats, fetal resorption, litter loss, decreases in the number of live pups at birth and the mean pup weights, and a delay in pup sexual maturation were observed at inhalation tiotropium doses of ≥ 0.078 mg/kg (approximately 35 times the RHDD on a mg/m^2 basis). In rabbits, an increase in post-implantation loss was observed at an inhalation dose of 0.4 mg/kg/day (approximately 360 times the RHDD on a mg/m^2 basis). Such effects were not observed at inhalation doses of 0.009 and up to 0.088 mg/kg/day in rats and rabbits, respectively. These doses correspond to approximately 4 and 80 times the RHDD on a mg/m^2 basis, respectively. These dose multiples may be over-estimated due to difficulties in measuring deposited doses in animal inhalation studies.
There are no adequate and well-controlled studies in pregnant women. SPIRIVA should be used during pregnancy only if the potential benefit justifies the potential risk to the fetus.

Use in Labor and Delivery

The safety and effectiveness of SPIRIVA has not been studied during labor and delivery.

Nursing Mothers

Clinical data from nursing women exposed to tiotropium are not available. Based on lactating rodent studies, tiotropium is excreted into breast milk. It is not known whether tiotropium is excreted in human milk, but because many drugs are excreted in human milk and given these findings in rats, caution should be exercised if SPIRIVA is administered to a nursing woman.

Pediatric Use

SPIRIVA HandiHaler is approved for use in the maintenance treatment of bronchospasm associated with chronic obstructive pulmonary disease, including chronic bronchitis and emphysema. This disease does not normally occur in children. The safety and effectiveness of SPIRIVA in pediatric patients have not been established.

Geriatric Use

Of the total number of patients who received SPIRIVA in the 1-year clinical trials, 426 were <65 years, 375 were 65–74 years and 105 were ≥75 years of age. Within each age subgroup, there were no differences between the proportion of patients with adverse events in the SPIRIVA and the comparator groups for most events. Dry mouth increased with age in the SPIRIVA group (differences from placebo were 9.0%, 17.1%, and 16.2% in the aforementioned age subgroups). A higher frequency of constipation and urinary tract infections with increasing age was observed in the SPIRIVA group in the placebo-controlled studies. The differences from placebo for constipation were 0%, 1.8%, and 7.8% for each of the age groups. The differences from placebo for urinary tract infections were −0.6%, 4.6% and 4.5%. No overall differences in effectiveness were observed among these groups. Based on available data, no adjustment of SPIRIVA dosage in geriatric patients is warranted.

Table 1: Adverse Experience Incidence (% Patients) in One-Year-COPD Clinical Trials

Body System (Event)	Placebo-Controlled Trials SPIRIVA [n=550]	Placebo-Controlled Trials Placebo [n=371]	Ipratropium-Controlled Trials SPIRIVA [n=356]	Ipratropium-Controlled Trials Ipratropium [n=179]
Body as a Whole				
Accidents	13	11	5	8
Chest Pain (non-specific)	7	5	5	2
Edema, Dependent	5	4	3	5
Gastrointestinal System Disorders				
Abdominal Pain	5	3	6	6
Constipation	4	2	1	1
Dry Mouth	16	3	12	6
Dyspepsia	6	5	1	1
Vomiting	4	2	1	2
Musculoskeletal System				
Myalgia	4	3	4	3
Resistance Mechanism Disorders				
Infection	4	3	1	3
Moniliasis	4	2	3	2
Respiratory System (upper)				
Epistaxis	4	2	1	1
Pharyngitis	9	7	7	3
Rhinitis	6	5	3	2
Sinusitis	11	9	3	2
Upper Respiratory Tract Infection	41	37	43	35
Skin and Appendage Disorders				
Rash	4	2	2	2
Urinary System				
Urinary Tract Infection	7	5	4	2

ADVERSE REACTIONS

Of the 2,663 patients in the four 1-year and two 6-month controlled clinical trials, 1,308 were treated with SPIRIVA at the recommended dose of 18 mcg once a day. Patients with narrow angle glaucoma, or symptomatic prostatic hypertrophy or bladder outlet obstruction were excluded from these trials.
The most commonly reported adverse drug reaction was dry mouth. Dry mouth was usually mild and often resolved during continued treatment. Other reactions reported in individual patients and consistent with possible anticholinergic effects included constipation, increased heart rate, blurred vision, glaucoma, urinary difficulty, and urinary retention.
Four multicenter, 1-year, controlled studies evaluated SPIRIVA in patients with COPD. Table 1 shows all adverse events that occurred with a frequency of ≥3% in the SPIRIVA group in the 1-year placebo-controlled trials where the rates in the SPIRIVA group exceeded placebo by ≥1%. The frequency of corresponding events in the ipratropium-controlled trials is included for comparison.
[See table 1 below]
Arthritis, coughing, and influenza-like symptoms occurred at a rate of ≥3% in the SPIRIVA treatment group, but were <1% in excess of the placebo group.
Other events that occurred in the SPIRIVA group at a frequency of 1–3% in the placebo-controlled trials where the rates exceeded that in the placebo group include: *Body as a Whole:* allergic reaction, leg pain; *Central and Peripheral Nervous System:* dysphonia, paresthesia; *Gastrointestinal System Disorders:* gastrointestinal disorder not otherwise specified (NOS), gastroesophageal reflux, stomatitis (including ulcerative stomatitis); *Metabolic and Nutritional Disorders:* hypercholesterolemia, hyperglycemia; *Musculoskeletal System Disorders:* skeletal pain: *Cardiac Events:* angina pectoris (including aggravated angina pectoris); *Psychiatric Disorder:* depression; *Infections:* herpes zoster; *Respiratory System Disorder (Upper):* laryngitis; *Vision Disorder:* cataract. In addition, among the adverse events observed in the clinical trials with an incidence of <1% were atrial fibrillation, supraventricular tachycardia, angioedema, and urinary retention.
In the 1-year trials, the incidence of dry mouth, constipation, and urinary tract infection increased with age. (See **PRECAUTIONS, Geriatric Use**)
Two multicenter, 6-month, controlled studies evaluated SPIRIVA in patients with COPD. The adverse events and the incidence rates were similar to those seen in the 1-year controlled trials.
In addition to adverse events identified during clinical trials, the following adverse reactions have been reported in the worldwide post-marketing experience: epistaxis, palpitations, pruritus, and urticaria.

OVERDOSAGE

High doses of tiotropium may lead to anticholinergic signs and symptoms. However, there were no systemic anticholinergic adverse effects following a single inhaled dose of up to 282 mcg tiotropium in 6 healthy volunteers. In a study of 12 healthy volunteers, bilateral conjunctivitis and dry mouth were seen following repeated once-daily inhalation of 141 mcg of tiotropium.
Acute intoxication by inadvertent oral ingestion of SPIRIVA capsules is unlikely since it is not well-absorbed systemically.
A case of overdose has been reported from post-marketing experience. A female patient was reported to have inhaled 30 capsules over a 2.5 day period, and developed altered mental status, tremors, abdominal pain, and severe constipation. The patient was hospitalized, SPIRIVA was discontinued, and the constipation was treated with an enema. The patient recovered and was discharged on the same day.
No mortality was observed at inhalation tiotropium doses up to 32.4 mg/kg in mice, 267.7 mg/kg in rats, and 0.6 mg/kg in dogs. These doses correspond to 7,3000, 120,000, and 850 times the recommended human daily dose on a mg/m^2 basis, respectively. These dose multiples may be over-estimated due to difficulties in measuring deposited doses in animal inhalation studies.

DOSAGE AND ADMINISTRATION

The recommended dosage of SPIRIVA HandiHaler is the inhalation of the contents of one SPIRIVA capsule, once-daily, with the HandiHaler inhalation device. (See **Patient's Instructions for Use**)
No dosage adjustment is required for geriatric, hepatically-impaired, or renally-impaired patients. However, patients with moderate to severe renal impairment given SPIRIVA should be monitored closely. (See **CLINICAL PHARMACOLOGY, Pharmacokinetics,** Special Populations and **PRECAUTIONS**)
SPIRIVA capsules are for inhalation only and must not be swallowed.

HOW SUPPLIED

SPIRIVA capsules, containing 18 mcg tiotropium, are light green, with TI01 printed on one side of the capsule and the Boehringer Ingelheim company logo on the other side.
The HandiHaler inhalation device is gray colored with a green button. It is imprinted with SPIRIVA HandiHaler (tiotropium bromide inhalation powder), the Boehringer Ingelheim company logo, and the Pfizer company logo. It is also imprinted to indicate that SPIRIVA capsules should not be stored in the HandiHaler device and that the HandiHaler device is only to be used with SPIRIVA capsules.
Six SPIRIVA capsules are packaged in an Aluminum/PVC/Aluminum blister card. One blister card consists of two blis-

ter strips, each containing 3 capsules and joined along a perforated-cut line. After using the first capsule, the 2 remaining capsules should be used over the next 2 consecutive days. Capsules should always be stored in the blister and only removed immediately before use. The foil lidding should only be peeled back as far as the *STOP* line printed on the blister foil to prevent exposure of more than one capsule. The drug should be used immediately after the packaging over an individual capsule is opened.

The following packages are available:
carton containing 6 SPIRIVA capsules (1 blister card) and 1 HandiHaler inhalation device (NDC 0597-0075-06)
carton containing 30 SPIRIVA capsules (5 blister cards) and 1 HandiHaler inhalation device (NDC 0597-0075-37)

Storage

Store at 25°C (77°F); excursions permitted to 15–30°C (59–86°F) [see USP Controlled Room Temperature].
The capsules should not be exposed to extreme temperature or moisture. Do not store capsules in the HandiHaler device.

℞ **only**

Manufactured by:
Boehringer Ingelheim Pharma GmbH & Co. KG
Ingelheim, Germany
Marketed by:
Boehringer Ingelheim Pharmaceuticals, Inc.
Ridgefield, CT 06877 USA
and
Pfizer Inc.
New York, NY 10017 USA
Address Medical Inquiries to:
www.Spiriva.com or (800) 542-6257
Licensed from Boehringer Ingelheim International GmbH.
SPIRIVA® and HandiHaler® are registered trademarks and are used under license from Boehringer Ingelheim International GmbH

Tiotropium bromide is covered by U.S. Patent No. 5,610,163 with other Patents Pending. The HandiHaler inhalation device is covered by U.S. Design Patient No. 355,029.
59873/US/1 January 2004

PATIENT'S INSTRUCTIONS FOR USE

Spiriva®
HandiHaler®
(tiotropium bromide
inhalation powder)

FOR ORAL INHALATION ONLY

Read all instructions before use.
This leaflet provides summary information about SPIRIVA capsules and the HandiHaler inhalation device. Before you start to take SPIRIVA or use the HandiHaler, read this leaflet carefully and keep it for future use. You should read the leaflet that comes with your prescription every time you refill it because there may be new information.
For more information, ask your health-care provider or pharmacist.

What should you know about SPIRIVA and HandiHaler?

Each SPIRIVA capsule contains a dry powder blend of active drug (18 mcg tiotropium) and lactose monohydrate as the carrier. The dry powder in the capsule is inhaled from the HandiHaler inhalation device. SPIRIVA capsules contain only a small amount of powder and as a result the capsule is only partially filled. When disposing of the capsule, you may notice that a tiny amount of this powder is left in the capsule. This is normal.
SPIRIVA is a once daily maintenance bronchodilator medicine that opens narrowed airways and helps keep them open for 24 hours. SPIRIVA HandiHaler should not be used for immediate relief of breathing problems, i.e., as a rescue medication.

SPIRIVA CAPSULES ARE INTENDED FOR ORAL INHALATION ONLY AND ARE TO BE USED ONLY WITH THE HANDIHALER INHALATION DEVICE.

SPIRIVA CAPSULES SHOULD NOT BE SWALLOWED.

The HandiHaler is an inhalation device that has been specially designed for use with SPIRIVA capsules. It must not be used to take any other medication.
Care must be taken not to allow the powder to enter into the eyes. If symptoms of eye pain, eye discomfort, blurred vision, visual halos, or colored images in association with red eyes occur, consult a physician immediately.

How do you take your dose of SPIRIVA using the HandiHaler?

Taking your dose of SPIRIVA, requires four main steps: Open the blister and the HandiHaler device, insert the SPIRIVA capsule, press the HandiHaler button, and inhale your medication. (See below for details.)

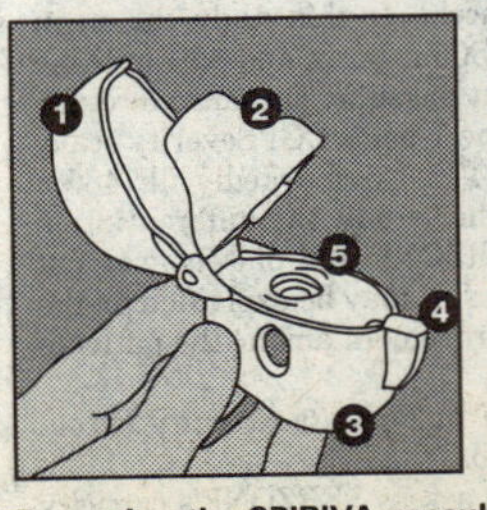

Become familiar with the components of the HandiHaler inhalation device:
1. dust cap
2. mouthpiece
3. base
4. piercing button
5. center chamber

Removing the SPIRIVA capsule from the blister.

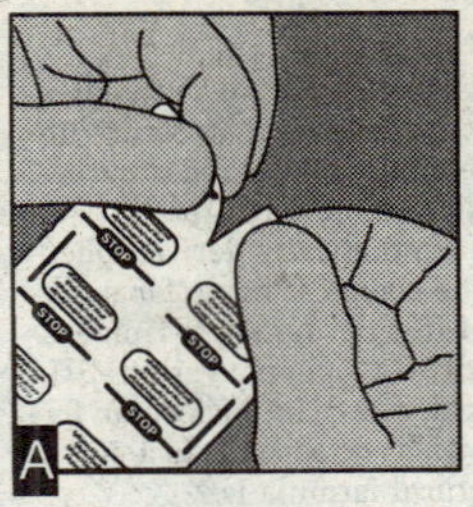

A) SPIRIVA capsules are packaged in a blister card. Each blister card consists of two blister strips, each containing 3 capsules and joined along a perforated-cut line. Prior to removing the first capsule from the blister card, separate the blister strips by tearing along the perforation. (Figure A)

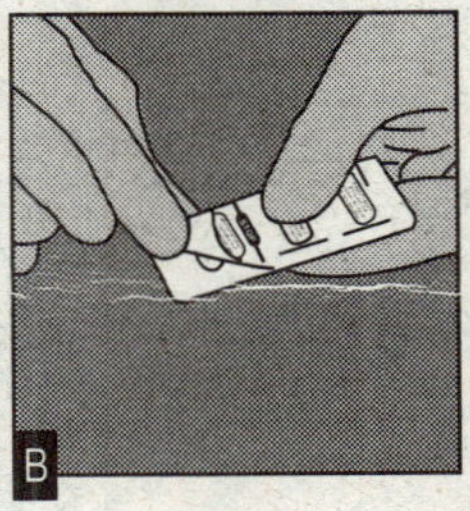

B) The blister should be carefully opened to expose only one capsule at a time. Immediately before you are ready to take your dose of SPIRIVA, peel back the aluminum foil using the tab until one capsule is fully visible. The foil lidding should only be peeled back as far as the ***STOP*** line printed on the blister foil to prevent exposure of more than one capsule. (Figure B)

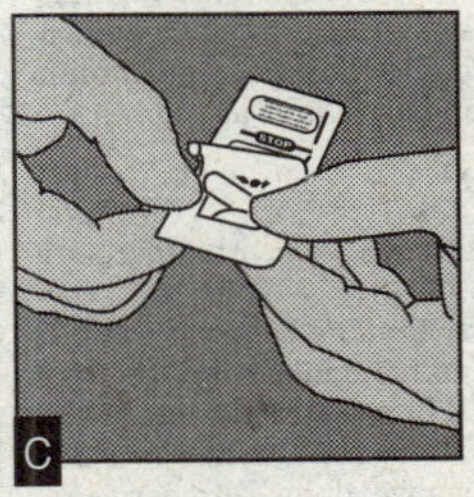

C) **Capsules should always be stored in the sealed blisters and only removed immediately before use. The drug should be used immediately after the packaging over an individual capsule is opened, or else its effectiveness may be reduced.** The blister strip should be carefully opened to expose one capsule at a time. After using the first capsule, the 2 remaining capsules should be used over the next 2 consecutive days. SPIRIVA capsules should always be stored in the blister. The blister should only be opened and the capsule removed immediately before use. If additional capsules are inadvertently exposed to air, they should not be used and should be discarded. (Figure C)

Do not store capsules in the HandiHaler device.

Opening the HandiHaler device and inserting the SPIRIVA capsule.

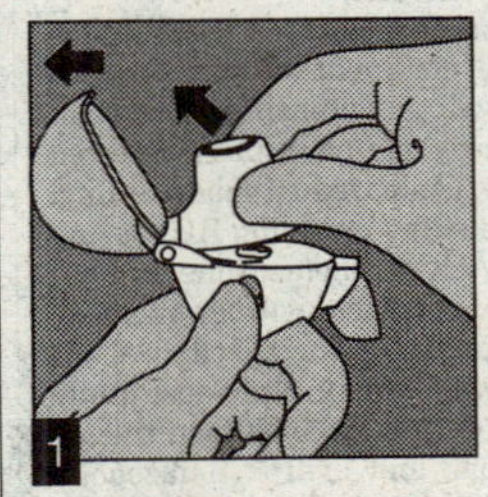

1) **OPEN:** Open the dust cap by pulling it upwards. Then open the mouthpiece. (Figure 1)

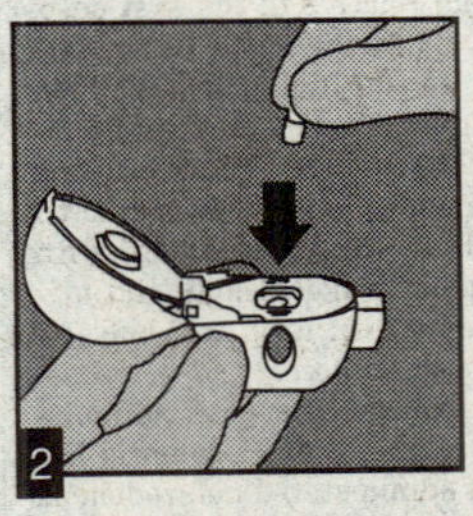

2) **INSERT:** Place the capsule in the center chamber. It does not matter which end of the capsule is placed in the chamber. (Figure 2)

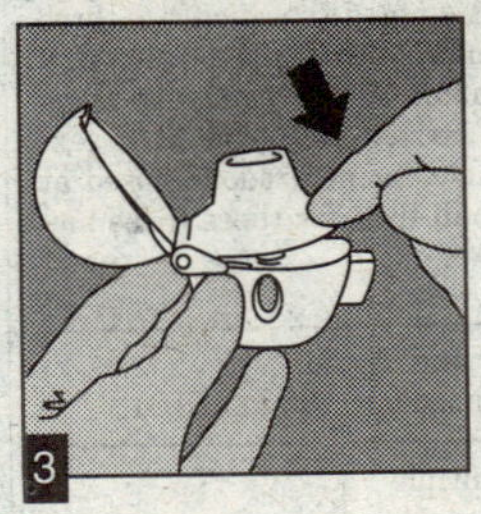

3) Close the mouthpiece **firmly until you hear a click,** leaving the dust cap open. (Figure 3)

Taking your dose of SPIRIVA.

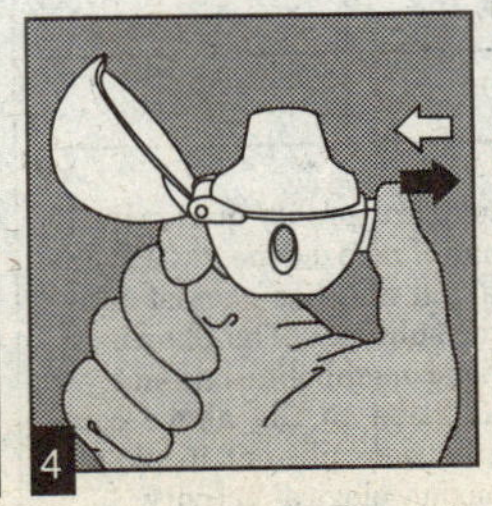

4) **PRESS: Hold the HandiHaler device with the mouthpiece upwards and press the piercing button completely in once, and release.** This makes holes in the capsule and allows the medication to be released when you breathe in. (Figure 4)

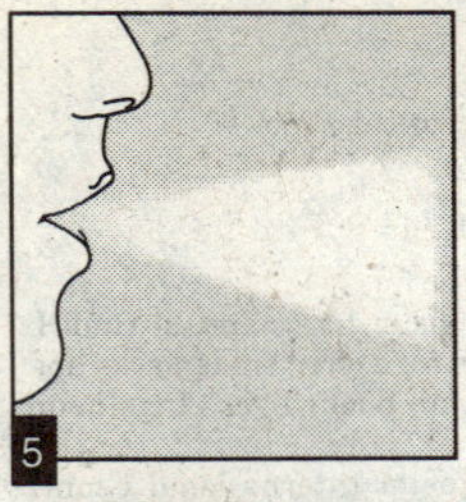

5) **Breathe out completely.** (Figure 5)
Important: Do not breathe into the mouthpiece at any time.

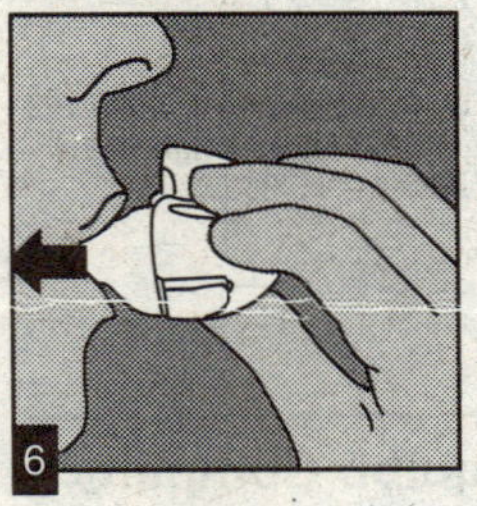

6) **INHALE:** Raise the HandiHaler device to your mouth and close your lips tightly around the mouthpiece. Keep your head in an upright position and breathe in slowly and deeply but at a rate **sufficient to hear the capsule vibrate.** Breathe in until your lungs are full; then hold your breath as long as is comfortable and at the same time take the HandiHaler device out of your mouth. Resume normal breathing. (Figure 6)

To ensure you get the full dose of SPIRIVA, you must repeat steps 5 and 6 once again.

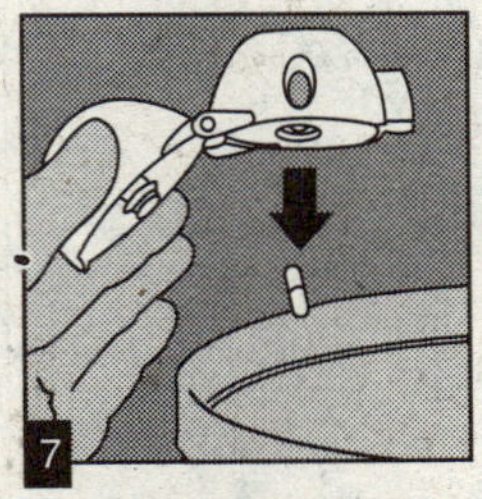

7) After you have finished taking your daily dose of SPIRIVA, open the mouthpiece again. Tip out the used capsule and dispose. (Figure 7)

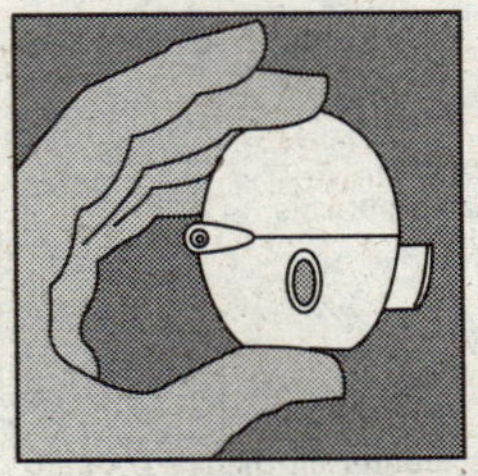

Close the mouthpiece and dust cap for storage of your HandiHaler device.

When and how should you clean your HandiHaler Device?

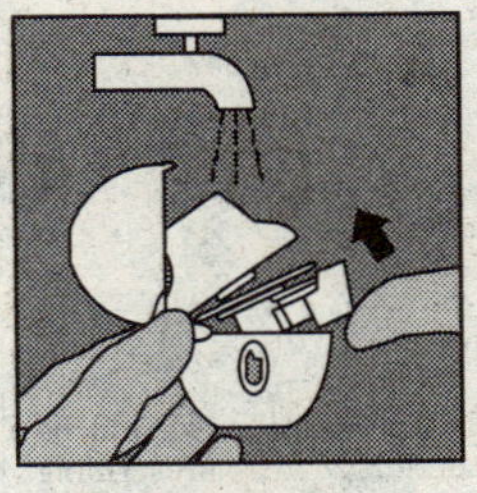

Normally, during a one-month period of use, the HandiHaler device does not need to be cleaned. However, if cleaning is needed the HandiHaler device can be cleaned as described below. Open the dust cap and mouthpiece. Open the base by lifting the piercing button. Rinse the complete inhaler with warm water to remove any powder. Do not use cleaning agents or detergents.
Dry the HandiHaler device thoroughly by tipping the excess water out on a paper towel and air-dry afterwards, leaving the dust cap, mouthpiece and base open. **It takes 24 hours to air dry, so clean it right after you use it and it will be ready for your next dose.** Do not use the HandiHaler device when it is wet.
If needed, the outside of the mouthpiece may be cleaned with a moist, but not wet tissue.
The HandiHaler device should not be placed in the dishwasher for cleaning.

Where should you store SPIRIVA capsules and the HandiHaler Device?

Store at 25°C (77°F); excursions permitted to 15–30°C (59–86°F) [see USP Controlled Room Temperature].
The capsules should not be exposed to extreme temperature or moisture. Do not store capsules in the HandiHaler.
As with all prescription medications, keep this out of the reach of children.

Tell your doctor before you use SPIRIVA HandiHaler:

if you may be pregnant or wish to become pregnant;
if you are a breastfeeding mother;
if you are taking any medications including eye drops, this includes those you can buy without a prescription;
if you have any other medical problems such as difficulty urinating or an enlarged prostate;
if you are allergic to any medications.

USE THIS PRODUCT AS DIRECTED, UNLESS INSTRUCTED TO DO OTHERWISE BY YOUR PHYSICIAN.

Manufactured by:
Boehringer Ingelheim Pharma GmbH & Co. KG
Ingelheim, Germany
Marketed by:

Continued on next page

Spiriva—Cont.

Boehringer Ingelheim Pharmaceuticals, Inc.
Ridgefield, CT 06877 USA
and
Pfizer Inc.
New York, NY 10017 USA
Licensed from Boehringer Ingelheim International GmbH.
SPIRIVA® and HandiHaler® are registered trademarks and are used under license from Boehringer Ingelheim International GmbH

Tiotropium bromide is covered by U.S. Patent No. 5,610,163 with other Patents Pending. The HandiHaler inhalation device is covered by U.S. Design Patient No. 355,029.
59873/US/1
January 2004

Bristol-Myers Squibb Company

P.O. BOX 4500
PRINCETON, NJ 08543-4500

For Medical Information Contact:

Generally:
Bristol-Myers Squibb Drug Information Department
P.O. Box 4500
Princeton, NJ 08543-4500
(800) 321-1335
(800) 426-7644 (Oncology/Virology)

Adverse Drug Experiences
and Product Defects Reporting call
between 8:30 AM–4:30 PM EST:
(609) 818-3737

Sales and Ordering:
Orders may be placed by:
1. Calling your purchase orders toll-free between 8:30 AM–5:00 PM EST:
(800) 631-5244
2. Mailing your purchase orders to:
Bristol-Myers Squibb U.S. Pharmaceuticals
Attn: Customer Service
P.O. Box 5250
Princeton, NJ 08543-5250
3. Faxing your purchase orders to:
(800) 523-2965
4. Transmitting computer-to-computer on the NWDA and UCS formats through Ordernet Services use: DEA#PE0048579

SERZONE® ℞

[*sər'zōn*]
(nefazodone hydrochloride) Tablets
Rx only
(Patient Information Included)

Before prescribing SERZONE, the physician should be thoroughly familiar with the details of this prescribing information.

WARNING

Cases of life-threatening hepatic failure have been reported in patients treated with SERZONE.

The reported rate in the United States is about 1 case of liver failure resulting in death or transplant per 250,000–300,000 patient-years of SERZONE treatment. The total patient-years is a summation of each patient's duration of exposure expressed in years. For example, 1 patient-year is equal to 2 patients each treated for 6 months, 3 patients each treated for 4 months, etc. (See WARNINGS.)

Ordinarily, treatment with SERZONE should not be initiated in individuals with active liver disease or with elevated baseline serum transaminases. There is no evidence that pre-existing liver disease increases the likelihood of developing liver failure, however, baseline abnormalities can complicate patient monitoring.

Patients should be advised to be alert for signs and symptoms of liver dysfunction (jaundice, anorexia, gastrointestinal complaints, malaise, etc.) and to report them to their doctor immediately if they occur.

SERZONE should be discontinued if clinical signs or symptoms suggest liver failure (see PRECAUTIONS: Information for Patients). Patients who develop evidence of hepatocellular injury such as increased serum AST or serum ALT levels ≥3 times the upper limit of NORMAL, while on SERZONE should be withdrawn from the drug. These patients should be presumed to be at increased risk for liver injury if SERZONE is reintroduced. Accordingly, such patients should not be considered for re-treatment.

DESCRIPTION

SERZONE® (nefazodone hydrochloride) is an antidepressant for oral administration with a chemical structure unrelated to selective serotonin reuptake inhibitors, tricyclics, tetracyclics, or monoamine oxidase inhibitors (MAOI).

Nefazodone hydrochloride is a synthetically derived phenylpiperazine antidepressant. The chemical name for nefazodone hydrochloride is 2-[3-[4-(3-chlorophenyl)-1-piperazinyl]propyl]-5-ethyl-2,4-dihydro-4-(2-phenoxyethyl)-3H-1,2,4-triazol-3-one monohydrochloride. The molecular formula is $C_{25}H_{32}ClN_5O_2$ • HCl, which corresponds to a molecular weight of 506.5. The structural formula is:

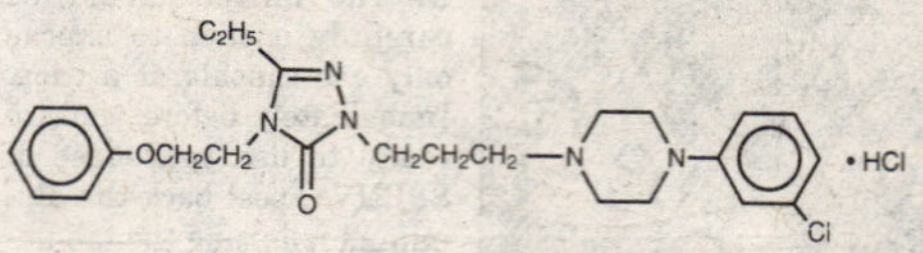

Nefazodone hydrochloride is a nonhygroscopic, white crystalline solid. It is freely soluble in chloroform, soluble in propylene glycol, and slightly soluble in polyethylene glycol and water.

SERZONE (nefazodone hydrochloride) is supplied as hexagonal tablets containing 50 mg, 100 mg, 150 mg, 200 mg, or 250 mg of nefazodone hydrochloride and the following inactive ingredients: microcrystalline cellulose, povidone, sodium starch glycolate, colloidal silicon dioxide, magnesium stearate, and iron oxides (red and/or yellow) as colorants.

CLINICAL PHARMACOLOGY

Pharmacodynamics

The mechanism of action of nefazodone, as with other antidepressants, is unknown.

Preclinical studies have shown that nefazodone inhibits neuronal uptake of serotonin and norepinephrine.

Nefazodone occupies central $5\text{-}HT_2$ receptors at nanomolar concentrations, and acts as an antagonist at this receptor. Nefazodone was shown to antagonize $alpha_1$-adrenergic receptors, a property which may be associated with postural hypotension. *In vitro* binding studies showed that nefazodone had no significant affinity for the following receptors: $alpha_2$ and beta adrenergic, $5\text{-}HT_{1A}$, cholinergic, dopaminergic, or benzodiazepine.

Pharmacokinetics

Nefazodone hydrochloride is rapidly and completely absorbed but is subject to extensive metabolism, so that its absolute bioavailability is low, about 20%, and variable. Peak plasma concentrations occur at about one hour and the half-life of nefazodone is 2–4 hours.

Both nefazodone and its pharmacologically similar metabolite, hydroxynefazodone, exhibit nonlinear kinetics for both dose and time, with AUC and C_{max} increasing more than proportionally with dose increases and more than expected upon multiple dosing over time, compared to single dosing. For example, in a multiple-dose study involving BID dosing with 50, 100, and 200 mg, the AUC for nefazodone and hydroxynefazodone increased by about 4-fold with an increase in dose from 200 to 400 mg per day; C_{max} increased by about 3-fold with the same dose increase. In a multiple-dose study involving BID dosing with 25, 50, 100, and 150 mg, the accumulation ratios for nefazodone and hydroxynefazodone AUC, after 5 days of BID dosing relative to the first dose, ranged from approximately 3 to 4 at the lower doses (50–100 mg/day) and from 5 to 7 at the higher doses (200–300 mg/day); there were also approximately 2- to 4-fold increases in C_{max} after 5 days of BID dosing relative to the first dose, suggesting extensive and greater than predicted accumulation of nefazodone and its hydroxy metabolite with multiple dosing. Steady-state plasma nefazodone and metabolite concentrations are attained within 4 to 5 days of initiation of BID dosing or upon dose increase or decrease.

Nefazodone is extensively metabolized after oral administration by n-dealkylation and aliphatic and aromatic hydroxylation, and less than 1% of administered nefazodone is excreted unchanged in urine. Attempts to characterize three metabolites identified in plasma, hydroxynefazodone (HO-NEF), meta-chlorophenylpiperazine (mCPP), and a triazoledione metabolite, have been carried out. The AUC (expressed as a multiple of the AUC for nefazodone dosed at 100 mg BID) and elimination half-lives for these three metabolites were as follows:

AUC Multiples and $T_{1/2}$ for Three Metabolites of Nefazodone (100 mg BID)

Metabolite	AUC Multiple	$T_{1/2}$
HO-NEF	0.4	1.5–4 h
mCPP	0.07	4–8 h
Triazole-dione	4.0	18 h

HO-NEF possesses a pharmacological profile qualitatively and quantitatively similar to that of nefazodone. mCPP has some similarities to nefazodone, but also has agonist activity at some serotonergic receptor subtypes. The pharmacological profile of the triazole-dione metabolite has not yet been well characterized. In addition to the above compounds, several other metabolites were present in plasma but have not been tested for pharmacological activity.

After oral administration of radiolabeled nefazodone, the mean half-life of total label ranged between 11 and 24 hours. Approximately 55% of the administered radioactivity was detected in urine and about 20–30% in feces.

Distribution—Nefazodone is widely distributed in body tissues, including the central nervous system (CNS). In humans the volume of distribution of nefazodone ranges from 0.22 to 0.87 L/kg.

Protein Binding—At concentrations of 25–2500 ng/mL nefazodone is extensively (>99%) bound to human plasma proteins *in vitro*. The administration of 200 mg BID of nefazodone for 1 week did not increase the fraction of unbound warfarin in subjects whose prothrombin times had been prolonged by warfarin therapy to 120–150% of the laboratory control (see **PRECAUTIONS: Drug Interactions**). While nefazodone did not alter the *in vitro* protein binding of chlorpromazine, desipramine, diazepam, diphenylhydantoin, lidocaine, prazosin, propranolol, or verapamil, it is unknown whether displacement of either nefazodone or these drugs occurs *in vivo*. There was a 5% decrease in the protein binding of haloperidol; this is probably of no clinical significance.

Effect of Food—Food delays the absorption of nefazodone and decreases the bioavailability of nefazodone by approximately 20%.

Renal Disease—In studies involving 29 renally impaired patients, renal impairment (creatinine clearances ranging from 7 to 60 mL/min/1.73m²) had no effect on steady-state nefazodone plasma concentrations.

Liver Disease—In a multiple-dose study of patients with liver cirrhosis, the AUC values for nefazodone and HO-NEF at steady state were approximately 25% greater than those observed in normal volunteers.

Age/Gender Effects—After single doses of 300 mg to younger (18–45 years) and older patients (>65 years), C_{max} and AUC for nefazodone and hydroxynefazodone were up to twice as high in the older patients. With multiple doses, however, differences were much smaller, 10–20%. A similar result was seen for gender, with a higher C_{max} and AUC in women after single doses but no difference after multiple doses.

Treatment with SERZONE (nefazodone hydrochloride) should be initiated at half the usual dose in elderly patients, especially women (see **DOSAGE AND ADMINISTRATION**), but the therapeutic dose range is similar in younger and older patients.

Clinical Efficacy Trial Results

Studies in Outpatients with Depression

During its premarketing development, the efficacy of SERZONE was evaluated at doses within the therapeutic range in five well-controlled, short-term (6–8 weeks) clinical investigations. These trials enrolled outpatients meeting DSM-III or DSM-IIIR criteria for major depression. Among these trials, two demonstrated the effectiveness of SERZONE, and two provided additional support for that conclusion.

One trial was a 6-week dose-titration study comparing SERZONE in two dose ranges (up to 300 mg/day and up to 600 mg/day [mean modal dose for this group was about 400 mg/day], on a BID schedule) and placebo. The second trial was an 8-week dose-titration study comparing SERZONE (up to 600 mg/day; mean modal dose was 375 mg/day), imipramine (up to 300 mg/day), and placebo, all on a BID schedule. Both studies demonstrated SERZONE, at doses titrated between 300 mg to 600 mg/day (therapeutic dose range), to be superior to placebo on at least three of the following four measures: 17-Item Hamilton Depression Rating Scale or HDRS (total score), Hamilton Depressed Mood item, Clinical Global Impressions (CGI) Severity score, and CGI Improvement score. Significant differences were also found for certain factors of the HDRS (e.g., anxiety factor, sleep disturbance factor, and retardation factor). In the two supportive studies, SERZONE was titrated up to 500 or 600 mg/day (mean modal doses of 462 mg/day and 363 mg/day). In the fifth study, the differentiation in response rates between SERZONE and placebo was not statistically significant. Three additional trials were conducted using subtherapeutic doses of SERZONE.

Overall, approximately two thirds of patients in these trials were women, and an analysis of the effects of gender on outcome did not suggest any differential responsiveness on the basis of sex. There were too few elderly patients in these trials to reveal possible age-related differences in response. Since its initial marketing as an antidepressant drug product, additional clinical investigations of SERZONE have been conducted. These studies explored SERZONE's use under conditions not evaluated fully at the time initial marketing approval was granted.

Studies in "Inpatients"

Two studies were conducted to evaluate SERZONE's effectiveness in hospitalized depressed patients. These were 6-week, dose-titration trials comparing SERZONE (up to 600 mg/day) and placebo, on a BID schedule. In one study, SERZONE was superior to placebo. In this study, the mean modal dose of SERZONE was 503 mg/day, and 85% of these inpatients were melancholic; at baseline, patients were distributed at the higher end of the 7-point CGI Severity scale, as follows: 4=moderately ill (17%); 5=markedly ill (48%); 6=severely ill (32%). In the other study, the differentiation in response rates between SERZONE and placebo was not statistically significant. This result may be explained by the "high" rate of spontaneous improvement among the patients randomized to placebo.

Studies of "Relapse Prevention in Patients Recently Recovered (Clinically) from Depression"

Two studies were conducted to assess SERZONE's capacity to maintain a clinical remission in acutely depressed patients who were judged to have responded adequately (HDRS total score ≤10) after a 16-week period of open treatment with SERZONE (titration up to 600 mg/day). In one study, SERZONE was superior to placebo. In this study, patients (n=131) were randomized to continuation on SERZONE or placebo for an additional 36 weeks (1 year total). This study demonstrated a significantly lower relapse rate (HDRS total score ≥18) for patients taking SERZONE compared to those on placebo. The second study was of appropriate design and power, but the sample of patients admitted for evaluation did not suffer relapses at a high enough incidence to provide a meaningful test of SERZONE's efficacy for this use.

Comparisons of Clinical Trial Results

Highly variable results have been seen in the clinical development of all antidepressant drugs. Furthermore, in those circumstances when the drugs have not been studied in the same controlled clinical trial(s), comparisons among the findings of studies evaluating the effectiveness of different antidepressant drug products are inherently unreliable. Because conditions of testing (e.g., patient samples, investigators, doses of the treatments administered and compared, outcome measures, etc.) vary among trials, it is virtually impossible to distinguish a difference in drug effect from a difference due to one or more of the confounding factors just enumerated.

INDICATIONS AND USAGE

SERZONE (nefazodone hydrochloride) is indicated for the treatment of depression.

The efficacy of SERZONE in the treatment of depression was established in 6–8 week controlled trials of outpatients and in a 6-week controlled trial of depressed inpatients whose diagnoses corresponded most closely to the DSM-III or DSM-IIIR category of major depressive disorder (see **CLINICAL PHARMACOLOGY**).

A major depressive episode implies a prominent and relatively persistent depressed or dysphoric mood that usually interferes with daily functioning (nearly every day for at least 2 weeks). It must include either depressed mood or loss of interest or pleasure and at least five of the following nine symptoms: depressed mood, loss of interest in usual activities, significant change in weight and/or appetite, insomnia or hypersomnia, psychomotor agitation or retardation, increased fatigue, feelings of guilt or worthlessness, slowed thinking or impaired concentration, a suicide attempt or suicidal ideation.

The efficacy of SERZONE in reducing relapse in patients with major depression who were judged to have had a satisfactory clinical response to 16 weeks of open-label SERZONE treatment for an acute depressive episode has been demonstrated in a randomized placebo-controlled trial (see **CLINICAL PHARMACOLOGY**). Although remitted patients were followed for as long as 36 weeks in the study cited (i.e., 52 weeks total), the physician who elects to use SERZONE for extended periods should periodically reevaluate the long-term usefulness of the drug for the individual patient.

CONTRAINDICATIONS

Coadministration of terfenadine, astemizole, cisapride, pimozide, or carbamazepine with SERZONE (nefazodone hydrochloride) is contraindicated (see **WARNINGS** and **PRECAUTIONS**).

SERZONE tablets are contraindicated in patients who were withdrawn from SERZONE because of evidence of liver injury (see **BOXED WARNING**). SERZONE tablets are also contraindicated in patients who have demonstrated hypersensitivity to nefazodone hydrochloride, its inactive ingredients, or other phenylpiperazine antidepressants.

The coadministration of triazolam and nefazodone causes a significant increase in the plasma level of triazolam (see **WARNINGS** and **PRECAUTIONS**), and a 75% reduction in the initial triazolam dosage is recommended if the two drugs are to be given together. Because not all commercially available dosage forms of triazolam permit a sufficient dosage reduction, the coadministration of triazolam and SERZONE should be avoided for most patients, including the elderly.

WARNINGS

Hepatotoxicity (See BOXED WARNING.)

Cases of life-threatening hepatic failure have been reported in patients treated with SERZONE.

The reported rate in the United States is about 1 case of liver failure resulting in death or transplant per 250,000–300,000 patient-years of use. This represents a rate of about 3–4 times the estimated background rate of liver failure. This rate is an underestimate because of under reporting, and the true risk could be considerably greater than this. A large cohort study of antidepressant users found no cases of liver failure leading to death or transplant among SERZONE users in about 30,000 patient-years of exposure. The spontaneous report data and the cohort study results provide estimates of the upper and lower limits of the risk of liver failure in nefazodone-treated patients, but are not capable of providing a precise risk estimate.

The time to liver injury for the reported liver failure cases resulting in death or transplant generally ranged from 2 weeks to 6 months on SERZONE therapy. Although some reports described dark urine and nonspecific prodromal symptoms (e.g., anorexia, malaise, and gastrointestinal symptoms), other reports did not describe the onset of clear prodromal symptoms prior to the onset of jaundice. The physician may consider the value of liver function testing. Periodic serum transaminase testing has not been proven to prevent serious injury but it is generally believed that early detection of drug-induced hepatic injury along with immediate withdrawal of the suspect drug enhances the likelihood for recovery.

Patients should be advised to be alert for signs and symptoms of liver dysfunction (jaundice, anorexia, gastrointestinal complaints, malaise, etc.) and to report them to their doctor immediately if they occur. Ongoing clinical assessment of patients should govern physician interventions, including diagnostic evaluations and treatment.

SERZONE (nefazodone hydrochloride) should be discontinued if clinical signs or symptoms suggest liver failure (see PRECAUTIONS: Information for Patients). Patients who develop evidence of hepatocellular injury such as increased serum AST or serum ALT levels ≥3 times the upper limit of NORMAL, while on SERZONE should be withdrawn from the drug. These patients should be presumed to be at increased risk for liver injury if SERZONE is reintroduced. Accordingly, such patients should not be considered for re-treatment.

Potential for Interaction with Monoamine Oxidase Inhibitors

In patients receiving antidepressants with pharmacological properties similar to nefazodone in combination with a monoamine oxidase inhibitor (MAOI), there have been reports of serious, sometimes fatal, reactions. For a selective serotonin reuptake inhibitor (SSRI), these reactions have included hyperthermia, rigidity, myoclonus, autonomic instability with possible rapid fluctuations of vital signs, and mental status changes that include extreme agitation progressing to delirium and coma. These reactions have also been reported in patients who have recently discontinued that drug and have been started on an MAOI. Some cases presented with features resembling neuroleptic malignant syndrome. Severe hyperthermia and seizures, sometimes fatal, have been reported in association with the combined use of tricyclic antidepressants and MAOIs. These reactions have also been reported in patients who have recently discontinued these drugs and have been started on an MAOI.

Although the effects of combined use of nefazodone and MAOI have not been evaluated in humans or animals, because nefazodone is an inhibitor of both serotonin and norepinephrine reuptake, it is recommended that nefazodone not be used in combination with an MAOI, or within 14 days of discontinuing treatment with an MAOI. At least 1 week should be allowed after stopping nefazodone before starting an MAOI.

Interaction with Triazolobenzodiazepines

Interaction studies of nefazodone with two triazolobenzodiazepines, i.e., triazolam and alprazolam, metabolized by cytochrome P450 3A4, have revealed substantial and clinically important increases in plasma concentrations of these compounds when administered concomitantly with nefazodone.

Triazolam

When a single oral 0.25-mg dose of triazolam was coadministered with nefazodone (200 mg BID) at steady state, triazolam half-life and AUC increased 4-fold and peak concentrations increased 1.7-fold. Nefazodone plasma concentrations were unaffected by triazolam. ***Coadministration of nefazodone potentiated the effects of triazolam on psychomotor performance tests.*** If triazolam is coadministered with SERZONE, a 75% reduction in the initial triazolam dosage is recommended. Because not all commercially available dosage forms of triazolam permit sufficient dosage reduction, coadministration of triazolam with SERZONE should be avoided for most patients, including the elderly. In the exceptional case where coadministration of triazolam with SERZONE may be considered appropriate, only the lowest possible dose of triazolam should be used (see **CONTRAINDICATIONS** and **PRECAUTIONS**).

Alprazolam

When alprazolam (1 mg BID) and nefazodone (200 mg BID) were coadministered, steady-state peak concentrations, AUC and half-life values for alprazolam increased by approximately 2-fold. Nefazodone plasma concentrations were unaffected by alprazolam. If alprazolam is coadministered with SERZONE, a 50% reduction in the initial alprazolam dosage is recommended. No dosage adjustment is required for SERZONE (nefazodone hydrochloride).

Potential Terfenadine, Astemizole, Cisapride, and Pimozide Interactions

Terfenadine, astemizole, cisapride, and pimozide are all metabolized by the cytochrome P450 3A4 (CYP3A4) isozyme, and it has been demonstrated that ketoconazole, erythromycin, and other inhibitors of CYP3A4 can block the metabolism of these drugs, which can result in increased plasma concentrations of parent drug. Increased plasma concentrations of terfenadine, astemizole, cisapride, and pimozide are associated with QT prolongation and with rare cases of serious cardiovascular adverse events, including death, due principally to ventricular tachycardia of the torsades de pointes type. Nefazodone has been shown *in vitro* to be an inhibitor of CYP3A4. Consequently, it is recommended that nefazodone not be used in combination with either terfenadine, astemizole, cisapride, or pimozide (see CONTRAINDICATIONS and PRECAUTIONS).

Interaction with Carbamazepine

The coadministration of carbamazepine 200 mg BID with nefazodone 200 mg BID, at steady state for both drugs, resulted in almost 95% reductions in AUCs for nefazodone and hydroxynefazodone, likely resulting in insufficient plasma nefazodone and hydroxynefazodone concentrations for achieving an antidepressant effect for SERZONE. Consequently, it is recommended that SERZONE not be used in combination with carbamazepine (see **CONTRAINDICATIONS** and **PRECAUTIONS**).

PRECAUTIONS

General

Hepatotoxicity (See **BOXED WARNING.**)

Postural Hypotension

A pooled analysis of the vital signs monitored during placebo-controlled premarketing studies revealed that 5.1% of nefazodone patients compared to 2.5% of placebo patients (p≤0.01) met criteria for a potentially important decrease in blood pressure at some time during treatment (systolic blood pressure ≤90 mmHg *and* a change from baseline of ≥20 mmHg). While there was no difference in the proportion of nefazodone and placebo patients having adverse events characterized as 'syncope' (nefazodone, 0.2%; placebo, 0.3%), the rates for adverse events characterized as 'postural hypotension' were as follows: nefazodone (2.8%), tricyclic antidepressants (10.9%), SSRI (1.1%), and placebo (0.8%). Thus, the prescriber should be aware that there is some risk of postural hypotension in association with nefazodone use. SERZONE (nefazodone hydrochloride) should be used with caution in patients with known cardiovascular or cerebrovascular disease that could be exacerbated by hypotension (history of myocardial infarction, angina, or ischemic stroke) and conditions that would predispose patients to hypotension (dehydration, hypovolemia, and treatment with antihypertensive medication).

Activation of Mania/Hypomania

During premarketing testing, hypomania or mania occurred in 0.3% of nefazodone-treated unipolar patients, compared to 0.3% of tricyclic- and 0.4% of placebo-treated patients. In patients classified as bipolar the rate of manic episodes was 1.6% for nefazodone, 5.1% for the combined tricyclic-treated groups, and 0% for placebo-treated patients. Activation of mania/hypomania is a known risk in a small proportion of patients with major affective disorder treated with other marketed antidepressants. As with all antidepressants, SERZONE should be used cautiously in patients with a history of mania.

Suicide

The possibility of a suicide attempt is inherent in depression and may persist until significant remission occurs. Close supervision of high-risk patients should accompany initial drug therapy. Prescriptions for SERZONE should be written for the smallest quantity of tablets consistent with good patient management in order to reduce the risk of overdose.

Seizures

During premarketing testing, a recurrence of a petit mal seizure was observed in a patient receiving nefazodone who had a history of such seizures. In addition, one nonstudy participant reportedly experienced a convulsion (type not documented) following a multiple-drug overdose (see **OVERDOSAGE**). Rare occurrences of convulsions (including grand mal seizures) following nefazodone administration have been reported since market introduction. A causal relationship to nefazodone has not been established (see **ADVERSE REACTIONS**).

Priapism

While priapism did not occur during premarketing experience with nefazodone, rare reports of priapism have been received since market introduction. A causal relationship to nefazodone has not been established (see **ADVERSE REACTIONS**). If patients present with prolonged or inappropriate erections, they should discontinue therapy immediately and consult their physicians. If the condition persists for more than 24 hours, a urologist should be consulted to determine appropriate management.

Use in Patients with Concomitant Illness

SERZONE (nefazodone hydrochloride) has not been evaluated or used to any appreciable extent in patients with a recent history of myocardial infarction or unstable heart disease. Patients with these diagnoses were systematically excluded from clinical studies during the product's premarketing testing. Evaluation of electrocardiograms of 1153 patients who received nefazodone in 6- to 8-week, double-blind, placebo-controlled trials did not indicate that nefazodone is associated with the development of clinically important ECG abnormalities. However, sinus bradycardia, defined as heart rate ≤50 bpm and a decrease of at least 15 bpm from baseline, was observed in 1.5% of nefazodone-treated patients compared to 0.4% of placebo-treated patients (p≤0.05). Because patients with a recent history of myocardial infarction or unstable heart disease were excluded from clinical trials, such patients should be treated with caution.

In patients with cirrhosis of the liver, the AUC values of nefazodone and HO-NEF were increased by approximately 25%.

Information for Patients (See Patient Information.)

Physicians are advised to discuss the following issues with patients for whom they prescribe SERZONE:

Hepatotoxicity

Patients should be informed that SERZONE therapy has been associated with liver abnormalities ranging from asymptomatic reversible serum transaminase increases to cases of liver failure resulting in transplant and/or death. At present, there is no way to predict who is likely to develop liver failure. Ordinarily, patients with active liver disease should not be treated with SERZONE. Patients should be

Continued on next page

Serzone—Cont.

advised to be alert for signs of liver dysfunction (jaundice, anorexia, gastrointestinal complaints, malaise, etc.) and to report them to their doctor immediately if they occur.

Time to Response/Continuation

As with all antidepressants, several weeks on treatment may be required to obtain the full antidepressant effect. Once improvement is noted, it is important for patients to continue drug treatment as directed by their physician.

Interference With Cognitive and Motor Performance

Since any psychoactive drug may impair judgment, thinking, or motor skills, patients should be cautioned about operating hazardous machinery, including automobiles, until they are reasonably certain that SERZONE therapy does not adversely affect their ability to engage in such activities.

Pregnancy

Patients should be advised to notify their physician if they become pregnant or intend to become pregnant during therapy.

Nursing

Patients should be advised to notify their physician if they are breast-feeding an infant (see **PRECAUTIONS: Nursing Mothers**).

Concomitant Medication

Patients should be advised to inform their physicians if they are taking, or plan to take, any prescription or over-the-counter drugs, since there is a potential for interactions. Significant caution is indicated if SERZONE is to be used in combination with XANAX®, concomitant use with HALCION® should be avoided for most patients including the elderly, and concomitant use with SELDANE®, HISMANAL®, PROPULSID®, ORAP®, or TEGRETOL® is contraindicated (see **CONTRAINDICATIONS** and **WARNINGS**).

Alcohol

Patients should be advised to avoid alcohol while taking SERZONE (nefazodone hydrochloride).

Allergic Reactions

Patients should be advised to notify their physician if they develop a rash, hives, or a related allergic phenomenon.

Visual Disturbances

There have been reports of visual disturbances associated with the use of nefazodone, including blurred vision, scotoma, and visual trails. Patients should be advised to notify their physician if they develop visual disturbances. (See **ADVERSE REACTIONS**.)

Laboratory Tests

There are no specific laboratory tests recommended.

Drug Interactions

Drugs Highly Bound to Plasma Protein

Because nefazodone is highly bound to plasma protein (see **CLINICAL PHARMACOLOGY: Pharmacokinetics**), administration of SERZONE (nefazodone hydrochloride) to a patient taking another drug that is highly protein bound may cause increased free concentrations of the other drug, potentially resulting in adverse events. Conversely, adverse effects could result from displacement of nefazodone by other highly bound drugs.

Warfarin—There were no effects on the prothrombin or bleeding times or upon the pharmacokinetics of R-warfarin when nefazodone (200 mg BID) was administered for 1 week to subjects who had been pretreated for 2 weeks with warfarin. Although the coadministration of nefazodone did decrease the subjects' exposure to S-warfarin by 12%, the lack of effects on the prothrombin and bleeding times indicates this modest change is not clinically significant. Although these results suggest no adjustments in warfarin dosage are required when nefazodone is administered to patients stabilized on warfarin, such patients should be monitored as required by standard medical practices.

CNS-Active Drugs

Monoamine Oxidase Inhibitors—See **WARNINGS**.

Haloperidol—When a single oral 5-mg dose of haloperidol was coadministered with nefazodone (200 mg BID) at steady state, haloperidol apparent clearance decreased by 35% with no significant increase in peak haloperidol plasma concentrations or time of peak. This change is of unknown clinical significance. Pharmacodynamic effects of haloperidol were generally not altered significantly. There were no changes in the pharmacokinetic parameters for nefazodone. Dosage adjustment of haloperidol may be necessary when coadministered with nefazodone.

Lorazepam—When lorazepam (2 mg BID) and nefazodone (200 mg BID) were coadministered to steady state, there was no change in any pharmacokinetic parameter for either drug compared to each drug administered alone. Therefore, dosage adjustment is not necessary for either drug when coadministered.

Triazolam/Alprazolam—See **CONTRAINDICATIONS** and **WARNINGS**.

Alcohol—Although nefazodone did not potentiate the cognitive and psychomotor effects of alcohol in experiments with normal subjects, the concomitant use of SERZONE (nefazodone hydrochloride) and alcohol in depressed patients is not advised.

Buspirone—In a study of steady-state pharmacokinetics in healthy volunteers, coadministration of buspirone (2.5 or 5 mg BID) with nefazodone (250 mg BID) resulted in marked increases in plasma buspirone concentrations (increases up to 20-fold in C_{max} and up to 50-fold in AUC) and statistically significant decreases (about 50%) in plasma concentrations of the buspirone metabolite 1-pyrimidinylpiperazine. With 5-mg BID doses of buspirone, slight increases in AUC were observed for nefazodone (23%) and its metabolites hydroxynefazodone (17%) and mCPP (9%). Subjects receiving nefazodone 250 mg BID and buspirone 5 mg b.i.d. experienced lightheadedness, asthenia, dizziness, and somnolence, adverse events also observed with either drug alone. If the two drugs are to be used in combination, a low dose of buspirone (eg, 2.5 mg q.d.) is recommended. Subsequent dose adjustment of either drug should be based on clinical assessment.

Pimozide—See **CONTRAINDICATIONS**, **WARNINGS**, and **PRECAUTIONS:** *Pharmacokinetics of Nefazodone in 'Poor Metabolizers' and Potential Interaction with Drugs that Inhibit and/or Are Metabolized by Cytochrome P450 Isozymes.*

Fluoxetine—When fluoxetine (20 mg QD) and nefazodone (200 mg BID) were administered at steady state there were no changes in the pharmacokinetic parameters for fluoxetine or its metabolite, norfluoxetine. Similarly, there were no changes in the pharmacokinetic parameters of nefazodone or HO-NEF; however, the mean AUC levels of the nefazodone metabolites mCPP and triazole-dione increased by 3- to 6-fold and 1.3-fold, respectively. When a 200-mg dose of nefazodone was administered to subjects who had been receiving fluoxetine for 1 week, there was an increased incidence of transient adverse events such as headache, lightheadedness, nausea, or paresthesia, possibly due to the elevated mCPP levels. Patients who are switched from fluoxetine to nefazodone without an adequate washout period may experience similar transient adverse events. The possibility of this happening can be minimized by allowing a washout period before initiating nefazodone therapy and by reducing the initial dose of nefazodone. Because of the long half-life of fluoxetine and its metabolites, this washout period may range from one to several weeks depending on the dose of fluoxetine and other individual patient variables.

Phenytoin—Pretreatment for 7 days with 200 mg BID of nefazodone had no effect on the pharmacokinetics of a single 300-mg oral dose of phenytoin. However, due to the nonlinear pharmacokinetics of phenytoin, the failure to observe a significant effect on the single-dose pharmacokinetics of phenytoin does not preclude the possibility of a clinically significant interaction with nefazodone when phenytoin is dosed chronically. However, no change in the initial dosage of phenytoin is considered necessary and any subsequent adjustment of phenytoin dosage should be guided by usual clinical practices.

Desipramine—When nefazodone (150 mg BID) and desipramine (75 mg QD) were administered together there were no changes in the pharmacokinetics of desipramine or its metabolite, 2-hydroxy desipramine. There were also no changes in the pharmacokinetics of nefazodone or its triazole-dione metabolite, but the AUC and C_{max} of mCPP increased by 44% and 48%, respectively, while the AUC of HO-NEF decreased by 19%. No changes in doses of either nefazodone or desipramine are necessary when the two drugs are given concomitantly. Subsequent dose adjustments should be made on the basis of clinical response.

Lithium—In 13 healthy subjects the coadministration of nefazodone (200 mg BID) with lithium (500 mg BID) for 5 days (steady-state conditions) was found to be well tolerated. When the two drugs were coadministered, there were no changes in the steady-state pharmacokinetics of either lithium, nefazodone, or its metabolite HO-NEF; however, there were small decreases in the steady-state plasma concentrations of two nefazodone metabolites, mCPP and triazole-dione, which are considered not to be of clinical significance. Therefore, no dosage adjustment of either lithium or nefazodone is required when they are coadministered.

Carbamazepine—The coadministration of nefazodone (200 mg BID) for 5 days to 12 healthy subjects on carbamazepine who had achieved steady state (200 mg BID) was found to be well tolerated. Steady-state conditions for carbamazepine, nefazodone, and several of their metabolites were achieved by day 5 of coadministration. With coadministration of the two drugs there were significant increases in the steady-state C_{max} and AUC of carbamazepine (23% and 23%, respectively), while the steady-state C_{max} and the AUC of the carbamazepine metabolite, 10,11 epoxycarbamazepine, decreased by 21% and 20%, respectively. The coadministration of the two drugs significantly reduced the steady-state C_{max} and AUC of nefazodone by 86% and 93%, respectively. Similar reductions in the C_{max} and AUC of HO-NEF were also observed (85% and 94%), while the reductions in C_{max} and AUC of mCPP and triazole-dione were more modest (13% and 44% for the former and 28% and 57% for the latter). Due to the potential for coadministration of carbamazepine to result in insufficient plasma nefazodone and hydroxynefazodone concentrations for achieving an antidepressant effect for SERZONE (nefazodone hydrochloride), it is recommended that SERZONE not be used in combination with carbamazepine (see **CONTRAINDICATIONS** and **WARNINGS**).

General Anesthetics—Little is known about the potential for interaction between nefazodone and general anesthetics; therefore, prior to elective surgery, SERZONE should be discontinued for as long as clinically feasible.

Other CNS-Active Drugs—The use of nefazodone in combination with other CNS-active drugs has not been systematically evaluated. Consequently, caution is advised if concomitant administration of SERZONE and such drugs is required.

Cimetidine

When nefazodone (200 mg BID) and cimetidine (300 mg QID) were coadministered for one week, no change in the steady-state pharmacokinetics of either nefazodone or cimetidine was observed compared to each dosed alone. Therefore, dosage adjustment is not necessary for either drug when coadministered.

Theophylline

When nefazodone (200 mg BID) was given to patients being treated with theophylline (600–1200 mg/day) for chronic obstructive pulmonary disease, there was no change in the steady-state pharmacokinetics of either nefazodone or theophylline. FEV_1 measurements taken when theophylline and nefazodone were coadministered did not differ from baseline dosage (i.e., when theophylline was administered alone). Therefore, dosage adjustment is not necessary for either drug when coadministered.

Cardiovascular-Active Drugs

Digoxin—When nefazodone (200 mg BID) and digoxin (0.2 mg QD) were coadministered for 9 days to healthy male volunteers (n=18) who were phenotyped as CYP2D6 extensive metabolizers, C_{max}, C_{min}, and AUC of digoxin were increased by 29%, 27%, and 15%, respectively. Digoxin had no effects on the pharmacokinetics of nefazodone and its active metabolites. Because of the narrow therapeutic index of digoxin, caution should be exercised when nefazodone and digoxin are coadministered; plasma level monitoring for digoxin is recommended.

Propranolol—The coadministration of nefazodone (200 mg BID) and propranolol (40 mg BID) for 5.5 days to healthy male volunteers (n=18), including 3 poor and 15 extensive CYP2D6 metabolizers, resulted in 30% and 14% reductions in C_{max} and AUC of propranolol, respectively, and a 14% reduction in C_{max} for the metabolite, 4-hydroxypropranolol. The kinetics of nefazodone, hydroxynefazodone, and triazole-dione were not affected by coadministration of propranolol. However, C_{max}, C_{min}, and AUC of m-chlorophenylpiperazine were increased by 23%, 54%, and 28%, respectively. No change in initial dose of either drug is necessary and dose adjustments should be made on the basis of clinical response.

HMG-CoA Reductase Inhibitors—When single 40-mg doses of simvastatin or atorvastatin, both substrates of CYP3A4, were given to healthy adult volunteers who had received SERZONE 200 mg BID for 6 days, approximately 20-fold increases in plasma concentrations of simvastatin and simvastatin acid and 3- to 4-fold increases in plasma concentrations of atorvastatin and atorvastatin lactone were seen. These effects appear to be due to the inhibition of CYP3A4 by SERZONE (nefazodone hydrochloride) because, in the same study, SERZONE had no significant effect on the plasma concentrations of pravastatin, which is not metabolized by CYP3A4 to a clinically significant extent.

There have been rare reports of rhabdomyolysis involving patients receiving the combination of SERZONE and either simvastatin or lovastatin, also a substrate of CYP3A4 (see **ADVERSE REACTIONS: Postintroduction Clinical Experience**). Rhabdomyolysis has been observed in patients receiving HMG-CoA reductase inhibitors administered alone (at recommended dosages) and in particular, for certain drugs in this class, when given in combination with inhibitors of the CYP3A4 isozyme.

Caution should be used if SERZONE is administered in combination with HMG-CoA reductase inhibitors that are metabolized by CYP3A4, such as simvastatin, atorvastatin, and lovastatin, and dosage adjustments of these HMG-CoA reductase inhibitors are recommended. Since metabolic interactions are unlikely between SERZONE (nefazodone hydrochloride) and HMG-CoA reductase inhibitors that undergo little or no metabolism by the CYP3A4 isozyme, such as pravastatin or fluvastatin, dosage adjustments should not be necessary.

Immunosuppressive Agents

There have been reports of increased blood concentrations of cyclosporine and tacrolimus into toxic ranges when patients received these drugs concomitantly with SERZONE. Both cyclosporine and tacrolimus are substrates of CYP3A4, and nefazodone is known to inhibit this enzyme. If either cyclosporine or tacrolimus is administered with SERZONE, blood concentrations of the immunosuppressive agent should be monitored and dosage adjusted accordingly.

Pharmacokinetics of Nefazodone in 'Poor Metabolizers' and Potential Interaction with Drugs that Inhibit and/or Are Metabolized by Cytochrome P450 Isozymes

CYP3A4 Isozyme—Nefazodone has been shown *in vitro* to be an inhibitor of CYP3A4. This is consistent with the interactions observed between nefazodone and triazolam, alprazolam, buspirone, atorvastatin, and simvastatin, drugs metabolized by this isozyme. Consequently, caution is indicated in the combined use of nefazodone with any drugs known to be metabolized by CYP3A4. In particular, the combined use of nefazodone with triazolam should be avoided for most patients, including the elderly. The combined use of nefazodone with terfenadine, astemizole, cisapride, or pimozide is contraindicated (see **CONTRAINDICATIONS** and **WARNINGS**).

CYP2D6 Isozyme—A subset (3% to 10%) of the population has reduced activity of the drug-metabolizing enzyme CYP2D6. Such individuals are referred to commonly as "poor metabolizers" of drugs such as debrisoquin, dextromethorphan, and the tricyclic antidepressants. The pharmacokinetics of nefazodone and its major metabolites are not altered in these "poor metabolizers." Plasma concentrations of one minor metabolite (mCPP) are increased in this population; the adjustment of SERZONE dosage is not required when administered to "poor metabolizers." Nefazodone and its metabolites have been shown *in vitro* to

be extremely weak inhibitors of CYP2D6. Thus, it is not likely that nefazodone will decrease the metabolic clearance of drugs metabolized by this isozyme.
CYP1A2 Isozyme—Nefazodone and its metabolites have been shown *in vitro* not to inhibit CYP1A2. Thus, metabolic interactions between nefazodone and drugs metabolized by this isozyme are unlikely.

Electroconvulsive Therapy (ECT)
There are no clinical studies of the combined use of ECT and nefazodone.

Carcinogenesis, Mutagenesis, Impairment of Fertility

Carcinogenesis
There is no evidence of carcinogenicity with nefazodone. The dietary administration of nefazodone to rats and mice for 2 years at daily doses of up to 200 mg/kg and 800 mg/kg, respectively, which are approximately 3 and 6 times, respectively, the maximum human daily dose on a mg/m^2 basis, produced no increase in tumors.

Mutagenesis
Nefazodone has been shown to have no genotoxic effects based on the following assays: bacterial mutation assays, a DNA repair assay in cultured rat hepatocytes, a mammalian mutation assay in Chinese hamster ovary cells, an *in vivo* cytogenetics assay in rat bone marrow cells, and a rat dominant lethal study.

Impairment of Fertility
A fertility study in rats showed a slight decrease in fertility at 200 mg/kg/day (approximately three times the maximum human daily dose on a mg/m^2 basis) but not at 100 mg/kg/day (approximately 1.5 times the maximum human daily dose on a mg/m^2 basis).

Pregnancy

Teratogenic Effects—Pregnancy Category C
Reproduction studies have been performed in pregnant rabbits and rats at daily doses up to 200 and 300 mg/kg, respectively (approximately 6 and 5 times, respectively, the maximum human daily dose on a mg/m^2 basis). No malformations were observed in the offspring as a result of nefazodone treatment. However, increased early pup mortality was seen in rats at a dose approximately five times the maximum human dose, and decreased pup weights were seen at this and lower doses, when dosing began during pregnancy and continued until weaning. The cause of these deaths is not known. The no-effect dose for rat pup mortality was 1.3 times the human dose on a mg/m^2 basis. There are no adequate and well-controlled studies in pregnant women. Nefazodone should be used during pregnancy only if the potential benefit justifies the potential risk to the fetus.

Labor and Delivery
The effect of SERZONE (nefazodone hydrochloride) on labor and delivery in humans is unknown.

Nursing Mothers
It is not known whether SERZONE or its metabolites are excreted in human milk. Because many drugs are excreted in human milk, caution should be exercised when SERZONE is administered to a nursing woman.

Pediatric Use
Safety and effectiveness in individuals below 18 years of age have not been established.

Geriatric Use
Of the approximately 7000 patients in clinical studies who received SERZONE for the treatment of depression, 18% were 65 years and older, while 5% were 75 years and older. Based on monitoring of adverse events, vital signs, electrocardiograms, and results of laboratory tests, no overall differences in safety between elderly and younger patients were observed in clinical studies. Efficacy in the elderly has not been demonstrated in placebo-controlled trials. Other reported clinical experience has not identified differences in responses between elderly and younger patients, but greater sensitivity of some older individuals cannot be ruled out.
Due to the increased systemic exposure to nefazodone seen in single-dose studies in elderly patients (see **CLINICAL PHARMACOLOGY: Pharmacokinetics**), treatment should be initiated at half the usual dose, but titration upward should take place over the same range as in younger patients (see **DOSAGE AND ADMINISTRATION**). The usual precautions should be observed in elderly patients who have concomitant medical illnesses or who are receiving concomitant drugs.

ADVERSE REACTIONS

Associated with Discontinuation of Treatment
Approximately 16% of the 3496 patients who received SERZONE (nefazodone hydrochloride) in worldwide premarketing clinical trials discontinued treatment due to an adverse experience. The more common (≥1%) events in clinical trials associated with discontinuation and considered to be drug related (i.e., those events associated with dropout at a rate approximately twice or greater for SERZONE compared to placebo) included: nausea (3.5%), dizziness (1.9%), insomnia (1.5%), asthenia (1.3%), and agitation (1.2%).

Incidence in Controlled Trials

Commonly Observed Adverse Events in Controlled Clinical Trials
The most commonly observed adverse events associated with the use of SERZONE (incidence of 5% or greater) and not seen at an equivalent incidence among placebo-treated patients (i.e., significantly higher incidence for SERZONE compared to placebo, p≤0.05), derived from the table below, were: somnolence, dry mouth, nausea, dizziness, constipation, asthenia, lightheadedness, blurred vision, confusion, and abnormal vision.

Treatment-Emergent Adverse Experience Incidence in 6- to 8-Week Placebo-Controlled Clinical Trials[1], SERZONE 300 to 600 mg/day Dose Range

Body System	Preferred Term	Percent of Patients SERZONE (n=393)	Placebo (n=394)
Body as a Whole	Headache	36	33
	Asthenia	11	5
	Infection	8	6
	Flu syndrome	3	2
	Chills	2	1
	Fever	2	1
	Neck rigidity	1	0
Cardiovascular	Postural hypotension	4	1
	Hypotension	2	1
Dermatological	Pruritus	2	1
	Rash	2	1
Gastrointestinal	Dry mouth	25	13
	Nausea	22	12
	Constipation	14	8
	Dyspepsia	9	7
	Diarrhea	8	7
	Increased appetite	5	3
	Nausea & vomiting	2	1
Metabolic	Peripheral edema	3	2
	Thirst	1	<1
Musculoskeletal	Arthralgia	1	<1
Nervous	Somnolence	25	14
	Dizziness	17	5
	Insomnia	11	9
	Lightheadedness	10	3
	Confusion	7	2
	Memory impairment	4	2
	Paresthesia	4	2
	Vasodilatation[2]	4	2
	Abnormal dreams	3	2
	Concentration decreased	3	1
	Ataxia	2	0
	Incoordination	2	1
	Psychomotor retardation	2	1
	Tremor	2	1
	Hypertonia	1	0
	Libido decreased	1	<1
Respiratory	Pharyngitis	6	5
	Cough increased	3	1
Special Senses	Blurred vision	9	3
	Abnormal vision[3]	7	1
	Tinnitus	2	1
	Taste perversion	2	1
	Visual field defect	2	0
Urogenital	Urinary frequency	2	1
	Urinary tract infection	2	1
	Urinary retention	2	1
	Vaginitis[4]	2	1
	Breast pain[4]	1	<1

[1] Events reported by at least 1% of patients treated with SERZONE and more frequent than the placebo group are included; incidence is rounded to the nearest 1% (<1% indicates an incidence less than 0.5%). Events for which the SERZONE (nefazodone hydrochloride) incidence was equal to or less than placebo are not listed in the table, but included the following: abdominal pain, pain, back pain, accidental injury, chest pain, neck pain, palpitation, migraine, sweating, flatulence, vomiting, anorexia, tooth disorder, weight gain, edema, myalgia, cramp, agitation, anxiety, depression, hypesthesia, CNS stimulation, dysphoria, emotional lability, sinusitis, rhinitis, dysmenorrhea[4], dysuria.
[2] Vasodilatation—flushing, feeling warm.
[3] Abnormal vision—scotoma, visual trails.
[4] Incidence adjusted for gender.

Adverse Events Occurring at an Incidence of 1% or More Among SERZONE-Treated Patients
The table that follows enumerates adverse events that occurred at an incidence of 1% or more, and were more frequent than in the placebo group, among SERZONE-treated patients who participated in short-term (6- to 8-week) placebo-controlled trials in which patients were dosed with SERZONE to ranges of 300 to 600 mg/day. This table shows the percentage of patients in each group who had at least one episode of an event at some time during their treatment. Reported adverse events were classified using standard COSTART-based Dictionary terminology.
The prescriber should be aware that these figures cannot be used to predict the incidence of side effects in the course of usual medical practice where patient characteristics and other factors differ from those which prevailed in the clinical trials. Similarly, the cited frequencies cannot be compared with figures obtained from other clinical investigations involving different treatments, uses, and investigators. The cited figures, however, do provide the prescribing physician with some basis for estimating the relative contribution of drug and nondrug factors to the side-effect incidence rate in the population studied.
[See table above]

Dose Dependency of Adverse Events
The table that follows enumerates adverse events that were more frequent in the SERZONE (nefazodone hydrochloride) dose range of 300 to 600 mg/day than in the SERZONE dose range of up to 300 mg/day. This table shows only those adverse events for which there was a statistically significant difference (p≤0.05) in incidence between the SERZONE dose ranges as well as a difference between the high dose range and placebo.
[See table at top of next page]

Visual Disturbances
In controlled clinical trials, blurred vision occurred in 9% of nefazodone-treated patients compared to 3% of placebo-treated patients. In these same trials abnormal vision, including scotomata and visual trails, occurred in 7% of nefazodone-treated patients compared to 1% of placebo-treated (see Treatment-Emergent Adverse Experience table, above). Dose-dependency was observed for these events in these trials, with none of the scotomata and visual trails at doses below 300 mg/day. However, scotomata and visual trails observed at doses below 300 mg/day have been reported in postmarketing experience with SERZONE. (See **PRECAUTIONS: Information for Patients.**)

Vital Sign Changes
(See **PRECAUTIONS**, *Postural Hypotension*.)

Weight Changes
In a pooled analysis of placebo-controlled premarketing studies, there were no differences between nefazodone and placebo groups in the proportions of patients meeting criteria for potentially important increases or decreases in body weight (a change of ≥7%).

Laboratory Changes
Of the serum chemistry, serum hematology, and urinalysis parameters monitored during placebo-controlled premarketing studies with nefazodone, a pooled analysis revealed a statistical trend between nefazodone and placebo for hematocrit, i.e., 2.8% of nefazodone patients met criteria for a potentially important decrease in hematocrit (≤37% male or ≤32% female) compared to 1.5% of placebo patients (0.05<p≤0.10). Decreases in hematocrit, presumably dilutional, have been reported with many other drugs that block alpha$_1$-adrenergic receptors. There was no apparent clinical significance of the observed changes in the few patients meeting these criteria.

ECG Changes
Of the ECG parameters monitored during placebo-controlled premarketing studies with nefazodone, a pooled analysis revealed a statistically significant difference between nefazodone and placebo for sinus bradycardia, i.e.,

Continued on next page

Serzone—Cont.

1.5% of nefazodone patients met criteria for a potentially important decrease in heart rate (≤50 bpm and a decrease of ≥15 bpm) compared to 0.4% of placebo patients ($p<0.05$). There was no obvious clinical significance of the observed changes in the few patients meeting these criteria.

Other Events Observed During the Premarketing Evaluation of SERZONE

During its premarketing assessment, multiple doses of SERZONE (nefazodone hydrochloride) were administered to 3496 patients in clinical studies, including more than 250 patients treated for at least one year. The conditions and duration of exposure to SERZONE varied greatly, and included (in overlapping categories) open and double-blind studies, uncontrolled and controlled studies, inpatient and outpatient studies, fixed-dose and titration studies. Untoward events associated with this exposure were recorded by clinical investigators using terminology of their own choosing. Consequently, it is not possible to provide a meaningful estimate of the proportion of individuals experiencing adverse events without first grouping similar types of untoward events into a smaller number of standardized event categories.

In the tabulations that follow, reported adverse events were classified using standard COSTART-based Dictionary terminology. The frequencies presented, therefore, represent the proportion of the 3496 patients exposed to multiple doses of SERZONE who experienced an event of the type cited on at least one occasion while receiving SERZONE. All reported events are included except those already listed in the Treatment-Emergent Adverse Experience Incidence table, those events listed in other safety-related sections of this insert, those adverse experiences subsumed under COSTART terms that are either overly general or excessively specific so as to be uninformative, those events for which a drug cause was very remote, and those events which were not serious and occurred in fewer than two patients.

It is important to emphasize that, although the events reported occurred during treatment with SERZONE (nefazodone hydrochloride), they were not necessarily caused by it.

Events are further categorized by body system and listed in order of decreasing frequency according to the following definitions: frequent adverse events are those occurring on one or more occasions in at least 1/100 patients (only those not already listed in the tabulated results from placebo-controlled trials appear in this listing); infrequent adverse events are those occurring in 1/100 to 1/1000 patients; rare events are those occurring in fewer than 1/1000 patients.

Body as a whole—Infrequent: allergic reaction, malaise, photosensitivity reaction, face edema, hangover effect, abdomen enlarged, hernia, pelvic pain, and halitosis. *Rare:* cellulitis.

Cardiovascular system—Infrequent: tachycardia, hypertension, syncope, ventricular extrasystoles, and angina pectoris. *Rare:* AV block, congestive heart failure, hemorrhage, pallor, and varicose vein.

Dermatological system—Infrequent: dry skin, acne, alopecia, urticaria, maculopapular rash, vesiculobullous rash, and eczema.

Gastrointestinal system—Frequent: gastroenteritis. *Infrequent:* eructation, periodontal abscess, abnormal liver function tests, gingivitis, colitis, gastritis, mouth ulceration, stomatitis, esophagitis, peptic ulcer, and rectal hemorrhage. *Rare:* glossitis, hepatitis, dysphagia, gastrointestinal hemorrhage, oral moniliasis, and ulcerative colitis.

Hemic and lymphatic system—Infrequent: ecchymosis, anemia, leukopenia, and lymphadenopathy.

Metabolic and nutritional system—Infrequent: weight loss, gout, dehydration, lactic dehydrogenase increased, SGOT increased, and SGPT increased. *Rare:* hypercholesteremia and hypoglycemia.

Musculoskeletal system—Infrequent: arthritis, tenosynovitis, muscle stiffness, and bursitis. *Rare:* tendinous contracture.

Nervous system—Infrequent: vertigo, twitching, depersonalization, hallucinations, suicide attempt, apathy, euphoria, hostility, suicidal thoughts, abnormal gait, thinking abnormal, attention decreased, derealization, neuralgia, paranoid reaction, dysarthria, increased libido, suicide, and myoclonus. *Rare:* hyperkinesia, increased salivation, cerebrovascular accident, hyperesthesia, hypotonia, ptosis, and neuroleptic malignant syndrome.

Respiratory system—Frequent: dyspnea and bronchitis. *Infrequent:* asthma, pneumonia, laryngitis, voice alteration, epistaxis, hiccup. *Rare:* hyperventilation and yawn.

Special senses—Frequent: eye pain. *Infrequent:* dry eye, ear pain, abnormality of accommodation, diplopia, conjunctivitis, mydriasis, keratoconjunctivitis, hyperacusis, and photophobia. *Rare:* deafness, glaucoma, night blindness, and taste loss.

Urogenital system—Frequent: impotence[a]. *Infrequent:* cystitis, urinary urgency, metrorrhagia[a], amenorrhea[a], polyuria, vaginal hemorrhage[a], breast enlargement[a], menorrhagia[a], urinary incontinence, abnormal ejaculation[a], hematuria, nocturia, and kidney calculus. *Rare:* uterine fibroids enlarged[a], uterine hemorrhage[a], anorgasmia, and oliguria.

[a]Adjusted for gender.

Postintroduction Clinical Experience

Postmarketing experience with SERZONE (nefazodone hydrochloride) has shown an adverse experience profile similar to that seen during the premarketing evaluation of nefazodone. Voluntary reports of adverse events temporally associated with SERZONE have been received since market introduction that are not listed above and for which a causal relationship has not been established. These include: Anaphylactic reactions; angioedema; convulsions (including grand mal seizures); galactorrhea; gynecomastia (male); hyponatremia; liver necrosis and liver failure, in some cases leading to liver transplantation and/or death (see **WARNINGS**); priapism (see **PRECAUTIONS**); prolactin increased; rhabdomyolysis involving patients receiving the combination of SERZONE and lovastatin or simvastatin (see **PRECAUTIONS**); serotonin syndrome; and Stevens-Johnson syndrome; and thrombocytopenia.

Dose Dependency of Adverse Events in Placebo-Controlled Trials[1]

Body System	Preferred Term	SERZONE 300–600 mg/day (n=209)	SERZONE ≤300 mg/day (n=211)	Placebo (n=212)
		Percent of Patients		
Gastrointestinal	Nausea	23	14	12
	Constipation	17	10	9
Nervous	Somnolence	28	16	13
	Dizziness	22	11	4
	Confusion	8	2	1
Special Senses	Abnormal vision	10	0	2
	Blurred vision	9	3	2
	Tinnitus	3	0	1

[1] Events for which there was a statistically significant difference ($p\leq0.05$) between the nefazodone dose groups.

DRUG ABUSE AND DEPENDENCE

Controlled Substance Class

SERZONE (nefazodone hydrochloride) is not a controlled substance.

Physical and Psychological Dependence

In animal studies, nefazodone did not act as a reinforcer for intravenous self-administration in monkeys trained to self-administer cocaine, suggesting no abuse liability. In a controlled study of abuse liability in human subjects, nefazodone showed no potential for abuse.

Nefazodone has not been systematically studied in humans for its potential for tolerance, physical dependence, or withdrawal. While the premarketing clinical experience with nefazodone did not reveal any tendency for a withdrawal syndrome or any drug-seeking behavior, it is not possible to predict on the basis of this limited experience the extent to which a CNS-active drug will be misused, diverted, and/or abused once marketed. Consequently, physicians should carefully evaluate patients for a history of drug abuse and follow such patients closely, observing them for signs of misuse or abuse of SERZONE (e.g., development of tolerance, dose escalation, drug-seeking behavior).

OVERDOSAGE

Human Experience

In premarketing clinical studies, there were seven reports of nefazodone overdose alone or in combination with other pharmacological agents. The amount of nefazodone ingested ranged from 1000 mg to 11,200 mg. Commonly reported symptoms from overdose of nefazodone included nausea, vomiting, and somnolence. One nonstudy participant took 2000–3000 mg of nefazodone with methocarbamol and alcohol; this person reportedly experienced a convulsion (type not documented). None of these patients died.

In postmarketing experience, overdose with SERZONE alone and in combination with alcohol and/or other substances has been reported. Commonly reported symptoms were similar to those reported from overdose in premarketing experience. While there have been rare reports of fatalities in patients taking overdoses of nefazodone, predominantly in combination with alcohol and/or other substances, no causal relationship to nefazodone has been established.

Overdosage Management

Treatment should consist of those general measures employed in the management of overdosage with any antidepressant.

Ensure an adequate airway, oxygenation, and ventilation. Monitor cardiac rhythm and vital signs. General supportive and symptomatic measures are also recommended. Induction of emesis is not recommended. Gastric lavage with a large-bore orogastric tube with appropriate airway protection, if needed, may be indicated if performed soon after ingestion, or in symptomatic patients.

Activated charcoal should be administered. Due to the wide distribution of nefazodone in body tissues, forced diuresis, dialysis, hemoperfusion, and exchange transfusion are unlikely to be of benefit. No specific antidotes for nefazodone are known.

In managing overdosage, consider the possibility of multiple drug involvement. The physician should consider contacting a poison control center for additional information on the treatment of any overdose. Telephone numbers for certified poison control centers are listed in the *Physicians' Desk Reference* (PDR).

DOSAGE AND ADMINISTRATION

Initial Treatment

The recommended starting dose for SERZONE (nefazodone hydrochloride) is 200 mg/day, administered in two divided doses (BID). In the controlled clinical trials establishing the antidepressant efficacy of SERZONE, the effective dose range was generally 300 to 600 mg/day. Consequently, most patients, depending on tolerability and the need for further clinical effect, should have their dose increased. Dose increases should occur in increments of 100 mg/day to 200 mg/day, again on a BID schedule, at intervals of no less than 1 week. As with all antidepressants, several weeks on treatment may be required to obtain a full antidepressant response.

Dosage for Elderly or Debilitated Patients

The recommended initial dose for elderly or debilitated patients is 100 mg/day, administered in two divided doses (BID). These patients often have reduced nefazodone clearance and/or increased sensitivity to the side effects of CNS-active drugs. It may also be appropriate to modify the rate of subsequent dose titration. As steady-state plasma levels do not change with age, the final target dose based on a careful assessment of the patient's clinical response may be similar in healthy younger and older patients.

Maintenance/Continuation/Extended Treatment

There is no body of evidence available from controlled trials to indicate how long the depressed patient should be treated with SERZONE. It is generally agreed, however, that pharmacological treatment for acute episodes of depression should continue for up to 6 months or longer. Whether the dose of antidepressant needed to induce remission is identical to the dose needed to maintain euthymia is unknown. Systematic evaluation of the efficacy of SERZONE has shown that efficacy is maintained for periods of up to 36 weeks following 16 weeks of open-label acute treatment (treated for 52 weeks total) at dosages that averaged 438 mg/day. For most patients, their maintenance dose was that associated with response during acute treatment. (See **CLINICAL PHARMACOLOGY**.) The safety of SERZONE in long-term use is supported by data from both double-blind and open-label trials involving more than 250 patients treated for at least one year.

Switching Patients to or from a Monoamine Oxidase Inhibitor

At least 14 days should elapse between discontinuation of an MAOI and initiation of therapy with SERZONE. In addition, at least 7 days should be allowed after stopping SERZONE before starting an MAOI.

HOW SUPPLIED

SERZONE® tablets are hexagonal tablets imprinted with BMS and the strength (i.e., 100 mg) on one side and the identification code number on the other. The 100 mg and 150 mg tablets are bisect scored on both tablet faces. The 50 mg, 200 mg, and 250 mg tablets are unscored.

NDC CODE	*DESCRIPTION*
NDC 0087-0031-47	50 mg light pink tablet, bottle of 60
NDC 0087-0032-31	100 mg white tablet, bottle of 60
NDC 0087-0039-31	150 mg peach tablet, bottle of 60
NDC 0087-0033-31	200 mg light yellow tablet, bottle of 60
NDC 0087-0041-31	250 mg white tablet, bottle of 60

Store at room temperature, below 40° C (104° F) and dispense in a tight container.

Bristol-Myers Squibb Company

Rx only

PATIENT INFORMATION SERZONE®

(nefazodone hydrochloride) Tablets

Read this information completely before using SERZONE. Read the information each time you get more medicine. There may be new information. This leaflet provides a summary about SERZONE and does not include everything there is to know about your medicine. This information is not meant to take the place of talking with your doctor.

Before taking this medication, be sure to check the tablets in the bottle to make sure they match one of the following descriptions:

- **50 mg** tablets are six-sided, **light pink** tablets imprinted with "BMS" and "50" on one face of the tablet;
- **100 mg** tablets are six-sided, **white** tablets imprinted with "BMS" and "100" on one face of the tablet;
- **150 mg** tablets are six-sided, **peach-colored** tablets imprinted with "BMS" and "150" on one face of the tablet;
- **200 mg** tablets are six-sided, **light yellow** tablets imprinted with "BMS" and "200" on one face of the tablet; and
- **250 mg** tablets are six-sided, **white** tablets imprinted with "BMS" and "250" on one face of the tablet.

What is the most important information that I should know about SERZONE?

Rarely, people who take SERZONE can develop serious liver problems. **If you get any of the following symptoms while taking SERZONE, call your doctor right away** because you may be developing a liver problem:

- Yellowing of the skin or whites of eyes (jaundice)

- Unusually dark urine
- Loss of appetite that lasts several days or longer
- Nausea
- Abdominal (lower stomach) pain

People who currently have liver problems should not take SERZONE.

What is SERZONE?

SERZONE (pronounced *sir-ZONE*) is a medicine used to treat depression. SERZONE is thought to treat depression by correcting an imbalance in the amounts of certain natural chemicals, such as serotonin and norepinephrine, which are in your brain.

Who should not take SERZONE?

Do ***not*** take SERZONE if you

- are allergic to SERZONE or the related medicine Desyrel® (trazodone).
- are taking Seldane® (terfenadine), an antihistamine; Hismanal® (astemizole), an antihistamine; Propulsid® (cisapride), used for heartburn; Halcion® (triazolam), used for insomnia; Orap® (pimozide), used to treat Tourette's syndrome; or Tegretol® (carbamazepine), used to control seizures.
- currently have liver problems.
- are taking or have taken within the last 14 days one of the medicines for depression known as monoamine oxidase inhibitors (MAOIs), such as Nardil® or Parnate®.

Be sure to tell your doctor if you

- have ever had liver problems;
- are taking ***any*** other medicine, vitamin supplement, or herbal remedy, including those sold without a prescription (over-the-counter);
- have heart problems or have had a heart attack or stroke;
- have had manic episodes (extreme agitation or excitability);
- have ever attempted suicide;
- have had convulsions (seizures);
- are pregnant or breast-feeding.

How should I take SERZONE?

- Take SERZONE at the same time every day exactly as prescribed by your doctor. You may take SERZONE with or without food.
- It may take a while for you to feel that SERZONE is working. You may not feel the full effect for several weeks. Once you feel better, it is important to keep taking SERZONE as directed by your doctor.
- If you miss a dose of SERZONE, skip that dose and continue with your regular schedule. Never take 2 doses at the same time.
- If you think that you have taken more SERZONE than prescribed, contact your doctor, local poison control center, or emergency room right away.

What should I avoid while taking SERZONE?

- Do not drive or operate possibly dangerous machinery (such as an automobile, power mower, or power tool) or participate in any hazardous activity that requires full mental alertness until you know how SERZONE affects you.
- Before taking SERZONE, tell your doctor about ***any*** medicines you are taking, including vitamin supplements, herbal remedies, and any non-prescription (over-the-counter) medicines. Some of these medicines may affect how SERZONE works and should not be used in combination without talking to your doctor.
- Do not drink alcoholic beverages while taking SERZONE.
- Tell your doctor if you are pregnant, planning to become pregnant, or become pregnant while taking SERZONE. It is not known whether SERZONE can harm your unborn baby.
- Talk with your doctor before taking SERZONE if you are breast-feeding. It is not known whether SERZONE can pass through your breast milk to the baby.

What are the possible side effects of SERZONE?

The most common side effects of SERZONE (nefazodone hydrochloride) are sleepiness, dry mouth, nausea, dizziness, constipation, weakness, lightheadedness, problems with vision, and confusion.

Call your doctor right away if you have any of the following side effects:

- Yellowing of the skin or whites of eyes (jaundice)
- Unusually dark urine
- Loss of appetite that lasts several days or longer
- Severe nausea
- Abdominal (lower stomach) pain
- Rash or hives
- Seizure (convulsion)
- Fainting
- Erection that lasts too long

Tell your doctor right away about any side effects that you have or discomfort that you experience. Do not change your dose or stop taking SERZONE without talking with your doctor first.

Medicines are sometimes prescribed for conditions that are not mentioned in patient information leaflets. Your doctor has prescribed SERZONE for you and you alone. Do not give SERZONE to other people, even if they have the same condition. It may harm them.

This leaflet provides a summary of the most important information about SERZONE. If you would like more information, talk with your doctor or pharmacist. You can ask for information about SERZONE that is written for healthcare professionals. You can also get more information by visiting *www.serzone.com*.

Serzone® (nefazodone hydrochloride) is a registered trademark of Bristol-Myers Squibb Company. Other brand names listed are trademarks of their respective owners and are not trademarks of Bristol-Myers Squibb Company.

Bristol-Myers Squibb Company
Princeton, NJ 08543 U.S.A.

This Patient Information Leaflet has been approved by the U.S. Food and Drug Administration.

Revised September 2003 0032DIM-23
D5-B0001-09-03

STADOL® Ⓒ ℞
(butorphanol tartrate)
Injection, USP

STADOL NS®
(butorphanol tartrate)
Nasal Spray

DESCRIPTION

Butorphanol tartrate is a synthetically derived opioid agonist-antagonist analgesic of the phenanthrene series. The chemical name is (-)-17-(cyclobutylmethyl) morphinan-3, 14-diol [S-(R*,R*)] - 2,3 - dihydroxybutanedioate (1:1) (salt). The molecular formula is $C_{21}H_{29}NO_2{,}C_4H_6O_6$, which corresponds to a molecular weight of 477.55 and the following structural formula:

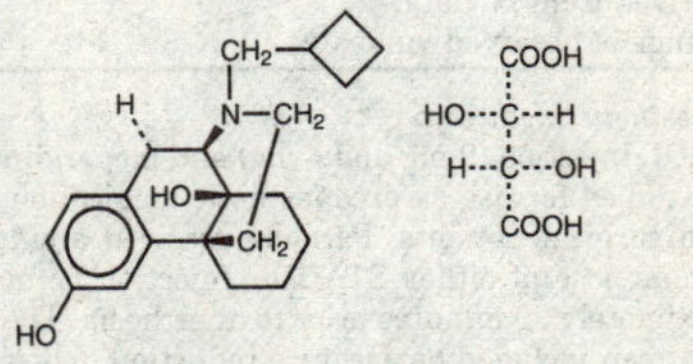

Butorphanol tartrate is a white crystalline substance. The dose is expressed as the tartrate salt. One milligram of the salt is equivalent to 0.68 mg of the free base. The n-octanol/aqueous buffer partition coefficient of butorphanol is 180:1 at pH 7.5.

STADOL (butorphanol tartrate) Injection, USP, is a sterile, parenteral, aqueous solution of butorphanol tartrate for intravenous or intramuscular administration. In addition to 1 or 2 mg of butorphanol tartrate, each mL of solution contains 3.3 mg of citric acid, 6.4 mg sodium citrate, and 6.4 mg sodium chloride, and 0.1 mg benzethonium chloride (in multiple dose vial only) as a preservative.

STADOL NS (butorphanol tartrate) Nasal Spray is an aqueous solution of butorphanol tartrate for administration as a metered spray to the nasal mucosa. Each bottle of STADOL NS contains 2.5 mL of a 10 mg/mL solution of butorphanol tartrate with sodium chloride, citric acid, and benzethonium chloride in purified water with sodium hydroxide and/or hydrochloric acid added to adjust the pH to 5.0. The pump reservoir must be fully primed (see **PATIENT INSTRUCTIONS**) prior to initial use. After initial priming, each metered spray delivers an average of 1.0 mg of butorphanol tartrate and the 2.5-mL bottle will deliver an average of 14–15 doses of STADOL NS. If not used for 48 hours or longer, the unit must be reprimed (see **PATIENT INSTRUCTIONS**). With intermittent use requiring repriming before each dose, the 2.5-mL bottle will deliver an average of 8–10 doses of STADOL NS depending on how much repriming is necessary.

CLINICAL PHARMACOLOGY

General Pharmacology and Mechanism of Action

Butorphanol is a mixed agonist-antagonist with low intrinsic activity at receptors of the μ-opioid type (morphine-like). It is also an agonist at κ-opioid receptors.

Its interactions with these receptors in the central nervous system apparently mediate most of its pharmacologic effects, including analgesia.

In addition to analgesia, CNS effects include depression of spontaneous respiratory activity and cough, stimulation of the emetic center, miosis, and sedation. Effects possibly mediated by non-CNS mechanisms include alteration in cardiovascular resistance and capacitance, bronchomotor tone, gastrointestinal secretory and motor activity, and bladder sphincter activity.

In an animal model, the dose of butorphanol tartrate required to antagonize morphine analgesia by 50% was similar to that for nalorphine, less than that for pentazocine and more than that for naloxone.

The pharmacological activity of butorphanol metabolites has not been studied in humans; in animal studies, butorphanol metabolites have demonstrated some analgesic activity.

In human studies of butorphanol (see **Clinical Trials**), sedation is commonly noted at doses of 0.5 mg or more. Narcosis is produced by 10–12 mg doses of butorphanol administered over 10–15 minutes intravenously.

Butorphanol, like other mixed agonist-antagonists with a high affinity for the κ-receptor, may produce unpleasant psychotomimetic effects in some individuals.

Nausea and/or vomiting may be produced by doses of 1 mg or more administered by any route.

In human studies involving individuals without significant respiratory dysfunction, 2 mg of butorphanol IV and 10 mg of morphine sulfate IV depressed respiration to a comparable degree. At higher doses, the magnitude of respiratory depression with butorphanol is not appreciably increased; however, the duration of respiratory depression is longer. Respiratory depression noted after administration of butorphanol to humans by any route is reversed by treatment with naloxone, a specific opioid antagonist (see **OVERDOSAGE: Treatment**).

Butorphanol tartrate demonstrates antitussive effects in animals at doses less than those required for analgesia.

Hemodynamic changes noted during cardiac catheterization in patients receiving single 0.025 mg/kg intravenous doses of butorphanol have included increases in pulmonary artery pressure, wedge pressure and vascular resistance, increases in left ventricular end diastolic pressure, and in systemic arterial pressure.

Pharmacodynamics

The analgesic effect of butorphanol is influenced by the route of administration. Onset of analgesia is within a few minutes for intravenous administration, within 15 minutes for intramuscular injection, and within 15 minutes for the nasal spray doses.

Peak analgesic activity occurs within 30–60 minutes following intravenous and intramuscular administration and within 1–2 hours following the nasal spray administration.

The duration of analgesia varies depending on the pain model as well as the route of administration, but is generally 3–4 hours with IM and IV doses as defined by the time 50% of patients required remedication. In postoperative studies, the duration of analgesia with IV or IM butorphanol was similar to morphine, meperidine, and pentazocine when administered in the same fashion at equipotent doses (see **Clinical Trials**). Compared to the injectable form and other drugs in this class, STADOL NS has a longer duration of action (4–5 hours) (see **Clinical Trials**).

Pharmacokinetics

STADOL Injection is rapidly absorbed after IM injection and peak plasma levels are reached in 20–40 minutes.

After nasal administration, mean peak blood levels of 0.9–1.04 ng/mL occur at 30–60 minutes after a 1 mg dose (see Table 1). The absolute bioavailability of STADOL NS is 60–70% and is unchanged in patients with allergic rhinitis. In patients using a nasal vasoconstrictor (oxymetazoline), the fraction of the dose absorbed was unchanged, but the rate of absorption was slowed. The peak plasma concentrations were approximately half those achieved in the absence of the vasoconstrictor.

Following its initial absorption/distribution phase, the single dose pharmacokinetics of butorphanol by the intravenous, intramuscular, and nasal routes of administration are similar (see Figure 1).

Figure 1—Butorphanol Plasma Levels After IV, IM, and Nasal Spray Administration of 2-mg Dose

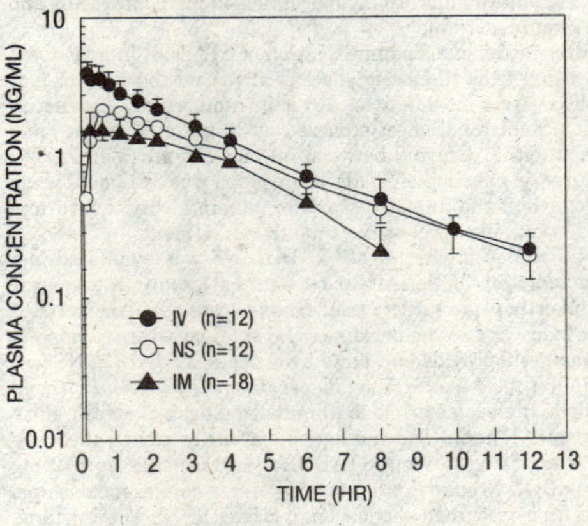

Serum protein binding is independent of concentration over the range achieved in clinical practice (up to 7 ng/mL) with a bound fraction of approximately 80%.

The volume of distribution of butorphanol varies from 305–901 liters and total body clearance from 52–154 liters/hour (see Table 1).

[See table 1 at top of next page]

Dose proportionality for STADOL NS has been determined at steady state in doses up to 4 mg at 6 hour intervals. Steady state is achieved within 2 days. The mean peak plasma concentration at steady state was 1.8-fold (maximal 3-fold) following a single dose.

The drug is transported across the blood brain and placental barriers and into human milk (see **PRECAUTIONS: Labor and Delivery** and **Nursing Mothers**).

Butorphanol is extensively metabolized in the liver. Metabolism is qualitatively and quantitatively similar following intravenous, intramuscular, or nasal administration. Oral bioavailability is only 5–17% because of extensive first pass metabolism of butorphanol.

The major metabolite of butorphanol is hydroxybutorphanol, while norbutorphanol is produced in small amounts. Both have been detected in plasma following administration of butorphanol, with norbutorphanol present at trace levels at most time points. The elimination half-life of hydroxybutorphanol is about 18 hours and, as a consequence, considerable accumulation (~5-fold) occurs when butorphanol is dosed to steady state (1 mg transnasally q6h for 5 days).

Continued on next page

Stadol—Cont.

Elimination occurs by urine and fecal excretion. When ^3H labeled butorphanol is administered to normal subjects, most (70–80%) of the dose is recovered in the urine, while approximately 15% is recovered in the feces.

About 5% of the dose is recovered in the urine as butorphanol. Forty-nine percent is eliminated in the urine as hydroxybutorphanol. Less than 5% is excreted in the urine as norbutorphanol.

Butorphanol pharmacokinetics in the elderly differ from younger patients (see Table 1). The mean absolute bioavailability of STADOL NS in elderly women (48%) was less than that in elderly men (75%), young men (68%), or young women (70%). Elimination half-life is increased in the elderly (6.6 hours as opposed to 4.7 hours in younger subjects).

In renally impaired patients with creatinine clearances <30 mL/min, the elimination half-life was approximately doubled and the total body clearance was approximately one half (10.5 hours [clearance 150 L/h] compared to 5.8 hours [clearance 260 L/h] in healthy subjects). No effect on C_{max} or T_{max} was observed after a single dose.

After intravenous administration to patients with hepatic impairment, the elimination half-life of butorphanol was approximately tripled and total body clearance was approximately one half (half-life 16.8 hours, clearance 92 L/h) compared to healthy subjects (half-life 4.8 hours, clearance 175 L/h). The exposure of hepatically impaired patients to butorphanol was significantly greater (about 2-fold) than that in healthy subjects. Similar results were seen after nasal administration. No effect on C_{max} or T_{max} was observed after a single intranasal dose.

For further recommendations, refer to **PRECAUTIONS: Hepatic and Renal Disease, Drug Interactions,** and **Geriatric Use** and **CLINICAL PHARMACOLOGY: Individualization of Dosage.**

Table 1—
Mean Pharmacokinetic Parameters of Butorphanol in Young and Elderly Subjects[a]

	Intravenous		Nasal	
Parameters	Young	Elderly	Young	Elderly
T_{max}[b] (h)			0.62 (0.32)[e] (0.15-1.50)[g]	1.03 (0.74) (0.25-3.00)
C_{max}[c] (ng/mL)			1.04 (0.40) (0.35-1.97)	0.90 (0.57) (0.10-2.68)
AUC (inf)[d] (h•ng/mL)	7.24 (1.57) (4.40-9.77)	8.71 (2.02) (4.76-13.03)	4.93 (1.24) (2.16-7.27)	5.24 (2.27) (0.30-10.34)
Half-life (h)	4.56 (1.67) (2.06-8.70)	5.61 (1.36) (3.25-8.79)	4.74 (1.57) (2.89-8.79)	6.56 (1.51) (3.75-9.17)
Absolute Bioavailability (%)			69 (16) (44-113)	61 (25) (3-121)
Volume of Distribution[f] (L)	487 (155) (305-901)	552 (124) (305-737)		
Total Body Clearance (L/h)	99 (23) (70-154)	82 (21) (52-143)		

(a) Young subjects (n = 24) are from 20 to 40 years old and elderly (n = 24) are greater than 65 years of age.
(b) Time to peak plasma concentration.
(c) Peak plasma concentration normalized to 1 mg dose.
(d) Area under the plasma concentration-time curve after a 1 mg dose.
(e) Mean (1 S.D.)
(f) Derived from IV data.
(g) (range of observed values)

Clinical Trials

The effectiveness of opioid analgesics varies in different pain syndromes. Studies with STADOL Injection have been performed in postoperative (primarily abdominal and orthopedic) pain and pain during labor and delivery, as preoperative and preanesthetic medication, and as a supplement to balanced anesthesia (see below).

Studies with STADOL NS have been performed in postoperative (general, orthopedic, oral, cesarean section) pain, in postepisiotomy pain, in pain of musculoskeletal origin, and in migraine headache pain (see below).

Use in the Management of Pain

Postoperative pain: The analgesic efficacy of STADOL Injection in postoperative pain was investigated in several double-blind active-controlled studies involving 958 butorphanol-treated patients. The following doses were found to have approximately equivalent analgesic effect: 2 mg butorphanol, 10 mg morphine, 40 mg pentazocine and 80 mg meperidine.

After intravenous administration of STADOL Injection, onset and peak analgesic effect occurred by the time of first observation (30 minutes). After intramuscular administration, pain relief onset occurred at 30 minutes or less, and peak effect occurred between 30 minutes and 1 hour. The duration of action of STADOL Injection was 3–4 hours when defined as the time necessary for pain intensity to return to pretreatment level or the time to retreatment.

The analgesic efficacy of STADOL NS was evaluated (approximately 35 patients per treatment group) in a general and orthopedic surgery trial. Single doses of STADOL NS (1 or 2 mg) and IM meperidine (37.5 or 75 mg) were compared. Analgesia provided by 1 and 2 mg doses of STADOL NS was similar to 37.5 and 75 mg meperidine, respectively, with onset of analgesia within 15 minutes and peak analgesic effect within 1 hour. The median duration of pain relief was 2.5 hours with 1 mg STADOL NS, 3.5 hours with 2 mg STADOL NS and 3.3 hours with either dose of meperidine.

In a postcesarean section trial, STADOL NS administered to 35 patients as two 1-mg doses 60 minutes apart was compared with a single 2-mg dose of STADOL NS or a single 2-mg IV dose of STADOL Injection (37 patients each). Onset of analgesia was within 15 minutes for all STADOL regimens. Peak analgesic effects of 2 mg intravenous STADOL Injection and STADOL NS were similar in magnitude.

The duration of pain relief provided by both 2-mg STADOL NS regimens was approximately 4.5 hours and was greater than intravenous STADOL Injection (2.6 hours).

Migraine headache pain: The analgesic efficacy of two 1-mg doses 1 hour apart of STADOL NS in migraine headache pain was compared with a single dose of 10 mg IM methadone (31 and 32 patients, respectively). Significant onset of analgesia occurred within 15 minutes for both STADOL NS and IM methadone. Peak analgesic effect occurred at 2 hours for STADOL NS and 1.5 hours for methadone. The median duration of pain relief was 6 hours with STADOL NS and 4 hours with methadone as judged by the time when approximately half of the patients remedicated.

In two other trials in patients with migraine headache pain, a 2-mg initial dose of STADOL NS followed by an additional 1-mg dose 1 hour later (76 patients) was compared with either 75 mg IM meperidine (24 patients) or placebo (72 patients). Onset, peak activity, and duration were similar with both active treatments; however, the incidence of adverse experiences (nausea, vomiting, dizziness) was higher in these two trials with the 2-mg initial dose of STADOL NS than in the trial with the 1-mg initial dose.

Preanesthetic Medication

STADOL Injection (2 mg and 4 mg) and meperidine (80 mg) were studied for use as preanesthetic medication in hospitalized surgical patients. Patients received a single intramuscular dose of either STADOL Injection or meperidine approximately 90 minutes prior to anesthesia. The anesthesia regimen included barbiturate induction, followed by nitrous oxide and oxygen with halothane or enflurane, with or without a muscle relaxant.

Anesthetic preparation was rated as satisfactory in all 42 STADOL Injection patients regardless of the type of surgery.

Balanced Anesthesia

STADOL Injection administered intravenously (mean dose 2 mg) was compared to intravenous morphine sulfate (mean dose 10 mg) as premedication shortly before thiopental induction, followed by balanced anesthesia in 50 ASA Class 1 and 2 patients. Anesthesia was then maintained by repeated intravenous doses, averaging 4.6 mg STADOL Injection and 22.8 mg morphine per patient.

Anesthetic induction and maintenance were generally rated as satisfactory with both STADOL Injection (25 patients) and morphine (25 patients) regardless of the type of surgery performed. Emergence from anesthesia was comparable with both agents.

Labor (see **PRECAUTIONS**)

The analgesic efficacy of intravenous STADOL Injection was studied in pain during labor. In a total of 145 patients, STADOL Injection (1 mg and 2 mg) was as effective as 40 mg and 80 mg of meperidine (144 patients) in the relief of pain in labor with no effect on the duration or progress of labor. Both drugs readily crossed the placenta and entered fetal circulation. The condition of the infants in these studies, determined by Apgar scores at 1 and 5 minutes (8 or above) and time to sustained respiration, showed that STADOL Injection had the same effects on the infants as meperidine.

In these studies, neurobehavioral testing in infants exposed to STADOL Injection at a mean of 18.6 hours after delivery showed no significant differences between treatment groups.

Individualization of Dosage

Use of butorphanol in geriatric patients, patients with renal impairment, patients with hepatic impairment, and during labor requires extra caution (see below and the appropriate sections in **PRECAUTIONS**).

STADOL Injection

For pain relief, the recommended initial dosage regimen of STADOL Injection is 1 mg IV or 2 mg IM with repeated doses every 3 to 4 hours, as necessary. This dosage regimen is likely to be effective for the majority of patients. Dosage adjustments of STADOL Injection should be based on observations of its beneficial and adverse effects. The initial dose in the elderly and in patients with renal or hepatic impairment should generally be half the recommended adult dose (0.5 mg IV and 1.0 mg IM). Repeat doses in these patients should be determined by the patient's response rather than at fixed intervals but will generally be no less than 6 hours (see **PRECAUTIONS**).

The usual preoperative dose is 2 mg IM given 60–90 minutes before surgery or 2 mg IV shortly before induction. This is approximately equivalent in sedative effect to 10 mg morphine or 80 mg of meperidine. This single preoperative dose should be individualized based on age, body weight, physical status, underlying pathological condition, use of other drugs, type of anesthesia to be used, and the surgical procedure involved.

During maintenance in balanced anesthesia, the usual incremental dose of STADOL Injection is 0.5 to 1.0 mg IV. The incremental dose may be higher, up to 0.06 mg/kg (4 mg/70 kg), depending on previous sedative, analgesic, and hypnotic drugs administered. The total dose of STADOL Injection will vary; however, patients seldom require less than 4 mg or more than 12.5 mg (approximately 0.06 to 0.18 mg/kg).

As with other opioids of this class, STADOL Injection may not provide adequate intraoperative analgesia in every patient or under all conditions. A failure to achieve successful analgesia during balanced anesthesia is commonly reflected by increases in general sympathetic tone. Consequently, if blood pressure or heart rate continues to rise, consideration should be given to adding a potent volatile liquid inhalation anesthetic or another intravenous medication.

In labor, the recommended initial dose of STADOL Injection is 1 or 2 mg IM or IV in mothers with fetuses of 37 weeks gestation or beyond and without signs of fetal distress. Dosage adjustments of STADOL Injection in labor should be based on initial response with consideration given to concomitant analgesic or sedative drugs and the expected time of delivery. A dose should not be repeated in less than 4 hours nor administered less than 4 hours prior to the anticipated delivery (see **PRECAUTIONS**).

STADOL NS

The usual recommended dose for initial nasal administration is 1 mg (1 spray in **one** nostril). If adequate pain relief is not achieved within 60–90 minutes, an additional 1-mg dose may be given.

The initial dose sequence outlined above may be repeated in 3–4 hours as required after the second dose of the sequence.

For the management of severe pain, an initial dose of 2 mg (1 spray in **each** nostril) may be used in patients who will be able to remain recumbent in the event drowsiness or dizziness occurs. In such patients, additional doses should not be given for 3–4 hours. The incidence of adverse events is higher with an initial 2-mg dose (see **Clinical Trials**).

The initial dose sequence in elderly patients and patients with renal or hepatic impairment should be limited to 1 mg followed, if needed, by 1 mg in 90–120 minutes. The repeat dose sequence in these patients should be determined by the patient's response rather than at fixed times but will generally be no less than at 6-hour intervals (see **PRECAUTIONS**).

INDICATIONS AND USAGE

STADOL (butorphanol tartrate) Injection and STADOL NS (butorphanol tartrate) Nasal Spray are indicated for the management of pain when the use of an opioid analgesic is appropriate.

STADOL Injection is also indicated as a preoperative or preanesthetic medication, as a supplement to balanced anesthesia, and for the relief of pain during labor.

CONTRAINDICATIONS

STADOL Injection and STADOL NS are contraindicated in patients hypersensitive to butorphanol tartrate or the preservative benzethonium chloride in STADOL NS or STADOL Injection in the multi-dose vial.

WARNINGS

Patients Dependent on Narcotics

Because of its opioid antagonist properties, butorphanol is not recommended for use in patients dependent on narcotics. Such patients should have an adequate period of withdrawal from opioid drugs prior to beginning butorphanol therapy. In patients taking opioid analgesics chronically, butorphanol has precipitated withdrawal symptoms such as anxiety, agitation, mood changes, hallucinations, dysphoria, weakness, and diarrhea.

Because of the difficulty in assessing opioid tolerance in patients who have recently received repeated doses of narcotic analgesic medication, caution should be used in the administration of butorphanol to such patients.

Drug Abuse and Dependence

Drug Abuse—Butorphanol tartrate, by all routes of administration, has been associated with episodes of abuse. Of the cases received, there were more reports of abuse with the nasal spray formulation than with the injectable formulation.

Physical Dependence, Tolerance, and Withdrawal—Prolonged, continuous use of butorphanol tartrate may result in physical dependence or tolerance (a decrease in response to a given dose). Abrupt cessation of use by patients with physical dependence may result in symptoms of withdrawal.

Note—Proper patient selection, dose and prescribing limitations, appropriate directions for use, and frequent monitoring are important to minimize the risk of abuse and physical dependence. (See **DRUG ABUSE AND DEPENDENCE**.)

PRECAUTIONS

General

Hypotension associated with syncope during the first hour of dosing with STADOL NS has been reported rarely, particularly in patients with past history of similar reactions to opioid analgesics. Therefore, patients should be advised to avoid activities with potential risks.

Head Injury and Increased Intracranial Pressure

As with other opioids, the use of butorphanol in patients with head injury may be associated with carbon dioxide retention and secondary elevation of cerebrospinal fluid pressure, drug-induced miosis, and alterations in mental state that would obscure the interpretation of the clinical course of patients with head injuries. In such patients, butorphanol should be used only if the benefits of use outweigh the potential risks.

Disorders of Respiratory Function or Control

Butorphanol may produce respiratory depression, especially in patients receiving other CNS active agents, or patients suffering from CNS diseases or respiratory impairment.

Hepatic and Renal Disease

In patients with hepatic or renal impairment, the initial dose of STADOL Injection should generally be half the recommended adult dose (0.5 mg IV and 1.0 mg IM). Repeat doses in these patients should be determined by the patient's response rather than at fixed intervals but will generally be no less than 6 hours apart. The initial dose sequence of STADOL NS should be limited to 1 mg followed, if needed, by 1 mg in 90–120 minutes. The repeat dose sequence in these patients should be determined by the patient's response rather than at fixed times but will generally be at intervals of no less than 6 hours (see **CLINICAL PHARMACOLOGY: Pharmacokinetics** and **Individualization of Dosage**).

Cardiovascular Effects

Because butorphanol may increase the work of the heart, especially the pulmonary circuit, the use of butorphanol in patients with acute myocardial infarction, ventricular dysfunction, or coronary insufficiency should be limited to those situations where the benefits clearly outweigh the risk (see **CLINICAL PHARMACOLOGY**).

Severe hypertension has been reported rarely during butorphanol therapy. In such cases, butorphanol should be discontinued and the hypertension treated with antihypertensive drugs. In patients who are not opioid dependent, naloxone has also been reported to be effective.

Use in Ambulatory Patients

1. Opioid analgesics, including butorphanol, impair the mental and physical abilities required for the performance of potentially dangerous tasks such as driving a car or operating machinery. Effects such as drowsiness or dizziness can appear, usually within the first hour after dosing. These effects may persist for varying periods of time after dosing. Patients who have taken butorphanol should not drive or operate dangerous machinery for at least 1 hour and until the effects of the drug are no longer present.
2. Alcohol should not be consumed while using butorphanol. Concurrent use of butorphanol with drugs that affect the central nervous system (eg, alcohol, barbiturates, tranquilizers, and antihistamines) may result in increased central nervous system depressant effects such as drowsiness, dizziness, and impaired mental function.
3. Butorphanol is one of a class of drugs known to be abused and thus should be handled accordingly (see **DRUG ABUSE AND DEPENDENCE**).
4. Patients should be instructed on the proper use of STADOL NS (see **PATIENT INSTRUCTIONS**).

Drug Interactions

Concurrent use of butorphanol with central nervous system depressants (eg, alcohol, barbiturates, tranquilizers, and antihistamines) may result in increased central nervous system depressant effects. When used concurrently with such drugs, the dose of butorphanol should be the smallest effective dose and the frequency of dosing reduced as much as possible when administered concomitantly with drugs that potentiate the action of opioids.

In healthy volunteers, the pharmacokinetics of a 1-mg dose of butorphanol administered as STADOL NS were not affected by the coadministration of a single 6-mg subcutaneous dose of sumatriptan. However, in another study in healthy volunteers, the pharmacokinetics of butorphanol were significantly altered (29% decrease in AUC and 38% decrease in C_{max}) when a 1-mg dose of STADOL NS was administered 1 minute after a 20-mg dose of sumatriptan nasal spray. (The two drugs were administered in opposite nostrils.) When the STADOL NS was administered 30 minutes after the sumatriptan nasal spray, the AUC of butorphanol increased 11% and C_{max} decreased 18%. In neither case were the pharmacokinetics of sumatriptan affected by coadministration with STADOL NS. These results suggest that the analgesic effect of STADOL NS may be diminished when it is administered shortly after sumatriptan nasal spray, but by 30 minutes any such reduction in effect should be minimal.

The safety of using STADOL NS and IMITREX® (sumatriptan) Nasal Spray during the same episode of migraine has not been established. However, it should be noted that both products are capable of producing transient increases in blood pressure.

The pharmacokinetics of a 1-mg dose of butorphanol administered as STADOL NS were not affected by the coadministration of cimetidine (300 mg QID). Conversely, the administration of STADOL NS (1 mg butorphanol QID) did not alter the pharmacokinetics of a 300-mg dose of cimetidine.

It is not known if the effects of butorphanol are altered by other concomitant medications that affect hepatic metabolism of drugs (erythromycin, theophylline, etc.), but physicians should be alert to the possibility that a smaller initial dose and longer intervals between doses may be needed.

The fraction of STADOL NS absorbed is unaffected by the concomitant administration of a nasal vasoconstrictor (oxymetazoline), but the rate of absorption is decreased. Therefore, a slower onset can be anticipated if STADOL NS is administered concomitantly with, or immediately following, a nasal vasoconstrictor.

No information is available about the use of butorphanol concurrently with MAO inhibitors.

Information for Patients (see **PRECAUTIONS: Use in Ambulatory Patients**).

Carcinogenesis, Mutagenesis, Impairment of Fertility

Two-year carcinogenicity studies were conducted in mice and rats given butorphanol tartrate in the diet up to 60 mg/kg/day (180 mg/m^2 for mice and 354 mg/m^2 for rats). There was no evidence of carcinogenicity in either species in these studies.

Butorphanol was not genotoxic in *S. typhimurium* or *E. coli* assays or in unscheduled DNA synthesis and repair assays conducted in cultured human fibroblast cells.

Rats treated orally with 160 mg/kg/day (944 mg/m^2) had a reduced pregnancy rate. However, a similar effect was not observed with a 2.5 mg/kg/day (14.75 mg/m^2) subcutaneous dose.

Pregnancy

Pregnancy Category C: Reproduction studies in mice, rats, and rabbits during organogenesis did not reveal any teratogenic potential to butorphanol. However, pregnant rats treated subcutaneously with butorphanol at 1 mg/kg (5.9 mg/m^2) had a higher frequency of stillbirths than controls. Butorphanol at 30 mg/kg/oral (360 mg/m^2) and 60 mg/kg/oral (720 mg/m^2) also showed higher incidences of post-implantation loss in rabbits.

There are no adequate and well-controlled studies of STADOL in pregnant women before 37 weeks of gestation. STADOL should be used during pregnancy only if the potential benefit justifies the potential risk to the infant.

Labor and Delivery

There have been rare reports of infant respiratory distress/apnea following the administration of STADOL Injection during labor. The reports of respiratory distress/apnea have been associated with administration of a dose within 2 hours of delivery, use of multiple doses, use with additional analgesic or sedative drugs, or use in preterm pregnancies (see **OVERDOSAGE: Treatment**).

In a study of 119 patients, the administration of 1 mg of IV STADOL Injection during labor was associated with transient (10–90 minutes) sinusoidal fetal heart rate patterns, but was not associated with adverse neonatal outcomes. In the presence of an abnormal fetal heart rate pattern, STADOL Injection should be used with caution.

STADOL NS is not recommended during labor or delivery because there is no clinical experience with its use in this setting.

Nursing Mothers

Butorphanol has been detected in milk following administration of STADOL Injection to nursing mothers. The amount an infant would receive is probably clinically insignificant (estimated 4 μg/L of milk in a mother receiving 2 mg IM four times a day).

Although there is no clinical experience with the use of STADOL NS in nursing mothers, it should be assumed that butorphanol will appear in the milk in similar amounts following the nasal route of administration.

Pediatric Use

Butorphanol is not recommended for use in patients below 18 years of age because safety and efficacy have not been established in this population.

Geriatric Use

Of the approximately 1500 patients treated with STADOL Injection in clinical studies, 15% were 61 years of age or older and 1% were 76 years or older. Of the approximately 1700 patients treated with STADOL NS in clinical studies, 8% were 65 years of age or older and 2% were 75 years or older.

Due to changes in clearance, the mean half-life of butorphanol is increased by 25% (to over 6 hours) in patients over the age of 65 years (see **CLINICAL PHARMACOLOGY: Pharmacokinetics**). Elderly patients may be more sensitive to the side effects of butorphanol. In clinical studies of STADOL NS, elderly patients had an increased frequency of headache, dizziness, drowsiness, vertigo, constipation, nausea and/or vomiting, and nasal congestion compared with younger patients. There are insufficient efficacy data for patients ≥65 years to determine whether they respond differently from younger patients.

The initial dose of STADOL Injection recommended for elderly patients should generally be half the recommended adult dose (0.5 mg IV and 1.0 mg IM). Repeat doses should be determined by the patient's response rather than at fixed intervals, but will generally be no less than 6 hours apart (see **CLINICAL PHARMACOLOGY: Individualization of Dosage**).

Initially a 1-mg dose of STADOL NS should generally be used in geriatric patients and 90–120 minutes should elapse before administering a second 1-mg dose, if needed (see **CLINICAL PHARMACOLOGY: Individualization of Dosage**).

Butorphanol and its metabolites are known to be substantially excreted by the kidney, and the risk of toxic reactions to this drug may be greater in patients with impaired renal function. Because elderly patients are more likely to have decreased renal function, care should be taken in dose selection.

ADVERSE REACTIONS

Clinical Trial Experience

A total of 2446 patients were studied in premarketing clinical trials of butorphanol. Approximately half received STADOL Injection with the remainder receiving STADOL NS. In nearly all cases the type and incidence of side effects with butorphanol by any route were those commonly observed with opioid analgesics.

The adverse experiences described below are based on data from short-term and long-term clinical trials in patients receiving butorphanol by any route. There has been no attempt to correct for placebo effect or to subtract the frequencies reported by placebo-treated patients in controlled trials.

The most frequently reported adverse experiences across all clinical trials with STADOL Injection and STADOL NS were somnolence (43%), dizziness (19%), nausea and/or vomiting (13%). In long-term trials with STADOL NS only, nasal congestion (13%) and insomnia (11%) were frequently reported.

The following adverse experiences were reported at a frequency of 1% or greater in clinical trials and were considered to be probably related to the use of butorphanol.

Body as a Whole: asthenia/lethargy, headache, sensation of heat.

Cardiovascular: vasodilation, palpitations.

Digestive: anorexia, constipation, dry mouth, nausea and/or vomiting, stomach pain.

Nervous: anxiety, confusion, dizziness, euphoria, floating feeling, insomnia, nervousness, paresthesia, somnolence, tremor.

Respiratory: bronchitis, cough, dyspnea, epistaxis, nasal congestion, nasal irritation, pharyngitis, rhinitis, sinus congestion, sinusitis, upper respiratory infection.

Skin and Appendages: sweating/clammy, pruritus.

Special Senses: blurred vision, ear pain, tinnitus, unpleasant taste.

The following adverse experiences were reported with a frequency of less than 1% in clinical trials and were considered to be probably related to the use of butorphanol.

Cardiovascular: hypotension, syncope.

Nervous: abnormal dreams, agitation, dysphoria, hallucinations, hostility, withdrawal symptoms.

Skin and Appendages: rash/hives.

Urogenital: impaired urination.

The following infrequent additional adverse experiences were reported in a frequency of less than 1% of the patients studied in short-term STADOL NS trials and under circumstances where the association between these events and butorphanol administration is unknown. They are being listed as alerting information for the physician.

Body as a Whole: edema.

Cardiovascular: chest pain, hypertension, tachycardia.

Nervous: depression.

Respiratory: shallow breathing.

Postmarketing Experience

Postmarketing experience with STADOL NS and STADOL Injection has shown an adverse event profile similar to that seen during the premarketing evaluation of butorphanol by all routes of administration. Adverse experiences that were associated with the use of STADOL NS or STADOL Injection and that are not listed above have been chosen for inclusion below because of their seriousness, frequency of reporting, or probable relationship to butorphanol. Because they are reported voluntarily from a population of unknown size, estimates of frequency cannot be made. These adverse experiences include apnea, convulsion, delusion, drug dependence, excessive drug effect associated with transient difficulty speaking and/or executing purposeful movements, overdose, and vertigo. Reports of butorphanol overdose with a fatal outcome have usually but not always been associated with ingestion of multiple drugs.

DRUG ABUSE AND DEPENDENCE

STADOL (butorphanol tartrate) Injection and STADOL NS (butorphanol tartrate) Nasal Spray are listed in Schedule IV of the Controlled Substances Act (CSA).

Proper patient selection, dose and prescribing limitations, appropriate directions for use, and frequent monitoring are important to minimize the risk of abuse and physical dependence with butorphanol tartrate. Special care should be ex-

Continued on next page

Stadol—Cont.

ercised in administering butorphanol to patients with a history of drug abuse or to patients receiving the drug on a continuous basis for an extended period.

Clinical Trial Experience

In all clinical trials, less than 1% of patients using STADOL NS had experiences that suggested the development of physical dependence or tolerance. Much of this information is based on experience with patients who did not have prolonged continuous exposure to STADOL NS. However, in one controlled clinical trial where patients with chronic pain from nonmalignant disease were treated with STADOL NS (n=303) or placebo (n=99) for up to 6 months, overuse (which may suggest the development of tolerance) was reported in nine (2.9%) patients receiving STADOL NS and no patients receiving placebo. Probable withdrawal symptoms were reported in eight (2.6%) patients using STADOL NS and no patients receiving placebo in the chronic nonmalignant pain study. Most of these patients abruptly discontinued STADOL NS after extended use or high doses. Symptoms suggestive of withdrawal included anxiety, agitation, tremulousness, diarrhea, chills, sweats, insomnia, confusion, incoordination, and hallucinations.

Postmarketing Experience

Butorphanol tartrate has been associated with episodes of abuse and dependence. Of the cases received, there were more reports of abuse with the nasal spray formulation than with the injectable formulation.

OVERDOSAGE

Clinical Manifestations

The clinical manifestations of butorphanol overdose are those of opioid drugs in general. Consequences of overdose vary with the amount of butorphanol ingested and individual response to the effects of opiates. The most serious symptoms are hypoventilation, cardiovascular insufficiency, coma, and death. Butorphanol overdose may be associated with ingestion of multiple drugs (see **ADVERSE REACTIONS: Postmarketing Experience**).

Overdose can occur due to accidental or intentional misuse of butorphanol, especially in young children who may gain access to the drug in the home.

Treatment

The management of suspected butorphanol overdosage includes maintenance of adequate ventilation, peripheral perfusion, normal body temperature, and protection of the airway. Patients should be under continuous observation with adequate serial measures of mental state, responsiveness, and vital signs. Oxygen and ventilatory assistance should be available with continual monitoring by pulse oximetry if indicated. In the presence of coma, placement of an artificial airway may be required. An adequate intravenous portal should be maintained to facilitate treatment of hypotension associated with vasodilation.

The use of a specific opioid antagonist such as naloxone should be considered. As the duration of butorphanol action usually exceeds the duration of action of naloxone, repeated dosing with naloxone may be required.

In managing cases of suspected butorphanol overdosage, the possibility of multiple drug ingestion should always be considered.

DOSAGE AND ADMINISTRATION

Factors to be considered in determining the dose are age, body weight, physical status, underlying pathological condition, use of other drugs, type of anesthesia to be used, and surgical procedure involved. Use in the elderly, in patients with hepatic or renal disease, or in labor requires extra caution (see **PRECAUTIONS** and **CLINICAL PHARMACOLOGY: Individualization of Dosage**). The following doses are for patients who do not have impaired hepatic or renal function and who are not on CNS active agents.

Use for Pain

STADOL Injection

Intravenous: The usual recommended single dose for IV administration is 1 mg repeated every 3 to 4 hours as necessary. The effective dosage range, depending on the severity of pain, is 0.5 to 2 mg repeated every 3 to 4 hours.

Intramuscular: The usual recommended single dose for IM administration is 2 mg in patients who will be able to remain recumbent, in the event drowsiness or dizziness occurs. This may be repeated every 3 to 4 hours, as necessary. The effective dosage range depending on the severity of pain is 1 to 4 mg repeated every 3 to 4 hours. There are insufficient clinical data to recommend single doses above 4 mg.

STADOL NS

The usual recommended dose for initial nasal administration is 1 mg (1 spray in **one** nostril). Adherence to this dose reduces the incidence of drowsiness and dizziness. If adequate pain relief is not achieved within 60–90 minutes, an additional 1-mg dose may be given.

The initial dose sequence outlined above may be repeated in 3–4 hours as required after the second dose of the sequence.

Depending on the severity of the pain, an initial dose of 2 mg (1 spray in **each** nostril) may be used in patients who will be able to remain recumbent in the event drowsiness or dizziness occurs. In such patients, single additional 2-mg doses should not be given for 3–4 hours.

Use as Preoperative/Preanesthetic Medication

The preoperative medication dosage of STADOL Injection should be individualized (see **CLINICAL PHARMACOLOGY: Individualization of Dosage**). The usual adult dose is 2 mg IM, administered 60–90 minutes before surgery. This is approximately equivalent in sedative effect to 10 mg morphine or 80 mg meperidine.

Use in Balanced Anesthesia

The usual dose of STADOL Injection is 2 mg IV shortly before induction and/or 0.5 to 1.0 mg IV in increments during anesthesia. The increment may be higher, up to 0.06 mg/kg (4 mg/70 kg), depending on previous sedative, analgesic, and hypnotic drugs administered. The total dose of STADOL Injection will vary; however, patients seldom require less than 4 mg or more than 12.5 mg (approximately 0.06 to 0.18 mg/kg).

The use of STADOL NS is not recommended because it has not been studied in induction or maintenance of anesthesia.

Labor

In patients at full term in early labor a 1–2 mg dose of STADOL Injection IV or IM may be administered and repeated after 4 hours. Alternative analgesia should be used for pain associated with delivery or if delivery is expected to occur within 4 hours.

If concomitant use of STADOL with drugs that may potentiate its effects is deemed necessary (see **PRECAUTIONS: Drug Interactions**), the lowest effective dose should be employed.

The use of STADOL NS is not recommended as it has not been studied in labor.

Safety and Handling

STADOL Injection is supplied in sealed delivery systems that have a low risk of accidental exposure to health care workers. Ordinary care should be taken to avoid aerosol generation while preparing a syringe for use. Following skin contact, rinsing with cool water is recommended.

STADOL NS is an open delivery system with increased risk of exposure to health care workers.

In the priming process, a certain amount of butorphanol may be aerosolized; therefore, the pump sprayer should be aimed away from the patient or other people or animals.

The disposal of Schedule IV controlled substances must be consistent with State and Federal Regulations. The unit should be disposed of by unscrewing the cap, rinsing the bottle, and placing the parts in a waste container.

HOW SUPPLIED

STADOL® (butorphanol tartrate) Injection, USP, for IM or IV use is available as follows:

NDC 0015-5644-20—2 mg per mL, 2-mL vial
NDC 0015-5645-20—1 mg per mL, 1-mL vial
NDC 0015-5646-20—2 mg per mL, 1-mL vial
NDC 0015-5648-20—2 mg per mL, 10-mL multi-dose vial

STADOL NS® (butorphanol tartrate) Nasal Spray

STADOL NS is supplied in a child-resistant prescription vial containing a metered-dose spray pump with protective clip and dust cover, a bottle of nasal spray solution, and a patient instruction leaflet. On average, one bottle will deliver 14–15 doses if no repriming is necessary.

NDC 0087-5650-41—10 mg per mL, 2.5-mL bottle.

U.S. Patent No. 4,464,378

PHARMACIST ASSEMBLY INSTRUCTIONS FOR STADOL NS NASAL SPRAY

The pharmacist will assemble STADOL NS prior to dispensing to the patient, according to the following instructions:

1. Open the child-resistant prescription vial and remove the spray pump and solution bottle.
2. Assemble STADOL NS by first unscrewing the white cap from the solution bottle and screwing the pump unit tightly onto the bottle. Make sure the clear cover is on the pump unit.
3. Return the STADOL NS bottle to the child-resistant prescription vial for dispensing to the patient.

Storage Conditions

Store at 25° C (77° F) controlled room temperature. See USP. Parenteral drug products should be inspected visually for particulate matter and discoloration prior to administration, whenever solution and container permit.

IMITREX® is the registered trademark of the GlaxoSmithKline Group of Companies.

Rx only

Bristol-Myers Squibb Company
Princeton, New Jersey 08543 USA
APOTHECON®
Distributed by Geneva Pharmaceuticals, Inc.
Dayton, NJ 08810 USA
565001DIL-8 1117206A2 Revised April 2002

PATIENT INSTRUCTIONS

Take medication as directed by your physician. For proper use of the nasal spray, read the following instructions carefully.

NOTE: VIALS DO NOT APPEAR "FULL." THEY ARE PREFILLED TO DELIVER ON AVERAGE 14–15 ONE (1) MG DOSES. (THE USUAL DOSE IS 1 MG—ONE SPRAY IN ONE NOSTRIL.)

THE UNIT MUST BE PRIMED WITH ONE OR TWO STROKES IF NOT USED FOR 48 HOURS OR LONGER.

Note: With intermittent use requiring repriming before each dose, the 2.5 mL bottle will deliver an average of 8–10 doses of STADOL NS.

When not in use, store spray unit in child-resistant container.

STADOL NS (butorphanol tartrate) Nasal Spray should not be used by anyone other than the person for whom it was prescribed. To prevent this, and to reduce the chance of children taking the drug it is important to dispose of any excess STADOL NS just as soon as it is no longer needed.

The best way to safely dispose of the unit is to unscrew the cap, rinse the bottle and spray assembly under the water faucet, and dispose of the parts in a waste can where children cannot easily get to them.

KEEP OUT OF THE REACH OF CHILDREN.

1. Blow nose gently to clear both nostrils. (Fig. 1)

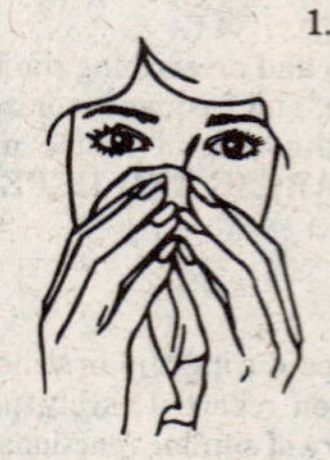

Fig. 1

2. Pull Clear cover off pump unit. Remove protective clip from neck of pump unit. (Fig. 2)

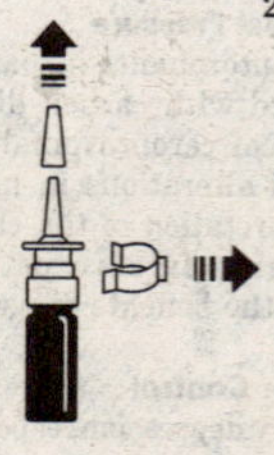

Fig. 2

3. Prime STADOL NS® by placing nozzle between first and second finger with thumb on the bottom of bottle. Pump sprayer unit FIRMLY and QUICKLY until a fine spray appears (up to 7–8 strokes). (Fig. 3)

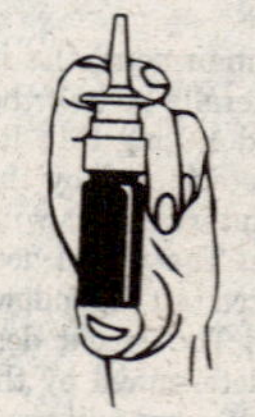

Fig. 3

4. Insert spray tip approximately 1 cm (width of small finger) into one nostril, pointing the tip toward the back of the nose. (Fig. 4)

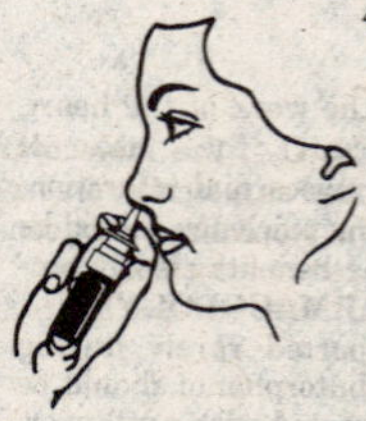

Fig. 4

5. Close other nostril with your forefinger and tilt head slightly forward. (Fig. 5)

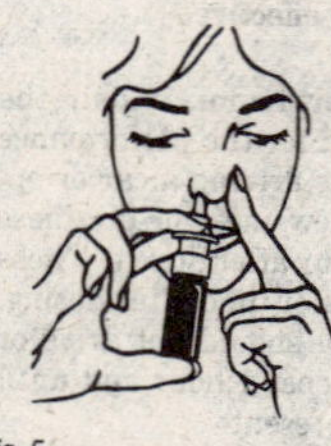

Fig. 5

6. Pump spray unit firmly and quickly by pushing down on the "finger grips" of the pump unit and against the thumb at the bottom of the bottle. Sniff gently with your mouth closed. (Fig. 6)

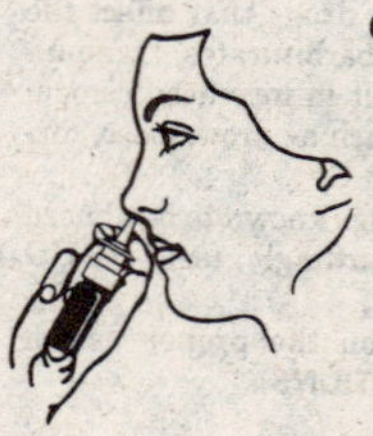

Fig. 6

7. After spraying, remove pump unit from nose. Tilt your head backwards and sniff gently a few more seconds. (Fig. 7)

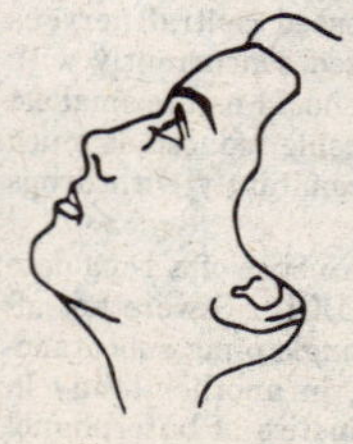

Fig. 7

8. Your doctor will tell you whether a two spray dose is needed. If needed, administer a second spray in the other nostril, following steps 4–7. Replace protective clip and clear cover, respectively, (Fig. 2) after each dose.

USUAL DOSE: One Spray. Spray ONLY ONCE into ONLY ONE nostril. DO NOT spray into both nostrils unless directed by your doctor. DO NOT repeat sooner than directed by your doctor.

Cubist Pharmaceuticals, Inc.

65 HAYDEN AVENUE
LEXINGTON, MA 02421

Direct Inquiries to:
1-866-RX-DAPTO
(phone) 866-793-2786
(fax) 866-305-2039

CUBICIN™ ℞

[kew-bĭ-sĭn]
(daptomycin for injection)
℞ only

To reduce the development of drug-resistant bacteria and maintain the effectiveness of CUBICIN and other antibacterial drugs, CUBICIN should be used only to treat or prevent infections caused by bacteria.

DESCRIPTION

CUBICIN contains daptomycin, a cyclic lipopeptide antibacterial agent derived from the fermentation of *Streptomyces roseosporus*. The chemical name is *N*-decanoyl-L-tryptophyl-L-asparaginyl-L-aspartyl-L-threonylglycyl-L-ornithyl-L-aspartyl-D-alanyl-L-aspartylglycyl-D-seryl-*threo*-3-methyl-L-glutamyl-3-anthraniloyl-L-alanine ϵ_1-lactone. The chemical structure is:

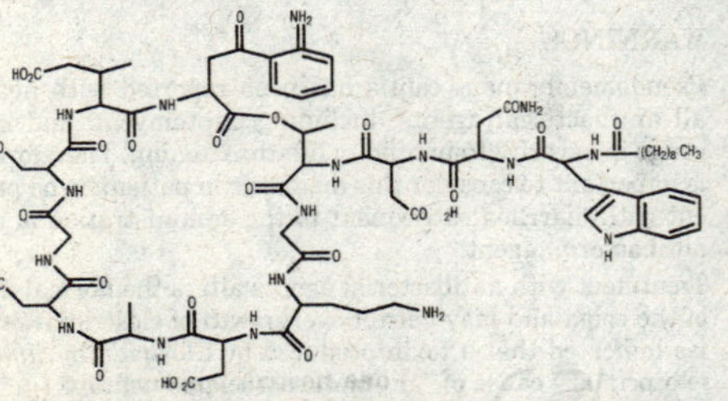

The empirical formula is $C_{72}H_{101}N_{17}O_{26}$; the molecular weight is 1620.67. CUBICIN is supplied as a sterile, preservative-free, pale yellow to light brown, lyophilized cake containing approximately 900 mg/g of daptomycin for intravenous use following reconstitution with 0.9% sodium chloride injection. The only inactive ingredient is sodium hydroxide, which is used in minimal quantities for pH adjustment. Freshly reconstituted solutions of CUBICIN range in color from pale yellow to light brown.

CLINICAL PHARMACOLOGY

Pharmacokinetics: The mean (SD) pharmacokinetic parameters of daptomycin on Day 7 following the intravenous administration of 4 mg/kg, 6 mg/kg, and 8 mg/kg q24h to healthy young adults (mean age 35.8 years) are summarized in Table 1.

[See table 1 above]

Daptomycin pharmacokinetics are nearly linear and time-independent at doses up to 6 mg/kg administered once daily for 7 days. Steady-state concentrations are achieved by the third daily dose. The mean (SD) steady-state trough concentrations (Days 4 to 8) attained following administration of 4, 6, and 8 mg/kg q24h are 5.9 (1.6), 9.4 (2.5), and 14.9 (2.9) μg/mL, respectively.

Distribution: Daptomycin is reversibly bound to human plasma proteins, primarily to serum albumin, in a concentration-independent manner. The mean serum protein binding of daptomycin was approximately 92% in healthy adults after the administration of 4 mg/kg or 6 mg/kg. Serum protein binding was not altered as a function of daptomycin concentration, dose, or number of doses received.

In clinical studies, mean serum protein binding in subjects with CL_{CR} ≥30 mL/min was comparable to that observed in healthy subjects with normal renal function. However, there was a trend toward decreasing serum protein binding among subjects with CL_{CR} <30 mL/min (87.6%), including hemodialysis patients (85.9%) and CAPD patients (83.5%). The protein binding of daptomycin in subjects with hepatic impairment (Child-Pugh B) was similar to healthy adult subjects. The apparent volume of distribution of daptomycin at steady-state in healthy adult subjects was approximately 0.09 L/kg.

Metabolism: *In vitro* studies with human hepatocytes indicate that daptomycin does not inhibit or induce the activities of the following human cytochrome (CYP) P450 isoforms: 1A2, 2A6, 2C9, 2C19, 2D6, 2E1, and 3A4. It is unlikely that daptomycin will inhibit or induce the metabolism of drugs metabolized by the CYP P450 system. It is unknown whether daptomycin is a substrate of the CYP P450 system.

In 5 healthy young adults, after infusion of radiolabeled ^{14}C-daptomycin, the plasma total radioactivity was similar

Table 1 Mean (SD) Daptomycin Pharmacokinetic Parameters in Healthy Volunteers on Day 7

Dose mg/kg	C_{max} (μg/mL)	T_{max}* (h)	AUC_{0-24} (μg•h/mL)	$t_{1/2}$ (h)	V_d (L/kg)	CL_T (mL/h/kg)	CL_R (mL/h/kg)	Ae_{24} %
4 (n=6)	57.8 (3.0)	0.8 (0.5,1.0)	494 (75)	8.1 (1.0)	0.096 (0.009)	8.3 (1.3)	4.8 (1.3)	53.0 (10.8)
6 (n=6)	98.6 (12)	0.5 (0.5,1.0)	747 (91)	8.9 (1.3)	0.104 (0.013)	8.1 (1.0)	4.4 (0.3)	47.4 (11.5)
8 (n=6)	133 (13.5)	0.5 (0.5,1.0)	1130 (117)	9.0 (1.2)	0.092 (0.012)	7.2 (0.8)	3.7 (0.5)	52.1 (5.19)

*Median (minimum, maximum)
C_{max} = Maximum plasma concentration; T_{max} = Time to C_{max}; AUC_{0-24} = Area under concentration-time curve from 0 to 24 hours; $t_{1/2}$ = Terminal elimination half-life; V_d = Apparent volume of distribution; CL_T = Systemic clearance; CL_R = Renal clearance; Ae_{24} = Percent of dose recovered in urine over 24 hours as unchanged daptomycin following the first dose.

Table 2 Mean (SD) Daptomycin Population Pharmacokinetic Parameters Following a Single 30-Minute Intravenous Infusion of 4 mg/kg to Infected Patients and Non-Infected Subjects with Varying Degrees of Renal Function

Renal Function	$AUC_{0-\infty}$ (μg•h/mL)	$t_{1/2}$ (h)	V_{SS} (L/kg)	CL_T (mL/h/kg)
Normal (CL_{CR} >80 mL/min) (N=165)	417 (155)	9.39 (4.74)	0.13 (0.05)	10.9 (4.0)
Mild Renal Impairment (CL_{CR} 50-80 mL/min) (N=64)	466 (177)	10.75 (8.36)	0.12 (0.05)	9.9 (4.0)
Moderate Renal Impairment (CL_{CR} 30-<50 mL/min) (N=24)	560 (258)	14.70 (10.50)	0.15 (0.06)	8.5 (3.4)
Severe Renal Impairment (CL_{CR} <30 mL/min) (N=8)	925 (467)	27.83 (14.85)	0.20 (0.15)	5.9 (3.9)
Hemodialysis and CAPD (N=21)	1244 (374)	29.81 (6.13)	0.15 (0.04)	3.7 (1.9)

Note: CL_{CR}= Creatinine clearance estimated using the Cockroft-Gault equation with actual body weight.

to the concentration determined by microbiological assay. Inactive metabolites of daptomycin have been detected in the urine, as determined by the difference in total radiolabeled concentrations and microbiologically active concentrations. The site of metabolism has not been identified.

Excretion: Daptomycin is excreted primarily by the kidney. In a mass balance study of 5 healthy subjects using radiolabeled daptomycin, approximately 78% of the administered dose was recovered from urine based on total radioactivity (approximately 52% of the dose based on microbiologically active concentrations) and 5.7% of the dose was recovered from feces (collected for up to 9 days), based on total radioactivity.

Because renal excretion is the primary route of elimination, dosing adjustment is necessary in patients with severe renal insufficiency (CL_{CR} <30 mL/min) (see **DOSAGE AND ADMINISTRATION**).

SPECIAL POPULATIONS

Renal Insufficiency: Population derived pharmacokinetic parameters were determined for patients with skin and skin structure infections and healthy non-infected subjects with varying degrees of renal function (n=282). Following the administration of a single 4 mg/kg IV dose of daptomycin, the plasma clearance (CL_T) was reduced and the systemic exposure ($AUC_{0-\infty}$) was increased with decreasing renal function (see Table 2). The mean $AUC_{0-\infty}$ was not markedly different for subjects and patients with CL_{CR} 30-80 mL/min as compared to those with normal renal function (CL_{CR} >80 mL/min). The mean $AUC_{0-\infty}$ values for subjects and patients with CL_{CR} <30 mL/min and hemodialysis (dosed post dialysis) / CAPD subjects were approximately 2- and 3-times higher, respectively, than the values in individuals with normal renal function. The mean C_{max} ranged from 59.6 μg/mL to 69.6 μg/mL in subjects with CL_{CR} ≥30 mL/min while those with CL_{CR} <30 mL/min ranged from 41.1 μg/mL to 57.7 μg/mL in 11 non-infected adult subjects undergoing dialysis, approximately 15% and 11% of the administered dose was removed by 4 hours of hemodialysis and 48 hours of CAPD, respectively. The recommended dosing regimens is 4 mg/kg once every 24 hours for patients with CL_{CR} ≥30 mL/min and 4 mg/kg once every 48 hours for CL_{CR} <30 mL/min, including those on hemodialysis and CAPD. Daptomycin should be administered following the completion of hemodialysis on hemodialysis days (see **DOSAGE AND ADMINISTRATION**).

[See table 2 above]

Hepatic Insufficiency: The pharmacokinetics of daptomycin were evaluated in 10 subjects with moderate hepatic impairment (Child-Pugh Class B) and compared with healthy volunteers (n=9) matched for gender, age, and weight. The pharmacokinetics of daptomycin were not altered in subjects with moderate hepatic impairment. No dosage adjustment is warranted when administering daptomycin to patients with mild to moderate hepatic impairment. The pharmacokinetics of daptomycin in patients with severe hepatic insufficiency have not been evaluated.

Gender: No clinically significant gender-related differences in daptomycin pharmacokinetics have been observed between healthy male and female subjects. No dosage adjustment is warranted based on gender when administering daptomycin.

Geriatric: The pharmacokinetics of daptomycin were evaluated in 12 healthy elderly subjects (≥75 years of age) and 11 healthy young matched controls (18-30 years of age). Following administration of a single intravenous 4 mg/kg dose, the mean total clearance of daptomycin was reduced approximately 35% and the mean $AUC_{0-\infty}$ increased approximately 58% in elderly subjects compared to young healthy subjects. There were no differences in C_{max}. No dosage adjustment is warranted for elderly patients with normal (for age) renal function.

Obesity: The pharmacokinetics of daptomycin were evaluated in six moderately obese (Body Mass Index [BMI] 25-39.9 kg/m^2) and six extremely dose (BMI ≥40 kg/m^2) subjects and controls matched for age, sex, and renal function. Following administration of a single intravenous 4 mg/kg dose based on total body weight, the plasma clearance of daptomycin increased approximately 18% in moderately obese subjects and 46% in extremely obese subjects compared with non-obese controls. The $AUC_{0-\infty}$ of daptomycin increased approximately 30% in moderately obese and 31% in extremely obese subjects compared with non-obese controls. The differences were most likely due to differences in the renal clearance of daptomycin. No dosage adjustment of daptomycin is warranted in obese subjects.

Pediatric: The pharmacokinetics of daptomycin in pediatric populations (<18 years of age) have not been established.

DRUG-DRUG INTERACTIONS

Drug-drug interaction studies were performed with daptomycin and other drugs that are likely to either be co-administered or associated with overlapping toxicity.

Aztreonam: In a study in which 15 healthy adult subjects received a single dose of daptomycin IV 6 mg/kg, aztreonam 1000 mg IV, and both in combination, the C_{max} and $AUC_{0-\infty}$ of daptomycin were not significantly altered by aztreonam; the C_{max} and $AUC_{0-\infty}$ of aztreonam were not significantly altered by daptomycin. No dosage adjustment of either antibiotic is warranted when co-administered.

Tobramycin: In a study in which 6 healthy adult males received a single dose of daptomycin IV 2 mg/kg, tobramycin IV 1 mg/kg, and both in combination, the mean C_{max} and $AUC_{0-\infty}$ of daptomycin increased 12.7% and 8.7%, respectively, when administered with tobramycin. The mean C_{max} and $AUC_{0-\infty}$ of tobramycin decreased 10.7% and 6.6%, respectively, when administered with daptomycin. None of these differences was statistically significant. The interaction between daptomycin and tobramycin with a clinical dose of daptomycin (4 mg/kg) is unknown. Caution is warranted when daptomycin is co-administered with tobramycin.

Warfarin: In 16 healthy subjects, concomitant administration of daptomycin 6 mg/kg once daily for 5 days followed by a single oral dose of warfarin (25 mg) had no significant effect on the pharmacokinetics of either drug and did not significantly alter the INR (International Normalized Ratio) (see **PRECAUTIONS, Drug Interactions**).

Simvastatin: In 20 healthy subjects on a stable daily dose of simvastatin 40 mg, administration of daptomycin IV 4 mg/kg once daily for 14 days (n=10) was not associated with a higher incidence of adverse events than subjects receiving placebo once daily (n=10) (see **PRECAUTIONS, Drug Interactions**).

Probenecid: Concomitant administration of probenecid (500 mg four times daily) and a single dose of daptomycin IV

Continued on next page

Cubicin—Cont.

4 mg/kg did not significantly alter the C_{max} and $AUC_{0-\infty}$ of daptomycin. No dosage adjustment of daptomycin is warranted when daptomycin is co-administered with probenecid.

MICROBIOLOGY

Daptomycin is an antibacterial agent of a new class of antibiotics, the cyclic lipopeptides. Daptomycin is a natural product which has clinical utility in the treatment of infections caused by aerobic Gram-positive bacteria. The *in vitro* spectrum of activity of daptomycin encompasses most clinically relevant Gram-positive pathogenic bacteria. Daptomycin retains potency against antibiotic-resistant Gram-positive bacteria, including isolates resistant to methicillin, vancomycin, and linezolid.

Daptomycin exhibits rapid, concentration-dependent bactericidal activity against Gram-positive organisms *in vitro*. This has been demonstrated both by time-kill curves and by MBC/MIC ratios using broth dilution methodology.

In vitro studies have demonstrated additive or indifferent interactions of daptomycin with other antibiotics. Antagonism, as determined by kill curve studies, has not been observed. *In vitro* synergistic interactions occurred with aminoglycosides and β-lactam antibiotics against some isolates of staphylococci and enterococci, including some MRSA isolates.

Mechanism of Action: The mechanism of action of daptomycin is distinct from any other antibiotic. Daptomycin binds to bacterial membranes and causes a rapid depolarization of membrane potential. The loss of membrane potential leads to inhibition of protein, DNA, and RNA synthesis, which results in bacterial cell death.

Resistance

Mechanisms of resistance: At this time, no mechanism of resistance to daptomycin has been identified. Currently, there are no known transferable elements that confer resistance to daptomycin.

Cross-resistance: Cross-resistance has not been observed with any other class of antibiotic.

Other: The emergence of resistance to daptomycin occurred in 2 of more than 1000 (<0.2%) infected subjects across the entire set of Phase 2 and 3 clinical trials. In one case, a resistant *S aureus* was isolated from a patient in a Phase 2 study who received daptomycin at less than the protocol-specified dose for the initial 5 days of therapy. In the second case, a resistant *E faecalis* was isolated from a patient with an infected chronic decubitus ulcer enrolled in a salvage trial.

Daptomycin has been shown to be active against most isolates of the following microorganisms both *in vitro* and in clinical infections, as described in the **INDICATIONS AND USAGE** section.

Aerobic and facultative Gram-positive microorganisms

Enterococcus faecalis (vancomycin-susceptible strains only)
Staphylococcus aureus (including methicillin-resistant strains)
Streptococcus agalactiae
Streptococcus dysgalactiae subsp *equisimilis*
Streptococcus pyogenes

The following *in vitro* data are available, but their clinical significance is unknown. Greater than 90% of the following microorganisms demonstrate an *in vitro* MIC less than or equal to the susceptible breakpoint for daptomycin versus the bacterial genus. The efficacy of daptomycin in treating clinical infections due to these microorganisms has not been established in adequate and well-controlled clinical trials.

Aerobic and facultative Gram-positive microorganisms

Corynebacterium jeikeium
Enterococcus faecalis (vancomycin-resistant strains)
Enterococcus faecium (including vancomycin-resistant strains)
Staphylococcus epidermidis (including methicillin-resistant strains)
Staphylococcus haemolyticus

Susceptibility Testing Methods

Susceptibility testing by dilution methods requires the use of daptomycin susceptibility powder. The testing also requires the presence of physiological levels of free calcium ions (50 mg/L calcium chloride) in Mueller-Hinton broth medium and a minimum of 28 mg/L calcium chloride in Mueller-Hinton agar medium.

Dilution technique: Quantitative methods are used to determine antimicrobial MICs. These MICs provide estimates of the susceptibility of bacteria to antimicrobial compounds. The MICs should be determined using a standardized procedure.[2,3] Standardized procedures are based on a dilution method (broth or agar) or equivalent with standardized inoculum concentrations and standardized concentrations of daptomycin powder. The MIC values should be interpreted according to the criteria in Table 3.

Diffusion technique: Quantitative methods that require measurement of zone diameters also provide reproducible estimates of the susceptibility of bacteria to antimicrobial compounds. One such standardized procedure requires the use of standardized inoculum concentrations.[1,3] This procedure uses paper disks impregnated with 30 µg of daptomycin to test the susceptibility of microorganisms to daptomycin. The disk diffusion interpretive criteria are provided in Table 3.

[See table 3 above]

Table 3 Susceptibility Interpretive Criteria for Daptomycin

Pathogen	Minimal inhibitory concentration (µg/mL)[a]			Disk diffusion zone diameter (mm)[b]		
	S	I	R	S	I	R
Staphylococcus aureus (methicillin-susceptible and methicillin-resistant)	≤1	(c)	(c)	≥16	(c)	(c)
Streptococcus pyogenes, *Streptococcus agalactiae*, and *Streptococcus dysgalactiae* subsp *equisimilis*	≤1	(c)	(c)	≥16	(c)	(c)
Enterococcus faecalis (vancomycin-susceptible only)	≤4	(c)	(c)	≥11	(c)	(c)

a. The MIC interpretive criteria for *S aureus* and *E faecalis* are applicable only to tests performed by broth microdilution using Mueller-Hinton broth adjusted to a calcium content of 50 mg/L; the MIC interpretive criteria for *Streptococcus* spp other than *S pneumoniae* are applicable only to tests performed by broth microdilution using Mueller-Hinton broth adjusted to a calcium content of 50 mg/L, supplemented with 2–5% lysed horse blood inoculated with a direct colony suspension and incubated in ambient air at 35°C for 20 to 24 hours.

b. The zone diameter interpretive criteria for *Streptococcus* spp other than *S pneumoniae* are applicable only to tests performed using Mueller-Hinton agar supplemented with 5% defibrinated sheep blood and incubated in 5% CO_2 at 35°C for 20 to 24 hours.

c. The current absence of data on daptomycin-resistant strains precludes defining any categories other than "Susceptible." Strains yielding test results suggestive of a "non-susceptible" category should be retested, and if the result is confirmed, the isolate should be submitted to a reference laboratory for further testing.

A report of "Susceptible" indicates that the pathogen is likely to be inhibited if the antimicrobial compound in the blood reaches the concentrations usually achievable.

Quality Control: Standardized susceptibility test procedures require the use of quality control microorganisms to control the technical aspects of the procedures. Standard daptomycin powder should provide the range of values noted in Table 4. Quality control microorganisms are specific strains of organisms with intrinsic biological properties relating to resistance mechanisms and their genetic expression within bacteria; the specific strains used for microbiological quality control are not clinically significant.

Table 4 Acceptable Quality Control Ranges for Daptomycin to Be Used in Validation of Susceptibility Test Results

QC Stain	Acceptable Quality Control Ranges: Minimum Inhibitory Concentration (MIC in µg/mL)[a]	Disk Diffusion (zone diameters in mm)[b]
Enterococcus faecalis ATCC 29212	1–8	Not applicable
Staphylococcus aureus ATCC 29213	0.25–1	Not applicable
Staphylococcus aureus ATCC 25923	Not applicable	18–23
Streptococcus pneumoniae ATCC 49619[c]	0.06–0.5[d]	19–26[e]

a. Quality control ranges reflect MICs obtained when Mueller-Hinton broth is supplemented with calcium to a final concentration of 50 mg/L.

b. Some lots of Mueller-Hinton agar are deficient in calcium and give small zone diameters.

c. This organism may be used for validation of susceptibility test results when testing *Streptococcus* spp other than *S pneumoniae*.

d. This quality control range for *S pneumoniae* is applicable only to tests performed by broth microdilution using cation adjusted Mueller-Hinton broth with 2–5% lysed horse blood inoculated with a direct colony suspension and incubated in ambient air at 35°C for 20 to 24 hours.

e. This quality control zone diameter range is applicable only to tests performed using Mueller-Hinton agar supplemented with 5% defibrinated sheep blood inoculated with a direct colony suspension and incubated in 5% CO_2 at 35°C for 20 to 24 hours.

INDICATIONS AND USAGE

CUBICIN (daptomycin for injection) is indicated for the treatment of complicated skin and skin structure infections caused by susceptible strains of the following Gram-positive microorganisms (see also **DOSAGE AND ADMINISTRATION**): *Staphylococcus aureus* (including methicillin-resistant strains), *Streptococcus pyogenes, Streptococcus agalactiae, Streptococcus dysgalactiae* subsp. *equisimilis* and *Enterococcus faecalis* (vancomycin-susceptible strains only). Combination therapy may be clinically indicated if the documented or presumed pathogens include Gram-negative or anaerobic organisms (see **CLINICAL STUDIES**).

Daptomycin is not indicated for the treatment of pneumonia.

Appropriate specimens for microbiological examination should be obtained in order to isolate and identify the causative pathogens and to determine their susceptibility to daptomycin. Empiric therapy may be initiated while awaiting test results. Antimicrobial therapy should be adjusted as needed based upon test results.

To reduce the development of drug-resistant bacteria and maintain the effectiveness of CUBICIN and other antibacterial drugs, CUBICIN should be used only to treat or prevent infections that are proven or strongly suspected to be caused by susceptible bacteria. When culture and susceptibility information are available, they should be considered in selecting or modifying antibacterial therapy. In the absence of such data, local epidemiology and susceptibility patterns may contribute to the empiric selection of therapy.

CONTRAINDICATIONS

CUBICIN is contraindicated in patients with known hypersensitivity to daptomycin.

WARNINGS

Pseudomembranous colitis has been reported with nearly all antibacterial agents, including daptomycin, and may range in severity from mild to life-threatening. Therefore, it is important to consider this diagnosis in patients who present with diarrhea subsequent to the administration of any antibacterial agent.

Treatment with antibacterial agents alters the normal flora of the colon and may permit overgrowth of clostridia. Studies indicated that a toxin produced by *Clostridium difficile* is a primary cause of "antibiotic-associated colitis."

If a diagnosis of pseudomembranous colitis has been established, appropriate therapeutic measures should be initiated. Mild cases of pseudomembranous colitis usually respond to drug discontinuation alone. In moderate to severe cases, consideration should be given to management with fluids and electrolytes, protein supplementation, and treatment with an antibacterial agent clinically effective against *C. difficile*.

PRECAUTIONS

General: The use of antibiotics may promote the overgrowth of nonsusceptible organisms. Should superinfection occur during therapy, appropriate measures should be taken.

Prescribing CUBICIN in the absence of a proven or strongly suspected bacterial infection or a prophylactic indication is unlikely to provide benefit to the patient and increases the risk of the development of drug-resistant bacteria.

Skeletal Muscle: In Phase 3 complicated skin and skin structure infection (cSSSI) trials, elevations in serum creatine phosphokinase (CPK) were reported as clinical adverse events in 15/534 (2.8%) daptomycin-treated patients, compared to 10/558 (1.8%) comparator-treated patients. Skeletal muscle effects associated with daptomycin were observed in animals (see **ANIMAL PHARMACOLOGY**).

Patients receiving CUBICIN should be monitored for the development of muscle pain or weakness, particularly of the distal extremities. CPK levels should be monitored weekly in patients who receive CUBICIN. Patients who develop unexplained elevations in CPK while receiving daptomycin should be monitored more frequently. Among patients with abnormal CPK (>500 U/L) at baseline, 2/19 (10.5%) treated with CUBICIN and 4/24 (16.7%) treated with comparator developed further increases in CPK while on therapy. In this same population, no patients developed myopathy. Daptomycin-treated patients with baseline CPK >500 U/L (n=19) did not experience an increased incidence of CPK elevations or myopathy relative to those treated with comparator (n=24).

CUBICIN should be discontinued in patients with unexplained signs and symptoms of myopathy in conjunction with CPK elevation >1000 U/L (~5× ULN), or in patients without reported symptoms who have marked elevations in CPK (≥10× ULN). In addition, consideration should be given to temporarily suspending agents associated with rhabdomyolysis, such as HMG-CoA reductase inhibitors, in patients receiving CUBICIN.

In a small number of patients in Phase 1 and Phase 2 studies, administration of CUBICIN was associated with decreases in nerve conduction velocity and with adverse events (eg, paresthesias, Bell's palsy), possibly reflective of peripheral or cranial neuropathy. Nerve conduction deficits were also detected in a similar number of comparator subjects in these studies.

In Phase 3 cSSSI and CAP studies, 7/989 (0.7%) daptomycin-treated patients and 7/1018 (0.7%) comparator-treated patients experienced paresthesias. New or worsening peripheral neuropathy was not diagnosed in any of these patients. In animals, effects of daptomycin on peripheral nerve were observed (see **ANIMAL PHARMACOLOGY**). Therefore, physicians should be alert to the possibility of signs and symptoms of neuropathy in patients receiving CUBICIN.

Drug Interactions: **Warfarin** Concomitant administration of daptomycin (6 mg/kg once every 24 hours for 5 days) and warfarin (25 mg single oral dose) had no significant effect on the pharmacokinetics of either drug, and the INR was not significantly altered. As experience with the concomitant administration of daptomycin and warfarin is limited to volunteer studies, anticoagulant activity in patients receiving daptomycin and warfarin should be monitored for the first several days after initiating therapy with CUBICIN (see **CLINICAL PHARMACOLOGY, Drug-Drug Interactions**).

HMG-CoA Reductase Inhibitors Inhibitors of HMG-CoA reductase may cause myopathy, which is manifested as muscle pain or weakness associated with elevated levels of CPK. There were no reports of skeletal myopathy in a placebo-controlled Phase I trial in which 10 healthy subjects on stable simvastatin therapy were treated concurrently with daptomycin (4 mg/kg once every 24 hours) for 14 days. Experience with co-administration of HMG-CoA reductase inhibitors and CUBICIN in patients is limited, therefore, consideration should be given to temporarily suspending use of HMG-CoA reductase inhibitors in patients receiving CUBICIN.

Drug-Laboratory Test Interactions: There are no reported drug-laboratory test interactions.

Carcinogenesis, Mutagenesis, Impairment of Fertility: Long-term carcinogenicity studies in animals have not been conducted to evaluate the carcinogenic potential of daptomycin. However, neither mutagenic nor clastogenic potential was found in a battery of genotoxicity tests, including the Ames assay, a mammalian cell gene mutation assay, a test for chromosomal aberrations in Chinese hamster ovary cells, an *in vivo* micronucleus assay, an *in vitro* DNA repair assay, and an *in vivo* sister chromatid exchange assay in Chinese hamsters.

Daptomycin did not affect the fertility or reproductive performance of male and female rats when administered intravenously at doses up to 150 mg/kg/day, which is approximately 9 times the estimated human exposure level based upon AUCs.

Pregnancy: **Teratogenic Effects: Pregnancy Category B** Reproductive and teratology studies performed in rats and rabbits at doses of up to 75 mg/kg, 3 and 6 times the human dose, respectively, on a body surface area basis, have revealed no evidence of harm to the fetus due to CUBICIN. There are, however, no adequate and well-controlled studies in pregnant women. Because animal reproduction studies are not always predictive of human response, this drug should be used during pregnancy only if clearly needed.

Nursing Mothers: It is not known if daptomycin is excreted in human milk. Caution should be exercised when CUBICIN is administered to nursing women.

Pediatric Use: Safety and efficacy of CUBICIN in patients under the age of 18 have not been established.

Geriatric Use: Of the 534 patients treated with CUBICIN in Phase 3 controlled clinical trials of complicated skin and skin structure infection, 27.0% were 65 years of age or older and 12.4% were 75 years or older. In the two Phase 3 clinical studies in patients with cSSSI, lower clinical success rates were seen in patients ≥65 years of age compared to those <65 years of age. In addition, treatment-emergent adverse events were more common in patients ≥65 years old than in patients <65 years of age in both cSSSI studies.

ANIMAL PHARMACOLOGY

In animals, daptomycin administration has been associated with effects on skeletal muscle with no changes in cardiac or smooth muscle. Skeletal muscle effects were characterized by degenerative/regenerative changes and variable elevations in CPK. No fibrosis or rhabdomyolysis was evident in repeat dose studies up to the highest doses tested in rats (150 mg/kg/day) and dogs (100 mg/kg/day). The degree of skeletal myopathy showed no increase when treatment was extended from 1 month to up to 6 months. Severity was dose dependent. All muscle effects, including microscopic changes, were fully reversible within 30 days following cessation of dosing.

In adult animals, effects on peripheral nerve (characterized by axonal degeneration and frequently accompanied by significant losses of patellar reflex, gag reflex, and pain perception) were observed at doses higher than those associated with skeletal myopathy. Deficits in the dogs' patellar reflexes were seen within 2 weeks of the start of treatment at 40 mg/kg (3.5 times the human AUC), with some clinical improvement noted within 2 weeks of the cessation of dosing. However, at 75 mg/kg daily for 1 month, 7/8 dogs failed to regain full patellar reflex responses within the duration of a 3 month recovery period. In a separate study in dogs receiving doses of 75 and 100 mg/kg/day for 2 weeks, minimal residual histological changes were noted at 6 months after cessation of dosing. However, recovery of peripheral nerve function was evident.

Tissue distribution studies in rats have shown that daptomycin is retained in the kidney but does not appear to penetrate across the blood-brain barrier following single and multiple doses.

Table 6 Incidence (%) of Creatine Phosphokinase (CPK) Elevations From Baseline While on Therapy in Either Daptomycin or Comparator Treatment Groups in Phase 3 cSSSI Studies

	All patients				Patients with normal CPK at baseline			
	Daptomycin (N=430)		Comparator (N=459)		Daptomycin (N=374)		Comparator (N=392)	
	%	n	%	n	%	n	%	n
No increase	90.7%	390	91.1%	418	91.2%	341	91.1%	357
Maximum Value >1× ULN*	9.3%	40	8.9%	41	8.8%	33	8.9%	35
>2× ULN	4.9%	21	4.8%	22	3.7%	14	3.1%	12
>4× ULN	1.4%	6	1.5%	7	1.1%	4	1.0%	4
>5× ULN	1.4%	6	0.4%	2	1.1%	4	0.0%	0
>10× ULN	0.5%	2	0.2%	1	0.2%	1	0.0%	0

* ULN (Upper Limit of Normal) is defined as 200 U/L.

Note: Elevations in CPK observed in patients treated with daptomycin or comparator were not clinically or statistically significantly different (P <0.05).

ADVERSE REACTIONS

Because clinical trials are conducted under widely varying conditions, adverse reaction rates observed in the clinical trials of a drug cannot be directly compared to rates in the clinical trials of another drug and may not reflect the rates observed in practice. The adverse reaction information from clinical trials does, however, provide a basis for identifying the adverse events that appear to be related to drug use and for approximating rates.

Clinical studies sponsored by Cubist enrolled 1409 patients treated with daptomycin and 1185 treated with comparator. Most adverse events reported in these clinical studies were described as mild or moderate in intensity. In Phase 3 cSSSI trials, daptomycin was discontinued in 15/534 (2.8%) patients due to an adverse event while comparator was discontinued in 17/558 (3.0%) patients.

The rates of most common adverse events, organized by body system, observed in cSSSI patients are displayed in Table 5.

Table 5 Incidence (%) of Adverse Events that Occurred in ≥ 2% of Patients in Either Daptomycin or Comparator Treatment Groups in Phase 3 cSSSI Studies

Adverse Event	Daptomycin (N=534)	Comparator* (N=558)
Gastrointestinal disorders		
Constipation	6.2%	6.8%
Nausea	5.8%	9.5%
Diarrhea	5.2%	4.3%
Vomiting	3.2%	3.8%
Dyspepsia	0.9%	2.5%
General disorders		
Injection site reactions	5.8%	7.7%
Fever	1.9%	2.5%
Nervous system disorders		
Headache	5.4%	5.4%
Insomnia	4.5%	5.4%
Dizziness	2.2%	2.0%
Skin/subcutaneous disorders		
Rash	4.3%	3.8%
Pruritis	2.8%	3.8%
Diagnostic investigations		
Abnormal liver function tests	3.0%	1.6%
Elevated CPK	2.8%	1.8%
Infections		
Fungal infections	2.6%	3.2%
Urinary tract infections	2.4%	0.5%
Vascular disorders		
Hypotension	2.4%	1.4%
Hypertension	1.1%	2.0%
Renal/urinary disorders		
Renal failure	2.2%	2.7%
Blood/lymphatic disorders		
Anemia	2.1%	2.3%
Respiratory disorders		
Dyspnea	2.1%	1.6%
Musculoskeletal disorders		
Limb pain	1.5%	2.0%
Arthralgia	0.9%	2.2%

* Comparators included vancomycin (1 g IV q12h) and semi-synthetic penicillins (ie, nafcillin, oxacillin, cloxacillin, flucloxacillin; 4-12 g/day in divided doses)

In Phase 3 studies of community-acquired pneumonia (CAP), the death rate and rates of serious cardiorespiratory adverse events were higher in daptomycin-treated patients than in comparator-treated patients. These differences were due to lack of therapeutic effectiveness of daptomycin in the treatment of CAP in patients experiencing these adverse events (see **INDICATIONS AND USAGE**). Additional adverse events that occurred in 1-2% of patients in either daptomycin- or comparator-treatment groups in the cSSSI studies are as follows: edema, cellulitis, hypoglycemia, elevated alkaline phosphatase, cough, back pain, abdominal pain, hypokalemia, hyperglycemia, decreased appetite, anxiety, chest pain, sore throat, cardiac failure, confusion, and Candida infections. These events occurred at rates ranging from 0.2-1.7% in daptomycin-treated patients and at rates of 0.4-1.8% in comparator-treated patients.

Additional drug-related adverse events (possibly or probably related) that occurred in <1% of patients receiving daptomycin in cSSSI trials are as follows:

Body as a Whole: fatigue, weakness, rigors, discomfort, jitteriness, flushing, hypersensitivity

Blood/Lymphatic System: leukocytosis, thrombocytopenia, thrombocytosis, eosinophilia, increased international normalized ratio

Cardiovascular System: supraventricular arrhythmia

Dermatologic System: eczema

Digestive System: abdominal distension, flatulence, stomatitis, jaundice, increased serum lactate dehydrogenase

Metabolic/Nutritional System: hypomagnesemia, increased serum bicarbonate, electrolyte disturbance

Musculoskeletal System: myalgia, muscle cramps, muscle weakness, osteomyelitis

Nervous System: vertigo, mental status change, paraesthesia

Special Senses: taste disturbance, eye irritation

Laboratory Changes

[See table 6 above]

In clinical trials, 0.2% of patients treated with CUBICIN had symptoms of muscle pain or weakness associated with CPK elevations to greater than 4 times the upper limit of normal. The symptoms resolved within 3 days and CPK returned to normal within 7-10 days after discontinuing treatment (see **PRECAUTIONS, Skeletal Muscle**). In Phase 3 comparator-controlled trials, there was no clinically or statistically significant difference (P <0.05) in the frequency of CPK elevations between patients treated with CUBICIN and those treated with comparator. CPK elevations in both groups were generally related to medical conditions, for example, skin and skin structure infection, surgical procedures, or intramuscular injections, and were not associated with muscle symptoms.

There were no substantial differences between CUBICIN and the comparators in the frequency or distribution of changes in other laboratory parameters, regardless of drug relationship.

OVERDOSAGE

In the event of overdosage, supportive care is advised with maintenance of glomerular filtration. Daptomycin is slowly cleared from the body by hemodialysis (approximately 15% recovered over 4 hours) or by peritoneal dialysis (approximately 11% recovered over 48 hours).

DOSAGE AND ADMINISTRATION

Complicated Skin and Skin Structure Infections: CUBICIN 4 mg/kg should be administered over a 30-minute period by intravenous infusion in 0.9% sodium chloride injection once every 24 hours for 7-14 days. Doses of CUBICIN higher than 4 mg/kg/day have not been studied in Phase 3 controlled clinical trials. In Phase 1 and 2 clinical studies, CPK elevations appeared to be more frequent when daptomycin was dosed more frequently than once daily. Therefore, CUBICIN should not be dosed more frequently than once a day.

Because daptomycin is eliminated primarily by the kidney, a dosage modification is recommended for patients with creatinine clearance <30 mL/min, including patients receiving hemodialysis or continuous ambulatory peritoneal dialysis (CAPD), as listed in Table 7. The recommended dosing regimen is 4 mg/kg once every 24 hours for patients with CL_{CR} ≥ 30 mL/min and 4 mg/kg once every 48 hours for CL_{CR}

Continued on next page

Cubicin—Cont.

<30 mL/min, including those on hemodialysis or CAPD. When possible, CUBICIN should be administered following hemodialysis on hemodialysis days (see **CLINICAL PHARMACOLOGY**).

Table 7 Recommended Dosage of CUBICIN (daptomycin for injection) in Adult Patients With Renal Impairment

Creatinine Clearance	Dosage Regimen
≥30 mL/min	4 mg/kg once every 24 hours
<30 mL/min, including hemodialysis or CAPD	4 mg/kg once every 48 hours

Preparation of Daptomycin for Administration: CUBICIN is supplied in single-use vials containing either 250 or 500 mg daptomycin as a sterile, lyophilized powder. The contents of a CUBICIN 250 mg vial should be reconstituted with 5 mL of 0.9% sodium chloride injection. The contents of a CUBICIN 500 mg vial should be reconstituted with 10 mL of 0.9% sodium chloride injection. Reconstituted CUBICIN should be further diluted with 0.9% sodium chloride injection to be administered by intravenous infusion over a period of 30 minutes.

Since no preservative or bacteriostatic agent is present in this product, aseptic technique must be used in preparation of final intravenous solution. Stability studies have shown that the reconstituted solution is stable in the vial for 12 hours at room temperature or up to 48 hours if stored under refrigeration at 2 to 8°C (36 to 46°F). The diluted solution is stable in the infusion bag for 12 hours at room temperature or 48 hours if stored under refrigeration. The combined time (vial and infusion bag) at room temperature should not exceed 12 hours; the combined time (vial and infusion bag) under refrigeration should not exceed 48 hours.

CUBICIN vials are for single-use only.

Parenteral drug products should be inspected visually for particulate matter prior to administration.

Because only limited data are available on the compatibility of CUBICIN with other intravenous substances, additives or other medications should not be added to daptomycin single-use vials or infused simultaneously through the same intravenous line. If the same intravenous line is used for sequential infusion of several different drugs, the line should be flushed with a compatible infusion solution before and after infusion with daptomycin.

Compatible Intravenous Solutions: CUBICIN is compatible with 0.9% sodium chloride injection and lactated Ringer's injection. CUBICIN is not compatible with dextrose-containing diluents.

HOW SUPPLIED

CUBICIN (daptomycin for injection) – Pale yellow to light brown lyophilized cake

Single-use 10 mL capacity vials:

500 mg/vial: Packages of 1 (NDC 67919-011-01)

250 mg/vial: Packages of 1 (NDC 67919-010-01)

STORAGE

Store original packages at refrigerated temperatures 2 to 8°C (36 to 46°F); avoid excessive heat.

CLINICAL STUDIES

Complicated Skin and Skin Structure Infections: Adult patients with clinically documented complicated skin and skin structure infections (Table 8) were enrolled in 2 randomized, multinational, multicenter, investigator-blinded studies comparing CUBICIN (4 mg/kg IV q24h) with either vancomycin (1 g IV q12h) or a semi-synthetic penicillin (ie, nafcillin, oxacillin, cloxacillin, or flucloxacillin; 4-12 g IV per day). Patients known to have bacteremia at baseline were excluded. Patients with creatinine clearance between 30-70 mL/min were to receive a lower dose of CUBICIN as specified in the protocol; however, the majority of patients in this subpopulation did not have the dose of daptomycin adjusted. Patients could switch to oral therapy after a minimum of 4 days of IV treatment if clinical improvement was demonstrated.

One study was conducted primarily in the United States and South Africa (study 9801), and the second (study 9901) was conducted at non–U.S. sites only. Both studies were similar in design but differed in patient characteristics, including history of diabetes and peripheral vascular disease. There were a total of 534 patients treated with CUBICIN and 558 treated with comparator in the 2 studies. The majority (89.7%) of patients received IV medication exclusively. The efficacy endpoints in both studies were the clinical success rates in the intent-to-treat (ITT) population and in the clinically evaluable (CE) population. In study 9801, clinical success rates in the ITT population were 62.5% (165/264) in patients treated with daptomycin and 60.9% (162/266) in patients treated with comparator drugs. Clinical success rates in the CE population were 76.0% (158/208) in patients treated with daptomycin and 76.7% (158/206) in patients treated with comparator drugs. In study 9901, clinical success rates in the ITT population were 80.4% (217/270) in patients treated with daptomycin and 80.5% (235/292) in patients treated with comparator drugs. Clinical success rates in the CE population were 89.9% (214/238) in patients treated with daptomycin and 90.4% (226/250) in patients treated with comparator drugs.

The success rates by pathogen for microbiologically evaluable patients are presented in Table 9.

[See table 8 below]

[See table 9 below]

℞ only

US Patent Nos. 6,468,967; 5,912,226; 4,885,243; 4,874,843

CUBICIN is a trademark of Cubist Pharmaceuticals, Inc.

Manufactured for:

Cubist Pharmaceuticals, Inc.

Lexington, MA 02421

Manufactured by:

Abbott Laboratories

Hospital Products Division

McPherson, KS 67460

For all medical inquiries, call 866-793-2786.

REFERENCES

1. National Committee for Clinical Laboratory Standards. Performance standards for antimicrobial disk susceptibility tests; approved standard–eighth edition. NCCLS document M2-A8, Villanova, (PA). 2003 January.
2. National Committee for Clinical Laboratory Standards. Methods for dilution antimicrobial susceptibility test for bacteria that grow aerobically; approved standard–sixth edition. NCCLS document M7-A6,Villanova, (PA). 2003 January.
3. National Committee for Clinical Laboratory Standards. Performance standards for antimicrobial susceptibility testing; thirteenth informational supplement. NCCLS document M100-S13, Villanova, (PA). 2003 January.

September 2003

Lexington, MA 02421

1109090803

Table 8 Investigator's Primary Diagnosis in the Complicated Skin and Skin Structure Infection Studies (Population: ITT)

Parameters	Study 9801 CUBICIN/Comparator[a] N=264/N=266	Study 9901 CUBICIN/Comparator[a] N=270/N=292	Pooled CUBICIN/Comparator[a] N=534/N=558
Wound Infection	99 (37.5%)/116 (43.6%)	102 (37.8%)/108 (37.0%)	201 (37.6%)/224 (40.1%)
Major Abscess	55 (20.8%)/43 (16.2%)	59 (21.9%)/65 (22.3%)	114 (21.3%)/108 (19.4%)
Ulcer Infection	71 (26.9%)/75 (28.2%)	53 (19.6%)/68 (23.3%)	124 (23.2%)/143 (25.6%)
Other Infection[b]	39 (14.8%)/32 (12.0%)	56 (20.7%)/51 (17.5%)	95 (17.8%)/83 (14.9%)

a. Vancomycin or semi-synthetic penicillins

b. The majority of cases were subsequently categorized as complicated cellulitis, major abscesses, or traumatic wound infections.

Table 9 Clinical Success Rates by Infecting Pathogen, Primary Comparative Complicated Skin and Skin Structure Infection Studies (Population: Microbiologically Evaluable)

Pathogen	Success Rate CUBICIN n/N (%)	Comparator[a] n/N (%)
Methicillin-susceptible *Staphylococcus aureus* (MSSA)[b]	170/198 (85.9)	180/207 (87.0)
Methicillin-resistant *Staphylococcus aureus* (MRSA)[b]	21/28 (75.0)	25/36 (69.4)
Streptococcus pyogenes	79/84 (94.0)	80/88 (90.9)
Streptococcus agalactiae	23/27 (85.2)	22/29 (75.9)
Streptococcus dysgalactiae subsp *equisimilis*	8/8 (100.0)	9/11 (81.8)
Enterococcus faecalis (vancomycin-susceptible only)[b]	27/37 (73.0)	40/53 (75.5)

a. Vancomycin or semi-synthetic penicillins

b. As determined by the central laboratory

Forest Pharmaceuticals, Inc.

(Subsidiary of Forest Laboratories, Inc.)
13600 SHORELINE DRIVE
ST. LOUIS, MO 63045

Direct Inquiries to:
Professional Affairs Department
13600 Shoreline Drive
St. Louis, MO 63045
(800) 678-1605

NAMENDA™ TABLETS ℞

[*nă-mĕn-dă*]

(memantine hydrochloride)

Rx Only

DESCRIPTION

NAMENDA™ (memantine hydrochloride) is an orally active NMDA receptor antagonist. The chemical name for memantine hydrochloride is 1-amino-3,5-dimethyladamantane hydrochloride with the following structural formula:

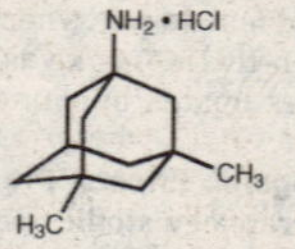

The molecular formula is $C_{12}H_{21}N \cdot HCl$ and the molecular weight is 215.76.

Memantine HCl occurs as a fine white to off-white powder and is soluble in water. NAMENDA is available for oral administration as capsule-shaped, film-coated tablets containing 5 mg and 10 mg of memantine hydrochloride. The tablets also contain the following inactive ingredients: microcrystalline cellulose, lactose monohydrate, colloidal silicon dioxide, talc and magnesium stearate. In addition the following inactive ingredients are also present as components of the film coat: hypromellose, triacetin, titanium dioxide, FD & C yellow #6 and FD & C blue #2 (5 mg tablets), iron oxide black (10 mg tablets).

CLINICAL PHARMACOLOGY

Mechanism of Action and Pharmacodynamics

Persistent activation of central nervous system N-methyl-D-aspartate (NMDA) receptors by the excitatory amino acid glutamate has been hypothesized to contribute to the symptomatology of Alzheimer's disease. Memantine is postulated to exert its therapeutic effect through its action as a low to moderate affinity uncompetitive (open-channel) NMDA receptor antagonist which binds preferentially to the NMDA receptor-operated cation channels. There is no evidence that memantine prevents or slows neurodegeneration in patients with Alzheimer's disease.

Memantine showed low to negligible affinity for GABA, benzodiazepine, dopamine, adrenergic, histamine and glycine receptors and for voltage-dependent Ca^{2+}, Na^{+} or K^{+} channels. Memantine also showed antagonistic effects at the $5HT_3$ receptor with a potency similar to that for the NMDA receptor and blocked nicotinic acetylcholine receptors with one-sixth to one-tenth the potency.

In vitro studies have shown that memantine does not affect the reversible inhibition of acetylcholinesterase by donepezil, galantamine, or tacrine.

Pharmacokinetics

Memantine is well absorbed after oral administration and has linear pharmacokinetics over the therapeutic dose range. It is excreted predominantly in the urine, unchanged, and has a terminal elimination half-life of about 60-80 hours.

Absorption and Distribution

Following oral administration memantine is highly absorbed with peak concentrations reached in about 3-7 hours. Food has no effect on the absorption of memantine. The mean volume of distribution of memantine is 9-11 L/kg and the plasma protein binding is low (45%).

Metabolism and Elimination

Memantine undergoes little metabolism, with the majority (57-82%) of an administered dose excreted unchanged in urine; the remainder is converted primarily to three polar metabolites: the N-gludantan conjugate, 6-hydroxy memantine, and 1-nitroso-deaminated memantine. These metabolites possess minimal NMDA receptor antagonist activity. The hepatic microsomal CYP450 enzyme system does not play a significant role in the metabolism of memantine. Memantine has a terminal elimination half-life of about 60-80 hours. Renal clearance involves active tubular secretion moderated by pH dependent tubular reabsorption.

Special Populations

Renal Impairment: Adequate information on the effect of renal impairment on the pharmacokinetics of memantine is not available. As the major route of elimination is renal, however, it is very likely that subjects with moderate and severe renal impairment will have significantly higher exposure than normal subjects.

Elderly: The pharmacokinetics of NAMENDA in young and elderly subjects are similar.

Gender: Following multiple dose administration of NAMENDA 20 mg b.i.d., females had about 45% higher exposure than males, but there was no difference in exposure when body weight was taken into account.

Drug-Drug Interactions

Substrates of Microsomal Enzymes: In vitro studies have shown that memantine produces minimal inhibition of CYP450 enzymes CYP1A2, CYP2A6, CYP2C9, CYP2D6, CYP2E1, and CYP3A4. These data indicate that no pharmacokinetic interactions with drugs metabolized by these enzymes are expected.

Inhibitors of Microsomal Enzymes: Since memantine undergoes minimal metabolism, with the majority of the dose excreted unchanged in urine, an interaction between memantine and drugs that are inhibitors of CYP450 enzymes is unlikely. Coadministration of NAMENDA with the AChE inhibitor donepezil HCl does not affect the pharmacokinetics of either compound.

Drugs Eliminated via Renal Mechanisms: Memantine is eliminated in part by tubular secretion. *In vivo* studies have shown that multiple doses of the diuretic hydrochlorothiazide/triamterene (HCTZ/TA) did not affect the AUC of memantine at steady state. Memantine did not affect the bioavailability of TA, and decreased AUC and C_{max} of HCTZ by about 20%.

Drugs that make the urine alkaline: The clearance of memantine was reduced by about 80% under alkaline urine conditions at pH 8. Therefore, alterations of urine pH towards the alkaline state may lead to an accumulation of the drug with a possible increase in adverse effects. Drugs that alkalinize the urine (e.g. carbonic anhydrase inhibitors, sodium bicarbonate) would be expected to reduce renal elimination of memantine.

Drugs highly bound to plasma proteins: Because the plasma protein binding of memantine is low (45%), an interaction with drugs that are highly bound to plasma proteins, such as warfarin and digoxin, is unlikely.

CLINICAL TRIALS

The effectiveness of NAMENDA (memantine hydrochloride) as a treatment for patients with moderate to severe Alzheimer's disease was demonstrated in 2 randomized, double-blind, placebo-controlled clinical studies (Studies 1 and 2) conducted in the United States that assessed both cognitive function and day to day function. The mean age of patients participating in these two trials was 76 with a range of 50-93 years. Approximately 66% of patients were female and 91% of patients were Caucasian.

A third study (Study 3), carried out in Latvia, enrolled patients with severe dementia, but did not assess cognitive function as a planned endpoint.

Study Outcome Measures: In each U.S. study, the effectiveness of NAMENDA was determined using both an instrument designed to evaluate overall function through caregiver-related assessment, and an instrument that measures cognition. Both studies showed that patients on NAMENDA experienced significant improvement on both measures compared to placebo.

Day-to-day function was assessed in both studies using the modified Alzheimer's disease Cooperative Study – Activities of Daily Living inventory (ADCS-ADL). The ADCS-ADL consists of a comprehensive battery of ADL questions used to measure the functional capabilities of patients. Each ADL item is rated from the highest level of independent performance to complete loss. The investigator performs the inventory by interviewing a caregiver familiar with the behavior of the patient. A subset of 19 items, including ratings of the patients' ability to eat, dress, bathe, telephone, travel, shop, and perform other household chores has been validated for the assessment of patients with moderate to severe dementia. This is the modified ADCS-ADL, which has a scoring range of 0 to 54, with the lower scores indicating greater functional impairment.

The ability of NAMENDA to improve cognitive performance was assessed in both studies with the Severe Impairment Battery (SIB), a multi-item instrument that has been validated for the evaluation of cognitive function in patients with moderate to severe dementia. The SIB examines selected aspects of cognitive performance, including elements of attention, orientation, language, memory, visuospatial ability, construction, praxis, and social interaction. The SIB scoring range is from 0 to 100, with lower scores indicating greater cognitive impairment.

Study 1 (Twenty-Eight-Week Study)

In a study of 28 weeks duration, 252 patients with moderate to severe probable Alzheimer's disease (diagnosed by DSM-IV and NINCDS-ADRDA criteria, with Mini-Mental State Examination scores ≥3 and ≤14 and Global Deterioration Scale Stages 5-6) were randomized to NAMENDA or placebo. For patients randomized to NAMENDA, treatment was initiated at 5 mg once daily and increased weekly by 5 mg/day in divided doses to a dose of 20 mg/day (10 mg twice a day).

Effects on the ADCS-ADL:

Figure 1 shows the time course for the change from baseline in the ADCS-ADL score for patients in the two treatment groups completing the 28 weeks of the study. At 28 weeks of treatment, the mean difference in the ADCS-ADL change scores for the NAMENDA-treated patients compared to the patients on placebo was 3.4 units. Using an analysis based on all patients and carrying their last study observation forward (LOCF analysis), NAMENDA treatment was statistically significantly superior to placebo.

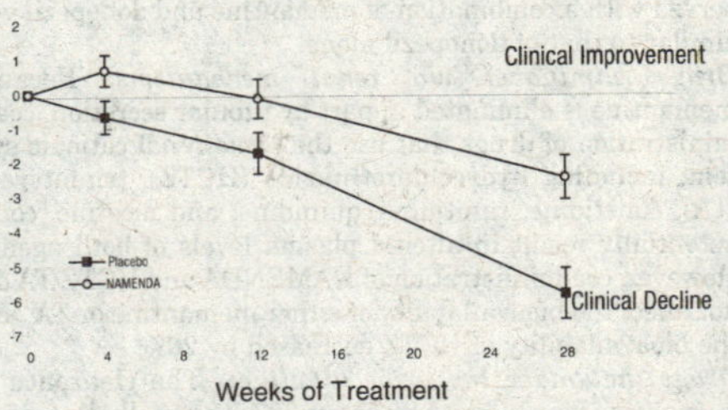

Figure 1: Time course of the change from baseline in ADCS-ADL score for patients completing 28 weeks of treatment.

Figure 2 shows the cumulative percentages of patients from each of the treatment groups who had attained at least the change in the ADCS-ADL shown on the X axis. The curves show that both patients assigned to NAMENDA and placebo have a wide range of responses and generally show deterioration (a negative change in ADCS-ADL compared to baseline), but that the NAMENDA group is more likely to show a smaller decline or an improvement. (In a cumulative distribution display, a curve for an effective treatment would be shifted to the left of the curve for placebo, while an ineffective or deleterious treatment would be superimposed upon or shifted to the right of the curve for placebo.)

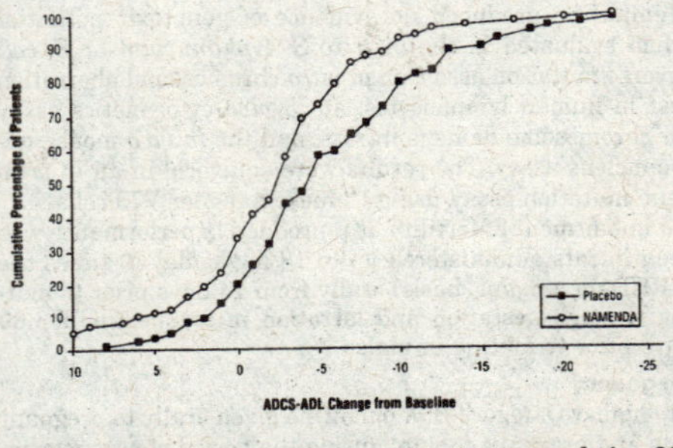

Figure 2: Cumulative percentage of patients completing 28 weeks of double-blind treatment with specified changes from baseline in ADCS-ADL scores.

Effects on the SIB:

Figure 3 shows the time course for the change from baseline in SIB score for the two treatment groups over the 28 weeks of the study. At 28 weeks of treatment, the mean difference in the SIB change scores for the NAMENDA-treated patients compared to the patients on placebo was 5.7 units. Using an LOCF analysis, NAMENDA treatment was statistically significantly superior to placebo.

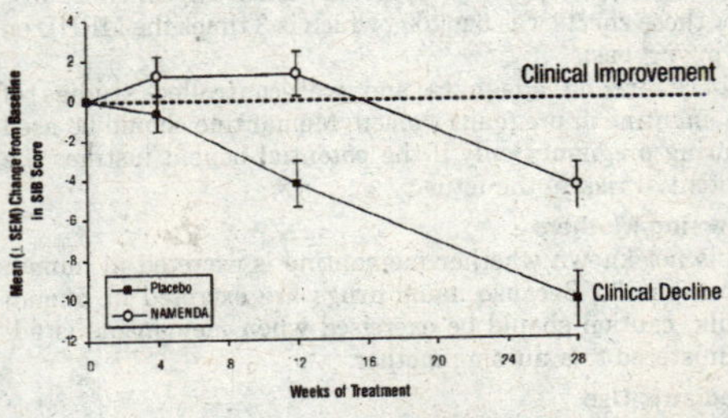

Figure 3: Time course of the change from baseline in SIB score for patients completing 28 weeks of treatment.

Figure 4 shows the cumulative percentages of patients from each treatment group who had attained at least the measure of change in SIB score shown on the X axis.

The curves show that both patients assigned to NAMENDA and placebo have a wide range of responses and generally show deterioration, but that the NAMENDA group is more likely to show a smaller decline or an improvement.

[See figure at top of next column]

Figure 4: Cumulative percentage of patients completing 28 weeks of double-blind treatment with specified changes from baseline in SIB scores.

Study 2 (Twenty-Four-Week Study)

In a study of 24 weeks duration, 404 patients with moderate to severe probable Alzheimer's disease (diagnosed by NINCDS-ADRDA criteria, with Mini-Mental State Examination scores ≥5 and ≤14) who had been treated with donepezil for at least 6 months and who had been on a stable dose of donepezil for the last 3 months were randomized to NAMENDA or placebo while still receiving donepezil. For

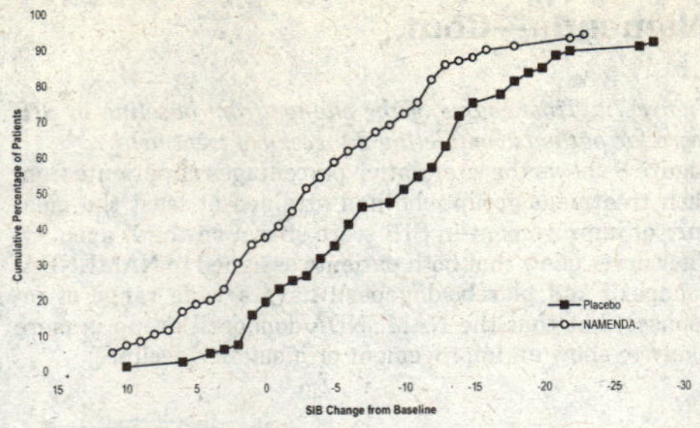

patients randomized to NAMENDA, treatment was initiated at 5 mg once daily and increased weekly by 5 mg/day in divided doses to a dose of 20 mg/day (10 mg twice a day).

Effects on the ADCS-ADL:

Figure 5 shows the time course for the change from baseline in the ADCS-ADL score for the two treatment groups over the 24 weeks of the study. At 24 weeks of treatment, the mean difference in the ADCS-ADL change scores for the NAMENDA/donepezil treated patients (combination therapy) compared to the patients on placebo/donepezil (monotherapy) was 1.6 units. Using an LOCF analysis, NAMENDA/donepezil treatment was statistically significantly superior to placebo/donepezil.

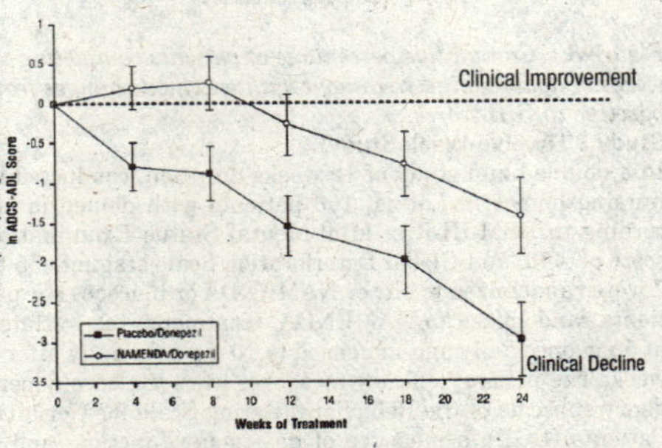

Figure 5: Time course of the change from baseline in ADCS-ADL score for patients completing 24 weeks of treatment.

Figure 6 shows the cumulative percentages of patients from each of the treatment groups who had attained at least the measure of improvement in the ADCS-ADL shown on the X axis.

The curves show that both patients assigned to NAMENDA/donepezil and placebo/donepezil have a wide range of responses and generally show deterioration, but that the NAMENDA/donepezil group is more likely to show a smaller decline or an improvement.

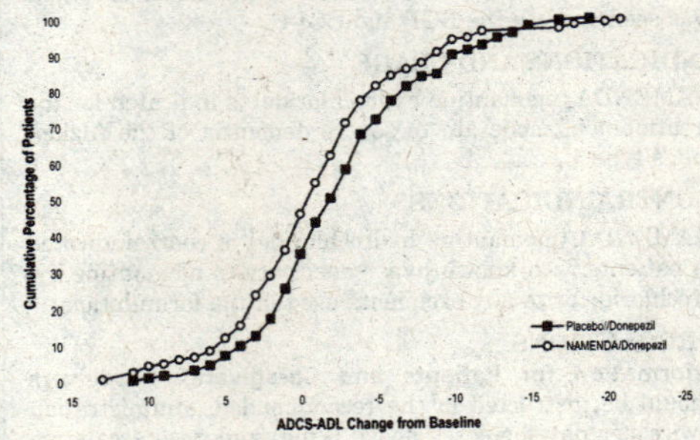

Figure 6: Cumulative percentage of patients completing 24 weeks of double-blind treatment with specified changes from baseline in ADCS-ADL scores.

Effects on the SIB:

Figure 7 shows the time course for the change from baseline in SIB score for the two treatment groups over the 24 weeks of the study. At 24 weeks of treatment, the mean difference in the SIB change scores for the NAMENDA/donepezil-treated patients compared to the patients on placebo/donepezil was 3.3 units. Using an LOCF analysis, NAMENDA/donepezil treatment was statistically significantly superior to placebo/donepezil.

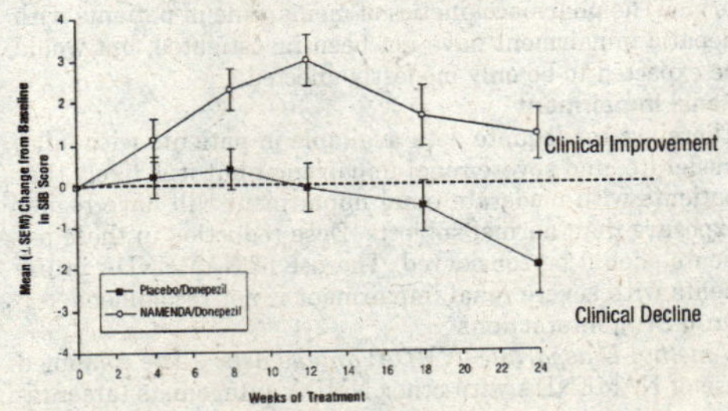

Continued on next page

Namenda—Cont.

Figure 7: Time course of the change from baseline in SIB score for patients completing 24 weeks of treatment.

Figure 8 shows the cumulative percentages of patients from each treatment group who had attained at least the measure of improvement in SIB score shown on the X axis. The curves show that both patients assigned to NAMENDA/donepezil and placebo/donepezil have a wide range of responses, but that the NAMENDA/donepezil group is more likely to show an improvement or a smaller decline.

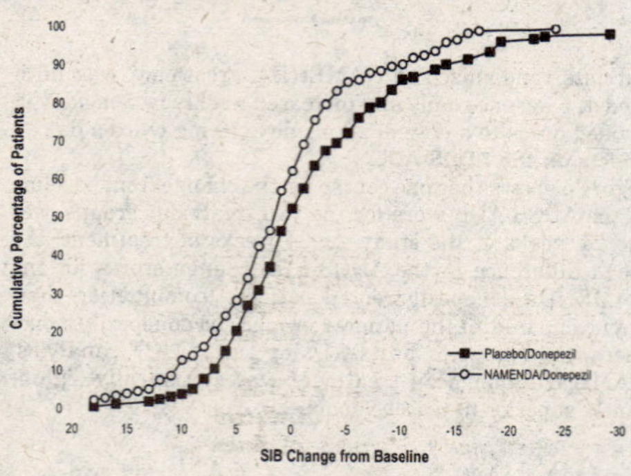

Figure 8: Cumulative percentage of patients completing 24 weeks of double-blind treatment with specified changes from baseline in SIB scores.

Study 3 (Twelve-Week Study)

In a double-blind study of 12 weeks duration, conducted in nursing homes in Latvia, 166 patients with dementia according to DSM-III-R, a Mini-Mental Status Examination score of <10, and Global Deterioration Scale staging of 5 to 7 were randomized to either NAMENDA or placebo. For patients randomized to NAMENDA, treatment was initiated at 5 mg once daily and increased to 10 mg once daily after 1 week. The primary efficacy measures were the care dependency subscale of the Behavioral Rating Scale for Geriatric Patients (BGP), a measure of day-to-day function, and a Clinical Global Impression of Change (CGI-C), a measure of overall clinical effect. No valid measure of cognitive function was used in this study. A statistically significant treatment difference at 12 weeks that favored NAMENDA over placebo was seen on both primary efficacy measures. Because the patients entered were a mixture of Alzheimer's disease and vascular dementia, an attempt was made to distinguish the two groups and all patients were later designated as having either vascular dementia or Alzheimer's disease, based on their scores on the Hachinski Ischemic Scale at study entry. Only about 50% of the patients had computerized tomography of the brain. For the subset designated as having Alzheimer's disease, a statistically significant treatment effect favoring NAMENDA over placebo at 12 weeks was seen on both the BGP and CGI-C.

INDICATIONS AND USAGE

NAMENDA (memantine hydrochloride) is indicated for the treatment of moderate to severe dementia of the Alzheimer's type.

CONTRAINDICATIONS

NAMENDA (memantine hydrochloride) is contraindicated in patients with known hypersensitivity to memantine hydrochloride or to any excipients used in the formulation.

PRECAUTIONS

Information for Patients and Caregivers: Caregivers should be instructed in the recommended administration (twice per day for doses above 5 mg) and dose escalation (minimum interval of one week between dose increases).

Neurological Conditions

Seizures: NAMENDA has not been systematically evaluated in patients with a seizure disorder. In clinical trials of NAMENDA, seizures occurred in 0.2% of patients treated with NAMENDA and 0.5% of patients treated with placebo.

Genitourinary Conditions

Conditions that raise urine pH may decrease the urinary elimination of memantine resulting in increased plasma levels of memantine.

Special Populations

Hepatic Impairment

NAMENDA undergoes partial hepatic metabolism, but the major fraction of a dose (57-82%) is excreted unchanged in urine. The pharmacokinetics of memantine in patients with hepatic impairment have not been investigated, but would be expected to be only modestly affected.

Renal Impairment

There are inadequate data available in patients with mild, moderate, and severe renal impairment but it is likely that patients with moderate renal impairment will have higher exposure than normal subjects. Dose reduction in these patients should be considered. The use of NAMENDA in patients with severe renal impairment is not recommended.

Drug-Drug Interactions

N-methyl-D-aspartate (NMDA) antagonists: The combined use of NAMENDA with other NMDA antagonists (amantadine, ketamine, and dextromethorphan) has not been systematically evaluated and such use should be approached with caution.

Effects of NAMENDA on substrates of microsomal enzymes: In vitro studies conducted with marker substrates of CYP450 enzymes (CYP1A2, -2A6, -2C9, -2D6, -2E1, -3A4) showed minimal inhibition of these enzymes by memantine. No pharmacokinetic interactions with drugs metabolized by these enzymes are expected.

Effects of inhibitors and/or substrates of microsomal enzymes on NAMENDA: Memantine is predominantly renally eliminated, and drugs that are substrates and/or inhibitors of the CYP450 system are not expected to alter the metabolism of memantine.

Acetylcholinesterase (AChE) inhibitors: Coadministration of NAMENDA with the AChE inhibitor donepezil HCl did not affect the pharmacokinetics of either compound. In a 24-week controlled clinical study in patients with moderate to severe Alzheimer's disease, the adverse event profile observed with a combination of memantine and donepezil was similar to that of donepezil alone.

Drugs eliminated via renal mechanisms: Because memantine is eliminated in part by tubular secretion, coadministration of drugs that use the same renal cationic system, including hydrochlorothiazide (HCTZ), triamterene (TA), cimetidine, ranitidine, quinidine, and nicotine, could potentially result in altered plasma levels of both agents. However, coadministration of NAMENDA and HCTZ/TA did not affect the bioavailability of either memantine or TA, and the bioavailability of HCTZ decreased by 20%.

Drugs that make the urine alkaline: The clearance of memantine was reduced by about 80% under alkaline urine conditions at pH 8. Therefore, alterations of urine pH towards the alkaline condition may lead to an accumulation of the drug with a possible increase in adverse effects. Urine pH is altered by diet, drugs (e.g. carbonic anhydrase inhibitors, sodium bicarbonate) and clinical state of the patient (e.g. renal tubular acidosis or severe infections of the urinary tract). Hence, memantine should be used with caution under these conditions.

Carcinogenesis, Mutagenesis and Impairment of Fertility

There was no evidence of carcinogenicity in a 113-week oral study in mice at doses up to 40 mg/kg/day (10 times the maximum recommended human dose [MRHD] on a mg/m^2 basis). There was also no evidence of carcinogenicity in rats orally dosed at up to 40 mg/kg/day for 71 weeks followed by 20 mg/kg/day (20 and 10 times the MRHD on a mg/m^2 basis, respectively) through 128 weeks.

Memantine produced no evidence of genotoxic potential when evaluated in the *in vitro S. typhimurium* or *E. coli* reverse mutation assay, an *in vitro* chromosomal aberration test in human lymphocytes, an *in vivo* cytogenetics assay for chromosome damage in rats, and the *in vivo* mouse micronucleus assay. The results were equivocal in an *in vitro* gene mutation assay using Chinese hamster V79 cells.

No impairment of fertility or reproductive performance was seen in rats administered up to 18 mg/kg/day (9 times the MRHD on a mg/m^2 basis) orally from 14 days prior to mating through gestation and lactation in females, or for 60 days prior to mating in males.

Pregnancy

Pregnancy Category B: Memantine given orally to pregnant rats and pregnant rabbits during the period of organogenesis was not teratogenic up to the highest doses tested (18 mg/kg/day in rats and 30 mg/kg/day in rabbits, which are 9 and 30 times, respectively, the maximum recommended human dose [MRHD] on a mg/m^2 basis).

Slight maternal toxicity, decreased pup weights and an increased incidence of nonossified cervical vertebrae were seen at an oral dose of 18 mg/kg/day in a study in which rats were given oral memantine beginning pre-mating and continuing through the postpartum period. Slight maternal toxicity and decreased pup weights were also seen at this dose in a study in which rats were treated from day 15 of gestation through the postpartum period. The no-effect dose for these effects was 6 mg/kg, which is 3 times the MRHD on a mg/m^2 basis.

There are no adequate and well-controlled studies of memantine in pregnant women. Memantine should be used during pregnancy only if the potential benefit justifies the potential risk to the fetus.

Nursing Mothers

It is not known whether memantine is excreted in human breast milk. Because many drugs are excreted in human milk, caution should be exercised when memantine is administered to a nursing mother.

Pediatric Use

There are no adequate and well-controlled trials documenting the safety and efficacy of memantine in any illness occurring in children.

ADVERSE REACTIONS

The experience described in this section derives from studies in patients with Alzheimer's disease and vascular dementia.

Adverse Events Leading to Discontinuation: In placebo-controlled trials in which dementia patients received doses of NAMENDA up to 20 mg/day, the likelihood of discontinuation because of an adverse event was the same in the NAMENDA group as in the placebo group. No individual adverse event was associated with the discontinuation of treatment in 1% or more of NAMENDA-treated patients and at a rate greater than placebo.

Adverse Events Reported in Controlled Trials: The reported adverse events in NAMENDA (memantine hydrochloride) trials reflect experience gained under closely monitored conditions in a highly selected patient population. In actual practice or in other clinical trials, these frequency estimates may not apply, as the conditions of use, reporting behavior and the types of patients treated may differ. Table 1 lists treatment-emergent signs and symptoms that were reported in at least 2% of patients in placebo-controlled dementia trials and for which the rate of occurrence was greater for patients treated with NAMENDA than for those treated with placebo. No adverse event occurred at a frequency of at least 5% and twice the placebo rate.

Table 1: Adverse Events Reported in Controlled Clinical Trials in at Least 2% of Patients Receiving NAMENDA and at a Higher Frequency than Placebo-treated Patients.

Body System Adverse Event	Placebo (N = 922) %	NAMENDA (N = 940) %
Body as a Whole		
Fatigue	1	2
Pain	1	3
Cardiovascular System		
Hypertension	2	4
Central and Peripheral Nervous System		
Dizziness	5	7
Headache	3	6
Gastrointestinal System		
Constipation	3	5
Vomiting	2	3
Musculoskeletal System		
Back pain	2	3
Psychiatric Disorders		
Confusion	5	6
Somnolence	2	3
Hallucination	2	3
Respiratory System		
Coughing	3	4
Dyspnea	1	2

Other adverse events occurring with an incidence of at least 2% in NAMENDA-treated patients but at a greater or equal rate on placebo were agitation, fall, inflicted injury, urinary incontinence, diarrhea, bronchitis, insomnia, urinary tract infection, influenza-like symptoms, gait abnormal, depression, upper respiratory tract infection, anxiety, peripheral edema, nausea, anorexia, and arthralgia.

The overall profile of adverse events and the incidence rates for individual adverse events in the subpopulation of patients with moderate to severe Alzheimer's disease were not different from the profile and incidence rates described above for the overall dementia population.

Vital Sign Changes: NAMENDA and placebo groups were compared with respect to (1) mean change from baseline in vital signs (pulse, systolic blood pressure, diastolic blood pressure, and weight) and (2) the incidence of patients meeting criteria for potentially clinically significant changes from baseline in these variables. There were no clinically important changes in vital signs in patients treated with NAMENDA. A comparison of supine and standing vital sign measures for NAMENDA and placebo in elderly normal subjects indicated that NAMENDA treatment is not associated with orthostatic changes.

Laboratory Changes: NAMENDA and placebo groups were compared with respect to (1) mean change from baseline in various serum chemistry, hematology, and urinalysis variables and (2) the incidence of patients meeting criteria for potentially clinically significant changes from baseline in these variables. These analyses revealed no clinically important changes in laboratory test parameters associated with NAMENDA treatment.

ECG Changes: NAMENDA and placebo groups were compared with respect to (1) mean change from baseline in various ECG parameters and (2) the incidence of patients meeting criteria for potentially clinically significant changes from baseline in these variables. These analyses revealed no clinically important changes in ECG parameters associated with NAMENDA treatment.

Other Adverse Events Observed During Clinical Trials

NAMENDA has been administered to approximately 1350 patients with dementia, of whom more than 1200 received the maximum recommended dose of 20 mg/day. Patients received NAMENDA treatment for periods of up to 884 days, with 862 patients receiving at least 24 weeks of treatment and 387 patients receiving 48 weeks or more of treatment. Treatment emergent signs and symptoms that occurred during 8 controlled clinical trials and 4 open-label trials were recorded as adverse events by the clinical investigators using terminology of their own choosing. To provide an overall estimate of the proportion of individuals having similar types of events, the events were grouped into a smaller number of standardized categories using WHO terminology, and event frequencies were calculated across all studies.

All adverse events occurring in at least two patients are included, except for those already listed in Table 1, WHO terms too general to be informative, minor symptoms or events unlikely to be drug-caused, e.g., because they are common in the study population. Events are classified by body system and listed using the following definitions: frequent adverse events – those occurring in at least 1/100 patients; infrequent adverse events – those occurring in 1/100 to 1/1000 patients. These adverse events are not necessarily related to NAMENDA treatment and in most cases were observed at a similar frequency in placebo-treated patients in the controlled studies.

Body as a Whole: *Frequent:* syncope. *Infrequent:* hypothermia, allergic reaction.

Cardiovascular System: *Frequent:* cardiac failure. *Infrequent:* angina pectoris, bradycardia, myocardial infarction, thrombophlebitis, atrial fibrillation, hypotension, cardiac arrest, postural hypotension, pulmonary embolism, pulmonary edema.

Central and Peripheral Nervous System: *Frequent:* transient ischemic attack, cerebrovascular accident, vertigo, ataxia, hypokinesia. *Infrequent:* paresthesia, convulsions, extrapyramidal disorder, hypertonia, tremor, aphasia, hypoesthesia, abnormal coordination, hemiplegia, hyperkinesia, involuntary muscle contractions, stupor, cerebral hemorrhage, neuralgia, ptosis, neuropathy.

Gastrointestinal System: *Infrequent:* gastroenteritis, diverticulitis, gastrointestinal hemorrhage, melena, esophageal ulceration.

Hemic and Lymphatic Disorders: *Frequent:* anemia. *Infrequent:* leukopenia.

Metabolic and Nutritional Disorders: *Frequent:* increased alkaline phosphatase, decreased weight. *Infrequent:* dehydration, hyponatremia, aggravated diabetes mellitus.

Psychiatric Disorders: *Frequent:* aggressive reaction. *Infrequent:* delusion, personality disorder, emotional lability, nervousness, sleep disorder, libido increased, psychosis, amnesia, apathy, paranoid reaction, thinking abnormal, crying abnormal, appetite increased, paroniria, delirium, depersonalization, neurosis, suicide attempt.

Respiratory System: *Frequent:* pneumonia. *Infrequent:* apnea, asthma, hemoptysis.

Skin and Appendages: *Frequent:* rash. *Infrequent:* skin ulceration, pruritus, cellulitis, eczema, dermatitis, erythematous rash, alopecia, urticaria

Special Senses: *Frequent:* cataract, conjunctivitis. *Infrequent:* macula lutea degeneration, decreased visual acuity, decreased hearing, tinnitus, blepharitis, blurred vision, corneal opacity, glaucoma, conjunctival hemorrhage, eye pain, retinal hemorrhage, xerophthalmia, diplopia, abnormal lacrimation, myopia, retinal detachment.

Urinary System: *Frequent:* frequent micturition. *Infrequent:* dysuria, hematuria, urinary retention

ADVERSE EVENTS FROM OTHER SOURCES

Memantine has been commercially available outside the United States since 1982, and has been evaluated in clinical trials including trials in patients with neuropathic pain, Parkinson's disease, organic brain syndrome, and spasticity. The following adverse events of possible importance for which there is inadequate data to determine the causal relationship have been reported to be temporally associated with memantine treatment in more than one patient and are not described elsewhere in labeling: acne, bone fracture, carpal tunnel syndrome, claudication, hyperlipidemia, impotence, otitis media, thrombocytopenia.

ANIMAL TOXICOLOGY

Memantine induced neuronal lesions (vacuolation and necrosis) in the multipolar and pyramidal cells in cortical layers III and IV of the posterior cingulate and retrosplenial neocortices in rats, similar to those which are known to occur in rodents administered other NMDA receptor antagonists. Lesions were seen after a single dose of memantine. In a study in which rats were given daily oral doses of memantine for 14 days, the no-effect dose for neuronal necrosis was 6 times the maximum recommended human dose on a mg/m^2 basis. The potential for induction of central neuronal vacuolation and necrosis by NMDA receptor antagonists in humans is unknown.

DRUG ABUSE AND DEPENDENCE

Controlled Substance Class: Memantine HCl is not a controlled substance.

Physical and Psychological Dependence: Memantine HCl is a low to moderate affinity uncompetitive NMDA antagonist that did not produce any evidence of drug-seeking behavior or withdrawal symptoms upon discontinuation in 2,504 patients who participated in clinical trials at therapeutic doses. Post marketing data, outside the U.S., retrospectively collected, has provided no evidence of drug abuse or dependence.

OVERDOSAGE

Because strategies for the management of overdose are continually evolving, it is advisable to contact a poison control center to determine the latest recommendations for the management of an overdose of any drug.

As in any cases of overdose, general supportive measures should be utilized, and treatment should be symptomatic. Elimination of memantine can be enhanced by acidification of urine. In a documented case of an overdosage with up to 400 mg of memantine, the patient experienced restlessness, psychosis, visual hallucinations, somnolence, stupor and loss of consciousness. The patient recovered without permanent sequelae.

DOSAGE AND ADMINISTRATION

The dosage of NAMENDA (memantine hydrochloride) shown to be effective in controlled clinical trials is 20 mg/day.

The recommended starting dose of NAMENDA is 5 mg once daily. The recommended target dose is 20 mg/day. The dose should be increased in 5 mg increments to 10 mg/day (5 mg twice a day), 15 mg/day (5 mg and 10 mg as separate doses), and 20 mg/day (10 mg twice a day). The minimum recommended interval between dose increases is one week.

NAMENDA can be taken with or without food.

Doses in Special Populations

Dose reduction in patients with moderate renal impairment should be considered. In patients with severe renal impairment the use of NAMENDA has not been systematically evaluated and is not recommended. (See Clinical Pharmacology-Pharmacokinetics)

HOW SUPPLIED

5 mg Tablet:

Bottle of 60 NDC #0456-3205-60
10 × 10 Unit Dose NDC #0456-3205-63

The capsule-shaped, film-coated tablets are tan, with the strength (5) debossed on one side and FL on the other.

10 mg Tablet:

Bottle of 60 NDC #0456-3210-60
10 × 10 Unit Dose NDC #0456-3210-63

The capsule-shaped, film-coated tablets are gray, with the strength (10) debossed on one side and FL on the other.

Titration Pak:

PVC/Aluminum Blister package containing 49 tablets. 28 × 5 mg and 21 × 10 mg tablets. NDC #0456-3200-14

The 5 mg capsule-shaped, film-coated tablets are tan, with the strength (5) debossed on one side and FL on the other. The 10 mg capsule-shaped, film-coated tablets are gray, with the strength (10) debossed on one side and FL on the other.

Store at 25°C (77°F); excursions permitted to 15-30°C (59-86°F)[see USP Controlled Room Temperature]

Forest Pharmaceuticals, Inc.
Subsidiary of Forest Laboratories, Inc.
St. Louis, MO 63045
Licensed from Merz Pharmaceuticals GmbH
10/03

Genentech, Inc.

1 DNA WAY
SOUTH SAN FRANCISCO, CA 94080-4990

For Medical Information Contact:

Medical Communications or Drug Safety Departments
(24 hours):
(800) 821-8590
(650) 225-1000
E-mail: medinfo@gene.com

Or write:
Medical Communications or Drug Safety Departments
Genentech, Inc.
1 DNA Way
South San Francisco, CA 94080-4990

RAPTIVA™ ℞

[răp-tē'vă]
(efalizumab)
For injection, subcutaneous

DESCRIPTION

RAPTIVA™ (efalizumab) is an immunosuppressive recombinant humanized IgG1 kappa isotype monoclonal antibody that binds to human CD11a (1). Efalizumab has a molecular weight of approximately 150 kilodaltons and is produced in a Chinese hamster ovary mammalian cell expression system in a nutrient medium containing the antibiotic gentamicin. Gentamicin is not detectable in the final product.

RAPTIVA is supplied as a sterile, white to off-white, lyophilized powder in single-use glass vials for subcutaneous (SC) injection. Reconstitution of the single-use vial with 1.3 mL of the supplied sterile water for injection (non-USP) yields approximately 1.5 mL of solution to deliver 125 mg per 1.25 mL (100 mg/mL) of RAPTIVA. The sterile water for injection supplied does not comply with USP requirement for pH. After reconstitution, RAPTIVA is a clear to pale yellow solution with a pH of approximately 6.2. Each single-use vial of RAPTIVA contains 150 mg of efalizumab, 123.2 mg of sucrose, 6.8 mg of L-histidine hydrochloride monohydrate, 4.3 mg of L-histidine and 3 mg of polysorbate 20 and is designed to deliver 125 mg of efalizumab in 1.25 mL.

CLINICAL PHARMACOLOGY

Mechanism of Action

RAPTIVA binds to CD11a, the α subunit of leukocyte function antigen-1 (LFA-1), which is expressed on all leukocytes, and decreases cell surface expression of CD11a. RAPTIVA inhibits the binding of LFA-1 to intercellular adhesion molecule-1 (ICAM-1), thereby inhibiting the adhesion of leukocytes to other cell types. Interaction between LFA-1 and ICAM-1 contributes to the initiation and maintenance of multiple processes, including activation of T lymphocytes, adhesion of T lymphocytes to endothelial cells, and migration of T lymphocytes to sites of inflammation including psoriatic skin. Lymphocyte activation and trafficking to skin play a role in the pathophysiology of chronic plaque psoriasis. In psoriatic skin, ICAM-1 cell surface expression is upregulated on endothelium and keratinocytes. CD11a is also expressed on the surface of B lymphocytes, monocytes, neutrophils, natural killer cells, and other leukocytes. Therefore, the potential exists for RAPTIVA to affect the activation, adhesion, migration, and numbers of cells other than T lymphocytes.

Pharmacokinetics

In patients with moderate to severe plaque psoriasis, following an initial SC RAPTIVA dose of 0.7 mg/kg followed by 11 weekly SC doses of 1 mg/kg/wk, serum concentrations reached a steady-state at 4 weeks with a mean trough concentration of approximately 9 μg/mL (n = 26). After the last dose, the mean peak concentration was approximately 12 μg/mL (n = 25). Mean steady-state clearance was 24 mL/kg/day (range = 5–76 mL/kg/day, n = 25). Mean time to eliminate RAPTIVA after the last steady-state dose was 25 days (range = 13–35 days, n = 17). The mean estimated RAPTIVA SC bioavailability was 50%. In a population pharmacokinetic analysis of 1088 patients, body weight was found to be the most significant covariate affecting RAPTIVA clearance. In patients receiving weekly SC doses of 1 mg/kg, RAPTIVA exposure was similar across body weight quartiles. RAPTIVA clearance was not significantly affected by gender or race. The pharmacokinetics of RAPTIVA in pediatric patients have not been studied. The effects of renal or hepatic impairment on the pharmacokinetics of RAPTIVA have not been studied.

Pharmacodynamics

At a dose of 1 mg/kg/wk SC, RAPTIVA reduced expression of CD11a on circulating T lymphocytes to approximately 15–25% of pre-dose values and reduced free CD11a binding sites to a mean of ≤5% of pre-dose values. These pharmacodynamic effects were seen 1–2 days after the first dose, and were maintained between weekly 1 mg/kg SC doses. Following discontinuation of RAPTIVA, CD11a expression returned to a mean of 74% of baseline at 5 weeks and stayed at comparable levels at 8 and 13 weeks. Following discontinuation of RAPTIVA, free CD11a binding sites returned to a mean of 86% of baseline at 8 weeks and stayed at comparable levels at 13 weeks. No assessments of CD11a expression or free CD11a binding sites were made after 13 weeks. In clinical trials, RAPTIVA treatment resulted in a mean increase (relative to baseline) in white blood cell (WBC) count of 34%, a doubling of mean lymphocyte counts and an increase in eosinophil counts of 29% due to decreased leukocyte adhesion to blood vessel walls and decreased trafficking from the vascular compartment to tissues. At Day 56 of 1 mg/kg/wk RAPTIVA treatment, 32% (213/676) of patients had a shift in total WBC from low or normal baseline value to above normal, 46% (324/701) had a shift to above normal absolute lymphocyte counts, and 5% (35/675) had a shift to above normal eosinophil counts. Following discontinuation of RAPTIVA treatment, the abnormal elevated lymphocyte counts took approximately 8 weeks to normalize among patients who had above normal lymphocyte counts. Plasma samples collected after first administration of 0.3 mg/kg IV RAPTIVA indicate that at 2 hours TNF-α and IL-6 plasma levels were elevated 9- and 90-fold, respectively, compared with baseline. Plasma samples collected after first administration of 0.7 mg/kg SC RAPTIVA indicate that at 2 days, IL-6 levels were elevated (10 pg/mL as compared with 5 pg/mL at baseline), whereas TNF-α was not detectable. In RAPTIVA-treated patients the mean levels of C reactive protein increased from baseline by 67% and the mean levels of fibrinogen increased by 15%.

CLINICAL STUDIES

RAPTIVA was evaluated in four randomized, double-blind, placebo-controlled studies in adults with chronic (>6 months), stable, plaque psoriasis, who had a minimum body surface area involvement of 10% and who were candidates for, or had previously received systemic therapy or phototherapy. In these studies 54–70% of patients had previously received systemic therapy or phototherapy (PUVA) for psoriasis. Patients with clinically significant flares and patients with guttate, erythrodermic, or pustular psoriasis as the sole form of psoriasis were excluded from the studies. Patients were randomized to receive doses of 1 mg/kg or 2 mg/kg of RAPTIVA or placebo administered once a week for 12 weeks. Patients randomized to RAPTIVA received 0.7 mg/kg as the first dose prior to receiving the full assigned dose in subsequent weeks. During the studies, patients could receive concomitant low potency topical steroids. No other concomitant psoriasis therapies were allowed during treatment or the follow-up period.

Patients were evaluated using the Psoriasis Area and Severity Index (PASI) during the study. The PASI is a composite score that takes into consideration both the fraction of body surface area affected and the nature and severity of the psoriatic changes within the affected regions (erythema, infiltration/plaque thickness, and desquamation). Both treatment groups in all four studies had baseline median PASI scores of 17. Both treatment groups across all four studies had baseline median body surface area involvement ranging between 22–28%. Compared with placebo, more pa-

Continued on next page

Raptiva—Cont.

tients randomized to RAPTIVA had at least a 75% reduction from baseline PASI score (PASI-75) 1 week after the 12-week treatment period (Table 1). RAPTIVA 2 mg/kg was not superior to RAPTIVA 1 mg/kg.

Table 1
Proportion of Patients with ≥75% Improvement in PASI after 12 Weeks of Treatment (PASI-75)

	Placebo	RAPTIVA 1 mg/kg/wk	Difference (95%CI)
Study 1	4% n = 187	27%[a] n = 369	22% (16%, 29%)
Study 2	2% n = 170	39%[a] n = 162	37% (28%, 46%)
Study 3	5% n = 122	22%[a] n = 232	17% (9%, 27%)
Study 4	3% n = 236	24%[a] n = 450	21% (15%, 27%)

[a] p<0.001 for comparison of RAPTIVA group with placebo group using Fisher's exact test within each study.

All three components of the PASI (plaque induration, scaling, and erythema) contributed comparably to the improvement in PASI. Other clinical responses evaluated (Table 2) included the proportion of patients who achieved minimal or clear status by a static Physician Global Assessment (sPGA) and the proportion of patients with a reduction in PASI of at least 50% from baseline (PASI-50) 1 week following the 12-week treatment period. The sPGA is a 6 category scale ranging from "very severe" to "clear" indicating the physician's overall assessment of the psoriasis severity focusing on plaque, scaling and erythema. Treatment success of minimal or clear consisted of none or slight elevation in plaque, none or minimal white color in scaling, and up to moderate definite red coloration in erythema. Across all four studies, the percentage of patients with baseline sPGA classifications of moderate was 48–56%, severe 33–43%, and 3–6% were classified as very severe.

[See table 2 below]

In Study 1, 12% of RAPTIVA-treated patients achieved a PASI-50 at Week 4 compared with 5% for placebo. The median time to PASI-50 among PASI-75 achievers was approximately 6 weeks. Similar results were observed in Studies 2, 3, and 4.

In Study 3, sustained response to extended RAPTIVA treatment was evaluated. RAPTIVA-treated patients who achieved a PASI-75 response at Week 12 were re-randomized to receive RAPTIVA or placebo for a second contiguous 12-week treatment period. Sixty-one of 79 patients (77%) re-randomized to a second 12-week treatment period with RAPTIVA maintained PASI-75 response compared with 8 of 40 patients (20%) re-randomized to placebo. Sustained responses to RAPTIVA have also been observed in uncontrolled, open-label extension treatment trials when patients received RAPTIVA without interruption for 24 weeks.

In Study 2, response to intermittent RAPTIVA treatment was evaluated among patients who achieved PASI-75 response with 12 weeks of RAPTIVA treatment and were followed off-treatment until relapse of psoriasis (50% loss of treatment response). In patients who resumed RAPTIVA treatment upon relapse of psoriasis, 31% (17/55) re-established a PASI-75 response (compared with the initial baseline). After 12 weeks of treatment, the median duration of a PASI-75 response after RAPTIVA discontinuation was between 1 and 2 months.

The safety and efficacy of RAPTIVA therapy beyond 1 year have not been established.

INDICATIONS AND USAGE

RAPTIVA™ (efalizumab) is indicated for the treatment of adult patients (18 years or older) with chronic moderate to severe plaque psoriasis who are candidates for systemic therapy or phototherapy.

CONTRAINDICATIONS

RAPTIVA should not be administered to patients with known hypersensitivity to RAPTIVA or any of its components.

WARNINGS

Serious Infections

RAPTIVA is an immunosuppressive agent and has the potential to increase the risk of infection and reactivate latent, chronic infections. RAPTIVA should not be administered to patients with clinically important infections. Caution should be exercised when considering the use of RAPTIVA in patients with a chronic infection or history of recurrent infections. If a patient develops a serious infection, RAPTIVA should be discontinued. New infections developing during RAPTIVA treatment should be monitored. During the first 12 weeks of controlled trials, serious infections occurred in 7 of 1620 (0.4 %) RAPTIVA-treated patients compared with 1 of 715 (0.1%) placebo-treated patients (see **ADVERSE REACTIONS, Infections**). Serious infections requiring hospitalization included cellulitis, pneumonia, abscess, sepsis, bronchitis, gastroenteritis, aseptic meningitis, Legionnaire's disease, and vertebral osteomyelitis (note some patients had more than one infection).

Malignancies

RAPTIVA is an immunosuppressive agent. Many immunosuppressive agents have the potential to increase the risk of malignancy. The role of RAPTIVA in the development of malignancies is not known. Caution should be exercised when considering the use of RAPTIVA in patients at high risk for malignancy or with a history of malignancy. If a patient develops a malignancy, RAPTIVA should be discontinued (see **ADVERSE REACTIONS, Malignancy**).

Thrombocytopenia

Platelet counts at or below 52,000 cells per µL were observed in 8 (0.3%) RAPTIVA-treated patients during clinical trials compared with none among the placebo-treated patients (see **ADVERSE REACTIONS, Thrombocytopenia**). Five of the 8 patients received a course of systemic steroids for thrombocytopenia. Thrombocytopenia resolved in the 7 patients receiving adequate follow-up (1 patient was lost to follow-up). Physicians should follow patients closely for signs and symptoms of thrombocytopenia. Assessment of platelet counts is recommended during treatment with RAPTIVA (see **PRECAUTIONS, Laboratory Tests**) and RAPTIVA should be discontinued if thrombocytopenia develops.

Psoriasis Worsening and Variants

Worsening of psoriasis can occur during or after discontinuation of RAPTIVA. During clinical studies, 19 of 2589 (0.7%) of RAPTIVA-treated patients had serious worsening of psoriasis during treatment (n = 5) or worsening past baseline after discontinuation of RAPTIVA (n = 14) (see **ADVERSE REACTIONS, Adverse Events of Psoriasis**). In some patients these events took the form of psoriatic erythroderma or pustular psoriasis. Some patients required hospitalization and alternative antipsoriatic therapy to manage the psoriasis worsening. Patients, including those not responding to RAPTIVA treatment, should be closely observed following discontinuation of RAPTIVA, and appropriate psoriasis treatment instituted as necessary.

PRECAUTIONS

Immunosuppression

The safety and efficacy of RAPTIVA in combination with other immunosuppressive agents or phototherapy have not been evaluated. Patients receiving other immunosuppressive agents should not receive concurrent therapy with RAPTIVA because of the possibility of increased risk of infections and malignancies.

Immunizations

The safety and efficacy of vaccines, administered to patients being treated with RAPTIVA have not been studied. In a small clinical study with IV administered RAPTIVA, a single dose of 0.3 mg/kg given before primary immunization with a neoantigen decreased the secondary immune response, and a dose of 1 mg/kg almost completely ablated it. A dose of 0.3 mg/kg IV has comparable pharmacodynamic effects to the recommended dose of 1 mg/kg SC. In chimpanzees exposed to RAPTIVA at ≥10 times the clinical exposure level (based on mean peak plasma levels) antibody responses were decreased following immunization with tetanus toxoid compared with untreated control animals. Acellular, live and live-attenuated vaccines should not be administered during RAPTIVA treatment.

First Dose Reactions

First dose reactions including headache, fever, nausea, and vomiting are associated with RAPTIVA treatment and are dose-level related in incidence and severity (see **ADVERSE REACTIONS**). Therefore, a conditioning dose of 0.7 mg/kg is recommended to reduce the incidence and severity of reactions associated with initial dosing (see **DOSAGE AND ADMINISTRATION**). One case of aseptic meningitis resulting in hospitalization has been observed in association with initial dosing (see **ADVERSE REACTIONS, Inflammatory/Immune-Mediated Reactions**).

Information for Patients

Patients should be informed that their physician may monitor platelet counts during therapy. Patients should be advised to seek immediate medical attention if they develop any of the signs and symptoms associated with severe thrombocytopenia, such as easy bleeding from the gums, bruising, or petechiae. Patients should also be informed that RAPTIVA is an immunosuppressant, and could increase their chances of developing an infection or a malignancy. Patients should be advised to promptly call the prescribing doctor's office if they develop any new signs of, or receive a new diagnosis of infection or malignancy while undergoing treatment with RAPTIVA.

Female patients should also be advised to notify their physicians if they become pregnant while taking RAPTIVA (or within 6 weeks of discontinuing RAPTIVA) and be advised of the existence of and encouraged to enroll in the RAPTIVA Pregnancy Registry.

If a patient or caregiver is to administer RAPTIVA, he/she should be instructed regarding injection techniques and how to measure the correct dose to ensure proper administration of RAPTIVA. Patients should be also referred to the RAPTIVA Patient Package Insert. In addition, patients should have available materials for and be instructed in the proper disposal of needles and syringes to comply with state and local laws. Patients should also be cautioned against reuse of syringes and needles.

Laboratory Tests

Assessment of platelet counts is recommended upon initiating and periodically while receiving RAPTIVA treatment. It is recommended that assessments be more frequent when initiating therapy (e.g., monthly) and may decrease in frequency with continued treatment (e.g., every 3 months). Severe thrombocytopenia has been observed (see **WARNINGS, Thrombocytopenia**).

Drug Interactions

No formal drug interaction studies have been performed with RAPTIVA. RAPTIVA should not be used with other immunosuppressive drugs (see **PRECAUTIONS, Immunosuppression**).

Acellular, live and live-attenuated vaccines should not be administered during RAPTIVA treatment (see **PRECAUTIONS, Immunizations**).

Drug/Laboratory Test Interactions

Increases in lymphocyte counts related to the pharmacologic mechanism of action are frequently observed during RAPTIVA treatment (see **CLINICAL PHARMACOLOGY, Pharmacodynamics**).

Carcinogenesis, Mutagenesis, Impairment of Fertility

Long-term animal studies have not been conducted to evaluate the carcinogenic potential of RAPTIVA.

Subcutaneous injections of male and female mice with an anti-mouse CD11a antibody at up to 30 times the equivalent of the 1 mg/kg clinical dose of RAPTIVA had no adverse effects on mating, fertility, or reproduction parameters. The clinical significance of this observation is uncertain.

Genotoxicity studies were not conducted.

Pregnancy (Category C)

Animal reproduction studies have not been conducted with RAPTIVA. It is also not known whether RAPTIVA can cause fetal harm when administered to a pregnant woman or can affect reproduction capacity. RAPTIVA should be given to a pregnant woman only if clearly needed.

In a developmental toxicity study conducted in mice using an anti-mouse CD11a antibody at up to 30 times the equivalent of the recommended clinical dose of RAPTIVA, no evidence of maternal toxicity, embryotoxicity, or teratogenicity was observed when administered during organogenesis. No adverse effects on behavioral, reproductive, or growth parameters were observed in offspring of female mice subcutaneously treated with an anti-mouse CD11a antibody during gestation and lactation using doses 3- to 30-times the equivalent of the recommended clinical dose of RAPTIVA. At 11 weeks of age, the offspring of these females exhibited a significant reduction in their ability to mount an antibody response, which showed evidence of partial reversibility by 25 weeks of age. Animal studies, however, are not always predictive of human response, and there are no adequate and well-controlled studies in pregnant women.

Since the effects of RAPTIVA on pregnant women and fetal development, including immune system development are not known, healthcare providers are encouraged to enroll patients who become pregnant while taking RAPTIVA (or within 6 weeks of discontinuing RAPTIVA) in the RAPTIVA Pregnancy Registry.

Nursing Mothers

It is not known whether RAPTIVA is excreted in human milk. An anti-mouse CD11a antibody was detected in milk samples of lactating mice exposed to anti-mouse CD11a antibody and the offspring of the exposed females exhibited significant reduction in antibody responses (see **PRECAUTIONS, Pregnancy**). Since maternal immunoglobulins are known to be present in the milk of lactating mothers, and animal data suggest the potential for adverse effects in nursing infants from RAPTIVA, a decision should be made whether to discontinue nursing while taking the drug or to discontinue the use of the drug, taking into account the importance of the drug to the mother.

Table 2
Percentage of Patients Responding after 12 Weeks of Treatment

Outcome Measurement	Study	Placebo	RAPTIVA 1 mg/kg/wk	Difference[a] (95% CI)
sPGA: Minimal or Clear	1	3%	26%	23% (16, 30)
	2	3%	32%	29% (21, 39)
	3	3%	19%	16% (8, 25)
	4	4%	20%	16% (11, 22)
>50% improvement in PASI (PASI-50)	1	14%	59%	45% (37, 53)
	2	15%	61%	46% (37, 56)
	3	16%	52%	36% (26, 47)
	4	14%	52%	38% (31, 45)

The number of patients in each study and treatment group is the same as listed in Table 1.
[a] p <0.001 for comparison of RAPTIVA group to placebo group using Fisher's exact test for all comparisons between groups.

Pediatric Use
The safety and efficacy of RAPTIVA in pediatric patients have not been studied.

Geriatric Use
Of the 1620 patients who received RAPTIVA in controlled trials, 128 were ≥65 years of age, and 2 were ≥75 years of age. Although no differences in safety or efficacy were observed between older and younger patients, the number of patients aged 65 and over is not sufficient to determine whether they respond differently from younger patients. Because the incidence of infections is higher in the elderly population, in general, caution should be used in treating the elderly.

ADVERSE REACTIONS

The most serious adverse reactions observed during treatment with RAPTIVA were serious infections, malignancies, thrombocytopenia and psoriasis worsening and variants (see **WARNINGS**).

The most common adverse reactions associated with RAPTIVA were a first dose reaction complex that included headache, chills, fever, nausea, and myalgia within two days following the first two injections. These reactions are dose-level related in incidence and severity and were largely mild to moderate in severity when a conditioning dose of 0.7 mg/kg was used as the first dose. In placebo-controlled trials, 29% of patients treated with RAPTIVA 1 mg/kg developed one or more of these symptoms following the first dose compared with 15% of patients receiving placebo. After the third dose, 4% and 3% of patients receiving RAPTIVA 1 mg/kg and placebo, respectively, experienced these symptoms. Less than 1% of patients discontinued RAPTIVA treatment because of these adverse events.

Other adverse events resulting in discontinuation of RAPTIVA treatment were psoriasis (0.6%), pain (0.4%), arthritis (0.4%), and arthralgia (0.3%).

Because clinical trials are conducted under widely varying conditions, adverse reaction rates observed in the clinical trials of one drug cannot be directly compared to rates in the clinical trials of another drug and may not reflect the rates observed in practice.

The data described below reflect RAPTIVA exposure for 2762 adult psoriasis patients (age range 18 to 75 years), including 2400 patients exposed for three months, 904 for six months, and 218 exposed for one year or more, in all controlled and uncontrolled studies. The median age of patients receiving RAPTIVA was 44 years, with 189 patients above the age of 65; 67% were men, and 89% were Caucasian. These data include patients treated at doses higher than the recommended dose of 1 mg/kg weekly.

Controlled clinical trials provide the most informative basis for estimating the frequency of RAPTIVA-related adverse drug reactions. Table 3 enumerates the adverse events occurring during controlled periods of the clinical trials where the frequency of the adverse events is at least 2% greater in the RAPTIVA-treated group than the placebo group.

Table 3
Adverse Events in Placebo Controlled Study Periods Reported at a ≥2% Higher Rate in the 1 mg/kg/wk RAPTIVA Treatment than Placebo Groups

	Placebo (n = 715)	RAPTIVA 1 mg/kg/wk (n = 1213)
Headache	159 (22%)	391 (32%)
Infection[a]	188 (26%)	350 (29%)
Chills	32 (4%)	154 (13%)
Nausea	51 (7%)	128 (11%)
Pain	38 (5%)	122 (10%)
Myalgia	35 (5%)	102 (8%)
Flu Syndrome	29 (4%)	83 (7%)
Fever	24 (3%)	80 (7%)
Back pain	14 (2%)	50 (4%)
Acne	4 (1%)	45 (4%)

[a] Includes diagnosed infections and other non-specific infections. Most common non-specific infection was upper respiratory infection.

Adverse events occurring at a rate between 1 and 2% greater in the RAPTIVA group compared with placebo were arthralgia, asthenia, peripheral edema, and psoriasis.

The following serious adverse reactions were observed in RAPTIVA-treated patients.

Infections
In the first 12 weeks of placebo-controlled studies, the proportion of patients with serious infection was 0.4% (7/1620) in the RAPTIVA-treated group (5 of these were hospitalized, 0.3%) and 0.1% (1/715) in the placebo group (see **WARNINGS, Serious Infections**). In the complete safety data from both controlled and uncontrolled studies, the overall incidence of hospitalization for infections was 1.6 per 100 patient-years for RAPTIVA-treated patients compared with 1.2 per 100 patient-years for placebo-treated patients. Including both controlled, uncontrolled, and follow-up study treatment periods there were 27 serious infections in 2475 RAPTIVA-treated patients. These infections included cellulitis, pneumonia, abscess, sepsis, sinusitis, bronchitis, gastroenteritis, aseptic meningitis, Legionnaire's disease, septic arthritis, and vertebral osteomyelitis. In controlled trials, the overall rate of infections in RAPTIVA-treated patients was 3% higher than in placebo-treated patients (Table 3).

Malignancies
Among the 2762 psoriasis patients who received RAPTIVA at any dose (median duration 8 months), 31 patients were diagnosed with 37 malignancies (see **WARNINGS, Malignancies**). The overall incidence of malignancies of any kind was 1.8 per 100 patient-years for RAPTIVA-treated patients compared with 1.6 per 100 patient-years for placebo-treated patients. Malignancies observed in the RAPTIVA-treated patients included non-melanoma skin cancer, non-cutaneous solid tumors, Hodgkin's lymphoma and non-Hodgkin's lymphoma, and malignant. The incidence of non-cutaneous solid tumors (8 in 1790 patient-years) and malignant melanoma were within the range expected for the general population.

The majority of the malignancies were non-melanoma skin cancers; 26 cases (13 basal, 13 squamous) in 20 patients (0.7% of 2762 RAPTIVA-treated patients). The incidence was comparable for RAPTIVA-treated and placebo-treated patients. However, the size of the placebo group and duration of follow-up were limited and a difference in rates of non-melanoma skin cancers cannot be excluded.

Thrombocytopenia
In the combined safety database of 2762 RAPTIVA-treated patients, there were eight occurrences (0.3%) of thrombocytopenia of <52,000 cells per µL reported (see **WARNINGS, Thrombocytopenia**). Three of the eight patients were hospitalized for thrombocytopenia, including one patient with heavy uterine bleeding; all cases were consistent with an immune mediated thrombocytopenia. Antiplatelet antibody was evaluated in one patient and was found to be positive. Each case resulted in discontinuation of RAPTIVA. Based on available platelet count measurements, the onset of platelet decline was between 8 and 12 weeks after the first dose of RAPTIVA in 5 of the patients. Onset was more delayed in 3 patients, occurring as late as one year in 1 patient. In these cases, the platelet count nadirs occurred between 12 and 72 weeks after the first dose of RAPTIVA.

Adverse Events of Psoriasis
In the combined safety database from all studies, serious psoriasis adverse events occurred in 19 RAPTIVA-treated patients (0.7%) including hospitalization in 17 patients (see **WARNINGS, Psoriasis Worsening/Variants**). Most of these events (14/19) occurred after discontinuation of study drug and occurred in both patients responding and not responding to RAPTIVA treatment. Serious adverse events of psoriasis included pustular, erythrodermic, and guttate subtypes. During the first 12 weeks of treatment within placebo-controlled studies, the rate of psoriasis adverse events (serious and non-serious) was 3.2% (52/1620) in the RAPTIVA-treated patients and 1.4% (10/715) in the placebo-treated patients.

Hypersensitivity Reactions
Symptoms associated with a hypersensitivity reaction (e.g., dyspnea, asthma, urticaria, angioedema, maculopapular rash) were evaluated by treatment group. In the first 12 weeks of the controlled clinical studies, the proportion of patients reporting at least one hypersensitivity reaction was 8% (95/1213) in the 1 mg/kg/wk group and 7% (49/715) patients in the placebo group. Urticaria was observed in 1% of patients (16/1213) receiving RAPTIVA and 0.4% of patients (3/715) receiving placebo during the initial 12-week treatment period. Other observed adverse events in patients receiving RAPTIVA that may be indicative of hypersensitivity included: laryngospasm, angioedema, erythema multiforme, asthma, and allergic drug eruption. One patient was hospitalized with a serum sickness-like reaction.

Inflammatory/Immune-Mediated Reactions
In the entire RAPTIVA clinical development program of 2762 RAPTIVA-treated patients, inflammatory, potentially immune-mediated adverse events resulting in hospitalization included inflammatory arthritis (12 cases, 0.4% of patients) and interstitial pneumonitis (2 cases). One case each of the following serious adverse reactions was observed: transverse myelitis, bronchiolitis obliterans, aseptic meningitis, idiopathic hepatitis, sialedenitis, and sensorineural hearing loss.

Laboratory Values
In RAPTIVA-treated patients, a mean elevation in alkaline phosphatase (5 Units/L) was observed; 4% of RAPTIVA-treated patients experienced a shift to above normal values compared with 0.6% of placebo-treated patients. The clinical significance of this change is unknown. Higher numbers of RAPTIVA-treated patients experienced elevations above normal in two or more liver function tests than placebo (3.1% vs. 1.5%).

Other laboratory adverse reactions that were observed included thrombocytopenia, (see **WARNINGS**, and **ADVERSE REACTIONS, Thrombocytopenia**), lymphocytosis (40%) (including three cases of transient atypical lymphocytosis), and leukocytosis (26%).

Immunogenicity
In patients evaluated for antibodies to RAPTIVA after RAPTIVA treatment ended, predominantly low-titer antibodies to RAPTIVA or other protein components of the RAPTIVA drug product were detected in 6.3% (67/1063) of patients. The long-term immunogenicity of RAPTIVA is unknown.

The data reflect the percentage of patients whose test results were considered positive for antibodies to RAPTIVA in the ELISA assay, and are highly dependent on the sensitivity and specificity of the assay. Additionally, the observed incidence of antibody positivity in an assay may be influenced by several factors including sample handling, timing of sample collection, concomitant medications, and underlying disease. For these reasons, comparison of the incidence of antibodies to RAPTIVA with the incidence of antibodies to other products may be misleading.

OVERDOSAGE

Doses up to 4 mg/kg/wk SC for 10 weeks following a conditioning (0.7 mg/kg) first dose have been administered without an observed increase in acute toxicity. The maximum administered single dose was 10 mg/kg IV. This was administered to one patient, who subsequently was admitted to the hospital for severe vomiting. In case of overdose, it is recommended that the patient be monitored for 24–48 hours for any acute signs or symptoms of adverse reactions or effects and appropriate treatment instituted.

DOSAGE AND ADMINISTRATION

The recommended dose of RAPTIVA is a single 0.7 mg/kg SC conditioning dose followed by weekly SC doses of 1 mg/kg (maximum single dose not to exceed a total of 200 mg).

RAPTIVA is intended for use under the guidance and supervision of a physician. If it is determined to be appropriate, patients may self-inject RAPTIVA after proper training in the preparation and injection technique and with medical follow-up.

Preparation for Administration
RAPTIVA should be administered using the sterile, disposable syringe and needles provided (see **HOW SUPPLIED** section). Remove the cap from the pre-filled syringe containing sterile water for injection (non-USP) and attach the needle to the syringe. Remove the plastic cap protecting the rubber stopper of the RAPTIVA vial and wipe the top of the rubber stopper with one of the provided alcohol swabs. After cleaning with the alcohol swab, do not touch the top of the vial. To prepare the RAPTIVA solution, using the provided pre-filled diluent syringe slowly inject the 1.3 mL of sterile water for injection (non-USP) into the RAPTIVA vial. Swirl the vial with a GENTLE rotary motion to dissolve the product. DO NOT SHAKE. Shaking will cause foaming of the RAPTIVA solution. Generally, dissolution of RAPTIVA takes less than 5 minutes. RAPTIVA is provided as a single-use vial and contains no antibacterial preservatives. Reconstitute immediately before use and use only once. If the reconstituted RAPTIVA is not used immediately, store the RAPTIVA vial at room temperature and use within 8 hours. The reconstituted solution should be clear to pale yellow and free of particulates.

Administration
Parenteral drug products should be inspected visually for particulate matter and discoloration prior to subcutaneous administration. If particulates or discolorations are noted, the product should not be used. Replace the needle on the syringe with a new needle. Insert the needle into the vial containing the RAPTIVA solution, invert the vial, and keeping the needle below the level of the liquid, withdraw the dose to be given into the syringe.

No other medications should be added to solutions containing RAPTIVA, and RAPTIVA should not be reconstituted with other diluents.

Sites for injection include thigh, abdomen, buttocks, or upper arm. Injection sites should be rotated.

Following administration, discard any unused reconstituted RAPTIVA solution.

Stability and Storage
Do not use a vial beyond the expiration date stamped on the carton or vial label. RAPTIVA (lyophilized powder) must be refrigerated at 2–8°C (36–46°F). Protect the vial from exposure to light. Store in original carton until time of use.

HOW SUPPLIED

RAPTIVA™ (efalizumab) is supplied as a lyophilized, sterile powder to deliver 125 mg of efalizumab per single-use vial. Each RAPTIVA carton contains four trays. Each tray contains one single-use vial designed to deliver 125 mg of efalizumab, one single-use prefilled diluent syringe containing 1.3 mL sterile water for injection (non-USP), two 25 gauge × 5/8 inch needles, two alcohol prep pads, a package insert with an accompanying patient information insert. The NDC number for the four administration dose pack carton is 50242-058-04.

REFERENCES

1. Werther WA, Gonzalez TN, O'Connor SJ, McCabe S, Chan B, Hotaling T, et al. Humanization of an anti-lymphocyte function-associated antigen (LFA)-1 monoclonal antibody and reengineering of the humanized antibody for binding to rhesus LFA-1. J Immunol 1996;157:4986–95.

Patient Information

RAPTIVA (Rap-TEE-vah)
(efalizumab)
for injection, subcutaneous

Read the Patient Information that comes with RAPTIVA™ (efalizumab) before you start using it and each time you get a refill. There may be new information. This information does not take the place of talking with your healthcare provider about your medical condition or treatment. It is important to remain under a healthcare provider's care while using RAPTIVA. **Do not change or stop treatment without first talking with your healthcare provider.** Talk to your healthcare provider or pharmacist if you have any questions about RAPTIVA.

Continued on next page

Raptiva—Cont.

WHAT IS THE MOST IMPORTANT INFORMATION I SHOULD KNOW ABOUT RAPTIVA?
RAPTIVA can decrease the activity of your immune system. Therefore, people using RAPTIVA may have an increased chance of getting:
- **Serious infections.** Some infections could become serious. If you have an infection, tell your healthcare provider before you start using RAPTIVA. If you get an infection that does not go away while taking RAPTIVA, tell your healthcare provider right away.
- **Cancers.** Many drugs that decrease the activity of the immune system can increase the risk of cancer. If you have had cancer you should tell your healthcare provider before you start taking RAPTIVA. The role of RAPTIVA in the development of cancer is not known.
- **Low platelet counts (thrombocytopenia).** Platelets help your blood clot. Low platelets give you a higher chance for bleeding. Call your doctor right away if you have increased bruising or bleeding. Your healthcare provider may do regular blood tests to check your platelets while you are taking RAPTIVA.
- **Worsening of psoriasis.** Some patients have had severe worsening or new forms of psoriasis while taking RAPTIVA or after stopping RAPTIVA. Tell your healthcare provider right away if your psoriasis gets worse or if you see any new rashes during or after treatment with RAPTIVA.

You should not receive vaccines while using RAPTIVA. RAPTIVA may prevent a vaccine from working. Talk to your healthcare provider if you need to receive a vaccine while using RAPTIVA.

WHAT IS RAPTIVA?
RAPTIVA is a medicine used to treat adult patients with moderate to severe plaque psoriasis who can be treated with medicines that affect the whole body (systemic therapy) or with phototherapy.
RAPTIVA is a man-made protein that is like proteins made in the body called antibodies. Antibodies fight disease in the human body. RAPTIVA may decrease the skin changes in the body that are the main problems of moderate to severe plaque psoriasis.
RAPTIVA has not been studied in children under 18 years of age.

WHO SHOULD NOT USE RAPTIVA?
Do not use RAPTIVA if you have ever had an allergic reaction to RAPTIVA.
Before using RAPTIVA, tell your healthcare provider
1. **about the following medical conditions:**
   - **If you are pregnant, planning to become pregnant, or become pregnant while using RAPTIVA.** It is not known if RAPTIVA can harm your unborn baby. If you become pregnant while taking RAPTIVA, notify your healthcare provider immediately. You and your healthcare provider will have to decide if RAPTIVA is right for you during pregnancy. If you use RAPTIVA when you are pregnant, ask your healthcare provider how you can be on the RAPTIVA pregnancy registry.
   - **If you are breast feeding.** It is not known if RAPTIVA passes into your milk. It may harm your baby. You will need to decide whether to use RAPTIVA or breast feed, but you may not do both.
   - **If you have any infections (see WHAT IS THE MOST IMPORTANT INFORMATION I SHOULD KNOW ABOUT RAPTIVA?).**
   - **If you have immune system problems**
2. **about all the medicines you take including prescription and nonprescription medicines, vitamins, and herbal supplements.** It is not known if RAPTIVA and other medicines affect each other. **Especially, tell your healthcare provider if you are using:**
   - **Other medicines or treatments for your psoriasis**
   - **Medicines called immunosuppressives or any medicine that affects your immune system.** Ask your healthcare provider or pharmacist if you are not sure if any of your medicines are immunosuppressives.

HOW SHOULD I USE RAPTIVA?
- RAPTIVA is an injection that you give yourself once a week.
- **See the end of this leaflet for instructions on how to prepare and inject RAPTIVA (HOW DO I PREPARE AND GIVE A RAPTIVA INJECTION?).** Ask your healthcare provider or pharmacist if you have any questions about using RAPTIVA.
- Use RAPTIVA exactly as prescribed by your healthcare provider. Your dose of RAPTIVA is based on your body weight. Tell your healthcare provider if your weight changes. Do not change your dose without talking to your healthcare provider. Do not stop using RAPTIVA without talking to your healthcare provider.
- RAPTIVA is injected under the skin (subcutaneous) of your upper leg (thigh), upper arm, abdomen, or buttocks once a week. Change (rotate) your skin injection site with each injection.
- Use RAPTIVA the same day each week. If you miss your dose of RAPTIVA contact your healthcare provider to find out when to take your next dose of RAPTIVA and what schedule to follow after that.
- If you take more than your regular dose of RAPTIVA, call your healthcare provider right away.
- See your healthcare provider regularly while using RAPTIVA. Do not miss your appointments. Your healthcare provider may do blood tests including platelet counts before and during treatment with RAPTIVA to check its affect on your body.

WHAT SHOULD I AVOID WHILE USING RAPTIVA?
Unless directed by your healthcare provider, do not:
- take other medicines called immunosuppressives.
- take treatments called phototherapy.

You should not receive vaccines while using RAPTIVA. Talk to your healthcare provider if you need to receive a vaccine while taking RAPTIVA (see **WHAT IS THE MOST IMPORTANT INFORMATION I SHOULD KNOW ABOUT RAPTIVA?**).

WHAT ARE THE POSSIBLE SIDE EFFECTS OF RAPTIVA?
RAPTIVA can cause serious side effects including the following (see WHAT IS THE MOST IMPORTANT INFORMATION I SHOULD KNOW ABOUT RAPTIVA?):
RAPTIVA can affect your immune system and might cause:
- **Serious infections**
- **Cancers**
- **Low platelet counts (thrombocytopenia)**
- **Worsening of psoriasis**

The most common side effects of RAPTIVA include headache, chills, fever, nausea, and muscle aches. These reactions usually happen within the first 48 hours following RAPTIVA injection, and often decrease after the first few weeks of use of RAPTIVA. Back pain, joint pain, and swelling of the arms or legs (peripheral edema) can also happen with RAPTIVA. Talk to your healthcare provider about any symptoms that bother you.
If you get any side effect that concerns you or if you get an infection, call your healthcare provider.
These are not all the side effects of RAPTIVA. For more information, ask your healthcare provider or pharmacist.

HOW SHOULD I STORE RAPTIVA?
- Store RAPTIVA vials in the refrigerator at 36° to 46°F (2° to 8°C) until you are ready to prepare your injection. **Do not freeze or store at room temperature.** Once RAPTIVA has been mixed with sterile water, you should use it right away to inject yourself. If you are unable to inject the drug after mixing, the mixture can stay at room temperature for up to 8 hours. Do not use RAPTIVA that was mixed more than 8 hours earlier.
  If you are traveling, be sure to store RAPTIVA at the right temperature. If you have any questions, ask your healthcare provider or pharmacist.
- Protect RAPTIVA vials from light while stored.
- Throw away RAPTIVA vials that are out of date.
- **Keep RAPTIVA and all medicines out of the reach of children.**

GENERAL INFORMATION ABOUT RAPTIVA
Medicines are sometimes prescribed for conditions that are not mentioned in patient information leaflets. Do not use RAPTIVA for a condition for which it was not prescribed. Do not give RAPTIVA to other people, even if they have the same symptoms you have. It may harm them.
This leaflet summarizes the most important information about RAPTIVA. If you would like more information, talk with your healthcare provider. You can ask your healthcare provider or pharmacist for information about RAPTIVA that is written for health professionals. For more information, you can also call 1-877-RAPTIVA (toll free).

HOW DO I PREPARE AND GIVE A RAPTIVA INJECTION?
If your dose amount is more than 1.25 mL, you will need to use 2 RAPTIVA blister trays, and you will give yourself 2 injections of RAPTIVA.

Setting Up the Equipment
1. Take the RAPTIVA blister tray out of the refrigerator, and place it on a flat, well-lit, clean work surface.
2. Wash your hands with soap and warm water before opening the blister tray.
3. Open the tray and lay out the contents. Allow the contents to come to room temperature.

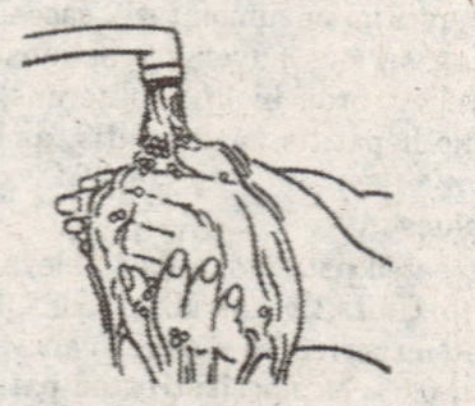

As shown below, the tray contains:
- One RAPTIVA vial
- One 1.3-mL prefilled syringe of sterile water
- Two 25-gauge needles
- Two alcohol prep pads

Contact your healthcare provider or pharmacist if you are missing any of the items listed above.

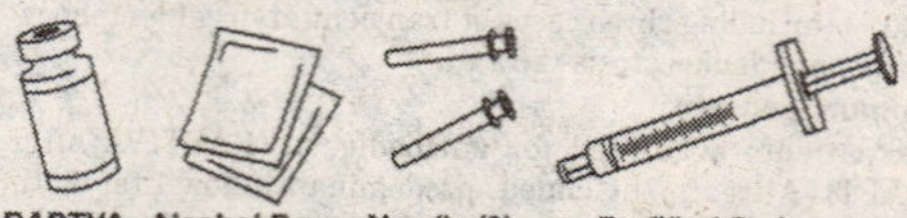

RAPTVA Vial **Alcohol Prep Pads (2)** **Needle (2)** **Prefilled Syringe**

4. Check the expiration (Exp.) date on the RAPTIVA vial label and prefilled syringe label. If the expiration date has passed, do not use the RAPTIVA vial or the prefilled syringe containing the sterile water. Contact your healthcare provider.
   [See figure at top of next column]
5. Remove the plastic cap protecting the rubber stopper of the RAPTIVA vial. Wipe the rubber stopper with an alcohol prep pad. Do not touch the top of the vial.

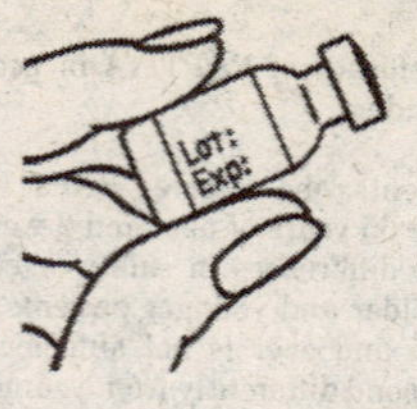

6. Remove one of the 25-gauge needles from its package. Remove the cap covering the prefilled syringe tip. Carefully place the capped 25-gauge needle onto the syringe tip. Remove the needle cap. Do not touch the needle.

Mixing RAPTIVA
If your RAPTIVA dose amount is greater than 1.25 mL, repeat Steps 1–3 of this section using a second RAPTIVA blister tray.
1. Keep the RAPTIVA vial upright on a firm surface, and slowly puncture the rubber stopper with the needle. Very slowly push down on the syringe plunger to inject all of the 1.3 mL of sterile water onto the side wall of the vial to cause less foaming. Some foaming may happen; this is normal.

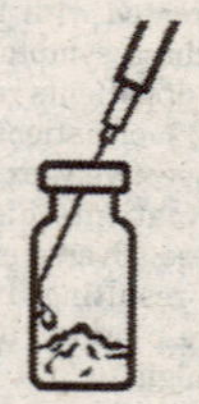

2. With the needle and syringe still in the vial stopper, gently swirl the vial to mix. Wait 5 minutes for the medicine to completely dissolve. To avoid excess foaming, **do not shake the vial.** Very slowly pull out the needle and syringe. Do not use the solution if it is discolored or cloudy or if particles (solid matter) are in the solution. The RAPTIVA solution should be clear to pale yellow.

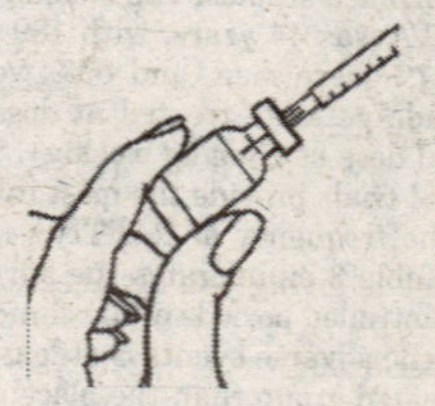

3. Slide the needle into the cap on a flat surface to pick up the cap. To lower the chance of a needlestick injury, do not touch the cap until it covers the needle all the way. Push the cap all the way down over the needle. Twist the capped needle off the syringe and discard it in a puncture-resistant container (see **DISPOSAL OF THE SYRINGE, NEEDLES, AND SUPPLIES). Never reuse a needle.**

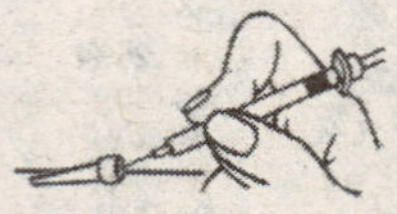

Preparing the RAPTIVA Dose for Injection
If your dose amount is more than 1.25 mL, split the dose evenly and follow Steps 1–8 of this section using the contents of two separate RAPTIVA blister trays.
1. Using an alcohol prep pad, wipe the rubber stopper of the vial containing the mixed RAPTIVA solution.

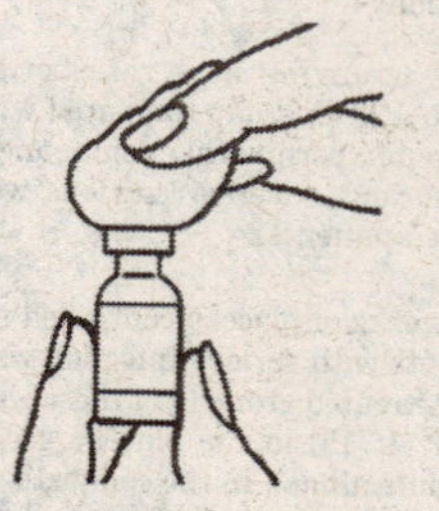

2. Remove the remaining unused needle from its package. Connect this needle to the syringe tip, and carefully remove the needle cap.
3. Keep the RAPTIVA vial in an upright position on a flat surface, and push the needle straight down through the rubber stopper on the vial.
4. Turn the vial upside down, keeping the needle in the vial (The needle will now be pointing upward.). Make sure the tip of the needle is covered all the way by the medicine in the vial. This will make it easier to get the medicine into the syringe.
5. Pull back on the plunger to fill the syringe. Remove the

correct dose of medicine by reading the numbers on the syringe.

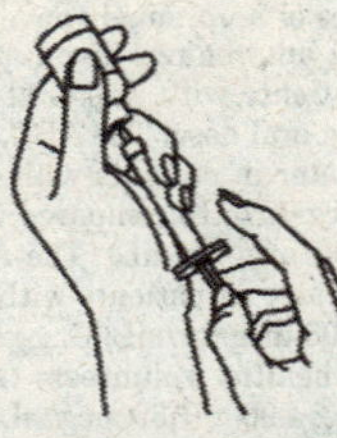

6. Hold the syringe upright and tap the side of the syringe to let air bubbles rise to the top. Gently push in the plunger of the syringe to push the air bubbles out.
7. After removing the bubbles, recheck the dose of medicine in the syringe. Make sure you have the right dose as instructed by your healthcare provider.
8. Slide the needle into the cap on a flat surface to pick up the syringe cap. Do not let the needle touch anything except the inside of the cap. Push the cap all the way down over the needle. Put the syringe down while preparing your skin for injection.

Selecting and Preparing the Injection Site

1. Wash your hands well with soap and water.

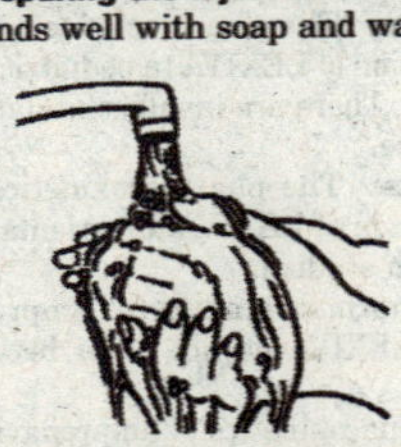

2. Choose an area of the body for the injection. Avoid, if possible, skin involved with psoriasis. Possible injection sites include the following:
   - Outer area of the upper legs (thighs)
   - Stomach area around the belly button

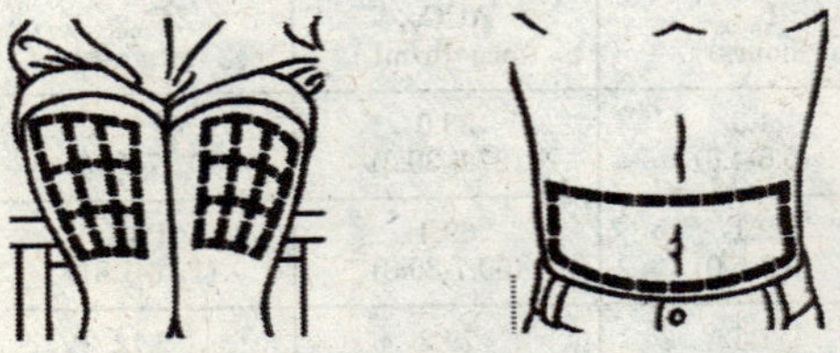

If someone else is giving you an injection, you can also use:
- Back of upper arms
- Buttocks

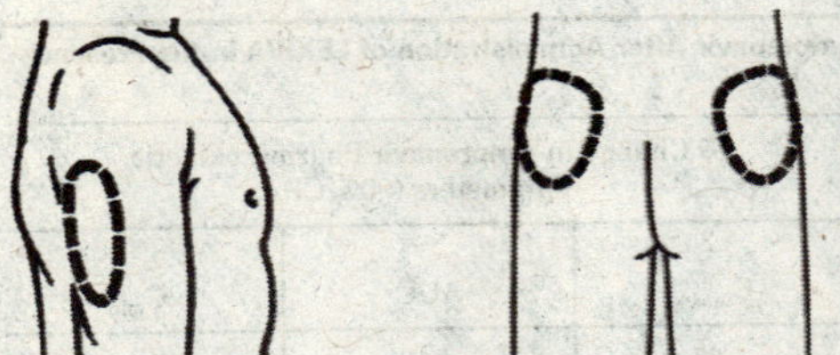

3. It is important to change (rotate) the injection site each time you take RAPTIVA to lower your chances of soreness and redness at the injection site. Changing the injection site will also improve absorption of the medication. Repeat injections given in the same area should be at least 1 inch apart. Do not give an injection close to a vein that you can see under the surface of your skin.
4. Wash the skin at the site of injection with soap and water. Let it air dry.
5. Cleanse the skin at the injection site with an alcohol-soaked cotton ball or pad using a circular motion. Let the area air dry all the way. **Do not touch this area again before giving the injection.**

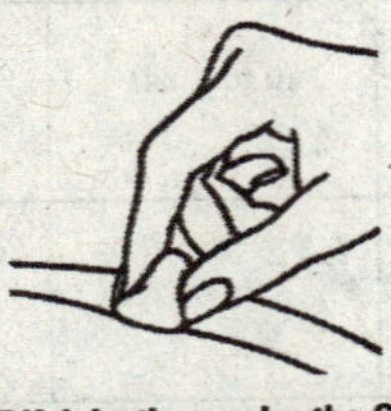

Giving the RAPTIVA Injection under the Skin

Your healthcare provider will teach you how to inject RAPTIVA. Do not inject RAPTIVA unless you have been taught the right way to give the injection.

1. Hold the syringe and remove the needle cover. Twisting the needle cover while pulling will help in the removal. **Do not** touch the needle or allow the needle to touch anything.
   [See figure at top of next column]
2. Hold the syringe in the hand you use to inject yourself. Use your other hand to pinch a patch of skin at the clean injection site. **Do not** lay the syringe down or allow the needle to touch anything.
3. Hold the syringe firmly between your thumb and fingers

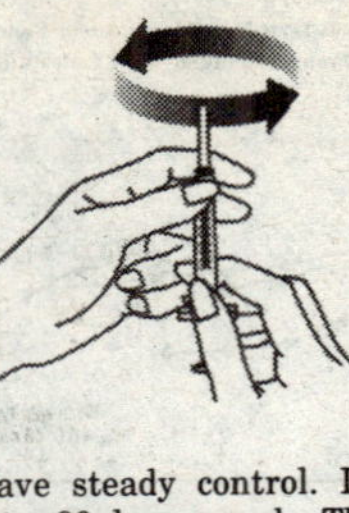

so that you have steady control. Insert the needle straight down at a 90-degree angle. This is important to make sure the medicine is injected into fatty tissue.

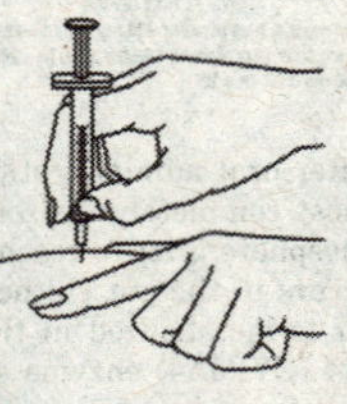

4. After the needle is inserted all the way into the skin, you can gently let go of the pinched skin. Be sure the needle stays in your skin. Slowly and smoothly push the plunger down into the syringe until it stops.
5. When all of the medicine has been injected, remove the needle and do not re-cap it. Press a dry, sterile gauze over the injection site. Do not use the alcohol prep pad. A small bandage may be put over the injection site.

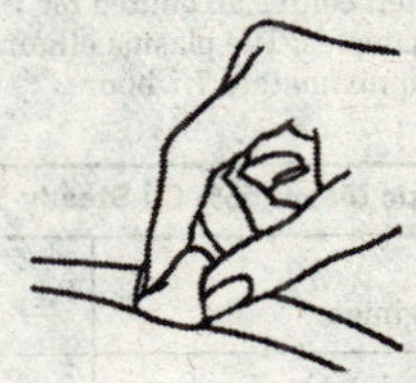

6. If your dose amount is more than 1.25 mL, you will need to give a second injection. Choose the second injection site at least 1 inch from the first injection site.

DISPOSAL OF THE SYRINGE, NEEDLES, AND SUPPLIES

1. Place the used syringe with the attached needle in a puncture-resistant container, like a sharps container. You can buy a sharps container at your local pharmacy.

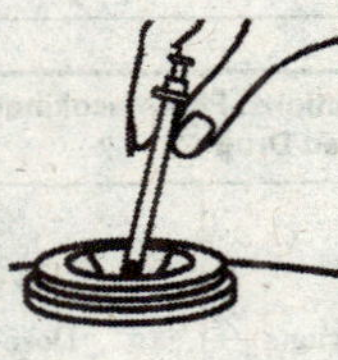

2. Talk to your healthcare provider about how to properly dispose of a filled container of your used syringes and needles. There may be special local and state laws for disposing of used needles and syringes. **Do not throw the filled container in the household trash and do not recycle.**
3. The needle cap, alcohol prep pads, and other used supplies can be thrown out with your regular trash.
4. **Always keep syringes, injection supplies, and disposal containers out of the reach of children.**
5. **Do not reuse these single-use syringes.**

Rx Only

RAPTIVA™ [efalizumab]

Manufactured by:
Genentech, Inc.
1 DNA Way
South San Francisco, CA 94080-4990
4826400
FDA Approval October 2003
©2003 Genentech, Inc.

In the PDR annual, the **Brand and Generic Name Index** (PINK section) alphabetizes drugs under both brand and generic names.

GlaxoSmithKline

FIVE MOORE DRIVE
RESEARCH TRIANGLE PARK, NC 27709

For Medical Emergencies, Medical Information for Healthcare Professionals, and Consumer Inquiries, Contact:
1-888-825-5249
www.druginfo.gsk.com

LEXIVA™ ℞

[lex-ē'-vah]
(fosamprenavir calcium)
Tablets

DESCRIPTION

LEXIVA (fosamprenavir calcium) is a prodrug of amprenavir, an inhibitor of human immunodeficiency virus (HIV) protease. The chemical name of fosamprenavir calcium is (3*S*)-tetrahydrofuran-3-yl (1*S*,2*R*)-3-[[(4-aminophenyl) sulfonyl](isobutyl)amino]-1-benzyl-2-(phosphonooxy) propylcarbamate monocalcium salt. Fosamprenavir calcium is a single stereoisomer with the (3*S*)(1*S*,2*R*) configuration. It has a molecular formula of $C_{25}H_{34}CaN_3O_9PS$ and a molecular weight of 623.7. It has the following structural formula:

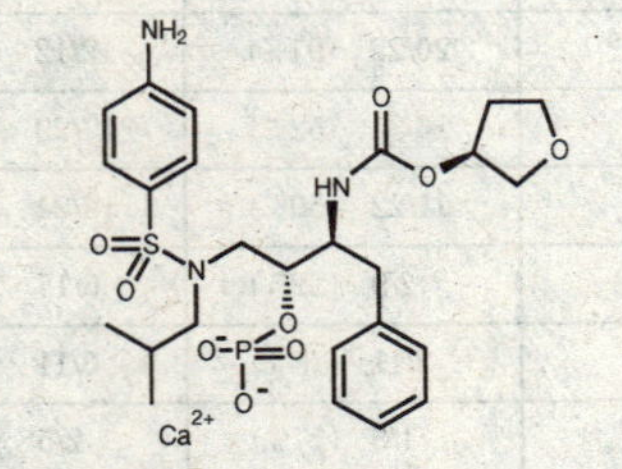

Fosamprenavir calcium is a white to cream-colored solid with a solubility of approximately 0.31 mg/mL in water at 25°C.

LEXIVA Tablets are available for oral administration in a strength of 700 mg of fosamprenavir as fosamprenavir calcium (equivalent to approximately 600 mg of amprenavir). Each 700-mg tablet contains the inactive ingredients colloidal silicon dioxide, croscarmellose sodium, magnesium stearate, microcrystalline cellulose, and povidone K30. The tablet film-coating contains the inactive ingredients hypromellose, iron oxide red, titanium dioxide, and triacetin.

MICROBIOLOGY

Mechanism of Action: Fosamprenavir is rapidly converted to amprenavir by cellular phosphatases in vivo. Amprenavir is an inhibitor of HIV-1 protease. Amprenavir binds to the active site of HIV-1 protease and thereby prevents the processing of viral Gag and Gag-Pol polyprotein precursors, resulting in the formation of immature non-infectious viral particles.

Antiviral Activity in Vitro: Fosamprenavir has little or no antiviral activity in vitro. The in vitro antiviral activity observed with fosamprenavir is not measurable due to trace amounts of amprenavir. The in vitro antiviral activity of amprenavir was evaluated against HIV-1 IIIB in both acutely and chronically infected lymphoblastic cell lines (MT-4, CEM-CCRF, H9) and in peripheral blood lymphocytes. The 50% inhibitory concentration (IC_{50}) of amprenavir ranged from 0.012 to 0.08 µM in acutely infected cells and was 0.41 µM in chronically infected cells (1 µM = 0.50 mcg/mL). Amprenavir exhibited synergistic anti-HIV-1 activity in combination with the nucleoside reverse transcriptase inhibitors (NRTIs) abacavir, didanosine, and zidovudine, and the protease inhibitor (PI) saquinavir, and additive anti-HIV-1 activity in combination with the non-nucleoside reverse transcriptase inhibitor (NNRTI) nevirapine and PIs indinavir, lopinavir, nelfinavir, and ritonavir in vitro. These drug combinations have not been adequately studied in humans. The relationship between in vitro anti-HIV-1 activity of amprenavir and the inhibition of HIV-1 replication in humans has not been defined.

Resistance: HIV-1 isolates with a decreased susceptibility to amprenavir have been selected in vitro and obtained from patients treated with fosamprenavir. Genotypic analysis of isolates from amprenavir-treated patients showed mutations in the HIV-1 protease gene resulting in amino acid substitutions primarily at positions V32I, M46I/L, I47V, I50V, I54L/M, and I84V, as well as mutations in the p7/p1 and p1/p6 Gag and Gag-Pol polyprotein precursor cleavage sites. Some of these amprenavir resistance-associated mutations have also been detected in HIV-1 isolates from antiretroviral-naive patients treated with LEXIVA. Of the 488 antiretroviral-naive patients treated with LEXIVA or LEXIVA/ritonavir, 61 patients (29 receiving LEXIVA and 32 receiving LEXIVA/ritonavir) with virological failure (plasma HIV-1 RNA>1,000 copies/mL on 2 occasions on or after Week 12) were genotyped. Five of the 29 antiretroviral-naive patients (17%) receiving LEXIVA without ritonavir had evidence of genotypic resistance to amprenavir: I54L/M

Continued on next page

Lexiva—Cont.

(n = 2), I54L + L33F (n = 1), V32I + I47V (n = 1), and M46I + I47V (n = 1). No amprenavir-associated mutations were detected in antiretroviral-naive patients treated with LEXIVA/ritonavir.

Cross-Resistance: Varying degrees of cross-resistance among HIV-1 protease inhibitors have been observed. An association between virologic response at 48 weeks (HIV-1 RNA level <400 copies/mL) and PI-resistance mutations detected in baseline HIV-1 isolates from PI-experienced patients receiving LEXIVA/ritonavir twice daily (n = 88), or lopinavir/ritonavir twice daily (n = 85) in study APV30003 is shown in Table 1. The majority of subjects had previously received either one (47%) or 2 PIs (36%), most commonly nelfinavir (57%) and indinavir (53%). Out of 102 subjects with baseline phenotypes receiving twice-daily LEXIVA/ritonavir, 54% (55) had resistance to at least one PI with 98% (54) of those having resistance to nelfinavir. Out of 97 subjects with baseline phenotypes in the lopinavir/ritonavir arm, 60% (58) had resistance to at least one PI with 97% (56) of those having resistance to nelfinavir.

Table 1. Responders at Study Week 48 by Presence of Baseline PI Resistance-Associated Mutations*

PI-mutations†	LEXIVA/Ritonavir b.i.d. (n = 88)	Lopinavir/ Ritonavir b.i.d. (n = 85)
D30N	21/22 (95%)	17/19 (89%)
N88D/S	20/22 (91%)	12/12 (100%)
L90M	16/31 (52%)	17/29 (59%)
M46I/L	11/22 (50%)	12/24 (50%)
V82A/F/T/S	2/9 (22%)	6/17 (35%)
I54V	2/11 (18%)	6/11 (55%)
I84V	1/6 (17%)	2/5 (40%)

*Results should be interpreted with caution because the subgroups were small.
† Most patients had >1 PI resistance-associated mutation at baseline.

The virologic response based upon baseline phenotype was assessed. Baseline isolates from PI-experienced patients responding to LEXIVA/ritonavir twice daily had a median shift in susceptibility to amprenavir relative to a standard wild-type reference strain of 0.7 (range: 0.1 to 5.4, n = 62), and baseline isolates from individuals failing therapy had a median shift in susceptibility of 1.9 (range: 0.2 to 14, n = 29). Because this was a select patient population, these data do not constitute definitive clinical susceptibility break points. Additional data are needed to determine clinically relevant break points for LEXIVA.

Isolates from 15 of the 20 patients receiving twice-daily LEXIVA/ritonavir and experiencing virologic failure/ongoing replication were subjected to genotypic analysis. The following amprenavir resistance-associated mutations were found either alone or in combination: V32I, M46I/L, I47V, I50V, I54L/M, and I84V.

CLINICAL PHARMACOLOGY

Pharmacokinetics in Adults: Fosamprenavir is a prodrug, which is rapidly hydrolyzed to amprenavir by enzymes in the gut epithelium as it is absorbed.

The pharmacokinetic properties of amprenavir after administration of LEXIVA with or without ritonavir, have been evaluated in both healthy adult volunteers and in HIV-infected patients; no substantial differences in steady-state amprenavir concentrations were observed between the 2 populations.

Absorption and Bioavailability: After administration of a single dose of LEXIVA to HIV-1-infected patients, the time to peak amprenavir concentration (T_{max}) occurred between 1.5 and 4 hours (median 2.5 hours). The absolute oral bioavailability of amprenavir after administration of LEXIVA in humans has not been established.

The pharmacokinetic parameters of amprenavir after administration of LEXIVA (with and without concomitant ritonavir) are shown in Table 2.

[See table 2 at right]

The median plasma amprenavir concentrations of the dosing regimens over the dosing intervals are displayed in Figure 1.

[See figure 1 at top of next column]

Effects of Food on Oral Absorption: LEXIVA Tablets may be taken with or without food (see DOSAGE AND ADMINISTRATION). Administration of a single 1,400-mg dose of LEXIVA in the fed state (standardized high-fat meal: 967 kcal, 67 grams fat, 33 grams protein, 58 grams carbohydrate) compared to the fasted state was associated with no significant changes in amprenavir C_{max}, T_{max}, or $AUC_{0-\infty}$.

Distribution: In vitro, amprenavir is approximately 90% bound to plasma proteins, primarily to alpha$_1$-acid glycoprotein. In vitro, concentration-dependent binding was observed over the concentration range of 1 to 10 ug/mL, with decreased binding at higher concentrations. The partitioning of amprenavir into erythrocytes is low, but increases as amprenavir concentrations increase, reflecting the higher amount of unbound drug at higher concentrations.

Figure 1. Mean (± SD) Steady-State Plasma Amprenavir Concentrations and Mean IC_{50} Values Against HIV from Protease Inhibitor-Naive Patients (in the Absence of Human Serum)

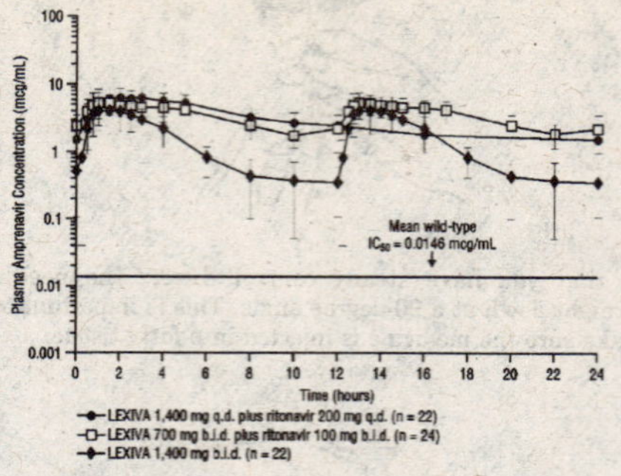

Metabolism: After oral administration, fosamprenavir is rapidly and almost completely hydrolyzed to amprenavir and inorganic phosphate prior to reaching the systemic circulation. This occurs in the gut epithelium during absorption. Amprenavir is metabolized in the liver by the cytochrome P450 3A4 (CYP3A4) enzyme system. The 2 major metabolites result from oxidation of the tetrahydrofuran and aniline moieties. Glucuronide conjugates of oxidized metabolites have been identified as minor metabolites in urine and feces.

Elimination: Excretion of unchanged amprenavir in urine and feces is minimal. Unchanged amprenavir in urine accounts for approximately 1% of the dose; unchanged amprenavir was not detectable in feces. Approximately 14% and 75% of an administered single dose of ^{14}C-amprenavir can be accounted for as metabolites in urine and feces, respectively. Two metabolites accounted for >90% of the radiocarbon in fecal samples. The plasma elimination half-life of amprenavir is approximately 7.7 hours.

Special Populations: ***Hepatic Insufficiency:*** The pharmacokinetics of amprenavir after administration of LEXIVA have not been studied in patients with hepatic insufficiency. The pharmacokinetics of amprenavir have been studied after administration of amprenavir given as AGENERASE® Capsules to adult patients with impaired hepatic function using a single 600-mg oral dose. The $AUC_{0-\infty}$ of amprenavir was significantly greater in patients with moderate cirrhosis (25.76 ± 14.68 mcg•hr/mL) compared with healthy volunteers (12.00 ± 4.38 mcg•hr/mL). The $AUC_{0-\infty}$ and C_{max} were significantly greater in patients with severe cirrhosis ($AUC_{0-\infty}$: 38.66 ± 16.08 mcg•hr/mL; C_{max}: 9.43 ± 2.61 mcg/mL) compared with healthy volunteers ($AUC_{0-\infty}$: 12.00 ± 4.38 mcg•hr/mL; C_{max}: 4.90 ± 1.39 mcg/mL). Based on these data, patients with impaired hepatic function receiving LEXIVA without concurrent ritonavir may require dosage reduction. There are no data on the use of LEXIVA in combination with ritonavir in patients with any degree of hepatic impairment (see PRECAUTIONS and DOSAGE AND ADMINISTRATION).

Renal Insufficiency: The impact of renal impairment on amprenavir elimination in adult patients has not been studied. The renal elimination of unchanged amprenavir represents approximately 1% of the administered dose; therefore, renal impairment is not expected to significantly impact the elimination of amprenavir.

Pediatric Patients: The pharmacokinetics of amprenavir after administration of LEXIVA to pediatric patients are under investigation. There are insufficient data at this time to recommend a dose.

Geriatric Patients: The pharmacokinetics of amprenavir after administration of LEXIVA to patients over 65 years of age have not been studied.

Gender: The pharmacokinetics of amprenavir after administration of LEXIVA do not differ between males and females.

Race: The pharmacokinetics of amprenavir after administration of LEXIVA do not differ between blacks and non-blacks.

Table 2. Geometric Mean (95% CI) Steady-State Plasma Amprenavir Pharmacokinetic Parameters

Regimen	C_{max} (mcg/mL)	T_{max} (hours)*	AUC_{24} (mcg•hr/mL)	C_{min} (mcg/mL)
LEXIVA 1,400 mg b.i.d.	4.82 (4.06-5.72)	1.3 (0.8-4.0)	33.0 (27.6-39.2)	0.35 (0.27-0.46)
LEXIVA 1,400 mg q.d. plus Ritonavir 200 mg q.d.	7.24 (6.32-8.28)	2.1 (0.8-5.0)	69.4 (59.7-80.8)	1.45 (1.16-1.81)
LEXIVA 700 mg b.i.d. plus Ritonavir 100 mg b.i.d.	6.08 (5.38-6.86)	1.5 (0.75-5.0)	79.2 (69.0-90.6)	2.12 (1.77-2.54)

*Data shown are median (range).

Table 3. Drug Interactions: Pharmacokinetic Parameters for Amprenavir After Administration of LEXIVA in the Presence of the Coadministered Drug

Coadministered Drug(s) and Dose(s)	Dose of LEXIVA*	n	% Change in Amprenavir Pharmacokinetic Parameters (90% CI)		
			C_{max}	AUC	C_{min}
Antacid (MAALOX TC®) 30 mL single dose	1,400 mg single dose	30	↓35 (↓24 to ↓42)	↓18 (↓9 to ↓26)	↑14 (↓7 to ↑39)
Atorvastatin 10 mg q.d. for 4 days	1,400 mg b.i.d. for 2 weeks	16	↓18 (↓34 to ↑1)	↓27 (↓41 to ↓12)	↓12 (↓27 to ↑6)
Atorvastatin 10 mg q.d. for 4 days	700 mg b.i.d. plus ritonavir 100 mg b.i.d. for 2 weeks	16	⇔	⇔	⇔
Efavirenz 600 mg q.d. for 2 weeks	1,400 mg q.d. plus ritonavir 200 mg q.d. for 2 weeks	16	⇔	↓13 (↓30 to ↑7)	↓36 (↓8 to ↓56)
Efavirenz 600 mg q.d. plus additional ritonavir 100 mg q.d for 2 weeks	1,400 mg q.d. plus ritonavir 200 mg q.d. for 2 weeks	16	↑18 (↑1 to ↑38)	↑11 (0 to ↑24)	⇔
Efavirenz 600 mg q.d. for 2 weeks	700 mg b.i.d. plus ritonavir 100 mg b.i.d. for 2 weeks	16	⇔	⇔	↓17 (↓4 to ↓29)
Lopinavir/ritonavir 533 mg/133 mg b.i.d.	1,400 mg b.i.d. for 2 weeks	18	See following section: **HIV Protease Inhibitors**		
Lopinavir/ritonavir 400 mg/100 mg b.i.d. for 2 weeks	700 mg b.i.d. plus ritonavir 100 mg b.i.d. for 2 weeks	18	↓58 (↓42 to ↓70)	↓63 (↓51 to ↓72)	↓65 (↓54 to ↓73)
Ranitidine 300 mg single dose	1,400 mg single dose	30	↓51 (↓43 to ↓58)	↓30 (↓22 to ↓37)	⇔ (↓19 to ↑21)

*Concomitant medication is also shown in this column where appropriate.
↑ = Increase; ↓ = Decrease; ⇔ = No change (↑ or ↓ <10%).

Table 4. Drug Interactions: Pharmacokinetic Parameters for Amprenavir After Administration of AGENERASE in the Presence of the Coadministered Drug

Coadministered Drug(s) and Dose(s)	Dose of **AGENERASE***	n	% Change in **Amprenavir** Pharmacokinetic Parameters (90% CI)		
			C_{max}	AUC	C_{min}
Clarithromycin 500 mg b.i.d. for 4 days	1,200 mg b.i.d. for 4 days	12	↑15 (↑1 to ↑31)	↑18 (↑8 to ↑29)	↑39 (↑31 to ↑47)
Delavirdine 600 mg b.i.d. for 10 days	600 mg b.i.d. for 10 days	9	↑40*	↑130*	↑125*
Ethinyl estradiol/ norethindrone 0.035 mg/1 mg for 1 cycle	1,200 mg b.i.d. for 28 days	10	⇔	↓22 (↓35 to ↓8)	↓20 (↓41 to ↑8)
Indinavir 800 mg t.i.d. for 2 weeks (fasted)	750 or 800 mg t.i.d. for 2 weeks (fasted)	9	↑18 (↓13 to ↑58)	↑33 (↑2 to ↑73)	↑25 (↓27 to ↑116)
Ketoconazole 400 mg single dose	1,200 mg single dose	12	↓16 (↓25 to ↓6)	↑31 (↑20 to ↑42)	NA
Lamivudine 150 mg single dose	600 mg single dose	11	⇔	⇔	NA
Nelfinavir 750 mg t.i.d. for 2 weeks (fed)	750 or 800 mg t.i.d. for 2 weeks (fed)	6	↓14 (↓38 to ↑20)	⇔	↑189 (↑52 to ↑448)
Rifabutin 300 mg q.d. for 10 days	1,200 mg b.i.d. for 10 days	5	⇔	↓15 (↓28 to 0)	↓15 (↓38 to ↑17)
Rifampin 300 mg q.d. for 4 days	1,200 mg b.i.d. for 4 days	11	↓70 (↓76 to ↓62)	↓82 (↓84 to ↓78)	↓92 (↓95 to ↓89)
Saquinavir 800 mg t.i.d. for 2 weeks (fed)	750 or 800 mg t.i.d. for 2 weeks (fed)	7	↓37 (↓54 to ↓14)	↓32 (↓49 to ↓9)	↓14 (↓52 to ↑54)
Zidovudine 300 mg single dose	600 single dose	12	⇔	↑13 (↓2 to ↑31)	NA

* Median percent change; confidence interval not reported.
↑ = Increase; ↓ = Decrease; ⇔ = No change (↑ or ↓ <10%); NA = C_{min} not calculated for single-dose study.

Table 5. Drug Interactions: Pharmacokinetic Parameters for Coadministered Drug in the Presence of Amprenavir After Administration of LEXIVA

Coadministered Drug(s) and Dose(s)	Dose of **LEXIVA***	n	% Change in Pharmacokinetic Parameters of **Coadministered Drug** (90% CI)		
			C_{max}	AUC	C_{min}
Atorvastatin 10 mg q.d. for 4 days	1,400 mg b.i.d. for 2 weeks	16	↑304 (↑205 to ↑437)	↑130 (↑100 to ↑164)	↓10 (↓ 27 to ↑12)
Atorvastatin 10 mg q.d. for 4 days	700 mg b.i.d. plus ritonavir 100 b.i.d. for 2 weeks	16	↑184 (↑126 to ↑257)	↑153 (↑115 to ↑199)	↑73 (↑45 to ↑108)
Lopinavir/ritonavir† 533 mg/133 mg b.i.d. for 2 weeks	1,400 mg b.i.d. for 2 weeks	18	See following section: **HIV Protease Inhibitors**		
Lopinavir/ritonavir† 400 mg/100 mg b.i.d. for 2 weeks	700 mg b.i.d. plus ritonavir 100 mg b.i.d. for 2 weeks	18	↑30 (↓15 to ↑47)	↑37 (↓20 to ↑55)	↑52 (↓28 to ↑82)

*Concomitant medication is also shown in this column where appropriate.
† Data represent lopinavir concentrations.
↑ = Increase; ↓ = Decrease; ⇔ = No change (↑ or ↓ <10%).

Drug Interactions: See also CONTRAINDICATIONS, WARNINGS, and PRECAUTIONS: Drug Interactions.
Amprenavir, the active metabolite of fosamprenavir, is metabolized in the liver by the cytochrome P450 enzyme system. Amprenavir inhibits CYP3A4. Data also suggest that amprenavir induces CYP3A4. Caution should be used when coadministering medications that are substrates, inhibitors, or inducers of CYP3A4, or potentially toxic medications that are metabolized by CYP3A4. Amprenavir does not inhibit CYP2D6, CYP1A2, CYP2C9, CYP2C19, CYP2E1, or uridine glucuronosyltransferase (UDPGT).
Drug interaction studies were performed with LEXIVA and other drugs likely to be coadministered or drugs commonly used as probes for pharmacokinetic interactions. The effects of coadministration on AUC, C_{max}, and C_{min} values are summarized in Table 3 (effect of other drugs on amprenavir) and Table 5 (effect of LEXIVA on other drugs). In addition, since LEXIVA delivers comparable amprenavir plasma concentrations as AGENERASE, drug interaction data derived from studies with AGENERASE are provided in Tables 4 and 6. For information regarding clinical recommendations, see PRECAUTIONS: Drug Interactions.
[See table 3 at bottom of previous page]
[See table 4 above]
[See table 5 above]
[See table 6 at bottom of next page]

Nucleoside Reverse Transcriptase Inhibitors: There was no clinically significant effect of amprenavir after administration of AGENERASE on abacavir in subjects receiving both agents based on historical data.
In a phase III clinical trial (APV30003), plasma amprenavir trough concentrations were similar for subjects receiving tenofovir disoproxil fumarate in combination with LEXIVA and ritonavir as compared to subjects not receiving tenofovir.
HIV Protease Inhibitors: In a 3-arm, randomized, crossover study involving healthy volunteers, amprenavir pharmacokinetics were compared after administration of LEXIVA 1,400 mg twice daily plus lopinavir/ritonavir 533 mg/133 mg twice daily for 2 weeks versus LEXIVA 700 mg twice daily plus ritonavir 100 mg twice daily for 2 weeks. Amprenavir concentrations were lower with the regimen containing lopinavir/ritonavir: C_{max} was 13% lower, AUC was 26% lower, and C_{min} was 42% lower. In the same study, lopinavir pharmacokinetics were compared after administration of LEXIVA 1,400 mg twice daily plus lopinavir/ritonavir 533 mg/133 mg twice daily for 2 weeks versus lopinavir/ritonavir 400 mg/100 mg twice daily for 2 weeks. Lopinavir concentrations were similar (less than 10% change in C_{max}, AUC, and C_{min} values) with these 2 regimens.
The effect of amprenavir after administration of AGENERASE Capsules on concentrations of other HIV protease inhibitors in subjects receiving both agents was evaluated using comparisons to historical data. Indinavir steady-state C_{max}, AUC, and C_{min} were decreased by 22%, 38%, and 27%, respectively, by concomitant amprenavir. Similar decreases in C_{max} and AUC were seen after the first dose. Saquinavir steady-state C_{max}, AUC, and C_{min} were increased 21%, decreased 19%, and decreased 48%, respectively, by concomitant amprenavir. Nelfinavir steady-state C_{max}, AUC, and C_{min} were increased by 12%, 15%, and 14%, respectively, by concomitant amprenavir.
Methadone: Coadministration of amprenavir and methadone can decrease plasma levels of methadone.
Coadministration of amprenavir and methadone as compared to a non-matched historical control group resulted in a 30%, 27%, and 25% decrease in serum amprenavir AUC, C_{max}, and C_{min}, respectively.

INDICATIONS AND USAGE

LEXIVA is indicated in combination with other antiretroviral agents for the treatment of HIV infection in adults.
The following points should be considered when initiating therapy with LEXIVA/ritonavir in protease inhibitor-experienced patients (see Description of Clinical Studies).

- **The protease inhibitor-experienced patient study was not large enough to reach a definitive conclusion that LEXIVA/ritonavir and lopinavir/ritonavir are clinically equivalent.**
- **Once-daily administration of LEXIVA plus ritonavir is not recommended for protease inhibitor-experienced patients.**

Description of Clinical Studies: ***Therapy-Naive Patients: Study APV30001:*** APV30001 was a randomized, open-label study, comparing treatment with LEXIVA Tablets (1,400 mg twice daily) versus nelfinavir (1,250 mg twice daily) in 249 antiretroviral treatment-naive patients. Both groups of patients also received abacavir (300 mg twice daily) and lamivudine (150 mg twice daily).
The mean age of the patients in this study was 37 years (range 17 to 70 years), 69% of the patients were males, 20% were CDC Class C (AIDS), 24% were Caucasian, 32% were black, and 44% were Hispanic. At baseline, the median CD4+ cell count was 212 cells/mm^3 (range: 2 to 1,136 cells/mm^3; 18% of patients had a CD4+ cell count of <50 cells/mm^3 and 30% were in the range of 50 to <200 cells/mm^3). Baseline median HIV-1 RNA was 4.83 $\log_{10}$ copies/mL (range: 1.69 to 7.41 $\log_{10}$ copies/mL; 45% of patients had >100,000 copies/mL).
The outcomes of randomized treatment are provided in Table 7.

Table 7. Outcomes of Randomized Treatment Through Week 48 (APV30001)

Outcome (Rebound or discontinuation = failure)	LEXIVA 1,400 mg b.i.d. (n = 166)	Nelfinavir 1,250 mg b.i.d. (n = 83)
Responder*	66% (57%)	52% (42%)
Virologic failure	19%	32%
Rebound	16%	19%
Never suppressed through Week 48	3%	13%
Clinical progression	1%	1%
Death	0%	1%
Discontinued due to adverse reactions	4%	2%
Discontinued due to other reasons†	10%	10%

*Patients achieved and maintained confirmed HIV-1 RNA <400 copies/mL (<50 copies/mL) through Week 48 (Roche AMPLICOR HIV-1 MONITOR Assay Version 1.5).
† Includes consent withdrawn, lost to follow up, protocol violations, those with missing data, and other reasons.

Treatment response by viral load strata is shown in Table 8.

Table 8. Proportions of Responders Through Week 48 by Screening Viral Load (APV30001)

Screening Viral Load HIV-1 RNA (copies/mL)	LEXIVA 1,400 mg b.i.d.		Nelfinavir 1,250 mg b.i.d.	
	<400 copies/mL	n	<400 copies/mL	n
≤100,000	65%	93	65%	46
>100,000	67%	73	36%	37

Through 48 weeks of therapy, the median increases from baseline in CD4+ cell counts were 201 cells/mm^3 in the group receiving LEXIVA and 216 cells/mm^3 in the nelfinavir group.
Study APV30002: APV30002 was a randomized, open-label study, comparing treatment with LEXIVA Tablets (1,400 mg once daily) plus ritonavir (200 mg once daily) versus nelfinavir (1,250 mg twice daily) in 649 treatment-naive patients. Both treatment groups also received abacavir (300 mg twice daily) and lamivudine (150 mg twice daily). The mean age of the patients in this study was 37 years (range 18 to 69 years), 73% of the patients were males, 22% were CDC Class C, 53% were Caucasian, 36% were black,

Continued on next page

Lexiva—Cont.

and 8% were Hispanic. At baseline, the median CD4+ cell count was 170 cells/mm^3 (range: 1 to 1,055 cells/mm^3; 20% of patients had a CD4+ cell count of <50 cells/mm^3 and 35% were in the range of 50 to <200 cells/mm^3). Baseline median HIV-1 RNA was 4.81 $\log_{10}$ copies/mL (range: 2.65 to 7.29 $\log_{10}$ copies/mL; 43% of patients had >100,000 copies/mL). The outcomes of randomized treatment are provided in Table 9.

Table 9. Outcomes of Randomized Treatment Through Week 48 (APV30002)

Outcome (Rebound or discontinuation = failure)	LEXIVA 1,400 mg q.d./ Ritonavir 200 mg q.d. (n = 322)	Nelfinavir 1,250 mg b.i.d. (n = 327)
Responder*	69% (58%)	68% (55%)
Virologic failure	6%	16%
Rebound	5%	8%
Never suppressed through Week 48	1%	8%
Death	1%	0%
Discontinued due to adverse reactions	9%	6%
Discontinued due to other reasons†	15%	10%

*Patients achieved and maintained confirmed HIV-1 RNA <400 copies/mL (<50 copies/mL) through Week 48 (Roche AMPLICOR HIV-1 MONITOR Assay Version 1.5).

† Includes consent withdrawn, lost to follow up, protocol violations, those with missing data, and other reasons.

Treatment response by viral load strata is shown in Table 10.

Table 10. Proportions of Responders Through Week 48 by Screening Viral Load (APV30002)

Screening Viral Load HIV-1 RNA (copies/mL)	LEXIVA 1,400 mg q.d./ Ritonavir 200 mg q.d.		Nelfinavir 1,250 mg b.i.d.	
	<400 copies/mL	n	<400 copies/mL	n
≤100,000	72%	197	73%	194
>100,000	66%	125	64%	133

Through 48 weeks of therapy, the median increases from baseline in CD4+ cell counts were 203 cells/mm^3 in the group receiving LEXIVA and 207 cells/mm^3 in the nelfinavir group.

Protease Inhibitor-Experienced Patients: Study APV30003: APV30003 was a randomized, open-label, multicenter study comparing 2 different regimens of LEXIVA plus ritonavir (LEXIVA Tablets 700 mg twice daily plus ritonavir 100 mg twice daily or LEXIVA Tablets 1,400 mg once daily plus ritonavir 200 mg once daily) versus lopinavir/ritonavir (400 mg/100 mg twice daily) in 315 patients who had experienced virologic failure to 1 or 2 prior protease inhibitor-containing regimens.

The mean age of the patients in this study was 42 years (range 24 to 72 years), 85% were male, 33% were CDC Class C, 67% were Caucasian, 24% were black, and 9% were Hispanic. The median CD4+ cell count at baseline was 263 cells/mm^3 (range: 2 to 1,171 cells/mm^3). Baseline median plasma HIV-1 RNA level was 4.14 $\log_{10}$ copies/mL (range: 1.69 to 6.41 $\log_{10}$ copies/mL).

The median durations of prior exposure to NRTIs were 257 weeks for patients receiving LEXIVA/ritonavir twice daily (79% had ≥3 prior NRTIs) and 210 weeks for patients receiving lopinavir/ritonavir (64% had ≥3 prior NRTIs). The median durations of prior exposure to protease inhibitors were 149 weeks for patients receiving LEXIVA/ritonavir twice daily (49% received ≥2 prior PIs) and 130 weeks for patients receiving lopinavir/ritonavir (40% received ≥2 prior PIs).

The time-averaged changes in plasma HIV-1 RNA from baseline (AAUCMB) at 48 weeks (the endpoint on which the study was powered) were –1.4 $\log_{10}$ copies/mL for twice-daily LEXIVA/ritonavir and –1.67 $\log_{10}$ copies/mL for the lopinavir/ritonavir group.

The proportions of patients who achieved and maintained confirmed HIV-1 RNA <400 copies/mL (secondary efficacy endpoint) were 58% with twice-daily LEXIVA/ritonavir and 61% with lopinavir/ritonavir (95% CI for the difference -16.6, 10.1). The proportions of patients with HIV-1 RNA <50 copies/mL with twice-daily LEXIVA/ritonavir and with lopinavir/ritonavir were 46% and 50%, respectively (95% CI for the difference -18.3, 8.9). The proportions of patients who were virologic failures were 29% with twice-daily LEXIVA/ritonavir and 27% with lopinavir/ritonavir.

The frequency of discontinuations due to adverse events and other reasons, and deaths were similar between treatment arms.

Through 48 weeks of therapy, the median increases from baseline in CD4+ cell counts were 81 cells/mm^3 with twice-daily LEXIVA/ritonavir and 91 cells/mm^3 with lopinavir/ritonavir.

This study was not large enough to reach a definitive conclusion that LEXIVA/ritonavir and lopinavir/ritonavir are clinically equivalent.

Once-daily administration of LEXIVA plus ritonavir is **not recommended** for protease inhibitor-experienced patients.

Table 6. Drug Interactions: Pharmacokinetic Parameters for Coadministered Drug in the Presence of Amprenavir After Administration of AGENERASE

Coadministered Drug(s) and Dose(s)	Dose of **AGENERASE**	n	% Change in Pharmacokinetic Parameters of **Coadministered Drug** (90% CI)		
			C_{max}	AUC	C_{min}
Clarithromycin 500 mg b.i.d. for 4 days	1,200 mg b.i.d. for 4 days	12	↓10 (↓24 to ↑7)	⇔	⇔
Delavirdine 600 mg b.i.d. for 10 days	600 mg b.i.d. for 10 days	9	↓47*	↓61*	↓88*
Ethinyl estradiol 0.035 mg for 1 cycle	1,200 mg b.i.d. for 28 days	10	⇔	⇔	↑32 (↓3 to ↑79)
Ketoconazole 400 mg single dose	1,200 mg single dose	12	↑19 (↑8 to ↑33)	↑44 (↑31 to ↑59)	NA
Lamivudine 150 mg single dose	600 mg single dose	11	⇔	⇔	NA
Methadone 44 to 100 mg q.d. for >30 days	1,200 mg b.i.d. for 10 days	16	R-Methadone (active)		
			↓25 (↓32 to ↓18)	↓13 (↓21 to ↓5)	↓21 (↓32 to ↓9)
			S-Methadone (inactive)		
			↓48 (↓55 to ↓40)	↓40 (↓46 to ↓32)	↓53 (↓60 to ↓43)
Norethindrone 1 mg for 1 cycle	1,200 mg b.i.d. for 28 days	10	⇔	↑18 (↑1 to ↑38)	↑45 (↑13 to ↑88)
Rifabutin 300 mg q.d. for 10 days	1,200 mg b.i.d. for 10 days	5	↑119 (↑82 to ↑164)	↑193 (↑156 to ↑235)	↑271 (↑171 to ↑409)
Rifampin 300 mg q.d. for 4 days	1,200 mg b.i.d. for 4 days	11	⇔	⇔	ND
Zidovudine 300 mg single dose	600 mg single dose	12	↑40 (↑14 to ↑71)	↑31 (↑19 to ↑45)	NA

* Median percent change; confidence interval not reported.

↑ = Increase; ↓ = Decrease; ⇔ = No change (↑ or ↓ <10%); NA = C_{min} not calculated for single-dose study; ND = Interaction cannot be determined as C_{min} was below the lower limit of quantitation.

Through Week 48, 50% and 37% of patients receiving LEXIVA/ritonavir once daily had plasma HIV-1 RNA <400 copies/mL and <50 copies/mL, respectively.

CONTRAINDICATIONS

LEXIVA is contraindicated in patients with previously demonstrated clinically significant hypersensitivity to any of the components of this product or to amprenavir.

Coadministration of LEXIVA with drugs that are highly dependent on CYP3A4 for clearance and for which elevated plasma concentrations are associated with serious and/or life-threatening events is contraindicated. These drugs are listed in Table 11.

Table 11. Drugs That Are Contraindicated with LEXIVA

Drug Class	Drugs Within Class That Are CONTRAINDICATED with LEXIVA
Ergot derivatives	Dihydroergotamine, ergonovine, ergotamine, methylergonovine
GI motility agent	Cisapride
Neuroleptic	Pimozide
Sedatives/hypnotics	Midazolam, triazolam

If LEXIVA is coadministered with ritonavir, the antiarrhythmic agents flecainide and propafenone are also contraindicated. Also, refer to the full prescribing information for NORVIR® (ritonavir) for other potential drug interactions.

WARNINGS

Serious and/or life-threatening drug interactions could occur between LEXIVA and amiodarone, lidocaine (systemic), tricyclic antidepressants, and quinidine. Concentration monitoring of these agents is recommended if these agents are used concomitantly with LEXIVA (see CONTRAINDICATIONS).

Severe and life-threatening skin reactions, including Stevens-Johnson syndrome, have occurred in patients treated with amprenavir (see ADVERSE REACTIONS). Acute hemolytic anemia has been reported in a patient treated with amprenavir.

Rifampin should not be used in combination with LEXIVA because it reduces plasma concentrations of amprenavir by about 90%. The effect of rifampin on amprenavir concentrations when rifampin is administered with LEXIVA plus ritonavir is not known.

Concomitant use of LEXIVA and St. John's wort (hypericum perforatum) or products containing St. John's wort is not recommended. Coadministration of protease inhibitors, including LEXIVA, with St. John's wort is expected to substantially decrease protease inhibitor concentrations and may result in suboptimal levels of amprenavir and lead to loss of virologic response and possible resistance to LEXIVA or to the class of protease inhibitors.

Concomitant use of LEXIVA with lovastatin or simvastatin is not recommended. Caution should be exercised if HIV protease inhibitors, including LEXIVA, are used concurrently with other HMG-CoA reductase inhibitors that are also metabolized by the CYP3A4 pathway (e.g., atorvastatin). The risk of myopathy, including rhabdomyolysis, may be increased when HIV protease inhibitors, including LEXIVA, are used in combination with these drugs.

Particular caution should be used when prescribing phosphodiesterase (PDE5) inhibitors for erectile dysfunction (e.g., sildenafil or vardenafil) in patients receiving protease inhibitors, including LEXIVA. Coadministration of a protease inhibitor with a PDE5 inhibitor is expected to substantially increase the PDE5 inhibitor concentration and may result in an increase in PDE5 inhibitor-associated adverse events, including hypotension, visual changes, and priapism (see PRECAUTIONS: Drug Interactions and Information for Patients, and the complete specific PDE5 inhibitor prescribing information).

New onset diabetes mellitus, exacerbation of pre-existing diabetes mellitus, and hyperglycemia have been reported during post-marketing surveillance in HIV-infected patients receiving protease inhibitor therapy. Some patients required either initiation or dose adjustments of insulin or oral hypoglycemic agents for treatment of these events. In some cases, diabetic ketoacidosis has occurred. In those patients who discontinued protease inhibitor therapy, hyperglycemia persisted in some cases. Because these events have been reported voluntarily during clinical practice, estimates of frequency cannot be made and causal relationships between protease inhibitor therapy and these events have not been established.

PRECAUTIONS

Sulfa Allergy: LEXIVA should be used with caution in patients with a known sulfonamide allergy. Fosamprenavir contains a sulfonamide moiety. The potential for cross-sensitivity between drugs in the sulfonamide class and fosamprenavir is unknown. In a clinical study of LEXIVA used as the sole protease inhibitor, rash occurred in 2 of 10 patients (20%) with a history of sulfonamide allergy compared with 42 of 126 patients (33%) with no history of sulfonamide allergy. In 2 clinical studies of LEXIVA plus low-dose ritonavir, rash occurred in 8 of 50 patients (16%) with a history of sulfonamide allergy compared with 50 of 412 patients (12%) with no history of sulfonamide allergy.

Hepatic Impairment and Toxicity: LEXIVA is principally metabolized by the liver; therefore, caution should be exercised when administering LEXIVA to patients with hepatic impairment because amprenavir concentrations may be increased (see CLINICAL PHARMACOLOGY: Special Populations: Hepatic Insufficiency). Patients with impaired hepatic function receiving LEXIVA without concurrent ritonavir may require dose reduction (see DOSAGE AND ADMINISTRATION). There are no data on the use of LEXIVA in combination with ritonavir in patients with any degree of hepatic impairment.

Patients with underlying hepatitis B or C or marked elevations in transaminases prior to treatment may be at increased risk for developing transaminase elevations. Appropriate laboratory testing should be conducted prior to initiating therapy with LEXIVA and patients should be monitored closely during treatment.

Patients with Hemophilia: There have been reports of spontaneous bleeding in patients with hemophilia A and B treated with protease inhibitors. In some patients, additional factor VIII was required. In many of the reported cases, treatment with protease inhibitors was continued or restarted. A causal relationship between protease inhibitor therapy and these episodes has not been established.

Immune Reconstitution: During the initial phase of treatment, patients responding to antiretroviral therapy may develop an inflammatory response to indolent or residual opportunistic infections (such as MAC, CMV, PCP, and TB), which may necessitate further evaluation and treatment.

Fat Redistribution: Redistribution/accumulation of body fat, including central obesity, dorsocervical fat enlargement (buffalo hump), peripheral wasting, facial wasting, breast enlargement, and "cushingoid appearance," have been observed in patients receiving antiretroviral therapy, including LEXIVA. The mechanism and long-term consequences of these events are currently unknown. A causal relationship has not been established.

Lipid Elevations: Treatment with LEXIVA plus ritonavir has resulted in increases in the concentration of triglycerides (see Tables 16 and 17). Triglyceride and cholesterol testing should be performed prior to initiating therapy with LEXIVA and at periodic intervals during therapy. Lipid disorders should be managed as clinically appropriate. (See PRECAUTIONS: Table 12. Drugs That Should Not Be Coadministered with LEXIVA and Table 13: Established and Other Potentially Significant Drug Interactions for additional information on potential drug interactions with LEXIVA and HMG-CoA reductase inhibitors).

Resistance/Cross-Resistance: Because the potential for HIV cross-resistance among protease inhibitors has not been fully explored, it is unknown what effect therapy with LEXIVA will have on the activity of subsequently administered protease inhibitors. LEXIVA has been studied in patients who have experienced treatment failure with protease inhibitors (see INDICATIONS AND USAGE: Description of Clinical Studies).

Information for Patients: A statement to patients and healthcare providers is included on the product's bottle label: ALERT: Find out about medicines that should NOT be taken with LEXIVA. **A Patient Information Sheet for LEXIVA Tablets is available for patient information.**

Patients should be informed that LEXIVA is not a cure for HIV infection and that they may continue to develop opportunistic infections and other complications associated with HIV disease. The long-term effects of LEXIVA are unknown at this time. Patients should be told that there are currently no data demonstrating that therapy with LEXIVA can reduce the risk of transmitting HIV to others.

Patients should be told that sustained decreases in plasma HIV-1 RNA have been associated with a reduced risk of progression to AIDS and death. Patients should remain under the care of a physician while using LEXIVA. Patients should be advised to take LEXIVA every day as prescribed. LEXIVA must always be used in combination with other antiretroviral drugs. Patients should not alter the dose or discontinue therapy without consulting their physician. If a dose is missed, patients should take the dose as soon as possible and then return to their normal schedule. However, if a dose is skipped, the patient should not double the next dose.

Patients should inform their healthcare provider if they have a sulfa allergy. The potential for cross-sensitivity between drugs in the sulfonamide class and fosamprenavir is unknown.

LEXIVA may interact with many drugs; therefore, patients should be advised to report to their healthcare provider the use of any other prescription or nonprescription medication or herbal products, particularly St. John's wort.

Patients receiving PDE5 inhibitors should be advised that they may be at an increased risk of PDE5 inhibitor-associated adverse events, including hypotension, visual changes, and priapism, and should promptly report any symptoms to their healthcare provider.

Patients receiving hormonal contraceptives should be instructed to use alternate contraceptive measures during therapy with LEXIVA because hormonal levels may be altered.

Patients should be informed that redistribution or accumulation of body fat may occur in patients receiving antiretroviral therapy, including LEXIVA, and that the cause and long-term health effects of these conditions are not known at this time.

Drug Interactions: See also CONTRAINDICATIONS, WARNINGS, and CLINICAL PHARMACOLOGY: Drug Interactions.

Amprenavir, the active metabolite of fosamprenavir, is an inhibitor of cytochrome P450 3A4 metabolism and therefore should not be administered concurrently with medications with narrow therapeutic windows that are substrates of CYP3A4. Data also suggest that amprenavir induces CYP3A4.

Amprenavir is metabolized by CYP3A4. Coadministration of LEXIVA and drugs that induce CYP3A4, such as rifampin, may decrease amprenavir concentrations and reduce its therapeutic effect. Coadministration of LEXIVA and drugs that inhibit CYP3A4 may increase amprenavir concentrations and increase the incidence of adverse effects.

The potential for drug interactions with LEXIVA changes when LEXIVA is coadministered with the potent CYP3A4 inhibitor ritonavir. The magnitude of CYP3A4 mediated drug interactions (effect on amprenavir or effect on coadministered drug) may change when LEXIVA is coadministered with ritonavir. Because ritonavir is a CYP2D6 inhibi-

Continued on next page

Table 12. Drugs That Should Not Be Coadministered with LEXIVA

Drug Class/Drug Name	Clinical Comment
Antiarrhythmics: Flecainide, propafenone	**CONTRAINDICATED** if LEXIVA is co-prescribed with **ritonavir** due to potential for serious and/or life-threatening reactions such as cardiac arrhythmias secondary to increases in plasma concentrations of antiarrhythmics.
Antimycobacterials: Rifampin*	May lead to loss of virologic response and possible resistance to LEXIVA or to the class of protease inhibitors.
Ergot derivatives: Dihydroergotamine, ergonovine, ergotamine, methylergonovine	**CONTRAINDICATED** due to potential for serious and/or life-threatening reactions such as acute ergot toxicity characterized by peripheral vasospasm and ischemia of the extremities and other tissues.
GI motility agents: Cisapride	**CONTRAINDICATED**due to potential for serious and/or life-threatening reactions such as cardiac arrhythmias.
Herbal products: St. John's wort (hypericum perforatum)	May lead to loss of virologic response and possible resistance to LEXIVA or to the class of protease inhibitors.
HMG co-reductase inhibitors: Lovastatin, simvastatin	Potential for serious reactions such as risk of myopathy including rhabdomyolysis.
Neuroleptic: Pimozide	**CONTRAINDICATED**due to potential for serious and/or life-threatening reactions such as cardiac arrhythmias.
Non-nucleoside reverse transcriptase inhibitor: Delavirdine*	May lead to loss of virologic response and possible resistance to delavirdine.
Sedative/hypnotics: Midazolam, triazolam	**CONTRAINDICATED** due to potential for serious and/or life-threatening reactions such as prolonged or increased sedation or respiratory depression.

*See CLINICAL PHARMACOLOGY Tables 3, 4, 5, or 6 for magnitude of interaction.

Table 13. Established and Other Potentially Significant Drug Interactions: Alteration in Dose or Regimen May Be Recommended Based on Drug Interaction Studies or Predicted Interaction (Information in the table applies to LEXIVA with or without ritonavir, unless otherwise indicated.)

Concomitant Drug Class: Drug Name	Effect on Concentration of Amprenavir or Concomitant Drug	Clinical Comment
	HIV-Antiviral Agents	
Non-nucleoside reverse transcriptase inhibitors: Efavirenz	**LEXIVA:** ↓ Amprenavir	Appropriate doses of the combinations with respect to safety and efficacy have not been established.
	LEXIVA/ritonavir: ↓ Amprenavir	An additional 100 mg/day (300 mg total) of ritonavir is recommended when efavirenz is administered with LEXIVA/ritonavir once daily. No change in the ritonavir dose is required when efavirenz is administered with LEXIVA plus ritonavir twice daily.
Non-nucleoside reverse transcriptase inhibitor: Nevirapine	↓ Amprenavir	Appropriate doses of the combinations with respect to safety and efficacy have not been established.
HIV protease inhibitors: Indinavir,* nelfinavir*	**LEXIVA:** ↑ Amprenavir Effect on indinavir and nelfinavir is not well established. **LEXIVA/ritonavir:** Interaction has not been evaluated.	Appropriate doses of the combinations with respect to safety and efficacy have not been established.
HIV protease inhibitors: Lopinavir/ritonavir*	↓ Amprenavir ↓ Lopinavir	An increased rate of adverse events has been observed with coadministration of these medications. Appropriate doses of the combinations with respect to safety and efficacy have not been established.
HIV protease inhibitor: Saquinavir*	**LEXIVA:** ↓ Amprenavir Effect on saquinavir is not well established. **LEXIVA/ritonavir:** Interaction has not been evaluated.	Appropriate doses of the combination with respect to safety and efficacy have not been established.
	Other Agents	
Antiarrhythmics: Amiodarone, lidocaine (systemic), and quinidine	↑ Antiarrhythmics	Caution is warranted and therapeutic concentration monitoring, if available, is recommended for antiarrhythmics when coadministered with LEXIVA.

(Table continued on next page)

Lexiva—Cont.

tor, clinically significant interactions with drugs metabolized by CYP2D6 are possible when coadministered with LEXIVA plus ritonavir.

There are other agents that may result in serious and/or life-threatening drug interactions (see CONTRAINDICATIONS and WARNINGS).

[See table 12 at top of previous page]
[See table 13 on previous page]

Carcinogenesis and Mutagenesis: Carcinogenicity studies of fosamprenavir in rats and mice are in progress; however, results are available from carcinogenicity studies with amprenavir. Amprenavir was evaluated for carcinogenic potential by oral gavage administration to mice and rats for up to 104 weeks. Results showed an increase in the incidence of benign hepatocellular adenomas and an increase in the combined incidence of hepatocellular adenomas plus carcinoma in males of both species at the highest doses tested. Female mice and rats were not affected. These observations were made at systemic exposures equivalent to approximately 2 times (mice) and 4 times (rats) the human exposure (based on $AUC_{0-24\ hr}$ measurement) at the recommended dose of 1,200 mg twice daily. Administration of amprenavir did not cause a statistically significant increase in the incidence of any other benign or malignant neoplasm in mice or rats. It is not known how predictive the results of rodent carcinogenicity studies may be for humans.

Fosamprenavir and amprenavir were not mutagenic or genotoxic in a battery of in vitro and in vivo assays. These assays included bacterial reverse mutation (Ames), mouse lymphoma, rat micronucleus and chromosome aberrations in human lymphocytes.

Impairment of Fertility: The effects of fosamprenavir on fertility and general reproductive performance were investigated in male (treated for 4 weeks before mating) and female rats (treated for 2 weeks before mating through postpartum day 6). Systemic exposures ($AUC_{0-24\ hr}$) to amprenavir in these studies were 3 (males) to 4 (females) times higher than exposures in humans following administration of the maximum recommended human dose (MRHD) of fosamprenavir alone or similar to those seen in humans following administration of fosamprenavir in combination with ritonavir. Fosamprenavir did not impair mating or fertility of male or female rats and did not affect the development and maturation of sperm from treated rats.

Pregnancy and Reproduction: Pregnancy Category C. Embryo/fetal development studies were conducted in rats (dosed from day 6 to day 17 of gestation) and rabbits (dosed from day 7 to day 20 of gestation). Administration of fosamprenavir to pregnant rats and rabbits produced no major effects on embryo-fetal development; however, the incidence of abortion was increased in rabbits that were administered fosamprenavir. Systemic exposures ($AUC_{0-24\ hr}$) to amprenavir at these dosages were 0.8 (rabbits) to 2 (rats) times the exposures in humans following administration of the MRHD of fosamprenavir alone or 0.3 (rabbits) to 0.7 (rats) times the exposures in humans following administration of the MRHD of fosamprenavir in combination with ritonavir. In contrast, administration of amprenavir was associated with abortions and an increased incidence of minor skeletal variations resulting from deficient ossification of the femur, humerus, and trochlea, in pregnant rabbits at the tested dose; approximately one twentieth the exposure seen at the recommended human dose.

The mating and fertility of the F_1 generation born to female rats given fosamprenavir was not different from control animals; however, fosamprenavir did cause a reduction in both pup survival and body weights. Surviving F_1 female rats showed an increased time to successful mating, an increased length of gestation, a reduced number of uterine implantation sites per litter, and reduced gestational body weights compared to control animals. Systemic exposure ($AUC_{0-24\ hr}$) to amprenavir in the F_0 pregnant rats was approximately 2 times higher than exposures in humans following administration of the MRHD of fosamprenavir alone or approximately the same as those seen in humans following administration of the MRHD of fosamprenavir in combination with ritonavir.

There are no adequate and well-controlled studies in pregnant women. LEXIVA should be used during pregnancy only if the potential benefit justifies the potential risk to the fetus.

Antiretroviral Pregnancy Registry: To monitor maternal-fetal outcomes of pregnant women exposed to LEXIVA, an Antiretroviral Pregnancy Registry has been established. Physicians are encouraged to register patients by calling 1-800-258-4263.

Nursing Mothers: **The Centers for Disease Control and Prevention recommend that HIV-infected mothers not breastfeed their infants to avoid risking postnatal transmission of HIV.** Although it is not known if amprenavir is excreted in human milk, amprenavir is secreted into the milk of lactating rats. Because of both the potential for HIV transmission and the potential for serious adverse reactions in nursing infants, **mothers should be instructed not to breastfeed if they are receiving LEXIVA.**

Pediatric Use: The safety and efficacy of LEXIVA Tablets have not been established in pediatric patients.

Geriatric Use: Clinical studies of LEXIVA did not include sufficient numbers of patients aged 65 and over to determine whether they respond differently from younger adults. In general, dose selection for an elderly patient should be cautious, reflecting the greater frequency of decreased he-

Table 13 *(cont.)*. Established and Other Potentially Significant Drug Interactions: Alteration in Dose or Regimen May Be Recommended Based on Drug Interaction Studies or Predicted Interaction (Information in the table applies to LEXIVA with or without ritonavir, unless otherwise indicated.)

Concomitant Drug Class: Drug Name	Effect on Concentration of Amprenavir or Concomitant Drug	Clinical Comment
	Other Agents (cont.)	
Antiarrhythmic: Bepridil	↑ Bepridil	Use with caution. Increased bepridil exposure may be associated with life-threatening reactions such as cardiac arrhythmias.
Anticoagulant: Warfarin		Concentrations of warfarin may be affected. It is recommended that INR (international normalized ratio) be monitored.
Anticonvulsants: Carbamazepine, phenobarbital, phenytoin	↓ Amprenavir	Use with caution. LEXIVA may be less effective due to decreased amprenavir plasma concentrations in patients taking these agents concomitantly.
Antifungals: Ketoconazole, itraconazole	↑ Ketoconazole ↑ Itraconazole	Increase monitoring for adverse events due to ketoconazole or itraconazole. **LEXIVA:** Dose reduction of ketoconazole or itraconazole may be needed for patients receiving more than 400 mg ketoconazole or itraconazole per day. **LEXIVA/ritonavir:** High doses of ketoconazole or itraconazole (>200 mg/day) are not recommended.
Antimycobacterial: Rifabutin*	↑ Rifabutin and rifabutin metabolite	A complete blood count should be performed weekly and as clinically indicated in order to monitor for neutropenia in patients receiving LEXIVA and rifabutin. **LEXIVA:** A dosage reduction of rifabutin by at least half the recommended dose is required. **LEXIVA/ritonavir:** Dosage reduction of rifabutin by at least 75% of the usual dose of 300 mg/day is recommended (a maximum dose of 150 mg every other day or three times per week).
Benzodiazepines: Alprazolam, clorazepate, diazepam, flurazepam	↑ Benzodiazepines	Clinical significance is unknown; however, a decrease in benzodiazepine dose may be needed.
Calcium channel blockers: Diltiazem, felodipine, nifedipine, nicardipine, nimodipine, verapamil, amlodipine, nisoldipine, isradipine	↑ Calcium channel blockers	Caution is warranted and clinical monitoring of patients is recommended.
Corticosteroid: Dexamethasone	↓ Amprenavir	Use with caution. LEXIVA may be less effective due to decreased amprenavir plasma concentrations in patients taking these agents concomitantly.
Histamine H_2-receptor antagonists, and proton-pump inhibitors	**LEXIVA:** ↓ Amprenavir **LEXIVA/ritonavir:** Interaction not evaluated	Use with caution. LEXIVA may be less effective due to decreased amprenavir plasma concentrations in patients taking these agents concomitantly.
HMG-CoA reductase inhibitor: Atorvastatin*	↑ Atorvastatin	Use ≤20 mg/day of atorvastatin with careful monitoring, or consider other HMG-CoA reductase inhibitors such as fluvastatin, pravastatin, or rosuvastatin in combination with LEXIVA.
Immunosuppressants: Cyclosporine, tacrolimus, rapamycin	↑ Immunosuppressants	Therapeutic concentration monitoring is recommended for immunosuppressant agents when coadministered with LEXIVA.
Narcotic analgesic: Methadone	↓ Methadone	Dosage of methadone may need to be increased when coadministered with LEXIVA.
Oral contraceptives: Ethinyl estradiol/ norethindrone	**LEXIVA:** ↑ Ethinyl estradiol/ norethindrone **LEXIVA/ritonavir:** Interaction not evaluated	Because hormonal levels may be altered, alternative methods of non-hormonal contraception are recommended.
PDE5 inhibitors: Sildenafil, vardenafil	↑ Sildenafil ↑ Vardenafil	Use sildenafil with caution at reduced doses of 25 mg every 48 hours with increased monitoring for adverse events. **LEXIVA:** Use vardenafil with caution at reduced doses of no more than 2.5 mg every 24 hours with increased monitoring for adverse events. **LEXIVA/ritonavir:** Use vardenafil with caution at reduced doses of no more than 2.5 mg every 72 hours with increased monitoring for adverse events.
Tricyclic antidepressants: Amitriptyline, imipramine	↑ Tricyclics	Therapeutic concentration monitoring is recommended for tricyclic antidepressants when coadministered with LEXIVA.

*See CLINICAL PHARMACOLOGY Tables 3, 4, 5, or 6 for magnitude of interaction.

Table 14. Selected Clinical Adverse Events Reported in Antiretroviral-Naive Patients

	APV30001*				APV30002*			
	LEXIVA 1,400 mg b.i.d. (n = 166)		Nelfinavir 1,250 mg b.i.d. (n = 83)		LEXIVA 1,400 mg q.d./Ritonavir 200 mg q.d. (n = 322)		Nelfinavir 1,250 mg b.i.d. (n = 327)	
Adverse Event	Moderate/ Severe Drug-Related	All Grades†	Moderate/ Severe Drug-Related	All Grades†	Moderate/ Severe Drug-Related	All Grades†	Moderate/ Severe Drug-Related	All Grades†
Gastrointestinal								
Diarrhea	5%	34%	18%	63%	10%	52%	18%	72%
Nausea	7%	39%	4%	24%	7%	37%	5%	27%
Vomiting	2%	16%	4%	17%	6%	20%	4%	13%
Abdominal pain	1%	5%	0%	8%	2%	11%	2%	11%
Skin								
Pruritus	0%	7%	0%	11%	<1%	7%	1%	9%
Rash	8%	35%	2%	19%	3%	17%	2%	21%
General disorders								
Fatigue	2%	10%	1%	7%	4%	18%	2%	13%
Nervous system								
Depressive/ mood disorders	1%	8%	0%	8%	<1%	8%	0%	6%
Headache	2%	19%	4%	20%	3%	21%	3%	27%
Paresthesia, oral	0%	2%	0%	0%	<1%	10%	0%	<1%

*All patients also received abacavir and lamivudine twice daily.
† Includes adverse events of all grades regardless of causality reported in >5% of patients.

Table 15. Selected Clinical Adverse Events Reported in Protease Inhibitor-Experienced Patients (Study APV30003)

	LEXIVA 700 mg b.i.d./ Ritonavir 100 mg b.i.d.* (n = 106)		Lopinavir 400 mg b.i.d./ Ritonavir 100 mg b.i.d.* (n = 103)	
Adverse Event	Moderate/Severe Drug-Related	All Grades†	Moderate/Severe Drug-Related	All Grades†
Gastrointestinal				
Diarrhea	13%	38%	11%	47%
Nausea	3%	20%	9%	31%
Vomiting	3%	10%	5%	17%
Abdominal pain	<1%	11%	2%	9%
Skin				
Pruritus	<1%	8%	0%	3%
Rash	3%	9%	0%	22%
General disorders				
Fatigue	<1%	9%	<1%	14%
Nervous system				
Depressive/mood disorders	<1%	11%	<1%	10%
Headache	4%	27%	2%	20%
Paresthesia, oral	0%	<1%	0%	0%

*All patients also received 2 reverse transcriptase inhibitors.
† Includes adverse events of all grades regardless of causality in >5% of patients.

Table 16. Grade 3/4 Laboratory Abnormalities Reported in ≥2% of Antiretroviral-Naive Adult Patients in Studies APV30001 and APV30002

	APV30001*		APV30002*	
Laboratory Abnormality	LEXIVA 1,400 mg b.i.d. (n = 166)	Nelfinavir 1,250 mg b.i.d. (n = 83)	LEXIVA 1,400 mg q.d./ Ritonavir 200 mg q.d. (n = 322)	Nelfinavir 1,250 mg b.i.d. (n = 327)
ALT (>5 × ULN)	6%	5%	8%	8%
AST (>5 × ULN)	6%	6%	6%	7%
Serum lipase (>2 × ULN)	8%	4%	6%	4%
Hypertriglyceridemia† (>750 mg/dL)	0%	1%	6%	2%
Neutropenia (<750 cells/mm^3)	3%	6%	3%	4%

*All patients also received abacavir and lamivudine twice daily.
† Fasting specimens.
ULN = Upper limit of normal.

Table 17. Grade 3/4 Laboratory Abnormalities Reported in ≥2% of Protease Inhibitor-Experienced Adult Patients in Study APV30003

Laboratory Abnormality	LEXIVA 700 mg b.i.d./ Ritonavir 100 mg b.i.d.* (n = 104)	Lopinavir 400 mg b.i.d./ Ritonavir 100 mg b.i.d.* (n = 103)
Hypertriglyceridemia† (>750 mg/dL)	11%‡	6%‡
Serum lipase (>2 × ULN)	5%	12%
ALT (>5 × ULN)	4%	4%
AST (>5 × ULN)	4%	2%
Hyperglycemia (>251 mg/dL)	2%‡	2%‡

*All patients also received 2 reverse transcriptase inhibitors.
† Fasting specimens.
‡ n = 100 for LEXIVA/ritonavir, n = 98 for lopinavir/ritonavir.
ULN = Upper limit of normal.

patic, renal, or cardiac function, and of concomitant disease or other drug therapy.

ADVERSE REACTIONS

LEXIVA was studied in 700 patients in Phase III controlled clinical studies. The most common treatment-emergent adverse events in clinical studies of LEXIVA were diarrhea, nausea, vomiting, headache, and rash and were generally mild to moderate in severity. Treatment discontinuation due to adverse events occurred in 6.4% of patients receiving LEXIVA and in 5.9% of patients receiving comparator treatments.

Severe or life-threatening skin reactions, including 1 case of Stevens-Johnson syndrome among 700 patients treated with LEXIVA, were reported in <1% of patients treated with LEXIVA in the clinical studies. Treatment with LEXIVA should be discontinued for severe or life-threatening rashes and for moderate rashes accompanied by systemic symptoms.

Skin rash (without regard to causality) occurred in approximately 19% of patients treated with LEXIVA in the pivotal efficacy studies. Rashes were usually maculopapular and of mild or moderate intensity, some with pruritus. Rash had a median onset of 11 days after initiation of LEXIVA and had a median duration of 13 days. Skin rash led to discontinuation of LEXIVA in <1% of patients. In some patients with mild or moderate rash, dosing with LEXIVA was often continued without interruption; if interrupted, reintroduction of LEXIVA generally did not result in rash recurrence.

Selected adverse events reported during the clinical efficacy studies of LEXIVA are shown in Tables 14 and 15. Each table presents drug-related adverse events of moderate or severe intensity and adverse events of all grades regardless of causality in patients treated with combination therapy for up to 48 weeks.

[See table 14 at left]
[See table 15 at left]

The percentages of patients with Grade 3 or 4 laboratory abnormalities in the clinical efficacy studies of LEXIVA are presented in Tables 16 and 17.

[See table 16 at left]

The incidence of Grade 3 or 4 hyperglycemia in antiretroviral-naive patients who received LEXIVA in the pivotal studies was <1%.

[See table 17 at left]

OVERDOSAGE

There is no known antidote for LEXIVA. It is not known whether amprenavir can be removed by peritoneal dialysis or hemodialysis. If overdosage occurs, the patient should be monitored for evidence of toxicity and standard supportive treatment applied as necessary.

DOSAGE AND ADMINISTRATION

LEXIVA Tablets may be taken with or without food.

The recommended oral dose of LEXIVA, alone or in combination with ritonavir, is as follows:

Therapy-Naive Patients:

- LEXIVA 1,400 mg twice daily (without ritonavir)
- LEXIVA 1,400 mg once daily plus ritonavir 200 mg once daily
- LEXIVA 700 mg twice daily plus ritonavir 100 mg twice daily

The twice-daily plus ritonavir dose is supported by pharmacokinetic and safety data (see CLINICAL PHARMACOLOGY and ADVERSE EVENTS).

Protease Inhibitor-Experienced Patients:

- LEXIVA 700 mg twice daily plus ritonavir 100 mg twice daily

Once-daily administration of LEXIVA plus ritonavir is not recommended in protease inhibitor-experienced patients (see Description of Clinical Studies).

Adjustment of Ritonavir Dose When LEXIVA plus Ritonavir are Administered with Efavirenz: An additional 100 mg/day (300 mg total) of ritonavir is recommended when efavirenz is administered with LEXIVA plus ritonavir once daily (see Table 13. Established and Other Potentially Significant Drug Interactions: Alteration in Dose or Regimen May Be Recommended Based on Drug Interaction Studies or Predicted Interaction).

Prescribers should consult the full prescribing information for NORVIR (ritonavir) when using this agent.

Patients with Hepatic Impairment: LEXIVA Tablets should be used with caution, at a reduced dosage of 700 mg twice daily in patients with mild or moderate hepatic impairment(Child-Pugh score ranging from 5 to 8) receiving LEXIVA without concurrent ritonavir (see CLINICAL PHARMACOLOGY: Hepatic Insufficiency). LEXIVA should not be used in patients with severe hepatic impairment (Child-Pugh score ranging from 9 to 12) because the dose cannot be reduced below 700 mg. There are no data on the use of LEXIVA in combination with ritonavir in patients with any degree of hepatic impairment.

HOW SUPPLIED

LEXIVA Tablets, 700 mg, are pink, film-coated, capsule-shaped, biconvex tablets, with "GX LL7" debossed on one face.

Bottles of 60 with child-resistant closures (NDC 0173-0721-00).

Store at controlled room temperature of 25°C (77°F); excursions permitted to 15° to 30°C (59° to 86°F) (see USP Controlled Room Temperature). Keep container tightly closed.

GlaxoSmithKline

Continued on next page

Lexiva—Cont.

Research Triangle Park, NC 27709
Vertex Pharmaceuticals Incorporated
Cambridge, MA 02139
LEXIVA is a trademark of the GlaxoSmithKline

October 2003/RL-2048

WELLBUTRIN XL™ ℞
[*wel'byū-trin*]
(bupropion hydrochloride extended-release tablets)

DESCRIPTION

WELLBUTRIN XL (bupropion hydrochloride), an antidepressant of the aminoketone class, is chemically unrelated to tricyclic, tetracyclic, selective serotonin re-uptake inhibitor, or other known antidepressant agents. Its structure closely resembles that of diethylpropion; it is related to phenylethylamines. It is designated as (±)-1-(3-chlorophenyl)-2-[(1,1-dimethylethyl)amino]-1-propanone hydrochloride. The molecular weight is 276.2. The molecular formula is $C_{13}H_{18}ClNO{\bullet}HCl$. Bupropion hydrochloride powder is white, crystalline, and highly soluble in water. It has a bitter taste and produces the sensation of local anesthesia on the oral mucosa. The structural formula is:

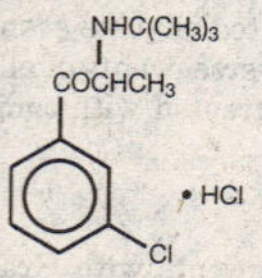

WELLBUTRIN XL Tablets are supplied for oral administration as 150-mg and 300-mg, creamy-white to pale yellow extended-release tablets. Each tablet contains the labeled amount of bupropion hydrochloride and the inactive ingredients: ethylcellulose aqueous dispersion (NF), glyceryl behenate, methacrylic acid copolymer dispersion (NF), polyvinyl alcohol, polyethylene glycol, povidone, silicon dioxide, and triethyl citrate. The tablets are printed with edible black ink.

The insoluble shell of the extended-release tablet may remain intact during gastrointestinal transit and is eliminated in the feces.

CLINICAL PHARMACOLOGY

Pharmacodynamics: Bupropion is a relatively weak inhibitor of the neuronal uptake of norepinephrine, serotonin, and dopamine, and does not inhibit monoamine oxidase. While the mechanism of action of bupropion, as with other antidepressants, is unknown, it is presumed that this action is mediated by noradrenergic and/or dopaminergic mechanisms.

Pharmacokinetics: Bupropion is a racemic mixture. The pharmacologic activity and pharmacokinetics of the individual enantiomers have not been studied. The mean elimination half-life (±SD) of bupropion after chronic dosing is 21 (±9) hours, and steady-state plasma concentrations of bupropion are reached within 8 days.

In a study comparing 14-day dosing with WELLBUTRIN XL Tablets 300 mg once daily to the immediate-release formulation of bupropion at 100 mg 3 times daily, equivalence was demonstrated for peak plasma concentration and area under the curve for bupropion and the 3 metabolites (hydroxybupropion, threohydrobupropion, and erythrohydrobupropion).

Absorption: Following oral administration of WELLBUTRIN XL Tablets to healthy volunteers, time to peak plasma concentrations for bupropion was approximately 5 hours and food did not affect the C_{max} or AUC of bupropion.

Distribution: In vitro tests show that bupropion is 84% bound to human plasma proteins at concentrations up to 200 mcg/mL. The extent of protein binding of the hydroxybupropion metabolite is similar to that for bupropion, whereas the extent of protein binding of the threohydrobupropion metabolite is about half that seen with bupropion.

Metabolism: Bupropion is extensively metabolized in humans. Three metabolites have been shown to be active: hydroxybupropion, which is formed via hydroxylation of the *tert*-butyl group of bupropion, and the amino-alcohol isomers threohydrobupropion and erythrohydrobupropion, which are formed via reduction of the carbonyl group. In vitro findings suggest that cytochrome P450IIB6 (CYP2B6) is the principal isoenzyme involved in the formation of hydroxybupropion, while cytochrome P450 isoenzymes are not involved in the formation of threohydrobupropion. Oxidation of the bupropion side chain results in the formation of a glycine conjugate of meta-chlorobenzoic acid, which is then excreted as the major urinary metabolite. The potency and toxicity of the metabolites relative to bupropion have not been fully characterized. However, it has been demonstrated in an antidepressant screening test in mice that hydroxybupropion is one half as potent as bupropion, while threohydrobupropion and erythrohydrobupropion are 5-fold less potent than bupropion. This may be of clinical importance because the plasma concentrations of the metabolites are as high or higher than those of bupropion.

Because bupropion is extensively metabolized, there is the potential for drug-drug interactions, particularly with those agents that are metabolized by the cytochrome P450IIB6 (CYP2B6) isoenzyme. Although bupropion is not metabolized by cytochrome P450IID6 (CYP2D6), there is the potential for drug-drug interactions when bupropion is co-administered with drugs metabolized by this isoenzyme (see PRECAUTIONS: Drug Interactions).

In humans, peak plasma concentrations of hydroxybupropion occur approximately 7 hours after administration of WELLBUTRIN XL. Following administration of WELLBUTRIN XL, peak plasma concentrations of hydroxybupropion are approximately 7 times the peak level of the parent drug at steady state. The elimination half-life of hydroxybupropion is approximately 20 (±5) hours, and its AUC at steady state is about 13 times that of bupropion. The times to peak concentrations for the erythrohydrobupropion and threohydrobupropion metabolites are similar to that of the hydroxybupropion metabolite. However, their elimination half-lives are longer, approximately 33 (±10) and 37 (±13) hours, respectively, and steady-state AUCs are 1.4 and 7 times that of bupropion, respectively.

Bupropion and its metabolites exhibit linear kinetics following chronic administration of 300 to 450 mg/day.

Elimination: Following oral administration of 200 mg of ^{14}C-bupropion in humans, 87% and 10% of the radioactive dose were recovered in the urine and feces, respectively. However, the fraction of the oral dose of bupropion excreted unchanged was only 0.5%, a finding consistent with the extensive metabolism of bupropion.

Population Subgroups: Factors or conditions altering metabolic capacity (e.g., liver disease, congestive heart failure [CHF], age, concomitant medications, etc.) or elimination may be expected to influence the degree and extent of accumulation of the active metabolites of bupropion. The elimination of the major metabolites of bupropion may be affected by reduced renal or hepatic function because they are moderately polar compounds and are likely to undergo further metabolism or conjugation in the liver prior to urinary excretion.

Hepatic: The effect of hepatic impairment on the pharmacokinetics of bupropion was characterized in 2 single-dose studies, one in patients with alcoholic liver disease and one in patients with mild to severe cirrhosis. The first study showed that the half-life of hydroxybupropion was significantly longer in 8 patients with alcoholic liver disease than in 8 healthy volunteers (32±14 hours versus 21±5 hours, respectively). Although not statistically significant, the AUCs for bupropion and hydroxybupropion were more variable and tended to be greater (by 53% to 57%) in patients with alcoholic liver disease. The differences in half-life for bupropion and the other metabolites in the 2 patient groups were minimal.

The second study showed no statistically significant differences in the pharmacokinetics of bupropion and its active metabolites in 9 patients with mild to moderate hepatic cirrhosis compared to 8 healthy volunteers. However, more variability was observed in some of the pharmacokinetic parameters for bupropion (AUC, C_{max}, and T_{max}) and its active metabolites ($t_{1/2}$) in patients with mild to moderate hepatic cirrhosis. In addition, in patients with severe hepatic cirrhosis, the bupropion C_{max} and AUC were substantially increased (mean difference: by approximately 70% and 3-fold, respectively) and more variable when compared to values in healthy volunteers; the mean bupropion half-life was also longer (29 hours in patients with severe hepatic cirrhosis vs 19 hours in healthy subjects). For the metabolite hydroxybupropion, the mean C_{max} was approximately 69% lower. For the combined amino-alcohol isomers threohydrobupropion and erythrohydrobupropion, the mean C_{max} was approximately 31% lower. The mean AUC increased by about 1½-fold for hydroxybupropion and about 2½-fold for threo/erythrohydrobupropion. The median T_{max} was observed 19 hours later for hydroxybupropion and 31 hours later for threo/erythrohydrobupropion. The mean half-lives for hydroxybupropion and threo/erythrohydrobupropion were increased 5- and 2-fold, respectively, in patients with severe hepatic cirrhosis compared to healthy volunteers (see WARNINGS, PRECAUTIONS, and DOSAGE AND ADMINISTRATION).

Renal: The effect of renal disease on the pharmacokinetics of bupropion has not been studied. The elimination of the major metabolites of bupropion may be affected by reduced renal function.

Left Ventricular Dysfunction: During a chronic dosing study with bupropion in 14 depressed patients with left ventricular dysfunction (history of CHF or an enlarged heart on x-ray), no apparent effect on the pharmacokinetics of bupropion or its metabolites was revealed, compared to healthy volunteers.

Age: The effects of age on the pharmacokinetics of bupropion and its metabolites have not been fully characterized, but an exploration of steady-state bupropion concentrations from several depression efficacy studies involving patients dosed in a range of 300 to 750 mg/day, on a 3 times daily schedule, revealed no relationship between age (18 to 83 years) and plasma concentration of bupropion. A single-dose pharmacokinetic study demonstrated that the disposition of bupropion and its metabolites in elderly subjects was similar to that of younger subjects. These data suggest there is no prominent effect of age on bupropion concentration; however, another pharmacokinetic study, single and multiple dose, has suggested that the elderly are at increased risk for accumulation of bupropion and its metabolites (see PRECAUTIONS: Geriatric Use).

Gender: A single-dose study involving 12 healthy male and 12 healthy female volunteers revealed no sex-related differences in the pharmacokinetic parameters of bupropion.

Smokers: The effects of cigarette smoking on the pharmacokinetics of bupropion were studied in 34 healthy male and female volunteers; 17 were chronic cigarette smokers and 17 were nonsmokers. Following oral administration of a single 150-mg dose of bupropion, there was no statistically significant difference in C_{max}, half-life, T_{max}, AUC, or clearance of bupropion or its active metabolites between smokers and nonsmokers.

CLINICAL TRIALS

The efficacy of bupropion as a treatment for major depressive disorder was established with the immediate-release formulation of bupropion in two 4-week, placebo-controlled trials in adult inpatients and in one 6-week, placebo-controlled trial in adult outpatients. In the first study, patients were titrated in a bupropion dose range of 300 to 600 mg/day of the immediate-release formulation on a 3 times daily schedule; 78% of patients received maximum doses of 450 mg/day or less. This trial demonstrated the effectiveness of bupropion on the Hamilton Depression Rating Scale (HDRS) total score, the depressed mood item (item 1) from that scale, and the Clinical Global Impressions (CGI) severity score. A second study included 2 fixed doses of the immediate-release formulation of bupropion (300 and 450 mg/day) and placebo. This trial demonstrated the effectiveness of bupropion, but only at the 450-mg/day dose of the immediate-release formulation; the results were positive for the HDRS total score and the CGI severity score, but not for HDRS item 1. In the third study, outpatients received 300 mg/day of the immediate-release formulation of bupropion. This study demonstrated the effectiveness of bupropion on the HDRS total score, HDRS item 1, the Montgomery-Asberg Depression Rating Scale, the CGI severity score, and the CGI improvement score.

Although there are no independent trials demonstrating the antidepressant effectiveness of WELLBUTRIN XL, studies have demonstrated similar bioavailability of the immediate-release and the extended-release formulations of bupropion under steady-state conditions, i.e., WELLBUTRIN XL 300 mg once daily was shown to have bioavailability that was similar to that of 100 mg 3 times daily of the immediate-release formulation of bupropion, with regard to both rate and extent of absorption, for parent drug and metabolites.

In a longer-term study, outpatients meeting DSM-IV criteria for major depressive disorder, recurrent type, who had responded during an 8-week open trial on bupropion (150 mg twice daily of the sustained-release formulation) were randomized to continuation of their same dose of bupropion or placebo, for up to 44 weeks of observation for relapse. Response during the open phase was defined as CGI Improvement score of 1 (very much improved) or 2 (much improved) for each of the final 3 weeks. Relapse during the double-blind phase was defined as the investigator's judgment that drug treatment was needed for worsening depressive symptoms. Patients receiving continued bupropion treatment experienced significantly lower relapse rates over the subsequent 44 weeks compared to those receiving placebo.

INDICATIONS AND USAGE

WELLBUTRIN XL is indicated for the treatment of major depressive disorder.

The efficacy of bupropion in the treatment of a major depressive episode was established in two 4-week controlled trials of inpatients and in one 6-week controlled trial of outpatients whose diagnoses corresponded most closely to the Major Depression category of the APA Diagnostic and Statistical Manual (DSM) (see CLINICAL PHARMACOLOGY).

A major depressive episode (DSM-IV) implies the presence of 1) depressed mood or 2) loss of interest or pleasure; in addition, at least 5 of the following symptoms have been present during the same 2-week period and represent a change from previous functioning: depressed mood, markedly diminished interest or pleasure in usual activities, significant change in weight and/or appetite, insomnia or hypersomnia, psychomotor agitation or retardation, increased fatigue, feelings of guilt or worthlessness, slowed thinking or impaired concentration, a suicide attempt, or suicidal ideation.

The efficacy of bupropion in maintaining an antidepressant response for up to 44 weeks following 8 weeks of acute treatment was demonstrated in a placebo-controlled trial with the sustained-release formulation of bupropion (see CLINICAL PHARMACOLOGY). Nevertheless, the physician who elects to use WELLBUTRIN XL for extended periods should periodically reevaluate the long-term usefulness of the drug for the individual patient.

CONTRAINDICATIONS

WELLBUTRIN XL is contraindicated in patients with a seizure disorder.

WELLBUTRIN XL is contraindicated in patients treated with ZYBAN® (bupropion hydrochloride) Sustained-Release Tablets, WELLBUTRIN (bupropion hydrochloride) the immediate-release formulation, WELLBUTRIN SR (bupropion hydrochloride) the sustained-release formulation, or any other medications that contain bupropion because the incidence of seizure is dose dependent.

WELLBUTRIN XL is contraindicated in patients with a current or prior diagnosis of bulimia or anorexia nervosa because of a higher incidence of seizures noted in patients treated for bulimia with the immediate-release formulation of bupropion.

WELLBUTRIN XL is contraindicated in patients undergoing abrupt discontinuation of alcohol or sedatives (including benzodiazepines).
The concurrent administration of WELLBUTRIN XL Tablets and a monoamine oxidase (MAO) inhibitor is contraindicated. At least 14 days should elapse between discontinuation of an MAO inhibitor and initiation of treatment with WELLBUTRIN XL Tablets.
WELLBUTRIN XL is contraindicated in patients who have shown an allergic response to bupropion or the other ingredients that make up WELLBUTRIN XL Tablets.

WARNINGS

Patients should be made aware that WELLBUTRIN XL contains the same active ingredient found in ZYBAN, used as an aid to smoking cessation treatment, and that WELLBUTRIN XL should not be used in combination with ZYBAN, or any other medications that contain bupropion, such as WELLBUTRIN SR (bupropion hydrochloride), the sustained-release formulation or WELLBUTRIN (bupropion hydrochloride), the immediate-release formulation.

Seizures: Bupropion is associated with a dose-related risk of seizures. The risk of seizures is also related to patient factors, clinical situations, and concomitant medications, which must be considered in selection of patients for therapy with WELLBUTRIN XL. WELLBUTRIN XL should be discontinued and not restarted in patients who experience a seizure while on treatment.

As both WELLBUTRIN XL and the sustained-release formulation of bupropion (WELLBUTRIN SR) are bioequivalent to the immediate-release formulation of bupropion, the seizure incidence with WELLBUTRIN XL, while not formally evaluated in clinical trials, may be similar to that presented below for the immediate-release and sustained-release formulations of bupropion.

- **Dose: At doses up to 300 mg/day of the sustained-release formulation of bupropion (WELLBUTRIN SR), the incidence of seizure is approximately 0.1% (1/1,000).**
  Data for the immediate-release formulation of bupropion revealed a seizure incidence of approximately 0.4% (i.e., 13 of 3,200 patients followed prospectively) in patients treated at doses in a range of 300 to 450 mg/day. This seizure incidence (0.4%) may exceed that of some other marketed antidepressants.
  Additional data accumulated for the immediate-release formulation of bupropion suggested that the estimated seizure incidence increases almost tenfold between 450 and 600 mg/day. The 600 mg dose is twice the usual adult dose and one and one-third the maximum recommended daily dose (450 mg) of WELLBUTRIN XL Tablets. This disproportionate increase in seizure incidence with dose incrementation calls for caution in dosing.
- **Patient factors: Predisposing factors that may increase the risk of seizure with bupropion use include history of head trauma or prior seizure, central nervous system (CNS) tumor, the presence of severe hepatic cirrhosis, and concomitant medications that lower seizure threshold.**
- **Clinical situations: Circumstances associated with an increased seizure risk include, among others, excessive use of alcohol or sedatives (including benzodiazepines); addiction to opiates, cocaine, or stimulants; use of over-the-counter stimulants and anorectics; and diabetes treated with oral hypoglycemics or insulin.**
- **Concomitant medications: Many medications (e.g., antipsychotics, antidepressants, theophylline, systemic steroids) are known to lower seizure threshold.**

Recommendations for Reducing the Risk of Seizure: **Retrospective analysis of clinical experience gained during the development of bupropion suggests that the risk of seizure may be minimized if**

- **the total daily dose of WELLBUTRIN XL Tablets does *not* exceed 450 mg,**
- **the rate of incrementation of dose is gradual.**

WELLBUTRIN XL should be administered with extreme caution to patients with a history of seizure, cranial trauma, or other predisposition(s) toward seizure, or patients treated with other agents (e.g., antipsychotics, other antidepressants, theophylline, systemic steroids, etc.) that lower seizure threshold.

Hepatic Impairment: WELLBUTRIN XL should be used with extreme caution in patients with severe hepatic cirrhosis. In these patients a reduced frequency and/or dose is required, as peak bupropion, as well as AUC, levels are substantially increased and accumulation is likely to occur in such patients to a greater extent than usual. The dose should not exceed 150 mg every other day in these patients (see CLINICAL PHARMACOLOGY, PRECAUTIONS, and DOSAGE AND ADMINISTRATION).

Potential for Hepatotoxicity: In rats receiving large doses of bupropion chronically, there was an increase in incidence of hepatic hyperplastic nodules and hepatocellular hypertrophy. In dogs receiving large doses of bupropion chronically, various histologic changes were seen in the liver, and laboratory tests suggesting mild hepatocellular injury were noted.

PRECAUTIONS

General: ***Agitation and Insomnia:*** Increased restlessness, agitation, anxiety, and insomnia, especially shortly after initiation of treatment, have been associated with treatment with bupropion. Patients in placebo-controlled trials with WELLBUTRIN SR, the sustained-release formulation of bupropion, experienced agitation, anxiety, and insomnia as shown in Table 1.
[See table 1 above]

Table 1. Incidence of Agitation, Anxiety, and Insomnia in Placebo-Controlled Trials

Adverse Event Term	WELLBUTRIN SR 300 mg/day (n = 376)	WELLBUTRIN SR 400 mg/day (n = 114)	Placebo (n = 385)
Agitation	3%	9%	2%
Anxiety	5%	6%	3%
Insomnia	11%	16%	6%

In clinical studies, these symptoms were sometimes of sufficient magnitude to require treatment with sedative/hypnotic drugs.
Symptoms were sufficiently severe to require discontinuation of treatment in 1% and 2.6% of patients treated with 300 and 400 mg/day, respectively, of bupropion sustained-release tablets and 0.8% of patients treated with placebo.

Psychosis, Confusion, and Other Neuropsychiatric Phenomena: Depressed patients treated with bupropion have been reported to show a variety of neuropsychiatric signs and symptoms, including delusions, hallucinations, psychosis, concentration disturbance, paranoia, and confusion. In some cases, these symptoms abated upon dose reduction and/or withdrawal of treatment.

Activation of Psychosis and/or Mania: Antidepressants can precipitate manic episodes in bipolar disorder patients during the depressed phase of their illness and may activate latent psychosis in other susceptible patients. WELLBUTRIN XL is expected to pose similar risks.

Altered Appetite and Weight: In placebo-controlled studies using WELLBUTRIN SR, the sustained-release formulation of bupropion, patients experienced weight gain or weight loss as shown in Table 2.
[See table 2 at top of next page]
In studies conducted with the immediate-release formulation of bupropion, 35% of patients receiving tricyclic antidepressants gained weight, compared to 9% of patients treated with the immediate-release formulation of bupropion. If weight loss is a major presenting sign of a patient's depressive illness, the anorectic and/or weight-reducing potential of WELLBUTRIN XL Tablets should be considered.

Suicide: The possibility of a suicide attempt is inherent in depression and may persist until significant remission occurs. Accordingly, prescriptions for WELLBUTRIN XL Tablets should be written for the smallest number of tablets consistent with good patient management.

Allergic Reactions: Anaphylactoid/anaphylactic reactions characterized by symptoms such as pruritus, urticaria, angioedema, and dyspnea requiring medical treatment have been reported in clinical trials with bupropion. In addition, there have been rare spontaneous postmarketing reports of erythema multiforme, Stevens-Johnson syndrome, and anaphylactic shock associated with bupropion. A patient should stop taking WELLBUTRIN XL and consult a doctor if experiencing allergic or anaphylactoid/anaphylactic reactions (e.g., skin rash, pruritus, hives, chest pain, edema, and shortness of breath) during treatment.
Arthralgia, myalgia, and fever with rash and other symptoms suggestive of delayed hypersensitivity have been reported in association with bupropion. These symptoms may resemble serum sickness.

Cardiovascular Effects: In clinical practice, hypertension, in some cases severe, requiring acute treatment, has been reported in patients receiving bupropion alone and in combination with nicotine replacement therapy. These events have been observed in both patients with and without evidence of pre-existing hypertension.
Data from a comparative study of the sustained-release formulation of bupropion (ZYBAN® Sustained-Release Tablets), nicotine transdermal system (NTS), the combination of sustained-release bupropion plus NTS, and placebo as an aid to smoking cessation suggest a higher incidence of treatment-emergent hypertension in patients treated with the combination of sustained-release bupropion and NTS. In this study, 6.1% of patients treated with the combination of sustained-release bupropion and NTS had treatment-emergent hypertension compared to 2.5%, 1.6%, and 3.1% of patients treated with sustained-release bupropion, NTS, and placebo, respectively. The majority of these patients had evidence of pre-existing hypertension. Three patients (1.2%) treated with the combination of ZYBAN and NTS and 1 patient (0.4%) treated with NTS had study medication discontinued due to hypertension compared to none of the patients treated with ZYBAN or placebo. Monitoring of blood pressure is recommended in patients who receive the combination of bupropion and nicotine replacement.
There is no clinical experience establishing the safety of WELLBUTRIN XL Tablets in patients with a recent history of myocardial infarction or unstable heart disease. Therefore, care should be exercised if it is used in these groups. Bupropion was well tolerated in depressed patients who had previously developed orthostatic hypotension while receiving tricyclic antidepressants, and was also generally well tolerated in a group of 36 depressed inpatients with stable congestive heart failure (CHF). However, bupropion was associated with a rise in supine blood pressure in the study of patients with CHF, resulting in discontinuation of treatment in 2 patients for exacerbation of baseline hypertension.

Hepatic Impairment: WELLBUTRIN XL should be used with extreme caution in patients with severe hepatic cirrhosis. In these patients, a reduced frequency and/or dose is required. WELLBUTRIN XL should be used with caution in patients with hepatic impairment (including mild to moderate hepatic cirrhosis) and reduced frequency and/or dose should be considered in patients with mild to moderate hepatic cirrhosis.
All patients with hepatic impairment should be closely monitored for possible adverse effects that could indicate high drug and metabolite levels (see CLINICAL PHARMACOLOGY, WARNINGS, and DOSAGE AND ADMINISTRATION).

Renal Impairment: No studies have been conducted in patients with renal impairment. Bupropion is extensively metabolized in the liver to active metabolites, which are further metabolized and subsequently excreted by the kidneys. WELLBUTRIN XL should be used with caution in patients with renal impairment and a reduced frequency and/or dose should be considered as bupropion and its metabolites may accumulate in such patients to a greater extent than usual. The patient should be closely monitored for possible adverse effects that could indicate high drug or metabolite levels.

Information for Patients: See the tear-off leaflet at the end of this labeling for Patient Information.
Patients should be made aware that WELLBUTRIN XL contains the same active ingredient found in ZYBAN, used as an aid to smoking cessation treatment, and that WELLBUTRIN XL should not be used in combination with ZYBAN or any other medications that contain bupropion hydrochloride (such as WELLBUTRIN SR, the sustained-release formulation, and WELLBUTRIN, the immediate-release formulation).
Physicians are advised to discuss the following issues with patients:
Patients should be told that WELLBUTRIN XL should be discontinued and not restarted if they experience a seizure while on treatment.
Patients should be told that any CNS-active drug like WELLBUTRIN XL Tablets may impair their ability to perform tasks requiring judgment or motor and cognitive skills. Consequently, until they are reasonably certain that WELLBUTRIN XL Tablets do not adversely affect their performance, they should refrain from driving an automobile or operating complex, hazardous machinery.
Patients should be told that the excessive use or abrupt discontinuation of alcohol or sedatives (including benzodiazepines) may alter the seizure threshold. Some patients have reported lower alcohol tolerance during treatment with WELLBUTRIN XL. Patients should be advised that the consumption of alcohol should be minimized or avoided.
Patients should be advised to inform their physicians if they are taking or plan to take any prescription or over-the-counter drugs. Concern is warranted because WELLBUTRIN XL Tablets and other drugs may affect each other's metabolism.
Patients should be advised to notify their physicians if they become pregnant or intend to become pregnant during therapy.
Patients should be advised to swallow WELLBUTRIN XL Tablets whole so that the release rate is not altered. Do not chew, divide, or crush tablets.
Patients should be advised that they may notice in their stool something that looks like a tablet. This is normal. The medication in WELLBUTRIN XL is contained in a nonabsorbable shell that has been specially designed to slowly release drug in the body. When this process is completed, the empty shell is eliminated from the body.

Laboratory Tests: There are no specific laboratory tests recommended.

Drug Interactions: Few systemic data have been collected on the metabolism of bupropion following concomitant administration with other drugs or, alternatively, the effect of concomitant administration of bupropion on the metabolism of other drugs.
Because bupropion is extensively metabolized, the coadministration of other drugs may affect its clinical activity. In vitro studies indicate that bupropion is primarily metabolized to hydroxybupropion by the CYP2B6 isoenzyme. Therefore, the potential exists for a drug interaction between WELLBUTRIN XL and drugs that are substrates or inhibitors of the CYP2B6 isoenzyme (e.g., orphenadrine, thiotepa, and cyclophosphamide). In addition, in vitro studies suggest that paroxetine, sertraline, norfluoxetine, and fluvoxamine as well as nelfinavir, ritonavir, and efavirenz inhibit the hydroxylation of bupropion. No clinical studies have been performed to evaluate this finding. The threohydrobupropion metabolite of bupropion does not appear to be produced by the cytochrome P450 isoenzymes. The effects of concomitant administration of cimetidine on the pharmacokinetics of bupropion and its active metabolites were studied in 24 healthy young male volunteers. Following oral administration of two 150-mg tablets of the sustained-release formulation of bupropion with and without 800 mg of cimetidine, the pharmacokinetics of bupropion and hydroxybupropion were unaffected. However, there were 16% and 32% increases in the AUC and C_{max}, respectively, of the combined moieties of threohydrobupropion and erythrohydrobupropion.

Continued on next page

Wellbutrin XL—Cont.

While not systematically studied, certain drugs may induce the metabolism of bupropion (e.g., carbamazepine, phenobarbital, phenytoin).

Animal data indicated that bupropion may be an inducer of drug-metabolizing enzymes in humans. In one study, following chronic administration of bupropion, 100 mg 3 times daily to 8 healthy male volunteers for 14 days, there was no evidence of induction of its own metabolism. Nevertheless, there may be the potential for clinically important alterations of blood levels of coadministered drugs.

Drugs Metabolized By Cytochrome P450IID6 (CYP2D6): Many drugs, including most antidepressants (SSRIs, many tricyclics), beta-blockers, antiarrhythmics, and antipsychotics are metabolized by the CYP2D6 isoenzyme. Although bupropion is not metabolized by this isoenzyme, bupropion and hydroxybupropion are inhibitors of CYP2D6 isoenzyme in vitro. In a study of 15 male subjects (ages 19 to 35 years) who were extensive metabolizers of the CYP2D6 isoenzyme, daily doses of bupropion given as 150 mg twice daily followed by a single dose of 50 mg desipramine increased the C_{max}, AUC, and $t_{½}$ of desipramine by an average of approximately 2-, 5-, and 2-fold, respectively. The effect was present for at least 7 days after the last dose of bupropion. Concomitant use of bupropion with other drugs metabolized by CYP2D6 has not been formally studied.

Therefore, co-administration of bupropion with drugs that are metabolized by CYP2D6 isoenzyme including certain antidepressants (e.g., nortriptyline, imipramine, desipramine, paroxetine, fluoxetine, sertraline), antipsychotics (e.g., haloperidol, risperidone, thioridazine), beta-blockers (e.g., metoprolol), and Type 1C antiarrhythmics (e.g., propafenone, flecainide), should be approached with caution and should be initiated at the lower end of the dose range of the concomitant medication. If bupropion is added to the treatment regimen of a patient already receiving a drug metabolized by CYP2D6, the need to decrease the dose of the original medication should be considered, particularly for those concomitant medications with a narrow therapeutic index.

MAO Inhibitors: Studies in animals demonstrate that the acute toxicity of bupropion is enhanced by the MAO inhibitor phenelzine (see CONTRAINDICATIONS).

Levodopa and Amantadine: Limited clinical data suggest a higher incidence of adverse experiences in patients receiving bupropion concurrently with either levodopa or amantadine. Administration of WELLBUTRIN XL Tablets to patients receiving either levodopa or amantadine concurrently should be undertaken with caution, using small initial doses and gradual dose increases.

Drugs That Lower Seizure Threshold: Concurrent administration of WELLBUTRIN XL Tablets and agents (e.g., antipsychotics, other antidepressants, theophylline, systemic steroids, etc.) that lower seizure threshold should be undertaken only with extreme caution (see WARNINGS). Low initial dosing and gradual dose increases should be employed.

Nicotine Transdermal System: (see PRECAUTIONS: Cardiovascular Effects).

Alcohol: In postmarketing experience, there have been rare reports of adverse neuropsychiatric events or reduced alcohol tolerance in patients who were drinking alcohol during treatment with bupropion. The consumption of alcohol during treatment with WELLBUTRIN XL should be minimized or avoided (also see CONTRAINDICATIONS).

Carcinogenesis, Mutagenesis, Impairment of Fertility: Lifetime carcinogenicity studies were performed in rats and mice at doses up to 300 and 150 mg/kg/day, respectively. These doses are approximately 7 and 2 times the maximum recommended human dose (MRHD), respectively, on a mg/m^2 basis. In the rat study there was an increase in nodular proliferative lesions of the liver at doses of 100 to 300 mg/kg/day (approximately 2 to 7 times the MRHD on a mg/m^2 basis); lower doses were not tested. The question of whether or not such lesions may be precursors of neoplasms of the liver is currently unresolved. Similar liver lesions were not seen in the mouse study, and no increase in malignant tumors of the liver and other organs was seen in either study.

Bupropion produced a positive response (2 to 3 times control mutation rate) in 2 of 5 strains in the Ames bacterial mutagenicity test and an increase in chromosomal aberrations in 1 of 3 in vivo rat bone marrow cytogenetic studies.

A fertility study in rats at doses up to 300 mg/kg/day revealed no evidence of impaired fertility.

Pregnancy: ***Teratogenic Effects:*** Pregnancy Category B. Teratology studies have been performed with bupropion immediate-release formulation at dosages up to 450 mg/kg in rats, and at doses up to 150 mg/kg in rabbits (approximately 7 to 11 and 7 times the MRHD, respectively, on a mg/m^2 basis), and have revealed no evidence of harm to the fetus due to bupropion. There are no adequate and well-controlled studies in pregnant women. Because animal reproduction studies are not always predictive of human response, this drug should be used during pregnancy only if clearly needed.

To monitor fetal outcomes of pregnant women exposed to WELLBUTRIN XL, GlaxoSmithKline maintains a Bupropion Pregnancy Registry. Health care providers are encouraged to register patients by calling (800) 336-2176.

Labor and Delivery: The effect of WELLBUTRIN XL Tablets on labor and delivery in humans is unknown.

Table 2. Incidence of Weight Gain and Weight Loss in Placebo-Controlled Trials

Weight Change	WELLBUTRIN SR 300 mg/day (n = 339)	WELLBUTRIN SR 400 mg/day (n = 112)	Placebo (n = 347)
Gained >5 lbs	3%	2%	4%
Lost >5 lbs	14%	19%	6%

Table 3. Treatment Discontinuations Due to Adverse Events in Placebo-Controlled Trials

Adverse Event Term	WELLBUTRIN SR 300 mg/day (n = 376)	WELLBUTRIN SR 400 mg/day (n = 114)	Placebo (n = 385)
Rash	2.4%	0.9%	0.0%
Nausea	0.8%	1.8%	0.3%
Agitation	0.3%	1.8%	0.3%
Migraine	0.0%	1.8%	0.3%

Nursing Mothers: Like many other drugs, bupropion and its metabolites are secreted in human milk. Because of the potential for serious adverse reactions in nursing infants from WELLBUTRIN XL Tablets, a decision should be made whether to discontinue nursing or to discontinue the drug, taking into account the importance of the drug to the mother.

Pediatric Use: The safety and effectiveness of WELLBUTRIN XL Tablets in pediatric patients below 18 years old have not been established. The immediate-release formulation of bupropion was studied in 104 pediatric patients (age range, 6 to 16) in clinical trials of the drug for other indications. Although generally well tolerated, the limited exposure is insufficient to assess the safety of bupropion in pediatric patients.

Geriatric Use: Of the approximately 6,000 patients who participated in clinical trials with bupropion sustained-release tablets (depression and smoking cessation studies), 275 were ≥65 years old and 47 were ≥75 years old. In addition, several hundred patients 65 and over participated in clinical trials using the immediate-release formulation of bupropion (depression studies). No overall differences in safety or effectiveness were observed between these subjects and younger subjects. Reported clinical experience has not identified differences in responses between the elderly and younger patients, but greater sensitivity of some older individuals cannot be ruled out.

A single-dose pharmacokinetic study demonstrated that the disposition of bupropion and its metabolites in elderly subjects was similar to that of younger subjects; however, another pharmacokinetic study, single and multiple dose, has suggested that the elderly are at increased risk for accumulation of bupropion and its metabolites (see CLINICAL PHARMACOLOGY).

Bupropion is extensively metabolized in the liver to active metabolites, which are further metabolized and excreted by the kidneys. The risk of toxic reaction to this drug may be greater in patients with impaired renal function. Because elderly patients are more likely to have decreased renal function, care should be taken in dose selection, and it may be useful to monitor renal function (see PRECAUTIONS: Renal Impairment and DOSAGE AND ADMINISTRATION).

ADVERSE REACTIONS (See also WARNINGS and PRECAUTIONS.)

WELLBUTRIN XL has been demonstrated to have similar bioavailability to the immediate-release formulation of bupropion (see CLINICAL PHARMACOLOGY). The information included under the Incidence in Controlled Trials subsection of ADVERSE REACTIONS is based primarily on data from controlled clinical trials with WELLBUTRIN SR Tablets, the sustained-release formulation of bupropion. WELLBUTRIN XL has not been studied in placebo-controlled trials, although it has been studied in non-placebo-controlled clinical bioavailability studies. Information on additional adverse events associated with the sustained-release formulation of bupropion in smoking cessation trials, as well as the immediate-release formulation of bupropion, is included in a separate section (see Other Events Observed During the Clinical Development and Postmarketing Experience of Bupropion).

Incidence in Controlled Trials With Bupropion: ***Adverse Events Associated With Discontinuation of Treatment Among Patients Treated With Bupropion:*** In placebo-controlled clinical trials, 9% and 11% of patients treated with 300 and 400 mg/day, respectively, of the sustained-release formulation of bupropion and 4% of patients treated with placebo discontinued treatment due to adverse events. The specific adverse events in these trials that led to discontinuation in at least 1% of patients treated with either 300 mg/day or 400 mg/day of WELLBUTRIN SR, the sustained-release formulation of bupropion, and at a rate at least twice the placebo rate are listed in Table 3.

[See table 3 above]

In clinical trials with the immediate-release formulation of bupropion, 10% of patients and volunteers discontinued due to an adverse event. Events resulting in discontinuation, in addition to those listed above for the sustained-release formulation of bupropion, include vomiting, seizures, and sleep disturbances.

Adverse Events Occurring at an Incidence of 1% or More Among Patients Treated With Bupropion: Table 4 enumerates treatment-emergent adverse events that occurred among patients treated with 300 and 400 mg/day of the sustained-release formulation of bupropion and with placebo in controlled trials. Events that occurred in either the 300- or 400-mg/day group at an incidence of 1% or more and were more frequent than in the placebo group are included. Reported adverse events were classified using a COSTART-based Dictionary.

Accurate estimates of the incidence of adverse events associated with the use of any drug are difficult to obtain. Estimates are influenced by drug dose, detection technique, setting, physician judgments, etc. The figures cited cannot be used to predict precisely the incidence of untoward events in the course of usual medical practice where patient characteristics and other factors differ from those that prevailed in the clinical trials. These incidence figures also cannot be compared with those obtained from other clinical studies involving related drug products as each group of drug trials is conducted under a different set of conditions.

Finally, it is important to emphasize that the tabulation does not reflect the relative severity and/or clinical importance of the events. A better perspective on the serious adverse events associated with the use of bupropion is provided in the WARNINGS and PRECAUTIONS sections.

[See table 4 on next page]

Additional events to those listed in Table 4 that occurred at an incidence of at least 1% in controlled clinical trials of the immediate-release formulation of bupropion (300 to 600 mg/day) and that were numerically more frequent than placebo were: cardiac arrhythmias (5% vs 4%), hypertension (4% vs 2%), hypotension (3% vs 2%), tachycardia (11% vs 9%), appetite increase (4% vs 2%), dyspepsia (3% vs 2%), menstrual complaints (5% vs 1%), akathisia (2% vs 1%), impaired sleep quality (4% vs 2%), sensory disturbance (4% vs 3%), confusion (8% vs 5%), decreased libido (3% vs 2%), hostility (6% vs 4%), auditory disturbance (5% vs 3%), and gustatory disturbance (3% vs 1%).

Incidence of Commonly Observed Adverse Events in Controlled Clinical Trials: Adverse events from Table 4 occurring in at least 5% of patients treated with the sustained-release formulation of bupropion and at a rate at least twice the placebo rate are listed below for the 300- and 400-mg/day dose groups.

300 mg/day of the Sustained-Release Formulation: Anorexia, dry mouth, rash, sweating, tinnitus, and tremor.

400 mg/day of the Sustained-Release Formulation: Abdominal pain, agitation, anxiety, dizziness, dry mouth, insomnia, myalgia, nausea, palpitation, pharyngitis, sweating, tinnitus, and urinary frequency.

Other Events Observed During the Clinical Development and Postmarketing Experience of Bupropion: In addition to the adverse events noted above, the following events have been reported in clinical trials and postmarketing experience with the sustained-release formulation of bupropion in depressed patients and in nondepressed smokers, as well as in clinical trials and postmarketing clinical experience with the immediate-release formulation of bupropion.

Adverse events for which frequencies are provided below occurred in clinical trials with the sustained-release formulation of bupropion. The frequencies represent the proportion of patients who experienced a treatment-emergent adverse event on at least one occasion in placebo-controlled studies for depression (n = 987) or smoking cessation (n = 1,013), or patients who experienced an adverse event requiring discontinuation of treatment in an open-label surveillance study with the sustained-release formulation of bupropion (n = 3,100). All treatment-emergent adverse events are included except those listed in Tables 1 through 4, those events listed in other safety-related sections, those adverse events subsumed under COSTART terms that are either overly general or excessively specific so as to be uninformative, those events not reasonably associated with the use of the drug, and those events that were not serious and occurred in fewer than 2 patients. Events of major clinical importance are described in the WARNINGS and PRECAUTIONS sections of the labeling.

Events are further categorized by body system and listed in order of decreasing frequency according to the following definitions of frequency: Frequent adverse events are defined as those occurring in at least 1/100 patients. Infrequent adverse events are those occurring in 1/100 to 1/1,000 patients, while rare events are those occurring in less than 1/1,000 patients.

Adverse events for which frequencies are not provided occurred in clinical trials or postmarketing experience with bupropion. Only those adverse events not previously listed for sustained-release bupropion are included. The extent to which these events may be associated with WELLBUTRIN XL is unknown.

Body (General): Infrequent were chills, facial edema, musculoskeletal chest pain, and photosensitivity. Rare was malaise. Also observed were arthralgia, myalgia, and fever with rash and other symptoms suggestive of delayed hypersensitivity. These symptoms may resemble serum sickness (see PRECAUTIONS).
Cardiovascular: Infrequent were postural hypotension, stroke, tachycardia, and vasodilation. Rare was syncope. Also observed were complete atrioventricular block, extrasystoles, hypotension, hypertension (in some cases severe, see PRECAUTIONS), myocardial infarction, phlebitis, and pulmonary embolism.
Digestive: Infrequent were abnormal liver function, bruxism, gastric reflux, gingivitis, glossitis, increased salivation, jaundice, mouth ulcers, stomatitis, and thirst. Rare was edema of tongue. Also observed were colitis, esophagitis, gastrointestinal hemorrhage, gum hemorrhage, hepatitis, intestinal perforation, liver damage, pancreatitis, and stomach ulcer.
Endocrine: Also observed were hyperglycemia, hypoglycemia, and syndrome of inappropriate antidiuretic hormone.
Hemic and Lymphatic: Infrequent was ecchymosis. Also observed were anemia, leukocytosis, leukopenia, lymphadenopathy, pancytopenia, and thrombocytopenia. Altered PT and/or INR, infrequently associated with hemorrhagic or thrombotic complications, were observed when bupropion was coadministered with warfarin.
Metabolic and Nutritional: Infrequent were edema and peripheral edema. Also observed was glycosuria.
Musculoskeletal: Infrequent were leg cramps. Also observed were muscle rigidity/fever/rhabdomyolysis and muscle weakness.
Nervous System: Infrequent were abnormal coordination, decreased libido, depersonalization, dysphoria, emotional lability, hostility, hyperkinesia, hypertonia, hypesthesia, suicidal ideation, and vertigo. Rare were amnesia, ataxia, derealization, and hypomania. Also observed were abnormal electroencephalogram (EEG), akinesia, aphasia, coma, delirium, dysarthria, dyskinesia, dystonia, euphoria, extrapyramidal syndrome, hallucinations, hypokinesia, increased libido, manic reaction, neuralgia, neuropathy, paranoid reaction, and unmasking tardive dyskinesia.
Respiratory: Rare was bronchospasm. Also observed was pneumonia.
Skin: Rare was maculopapular rash. Also observed were alopecia, angioedema, exfoliative dermatitis, and hirsutism.
Special Senses: Infrequent were accommodation abnormality and dry eye. Also observed were deafness, diplopia, and mydriasis.
Urogenital: Infrequent were impotence, polyuria, and prostate disorder. Also observed were abnormal ejaculation, cystitis, dyspareunia, dysuria, gynecomastia, menopause, painful erection, salpingitis, urinary incontinence, urinary retention, and vaginitis.

Table 4. Treatment-Emergent Adverse Events in Placebo-Controlled Trials*

Body System/ Adverse Event	WELLBUTRIN SR 300 mg/day (n = 376)	WELLBUTRIN SR 400 mg/day (n = 114)	Placebo (n = 385)
Body (General)			
Headache	26%	25%	23%
Infection	8%	9%	6%
Abdominal pain	3%	9%	2%
Asthenia	2%	4%	2%
Chest pain	3%	4%	1%
Pain	2%	3%	2%
Fever	1%	2%	—
Cardiovascular			
Palpitation	2%	6%	2%
Flushing	1%	4%	—
Migraine	1%	4%	1%
Hot flashes	1%	3%	1%
Digestive			
Dry mouth	17%	24%	7%
Nausea	13%	18%	8%
Constipation	10%	5%	7%
Diarrhea	5%	7%	6%
Anorexia	5%	3%	2%
Vomiting	4%	2%	2%
Dysphagia	0%	2%	0%
Musculoskeletal			
Myalgia	2%	6%	3%
Arthralgia	1%	4%	1%
Arthritis	0%	2%	0%
Twitch	1%	2%	—
Nervous system			
Insomnia	11%	16%	6%
Dizziness	7%	11%	5%
Agitation	3%	9%	2%
Anxiety	5%	6%	3%
Tremor	6%	3%	1%
Nervousness	5%	3%	3%
Somnolence	2%	3%	2%
Irritability	3%	2%	2%
Memory decreased	—	3%	1%
Paresthesia	1%	2%	1%
Central nervous system stimulation	2%	1%	1%
Respiratory			
Pharyngitis	3%	11%	2%
Sinusitis	3%	1%	2%
Increased cough	1%	2%	1%
Skin			
Sweating	6%	5%	2%
Rash	5%	4%	1%
Pruritus	2%	4%	2%
Urticaria	2%	1%	0%
Special senses			
Tinnitus	6%	6%	2%
Taste perversion	2%	4%	—
Amblyopia	3%	2%	2%
Urogenital			
Urinary frequency	2%	5%	2%
Urinary urgency	—	2%	0%
Vaginal hemorrhage†	0%	2%	—
Urinary tract infection	1%	0%	—

*Adverse events that occurred in at least 1% of patients treated with either 300 or 400 mg/day of the sustained-release formulation of bupropion, but equally or more frequently in the placebo group, were: abnormal dreams, accidental injury, acne, appetite increased, back pain, bronchitis, dysmenorrhea, dyspepsia, flatulence, flu syndrome, hypertension, neck pain, respiratory disorder, rhinitis, and tooth disorder.
† Incidence based on the number of female patients.
— Hyphen denotes adverse events occurring in greater than 0 but less than 0.5% of patients.

DRUG ABUSE AND DEPENDENCE

Controlled Substance Class: Bupropion is not a controlled substance.
Humans: Controlled clinical studies of bupropion (immediate-release formulation) conducted in normal volunteers, in subjects with a history of multiple drug abuse, and in depressed patients showed some increase in motor activity and agitation/excitement.
In a population of individuals experienced with drugs of abuse, a single dose of 400 mg of bupropion produced mild amphetamine-like activity as compared to placebo on the Morphine-Benzedrine Subscale of the Addiction Research Center Inventories (ARCI), and a score intermediate between placebo and amphetamine on the Liking Scale of the ARCI. These scales measure general feelings of euphoria and drug desirability.
Findings in clinical trials, however, are not known to reliably predict the abuse potential of drugs. Nonetheless, evidence from single-dose studies does suggest that the recommended daily dosage of bupropion when administered in divided doses is not likely to be especially reinforcing to amphetamine or stimulant abusers. However, higher doses that could not be tested because of the risk of seizure might be modestly attractive to those who abuse stimulant drugs.
Animals: Studies in rodents and primates have shown that bupropion exhibits some pharmacologic actions common to psychostimulants. In rodents, it has been shown to increase locomotor activity, elicit a mild stereotyped behavioral response, and increase rates of responding in several schedule-controlled behavior paradigms. In primate models to assess the positive reinforcing effects of psychoactive drugs, bupropion was self-administered intravenously. In rats, bupropion produced amphetamine-like and cocaine-like discriminative stimulus effects in drug discrimination paradigms used to characterize the subjective effects of psychoactive drugs.

OVERDOSAGE

Human Overdose Experience: There has been very limited experience with overdosage of the sustained-release formulation of bupropion (WELLBUTRIN SR Tablets); 3 cases were reported during clinical trials. One patient ingested 3,000 mg of the sustained-release formulation of bupropion and vomited quickly after the overdose; the patient experienced blurred vision and lightheadedness. A second patient ingested a "handful" of WELLBUTRIN SR Tablets (the sustained-release formulation) and experienced confusion, lethargy, nausea, jitteriness, and seizure. A third patient ingested 3,600 mg of the sustained-release formulation of bupropion and a bottle of wine; the patient experienced nausea, visual hallucinations, and "grogginess." None of the patients experienced further sequelae.
There has been extensive experience with overdosage of the immediate-release formulation of bupropion. Thirteen overdoses occurred during clinical trials. Twelve patients ingested 850 to 4,200 mg and recovered without significant sequelae. Another patient who ingested 9,000 mg of the immediate-release formulation of bupropion and 300 mg of tranylcypromine experienced a grand mal seizure and recovered without further sequelae.
Since introduction, overdoses of up to 17,500 mg of the immediate-release formulation of bupropion have been reported. Seizure was reported in approximately one third of all cases. Other serious reactions reported with overdoses of the immediate-release formulation of bupropion alone included hallucinations, loss of consciousness, and sinus tachycardia. Fever, muscle rigidity, rhabdomyolysis, hypotension, stupor, coma, and respiratory failure have been reported when the immediate-release formulation of bupropion was part of multiple drug overdoses.
Although most patients recovered without sequelae, deaths associated with overdoses of the immediate-release formulation of bupropion alone have been reported rarely in patients ingesting massive doses of the drug. Multiple uncontrolled seizures, bradycardia, cardiac failure, and cardiac arrest prior to death were reported in these patients.
Overdosage Management: Ensure an adequate airway, oxygenation, and ventilation. Monitor cardiac rhythm and vital signs. EEG monitoring is also recommended for the first 48 hours post-ingestion. General supportive and symptomatic measures are also recommended. Induction of emesis is not recommended. Gastric lavage with a large-bore orogastric tube with appropriate airway protection, if needed, may be indicated if performed soon after ingestion or in symptomatic patients.
Activated charcoal should be administered. There is no experience with the use of forced diuresis, dialysis, hemoperfusion, or exchange transfusion in the management of bupropion overdoses. No specific antidotes for bupropion are known.
Due to the dose-related risk of seizures with WELLBUTRIN XL, hospitalization following suspected overdose should be considered. Based on studies in animals, it is recommended that seizures be treated with intravenous benzodiazepine administration and other supportive measures, as appropriate.
In managing overdosage, consider the possibility of multiple drug involvement. The physician should consider contacting a poison control center for additional information on the treatment of any overdose. Telephone numbers for certified poison control centers are listed in the *Physicians' Desk Reference* (PDR).

Continued on next page

Wellbutrin XL—Cont.

DOSAGE AND ADMINISTRATION

General Dosing Considerations: It is particularly important to administer WELLBUTRIN XL Tablets in a manner most likely to minimize the risk of seizure (see WARNINGS). Gradual escalation in dosage is also important if agitation, motor restlessness, and insomnia, often seen during the initial days of treatment, are to be minimized. If necessary, these effects may be managed by temporary reduction of dose or the short-term administration of an intermediate to long-acting sedative hypnotic. A sedative hypnotic usually is not required beyond the first week of treatment. Insomnia may also be minimized by avoiding bedtime doses. If distressing, untoward effects supervene, dose escalation should be stopped. WELLBUTRIN XL should be swallowed whole and not crushed, divided, or chewed. WELLBUTRIN XL may be taken without regard to meals.

Initial Treatment: The usual adult target dose for WELLBUTRIN XL Tablets is 300 mg/day, given once daily in the morning. Dosing with WELLBUTRIN XL Tablets should begin at 150 mg/day given as a single daily dose in the morning. If the 150-mg initial dose is adequately tolerated, an increase to the 300-mg/day target dose, given as once daily, may be made as early as day 4 of dosing. There should be an interval of at least 24 hours between successive doses.

Increasing the Dosage Above 300 mg/day: As with other antidepressants, the full antidepressant effect of WELLBUTRIN XL Tablets may not be evident until 4 weeks of treatment or longer. An increase in dosage to the maximum of 450 mg/day, given as a single dose, may be considered for patients in whom no clinical improvement is noted after several weeks of treatment at 300 mg/day.

Switching Patients from WELLBUTRIN Tablets or from WELLBUTRIN SR Sustained-Release Tablets: When switching patients from WELLBUTRIN Tablets to WELLBUTRIN XL or from WELLBUTRIN SR Sustained-Release Tablets to WELLBUTRIN XL, give the same total daily dose when possible. Patients who are currently being treated with WELLBUTRIN Tablets at 300 mg/day (for example, 100 mg 3 times a day) may be switched to WELLBUTRIN XL 300 mg once daily. Patients who are currently being treated with WELLBUTRIN SR Sustained-Release Tablets at 300 mg/day (for example, 150 mg twice daily) may be switched to WELLBUTRIN XL 300 mg once daily.

Maintenance Treatment: It is generally agreed that acute episodes of depression require several months or longer of sustained pharmacological therapy beyond response to the acute episode. It is unknown whether or not the dose of WELLBUTRIN XL needed for maintenance treatment is identical to the dose needed to achieve an initial response. Patients should be periodically reassessed to determine the need for maintenance treatment and the appropriate dose for such treatment.

Dosage Adjustment for Patients With Impaired Hepatic Function: WELLBUTRIN XL should be used with extreme caution in patients with severe hepatic cirrhosis. The dose should not exceed 150 mg every other day in these patients. WELLBUTRIN XL should be used with caution in patients with hepatic impairment (including mild to moderate hepatic cirrhosis) and a reduced frequency and/or dose should be considered in patients with mild to moderate hepatic cirrhosis (see CLINICAL PHARMACOLOGY, WARNINGS, and PRECAUTIONS).

Dosage Adjustment for Patients With Impaired Renal Function: WELLBUTRIN XL should be used with caution in patients with renal impairment and a reduced frequency and/or dose should be considered (see CLINICAL PHARMACOLOGY and PRECAUTIONS).

HOW SUPPLIED

WELLBUTRIN XL Extended-Release Tablets, 150 mg of bupropion hydrochloride, are creamy-white to pale yellow, round, tablets printed with "WELLBUTRIN XL 150" in bottles of 30 tablets (NDC 0173-0730-01).

WELLBUTRIN XL Extended-Release Tablets, 300 mg of bupropion hydrochloride, are creamy-white to pale yellow, round, tablets printed with "WELLBUTRIN XL 300" in bottles of 30 tablets (NDC 0173-0731-01).

Store at 25°C (77°F); excursions permitted to 15-30°C (59-86°F) [see USP Controlled Room Temperature].

Manufactured by: Biovail Corporation
Mississauga, ON L5N 8M5, Canada
for GlaxoSmithKline, Research Triangle Park, NC 27709

September 2003/RL-2017

Janssen Pharmaceutica Products, L.P.

1125 TRENTON-HARBOURTON ROAD
P.O. BOX 200
TITUSVILLE, NJ 08560-0200

For Medical Information Monday through Friday 9 am-5 pm EST Contact:
(800) JANSSEN
FAX: (609) 730-3138
After Hours and Weekends:
(800) JANSSEN

RISPERDAL® CONSTA™ ℞

[*rĭs-pər-dăl cŏn-stă*]
(RISPERIDONE)
LONG-ACTING INJECTION

Rx Only

DESCRIPTION

RISPERDAL® (risperidone) is a psychotropic agent belonging to the chemical class of benzisoxazole derivatives. The chemical designation is 3-[2-[4-(6-fluoro-1,2-benzisoxazol-3-yl)-1-piperidinyl]ethyl]-6,7,8,9-tetrahydro-2-methyl-4H-pyrido[1,2-a]pyrimidin-4-one. Its molecular formula is $C_{23}H_{27}FN_4O_2$ and its molecular weight is 410.49. The structural formula is:

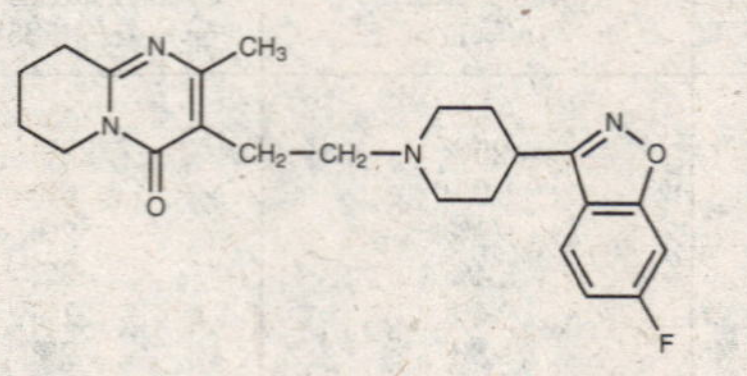

Risperidone is practically insoluble in water, freely soluble in methylene chloride, and soluble in methanol and 0.1 N HCl.

RISPERDAL® CONSTA™ (risperidone) Long-Acting Injection is a combination of extended release microspheres for injection and diluent for parenteral use.

The extended release microspheres formulation is a white to off-white, free-flowing powder that is available in dosage strengths of 25, 37.5, or 50 mg risperidone per vial. Risperidone is micro-encapsulated in 7525 polylactide-co-glycolide (PLG) at a concentration of 381 mg risperidone per gram of microspheres.

The diluent for parenteral use is a clear, colorless solution. Composition of the diluent includes polysorbate 20, sodium carboxymethyl cellulose, disodium hydrogen phosphate dihydrate, citric acid anhydrous, sodium chloride, sodium hydroxide, and water for injection. The microspheres are suspended in the diluent prior to injection.

RISPERDAL® CONSTA™ is provided as a dose pack, consisting of a vial containing the microspheres, a pre-filled syringe containing the diluent, a SmartSite® Needle-Free Vial Access Device, and one Needle-Pro® 20 G TW safety needle.

CLINICAL PHARMACOLOGY

Pharmacodynamics

The mechanism of action of RISPERDAL® (risperidone), as with other drugs used to treat schizophrenia, is unknown. However, it has been proposed that the drug's therapeutic activity in schizophrenia is mediated through a combination of dopamine Type 2 (D_2) and serotonin Type 2 ($5HT_2$) receptor antagonism. Antagonism at receptors other than D_2 and $5HT_2$ may explain some of the other effects of RISPERDAL®.

RISPERDAL® is a selective monoaminergic antagonist with high affinity (Ki of 0.12 to 7.3 nM) for the serotonin Type 2 ($5HT_2$), dopamine Type 2 (D_2), α_1 and α_2 adrenergic, and H_1 histaminergic receptors. RISPERDAL® acts as an antagonist at other receptors, but with lower potency. RISPERDAL® has low to moderate affinity (Ki of 47 to 253 nM) for the serotonin $5HT_{1C}$, $5HT_{1D}$, and $5HT_{1A}$ receptors, weak affinity (Ki of 620 to 800 nM) for the dopamine D_1 and haloperidol-sensitive sigma site, and no affinity (when tested at concentrations $>10^{-5}$ M) for cholinergic muscarinic or β_1 and β_2 adrenergic receptors.

Pharmacokinetics

Absorption

After a single intramuscular (gluteal) injection of RISPERDAL® CONSTA™ (risperidone), there is a small initial release of the drug (<about 1% of the dose), followed by a lag time of 3 weeks. The main release of the drug starts from 3 weeks onward, is maintained from 4 to 6 weeks, and subsides by 7 weeks following the intramuscular (IM) injection. Therefore, oral antipsychotic supplementation should be given during the first 3 weeks of treatment with RISPERDAL® CONSTA™ to maintain therapeutic levels until the main release of risperidone from the injection site has begun (see DOSAGE AND ADMINISTRATION).

The combination of the release profile and the dosage regimen (IM injections every 2 weeks) of RISPERDAL® CONSTA™ results in sustained therapeutic concentrations. Steady-state plasma concentrations are reached after 4 injections and are maintained for 4 to 6 weeks after the last injection. Plasma concentrations of risperidone, 9-hydroxyrisperidone (the major metabolite), and risperidone plus 9-hydroxyrisperidone are linear over the dosing range of 25 mg to 50 mg.

Distribution

Once absorbed, risperidone is rapidly distributed. The volume of distribution is 1-2 L/kg. In plasma, risperidone is bound to albumin and α_1-acid glycoprotein. The plasma protein binding of risperidone is approximately 90%, and that of its major metabolite, 9-hydroxyrisperidone, is 77%. Neither risperidone nor 9-hydroxyrisperidone displaces each other from plasma binding sites. High therapeutic concentrations of sulfamethazine (100 mcg/mL), warfarin (10 mcg/mL), and carbamazepine (10 mcg/mL) caused only a slight increase in the free fraction of risperidone at 10 ng/mL and of 9-hydroxyrisperidone at 50 ng/mL, changes of unknown clinical significance.

Metabolism

Risperidone is extensively metabolized in the liver. The main metabolic pathway is through hydroxylation of risperidone to 9-hydroxyrisperidone by the enzyme, CYP 2D6. A minor metabolic pathway is through N-dealkylation. The main metabolite, 9-hydroxyrisperidone, has similar pharmacological activity as risperidone. Consequently, the clinical effect of the drug (i.e., the active moiety) results from the combined concentrations of risperidone plus 9-hydroxyrisperidone.

CYP 2D6, also called debrisoquin hydroxylase, is the enzyme responsible for metabolism of many neuroleptics, antidepressants, antiarrhythmics, and other drugs. CYP 2D6 is subject to genetic polymorphism (about 6%-8% of Caucasians, and a very low percentage of Asians, have little or no activity and are "poor metabolizers") and to inhibition by a variety of substrates and some non-substrates, notably quinidine. Extensive CYP 2D6 metabolizers convert risperidone rapidly into 9-hydroxyrisperidone, whereas poor CYP 2D6 metabolizers convert it much more slowly. Although extensive metabolizers have lower risperidone and higher 9-hydroxyrisperidone concentrations than poor metabolizers, the pharmacokinetics of the active moiety, after single and multiple doses, are similar in extensive and poor metabolizers.

The interactions of RISPERDAL® CONSTA™ and other drugs have not been systematically evaluated in human subjects. Risperidone could be subject to two kinds of drug-drug interactions (see PRECAUTIONS – Drug Interactions). First, inhibitors of CYP 2D6 interfere with conversion of risperidone to 9-hydroxyrisperidone. This occurs with quinidine, giving essentially all recipients a risperidone pharmacokinetic profile typical of poor metabolizers. The therapeutic benefits and adverse effects of risperidone in patients receiving quinidine have not been evaluated, but observations in a modest number (n≅70) of poor metabolizers given risperidone do not suggest important differences between poor and extensive metabolizers. Second, co-administration of carbamazepine and other known enzyme inducers (e.g., phenytoin, rifampin, and phenobarbital) with risperidone cause a decrease in the combined plasma concentrations of risperidone and 9-hydroxyrisperidone (see PRECAUTIONS – Drug Interactions). It would also be possible for risperidone to interfere with metabolism of other drugs metabolized by CYP 2D6. Relatively weak binding of risperidone to the enzyme suggests this is unlikely.

In a drug interaction study in schizophrenic patients, 11 subjects received oral risperidone titrated to 6 mg/day for 3 weeks, followed by concurrent administration of carbamazepine for an additional 3 weeks. During co-administration, the plasma concentrations of risperidone and its pharmacologically active metabolite, 9-hydroxyrisperidone, were decreased by about 50%. Plasma concentrations of carbamazepine did not appear to be affected. Co-administration of other known 4 enzyme inducers (e.g., phenytoin, rifampin, and phenobarbital) with risperidone may cause similar decreases in the combined plasma concentrations of risperidone and 9-hydroxyrisperidone, which could lead to decreased efficacy of risperidone treatment (see PRECAUTIONS – Drug Interactions and DOSAGE AND ADMINISTRATION – Co-Administration of RISPERDAL® CONSTA™ with Certain Other Medications).

Fluoxetine (20 mg QD) and paroxetine (20 mg QD) have been shown to increase the plasma concentration of risperidone 2.5–2.8 fold and 3–9 fold respectively. Fluoxetine did not affect the plasma concentration of 9-hydroxyrisperidone. Paroxetine lowered the concentration of 9-hydroxyrisperidone an average of 13% (see PRECAUTIONS – Drug Interactions and DOSAGE AND ADMINISTRATION – Co-Administration of RISPERDAL® CONSTA™ with Certain Other Medications).

Repeated oral doses of risperidone (3 mg BID) did not affect the exposure (AUC) or peak plasma concentrations (C_{max}) of lithium (n=13) (see PRECAUTIONS – Drug Interactions).

Repeated oral doses of risperidone (4 mg QD) did not affect the pre-dose or average plasma concentrations and exposure (AUC) of valproate (1000 mg/day in three divided doses) compared to placebo (n=21). However, there was a 20% increase in valproate peak plasma concentration (C_{max}) after concomitant administration of risperidone (see PRECAUTIONS – Drug Interactions).

There were no significant interactions between oral risperidone (1 mg QD) and erythromycin (500 mg QID) (see PRECAUTIONS – Drug Interactions).

Excretion

Risperidone and its metabolites are eliminated via the urine and, to a much lesser extent, via the feces. As illustrated by a mass balance study of a single 1 mg oral dose of ^{14}C-risperidone administered as solution to three healthy male volunteers, total recovery of radioactivity at 1 week was 84%, including 70% in the urine and 14% in the feces.

The apparent half-life of risperidone plus 9-hydroxyrisperidone following RISPERDAL® CONSTA™ administration is 3 to 6 days, and is associated with a monoexponential decline in plasma concentrations. This half-life of 3-6 days is related to the erosion of the microspheres and subsequent absorption of risperidone. The clearance of risperidone and risperidone plus 9-hydroxyrisperidone was 13.7 L/h and 5.0 L/h in extensive CYP 2D6 metabolizers, and 3.3 L/h and 3.2 L/h in poor CYP 2D6 metabolizers, respectively. No accumulation of risperidone was observed during long-term use (up to 12 months) in patients treated every 2 weeks with 25 mg or 50 mg RISPERDAL® CONSTA™. The elimination phase is complete approximately 7 to 8 weeks after the last injection.

Special Populations

Renal Impairment

In patients with moderate to severe renal disease treated with oral RISPERDAL®, clearance of the sum of risperidone and its active metabolite decreased by 60% compared with young healthy subjects. Although patients with renal impairment were not studied with RISPERDAL® CONSTA™, it is recommended that patients with renal impairment be carefully titrated on oral RISPERDAL® before treatment with RISPERDAL® CONSTA™ is initiated (see PRECAUTIONS and DOSAGE AND ADMINISTRATION).

Hepatic Impairment

While the pharmacokinetics of oral RISPERDAL® in subjects with liver disease were comparable to those in young healthy subjects, the mean free fraction of risperidone in plasma was increased by about 35% because of the diminished concentration of both albumin and α_1-acid glycoprotein. Although patients with hepatic impairment were not studied with RISPERDAL® CONSTA™, it is recommended that patients with hepatic impairment be carefully titrated on oral RISPERDAL® before treatment with RISPERDAL® CONSTA™ is initiated (see PRECAUTIONS and DOSAGE AND ADMINISTRATION).

Elderly

In an open-label trial, steady-state concentrations of risperidone plus 9-hydroxyrisperidone in otherwise healthy elderly patients (≥65 years old) treated with RISPERDAL® CONSTA™ for up to 12 months fell within the range of values observed in otherwise healthy nonelderly patients. Dosing recommendations are the same for otherwise healthy elderly patients and nonelderly patients (see DOSAGE AND ADMINISTRATION).

Race and Gender Effects

No specific pharmacokinetic study was conducted to investigate race and gender effects, but a population pharmacokinetic analysis did not identify important differences in the disposition of risperidone due to gender (whether or not corrected for body weight) or race.

Clinical Trials

The effectiveness of RISPERDAL® CONSTA™ (risperidone) in the treatment of schizophrenia was established, in part, on the basis of extrapolation from the established effectiveness of the oral formulation of risperidone. In addition, the effectiveness of RISPERDAL® CONSTA™ in the treatment of schizophrenia was established in a 12-week, placebo-controlled trial in adult psychotic inpatients and outpatients who met the DSM-IV criteria for schizophrenia.

Efficacy data were obtained from 400 patients with schizophrenia who were randomized to receive injections of 25, 50, or 75 mg RISPERDAL® CONSTA™ or placebo every 2 weeks. During a 1-week run-in period, patients were discontinued from other antipsychotics and were titrated to a dose of 4 mg oral RISPERDAL®. Patients who received RISPERDAL® CONSTA™ were given doses of oral RISPERDAL® (2 mg for patients in the 25-mg group, 4 mg for patients in the 50-mg group, and 6 mg for patients in the 75-mg group) for the 3 weeks after the first injection to provide therapeutic plasma concentrations until the main release phase of risperidone from the injection site had begun. Patients who received placebo injections were given placebo tablets.

Efficacy was evaluated using the Positive and Negative Syndrome Scale (PANSS), a validated, multi-item inventory, composed of five subscales to evaluate positive symptoms, negative symptoms, disorganized thoughts, uncontrolled hostility/excitement, and anxiety/depression.

The primary efficacy variable in this trial was change from baseline to endpoint in the total PANSS score. The mean total PANSS score at baseline for schizophrenic patients in this study was 81.5.

Total PANSS scores showed significant improvement in the change from baseline to endpoint in schizophrenic patients treated with each dose of RISPERDAL® CONSTA™ (25 mg, 50 mg, or 75 mg) compared with patients treated with placebo. While there were no statistically significant differences between the treatment effects for the three dose groups, the effect size for the 75 mg dose group was actually numerically less than that observed for the 50 mg dose group.

Subgroup analyses did not indicate any differences in treatment outcome as a function of age, race, or gender.

INDICATIONS AND USAGE

RISPERDAL® CONSTA™ (risperidone) is indicated for the treatment of schizophrenia.

The efficacy of RISPERDAL® CONSTA™ is based in part on a 12-week, placebo-controlled trial in schizophrenic inpatients or outpatients, along with extrapolation from the established efficacy of oral RISPERDAL® in this population.

The effectiveness of RISPERDAL® CONSTA™ in longer-term use, that is, more than 12 weeks, has not been systematically evaluated in controlled trials. However, oral risperidone has been shown to be effective in delaying time to relapse in longer-term use. Patients should be periodically reassessed to determine the need for continued treatment (see DOSAGE AND ADMINISTRATION).

CONTRAINDICATIONS

RISPERDAL® CONSTA™ (risperidone) is contraindicated in patients with a known hypersensitivity to the product or any of its components.

WARNINGS

Neuroleptic Malignant Syndrome (NMS)

A potentially fatal symptom complex sometimes referred to as Neuroleptic Malignant Syndrome (NMS) has been reported in association with antipsychotic drugs. Clinical manifestations of NMS are hyperpyrexia, muscle rigidity, altered mental status, and evidence of autonomic instability (irregular pulse or blood pressure, tachycardia, diaphoresis, and cardiac dysrhythmia). Additional signs may include elevated creatine phosphokinase, myoglobinuria (rhabdomyolysis), and acute renal failure.

The diagnostic evaluation of patients with this syndrome is complicated. In arriving at a diagnosis, it is important to identify cases in which the clinical presentation includes both serious medical illness (e.g., pneumonia, systemic infection, etc.) and untreated or inadequately treated extrapyramidal signs and symptoms (EPS). Other important considerations in the differential diagnosis include central anticholinergic toxicity, heat stroke, drug fever, and primary central nervous system pathology.

The management of NMS should include: (1) immediate discontinuation of antipsychotic drugs and other drugs not essential to concurrent therapy; (2) intensive symptomatic treatment and medical monitoring; and (3) treatment of any concomitant serious medical problems for which specific treatments are available. There is no general agreement about specific pharmacological treatment regimens for uncomplicated NMS.

If a patient requires antipsychotic drug treatment after recovery from NMS, the potential reintroduction of drug therapy should be carefully considered. The patient should be carefully monitored, since recurrences of NMS have been reported.

Tardive Dyskinesia

A syndrome of potentially irreversible, involuntary, dyskinetic movements may develop in patients treated with antipsychotic drugs. Although the prevalence of the syndrome appears to be highest among the elderly, especially elderly women, it is impossible to rely upon prevalence estimates to predict, at the inception of antipsychotic treatment, which patients are likely to develop the syndrome. Whether antipsychotic drug products differ in their potential to cause tardive dyskinesia is unknown.

The risk of developing tardive dyskinesia and the likelihood that it will become irreversible are believed to increase as the duration of treatment and the total cumulative dose of antipsychotic drugs administered to the patient increase. However, the syndrome can develop, although much less commonly, after relatively brief treatment periods at low doses.

There is no known treatment for established cases of tardive dyskinesia, although the syndrome may remit, partially or completely, if antipsychotic treatment is withdrawn. Antipsychotic treatment, itself, however, may suppress (or partially suppress) the signs and symptoms of the syndrome and thereby may possibly mask the underlying process. The effect that symptomatic suppression has upon the long-term course of the syndrome is unknown.

Given these considerations, RISPERDAL® CONSTA™ should be prescribed in a manner that is most likely to minimize the occurrence of tardive dyskinesia. Chronic antipsychotic treatment should generally be reserved for patients who suffer from a chronic illness that (1) is known to respond to antipsychotic drugs, and (2) for whom alternative, equally effective, but potentially less harmful treatments are not available or appropriate. In patients who do require chronic treatment, the smallest dose and the shortest duration of treatment producing a satisfactory clinical response should be sought. The need for continued treatment should be reassessed periodically.

If signs and symptoms of tardive dyskinesia appear in a patient treated with RISPERDAL® CONSTA™, drug discontinuation should be considered. However, some patients may require treatment with RISPERDAL® CONSTA™ despite the presence of the syndrome.

Cerebrovascular Adverse Events, Including Stroke, in Elderly Patients with Dementia

Cerebrovascular adverse events (e.g., stroke, transient ischemic attack), including fatalities, were reported in patients (mean age 85 years; range 73-97) in trials of oral risperidone in elderly patients with dementia-related psychosis. In placebo-controlled trials, there was a significantly higher incidence of cerebrovascular adverse events in patients treated with oral risperidone compared to patients treated with placebo. RISPERDAL® CONSTA™ is not approved for the treatment of patients with dementia-related psychosis.

Hyperglycemia and Diabetes Mellitus

Hyperglycemia, in some cases extreme and associated with ketoacidosis or hyperosmolar coma or death, has been reported in patients treated with atypical antipsychotics including RISPERDAL®. Assessment of the relationship between atypical antipsychotic use and glucose abnormalities is complicated by the possibility of an increased background risk of diabetes mellitus in patients with schizophrenia and the increasing incidence of diabetes mellitus in the general population. Given these confounders, the relationship between atypical antipsychotic use and hyperglycemia-related adverse events is not completely understood. However, epidemiological studies suggest an increased risk of treatment-emergent hyperglycemia-related adverse events in patients treated with the atypical antipsychotics. Precise risk estimates for hyperglycemia-related adverse events in patients treated with atypical antipsychotics are not available.

Patients with an established diagnosis of diabetes mellitus who are started on atypical antipsychotics should be monitored regularly for worsening of glucose control. Patients with risk factors for diabetes mellitus (e.g., obesity, family history of diabetes) who are starting treatment with atypical antipsychotics should undergo fasting blood glucose testing at the beginning of treatment and periodically during treatment. Any patient treated with atypical antipsychotics should be monitored for symptoms of hyperglycemia including polydipsia, polyuria, polyphagia, and weakness. Patients who develop symptoms of hyperglycemia during treatment with atypical antipsychotics should undergo fasting blood glucose testing. In some cases, hyperglycemia has resolved when the atypical antipsychotic was discontinued; however, some patients required continuation of anti-diabetic treatment despite discontinuation of the suspect drug.

PRECAUTIONS

General

Orthostatic Hypotension

RISPERDAL® CONSTA™ (risperidone) may induce orthostatic hypotension associated with dizziness, tachycardia, and in some patients, syncope, probably reflecting its alpha-adrenergic antagonistic properties. Syncope was reported in 0.8% (12/1499 patients) of patients treated with RISPERDAL® CONSTA™ in multiple-dose studies. Patients should be instructed in nonpharmacologic interventions that help to reduce the occurrence of orthostatic hypotension (e.g., sitting on the edge of the bed for several minutes before attempting to stand in the morning and slowly rising from a seated position).

RISPERDAL® CONSTA™ should be used with particular caution in (1) patients with known cardiovascular disease (history of myocardial infarction or ischemia, heart failure, or conduction abnormalities), cerebrovascular disease, and conditions which would predispose patients to hypotension, e.g., dehydration and hypovolemia, and (2) in the elderly and patients with renal or hepatic impairment. Monitoring of orthostatic vital signs should be considered in all such patients, and a dose reduction should be considered if hypotension occurs. Clinically significant hypotension has been observed with concomitant use of oral RISPERDAL® and antihypertensive medication.

Seizures

During premarketing testing, seizures occurred in 0.3% (5/1499 patients) of patients treated with RISPERDAL® CONSTA™. Therefore, RISPERDAL® CONSTA™ should be used cautiously in patients with a history of seizures.

Dysphagia

Esophageal dysmotility and aspiration have been associated with antipsychotic drug use. Aspiration pneumonia is a common cause of morbidity and mortality in patients with advanced Alzheimer's dementia. RISPERDAL® CONSTA™ and other antipsychotic drugs should be used cautiously in patients at risk for aspiration pneumonia.

Osteodystrophy and Tumors in Animals

RISPERDAL® CONSTA™ produced osteodystrophy in male and female rats in a 1-year toxicity study and a 2-year carcinogenicity study at a dose of 40 mg/kg administered IM every 2 weeks.

RISPERDAL® CONSTA™ produced renal tubular tumors (adenoma, adenocarcinoma) and adrenomedullary pheochromocytomas in male rats in the 2-year carcinogenicity study at 40 mg/kg administered IM every 2 weeks. In addition, RISPERDAL® CONSTA™ produced an increase in a marker of cellular proliferation in renal tissue in males in the 1-year toxicity study and in renal tumor-bearing males in the 2-year carcinogenicity study at 40 mg/kg administered IM every 2 weeks. (Cellular proliferation was not measured at the low dose or in females in either study.)

The effect dose for osteodystrophy and the tumor findings is 8 times the IM maximum recommended human dose (MRHD) (50 mg) on a mg/m^2 basis and is associated with a plasma exposure (AUC) 2 times the expected plasma exposure (AUC) at the IM MRHD. The no-effect dose for these findings was 5 mg/kg (equal to the IM MRHD on a mg/m^2 basis). Plasma exposure (AUC) at the no-effect dose was one third the expected plasma exposure (AUC) at the IM MRHD.

Neither the renal or adrenal tumors, nor osteodystrophy, were seen in studies of orally administered risperidone. Osteodystrophy was not observed in dogs at doses up to 14 times (based on AUC) the IM MRHD in a 1-year toxicity study.

The renal tubular and adrenomedullary tumors in male rats and other tumor findings are described in more detail under PRECAUTIONS, Carcinogenicity, Mutagenesis, Impairment of Fertility.

The relevance of these findings to human risk is unknown.

Continued on next page

Risperdal Consta—Cont.

Hyperprolactinemia

As with other drugs that antagonize dopamine D_2 receptors, risperidone elevates prolactin levels and the elevation persists during chronic administration. Tissue culture experiments indicate that approximately one-third of human breast cancers are prolactin-dependent *in vitro*, a factor of potential importance if the prescription of these drugs is contemplated in a patient with previously detected breast cancer. Although disturbances such as galactorrhea, amenorrhea, gynecomastia, and impotence have been reported with prolactin-elevating compounds, the clinical significance of elevated serum prolactin levels is unknown for most patients.

As has been observed with other compounds that increase prolactin release, an increase in the incidence of pituitary gland, mammary gland, and endocrine pancreatic islet cell hyperplasias and/or neoplasias, was observed in rodent carcinogenicity studies with RISPERDAL® Tablets and RISPERDAL® CONSTA™ (see PRECAUTIONS – Carcinogenicity, Mutagenesis, Impairment of Fertility). Neither clinical studies nor epidemiologic studies conducted to date have shown an association between chronic administration of this class of drugs and tumorigenesis in humans; the available evidence is considered too limited to be conclusive at this time.

Potential for Cognitive and Motor Impairment

Somnolence was reported by 5% of patients treated with RISPERDAL® CONSTA™ in multiple-dose trials. Since risperidone has the potential to impair judgment, thinking, or motor skills, patients should be cautioned about operating hazardous machinery, including automobiles, until they are reasonably certain that treatment with RISPERDAL® CONSTA™ does not affect them adversely.

Priapism

No cases of priapism have been reported in patients treated with RISPERDAL® CONSTA™. However, rare cases of priapism have been reported in patients treated with oral RISPERDAL®. While the relationship of these events to oral RISPERDAL® use has not been established, other drugs with alpha-adrenergic blocking effects have been reported to induce priapism, and it is possible that RISPERDAL® may share this capacity. Severe priapism may require surgical intervention.

Thrombotic Thrombocytopenic Purpura (TTP)

A single case of TTP was reported in a 28 year-old female patient receiving oral RISPERDAL® in a large, open premarketing experience (approximately 1300 patients). She experienced jaundice, fever, and bruising, but eventually recovered after receiving plasmapheresis. The relationship to RISPERDAL® therapy is unknown.

Antiemetic Effect

Risperidone has an antiemetic effect in animals; this effect may also occur in humans, and may mask signs and symptoms of overdosage with certain drugs or of conditions such as intestinal obstruction, Reye's syndrome, and brain tumor.

Body Temperature Regulation

Disruption of body temperature regulation has been attributed to antipsychotic agents. Both hyperthermia and hypothermia have been reported in association with oral RISPERDAL® use. Caution is advised when prescribing RISPERDAL® CONSTA™ for patients who will be exposed to temperature extremes.

Suicide

The possibility of a suicide attempt is inherent in schizophrenia, and close supervision of high-risk patients should accompany drug therapy. RISPERDAL® CONSTA™ is to be administered by a health care professional (see DOSAGE and ADMINISTRATION); therefore, suicide due to an overdose is unlikely.

Use in Patients with Concomitant Illness

Clinical experience with RISPERDAL® CONSTA™ in patients with certain concomitant systemic illnesses is limited. Caution is advisable when using RISPERDAL® CONSTA™ in patients with diseases or conditions that could affect metabolism or hemodynamic responses.

RISPERDAL® CONSTA™ has not been evaluated or used to any appreciable extent in patients with a recent history of myocardial infarction or unstable heart disease. Patients with these diagnoses were excluded from clinical studies during the product's premarket testing.

Increased plasma concentrations of risperidone and 9-hydroxyrisperidone occur in patients with severe renal impairment (creatinine clearance <30 mL/min/1.73 m^2) treated with oral RISPERDAL®; an increase in the free fraction of risperidone is also seen in patients with severe hepatic impairment. Patients with renal or hepatic impairment should be carefully titrated on oral RISPERDAL® before treatment with RISPERDAL® CONSTA™ is initiated (see DOSAGE AND ADMINISTRATION).

Information for Patients

Physicians are advised to discuss the following issues with patients for whom they prescribe RISPERDAL® CONSTA™.

Orthostatic Hypotension

Patients should be advised of the risk of orthostatic hypotension and instructed in nonpharmacologic interventions that help to reduce the occurrence of orthostatic hypotension (e.g., sitting on the edge of the bed for several minutes before attempting to stand in the morning and slowly rising from a seated position).

Interference With Cognitive and Motor Performance

Because RISPERDAL® CONSTA™ has the potential to impair judgment, thinking, or motor skills, patients should be cautioned about operating hazardous machinery, including automobiles, until they are reasonably certain that treatment with RISPERDAL® CONSTA™ does not affect them adversely.

Pregnancy

Patients should be advised to notify their physician if they become pregnant or intend to become pregnant during therapy and for at least 12 weeks after the last injection of RISPERDAL® CONSTA™.

Nursing

Patients should be advised not to breast-feed an infant during treatment and for at least 12 weeks after the last injection of RISPERDAL® CONSTA™.

Concomitant Medication

Patients should be advised to inform their physicians if they are taking, or plan to take, any prescription or over-the-counter drugs, since there is a potential for interactions.

Alcohol

Patients should be advised to avoid alcohol during treatment with RISPERDAL® CONSTA™.

Laboratory Tests

No specific laboratory tests are recommended.

Drug Interactions

The interactions of RISPERDAL® CONSTA™ and other drugs have not been systematically evaluated. Given the primary CNS effects of risperidone, caution should be used when RISPERDAL® CONSTA™ is administered in combination with other centrally-acting drugs or alcohol.

Because of its potential for inducing hypotension, RISPERDAL® CONSTA™ may enhance the hypotensive effects of other therapeutic agents with this potential.

RISPERDAL® CONSTA™ may antagonize the effects of levodopa and dopamine agonists.

Amytriptyline does not affect the pharmacokinetics of risperidone or the active antipsychotic fraction. Cimetidine and ranitidine increased the bioavailability of risperidone, but only marginally increased the plasma concentration of the active antipsychotic fraction.

Chronic administration of clozapine with risperidone may decrease the clearance of risperidone.

Carbamazepine and Other Enzyme Inducers

In a drug interaction study in schizophrenic patients, 11 subjects received oral risperidone titrated to 6 mg/day for 3 weeks, followed by concurrent administration of carbamazepine for an additional 3 weeks. During co-administration, the plasma concentrations of risperidone and its pharmacologically active metabolite, 9-hydroxyrisperidone, were decreased by about 50%. Plasma concentrations of carbamazepine did not appear to be affected. Co-administration of other known enzyme inducers (e.g., phenytoin, rifampin, and phenobarbital) with risperidone may cause similar decreases in the combined plasma concentrations of risperidone and 9-hydroxyrisperidone, which could lead to decreased efficacy of risperidone treatment. At the initiation of therapy with carbamazepine or other known hepatic enzyme inducers, patients should be closely monitored during the first 4-8 weeks, since the dose of RISPERDAL® CONSTA™ may need to be adjusted. A dose increase, or additional oral RISPERDAL®, may need to be considered. On discontinuation of carbamazepine or other hepatic enzyme inducers, the dosage of RISPERDAL® CONSTA™ should be re-evaluated and, if necessary, decreased. Patients may be placed on a lower dose of RISPERDAL® CONSTA™ between 2 to 4 weeks before the planned discontinuation of carbamazepine therapy to adjust for the expected increase in plasma concentrations of risperidone plus 9-hydroxyrisperidone. For patients treated with the lowest available dose (25 mg) of RISPERDAL® CONSTA™, it is recommended to continue treatment with the 25-mg dose unless clinical judgment necessitates interruption of treatment with RISPERDAL® CONSTA™.

Fluoxetine and Paroxetine

Fluoxetine (20 mg QD) and paroxetine (20 mg QD), which inhibit CYP 2D6, have been shown to increase the plasma concentration of risperidone 2.5-2.8 fold and 3-9 fold respectively. Fluoxetine did not affect the plasma concentration of 9-hydroxyrisperidone. Paroxetine lowered the concentration of 9-hydroxyrisperidone an average of 13%. When either concomitant fluoxetine or paroxetine is initiated or discontinued, the physician should re-evaluate the dosage of RISPERDAL® CONSTA™. When initiation of fluoxetine or paroxetine is considered, patients may be placed on a lower dose of RISPERDAL® CONSTA™ between 2 to 4 weeks before the planned start of fluoxetine or paroxetine therapy to adjust for the expected increase in plasma concentrations of risperidone. For patients treated with the lowest available dose (25 mg), it is recommended to continue treatment with the 25-mg dose unless clinical judgment necessitates interruption of treatment with RISPERDAL® CONSTA™. The effects of discontinuation of concomitant fluoxetine or paroxetine therapy on the pharmacokinetics of risperidone and 9-hydroxyrisperidone have not been studied.

Lithium

Repeated oral doses of risperidone (3 mg BID) did not affect the exposure (AUC) or peak plasma concentrations (C_{max}) of lithium (n=13).

Valproate

Repeated oral doses of risperidone (4 mg QD) did not affect the pre-dose or average plasma concentrations and exposure (AUC) of valproate (1000 mg/day in three divided doses) compared to placebo (n=21). However, there was a 20% increase in valproate peak plasma concentration (C_{max}) after concomitant administration of risperidone.

Digoxin

RISPERDAL® (0.25 mg BID) did not show a clinically relevant effect on the pharmacokinetics of digoxin.

Drugs that Inhibit CYP 2D6 and Other CYP Isozymes

Risperidone is metabolized to 9-hydroxyrisperidone by CYP 2D6, an enzyme that is polymorphic in the population and that can be inhibited by a variety of psychotropic and other drugs (see CLINICAL PHARMACOLOGY). Drug interactions that reduce the metabolism of risperidone to 9-hydroxyrisperidone would increase the plasma concentrations of risperidone and lower the concentrations of 9-hydroxyrisperidone. Analysis of clinical studies involving a modest number of poor metabolizers (n≅70 patients) does not suggest that poor and extensive metabolizers have different rates of adverse effects. No comparison of effectiveness in the two groups has been made.

In vitro studies showed that drugs metabolized by other CYP isozymes, including 1A1, 1A2, 2C9, 2C19, and 3A4, are only weak inhibitors of risperidone metabolism.

There were no significant interactions between risperidone and erythromycin (see CLINICAL PHARMACOLOGY).

Drugs Metabolized by CYP 2D6

In vitro studies indicate that risperidone is a relatively weak inhibitor of CYP 2D6. Therefore, RISPERDAL® CONSTA™ is not expected to substantially inhibit the clearance of drugs that are metabolized by this enzymatic pathway. In drug interaction studies, oral risperidone did not significantly affect the pharmacokinetics of donepezil and galantamine, which are metabolized by CYP 2D6.

Carcinogenesis, Mutagenesis, Impairment of Fertility

Carcinogenesis - Oral

Carcinogenicity studies were conducted in Swiss albino mice and Wistar rats. Risperidone was administered in the diet at doses of 0.63, 2.5, and 10 mg/kg for 18 months to mice and for 25 months to rats. These doses are equivalent to 2.4, 9.4, and 37.5 times the oral maximum recommended human dose (MRHD) (16 mg/day) on a mg/kg basis, or 0.2, 0.75, and 3 times the oral MRHD (mice) or 0.4, 1.5, and 6 times the oral MRHD (rats) on a mg/m^2 basis. A maximum tolerated dose was not achieved in male mice. There was a significant increase in pituitary gland adenomas in female mice at doses 0.75 and 3 times the oral MRHD on a mg/m^2 basis. There was a significant increase in endocrine pancreatic adenomas in male rats at doses 1.5 and 6 times the oral MRHD on a mg/m^2 basis. Mammary gland adenocarcinomas were significantly increased in female mice at all doses tested (0.2, 0.75, and 3 times the oral MRHD on a mg/m^2 basis), in female rats at all doses tested (0.4, 1.5, and 6 times the oral MRHD on a mg/m^2 basis), and in male rats at a dose 6 times the oral MRHD on a mg/m^2 basis.

Carcinogenesis - IM

RISPERDAL® CONSTA™ was evaluated in a 24-month carcinogenicity study in which SPF Wistar rats were treated every 2 weeks with IM injections of either 5 mg/kg or 40 mg/kg of risperidone. These doses are 1 and 8 times the MRHD (50 mg) on a mg/m^2 basis. A control group received injections of 0.9% NaCl, and a vehicle control group was injected with placebo microspheres. There was a significant increase in pituitary gland adenomas, endocrine pancreas adenomas, and adrenomedullary pheochromocytomas at 8 times the IM MRHD on a mg/m^2 basis. The incidence of mammary gland adenocarcinomas was significantly increased in female rats at both doses (1 and 8 times the IM MRHD on a mg/m^2 basis). A significant increase in renal tubular tumors (adenoma, adenocarcinomas) was observed in male rats at 8 times the IM MRHD on a mg/m^2 basis. Plasma exposures (AUC) in rats were 0.3 and 2 times (at 5 and 40 mg/kg, respectively) the expected plasma exposure (AUC) at the IM MRHD.

Dopamine D_2 receptor antagonists have been shown to chronically elevate prolactin levels in rodents. Serum prolactin levels were not measured during the carcinogenicity studies of oral risperidone; however, measurements taken during subchronic toxicity studies showed that oral risperidone elevated serum prolactin levels 5- to 6-fold in mice and rats at the same doses used in the oral carcinogenicity studies. Serum prolactin levels increased in a dose-dependent manner up to 6- and 1.5-fold in male and female rats, respectively, at the end of the 24-month treatment with RISPERDAL® CONSTA™ every 2 weeks. Increases in the incidence of pituitary gland, endocrine pancreas, and mammary gland neoplasms have been found in rodents after chronic administration of other antipsychotic drugs and may be prolactin-mediated.

The relevance for human risk of the findings of prolactin-mediated endocrine tumors in rodents is unknown (see PRECAUTIONS - Hyperprolactinemia).

Mutagenesis

No evidence of mutagenic potential for oral risperidone was found in the *in vitro* Ames reverse mutation test, *in vitro* mouse lymphoma assay, *in vitro* rat hepatocyte DNA-repair assay, *in vivo* oral micronucleus test in mice, the sex-linked recessive lethal test in *Drosophila*, or the *in vitro* chromosomal aberration test in human lymphocytes or in Chinese hamster cells.

In addition, no evidence of mutagenic potential was found in the *in vitro* Ames reverse mutation test for RISPERDAL® CONSTA™.

Impairment of Fertility

Oral risperidone (0.16 to 5 mg/kg) was shown to impair mating, but not fertility, in Wistar rats in three reproductive studies (two mating and fertility studies and a multigenerational study) at doses 0.1 to 3 times the oral maximum recommended human dose (MRHD) (16 mg/day) on a mg/m^2 basis. The effect appeared to be in females, since impaired mating behavior was not noted in the mating and fertility study in which males only were treated. In a subchronic study in Beagle dogs in which oral risperidone was administered at doses of 0.31 to 5 mg/kg, sperm motility and concentration were decreased at doses 0.6 to 10 times the oral MRHD on a mg/m^2 basis. Dose-related decreases were also noted in serum testosterone at the same doses. Serum testosterone and sperm values partially recovered, but remained decreased after treatment was discontinued. No no-effect doses were noted in either rat or dog.

No mating and fertility studies were conducted with RISPERDAL® CONSTA™.

Pregnancy

Pregnancy Category C

The teratogenic potential of oral risperidone was studied in three embryofetal development studies in Sprague-Dawley and Wistar rats (0.63-10 mg/kg or 0.4 to 6 times the oral maximum recommended human dose [MRHD] on a mg/m^2 basis) and in one embryofetal development study in New Zealand rabbits (0.31-5 mg/kg or 0.4 to 6 times the oral MRHD on a mg/m^2 basis). The incidence of malformations was not increased compared to control in offspring of rats or rabbits given 0.4 to 6 times the oral MRHD on a mg/m^2 basis. In three reproductive studies in rats (two peri/post-natal development studies and a multigenerational study), there was an increase in pup deaths during the first 4 days of lactation at doses of 0.16-5 mg/kg or 0.1 to 3 times the oral MRHD on a mg/m^2 basis. It is not known whether these deaths were due to a direct effect on the fetuses or pups or to effects on the dams.

There was no no-effect dose for increased rat pup mortality. In one peri/post-natal development study, there was an increase in stillborn rat pups at a dose of 2.5 mg/kg or 1.5 times the oral MRHD on a mg/m^2 basis. In a cross-fostering study in Wistar rats, toxic effects on the fetus or pups, as evidenced by a decrease in the number of live pups and an increase in the number of dead pups at birth (Day 0), and a decrease in birth weight in pups of drug-treated dams were observed. In addition, there was an increase in deaths by Day 1 among pups of drug-treated dams, regardless of whether or not the pups were cross-fostered. Risperidone also appeared to impair maternal behavior in that pup body weight gain and survival (from Days 1 to 4 of lactation) were reduced in pups born to control but reared by drug-treated dams. These effects were all noted at the one dose of risperidone tested, i.e., 5 mg/kg or 3 times the oral MRHD on a mg/m^2 basis.

No studies were conducted with RISPERDAL® CONSTA™. Placental transfer of risperidone occurs in rat pups. There are no adequate and well-controlled studies in pregnant women. However, there was one report of a case of agenesis of the corpus callosum in an infant exposed to risperidone *in utero*. The causal relationship to oral RISPERDAL® therapy is unknown.

RISPERDAL® CONSTA™ should be used during pregnancy only if the potential benefit justifies the potential risk to the fetus.

Labor and Delivery

The effect of RISPERDAL® CONSTA™ on labor and delivery in humans is unknown.

Nursing Mothers

In animal studies, risperidone and 9-hydroxyrisperidone are excreted in milk. Risperidone and 9-hydroxyrisperidone are also excreted in human breast milk. Therefore, women should not breast-feed during treatment with RISPERDAL® CONSTA™ and for at least 12 weeks after the last injection.

Pediatric Use

RISPERDAL® CONSTA™ has not been studied in children younger than 18 years old.

Geriatric Use

In an open-label study, 57 clinically stable, elderly patients (≥65 years old) with schizophrenia or schizoaffective disorder received RISPERDAL® CONSTA™ every 2 weeks for up to 12 months. In general, no differences in the tolerability of RISPERDAL® CONSTA™ were observed between otherwise healthy elderly and nonelderly patients. Therefore, dosing recommendations for otherwise healthy elderly patients are the same as for nonelderly patients. Because elderly patients exhibit a greater tendency to orthostatic hypotension than nonelderly patients, elderly patients should be instructed in nonpharmacologic interventions that help to reduce the occurrence of orthostatic hypotension (e.g., sitting on the edge of the bed for several minutes before attempting to stand in the morning and slowly rising from a seated position). In addition, monitoring of orthostatic vital signs should be considered in elderly patients for whom orthostatic hypotension is of concern (see CLINICAL PHARMACOLOGY, PRECAUTIONS, and DOSAGE AND ADMINISTRATION).

ADVERSE REACTIONS

Adverse findings were assessed by spontaneous reports of adverse events, laboratory tests, vital signs, body weight, and ECGs. Adverse events were classified using the World Health Organization preferred terms. Treatment-emergent adverse events were defined as those events with an onset between the first dose and 49 days after the last dose.

The prescriber should be aware that these figures cannot be used to predict the incidence of side effects in the course of usual medical practice where patient characteristics and other factors differ from those which prevailed in this clinical trial. Similarly, the cited frequencies cannot be compared with figures obtained from other clinical investigations involving different treatments, uses, and investigators. The cited figures, however, do provide the prescribing physician with some basis for estimating the relative contribution of drug and nondrug factors to the side effect incidence rate in the population studied.

Associated with Discontinuation of Treatment

In the 12-week, placebo-controlled trial, the incidence of schizophrenic patients who discontinued treatment due to an adverse event was lower with RISPERDAL® CONSTA™ (11%; 22/202 patients) than with placebo (13%; 13/98 patients).

Incidence in Controlled Trials

The incidence of adverse reactions in the placebo-controlled trial was based on 202 schizophrenic patients treated with 25 or 50 mg RISPERDAL® CONSTA™ and 98 schizophrenic patients treated with placebo for up to 12 weeks.

Commonly Observed Adverse Events in Controlled Clinical Trials

Spontaneously reported, treatment-emergent adverse events with an incidence of 5% or greater in at least one of the RISPERDAL® CONSTA™ groups (25 mg or 50 mg) and at least twice that of placebo were: somnolence, akathisia, parkinsonism, dyspepsia, constipation, dry mouth, fatigue, weight increase.

Adverse Events Occurring at an Incidence of 2% or More in Patients Treated with RISPERDAL® CONSTA™:

Table 1 enumerates adverse events that occurred at an incidence of 2% or more, and were at least as frequent among patients treated with 25 mg or 50 mg RISPERDAL® CONSTA™ as patients treated with placebo in the 12-week, placebo-controlled trial. This table shows the percentage of patients in each dose group who spontaneously reported at least one episode of an event at some time during double-blind treatment. All patients were titrated to a dose of 4 mg oral RISPERDAL® during a 1-week run-in period. Patients who received RISPERDAL® CONSTA™ were given doses of oral RISPERDAL® (2 mg for patients in the 25-mg group, and 4 mg for patients in the 50-mg group) during the 3 weeks after the first injection to provide therapeutic levels until the main release phase of risperidone from the injection site had begun. Patients who received placebo injections were given placebo tablets.

Table 1. Incidence (% of Patients) of Treatment-Emergent Adverse Events in a 12-Week, Placebo-Controlled Clinical Trial

WHO Body System Disorder/ Preferred Term	RISPERDAL® CONSTA™ 25 mg (N=99)	RISPERDAL® CONSTA™ 50 mg (N=103)	Placebo (N=98)
Psychiatric			
Insomnia	16	13	14
Hallucination	7	6	5
Somnolence	5	6	3
Suicide attempt	1	4	3
Abnormal thinking	0	3	2
Abnormal dreaming	2	0	0
Central & peripheral nervous system			
Headache	15	22	12
Dizziness	8	11	6
Akathisia	2	9	4
Parkinsonism[a]	4	10	3
Tremor	0	3	0
Hypoasthesia	2	0	0
Gastrointestinal			
Dyspepsia	7	7	2
Constipation	5	7	1
Mouth dry	0	7	1
Toothache	1	3	0
Saliva increased	6	2	1
Tooth disorder	4	2	0
Diarrhea	5	1	3
Body as a whole - general			
Fatigue	3	7	0
Pain	10	3	4
Peripheral edema	2	3	1
Leg pain	4	1	1
Fever	2	1	0
Syncope	2	0	0
Respiratory system			
Rhinitis	14	4	8
Coughing	5	2	4
Sinusitis	3	1	0
Upper respiratory tract infection	2	0	1
Metabolic & nutritional			
Weight increase	5	4	2
Weight decrease	4	1	1
Cardiovascular			
Hypertension	3	3	2
Hearing & vestibular			
Ear disorder (NOS)	0	3	0
Vision			
Vision abnormal	2	3	0
Skin & appendage			
Acne	2	2	0
Skin dry	2	0	0
Musculo-Skeletal			
Myalgia	4	2	1

[a] Includes adverse events of bradykinesia, extrapyramidal disorder, and hypokinesia.

Dose Dependency of Adverse Events

Extrapyramidal Symptoms:

Two methods were used to measure extrapyramidal symptoms (EPS) in the 12-week, placebo-controlled trial comparing three doses of RISPERDAL® CONSTA™ (25 mg, 50 mg, and 75 mg) with placebo, including: (1) the incidence of spontaneous reports of EPS symptoms; and (2) the change from baseline to endpoint on the total score (sum of the subscale scores for parkinsonism, dystonia, and dyskinesia) of the Extrapyramidal Symptom Rating Scale (ESRS).

As shown in Table 1, the overall incidence of EPS-related adverse events (akathisia, dystonia, parkinsonism, and tremor) in patients treated with 25 mg RISPERDAL® CONSTA™ was comparable to that of patients treated with placebo; the incidence of EPS-related adverse events was higher in patients treated with 50 mg RISPERDAL® CONSTA™.

The median change from baseline to endpoint in total ESRS score showed no worsening in patients treated with RISPERDAL® CONSTA™ compared with patients treated with placebo: 0 (placebo group); -1 (25-mg group, significantly less than the placebo group); and 0 (50-mg group).

Vital Sign Changes:

RISPERDAL® is associated with orthostatic hypotension and tachycardia (see PRECAUTIONS). In the placebo-controlled trial, orthostatic hypotension was observed in 2% of patients treated with 25 mg or 50 mg RISPERDAL® CONSTA™ (see PRECAUTIONS).

Weight Changes:

In the 12-week, placebo-controlled trial, 9% of patients treated with RISPERDAL® CONSTA™, compared with 6% of patients treated with placebo, experienced a weight gain of >7% of body weight at endpoint.

Laboratory Changes:

The percentage of patients treated with RISPERDAL® CONSTA™ who experienced potentially important changes in routine serum chemistry, hematology, or urinalysis parameters was similar to or less than that of placebo patients. Additionally, no patients discontinued treatment due to changes in serum chemistry, hematology, or urinalysis parameters.

ECG Changes:

The electrocardiograms of 202 schizophrenic patients treated with 25 mg or 50 mg RISPERDAL® CONSTA™ and 98 schizophrenic patients treated with placebo in a 12-week, double-blind, placebo-controlled trial were evaluated. Compared with placebo, there were no statistically significant differences in QTc intervals (using Fridericia's and linear correction factors) during treatment with RISPERDAL® CONSTA™.

Between-group comparisons for pooled placebo-controlled trials with oral RISPERDAL® revealed no statistically significant differences between risperidone and placebo in mean changes from baseline in ECG parameters, including QT, QTc, and PR intervals, and heart rate. When all oral RISPERDAL® doses were pooled from randomized controlled trials in several indications, there was a mean increase in heart rate of 1 beat per minute compared to no change for placebo patients. In short-term schizophrenia trials, higher doses of oral risperidone (8-16 mg/day) were associated with a higher mean increase in heart rate compared to placebo (4-6 beats per minute).

Pain assessment and local injection site reactions:

The mean intensity of injection pain reported by patients using a visual analog scale (0 = no pain to 100 = unbearably painful) decreased in all treatment groups from the first to the last injection (placebo: 16.7 to 12.6; 25 mg: 12.0 to 9.0; 50 mg: 18.2 to 11.8). After the sixth injection (Week 10), investigator ratings indicated that 1% of patients treated with 25 mg or 50 mg RISPERDAL® CONSTA™ experienced redness, swelling, or induration at the injection site.

Other Events Observed During the Premarketing Evaluation of RISPERDAL® CONSTA™

During its premarketing assessment, RISPERDAL® CONSTA™ was administered to 1499 patients in multiple-dose studies. The conditions and duration of exposure to RISPERDAL® CONSTA™ varied greatly, and included (in overlapping categories) open-label and double-blind studies, uncontrolled and controlled studies, inpatient and outpatient studies, fixed-dose and titration studies, and short-term and long-term exposure studies. In all studies, untoward events associated with this exposure were obtained by spontaneous report and were recorded by clinical investigators using terminology of their own choosing. Consequently, it is not possible to provide a meaningful estimate of the proportion of individuals experiencing adverse events without first grouping similar types of untoward events into a smaller number of standardized event categories.

In the listings that follow, spontaneously reported adverse events were classified using World Health Organization (WHO) preferred terms. The frequencies presented, therefore, represent the proportion of the 1499 patients exposed to multiple doses of RISPERDAL® CONSTA™ who experienced an event of the type cited on at least one occasion while receiving RISPERDAL® CONSTA™. All reported events are included except those already listed in Table 1, those events for which a drug cause was remote, those event terms which were so general as to be uninformative, and those events reported only once which did not have a sub-

Continued on next page

Risperdal Consta—Cont.

stantial probability of being acutely life-threatening. It is important to emphasize that, although the reported events occurred during treatment with RISPERDAL® CONSTA™, they were not necessarily caused by it.

Events are further categorized by body system and listed in order of decreasing frequency according to the following definitions: frequent adverse events are those occurring in at least 1/100 patients (only those not already listed in the tabulated results from the placebo-controlled trial appear in this listing); infrequent adverse events are those occurring in 1/100 to 1/1000 patients; and rare events are those occurring in fewer than 1/1000 patients.

Psychiatric Disorders

Frequent: anxiety, psychosis, depression, agitation, nervousness, paranoid reaction, delusion, apathy. *Infrequent:* anorexia, impaired concentration, impotence, emotional lability, manic reaction, decreased libido, increased appetite, amnesia, confusion, euphoria, depersonalization, paroniria, delirium, psychotic depression.

Central and Peripheral Nervous System Disorders

Frequent: hypertonia, dystonia. *Infrequent:* dyskinesia, vertigo, leg cramps, tardive dyskinesia[a], involuntary muscle contractions, paraesthesia, abnormal gait, bradykinesia, convulsions, hypokinesia, ataxia, fecal incontinence, oculogyric crisis, tetany, apraxia, dementia, migraine. *Rare:* neuroleptic malignant syndrome.

[a] In the integrated database of multiple-dose studies (1499 patients with schizophrenia or schizoaffective disorder), 9 patients (0.6%) treated with RISPERDAL® CONSTA™ (all dosages combined) experienced an adverse event of tardive dyskinesia.

Body as a Whole/General Disorders

Frequent: back pain, chest pain, asthenia. *Infrequent:* malaise, choking.

Gastrointestinal Disorders

Frequent: nausea, vomiting, abdominal pain. *Infrequent:* gastritis, gastroesophageal reflux, flatulence, hemorrhoids, melena, dysphagia, rectal hemorrhage, stomatitis, colitis, gastric ulcer, gingivitis, irritable bowel syndrome, ulcerative stomatitis.

Respiratory System Disorders

Frequent: dyspnea. *Infrequent:* pneumonia, stridor, hemoptysis. *Rare:* pulmonary edema.

Skin and Appendage Disorders

Frequent: rash. *Infrequent:* eczema, pruritus, erythematous rash, dermatitis, alopecia, seborrhea, photosensitivity reaction, increased sweating.

Metabolic and Nutritional Disorders

Infrequent: hyperuricemia, hyperglycemia, hyperlipemia, hypokalemia, glycosuria, hypercholesterolemia, obesity, dehydration, diabetes mellitus, hyponatremia.

Musculo-Skeletal System Disorders

Frequent: arthralgia, skeletal pain. *Infrequent:* torticollis, arthrosis, muscle weakness, tendinitis, arthritis, arthropathy.

Heart Rate and Rhythm Disorders

Frequent: tachycardia. *Infrequent:* bradycardia, AV block, palpitation, bundle branch block. *Rare:* T-wave inversion.

Cardiovascular Disorders

Frequent: hypotension. *Infrequent:* postural hypotension.

Urinary System Disorders

Frequent: urinary incontinence. *Infrequent:* hematuria, micturition frequency, renal pain, urinary retention.

Vision Disorders

Infrequent: conjunctivitis, eye pain, abnormal accommodation.

Reproductive Disorders, Female

Frequent: amenorrhea. *Infrequent:* nonpuerperal lactation, vaginitis, dysmenorrhea, breast pain, leukorrhea.

Resistance Mechanism Disorders

Infrequent: abscess.

Liver and Biliary System Disorders

Frequent: increased hepatic enzymes. *Infrequent:* hepatomegaly, increased SGPT.

Rare: bilirubinemia, increased GGT, hepatitis, hepatocellular damage, jaundice, fatty liver, increased SGOT.

Reproductive Disorders, Male

Infrequent: ejaculation failure.

Application Site Disorders

Frequent: injection site pain. *Infrequent:* injection site reaction.

Hearing and Vestibular Disorders

Infrequent: earache, deafness, hearing decreased.

Red Blood Cell Disorders

Frequent: anemia.

White Cell and Resistance Disorders

Infrequent: lymphadenopathy, leucopenia, cervical lymphadenopathy.

Rare: granulocytopenia, leukocytosis, lymphopenia.

Endocrine Disorders

Infrequent: hyperprolactinemia, gynecomastia, hypothyroidism.

Platelet, Bleeding and Clotting Disorders

Infrequent: purpura, epistaxis. *Rare:* pulmonary embolism, hematoma, thrombocytopenia.

Myo-, Endo-, and Pericardial and Valve Disorders

Infrequent: myocardial ischemia, angina pectoris, myocardial infarction.

Vascular (Extracardiac) Disorders

Infrequent: phlebitis. *Rare:* intermittent claudication, flushing, thrombophlebitis.

Postintroduction Reports

Adverse events reported since market introduction which were temporally (but not necessarily causally) related to oral RISPERDAL® therapy include the following: anaphylactic reaction, angioedema, apnea, atrial fibrillation, cerebrovascular disorder, including cerebrovascular accident, hyperglycemia, diabetes mellitus aggravated, including diabetic ketoacidosis, intestinal obstruction, jaundice, mania, pancreatitis, Parkinson's disease aggravated, pulmonary embolism. There have been rare reports of sudden death and/or cardiopulmonary arrest in patients receiving oral RISPERDAL®. A causal relationship with oral RISPERDAL® has not been established. It is important to note that sudden and unexpected death may occur in psychotic patients whether they remain untreated or whether they are treated with other antipsychotic drugs.

DRUG ABUSE AND DEPENDENCE

Controlled Substance Class

RISPERDAL® CONSTA™ (risperidone) is not a controlled substance.

Physical and Psychological Dependence

RISPERDAL® CONSTA™ has not been systematically studied in animals or humans for its potential for abuse, tolerance, or physical dependence. Because RISPERDAL® CONSTA™ is to be administered by health care professionals, the potential for misuse or abuse by patients is low.

OVERDOSAGE

Human Experience

No cases of overdose were reported in premarketing studies with RISPERDAL® CONSTA™ (risperidone). Because RISPERDAL® CONSTA™ is to be administered by health care professionals, the potential for overdosage by patients is low.

In premarketing experience with oral RISPERDAL® (risperidone), there were eight reports of acute RISPERDAL® overdosage, with estimated doses ranging from 20 to 300 mg and no fatalities. In general, reported signs and symptoms were those resulting from an exaggeration of the drug's known pharmacological effects, i.e., drowsiness and sedation, tachycardia and hypotension, and extrapyramidal symptoms. One case, involving an estimated overdose of 240 mg, was associated with hyponatremia, hypokalemia, prolonged QT, and widened QRS. Another case, involving an estimated overdose of 36 mg, was associated with a seizure.

Postmarketing experience with oral RISPERDAL® includes reports of acute overdose, with estimated doses of up to 360 mg. In general, the most frequently reported signs and symptoms are those resulting from an exaggeration of the drug's known pharmacological effects, i.e., drowsiness, sedation, tachycardia, hypotension, and extrapyramidal symptoms. Other adverse events reported since market introduction which were temporally (but not necessarily causally) related to oral RISPERDAL® overdose include torsades de pointes, prolonged QT interval, convulsions, cardiopulmonary arrest, and rare fatality associated with multiple drug overdose.

Management of Overdosage

In case of acute overdosage, establish and maintain an airway and ensure adequate oxygenation and ventilation. Cardiovascular monitoring should commence immediately and should include continuous electrocardiographic monitoring to detect possible arrhythmias. If antiarrhythmic therapy is administered, disopyramide, procainamide, and quinidine carry a theoretical hazard of QT prolonging effects that might be additive to those of risperidone. Similarly, it is reasonable to expect that the alpha-blocking properties of bretylium might be additive to those of risperidone, resulting in problematic hypotension.

There is no specific antidote to oral RISPERDAL®. Therefore, appropriate supportive measures should be instituted. The possibility of multiple drug involvement should be considered. Hypotension and circulatory collapse should be treated with appropriate measures, such as intravenous fluids and/or sympathomimetic agents (epinephrine and dopamine should not be used, since beta stimulation may worsen hypotension in the setting of risperidone-induced alpha blockade). In cases of severe extrapyramidal symptoms, anticholinergic medication should be administered. Close medical supervision and monitoring should continue until the patient recovers.

DOSAGE AND ADMINISTRATION

For patients who have never taken oral RISPERDAL®, it is recommended to establish tolerability with oral RISPERDAL® prior to initiating treatment with RISPERDAL® CONSTA™ (risperidone).

RISPERDAL® CONSTA™ should be administered every 2 weeks by deep intramuscular (IM) gluteal injection. Each injection should be administered by a health care professional using the enclosed safety needle (see HOW SUPPLIED). Injections should alternate between the two buttocks. Do not administer intravenously.

The recommended dose is 25 mg IM every 2 weeks. Although dose response for effectiveness has not been established for RISPERDAL® CONSTA™, some patients not responding to 25 mg may benefit from a higher dose of 37.5 mg or 50 mg. The maximum dose should not exceed 50 mg RISPERDAL® CONSTA™ every 2 weeks. No additional benefit was observed with dosages greater than 50 mg RISPERDAL® CONSTA™; however, a higher incidence of adverse effects was observed.

Oral RISPERDAL® (or another antipsychotic medication) should be given with the first injection of RISPERDAL® CONSTA™ and continued for 3 weeks (and then discontinued) to ensure that adequate therapeutic plasma concentrations are maintained prior to the main release phase of risperidone from the injection site (see CLINICAL PHARMACOLOGY).

Upward dosage adjustment should not be made more frequently than every 4 weeks. The clinical effects of this dose adjustment should not be anticipated earlier than 3 weeks after the first injection with the higher dose.

Do not combine two different dosage strengths of RISPERDAL® CONSTA™ in a single administration.

Pediatric Use

RISPERDAL® CONSTA™ has not been studied in children younger than 18 years old.

Dosage in Special Populations

For elderly patients treated with RISPERDAL® CONSTA™, the recommended dosage is 25 mg IM every 2 weeks. Oral RISPERDAL® (or another antipsychotic medication) should be given with the first injection of RISPERDAL® CONSTA™ and should be continued for 3 weeks to ensure that adequate therapeutic plasma concentrations are maintained prior to the main release phase of risperidone from the injection site (see CLINICAL PHARMACOLOGY).

Patients with renal or hepatic impairment should be treated with titrated doses of oral RISPERDAL® prior to initiating treatment with RISPERDAL® CONSTA™. The recommended starting dose is 0.5 mg oral RISPERDAL® b.i.d. during the first week, which can be increased to 1 mg b.i.d. or 2 mg once daily during the second week. If a dose of at least 2 mg oral RISPERDAL® is well tolerated, an injection of 25 mg RISPERDAL® CONSTA™ can be administered every 2 weeks. Oral supplementation should be continued for 3 weeks after the first injection until the main release of risperidone from the injection site has begun. In some patients, slower titration may be medically appropriate.

Patients with renal impairment may have less ability to eliminate risperidone than normal adults. Patients with impaired hepatic function may have an increase in the free fraction of the risperidone, possibly resulting in an enhanced effect (see CLINICAL PHARMACOLOGY). Elderly patients and patients with a predisposition to hypotensive reactions or for whom such reactions would pose a particular risk should be instructed in nonpharmacologic interventions that help to reduce the occurrence of orthostatic hypotension (e.g., sitting on the edge of the bed for several minutes before attempting to stand in the morning and slowly rising from a seated position). These patients should avoid sodium depletion or dehydration, and circumstances that accentuate hypotension (alcohol intake, high ambient temperature, etc.). Monitoring of orthostatic vital signs should be considered (see PRECAUTIONS).

Maintenance Therapy

Although no controlled studies have been conducted to answer the question of how long patients should be treated with RISPERDAL® CONSTA™, oral risperidone has been shown to be effective in delaying time to relapse in longer-term use. It is recommended that responding patients be continued on treatment with RISPERDAL® CONSTA™ at the lowest dose needed. Patients should be periodically reassessed to determine the need for continued treatment.

Reinitiation of Treatment in Patients Previously Discontinued

There are no data to specifically address reinitiation of treatment. When restarting patients who have had an interval off treatment with RISPERDAL® CONSTA™, supplementation with oral RISPERDAL® (or another antipsychotic medication) should be administered.

Switching from Other Antipsychotics

There are no systematically collected data to specifically address switching schizophrenic patients from other antipsychotics to RISPERDAL® CONSTA™, or concerning concomitant administration with other antipsychotics. Previous antipsychotics should be continued for 3 weeks after the first injection of RISPERDAL® CONSTA™ to ensure that therapeutic concentrations are maintained until the main release phase of risperidone from the injection site has begun (see CLINICAL PHARMACOLOGY). For schizophrenic patients who have never taken oral RISPERDAL®, it is recommended to establish tolerability with oral RISPERDAL® prior to initiating treatment with RISPERDAL® CONSTA™. As recommended with other antipsychotic medications, the need for continuing existing EPS medication should be re-evaluated periodically.

Co-Administration of RISPERDAL® CONSTA™ with Certain Other Medications

Co-administration of carbamazepine and other enzyme inducers (e.g., phenytoin, rifampin, phenobarbital) with risperidone would be expected to cause decreases in the plasma concentrations of active moiety (the sum of risperidone and 9-hydroxyrisperidone), which could lead to decreased efficacy of risperidone treatment. The dose of risperidone needs to be titrated accordingly for patients receiving these enzyme inducers, especially during initiation or discontinuation of therapy with these inducers (see CLINICAL PHARMACOLOGY and PRECAUTIONS). At the initiation of therapy with carbamazepine or other known hepatic enzyme inducers, patients should be closely monitored during the first 4-8 weeks, since the dose of RISPERDAL® CONSTA™ may need to be adjusted. A dose increase, or additional oral RISPERDAL®, may need to be considered. On discontinuation of carbamazepine or other hepatic enzyme inducers, the dosage of RISPERDAL® CONSTA™ should be re-evaluated and, if necessary, decreased. Patients may be placed on a lower dose of

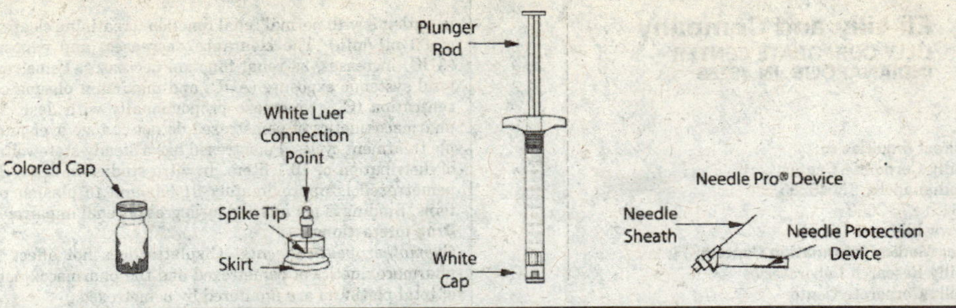

RISPERDAL® CONSTA™ between 2 to 4 weeks before the planned discontinuation of carbamazepine therapy to adjust for the expected increase in plasma concentrations of risperidone plus 9-hydroxyrisperidone. For patients treated with the lowest available dose (25 mg) of RISPERDAL® CONSTA™, it is recommended to continue treatment with the 25-mg dose unless clinical judgment necessitates interruption of treatment with RISPERDAL® CONSTA™.

Fluoxetine and paroxetine have been shown to increase the plasma concentration of risperidone 2.5-2.8 fold and 3-9 fold respectively. Fluoxetine did not affect the plasma concentration of 9-hydroxyrisperidone. Paroxetine lowered the concentration of 9-hydroxyrisperidone an average of 13%. The dose of risperidone needs to be titrated accordingly when fluoxetine or paroxetine is co-administered. When either concomitant fluoxetine or paroxetine is initiated or discontinued, the physician should re-evaluate the dosage of RISPERDAL® CONSTA™. When initiation of fluoxetine or paroxetine is considered, patients may be placed on a lower dose of RISPERDAL® CONSTA™ between 2 to 4 weeks before the planned start of fluoxetine or paroxetine therapy to adjust for the expected increase in plasma concentrations of risperidone. For patients treated with the lowest available dose (25 mg), it is recommended to continue treatment with the 25-mg dose unless clinical judgment necessitates interruption of treatment with RISPERDAL® CONSTA™. The effects of discontinuation of concomitant fluoxetine or paroxetine therapy on the pharmacokinetics of risperidone and 9-hydroxyrisperidone have not been studied.

Instructions for Use

RISPERDAL® CONSTA™ must be suspended **only** in the diluent supplied in the dose pack, and must be administered with the needle supplied in the dose pack. All components are required for administration. Do not substitute any components of the dose pack.

[See figure above]
Remove the dose pack of RISPERDAL® CONSTA™ from the refrigerator and allow it to come to room temperature prior to reconstitution.

1. Flip off the plastic colored cap from the vial.

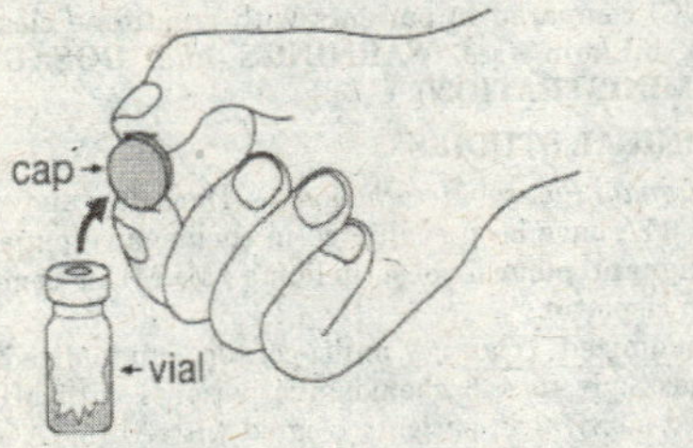

2. Peel back the blister pouch and remove the SmartSite® Needle-Free Vial Access Device by holding the white luer cap. Do **not** touch the spike tip of the access device at any time.

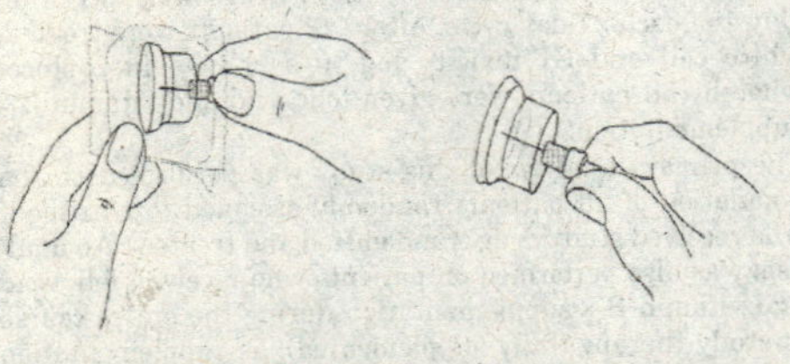

3. Press the spike tip of the SmartSite® Access Device through the vial's rubber stopper until the device clicks into place.
[See first figure at top of next column]
4. Swab the syringe connection point (blue circle) of the SmartSite® Access Device with preferred antiseptic prior to attaching the syringe to the SmartSite® Access Device.
[See second figure in next column]
5. Twist off the white cap from the pre-filled syringe and remove together with the rubber tip cap inside.
[See third figure in next column]
6. **Press** the syringe tip into the blue circle of the SmartSite® Access Device and **Twist** in a clockwise motion to ensure that the syringe is securely attached to the white luer cap of the access device. Keep the syringe

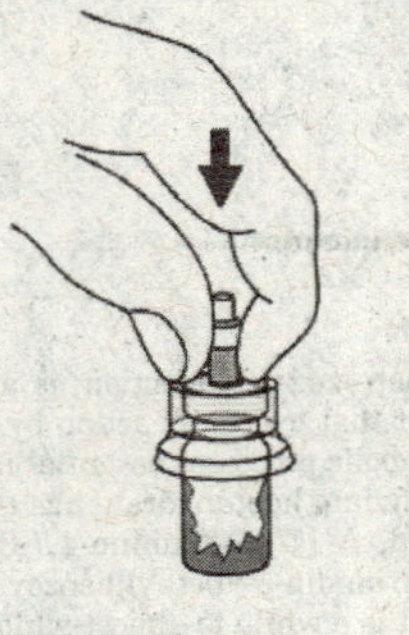

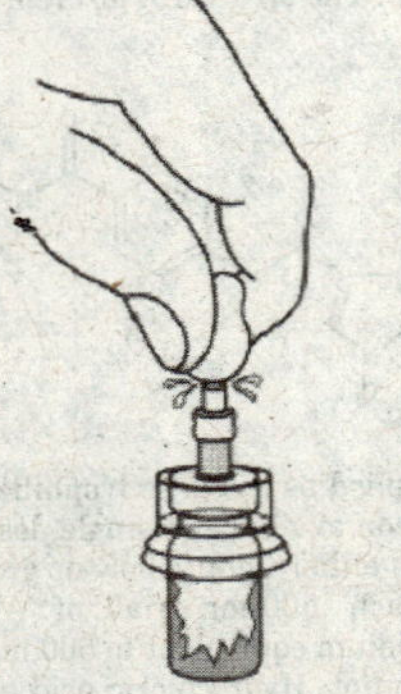

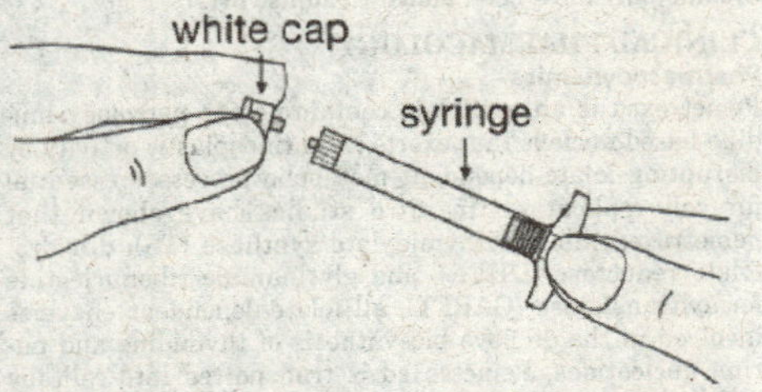

and SmartSite® Access Device aligned, and hold the skirt of the access device during attachment to prevent spinning.

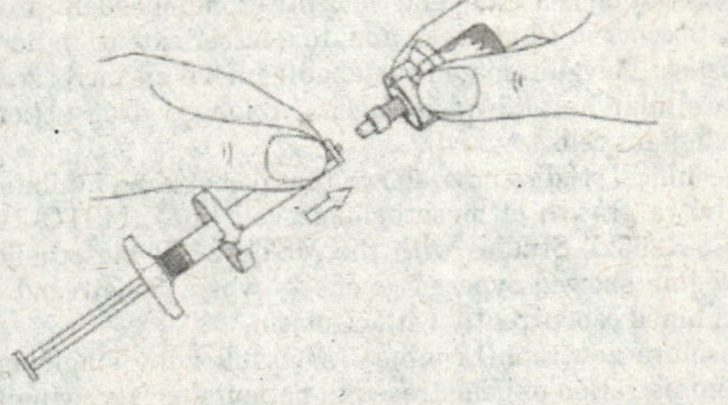

7. Inject the entire contents of the syringe containing the diluent into the vial.

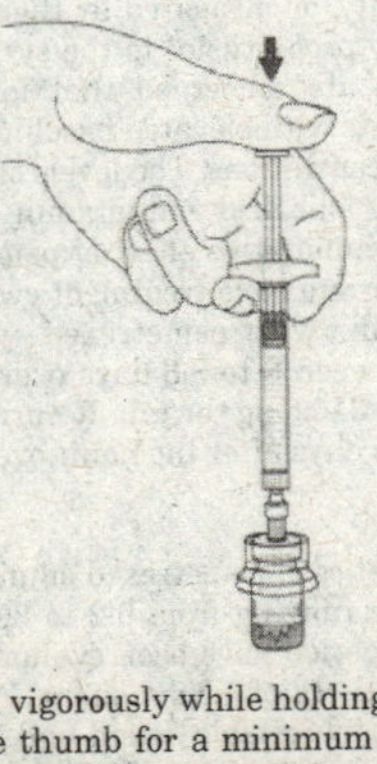

8. Shake the vial vigorously while holding the plunger rod down with the thumb for a minimum of 10 seconds to ensure a homogeneous suspension. When properly mixed, the suspension appears uniform, thick, and milky in color. The particles will be visible in liquid, but no dry particles remain.

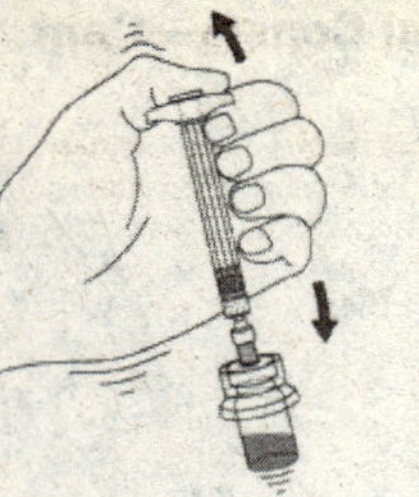

9. Do not store the vial after reconstitution or the suspension may settle. *If 2 minutes pass before injection, reconstitute by shaking vigorously.*
10. Invert the vial completely and slowly withdraw the suspension from the vial. Tear section of the vial label at the perforation and apply detached label to syringe for identification purposes.

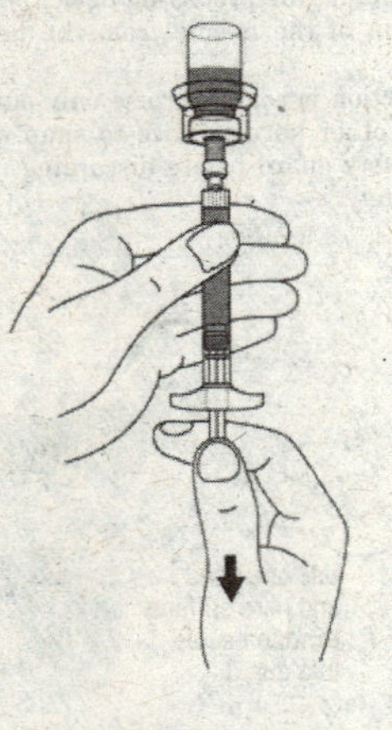

11. Unscrew the syringe from the SmartSite® access device and discard both the vial and access device appropriately.

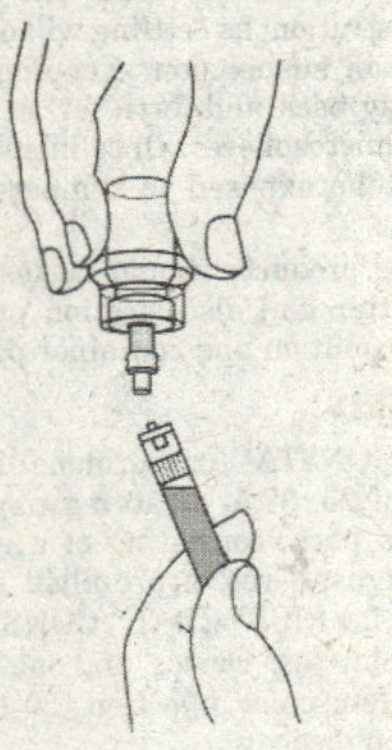

12. Peel the blister pouch of the Needle-Pro® device open halfway. Grasp sheath using the plastic peel pouch.

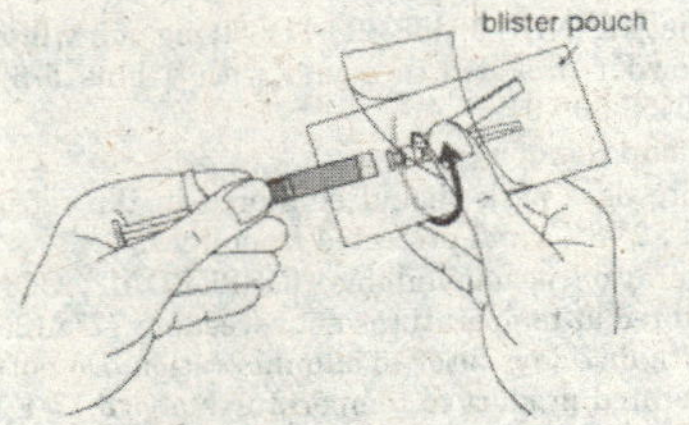

13. Attach the luer connection of the Needle-Pro® device to the syringe with an easy clockwise twisting motion. Seat the needle firmly on the Needle-Pro® device with a push and clockwise twist.
14. *If 2 minutes pass before injection, reconstitute by shaking vigorously.*
15. Pull sheath away from the needle. Do not twist sheath, as needle may be loosened from Needle-Pro® device. Tap the syringe gently to make any air bubbles rise to the top. De-aerate syringe by moving plunger rod carefully forward, with needle in an upward position. Inject entire contents intramuscularly (IM) into the upper-outer quadrant of the gluteal area within 2 minutes to avoid settling. **DO NOT ADMINISTER INTRAVENOUSLY.**

Continued on next page

Risperdal Consta—Cont.

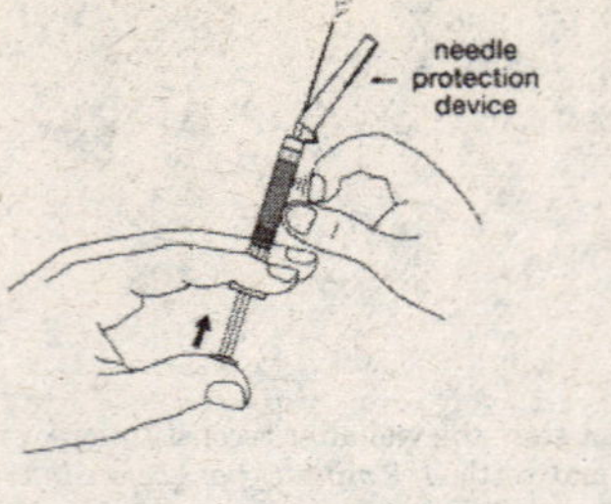

WARNING: To avoid a needle stick injury with a contaminated needle, do not:
- intentionally disengage the Needle-Pro® device
- attempt to straighten the needle or engage Needle-Pro® device if the needle is bent or damaged
- mishandle the needle protection device which could lead to protrusion of the needle from the needle protector sheath

16. After injection is complete, use only one hand and tabletop or other hard surface to snap needle into the orange safety guard before discarding. Discard needle appropriately.

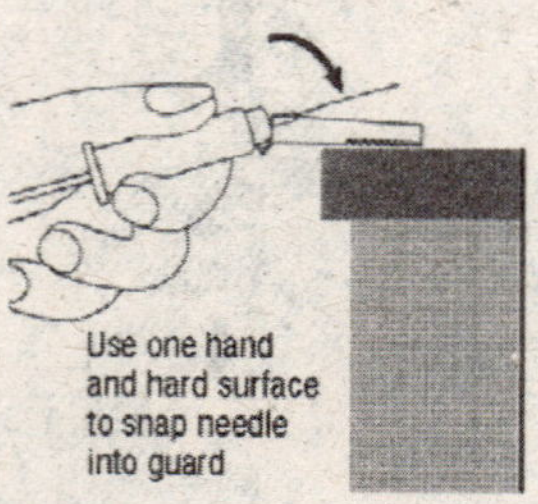

Upon suspension in the diluent, it is recommended to use RISPERDAL® CONSTA™ immediately. RISPERDAL® CONSTA™ must be used within 6 hours of suspension. Resuspension of RISPERDAL® CONSTA™ will be necessary prior to administration, as settling will occur over time once the product is in suspension. Keeping the vial upright, shake vigorously back and forth for as long as it takes to resuspend the microspheres. Once in suspension, the product should not be exposed to temperatures above 77°F (25°C).

Parenteral drug products should be inspected visually for particulate matter and discoloration prior to administration, whenever solution and container permit.

HOW SUPPLIED

RISPERDAL® CONSTA™ (risperidone) is available in dosage strengths of 25, 37.5, or 50 mg risperidone. It is provided as a dose pack, consisting of a vial containing the risperidone microspheres, a pre-filled syringe containing 2 mL of diluent for RISPERDAL® CONSTA™, a SmartSite® Needle-Free Vial Access Device, and one Needle-Pro® safety needle for intramuscular injection (20 G TW needle with needle protection device).

25-mg vial/kit (NDC 50458-306-11): 25 mg of a white to off-white powder provided in a vial with a pink flip-off cap (NDC 50458-306-01).

37.5-mg vial/kit (NDC 50458-307-11): 37.5 mg of a white to off-white powder provided in a vial with a green flip-off cap (NDC 50458-307-01).

50-mg vial/kit (NDC 50458-308-11): 50 mg of a white to off-white powder provided in a vial with a blue flip-off cap (NDC 50458-308-01).

Storage and Handling

The entire dose pack should be stored in the refrigerator (36°-46°F; 2°-8°C) and protected from light.

If refrigeration is unavailable, RISPERDAL® CONSTA™ can be stored at temperatures not exceeding 77°F (25°C) for no more than 7 days prior to administration. Do not expose unrefrigerated product to temperatures above 77°F (25°C).

Keep out of reach of children.

7519501
US Patent 4,804,663
January 2004

Risperidone is manufactured by:
Janssen Pharmaceutical Ltd.
Wallingstown, Little Island, County Cork, Ireland
Microspheres are manufactured by:
Alkermes Controlled Therapeutics II
Wilmington, Ohio
Diluent is manufactured by:
Vetter Pharma Fertigung GmbH & Co. KG
Ravensburg, Germany
RISPERDAL® CONSTA™ is distributed by:
Janssen Pharmaceutica Products, L.P.
Titusville, NJ 08560

Eli Lilly and Company

LILLY CORPORATE CENTER
INDIANAPOLIS, IN 46285

Direct Inquiries to:
Lilly Corporate Center
Indianapolis, IN 46285
(317) 276-2000
www.lilly.com
For Medical Information Contact:
Lilly Research Laboratories
Lilly Corporate Center
Indianapolis, IN 46285
(800) 545-5979

ALIMTA® ℞

[*ā-lĭm-tă*]
pemetrexed for injection

DESCRIPTION

ALIMTA®, pemetrexed for injection, is an antifolate antineoplastic agent that exerts its action by disrupting folate-dependent metabolic processes essential for cell replication. Pemetrexed disodium heptahydrate has the chemical name L-Glutamic acid, *N*-[4-[2-(2-amino-4,7-dihydro-4-oxo-1*H*-pyrrolo[2,3-*d*]pyrimidin-5-yl)ethyl]benzoyl]-, disodium salt, heptahydrate. It is a white to almost-white solid with a molecular formula of $C_{20}H_{19}N_5Na_2O_6 \bullet 7H_2O$ and a molecular weight of 597.49. The structural formula is as follows:

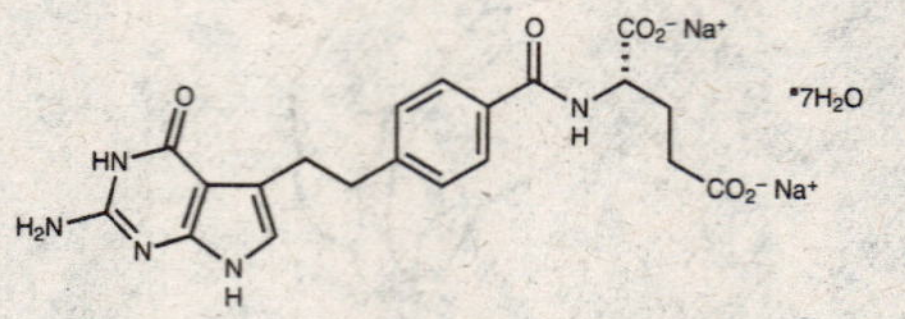

ALIMTA is supplied as a sterile lyophilized powder for intravenous infusion available in single-dose vials. The product is a white to either light yellow or green-yellow lyophilized solid. Each 500-mg vial of ALIMTA contains pemetrexed disodium equivalent to 500 mg pemetrexed and 500 mg of mannitol. Hydrochloric acid and/or sodium hydroxide may have been added to adjust pH.

CLINICAL PHARMACOLOGY

Pharmacodynamics

Pemetrexed is an antifolate containing the pyrrolopyrimidine-based nucleus that exerts its antineoplastic activity by disrupting folate-dependent metabolic processes essential for cell replication. In vitro studies have shown that pemetrexed inhibits thymidylate synthase (TS), dihydrofolate reductase (DHFR), and glycinamide ribonucleotide formyltransferase (GARFT), all folate-dependent enzymes involved in the de novo biosynthesis of thymidine and purine nucleotides. Pemetrexed is transported into cells by both the reduced folate carrier and membrane folate binding protein transport systems. Once in the cell, pemetrexed is converted to polyglutamate forms by the enzyme folyl polyglutamate synthase. The polyglutamate forms are retained in cells and are inhibitors of TS and GARFT. Polyglutamation is a time- and concentration-dependent process that occurs in tumor cells and, to a lesser extent, in normal tissues. Polyglutamated metabolites have an increased intracellular half-life resulting in prolonged drug action in malignant cells.

Preclinical studies have shown that pemetrexed inhibits the in vitro growth of mesothelioma cell lines (MSTO-211H, NCI-H2052). Studies with the MSTO-211H mesothelioma cell line showed synergistic effects when pemetrexed was combined concurrently with cisplatin.

Absolute neutrophil counts (ANC) following single-agent administration of pemetrexed to patients not receiving folic acid and vitamin B_{12} supplementation were characterized using population pharmacodynamic analyses. Severity of hematologic toxicity, as measured by the depth of the ANC nadir, is inversely proportional to the systemic exposure of ALIMTA. It was also observed that lower ANC nadirs occurred in patients with elevated baseline cystathionine or homocysteine concentrations. The levels of these substances can be reduced by folic acid and vitamin B_{12} supplementation. There is no cumulative effect of pemetrexed exposure on ANC nadir over multiple treatment cycles.

Time to ANC nadir with pemetrexed systemic exposure (AUC), varied between 8 to 9.6 days over a range of exposures from 38.3 to 316.8 μg•hr/mL. Return to baseline ANC occurred 4.2 to 7.5 days after the nadir over the same range of exposures.

Pharmacokinetics

The pharmacokinetics of pemetrexed administered as a single agent in doses ranging from 0.2 to 838 mg/m² infused over a 10-minute period have been evaluated in 426 cancer patients with a variety of solid tumors. Pemetrexed is not metabolized to an appreciable extent and is primarily eliminated in the urine, with 70% to 90% of the dose recovered unchanged within the first 24 hours following administration. The total systemic clearance of pemetrexed is 91.8 mL/min and the elimination half-life of pemetrexed is 3.5 hours in patients with normal renal function (creatinine clearance of 90 mL/min). The clearance decreases, and exposure (AUC) increases, as renal function decreases. Pemetrexed total systemic exposure (AUC) and maximum plasma concentration (C_{max}) increase proportionally with dose. The pharmacokinetics of pemetrexed do not change over multiple treatment cycles. Pemetrexed has a steady-state volume of distribution of 16.1 liters. In vitro studies indicate that pemetrexed is approximately 81% bound to plasma proteins. Binding is not affected by degree of renal impairment.

Drug Interactions

Chemotherapeutic Agents—Cisplatin does not affect the pharmacokinetics of pemetrexed and the pharmacokinetics of total platinum are unaltered by pemetrexed.

Vitamins—Coadministration of oral folic acid or intramuscular vitamin B_{12} does not affect the pharmacokinetics of pemetrexed.

Drugs Metabolized by Cytochrome P450 Enzymes—Results from in vitro studies with human liver microsomes predict that pemetrexed would not cause clinically significant inhibition of metabolic clearance of drugs metabolized by CYP3A, CYP2D6, CYP2C9, and CYP1A2. No studies were conducted to determine the cytochrome P450 isozyme induction potential of pemetrexed, because ALIMTA used as recommended (once every 21 days) would not be expected to cause any significant enzyme induction.

Aspirin—Aspirin, administered in low to moderate doses (325 mg every 6 hours), does not affect the pharmacokinetics of pemetrexed. The effect of greater doses of aspirin on pemetrexed pharmacokinetics is unknown.

Ibuprofen—Daily ibuprofen doses of 400 mg qid reduce pemetrexed's clearance by about 20% (and increase AUC by 20%) in patients with normal renal function. The effect of greater doses of ibuprofen on pemetrexed pharmacokinetics is unknown (*see* **Drug Interactions** *under* **PRECAUTIONS**).

Special Populations

The pharmacokinetics of pemetrexed in special populations were examined in about 400 patients in controlled and single arm studies.

Geriatric—No effect of age on the pharmacokinetics of pemetrexed was observed over a range of 26 to 80 years.

Pediatric—Pediatric patients were not included in clinical trials.

Gender—The pharmacokinetics of pemetrexed were not different in male and female patients.

Race—The pharmacokinetics of pemetrexed were similar in Caucasians and patients of African descent. Insufficient data are available to compare pharmacokinetics for other ethnic groups.

Hepatic Insufficiency—There was no effect of elevated AST (SGOT), ALT (SGPT), or total bilirubin on the pharmacokinetics of pemetrexed. However, studies of hepatically impaired patients have not been conducted (*see* **PRECAUTIONS**).

Renal Insufficiency—Pharmacokinetic analyses of pemetrexed included 127 patients with reduced renal function. Plasma clearance of pemetrexed in the presence of cisplatin decreases as renal function decreases, with increase in systemic exposure. Patients with creatinine clearances of 45, 50, and 80 mL/min had 65%, 54%, and 13% increases, respectively in pemetrexed total systemic exposure (AUC) compared to patients with creatinine clearance of 100 mL/min (*see* **WARNINGS** *and* **DOSAGE AND ADMINISTRATION**).

CLINICAL STUDIES

Malignant Pleural Mesothelioma—The safety and efficacy of ALIMTA have been evaluated in chemonaive patients with malignant pleural mesothelioma (MPM) in combination with cisplatin.

Randomized Trial: A multi-center, randomized, single-blind study in 448 chemonaive patients with MPM compared survival in patients treated with ALIMTA in combination with cisplatin to survival in patients receiving cisplatin alone. ALIMTA was administered intravenously over 10 minutes at a dose of 500 mg/m² and cisplatin was administered intravenously over 2 hours at a dose of 75 mg/m² beginning approximately 30 minutes after the end of administration of ALIMTA. Both drugs were given on Day 1 of each 21-day cycle. After 112 patients were treated, white cell and GI toxicity led to a change in protocol whereby all patients were given folic acid and vitamin B_{12} supplementation.

The primary analysis of this study was performed on the population of all patients randomly assigned to treatment who received study drug (randomized and treated). An analysis was also performed on patients who received folic acid and vitamin B_{12} supplementation during the entire course of study therapy (fully supplemented), as supplementation is recommended (*see* **DOSAGE AND ADMINISTRATION**). Results in all patients and those fully supplemented were similar. Patient demographics are shown in Table 1.

[See table 1 on next page]

Table 2 summarizes the survival results for all randomized and treated patients regardless of vitamin supplementation status and those patients receiving vitamin supplementation from the time of enrollment in the trial.

[See table 2 at bottom of next page]

Similar results were seen in the analysis of patients (N=303) with confirmed histologic diagnosis of malignant pleural mesothelioma. Exploratory demographic analyses showed no apparent differences in patients over or under 65. There were too few non-white patients to assess possible ethnic differences. The effect in women (median survival 15.7 months with the combination vs. 7.5 months on cisplatin alone), however, was larger than the effect in males (median survival 11 vs. 9.4 respectively). As with any exploratory analysis, it is not clear whether this difference is real or is a chance finding.

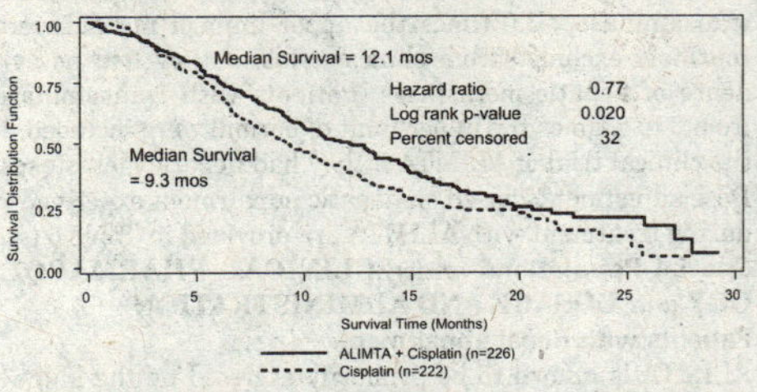

Figure 1: Kaplan-Meier Estimates of Survival Time for ALIMTA plus Cisplatin and Cisplatin Alone in all Randomized and Treated Patients.

Objective tumor response for malignant pleural mesothelioma is difficult to measure and response criteria are not universally agreed upon. However, based upon prospectively defined criteria, the objective tumor response rate for ALIMTA plus cisplatin was greater than the objective tumor response rate for cisplatin alone. There was also improvement in lung function (forced vital capacity) in the ALIMTA plus cisplatin arm compared to the control arm.

Patients who received full supplementation with folic acid and vitamin B_{12} during study therapy received a median of 6 and 4 cycles in the ALIMTA/cisplatin (N=168) and cisplatin (N=163) arms, respectively. Patients who never received folic acid and vitamin B_{12} during study therapy received a median of 2 cycles in both treatment arms (N=32 and N=38 for the ALIMTA/cisplatin and cisplatin arm, respectively). Patients receiving ALIMTA in the fully supplemented group received a relative dose intensity of 93% of the protocol specified ALIMTA dose intensity; patients treated with cisplatin in the same group received 94% of the projected dose intensity. Patients treated with cisplatin alone had a dose intensity of 96%.

INDICATIONS AND USAGE

ALIMTA in combination with cisplatin is indicated for the treatment of patients with malignant pleural mesothelioma whose disease is unresectable or who are otherwise not candidates for curative surgery.

CONTRAINDICATIONS

ALIMTA is contraindicated in patients who have a history of severe hypersensitivity reaction to pemetrexed or to any other ingredient used in the formulation.

WARNINGS

Decreased Renal Function

ALIMTA is primarily eliminated unchanged by renal excretion. No dosage adjustment is needed in patients with creatinine clearance ≥45 mL/min. Insufficient numbers of patients have been studied with creatinine clearance <45 mL/min to give a dose recommendation. Therefore, ALIMTA should not be administered to patients whose creatinine clearance is <45 mL/min (*see* **Dose Reduction Recommendations** *under* **DOSAGE AND ADMINISTRATION**).

One patient with severe renal impairment (creatinine clearance 19 mL/min) who did not receive folic acid and vitamin B_{12} died of drug-related toxicity following administration of ALIMTA alone.

Bone Marrow Suppression

ALIMTA can suppress bone marrow function, manifested by neutropenia, thrombocytopenia, and anemia (*see* **ADVERSE REACTIONS**); myelosuppression is usually the dose-limiting toxicity. Dose reductions for subsequent cycles are based on nadir ANC, platelet count, and maximum nonhematologic toxicity seen in the previous cycle (*see* **Dose Reduction Recommendations** *under* **DOSAGE AND ADMINISTRATION**).

Need for Folate and Vitamin B_{12} Supplementation

Patients treated with ALIMTA must be instructed to take folic acid and vitamin B_{12} as a prophylactic measure to reduce treatment-related hematologic and GI toxicity (*see* **DOSAGE AND ADMINISTRATION**). In clinical studies, less overall toxicity and reductions in Grade 3/4 hematologic and nonhematologic toxicities such as neutropenia, febrile neutropenia, and infection with Grade 3/4 neutropenia were reported when pretreatment with folic acid and vitamin B_{12} was administered.

Pregnancy Category D

ALIMTA may cause fetal harm when administered to a pregnant woman. Pemetrexed was fetotoxic and teratogenic in mice at i.v. doses of 0.2 mg/kg (0.6 mg/m^2) or 5 mg/kg (15 mg/m^2) when given on gestation days 6 through 15. Pemetrexed caused fetal malformations (incomplete ossification of talus and skull bone) at 0.2 mg/kg (about 1/833 the recommended i.v. human dose on a mg/m^2 basis), and cleft palate at 5 mg/kg (about 1/33 the recommended i.v. human dose on a mg/m^2 basis). Embryotoxicity was characterized by increased embryo-fetal deaths and reduced litter sizes. There are no studies of ALIMTA in pregnant women. Patients should be advised to avoid becoming pregnant. If ALIMTA is used during pregnancy, or if the patient becomes pregnant while taking ALIMTA, the patient should be apprised of the potential hazard to the fetus.

PRECAUTIONS

General

ALIMTA should be administered under the supervision of a qualified physician experienced in the use of antineoplastic agents. Appropriate management of complications is possible only when adequate diagnostic and treatment facilities are readily available. Treatment-related adverse events of ALIMTA seen in clinical trials have been reversible. Skin rash has been reported more frequently in patients not pretreated with a corticosteroid in clinical trials. Pretreatment with dexamethasone (or equivalent) reduces the incidence and severity of cutaneous reaction (*see* **DOSAGE AND ADMINISTRATION**).

The effect of third space fluid, such as pleural effusion and ascites, on ALIMTA is unknown. In patients with clinically significant third space fluid, consideration should be given to draining the effusion prior to ALIMTA administration.

Laboratory Tests

Complete blood cell counts, including platelet counts and periodic chemistry tests, should be performed on all patients receiving ALIMTA. Patients should be monitored for nadir and recovery, which were tested in the clinical study before each dose and on days 8 and 15 of each cycle. Patients should not begin a new cycle of treatment unless the ANC is ≥1500 cells/mm^3, the platelet count is ≥100,000 cells/mm^3, and creatinine clearance is ≥45 mL/min.

Drug Interactions

ALIMTA is primarily eliminated unchanged renally as a result of glomerular filtration and tubular secretion. Concomitant administration of nephrotoxic drugs could result in delayed clearance of ALIMTA. Concomitant administration of substances that are also tubularly secreted (e.g., probenecid) could potentially result in delayed clearance of ALIMTA.

Although ibuprofen (400 mg qid) can be administered with ALIMTA in patients with normal renal function (creatinine clearance ≥80 mL/min), caution should be used when administering ibuprofen concurrently with ALIMTA to patients with mild to moderate renal insufficiency (creatinine clearance from 45 to 79 mL/min). Patients with mild to moderate renal insufficiency should avoid taking NSAIDs with short elimination half-lives for a period of 2 days before, the day of, and 2 days following administration of ALIMTA.

In the absence of data regarding potential interaction between ALIMTA and NSAIDs with longer half-lives, all patients taking these NSAIDs should interrupt dosing for at least 5 days before, the day of, and 2 days following ALIMTA administration. If concomitant administration of an NSAID is necessary, patients should be monitored closely for toxicity, especially myelosuppression, renal, and gastrointestinal toxicity.

Drug/Laboratory Test Interactions

None known.

Carcinogenesis, Mutagenesis, Impairment of Fertility

No carcinogenicity studies have been conducted with pemetrexed. Pemetrexed was clastogenic in the in vivo micronucleus assay in mouse bone marrow but was not mutagenic in multiple in vitro tests (Ames assay, CHO cell assay). Pemetrexed administered at i.v. doses of 0.1 mg/kg/day or greater to male mice (about 1/1666 the recommended human dose on a mg/m^2 basis) resulted in reduced fertility, hypospermia, and testicular atrophy.

Pregnancy

Pregnancy Category D (*see* **WARNINGS**).

Nursing Mothers

It is not known whether ALIMTA or its metabolites are excreted in human milk. Because many drugs are excreted in human milk, and because of the potential for serious ad-

Continued on next page

Table 1: Summary of Patient Characteristics

Patient characteristic	Randomized and Treated Patients		Fully Supplemented Patients	
	ALIMTA/cis (N=226)	Cisplatin (N=222)	ALIMTA/cis (N=168)	Cisplatin (N=163)
Age (yrs)				
Median (range)	61 (29-85)	60 (19-84)	60 (29-85)	60 (19–82)
Gender (%)				
Male	184 (81.4)	181 (81.5)	136 (81.0)	134 (82.2)
Female	42 (18.6)	41 (18.5)	32 (19.0)	29 (17.8)
Origin (%)				
Caucasian	204 (90.3)	206 (92.8)	150 (89.3)	153 (93.9)
Hispanic	11 (4.9)	12 (5.4)	10 (6.0)	7 (4.3)
Asian	10 (4.4)	4 (1.9)	7 (4.2)	3 (1.8)
African descent	1 (0.4)	0	1 (0.6)	0
Stage at Entry (%)				
I	16 (7.1)	14 (6.3)	15 (8.9)	12 (7.4)
II	35 (15.6)	33 (15.0)	27 (16.2)	27 (16.8)
III	73 (32.4)	68 (30.6)	51 (30.5)	49 (30.4)
IV	101 (44.9)	105 (47.2)	74 (44.3)	73 (45.3)
Unspecified	1 (0.4)	2 (0.9)	1 (0.6)	2 (1.2)
Diagnosis/Histology[a] (%)				
Epithelial	154 (68.1)	152 (68.5)	117 (69.6)	113 (69.3)
Mixed	37 (16.4)	36 (16.2)	25 (14.9)	25 (15.3)
Sarcomatoid	18 (8.0)	25 (11.3)	14 (8.3)	17 (10.4)
Other	17 (7.5)	9 (4.1)	12 (7.1)	8 (4.9)
Baseline KPS[b] (%)				
70-80	109 (48.2)	97 (43.7)	83 (49.4)	69 (42.3)
90-100	117 (51.8)	125 (56.3)	85 (50.6)	94 (57.7)

[a] Only 67% of the patients had the histologic diagnosis of malignant mesothelioma confirmed by independent review.
[b] Karnofsky Performance Scale.

Table 2: Efficacy of ALIMTA plus Cisplatin vs. Cisplatin in Malignant Pleural Mesothelioma

Efficacy Parameter	Randomized and Treated Patients		Fully Supplemented Patients	
	ALIMTA/cis (N=226)	Cisplatin (N=222)	ALIMTA/cis (N=168)	Cisplatin (N=163)
Median overall survival (95% CI)	12.1 mos (10.0-14.4)	9.3 mos (7.8-10.7)	13.3 mos (11.4-14.9)	10.0 mos (8.4-11.9)
Hazard ratio Log rank p-value*	0.77 0.020		0.75 0.051	

*p-value refers to comparison between arms.

Alimta—Cont.

verse reactions in nursing infants from ALIMTA, it is recommended that nursing be discontinued if the mother is treated with ALIMTA.

Pediatric Use

The safety and effectiveness of ALIMTA in pediatric patients have not been established.

Geriatric Use

Dose adjustments based on age other than those recommended for all patients have not been necessary (*see* **Special Populations** *under* CLINICAL PHARMACOLOGY *and* DOSAGE AND ADMINISTRATION).

Gender

Dose adjustments based on gender other than those recommended for all patients have not been necessary (*see* **Special Populations** *under* CLINICAL PHARMACOLOGY *and* DOSAGE AND ADMINISTRATION).

Patients with Hepatic Impairment

Patients with bilirubin >1.5 times the upper limit of normal were excluded from clinical trials of ALIMTA. Patients with transaminase >3.0 times the upper limit of normal were routinely excluded from clinical trials if they had no evidence of hepatic metastases. Patients with transaminase from 3 to 5 times the upper limit of normal were included in the clinical trial of ALIMTA if they had hepatic metastases. Dose adjustments based on hepatic impairment experienced during treatment with ALIMTA are provided in Table 6 (*see* **Special Populations** *under* CLINICAL PHARMACOLOGY *and* DOSAGE AND ADMINISTRATION).

Patients with Renal Impairment

ALIMTA is known to be primarily excreted by the kidney. Decreased renal function will result in reduced clearance and greater exposure (AUC) to ALIMTA compared with patients with normal renal function. Cisplatin coadministration with ALIMTA has not been studied in patients with moderate renal impairment (*see* **Special Populations** *under* CLINICAL PHARMACOLOGY).

ADVERSE REACTIONS

In Table 3 adverse events occurring in at least 5% of patients are shown along with important effects (renal failure, infection) occurring at lower rates. Adverse events equally or more common in the cisplatin group are not included. The adverse effects more common in the ALIMTA group were primarily hematologic effects, fever and infection, stomatitis/pharyngitis, and rash/desquamation.

[See table 3 at left]

Table 3: Adverse Events* in Fully Supplemented Patients Receiving ALIMTA plus Cisplatin in MPM CTC Grades (% incidence)

	All Reported Adverse Events Regardless of Causality					
	ALIMTA/cis (N=168)			Cisplatin (N=163)		
	All Grades	Grade 3	Grade 4	All Grades	Grade 3	Grade 4
Laboratory						
Hematologic						
Neutropenia	58	19	5	16	3	1
Leukopenia	55	14	2	20	1	0
Anemia	33	5	1	14	0	0
Thrombocytopenia	27	4	1	10	0	0
Renal						
Creatinine elevation	16	1	0	12	1	0
Renal failure	2	0	1	1	0	0
Clinical						
Constitutional Symptoms						
Fatigue	80	17	0	74	12	1
Fever	17	0	0	9	0	0
Other constitutional symptoms	11	2	1	8	1	1
Cardiovascular General						
Thrombosis/embolism	7	4	2	4	3	1
Gastrointestinal						
Nausea	84	11	1	79	6	0
Vomiting	58	10	1	52	4	1
Constipation	44	2	1	39	1	0
Anorexia	35	2	0	25	1	0
Stomatitis/pharyngitis	28	2	1	9	0	0
Diarrhea without colostomy	26	4	0	16	1	0
Dehydration	7	3	1	1	1	0
Dysphagia/esophagitis/ odynophagia	6	1	0	6	0	0
Pulmonary						
Dyspnea	66	10	1	62	5	2
Pain						
Chest pain	40	8	1	30	5	1
Neurology						
Neuropathy/sensory	17	0	0	15	1	0
Mood alteration/depression	14	1	0	9	1	0
Infection/Febrile Neutropenia						
Infection without neutropenia	11	1	1	4	0	0
Infection with Grade 3 or Grade 4 neutropenia	6	1	0	4	0	0
Infection/febrile neutropenia-other	3	1	0	2	0	0
Febrile neutropenia	1	1	0	1	0	0
Immune						
Allergic reaction/hypersensitivity	2	0	0	1	0	0
Dermatology/Skin						
Rash/desquamation	22	1	0	9	0	0

* Refer to NCI CTC Version 2.0.

Table 4 compares the incidence (percentage of patients) of CTC Grade 3/4 toxicities in patients who received vitamin supplementation with daily folic acid and vitamin B_{12} from the time of enrollment in the study (fully supplemented) with the incidence in patients who never received vitamin supplementation (never supplemented) during the study in the ALIMTA plus cisplatin arm.

Table 4: Selected Grade 3/4 Adverse Events Comparing Fully Supplemented versus Never Supplemented Patients in the ALIMTA plus Cisplatin arm (% incidence)

Adverse Event Regardless of Causality[a](%)	**Fully Supplemented Patients** (N=168)	**Never Supplemented Patients** (N=32)
Neutropenia	24	38
Thrombocytopenia	5	9
Nausea	12	31
Vomiting	11	34
Anorexia	2	9
Diarrhea without colostomy	4	9
Dehydration	4	9
Fever	0	6
Febrile neutropenia	1	9
Infection with Grade 3/4 neutropenia	1	6
Fatigue	17	25

[a] Refer to NCI CTC criteria for lab and non-laboratory values for each grade of toxicity (Version 2.0).

The following adverse events were greater in the fully supplemented group compared to the never supplemented group: hypertension (11%, 3%), chest pain (8%, 6%), and thrombosis/embolism (6%, 3%).

For fully supplemented patients treated with ALIMTA plus cisplatin, the incidence of CTC Grade 3/4 fatigue, leukopenia, neutropenia, and thrombocytopenia were greater in patients 65 years or older as compared to patients younger than 65. No relevant effect for ALIMTA safety due to gender or race was identified, except an increased incidence of rash in men (24%) compared to women (16%).

OVERDOSAGE

There have been few cases of ALIMTA overdose. Reported toxicities included neutropenia, anemia, thrombocytopenia, mucositis, and rash. Anticipated complications of overdose include bone marrow suppression as manifested by neutropenia, thrombocytopenia, and anemia. In addition, infection with or without fever, diarrhea, and mucositis may be seen. If an overdose occurs, general supportive measures should be instituted as deemed necessary by the treating physician.

In clinical trials, leucovorin was permitted for CTC Grade 4 leukopenia lasting ≥3 days, CTC Grade 4 neutropenia lasting ≥3 days, and immediately for CTC Grade 4 thrombocytopenia, bleeding associated with Grade 3 thrombocytopenia, or Grade 3 or 4 mucositis. The following intravenous doses and schedules of leucovorin were recommended for intravenous use: 100 mg/m^2, intravenously once, followed by leucovorin, 50 mg/m^2, intravenously every 6 hours for 8 days.

The ability of ALIMTA to be dialyzed is unknown.

DOSAGE AND ADMINISTRATION

ALIMTA is for Intravenous Infusion Only

Combination Use With Cisplatin

Malignant Pleural Mesothelioma—The recommended dose of ALIMTA is 500 mg/m^2 administered as an intravenous infusion over 10 minutes on Day 1 of each 21-day cycle. The recommended dose of cisplatin is 75 mg/m^2 infused over 2 hours beginning approximately 30 minutes after the end of ALIMTA administration. Patients should receive hydration consistent with local practice prior to and/or after receiving cisplatin. See cisplatin package insert for more information.

Premedication Regimen

Corticosteroid—Skin rash has been reported more frequently in patients not pretreated with a corticosteroid. Pretreatment with dexamethasone (or equivalent) reduces the incidence and severity of cutaneous reaction. In clinical trials, dexamethasone 4 mg was given by mouth twice daily the day before, the day of, and the day after ALIMTA administration.

Vitamin Supplementation—To reduce toxicity, patients treated with ALIMTA must be instructed to take a low-dose oral folic acid preparation or multivitamin with folic acid on a daily basis. At least 5 daily doses of folic acid must be taken during the 7-day period preceding the first dose of ALIMTA; and dosing should continue during the full course of therapy and for 21 days after the last dose of ALIMTA. Patients must also receive one (1) intramuscular injection of vitamin B_{12} during the week preceding the first dose of ALIMTA and every 3 cycles thereafter. Subsequent vitamin B_{12} injections may be given the same day as ALIMTA. In clinical trials, the dose of folic acid studied ranged from 350 to 1000 µg, and the dose of vitamin B_{12} was 1000 µg. The most commonly used dose of oral folic acid in clinical trials was 400 µg (*see* **WARNINGS**).

Laboratory Monitoring and Dose Reduction Recommendations

Monitoring—Complete blood cell counts, including platelet counts, should be performed on all patients receiving ALIMTA. Patients should be monitored for nadir and recovery, which were tested in the clinical study before each dose and on days 8 and 15 of each cycle. Patients should not begin a new cycle of treatment unless the ANC is ≥1500 cells/mm^3, the platelet count is ≥100,000 cells/mm^3, and creatinine clearance is ≥45 mL/min. Periodic chemistry tests should be performed to evaluate renal and hepatic function.

Dose Reduction Recommendations—Dose adjustments at the start of a subsequent cycle should be based on nadir hematologic counts or maximum nonhematologic toxicity from the preceding cycle of therapy. Treatment may be delayed to allow sufficient time for recovery. Upon recovery, patients should be retreated using the guidelines in Tables 5–7.

Table 5: Dose Reduction for ALIMTA and Cisplatin - Hematologic Toxicities

Nadir ANC <500/mm^3 and nadir platelets ≥50,000/mm^3.	75% of previous dose (both drugs).
Nadir platelets <50,000/mm^3 regardless of nadir ANC.	50% of previous dose (both drugs).

If patients develop nonhematologic toxicities (excluding neurotoxicity) ≥Grade 3 (except Grade 3 transaminase elevations), ALIMTA should be withheld until resolution to less than or equal to the patient's pre-therapy value. Treatment should be resumed according to guidelines in Table 6.

Table 6: Dose Reduction - Nonhematologic Toxicities[a,b]

	Dose of ALIMTA (mg/m^2)	Dose of Cisplatin (mg/m^2)
Any Grade 3[c] or 4 toxicities except mucositis	75% of previous dose	75% of previous dose
Any diarrhea requiring hospitalization	75% of previous dose	75% of previous dose
Grade 3 or 4 mucositis	50% of previous dose	100% of previous dose

[a] NCI Common Toxicity Criteria (CTC).
[b] Excluding neurotoxicity.
[c] Except Grade 3 transaminase elevation.

In the event of neurotoxicity, the recommended dose adjustments for ALIMTA and cisplatin are described in Table 7. Patients should discontinue therapy if Grade 3 or 4 neurotoxicity is experienced.

Table 7: Dose Reduction for ALIMTA and Cisplatin - Neurotoxicity

CTC Grade	Dose of ALIMTA (mg/m^2)	Dose of Cisplatin (mg/m^2)
0-1	100% of previous dose	100% of previous dose
2	100% of previous dose	50% of previous dose

ALIMTA therapy should be discontinued if a patient experiences any hematologic or nonhematologic Grade 3 or 4 toxicity after 2 dose reductions (except Grade 3 transaminase elevations) or immediately if Grade 3 or 4 neurotoxicity is observed.

Elderly Patients—No dose reductions other than those recommended for all patients are necessary for patients ≥65 years of age.

Children—ALIMTA is not recommended for use in children, as safety and efficacy have not been established in children.

Renally Impaired Patients—In clinical studies, patients with creatinine clearance ≥45 mL/min required no dose adjustments other than those recommended for all patients. Insufficient numbers of patients with creatinine clearance below 45 mL/min have been treated to make dosage recommendations for this group of patients. Therefore, ALIMTA should not be administered to patients whose creatinine clearance is <45 mL/min using the standard Cockcroft and Gault formula (below) or GFR measured by Tc99m-DPTA serum clearance method:

[See table below]

Caution should be exercised when administering ALIMTA concurrently with NSAIDs to patients whose creatinine clearance is <80 mL/min (*see* **Drug Interactions** *under* **PRECAUTIONS**).

Hepatically Impaired Patients—ALIMTA is not extensively metabolized by the liver. Dose adjustments based on hepatic impairment experienced during treatment with ALIMTA are provided in Table 6 (*see* **Patients with Hepatic Impairment** *under* **PRECAUTIONS**).

Preparation and Administration Precautions

As with other potentially toxic anticancer agents, care should be exercised in the handling and preparation of infusion solutions of ALIMTA. The use of gloves is recommended. If a solution of ALIMTA contacts the skin, wash the skin immediately and thoroughly with soap and water. If ALIMTA contacts the mucous membranes, flush thoroughly with water. Several published guidelines for handling and disposal of anticancer agents are available.[1–8] There is no general agreement that all of the procedures recommended in the guidelines are necessary or appropriate.

ALIMTA is not a vesicant. There is no specific antidote for extravasation of ALIMTA. To date, there have been few reported cases of ALIMTA extravasation, which were not assessed as serious by the investigator. ALIMTA extravasation should be managed with local standard practice for extravasation as with other non-vesicants.

Preparation for Intravenous Infusion Administration

1. Use aseptic technique during the reconstitution and further dilution of ALIMTA for intravenous infusion administration.
2. Calculate the dose and the number of ALIMTA vials needed. Each vial contains 500 mg of ALIMTA. The vial contains an excess of ALIMTA to facilitate delivery of label amount.
3. Reconstitute 500-mg vials with 20 mL of 0.9% Sodium Chloride Injection (preservative free) to give a solution containing 25 mg/mL ALIMTA. Gently swirl each vial until the powder is completely dissolved. The resulting solution is clear and ranges in color from colorless to yellow or green-yellow without adversely affecting product quality. The pH of the reconstituted ALIMTA solution is between 6.6 and 7.8. FURTHER DILUTION IS REQUIRED.
4. Parenteral drug products should be inspected visually for particulate matter and discoloration prior to administration. If particulate matter is observed, do not administer.
5. The appropriate volume of reconstituted ALIMTA solution should be further diluted to 100 mL with 0.9% Sodium Chloride Injection (preservative free) and administered as an intravenous infusion over 10 minutes.
6. Chemical and physical stability of reconstituted and infusion solutions of ALIMTA were demonstrated for up to 24 hours following initial reconstitution, when stored at refrigerated or ambient room temperature [see USP Controlled Room Temperature] and lighting. When prepared as directed, reconstitution and infusion solutions of ALIMTA contain no antimicrobial preservatives. Discard any unused portion.

Reconstitution and further dilution prior to intravenous infusion is only recommended with 0.9% Sodium Chloride Injection (preservative free). ALIMTA is physically incompatible with diluents containing calcium, including Lactated Ringer's Injection, USP and Ringer's Injection, USP and therefore these should not be used. Coadministration of ALIMTA with other drugs and diluents has not been studied, and therefore is not recommended.

HOW SUPPLIED

ALIMTA®, pemetrexed for injection is available in sterile single-use vials containing 500 mg pemetrexed.

NDC 0002-7623-01 (VL7623): single-use vial with flip-off cap individually packaged in a carton.

Storage

ALIMTA, pemetrexed for injection, should be stored at 25°C (77°F); excursions permitted to 15-30°C (59-86°F) [see USP Controlled Room Temperature].

Chemical and physical stability of reconstituted and infusion solutions of ALIMTA were demonstrated for up to 24 hours following initial reconstitution, when stored refrigerated, 2-8°C (36-46°F), or at 25°C (77°F), excursions permitted to 15-30°C (59-86°F) [see USP Controlled Room Temperature]. When prepared as directed, reconstituted and infusion solutions of ALIMTA contain no antimicrobial preservatives. Discard unused portion.

ALIMTA is not light sensitive.

REFERENCES

1. ONS Clinical Practice Committee. Cancer Chemotherapy Guidelines and Recommendations for Practice. Pittsburgh, PA: Oncology Nursing Society; 1999:32-41.
2. Recommendations for the Safe Handling of Parenteral Antineoplastic Drugs. Washington, DC: Division of Safety, Clinical Center Pharmacy Department and Cancer Nursing Services, National Institutes of Health; 1992. US Dept of Health and Human Services, Public Health Service Publication NIH 92-2621.
3. AMA Council on Scientific Affairs. Guidelines for Handling Parenteral Antineoplastics. *JAMA*. 1985;253:1590-1591.
4. National Study Commission on Cytotoxic Exposure-Recommendations for Handling Cytotoxic Agents. 1987. Available from Louis P. Jeffrey, ScD, Chairman, National Study Commission on Cytotoxic Exposure. Massachusetts College of Pharmacy and Allied Health Sciences, 179 Longwood Avenue, Boston, MA 02115.
5. Clinical Oncological Society of Australia. Guidelines and Recommendations for Safe Handling of Antineoplastic Agents. *Med J Australia*. 1983;1:426-428.
6. Jones RB, Frank R, Mass T. Safe Handling of Chemotherapeutic Agents: A Report from the Mount Sinai Medical Center. CA — *A Cancer J for Clin*. 1983;33:258-263.
7. American Society of Hospital Pharmacists. ASHP Technical Assistance Bulletin on Handling Cytotoxic and Hazardous Drugs. *Am J Hosp Pharm*. 1990;47:1033-1049.
8. Controlling Occupational Exposure to Hazardous Drugs. (OSHA Work-Practice Guidelines). *Am J Health-Syst Pharm*. 1996;53:1669-1685.

Literature issued February 5, 2004

Manufactured by Lilly France S.A.S.
F-67640 Fegersheim, France
for Eli Lilly and Company
Indianapolis, IN 46285, USA
www.ALIMTA.com

PA 9301 FSAMP

INFORMATION FOR PATIENTS AND CAREGIVERS

ALIMTA® (uh-LIM-tuh)
(pemetrexed for injection)

Read the Patient Information that comes with ALIMTA before you start treatment and each time you get treated with ALIMTA. There may be new information. This leaflet does not take the place of talking to your doctor about your medical condition or treatment. Talk to your doctor if you have any questions about ALIMTA.

What is ALIMTA?

ALIMTA is a treatment for a type of cancer called malignant pleural mesothelioma. This cancer affects the inside lining of the chest cavity. ALIMTA is given with cisplatin, another anti-cancer medicine (chemotherapy). **To lower your chances of side effects of ALIMTA, you must also take folic acid and vitamin B_{12} prior to and during your treatment with ALIMTA.** Your doctor will prescribe a medicine called a "corticosteroid" to take for 3 days during your treatment with ALIMTA. Corticosteroid medicines lower your chances of getting skin reactions with ALIMTA.

ALIMTA has not been studied in children.

What should I tell my doctor before taking ALIMTA?

Tell your doctor about all of your medical conditions, including if you:

- **are pregnant or planning to become pregnant.** ALIMTA may harm your unborn baby.
- **are breastfeeding.** It is not known if ALIMTA passes into breast milk. You should stop breastfeeding once you start treatment with ALIMTA.
- **are taking other medicines,** including prescription and nonprescription medicines, vitamins, and herbal supplements. ALIMTA and other medicines may affect each other causing serious side effects. Especially, tell your doctor if you are taking medicines called "nonsteroidal anti-inflammatory drugs" (NSAIDs) for pain or swelling. There are many NSAID medicines. If you are not sure, ask your doctor or pharmacist if any of your medicines are NSAIDs.

How is ALIMTA given?

- ALIMTA is slowly infused (injected) into a vein. The injection or infusion will last about 10 minutes. You will usually receive ALIMTA once every 21 days (3 weeks).

$$\text{Males: } \frac{[140 - \text{Age in years}] \times \text{Actual Body Weight (kg)}}{72 \times \text{Serum Creatinine (mg/dL)}} = \text{mL/min}$$

Females: Estimated creatinine clearance for males × 0.85

Continued on next page

Alimta—Cont.

- Cisplatin is infused in your vein for about 2 hours starting about 30 minutes after your treatment with ALIMTA.
- Your doctor will prescribe a medicine called a "corticosteroid" to take for 3 days during your treatment with ALIMTA. Corticosteroid medicines lower your chances for getting skin reactions with ALIMTA.
- **It is very important to take folic acid and vitamin B_{12} during your treatment with ALIMTA to lower your chances of harmful side effects.** You must start taking 350–1000 micrograms of folic acid every day for at least 5 days out of the 7 days before your first dose of ALIMTA. You must keep taking folic acid every day during the time you are getting treatment with ALIMTA, and for 21 days after your last treatment. You can get folic acid vitamins over-the-counter. Folic acid is also found in many multivitamin pills. Ask your doctor or pharmacist for help if you are not sure how to choose a folic acid product. Your doctor will give you vitamin B_{12} injections while you are getting treatment with ALIMTA. You will get your first vitamin B_{12} injection during the week before your first dose of ALIMTA, and then about every 9 weeks during treatment.
- You will have regular blood tests before and during your treatment with ALIMTA. Your doctor may adjust your dose of ALIMTA or delay treatment based on the results of your blood tests and on your general condition.

What should I avoid while taking ALIMTA?

- **Women who can become pregnant should not become pregnant during treatment with ALIMTA.** ALIMTA may harm the unborn baby.
- **Ask your doctor before taking medicines called NSAIDs.** There are many NSAID medicines. If you are not sure, ask your doctor or pharmacist if any of your medicines are NSAIDs.

What are the possible side effects of ALIMTA?

Most patients taking ALIMTA will have side effects. Sometimes it is not always possible to tell whether ALIMTA, another medicine, or the cancer itself is causing these side effects. **Call your doctor right away if you have a fever, chills, diarrhea, or mouth sores.** These symptoms could mean you have an infection.

The most common side effects of ALIMTA when taken with cisplatin are:

- **Stomach upset, including nausea, vomiting, and diarrhea.** You can obtain medicines to help control some of these symptoms. Call your doctor if you get any of these symptoms.
- **Low blood cell counts:**
  - **Low red blood cells.** Low red blood cells may make you feel tired, get tired easily, appear pale, and become short of breath.
  - **Low white blood cells.** Low white blood cells may give you a greater chance for infection. If you have a fever (temperature above 100.4°F) or other signs of infection, call your doctor right away.
  - **Low platelets.** Low platelets give you a greater chance for bleeding. Your doctor will do blood tests to check your blood counts before and during treatment with ALIMTA.
- **Tiredness.** You may feel tired or weak for a few days after your ALIMTA treatments. If you have severe weakness or tiredness, call your doctor.
- **Mouth, throat, or lip sores** (stomatitis, pharyngitis). You may get redness or sores in your mouth, throat, or on your lips. These symptoms may happen a few days after ALIMTA treatment. Talk with your doctor about proper mouth and throat care.
- **Loss of appetite.** You may lose your appetite and lose weight during your treatment. Talk to your doctor if this is a problem for you.
- **Rash.** You may get a rash or itching during treatment. These usually appear between treatments with ALIMTA and usually go away before the next treatment. Call your doctor if you get a severe rash or itching.

Talk with your doctor, nurse or pharmacist about any side effect that bothers you or that doesn't go away.

These are not all the side effects of ALIMTA. For more information, ask your doctor, nurse or pharmacist.

General information about ALIMTA

Medicines are sometimes prescribed for conditions other than those listed in patient information leaflets. ALIMTA was prescribed for your medical condition.

This leaflet summarizes the most important information about ALIMTA. If you would like more information, talk with your doctor. You can ask your doctor or pharmacist for information about ALIMTA that is written for health professionals. You can also call 1-800-LILLY-RX (1-800-545-5979) or visit www.ALIMTA.com.

Literature issued February 5, 2004

Manufactured by Lilly France S.A.S.
F-67640 Fegersheim, France
for Eli Lilly and Company
Indianapolis, IN 46285, USA
www.ALIMTA.com

PA 9301 FSAMP

SYMBYAX™ ℞

[sim-bee-ax]

(olanzapine and fluoxetine HCl capsules)

DESCRIPTION

SYMBYAX™ (olanzapine and fluoxetine HCl capsules) combines 2 psychotropic agents, olanzapine (the active ingredient in Zyprexa®, and Zyprexa Zydis®) and fluoxetine hydrochloride (the active ingredient in Prozac®, Prozac Weekly™, and Sarafem®).

Olanzapine belongs to the thienobenzodiazepine class. The chemical designation is 2-methyl-4-(4-methyl-1-piperazinyl)-10*H*-thieno[2,3-b] [1,5]benzodiazepine. The molecular formula is $C_{17}H_{20}N_4S$, which corresponds to a molecular weight of 312.44.

Fluoxetine hydrochloride is a selective serotonin reuptake inhibitor (SSRI). The chemical designation is (±)-N-methyl-3-phenyl-3-[(α,α,α-trifluoro-*p*-tolyl)oxy]propylamine hydrochloride. The molecular formula is $C_{17}H_{18}F_3NO \bullet HCl$, which corresponds to a molecular weight of 345.79.

The chemical structures are:

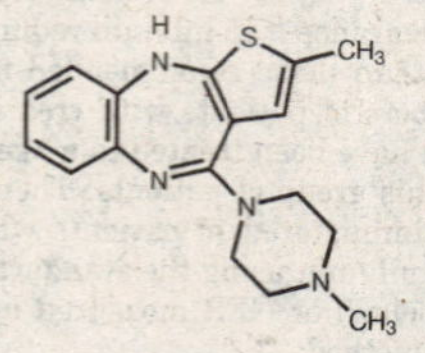

olanzapine

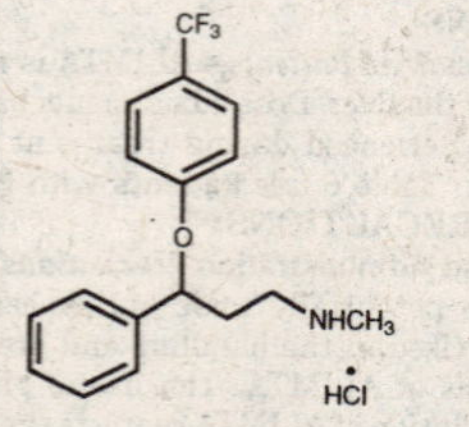

fluoxetine hydrochloride

Olanzapine is a yellow crystalline solid, which is practically insoluble in water.

Fluoxetine hydrochloride is a white to off-white crystalline solid with a solubility of 14 mg/mL in water.

SYMBYAX capsules are available for oral administration in the following strength combinations:

	6 mg/ 25 mg	6 mg/ 50 mg	12 mg/ 25 mg	12 mg/ 50 mg
olanzapine equivalent	6	6	12	12
fluoxetine base equivalent	25	50	25	50

Each capsule also contains pregelatinized starch, gelatin, dimethicone, titanium dioxide, sodium lauryl sulfate, edible black ink, red iron oxide, yellow iron oxide, and/or black iron oxide.

CLINICAL PHARMACOLOGY

Pharmacodynamics

Although the exact mechanism of SYMBYAX is unknown, it has been proposed that the activation of 3 monoaminergic neural systems (serotonin, norepinephrine, and dopamine) is responsible for its enhanced antidepressant effect. This is supported by animal studies in which the olanzapine/fluoxetine combination has been shown to produce synergistic increases in norepinephrine and dopamine release in the prefrontal cortex compared with either component alone, as well as increases in serotonin.

Olanzapine is a psychotropic agent with high affinity binding to the following receptors: serotonin $5HT_{2A/2C}$ (K_i=4 and 11 nM, respectively), dopamine D_{1-4} (K_i=11 to 31 nM), muscarinic M_{1-5} (K_i=1.9 to 25 nM), histamine H_1 (K_i=7 nM), and adrenergic α_1 receptors (K_i=19 nM). Olanzapine binds weakly to $GABA_A$, BZD, and β-adrenergic receptors (K_i>10 μM). Fluoxetine is an inhibitor of the serotonin transporter and is a weak inhibitor of the norepinephrine and dopamine transporters.

Antagonism at receptors other than dopamine and $5HT_2$ with similar receptor affinities may explain some of the other therapeutic and side effects of olanzapine. Olanzapine's antagonism of muscarinic M_{1-5} receptors may explain its anticholinergic effects. The antagonism of histamine H_1 receptors by olanzapine may explain the somnolence observed with this drug. The antagonism of α_1-adrenergic receptors by olanzapine may explain the orthostatic hypotension observed with this drug. Fluoxetine has relatively low affinity for muscarinic, α_1-adrenergic, and histamine H_1 receptors.

Pharmacokinetics

Fluoxetine (administered as a 60-mg single dose or 60 mg daily for 8 days) caused a small increase in the mean maximum concentration of olanzapine (16%) following a 5-mg dose, an increase in the mean area under the curve (17%) and a small decrease in mean apparent clearance of olanzapine (16%). In another study, a similar decrease in apparent clearance of olanzapine of 14% was observed following olanzapine doses of 6 or 12 mg with concomitant fluoxetine doses of 25 mg or more. The decrease in clearance reflects an increase in bioavailability. The terminal half-life is not affected, and therefore the time to reach steady state should not be altered. The overall steady-state plasma concentrations of olanzapine and fluoxetine when given as the combination in the therapeutic dose ranges were comparable with those typically attained with each of the monotherapies. The small change in olanzapine clearance, observed in both studies, likely reflects the inhibition of a minor metabolic pathway for olanzapine via CYP2D6 by fluoxetine, a potent CYP2D6 inhibitor, and was not deemed clinically significant. Therefore, the pharmacokinetics of the individual components is expected to reasonably characterize the overall pharmacokinetics of the combination.

Absorption and Bioavailability

SYMBYAX — Following a single oral 12-mg/50-mg dose of SYMBYAX, peak plasma concentrations of olanzapine and fluoxetine occur at approximately 4 and 6 hours, respectively. The effect of food on the absorption and bioavailability of SYMBYAX has not been evaluated. The bioavailability of olanzapine given as Zyprexa, and the bioavailability of fluoxetine given as Prozac were not affected by food. It is unlikely that there would be a significant food effect on the bioavailability of SYMBYAX.

Olanzapine — Olanzapine is well absorbed and reaches peak concentration approximately 6 hours following an oral dose. Food does not affect the rate or extent of olanzapine absorption when olanzapine is given as Zyprexa. It is eliminated extensively by first pass metabolism, with approximately 40% of the dose metabolized before reaching the systemic circulation.

Fluoxetine — Following a single oral 40-mg dose, peak plasma concentrations of fluoxetine from 15 to 55 ng/mL are observed after 6 to 8 hours. Food does not appear to affect the systemic bioavailability of fluoxetine given as Prozac, although it may delay its absorption by 1 to 2 hours, which is probably not clinically significant.

Distribution

SYMBYAX — The in vitro binding to human plasma proteins of the olanzapine/fluoxetine combination is similar to the binding of the individual components.

Olanzapine — Olanzapine is extensively distributed throughout the body, with a volume of distribution of approximately 1000 L. It is 93% bound to plasma proteins over the concentration range of 7 to 1100 ng/mL, binding primarily to albumin and α_1-acid glycoprotein.

Fluoxetine — Over the concentration range from 200 to 1000 ng/mL, approximately 94.5% of fluoxetine is bound in vitro to human serum proteins, including albumin and α_1-glycoprotein. The interaction between fluoxetine and other highly protein-bound drugs has not been fully evaluated (*see* PRECAUTIONS, Drugs tightly bound to plasma proteins).

Metabolism and Elimination

SYMBYAX — SYMBYAX therapy yielded steady-state concentrations of norfluoxetine similar to those seen with fluoxetine in the therapeutic dose range.

Olanzapine — Olanzapine displays linear pharmacokinetics over the clinical dosing range. Its half-life ranges from 21 to 54 hours (5th to 95th percentile; mean of 30 hr), and apparent plasma clearance ranges from 12 to 47 L/hr (5th to 95th percentile; mean of 25 L/hr). Administration of olanzapine once daily leads to steady-state concentrations in about 1 week that are approximately twice the concentrations after single doses. Plasma concentrations, half-life, and clearance of olanzapine may vary between individuals on the basis of smoking status, gender, and age (*see* Special Populations).

Following a single oral dose of ^{14}C-labeled olanzapine, 7% of the dose of olanzapine was recovered in the urine as unchanged drug, indicating that olanzapine is highly metabolized. Approximately 57% and 30% of the dose was recovered in the urine and feces, respectively. In the plasma, olanzapine accounted for only 12% of the AUC for total radioactivity, indicating significant exposure to metabolites. After multiple dosing, the major circulating metabolites were the 10-N-glucuronide, present at steady state at 44% of the concentration of olanzapine, and 4′-N-desmethyl olanzapine, present at steady state at 31% of the concentration of olanzapine. Both metabolites lack pharmacological activity at the concentrations observed.

Direct glucuronidation and CYP450-mediated oxidation are the primary metabolic pathways for olanzapine. In vitro studies suggest that CYP1A2, CYP2D6, and the flavin-containing monooxygenase system are involved in olanzapine oxidation. CYP2D6-mediated oxidation appears to be a minor metabolic pathway in vivo, because the clearance of olanzapine is not reduced in subjects who are deficient in this enzyme.

Fluoxetine — Fluoxetine is a racemic mixture (50/50) of *R*-fluoxetine and *S*-fluoxetine enantiomers. In animal models, both enantiomers are specific and potent serotonin uptake inhibitors with essentially equivalent pharmacologic activity. The *S*-fluoxetine enantiomer is eliminated more slowly and is the predominant enantiomer present in plasma at steady state.

Fluoxetine is extensively metabolized in the liver to its only identified active metabolite, norfluoxetine, via the CYP2D6 pathway. A number of unidentified metabolites exist.

In animal models, *S*-norfluoxetine is a potent and selective inhibitor of serotonin uptake and has activity essentially equivalent to *R*- or *S*-fluoxetine. *R*-norfluoxetine is significantly less potent than the parent drug in the inhibition of serotonin uptake. The primary route of elimination appears to be hepatic metabolism to inactive metabolites excreted by the kidney.

Clinical issues related to metabolism and elimination — The complexity of the metabolism of fluoxetine has several consequences that may potentially affect the clinical use of SYMBYAX.

Variability in metabolism — A subset (about 7%) of the population has reduced activity of the drug metabolizing enzyme CYP2D6. Such individuals are referred to as "poor metabolizers" of drugs such as debrisoquin, dextromethorphan, and the tricyclic antidepressants (TCAs). In a study involving labeled and unlabeled enantiomers administered as a racemate, these individuals metabolized *S*-fluoxetine at a slower rate and thus achieved higher concentrations of *S*-fluoxetine. Consequently, concentrations of *S*-norfluoxetine at steady state were lower. The metabolism of *R*-fluoxetine in these poor metabolizers appears normal. When compared with normal metabolizers, the total sum at steady state of the plasma concentrations of the 4 enantiomers was not significantly greater among poor metabolizers. Thus, the net pharmacodynamic activities were essentially the same. Alternative nonsaturable pathways (non-CYP2D6) also contribute to the metabolism of fluoxetine. This explains how fluoxetine achieves a steady-state concentration rather than increasing without limit.

Because the metabolism of fluoxetine, like that of a number of other compounds including TCAs and other selective serotonin antidepressants, involves the CYP2D6 system, concomitant therapy with drugs also metabolized by this enzyme system (such as the TCAs) may lead to drug interactions (*see* PRECAUTIONS, Drug Interactions).

Accumulation and slow elimination — The relatively slow elimination of fluoxetine (elimination half-life of 1 to 3 days after acute administration and 4 to 6 days after chronic administration) and its active metabolite, norfluoxetine (elimination half-life of 4 to 16 days after acute and chronic administration), leads to significant accumulation of these active species in chronic use and delayed attainment of steady state, even when a fixed dose is used. After 30 days of dosing at 40 mg/day, plasma concentrations of fluoxetine in the range of 91 to 302 ng/mL and norfluoxetine in the range of 72 to 258 ng/mL have been observed. Plasma concentrations of fluoxetine were higher than those predicted by single-dose studies, because the metabolism of fluoxetine is not proportional to dose. However, norfluoxetine appears to have linear pharmacokinetics. Its mean terminal half-life after a single dose was 8.6 days and after multiple dosing was 9.3 days. Steady-state levels after prolonged dosing are similar to levels seen at 4 to 5 weeks.

The long elimination half-lives of fluoxetine and norfluoxetine assure that, even when dosing is stopped, active drug substance will persist in the body for weeks (primarily depending on individual patient characteristics, previous dosing regimen, and length of previous therapy at discontinuation). This is of potential consequence when drug discontinuation is required or when drugs are prescribed that might interact with fluoxetine and norfluoxetine following the discontinuation of fluoxetine.

Special Populations

Geriatric — Based on the individual pharmacokinetic profiles of olanzapine and fluoxetine, the pharmacokinetics of SYMBYAX may be altered in geriatric patients. Caution should be used in dosing the elderly, especially if there are other factors that might additively influence drug metabolism and/or pharmacodynamic sensitivity.

In a study involving 24 healthy subjects, the mean elimination half-life of olanzapine was about 1.5 times greater in elderly subjects (>65 years of age) than in non-elderly subjects (≤65 years of age).

The disposition of single doses of fluoxetine in healthy elderly subjects (>65 years of age) did not differ significantly from that in younger normal subjects. However, given the long half-life and nonlinear disposition of the drug, a single-dose study is not adequate to rule out the possibility of altered pharmacokinetics in the elderly, particularly if they have systemic illness or are receiving multiple drugs for concomitant diseases. The effects of age upon the metabolism of fluoxetine have been investigated in 260 elderly but otherwise healthy depressed patients (≥60 years of age) who received 20 mg fluoxetine for 6 weeks. Combined fluoxetine plus norfluoxetine plasma concentrations were 209.3 ± 85.7 ng/mL at the end of 6 weeks. No unusual age-associated pattern of adverse events was observed in those elderly patients.

Renal impairment — The pharmacokinetics of SYMBYAX has not been studied in patients with renal impairment. However, olanzapine and fluoxetine individual pharmacokinetics do not differ significantly in patients with renal impairment. SYMBYAX dosing adjustment based upon renal impairment is not routinely required.

Because olanzapine is highly metabolized before excretion and only 7% of the drug is excreted unchanged, renal dysfunction alone is unlikely to have a major impact on the pharmacokinetics of olanzapine. The pharmacokinetic characteristics of olanzapine were similar in patients with severe renal impairment and normal subjects, indicating that dosage adjustment based upon the degree of renal impairment is not required. In addition, olanzapine is not removed by dialysis. The effect of renal impairment on olanzapine metabolite elimination has not been studied.

In depressed patients on dialysis (N=12), fluoxetine administered as 20 mg once daily for 2 months produced steady-state fluoxetine and norfluoxetine plasma concentrations comparable with those seen in patients with normal renal function. While the possibility exists that renally excreted metabolites of fluoxetine may accumulate to higher levels in patients with severe renal dysfunction, use of a lower or less frequent dose is not routinely necessary in renally impaired patients.

Hepatic impairment — Based on the individual pharmacokinetic profiles of olanzapine and fluoxetine, the pharmacokinetics of SYMBYAX may be altered in patients with hepatic impairment. The lowest starting dose should be considered for patients with hepatic impairment (*see* PRECAUTIONS, Use in patients with concomitant illness *and* DOSAGE AND ADMINISTRATION, Special Populations).

Although the presence of hepatic impairment may be expected to reduce the clearance of olanzapine, a study of the effect of impaired liver function in subjects (N=6) with clinically significant cirrhosis (Childs-Pugh Classification A and B) revealed little effect on the pharmacokinetics of olanzapine.

As might be predicted from its primary site of metabolism, liver impairment can affect the elimination of fluoxetine. The elimination half-life of fluoxetine was prolonged in a study of cirrhotic patients, with a mean of 7.6 days compared with the range of 2 to 3 days seen in subjects without liver disease; norfluoxetine elimination was also delayed, with a mean duration of 12 days for cirrhotic patients compared with the range of 7 to 9 days in normal subjects.

Gender — Clearance of olanzapine is approximately 30% lower in women than in men. There were, however, no apparent differences between men and women in effectiveness or adverse effects. Dosage modifications based on gender should not be needed.

Smoking status — Olanzapine clearance is about 40% higher in smokers than in nonsmokers, although dosage modifications are not routinely required.

Race — No SYMBYAX pharmacokinetic study was conducted to investigate the effects of race. Results from an olanzapine cross-study comparison between data obtained in Japan and data obtained in the US suggest that exposure to olanzapine may be about 2-fold greater in the Japanese when equivalent doses are administered. Olanzapine clinical study safety and efficacy data, however, did not suggest clinically significant differences among Caucasian patients, patients of African descent, and a 3rd pooled category including Asian and Hispanic patients. Dosage modifications for race, therefore, are not routinely required.

Combined effects — The combined effects of age, smoking, and gender could lead to substantial pharmacokinetic differences in populations. The clearance of olanzapine in young smoking males, for example, may be 3 times higher than that in elderly nonsmoking females. SYMBYAX dosing modification may be necessary in patients who exhibit a combination of factors that may result in slower metabolism of the olanzapine component (*see* DOSAGE AND ADMINISTRATION, Special Populations).

CLINICAL STUDIES

The efficacy of SYMBYAX for the treatment of depressive episodes associated with bipolar disorder was established in 2 identically designed, 8-week, randomized, double-blind, controlled studies of patients who met Diagnostic and Statistical Manual 4th edition (DSM-IV) criteria for Bipolar I Disorder, Depressed utilizing flexible dosing of SYMBYAX (6/25, 6/50, or 12/50 mg/day), olanzapine (5 to 20 mg/day), and placebo. These studies included patients (≥18 years of age) with or without psychotic symptoms and with or without a rapid cycling course.

The primary rating instrument used to assess depressive symptoms in these studies was the Montgomery-Asberg Depression Rating Scale (MADRS), a 10-item clinician-rated scale with total scores ranging from 0 to 60. The primary outcome measure of these studies was the change from baseline to endpoint in the MADRS total score. In both studies, SYMBYAX was statistically significantly superior to both olanzapine monotherapy and placebo in reduction of the MADRS total score. The results of the studies are summarized below (Table 1).

Table 1: MADRS Total Score Mean Change from Baseline to Endpoint

	Treatment Group	Baseline Mean	Change to Endpoint Mean[1]
Study 1	SYMBYAX (N=40)	30	-16[a]
	Olanzapine (N=182)	32	-12
	Placebo (N=181)	31	-10
Study 2	SYMBYAX (N=42)	32	-18[a]
	Olanzapine (N=169)	33	-14
	Placebo (N=174)	31	-9

[1] Negative number denotes improvement from baseline.

[a] Statistically significant compared to both olanzapine and placebo.

INDICATIONS AND USAGE

SYMBYAX is indicated for the treatment of depressive episodes associated with bipolar disorder. The efficacy of SYMBYAX was established in 2 identically designed, 8-week, randomized, double-blind clinical studies.

Unlike with unipolar depression, there are no established guidelines for the length of time patients with bipolar disorder experiencing a major depressive episode should be treated with agents containing antidepressant drugs.

The effectiveness of SYMBYAX for maintaining antidepressant response in this patient population beyond 8 weeks has not been established in controlled clinical studies. Physicians who elect to use SYMBYAX for extended periods should periodically reevaluate the benefits and long-term risks of the drug for the individual patient.

CONTRAINDICATIONS

Hypersensitivity — SYMBYAX is contraindicated in patients with a known hypersensitivity to the product or any component of the product.

Monoamine oxidase inhibitors (MAOI) — There have been reports of serious, sometimes fatal reactions (including hyperthermia, rigidity, myoclonus, autonomic instability with possible rapid fluctuations of vital signs, and mental status changes that include extreme agitation progressing to delirium and coma) in patients receiving fluoxetine in combination with an MAOI, and in patients who have recently discontinued fluoxetine and are then started on an MAOI. Some cases presented with features resembling neuroleptic malignant syndrome. Therefore, SYMBYAX should not be used in combination with an MAOI, or within a minimum of 14 days of discontinuing therapy with an MAOI. Since fluoxetine and its major metabolite have very long elimination half-lives, at least 5 weeks [perhaps longer, especially if fluoxetine has been prescribed chronically and/or at higher doses (*see* CLINICAL PHARMACOLOGY, Accumulation and slow elimination)] should be allowed after stopping SYMBYAX before starting an MAOI.

Thioridazine — Thioridazine should not be administered with SYMBYAX or administered within a minimum of 5 weeks after discontinuation of SYMBYAX (*see* WARNINGS, Thioridazine).

WARNINGS

Hyperglycemia and Diabetes Mellitus — Hyperglycemia, in some cases extreme and associated with ketoacidosis or hyperosmolar coma or death, has been reported in patients treated with atypical antipsychotics, including olanzapine alone, as well as olanzapine taken concomitantly with fluoxetine. Assessment of the relationship between atypical antipsychotic use and glucose abnormalities is complicated by the possibility of an increased background risk of diabetes mellitus in patients with schizophrenia and the increasing incidence of diabetes mellitus in the general population. Given these confounders, the relationship between atypical antipsychotic use and hyperglycemia-related adverse events is not completely understood. However, epidemiological studies suggest an increased risk of treatment-emergent hyperglycemia-related adverse events in patients treated with the atypical antipsychotics. Precise risk estimates for hyperglycemia-related adverse events in patients treated with atypical antipsychotics are not available.

Patients with an established diagnosis of diabetes mellitus who are started on atypical antipsychotics should be monitored regularly for worsening of glucose control. Patients with risk factors for diabetes mellitus (e.g., obesity, family history of diabetes) who are starting treatment with atypical antipsychotics should undergo fasting blood glucose testing at the beginning of treatment and periodically during treatment. Any patient treated with atypical antipsychotics should be monitored for symptoms of hyperglycemia including polydipsia, polyuria, polyphagia, and weakness. Patients who develop symptoms of hyperglycemia during treatment with atypical antipsychotics should undergo fasting blood glucose testing. In some cases, hyperglycemia has resolved when the atypical antipsychotic was discontinued; however, some patients required continuation of anti-diabetic treatment despite discontinuation of the suspect drug.

Cerebrovascular adverse events (CVAE), including stroke, in elderly patients with dementia — Cerebrovascular adverse events (e.g., stroke, transient ischemic attack), including fatalities, were reported in patients in trials of olanzapine in elderly patients with dementia-related psychosis. In placebo-controlled trials, there was a significantly higher incidence of cerebrovascular adverse events in patients treated with olanzapine compared to patients treated with placebo. Olanzapine is not approved for the treatment of patients with dementia-related psychosis.

Orthostatic hypotension — SYMBYAX may induce orthostatic hypotension associated with dizziness, tachycardia, bradycardia, and in some patients, syncope, especially during the initial dose-titration period.

In the bipolar depression studies, statistically significantly more orthostatic changes occurred with the SYMBYAX group compared to placebo and olanzapine groups. Orthostatic systolic blood pressure decrease of at least 30 mm Hg occurred in 7.3% (6/82), 1.4% (5/346), and 1.4% (5/352) of the SYMBYAX, olanzapine and placebo groups, respectively. Among the group of controlled clinical studies with SYMBYAX, an orthostatic systolic blood pressure decrease of ≥30 mm Hg occurred in 4% (21/512) of SYMBYAX-

Continued on next page

Symbyax—Cont.

treated patients, 5% (10/204) of fluoxetine-treated patients, 2% (16/644) of olanzapine-treated patients, and 2% (8/445) of placebo-treated patients. In this group of studies, the incidence of syncope in SYMBYAX-treated patients was 0.4% (2/571) compared to placebo 0.2% (1/477).

In a clinical pharmacology study of SYMBYAX, three healthy subjects were discontinued from the trial after experiencing severe, but self-limited, hypotension and bradycardia that occurred 2 to 9 hours following a single 12-mg/50-mg dose of SYMBYAX. Reactions consisting of this combination of hypotension and bradycardia (and also accompanied by sinus pause) have been observed in at least three other healthy subjects treated with various formulations of olanzapine (one oral, two intramuscular). In controlled clinical studies, the incidence of patients with a ≥20 bpm decrease in orthostatic pulse concomitantly with a ≥20 mm Hg decrease in orthostatic systolic blood pressure was 0.4% (2/549) in the SYMBYAX group, 0.2% (1/455) in the placebo group, 0.8% (5/659) in the olanzapine group, and 0% (0/241) in the fluoxetine group.

SYMBYAX should be used with particular caution in patients with known cardiovascular disease (history of myocardial infarction or ischemia, heart failure, or conduction abnormalities), cerebrovascular disease, or conditions that would predispose patients to hypotension (dehydration, hypovolemia, and treatment with antihypertensive medications).

Allergic events and rash — In SYMBYAX premarketing controlled clinical studies, the overall incidence of rash or allergic events in SYMBYAX-treated patients [4.6% (26/571)] was similar to that of placebo [5.2% (25/477)]. The majority of the cases of rash and/or urticaria were mild; however, three patients discontinued (one due to rash, which was moderate in severity, and two due to allergic events, one of which included face edema).

In fluoxetine US clinical studies, 7% of 10,782 fluoxetine-treated patients developed various types of rashes and/or urticaria. Among the cases of rash and/or urticaria reported in premarketing clinical studies, almost a third were withdrawn from treatment because of the rash and/or systemic signs or symptoms associated with the rash. Clinical findings reported in association with rash include fever, leukocytosis, arthralgias, edema, carpal tunnel syndrome, respiratory distress, lymphadenopathy, proteinuria, and mild transaminase elevation. Most patients improved promptly with discontinuation of fluoxetine and/or adjunctive treatment with antihistamines or steroids, and all patients experiencing these events were reported to recover completely.

In fluoxetine premarketing clinical studies, 2 patients are known to have developed a serious cutaneous systemic illness. In neither patient was there an unequivocal diagnosis, but 1 was considered to have a leukocytoclastic vasculitis, and the other, a severe desquamating syndrome that was considered variously to be a vasculitis or erythema multiforme. Other patients have had systemic syndromes suggestive of serum sickness.

Since the introduction of fluoxetine, systemic events, possibly related to vasculitis, have developed in patients with rash. Although these events are rare, they may be serious, involving the lung, kidney, or liver. Death has been reported to occur in association with these systemic events.

Anaphylactoid events, including bronchospasm, angioedema, and urticaria alone and in combination, have been reported.

Pulmonary events, including inflammatory processes of varying histopathology and/or fibrosis, have been reported rarely. These events have occurred with dyspnea as the only preceding symptom.

Whether these systemic events and rash have a common underlying cause or are due to different etiologies or pathogenic processes is not known. Furthermore, a specific underlying immunologic basis for these events has not been identified. Upon the appearance of rash or of other possible allergic phenomena for which an alternative etiology cannot be identified, SYMBYAX should be discontinued.

Neuroleptic malignant syndrome (NMS) — A potentially fatal symptom complex sometimes referred to as NMS has been reported in association with administration of antipsychotic drugs, including olanzapine. Clinical manifestations of NMS are hyperpyrexia, muscle rigidity, altered mental status, and evidence of autonomic instability (irregular pulse or blood pressure, tachycardia, diaphoresis, and cardiac dysrhythmia). Additional signs may include elevated creatinine phosphokinase, myoglobinuria (rhabdomyolysis), and acute renal failure.

The diagnostic evaluation of patients with this syndrome is complicated. In arriving at a diagnosis, it is important to exclude cases where the clinical presentation includes both serious medical illness (e.g., pneumonia, systemic infection, etc.) and untreated or inadequately treated extrapyramidal signs and symptoms (EPS). Other important considerations in the differential diagnosis include central anticholinergic toxicity, heat stroke, drug fever, and primary central nervous system pathology.

The management of NMS should include: 1) immediate discontinuation of antipsychotic drugs and other drugs not essential to concurrent therapy, 2) intensive symptomatic treatment and medical monitoring, and 3) treatment of any concomitant serious medical problems for which specific treatments are available. There is no general agreement about specific pharmacological treatment regimens for NMS.

If after recovering from NMS, a patient requires treatment with an antipsychotic, the patient should be carefully monitored, since recurrences of NMS have been reported.

Tardive dyskinesia — A syndrome of potentially irreversible, involuntary, dyskinetic movements may develop in patients treated with antipsychotic drugs. Although the prevalence of the syndrome appears to be highest among the elderly, especially elderly women, it is impossible to rely upon prevalence estimates to predict, at the inception of antipsychotic treatment, which patients are likely to develop the syndrome. Whether antipsychotic drug products differ in their potential to cause tardive dyskinesia is unknown.

The risk of developing tardive dyskinesia and the likelihood that it will become irreversible are believed to increase as the duration of treatment and the total cumulative dose of antipsychotic drugs administered to the patient increase. However, the syndrome can develop, although much less commonly, after relatively brief treatment periods at low doses or may even arise after discontinuation of treatment. There is no known treatment for established cases of tardive dyskinesia, although the syndrome may remit, partially or completely, if antipsychotic treatment is withdrawn. Antipsychotic treatment itself, however, may suppress (or partially suppress) the signs and symptoms of the syndrome and thereby may possibly mask the underlying process. The effect that symptomatic suppression has upon the long-term course of the syndrome is unknown.

The incidence of dyskinetic movement in SYMBYAX-treated patients was infrequent. The mean score on the Abnormal Involuntary Movement Scale (AIMS) across clinical studies involving SYMBYAX-treated patients decreased from baseline. Nonetheless, SYMBYAX should be prescribed in a manner that is most likely to minimize the risk of tardive dyskinesia. If signs and symptoms of tardive dyskinesia appear in a patient on SYMBYAX, drug discontinuation should be considered. However, some patients may require treatment with SYMBYAX despite the presence of the syndrome. The need for continued treatment should be reassessed periodically.

Thioridazine — In a study of 19 healthy male subjects, which included 6 slow and 13 rapid hydroxylators of debrisoquin, a single 25-mg oral dose of thioridazine produced a 2.4-fold higher C_{max} and a 4.5-fold higher AUC for thioridazine in the slow hydroxylators compared with the rapid hydroxylators. The rate of debrisoquin hydroxylation is felt to depend on the level of CYP2D6 isozyme activity. Thus, this study suggests that drugs that inhibit CYP2D6, such as certain SSRIs, including fluoxetine, will produce elevated plasma levels of thioridazine (*see* PRECAUTIONS).

Thioridazine administration produces a dose-related prolongation of the QT_c interval, which is associated with serious ventricular arrhythmias, such as torsades de pointes-type arrhythmias and sudden death. This risk is expected to increase with fluoxetine-induced inhibition of thioridazine metabolism (*see* CONTRAINDICATIONS, Thioridazine).

PRECAUTIONS

General

Concomitant use of olanzapine and fluoxetine products — SYMBYAX contains the same active ingredients that are in Zyprexa and Zyprexa Zydis (olanzapine) and in Prozac, Prozac Weekly, and Sarafem (fluoxetine HCl). Caution should be exercised when prescribing these medications concomitantly with SYMBYAX.

Abnormal bleeding — Published case reports have documented the occurrence of bleeding episodes in patients treated with psychotropic drugs that interfere with serotonin reuptake. Subsequent epidemiological studies, both of the case-control and cohort design, have demonstrated an association between use of psychotropic drugs that interfere with serotonin reuptake and the occurrence of upper gastrointestinal bleeding. In two studies, concurrent use of a nonsteroidal anti-inflammatory drug (NSAID) or aspirin potentiated the risk of bleeding (*see* DRUG INTERACTIONS). Although these studies focused on upper gastrointestinal bleeding, there is reason to believe that bleeding at other sites may be similarly potentiated. Patients should be cautioned regarding the risk of bleeding associated with the concomitant use of SYMBYAX with NSAIDs, aspirin, or other drugs that affect coagulation.

Mania/Hypomania — In the two controlled bipolar depression studies there was no statistically significant difference in the incidence of manic events (manic reaction or manic depressive reaction) between SYMBYAX- and placebo-treated patients. In one of the studies, the incidence of manic events was (7% [3/43]) in SYMBYAX-treated patients compared to (3% [5/184]) in placebo-treated patients. In the other study, the incidence of manic events was (2% [1/43]) in SYMBYAX-treated patients compared to (8% [15/193]) in placebo-treated patients. This limited controlled trial experience of SYMBYAX in the treatment of bipolar depression makes it difficult to interpret these findings until additional data is obtained. Because of this and the cyclical nature of bipolar disorder, patients should be monitored closely for the development of symptoms of mania/hypomania during treatment with SYMBYAX.

Body temperature regulation — Disruption of the body's ability to reduce core body temperature has been attributed to antipsychotic drugs. Appropriate care is advised when prescribing SYMBYAX for patients who will be experiencing conditions which may contribute to an elevation in core body temperature, e.g., exercising strenuously, exposure to extreme heat, receiving concomitant medication with anticholinergic activity, or being subject to dehydration.

Cognitive and motor impairment — Somnolence was a commonly reported adverse event associated with SYMBYAX treatment, occurring at an incidence of 22% in SYMBYAX patients compared with 11% in placebo patients. Somnolence led to discontinuation in 2% (10/571) of patients in the premarketing controlled clinical studies.

As with any CNS-active drug, SYMBYAX has the potential to impair judgment, thinking, or motor skills. Patients should be cautioned about operating hazardous machinery, including automobiles, until they are reasonably certain that SYMBYAX therapy does not affect them adversely.

Dysphagia — Dysphagia was observed infrequently in SYMBYAX-treated patients in premarketing clinical studies. Nonetheless, like other psychotropic drugs, SYMBYAX should be used cautiously in patients at risk for aspiration pneumonia.

Esophageal dysmotility and aspiration have been associated with antipsychotic drug use. Two olanzapine-treated patients (2/407) in 2 olanzapine studies in patients with Alzheimer's disease died from aspiration pneumonia during or within 30 days of the termination of the double-blind portion of their respective studies; there were no deaths in the placebo-treated patients. One of these patients had experienced dysphagia prior to the development of aspiration pneumonia. Aspiration pneumonia is a common cause of morbidity and mortality in patients with advanced Alzheimer's disease.

Half-life — Because of the long elimination half-lives of fluoxetine and its major active metabolite, changes in dose will not be fully reflected in plasma for several weeks, affecting both strategies for titration to final dose and withdrawal from treatment (*see* CLINICAL PHARMACOLOGY, Accumulation and slow elimination).

Hyperprolactinemia — As with other drugs that antagonize dopamine D_2 receptors, SYMBYAX elevates prolactin levels, and a modest elevation persists during administration; however, possibly associated clinical manifestations (e.g., galactorrhea and breast enlargement) were infrequently observed.

Tissue culture experiments indicate that approximately one-third of human breast cancers are prolactin dependent in vitro, a factor of potential importance if the prescription of these drugs is contemplated in a patient with previously detected breast cancer of this type. Although disturbances such as galactorrhea, amenorrhea, gynecomastia, and impotence have been reported with prolactin-elevating compounds, the clinical significance of elevated serum prolactin levels is unknown for most patients. As is common with compounds that increase prolactin release, an increase in mammary gland neoplasia was observed in the olanzapine carcinogenicity studies conducted in mice and rats (*see* Carcinogenesis). However, neither clinical studies nor epidemiologic studies have shown an association between chronic administration of this class of drugs and tumorigenesis in humans; the available evidence is considered too limited to be conclusive.

Hyponatremia — Hyponatremia has been observed in SYMBYAX premarketing clinical studies. In controlled trials, no SYMBYAX-treated patients had a treatment-emergent serum sodium below 130 mmol/L; however, a lowering of serum sodium below the reference range occurred at an incidence of 2% (10/500) of SYMBYAX patients compared with 0.5% (2/380) of placebo patients. In open label studies, 0.3% (5/1889) of these SYMBYAX-treated patients had a treatment-emergent serum sodium below 130 mmol/L.

Cases of hyponatremia (some with serum sodium lower than 110 mmol/L) have been reported with fluoxetine. The hyponatremia appeared to be reversible when fluoxetine was discontinued. Although these cases were complex with varying possible etiologies, some were possibly due to the syndrome of inappropriate antidiuretic hormone secretion (SIADH). The majority of these occurrences have been in older patients and in patients taking diuretics or who were otherwise volume depleted. In two 6-week controlled studies in patients ≥60 years of age, 10 of 323 fluoxetine patients and 6 of 327 placebo recipients had a lowering of serum sodium below the reference range; this difference was not statistically significant. The lowest observed concentration was 129 mmol/L. The observed decreases were not clinically significant.

Seizures — Seizures occurred in 0.2% (4/2066) of SYMBYAX-treated patients during open-label premarketing clinical studies. No seizures occurred in the premarketing controlled SYMBYAX studies. Seizures have also been reported with both olanzapine and fluoxetine monotherapy. Therefore, SYMBYAX should be used cautiously in patients with a history of seizures or with conditions that potentially lower the seizure threshold. Conditions that lower the seizure threshold may be more prevalent in a population of ≥65 years of age.

Suicide — The possibility of a suicide attempt is inherent in bipolar disorder and may persist until significant remission occurs. Close supervision of high-risk patients should accompany drug therapy. Prescriptions for SYMBYAX should be written for the smallest quantity consistent with good patient management in order to reduce the risk of overdose.

Transaminase elevations — As with olanzapine, asymptomatic elevations of hepatic transaminases [ALT (SGPT), AST (SGOT), and GGT] and alkaline phosphatase have been observed with SYMBYAX. In the SYMBYAX-controlled database, ALT (SGPT) elevations (≥3 times the upper limit of the normal range) were observed in 6.3% (31/495) of patients exposed to SYMBYAX compared with 0.5% (2/384) of the placebo patients and 4.5% (25/560) of olanzapine-treated patients. The difference between SYMBYAX and placebo was statistically significant. None of these 31 SYMBYAX-treated patients experienced jaundice and three had transient elevations >200 IU/L.

In olanzapine placebo-controlled studies, clinically significant ALT (SGPT) elevations (≥3 times the upper limit of the normal range) were observed in 2% (6/243) of patients exposed to olanzapine compared with 0% (0/115) of the placebo patients. None of these patients experienced jaundice. In 2 of these patients, liver enzymes decreased toward normal despite continued treatment, and in 2 others, enzymes decreased upon discontinuation of olanzapine. In the remaining 2 patients, 1, seropositive for hepatitis C, had persistent enzyme elevations for 4 months after discontinuation, and the other had insufficient follow-up to determine if enzymes normalized.

Within the larger olanzapine premarketing database of about 2400 patients with baseline SGPT ≤90 IU/L, the incidence of SGPT elevation to >200 IU/L was 2% (50/2381). Again, none of these patients experienced jaundice or other symptoms attributable to liver impairment and most had transient changes that tended to normalize while olanzapine treatment was continued. Among all 2500 patients in olanzapine clinical studies, approximately 1% (23/2500) discontinued treatment due to transaminase increases.

Caution should be exercised in patients with signs and symptoms of hepatic impairment, in patients with pre-existing conditions associated with limited hepatic functional reserve, and in patients who are being treated with potentially hepatotoxic drugs. Periodic assessment of transaminases is recommended in patients with significant hepatic disease (*see* Laboratory Tests).

Weight gain — In clinical studies, the mean weight increase for SYMBYAX-treated patients was statistically significantly greater than placebo-treated (3.6 kg vs -0.3 kg) and fluoxetine-treated (3.6 kg vs -0.7 kg) patients, but was not statistically significantly different from olanzapine-treated patients (3.6 kg vs 3.0 kg). Fourteen percent of SYMBYAX-treated patients met criterion for having gained >10% of their baseline weight. This was statistically significantly greater than placebo-treated (<1%) and fluoxetine-treated patients (<1%) but was not statistically significantly different than olanzapine-treated patients (11%).

Use in Patients with Concomitant Illness

Clinical experience with SYMBYAX in patients with concomitant systemic illnesses is limited (*see* CLINICAL PHARMACOLOGY, Renal impairment *and* Hepatic impairment). The following precautions for the individual components may be applicable to SYMBYAX.

Olanzapine exhibits in vitro muscarinic receptor affinity. In premarketing clinical studies, SYMBYAX was associated with constipation, dry mouth, and tachycardia, all adverse events possibly related to cholinergic antagonism. Such adverse events were not often the basis for study discontinuations; SYMBYAX should be used with caution in patients with clinically significant prostatic hypertrophy, narrow angle glaucoma, a history of paralytic ileus, or related conditions.

In a fixed-dose study of olanzapine (olanzapine at doses of 5, 10, and 15 mg/day) and placebo in nursing home patients (mean age: 83 years, range: 61 to 97; median Mini-Mental State Examination (MMSE): 5, range: 0 to 22) having various psychiatric symptoms in association with Alzheimer's disease, the following treatment-emergent adverse events were reported in all (each and every) olanzapine-treated groups at an incidence of either (1) 2-fold or more in excess of the placebo-treated group, where at least 1 placebo-treated patient was reported to have experienced the event, or (2) at least 2 cases if no placebo-treated patient was reported to have experienced the event: somnolence, abnormal gait, fever, dehydration, and back pain. The rate of discontinuation in this study for olanzapine was 12% vs 4% with placebo. Discontinuations due to abnormal gait (1% for olanzapine vs 0% for placebo), accidental injury (1% for olanzapine vs 0% for placebo), and somnolence (3% for olanzapine vs 0% for placebo) were considered to be drug related.

As with other CNS-active drugs, SYMBYAX should be used with caution in elderly patients with dementia.

SYMBYAX has not been evaluated or used to any appreciable extent in patients with a recent history of myocardial infarction or unstable heart disease. Patients with these diagnoses were excluded from clinical studies during the premarket testing.

Caution is advised when using SYMBYAX in cardiac patients and in patients with diseases or conditions that could affect hemodynamic responses (*see* WARNINGS, Orthostatic hypotension).

In subjects with cirrhosis of the liver, the clearances of fluoxetine and its active metabolite, norfluoxetine, were decreased, thus increasing the elimination half-lives of these substances. A lower dose of the fluoxetine-component of SYMBYAX should be used in patients with cirrhosis. Caution is advised when using SYMBYAX in patients with diseases or conditions that could affect its metabolism (*see* CLINICAL PHARMACOLOGY, Hepatic impairment *and* DOSING AND ADMINISTRATION, Special Populations).

Olanzapine and fluoxetine individual pharmacokinetics do not differ significantly in patients with renal impairment. SYMBYAX dosing adjustment based upon renal impairment is not routinely required (*see* CLINICAL PHARMACOLOGY, Renal impairment).

Information for Patients

Physicians are advised to discuss the following issues with patients for whom they prescribe SYMBYAX:

Abnormal bleeding — Patients should be cautioned about the concomitant use of SYMBYAX and NSAIDs, aspirin, or other drugs that affect coagulation since the combined use of psychotropic drugs that interfere with serotonin reuptake and these agents has been associated with an increased risk of bleeding (*see* PRECAUTIONS, Abnormal bleeding).

Alcohol — Patients should be advised to avoid alcohol while taking SYMBYAX.

Cognitive and motor impairment — As with any CNS-active drug, SYMBYAX has the potential to impair judgment, thinking, or motor skills. Patients should be cautioned about operating hazardous machinery, including automobiles, until they are reasonably certain that SYMBYAX therapy does not affect them adversely.

Concomitant medication — Patients should be advised to inform their physician if they are taking Prozac®, Prozac Weekly™, Sarafem®, fluoxetine, Zyprexa®, or Zyprexa Zydis®. Patients should also be advised to inform their physicians if they are taking or plan to take any prescription or over-the-counter drugs, including herbal supplements, since there is a potential for interactions.

Heat exposure and dehydration — Patients should be advised regarding appropriate care in avoiding overheating and dehydration.

Nursing — Patients, if taking SYMBYAX, should be advised not to breast-feed.

Orthostatic hypotension — Patients should be advised of the risk of orthostatic hypotension, especially during the period of initial dose titration and in association with the use of concomitant drugs that may potentiate the orthostatic effect of olanzapine, e.g., diazepam or alcohol (*see* WARNINGS *and* Drug Interactions).

Pregnancy — Patients should be advised to notify their physician if they become pregnant or intend to become pregnant during SYMBYAX therapy.

Rash — Patients should be advised to notify their physician if they develop a rash or hives while taking SYMBYAX.

Treatment adherence — Patients should be advised to take SYMBYAX exactly as prescribed, and to continue taking SYMBYAX as prescribed even after their mood symptoms improve. Patients should be advised that they should not alter their dosing regimen, or stop taking SYMBYAX, without consulting their physician.

Patient information is printed at the end of this insert. Physicians should discuss this information with their patients and instruct them to read the patient package insert before starting therapy with SYMBYAX and each time their prescription is refilled.

Laboratory Tests

Periodic assessment of transaminases is recommended in patients with significant hepatic disease (*see* Transaminase elevations).

Drug Interactions

The risks of using SYMBYAX in combination with other drugs have not been extensively evaluated in systematic studies. The drug-drug interactions of the individual components are applicable to SYMBYAX. As with all drugs, the potential for interaction by a variety of mechanisms (e.g., pharmacodynamic, pharmacokinetic drug inhibition or enhancement, etc.) is a possibility. Caution is advised if the concomitant administration of SYMBYAX and other CNS-active drugs is required. In evaluating individual cases, consideration should be given to using lower initial doses of the concomitantly administered drugs, using conservative titration schedules, and monitoring of clinical status (*see* CLINICAL PHARMACOLOGY, Accumulation and slow elimination).

Antihypertensive agents — Because of the potential for olanzapine to induce hypotension, SYMBYAX may enhance the effects of certain antihypertensive agents (*see* WARNINGS, Orthostatic hypotension).

Anti-Parkinsonian — The olanzapine component of SYMBYAX may antagonize the effects of levodopa and dopamine agonists.

Benzodiazepines — Multiple doses of olanzapine did not influence the pharmacokinetics of diazepam and its active metabolite N-desmethyldiazepam. However, the coadministration of diazepam with olanzapine potentiated the orthostatic hypotension observed with olanzapine.

When concurrently administered with fluoxetine, the half-life of diazepam may be prolonged in some patients (*see* CLINICAL PHARMACOLOGY, Accumulation and slow elimination). Coadministration of alprazolam and fluoxetine has resulted in increased alprazolam plasma concentrations and in further psychomotor performance decrement due to increased alprazolam levels.

Biperiden — Multiple doses of olanzapine did not influence the pharmacokinetics of biperiden.

Carbamazepine — Carbamazepine therapy (200 mg BID) causes an approximate 50% increase in the clearance of olanzapine. This increase is likely due to the fact that carbamazepine is a potent inducer of CYP1A2 activity. Higher daily doses of carbamazepine may cause an even greater increase in olanzapine clearance.

Patients on stable doses of carbamazepine have developed elevated plasma anticonvulsant concentrations and clinical anticonvulsant toxicity following initiation of concomitant fluoxetine treatment.

Clozapine — Elevation of blood levels of clozapine has been observed in patients receiving concomitant fluoxetine.

Electroconvulsive therapy (ECT) — There are no clinical studies establishing the benefit of the combined use of ECT and fluoxetine. There have been rare reports of prolonged seizures in patients on fluoxetine receiving ECT treatment (*see* Seizures).

Ethanol — Ethanol (45 mg/70 kg single dose) did not have an effect on olanzapine pharmacokinetics. The coadministration of ethanol with SYMBYAX may potentiate sedation and orthostatic hypotension.

Fluvoxamine — Fluvoxamine, a CYP1A2 inhibitor, decreases the clearance of olanzapine. This results in a mean increase in olanzapine C_{max} following fluvoxamine administration of 54% in female nonsmokers and 77% in male smokers. The mean increase in olanzapine AUC is 52% and 108%, respectively. Lower doses of the olanzapine component of SYMBYAX should be considered in patients receiving concomitant treatment with fluvoxamine.

Haloperidol — Elevation of blood levels of haloperidol has been observed in patients receiving concomitant fluoxetine.

Lithium — Multiple doses of olanzapine did not influence the pharmacokinetics of lithium.

There have been reports of both increased and decreased lithium levels when lithium was used concomitantly with fluoxetine. Cases of lithium toxicity and increased serotonergic effects have been reported. Lithium levels should be monitored in patients taking SYMBYAX concomitantly with lithium.

Monoamine oxidase inhibitors — See CONTRAINDICATIONS.

Phenytoin — Patients on stable doses of phenytoin have developed elevated plasma levels of phenytoin with clinical phenytoin toxicity following initiation of concomitant fluoxetine.

Pimozide — A single case report has suggested possible additive effects of pimozide and fluoxetine leading to bradycardia.

Sumatriptan — There have been rare postmarketing reports describing patients with weakness, hyperreflexia, and incoordination following the use of an SSRI and sumatriptan. If concomitant treatment with sumatriptan and an SSRI (e.g., fluoxetine, fluvoxamine, paroxetine, sertraline, or citalopram) is clinically warranted, appropriate observation of the patient is advised.

Theophylline — Multiple doses of olanzapine did not affect the pharmacokinetics of theophylline or its metabolites.

Thioridazine — See CONTRAINDICATIONS and WARNINGS, Thioridazine.

Tricyclic antidepressants (TCAs) — Single doses of olanzapine did not affect the pharmacokinetics of imipramine or its active metabolite desipramine.

In two fluoxetine studies, previously stable plasma levels of imipramine and desipramine have increased >2- to 10-fold when fluoxetine has been administered in combination. This influence may persist for three weeks or longer after fluoxetine is discontinued. Thus, the dose of TCA may need to be reduced and plasma TCA concentrations may need to be monitored temporarily when SYMBYAX is coadministered or has been recently discontinued (*see* Drugs metabolized by CYP2D6 *and* CLINICAL PHARMACOLOGY, Accumulation and slow elimination).

Tryptophan — Five patients receiving fluoxetine in combination with tryptophan experienced adverse reactions, including agitation, restlessness, and gastrointestinal distress.

Valproate — In vitro studies using human liver microsomes determined that olanzapine has little potential to inhibit the major metabolic pathway, glucuronidation, of valproate. Further, valproate has little effect on the metabolism of olanzapine in vitro. Thus, a clinically significant pharmacokinetic interaction between olanzapine and valproate is unlikely.

Warfarin — Warfarin (20-mg single dose) did not affect olanzapine pharmacokinetics. Single doses of olanzapine did not affect the pharmacokinetics of warfarin.

Altered anticoagulant effects, including increased bleeding, have been reported when fluoxetine is coadministered with warfarin (*see* PRECAUTIONS, Abnormal bleeding). Patients receiving warfarin therapy should receive careful coagulation monitoring when SYMBYAX is initiated or stopped.

Drugs that interfere with hemostasis (NSAIDs, aspirin, warfarin, etc.) — Serotonin release by platelets plays an important role in hemostasis. Epidemiological studies of the case-control and cohort design that have demonstrated an association between use of psychotropic drugs that interfere with serotonin reuptake and the occurrence of upper gastrointestinal bleeding have also shown that concurrent use of an NSAID or aspirin potentiated the risk of bleeding (*see* PRECAUTIONS, Abnormal bleeding). Thus, patients should be cautioned about the use of such drugs concurrently with SYMBYAX.

Drugs metabolized by CYP2D6 — In vitro studies utilizing human liver microsomes suggest that olanzapine has little potential to inhibit CYP2D6. Thus, olanzapine is unlikely to cause clinically important drug interactions mediated by this enzyme.

Approximately 7% of the normal population has a genetic variation that leads to reduced levels of activity of CYP2D6. Such individuals have been referred to as poor metabolizers of drugs such as debrisoquin, dextromethorphan, and TCAs. Many drugs, such as most antidepressants, including fluoxetine and other selective uptake inhibitors of serotonin, are metabolized by this isoenzyme; thus, both the pharmacokinetic properties and relative proportion of metabolites are altered in poor metabolizers. However, for fluoxetine and its metabolite, the sum of the plasma concentrations of

Continued on next page

Symbyax—Cont.

the 4 enantiomers is comparable between poor and extensive metabolizers (*see* CLINICAL PHARMACOLOGY, Variability in metabolism).
Fluoxetine, like other agents that are metabolized by CYP2D6, inhibits the activity of this isoenzyme, and thus may make normal metabolizers resemble poor metabolizers. Therapy with medications that are predominantly metabolized by the CYP2D6 system and that have a relatively narrow therapeutic index should be initiated at the low end of the dose range if a patient is receiving fluoxetine concurrently or has taken it in the previous five weeks. If fluoxetine is added to the treatment regimen of a patient already receiving a drug metabolized by CYP2D6, the need for a decreased dose of the original medication should be considered. Drugs with a narrow therapeutic index represent the greatest concern (including but not limited to, flecainide, vinblastine, and TCAs). Due to the risk of serious ventricular arrhythmias and sudden death potentially associated with elevated thioridazine plasma levels, thioridazine should not be administered with fluoxetine or within a minimum of five weeks after fluoxetine has been discontinued (*see* CONTRAINDICATIONS, Monoamine oxidase inhibitors (MAOI) *and* WARNINGS, Thioridazine).
Drugs metabolized by CYP3A — In vitro studies utilizing human liver microsomes suggest that olanzapine has little potential to inhibit CYP3A. Thus, olanzapine is unlikely to cause clinically important drug interactions mediated by these enzymes.
In an in vivo interaction study involving the coadministration of fluoxetine with single doses of terfenadine (a CYP3A substrate), no increase in plasma terfenadine concentrations occurred with concomitant fluoxetine. In addition, in vitro studies have shown ketoconazole, a potent inhibitor of CYP3A activity, to be at least 100 times more potent than fluoxetine or norfluoxetine as an inhibitor of the metabolism of several substrates for this enzyme, including astemizole, cisapride, and midazolam. These data indicate that fluoxetine's extent of inhibition of CYP3A activity is not likely to be of clinical significance.
Effect of olanzapine on drugs metabolized by other CYP enzymes — In vitro studies utilizing human liver microsomes suggest that olanzapine has little potential to inhibit CYP1A2, CYP2C9, and CYP2C19. Thus, olanzapine is unlikely to cause clinically important drug interactions mediated by these enzymes.
The effect of other drugs on olanzapine — Fluoxetine, an inhibitor of CYP2D6, decreases olanzapine clearance a small amount (*see* CLINICAL PHARMACOLOGY, Pharmacokinetics). Agents that induce CYP1A2 or glucuronyl transferase enzymes, such as omeprazole and rifampin, may cause an increase in olanzapine clearance. Fluvoxamine, an inhibitor of CYP1A2, decreases olanzapine clearance (*see* Drug Interactions, Fluvoxamine). The effect of CYP1A2 inhibitors, such as fluvoxamine and some fluoroquinolone antibiotics, on SYMBYAX has not been evaluated. Although olanzapine is metabolized by multiple enzyme systems, induction or inhibition of a single enzyme may appreciably alter olanzapine clearance. Therefore, a dosage increase (for induction) or a dosage decrease (for inhibition) may need to be considered with specific drugs.
Drugs tightly bound to plasma proteins — The in vitro binding of SYMBYAX to human plasma proteins is similar to the individual components. The interaction between SYMBYAX and other highly protein-bound drugs has not been fully evaluated. Because fluoxetine is tightly bound to plasma protein, the administration of fluoxetine to a patient taking another drug that is tightly bound to protein (e.g., Coumadin, digitoxin) may cause a shift in plasma concentrations potentially resulting in an adverse effect. Conversely, adverse effects may result from displacement of protein-bound fluoxetine by other tightly bound drugs (*see* CLINICAL PHARMACOLOGY, Distribution *and* PRECAUTIONS, Drug Interactions).

Carcinogenesis, Mutagenesis, Impairment of Fertility

No carcinogenicity, mutagenicity, or fertility studies were conducted with SYMBYAX. The following data are based on findings in studies performed with the individual components.
Carcinogenesis
Olanzapine — Oral carcinogenicity studies were conducted in mice and rats. Olanzapine was administered to mice in two 78-week studies at doses of 3, 10, and 30/20 mg/kg/day [equivalent to 0.8 to 5 times the maximum recommended human daily dose (MRHD) on a mg/m² basis] and 0.25, 2, and 8 mg/kg/day (equivalent to 0.06 to 2 times the MRHD on a mg/m² basis). Rats were dosed for 2 years at doses of 0.25, 1, 2.5, and 4 mg/kg/day (males) and 0.25, 1, 4, and 8 mg/kg/day (females) (equivalent to 0.1 to 2 and 0.1 to 4 times the MRHD on a mg/m² basis, respectively). The incidence of liver hemangiomas and hemangiosarcomas was significantly increased in one mouse study in females dosed at 8 mg/kg/day (2 times the MRHD on a mg/m² basis). These tumors were not increased in another mouse study in females dosed at 10 or 30/20 mg/kg/day (2 to 5 times the MRHD on a mg/m² basis); in this study, there was a high incidence of early mortalities in males of the 30/20 mg/kg/day group. The incidence of mammary gland adenomas and adenocarcinomas was significantly increased in female mice dosed at ≥2 mg/kg/day and in female rats dosed at ≥4 mg/kg/day (0.5 and 2 times the MRHD on a mg/m² basis, respectively). Antipsychotic drugs have been shown to chronically elevate prolactin levels in rodents. Serum prolactin levels were not measured during the olanzapine carcinogenicity studies; however, measurements during subchronic toxicity studies showed that olanzapine elevated serum prolactin levels up to 4-fold in rats at the same doses used in the carcinogenicity study. An increase in mammary gland neoplasms has been found in rodents after chronic administration of other antipsychotic drugs and is considered to be prolactin-mediated. The relevance for human risk of the finding of prolactin-mediated endocrine tumors in rodents is unknown (*see* PRECAUTIONS, Hyperprolactinemia).
Fluoxetine — The dietary administration of fluoxetine to rats and mice for two years at doses of up to 10 and 12 mg/kg/day, respectively (approximately 1.2 and 0.7 times, respectively, the MRHD on a mg/m² basis), produced no evidence of carcinogenicity.
Mutagenesis
Olanzapine — No evidence of mutagenic potential for olanzapine was found in the Ames reverse mutation test, in vivo micronucleus test in mice, the chromosomal aberration test in Chinese hamster ovary cells, unscheduled DNA synthesis test in rat hepatocytes, induction of forward mutation test in mouse lymphoma cells, or in vivo sister chromatid exchange test in bone marrow of Chinese hamsters.
Fluoxetine — Fluoxetine and norfluoxetine have been shown to have no genotoxic effects based on the following assays: bacterial mutation assay, DNA repair assay in cultured rat hepatocytes, mouse lymphoma assay, and in vivo sister chromatid exchange assay in Chinese hamster bone marrow cells.
Impairment of Fertility
SYMBYAX — Fertility studies were not conducted with SYMBYAX. However in a repeat-dose rat toxicology study of three months duration, ovary weight was decreased in females treated with the low-dose [2 and 4 mg/kg/day (1 and 0.5 times the MRHD on a mg/m² basis), respectively] and high-dose [4 and 8 mg/kg/day (2 and 1 times the MRHD on a mg/m² basis), respectively] combinations of olanzapine and fluoxetine. Decreased ovary weight, and corpora luteal depletion and uterine atrophy were observed to a greater extent in the females receiving the high-dose combination than in females receiving either olanzapine or fluoxetine alone. In a 3-month repeat-dose dog toxicology study, reduced epididymal sperm and reduced testicular and prostate weights were observed with the high-dose combination of olanzapine and fluoxetine (5 and 5 mg/kg/day (9 and 2 times the MRHD on a mg/m² basis, respectively) and with olanzapine alone (5 mg/kg/day or 9 times the MRHD on a mg/m² basis).
Olanzapine — In a fertility and reproductive performance study in rats, male mating performance, but not fertility, was impaired at a dose of 22.4 mg/kg/day and female fertility was decreased at a dose of 3 mg/kg/day (11 and 1.5 times the MRHD on a mg/m² basis, respectively). Discontinuance of olanzapine treatment reversed the effects on male-mating performance. In female rats, the precoital period was increased and the mating index reduced at 5 mg/kg/day (2.5 times the MRHD on a mg/m² basis). Diestrous was prolonged and estrous was delayed at 1.1 mg/kg/day (0.6 times the MRHD on a mg/m² basis); therefore, olanzapine may produce a delay in ovulation.
Fluoxetine — Two fertility studies conducted in rats at doses of up to 7.5 and 12.5 mg/kg/day (approximately 0.9 and 1.5 times the MRHD on a mg/m² basis) indicated that fluoxetine had no adverse effects on fertility.

Pregnancy — Pregnancy Category C

SYMBYAX
Embryo fetal development studies were conducted in rats and rabbits with olanzapine and fluoxetine in low-dose and high-dose combinations. In rats, the doses were: 2 and 4 mg/kg/day (low-dose) [1 and 0.5 times the MRHD on a mg/m² basis, respectively], and 4 and 8 mg/kg/day (high-dose) [2 and 1 times the MRHD on a mg/m² basis, respectively]. In rabbits, the doses were 4 and 4 mg/kg/day (low-dose) [4 and 1 times the MRHD on a mg/m² basis, respectively], and 8 and 8 mg/kg/day (high-dose) [9 and 2 times the MRHD on a mg/m² basis, respectively]. In these studies, olanzapine and fluoxetine were also administered alone at the high-doses (4 and 8 mg/kg/day, respectively, in the rat; 8 and 8 mg/kg/day, respectively, in the rabbit). In the rabbit, there was no evidence of teratogenicity; however, the high-dose combination produced decreases in fetal weight and retarded skeletal ossification in conjunction with maternal toxicity. Similarly, in the rat there was no evidence of teratogenicity; however, a decrease in fetal weight was observed with the high-dose combination.
In a pre- and postnatal study conducted in rats, olanzapine and fluoxetine were administered during pregnancy and throughout lactation in combination (low-dose: 2 and 4 mg/kg/day [1 and 0.5 times the MRHD on a mg/m² basis], respectively, high-dose: 4 and 8 mg/kg/day [2 and 1 times the MRHD on a mg/m² basis], respectively, and alone: 4 and 8 mg/kg/day [2 and 1 times the MRHD on a mg/m² basis], respectively). Administration of the high-dose combination resulted in a marked elevation in offspring mortality and growth retardation in comparison to the same doses of olanzapine and fluoxetine administered alone. These effects were not observed with the low-dose combination; however, there were a few cases of testicular degeneration and atrophy, depletion of epididymal sperm and infertility in the male progeny. The effects of the high-dose combination on postnatal endpoints could not be assessed due to high progeny mortality.
There are no adequate and well-controlled studies with SYMBYAX in pregnant women. SYMBYAX should be used during pregnancy only if the potential benefit justifies the potential risk to the fetus.
Olanzapine
In reproduction studies in rats at doses up to 18 mg/kg/day and in rabbits at doses up to 30 mg/kg/day (9 and 30 times the MRHD on a mg/m² basis, respectively), no evidence of teratogenicity was observed. In a rat teratology study, early resorptions and increased numbers of nonviable fetuses were observed at a dose of 18 mg/kg/day (9 times the MRHD on a mg/m² basis). Gestation was prolonged at 10 mg/kg/day (5 times the MRHD on a mg/m² basis). In a rabbit teratology study, fetal toxicity (manifested as increased resorptions and decreased fetal weight) occurred at a maternally toxic dose of 30 mg/kg/day (30 times the MRHD on a mg/m² basis).
Placental transfer of olanzapine occurs in rat pups.
There are no adequate and well-controlled clinical studies with olanzapine in pregnant women. Seven pregnancies were observed during premarketing clinical studies with olanzapine, including two resulting in normal births, one resulting in neonatal death due to a cardiovascular defect, three therapeutic abortions, and one spontaneous abortion.
Fluoxetine
In embryo fetal development studies in rats and rabbits, there was no evidence of teratogenicity following administration of up to 12.5 and 15 mg/kg/day, respectively (1.5 and 3.6 times the MRHD on a mg/m² basis, respectively) throughout organogenesis. However, in rat reproduction studies, an increase in stillborn pups, a decrease in pup weight, and an increase in pup deaths during the first 7 days postpartum occurred following maternal exposure to 12 mg/kg/day (1.5 times the MRHD on a mg/m² basis) during gestation or 7.5 mg/kg/day (0.9 times the MRHD on a mg/m² basis) during gestation and lactation. There was no evidence of developmental neurotoxicity in the surviving offspring of rats treated with 12 mg/kg/day during gestation. The no-effect dose for rat pup mortality was 5 mg/kg/day (0.6 times the MRHD on a mg/m² basis).

Labor and Delivery

SYMBYAX
The effect of SYMBYAX on labor and delivery in humans is unknown. Parturition in rats was not affected by SYMBYAX. SYMBYAX should be used during labor and delivery only if the potential benefit justifies the potential risk.
Olanzapine
Parturition in rats was not affected by olanzapine. The effect of olanzapine on labor and delivery in humans is unknown.
Fluoxetine
The effect of fluoxetine on labor and delivery in humans is unknown. Fluoxetine crosses the placenta; therefore, there is a possibility that fluoxetine may have adverse effects on the newborn.

Nursing Mothers

SYMBYAX
There are no adequate and well-controlled studies with SYMBYAX in nursing mothers or infants. No studies have been conducted to examine the excretion of olanzapine or fluoxetine in breast milk following SYMBYAX treatment. It is recommended that women not breast-feed when receiving SYMBYAX.
Olanzapine
Olanzapine was excreted in milk of treated rats during lactation.
Fluoxetine
Fluoxetine is excreted in human breast milk. In one breast milk sample, the concentration of fluoxetine plus norfluoxetine was 70.4 ng/mL. The concentration in the mother's plasma was 295.0 ng/mL. No adverse effects on the infant were reported. In another case, an infant nursed by a mother on fluoxetine developed crying, sleep disturbance, vomiting, and watery stools. The infant's plasma drug levels were 340 ng/mL of fluoxetine and 208 ng/mL of norfluoxetine on the 2nd day of feeding.

Pediatric Use

Safety and effectiveness of SYMBYAX in pediatric patients have not been established.

Geriatric Use

SYMBYAX
Clinical studies of SYMBYAX did not include sufficient numbers of patients ≥65 years of age to determine whether they respond differently from younger patients. Other reported clinical experience has not identified differences in responses between the elderly and younger patients. In general, dose selection for an elderly patient should be cautious, usually starting at the low end of the dosing range, reflecting the greater frequency of decreased hepatic, renal, or cardiac function, and of concomitant disease or other drug therapy (*see* DOSAGE AND ADMINISTRATION).
Olanzapine
Of the 2500 patients in premarketing clinical studies with olanzapine, 11% (263 patients) were ≥65 years of age. In patients with schizophrenia, there was no indication of any different tolerability of olanzapine in the elderly compared with younger patients. Studies in patients with various psychiatric symptoms in association with Alzheimer's disease have suggested that there may be a different tolerability profile in this population compared with younger patients with schizophrenia. In placebo-controlled studies of olanzapine in elderly patients with dementia-related psychosis, there was a significantly higher incidence of cerebrovascular adverse events (e.g., stroke, transient ischemic attack) in patients treated with olanzapine compared to

patients treated with placebo. Olanzapine is not approved for the treatment of patients with dementia-related psychosis (*see* WARNINGS, Cerebrovascular adverse events).

As with other CNS-active drugs, olanzapine should be used with caution in elderly patients with dementia. Also, the presence of factors that might decrease pharmacokinetic clearance or increase the pharmacodynamic response to olanzapine should lead to consideration of a lower starting dose for any geriatric patient.

Fluoxetine

US fluoxetine clinical studies (10,782 patients) included 687 patients ≥65 years of age and 93 patients ≥75 years of age. No overall differences in safety or effectiveness were observed between these subjects and younger subjects, and other reported clinical experience has not identified differences in responses between the elderly and younger patients, but greater sensitivity of some older individuals cannot be ruled out. As with other SSRIs, fluoxetine has been associated with cases of clinically significant hyponatremia in elderly patients.

ADVERSE REACTIONS

The information below is derived from a premarketing clinical study database for SYMBYAX consisting of 2066 patients with various diagnoses with approximately 1061 patient-years of exposure. The conditions and duration of treatment with SYMBYAX varied greatly and included (in overlapping categories) open-label and double-blind phases of studies, inpatients and outpatients, fixed-dose and dose-titration studies, and short-term or long-term exposure.

Adverse events were recorded by clinical investigators using descriptive terminology of their own choosing. Consequently, it is not possible to provide a meaningful estimate of the proportion of individuals experiencing adverse events without first grouping similar types of events into a limited (i.e., reduced) number of standardized event categories.

In the tables and tabulations that follow, COSTART Dictionary terminology has been used to classify reported adverse events. The data in the tables represent the proportion of individuals who experienced, at least once, a treatment-emergent adverse event of the type listed. An event was considered treatment-emergent if it occurred for the first time or worsened while receiving therapy following baseline evaluation. It is possible that events reported during therapy were not necessarily related to drug exposure.

The prescriber should be aware that the figures in the tables and tabulations cannot be used to predict the incidence of side effects in the course of usual medical practice where patient characteristics and other factors differ from those that prevailed in the clinical studies. Similarly, the cited frequencies cannot be compared with figures obtained from other clinical investigations involving different treatments, uses, and investigators. The cited figures, however, do provide the prescribing clinician with some basis for estimating the relative contribution of drug and non-drug factors to the side effect incidence rate in the population studied.

Incidence in Controlled Clinical Studies

The following findings are based on the short-term, controlled premarketing studies in various diagnoses including bipolar depression.

Adverse events associated with discontinuation of treatment — Overall, 10% of the patients in the SYMBYAX group discontinued due to adverse events compared with 4.6% for placebo. Table 2 enumerates the adverse events leading to discontinuation associated with the use of SYMBYAX (incidence of at least 1% for SYMBYAX and greater than that for placebo). The bipolar depression column shows the incidence of adverse events with SYMBYAX in the bipolar depression studies and the "SYMBYAX-Controlled" column shows the incidence in the controlled SYMBYAX studies; the placebo column shows the incidence in the pooled controlled studies that included a placebo arm.

Table 2: Adverse Events Associated with Discontinuation*

Adverse Event	Percentage of Patients Reporting Event		
	SYMBYAX		Placebo
	Bipolar Depression (N=86)	SYMBYAX-Controlled (N=571)	(N=477)
Asthenia	0	1	0
Somnolence	0	2	0
Weight gain	0	2	0
Chest pain	1	0	0

* Table includes events associated with discontinuation of at least 1% and greater than placebo

Commonly observed adverse events in controlled clinical studies — The most commonly observed adverse events associated with the use of SYMBYAX (incidence of ≥5% and at least twice that for placebo in the SYMBYAX-controlled database) were: asthenia, edema, increased appetite, peripheral edema, pharyngitis, somnolence, thinking abnormal, tremor, and weight gain.

Adverse events occurring at an incidence of 2% or more in controlled clinical studies — Table 3 enumerates the treatment-emergent adverse events associated with the use of SYMBYAX (incidence of at least 2% for SYMBYAX and twice or more that for placebo).

Table 3: Treatment-Emergent Adverse Events: Incidence in Controlled Clinical Studies

Body System/ Adverse Event[1]	Percentage of Patients Reporting Event		
	SYMBYAX		Placebo
	Bipolar Depression (N=86)	SYMBYAX-Controlled (N=571)	(N=477)
Body as a Whole			
Asthena	13	15	3
Accidental injury	5	3	2
Fever	4	3	1
Cardiovascular System			
Hypertension	2	2	1
Tachycardia	2	2	0
Digestive System			
Diarrhea	19	8	7
Dry Mouth	16	11	6
Increased appetite	13	16	4
Tooth disorder	1	2	1
Metabolic and Nutritional Disorders			
Weight gain	17	21	3
Peripheral edema	4	8	1
Edema	0	5	0
Musculoskeletal System			
Joint disorder	1	2	1
Twitching	6	2	1
Arthralgia	5	3	1
Nervous System			
Somnolence	21	22	11
Tremor	9	8	3
Thinking abnormal	6	6	3
Libido decreased	4	2	1
Hyperkinesia	2	1	1
Personality disorder	2	1	1
Sleep disorder	2	1	1
Amnesia	1	3	0
Respiratory System			
Pharyngitis	4	6	3
Dyspnea	1	2	1
Special Senses			
Ambylopia	5	4	2
Ear pain	2	1	1
Otitis media	2	0	0
Speech disorder	0	2	0
Urogenital System			
Abnormal ejaculation[2]	7	2	1
Impotence[2]	4	2	1
Anorgasmia	3	1	0

[1] Included are events reported by at least 2% of patients taking SYMBYAX except the following events, which had an incidence on placebo ≥SYMBYAX: abdominal pain, abnormal dreams, agitation, akathisia, anorexia, anxiety, apathy, back pain, chest pain, constipation, cough increased, depression, dizziness, dysmenorrhea[2], dyspepsia, flatulence, flu syndrome, headache, hypertonia, insomnia, manic reaction, myalgia, nausea, nervousness, pain, palpitation, paresthesia, rash, rhinitis, sinusitis, sweating, vomiting.

[2] Adjusted for gender.

Additional Findings Observed in Clinical Studies

The following findings are based on clinical studies.

Effect on cardiac repolarization — The mean increase in QT_c interval for SYMBYAX-treated patients (4.9 msec) in clinical studies was significantly greater than that for placebo-treated (-0.9 msec) and olanzapine-treated (0.6 msec) patients, but was not significantly different from fluoxetine-treated (3.7 msec) patients. There were no differences between patients treated with SYMBYAX, placebo, olanzapine, or fluoxetine in the incidence of QT_c outliers (>500 msec).

Laboratory changes — In clinical studies, SYMBYAX was associated with asymptomatic mean increases in alkaline phosphatase, cholesterol, GGT, and uric acid compared with placebo (*see* PRECAUTIONS, Transaminase elevations).

SYMBYAX was associated with a slight decrease in hemoglobin that was statistically significantly greater than that seen with placebo, olanzapine, and fluoxetine.

An elevation in serum prolactin was observed with SYMBYAX. This elevation was not statistically different than that seen with olanzapine (*see* PRECAUTIONS, Hyperprolactinemia).

Sexual dysfunction — In the pool of controlled SYMBYAX studies, there were higher rates of the treatment-emergent adverse events decreased libido, anorgasmia, impotence and abnormal ejaculation in the SYMBYAX group than in the placebo group. One case of decreased libido led to discontinuation in the SYMBYAX group. In the controlled studies that contained a fluoxetine arm, the rates of decreased libido and abnormal ejaculation in the SYMBYAX group were less than the rates in the fluoxetine group. None of the differences were statistically significant.

Sexual dysfunction, including priapism, has been reported with all SSRIs. While it is difficult to know the precise risk of sexual dysfunction associated with the use of SSRIs, physicians should routinely inquire about such possible side effects.

Vital signs — Tachycardia, bradycardia, and orthostatic hypotension have occurred in SYMBYAX-treated patients (*see* WARNINGS, Orthostatic hypotension). The mean pulse of SYMBYAX-treated patients was reduced by 1.6 beats/min.

Other Events Observed in Clinical Studies

Following is a list of all treatment-emergent adverse events reported at anytime by individuals taking SYMBYAX in clinical studies except (1) those listed in the body or footnotes of Tables 2 and 3 above or elsewhere in labeling, (2) those for which the COSTART terms were uninformative or misleading, (3) those events for which a causal relationship to SYMBYAX use was considered remote, and (4) events occurring in only 1 patient treated with SYMBYAX and which did not have a substantial probability of being acutely life-threatening.

Events are classified within body system categories using the following definitions: frequent adverse events are defined as those occurring on 1 or more occasions in at least 1/100 patients, infrequent adverse events are those occurring in 1/100 to 1/1000 patients, and rare events are those occurring in <1/1000 patients.

Body as a Whole — *Frequent:* chills, infection, neck pain, neck rigidity, photosensitivity reaction; *Infrequent:* cellulitis, cyst, hernia, intentional injury, intentional overdose, malaise, moniliasis, overdose, pelvic pain, suicide attempt; *Rare:* death, tolerance decreased.

Cardiovascular System — *Frequent:* migraine, vasodilatation; *Infrequent:* arrhythmia, bradycardia, cerebral ischemia, electrocardiogram abnormal, hypotension, QT-interval prolonged; *Rare:* angina pectoris, atrial arrhythmia, atrial fibrillation, bundle branch block, congestive heart failure, myocardial infarct, peripheral vascular disorder, T-wave inverted.

Digestive System — *Frequent:* increased salivation, thirst; *Infrequent:* cholelithiasis, colitis, eructation, esophagitis, gastritis, gastroenteritis, gingivitis, hepatomegaly, nausea and vomiting, peptic ulcer, periodontal abscess, stomatitis, tooth caries; *Rare:* aphthous stomatitis, fecal incontinence, gastrointestinal hemorrhage, gum hemorrhage, intestinal obstruction, liver fatty deposit, pancreatitis.

Endocrine System — *Infrequent:* hypothyroidism.

Hemic and Lymphatic System — *Frequent:* ecchymosis; *Infrequent:* anemia, leukocytosis, lymphadenopathy; *Rare:* coagulation disorder, leukopenia, purpura, thrombocythemia.

Metabolic and Nutritional — *Frequent:* generalized edema, weight loss; *Infrequent:* alcohol intolerance, dehydration, glycosuria, hyperlipemia, hypoglycemia, hypokalemia, obesity; *Rare:* acidosis, bilirubinemia, creatinine increased, gout, hyperkalemia, hypoglycemic reaction.

Musculoskeletal System — *Infrequent:* arthritis, bone disorder, generalized spasm, leg cramps, tendinous contracture, tenosynovitis; *Rare:* arthrosis, bursitis, myasthenia, myopathy, osteoporosis, rheumatoid arthritis.

Nervous System — *Infrequent:* abnormal gait, ataxia, buccoglossal syndrome, cogwheel rigidity, coma, confusion, depersonalization, dysarthria, emotional lability, euphoria, extrapyramidal syndrome, hostility, hypesthesia, hypokinesia, incoordination, movement disorder, myoclonus, neuralgia, neurosis, vertigo; *Rare:* acute brain syndrome, aphasia, dystonia, libido increased, subarachnoid hemorrhage, withdrawal syndrome.

Continued on next page

Symbyax—Cont.

Respiratory System — *Frequent:* bronchitis, lung disorder; *Infrequent:* apnea, asthma, epistaxis, hiccup, hyperventilation, laryngitis, pneumonia, voice alteration, yawn; *Rare:* emphysema, hemoptysis, laryngismus.

Skin and Appendages — *Infrequent:* acne, alopecia, contact dermatitis, dry skin, eczema, pruritis, psoriasis, skin discoloration, vesiculobullous rash; *Rare:* exfoliative dermatitis, maculopapular rash, seborrhea, skin ulcer.

Special Senses — *Frequent:* abnormal vision, taste perversion, tinnitus; *Infrequent:* abnormality of accommodation, conjunctivitis, deafness, diplopia, dry eyes, eye pain, miosis; *Rare:* eye hemorrhage.

Urogenital System — *Frequent:* breast pain, menorrhagia[1], urinary frequency, urinary incontinence, urinary tract infection; *Infrequent:* amenorrhea[1], breast enlargement, breast neoplasm, cystitis, dysuria, female lactation[1], fibrocystic breast[1], hematuria, hypomenorrhea[1], leukorrhea[1], menopause[1], metrorrhagia[1], oliguria, ovarian disorder[1], polyuria, urinary retention, urinary urgency, urination impaired, vaginal hemorrhage[1], vaginal moniliasis[1], vaginitis[1]; *Rare:* breast carcinoma, breast engorgement, endometrial disorder[1], gynecomastia[1], kidney calculus, uterine fibroids enlarged[1].

[1] Adjusted for gender.

Other Events Observed with Olanzapine or Fluoxetine Monotherapy

The following adverse events were not observed in SYMBYAX-treated patients during premarketing clinical studies but have been reported with olanzapine or fluoxetine monotherapy: aplastic anemia, cholestatic jaundice, diabetic coma, dyskinesia, eosinophilic pneumonia, hepatitis, idiosyncratic hepatitis, priapism, pulmonary embolism, serotonin syndrome, serum sickness-like reaction, sudden unexpected death, suicidal ideation, vasculitis, violent behaviors.

DRUG ABUSE AND DEPENDENCE

Controlled substance class — SYMBYAX is not a controlled substance.

Physical and psychological dependence — SYMBYAX, as with fluoxetine and olanzapine, has not been systematically studied in humans for its potential for abuse, tolerance, or physical dependence. While the clinical studies did not reveal any tendency for any drug-seeking behavior, these observations were not systematic, and it is not possible to predict on the basis of this limited experience the extent to which a CNS-active drug will be misused, diverted, and/or abused once marketed. Consequently, physicians should carefully evaluate patients for history of drug abuse and follow such patients closely, observing them for signs of misuse or abuse of SYMBYAX (e.g., development of tolerance, incrementation of dose, drug-seeking behavior).

In studies in rats and Rhesus monkeys designed to assess abuse and dependence potential, olanzapine alone was shown to have acute depressive CNS effects but little or no potential of abuse or physical dependence at oral doses up to 15 (rat) and 8 (monkey) times the MRHD (20 mg) on a mg/m^2 basis.

OVERDOSAGE

SYMBYAX

During premarketing clinical studies of the olanzapine/fluoxetine combination, overdose of both fluoxetine and olanzapine were reported in five study subjects. Four of the five subjects experienced loss of consciousness (3) or coma (1). No fatalities occurred.

Since the market introduction of olanzapine in October 1996, adverse event cases involving combination use of fluoxetine and olanzapine have been reported to Eli Lilly and Company. An overdose of combination therapy is defined as confirmed or suspected ingestion of a dose of olanzapine 20 mg or greater in combination with a dose of fluoxetine 80 mg or greater. As of 1 February 2002, 12 cases of combination therapy overdose were reported, most of which involved additional substances. Adverse events associated with these reports included somnolence; impaired consciousness (coma, lethargy); impaired neurologic function (ataxia, confusion, convulsions, dysarthria); arrhythmias; and fatality. Fatalities have been confounded by exposure to additional substances including alcohol, thioridazine, oxycodone, and propoxyphene.

Olanzapine

In postmarketing reports of overdose with olanzapine alone, symptoms have been reported in the majority of cases. In symptomatic patients, symptoms with ≥10% incidence included agitation/aggressiveness, dysarthria, tachycardia, various extrapyramidal symptoms, and reduced level of consciousness ranging from sedation to coma. Among less commonly reported symptoms were the following potentially medically serious events: aspiration, cardiopulmonary arrest, cardiac arrhythmias (such as supraventricular tachycardia as well as a patient that experienced sinus pause with spontaneous resumption of normal rhythm), delirium, possible neuroleptic malignant syndrome, respiratory depression/arrest, convulsion, hypertension, and hypotension. Eli Lilly and Company has received reports of fatality in association with overdose of olanzapine alone. In 1 case of death, the amount of acutely ingested olanzapine was reported to be possibly as low as 450 mg; however, in another case, a patient was reported to survive an acute olanzapine ingestion of 1500 mg.

Fluoxetine

Worldwide exposure to fluoxetine is estimated to be over 38 million patients (circa 1999). Of the 1578 cases of overdose involving fluoxetine, alone or with other drugs, reported from this population, there were 195 deaths.

Among 633 adult patients who overdosed on fluoxetine alone, 34 resulted in a fatal outcome, 378 completely recovered, and 15 patients experienced sequelae after overdose, including abnormal accommodation, abnormal gait, confusion, unresponsiveness, nervousness, pulmonary dysfunction, vertigo, tremor, elevated blood pressure, impotence, movement disorder, and hypomania. The remaining 206 patients had an unknown outcome. The most common signs and symptoms associated with non-fatal overdose were seizures, somnolence, nausea, tachycardia, and vomiting. The largest known ingestion of fluoxetine in adult patients was 8 grams in a patient who took fluoxetine alone and who subsequently recovered. However, in an adult patient who took fluoxetine alone, an ingestion as low as 520 mg has been associated with lethal outcome, but causality has not been established.

Among pediatric patients (ages 3 months to 17 years), there were 156 cases of overdose involving fluoxetine alone or in combination with other drugs. Six patients died, 127 patients completely recovered, 1 patient experienced renal failure, and 22 patients had an unknown outcome. One of the 6 fatalities was a 9-year-old boy who had a history of OCD, Tourette's Syndrome with tics, attention deficit disorder, and fetal alcohol syndrome. He had been receiving 100 mg of fluoxetine daily for 6 months in addition to clonidine, methylphenidate, and promethazine. Mixed-drug ingestion or other methods of suicide complicated all 6 overdoses in children that resulted in fatalities. The largest ingestion in pediatric patients was 3 grams, which was nonlethal.

Other important adverse events reported with fluoxetine overdose (single or multiple drugs) included coma, delirium, ECG abnormalities (such as QT-interval prolongation and ventricular tachycardia, including torsades de pointes-type arrhythmias), hypotension, mania, neuroleptic malignant syndrome-like events, pyrexia, stupor, and syncope.

Management of overdose — In managing overdose, the possibility of multiple drug involvement should be considered. In case of acute overdose, establish and maintain an airway and ensure adequate ventilation, which may include intubation. Induction of emesis is not recommended as the possibility of obtundation, seizures, or dystonic reactions of the head and neck following overdose may create a risk for aspiration. Gastric lavage (after intubation, if patient is unconscious) and administration of activated charcoal together with a laxative should be considered. Cardiovascular monitoring should commence immediately and should include continuous electrocardiographic monitoring to detect possible arrhythmias.

A specific precaution involves patients who are taking or have recently taken SYMBYAX and may have ingested excessive quantities of a TCA (tricyclic antidepressant). In such cases, accumulation of the parent TCA and/or an active metabolite may increase the possibility of serious sequelae and extend the time needed for close medical observation.

Due to the large volume of distribution of olanzapine and fluoxetine, forced diuresis, dialysis, hemoperfusion, and exchange transfusion are unlikely to be of benefit. No specific antidote for either fluoxetine or olanzapine overdose is known. Hypotension and circulatory collapse should be treated with appropriate measures such as intravenous fluids and/or sympathomimetic agents. Do not use epinephrine, dopamine, or other sympathomimetics with β-agonist activity, since beta stimulation may worsen hypotension in the setting of olanzapine-induced alpha blockade.

The physician should consider contacting a poison control center for additional information on the treatment of any overdose. Telephone numbers for certified poison control centers are listed in the *Physicians' Desk Reference (PDR).*

DOSAGE AND ADMINISTRATION

SYMBYAX should be administered once daily in the evening, generally beginning with the 6-mg/25-mg capsule. While food has no appreciable effect on the absorption of olanzapine and fluoxetine given individually, the effect of food on the absorption of SYMBYAX has not been studied. Dosage adjustments, if indicated, can be made according to efficacy and tolerability. Antidepressant efficacy was demonstrated with SYMBYAX in a dose range of olanzapine 6 to 12 mg and fluoxetine 25 to 50 mg (*see* CLINICAL STUDIES).

The safety of doses above 18 mg/75 mg has not been evaluated in clinical studies.

Special Populations

The starting dose of SYMBYAX 6 mg/25 mg should be used for patients with a predisposition to hypotensive reactions, patients with hepatic impairment, or patients who exhibit a combination of factors that may slow the metabolism of SYMBYAX (female gender, geriatric age, nonsmoking status). When indicated, dose escalation should be performed with caution in these patients. SYMBYAX has not been systematically studied in patients over 65 years of age or in patients <18 years of age (*see* WARNINGS, Orthostatic Hypotension, PRECAUTIONS, Pediatric Use, *and* Geriatric Use, *and* CLINICAL PHARMACOLOGY, Pharmacokinetics).

HOW SUPPLIED

SYMBYAX capsules are supplied in 6/25-, 6/50-, 12/25-, and 12/50-mg (mg equivalent olanzapine/mg equivalent fluoxetine[a]) strengths.

[See table below]

Store at 25°C (77°F); excursions permitted to 15–30°C (59–86°F) [see USP Controlled Room Temperature].

Keep tightly closed and protect from moisture.

SYMBYAX	CAPSULE STRENGTH			
	6 mg/25 mg	6 mg/50 mg	12 mg/25 mg	12 mg/50 mg
Color	Mustard Yellow & Light Yellow	Mustard Yellow & Light Grey	Red & Light Yellow	Red & Light Grey
Capsule No.	PU3231	PU3233	PU3232	PU3234
Identification	Lilly 3231 6/25	Lilly 3233 6/50	Lilly 3232 12/25	Lilly 3234 12/50
NDC Codes				
Bottles 30	0002-3231-30	0002-3233-30	0002-3232-30	0002-3234-30
Bottles 100	0002-3231-02	0002-3233-02	0002-3232-02	0002-3234-02
Bottles 1000	0002-3231-04	0002-3233-04	0002-3232-04	0002-3234-04
Blisters ID[b] 100	0002-3231-33	0002-3233-33	0002-3232-33	0002-3234-33

[a] Fluoxetine base equivalent.
[b] IDENTI-DOSE®, Unit Dose Medication, Lilly.

Patient Information

SYMBYAX™ (SIM-bee-ax)
(olanzapine and fluoxetine HCl capsules)

Read the Patient Information that comes with SYMBYAX before you start using it and each time you get a refill. There may be new information. This information does not take the place of talking with your doctor about your medical condition or treatment. It is important to stay under a doctor's care while taking SYMBYAX. **Do not change or stop treatment without first talking with your doctor.** Talk to your doctor or pharmacist if you have any questions about SYMBYAX.

What is SYMBYAX?

SYMBYAX is a prescription medicine used to treat adults who have depression with bipolar disorder. SYMBYAX contains two medicines, olanzapine and fluoxetine hydrochloride.

Olanzapine is also the active ingredient in Zyprexa® and Zyprexa Zydis®. Fluoxetine hydrochloride is also the active ingredient in Prozac®, Prozac Weekly™, and Sarafem®. SYMBYAX has not been studied in children.

What is bipolar disorder?

Bipolar disorder, once called manic-depressive illness, is a brain disorder that causes unusual changes in a person's mood, energy level, and ability to function. Bipolar disorder is a long-term illness that can be treated with medicines, but it usually requires life-long treatment.

Who should not take SYMBYAX?

Do not take SYMBYAX if you are:

- **Taking a medicine known as a monoamine oxidase inhibitor (MAOI) or have stopped taking a MAOI within the last 2 weeks.** An MAOI is a medicine sometimes used for depression and other mental problems. Examples of MAOI medicines are Nardil® (phenylzine sulfate) and Parnate® (tranylcypromine sulfate). Taking SYMBYAX with a MAOI may cause serious side effects that can be life threatening. Do not take a MAOI for at least 5 weeks after you stop taking SYMBYAX.
- **Taking Mellaril® (thioridazine) for mental problems.** Mellaril® (thioridazine) can cause a heart problem (prolongation of the QT_c interval) **that can cause death.** Taking SYMBYAX with Mellaril® (thioridazine) can increase your chances of having this serious and life-threatening heart problem. Do not take Mellaril® (thioridazine) for at least 5 weeks after you stop taking SYMBYAX.
- **Allergic to SYMBYAX or any of its ingredients.** The active ingredients are olanzapine and fluoxetine hydrochloride. See the end of this leaflet for a complete list of ingredients in SYMBYAX.

What should I tell my doctor before taking SYMBYAX?

- **Tell your doctor if you are taking fluoxetine, Prozac,**

Prozac Weekly, Sarafem, olanzapine, Zyprexa, or Zyprexa Zydis. These medicines each contain an active ingredient that is also found in SYMBYAX.

- **Tell your doctor about all the medicines you take, including prescription and non-prescription medicines, vitamins and herbal supplements. SYMBYAX can interact with many other medicines, causing serious or life-threatening side effects.** Your doctor will decide if you can take SYMBYAX with your other medicines, or if your dose should be adjusted. Keep a list of your medicines with you and show it to your doctor and pharmacist every time you are prescribed a new medicine or start a new non-prescription medicine, vitamin, or herbal supplement.
- **Tell your doctor if you are taking SYMBYAX and are taking or plan to take nonsteroidal anti-inflammatory drugs or aspirin** since combined use of these drug products has been associated with an increased risk of bleeding.

Before taking SYMBYAX, tell your doctor if you have or had the following medical conditions:

- **Are pregnant or plan to become pregnant.** It is not known if SYMBYAX can harm your unborn baby. You and your doctor should decide if SYMBYAX is right for you during pregnancy.
- **Are breast-feeding or plan to breast-feed.** SYMBYAX may pass into your milk and may harm your baby. You should choose either to breast-feed or take SYMBYAX, but not both.
- **Are older than age 65 and have a mental problem called dementia** (slow loss of mental function)
- **High blood sugar, diabetes or family history of diabetes**
- **Liver problems.** You may need a lower dose of SYMBYAX.
- **Seizures** (convulsions or fits)
- **Low blood pressure.** SYMBYAX may cause dizziness or fainting in people with low blood pressure.
- **Heart problems including heart attacks**
- **Strokes, or mini-strokes called transient ischemic attacks (TIA)**
- **High blood pressure**
- **An enlarged prostate** (men)
- **An eye problem called narrow angle glaucoma**
- **A stomach problem called a paralytic ileus**

Also, tell your doctor if you

- **Currently smoke**
- **Drink alcohol,** especially if you drink a lot
- **Exercise a lot** or are often in **hot places**

How should I take SYMBYAX?

- Take SYMBYAX exactly as instructed by your doctor. Your doctor will usually start you on a low dose of SYMBYAX. Your dose may be adjusted depending on your body's response to SYMBYAX. Your dose will also depend on certain medical problems you have. **Do not stop taking SYMBYAX or change your dose even if you feel better, without talking with your doctor.**
- SYMBYAX is usually taken once a day in the evening. Take SYMBYAX at the same time each day. SYMBYAX may be taken with or without food.
- If you miss a dose, take it as soon as you remember. However, if it is almost time for your next dose, skip the missed dose and take only your regularly scheduled dose. Do not take more than your doctor has prescribed for you.
- Tell your doctor if your depression does not get better while taking SYMBYAX. Your doctor may adjust your dose or give you a different medicine.
- If you take too much SYMBYAX or overdose, call your doctor or poison control center right away, or go to the nearest emergency room.

What should I avoid while taking SYMBYAX?

- Do not drive or operate other dangerous machinery until you know how SYMBYAX affects you. SYMBYAX can impair your judgment, thinking, and motor skills.
- Do not take medicines, including prescription and non-prescription medicines, vitamins and herbal supplements unless you have talked to your doctor about them.
- Do not get pregnant.
- Do not breast-feed.
- Do not drink alcohol.
- Do not get over-heated or dehydrated (loss of body fluids) during hot weather or exercise, or when using a hot tub.
- Do not take a MAOI medicine or Mellaril® (thioridazine) for at least 5 weeks after you stop taking SYMBYAX.

What are the possible side effects of SYMBYAX?

All medicines may cause side effects in some patients. Serious side effects reported by patients treated with SYMBYAX follow below:

- **Severe allergic reactions** that cause hives, swelling of your face, eyes, mouth, or tongue, trouble breathing or a rash with fever and joint pain. Tell your doctor right away if you get these symptoms. Your doctor may stop SYMBYAX and prescribe medicines to treat your allergic reaction.
- **Strokes and "mini-strokes" called transient ischemic attacks (TIAs).** These are more common in elderly patients with dementia. As with other mental health drugs, SYMBYAX should be used with caution in elderly patients with dementia. SYMBYAX is not approved for the treatment of elderly patients with dementia.
- **High blood sugar or diabetes.** Patients who already have diabetes should have their blood sugar checked regularly during treatment with SYMBYAX. Patients at risk for diabetes (for example, those who are overweight or have a family history of diabetes) who are starting treatment with SYMBYAX should undergo blood sugar testing on an empty stomach at the beginning of treatment and regularly during treatment. Any patient treated with SYMBYAX should be monitored for signs of high blood sugar including being thirsty, going to the bathroom a lot, eating a lot, and feeling weak. Patients who develop signs of high blood sugar during treatment with SYMBYAX should undergo blood sugar testing on an empty stomach. In some cases, high blood sugar has gone away when SYMBYAX was stopped; however, some patients had to keep taking medicine for diabetes even though they stopped taking SYMBYAX.
- **Neuroleptic malignant syndrome (NMS).** NMS is a rare, but life-threatening reaction to certain medicines for mental problems, including SYMBYAX. Stop taking SYMBYAX and call your doctor right away if you get any of the following symptoms of NMS, such as a high fever, sweating, muscle stiffness, trouble thinking clearly, a change in mental functioning, sleepiness, or changes in your breathing, heartbeat, and blood pressure. NMS can cause death and must be treated in a hospital.
- **Tardive dyskinesia.** This is a condition caused by certain medicines for mental problems, including SYMBYAX. It causes body movements, mostly in your face or tongue, that keep happening and that you cannot control. It may start after you stop taking SYMBYAX. Tardive dyskinesia may not go away, even if you stop taking SYMBYAX. Tell your doctor if you get body movements that you can't control.
- **Low blood pressure.** SYMBYAX may cause low blood pressure in some patients. Low blood pressure is more likely in patients who have heart problems, who have brain problems such as strokes, who take certain medicines, or who drink alcohol. Signs of low blood pressure include dizziness, fast heartbeat, and fainting. To lower your chances of fainting while taking SYMBYAX, stand up slowly if you have been sitting or lying down.
- **Seizures.** SYMBYAX should be used cautiously in people who have had seizures in the past or who have conditions that increase their risk for seizures.
- **Impaired judgment, thinking, and motor skills**
- **Trouble swallowing**
- **Abnormal bleeding.** When SYMBYAX is used alone, and especially with certain other medicines that can increase bleeding risk (for example; ibuprofen or aspirin), your risk of bleeding can increase. If you notice increased or unusual bruising or other bleeding, contact your doctor.
- **Low salt levels in the blood.** SYMBYAX can cause a low salt level in the blood. Weakness, confusion, or trouble thinking can be caused by low salt levels in the blood. If you develop any of these symptoms, contact your doctor.
- **Body temperature problems.** SYMBYAX can cause problems in keeping your body temperature regular. Do not become overheated or dehydrated during hot weather or exercise, or when using a hot tub.

Common side effects of SYMBYAX are:

- Weight gain
- Sleepiness
- Diarrhea
- Dry mouth
- Increased appetite
- Feeling weak
- Swelling of your hands and feet
- Tremors (shakes)
- Sore throat
- Trouble concentrating
- SYMBYAX can cause problems in keeping your body temperature regulated.

Tell your doctor about any side effect that bothers you or won't go away. Your doctor may be able to help you manage the side effect.

These are not all the side effects of SYMBYAX. For more information ask your doctor or pharmacist.

Other important safety information about SYMBYAX

- The symptoms of bipolar disorder may include thoughts of harming yourself or others or committing suicide. Tell your doctor immediately or go to an emergency center if you have any of these thoughts.
- Symptoms of bipolar disorder may include mania. If you experience manic symptoms (for example; racing thoughts, poor sleep, irritability, mood swings, extra energy), contact your doctor.
- If your depression becomes worse, contact your doctor.
- Rarely, people taking medicines of this type have started to leak milk from their breasts, and women have missed periods or had irregular periods. If these symptoms occur, contact your doctor.
- If you gain weight while taking SYMBYAX, contact your doctor to discuss changes you can make in your activities or eating habits to help manage your weight.
- Problems with sexual functioning have commonly occurred in patients taking SYMBYAX. If these symptoms occur, contact your doctor.

How do I store SYMBYAX?

- Store SYMBYAX at room temperature, 59° to 86°F (15° to 30°C).
- Keep the container tightly closed and protect from moisture.
- **Keep SYMBYAX and all medicines away from children.**

General information about SYMBYAX

Medicines are sometimes prescribed for conditions that are not mentioned in patient information leaflets. Do not take SYMBYAX for a condition for which it was not prescribed. Do not give SYMBYAX to other people, even if they have the same symptoms that you have. It may harm them.

This leaflet summarizes important information about SYMBYAX. If you would like more information, talk with your doctor. You can ask your doctor or pharmacist for information that is written for health professionals. You can also call 1-800-Lilly-Rx (1-800-545-5979) or visit our website at www.SYMBYAX.com.

What are the ingredients in SYMBYAX?

Active ingredients: olanzapine and fluoxetine hydrochloride

Inactive ingredients: pregelatinized starch, gelatin, dimethicone, titanium dioxide, sodium lauryl sulfate, edible black ink, red iron oxide, yellow iron oxide, and/or black iron oxide.

Rx Only

This patient information has been approved by the US Food and Drug Administration.

Literature revised December 30, 2003

Eli Lilly and Company
Indianapolis, IN 46285
www.SYMBYAX.com

PV 4201 AMP

ZYPREXA® ℞

[*zī-prex-ah*]

Olanzapine Tablets

ZYPREXA® ZYDIS®

Olanzapine Orally Disintegrating Tablets

ZYPREXA® IntraMuscular

Olanzapine for Injection

DESCRIPTION

ZYPREXA (olanzapine) is a psychotropic agent that belongs to the thienobenzodiazepine class. The chemical designation is 2-methyl-4-(4-methyl-1-piperazinyl)-10*H*-thieno[2,3-*b*][1,5]benzodiazepine. The molecular formula is $C_{17}H_{20}N_4S$, which corresponds to a molecular weight of 312.44. The chemical structure is:

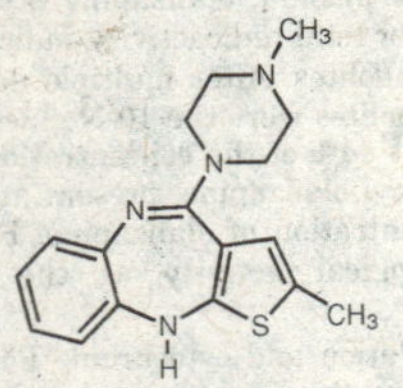

Olanzapine is a yellow crystalline solid, which is practically insoluble in water.

ZYPREXA tablets are intended for oral administration only. Each tablet contains olanzapine equivalent to 2.5 mg (8 μmol), 5 mg (16 μmol), 7.5 mg (24 μmol), 10 mg (32 μmol), 15 mg (48 μmol), or 20 mg (64 μmol). Inactive ingredients are carnauba wax, crospovidone, hydroxypropyl cellulose, hypromellose, lactose, magnesium stearate, microcrystalline cellulose, and other inactive ingredients. The color coating contains Titanium Dioxide (all strengths), FD&C Blue No. 2 Aluminum Lake (15 mg), or Synthetic Red Iron Oxide (20 mg). The 2.5, 5.0, 7.5, and 10 mg tablets are imprinted with edible ink which contains FD&C Blue No. 2 Aluminum Lake.

ZYPREXA ZYDIS (olanzapine orally disintegrating tablets) is intended for oral administration only.

Each orally disintegrating tablet contains olanzapine equivalent to 5 mg (16 μmol), 10 mg (32 μmol), 15 mg (48 μmol) or 20 mg (64 μmol). It begins disintegrating in the mouth within seconds, allowing its contents to be subsequently swallowed with or without liquid. ZYPREXA ZYDIS (olanzapine orally disintegrating tablets) also contains the following inactive ingredients: gelatin, mannitol, aspartame, sodium methyl paraben and sodium propyl paraben.

ZYPREXA IntraMuscular (olanzapine for injection) is intended for intramuscular use only. Each vial provides for the administration of 10 mg (32 μmol) olanzapine with inactive ingredients 50 mg lactose monohydrate and 3.5 mg tartaric acid. Hydrochloric acid and/or sodium hydroxide may have been added during manufacturing to adjust pH.

CLINICAL PHARMACOLOGY

Pharmacodynamics

Olanzapine is a selective monoaminergic antagonist with high affinity binding to the following receptors: serotonin $5HT_{2A/2C}$ (K_i=4 and 11 nM, respectively), dopamine $D_{1\text{-}4}$ (K_i=11-31 nM), muscarinic $M_{1\text{-}5}$ (K_i=1.9-25 nM), histamine H_1 (K_i=7 nM), and adrenergic α_1 receptors (K_i=19 nM). Olanzapine binds weakly to $GABA_A$, BZD, and β adrenergic receptors (K_i>10 μM).

The mechanism of action of olanzapine, as with other drugs having efficacy in schizophrenia, is unknown. However, it

Continued on next page

Zyprexa—Cont.

has been proposed that this drug's efficacy in schizophrenia is mediated through a combination of dopamine and serotonin type 2 ($5HT_2$) antagonism. The mechanism of action of olanzapine in the treatment of acute manic episodes associated with Bipolar I Disorder is unknown.

Antagonism at receptors other than dopamine and $5HT_2$ with similar receptor affinities may explain some of the other therapeutic and side effects of olanzapine. Olanzapine's antagonism of muscarinic M_{1-5} receptors may explain its anticholinergic effects. Olanzapine's antagonism of histamine H_1 receptors may explain the somnolence observed with this drug. Olanzapine's antagonism of adrenergic α_1 receptors may explain the orthostatic hypotension observed with this drug.

Pharmacokinetics

Oral Administration

Olanzapine is well absorbed and reaches peak concentrations in approximately 6 hours following an oral dose. It is eliminated extensively by first pass metabolism, with approximately 40% of the dose metabolized before reaching the systemic circulation. Food does not affect the rate or extent of olanzapine absorption. Pharmacokinetic studies showed that ZYPREXA tablets and ZYPREXA ZYDIS (olanzapine orally disintegrating tablets) dosage forms of olanzapine are bioequivalent.

Olanzapine displays linear kinetics over the clinical dosing range. Its half-life ranges from 21 to 54 hours (5th to 95th percentile; mean of 30 hr), and apparent plasma clearance ranges from 12 to 47 L/hr (5th to 95th percentile; mean of 25 L/hr).

Administration of olanzapine once daily leads to steady-state concentrations in about one week that are approximately twice the concentrations after single doses. Plasma concentrations, half-life, and clearance of olanzapine may vary between individuals on the basis of smoking status, gender, and age (*see* Special Populations).

Olanzapine is extensively distributed throughout the body, with a volume of distribution of approximately 1000 L. It is 93% bound to plasma proteins over the concentration range of 7 to 1100 ng/mL, binding primarily to albumin and α_1-acid glycoprotein.

Metabolism and Elimination — Following a single oral dose of ^{14}C labeled olanzapine, 7% of the dose of olanzapine was recovered in the urine as unchanged drug, indicating that olanzapine is highly metabolized. Approximately 57% and 30% of the dose was recovered in the urine and feces, respectively. In the plasma, olanzapine accounted for only 12% of the AUC for total radioactivity, indicating significant exposure to metabolites. After multiple dosing, the major circulating metabolites were the 10-N-glucuronide, present at steady state at 44% of the concentration of olanzapine, and 4'-N-desmethyl olanzapine, present at steady state at 31% of the concentration of olanzapine. Both metabolites lack pharmacological activity at the concentrations observed.

Direct glucuronidation and cytochrome P450 (CYP) mediated oxidation are the primary metabolic pathways for olanzapine. In vitro studies suggest that CYPs 1A2 and 2D6, and the flavin-containing monooxygenase system are involved in olanzapine oxidation. CYP2D6 mediated oxidation appears to be a minor metabolic pathway in vivo, because the clearance of olanzapine is not reduced in subjects who are deficient in this enzyme.

Intramuscular Administration

ZYPREXA IntraMuscular results in rapid absorption with peak plasma concentrations occurring within 15 to 45 minutes. Based upon a pharmacokinetic study in healthy volunteers, a 5 mg dose of intramuscular olanzapine for injection produces, on average, a maximum plasma concentration approximately 5 times higher than the maximum plasma concentration produced by a 5 mg dose of oral olanzapine. Area under the curve achieved after an intramuscular dose is similar to that achieved after oral administration of the same dose. The half-life observed after intramuscular administration is similar to that observed after oral dosing. The pharmacokinetics are linear over the clinical dosing range. Metabolic profiles after intramuscular administration are qualitatively similar to metabolic profiles after oral administration.

Special Populations

Renal Impairment — Because olanzapine is highly metabolized before excretion and only 7% of the drug is excreted unchanged, renal dysfunction alone is unlikely to have a major impact on the pharmacokinetics of olanzapine. The pharmacokinetic characteristics of olanzapine were similar in patients with severe renal impairment and normal subjects, indicating that dosage adjustment based upon the degree of renal impairment is not required. In addition, olanzapine is not removed by dialysis. The effect of renal impairment on metabolite elimination has not been studied.

Hepatic Impairment — Although the presence of hepatic impairment may be expected to reduce the clearance of olanzapine, a study of the effect of impaired liver function in subjects (n=6) with clinically significant (Childs Pugh Classification A and B) cirrhosis revealed little effect on the pharmacokinetics of olanzapine.

Age — In a study involving 24 healthy subjects, the mean elimination half-life of olanzapine was about 1.5 times greater in elderly (>65 years) than in non-elderly subjects (≤65 years). Caution should be used in dosing the elderly, especially if there are other factors that might additively influence drug metabolism and/or pharmacodynamic sensitivity (*see* DOSAGE AND ADMINISTRATION).

Gender — Clearance of olanzapine is approximately 30% lower in women than in men. There were, however, no apparent differences between men and women in effectiveness or adverse effects. Dosage modifications based on gender should not be needed.

Smoking Status — Olanzapine clearance is about 40% higher in smokers than in nonsmokers, although dosage modifications are not routinely recommended.

Race — In vivo studies have shown that exposures are similar among Japanese, Chinese and Caucasians, especially after normalization for body weight differences. Dosage modifications for race are, therefore, not recommended.

Combined Effects — The combined effects of age, smoking, and gender could lead to substantial pharmacokinetic differences in populations. The clearance in young smoking males, for example, may be 3 times higher than that in elderly nonsmoking females. Dosing modification may be necessary in patients who exhibit a combination of factors that may result in slower metabolism of olanzapine (*see* DOSAGE AND ADMINISTRATION).

For specific information about the pharmacology of lithium or valproate, refer to the CLINICAL PHARMACOLOGY section of the package inserts for these other products.

Clinical Efficacy Data

Schizophrenia

The efficacy of oral olanzapine in the treatment of schizophrenia was established in 2 short-term (6-week) controlled trials of inpatients who met DSM III-R criteria for schizophrenia. A single haloperidol arm was included as a comparative treatment in one of the two trials, but this trial did not compare these two drugs on the full range of clinically relevant doses for both.

Several instruments were used for assessing psychiatric signs and symptoms in these studies, among them the Brief Psychiatric Rating Scale (BPRS), a multi-item inventory of general psychopathology traditionally used to evaluate the effects of drug treatment in schizophrenia. The BPRS psychosis cluster (conceptual disorganization, hallucinatory behavior, suspiciousness, and unusual thought content) is considered a particularly useful subset for assessing actively psychotic schizophrenic patients. A second traditional assessment, the Clinical Global Impression (CGI), reflects the impression of a skilled observer, fully familiar with the manifestations of schizophrenia, about the overall clinical state of the patient. In addition, two more recently developed scales were employed; these included the 30-item Positive and Negative Symptoms Scale (PANSS), in which are embedded the 18 items of the BPRS, and the Scale for Assessing Negative Symptoms (SANS). The trial summaries below focus on the following outcomes: PANSS total and/or BPRS total; BPRS psychosis cluster; PANSS negative subscale or SANS; and CGI Severity. The results of the trials follow:

(1) In a 6-week, placebo-controlled trial (n=149) involving two fixed olanzapine doses of 1 and 10 mg/day (once daily schedule), olanzapine, at 10 mg/day (but not at 1 mg/day), was superior to placebo on the PANSS total score (also on the extracted BPRS total), on the BPRS psychosis cluster, on the PANSS Negative subscale, and on CGI Severity.

(2) In a 6-week, placebo-controlled trial (n=253) involving 3 fixed dose ranges of olanzapine (5.0 ± 2.5 mg/day, 10.0 ± 2.5 mg/day, and 15.0 ± 2.5 mg/day) on a once daily schedule, the two highest olanzapine dose groups (actual mean doses of 12 and 16 mg/day, respectively) were superior to placebo on BPRS total score, BPRS psychosis cluster, and CGI severity score; the highest olanzapine dose group was superior to placebo on the SANS. There was no clear advantage for the high dose group over the medium dose group.

Examination of population subsets (race and gender) did not reveal any differential responsiveness on the basis of these subgroupings.

In a longer-term trial, adult outpatients (n=326) who predominantly met DSM-IV criteria for schizophrenia and who remained stable on olanzapine during open label treatment for at least 8 weeks were randomized to continuation on their current olanzapine doses (ranging from 10 to 20 mg/day) or to placebo. The follow-up period to observe patients for relapse, defined in terms of increases in BPRS positive symptoms or hospitalization, was planned for 12 months, however, criteria were met for stopping the trial early due to an excess of placebo relapses compared to olanzapine relapses, and olanzapine was superior to placebo on time to relapse, the primary outcome for this study. Thus, olanzapine was more effective than placebo at maintaining efficacy in patients stabilized for approximately 8 weeks and followed for an observation period of up to 8 months.

Bipolar Disorder

Monotherapy — The efficacy of oral olanzapine in the treatment of acute manic or mixed episodes was established in 2 short-term (one 3-week and one 4-week) placebo-controlled trials in patients who met the DSM-IV criteria for Bipolar I Disorder with manic or mixed episodes. These trials included patients with or without psychotic features and with or without a rapid-cycling course.

The primary rating instrument used for assessing manic symptoms in these trials was the Young Mania Rating Scale (Y-MRS), an 11-item clinician-rated scale traditionally used to assess the degree of manic symptomatology (irritability, disruptive/aggressive behavior, sleep, elevated mood, speech, increased activity, sexual interest, language/thought disorder, thought content, appearance, and insight) in a range from 0 (no manic features) to 60 (maximum score). The primary outcome in these trials was change from baseline in the Y-MRS total score. The results of the trials follow:

(1) In one 3-week placebo-controlled trial (n=67) which involved a dose range of olanzapine (5-20 mg/day, once daily, starting at 10 mg/day), olanzapine was superior to placebo in the reduction of Y-MRS total score. In an identically designed trial conducted simultaneously with the first trial, olanzapine demonstrated a similar treatment difference, but possibly due to sample size and site variability, was not shown to be superior to placebo on this outcome.

(2) In a 4-week placebo-controlled trial (n=115) which involved a dose range of olanzapine (5-20 mg/day, once daily, starting at 15 mg/day), olanzapine was superior to placebo in the reduction of Y-MRS total score.

(3) In another trial, 361 patients meeting DSM-IV criteria for a manic or mixed episode of bipolar disorder who had responded during an initial open-label treatment phase for about two weeks, on average, to olanzapine 5 to 20 mg/day were randomized to either continuation of olanzapine at their same dose (n=225) or to placebo (n=136), for observation of relapse. Approximately 50% of the patients had discontinued from the olanzapine group by day 59 and 50% of the placebo group had discontinued by day 23 of double-blind treatment. Response during the open-label phase was defined by having a decrease of the Y-MRS total score to ≤12 and HAM-D 21 to ≤8. Relapse during the double-blind phase was defined as an increase of the Y-MRS or HAM-D 21 total score to ≥15, or being hospitalized for either mania or depression. In the randomized phase, patients receiving continued olanzapine experienced a significantly longer time to relapse.

Combination Therapy — The efficacy of oral olanzapine with concomitant lithium or valproate in the treatment of acute manic episodes was established in two controlled trials in patients who met the DSM-IV criteria for Bipolar I Disorder with manic or mixed episodes. These trials included patients with or without psychotic features and with or without a rapid-cycling course. The results of the trials follow:

(1) In one 6-week placebo-controlled combination trial, 175 outpatients on lithium or valproate therapy with inadequately controlled manic or mixed symptoms (Y-MRS ≥16) were randomized to receive either olanzapine or placebo, in combination with their original therapy. Olanzapine (in a dose range of 5-20 mg/day, once daily, starting at 10 mg/day) combined with lithium or valproate (in a therapeutic range of 0.6 mEq/L to 1.2 mEq/L or 50 µg/mL to 125 µg/mL, respectively) was superior to lithium or valproate alone in the reduction of Y-MRS total score.

(2) In a second 6-week placebo-controlled combination trial, 169 outpatients on lithium or valproate therapy with inadequately controlled manic or mixed symptoms (Y-MRS ≥16) were randomized to receive either olanzapine or placebo, in combination with their original therapy. Olanzapine (in a dose range of 5-20 mg/day, once daily, starting at 10 mg/day) combined with lithium or valproate (in a therapeutic range of 0.6 mEq/L to 1.2 mEq/L or 50 µg/mL to 125 µg/mL, respectively) was superior to lithium or valproate alone in the reduction of Y-MRS total score.

Agitation Associated with Schizophrenia and Bipolar I Mania

The efficacy of intramuscular olanzapine for injection for the treatment of agitation was established in 3 short-term (24 hours of IM treatment) placebo-controlled trials in agitated inpatients from two diagnostic groups: schizophrenia and Bipolar I Disorder (manic or mixed episodes). Each of the trials included a single active comparator treatment arm of either haloperidol injection (schizophrenia studies) or lorazepam injection (bipolar mania study). Patients enrolled in the trials needed to be: (1) judged by the clinical investigators as clinically agitated and clinically appropriate candidates for treatment with intramuscular medication, and (2) exhibiting a level of agitation that met or exceeded a threshold score of ≥14 on the five items comprising the Positive and Negative Syndrome Scale (PANSS) Excited Component (i.e., poor impulse control, tension, hostility, uncooperativeness and excitement items) with at least one individual item score ≥4 using a 1-7 scoring system (1=absent, 4=moderate, 7=extreme). In the studies, the mean baseline PANSS Excited Component score was 18.4, with scores ranging from 13 to 32 (out of a maximum score of 35), thus suggesting predominantly moderate levels of agitation with some patients experiencing mild or severe levels of agitation. The primary efficacy measure used for assessing agitation signs and symptoms in these trials was the change from baseline in the PANSS Excited Component at 2 hours post-injection. Patients could receive up to three injections during the 24 hour IM treatment periods; however, patients could not receive the second injection until after the initial 2 hour period when the primary efficacy measure was assessed. The results of the trials follow:

(1) In a placebo-controlled trial in agitated inpatients meeting DSM-IV criteria for schizophrenia (n=270), four fixed intramuscular olanzapine for injection doses of 2.5 mg, 5 mg, 7.5 mg and 10 mg were evaluated. All doses were statistically superior to placebo on the PANSS Excited Component at 2 hours post-injection. However, the effect was larger and more consistent for the three highest doses. There were no significant pairwise differences for the 7.5 and 10 mg doses over the 5 mg dose.

(2) In a second placebo-controlled trial in agitated inpatients meeting DSM-IV criteria for schizophrenia (n=311), one fixed intramuscular olanzapine for injection dose of

10 mg was evaluated. Olanzapine for injection was statistically superior to placebo on the PANSS Excited Component at 2 hours post-injection.

(3) In a placebo-controlled trial in agitated inpatients meeting DSM-IV criteria for Bipolar I Disorder (and currently displaying an acute manic or mixed episode with or without psychotic features) (n=201), one fixed intramuscular olanzapine for injection dose of 10 mg was evaluated. Olanzapine for injection was statistically superior to placebo on the PANSS Excited Component at 2 hours post-injection.

Examination of population subsets (age, race, and gender) did not reveal any differential responsiveness on the basis of these subgroupings.

INDICATIONS AND USAGE

Schizophrenia

Oral ZYPREXA is indicated for the treatment of schizophrenia.

The efficacy of ZYPREXA was established in short-term (6-week) controlled trials of schizophrenic inpatients (*see* CLINICAL PHARMACOLOGY).

The effectiveness of oral ZYPREXA at maintaining a treatment response in schizophrenic patients who had been stable on ZYPREXA for approximately 8 weeks and were then followed for a period of up to 8 months has been demonstrated in a placebo-controlled trial (*see* CLINICAL PHARMACOLOGY). Nevertheless, the physician who elects to use ZYPREXA for extended periods should periodically re-evaluate the long-term usefulness of the drug for the individual patient (*see* DOSAGE AND ADMINISTRATION).

Bipolar Disorder

Acute Monotherapy — Oral ZYPREXA is indicated for the treatment of acute mixed or manic episodes associated with Bipolar I Disorder.

The efficacy of ZYPREXA was established in two placebo-controlled trials (one 3-week and one 4-week) with patients meeting DSM-IV criteria for Bipolar I Disorder who currently displayed an acute manic or mixed episode with or without psychotic features (*see* CLINICAL PHARMACOLOGY).

Maintenance Monotherapy — The benefit of maintaining bipolar patients on monotherapy with oral ZYPREXA after achieving a responder status for an average duration of two weeks was demonstrated in a controlled trial (*see* Clinical Efficacy Data *under* CLINICAL PHARMACOLOGY). The physician who elects to use ZYPREXA for extended periods should periodically re-evaluate the long-term usefulness of the drug for the individual patient (*see* DOSAGE AND ADMINISTRATION).

Combination Therapy — The combination of oral ZYPREXA with lithium or valproate is indicated for the short-term treatment of acute manic episodes associated with Bipolar I Disorder.

The efficacy of ZYPREXA in combination with lithium or valproate was established in two placebo-controlled (6-week) trials with patients meeting DSM-IV criteria for Bipolar I Disorder who currently displayed an acute manic or mixed episode with or without psychotic features (*see* CLINICAL PHARMACOLOGY).

Agitation Associated with Schizophrenia and Bipolar I Mania

ZYPREXA IntraMuscular is indicated for the treatment of agitation associated with schizophrenia and bipolar I mania. "Psychomotor agitation" is defined in DSM-IV as "excessive motor activity associated with a feeling of inner tension." Patients experiencing agitation often manifest behaviors that interfere with their diagnosis and care, e.g., threatening behaviors, escalating or urgently distressing behavior, or self-exhausting behavior, leading clinicians to the use of intramuscular antipsychotic medications to achieve immediate control of the agitation.

The efficacy of ZYPREXA IntraMuscular for the treatment of agitation associated with schizophrenia and bipolar I mania was established in 3 short-term (24 hours) placebo-controlled trials in agitated inpatients with schizophrenia or Bipolar I Disorder (manic or mixed episodes) (*see* CLINICAL PHARMACOLOGY).

CONTRAINDICATIONS

ZYPREXA is contraindicated in patients with a known hypersensitivity to the product.

For specific information about the contraindications of lithium or valproate, refer to the CONTRAINDICATIONS section of the package inserts for these other products.

WARNINGS

Hyperglycemia and Diabetes Mellitus — Hyperglycemia, in some cases extreme and associated with ketoacidosis or hyperosmolar coma or death, has been reported in patients treated with atypical antipsychotics including olanzapine. Assessment of the relationship between atypical antipsychotic use and glucose abnormalities is complicated by the possibility of an increased background risk of diabetes mellitus in patients with schizophrenia and the increasing incidence of diabetes mellitus in the general population. Given these confounders, the relationship between atypical antipsychotic use and hyperglycemia-related adverse events is not completely understood. However, epidemiological studies suggest an increased risk of treatment-emergent hyperglycemia-related adverse events in patients treated with the atypical antipsychotics. Precise risk estimates for hyperglycemia-related adverse events in patients treated with atypical antipsychotics are not available.

Patients with an established diagnosis of diabetes mellitus who are started on atypical antipsychotics should be monitored regularly for worsening of glucose control. Patients with risk factors for diabetes mellitus (e.g., obesity, family history of diabetes) who are starting treatment with atypical antipsychotics should undergo fasting blood glucose testing at the beginning of treatment and periodically during treatment. Any patient treated with atypical antipsychotics should be monitored for symptoms of hyperglycemia including polydipsia, polyuria, polyphagia, and weakness. Patients who develop symptoms of hyperglycemia during treatment with atypical antipsychotics should undergo fasting blood glucose testing. In some cases, hyperglycemia has resolved when the atypical antipsychotic was discontinued; however, some patients required continuation of anti-diabetic treatment despite discontinuation of the suspect drug.

Cerebrovascular Adverse Events, Including Stroke, in Elderly Patients with Dementia — Cerebrovascular adverse events (e.g., stroke, transient ischemic attack), including fatalities, were reported in patients in trials of olanzapine in elderly patients with dementia-related psychosis. In placebo-controlled trials, there was a significantly higher incidence of cerebrovascular adverse events in patients treated with olanzapine compared to patients treated with placebo. Olanzapine is not approved for the treatment of patients with dementia-related psychosis.

Neuroleptic Malignant Syndrome (NMS) — A potentially fatal symptom complex sometimes referred to as Neuroleptic Malignant Syndrome (NMS) has been reported in association with administration of antipsychotic drugs, including olanzapine. Clinical manifestations of NMS are hyperpyrexia, muscle rigidity, altered mental status and evidence of autonomic instability (irregular pulse or blood pressure, tachycardia, diaphoresis and cardiac dysrhythmia). Additional signs may include elevated creatinine phosphokinase, myoglobinuria (rhabdomyolysis), and acute renal failure.

The diagnostic evaluation of patients with this syndrome is complicated. In arriving at a diagnosis, it is important to exclude cases where the clinical presentation includes both serious medical illness (e.g., pneumonia, systemic infection, etc.) and untreated or inadequately treated extrapyramidal signs and symptoms (EPS). Other important considerations in the differential diagnosis include central anticholinergic toxicity, heat stroke, drug fever, and primary central nervous system pathology.

The management of NMS should include: 1) immediate discontinuation of antipsychotic drugs and other drugs not essential to concurrent therapy; 2) intensive symptomatic treatment and medical monitoring; and 3) treatment of any concomitant serious medical problems for which specific treatments are available. There is no general agreement about specific pharmacological treatment regimens for NMS.

If a patient requires antipsychotic drug treatment after recovery from NMS, the potential reintroduction of drug therapy should be carefully considered. The patient should be carefully monitored, since recurrences of NMS have been reported.

Tardive Dyskinesia — A syndrome of potentially irreversible, involuntary, dyskinetic movements may develop in patients treated with antipsychotic drugs. Although the prevalence of the syndrome appears to be highest among the elderly, especially elderly women, it is impossible to rely upon prevalence estimates to predict, at the inception of antipsychotic treatment, which patients are likely to develop the syndrome. Whether antipsychotic drug products differ in their potential to cause tardive dyskinesia is unknown.

The risk of developing tardive dyskinesia and the likelihood that it will become irreversible are believed to increase as the duration of treatment and the total cumulative dose of antipsychotic drugs administered to the patient increase. However, the syndrome can develop, although much less commonly, after relatively brief treatment periods at low doses.

There is no known treatment for established cases of tardive dyskinesia, although the syndrome may remit, partially or completely, if antipsychotic treatment is withdrawn. Antipsychotic treatment, itself, however, may suppress (or partially suppress) the signs and symptoms of the syndrome and thereby may possibly mask the underlying process. The effect that symptomatic suppression has upon the long-term course of the syndrome is unknown.

Given these considerations, olanzapine should be prescribed in a manner that is most likely to minimize the occurrence of tardive dyskinesia. Chronic antipsychotic treatment should generally be reserved for patients (1) who suffer from a chronic illness that is known to respond to antipsychotic drugs, and (2) for whom alternative, equally effective, but potentially less harmful treatments are not available or appropriate. In patients who do require chronic treatment, the smallest dose and the shortest duration of treatment producing a satisfactory clinical response should be sought. The need for continued treatment should be reassessed periodically.

If signs and symptoms of tardive dyskinesia appear in a patient on olanzapine, drug discontinuation should be considered. However, some patients may require treatment with olanzapine despite the presence of the syndrome.

For specific information about the warnings of lithium or valproate, refer to the WARNINGS section of the package inserts for these other products.

PRECAUTIONS

General

Hemodynamic Effects — Olanzapine may induce orthostatic hypotension associated with dizziness, tachycardia, and in some patients, syncope, especially during the initial dose-titration period, probably reflecting its α_1-adrenergic antagonistic properties. Hypotension, bradycardia with or without hypotension, tachycardia, and syncope were also reported during the clinical trials with intramuscular olanzapine for injection. In an open-label clinical pharmacology study in non-agitated patients with schizophrenia in which the safety and tolerability of intramuscular olanzapine were evaluated under a maximal dosing regimen (three 10 mg doses administered 4 hours apart), approximately one-third of these patients experienced a significant orthostatic decrease in systolic blood pressure (i.e., decrease ≥30 mmHg) (*see* DOSAGE AND ADMINISTRATION). Syncope was reported in 0.6% (15/2500) of olanzapine-treated patients in phase 2-3 oral olanzapine studies and in 0.3% (2/722) of olanzapine-treated patients with agitation in the intramuscular olanzapine for injection studies. Three normal volunteers in phase 1 studies with intramuscular olanzapine experienced hypotension, bradycardia, and sinus pauses of up to 6 seconds that spontaneously resolved (in 2 cases the events occurred on intramuscular olanzapine, and in 1 case, on oral olanzapine). The risk for this sequence of hypotension, bradycardia, and sinus pause may be greater in nonpsychiatric patients compared to psychiatric patients who are possibly more adapted to certain effects of psychotropic drugs.

For oral olanzapine therapy, the risk of orthostatic hypotension and syncope may be minimized by initiating therapy with 5 mg QD (*see* DOSAGE AND ADMINISTRATION). A more gradual titration to the target dose should be considered if hypotension occurs.

For intramuscular olanzapine for injection therapy, patients should remain recumbent if drowsy or dizzy after injection until examination has indicated that they are not experiencing postural hypotension and/or bradycardia.

Olanzapine should be used with particular caution in patients with known cardiovascular disease (history of myocardial infarction or ischemia, heart failure, or conduction abnormalities), cerebrovascular disease, and conditions which would predispose patients to hypotension (dehydration, hypovolemia, and treatment with antihypertensive medications) where the occurrence of syncope, or hypotension and/or bradycardia might put the patient at increased medical risk.

Seizures — During premarketing testing, seizures occurred in 0.9% (22/2500) of olanzapine-treated patients. There were confounding factors that may have contributed to the occurrence of seizures in many of these cases. Olanzapine should be used cautiously in patients with a history of seizures or with conditions that potentially lower the seizure threshold, e.g., Alzheimer's dementia. Conditions that lower the seizure threshold may be more prevalent in a population of 65 years or older.

Hyperprolactinemia — As with other drugs that antagonize dopamine D_2 receptors, olanzapine elevates prolactin levels, and a modest elevation persists during chronic administration. Tissue culture experiments indicate that approximately one-third of human breast cancers are prolactin dependent in vitro, a factor of potential importance if the prescription of these drugs is contemplated in a patient with previously detected breast cancer of this type. Although disturbances such as galactorrhea, amenorrhea, gynecomastia, and impotence have been reported with prolactin-elevating compounds, the clinical significance of elevated serum prolactin levels is unknown for most patients. As is common with compounds which increase prolactin release, an increase in mammary gland neoplasia was observed in the olanzapine carcinogenicity studies conducted in mice and rats (*see* Carcinogenesis). However, neither clinical studies nor epidemiologic studies have shown an association between chronic administration of this class of drugs and tumorigenesis in humans; the available evidence is considered too limited to be conclusive.

Transaminase Elevations — In placebo-controlled studies, clinically significant ALT (SGPT) elevations (≥3 times the upper limit of the normal range) were observed in 2% (6/243) of patients exposed to olanzapine compared to none (0/115) of the placebo patients. None of these patients experienced jaundice. In two of these patients, liver enzymes decreased toward normal despite continued treatment and in two others, enzymes decreased upon discontinuation of olanzapine. In the remaining two patients, one, seropositive for hepatitis C, had persistent enzyme elevation for four months after discontinuation, and the other had insufficient follow-up to determine if enzymes normalized.

Within the larger premarketing database of about 2400 patients with baseline SGPT ≤90 IU/L, the incidence of SGPT elevation to >200 IU/L was 2% (50/2381). Again, none of these patients experienced jaundice or other symptoms attributable to liver impairment and most had transient changes that tended to normalize while olanzapine treatment was continued.

Among 2500 patients in oral olanzapine clinical trials, about 1% (23/2500) discontinued treatment due to transaminase increases.

Caution should be exercised in patients with signs and symptoms of hepatic impairment, in patients with pre-existing conditions associated with limited hepatic functional reserve, and in patients who are being treated with potentially hepatotoxic drugs. Periodic assessment of transaminases is recommended in patients with significant hepatic disease (*see* Laboratory Tests).

Continued on next page

Zyprexa—Cont.

Potential for Cognitive and Motor Impairment — Somnolence was a commonly reported adverse event associated with olanzapine treatment, occurring at an incidence of 26% in olanzapine patients compared to 15% in placebo patients. This adverse event was also dose related. Somnolence led to discontinuation in 0.4% (9/2500) of patients in the premarketing database.

Since olanzapine has the potential to impair judgment, thinking, or motor skills, patients should be cautioned about operating hazardous machinery, including automobiles, until they are reasonably certain that olanzapine therapy does not affect them adversely.

Body Temperature Regulation — Disruption of the body's ability to reduce core body temperature has been attributed to antipsychotic agents. Appropriate care is advised when prescribing olanzapine for patients who will be experiencing conditions which may contribute to an elevation in core body temperature, e.g., exercising strenuously, exposure to extreme heat, receiving concomitant medication with anticholinergic activity, or being subject to dehydration.

Dysphagia — Esophageal dysmotility and aspiration have been associated with antipsychotic drug use. Two olanzapine-treated patients (2/407) in two studies in patients with Alzheimer's disease died from aspiration pneumonia during or within 30 days of the termination of the double-blind portion of their respective studies; there were no deaths in the placebo-treated patients. One of these patients had experienced dysphagia prior to the development of aspiration pneumonia. Aspiration pneumonia is a common cause of morbidity and mortality in patients with advanced Alzheimer's disease. Olanzapine and other antipsychotic drugs should be used cautiously in patients at risk for aspiration pneumonia.

Suicide — The possibility of a suicide attempt is inherent in schizophrenia and in bipolar disorder, and close supervision of high-risk patients should accompany drug therapy. Prescriptions for olanzapine should be written for the smallest quantity of tablets consistent with good patient management, in order to reduce the risk of overdose.

Use in Patients with Concomitant Illness — Clinical experience with olanzapine in patients with certain concomitant systemic illnesses (*see* Renal Impairment and Hepatic Impairment *under* CLINICAL PHARMACOLOGY, Special Populations) is limited.

Olanzapine exhibits in vitro muscarinic receptor affinity. In premarketing clinical trials with olanzapine, olanzapine was associated with constipation, dry mouth, and tachycardia, all adverse events possibly related to cholinergic antagonism. Such adverse events were not often the basis for discontinuations from olanzapine, but olanzapine should be used with caution in patients with clinically significant prostatic hypertrophy, narrow angle glaucoma, or a history of paralytic ileus.

In a fixed-dose study of oral olanzapine (olanzapine at doses of 5, 10, and 15 mg/day) and placebo in nursing home patients (mean age: 83 years, range: 61-97; median Mini-Mental State Examination (MMSE): 5, range: 0-22) having various psychiatric symptoms in association with Alzheimer's disease, the following treatment-emergent adverse events were reported in all (each and every) olanzapine-treated groups at an incidence of either (1) two-fold or more in excess of the placebo-treated group, where at least 1 placebo-treated patient was reported to have experienced the event, or (2) at least 2 cases if no placebo-treated patient was reported to have experienced the event: somnolence, abnormal gait, fever, dehydration, and back pain. The rate of discontinuation in this study for olanzapine was 12% vs 4% with placebo. Discontinuations due to abnormal gait (1% for olanzapine vs 0% for placebo), accidental injury (1% for olanzapine vs 0% for placebo), and somnolence (3% for olanzapine vs 0% for placebo) were considered to be drug related. As with other CNS-active drugs, olanzapine should be used with caution in elderly patients with dementia (*see* PRECAUTIONS).

Olanzapine has not been evaluated or used to any appreciable extent in patients with a recent history of myocardial infarction or unstable heart disease. Patients with these diagnoses were excluded from premarketing clinical studies. Because of the risk of orthostatic hypotension with olanzapine, caution should be observed in cardiac patients (*see* Hemodynamic Effects).

For specific information about the precautions of lithium or valproate, refer to the PRECAUTIONS section of the package inserts for these other products.

Information for Patients

Physicians are advised to discuss the following issues with patients for whom they prescribe olanzapine:

Orthostatic Hypotension — Patients should be advised of the risk of orthostatic hypotension, especially during the period of initial dose titration and in association with the use of concomitant drugs that may potentiate the orthostatic effect of olanzapine, e.g., diazepam or alcohol (*see* Drug Interactions).

Interference with Cognitive and Motor Performance — Because olanzapine has the potential to impair judgment, thinking, or motor skills, patients should be cautioned about operating hazardous machinery, including automobiles, until they are reasonably certain that olanzapine therapy does not affect them adversely.

Pregnancy — Patients should be advised to notify their physician if they become pregnant or intend to become pregnant during therapy with olanzapine.

Nursing — Patients should be advised not to breast-feed an infant if they are taking olanzapine.

Concomitant Medication — Patients should be advised to inform their physicians if they are taking, or plan to take, any prescription or over-the-counter drugs, since there is a potential for interactions.

Alcohol — Patients should be advised to avoid alcohol while taking olanzapine.

Heat Exposure and Dehydration — Patients should be advised regarding appropriate care in avoiding overheating and dehydration.

Phenylketonurics — ZYPREXA ZYDIS (olanzapine orally disintegrating tablets) contains phenylalanine (0.34, 0.45, 0.67, or 0.90 mg per 5, 10, 15, or 20 mg tablet, respectively).

Laboratory Tests

Periodic assessment of transaminases is recommended in patients with significant hepatic disease (*see* Transaminase Elevations).

Drug Interactions

The risks of using olanzapine in combination with other drugs have not been extensively evaluated in systematic studies. Given the primary CNS effects of olanzapine, caution should be used when olanzapine is taken in combination with other centrally acting drugs and alcohol.

Because of its potential for inducing hypotension, olanzapine may enhance the effects of certain antihypertensive agents.

Olanzapine may antagonize the effects of levodopa and dopamine agonists.

The Effect of Other Drugs on Olanzapine — Agents that induce CYP1A2 or glucuronyl transferase enzymes, such as omeprazole and rifampin, may cause an increase in olanzapine clearance. Inhibitors of CYP1A2 could potentially inhibit olanzapine clearance. Although olanzapine is metabolized by multiple enzyme systems, induction or inhibition of a single enzyme may appreciably alter olanzapine clearance. Therefore, a dosage increase (for induction) or a dosage decrease (for inhibition) may need to be considered with specific drugs.

Charcoal — The administration of activated charcoal (1 g) reduced the Cmax and AUC of oral olanzapine by about 60%. As peak olanzapine levels are not typically obtained until about 6 hours after dosing, charcoal may be a useful treatment for olanzapine overdose.

Cimetidine and Antacids — Single doses of cimetidine (800 mg) or aluminum- and magnesium-containing antacids did not affect the oral bioavailability of olanzapine.

Carbamazepine — Carbamazepine therapy (200 mg bid) causes an approximately 50% increase in the clearance of olanzapine. This increase is likely due to the fact that carbamazepine is a potent inducer of CYP1A2 activity. Higher daily doses of carbamazepine may cause an even greater increase in olanzapine clearance.

Ethanol — Ethanol (45 mg/70 kg single dose) did not have an effect on olanzapine pharmacokinetics.

Fluoxetine — Fluoxetine (60 mg single dose or 60 mg daily for 8 days) causes a small (mean 16%) increase in the maximum concentration of olanzapine and a small (mean 16%) decrease in olanzapine clearance. The magnitude of the impact of this factor is small in comparison to the overall variability between individuals, and therefore dose modification is not routinely recommended.

Fluvoxamine — Fluvoxamine, a CYP1A2 inhibitor, decreases the clearance of olanzapine. This results in a mean increase in olanzapine Cmax following fluvoxamine of 54% in female nonsmokers and 77% in male smokers. The mean increase in olanzapine AUC is 52% and 108%, respectively. Lower doses of olanzapine should be considered in patients receiving concomitant treatment with fluvoxamine.

Warfarin — Warfarin (20 mg single dose) did not affect olanzapine pharmacokinetics.

Effect of Olanzapine on Other Drugs — In vitro studies utilizing human liver microsomes suggest that olanzapine has little potential to inhibit CYP1A2, CYP2C9, CYP2C19, CYP2D6, and CYP3A. Thus, olanzapine is unlikely to cause clinically important drug interactions mediated by these enzymes.

Lithium — Multiple doses of olanzapine (10 mg for 8 days) did not influence the kinetics of lithium. Therefore, concomitant olanzapine administration does not require dosage adjustment of lithium.

Valproate — Studies in vitro using human liver microsomes determined that olanzapine has little potential to inhibit the major metabolic pathway, glucuronidation, of valproate. Further, valproate has little effect on the metabolism of olanzapine in vitro. In vivo administration of olanzapine (10 mg daily for 2 weeks) did not affect the steady state plasma concentrations of valproate. Therefore, concomitant olanzapine administration does not require dosage adjustment of valproate.

Single doses of olanzapine did not affect the pharmacokinetics of imipramine or its active metabolite desipramine, and warfarin. Multiple doses of olanzapine did not influence the kinetics of diazepam and its active metabolite N-desmethyldiazepam, ethanol, or biperiden. However, the co-administration of either diazepam or ethanol with olanzapine potentiated the orthostatic hypotension observed with olanzapine. Multiple doses of olanzapine did not affect the pharmacokinetics of theophylline or its metabolites.

Lorazepam — Administration of intramuscular lorazepam (2 mg) 1 hour after intramuscular olanzapine for injection (5 mg) did not significantly affect the pharmacokinetics of olanzapine, unconjugated lorazepam, or total lorazepam. However, this co-administration of intramuscular lorazepam and intramuscular olanzapine for injection added to the somnolence observed with either drug alone.

Carcinogenesis, Mutagenesis, Impairment of Fertility

Carcinogenesis — Oral carcinogenicity studies were conducted in mice and rats. Olanzapine was administered to mice in two 78-week studies at doses of 3, 10, 30/20 mg/kg/day (equivalent to 0.8-5 times the maximum recommended human daily oral dose on a mg/m² basis) and 0.25, 2, 8 mg/kg/day (equivalent to 0.06-2 times the maximum recommended human daily oral dose on a mg/m² basis). Rats were dosed for 2 years at doses of 0.25, 1, 2.5, 4 mg/kg/day (males) and 0.25, 1, 4, 8 mg/kg/day (females) (equivalent to 0.13-2 and 0.13-4 times the maximum recommended human daily oral dose on a mg/m² basis, respectively). The incidence of liver hemangiomas and hemangiosarcomas was significantly increased in one mouse study in female mice dosed at 8 mg/kg/day (2 times the maximum recommended human daily oral dose on a mg/m² basis). These tumors were not increased in another mouse study in females dosed at 10 or 30/20 mg/kg/day (2-5 times the maximum recommended human daily oral dose on a mg/m² basis); in this study, there was a high incidence of early mortalities in males of the 30/20 mg/kg/day group. The incidence of mammary gland adenomas and adenocarcinomas was significantly increased in female mice dosed at ≥2 mg/kg/day and in female rats dosed at ≥4 mg/kg/day (0.5 and 2 times the maximum recommended human daily oral dose on a mg/m² basis, respectively). Antipsychotic drugs have been shown to chronically elevate prolactin levels in rodents. Serum prolactin levels were not measured during the olanzapine carcinogenicity studies; however, measurements during subchronic toxicity studies showed that olanzapine elevated serum prolactin levels up to 4-fold in rats at the same doses used in the carcinogenicity study. An increase in mammary gland neoplasms has been found in rodents after chronic administration of other antipsychotic drugs and is considered to be prolactin mediated. The relevance for human risk of the finding of prolactin mediated endocrine tumors in rodents is unknown (*see* Hyperprolactinemia *under* PRECAUTIONS, General).

Mutagenesis — No evidence of mutagenic potential for olanzapine was found in the Ames reverse mutation test, in vivo micronucleus test in mice, the chromosomal aberration test in Chinese hamster ovary cells, unscheduled DNA synthesis test in rat hepatocytes, induction of forward mutation test in mouse lymphoma cells, or in vivo sister chromatid exchange test in bone marrow of Chinese hamsters.

Impairment of Fertility — In an oral fertility and reproductive performance study in rats, male mating performance, but not fertility, was impaired at a dose of 22.4 mg/kg/day and female fertility was decreased at a dose of 3 mg/kg/day (11 and 1.5 times the maximum recommended human daily oral dose on a mg/m² basis, respectively). Discontinuance of olanzapine treatment reversed the effects on male mating performance. In female rats, the precoital period was increased and the mating index reduced at 5 mg/kg/day (2.5 times the maximum recommended human daily oral dose on a mg/m² basis). Diestrous was prolonged and estrous delayed at 1.1 mg/kg/day (0.6 times the maximum recommended human daily oral dose on a mg/m² basis); therefore olanzapine may produce a delay in ovulation.

Pregnancy

Pregnancy Category C — In oral reproduction studies in rats at doses up to 18 mg/kg/day and in rabbits at doses up to 30 mg/kg/day (9 and 30 times the maximum recommended human daily oral dose on a mg/m² basis, respectively) no evidence of teratogenicity was observed. In an oral rat teratology study, early resorptions and increased numbers of nonviable fetuses were observed at a dose of 18 mg/kg/day (9 times the maximum recommended human daily oral dose on a mg/m² basis). Gestation was prolonged at 10 mg/kg/day (5 times the maximum recommended human daily oral dose on a mg/m² basis). In an oral rabbit teratology study, fetal toxicity (manifested as increased resorptions and decreased fetal weight) occurred at a maternally toxic dose of 30 mg/kg/day (30 times the maximum recommended human daily oral dose on a mg/m² basis).

Placental transfer of olanzapine occurs in rat pups.

There are no adequate and well-controlled trials with olanzapine in pregnant females. Seven pregnancies were observed during clinical trials with olanzapine, including 2 resulting in normal births, 1 resulting in neonatal death due to a cardiovascular defect, 3 therapeutic abortions, and 1 spontaneous abortion. Because animal reproduction studies are not always predictive of human response, this drug should be used during pregnancy only if the potential benefit justifies the potential risk to the fetus.

Labor and Delivery

Parturition in rats was not affected by olanzapine. The effect of olanzapine on labor and delivery in humans is unknown.

Nursing Mothers

Olanzapine was excreted in milk of treated rats during lactation. It is not known if olanzapine is excreted in human milk. It is recommended that women receiving olanzapine should not breast-feed.

Pediatric Use

Safety and effectiveness in pediatric patients have not been established.

Geriatric Use

Of the 2500 patients in premarketing clinical studies with oral olanzapine, 11% (263) were 65 years of age or over. In patients with schizophrenia, there was no indication of any different tolerability of olanzapine in the elderly compared to younger patients. Studies in patients with various psychiatric symptoms in association with Alzheimer's disease have suggested that there may be a different tolerability profile in this population compared to younger patients with schizophrenia. As with other CNS-active drugs, olanzapine should be used with caution in elderly patients with dementia. Also, the presence of factors that might decrease pharmacokinetic clearance or increase the pharmacodynamic response to olanzapine should lead to consideration of a lower starting dose for any geriatric patient (*see* PRECAUTIONS *and* DOSAGE AND ADMINISTRATION).

ADVERSE REACTIONS

The information below is derived from a clinical trial database for olanzapine consisting of 8661 patients with approximately 4165 patient-years of exposure to oral olanzapine and 722 patients with exposure to intramuscular olanzapine for injection. This database includes: (1) 2500 patients who participated in multiple-dose oral olanzapine premarketing trials in schizophrenia and Alzheimer's disease representing approximately 1122 patient-years of exposure as of February 14, 1995; (2) 182 patients who participated in oral olanzapine premarketing bipolar mania trials representing approximately 66 patient-years of exposure; (3) 191 patients who participated in an oral olanzapine trial of patients having various psychiatric symptoms in association with Alzheimer's disease representing approximately 29 patient-years of exposure; (4) 5788 patients from 88 additional oral olanzapine clinical trials as of December 31, 2001; and (5) 722 patients who participated in intramuscular olanzapine for injection premarketing trials in agitated patients with schizophrenia, Bipolar I Disorder (manic or mixed episodes), or dementia. In addition, information from the premarketing 6-week clinical study database for olanzapine in combination with lithium or valproate, consisting of 224 patients who participated in bipolar mania trials with approximately 22 patient-years of exposure, is included below.

The conditions and duration of treatment with olanzapine varied greatly and included (in overlapping categories) open-label and double-blind phases of studies, inpatients and outpatients, fixed-dose and dose-titration studies, and short-term or longer-term exposure. Adverse reactions were assessed by collecting adverse events, results of physical examinations, vital signs, weights, laboratory analytes, ECGs, chest x-rays, and results of ophthalmologic examinations.

Certain portions of the discussion below relating to objective or numeric safety parameters, namely, dose-dependent adverse events, vital sign changes, weight gain, laboratory changes, and ECG changes are derived from studies in patients with schizophrenia and have not been duplicated for bipolar mania or agitation. However, this information is also generally applicable to bipolar mania and agitation.

Adverse events during exposure were obtained by spontaneous report and recorded by clinical investigators using terminology of their own choosing. Consequently, it is not possible to provide a meaningful estimate of the proportion of individuals experiencing adverse events without first grouping similar types of events into a smaller number of standardized event categories. In the tables and tabulations that follow, standard COSTART dictionary terminology has been used initially to classify reported adverse events.

The stated frequencies of adverse events represent the proportion of individuals who experienced, at least once, a treatment-emergent adverse event of the type listed. An event was considered treatment emergent if it occurred for the first time or worsened while receiving therapy following baseline evaluation. The reported events do not include those event terms that were so general as to be uninformative. Events listed elsewhere in labeling may not be repeated below. It is important to emphasize that, although the events occurred during treatment with olanzapine, they were not necessarily caused by it. The entire label should be read to gain a complete understanding of the safety profile of olanzapine.

The prescriber should be aware that the figures in the tables and tabulations cannot be used to predict the incidence of side effects in the course of usual medical practice where patient characteristics and other factors differ from those that prevailed in the clinical trials. Similarly, the cited frequencies cannot be compared with figures obtained from other clinical investigations involving different treatments, uses, and investigators. The cited figures, however, do provide the prescribing physician with some basis for estimating the relative contribution of drug and nondrug factors to the adverse event incidence in the population studied.

Incidence of Adverse Events in Short-Term, Placebo-Controlled and Combination Trials

The following findings are based on premarketing trials of (1) oral olanzapine for schizophrenia, bipolar mania, a subsequent trial of patients having various psychiatric symptoms in association with Alzheimer's disease, and premarketing combination trials, and (2) intramuscular olanzapine for injection in agitated patients with schizophrenia or bipolar mania.

Adverse Events Associated with Discontinuation of Treatment in Short-Term, Placebo-Controlled Trials

Schizophrenia — Overall, there was no difference in the incidence of discontinuation due to adverse events (5% for oral olanzapine vs 6% for placebo). However, discontinuations due to increases in SGPT were considered to be drug related (2% for oral olanzapine vs 0% for placebo) (*see* PRECAUTIONS).

Bipolar Mania Monotherapy — Overall, there was no difference in the incidence of discontinuation due to adverse events (2% for oral olanzapine vs 2% for placebo).

Agitation — Overall, there was no difference in the incidence of discontinuation due to adverse events (0.4% for intramuscular olanzapine for injection vs 0% for placebo).

Adverse Events Associated with Discontinuation of Treatment in Short-Term Combination Trials

Bipolar Mania Combination Therapy — In a study of patients who were already tolerating either lithium or valproate as monotherapy, discontinuation rates due to adverse events were 11% for the combination of oral olanzapine with lithium or valproate compared to 2% for patients who remained on lithium or valproate monotherapy. Discontinuations with the combination of oral olanzapine and lithium or valproate that occurred in more than 1 patient were: somnolence (3%), weight gain (1%), and peripheral edema (1%).

Commonly Observed Adverse Events in Short-Term, Placebo-Controlled Trials

The most commonly observed adverse events associated with the use of oral olanzapine (incidence of 5% or greater) and not observed at an equivalent incidence among placebo-treated patients (olanzapine incidence at least twice that for placebo) were:

Common Treatment-Emergent Adverse Events Associated with the Use of Oral Olanzapine in 6-Week Trials — SCHIZOPHRENIA

Adverse Event	Percentage of Patients Reporting Event	
	Olanzapine (N=248)	Placebo (N=118)
Postural hypotension	5	2
Constipation	9	3
Weight gain	6	1
Dizziness	11	4
Personality disorder[1]	8	4
Akathisia	5	1

[1] Personality disorder is the COSTART term for designating non-aggressive objectionable behavior.

Common Treatment-Emergent Adverse Events Associated with the Use of Oral Olanzapine in 3-Week and 4-Week Trials — BIPOLAR MANIA

Adverse Event	Percentage of Patients Reporting Event	
	Olanzapine (N=125)	Placebo (N=129)
Asthenia	15	6
Dry mouth	22	7
Constipation	11	5
Dyspepsia	11	5
Increased appetite	6	3
Somnolence	35	13
Dizziness	18	6
Tremor	6	3

There was one adverse event (somnolence) observed at an incidence of 5% or greater among intramuscular olanzapine for injection-treated patients and not observed at an equivalent incidence among placebo-treated patients (olanzapine incidence at least twice that for placebo) during the placebo-controlled premarketing studies. The incidence of somnolence during the 24 hour IM treatment period in clinical trials in agitated patients with schizophrenia or bipolar mania was 6% for intramuscular olanzapine for injection and 3% for placebo.

Adverse Events Occurring at an Incidence of 2% or More Among Oral Olanzapine-Treated Patients in Short-Term, Placebo-Controlled Trials

Table 1 enumerates the incidence, rounded to the nearest percent, of treatment-emergent adverse events that occurred in 2% or more of patients treated with oral olanzapine (doses ≥2.5 mg/day) and with incidence greater than placebo who participated in the acute phase of placebo-controlled trials.

Table 1
Treatment-Emergent Adverse Events: Incidence in Short-Term, Placebo-Controlled Clinical Trials[1] with Oral Olanzapine

Body System/Adverse Event	Percentage of Patients Reporting Event	
	Olanzapine (N=532)	Placebo (N=294)
Body as a Whole		
Accidental injury	12	8
Asthenia	10	9
Fever	6	2
Back pain	5	2
Chest pain	3	1
Cardiovascular System		
Postural hypotension	3	1
Tachycardia	3	1
Hypertension	2	1
Digestive System		
Dry mouth	9	5
Constipation	9	4
Dyspepsia	7	5
Vomiting	4	3
Increased appetite	3	2
Hemic and Lymphatic System		
Ecchymosis	5	3
Metabolic and Nutritional Disorders		
Weight gain	5	3
Peripheral edema	3	1
Musculoskeletal System		
Extremity pain (other than joint)	5	3
Joint pain	5	3
Nervous System		
Somnolence	29	13
Insomnia	12	11
Dizziness	11	4
Abnormal gait	6	1
Tremor	4	3
Akathisia	3	2
Hypertonia	3	2
Articulation impairment	2	1
Respiratory System		
Rhinitis	7	6
Cough increased	6	3
Pharyngitis	4	3
Special Senses		
Amblyopia	3	2
Urogenital System		
Urinary incontinence	2	1
Urinary tract infection	2	1

[1] Events reported by at least 2% of patients treated with olanzapine, except the following events which had an incidence equal to or less than placebo: abdominal pain, agitation, anorexia, anxiety, apathy, confusion, depression, diarrhea, dysmenorrhea[2], hallucinations, headache, hostility, hyperkinesia, myalgia, nausea, nervousness, paranoid reaction, personality disorder[3], rash, thinking abnormal, weight loss.

[2] Denominator used was for females only (olanzapine, N=201; placebo, N=114).

[3] Personality disorder is the COSTART term for designating non-aggressive objectionable behavior.

Commonly Observed Adverse Events in Short-Term Combination Trials

In the bipolar mania combination placebo-controlled trials, the most commonly observed adverse events associated with the combination of olanzapine and lithium or valproate (incidence of ≥5% and at least twice placebo) were:

Common Treatment-Emergent Adverse Events Associated with the Use of Oral Olanzapine in 6-Week Combination Trials — BIPOLAR MANIA

Adverse Event	Percentage of Patients Reporting Event	
	Olanzapine with lithium or valproate (N=229)	Placebo with lithium or valproate (N=115)
Dry mouth	32	9
Weight gain	26	7
Increased appetite	24	8

Continued on next page

Zyprexa—Cont.

Dizziness	14	7
Back pain	8	4
Constipation	8	4
Speech disorder	7	1
Increased salivation	6	2
Amnesia	5	2
Paresthesia	5	2

Adverse Events Occurring at an Incidence of 2% or More Among Oral Olanzapine-Treated Patients in Short-Term Combination Trials
Table 2 enumerates the incidence, rounded to the nearest percent, of treatment-emergent adverse events that occurred in 2% or more of patients treated with the combination of olanzapine (doses ≥5 mg/day) and lithium or valproate and with incidence greater than lithium or valproate alone who participated in the acute phase of placebo-controlled combination trials.

Table 2
Treatment-Emergent Adverse Events: Incidence in Short-Term, Placebo-Controlled Combination Clinical Trials[1] with Oral Olanzapine

Body System/Adverse Event	Percentage of Patients Reporting Event: Olanzapine with lithium or valproate (N=229)	Placebo with lithium or valproate (N=115)
Body as a Whole		
Asthenia	18	13
Back pain	8	4
Accidental injury	4	2
Chest pain	3	2
Cardiovascular System		
Hypertension	2	1
Digestive System		
Dry mouth	32	9
Increased appetite	24	8
Thirst	10	6
Constipation	8	4
Increased salivation	6	2
Metabolic and Nutritional Disorders		
Weight gain	26	7
Peripheral edema	6	4
Edema	2	1
Nervous System		
Somnolence	52	27
Tremor	23	13
Depression	18	17
Dizziness	14	7
Speech disorder	7	1
Amnesia	5	2
Paresthesia	5	2
Apathy	4	3
Confusion	4	1
Euphoria	3	2
Incoordination	2	0
Respiratory System		
Pharyngitis	4	1
Dyspnea	3	1
Skin and Appendages		
Sweating	3	1
Acne	2	0
Dry skin	2	0
Special Senses		
Amblyopia	9	5
Abnormal vision	2	0
Urogenital System		
Dysmenorrhea[2]	2	0
Vaginitis[2]	2	0

[1] Events reported by at least 2% of patients treated with olanzapine, except the following events which had an incidence equal to or less than placebo: abdominal pain, abnormal dreams, abnormal ejaculation, agitation, akathisia, anorexia, anxiety, arthralgia, cough increased, diarrhea, dyspepsia, emotional lability, fever, flatulence, flu syndrome, headache, hostility, insomnia, libido decreased, libido increased, menstrual disorder[2], myalgia, nausea, nervousness, pain, paranoid reaction, personality disorder, rash, rhinitis, sleep disorder, thinking abnormal, vomiting.
[2] Denominator used was for females only (olanzapine, N=128; placebo, N=51).

For specific information about the adverse reactions observed with lithium or valproate, refer to the ADVERSE REACTIONS section of the package inserts for these other products.
Adverse Events Occurring at an Incidence of 1% or More Among Intramuscular Olanzapine for Injection-Treated Patients in Short-Term, Placebo-Controlled Trials
Table 3 enumerates the incidence, rounded to the nearest percent, of treatment-emergent adverse events that occurred in 1% or more of patients treated with intramuscular olanzapine for injection (dose range of 2.5-10.0 mg/injection) and with incidence greater than placebo who participated in the short-term, placebo-controlled trials in agitated patients with schizophrenia or bipolar mania.

Table 3
Treatment-Emergent Adverse Events: Incidence in Short-Term (24 Hour), Placebo-Controlled Clinical Trials with Intramuscular Olanzapine for Injection in Agitated Patients with Schizophrenia or Bipolar Mania[1]

Body System/Adverse Event	Percentage of Patients Reporting Event: Olanzapine (N=415)	Placebo (N=150)
Body as a Whole		
Asthenia	2	1
Cardiovascular System		
Hypotension	2	0
Postural hypotension	1	0
Nervous System		
Somnolence	6	3
Dizziness	4	2
Tremor	1	0

[1] Events reported by at least 1% of patients treated with olanzapine for injection, except the following events which had an incidence equal to or less than placebo: agitation, anxiety, dry mouth, headache, hypertension, insomnia, nervousness.

Additional Findings Observed in Clinical Trials
The following findings are based on clinical trials.
Dose Dependency of Adverse Events in Short-Term, Placebo-Controlled Trials
Extrapyramidal Symptoms — The following table enumerates the percentage of patients with treatment-emergent extrapyramidal symptoms as assessed by categorical analyses of formal rating scales during acute therapy in a controlled clinical trial comparing oral olanzapine at 3 fixed doses with placebo in the treatment of schizophrenia.
[See table below]
The following table enumerates the percentage of patients with treatment-emergent extrapyramidal symptoms as assessed by spontaneously reported adverse events during acute therapy in the same controlled clinical trial comparing olanzapine at 3 fixed doses with placebo in the treatment of schizophrenia.
[See first table at top of next page]
The following table enumerates the percentage of patients with treatment-emergent extrapyramidal symptoms as assessed by categorical analyses of formal rating scales during controlled clinical trials comparing fixed doses of intramuscular olanzapine for injection with placebo in agitation. Patients in each dose group could receive up to three injections during the trials (*see* CLINICAL PHARMACOLOGY). Patient assessments were conducted during the 24 hours following the initial dose of intramuscular olanzapine for injection. There were no statistically significant differences from placebo.
[See second table on next page]
The following table enumerates the percentage of patients with treatment-emergent extrapyramidal symptoms as assessed by spontaneously reported adverse events in the same controlled clinical trial comparing fixed doses of intramuscular olanzapine for injection with placebo in agitated patients with schizophrenia. There were no statistically significant differences from placebo.
[See third table on next page]
Other Adverse Events — The following table addresses dose relatedness for other adverse events using data from a schizophrenia trial involving fixed dosage ranges of oral olanzapine. It enumerates the percentage of patients with treatment-emergent adverse events for the three fixed-dose range groups and placebo. The data were analyzed using the Cochran-Armitage test, excluding the placebo group, and the table includes only those adverse events for which there was a statistically significant trend.
[See fourth table at bottom of next page]
Vital Sign Changes — Oral olanzapine was associated with orthostatic hypotension and tachycardia in clinical trials. Intramuscular olanzapine for injection was associated with bradycardia, hypotension, and tachycardia in clinical trials (*see* PRECAUTIONS).
Weight Gain — In placebo-controlled, 6-week studies, weight gain was reported in 5.6% of olanzapine patients compared to 0.8% of placebo patients. Olanzapine patients gained an average of 2.8 kg, compared to an average 0.4 kg weight loss in placebo patients; 29% of olanzapine patients gained greater than 7% of their baseline weight, compared to 3% of placebo patients. A categorization of patients at baseline on the basis of body mass index (BMI) revealed a significantly greater effect in patients with low BMI compared to normal or overweight patients; nevertheless, weight gain was greater in all 3 olanzapine groups compared to the placebo group. During long-term continuation therapy with olanzapine (238 median days of exposure), 56% of olanzapine patients met the criterion for having gained greater than 7% of their baseline weight. Average weight gain during long-term therapy was 5.4 kg.
Laboratory Changes — An assessment of the premarketing experience for olanzapine revealed an association with asymptomatic increases in SGPT, SGOT, and GGT (*see* PRECAUTIONS). Olanzapine administration was also associated with increases in serum prolactin (*see* PRECAUTIONS), with an asymptomatic elevation of the eosinophil count in 0.3% of patients, and with an increase in CPK.
Given the concern about neutropenia associated with other psychotropic compounds and the finding of leukopenia associated with the administration of olanzapine in several animal models (*see* ANIMAL TOXICOLOGY), careful attention was given to examination of hematologic parameters in premarketing studies with olanzapine. There was no indication of a risk of clinically significant neutropenia associated with olanzapine treatment in the premarketing database for this drug.
ECG Changes — Between-group comparisons for pooled placebo-controlled trials revealed no statistically significant olanzapine/placebo differences in the proportions of patients experiencing potentially important changes in ECG parameters, including QT, QTc, and PR intervals. Olanzapine use was associated with a mean increase in heart rate of 2.4 beats per minute compared to no change among placebo patients. This slight tendency to tachycardia may be related to olanzapine's potential for inducing orthostatic changes (*see* PRECAUTIONS).

Other Adverse Events Observed During the Clinical Trial Evaluation of Olanzapine
Following is a list of terms that reflect treatment-emergent adverse events reported by patients treated with oral olanzapine (at multiple doses ≥1 mg/day) in clinical trials (8661 patients, 4165 patient-years of exposure). This listing may not include those events already listed in previous tables or elsewhere in labeling, those events for which a drug cause was remote, those event terms which were so general as to be uninformative, and those events reported only once or twice which did not have a substantial probability of being acutely life-threatening.
Events are further categorized by body system and listed in order of decreasing frequency according to the following definitions: frequent adverse events are those occurring in at least 1/100 patients (only those not already listed in the tabulated results from placebo-controlled trials appear in this listing); infrequent adverse events are those occurring in 1/100 to 1/1000 patients; rare events are those occurring in fewer than 1/1000 patients.
Body as a Whole — *Frequent:* dental pain and flu syndrome; *Infrequent:* abdomen enlarged, chills, face edema, intentional injury, malaise, moniliasis, neck pain, neck rigidity, pelvic pain, photosensitivity reaction, and suicide attempt; *Rare:* chills and fever, hangover effect, and sudden death.
Cardiovascular System — *Frequent:* hypotension; *Infrequent:* atrial fibrillation, bradycardia, cerebrovascular accident, congestive heart failure, heart arrest, hemorrhage, migraine, pallor, palpitation, vasodilatation, and ventricular extrasystoles; *Rare:* arteritis, heart failure, and pulmonary embolus.
Digestive System — *Frequent:* flatulence, increased salivation, and thirst; *Infrequent:* dysphagia, esophagitis, fecal impaction, fecal incontinence, gastritis, gastroenteritis, gingivitis, hepatitis, melena, mouth ulceration, nausea and

TREATMENT-EMERGENT EXTRAPYRAMIDAL SYMPTOMS ASSESSED BY RATING SCALES INCIDENCE IN A FIXED DOSAGE RANGE, PLACEBO-CONTROLLED CLINICAL TRIAL OF ORAL OLANZAPINE IN SCHIZOPHRENIA — ACUTE PHASE*

	Percentage of Patients Reporting Event: Placebo	Olanzapine 5± 2.5 mg/day	Olanzapine 10 ± 2.5 mg/day	Olanzapine 15 ± 2.5 mg/day
Parkinsonism[1]	15	14	12	14
Akathisia[2]	23	16	19	27

* No statistically significant differences.
[1] Percentage of patients with a Simpson-Angus Scale total score >3.
[2] Percentage of patients with a Barnes Akathisia Scale global score ≥2.

vomiting, oral moniliasis, periodontal abscess, rectal hemorrhage, stomatitis, tongue edema, and tooth caries; *Rare:* aphthous stomatitis, enteritis, eructation, esophageal ulcer, glossitis, ileus, intestinal obstruction, liver fatty deposit, and tongue discoloration.
Endocrine System — *Infrequent:* diabetes mellitus; *Rare:* diabetic acidosis and goiter.
Hemic and Lymphatic System — *Infrequent:* anemia, cyanosis, leukocytosis, leukopenia, lymphadenopathy, and thrombocytopenia; *Rare:* normocytic anemia and thrombocythemia.
Metabolic and Nutritional Disorders — *Infrequent:* acidosis, alkaline phosphatase increased, bilirubinemia, dehydration, hypercholesteremia, hyperglycemia, hyperlipemia, hyperuricemia, hypoglycemia, hypokalemia, hyponatremia, lower extremity edema, and upper extremity edema; *Rare:* gout, hyperkalemia, hypernatremia, hypoproteinemia, ketosis, and water intoxication.
Musculoskeletal System — *Frequent:* joint stiffness and twitching; *Infrequent:* arthritis, arthrosis, leg cramps, and myasthenia; *Rare:* bone pain, bursitis, myopathy, osteoporosis, and rheumatoid arthritis.
Nervous System — *Frequent:* abnormal dreams, amnesia, delusions, emotional lability, euphoria, manic reaction, paresthesia, and schizophrenic reaction; *Infrequent:* akinesia, alcohol misuse, antisocial reaction, ataxia, CNS stimulation, cogwheel rigidity, delirium, dementia, depersonalization, dysarthria, facial paralysis, hypesthesia, hypokinesia, hypotonia, incoordination, libido decreased, libido increased, obsessive compulsive symptoms, phobias, somatization, stimulant misuse, stupor, stuttering, tardive dyskinesia, vertigo, and withdrawal syndrome; *Rare:* circumoral paresthesia, coma, encephalopathy, neuralgia, neuropathy, nystagmus, paralysis, subarachnoid hemorrhage, and tobacco misuse.
Respiratory System — *Frequent:* dyspnea; *Infrequent:* apnea, asthma, epistaxis, hemoptysis, hyperventilation, hypoxia, laryngitis, and voice alteration; *Rare:* atelectasis, hiccup, hypoventilation, lung edema, and stridor.
Skin and Appendages — *Frequent:* sweating; *Infrequent:* alopecia, contact dermatitis, dry skin, eczema, maculopapular rash, pruritus, seborrhea, skin discoloration, skin ulcer, urticaria, and vesiculobullous rash; *Rare:* hirsutism and pustular rash.
Special Senses — *Frequent:* conjunctivitis; *Infrequent:* abnormality of accommodation, blepharitis, cataract, deafness, diplopia, dry eyes, ear pain, eye hemorrhage, eye inflammation, eye pain, ocular muscle abnormality, taste perversion, and tinnitus; *Rare:* corneal lesion, glaucoma, keratoconjunctivitis, macular hypopigmentation, miosis, mydriasis, and pigment deposits lens.
Urogenital System — *Frequent:* vaginitis*; *Infrequent:* abnormal ejaculation*, amenorrhea*, breast pain, cystitis, decreased menstruation*, dysuria, female lactation*, glycosuria, gynecomastia, hematuria, impotence*, increased menstruation*, menorrhagia*, metrorrhagia*, polyuria, premenstrual syndrome*, pyuria, urinary frequency, urinary retention, urinary urgency, urination impaired, uterine fibroids enlarged*, and vaginal hemorrhage*; *Rare:* albuminuria, breast enlargement, mastitis, and oliguria.

*Adjusted for gender.

TREATMENT-EMERGENT EXTRAPYRAMIDAL SYMPTOMS ASSESSED BY ADVERSE EVENTS INCIDENCE IN A FIXED DOSAGE RANGE, PLACEBO-CONTROLLED CLINICAL TRIAL OF ORAL OLANZAPINE IN SCHIZOPHRENIA — ACUTE PHASE

	Percentage of Patients Reporting Event			
	Placebo (N=68)	Olanzapine 5 ± 2.5 mg/day (N=65)	Olanzapine 10± 2.5 mg/day (N=64)	Olanzapine 15 ± 2.5 mg/day (N=69)
Dystonic events[1]	1	3	2	3
Parkinsonism events[2]	10	8	14	20
Akathisia events[3]	1	5	11*	10*
Dyskinetic events[4]	4	0	2	1
Residual events[5]	1	2	5	1
Any extrapyramidal event	16	15	25	32*

* Statistically significantly different from placebo.
[1] Patients with the following COSTART terms were counted in this category: dystonia, generalized spasm, neck rigidity, oculogyric crisis, opisthotonos, torticollis.
[2] Patients with the following COSTART terms were counted in this category: akinesia, cogwheel rigidity, extrapyramidal syndrome, hypertonia, hypokinesia, masked facies, tremor.
[3] Patients with the following COSTART terms were counted in this category: akathisia, hyperkinesia.
[4] Patients with the following COSTART terms were counted in this category: buccoglossal syndrome, choreoathetosis, dyskinesia, tardive dyskinesia.
[5] Patients with the following COSTART terms were counted in this category: movement disorder, myoclonus, twitching.

TREATMENT-EMERGENT EXTRAPYRAMIDAL SYMPTOMS ASSESSED BY RATING SCALES INCIDENCE IN A FIXED DOSE, PLACEBO-CONTROLLED CLINICAL TRIAL OF INTRAMUSCULAR OLANZAPINE FOR INJECTION IN AGITATED PATIENTS WITH SCHIZOPHRENIA*

	Percentage of Patients Reporting Event				
	Placebo	Olanzapine IM 2.5 mg	Olanzapine IM 5 mg	Olanzapine IM 7.5 mg	Olanzapine IM 10 mg
Parkinsonism[1]	0	0	0	0	3
Akathisia[2]	0	0	5	0	0

* No statistically significant differences.
[1] Percentage of patients with a Simpson-Angus total score >3.
[2] Percentage of patients with a Barnes Akathisia Scale global score ≥2.

TREATMENT-EMERGENT EXTRAPYRAMIDAL SYMPTOMS ASSESSED BY ADVERSE EVENTS INCIDENCE IN A FIXED DOSE, PLACEBO-CONTROLLED CLINICAL TRIAL OF INTRAMUSCULAR OLANZAPINE FOR INJECTION IN AGITATED PATIENTS WITH SCHIZOPHRENIA*

	Percentage of Patients Reporting Event				
	Placebo (N=45)	Olanzapine IM 2.5 mg (N=48)	Olanzapine IM 5 mg (N=45)	Olanzapine IM 7.5 mg (N=46)	Olanzapine IM 10 mg (N=46)
Dystonic events[1]	0	0	0	0	0
Parkinsonism events[2]	0	4	2	0	0
Akathisia events[3]	0	2	0	0	0
Dyskinetic events[4]	0	0	0	0	0
Residual events[5]	0	0	0	0	0
Any extrapyramidal event	0	4	2	0	0

* No statistically significant differences.
[1] Patients with the following COSTART terms were counted in this category: dystonia, generalized spasm, neck rigidity, oculogyric crisis, opisthotonos, torticollis.
[2] Patients with the following COSTART terms were counted in this category: akinesia, cogwheel rigidity, extrapyramidal syndrome, hypertonia, hypokinesia, masked facies, tremor.
[3] Patients with the following COSTART terms were counted in this category: akathisia, hyperkinesia.
[4] Patients with the following COSTART terms were counted in this category: buccoglossal syndrome, choreoathetosis, dyskinesia, tardive dyskinesia.
[5] Patients with the following COSTART terms were counted in this category: movement disorder, myoclonus, twitching.

	Percentage of Patients Reporting Event			
Adverse Event	Placebo (N=68)	Olanzapine 5 ± 2.5 mg/day (N=65)	Olanzapine 10 ± 2.5 mg/day (N=64)	Olanzapine 15 ± 2.5 mg/day (N=69)
Asthenia	15	8	9	20
Dry mouth	4	3	5	13
Nausea	9	0	2	9
Somnolence	16	20	30	39
Tremor	3	0	5	7

Following is a list of terms that reflect treatment-emergent adverse events reported by patients treated with intramuscular olanzapine for injection (at one or more doses ≥2.5 mg/injection) in clinical trials (722 patients). This listing may not include those events already listed in previous tables or elsewhere in labeling, those events for which a drug cause was remote, those event terms which were so general as to be uninformative, and those events reported only once which did not have a substantial probability of being acutely life-threatening.
Events are further categorized by body system and listed in order of decreasing frequency according to the following definitions: frequent adverse events are those occurring in at least 1/100 patients (only those not already listed in the tabulated results from placebo-controlled trials appear in this listing); infrequent adverse events are those occurring in 1/100 to 1/1000 patients.
Body as a Whole — *Frequent:* injection site pain; *Infrequent:* abdominal pain and fever.
Cardiovascular System — *Infrequent:* AV block, heart block, and syncope.
Digestive System — *Infrequent:* diarrhea and nausea.
Hemic and Lymphatic System — *Infrequent:* anemia.
Metabolic and Nutritional Disorders — *Infrequent:* creatine phosphokinase increased, dehydration, and hyperkalemia.
Musculoskeletal System — *Infrequent:* twitching.
Nervous System — *Infrequent:* abnormal gait, akathisia, articulation impairment, confusion, and emotional lability.
Skin and Appendages — *Infrequent:* sweating.
Postintroduction Reports
Adverse events reported since market introduction that were temporally (but not necessarily causally) related to ZYPREXA therapy include the following: allergic reaction (e.g., anaphylactoid reaction, angioedema, pruritus or urticaria), diabetic coma, pancreatitis, and priapism.

DRUG ABUSE AND DEPENDENCE

Controlled Substance Class
Olanzapine is not a controlled substance.
Physical and Psychological Dependence
In studies prospectively designed to assess abuse and dependence potential, olanzapine was shown to have acute depressive CNS effects but little or no potential of abuse or physical dependence in rats administered oral doses up to 15 times the maximum recommended human daily oral dose (20 mg) and rhesus monkeys administered oral doses up to 8 times the maximum recommended human daily oral dose on a mg/m^2 basis.
Olanzapine has not been systematically studied in humans for its potential for abuse, tolerance, or physical dependence. While the clinical trials did not reveal any tendency for any drug-seeking behavior, these observations were not systematic, and it is not possible to predict on the basis of this limited experience the extent to which a CNS-active drug will be misused, diverted, and/or abused once mar-

Continued on next page

Zyprexa—Cont.

keted. Consequently, patients should be evaluated carefully for a history of drug abuse, and such patients should be observed closely for signs of misuse or abuse of olanzapine (e.g., development of tolerance, increases in dose, drug-seeking behavior).

OVERDOSAGE

Human Experience

In premarketing trials involving more than 3100 patients and/or normal subjects, accidental or intentional acute overdosage of olanzapine was identified in 67 patients. In the patient taking the largest identified amount, 300 mg, the only symptoms reported were drowsiness and slurred speech. In the limited number of patients who were evaluated in hospitals, including the patient taking 300 mg, there were no observations indicating an adverse change in laboratory analytes or ECG. Vital signs were usually within normal limits following overdoses.

In postmarketing reports of overdose with olanzapine alone, symptoms have been reported in the majority of cases. In symptomatic patients, symptoms with ≥10% incidence included agitation/aggressiveness, dysarthria, tachycardia, various extrapyramidal symptoms, and reduced level of consciousness ranging from sedation to coma. Among less commonly reported symptoms were the following potentially medically serious events: aspiration, cardiopulmonary arrest, cardiac arrhythmias (such as supraventricular tachycardia and one patient experiencing sinus pause with spontaneous resumption of normal rhythm), delirium, possible neuroleptic malignant syndrome, respiratory depression/arrest, convulsion, hypertension, and hypotension. Eli Lilly and Company has received reports of fatality in association with overdose of olanzapine alone. In one case of death, the amount of acutely ingested olanzapine was reported to be possibly as low as 450 mg; however, in another case, a patient was reported to survive an acute olanzapine ingestion of 1500 mg.

Overdosage Management

The possibility of multiple drug involvement should be considered. In case of acute overdosage, establish and maintain an airway and ensure adequate oxygenation and ventilation, which may include intubation. Gastric lavage (after intubation, if patient is unconscious) and administration of activated charcoal together with a laxative should be considered. The possibility of obtundation, seizures, or dystonic reaction of the head and neck following overdose may create a risk of aspiration with induced emesis. Cardiovascular monitoring should commence immediately and should include continuous electrocardiographic monitoring to detect possible arrhythmias.

There is no specific antidote to olanzapine. Therefore, appropriate supportive measures should be initiated. Hypotension and circulatory collapse should be treated with appropriate measures such as intravenous fluids and/or sympathomimetic agents. (Do not use epinephrine, dopamine, or other sympathomimetics with beta-agonist activity, since beta stimulation may worsen hypotension in the setting of olanzapine-induced alpha blockade.) Close medical supervision and monitoring should continue until the patient recovers.

DOSAGE AND ADMINISTRATION

Schizophrenia

Usual Dose — Oral olanzapine should be administered on a once-a-day schedule without regard to meals, generally beginning with 5 to 10 mg initially, with a target dose of 10 mg/day within several days. Further dosage adjustments, if indicated, should generally occur at intervals of not less than 1 week, since steady state for olanzapine would not be achieved for approximately 1 week in the typical patient. When dosage adjustments are necessary, dose increments/decrements of 5 mg QD are recommended.

Efficacy in schizophrenia was demonstrated in a dose range of 10 to 15 mg/day in clinical trials. However, doses above 10 mg/day were not demonstrated to be more efficacious than the 10 mg/day dose. An increase to a dose greater than the target dose of 10 mg/day (i.e., to a dose of 15 mg/day or greater) is recommended only after clinical assessment. The safety of doses above 20 mg/day has not been evaluated in clinical trials.

Dosing in Special Populations — The recommended starting dose is 5 mg in patients who are debilitated, who have a predisposition to hypotensive reactions, who otherwise exhibit a combination of factors that may result in slower metabolism of olanzapine (e.g., nonsmoking female patients ≥65 years of age), or who may be more pharmacodynamically sensitive to olanzapine (*see* CLINICAL PHARMACOLOGY; also *see* Use in Patients with Concomitant Illness and Drug Interactions *under* PRECAUTIONS). When indicated, dose escalation should be performed with caution in these patients.

Maintenance Treatment — While there is no body of evidence available to answer the question of how long the patient treated with olanzapine should remain on it, the effectiveness of oral olanzapine, 10 mg/day to 20 mg/day, in maintaining treatment response in schizophrenic patients who had been stable on ZYPREXA for approximately 8 weeks and were then followed for a period of up to 8 months has been demonstrated in a placebo-controlled trial (*see* CLINICAL PHARMACOLOGY). Patients should be periodically reassessed to determine the need for maintenance treatment with appropriate dose.

	TABLET STRENGTH					
	2.5 mg	5 mg	7.5 mg	10 mg	15 mg	20 mg
Tablet No.	4112	4115	4116	4117	4415	4420
Identification	LILLY 4112	LILLY 4115	LILLY 4116	LILLY 4117	LILLY 4415	LILLY 4420
NDC Codes:						
Bottles 60	NDC 0002-4112-60	NDC 0002-4115-60	NDC 0002-4116-60	NDC 0002-4117-60	NDC 0002-4415-60	NDC 0002-4420-60
Blisters - ID* 100	NDC 0002-4112-33	NDC 0002-4115-33	NDC 0002-4116-33	NDC 0002-4117-33	NDC 0002-4415-33	NDC 0002-4420-33
Bottles 1000	NDC 0002-4112-04	NDC 0002-4115-04	NDC 0002-4116-04	NDC 0002-4117-04	NDC 0002-4415-04	NDC 0002-4420-04

*Identi-Dose® (unit dose medication, Lilly)

ZYPREXA ZYDIS Tablets*	TABLET STRENGTH			
	5 mg	10 mg	15 mg	20 mg
Tablet No.	4453	4454	4455	4456
Debossed	5	10	15	20
NDC Codes:				
Dose Pack 30 (Child-Resistant)	NDC 0002-4453-85	NDC 0002-4454-85	NDC 0002-4455-85	NDC 0002-4456-85

ZYPREXA is a registered trademark of Eli Lilly and Company.
ZYDIS is a registered trademark of R. P. Scherer Corporation.
*ZYPREXA ZYDIS (olanzapine orally disintegrating tablets) is manufactured for Eli Lilly and Company by Scherer DDS Limited, United Kingdom, SN5 8RU.

Bipolar Disorder

Usual Monotherapy Dose — Oral olanzapine should be administered on a once-a-day schedule without regard to meals, generally beginning with 10 or 15 mg. Dosage adjustments, if indicated, should generally occur at intervals of not less than 24 hours, reflecting the procedures in the placebo-controlled trials. When dosage adjustments are necessary, dose increments/decrements of 5 mg QD are recommended.

Short-term (3-4 weeks) antimanic efficacy was demonstrated in a dose range of 5 mg to 20 mg/day in clinical trials. The safety of doses above 20 mg/day has not been evaluated in clinical trials.

Maintenance Monotherapy — The benefit of maintaining bipolar patients on monotherapy with oral ZYPREXA at a dose of 5 to 20 mg/day, after achieving a responder status for an average duration of two weeks, was demonstrated in a controlled trial (*see* Clinical Efficacy Data *under* CLINICAL PHARMACOLOGY). The physician who elects to use ZYPREXA for extended periods should periodically re-evaluate the long-term usefulness of the drug for the individual patient.

Bipolar Mania Usual Dose in Combination with Lithium or Valproate — When administered in combination with lithium or valproate, oral olanzapine dosing should generally begin with 10 mg once-a-day without regard to meals.

Short-term (6 weeks) antimanic efficacy was demonstrated in a dose range of 5 mg to 20 mg/day in clinical trials. The safety of doses above 20 mg/day has not been evaluated in clinical trials.

Dosing in Special Populations — *See* Dosing in Special Populations *under* DOSAGE AND ADMINISTRATION, Schizophrenia.

Administration of ZYPREXA ZYDIS (olanzapine orally disintegrating tablets) After opening sachet, peel back foil on blister. Do not push tablet through foil. Immediately upon opening the blister, using dry hands, remove tablet and place entire ZYPREXA ZYDIS in the mouth. Tablet disintegration occurs rapidly in saliva so it can be easily swallowed with or without liquid.

Agitation Associated with Schizophrenia and Bipolar I Mania

Usual Dose for Agitated Patients with Schizophrenia or Bipolar Mania — The efficacy of intramuscular olanzapine for injection in controlling agitation in these disorders was demonstrated in a dose range of 2.5 mg to 10 mg. The recommended dose in these patients is 10 mg. A lower dose of 5 or 7.5 mg may be considered when clinical factors warrant (*see* CLINICAL PHARMACOLOGY). If agitation warranting additional intramuscular doses persists following the initial dose, subsequent doses up to 10 mg may be given. However, the efficacy of repeated doses of intramuscular olanzapine for injection in agitated patients has not been systematically evaluated in controlled clinical trials. Also, the safety of total daily doses greater than 30 mg, or 10 mg injections given more frequently than 2 hours after the initial dose, and 4 hours after the second dose have not been evaluated in clinical trials. Maximal dosing of intramuscular olanzapine (e.g., three doses of 10 mg administered 2-4 hours apart) may be associated with a substantial occurrence of significant orthostatic hypotension (*see* PRECAUTIONS, Hemodynamic Effects). Thus, it is recommended that patients requiring subsequent intramuscular injections be assessed for orthostatic hypotension prior to the administration of any subsequent doses of intramuscular olanzapine for injection. The administration of an additional dose to a patient with a clinically significant postural change in systolic blood pressure is not recommended.

If ongoing olanzapine therapy is clinically indicated, oral olanzapine may be initiated in a range of 5-20 mg/day as soon as clinically appropriate (*see* Schizophrenia or Bipolar Disorder *under* DOSAGE AND ADMINISTRATION).

Intramuscular Dosing in Special Populations — A dose of 5 mg per injection should be considered for geriatric patients or when other clinical factors warrant. A lower dose of 2.5 mg per injection should be considered for patients who otherwise might be debilitated, be predisposed to hypotensive reactions, or be more pharmacodynamically sensitive to olanzapine (*see* CLINICAL PHARMACOLOGY; also *see* Use in Patients with Concomitant Illness and Drug Interactions *under* PRECAUTIONS).

Administration of ZYPREXA IntraMuscular

ZYPREXA IntraMuscular is intended for intramuscular use only. Do not administer intravenously or subcutaneously. Inject slowly, deep into the muscle mass.

Parenteral drug products should be inspected visually for particulate matter and discoloration prior to administration, whenever solution and container permit.

Directions for preparation of ZYPREXA IntraMuscular with Sterile Water for Injection

Dissolve the contents of the vial using 2.1 mL of Sterile Water for Injection to provide a solution containing approximately 5 mg/mL of olanzapine. The resulting solution should appear clear and yellow. ZYPREXA IntraMuscular reconstituted with Sterile Water for Injection should be used immediately (within 1 hour) after reconstitution. **Discard any unused portion.**

The following table provides injection volumes for delivering various doses of intramuscular olanzapine for injection reconstituted with Sterile Water for Injection.

Dose, mg Olanzapine	Volume of Injection, mL
10.0	Withdraw total contents of vial
7.5	1.5
5.0	1.0
2.5	0.5

HOW SUPPLIED

The ZYPREXA 2.5 mg, 5 mg, 7.5 mg, and 10 mg tablets are white, round, and imprinted in blue ink with LILLY and tablet number. The 15 mg tablets are elliptical, blue, and debossed with LILLY and tablet number. The 20 mg tablets are elliptical, pink, and debossed with LILLY and tablet number. The tablets are available as follows:

[See first table above]

ZYPREXA ZYDIS (olanzapine orally disintegrating tablets) are yellow, round, and debossed with the tablet strength. The tablets are available as follows:

[See second table above]

ZYPREXA IntraMuscular is available in:

NDC 0002-7597-01 (No. VL7597) – 10 mg vial (1s)

Store ZYPREXA tablets, ZYPREXA ZYDIS, and ZYPREXA IntraMuscular vials (before reconstitution) at controlled room temperature, 20° to 25°C (68° to 77°F) [*see* USP]. Reconstituted ZYPREXA IntraMuscular may be stored at controlled room temperature, 20° to 25°C (68° to 77°F) [*see* USP] for up to 1 hour if necessary. **Discard any unused portion of reconstituted ZYPREXA IntraMuscular.** The USP defines controlled room temperature as a temperature maintained thermostatically that encompasses the usual and customary working environment of 20° to 25°C (68° to 77°F); that results in a mean kinetic temperature calculated to be not more than 25°C; and that allows for excursions between 15° and 30°C (59° and 86°F) that are experienced in pharmacies, hospitals, and warehouses.

Protect ZYPREXA tablets and ZYPREXA ZYDIS from light and moisture. Protect ZYPREXA IntraMuscular from light, do not freeze.

ANIMAL TOXICOLOGY

In animal studies with olanzapine, the principal hematologic findings were reversible peripheral cytopenias in individual dogs dosed at 10 mg/kg (17 times the maximum recommended human daily oral dose on a mg/m^2 basis), dose-related decreases in lymphocytes and neutrophils in mice, and lymphopenia in rats. A few dogs treated with 10 mg/kg developed reversible neutropenia and/or reversible hemolytic anemia between 1 and 10 months of treatment. Dose-related decreases in lymphocytes and neutrophils were seen in mice given doses of 10 mg/kg (equal to 2 times the maximum recommended human daily oral dose on a mg/m² basis) in studies of 3 months' duration. Nonspecific lymphopenia, consistent with decreased body weight gain, occurred in rats receiving 22.5 mg/kg (11 times the maximum recommended human daily oral dose on a mg/m² basis) for 3 months or 16 mg/kg (8 times the maximum recommended human daily oral dose on a mg/m² basis) for 6 or 12 months. No evidence of bone marrow cytotoxicity was found in any of the species examined. Bone marrows were normocellular or hypercellular, indicating that the reductions in circulating blood cells were probably due to peripheral (non-marrow) factors.

Literature revised March 29, 2004

Eli Lilly and Company
Indianapolis, IN 46285, USA
www.ZYPREXA.com
PA 3091 AMP

Lilly ICOS LLC

c/o ELI LILLY AND COMPANY
LILLY CORPORATE CENTER
INDIANAPOLIS, IN 46285

Direct Inquiries to:
Lilly ICOS LLC
c/o Eli Lilly and Company
Lilly Corporate Center
Indianapolis, IN 46285
(317) 276-2000
www.cialis.com

For Medical Information Contact:
Lilly ICOS LLC
1-877-Cialis-1

CIALIS® ℞

[see-al-iss]
(tadalafil)
tablets

DESCRIPTION

CIALIS® (tadalafil), an oral treatment for erectile dysfunction, is a selective inhibitor of cyclic guanosine monophosphate (cGMP)-specific phosphodiesterase type 5 (PDE5). Tadalafil has the empirical formula $C_{22}H_{19}N_3O_4$ representing a molecular weight of 389.41. The structural formula is:

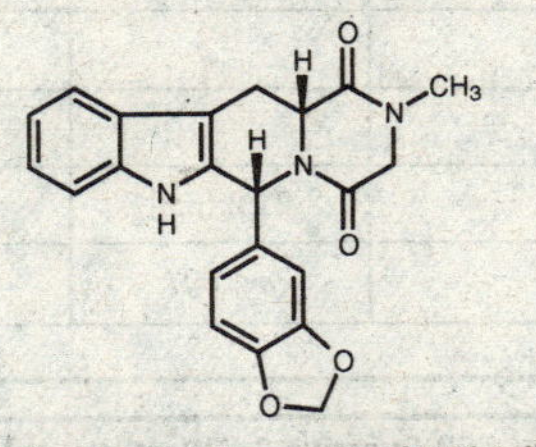

The chemical designation is pyrazino[1',2':1,6]pyrido[3,4-b]indole-1,4-dione, 6-(1,3-benzodioxol-5-yl)-2,3,6,7,12,12a-hexahydro-2-methyl-, (6R,12aR)-. It is a crystalline solid that is practically insoluble in water and very slightly soluble in ethanol.

CIALIS is available as film-coated, almond-shaped tablets for oral administration. Each tablet contains 5, 10, or 20 mg of tadalafil and the following inactive ingredients: croscarmellose sodium, hydroxypropyl cellulose, hypromellose, iron oxide, lactose monohydrate, magnesium stearate, microcrystalline cellulose, sodium lauryl sulfate, talc, titanium dioxide, and triacetin.

CLINICAL PHARMACOLOGY

Mechanism of Action

Penile erection during sexual stimulation is caused by increased penile blood flow resulting from the relaxation of penile arteries and corpus cavernosal smooth muscle. This response is mediated by the release of nitric oxide (NO) from nerve terminals and endothelial cells, which stimulates the synthesis of cGMP in smooth muscle cells. Cyclic GMP causes smooth muscle relaxation and increased blood flow into the corpus cavernosum. The inhibition of phosphodiesterase type 5 (PDE5) enhances erectile function by increasing the amount of cGMP. Tadalafil inhibits PDE5. Because sexual stimulation is required to initiate the local release of nitric oxide, the inhibition of PDE5 by tadalafil has no effect in the absence of sexual stimulation.

Studies *in vitro* have demonstrated that tadalafil is a selective inhibitor of PDE5. PDE5 is found in corpus cavernosum smooth muscle, vascular and visceral smooth muscle, skeletal muscle, platelets, kidney, lung, cerebellum, and pancreas.

In vitro studies have shown that the effect of tadalafil is more potent on PDE5 than on other phosphodiesterases. These studies have shown that tadalafil is >10,000-fold more potent for PDE5 than for PDE1, PDE2, PDE4, and PDE7 enzymes, which are found in the heart, brain, blood vessels, liver, leukocytes, skeletal muscle, and other organs. Tadalafil is >10,000-fold more potent for PDE5 than for PDE3, an enzyme found in the heart and blood vessels. Additionally, tadalafil is 700-fold more potent for PDE5 than for PDE6, which is found in the retina and is responsible for phototransduction. Tadalafil is >9,000-fold more potent for PDE5 than for PDE8, PDE9, and PDE10 and 14-fold more potent for PDE5 than for PDE11A1, an enzyme found in human skeletal muscle. Tadalafil inhibits human recombinant PDE11A1 activity at concentrations within the therapeutic range. The physiological role and clinical consequence of PDE11 inhibition in humans have not been defined.

Pharmacokinetics

Over a dose range of 2.5 to 20 mg, tadalafil exposure (AUC) increases proportionally with dose in healthy subjects. Steady-state plasma concentrations are attained within 5 days of once-daily dosing, and exposure is approximately 1.6-fold greater than after a single dose. Tadalafil is eliminated predominantly by hepatic metabolism, mainly by cytochrome P450 3A4 (CYP3A4). The concomitant use of potent CYP3A4 inhibitors such as ritonavir or ketoconazole resulted in significant increases in tadalafil AUC values (*see* **PRECAUTIONS** *and* **DOSAGE AND ADMINISTRATION**). Mean tadalafil concentrations measured after the administration of a single oral dose of 20 mg to healthy male subjects are depicted in Figure 1.

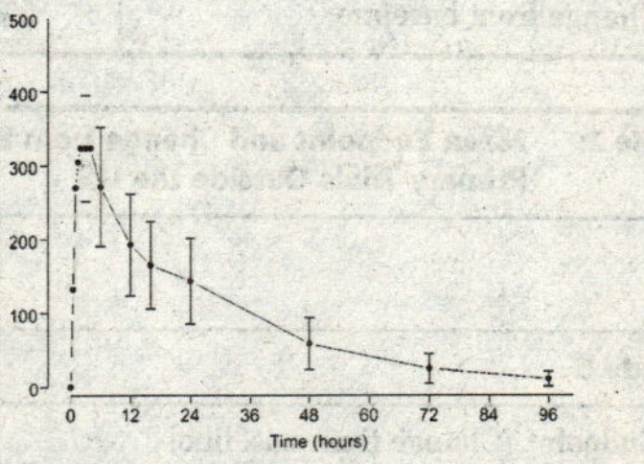

Figure 1: **Plasma tadalafil concentrations (mean ± SD) following a single 20-mg tadalafil dose**

Absorption — After single oral-dose administration, the maximum observed plasma concentration (C_{max}) of tadalafil is achieved between 30 minutes and 6 hours (median time of 2 hours). Absolute bioavailability of tadalafil following oral dosing has not been determined.

The rate and extent of absorption of tadalafil are not influenced by food; thus CIALIS may be taken with or without food.

Distribution — The mean apparent volume of distribution following oral administration is approximately 63 L, indicating that tadalafil is distributed into tissues. At therapeutic concentrations, 94% of tadalafil in plasma is bound to proteins.

Less than 0.0005% of the administered dose appeared in the semen of healthy subjects.

Metabolism — Tadalafil is predominantly metabolized by CYP3A4 to a catechol metabolite. The catechol metabolite undergoes extensive methylation and glucuronidation to form the methylcatechol and methylcatechol glucuronide conjugate, respectively. The major circulating metabolite is the methylcatechol glucuronide. Methylcatechol concentrations are less than 10% of glucuronide concentrations. *In vitro* data suggests that metabolites are not expected to be pharmacologically active at observed metabolite concentrations.

Elimination — The mean oral clearance for tadalafil is 2.5 L/hr and the mean terminal half-life is 17.5 hours in healthy subjects. Tadalafil is excreted predominantly as metabolites, mainly in the feces (approximately 61% of the dose) and to a lesser extent in the urine (approximately 36% of the dose).

Pharmacokinetics in Special Populations

Geriatric — Healthy male elderly subjects (65 years or over) had a lower oral clearance of tadalafil, resulting in 25% higher exposure (AUC) with no effect on C_{max} relative to that observed in healthy subjects 19 to 45 years of age. No dose adjustment is warranted based on age alone. However, greater sensitivity to medications in some older individuals should be considered (*see* **Geriatric Use** *under* **PRECAUTIONS**).

Pediatric — Tadalafil has not been evaluated in individuals less than 18 years old.

Hepatic Impairment — In clinical pharmacology studies, tadalafil exposure (AUC) in subjects with mild or moderate hepatic impairment (Child-Pugh Class A or B) was comparable to exposure in healthy subjects when a dose of 10 mg was administered. There are no available data for doses higher than 10 mg of tadalafil in patients with hepatic impairment. Insufficient data are available for subjects with severe hepatic impairment (Child-Pugh Class C). Therefore, for patients with mild or moderate hepatic impairment, the maximum dose should not exceed 10 mg, and use in patients with severe hepatic impairment is not recommended (*see* **DOSAGE AND ADMINISTRATION**).

Renal Insufficiency — In clinical pharmacology studies using single-dose tadalafil (5 to 10 mg), tadalafil exposure (AUC) doubled in subjects with mild (creatinine clearance 51 to 80 mL/min) or moderate (creatinine clearance 31 to 50 mL/min) renal insufficiency. In subjects with end-stage renal disease on hemodialysis, there was a two-fold increase in C_{max} and 2.7- to 4.1-fold increase in AUC following single-dose administration of 10 or 20 mg tadalafil. Exposure to total methylcatechol (unconjugated plus glucuronide) was 2- to 4-fold higher in subjects with renal impairment, compared to those with normal renal function. Hemodialysis (performed between 24 and 30 hours post-dose) contributed negligibly to tadalafil or metabolite elimination. In a clinical pharmacology study (N=28) at a dose of 10 mg, back pain was reported as a limiting adverse event in male patients with moderate renal impairment. At a dose of 5 mg, the incidence and severity of back pain was not significantly different than in the general population. In patients on hemodialysis taking 10- or 20-mg tadalafil, there were no reported cases of back pain. The dose of tadalafil should be limited to 5 mg not more than once daily in patients with severe renal insufficiency or end-stage renal disease. A starting dose of 5 mg not more than once daily is recommended for patients with moderate renal insufficiency; the maximum recommended dose is 10 mg not more than once in every 48 hours. No dose adjustment is required in patients with mild renal insufficiency (*see* **DOSAGE AND ADMINISTRATION**).

Patients with Diabetes Mellitus — In male patients with diabetes mellitus after a 10 mg tadalafil dose, exposure (AUC) was reduced approximately 19% and C_{max} was 5% lower than that observed in healthy subjects. No dose adjustment is warranted.

Pharmacodynamics

Effects on Blood Pressure — Tadalafil 20 mg administered to healthy male subjects produced no significant difference compared to placebo in supine systolic and diastolic blood pressure (difference in the mean maximal decrease of 1.6/0.8 mm Hg, respectively) and in standing systolic and diastolic blood pressure (difference in the mean maximal decrease of 0.2/4.6 mm Hg, respectively). In addition, there was no significant effect on heart rate.

Effects on Blood Pressure when CIALIS is Administered with Nitrates — In clinical pharmacology studies, tadalafil (5 to 20 mg) was shown to potentiate the hypotensive effect of nitrates. Therefore, the use of CIALIS in patients taking any form of nitrates is contraindicated (*see* **CONTRAINDICATIONS**).

A study was conducted to assess the degree of interaction between nitroglycerin and tadalafil, should nitroglycerin be required in an emergency situation after tadalafil was taken. This was a double-blind, placebo-controlled, crossover study in 150 male subjects at least 40 years of age (including subjects with diabetes mellitus and/or controlled hypertension) and receiving daily doses of tadalafil 20 mg or matching placebo for 7 days. Subjects were administered a single dose of 0.4 mg sublingual nitroglycerin (NTG) at prespecified timepoints, following their last dose of tadalafil (2, 4, 8, 24, 48, 72, and 96 hours after tadalafil). The objective of the study was to determine when, after tadalafil dosing, no apparent blood pressure interaction was observed. In this study, a significant interaction between tadalafil and NTG was observed at each timepoint up to and including 24 hours. At 48 hours, by most hemodynamic measures, the interaction between tadalafil and NTG was not observed, although a few more tadalafil subjects compared to placebo experienced greater blood-pressure lowering at this timepoint. After 48 hours, the interaction was not detectable (*see* Figure 2).

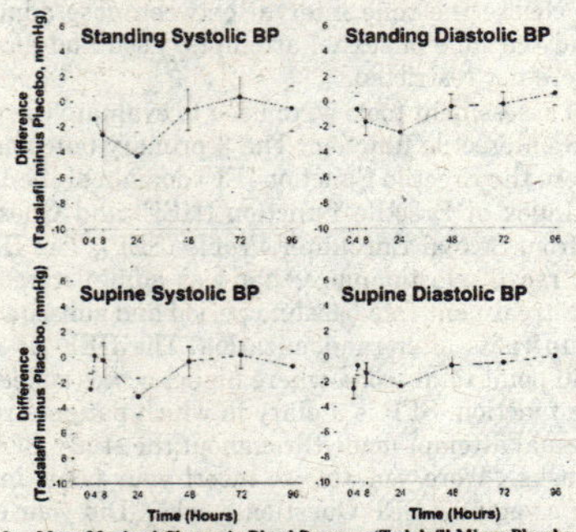

Figure 2: **Mean Maximal Change in Blood Pressure (Tadalafil Minus Placebo, Point Estimate with 90% CI) in Response to Sublingual Nitroglycerin at 2 (Supine Only), 4, 8, 24, 48, 72, and 96 Hours after the Last Dose of Tadalafil 20 mg or Placebo**

Therefore, CIALIS administration with nitrates is contraindicated. In a patient who has taken CIALIS, where nitrate administration is deemed medically necessary in a life-threatening situation, at least 48 hours should elapse after the last dose of CIALIS before nitrate administration is considered. In such circumstances, nitrates should still only be administered under close medical supervision with appropriate hemodynamic monitoring (*see* **CONTRAINDICATIONS**).

Effects on Exercise Stress Testing — The effects of tadalafil on cardiac function, hemodynamics, and exercise tolerance were investigated in a single clinical pharmacology study. In this blinded crossover trial, 23 subjects with stable coronary artery disease and evidence of exercise-induced cardiac ischemia were enrolled. The primary endpoint was time to cardiac ischemia. The mean difference in total exercise time was 3 seconds (tadalafil 10 mg minus placebo), which represented no clinically meaningful difference. Further statistical analysis demonstrated that tadalafil was non-inferior to placebo with respect to time to ischemia. Of note, in this study, in some subjects who received tadalafil followed by sublingual nitroglycerin in the post-exercise period, clinically significant reductions in blood pressure were observed,

Continued on next page

Cialis—Cont.

consistent with the augmentation by tadalafil of the blood-pressure-lowering effects of nitrates.

Effects on Vision — Single oral doses of phosphodiesterase inhibitors have demonstrated transient dose-related impairment of color discrimination (blue/green), using the Farnsworth-Munsell 100-hue test, with peak effects near the time of peak plasma levels. This finding is consistent with the inhibition of PDE6, which is involved in phototransduction in the retina. In a study to assess the effects of a single dose of tadalafil 40 mg on vision (N=59), no effects were observed on visual acuity, intraocular pressure, or pupillometry. Across all clinical studies with CIALIS, reports of changes in color vision were rare (<0.1% of patients).

Effects on Sperm Characteristics — There were no clinically relevant effects on sperm concentration, sperm count, motility, or morphology in humans in placebo-controlled studies of daily doses of tadalafil 10 mg (N=204) or 20 mg (N=217) for 6 months. In addition, tadalafil had no effect on serum levels of testosterone, luteinizing hormone, or follicle stimulating hormone.

Effects on Cardiac Electrophysiology — The effect of a single 100-mg dose of tadalafil on the QT interval was evaluated at the time of peak tadalafil concentration in a randomized, double-blinded, placebo, and active (intravenous ibutilide)-controlled crossover study in 90 healthy males aged 18 to 53 years. The mean change in QT_c (Fridericia QT correction) for tadalafil, relative to placebo, was 3.5 milliseconds (two-sided 90% CI=1.9, 5.1). The mean change in QT_c (Individual QT correction) for tadalafil, relative to placebo, was 2.8 milliseconds (two-sided 90% CI=1.2, 4.4). A 100-mg dose of tadalafil (5 times the highest recommended dose) was chosen because this dose yields exposures covering those observed upon coadministration of tadalafil with potent CYP3A4 inhibitors or those observed in renal impairment. In this study, the mean increase in heart rate associated with a 100-mg dose of tadalafil compared to placebo was 3.1 beats per minute.

Clinical Studies

The efficacy and safety of tadalafil in the treatment of erectile dysfunction has been evaluated in 22 clinical trials of up to 24-weeks duration, involving over 4000 patients. CIALIS, when taken as needed up to once daily, was shown to be effective in improving erectile function in men with erectile dysfunction (ED).

Study Design — CIALIS was studied in the general ED population in 7 randomized, multicenter, double-blinded, placebo-controlled, parallel-arm design, primary efficacy and safety studies of 12-weeks duration. Two of these studies were conducted in the United States and 5 were conducted in centers outside the US. Additional efficacy and safety studies were performed in ED patients with diabetes mellitus and in patients who developed ED status post bilateral nerve-sparing radical prostatectomy.

In these 7 trials, CIALIS was taken as needed, at doses ranging from 2.5 to 20 mg, up to once daily. Patients were free to choose the time interval between dose administration and the time of sexual attempts. Food and alcohol intake were not restricted.

Several assessment tools were used to evaluate the effect of CIALIS on erectile function. The 3 primary outcome measures were the Erectile Function (EF) domain of the International Index of Erectile Function (IIEF) and Questions 2 and 3 from Sexual Encounter Profile (SEP). The IIEF is a 4-week recall questionnaire that was administered at the end of a treatment-free baseline period and subsequently at follow-up visits after randomization. The IIEF EF domain has a 30-point total score, where higher scores reflect better erectile function. SEP is a diary in which patients recorded each sexual attempt made throughout the study. SEP Question 2 asks, "Were you able to insert your penis into your partner's vagina?" SEP Question 3 asks, "Did your erection last long enough for you to have successful intercourse?" The overall percentage of successful attempts to insert the penis into the vagina (SEP2) and to maintain the erection for successful intercourse (SEP3) is derived for each patient.

Study Results —

ED Population in US Trials — The 2 primary US efficacy and safety trials included a total of 402 men with erectile dysfunction, with a mean age of 59 years (range 27 to 87 years). The population was 78% White, 14% Black, 7% Hispanic, and 1% of other ethnicities, and included patients with ED of various severities, etiologies (organic, psychogenic, mixed), and with multiple co-morbid conditions, including diabetes mellitus, hypertension, and other cardiovascular disease. Most (>90%) patients reported ED of at least 1-year duration. Study A was conducted primarily in academic centers. Study B was conducted primarily in community-based urology practices. In each of these 2 trials, CIALIS 20 mg showed clinically meaningful and statistically significant improvements in all 3 primary efficacy variables (*see* Table 1). The treatment effect of CIALIS did not diminish over time.

[See table 1 above]

General ED Population in Trials Outside the US — The 5 primary efficacy and safety studies conducted in the general ED population outside the US included 1112 patients, with a mean age of 59 years (range 21 to 82 years). The population was 76% White, 1% Black, 3% Hispanic, and 20% of other ethnicities, and included patients with ED of various severities, etiologies (organic, psychogenic, mixed), and with multiple co-morbid conditions, including diabetes mellitus, hypertension, and other cardiovascular disease. Most (90%) patients reported ED of at least 1-year duration. In these 5 trials, CIALIS 5, 10, and 20 mg showed clinically meaningful and statistically significant improvements in all 3 primary efficacy variables (*see* Tables 2, 3, and 4). The treatment effect of CIALIS did not diminish over time.

[See table 2 above]
[See table 3 above]

Table 1: Mean Endpoint and Change from Baseline for the Primary Efficacy Variables in the Two Primary US Trials

	Study A			Study B		
	Placebo	CIALIS 20 mg		Placebo	CIALIS 20 mg	
	(N=49)	(N=146)	p-value	(N=48)	(N=159)	p-value
EF Domain Score						
Endpoint	13.5	19.5		13.6	22.5	
Change from baseline	-0.2	6.9	<.001	0.3	9.3	<.001
Insertion of Penis (SEP2)						
Endpoint	39%	62%		43%	77%	
Change from baseline	2%	26%	<.001	2%	32%	<.001
Maintenance of Erection (SEP3)						
Endpoint	25%	50%		23%	64%	
Change from baseline	5%	34%	<.001	4%	44%	<.001

Table 2: Mean Endpoint and Change from Baseline for the EF Domain of the IIEF in the General ED Population in Five Primary Trials Outside the US

	Placebo	CIALIS 5 mg	CIALIS 10 mg	CIALIS 20 mg
Study C				
Endpoint [Change from baseline]	15.0 [0.7]	17.9 [4.0]	20.0 [5.6]	
		p=.006	*p*<.001	
Study D				
Endpoint [Change from baseline]	14.4 [1.1]	17.5 [5.1]	20.6 [6.0]	
		p=.002	*p*<.001	
Study E				
Endpoint [Change from baseline]	18.1 [2.6]		22.6 [8.1]	25.0 [8.0]
			p<.001	*p*<.001
Study F*				
Endpoint [Change from baseline]	12.7 [-1.6]			22.8 [6.8]
				p<.001
Study G				
Endpoint [Change from baseline]	14.5 [-0.9]		21.2 [6.6]	23.3 [8.0]
			p<.001	*p*<.001

* Treatment duration in Study F was 6 months

Table 3: Mean Post-Baseline Success Rate and Change from Baseline for SEP Question 2 ("Were you able to insert your penis into the partner's vagina?") in the General ED Population in Five Pivotal Trials Outside the US

	Placebo	CIALIS 5 mg	CIALIS 10 mg	CIALIS 20 mg
Study C				
Endpoint [Change from baseline]	49% [6%]	57% [15%]	73% [29%]	
		p=.063	*p*<.001	
Study D				
Endpoint [Change from baseline]	46% [2%]	56% [18%]	68% [15%]	
		p=.008	*p*<.001	
Study E				
Endpoint [Change from baseline]	55% [10%]		77% [35%]	85% [35%]
			p<.001	*p*<.001
Study F*				
Endpoint [Change from baseline]	42% [-8%]			81% [27%]
				p<.001
Study G				
Endpoint [Change from baseline]	45% [-6%]		73% [21%]	76% [21%]
			p<.001	*p*<.001

* Treatment duration in Study F was 6 months

[See table 4 at right]
In addition, there were improvements in EF domain scores, success rates based upon SEP Questions 2 and 3, and patient-reported improvement in erections across patients with ED of all degrees of disease severity while taking CIALIS, compared to patients on placebo.
Therefore, in all 7 primary efficacy and safety studies, CIALIS showed statistically significant improvement in patients' ability to achieve an erection sufficient for vaginal penetration and to maintain the erection long enough for successful intercourse, as measured by the IIEF questionnaire and by SEP diaries.
Efficacy in ED Patients with Diabetes Mellitus — CIALIS was shown to be effective in treating ED in patients with diabetes mellitus. Patients with diabetes were included in all 7 primary efficacy studies in the general ED population (N=235) and in 1 study that specifically assessed CIALIS in ED patients with type 1 or type 2 diabetes (N=216). In this randomized, placebo-controlled, double-blinded, parallel-arm design prospective trial, CIALIS demonstrated clinically meaningful and statistically significant improvement in erectile function, as measured by the EF domain of the IIEF questionnaire and Questions 2 and 3 of the SEP diary (*see* Table 5).
[See table 5 at right]
Efficacy in ED Patients following Radical Prostatectomy — CIALIS was shown to be effective in treating patients who developed ED following bilateral nerve-sparing radical prostatectomy. In 1 randomized, placebo-controlled, double-blinded, parallel-arm design prospective trial in this population (N=303), CIALIS demonstrated clinically meaningful and statistically significant improvement in erectile function, as measured by the EF domain of the IIEF questionnaire and Questions 2 and 3 of the SEP diary (*see* Table 6).
[See table 6 at right]
Studies to Determine the Optimal Use of CIALIS — Several studies were conducted with the objective of determining the optimal use of CIALIS in the treatment of ED. In 1 of these studies, the percentage of patients reporting successful erections within 30 minutes of dosing was determined. In this randomized, placebo-controlled, double-blinded trial, 223 patients were randomized to placebo, CIALIS 10, or 20 mg. Using a stopwatch, patients recorded the time following dosing at which a successful erection was obtained. A successful erection was defined as at least 1 erection in 4 attempts that led to successful intercourse. At or prior to 30 minutes, 35% (26/74), 38% (28/74), and 52% (39/75) of patients in the placebo, 10-, and 20-mg groups, respectively, reported successful erections as defined above.
Two studies were conducted to assess the efficacy of CIALIS at a given timepoint after dosing, specifically at 24 hours and at 36 hours after dosing.
In the first of these studies, 348 patients with ED were randomized to placebo or CIALIS 20 mg. Patients were encouraged to make 4 total attempts at intercourse; 2 attempts were to occur at 24 hours after dosing and 2 completely separate attempts were to occur at 36 hours after dosing. The results demonstrated a difference between the placebo group and the CIALIS group at each of the pre-specified timepoints. At the 24-hour timepoint, (more specifically, 22 to 26 hours), 53/144 (37%) patients reported at least 1 successful intercourse in the placebo group versus 84/138 (61%) in the CIALIS 20-mg group. At the 36-hour timepoint (more specifically, 33 to 39 hours), 49/133 (37%) of patients reported at least 1 successful intercourse in the placebo group versus 88/137 (64%) in the CIALIS 20-mg group.
In the second of these studies, a total of 483 patients were evenly randomized to 1 of 6 groups: 3 different dosing groups (placebo, CIALIS 10, or 20 mg) that were instructed to attempt intercourse at 2 different times (24 and 36 hours post-dosing). Patients were encouraged to make 4 separate attempts at their assigned dose and assigned timepoint. In this study, the results demonstrated a statistically significant difference between the placebo group and the CIALIS groups at each of the pre-specified timepoints. At the 24-hour timepoint, the mean, per-patient percentage of attempts resulting in successful intercourse were 42, 56, and 67% for the placebo, CIALIS 10-, and 20-mg groups, respectively. At the 36-hour timepoint, the mean, per-patient percentage of attempts resulting in successful intercourse were 33, 56, and 62% for placebo, CIALIS 10-, and 20-mg groups, respectively.

Table 4: Mean Post-Baseline Success Rate and Change from Baseline for SEP Question 3 ("Did your erection last long enough for you to have successful intercourse?") in the General ED Population in Five Pivotal Trials Outside the US

	Placebo	CIALIS 5 mg	CIALIS 10 mg	CIALIS 20 mg
Study C				
Endpoint [Change from baseline]	26% [4%]	38% [19%]	58% [32%]	
		p=.040	*p<.001*	
Study D				
Endpoint [Change from baseline]	28% [4%]	42% [24%]	51% [26%]	
		p<.001	*p<.001*	
Study E				
Endpoint [Change from baseline]	43% [15%]		70% [48%]	78% [50%]
			p<.001	*p<.001*
Study F*				
Endpoint [Change from baseline]	27% [1%]			74% [40%]
				p<.001
Study G				
Endpoint [Change from baseline]	32% [5%]		57% [33%]	62% [29%]
			p<.001	*p<.001*

* Treatment duration in Study F was 6 months

Table 5: Mean Endpoint and Change from Baseline for the Primary Efficacy Variables in a Study in ED Patients with Diabetes

	Placebo	CIALIS 10 mg	CIALIS 20 mg	
	(N=71)	(N=73)	(N=72)	p-value
EF Domain Score				
Endpoint [Change from baseline]	12.2 [0.1]	19.3 [6.4]	18.7 [7.3]	<.001
Insertion of Penis (SEP2)				
Endpoint [Change from baseline]	30% [-4%]	57% [22%]	54% [23%]	<.001
Maintenance of Erection (SEP3)				
Endpoint [Change from baseline]	20% [2%]	48% [28%]	42% [29%]	<.001

Table 6: Mean Endpoint and Change from Baseline for the Primary Efficacy Variables in a Study in Patients who Developed ED Following Bilateral Nerve-Sparing Radical Prostatectomy

	Placebo	CIALIS 20 mg	
	(N=102)	(N=201)	p-value
EF Domain Score			
Endpoint [Change from baseline]	13.3 [1.1]	17.7 [5.3]	<.001
Insertion of Penis (SEP2)			
Endpoint [Change from baseline]	32% [2%]	54% [22%]	<.001
Maintenance of Erection (SEP3)			
Endpoint [Change from baseline]	19% [4%]	41% [23%]	<.001

INDICATIONS AND USAGE

CIALIS is indicated for the treatment of erectile dysfunction.

CONTRAINDICATIONS

Nitrates — Administration of CIALIS to patients who are using any form of organic nitrate, either regularly and/or intermittently, is contraindicated. In clinical pharmacology studies, tadalafil was shown to potentiate the hypotensive effect of nitrates. This is thought to result from the combined effects of nitrates and tadalafil on the nitric oxide/cGMP pathway (*see* **Pharmacodynamics, Effects on Blood Pressure when CIALIS is Administered with Nitrates** *under* **CLINICAL PHARMACOLOGY**).

Alpha Blockers — Administration of CIALIS to patients taking any alpha-adrenergic antagonist other than 0.4 mg once-daily tamsulosin is contraindicated. In a drug-drug interaction study, when tadalafil 20 mg was administered to healthy subjects taking doxazosin (8 mg daily), there was a significant augmentation of the blood-pressure-lowering effect of doxazosin (*see* **Drug Interactions** *under* **PRECAUTIONS**).

Hypersensitivity — CIALIS is contraindicated for patients with a known hypersensitivity to tadalafil or any component of the tablet.

WARNINGS

Cardiovascular

General — Physicians should consider the cardiovascular status of their patients, since there is a degree of cardiac risk associated with sexual activity. Therefore, treatments for erectile dysfunction, including CIALIS, should not be used in men for whom sexual activity is inadvisable as a result of their underlying cardiovascular status.

Left Ventricular Outflow Obstruction — Patients with left ventricular outflow obstruction, (e.g., aortic stenosis and idiopathic hypertrophic subaortic stenosis) can be sensitive to the action of vasodilators, including PDE5 inhibitors.

Patients Not Studied in Clinical Trials

The following groups of patients with cardiovascular disease were not included in clinical safety and efficacy trials for CIALIS, and, therefore, the use of CIALIS is not recommended in these groups until further information is available:

— patients with a myocardial infarction within the last 90 days
— patients with unstable angina or angina occurring during sexual intercourse
— patients with New York Heart Association Class 2 or greater heart failure in the last 6 months
— patients with uncontrolled arrhythmias, hypotension (<90/50 mm Hg), or uncontrolled hypertension (>170/100 mm Hg)
— patients with a stroke within the last 6 months

In addition, patients with known hereditary degenerative retinal disorders, including retinitis pigmentosa, were not included in the clinical trials, and use in these patients is not recommended.

Prolonged Erection

There have been rare reports of prolonged erections greater than 4 hours and priapism (painful erections greater than 6 hours in duration) for this class of compounds. Priapism, if not treated promptly, can result in irreversible damage to the erectile tissue. Patients who have an erection lasting greater than 4 hours, whether painful or not, should seek emergency medical attention.

PRECAUTIONS

Evaluation of erectile dysfunction should include an appropriate medical assessment to identify potential underlying causes, as well as treatment options.

Continued on next page

Cialis—Cont.

Before prescribing CIALIS, it is important to note the following:

Renal Insufficiency

CIALIS should be limited to 5 mg not more than once daily in patients with severe renal insufficiency or end-stage renal disease. The starting dose of CIALIS in patients with a moderate degree of renal insufficiency should be 5 mg not more than once daily, and the maximum dose should be limited to 10 mg not more than once in every 48 hours. No dose adjustment is required in patients with mild renal insufficiency (*see* **Pharmacokinetics in Special Populations** *under* **CLINICAL PHARMACOLOGY**).

Hepatic Impairment

In patients with mild or moderate hepatic impairment, the dose of CIALIS should not exceed 10 mg. Because of insufficient information in patients with severe hepatic impairment, use of CIALIS in this group is not recommended (*see* **Pharmacokinetics in Special Populations** *under* **CLINICAL PHARMACOLOGY**).

Concomitant Use of Potent Inhibitors of Cytochrome P450 3A4 (CYP3A4)

CIALIS is metabolized predominantly by CYP3A4 in the liver. The dose of CIALIS should be limited to 10 mg no more than once every 72 hours in patients taking potent inhibitors of CYP3A4 such as ritonavir, ketoconazole, and itraconazole (*see* Effects of Other Drugs on CIALIS *under* **Drug Interactions**).

General

As with other PDE5 inhibitors, tadalafil has mild systemic vasodilatory properties that may result in transient decreases in blood pressure. In a clinical pharmacology study, tadalafil 20 mg resulted in a mean maximal decrease in supine blood pressure, relative to placebo, of 1.6/0.8 mm Hg in healthy subjects (*see* **Clinical Studies** *under* **CLINICAL PHARMACOLOGY**). While this effect should not be of consequence in most patients, prior to prescribing CIALIS, physicians should carefully consider whether their patients with underlying cardiovascular disease could be affected adversely by such vasodilatory effects. Patients with significant left ventricular outflow obstruction or severely impaired autonomic control of blood pressure may be particularly sensitive to the actions of vasodilators.

The safety and efficacy of combinations of CIALIS and other treatments for erectile dysfunction have not been studied. Therefore, the use of such combinations is not recommended.

CIALIS should be used with caution in patients who have conditions that might predispose them to priapism (such as sickle cell anemia, multiple myeloma, or leukemia), or in patients with anatomical deformation of the penis (such as angulation, cavernosal fibrosis, or Peyronie's disease).

When administered in combination with aspirin, tadalafil 20 mg did not prolong bleeding time, relative to aspirin alone. CIALIS has not been administered to patients with bleeding disorders or significant active peptic ulceration. Although CIALIS has not been shown to increase bleeding times in healthy subjects, use in patients with bleeding disorders or significant active peptic ulceration should be based upon a careful risk-benefit assessment and caution.

Information for Patients

Physicians should discuss with patients the contraindication of CIALIS with regular and/or intermittent use of organic nitrates. Patients should be counseled that concomitant use of CIALIS with nitrates could cause blood pressure to suddenly drop to an unsafe level, resulting in dizziness, syncope, or even heart attack or stroke.

Physicians should discuss with patients the appropriate action in the event that they experience anginal chest pain requiring nitroglycerin following intake of CIALIS. In such a patient, who has taken CIALIS, where nitrate administration is deemed medically necessary for a life-threatening situation, at least 48 hours should have elapsed after the last dose of CIALIS before nitrate administration is considered. In such circumstances, nitrates should still only be administered under close medical supervision with appropriate hemodynamic monitoring. Therefore, patients who experience anginal chest pain after taking CIALIS should seek immediate medical attention.

Physicians should inform their patients that concomitant use of CIALIS with alpha-adrenergic antagonists (other than 0.4 mg once-daily tamsulosin) is contraindicated because coadministration can lead to significant reductions in blood pressure.

Physicians should discuss with patients the potential for CIALIS to augment the blood-pressure-lowering effect of other anti-hypertensive medications.

Patients should be made aware that both alcohol and CIALIS, a PDE5 inhibitor, act as mild vasodilators. When mild vasodilators are taken in combination, blood-pressure-lowering effects of each individual compound may be increased. Therefore, physicians should inform patients that substantial consumption of alcohol (e.g., 5 units or greater) in combination with CIALIS can increase the potential for orthostatic signs and symptoms, including increase in heart rate, decrease in standing blood pressure, dizziness, and headache.

Physicians should consider the potential cardiac risk of sexual activity in patients with preexisting cardiovascular disease. Patients who experience symptoms upon initiation of sexual activity should be advised to refrain from further sexual activity and seek immediate medical attention.

There have been rare reports of prolonged erections greater than 4 hours and priapism (painful erections greater than 6 hours in duration) for this class of compounds. Priapism, if not treated promptly, can result in irreversible damage to the erectile tissue. Patients who have an erection lasting greater than 4 hours, whether painful or not, should seek emergency medical attention.

The use of CIALIS offers no protection against sexually transmitted diseases. Counseling of patients about the protective measures necessary to guard against sexually transmitted diseases, including Human Immunodeficiency Virus (HIV) should be considered.

Patients should read the patient leaflet entitled "INFORMATION FOR THE PATIENT" before starting therapy with CIALIS and each time the prescription is renewed or refilled.

Drug Interactions

Effects of Other Drugs on CIALIS

Cytochrome P450 Inhibitors

CIALIS is a substrate of and predominantly metabolized by CYP3A4. Studies have shown that drugs that inhibit CYP3A4 can increase tadalafil exposure (*see* **PRECAUTIONS** *and* **DOSAGE AND ADMINISTRATION**).

Ketoconazole — Ketoconazole (400 mg daily), a selective and potent inhibitor of CYP3A4, increased tadalafil 20-mg single-dose exposure (AUC) by 312% and C_{max} by 22%, relative to the values for tadalafil 20 mg alone. Ketoconazole (200 mg daily) increased tadalafil 10-mg single-dose exposure (AUC) by 107% and C_{max} by 15%, relative to the values for tadalafil 10 mg alone.

HIV Protease inhibitor — Ritonavir (200 mg twice daily), an inhibitor of CYP3A4, CYP2C9, CYP2C19, and CYP2D6, increased tadalafil 20-mg single-dose exposure (AUC) by 124% with no change in C_{max}, relative to the values for tadalafil 20 mg alone. Although specific interactions have not been studied, other HIV protease inhibitors would likely increase tadalafil exposure (*see* **DOSAGE AND ADMINISTRATION**).

Based upon these results, in patients taking concomitant potent CYP3A4 inhibitors, the dose of CIALIS should not exceed 10 mg, and CIALIS should not be taken more frequently than once in every 72 hours (*see* **DOSAGE AND ADMINISTRATION**).

Other cytochrome P450 inhibitors — Although specific interactions have not been studied, other CYP3A4 inhibitors, such as erythromycin, itraconazole, and grapefruit juice, would likely increase tadalafil exposure.

Cytochrome P450 Inducers

Studies have shown that drugs that induce CYP3A4 can decrease tadalafil exposure.

Rifampin — Rifampin (600 mg daily), a CYP3A4 inducer, reduced tadalafil 10-mg single-dose exposure (AUC) by 88% and C_{max} by 46%, relative to the values for tadalafil 10 mg alone. Although specific interactions have not been studied, other CYP3A4 inducers, such as carbamazepine, phenytoin, and phenobarbitol, would likely decrease tadalafil exposure. No dose adjustment is warranted.

Gastrointestinal Drugs

H_2 antagonists — An increase in gastric pH resulting from administration of nizatidine had no significant effect on tadalafil pharmacokinetics.

Antacids — Simultaneous administration of an antacid (magnesium hydroxide/aluminum hydroxide) and tadalafil reduced the apparent rate of absorption of tadalafil without altering exposure (AUC) to tadalafil.

Effects of CIALIS on Other Drugs

Drugs Metabolized by Cytochrome P450

CIALIS is not expected to cause clinically significant inhibition or induction of the clearance of drugs metabolized by cytochrome P450 (CYP) isoforms. Studies have shown that tadalafil does not inhibit or induce P450 isoforms CYP1A2, CYP3A4, CYP2C9, CYP2C19, CYP2D6, and CYP2E1.

CYP1A2 substrate — Tadalafil had no clinically significant effect on the pharmacokinetics of theophylline. When tadalafil was administered to subjects taking theophylline, a small augmentation (3 beats per minute) of the increase in heart rate associated with theophylline was observed.

CYP3A4 substrates — Tadalafil had no clinically significant effect on exposure (AUC) to midazolam or lovastatin.

CYP2C9 substrate — Tadalafil had no clinically significant effect on exposure (AUC) to S-warfarin or R-warfarin, nor did tadalafil affect changes in prothrombin time induced by warfarin.

Alcohol

Alcohol and PDE5 inhibitors, including tadalafil, are mild systemic vasodilators. The interaction of tadalafil with alcohol was evaluated in 3 clinical pharmacology studies. In 2 of these, alcohol was administered at a dose of 0.7 g/kg, which is equivalent to approximately 6 ounces of 80-proof vodka in an 80-kg male, and tadalafil was administered at a dose of 10 mg in 1 study and 20 mg in another. In both these studies, all patients imbibed the entire alcohol dose within 10 minutes of starting. In one of these two studies, blood alcohol levels of 0.08% were confirmed. In these two studies, more patients had clinically significant decreases in blood pressure on the combination of tadalafil and alcohol as compared to alcohol alone. Some subjects reported postural dizziness, and orthostatic hypotension was observed in some subjects. When tadalafil 20 mg was administered with a lower dose of alcohol (0.6 g/kg, which is equivalent to approximately 4 ounces of 80-proof vodka, administered in less than 10 minutes), orthostatic hypotension was not observed, dizziness occurred with similar frequency to alcohol alone, and the hypotensive effects of alcohol were not potentiated.

Tadalafil did not affect alcohol plasma concentrations and alcohol did not affect tadalafil plasma concentrations.

Both alcohol and CIALIS, a PDE5 inhibitor, act as mild vasodilators. When mild vasodilators are taken in combination, blood-pressure-lowering effects of each individual compound may be increased. Substantial consumption of alcohol (e.g., 5 units or greater) in combination with CIALIS can increase the potential for orthostatic signs and symptoms, including increase in heart rate, decrease in standing blood pressure, dizziness, and headache.

Anti-Hypertensives

PDE5 inhibitors, including tadalafil, are mild systemic vasodilators. Clinical pharmacology studies were conducted to assess the effect of tadalafil on the potentiation of the blood-pressure-lowering effects of selected anti-hypertensive medications.

Alpha Blockers

Doxazosin — When tadalafil 20 mg was administered to healthy subjects taking doxazosin (8 mg daily), an alpha[1]-adrenergic blocker, there was significant augmentation of the blood-pressure-lowering effect of doxazosin.

Tamsulosin — In a clinical pharmacology study, when a single dose of tadalafil 20 mg was administered to healthy subjects taking 0.4 mg once-daily tamsulosin, a selective alpha[1A]-adrenergic blocker, no significant decreases in blood pressure were observed.

Therefore, based upon significant augmentation of the blood-pressure-lowering effect of doxazosin, an alpha[1]-adrenergic blocker, and no significant effect seen with 0.4 mg once-daily tamsulosin, a selective alpha[1A]-adrenergic blocker, administration of CIALIS to patients taking any alpha-adrenergic blocker other than 0.4 mg once-daily tamsulosin is contraindicated.

Other Anti-Hypertensive Agents

Amlodipine — A study was conducted to assess the interaction of amlodipine (5 mg daily) and tadalafil 10 mg. There was no effect of tadalafil on amlodipine blood levels and no effect of amlodipine on tadalafil blood levels. The mean reduction in supine systolic/diastolic blood pressure due to tadalafil 10 mg in subjects taking amlodipine was 3/2 mm Hg, compared to placebo. In a similar study using tadalafil 20 mg, there were no clinically significant differences between tadalafil and placebo in subjects taking amlodipine.

Metoprolol — A study was conducted to assess the interaction of sustained-release metoprolol (25 to 200 mg daily) and tadalafil 10 mg. Following dosing, the mean reduction in supine systolic/diastolic blood pressure due to tadalafil 10 mg in subjects taking metoprolol was 5/3 mm Hg, compared to placebo.

Bendrofluazide — A study was conducted to assess the interaction of bendrofluazide (2.5 mg daily) and tadalafil 10 mg. Following dosing, the mean reduction in supine systolic/diastolic blood pressure due to tadalafil 10 mg in subjects taking bendrofluazide was 6/4 mm Hg, compared to placebo.

Enalapril — A study was conducted to assess the interaction of enalapril (10 to 20 mg daily) and tadalafil 10 mg. Following dosing, the mean reduction in supine systolic/diastolic blood pressure due to tadalafil 10 mg in subjects taking enalapril was 4/1 mm Hg, compared to placebo.

Angiotensin II receptor blocker (and other anti-hypertensives) — A study was conducted to assess the interaction of angiotensin II receptor blockers and tadalafil 20 mg. Subjects in the study were taking any marketed angiotensin II receptor blocker, either alone, as a component of a combination product, or as part of a multiple anti-hypertensive regimen. Following dosing, ambulatory measurements of blood pressure revealed differences between tadalafil and placebo of 8/4 mm Hg in systolic/diastolic blood pressure.

Aspirin

Tadalafil did not potentiate the increase in bleeding time caused by aspirin.

Carcinogenesis, Mutagenesis, Impairment of Fertility

Tadalafil was not carcinogenic to rats or mice when administered daily for 2 years at doses up to 400 mg/kg/day. Systemic drug exposures, as measured by AUC of unbound tadalafil, were approximately 10-fold for mice, and 14- and 26-fold for male and female rats, respectively, the exposures in human males given Maximum Recommended Human Dose (MRHD) of 20 mg.

Tadalafil was not mutagenic in the *in vitro* bacterial Ames assays or the forward mutation test in mouse lymphoma cells. Tadalafil was not clastogenic in the *in vitro* chromosomal aberration test in human lymphocytes or the *in vivo* rat micronucleus assays.

There were no effects on fertility, reproductive performance or reproductive organ morphology in male or female rats given oral doses of tadalafil up to 400 mg/kg/day, a dose producing AUCs for unbound tadalafil of 14-fold for males or 26-fold for females the exposures observed in human males given the MRHD of 20 mg. In beagle dogs given tadalafil daily for 3 to 12 months, there was treatment-related non-reversible degeneration and atrophy of the seminiferous tubular epithelium in the testes in 20-100% of the dogs that resulted in a decrease in spermatogenesis in 40-75% of the dogs at doses of ≥10 mg/kg/day. Systemic exposure (based on AUC) at no-observed-adverse-effect-level (NOAEL) (10 mg/kg/day) for unbound tadalafil was similar to that expected in humans at the MRHD of 20 mg.

There were no treatment-related testicular findings in rats or mice treated with doses up to 400 mg/kg/day for 2 years.

In men, there were no clinically relevant effects on sperm concentration, sperm count, motility, or morphology in placebo-controlled studies of daily doses of tadalafil 10 mg

Table 7: Treatment-Emergent Adverse Events Reported by ≥2% of Patients Treated with Tadalafil (10 or 20 mg) and More Frequent on Drug than Placebo in the Eight Primary Placebo-Controlled Phase 3 Studies (Including a Study in Patients with Diabetes)

	Placebo	Tadalafil 5 mg	Tadalafil 10 mg	Tadalafil 20 mg
Adverse Event	**(N=476)**	**(N=151)**	**(N=394)**	**(N=635)**
Headache	5%	11%	11%	15%
Dyspepsia	1%	4%	8%	10%
Back pain	3%	3%	5%	6%
Myalgia	1%	1%	4%	3%
Nasal congestion	1%	2%	3%	3%
Flushing*	1%	2%	3%	3%
Pain in limb	1%	1%	3%	3%

* The term flushing includes: facial flushing and flushing

(N=204) or 20 mg (N=217) for 6 months. In addition, tadalafil had no effect on serum levels of testosterone, luteinizing hormone, or follicle stimulating hormone in males.

Animal Toxicology

Animal studies showed vascular inflammation in tadalafil-treated mice, rats, and dogs. In mice and rats, lymphoid necrosis and hemorrhage were seen in the spleen, thymus, and mesenteric lymph nodes at unbound tadalafil exposure of 2- to 33-fold above the human exposure (AUCs) at the MRHD of 20 mg. In dogs, an increased incidence of disseminated arteritis was observed in 1- and 6-month studies at unbound tadalafil exposure of 1- to 54-fold above the human exposure (AUC) at the MRHD of 20 mg. In a 12-month dog study, no disseminated arteritis was observed, but 2 dogs exhibited marked decreases in white blood cells (neutrophils) and moderate decreases in platelets with inflammatory signs at unbound tadalafil exposures of approximately 14- to 18-fold the human exposure at the MRHD of 20 mg. The abnormal blood-cell findings were reversible within 2 weeks upon removal of the drug.

Pregnancy, Nursing Mothers, and Pediatric Use

CIALIS is not indicated for use in newborns, children, or women.

Tadalafil and/or its metabolites cross the placenta, resulting in fetal exposure in rats. Tadalafil and/or its metabolites were secreted into the milk in lactating rats at concentrations approximately 2.4-fold greater than found in the plasma. Following a single-oral dose of 10 mg/kg, approximately 0.1% of the total radioactive dose was excreted into the milk within 3 hours. It is not known if tadalafil and/or its metabolites is excreted in human breast milk. Use of tadalafil in nursing mothers is not recommended.

Pregnancy Category B — There was no evidence of teratogenicity, embryotoxicity, or fetotoxicity in rat or mouse fetuses that received up to 1000 mg/kg/day during the major organ development. Plasma exposure at this dose is approximately 11-fold greater than the AUC values for unbound tadalafil in humans given the MRHD of 20 mg. In a rat prenatal and postnatal development study at doses of 60, 200, and 1000 mg/kg, there was a reduction in postnatal survival of pups. The no-observed-effect-level (NOEL) for maternal toxicity was 200 mg/kg/day and for developmental toxicity was 30 mg/kg/day, which gives approximately 16- and 10-fold exposure multiples, respectively, of the human AUC for the MRHD dose of 20 mg. There are no adequate and well-controlled studies of tadalafil in pregnant women.

Geriatric Use

Approximately 25% of patients in the primary efficacy and safety studies of tadalafil were greater than 65 years of age. No overall differences in efficacy and safety were observed between older and younger patients. No dose adjustment is warranted based on age alone. However, greater sensitivity to medications in some older individuals should be considered (*see* **Special Populations** *under* **CLINICAL PHARMACOLOGY**).

ADVERSE REACTIONS

Tadalafil was administered to over 5700 men (mean age 59, range 19 to 87 years) during clinical trials worldwide. Over 1000 patients were treated for 1 year or longer and over 1300 patients were treated for 6 months or more.

In placebo-controlled Phase 3 clinical trials, the discontinuation rate due to adverse events in patients treated with tadalafil 10 or 20 mg was 3.1%, compared to 1.4% in placebo-treated patients.

When tadalafil was taken as recommended in the placebo-controlled clinical trials, the following adverse events were reported (*see* Table 7):

[See table 7 above]

Back pain or myalgia was reported at incidence rates described in Table 7. In tadalafil clinical pharmacology trials, back pain or myalgia generally occurred 12 to 24 hours after dosing and typically resolved within 48 hours. The back pain/myalgia associated with tadalafil treatment was characterized by diffuse bilateral lower lumbar, gluteal, thigh, or thoracolumbar muscular discomfort and was exacerbated by recumbancy. In general, pain was reported as mild or moderate in severity and resolved without medical treatment, but severe back pain was reported infrequently (<5% of all reports). When medical treatment was necessary, acetaminophen or non-steroidal anti-inflammatory drugs were generally effective; however, in a small percentage of subjects who required treatment, a mild narcotic (e.g. codeine) was used. Overall, approximately 0.5% of all tadalafil-treated subjects discontinued treatment as a consequence of back pain/myalgia. Diagnostic testing, including measures for inflammation, muscle injury, or renal damage revealed no evidence of medically significant underlying pathology.

Across all studies with any tadalafil dose, reports of changes in color vision were rare (<0.1% of patients).

The following section identifies additional, less frequent events (<2%) reported in controlled clinical trials; a causal relationship of these events to CIALIS is uncertain. Excluded from this list are those events that were minor, those with no plausible relation to drug use, and reports too imprecise to be meaningful:

Body as a whole: asthenia, face edema, fatigue, pain

Cardiovascular: angina pectoris, chest pain, hypotension, hypertension, myocardial infarction, postural hypotension, palpitations, syncope, tachycardia

Digestive: abnormal liver function tests, diarrhea, dry mouth, dysphagia, esophagitis, gastroesophageal reflux, gastritis, GGTP increased, loose stools, nausea, upper abdominal pain, vomiting

Musculoskeletal: arthralgia, neck pain

Nervous: dizziness, hypesthesia, insomnia, paresthesia, somnolence, vertigo

Respiratory: dyspnea, epistaxis, pharyngitis

Skin and Appendages: pruritus, rash, sweating

Ophthalmologic: blurred vision, changes in color vision, conjunctivitis (including conjunctival hyperemia), eye pain, lacrimation increase, swelling of eyelids

Urogenital: erection increased, spontaneous penile erection

OVERDOSAGE

Single doses up to 500 mg have been given to healthy subjects, and multiple daily doses up to 100 mg have been given to patients. Adverse events were similar to those seen at lower doses. In cases of overdose, standard supportive measures should be adopted as required. Hemodialysis contributes negligibly to tadalafil elimination.

DOSAGE AND ADMINISTRATION

The recommended starting dose of CIALIS in most patients is 10 mg, taken prior to anticipated sexual activity. The dose may be increased to 20 mg or decreased to 5 mg, based on individual efficacy and tolerability. The maximum recommended dosing frequency is once per day in most patients. CIALIS was shown to improve erectile function compared to placebo up to 36 hours following dosing. Therefore, when advising patients on optimal use of CIALIS, this should be taken into consideration.

CIALIS may be taken without regard to food.

Renal Insufficiency — No dose adjustment is required in patients with mild renal insufficiency. For patients with moderate (creatinine clearance 31 to 50 mL/min) renal insufficiency, a starting dose of 5 mg not more than once daily is recommended, and the maximum dose should be limited to 10 mg not more than once in every 48 hours. For patients with severe (creatinine clearance <30 mL/min) renal insufficiency on hemodialysis, the maximum recommended dose is 5 mg (*see* **General** *and* **Patients with Renal Insufficiency** *under* **PRECAUTIONS** *and* **Pharmacokinetics in Special Populations** *under* **CLINICAL PHARMACOLOGY**).

Hepatic Impairment — For patients with mild or moderate degrees of hepatic impairment (Child-Pugh Class A or B), the dose of CIALIS should not exceed 10 mg once daily. In patients with severe hepatic impairment (Child-Pugh Class C), the use of CIALIS is not recommended (*see* **Patients with Hepatic Impairment** *under* **PRECAUTIONS** *and* **Pharmacokinetics in Special Populations** *under* **CLINICAL PHARMACOLOGY**).

Concomitant Medications — For patients taking concomitant potent inhibitors of CYP3A4, such as ketoconazole or ritonavir, the maximum recommended dose of CIALIS is 10 mg, not to exceed once every 72 hours (*see* **General** *and* **Drug Interactions** *under* **PRECAUTIONS**).

Concomitant use of nitrates in any form and alpha-adrenergic blockers (other than 0.4 mg once-daily tamsulosin) is contraindicated (*see* **CONTRAINDICATIONS** *and* **Drug Interactions** *under* **PRECAUTIONS**).

Geriatrics — No dose adjustment is required in patients >65 years of age.

HOW SUPPLIED

CIALIS® (tadalafil) is supplied as follows:

Three strengths of film-coated, almond-shaped tablets are available in different sizes and different shades of yellow, and supplied in the following package sizes:

5-mg tablets debossed with "C 5"
Bottles of 30 NDC 0002-4462-30
10-mg tablets debossed with "C 10"
Bottles of 30 NDC 0002-4463-30
20-mg tablets debossed with "C 20"
Bottles of 30 NDC 0002-4464-30

Store at 25°C (77°F); excursions permitted to 15-30°C (59-86°F) [see USP Controlled Room Temperature].

Keep out of reach of children.

Literature issued November, 2003

Manufactured for Lilly ICOS LLC
by Eli Lilly and Company
Indianapolis, IN 46285, USA

PV 3530 AMP

MedPointe Pharmaceuticals
MedPointe Healthcare Inc.
SOMERSET, NJ 08873

For Medical Information, Contact:
Generally:
Medical Information
800-526-3840
After Hours and Weekend Emergencies:
800-526-3840

MedPointe Pharmaceuticals
MedPointe Healthcare Inc.
Sales and Ordering
Somerset, NJ 08873

ZOMIG® NASAL SPRAY ℞
[*zō-mĭg*]
(zolmitriptan)
FOR NASAL USE ONLY

DESCRIPTION

ZOMIG® (zolmitriptan) Nasal Spray contains zolmitriptan, which is a selective 5-hydroxytryptamine $_{1B/1D}$ (5-$HT_{1B/1D}$) receptor agonist. Zolmitriptan is chemically designated as (S)-4-[[3-[2-(dimethylamino)ethyl]-1H-indol-5-yl]methyl]-2-oxazolidinone and has the following chemical structure:

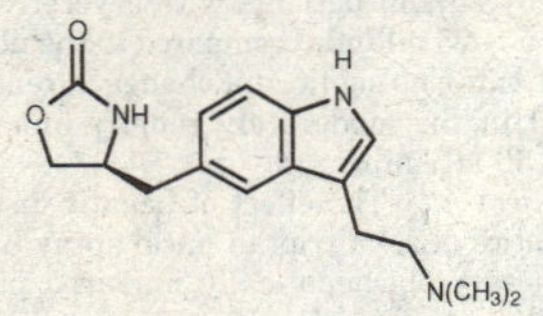

The empirical formula is $C_{16}H_{21}N_3O_2$, representing a molecular weight of 287.36. Zolmitriptan is a white to almost white powder that is readily soluble in water. ZOMIG Nasal Spray is supplied as a clear to pale yellow solution of zolmitriptan, buffered to a pH 5.0. Each ZOMIG Nasal Spray contains 5 mg of zolmitriptan in a 100-μL unit dose aqueous buffered solution containing citric acid, anhydrous, USP, disodium phosphate dodecahydrate USP and purified water USP.

ZOMIG Nasal Spray is hypertonic. The osmolarity of ZOMIG Nasal Spray 5 mg is 420 to 470 mOsmol.

CLINICAL PHARMACOLOGY

Mechanism of Action: Zolmitriptan binds with high affinity to human recombinant 5-HT_{1D} and 5-HT_{1B} receptors. Zolmitriptan exhibits modest affinity for 5-HT_{1A} receptors, but has no significant affinity (as measured by radioligand binding assays) or pharmacological activity at 5-HT_2, 5-HT_3, 5-HT_4, alpha$_1$, alpha$_2$, or beta$_1$ adrenergic; H_1, H_2, histaminic; muscarinic; dopamine$_1$, or dopamine$_2$ receptors. The N-desmethyl metabolite also has high affinity for 5-$HT_{1B/1D}$ and modest affinity for 5-HT_{1A} receptors.

Current theories proposed to explain the etiology of migraine headache suggest that symptoms are due to local cranial vasodilatation and/or to the release of sensory neuropeptides (vasoactive intestinal peptide, substance P and calcitonin gene-related peptide) through nerve endings in the trigeminal system. The therapeutic activity of zolmitriptan for the treatment of migraine headache can most likely be attributed to the agonist effects at the 5-$HT_{1B/1D}$ receptors on intracranial blood vessels (including the arterio-venous anastomoses) and sensory nerves of the trigeminal system which result in cranial vessel constriction and inhibition of pro-inflammatory neuropeptide release.

Clinical Pharmacokinetics and Bioavailability:

Absorption: Zolmitriptan nasal spray is rapidly absorbed via the nasopharynx as detected in a Photon Emission Tomography (PET) study using ^{11}C zolmitriptan. Zolmitriptan was detected in plasma by 5 minutes and peak plasma concentration generally was achieved by 3 hours. The time at

Continued on next page

Zomig Nasal Spray—Cont.

which maximum plasma concentrations were observed was similar after single (1 day) or multiple (4 day) nasal dosing. Plasma concentrations of zolmitriptan are sustained for 4 to 6 hours after dosing. Zolmitriptan displays linear kinetics after multiple doses of 2.5 mg, 5 mg, or 10 mg. The mean relative bioavailability of the nasal spray formulation is 102%, compared to the oral tablet.

Zolmitriptan and its active metabolite display dose proportionality after single or multiple dosing. Dose proportional increases in zolmitriptan and N-desmethyl metabolite C_{max} and AUC were observed for 2.5 and 5 mg nasal spray doses. The pharmacokinetics for elimination of zolmitriptan and its active N-desmethyl metabolite are similar for all nasal spray dosages. The N-desmethyl metabolite is detected in plasma by 15 minutes and peak plasma concentration is generally achieved by 3 hours after administration.

Food has no significant effect on the bioavailability of zolmitriptan.

Distribution: Plasma protein binding of zolmitriptan is 25% over the concentration range of 10 - 1000 ng/mL. The mean (±SD) apparent volume of distribution for zolmitriptan nasal spray formulation is 8.6±3.3 L/kg.

Metabolism: Zolmitriptan is converted to an active N-desmethyl metabolite such that the metabolite concentrations are about two- thirds that of zolmitriptan. Because the $5HT_{1B/1D}$ potency of the metabolite is 2 to 6 times that of the parent compound, the metabolite may contribute a substantial portion of the overall effect after zolmitriptan administration.

Excretion: The mean elimination half-life for zolmitriptan and its active N-desmethyl metabolite following nasal spray administration are approximately 3 hours, which is similar to the half-life values seen after oral tablet administration. The half-life values were similar for zolmitriptan and the N-desmethyl metabolite after single (1 day) and multiple (4 day) nasal dosing.

Mean total plasma clearance is 25.9 mL/min/kg, of which one-sixth is renal clearance. The renal clearance is greater than the glomerular filtration rate suggesting renal tubular secretion.

Special Populations

Age: The pharmacokinetics of oral zolmitriptan in healthy elderly non-migraineur volunteers (age 65 - 76 yrs) was similar to those in younger non-migraineur volunteers (age 18-39 yrs).

Gender: Mean plasma concentrations of orally administered zolmitriptan were up to 1.5-fold higher in females than males.

Renal Impairment: The effect of renal impairment on the pharmacokinetics of zolmitriptan nasal spray has not been evaluated. After orally dosing zolmitriptan, renal clearance was reduced by 25% in patients with severe renal impairment (Clcr ≥ 5 ≤ 25 mL/min) compared to the normal group (Clcr ≥ 70 mL/min); no significant change in renal clearance was observed in the moderately renally impaired group (Clcr ≥ 26 ≤ 50 mL/min).

Hepatic Impairment: The effect of hepatic disease on the pharmacokinetics of zolmitriptan nasal spray has not been evaluated. In severely hepatically impaired patients, the mean C_{max}, T_{max}, and $AUC_{0-\infty}$ of zolmitriptan dosed orally were increased 1.5, 2, and 3-fold, respectively, compared to normals. Seven out of 27 patients experienced 20 to 80 mm Hg elevations in systolic and/or diastolic blood pressure after a 10 mg dose. Because of the similarity in exposure, zolmitriptan tablets and nasal spray should have similar dosage adjustments and should be administered with caution in subjects with liver disease, generally using doses less than 2.5 mg. Doses lower than 5 mg can only be achieved through the use of an oral formulation. (see WARNINGS and PRECAUTIONS).

Hypertensive Patients: No differences in the pharmacokinetics of oral zolmitriptan or its effects on blood pressure were seen in mild to moderate hypertensive volunteers compared to normotensive controls.

Race: Retrospective analysis of pharmacokinetic data between Japanese and Caucasians revealed no significant differences for orally dosed zolmitriptan.

Drug Interactions: All drug interaction studies were performed in healthy volunteers using a single 10 mg dose of zolmitriptan and a single dose of the other drug except where otherwise noted. Eight drug interaction studies have been performed with zolmitriptan tablets and one study (xylometazoline) was performed with nasal spray.

Xylometazoline: An in vivo drug interaction study with ZOMIG Nasal Spray indicated that 1 spray (100µL dose) of xylometazoline (0.1% w/v), a decongestant, administered 30 minutes prior to a 5 mg nasal dose of zolmitriptan did not alter the pharmacokinetics of zolmitriptan.

Fluoxetine: The pharmacokinetics of zolmitriptan, as well as its effect on blood pressure, were unaffected by 4 weeks of pretreatment with oral fluoxetine (20 mg/day).

MAO Inhibitors: Following one week of administration of 150 mg bid moclobemide, a specific MAO-A inhibitor, there was an increase of about 25% in both C_{max} and AUC for zolmitriptan and a 3-fold increase in the C_{max} and AUC of the active N-desmethyl metabolite of zolmitriptan (see CONTRAINDICATIONS and PRECAUTIONS).

Selegiline, a selective MAO-B inhibitor, at a dose of 10 mg/day for 1 week, had no effect on the pharmacokinetics of zolmitriptan and its metabolite.

Propranolol: C_{max} and AUC of zolmitriptan increased 1.5-fold after one week of dosing with propranolol (160 mg/day). C_{max} and AUC of the N-desmethyl metabolite were reduced by 30% and 15%, respectively. There were no interactive effects on blood pressure or pulse rate following administration of propranolol with zolmitriptan.

Acetaminophen: A single 1 g dose of acetaminophen does not alter the pharmacokinetics of zolmitriptan and its N-desmethyl metabolite. However, zolmitriptan delayed the T_{max} of acetaminophen by one hour.

Metoclopramide: A single 10 mg dose of metoclopramide had no effect on the pharmacokinetics of zolmitriptan or its metabolites.

Oral Contraceptives: Retrospective analysis of pharmacokinetic data across studies indicated that mean plasma concentrations of zolmitriptan were generally higher in females taking oral contraceptives compared to those not taking oral contraceptives. Mean C_{max} and AUC of zolmitriptan were found to be higher by 30% and 50%, respectively, and T_{max} was delayed by one-half hour in females taking oral contraceptives. The effect of zolmitriptan on the pharmacokinetics of oral contraceptives has not been studied.

Cimetidine: Following the administration of cimetidine, the half-life and AUC of a 5 mg dose of zolmitriptan and its active metabolite were approximately doubled (see PRECAUTIONS).

Clinical Studies: The efficacy of ZOMIG Nasal Spray 5 mg in the acute treatment of migraine headache with or without aura was demonstrated in a randomized, outpatient, double-blind, placebo-controlled trial.

Patients were instructed to treat a moderate to severe headache. Headache response, defined as a reduction in headache severity from moderate or severe pain to mild or no pain, was assessed 15, 30, 45 minutes and 1, 2, and 4 hours after dosing. Pain free response rates and associated symptoms such as nausea, photophobia, and phonophobia were also assessed. A dose of escape medication was allowed 4 to 24 hours after the initial treatment for persistent and recurrent headache.

Of the 1372 patients treated in the study, 83% were female and 99% were Caucasian, with a mean age of 40.6 years (range 18 to 65 years).

The two hour headache response rates in patients treated with ZOMIG Nasal Spray were statistically significant among patients receiving ZOMIG Nasal Spray compared to placebo. There was a greater percentage of patients with a headache response at 2 hours in the higher dose groups. The headache response efficacy endpoints of the controlled clinical study, analyzed from the first attack data, are shown in Table 1.

Table 1
First Attack Data: Percentage of Patients with Headache Response to ZOMIG Nasal Spray (Mild or No Headache) 2 Hours Following Treatment (N = number of randomized patients treating a migraine attack)
The 2 hour headache response was the primary end-point

N	PLACEBO (226)	ZOMIG 5 mg (235)
2 hours	31%	69%†

†p <0.0001 in comparison with placebo

The estimated probability of achieving an initial headache response by 4 hours following treatment with ZOMIG Nasal Spray is depicted in Figure 1.

Figure 1
Estimated probability of achieving an initial headache response within 4 hours of initial treatment

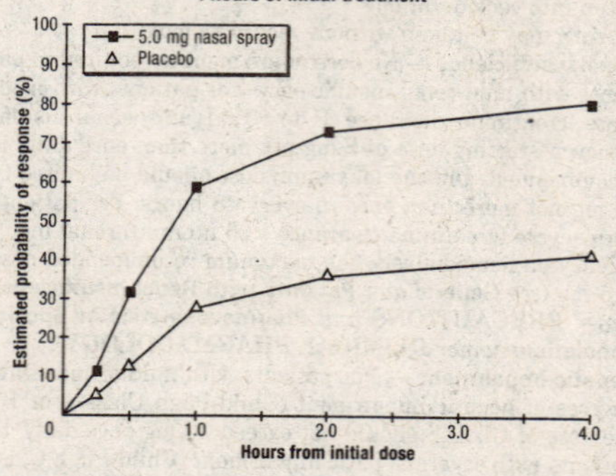

Note: Figure 1 shows the Kaplan-Meier plot of the probability over time of obtaining headache response (moderate or severe headache improving to mild or no pain) following treatment with zolmitriptan nasal spray. The averages displayed are based on a placebo controlled, outpatient trial providing evidence of efficacy. Patients not achieving headache response or taking additional treatment prior to 4 hours were censored to 4 hours.

For patients with migraine associated photophobia, phonophobia, and nausea at baseline, there was a decreased incidence of these symptoms following administration of ZOMIG Nasal Spray as compared to placebo.

Four to 24 hours following the initial dose of study treatment, patients were allowed to use additional treatment for pain relief in the form of a second dose of study treatment or other medication. The estimated probability of patients taking a second dose or other medication for migraine over the 24 hours following the initial dose of study treatment is summarized in Figure 2.

Figure 2: Estimated probability of patients taking an escape medication within the 24 hours following the initial dose of study treatment

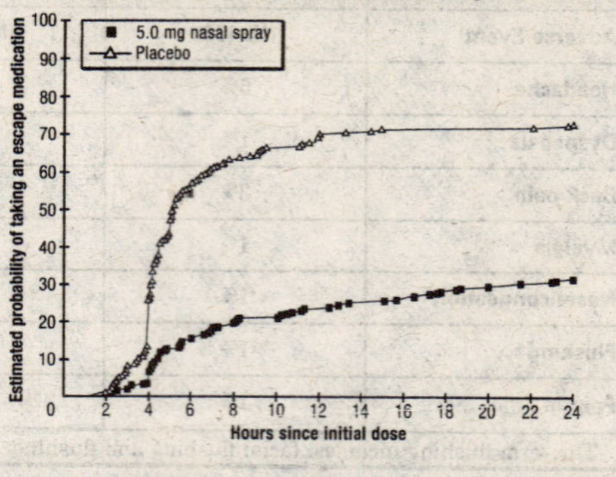

*This Kaplan-Meier plot is based on data obtained from the placebo controlled clinical trial. Patients not using additional treatments were censored at 24 hours. The plot includes both patients who had headache response at 2 hours and those who had no response to the initial dose. It should be noted that the protocol did not allow remedication within 4 hours post dose.

The efficacy of ZOMIG was unaffected by presence of aura; presence of headache upon awakening, relationship to menses; gender, age or weight of the patient; or presence of pretreatment nausea.

The efficacy of ZOMIG Nasal Spray 5 mg was further supported by an interim analysis of another similarly designed trial. The 2 hour headache response rates for the first 210 subjects in that study for ZOMIG 5 mg and placebo were 70% and 47%, respectively (N=108 and 102, respectively, p=0.0006).

INDICATIONS AND USAGE

ZOMIG Nasal Spray is indicated for the acute treatment of migraine with or without aura in adults.

ZOMIG is not intended for the prophylactic therapy of migraine or for use in the management of hemiplegic or basilar migraine (see CONTRAINDICATIONS). Safety and effectiveness of ZOMIG have not been established for cluster headache, which is present in an older, predominantly male population.

CONTRAINDICATIONS

ZOMIG should not be given to patients with ischemic heart disease (angina pectoris, history of myocardial infarction, or documented silent ischemia) or to patients who have symptoms or findings consistent with ischemic heart disease, coronary artery vasospasm, including Prinzmetal's variant angina, or other significant underlying cardiovascular disease (see WARNINGS).

ZOMIG should not be given to patients with cerebrovascular syndromes including (but not limited to) stroke of any type as well as transient ischemic attacks.

Because ZOMIG may increase blood pressure, it should not be given to patients with uncontrolled hypertension (see WARNINGS).

ZOMIG should not be used within 24 hours of treatment with another $5\text{-}HT_1$ agonist, or an ergotamine-containing or ergot-type medication like dihydroergotamine or methysergide.

ZOMIG should not be administered to patients with hemiplegic or basilar migraine.

Concurrent administration of MAO-A inhibitors or use of zolmitriptan within 2 weeks of discontinuation of MAO-A inhibitor therapy is contraindicated (see CLINICAL PHARMACOLOGY: Drug Interactions and PRECAUTIONS: Drug Interactions).

ZOMIG is contraindicated in patients who are hypersensitive to zolmitriptan or any of its inactive ingredients.

WARNINGS

ZOMIG should only be used where a clear diagnosis of migraine has been established.

Risk of Myocardial Ischemia and/or Infarction and Other Adverse Cardiac Events:

ZOMIG should not be given to patients with documented ischemic or vasospastic coronary artery disease (see CONTRAINDICATIONS). It is strongly recommended that zolmitriptan not be given to patients in whom unrecognized coronary artery disease (CAD) is predicted by the presence of risk factors (eg, hypertension, hypercholesterolemia, smoker, obesity, diabetes, strong family history of CAD, female with surgical or physiological menopause, or male over 40 years of age) unless a cardiovascular evaluation provides satisfactory clinical evidence that the patient is reasonably free of coronary artery and ischemic myocardial disease or other significant underlying cardiovascular disease. The sensitivity of cardiac diagnostic procedures to detect cardiovascular disease or predisposition to coronary artery vasospasm is modest, at best. If, during the cardiovascular evaluation, the patient's medical history, electrocardiographic or other investigations reveal findings indicative of, or consistent with, coronary artery vasospasm or myocardial ischemia, zolmitriptan should not be administered (see CONTRAINDICATIONS). For patients with risk factors predictive of CAD, who are determined to have a satisfactory cardiovascular evaluation, it is strongly

recommended that administration of the first dose of zolmitriptan take place in the setting of a physician's office or similar medically staffed and equipped facility unless the patient has previously received zolmitriptan.

Because cardiac ischemia can occur in the absence of clinical symptoms, consideration should be given to obtaining on the first occasion of use an electrocardiogram (ECG) during the interval immediately following ZOMIG, in these patients with risk factors.

It is recommended that patients who are intermittent long-term users of ZOMIG and who have or acquire risk factors predictive of CAD, as described above, undergo periodic interval cardiovascular evaluation as they continue to use ZOMIG.

The systematic approach described above is intended to reduce the likelihood that patients with unrecognized cardiovascular disease will be inadvertently exposed to zolmitriptan.

Cardiac Events and Fatalities: Serious adverse cardiac events, including acute myocardial infarction, have been reported within a few hours following administration of zolmitriptan. Life-threatening disturbances of cardiac rhythm, and death have been reported within a few hours following the administration of other $5\text{-}HT_1$ agonists. Considering the extent of use of $5\text{-}HT_1$ agonists in patients with migraine, the incidence of these events is extremely low.

ZOMIG can cause coronary vasospasm; at least one of these events occurred in a patient with no cardiac disease history and with documented absence of coronary artery disease. Because of the close proximity of the events to ZOMIG use, a causal relationship cannot be excluded. In the cases where there has been known underlying coronary artery disease, the relationship is uncertain.

Patients with symptomatic Wolff-Parkinson-White syndrome or arrhythmias associated with other cardiac accessory conduction pathway disorders should not receive ZOMIG.

Premarketing experience with zolmitriptan: Among the more than 2500 patients with migraine who participated in premarketing controlled clinical trials of ZOMIG Tablets, no deaths or serious cardiac events were reported. In premarketing controlled clinical trial of ZOMIG Nasal Spray, more than 1300 patients participated and there were no deaths or serious cardiac events to report.

Postmarketing experience with zolmitriptan: Serious cardiovascular events have been reported in association with the use of ZOMIG Tablets, and in very rare cases, these events have occurred in the absence of known cardiovascular disease. The uncontrolled nature of postmarketing surveillance, however, makes it impossible to determine definitively the proportion of the reported cases that were actually caused by zolmitriptan or to reliably assess causation in individual cases.

Cerebrovascular Events and Fatalities with $5\text{-}HT_1$ agonists: Cerebral hemorrhage, subarachnoid hemorrhage, stroke, and other cerebrovascular events have been reported in patients treated with $5\text{-}HT_1$ agonists; and some have resulted in fatalities. In a number of cases, it appears possible that the cerebrovascular events were primary, the agonist having been administered in the incorrect belief that the symptoms experienced were a consequence of migraine, when they were not. It should be noted that patients with migraine may be at increased risk of certain cerebrovascular events (eg, stroke, hemorrhage, transient ischemic attack).

Other Vasospasm-Related Events: $5\text{-}HT_1$ agonists may cause vasospastic reactions other than coronary artery vasospasm such as peripheral and gastrointestinal vascular ischemia. As with other serotonin $5HT_1$ agonists, very rare gastrointestinal ischemic events including ischemic colitis and gastrointestinal infarction or necrosis have been reported with ZOMIG Tablets; these may present as bloody diarrhea or abdominal pain.

Increase in Blood Pressure: As with other $5\text{-}HT_1$ agonists, significant elevations in systemic blood pressure have been reported on rare occasions with ZOMIG Tablet use, in patients with and without a history of hypertension; very rarely these increases in blood pressure have been associated with significant clinical events. Zolmitriptan is contraindicated in patients with uncontrolled hypertension. In volunteers, an increase of 1 and 5 mm Hg in the systolic and diastolic blood pressure, respectively, was seen at 5 mg. In the headache trials, vital signs were measured only in the small inpatient study and no effect on blood pressure was seen. In a study of patients with moderate to severe liver disease, 7 of 27 experienced 20 to 80 mm Hg elevations in systolic and/or diastolic blood pressure after a dose of 10 mg of zolmitriptan (see CONTRAINDICATIONS).

An 18% increase in mean pulmonary artery pressure was seen following dosing with another $5\text{-}HT_1$ agonist in a study evaluating subjects undergoing cardiac catheterization.

Local Adverse Reactions: Among 922 patients using the zolmitriptan nasal spray to treat 2311 attacks in the controlled clinical study who were exposed, across all doses (0.5 to 5 mg), approximately 3% noted local irritation or soreness at the site of administration. Adverse events of any kind, perceived in the nasopharynx (which may include systemic effects of triptans) were severe in about 1% of patients and approximately 60% resolved in 1 hour. Nasopharyngeal examinations, in a subset of patients participating in two long term trials of up to one year duration, failed to demonstrate any clinically significant changes with repeated use of ZOMIG Nasal Spray.

All nasopharyngeal adverse events with an incidence of ≥ 2% of patients in any zolmitriptan nasal spray dose groups are included in ADVERSE REACTIONS Table 2.

PRECAUTIONS

General: As with other $5\text{-}HT_{1B/1D}$ agonists, sensations of tightness, pain, pressure, and heaviness have been reported after treatment with ZOMIG Tablets in the precordium, throat, neck, and jaw. Because zolmitriptan may cause coronary artery vasospasm, patients who experience signs or symptoms suggestive of angina following dosing should be evaluated for the presence of CAD or a predisposition to Prinzmetal's variant angina before receiving additional doses of medication, and should be monitored electrocardiographically if dosing is resumed and similar symptoms recur. Similarly, patients who experience other symptoms or signs suggestive of decreased arterial flow following the use of any 5-HT agonist, such as ischemic bowel syndrome or Raynaud's syndrome, are candidates for further evaluation. (see WARNINGS).

Zolmitriptan should also be administered with caution to patients with diseases that may alter the absorption, metabolism, or excretion of drugs, such as impaired hepatic function (see CLINICAL PHARMACOLOGY).

For a given attack, if a patient does not respond to the first dose of zolmitriptan, the diagnosis of migraine headache should be reconsidered before administration of a second dose.

Binding to Melanin-Containing Tissues: When pigmented rats were given a single oral dose of 10 mg/kg of radiolabeled zolmitriptan, the radioactivity in the eye after 7 days, the latest time point examined, was still 75% of the value measured after 4 hours. This suggests that zolmitriptan and/or its metabolites may bind to the melanin of the eye. Because there could be accumulation in melanin rich tissues over time, this raises the possibility that zolmitriptan could cause toxicity in these tissues after extended use. However, no effects on the retina related to treatment with zolmitriptan were noted in any of the toxicity studies including those conducted by the nasal route. Although no systematic monitoring of ophthalmologic function was undertaken in clinical trials, and no specific recommendations for ophthalmologic monitoring are offered, prescribers should be aware of the possibility of long-term ophthalmologic effects.

Information for Patients: See PATIENT INFORMATION at the end of this labeling for the figures and text of the separate leaflet provided for patients.

The ZOMIG Nasal Spray device is packaged in a carton and is a blue colored plastic device with a gray protection cap, labeled to indicate the nominal dose. Patients should be cautioned to not remove the gray protection cap until prior to dosing. The ZOMIG Nasal Spray device is placed in a nostril and actuated to deliver a single dose. **Patients should be cautioned to avoid spraying the contents of the device in their eyes.**

Laboratory Tests: No monitoring of specific laboratory tests is recommended.

Drug Interactions: Ergot-containing drugs have been reported to cause prolonged vasospastic reactions. Because there is a theoretical basis that these effects may be additive, use of ergotamine-containing or ergot-type medications (like dihydroergotamine or methysergide) and zolmitriptan within 24 hours of each other should be avoided (see CONTRAINDICATIONS).

MAO-A inhibitors increase the systemic exposure of zolmitriptan.

Therefore, the use of zolmitriptan in patients receiving MAO-A inhibitors is contraindicated (see CLINICAL PHARMACOLOGY and CONTRAINDICATIONS).

Concomitant use of other $5\text{-}HT_{1B/1D}$ agonists within 24 hours of ZOMIG treatment is not recommended. (see CONTRAINDICATIONS).

Following administration of cimetidine, the half-life and AUC of zolmitriptan and its active metabolites were approximately doubled (see CLINICAL PHARMACOLOGY).

Selective serotonin reuptake inhibitors (SSRIs) (eg, fluoxetine, fluvoxamine, paroxetine, sertraline) have been reported, rarely, to cause weakness, hyperreflexia, and incoordination when coadministered with $5\text{-}HT_1$ agonists. If concomitant treatment with zolmitriptan and an SSRI is clinically warranted, appropriate observation of the patient is advised.

Drug/Laboratory Test Interactions: Zolmitriptan is not known to interfere with commonly employed clinical laboratory tests.

Carcinogenesis, Mutagenesis, Impairment of Fertility:

Carcinogenesis: Carcinogenicity studies by oral gavage were carried out in mice and rats at doses up to 400 mg/kg/day. Mice were dosed for 85 weeks (males) and 92 weeks (females). The exposure (plasma AUC of parent drug) at the highest dose level was approximately 800 times that seen in humans after a single 10 mg dose (the maximum recommended total daily dose). There was no effect of zolmitriptan on tumor incidence. Control, low dose, and middle dose rats were dosed for 104-105 weeks; the high dose group was sacrificed after 101 weeks (males) and 86 weeks (females) due to excess mortality. Aside from an increase in the incidence of thyroid follicular cell hyperplasia and thyroid follicular cell adenomas seen in male rats receiving 400 mg/kg/day, an exposure approximately 3000 times that seen in humans after dosing with 10 mg, no tumors were noted.

Mutagenesis: Zolmitriptan was mutagenic in an Ames test, in 2 of 5 strains of S. typhimurium tested, in the presence of, but not in the absence of, metabolic activation. It was not mutagenic in an *in vitro* mammalian gene cell mutation (CHO/HGPRT) assay. Zolmitriptan was clastogenic in an *in vitro* human lymphocyte assay both in the absence of and the presence of metabolic activation. Zolmitriptan was not clastogenic in *in vivo* mouse and rat micronucleus assays. Zolmitriptan was not genotoxic in an unscheduled DNA synthesis study.

Impairment of Fertility: Studies of male and female rats administered zolmitriptan prior to and during mating and up to implantation have shown no impairment of fertility at doses up to 400 mg/kg/day. Exposure at this dose was approximately 3000 times exposure at the maximum recommended human dose of 10 mg/day.

Pregnancy: Pregnancy Category C: There are no adequate and well controlled studies in pregnant women; therefore, zolmitriptan should be used during pregnancy only if the potential benefit justifies the potential risk to the fetus.

In reproductive toxicity studies in rats and rabbits, oral administration of zolmitriptan to pregnant animals was associated with embryolethality and fetal abnormalities. When pregnant rats were administered oral zolmitriptan during the period of organogenesis at doses of 100, 400, and 1200 mg/kg/day, there was a dose-related increase in embryolethality which became statistically significant at the high dose. The maternal plasma exposures at these doses were approximately 280, 1100, and 5000 times the exposure in humans receiving the maximum recommended total daily dose of 10 mg. The high dose was maternally toxic, as evidenced by a decreased maternal body weight gain during gestation. In a similar study in rabbits, embryolethality was increased at the maternally toxic doses of 10 and 30 mg/kg/day (maternal plasma exposures equivalent to 11 and 42 times exposure in humans receiving the maximum recommended total daily dose of 10 mg), and increased incidences of fetal malformations (fused sternebrae, rib anomalies) and variations (major blood vessel variations, irregular ossification pattern of ribs) were observed at 30 mg/kg/day. Three mg/kg/day was a no effect dose (equivalent to human exposure at a dose of 10 mg). When female rats were given zolmitriptan during gestation, parturition, and lactation, an increased incidence of hydronephrosis was found in the offspring at the maternally toxic dose of 400 mg/kg/day (1100 times human exposure).

Nursing Mothers: It is not known whether zolmitriptan is excreted in human milk. Because many drugs are excreted in human milk, caution should be exercised when zolmitriptan is administered to a nursing woman. Lactating rats dosed with zolmitriptan had levels in milk equivalent to maternal plasma levels at 1 hour and 4 times higher than plasma levels at 4 hours.

Pediatric Use: Safety and effectiveness of ZOMIG in pediatric patients have not been established therefore ZOMIG is not recommended for use in patients under 18 years of age. Postmarketing experience with other triptans includes a limited number of reports that describe pediatric patients who have experienced clinically serious adverse events that are similar in nature to those reported rarely in adults.

Geriatric Use: Although the pharmacokinetic disposition of the drug in the elderly is similar to that seen in younger adults, there is no information about the safety and effectiveness of zolmitriptan in this population because patients over age 65 were excluded from the controlled clinical trials. (see CLINICAL PHARMACOLOGY: Special Populations).

ADVERSE REACTIONS

Serious cardiac events, including myocardial infarction, have occurred following the use of ZOMIG Tablets. These events are extremely rare and most have been reported in patients with risk factors predictive of CAD. Events reported, in association with drugs of this class, have included coronary artery vasospasm, transient myocardial ischemia, myocardial infarction, ventricular tachycardia, and ventricular fibrillation (see CONTRAINDICATIONS, WARNINGS, and PRECAUTIONS).

Incidence in Controlled Clinical Trials: Among 464 patients treating single attacks with zolmitriptan nasal spray in a blinded placebo controlled trial, there was a low withdrawal rate related to adverse events: 5 mg (1.3%), and placebo (0.4%). None of the withdrawals were due to a serious event. One patient was withdrawn due to abnormal ECG changes from baseline that were incidentally found 23 days after the last dose of ZOMIG Nasal Spray. The most common adverse events in clinical trials for ZOMIG Nasal Spray were: unusual taste, paresthesia, hyperesthesia, and dizziness. Table 2 lists the adverse events that occurred in ≥ 2% of the 236 patients in the 5 mg dose group of the controlled clinical trial.

Table 2
Adverse events with an incidence of ≥ 2% of patients in the zolmitriptan 5 mg nasal spray treatment group by body system and greater than placebo.

Body System and Adverse event	Placebo (N=228)	Zolmitriptan nasal spray 5.0 mg (N=236)
ATYPICAL SENSATIONS		
Hyperesthesia	0%	5%
Paraesthesia	6%	10%
EAR/NOSE/THROAT		
Disorder/Discomfort of nasal cavity	2%	3%
PAIN AND PRESSURE SENSATIONS		
Pain Location Specified	1%	4%
Pain Throat	1%	4%
Tightness Throat	1%	2%

Continued on next page

Zomig Nasal Spray—Cont.

DIGESTIVE		
Dry Mouth	0%	2%
Nausea	1%	4%
NEUROLOGICAL		
Dizziness	4%	3%
Somnolence	2%	4%
Unusual Taste	3%	21%
OTHER		
Asthenia	1%	3%

Adverse clinical events occurring in $\geq$ 1% and < 2% of patients in all attacks of the controlled clinical trial were pain abdominal, pressure throat, vomiting, headache, tightness chest, dysphagia, insomnia, palpitation and reaction aggravation.

ZOMIG is generally well tolerated. Across all doses, most adverse reactions were mild and transient and did not lead to long-lasting effects. The incidence of adverse events in controlled clinical trials was not affected by gender, weight, or age of the patients (18-39 vs. 40-65 years of age), or presence of aura. There were insufficient data to assess the impact of race on the incidence of adverse events.

Other Events: In the paragraphs that follow, the frequencies of less commonly reported adverse clinical events are presented. Because the reports include events observed in open and uncontrolled studies, the role of ZOMIG in their causation cannot be reliably determined. Furthermore, variability associated with adverse event reporting, the terminology used to describe adverse events, etc., limit the value of the quantitative frequency estimates provided. Event frequencies are calculated as the number of patients who used ZOMIG Nasal Spray and reported an event divided by the total number of patients exposed to ZOMIG Nasal Spray (n=3059). All reported events are included except those already listed in the previous table, those too general to be informative, and those not reasonably associated with the use of the drug. Events are further classified within body system categories and enumerated in order of decreasing frequency using the following definitions: infrequent adverse events are those occurring in 1/100 to 1/1000 patients and rare adverse events are those occurring in fewer than 1/1000 patients.

Body: Infrequent was allergic reaction, back pain, chills, cyst, flu syndrome, infection, jaw pain, pressure other, jaw tightening, edema of the face, abnormal laboratory test, neck pain, neoplasm, and neck tightness, chest heaviness, chest pain, and chest pressure. Rare were cellulitis, fever, jaw pressure, and neck heaviness.

Cardiovascular: Infrequent were arrhythmias, hypertension, syncope, thrombophlebitis, and tachycardia. Rare were angina pectoris, bradycardia, atrial fibrillation, myocardial infarct, vasodilation, and vascular disorder.

Digestive: Infrequent were diarrhea, dyspepsia, tongue edema, gastrointestinal disorder, increased saliva, and thirst. Rare were increased appetite, colitis, constipation, eructation, gastritis, gastrointestinal carcinoma, gingivitis, hepatic neoplasia, intestinal obstruction, jaundice, sialadenitis, and stomatitis.

Endocrine System: Rare were hyperthyroidism and thyroid edema.

Hemic: Infrequent was cyanosis. Rare were ecchymosis, lymphadenopathy and leukopenia.

Metabolic Nutritional: Rare were increased weight, dehydration, and peripheral edema.

Musculoskeletal: Infrequent were arthralgia, joint disorder, and myalgia. Rare were bone pain, osteoporosis, tenosynovitis and twitching.

Nervous System: Infrequent were agitation, amnesia, anxiety, ataxia, abnormal coordination, confusion, depersonalization, depression, hypertonia, insomnia, nervousness, speech disorder, abnormal thinking, tremor, vertigo, and circumoral paresthesia.

Rare were apathy, convulsions, abnormal dreams, euphoria, hypertonia, irritability tardive dyskinesia, manic reaction, neuropathy, and psychosis.

Respiratory: Infrequent were bronchitis, increased cough, dyspnea, epistasis, laryngeal edema, pharyngitis, rhinitis, sinusitis, throat discomfort, and voice alteration. Rare was hiccup, hyperventilation, laryngitis, pneumonia, increased sputum, and yawning.

Skin: Infrequent was pruritus, rash, skin disorder, and sweating. Rare were eczema, erythema, erythema multiform, hair disorder, and neoplasm.

Special Senses: Infrequent were amblyopia, disorder of lacrimation, ear pain, eye pain, parosmia and tinnitus. Rare were conjunctivitis, dry eye, photophobia, and visual field defect.

Urogenital: Infrequent was polyuria and menorrhagia. Rare were breast carcinoma, dysmenorrhea, metrorrhagia, breast neoplasm, unintended pregnancy, suspicious PAP smear, uterine disorder, enlarged uterine fibroids, fibrocytic breast, vaginitis, urogenital neoplasm, cystitis, urinary tract infection, kidney pain, pyelonephritis, urinary frequency, urine impaired, and urinary tract disorder.

The adverse experience profile seen with ZOMIG Nasal Spray is similar to that seen with ZOMIG tablets and Zomig-ZMT tablets except for the occurrence of local adverse effects from the nasal spray (see ZOMIG Tablet Prescribing information).

Postmarketing Experience with ZOMIG Tablets: The following section enumerates potentially important adverse events that have occurred in clinical practice and which have been reported spontaneously to various surveillance systems. The events enumerated represent reports arising from both domestic and non-domestic use of oral zolmitriptan. The events enumerated include all except those already listed in the ADVERSE REACTIONS section above or those too general to be informative. Because the reports cite events reported spontaneously from worldwide postmarketing experience, frequency of events and the role of zolmitriptan in their causation cannot be reliably determined.

Cardiovascular: Coronary artery vasospasm, transient myocardial ischemia, angina pectoris, and myocardial infarction.

Digestive: Very rare gastrointestinal ischemic events including ischemic colitis and gastrointestinal infarction or necrosis have been reported; these may present as bloody diarrhea or abdominal pain. (See WARNINGS.)

Neurological: As with other acute migraine treatments including other $5HT_1$ agonists, there have been rare reports of headache.

General: As with other 5-$HT_{1B/1D}$ agonists, there have been very rare reports of anaphylaxis or anaphylactoid reactions in patients receiving ZOMIG. There have been rare reports of hypersensitivity reactions, including angioedema.

DRUG ABUSE AND DEPENDENCE

The abuse potential of ZOMIG has not been assessed in clinical trials.

OVERDOSAGE

There is no experience with clinical overdose. Volunteers receiving single 50 mg oral doses of zolmitriptan commonly experienced sedation.

The elimination half-life of ZOMIG is 3 hours (see CLINICAL PHARMACOLOGY) and therefore monitoring of patients after overdose with ZOMIG should continue for at least 15 hours or while symptoms or signs persist.

There is no specific antidote to zolmitriptan. In cases of severe intoxication, intensive care procedures are recommended, including establishing and maintaining a patent airway, ensuring adequate oxygenation and ventilation, and monitoring and support of the cardiovascular system.

It is unknown what effect hemodialysis or peritoneal dialysis has on the plasma concentrations of zolmitriptan.

DOSAGE AND ADMINISTRATION

Administer one dose of ZOMIG Nasal Spray 5 mg for the treatment of acute migraine. If the headache returns the dose may be repeated after 2 hours. The maximum daily dose should not exceed 10 mg in any 24-hour period.

In controlled clinical trials, single doses of 5 mg zolmitriptan nasal spray were administered into one nostril and were effective for the treatment of acute migraines in adults.

Individuals may vary in response to ZOMIG Nasal Spray. The pharmacokinetics of a 5 mg nasal spray dose is similar to the 5 mg oral formulations. Doses lower than 5 mg can only be achieved through the use of an oral formulation. The choice of dose, and route of administration should therefore be made on an individual basis. The effectiveness of a second dose has not been established in placebo-controlled trials.

The safety of treating an average of more than four headaches in a 30 day period has not been established.

Hepatic Impairment: Patients with moderate to severe hepatic impairment have decreased clearance of zolmitriptan and significant elevation in blood pressure was observed in some patients. Use of a lower dose of an alternate formulation with blood pressure monitoring is recommended (see CLINICAL PHARMACOLOGY AND WARNINGS).

HOW SUPPLIED

The ZOMIG Nasal Spray device is a blue colored plastic device with a gray protection cap, labeled to indicate the nominal dose. Each ZOMIG Nasal Spray device administers a single dose of ZOMIG.

ZOMIG Nasal Spray is supplied as a clear to pale yellow solution of zolmitriptan, buffered to a pH 5.0. Each ZOMIG Nasal Spray device contains 5 mg of zolmitriptan in a 100-μL unit dose aqueous buffered solution containing citric acid, anhydrous, USP, disodium phosphate dodecahydrate USP and purified water USP.

5 mg ZOMIG® Nasal Spray is supplied in boxes of 6 single use nasal spray units. (NDC 310-0208-60).

Each ZOMIG® Nasal Spray single dose unit spray supplies 5 mg of zolmitriptan. The ZOMIG® Nasal Spray unit must be discarded after use.

Store at controlled room temperature, 20-25°C (68-77°F) [see USP].

PATIENT SUMMARY OF INFORMATION

Zomig® Nasal Spray
ZOLMITRIPTAN

Please read this information before you start taking ZOMIG® Nasal Spray and each time you renew your prescription just in case anything has changed. Remember, this summary does not take the place of discussions with your doctor. You and your doctor should discuss ZOMIG Nasal Spray when you start taking your medication and at regular checkups.

What is ZOMIG Nasal Spray?

ZOMIG Nasal Spray is a prescription medication used to treat migraine headaches in adults. ZOMIG Nasal Spray is not for other types of headaches. The safety and efficacy of ZOMIG in patients under 18 have not been established.

What is a Migraine Headache?

Migraine is an intense, throbbing headache. You may have pain on one or both sides of your head. You may have nausea and vomiting, and be sensitive to light and noise. The pain and symptoms of a migraine headache can be worse than a common headache. Some women get migraines around the time of their menstrual period. Some people have visual symptoms before the headache, such as flashing lights or wavy lines, called an aura.

How does ZOMIG Nasal Spray work?

Treatment with ZOMIG Nasal Spray reduces swelling of blood vessels surrounding the brain. This swelling is associated with the headache pain of a migraine attack. ZOMIG Nasal Spray blocks the release of substances from nerve endings that cause more pain and other symptoms like nausea, and sensitivity to light and sound.

It is thought that these actions contribute to relief of your symptoms by ZOMIG Nasal Spray.

Who should not take ZOMIG Nasal Spray?

Do not take ZOMIG Nasal Spray if you:

- Have heart disease or a history of heart disease
- Have uncontrolled high blood pressure
- Have hemiplegic or basilar migraine (if you are not sure about this, ask your doctor)
- Have or had a stroke or problems with your blood circulation
- Have serious liver problems
- Have taken any of the following medicines in the last 24 hours: other "triptans" like almotriptan (Axert®), eletriptan (Relpax®), frovatriptan (Frova™), naratriptan (Amerge®), rizatriptan (Maxalt®), sumatriptan (Imitrex®); ergotamines like Bellergal-S®, Cafergot®, Ergomar®, Wigraine®; dihydroergotamine like D.H.E. 45® or Migranal®; or methysergide (Sansert®). These medications have side effects similar to ZOMIG Nasal Spray.
- Have taken monoamine oxidase (MAO) inhibitors such as phenelzine sulfate (Nardil®) or tranylcypromaine sulfate (Parnate®) for depression or other conditions, or if it has been less than 2 weeks since you stopped taking a MAO inhibitor.
- Are allergic to ZOMIG Nasal Spray or any of its ingredients. The active ingredient is zolmitriptan. The inactive ingredients are listed at the end of this leaflet.

Tell your doctor about all the medicines you take or plan to take, including prescription and nonprescription medicines, supplements, and herbal remedies. Your doctor will decide if you can take ZOMIG Nasal Spray with your other medicines.

Tell your doctor if you know that you have any of the following: risk factors for heart disease like high cholesterol, diabetes, smoking, obesity (overweight), menopause, or a family history of heart disease or stroke.

Tell your doctor if you are pregnant, planning to become pregnant, breast feeding, planning to breast feed, or not using effective birth control.

How should I take ZOMIG Nasal Spray?

The ZOMIG Nasal Spray device is a blue colored plastic sprayer device with a gray protection cap, labeled to indicate the dose. For adults, the usual dose is a single nasal spray taken into one nostril. If your headache comes back after your first dose, you may take a second dose anytime after 2 hours of taking the first dose. For any attack where the first dose didn't work, do not take a second dose without talking with your doctor. Do not take more than a total of 10 mg of ZOMIG (tablets or spray combined) in any 24-hour period. If you take too much medicine, contact your doctor, hospital emergency department, or poison control center right away.

The ZOMIG Nasal Spray device consists of the following parts:

A) The Tip: This is the part that you put into your nostril. The medicine comes out of a tiny hole in the top.

B) The Protective Cap: This covers the tip to protect it. Do not remove the protective cap until just before you are ready to take your ZOMIG Nasal Spray.

C) The Finger-grip: This is the part that you hold when you use the sprayer.

D) The Plunger: This is the part that you press when you put the tip into your nostril. This sprayer works only once.

Steps for using ZOMIG Nasal Spray

(Please read all steps before using for the first time):

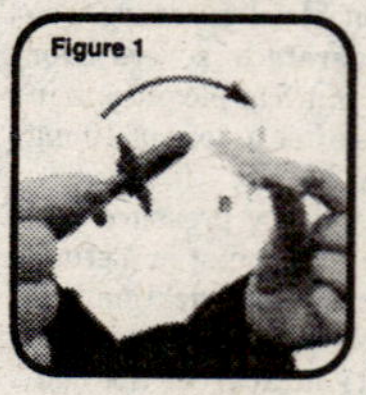

1. Blow your nose gently before use. Remove the protective cap (B) (Figure 1).

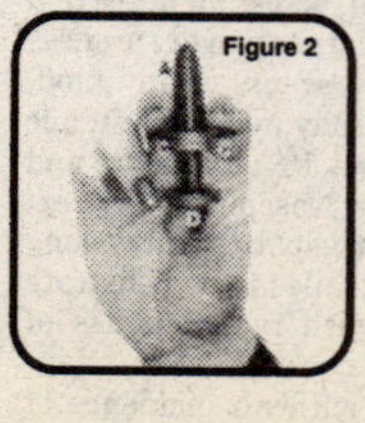

Hold the nasal sprayer device gently with your fingers and thumb as shown in the picture to the right (Figure 2). Do not press the plunger until you have put the tip into your nostril or you will lose the dose.

2. Block one nostril by pressing firmly on the side of your nose (Figure 3). Either nostril can be used.

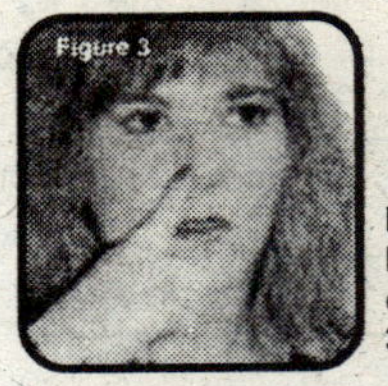

Put the tip (A) of the sprayer device into the other nostril as far as feels comfortable and tilt your head slightly as shown in the picture to the right (Figure 4).

Do not press the plunger yet.

Do not spray the contents of the device in your eyes.

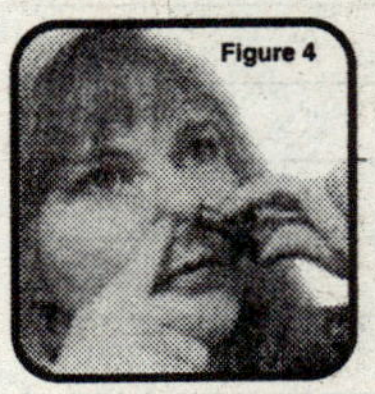

3. Breathe in gently through your nose and at the same time press the plunger (D) firmly with your thumb. The plunger may feel stiff and you may hear a click. Keep your head slightly tilted back and remove the tip from your nose. Breathe gently through your mouth for 5-10 seconds. You may feel liquid in your nose or the back of your throat. This is normal and will soon pass.

What are the possible side effects of ZOMIG Nasal Spray?
ZOMIG Nasal Spray is generally well tolerated. As with any medicine, people taking ZOMIG Nasal Spray may have side effects. The side effects are usually mild and do not last long.
The most common side effects of ZOMIG Nasal Spray are:
- unusual taste, dry mouth
- tingling sensation, skin sensitivity, especially around the nose
- pain, pressure, and tightness sensations (eg, in the nose, throat, or chest)
- drowsiness, weakness, dizziness
- nausea

In very rare cases, patients taking triptans may experience serious side effects, such as heart attacks, high blood pressure, stroke, or serious allergic reactions. Extremely rarely, patients have died. **Call your doctor right away if you have any of the following problems after taking ZOMIG Nasal Spray:**
- **severe tightness, pain, pressure or heaviness in your chest, throat, neck, or jaw**
- **shortness of breath or wheezing**
- **sudden or severe stomach pain**
- **hives; tongue, mouth, or throat swelling**
- **problems seeing**
- **unusual weakness or numbness**

This is not a complete list of side effects. Talk to your doctor if you develop any symptoms that concern you.

What to do in case of an overdose?
Call your doctor or poison control center or go to the ER.

General advice about ZOMIG Nasal Spray
Medicines are sometimes prescribed for conditions that are not mentioned in patient information leaflets. Do not use ZOMIG Nasal Spray for a condition for which it was not prescribed. Do not give ZOMIG Nasal Spray to other people, even if they have the same symptoms as you. People may be harmed if they take medicines that have not been prescribed for them.
This leaflet summarizes the most important information about ZOMIG Nasal Spray. If you would like more information about ZOMIG Nasal Spray, talk to your doctor. You can ask your doctor or pharmacist for information on ZOMIG Nasal Spray that is written for health professionals. You can also call **1-800-236-9933** or visit our web site at **www.ZOMIG.com.**

What are the ingredients in ZOMIG Nasal Spray?
Active ingredient: zolmitriptan
Inactive ingredients: anhydrous citric acid, dibasic sodium phosphate, and purified water
Store your medication at controlled room temperature, 20–25°C (68–77°F), and away from children. Discard after use or when it expires.
ZOMIG is a trademark of the AstraZeneca group of companies.

Manufactured for:
AstraZeneca Pharmaceuticals LP,
Wilmington, Delaware 19850
By: AstraZeneca UK Limited,
Macclesfield, Cheshire, UK
Made in the United Kingdom
Rev. 09/03

To keep your **PDR** up to date throughout the year, note these revisions on the corresponding pages of the annual volume. Simply write **"See Supplement A"** next to the product heading.

Ortho Biotech Products, L.P.

430 ROUTE 22 EAST
P.O. BOX 6914
BRIDGEWATER, NJ 08807-0914

Direct Inquiries to:
(800) 325-7504
Prompt #1, Customer Service
Prompt #2, Medical Information
FAX: (908) 526-9230

ORTHOVISC® ℞
High Molecular Weight Hyaluronan

CAUTION
Federal law restricts this device to sale by or on the order of a physician (or properly licensed practitioner).

DESCRIPTION
ORTHOVISC® is a sterile, non-pyrogenic, clear, viscoelastic solution of hyaluronan contained in a single-use syringe. ORTHOVISC® consists of high molecular weight (1.0-2.9 million daltons), ultra-pure natural hyaluronan dissolved in physiological saline. Hyaluronan is a natural complex sugar of the glycosaminoglycan family. The hyaluronan is extracted from rooster combs.

INDICATIONS
ORTHOVISC® is indicated in the treatment of pain in osteoarthritis (OA) of the knee in patients who have failed to respond adequately to conservative non-pharmacologic therapy and to simple analgesics, e.g. acetaminophen.

CONTRAINDICATIONS
- Do not administer to patients with known hypersensitivity (allergy) to hyaluronate preparations.
- Do not administer to patients with known allergies to avian or avian-derived products (including eggs, feathers, or poultry).
- Do not inject ORTHOVISC® in the knees of patients with infections or skin diseases in the area of the injection site or joint.

WARNINGS
- Do not concomitantly use disinfectants containing quarternary ammonium salts for skin preparation as hyaluronic acid can precipitate in their presence.
- Transient increases in inflammation in the injected knee following ORTHOVISC® injection have been reported in some patients with inflammatory osteoarthritis.

PRECAUTIONS
General
- Strict aseptic injection technique should be used during the application of ORTHOVISC®.
- The safety and effectiveness of the use of ORTHOVISC® in joints other than the knee have not been demonstrated.
- The effectiveness of a single treatment cycle of less than 3 injections has not been established. Pain relief may not be seen until after the third injection.
- The safety and effectiveness has not been established for more than one course of treatment.
- STERILE CONTENTS. The pre-filled syringe is intended for single use only. The contents of the syringe should be used immediately after opening. Discard any unused ORTHOVISC®. Do not resterilize.
- Do not use ORTHOVISC® if the package has been opened or damaged.
- Store ORTHOVISC® in its original package at room temperature (below 77°F/25°C). DO NOT FREEZE.
- Remove joint effusion, if present, before injecting ORTHOVISC®.
- Only medical professionals trained in accepted injection techniques for delivering agents into the knee joint should inject ORTHOVISC® for the indicated use.

Information for Patients
- Transient pain or swelling may occur after the intraarticular (IA) injection.
- As with any invasive joint procedure, it is recommended that patients avoid strenuous activity or prolonged (i.e., more than one hour) weight-bearing activities such as running or tennis within 48 hours following the intraarticular injection.

Use in Specific Populations
- **Pregnancy:** The safety and effectiveness of the use of ORTHOVISC® in pregnant women has not been tested.
- **Nursing Mothers:** It is not known if ORTHOVISC® is excreted in human milk. The safety and effectiveness of the use of the product in lactating women has not been tested.
- **Children:** The safety and effectiveness of the use of ORTHOVISC® in children has not been tested.

ADVERSE EVENTS
ORTHOVISC® was investigated in 3 randomized, controlled clinical studies conducted in the U.S. An integrated safety analysis was conducted, pooling the ORTHOVISC® groups from the 3 studies and pooling the control groups, which were either intraarticular saline injections or arthrocentesis. In the integrated analysis, there were 562 patients in the groups treated with ORTHOVISC® (434 receiving 3 injections and 128 receiving 4 injections), 296 in the group treated with physiological saline, and 123 in the group treated with arthrocentesis.

Adverse events occurring at >5% of the overall integrated population included: arthralgia (12.6% in the ORTHOVISC® group, 17.2% in the saline group, and 0.8% in the arthrocentesis group); back pain (6.9% in the ORTHOVISC® group, 12.2% in the saline group, 2 and 4.9% in the arthrocentesis group); and headache NOS (12.1% in the ORTHOVISC® group, 16.6% in the saline group, and 17.9% in the arthrocentesis group). Injection site adverse events (including erythema, edema, pain and reaction NOS) occurred at rates of 0.4%, 0.9%, 2.5% and 0.2%, respectively, in the ORTHOVISC® group, compared to 0.0%, 0.3%, 2.0%, and 0.7% in the saline group and 0.0%, 0.0%, 0.8% and 0.8% in the arthrocentesis group.
Local adverse events reported on a by-patient basis for the combined ITT populations of the three studies are presented in Table 1.
[See table 1 at top of next page]

CLINICAL STUDIES
The effectiveness of ORTHOVISC® for the treatment of osteoarthritis of the knee was evaluated in three main studies; two randomized, controlled, double-blind multicenter studies (OAK9501 and OAK2001) that involved unilateral treatment, and one study (OAK9801) that involved bilateral treatment. Because bilateral treatment confounded the assessment of effectiveness of the OAK9801 study, the effectiveness data are summarized for the OAK9501 and OAK2001 studies. Safety data for all three studies are reported in "Adverse Events."

Study Design/Analysis
The objective of the randomized studies was to assess the effectiveness of ORTHOVISC® for the treatment of joint pain of patients with idiopathic osteoarthritis of the knee. The OAK9501 study randomized patients to 3 weekly injections of either ORTHOVISC® (O3) or saline. The OAK2001 study randomized patients to one of three treatments: 4 ORTHOVISC® injections (O4), 3 ORTHOVISC® injections + 1 arthrocentesis (O3A1) procedure, or 4 arthrocentesis (A4) procedures. Follow-up occurred at weeks 7/8, 11/12, 15/16 and 21/22, with final follow-up at week 27/28. When each study was analyzed individually, the primary analyses for each study did not show statistical significance. A combined analysis was additionally performed. The combined data consisted of data obtained from a subgroup of patients from each of the studies (the "ITT Subgroup" from OAK9501 and the "Evaluable Subgroup" from OAK2001) who had Kellgren-Lawrence radiographic grades of II or III at baseline and WOMAC pain in the contralateral knee of <175mm (out of 500) and is referred to as the effectiveness subgroup population. For the effectiveness subgroup population, the primary effectiveness analysis performed was to determine the proportion of patients achieving a 20% improvement from baseline in the WOMAC Pain Score in conjunction with a minimum absolute improvement of 50 mm from baseline in the WOMAC Pain Score, and a 40% and 50% improvement from baseline in WOMAC Pain Score at four assessment points between Weeks 7/8 to 21/22 for the index knee.

Study Population
OAK9501 included 226 patients at 10 centers, and OAK2001 involved 373 patients at 24 centers. Within the individual studies, baseline and demographic variables were similar among groups. Table 2 below summarizes the baseline and patient demographic characteristics for the combined effectiveness subgroup.
[See table 2 on next page]

Combined Study Results
In the combined analysis of OAK9501 and OAK2001, two subgroup populations (representing patients with baseline Kellgren-Lawrence grade II or III radiographic findings and contralateral knee pain <175 mm on the WOMAC Pain Score) were analyzed together, comprising 5 treatment groups (4 ORTHOVISC® injections [O4], 3 ORTHOVISC® injections followed by 1 arthrocentesis [O3A1], 3 ORTHOVISC® injections [O3], 4 arthrocentesis procedures [A4] and 3 saline injections [Saline]). For the GEE analyses, the O3A1 and O3 groups were also pooled to form a sixth group [O3A1/O3].
The primary effectiveness analysis was performed to determine the proportion of patients achieving a 20% improvement from baseline in WOMAC Pain Score in conjunction with a minimum absolute improvement of 50 mm from baseline in the WOMAC Pain Score, and a 40% and 50% improvement from baseline in WOMAC Pain Score at four assessment points between Weeks 8 to 22 for the index knee. A significantly larger proportion of O4 patients achieved 40% and 50% improvements from baseline in WOMAC Pain Score compared to both A4 and Saline over 7-22 weeks (based on GEE analysis). Similarly, a significantly larger proportion of O3 and O3A1/O3 patients achieved 40% and 50% improvements from baseline in WOMAC Pain Score than Saline patients (based on GEE analysis) (Table 3). Table 4 presents the mean number of patients from the effectiveness subgroup over the four follow-up visits that achieved improvement over weeks 8 through 22.

Continued on next page

Orthovisc—Cont.

Table 3
GEE Results (P-Values) for the Effectiveness Subgroups for the Primary Endpoints

Endpoint	O4 vs. A4	O4 vs. Saline	O3 vs. Saline
20% improvement from baseline and 50 mm absolute improvement in WOMAC Pain	0.0738	0.1116	0.0789
40% improvement in WOMAC Pain Score from baseline	**0.0094***	**0.0015***	**0.0166***
50% improvement in WOMAC Pain Score from baseline	**0.0360***	**0.0015***	**0.0274***

O4 4 weekly ORTHOVISC® injections—OAK2001 Study
O3 3 weekly ORTHOVISC® injections—OAK9501 Study
A4 4 control [arthrocentesis only] procedures—OAK2001 Study
Saline 3 control [saline injection] procedures—OAK9501 Study
* Statistically significant

[See table 4 at right]

O4 4 weekly ORTHOVISC® injections—OAK2001 Study
O3A1 3 weekly ORTHOVISC® injections + 1 control [arthrocentesis only] procedure—OAK2001 Study
O3 3 weekly ORTHOVISC® injections—OAK9501 Study
A4 4 control [arthrocentesis only] procedures—OAK2001 Study
Saline 3 control [saline injection] procedures—OAK9501 Study

Summary

In summary, with respect to patients achieving ≥40% and ≥50% improvement compared to baseline, the four injection ORTHOVISC® regimen demonstrated effectiveness compared to both Saline and Arthrocentesis control procedures, and the three-weekly injection regimen demonstrated effectiveness compared to Saline in the indicated patient population.

Table 1
Local individual adverse events reported on a by-patient basis for the combined ITT populations of the three studies.

Adverse Event	ORTHOVISC N = 562		Saline N = 296		Arthrocentesis N = 123	
Any Adverse Event	349	(62.1%)	204	(68.9%)	65	(52.8%)
Injection site erythema	2	(0.4%)	0	(0%)	0	(0%)
Injection site edema	5	(0.9%)	1	(0.3%)	0	(0%)
Injection site pain	14	(2.5%)	6	(2.0%)	1	(0.8%)
Injection site reaction NOS[1]	1	(0.2%)	2	(0.7%)	1	(0.8%)
Pain NOS[1]	14	(2.5%)	11	(3.7%)	1	(0.8%)
Arthralgia	71	(12.6%)	51	(17.2%)	1	(0.8%)
Arthritis NOS[1]	4	(0.7%)	5	(1.7%)	0	(0%)
Arthropathy NOS[1]	5	(0.9%)	3	(1.0%)	0	(0%)
Baker's cyst	2	(0.4%)	2	(0.7%)	0	(0%)
Bursitis	6	(1.1%)	6	(2.0%)	2	(1.6%)
Joint disorder NOS[1]	2	(0.4%)	0	(0%)	0	(0%)
Joint effusion	2	(0.4%)	1	(0.3%)	1	(0.8%)
Joint stiffness	3	(0.5%)	2	(0.7%)	0	(0%)
Joint swelling	4	(0.7%)	2	(0.7%)	1	(0.8%)
Localized osteoarthritis	5	(0.9%)	1	(0.3%)	1	(0.8%)
Aggravated osteoarthritis	2	(0.4%)	0	(0%)	1	(0.8%)
Knee arthroplasty	3	(0.5%)	2	(0.7%)	0	(0%)

Notes: [1]NOS = Not otherwise specified.

Table 2
Baseline and patient demographics summary—effectiveness subgroup.[1]

Characteristic	O3 N = 83	Saline × 3 N = 81	O4 N = 104	O3A1 N = 90	A4 N = 100
No. (%) female	51 (61.4%)	49 (60.5%)	46 (44.2%)	59 (65.5%)	50 (50.0%)
Mean ±SD age (years)	65 ± 8	68 ± 9	59 ± 9	59 ± 9	59 ± 8
Mean ±SD BMI (kg/m²)	32 ± 7	30 ± 6	29 ± 4	30 ± 4	30 ± 4
Mean ±SD WOMAC Pain (0-500mm) Study Knee	274 ± 65	268 ± 70	288 ± 60	290 ± 50	293 ± 59
Mean ±SD WOMAC Pain (0-500mm) Contralateral	83 ± 57	87 ± 54	69 ± 47	70 ± 47	68 ± 48
Mean ±SD Investigator Global (0-100mm)	53 ± 19	51 ± 19	59 ± 14	58 ± 14	58 ± 15
Mean ±SD Patient Global (0-100mm)	56 ± 20	53 ± 22	67 ± 15	62 ± 17	64 ± 15

Notes: [1]Patients with Kellgren-Lawrence radiographic grades of II or III at baseline and WOMAC pain in the contralateral knee of <175mm (out of 500).

Table 4
Summary of mean number patients achieving primary individual patient success criteria—effectiveness subgroups from OAK9501 and OAK2001—over weeks 8 through 22 (4 visits).

	O4 N = 104	O3A1 N =90	A4 N = 100	O3 N = 83	Saline × 3 N = 81
Mean No. (%) patients achieving ≥20% improvement from baseline and absolute improvement of 50 mm in WOMAC Pain	77.5 (74.5%)	58.3 (64.7%)	64.5 (64.5%)	59.3 (71.4%)	50.8 (62.7%)
Mean No. (%) patients achieving ≥40% improvement from baseline	68.0 (65.4%)	47.0 (52.2%)	48.8 (48.8%)	45.8 (55.1%)	34.3 (42.3%)
Mean No. (%) patients achieving ≥50% improvement from baseline	59.3 (57.0%)	40.5 (45.0%)	43.5 (43.5%)	38.5 (46.4%)	28.3 (34.9%)

DETAILED DEVICE DESCRIPTION

Hyaluronan is a high molecular weight polysaccharide composed of repeating disaccharide units of sodium glucuronate and N-acetylglucosamine.

Each syringe contains the following in a 2 ml dose sterile-filled into a syringe:

Hyaluronan	30 mg
Sodium Chloride	18 mg
Water for Injection	q.s. up to 2.0 ml

ORTHOVISC® does not contain any synthetic additives.

HOW SUPPLIED

ORTHOVISC® is supplied as a sterile-filled solution, in a single-use syringe, sealed in a sterile pouch inside a carton. The product is presented as a sterile, non-pyrogenic solution in a 2 ml syringe. Each syringe is labeled "ORTHOVISC®" for ready identification. A rubber cap is provided on the syringe tip to prevent leakage and protect sterility of the product.

DIRECTIONS FOR USE

ORTHOVISC® is injected into the knee joint in a series of intra-articular injections one week apart for a total of three or four injections. Standard intra-articular injection site preparation, aseptic technique and precautions should be used.

- After removal of the protective rubber cap on the tip of the syringe, securely attach a small gauge needle (18-21 gauge) to the tip.
- Inject ORTHOVISC® into the knee joint using proper injection technique.
- Inject the full contents of the syringe into one knee only.
- If treatment is bilateral, a separate syringe should be used for each knee.

ORTHOVISC® is a registered trademark of Anika Therapeutics, Inc.

Manufactured by:
Anika Therapeutics, Inc.
236 West Cummings Park
Woburn, Massachusetts USA 01801
Distributed by:
ORTHO BIOTECH
Ortho Biotech Products, L.P.
Raritan, NJ 08869-0670 USA
AML 530-220 01/04 Product Code 59676-360-01

Patient Information

ORTHOVISC® High Molecular Weight Hyaluronan

What is ORTHOVISC®?

ORTHOVISC® is a viscous (thick) sterile mixture made from highly purified hyaluronan from rooster combs. Hyaluronan is a natural chemical found in the body. High amounts of hyaluronan are found in the joint tissues and in the fluid that fills the joints. The body's own hyaluronan acts like a lubricant and a shock absorber in the joint. It is needed for the joint to work properly. When you have osteoarthritis, there may not be enough natural hyaluronan in the joint, and the quality of that hyaluronan may be poorer than normal. ORTHOVISC® is given in a shot (injection) directly into the knee joint.

What is ORTHOVISC® used for?

ORTHOVISC® is used to relieve knee pain due to osteoarthritis. It is used for patients who do not get adequate pain relief from simple pain relievers like acetaminophen or from exercise and physical therapy.

What are the benefits of ORTHOVISC®?

Clinical trials conducted in the U.S. have shown that ORTHOVISC® provides pain relief to patients who have not been able to find pain relief with simple pain medication or exercise compared to saline placebo injections.

What other treatments are available for osteoarthritis?

If you have pain due to osteoarthritis of the knee, there are things you can do that do not involve ORTHOVISC® injections. These include:

Non-drug treatments:
- Avoiding activities that cause pain in your knee
- Exercise
- Physical therapy
- Removal of excess fluid from the knee

Drug therapy:
- Pain medication such as acetaminophen and narcotics
- Drugs that reduce inflammation, such as aspirin and other "nonsteroidal anti-inflammatory" agents (NSAIDs) (such as ibuprofen and naproxen)
- Corticosteroids that are injected directly into the knee joint

Are there any reasons why you should not take ORTHOVISC®?
- You should not take this product if you are allergic to hyaluronate products.
- You should not take this product if you are allergic to products from birds (poultry, feathers, eggs, etc.). If you are injected with ORTHOVISC® and are allergic to bird products, you could develop an allergic reaction to the injections.
- You should not have an injection into the knee if you have infections or skin diseases around the injection site.

Things you should know about ORTHOVISC®
- ORTHOVISC® should be injected by a qualified physician.
- Tell your physician if you are allergic to products from birds, such as feathers, eggs and poultry. If you are allergic to bird products and you have ORTHOVISC® injections, you may have a severe reaction and even die from the injection.
- For 48 hours after you receive the injection, you should avoid activities such as jogging, tennis, heavy lifting or standing on your feet for a long time (more than one hour).
- The safety and effectiveness of ORTHOVISC® in joints other than the knee has not been demonstrated in U.S. studies.
- The safety and effectiveness of ORTHOVISC® has not been shown in pregnant or nursing women. You should tell your doctor if you are pregnant or nursing.
- The safety and effectiveness of ORTHOVISC® has not been shown in children.
- The safety and effectiveness has not been established for more than one course of treatment.

Possible complications
- Side effects are sometimes seen when ORTHOVISC® is injected into the knee joint. These can include: pain, swelling, heat, rash, itching, bruising and/or redness. You may also feel achy. These reactions are generally mild and do not last long.
- If any of these symptoms or signs appear after you are given ORTHOVISC® or if you have any other problems, you should call your doctor.

How is ORTHOVISC® given?
Your doctor will inject ORTHOVISC® (30 mg/2 mL) into your knee once a week, for a total of 3 or 4 injections.

Distributed by:
ORTHO BIOTECH
Ortho Biotech Products, L.P.
Raritan, NJ 08869
Manufactured by:
Anika Therapeutics, Inc.
236 West Cummings Park
Woburn, MA 01890
AML 530-220 01/04 PI
Distributed By:
ORTHO BIOTECH
Ortho Biotech Products, L.P. Bridgewater, NJ 08807-0914 USA

Printed in U.S.A 2/04 08VSC1001
Manufactured By:
Anika Therapeutics, Inc. Woburn, MA 01801 USA

In the PDR annual,
the **Brand and Generic Name Index**
(PINK section)
alphabetizes drugs under both
brand and generic names.

Pfizer Inc.

235 EAST 42ND STREET
NEW YORK, NY 10017-5755

For Medical Information Contact:
(800) 438-1985
24 hours a day, 7 days a week
Pfizer Labs and Roerig Division:
For Medical Information Contact:
24 hours a day, seven days a week:
(800) 438-1985
Distribution:
1855 Shelby Oaks Drive North
Memphis, TN 38134
(901) 387-5200
Customer Service:
(800) 533-4535
EXPORT INQUIRIES:
Pfizer International Inc.
(212) 573-2323

CADUET® ℞
[kă-dew-ĕt]
(amlodipine besylate/atorvastatin calcium)
Tablets

DESCRIPTION
CADUET® (amlodipine besylate and atorvastatin calcium) tablets combine the long-acting calcium channel blocker amlodipine besylate with the synthetic lipid-lowering agent atorvastatin calcium.
The amlodipine besylate component of CADUET is chemically described as 3-Ethyl-5-methyl (±)-2-[(2-aminoethoxy)methyl]-4-(o-chlorophenyl)-1,4-dihydro-6-methyl-3,5-pyridinedicarboxylate, monobenzenesulphonate. Its empirical formula is $C_{20}H_{25}ClN_2O_5 \bullet C_6H_6O_3S$.
The atorvastatin calcium component of CADUET is chemically described as [R-(R*, R*)]-2-(4-fluorophenyl)-ß, δ-dihydroxy-5-(1-methylethyl)-3-phenyl-4-[(phenylamino)carbonyl]-1H-pyrrole-1-heptanoic acid, calcium salt (2:1) trihydrate. Its empirical formula is $(C_{33}H_{34}FN_2O_5)_2Ca \bullet 3H_2O$.
The structural formulae for amlodipine besylate and atorvastatin calcium are shown below.

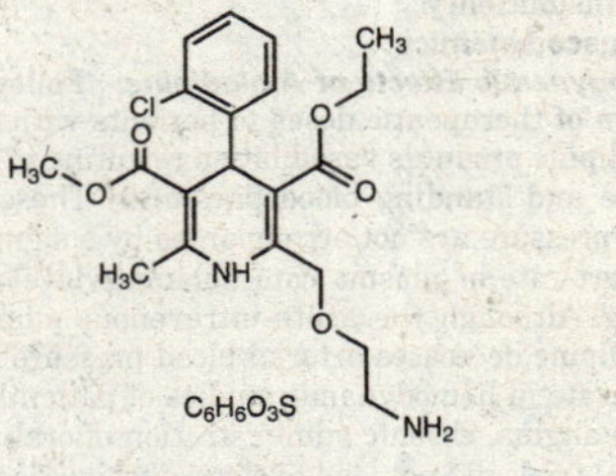

Amlodipine besylate

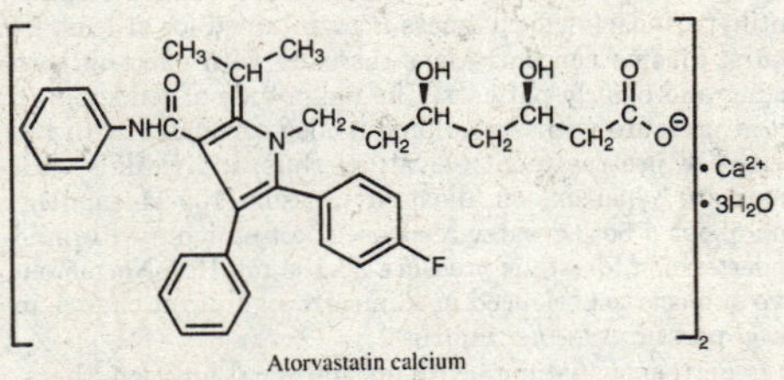

Atorvastatin calcium

CADUET contains amlodipine besylate, a white to off-white crystalline powder, and atorvastatin calcium, also a white to off-white crystalline powder. Amlodipine besylate has a molecular weight of 567.1 and atorvastatin calcium has a molecular weight of 1209.42. Amlodipine besylate is slightly soluble in water and sparingly soluble in ethanol. Atorvastatin calcium is insoluble in aqueous solutions of pH 4 and below. Atorvastatin calcium is very slightly soluble in distilled water, pH 7.4 phosphate buffer, and acetonitrile; slightly soluble in ethanol, and freely soluble in methanol.
CADUET tablets are formulated for oral administration in the following strength combinations:
[See table 1 at top of next page]
Each tablet also contains calcium carbonate, croscarmellose sodium, microcrystalline cellulose, pregelatinized starch, polysorbate 80, hydroxypropyl cellulose, purified water, colloidal silicon dioxide (anhydrous), magnesium stearate, Opadry® II White 85F28751 (polyvinyl alcohol, titanium dioxide, PEG 3000 and talc) or Opadry® II Blue 85F10919 (polyvinyl alcohol, titanium dioxide, PEG 3000, talc and FD&C blue #2). Combinations of atorvastatin with 5 mg amlodipine are film coated white, and combinations of atorvastatin with 10 mg amlodipine are film coated blue.

CLINICAL PHARMACOLOGY
Mechanism of Action
CADUET
CADUET is a combination of two drugs, a dihydropyridine calcium antagonist (calcium ion antagonist or slow-channel blocker) amlodipine (antihypertensive/antianginal agent) and an HMG-CoA reductase inhibitor atorvastatin (cholesterol lowering agent). The amlodipine component of CADUET inhibits the transmembrane influx of calcium ions into vascular smooth muscle and cardiac muscle. The atorvastatin component of CADUET is a selective, competitive inhibitor of HMG-CoA reductase, the rate-limiting enzyme that converts 3-hydroxy-3-methylglutaryl-coenzyme A to mevalonate, a precursor of sterols, including cholesterol.

The Amlodipine Component of CADUET
Experimental data suggest that amlodipine binds to both dihydropyridine and nondihydropyridine binding sites. The contractile processes of cardiac muscle and vascular smooth muscle are dependent upon the movement of extracellular calcium ions into these cells through specific ion channels. Amlodipine inhibits calcium ion influx across cell membranes selectively, with a greater effect on vascular smooth muscle cells than on cardiac muscle cells. Negative inotropic effects can be detected *in vitro* but such effects have not been seen in intact animals at therapeutic doses. Serum calcium concentration is not affected by amlodipine. Within the physiologic pH range, amlodipine is an ionized compound (pKa=8.6), and its kinetic interaction with the calcium channel receptor is characterized by a gradual rate of association and dissociation with the receptor binding site, resulting in a gradual onset of effect.
Amlodipine is a peripheral arterial vasodilator that acts directly on vascular smooth muscle to cause a reduction in peripheral vascular resistance and reduction in blood pressure.
The precise mechanisms by which amlodipine relieves angina have not been fully delineated, but are thought to include the following:
Exertional Angina: In patients with exertional angina, amlodipine reduces the total peripheral resistance (afterload) against which the heart works and reduces the rate pressure product, and thus myocardial oxygen demand, at any given level of exercise.
Vasospastic Angina: Amlodipine has been demonstrated to block constriction and restore blood flow in coronary arteries and arterioles in response to calcium, potassium epinephrine, serotonin, and thromboxane A_2 analog in experimental animal models and in human coronary vessels *in vitro*. This inhibition of coronary spasm is responsible for the effectiveness of amlodipine in vasospastic (Prinzmetal's or variant) angina.

The Atorvastatin Component of CADUET
Cholesterol and triglycerides circulate in the bloodstream as part of lipoprotein complexes. With ultracentrifugation, these complexes separate into HDL (high-density lipoprotein), IDL (intermediate-density lipoprotein), LDL (low-density lipoprotein), and VLDL (very-low-density lipoprotein) fractions. Triglycerides (TG) and cholesterol in the liver are incorporated into VLDL and released into the plasma for delivery to peripheral tissues. LDL is formed from VLDL and is catabolized primarily through the high-affinity LDL receptor.
Clinical and pathologic studies show that elevated plasma levels of total cholesterol (total-C), LDL-cholesterol (LDL-C), and apolipoprotein B (apo B) promote human atherosclerosis and are risk factors for developing cardiovascular disease, while increased levels of HDL-C are associated with a decreased cardiovascular risk.
Epidemiologic investigations have established that cardiovascular morbidity and mortality vary directly with the level of total-C and LDL-C, and inversely with the level of HDL-C.
In animal models, atorvastatin lowers plasma cholesterol and lipoprotein levels by inhibiting HMG-CoA reductase and cholesterol synthesis in the liver and by increasing the number of hepatic LDL receptors on the cell-surface to enhance uptake and catabolism of LDL; atorvastatin also reduces LDL production and the number of LDL particles.
Atorvastatin reduces total-C, LDL-C, and apo B in patients with homozygous and heterozygous familial hypercholesterolemia (FH), nonfamilial forms of hypercholesterolemia, and mixed dyslipidemia. Atorvastatin also reduces VLDL-C and TG and produces variable increases in HDL-C and apolipoprotein A-1. Atorvastatin reduces total-C, LDL-C, VLDL-C, apo B, TG, and non-HDL-C, and increases HDL-C in patients with isolated hypertriglyceridemia. Atorvastatin reduces intermediate density lipoprotein cholesterol (IDL-C) in patients with dysbetalipoproteinemia.
The effect of atorvastatin on cardiovascular morbidity and mortality has not been determined.
Like LDL, cholesterol-enriched triglyceride-rich lipoproteins, including VLDL, intermediate density lipoprotein (IDL), and remnants, can also promote atherosclerosis. Elevated plasma triglycerides are frequently found in a triad with low HDL-C levels and small LDL particles, as well as in association with non-lipid metabolic risk factors for coronary heart disease. As such, total plasma TG has not consistently been shown to be an independent risk factor for CHD. Furthermore, the independent effect of raising HDL or lowering TG on the risk of coronary and cardiovascular morbidity and mortality has not been determined.

Pharmacokinetics and Metabolism
Absorption
Studies with amlodipine: After oral administration of therapeutic doses of amlodipine alone, absorption produces peak plasma concentrations between 6 and 12 hours. Abso-

Continued on next page

Caduet—Cont.

lute bioavailability has been estimated to be between 64 and 90%. The bioavailability of amlodipine when administered alone is not altered by the presence of food.

Studies with atorvastatin: After oral administration alone, atorvastatin is rapidly absorbed; maximum plasma concentrations occur within 1 to 2 hours. Extent of absorption increases in proportion to atorvastatin dose. The absolute bioavailability of atorvastatin (parent drug) is approximately 14% and the systemic availability of HMG-CoA reductase inhibitory activity is approximately 30%. The low systemic availability is attributed to presystemic clearance in gastrointestinal mucosa and/or hepatic first-pass metabolism. Although food decreases the rate and extent of drug absorption by approximately 25% and 9%, respectively, as assessed by Cmax and AUC, LDL-C reduction is similar whether atorvastatin is given with or without food. Plasma atorvastatin concentrations are lower (approximately 30% for Cmax and AUC) following evening drug administration compared with morning. However, LDL-C reduction is the same regardless of the time of day of drug administration (see **DOSAGE AND ADMINISTRATION**).

Studies with CADUET: Following oral administration of CADUET peak plasma concentrations of amlodipine and atorvastatin are seen at 6 to 12 hours and 1 to 2 hours post dosing, respectively. The rate and extent of absorption (bioavailability) of amlodipine and atorvastatin from CADUET are not significantly different from the bioavailability of amlodipine and atorvastatin administered separately (see above).

The bioavailability of amlodipine from CADUET was not affected by food. Although food decreases the rate and extent of absorption of atorvastatin from CADUET by approximately 32% and 11%, respectively, as it does with atorvastatin when given alone. LDL-C reduction is similar whether atorvastatin is given with or without food.

Distribution

Studies with amlodipine: *Ex vivo* studies have shown that approximately 93% of the circulating amlodipine drug is bound to plasma proteins in hypertensive patients. Steady-state plasma levels of amlodipine are reached after 7 to 8 days of consecutive daily dosing.

Studies with atorvastatin: Mean volume of distribution of atorvastatin is approximately 381 liters. Atorvastatin is ≥98% bound to plasma proteins. A blood/plasma ratio of approximately 0.25 indicates poor drug penetration into red blood cells. Based on observations in rats, atorvastatin calcium is likely to be secreted in human milk (see **CONTRAINDICATIONS, Pregnancy and Lactation**, and **PRECAUTIONS, Nursing Mothers**).

Metabolism

Studies with amlodipine: Amlodipine is extensively (about 90%) converted to inactive metabolites via hepatic metabolism.

Studies with atorvastatin: Atorvastatin is extensively metabolized to ortho- and parahydroxylated derivatives and various beta-oxidation products. *In vitro* inhibition of HMG-CoA reductase by ortho- and parahydroxylated metabolites is equivalent to that of atorvastatin. Approximately 70% of circulating inhibitory activity for HMG-CoA reductase is attributed to active metabolites. *In vitro* studies suggest the importance of atorvastatin metabolism by cytochrome P450 3A4, consistent with increased plasma concentrations of atorvastatin in humans following coadministration with erythromycin, a known inhibitor of this isozyme (see **PRECAUTIONS, Drug Interactions**). In animals, the ortho-hydroxy metabolite undergoes further glucuronidation.

Excretion

Studies with amlodipine: Elimination from the plasma is biphasic with a terminal elimination half-life of about 30-50 hours. Ten percent of the parent amlodipine compound and 60% of the metabolites of amlodipine are excreted in the urine.

Studies with atorvastatin: Atorvastatin and its metabolites are eliminated primarily in bile following hepatic and/or extra-hepatic metabolism; however, the drug does not appear to undergo enterohepatic recirculation. Mean plasma elimination half-life of atorvastatin in humans is approximately 14 hours, but the half-life of inhibitory activity for HMG-CoA reductase is 20 to 30 hours due to the contribution of active metabolites. Less than 2% of a dose of atorvastatin is recovered in urine following oral administration.

Special Populations

Geriatric

Studies with amlodipine: Elderly patients have decreased clearance of amlodipine with a resulting increase in AUC of approximately 40-60%, and a lower initial dose of amlodipine may be required.

Studies with atorvastatin: Plasma concentrations of atorvastatin are higher (approximately 40% for Cmax and 30% for AUC) in healthy elderly subjects (age ≥65 years) than in young adults. Clinical data suggest a greater degree of LDL-lowering at any dose of atorvastatin in the elderly population compared to younger adults (see **PRECAUTIONS** section, **Geriatric Use**).

Pediatric

Studies with amlodipine: Sixty-two hypertensive patients aged 6 to 17 years received doses of amlodipine between 1.25 mg and 20 mg. Weight-adjusted clearance and volume of distribution were similar to values in adults.

Studies with atorvastatin: Pharmacokinetic data in the pediatric population are not available.

Table 1. CADUET Tablet Strengths

	5 mg/ 10 mg	5 mg/ 20 mg	5 mg/ 40 mg	5 mg/ 80 mg	10 mg/ 10 mg	10 mg/ 20 mg	10 mg/ 40 mg	10 mg/ 80 mg
amlodipine equivalent (mg)	5	5	5	5	10	10	10	10
atorvastatin equivalent (mg)	10	20	40	80	10	20	40	80

Gender

Studies with atorvastatin: Plasma concentrations of atorvastatin in women differ from those in men (approximately 20% higher for Cmax and 10% lower for AUC); however, there is no clinically significant difference in LDL-C reduction with atorvastatin between men and women.

Renal Insufficiency

Studies with amlodipine: The pharmacokinetics of amlodipine are not significantly influenced by renal impairment. Patients with renal failure may therefore receive the usual initial amlodipine dose.

Studies with atorvastatin: Renal disease has no influence on the plasma concentrations or LDL-C reduction of atorvastatin; thus, dose adjustment of atorvastatin in patients with renal dysfunction is not necessary (see **DOSAGE AND ADMINISTRATION**).

Hemodialysis

While studies have not been conducted in patients with end-stage renal disease, hemodialysis is not expected to significantly enhance clearance of atorvastatin and/or amlodipine since both drugs are extensively bound to plasma proteins.

Hepatic Insufficiency

Studies with amlodipine: Elderly patients and patients with hepatic insufficiency have decreased clearance of amlodipine with a resulting increase in AUC of approximately 40-60%, and a lower initial dose may be required.

Studies with atorvastatin: In patients with chronic alcoholic liver disease, plasma concentrations of atorvastatin are markedly increased. Cmax and AUC are each 4-fold greater in patients with Childs-Pugh A disease. Cmax and AUC of atorvastatin are approximately 16-fold and 11-fold increased, respectively, in patients with Childs-Pugh B disease (see **CONTRAINDICATIONS**).

Heart Failure

Studies with amlodipine: In patients with moderate to severe heart failure, the increase in AUC for amlodipine was similar to that seen in the elderly and in patients with hepatic insufficiency.

Pharmacodynamics

Hemodynamic Effects of Amlodipine: Following administration of therapeutic doses to patients with hypertension, amlodipine produces vasodilation resulting in a reduction of supine and standing blood pressures. These decreases in blood pressure are not accompanied by a significant change in heart rate or plasma catecholamine levels with chronic dosing. Although the acute intravenous administration of amlodipine decreases arterial blood pressure and increases heart rate in hemodynamic studies of patients with chronic stable angina, chronic administration of oral amlodipine in clinical trials did not lead to clinically significant changes in heart rate or blood pressures in normotensive patients with angina.

With chronic once daily oral administration of amlodipine, antihypertensive effectiveness is maintained for at least 24 hours. Plasma concentrations correlate with effect in both young and elderly patients. The magnitude of reduction in blood pressure with amlodipine is also correlated with the height of pretreatment elevation; thus, individuals with moderate hypertension (diastolic pressure 105-114 mmHg) had about a 50% greater response than patients with mild hypertension (diastolic pressure 90-104 mmHg). Normotensive subjects experienced no clinically significant change in blood pressures (+1/−2 mmHg).

In hypertensive patients with normal renal function, therapeutic doses of amlodipine resulted in a decrease in renal vascular resistance and an increase in glomerular filtration rate and effective renal plasma flow without change in filtration fraction or proteinuria.

As with other calcium channel blockers, hemodynamic measurements of cardiac function at rest and during exercise (or pacing) in patients with normal ventricular function treated with amlodipine have generally demonstrated a small increase in cardiac index without significant influence on dP/dt or on left ventricular end diastolic pressure or volume. In hemodynamic studies, amlodipine has not been associated with a negative inotropic effect when administered in the therapeutic dose range to intact animals and man, even when co-administered with beta-blockers to man. Similar findings, however, have been observed in normals or well-compensated patients with heart failure with agents possessing significant negative inotropic effects.

Electrophysiologic Effects of Amlodipine: Amlodipine does not change sinoatrial nodal function or atrioventricular conduction in intact animals or man. In patients with chronic stable angina, intravenous administration of 10 mg did not significantly alter A-H and H-V conduction and sinus node recovery time after pacing. Similar results were obtained in patients receiving amlodipine and concomitant beta blockers. In clinical studies in which amlodipine was administered in combination with beta-blockers to patients with either hypertension or angina, no adverse effects on electrocardiographic parameters were observed. In clinical trials with angina patients alone, amlodipine therapy did not alter electrocardiographic intervals or produce higher degrees of AV blocks.

LDL-C Reduction with Atorvastatin: Atorvastatin as well as some of its metabolites are pharmacologically active in humans. The liver is the primary site of action and the principal site of cholesterol synthesis and LDL clearance. Drug dosage rather than systemic drug concentration correlates better with LDL-C reduction. Individualization of drug dosage should be based on therapeutic response (see **DOSAGE AND ADMINISTRATION**).

Clinical Studies

Clinical Studies with Amlodipine

Amlodipine Effects in Hypertension

Adult Patients: The antihypertensive efficacy of amlodipine has been demonstrated in a total of 15 double-blind, placebo-controlled, randomized studies involving 800 patients on amlodipine and 538 on placebo. Once daily administration produced statistically significant placebo-corrected reductions in supine and standing blood pressures at 24 hours postdose, averaging about 12/6 mmHg in the standing position and 13/7 mmHg in the supine position in patients with mild to moderate hypertension. Maintenance of the blood pressure effect over the 24-hour dosing interval was observed, with little difference in peak and trough effect. Tolerance was not demonstrated in patients studied for up to 1 year. The 3 parallel, fixed doses, dose response studies showed that the reduction in supine and standing blood pressures was dose-related within the recommended dosing range. Effects on diastolic pressure were similar in young and older patients. The effect on systolic pressure was greater in older patients, perhaps because of greater baseline systolic pressure. Effects were similar in black patients and in white patients.

Pediatric Patients: Two-hundred sixty-eight hypertensive patients aged 6 to 17 years were randomized first to amlodipine 2.5 or 5 mg once daily for 4 weeks and then randomized again to the same dose or to placebo for another 4 weeks. Patients receiving 5 mg amlodipine at the end of 8 weeks had lower blood pressure than those secondarily randomized to placebo. The magnitude of the treatment effect is difficult to interpret, but it is probably less than 5 mmHg systolic on the 5 mg dose. Adverse events were similar to those seen in adults.

Amlodipine Effects in Chronic Stable Angina: The effectiveness of 5–10 mg/day of amlodipine in exercise-induced angina has been evaluated in 8 placebo-controlled, double-blind clinical trials of up to 6 weeks duration involving 1038 patients (684 amlodipine, 354 placebo) with chronic stable angina. In 5 of the 8 studies, significant increases in exercise time (bicycle or treadmill) were seen with the 10 mg dose. Increases in symptom-limited exercise time averaged 12.8% (63 sec) for amlodipine 10 mg, and averaged 7.9% (38 sec) for amlodipine 5 mg. Amlodipine 10 mg also increased time to 1 mm ST segment deviation in several studies and decreased angina attack rate. The sustained efficacy of amlodipine in angina patients has been demonstrated over long-term dosing. In patients with angina, there were no clinically significant reductions in blood pressures (4/1 mmHg) or changes in heart rate (+0.3 bpm).

Amlodipine Effects in Vasospastic Angina: In a double-blind, placebo-controlled clinical trial of 4 weeks duration in 50 patients, amlodipine therapy decreased attacks by approximately 4/week compared with a placebo decrease of approximately 1/week ($p<0.01$). Two of 23 amlodipine and 7 of 27 placebo patients discontinued from the study due to lack of clinical improvement.

Amlodipine Effects in Patients with Congestive Heart Failure: Amlodipine has been compared to placebo in four 8–12 week studies of patients with NYHA class II/III heart failure, involving a total of 697 patients. In these studies, there was no evidence of worsened heart failure based on measures of exercise tolerance, NYHA classification, symptoms, or LVEF. In a long-term (follow-up at least 6 months, mean 13.8 months) placebo-controlled mortality/morbidity study of amlodipine 5–10 mg in 1153 patients with NYHA classes III (n=931) or IV (n=222) heart failure on stable doses of diuretics, digoxin, and ACE inhibitors, amlodipine had no effect on the primary endpoint of the study which was the combined endpoint of all-cause mortality and cardiac morbidity (as defined by life-threatening arrhythmia, acute myocardial infarction, or hospitalization for worsened heart failure), or on NYHA classification, or symptoms of heart failure. Total combined all-cause mortality and cardiac morbidity events were 222/571 (39%) for patients on amlodipine and 246/583 (42%) for patients on placebo; the cardiac morbid events represented about 25% of the endpoints in the study.

Another study (PRAISE-2) randomized patients with NYHA class III (80%) or IV (20%) heart failure without clinical symptoms or objective evidence of underlying ischemic disease, on stable doses of ACE inhibitor (99%), digitalis (99%) and diuretics (99%), to placebo (n=827) or amlodipine (n=827) and followed them for a mean of 33 months.

There was no statistically significant difference between amlodipine and placebo in the primary endpoint of all cause mortality (95% confidence limits from 8% reduction to 29% increase on amlodipine). With amlodipine there were more reports of pulmonary edema.

Clinical Studies with Atorvastatin

Atorvastatin Studies in Hypercholesterolemia (Heterozygous Familial and Nonfamilial) and Mixed Dyslipidemia (Fredrickson Types IIa and IIb): Atorvastatin reduces total-C, LDL-C, VLDL-C, apo B, and TG, and increases HDL-C in patients with hypercholesterolemia and mixed dyslipidemia. Therapeutic response is seen within 2 weeks, and maximum response is usually achieved within 4 weeks and maintained during chronic therapy.

Atorvastatin is effective in a wide variety of patient populations with hypercholesterolemia, with and without hypertriglyceridemia, in men and women, and in the elderly.

In two multicenter, placebo-controlled, dose-response studies in patients with hypercholesterolemia, atorvastatin given as a single dose over 6 weeks significantly reduced total-C, LDL-C, apo B, and TG (pooled results are provided in Table 2).

[See table 2 at right]

In patients with *Fredrickson* Types IIa and IIb hyperlipoproteinemia pooled from 24 controlled trials, the median (25th and 75th percentile) percent changes from baseline in HDL-C for atorvastatin 10, 20, 40, and 80 mg were 6.4 (-1.4, 14), 8.7 (0, 17), 7.8 (0, 16), and 5.1 (-2.7, 15), respectively. Additionally, analysis of the pooled data demonstrated consistent and significant decreases in total-C, LDL-C, TG, total-C/HDL-C, and LDL-C/HDL-C.

In three multicenter, double-blind studies in patients with hypercholesterolemia, atorvastatin was compared to other HMG-CoA reductase inhibitors. After randomization, patients were treated for 16 weeks with either atorvastatin 10 mg per day or a fixed dose of the comparative agent (Table 3).

[See table 3 at right]

The impact on clinical outcomes of the differences in lipid-altering effects between treatments shown in Table 3 is not known. Table 3 does not contain data comparing the effects of atorvastatin 10 mg and higher doses of lovastatin, pravastatin, and simvastatin. The drugs compared in the studies summarized in the table are not necessarily interchangeable.

Atorvastatin Effects in Hypertriglyceridemia (Fredrickson Type IV): The response to atorvastatin in 64 patients with isolated hypertriglyceridemia treated across several clinical trials is shown in the table below. For the atorvastatin-treated patients, median (min, max) baseline TG level was 565 (267–1502).

[See table 4 at right]

Atorvastatin Effects in Dysbetalipoproteinemia (Fredrickson Type III): The results of an open-label crossover study of atorvastatin in 16 patients (genotypes: 14 apo E2/E2 and 2 apo E3/E2) with dysbetalipoproteinemia (*Fredrickson* Type III) are shown in the table below.

[See table 5 at right]

Atorvastatin Effects in Homozygous Familial Hypercholesterolemia: In a study without a concurrent control group, 29 patients ages 6 to 37 years with homozygous FH received maximum daily doses of 20 to 80 mg of atorvastatin. The mean LDL-C reduction in this study was 18%. Twenty-five patients with a reduction in LDL-C had a mean response of 20% (range of 7% to 53%, median of 24%); the remaining 4 patients had 7% to 24% increases in LDL-C. Five of the 29 patients had absent LDL-receptor function. Of these, 2 patients also had a portacaval shunt and had no significant reduction in LDL-C. The remaining 3 receptor-negative patients had a mean LDL-C reduction of 22%.

Atorvastatin Effects in Heterozygous Familial Hypercholesterolemic Pediatric Patients: In a double-blind, placebo-controlled study followed by an open-label phase, 187 boys and postmenarchal girls 10–17 years of age (mean age 14.1 years) with heterozygous FH or severe hypercholesterolemia were randomized to atorvastatin (n=140) or placebo (n=47) for 26 weeks and then all received atorvastatin for 26 weeks. Inclusion in the study required 1) a baseline LDL-C level ≥ 190 mg/dL or 2) a baseline LDL-C ≥ 160 mg/dL and positive family history of FH or documented premature cardiovascular disease in a first- or second-degree relative. The mean baseline LDL-C value was 218.6 mg/dL (range: 138.5-385.0 mg/dL) in the atorvastatin group compared to 230.0 mg/dL (range: 160.0-324.5 mg/dL) in placebo group. The dosage of atorvastatin (once daily) was 10 mg for the first 4 weeks and up-titrated to 20 mg if the LDL-C level was > 130 mg/dL. The number of atorvastatin-treated patients who required up-titration to 20 mg after Week 4 during the double-blind phase was 80 (57.1%).

Atorvastatin significantly decreased plasma levels of total-C, LDL-C, triglycerides, and apolipoprotein B during the 26 week double-blind phase (see Table 6).

[See table 6 at right]

The mean achieved LDL-C value was 130.7 mg/dL (range: 70.0–242.0 mg/dL) in the atorvastatin group compared to 228.5 mg/dL (range: 152.0–385.0 mg/dL) in the placebo group during the 26 week double-blind phase.

The safety and efficacy of atorvastatin doses above 20 mg have not been studied in controlled trials in children. The long-term efficacy of atorvastatin therapy in childhood to reduce morbidity and mortality in adulthood has not been established.

Clinical Study of Combined Amlodipine and Atorvastatin in Patients with Hypertension and Dyslipidemia

In a double-blind, placebo-controlled study, a total of 1660 patients with co-morbid hypertension and dyslipidemia received once daily treatment with eight dose combinations of amlodipine and atorvastatin (5/10, 10/10, 5/20, 10/20, 5/40, 10/40, 5/80, or 10/80 mg), amlodipine alone (5 mg or 10 mg), atorvastatin alone (10 mg, 20 mg, 40 mg, or 80 mg) or placebo. In addition to concomitant hypertension and dyslipidemia, 15% of the patients had diabetes mellitus, 22% were smokers and 14% had a positive family history of cardiovascular disease. At eight weeks, all eight combination-treatment groups of amlodipine and atorvastatin demonstrated statistically significant dose-related reductions in systolic blood pressure (SBP), diastolic blood pressure (DBP) and LDL-C compared to placebo, with no overall modification of effect of either component on SBP, DBP and LDL-C (Table 7).

[See table 7 on next page]

Table 2. Dose-Response in Patients With Primary Hypercholesterolemia (Adjusted Mean % Change From Baseline)[a]

DOSE	N	TC	LDL-C	ApoB	TG	HDL-C	Non-HDL-C/ HDL-C
Placebo	21	4	4	3	10	-3	7
10	22	-29	-39	-32	-19	6	-34
20	20	-33	-43	-35	-26	9	-41
40	21	-37	-50	-42	-29	6	-45
80	23	-45	-60	-50	-37	5	-53

[a]Results are pooled from 2 dose-response studies.

Table 3. Mean Percent Change From Baseline at Endpoint (Double-Blind, Randomized, Active-Controlled Trials)

Treatment (Daily Dose)	N	Total-C	LDL-C	Apo B	TG	HDL-C	Non-HDL-C/ HDL-C
Study 1							
Atorvastatin 10 mg	707	-27[a]	-36[a]	-28[a]	-17[a]	+7	-37[a]
Lovastatin 20 mg	191	-19	-27	-20	- 6	+7	-28
95% CI for Diff[1]		-9.2, -6.5	-10.7, -7.1	-10.0, -6.5	-15.2, -7.1	-1.7, 2.0	-11.1, -7.1
Study 2							
Atorvastatin 10 mg	222	-25[b]	-35[b]	-27[b]	-17[b]	+6	-36[b]
Pravastatin 20 mg	77	-17	-23	-17	-9	+8	-28
95% CI for Diff[1]		-10.8, -6.1	-14.5, -8.2	-13.4, -7.4	-14.1, -0.7	-4.9, 1.6	-11.5, -4.1
Study 3							
Atorvastatin 10 mg	132	-29[c]	-37[c]	-34[c]	-23[c]	+7	-39[c]
Simvastatin 10 mg	45	-24	-30	-30	-15	+7	-33
95% CI for Diff[1]		-8.7, -2.7	-10.1, -2.6	-8.0, -1.1	-15.1, -0.7	-4.3, 3.9	-9.6, -1.9

[1] A negative value for the 95% CI for the difference between treatments favors atorvastatin for all except HDL-C, for which a positive value favors atorvastatin. If the range does not include 0, this indicates a statistically significant difference.
[a] Significantly different from lovastatin, ANCOVA, p ≤0.05
[b] Significantly different from pravastatin, ANCOVA, p ≤0.05
[c] Significantly different from simvastatin, ANCOVA, p ≤0.05

Table 4. Combined Patients With Isolated Elevated TG: Median (min, max) Percent Changes From Baseline

	Placebo (N=12)	Atorvastatin 10 mg (N=37)	Atorvastatin 20 mg (N=13)	Atorvastatin 80 mg (N=14)
Triglycerides	-12.4 (-36.6, 82.7)	-41.0 (-76.2, 49.4)	-38.7 (-62.7, 29.5)	-51.8 (-82.8, 41.3)
Total-C	-2.3 (-15.4, 24.4)	-28.2 (-44.9, -6.8)	-34.9 (-49.6, -15.2)	-44.4 (-63.5, -3.8)
LDL-C	3.6 (-31.3, 31.6)	-26.5 (-57.7, 9.8)	-30.4 (-53.9, 0.3)	-40.5 (-60.6, -13.8)
HDL-C	3.8 (-18.6, 13.4)	13.8 (-9.7, 61.5)	11.0 (-3.2, 25.2)	7.5 (-10.8, 37.2)
VLDL-C	-1.0 (-31.9, 53.2)	-48.8 (-85.8, 57.3)	-44.6 (-62.2, -10.8)	-62.0 (-88.2, 37.6)
non-HDL-C	-2.8 (-17.6, 30.0)	-33.0 (-52.1, -13.3)	-42.7 (-53.7, -17.4)	-51.5 (-72.9, -4.3)

Table 5. Open-Label Crossover Study of 16 Patients With Dysbetalipoproteinemia (*Fredrickson* Type III)

		Median % Change (min, max)	
	Median (min, max) at Baseline (mg/dL)	Atorvastatin 10 mg	Atorvastatin 80 mg
Total-C	442 (225, 1320)	-37 (-85, 17)	-58 (-90, -31)
Triglycerides	678 (273, 5990)	-39 (-92, -8)	-53 (-95, -30)
IDL-C + VLDL-C	215 (111, 613)	-32 (-76, 9)	-63 (-90, -8)
non-HDL-C	411 (218, 1272)	-43 (-87, -19)	-64 (-92, -36)

Table 6. Lipid-altering Effects of Atorvastatin in Adolescent Boys and Girls with Heterozygous Familial Hypercholesterolemia or Severe Hypercholesterolemia (Mean Percent Change from Baseline at Endpoint in Intention-to-Treat Population)

DOSAGE	N	Total-C	LDL-C	HDL-C	TG	Apolipoprotein B
Placebo	47	-1.5	-0.4	-1.9	1.0	0.7
Atorvastatin	140	-31.4	-39.6	2.8	-12.0	-34.0

INDICATIONS AND USAGE

CADUET (amlodipine and atorvastatin) is indicated in patients for whom treatment with both amlodipine and atorvastatin is appropriate.

Amlodipine

1. ***Hypertension***: Amlodipine is indicated for the treatment of hypertension. It may be used alone or in combination with other antihypertensive agents;
2. ***Chronic Stable Angina***: Amlodipine is indicated for the treatment of chronic stable angina, for the treatment of confirmed or suspected vasospastic angina and for the treatment of hypertension. Amlodipine may be used alone or in combination with other antianginal or antihypertensive agents;
3. ***Vasospastic Angina (Prinzmetal's or Variant Angina)***: Amlodipine is indicated for the treatment of confirmed or suspected vasospastic angina. Amlodipine may be used as monotherapy or in combination with other antianginal drugs.

AND

Atorvastatin

1. ***Heterozygous Familial and Nonfamilial***: Atorvastatin is indicated as an adjunct to diet to reduce elevated total-C,

Continued on next page

Caduet—Cont.

LDL-C, apo B, and TG levels and to increase HDL-C in patients with primary hypercholesterolemia (heterozygous familial and nonfamilial) and mixed dyslipidemia (*Fredrickson* Types IIa and IIb);

2. ***Elevated Serum TG Levels***: Atorvastatin is indicated as an adjunct to diet for the treatment of patients with elevated serum TG levels (*Fredrickson* Type IV);
3. ***Primary Dysbetalipoproteinemia***: Atorvastatin is indicated for the treatment of patients with primary dysbetalipoproteinemia (*Fredrickson* Type III) who do not respond adequately to diet;
4. ***Homozygous Familial Hypercholesterolemia***: Atorvastatin is indicated to reduce total-C and LDL-C in patients with homozygous familial hypercholesterolemia as an adjunct to other lipid-lowering treatments (e.g., LDL apheresis) or if such treatments are unavailable;
5. ***Pediatric Patients***: Atorvastatin is indicated as an adjunct to diet to reduce total-C, LDL-C, and apo B levels in boys and postmenarchal girls, 10 to 17 years of age, with heterozygous familial hypercholesterolemia if after an adequate trial of diet therapy the following findings are present:

a. LDL-C remains ≥ 190 mg/dL or

b. LDL-C remains ≥ 160 mg/dL and:

- there is a positive family history of premature cardiovascular disease or
- two or more other CVD risk factors are present in the pediatric patients.

Therapy with lipid-altering agents should be a component of multiple-risk-factor intervention in individuals at increased risk for atherosclerotic vascular disease due to hypercholesterolemia. Lipid-altering agents should be used, in addition to a diet restricted in saturated fat and cholesterol, only when the response to diet and other nonpharmacological measures has been inadequate (see *National Cholesterol Education Program (NCEP) Guidelines,* summarized in Table 8).

[See table 8 below]

Table 7. Efficacy in Terms of Reduction in Blood Pressure and LDL-C
Efficacy of the Combined Treatments in Reducing Systolic BP

Parameter / Analysis		ATO 0 mg	ATO 10 mg	ATO 20 mg	ATO 40 mg	ATO 80 mg
AML 0 mg	Mean Change (mmHg)	-3.0	-4.5	-6.2	-6.2	-6.4
	Difference versus placebo (mmHg)	-	-1.5	-3.2	-3.2	-3.4
AML 5 mg	Mean change (mmHg)	-12.8	-13.7	-15.3	-12.7	-12.2
	Difference versus placebo (mmHg)	-9.8	-10.7	-12.3	-9.7	-9.2
AML 10 mg	Mean change (mmHg)	-16.2	-15.9	-16.1	-16.3	-17.6
	Difference versus placebo (mmHg)	-13.2	-12.9	-13.1	-13.3	-14.6

Efficacy of the Combined Treatments in Reducing Diastolic BP

Parameter / Analysis		ATO 0 mg	ATO 10 mg	ATO 20 mg	ATO 40 mg	ATO 80 mg
AML 0 mg	Mean change (mmHg)	-3.3	-4.1	-3.9	-5.1	-4.1
	Difference versus placebo (mmHg)	-	-0.8	-0.6	-1.8	-0.8
AML 5 mg	Mean change (mmHg)	-7.6	-8.2	-9.4	-7.3	-8.4
	Difference versus placebo (mmHg)	-4.3	-4.9	-6.1	-4.0	-5.1
AML 10 mg	Mean change (mmHg)	-10.4	-9.1	-10.6	-9.8	-11.1
	Difference versus placebo (mmHg)	-7.1	-5.8	-7.3	-6.5	-7.8

Efficacy of the Combined Treatments in Reducing LDL-C (% change)

Parameter / Analysis		ATO 0 mg	AT010 mg	AT0 20 mg	ATO 40 mg	ATO 80 mg
AML 0 mg	Mean % chg	-1.1	-33.4	-39.5	-43.1	-47.2
AML 5 mg	Mean % chg	-0.1	-38.7	-42.3	-44.9	-48.4
AML 10 mg	Mean % chg	-2.5	-36.6	-38.6	-43.2	-49.1

Table 8. NCEP Treatment Guidelines: LDL-C Goals and Cutpoints for Therapeutic Lifestyle Changes and Drug Therapy in Different Risk Categories

Risk Category	LDL Goal (mg/dL)	LDL Level at Which to Initiate Therapeutic Lifestyle Changes (mg/dL)	LDL Level at Which to Consider Drug Therapy (mg/dL)
CHD[a] or CHD risk equivalents (10-year risk >20%)	<100	≥100	≥130 (100-129: drug optional)[b]
2+ Risk Factors (10-year risk ≤20%)	<130	≥130	10-year risk 10%-20%: ≥130 10-year risk <10%: ≥ 160
0-1 Risk Factor[c]	<160	≥160	≥190 (160-189: LDL-lowering drug optional)

[a] CHD, coronary heart disease

[b] Some authorities recommend use of LDL-lowering drugs in this category if an LDL-C level of < 100 mg/dL cannot be achieved by therapeutic lifestyle changes. Others prefer use of drugs that primarily modify triglycerides and HDL-C, e.g., nicotinic acid or fibrate. Clinical judgement also may call for deferring drug therapy in this subcategory.

[c] Almost all people with 0-1 risk factor have 10-year risk <10%; thus, 10-year risk assessment in people with 0-1 risk factor is not necessary.

After the LDL-C goal has been achieved, if the TG is still ≥ 200 mg/dL, non-HDL-C (total-C minus HDL-C) becomes a secondary target of therapy. Non-HDL-C goals are set 30 mg/dL higher than LDL-C goals for each risk category.

Prior to initiating therapy with atorvastatin, secondary causes for hypercholesterolemia (e.g., poorly controlled diabetes mellitus, hypothyroidism, nephrotic syndrome, dysproteinemias, obstructive liver disease, other drug therapy, and alcoholism) should be excluded, and a lipid profile performed to measure total-C, LDL-C, HDL-C, and TG. For patients with TG <400 mg/dL (<4.5 mmol/L), LDL-C can be estimated using the following equation: LDL-C = total-C - (0.20 x [TG] + HDL-C). For TG levels >400 mg/dL (>4.5 mmol/L), this equation is less accurate and LDL-C concentrations should be determined by ultracentrifugation.

The antidyslipidemic component of CADUET has not been studied in conditions where the major lipoprotein abnormality is elevation of chylomicrons (*Fredrickson* Types I and V).

The NCEP classification of cholesterol levels in pediatric patients with a familial history of hypercholesterolemia or premature cardiovascular disease is summarized below:

Table 9. NCEP Classification of Cholesterol Levels in Pediatric Patients

Category	Total-C (mg/dL)	LDL-C (mg/dL)
Acceptable	<170	<110
Borderline	170-199	110-129
High	≥200	≥130

CONTRAINDICATIONS

CADUET contains atorvastatin and is therefore contraindicated in patients with active liver disease or unexplained persistent elevations of serum transaminases.

CADUET is contraindicated in patients with known hypersensitivity to any component of this medication.

Pregnancy and Lactation

Atherosclerosis is a chronic process and discontinuation of lipid-lowering drugs during pregnancy should have little impact on the outcome of long-term therapy of primary hypercholesterolemia. Cholesterol and other products of cholesterol biosynthesis are essential components for fetal development (including synthesis of steroids and cell membranes). Since HMG-CoA reductase inhibitors decrease cholesterol synthesis and possibly the synthesis of other biologically active substances derived from cholesterol, they may cause fetal harm when administered to pregnant women. Therefore, HMG-CoA reductase inhibitors are contraindicated during pregnancy and in nursing mothers. CADUET, WHICH INCLUDES ATORVASTATIN, SHOULD BE ADMINISTERED TO WOMEN OF CHILDBEARING AGE ONLY WHEN SUCH PATIENTS ARE HIGHLY UNLIKELY TO CONCEIVE AND HAVE BEEN INFORMED OF THE POTENTIAL HAZARDS. If the patient becomes pregnant while taking this drug, therapy should be discontinued and the patient apprised of the potential hazard to the fetus.

WARNINGS

Increased Angina and/or Myocardial Infarction

Rarely, patients, particularly those with severe obstructive coronary artery disease, have developed documented increased frequency, duration and/or severity of angina or acute myocardial infarction on starting calcium channel blocker therapy or at the time of dosage increase. The mechanism of this effect has not been elucidated.

Liver Dysfunction

HMG-CoA reductase inhibitors, like some other lipid-lowering therapies, have been associated with biochemical abnormalities of liver function. **Persistent elevations (>3 times the upper limit of normal [ULN] occurring on 2 or more occasions) in serum transaminases occurred in 0.7% of patients who received atorvastatin in clinical trials. The incidence of these abnormalities was 0.2%, 0.2%, 0.6%, and 2.3% for 10, 20, 40, and 80 mg, respectively.**

In clinical trials in patients taking atorvastatin the following has been observed. One patient in clinical trials developed jaundice. Increases in liver function tests (LFT) in other patients were not associated with jaundice or other clinical signs or symptoms. Upon dose reduction, drug interruption, or discontinuation, transaminase levels returned to or near pretreatment levels without sequelae. Eighteen of 30 patients, with persistent LFT elevations continued treatment with a reduced dose of atorvastatin.

It is recommended that liver function tests be performed prior to and at 12 weeks following both the initiation of therapy and any elevation of dose, and periodically (e.g., semiannually) thereafter. Liver enzyme changes generally occur in the first 3 months of treatment with atorvastatin. Patients who develop increased transaminase levels should be monitored until the abnormalities resolve. Should an increase in ALT or AST of >3 times ULN persist, reduction of dose or withdrawal of CADUET is recommended.

CADUET should be used with caution in patients who consume substantial quantities of alcohol and/or have a history of liver disease. Active liver disease or unexplained persistent transaminase elevations are contraindications to the use of CADUET (see **CONTRAINDICATIONS**).

Skeletal Muscle

Rare cases of rhabdomyolysis with acute renal failure secondary to myoglobinuria have been reported with the atorvastatin component of CADUET and with other drugs in the HMG-CoA reductase inhibitor class.

Uncomplicated myalgia has been reported in atorvastatin-treated patients (see **ADVERSE REACTIONS**). Myopathy, defined as muscle aches or muscle weakness in conjunction with increases in creatine phosphokinase (CPK) values >10 times ULN, should be considered in any patient with diffuse myalgias, muscle tenderness or weakness, and/or marked elevation of CPK. Patients should be advised to report promptly unexplained muscle pain, tenderness or weakness, particularly if accompanied by malaise or fever. CADUET therapy should be discontinued if markedly elevated CPK levels occur or myopathy is diagnosed or suspected.

The risk of myopathy during treatment with drugs in the HMG-CoA reductase inhibitor class is increased with concurrent administration of cyclosporine, fibric acid derivatives, erythromycin, niacin, or azole antifungals. Physicians considering combined therapy with CADUET and fibric acid derivatives, erythromycin, immunosuppressive drugs, azole antifungals, or lipid-lowering doses of niacin should carefully weigh the potential benefits and risks and should carefully monitor patients for any signs or symptoms of muscle pain, tenderness, or weakness, particularly during the initial months of therapy and during any periods of upward dosage titration of either drug. Periodic creatine phosphokinase (CPK) determinations may be considered in such situations, but there is no assurance that such monitoring will prevent the occurrence of severe myopathy.

In patients taking CADUET, therapy should be temporarily withheld or discontinued in any patient with an acute, serious condition suggestive of a myopathy or having a risk factor predisposing to the development of renal failure secondary to rhabdomyolysis (e.g., severe acute infection, hypotension, major surgery, trauma, severe metabolic, endocrine and electrolyte disorders, and uncontrolled seizures).

PRECAUTIONS

General

Since the vasodilation induced by the amlodipine component of CADUET is gradual in onset, acute hypotension has rarely been reported after oral administration of amlodipine. Nonetheless, caution should be exercised when administering CADUET as with any other peripheral vasodilator particularly in patients with severe aortic stenosis.

Before instituting therapy with CADUET, an attempt should be made to control hypercholesterolemia with appropriate diet, exercise, and weight reduction in obese patients, and to treat other underlying medical problems (see **INDICATIONS AND USAGE**).

Use in Patients with Congestive Heart Failure

In general, calcium channel blockers should be used with caution in patients with heart failure. The amlodipine component of CADUET (5–10 mg per day) has been studied in a placebo-controlled trial of 1153 patients with NYHA Class III or IV heart failure (see **CLINICAL PHARMACOLOGY**) on stable doses of ACE inhibitor, digoxin, and diuretics. Follow-up was at least 6 months, with a mean of about 14 months. There was no overall adverse effect on survival or cardiac morbidity (as defined by life-threatening arrhythmia, acute myocardial infarction, or hospitalization for worsened heart failure). Amlodipine has been compared to placebo in four 8–12 week studies of patients with NYHA class II/III heart failure, involving a total of 697 patients. In these studies, there was no evidence of worsened heart failure based on measures of exercise tolerance, NYHA classification, symptoms, or LVEF.

Beta-Blocker Withdrawal

The amlodipine component of CADUET is not a beta-blocker and therefore gives no protection against the dangers of abrupt beta-blocker withdrawal; any such withdrawal should be by gradual reduction of the dose of beta-blocker.

Endocrine Function

HMG-CoA reductase inhibitors, such as the atorvastatin component of CADUET interfere with cholesterol synthesis and theoretically might blunt adrenal and/or gonadal steroid production. Clinical studies have shown that atorvastatin does not reduce basal plasma cortisol concentration or impair adrenal reserve. The effects of HMG-CoA reductase inhibitors on male fertility have not been studied in adequate numbers of patients. The effects, if any, on the pituitary-gonadal axis in premenopausal women are unknown. Caution should be exercised if an HMG-CoA reductase inhibitor is administered concomitantly with drugs that may decrease the levels or activity of endogenous steroid hormones, such as ketoconazole, spironolactone, and cimetidine.

CNS Toxicity

Studies with atorvastatin: Brain hemorrhage was seen in a female dog treated with atorvastatin calcium for 3 months at a dose equivalent to 120 mg atorvastatin/kg/day. Brain hemorrhage and optic nerve vacuolation were seen in another female dog that was sacrificed in moribund condition after 11 weeks of escalating doses of atorvastatin calcium equivalent to up to 280 mg atorvastatin/kg/day. The 120 mg/kg dose of atorvastatin resulted in a systemic exposure approximately 16 times the human plasma area-under-the-curve (AUC, 0–24 hours) based on the maximum human dose of 80 mg/day. A single tonic convulsion was seen in each of 2 male dogs (one treated with atorvastatin calcium at a dose equivalent to 10 mg atorvastatin/kg/day and one at a dose equivalent to 120 mg atorvastatin/kg/day) in a 2-year study. No CNS lesions have been observed in mice after chronic treatment for up to 2 years at doses of atorvastatin calcium equivalent to up to 400 mg atorvastatin/kg/day or in rats at doses equivalent to up to 100 mg atorvastatin/kg/day. These doses were 6 to 11 times (mouse) and 8 to 16 times (rat) the human AUC (0–24) based on the maximum recommended human dose of 80 mg atorvastatin/day.

CNS vascular lesions, characterized by perivascular hemorrhages, edema, and mononuclear cell infiltration of perivascular spaces, have been observed in dogs treated with other members of the HMG-CoA reductase class. A chemically similar drug in this class produced optic nerve degeneration (Wallerian degeneration of retinogeniculate fibers) in clinically normal dogs in a dose-dependent fashion at a dose that produced plasma drug levels about 30 times higher than the mean drug level in humans taking the highest recommended dose.

Information for Patients

Due to the risk of myopathy with drugs of the HMG-CoA reductase class, to which the atorvastatin component of CADUET belongs, patients should be advised to report promptly unexplained muscle pain, tenderness, or weakness, particularly if accompanied by malaise or fever.

Drug Interactions

Data from a drug-drug interaction study involving 10 mg of amlodipine and 80 mg of atorvastatin in healthy subjects indicate that the pharmacokinetics of amlodipine are not altered when the drugs are coadministered. The effect of amlodipine on the pharmacokinetics of atorvastatin showed no effect on the Cmax: 91% (90% confidence interval: 80 to 103%), but the AUC of atorvastatin increased by 18% (90% confidence interval: 109 to 127%) in the presence of amlodipine.

No drug interaction studies have been conducted with CADUET and other drugs, although studies have been conducted in the individual amlodipine and atorvastatin components, as described below:

Studies with Amlodipine:

In vitro data in human plasma indicate that amlodipine has no effect on the protein binding of drugs tested (digoxin, phenytoin, warfarin, and indomethacin).

Cimetidine: Co-administration of amlodipine with cimetidine did not alter the pharmacokinetics of amlodipine.

Maalox® (antacid): Co-administration of the antacid Maalox with a single dose of amlodipine had no significant effect on the pharmacokinetics of amlodipine.

Sildenafil: A single 100 mg dose of sildenafil (Viagra®) in subjects with essential hypertension had no effect on the pharmacokinetic parameters of amlodipine. When amlodipine and sildenafil were used in combination, each agent independently exerted its own blood pressure lowering effect.

Digoxin: Co-administration of amlodipine with digoxin did not change serum digoxin levels or digoxin renal clearance in normal volunteers.

Ethanol (alcohol): Single and multiple 10 mg doses of amlodipine had no significant effect on the pharmacokinetics of ethanol.

Warfarin: Co-administration of amlodipine with warfarin did not change the warfarin prothrombin response time.

In clinical trials, amlodipine has been safely administered with thiazide diuretics, beta-blockers, angiotensin-converting enzyme inhibitors, long-acting nitrates, sublingual nitroglycerin, digoxin, warfarin, non-steroidal anti-inflammatory drugs, antibiotics, and oral hypoglycemic drugs.

Studies with Atorvastatin:

The risk of myopathy during treatment with drugs of the HMG-CoA reductase class is increased with concurrent administration of cyclosporine, fibric acid derivatives, niacin (nicotinic acid), erythromycin, or azole antifungals (see **WARNINGS, Skeletal Muscle**).

Antacid: When atorvastatin and Maalox TC suspension were coadministered, plasma concentrations of atorvastatin decreased approximately 35%. However, LDL-C reduction was not altered.

Antipyrine: Because atorvastatin does not affect the pharmacokinetics of antipyrine, interactions with other drugs metabolized via the same cytochrome isozymes are not expected.

Colestipol: Plasma concentrations of atorvastatin decreased approximately 25% when colestipol and atorvastatin were coadministered. However, LDL-C reduction was greater when atorvastatin and colestipol were coadministered than when either drug was given alone.

Cimetidine: Atorvastatin plasma concentrations and LDL-C reduction were not altered by coadministration of cimetidine.

Digoxin: When multiple doses of atorvastatin and digoxin were coadministered, steady-state plasma digoxin concentrations increased by approximately 20%. Patients taking digoxin should be monitored appropriately.

Erythromycin: In healthy individuals, plasma concentrations of atorvastatin increased approximately 40% with coadministration of atorvastatin and erythromycin, a known inhibitor of cytochrome P450 3A4 (see **WARNINGS, Skeletal Muscle**).

Oral Contraceptives: Coadministration of atorvastatin and an oral contraceptive increased AUC values for norethindrone and ethinyl estradiol by approximately 30% and 20%. These increases should be considered when selecting an oral contraceptive for a woman taking CADUET.

Warfarin: Atorvastatin had no clinically significant effect on prothrombin time when administered to patients receiving chronic warfarin treatment.

Drug/Laboratory Test Interactions

None known.

Carcinogenesis, Mutagenesis, Impairment of Fertility

Studies with amlodipine: Rats and mice treated with amlodipine maleate in the diet for up to two years, at concentrations calculated to provide daily dosage levels of 0.5, 1.25, and 2.5 mg amlodipine/kg/day, showed no evidence of a carcinogenic effect of the drug. For the mouse, the highest dose was, on a mg/m^2 basis, similar to the maximum recommended human dose of 10 mg amlodipine/day*. For the rat, the highest dose level was, on a mg/m^2 basis, about twice the maximum recommended human dose*.

Mutagenicity studies conducted with amlodipine maleate revealed no drug related effects at either the gene or chromosome levels.

There was no effect on the fertility of rats treated orally with amlodipine maleate (males for 64 days and females for 14 days prior to mating) at doses up to 10 mg amlodipine/kg/day (8 times* the maximum recommended human dose of 10 mg/day on a mg/m^2 basis).

*Based on patient weight of 50 kg.

Studies with atorvastatin: In a 2-year carcinogenicity study with atorvastatin calcium in rats at dose levels equivalent to 10, 30, and 100 mg atorvastatin/kg/day, 2 rare tumors were found in muscle in high-dose females: in one, there was a rhabdomyosarcoma and, in another, there was a fibrosarcoma. This dose represents a plasma AUC (0-24) value of approximately 16 times the mean human plasma drug exposure after an 80 mg oral dose.

A 2-year carcinogenicity study in mice given atorvastatin calcium at dose levels equivalent to 100, 200, and 400 mg atorvastatin/kg/day resulted in a significant increase in liver adenomas in high-dose males and liver carcinomas in high-dose females. These findings occurred at plasma AUC (0-24) values of approximately 6 times the mean human plasma drug exposure after an 80 mg oral dose.

In vitro, atorvastatin was not mutagenic or clastogenic in the following tests with and without metabolic activation: the Ames test with *Salmonella typhimurium* and *Escherichia coli*, the HGPRT forward mutation assay in Chinese hamster lung cells, and the chromosomal aberration assay in Chinese hamster lung cells. Atorvastatin was negative in the *in vivo* mouse micronucleus test.

There were no effects on fertility when rats were given atorvastatin calcium at doses equivalent to up to 175 mg atorvastatin/kg/day (15 times the human exposure). There was aplasia and aspermia in the epididymides of 2 of 10 rats treated with atorvastatin calcium at a dose equivalent to 100 mg atorvastatin/kg/day for 3 months (16 times the human AUC at the 80 mg dose); testis weights were significantly lower at 30 and 100 mg/kg/day and epididymal weight was lower at 100 mg/kg/day. Male rats given the equivalent of 100 mg atorvastatin/kg/day for 11 weeks prior to mating had decreased sperm motility, spermatid head concentration, and increased abnormal sperm. Atorvastatin caused no adverse effects on semen parameters, or reproductive organ histopathology in dogs given doses of atorvastatin calcium equivalent to 10, 40, or 120 mg atorvastatin/kg/day for two years.

Pregnancy

Pregnancy Category X (see CONTRAINDICATIONS)

Safety in pregnant women has not been established with CADUET. CADUET should be administered to women of child-bearing potential only when such patients are highly unlikely to conceive and have been informed of the potential hazards. If the woman becomes pregnant while taking CADUET, it should be discontinued and the patient advised again as to the potential hazards to the fetus.

Studies with amlodipine: No evidence of teratogenicity or other embryo/fetal toxicity was found when pregnant rats and rabbits were treated orally with amlodipine maleate at doses up to 10 mg amlodipine/kg/day (respectively 8 times* and 23 times* the maximum recommended human dose of 10 mg/day on a mg/m^2 basis) during their respective periods of major organogenesis. However, litter size was significantly decreased (by about 50%) and the number of intrauterine deaths was significantly increased (about 5-fold) in rats receiving amlodipine maleate at 10 mg amlodipine/kg/day for 14 days before mating and throughout mating and gestation. Amlodipine maleate has been shown to prolong both the gestation period and the duration of labor in rats at this dose. There are no adequate and well-controlled studies in pregnant women.

*Based on patient weight of 50 kg.

Studies with atorvastatin: Atorvastatin crosses the rat placenta and reaches a level in fetal liver equivalent to that of maternal plasma. Atorvastatin was not teratogenic in rats at doses of atorvastatin calcium equivalent to up to 300 mg atorvastatin/kg/day or in rabbits at doses of atorvastatin calcium equivalent to up to 100 mg atorvastatin/kg/day. These doses resulted in multiples of about 30 times (rat) or 20 times (rabbit) the human exposure based on surface area (mg/m^2).

In a study in rats given atorvastatin calcium at doses equivalent to 20, 100, or 225 mg atorvastatin/kg/day, from gestation day 7 through to lactation day 21 (weaning), there was decreased pup survival at birth, neonate, weaning, and maturity for pups of mothers dosed with 225 mg/kg/day. Body weight was decreased on days 4 and 21 for pups of mothers dosed at 100 mg/kg/day; pup body weight was decreased at birth and at days 4, 21, and 91 at 225 mg/kg/day. Pup development was delayed (rotorod performance at 100 mg/kg/

Continued on next page

Caduet—Cont.

day and acoustic startle at 225 mg/kg/day; pinnae detachment and eye opening at 225 mg/kg/day). These doses of atorvastatin correspond to 6 times (100 mg/kg) and 22 times (225 mg/kg) the human AUC at 80 mg/day.

Rare reports of congenital anomalies have been received following intrauterine exposure to HMG-CoA reductase inhibitors. There has been one report of severe congenital bony deformity, tracheo-esophageal fistula, and anal atresia (VATER association) in a baby born to a woman who took lovastatin with dextroamphetamine sulfate during the first trimester of pregnancy.

Labor and Delivery

No studies have been conducted in pregnant women on the effect of CADUET, amlodipine or atorvastatin on the mother or the fetus during labor or delivery, or on the duration of labor or delivery. Amlodipine has been shown to prolong the duration of labor in rats.

Nursing Mothers

It is not known whether the amlodipine component of CADUET is excreted in human milk. Nursing rat pups taking atorvastatin had plasma and liver drug levels of 50% and 40%, respectively, of that in their mother's milk. Because of the potential for adverse reactions in nursing infants, women taking CADUET should not breast-feed (see **CONTRAINDICATIONS**).

Pediatric Use

There have been no studies conducted to determine the safety or effectiveness of CADUET in pediatric populations.

Studies with amlodipine: The effect of amlodipine on blood pressure in patients less than 6 years of age is not known.

Studies with atorvastatin: Safety and effectiveness in patients 10–17 years of age with heterozygous familial hypercholesterolemia have been evaluated in controlled clinical trials of 6 months duration in adolescent boys and postmenarchal girls. Patients treated with atorvastatin had an adverse experience profile generally similar to that of patients treated with placebo, the most common adverse experiences observed in both groups, regardless of causality assessment, were infections. **Doses greater than 20 mg have not been studied in this patient population.** In this limited controlled study, there was no detectable effect on growth or sexual maturation in boys or on menstrual cycle length in girls. See **CLINICAL PHARMACOLOGY, Clinical Studies** section; **ADVERSE REACTIONS,** *Pediatric Patients*; and **DOSAGE AND ADMINISTRATION,** *Pediatric Patients (10-17 years of age) with Heterozygous Familial Hypercholesterolemia*. Adolescent females should be counseled on appropriate contraceptive methods while on atorvastatin therapy (see **CONTRAINDICATIONS** and **PRECAUTIONS, Pregnancy**). **Atorvastatin has not been studied in controlled clinical trials involving pre-pubertal patients or patients younger than 10 years of age.**

Clinical efficacy with doses of atorvastatin up to 80 mg/day for 1 year have been evaluated in an uncontrolled study of patients with homozygous FH including 8 pediatric patients. See **CLINICAL PHARMACOLOGY, Clinical Studies,** *Atorvastatin Effects in Homozygous Familial Hypercholesterolemia*.

Geriatric Use

There have been no studies conducted to determine the safety or effectiveness of CADUET in geriatric populations.

In studies with amlodipine: Clinical studies of amlodipine did not include sufficient numbers of subjects aged 65 and over to determine whether they respond differently from younger subjects. Other reported clinical experience has not identified differences in responses between the elderly and younger patients. In general, dose selection of the amlodipine component of CADUET for an elderly patient should be cautious, usually starting at the low end of the dosing range, reflecting the greater frequency of decreased hepatic, renal, or cardiac function, and of concomitant disease or other drug therapy. Elderly patients have decreased clearance of amlodipine with a resulting increase of AUC of approximately 40-60%, and a lower initial dose may be required (see **DOSAGE AND ADMINISTRATION**).

In studies with atorvastatin: The safety and efficacy of atorvastatin (10-80 mg) in the geriatric population (≥65 years of age) was evaluated in the ACCESS study. In this 54-week open-label trial 1,958 patients initiated therapy with atorvastatin calcium 10 mg. Of these, 835 were elderly (≥65 years) and 1,123 were non-elderly. The mean change in LDL-C from baseline after 6 weeks of treatment with atorvastatin calcium 10 mg was –38.2% in the elderly patients versus –34.6% in the non-elderly group.

The rates of discontinuation in patients on atorvastatin due to adverse events were similar between the two age groups. There were no differences in clinically relevant laboratory abnormalities between the age groups.

ADVERSE REACTIONS

CADUET

CADUET (amlodipine besylate/atorvastatin calcium) has been evaluated for safety in 1092 patients in double-blind placebo controlled studies treated for co-morbid hypertension and dyslipidemia. In general, treatment with CADUET was well tolerated. For the most part, adverse experiences have been mild or moderate in severity. In clinical trials with CADUET, no adverse experiences peculiar to this combination have been observed. Adverse experiences are similar in terms of nature, severity, and frequency to those reported previously with amlodipine and atorvastatin.

The following information is based on the clinical experience with amlodipine and atorvastatin.

Table 10. Adverse Events in Placebo-Controlled Studies (% of Patients)

		atorvastatin			
Body System/ Adverse Event	**Placebo N=270**	**10 mg N=863**	**20 mg N=36**	**40 mg N=79**	**80 mg N=94**
BODY AS A WHOLE					
Infection	10.0	10.3	2.8	10.1	7.4
Headache	7.0	5.4	16.7	2.5	6.4
Accidental Injury	3.7	4.2	0.0	1.3	3.2
Flu Syndrome	1.9	2.2	0.0	2.5	3.2
Abdominal Pain	0.7	2.8	0.0	3.8	2.1
Back Pain	3.0	2.8	0.0	3.8	1.1
Allergic Reaction	2.6	0.9	2.8	1.3	0.0
Asthenia	1.9	2.2	0.0	3.8	0.0
DIGESTIVE SYSTEM					
Constipation	1.8	2.1	0.0	2.5	1.1
Diarrhea	1.5	2.7	0.0	3.8	5.3
Dyspepsia	4.1	2.3	2.8	1.3	2.1
Flatulence	3.3	2.1	2.8	1.3	1.1
RESPIRATORY SYSTEM					
Sinusitis	2.6	2.8	0.0	2.5	6.4
Pharyngitis	1.5	2.5	0.0	1.3	2.1
SKIN AND APPENDAGES					
Rash	0.7	3.9	2.8	3.8	1.1
MUSCULOSKELETAL SYSTEM					
Arthralgia	1.5	2.0	0.0	5.1	0.0
Myalgia	1.1	3.2	5.6	1.3	0.0

The Amlodipine Component of CADUET

Amlodipine has been evaluated for safety in more than 11,000 patients in U.S. and foreign clinical trials. In general, treatment with amlodipine was well tolerated at doses up to 10 mg daily. Most adverse reactions reported during therapy with amlodipine were of mild or moderate severity. In controlled clinical trials directly comparing amlodipine (N=1730) in doses up to 10 mg to placebo (N=1250), discontinuation of amlodipine due to adverse reactions was required in only about 1.5% of patients and was not significantly different from placebo (about 1%). The most common side effects are headache and edema. The incidence (%) of side effects which occurred in a dose related manner are as follows:

Adverse Event		amlodipine		
	2.5 mg N=275	5.0 mg N=296	10.0 mg N=268	Placebo N=520
Edema	1.8	3.0	10.8	0.6
Dizziness	1.1	3.4	3.4	1.5
Flushing	0.7	1.4	2.6	0.0
Palpitation	0.7	1.4	4.5	0.6

Other adverse experiences which were not clearly dose related but which were reported with an incidence greater than 1.0% in placebo-controlled clinical trials include the following:

Placebo-Controlled Studies

	amlodipine (%) (N=1730)	Placebo (%) (N=1250)
Headache	7.3	7.8
Fatigue	4.5	2.8
Nausea	2.9	1.9
Abdominal Pain	1.6	0.3
Somnolence	1.4	0.6

For several adverse experiences that appear to be drug and dose related, there was a greater incidence in women than men associated with amlodipine treatment as shown in the following table:

ADR	amlodipine		Placebo	
	M=% (N=1218)	F=% (N=512)	M=% (N=914)	F=% (N=336)
Edema	5.6	14.6	1.4	5.1
Flushing	1.5	4.5	0.3	0.9
Palpitations	1.4	3.3	0.9	0.9
Somnolence	1.3	1.6	0.8	0.3

The following events occurred in ≤1% but >0.1% of patients treated with amlodipine in controlled clinical trials or under conditions of open trials or marketing experience where a causal relationship is uncertain; they are listed to alert the physician to a possible relationship:

Cardiovascular: arrhythmia (including ventricular tachycardia and atrial fibrillation), bradycardia, chest pain, hypotension, peripheral ischemia, syncope, tachycardia, postural dizziness, postural hypotension, vasculitis.

Central and Peripheral Nervous System: hypoesthesia, neuropathy peripheral, paresthesia, tremor, vertigo.

Gastrointestinal: anorexia, constipation, dyspepsia,** dysphagia, diarrhea, flatulence, pancreatitis, vomiting, gingival hyperplasia.

General: allergic reaction, asthenia,** back pain, hot flushes, malaise, pain, rigors, weight gain, weight decrease.

Musculoskeletal System: arthralgia, arthrosis, muscle cramps,** myalgia.

Psychiatric: sexual dysfunction (male** and female), insomnia, nervousness, depression, abnormal dreams, anxiety, depersonalization.

Respiratory System: dyspnea,** epistaxis.

Skin and Appendages: angioedema, erythema multiforme, pruritus,** rash,** rash erythematous, rash maculopapular.

**These events occurred in less than 1% in placebo-controlled trials, but the incidence of these side effects was between 1% and 2% in all multiple dose studies.

Special Senses: abnormal vision, conjunctivitis, diplopia, eye pain, tinnitus.

Urinary System: micturition frequency, micturition disorder, nocturia.

Autonomic Nervous System: dry mouth, sweating increased.

Metabolic and Nutritional: hyperglycemia, thirst.

Hemopoietic: leukopenia, purpura, thrombocytopenia.

The following events occurred in ≤0.1% of patients treated with amlodipine in controlled clinical trials or under conditions of open trials or marketing experience: cardiac failure, pulse irregularity, extrasystoles, skin discoloration, urticaria, skin dryness, alopecia, dermatitis, muscle weakness, twitching, ataxia, hypertonia, migraine, cold and clammy skin, apathy, agitation, amnesia, gastritis, increased appetite, loose stools, coughing, rhinitis, dysuria, polyuria, parosmia, taste perversion, abnormal visual accommodation, and xerophthalmia.

Other reactions occurred sporadically and cannot be distinguished from medications or concurrent disease states such as myocardial infarction and angina.

Amlodipine therapy has not been associated with clinically significant changes in routine laboratory tests. No clinically relevant changes were noted in serum potassium, serum glucose, total triglycerides, total cholesterol, HDL cholesterol, uric acid, blood urea nitrogen, or creatinine.

The following postmarketing event has been reported infrequently with amlodipine treatment where a causal relationship is uncertain: gynecomastia. In postmarketing experience, jaundice and hepatic enzyme elevations (mostly consistent with cholestasis or hepatitis) in some cases severe enough to require hospitalization have been reported in association with use of amlodipine.

Amlodipine has been used safely in patients with chronic obstructive pulmonary disease, well-compensated congestive heart failure, peripheral vascular disease, diabetes mellitus, and abnormal lipid profiles.

The Atorvastatin Component of CADUET

Atorvastatin is generally well-tolerated. Adverse reactions have usually been mild and transient. In controlled clinical studies of 2502 patients, <2% of patients were discontinued due to adverse experiences attributable to atorvastatin calcium. The most frequent adverse events thought to be related to atorvastatin calcium were constipation, flatulence, dyspepsia, and abdominal pain.

Clinical Adverse Experiences

Adverse experiences reported in ≥2% of patients in placebo-controlled clinical studies of atorvastatin, regardless of causality assessment, are shown in Table 10.

[See table 10 above]

The following adverse events were reported, regardless of causality assessment, in patients treated with atorvastatin in clinical trials. The events in italics occurred in ≥2% of patients and the events in plain type occurred in <2% of patients.

Body as a Whole: *Chest pain*, face edema, fever, neck rigidity, malaise, photosensitivity reaction, generalized edema.

Digestive System: *Nausea*, gastroenteritis, liver function tests abnormal, colitis, vomiting, gastritis, dry mouth, rectal hemorrhage, esophagitis, eructation, glossitis, mouth ulceration, anorexia, increased appetite, stomatitis, biliary pain, cheilitis, duodenal ulcer, dysphagia, enteritis, melena, gum hemorrhage, stomach ulcer, tenesmus, ulcerative stomatitis, hepatitis, pancreatitis, cholestatic jaundice.

Respiratory System: *Bronchitis, rhinitis*, pneumonia, dyspnea, asthma, epistaxis.

Nervous System: *Insomnia, dizziness*, paresthesia, somnolence, amnesia, abnormal dreams, libido decreased, emotional lability, incoordination, peripheral neuropathy, torticollis, facial paralysis, hyperkinesia, depression, hypesthesia, hypertonia.

Musculoskeletal System: *Arthritis*, leg cramps, bursitis, tenosynovitis, myasthenia, tendinous contracture, myositis.

Skin and Appendages: Pruritus, contact dermatitis, alopecia, dry skin, sweating, acne, urticaria, eczema, seborrhea, skin ulcer.

Urogenital System: *Urinary tract infection*, urinary frequency, cystitis, hematuria, impotence, dysuria, kidney cal-

culus, nocturia, epididymitis, fibrocystic breast, vaginal hemorrhage, albuminuria, breast enlargement, metrorrhagia, nephritis, urinary incontinence, urinary retention, urinary urgency, abnormal ejaculation, uterine hemorrhage.
Special Senses: Amblyopia, tinnitus, dry eyes, refraction disorder, eye hemorrhage, deafness, glaucoma, parosmia, taste loss, taste perversion.
Cardiovascular System: Palpitation, vasodilatation, syncope, migraine, postural hypotension, phlebitis, arrhythmia, angina pectoris, hypertension.
Metabolic and Nutritional Disorders: *Peripheral edema*, hyperglycemia, creatine phosphokinase increased, gout, weight gain, hypoglycemia.
Hemic and Lymphatic System: Ecchymosis, anemia, lymphadenopathy, thrombocytopenia, petechia.
Postintroduction Reports with Atorvastatin
Adverse events associated with atorvastatin therapy reported since market introduction, that are not listed above, regardless of causality assessment, include the following: anaphylaxis, angioneurotic edema, bullous rashes (including erythema multiforme, Stevens-Johnson syndrome, and toxic epidermal necrolysis), and rhabdomyolysis.
Pediatric Patients (ages 10–17 years)
In a 26-week controlled study in boys and postmenarchal girls (n=140), the safety and tolerability profile of atorvastatin 10 to 20 mg daily was generally similar to that of placebo (see **CLINICAL PHARMACOLOGY, Clinical Studies** section and **PRECAUTIONS, Pediatric Use**).

OVERDOSAGE

There is no information on overdosage with CADUET in humans.
Information on Amlodipine
Single oral doses of amlodipine maleate equivalent to 40 mg amlodipine/kg and 100 mg amlodipine/kg in mice and rats, respectively, caused deaths. Single oral amlodipine maleate doses equivalent to 4 or more mg amlodipine/kg in dogs (11 or more times the maximum recommended clinical dose on a mg/m^2 basis) caused a marked peripheral vasodilation and hypotension.
Overdosage might be expected to cause excessive peripheral vasodilation with marked hypotension and possibly a reflex tachycardia. In humans, experience with intentional overdosage of amlodipine is limited. Reports of intentional overdosage include a patient who ingested 250 mg and was asymptomatic and was not hospitalized; another (120 mg) was hospitalized, underwent gastric lavage and remained normotensive; the third (105 mg) was hospitalized and had hypotension (90/50 mmHg) which normalized following plasma expansion. A patient who took 70 mg amlodipine and an unknown quantity of benzodiazepine in a suicide attempt developed shock which was refractory to treatment and died the following day with abnormally high benzodiazepine plasma concentration. A case of accidental drug overdose has been documented in a 19-month-old male who ingested 30 mg amlodipine (about 2 mg/kg). During the emergency room presentation, vital signs were stable with no evidence of hypotension, but a heart rate of 180 bpm. Ipecac was administered 3.5 hours after ingestion and on subsequent observation (overnight) no sequelae were noted.
If massive overdose should occur, active cardiac and respiratory monitoring should be instituted. Frequent blood pressure measurements are essential. Should hypotension occur, cardiovascular support including elevation of the extremities and the judicious administration of fluids should be initiated. If hypotension remains unresponsive to these conservative measures, administration of vasopressors (such as phenylephrine) should be considered with attention to circulating volume and urine output. Intravenous calcium gluconate may help to reverse the effects of calcium entry blockade. As amlodipine is highly protein bound, hemodialysis is not likely to be of benefit.
Information on Atorvastatin
There is no specific treatment for atorvastatin overdosage. In the event of an overdose, the patient should be treated symptomatically, and supportive measures instituted as required. Due to extensive drug binding to plasma proteins, hemodialysis is not expected to significantly enhance atorvastatin clearance.

DOSAGE AND ADMINISTRATION

Dosage of CADUET must be individualized on the basis of both effectiveness and tolerance for each individual component in the treatment of hypertension/angina and hyperlipidemia.
Amlodipine (Hypertension or angina)
Adults: The usual initial antihypertensive oral dose of amlodipine is 5 mg once daily with a maximum dose of 10 mg once daily. Small, fragile, or elderly individuals, or patients with hepatic insufficiency may be started on 2.5 mg once daily and this dose may be used when adding amlodipine to other antihypertensive therapy. Management of patients needing 2.5 mg amlodipine requires individual assessments of hypertension and therapy with the individual amlodipine component, since an amlodipine 2.5 mg CADUET tablet is not available.
Dosage should be adjusted according to each patient's need. In general, titration should proceed over 7 to 14 days so that the physician can fully assess the patient's response to each dose level. Titration may proceed more rapidly, however, if clinically warranted, provided the patient is assessed frequently.
The recommended dose of amlodipine for chronic stable or vasospastic angina is 5–10 mg, with the lower dose suggested in the elderly and in patients with hepatic insufficiency. Most patients will require 10 mg for adequate effect. See **ADVERSE REACTIONS** section for information related to dosage and side effects.
Children: The effective antihypertensive oral dose of amlodipine in pediatric patients ages 6-17 years is 2.5 mg to 5 mg once daily. Doses in excess of 5 mg daily have not been studied in pediatric patients. See **CLINICAL PHARMACOLOGY**.
Atorvastatin (Hyperlipidemia)
The patient should be placed on a standard cholesterol-lowering diet before receiving atorvastatin and should continue on this diet during treatment with atorvastatin.
Hypercholesterolemia (Heterozygous Familial and Nonfamilial) and Mixed Dyslipidemia (Fredrickson Types IIa and IIb)
The recommended starting dose of atorvastatin is 10 or 20 mg once daily. Patients who require a large reduction in LDL-C (more than 45%) may be started at 40 mg once daily. The dosage range of atorvastatin is 10 to 80 mg once daily. Atorvastatin can be administered as a single dose at any time of the day, with or without food. The starting dose and maintenance doses of atorvastatin should be individualized according to patient characteristics such as goal of therapy and response (see *NCEP Guidelines*, summarized in Table 8). After initiation and/or upon titration of atorvastatin, lipid levels should be analyzed within 2 to 4 weeks and dosage adjusted accordingly.
Since the goal of treatment is to lower LDL-C, the NCEP recommends that LDL-C levels be used to initiate and assess treatment response. Only if LDL-C levels are not available, should total-C be used to monitor therapy.
Heterozygous Familial Hypercholesterolemia in Pediatric Patients (10-17 years of age)
The recommended starting dose of atorvastatin is 10 mg/day; the maximum recommended dose is 20 mg/day (doses greater than 20 mg have not been studied in this patient population). Doses should be individualized according to the recommended goal of therapy (see NCEP Pediatric Panel Guidelines[1], **CLINICAL PHARMACOLOGY,** and **INDICATIONS AND USAGE**). Adjustments should be made at intervals of 4 weeks or more.
Homozygous Familial Hypercholesterolemia
The dosage of atorvastatin in patients with homozygous FH is 10 to 80 mg daily. Atorvastatin should be used as an adjunct to other lipid-lowering treatments (e.g., LDL apheresis) in these patients or if such treatments are unavailable.
Note: a 2.5/80 mg CADUET tablet is not available. Management of patients needing a 2.5/80 mg combination requires individual assessments of dyslipidemia and therapy with the individual components as a 2.5/80 mg CADUET tablet is not available.
Concomitant Therapy
Atorvastatin may be used in combination with a bile acid binding resin for additive effect. The combination of HMG-CoA reductase inhibitors and fibrates should generally be avoided (see **WARNINGS, Skeletal Muscle,** and **PRECAUTIONS, Drug Interactions** for other drug-drug interactions).
Dosage in Patients With Renal Insufficiency
Renal disease does not affect the plasma concentrations nor LDL-C reduction of atorvastatin; thus, dosage adjustment in patients with renal dysfunction is not necessary (see **CLINICAL PHARMACOLOGY, Pharmacokinetics**).
CADUET
CADUET may be substituted for its individually titrated components. Patients may be given the equivalent dose of CADUET or a dose of CADUET with increased amounts of amlodipine, atorvastatin or both for additional antianginal effects, blood pressure lowering, or lipid lowering effect.
CADUET may be used to provide additional therapy for patients already on one of its components. As initial therapy for one indication and continuation of treatment of the other, the recommended starting dose of CADUET should be selected based on the continuation of the component being used and the recommended starting dose for the added monotherapy.
CADUET may be used to initiate treatment in patients with hyperlipidemia and either hypertension or angina. The recommended starting dose of CADUET should be based on the appropriate combination of recommendations for the monotherapies. The maximum dose of the amlodipine component of CADUET is 10 mg once daily. The maximum dose of the atorvastatin component of CADUET is 80 mg once daily.
See above for detailed information related to the dosing and administration of amlodipine and atorvastatin.

[1] National Cholesterol Education Program (NCEP): Highlights of the Report of the Expert Panel on Blood Cholesterol Levels in Children Adolescents. *Pediatrics*. 89(3):495-501. 1992.

HOW SUPPLIED

CADUET® tablets contain amlodipine besylate and atorvastatin calcium equivalent to amlodipine and atorvastatin in the dose strengths described below.
CADUET tablets are differentiated by tablet color/size and are engraved with "Pfizer" on one side and a unique number on the other side. CADUET tablets are supplied for oral administration in the following strengths and package configurations:
[See table 11 above]

Table 11. CADUET Packaging Configurations

CADUET				
Package Configuration	Tablet Strength (amlodipine besylate/ atorvastatin calcium) mg	NDC #	Engraving	Tablet Color
Bottle of 30	5/10	0069-2150-30	CDT 051	White
Bottle of 30	5/20	0069-2170-30	CDT 052	White
Bottle of 30	5/40	0069-2190-30	CDT 054	White
Bottle of 30	5/80	0069-2260-30	CDT 058	White
Bottle of 30	10/10	0069-2160-30	CDT 101	Blue
Bottle of 30	10/20	0069-2180-30	CDT 102	Blue
Bottle of 30	10/40	0069-2250-30	CDT 104	Blue
Bottle of 30	10/80	0069-2270-30	CDT 108	Blue

Store at 25°C (77°F); excursions permitted to 15-30°C (59-86°F) [see USP Controlled Room Temperature].
Rx only
Manufactured by:
Pfizer Ireland Pharmaceuticals
Dublin, Ireland
Distributed by
Pfizer Labs
Division of Pfizer Inc, NY, NY 10017
69-6113-00-0 **Issued January 2004**

INSPRA™ ℞

[*ĭn-sprä*]
(eplerenone) tablets

DESCRIPTION

INSPRA™ contains eplerenone, a blocker of aldosterone binding at the mineralocorticoid receptor.
Eplerenone is chemically described as Pregn-4-ene-7,21-dicarboxylic acid, 9,11-epoxy-17-hydroxy-3-oxo-, γ-lactone, methyl ester, (7α,11α,17α)-. Its empirical formula is $C_{24}H_{30}O_6$ and it has a molecular weight of 414.50. The structural formula of eplerenone is represented below:

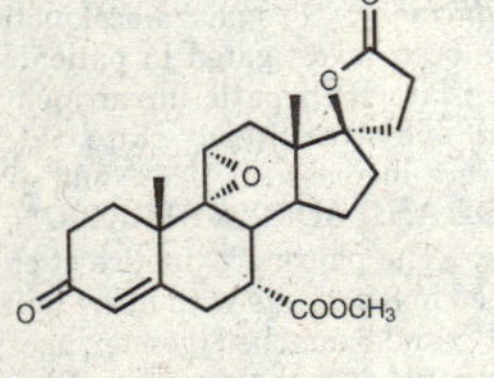

eplerenone

Eplerenone is an odorless, white to off-white crystalline powder. It is very slightly soluble in water, with its solubility essentially pH independent. The octanol/water partition coefficient of eplerenone is approximately 7.1 at pH 7.0.
INSPRA for oral administration contains 25 mg or 50 mg of eplerenone and the following inactive ingredients: lactose, microcrystalline cellulose, croscarmellose sodium, hypromellose, sodium lauryl sulfate, talc, magnesium stearate, titanium dioxide, polyethylene glycol, polysorbate 80, and iron oxide yellow and iron oxide red.

CLINICAL PHARMACOLOGY

Mechanism of Action
Eplerenone binds to the mineralocorticoid receptor and blocks the binding of aldosterone, a component of the renin-angiotensin-aldosterone-system (RAAS). Aldosterone synthesis, which occurs primarily in the adrenal gland, is modulated by multiple factors, including angiotensin II and non-RAAS mediators such as adrenocorticotropic hormone (ACTH) and potassium. Aldosterone binds to mineralocorticoid receptors in both epithelial (e.g., kidney) and nonepi-

Continued on next page

Inspra—Cont.

thelial (e.g., heart, blood vessels, and brain) tissues and increases blood pressure through induction of sodium reabsorption and possibly other mechanisms.

Eplerenone has been shown to produce sustained increases in plasma renin and serum aldosterone, consistent with inhibition of the negative regulatory feedback of aldosterone on renin secretion. The resulting increased plasma renin activity and aldosterone circulating levels do not overcome the effects of eplerenone.

Eplerenone selectively binds to recombinant human mineralocorticoid receptors relative to its binding to recombinant human glucocorticoid, progesterone and androgen receptors.

Pharmacokinetics

General: Eplerenone is cleared predominantly by cytochrome P450 (CYP) 3A4 metabolism, with an elimination half-life of 4 to 6 hours. Steady state is reached within 2 days. Absorption is not affected by food. Inhibitors of CYP3A4 (e.g., ketoconazole, saquinavir) increase blood levels of eplerenone.

Absorption and Distribution: Mean peak plasma concentrations of eplerenone are reached approximately 1.5 hours following oral administration. The absolute bioavailability of eplerenone is unknown. Both peak plasma levels (C_{max}) and area under the curve (AUC) are dose proportional for doses of 25 to 100 mg and less than proportional at doses above 100 mg.

The plasma protein binding of eplerenone is about 50% and it is primarily bound to alpha 1-acid glycoproteins. The apparent volume of distribution at steady state ranged from 43 to 90 L. Eplerenone does not preferentially bind to red blood cells.

Metabolism and Excretion: Eplerenone metabolism is primarily mediated via CYP3A4. No active metabolites of eplerenone have been identified in human plasma.

Less than 5% of an eplerenone dose is recovered as unchanged drug in the urine and feces. Following a single oral dose of radiolabeled drug, approximately 32% of the dose was excreted in the feces and approximately 67% was excreted in the urine. The elimination half-life of eplerenone is approximately 4 to 6 hours. The apparent plasma clearance is approximately 10 L/hr.

Special Populations

Age, Gender, and Race: The pharmacokinetics of eplerenone at a dose of 100 mg once daily have been investigated in the elderly (≥65 years), in males and females, and in blacks. The pharmacokinetics of eplerenone did not differ significantly between males and females. At steady state, elderly subjects had increases in C_{max} (22%) and AUC (45%) compared with younger subjects (18 to 45 years). At steady state, C_{max} was 19% lower and AUC was 26% lower in blacks. (See **PRECAUTIONS, Congestive Heart Failure Post-Myocardial Infarction and Hypertension, Geriatric Use** and **DOSAGE AND ADMINISTRATION, Hypertension.**)

Renal Insufficiency: The pharmacokinetics of eplerenone were evaluated in patients with varying degrees of renal insufficiency and in patients undergoing hemodialysis. Compared with control subjects, steady-state AUC and C_{max} were increased by 38% and 24%, respectively, in patients with severe renal impairment and were decreased by 26% and 3%, respectively, in patients undergoing hemodialysis. No correlation was observed between plasma clearance of eplerenone and creatinine clearance. Eplerenone is not removed by hemodialysis. (See **WARNINGS, Hyperkalemia in Patients Treated for Hypertension** and **PRECAUTIONS, Hyperkalemia in Patients Treated for Congestive Heart Failure Post-Myocardial Infarction and Congestive Heart Failure Post-Myocardial Infarction and Hypertension.**)

Hepatic Insufficiency: The pharmacokinetics of eplerenone 400 mg have been investigated in patients with moderate (Child-Pugh Class B) hepatic impairment and compared with normal subjects. Steady-state C_{max} and AUC of eplerenone were increased by 3.6% and 42%, respectively. (See **DOSAGE AND ADMINISTRATION, Hypertension.**)

Heart Failure: The pharmacokinetics of eplerenone 50 mg were evaluated in 8 patients with heart failure (NYHA classification II-IV) and 8 matched (gender, age, weight) healthy controls. Compared with the controls, steady state AUC and C_{max} in patients with stable heart failure were 38% and 30% higher, respectively.

Drug-Drug Interactions

(See **PRECAUTIONS, Congestive Heart Failure Post-Myocardial Infarction and Hypertension, Drug Interactions.**)

Drug-drug interaction studies were conducted with a 100 mg dose of eplerenone.

Eplerenone is metabolized primarily by CYP3A4. A potent inhibitor of CYP3A4 (ketoconazole) caused increased exposure of about 5-fold while less potent CYP3A4 inhibitors (erythromycin, saquinavir, verapamil, and fluconazole) gave approximately 2-fold increases. Grapefruit juice caused only a small increase (about 25%) in exposure. (See **PRECAUTIONS, Congestive Heart Failure Post-Myocardial Infarction and Hypertension,** Drug Interactions and **DOSAGE AND ADMINISTRATION, Hypertension.**)

Eplerenone is not an inhibitor of CYP1A2, CYP3A4, CYP2C19, CYP2C9, or CYP2D6. Eplerenone did not inhibit the metabolism of chlorzoxazone, diclofenac, methylphenidate, losartan, amiodarone, dexamethasone, mephobarbital, phenytoin, phenacetin, dextromethorphan, metoprolol, tolbutamide, amlodipine, astemizole, cisapride, 17α-ethinyl estradiol, fluoxetine, lovastatin, methylprednisolone, midazolam, nifedipine, simvastatin, triazolam, verapamil, and warfarin in vitro. Eplerenone is not a substrate or an inhibitor of P-Glycoprotein at clinically relevant doses.

No clinically significant drug-drug pharmacokinetic interactions were observed when eplerenone was administered with digoxin, warfarin, midazolam, cisapride, cyclosporine, simvastatin, glyburide, or oral contraceptives (norethindrone/ethinyl estradiol). St. Johns Wort (a CYP3A4 inducer) caused a small (about 30%) decrease in eplerenone AUC.

No significant changes in eplerenone pharmacokinetics were observed when eplerenone was administered with aluminum and magnesium-containing antacids.

CLINICAL STUDIES

Congestive Heart Failure Post-Myocardial Infarction

The eplerenone post-acute myocardial infarction heart failure efficacy and survival study (EPHESUS) was a multinational, multicenter, double-blind, randomized, placebo-controlled study in patients clinically stable 3-14 days after an acute myocardial infarction (MI) with left ventricular dysfunction (as measured by left ventricular ejection fraction [LVEF] ≤40%) and either diabetes or clinical evidence of congestive heart failure (CHF) (pulmonary congestion by exam or chest x-ray or S_3). Patients with CHF of valvular or congenital etiology, patients with unstable post-infarct angina, and patients with serum potassium >5.0 mEq/L or serum creatinine >2.5 mg/dL were to be excluded. Patients were allowed to receive standard post-MI drug therapy and to undergo revascularization by angioplasty or coronary artery bypass graft surgery.

Patients randomized to INSPRA were given an initial dose of 25 mg once daily and titrated to the target dose of 50 mg once daily after 4 weeks if serum potassium was < 5.0 mEq/L. Dosage was reduced or suspended anytime during the study if serum potassium levels were ≥ 5.5 mEq/L. (See **DOSAGE AND ADMINISTRATION, Congestive Heart Failure Post-Myocardial Infarction.**)

EPHESUS randomized 6,632 patients (9.3% U.S.) at 671 centers in 27 countries. The study population was primarily white (90%, with 1% black, 1% Asian, 6% Hispanic, 2% other) and male (71%). The mean age was 64 years (range, 22-94 years). The majority of patients had pulmonary congestion (75%) by exam or x-ray and were Killip Class II (64%). The mean ejection fraction was 33%. The average time to enrollment was 7 days post-MI. Medical histories prior to the index MI included hypertension (60%), coronary artery disease (62%), dyslipidemia (48%), angina (41%), type 2 diabetes (30%), previous MI (27%), and HF (15%).

The mean dose of INSPRA was 43 mg/day. Patients also received standard care including aspirin (92%), ACE inhibitors (90%), β-blockers (83%), nitrates (72%), loop diuretics (66%), or HMG-CoA reductase inhibitors (60%).

Patients were followed for an average of 16 months (range, 0-33 months). The ascertainment rate for vital status was 99.7%.

The co-primary endpoints for EPHESUS were (1) the time to death from any cause, and (2) the time to first occurrence of either cardiovascular (CV) mortality [defined as sudden cardiac death or death due to progression of congestive heart failure (CHF), stroke, or other CV causes] or CV hospitalization (defined as hospitalization for progression of CHF, ventricular arrhythmias, acute myocardial infarction, or stroke). For the co-primary endpoint for death from any cause, there were 478 deaths in the INSPRA group (14.4%) and 554 deaths in the placebo group (16.7%). The risk of death with INSPRA was reduced by 15% [hazard ratio equal to 0.85 (95% confidence interval 0.75 to 0.96; p = 0.008 by log rank test)]. Kaplan-Meier estimates of all-cause mortality are shown in Figure 1 and the components of mortality are provided in Table 1.

Figure 1. Kaplan-Meier Estimates of All-Cause Mortality

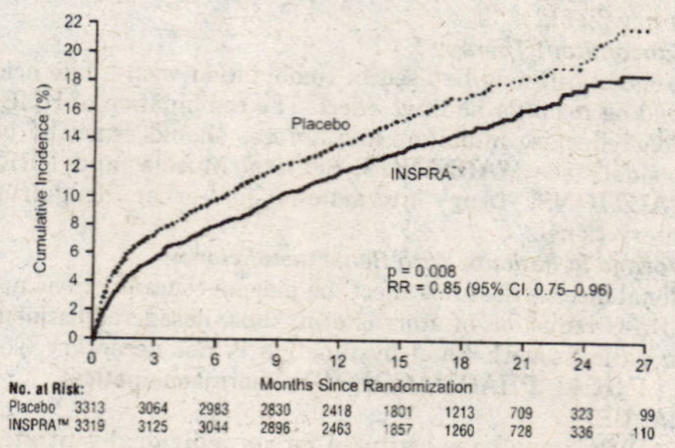

Table 1. Components of All-Cause Mortality in EPHESUS

	INSPRA™ (N=3319) n (%)	Placebo (N=3313) n (%)	Hazard Ratio	p-value
Death from any cause	478 (14.4)	554 (16.7)	0.85	0.008
CV Death	407 (12.3)	483 (14.6)	0.83	0.005
Non-CV Death	60 (1.8)	54 (1.6)		
Unknown or unwitnessed death	11 (0.3)	17 (0.5)		

Most CV deaths were attributed to sudden death, acute MI, and CHF.

The time to first event for the co-primary endpoint of CV death or hospitalization as defined above, was longer in the INSPRA group (hazard ratio 0.87, 95% confidence interval 0.79 to 0.95, p = 0.002). An analysis that included the time to first occurrence of CV mortality and all CV hospitalizations (atrial arrhythmia, angina, CV procedures, progression of CHF, MI, stroke, ventricular arrhythmia, or other CV causes) showed a smaller effect with a hazard ratio of 0.92 (95% confidence interval 0.86 to 0.99; p = 0.028). The combined endpoints, including combined all-cause hospitalization and mortality were driven primarily by CV mortality. The combined endpoints in EPHESUS, including all-cause hospitalization and all-cause mortality, are presented in Table 2.

Table 2. Rates of Death or Hospitalization in EPHESUS

Event	INSPRA™ n (%)	Placebo n (%)
CV death or hospitalization for progression of CHF, stroke, MI or ventricular arrhythmia[1]	885 (26.7)	993 (30.0)
Death	407 (12.3)	483 (14.6)
Hospitalization	606 (18.3)	649 (19.6)
CV death or hospitalization for progression of CHF, stroke, MI, ventricular arrhythmia, atrial arrhythmia, angina, CV procedures, or other CV causes (PVD; Hypotension)	1516 (45.7)	1610 (48.6)
Death	407 (12.3)	483 (14.6)
Hospitalization	1281 (38.6)	1307 (39.5)
All-cause death or hospitalization	1734 (52.2)	1833 (55.3)
Death[1]	478 (14.4)	554 (16.7)
Hospitalization	1497 (45.1)	1530 (46.2)

[1]Co-Primary Endpoint.

Mortality hazard ratios varied for some subgroups as shown in Figure 2. Mortality hazard ratios appeared favorable for INSPRA for both genders and for all races or ethnic groups, although the numbers of non-caucasians were low (648, 10%). Patients with diabetes without clinical evidence of CHF and patients greater than 75 years did not appear to benefit from the use of INSPRA. Such subgroup analyses must be interpreted cautiously.

[See figure 2 at top of next page]

Analyses conducted for a variety of CV biomarkers did not confirm a mechanism of action by which mortality was reduced.

Hypertension

The safety and efficacy of INSPRA have been evaluated alone and in combination with other antihypertensive agents in clinical studies of 3091 hypertensive patients. The studies included 46% women, 14% blacks, and 22% elderly (age ≥65). The studies excluded patients with elevated baseline serum potassium (>5.0 mEq/L) and elevated baseline serum creatinine (generally >1.5 mg/dL in males and >1.3 mg/dL in females).

Two fixed-dose, placebo-controlled, 8- to 12-week monotherapy studies in patients with baseline diastolic blood pressures of 95 to 114 mm Hg were conducted to assess the antihypertensive effect of INSPRA. In these two studies, 611 patients were randomized to INSPRA and 140 patients to placebo. Patients received INSPRA in doses of 25 to 400 mg daily as either a single daily dose or divided into two daily doses. The mean placebo-subtracted reductions in trough cuff blood pressure achieved by INSPRA in these studies at doses up to 200 mg are shown in Figures 3 and 4.

Figure 3. INSPRA™ Dose Response – Trough Cuff SBP Placebo-Subtracted Adjusted Mean Change from Baseline in Hypertension Studies

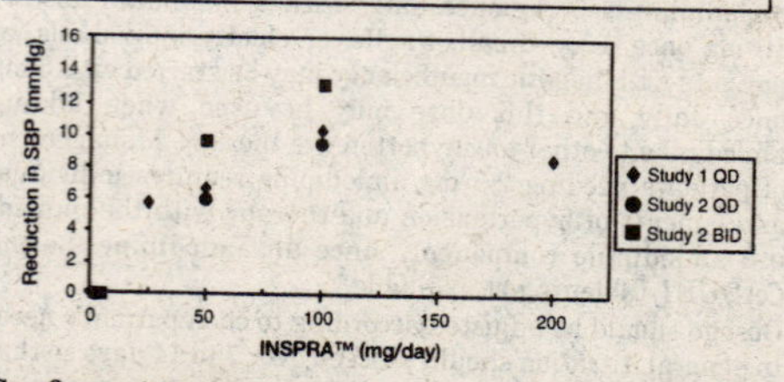

[See figure 4 on next page]

Patients treated with INSPRA 50 to 200 mg daily experienced significant decreases in sitting systolic and diastolic blood pressure at trough with differences from placebo of 6-13 mm Hg (systolic) and 3-7 mm Hg (diastolic). These effects were confirmed by assessments with 24-hour ambulatory blood pressure monitoring (ABPM). In these studies,

Figure 2. Hazard Ratios of All-Cause Mortality by Subgroups

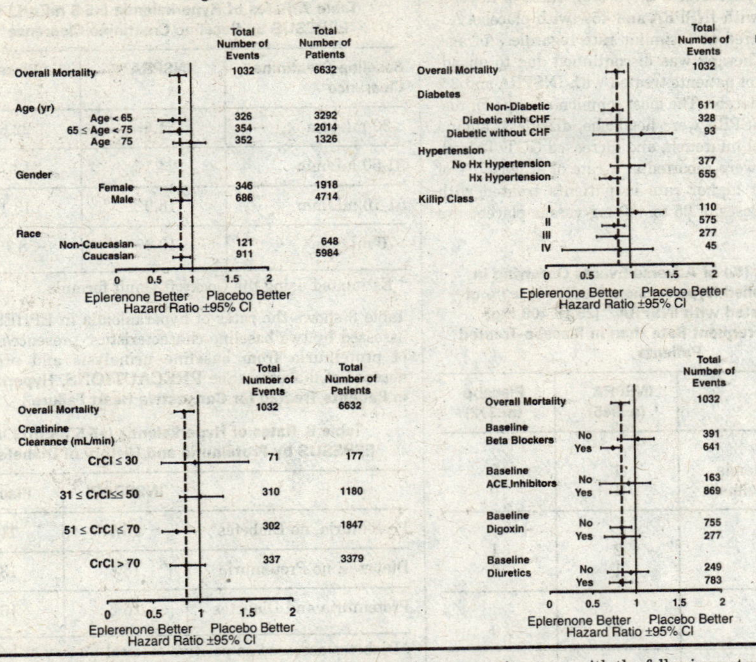

Figure 4. INSPRA™ Dose Response – Trough Cuff DBP Placebo-Subtracted Adjusted Mean Change from Baseline in Hypertension Studies

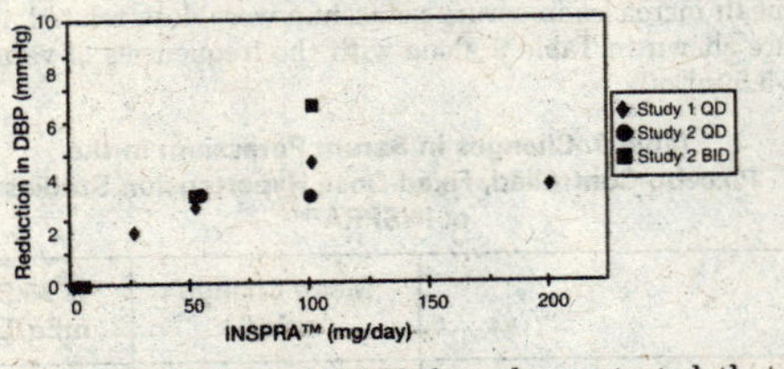

assessments of 24-hour ABPM data demonstrated that INSPRA, administered once or twice daily, maintained antihypertensive efficacy over the entire dosing interval. However, at a total daily dose of 100 mg, INSPRA administered as 50 mg twice per day produced greater trough cuff (4/3 mm Hg) and ABPM (2/1 mm Hg) blood pressure reductions than 100 mg given once daily.

Blood pressure lowering was apparent within 2 weeks from the start of therapy with INSPRA, with maximal antihypertensive effects achieved within 4 weeks. Stopping INSPRA following treatment for 8 to 24 weeks in six studies did not lead to adverse event rates in the week following withdrawal of INSPRA greater than following placebo or active control withdrawal. Blood pressures in patients not taking other antihypertensives rose 1 week after withdrawal of INSPRA by about 6/3 mm Hg, suggesting that the antihypertensive effect of INSPRA was maintained through 8 to 24 weeks.

Blood pressure reductions with INSPRA in the two fixed-dose monotherapy studies and other studies using titrated doses, as well as concomitant treatments, were not significantly different when analyzed by age, gender, or race with one exception. In a study in patients with low renin hypertension, blood pressure reductions in blacks were smaller than those in whites during the initial titration period with INSPRA.

INSPRA has been studied concomitantly with treatment with ACE inhibitors, angiotensin II receptor antagonists, calcium channel blockers, beta blockers, and hydrochlorothiazide. When administered concomitantly with one of these drugs INSPRA usually produced its expected antihypertensive effects.

There was no significant change in average heart rate among patients treated with INSPRA in the combined clinical studies. No consistent effects of INSPRA on heart rate, QRS duration, or PR or QT interval were observed in 147 normal subjects evaluated for electrocardiographic changes during pharmacokinetic studies.

INDICATIONS AND USAGE

Congestive Heart Failure Post-Myocardial Infarction

INSPRA is indicated to improve survival of stable patients with left ventricular systolic dysfunction (ejection fraction ≤40%) and clinical evidence of congestive heart failure after an acute myocardial infarction. (See **CLINICAL STUDIES, Congestive Heart Failure Post-Myocardial Infarction).**

Hypertension

INSPRA is indicated for the treatment of hypertension. INSPRA may be used alone or in combination with other antihypertensive agents. (See **CLINICAL STUDIES, Hypertension.**)

CONTRAINDICATIONS

INSPRA is contraindicated in all patients with the following:

- serum potassium >5.5 mEq/L at initiation
- creatinine clearance ≤30 mL/min
- concomitant use with the following potent CYP3A4 inhibitors: ketoconazole, itraconazole, nefazodone, troleandomycin, clarithromycin, ritonavir, and nelfinavir. Inspra should also not be used with other drugs noted in the **CONTRAINDICATIONS, WARNINGS** or **PRECAUTIONS** sections of their labeling to be potent CYP3A4 inhibitors. (See **CLINICAL PHARMACOLOGY, Drug-Drug Interactions; PRECAUTIONS, Congestive Heart Failure Post-Myocardial Infarction and Hypertension, Drug Interactions** and **DOSAGE AND ADMINISTRATION, Hypertension.**)

Hypertension

INSPRA is also contraindicated for the treatment of hypertension in patients with the following:

- type 2 diabetes with microalbuminuria
- serum creatinine >2.0 mg/dL in males or >1.8 mg/dL in females
- creatinine clearance <50 mL/min
- concomitant use of potassium supplements or potassium-sparing diuretics (amiloride, spironolactone, or triamterene)

(See **CLINICAL PHARMACOLOGY, Pharmacokinetics, Drug-Drug Interactions; WARNINGS, Hyperkalemia in Patients Treated for Hypertension; PRECAUTIONS, Congestive Heart Failure Post-Myocardial Infarction and Hypertension, Drug Interactions;** and **ADVERSE REACTIONS, Clinical Laboratory Test Findings, Hypertension, Potassium.**)

WARNINGS

Hyperkalemia in Patients Treated for Hypertension

The principal risk of INSPRA is hyperkalemia. Hyperkalemia can cause serious, sometimes fatal, arrhythmias. This risk can be minimized by patient selection, avoidance of certain concomitant treatments, and monitoring. For patient selection and avoidance of certain concomitant medications, see **CONTRAINDICATIONS; PRECAUTIONS, Congestive Heart Failure Post-Myocardial Infarction and Hypertension, Drug Interactions;** and **ADVERSE REACTIONS, Clinical Laboratory Test Findings, Congestive Heart Failure Post-Myocardial Infarction and Hypertension, Potassium.** Periodic monitoring is recommended in patients at risk for the development of hyperkalemia (including patients receiving concomitant ACE inhibitors or angiotensin II receptor antagonists) until the effect of INSPRA is established. Dose reduction of INSPRA has been shown to decrease potassium levels. (See **DOSAGE AND ADMINISTRATION, Congestive Heart Failure Post-Myocardial Infarction and Hypertension.**)

PRECAUTIONS

Hyperkalemia in Patients Treated for Congestive Heart Failure Post-Myocardial Infarction

The principal risk of INSPRA is hyperkalemia. Hyperkalemia can cause serious, sometimes fatal, arrhythmias. Patients who develop hyperkalemia (>5.5 mEq/L) may still benefit from INSPRA with proper dose adjustment. Hyperkalemia can be minimized by patient selection, avoidance of certain concomitant treatments, and periodic monitoring until the effect of INSPRA has been established. For patient selection and avoidance of certain concomitant medications, see **CONTRAINDICATIONS; PRECAUTIONS, Congestive Heart Failure Post-Myocardial Infarction and Hypertension, Drug Interactions;** and **ADVERSE REACTIONS, Clinical Laboratory Test Findings, Congestive Heart Failure Post-Myocardial Infarction, Potassium.** Dose reduction of INSPRA has been shown to decrease potassium levels. (See **DOSAGE AND ADMINISTRATION, Congestive Heart Failure Post-Myocardial Infarction.**)

Patients with CHF post MI who have serum creatinine levels >2.0 mg/dL (males) or >1.8 mg/dL (females) or creatinine clearance ≤50 mL/min should be treated with caution. The rates of hyperkalemia increased with declining renal function. (See **ADVERSE REACTIONS, Clinical Laboratory Test Findings, Congestive Heart Failure Post-Myocardial Infarction, Potassium.**)

Diabetic patients with CHF post-MI, including those with proteinuria, should also be treated with caution. The subset of patients in EPHESUS with both diabetes and proteinuria on the baseline urinalysis had increased rates of hyperkalemia. (See **ADVERSE REACTIONS Clinical Laboratory Test Findings, Congestive Heart Failure Post-Myocardial Infarction, Potassium.**)

Congestive Heart Failure Post-Myocardial Infarction and Hypertension

Impaired Hepatic Function: In 16 subjects with mild-to-moderate hepatic impairment who received 400 mg of eplerenone no elevations of serum potassium above 5.5 mEq/L were observed. The mean increase in serum potassium was 0.12 mEq/L in patients with hepatic impairment and 0.13 mEq/L in normal controls. The use of INSPRA in patients with severe hepatic impairment has not been evaluated. (See **DOSAGE AND ADMINISTRATION** and **CLINICAL PHARMACOLOGY, Special Populations.**)

Impaired Renal Function: (See **CONTRAINDICATIONS; WARNINGS;** and **PRECAUTIONS.**)

Information for Patients: Patients receiving INSPRA should be informed not to use potassium supplements, salt substitutes containing potassium, or contraindicated drugs without consulting the prescribing physician. (See **CONTRAINDICATIONS; WARNINGS;** and **PRECAUTIONS.**)

Drug Interactions:

Inhibitors of CYP3A4- Eplerenone metabolism is predominantly mediated via CYP3A4. A pharmacokinetic study evaluating the administration of a single dose of INSPRA 100 mg with ketoconazole 200 mg BID, a potent inhibitor of the CYP3A4 pathway, showed a 1.7-fold increase in C_{max} of eplerenone and a 5.4-fold increase in AUC of eplerenone. INSPRA should not be used with drugs described as strong inhibitors of CYP3A4 in their labeling. (See **CONTRAINDICATIONS.**)

Administration of eplerenone with other CYP3A4 inhibitors (e.g., erythromycin 500 mg BID, verapamil 240 mg QD, saquinavir 1200 mg TID, fluconazole 200 mg QD) resulted in increases in C_{max} of eplerenone ranging from 1.4- to 1.6-fold and AUC from 2.0- to 2.9-fold. (See **CLINICAL PHARMACOLOGY, Pharmacokinetics, Drug-Drug Interactions** and **DOSAGE AND ADMINISTRATION, Hypertension.**)

ACE Inhibitors and Angiotensin II Receptor Antagonists (Congestive Heart Failure Post-Myocardial Infarction)- In EPHESUS, 3020 (91%) patients receiving INSPRA 25 to 50 mg also received ACE inhibitors or angiotensin II receptor antagonists (ACEI/ARB). Rates of patients with maximum potassium levels >5.5 mEq/L were similar regardless of the use of ACEI/ARB.

ACE Inhibitors and Angiotensin II Receptor Antagonists (Hypertension)- In clinical studies of patients with hypertension, the addition of INSPRA 50 to 100 mg to ACE inhibitors and angiotensin II receptor antagonists increased mean serum potassium slightly (about 0.09-0.13 mEq/L). In a study in diabetics with microalbuminuria INSPRA 200 mg combined with the ACE inhibitor enalapril 10 mg increased the frequency of hyperkalemia (serum potassium >5.5 mEq/L) from 17% on enalapril alone to 38%. (See **CONTRAINDICATIONS.**)

Lithium- A drug interaction study of eplerenone with lithium has not been conducted. Lithium toxicity has been reported in patients receiving lithium concomitantly with diuretics and ACE inhibitors. Serum lithium levels should be monitored frequently if INSPRA is administered concomitantly with lithium.

Nonsteroidal Anti-Inflammatory Drugs (NSAIDs)- A drug interaction study of eplerenone with an NSAID has not been conducted. The administration of other potassium-sparing antihypertensives with NSAIDs has been shown to reduce the antihypertensive effect in some patients and result in severe hyperkalemia in patients with impaired renal function. Therefore, when INSPRA and NSAIDs are used concomitantly, patients should be observed to determine whether the desired effect on blood pressure is obtained.

Pregnancy:

Pregnancy Category B- There are no adequate and well-controlled studies in pregnant women. INSPRA should be used during pregnancy only if the potential benefit justifies the potential risk to the fetus.

Teratogenic Effects- Embryo-fetal development studies were conducted with doses up to 1000 mg/kg/day in rats and 300 mg/kg/day in rabbits (exposures up to 32 and 31 times the human AUC for the 100-mg/day therapeutic dose, respectively). No teratogenic effects were seen in rats or rabbits, although decreased body weight in maternal rabbits and increased rabbit fetal resorptions and post-implantation loss were observed at the highest administered dosage. Because animal reproduction studies are not always predictive of human response, INSPRA should be used during pregnancy only if clearly needed.

Nursing Mothers: The concentration of eplerenone in human breast milk after oral administration is unknown. However preclinical data show that eplerenone and/or metabolites are present in rat breast milk (0.85:1 [milk:plasma] AUC ratio) obtained after a single oral dose. Peak concentrations in plasma and milk were obtained from 0.5 to 1 hour after dosing. Rat pups exposed by this route

Continued on next page

Inspra—Cont.

developed normally. Because many drugs are excreted in human milk and because of the unknown potential for adverse effects on the nursing infant, a decision should be made whether to discontinue nursing or discontinue the drug, taking into account the importance of the drug to the mother.

Pediatric Use: The safety and effectiveness of INSPRA has not been established in pediatric patients.

Geriatric Use:

Congestive Heart Failure Post-Myocardial Infarction- Of the total number of patients in EPHESUS, 3340 (50%) were 65 and over, while 1326 (20%) were 75 and over. Patients greater than 75 years did not appear to benefit from the use of INSPRA. (See **CLINICAL STUDIES, Congestive Heart Failure Post-Myocardial Infarction.**) No differences in overall incidence of adverse events were observed between elderly and younger patients. However, due to age-related decreases in creatinine clearance, the incidence of laboratory-documented hyperkalemia was increased in patients 65 and older. (See **PRECAUTIONS, Hyperkalemia in Patients Treated for Congestive Heart Failure.**)

Hypertension- Of the total number of subjects in clinical hypertension studies of INSPRA, 1123 (23%) were 65 and over, while 212 (4%) were 75 and over. No overall differences in safety or effectiveness were observed between elderly subjects and younger subjects.

Carcinogenesis, Mutagenesis, Impairment of Fertility: Eplerenone was non-genotoxic in a battery of assays including in vitro bacterial mutagenesis (Ames test in *Salmonella* spp. and *E. Coli*), in vitro mammalian cell mutagenesis (mouse lymphoma cells), in vitro chromosomal aberration (Chinese hamster ovary cells), in vivo rat bone marrow micronucleus formation, and in vivo/ex vivo unscheduled DNA synthesis in rat liver.

There was no drug-related tumor response in heterozygous P53 deficient mice when tested for 6 months at dosages up to 1000 mg/kg/day (systemic AUC exposures up to 9 times the exposure in humans receiving the 100-mg/day therapeutic dose). Statistically significant increases in benign thyroid tumors were observed after 2 years in both male and female rats when administered eplerenone 250 mg/kg/day (highest dose tested) and in male rats only at 75 mg/kg/day. These dosages provided systemic AUC exposures approximately 2 to 12 times higher than the average human therapeutic exposure at 100 mg/day. Repeat dose administration of eplerenone to rats increases the hepatic conjugation and clearance of thyroxin, which results in increased levels of TSH by a compensatory mechanism. Drugs that have produced thyroid tumors by this rodent-specific mechanism have not shown a similar effect in humans.

Male rats treated with eplerenone at 1000 mg/kg/day for 10 weeks (AUC 17 times that at the 100-mg/day human therapeutic dose) had decreased weights of seminal vesicles and epididymides and slightly decreased fertility. Dogs administered eplerenone at dosages of 15 mg/kg/day and higher (AUC 5 times that at the 100-mg/day human therapeutic dose) had dose-related prostate atrophy. The prostate atrophy was reversible after daily treatment for 1 year at 100 mg/kg/day. Dogs with prostate atrophy showed no decline in libido, sexual performance, or semen quality. Testicular weight and histology were not affected by eplerenone in any test animal species at any dosage.

ADVERSE REACTIONS

Congestive Heart Failure Post-Myocardial Infarction

In EPHESUS, safety was evaluated in 3307 patients treated with INSPRA and 3301 placebo-treated patients. The overall incidence of adverse events reported with INSPRA (78.9%) was similar to placebo (79.5%). Adverse events occurred at a similar rate regardless of age, gender, or race. Patients discontinued treatment due to an adverse event at similar rates in either treatment group (4.4% INSPRA vs. 4.3% placebo).

Adverse events that occurred more frequently in patients treated with INSPRA than placebo were hyperkalemia (3.4% vs 2.0%) and increased creatinine (2.4% vs 1.5%). Discontinuations due to hyperkalemia or abnormal renal function were less than 1.0% in both groups. Hypokalemia occurred less frequently in patients treated with INSPRA (0.6% vs. 1.6%).

The rates of sex hormone related adverse events are shown in Table 3.

Table 3. Rates of Sex Hormone Related Adverse Events in EPHESUS

	Rates in Males			Rates in Females
	Gynecomastia	Mastodynia	Either	Abnormal Vaginal Bleeding
INSPRA™	0.4%	0.1%	0.5%	0.4%
Placebo	0.5%	0.1%	0.6%	0.4%

Hypertension

INSPRA has been evaluated for safety in 3091 patients treated for hypertension. A total of 690 patients were treated for over 6 months and 106 patients were treated for over 1 year.

In placebo-controlled studies, the overall rates of adverse events were 47% with INSPRA and 45% with placebo. Adverse events occurred at a similar rate regardless of age, gender, or race. Therapy was discontinued due to an adverse event in 3% of patients treated with INSPRA and 3% of patients given placebo. The most common reasons for discontinuation of INSPRA were headache, dizziness, angina pectoris/myocardial infarction, and increased GGT. The adverse events that were reported at a rate of at least 1% of patients and at a higher rate in patients treated with INSPRA in daily doses of 25 to 400 mg versus placebo are shown in Table 4.

Table 4. Rates (%) of Adverse Events Occurring in Placebo-Controlled Hypertension Studies in ≥1% of Patients Treated with INSPRA™ (25 to 400 mg) and at a More Frequent Rate than in Placebo-Treated Patients

	INSPRA™ (n=945)	Placebo (n=372)
Metabolic		
Hypercholesterolemia	1	0
Hypertriglyceridemia	1	0
Digestive		
Diarrhea	2	1
Abdominal pain	1	0
Urinary		
Albuminuria	1	0
Respiratory		
Coughing	2	1
Central/Peripheral Nervous System		
Dizziness	3	2
Body as a Whole		
Fatigue	2	1
Influenza-like symptoms	2	1

Note: Adverse events that are too general to be informative or are very common in the treated population are excluded.

Gynecomastia and abnormal vaginal bleeding were reported with INSPRA but not with placebo. The rates of these sex hormone related adverse events are shown in Table 5. The rates increased slightly with increasing duration of therapy. In females, abnormal vaginal bleeding was also reported in 0.8% of patients on antihypertensive medications (other than spironolactone) in active control arms of the studies with INSPRA.

Table 5. Rates of Sex Hormone Related Adverse Events with INSPRA™ in Hypertension Clinical Studies

	Rates in Males			Rates in Females
	Gynecomastia	Mastodynia	Either	Abnormal Vaginal Bleeding
All controlled studies	0.5%	0.8%	1.0%	0.6%
Controlled studies lasting ≥ 6 months	0.7%	1.3%	1.6%	0.8%
Open label, long-term study	1.0%	0.3%	1.0%	2.1%

Clinical Laboratory Test Findings

Congestive Heart Failure Post-Myocardial Infarction:

Creatinine- Increases of more than 0.5 mg/dL were reported for 6.5% of patients administered INSPRA and for 4.9% of placebo-treated patients.

Potassium- In EPHESUS, the frequency of patients with changes in potassium (<3.5 mEq/L or >5.5 mEq/L or ≥6.0 mEq/L) receiving INSPRA compared with placebo are displayed in Table 6.

Table 6. Hypokalemia (<3.5 mEq/L) or Hyperkalemia (>5.5 or ≥6.0 mEq/L) in EPHESUS

Potassium (mEq/L)	INSPRA™ (N=3251) n (%)	Placebo (N=3237) n (%)
< 3.5	273 (8.4)	424 (13.1)
>5.5	508 (15.6)	363 (11.2)
≥ 6.0	180 (5.5)	126 (3.9)

Table 7 shows the rates of hyperkalemia in EPHESUS as assessed by baseline renal function (creatinine clearance).

Table 7. Rates of Hyperkalemia (>5.5 mEq/L) in EPHESUS by Baseline Creatinine Clearance*

Baseline Creatinine Clearance	INSPRA™	Placebo
≤30 mL/min	31.5%	22.6%
31-50 mL/min	24.1%	12.7%
51-70 mL/min	16.9%	13.1%
>70 mL/min	10.8%	8.7%

* Estimated using the Cockroft-Gault formula.

Table 8 shows the rates of hyperkalemia in EPHESUS as assessed by two baseline characteristics: presence/absence of proteinuria from baseline urinalysis and presence/absence of diabetes. (See **PRECAUTIONS, Hyperkalemia in Patients Treated for Congestive Heart Failure.**)

Table 8. Rates of Hyperkalemia (>5.5 mEq/L) in EPHESUS by Proteinuria and History of Diabetes*

	INSPRA™	Placebo
Proteinuria, no Diabetes	16%	11%
Diabetes, no Proteinuria	18%	13%
Proteinuria and Diabetes	26%	16%

*Diabetes assessed as positive medical history at baseline; proteinuria assessed by positive dipstick urinalysis at baseline.

Hypertension:

Potassium- In placebo-controlled fixed-dose studies, the mean increases in serum potassium were dose related and are shown in Table 9 along with the frequencies of values >5.5 mEq/L.

Table 9. Changes in Serum Potassium in the Placebo-Controlled, Fixed-Dose Hypertension Studies of INSPRA™

Daily Dosage	n	Mean Change mEq/L	% >5.5 mEq/L
Placebo	194	0	1
25	97	0.08	0
50	245	0.14	0
100	193	0.09	1
200	139	0.19	1
400	104	0.36	8.7

Patients with both type 2 diabetes and microalbuminuria are at increased risk of developing persistent hyperkalemia. In a study in such patients taking INSPRA 200 mg, the frequencies of maximum serum potassium levels >5.5 mEq/L were 33% with INSPRA given alone and 38% when INSPRA was given with enalapril.

Rates of hyperkalemia increased with decreasing renal function. In all studies serum potassium elevations >5.5 mEq/L were observed in 10.4% of patients treated with INSPRA with baseline calculated creatinine clearance <70 mL/min, 5.6% of patients with baseline creatinine clearance of 70 to 100 mL/min, and 2.6% of patients with baseline creatinine clearance of >100 mL/min. (See **WARNINGS, Hyperkalemia in Patients Treated for Hypertension.**)

Sodium- Serum sodium decreased in a dose-related manner. Mean decreases ranged from 0.7 mEq/L at 50 mg daily to 1.7 mEq/L at 400 mg daily. Decreases in sodium (<135 mEq/L) were reported for 2.3% of patients administered INSPRA and 0.6% of placebo-treated patients.

Triglycerides- Serum triglycerides increased in a dose-related manner. Mean increases ranged from 7.1 mg/dL at 50 mg daily to 26.6 mg/dL at 400 mg daily. Increases in triglycerides (above 252 mg/dL) were reported for 15% of patients administered INSPRA and 12% of placebo-treated patients.

Cholesterol- Serum cholesterol increased in a dose-related manner. Mean changes ranged from a decrease of 0.4 mg/dL at 50 mg daily to an increase of 11.6 mg/dL at 400 mg daily. Increases in serum cholesterol values greater than 200 mg/dL were reported for 0.3% of patients administered INSPRA and 0% of placebo-treated patients.

Liver Function Tests- Serum alanine aminotransferase (ALT) and gamma glutamyl transpeptidase (GGT) increased in a dose-related manner. Mean increases ranged from 0.8 U/L at 50 mg daily to 4.8 U/L at 400 mg daily for ALT and 3.1 U/L at 50 mg daily to 11.3 U/L at 400 mg daily for GGT. Increases in ALT levels greater than 120 U/L (3 times upper limit of normal) were reported for 15/2259 patients administered INSPRA and 1/351 placebo-treated patients. Increases in ALT levels greater than 200 U/L (5 times upper limit of normal) were reported for 5/2259 of patients administered INSPRA and 1/351 placebo-treated patients. Increases of ALT greater than 120 U/L and bilirubin greater than 1.2 mg/dL were reported 1/2259 patients administered INSPRA and 0/351 placebo-treated patients. Hepatic failure was not reported in patients receiving INSPRA.

BUN/Creatinine- Serum creatinine increased in a dose-related manner. Mean increases ranged from 0.01 mg/dL at 50 mg daily to 0.03 mg/dL at 400 mg daily. Increases in blood urea nitrogen to greater than 30 mg/dL and serum creatinine to greater than 2 mg/dL were reported for 0.5% and 0.2%, respectively, of patients administered INSPRA and 0% of placebo-treated patients.

Uric Acid- Increases in uric acid to greater than 9 mg/dL were reported in 0.3% of patients administered INSPRA and 0% of placebo-treated patients.

OVERDOSAGE

No cases of human overdosage with eplerenone have been reported. Lethality was not observed in mice, rats, or dogs after single oral doses that provided C_{max} exposures at least 25 times higher than in humans receiving eplerenone 100 mg/day. Dogs showed emesis, salivation, and tremors at a C_{max} 41 times the human therapeutic C_{max}, progressing to sedation and convulsions at higher exposures.

The most likely manifestation of human overdosage would be anticipated to be hypotension or hyperkalemia. Eplerenone cannot be removed by hemodialysis. Eplerenone has been shown to bind extensively to charcoal. If symptomatic hypotension should occur, supportive treatment should be instituted. If hyperkalemia develops, standard treatment should be initiated.

DOSAGE AND ADMINISTRATION

Congestive Heart Failure Post-Myocardial Infarction

The recommended dose of INSPRA is 50 mg once daily. Treatment should be initiated at 25 mg once daily and titrated to the target dose of 50 mg once daily preferably within 4 weeks as tolerated by the patient. INSPRA may be administered with or without food.

Serum potassium should be measured before initiating INSPRA therapy, within the first week and at one month after the start of treatment or dose adjustment. Serum potassium should be assessed periodically thereafter. Factors such as patient characteristics and serum potassium levels may indicate that additional monitoring is appropriate. (See **PRECAUTIONS, Hyperkalemia in Patients Treated for Congestive Heart Failure** and **ADVERSE REACTIONS, Clinical Laboratory Test Findings, Congestive Heart Failure Post-Myocardial Infarction, Potassium.**) In EPHESUS, the majority of hyperkalemia was observed within the first three months after randomization. The dose should be adjusted based on the serum potassium level and the dose adjustment table shown in Table 10.

Table 10. Dose Adjustment in Congestive Heart Failure

Serum Potassium (mEq/L)	Action	Dose Adjustment
< 5.0	Increase	25mg QOD to 25mg QD 25mg QD to 50mg QD
5.0-5.4	Maintain	No adjustment
5.5-5.9	Decrease	50mg QD to 25mg QD 25mg QD to 25mg QOD 25mg QOD to withhold
≥ 6.0	Withhold	

Following withholding INSPRA due to serum potassium ≥6.0 mEq/L, INSPRA can be restarted at a dose of 25 mg QOD when serum potassium levels have fallen below 5.5 mEq/L.

Hypertension

INSPRA may be used alone or in combination with other antihypertensive agents. The recommended starting dose of INSPRA is 50 mg administered once daily. The full therapeutic effect of INSPRA is apparent within 4 weeks. For patients with an inadequate blood pressure response to 50 mg once daily the dosage of INSPRA should be increased to 50 mg twice daily. Higher dosages of INSPRA are not recommended either because they have no greater effect on blood pressure than 100 mg or because they are associated with an increased risk of hyperkalemia. (See **CLINICAL STUDIES, Hypertension.**)

No adjustment of the starting dose is recommended for the elderly or for patients with mild-to-moderate hepatic impairment. For patients receiving weak CYP3A4 inhibitors, such as erythromycin, saquinavir, verapamil, and fluconazole the starting dose should be reduced to 25 mg once daily. (See **CONTRAINDICATIONS** and **PRECAUTIONS, Congestive Heart Failure Post-Myocardial Infarction and Hypertension, Drug Interactions.**)

HOW SUPPLIED

INSPRA Tablets, 25 mg, are yellow diamond biconvex film-coated tablets. They are debossed with *Pfizer* on one side and *NSR* over *25* on the other. They are supplied as follows:

NDC Number	Size
0025-1710-01	Bottle of 30 tablets
0025-1710-02	Bottle of 90 tablets
0025-1710-03	Hospital Unit Dose

INSPRA Tablets, 50 mg, are yellow diamond biconvex film-coated tablets. They are debossed with *Pfizer* on one side and *NSR* over *50* on the other. They are supplied as follows:

NDC Number	Size
0025-1720-03	Bottle of 30 tablets
0025-1720-01	Bottle of 90 tablets

Store at 25°C (77°F); excursions permitted to 15-30°C (59-86°F) [See USP Controlled Room Temperature].

Rx only

U.S. Patent No. 4,559,332

INSPRA Tablets are manufactured for:
G.D. Searle LLC
October 2003
Distributed by
Pfizer
G.D. Searle LLC
Subsidiary of Pfizer Inc, NY, NY 10017
819 570 103A P04036-4

Schwarz Pharma, Inc.
6140 W. EXECUTIVE DRIVE
MEQUON, WI 53092

For Medical Information Contact:
Schwarz Pharma, Inc.
Medical and Drug Information
(262) 238-9994
(800) 558-5114

TRILYTE™ with flavor packs ℞
[*trī-līt*]
(PEG-3350, sodium chloride, sodium bicarbonate and potassium chloride for oral solution)
Rx Only

DESCRIPTION

TriLyte is a white powder for reconstitution containing 420 g polyethylene glycol 3350, 5.72 g sodium bicarbonate, 11.2 g sodium chloride, 1.48 g potassium chloride. Flavor packs, each containing 3.22 g of flavoring ingredients, are attached to the 4 liter bottle. See individual flavor packs for complete listing of ingredients. When dissolved in water to a volume of 4 liters, TriLyte™ with flavor packs (PEG-3350, sodium chloride, sodium bicarbonate and potassium chloride for oral solution) is an isosmotic solution, for oral administration, having a pleasant mineral water taste. One flavor pack can be added before reconstitution to flavor the solution. TriLyte™ with flavor packs is administered orally or via nasogastric tube as a gastrointestinal lavage.

CLINICAL PHARMACOLOGY

TriLyte™ with flavor packs induces a diarrhea which rapidly cleanses the bowel, usually within 4 hours. The osmotic activity of polyethylene glycol 3350 and the electrolyte concentration result in virtually no net absorption or excretion of ions or water. Accordingly, large volumes may be administered without significant changes in fluid or electrolyte balance.

INDICATIONS AND USAGE

TriLyte™ with flavor packs is indicated for bowel cleansing prior to colonoscopy.

CONTRAINDICATIONS

TriLyte™ with flavor packs is contraindicated in patients known to be hypersensitive to any of the components. TriLyte™ with flavor packs is contraindicated in patients with ileus, gastrointestinal obstruction, gastric retention, bowel perforation, toxic colitis or toxic megacolon.

WARNINGS

The flavor packs are for use only with the accompanying 4 liter bottle. No additional ingredients, e.g. flavorings, should be added to the solution. TriLyte™ with flavor packs should be used with caution in patients with severe ulcerative colitis. Use of TriLyte™ with flavor packs in children younger than 2 years of age should be carefully monitored for occurrence of possible hypoglycemia, as this solution has no caloric substrate. Dehydration has been reported in 1 child and hypokalemia has been reported in 3 children.

PRECAUTIONS

General: Patients with impaired gag reflex, unconscious, or semiconscious patients, and patients prone to regurgitation or aspiration should be observed during the administration of TriLyte™ with flavor packs, especially if it is administered via nasogastric tube. If a patient experiences severe bloating, distention or abdominal pain, administration should be slowed or temporarily discontinued until the symptoms abate. If gastrointestinal obstruction or perforation is suspected, appropriate studies should be performed to rule out these conditions before administration of TriLyte™ with flavor packs.

Information for Patients: TriLyte™ with flavor packs produces a watery stool which cleanses the bowel before examination. Prepare the solution according to the instructions on the bottle. It is more palatable if chilled. For best results, no solid food should be consumed during the 3 to 4 hour period before drinking the solution, but in no case should solid foods be eaten within 2 hours of taking TriLyte™ with flavor packs.

Adults drink 240 mL (8 oz.) every 10 minutes. Pediatric patients (aged 6 months or greater) drink 25 mL/kg/hour. Rapid drinking of each portion is better than drinking small amounts continuously. The first bowel movement should occur approximately one hour after the start of TriLyte™ with flavor packs administration. You may experience some abdominal bloating and distention before the bowels start to move. If severe discomfort or distention occur, stop drinking temporarily or drink each portion at longer intervals until these symptoms disappear. Continue drinking until the watery stool is clear and free of solid matter. This usually requires at least 3 liters. Any unused portion should be discarded.

Use of TriLyte™ with flavor packs in children younger than 2 years of age should be carefully monitored for occurrence of possible hypoglycemia, as this solution has no caloric substrate. Dehydration has been reported in 1 child and hypokalemia has been reported in 3 children.

Drug Interactions: Oral medication administered within one hour of the start of administration of TriLyte™ with flavor packs may be flushed from the gastrointestinal tract and not absorbed.

Carcinogenesis, Mutagenesis, Impairment of Fertility: Carcinogenic and reproductive studies with animals have not been performed.

Pregnancy: Category C. Animal reproduction studies have not been conducted with TriLyte™ with flavor packs. It is also not known whether TriLyte™ with flavor packs can cause fetal harm when administered to a pregnant woman or can affect reproductive capacity. TriLyte™ with flavor packs should be given to a pregnant woman only if clearly needed.

Pediatric Use: Safety and effectiveness of TriLyte™ with flavor packs in pediatric patients aged 6 months and older is supported by evidence from adequate and well-controlled clinical trials of a similar product in adults with additional safety and efficacy data from published studies of similar formulations.

ADVERSE REACTIONS

Nausea, abdominal fullness and bloating are the most common adverse reactions (occurring in up to 50% of patients) to administration of TriLyte™ with flavor packs. Abdominal cramps, vomiting and anal irritation occur less frequently. These adverse reactions are transient and subside rapidly. Isolated cases of urticaria, rhinorrhea, dermatitis and (rarely) anaphylactic reaction have been reported which may represent allergic reactions.

Published literature contains isolated reports of serious adverse reactions following the administration of PEG-ELS products in patients over 60 years of age. These adverse events include upper GI bleeding from Mallory-Weiss Tear, esophageal perforation, asystole, sudden dyspnea with pulmonary edema, and "butterfly-like" infiltrate on chest X-ray after vomiting and aspirating PEG.

DOSAGE AND ADMINISTRATION

TriLyte™ with flavor packs is usually administered orally, but may be given via nasogastric tube to patients who are unwilling or unable to drink the solution. Ideally, the patient should fast for approximately three or four hours prior to TriLyte™ with flavor packs administration, but in no case should solid food be given for at least two hours before the solution is given.

Oral Administration: Adults: At a rate of 240 mL (8 oz.) every 10 minutes, until the rectal effluent is clear or 4 liters are consumed. **Pediatric Patients (aged 6 months or greater):** At a rate of 25 mL/kg/hour, until the rectal effluent is clear or 4 liters are consumed. Rapid drinking of each portion is preferred to drinking small amounts continuously.

Nasogastric Tube Administration: Adults: At a rate of 20-30 mL per minute (1.2-1.8 liters per hour). **Pediatric Patients (aged 6 months or greater):** At a rate of 25 mL/kg/hour, until the rectal effluent is clear or 4 liters are consumed.

The first bowel movement should occur approximately one hour after the start of TriLyte™ with flavor packs administration. Ingestion of 4 liters of TriLyte™ with flavor packs solution prior to gastrointestinal examination produces satisfactory preparation in over 95% of patients.

Various regimens have been used. One method is to schedule patients for examination in midmorning or later, allowing the patients 3 hours for drinking and an additional 1 hour period for complete bowel evacuation. Another method is to administer TriLyte™ with flavor packs on the evening before the examination.

Preparation of the Solution: This preparation can be used with or without the flavor packs. The pharmacist should dispense the bottle and the attached flavor packs to the patient.

1. To add flavor, tear open one flavor pack at the indicated marking and pour contents into the bottle BEFORE reconstitution. Discard unused flavor packs.
2. SHAKE WELL to incorporate flavoring into the powder.
3. Add tap water to the top of the FILL line marked 4 liters. Replace cap tightly and SHAKE WELL until all ingredients have dissolved. No additional ingredients, e.g. flavorings, should be added to the solution.

Note: If not using a flavor pack, omit steps 1 and 2 above. Dissolution is facilitated by using lukewarm water. The solution is more palatable if chilled before administration. However, chilled solution is not recommended for infants. The reconstituted solution should be refrigerated and used within 48 hours. Discard any unused portion.

Continued on next page

TriLyte—Cont.

HOW SUPPLIED

TriLyte™ with flavor packs (PEG-3350, sodium chloride, sodium bicarbonate and potassium chloride for oral solution) is supplied in a 4 liter bottle with an attached package containing flavor packs. This preparation is supplied in powdered form (white to off-white powder) for oral administration as a solution following reconstitution. Each 4 liter bottle contains polyethylene glycol 3350 420 g, sodium bicarbonate 5.72 g, sodium chloride 11.2 g, potassium chloride 1.48 g. Each flavor pack contains 3.22 g of flavoring ingredients. When made up to 4 liters volume with water, the solution contains PEG-3350 31.3 mmol/L, sodium 65 mmol/L, chloride 53 mmol/L, bicarbonate 17 mmol/L and potassium 5 mmol/L.

TriLyte™ with flavor packs 4 liter NDC 0091-0447-23

Rx Only

STORAGE: Store in sealed container at 25°C (77°F); excursions permitted between 15° - 30° C (59° - 86°F). When reconstituted, keep solution refrigerated. Use within 48 hours. Discard unused portion.

SCHWARZ PHARMA, Inc.
Milwaukee, WI 53201, USA

TAP Pharmaceuticals Inc.
LAKE FOREST, IL 60045

For Medical Information Contact:
(800) 622-2011
(LUPRON, PREVACID, PREVPAC and PREVACID NAPRAPAC)

PREVACID® NapraPAC™ 375 ℞
[*pre'-va-sid*]
(lansoprazole delayed-release 15 mg capsules and naproxen 375 mg tablets kit)

PREVACID® NapraPAC™ 500 ℞
(lansoprazole delayed-release 15 mg capsules and naproxen 500 mg tablets kit)

PREVACID® NapraPAC™ (375 or 500) is a combination package containing NAPROSYN® (naproxen) Tablets, a nonsteroidal anti-inflammatory drug (NSAID) with analgesic and antipyretic properties, and PREVACID® (lansoprazole) Delayed-Release Capsules, a proton pump inhibitor (PPI). The information described in this labeling concerns only the use of these products as indicated in this combination package and does not include all individual use information. For information on use of the components when dispensed as individual medications outside this combination package, please see the package inserts for NAPROSYN Tablets and PREVACID Delayed-Release Capsules.

DESCRIPTION

PREVACID® NapraPAC™ 375 is a combination package containing NAPROSYN 375 mg tablets and PREVACID 15 mg capsules. PREVACID® NapraPAC™ 500 is a combination package containing NAPROSYN 500 mg tablets and PREVACID 15 mg capsules.

NAPROSYN

Naproxen is a member of the arylacetic acid group of nonsteroidal anti-inflammatory drugs (NSAID).

The chemical name for naproxen is (S)-6-methoxy-α-methyl-2-naphthaleneacetic acid. Its empirical formula is $C_{14}H_{14}O_3$ with a molecular weight of 230.26. Naproxen has the following structure:

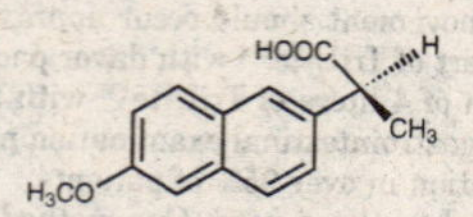

Naproxen is an odorless, white to off-white crystalline substance. It is lipid-soluble, practically insoluble in water at low pH and freely soluble in water at high pH. The octanol/water partition coefficient of naproxen at pH 7.4 is 1.6 to 1.8.

NAPROSYN tablets contain 250 mg, 375 mg or 500 mg of naproxen (active ingredient) and croscarmellose sodium, iron oxides, povidone and magnesium stearate (inactive ingredients).

PREVACID

The active ingredient in PREVACID capsules is a substituted benzimidazole, 2-[[[3-methyl-4-(2,2,2-trifluoroethoxy)-2-pyridyl]methyl] sulfinyl] benzimidazole, a compound that inhibits gastric acid secretion. Its empirical formula is $C_{16}H_{14}F_3N_3O_2S$ with a molecular weight of 369.37. The structural formula is:

[See chemical structure at top of next column]

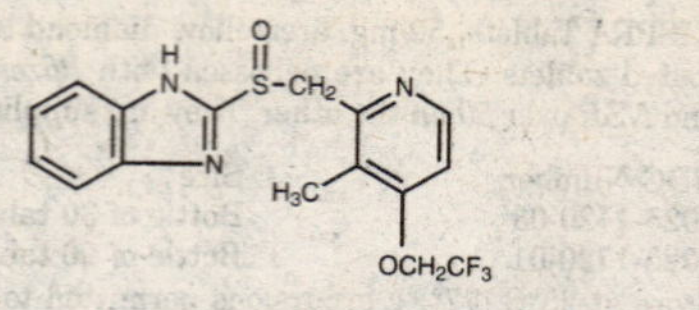

Lansoprazole is a white to brownish-white odorless crystalline powder which melts with decomposition at approximately 166°C. Lansoprazole is freely soluble in dimethylformamide; soluble in methanol; sparingly soluble in ethanol; slightly soluble in ethyl acetate, dichloromethane and acetonitrile; very slightly soluble in ether; and practically insoluble in hexane and water.

Lansoprazole is stable when exposed to light for up to two months. The rate of degradation of the compound in aqueous solution increases with decreasing pH. The degradation half-life of the drug substance in aqueous solution at 25°C is approximately 0.5 hour at pH 5.0 and approximately 18 hours at pH 7.0.

PREVACID capsules contain enteric-coated granules consisting of lansoprazole (15 mg) [active ingredient], hydroxypropyl cellulose, low substituted hydroxypropyl cellulose, colloidal silicon dioxide, magnesium carbonate, methacrylic acid copolymer, starch, talc, sugar sphere, sucrose, polyethylene glycol, polysorbate 80, and titanium dioxide [inactive ingredients]. Components of the gelatin capsule include gelatin, titanium dioxide, D&C Red No. 28, FD&C Blue No. 1, FD&C Green No. 3, and FD&C Red No. 40 [inactive ingredients].

CLINICAL PHARMACOLOGY

Pharmacokinetics

NAPROSYN

Absorption

Naproxen is rapidly and completely absorbed from the gastrointestinal tract, with an *in vivo* bioavailability of 95%. After administration of naproxen tablets, peak plasma levels are attained in 2 to 4 hours. The elimination half-life of naproxen ranges from 12 to 17 hours. Steady-state levels of naproxen are reached in 4 to 5 days, and the degree of naproxen accumulation is consistent with this half-life.

Distribution

Naproxen has a volume of distribution of 0.16 L/kg. At therapeutic levels, naproxen is greater than 99% albumin-bound. At doses of naproxen greater than 500 mg/day, there is a less than dose-proportional increase in plasma levels due to an increase in clearance caused by saturation of plasma protein binding at higher doses (average trough C_{ss} 36.5, 49.2 and 56.4 mg/L with 500, 1000 and 1500 mg daily doses of naproxen). However, the concentration of unbound naproxen continues to increase proportionally to dose.

Metabolism

Naproxen is extensively metabolized to 6-O-desmethyl naproxen, and both parent and metabolites do not induce metabolizing enzymes.

Elimination

The clearance of naproxen is 0.13 mL/min/kg. Approximately 95% of the naproxen from any dose is excreted in the urine, primarily as naproxen (less than 1%), 6-O-desmethyl naproxen (less than 1%) or their conjugates (66% to 92%). The plasma half-life of the naproxen anion in humans ranges from 12 to 17 hours. The corresponding half-lives of both naproxen's metabolites and conjugates are shorter than 12 hours, and their rates of excretion have been found to coincide closely with the rate of naproxen disappearance from the plasma. In patients with renal failure metabolites may accumulate.

Special Populations

Pediatric Use

The combination of naproxen and lansoprazole has not been studied in pediatric patients. (See **CLINICAL PHARMACOLOGY**, PREVACID Special Populations – *Pediatric Use.)*

Renal Insufficiency

Naproxen pharmacokinetics has not been determined in subjects with renal insufficiency. Given that naproxen, its metabolites and conjugates are primarily excreted by the kidney, the potential exists for naproxen to accumulate in the presence of renal insufficiency. (See **CLINICAL PHARMACOLOGY**, PREVACID Special Populations -*Renal Insufficiency.)*

PREVACID

PREVACID capsules contain an enteric-coated granule formulation of lansoprazole. Absorption of lansoprazole begins only after the granules leave the stomach. Absorption is rapid, with mean peak plasma levels of lansoprazole occurring after approximately 1.7 hours. Peak plasma concentrations of lansoprazole (C_{max}) and the area under the plasma concentration curve (AUC) of lansoprazole are approximately proportional in doses from 15 mg to 60 mg after single-dose oral administration. Lansoprazole does not accumulate and its pharmacokinetics are unaltered by multiple dosing.

Absorption

The absorption of lansoprazole is rapid, with mean C_{max} occurring approximately 1.7 hours after oral dosing, and relatively complete with absolute bioavailability over 80%. In healthy subjects, the mean (± SD) plasma half-life was 1.5 (± 1.0) hours. Both C_{max} and AUC are diminished by about 50–70% if the drug is given 30 minutes after food as opposed to the fasting condition. There is no significant food effect if the drug is given before meals.

Distribution

Lansoprazole is 97% bound to plasma proteins. Plasma protein binding is consistent over the concentration range of 0.05 to 5.0 µg/mL.

Metabolism

Lansoprazole is extensively metabolized in the liver. Two metabolites have been identified in measurable quantities in plasma (the hydroxylated sulfinyl and sulfone derivatives of lansoprazole). These metabolites have very little or no antisecretory activity. Lansoprazole is thought to be transformed into two active species which inhibit acid secretion by (H^+,K^+)-ATPase within the parietal cell canaliculus, but are not present in the systemic circulation. The plasma elimination half-life of lansoprazole does not reflect its duration of suppression of gastric acid secretion. Thus, the plasma elimination half-life is less than 2 hours while the acid inhibitory effect lasts more than 24 hours.

Elimination

Following single-dose oral administration of PREVACID, virtually no unchanged lansoprazole was excreted in the urine. In one study, after a single oral dose of ^{14}C-lansoprazole, approximately one-third of the administered radiation was excreted in the urine and two-thirds was recovered in the feces. This implies a significant biliary excretion of the metabolites of lansoprazole.

Special Populations

Pediatric Use

The combination of lansoprazole and naproxen has not been studied in pediatric patients. (See **CLINICAL PHARMACOLOGY**, NAPROSYN Special Populations – *Pediatric Use.)*

Geriatric Use

The clearance of lansoprazole is decreased in the elderly, with elimination half-life increased approximately 50% to 100%. Because the mean half-life in the elderly remains between 1.9 to 2.9 hours, repeated once daily dosing does not result in accumulation of lansoprazole. Peak plasma levels were not increased in the elderly.

Gender

In a study comparing 12 male and 6 female human subjects, no gender differences were found in pharmacokinetics and intragastric pH results. (See **PRECAUTIONS**, PREVACID **Use in Women**.)

Renal Insufficiency

In patients with severe renal insufficiency, plasma protein binding decreased by 1.0%-1.5% after administration of 60 mg of lansoprazole. Patients with renal insufficiency had a shortened elimination half-life and decreased total AUC (free and bound). AUC for free lansoprazole in plasma, however, was not related to the degree of renal impairment, and C_{max} and T_{max} were not different from subjects with healthy kidneys. (See **CLINICAL PHARMACOLOGY**, NAPROSYN Special Populations—*Renal Insufficiency.)*

Hepatic Insufficiency

In patients with various degrees of chronic hepatic disease, the mean plasma half-life of the drug was prolonged from 1.5 hours to 3.2–7.2 hours. An increase in mean AUC of up to 500% was observed at steady state in hepatically-impaired patients compared to healthy subjects. Dose reduction in patients with severe hepatic disease should be considered.

Race

The pooled pharmacokinetic parameters of PREVACID from twelve U.S. Phase I studies (N=513) were compared to the mean pharmacokinetic parameters from two Asian studies (N=20). The mean AUCs of PREVACID in Asian subjects are approximately twice that seen in pooled U.S. data; however, the inter-individual variability is high. The C_{max} values are comparable.

Pharmacodynamics

NAPROSYN

Naproxen is an NSAID with analgesic and antipyretic properties. The naproxen anion inhibits prostaglandin synthesis but beyond this its mode of action is unknown.

PREVACID

Mechanism of Action

Lansoprazole belongs to a class of antisecretory compounds, the substituted benzimidazoles, that do not exhibit anticholinergic or histamine H2-receptor antagonist properties, but that suppress gastric acid secretion by specific inhibition of the (H^+,K^+)-ATPase enzyme system at the secretory surface of the gastric parietal cell. Because this enzyme system is regarded as the acid (proton) pump within the parietal cell, lansoprazole has been characterized as a gastric acid-pump inhibitor, in that it blocks the final step of acid production. This effect is dose-related and leads to inhibition of both basal and stimulated gastric acid secretion irrespective of the stimulus.

Antisecretory Activity

After oral administration, lansoprazole was shown to significantly decrease the basal acid output and significantly increase the mean gastric pH and percent of time the gastric pH was >3 and >4. Lansoprazole also significantly reduced meal-stimulated gastric acid output and secretion volume, as well as pentagastrin-stimulated acid output. In patients with hypersecretion of acid, lansoprazole significantly reduced basal and pentagastrin- stimulated gastric acid secretion. Lansoprazole inhibited the normal increases in secretion volume, acidity and acid output induced by insulin.

In a crossover study that included lansoprazole 15 and 30 mg for five days, the following effects on intragastric pH were noted:

[See table 1 at top of next page]

After the initial dose in this study, increased gastric pH was seen within 1-2 hours with lansoprazole 30 mg and 2-3 hours with lansoprazole 15 mg. After multiple daily dosing, increased gastric pH was seen within the first hour postdosing with lansoprazole 30 mg and within 1-2 hours postdosing with lansoprazole 15 mg.

The inhibition of gastric acid secretion as measured by intragastric pH returns gradually to normal over two to four days after multiple doses. There is no indication of rebound gastric acidity.

Table 1 Mean Antisecretory Effects After Single and Multiple Daily Dosing

Parameter	Baseline Value	PREVACID 15 mg Day 1	PREVACID 15 mg Day 5	PREVACID 30 mg Day 1	PREVACID 30 mg Day 5
Mean 24-Hour pH	2.1	2.7⁺	4.0⁺	3.6*	4.9*
Mean Nighttime pH	1.9	2.4	3.0⁺	2.6	3.8*
% Time Gastric pH>3	18	33⁺	59⁺	51*	72*
% Time Gastric pH>4	12	22⁺	49⁺	41*	66*

NOTE: An intragastric pH of >4 reflects a reduction in gastric acid by 99%.
*(p<0.05) versus baseline and lansoprazole 15 mg.
⁺(p<0.05) versus baseline only.

Table 2 NSAID-Associated Gastric Ulcer Risk Reduction Rates

% of Patients Remaining Gastric Ulcer-Free[1]

Week	PREVACID 15 mg QD (N=121)	PREVACID 30 mg QD (N=116)	Misoprostol 200 µg QID (N=106)	Placebo (N=112)
4	90 %	92 %	96 %	66 %
8	86 %	88 %	95 %	60 %
12	80 %	82 %	93 %	51 %

[1] % = Life Table Estimate
(p<0.001) PREVACID 15 mg QD versus placebo; PREVACID 30 mg QD versus placebo; and misoprostol 200 µg QID versus placebo.
(p<0.05) Misoprostol 200 µg QID versus PREVACID 15 mg QD; and misoprostol 200 µg QID versus PREVACID 30 mg QD

Table 3 Gastric Ulcer Risk Reduction Rates in Patients whose NSAID was Naproxen Only or Naproxen and Aspirin Only

% of Patients Remaining Gastric Ulcer-Free[1]

Week	PREVACID 15 mg QD (N=37)	PREVACID 30 mg QD (N=24)	Misoprostol 200 µg QID (N=28)	Placebo (N=30)
4	91%	83%	88%	52%
8	89%	83%	88%	52%
12	89%	83%	83%	33%

[1] % = Life Table Estimate
(p<0.001) PREVACID 15 mg QD versus placebo; PREVACID 30 mg QD versus placebo; and misoprostol 200 µg QID versus placebo.

Enterochromaffin-like (ECL) Cell Effects

During lifetime exposure of rats with up to 150 mg/kg/day of lansoprazole dosed 7 days per week, marked hypergastrinemia was observed followed by ECL cell proliferation and formation of carcinoid tumors, especially in female rats. (See **PRECAUTIONS**, PREVACID **Carcinogenesis, Mutagenesis, Impairment of Fertility**.)

Gastric biopsy specimens from the body of the stomach from approximately 150 patients treated continuously with lansoprazole for at least one year did not show evidence of ECL cell effects similar to those seen in rat studies. Longer term data are needed to rule out the possibility of an increased risk of the development of gastric tumors in patients receiving long-term therapy with lansoprazole.

Other Gastric Effects in Humans

Lansoprazole did not significantly affect mucosal blood flow in the fundus of the stomach. Due to the normal physiologic effect caused by the inhibition of gastric acid secretion, a decrease of about 17% in blood flow in the antrum, pylorus, and duodenal bulb was seen. Lansoprazole significantly slowed the gastric emptying of digestible solids. Lansoprazole increased serum pepsinogen levels and decreased pepsin activity under basal conditions and in response to meal stimulation or insulin injection. As with other agents that elevate intragastric pH, increases in gastric pH were associated with increases in nitrate-reducing bacteria and elevation of nitrite concentration in gastric juice in patients with gastric ulcer. No significant increase in nitrosamine concentrations was observed.

Serum Gastrin Effects

In over 2100 patients, median fasting serum gastrin levels increased 50% to 100% from baseline but remained within normal range after treatment with lansoprazole given orally in doses of 15 mg to 60 mg. These elevations reached a plateau within two months of therapy and returned to pretreatment levels within four weeks after discontinuation of therapy.

Endocrine Effects

Human studies for up to one year have not detected any clinically significant effects on the endocrine system. Hormones studied include testosterone, luteinizing hormone (LH), follicle stimulating hormone (FSH), sex hormone binding globulin (SHBG), dehydroepiandrosterone sulfate (DHEA-S), prolactin, cortisol, estradiol, insulin, aldosterone, parathormone, glucagon, thyroid stimulating hormone (TSH), triiodothyronine (T_3), thyroxine (T_4), and somatotropic hormone (STH). Lansoprazole in oral doses of 15 to 60 mg for up to one year had no clinically significant effect on sexual function. In addition, lansoprazole in oral doses of 15 to 60 mg for two to eight weeks had no clinically significant effect on thyroid function.

In 24-month carcinogenicity studies in Sprague-Dawley rats with daily dosages up to 150 mg/kg, proliferative changes in the Leydig cells of the testes, including benign neoplasm, were increased compared to control rates.

Other Effects

No systemic effects of lansoprazole on the central nervous system, lymphoid, hematopoietic, renal, hepatic, cardiovascular or respiratory systems have been found in humans. No visual toxicity was observed among 56 patients who had extensive baseline eye evaluations, were treated with up to 180 mg/day of lansoprazole and were observed for up to 58 months. Other rat-specific findings after lifetime exposure included focal pancreatic atrophy, diffuse lymphoid hyperplasia in the thymus, and spontaneous retinal atrophy.

CLINICAL STUDIES

PREVACID® NapraPAC™ (375 or 500)

Risk Reduction of NSAID-Associated Gastric Ulcer

A large U.S., multicenter, double-blind, placebo- and misoprostol-controlled (misoprostol blinded only to the endoscopist) study was conducted in patients who required chronic use of an NSAID and had a history of an endoscopically documented gastric ulcer. Patients took one or more NSAIDs during the study. Concomitant aspirin use (≤ 325 mg) was allowed. The proportion of patients remaining free from gastric ulcer at 4, 8, and 12 weeks was significantly higher with 15 or 30 mg of PREVACID than placebo (see Table 2). A total of 537 patients were enrolled in the study, and 535 patients were treated. Patients ranged in age from 23 to 89 years (median age 60 years), with 65% female patients and 35% male patients. Race was distributed as follows: 90% Caucasian, 6% Black, 4% other. Concomitant aspirin was used in 20% of the patients. The 30 mg dose of PREVACID demonstrated no additional benefit in risk reduction of the NSAID-associated gastric ulcer than the 15 mg dose.

[See table 2 above]

A retrospective subset analysis of 119 patients whose NSAID was naproxen only or naproxen and aspirin only, was performed. Again, the proportion of patients remaining free from gastric ulcer at 4, 8, and 12 weeks was significantly higher with 15 or 30 mg of PREVACID than placebo (see Table 3). Patients ranged in age from 37 to 84 years (median age 58 years) with 61% female patients and 39% male patients. Race was distributed as follows: 88% Caucasian, 8% Black, 4% other. Concomitant aspirin was used in 15% of the patients. The 30 mg dose of PREVACID demonstrated no additional benefit in risk reduction of the NSAID-associated gastric ulcer than the 15 mg dose.

[See table 3 above]

For patients who received PREVACID the highest total daily dose of naproxen was as follows: 5 patients took < 750 mg/daily, 54 patients took 750 - 1000 mg daily. Only 2 patients who received PREVACID took greater than 1000 mg of naproxen.

NAPROSYN

General Information

Naproxen has been studied in patients with rheumatoid arthritis, osteoarthritis and ankylosing spondylitis. Improvement in patients treated for rheumatoid arthritis was demonstrated by a reduction in joint swelling, a reduction in duration of morning stiffness, a reduction in disease activity as assessed by both the investigator and patient, and by increased mobility as demonstrated by a reduction in walking time. Generally, response to naproxen has not been found to be dependent on age, sex, severity or duration of rheumatoid arthritis.

In patients with osteoarthritis, the therapeutic action of naproxen has been shown by a reduction in joint pain or tenderness, an increase in range of motion in knee joints, increased mobility as demonstrated by a reduction in walking time, and improvement in capacity to perform activities of daily living impaired by the disease.

In a clinical trial comparing standard formulations of naproxen 375 mg bid (750 mg a day) vs 750 mg bid (1500 mg/day), 9 patients in the 750 mg group terminated prematurely because of adverse events. Nineteen patients in the 1500 mg group terminated prematurely because of adverse events. Most of these adverse events were gastrointestinal events.

In clinical studies in patients with rheumatoid arthritis or osteoarthritis, naproxen has been shown to be comparable to aspirin and indomethacin in controlling the aforementioned measures of disease activity, but the frequency and severity of the milder gastrointestinal adverse effects (nausea, dyspepsia, heartburn) and nervous system adverse effects (tinnitus, dizziness, lightheadedness) were less in naproxen-treated patients than in those treated with aspirin or indomethacin.

In patients with ankylosing spondylitis, naproxen has been shown to decrease night pain, morning stiffness and pain at rest. In double-blind studies the drug was shown to be as effective as aspirin, but with fewer side effects.

Naproxen may be used safely in combination with gold salts and/or corticosteroids; however, in controlled clinical trials, when added to the regimen of patients receiving corticosteroids, it did not appear to cause greater improvement over that seen with corticosteroids alone. Whether naproxen has a "steroid-sparing" effect has not been adequately studied. When added to the regimen of patients receiving gold salts, naproxen did result in greater improvement. Its use in combination with salicylates is not recommended because there is evidence that aspirin increases the rate of excretion of naproxen and data are inadequate to demonstrate that naproxen and aspirin produce greater improvement over that achieved with aspirin alone. In addition, as with other NSAIDs, the combination may result in higher frequency of adverse events than demonstrated for either product alone.

In ^{51}Cr blood loss and gastroscopy studies with normal volunteers, daily administration of 1000 mg of naproxen has been demonstrated to cause statistically significantly less gastric bleeding and erosion than 3250 mg of aspirin.

INDICATIONS AND USAGE

PREVACID® NapraPAC™ (375 or 500) is indicated for reducing the risk of NSAID-associated gastric ulcers in patients with a history of documented gastric ulcer who require the use of an NSAID for treatment of the signs and symptoms of rheumatoid arthritis, osteoarthritis, and ankylosing spondylitis. (See **CLINICAL STUDIES** and **DOSAGE AND ADMINISTRATION**.) Controlled studies did not extend beyond 12 weeks.

CONTRAINDICATIONS

PREVACID® NapraPAC™ (375 or 500) is contraindicated in patients with known hypersensitivity or allergic reactions to any component of the formulations of PREVACID, NAPROSYN, or over-the-counter products containing naproxen.

Naproxen is also contraindicated in patients in whom aspirin or other nonsteroidal anti-inflammatory/analgesic drugs induce the syndrome of asthma, rhinitis, and nasal polyps. Both types of reactions have the potential of being fatal. Anaphylactoid reactions to naproxen, whether of the true allergic type or the pharmacologic idiosyncratic (eg, aspirin hypersensitivity syndrome) type, usually but not always occur in patients with a known history of such reactions. Therefore, careful questioning of patients for such things as asthma, nasal polyps, urticaria, and hypotension associated with nonsteroidal anti-inflammatory drugs before starting therapy is important. In addition, if such symptoms occur during therapy, treatment should be discontinued.

WARNINGS

NAPROSYN

Risk of GI Ulceration, Bleeding and Perforation With NSAID Therapy

Serious gastrointestinal toxicity such as bleeding, ulceration and perforation can occur at any time, with or without warning symptoms, in patients treated chronically with NSAID therapy. Although minor upper gastrointestinal problems, such as dyspepsia, are common, usually developing early in therapy, physicians should remain alert for ulceration and bleeding in patients treated chronically with NSAIDs even in the absence of previous GI tract symptoms. In patients observed in clinical trials of several months to 2 years' duration, symptomatic upper GI ulcers, gross bleeding or perforation appear to occur in approximately 1% of patients treated for 3 to 6 months and in about 2% to 4% of patients treated for 1 year.

Physicians should inform patients about the signs and/or symptoms of serious GI toxicity and what steps to take if they occur.

Continued on next page

Prevacid NapraPAC—Cont.

Studies to date with naproxen have not identified any subset of patients not at risk of developing peptic ulceration and bleeding. Except for a prior history of serious GI events and other risk factors known to be associated with peptic ulcer disease, such as alcoholism, smoking, etc., no risk factors (e.g., age, sex) have been associated with increased risk. Elderly or debilitated patients seem to tolerate ulceration or bleeding less well than other individuals and most spontaneous reports of fatal GI events are in this population. Studies to date are inconclusive concerning the relative risk of various NSAIDs in causing such reactions. High doses of any NSAID probably carry a greater risk of these reactions, although controlled clinical trials showing this do not exist in most cases. In considering the use of relatively large doses (within the recommended dosage range), sufficient benefit should be anticipated to offset the potential increased risk of GI toxicity.

Physicians should consider alternative treatment to NSAIDs in patients who have experienced a serious gastrointestinal toxicity associated with NSAID use. For patients who require the use of an NSAID, coadministration of PREVACID 15 mg Delayed-Release Capsules with NSAIDs has been proven effective to reduce the risk of gastric ulcers associated with NSAID use in patients with a previous history of documented gastric ulcers. (See **CLINICAL STUDIES**, PREVACID® NapraPAC™ (375 or 500), **Risk Reduction of NSAID-Associated Gastric Ulcer**.)

PRECAUTIONS

General

NAPROSYN

NAPROXEN-CONTAINING PRODUCTS SUCH AS NAPROSYN® (NAPROXEN) TABLETS, EC-NAPROSYN® (NAPROXEN) DELAYED-RELEASE TABLETS, ANAPROX®/ANAPROX DS® (NAPROXEN SODIUM) TABLETS, NAPROSYN® (NAPROXEN) SUSPENSION, ALEVE® (NAPROXEN SODIUM), AND OTHER NAPROXEN PRODUCTS INCLUDING PREVACID® NapraPAC™ (375 or 500), SHOULD NOT BE USED CONCOMITANTLY SINCE THEY ALL CIRCULATE IN THE PLASMA AS THE NAPROXEN ANION.

NAPROSYN cannot be expected to substitute for corticosteroids or to treat corticosteroid insufficiency. If the steroid dose is reduced or eliminated during therapy, the steroid dosage should be reduced slowly and the patient should be observed closely for any evidence of adverse effects, including adrenal insufficiency and exacerbation of symptoms of arthritis.

Patients with initial hemoglobin values of 10 grams or less who are to receive long-term therapy should have hemoglobin values determined periodically.

The antipyretic and anti-inflammatory activities of the drug may reduce fever and inflammation, thus diminishing their utility as diagnostic signs in detecting complications of presumed noninfectious, noninflammatory painful conditions.

Because of adverse eye findings in animal studies with drugs of this class, it is recommended that ophthalmic studies be carried out if any change or disturbance in vision occurs.

PREVACID

Symptomatic response to therapy with lansoprazole does not preclude the presence of gastric malignancy.

Information for Patients

Each convenience package of PREVACID® NapraPAC™ (375 or 500) contains sufficient product for seven days of treatment. Each daily dose consists of one PREVACID 15 mg capsule and two NAPROSYN tablets, either 375 mg or 500 mg. Take the PREVACID capsule and one NAPROSYN tablet in the morning before eating with a glass of water. Take the second NAPROSYN tablet in the evening with a glass of water.

NAPROSYN, like other drugs of this class, is not free of side effects. The side effects of this formulation can cause discomfort and, rarely, there are more serious side effects, such as gastrointestinal bleeding, which may result in hospitalization and even fatal outcomes. PREVACID when taken with naproxen has been shown to reduce the risk of NSAID-associated gastric ulcers in patients with a history of ulcer.

NSAIDs (Nonsteroidal Anti-Inflammatory Drugs) are often essential agents in the management of arthritis and have a major role in the treatment of pain. Naproxen as NAPROSYN is indicated for the treatment of rheumatoid arthritis, osteoarthritis, and ankylosing spondylitis.

Physicians may wish to discuss with their patients the potential risks (see **WARNINGS, PRECAUTIONS** and **ADVERSE REACTIONS**) and likely benefits of naproxen treatment, particularly when it is used for less serious conditions where treatment without NSAIDs may represent an acceptable alternative to both the patient and physician.

Caution should be exercised by patients whose activities require alertness if they experience drowsiness, dizziness, vertigo or depression during therapy with naproxen.

Renal Effects

NAPROSYN

As with other nonsteroidal anti-inflammatory drugs, long-term administration of naproxen to animals has resulted in renal papillary necrosis and other abnormal renal pathology. In humans, there have been reports of acute interstitial nephritis, hematuria, proteinuria and occasionally nephrotic syndrome associated with naproxen-containing products and other NSAIDs since they have been marketed.

A second form of renal toxicity has been seen in patients taking naproxen as well as other nonsteroidal anti-inflammatory drugs. In patients with prerenal conditions leading to a reduction in renal blood flow or blood volume, where the renal prostaglandins have a supportive role in the maintenance of renal perfusion, administration of a nonsteroidal anti-inflammatory drug may cause a dose-dependent reduction in prostaglandin formation and precipitate overt renal decompensation. Patients at greatest risk of this reaction are those with impaired renal function, heart failure, liver dysfunction, those taking diuretics and the elderly. Discontinuation of nonsteroidal anti- inflammatory therapy is typically followed by recovery to the pretreatment state.

Naproxen and its metabolites are eliminated primarily by the kidneys; therefore, the drug should be used with caution in patients with significantly impaired renal function, and the monitoring of serum creatinine and/or creatinine clearance is advised in these patients. Caution should be used if the drug is given to patients with creatinine clearance of less than 20 mL/minute because accumulation of naproxen metabolites has been seen in such patients.

Chronic alcoholic liver disease and probably other diseases with decreased or abnormal plasma proteins (albumin) reduce the total plasma concentration of naproxen, but the plasma concentration of unbound naproxen is increased. Caution is advised when high doses are required and some adjustment of dosage may be required in these patients. It is prudent to use the lowest effective dose.

Studies indicate that although total plasma concentration of naproxen is unchanged, the unbound plasma fraction of naproxen is increased in the elderly. Caution is advised when high doses are required and some adjustment of dosage may be required in elderly patients. As with other drugs used in the elderly, it is prudent to use the lowest effective dose.

Hepatic Function

NAPROSYN

As with other nonsteroidal anti-inflammatory drugs, borderline elevations of one or more liver tests may occur in up to 15% of patients. These abnormalities may progress, may remain essentially unchanged, or may be transient with continued therapy. The SGPT (ALT) test is probably the most sensitive indicator of liver dysfunction. Meaningful (3 times the upper limit of normal) elevations of SGPT or SGOT (AST) occurred in controlled clinical trials in less than 1% of patients. A patient with symptoms and/or signs suggesting liver dysfunction or in whom an abnormal liver test has occurred, should be evaluated for evidence of the development of more severe hepatic reaction while on therapy with naproxen. Severe hepatic reactions, including jaundice and cases of fatal hepatitis, have been reported with naproxen as with other nonsteroidal anti-inflammatory drugs. Although such reactions are rare, if abnormal liver tests persist or worsen, if clinical signs and symptoms consistent with liver disease develop, or if systemic manifestations occur (eg, eosinophilia, rash, etc.), naproxen should be discontinued.

Fluid Retention and Edema

NAPROSYN

Peripheral edema has been observed in some patients receiving naproxen.

Laboratory Tests

NAPROSYN

Because serious GI tract ulceration and bleeding can occur without warning symptoms, physicians should follow patients chronically treated with naproxen for signs and symptoms of ulceration and bleeding and should inform them of the importance of this follow-up and what they should do if certain signs and symptoms do appear (see **WARNINGS**, NAPROSYN **Risk of GI Ulcerations, Bleeding and Perforation With NSAID Therapy**).

Drug Interactions

NAPROSYN

The use of NSAIDs in patients who are receiving ACE inhibitors may potentiate renal disease states (see **PRECAUTIONS**, NAPROSYN **Renal Effects**).

In vitro studies have shown that naproxen anion, because of its affinity for protein, may displace from their binding sites other drugs that are also albumin-bound (see **CLINICAL PHARMACOLOGY**, NAPROSYN **Pharmacokinetics**).

Theoretically, the naproxen anion itself could likewise be displaced. Short-term controlled studies failed to show that taking the drug significantly affects prothrombin times when administered to individuals on coumarin-type anticoagulants. Caution is advised nonetheless, since interactions have been seen with other nonsteroidal agents of this class. Similarly, patients receiving the drug and a hydantoin, sulfonamide or sulfonylurea should be observed for signs of toxicity to these drugs (see **CLINICAL STUDIES**, NAPROSYN **General Information**).

Concomitant administration of naproxen and aspirin is not recommended because naproxen is displaced from its binding sites during the concomitant administration of aspirin, resulting in lower plasma concentrations and peak plasma levels.

The natriuretic effect of furosemide has been reported to be inhibited by some drugs of this class. Inhibition of renal lithium clearance leading to increases in plasma lithium concentrations has also been reported. Naproxen and other nonsteroidal anti-inflammatory drugs can reduce the antihypertensive effect of propranolol and other beta-blockers.

Probenecid given concurrently increases naproxen anion plasma levels and extends its plasma half-life significantly.

Caution should be used if naproxen is administered concomitantly with methotrexate. Naproxen, and other nonsteroidal anti-inflammatory drugs have been reported to reduce the tubular secretion of methotrexate in an animal model, possibly increasing the toxicity of methotrexate.

PREVACID

Lansoprazole is metabolized through the cytochrome P_{450} system, specifically through the CYP3A and CYP2C19 isozymes. Studies have shown that lansoprazole does not have clinically significant interactions with other drugs metabolized by the cytochrome P_{450} system, such as warfarin, antipyrine, indomethacin, ibuprofen, phenytoin, propranolol, prednisone, diazepam, or clarithromycin in healthy subjects. These compounds are metabolized through various cytochrome P_{450} isozymes including CYP1A2, CYP2C9, CYP2C19, CYP2D6, and CYP3A. When lansoprazole was administered concomitantly with theophylline (CYP1A2, CYP3A), a minor increase (10%) in the clearance of theophylline was seen. Because of the small magnitude and the direction of the effect on theophylline clearance, this interaction is unlikely to be of clinical concern. Nonetheless, individual patients may require additional titration of their theophylline dosage when lansoprazole is started or stopped to ensure clinically effective blood levels.

In a study of healthy subjects neither the pharmacokinetics of warfarin enantiomers nor prothrombin time were affected following single or multiple 60 mg doses of lansoprazole. However, there have been reports of increased International Normalized Ratio (INR) and prothrombin time in patients receiving proton pump inhibitors, including lansoprazole, and warfarin concomitantly. Increases in INR and prothrombin time may lead to abnormal bleeding and even death. Patients treated with proton pump inhibitors and warfarin concomitantly may need to be monitored for increases in INR and prothrombin time.

Lansoprazole has also been shown to have no clinically significant interaction with amoxicillin.

In a single-dose crossover study examining lansoprazole 30 mg and omeprazole 20 mg each administered alone and concomitantly with sucralfate 1 gram, absorption of the proton pump inhibitors was delayed and their bioavailability was reduced by 17% and 16%, respectively, when administered concomitantly with sucralfate. Therefore, proton pump inhibitors should be taken at least 30 minutes prior to sucralfate. In clinical trials, antacids were administered concomitantly with PREVACID Delayed-Release Capsules; this did not interfere with its effect.

Lansoprazole causes a profound and long-lasting inhibition of gastric acid secretion; therefore, it is theoretically possible that lansoprazole may interfere with the absorption of drugs where gastric pH is an important determinant of bioavailability (e.g., ketoconazole, ampicillin esters, iron salts, digoxin).

Drug/Laboratory Test Interactions

NAPROSYN

Naproxen may decrease platelet aggregation and prolong bleeding time. This effect should be kept in mind when bleeding times are determined.

The administration of naproxen may result in increased urinary values for 17-ketogenic steroids because of an interaction between the drug and/or its metabolites with m-dinitrobenzene used in this assay. Although 17-hydroxy-corticosteroid measurements (Porter-Silber test) do not appear to be artifactually altered, it is suggested that therapy with naproxen be temporarily discontinued 72 hours before adrenal function tests are performed if the Porter-Silber test is to be used.

Naproxen may interfere with some urinary assays of 5-hydroxy indoleacetic acid (5HIAA).

Carcinogenesis, Mutagenesis, Impairment of Fertility

NAPROSYN

A 2-year study was performed in rats to evaluate the carcinogenic potential of naproxen at rat doses of 8, 16, and 24 mg/kg/day (50, 100, and 150 mg/m^2). The maximum dose used was 0.28 times the systemic exposure to humans at the recommended dose. No evidence of tumorigenicity was found.

PREVACID

In two 24-month carcinogenicity studies, Sprague-Dawley rats were treated orally with doses of 5 to 150 mg/kg/day, about 1 to 40 times the exposure on a body surface (mg/m^2) basis, of a 50-kg person of average height (1.46 m^2 body surface area) given the recommended human dose of 30 mg/day (22.2 mg/m^2). Lansoprazole produced dose-related gastric enterochromaffin-like (ECL) cell hyperplasia and ECL cell carcinoids in both male and female rats. It also increased the incidence of intestinal metaplasia of the gastric epithelium in both sexes. In male rats, lansoprazole produced a dose-related increase of testicular interstitial cell adenomas. The incidence of these adenomas in rats receiving doses of 15 to 150 mg/kg/day (4 to 40 times the recommended human dose based on body surface area) exceeded the low background incidence (range = 1.4 to 10%) for this strain of rat. Testicular interstitial cell adenoma also occurred in 1 of 30 rats treated with 50 mg/kg/day (13 times the recommended human dose based on body surface area) in a 1-year toxicity study.

In a 24-month carcinogenicity study, CD-1 mice were treated orally with doses of 15 to 600 mg/kg/day, 2 to 80 times the recommended human dose based on body surface area. Lansoprazole produced a dose-related increased incidence of gastric ECL cell hyperplasia. It also produced an increased incidence of liver tumors (hepatocellular adenoma plus carcinoma). The tumor incidences in male mice treated with 300 and 600 mg/kg/day (40 to 80 times the recommended human dose based on body surface area) and female mice treated with 150 to 600 mg/kg/day (20 to 80 times the recommended human dose based on body surface area) exceeded the ranges of background incidences in historical controls for this strain of mice. Lansoprazole treatment produced adenoma of rete testis in male mice receiving 75 to 600 mg/kg/day (10 to 80 times the recommended human dose based on body surface area).

Lansoprazole was not genotoxic in the Ames test, the *ex vivo* rat hepatocyte unscheduled DNA synthesis (UDS) test, the *in vivo* mouse micronucleus test or the rat bone marrow cell chromosomal aberration test. It was positive in *in vitro* human lymphocyte chromosomal aberration assays.

Lansoprazole at oral doses up to 150 mg/kg/day (40 times the recommended human dose based on body surface area) was found to have no effect on fertility and reproductive performance of male and female rats.

Pregnancy: Teratogenic Effects

Pregnancy Category B

PREVACID® NapraPAC™ (375 or 500)

There are no adequate and well-controlled studies in pregnant women. Because animal reproduction studies are not always predictive of human response, PREVACID® NapraPAC™ (375 or 500) should not be used during pregnancy unless clearly needed.

NAPROSYN

Reproduction studies have been performed in rats at 20 mg/kg/day (125 mg/m^2/day, 0.23 times the human systemic exposure), rabbits at 20 mg/kg/day (220 mg/m^2/day, 0.27 times the human systemic exposure), and mice at 170 mg/kg/day (510 mg/m^2/day, 0.28 times the human systemic exposure) with no evidence of impaired fertility or harm to the fetus due to the drug. There are no adequate and well-controlled studies in pregnant women. Because animal reproduction studies are not always predictive of human response, naproxen should not be used during pregnancy unless clearly needed.

PREVACID

Teratology studies have been performed in pregnant rats at oral doses up to 150 mg/kg/day (40 times the recommended human dose based on body surface area) and pregnant rabbits at oral doses up to 30 mg/kg/day (16 times the recommended human dose based on body surface area) and have revealed no evidence of impaired fertility or harm to the fetus due to lansoprazole.

Nonteratogenic Effects

NAPROSYN

There is some evidence to suggest that when inhibitors of prostaglandin synthesis are used to delay preterm labor there is an increased risk of neonatal complications such as necrotizing enterocolitis, patent ductus arteriosus and intracranial hemorrhage. Naproxen treatment given in late pregnancy to delay parturition has been associated with persistent pulmonary hypertension, renal dysfunction and abnormal prostaglandin E levels in preterm infants. Because of the known effect of drugs of this class on the human fetal cardiovascular system (closure of ductus arteriosus), use during third trimester should be avoided.

Nursing Mothers

PREVACID® NapraPAC™ (375 or 500)

No studies were conducted in this population with PREVACID® NapraPAC™, however, because of the possible adverse effects of prostaglandin-inhibiting drugs on neonates, use of PREVACID® NapraPAC™ (375 or 500) in nursing mothers should be avoided.

NAPROSYN

The naproxen anion has been found in the milk of lactating women at a concentration of approximately 1% of that found in plasma. Because of the possible adverse effects of prostaglandin-inhibiting drugs on neonates, use in nursing mothers should be avoided.

PREVACID

Lansoprazole or its metabolites are excreted in the milk of rats. It is not known whether lansoprazole is excreted in human milk. Because many drugs are excreted in human milk, because of the potential for serious adverse reactions in nursing infants from lansoprazole, and because of the potential for tumorigenicity shown for lansoprazole in rat carcinogenicity studies, a decision should be made whether to discontinue nursing or to discontinue the drug, taking into account the importance of the drug to the mother.

Pediatric Use

PREVACID® NapraPAC™ (375 or 500)

The safety and effectiveness of PREVACID® NapraPAC™ (375 or 500) in pediatric patients have not been established.

Geriatric Use

NAPROSYN

Studies indicate that although total plasma concentration of naproxen is unchanged, the unbound plasma fraction of naproxen is increased in the elderly. Caution is advised when high doses are required and some adjustment of dosage may be required in elderly patients. As with other drugs used in the elderly, it is prudent to use the lowest effective dose.

PREVACID

The incidence rates of adverse events and laboratory test abnormalities are also similar to those seen in younger patients. For elderly patients, dosage and administration of lansoprazole need not be altered.

Use in Women

PREVACID

Over 4,000 women were treated with lansoprazole. Ulcer healing rates in females were similar to those in males. The incidence rates of adverse events were also similar to those seen in males.

ADVERSE REACTIONS

NAPROSYN

The following adverse reactions are divided into three parts based on frequency and whether or not the possibility exists of a causal relationship between naproxen and these adverse events. In those reactions listed as "Probable Causal Relationship" there is at least 1 case for each adverse reaction where there is evidence to suggest that there is a causal relationship between drug usage and the reported event.

Adverse reactions reported in controlled clinical trials in 960 patients treated for rheumatoid arthritis or osteoarthritis are listed below. In general, reactions in patients treated chronically were reported 2 to 10 times more frequently than they were in short- term studies in the 962 patients treated for mild to moderate pain or for dysmenorrhea. The most frequent complaints reported related to the gastrointestinal tract.

A clinical study found gastrointestinal reactions to be more frequent and more severe in rheumatoid arthritis patients taking daily doses of 1500 mg naproxen compared to those taking 750 mg naproxen.

The following adverse reactions are divided into three parts based on frequency and causal relationship.

Incidence greater than 1% (Probable Causal Relationship): *Gastrointestinal* - constipation*, heartburn*, abdominal pain*, nausea*, dyspepsia, diarrhea, stomatitis; *Central Nervous System* - headache*, dizziness*, drowsiness*, lightheadedness, vertigo; *Dermatologic* - itching (pruritus)*, skin eruptions*, ecchymoses*, sweating, purpura; *Special Senses*- tinnitus*, hearing disturbances, visual disturbances; *Cardiovascular* - edema*, dyspnea*, palpitations; *General* - thirst

*Incidence of reported reaction between 3% and 9%. Those reactions occurring in less than 3% of the patients are unmarked.

Incidence less than 1% (Probable Causal Relationship): The following adverse reactions were reported less frequently than 1% during controlled clinical trials and through voluntary reports since marketing. Those reactions observed through voluntary reporting since marketing of NAPROSYN are underlined.

Gastrointestinal - abnormal liver function tests, colitis, gastrointestinal bleeding and/or perforation, hematemesis, jaundice, pancreatitis, melena, vomiting; *Renal* - glomerular nephritis, hematuria, hyperkalemia, interstitial nephritis, nephrotic syndrome, renal disease, renal failure, renal papillary necrosis; *Hematologic* - agranulocytosis, eosinophilia, granulocytopenia, leukopenia, thrombocytopenia; *Central Nervous System* - depression, dream abnormalities, inability to concentrate, insomnia, malaise, myalgia, muscle weakness; *Dermatologic* - alopecia, photosensitive dermatitis, urticaria, skin rashes, photosensitivity reactions resembling porphyria cutanea tarda, epidermolysis bullosa; *Special Senses* - hearing impairment; *Cardiovascular* - congestive heart failure; *Respiratory* - eosinophilic pneumonitis; *General* - anaphylactoid reactions, angioneurotic edema, menstrual disorders, pyrexia (chills and fever)

Incidence less than 1% (Causal Relationship Unknown): These observations are being listed to serve as alerting information to the physician. *Hematologic* - aplastic anemia, hemolytic anemia; *Central Nervous System* - aseptic meningitis, cognitive dysfunction; *Dermatologic* - epidermal necrolysis, erythema multiforme, Stevens-Johnson syndrome; *Gastrointestinal* - nonpeptic gastrointestinal ulceration, ulcerative stomatitis; *Cardiovascular* - vasculitis; *General* - hyperglycemia, hypoglycemia

PREVACID

Clinical

Worldwide, over 10,000 patients have been treated with lansoprazole in Phase 2-3 clinical trials involving various dosages and durations of treatment. The adverse reaction profiles for PREVACID Delayed-Release Capsules and PREVACID for Delayed-Release Oral Suspension are similar. In general, lansoprazole treatment has been well-tolerated in both short-term and long-term trials.

The following adverse events were reported by the treating physician to have a possible or probable relationship to drug in 1% or more of PREVACID-treated patients and occurred at a greater rate in PREVACID-treated patients than placebo-treated patients in Table 4.

Table 4 Incidence of Possibly or Probably Treatment-Related Adverse Events in Short-Term, Placebo-Controlled Studies

Body System/Adverse Event	PREVACID (N= 2768) %	Placebo (N= 1023) %
Body as a Whole		
Abdominal Pain	2.1	1.2
Digestive System		
Constipation	1.0	0.4
Diarrhea	3.8	2.3
Nausea	1.3	1.2

Headache was also seen at greater than 1% incidence but was more common on placebo. The incidence of diarrhea was similar between patients who received placebo and patients who received lansoprazole 15 mg and 30 mg, but higher in the patients who received lansoprazole 60 mg (2.9%, 1.4%, 4.2%, and 7.4%, respectively).

The most commonly reported possibly or probably treatment-related adverse event during maintenance therapy was diarrhea.

In the risk reduction study of PREVACID for NSAID-associated gastric ulcers, the incidence of diarrhea for patients treated with PREVACID was 5%, misoprostol 22%, and placebo 3%.

Additional adverse experiences occurring in <1% of patients or subjects in domestic trials are shown below. Refer to **Postmarketing** for adverse reactions occurring since the drug was marketed.

Body as a Whole—abdomen enlarged, allergic reaction, asthenia, back pain, candidiasis, carcinoma, chest pain (not otherwise specified), chills, edema, fever, flu syndrome, halitosis, infection (not otherwise specified), malaise, neck pain, neck rigidity, pain, pelvic pain; *Cardiovascular System* - angina, arrhythmia, bradycardia, cerebrovascular accident/cerebral infarction, hypertension/hypotension, migraine, myocardial infarction, palpitations, shock (circulatory failure), syncope, tachycardia, vasodilation; *Digestive System* – abnormal stools, anorexia, bezoar, cardiospasm, cholelithiasis, colitis, dry mouth, dyspepsia, dysphagia, enteritis, eructation, esophageal stenosis, esophageal ulcer, esophagitis, fecal discoloration, flatulence, gastric nodules/fundic gland polyps, gastritis, gastroenteritis, gastrointestinal anomaly, gastrointestinal disorder, gastrointestinal hemorrhage, glossitis, gum hemorrhage, hematemesis, increased appetite, increased salivation, melena, mouth ulceration, nausea and vomiting, nausea and vomiting and diarrhea, oral moniliasis, rectal disorder, rectal hemorrhage, stomatitis, tenesmus, thirst, tongue disorder, ulcerative colitis, ulcerative stomatitis; *Endocrine System* - diabetes mellitus, goiter, hypothyroidism; *Hemic and Lymphatic System* - anemia, hemolysis, lymphadenopathy; *Metabolic and Nutritional Disorders* - gout, dehydration, hyperglycemia/hypoglycemia, peripheral edema, weight gain/loss; *Musculoskeletal System* - arthralgia, arthritis, bone disorder, joint disorder, leg cramps, musculoskeletal pain, myalgia, myasthenia, synovitis; *Nervous System* - abnormal dreams, agitation, amnesia, anxiety, apathy, confusion, convulsion, depersonalization, depression, diplopia, dizziness, emotional lability, hallucinations, hemiplegia, hostility aggravated, hyperkinesia, hypertonia, hypesthesia, insomnia, libido decreased/increased, nervousness, neurosis, paresthesia, sleep disorder, somnolence, thinking abnormality, tremor, vertigo; *Respiratory System* - asthma, bronchitis, cough increased, dyspnea, epistaxis, hemoptysis, hiccup, laryngeal neoplasia, pharyngitis, pleural disorder, pneumonia, respiratory disorder, upper respiratory inflammation/infection, rhinitis, sinusitis, stridor; *Skin and Appendages* - acne, alopecia, contact dermatitis, dry skin, fixed eruption, hair disorder, maculopapular rash, nail disorder, pruritus, rash, skin carcinoma, skin disorder, sweating, urticaria; *Special Senses* - abnormal vision, blurred vision, conjunctivitis, deafness, dry eyes, ear disorder, eye pain, otitis media, parosmia, photophobia, retinal degeneration, taste loss, taste perversion, tinnitus, visual field defect; *Urogenital System* - abnormal menses, breast enlargement, breast pain, breast tenderness, dysmenorrhea, dysuria, gynecomastia, impotence, kidney calculus, kidney pain, leukorrhea, menorrhagia, menstrual disorder, penis disorder, polyuria, testis disorder, urethral pain, urinary frequency, urinary tract infection, urinary urgency, urination impaired, vaginitis.

Postmarketing

On-going Safety Surveillance: Additional adverse experiences have been reported since lansoprazole has been marketed. The majority of these cases are foreign-sourced and a relationship to lansoprazole has not been established. Because these events were reported voluntarily from a population of unknown size, estimates of frequency cannot be made. These events are listed below by COSTART body system.

Body as a Whole—anaphylactoid-like reaction; *Digestive System* - hepatotoxicity, pancreatitis, vomiting; *Hemic and Lymphatic System* - agranulocytosis, aplastic anemia, hemolytic anemia, leukopenia, neutropenia, pancytopenia, thrombocytopenia, and thrombotic thrombocytopenic purpura; *Skin and Appendages* – severe dermatologic reactions including erythema multiforme, Stevens-Johnson syndrome, toxic epidermal necrolysis (some fatal); *Special Senses* - speech disorder; *Urogenital System* - urinary retention.

Laboratory Values

The following changes in laboratory parameters for lansoprazole were reported as adverse events:

Abnormal liver function tests, increased SGOT (AST), increased SGPT (ALT), increased creatinine, increased alkaline phosphatase, increased globulins, increased GGTP, increased/decreased/abnormal WBC, abnormal AG ratio, abnormal RBC, bilirubinemia, eosinophilia, hyperlipemia, increased/decreased electrolytes, increased/decreased cholesterol, increased glucocorticoids, increased LDH, increased/decreased/abnormal platelets, and increased gastrin levels. Urine abnormalities such as albuminuria, glycosuria, and hematuria were also reported. Additional isolated laboratory abnormalities were reported.

In the placebo controlled studies, when SGOT (AST) and SGPT (ALT) were evaluated, 0.4% (4/978) placebo patients and 0.4% (11/2677) lansoprazole patients had enzyme elevations greater than three times the upper limit of normal range at the final treatment visit. None of these lansoprazole patients reported jaundice at any time during the study.

Continued on next page

Prevacid NapraPAC—Cont.

OVERDOSAGE

PREVACID® NapraPAC™ (375 or 500)

In case of an overdose, patients should contact a physician, poison control center, or emergency room. There are no data suggesting increased toxicity of the combination of naproxen and lansoprazole compared with individual components.

NAPROSYN

Significant naproxen overdosage may be characterized by drowsiness, heartburn, indigestion, nausea or vomiting. In the event that ANAPROX/ANAPROX-DS, ALEVE, or naproxen sodium is taken with PREVACID® NapraPAC™ (375 or 500), earlier and higher blood levels may be anticipated due to the rapid absorption of naproxen sodium. A few patients have experienced seizures, but it is not clear whether or not these were drug-related. It is not known what dose of the drug would be life-threatening. The oral LD_{50} of the drug is 543 mg/kg in rats, 1234 mg/kg in mice, 4110 mg/kg in hamsters, and greater than 1000 mg/kg in dogs.

Should a patient ingest a large number of tablets, accidentally or purposefully, the stomach may be emptied and usual supportive measures employed. In animals 0.5 g/kg of activated charcoal was effective in reducing plasma levels of naproxen. Hemodialysis does not decrease the plasma concentration of naproxen because of the high degree of its protein binding.

PREVACID

Oral doses up to 5000 mg/kg in rats (approximately 1300 times the 30 mg human dose based on body surface area) and mice (about 675.7 times the 30 mg human dose based on body surface area) did not produce deaths or any clinical signs.

Lansoprazole is not removed from the circulation by hemodialysis. In one reported case of overdose, the patient consumed 600 mg of lansoprazole with no adverse reaction.

DOSAGE AND ADMINISTRATION

Risk Reduction of NSAID-Associated Gastric Ulcers in the Treatment of Osteoarthritis, Rheumatoid Arthritis, Ankylosing Spondylitis

Each convenience package of PREVACID® NapraPAC™ (375 or 500) contains sufficient product for seven days of treatment. Each daily dose consists of one PREVACID 15 mg capsule and two NAPROSYN tablets, either 375 mg or 500 mg. Take the PREVACID capsule and one NAPROSYN tablet in the morning before eating with a glass of water. Take the second NAPROSYN tablet in the evening with a glass of water.

The maximum daily naproxen dose of PREVACID® NapraPAC™ (375 or 500) is 1000 mg. Controlled studies for PREVACID® NapraPAC™ did not extend beyond 12 weeks. For PREVACID® NapraPAC™ (375 or 500), no adjustment of the 15 mg PREVACID component is necessary in patients with renal insufficiency or for the elderly. Dosage adjustment for the NAPROSYN component should be considered for patients with renal insufficiency, liver disease or the elderly (see **PRECAUTIONS - Renal Effects** and **Hepatic Function**).

PREVACID Delayed-Release Capsules should be swallowed whole. The capsule should not be chewed or crushed.

HOW SUPPLIED

PREVACID® NapraPAC™ 375 is supplied as a weekly blister card packaged as a monthly (28 days) course of therapy. Each weekly blister card contains:

NAPROSYN

— fourteen pink, biconvex oval tablets, engraved with NPR LE 375 on one side.

PREVACID

— seven opaque, hard gelatin, pink and green PREVACID 15 mg capsules, with the TAP logo and "PREVACID 15" imprinted on the capsules.

PREVACID® NapraPAC™ 500 is supplied as a weekly blister card packaged as a monthly (28 days) course of therapy. Each weekly blister card contains:

NAPROSYN

— fourteen yellow, capsule-shaped tablets, engraved with NPR LE 500 on one side and scored on the other.

PREVACID

— seven opaque, hard gelatin, pink and green PREVACID 15 mg capsules, with the TAP logo and "PREVACID 15" imprinted on the capsules.

NDC 0300-1545-07 Weekly Blister Card, 375 mg
NDC 0300-1546-07 Weekly Blister Card, 500 mg
NDC 0300-1545-30 One Month Administration Pack, 375 mg
NDC 0300-1546-30 One Month Administration Pack, 500 mg

Storage: Protect from light and moisture.
Store at 25°C (77°F), excursions permitted to 15-30°C (59-86°F). [See USP Controlled Room Temperature]
Store and dispense in original container.

Rx only

U.S. Patent No. 6,047,829

Distributed by TAP Pharmaceuticals Inc.
Lake Forest, Illinois 60045, U.S.A.

ALEVE® is a registered trademark of Bayer-Roche L.L.C. ANAPROX®/ANAPROX DS®, EC-NAPROSYN®, NAPROSYN®, and NAPROSYN® SUSPENSION are registered trademarks of and NapraPAC™ is a trademark of Syntex Pharmaceuticals International Ltd., A Bermuda Corporation

PREVACID® is a registered trademark of TAP Pharmaceuticals Inc.

3646-R3, Rev. November, 2003

REVISED INFORMATION

As new research data and clinical findings become available, the product information in *PDR* is revised accordingly. Revisions submitted since the 2004 edition went to press can be found below. To remind yourself of a revision, write "See Supplement A" next to the product's heading in the book.

AstraZeneca LP

WILMINGTON, DE 19850-5437

For Medical Information, Adverse Drug Experiences, and Customer Service Contact: (800) 236-9933

ENTOCORT™ EC ℞

[*ĕn'tō-kōrt*]
(budesonide)
Capsules

Prescribing information for this product, which appears on pages 608–610 of the 2004 PDR, has been revised as follows. Please write "See Supplement A" next to the product heading.

How Supplied section revised to reflect the new capsule identifier. Capsules now read "Entocort EC 3 mg".

65006-00
Rev. 10/02

NEXIUM® ℞

[*nĕk-sē-um*]
(esomeprazole magnesium)
delayed release capsules

Prescribing information for this product, which appears on pages 624–628 of the 2004 PDR, has been revised as follows. Please write "See Supplement A" next to the product heading.

How supplied section revised to reflect the new capsule identifier. Capsules now read "NEXIUM 20 mg" and "NEXIUM 40 mg"

620514-05
Rev. 08/03

PRILOSEC® ℞

[*prī-lō-sĕk*]
(omeprazole)
Delayed release capsules

Prescribing information for this product, which appears on pages 633–638 of the 2004 PDR, has been revised as follows. Please write "See Supplement A" next to the product heading.

"hydroxypropyl methylcellulose" revised to "hypromellose" DESCRIPTION section

"blurred vision" and "eye irritation" added to the ADVERSE REACTIONS section

Precautions, Drug Interactions, added drug interaction related to warfarin. "There have been reports of increased INR and prothrombin time in patients receiving proton pump inhibitors, including omeprazole, and warfarin concomitantly. Increases in INR and prothrombin time may lead to abnormal bleeding and even death. Patients treated with proton pump inhibitors and warfarin may need to be monitored for increases in INR and prothrombin time."

Deleted the following NDCs from the HOW SUPPLIED section:

0186-0606-68 10 mg 100 count Bottle
0186-0606-28 10 mg HUD
0186-0742-28 20 mg HUD
0186-0743-28 40 mg HUD

640004-39
Rev. 10/03

AstraZeneca Pharmaceuticals LP

1800 CONCORD PIKE
WILMINGTON, DE 19850-5437 USA

For Product and Business Information, and Adverse Drug Experiences:
Information Center
1-800-236-9933

For Product Ordering:
Trade Customer Service
1-800-842-9920

Internet: www.astrazeneca-us.com

MERREM® I.V. ℞

(meropenem for injection)
For Intravenous Use Only

Prescribing information for this product, which appears on pages 674–678 of the 2004 PDR, has been completely revised as follows. Please write "See Supplement A" next to the product heading.

To reduce the development of drug-resistant bacteria and maintain the effectiveness of MERREM® I.V. (meropenem for injection) and other antibacterial drugs, MERREM I.V. should be used only to treat or prevent infections that are proven or strongly suspected to be caused by bacteria.

DESCRIPTION

MERREM® I.V. (meropenem for injection) is a sterile, pyrogen-free, synthetic, broad-spectrum, carbapenem antibiotic for intravenous administration. It is (4R,5S,6S)-3-[[(3S,5S)-5-(Dimethylcarbamoyl)-3-pyrrolidinyl]thio]-6-[(1R)-1-hydroxyethyl]-4-methyl-7-oxo-1-azabicyclo[3.2.0]hept-2-ene-2-carboxylic acid trihydrate. Its empirical formula is $C_{17}H_{25}N_3O_5S \cdot 3H_2O$ with a molecular weight of 437.52. Its structural formula is:

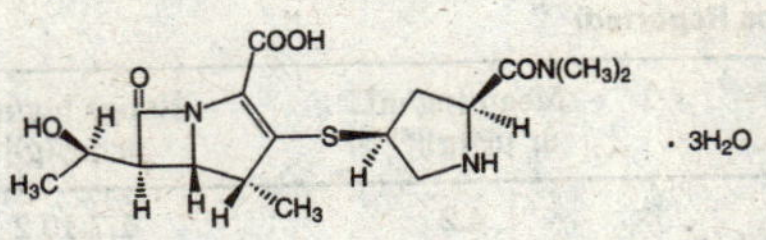

MERREM I.V. is a white to pale yellow crystalline powder. The solution varies from colorless to yellow depending on the concentration. The pH of freshly constituted solutions is between 7.3 and 8.3. Meropenem is soluble in 5% monobasic potassium phosphate solution, sparingly soluble in water, very slightly soluble in hydrated ethanol, and practically insoluble in acetone or ether.

When constituted as instructed (see **DOSAGE AND ADMINISTRATION; PREPARATION OF SOLUTION**), each 1 g MERREM I.V. vial will deliver 1 g of meropenem and 90.2 mg of sodium as sodium carbonate (3.92 mEq). Each 500 mg MERREM I.V. vial will deliver 500 mg meropenem and 45.1 mg of sodium as sodium carbonate (1.96 mEq).

MERREM I.V. in the ADD-Vantage† vial is intended for intravenous use only after dilution with the appropriate volume of diluent solution in the Abbott ADD-Vantage® diluent container. (See **DOSAGE AND ADMINISTRATION; PREPARATION OF SOLUTION.**) MERREM I.V. in the ADD-Vantage vial is available in two strengths. Each 1 g ADD-Vantage vial of MERREM I.V. will deliver 90.2 mg of sodium as sodium carbonate (3.92 mEq), and each 500 mg ADD-Vantage vial will deliver 45.1 mg of sodium as sodium carbonate (1.96 mEq).

CLINICAL PHARMACOLOGY

At the end of a 30-minute intravenous infusion of a single dose of MERREM I.V. in normal volunteers, mean peak plasma concentrations are approximately 23 μg/mL (range 14-26) for the 500 mg dose and 49 μg/mL (range 39-58) for the 1 g dose. A 5-minute intravenous bolus injection of MERREM I.V. in normal volunteers results in mean peak plasma concentrations of approximately 45 μg/mL (range 18-65) for the 500 mg dose and 112 μg/mL (range 83-140) for the 1 g dose.

Following intravenous doses of 500 mg, mean plasma concentrations of meropenem usually decline to approximately 1 μg/mL at 6 hours after administration.

In subjects with normal renal function, the elimination half-life of MERREM I.V. is approximately 1 hour. Approximately 70% of the intravenously administered dose is recovered as unchanged meropenem in the urine over 12 hours, after which little further urinary excretion is detectable. Urinary concentrations of meropenem in excess of 10 μg/mL are maintained for up to 5 hours after a 500 mg dose. No accumulation of meropenem in plasma or urine was observed with regimens using 500 mg administered every 8 hours or 1 g administered every 6 hours in volunteers with normal renal function.

Plasma protein binding of meropenem is approximately 2%. There is one metabolite which is microbiologically inactive. Meropenem penetrates well into most body fluids and tissues including cerebrospinal fluid, achieving concentrations matching or exceeding those required to inhibit most susceptible bacteria. After a single intravenous dose of MERREM I.V., the highest mean concentrations of meropenem were found in tissues and fluids at 1 hour (0.5 to 1.5 hours) after the start of infusion, except where indicated in the tissues and fluids listed in the table below.

[See table at bottom of next page]

The pharmacokinetics of MERREM I.V. in pediatric patients 2 years of age or older are essentially similar to those in adults. The elimination half-life for meropenem was approximately 1.5 hours in pediatric patients of age 3 months to 2 years. The pharmacokinetics are linear over the dose range from 10 to 40 mg/kg.

Pharmacokinetic studies with MERREM I.V. in patients with renal insufficiency have shown that the plasma clearance of meropenem correlates with creatinine clearance. Dosage adjustments are necessary in subjects with renal impairment. (See **DOSAGE AND ADMINISTRATION-Use in Adults with Renal Impairment.**) A pharmacokinetic study with MERREM I.V. in elderly patients with renal insufficiency has shown a reduction in plasma clearance of meropenem that correlates with age-associated reduction in creatinine clearance.

Meropenem I.V. is hemodialyzable. However, there is no information on the usefulness of hemodialysis to treat overdosage. (See **OVERDOSAGE.**)

A pharmacokinetic study with MERREM I.V. in patients with hepatic impairment has shown no effects of liver disease on the pharmacokinetics of meropenem.

Microbiology

The bactericidal activity of meropenem results from the inhibition of cell wall synthesis. Meropenem readily penetrates the cell wall of most gram-positive and gram-negative bacteria to reach penicillin-binding-protein (PBP) targets. Its strongest affinities are toward PBPs 2, 3 and 4 of *Escherichia coli* and *Pseudomonas aeruginosa;* and PBPs 1, 2, and 4 of *Staphylococcus aureus.* Bactericidal concentrations (defined as a 3 $\log_{10}$ reduction in cell counts within 12 to 24 hours) are typically 1-2 times the bacteriostatic concentrations of meropenem, with the exception of *Listeria monocytogenes,* against which lethal activity is not observed.

Meropenem has significant stability to hydrolysis by β-lactamases of most categories, both penicillinases and

Continued on next page

Merrem I.V.—Cont.

cephalosporinases produced by gram-positive and gram-negative bacteria, with the exception of metallo-β-lactamases. Meropenem should not be used to treat methicillin-resistant staphylococci. Cross resistance is sometimes observed with strains resistant to other carbapenems.
In vitro tests show meropenem to act synergistically with aminoglycoside antibiotics against some isolates of *Pseudomonas aeruginosa*.
Meropenem has been shown to be active against most strains of the following microorganisms, both *in vitro* and in clinical infections as described in the **INDICATIONS AND USAGE** section.

Gram-Positive Aerobes
Streptococcus pneumoniae (excluding penicillin-resistant strains)
Viridans group streptococci

NOTE: Penicillin-resistant strains had meropenem MIC_{90} values of 1 or 2 μg/mL, which is above the 0.12 μg/mL susceptible breakpoint for this species.

Gram-Negative Aerobes
Escherichia coli
Haemophilus influenzae (β-lactamase and non-β-lactamase producing)
Klebsiella pneumoniae
Neisseria meningitidis
Pseudomonas aeruginosa

Anaerobes
Bacteroides fragilis
Bacteroides thetaiotaomicron
Peptostreptococcus species

The following in vitro data are available, **but their clinical significance is unknown.**
Meropenem exhibits *in vitro* minimum inhibitory concentrations (MIC's) of 0.12 μg/mL against most (≥ 90%) strains of *Streptococcus pneumoniae* 0.5 μg/mL or less against most (≥ 90%) strains of *Haemophilus influenzae*, and 4 μg/mL or less against most (≥ 90%) strains of the other microorganisms in the following list; however, the safety and effectiveness of meropenem in treating clinical infections due to these microorganisms have not been established in adequate and well-controlled clinical trials.

Gram-Positive Aerobes
Staphylococcus aureus (β-lactamase and non-β-lactamase producing)
Staphylococcus epidermidis (β-lactamase and non-β-lactamase-producing)

NOTE: Staphylococci which are resistant to methicillin/oxacillin must be considered resistant to meropenem.

Gram-Negative Aerobes
Acinetobacter species
Aeromonas hydrophila
Campylobacter jejuni
Citrobacter diversus
Citrobacter freundii
Enterobacter cloacae
Haemophilus influenzae (ampicillin-resistant, non-β-lactamase-producing strains [BLNAR strains])
Hafnia alvei
Klebsiella oxytoca
Moraxella catarrhalis (β-lactamase and non-β-lactamase-producing strains)
Morganella morganii
Pasteurella multocida
Proteus mirabilis
Proteus vulgaris
Salmonella species
Serratia marcescens
Shigella species
Yersinia enterocolitica

Anaerobes
Bacteroides distasonis
Bacteroides ovatus
Bacteroides uniformis
Bacteroides ureolyticus
Bacteroides vulgatus
Clostridium difficile
Clostridium perfringens
Eubacterium lentum
Fusobacterium species
Prevotella bivia
Prevotella intermedia
Prevotella melaninogenica
Porphyromonas asaccharolytica
Propionibacterium acnes

Susceptibility Tests

Dilution Techniques:
Quantitative methods are used to determine antimicrobial minimum inhibitory concentrations (MIC's). These MIC's provide estimates of the susceptibility of bacteria to antimicrobial compounds. The MIC's should be determined using a standardized procedure. Standardized procedures are based on a dilution method[1] (broth or agar) or equivalent with standardized inoculum concentrations and standardized concentrations of meropenem powder. The MIC values should be interpreted according to the following criteria for indicated aerobic organisms other than *Haemophilus* species and streptococci:

MIC (μg/mL)	Interpretation
≤ 4	(S) Susceptible
8	(I) Intermediate
≥ 16	(R) Resistant

Haemophilus Test Media (HTM) and the following interpretive criteria should be used when testing *Haemophilus* species:

MIC (μg/mL)	Interpretation
≤ 0.5	(S) Susceptible

The current absence of resistant strains precludes defining any categories other than "Susceptible". Strains yielding results suggestive of a "Nonsusceptible" category should be submitted to a reference laboratory for further testing.
The following criteria should be used when testing streptococci including *Streptococcus pneumoniae*:
When testing *S. pneumoniae*:

MIC (μg/mL)	Interpretation
≤ 0.12	(S) Susceptible

When testing viridans group streptococci:

MIC (μg/mL)	Interpretation
≤ 0.5	(S) Susceptible

The current absence of resistant strains precludes defining any categories other than "Susceptible". Strains yielding results suggestive of a "Nonsusceptible" category should be submitted to a reference laboratory for further testing.
A report of 'Susceptible' indicates that the pathogen is likely to be inhibited if the antimicrobial compound in the blood reaches the concentrations usually achievable. A report of 'Intermediate' indicates that the result should be considered equivocal, and, if the microorganism is not fully susceptible to alternative, clinically feasible drugs, the test should be repeated. This category implies possible clinical applicability in body sites where the drug is physiologically concentrated or in situations where high dosage of drug can be used. This category also provides a buffer zone which prevents small uncontrolled technical factors from causing major discrepancies in interpretation. A report of 'Resistant' indicates that the pathogen is not likely to be inhibited if the antimicrobial compound in the blood reaches the concentrations usually achievable; other therapy should be selected.

Meropenem Concentrations in Selected Tissues
(Highest Concentrations Reported)

Tissue	I.V. Dose (g)	Number of Samples	Mean [μg/mL or μg/(g)]***	Range [μg/mL or μg/(g)]
Endometrium	0.5	7	4.2	1.7-10.2
Myometrium	0.5	15	3.8	0.4-8.1
Ovary	0.5	8	2.8	0.8-4.8
Cervix	0.5	2	7.0	5.4-8.5
Fallopian tube	0.5	9	1.7	0.3-3.4
Skin	0.5	22	3.3	0.5-12.6
Skin	1.0	10	5.3	1.3-16.7
Colon	1.0	2	2.6	2.5-2.7
Bile	1.0	7	14.6 (3 h)	4.0-25.7
Gall bladder	1.0	1	—	3.9
Interstitial fluid	1.0	5	26.3	20.9-37.4
Peritoneal fluid	1.0	9	30.2	7.4-54.6
Lung	1.0	2	4.8 (2 h)	1.4-8.2
Bronchial mucosa	1.0	7	4.5	1.3-11.1
Muscle	1.0	2	6.1 (2 h)	5.3-6.9
Fascia	1.0	9	8.8	1.5-20
Heart valves	1.0	7	9.7	6.4-12.1
Myocardium	1.0	10	15.5	5.2-25.5
CSF (inflamed)	20 mg/kg*	8	1.1 (2 h)	0.2-2.8
	40 mg/kg**	5	3.3 (3 h)	0.9-6.5
CSF (uninflamed)	1.0	4	0.2 (2 h)	0.1-0.3

* in pediatric patients of age 5 months to 8 years
** in pediatric patients of age 1 month to 15 years
*** at 1 hour unless otherwise noted

Standardized susceptibility test procedures require the use of laboratory control microorganisms to control the technical aspects of the laboratory procedures. Standard meropenem powder should provide the following MIC values:

Microorganism	ATCC	MIC (μg/mL)
Enterococcus faecalis	29212	2.0-8.0
Escherichia coli	25922	0.008-0.06
Haemophilus influenzae	49766	0.03-0.12
Pseudomonas aeruginosa	27853	0.25-1.0
Streptococcus pneumoniae	49619	0.06-0.25

Diffusion Techniques:
Quantitative methods that require measurement of zone diameters also provide reproducible estimates of the susceptibility of bacteria to antimicrobial compounds. One such standardized procedure[2] requires the use of standardized inoculum concentrations. This procedure uses paper disks impregnated with 10-μg of meropenem to test the susceptibility of microorganisms to meropenem.
Reports from the laboratory providing results of the standard single-disk susceptibility test with a 10-μg disk should be interpreted according to the following criteria for indicated aerobic organisms other than *Haemophilus* species and streptococci:

Zone Diameter (mm)	Interpretation
≥ 16	(S) Susceptible
14-15	(I) Intermediate
≤ 13	(R) Resistant

Haemophilus Test Media and the following criteria should be used when testing *Haemophilus* species:

Zone Diameter (mm)	Interpretation
≥ 20	(S) Susceptible

The current absence of resistant strains precludes defining any categories other than "Susceptible". Strains yielding results suggestive of a "Nonsusceptible" category should be submitted to a reference laboratory for further testing.
Streptococcus pneumoniae isolates should be tested using 1-μg/mL oxacillin disk. Isolates with oxacillin zone sizes of ≥ 20 mm are susceptible (MIC ≤ 0.06 μg/mL) to penicillin and can be considered susceptible to meropenem for approved indications, and meropenem need not be tested. A meropenem MIC should be determined on isolates of *S. pneumoniae* with oxacillin zone sizes of ≤ 19 mm. The disk test does not distinguish penicillin intermediate strains (i.e., MIC's = 0.12-1.0 μg/mL) from strains that are penicillin resistant (i.e. MIC's ≥ 2 μg/mL). Viridans group streptococci should be tested for meropenem susceptibility using an MIC method. Reliable disk diffusion tests for meropenem do not yet exist for testing streptococci.
Interpretation should be as stated above for results using dilution techniques. Interpretation involves correlation of the diameter obtained in the disk test with the MIC for meropenem.
As with standardized dilution techniques, diffusion methods require the use of laboratory control microorganisms that are used to control the technical aspects of the laboratory procedures. For the diffusion technique, the 10-μg meropenem disk should provide the following zone diameters in these laboratory test quality control strains:

Microorganism	ATCC	Zone Diameter (mm)
Escherichia coli	25922	28-34
Haemophilus influenzae	49247	20-28
Pseudomonas aeruginosa	27853	27-33

Anaerobic Techniques:
For anaerobic bacteria, susceptibility to meropenem as MIC's can be determined by standardized test methods.[3] The MIC values obtained should be interpreted according to the following criteria:

MIC (μg/mL)	Interpretation
≤ 4	(S) Susceptible
8	(I) Intermediate
≥ 16	(R) Resistant

Interpretation is identical to that stated above for results using dilution techniques.
As with other susceptibility techniques, the use of laboratory control microorganisms is required to control the technical aspects of the laboratory standardized procedures. Standardized meropenem powder should provide the following MIC values:

Microorganism	ATCC	MIC (μg/mL)
Bacteroides fragilis	25285	0.06-0.25
Bacteroides thetaiotaomicron	29741	0.125-0.5

INDICATIONS AND USAGE

To reduce the development of drug-resistant bacteria and maintain the effectiveness of MERREM I.V. and other antibacterial drugs, MERREM I.V. should only be used to treat or prevent infections that are proven or strongly suspected to be caused by susceptible bacteria. When culture and susceptibility information are available, they should be considered in selecting or modifying antibacterial therapy. In the absence of such data, local epidemiology and susceptibility patterns may contribute to the empiric selection of therapy.
MERREM I.V. is indicated as single agent therapy for the treatment of the following infections when caused by susceptible strains of the designated microorganisms:

Intra-abdominal Infections
Complicated appendicitis and peritonitis caused by viridans group streptococci, *Escherichia coli, Klebsiella pneumoniae, Pseudomonas aeruginosa, Bacteroides fragilis, B. thetaiotaomicron,* and *Peptostreptococcus* species.

Bacterial Meningitis (Pediatric patients ≥ 3 months only)
Bacterial meningitis caused by *Streptococcus pneumoniae*‡, *Haemophilus influenzae* (β-lactamase and non-β-lactamase-producing strains), and *Neisseria meningitidis*.

‡The efficacy of meropenem as monotherapy in the treatment of meningitis caused by penicillin nonsusceptible strains of *Streptococcus pneumoniae* has not been established.

MERREM I.V. has been found to be effective in eliminating concurrent bacteremia in association with bacterial meningitis.
For information regarding use in pediatric patients (3 months of age and older) see **PRECAUTIONS-Pediatrics, ADVERSE REACTIONS,** and **DOSAGE AND ADMINISTRATION** sections.
Appropriate cultures should usually be performed before initiating antimicrobial treatment in order to isolate and identify the organisms causing infection and determine their susceptibility to MERREM I.V.
MERREM I.V. is useful as presumptive therapy in the indicated condition (i.e., intra-abdominal infections) prior to the identification of the causative organisms because of its broad spectrum of bactericidal activity.
Antimicrobial therapy should be adjusted, if appropriate, once the results of culture(s) and antimicrobial susceptibility testing are known.

CONTRAINDICATIONS

MERREM I.V. is contraindicated in patients with known hypersensitivity to any component of this product or to other drugs in the same class or in patients who have demonstrated anaphylactic reactions to β-lactams.

WARNINGS

SERIOUS AND OCCASIONALLY FATAL HYPERSENSITIVITY (ANAPHYLACTIC) REACTIONS HAVE BEEN REPORTED IN PATIENTS RECEIVING THERAPY WITH β-LACTAMS. THESE REACTIONS ARE MORE LIKELY TO OCCUR IN INDIVIDUALS WITH A HISTORY OF SENSITIVITY TO MULTIPLE ALLERGENS.
THERE HAVE BEEN REPORTS OF INDIVIDUALS WITH A HISTORY OF PENICILLIN HYPERSENSITIVITY WHO HAVE EXPERIENCED SEVERE HYPERSENSITIVITY REACTIONS WHEN TREATED WITH ANOTHER β-LACTAM. BEFORE INITIATING THERAPY WITH MERREM I.V., CAREFUL INQUIRY SHOULD BE MADE CONCERNING PREVIOUS HYPERSENSITIVITY REACTIONS TO PENICILLINS, CEPHALOSPORINS, OTHER β-LACTAMS, AND OTHER ALLERGENS. IF AN ALLERGIC REACTION TO MERREM I.V. OCCURS, DISCONTINUE THE DRUG IMMEDIATELY. **SERIOUS ANAPHYLACTIC REACTIONS REQUIRE IMMEDIATE EMERGENCY TREATMENT WITH EPINEPHRINE, OXYGEN, INTRAVENOUS STEROIDS, AND AIRWAY MANAGEMENT, INCLUDING INTUBATION. OTHER THERAPY MAY ALSO BE ADMINISTERED AS INDICATED.**
Seizures and other CNS adverse experiences have been reported during treatment with MERREM I.V. (See **PRECAUTIONS** and **ADVERSE REACTIONS.**)
Pseudomembranous colitis has been reported with nearly all antibacterial agents, including meropenem, and may range in severity from mild to life-threatening. Therefore, it is important to consider this diagnosis in patients who present with diarrhea subsequent to the administration of antibacterial agents.
Treatment with antibacterial agents alters the normal flora of the colon and may permit overgrowth of clostridia. Studies indicate that a toxin produced by *Clostridium difficile* is a primary cause of "antibiotic-associated colitis".
After the diagnosis of pseudomembranous colitis has been established, therapeutic measures should be initiated. Mild cases of pseudomembranous colitis usually respond to drug discontinuation alone. In moderate-to-severe cases, consideration should be given to management with fluids and electrolytes, protein supplementation, and treatment with an antibacterial drug clinically effective against *Clostridium difficile* colitis.

PRECAUTIONS

General: Prescribing MERREM I.V. in the absence of a proven or strongly suspected bacterial infection or a prophylactic indication is unlikely to provide benefit to the patient and increases the risk of the development of drug-resistant bacteria.
Seizures and other CNS adverse experiences have been reported during treatment with MERREM I.V. These experiences have occurred most commonly in patients with CNS disorders (e.g., brain lesions or history of seizures) or with bacterial meningitis and/or compromised renal function.
During the initial clinical investigations, 2904 immunocompetent adult patients were treated for infections outside the CNS, with the overall seizure rate being 0.7% (based on 20 patients with this adverse event). All meropenem-treated patients with seizures had pre-existing contributing factors. Among these are included prior history of seizures or CNS abnormality and concomitant medications with seizure potential. Dosage adjustment is recommended in patients with advanced age and/or reduced renal function. (See **DOSAGE AND ADMINISTRATION - Use in Adults with Renal Impairment.**)
Close adherence to the recommended dosage regimens is urged, especially in patients with known factors that predispose to convulsive activity. Anticonvulsant therapy should be continued in patients with known seizure disorders. If focal tremors, myoclonus, or seizures occur, patients should be evaluated neurologically, placed on anticonvulsant therapy if not already instituted, and the dosage of MERREM I.V. re-examined to determine whether it should be decreased or the antibiotic discontinued.
In patients with renal dysfunction, thrombocytopenia has been observed but no clinical bleeding reported. (See **DOSAGE AND ADMINISTRATION - Use in Adults with Renal Impairment.**)
There is inadequate information regarding the use of MERREM I.V. in patients on hemodialysis.
As with other broad-spectrum antibiotics, prolonged use of meropenem may result in overgrowth of nonsusceptible organisms. Repeated evaluation of the patient is essential. If superinfection does occur during therapy, appropriate measures should be taken.
Laboratory Tests: While MERREM I.V. possesses the characteristic low toxicity of the beta-lactam group of antibiotics, periodic assessment of organ system functions, including renal, hepatic, and hematopoietic, is advisable during prolonged therapy.
Drug Interactions: Probenecid competes with meropenem for active tubular secretion and thus inhibits the renal excretion of meropenem. This led to statistically significant increases in the elimination half-life (38%) and in the extent of systemic exposure (56%). Therefore, the coadministration of probenecid with meropenem is not recommended.
There is evidence that meropenem may reduce serum levels of valproic acid to subtherapeutic levels (therapeutic range considered to be 50 to 100 μg/mL total valproate).
Carcinogenesis, Mutagenesis, Impairment of Fertility:
Carcinogenesis: Carcinogenesis studies have not been performed.
Mutagenesis: Genetic toxicity studies were performed with meropenem using the bacterial reverse mutation test, the Chinese hamster ovary HGPRT assay, cultured human lymphocytes cytogenic assay, and the mouse micronucleus test. There was no evidence of mutagenic potential found in any of these tests.
Impairment of fertility: Reproductive studies were performed with meropenem in rats at doses up to 1000 mg/kg/day, and cynomolgus monkeys at doses up to 360 mg/kg/day (on the basis of AUC comparisons, approximately 1.8 times and 3.7 times, respectively, to the human exposure at the usual dose of 1 g every 8 hours). There was no reproductive toxicity seen.
Pregnancy Category B: Reproductive studies have been performed with meropenem in rats at doses of up to 1000 mg/kg/day, and cynomolgus monkeys at doses of up to 360 mg/kg/day (on the basis of AUC comparisons, approximately 1.8 times and 3.7 times, respectively, to the human exposure at the usual dose of 1 g every 8 hours). These studies revealed no evidence of impaired fertility or harm to the fetus due to meropenem, although there were slight changes in fetal body weight at doses of 250 mg/kg/day (on the basis of AUC comparisons, 0.4 times the human exposure at a dose of 1 g every 8 hours) and above in rats. There are, however, no adequate and well-controlled studies in pregnant women. Because animal reproduction studies are not always predictive of human response, this drug should be used during pregnancy only if clearly needed.
Pediatric Use: The safety and effectiveness of MERREM I.V. have been established for pediatric patients ≥ 3 months of age. Use of MERREM I.V. in pediatric patients with bacterial meningitis is supported by evidence from adequate and well-controlled studies in the pediatric population. Use of MERREM I.V. in pediatric patients with intra-abdominal infections is supported by evidence from adequate and well-controlled studies with adults with additional data from pediatric pharmacokinetics studies and controlled clinical trials in pediatric patients. (See **CLINICAL PHARMACOLOGY, INDICATIONS AND USAGE, ADVERSE REACTIONS, DOSAGE AND ADMINISTRATION,** and **CLINICAL STUDIES** sections.)
Nursing Mothers: It is not known whether this drug is excreted in human milk. Because many drugs are excreted in human milk, caution should be exercised when MERREM I.V. is administered to a nursing woman.
Geriatric Use: Of the total number of subjects in clinical studies of MERREM I.V., approximately 1100 (30%) were 65 years of age and older, while 400 (11%) were 75 years and older. No overall differences in safety or effectiveness were observed between these subjects and younger subjects; spontaneous reports and other reported clinical experience have not identified differences in responses between the elderly and younger patients, but greater sensitivity of some older individuals cannot be ruled out.
A pharmacokinetic study with MERREM I.V. in elderly patients with renal insufficiency has shown a reduction in plasma clearance of meropenem that correlates with age-associated reduction in creatinine clearance. (See **DOSAGE AND ADMINISTRATION; Use in Adults with Renal Impairment.**)
MERREM I.V. is known to be substantially excreted by the kidney, and the risk of toxic reactions to this drug may be greater in patients with impaired renal function. Because elderly patients are more likely to have decreased renal function, care should be taken in dose selection, and it may be useful to monitor renal function.
Information For Patients: Patients should be counseled that antibacterial drugs including MERREM I.V. should only be used to treat bacterial infections. They do not treat viral infections (eg, the common cold). When MERREM I.V. is prescribed to treat a bacterial infection, patients should be told that although it is common to feel better early in the course of therapy, the medication should be taken exactly as directed. Skipping doses or not completing the full course of therapy may (1) decrease the effectiveness of the immediate treatment and (2) increase the likelihood that bacteria will develop resistance and will not be treatable by MERREM I.V. or other antibacterial drugs in the future.

ADVERSE REACTIONS

Adult Patients:
During clinical investigations, 2904 immunocompetent adult patients were treated for infections outside the CNS with MERREM I.V. (500 mg or 1000 mg q 8 hours). Deaths in 5 patients were assessed as possibly related to meropenem; 36 (1.2%) patients had meropenem discontinued because of adverse events. Many patients in these trials were severely ill and had multiple background diseases, physiological impairments and were receiving multiple other drug therapies. In the seriously ill patient population, it was not possible to determine the relationship between observed adverse events and therapy with MERREM I.V.
The following adverse reaction frequencies were derived from the clinical trials in the 2904 patients treated with MERREM I.V.

Local Adverse Reactions
Local adverse reactions that were reported irrespective of the relationship to therapy with MERREM I.V. were as follows:

Inflammation at the injection site	2.4%
Injection site reaction	0.9%
Phlebitis/thrombophlebitis	0.8%
Pain at the injection site	0.4%
Edema at the injection site	0.2%

Systemic Adverse Reactions
Systemic adverse clinical reactions that were reported irrespective of the relationship to MERREM I.V. occurring in greater than 1.0% of the patients were diarrhea (4.8%), nausea/vomiting (3.6%), headache (2.3%), rash (1.9%), sepsis (1.6%), constipation (1.4%), apnea (1.3%), shock (1.2%), and pruritus (1.2%).
Additional adverse systemic clinical reactions that were reported irrespective of relationship to therapy with MERREM I.V. and occurring in less than or equal to 1.0% but greater than 0.1% of the patients are listed below within each body system in order of decreasing frequency:
Bleeding events were seen as follows: gastrointestinal hemorrhage (0.5%), melena (0.3%), epistaxis (0.2%), hemoperitoneum (0.2%), summing to 1.2%.
Body as a Whole: pain, abdominal pain, chest pain, fever, back pain, abdominal enlargement, chills, pelvic pain
Cardiovascular: heart failure, heart arrest, tachycardia, hypertension, myocardial infarction, pulmonary embolus, bradycardia, hypotension, syncope
Digestive System: oral moniliasis, anorexia, cholestatic jaundice/jaundice, flatulence, ileus, hepatic failure, dyspepsia, intestinal obstruction
Hemic/Lymphatic: anemia, hypochromic anemia, hypervolemia
Metabolic/Nutritional: peripheral edema, hypoxia
Nervous System: insomnia, agitation/delirium, confusion, dizziness, seizure (see **PRECAUTIONS**), nervousness, paresthesia, hallucinations, somnolence, anxiety, depression, asthenia
Respiratory: respiratory disorder, dyspnea, pleural effusion, asthma, cough increased, lung edema
Skin and Appendages: urticaria, sweating, skin ulcer
Urogenital System: dysuria, kidney failure, vaginal moniliasis, urinary incontinence

Adverse Laboratory Changes
Adverse laboratory changes that were reported irrespective of relationship to MERREM I.V. and occurring in greater than 0.2% of the patients were as follows:
Hepatic: increased SGPT (ALT), SGOT (AST), alkaline phosphatase, LDH, and bilirubin
Hematologic: increased platelets, increased eosinophils, decreased platelets, decreased hemoglobin, decreased hematocrit, decreased WBC, shortened prothrombin time and shortened partial thromboplastin time, leukocytosis, hypokalemia
Renal: increased creatinine and increased BUN
NOTE: For patients with varying degrees of renal impairment, the incidence of heart failure, kidney failure, seizure and shock reported irrespective of relationship to MERREM I.V., increased in patients with moderately severe renal impairment (creatinine clearance >10 to 26 mL/min).
Urinalysis: presence of urine red blood cells

Pediatric Patients:
Clinical Adverse Reactions
MERREM I.V. was studied in 515 pediatric patients (≥ 3 months to < 13 years of age) with serious bacterial infections (excluding meningitis. See next section.) at dosages of 10 to 20 mg/kg every 8 hours. The types of clinical adverse events seen in these patients are similar to the adults, with the most common adverse events reported as possibly, probably, or definitely related to MERREM I.V. and their rates of occurrence as follows:

Diarrhea	3.5%

Continued on next page

Merrem I.V.—Cont.

Rash	1.6%
Nausea and Vomiting	0.8%

MERREM I.V. was studied in 321 pediatric patients (≥ 3 months to < 17 years of age) with meningitis at a dosage of 40 mg/kg every 8 hours. The types of clinical adverse events seen in these patients are similar to the adults, with the most common adverse events reported as possibly, probably, or definitely related to MERREM I.V. and their rates of occurrence as follows:

Diarrhea	4.7%
Rash (mostly diaper area moniliasis)	3.1%
Oral Moniliasis	1.9%
Glossitis	1.0%

In the meningitis studies the rates of seizure activity during therapy were comparable between patients with no CNS abnormalities who received meropenem and those who received comparator agents (either cefotaxime or ceftriaxone). In the MERREM I.V. treated group, 12/15 patients with seizures had late onset seizures (defined as occurring on day 3 or later) versus 7/20 in the comparator arm.

Adverse Laboratory Changes:
Laboratory abnormalities seen in the pediatric-aged patients in both the pediatric and the meningitis studies are similar to those reported in adult patients.
There is no experience in pediatric patients with renal impairment.

Post-marketing Experience:
Worldwide post-marketing adverse events not previously listed in the product label and reported as possibly, probably, or definitely drug related are listed within each body system in order of decreasing severity. Hematologic - agranulocytosis, neutropenia, and leukopenia. Skin - toxic epidermal necrolysis, Stevens-Johnson Syndrome, angioedema, and erythema multiform.

OVERDOSAGE

In mice and rats, large intravenous doses of meropenem (2200-4000 mg/kg) have been associated with ataxia, dyspnea, convulsions, and mortalities.
Intentional overdosing of MERREM I.V. is unlikely, although accidental overdosing might occur if large doses are given to patients with reduced renal function. The largest dose of meropenem administered in clinical trials has been 2 g given intravenously every 8 hours. At this dosage, no adverse pharmacological effects or increased safety risks have been observed.
No specific information is available for the treatment of MERREM I.V. overdosage. In the event of an overdose, MERREM I.V. should be discontinued and general supportive treatment given until renal elimination takes place. Meropenem and its metabolite are readily dialyzable and effectively removed by hemodialysis; however, no information is available on the use of hemodialysis to treat overdosage.

CLINICAL STUDIES

Intra-abdominal:
One controlled clinical study of complicated intra-abdominal infection was performed in the United States where meropenem was compared to clindamycin/tobramycin. Three controlled clinical studies of complicated intra-abdominal infections were performed in Europe; meropenem was compared to imipenem (two trials) and cefotaxime/metronidazole (one trial).
Using strict evaluability criteria and microbiologic eradication and clinical cures at follow-up which occurred 7 or more days after completion of therapy, the following presumptive microbiologic eradication/clinical cure rates and statistical findings were obtained:
[See table below]

Treatment Arm	No. evaluable/ No. enrolled (%)	Microbiologic Eradication Rate	Clinical Cure Rate	Outcome
meropenem	146/516 (28%)	98/146 (67%)	101/146 (69%)	
imipenem	65/220 (30%)	40/65 (62%)	42/65 (65%)	Meropenem equivalent to control
cefotaxime/ metronidazole	26/85 (30%)	22/26 (85%)	22/26 (85%)	Meropenem not equivalent to control
clindamycin/ tobramycin	50/212 (24%)	38/50 (76%)	38/50 (76%)	Meropenem equivalent to control

The finding that meropenem was not statistically equivalent to cefotaxime/metronidazole may have been due to uneven assignment of more seriously ill patients to the meropenem arm. Currently there is no additional information available to further interpret this observation.

Bacterial Meningitis:
Four hundred forty-six patients (397 pediatric patients ≥ 3 months to < 17 years of age) were enrolled in 4 separate clinical trials and randomized to treatment with meropenem (n=225) at a dose of 40 mg/kg q 8 hours or a comparator drug, i.e., cefotaxime (n=187) or ceftriaxone (n=34), at the approved dosing regimens. A comparable number of patients were found to be clinically evaluable (ranging from 61-68%) and with a similar distribution of pathogens isolated on initial CSF culture.

Patients were defined as clinically not cured if any one of the following three criteria were met:

1. At the 5-7 week post-completion of therapy visit, the patient had any one of the following: moderate to severe motor, behavior or development deficits, hearing loss of >60 decibels in one or both ears, or blindness.
2. During therapy the patient's clinical status necessitated the addition of other antibiotics.
3. Either during or post-therapy, the patient developed a large subdural effusion needing surgical drainage, or a cerebral abscess, or a bacteriologic relapse.

Using the definition, the following efficacy rates were obtained, per organism. The values represent the number of patients clinically cured/number of clinically evaluable patients, with the percent cure in parentheses.
[See first table at bottom ofnext page]
Sequelae were the most common reason patients were assessed as clinically not cured.
Five patients were found to be bacteriologically not cured, 3 in the comparator group (1 relapse and 2 patients with cerebral abscesses) and 2 in the meropenem group (1 relapse and 1 with continued growth of *Pseudomonas aeruginosa*).
The adverse events seen were comparable between the two treatment groups both in type and frequency. The meropenem group did have a statistically higher number of patients with transient elevation of liver enzymes. (See **ADVERSE REACTIONS**.) Rates of seizure activity during therapy were comparable between patients with no CNS abnormalities who received meropenem and those who received comparator agents. In the MERREM I.V. treated group, 12/15 patients with seizures had late onset seizures (defined as occurring on day 3 or later) versus 7/20 in the comparator arm.
With respect to hearing loss, 263 of the 271 evaluable patients had at least one hearing test performed post-therapy. The following table shows the degree of hearing loss between the meropenem-treated patients and the comparator-treated patients.

Degree of Hearing Loss (in one or both ears)	Meropenem n = 128	Comparator n = 135
No loss	61%	56%
20-40 decibels	20%	24%
>40-60 decibels	8%	7%
>60 decibels	9%	10%

DOSAGE AND ADMINISTRATION

Adults: One gram (1 g) by intravenous administration every 8 hours. MERREM I.V. should be given by intravenous infusion, over approximately 15 to 30 minutes or as an intravenous bolus injection (5 to 20 mL) over approximately 3-5 minutes.

Use in Adults with Renal Impairment: Dosage should be reduced in patients with creatinine clearance less than 51 mL/min. (see dosing table below.)
[See second table at bottom of next page]
When only serum creatinine is available, the following formula (Cockcroft and Gault equation)[4] may be used to estimate creatinine clearance.
[See third table at bottom of next page]
There is inadequate information regarding the use of MERREM I.V. in patients on hemodialysis.
There is no experience with peritoneal dialysis.

Use in Adults With Hepatic Insufficiency: No dosage adjustment is necessary in patients with impaired hepatic function.

Use in Elderly Patients: No dosage adjustment is required for elderly patients with creatinine clearance values above 50 mL/min.

Use in Pediatric Patients: For pediatric patients from 3 months of age and older, the MERREM I.V. dose is 20 or 40 mg/kg every 8 hours (maximum dose is 2 g every 8 hours), depending on the type of infection (intra-abdominal or meningitis). (See dosing table below.) Pediatric patients weighing over 50 kg should be administered MERREM I.V. at a dose of 1 g every 8 hours for intra-abdominal infections and 2 g every 8 hours for meningitis. MERREM I.V. should be given as intravenous infusion over approximately 15 to 30 minutes or as an intravenous bolus injection (5 to 20 mL) over approximately 3-5 minutes.

Recommended MERREM I.V. Dosage Schedule for Pediatrics With Normal Renal Function

Type of Infection	Dose(mg/kg)	Dosing Interval
Intra-abdominal	20	every 8 hours
Meningitis	40	every 8 hours

There is no experience in pediatric patients with renal impairment.

PREPARATION OF SOLUTION

For Intravenous Bolus Administration
Constitute injection vials (500 mg and 1 g) with sterile Water for Injection. (See table below.) Shake to dissolve and let stand until clear.

Vial Size	Amount of Diluent Added (mL)	Approximate Withdrawable Volume (mL)	Approximate Average Concentration (mg/mL)
500 mg	10	10	50
1 g	20	20	50

For Infusion
Infusion vials (500 mg and 1 g) may be directly constituted with a compatible infusion fluid. (See **COMPATIBILITY AND STABILITY.**) Alternatively, an injection vial may be constituted, then the resulting solution added to an I.V. container and further diluted with an appropriate infusion fluid. (See **COMPATIBILITY AND STABILITY.**)

NOTE: ADD-VANTAGE VIALS ARE NOT TO BE USED IN THIS MANNER.

For ADD-Vantage Vials
ADD-Vantage vials of MERREM I.V. are to be constituted only with Sodium Chloride Injection 0.45%, Sodium Chloride Injection 0.9% or Dextrose Injection 5% in the 50, 100, and 250 mL Abbott ADD-Vantage® flexible diluent containers. MERREM I.V. supplied in single-use ADD-Vantage vials should be prepared as directed.

DIRECTIONS FOR USE OF MERREM I.V. (meropenem for injection) IN ADD-VANTAGE VIALS:

To Open Diluent Container: Peel overwrap from the corner and remove container. Some opacity of the plastic due to moisture absorption during the sterilization process may be observed. This is normal and does not affect the solution quality or safety. The opacity will diminish gradually.

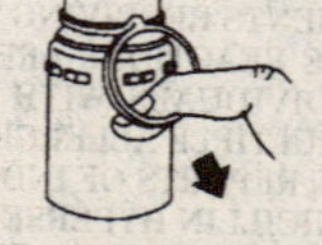

Figure 1

To Assemble ADD-Vantage Vial and Flexible Diluent Container: (Use Aseptic Technique)

1. Remove the protective covers from the top of the vial and the vial port on the diluent container as follows:

a. To remove the breakaway vial cap, swing the pull ring over the top of the vial and pull down far enough to start the opening (see Figure 1), then pull straight up to remove the cap. (See Figure 2.)

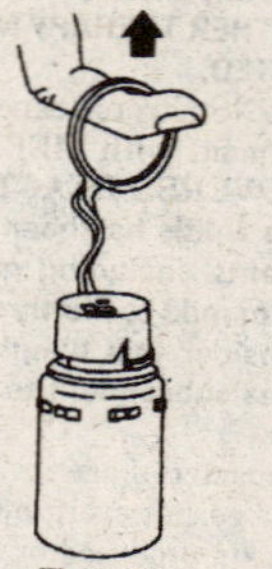

Figure 2

NOTE: Once the breakaway cap has been removed, do not access vial with syringe.

b. To remove the vial port cover, grasp the tab on the pull ring, pull up to break the three tie strings, then pull back to remove the cover. (See Figure 3.)

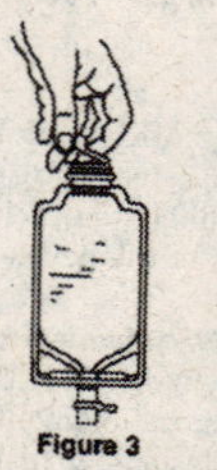

Figure 3

2. Screw the vial into the vial port until it will go no further. THE VIAL MUST BE SCREWED IN TIGHTLY TO ASSURE A SEAL. This occurs approximately 1/2 turn (180°) after the first audible click. (See Figure 4.) The clicking sound does not assure a seal; the vial must be turned as far as it will go.
NOTE: ONCE VIAL IS SEATED, DO NOT ATTEMPT TO REMOVE.
[See figure at top of next column]
3. Recheck the vial to assure that it is tight by trying to turn it further in the direction of assembly.
4. Label appropriately.

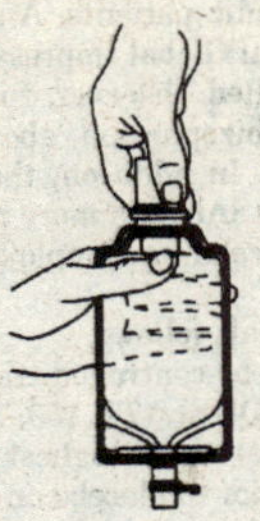

Figure 4

To Prepare Admixture:

1. Squeeze the bottom of the diluent container gently to inflate the portion of the container surrounding the end of the drug vial.
2. With the other hand, push the drug vial down into the container telescoping the walls of the container. Grasp the inner cap of the vial through the walls of the container. (See Figure 5.)

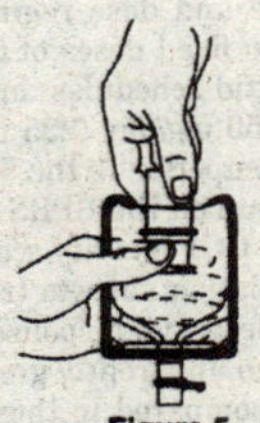

Figure 5

3. Pull the inner cap from the drug vial. (See Figure 6.) Verify that the rubber stopper has been pulled out and invert the system several times, allowing the drug and diluent to mix.

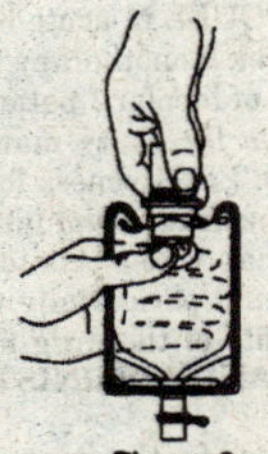

Figure 6

4. Mix contents thoroughly and use within the specified time.

Preparation For Administration: (Use Aseptic Technique)

1. Confirm the activation and admixture of vial contents.
2. Check for leaks by squeezing container firmly. If leaks are found, discard unit as sterility may be impaired.
3. Close flow control clamp of administration set.
4. Remove cover from outlet port at bottom of container.
5. Insert piercing pin of administration set into port with a twisting motion until the pin is firmly seated.
   NOTE: See full directions on administration set carton.
6. Lift the free end of the hanger loop on the bottom of the vial, breaking the two tie strings. Bend the loop outward to lock it in the upright position, then suspend container from hanger.
7. Squeeze and release drip chamber to establish proper fluid level in chamber.
8. Open flow control clamp and clear air from set. Close clamp.
9. Attach set to venipuncture device. If device is not indwelling, prime and make venipuncture.
10. Regulate rate of administration with flow control clamp.

	Number of Hours Stable at Controlled Room Temperature 15-25°C (59-77°F)	Number of Hours Stable at 4°C (39°F)
Sodium Chloride Injection 0.9%	4	24
Dextrose Injection 5.0%	1	4
Dextrose Injection 10.0%	1	2
Dextrose and Sodium Chloride Injection 5.0%/0.9%	1	2
Dextrose and Sodium Chloride Injection 5.0%/0.2%	1	4
Potassium Chloride in Dextrose Injection 0.15%/5.0%	1	6
Sodium Bicarbonate in Dextrose Injection 0.02%/5.0%	1	6
Dextrose Injection 5.0% in Normosol®-M	1	8
Dextrose Injection 5.0% in Ringers Lactate Injection	1	4
Dextrose and Sodium Chloride Injection 2.5%/0.45%	3	12
Mannitol Injection 2.5%	2	16
Ringers Injection	4	24
Ringers Lactate Injection	4	12
Sodium Lactate Injection 1/6 N	2	24
Sodium Bicarbonate Injection 5.0%	1	4

WARNING: Do not use flexible container in series connections.

COMPATIBILITY AND STABILITY

Compatibility of MERREM I.V. with other drugs has not been established. MERREM I.V. should not be mixed with or physically added to solutions containing other drugs.

Freshly prepared solutions of MERREM I.V. should be used whenever possible. However, constituted solutions of MERREM I.V. maintain satisfactory potency at controlled room temperature 15-25°C (59-77°F) or under refrigeration at 4°C (39°F) as described below. Solutions of intravenous MERREM I.V. should not be frozen.

Intravenous Bolus Administration

MERREM I.V. injection vials constituted with sterile Water for Injection for bolus administration (up to 50 mg/mL of MERREM I.V.) may be stored for up to 2 hours at controlled room temperature 15-25°C (59-77°F) or for up to 12 hours at 4°C (39°F).

Intravenous Infusion Administration

Stability in Infusion Vials: MERREM I.V. infusion vials constituted with Sodium Chloride Injection 0.9% (MERREM I.V. concentrations ranging from 2.5 to 50 mg/mL) are stable for up to 2 hours at controlled room temperature 15-25°C (55-77°F) or for up to 18 hours at 4°C (39°F). Infusion vials of MERREM I.V. constituted with Dextrose Injection 5% (MERREM I.V. concentrations ranging from 2.5 to 50 mg/mL) are stable for up to 1 hour at controlled room temperature 15-25°C (59-77°F) or for up to 8 hours at 4°C (39°F).

Stability in Plastic I.V. Bags: Solutions prepared for infusion (MERREM I.V. concentrations ranging from 1 to 20 mg/mL) may be stored in plastic intravenous bags with diluents as shown below:

[See table above]

Stability in Baxter Minibag Plus: Solutions of MERREM I.V. (MERREM I.V. concentrations ranging from 2.5 to 20 mg/mL) in Baxter Minibag Plus bags with Sodium Chloride Injection 0.9% may be stored for up to 4 hours at controlled room temperatures 15-25°C (59-77°F) or for up to 24 hours at 4°C (39°F). Solutions of MERREM I.V. (MERREM I.V. concentrations ranging from 2.5 to 20 mg/mL) in Baxter Minibag Plus bags with Dextrose Injection 5.0% may be stored up to 1 hour at controlled room temperatures 15-25°C (59-77°F) or for up to 6 hours at 4°C (39°F).

Stability in Plastic Syringes, Tubing and Intravenous Infusion Sets: Solutions of MERREM I.V. (MERREM I.V. concentrations ranging from 1 to 20 mg/mL) in Water for Injection or Sodium Chloride Injection 0.9% (for up to 4 hours) or in Dextrose Injection 5.0% (for up to 2 hours) at controlled room temperatures 15-25°C (59-77°F) are stable in plastic tubing and volume control devices of common intravenous infusion sets.

Solutions of MERREM I.V. (MERREM I.V. concentrations ranging from 1 to 20 mg/mL) in Water for Injection or Sodium Chloride Injection 0.9% (for up to 48 hours) or in Dextrose Injection 5% (for up to 6 hours) are stable at 4°C (39°F) in plastic syringes.

MICROORGANISM	MERREM I.V.	COMPARATOR
S. pneumoniae	17/24 (71)	19/30 (63)
H. influenzae (+)	8/10 (80)	6/6 (100)
H. influenzae (−/NT)	44/59 (75)	44/60 (73)
N. meningitidis	30/35 (86)	35/39 (90)
TOTAL (including others)	102/131 (78)	108/140 (77)

(+) β-lactamase-producing; (−/NT) non-β-lactamase-producing or not tested

Recommended MERREM I.V. Dosage Schedule for Adults With Impaired Renal Function

Creatinine Clearance (mL/min)	Dose (dependent on type of infection)	Dosing Interval
26-50	recommended dose (1000 mg)	every 12 hours
10-25	one-half recommended dose	every 12 hours
<10	one-half recommended dose	every 24 hours

Males: Creatinine Clearance (mL/min) = $\frac{\text{Weight (kg)} \times (140 - \text{age})}{72 \times \text{serum creatinine (mg/dL)}}$

Females: 0.85 × above value

ADD-Vantage Vials: ADD-Vantage vials diluted in Sodium Chloride Injection 0.45% (MERREM I.V. concentrations ranging from 5 to 20 mg/mL) may be stored for up to 6 hours at controlled room temperature 15-25°C (59-77°F) or for 24 hours at 4°C (39°F). ADD-Vantage vials diluted in Sodium Chloride Injection 0.9% (MERREM I.V. concentrations ranging from 1-20 mg/mL) may be stored for up to 4 hours at controlled room temperature 15-25°C (59-77°F) or for 24 hours at 4°C (39°F). ADD-Vantage vials diluted with Dextrose Injection 5.0% (MERREM I.V. concentrations ranging from 1-20 mg/mL) may be stored for up to 1 hour at controlled room temperature 15-25°C (59-77°F) or for 8 hours at 4°C (39°F).

NOTE: Parenteral drug products should be inspected visually for particulate matter and discoloration prior to administration, whenever solution and container permit.

HOW SUPPLIED

MERREM I.V. is supplied in 20 mL and 30 mL injection vials containing sufficient meropenem to deliver 500 mg or 1 g for intravenous administration, respectively. MERREM I.V. is supplied in 100 mL infusion vials containing sufficient meropenem to deliver 500 mg or 1 g for intravenous administration. The dry powder should be stored at controlled room temperature 20-25°C (68-77°F) [see USP].

MERREM I.V. is also supplied as ADD-Vantage Vials containing sufficient meropenem to deliver 500 mg or 1 g for intravenous administration.

500 mg Injection Vial	(NDC 0310-0325-20)
1 g Injection Vial	(NDC 0310-0321-30)
500 mg ADD-Vantage	(NDC 0310-0325-15)
1 g ADD-Vantage	(NDC 0310-0321-15)

REFERENCES

1. National Committee for Clinical Laboratory Standards. Methods for Dilution Antimicrobial Susceptibility Tests for Bacteria that Grow Aerobically—Third Edition. Approved Standard NCCLS Document M7-A3, Vol. 13, No. 25, NCCLS, Villanova, PA; December, 1993.
2. National Committee for Clinical Laboratory Standards. Performance Standards for Antimicrobial Disk Susceptibility Tests—Fifth Edition. Approved Standard NCCLS Document M2-A5, Vol. 13, No. 24, NCCLS, Villanova, PA; December 1993.
3. National Committee for Clinical Laboratory Standards. Methods for Antimicrobial Susceptibility Testing of Anaerobic Bacteria—Third Edition. Approved Standard NCCLS Document M11-A3, Vol. 13, No. 26, NCCLS, Villanova, PA; December 1993.
4. Cockcroft DW, Gault MH. Prediction of creatinine clearance from serum creatinine. Nephron. 1976; 16:31-41.

† ADD-Vantage is a registered trademark of Abbott Laboratories Inc.

All other trademarks are the property of the AstraZeneca group of companies.

Manufactured for:
AstraZeneca Pharmaceuticals LP
Wilmington, DE 19850
By: ACS Dobfar SpA
Viale Addetta, 4/12
20067 Tribiano, Milano, Italy
Made in Italy
64213-01
Rev 01/04

NOLVADEX® ℞
[*nōl-vă-dĕks*]
(tamoxifen citrate)

Prescribing information for this product, which appears on pages 678–685 of the 2004 PDR, has been revised. **Please visit www.NOLVADEX.com or call the AstraZeneca Information Center at 1-800-236-9933 for the most current full prescribing information.**

SEROQUEL® ℞
(quetiapine fumarate)

Prescribing information for this product, which appears on pages 685–689 of the 2004 PDR, has been completely revised as follows. Please write "See Supplement A" next to the product heading.

DESCRIPTION

SEROQUEL (quetiapine fumarate) is a psychotropic agent belonging to a new chemical class, the dibenzothiazepine derivatives. The chemical designation is 2-[2-(4-dibenzo [*b,f*] [1,4]thiazepin-11-yl-1-piperazinyl)ethoxy]-ethanol fumarate (2:1) (salt). It is present in tablets as the fumarate salt. All doses and tablet strengths are expressed as milligrams of base, not as fumarate salt. Its molecular formula is $C_{42}H_{50}N_6O_4S_2 \bullet C_4H_4O_4$ and it has a molecular weight of 883.11 (fumarate salt). The structural formula is:

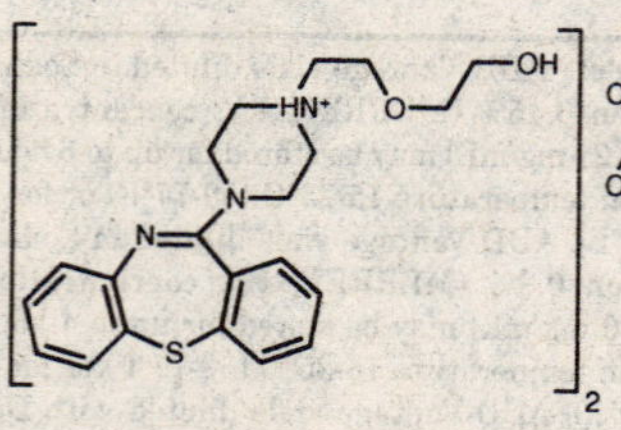

Quetiapine fumarate is a white to off-white crystalline powder which is moderately soluble in water.

SEROQUEL is supplied for oral administration as 25 mg (round, peach), 100 mg (round, yellow), 200 mg (round, white), and 300 mg (capsule-shaped, white) tablets.

Inactive ingredients are povidone, dibasic dicalcium phosphate dihydrate, microcrystalline cellulose, sodium starch glycolate, lactose monohydrate, magnesium stearate, hypromellose, polyethylene glycol and titanium dioxide.

The 25 mg tablets contain red ferric oxide and yellow ferric oxide and the 100 mg tablets contain only yellow ferric oxide.

CLINICAL PHARMACOLOGY

Pharmacodynamics

SEROQUEL is an antagonist at multiple neurotransmitter receptors in the brain: serotonin $5HT_{1A}$ and $5HT_2$ (IC_{50s}=717 & 148nM respectively), dopamine D_1 and D_2 (IC_{50s}=1268 & 329nM respectively), histamine H_1 (IC_{50}=30nM), and adrenergic α_1 and α_2 receptors (IC_{50s}=94 & 271nM, respectively). SEROQUEL has no appreciable affinity at cholinergic muscarinic and benzodiazepine receptors (IC_{50s}>5000 nM).

The mechanism of action of SEROQUEL, as with other drugs having efficacy in the treatment of schizophrenia and acute manic episodes associated with bipolar disorder, is unknown. However, it has been proposed that this drug's efficacy in schizophrenia is mediated through a combination of dopamine type 2 (D_2) and serotonin type 2 ($5HT_2$) antagonism. Antagonism at receptors other than dopamine and $5HT_2$ with similar receptor affinities may explain some of the other effects of SEROQUEL.

SEROQUEL's antagonism of histamine H_1 receptors may explain the somnolence observed with this drug.

SEROQUEL's antagonism of adrenergic α_1 receptors may explain the orthostatic hypotension observed with this drug.

Pharmacokinetics

Quetiapine fumarate activity is primarily due to the parent drug. The multiple-dose pharmacokinetics of quetiapine are dose-proportional within the proposed clinical dose range, and quetiapine accumulation is predictable upon multiple dosing. Elimination of quetiapine is mainly via hepatic metabolism with a mean terminal half-life of about 6 hours within the proposed clinical dose range. Steady-state concentrations are expected to be achieved within two days of dosing. Quetiapine is unlikely to interfere with the metabolism of drugs metabolized by cytochrome P450 enzymes.

Absorption: Quetiapine fumarate is rapidly absorbed after oral administration, reaching peak plasma concentrations in 1.5 hours. The tablet formulation is 100% bioavailable relative to solution. The bioavailability of quetiapine is marginally affected by administration with food, with C_{max} and AUC values increased by 25% and 15%, respectively.

Distribution: Quetiapine is widely distributed throughout the body with an apparent volume of distribution of 10±4 L/kg. It is 83% bound to plasma proteins at therapeutic concentrations. *In vitro*, quetiapine did not affect the binding of warfarin or diazepam to human serum albumin. In turn, neither warfarin nor diazepam altered the binding of quetiapine.

Metabolism and Elimination: Following a single oral dose of ^{14}C-quetiapine, less than 1% of the administered dose was excreted as unchanged drug, indicating that quetiapine is highly metabolized. Approximately 73% and 20% of the dose was recovered in the urine and feces, respectively.

Quetiapine is extensively metabolized by the liver. The major metabolic pathways are sulfoxidation to the sulfoxide metabolite and oxidation to the parent acid metabolite; both metabolites are pharmacologically inactive. *In vitro* studies using human liver microsomes revealed that the cytochrome P450 3A4 isoenzyme is involved in the metabolism of quetiapine to its major, but inactive, sulfoxide metabolite.

Population Subgroups

Age: Oral clearance of quetiapine was reduced by 40% in elderly patients (≥ 65 years, n=9) compared to young patients (n=12), and dosing adjustment may be necessary (See **DOSAGE AND ADMINISTRATION**).

Gender: There is no gender effect on the pharmacokinetics of quetiapine.

Race: There is no race effect on the pharmacokinetics of quetiapine.

Smoking: Smoking has no effect on the oral clearance of quetiapine.

Renal Insufficiency: Patients with severe renal impairment (Clcr=10–30 mL/min/1.73 m^2, n=8) had a 25% lower mean oral clearance than normal subjects (Clcr > 80 mL/min/1.73 m^2, n=8), but plasma quetiapine concentrations in the subjects with renal insufficiency were within the range of concentrations seen in normal subjects receiving the same dose. Dosage adjustment is therefore not needed in these patients.

Hepatic Insufficiency: Hepatically impaired patients (n=8) had a 30% lower mean oral clearance of quetiapine than normal subjects. In two of the 8 hepatically impaired patients, AUC and C_{max} were 3-times higher than those observed typically in healthy subjects. Since quetiapine is extensively metabolized by the liver, higher plasma levels are expected in the hepatically impaired population, and dosage adjustment may be needed (See **DOSAGE AND ADMINISTRATION**).

Drug-Drug Interactions: *In vitro* enzyme inhibition data suggest that quetiapine and 9 of its metabolites would have little inhibitory effect on *in vivo* metabolism mediated by cytochromes P450 1A2, 2C9, 2C19, 2D6 and 3A4.

Quetiapine oral clearance is increased by the prototype cytochrome P450 3A4 inducer, phenytoin, and decreased by the prototype cytochrome P450 3A4 inhibitor, ketoconazole. Dose adjustment of quetiapine will be necessary if it is coadministered with phenytoin or ketoconazole (See **Drug Interactions** under **PRECAUTIONS** and **DOSAGE AND ADMINISTRATION**).

Quetiapine oral clearance is not inhibited by the nonspecific enzyme inhibitor, cimetidine.

Quetiapine at doses of 750 mg/day did not affect the single dose pharmacokinetics of antipyrine, lithium or lorazepam (See **Drug Interactions** under **PRECAUTIONS**).

Clinical Efficacy Data

Bipolar Mania

The efficacy of SEROQUEL in the treatment of acute manic episodes was established in 3 short-term (3-week) placebo-controlled trials in patients who met DSM-IV criteria for Bipolar I disorder with manic episodes. These trials included patients with or without psychotic features and excluded patients with rapid cycling and mixed episodes. Of these trials, 2 were monotherapy and 1 was adjunct therapy to either lithium or divalproex. Adjunct therapy is defined as the simultaneous initiation or subsequent administration of SEROQUEL with lithium or divalproex.

The primary rating instrument used for assessing manic symptoms in these trials was the Young Mania Rating Scale (YMRS), an 11-item clinician-rated scale traditionally used to assess the degree of manic symptomatology (irritability, disruptive/aggressive behavior, sleep, elevated mood, speech, increased activity, sexual interest, language/thought disorder, thought content, appearance, and insight) in a range from 0 (no manic features) to 60 (maximum score). The primary outcome in these trials was change from baseline in the YMRS total score at Day 21.

The results of the trials follow:

Monotherapy

In two 3-week trials (n=300, n=299) comparing SEROQUEL to placebo, SEROQUEL was superior to placebo in the reduction of the YMRS total score. The majority of patients in these trials taking SEROQUEL were dosed in a range of 400 and 800 mg per day.

Adjunct Therapy

In this 3-week placebo-controlled trial, 170 patients with acute bipolar mania (YMRS ≥ 20) were randomized to receive SEROQUEL or placebo as adjunct treatment to lithium or divalproex. Patients may or may not have received an adequate treatment course of lithium or divalproex prior to randomization. SEROQUEL was superior to placebo when added to lithium or divalproex alone in the reduction of YMRS total score.

The majority of patients in this trial taking SEROQUEL were dosed in a range between 400 and 800 mg per day. In a similarly designed trial (n=200), SEROQUEL was associated with an improvement in YMRS scores but did not demonstrate superiority to placebo, possibly due to a higher placebo effect.

Schizophrenia

The efficacy of SEROQUEL in the treatment of schizophrenia was established in 3 short-term (6-week) controlled trials of inpatients with schizophrenia who met DSM III-R criteria for schizophrenia. Although a single fixed dose haloperidol arm was included as a comparative treatment in one of the three trials, this single haloperidol dose group was inadequate to provide a reliable and valid comparison of SEROQUEL and haloperidol.

Several instruments were used for assessing psychiatric signs and symptoms in these studies, among them the Brief Psychiatric Rating Scale (BPRS), a multi-item inventory of general psychopathology traditionally used to evaluate the effects of drug treatment in schizophrenia. The BPRS psychosis cluster (conceptual disorganization, hallucinatory behavior, suspiciousness, and unusual thought content) is considered a particularly useful subset for assessing actively psychotic schizophrenic patients. A second traditional assessment, the Clinical Global Impression (CGI), reflects the impression of a skilled observer, fully familiar with the manifestations of schizophrenia, about the overall clinical state of the patient. In addition, the Scale for Assessing Negative Symptoms (SANS), a more recently developed but less well evaluated scale, was employed for assessing negative symptoms.

The results of the trials follow:

(1) In a 6-week, placebo-controlled trial (n=361) involving 5 fixed doses of SEROQUEL (75, 150, 300, 600 and 750 mg/day on a tid schedule), the 4 highest doses of SEROQUEL were generally superior to placebo on the BPRS total score, the BPRS psychosis cluster and the CGI severity score, with the maximal effect seen at 300 mg/day, and the effects of doses of 150 to 750 were generally indistinguishable. SEROQUEL, at a dose of 300 mg/day, was superior to placebo on the SANS.

(2) In a 6-week, placebo-controlled trial (n=286) involving titration of SEROQUEL in high (up to 750 mg/day on a tid schedule) and low (up to 250 mg/day on a tid schedule) doses, only the high dose SEROQUEL group (mean dose, 500 mg/day) was generally superior to placebo on the BPRS total score, the BPRS psychosis cluster, the CGI severity score, and the SANS.

(3) In a 6-week dose and dose regimen comparison trial (n=618) involving two fixed doses of SEROQUEL (450 mg/day on both bid and tid schedules and 50 mg/day on a bid schedule), only the 450 mg/day (225 mg bid schedule) dose group was generally superior to the 50 mg/day (25 mg bid) SEROQUEL dose group on the BPRS total score, the BPRS psychosis cluster, the CGI severity score, and on the SANS.

Examination of population subsets (race, gender, and age) did not reveal any differential responsiveness on the basis of race or gender, with an apparently greater effect in patients under the age of 40 compared to those older than 40. The clinical significance of this finding is unknown.

INDICATIONS AND USAGE

Bipolar Mania

SEROQUEL is indicated for the short-term treatment of acute manic episodes associated with bipolar I disorder, as either monotherapy or adjunct therapy to lithium or divalproex.

The efficacy of SEROQUEL in acute bipolar mania was established in two 3-week monotherapy trials and one 3-week adjunct therapy trial of bipolar I patients initially hospitalized for up to 7 days for acute mania (See **CLINICAL PHARMACOLOGY**). Effectiveness for more than 3 weeks has not been systematically evaluated in clinical trials. Therefore, the physician who elects to use SEROQUEL for extended periods should periodically re-evaluate the long-term risks and benefits of the drug for the individual patient (See **DOSAGE AND ADMINISTRATION**).

Schizophrenia

SEROQUEL is indicated for the treatment of schizophrenia.

The efficacy of SEROQUEL in schizophrenia was established in short-term (6-week) controlled trials of schizophrenic inpatients (See **CLINICAL PHARMACOLOGY**).

The effectiveness of SEROQUEL in long-term use, that is, for more than 6 weeks, has not been systematically evaluated in controlled trials. Therefore, the physician who elects to use SEROQUEL for extended periods should periodically re-evaluate the long-term usefulness of the drug for the individual patient (See **DOSAGE AND ADMINISTRATION**).

CONTRAINDICATIONS

SEROQUEL is contraindicated in individuals with a known hypersensitivity to this medication or any of its ingredients.

WARNINGS

Neuroleptic Malignant Syndrome (NMS)

A potentially fatal symptom complex sometimes referred to as Neuroleptic Malignant Syndrome (NMS) has been reported in association with administration of antipsychotic drugs, including SEROQUEL. Rare cases of NMS have been reported with SEROQUEL. Clinical manifestations of NMS are hyperpyrexia, muscle rigidity, altered mental status, and evidence of autonomic instability (irregular pulse or blood pressure, tachycardia, diaphoresis, and cardiac dysrhythmia). Additional signs may include elevated creatine phosphokinase, myoglobinuria (rhabdomyolysis) and acute renal failure.

The diagnostic evaluation of patients with this syndrome is complicated. In arriving at a diagnosis, it is important to exclude cases where the clinical presentation includes both serious medical illness (e.g., pneumonia, systemic infection, etc.) and untreated or inadequately treated extrapyramidal signs and symptoms (EPS). Other important considerations in the differential diagnosis include central anticholinergic toxicity, heat stroke, drug fever and primary central nervous system (CNS) pathology.

The management of NMS should include: 1) immediate discontinuation of antipsychotic drugs and other drugs not essential to concurrent therapy; 2) intensive symptomatic treatment and medical monitoring; and 3) treatment of any concomitant serious medical problems for which specific treatments are available. There is no general agreement about specific pharmacological treatment regimens for NMS.

If a patient requires antipsychotic drug treatment after recovery from NMS, the potential reintroduction of drug therapy should be carefully considered. The patient should be carefully monitored since recurrences of NMS have been reported.

Tardive Dyskinesia

A syndrome of potentially irreversible, involuntary, dyskinetic movements may develop in patients treated with antipsychotic drugs. Although the prevalence of the syndrome appears to be highest among the elderly, especially elderly women, it is impossible to rely upon prevalence estimates to predict, at the inception of antipsychotic treatment, which patients are likely to develop the syndrome. Whether antipsychotic drug products differ in their potential to cause tardive dyskinesia is unknown.

The risk of developing tardive dyskinesia and the likelihood that it will become irreversible are believed to increase as the duration of treatment and the total cumulative dose of antipsychotic drugs administered to the patient increase. However, the syndrome can develop, although much less commonly, after relatively brief treatment periods at low doses.

There is no known treatment for established cases of tardive dyskinesia, although the syndrome may remit, partially or completely, if antipsychotic treatment is withdrawn. Antipsychotic treatment, itself, however, may suppress (or partially suppress) the signs and symptoms of the syndrome and thereby may possibly mask the underlying process. The effect that symptomatic suppression has upon the long-term course of the syndrome is unknown.

Given these considerations, SEROQUEL should be prescribed in a manner that is most likely to minimize the occurrence of tardive dyskinesia. Chronic antipsychotic treatment should generally be reserved for patients who appear to suffer from a chronic illness that (1) is known to respond to antipsychotic drugs, and (2) for whom alternative, equally effective, but potentially less harmful treatments are not available or appropriate. In patients who do require chronic treatment, the smallest dose and the shortest duration of treatment producing a satisfactory clinical response should be sought. The need for continued treatment should be reassessed periodically.

If signs and symptoms of tardive dyskinesia appear in a patient on SEROQUEL, drug discontinuation should be considered. However, some patients may require treatment with SEROQUEL despite the presence of the syndrome.

Hyperglycemia and Diabetes Mellitus

Hyperglycemia, in some cases extreme and associated with ketoacidosis or hyperosmolar coma or death, has been reported in patients treated with atypical antipsychotics, including Seroquel. Assessment of the relationship between atypical antipsychotic use and glucose abnormalities is complicated by the possibility of an increased background risk of diabetes mellitus in patients with schizophrenia and the increasing incidence of diabetes mellitus in the general population. Given these confounders, the relationship between atypical antipsychotic use and hyperglycemia-related adverse events is not completely understood. However, epidemiological studies suggest an increased risk of treatment-emergent hyperglycemia-related adverse events in patients treated with the atypical antipsychotics. Precise risk estimates for hyperglycemia-related adverse events in patients treated with atypical antipsychotics are not available.

Patients with an established diagnosis of diabetes mellitus who are started on atypical antipsychotics should be monitored regularly for worsening of glucose control. Patients with risk factors for diabetes mellitus (eg, obesity, family history of diabetes) who are starting treatment with atypical antipsychotics should undergo fasting blood glucose testing at the beginning of treatment and periodically during treatment. Any patient treated with atypical antipsychotics should be monitored for symptoms of hyperglycemia including polydipsia, polyuria, polyphagia, and weakness. Patients who develop symptoms of hyperglycemia during treatment with atypical antipsychotics should undergo fasting blood glucose testing. In some cases, hyperglycemia has resolved when the atypical antipsychotic was discontinued; however, some patients required continuation of anti-diabetic treatment despite discontinuation of the suspect drug.

PRECAUTIONS

General

Orthostatic Hypotension: SEROQUEL may induce orthostatic hypotension associated with dizziness, tachycardia and, in some patients, syncope, especially during the initial dose-titration period, probably reflecting its α_1-adrenergic antagonist properties. Syncope was reported in 1% (23/2567) of the patients treated with SEROQUEL, compared with 0% (0/607) on placebo and about 0.4% (2/527) on active control drugs.

SEROQUEL should be used with particular caution in patients with known cardiovascular disease (history of myocardial infarction or ischemic heart disease, heart failure or conduction abnormalities), cerebrovascular disease or conditions which would predispose patients to hypotension (dehydration, hypovolemia and treatment with antihypertensive medications). The risk of orthostatic hypotension and syncope may be minimized by limiting the initial dose to 25 mg bid (See **DOSAGE AND ADMINISTRATION**). If hypotension occurs during titration to the target dose, a return to the previous dose in the titration schedule is appropriate.

Cataracts: The development of cataracts was observed in association with quetiapine treatment in chronic dog studies (see Animal Toxicology). Lens changes have also been observed in patients during long-term SEROQUEL treatment, but a causal relationship to SEROQUEL use has not been established. Nevertheless, the possibility of lenticular changes cannot be excluded at this time. Therefore, examination of the lens by methods adequate to detect cataract formation, such as slit lamp exam or other appropriately sensitive methods, is recommended at initiation of treatment or shortly thereafter, and at 6 month intervals during chronic treatment.

Seizures: During clinical trials, seizures occurred in 0.6% (18/2792) of patients treated with SEROQUEL compared to 0.2% (1/607) on placebo and 0.7% (4/527) on active control drugs. As with other antipsychotics SEROQUEL should be used cautiously in patients with a history of seizures or with conditions that potentially lower the seizure threshold, e.g., Alzheimer's dementia. Conditions that lower the seizure threshold may be more prevalent in a population of 65 years or older.

Hypothyroidism: Clinical trials with SEROQUEL demonstrated a dose-related decrease in total and free thyroxine (T4) of approximately 20% at the higher end of the therapeutic dose range and was maximal in the first two to four weeks of treatment and maintained without adaptation or progression during more chronic therapy. Generally, these changes were of no clinical significance and TSH was unchanged in most patients, and levels of TBG were unchanged. In nearly all cases, cessation of SEROQUEL treatment was associated with a reversal of the effects on total and free T4, irrespective of the duration of treatment. About 0.4% (12/2791) of SEROQUEL patients did experience TSH increases in monotherapy studies. Six of the patients with TSH increases needed replacement thyroid treatment. In the mania adjunct studies, where SEROQUEL was added to lithium or divalproate, 12% (24/196) of SEROQUEL treated patients compared to 7% (15/203) of placebo treated patients had elevated TSH levels. Of the SEROQUEL treated patients with elevated TSH levels, 3 had simultaneous low free T4 levels.

Cholesterol and Triglyceride Elevations: In schizophrenia trials, SEROQUEL-treated patients had increases from baseline in cholesterol and triglyceride of 11% and 17%, respectively, compared to slight decreases for placebo patients. These changes were only weakly related to the increases in weight observed in SEROQUEL-treated patients.

Hyperprolactinemia: Although an elevation of prolactin levels was not demonstrated in clinical trials with SEROQUEL, increased prolactin levels were observed in rat studies with this compound, and were associated with an increase in mammary gland neoplasia in rats (see **Carcinogenesis**). Tissue culture experiments indicate that approximately one-third of human breast cancers are prolactin dependent *in vitro*, a factor of potential importance if the prescription of these drugs is contemplated in a patient with previously detected breast cancer. Although disturbances such as galactorrhea, amenorrhea, gynecomastia, and impotence have been reported with prolactin-elevating compounds, the clinical significance of elevated serum prolactin levels is unknown for most patients. Neither clinical studies nor epidemiologic studies conducted to date have shown an association between chronic administration of this class of drugs and tumorigenesis in humans; the available evidence is considered too limited to be conclusive at this time.

Transaminase Elevations: Asymptomatic, transient and reversible elevations in serum transaminases (primarily ALT) have been reported. In schizophrenia trials, the proportions of patients with transaminase elevations of > 3 times the upper limits of the normal reference range in a pool of 3- to 6-week placebo-controlled trials were approximately 6% for SEROQUEL compared to 1% for placebo. In acute bipolar mania trials, the proportions of patients with transaminase elevations of > 3 times the upper limits of the normal reference range in a pool of 3- to 12-week placebo-controlled trials were approximately 1% for both SEROQUEL and placebo. These hepatic enzyme elevations usually occurred within the first 3 weeks of drug treatment and promptly returned to pre-study levels with ongoing treatment with SEROQUEL.

Potential for Cognitive and Motor Impairment: Somnolence was a commonly reported adverse event reported in patients treated with SEROQUEL especially during the 3–5 day period of initial dose-titration. In schizophrenia trials, somnolence was reported in 18% of patients on SEROQUEL compared to 11% of placebo patients. In acute bipolar mania trials using SEROQUEL as monotherapy, somnolence was reported in 16% of patients on SEROQUEL compared to 4% of placebo patients. In acute bipolar mania trials using SEROQUEL as adjunct therapy, somnolence was reported in 34% of patients on SEROQUEL compared to 9% of placebo patients. Since SEROQUEL has the potential to impair judgment, thinking, or motor skills, patients should be cautioned about performing activities requiring mental alertness, such as operating a motor vehicle (including automobiles) or operating hazardous machinery until they are reasonably certain that SEROQUEL therapy does not affect them adversely.

Priapism: One case of priapism in a patient receiving SEROQUEL has been reported prior to market introduction. While a causal relationship to use of SEROQUEL has not been established, other drugs with alpha-adrenergic blocking effects have been reported to induce priapism, and it is possible that SEROQUEL may share this capacity. Severe priapism may require surgical intervention.

Body Temperature Regulation: Although not reported with SEROQUEL, disruption of the body's ability to reduce core body temperature has been attributed to antipsychotic agents. Appropriate care is advised when prescribing SEROQUEL for patients who will be experiencing conditions which may contribute to an elevation in core body temperature, e.g., exercising strenuously, exposure to extreme heat, receiving concomitant medication with anticholinergic activity, or being subject to dehydration.

Dysphagia: Esophageal dysmotility and aspiration have been associated with antipsychotic drug use. Aspiration pneumonia is a common cause of morbidity and mortality in elderly patients, in particular those with advanced Alzheimer's dementia. SEROQUEL and other antipsychotic drugs should be used cautiously in patients at risk for aspiration pneumonia.

Suicide: The possibility of a suicide attempt is inherent in bipolar disorder and schizophrenia: close supervision of high risk patients should accompany drug therapy. Prescriptions for SEROQUEL should be written for the smallest quantity of tablets consistent with good patient management in order to reduce the risk of overdose.

Use in Patients with Concomitant Illness: Clinical experience with SEROQUEL in patients with certain concomitant systemic illnesses (see Renal Impairment and Hepatic Impairment under **CLINICAL PHARMACOLOGY**, Special Populations) is limited. SEROQUEL has not been evaluated or used to any appreciable extent in patients with a recent history of myocardial infarction or unstable heart disease. Patients with these diagnoses were excluded from premarketing clinical studies. Because of the risk of orthostatic hypotension with SEROQUEL, caution should be observed in cardiac patients (see **Orthostatic Hypotension**).

Information for Patients

Physicians are advised to discuss the following issues with patients for whom they prescribe SEROQUEL.

Orthostatic Hypotension: Patients should be advised of the risk of orthostatic hypotension, especially during the 3–5 day period of initial dose titration, and also at times of re-initiating treatment or increases in dose.

Interference with Cognitive and Motor Performance: Since somnolence was a commonly reported adverse event associated with SEROQUEL treatment, patients should be advised of the risk of somnolence, especially during the 3–5 day period of initial dose titration. Patients should be cautioned about performing any activity requiring mental alertness, such as operating a motor vehicle (including automobiles) or operating hazardous machinery, until they are reasonably certain that SEROQUEL therapy does not affect them adversely.

Pregnancy: Patients should be advised to notify their physician if they become pregnant or intend to become pregnant during therapy.

Nursing: Patients should be advised not to breast feed if they are taking SEROQUEL.

Concomitant Medication: As with other medications, patients should be advised to notify their physicians if they are taking, or plan to take, any prescription or over-the-counter drugs.

Alcohol: Patients should be advised to avoid consuming alcoholic beverages while taking SEROQUEL.

Heat Exposure and Dehydration: Patients should be advised regarding appropriate care in avoiding overheating and dehydration.

Laboratory Tests

No specific laboratory tests are recommended.

Drug Interactions

The risks of using SEROQUEL in combination with other drugs have not been extensively evaluated in systematic studies. Given the primary CNS effects of SEROQUEL, caution should be used when it is taken in combination with other centrally acting drugs. SEROQUEL potentiated the cognitive and motor effects of alcohol in a clinical trial in subjects with selected psychotic disorders, and alcoholic beverages should be avoided while taking SEROQUEL.

Because of its potential for inducing hypotension, SEROQUEL may enhance the effects of certain antihypertensive agents.

SEROQUEL may antagonize the effects of levodopa and dopamine agonists.

The Effect of Other Drugs on Quetiapine

Phenytoin: Coadministration of quetiapine (250 mg tid) and phenytoin (100 mg tid) increased the mean oral clearance of quetiapine by 5-fold. Increased doses of SEROQUEL may be required to maintain control of symptoms of schizophrenia in patients receiving quetiapine and phenytoin, or other hepatic enzyme inducers (e.g., carbamazepine, barbiturates, rifampin, glucocorticoids). Caution should be taken if phenytoin is withdrawn and replaced with a non-inducer (e.g., valproate) (see **DOSAGE AND ADMINISTRATION**).

Divalproex: Coadministration of quetiapine (150 mg bid) and divalproex (500 mg bid) increased the mean maximum plasma concentration of quetiapine at steady state by 17% without affecting the extent of absorption or mean oral clearance.

Thioridazine: Thioridazine (200 mg bid) increased the oral clearance of quetiapine (300 mg bid) by 65%.

Cimetidine: Administration of multiple daily doses of cimetidine (400 mg tid for 4 days) resulted in a 20% decrease in the mean oral clearance of quetiapine (150 mg tid). Dosage adjustment for quetiapine is not required when it is given with cimetidine.

P450 3A Inhibitors: Coadministration of ketoconazole (200 mg once daily for 4 days), a potent inhibitor of cytochrome P450 3A, reduced oral clearance of quetiapine by 84%, resulting in a 335% increase in maximum plasma concentration of quetiapine. Caution is indicated when

Continued on next page

Seroquel—Cont.

SEROQUEL is administered with ketoconazole and other inhibitors of cytochrome P450 3A (e.g., itraconazole, fluconazole, and erythromycin).

Fluoxetine, Imipramine, Haloperidol, and Risperidone: Coadministration of fluoxetine (60 mg once daily); imipramine (75 mg bid), haloperidol (7.5 mg bid), or risperidone (3 mg bid) with quetiapine (300 mg bid) did not alter the steady-state pharmacokinetics of quetiapine.

Effect of Quetiapine on Other Drugs

Lorazepam: The mean oral clearance of lorazepam (2 mg, single dose) was reduced by 20% in the presence of quetiapine administered as 250 mg tid dosing.

Divalproex: The mean maximum concentration and extent of absorption of total and free valproic acid at steady state were decreased by 10 to 12% when divalproex (500 mg bid) was administered with quetiapine (150 mg bid). The mean oral clearance of total valproic acid (administered as divalproex 500 mg bid) was increased by 11% in the presence of quetiapine (150 mg bid). The changes were not significant

Lithium: Concomitant administration of quetiapine (250 mg tid) with lithium had no effect on any of the steady-state pharmacokinetic parameters of lithium.

Antipyrine: Administration of multiple daily doses up to 750 mg/day (on a tid schedule) of quetiapine to subjects with selected psychotic disorders had no clinically relevant effect on the clearance of antipyrine or urinary recovery of antipyrine metabolites. These results indicate that quetiapine does not significantly induce hepatic enzymes responsible for cytochrome P450 mediated metabolism of antipyrine.

Carcinogenesis, Mutagenesis, Impairment of Fertility

Carcinogenesis: Carcinogenicity studies were conducted in C57BL mice and Wistar rats. Quetiapine was administered in the diet to mice at doses of 20, 75, 250, and 750 mg/kg and to rats by gavage at doses of 25, 75, and 250 mg/kg for two years. These doses are equivalent to 0.1, 0.5, 1.5, and 4.5 times the maximum human dose (800 mg/day) on a mg/m^2 basis (mice) or 0.3, 0.9, and 3.0 times the maximum human dose on a mg/m^2 basis (rats). There were statistically significant increases in thyroid gland follicular adenomas in male mice at doses of 250 and 750 mg/kg or 1.5 and 4.5 times the maximum human dose on a mg/m^2 basis and in male rats at a dose of 250 mg/kg or 3.0 times the maximum human dose on a mg/m^2 basis. Mammary gland adenocarcinomas were statistically significantly increased in female rats at all doses tested (25, 75, and 250 mg/kg or 0.3, 0.9, and 3.0 times the maximum recommended human dose on a mg/m^2 basis).

Thyroid follicular cell adenomas may have resulted from chronic stimulation of the thyroid gland by thyroid stimulating hormone (TSH) resulting from enhanced metabolism and clearance of thyroxine by rodent liver. Changes in TSH, thyroxine, and thyroxine clearance consistent with this mechanism were observed in subchronic toxicity studies in rat and mouse and in a 1-year toxicity study in rat; however, the results of these studies were not definitive. The relevance of the increases in thyroid follicular cell adenomas to human risk, through whatever mechanism, is unknown.

Antipsychotic drugs have been shown to chronically elevate prolactin levels in rodents. Serum measurements in a 1-yr toxicity study showed that quetiapine increased median serum prolactin levels a maximum of 32- and 13-fold in male and female rats, respectively. Increases in mammary neoplasms have been found in rodents after chronic administration of other antipsychotic drugs and are considered to be prolactin-mediated. The relevance of this increased incidence of prolactin-mediated mammary gland tumors in rats to human risk is unknown (see Hyperprolactinemia in **PRECAUTIONS, General**).

Mutagenesis: The mutagenic potential of quetiapine was tested in six *in vitro* bacterial gene mutation assays and in an *in vitro* mammalian gene mutation assay in Chinese Hamster Ovary cells. However, sufficiently high concentrations of quetiapine may not have been used for all tester strains. Quetiapine did produce a reproducible increase in mutations in one *Salmonella typhimurium* tester strain in the presence of metabolic activation. No evidence of clastogenic potential was obtained in an *in vitro* chromosomal aberration assay in cultured human lymphocytes or in the *in vivo* micronucleus assay in rats.

Impairment of Fertility: Quetiapine decreased mating and fertility in male Sprague-Dawley rats at oral doses of 50 and 150 mg/kg or 0.6 and 1.8 times the maximum human dose on a mg/m^2 basis. Drug-related effects included increases in interval to mate and in the number of matings required for successful impregnation. These effects continued to be observed at 150 mg/kg even after a two-week period without treatment. The no-effect dose for impaired mating and fertility in male rats was 25 mg/kg, or 0.3 times the maximum human dose on a mg/m^2 basis. Quetiapine adversely affected mating and fertility in female Sprague-Dawley rats at an oral dose of 50 mg/kg, or 0.6 times the maximum human dose on a mg/m^2 basis. Drug-related effects included decreases in matings and in matings resulting in pregnancy, and an increase in the interval to mate. An increase in irregular estrus cycles was observed at doses of 10 and 50 mg/kg, or 0.1 and 0.6 times the maximum human dose on a mg/m^2 basis. The no-effect dose in female rats was 1 mg/kg, or 0.01 times the maximum human dose on a mg/m^2 basis.

Pregnancy

Pregnancy Category C

The teratogenic potential of quetiapine was studied in Wistar rats and Dutch Belted rabbits dosed during the period of organogenesis. No evidence of a teratogenic effect was detected in rats at doses of 25 to 200 mg/kg or 0.3 to 2.4 times the maximum human dose on a mg/m^2 basis or in rabbits at 25 to 100 mg/kg or 0.6 to 2.4 times the maximum human dose on a mg/m^2 basis. There was, however, evidence of embryo/fetal toxicity. Delays in skeletal ossification were detected in rat fetuses at doses of 50 and 200 mg/kg (0.6 and 2.4 times the maximum human dose on a mg/m^2 basis) and in rabbits at 50 and 100 mg/kg (1.2 and 2.4 times the maximum human dose on a mg/m^2 basis). Fetal body weight was reduced in rat fetuses at 200 mg/kg and rabbit fetuses at 100 mg/kg (2.4 times the maximum human dose on a mg/m^2 basis for both species). There was an increased incidence of a minor soft tissue anomaly (carpal/tarsal flexure) in rabbit fetuses at a dose of 100 mg/kg (2.4 times the maximum human dose on a mg/m^2 basis). Evidence of maternal toxicity (i.e., decreases in body weight gain and/or death) was observed at the high dose in the rat study and at all doses in the rabbit study. In a peri/postnatal reproductive study in rats, no drug-related effects were observed at doses of 1, 10, and 20 mg/kg or 0.01, 0.12, and 0.24 times the maximum human dose on a mg/m^2 basis. However, in a preliminary peri/postnatal study, there were increases in fetal and pup death, and decreases in mean litter weight at 150 mg/kg, or 3.0 times the maximum human dose on a mg/m^2 basis.

There are no adequate and well-controlled studies in pregnant women and quetiapine should be used during pregnancy only if the potential benefit justifies the potential risk to the fetus.

Labor and Delivery: The effect of SEROQUEL on labor and delivery in humans is unknown.

Nursing Mothers: SEROQUEL was excreted in milk of treated animals during lactation. It is not known if SEROQUEL is excreted in human milk. It is recommended that women receiving SEROQUEL should not breast feed.

Pediatric Use: The safety and effectiveness of SEROQUEL in pediatric patients have not been established.

Geriatric Use: Of the approximately 3400 patients in clinical studies with SEROQUEL, 7% (232) were 65 years of age or over. In general, there was no indication of any different tolerability of SEROQUEL in the elderly compared to younger adults. Nevertheless, the presence of factors that might decrease pharmacokinetic clearance, increase the pharmacodynamic response to SEROQUEL, or cause poorer tolerance or orthostasis, should lead to consideration of a lower starting dose, slower titration, and careful monitoring during the initial dosing period in the elderly. The mean plasma clearance of SEROQUEL was reduced by 30% to 50% in elderly patients when compared to younger patients (see Pharmacokinetics under **CLINICAL PHARMACOLOGY** and **DOSAGE AND ADMINISTRATION**).

ADVERSE REACTIONS

The information below is derived from a clinical trial database for SEROQUEL consisting of over 3000 patients. This database includes 405 patients exposed to SEROQUEL for the treatment of acute bipolar mania (monotherapy and adjunct therapy) and approximately 2600 patients and/or normal subjects exposed to 1 or more doses of SEROQUEL for the treatment of schizophrenia.

Of these approximately 3000 subjects, approximately 2700 (2300 in schizophrenia and 405 in acute bipolar mania) were patients who participated in multiple dose effectiveness trials, and their experience corresponded to approximately 914.3 patient-years. The conditions and duration of treatment with SEROQUEL varied greatly and included (in overlapping categories) open-label and double-blind phases of studies, inpatients and outpatients, fixed-dose and dose-titration studies, and short-term or longer-term exposure. Adverse reactions were assessed by collecting adverse events, results of physical examinations, vital signs, weights, laboratory analyses, ECGs, and results of ophthalmologic examinations.

Adverse events during exposure were obtained by general inquiry and recorded by clinical investigators using terminology of their own choosing. Consequently, it is not possible to provide a meaningful estimate of the proportion of individuals experiencing adverse events without first grouping similar types of events into a smaller number of standardized event categories. In the tables and tabulations that follow, standard COSTART terminology has been used to classify reported adverse events.

The stated frequencies of adverse events represent the proportion of individuals who experienced, at least once, a treatment-emergent adverse event of the type listed. An event was considered treatment emergent if it occurred for the first time or worsened while receiving therapy following baseline evaluation.

Adverse Findings Observed in Short-Term, Controlled Trials

Adverse Events Associated with Discontinuation of Treatment in Short-Term, Placebo-Controlled Trials

Acute Bipolar Mania: Overall, discontinuations due to adverse events were 5.7 % for SEROQUEL vs. 5.1% for placebo in monotherapy and 3.6% for SEROQUEL vs. 5.9% for placebo in adjunct therapy.

Schizophrenia: Overall, there was little difference in the incidence of discontinuation due to adverse events (4% for SEROQUEL vs. 3% for placebo) in a pool of controlled trials. However, discontinuations due to somnolence and hypotension were considered to be drug related (see **PRECAUTIONS**):

Adverse Event	SEROQUEL	Placebo
Somnolence	0.8%	0%
Hypotension	0.4%	0%

Adverse Events Occurring at an Incidence of 1% or More Among SEROQUEL Treated Patients in Short-Term, Placebo-Controlled Trials: The prescriber should be aware that the figures in the tables and tabulations cannot be used to predict the incidence of side effects in the course of usual medical practice where patient characteristics and other factors differ from those that prevailed in the clinical trials. Similarly, the cited frequencies cannot be compared with figures obtained from other clinical investigations involving different treatments, uses, and investigators. The cited figures, however, do provide the prescribing physician with some basis for estimating the relative contribution of drug and nondrug factors to the side effect incidence in the population studied.

Table 1 enumerates the incidence, rounded to the nearest percent, of treatment-emergent adverse events that occurred during acute therapy of schizophrenia (up to 6 weeks) and bipolar mania (up to 12 weeks) in 1% or more of patients treated with SEROQUEL (doses ranging from 75 to 800 mg/day) where the incidence in patients treated with SEROQUEL was greater than the incidence in placebo-treated patients.

Table 1. Treatment-Emergent Adverse Experience Incidence in 3- to 12-Week Placebo-Controlled Clinical Trials[1] for the Treatment of Schizophrenia and Acute Bipolar Mania (monotherapy)

Body System/ Preferred Term	SEROQUEL (n=719)	Placebo (n=404)
Body as a Whole		
Headache	21%	14%
Pain	7%	5%
Asthenia	5%	3%
Abdominal pain	4%	1%
Back pain	3%	1%
Fever	2%	1%
Cardiovascular		
Tachycardia	6%	4%
Postural Hypotension	4%	1%
Digestive		
Dry Mouth	9%	3%
Constipation	8%	3%
Vomiting	6%	5%
Dyspepsia	5%	1%
Gastroenteritis	2%	0%
Gamma Glutamyl Transpeptidase Increased	1%	0%
Metabolic and Nutritional		
Weight Gain	5%	1%
SGPT Increased	5%	1%
SGOT Increased	3%	1%
Nervous		
Agitation	20%	17%
Somnolence	18%	8%
Dizziness	11%	5%
Anxiety	4%	3%
Respiratory System		
Pharyngitis	4%	3%
Rhinitis	3%	1%
Skin and Appendages		
Rash	4%	2%
Special Senses		
Amblyopia	2%	1%

[1] Events for which the SEROQUEL incidence was equal to or less than placebo are not listed in the table, but included the following: accidental injury, akathisia, chest pain, cough increased, depression, diarrhea, extrapyramidal syndrome, hostility, hypertension, hypertonia, hypotension, increased appetite, infection, insomnia, leukopenia, malaise, nausea, nervousness, paresthesia, peripheral edema, sweating, tremor, and weight loss.

In these studies, the most commonly observed adverse events associated with the use of SEROQUEL (incidence of 5% or greater) and observed at a rate on SEROQUEL at least twice that of placebo were somnolence (18%), dizziness (11%), dry mouth (9%), constipation (8%), SGPT increased (5%), weight gain (5%), and dyspepsia (5%).

Table 2 enumerates the incidence, rounded to the nearest percent, of treatment-emergent adverse events that occurred during therapy (up to 3-weeks) of acute mania in 5% or more of patients treated with SEROQUEL (doses ranging from 100 to 800 mg/day) used as adjunct therapy to lithium and divalproex where the incidence in patients treated with SEROQUEL was greater than the incidence in placebo-treated patients.

Table 2. Treatment-Emergent Adverse Experience Incidence in 3-Week Placebo-Controlled Clinical Trials[1] for the Treatment of Acute Bipolar Mania (Adjunct Therapy)

Body System/ Preferred Term	SEROQUEL (n=196)	Placebo (n=203)
Body as a Whole		
Headache	17%	13%
Asthenia	10%	4%
Abdominal pain	7%	3%
Back pain	5%	3%

Cardiovascular		
Postural Hypotension	7%	2%
Digestive		
Dry Mouth	19%	3%
Constipation	10%	5%
Metabolic and Nutritional		
Weight gain	6%	3%
Nervous		
Somnolence	34%	9%
Dizziness	9%	6%
Tremor	8%	7%
Agitation	6%	4%
Respiratory		
Pharyngitis	6%	3%

[1] Events for which the SEROQUEL incidence was equal to or less than placebo are not listed in the table, but included the following: akathisia, diarrhea, insomnia, and nausea.

In these studies, the most commonly observed adverse events associated with the use of SEROQUEL (incidence of 5% or greater) and observed at a rate on SEROQUEL at least twice that of placebo were somnolence (34%), dry mouth (19%), asthenia (10%), constipation (10%), abdominal pain (7%), postural hypotension (7%), pharyngitis (6%), and weight gain (6%).

Explorations for interactions on the basis of gender, age, and race did not reveal any clinically meaningful differences in the adverse event occurrence on the basis of these demographic factors.

Dose Dependency of Adverse Events in Short-Term, Placebo-Controlled Trials

Dose-related Adverse Events: Spontaneously elicited adverse event data from a study of schizophrenia comparing five fixed doses of SEROQUEL (75 mg, 150 mg, 300 mg, 600 mg, and 750 mg/day) to placebo were explored for dose-relatedness of adverse events. Logistic regression analyses revealed a positive dose response ($p<0.05$) for the following adverse events: dyspepsia, abdominal pain, and weight gain.

Extrapyramidal Symptoms: Data from one 6-week clinical trial of schizophrenia comparing five fixed doses of SEROQUEL (75, 150, 300, 600, 750 mg/day) provided evidence for the lack of treatment-emergent extrapyramidal symptoms (EPS) and dose-relatedness for EPS associated with SEROQUEL treatment. Three methods were used to measure EPS: (1) Simpson-Angus total score (mean change from baseline) which evaluates parkinsonism and akathisia, (2) incidence of spontaneous complaints of EPS (akathisia, akinesia, cogwheel rigidity, extrapyramidal syndrome, hypertonia, hypokinesia, neck rigidity, and tremor), and (3) use of anticholinergic medications to treat emergent EPS.

Dose Groups	Placebo	SEROQUEL 75mg	150mg	300mg	600mg	750mg
Parkinsonism	0.6	-1.0	-1.2	-1.6	-1.8	-1.8
EPS incidence	16%	6%	6%	4%	8%	6%
Anticholinergic Medications	14%	11%	10%	8%	12%	11%

In six additional placebo-controlled clinical trials (3 in acute mania and 3 in schizophrenia) using variable doses of SEROQUEL, there were no differences between the SEROQUEL and placebo treatment groups in the incidence of EPS, as assessed by Simpson-Angus total scores, spontaneous complaints of EPS and the use of concomitant anticholinergic medications to treat EPS.

Vital Signs and Laboratory Studies

Vital Sign Changes: SEROQUEL is associated with orthostatic hypotension (see **PRECAUTIONS**).

Weight Gain: In schizophrenia trials the proportions of patients meeting a weight gain criterion of ≥7% of body weight were compared in a pool of four 3- to 6-week placebo-controlled clinical trials, revealing a statistically significantly greater incidence of weight gain for SEROQUEL (23%) compared to placebo (6%). In mania monotherapy trials the proportions of patients meeting the same weight gain criterion were 21% compared to 7% for placebo and in mania adjunct therapy trials the proportion of patients meeting the same weight criterion were 13% compared to 4% for placebo.

Laboratory Changes: An assessment of the premarketing experience for SEROQUEL suggested that it is associated with asymptomatic increases in SGPT and increases in both total cholesterol and triglycerides (see **PRECAUTIONS**).

An assessment of hematological parameters in short-term, placebo-controlled trials revealed no clinically important differences between SEROQUEL and placebo.

ECG Changes: Between group comparisons for pooled placebo-controlled trials revealed no statistically significant SEROQUEL/placebo differences in the proportions of patients experiencing potentially important changes in ECG parameters, including QT, QTc, and PR intervals. However, the proportions of patients meeting the criteria for tachycardia were compared in four 3- to 6-week placebo-controlled clinical trials for the treatment of schizophrenia revealing a 1% (4/399) incidence for SEROQUEL compared to 0.6% (1/156) incidence for placebo. In acute (monotherapy) bipolar mania trials the proportions of patients meeting the criteria for tachycardia was 0.5% (1/192) for SEROQUEL compared to 0% (0/178) incidence for placebo. In acute bipolar mania (adjunct) trials the proportions of patients meeting the same criteria was 0.6% (1/166) for SEROQUEL compared to 0% (0/171) incidence for placebo. SEROQUEL use was associated with a mean increase in heart rate, assessed by ECG, of 7 beats per minute compared to a mean increase of 1 beat per minute among placebo patients. This slight tendency to tachycardia may be related to SEROQUEL's potential for inducing orthostatic changes (see **PRECAUTIONS**).

Other Adverse Events Observed During the Pre-Marketing Evaluation of SEROQUEL

Following is a list of COSTART terms that reflect treatment-emergent adverse events as defined in the introduction to the ADVERSE REACTIONS section reported by patients treated with SEROQUEL at multiple doses ≥ 75 mg/day during any phase of a trial within the premarketing database of approximately 2200 patients treated for schizophrenia. All reported events are included except those already listed in Table 1 or elsewhere in labeling, those events for which a drug cause was remote, and those event terms which were so general as to be uninformative. It is important to emphasize that, although the events reported occurred during treatment with SEROQUEL, they were not necessarily caused by it.

Events are further categorized by body system and listed in order of decreasing frequency according to the following definitions: frequent adverse events are those occurring in at least 1/100 patients (only those not already listed in the tabulated results from placebo-controlled trials appear in this listing); infrequent adverse events are those occurring in 1/100 to 1/1000 patients; rare events are those occurring in fewer than 1/1000 patients.

Nervous System: ***Frequent:*** hypertonia, dysarthria; ***Infrequent:*** abnormal dreams, dyskinesia, thinking abnormal, tardive dyskinesia, vertigo, involuntary movements, confusion, amnesia, psychosis, hallucinations, hyperkinesia, libido increased*, urinary retention, incoordination, paranoid reaction, abnormal gait, myoclonus, delusions, manic reaction, apathy, ataxia, depersonalization, stupor, bruxism, catatonic reaction, hemiplegia; ***Rare:*** aphasia, buccoglossal syndrome, choreoathetosis, delirium, emotional lability, euphoria, libido decreased*, neuralgia, stuttering, subdural hematoma.

Body as a Whole: ***Frequent:*** flu syndrome; ***Infrequent:*** neck pain, pelvic pain*, suicide attempt, malaise, photosensitivity reaction, chills, face edema, moniliasis; ***Rare:*** abdomen enlarged.

Digestive System: ***Frequent:*** anorexia; ***Infrequent:*** increased salivation, increased appetite, gamma glutamyl transpeptidase increased, gingivitis, dysphagia, flatulence, gastroenteritis, gastritis, hemorrhoids, stomatitis, thirst, tooth caries, fecal incontinence, gastroesophageal reflux, gum hemorrhage, mouth ulceration, rectal hemorrhage, tongue edema; ***Rare:*** glossitis, hematemesis, intestinal obstruction, melena, pancreatitis.

Cardiovascular System: ***Frequent:*** palpitation; ***Infrequent:*** vasodilatation, QT interval prolonged, migraine, bradycardia, cerebral ischemia, irregular pulse, T wave abnormality, bundle branch block, cerebrovascular accident, deep thrombophlebitis, T wave inversion; ***Rare:*** angina pectoris, atrial fibrillation, AV block first degree, congestive heart failure, ST elevated, thrombophlebitis, T wave flattening, ST abnormality, increased QRS duration.

Respiratory System: ***Frequent:*** pharyngitis, rhinitis, cough increased, dyspnea; ***Infrequent:*** pneumonia, epistaxis, asthma; ***Rare:*** hiccup, hyperventilation.

Metabolic and Nutritional System: ***Frequent:*** peripheral edema; ***Infrequent:*** weight loss, alkaline phosphatase increased, hyperlipemia, alcohol intolerance, dehydration, hyperglycemia, creatinine increased, hypoglycemia; ***Rare:*** glycosuria, gout, hand edema, hypokalemia, water intoxication.

Skin and Appendages System: ***Frequent:*** sweating; ***Infrequent:*** pruritis, acne, eczema, contact dermatitis, maculopapular rash, seborrhea, skin ulcer; ***Rare:*** exfoliative dermatitis, psoriasis, skin discoloration.

Urogenital System: ***Infrequent:*** dysmenorrhea*, vaginitis*, urinary incontinence, metrorrhagia*, impotence*, dysuria, vaginal moniliasis*, abnormal ejaculation*, cystitis, urinary frequency, amenorrhea*, female lactation*, leukorrhea*, vaginal hemorrhage*, vulvo-vaginitis* orchitis*; ***Rare:*** gynecomastia*, nocturia, polyuria, acute kidney failure.

Special Senses: ***Infrequent:*** conjunctivitis, abnormal vision, dry eyes, tinnitus, taste perversion, blepharitis, eye pain; ***Rare:*** abnormality of accommodation, deafness, glaucoma.

Musculoskeletal System: ***Infrequent:*** pathological fracture, myasthenia, twitching, arthralgia, arthritis, leg cramps, bone pain.

Hemic and Lymphatic System: ***Frequent:*** leukopenia; ***Infrequent:*** leukocytosis, anemia, ecchymosis, eosinophilia, hypochromic anemia; lymphadenopathy, cyanosis; ***Rare:*** hemolysis, thrombocytopenia.

Endocrine System: ***Infrequent:*** hypothyroidism, diabetes mellitus; ***Rare:*** hyperthyroidism.

*adjusted for gender

Post Marketing Experience: Adverse events reported since market introduction which were temporally related to SEROQUEL therapy include: leukopenia/neutropenia. If a patient develops a low white cell count consider discontinuation of therapy. Possible risk factors for leukopenia/neutropenia include pre-existing low white cell count and history of drug induced leukopenia/neutropenia.

Other adverse events reported since market introduction, which were temporally related to SEROQUEL therapy, but not necessarily causally related, include the following: agranulocytosis, anaphylaxis, hyponatremia, rhabdomyolysis, syndrome of inappropriate antidiuretic hormone secretion (SIADH), and Steven Johnson syndrome (SJS).

DRUG ABUSE AND DEPENDENCE

Controlled Substance Class: SEROQUEL is not a controlled substance.

Physical and Psychologic dependence: SEROQUEL has not been systematically studied, in animals or humans, for its potential for abuse, tolerance or physical dependence. While the clinical trials did not reveal any tendency for any drug-seeking behavior, these observations were not systematic and it is not possible to predict on the basis of this limited experience the extent to which a CNS-active drug will be misused, diverted, and/or abused once marketed. Consequently, patients should be evaluated carefully for a history of drug abuse, and such patients should be observed closely for signs of misuse or abuse of SEROQUEL, e.g., development of tolerance, increases in dose, drug-seeking behavior.

OVERDOSAGE

Human experience: Experience with SEROQUEL (quetiapine fumarate) in acute overdosage was limited in the clinical trial database (6 reports) with estimated doses ranging from 1200 mg to 9600 mg and no fatalities. In general, reported signs and symptoms were those resulting from an exaggeration of the drug's known pharmacological effects, i.e., drowsiness and sedation, tachycardia and hypotension. One case, involving an estimated overdose of 9600 mg, was associated with hypokalemia and first degree heart block. In post-marketing experience, there have been very rare reports of overdose of SEROQUEL alone resulting in death, coma or QTc prolongation.

Management of Overdosage: In case of acute overdosage, establish and maintain an airway and ensure adequate oxygenation and ventilation. Gastric lavage (after intubation, if patient is unconscious) and administration of activated charcoal together with a laxative should be considered. The possibility of obtundation, seizure or dystonic reaction of the head and neck following overdose may create a risk of aspiration with induced emesis. Cardiovascular monitoring should commence immediately and should include continuous electro-cardiographic monitoring to detect possible arrhythmias. If antiarrhythmic therapy is administered, disopyramide, procainamide and quinidine carry a theoretical hazard of additive QT-prolonging effects when administered in patients with acute overdosage of SEROQUEL. Similarly it is reasonable to expect that the alpha-adrenergic-blocking properties of bretylium might be additive to those of quetiapine, resulting in problematic hypotension.

There is no specific antidote to SEROQUEL. Therefore appropriate supportive measures should be instituted. The possibility of multiple drug involvement should be considered. Hypotension and circulatory collapse should be treated with appropriate measures such as intravenous fluids and/or sympathomimetic agents (epinephrine and dopamine should not be used, since beta stimulation may worsen hypotension in the setting of quetiapine-induced alpha blockade). In cases of severe extrapyramidal symptoms, anticholinergic medication should be administered. Close medical supervision and monitoring should continue until the patient recovers.

DOSAGE AND ADMINISTRATION

Acute Bipolar Mania

Usual Dose: When used as monotherapy or adjunct therapy (with lithium or divalproex), SEROQUEL should be initiated in BID doses totaling 100 mg/day on Day 1, increased to 400 mg/day on Day 4 in increments of up to 100 mg/day in BID divided doses. Further dosage adjustments up to 800 mg/day by Day 6 should be in increments of no greater than 200 mg/day. Data indicates that the majority of patients responded between 400 to 800 mg/day. The safety of doses above 800 mg/day has not been evaluated in clinical trials.

Schizophrenia

Usual Dose: SEROQUEL should generally be administered with an initial dose of 25 mg bid, with increases in increments of 25–50 mg bid or tid on the second and third day, as tolerated, to a target dose range of 300 to 400 mg daily by the fourth day, given bid or tid. Further dosage adjustments, if indicated, should generally occur at intervals of not less than 2 days, as steady state for SEROQUEL would not be achieved for approximately 1–2 days in the typical patient. When dosage adjustments are necessary, dose increments/decrements of 25–50 mg bid are recommended. Most efficacy data with SEROQUEL were obtained using tid regimens, but in one controlled trial 225 mg bid was also effective.

Efficacy in schizophrenia was demonstrated in a dose range of 150 to 750 mg/day in the clinical trials supporting the effectiveness of SEROQUEL. In a dose response study, doses above 300 mg/day were not demonstrated to be more efficacious than the 300 mg/day dose. In other studies, however, doses in the range of 400–500 mg/day appeared to be needed. The safety of doses above 800 mg/day has not been evaluated in clinical trials.

Dosing in Special Populations

Consideration should be given to a slower rate of dose titration and a lower target dose in the elderly, and in patients who are debilitated or who have a predisposition to hypotensive reactions (see **CLINICAL PHARMACOLOGY**). When indicated, dose escalation should be performed with caution in these patients.

Continued on next page

Seroquel—Cont.

Patients with hepatic impairment should be started on 25 mg/day. The dose should be increased daily in increments of 25–50 mg/day to an effective dose, depending on the clinical response and tolerability of the patient.

The elimination of quetiapine was enhanced in the presence of phenytoin. Higher maintenance doses of quetiapine may be required when it is coadministered with phenytoin and other enzyme inducers such as carbamazepine and phenobarbital (See Drug Interactions under **PRECAUTIONS**).

Maintenance Treatment: While there is no body of evidence available to answer the question of how long the patient treated with SEROQUEL should remain on it, the effectiveness of maintenance treatment is well established for many other drugs used to treat schizophrenia. It is recommended that responding patients be continued on SEROQUEL, but at the lowest dose needed to maintain remission. Patients should be periodically reassessed to determine the need for maintenance treatment.

Reinitiation of Treatment in Patients Previously Discontinued: Although there are no data to specifically address reinitiation of treatment, it is recommended that when restarting patients who have had an interval of less than one week off SEROQUEL, titration of SEROQUEL is not required and the maintenance dose may be reinitiated. When restarting therapy of patients who have been off SEROQUEL for more than one week, the initial titration schedule should be followed.

Switching from Antipsychotics: There are no systematically collected data to specifically address switching patients with schizophrenia from antipsychotics to SEROQUEL, or concerning concomitant administration with antipsychotics. While immediate discontinuation of the previous antipsychotic treatment may be acceptable for some patients with schizophrenia, more gradual discontinuation may be most appropriate for others. In all cases, the period of overlapping antipsychotic administration should be minimized. When switching patients with schizophrenia from depot antipsychotics, if medically appropriate, initiate SEROQUEL therapy in place of the next scheduled injection. The need for continuing existing EPS medication should be reevaluated periodically.

HOW SUPPLIED

25 mg Tablets (NDC 0310-0275) peach, round, biconvex, film coated tablets, identified with 'SEROQUEL' and '25' on one side and plain on the other side, are supplied in bottles of 100 tablets and 1000 tablets, and hospital unit dose packages of 100 tablets.

100 mg Tablets (NDC 0310-0271) yellow, round, biconvex film coated tablets, identified with 'SEROQUEL' and '100' on one side and plain on the other side, are supplied in bottles of 100 tablets and hospital unit dose packages of 100 tablets.

200 mg Tablets (NDC 0310-0272) white, round, biconvex, film coated tablets, identified with 'SEROQUEL' and '200' on one side and plain on the other side, are supplied in bottles of 100 tablets and hospital unit dose packages of 100 tablets.

300 mg Tablets (NDC 0310-0274) white, capsule-shaped, biconvex, film coated tablets, intagliated with 'SEROQUEL' on one side and '300' on the other side, are supplied in bottles of 60 tablets and hospital unit dose packages of 100 tablets.

Store at 25°C (77°F); excursions permitted to 15–30°C (59–86°F) [See USP].

ANIMAL TOXICOLOGY

Quetiapine caused a dose-related increase in pigment deposition in thyroid gland in rat toxicity studies which were 4 weeks in duration or longer and in a mouse 2 year carcinogenicity study. Doses were 10–250 mg/kg in rats, 75–750 mg/kg in mice; these doses are 0.1–3.0, and 0.1–4.5 times the maximum recommended human dose (on a mg/m^2 basis), respectively. Pigment deposition was shown to be irreversible in rats. The identity of the pigment could not be determined, but was found to be co-localized with quetiapine in thyroid gland follicular epithelial cells. The functional effects and the relevance of this finding to human risk are unknown.

In dogs receiving quetiapine for 6 or 12 months, but not for 1 month, focal triangular cataracts occurred at the junction of posterior sutures in the outer cortex of the lens at a dose of 100 mg/kg, or 4 times the maximum recommended human dose on a mg/m^2 basis. This finding may be due to inhibition of cholesterol biosynthesis by quetiapine. Quetiapine caused a dose related reduction in plasma cholesterol levels in repeat-dose dog and monkey studies; however, there was no correlation between plasma cholesterol and the presence of cataracts in individual dogs. The appearance of delta-8-cholestanol in plasma is consistent with inhibition of a late stage in cholesterol biosynthesis in these species. There also was a 25% reduction in cholesterol content of the outer cortex of the lens observed in a special study in quetiapine treated female dogs. Drug-related cataracts have not been seen in any other species; however, in a 1-year study in monkeys, a striated appearance of the anterior lens surface was detected in 2/7 females at a dose of 225 mg/kg or 5.5 times the maximum recommended human dose on a mg/m^2 basis.

AstraZeneca Pharmaceuticals LP
Wilmington, DE 19850
Made in USA
217460
64245-01
Rev 01/04
AstraZeneca

ZOLADEX® 3.6 MG ℞

[*zōl'-ă-dĕx*]
(goserelin acetate implant)

Prescribing information for this product, which appears on pages 701–704 of the 2004 PDR, has been revised as follows. Please write "See Supplement A" next to the product heading.

Revise PI to incorporate changes to steps 4 and 6 of the Administration Technique.

Revise step #4 to:

Holding the syringe around the protective sleeve, using an aseptic technique, pinch the skin of the patient's anterior abdominal wall below the navel line. With the bevel of the needle facing up, insert the needle at a 30 to 45 degree angle to the skin in one continuous deliberate motion until the protective sleeve touches the patient's skin (Figure 3).

Revise step #6 to:

To administer the ZOLADEX implant and to activate the protective sleeve, grasp the barrel at the finger grip and depress the plunger until you cannot depress it any further. If the plunger is not depressed **fully** the protective sleeve will **NOT** activate. When the protective sleeve 'clicks', the protective sleeve will automatically begin to slide to cover the needle.

NOTE: The needle does not retract.
64216-00
Rev. 12/03

ZOLADEX® 10.8 mg 3-month ℞

[*zōl'-ă-dĕx*]
(goserelin acetate implant)

Prescribing information for this product, which appears on pages 704–707 of the 2004 PDR, has been revised as follows. Please write "See Supplement A" next to the product heading.

Revise PI to incorporate changes to steps 4 and 6 of the Administration Technique.

Revise step #4 to:

Holding the syringe around the protective sleeve, using an aseptic technique, pinch the skin of the patient's anterior abdominal wall below the navel line. With the bevel of the needle facing up, insert the needle at a 30 to 45 degree angle to the skin in one continuous deliberate motion until the protective sleeve touches the patient's skin (Figure 3).

Revise step #6 to:

To administer the ZOLADEX implant and to activate the protective sleeve, grasp the barrel at the finger grip and depress the plunger until you cannot depress it any further. If the plunger is not depressed **fully** the protective sleeve will **NOT** activate. When the protective sleeve 'clicks', the protective sleeve will automatically begin to slide to cover the needle.

NOTE: The needle does not retract.
64225-00
Rev 12/03

Bayer Pharmaceuticals Corporation

400 MORGAN LANE
WEST HAVEN, CT 06516

For Medical Information Contact:
Director, Medical Services
(800) 468-0894
(203) 812-2000

AVELOX® ℞

[*ă'vĕ-lŏks*]
(moxifloxacin hydrochloride) Tablets
AVELOX® I.V.
(moxifloxacin hydrochloride in sodium chloride injection)

Prescribing information for this product, which appears on pages 834–839 of the 2004 PDR, has been completely revised as follows. Please write "See Supplement A" next to the product heading.

To reduce the development of drug-resistant bacteria and maintain the effectiveness of AVELOX® and other antibacterial drugs, AVELOX should be used only to treat or prevent infections that are proven or strongly suspected to be caused by bacteria.

DESCRIPTION

AVELOX (moxifloxacin hydrochloride) is a synthetic broad spectrum antibacterial agent and is available as AVELOX Tablets for oral administration and as AVELOX I.V. for intravenous administration. Moxifloxacin, a fluoroquinolone, is available as the monohydrochloride salt of 1-cyclopropyl-7-[(S,S)-2,8-diazabicyclo[4.3.0]non-8-yl]-6-fluoro-8-methoxy-1,4-dihydro-4-oxo-3 quinoline carboxylic acid. It is a slightly yellow to yellow crystalline substance with a molecular weight of 437.9. Its empirical formula is $C_{21}H_{24}FN_3O_4$ *HCl and its chemical structure is as follows:

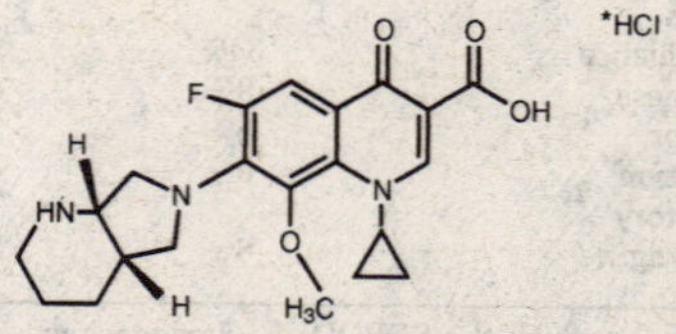

AVELOX Tablets are available as film-coated tablets containing moxifloxacin hydrochloride (equivalent to 400 mg moxifloxacin). The inactive ingredients are microcrystalline cellulose, lactose monohydrate, croscarmellose sodium, magnesium stearate, hypromellose, titanium dioxide, polyethylene glycol and ferric oxide.

AVELOX I.V. is available in ready-to-use 250 mL latex-free flexibags as a sterile, preservative free, 0.8% sodium chloride aqueous solution of moxifloxacin hydrochloride (containing 400 mg moxifloxacin) with pH ranging from 4.1 to 4.6. The appearance of the intravenous solution is yellow. The color does not affect, nor is it indicative of, product stability. The inactive ingredients are sodium chloride, USP, water for Injection, USP, and may include hydrochloric acid and/or sodium hydroxide for pH adjustment.

CLINICAL PHARMACOLOGY

Absorption

Moxifloxacin, given as an oral tablet, is well absorbed from the gastrointestinal tract. The absolute bioavailability of moxifloxacin is approximately 90 percent. Co-administration with a high fat meal (i.e., 500 calories from fat) does not affect the absorption of moxifloxacin.

Consumption of 1 cup of yogurt with moxifloxacin does not significantly affect the extent or rate of systemic absorption (AUC).

The mean (± SD) C_{max} and AUC values following single and multiple doses of 400 mg moxifloxacin given orally are summarized below.

[See first table at bottom of next page]

The mean (± SD) C_{max} and AUC values following single and multiple doses of 400 mg moxifloxacin given by 1 hour I.V. infusion are summarized below.

[See second table at bottom of next page]

Plasma concentrations increase proportionately with dose up to the highest dose tested (1200 mg single oral dose). The mean (± SD) elimination half-life from plasma is 12 ± 1.3 hours; steady-state is achieved after at least three days with a 400 mg once daily regimen.

Mean Steady-State Plasma Concentrations of Moxifloxacin Obtained With Once Daily Dosing of 400 mg Either Orally (n=10) or by I.V. Infusion (n=12)

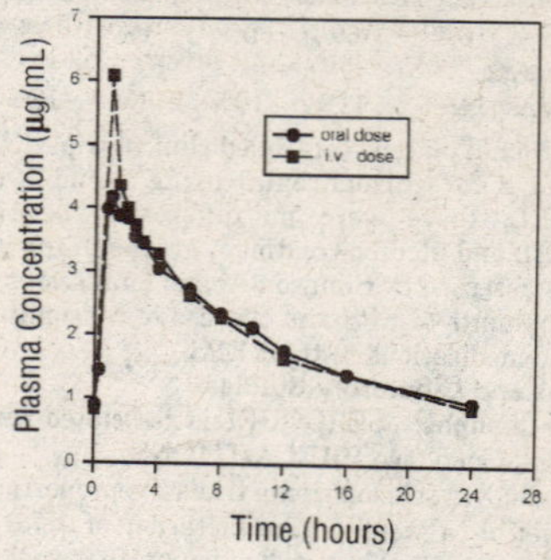

Distribution

Moxifloxacin is approximately 50% bound to serum proteins, independent of drug concentration. The volume of distribution of moxifloxacin ranges from 1.7 to 2.7 L/kg. Moxifloxacin is widely distributed throughout the body, with tissue concentrations often exceeding plasma concentrations. Moxifloxacin has been detected in the saliva, nasal and bronchial secretions, mucosa of the sinuses, skin blister fluid, and subcutaneous tissue, and skeletal muscle following oral or intravenous administration of 400 mg. Concentrations measured at 3 hours post-dose are summarized in the following table. The rates of elimination of moxifloxacin from tissues generally parallel the elimination from plasma.

[See table at top of next page]

Metabolism

Approximately 52% of an oral or intravenous dose of moxifloxacin is metabolized via glucuronide and sulfate conjugation. The cytochrome P450 system is not involved in moxifloxacin metabolism, and is not affected by moxifloxacin. The sulfate conjugate (M1) accounts for approximately 38% of the dose, and is eliminated primarily in the feces. Approximately 14% of an oral or intravenous dose is converted to a glucuronide conjugate (M2), which is excreted exclusively in the urine. Peak plasma concentrations of M2 are approximately 40% those of the parent drug, while plasma concentrations of M1 are generally less than 10% those of moxifloxacin.

In vitro studies with cytochrome (CYP) P450 enzymes indicate that moxifloxacin does not inhibit CYP3A4, CYP2D6,

CYP2C9, CYP2C19, or CYP1A2, suggesting that moxifloxacin is unlikely to alter the pharmacokinetics of drugs metabolized by these enzymes.

Excretion
Approximately 45% of an oral or intravenous dose of moxifloxacin is excreted as unchanged drug (~20% in urine and ~25% in feces). A total of 96% ± 4% of an oral dose is excreted as either unchanged drug or known metabolites. The mean (± SD) apparent total body clearance and renal clearance are 12 ± 2.0 L/hr and 2.6 ± 0.5 L/hr, respectively.

Special Populations
Geriatric
Following oral administration of 400 mg moxifloxacin for 10 days in 16 elderly (8 male; 8 female) and 17 young (8 male; 9 female) healthy volunteers, there were no age-related changes in moxifloxacin pharmacokinetics. In 16 healthy male volunteers (8 young; 8 elderly) given a single 200 mg dose of oral moxifloxacin, the extent of systemic exposure (AUC and C_{max}) was not statistically different between young and elderly males and elimination half-life was unchanged. No dosage adjustment is necessary based on age. In large phase III studies, the concentrations around the time of the end of the infusion in elderly patients following intravenous infusion of 400 mg were similar to those observed in young patients.

Pediatric
The pharmacokinetics of moxifloxacin in pediatric subjects have not been studied.

Gender
Following oral administration of 400 mg moxifloxacin daily for 10 days to 23 healthy males (19-75 years) and 24 healthy females (19-70 years), the mean AUC and C_{max} were 8% and 16% higher, respectively, in females compared to males. There are no significant differences in moxifloxacin pharmacokinetics between male and female subjects when differences in body weight are taken into consideration.
A 400 mg single dose study was conducted in 18 young males and females. The comparison of moxifloxacin pharmacokinetics in this study (9 young females and 9 young males) showed no differences in AUC or C_{max} due to gender. Dosage adjustments based on gender are not necessary.

Race
Steady-state moxifloxacin pharmacokinetics in male Japanese subjects were similar to those determined in Caucasians, with a mean C_{max} of 4.1 μg/mL, an AUC_{24} of 47 μg•h/mL, and an elimination half-life of 14 hours, following 400 mg p.o. daily.

Renal Insufficiency
The pharmacokinetic parameters of moxifloxacin are not significantly altered in mild, moderate, severe, or end-stage renal disease. No dosage adjustment is necessary in patients with renal impairment, including those patients requiring hemodialysis (HD) or continuous ambulatory peritoneal dialysis (CAPD).
In a single oral dose study of 24 patients with varying degrees of renal function from normal to severely impaired, the mean peak concentrations (C_{max}) of moxifloxacin were reduced by 21% and 28% in the patients with moderate ($CL_{CR} \geq 30$ and ≤ 60 mL/min) and severe ($CL_{CR} < 30$ mL/min) renal impairment, respectively. The mean systemic exposure (AUC) in these patients was increased by 13%. In the moderate and severe renally impaired patients, the mean AUC for the sulfate conjugate (M1) increased by 1.7-fold (ranging up to 2.8-fold) and mean AUC and C_{max} for the glucuronide conjugate (M2) increased by 2.8-fold (ranging up to 4.8-fold) and 1.4-fold (ranging up to 2.5-fold), respectively.
The pharmacokinetics of single dose and multiple dose moxifloxacin were studied in patients with $CL_{CR} < 20$ mL/min on either hemodialysis or continuous ambulatory peritoneal dialysis (8 HD, 8 CAPD). Following a single 400 mg oral dose, the AUC of moxifloxacin in these HD and CAPD patients did not vary significantly from the AUC generally found in healthy volunteers. C_{max} values of moxifloxacin were reduced by about 45% and 33% in HD and CAPD patients, respectively, compared to healthy, historical controls. The exposure (AUC) to the sulfate conjugate (M1) increased by 1.4- to 1.5-fold in these patients. The mean AUC of the glucuronide conjugate (M2) increased by a factor of 7.5, whereas the mean C_{max} values of the glucuronide conjugate (M2) increased by a factor of 2.5 to 3, compared to healthy subjects. The sulfate and the glucuronide conjugates of moxifloxacin are not microbiologically active, and the clinical implication of increased exposure to these metabolites in patients with renal disease including those undergoing HD and CAPD has not been studied.
Oral administration of 400 mg QD moxifloxacin for 7 days to patients on HD or CAPD produced mean systemic exposure (AUC_{ss}) to moxifloxacin similar to that generally seen in healthy volunteers. Steady-state C_{max} values were about 22% lower in HD patients but were comparable between CAPD patients and healthy volunteers. Both HD and CAPD removed only small amounts of moxifloxacin from the body (approximately 9% by HD, and 3% by CAPD). HD and CAPD also removed about 4% and 2% of the glucuronide metabolite (M2), respectively.

Hepatic Insufficiency
In 400 mg single oral dose studies in 6 patients with mild (Child Pugh Class A), and 10 patients with moderate (Child Pugh Class B), hepatic insufficiency, moxifloxacin mean systemic exposure (AUC) was 78% and 102%, respectively, of 18 healthy controls and mean peak concentration (C_{max}) was 79% and 84% of controls.
The mean AUC of the sulfate conjugate of moxifloxacin (M1) increased by 3.9-fold (ranging up to 5.9-fold) and 5.7-fold (ranging up to 8.0-fold) in the mild and moderate groups, respectively. The mean C_{max} of M1 increased by approximately 3-fold in both groups (ranging up to 4.7- and 3.9-fold). The mean AUC of the glucuronide conjugate of moxifloxacin (M2) increased by 1.5-fold (ranging up to 2.5-fold) in both groups. The mean C_{max} of M2 increased by 1.6- and 1.3-fold (ranging up to 2.7- and 2.1-fold), respectively. The clinical significance of increased exposure to the sulfate and glucuronide conjugates has not been studied. No dosage adjustment is recommended for mild or moderate hepatic insufficiency (Child Pugh Classes A and B). The pharmacokinetics of moxifloxacin in severe hepatic insufficiency (Child Pugh Class C) have not been studied. (See **DOSAGE AND ADMINISTRATION**.)

Moxifloxacin Concentrations (mean ± SD) After Oral Dosing in Plasma and Tissues Measured 3 Hours After Dosing with 400 mg§

Tissue or Fluid	N	Plasma Concentration (μg/mL)	Tissue or Fluid Concentration (μg/mL or μg/g)	Tissue Plasma Ratio:
Respiratory				
Alveolar Macrophages	5	3.3 ± 0.7	61.8 ± 27.3	21.2 ± 10.0
Bronchial Mucosa	8	3.3 ± 0.7	5.5 ± 1.3	1.7 ± 0.3
Epithelial Lining Fluid	5	3.3 ± 0.7	24.4 ± 14.7	8.7 ± 6.1
Sinus				
Maxillary Sinus Mucosa	4	3.7 ± 1.1†	7.6 ± 1.7	2.0 ± 0.3
Anterior Ethmoid Mucosa	3	3.7 ± 1.1†	8.8 ± 4.3	2.2 ± 0.6
Nasal Polyps	4	3.7 ± 1.1†	9.8 ± 4.5	2.6 ± 0.6

§ all moxifloxacin concentrations were measured after a single 400 mg dose, except the sinus concentrations which were measured after 5 days of dosing.
†N = 5

Photosensitivity Potential
A study of the skin response to ultraviolet (UVA and UVB) and visible radiation conducted in 32 healthy volunteers (8 per group) demonstrated that moxifloxacin does not show phototoxicity in comparison to placebo. The minimum erythematous dose (MED) was measured before and after treatment with moxifloxacin (200 mg or 400 mg once daily), lomefloxacin (400 mg once daily), or placebo. In this study, the MED measured for both doses of moxifloxacin were not significantly different from placebo, while lomefloxacin significantly lowered the MED. (See **PRECAUTIONS, Information for Patients.**)

Drug-drug Interactions
The potential for pharmacokinetic drug interactions between moxifloxacin and itraconazole, theophylline, warfarin, digoxin, atenolol, probenecid, morphine, oral contraceptives, ranitidine, glyburide, calcium, iron, and antacids has been evaluated. There was no clinically significant effect of moxifloxacin on itraconazole, theophylline, warfarin, digoxin, atenolol, oral contraceptives, or glyburide kinetics. Itraconazole, theophylline, warfarin, digoxin, probenecid, morphine, ranitidine, and calcium did not significantly affect the pharmacokinetics of moxifloxacin. These results and the data from *in vitro* studies suggest that moxifloxacin is unlikely to significantly alter the metabolic clearance of drugs metabolized by CYP3A4, CYP2D6, CYP2C9, CYP2C19, or CYP1A2 enzymes.
As with all other quinolones, iron and antacids significantly reduced bioavailability of moxifloxacin.
Itraconazole: In a study involving 11 healthy volunteers, there was no significant effect of itraconazole (200 mg once daily for 9 days), a potent inhibitor of cytochrome P4503A4, on the pharmacokinetics of moxifloxacin (a single 400 mg dose given on the 7th day of itraconazole dosing). In addition, moxifloxacin was shown not to affect the pharmacokinetics of itraconazole.
Theophylline: No significant effect of moxifloxacin (200 mg every twelve hours for 3 days) on the pharmacokinetics of theophylline (400 mg every twelve hours for 3 days) was detected in a study involving 12 healthy volunteers. In addition, theophylline was not shown to affect the pharmacokinetics of moxifloxacin. The effect of co-administration of a 400 mg dose of moxifloxacin with theophylline has not been studied, but it is not expected to be clinically significant based on *in vitro* metabolic data showing that moxifloxacin does not inhibit the CYP1A2 isoenzyme.
Warfarin: No significant effect of moxifloxacin (400 mg once daily for eight days) on the pharmacokinetics of R- and S-warfarin (25 mg single dose of warfarin sodium on the fifth day) was detected in a study involving 24 healthy volunteers. No significant change in prothrombin time was observed. (See **PRECAUTIONS, Drug Interactions.**)
Digoxin: No significant effect of moxifloxacin (400 mg once daily for two days) on digoxin (0.6 mg as a single dose) AUC was detected in a study involving 12 healthy volunteers. The mean digoxin C_{max} increased by about 50% during the distribution phase of digoxin. This transient increase in digoxin C_{max} is not viewed to be clinically significant. Moxifloxacin pharmacokinetics were similar in the presence or absence of digoxin. No dosage adjustment for moxifloxacin

Continued on next page

	C_{max} (mg/L)	AUC (mg•h/L)	Half-life (hr)
Single Dose Oral			
Healthy (n = 372)	3.1 ± 1.0	36.1 ± 9.1	11.5 - 15.6*
Multiple Dose Oral			
Healthy young male/female (n = 15)	4.5 ± 0.5	48.0 ± 2.7	12.7 ± 1.9
Healthy elderly male (n = 8)	3.8 ± 0.3	51.8 ± 6.7	
Healthy elderly female (n = 8)	4.6 ± 0.6	54.6 ± 6.7	
Healthy young male (n = 8)	3.6 ± 0.5	48.2 ± 9.0	
Healthy young female (n = 9)	4.2 ± 0.5	49.3 ± 9.5	

*Range of means from different studies

	C_{max} (mg/L)	AUC (mg•h/L)	Half-life (hr)
Single Dose I.V.			
Healthy young male/female (n = 56)	3.9 ± 0.9	39.3 ± 8.6	8.2 - 15.4*
Patients (n = 118)			
Male (n = 64)	4.4 ± 3.7		
Female (n = 54)	4.5 ± 2.0		
< 65 years (n = 58)	4.6 ± 4.2		
≥ 65 years (n = 60)	4.3 ± 1.3		
Multiple Dose I.V.			
Healthy young male (n = 8)	4.2 ± 0.8	38.0 ± 4.7	14.8 ± 2.2
Healthy elderly (n = 12; 8 male, 4 female)	6.1 ± 1.3	48.2 ± 0.9	10.1 ± 1.6
Patients** (n = 107)			
Male (n = 58)	4.2 ± 2.6		
Female (n = 49)	4.6 ± 1.5		
< 65 years (n = 52)	4.1 ± 1.4		
≥ 65 years (n = 55)	4.7 ± 2.7		

* Range of means from different studies
**Expected C_{max} (concentration obtained around the time of the end of the infusion)

Avelox—Cont.

or digoxin is required when these drugs are administered concomitantly.

Atenolol: In a crossover study involving 24 healthy volunteers (12 male; 12 female), the mean atenolol AUC following a single oral dose of 50 mg atenolol with placebo was similar to that observed when atenolol was given concomitantly with a single 400 mg oral dose of moxifloxacin. The mean C_{max} of single dose atenolol decreased by about 10% following co-administration with a single dose of moxifloxacin.

Morphine: No significant effect of morphine sulfate (a single 10 mg intramuscular dose) on the mean AUC and C_{max} of moxifloxacin (400 mg single dose) was observed in a study of 20 healthy male and female volunteers.

Oral Contraceptives: A placebo-controlled study in 29 healthy female subjects showed that moxifloxacin 400 mg daily for 7 days did not interfere with the hormonal suppression of oral contraception with 0.15 mg levonorgestrel/0.03 mg ethinylestradiol (as measured by serum progesterone, FSH, estradiol, and LH), or with the pharmacokinetics of the administered contraceptive agents.

Probenecid: Probenecid (500 mg twice daily for two days) did not alter the renal clearance and total amount of moxifloxacin (400 mg single dose) excreted renally in a study of 12 healthy volunteers.

Ranitidine: No significant effect of ranitidine (150 mg twice daily for three days as pretreatment) on the pharmacokinetics of moxifloxacin (400 mg single dose) was detected in a study involving 10 healthy volunteers.

Antidiabetic agents: In diabetics, glyburide (2.5 mg once daily for two weeks pretreatment and for five days concurrently) mean AUC and C_{max} were 12% and 21% lower, respectively, when taken with moxifloxacin (400 mg once daily for five days) in comparison to placebo. Nonetheless, blood glucose levels were decreased slightly in patients taking glyburide and moxifloxacin in comparison to those taking glyburide alone, suggesting no interference by moxifloxacin on the activity of glyburide. These interaction results are not viewed as clinically significant.

Calcium: Twelve healthy volunteers were administered concomitant moxifloxacin (single 400 mg dose) and calcium (single dose of 500 mg Ca^{++} dietary supplement) followed by an additional two doses of calcium 12 and 24 hours after moxifloxacin administration. Calcium had no significant effect on the mean AUC of moxifloxacin. The mean C_{max} was slightly reduced and the time to maximum plasma concentration was prolonged when moxifloxacin was given with calcium compared to when moxifloxacin was given alone (2.5 hours versus 0.9 hours). These differences are not considered to be clinically significant.

Antacids: When moxifloxacin (single 400 mg tablet dose) was administered two hours before, concomitantly, or 4 hours after an aluminum/magnesium-containing antacid (900 mg aluminum hydroxide and 600 mg magnesium hydroxide as a single oral dose) to 12 healthy volunteers there was a 26%, 60% and 23% reduction in the mean AUC of moxifloxacin, respectively. Moxifloxacin should be taken at least 4 hours before or 8 hours after antacids containing magnesium or aluminum, as well as sucralfate, metal cations such as iron, and multivitamin preparations with zinc, or VIDEX® (didanosine) chewable/buffered tablets or the pediatric powder for oral solution. (See **PRECAUTIONS, Drug Interactions** and **DOSAGE AND ADMINISTRATION.**)

Iron: When moxifloxacin tablets were administered concomitantly with iron (ferrous sulfate 100 mg once daily for two days), the mean AUC and C_{max} of moxifloxacin was reduced by 39% and 59%, respectively. Moxifloxacin should only be taken more than 4 hours before or 8 hours after iron products. (See **PRECAUTIONS, Drug Interactions** and **DOSAGE AND ADMINISTRATION.**)

Electrocardiogram: Prolongation of the QT interval in the ECG has been observed in some patients receiving moxifloxacin. Following oral dosing with 400 mg of moxifloxacin the mean (± SD) change in QTc from the pre-dose value at the time of maximum drug concentration was 6 msec (± 26) (n = 787). Following a course of daily intravenous dosing (400 mg; 1 hour infusion each day) the mean change in QTc from the Day 1 pre-dose value was 9 msec (± 24) on Day 1 (n = 69) and 3 msec (± 29) on Day 3 (n = 290). (See **WARNINGS.**)

There is limited information available on the potential for a pharmacodynamic interaction in humans between moxifloxacin and other drugs that prolong the QTc interval of the electrocardiogram. Sotalol, a Class III antiarrhythmic, has been shown to further increase the QTc interval when combined with high doses of intravenous (I.V.) moxifloxacin in dogs. Therefore, moxifloxacin should be avoided with Class IA and Class III antiarrhythmics. (See **ANIMAL PHARMACOLOGY, WARNINGS,** and **PRECAUTIONS.**)

MICROBIOLOGY

Moxifloxacin has *in vitro* activity against a wide range of Gram-positive and Gram-negative microorganisms. The bactericidal action of moxifloxacin results from inhibition of the topoisomerase II (DNA gyrase) and topoisomerase IV required for bacterial DNA replication, transcription, repair, and recombination. It appears that the C8-methoxy moiety contributes to enhanced activity and lower selection of resistant mutants of Gram-positive bacteria compared to the C8-H moiety. The presence of the bulky bicycloamine substituent at the C-7 position prevents active efflux, associated with the *NorA* or *pmrA* genes seen in certain Gram-positive bacteria.

The mechanism of action for quinolones, including moxifloxacin, is different from that of macrolides, beta-lactams, aminoglycosides, or tetracyclines; therefore, microorganisms resistant to these classes of drugs may be susceptible to moxifloxacin and other quinolones. There is no known cross-resistance between moxifloxacin and other classes of antimicrobials.

In vitro resistance to moxifloxacin develops slowly via multiple-step mutations. Resistance to moxifloxacin occurs *in vitro* at a general frequency of between 1.8×10^{-9} to $< 1 \times 10^{-11}$ for Gram-positive bacteria.

Cross-resistance has been observed between moxifloxacin and other fluoroquinolones against Gram-negative bacteria. Gram-positive bacteria resistant to other fluoroquinolones may, however, still be susceptible to moxifloxacin.

Moxifloxacin has been shown to be active against most strains of the following microorganisms, both *in vitro* and in clinical infections as described in the **INDICATIONS AND USAGE** section.

Aerobic Gram-positive microorganisms

Staphylococcus aureus (methicillin-susceptible strains only)

Streptococcus pneumoniae (including penicillin-resistant strains*)

Streptococcus pyogenes

* Note: penicillin-resistant *S. pneumoniae* are those strains with a penicillin MIC value of ≥ 2μg/mL

Aerobic Gram-negative microorganisms

Haemophilus influenzae

Haemophilus parainfluenzae

Klebsiella pneumoniae

Moraxella catarrhalis

Other microorganisms

Chlamydia pneumoniae

Mycoplasma pneumoniae

The following *in vitro* data are available, **but their clinical significance is unknown.**

Moxifloxacin exhibits *in vitro* minimum inhibitory concentrations (MICs) of 2 μg/mL or less against most (≥ 90%) strains of the following microorganisms; however, the safety and effectiveness of moxifloxacin in treating clinical infections due to these microorganisms have not been established in adequate and well-controlled clinical trials.

Aerobic Gram-positive microorganisms

Staphylococcus epidermidis (methicillin-susceptible strains only)

Streptococcus agalactiae

Streptococcus viridans group

Aerobic Gram-negative microorganisms

Citrobacter freundii

Enterobacter cloacae

Escherichia coli

Klebsiella oxytoca

Legionella pneumophila

Proteus mirabilis

Anaerobic microorganisms

Fusobacterium species

Peptostreptococcus species

Prevotella species

Susceptibility Tests

Dilution Techniques: Quantitative methods are used to determine antimicrobial minimum inhibitory concentrations (MICs). These MICs provide estimates of the susceptibility of bacteria to antimicrobial compounds. The MICs should be determined using a standardized procedure. Standardized procedures are based on a dilution method[1] (broth or agar) or equivalent with standardized inoculum concentrations and standardized concentrations of moxifloxacin powder. The MIC values should be interpreted according to the following criteria:

For testing Enterobacteriaceae and *Staphylococcus* species:

MIC (μg/mL)	Interpretation	
≤ 2.0	Susceptible	(S)
4.0	Intermediate	(I)
≥ 8.0	Resistant	(R)

For testing *Haemophilus influenzae* and *Haemophilus parainfluenzae*[a]:

MIC (μg/mL)	Interpretation	
≤ 1.0	Susceptible	(S)

[a] This interpretive standard is applicable only to broth microdilution susceptibility tests with *Haemophilus influenzae* and *Haemophilus parainfluenzae* using *Haemophilus* Test Medium[1].

The current absence of data on resistant strains precludes defining any results other than "Susceptible". Strains yielding MIC results suggestive of a "nonsusceptible" category should be submitted to a reference laboratory for further testing.

For testing *Streptococcus* species including *Streptococcus pneumoniae*[b]:

MIC (μg/mL)	Interpretation	
≤ 1.0	Susceptible	(S)
2.0	Intermediate	(I)
≥ 4.0	Resistant	(R)

[b] This interpretive standard is applicable only to broth microdilution susceptibility tests using cation-adjusted Mueller-Hinton broth with 2 - 5% lysed horse blood.

A report of "Susceptible" indicates that the pathogen is likely to be inhibited if the antimicrobial compound in the blood reaches the concentrations usually achievable. A report of "Intermediate" indicates that the result should be considered equivocal, and, if the microorganism is not fully susceptible to alternative, clinically feasible drugs, the test should be repeated. This category implies possible clinical applicability in body sites where the drug is physiologically concentrated or in situations where a high dosage of drug can be used. This category also provides a buffer zone which prevents small uncontrolled technical factors from causing major discrepancies in interpretation. A report of "Resistant" indicates that the pathogen is not likely to be inhibited if the antimicrobial compound in the blood reaches the concentrations usually achievable; other therapy should be selected.

Standardized susceptibility test procedures require the use of laboratory control microorganisms to control the technical aspects of the laboratory procedures. Standard moxifloxacin powder should provide the following MIC values:

Microorganism		MIC (μg/mL)
Enterococcus faecalis	ATCC 29212	0.06 - 0.5
Escherichia coli	ATCC 25922	0.008 - 0.06
Haemophilus influenzae	ATCC 49247[c]	0.008 - 0.03
Staphylococcus aureus	ATCC 29213	0.015 - 0.06
Streptococcus pneumoniae	ATCC 49619[d]	0.06 - 0.25

[c] This quality control range is applicable to only *H. influenzae* ATCC 49247 tested by a broth microdilution procedure using *Haemophilus* Test Medium (HTM)[1].

[d] This quality control range is applicable to only *S. pneumoniae* ATCC 49619 tested by a broth microdilution procedure using cation-adjusted Mueller-Hinton broth with 2 - 5% lysed horse blood.

Diffusion Techniques: Quantitative methods that require measurement of zone diameters also provide reproducible estimates of the susceptibility of bacteria to antimicrobial compounds. One such standardized procedure[2] requires the use of standardized inoculum concentrations. This procedure uses paper disks impregnated with 5-μg moxifloxacin to test the susceptibility of microorganisms to moxifloxacin. Reports from the laboratory providing results of the standard single-disk susceptibility test with a 5-μg moxifloxacin disk should be interpreted according to the following criteria:

The following zone diameter interpretive criteria should be used for testing Enterobacteriaceae and *Staphylococcus* species:

Zone Diameter (mm)	Interpretation	
≥ 19	Susceptible	(S)
16 – 18	Intermediate	(I)
≤ 15	Resistant	(R)

For testing *Haemophilus influenzae* and *Haemophilus parainfluenzae*[e]:

Zone Diameter (mm)	Interpretation	
≥ 18	Susceptible	(S)

[e] This zone diameter standard is applicable only to tests with *Haemophilus influenzae* and *Haemophilus parainfluenzae* using *Haemophilus* Test Medium (HTM)[2].

The current absence of data on resistant strains precludes defining any results other than "Susceptible". Strains yielding zone diameter results suggestive of a "nonsusceptible" category should be submitted to a reference laboratory for further testing.

For testing *Streptococcus* species including *Streptococcus pneumoniae*[f]:

Zone Diameter (mm)	Interpretation	
≥ 18	Susceptible	(S)
15 – 17	Intermediate	(I)
≤ 14	Resistant	(R)

[f] These interpretive standards are applicable only to disk diffusion tests using Mueller-Hinton agar supplemented with 5% sheep blood incubated in 5% CO_2.

Interpretation should be as stated above for results using dilution techniques. Interpretation involves correlation of the diameter obtained in the disk test with the MIC for moxifloxacin.

As with standardized dilution techniques, diffusion methods require the use of laboratory control microorganisms that are used to control the technical aspects of the laboratory procedures. For the diffusion technique, the 5-μg moxifloxacin disk should provide the following zone diameters in these laboratory test quality control strains:

Microorganism		Zone Diameter (mm)
Escherichia coli	ATCC 25922	28 - 35
Haemophilus influenzae	ATCC 49247[g]	31 - 39
Staphylococcus aureus	ATCC 25923	28 - 35
Streptococcus pneumoniae	ATCC 49619[h]	25 - 31

[g] These quality control limits are applicable to only *H. influenzae* ATCC 49247 testing using *Haemophilus* Test Medium (HTM)[2].

[h] These quality control limits are applicable only to tests conducted with *S. pneumoniae* ATCC 49619 performed by disk diffusion using Mueller-Hinton agar supplemented with 5% defibrinated sheep blood.

INDICATIONS AND USAGE

AVELOX Tablets and I.V. are indicated for the treatment of adults (≥ 18 years of age) with infections caused by susceptible strains of the designated microorganisms in the conditions listed below. (See **DOSAGE AND ADMINISTRATION** for specific recommendations. In addition, for I.V. use see **PRECAUTIONS, Geriatric Use.**)

Acute Bacterial Sinusitis caused by *Streptococcus pneumoniae, Haemophilus influenzae,* or *Moraxella catarrhalis.*

Acute Bacterial Exacerbation of Chronic Bronchitis caused by *Streptococcus pneumoniae, Haemophilus influenzae, Haemophilus parainfluenzae, Klebsiella pneumoniae, Staphylococcus aureus,* or *Moraxella catarrhalis.*

Community Acquired Pneumonia caused by *Streptococcus pneumoniae* (including penicillin-resistant strains, MIC value for penicillin ≥ 2 µg/mL), *Haemophilus influenzae, Moraxella catarrhalis, Staphylococcus aureus, Klebsiella pneumoniae, Mycoplasma pneumoniae,* or *Chlamydia pneumoniae.*

Uncomplicated Skin and Skin Structure Infections caused by *Staphylococcus aureus* or *Streptococcus pyogenes.*

Appropriate culture and susceptibility tests should be performed before treatment in order to isolate and identify organisms causing infection and to determine their susceptibility to moxifloxacin. Therapy with AVELOX may be initiated before results of these tests are known; once results become available, appropriate therapy should be continued.

To reduce the development of drug-resistant bacteria and maintain the effectiveness of AVELOX and other antibacterial drugs, AVELOX should be used only to treat or prevent infections that are proven or strongly suspected to be caused by susceptible bacteria. When culture and susceptibility information are available, they should be considered in selecting or modifying antibacterial therapy. In the absence of such data, local epidemiology and susceptibility patterns may contribute to the empiric selection of therapy.

CONTRAINDICATIONS

Moxifloxacin is contraindicated in persons with a history of hypersensitivity to moxifloxacin or any member of the quinolone class of antimicrobial agents.

WARNINGS

THE SAFETY AND EFFECTIVENESS OF MOXIFLOXACIN IN PEDIATRIC PATIENTS, ADOLESCENTS (LESS THAN 18 YEARS OF AGE), PREGNANT WOMEN, AND LACTATING WOMEN HAVE NOT BEEN ESTABLISHED. (SEE PRECAUTIONS-PEDIATRIC USE, PREGNANCY AND NURSING MOTHERS SUBSECTIONS.)

Moxifloxacin has been shown to prolong the QT interval of the electrocardiogram in some patients. The drug should be avoided in patients with known prolongation of the QT interval, patients with uncorrected hypokalemia and patients receiving Class IA (e.g. quinidine, procainamide) or Class III (e.g. amiodarone, sotalol) antiarrhythmic agents, due to the lack of clinical experience with the drug in these patient populations.

Pharmacokinetic studies between moxifloxacin and other drugs that prolong the QT interval such as cisapride, erythromycin, antipsychotics, and tricyclic antidepressants have not been performed. An additive effect of moxifloxacin and these drugs cannot be excluded, therefore caution should be exercised when moxifloxacin is given concurrently with these drugs. In premarketing clinical trials, the rate of cardiovascular adverse events was similar in 798 moxifloxacin and 702 comparator treated patients who received concomitant therapy with drugs known to prolong the QTc interval. Moxifloxacin should be used with caution in patients with ongoing proarrhythmic conditions, such as clinically significant bradycardia, acute myocardial ischemia. The magnitude of QT prolongation may increase with increasing concentrations of the drug or increasing rates of infusion of the intravenous formulation. Therefore the recommended dose or infusion rate should not be exceeded. QT prolongation may lead to an increased risk for ventricular arrhythmias including torsade de pointes. No cardiovascular morbidity or mortality attributable to QTc prolongation occurred with moxifloxacin treatment in over 7,900 patients in controlled clinical studies, including 223 patients who were hypokalemic at the start of treatment, and there was no increase in mortality in over 18,000 moxifloxacin tablet treated patients in a post-marketing observational study in which ECGs were not performed. (See **CLINICAL PHARMACOLOGY, Electrocardiogram.** For I.V. use see **DOSAGE AND ADMINISTRATION** and **PRECAUTIONS, Geriatric Use.**)

The oral administration of moxifloxacin caused lameness in immature dogs. Histopathological examination of the weight-bearing joints of these dogs revealed permanent lesions of the cartilage. Related quinolone-class drugs also produce erosions of cartilage of weight-bearing joints and other signs of arthropathy in immature animals of various species. (See **ANIMAL PHARMACOLOGY.**)

Convulsions have been reported in patients receiving quinolones. Quinolones may also cause central nervous system (CNS) events including: dizziness, confusion, tremors, hallucinations, depression, and, rarely, suicidal thoughts or acts. These reactions may occur following the first dose. If these reactions occur in patients receiving moxifloxacin, the drug should be discontinued and appropriate measures instituted. As with all quinolones, moxifloxacin should be used with caution in patients with known or suspected CNS disorders (e.g. severe cerebral arteriosclerosis, epilepsy) or in the presence of other risk factors that may predispose to seizures or lower the seizure threshold. (See **PRECAUTIONS: General, Information for Patients,** and **ADVERSE REACTIONS.**)

Serious anaphylactic reactions, some following the first dose, have been reported in patients receiving quinolone therapy, including moxifloxacin. Some reactions were accompanied by cardiovascular collapse, loss of consciousness, tingling, pharyngeal or facial edema, dyspnea, urticaria, and itching. Serious anaphylactic reactions require immediate emergency treatment with epinephrine. Moxifloxacin should be discontinued at the first appearance of a skin rash or any other sign of hypersensitivity. Oxygen, intravenous steroids, and airway management, including intubation, may be administered as indicated.

Severe and sometimes fatal events, some due to hypersensitivity, and some of uncertain etiology, have been reported in patients receiving therapy with all antibiotics. These events may be severe and generally occur following the administration of multiple doses. Clinical manifestations may include one or more of the following: rash, fever, eosinophilia, jaundice, and hepatic necrosis.

Pseudomembranous colitis has been reported with nearly all antibacterial agents and may range in severity from mild to life-threatening. Therefore, it is important to consider this diagnosis in patients who present with diarrhea subsequent to the administration of antibacterial agents.

Treatment with antibacterial agents alters the normal flora of the colon and may permit overgrowth of clostridia. Studies indicate that a toxin produced by *Clostridium difficile* is one primary cause of "antibiotic-associated colitis." After the diagnosis of pseudomembranous colitis has been established, therapeutic measures should be initiated. Mild cases of pseudomembranous colitis usually respond to drug discontinuation alone. In moderate to severe cases, consideration should be given to management with fluids and electrolytes, protein supplementation, and treatment with an antibacterial drug clinically effective against *C. difficile* colitis.

Peripheral neuropathy: Rare cases of sensory or sensorimotor axonal polyneuropathy affecting small and/or large axons resulting in paresthesias, hypoesthesias, dysesthesias and weakness have been reported in patients receiving quinolones.

Tendon Effects: Ruptures of the shoulder, hand, Achilles tendon or other tendons that required surgical repair or resulted in prolonged disability have been reported in patients receiving quinolones, including moxifloxacin. Post-marketing surveillance reports indicate that this risk may be increased in patients receiving concomitant corticosteroids, especially the elderly. Moxifloxacin should be discontinued if the patient experiences pain, inflammation, or rupture of a tendon. Patients should rest and refrain from exercise until the diagnosis of tendonitis or tendon rupture has been excluded. Tendon rupture can occur during or after therapy with quinolones, including moxifloxacin.

PRECAUTIONS

General: Quinolones may cause central nervous system (CNS) events, including: nervousness, agitation, insomnia, anxiety, nightmares or paranoia. (See **WARNINGS** and **Information for Patients.**)

Prescribing AVELOX in the absence of a proven or strongly suspected bacterial infection or a prophylactic indication is unlikely to provide benefit to the patient and increases the risk of the development of drug-resistant bacteria.

Information for Patients:

To assure safe and effective use of moxifloxacin, the following information and instructions should be communicated to the patient when appropriate:

Patients should be advised:

- that antibacterial drugs including AVELOX should only be used to treat bacterial infections. They do not treat viral infections (e.g., the common cold). When AVELOX is prescribed to treat a bacterial infection, patients should be told that although it is common to feel better early in the course of therapy, the medication should be taken exactly as directed. Skipping doses or not completing the full course of therapy may (1) decrease the effectiveness of the immediate treatment and (2) increase the likelihood that bacteria will develop resistance and will not be treatable by AVELOX or other antibacterial drugs in the future.
- that moxifloxacin may produce changes in the electrocardiogram (QTc interval prolongation).
- that moxifloxacin should be avoided in patients receiving Class IA (e.g. quinidine, procainamide) or Class III (e.g. amiodarone, sotalol) antiarrhythmic agents.
- that moxifloxacin may add to the QTc prolonging effects of other drugs such as cisapride, erythromycin, antipsychotics, and tricyclic antidepressants.
- to inform their physician of any personal or family history of QTc prolongation or proarrhythmic conditions such as recent hypokalemia, significant bradycardia, acute myocardial ischemia.
- to inform their physician of any other medications when taken concurrently with moxifloxacin, including over-the-counter medications.
- to contact their physician if they experience palpitations or fainting spells while taking moxifloxacin.
- that moxifloxacin tablets may be taken with or without meals, and to drink fluids liberally.
- that moxifloxacin tablets should be taken at least 4 hours before or 8 hours after multivitamins (containing iron or zinc), antacids (containing magnesium or aluminum), sucralfate, or VIDEX® (didanosine) chewable/buffered tablets or the pediatric powder for oral solution. (See **CLINICAL PHARMACOLOGY, Drug Interactions** and **PRECAUTIONS, Drug Interactions.**)
- that moxifloxacin may be associated with hypersensitivity reactions, including anaphylactic reactions, even following a single dose, and to discontinue the drug at the first sign of a skin rash or other signs of an allergic reaction.
- to discontinue treatment; rest and refrain from exercise; and inform their physician if they experience pain, inflammation, or rupture of a tendon.
- that moxifloxacin may cause dizziness and lightheadedness; therefore, patients should know how they react to this drug before they operate an automobile or machinery or engage in activities requiring mental alertness or coordination.
- that phototoxicity has been reported in patients receiving certain quinolones. There was no phototoxicity seen with moxifloxacin at the recommended dose. In keeping with good medical practice, avoid excessive sunlight or artificial ultraviolet light (e.g. tanning beds). If sunburn-like reaction or skin eruptions occur, contact your physician. (See **CLINICAL PHARMACOLOGY, Photosensitivity Potential.**)
- that convulsions have been reported in patients receiving quinolones, and they should notify their physician before taking this drug if there is a history of this condition.

Drug Interactions:

Antacids, Sucralfate, Metal Cations, Multivitamins: Quinolones form chelates with alkaline earth and transition metal cations. Oral administration of quinolones with antacids containing aluminum or magnesium, with sucralfate, with metal cations such as iron, or with multivitamins containing iron or zinc, or with formulations containing divalent and trivalent cations such as VIDEX® (didanosine) chewable/buffered tablets or the pediatric powder for oral solution, may substantially interfere with the absorption of quinolones, resulting in systemic concentrations considerably lower than desired. Therefore, moxifloxacin should be taken at least 4 hours before or 8 hours after these agents. (See **CLINICAL PHARMACOLOGY, Drug Interactions** and **DOSAGE AND ADMINISTRATION.**)

No clinically significant drug-drug interactions between itraconazole, theophylline, warfarin, digoxin, atenolol, oral contraceptives or glyburide have been observed with moxifloxacin. Itraconazole, theophylline, digoxin, probenecid, morphine, ranitidine, and calcium have been shown not to significantly alter the pharmacokinetics of moxifloxacin. (See **CLINICAL PHARMACOLOGY.**)

Warfarin: No significant effect of moxifloxacin on R- and S-warfarin was detected in a clinical study involving 24 healthy volunteers. No significant changes in prothrombin time were noted in the presence of moxifloxacin. Quinolones, including moxifloxacin, have been reported to enhance the anticoagulant effects of warfarin or its derivatives in the patient population. In addition, infectious disease and its accompanying inflammatory process, age, and general status of the patient are risk factors for increased anticoagulant activity. Therefore the prothrombin time, International Normalized Ratio (INR), or other suitable anticoagulation tests should be closely monitored if a quinolone is administered concomitantly with warfarin or its derivatives.

Drugs metabolized by Cytochrome P450 enzymes: *In vitro* studies with cytochrome P450 isoenzymes (CYP) indicate that moxifloxacin does not inhibit CYP3A4, CYP2D6, CYP2C9, CYP2C19, or CYP1A2, suggesting that moxifloxacin is unlikely to alter the pharmacokinetics of drugs metabolized by these enzymes (e.g. midazolam, cyclosporine, warfarin, theophylline).

Nonsteroidal anti-inflammatory drugs (NSAIDs): Although not observed with moxifloxacin in preclinical and clinical trials, the concomitant administration of a nonsteroidal anti-inflammatory drug with a quinolone may increase the risks of CNS stimulation and convulsions. (See **WARNINGS.**)

Carcinogenesis, Mutagenesis, Impairment of Fertility:

Long term studies in animals to determine the carcinogenic potential of moxifloxacin have not been performed.

Moxifloxacin was not mutagenic in 4 bacterial strains (TA 98, TA 100, TA 1535, TA 1537) used in the Ames *Salmonella* reversion assay. As with other quinolones, the positive response observed with moxifloxacin in strain TA 102 using the same assay may be due to the inhibition of DNA gyrase. Moxifloxacin was not mutagenic in the CHO/HGPRT mammalian cell gene mutation assay. An equivocal result was obtained in the same assay when v79 cells were used. Moxifloxacin was clastogenic in the v79 chromosome aberration assay, but it did not induce unscheduled DNA synthesis in cultured rat hepatocytes. There was no evidence of genotoxicity *in vivo* in a micronucleus test or a dominant lethal test in mice.

Moxifloxacin had no effect on fertility in male and female rats at oral doses as high as 500 mg/kg/day, approximately 12 times the maximum recommended human dose based on body surface area (mg/m^2), or at intravenous doses as high as 45 mg/kg/day, approximately equal to the maximum recommended human dose based on body surface area (mg/m^2). At 500 mg/kg orally there were slight effects on sperm morphology (head-tail separation) in male rats and on the estrous cycle in female rats.

Pregnancy: Teratogenic Effects. Pregnancy Category C: Moxifloxacin was not teratogenic when administered to pregnant rats during organogenesis at oral doses as high as

Continued on next page

Avelox—Cont.

500 mg/kg/day or 0.24 times the maximum recommended human dose based on systemic exposure (AUC), but decreased fetal body weights and slightly delayed fetal skeletal development (indicative of fetotoxicity) were observed. Intravenous administration of 80 mg/kg/day (approximately 2 times the maximum recommended human dose based on body surface area (mg/m^2)) to pregnant rats resulted in maternal toxicity and a marginal effect on fetal and placental weights and the appearance of the placenta. There was no evidence of teratogenicity at intravenous doses as high as 80 mg/kg/day. Intravenous administration of 20 mg/kg/day (approximately equal to the maximum recommended human oral dose based upon systemic exposure) to pregnant rabbits during organogenesis resulted in decreased fetal body weights and delayed fetal skeletal ossification. When rib and vertebral malformations were combined, there was an increased fetal and litter incidence of these effects. Signs of maternal toxicity in rabbits at this dose included mortality, abortions, marked reduction of food consumption, decreased water intake, body weight loss and hypoactivity. There was no evidence of teratogenicity when pregnant Cynomolgus monkeys were given oral doses as high as 100 mg/kg/day (2.5 times the maximum recommended human dose based upon systemic exposure). An increased incidence of smaller fetuses was observed at 100 mg/kg/day. In an oral pre- and postnatal development study conducted in rats, effects observed at 500 mg/kg/day included slight increases in duration of pregnancy and prenatal loss, reduced pup birth weight and decreased neonatal survival. Treatment-related maternal mortality occurred during gestation at 500 mg/kg/day in this study.

Since there are no adequate or well-controlled studies in pregnant women, moxifloxacin should be used during pregnancy only if the potential benefit justifies the potential risk to the fetus.

Nursing Mothers:

Moxifloxacin is excreted in the breast milk of rats. Moxifloxacin may also be excreted in human milk. Because of the potential for serious adverse reactions in infants nursing from mothers taking moxifloxacin, a decision should be made whether to discontinue nursing or to discontinue the drug, taking into account the importance of the drug to the mother.

Pediatric Use:

Safety and effectiveness in pediatric patients and adolescents less than 18 years of age have not been established. Moxifloxacin causes arthropathy in juvenile animals. (See **WARNINGS.**)

Geriatric Use:

In controlled multiple-dose clinical trials, 23% of patients receiving oral moxifloxacin were greater than or equal to 65 years of age and 9% were greater than or equal to 75 years of age. The clinical trial data demonstrate that there is no difference in the safety and efficacy of oral moxifloxacin in patients aged 65 or older compared to younger adults.

In intravenous trials in community acquired pneumonia, 45% of moxifloxacin patients were greater than or equal to 65 years of age, and 24% were greater than or equal to 75 years of age. In the pool of 491 elderly (> 65 years) patients, the following ECG abnormalities were reported in moxifloxacin vs. comparator patients: ST-T wave changes (2 events vs. 0 events), QT prolongation (2 vs. 0), ventricular tachycardia (1 vs. 0), atrial flutter (1 vs. 0), tachycardia (2 vs. 1), atrial fibrillation (1 vs. 0), supraventricular tachycardia (1 vs. 0), ventricular extrasystoles (2 vs. 0), and arrhythmia (0 vs. 1). None of the abnormalities was associated with a fatal outcome and a majority of these patients completed a full course of therapy.

ADVERSE REACTIONS

Clinical efficacy trials enrolled over 7,900 moxifloxacin orally and intravenously treated patients, of whom over 6,700 patients received the 400 mg dose. Most adverse events reported in moxifloxacin trials were described as mild to moderate in severity and required no treatment. Moxifloxacin was discontinued due to adverse reactions thought to be drug-related in 3.6% of orally treated patients and 5.7 % of sequentially (intravenous followed by oral) treated patients. The latter studies were conducted in community acquired pneumonia with, in general, a sicker patient population compared to the tablet studies.

Adverse reactions, judged by investigators to be at least possibly drug-related, occurring in greater than or equal to 3% of moxifloxacin treated patients were: nausea (7%), diarrhea (6%), dizziness (3%).

Additional clinically relevant uncommon events, judged by investigators to be at least possibly drug-related, that occurred in greater than or equal to 0.1% and less than 3% of moxifloxacin treated patients were:

BODY AS A WHOLE: headache, abdominal pain, injection site reaction, asthenia, moniliasis, pain, malaise, lab test abnormal (not specified), allergic reaction, leg pain, back pain, chest pain

CARDIOVASCULAR: palpitation, tachycardia, hypertension, peripheral edema, QT interval prolonged

CENTRAL NERVOUS SYSTEM: insomnia, nervousness, anxiety, confusion, somnolence, tremor, vertigo, paresthesia

DIGESTIVE: vomiting, abnormal liver function test, dyspepsia, dry mouth, constipation, oral moniliasis, anorexia, stomatitis, glossitis, flatulence, gastrointestinal disorder, GGTP increased

HEMIC AND LYMPHATIC: prothrombin decrease (prothrombin time prolonged/International Normalized Ratio (INR) increased), thrombocythemia, thrombocytopenia, eosinophilia, leukopenia

METABOLIC AND NUTRITIONAL: amylase increased, lactic dehydrogenase increased

MUSCULOSKELETAL: arthralgia, myalgia

RESPIRATORY: dyspnea

SKIN/APPENDAGES: rash (maculopapular, purpuric, pustular), pruritus, sweating

SPECIAL SENSES: taste perversion

UROGENITAL: vaginal moniliasis, vaginitis

Additional clinically relevant rare events, judged by investigators to be at least possibly drug-related, that occurred in less than 0.1% of moxifloxacin treated patients were: abnormal dreams, abnormal vision, agitation, amblyopia, amnesia, anemia, aphasia, arthritis, asthma, atrial fibrillation, convulsions, depersonalization, depression, diarrhea (*Clostridium difficile*), dysphagia, ECG abnormal, emotional lability, face edema, gastritis, hallucinations, hyperglycemia, hyperlipidemia, hypertonia, hyperuricemia, hypesthesia, hypotension, incoordination, jaundice (predominantly cholestatic), kidney function abnormal, parosmia, pelvic pain, prothrombin increase (prothrombin time decreased/International Normalized Ratio (INR) decreased), sleep disorders, speech disorders, supraventricular tachycardia, taste loss, tendon disorder, thinking abnormal, thromboplastin decrease, tinnitus, tongue discoloration, urticaria, vasodilatation, ventricular tachycardia

Post-Marketing Adverse Event Reports:

Additional adverse events have been reported from worldwide post-marketing experience with moxifloxacin. Because these events are reported voluntarily from a population of uncertain size, it is not always possible to reliably estimate their frequency or establish a causal relationship to drug exposure. These events, some of them life-threatening, include anaphylactic reaction, anaphylactic shock, angioedema (including laryngeal edema), hepatitis (predominantly cholestatic), pseudomembranous colitis, psychotic reaction, Stevens-Johnson syndrome, syncope, tendon rupture, and ventricular tachyarrhythmias (including in very rare cases cardiac arrest and torsade de pointes, and usually in patients with concurrent severe underlying proarrhythmic conditions).

LABORATORY CHANGES

Changes in laboratory parameters, without regard to drug relationship, which are not listed above and which occurred in ≥ 2% of patients and at an incidence greater than in controls included: increases in MCH, neutrophils, WBCs, PT ratio, ionized calcium, chloride, albumin, globulin, bilirubin; decreases in hemoglobin, RBCs, neutrophils, eosinophils, basophils, PT ratio, glucose, pO_2, bilirubin and amylase. It cannot be determined if any of the above laboratory abnormalities were caused by the drug or the underlying condition being treated.

OVERDOSAGE

Single oral overdoses up to 2.8 g were not associated with any serious adverse events. In the event of acute overdose, the stomach should be emptied and adequate hydration maintained. ECG monitoring is recommended due to the possibility of QT interval prolongation. The patient should be carefully observed and given supportive treatment. The administration of activated charcoal as soon as possible after oral overdose may prevent excessive increase of systemic moxifloxacin exposure. About 3% and 9% of the dose of moxifloxacin, as well as about 2% and 4.5% of its glucuronide metabolite are removed by continuous ambulatory peritoneal dialysis and hemodialysis, respectively.

Single oral moxifloxacin doses of 2000, 500, and 1500 mg/kg were lethal to rats, mice, and Cynomolgus monkeys, respectively. The minimum lethal intravenous dose in mice and rats was 100 mg/kg. Toxic signs after administration of a single high dose of moxifloxacin to these animals included CNS and gastrointestinal effects such as decreased activity, somnolence, tremor, convulsions, vomiting and diarrhea.

DOSAGE AND ADMINISTRATION

The dose of AVELOX is 400 mg (orally or as an intravenous infusion) once every 24 hours. The duration of therapy depends on the type of infection as described below.

Infection*	Daily Dose	Duration
Acute Bacterial Sinusitis	400 mg	10 days
Acute Bacterial Exacerbation of Chronic Bronchitis	400 mg	5 days
Community Acquired Pneumonia	400 mg	7-14 days
Uncomplicated Skin and Skin Structure Infections	400 mg	7 days

*due to the designated pathogens (See **INDICATIONS AND USAGE.**). For I.V. use see **Precautions, Geriatric Use.**

Oral doses of moxifloxacin should be administered at least 4 hours before or 8 hours after antacids containing magnesium or aluminum, as well as sucralfate, metal cations such as iron, and multivitamin preparations with zinc, or VIDEX® (didanosine) chewable/buffered tablets or the pediatric powder for oral solution. (See **CLINICAL PHARMACOLOGY, Drug Interactions** and **PRECAUTIONS, Drug Interactions.**)

Impaired Renal Function

No dosage adjustment is required in renally impaired patients, including those on either hemodialysis or continuous ambulatory peritoneal dialysis.

Impaired Hepatic Function

No dosage adjustment is required in patients with mild or moderate hepatic insufficiency (Child Pugh Classes A and B). The pharmacokinetics of moxifloxacin in patients with severe hepatic insufficiency (Child Pugh Class C) have not been studied. (See **CLINICAL PHARMACOLOGY, Hepatic Insufficiency.**)

When switching from intravenous to oral dosage administration, no dosage adjustment is necessary. Patients whose therapy is started with AVELOX I.V. may be switched to AVELOX Tablets when clinically indicated at the discretion of the physician.

AVELOX I.V. should be administered by INTRAVENOUS infusion only. It is not intended for intra-arterial, intramuscular, intrathecal, intraperitoneal, or subcutaneous administration.

AVELOX I.V. should be administered by intravenous infusion over a period of 60 minutes by direct infusion or through a Y-type intravenous infusion set which may already be in place. CAUTION: RAPID OR BOLUS INTRAVENOUS INFUSION MUST BE AVOIDED.

Since only limited data are available on the compatibility of moxifloxacin intravenous injection with other intravenous substances, additives or other medications should not be added to AVELOX I.V. or infused simultaneously through the same intravenous line. If the same intravenous line or a Y-type line is used for sequential infusion of other drugs, or if the "piggyback" method of administration is used, the line should be flushed before and after infusion of AVELOX I.V. with an infusion solution compatible with AVELOX I.V. as well as with other drug(s) administered via this common line.

AVELOX I.V. is compatible with the following intravenous solutions at ratios from 1:10 to 10:1:

0.9% Sodium Chloride Injection, USP
1M Sodium Chloride Injection
5% Dextrose Injection, USP
Sterile Water for Injection, USP
10% Dextrose for Injection, USP
Lactated Ringer's for Injection

Preparation for administration of AVELOX I.V. injection premix in flexible containers:

1. Close flow control clamp of administration set.
2. Remove cover from port at bottom of container.
3. Insert piercing pin from an appropriate transfer set (e.g. one that does not require excessive force, such as ISO compatible administration set) into port with a gentle twisting motion until pin is firmly seated.

NOTE: Refer to complete directions that have been provided with the administration set.

HOW SUPPLIED

Tablets

AVELOX (moxifloxacin hydrochloride) Tablets are available as oblong, dull red film-coated tablets containing 400 mg moxifloxacin.

The tablet is coded with the word "BAYER" on one side and "M400" on the reverse side.

Package	NDC Code
Bottles of 30:	0026-8581-69
Unit Dose Pack of 50:	0026-8581-88
ABC Pack of 5:	0026-8581-41

Store at 25°C (77°F); excursions permitted to 15-30°C (59-86°F) [see USP Controlled Room Temperature]. Avoid high humidity.

Intravenous Solution – Premix Bags

AVELOX I.V. (moxifloxacin hydrochloride in sodium chloride injection) is available in ready-to-use 250 mL latex-free flexible bags containing 400 mg of moxifloxacin in 0.8% saline. NO FURTHER DILUTION OF THIS PREPARATION IS NECESSARY.

Package	NDC Code
250 mL flexible container	0026-8582-31

Parenteral drug products should be inspected visually for particulate matter prior to administration. Samples containing visible particulates should not be used.

Since the premix flexible containers are for single-use only, any unused portion should be discarded.

Store at 25°C (77°F); excursions permitted to 15-30°C (59-86°F) [see USP Controlled Room Temperature]. **DO NOT REFRIGERATE – PRODUCT PRECIPITATES UPON REFRIGERATION.**

ANIMAL PHARMACOLOGY

Quinolones have been shown to cause arthropathy in immature animals. In studies in juvenile dogs oral doses of moxifloxacin ≥ 30 mg/kg/day (approximately 1.5 times the maximum recommended human dose based upon systemic exposure) for 28 days resulted in arthropathy. There was no evidence of arthropathy in mature monkeys and rats at oral doses up to 135 and 500 mg/kg, respectively.

Unlike some other members of the quinolone class, crystalluria was not observed in 6 month repeat dose studies in rats and monkeys with moxifloxacin.

No ocular toxicity was observed in a 13 week oral repeat dose study in dogs with a moxifloxacin dose of 60 mg/kg. Ocular toxicity was not observed in 6 month repeat dose studies in rats and monkeys (daily oral doses up to 500 mg/kg and 135 mg/kg, respectively). In beagle dogs, electroretinographic (ERG) changes were observed in a 2 week study at oral doses of 60 and 90 mg/kg. Histopathological changes were observed in the retina from one of four dogs at 90 mg/kg, a dose associated with mortality in this study.

Some quinolones have been reported to have proconvulsant activity that is exacerbated with concomitant use of non-steroidal anti-inflammatory drugs (NSAIDs). Moxifloxacin at an oral dose of 300 mg/kg did not show an increase in acute toxicity or potential for CNS toxicity (e.g. seizures) in mice when used in combination with NSAIDs such as diclofenac, ibuprofen, or fenbufen.

In dog studies, at plasma concentrations about five times the human therapeutic level, a QT-prolonging effect of moxifloxacin was found. Electrophysiological *in vitro* studies suggested an inhibition of the rapid activating component of the delayed rectifier potassium current (I_{Kr}) as an underlying mechanism. In dogs, the combined infusion of sotalol, a Class III antiarrhythmic agent, with moxifloxacin induced a higher degree of QTc prolongation than that induced by the same dose (30 mg/kg) of moxifloxacin alone.

In a local tolerability study performed in dogs, no signs of local intolerability were seen when moxifloxacin was administered intravenously. After intra-arterial injection, inflammatory changes involving the peri-arterial soft tissue were observed suggesting that intra-arterial administration of moxifloxacin should be avoided.

CLINICAL STUDIES

Acute Bacterial Exacerbation of Chronic Bronchitis

AVELOX Tablets (400 mg once daily for five days) were evaluated for the treatment of acute bacterial exacerbation of chronic bronchitis in a large, randomized, double-blind, controlled clinical trial conducted in the US. This study compared AVELOX with clarithromycin (500 mg twice daily for 10 days) and enrolled 629 patients. The primary endpoint for this trial was clinical success at 7-17 days post-therapy. The clinical success for AVELOX was 89% (222/250) compared to 89% (224/251) for clarithromycin.

The following outcomes are the clinical success rates at the follow-up visit for the clinically evaluable patient groups by pathogen:

PATHOGEN	AVELOX	Clarithromycin
Streptococcus pneumoniae	100% (16/16)	87% (20/23)
Haemophilus influenzae	89% (33/37)	88% (36/41)
Haemophilus parainfluenzae	100% (16/16)	100% (14/14)
Moraxella catarrhalis	85% (29/34)	100% (24/24)
Staphylococcus aureus	94% (15/16)	75% (6/8)
Klebsiella pneumoniae	90% (18/20)	91% (10/11)

The microbiological eradication rates (eradication plus presumed eradication) in AVELOX treated patients were *Streptococcus pneumoniae* 100%, *Haemophilus influenzae* 89%, *Haemophilus parainfluenzae* 100%, *Moraxella catarrhalis* 85%, *Staphylococcus aureus* 94%, and *Klebsiella pneumoniae* 85%.

Community Acquired Pneumonia

A large, randomized, double-blind, controlled clinical trial was conducted in the US to compare the efficacy of AVELOX Tablets (400 mg once daily) to that of high-dose clarithromycin (500 mg twice daily) in the treatment of patients with clinically and radiologically documented community acquired pneumonia. This study enrolled 474 patients (382 of which were valid for the primary efficacy analysis conducted at the 14 - 35 day follow-up visit). Clinical success for clinically evaluable patients was 95% (184/194) for AVELOX and 95% (178/188) for high dose clarithromycin.

A large, randomized, double-blind, controlled trial was conducted in the US and Canada to compare the efficacy of sequential IV/PO AVELOX 400 mg QD for 7-14 days to an IV/PO fluoroquinolone control (trovafloxacin or levofloxacin) in the treatment of patients with clinically and radiologically documented community acquired pneumonia. This study enrolled 516 patients, 362 of which were valid for the primary efficacy analysis conducted at the 7-30 day post-therapy visit. The clinical success rate was 86% (157/182) for AVELOX therapy and 89% (161/180) for the fluoroquinolone comparators.

An open-label ex-US study that enrolled 628 patients compared AVELOX to sequential IV/PO amoxicillin/clavulanate (1.2 g IV q8h/625 mg PO q8h) with or without high-dose IV/PO clarithromycin (500 mg BID). The intravenous formulations of the comparators are not FDA approved. The clinical success rate at Day 5-7 (the primary efficacy timepoint) for AVELOX therapy was 93% (241/258) and demonstrated superiority to amoxicillin/clavulanate ± clarithromycin (85%, 239/280) [95% C.I. 2.9%, 13.2%]. The clinical success rate at the 21-28 days post-therapy visit for AVELOX was 84% (216/258), which also demonstrated superiority to the comparators (74%, 208/280) [95% C.I. 2.6%, 16.3%].

The clinical success rates by pathogen across four CAP studies are presented below:

Clinical Success Rates By Pathogen (Pooled CAP Studies)

PATHOGEN	AVELOX
Streptococcus pneumoniae	94% (80/85)
Staphylococcus aureus	85% (17/20)
Klebsiella pneumoniae	92% (11/12)
Haemophilus influenzae	92% (56/61)
Chlamydia pneumoniae	93% (119/128)
Mycoplasma pneumoniae	96% (73/76)
Moraxella catarrhalis	92% (11/12)

Community Acquired Pneumonia due to Penicillin-Resistant *Streptococcus pneumoniae* (PRSP)

The clinical and bacteriological efficacy of AVELOX in the treatment of community acquired pneumonia due to penicillin-resistant *Streptococcus pneumoniae* (penicillin MIC ≥ 2 μg/mL) was evaluated in 9 clinical studies: 4 comparative, double-blind tablet studies; 2 non-comparative, open-label tablet studies; 1 comparative, double-blind sequential intravenous to oral study; and 2 comparative, open-label, sequential intravenous to oral studies. All studies required strict assessment criteria with investigator assessment of treatment outcome as success or failure only. The primary efficacy parameter in these studies was clinical cure at the test-of-cure visit, which ranged from Day 6 to 44 post-treatment. Of the 21 AVELOX-treated broth microdilution-confirmed valid for efficacy PRSP patients, 7 had PRSP bacteremia, 12 had severe pneumonia (by the Original American Thoracic Society criteria). The clinical success rates of *S. pneumoniae* and PRSP valid for efficacy patients are summarized in the following table.

Pathogen	AVELOX		Comparators	
	n/N	%	n/N	%
All *S. pneumoniae*	230/244	94	138/162	85
S. pneumoniae bacteremia	53/58	91	35/41	85
S. pneumoniae with Penicillin MIC ≥ 2 μg/mL	21/21*	100	5/5	100
S. pneumoniae bacteremia with Penicillin MIC ≥ 2 μg/mL	7/7	100	2/2	100

*All of these patients were bacteriologic successes at the test-of-cure visit, and 7 of the 21 patients had MIC = 4 μg/mL

Acute Bacterial Sinusitis

In a large, controlled double-blind study conducted in the US, AVELOX Tablets (400 mg once daily for ten days) were compared with cefuroxime axetil (250 mg twice daily for ten days) for the treatment of acute bacterial sinusitis. The trial included 457 patients valid for the primary efficacy determination. Clinical success (cure plus improvement) at the 7 to 21 day post-therapy test of cure visit was 90% for AVELOX and 89% for cefuroxime.

An additional non-comparative study was conducted to gather bacteriological data and to evaluate microbiological eradication in adult patients treated with AVELOX 400 mg once daily for seven days. All patients (n = 336) underwent antral puncture in this study. Clinical success rates and eradication/presumed eradication rates at the 21 to 37 day follow-up visit were 97% (29 out of 30) for *Streptococcus pneumoniae*, 83% (15 out of 18) for *Moraxella catarrhalis*, and 80% (24 out of 30) for *Haemophilus influenzae*.

Uncomplicated Skin and Skin Structure Infections

A randomized, double-blind, controlled clinical trial conducted in the US compared the efficacy of AVELOX 400 mg once daily for seven days with cephalexin HCl 500 mg three times daily for seven days. The percentage of patients treated for uncomplicated abscesses was 30%, furuncles 8%, cellulitis 16%, impetigo 20%, and other skin infections 26%. Adjunctive procedures (incision and drainage or debridement) were performed on 17% of the AVELOX treated patients and 14% of the comparator treated patients. Clinical success rates in evaluable patients were 89% (108/122) for AVELOX and 91% (110/121) for cephalexin HCl.

REFERENCES

1. National Committee for Clinical Laboratory Standards, Methods for Dilution Antimicrobial Susceptibility Tests for Bacteria That Grow Aerobically-Sixth Edition. Approved Standard NCCLS Document M7-A6, Vol. 23, No. 2, NCCLS, Wayne, PA, January, 2003.

2. National Committee for Clinical Laboratory Standards, Performance Standards for Antimicrobial Disk Susceptibility Tests-Eighth Edition. Approved Standard NCCLS Document M2-A8, Vol. 23, No. 1, NCCLS, Wayne, PA, January, 2003.

Patient Information About:
AVELOX®
(moxifloxacin hydrochloride)
400 mg Tablets

This section contains important information about AVELOX (moxifloxacin hydrochloride), and should be read completely before you begin treatment. This section does not take the place of discussions with your doctor or health care professional about your medical condition or your treatment. This section does not list all benefits and risks of AVELOX. The medicine described here can be prescribed only by a licensed health care professional. If you have any questions about AVELOX talk with your health care professional. Only your health care professional can determine if AVELOX is right for you.

What is AVELOX?

AVELOX is an antibiotic used to treat lung, sinus, or skin infections caused by certain germs called bacteria. AVELOX kills many of the types of bacteria that can infect the lungs and sinuses and has been shown in a large number of clinical trials to be safe and effective for the treatment of bacterial infections.

Sometimes viruses rather than bacteria may infect the lungs and sinuses (for example the common cold). AVELOX, like all other antibiotics, does not kill viruses.

You should contact your doctor if you think your condition is not improving while taking AVELOX.

AVELOX Tablets are red and contain 400 mg of active drug.

How and when should I take AVELOX?

AVELOX should be taken once a day for 5-14 days depending on your prescription. It should be swallowed and may be taken with or without food. Try to take the tablet at the same time each day.

You may begin to feel better quickly; however, in order to make sure that all bacteria are killed, you should complete the full course of medication. Do not take more than the prescribed dose of AVELOX even if you missed a dose by mistake. You should not take a double dose.

Who should not take AVELOX?

You should not take AVELOX if you have ever had a severe allergic reaction to any of the group of antibiotics known as "quinolones" such as ciprofloxacin or levofloxacin. If you develop hives, difficulty breathing, or other symptoms of a severe allergic reaction, seek emergency treatment right away. If you develop a skin rash, you should stop taking AVELOX and call your health care professional.

You should avoid AVELOX if you have a rare condition known as congenital prolongation of the QT interval. If you or any of your family members have this condition you should inform your health care professional. You should avoid AVELOX if you are being treated for heart rhythm disturbances with certain medicines such as quinidine, procainamide, amiodarone or sotalol. Inform your health care professional if you are taking a heart rhythm drug.

You should also avoid AVELOX if the amount of potassium in your blood is low. Low potassium can sometimes be caused by medicines called diuretics such as furosemide and hydrochlorothiazide. If you are taking a diuretic medicine you should speak with your health care professional.

If you are pregnant or planning to become pregnant while taking AVELOX, talk to your doctor before taking this medication. AVELOX is not recommended for use during pregnancy or nursing, as the effects on the unborn child or nursing infant are unknown.

AVELOX is not recommended for children.

What are the possible side effects of AVELOX?

AVELOX is generally well tolerated. The most common side effects caused by AVELOX, which are usually mild, include dizziness, nausea, and diarrhea. If diarrhea persists call your health care provider. You should be careful about driving or operating machinery until you are sure AVELOX is not causing dizziness. If you notice any side effects not mentioned in this section or you have any concerns about the side effects you are experiencing, please inform your health care professional.

In some people, AVELOX, as with some other antibiotics, may produce a small effect on the heart that is seen on an electrocardiogram test. Although this has not caused any serious problems in more than 7,900 patients who have already taken the medication in clinical studies, in theory it could result in extremely rare cases of abnormal heartbeat which may be dangerous. Contact your health care professional if you develop heart palpitations (fast beating), or have fainting spells.

Convulsions have been reported in patients receiving quinolone antibiotics. Be sure to let your physician know if you have a history of convulsions. Quinolones, including AVELOX, have been rarely associated with other central nervous system events including confusion, tremors, hallucinations, and depression.

Quinolones, including AVELOX, have been rarely associated with inflammation of tendons. If you experience pain, swelling or rupture of a tendon, you should stop taking AVELOX and call your health care professional.

What about other medicines I am taking?

Tell your doctor about all other prescription and non-prescription medicines or supplements you are taking. You should avoid taking AVELOX with certain medicines used to treat an abnormal heartbeat. These include quinidine, procainamide, amiodarone, and sotalol.

Some medicines also produce an effect on the electrocardiogram test, including cisapride, erythromycin, some antidepressants and some antipsychotic drugs. These may increase the risk of heart beat problems when taken with AVELOX.

Many antacids and multivitamins may interfere with the absorption of AVELOX and may prevent it from working properly. You should take AVELOX either 4 hours before or 8 hours after taking these products.

Remember

Take your dose of AVELOX once a day.

Complete the course of medication even if you are feeling better.

Keep this medication out of the reach of children.

This information does not take the place of discussions with your doctor or health care professional about your medical condition or your treatment.

For more complete information about AVELOX request full prescribing information from your health care professional, pharmacist, or visit our website at www.aveloxusa.com.

Bayer HealthCare
Bayer Pharmaceuticals Corporation
400 Morgan Lane
West Haven, CT 06516
Made in Germany
℞ Only
08753736, R.5 4/04 12315

Printed in U.S.A.

CIPRO® ℞
[*sī'prō*]
(ciprofloxacin hydrochloride)
TABLETS
CIPRO® ℞
(ciprofloxacin*)
ORAL SUSPENSION

Prescribing information for this product, which appears on pages 839–845 of the 2004 PDR, has been completely revised as follows. Please write "See Supplement A" next to the product heading.

To reduce the development of drug-resistant bacteria and maintain the effectiveness of CIPRO® Tablets and CIPRO Oral Suspension and other antibacterial drugs, CIPRO Tablets and CIPRO Oral Suspension should be used only to treat or prevent infections that are proven or strongly suspected to be caused by bacteria.

DESCRIPTION

CIPRO (ciprofloxacin hydrochloride) Tablets and CIPRO (ciprofloxacin*) Oral Suspension are synthetic broad spectrum antimicrobial agents for oral administration. Ciprofloxacin hydrochloride, USP, a fluoroquinolone, is the monohydrochloride monohydrate salt of 1-cyclopropyl-6-fluoro-1, 4-dihydro-4-oxo-7-(1-piperazinyl)-3-quinolinecarboxylic acid. It is a faintly yellowish to light yellow crystalline substance with a molecular weight of 385.8. Its empirical formula is $C_{17}H_{18}FN_3O_3 \cdot HCl \cdot H_2O$ and its chemical structure is as follows:

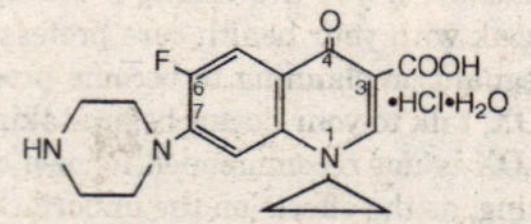

Ciprofloxacin is 1-cyclopropyl-6-fluoro-1,4-dihydro-4-oxo-7-(1-piperazinyl)-3-quinolinecarboxylic acid. Its empirical formula is $C_{17}H_{18}FN_3O_3$ and its molecular weight is 331.4. It is a faintly yellowish to light yellow crystalline substance and its chemical structure is as follows:

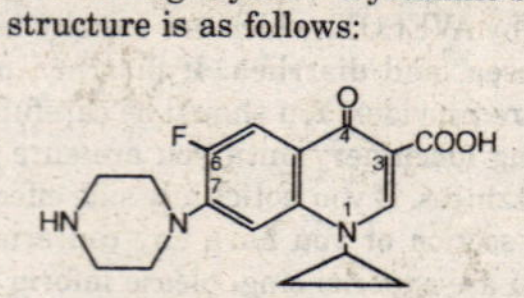

CIPRO film-coated tablets are available in 100 mg, 250 mg, 500 mg and 750 mg (ciprofloxacin equivalent) strengths. Ciprofloxacin tablets are white to slightly yellowish. The inactive ingredients are cornstarch, microcrystalline cellulose, silicon dioxide, crospovidone, magnesium stearate, hypromellose, titanium dioxide, polyethylene glycol and water.

Ciprofloxacin Oral Suspension is available in 5% (5 g ciprofloxacin in 100 mL) and 10% (10 g ciprofloxacin in 100 mL) strengths. Ciprofloxacin Oral Suspension is a white to slightly yellowish suspension with strawberry flavor which may contain yellow-orange droplets. It is composed of ciprofloxacin microcapsules and diluent which are mixed prior to dispensing (See instructions for USE/HANDLING). The components of the suspension have the following compositions:

Microcapsules - ciprofloxacin, povidone, methacrylic acid copolymer, hypromellose, magnesium stearate, and Polysorbate 20.

Diluent - medium-chain triglycerides, sucrose, lecithin, water, and strawberry flavor.

* Does not comply with USP with regards to "loss on drying" and "residue on ignition".

CLINICAL PHARMACOLOGY

Absorption: Ciprofloxacin given as an oral tablet is rapidly and well absorbed from the gastrointestinal tract after oral administration. The absolute bioavailability is approximately 70% with no substantial loss by first pass metabolism. Ciprofloxacin maximum serum concentrations and area under the curve are shown in the chart for the 250 mg to 1000 mg dose range.

Dose (mg)	Maximum Serum Concentration (µg/mL)	Area Under Curve (AUC) (µg•hr/mL)
250	1.2	4.8
500	2.4	11.6
750	4.3	20.2
1000	5.4	30.8

Maximum serum concentrations are attained 1 to 2 hours after oral dosing. Mean concentrations 12 hours after dosing with 250, 500, or 750 mg are 0.1, 0.2, and 0.4 µg/mL, respectively. The serum elimination half-life in subjects with normal renal function is approximately 4 hours. Serum concentrations increase proportionately with doses up to 1000 mg.

A 500 mg oral dose given every 12 hours has been shown to produce an area under the serum concentration time curve (AUC) equivalent to that produced by an intravenous infusion of 400 mg ciprofloxacin given over 60 minutes every 12 hours. A 750 mg oral dose given every 12 hours has been shown to produce an AUC at steady-state equivalent to that produced by an intravenous infusion of 400 mg given over 60 minutes every 8 hours. A 750 mg oral dose results in a C_{max} similar to that observed with a 400 mg I.V. dose. A 250 mg oral dose given every 12 hours produces an AUC equivalent to that produced by an infusion of 200 mg ciprofloxacin given every 12 hours.

[See table below]

Steady-state Pharmacokinetic Parameters Following Multiple Oral and I.V. Doses

Parameters	500 mg q12h, P.O.	400 mg q12h, I.V.	750 mg q12h, P.O.	400 mg q8h, I.V.
AUC (µg•hr/mL)	13.7[a]	12.7[a]	31.6[b]	32.9[c]
C_{max} (µg/mL)	2.97	4.56	3.59	4.07

[a]AUC $_{0\text{-}12h}$
[b]AUC 24h=AUC$_{0\text{-}12h}$ × 2
[c]AUC 24h=AUC$_{0\text{-}8h}$ × 3

Distribution: The binding of ciprofloxacin to serum proteins is 20 to 40% which is not likely to be high enough to cause significant protein binding interactions with other drugs.

After oral administration, ciprofloxacin is widely distributed throughout the body. Tissue concentrations often exceed serum concentrations in both men and women, particularly in genital tissue including the prostate. Ciprofloxacin is present in active form in the saliva, nasal and bronchial secretions, mucosa of the sinuses, sputum, skin blister fluid, lymph, peritoneal fluid, bile, and prostatic secretions. Ciprofloxacin has also been detected in lung, skin, fat, muscle, cartilage, and bone. The drug diffuses into the cerebrospinal fluid (CSF); however, CSF concentrations are generally less than 10% of peak serum concentrations. Low levels of the drug have been detected in the aqueous and vitreous humors of the eye.

Metabolism: Four metabolites have been identified in human urine which together account for approximately 15% of an oral dose. The metabolites have antimicrobial activity, but are less active than unchanged ciprofloxacin.

Excretion: The serum elimination half-life in subjects with normal renal function is approximately 4 hours. Approximately 40 to 50% of an orally administered dose is excreted in the urine as unchanged drug. After a 250 mg oral dose, urine concentrations of ciprofloxacin usually exceed 200 µg/mL during the first two hours and are approximately 30 µg/mL at 8 to 12 hours after dosing. The urinary excretion of ciprofloxacin is virtually complete within 24 hours after dosing. The renal clearance of ciprofloxacin, which is approximately 300 mL/minute, exceeds the normal glomerular filtration rate of 120 mL/minute. Thus, active tubular secretion would seem to play a significant role in its elimination. Co-administration of probenecid with ciprofloxacin results in about a 50% reduction in the ciprofloxacin renal clearance and a 50% increase in its concentration in the systemic circulation. Although bile concentrations of ciprofloxacin are several fold higher than serum concentrations after oral dosing, only a small amount of the dose administered is recovered from the bile as unchanged drug. An additional 1 to 2% of the dose is recovered from the bile in the form of metabolites. Approximately 20 to 35% of an oral dose is recovered from the feces within 5 days after dosing. This may arise from either biliary clearance or transintestinal elimination.

With oral administration, a 500 mg dose, given as 10 mL of the 5% CIPRO Suspension (containing 250 mg ciprofloxacin/5mL) is bioequivalent to the 500 mg tablet. A 10 mL volume of the 5% CIPRO Suspension (containing 250 mg ciprofloxacin/5mL) is bioequivalent to a 5 mL volume of the 10% CIPRO Suspension (containing 500 mg ciprofloxacin/5mL).

Drug-drug Interactions: When CIPRO Tablet is given concomitantly with food, there is a delay in the absorption of the drug, resulting in peak concentrations that occur closer to 2 hours after dosing rather than 1 hour whereas there is no delay observed when CIPRO Suspension is given with food. The overall absorption of CIPRO Tablet or CIPRO Suspension, however, is not substantially affected. The pharmacokinetics of ciprofloxacin given as the suspension are also not affected by food. Concurrent administration of antacids containing magnesium hydroxide or aluminum hydroxide may reduce the bioavailability of ciprofloxacin by as much as 90%. (See **PRECAUTIONS.**)

The serum concentrations of ciprofloxacin and metronidazole were not altered when these two drugs were given concomitantly.

Concomitant administration of ciprofloxacin with theophylline decreases the clearance of theophylline resulting in elevated serum theophylline levels and increased risk of a patient developing CNS or other adverse reactions. Ciprofloxacin also decreases caffeine clearance and inhibits the formation of paraxanthine after caffeine administration. (See **PRECAUTIONS.**)

Special Populations: Pharmacokinetic studies of the oral (single dose) and intravenous (single and multiple dose) forms of ciprofloxacin indicate that plasma concentrations of ciprofloxacin are higher in elderly subjects (> 65 years) as compared to young adults. Although the C_{max} is increased 16-40%, the increase in mean AUC is approximately 30%, and can be at least partially attributed to decreased renal clearance in the elderly. Elimination half-life is only slightly (~20%) prolonged in the elderly. These differences are not considered clinically significant. (See **PRECAUTIONS: Geriatric Use.**)

In patients with reduced renal function, the half-life of ciprofloxacin is slightly prolonged. Dosage adjustments may be required. (See **DOSAGE AND ADMINISTRATION.**)

In preliminary studies in patients with stable chronic liver cirrhosis, no significant changes in ciprofloxacin pharmacokinetics have been observed. The kinetics of ciprofloxacin in patients with acute hepatic insufficiency, however, have not been fully elucidated.

Following a single oral dose of 10 mg/kg ciprofloxacin suspension to 16 children ranging in age from 4 months to 7 years, the mean C_{max} was 2.4 µg/mL (range: 1.5 – 3.4 µg/mL) and the mean AUC was 9.2 µg*h/mL (range: 5.8 – 14.9 µg*h/mL). There was no apparent age-dependence, and no notable increase in C_{max} or AUC upon multiple dosing (10 mg/kg TID). In children with severe sepsis who were given intravenous ciprofloxacin (10 mg/kg as a 1-hour infusion), the mean C_{max} was 6.1 µg/mL (range: 4.6 – 8.3 µg/mL) in 10 children less than 1 year of age; and 7.2 µg/mL (range: 4.7 – 11.8 µg/mL) in 10 children between 1 and 5 years of age. The AUC values were 17.4 µg*h/mL (range: 11.8 – 32.0 µg*h/mL) and 16.5 µg*h/mL (range: 11.0 – 23.8 µg*h/mL) in the respective age groups. These values are within the range reported for adults at therapeutic doses. Based on population pharmacokinetic analysis of pediatric patients with various infections, the predicted mean half-life in children is approximately 4 - 5 hours, and the bioavailability of the oral suspension is approximately 60%.

MICROBIOLOGY

Ciprofloxacin has *in vitro* activity against a wide range of gram-negative and gram-positive microorganisms. The bactericidal action of ciprofloxacin results from inhibition of the enzymes topoisomerase II (DNA gyrase) and topoisomerase IV, which are required for bacterial DNA replication, transcription, repair, and recombination. The mechanism of action of fluoroquinolones, including ciprofloxacin, is different from that of penicillins, cephalosporins, aminoglycosides, macrolides, and tetracyclines; therefore, microorganisms resistant to these classes of drugs may be susceptible to ciprofloxacin and other quinolones. There is no known cross-resistance between ciprofloxacin and other classes of antimicrobials. *In vitro* resistance to ciprofloxacin develops slowly by multiple step mutations.

Ciprofloxacin is slightly less active when tested at acidic pH. The inoculum size has little effect when tested *in vitro*. The minimal bactericidal concentration (MBC) generally does not exceed the minimal inhibitory concentration (MIC) by more than a factor of 2.

Ciprofloxacin has been shown to be active against most strains of the following microorganisms, both *in vitro* and in clinical infections as described in the **INDICATIONS AND USAGE** section of the package insert for CIPRO (ciprofloxacin hydrochloride) Tablets and CIPRO (ciprofloxacin*) 5% and 10% Oral Suspension.

Aerobic gram-positive microorganisms
Enterococcus faecalis (Many strains are only moderately susceptible.)
Staphylococcus aureus (methicillin-susceptible strains only)
Staphylococcus epidermidis (methicillin-susceptible strains only)
Staphylococcus saprophyticus
Streptococcus pneumoniae (penicillin-susceptible strains only)
Streptococcus pyogenes

Aerobic gram-negative microorganisms
Campylobacter jejuni
Citrobacter diversus
Citrobacter freundii
Enterobacter cloacae
Escherichia coli
Haemophilus influenzae
Haemophilus parainfluenzae
Klebsiella pneumoniae
Moraxella catarrhalis
Morganella morganii
Neisseria gonorrhoeae
Proteus mirabilis
Proteus vulgaris
Providencia rettgeri
Providencia stuartii
Pseudomonas aeruginosa
Salmonella typhi
Serratia marcescens
Shigella boydii
Shigella dysenteriae
Shigella flexneri
Shigella sonnei

Ciprofloxacin has been shown to be active against *Bacillus anthracis* both *in vitro* and by use of serum levels as a surrogate marker (see **INDICATIONS AND USAGE** and **INHALATIONAL ANTHRAX – ADDITIONAL INFORMATION**).

The following *in vitro* data are available, **but their clinical significance is unknown.**

Ciprofloxacin exhibits *in vitro* minimum inhibitory concentrations (MICs) of 1 µg/mL or less against most (≥ 90%)

strains of the following microorganisms; however, the safety and effectiveness of ciprofloxacin in treating clinical infections due to these microorganisms have not been established in adequate and well-controlled clinical trials.

Aerobic gram-positive microorganisms

Staphylococcus haemolyticus
Staphylococcus hominis
Streptococcus pneumoniae (penicillin-resistant strains only)

Aerobic gram-negative microorganisms

Acinetobacter lwoffi
Aeromonas hydrophila
Edwardsiella tarda
Enterobacter aerogenes
Klebsiella oxytoca
Legionella pneumophila
Pasteurella multocida
Salmonella enteritidis
Vibrio cholerae
Vibrio parahaemolyticus
Vibrio vulnificus
Yersinia enterocolitica

Most strains of *Burkholderia cepacia* and some strains of *Stenotrophomonas maltophilia* are resistant to ciprofloxacin as are most anaerobic bacteria, including *Bacteroides fragilis* and *Clostridium difficile*.

Susceptibility Tests

Dilution Techniques: Quantitative methods are used to determine antimicrobial minimum inhibitory concentrations (MICs). These MICs provide estimates of the susceptibility of bacteria to antimicrobial compounds. The MICs should be determined using a standardized procedure. Standardized procedures are based on a dilution method[1] (broth or agar) or equivalent with standardized inoculum concentrations and standardized concentrations of ciprofloxacin powder. The MIC values should be interpreted according to the following criteria:

For testing aerobic microorganisms other than *Haemophilus influenzae*, *Haemophilus parainfluenzae*, and *Neisseria gonorrhoeae*[a]:

MIC (μg/mL)	Interpretation
≤1	Susceptible (S)
2	Intermediate (I)
≥4	Resistant (R)

[a] These interpretive standards are applicable only to broth microdilution susceptibility tests with streptococci using cation-adjusted Mueller-Hinton broth with 2-5% lysed horse blood.

For testing *Haemophilus influenzae* and *Haemophilus parainfluenzae*[b]:

MIC (μg/mL)	Interpretation
≤1	Susceptible (S)

[b] This interpretive standard is applicable only to broth microdilution susceptibility tests with *Haemophilus influenzae* and *Haemophilus parainfluenzae* using *Haemophilus* Test Medium[1].

The current absence of data on resistant strains precludes defining any results other than "Susceptible". Strains yielding MIC results suggestive of a "nonsusceptible" category should be submitted to a reference laboratory for further testing.

For testing *Neisseria gonorrhoeae*[c]:

MIC (μg/mL)	Interpretation
≤ 0.06	Susceptible (S)
0.12–0.5	Intermediate (I)
≥1	Resistant (R)

[c] This interpretive standard is applicable only to agar dilution test with GC agar base and 1% defined growth supplement.

A report of "Susceptible" indicates that the pathogen is likely to be inhibited if the antimicrobial compound in the blood reaches the concentrations usually achievable. A report of "Intermediate" indicates that the result should be considered equivocal, and, if the microorganism is not fully susceptible to alternative, clinically feasible drugs, the test should be repeated. This category implies possible clinical applicability in body sites where the drug is physiologically concentrated or in situations where high dosage of drug can be used. This category also provides a buffer zone, which prevents small uncontrolled technical factors from causing major discrepancies in interpretation. A report of "Resistant" indicates that the pathogen is not likely to be inhibited if the antimicrobial compound in the blood reaches the concentrations usually achievable; other therapy should be selected.

Standardized susceptibility test procedures require the use of laboratory control microorganisms to control the technical aspects of the laboratory procedures. Standard ciprofloxacin powder should provide the following MIC values:

Organism		MIC (μg/mL)
E. faecalis	ATCC 29212	0.25 – 2.0
E. coli	ATCC 25922	0.004 – 0.015
H. influenzae[a]	ATCC 49247	0.004 – 0.03
N. gonorrhoeae[b]	ATCC 49226	0.001 – 0.008
P. aeruginosa	ATCC 27853	0.25 – 1.0
S. aureus	ATCC 29213	0.12 – 0.5

[a] This quality control range is applicable to only *H. influenzae* ATCC 49247 tested by a broth microdilution procedure using *Haemophilus* Test Medium (HTM)[1].

[b] This quality control range is applicable to only *N. gonorrhoeae* ATCC 49226 tested by an agar dilution procedure using GC agar base and 1% defined growth supplement.

Diffusion Techniques: Quantitative methods that require measurement of zone diameters also provide reproducible estimates of the susceptibility of bacteria to antimicrobial compounds. One such standardized procedure[2] requires the use of standardized inoculum concentrations. This procedure uses paper disks impregnated with 5-μg ciprofloxacin to test the susceptibility of microorganisms to ciprofloxacin. Reports from the laboratory providing results of the standard single-disk susceptibility test with a 5-μg ciprofloxacin disk should be interpreted according to the following criteria:

For testing aerobic microorganisms other than *Haemophilus influenzae*, *Haemophilus parainfluenzae*, and *Neisseria gonorrhoeae*[a]:

Zone Diameter (mm)	Interpretation
≥ 21	Susceptible (S)
16 – 20	Intermediate (I)
≤ 15	Resistant (R)

[a] These zone diameter standards are applicable only to tests performed for streptococci using Mueller-Hinton agar supplemented with 5% sheep blood incubated in 5% CO_2.

For testing *Haemophilus influenzae* and *Haemophilus parainfluenzae*[b]:

Zone Diameter (mm)	Interpretation
≥ 21	Susceptible (S)

[b] This zone diameter standard is applicable only to tests with *Haemophilus influenzae* and *Haemophilus parainfluenzae* using *Haemophilus* Test Medium (HTM)[2].

The current absence of data on resistant strains precludes defining any results other than "Susceptible". Strains yielding zone diameter results suggestive of a "nonsusceptible" category should be submitted to a reference laboratory for further testing.

For testing *Neisseria gonorrhoeae*[c]:

Zone Diameter (mm)	Interpretation
≥ 41	Susceptible (S)
28 – 40	Intermediate (I)
≤ 27	Resistant (R)

[c] This zone diameter standard is applicable only to disk diffusion tests with GC agar base and 1% defined growth supplement.

Interpretation should be as stated above for results using dilution techniques. Interpretation involves correlation of the diameter obtained in the disk test with the MIC for ciprofloxacin.

As with standardized dilution techniques, diffusion methods require the use of laboratory control microorganisms that are used to control the technical aspects of the laboratory procedures. For the diffusion technique, the 5-μg ciprofloxacin disk should provide the following zone diameters in these laboratory test quality control strains:

Organism		Zone Diameter (mm)
E. coli	ATCC 25922	30 – 40
H. influenzae[a]	ATCC 49247	34 – 42
N. gonorrhoeae[b]	ATCC 49226	48 – 58
P. aeruginosa	ATCC 27853	25 – 33
S. aureus	ATCC 25923	22 – 30

[a] These quality control limits are applicable to only *H. influenzae* ATCC 49247 testing using *Haemophilus* Test Medium (HTM)[2].

[b] These quality control limits are applicable only to tests conducted with *N. gonorrhoeae* ATCC 49226 performed by disk diffusion using GC agar base and 1% defined growth supplement.

INDICATIONS AND USAGE

CIPRO is indicated for the treatment of infections caused by susceptible strains of the designated microorganisms in the conditions and patient populations listed below. Please see **DOSAGE AND ADMINISTRATION** for specific recommendations.

Adult Patients:

Urinary Tract Infections caused by *Escherichia coli, Klebsiella pneumoniae, Enterobacter cloacae, Serratia marcescens, Proteus mirabilis, Providencia rettgeri, Morganella morganii, Citrobacter diversus, Citrobacter freundii, Pseudomonas aeruginosa, Staphylococcus epidermidis, Staphylococcus saprophyticus,* or *Enterococcus faecalis.*

Acute Uncomplicated Cystitis in females caused by *Escherichia coli* or *Staphylococcus saprophyticus.*

Chronic Bacterial Prostatitis caused by *Escherichia coli* or *Proteus mirabilis.*

Lower Respiratory Tract Infections caused by *Escherichia coli, Klebsiella pneumoniae, Enterobacter cloacae, Proteus mirabilis, Pseudomonas aeruginosa, Haemophilus influenzae, Haemophilus parainfluenzae,* or *Streptococcus pneumoniae.* Also, *Moraxella catarrhalis* for the treatment of acute exacerbations of chronic bronchitis.

NOTE: Although effective in clinical trials, ciprofloxacin is not a drug of first choice in the treatment of presumed or confirmed pneumonia secondary to *Streptococcus pneumoniae.*

Acute Sinusitis caused by *Haemophilus influenzae, Streptococcus pneumoniae,* or *Moraxella catarrhalis.*

Skin and Skin Structure Infections caused by *Escherichia coli, Klebsiella pneumoniae, Enterobacter cloacae, Proteus mirabilis, Proteus vulgaris, Providencia stuartii, Morganella morganii, Citrobacter freundii, Pseudomonas aeruginosa, Staphylococcus aureus* (methicillin-susceptible), *Staphylococcus epidermidis,* or *Streptococcus pyogenes.*

Bone and Joint Infections caused by *Enterobacter cloacae, Serratia marcescens,* or *Pseudomonas aeruginosa.*

Complicated Intra-Abdominal Infections (used in combination with metronidazole) caused by *Escherichia coli, Pseudomonas aeruginosa, Proteus mirabilis, Klebsiella pneumoniae,* or *Bacteroides fragilis.*

Infectious Diarrhea caused by *Escherichia coli* (enterotoxigenic strains), *Campylobacter jejuni, Shigella boydii*[†], *Shigella dysenteriae, Shigella flexneri* or *Shigella sonnei*[†] when antibacterial therapy is indicated.

Typhoid Fever (Enteric Fever) caused by *Salmonella typhi.*

NOTE: The efficacy of ciprofloxacin in the eradication of the chronic typhoid carrier state has not been demonstrated.

Uncomplicated cervical and urethral gonorrhea due to *Neisseria gonorrhoeae.*

Pediatric patients (1 to 17 years of age):

Complicated Urinary Tract Infections and Pyelonephritis due to *Escherichia coli.*

NOTE: Although effective in clinical trials, ciprofloxacin is not a drug of first choice in the pediatric population due to an increased incidence of adverse events compared to controls, including events related to joints and/or surrounding tissues. (See **WARNINGS, PRECAUTIONS, Pediatric Use, ADVERSE REACTIONS** and **CLINICAL STUDIES**.) Ciprofloxacin, like other fluoroquinolones, is associated with arthropathy and histopathological changes in weight-bearing joints of juvenile animals. (See **ANIMAL PHARMACOLOGY**.)

Adult and Pediatric Patients:

Inhalational anthrax (post-exposure): To reduce the incidence or progression of disease following exposure to aerosolized *Bacillus anthracis.*

Ciprofloxacin serum concentrations achieved in humans serve as a surrogate endpoint reasonably likely to predict clinical benefit and provide the basis for this indication.[4] (See also, **INHALATIONAL ANTHRAX – ADDITIONAL INFORMATION**).

[†]Although treatment of infections due to this organism in this organ system demonstrated a clinically significant outcome, efficacy was studied in fewer than 10 patients.

If anaerobic organisms are suspected of contributing to the infection, appropriate therapy should be administered. Appropriate culture and susceptibility tests should be performed before treatment in order to isolate and identify organisms causing infection and to determine their susceptibility to ciprofloxacin. Therapy with CIPRO may be initiated before results of these tests are known; once results become available appropriate therapy should be continued. As with other drugs, some strains of *Pseudomonas aeruginosa* may develop resistance fairly rapidly during treatment with ciprofloxacin. Culture and susceptibility testing performed periodically during therapy will provide information not only on the therapeutic effect of the antimicrobial agent but also on the possible emergence of bacterial resistance.

To reduce the development of drug-resistant bacteria and maintain the effectiveness of CIPRO Tablets and CIPRO Oral Suspension and other antibacterial drugs, CIPRO Tablets and CIPRO Oral Suspension should be used only to treat or prevent infections that are proven or strongly suspected to be caused by susceptible bacteria. When culture and susceptibility information are available, they should be considered in selecting or modifying antibacterial therapy. In the absence of such data, local epidemiology and susceptibility patterns may contribute to the empiric selection of therapy.

CONTRAINDICATIONS

CIPRO (ciprofloxacin hydrochloride) is contraindicated in persons with a history of hypersensitivity to ciprofloxacin or any member of the quinolone class of antimicrobial agents.

WARNINGS

Pregnant Women: THE SAFETY AND EFFECTIVENESS OF CIPROFLOXACIN IN PREGNANT AND LACTATING WOMEN HAVE NOT BEEN ESTABLISHED. (See **PRECAUTIONS: Pregnancy,** and **Nursing Mothers** subsections.)

Pediatrics: Ciprofloxacin should be used in pediatric patients (less than 18 years of age) only for infections listed in the **INDICATIONS AND USAGE** section. An increased incidence of adverse events compared to controls, including events related to joints and/or surrounding tissues, has been observed. (See **ADVERSE REACTIONS.**)

Continued on next page

Cipro—Cont.

In pre-clinical studies, oral administration of ciprofloxacin caused lameness in immature dogs. Histopathological examination of the weight-bearing joints of these dogs revealed permanent lesions of the cartilage. Related quinolone-class drugs also produce erosions of cartilage of weight-bearing joints and other signs of arthropathy in immature animals of various species. (See **ANIMAL PHARMACOLOGY**.)

Central Nervous System Disorders: Convulsions, increased intracranial pressure, and toxic psychosis have been reported in patients receiving quinolones, including ciprofloxacin. Ciprofloxacin may also cause central nervous system (CNS) events including: dizziness, confusion, tremors, hallucinations, depression, and, rarely, suicidal thoughts or acts. These reactions may occur following the first dose. If these reactions occur in patients receiving ciprofloxacin, the drug should be discontinued and appropriate measures instituted. As with all quinolones, ciprofloxacin should be used with caution in patients with known or suspected CNS disorders that may predispose to seizures or lower the seizure threshold (e.g. severe cerebral arteriosclerosis, epilepsy), or in the presence of other risk factors that may predispose to seizures or lower the seizure threshold (e.g. certain drug therapy, renal dysfunction). (See **PRECAUTIONS: General, Information for Patients, Drug Interactions** and **ADVERSE REACTIONS**.)

Theophylline: SERIOUS AND FATAL REACTIONS HAVE BEEN REPORTED IN PATIENTS RECEIVING CONCURRENT ADMINISTRATION OF CIPROFLOXACIN AND THEOPHYLLINE. These reactions have included cardiac arrest, seizure, status epilepticus, and respiratory failure. Although similar serious adverse effects have been reported in patients receiving theophylline alone, the possibility that these reactions may be potentiated by ciprofloxacin cannot be eliminated. If concomitant use cannot be avoided, serum levels of theophylline should be monitored and dosage adjustments made as appropriate.

Hypersensitivity Reactions: Serious and occasionally fatal hypersensitivity (anaphylactic) reactions, some following the first dose, have been reported in patients receiving quinolone therapy. Some reactions were accompanied by cardiovascular collapse, loss of consciousness, tingling, pharyngeal or facial edema, dyspnea, urticaria, and itching. Only a few patients had a history of hypersensitivity reactions. Serious anaphylactic reactions require immediate emergency treatment with epinephrine. Oxygen, intravenous steroids, and airway management, including intubation, should be administered as indicated.

Severe hypersensitivity reactions characterized by rash, fever, eosinophilia, jaundice, and hepatic necrosis with fatal outcome have also been rarely reported in patients receiving ciprofloxacin along with other drugs. The possibility that these reactions were related to ciprofloxacin cannot be excluded. Ciprofloxacin should be discontinued at the first appearance of a skin rash or any other sign of hypersensitivity.

Pseudomembranous Colitis: Pseudomembranous colitis has been reported with nearly all antibacterial agents, including ciprofloxacin, and may range in severity from mild to life-threatening. Therefore, it is important to consider this diagnosis in patients who present with diarrhea subsequent to the administration of antibacterial agents.

Treatment with antibacterial agents alters the normal flora of the colon and may permit overgrowth of clostridia. Studies indicate that a toxin produced by *Clostridium difficile* is one primary cause of "antibiotic-associated colitis."

After the diagnosis of pseudomembranous colitis has been established, therapeutic measures should be initiated. Mild cases of pseudomembranous colitis usually respond to drug discontinuation alone. In moderate to severe cases, consideration should be given to management with fluids and electrolytes, protein supplementation, and treatment with an antibacterial drug clinically effective against *C. difficile* colitis. Drugs that inhibit peristalsis should be avoided.

Peripheral neuropathy: Rare cases of sensory or sensorimotor axonal polyneuropathy affecting small and/or large axons resulting in paresthesias, hypoesthesias, dysesthesias and weakness have been reported in patients receiving quinolones, including ciprofloxacin. Ciprofloxacin should be discontinued if the patient experiences symptoms of neuropathy including pain, burning, tingling, numbness, and/or weakness, or is found to have deficits in light touch, pain, temperature, position sense, vibratory sensation, and/or motor strength in order to prevent the development of an irreversible condition.

Tendon Effects: Ruptures of the shoulder, hand, Achilles tendon or other tendons that required surgical repair or resulted in prolonged disability have been reported in patients receiving quinolones, including ciprofloxacin. Post-marketing surveillance reports indicate that this risk may be increased in patients receiving concomitant corticosteroids, especially the elderly. Ciprofloxacin should be discontinued if the patient experiences pain, inflammation, or rupture of a tendon. Patients should rest and refrain from exercise until the diagnosis of tendinitis or tendon rupture has been excluded. Tendon rupture can occur during or after therapy with quinolones, including ciprofloxacin.

Syphilis: Ciprofloxacin has not been shown to be effective in the treatment of syphilis. Antimicrobial agents used in high dose for short periods of time to treat gonorrhea may mask or delay the symptoms of incubating syphilis. All patients with gonorrhea should have a serologic test for syphilis at the time of diagnosis. Patients treated with ciprofloxacin should have a follow-up serologic test for syphilis after three months.

PRECAUTIONS

General: Crystals of ciprofloxacin have been observed rarely in the urine of human subjects but more frequently in the urine of laboratory animals, which is usually alkaline. (See **ANIMAL PHARMACOLOGY**.) Crystalluria related to ciprofloxacin has been reported only rarely in humans because human urine is usually acidic. Alkalinity of the urine should be avoided in patients receiving ciprofloxacin. Patients should be well hydrated to prevent the formation of highly concentrated urine.

Central Nervous System: Quinolones, including ciprofloxacin, may also cause central nervous system (CNS) events, including: nervousness, agitation, insomnia, anxiety, nightmares or paranoia. (See **WARNINGS, Information for Patients**, and **Drug Interactions**.)

Renal Impairment: Alteration of the dosage regimen is necessary for patients with impairment of renal function. (See **DOSAGE AND ADMINISTRATION**.)

Phototoxicity: Moderate to severe phototoxicity manifested as an exaggerated sunburn reaction has been observed in patients who are exposed to direct sunlight while receiving some members of the quinolone class of drugs. Excessive sunlight should be avoided. Therapy should be discontinued if phototoxicity occurs.

As with any potent drug, periodic assessment of organ system functions, including renal, hepatic, and hematopoietic function, is advisable during prolonged therapy.

Prescribing CIPRO Tablets and CIPRO Oral Suspension in the absence of a proven or strongly suspected bacterial infection or a prophylactic indication is unlikely to provide benefit to the patient and increases the risk of the development of drug-resistant bacteria.

Information for Patients:

Patients should be advised:

- that antibacterial drugs including CIPRO Tablets and CIPRO Oral Suspension should only be used to treat bacterial infections. They do not treat viral infections (e.g., the common cold). When CIPRO Tablets and CIPRO Oral Suspension is prescribed to treat a bacterial infection, patients should be told that although it is common to feel better early in the course of therapy, the medication should be taken exactly as directed. Skipping doses or not completing the full course of therapy may (1) decrease the effectiveness of the immediate treatment and (2) increase the likelihood that bacteria will develop resistance and will not be treatable by CIPRO Tablets and CIPRO Oral Suspension or other antibacterial drugs in the future.
- that ciprofloxacin may be taken with or without meals and to drink fluids liberally. As with other quinolones, concurrent administration of ciprofloxacin with magnesium/aluminum antacids, or sucralfate, Videx® (didanosine) chewable/buffered tablets or pediatric powder, or with other products containing calcium, iron or zinc should be avoided. Ciprofloxacin may be taken two hours before or six hours after taking these products. Ciprofloxacin should not be taken with dairy products (like milk or yogurt) or calcium-fortified juices alone since absorption of ciprofloxacin may be significantly reduced; however, ciprofloxacin may be taken with a meal that contains these products.
- that ciprofloxacin may be associated with hypersensitivity reactions, even following a single dose, and to discontinue the drug at the first sign of a skin rash or other allergic reaction.
- to avoid excessive sunlight or artificial ultraviolet light while receiving ciprofloxacin and to discontinue therapy if phototoxicity occurs.
- that peripheral neuropathies have been associated with ciprofloxacin use. If symptoms of peripheral neuropathy including pain, burning, tingling, numbness and/or weakness develop, they should discontinue treatment and contact their physicians.
- to discontinue treatment; rest and refrain from exercise; and inform their physician if they experience pain, inflammation, or rupture of a tendon.
- that ciprofloxacin may cause dizziness and lightheadedness; therefore, patients should know how they react to this drug before they operate an automobile or machinery or engage in activities requiring mental alertness or coordination.
- that ciprofloxacin may increase the effects of theophylline and caffeine. There is a possibility of caffeine accumulation when products containing caffeine are consumed while taking quinolones.
- that convulsions have been reported in patients receiving quinolones, including ciprofloxacin, and to notify their physician before taking this drug if there is a history of this condition.
- that ciprofloxacin has been associated with an increased rate of adverse events involving joints and surrounding tissue structures (like tendons) in pediatric patients (less than 18 years of age). Parents should inform their child's physician if the child has a history of joint-related problems before taking this drug. Parents of pediatric patients should also notify their child's physician of any joint-related problems that occur during or following ciprofloxacin therapy. (See **WARNINGS, PRECAUTIONS, Pediatric Use** and **ADVERSE REACTIONS**.)

Drug Interactions: As with some other quinolones, concurrent administration of ciprofloxacin with theophylline may lead to elevated serum concentrations of theophylline and prolongation of its elimination half-life. This may result in increased risk of theophylline-related adverse reactions. (See **WARNINGS**.) If concomitant use cannot be avoided, serum levels of theophylline should be monitored and dosage adjustments made as appropriate.

Some quinolones, including ciprofloxacin, have also been shown to interfere with the metabolism of caffeine. This may lead to reduced clearance of caffeine and a prolongation of its serum half-life.

Concurrent administration of a quinolone, including ciprofloxacin, with multivalent cation-containing products such as magnesium/aluminum antacids, sucralfate, Videx® (didanosine) chewable/buffered tablets or pediatric powder, or products containing calcium, iron, or zinc may substantially decrease its absorption, resulting in serum and urine levels considerably lower than desired. (See **DOSAGE AND ADMINISTRATION** for concurrent administration of these agents with ciprofloxacin.)

Histamine H_2-receptor antagonists appear to have no significant effect on the bioavailability of ciprofloxacin.

Altered serum levels of phenytoin (increased and decreased) have been reported in patients receiving concomitant ciprofloxacin.

The concomitant administration of ciprofloxacin with the sulfonylurea glyburide has, on rare occasions, resulted in severe hypoglycemia.

Some quinolones, including ciprofloxacin, have been associated with transient elevations in serum creatinine in patients receiving cyclosporine concomitantly.

Quinolones, including ciprofloxacin, have been reported to enhance the effects of the oral anticoagulant warfarin or its derivatives. When these products are administered concomitantly, prothrombin time or other suitable coagulation tests should be closely monitored.

Probenecid interferes with renal tubular secretion of ciprofloxacin and produces an increase in the level of ciprofloxacin in the serum. This should be considered if patients are receiving both drugs concomitantly.

Renal tubular transport of methotrexate may be inhibited by concomitant administration of ciprofloxacin potentially leading to increased plasma levels of methotrexate. This might increase the risk of methotrexate associated toxic reactions. Therefore, patients under methotrexate therapy should be carefully monitored when concomitant ciprofloxacin therapy is indicated.

Metoclopramide significantly accelerates the absorption of oral ciprofloxacin resulting in shorter time to reach maximum plasma concentrations. No significant effect was observed on the bioavailability of ciprofloxacin.

Non-steroidal anti-inflammatory drugs (but not acetyl salicylic acid) in combination of very high doses of quinolones have been shown to provoke convulsions in pre-clinical studies.

Carcinogenesis, Mutagenesis, Impairment of Fertility: Eight *in vitro* mutagenicity tests have been conducted with ciprofloxacin, and the test results are listed below:

Salmonella/Microsome Test (Negative)
E. coli DNA Repair Assay (Negative)
Mouse Lymphoma Cell Forward Mutation Assay (Positive)
Chinese Hamster V_{79} Cell HGPRT Test (Negative)
Syrian Hamster Embryo Cell Transformation Assay (Negative)
Saccharomyces cerevisiae Point Mutation Assay (Negative)
Saccharomyces cerevisiae Mitotic Crossover and Gene Conversion Assay (Negative)
Rat Hepatocyte DNA Repair Assay (Positive)

Thus, 2 of the 8 tests were positive, but results of the following 3 *in vivo* test systems gave negative results:

Rat Hepatocyte DNA Repair Assay
Micronucleus Test (Mice)
Dominant Lethal Test (Mice)

Long-term carcinogenicity studies in rats and mice resulted in no carcinogenic or tumorigenic effects due to ciprofloxacin at daily oral dose levels up to 250 and 750 mg/kg to rats and mice, respectively (approximately 1.7- and 2.5- times the highest recommended therapeutic dose based upon mg/m^2).

Results from photo co-carcinogenicity testing indicate that ciprofloxacin does not reduce the time to appearance of UV-induced skin tumors as compared to vehicle control. Hairless (Skh-1) mice were exposed to UVA light for 3.5 hours five times every two weeks for up to 78 weeks while concurrently being administered ciprofloxacin. The time to development of the first skin tumors was 50 weeks in mice treated concomitantly with UVA and ciprofloxacin (mouse dose approximately equal to maximum recommended human dose based upon mg/m^2), as opposed to 34 weeks when animals were treated with both UVA and vehicle. The times to development of skin tumors ranged from 16-32 weeks in mice treated concomitantly with UVA and other quinolones.[3]

In this model, mice treated with ciprofloxacin alone did not develop skin or systemic tumors. There are no data from similar models using pigmented mice and/or fully haired mice. The clinical significance of these findings to humans is unknown.

Fertility studies performed in rats at oral doses of ciprofloxacin up to 100 mg/kg (approximately 0.7-times the highest recommended therapeutic dose based upon mg/m^2) revealed no evidence of impairment.

Pregnancy: Teratogenic Effects. Pregnancy Category C: There are no adequate and well-controlled studies in pregnant women. An expert review of published data on experiences with ciprofloxacin use during pregnancy by TERIS –

the Teratogen Information System – concluded that therapeutic doses during pregnancy are unlikely to pose a substantial teratogenic risk (quantity and quality of data=fair), but the data are insufficient to state that there is no risk.[7] A controlled prospective observational study followed 200 women exposed to fluoroquinolones (52.5% exposed to ciprofloxacin and 68% first trimester exposures) during gestation.[8] In utero exposure to fluoroquinolones during embryogenesis was not associated with increased risk of major malformations. The reported rates of major congenital malformations were 2.2% for the fluoroquinolone group and 2.6% for the control group (background incidence of major malformations is 1-5%). Rates of spontaneous abortions, prematurity and low birth weight did not differ between the groups and there were no clinically significant musculoskeletal dysfunctions up to one year of age in the ciprofloxacin exposed children.
Another prospective follow-up study reported on 549 pregnancies with fluoroquinolone exposure (93% first trimester exposures).[9] There were 70 ciprofloxacin exposures, all within the first trimester. The malformation rates among live-born babies exposed to ciprofloxacin and to fluoroquinolones overall were both within background incidence ranges. No specific patterns of congenital abnormalities were found. The study did not reveal any clear adverse reactions due to in utero exposure to ciprofloxacin.
No differences in the rates of prematurity, spontaneous abortions, or birth weight were seen in women exposed to ciprofloxacin during pregnancy.[7,8] However, these small postmarketing epidemiology studies, of which most experience is from short term, first trimester exposure, are insufficient to evaluate the risk for less common defects or to permit reliable and definitive conclusions regarding the safety of ciprofloxacin in pregnant women and their developing fetuses. Ciprofloxacin should not be used during pregnancy unless the potential benefit justifies the potential risk to both fetus and mother (see **WARNINGS**).
Reproduction studies have been performed in rats and mice using oral doses up to 100 mg/kg (0.6 and 0.3 times the maximum daily human dose based upon body surface area, respectively) and have revealed no evidence of harm to the fetus due to ciprofloxacin. In rabbits, oral ciprofloxacin dose levels of 30 and 100 mg/kg (approximately 0.4- and 1.3-times the highest recommended therapeutic dose based upon mg/m^2) produced gastrointestinal toxicity resulting in maternal weight loss and an increased incidence of abortion, but no teratogenicity was observed at either dose level. After intravenous administration of doses up to 20 mg/kg (approximately 0.3- times the highest recommended therapeutic dose based upon mg/m^2) no maternal toxicity was produced and no embryotoxicity or teratogenicity was observed. (See **WARNINGS**.)
Nursing Mothers: Ciprofloxacin is excreted in human milk. The amount of ciprofloxacin absorbed by the nursing infant is unknown. Because of the potential for serious adverse reactions in infants nursing from mothers taking ciprofloxacin, a decision should be made whether to discontinue nursing or to discontinue the drug, taking into account the importance of the drug to the mother.
Pediatric Use: Ciprofloxacin, like other quinolones, causes arthropathy and histological changes in weight-bearing joints of juvenile animals resulting in lameness. (See **ANIMAL PHARMACOLOGY**.)
Inhalational Anthrax (Post-Exposure)
Ciprofloxacin is indicated in pediatric patients for inhalational anthrax (post-exposure). The risk-benefit assessment indicates that administration of ciprofloxacin to pediatric patients is appropriate. For information regarding pediatric dosing in inhalational anthrax (post-exposure), see **DOSAGE AND ADMINISTRATION** and **INHALATIONAL ANTHRAX – ADDITIONAL INFORMATION.**
Complicated Urinary Tract Infection and Pyelonephritis
Ciprofloxacin is indicated for the treatment of complicated urinary tract infections and pyelonephritis due to *Escherichia coli*. Although effective in clinical trials, ciprofloxacin is not a drug of first choice in the pediatric population due to an increased incidence of adverse events compared to the controls, including events related to joints and/or surrounding tissues. The rates of these events in pediatric patients with complicated urinary tract infection and pyelonephritis within six weeks of follow-up were 9.3% (31/335) versus 6.0% (21/349) for control agents. The rates of these events occurring at any time up to the one year follow-up were 13.7% (46/335) and 9.5% (33/349), respectively. The rate of all adverse events regardless of drug relationship at six weeks was 41% (138/335) in the ciprofloxacin arm compared to 31% (109/349) in the control arm. (See **ADVERSE REACTIONS** and **CLINICAL STUDIES**.)
Cystic Fibrosis
Short-term safety data from a single trial in pediatric cystic fibrosis patients are available. In a randomized, double-blind clinical trial for the treatment of acute pulmonary exacerbations in cystic fibrosis patients (ages 5-17 years), 67 patients received ciprofloxacin I.V. 10 mg/kg/dose q8h for one week followed by ciprofloxacin tablets 20 mg/kg/dose q12h to complete 10-21 days treatment and 62 patients received the combination of ceftazidime I.V. 50 mg/kg/dose q8h and tobramycin I.V. 3 mg/kg/dose q8h for a total of 10-21 days. Patients less than 5 years of age were not studied. Safety monitoring in the study included periodic range of motion examinations and gait assessments by treatment-blinded examiners. Patients were followed for an average of 23 days after completing treatment (range 0-93 days). This study was not designed to determine long term effects and the safety of repeated exposure to ciprofloxacin.

Findings Involving Joint or Peri-articular Tissues as Assessed by the IPSC

	Ciprofloxacin	Comparator
All Patients (within 6 weeks)	31/335 (9.3%)	21/349 (6.0%)
95% Confidence Interval*	(-0.8%, +7.2%)	
Age Group		
≥12 months < 24 months	1/36 (2.8%)	0/41
≥ 2 years < 6 years	5/124 (4.0%)	3/118 (2.5%)
≥ 6 years < 12 years	18/143 (12.6%)	12/153 (7.8%)
≥ 12 years to 17 years	7/32 (21.9%)	6/37 (16.2%)
All Patients (within 1 year)	46/335 (13.7%)	33/349 (9.5%)
95% Confidence Interval*	(-0.6%, +9.1%)	

*The study was designed to demonstrate that the arthropathy rate for the ciprofloxacin group did not exceed that of the control group by more than + 6%. At both the 6 week and 1 year evaluations, the 95% confidence interval indicated that it could not be concluded that ciprofloxacin group had findings comparable to the control group.

Musculoskeletal adverse events in patients with cystic fibrosis were reported in 22% of the patients in the ciprofloxacin group and 21% in the comparison group. Decreased range of motion was reported in 12% of the subjects in the ciprofloxacin group and 16% in the comparison group. Arthralgia was reported in 10% of the patients in the ciprofloxacin group and 11% in the comparison group. Other adverse events were similar in nature and frequency between treatment arms. One of sixty-seven patients developed arthritis of the knee nine days after a ten day course of treatment with ciprofloxacin. Clinical symptoms resolved, but an MRI showed knee effusion without other abnormalities eight months after treatment. However, the relationship of this event to the patient's course of ciprofloxacin can not be definitively determined, particularly since patients with cystic fibrosis may develop arthralgias/arthritis as part of their underlying disease process.
Geriatric Use: In a retrospective analysis of 23 multiple-dose controlled clinical trials of ciprofloxacin encompassing over 3500 ciprofloxacin treated patients, 25% of patients were greater than or equal to 65 years of age and 10% were greater than or equal to 75 years of age. No overall differences in safety or effectiveness were observed between these subjects and younger subjects, and other reported clinical experience has not identified differences in responses between the elderly and younger patients, but greater sensitivity of some older individuals on any drug therapy cannot be ruled out. Ciprofloxacin is known to be substantially excreted by the kidney, and the risk of adverse reactions may be greater in patients with impaired renal function. No alteration of dosage is necessary for patients greater than 65 years of age with normal renal function. However, since some older individuals experience reduced renal function by virtue of their advanced age, care should be taken in dose selection for elderly patients, and renal function monitoring may be useful in these patients. (See **CLINICAL PHARMACOLOGY** and **DOSAGE AND ADMINISTRATION**.)

ADVERSE REACTIONS

Adverse Reactions in Adult Patients: During clinical investigations with oral and parenteral ciprofloxacin, 49,038 patients received courses of the drug. Most of the adverse events reported were described as only mild or moderate in severity, abated soon after the drug was discontinued, and required no treatment. Ciprofloxacin was discontinued because of an adverse event in 1.0% of orally treated patients. The most frequently reported drug related events, from clinical trials of all formulations, all dosages, all drug-therapy durations, and for all indications of ciprofloxacin therapy were nausea (2.5%), diarrhea (1.6%), liver function tests abnormal (1.3%), vomiting (1.0%), and rash (1.0%).
Additional medically important events that occurred in less than 1% of ciprofloxacin patients are listed below.

BODY AS A WHOLE: headache, abdominal pain/discomfort, foot pain, pain, pain in extremities, injection site reaction (ciprofloxacin intravenous)
CARDIOVASCULAR: palpitation, atrial flutter, ventricular ectopy, syncope, hypertension, angina pectoris, myocardial infarction, cardiopulmonary arrest, cerebral thrombosis, phlebitis, tachycardia, migraine, hypotension
CENTRAL NERVOUS SYSTEM: restlessness, dizziness, lightheadedness, insomnia, nightmares, hallucinations, manic reaction, irritability, tremor, ataxia, convulsive seizures, lethargy, drowsiness, weakness, malaise, anorexia, phobia, depersonalization, depression, paresthesia, abnormal gait, grand mal convulsion
GASTROINTESTINAL: painful oral mucosa, oral candidiasis, dysphagia, intestinal perforation, gastrointestinal bleeding, cholestatic jaundice, hepatitis
HEMIC/LYMPHATIC: lymphadenopathy, petechia
METABOLIC/NUTRITIONAL: amylase increase, lipase increase
MUSCULOSKELETAL: arthralgia or back pain, joint stiffness, achiness, neck or chest pain, flare up of gout
RENAL/UROGENITAL: interstitial nephritis, nephritis, renal failure, polyuria, urinary retention, urethral bleeding, vaginitis, acidosis, breast pain
RESPIRATORY: dyspnea, epistaxis, laryngeal or pulmonary edema, hiccough, hemoptysis, bronchospasm, pulmonary embolism
SKIN/HYPERSENSITIVITY: allergic reaction, pruritus, urticaria, photosensitivity, flushing, fever, chills, angioedema, edema of the face, neck, lips, conjunctivae or hands, cutaneous candidiasis, hyperpigmentation, erythema nodosum, sweating
SPECIAL SENSES: blurred vision, disturbed vision (change in color perception, overbrightness of lights), decreased visual acuity, diplopia, eye pain, tinnitus, hearing loss, bad taste, chromatopsia

In several instances nausea, vomiting, tremor, irritability, or palpitation were judged by investigators to be related to elevated serum levels of theophylline possibly as a result of drug interaction with ciprofloxacin.
In randomized, double-blind controlled clinical trials comparing ciprofloxacin tablets (500 mg BID) to cefuroxime axetil (250 mg - 500 mg BID) and to clarithromycin (500 mg BID) in patients with respiratory tract infections, ciprofloxacin demonstrated a CNS adverse event profile comparable to the control drugs.
Adverse Reactions in Pediatric Patients: Ciprofloxacin, administered I.V. and/or orally, was compared to a cephalosporin for treatment of complicated urinary tract infections (cUTI) or pyelonephritis in pediatric patients 1 to 17 years of age (mean age of 6 ± 4 years). The trial was conducted in the US, Canada, Argentina, Peru, Costa Rica, Mexico, South Africa, and Germany. The duration of therapy was 10 to 21 days (mean duration of treatment was 11 days with a range of 1 to 88 days). The primary objective of the study was to assess musculoskeletal and neurological safety within 6 weeks of therapy and through one year of follow-up in the 335 ciprofloxacin- and 349 comparator-treated patients enrolled.
An Independent Pediatric Safety Committee (IPSC) reviewed all cases of musculoskeletal adverse events as well as all patients with an abnormal gait or abnormal joint exam (baseline or treatment-emergent). These events were evaluated in a comprehensive fashion and included such conditions as arthralgia, abnormal gait, abnormal joint exam, sprains, leg pain, back pain, arthrosis, bone pain, pain, myalgia, arm pain, and decreased range of motion in a joint. The affected joints included: knee, elbow, ankle, hip, wrist, and shoulder. Within 6 weeks of treatment initiation, the rates of these events were 9.3% (31/335) in the ciprofloxacin-treated group versus 6.0 % (21/349) in comparator-treated patients. The majority of these events were mild or moderate in intensity. All musculoskeletal events occurring by 6 weeks resolved (clinical resolution of signs and symptoms), usually within 30 days of end of treatment. Radiological evaluations were not routinely used to confirm resolution of the events. The events occurred more frequently in ciprofloxacin-treated patients than control patients, regardless of whether they received I.V. or oral therapy. Ciprofloxacin-treated patients were more likely to report more than one event and on more than one occasion compared to control patients. These events occurred in all age groups and the rates were consistently higher in the ciprofloxacin group compared to the control group. At the end of 1 year, the rate of these events reported at any time during that period was 13.7% (46/335) in the ciprofloxacin-treated group versus 9.5% (33/349) comparator-treated patients.
An adolescent female discontinued ciprofloxacin for wrist pain that developed during treatment. An MRI performed 4 weeks later showed a tear in the right ulnar fibrocartilage. A diagnosis of overuse syndrome secondary to sports activity was made, but a contribution from ciprofloxacin cannot be excluded. The patient recovered by 4 months without surgical intervention.
[See table above]
The incidence rates of neurological events within 6 weeks of treatment initiation were 3% (9/335) in the ciprofloxacin group versus 2% (7/349) in the comparator group and included dizziness, nervousness, insomnia, and somnolence.

Continued on next page

Cipro—Cont.

In this trial, the overall incidence rates of adverse events regardless of relationship to study drug and within 6 weeks of treatment initiation were 41% (138/335) in the ciprofloxacin group versus 31% (109/349) in the comparator group. The most frequent events were gastrointestinal: 15% (50/335) of ciprofloxacin patients compared to 9% (31/349) of comparator patients. Serious adverse events were seen in 7.5% (25/335) of ciprofloxacin-treated patients compared to 5.7% (20/349) of control patients. Discontinuation of drug due to an adverse event was observed in 3% (10/335) of ciprofloxacin-treated patients versus 1.4% (5/349) of comparator patients. Other adverse events that occurred in at least 1% of ciprofloxacin patients were diarrhea 4.8%, vomiting 4.8%, abdominal pain 3.3%, accidental injury 3.0%, rhinitis 3.0%, dyspepsia 2.7%, nausea 2.7%, fever 2.1%, asthma 1.8% and rash 1.8%.

In addition to the events reported in pediatric patients in clinical trials, it should be expected that events reported in adults during clinical trials or post-marketing experience may also occur in pediatric patients.

Post-Marketing Adverse Events: The following adverse events have been reported from worldwide marketing experience with quinolones, including ciprofloxacin. Because these events are reported voluntarily from a population of uncertain size, it is not always possible to reliably estimate their frequency or establish a causal relationship to drug exposure. Decisions to include these events in labeling are typically based on one or more of the following factors: (1) seriousness of the event, (2) frequency of the reporting, or (3) strength of causal connection to the drug.

Agitation, agranulocytosis, albuminuria, anaphylactic reactions, anosmia, candiduria, cholesterol elevation (serum), confusion, constipation, delirium, dyspepsia, dysphagia, erythema multiforme, exfoliative dermatitis, fixed eruption, flatulence, glucose elevation (blood), hemolytic anemia, hepatic failure, hepatic necrosis, hyperesthesia, hypertonia, hypesthesia, hypotension (postural), jaundice, marrow depression (life threatening), methemoglobinemia, moniliasis (oral, gastrointestinal, vaginal), myalgia, myasthenia, myasthenia gravis (possible exacerbation), myoclonus, nystagmus, pancreatitis, pancytopenia (life threatening or fatal outcome), peripheral neuropathy, phenytoin alteration (serum), potassium elevation (serum), prothrombin time prolongation or decrease, pseudomembranous colitis (The onset of pseudomembranous colitis symptoms may occur during or after antimicrobial treatment.), psychosis (toxic), renal calculi, serum sickness like reaction, Stevens-Johnson syndrome, taste loss, tendinitis, tendon rupture, torsade de pointes, toxic epidermal necrolysis, triglyceride elevation (serum), twitching, vaginal candidiasis, and vasculitis. (See **PRECAUTIONS**.)

Adverse Laboratory Changes: Changes in laboratory parameters listed as adverse events without regard to drug relationship are listed below:

Hepatic	–Elevations of ALT (SGPT) (1.9%), AST (SGOT) (1.7%), alkaline phosphatase (0.8%), LDH (0.4%), serum bilirubin (0.3%).
Hematologic	–Eosinophilia (0.6%), leukopenia (0.4%), decreased blood platelets (0.1%), elevated blood platelets (0.1%), pancytopenia (0.1%).
Renal	–Elevations of serum creatinine (1.1%), BUN (0.9%), CRYSTALLURIA, CYLINDRURIA, AND HEMATURIA HAVE BEEN REPORTED.

Other changes occurring in less than 0.1% of courses were: elevation of serum gammaglutamyl transferase, elevation of serum amylase, reduction in blood glucose, elevated uric acid, decrease in hemoglobin, anemia, bleeding diathesis, increase in blood monocytes, leukocytosis.

OVERDOSAGE

In the event of acute overdosage, reversible renal toxicity has been reported in some cases. The stomach should be emptied by inducing vomiting or by gastric lavage. The patient should be carefully observed and given supportive treatment, including monitoring of renal function and administration of magnesium, aluminum, or calcium containing antacids which can reduce the absorption of ciprofloxacin. Adequate hydration must be maintained. Only a small amount of ciprofloxacin (< 10%) is removed from the body after hemodialysis or peritoneal dialysis.

Single doses of ciprofloxacin were relatively non-toxic via the oral route of administration in mice, rats, and dogs. No deaths occurred within a 14-day post treatment observation period at the highest oral doses tested; up to 5000 mg/kg in either rodent species, or up to 2500 mg/kg in the dog. Clinical signs observed included hypoactivity and cyanosis in both rodent species and severe vomiting in dogs. In rabbits, significant mortality was seen at doses of ciprofloxacin > 2500 mg/kg. Mortality was delayed in these animals, occurring 10-14 days after dosing.

In mice, rats, rabbits and dogs, significant toxicity including tonic/clonic convulsions was observed at intravenous doses of ciprofloxacin between 125 and 300 mg/kg.

DOSAGE AND ADMINISTRATION - ADULTS

CIPRO Tablets and Oral Suspension should be administered orally to adults as described in the Dosage Guidelines table.

The determination of dosage for any particular patient must take into consideration the severity and nature of the infection, the susceptibility of the causative organism, the integrity of the patient's host-defense mechanisms, and the status of renal function and hepatic function.

The duration of treatment depends upon the severity of infection. The usual duration is 7 to 14 days; however, for severe and complicated infections more prolonged therapy may be required. Ciprofloxacin should be administered at least 2 hours before or 6 hours after magnesium/aluminum antacids, or sucralfate, Videx® (didanosine) chewable/buffered tablets or pediatric powder for oral solution, or other products containing calcium, iron or zinc.

[See table below]

Conversion of I.V. to Oral Dosing in Adults: Patients whose therapy is started with CIPRO I.V. may be switched to CIPRO Tablets or Oral Suspension when clinically indicated at the discretion of the physician (See **CLINICAL PHARMACOLOGY** and table below for the equivalent dosing regimens).

Equivalent AUC Dosing Regimens

Cipro Oral Dosage	Equivalent Cipro I.V. Dosage
250 mg Tablet q 12 h	200 mg I.V. q 12 h
500 mg Tablet q 12 h	400 mg I.V. q 12 h
750 mg Tablet q 12 h	400 mg I.V. q 8 h

ADULT DOSAGE GUIDELINES

Infection	Severity	Dose	Frequency	Usual Durations†
Urinary Tract	Acute Uncomplicated Mild/Moderate Severe/Complicated	100 mg or 250 mg 250 mg 500 mg	q 12 h q 12 h q 12 h	3 Days 7 to 14 Days 7 to 14 Days
Chronic Bacterial Prostatitis	Mild/Moderate	500 mg	q 12 h	28 Days
Lower Respiratory Tract	Mild/Moderate Severe/Complicated	500 mg 750 mg	q 12 h q 12 h	7 to 14 Days 7 to 14 Days
Acute Sinusitis	Mild/Moderate	500 mg	q 12 h	10 Days
Skin and Skin Structure	Mild/Moderate Severe/Complicated	500 mg 750 mg	q 12 h q 12 h	7 to 14 Days 7 to 14 Days
Bone and Joint	Mild/Moderate Severe/Complicated	500 mg 750 mg	q 12 h q 12 h	≥ 4 to 6 weeks ≥ 4 to 6 weeks
Intra-Abdominal*	Complicated	500 mg	q 12 h	7 to 14 Days
Infectious Diarrhea	Mild/Moderate/Severe	500 mg	q 12 h	5 to 7 Days
Typhoid Fever	Mild/Moderate	500 mg	q 12 h	10 Days
Urethral and Cervical Gonococcal Infections	Uncomplicated	250 mg	single dose	single dose
Inhalational anthrax (post-exposure)**		500 mg	q 12 h	60 Days

* used in conjunction with metronidazole

† Generally ciprofloxacin should be continued for at least 2 days after the signs and symptoms of infection have disappeared, except for inhalational anthrax (post-exposure).

** Drug administration should begin as soon as possible after suspected or confirmed exposure. This indication is based on a surrogate endpoint, ciprofloxacin serum concentrations achieved in humans, reasonably likely to predict clinical benefit.[4] For a discussion of ciprofloxacin serum concentrations in various human populations, see **INHALATIONAL ANTHRAX – ADDITIONAL INFORMATION.**

Adults with Impaired Renal Function: Ciprofloxacin is eliminated primarily by renal excretion; however, the drug is also metabolized and partially cleared through the biliary system of the liver and through the intestine. These alternative pathways of drug elimination appear to compensate for the reduced renal excretion in patients with renal impairment. Nonetheless, some modification of dosage is recommended, particularly for patients with severe renal dysfunction. The following table provides dosage guidelines for use in patients with renal impairment:

RECOMMENDED STARTING AND MAINTENANCE DOSES FOR PATIENTS WITH IMPAIRED RENAL FUNCTION

Creatinine Clearance (mL/min)	Dose
> 50	See Usual Dosage.
30 – 50	250 – 500 mg q 12 h
5 – 29	250 – 500 mg q 18 h
Patients on hemodialysis or Peritoneal dialysis	250 – 500 mg q 24 h (after dialysis)

When only the serum creatinine concentration is known, the following formula may be used to estimate creatinine clearance.

[See first table at top of next page]

The serum creatinine should represent a steady state of renal function.

In patients with severe infections and severe renal impairment, a unit dose of 750 mg may be administered at the intervals noted above. Patients should be carefully monitored.

DOSAGE AND ADMINISTRATION – PEDIATRICS

CIPRO Tablets and Oral Suspension should be administered orally as described in the Dosage Guidelines table. An increased incidence of adverse events compared to controls, including events related to joints and/or surrounding tissues, has been observed. (See **ADVERSE REACTIONS** and **CLINICAL STUDIES**.)

Dosing and initial route of therapy (i.e., I.V. or oral) for complicated urinary tract infection or pyelonephritis should be determined by the severity of the infection. In the clinical trial, pediatric patients with moderate to severe infection were initiated on 6 to 10 mg/kg I.V. every 8 hours and allowed to switch to oral therapy (10 to 20 mg/kg every 12 hours), at the discretion of the physician.

[See second table at top of next page]

Pediatric patients with moderate to severe renal insufficiency were excluded from the clinical trial of complicated urinary tract infection and pyelonephritis. No information is available on dosing adjustments necessary for pediatric patients with moderate to severe renal insufficiency (i.e., creatinine clearance of < 50 mL/min/1.73m²).

HOW SUPPLIED

CIPRO (ciprofloxacin hydrochloride) Tablets are available as round, slightly yellowish film-coated tablets containing 100 mg or 250 mg ciprofloxacin. The 100 mg tablet is coded with the word "CIPRO" on one side and "100" on the reverse side. The 250 mg tablet is coded with the word "CIPRO" on one side and "250" on the reverse side. CIPRO is also available as capsule shaped, slightly yellowish film-coated tablets containing 500 mg or 750 mg ciprofloxacin. The 500 mg tablet is coded with the word "CIPRO" on one side and "500" on the reverse side. The 750 mg tablet is coded with the word "CIPRO" on one side and "750" on the reverse side. CIPRO 250 mg, 500 mg, and 750 mg are available in bottles of 50, 100, and Unit Dose packages of 100. The 100 mg strength is available only as CIPRO Cystitis pack containing 6 tablets for use only in female patients with acute uncomplicated cystitis.

[See third table on next page]

Store below 30°C (86°F).

CIPRO Oral Suspension is supplied in 5% and 10% strengths. The drug product is composed of two components (microcapsules containing the active ingredient and diluent) which must be mixed by the pharmacist. See Instructions To The Pharmacist For Use/Handling.

[See fourth table on next page]

Microcapsules and diluent should be stored below 25°C (77°F) and protected from freezing.

Reconstituted product may be stored below 30°C (86°F) for 14 days. Protect from freezing. A teaspoon is provided for the patient.

ANIMAL PHARMACOLOGY

Ciprofloxacin and other quinolones have been shown to cause arthropathy in immature animals of most species tested. (See **WARNINGS**.) Damage of weight bearing joints was observed in juvenile dogs and rats. In young beagles, 100 mg/kg ciprofloxacin, given daily for 4 weeks, caused degenerative articular changes of the knee joint. At 30 mg/kg, the effect on the joint was minimal. In a subsequent study in young beagle dogs, oral ciprofloxacin doses of 30 mg/kg and 90 mg/kg ciprofloxacin (approximately 1.3- and 3.5-times the pediatric dose based upon comparative plasma AUCs) given daily for 2 weeks caused articular changes which were still observed by histopathology after a treatment-free period of 5 months. At 10 mg/kg (approximately 0.6-times the pediatric dose based upon comparative plasma AUCs), no effects on joints were observed. This dose was also not associated with arthrotoxicity after an additional treatment-free period of 5 months. In another study, removal of weight bearing from the joint reduced the lesions but did not totally prevent them.

Crystalluria, sometimes associated with secondary nephropathy, occurs in laboratory animals dosed with ciprofloxacin. This is primarily related to the reduced solu-

Men: Creatinine clearance (mL/min) = $\frac{\text{Weight (kg)} \times (140 - \text{age})}{72 \times \text{serum creatinine (mg/dL)}}$

Women: 0.85 × the value calculated for men.

PEDIATRIC DOSAGE GUIDELINES

Infection	Route of Administration	Dose (mg/kg)	Frequency	Total Duration
Complicated Urinary Tract or Pyelonephritis (patients from 1 to 17 years of age)	Intravenous	6 to 10 mg/kg (maximum 400 mg per dose; not to be exceeded even in patients weighing >51 kg)	Every 8 hours	10-21 days*
	Oral	10 mg/kg to 20 mg/kg (maximum 750 mg per dose; not to be exceeded even in patients weighing >51 kg)	Every 12 hours	
Inhalational Anthrax (Post-Exposure)**	Intravenous	10 mg/kg (maximum 400 mg per dose)	Every 12 hours	60 days
	Oral	15 mg/kg (maximum 500 mg per dose)	Every 12 hours	

*The total duration of therapy for complicated urinary tract infection and pyelonephritis in the clinical trial was determined by the physician. The mean duration of treatment was 11 days (range 10 to 21 days).
Drug administration should begin as soon as possible after suspected or confirmed exposure to *Bacillus anthracis* spores. This indication is based on a surrogate endpoint, ciprofloxacin serum concentrations achieved in humans, reasonably likely to predict clinical benefit.[4] For a discussion of ciprofloxacin serum concentrations in various human populations, see **INHALATIONAL ANTHRAX – ADDITIONAL INFORMATION.

	Strength	NDC Code	Tablet Identification
Bottles of 50:	750 mg	NDC 0026-8514-50	CIPRO 750
Bottles of 100:	250 mg	NDC 0026-8512-51	CIPRO 250
	500 mg	NDC 0026-8513-51	CIPRO 500
Unit Dose Package of 100:	250 mg	NDC 0026-8512-48	CIPRO 250
	500 mg	NDC 0026-8513-48	CIPRO 500
	750 mg	NDC 0026-8514-48	CIPRO 750
Cystitis Package of 6:	100 mg	NDC 0026-8511-06	CIPRO 100

Strengths	Total volume after reconstitution	Ciprofloxacin Concentration	Ciprofloxacin contents per bottle	NDC Code
5%	100 mL	250 mg/5 mL	5,000 mg	0026-8551-36
10%	100 mL	500 mg/5 mL	10,000 mg	0026-8553-36

Clinical Success and Bacteriologic Eradication at Test of Cure (5 to 9 Days Post-Therapy)

	CIPRO	Comparator
Randomized Patients	337	352
Per Protocol Patients	211	231
Clinical Response at 5 to 9 Days Post-Treatment	95.7% (202/211)	92.6% (214/231)
	95% CI [-1.3%, 7.3%]	
Bacteriologic Eradication by Patient at 5 to 9 Days Post-Treatment*	84.4% (178/211)	78.3% (181/231)
	95% CI [-1.3%, 13.1%]	
Bacteriologic Eradication of the Baseline Pathogen at 5 to 9 Days Post-Treatment		
Escherichia coli	156/178 (88%)	161/179 (90%)

*Patients with baseline pathogen(s) eradicated and no new infections or superinfections/total number of patients. There were 5.5% (6/211) ciprofloxacin and 9.5% (22/231) comparator patients with superinfections or new infections.

bility of ciprofloxacin under alkaline conditions, which predominate in the urine of test animals; in man, crystalluria is rare since human urine is typically acidic. In rhesus monkeys, crystalluria without nephropathy was noted after single oral doses as low as 5 mg/kg. (approximately 0.07-times the highest recommended therapeutic dose based upon mg/m^2). After 6 months of intravenous dosing at 10 mg/kg/day, no nephropathological changes were noted; however, nephropathy was observed after dosing at 20 mg/kg/day for the same duration (approximately 0.2-times the highest recommended therapeutic dose based upon mg/m^2).

In dogs, ciprofloxacin at 3 and 10 mg/kg by rapid I.V. injection (15 sec.) produces pronounced hypotensive effects. These effects are considered to be related to histamine release, since they are partially antagonized by pyrilamine, an antihistamine. In rhesus monkeys, rapid I.V. injection also produces hypotension but the effect in this species is inconsistent and less pronounced.

In mice, concomitant administration of nonsteroidal anti-inflammatory drugs such as phenylbutazone and indomethacin with quinolones has been reported to enhance the CNS stimulatory effect of quinolones.

Ocular toxicity seen with some related drugs has not been observed in ciprofloxacin-treated animals.

CLINICAL STUDIES

Complicated Urinary Tract Infection and Pyelonephritis – Efficacy in Pediatric Patients:

NOTE: Although effective in clinical trials, ciprofloxacin is not a drug of first choice in the pediatric population due to an increased incidence of adverse events compared to controls, including events related to joints and/or surrounding tissues.

Ciprofloxacin, administered I.V. and/or orally, was compared to a cephalosporin for treatment of complicated urinary tract infections (cUTI) and pyelonephritis in pediatric patients 1 to 17 years of age (mean age of 6 ± 4 years). The trial was conducted in the US, Canada, Argentina, Peru, Costa Rica, Mexico, South Africa, and Germany. The duration of therapy was 10 to 21 days (mean duration of treatment was 11 days with a range of 1 to 88 days). The primary objective of the study was to assess musculoskeletal and neurological safety.

Patients were evaluated for clinical success and bacteriological eradication of the baseline organism(s) with no new infection or superinfection at 5 to 9 days post-therapy (Test of Cure or TOC). The Per Protocol population had a causative organism(s) with protocol specified colony count(s) at baseline, no protocol violation, and no premature discontinuation or loss to follow-up (among other criteria).

The clinical success and bacteriologic eradication rates in the Per Protocol population were similar between ciprofloxacin and the comparator group as shown below.
[See fifth table at left]

INHALATIONAL ANTHRAX IN ADULTS AND PEDIATRICS – ADDITIONAL INFORMATION

The mean serum concentrations of ciprofloxacin associated with a statistically significant improvement in survival in the rhesus monkey model of inhalational anthrax are reached or exceeded in adult and pediatric patients receiving oral and intravenous regimens. (See **DOSAGE AND ADMINISTRATION.**) Ciprofloxacin pharmacokinetics have been evaluated in various human populations. The mean peak serum concentration achieved at steady-state in human adults receiving 500 mg orally every 12 hours is 2.97 μg/mL, and 4.56 μg/mL following 400 mg intravenously every 12 hours. The mean trough serum concentration at steady-state for both of these regimens is 0.2 μg/mL. In a study of 10 pediatric patients between 6 and 16 years of age, the mean peak plasma concentration achieved is 8.3 μg/mL and trough concentrations range from 0.09 to 0.26 μg/mL, following two 30-minute intravenous infusions of 10 mg/kg administered 12 hours apart. After the second intravenous infusion patients switched to 15 mg/kg orally every 12 hours achieve a mean peak concentration of 3.6 μg/mL after the initial oral dose. Long-term safety data, including effects on cartilage, following the administration of ciprofloxacin to pediatric patients are limited. (For additional information, see **PRECAUTIONS, Pediatric Use.**) Ciprofloxacin serum concentrations achieved in humans serve as a surrogate endpoint reasonably likely to predict clinical benefit and provide the basis for this indication.[4]

A placebo-controlled animal study in rhesus monkeys exposed to an inhaled mean dose of 11 LD_{50} (~5.5 × 10^5 spores (range 5-30 LD_{50}) of *B. anthracis* was conducted. The minimal inhibitory concentration (MIC) of ciprofloxacin for the anthrax strain used in this study was 0.08 μg/mL. In the animals studied, mean serum concentrations of ciprofloxacin achieved at expected T_{max} (1 hour post-dose) following oral dosing to steady-state ranged from 0.98 to 1.69 μg/mL. Mean steady-state trough concentrations at 12 hours post-dose ranged from 0.12 to 0.19 μg/mL[5]. Mortality due to anthrax for animals that received a 30-day regimen of oral ciprofloxacin beginning 24 hours post-exposure was significantly lower (1/9), compared to the placebo group (9/10) [p= 0.001]. The one ciprofloxacin-treated animal that died of anthrax did so following the 30-day drug administration period.[6]

Instructions To The Pharmacist For Use/Handling Of CIPRO Oral Suspension:

CIPRO Oral Suspension is supplied in 5% (5 g ciprofloxacin in 100 mL) and 10% (10 g ciprofloxacin in 100 mL) strengths. The drug product is composed of two components (microcapsules and diluent) which must be combined prior to dispensing.

One teaspoonful (5 mL) of 5% ciprofloxacin oral suspension = 250 mg of ciprofloxacin.

One teaspoonful (5 mL) of 10% ciprofloxacin oral suspension = 500 mg of ciprofloxacin.

Appropriate Dosing Volumes of the Oral Suspensions:

Dose	5%	10%
250 mg	5 mL	2.5 mL
500 mg	10 mL	5 mL
750 mg	15 mL	7.5 mL

Preparation of the suspension:

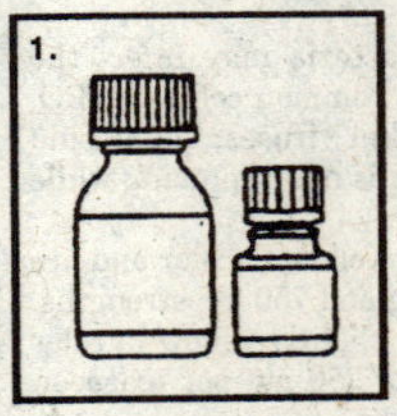

1. The small bottle contains the microcapsules, the large bottle contains the diluent.

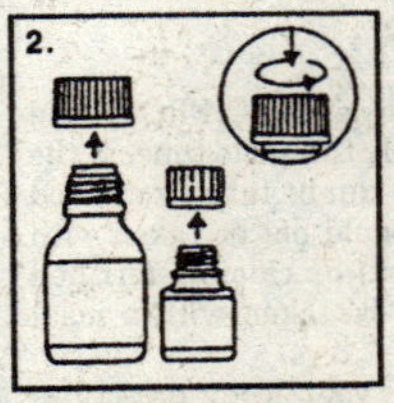

2. Open both bottles. Child-proof cap: Press down according to instructions on the cap while turning to the left.

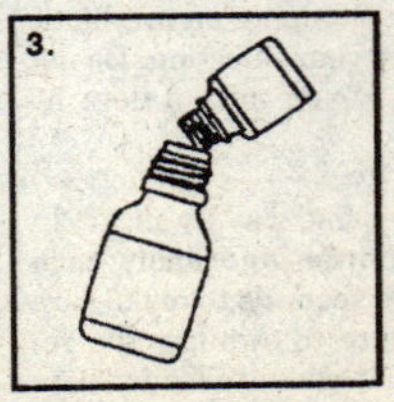

3. Pour the microcapsules completely into the larger bottle of diluent. **Do not add water to the suspension.**

Continued on next page

Cipro—Cont.

4.

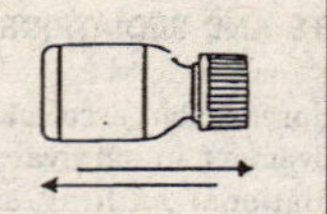

4. Remove the top layer of the diluent bottle label (to reveal the CIPRO Oral Suspension label). Close the large bottle completely according to the directions on the cap and shake vigorously for about 15 seconds. The suspension is ready for use.

CIPRO Oral Suspension should not be administered through feeding tubes due to its physical characteristics. Instruct the patient to shake CIPRO Oral Suspension vigorously each time before use for approximately 15 seconds and not to chew the microcapsules.

References:

1. National Committee for Clinical Laboratory Standards, Methods for Dilution Antimicrobial Susceptibility Tests for Bacteria That Grow Aerobically-Fifth Edition. Approved Standard NCCLS Document M7-A5, Vol. 20, No. 2, NCCLS, Wayne, PA, January, 2000. 2. National Committee for Clinical Laboratory Standards, Performance Standards for Antimicrobial Disk Susceptibility Tests-Seventh Edition. Approved Standard NCCLS Document M2-A7, Vol. 20, No. 1, NCCLS, Wayne, PA, January, 2000. 3. Report presented at the FDA's Anti-Infective Drug and Dermatological Drug Product's Advisory Committee meeting, March 31, 1993, Silver Spring, MD. Report available from FDA, CDER, Advisors and Consultants Staff, HFD-21, 1901 Chapman Avenue, Room 200, Rockville, MD 20852, USA. 4. 21 CFR 314.510 (Subpart H – Accelerated Approval of New Drugs for Life-Threatening Illnesses). 5. Kelly DJ, et al. Serum concentrations of penicillin, doxycycline, and ciprofloxacin during prolonged therapy in rhesus monkeys. J Infect Dis 1992; 166:1184-7. 6. Friedlander AM, et al. Postexposure prophylaxis against experimental inhalational anthrax. J Infect Dis 1993; 167:1239-42. 7. Friedman J, Polifka J. Teratogenic effects of drugs: a resource for clinicians (TERIS). Baltimore, Maryland: Johns Hopkins University Press, 2000:149-195. 8. Loebstein R, Addis A, Ho E, et al. Pregnancy outcome following gestational exposure to fluoroquinolones: a multicenter prospective controlled study. Antimicrob Agents Chemother. 1998;42(6):1336-1339. 9. Schaefer C, Amoura-Elefant E, Vial T, et al. Pregnancy outcome after prenatal quinolone exposure. Evaluation of a case registry of the European network of teratology information services (ENTIS). Eur J Obstet Gynecol Reprod Biol. 1996;69:83-89.

Patient Information About:
CIPRO®
(ciprofloxacin hydrochloride) TABLETS
CIPRO®
(ciprofloxacin*) ORAL SUSPENSION

This section contains important patient information about CIPRO (ciprofloxacin hydrochloride) Tablets and CIPRO (ciprofloxacin*) Oral Suspension and should be read completely before you begin treatment. This section does not take the place of discussion with your doctor or health care professional about your medical condition or your treatment. This section does not list all benefits and risks of CIPRO. If you have any concerns about your condition or your medicine, ask your doctor. Only your doctor can determine if CIPRO is right for you.

What is CIPRO?

CIPRO is an antibiotic used to treat bladder, kidney, prostate, cervix, stomach, intestine, lung, sinus, bone, and skin infections caused by certain germs called bacteria. CIPRO kills many types of bacteria that can infect these areas of the body. CIPRO has been shown in a large number of clinical trials to be safe and effective for the treatment of bacterial infections.

Sometimes viruses rather than bacteria may infect the lungs and sinuses (for example the common cold). CIPRO, like all other antibiotics, does not kill viruses. You should contact your doctor if your condition is not improving while taking CIPRO.

CIPRO Tablets are white to slightly yellow in color and are available in 100 mg, 250 mg, 500 mg and 750 mg strengths. CIPRO Oral Suspension is white to slightly yellow in color and is available in concentrations of 250 mg per teaspoon (5%) and 500 mg per teaspoon (10%).

How and when should I take CIPRO?

CIPRO Tablets:

Unless directed otherwise by your physician, CIPRO should be taken twice a day at approximately the same time, in the morning and in the evening. CIPRO can be taken with food or on an empty stomach. CIPRO should not be taken with dairy products (like milk or yogurt) or calcium-fortified juices alone; however, CIPRO may be taken with a meal that contains these products.

You should take CIPRO for as long as your doctor prescribes it, even after you start to feel better. Stopping an antibiotic too early may result in failure to cure your infection. Do not take a double dose of CIPRO even if you miss a dose by mistake.

CIPRO Oral Suspension:

Take CIPRO Oral Suspension in the same way as above. In addition, remember to **shake the bottle vigorously each time before use for approximately 15 seconds** to make sure the suspension is mixed well. Be sure to swallow the required amount of suspension. Do not chew the microcapsules. Close the bottle completely after use. The product can be used for 14 days when stored in a refrigerator or at room temperature. After treatment has been completed, any remaining suspension should be discarded.

Who should not take CIPRO?

You should not take CIPRO if you have ever had a severe reaction to any of the group of antibiotics known as "quinolones".

CIPRO is not recommended during pregnancy or nursing, as the effects of CIPRO on the unborn child or nursing infant are unknown. If you are pregnant or plan to become pregnant while taking CIPRO talk to your doctor before taking this medication.

Due to possible side effects, CIPRO is not recommended for persons less than 18 years of age except for specific serious infections, such as complicated urinary tract infections.

What are the possible side effects of CIPRO?

CIPRO is generally well tolerated. The most common side effects, which are usually mild, include nausea, diarrhea, vomiting, and abdominal pain/discomfort. If diarrhea persists, call your health care professional.

Rare cases of allergic reactions have been reported in patients receiving quinolones, including CIPRO, even after just one dose. If you develop hives, difficulty breathing, or other symptoms of a severe allergic reaction, seek emergency treatment right away. If you develop a skin rash, you should stop taking CIPRO and call your health care professional.

Some patients taking quinolone antibiotics may become more sensitive to sunlight or ultraviolet light such as that used in tanning salons. You should avoid excessive exposure to sunlight or ultraviolet light while you are taking CIPRO. You should be careful about driving or operating machinery until you are sure CIPRO is not causing dizziness. Convulsions have been reported in patients receiving quinolone antibiotics including ciprofloxacin. Be sure to let your physician know if you have a history of convulsions. Quinolones, including ciprofloxacin, have been rarely associated with other central nervous system events including confusion, tremors, hallucinations, and depression.

CIPRO has been rarely associated with inflammation of tendons. If you experience pain, swelling or rupture of a tendon, you should stop taking CIPRO and call your health care professional.

CIPRO has been associated with an increased rate of side effects with joints and surrounding structures (like tendons) in pediatric patients (less than 18 years of age). Parents should inform their child's physician if the child has a history of joint-related problems before taking this drug. Parents of pediatric patients should also notify their child's physician of any joint related problems that occur during or following CIPRO therapy.

If you notice any side effects not mentioned in this section, or if you have any concerns about side effects you may be experiencing, please inform your health care professional.

What about other medications I am taking?

CIPRO can affect how other medicines work. Tell your doctor about all other prescription and non-prescription medicines or supplements you are taking. This is especially important if you are taking theophylline. Other medications including warfarin, glyburide, and phenytoin may also interact with CIPRO.

Many antacids, multivitamins, and other dietary supplements containing magnesium, calcium, aluminum, iron or zinc can interfere with the absorption of CIPRO and may prevent it from working. Other medications such as sulcrafate and Videx® (didanosine) chewable/buffered tablets or pediatric powder may also stop CIPRO from working. You should take CIPRO either 2 hours before or 6 hours after taking these products.

What if I have been prescribed CIPRO for possible anthrax exposure?

CIPRO has been approved to reduce the chance of developing anthrax infection following exposure to the anthrax bacteria. In general, CIPRO is not recommended for children; however, it is approved for use in patients younger than 18 years old for anthrax exposure. If you are pregnant, or plan to become pregnant while taking CIPRO, you and your doctor should discuss if the benefits of taking CIPRO for anthrax outweigh the risks.

CIPRO is generally well tolerated. Side effects that may occur during treatment to prevent anthrax might be acceptable due to the seriousness of the disease. You and your doctor should discuss the risks of not taking your medicine against the risks of experiencing side effects.

CIPRO can cause dizziness, confusion, or other similar side effects in some people. Therefore, it is important to know how CIPRO affects you before driving a car or performing other activities that require you to be alert and coordinated such as operating machinery.

Your doctor has prescribed CIPRO only for you. Do not give it to other people. Do not use it for a condition for which it was not prescribed. You should take your CIPRO for as long as your doctor prescribes it; stopping CIPRO too early may result in failure to prevent anthrax.

Remember:

Do not give CIPRO to anyone other than the person for whom it was prescribed.

Take your dose of CIPRO in the morning and in the evening. Complete the course of CIPRO even if you are feeling better. Keep CIPRO and all medications out of reach of children.

* Does not comply with USP with regards to "loss on drying" and "residue on ignition".

Bayer HealthCare
Bayer Pharmaceuticals Corporation
400 Morgan Lane
West Haven, CT 06516 USA

℞ Only
08753744, R.4 4/04 Bay o 9867 5202-2-A-U.S.-16
12320

Printed in U.S.A.

CIPRO (ciprofloxacin*) 5% and 10% Oral Suspension Made in Italy.
Cipro (ciprofloxacin HCl) Tablets Made in U.S.A. and Germany

CIPRO® I.V. ℞

[sĭprō]
(ciprofloxacin)
For Intravenous Infusion

Prescribing information for this product, which appears on page(s) 845-849 of the 2004 PDR, has been completely revised as follows. Please write "See Supplement A" next to the product heading.

To reduce the development of drug-resistant bacteria and maintain the effectiveness of CIPRO® I.V. and other antibacterial drugs, CIPRO I.V. should be used only to treat or prevent infections that are proven or strongly suspected to be caused by bacteria.

DESCRIPTION

CIPRO I.V. (ciprofloxacin) is a synthetic broad-spectrum antimicrobial agent for intravenous (I.V.) administration. Ciprofloxacin, a fluoroquinolone, is 1-cyclopropyl-6-fluoro-1,4-dihydro-4-oxo-7-(1-piperazinyl)-3-quinolinecarboxylic acid. Its empirical formula is $C_{17}H_{18}FN_3O_3$ and its chemical structure is:

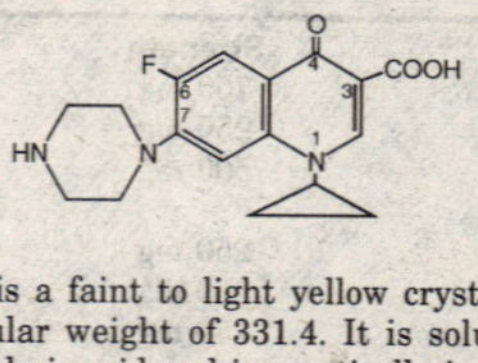

Ciprofloxacin is a faint to light yellow crystalline powder with a molecular weight of 331.4. It is soluble in dilute (0.1N) hydrochloric acid and is practically insoluble in water and ethanol. CIPRO I.V. solutions are available as sterile 1.0% aqueous concentrates, which are intended for dilution prior to administration, and as 0.2% ready-for-use infusion solutions in 5% Dextrose Injection. All formulas contain lactic acid as a solubilizing agent and hydrochloric acid for pH adjustment. The pH range for the 1.0% aqueous concentrates in vials is 3.3 to 3.9. The pH range for the 0.2% ready-for-use infusion solutions is 3.5 to 4.6.

The plastic container is latex-free and is fabricated from a specially formulated polyvinyl chloride. Solutions in contact with the plastic container can leach out certain of its chemical components in very small amounts within the expiration period, e.g., di(2-ethylhexyl) phthalate (DEHP), up to 5 parts per million. The suitability of the plastic has been confirmed in tests in animals according to USP biological tests for plastic containers as well as by tissue culture toxicity studies.

CLINICAL PHARMACOLOGY

Absorption

Following 60-minute intravenous infusions of 200 mg and 400 mg ciprofloxacin to normal volunteers, the mean maximum serum concentrations achieved were 2.1 and 4.6 μg/mL, respectively; the concentrations at 12 hours were 0.1 and 0.2 μg/mL, respectively.

Steady-state Ciprofloxacin Serum Concentrations (μg/mL) After 60-minute I.V. Infusions q 12 h.

	Time after starting the infusion					
Dose	**30 min**	**1 hr**	**3 hr**	**6 hr**	**8 hr**	**12 hr**
200 mg	1.7	2.1	0.6	0.3	0.2	0.1
400 mg	3.7	4.6	1.3	0.7	0.5	0.2

The pharmacokinetics of ciprofloxacin are linear over the dose range of 200 to 400 mg administered intravenously. Comparison of the pharmacokinetic parameters following the 1st and 5th I.V. dose on a q 12 h regimen indicates no evidence of drug accumulation.

The absolute bioavailability of oral ciprofloxacin is within a range of 70–80% with no substantial loss by first pass metabolism. An intravenous infusion of 400-mg ciprofloxacin given over 60 minutes every 12 hours has been shown to produce an area under the serum concentration time curve (AUC) equivalent to that produced by a 500-mg oral dose given every 12 hours. An intravenous infusion of 400 mg ciprofloxacin given over 60 minutes every 8 hours has been shown to produce an AUC at steady-state equivalent to that produced by a 750-mg oral dose given every 12 hours. A 400-mg I.V. dose results in a C_{max} similar to that observed with a 750-mg oral dose. An infusion of 200 mg ciprofloxacin given every 12 hours produces an AUC equivalent to that produced by a 250-mg oral dose given every 12 hours.

[See table at bottom of next page]

Distribution

After intravenous administration, ciprofloxacin is present in saliva, nasal and bronchial secretions, sputum, skin blister fluid, lymph, peritoneal fluid, bile, and prostatic secretions. It has also been detected in the lung, skin, fat, muscle, cartilage, and bone. Although the drug diffuses into cerebrospinal fluid (CSF), CSF concentrations are generally less than 10% of peak serum concentrations. Levels of the drug in the aqueous and vitreous chambers of the eye are lower than in serum.

Metabolism

After I.V. administration, three metabolites of ciprofloxacin have been identified in human urine which together account for approximately 10% of the intravenous dose. The binding of ciprofloxacin to serum proteins is 20 to 40%.

Excretion

The serum elimination half-life is approximately 5–6 hours and the total clearance is around 35 L/hr. After intravenous administration, approximately 50% to 70% of the dose is excreted in the urine as unchanged drug. Following a 200-mg I.V. dose, concentrations in the urine usually exceed 200 μg/mL 0–2 hours after dosing and are generally greater than 15 μg/mL 8–12 hours after dosing. Following a 400-mg I.V. dose, urine concentrations generally exceed 400 μg/mL 0–2 hours after dosing and are usually greater than 30 μg/mL 8–12 hours after dosing. The renal clearance is approximately 22 L/hr. The urinary excretion of ciprofloxacin is virtually complete by 24 hours after dosing. Although bile concentrations of ciprofloxacin are several fold higher than serum concentrations after intravenous dosing, only a small amount of the administered dose (< 1%) is recovered from the bile as unchanged drug. Approximately 15% of an I.V. dose is recovered from the feces within 5 days after dosing.

Special Populations

Pharmacokinetic studies of the oral (single dose) and intravenous (single and multiple dose) forms of ciprofloxacin indicate that plasma concentrations of ciprofloxacin are higher in elderly subjects (> 65 years) as compared to young adults. Although the C_{max} is increased 16–40%, the increase in mean AUC is approximately 30%, and can be at least partially attributed to decreased renal clearance in the elderly. Elimination half-life is only slightly (~20%) prolonged in the elderly. These differences are not considered clinically significant. (See **PRECAUTIONS: Geriatric Use.**)

In patients with reduced renal function, the half-life of ciprofloxacin is slightly prolonged and dosage adjustments may be required. (See **DOSAGE AND ADMINISTRATION.**)

In preliminary studies in patients with stable chronic liver cirrhosis, no significant changes in ciprofloxacin pharmacokinetics have been observed. However, the kinetics of ciprofloxacin in patients with acute hepatic insufficiency have not been fully elucidated.

Following a single oral dose of 10 mg/kg ciprofloxacin suspension to 16 children ranging in age from 4 months to 7 years, the mean C_{max} was 2.4 μg/mL (range: 1.5–3.4 μg/mL) and the mean AUC was 9.2 μg*h/mL (range: 5.8–14.9 μg*h/mL). There was no apparent age-dependence, and no notable increase in C_{max} or AUC upon multiple dosing (10 mg/kg TID). In children with severe sepsis who were given intravenous ciprofloxacin (10 mg/kg as a 1-hour infusion), the mean C_{max} was 6.1 μg/mL (range: 4.6–8.3 μg/mL) in 10 children less than 1 year of age; and 7.2 μg/mL (range: 4.7–11.8 μg/mL) in 10 children between 1 and 5 years of age. The AUC values were 17.4 μg*h/mL (range: 11.8–32.0 μg*h/mL) and 16.5 μg*h/mL (range: 11.0–23.8 μg*h/mL) in the respective age groups. These values are within the range reported for adults at therapeutic doses. Based on population pharmacokinetic analysis of pediatric patients with various infections, the predicted mean half-life in children is approximately 4–5 hours, and the bioavailability of the oral suspension is approximately 60%.

Drug-drug Interactions: The potential for pharmacokinetic drug interactions between ciprofloxacin and theophylline, caffeine, cyclosporins, phenytoin, sulfonylurea glyburide, metronidazole, warfarin, probenecid, and piperacillin sodium has been evaluated. (See **PRECAUTIONS: Drug Interactions.**)

MICROBIOLOGY

Ciprofloxacin has *in vitro* activity against a wide range of gram-negative and gram-positive microorganisms. The bactericidal action of ciprofloxacin results from inhibition of the enzymes topoisomerase II (DNA gyrase) and topoisomerase IV, which are required for bacterial DNA replication, transcription, repair, and recombination. The mechanism of action of fluoroquinolones, including ciprofloxacin, is different from that of penicillins, cephalosporins, aminoglycosides, macrolides, and tetracyclines; therefore, microorganisms resistant to these classes of drugs may be susceptible to ciprofloxacin and other quinolones. There is no known cross-resistance between ciprofloxacin and other classes of antimicrobials. *In vitro* resistance to ciprofloxacin develops slowly by multiple step mutations.

Ciprofloxacin is slightly less active when tested at acidic pH. The inoculum size has little effect when tested *in vitro*. The minimal bactericidal concentration (MBC) generally does not exceed the minimal inhibitory concentration (MIC) by more than a factor of 2.

Ciprofloxacin has been shown to be active against most strains of the following microorganisms, both *in vitro* and in clinical infections as described in the **INDICATIONS AND USAGE** section of the package insert for CIPRO I.V. (ciprofloxacin for intravenous infusion).

Aerobic gram-positive microorganisms

Enterococcus faecalis (Many strains are only moderately susceptible.)
Staphylococcus aureus (methicillin-susceptible strains only)
Staphylococcus epidermidis (methicillin-susceptible strains only)
Staphylococcus saprophyticus
Streptococcus pneumoniae (penicillin-susceptible strains)
Streptococcus pyogenes

Aerobic gram-negative microorganisms

Citrobacter diversus
Citrobacter freundii
Enterobacter cloacae
Escherichia coli
Haemophilus influenzae
Haemophilus parainfluenzae
Klebsiella pneumoniae
Moraxella catarrhalis
Morganella morganii
Proteus mirabilis
Proteus vulgaris
Providencia rettgeri
Providencia stuartii
Pseudomonas aeruginosa
Serratia marcescens

Ciprofloxacin has been shown to be active against *Bacillus anthracis* both *in vitro* and by use of serum levels as a surrogate marker (see **INDICATIONS AND USAGE** and **INHALATIONAL ANTHRAX — ADDITIONAL INFORMATION**).

The following *in vitro* data are available, **but their clinical significance is unknown.**

Ciprofloxacin exhibits *in vitro* minimum inhibitory concentrations (MICs) of 1 μg/mL or less against most (≥ 90%) strains of the following microorganisms; however, the safety and effectiveness of ciprofloxacin intravenous formulations in treating clinical infections due to these microorganisms have not been established in adequate and well-controlled clinical trials.

Aerobic gram-positive microorganisms

Staphylococcus haemolyticus
Staphylococcus hominis
Streptococcus pneumoniae (penicillin-resistant strains)

Aerobic gram-negative microorganisms

Acinetobacter lwoffi
Aeromonas hydrophila
Campylobacter jejuni
Edwardsiella tarda
Enterobacter aerogenes
Klebsiella oxytoca
Legionella pneumophila
Neisseria gonorrhoeae
Pasteurella multocida
Salmonella enteritidis
Salmonella typhi
Shigella boydii
Shigella dysenteriae
Shigella flexneri
Shigella sonnei
Vibrio cholerae
Vibrio parahaemolyticus
Vibrio vulnificus
Yersinia enterocolitica

Most strains of *Burkholderia cepacia* and some strains of *Stenotrophomonas maltophilia* are resistant to ciprofloxacin as are most anaerobic bacteria, including *Bacteroides fragilis* and *Clostridium difficile.*

Susceptibility Tests

Dilution Techniques: Quantitative methods are used to determine antimicrobial minimum inhibitory concentrations (MICs). These MICs provide estimates of the susceptibility of bacteria to antimicrobial compounds. The MICs should be determined using a standardized procedure. Standardized procedures are based on a dilution method[1] (broth or agar) or equivalent with standardized inoculum concentrations and standardized concentrations of ciprofloxacin powder. The MIC values should be interpreted according to the following criteria:

For testing aerobic microorganisms other than *Haemophilus influenzae*, and *Haemophilus parainfluenzae*[a]:

Steady-state Pharmacokinetic Parameter Following Multiple Oral and I.V. Doses

Parameters	500 mg q12h, P.O.	400 mg q12h, I.V.	750 mg q12h, P.O.	400 mg q8h, I.V.
AUC (μg•hr/mL)	13.7[a]	12.7[a]	31.6[b]	32.9[c]
C_{max} (μg/mL)	2.97	4.56	3.59	4.07

[a] AUC_{0-12h}
[b] AUC 24h=AUC_{0-12h} × 2
[c] AUC 24h=AUC_{0-8h} × 3

MIC (μg/mL)	Interpretation
≤ 1	Susceptible (S)
2	Intermediate (I)
≥ 4	Resistant (R)

[a]These interpretive standards are applicable only to broth microdilution susceptibility tests with streptococci using cation-adjusted Mueller-Hinton broth with 2–5% lysed horse blood.

For testing *Haemophilus influenzae* and *Haemophilus parainfluenzae*[b]:

MIC (μg/mL)	Interpretation
≤ 1	Susceptible (S)

[b]This interpretive standard is applicable only to broth microdilution susceptibility tests with *Haemophilus influenzae* and *Haemophilus parainfluenzae* using *Haemophilus* Test Medium [1].

The current absence of data on resistant strains precludes defining any results other than "Susceptible". Strains yielding MIC results suggestive of a "nonsusceptible" category should be submitted to a reference laboratory for further testing.

A report of "Susceptible" indicates that the pathogen is likely to be inhibited if the antimicrobial compound in the blood reaches the concentrations usually achievable. A report of "Intermediate" indicates that the result should be considered equivocal, and, if the microorganism is not fully susceptible to alternative, clinically feasible drugs, the test should be repeated. This category implies possible clinical applicability in body sites where the drug is physiologically concentrated or in situations where high dosage of drug can be used. This category also provides a buffer zone, which prevents small uncontrolled technical factors from causing major discrepancies in interpretation. A report of "Resistant" indicates that the pathogen is not likely to be inhibited if the antimicrobial compound in the blood reaches the concentrations usually achievable; other therapy should be selected.

Standardized susceptibility test procedures require the use of laboratory control microorganisms to control the technical aspects of the laboratory procedures. Standard ciprofloxacin powder should provide the following MIC values:

Organism		MIC (μg/mL)
E. faecalis	ATCC 29212	0.25 – 2.0
E. coli	ATCC 25922	0.004 – 0.015
H. influenzae[a]	ATCC 49247	0.004 – 0.03
P. aeruginosa	ATCC 27853	0.25 – 1.0
S. aureus	ATCC 29213	0.12 – 0.5

[a] This quality control range is applicable to only *H. influenzae* ATCC 49247 tested by a broth microdilution procedure using *Haemophilus* Test Medium (HTM)[1].

Diffusion Techniques: Quantitative methods that require measurement of zone diameters also provide reproducible estimates of the susceptibility of bacteria to antimicrobial compounds. One such standardized procedure[2] requires the use of standardized inoculum concentrations. This procedure uses paper disks impregnated with 5-μg ciprofloxacin to test the susceptibility of microorganisms to ciprofloxacin. Reports from the laboratory providing results of the standard single-disk susceptibility test with a 5-μg ciprofloxacin disk should be interpreted according to the following criteria:

For testing aerobic microorganisms other than *Haemophilus influenzae*, and *Haemophilus parainfluenzae*[a]:

Zone Diameter (mm)	Interpretation
≥ 21	Susceptible (S)
16–20	Intermediate (I)
≤ 15	Resistant (R)

[a]These zone diameter standards are applicable only to tests performed for streptococci using Mueller-Hinton agar supplemented with 5% sheep blood incubated in 5% CO_2.

For testing *Haemophilus influenzae* and *Haemophilus parainfluenzae*[b]:

Zone Diameter (mm)	Interpretation
≥ 21	Susceptible (S)

[b]This zone diameter standard is applicable only to tests with *Haemophilus influenzae* and *Haemophilus parainfluenzae*using *Haemophilus* Test Medium (HTM)[2].

The current absence of data on resistant strains precludes defining any results other than "Susceptible". Strains yielding zone diameter results suggestive of a "nonsusceptible" category should be submitted to a reference laboratory for further testing. Interpretation should be as stated above for results using dilution techniques. Interpretation involves correlation of the diameter obtained in the disk test with the MIC for ciprofloxacin.

As with standardized dilution techniques, diffusion methods require the use of laboratory control microorganisms that are used to control the technical aspects of the laboratory procedures. For the diffusion technique, the 5-μg ciprofloxacin disk should provide the following zone diameters in these laboratory test quality control strains:

Continued on next page

Cipro I.V.—Cont.

Organism		Zone Diameter (mm)
E. coli	ATCC 25922	30–40
H. influenzae[a]	ATCC 49247	34–42
P. aeruginosa	ATCC 27853	25–33
S. aureus	ATCC 25923	22–30

[a] These quality control limits are applicable to only *H. influenzae* ATCC 49247 testing using *Haemophilus* Test Medium (HTM)[2].

INDICATIONS AND USAGE

CIPRO I.V. is indicated for the treatment of infections caused by susceptible strains of the designated microorganisms in the conditions and patient populations listed below when the intravenous administration offers a route of administration advantageous to the patient. Please see **DOSAGE AND ADMINISTRATION** for specific recommendations.

Adult Patients:

Urinary Tract Infections caused by *Escherichia coli* (including cases with secondary bacteremia), *Klebsiella pneumoniae* subspecies *pneumoniae, Enterobacter cloacae, Serratia marcescens, Proteus mirabilis, Providencia rettgeri, Morganella morganii, Citrobacter diversus, Citrobacter freundii, Pseudomonas aeruginosa, Staphylococcus epidermidis, Staphylococcus saprophyticus,* or *Enterococcus faecalis.*

Lower Respiratory Infections caused by *Escherichia coli, Klebsiella pneumoniae* subspecies *pneumoniae, Enterobacter cloacae, Proteus mirabilis, Pseudomonas aeruginosa, Haemophilus influenzae, Haemophilus parainfluenzae,* or *Streptococcus pneumoniae.* Also, *Moraxella catarrhalis* for the treatment of acute exacerbations of chronic bronchitis.

NOTE: Although effective in clinical trials, ciprofloxacin is not a drug of first choice in the treatment of presumed or confirmed pneumonia secondary to *Streptococcus pneumoniae.*

Nosocomial Pneumonia caused by *Haemophilus influenzae* or *Klebsiella pneumoniae.*

Skin and Skin Structure Infections caused by *Escherichia coli, Klebsiella pneumoniae* subspecies *pneumoniae, Enterobacter cloacae, Proteus mirabilis, Proteus vulgaris, Providencia stuartii, Morganella morganii, Citrobacter freundii, Pseudomonas aeruginosa, Staphylococcus aureus* (methicillin susceptible), *Staphylococcus epidermidis,* or *Streptococcus pyogenes.*

Bone and Joint Infections caused by *Enterobacter cloacae, Serratia marcescens,* or *Pseudomonas aeruginosa.*

Complicated Intra-Abdominal Infections (used in conjunction with metronidazole) caused by *Escherichia coli, Pseudomonas aeruginosa, Proteus mirabilis, Klebsiella pneumoniae,* or *Bacteroides fragilis.*

Acute Sinusitis caused by *Haemophilus influenzae, Streptococcus pneumoniae,* or *Moraxella catarrhalis.*

Chronic Bacterial Prostatitis caused by *Escherichia coli* or *Proteus mirabilis.*

Empirical Therapy for Febrile Neutropenic Patients in combination with piperacillin sodium. (See **CLINICAL STUDIES.**)

Pediatric patients (1 to 17 years of age):

Complicated Urinary Tract Infections and Pyelonephritis due to *Escherichia coli.*

NOTE: Although effective in clinical trials, ciprofloxacin is not a drug of first choice in the pediatric population due to an increased incidence of adverse events compared to controls, including events related to joints and/or surrounding tissues. (See **WARNINGS, PRECAUTIONS, Pediatric Use, ADVERSE REACTIONS** and **CLINICAL STUDIES.**) Ciprofloxacin, like other fluoroquinolones, is associated with arthropathy and histopathological changes in weight-bearing joints of juvenile animals. (See **ANIMAL PHARMACOLOGY.**)

Adult and Pediatric Patients:

Inhalational anthrax (post-exposure): To reduce the incidence or progression of disease following exposure to aerosolized *Bacillus anthracis.*

Ciprofloxacin serum concentrations achieved in humans serve as a surrogate endpoint reasonably likely to predict clinical benefit and provide the basis for this indication.[4] (See also, **INHALATIONAL ANTHRAX – ADDITIONAL INFORMATION**).

If anaerobic organisms are suspected of contributing to the infection, appropriate therapy should be administered.

Appropriate culture and susceptibility tests should be performed before treatment in order to isolate and identify organisms causing infection and to determine their susceptibility to ciprofloxacin. Therapy with CIPRO I.V. may be initiated before results of these tests are known; once results become available, appropriate therapy should be continued.

As with other drugs, some strains of *Pseudomonas aeruginosa* may develop resistance fairly rapidly during treatment with ciprofloxacin. Culture and susceptibility testing performed periodically during therapy will provide information not only on the therapeutic effect of the antimicrobial agent but also on the possible emergence of bacterial resistance.

To reduce the development of drug-resistant bacteria and maintain the effectiveness of CIPRO I.V. and other antibacterial drugs, CIPRO I.V. should be used only to treat or prevent infections that are proven or strongly suspected to be caused by susceptible bacteria. When culture and susceptibility information are available, they should be considered in selecting or modifying antibacterial therapy. In the absence of such data, local epidemiology and susceptibility patterns may contribute to the empiric selection of therapy.

CONTRAINDICATIONS

CIPRO I.V. (ciprofloxacin) is contraindicated in persons with history of hypersensitivity to ciprofloxacin or any member of the quinolone class of antimicrobial agents.

WARNINGS

Pregnant Women: THE SAFETY AND EFFECTIVENESS OF CIPROFLOXACIN IN PREGNANT AND LACTATING WOMEN HAVE NOT BEEN ESTABLISHED. (See PRECAUTIONS: Pregnancy, and **Nursing Mothers** subsections.)

Pediatrics: Ciprofloxacin should be used in pediatric patients (less than 18 years of age) only for infections listed in the **INDICATIONS AND USAGE** section. An increased incidence of adverse events compared to controls, including events related to joints and/or surrounding tissues, has been observed. (See **ADVERSE REACTIONS.**)

In pre-clinical studies, oral administration of ciprofloxacin caused lameness in immature dogs. Histopathological examination of the weight-bearing joints of these dogs revealed permanent lesions of the cartilage. Related quinolone-class drugs also produce erosions of cartilage of weight-bearing joints and other signs of arthropathy in immature animals of various species. (See **ANIMAL PHARMACOLOGY.**)

Central Nervous System Disorders: Convulsions, increased intracranial pressure and toxic psychosis have been reported in patients receiving quinolones, including ciprofloxacin. Ciprofloxacin may also cause central nervous system (CNS) events including: dizziness, confusion, tremors, hallucinations, depression, and, rarely, suicidal thoughts or acts. These reactions may occur following the first dose. If these reactions occur in patients receiving ciprofloxacin, the drug should be discontinued and appropriate measures instituted. As with all quinolones, ciprofloxacin should be used with caution in patients with known or suspected CNS disorders that may predispose to seizures or lower the seizure threshold (e.g. severe cerebral arteriosclerosis, epilepsy), or in the presence of other risk factors that may predispose to seizures or lower the seizure threshold (e.g. certain drug therapy, renal dysfunction). (**See PRECAUTIONS: General, Information for Patients, Drug Interaction** and **ADVERSE REACTIONS.**)

Theophylline: SERIOUS AND FATAL REACTIONS HAVE BEEN REPORTED IN PATIENTS RECEIVING CONCURRENT ADMINISTRATION OF INTRAVENOUS CIPROFLOXACIN AND THEOPHYLLINE. These reactions have included cardiac arrest, seizure, status epilepticus, and respiratory failure. Although similar serious adverse events have been reported in patients receiving theophylline alone, the possibility that these reactions may be potentiated by ciprofloxacin cannot be eliminated. If concomitant use cannot be avoided, serum levels of theophylline should be monitored and dosage adjustments made as appropriate.

Hypersensitivity Reactions: Serious and occasionally fatal hypersensitivity (anaphylactic) reactions, some following the first dose, have been reported in patients receiving quinolone therapy. Some reactions were accompanied by cardiovascular collapse, loss of consciousness, tingling, pharyngeal or facial edema, dyspnea, urticaria, and itching. Only a few patients had a history of hypersensitivity reactions. Serious anaphylactic reactions require immediate emergency treatment with epinephrine and other resuscitation measures, including oxygen, intravenous fluids, intravenous antihistamines, corticosteroids, pressor amines, and airway management, as clinically indicated.

Severe hypersensitivity reactions characterized by rash, fever, eosinophilia, jaundice, and hepatic necrosis with fatal outcome have also been reported extremely rarely in patients receiving ciprofloxacin along with other drugs. The possibility that these reactions were related to ciprofloxacin cannot be excluded. Ciprofloxacin should be discontinued at the first appearance of a skin rash or any other sign of hypersensitivity.

Pseudomembranous Colitis: Pseudomembranous colitis has been reported with nearly all antibacterial agents, including ciprofloxacin, and may range in severity from mild to life-threatening. Therefore, it is important to consider this diagnosis in patients who present with diarrhea subsequent to the administration of antibacterial agents.

Treatment with antibacterial agents alters the normal flora of the colon and may permit overgrowth of clostridia. Studies indicate that a toxin produced by *Clostridium difficile* is one primary cause of "antibiotic-associated colitis."

After the diagnosis of pseudomembranous colitis has been established, therapeutic measures should be initiated. Mild cases of pseudomembranous colitis usually respond to drug discontinuation alone. In moderate to severe cases, consideration should be given to management with fluids and electrolytes, protein supplementation, and treatment with an antibacterial drug clinically effective against *C. difficile* colitis. Drugs that inhibit peristalsis should be avoided.

Peripheral neuropathy: Rare cases of sensory or sensorimotor axonal polyneuropathy affecting small and/or large axons resulting in paresthesias, hypoesthesias, dysesthesias and weakness have been reported in patients receiving quinolones, including ciprofloxacin. Ciprofloxacin should be discontinued if the patient experiences symptoms of neuropathy including pain, burning, tingling, numbness, and/or weakness, or is found to have deficits in light touch, pain, temperature, position sense, vibratory sensation, and/or motor strength in order to prevent the development of an irreversible condition.

Tendon Effects: Ruptures of the shoulder, hand, Achilles tendon or other tendons that required surgical repair or resulted in prolonged disability have been reported in patients receiving quinolones, including ciprofloxacin. Post-marketing surveillance reports indicate that this risk may be increased in patients receiving concomitant corticosteroids, especially the elderly. Ciprofloxacin should be discontinued if the patient experiences pain, inflammation, or rupture of a tendon. Patients should rest and refrain from exercise until the diagnosis of tendonitis or tendon rupture has been excluded. Tendon rupture can occur during or after therapy with quinolones, including ciprofloxacin.

PRECAUTIONS

General: INTRAVENOUS CIPROFLOXACIN SHOULD BE ADMINISTERED BY SLOW INFUSION OVER A PERIOD OF 60 MINUTES. Local I.V. site reactions have been reported with the intravenous administration of ciprofloxacin. These reactions are more frequent if infusion time is 30 minutes or less or if small veins of the hand are used. (See **ADVERSE REACTIONS.**)

Central Nervous System: Quinolones, including ciprofloxacin, may also cause central nervous system (CNS) events, including: nervousness, agitation, insomnia, anxiety, nightmares or paranoia. (See **WARNINGS, Information for Patients,** and **Drug Interactions.**)

Crystals of ciprofloxacin have been observed rarely in the urine of human subjects but more frequently in the urine of laboratory animals, which is usually alkaline. (See **ANIMAL PHARMACOLOGY.**) Crystalluria related to ciprofloxacin has been reported only rarely in humans because human urine is usually acidic. Alkalinity of the urine should be avoided in patients receiving ciprofloxacin. Patients should be well hydrated to prevent the formation of highly concentrated urine.

Renal Impairment: Alteration of the dosage regimen is necessary for patients with impairment of renal function. (See **DOSAGE AND ADMINISTRATION.**)

Phototoxicity: Moderate to severe phototoxicity manifested as an exaggerated sunburn reaction has been observed in some patients who were exposed to direct sunlight while receiving some members of the quinolone class of drugs. Excessive sunlight should be avoided.

As with any potent drug, periodic assessment of organ system functions, including renal, hepatic, and hematopoietic, is advisable during prolonged therapy.

Prescribing CIPRO I.V. in the absence of a proven or strongly suspected bacterial infection or a prophylactic indication is unlikely to provide benefit to the patient and increases the risk of the development of drug-resistant bacteria.

Information For Patients:

Patients should be advised:

- that antibacterial drugs including CIPRO I.V. should only be used to treat bacterial infections. They do not treat viral infections (e.g., the common cold). When CIPRO I.V. is prescribed to treat a bacterial infection, patients should be told that although it is common to feel better early in the course of therapy, the medication should be taken exactly as directed. Skipping doses or not completing the full course of therapy may (1) decrease the effectiveness of the immediate treatment and (2) increase the likelihood that bacteria will develop resistance and will not be treatable by CIPRO I.V. or other antibacterial drugs in the future.
- that ciprofloxacin may be associated with hypersensitivity reactions, even following a single dose, and to discontinue the drug at the first sign of a skin rash or other allergic reaction.
- that ciprofloxacin may cause dizziness and lightheadedness; therefore, patients should know how they react to this drug before they operate an automobile or machinery or engage in activities requiring mental alertness or coordination.
- that ciprofloxacin may increase the effects of theophylline and caffeine. There is a possibility of caffeine accumulation when products containing caffeine are consumed while taking ciprofloxacin.
- that peripheral neuropathies have been associated with ciprofloxacin use. If symptoms of peripheral neuropathy including pain, burning, tingling, numbness and/or weakness develop, they should discontinue treatment and contact their physicians.
- to discontinue treatment; rest and refrain from exercise; and inform their physician if they experience pain, inflammation, or rupture of a tendon.
- that convulsions have been reported in patients taking quinolones, including ciprofloxacin, and to notify their physician before taking this drug if there is a history of this condition.
- that ciprofloxacin has been associated with an increased rate of adverse events involving joints and surrounding tissue structures (like tendons) in pediatric patients (less than 18 years of age). Parents should inform their child's physician if the child has a history of joint-related problems before taking this drug. Parents of pediatric patients should also notify their child's physician of any joint-related problems that occur during or following ciprofloxacin therapy. (See **WARNINGS, PRECAUTIONS, Pediatric Use** and **ADVERSE REACTIONS.**)

Drug Interactions: As with some other quinolones, concurrent administration of ciprofloxacin with theophylline may lead to elevated serum concentrations of theophylline and prolongation of its elimination half-life. This may result in increased risk of theophylline-related adverse reactions.

(See **WARNINGS.**) If concomitant use cannot be avoided, serum levels of theophylline should be monitored and dosage adjustments made as appropriate.
Some quinolones, including ciprofloxacin, have also been shown to interfere with the metabolism of caffeine. This may lead to reduced clearance of caffeine and prolongation of its serum half-life.
Some quinolones, including ciprofloxacin, have been associated with transient elevations in serum creatinine in patients receiving cyclosporine concomitantly.
Altered serum levels of phenytoin (increased and decreased) have been reported in patients receiving concomitant ciprofloxacin.
The concomitant administration of ciprofloxacin with the sulfonylurea glyburide has, in some patients, resulted in severe hypoglycemia. Fatalities have been reported.
The serum concentrations of ciprofloxacin and metronidazole were not altered when these two drugs were given concomitantly. Quinolones, including ciprofloxacin, have been reported to enhance the effects of the oral anticoagulant warfarin or its derivatives. When these products are administered concomitantly, prothrombin time or other suitable coagulation tests should be closely monitored.
Probenecid interferes with renal tubular secretion of ciprofloxacin and produces an increase in the level of ciprofloxacin in the serum. This should be considered if patients are receiving both drugs concomitantly.
Renal tubular transport of methotrexate may be inhibited by concomitant administration of ciprofloxacin potentially leading to increased plasma levels of methotrexate. This might increase the risk of methotrexate associated toxic reactions. Therefore, patients under methotrexate therapy should be carefully monitored when concomitant ciprofloxacin therapy is indicated.
Non-steroidal anti-inflammatory drugs (but not acetyl salicylic acid) in combination of very high doses of quinolones have been shown to provoke convulsions in pre-clinical studies.
Following infusion of 400 mg I.V. ciprofloxacin every eight hours in combination with 50 mg/kg I.V. piperacillin sodium every four hours, mean serum ciprofloxacin concentrations were 3.02 µg/mL 1/2 hour and 1.18 µg/mL between 6–8 hours after the end of infusion.

Carcinogenesis, Mutagenesis, Impairment of Fertility: Eight *in vitro* mutagenicity tests have been conducted with ciprofloxacin. Test results are listed below:

- Salmonella/Microsome Test (Negative)
- *E. coli* DNA Repair Assay (Negative)
- Mouse Lymphoma Cell Forward Mutation Assay (Positive)
- Chinese Hamster V_{79} Cell HGPRT Test (Negative)
- Syrian Hamster Embryo Cell Transformation Assay (Negative)
- *Saccharomyces cerevisiae* Point Mutation Assay (Negative)
- *Saccharomyces cerevisiae* Mitotic Crossover and Gene Conversion Assay (Negative)
- Rat Hepatocyte DNA Repair Assay (Positive)

Thus, two of the eight tests were positive, but results of the following three *in vivo* test systems gave negative results:

- Rat Hepatocyte DNA Repair Assay
- Micronucleus Test (Mice)
- Dominant Lethal Test (Mice)

Long-term carcinogenicity studies in rats and mice resulted in no carcinogenic or tumorigenic effects due to ciprofloxacin at daily oral dose levels up to 250 and 750 mg/kg to rats and mice, respectively (approximately 1.7- and 2.5- times the highest recommended therapeutic dose based upon mg/m^2).
Results from photo co-carcinogenicity testing indicate that ciprofloxacin does not reduce the time to appearance of UV-induced skin tumors as compared to vehicle control. Hairless (Skh-1) mice were exposed to UVA light for 3.5 hours five times every two weeks for up to 78 weeks while concurrently being administered ciprofloxacin. The time to development of the first skin tumors was 50 weeks in mice treated concomitantly with UVA and ciprofloxacin (mouse dose approximately equal to maximum recommended human dose based upon mg/m^2), as opposed to 34 weeks when animals were treated with both UVA and vehicle. The times to development of skin tumors ranged from 16–32 weeks in mice treated concomitantly with UVA and other quinolones.[3]
In this model, mice treated with ciprofloxacin alone did not develop skin or systemic tumors. There are no data from similar models using pigmented mice and/or fully haired mice. The clinical significance of these findings to humans is unknown.
Fertility studies performed in rats at oral doses of ciprofloxacin up to 100 mg/kg (approximately 0.7-times the highest recommended therapeutic dose based upon mg/m^2) revealed no evidence of impairment.

Pregnancy: Teratogenic Effects. Pregnancy Category C: There are no adequate and well-controlled studies in pregnant women. An expert review of published data on experiences with ciprofloxacin use during pregnancy by TERIS – the Teratogen Information System - concluded that therapeutic doses during pregnancy are unlikely to pose a substantial teratogenic risk (quantity and quality of data=fair), but the data are insufficient to state that there is no risk.[7]
A controlled prospective observational study followed 200 women exposed to fluoroquinolones (52.5% exposed to ciprofloxacin and 68% first trimester exposures) during gestation.[8] In utero exposure to fluoroquinolones during embryogenesis was not associated with increased risk of major malformations. The reported rates of major congenital malformations were 2.2% for the fluoroquinolone group and 2.6% for the control group (background incidence of major malformations is 1–5%). Rates of spontaneous abortions, prematurity and low birth weight did not differ between the groups and there were no clinically significant musculoskeletal dysfunctions up to one year of age in the ciprofloxacin exposed children.
Another prospective follow-up study reported on 549 pregnancies with fluoroquinolone exposure (93% first trimester exposures).[9] There were 70 ciprofloxacin exposures, all within the first trimester. The malformation rates among live-born babies exposed to ciprofloxacin and to fluoroquinolones overall were both within background incidence ranges. No specific patterns of congenital abnormalities were found. The study did not reveal any clear adverse reactions due to in utero exposure to ciprofloxacin.
No differences in the rates of prematurity, spontaneous abortions, or birth weight were seen in women exposed to ciprofloxacin during pregnancy.[7,8] However, these small postmarketing epidemiology studies, of which most experience is from short term, first trimester exposure, are insufficient to evaluate the risk for less common defects or to permit reliable and definitive conclusions regarding the safety of ciprofloxacin in pregnant women and their developing fetuses. Ciprofloxacin should not be used during pregnancy unless the potential benefit justifies the potential risk to both fetus and mother (see **WARNINGS**).
Reproduction studies have been performed in rats and mice using oral doses up to 100 mg/kg (0.6 and 0.3 times the maximum daily human dose based upon body surface area, respectively) and have revealed no evidence of harm to the fetus due to ciprofloxacin. In rabbits, oral ciprofloxacin dose levels of 30 and 100 mg/kg (approximately 0.4- and 1.3-times the highest recommended therapeutic dose based upon mg/m^2) produced gastrointestinal toxicity resulting in maternal weight loss and an increased incidence of abortion, but no teratogenicity was observed at either dose level. After intravenous administration of doses up to 20 mg/kg (approximately 0.3-times the highest recommended therapeutic dose based upon mg/m^2) no maternal toxicity was produced and no embryotoxicity or teratogenicity was observed. (See **WARNINGS.**)

Nursing Mothers: Ciprofloxacin is excreted in human milk. The amount of ciprofloxacin absorbed by the nursing infant is unknown. Because of the potential for serious adverse reactions in infants nursing from mothers taking ciprofloxacin, a decision should be made whether to discontinue nursing or to discontinue the drug, taking into account the importance of the drug to the mother.

Pediatric Use: Ciprofloxacin, like other quinolones, causes arthropathy and histological changes in weight-bearing joints of juvenile animals resulting in lameness. (See **ANIMAL PHARMACOLOGY.**)

Inhalational Anthrax (Post-Exposure)
Ciprofloxacin is indicated in pediatric patients for inhalational anthrax (post-exposure). The risk-benefit assessment indicates that administration of ciprofloxacin to pediatric patients is appropriate. For information regarding pediatric dosing in inhalational anthrax (post-exposure), see **DOSAGE AND ADMINISTRATION** and **INHALATIONAL ANTHRAX – ADDITIONAL INFORMATION.**

Complicated Urinary Tract Infection and Pyelonephritis
Ciprofloxacin is indicated for the treatment of complicated urinary tract infections and pyelonephritis due to *Escherichia coli.* Although effective in clinical trials, ciprofloxacin is not a drug of first choice in the pediatric population due to an increased incidence of adverse events compared to the controls, including those related to joints and/or surrounding tissues. The rates of these events in pediatric patients with complicated urinary tract infection and pyelonephritis within six weeks of follow-up were 9.3% (31/335) versus 6.0% (21/349) for control agents. The rates of these events occurring at any time up to the one year follow-up were 13.7% (46/335) and 9.5% (33/349), respectively. The rate of all adverse events regardless of drug relationship at six weeks was 41% (138/335) in the ciprofloxacin arm compared to 31% (109/349) in the control arm. (See **ADVERSE REACTIONS** and **CLINICAL STUDIES.**)

Cystic Fibrosis
Short-term safety data from a single trial in pediatric cystic fibrosis patients are available. In a randomized, double-blind clinical trial for the treatment of acute pulmonary exacerbations in cystic fibrosis patients (ages 5–17 years), 67 patients received ciprofloxacin I.V. 10 mg/kg/dose q8h for one week followed by ciprofloxacin tablets 20 mg/kg/dose q12h to complete 10–21 days treatment and 62 patients received the combination of ceftazidime I.V. 50 mg/kg/dose q8h and tobramycin I.V. 3 mg/kg/dose q8h for a total of 10–21 days. Patients less than 5 years of age were not studied. Safety monitoring in the study included periodic range of motion examinations and gait assessments by treatment-blinded examiners. Patients were followed for an average of 23 days after completing treatment (range 0-93 days). This study was not designed to determine long term effects and the safety of repeated exposure to ciprofloxacin.
Musculoskeletal adverse events in patients with cystic fibrosis were reported in 22% of the patients in the ciprofloxacin group and 21% in the comparison group. Decreased range of motion was reported in 12% of the subjects in the ciprofloxacin group and 16% in the comparison group. Arthralgia was reported in 10% of the patients in the ciprofloxacin group and 11% in the comparison group. Other adverse events were similar in nature and frequency between treatment arms. One of sixty-seven patients developed arthritis of the knee nine days after a ten day course of treatment with ciprofloxacin. Clinical symptoms resolved, but an MRI showed knee effusion without other abnormalities eight months after treatment. However, the relationship of this event to the patient's course of ciprofloxacin can not be definitively determined, particularly since patients with cystic fibrosis may develop arthralgias/arthritis as part of their underlying disease process.

Geriatric Use: In a retrospective analysis of 23 multiple-dose controlled clinical trials of ciprofloxacin encompassing over 3500 ciprofloxacin treated patients, 25% of patients were greater than or equal to 65 years of age and 10% were greater than or equal to 75 years of age. No overall differences in safety or effectiveness were observed between these subjects and younger subjects, and other reported clinical experience has not identified differences in responses between the elderly and younger patients, but greater sensitivity of some older individuals on any drug therapy cannot be ruled out. Ciprofloxacin is known to be substantially excreted by the kidney, and the risk of adverse reactions may be greater in patients with impaired renal function. No alteration of dosage is necessary for patients greater than 65 years of age with normal renal function. However, since some older individuals experience reduced renal function by virtue of their advanced age, care should be taken in dose selection for elderly patients, and renal function monitoring may be useful in these patients. (See **CLINICAL PHARMACOLOGY** and **DOSAGE AND ADMINISTRATION.**)

ADVERSE REACTIONS

Adverse Reactions in Adult Patients: During clinical investigations with oral and parenteral ciprofloxacin, 49,038 patients received courses of the drug. Most of the adverse events reported were described as only mild or moderate in severity, abated soon after the drug was discontinued, and required no treatment. Ciprofloxacin was discontinued because of an adverse event in 1.8% of intravenously treated patients.
The most frequently reported drug related events, from clinical trials of all formulations, all dosages, all drug-therapy durations, and for all indications of ciprofloxacin therapy were nausea (2.5%), diarrhea (1.6%), liver function tests abnormal (1.3%), vomiting (1.0%), and rash (1.0%).
In clinical trials the following events were reported, regardless of drug relationship, in greater than 1% of patients treated with intravenous ciprofloxacin: nausea, diarrhea, central nervous system disturbance, local I.V. site reactions, liver function tests abnormal, eosinophilia, headache, restlessness, and rash. Many of these events were described as only mild or moderate in severity, abated soon after the drug was discontinued, and required no treatment. Local I.V. site reactions are more frequent if the infusion time is 30 minutes or less. These may appear as local skin reactions which resolve rapidly upon completion of the infusion. Subsequent intravenous administration is not contraindicated unless the reactions recur or worsen.
Additional medically important events, without regard to drug relationship or route of administration, that occurred in 1% or less of ciprofloxacin patients are listed below:
BODY AS A WHOLE: abdominal pain/discomfort, foot pain, pain, pain in extremities
CARDIOVASCULAR: cardiovascular collapse, cardiopulmonary arrest, myocardial infarction, arrhythmia, tachycardia, palpitation, cerebral thrombosis, syncope, cardiac murmur, hypertension, hypotension, angina pectoris, atrial flutter, ventricular ectopy, (thrombo)-phlebitis, vasodilation, migraine
CENTRAL NERVOUS SYSTEM: convulsive seizures, paranoia, toxic psychosis, depression, dysphasia, phobia, depersonalization, manic reaction, unresponsiveness, ataxia, confusion, hallucinations, dizziness, lightheadedness, paresthesia, anxiety, tremor, insomnia, nightmares, weakness, drowsiness, irritability, malaise, lethargy, abnormal gait, grand mal convulsion, anorexia
GASTROINTESTINAL: ileus, jaundice, gastrointestinal bleeding, *C. difficile* associated diarrhea, pseudomembranous colitis, pancreatitis, hepatic necrosis, intestinal perforation, dyspepsia, epigastric pain, constipation, oral ulceration, oral candidiasis, mouth dryness, anorexia, dysphagia, flatulence, hepatitis, painful oral mucosa
HEMIC/LYMPHATIC: agranulocytosis, prolongation of prothrombin time, lymphadenopathy, petechia
METABOLIC/NUTRITIONAL: amylase increase, lipase increase
MUSCULOSKELETAL: arthralgia, jaw, arm or back pain, joint stiffness, neck and chest pain, achiness, flare up of gout, myasthenia gravis
RENAL/UROGENITAL: renal failure, interstitial nephritis, nephritis, hemorrhagic cystitis, renal calculi, frequent urination, acidosis, urethral bleeding, polyuria, urinary retention, gynecomastia, candiduria, vaginitis, breast pain. Crystalluria, cylindruria, hematuria and albuminuria have also been reported.
RESPIRATORY: respiratory arrest, pulmonary embolism, dyspnea, laryngeal or pulmonary edema, respiratory distress, pleural effusion, hemoptysis, epistaxis, hiccough, bronchospasm
SKIN/HYPERSENSITIVITY: allergic reactions, anaphylactic reactions, erythema multiforme/Stevens-Johnson syndrome, exfoliative dermatitis, toxic epidermal necrolysis, vasculitis, angioedema, edema of the lips, face, neck, conjunctivae, hands or lower extremities, purpura, fever, chills, flushing, pruritus, urticaria, cutaneous candidiasis, vesi-

Continued on next page

Cipro I.V.—Cont.

cles, increased perspiration, hyperpigmentation, erythema nodosum, thrombophlebitis, burning, paresthesia, erythema, swelling, photosensitivity (See **WARNINGS**.)
SPECIAL SENSES: decreased visual acuity, blurred vision, disturbed vision (flashing lights, change in color perception, overbrightness of lights, diplopia), eye pain, anosmia, hearing loss, tinnitus, nystagmus, chromatopsia, a bad taste. In several instances, nausea, vomiting, tremor, irritability, or palpitation were judged by investigators to be related to elevated serum levels of theophylline possibly as a result of drug interaction with ciprofloxacin.
In randomized, double-blind controlled clinical trials comparing ciprofloxacin (I.V. and I.V./P.O. sequential) with intravenous beta-lactam control antibiotics, the CNS adverse event profile of ciprofloxacin was comparable to that of the control drugs.

Adverse Reactions in Pediatric Patients: Ciprofloxacin, administered I.V. and/or orally, was compared to a cephalosporin for treatment of complicated urinary tract infections (cUTI) or pyelonephritis in pediatric patients 1 to 17 years of age (mean age of 6 ± 4 years). The trial was conducted in the US, Canada, Argentina, Peru, Costa Rica, Mexico, South Africa, and Germany. The duration of therapy was 10 to 21 days (mean duration of treatment was 11 days with a range of 1 to 88 days). The primary objective of the study was to assess musculoskeletal and neurological safety within 6 weeks of therapy and through one year of follow-up in the 335 ciprofloxacin- and 349 comparator-treated patients enrolled.
An Independent Pediatric Safety Committee (IPSC) reviewed all cases of musculoskeletal adverse events as well as all patients with an abnormal gait or abnormal joint exam (baseline or treatment-emergent). These events were evaluated in a comprehensive fashion and included such conditions as arthralgia, abnormal gait, abnormal joint exam, joint sprains, leg pain, back pain, arthrosis, bone pain, pain, myalgia, arm pain, and decreased range of motion in a joint. The affected joints included: knee, elbow, ankle, hip, wrist, and shoulder. Within 6 weeks of treatment initiation, the rates of these events were 9.3% (31/335) in the ciprofloxacin-treated group versus 6.0 % (21/349) in comparator-treated patients. The majority of these events were mild or moderate in intensity. All musculoskeletal events occurring by 6 weeks resolved (clinical resolution of signs and symptoms), usually within 30 days of end of treatment. Radiological evaluations were not routinely used to confirm resolution of the events. The events occurred more frequently in ciprofloxacin-treated patients than control patients, regardless of whether they received I.V. or oral therapy. Ciprofloxacin-treated patients were more likely to report more than one event and on more than one occasion compared to control patients. These events occurred in all age groups and the rates were consistently higher in the ciprofloxacin group compared to the control group. At the end of 1 year, the rate of these events reported at any time during that period was 13.7% (46/335) in the ciprofloxacin-treated group versus 9.5% (33/349) comparator-treated patients.
An adolescent female discontinued ciprofloxacin for wrist pain that developed during treatment. An MRI performed 4 weeks later showed a tear in the right ulnar fibrocartilage. A diagnosis of overuse syndrome secondary to sports activity was made, but a contribution from ciprofloxacin cannot be excluded. The patient recovered by 4 months without surgical intervention.

Findings Involving Joint or Peri-articular Tissues as Assessed by the IPSC

	Ciprofloxacin	Comparator
All Patients (within 6 weeks)	31/335 (9.3%)	21/349 (6.0%)
95% Confidence Interval*	(−0.8%, +7.2%)	
Age Group		
≥ 12 months < 24 months	1/36 (2.8%)	0/41
≥ 2 years < 6 years	5/124 (4.0%)	3/118 (2.5%)
≥ 6 years < 12 years	18/143 (12.6%)	12/153 (7.8%)
≥ 12 years to 17 years	7/32 (21.9%)	6/37 (16.2 %)
All Patients (within 1 year)	46/335 (13.7%)	33/349 (9.5%)
95% Confidence Interval*	(−0.6%, +9.1%)	

*The study was designed to demonstrate that the arthropathy rate for the ciprofloxacin group did not exceed that of the control group by more than + 6%. At both the 6 week and 1 year evaluations, the 95% confidence interval indicated that it could not be concluded that the ciprofloxacin group had findings comparable to the control group.

The incidence rates of neurological events within 6 weeks of treatment initiation were 3% (9/335) in the ciprofloxacin group versus 2% (7/349) in the comparator group and included dizziness, nervousness, insomnia, and somnolence.
In this trial, the overall incidence rates of adverse events regardless of relationship to study drug and within 6 weeks of treatment initiation were 41% (138/335) in the ciprofloxacin group versus 31% (109/349) in the comparator group. The most frequent events were gastrointestinal: 15% (50/335) of ciprofloxacin patients compared to 9% (31/349) of comparator patients. Serious adverse events were seen in 7.5% (25/335) of ciprofloxacin-treated patients compared to 5.7% (20/349) of control patients. Discontinuation of drug due to an adverse event was observed in 3% (10/335) of ciprofloxacin-treated patients versus 1.4% (5/349) of comparator patients. Other adverse events that occurred in at least 1% of ciprofloxacin patients were diarrhea 4.8%, vomiting 4.8%, abdominal pain 3.3%, accidental injury 3.0%, rhinitis 3.0%, dyspepsia 2.7%, nausea 2.7%, fever 2.1%, asthma 1.8% and rash 1.8%.
In addition to the events reported in pediatric patients in clinical trials, it should be expected that events reported in adults during clinical trials or post-marketing experience may also occur in pediatric patients.

Post-Marketing Adverse Events: The following adverse events have been reported from worldwide marketing experience with quinolones, including ciprofloxacin. Because these events are reported voluntarily from a population of uncertain size, it is not always possible to reliably estimate their frequency or establish a causal relationship to drug exposure. Decisions to include these events in labeling are typically based on one or more of the following factors: (1) seriousness of the event, (2) frequency of the reporting, or (3) strength of causal connection to the drug.
Agitation, agranulocytosis, albuminuria, anosmia, candiduria, cholesterol elevation (serum), confusion, constipation, delirium, dyspepsia, dysphagia, erythema multiforme, exfoliative dermatitis, fixed eruption, flatulence, glucose elevation (blood), hemolytic anemia, hepatic failure, hepatic necrosis, hyperesthesia, hypertonia, hypesthesia, hypotension (postural), jaundice, marrow depression (life threatening), methemoglobinemia, moniliasis (oral, gastrointestinal, vaginal), myalgia, myasthenia, myasthenia gravis (possible exacerbation), myoclonus, nystagmus, pancreatitis, pancytopenia (life threatening or fatal outcome), peripheral neuropathy, phenytoin alteration (serum), potassium elevation (serum), prothrombin time prolongation or decrease, pseudomembranous colitis (The onset of pseudomembranous colitis symptoms may occur during or after antimicrobial treatment.), psychosis (toxic), renal calculi, serum sickness like reaction, Stevens-Johnson syndrome, taste loss, tendinitis, tendon rupture, torsade de pointes, toxic epidermal necrolysis, triglyceride elevation (serum), twitching, vaginal candidiasis, and vasculitis. (See **PRECAUTIONS**.)

Adverse Laboratory Changes: The most frequently reported changes in laboratory parameters with intravenous ciprofloxacin therapy, without regard to drug relationship are listed below:

Hepatic	—	elevations of AST (SGOT), ALT (SGPT), alkaline phosphatase, LDH, and serum bilirubin
Hematologic	—	elevated eosinophil and platelet counts, decreased platelet counts, hemoglobin and/or hematocrit
Renal	—	elevations of serum creatinine, BUN, and uric acid
Other	—	elevations of serum creatine phosphokinase, serum theophylline (in patients receiving theophylline concomitantly), blood glucose, and triglycerides

Other changes occurring infrequently were: decreased leukocyte count, elevated atypical lymphocyte count, immature WBCs, elevated serum calcium, elevation of serum gamma-glutamyl transpeptidase (γ GT), decreased BUN, decreased uric acid, decreased total serum protein, decreased serum albumin, decreased serum potassium, elevated serum potassium, elevated serum cholesterol. Other changes occurring rarely during administration of ciprofloxacin were: elevation of serum amylase, decrease of blood glucose, pancytopenia, leukocytosis, elevated sedimentation rate, change in serum phenytoin, decreased prothrombin time, hemolytic anemia, and bleeding diathesis.

OVERDOSAGE

In the event of acute overdosage, the patient should be carefully observed and given supportive treatment. Adequate hydration must be maintained. Only a small amount of ciprofloxacin (< 10%) is removed from the body after hemodialysis or peritoneal dialysis.
In mice, rats, rabbits and dogs, significant toxicity including tonic/clonic convulsions was observed at intravenous doses of ciprofloxacin between 125 and 300 mg/kg.

DOSAGE AND ADMINISTRATION - ADULTS

CIPRO I.V. should be administered to adults by intravenous infusion over a period of 60 minutes at dosages described in the Dosage Guidelines table. Slow infusion of a dilute solution into a larger vein will minimize patient discomfort and reduce the risk of venous irritation. (See **Preparation of CIPRO I.V. for Administration** section.)
The determination of dosage for any particular patient must take into consideration the severity and nature of the infection, the susceptibility of the causative microorganism, the integrity of the patient's host-defense mechanisms, and the status of renal and hepatic function.
[See table below]

CIPRO I.V. should be administered by intravenous infusion over a period of 60 minutes.

Conversion of I.V. to Oral Dosing in Adults: CIPRO Tablets and CIPRO Oral Suspension for oral administration are available. Parenteral therapy may be switched to oral CIPRO when the condition warrants, at the discretion of the physician. (See **CLINICAL PHARMACOLOGY** and table below for the equivalent dosing regimens.)

Equivalent AUC Dosing Regimens

CIPRO Oral Dosage	Equivalent CIPRO I.V. Dosage
250 mg Tablet q 12 h	200 mg I.V. q 12 h
500 mg Tablet q 12 h	400 mg I.V. q 12 h
750 mg Tablet q 12 h	400 mg I.V. q 8 h

Parenteral drug products should be inspected visually for particulate matter and discoloration prior to administration.

Adults with Impaired Renal Function: Ciprofloxacin is eliminated primarily by renal excretion; however, the drug is also metabolized and partially cleared through the biliary system of the liver and through the intestine. These alternative pathways of drug elimination appear to compensate

ADULT DOSAGE GUIDELINES

Infection†	Severity	Dose	Frequency	Usual Duration
Urinary Tract	Mild/Moderate Severe/Complicated	200 mg 400 mg	q12h q12h	7–14 Days 7–14 Days
Lower Respiratory Tract	Mild/Moderate Severe/Complicated	400 mg 400 mg	q12h q8h	7–14 Days 7–14 Days
Nosocomial Pneumonia	Mild/Moderate/Severe	400 mg	q8h	10–14 Days
Skin and Skin Structure	Mild/Moderate Severe/Complicated	400 mg 400 mg	q12h q8h	7–14 Days 7–14 Days
Bone and Joint	Mild/Moderate Severe/Complicated	400 mg 400 mg	q12h q8h	≥ 4–6 Weeks ≥ 4–6 Weeks
Intra-Abdominal*	Complicated	400 mg	q12h	7–14 Days
Acute Sinusitis	Mild/Moderate	400 mg	q12h	10 Days
Chronic Bacterial Prostatitis	Mild/Moderate	400 mg	q12h	28 Days
Empirical Therapy in Febrile Neutropenic Patients	Severe Ciprofloxacin + Piperacillin	 400 mg 50 mg/kg Not to exceed 24 g/day	 q8h q4h	7–14 Days
Inhalational anthrax (post-exposure)**		400 mg	q12h	60 Days

* used in conjunction with metronidazole. (See product labeling for prescribing information.)
† DUE TO THE DESIGNATED PATHOGENS (See **INDICATIONS AND USAGE**.)
** Drug administration should begin as soon as possible after suspected or confirmed exposure. This indication is based on a surrogate endpoint, ciprofloxacin serum concentrations achieved in humans, reasonably likely to predict clinical benefit.[4] For a discussion of ciprofloxacin serum concentrations in various human populations, see **INHALATIONAL ANTHRAX — ADDITIONAL INFORMATION**. Total duration of ciprofloxacin administration (I.V. or oral) for inhalational anthrax (post-exposure) is 60 days.

for the reduced renal excretion in patients with renal impairment. Nonetheless, some modification of dosage is recommended for patients with severe renal dysfunction. The following table provides dosage guidelines for use in patients with renal impairment:

RECOMMENDED STARTING AND MAINTENANCE DOSES FOR PATIENTS WITH IMPAIRED RENAL FUNCTION

Creatinine Clearance (mL/min)	Dosage
> 30	See usual dosage.
5–29	200–400 mg q 18–24 hr

When only the serum creatinine concentration is known, the following formula may be used to estimate creatinine clearance:

[See first table at right]

The serum creatinine should represent a steady state of renal function.

For patients with changing renal function or for patients with renal impairment and hepatic insufficiency, careful monitoring is suggested.

DOSAGE AND ADMINISTRATION - PEDIATRICS

CIPRO I.V. should be administered as described in the Dosage Guidelines table. An increased incidence of adverse events compared to controls, including events related to joints and/or surrounding tissues, has been observed. (See **ADVERSE REACTIONS** and **CLINICAL STUDIES**.)

Dosing and initial route of therapy (i.e., I.V. or oral) for complicated urinary tract infection or pyelonephritis should be determined by the severity of the infection. In the clinical trial, pediatric patients with moderate to severe infection were initiated on 6 to 10 mg/kg I.V. every 8 hours and allowed to switch to oral therapy (10 to 20 mg/kg every 12 hours), at the discretion of the physician.

[See second table at right]

Pediatric patients with moderate to severe renal insufficiency were excluded from the clinical trial of complicated urinary tract infection and pyelonephritis. No information is available on dosing adjustments necessary for pediatric patients with moderate to severe renal insufficiency (i.e., creatinine clearance of < 50 mL/min/1.73m^2).

Preparation of CIPRO I.V. for Administration

Vials (Injection Concentrate): THIS PREPARATION MUST BE DILUTED BEFORE USE. The intravenous dose should be prepared by aseptically withdrawing the concentrate from the vial of CIPRO I.V. This should be diluted with a suitable intravenous solution to a final concentration of 1–2mg/mL. (See **COMPATIBILITY AND STABILITY**.) The resulting solution should be infused over a period of 60 minutes by direct infusion or through a Y-type intravenous infusion set which may already be in place.

If the Y-type or "piggyback" method of administration is used, it is advisable to discontinue temporarily the administration of any other solutions during the infusion of CIPRO I.V. If the concomitant use of CIPRO I.V. and another drug is necessary each drug should be given separately in accordance with the recommended dosage and route of administration for each drug.

Flexible Containers: CIPRO I.V. is also available as a 0.2% premixed solution in 5% dextrose in flexible containers of 100 mL or 200 mL. The solutions in flexible containers do not need to be diluted and may be infused as described above.

COMPATIBILITY AND STABILITY

Ciprofloxacin injection 1% (10 mg/mL), when diluted with the following intravenous solutions to concentrations of 0.5 to 2.0 mg/mL, is stable for up to 14 days at refrigerated or room temperature storage.

- 0.9% Sodium Chloride Injection, USP
- 5% Dextrose Injection, USP
- Sterile Water for Injection
- 10% Dextrose for Injection
- 5% Dextrose and 0.225% Sodium Chloride for Injection
- 5% Dextrose and 0.45% Sodium Chloride for Injection
- Lactated Ringer's for Injection

HOW SUPPLIED

CIPRO I.V. (ciprofloxacin) is available as a clear, colorless to slightly yellowish solution. CIPRO I.V. is available in 200 mg and 400 mg strengths. The concentrate is supplied in vials while the premixed solution is supplied in latex-free flexible containers as follows:

[See third table at right]

STORAGE

Vial: Store between 5–30°C (41–86°F).

Flexible Container: Store between 5–25°C (41–77°F).

Protect from light, avoid excessive heat, protect from freezing.

CIPRO I.V. (ciprofloxacin) is also available in a 120 mL Pharmacy Bulk Package.

Ciprofloxacin is also available as CIPRO (ciprofloxacin HCl) Tablets 100, 250, 500, and 750 mg and CIPRO (ciprofloxacin*) 5% and 10% Oral Suspension.

*Does not comply with USP with regards to "loss on drying" and "residue on ignition".

ANIMAL PHARMACOLOGY

Ciprofloxacin and other quinolones have been shown to cause arthropathy in immature animals of most species tested. (See **WARNINGS**.) Damage of weight bearing joints was observed in juvenile dogs and rats. In young beagles, 100 mg/kg ciprofloxacin, given daily for 4 weeks, caused degenerative articular changes of the knee joint. At 30 mg/kg, the effect on the joint was minimal. In a subsequent study in young beagle dogs, oral ciprofloxacin doses of 30 mg/kg and 90 mg/kg ciprofloxacin (approximately 1.3- and 3.5-times the pediatric dose based upon comparative plasma AUCs) given daily for 2 weeks caused articular changes which were still observed by histopathology after a treatment-free period of 5 months. At 10 mg/kg (approximately 0.6-times the pediatric dose based upon comparative plasma AUCs), no effects on joints were observed. This dose was also not associated with arthrotoxicity after an additional treatment-free period of 5 months. In another study, removal of weight bearing from the joint reduced the lesions but did not totally prevent them.

Crystalluria, sometimes associated with secondary nephropathy, occurs in laboratory animals dosed with ciprofloxacin. This is primarily related to the reduced solubility of ciprofloxacin under alkaline conditions, which predominate in the urine of test animals; in man, crystalluria is rare since human urine is typically acidic. In rhesus monkeys, crystalluria without nephropathy was noted after single oral doses as low as 5 mg/kg (approximately 0.07-times the highest recommended therapeutic dose based upon mg/m^2). After 6 months of intravenous dosing at 10 mg/kg/day,

$$\text{Men: Creatinine clearance (mL/min)} = \frac{\text{Weight (kg)} \times (140 - \text{age})}{72 \times \text{serum creatinine (mg/dL)}}$$

Women: 0.85 × the value calculated for men.

PEDIATRIC DOSAGE GUIDELINES

Infection	Route of Administration	Dose (mg/kg)	Frequency	Total Duration
Complicated Urinary Tract or Pyelonephritis (patients from 1 to 17 years of age)	Intravenous	6 to 10 mg/kg (maximum 400 mg per dose; not to be exceeded even in patients weighing > 51 kg)	Every 8 hours	10–21 days*
	Oral	10 mg/kg to 20 mg/kg (maximum 750 mg per dose; not to be exceeded even in patients weighing > 51 kg)	Every 12 hours	
Inhalational Anthrax (Post-Exposure)**	Intravenous	10 mg/kg (maximum 400 mg per dose)	Every 12 hours	60 days
	Oral	15 mg/kg (maximum 500 mg per dose)	Every 12 hours	

* The total duration of therapy for complicated urinary tract infection and pyelonephritis in the clinical trial was determined by the physician. The mean duration of treatment was 11 days (range 10 to 21 days).

** Drug administration should begin as soon as possible after suspected or confirmed exposure to *Bacillus anthracis* spores. This indication is based on a surrogate endpoint, ciprofloxacin serum concentrations achieved in humans, reasonably likely to predict clinical benefit.[4] For a discussion of ciprofloxacin serum concentrations in various human populations, see **INHALATIONAL ANTHRAX – ADDITIONAL INFORMATION**.

VIAL: manufactured by Bayer Healthcare LLC and Hollister-Stier, Spokane, WA 99220.

SIZE	STRENGTH	NDC NUMBER
20 mL	200 mg, 1%	0026-8562-20
40 mL	400 mg, 1%	0026-8564-64

FLEXIBLE CONTAINER: manufactured for Bayer Pharmaceuticals Corporation by Abbott Laboratories, North Chicago, IL 60064.

SIZE	STRENGTH	NDC NUMBER
100 mL 5% Dextrose	200 mg, 0.2%	0026-8552-36
200 mL 5% Dextrose	400 mg, 0.2%	0026-8554-63

FLEXIBLE CONTAINER: manufactured for Bayer Pharmaceuticals Corporation by Baxter Healthcare Corporation, Deerfield, IL 60015.

SIZE	STRENGTH	NDC NUMBER
100 mL 5% Dextrose	200 mg, 0.2%	0026-8527-36
200 mL 5% Dextrose	400 mg, 0.2%	0026-8527-63

Outcomes	Ciprofloxacin/Piperacillin N = 233 Success (%)	Tobramycin/Piperacillin N = 237 Success (%)
Clinical Resolution of Initial Febrile Episode with No Modifications of Empirical Regimen*	63 (27.0%)	52 (21.9%)
Clinical Resolution of Initial Febrile Episode Including Patients with Modifications of Empirical Regimen	187 (80.3%)	185 (78.1%)
Overall Survival	224 (96.1%)	223 (94.1%)

* To be evaluated as a clinical resolution, patients had to have: (1) resolution of fever; (2) microbiological eradication of infection (if an infection was microbiologically documented); (3) resolution of signs/symptoms of infection; and (4) no modification of empirical antibiotic regimen.

Clinical Success and Bacteriologic Eradication at Test of Cure (5 to 9 Days Post-Therapy)

	CIPRO	Comparator
Randomized Patients	337	352
Per Protocol Patients	211	231
Clinical Response at 5 to 9 Days Post-Treatment	95.7% (202/211)	92.6% (214/231)
	95% CI [−1.3%, 7.3%]	
Bacteriologic Eradication by Patient at 5 to 9 Days Post-Treatment*	84.4% (178/211)	78.3% (181/231)
	95% CI [−1.3%, 13.1%]	
Bacteriologic Eradication of the Baseline Pathogen at 5 to 9 Days Post-Treatment		
Escherichia coli	156/178 (88%)	161/179 (90%)

* Patients with baseline pathogen(s) eradicated and no new infections or superinfections/total number of patients. There were 5.5% (6/211) ciprofloxacin and 9.5% (22/231) comparator patients with superinfections or new infections.

Continued on next page

Cipro I.V.—Cont.

no nephropathological changes were noted; however, nephropathy was observed after dosing at 20 mg/kg/day for the same duration (approximately 0.2-times the highest recommended therapeutic dose based upon mg/m²).

In dogs, ciprofloxacin administered at 3 and 10 mg/kg by rapid intravenous injection (15 sec.) produces pronounced hypotensive effects. These effects are considered to be related to histamine release because they are partially antagonized by pyrilamine, an antihistamine. In rhesus monkeys, rapid intravenous injection also produces hypotension, but the effect in this species is inconsistent and less pronounced. In mice, concomitant administration of nonsteroidal anti-inflammatory drugs, such as phenylbutazone and indomethacin, with quinolones has been reported to enhance the CNS stimulatory effect of quinolones.

Ocular toxicity, seen with some related drugs, has not been observed in ciprofloxacin-treated animals.

INHALATIONAL ANTHRAX – ADDITIONAL INFORMATION

The mean serum concentrations of ciprofloxacin associated with a statistically significant improvement in survival in the rhesus monkey model of inhalational anthrax are reached or exceeded in adult and pediatric patients receiving oral and intravenous regimens. (See **DOSAGE AND ADMINISTRATION**.) Ciprofloxacin pharmacokinetics have been evaluated in various human populations.The mean peak serum concentration achieved at steady-state in human adults receiving 500 mg orally every 12 hours is 2.97 µg/mL, and 4.56 µg/mL following 400 mg intravenously every 12 hours. The mean trough serum concentration at steady-state for both of these regimens is 0.2 µg/mL. In a study of 10 pediatric patients between 6 and 16 years of age, the mean peak plasma concentration achieved is 8.3 µg/mL and trough concentrations range from 0.09 to 0.26 µg/mL, following two 30-minute intravenous infusions of 10 mg/kg administered 12 hours apart. After the second intravenous infusion patients switched to 15 mg/kg orally every 12 hours achieve a mean peak concentration of 3.6 µg/mL after the initial oral dose. Long-term safety data, including effects on cartilage, following the administration of ciprofloxacin to pediatric patients are limited. (For additional information, see **PRECAUTIONS, Pediatric Use**.) Ciprofloxacin serum concentrations achieved in humans serve as a surrogate endpoint reasonably likely to predict clinical benefit and provide the basis for this indication.[4]

A placebo-controlled animal study in rhesus monkeys exposed to an inhaled mean dose of 11 LD_{50} (~5.5 × 10^5) spores (range 5–30 LD_{50}) of *B. anthracis* was conducted. The minimal inhibitory concentration (MIC) of ciprofloxacin for the anthrax strain used in this study was 0.08 µg/mL. In the animals studied, mean serum concentrations of ciprofloxacin achieved at expected T_{max} (1 hour post-dose) following oral dosing to steady-state ranged from 0.98 to 1.69 µg/mL. Mean steady-state trough concentrations at 12 hours post-dose ranged from 0.12 to 0.19 µg/mL[5]. Mortality due to anthrax for animals that received a 30-day regimen of oral ciprofloxacin beginning 24 hours post-exposure was significantly lower (1/9), compared to the placebo group (9/10) [p=0.001]. The one ciprofloxacin-treated animal that died of anthrax did so following the 30-day drug administration period.[6]

CLINICAL STUDIES

EMPIRICAL THERAPY IN ADULT FEBRILE NEUTROPENIC PATIENTS

The safety and efficacy of ciprofloxacin, 400 mg I.V. q 8h, in combination with piperacillin sodium, 50 mg/kg I.V. q 4h, for the empirical therapy of febrile neutropenic patients were studied in one large pivotal multicenter, randomized trial and were compared to those of tobramycin, 2 mg/kg I.V. q 8h, in combination with piperacillin sodium, 50 mg/kg I.V. q 4h.

Clinical response rates observed in this study were as follows:

[See fourth table on previous page]

Complicated Urinary Tract Infection and Pyelonephritis – Efficacy in Pediatric Patients:

NOTE: Although effective in clinical trials, ciprofloxacin is not a drug of first choice in the pediatric population due to an increased incidence of adverse events compared to controls, including events related to joints and/or surrounding tissues.

Ciprofloxacin, administered I.V. and/or orally, was compared to a cephalosporin for treatment of complicated urinary tract infections (cUTI) and pyelonephritis in pediatric patients 1 to 17 years of age (mean age of 6 ± 4 years). The trial was conducted in the US, Canada, Argentina, Peru, Costa Rica, Mexico, South Africa, and Germany. The duration of therapy was 10 to 21 days (mean duration of treatment was 11 days with a range of 1 to 88 days). The primary objective of the study was to assess musculoskeletal and neurological safety.

Patients were evaluated for clinical success and bacteriological eradication of the baseline organism(s) with no new infection or superinfection at 5 to 9 days post-therapy (Test of Cure or TOC). The Per Protocol population had a causative organism(s) with protocol specified colony count(s) at baseline, no protocol violation, and no premature discontinuation or loss to follow-up (among other criteria).

The clinical success and bacteriologic eradication rates in the Per Protocol population were similar between ciprofloxacin and the comparator group as shown below.

[See fifth table on previous page]

REFERENCES

1. National Committee for Clinical Laboratory Standards, Methods for Dilution Antimicrobial Susceptibility Tests for Bacteria That Grow Aerobically - Fifth Edition. Approved Standard NCCLS Document M7-A5, Vol. 20, No. 2, NCCLS, Wayne, PA, January, 2000. 2. National Committee for Clinical Laboratory Standards, Performance Standards for Antimicrobial Disk Susceptibility Tests - Seventh Edition. Approved Standard NCCLS Document M2-A7, Vol. 20, No. 1, NCCLS, Wayne, PA, January, 2000. 3. Report presented at the FDA's Anti-Infective Drug and Dermatological Drug Products Advisory Committee Meeting, March 31, 1993, Silver Spring, MD. Report available from FDA, CDER, Advisors and Consultants Staff, HFD-21, 1901 Chapman Avenue, Room 200, Rockville, MD 20852, USA. 4. 21 CFR 314.510 (Subpart H – Accelerated Approval of New Drugs for Life-Threatening Illnesses). 5. Kelly DJ, et al. Serum concentrations of penicillin, doxycycline, and ciprofloxacin during prolonged therapy in rhesus monkeys. J Infect Dis 1992; 166: 1184–7. 6. Friedlander AM, et al. Postexposure prophylaxis against experimental inhalational anthrax. J Infect Dis 1993; 167: 1239–42. 7. Friedman J, Polifka J. Teratogenic effects of drugs: a resource for clinicians (TERIS). Baltimore, Maryland: Johns Hopkins University Press, 2000:149–195. 8. Loebstein R, Addis A, Ho E, et al. Pregnancy outcome following gestational exposure to fluoroquinolones: a multicenter prospective controlled study. Antimicrob Agents Chemother. 1998;42(6): 1336–1339. 9. Schaefer C, Amoura-Elefant E, Vial T, et al. Pregnancy outcome after prenatal quinolone exposure. Evaluation of a case registry of the European network of teratology information services (ENTIS). Eur J Obstet Gynecol Reprod Biol. 1996;69:83–89.

Bayer HealthCare
Bayer Pharmaceuticals Corporation
400 Morgan Lane
West Haven, CT 06516 USA
℞ Only
08724752, R.6 4/04

EN-0050 BAY q 3939 5202-4-A-U.S.-12
Printed In U.S.A.

CIPRO® XR ℞

[sĭ'prō]

(ciprofloxacin* extended-release tablets)

Prescribing information for this product, which appears on pages 853–857 of the 2004 PDR, has been completely revised as follows. Please write "See Supplement A" next to the product heading.

To reduce the development of drug-resistant bacteria and maintain the effectiveness of CIPRO® XR and other antibacterial drugs, CIPRO XR should be used only to treat or prevent infections that are proven or strongly suspected to be caused by bacteria.

DESCRIPTION

CIPRO XR (ciprofloxacin* extended-release tablets) contains ciprofloxacin, a synthetic broad-spectrum antimicrobial agent for oral administration. CIPRO XR tablets are coated, bilayer tablets consisting of an immediate-release layer and an erosion-matrix type controlled-release layer. The tablets contain a combination of two types of ciprofloxacin drug substance, ciprofloxacin hydrochloride and ciprofloxacin betaine (base). Ciprofloxacin hydrochloride is 1-cyclopropyl-6-fluoro-1, 4-dihydro-4-oxo-7-(1-piperazinyl)-3-quinolinecarboxylic acid hydrochloride. It is provided as a mixture of the monohydrate and the sesquihydrate. The empirical formula of the monohydrate is $C_{17}H_{18}FN_3O_3 \bullet HCl \bullet H_2O$ and its molecular weight is 385.8. The empirical formula of the sesquihydrate is $C_{17}H_{18}FN_3O_3 \bullet HCl \bullet 1.5\ H_2O$ and its molecular weight is 394.8. The drug substance is a faintly yellowish to light yellow crystalline substance. The chemical structure of the monohydrate is as follows:

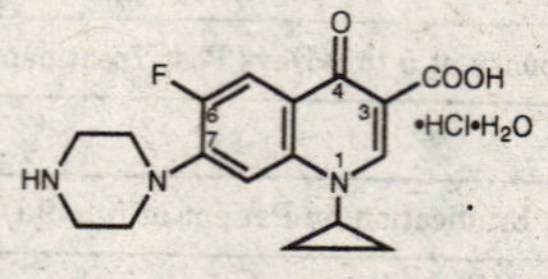

Ciprofloxacin betaine is 1-cyclopropyl-6-fluoro-1, 4-dihydro-4-oxo-7-(1-piperazinyl)-3-quinolinecarboxylic acid. As a hydrate, its empirical formula is $C_{17}H_{18}FN_3O_3 \bullet 3.5\ H_2O$ and its molecular weight is 394.3. It is a pale yellowish to light yellow crystalline substance and its chemical structure is as follows:

[See chemical structure at top of next column]

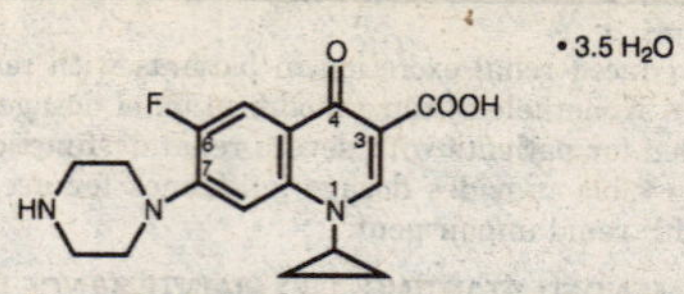

CIPRO XR is available in 500 mg and 1000 mg (ciprofloxacin equivalent) tablet strengths. CIPRO XR tablets are nearly white to slightly yellowish, film-coated, oblong-shaped tablets. Each CIPRO XR 500 mg tablet contains 500 mg of ciprofloxacin as ciprofloxacin HCl (287.5 mg, calculated as ciprofloxacin on the dried basis) and ciprofloxacin† (212.6 mg, calculated on the dried basis). Each CIPRO XR 1000 mg tablet contains 1000 mg of ciprofloxacin as ciprofloxacin HCl (574.9 mg, calculated as ciprofloxacin on the dried basis) and ciprofloxacin† (425.2 mg, calculated on the dried basis). The inactive ingredients are crospovidone, hypromellose, magnesium stearate, polyethylene glycol, silica colloidal anhydrous, succinic acid, and titanium dioxide.

* as ciprofloxacin † and ciprofloxacin hydrochloride
† does not comply with the loss on drying test and residue on ignition test of the USP monograph.

CLINICAL PHARMACOLOGY

Absorption

CIPRO XR tablets are formulated to release drug at a slower rate compared to immediate-release tablets. Approximately 35% of the dose is contained within an immediate-release component, while the remaining 65% is contained in a slow-release matrix.

Maximum plasma ciprofloxacin concentrations are attained between 1 and 4 hours after dosing with CIPRO XR. In comparison to the 250 mg and 500 mg ciprofloxacin immediate-release BID treatment, the C_{max} of CIPRO XR 500 mg and 1000 mg once daily are higher than the corresponding BID doses, while the AUCs over 24 hours are equivalent.

The following table compares the pharmacokinetic parameters obtained at steady state for these four treatment regimens (500 mg QD CIPRO XR versus 250 mg BID ciprofloxacin immediate-release tablets and 1000 mg QD CIPRO XR versus 500 mg BID ciprofloxacin immediate-release).

[See table below]

Results of the pharmacokinetic studies demonstrate that CIPRO XR may be administered with or without food (e.g. high-fat and low-fat meals or under fasted conditions).

Distribution

The volume of distribution calculated for intravenous ciprofloxacin is approximately 2.1–2.7 L/kg. Studies with the oral and intravenous forms of ciprofloxacin have demonstrated penetration of ciprofloxacin into a variety of tissues. The binding of ciprofloxacin to serum proteins is 20% to 40%, which is not likely to be high enough to cause significant protein binding interactions with other drugs. Following administration of a single dose of CIPRO XR, ciprofloxacin concentrations in urine collected up to 4 hours after dosing averaged over 300 mg/L for both the 500 mg and 1000 mg tablets; in urine excreted from 12 to 24 hours after dosing, ciprofloxacin concentration averaged 27 mg/L for the 500 mg tablet, and 58 mg/L for the 1000 mg tablet.

Metabolism

Four metabolites of ciprofloxacin were identified in human urine. The metabolites have antimicrobial activity, but are less active than unchanged ciprofloxacin. The primary metabolites are oxociprofloxacin (M3) and sulfociprofloxacin (M2), each accounting for roughly 3% to 8% of the total dose. Other minor metabolites are desethylene ciprofloxacin (M1), and formylciprofloxacin (M4). The relative proportion of drug and metabolite in serum corresponds to the composition found in urine. Excretion of these metabolites was essentially complete by 24 hours after dosing.

Elimination

The elimination kinetics of ciprofloxacin are similar for the immediate-release and the CIPRO XR tablet. In studies comparing the CIPRO XR and immediate-release ciprofloxacin, approximately 35% of an orally administered dose was excreted in the urine as unchanged drug for both formulations. The urinary excretion of ciprofloxacin is virtually complete within 24 hours after dosing. The renal clearance of ciprofloxacin, which is approximately 300 mL/minute, exceeds the normal glomerular filtration rate of 120 mL/minute. Thus, active tubular secretion would seem to play a significant role in its elimination. Co-administration of probenecid with immediate-release ciprofloxacin results in about a 50% reduction in the ciprofloxacin renal clearance and a 50% increase in its concentration in the systemic circulation. Although bile concentrations of ciprofloxacin are several fold higher than serum concentrations after oral dosing with the immediate-release tablet, only a small amount of the dose administered is recovered

Ciprofloxacin Pharmacokinetics (Mean ± SD) Following CIPRO® and CIPRO XR Administration

	C_{max} (mg/L)	AUC_{0-24h} (mg•h/L)	$T_{1/2}$(hr)	T_{max}(hr)§
CIPRO XR 500 mg QD	1.59 ± 0.43	7.97 ± 1.87	6.6 ± 1.4	1.5 (1.0–2.5)
CIPRO 250 mg BID	1.14 ± 0.23	8.25 ± 2.15	4.8 ± 0.6	1.0 (0.5–2.5)
CIPRO XR 1000 mg QD	3.11 ± 1.08	16.83 ± 5.65	6.31 ± 0.72	2.0 (1–4)
CIPRO 500 mg BID	2.06 ± 0.41	17.04 ± 4.79	5.66 ± 0.89	2.0 (0.5–3.5)

§ median (range)

from the bile as unchanged drug. An additional 1% to 2% of the dose is recovered from the bile in the form of metabolites. Approximately 20% to 35% of an oral dose of immediate-release ciprofloxacin is recovered from the feces within 5 days after dosing. This may arise from either biliary clearance or transintestinal elimination.

Special Populations

Pharmacokinetic studies of the immediate-release oral tablet (single dose) and intravenous (single and multiple dose) forms of ciprofloxacin indicate that plasma concentrations of ciprofloxacin are higher in elderly subjects (> 65 years) as compared to young adults. C_{max} is increased 16% to 40%, and mean AUC is increased approximately 30%, which can be at least partially attributed to decreased renal clearance in the elderly. Elimination half-life is only slightly (~20%) prolonged in the elderly. These differences are not considered clinically significant. (See **PRECAUTIONS, Geriatric Use.**)

In patients with reduced renal function, the half-life of ciprofloxacin is slightly prolonged. No dose adjustment is required for patients with uncomplicated urinary tract infections receiving 500 mg CIPRO XR. For complicated urinary tract infection and acute uncomplicated pyelonephritis, where 1000 mg is the appropriate dose, the dosage of CIPRO XR should be reduced to CIPRO XR 500 mg q24h in patients with creatinine clearance below 30 mL/min. (See **DOSAGE AND ADMINISTRATION.**)

In studies in patients with stable chronic cirrhosis, no significant changes in ciprofloxacin pharmacokinetics have been observed. The kinetics of ciprofloxacin in patients with acute hepatic insufficiency, however, have not been fully elucidated. (See **DOSAGE AND ADMINISTRATION.**)

Drug-drug Interactions

Previous studies with immediate-release ciprofloxacin have shown that concomitant administration of ciprofloxacin with theophylline decreases the clearance of theophylline resulting in elevated serum theophylline levels and increased risk of a patient developing CNS or other adverse reactions. Ciprofloxacin also decreases caffeine clearance and inhibits the formation of paraxanthine after caffeine administration. Absorption of ciprofloxacin is significantly reduced by concomitant administration of multivalent cation-containing products such as magnesium/aluminum antacids, sucralfate, VIDEX® (didanosine) chewable/buffered tablets or pediatric powder, or products containing calcium, iron, or zinc. (See **PRECAUTIONS, Drug Interactions** and **Information for Patients,** and **DOSAGE AND ADMINISTRATION.**)

Antacids: When CIPRO XR given as a single 1000 mg dose was administered two hours before, or four hours after a magnesium/aluminum-containing antacid (900 mg aluminum hydroxide and 600 mg magnesium hydroxide as a single oral dose) to 18 healthy volunteers, there was a 4% and 19% reduction, respectively, in the mean C_{max} of ciprofloxacin. The reduction in the mean AUC was 24% and 26%, respectively. CIPRO XR should be administered at least 2 hours before or 6 hours after antacids containing magnesium or aluminum, as well as sucralfate, VIDEX® (didanosine) chewable/buffered tablets or pediatric powder, metal cations such as iron, and multivitamin preparations with zinc. Although CIPRO XR may be taken with meals that include milk, concomitant administration with dairy products or with calcium-fortified juices alone should be avoided, since decreased absorption is possible. (See **PRECAUTIONS, Information for Patients** and **Drug Interactions,** and **DOSAGE AND ADMINISTRATION.**)

Omeprazole: When CIPRO XR was administered as a single 1000 mg dose concomitantly with omeprazole (40 mg once daily for three days) to 18 healthy volunteers, the mean AUC and C_{max} of ciprofloxacin were reduced by 20% and 23%, respectively. The clinical significance of this interaction has not been determined. (See **PRECAUTIONS, Drug Interactions.**)

MICROBIOLOGY

Ciprofloxacin has *in vitro* activity against a wide range of gram-negative and gram-positive organisms. The bactericidal action of ciprofloxacin results from inhibition of topoisomerase II (DNA gyrase) and topoisomerase IV (both Type II topoisomerases), which are required for bacterial DNA replication, transcription, repair, and recombination. The mechanism of action of quinolones, including ciprofloxacin, is different from that of other antimicrobial agents such as beta-lactams, macrolides, tetracyclines, or aminoglycosides; therefore, organisms resistant to these drugs may be susceptible to ciprofloxacin. There is no known cross-resistance between ciprofloxacin and other classes of antimicrobials. Resistance to ciprofloxacin *in vitro* develops slowly (multiple-step mutation). Resistance to ciprofloxacin due to spontaneous mutations occurs at a general frequency of between $< 10^{-9}$ to 1×10^{-6}.

Ciprofloxacin is slightly less active when tested at acidic pH. The inoculum size has little effect when tested *in vitro*. The minimal bactericidal concentration (MBC) generally does not exceed the minimal inhibitory concentration (MIC) by more than a factor of 2.

Ciprofloxacin has been shown to be active against most strains of the following microorganisms, both *in vitro* and in clinical infections as described in the **INDICATIONS AND USAGE** section.

Aerobic gram-positive microorganisms
Enterococcus faecalis (Many strains are only moderately susceptible.)
Staphylococcus saprophyticus

Aerobic gram-negative microorganisms
Escherichia coli
Klebsiella pneumoniae
Proteus mirabilis
Pseudomonas aeruginosa

The following *in vitro* data are available, but their clinical significance is unknown.

Ciprofloxacin exhibits *in vitro* minimum inhibitory concentrations (MICs) of 1 μg/mL or less against most (≥ 90%) strains of the following microorganisms; however, the safety and effectiveness of CIPRO XR in treating clinical infections due to these microorganisms have not been established in adequate and well-controlled clinical trials.

Aerobic gram-negative microorganisms
Citrobacter koseri
Citrobacter freundii
Edwardsiella tarda
Enterobacter aerogenes
Enterobacter cloacae
Klebsiella oxytoca
Morganella morganii
Proteus vulgaris
Providencia rettgeri
Providencia stuartii
Serratia marcescens

Susceptibility Tests

Dilution Techniques: Quantitative methods are used to determine antimicrobial minimal inhibitory concentrations (MICs). These MICs provide estimates of the susceptibility of bacteria to antimicrobial compounds. The MICs should be determined using a standardized procedure. Standardized procedures are based on a dilution method[1] (broth or agar) or equivalent with standardized inoculum concentrations and standardized concentrations of ciprofloxacin. The MIC values should be interpreted according to the following criteria:

For testing *Enterobacteriaceae, Enterococcus* species, *Pseudomonas aeruginosa,* and *Staphylococcus* species:

MIC (μg/mL)	Interpretation
≤ 1	Susceptible (S)
2	Intermediate (I)
≥ 4	Resistant (R)

A report of "Susceptible" indicates that the pathogen is likely to be inhibited if the antimicrobial compound in the blood reaches the concentrations usually achievable. A report of "Intermediate" indicates that the result should be considered equivocal, and, if the microorganism is not fully susceptible to alternative, clinically feasible drugs, the test should be repeated. This category implies possible clinical applicability in body sites where the drug is physiologically concentrated or in situations where high dosage of drug can be used. This category also provides a buffer zone which prevents small uncontrolled technical factors from causing major discrepancies in interpretation. A report of "Resistant" indicates that the pathogen is not likely to be inhibited if the antimicrobial compound in the blood reaches the concentrations usually achievable; other therapy should be selected.

Standardized susceptibility test procedures require the use of laboratory control microorganisms to control the technical aspects of the laboratory procedures. Standard ciprofloxacin powder should provide the following MIC values:

Microorganism		MIC Range (μg/mL)
Enterococcus faecalis	ATCC 29212	0.25 – 2.0
Escherichia coli	ATCC 25922	0.004 – 0.015
Staphylococcus aureus	ATCC 29213	0.12 – 0.5
Pseudomonas aeruginosa	ATCC 27853	0.25 – 1

Diffusion Techniques: Quantitative methods that require measurement of zone diameters also provide reproducible estimates of the susceptibility of bacteria to antimicrobial compounds. One such standardized procedure[2] requires the use of standardized inoculum concentrations. This procedure uses paper disks impregnated with 5-μg ciprofloxacin to test the susceptibility of microorganisms to ciprofloxacin. Reports from the laboratory providing results of the standard single-disk susceptibility test with a 5-μg ciprofloxacin disk should be interpreted according to the following criteria:

For testing *Enterobacteriaceae, Enterococcus* species, *Pseudomonas aeruginosa,* and *Staphylococcus* species:

Zone Diameter (mm)	Interpretation
≥ 21	Susceptible (S)
16–20	Intermediate (I)
≤ 15	Resistant (R)

Interpretation should be as stated above for results using dilution techniques. Interpretation involves correlation of the diameter obtained in the disk test with the MIC for ciprofloxacin.

As with standardized dilution techniques, diffusion methods require the use of laboratory control microorganisms that are used to control the technical aspects of the laboratory procedures. For the diffusion technique, the 5-μg ciprofloxacin disk should provide the following zone diameters in these laboratory test quality control strains:

Microorganism		Zone Diameter (mm)
Escherichia coli	ATCC 25922	30 – 40
Staphylococcus aureus	ATCC 25923	22 – 30
Pseudomonas aeruginosa	ATCC 27853	25 – 33

INDICATIONS AND USAGE

CIPRO XR is indicated only for the treatment of urinary tract infections, including acute uncomplicated pyelonephritis, caused by susceptible strains of the designated microorganisms as listed below. CIPRO XR and ciprofloxacin immediate-release tablets are not interchangeable. Please see **DOSAGE AND ADMINISTRATION** for specific recommendations.

Uncomplicated Urinary Tract Infections (Acute Cystitis) caused by *Escherichia coli, Proteus mirabilis, Enterococcus faecalis,* or *Staphylococcus saprophyticus*[a].

Complicated Urinary Tract Infections caused by *Escherichia coli, Klebsiella pneumoniae, Enterococcus faecalis, Proteus mirabilis,* or *Pseudomonas aeruginosa* [a].

Acute Uncomplicated Pyelonephritis caused by *Escherichia coli.*

[a] Treatment of infections due to this organism in the organ system was studied in fewer than 10 patients.

THE SAFETY AND EFFICACY OF CIPRO XR IN TREATING INFECTIONS OTHER THAN URINARY TRACT INFECTIONS HAS NOT BEEN DEMONSTRATED.

Appropriate culture and susceptibility tests should be performed before treatment in order to isolate and identify organisms causing infection and to determine their susceptibility to ciprofloxacin. Therapy with CIPRO XR may be initiated before results of these tests are known; once results become available appropriate therapy should be continued. Culture and susceptibility testing performed periodically during therapy will provide information not only on the therapeutic effect of the antimicrobial agent but also on the possible emergence of bacterial resistance.

To reduce the development of drug-resistant bacteria and maintain the effectiveness of CIPRO XR and other antibacterial drugs, CIPRO XR should be used only to treat or prevent infections that are proven or strongly suspected to be caused by susceptible bacteria. When culture and susceptibility information are available, they should be considered in selecting or modifying antibacterial therapy. In the absence of such data, local epidemiology and susceptibility patterns may contribute to the empiric selection of therapy.

CONTRAINDICATIONS

CIPRO XR is contraindicated in persons with a history of hypersensitivity to ciprofloxacin or any member of the quinolone class of antimicrobial agents.

WARNINGS

THE SAFETY AND EFFECTIVENESS OF CIPRO XR IN PEDIATRIC PATIENTS AND ADOLESCENTS (UNDER THE AGE OF 18 YEARS), PREGNANT WOMEN, AND NURSING WOMEN HAVE NOT BEEN ESTABLISHED. (See **PRECAUTIONS: Pediatric Use, Pregnancy,** and **Nursing Mothers** subsections.) The oral administration of ciprofloxacin caused lameness in immature dogs. Histopathological examination of the weight-bearing joints of these dogs revealed permanent lesions of the cartilage. Related quinolone-class drugs also produce erosions of cartilage of weight-bearing joints and other signs of arthropathy in immature animals of various species. (See **ANIMAL PHARMACOLOGY.**)

Convulsions, increased intracranial pressure, and toxic psychosis have been reported in patients receiving quinolones, including ciprofloxacin. Ciprofloxacin may also cause central nervous system (CNS) events including: dizziness, confusion, tremors, hallucinations, depression, and, rarely, suicidal thoughts or acts. These reactions may occur following the first dose. If these reactions occur in patients receiving ciprofloxacin, the drug should be discontinued and appropriate measures instituted. As with all quinolones, ciprofloxacin should be used with caution in patients with known or suspected CNS disorders that may predispose to seizures or lower the seizure threshold (e.g. severe cerebral arteriosclerosis, epilepsy), or in the presence of other risk factors that may predispose to seizures or lower the seizure threshold (e.g. certain drug therapy, renal dysfunction). (See **PRECAUTIONS: General, Information for Patients, Drug Interactions** and **ADVERSE REACTIONS.**)

SERIOUS AND FATAL REACTIONS HAVE BEEN REPORTED IN PATIENTS RECEIVING CONCURRENT ADMINISTRATION OF CIPROFLOXACIN AND THEOPHYLLINE. These reactions have included cardiac arrest, seizure, status epilepticus, and respiratory failure. Although similar serious adverse effects have been reported in patients receiving theophylline alone, the possibility that these reactions may be potentiated by ciprofloxacin cannot be eliminated. If concomitant use cannot be avoided, serum levels of theophylline should be monitored and dosage adjustments made as appropriate.

Serious and occasionally fatal hypersensitivity (anaphylactic) reactions, some following the first dose, have been reported in patients receiving quinolone therapy. Some reactions were accompanied by cardiovascular collapse, loss of consciousness, tingling, pharyngeal or facial edema, dyspnea, urticaria, and itching. Only a few patients had a history of hypersensitivity reactions. Serious anaphylactic reactions require immediate emergency treatment with epinephrine. Oxygen, intravenous steroids, and airway management, including intubation, should be administered as indicated.

Continued on next page

Cipro XR—Cont.

Severe hypersensitivity reactions characterized by rash, fever, eosinophilia, jaundice, and hepatic necrosis with fatal outcome have also been rarely reported in patients receiving ciprofloxacin along with other drugs. The possibility that these reactions were related to ciprofloxacin cannot be excluded. Ciprofloxacin should be discontinued at the first appearance of a skin rash or any other sign of hypersensitivity.

Pseudomembranous colitis has been reported with nearly all antibacterial agents, including ciprofloxacin, and may range in severity from mild to life-threatening. Therefore, it is important to consider this diagnosis in patients who present with diarrhea subsequent to the administration of antibacterial agents.

Treatment with antibacterial agents alters the normal flora of the colon and may permit overgrowth of clostridia. Studies indicate that a toxin produced by *Clostridium difficile* is one primary cause of "antibiotic-associated colitis."

If a diagnosis of pseudomembranous colitis is established, therapeutic measures should be initiated. Mild cases of pseudomembranous colitis usually respond to drug discontinuation alone. In moderate to severe cases, consideration should be given to management with fluids and electrolytes, protein supplementation, and treatment with an antibacterial drug clinically effective against *C difficile* colitis. Drugs that inhibit peristalsis should be avoided.

Peripheral neuropathy: Rare cases of sensory or sensorimotor axonal polyneuropathy affecting small and/or large axons resulting in paresthesias, hypoesthesias, dysesthesias and weakness have been reported in patients receiving quinolones, including ciprofloxacin. Ciprofloxacin should be discontinued if the patient experiences symptoms of neuropathy including pain, burning, tingling, numbness, and/or weakness, or is found to have deficits in light touch, pain, temperature, position sense, vibratory sensation, and/or motor strength in order to prevent the development of an irreversible condition.

Tendon Effects: Ruptures of the shoulder, hand, Achilles tendon or other tendons that required surgical repair or resulted in prolonged disability have been reported in patients receiving quinolones, including ciprofloxacin. Post-marketing surveillance reports indicate that this risk may be increased in patients receiving concomitant corticosteroids, especially the elderly. Ciprofloxacin should be discontinued if the patient experiences pain, inflammation, or rupture of a tendon. Patients should rest and refrain from exercise until the diagnosis of tendonitis or tendon rupture has been excluded. Tendon rupture can occur during or after therapy with quinolones, including ciprofloxacin.

PRECAUTIONS

General: Crystals of ciprofloxacin have been observed rarely in the urine of human subjects but more frequently in the urine of laboratory animals, which is usually alkaline. (See **ANIMAL PHARMACOLOGY.**) Crystalluria related to ciprofloxacin has been reported only rarely in humans because human urine is usually acidic. Alkalinity of the urine should be avoided in patients receiving ciprofloxacin. Patients should be well hydrated to prevent the formation of highly concentrated urine.

Quinolones, including ciprofloxacin, may also cause central nervous system (CNS) events, including: nervousness, agitation, insomnia, anxiety, nightmares or paranoia. (See **WARNINGS Information for Patients**, and **Drug Interactions.**)

Moderate to severe phototoxicity manifested as an exaggerated sunburn reaction has been observed in patients who are exposed to direct sunlight while receiving some members of the quinolone class of drugs. Excessive sunlight should be avoided. Therapy should be discontinued if phototoxicity occurs.

Prescribing CIPRO XR in the absence of a proven or strongly suspected bacterial infection or a prophylactic indication is unlikely to provide benefit to the patient and increases the risk of the development of drug-resistant bacteria.

Information for Patients:

Patients should be advised:

- that antibacterial drugs including CIPRO XR should only be used to treat bacterial infections. They do not treat viral infections (e.g., the common cold). When CIPRO XR is prescribed to treat a bacterial infection, patients should be told that although it is common to feel better early in the course of therapy, the medication should be taken exactly as directed. Skipping doses or not completing the full course of therapy may (1) decrease the effectiveness of the immediate treatment and (2) increase the likelihood that bacteria will develop resistance and will not be treatable by CIPRO XR or other antibacterial drugs in the future.
- that CIPRO XR may be taken with or without meals and to drink fluids liberally. As with other quinolones, concurrent administration with magnesium/aluminum antacids, or sucralfate, VIDEX® (didanosine) chewable/buffered tablets or pediatric powder, or with other products containing calcium, iron, or zinc should be avoided. CIPRO XR may be taken two hours before or six hours after taking these products. (See **CLINICAL PHARMACOLOGY, Drug-drug Interactions, DOSAGE AND ADMINISTRATION**, and **PRECAUTIONS, Drug Interactions.**) CIPRO XR should not be taken with dairy products (like milk or yogurt) or calcium-fortified juices alone since absorption of ciprofloxacin may be significantly reduced; however, CIPRO XR may be taken with a meal that contains these products. (See **CLINICAL PHARMACOLOGY, Drug-drug Interactions, DOSAGE AND ADMINISTRATION**, and **PRECAUTIONS, Drug Interactions.**)
- If the patient should forget to take CIPRO XR at the usual time, he/she may take the dose later in the day. Do not take more than one CIPRO XR tablet per day even if a patient misses a dose. Swallow the CIPRO XR tablet whole. **DO NOT SPLIT, CRUSH, OR CHEW THE TABLET.**
- that ciprofloxacin may be associated with hypersensitivity reactions, even following a single dose, and to discontinue CIPRO XR at the first sign of a skin rash or other allergic reaction.
- to avoid excessive sunlight or artificial ultraviolet light while receiving CIPRO XR and to discontinue therapy if phototoxicity occurs.
- that peripheral neuropathies have been associated with ciprofloxacin use. If symptoms of peripheral neuropathy including pain, burning, tingling, numbness and/or weakness develop, they should discontinue treatment and contact their physicians.
- that if they experience pain, inflammation, or rupture of a tendon to discontinue treatment, to inform their physician, and to rest and refrain from exercise.
- that CIPRO XR may cause dizziness and lightheadedness; therefore, patients should know how they react to this drug before they operate an automobile or machinery or engage in activities requiring mental alertness or coordination.
- that CIPRO XR may increase the effects of theophylline and caffeine. There is a possibility of caffeine accumulation when products containing caffeine are consumed while taking quinolones.
- that convulsions have been reported in patients receiving quinolones, including ciprofloxacin, and to notify their physician before taking CIPRO XR if there is a history of this condition.

Drug Interactions: As with some other quinolones, concurrent administration of ciprofloxacin with theophylline may lead to elevated serum concentrations of theophylline and prolongation of its elimination half-life. This may result in increased risk of theophylline-related adverse reactions. (See **WARNINGS.**) If concomitant use cannot be avoided, serum levels of theophylline should be monitored and dosage adjustments made as appropriate.

Some quinolones, including ciprofloxacin, have also been shown to interfere with the metabolism of caffeine. This may lead to reduced clearance of caffeine and a prolongation of its serum half-life.

Concurrent administration of a quinolone, including ciprofloxacin, with multivalent cation-containing products such as magnesium/aluminum antacids, sucralfate, VIDEX® (didanosine) chewable/buffered tablets or pediatric powder, or products containing calcium, iron, or zinc may substantially interfere with the absorption of the quinolone, resulting in serum and urine levels considerably lower than desired. CIPRO XR should be administered at least 2 hours before or 6 hours after antacids containing magnesium or aluminum, as well as sucralfate, VIDEX® (didanosine) chewable/buffered tablets or pediatric powder, metal cations such as iron, and multivitamin preparations with zinc. (See **CLINICAL PHARMACOLOGY, Drug-drug Interactions, PRECAUTIONS, Information for Patients**, and **DOSAGE AND ADMINISTRATION.**)

Histamine H_2-receptor antagonists appear to have no significant effect on the bioavailability of ciprofloxacin.

Absorption of the CIPRO XR tablet was slightly diminished (20%) when given concomitantly with omeprazole. (See **CLINICAL PHARMACOLOGY, Drug-drug Interactions.**)

Altered serum levels of phenytoin (increased and decreased) have been reported in patients receiving concomitant ciprofloxacin.

The concomitant administration of ciprofloxacin with the sulfonylurea glyburide has, on rare occasions, resulted in severe hypoglycemia.

Some quinolones, including ciprofloxacin, have been associated with transient elevations in serum creatinine in patients receiving cyclosporine concomitantly.

Quinolones, including ciprofloxacin, have been reported to enhance the effects of the oral anticoagulant warfarin or its derivatives. When these products are administered concomitantly, prothrombin time or other suitable coagulation tests should be closely monitored.

Probenecid interferes with renal tubular secretion of ciprofloxacin and produces an increase in the level of ciprofloxacin in the serum. This should be considered if patients are receiving both drugs concomitantly.

Renal tubular transport of methotrexate may be inhibited by concomitant administration of ciprofloxacin potentially leading to increased plasma levels of methotrexate. This might increase the risk of methotrexate associated toxic reactions. Therefore, patients under methotrexate therapy should be carefully monitored when concomitant ciprofloxacin therapy is indicated.

Metoclopramide significantly accelerates the absorption of oral ciprofloxacin resulting in a shorter time to reach maximum plasma concentrations. No significant effect was observed on the bioavailability of ciprofloxacin.

Non-steroidal anti-inflammatory drugs (but not acetyl salicylic acid) in combination of very high doses of quinolones have been shown to provoke convulsions in pre-clinical studies.

Carcinogenesis, Mutagenesis, Impairment of Fertility: Eight *in vitro* mutagenicity tests have been conducted with ciprofloxacin, and the test results are listed below:

Salmonella/Microsome Test (Negative)
E. coli DNA Repair Assay (Negative)
Mouse Lymphoma Cell Forward Mutation Assay (Positive)
Chinese Hamster V_{79} Cell HGPRT Test (Negative)
Syrian Hamster Embryo Cell Transformation Assay (Negative)
Saccharomyces cerevisiae Point Mutation Assay (Negative)
Saccharomyces cerevisiae Mitotic Crossover and Gene Conversion Assay (Negative)
Rat Hepatocyte DNA Repair Assay (Positive)

Thus, 2 of the 8 tests were positive, but results of the following 3 *in vivo* test systems gave negative results:

Rat Hepatocyte DNA Repair Assay
Micronucleus Test (Mice)
Dominant Lethal Test (Mice)

Ciprofloxacin was not carcinogenic or tumorigenic in 2-year carcinogenicity studies with rats and mice at daily oral dose levels of 250 and 750 mg/kg, respectively (approximately 2 and 3 -fold greater than the 1000 mg daily human dose based upon body surface area).

Results from photo co-carcinogenicity testing indicate that ciprofloxacin does not reduce the time to appearance of UV-induced skin tumors as compared to vehicle control. Hairless (Skh-1) mice were exposed to UVA light for 3.5 hours five times every two weeks for up to 78 weeks while concurrently being administered ciprofloxacin. The time to development of the first skin tumors was 50 weeks in mice treated concomitantly with UVA and ciprofloxacin (mouse dose approximately equal to the maximum recommended daily human dose of 1000 mg based upon mg/m^2), as opposed to 34 weeks when animals were treated with both UVA and vehicle. The times to development of skin tumors ranged from 16–32 weeks in mice treated concomitantly with UVA and other quinolones.

In this model, mice treated with ciprofloxacin alone did not develop skin or systemic tumors. There are no data from similar models using pigmented mice and/or fully haired mice. The clinical significance of these findings to humans is unknown.

Fertility studies performed in rats at oral doses of ciprofloxacin up to 100 mg/kg (1.0 times the highest recommended daily human dose of 1000 mg based upon body surface area) revealed no evidence of impairment.

Pregnancy: Teratogenic Effects. Pregnancy Category C: There are no adequate and well-controlled studies in pregnant women. An expert review of published data on experiences with ciprofloxacin use during pregnancy by TERIS - the Teratogen Information System – concluded that therapeutic doses during pregnancy are unlikely to pose a substantial teratogenic risk (quantity and quality of data=fair), but the data are insufficient to state there is no risk.

A controlled prospective observational study followed 200 women exposed to fluoroquinolones (52.5% exposed to ciprofloxacin and 68% first trimester exposures) during gestation. In utero exposure to fluoroquinolones during embryogenesis was not associated with increased risk of major malformations. The reported rates of major congenital malformations were 2.2% for the fluoroquinolone group and 2.6% for the control group (background incidence of major malformations is 1–5%). Rates of spontaneous abortions, prematurity and low birth weight did not differ between the groups and there were no clinically significant musculoskeletal dysfunctions up to one year of age in the ciprofloxacin exposed children.

Another prospective follow-up study reported on 549 pregnancies with fluoroquinolone exposure (93% first trimester exposures). There were 70 ciprofloxacin exposures, all within the first trimester. The malformation rates among live-born babies exposed to ciprofloxacin and to fluoroquinolones overall were both within background incidence ranges. No specific patterns of congenital abnormalities were found. The study did not reveal any clear adverse reactions due to in utero exposure to ciprofloxacin.

No differences in the rates of prematurity, spontaneous abortions, or birth weight were seen in women exposed to ciprofloxacin during pregnancy. However, these small postmarketing epidemiology studies, of which most experience is from short term, first trimester exposure, are insufficient to evaluate the risk for the less common defects or to permit reliable and definitive conclusions regarding the safety of ciprofloxacin in pregnant women and their developing fetuses. Ciprofloxacin should not be used during pregnancy unless potential benefit justifies the potential risk to both fetus and mother (see **WARNINGS**).

Reproduction studies have been performed in rats and mice using oral doses up to 100 mg/kg (0.7 and 0.4 times the maximum daily human dose of 1000 mg based upon body surface area, respectively) and have revealed no evidence of harm to the fetus due to ciprofloxacin. In rabbits, ciprofloxacin (30 and 100 mg/kg orally) produced gastrointestinal disturbances resulting in maternal weight loss and an increased incidence of abortion, but no teratogenicity was observed at either dose. After intravenous administration of doses up to 20 mg/kg, no maternal toxicity was produced in the rabbit, and no embryotoxicity or teratogenicity was observed.

Nursing Mothers: Ciprofloxacin is excreted in human milk. The amount of ciprofloxacin absorbed by the nursing infant is unknown. Because of the potential for serious adverse reactions in infants nursing from mothers taking ciprofloxacin, a decision should be made whether to discontinue nursing or to discontinue the drug, taking into account the importance of the drug to the mother.

Pediatric Use: Safety and effectiveness of CIPRO XR in pediatric patients and adolescents less than 18 years of age have not been established. Ciprofloxacin causes arthropathy in juvenile animals. (See **WARNINGS.**)

Geriatric Use: In a large, prospective, randomized CIPRO XR clinical trial in complicated urinary tract infections, 49% (509/1035) of the patients were 65 and over, while 30% (308/1035) were 75 and over. No overall differences in safety or effectiveness were observed between these subjects and younger subjects, and clinical experience with other formulations of ciprofloxacin has not identified differences in responses between the elderly and younger patients, but greater sensitivity of some older individuals cannot be ruled out. Ciprofloxacin is known to be substantially excreted by the kidney, and the risk of adverse reactions may be greater in patients with impaired renal function. No alteration of dosage is necessary for patients greater than 65 years of age with normal renal function. However, since some older individuals experience reduced renal function by virtue of their advanced age, care should be taken in dose selection for elderly patients, and renal function monitoring may be useful in these patients. (See **CLINICAL PHARMACOLOGY** and **DOSAGE AND ADMINISTRATION.**)

ADVERSE REACTIONS

Clinical trials in patients with urinary tract infections enrolled 961 patients treated with 500 mg or 1000 mg CIPRO XR. Most adverse events reported were described as mild to moderate in severity and required no treatment. The overall incidence, type and distribution of adverse events were similar in patients receiving both 500 mg and 1000 mg of CIPRO XR. Because clinical trials are conducted under widely varying conditions, adverse reaction rates observed in clinical trials of a drug cannot be directly compared to rates observed in clinical trials of another drug and may not reflect the rates observed in practice. The adverse reaction information from clinical studies does, however, provide a basis for identifying the adverse events that appear to be related to drug use and for approximating rates.

In the clinical trial of uncomplicated urinary tract infection, CIPRO XR (500 mg once daily) in 444 patients was compared to ciprofloxacin immediate-release tablets (250 mg twice daily) in 447 patients for 3 days. Discontinuations due to adverse reactions thought to be drug-related occurred in 0.2% (1/444) of patients in the CIPRO XR arm and in 0% (0/447) of patients in the control arm.

In the clinical trial of complicated urinary tract infection and acute uncomplicated pyelonephritis, CIPRO XR (1000 mg once daily) in 517 patients was compared to ciprofloxacin immediate-release tablets (500 mg twice daily) in 518 patients for 7 to 14 days. Discontinuations due to adverse reactions thought to be drug-related occurred in 3.1% (16/517) of patients in the CIPRO XR arm and in 2.3% (12/518) of patients in the control arm. The most common reasons for discontinuation in the CIPRO XR arm were nausea/vomiting (4 patients) and dizziness (3 patients). In the control arm the most common reason for discontinuation was nausea/vomiting (3 patients).

In these clinical trials, the following events occurred in ≥2% of all CIPRO XR patients, regardless of drug relationship: nausea (4%), headache (3%), dizziness (2%), diarrhea (2%), vomiting (2%) and vaginal moniliasis (2%).

Adverse events, judged by investigators to be at least possibly drug-related, occurring in greater than or equal to 1% of all CIPRO XR treated patients were: nausea (3%), diarrhea (2%), headache (1%), dyspepsia (1%), dizziness (1%), and vaginal moniliasis (1%). Vomiting (1%) occurred in the 1000 mg group.

Additional uncommon events, judged by investigators to be at least possibly drug-related, that occurred in less than 1% of CIPRO XR treated patients were:

BODY AS A WHOLE: abdominal pain, asthenia, malaise, photosensitivity reaction
CARDIOVASCULAR: bradycardia, migraine, syncope
DIGESTIVE: anorexia, constipation, dry mouth, flatulence, liver function tests abnormal, thirst
HEMIC/LYMPHATIC: prothrombin decrease
CENTRAL NERVOUS SYSTEM: abnormal dreams, depersonalization, depression, hypertonia, incoordination, insomnia, somnolence, tremor, vertigo
METABOLIC: hyperglycemia
SKIN/APPENDAGES: dry skin, maculopapular rash, pruritus, rash, skin disorder, urticaria, vesiculobullous rash
SPECIAL SENSES: diplopia, taste perversion
UROGENITAL: dysmenorrhea, hematuria, kidney function abnormal, vaginitis

The following additional adverse events, some of them life threatening, regardless of incidence or relationship to drug, have been reported during clinical trials and from worldwide post-marketing experience in patients given ciprofloxacin (includes all formulations, all dosages, all drug-therapy durations, and all indications). Because these reactions have been reported voluntarily from a population of uncertain size, it is not always possible to reliably estimate their frequency or a causal relationship to drug exposure. The events in alphabetical order are:

abnormal gait,achiness, acidosis, agitation, agranulocytosis, allergic reactions (ranging from urticaria to anaphylactic reactions), amylase increase, anemia, angina pectoris, angioedema, anosmia, anxiety, arrhythmia, arthralgia, ataxia, atrial flutter, bleeding diathesis, blurred vision, bronchospasm, *C difficile* associated diarrhea, candidiasis (cutaneous, oral), candiduria, cardiac murmur, cardiopulmonary arrest, cardiovascular collapse, cerebral thrombosis, chills, cholestatic jaundice, chromatopsia, confusion, convulsion, delirium, drowsiness, dysphagia, dysphasia, dyspnea, edema (conjunctivae, face, hands, laryngeal, lips, lower extremities, neck, pulmonary), epistaxis, erythema multiforme, erythema nodosum, exfoliative dermatitis, fever, fixed eruptions, flushing, gastrointestinal bleeding, gout (flare up), grand mal convulsion, gynecomastia, hallucinations, hearing loss, hemolytic anemia, hemoptysis, hemorrhagic cystitis, hepatic failure, hepatic necrosis, hepatitis, hiccup, hyperesthesia, hyperpigmentation, hypertension, hypertonia, hypesthesia, hypotension, ileus, interstitial nephritis, intestinal perforation, jaundice, joint stiffness, lethargy, lightheadedness, lipase increase, lymphadenopathy, manic reaction, marrow depression, migraine, moniliasis (oral, gastrointestinal, vaginal), myalgia, myasthenia, myasthenia gravis (possible exacerbation), myocardial infarction, myoclonus, nephritis, nightmares, nystagmus, oral ulceration, pain (arm, back, breast, chest, epigastric, eye, extremities, foot, jaw, neck, oral mucosa), palpitation, pancreatitis, pancytopenia, paranoia, paresthesia, peripheral neuropathy, perspiration (increased), petechia, phlebitis, phobia, pleural effusion, polyuria, postural hypotension, prothrombin time prolongation, pseudomembranous colitis (the onset of symptoms may occur during or after antimicrobial treatment), pulmonary embolism, purpura, renal calculi, renal failure, respiratory arrest, respiratory distress, restlessness, serum sickness-like reaction, Stevens-Johnson syndrome, sweating, tachycardia, taste loss, tendinitis, tendon rupture, tinnitus, torsade de pointes, toxic epidermal necrolysis, toxic psychosis, twitching, unresponsiveness, urethral bleeding, urinary retention, urination (frequent), vaginal pruritus, vasculitis, ventricular ectopy, vesicles, visual acuity (decreased), visual disturbances (flashing lights, change in color perception, overbrightness of lights).

Laboratory Changes:

The following adverse laboratory changes, in alphabetical order, regardless of incidence or relationship to drug, have been reported in patients given ciprofloxacin (includes all formulations, all dosages, all drug-therapy durations, and all indications):

Decreases in blood glucose, BUN, hematocrit, hemoglobin, leukocyte counts, platelet counts, prothrombin time, serum albumin, serum potassium, total serum protein, uric acid.

Increases in alkaline phosphatase, ALT (SGPT), AST (SGOT), atypical lymphocyte counts, blood glucose, blood monocytes, BUN, cholesterol, eosinophil counts, LDH, platelet counts, prothrombin time, sedimentation rate, serum amylase, serum bilirubin, serum calcium, serum cholesterol, serum creatine phosphokinase, serum creatinine, serum gamma-glutamyl transpeptidase (GGT), serum potassium, serum theophylline (in patients receiving theophylline concomitantly), serum triglycerides, uric acid.

Others: albuminuria, change in serum phenytoin, crystalluria, cylindruria, immature WBCs, leukocytosis, methemoglobinemia, pancytopenia.

OVERDOSAGE

In the event of acute excessive overdosage, reversible renal toxicity has been reported in some cases. The stomach should be emptied by inducing vomiting or by gastric lavage. The patient should be carefully observed and given supportive treatment, including administration of magnesium or calcium containing antacids which can reduce the absorption of ciprofloxacin. Adequate hydration must be maintained. Only a small amount of ciprofloxacin (< 10%) is removed from the body after hemodialysis or peritoneal dialysis.

In mice, rats, rabbits and dogs, significant toxicity including tonic/clonic convulsions was observed at intravenous doses of ciprofloxacin between 125 and 300 mg/kg.

Single doses of ciprofloxacin were relatively non-toxic via the oral route of administration in mice, rats, and dogs. No deaths occurred within a 14-day post treatment observation period at the highest oral doses tested; up to 5000 mg/kg in either rodent species, or up to 2500 mg/kg in the dog. Clinical signs observed included hypoactivity and cyanosis in both rodent species and severe vomiting in dogs. In rabbits, significant mortality was seen at doses of ciprofloxacin > 2500 mg/kg. Mortality was delayed in these animals, occurring 10–14 days after dosing.

DOSAGE AND ADMINISTRATION

CIPRO XR and ciprofloxacin immediate-release tablets are not interchangeable. Cipro XR should be administered orally once daily as described in the following Dosage Guidelines table:

[See table above]

DOSAGE GUIDELINES

Indication	Unit Dose	Frequency	Usual Duration
Uncomplicated Urinary Tract Infection (Acute Cystitis)	500 mg	Q24h	3 Days
Complicated Urinary Tract Infection	1000 mg	Q24h	7–14 Days
Acute Uncomplicated Pyelonephritis	1000 mg	Q24h	7–14 Days

Patients whose therapy is started with CIPRO I.V. for urinary tract infections may be switched to CIPRO XR when clinically indicated at the discretion of the physician.

CIPRO XR should be administered at least 2 hours before or 6 hours after antacids containing magnesium or aluminum, as well as sucralfate, VIDEX® (didanosine) chewable/buffered tablets or pediatric powder, metal cations such as iron, and multivitamin preparations with zinc. Although CIPRO XR may be taken with meals that include milk, concomitant administration with dairy products alone, or with calcium-fortified products should be avoided, since decreased absorption is possible. A 2-hour window between substantial calcium intake (> 800 mg) and dosing with CIPRO XR is recommended. CIPRO XR should be swallowed whole. **DO NOT SPLIT, CRUSH, OR CHEW THE TABLET.** (See **CLINICAL PHARMACOLOGY, Drug-drug Interactions, PRECAUTIONS, Drug Interactions** and **Information for Patients.**)

Impaired Renal Function:

Ciprofloxacin is eliminated primarily by renal excretion; however, the drug is also metabolized and partially cleared through the biliary system of the liver and through the intestine. These alternate pathways of drug elimination appear to compensate for the reduced renal excretion in patients with renal impairment. No dosage adjustment is required for patients with uncomplicated urinary tract infections receiving 500 mg CIPRO XR. In patients with complicated urinary tract infections and acute uncomplicated pyelonephritis, who have a creatinine clearance of < 30 mL/min, the dose of CIPRO XR should be reduced from 1000 mg to 500 mg daily. For patients on hemodialysis or peritoneal dialysis, administer CIPRO XR after the dialysis procedure is completed. (See **CLINICAL PHARMACOLOGY Special Populations,** and **PRECAUTIONS, Geriatric Use.**)

Impaired Hepatic Function:

No dosage adjustment is required with CIPRO XR in patients with stable chronic cirrhosis. The kinetics of ciprofloxacin in patients with acute hepatic insufficiency, however, have not been fully elucidated. (See **CLINICAL PHARMACOLOGY, Special Populations.**)

HOW SUPPLIED

CIPRO XR is available as nearly white to slightly yellowish, film-coated, oblong-shaped tablets containing 500 mg or 1000 mg ciprofloxacin. The 500 mg tablet is coded with the word "BAYER" on one side and "C500 QD" on the reverse side. The 1000 mg tablet is coded with the word "BAYER" on one side and "C1000 QD" on the reverse side.

	Strength	NDC Code
Bottles of 30	500 mg	0026-8889-69
Bottles of 50	500 mg	0026-8889-50
Bottles of 100	500 mg	0026-8889-51
Bottles of 50	1000 mg	0026-8897-50
Bottles of 100	1000 mg	0026-8897-51
Unit Dose Pack of 30	1000 mg	0026-8897-69

Store at 25°C (77°F); excursions permitted to 15–30°C (59–86°F) [see USP Controlled Room Temperature].

ANIMAL PHARMACOLOGY

Ciprofloxacin and other quinolones have been shown to cause arthropathy in immature animals of most species tested. (See **WARNINGS.**) Damage of weight bearing joints was observed in juvenile dogs and rats. In young beagles, 100 mg/kg ciprofloxacin, given daily for 4 weeks, caused degenerative articular changes of the knee joint. At 30 mg/kg, the effect on the joint was minimal. In a subsequent study in beagles, removal of weight bearing from the joint reduced the lesions but did not totally prevent them.

Crystalluria, sometimes associated with secondary nephropathy, occurs in laboratory animals dosed with ciprofloxacin. This is primarily related to the reduced solubility of ciprofloxacin under alkaline conditions, which predominate in the urine of test animals; in man, crystalluria is rare since human urine is typically acidic. In rhesus monkeys, crystalluria without nephropathy has been noted after single oral doses as low as 5 mg/kg. After 6 months of intravenous dosing at 10 mg/kg/day, no nephropathological changes were noted; however, nephropathy was observed after dosing at 20 mg/kg/day for the same duration.

In mice, concomitant administration of nonsteroidal anti-inflammatory drugs such as phenylbutazone and indomethacin with quinolones has been reported to enhance the CNS stimulatory effect of quinolones.

Ocular toxicity seen with some related drugs has not been observed in ciprofloxacin-treated animals.

CLINICAL STUDIES

Uncomplicated Urinary Tract Infections (acute cystitis)

CIPRO XR was evaluated for the treatment of uncomplicated urinary tract infections (acute cystitis) in a randomized, double-blind, controlled clinical trial conducted in the US. This study compared CIPRO XR (500 mg once daily for three days) with ciprofloxacin immediate-release tablets (CIPRO® 250 mg BID for three days). Of the 905 patients enrolled, 452 were randomly assigned to the CIPRO XR treatment group and 453 were randomly assigned to the control group. The primary efficacy variable was bacteriologic eradication of the baseline organism(s) with no new infection or superinfection at test-of-cure (Day 4–11 Post-therapy).

The bacteriologic eradication and clinical success rates were similar between CIPRO XR and the control group. The eradication and clinical success rates and their corresponding

Continued on next page

Cipro XR—Cont.

95% confidence intervals for the differences between rates (CIPRO XR minus control group) are given in the following table:
[See first table at right]

Complicated Urinary Tract Infections and Acute Uncomplicated Pyelonephritis

CIPRO XR was evaluated for the treatment of complicated urinary tract infections (cUTI) and acute uncomplicated pyelonephritis (AUP) in a randomized, double-blind, controlled clinical trial conducted in the US and Canada. The study enrolled 1,042 patients (521 patients per treatment arm) and compared CIPRO XR (1000 mg once daily for 7 to 14 days) with immediate-release ciprofloxacin (500 mg BID for 7 to 14 days). The primary efficacy endpoint for this trial was bacteriologic eradication of the baseline organism(s) with no new infection or superinfection at 5 to 11 days post-therapy (test-of-cure or TOC) for the Per Protocol and Modified Intent-To-Treat (MITT) populations.

The Per Protocol population was defined as patients with a diagnosis of cUTI or AUP, a causative organism(s) at baseline present at ≥ 10^5 CFU/mL, no inclusion criteria violation, a valid test-of-cure urine culture within the TOC window, an organism susceptible to study drug, no premature discontinuation or loss to follow-up, and compliance with the dosage regimen (among other criteria). More patients in the CIPRO XR arm than in the control arm were excluded from the Per Protocol population and this should be considered in the interpretation of the study results. Reasons for exclusion with the greatest discrepancy between the two arms were no valid test-of-cure urine culture, an organism resistant to the study drug, and premature discontinuation due to adverse events.

An analysis of all patients with a causative organism(s) isolated at baseline and who received study medication, defined as the MITT population, included 342 patients in the CIPRO XR arm and 324 patients in the control arm. Patients with missing responses were counted as failures in this analysis. In the MITT analysis of cUTI patients, bacteriologic eradication was 160/271 (59.0%) versus 156/248 (62.9%) in CIPRO XR and control arm, respectively [97.5% CI* (-13.5%, 5.7%)]. Clinical cure was 184/271 (67.9%) for CIPRO XR and 182/248 (73.4%) for control arm, respectively [97.5% CI* (-14.4%, 3.5%)]. Bacterial eradication in the MITT analysis of patients with AUP at TOC was 47/71 (66.2%) and 58/76 (76.3%) for CIPRO XR and control arm, respectively [97.5% CI* (-26.8%, 6.5%)]. Clinical cure at TOC was 50/71 (70.4%) for CIPRO XR and 58/76 (76.3%) for the control arm [97.5% CI* (-22.0%, 10.4%)].

* confidence interval of the difference in rates (CIPRO XR minus control).

In the Per Protocol population, the differences between CIPRO XR and the control arm in bacteriologic eradication rates at the TOC visit were not consistent between AUP and cUTI patients. The bacteriologic eradication rate for cUTI patients was higher in the CIPRO XR arm than in the control arm. For AUP patients, the bacteriologic eradication rate was lower in the CIPRO XR arm than in the control arm. This inconsistency was not observed between the two treatment groups for clinical cure rates. Clinical cure rates were 96.1% (198/206) and 92.1% (211/229) for CIPRO XR and the control arm, respectively.

The bacterial eradication and clinical cure rates by infection type for CIPRO XR and the control arm at the TOC visit and their corresponding 97.5% confidence intervals for the differences between rates (CIPRO XR minus control arm) are given below for the Per Protocol population analysis:
[See second table at right]

Of the 166 cUTI patients treated with CIPRO XR, 148 (89%) had the causative organism(s) eradicated, 8 (5%) had persistence, 5 (3%) patients developed superinfections and 5 (3%) developed new infections. Of the 177 cUTI patients treated in the control arm, 144 (81%) had the causative organism(s) eradicated, 16 (9%) patients had persistence, 3 (2%) developed superinfections and 14 (8%) developed new infections. Of the 40 patients with AUP treated with CIPRO XR, 35 (87.5%) had the causative organism(s) eradicated, 2 (5%) patients had persistence and 3 (7.5%) developed new infections. Of the 5 CIPRO XR AUP patients without eradication at TOC, 4 were considered clinical cures and did not receive alternative antibiotic therapy. Of the 52 patients with AUP treated in the control arm, 51 (98%) had the causative organism(s) eradicated. One patient (2%) had persistence.

	CIPRO XR 500 mg QD × 3 Days	CIPRO 250 mg BID × 3 Days
Randomized Patients	452	453
Per Protocol Patients†	199	223
Bacteriologic Eradication at TOC (n/N)*	188/199 (94.5%)	209/223 (93.7%)
	CI [−3.5%, 5.1%]	
Bacteriologic Eradication (by organism) at TOC (n/N)**		
E. coli	156/160 (97.5%)	176/181 (97.2%)
E. faecalis	10/11 (90.9%)	17/21 (81.0%)
P. mirabilis	11/12 (91.7%)	7/7 (100%)
S. saprophyticus	6/7 (85.7%)	9/9 (100%)
Clinical Response at TOC (n/N)***	189/199 (95.0%)	204/223 (91.5%)
	CI [−1.1%, 8.1%]	

* n/N = patients with baseline organism(s) eradicated and no new infections or superinfections/total number of patients
** n/N = patients with specified baseline organism eradicated/patients with specified baseline organism
*** n/N = patients with clinical success/total number of patients
† The presence of a pathogen at a level of ≥ 10^5 CFU/mL was required for microbiological evaluability criteria, except for *S. saprophyticus* (≥ 10^4 CFU/mL).

	CIPRO XR 1000 mg QD	CIPRO 500 mg BID
Randomized Patients	521	521
Per Protocol Patient^	206	229
cUTI Patients		
Bacteriologic Eradication at TOC (n/N)*	148/166 (89.2%)	144/177 (81.4%)
	CI [−0.7%, 16.3%]	
Bacteriologic Eradication (by organism) at TOC (n/N)**		
E. coli	91/94 (96.8%)	90/92 (97.8%)
K. pneumoniae	20/21 (95.2%)	19/23 (82.6%)
E. faecalis	17/17 (100%)	14/21 (66.7%)
P. mirabilis	11/12 (91.6%)	10/10 (100%)
P. aeruginosa	3/3 (100%)	3/3 (100%)
Clinical Cure at TOC (n/N)***	159/166 (95.8%)	161/177 (91.0%)
	CI [−1.1%, 10.8%]	
AUP Patients		
Bacteriologic Eradication at TOC (n/N)*	35/40 (87.5%)	51/52 (98.1%)
	CI [−34.8%, 6.2%]	
Bacteriologic Eradication of *E. coli* at TOC (n/N)**	35/36 (97.2%)	41/41 (100%)
Clinical Cure at TOC (n/N)***	39/40 (97.5%)	50/52 (96.2%)
	CI [−15.3%, 21.1%]	

^Patients excluded from the Per Protocol population were primarily those with no causative organism(s) at baseline or no organism present at ≥ 10^5 CFU/mL at baseline, inclusion criteria violation, no valid test-of-cure urine culture within the TOC window, an organism resistant to study drug, premature discontinuation due to an adverse event, lost to follow-up, or non-compliance with dosage regimen (among other criteria).
* n/N = patients with baseline organism(s) eradicated and no new infections or superinfections/total number of patients
**n/N = patients with specified baseline organism eradicated/patients with specified baseline organism
***n/N = patients with clinical success/total number of patients

REFERENCES

1. NCCLS, Methods for Dilution Antimicrobial Susceptibility Tests for Bacteria That Grow Aerobically-Sixth Edition. Approved Standard NCCLS Document M7-A6, Vol. 23, No. 2, NCCLS, Wayne, PA, January, 2003.
2. NCCLS, Performance Standards for Antimicrobial Disk Susceptibility Tests-Eighth Edition. Approved Standard NCCLS Document M2-A8, Vol. 23, No. 1, NCCLS, Wayne, PA, January, 2003.

PATIENT INFORMATION ABOUT CIPRO® XR

(ciprofloxacin extended-release tablets)

This section contains important patient information about CIPRO XR and should be read completely before you begin treatment. This section does not take the place of discussion with your doctor or health care professional about your medical condition or your treatment. This section does not list all benefits and risks of CIPRO XR. CIPRO XR can be prescribed only by a licensed health care professional. Your doctor has prescribed CIPRO XR only for you.

CIPRO XR is intended only to treat urinary tract infections and acute uncomplicated pyelonephritis (also known as a kidney infection). It should not be used to treat other infections. Do not give it to other people even if they have a similar condition. Do not use it for a condition for which it was not prescribed. If you have any concerns about your condition or your medicine, ask your doctor. Only your doctor can determine if CIPRO XR is right for you.

What is CIPRO XR?

CIPRO XR is an antibiotic in the quinolone class that contains the active ingredient ciprofloxacin. CIPRO XR is specifically formulated to be taken just once daily to kill bacteria causing infection in the urinary tract. CIPRO XR has been shown in clinical trials to be effective in the treatment of urinary tract infections. You should contact your doctor if your condition is not improving while taking CIPRO XR.

CIPRO XR tablets are nearly white to slightly yellowish, film-coated, oblong-shaped tablets. CIPRO XR is available in 500 mg and 1000 mg tablet strengths.

How and when should I take CIPRO XR?

CIPRO XR should be taken once a day for three (3) to fourteen (14) days depending on your infection. Take CIPRO XR at approximately the same time each day with food or on an empty stomach. CIPRO XR should not be taken with dairy products (like milk or yogurt) or calcium-fortified juices alone; however, CIPRO XR may be taken with a meal that contains these products. Should you forget to take it at the usual time, you may take your dose later in the day. Do not take more than one CIPRO XR tablet per day even if you missed a dose. Swallow the CIPRO XR tablet whole. **DO NOT SPLIT, CRUSH, OR CHEW THE TABLET.**

You should take CIPRO XR for as long as your doctor prescribes it, even after you start to feel better. Stopping an antibiotic too early may result in failure to cure your infection.

Who should not take CIPRO XR?

You should not take CIPRO XR if you have ever had a severe reaction to any of the group of antibiotics known as "quinolones."

CIPRO XR is not recommended for use during pregnancy or nursing, as the effects on the unborn child or nursing infant are unknown. If you are pregnant or plan to become pregnant while taking CIPRO XR, talk to your doctor before taking this medication.

CIPRO XR is not recommended for persons less than 18 years of age.

What are the possible side effects of CIPRO XR?

CIPRO XR is generally well tolerated. The most common side effects, which are usually mild, include nausea, headache, dyspepsia, dizziness, vaginal yeast infection and diarrhea. If diarrhea persists, call your health care professional. Antibiotics of the quinolone class may also cause vomiting, rash, and abdominal pain/discomfort.

You should be careful about driving or operating machinery until you are sure CIPRO XR is not causing dizziness.

Rare cases of allergic reactions have been reported in patients receiving quinolones, including ciprofloxacin, even after just one dose. If you develop hives, difficulty breathing, or other symptoms of a severe allergic reaction, seek emergency treatment right away. If you develop a skin rash, you should stop taking CIPRO XR and call your health care professional.

Some patients taking quinolone antibiotics may become more sensitive to sunlight or ultraviolet light such as that used in tanning salons. You should avoid excessive exposure to sunlight or ultraviolet light while you are taking CIPRO XR.

Ciprofloxacin has been rarely associated with inflammation of tendons. If you experience pain, swelling or rupture of a tendon, you should stop taking CIPRO XR and call your health care professional.

Convulsions have been reported in patients receiving quinolone antibiotics including ciprofloxacin. If you have experienced convulsions in the past, be sure to let your physician know that you have a history of convulsions. Quinolones, including ciprofloxacin, have been rarely associated with other central nervous system events including confusion, tremors, hallucinations, and depression.

If you notice any side effects not mentioned in this section, or if you have any concerns about side effects you may be experiencing, please inform your health care professional.

What about other medications I am taking?

CIPRO XR can affect how other medicines work. Tell your doctor about all other prescriptions and nonprescription medicines or supplements you are taking. This is especially important if you are taking theophylline or VIDEX® (didanosine) chewable/buffered tablets or pediatric powder. Other medications including warfarin, glyburide, and phenytoin may also interact with CIPRO XR.

Many antacids, multivitamins, and other dietary supplements containing magnesium, calcium, aluminum, iron or zinc can interfere with the absorption of CIPRO XR and may prevent it from working. You should take CIPRO XR either 2 hours before or 6 hours after taking these products.

Remember:

Do not give CIPRO XR to anyone other than the person for whom it was prescribed.

Complete the course of CIPRO XR even if you are feeling better.

Keep CIPRO XR and all medications out of reach of children.

This information does not take the place of discussions with your doctor or health care professional about your medication or treatment.

℞Only

Bayer HealthCare
Bayer Pharmaceuticals Corporation
400 Morgan Lane
West Haven, CT 06516
Made in Germany

08852106, R.4 Bay o 9867/q 3939 4/04 12313

Printed in U.S.A.

To keep your **PDR** up to date throughout the year, note these revisions on the corresponding pages of the annual volume. Simply write **"See Supplement A"** next to the product heading.

Boehringer Ingelheim Pharmaceuticals, Inc.

A subsidiary of Boehringer Ingelheim Corporation
900 RIDGEBURY ROAD
POST OFFICE BOX 368
RIDGEFIELD, CT 06877-0368

For Medical Information Contact:
1-800-542-6257
or email:
druginfo@rdg.boehringer-ingelheim.com

AGGRENOX® ℞

(aspirin/extended-release dipyridamole)
25 mg/200 mg capsules
Prescribing Information

Prescribing information for this product, which appears on pages 991–994 of the 2004 PDR, has been completely revised as follows. Please write "See Supplement A" next to the product heading.

DESCRIPTION

AGGRENOX® (aspirin/extended-release dipyridamole) is a combination antiplatelet agent intended for oral administration. Each hard gelatin capsule contains 200 mg dipyridamole in an extended-release form and 25 mg aspirin, as an immediate-release sugar-coated tablet. In addition, each capsule contains the following inactive ingredients: acacia, aluminum stearate, colloidal silicon dioxide, corn starch, dimethicone, hydroxypropyl methylcellulose, hydroxypropyl methylcellulose phthalate, lactose monohydrate, methacrylic acid copolymer, microcrystalline cellulose, povidone, stearic acid, sucrose, talc, tartaric acid, titanium dioxide and triacetin.

Each capsule shell contains gelatin, red iron oxide and yellow iron oxide, titanium dioxide and water.

Dipyridamole

Dipyridamole is an antiplatelet agent chemically described as 2,2′,2″,2‴-[(4,8-Dipiperidinopyrimido[5,4-*d*]pyrimidine-2,6-diyl)dinitrilo]-tetraethanol. It has the following structural formula:

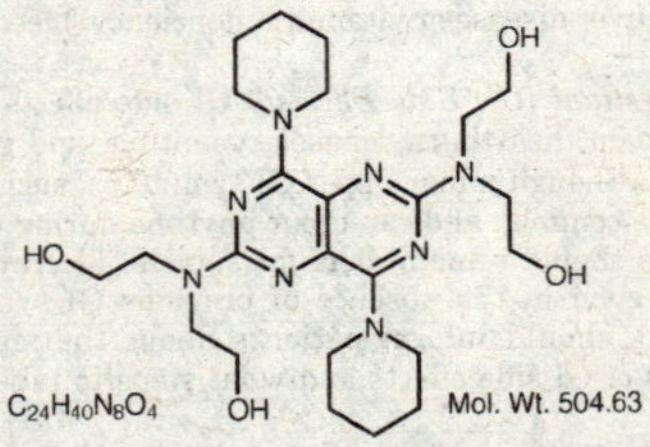

$C_{24}H_{40}N_8O_4$ Mol. Wt. 504.63

Dipyridamole is an odorless yellow crystalline substance, having a bitter taste. It is soluble in dilute acids, methanol and chloroform, and is practically insoluble in water.

Aspirin

The antiplatelet agent aspirin (acetylsalicylic acid) is chemically known as benzoic acid, 2-(acetyloxy)-, and has the following structural formula:

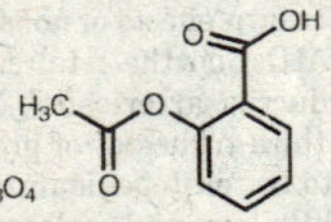

$C_9H_8O_4$ Mol. Wt. 180.16

Aspirin is an odorless white needle-like crystalline or powdery substance. When exposed to moisture, aspirin hydrolyzes into salicylic and acetic acids, and gives off a vinegary odor. It is highly lipid soluble and slightly soluble in water.

CLINICAL PHARMACOLOGY

Mechanism of Action

The antithrombotic action of AGGRENOX (aspirin/extended-release dipyridamole) is the result of the additive antiplatelet effects of dipyridamole and aspirin.

Dipyridamole

Dipyridamole inhibits the uptake of adenosine into platelets, endothelial cells and erythrocytes *in vitro* and *in vivo*; the inhibition occurs in a dose-dependent manner at therapeutic concentrations (0.5–1.9 µg/mL). This inhibition results in an increase in local concentrations of adenosine which acts on the platelet A_2-receptor thereby stimulating platelet adenylate cyclase and increasing platelet cyclic-3′,5′-adenosine monophosphate (cAMP) levels. Via this mechanism, platelet aggregation is inhibited in response to various stimuli such as platelet activating factor (PAF), collagen and adenosine diphosphate (ADP).

Dipyridamole inhibits phosphodiesterase (PDE) in various tissues. While the inhibition of cAMP-PDE is weak, therapeutic levels of dipyridamole inhibit cyclic-3′,5′-guanosine monophosphate-PDE (cGMP-PDE), thereby augmenting the increase in cGMP produced by EDRF (endothelium-derived relaxing factor, now identified as nitric oxide).

Aspirin

Aspirin inhibits platelet aggregation by irreversible inhibition of platelet cyclooxygenase and thus inhibits the generation of thromboxane A_2, a powerful inducer of platelet aggregation and vasoconstriction.

Pharmacokinetics

There are no significant interactions between aspirin and dipyridamole. The kinetics of the components are unchanged by their co-administration as AGGRENOX.

Dipyridamole

Absorption: Peak plasma levels of dipyridamole are achieved 2 hours (range 1–6 hours) after administration of a daily dose of 400 mg AGGRENOX (given as 200 mg b.i.d.). The peak plasma concentration at steady-state is 1.98 µg/mL (1.01–3.99 µg/mL) and the steady-state trough concentration is 0.53 µg/mL (0.18–1.01 µg/mL).

Effect of Food: When AGGRENOX capsules were taken with a high fat meal, dipyridamole peak plasma levels (C_{max}) and total absorption (AUC) were decreased at steady-state by 20–30% compared to fasting. Due to the similar degree of inhibition of adenosine uptake at these plasma concentrations, this food effect is not considered clinically relevant.

Distribution: Dipyridamole is highly lipophilic (log P=3.71, pH=7); however, it has been shown that the drug does not cross the blood-brain barrier to any significant extent in animals. The steady-state volume of distribution of dipyridamole is about 92 L. Approximately 99% of dipyridamole is bound to plasma proteins, predominantly to alpha 1-acid glycoprotein and albumin.

Metabolism and Elimination: Dipyridamole is metabolized in the liver, primarily by conjugation with glucuronic acid, of which monoglucuronide which has low pharmacodynamic activity is the primary metabolite. In plasma, about 80% of the total amount is present as parent compound and 20% as monoglucuronide. Most of the glucuronide metabolite (about 95%) is excreted via bile into the feces, with some evidence of enterohepatic circulation. Renal excretion of parent compound is negligible and urinary excretion of the glucuronide metabolite is low (about 5%). With intravenous (i.v.) treatment of dipyridamole, a triphasic profile is obtained: a rapid alpha phase, with a half-life of about 3.4 minutes, a beta phase, with a half-life of about 39 minutes, (which, together with the alpha phase accounts for about 70% of the total area under the curve, AUC) and a prolonged elimination phase λ_z with a half-life of about 15.5 hours. Due to the extended absorption phase of the dipyridamole component, only the terminal phase is apparent from oral treatment with AGGRENOX which, in trial 9.123 was 13.6 hours.

Special Populations:

Geriatric Patients: In ESPS2 (See **CLINICAL PHARMACOLOGY, Clinical Trials**), plasma concentrations (determined as AUC) of dipyridamole in healthy elderly subjects (>65 years) were about 40% higher than in subjects younger than 55 years receiving treatment with AGGRENOX.

Hepatic Dysfunction: No study has been conducted with the AGGRENOX formulation in patients with hepatic dysfunction.

In a study conducted with an intravenous formulation of dipyridamole, patients with mild to severe hepatic insufficiency showed no change in plasma concentrations of dipyridamole but showed an increase in the pharmacologically inactive monoglucuronide metabolite. Dipyridamole can be dosed without restriction as long as there is no evidence of hepatic failure.

Renal Dysfunction: No study has been conducted with the AGGRENOX formulation in patients with renal dysfunction.

In ESPS2 patients (See **CLINICAL PHARMACOLOGY, Clinical Trials**), with creatinine clearances ranging from about 15 mL/min to >100 mL/min, no changes were observed in the pharmacokinetics of dipyridamole or its glucuronide metabolite if data were corrected for differences in age.

Aspirin

Absorption: Peak plasma levels of aspirin are achieved 0.63 hours (0.5–1 hour) after administration of a 50 mg aspirin daily dose from AGGRENOX (given as 25 mg b.i.d.). The peak plasma concentration at steady-state is 319 ng/mL (175–463 ng/mL). Aspirin undergoes moderate hydrolysis to salicylic acid in the liver and the gastrointestinal wall, with 50%–75% of an administered dose reaching the systemic circulation as intact aspirin.

Effect of Food: When AGGRENOX capsules were taken with a high fat meal, there was no difference for aspirin in AUC at steady-state, and the approximately 50% decrease in C_{max} was not considered clinically relevant based on a similar degree of cyclooxygenase inhibition comparing the fed and fasted state.

Distribution: Aspirin is poorly bound to plasma proteins and its apparent volume of distribution is low (10 L). Its metabolite, salicylic acid, is highly bound to plasma proteins, but its binding is concentration-dependent (nonlinear). At low concentrations (<100 µg/mL), approximately 90% of salicylic acid is bound to albumin. Salicylic acid is widely distributed to all tissues and fluids in the body, including the central nervous system, breast milk, and fetal tissues. Early signs of salicylate overdose (salicylism), including tinnitus (ringing in the ears), occur at plasma concentrations approximating 200 µg/mL (See **ADVERSE REACTIONS; OVERDOSAGE**).

Metabolism and Elimination: Aspirin is rapidly hydrolyzed in plasma to salicylic acid, with a half-life of 20 minutes. Plasma levels of aspirin are essentially undetectable 2–2.5 hours after dosing and peak salicylic acid concentrations occur 1 hour (range: 0.5–2 hours) after administration of aspirin. Salicylic acid is primarily conjugated in the liver to form salicyluric acid, a phenolic glucuronide, an acyl glucuronide, and a number of minor metabolites. Salicylate

Continued on next page

Aggrenox—Cont.

metabolism is saturable and total body clearance decreases at higher serum concentrations due to the limited ability of the liver to form both salicyluric acid and phenolic glucuronide. Following toxic doses (10–20 g), the plasma half-life may be increased to over 20 hours.
The elimination of acetylsalicylic acid follows first-order kinetics with AGGRENOX and has a half-life of 0.33 hours. The half-life of salicylic acid is 1.71 hours. Both values correspond well with data from the literature at lower doses which state a resultant half-life of approximately 2–3 hours. At higher doses, the elimination of salicylic acid follows zero-order kinetics (i.e., the rate of elimination is constant in relation to plasma concentration), with an apparent half-life of 6 hours or higher. Renal excretion of unchanged drug depends upon urinary pH. As urinary pH rises above 6.5, the renal clearance of free salicylate increases from <5% to >80%. Alkalinization of the urine is a key concept in the management of salicylate overdose (See **OVERDOSAGE**). Following therapeutic doses, about 10% is excreted as salicylic acid and 75% as salicyluric acid, as the phenolic and acyl glucuronides, in urine.

Special Populations:

Hepatic Dysfunction: Aspirin is to be avoided in patients with severe hepatic insufficiency.
Renal Dysfunction: Aspirin is to be avoided in patients with severe renal failure (glomerular filtration rate less than 10 mL/min).

Clinical Trials

AGGRENOX® was studied in a double-blind, placebo-controlled, 24-month study (European Stroke Prevention Study 2, ESPS2) in which 6602 patients had an ischemic stroke (76%) or transient ischemic attack (TIA, 24%) within three months prior to entry. Patients were randomized to one of four treatment groups: AGGRENOX (aspirin/extended-release dipyridamole) 25 mg/200 mg; extended-release dipyridamole (ER-DP) 200 mg alone; aspirin (ASA) 25 mg alone; or placebo. Patients received one capsule twice daily (morning and evening). Efficacy assessments included analyses of stroke (fatal or nonfatal) and death (from all causes) as confirmed by a blinded morbidity and mortality assessment group.

Stroke Endpoint:

AGGRENOX reduced the risk of stroke by 22.1% compared to aspirin 50 mg/day alone (p =0.008) and reduced the risk of stroke by 24.4% compared to extended-release dipyridamole 400 mg/day alone (p = 0.002) (Table 1). AGGRENOX reduced the risk of stroke by 36.8% compared to placebo (p <0.001).
[See table below]
[See figure 1 at top of next column]

Combined Stroke or Death Endpoint

In ESPS2, AGGRENOX reduced the risk of stroke or death by 12.1% compared to aspirin alone and by 10.3% compared to extended-release dipyridamole alone. These results were not statistically significant. AGGRENOX reduced the risk of stroke or death by 24.2% compared to placebo.

Death Endpoint

The incidence rate of all cause mortality was 11.3% for AGGRENOX, 11.0% for aspirin alone, 11.4% for extended-release dipyridamole alone and 12.3% for placebo alone. The differences between the AGGRENOX, aspirin alone and extended-release dipyridamole alone treatment groups were not statistically significant. These incidence rates for AGGRENOX and aspirin alone are consistent with previous aspirin studies in stroke and TIA patients.

INDICATIONS AND USAGE

AGGRENOX (aspirin/extended-release dipyridamole) is indicated to reduce the risk of stroke in patients who have had transient ischemia of the brain or completed ischemic stroke due to thrombosis.

ESPS2: Cumulative Stroke Rate (Fatal or Nonfatal) Over 24 Months Of Follow-Up

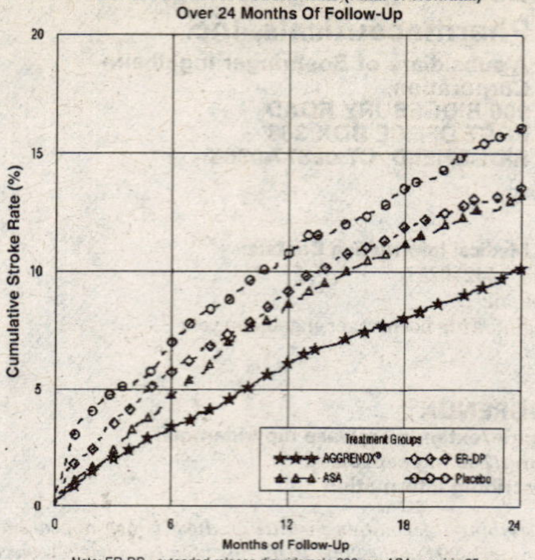

Note: ER-DP - extended-release dipyridamole 200 mg; ASA - aspirin 25 mg.
Note: The dosage regimen for all treatment groups is b.i.d.

CONTRAINDICATIONS

AGGRENOX (aspirin/extended-release dipyridamole) is contraindicated in patients with hypersensitivity to dipyridamole, aspirin or any of the other product components.
Allergy: Aspirin is contraindicated in patients with known allergy to nonsteroidal anti-inflammatory drug products and in patients with the syndrome of asthma, rhinitis, and nasal polyps. Aspirin may cause severe urticaria, angioedema or bronchospasm (asthma).
Reye's Syndrome: Aspirin should not be used in children or teenagers for viral infections, with or without fever, because of the risk of Reye's syndrome with concomitant use of aspirin in certain viral illnesses.

WARNINGS

Alcohol Warning: Patients who consume three or more alcoholic drinks every day should be counseled about the bleeding risks involved with chronic, heavy alcohol use while taking aspirin.
Coagulation Abnormalities: Even low doses of aspirin can inhibit platelet function leading to an increase in bleeding time. This can adversely affect patients with inherited or acquired (liver disease or vitamin K deficiency) bleeding disorders.
Gastrointestinal (GI) Side Effects: GI side effects include stomach pain, heartburn, nausea, vomiting, and gross GI bleeding. Although minor upper GI symptoms, such as dyspepsia, are common and can occur anytime during therapy, physicians should remain alert for signs of ulceration and bleeding, even in the absence of previous GI symptoms. Physicians should inform patients about the signs and symptoms of GI side effects and what steps to take if they occur.
Peptic Ulcer Disease: Patients with a history of active peptic ulcer disease should avoid using aspirin, which can cause gastric mucosal irritation, and bleeding.
Pregnancy: AGGRENOX can cause fetal harm when administered to a pregnant woman. Maternal aspirin use during later stages of pregnancy may cause low birth weight, increased incidence for intracranial hemorrhage in premature infants, stillbirths and neonatal death. Because of the above and because of the known effects of nonsteroidal anti-inflammatory drugs (NSAIDs) on the fetal cardiovascular system (closure of the ductus arteriosus), AGGRENOX should be avoided in the third trimester of pregnancy.
Aspirin has been shown to be teratogenic in rats (spina bifida, exencephaly, microphthalmia and coelosomia) and rabbits (congested fetuses, agenesis of skull and upper jaw, generalized edema with malformation of the head, and diaphanous skin) at oral doses of 330 mg/kg/day and 110 mg/kg/day, respectively. These doses, which also resulted in a high resorption rate in rats (63% of implantations versus 5% in controls), are, on a mg/m^2 basis, about 66 and 44 times, respectively, the dose of aspirin contained in the maximum recommended daily human dose of AGGRENOX. Reproduction studies with dipyridamole have been performed in mice, rabbits and rats at oral doses of up to 125 mg/kg, 40 mg/kg and 1000 mg/kg, respectively about 1 ½, 2 and 25 times the maximum recommended daily human oral dose, respectively, on a mg/m^2 basis) and have revealed no evidence of harm to the fetus due to dipyridamole. When 330 mg aspirin/kg/day was combined with 75 mg dipyridamole/kg/day in the rat, the resorption rate approached 100%, indicating potentiation of aspirin-related fetal toxicity. There are no adequate and well-controlled studies in pregnant women. If AGGRENOX is used during pregnancy, or if the patient becomes pregnant while taking AGGRENOX, the patient should be apprised of the potential hazard to the fetus.

PRECAUTIONS

General

AGGRENOX (aspirin/extended-release dipyridamole) is not interchangeable with the individual components of aspirin and Persantine® Tablets.
Coronary Artery Disease: Dipyridamole has a vasodilatory effect and should be used with caution in patients with severe coronary artery disease (e.g., unstable angina or recently sustained myocardial infarction). Chest pain may be aggravated in patients with underlying coronary artery disease who are receiving dipyridamole.
For stroke or TIA patients for whom aspirin is indicated to prevent recurrent myocardial infarction (MI) or angina pectoris, the aspirin in this product may not provide adequate treatment for the cardiac indications.
Hepatic Insufficiency: Elevations of hepatic enzymes and hepatic failure have been reported in association with dipyridamole administration.
Hypotension: Dipyridamole should be used with caution in patients with hypotension since it can produce peripheral vasodilation.
Renal Failure: Avoid aspirin in patients with severe renal failure (glomerular filtration rate less than 10 mL/minute).
Risk of Bleeding: In ESPS2 the incidence of gastrointestinal bleeding was 68 patients (4.1%) in the AGGRENOX group, 36 patients (2.2%) in the extended-release dipyridamole group, 52 patients (3.2%) in the aspirin group, and 34 patients (2.1%) in the placebo groups.
The incidence of intracranial hemorrhage was 9 patients (0.6%) in the AGGRENOX group, 6 patients (0.5%) in the extended-release dipyridamole group, 6 patients (0.4%) in the aspirin group and 7 patients (0.4%) in the placebo groups.

Laboratory Tests

Aspirin has been associated with elevated hepatic enzymes, blood urea nitrogen and serum creatinine, hyperkalemia, proteinuria and prolonged bleeding time.
Dipyridamole has been associated with elevated hepatic enzymes.

Drug Interactions

No pharmacokinetic drug-drug interaction studies were conducted with the AGGRENOX formulation. The following information was obtained from the literature.
Adenosine: Dipyridamole has been reported to increase the plasma levels and cardiovascular effects of adenosine. Adjustment of adenosine dosage may be necessary.
Angiotensin Converting Enzyme (ACE) Inhibitors: Due to the indirect effect of aspirin on the renin-angiotensin conversion pathway, the hyponatremic and hypotensive effects of ACE inhibitors may be diminished by concomitant administration of aspirin.
Acetazolamide: Concurrent use of aspirin and acetazolamide can lead to high serum concentrations of acetazolamide (and toxicity) due to competition at the renal tubule for secretion.

Table 1: Summary of First Stroke (Fatal or Nonfatal): ESPS2: Intent-to-Treat Population

	Total Number of Patients n	Number of Patients With Stroke Within 2 Years n (%)	Kaplan-Meier Estimate of Survival at 2 Years (95% C.I.)	Gehan-Wilcoxon Test P-value	Risk Reduction at 2 Years	Odds Ratio (95% C.I.)
Individual Treatment Group						
AGGRENOX	1650	157 (9.5%)	89.9% (88.4%, 91.4%)	-	-	-
ER-DP	1654	211 (12.8%)	86.7% (85.0%, 88.4%)	-	-	-
ASA	1649	206 (12.5%)	87.1% (85.4%, 88.7%)	-	-	-
Placebo	1649	250 (15.2%)	84.1% (82.2%, 85.9%)	-	-	-
Pairwise Treatment Group Comparisons						
AGGRENOX vs. ER-DP	-	-	-	0.002**	24.4%	0.72 (0.58, 0.90)
AGGRENOX vs. ASA	-	-	-	0.008**	22.1%	0.74 (0.59, 0.92)
AGGRENOX vs. Placebo	-	-	-	<0.001**	36.8%	0.59 (0.48, 0.73)
ER-DP vs. Placebo	-	-	-	0.036*	16.5%	0.82 (0.67, 1.00)
ASA vs. Placebo	-	-	-	0.009**	18.9%	0.80 (0.66, 0.97)

*0.010 < p-value ≤0.050; **p-value ≤0.010.
Note: ER-DP = extended-release dipyridamole 200 mg; ASA = aspirin 25 mg. The dosage regimen for all treatment groups is b.i.d.

Anticoagulant Therapy (heparin and warfarin): Patients on anticoagulation therapy are at increased risk for bleeding because of drug-drug interactions and effects on platelets. Aspirin can displace warfarin from protein binding sites, leading to prolongation of both the prothrombin time and the bleeding time. Aspirin can increase the anticoagulant activity of heparin, increasing bleeding risk.
Anticonvulsants: Salicylic acid can displace protein-bound phenytoin and valproic acid, leading to a decrease in the total concentration of phenytoin and an increase in serum valproic acid levels.
Beta Blockers: The hypotensive effects of beta blockers may be diminished by the concomitant administration of aspirin due to inhibition of renal prostaglandins, leading to decreased renal blood flow and salt and fluid retention.
Cholinesterase Inhibitors: Dipyridamole may counteract the anticholinesterase effect of cholinesterase inhibitors, thereby potentially aggravating myasthenia gravis.
Diuretics: The effectiveness of diuretics in patients with underlying renal or cardiovascular disease may be diminished by the concomitant administration of aspirin due to inhibition of renal prostaglandins, leading to decreased renal blood flow and salt and fluid retention.
Methotrexate: Salicylate can inhibit renal clearance of methotrexate, leading to bone marrow toxicity, especially in the elderly or renal impaired.
Nonsteroidal Anti-Inflammatory Drugs (NSAIDs): The concurrent use of aspirin with other NSAIDs may increase bleeding or lead to decreased renal function.
Oral Hypoglycemics: Moderate doses of aspirin may increase the effectiveness of oral hypoglycemic drugs, leading to hypoglycemia.
Uricosuric Agents (probenecid and sulfinpyrazone): Salicylates antagonize the uricosuric action of uricosuric agents.

Carcinogenesis, Mutagenesis, Impairment of Fertility

In studies in which dipyridamole was administered in the feed to mice (up to 111 weeks in males and females) and rats (up to 128 weeks in males and up to 142 weeks in females), there was no evidence of drug-related carcinogenesis. The highest dose administered in these studies (75 mg/kg/day) was, on a mg/m^2 basis, about equivalent to the maximum recommended daily human oral dose (MRHD) in mice and about twice the MRHD in rats.

Combinations of dipyridamole and aspirin (1:5 ratio) tested negative in the Ames test, *in vivo* chromosome aberration tests (in mice and hamsters), oral micronucleus tests (in mice and hamsters) and oral dominant lethal test (in mice). Aspirin, alone, induced chromosome aberrations in cultured human fibroblasts. Mutagenicity tests of dipyridamole alone with bacterial and mammalian cell systems were negative.

Combinations of dipyridamole and aspirin have not been evaluated for effects on fertility and reproductive performance. There was no evidence of impaired fertility when dipyridamole was administered to male and female rats at oral doses up to 500 mg/kg/day (about 12 times the MRHD on a mg/m^2 basis). A significant reduction in number of corpora lutea with consequent reduction in implantations and live fetuses was, however, observed at 1250 mg/kg (more than 30 times the MRHD on a mg/m^2 basis). Aspirin inhibits ovulation in rats.

Pregnancy

Teratogenic Effects: PREGNANCY CATEGORY D. See **WARNINGS**

Labor and Delivery

Aspirin can result in excessive blood loss at delivery as well as prolonged gestation and prolonged labor. Because of these effects on the mother and because of adverse fetal effects seen with aspirin during the later stages of pregnancy (see **WARNINGS/Pregnancy** subsection), AGGRENOX should be avoided in the third trimester of pregnancy and during labor and delivery.

Nursing Mothers

Both dipyridamole and aspirin are excreted in human milk. Caution should be exercised when AGGRENOX is administered to a nursing woman.

Pediatric Use

Safety and effectiveness of AGGRENOX in pediatric patients have not been studied. Due to the aspirin component, use of this product in the pediatric population is not recommended (See **CONTRAINDICATIONS**).

ADVERSE REACTIONS

A 24-month, multicenter, double-blind, randomized study (ESPS2) was conducted to compare the efficacy and safety of AGGRENOX (aspirin/extended-release dipyridamole) with placebo, extended-release dipyridamole alone and aspirin alone. The study was conducted in a total of 6602 male and female patients who had experienced a previous ischemic stroke or transient ischemia of the brain within three months prior to randomization.

Table 2 presents the incidence of adverse events that occurred in 1% or more of patients treated with AGGRENOX where the incidence was also greater than in those patients treated with placebo. There is no clear benefit of the dipyridamole/aspirin combination over aspirin with respect to safety.

[See table 2 above]

Discontinuation due to adverse events in ESPS2 was 25% for AGGRENOX, 25% for extended-release dipyridamole, 19% for aspirin, and 21% for placebo (refer to Table 3).

[See table 3 at bottom of next page]

Other adverse events:

Adverse reactions that occurred in less than 1% of patients treated with AGGRENOX in the ESPS2 study and that were medically judged to be possibly related to either dipyridamole or aspirin are listed below (See **WARNINGS**). *Body as a Whole:* Allergic reaction, fever. *Cardiovascular:* Hypotension. *Central Nervous System:* Coma, dizziness, paresthesia, cerebral hemorrhage, intracranial hemorrhage, subarachnoid hemorrhage. *Gastrointestinal:* Gastritis, ulceration and perforation. *Hearing & Vestibular Disorders:* Tinnitus, and deafness. Patients with high frequency hearing loss may have difficulty perceiving tinnitus. In these patients, tinnitus cannot be used as a clinical indicator of salicylism. *Heart Rate and Rhythm Disorders:* Tachycardia, palpitation, arrhythmia, supraventricular tachycardia. *Liver and Biliary System Disorders:* Cholelithiasis, jaundice, hepatic function abnormal. *Metabolic & Nutritional Disorders:* Hyperglycemia, thirst. *Platelet, Bleeding and Clotting Disorders:* Hematoma, gingival bleeding. *Psychiatric Disorders:* Agitation. *Reproductive:* Uterine hemorrhage. *Respiratory:* Hyperpnea, asthma, bronchospasm, hemoptysis, pulmonary edema. *Special Senses Other Disorders:* Taste loss. *Skin and Appendages Disorders:* Pruritus, urticaria. *Urogenital:* Renal insufficiency and failure, hematuria. *Vascular (Extracardiac) Disorders:* Flushing.

The following is a list of additional adverse reactions that have been reported either in the literature or are from postmarketing spontaneous reports for either dipyridamole or aspirin. *Body as a Whole:* Hypothermia, chest pain. *Cardiovascular:* Angina pectoris. *Central Nervous System:* Cerebral edema. *Fluid and Electrolyte:* Hyperkalemia, metabolic acidosis, respiratory alkalosis, hypokalemia. *Gastrointestinal:* Pancreatitis, Reye's syndrome, hematemesis. *Hearing*

Continued on next page

Table 2: Incidence of Adverse Events in ESPS2*

	Indivdual Treatment Group			
Body System/Preferred Term	**AGGRENOX**	**ER-DP Alone**	**ASA Alone**	**Placebo**
Total Number of Patients	1650	1654	1649	1649
Total Number (%) of Patients With at Least One On-Treatment Adverse Event	1319 (79.9%)	1305 (78.9%)	1323 (80.2%)	1304 (79.1%)
Central & Peripheral Nervous System Disorders				
Headache	647 (39.2%)	634 (38.3%)	558 (33.8%)	543 (32.9%)
Convulsions	28 (1.7%)	15 (0.9%)	28 (1.7%)	26 (1.6%)
Gastro-Intestinal System Disorders				
Dyspepsia	303 (18.4%)	288 (17.4%)	299 (18.1%)	275 (16.7%)
Abdominal Pain	289 (17.5%)	255 (15.4%)	262 (15.9%)	239 (14.5%)
Nausea	264 (16.0%)	254 (15.4%)	210 (12.7%)	232 (14.1%)
Diarrhea	210 (12.7%)	257 (15.5%)	112 (6.8%)	161 (9.8%)
Vomiting	138 (8.4%)	129 (7.8%)	101 (6.1%)	118 (7.2%)
Hemorrhage Rectum	26 (1.6%)	22 (1.3%)	16 (1.0%)	13 (0.8%)
Melena	31 (1.9%)	10 (0.6%)	20 (1.2%)	13 (0.8%)
Hemorrhoids	16 (1.0%)	13 (0.8%)	10 (0.6%)	10 (0.6%)
GI Hemorrhage	20 (1.2%)	5 (0.3%)	15 (0.9%)	7 (0.4%)
Body as a Whole - General Disorders				
Pain	105 (6.4%)	88 (5.3%)	103 (6.2%)	99 (6.0%)
Fatigue	95 (5.8%)	93 (5.6%)	97 (5.9%)	90 (5.5%)
Back Pain	76 (4.6%)	77 (4.7%)	74 (4.5%)	65 (3.9%)
Accidental Injury	42 (2.5%)	24 (1.5%)	51 (3.1%)	37 (2.2%)
Malaise	27 (1.6%)	23 (1.4%)	26 (1.6%)	22 (1.3%)
Asthenia	29 (1.8%)	19 (1.1%)	17 (1.0%)	18 (1.1%)
Syncope	17 (1.0%)	13 (0.8%)	16 (1.0%)	8 (0.5%)
Psychiatric Disorders				
Amnesia	39 (2.4%)	40 (2.4%)	57 (3.5%)	34 (2.1%)
Confusion	18 (1.1%)	9 (0.5%)	22 (1.3%)	15 (0.9%)
Anorexia	19 (1.2%)	17 (1.0%)	10 (0.6%)	15 (0.9%)
Somnolence	20 (1.2%)	13 (0.8%)	18 (1.1%)	9 (0.5%)
Musculoskeletal System Disorders				
Arthralgia	91 (5.5%)	75 (4.5%)	91 (5.5%)	76 (4.6%)
Arthritis	34 (2.1%)	25 (1.5%)	17 (1.0%)	19 (1.2%)
Arthrosis	18 (1.1%)	22 (1.3%)	13 (0.8%)	14 (0.8%)
Myalgia	20 (1.2%)	16 (1.0%)	11 (0.7%)	11 (0.7%)
Respiratory System Disorders				
Coughing	25 (1.5%)	18 (1.1%)	32 (1.9%)	21 (1.3%)
Upper Respiratory Tract Infection	16 (1.0%)	9 (0.5%)	16 (1.0%)	14 (0.8%)
Cardiovascular Disorders, General				
Cardiac Failure	26 (1.6%)	17 (1.0%)	30 (1.8%)	25 (1.5%)
Platelet, Bleeding & Clotting Disorders				
Hemorrhage NOS	52 (3.2%)	24 (1.5%)	46 (2.8%)	24 (1.5%)
Epistaxis	39 (2.4%)	16 (1.0%)	45 (2.7%)	25 (1.5%)
Purpura	23 (1.4%)	8 (0.5%)	9 (0.5%)	7 (0.4%)
Neoplasm				
Neoplasm NOS	28 (1.7%)	16 (1.0%)	23 (1.4%)	20 (1.2%)
Red Blood Cell Disorders				
Anemia	27 (1.6%)	16 (1.0%)	19 (1.2%)	9 (0.5%)

*Reported by ≥1% of patients during AGGRENOX treatment where the incidence was greater than in those treated with placebo.

Note: ER-DP = extended-release dipyridamole 200 mg; ASA = aspirin 25 mg. The dosage regimen for all treatment groups is b.i.d. NOS = not otherwise specified.

Aggrenox—Cont.

and Vestibular Disorders: Hearing loss. *Hypersensitivity:* Acute anaphylaxis, laryngeal edema. *Liver and Biliary System Disorders:* Hepatitis, hepatic failure. *Musculoskeletal:* Rhabdomyolysis. *Metabolic & Nutritional Disorders:* Hypoglycemia, dehydration. *Platelet, Bleeding and Clotting Disorders:* Prolongation of the prothrombin time, disseminated intravascular coagulation, coagulopathy, thrombocytopenia. *Reproductive:* Prolonged pregnancy and labor, stillbirths, lower birth weight infants, antepartum and postpartum bleeding. *Respiratory:* Tachypnea, dyspnea. *Skin and Appendages Disorders:* Rash, alopecia, angioedema, Stevens-Johnson syndrome. *Urogenital:* Interstitial nephritis, papillary necrosis, proteinuria. *Vascular (Extracardiac Disorders):* Allergic vasculitis.

The following is a list of additional adverse events that have been reported either in the literature or are from post-marketing spontaneous reports for either dipyridamole or aspirin. The causal relationship of these adverse events has not been established: anorexia, aplastic anemia, pancytopenia, thrombocytosis.

Laboratory Changes

Over the course of the 24-month study (ESPS2), patients treated with AGGRENOX showed a decline (mean change from baseline) in hemoglobin of 0.25 g/dL, hematocrit of 0.75%, and erythrocyte count of $0.13 \times 10^6/mm^3$.

OVERDOSAGE

Because of the dose ratio of dipyridamole to aspirin, overdosage of AGGRENOX (aspirin/extended-release dipyridamole) is likely to be dominated by signs and symptoms of dipyridamole overdose. In case of real or suspected overdose, seek medical attention or contact a Poison Control Center immediately. Careful medical management is essential.

Dipyridamole

Based upon the known hemodynamic effects of dipyridamole, symptoms such as warm feeling, flushes, sweating, restlessness, feeling of weakness and dizziness may occur. A drop in blood pressure and tachycardia might also be observed.

Symptomatic treatment is recommended, possibly including a vasopressor drug. Gastric lavage should be considered. Administration of xanthine derivatives (e.g. aminophylline) may reverse the hemodynamic effects of dipyridamole overdose. Since dipyridamole is highly protein bound, dialysis is not likely to be of benefit.

Aspirin

Salicylate toxicity may result from acute ingestion (overdose) or chronic intoxication. The early signs of salicylic overdose (salicylism), including tinnitus (ringing in the ears), occur at plasma concentrations approaching 200 µg/mL. Plasma concentrations of aspirin above 300 µg/mL are clearly toxic. Severe toxic effects are associated with levels above 400 µg/mL. A single lethal dose of aspirin in adults is not known with certainty but death may be expected at 30 g.

Treatment consists primarily of supporting vital functions, increasing salicylate elimination, and correcting the acid-base disturbance. Gastric emptying and/or lavage are recommended as soon as possible after ingestion, even if the patient has vomited spontaneously. After lavage and/or emesis, administration of activated charcoal, as a slurry, is beneficial, if less than 3 hours have passed since ingestion. Charcoal absorption should not be employed prior to emesis and lavage.

Severity of aspirin intoxication is determined by measuring the blood salicylate level. Acid-base status should be closely followed with serial blood gas and serum pH measurements. Fluid and electrolyte balance should also be maintained.

In severe cases, hyperthermia and hypovolemia are the major immediate threats to life. Children should be sponged with tepid water. Replacement fluid should be administered intravenously and augmented with correction of acidosis. Plasma electrolytes and pH should be monitored to promote alkaline diuresis of salicylate if renal function is normal. Infusion of glucose may be required to control hypoglycemia. Hemodialysis and peritoneal dialysis can be performed to reduce the body drug content. In patients with renal insufficiency or in cases of life-threatening intoxication, dialysis is usually required. Exchange transfusion may be indicated in infants and young children.

DOSAGE AND ADMINISTRATION

The recommended dose of AGGRENOX (aspirin/extended-release dipyridamole) is one capsule given orally twice daily, one in the morning and one in the evening. The capsules should be swallowed whole without chewing. AGGRENOX capsules may be administered with or without food.

AGGRENOX is not interchangeable with the individual components of aspirin and Persantine® Tablets.

HOW SUPPLIED

AGGRENOX (aspirin/extended-release dipyridamole) is available as a hard gelatin capsule, with a red cap and an ivory-colored body, 24.0 mm in length, containing yellow extended-release pellets incorporating dipyridamole and a round white tablet incorporating immediate-release aspirin. The capsule body is imprinted in red with the Boehringer Ingelheim logo and with "01A".

AGGRENOX is supplied in unit-of-use bottles of 60 capsules (NDC 0597-0001-60).

Store at 25°C (77°F); excursions permitted to 15-30°C (59-86°F) [see USP Controlled Room Temperature]. Protect from excessive moisture.

℞ only

Marketed by: Boehringer Ingelheim Pharmaceuticals Inc., Ridgefield, CT 06877 USA

Manufactured by: Boehringer Ingelheim Pharma GmbH & Co KG, Biberach, Germany

Licensed from: Boehringer Ingelheim International GmbH

Patent No. 6,015,577

Revised:05/08/03

42633/US/4

VIRAMUNE® ℞
(nevirapine) Tablets
VIRAMUNE®
(nevirapine) Oral Suspension
℞ only

Prescribing information for this product, which appears on pages 1023–1029 of the 2004 PDR, has been completely revised as follows. Please write "See Supplement A" next to the product heading.

WARNING

Severe, life-threatening, and in some cases fatal hepatotoxicity, including fulminant and cholestatic hepatitis, hepatic necrosis and hepatic failure, has been reported in patients treated with VIRAMUNE®. In some cases, patients presented with non-specific prodromal signs or symptoms of hepatitis and progressed to hepatic failure. These events are often associated with rash. Women, and patients with higher CD4 counts, are at increased risk of these hepatic events. Women with CD4 counts >250 cells/mm³, including pregnant women receiving chronic treatment for HIV infection, are at considerably higher risk of these events. Patients with signs or symptoms of hepatitis must discontinue VIRAMUNE and seek medical evaluation immediately. (See WARNINGS)

Severe, life-threatening skin reactions, including fatal cases, have occurred in patients treated with VIRAMUNE. These have included cases of Stevens-Johnson syndrome, toxic epidermal necrolysis, and hypersensitivity reactions characterized by rash, constitutional findings, and organ dysfunction. Patients developing signs or symptoms of severe skin reactions or hypersensitivity reactions must discontinue VIRAMUNE and seek medical evaluation immediately. (See WARNINGS)

It is essential that patients be monitored intensively during the first 18 weeks of therapy with VIRAMUNE to detect potentially life-threatening hepatotoxicity or skin reactions. The greatest risk of severe rash or hepatic events (often associated with rash) occurs in the first 6 weeks of therapy. However, the risk of any hepatic event, with or without rash, continues past this period and monitoring should continue at frequent intervals. In some cases, hepatic injury has progressed despite discontinuation of treatment. VIRAMUNE should not be restarted following severe hepatic, skin or hypersensitivity reactions. In addition, the 14-day lead-in period with VIRAMUNE 200 mg daily dosing must be strictly followed. (See WARNINGS)

DESCRIPTION

VIRAMUNE is the brand name for nevirapine (NVP), a non-nucleoside reverse transcriptase inhibitor with activity against Human Immunodeficiency Virus Type 1 (HIV-1). Nevirapine is structurally a member of the dipyridodiazepinone chemical class of compounds.

VIRAMUNE Tablets are for oral administration. Each tablet contains 200 mg of nevirapine and the inactive ingredients microcrystalline cellulose, lactose monohydrate, povidone, sodium starch glycolate, colloidal silicon dioxide and magnesium stearate.

VIRAMUNE Oral Suspension is for oral administration. Each 5 mL of VIRAMUNE suspension contains 50 mg of nevirapine (as nevirapine hemihydrate). The suspension also contains the following excipients: carbomer 934P, methylparaben, propylparaben, sorbitol, sucrose, polysorbate 80, sodium hydroxide and purified water.

The chemical name of nevirapine is 11-cyclopropyl-5,11-dihydro-4-methyl-6H-dipyrido [3,2-b:2′,3′-e][1,4] diazepin-6-one. Nevirapine is a white to off-white crystalline powder with the molecular weight of 266.30 and the molecular formula $C_{15}H_{14}N_4O$. Nevirapine has the following structural formula:

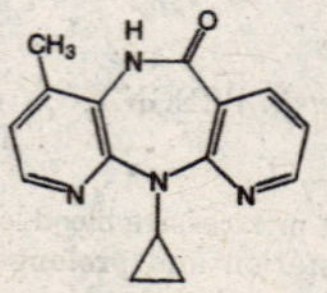

MICROBIOLOGY

Mechanism of Action:

Nevirapine is a non-nucleoside reverse transcriptase inhibitor (NNRTI) of HIV-1. Nevirapine binds directly to reverse transcriptase (RT) and blocks the RNA-dependent and DNA-dependent DNA polymerase activities by causing a disruption of the enzyme's catalytic site. The activity of nevirapine does not compete with template or nucleoside triphosphates. HIV-2 RT and eukaryotic DNA polymerases (such as human DNA polymerases α, β, γ, or δ) are not inhibited by nevirapine.

In Vitro HIV Susceptibility:

The *in vitro* antiviral activity of nevirapine was measured in peripheral blood mononuclear cells, monocyte derived macrophages, and lymphoblastoid cell lines. IC_{50} values (50% inhibitory concentration) ranged from 10-100 nM against laboratory and clinical isolates of HIV-1. In cell culture, nevirapine demonstrated additive to synergistic activity against HIV-1 in drug combination regimens with zidovudine (ZDV), didanosine (ddI), stavudine (d4T), lamivudine (3TC), saquinavir, and indinavir. The relationship between *in vitro* susceptibility of HIV-1 to nevirapine and the inhibition of HIV-1 replication in humans has not been established.

Resistance:

HIV-1 isolates with reduced susceptibility (100-250-fold) to nevirapine emerge *in vitro*. Genotypic analysis showed mutations in the HIV-1 RT gene Y181C and/or V106A depending upon the virus strain and cell line employed. Time to emergence of nevirapine resistance *in vitro* was not altered when selection included nevirapine in combination with several other NNRTIs.

Phenotypic and genotypic changes in HIV-1 isolates from patients treated with either nevirapine (n=24) or nevirapine and ZDV (n=14) were monitored in Phase I/II trials over 1 to

Table 3: Incidence of Adverse Events that Led to the Discontinuation of Treatment: Adverse Events with an Incidence of ≥1% in the AGGRENOX group

	Treatment Groups			
	AGGRENOX®	ER-DP	ASA	Placebo
Total Number of Patients	1650	1654	1649	1649
Patients with at least one Adverse Event that led to treatment discontinuation	417 (25%)	419 (25%)	318 (19%)	352 (21%)
Headache	165 (10%)	166 (10%)	57 (3%)	69 (4%)
Dizziness	85 (5%)	97 (6%)	69 (4%)	68 (4%)
Nausea	91 (6%)	95 (6%)	51 (3%)	53 (3%)
Abdominal Pain	74 (4%)	64 (4%)	56 (3%)	52 (3%)
Dyspepsia	59 (4%)	61 (4%)	49 (3%)	46 (3%)
Vomiting	53 (3%)	52 (3%)	28 (2%)	24 (1%)
Diarrhea	35 (2%)	41 (2%)	9 (<1%)	16 (<1%)
Stroke	39 (2%)	48 (3%)	57 (3%)	73 (4%)
Transient Ischemic Attack	35 (2%)	40 (2%)	26 (2%)	48 (3%)
Angina Pectoris	23 (1%)	20 (1%)	16 (<1%)	26 (2%)

Note: ER-DP = extended-release dipyridamole 200 mg; ASA = aspirin 25 mg. The dosage regimen for all treatment groups is b.i.d.

≥12 weeks. After 1 week of nevirapine monotherapy, isolates from 3/3 patients had decreased susceptibility to nevirapine *in vitro*; one or more of the RT mutations K103N, V106A, V108I, Y181C, Y188C and G190A were detected in HIV-1 isolates from some patients as early as 2 weeks after therapy initiation. By week eight of nevirapine monotherapy, 100% of the patients tested (n=24) had HIV-1 isolates with a >100-fold decrease in susceptibility to nevirapine *in vitro* compared to baseline, and had one or more of the nevirapine-associated RT resistance mutations; 19 of 24 patients (80%) had isolates with Y181C mutations regardless of dose. Nevirapine+ZDV combination therapy did not alter the emergence rate of nevirapine-resistant virus or the magnitude of nevirapine resistance *in vitro*. The clinical relevance of phenotypic and genotypic changes associated with nevirapine therapy has not been established.

Cross-resistance:
Rapid emergence of HIV-1 strains which are cross-resistant to NNRTIs has been observed *in vitro*. Nevirapine-resistant HIV-1 isolates were cross-resistant to the NNRTIs efavirenz and delavirdine. However, nevirapine-resistant isolates were susceptible to the nucleoside analogues ZDV and ddI. Similarly, ZDV-resistant isolates were susceptible to nevirapine *in vitro*.

ANIMAL PHARMACOLOGY

Animal studies have shown that nevirapine is widely distributed to nearly all tissues and readily crosses the blood-brain barrier.

CLINICAL PHARMACOLOGY

Pharmacokinetics in Adults:

Absorption and Bioavailability: Nevirapine is readily absorbed (>90%) after oral administration in healthy volunteers and in adults with HIV-1 infection. Absolute bioavailability in 12 healthy adults following single-dose administration was 93 ± 9% (mean ± SD) for a 50 mg tablet and 91 ± 8% for an oral solution. Peak plasma nevirapine concentrations of 2 ± 0.4 μg/mL (7.5 μM) were attained by 4 hours following a single 200 mg dose. Following multiple doses, nevirapine peak concentrations appear to increase linearly in the dose range of 200 to 400 mg/day. Steady state trough nevirapine concentrations of 4.5 ± 1.9 μg/mL (17 ± 7 μM), (n = 242) were attained at 400 mg/day. Nevirapine tablets and suspension have been shown to be comparably bioavailable and interchangeable at doses up to 200 mg. When VIRAMUNE (200 mg) was administered to 24 healthy adults (12 female, 12 male), with either a high fat breakfast (857 kcal, 50 g fat, 53% of calories from fat) or antacid (Maalox® 30 mL), the extent of nevirapine absorption (AUC) was comparable to that observed under fasting conditions. In a separate study in HIV-1 infected patients (n=6), nevirapine steady-state systemic exposure (AUC_τ) was not significantly altered by didanosine, which is formulated with an alkaline buffering agent. VIRAMUNE may be administered with or without food, antacid or didanosine.

Distribution: Nevirapine is highly lipophilic and is essentially nonionized at physiologic pH. Following intravenous administration to healthy adults, the apparent volume of distribution (Vdss) of nevirapine was 1.21 ± 0.09 L/kg, suggesting that nevirapine is widely distributed in humans. Nevirapine readily crosses the placenta and is also found in breast milk. (See PRECAUTIONS, *Nursing Mothers*) Nevirapine is about 60% bound to plasma proteins in the plasma concentration range of 1–10 μg/mL. Nevirapine concentrations in human cerebrospinal fluid (n=6) were 45% (± 5%) of the concentrations in plasma; this ratio is approximately equal to the fraction not bound to plasma protein.

Metabolism/Elimination: *In vivo* studies in humans and *in vitro* studies with human liver microsomes have shown that nevirapine is extensively biotransformed via cytochrome P450 (oxidative) metabolism to several hydroxylated metabolites. *In vitro* studies with human liver microsomes suggest that oxidative metabolism of nevirapine is mediated primarily by cytochrome P450 (CYP) isozymes from the CYP3A4 and CYP2B6 families, although other isozymes may have a secondary role. In a mass balance/excretion study in eight healthy male volunteers dosed to steady state with nevirapine 200 mg given twice daily followed by a single 50 mg dose of ^{14}C-nevirapine, approximately 91.4 ± 10.5% of the radiolabeled dose was recovered, with urine (81.3 ± 11.1%) representing the primary route of excretion compared to feces (10.1 ± 1.5%). Greater than 80% of the radioactivity in urine was made up of glucuronide conjugates of hydroxylated metabolites. Thus cytochrome P450 metabolism, glucuronide conjugation, and urinary excretion of glucuronidated metabolites represent the primary route of nevirapine biotransformation and elimination in humans. Only a small fraction (<5%) of the radioactivity in urine (representing <3% of the total dose) was made up of parent compound; therefore, renal excretion plays a minor role in elimination of the parent compound.

Nevirapine is an inducer of hepatic cytochrome P450 (CYP) metabolic enzymes 3A4 and 2B6. Nevirapine induces CYP3A4 and CYP2B6 by approximately 20–25%, as indicated by erythromycin breath test results and urine metabolites. Autoinduction of CYP3A4 and CYP2B6 mediated metabolism leads to an approximately 1.5 to 2 fold increase in the apparent oral clearance of nevirapine as treatment continues from a single dose to two-to-four weeks of dosing with 200–400 mg/day. Autoinduction also results in a corresponding decrease in the terminal phase half-life of nevirapine in plasma, from approximately 45 hours (single dose) to approximately 25–30 hours following multiple dosing with 200–400 mg/day.

Table 1: Drug Interactions:
Changes in Pharmacokinetic Parameters for Co-administered Drug in the Presence of VIRAMUNE
(All interaction studies were conducted in HIV-1 positive patients)

Co-administered Drug	Dose of Co-administered Drug	Dose Regimen of VIRAMUNE	n	% Change of Co-administered Drug Pharmacokinetic Parameters (90% CI)		
Antiretrovirals				AUC	C_{max}	C_{min}
Didanosine	100–150 mg BID	200 mg QD × 14 days; 200 mg BID × 14 days	18	↔	↔	§
Efavirenz[a]	600 mg QD	200 mg QD × 14 days; 400 mg QD × 14 days	17	↓28 (↓34 to ↓14)	↓12 (↓23 to ↑1)	↓32 (↓35 to ↓19)
Indinavir[a]	800 mg q8H	200 mg QD × 14 days; 200 mg BID × 14 days	19	↓31 (↓39 to ↓22)	↓15 (↓24 to ↓4)	↓44 (↓53 to ↓33)
Lopinavir[a,b]	300/75 mg/m² (lopinavir/ritonavir)[b]	7 mg/kg or 4 mg/kg QD × 2 weeks; BID × 1 week	12, 15[c]	↓14 (↓36 to ↑16)	↓22 (↓44 to ↑9)	↓55 (↓75 to ↓9)
Lopinavir[a]	400/100 mg BID (lopinavir/ritonavir)	200 mg QD × 14 days; 200 mg BID > 1 year	22, 19[c]	↓27 (↓47 to ↓2)	↓19 (↓38 to ↑5)	↓51 (↓72 to ↓26)
Nelfinavir[a]	750 mg TID	200 mg QD × 14 days; 200 mg BID × 14 days	23	↔	↔	↓32 (↓50 to ↑5)
Nelfinavir-M8 metabolite				↓62 (↓70 to ↓53)	↓59 (↓68 to ↓48)	↓66 (↓74 to ↓55)
Ritonavir	600 mg BID	200 mg QD × 14 days; 200 mg BID × 14 days	18	↔	↔	↔
Saquinavir[a]	600 mg TID	200 mg QD × 14 days; 200 mg BID × 21 days	23	↓38 (↓47 to ↓11)	↓32 (↓44 to ↓6)	§
Stavudine	30–40 mg BID	200 mg QD × 14 days; 200 mg BID × 14 days	22	↔	↔	§
Zalcitabine	0,125–0.25 mg TID	200 mg QD × 14 days; 200 mg BID × 14 days	6	↔	↔	§
Zidovudine	100–200 mg TID	200 mg QD × 14 days; 200 mg BID × 14 days	11	↓28 (↓40 to ↓4)	↓30 (↓51 to ↑14)	§
Other Medications				AUC	C_{max}	C_{min}
Clarithromycin[a]	500 mg BID	200 mg QD × 14 days; 200 mg BID × 14 days	15	↓31 (↓38 to ↓24)	↓23 (↓31 to ↓14)	↓57 (↓70 to ↓36)
Metabolite 14-OH-clarithromycin				↑42 (↑16 to ↑73)	↑47 (↑21 to ↑80)	↔
Ethinyl estradiol[a] and	0.035 mg (as Ortho-Novum® 1/35)	200 mg QD × 14 days; 200 mg BID × 14 days	10	↓20 (↓33 to ↓3)	↔	§
Norethindrone[a]	1 mg (as Ortho-Novum® 1/35)			↓19 (↓30 to ↓7)	↓16 (↓27 to ↓3)	§
Fluconazole	200 mg QD	200 mg QD × 14 days; 200 mg BID × 14 days	19	↔	↔	↔
Ketoconazole[a]	400 mg QD	200 mg QD × 14 days; 200 mg BID × 14 days	21	↓72 (↓80 to ↓60)	↓44 (↓58 to ↓27)	§
Rifabutin[a]	150 or 300 mg QD	200 mg QD × 14 days; 200 mg BID × 14 days	19	↑17 (↓2 to ↑40)	↑28 (↑9 to ↑51)	↔
Metabolite 25-O-desacetyl-rifabutin				↑24 (↓16 to ↑84)	↑29 (↓2 to ↑68)	↑22 (↓14 to ↑74)
Rifampin[a]	600 mg QD	200 mg QD × 14 days; 200 mg BID × 14 days	14	↑11 (↓4 to ↑28)	↔	§

§ = C_{min} below detectable level of the assay
↑ = Increase, ↓ = Decrease, ↔ = No Effect
[a]For information regarding clinical recommendations see PRECAUTIONS, *Drug Interactions*, Table 3
[b]Pediatric subjects ranging in age from 6 months to 12 years
[c]Parallel group design; n for VIRAMUNE +lopinavir/ritonavir, n for lopinavir/ritonavir alone

Pharmacokinetics in Special Populations:

Renal Impairment: HIV seronegative adults with mild (CrCL 50-79 mL/min; n=7), moderate (CrCL 30-49 mL/min; n=6), or severe (CrCL <30 mL/min; n=4) renal impairment received a single 200 mg dose of nevirapine in a pharmacokinetic study. These subjects did not require dialysis. The study included six additional subjects with renal failure requiring dialysis.

In subjects with renal impairment (mild, moderate or severe), there were no significant changes in the pharmacokinetics of nevirapine. However, subjects requiring dialysis exhibited a 44% reduction in nevirapine AUC over a one-week exposure period. There was also evidence of accumulation of nevirapine hydroxy-metabolites in plasma in subjects requiring dialysis. An additional 200 mg dose following each dialysis treatment is indicated. (See DOSAGE and ADMINISTRATION; PRECAUTIONS)

Hepatic Impairment: HIV seronegative adults with mild (Child-Pugh Class A; n=6) or moderate (Child-Pugh Class B; n=4) hepatic impairment received a single 200 mg dose of nevirapine in a pharmacokinetic study.

In the majority of patients with mild or moderate hepatic impairment, no significant changes were seen in the pharmacokinetics of nevirapine. However, a significant increase in the AUC of nevirapine observed in one patient with Child-Pugh Class B and ascites suggests that patients with worsening hepatic function and ascites may be at risk of accumulating nevirapine in the systemic circulation. Because nevirapine induces its own metabolism with multiple dosing, a single dose study may not reflect the impact of hepatic impairment on multiple dose pharmacokinetics. (See PRECAUTIONS) Nevirapine should not be administered to patients with severe hepatic impairment. (See WARNINGS)

Gender: In one Phase I study in healthy volunteers (15 females, 15 males), the weight-adjusted apparent volume of distribution (Vdss/F) of nevirapine was higher in the female subjects (1.54 L/kg) compared to the males (1.38 L/kg), suggesting that nevirapine was distributed more extensively in the female subjects. However, this difference was offset by a slightly shorter terminal-phase half-life in the females re-

Continued on next page

Viramune—Cont.

sulting in no significant gender difference in nevirapine oral clearance (24.6±7.7 mL/kg/hr in females vs. 19.9±3.9 mL/kg/hr in males after single dose) or plasma concentrations following either single- or multiple-dose administration(s).

Race: An evaluation of nevirapine plasma concentrations (pooled data from several clinical trials) from HIV-1-infected patients (27 Black, 24 Hispanic, 189 Caucasian) revealed no marked difference in nevirapine steady-state trough concentrations (median C_{minss} = 4.7 µg/mL Black, 3.8 µg/mL Hispanic, 4.3 µg/mL Caucasian) with long-term nevirapine treatment at 400 mg/day. However, the pharmacokinetics of nevirapine have not been evaluated specifically for the effects of ethnicity.

Geriatric Patients: Nevirapine pharmacokinetics in HIV-1 infected adults do not appear to change with age (range 18–68 years); however, nevirapine has not been extensively evaluated in patients beyond the age of 55 years.

Pediatric Patients: The pharmacokinetics of nevirapine have been studied in two open-label studies in children with HIV-1 infection. In one study (BI 853; ACTG 165), nine HIV-1-infected children ranging in age from 9 months to 14 years were administered a single dose (7.5 mg, 30 mg, or 120 mg per m^2; n=3 per dose) of nevirapine suspension after an overnight fast. The mean nevirapine apparent clearance adjusted for body weight was greater in children compared to adults.

In a multiple dose study (BI 882; ACTG 180), nevirapine suspension or tablets (240 or 400 mg/m^2/day) were administered as monotherapy or in combination with ZDV or ZDV+ddI to 37 HIV-1-infected pediatric patients with the following demographics: male (54%), racial minority groups (73%), median age of 11 months (range: 2 months–15 years). The majority of these patients received 120 mg/m^2/day of nevirapine for approximately 4 weeks followed by 120 mg/m^2/b.i.d. (patients > 9 years of age) or 200 mg/m^2/b.i.d. (patients ≤ 9 years of age). Nevirapine apparent clearance adjusted for body weight reached maximum values by age 1 to 2 years and then decreased with increasing age. Nevirapine apparent clearance adjusted for body weight was at least two-fold greater in children younger than 8 years compared to adults. The relationship between nevirapine clearance with long term drug administration and age is shown in Figure 1. The pediatric dosing regimens were selected in order to achieve steady-state plasma concentrations in pediatric patients that approximate those in adults. (See DOSAGE AND ADMINISTRATION, *Pediatric Patients*)

Figure 1: Nevirapine Apparent Clearance (mL/kg/hr) in Pediatric Patients

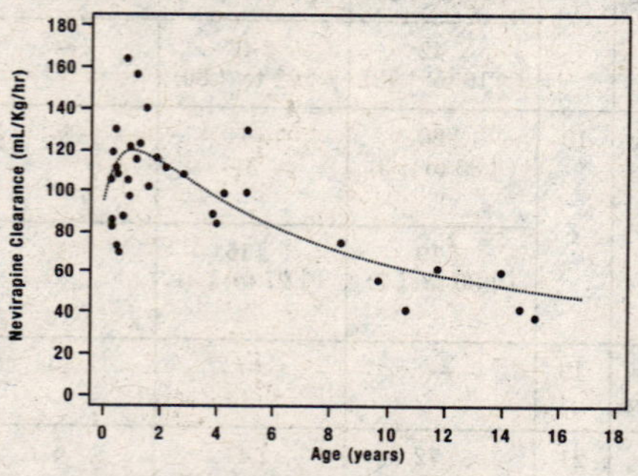

Drug Interactions: (See PRECAUTIONS, *Drug Interactions*) Nevirapine induces hepatic cytochrome P450 metabolic isoenzymes 3A4 and 2B6. Co-administration of VIRAMUNE and drugs primarily metabolized by CYP3A4 or CYP2B6 may result in decreased plasma concentrations of these drugs and attenuate their therapeutic effects.

While primarily an inducer of cytochrome P450 3A4 and 2B6 enzymes, nevirapine may also inhibit this system. Among human hepatic cytochrome P450s, nevirapine was capable in vitro of inhibiting the 10-hydroxylation of (R)-warfarin (CYP3A4). The estimated K_i for the inhibition of CYP3A4 was 270 µM, a concentration that is unlikely to be achieved in patients as the therapeutic range is <25 µM. Therefore, nevirapine may have minimal inhibitory effect on other substrates of CYP3A4.

Nevirapine does not appear to affect the plasma concentrations of drugs that are substrates of other CYP450 enzyme systems, such as 1A2, 2D6, 2A6, 2E1, 2C9 or 2C19.

Table 1 (see below) contains the results of drug interaction studies performed with VIRAMUNE and other drugs likely to be co-administered. The effects of VIRAMUNE on the AUC, C_{max}, and C_{min} of co-administered drugs are summarized. To measure the full potential pharmacokinetic interaction effect following induction, patients on the concomitant drug at steady state were administered 28 days of VIRAMUNE (200 mg QD for 14 days followed by 200 mg BID for 14 days) followed by a steady state reassessment of the concomitant drug.

[See table 1 at top of previous page]

Because of the design of the drug interaction trials (addition of 28 days of VIRAMUNE therapy to existing HIV therapy) the effect of the concomitant drug on plasma nevirapine steady state concentrations was estimated by comparison to historical controls.

Administration of rifampin had a clinically significant effect on nevirapine pharmacokinetics, decreasing AUC and C_{max} by greater than 50%. Administration of fluconazole resulted in an approximate 100% increase in nevirapine exposure, based on a comparison to historic data. (See PRECAUTIONS, *Drug Interactions*, Table 3). The effect of other drugs listed in Table 1 on nevirapine pharmacokinetics was not significant.

INDICATIONS AND USAGE

VIRAMUNE (nevirapine) is indicated for use in combination with other antiretroviral agents for the treatment of HIV-1 infection. This indication is based on one principal clinical trial that demonstrated prolonged suppression of HIV-RNA and two smaller supportive studies, one of which is described below.

Description of Clinical Studies:

Trial BI 1090, was a placebo-controlled, double-blind, randomized trial in 2249 HIV-1 infected patients with <200 CD4+ cells at screening. Initiated in 1995, BI 1090 compared treatment with VIRAMUNE + lamivudine + background therapy versus lamivudine + background therapy in NNRTI naïve patients. Treatment doses were VIRAMUNE, 200 mg daily for two weeks followed by 200 mg twice daily or placebo, and lamivudine 150 mg twice daily. Other antiretroviral agents were given at approved doses. Initial background therapy (in addition to lamivudine) was one NRTI in 1309 patients (58%), two or more NRTIs in 771 (34%), and PIs and NRTIs in 169 (8%). The patients (median age 36.5 years, 70% Caucasian, 79% male) had advanced HIV infection, with a median baseline CD4+ cell count of 96 cells/mm^3 and a baseline HIV RNA of 4.58 log_{10} copies/mL (38,291 copies/mL). Prior to entering the trial, 45% had previously experienced an AIDS-defining clinical event. Eighty-nine percent had antiretroviral treatment prior to entering the trial. BI 1090 was originally designed as a clinical endpoint study. Prior to unblinding the trial, the primary endpoint was changed to proportion of patients with HIV RNA <50 copies/mL and not previously failed at 48 weeks. Treatment response and outcomes are shown in Figure 2 and Table 2.

Figure 2: BI 1090: Percent Responders by Visit (LOQ=50 copies/mL)

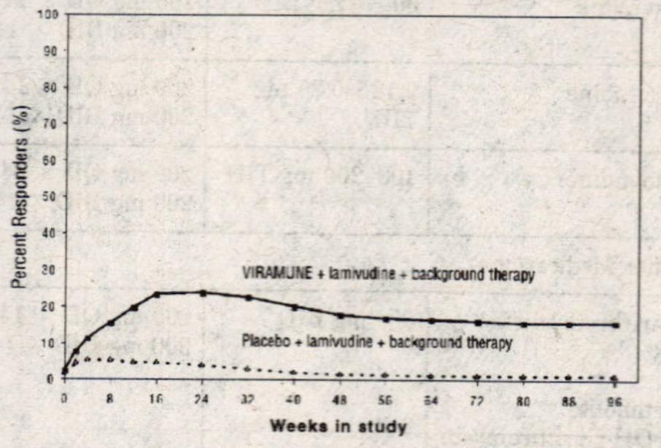

Total number of patients with HIV-RNA data at specified time point, plus number of patients who previously reached a failure endpoint:

	8 Weeks	48 Weeks	96 Weeks
VIRAMUNE:	1120	1097	941
Placebo:	1128	1120	1105

Table 2: BI 1090 Outcomes through 48 weeks

Outcome	VIRAMUNE (N=1121) %	Placebo (N=1128) %
Responders at 48 weeks: HIV RNA <50 copies/mL	18.0	1.6
Treatment Failure	82.0	98.4
Never suppressed viral load	44.6	66.4
Virologic failure after response	7.2	4.3
CDC category C event or death	9.6	11.2
Added antiretroviral therapy[1] while <50 copies/mL	5.0	0.9
Discontinued trial therapy due to AE	7.0	5.9
Discontinued trial <48 weeks[2]	8.5	9.8

[1] including change to open-label NVP

[2] includes withdrawal of consent, lost to follow-up, non-compliance with protocol, other administrative reasons

The change from baseline in CD4+ cell count through one year of therapy was significantly greater for the VIRAMUNE group compared to the placebo group for the overall study population (64 cells/mm^3 vs 22 cells/mm^3, respectively), as well as for patients who entered the trial as treatment naïve or having received only ZDV (85 cells/mm^3 vs 25 cells/mm^3, respectively).

At two years into the study, 16% of subjects on VIRAMUNE had experienced class C CDC events as compared to 21% of subjects on the control arm.

Trial BI 1046 (INCAS) was a double-blind, placebo-controlled, randomized, three arm trial with 151 HIV-1 infected patients with CD4+ cell counts of 200–600 at baseline. BI 1046 compared treatment with VIRAMUNE+zidovudine+didanosine to VIRAMUNE+zidovudine and zidovudine+didanosine. Treatment doses were VIRAMUNE at 200 mg daily for two weeks followed by 200 mg twice daily or placebo, zidovudine at 200 mg three times daily, and didanosine at 125 or 200 mg twice daily (depending on body weight). The patients had mean baseline HIV RNA of 4.41 log_{10} copies/mL (25,704 copies/mL) and mean baseline CD4+ cell count of 376 cells/mm^3. The primary endpoint was the proportion of patients with HIV-RNA < 400 copies/mL and not previously failed at 48 weeks. The virologic responder rates at 48 weeks were 45% for patients treated with VIRAMUNE+zidovudine+didanosine, 19% for patients treated with zidovudine+didanosine, and 0% for patients treated with VIRAMUNE+zidovudine.

CD4+ cell counts in the VIRAMUNE+ZDV+ddI group increased above baseline by a mean of 139 cells/mm^3 at one year, significantly greater than the increase of 87 cells/mm^3 in the ZDV+ddI patients. The VIRAMUNE+ZDV group mean decreased by 6 cells/mm^3 below baseline.

CONTRAINDICATIONS

VIRAMUNE (nevirapine) is contraindicated in patients with clinically significant hypersensitivity to any of the components contained in the tablet or the oral suspension.

WARNINGS

General:

The first 18 weeks of therapy with VIRAMUNE are a critical period during which intensive monitoring of patients is required to detect potentially life-threatening hepatic events and skin reactions. The optimal frequency of monitoring during this time period has not been established. Some experts recommend clinical and laboratory monitoring more often than once per month, and in particular, would include monitoring of liver function tests at baseline, prior to dose escalation and at two weeks post-dose escalation. After the initial 18 week period, frequent clinical and laboratory monitoring should continue throughout VIRAMUNE treatment. In addition, the 14-day lead-in period with VIRAMUNE 200 mg daily dosing has been demonstrated to reduce the frequency of rash.

Resistant virus emerges rapidly and uniformly when VIRAMUNE is administered as monotherapy. Therefore, VIRAMUNE should always be administered in combination with other antiretroviral agents for the treatment of HIV-1 infection.

Hepatic Events:

Severe, life-threatening, and in some cases fatal hepatotoxicity, including fulminant and cholestatic hepatitis, hepatic necrosis and hepatic failure, have been reported in patients treated with VIRAMUNE. In clinical trials, the risk of hepatic events regardless of severity was greatest in the first 6 weeks of therapy. The risk continued to be greater in the VIRAMUNE groups compared to controls through 18 weeks of treatment. However, hepatic events may occur at any time during treatment. In some cases, patients presented with non-specific, prodromal signs or symptoms of fatigue, malaise, anorexia, nausea, jaundice, liver tenderness or hepatomegaly, with or without initially abnormal serum transaminase levels. Some of these events have progressed to hepatic failure with transaminase elevation, with or without hyperbilirubinemia, prolonged partial thromboplastin time, or eosinophilia. Rash and fever accompanied some of these hepatic events. Patients with signs or symptoms of hepatitis must be advised to discontinue VIRAMUNE and immediately seek medical evaluation, which should include liver function tests.

The patients at greatest risk of hepatic events, including potentially fatal events, are women with high CD4 counts.

In addition, serious hepatotoxicity (including liver failure requiring transplantation in one instance) has been reported in HIV-uninfected individuals receiving multiple doses of VIRAMUNE in the setting of post-exposure prophylaxis, an unapproved use.

Increased AST or ALT levels and/or co-infection with hepatitis B or C at the start of antiretroviral therapy are associated with a greater risk of hepatic adverse events.

In general, women have a three fold higher risk than men for symptomatic, often rash-associated, hepatic events (5.8% versus 2.2%), and patients with higher CD4 counts at initiation of VIRAMUNE therapy are at higher risk for symptomatic hepatic events with VIRAMUNE. In a retrospective review, women with CD4 counts >250 cells/mm^3 had a 12 fold higher risk of symptomatic hepatic adverse events compared to women with CD4 counts <250 cells/mm^3 (11.0% versus 0.9%). An increased risk was observed in men with CD4 counts >400 cells/mm^3 (6.3% versus 2.3% for men with CD4 counts <400 cells/mm^3).

Because increased nevirapine levels and nevirapine accumulation may be observed in patients with serious liver disease, VIRAMUNE should not be administered to patients with severe hepatic impairment. (See CLINICAL PHARMACOLOGY, *Pharmacokinetics in Special Populations: Hepatic Impairment*; PRECAUTIONS, *General*).

Intensive clinical and laboratory monitoring, including liver function tests, is essential at baseline and during the first 18 weeks of treatment. (See WARNINGS, *General*) Monitoring should continue at frequent intervals thereafter. Liver function tests should be performed immediately if a patient experiences signs or symptoms suggestive of hepatitis and/or hypersensitivity reaction. Liver function tests should also be obtained for all patients who develop a rash in the first 18 weeks of treatment. Physicians and patients

should be vigilant for the appearance of signs or symptoms of hepatitis, such as fatigue, malaise, anorexia, nausea, jaundice, bilirubinuria, acholic stools, liver tenderness or hepatomegaly. The diagnosis of hepatotoxicity should be considered in this setting, even if liver function tests are initially normal or alternative diagnoses are possible. (See PRECAUTIONS, *Information for Patients*; ADVERSE REACTIONS; DOSAGE AND ADMINISTRATION).

If clinical hepatitis occurs, VIRAMUNE should be permanently discontinued and not restarted after recovery. In some cases, hepatic injury progresses despite discontinuation of treatment.

Skin Reactions:

Severe, life-threatening skin reactions, including fatal cases, have been reported with VIRAMUNE treatment, occurring most frequently during the first 6 weeks of therapy. These have included cases of Stevens-Johnson syndrome, toxic epidermal necrolysis, and hypersensitivity reactions characterized by rash, constitutional findings, and organ dysfunction. Patients developing signs or symptoms of severe skin reactions or hypersensitivity reactions (including, but not limited to, severe rash or rash accompanied by fever, general malaise, fatigue, muscle or joint aches, blisters, oral lesions, conjunctivitis, facial edema, and/or hepatitis, eosinophilia, granulocytopenia, lymphadenopathy, and renal dysfunction) must permanently discontinue VIRAMUNE and seek medical evaluation immediately. (See PRECAUTIONS, *Information for Patients*; ADVERSE REACTIONS) VIRAMUNE should not be restarted following severe skin rash or hypersensitivity reaction. Some of the risk factors for developing serious cutaneous reactions include failure to follow the initial dosing of 200 mg daily during the 14-day lead-in period and delay in stopping the VIRAMUNE treatment after the onset of the initial symptoms.

If patients present with a suspected VIRAMUNE-associated rash, liver function tests should be performed. Patients with rash-associated AST or ALT elevations should be permanently discontinued from VIRAMUNE.

Therapy with VIRAMUNE must be initiated with a 14-day lead-in period of 200 mg/day (4 mg/kg/day in pediatric patients), which has been shown to reduce the frequency of rash. If rash is observed during this lead-in period, dose escalation should not occur until the rash has resolved. (See DOSAGE AND ADMINISTRATION) Patients should be monitored closely if isolated rash of any severity occurs. Women appear to be at higher risk than men of developing rash with VIRAMUNE.

In a clinical trial, concomitant prednisone use (40 mg/day for the first 14 days of VIRAMUNE administration) was associated with an increase in incidence and severity of rash during the first 6 weeks of VIRAMUNE therapy. Therefore, use of prednisone to prevent VIRAMUNE-associated rash is not recommended.

St. John's wort:

Concomitant use of St. John's wort (hypericum perforatum) or St. John's wort containing products and VIRAMUNE is not recommended. Co-administration of Non-Nucleoside Reverse Transcriptase Inhibitors (NNRTIs), including VIRAMUNE, with St. John's wort is expected to substantially decrease NNRTI concentrations and may result in sub-optimal levels of VIRAMUNE and lead to loss of virologic response and possible resistance to VIRAMUNE or to the class of NNRTIs.

PRECAUTIONS

General:

Nevirapine is extensively metabolized by the liver and nevirapine metabolites are extensively eliminated by the kidney. No adjustment in nevirapine dosing is required in patients with CrCL ≥20 mL/min. In patients undergoing chronic hemodialysis, an additional 200 mg dose following each dialysis treatment is indicated. Nevirapine metabolites may accumulate in patients receiving dialysis; however, the clinical significance of this accumulation is not known. (See CLINICAL PHARMACOLOGY, *Pharmacokinetics in Special Populations: Renal Impairment*; DOSAGE AND ADMINISTRATION, *Dosage Adjustment*)

It is not clear whether a dosing adjustment is needed for patients with mild to moderate hepatic impairment, because multiple dose pharmacokinetic data are not available for this population. However, patients with moderate hepatic impairment and ascites may be at risk of accumulating nevirapine in the systemic circulation. Caution should be exercised when nevirapine is administered to patients with moderate hepatic impairment. Nevirapine should not be administered to patients with severe hepatic impairment. (See WARNINGS; CLINICAL PHARMACOLOGY, *Pharmacokinetics in Special Populations: Hepatic Impairment*)

The duration of clinical benefit from antiretroviral therapy may be limited. Patients receiving VIRAMUNE or any other antiretroviral therapy may continue to develop opportunistic infections and other complications of HIV infection, and therefore should remain under close clinical observation by physicians experienced in the treatment of patients with associated HIV diseases.

When administering VIRAMUNE as part of an antiretroviral regimen, the complete product information for each therapeutic component should be consulted before initiation of treatment.

Drug Interactions:

Nevirapine is principally metabolized by the liver via the cytochrome P450 isoenzymes, 3A4 and 2B6. Nevirapine is known to be an inducer of these enzymes. As a result, drugs that are metabolized by these enzyme systems may have lower than expected plasma levels when co-administered with nevirapine.

The specific pharmacokinetic changes that occur with co-administration of nevirapine and other drugs are listed in CLINICAL PHARMACOLOGY, Table 1. Clinical comments about possible dosage modifications based on these pharmacokinetic changes are listed in Table 3. The data in Tables 1 and 3 are based on the results of drug interaction studies conducted in HIV-1 seropositive subjects unless otherwise indicated.

In addition to established drug interactions, there may be potential pharmacokinetic interactions between nevirapine and other drug classes that are metabolized by the cytochrome P450 system. These potential drug interaction studies are listed in Table 4. Although specific drug interaction studies in HIV-1 seropositive subjects have not been conducted for the classes of drugs listed in Table 4, additional clinical monitoring may be warranted when co-administering these drugs.

The *in vitro* interaction between nevirapine and the antithrombotic agent warfarin is complex. As a result, when giving these drugs concomitantly, plasma warfarin levels may change with the potential for increases in coagulation time. When warfarin is co-administered with nevirapine, anticoagulation levels should be monitored frequently.

[See table 3 above]

Table 3

***Established* Drug Interactions: Alteration in Dose or Regimen May Be Recommended Based on Drug Interaction Studies (See CLINICAL PHARMACOLOGY, Table 1 for Magnitude of Interaction)**

Drug Name	Effect on Concentration of Nevirapine or Concomitant Drug	Clinical Comment
Clarithromycin	↓ Clarithromycin ↑ 14-OH clarithromycin	Clarithromycin exposure was significantly decreased by nevirapine; however, 14-OH metabolite concentrations were increased. Because clarithromycin active metabolite has reduced activity against *Mycobacterium avium-intracellulare complex*, overall activity against this pathogen may be altered. Alternatives to clarithromycin, such as azithromycin, should be considered.
Efavirenz	↓ Efavirenz	Appropriate doses for this combination are not established.
Ethinyl estradiol and Norethindrone	↓ Ethinyl estradiol ↓ Norethindrone	Oral contraceptives and other hormonal methods of birth control should not be used as the sole method of contraception in women taking nevirapine, since nevirapine may lower the plasma levels of these medications. An alternative or additional method of contraception is recommended.
Fluconazole	↑ Nevirapine	Because of the risk of increased exposure to nevirapine, caution should be used in concomitant administration, and patients should be monitored closely for nevirapine-associated adverse events.
Indinavir	↓ Indinavir	Appropriate doses for this combination are not established, but an increase in the dosage of indinavir may be required.
Ketoconazole	↓ Ketoconazole	Nevirapine and ketoconazole should not be administered concomitantly because decreases in ketoconazole plasma concentrations may reduce the efficacy of the drug.
Lopinavir/Ritonavir	↓ Lopinavir	A dose increase of lopinavir/ritonavir to 533/133 mg twice daily with food is recommended in combination with nevirapine.
Methadone	↓ Methadone[a]	Methadone levels may be decreased; increased dosages may be required to prevent symptoms of opiate withdrawal. Methadone maintained patients beginning nevirapine therapy should be monitored for evidence of withdrawal and methadone dose should be adjusted accordingly.
Nelfinavir	↓ Nelfinavir M8 Metabolite ↓ Nelfinavir C_{min}	The appropriate dose for nelfinavir in combination with nevirapine, with respect to safety and efficacy, has not been established.
Rifabutin	↑ Rifabutin	Rifabutin and its metabolite concentrations were moderately increased. Due to high intersubject variability, however, some patients may experience large increases in rifabutin exposure and may be at higher risk for rifabutin toxicity. Therefore, caution should be used in concomitant administration.
Rifampin	↓ Nevirapine	Nevirapine and rifampin should not be administered concomitantly because decreases in nevirapine plasma concentrations may reduce the efficacy of the drug. Physicians needing to treat patients co-infected with tuberculosis and using a nevirapine containing regimen may use rifabutin instead.
Saquinavir	↓ Saquinavir	Appropriate doses for this combination are not established, but an increase in the dosage of saquinavir may be required.

[a]Based on reports of narcotic withdrawal syndrome in patients treated with nevirapine and methadone concurrently, and evidence of decreased plasma concentrations of methadone.

Table 4

***Potential* Drug Interactions: Use With Caution, Dose Adjustment of Co-administered Drug May Be Needed due to Possible Decrease in Clinical Effect**

Examples of Drugs in Which Plasma Concentrations May Be Decreased By Co-administration With Nevirapine

Drug Class	Examples of Drugs
Antiarrhythmics	Amiodarone, disopyramide, lidocaine

Continued on next page

Viramune—Cont.

Anticonvulsants	Carbamazepine, clonazepam, ethosuximide
Antifungals	Itraconazole
Calcium channel blockers	Diltiazem, nifedipine, verapamil
Cancer chemotherapy	Cyclophosphamide
Ergot alkaloids	Ergotamine
Immunosuppressants	Cyclosporin, tacrolimus, sirolimus
Motility agents	Cisapride
Opiate agonists	Fentanyl

Examples of Drugs in Which Plasma Concentrations May Be Increased By Co-administration With Nevirapine

Antithrombotics	Warfarin Potential effect on anticoagulation. Monitoring of anticoagulation levels is recommended.

Fat redistribution: Redistribution/accumulation of body fat including central obesity, dorsocervical fat enlargement (buffalo hump), peripheral wasting, facial wasting, breast enlargement, and "cushingoid appearance" have been observed in patients receiving antiretroviral therapy. The mechanism and long-term consequences of these events are currently unknown. A causal relationship has not been established.

Information for Patients:

Patients should be informed of the possibility of severe liver disease or skin reactions associated with VIRAMUNE that may result in death. Patients developing signs or symptoms of liver disease or severe skin reactions should be instructed to discontinue VIRAMUNE and seek medical attention immediately, including performance of laboratory monitoring. Symptoms of liver disease include fatigue, malaise, anorexia, nausea, jaundice, acholic stools, liver tenderness or hepatomegaly. Symptoms of severe skin or hypersensitivity reactions include rash accompanied by fever, general malaise, fatigue, muscle or joint aches, blisters, oral lesions, conjunctivitis, facial edema and/or hepatitis.

Intensive clinical and laboratory monitoring, including liver function tests, is essential during the first 18 weeks of therapy with VIRAMUNE to detect potentially life-threatening hepatotoxicity. However, liver disease can occur after this period, therefore monitoring should continue at frequent intervals throughout VIRAMUNE treatment. Extra vigilance is warranted during the first 6 weeks of therapy, which is the period of greatest risk of hepatic events and skin reactions. Patients with signs and symptoms of hepatitis should discontinue VIRAMUNE and seek medical evaluation immediately. If VIRAMUNE is discontinued due to hepatitis, it should not be restarted. Patients should be advised that co-infection with hepatitis B or C and/or increased liver function tests at the start of antiretroviral therapy are associated with a greater risk of hepatic events with VIRAMUNE. Patients, particularly women, with increased CD4+ cell count at initiation of VIRAMUNE therapy (>250 cells/mm^3 in women and >400 cells/mm^3 in men) may be at substantially higher risk for development of hepatic events, often associated with rash. (See WARNINGS, *Hepatic Events*)

The majority of rashes associated with VIRAMUNE occur within the first 6 weeks of initiation of therapy. Patients should be instructed that if any rash occurs during the two-week lead-in period, the VIRAMUNE dose should not be escalated until the rash resolves. Any patient experiencing severe rash or hypersensitivity reactions should discontinue VIRAMUNE and consult a physician. VIRAMUNE should not be restarted following severe skin rash or hypersensitivity reaction. Women tend to be at higher risk for development of VIRAMUNE associated rash.

Oral contraceptives and other hormonal methods of birth control should not be used as the sole method of contraception in women taking VIRAMUNE, since nevirapine may lower the plasma levels of these medications. Additionally, when oral contraceptives are used for hormonal regulation during VIRAMUNE therapy, the therapeutic effect of the hormonal therapy should be monitored. (See PRECAUTIONS, *Drug Interactions*)

Patients should be informed that VIRAMUNE therapy has not been shown to reduce the risk of transmission of HIV-1 to others through sexual contact or blood contamination. The long-term effects of VIRAMUNE are unknown at this time.

VIRAMUNE is not a cure for HIV-1 infection; patients may continue to experience illnesses associated with advanced HIV-1 infection, including opportunistic infections. Patients should be advised to remain under the care of a physician when using VIRAMUNE.

Patients should be informed to take VIRAMUNE every day as prescribed. Patients should not alter the dose without consulting their doctor. If a dose is missed, patients should take the next dose as soon as possible. However, if a dose is skipped, the patient should not double the next dose. Patients should be advised to report to their doctor the use of any other medications. Based on the known metabolism of methadone, nevirapine may decrease plasma concentrations of methadone by increasing its hepatic metabolism. Narcotic withdrawal syndrome has been reported in patients treated with VIRAMUNE and methadone concomitantly. Methadone-maintained patients beginning nevirapine therapy should be monitored for evidence of withdrawal and methadone dose should be adjusted accordingly.

VIRAMUNE may interact with some drugs, therefore, patients should be advised to report to their doctor the use of any other prescription, non-prescription medication or herbal products, particularly St. John's wort.

Patients should be informed that redistribution or accumulation of body fat may occur in patients receiving antiretroviral therapy and that the cause and long term health effects of these conditions are not known at this time.

The Patient Package Insert provides written information for the patient, and should be dispensed with each new prescription and refill.

Carcinogenesis, Mutagenesis, Impairment of Fertility:

Long-term carcinogenicity studies in mice and rats were carried out with nevirapine. Mice were dosed with 0, 50, 375 or 750 mg/kg/day for two years. Hepatocellular adenomas and carcinomas were increased at all doses in males and at the two high doses in females. In studies in which rats were administered nevirapine at doses of 0, 3.5, 17.5 or 35 mg/kg/day for two years, an increase in hepatocellular adenomas was seen in males at all doses and in females at the high dose. The systemic exposure (based on AUCs) at all doses in the two animal studies were lower than that measured in humans at the 200 mg bid dose. The mechanism of the carcinogenic potential is unknown. However, in genetic toxicology assays, nevirapine showed no evidence of mutagenic or clastogenic activity in a battery of *in vitro* and *in vivo* studies. These included microbial assays for gene mutation (Ames: Salmonella strains and *E. coli*), mammalian cell gene mutation assay (CHO/HGPRT), cytogenetic assays using a Chinese hamster ovary cell line and a mouse bone marrow micronucleus assay following oral administration. Given the lack of genotoxic activity of nevirapine, the relevance to humans of hepatocellular neoplasms in nevirapine treated mice and rats is not known. In reproductive toxicology studies, evidence of impaired fertility was seen in female rats at doses providing systemic exposure, based on AUC, approximately equivalent to that provided with the recommended clinical dose of VIRAMUNE.

Pregnancy: Pregnancy Category C

No observable teratogenicity was detected in reproductive studies performed in pregnant rats and rabbits. In rats, a significant decrease in fetal body weight occurred at doses providing systemic exposure approximately 50% higher, based on AUC, than that seen at the recommended human clinical dose.

The maternal and developmental no-observable-effect level dosages in rats and rabbits produced systemic exposures approximately equivalent to or approximately 50% higher, respectively, than those seen at the recommended daily human dose, based on AUC. There are no adequate and well-controlled studies in pregnant women. VIRAMUNE should be used during pregnancy only if the potential benefit justifies the potential risk to the fetus. Severe hepatic events, including fatalities, have been reported in pregnant women receiving chronic VIRAMUNE therapy as part of combination treatment of HIV infection. It is unclear if pregnancy augments the already increased risk observed in non-pregnant women. (see Boxed WARNING)

Antiretroviral Pregnancy Registry:

To monitor maternal-fetal outcomes of pregnant women exposed to VIRAMUNE, an Antiretroviral Pregnancy Registry has been established. Physicians are encouraged to register patients by calling (800) 258-4263.

Nursing Mothers:

The Centers for Disease Control and Prevention recommend that HIV-infected mothers not breast-feed their infants to avoid risking postnatal transmission of HIV. Nevirapine is excreted in breast milk. Because of both the potential for HIV transmission and the potential for serious adverse reactions in nursing infants, mothers should be instructed not to breast-feed if they are receiving VIRAMUNE.

Pediatric Use:

The pharmacokinetics of nevirapine have been studied in two open-label studies in children with HIV-1 infection. (See CLINICAL PHARMACOLOGY, *Pharmacokinetics in Special Populations*) For dose recommendations for pediatric patients see DOSAGE AND ADMINISTRATION. The most frequently reported adverse events related to VIRAMUNE in pediatric patients were similar to those observed in adults, with the exception of granulocytopenia, which was more commonly observed in children. (See ADVERSE REACTIONS, *Pediatric Patients*) The evaluation of the antiviral activity of VIRAMUNE in pediatric patients is ongoing.

Geriatric Use:

Clinical studies of VIRAMUNE did not include sufficient numbers of subjects aged 65 and older to determine whether elderly subjects respond differently from younger subjects. In general, dose selection for an elderly patient should be cautious, reflecting the greater frequency of decreased hepatic, renal or cardiac function, and of concomitant disease or other drug therapy.

ADVERSE REACTIONS

Adults:

Clinical practice has shown that the most serious adverse reactions associated with VIRAMUNE are clinical hepatitis/hepatic failure, Stevens-Johnson syndrome, toxic epidermal necrolysis, and hypersensitivity reactions. Clinical hepatitis/hepatic failure may be isolated or associated with signs of hypersensitivity which may include severe rash or rash accompanied by fever, general malaise, fatigue, muscle or joint aches, blisters, oral lesions, conjunctivitis, facial edema, and/or hepatitis, eosinophilia, granulocytopenia, lymphadenopathy, and renal dysfunction.

Severe and life-threatening hepatotoxicity, and fatal fulminant hepatitis have been reported in patients treated with VIRAMUNE. Hepatic adverse events have been reported to occur more frequently during the first 18 weeks of treatment, but such events may occur at any time during treatment.

In controlled clinical trials, clinical hepatic events regardless of severity occurred in 4.0% (range 2.5% to 11.0%) of patients who received VIRAMUNE and 1.2% of patients in control groups. Transaminase elevations (ALT or AST > 5× ULN) were observed in 8.8% of patients receiving VIRAMUNE and 6.2% of patients in control groups in clinical trials. In a retrospective analysis of controlled and uncontrolled clinical trials, patients with higher CD4 counts at initiation of VIRAMUNE therapy, particularly women, were at greater risk for acute symptomatic hepatic events, including death, especially in the first six weeks of therapy. Patients with chronic hepatitis B or C infection were at higher risk for later hepatic events. (See WARNINGS)

The most common clinical toxicity of VIRAMUNE is rash. Severe or life-threatening rash occurred in approximately 2% of VIRAMUNE-treated patients, most frequently within the first 6 weeks of therapy. (See Table 5) Rashes are usually mild to moderate, maculopapular erythematous cutaneous eruptions, with or without pruritus, located on the trunk, face and extremities. Women tend to be at higher risk for development of VIRAMUNE associated rash.

[See table 5 at bottom of next page]

Treatment related, adverse experiences of moderate or severe intensity observed in >2% of patients receiving VIRAMUNE in placebo-controlled trials are shown in Table 6.

[See table 6 at bottom of next page]

Laboratory Abnormalities: Liver function test abnormalities (AST, ALT) were observed more frequently in patients receiving VIRAMUNE than in controls. (Table 7) Asymptomatic elevations in GGT occur frequently but are not a contraindication to continue VIRAMUNE therapy in the absence of elevations in other liver function tests. Other laboratory abnormalities (bilirubin, anemia, neutropenia, thrombocytopenia) were observed with similar frequencies in clinical trials comparing VIRAMUNE and control regimens. (See Table 7)

[See table 7 at bottom of next page]

Because clinical hepatitis has been reported in VIRAMUNE-treated patients, intensive clinical and laboratory monitoring, including liver function tests, is essential at baseline and during the first 18 weeks of treatment. Monitoring should continue at frequent intervals thereafter, depending on the patient's clinical status. (See WARNINGS)

Post Marketing Surveillance: In addition to the adverse events identified during clinical trials, the following events have been reported with the use of VIRAMUNE in clinical practice:

Body as a Whole: fever, somnolence, drug withdrawal (See PRECAUTIONS: *Drug Interactions*), redistribution/accumulation of body fat (see PRECAUTIONS, Fat redistribution).

Gastrointestinal: vomiting

Liver and Biliary: jaundice, fulminant and cholestatic hepatitis, hepatic necrosis, hepatic failure

Hematology: anemia, eosinophilia, neutropenia

Musculoskeletal: arthralgia

Neurologic: paraesthesia

Skin and Appendages: allergic reactions including anaphylaxis, angioedema, bullous eruptions, ulcerative stomatitis and urticaria have all been reported. In addition, hypersensitivity syndrome and hypersensitivity reactions with rash associated with constitutional findings such as fever, blistering, oral lesions, conjunctivitis, facial edema, muscle or joint aches, general malaise, fatigue or significant hepatic abnormalities (See WARNINGS) plus one or more of the following: hepatitis, eosinophilia, granulocytopenia, lymphadenopathy and/or renal dysfunction have been reported with the use of VIRAMUNE.

Pediatric Patients:

Safety was assessed in trial BI 882 in which patients were followed for a mean duration of 33.9 months (range: 6.8 months to 5.3 years, including long-term follow-up in 29 of these patients in trial BI 892). The most frequently reported adverse events related to VIRAMUNE in pediatric patients were similar to those observed in adults, with the exception of granulocytopenia, which was more commonly observed in children. Serious adverse events were assessed in ACTG 245, a double-blind, placebo-controlled trial of VIRAMUNE (n = 305) in which pediatric patients received combination treatment with VIRAMUNE. In this trial two patients were reported to experience Stevens-Johnson syndrome or

Stevens-Johnson/toxic epidermal necrolysis transition syndrome. Cases of allergic reaction, including one case of anaphylaxis, were also reported.

Table 8 summarizes the marked laboratory abnormalities occurring in pediatric patients in Trial BI 882 and in follow-up Trial BI 892.

Table 5: Risk of Rash (%) in Adult Placebo Controlled Trials[1] – Regardless of Causality

		VIRAMUNE	Placebo
		n=1374 %	n=1331 %
Through 6 weeks of treatment[2]			
Rash events of all grades[3]		14.8	5.9
Grade 1	Erythema, pruritus	8.5	4.2
Grade 2	Diffuse maculopapular rash, dry desquamation	4.8	1.6
Grade 3 or 4	Grade 3: vesiculation, moist desquamation, ulceration; Grade 4: erythema multiforme, Stevens Johnson syndrome, toxic epidermal necrolysis, necrosis requiring surgery, exfoliative dermatitis	1.5	0.1
Through 52 weeks of treatment[2]			
Rash events of all grades[3]		24.0	14.9
Grade 1	See above	15.5	10.8
Grade 2	See above	7.1	3.9
Grade 3 or 4	See above	1.7	0.2
Proportion of Patients who Discontinued Treatment Due to Rash			
		4.3	1.2

[1] Trials 1037, 1038, 1046 and 1090
[2] % based on Kaplan-Meier probability estimates
[3] NCI grading system

Table 6: Percentage of Patients with Moderate or Severe Drug Related Events in Adult Placebo Controlled Trials

	Trial 1090[1]		Trials 1037, 1038, 1046[2]	
	VIRAMUNE (n=1121)	Placebo (n=1128)	VIRAMUNE (n=253)	Placebo (n=203)
Median exposure (weeks)	58	52	28	28
Any adverse event	14.5%	11.1%	31.6%	13.3%
Rash	5.1	1.8	6.7	1.5
Abnormal LFTs	1.2	0.9	6.7	1.5
Nausea	0.5	1.1	8.7	3.9
Granulocytopenia	1.8	2.8	0.4	0
Headache	0.7	0.4	3.6	0.5
Fatigue	0.2	0.3	4.7	3.9
Diarrhea	0.2	0.8	2.0	0.5
Abdominal pain	0.1	0.4	2.0	0
Myalgia	0.2	0	1.2	2.0

[1] Background therapy included 3TC for all patients and combinations of NRTIs and PIs. Patients had CD4+ cell counts <200 cells/mm^3.
[2] Background therapy included ZDV and ZDV+ddI; VIRAMUNE monotherapy was administered in some patients. Patients had CD4+ cell count ≥200 cells/mm^3.

Table 7: Percentage of Adult Patients with Laboratory Abnormalities

	Trial 1090[1]		Trials,1037, 1038, 1046[2]	
	VIRAMUNE	Placebo	VIRAMUNE	Placebo
Laboratory Abnormality	n=1121	n=1128	n=253	n=203
Blood Chemistry				
SGPT (ALT) >250 U/L	5.3%	4.4%	14.0%	4.0%
SGOT (AST) >250 U/L	3.7	2.5	7.6	1.5
Bilirubin >2.5 mg/dL	1.7	2.2	1.7	1.5
Hematology				
Hemoglobin <8.0 g/dL	3.2	4.1	0	0
Platelets <50,000/mm^3	1.3	1.0	0.4	1.5
Neutrophils <750/mm^3	13.3	13.5	3.6	1.0

[1] Background therapy included 3TC for all patients and combinations of NRTIs and PIs. Patients had CD4+ cell counts <200 cells/mm^3.
[2] Background therapy included ZDV and ZDV+ddI; VIRAMUNE monotherapy was administered in some patients. Patients had CD4+ cell count ≥200 cells/mm^3.

Table 8: Number of Pediatric Patients (%) with Laboratory Abnormalities in Trials BI 882 and BI 892 Combined

	No. (%) of Patients n=37
Blood Chemistry	
Increased ALT (>250 U/L)	4 (11)
Increased AST (>250 U/L)	5 (14)
Increased GGT (>450 U/L)	4 (11)
Increased total bilirubin (>2.5 mg/dL)	1 (3)
Increased alkaline phosphatase (>2× ULN)	19 (51)
Increased amylase (>2× ULN)	6 (16)
Hematology	
Decreased Hg (<8.0 g/dL)	7 (19)
Decreased platelets (<50,000/mm^3)	4 (11)
Decreased neutrophils (<750/mm^3)	14 (38)
Increased MCV (>100 F/L)	13 (35)

OVERDOSAGE

There is no known antidote for VIRAMUNE overdosage. Cases of VIRAMUNE overdose at doses ranging from 800 to 1800 mg per day for up to 15 days have been reported. Patients have experienced events including edema, erythema nodosum, fatigue, fever, headache, insomnia, nausea, pulmonary infiltrates, rash, vertigo, vomiting and weight decrease. All events subsided following discontinuation of VIRAMUNE.

DOSAGE AND ADMINISTRATION

Adults:

The recommended dose for VIRAMUNE is one 200 mg tablet daily for the first 14 days **(this lead-in period should be used because it has been found to lessen the frequency of rash)**, followed by one 200 mg tablet twice daily, in combination with other antiretroviral agents. For concomitantly administered antiretroviral therapy, the manufacturer's recommended dosage and monitoring should be followed.

Pediatric Patients:

The recommended oral dose of VIRAMUNE for pediatric patients 2 months up to 8 years of age is 4 mg/kg once daily for the first 14 days followed by 7 mg/kg twice daily thereafter. For patients 8 years and older the recommended dose is 4 mg/kg once daily for two weeks followed by 4 mg/kg twice daily thereafter. The total daily dose should not exceed 400 mg for any patient.

VIRAMUNE suspension should be shaken gently prior to administration. It is important to administer the entire measured dose of suspension by using an oral dosing syringe or dosing cup. An oral dosing syringe is recommended, particularly for volumes of 5 mL or less. If a dosing cup is used, it should be thoroughly rinsed with water and the rinse should also be administered to the patient.

Monitoring of Patients:

Intensive clinical and laboratory monitoring, including liver function tests, is essential at baseline and during the first 18 weeks of treatment with VIRAMUNE. The optimal frequency of monitoring during this period has not been established. Some experts recommend clinical and laboratory monitoring more often than once per month, and in particular, would include monitoring of liver function tests at baseline, prior to dose escalation, and at two weeks post dose escalation. After the initial 18 week period, frequent clinical and laboratory monitoring should continue throughout VIRAMUNE treatment. (See WARNINGS) In some cases, hepatic injury has progressed despite discontinuation of treatment.

Dosage Adjustment:

VIRAMUNE should be discontinued if patients experience severe rash or a rash accompanied by constitutional findings. (See WARNINGS) Patients experiencing rash during the 14-day lead-in period of 200 mg/day (4 mg/kg/day in pediatric patients) should not have their VIRAMUNE dose increased until the rash has resolved. (See PRECAUTIONS, *Information for Patients*)

If clinical hepatitis occurs, VIRAMUNE should be permanently discontinued and not restarted after recovery.

Patients who interrupt VIRAMUNE dosing for more than 7 days should restart the recommended dosing, using one 200 mg tablet daily (4 mg/kg/day in pediatric patients) for the first 14 days (lead-in) followed by one 200 mg tablet twice daily (4 or 7 mg/kg twice daily, according to age, for pediatric patients).

An additional 200 mg dose of VIRAMUNE following each dialysis treatment is indicated in patients requiring dialysis. Nevirapine metabolites may accumulate in patients receiving dialysis; however, the clinical significance of this accumulation is not known. (See CLINICAL PHARMACOL-

Continued on next page

Viramune—Cont.

OGY, *Pharmacokinetics in Special Populations*: Renal Impairment) Patients with CrCL ≥20 mL/min do not require an adjustment in VIRAMUNE dosing.

HOW SUPPLIED

VIRAMUNE (nevirapine) Tablets, 200 mg, are white, oval, biconvex tablets, 9.3 mm × 19.1 mm. One side is embossed with "54 193", with a single bisect separating the "54" and "193". The opposite side has a single bisect.

VIRAMUNE Tablets are supplied in bottles of 60 (NDC 0597-0046-60).

VIRAMUNE (nevirapine) Oral Suspension is a white to off-white preserved suspension containing 50 mg nevirapine (as nevirapine hemihydrate) in each 5 mL. VIRAMUNE suspension is supplied in plastic bottles with child-resistant closures containing 240 mL of suspension (NDC 0597-0047-24).

VIRAMUNE Tablets and VIRAMUNE Oral Suspension should be stored at 25°C (77°F); excursions permitted to 15°–30°C (59°F–86°F). [see USP Controlled Room Temperature] Store in a safe place out of the reach of children.

Boehringer Ingelheim Pharmaceuticals, Inc.
Ridgefield, CT 06877 USA
Boehringer Ingelheim

(01/04)
Revised 01/23/04
4077435/US/11

Cephalon, Inc.

**145 BRANDYWINE PARKWAY
WEST CHESTER, PA 19380**

For Medical Information/Adverse Drug Experience Reporting Contact:
(800) 896-5855
Fax 610-738-6669

PROVIGIL® ℞
[*prō-vĭ-jĭl*]
(modafinil) Tablets [C-IV]
Rx Only

Prescribing information for this product, which appears on pages 1160–1163 of the 2004 PDR, has been completely revised as follows. Please write "See Supplement A" next to the product heading.

DESCRIPTION

PROVIGIL (modafinil) is a wakefulness-promoting agent for oral administration. Modafinil is a racemic compound. The chemical name for modafinil is 2-[(diphenylmethyl) sulfinyl]acetamide. The molecular formula is $C_{15}H_{15}NO_2S$ and the molecular weight is 273.36.

The chemical structure is:

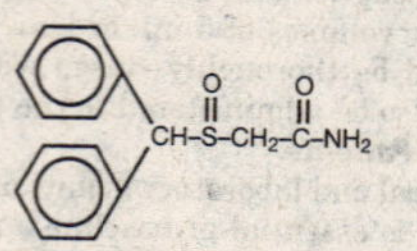

Modafinil is a white to off-white, crystalline powder that is practically insoluble in water and cyclohexane. It is sparingly to slightly soluble in methanol and acetone. PROVIGIL tablets contain 100 mg or 200 mg of modafinil and the following inactive ingredients: lactose, microcrystalline cellulose, pregelatinized starch, croscarmellose sodium, povidone, and magnesium stearate.

CLINICAL PHARMACOLOGY

Mechanism of Action and Pharmacology

The precise mechanism(s) through which modafinil promotes wakefulness is unknown. Modafinil has wake-promoting actions like sympathomimetic agents including amphetamine and methylphenidate, although the pharmacologic profile is not identical to that of sympathomimetic amines.

At pharmacologically relevant concentrations, modafinil does not bind to most potentially relevant receptors for sleep/wake regulation, including those for norepinephrine, serotonin, dopamine, GABA, adenosine, histamine-3, melatonin, or benzodiazepines. Modafinil also does not inhibit the activities of MAO-B or phosphodiesterases II-V.

Modafinil is not a direct- or indirect-acting dopamine receptor agonist and is inactive in several *in vivo* preclinical models capable of detecting enhanced dopaminergic activity. *In vitro*, modafinil binds to the dopamine reuptake site and causes an increase in extracellular dopamine, but no increase in dopamine release. In a preclinical model, the wakefulness induced by amphetamine, but not modafinil, is antagonized by the dopamine receptor antagonist haloperidol.

Modafinil does not appear to be a direct or indirect α_1-adrenergic agonist. Although modafinil-induced wakefulness can be attenuated by the α_1-adrenergic receptor antagonist, prazosin, in assay systems known to be responsive to α-adrenergic agonists, modafinil has no activity. Modafinil does not display sympathomimetic activity in the rat vas deferens preparations (agonist-stimulated or electrically stimulated) nor does it increase the formation of the adrenergic receptor-mediated second messenger phosphatidyl inositol in *in vitro* models. Unlike sympathomimetic agents, modafinil does not reduce cataplexy in narcoleptic canines and has minimal effects on cardiovascular and hemodynamic parameters.

In the cat, equal wakefulness-promoting doses of methylphenidate and amphetamine increased neuronal activation throughout the brain. Modafinil at an equivalent wakefulness-promoting dose selectively and prominently increased neuronal activation in more discrete regions of the brain. The relationship of this finding in cats to the effects of modafinil in humans is unknown.

In addition to its wakefulness-promoting effects and increased locomotor activity in animals, in humans, PROVIGIL produces psychoactive and euphoric effects, alterations in mood, perception, thinking, and feelings typical of other CNS stimulants. Modafinil is reinforcing, as evidenced by its self-administration in monkeys previously trained to self-administer cocaine; modafinil was also partially discriminated as stimulant-like.

The optical enantiomers of modafinil have similar pharmacological actions in animals. Two major metabolites of modafinil, modafinil acid and modafinil sulfone, do not appear to contribute to the CNS-activating properties of modafinil.

Pharmacokinetics

Modafinil is a racemic compound, whose enantiomers have different pharmacokinetics (e.g., the half-life of the *l*-isomer is approximately three times that of the *d*-isomer in humans). The enantiomers do not interconvert. At steady state, total exposure to the *l*-isomer is approximately three times that for the *d*-isomer. The trough concentration (C_{minss}) of circulating modafinil after once daily dosing consists of 90% of the *l*-isomer and 10% of the *d*-isomer. The effective elimination half-life of modafinil after multiple doses is about 15 hours. The enantiomers of modafinil exhibit linear kinetics upon multiple dosing of 200-600 mg/day once daily in healthy volunteers. Apparent steady states of total modafinil and *l*-(-)-modafinil are reached after 2-4 days of dosing.

Absorption and Distribution

Absorption of PROVIGIL tablets is rapid, with peak plasma concentrations occurring at 2-4 hours. The bioavailability of PROVIGIL tablets is approximately equal to that of an aqueous suspension. The absolute oral bioavailability was not determined due to the aqueous insolubility (<1 mg/mL) of modafinil, which precluded intravenous administration. Food has no effect on overall PROVIGIL bioavailability; however, its absorption (t_{max}) may be delayed by approximately one hour if taken with food.

Modafinil is well distributed in body tissue with an apparent volume of distribution (~0.9 L/kg) larger than the volume of total body water (0.6 L/kg). In human plasma, *in vitro*, modafinil is moderately bound to plasma protein (~60%, mainly to albumin). At serum concentrations obtained at steady state after doses of 200 mg/day, modafinil exhibits no displacement of protein binding of warfarin, diazepam, or propranolol. Even at much larger concentrations (1000μM; >25 times the C_{max} of 40μM at steady state at 400 mg/day), modafinil has no effect on warfarin binding. Modafinil acid at concentrations >500μM decreases the extent of warfarin binding, but these concentrations are >35 times those achieved therapeutically.

Metabolism and Elimination

The major route of elimination (~90%) is metabolism, primarily by the liver, with subsequent renal elimination of the metabolites. Urine alkalinization has no effect on the elimination of modafinil.

Metabolism occurs through hydrolytic deamidation, S-oxidation, aromatic ring hydroxylation, and glucuronide conjugation. Less than 10% of an administered dose is excreted as the parent compound. In a clinical study using radiolabeled modafinil, a total of 81% of the administered radioactivity was recovered in 11 days post-dose, predominantly in the urine (80% vs. 1.0% in the feces). The largest fraction of the drug in urine was modafinil acid, but at least six other metabolites were present in lower concentrations. Only two metabolites reach appreciable concentrations in plasma, i.e., modafinil acid and modafinil sulfone. In preclinical models, modafinil acid, modafinil sulfone, 2-[(diphenylmethyl)-sulfonyl]acetic acid and 4-hydroxy modafinil, were inactive or did not appear to mediate the arousal effects of modafinil.

In humans, decreases in trough levels of modafinil have sometimes been observed after multiple weeks of dosing, suggesting auto-induction, but the magnitude of the decreases and the inconsistency of their occurrence suggest that their clinical significance is minimal. Significant accumulation of modafinil sulfone has been observed after multiple doses due to its long elimination half-life of 40 hours. Induction of metabolizing enzymes, most importantly cytochrome P-450 (CYP) 3A4, has also been observed *in vitro* after incubation of primary cultures of human hepatocytes with modafinil and *in vivo* after extended administration of modafinil at 400 mg/day. (For further discussion of the effects of modafinil on CYP enzyme activities see **PRECAUTIONS, Drug Interactions**).

Drug-Drug Interactions: Because modafinil and modafinil sulfone are reversible inhibitors of the drug-metabolizing enzyme CYP2C19, co-administration of modafinil with drugs such as diazepam, phenytoin and propranolol, which are largely eliminated via that pathway, may increase the circulating levels of those compounds. In addition, in individuals deficient in the enzyme CYP2D6 (i.e., 7-10% of the Caucasian population; similar or lower in other populations), the levels of CYP2D6 substrates such as tricyclic antidepressants and selective serotonin reuptake inhibitors, which have ancillary routes of elimination through CYP2C19, may be increased by co-administration of modafinil. Dose adjustments may be necessary for patients being treated with these and similar medications (See **PRECAUTIONS, Drug Interactions**).

Coadministration of modafinil with other CNS active drugs such as methylphenidate and dextroamphetamine did not significantly alter the pharmacokinetics of either drug.

Chronic administration of modafinil 400 mg was found to decrease the systemic exposure to two CYP3A4 substrates, ethinyl estradiol and triazolam, after oral administration suggesting that CYP3A4 had been induced. Chronic administration of modafinil can increase the elimination of substrates of CYP3A4. Dose adjustments may be necessary for patients being treated with these and similar medications (See **PRECAUTIONS, Drug Interactions**).

An apparent concentration-related suppression of CYP2C9 activity was observed in human hepatocytes after exposure to modafinil *in vitro* suggesting that there is a potential for a metabolic interaction between modafinil and the substrates of this enzyme (e.g., S-warfarin, phenytoin). However, in an interaction study in healthy volunteers, chronic modafinil treatment did not show a significant effect on the pharmacokinetics of warfarin when compared to placebo. (See **PRECAUTIONS, Drug Interactions,** *Other Drugs*, Warfarin).

Special Populations

Gender Effect: The pharmacokinetics of modafinil are not affected by gender.

Age Effect: A slight decrease (~20%) in the oral clearance (CL/F) of modafinil was observed in a single dose study at 200 mg in 12 subjects with a mean age of 63 years (range 53 - 72 years), but the change was considered not likely to be clinically significant. In a multiple dose study (300 mg/day) in 12 patients with a mean age of 82 years (range 67 - 87 years), the mean levels of modafinil in plasma were approximately two times those historically obtained in matched younger subjects. Due to potential effects from the multiple concomitant medications with which most of the patients were being treated, the apparent difference in modafinil pharmacokinetics may not be attributable solely to the effects of aging. However, the results suggest that the clearance of modafinil may be reduced in the elderly (See **DOSAGE AND ADMINISTRATION**).

Race Effect: The influence of race on the pharmacokinetics of modafinil has not been studied.

Renal Impairment: In a single dose 200 mg modafinil study, severe chronic renal failure (creatinine clearance ≤20 mL/min) did not significantly influence the pharmacokinetics of modafinil, but exposure to modafinil acid (an inactive metabolite) was increased 9 fold (See **PRECAUTIONS**).

Hepatic Impairment: Pharmacokinetics and metabolism were examined in patients with cirrhosis of the liver (6 M and 3 F). Three patients had stage B or B+ cirrhosis (per the Child criteria) and 6 patients had stage C or C+ cirrhosis. Clinically 8 of 9 patients were icteric and all had ascites. In these patients, the oral clearance of modafinil was decreased by about 60% and the steady state concentration was doubled compared to normal patients. The dose of PROVIGIL should be reduced in patients with severe hepatic impairment (See **PRECAUTIONS** and **DOSAGE AND ADMINISTRATION**).

CLINICAL TRIALS

The effectiveness of PROVIGIL in reducing excessive sleepiness has been established in the following sleep disorders: narcolepsy, obstructive sleep apnea/hypopnea syndrome (OSAHS), and shift work sleep disorder (SWSD).

Narcolepsy

The effectiveness of PROVIGIL in reducing the excessive sleepiness (ES) associated with narcolepsy was established in two US 9-week, multicenter, placebo-controlled, two-dose (200 mg per day and 400 mg per day) parallel-group, double-blind studies of outpatients who met the ICD-9 and American Sleep Disorders Association criteria for narcolepsy (which are also consistent with the American Psychiatric Association DSM-IV criteria). These criteria include either 1) recurrent daytime naps or lapses into sleep that occur almost daily for at least three months, plus sudden bilateral loss of postural muscle tone in association with intense emotion (cataplexy) or 2) a complaint of excessive sleepiness or sudden muscle weakness with associated features: sleep paralysis, hypnagogic hallucinations, automatic behaviors, disrupted major sleep episode; and polysomnography demonstrating one of the following: sleep latency less than 10 minutes or rapid eye movement (REM) sleep latency less than 20 minutes. In addition, for entry into these studies, all patients were required to have objectively documented excessive daytime sleepiness, a Multiple Sleep Latency Test (MSLT) with two or more sleep onset REM periods, and the absence of any other clinically significant active medical or psychiatric disorder. The MSLT, an objective daytime polysomnographic assessment of the patient's ability to fall asleep in an unstimulating environment, measures latency (in minutes) to sleep onset averaged over 4 test sessions at 2-hour intervals following nocturnal polysomnography. For each test session, the subject was told to lie quietly

Table 1. Average Baseline Sleep Latency and Change from Baseline at Final Visit (MWT and MSLT in minutes)

Disorder	Measure	PROVIGIL 200 mg*		PROVIGIL 400 mg*		Placebo	
		Baseline	Change from baseline	Baseline	Change from baseline	Baseline	Change from baseline
Narcolepsy I	MWT	5.8	2.3	6.6	2.3	5.8	-0.7
Narcolepsy II	MWT	6.1	2.2	5.9	2.0	6.0	-0.7
OSAHS	MWT	13.1	1.6	13.6	1.5	13.8	-1.1
SWSD	MSLT	2.1	1.7	–	–	2.0	0.3

*Significantly different than placebo for all trials ($p<0.01$) for all trials but SWSD, which was $p<0.05$)

and attempt to sleep. Each test session was terminated after 20 minutes if no sleep occurred or 15 minutes after sleep onset.

In both studies, the primary measures of effectiveness were 1) sleep latency, as assessed by the Maintenance of Wakefulness Test (MWT) and 2) the change in the patient's overall disease status, as measured by the Clinical Global Impression of Change (CGI-C). For a successful trial, both measures had to show significant improvement.

The MWT measures latency (in minutes) to sleep onset averaged over 4 test sessions at 2 hour intervals following nocturnal polysomnography. For each test session, the subject was asked to attempt to remain awake without using extraordinary measures. Each test session was terminated after 20 minutes if no sleep occurred or 10 minutes after sleep onset. The CGI-C is a 7-point scale, centered at *No Change*, and ranging from *Very Much Worse* to *Very Much Improved*. Patients were rated by evaluators who had no access to any data about the patients other than a measure of their baseline severity. Evaluators were not given any specific guidance about the criteria they were to apply when rating patients.

Other assessments of effect included the Multiple Sleep Latency Test (MSLT), Epworth Sleepiness Scale (ESS; a series of questions designed to assess the degree of sleepiness in everyday situations) the Steer Clear Performance Test (SCPT; a computer-based evaluation of a patient's ability to avoid hitting obstacles in a simulated driving situation), standard nocturnal polysomnography, and patient's daily sleep log. Patients were also assessed with the Quality of Life in Narcolepsy (QOLIN) scale, which contains the validated SF-36 health questionnaire.

Both studies demonstrated improvement in objective and subjective measures of excessive daytime sleepiness for both the 200 mg and 400 mg doses compared to placebo. Patients treated with either dose of PROVIGIL showed a statistically significantly enhanced ability to remain awake on the MWT (all p values <0.001) at weeks 3, 6, 9, and final visit compared to placebo and a statistically significantly greater global improvement, as rated on the CGI-C scale (all p values <0.05).

The average sleep latencies (in minutes) on the MWT at baseline for the 2 controlled trials are shown in Table 1 below, along with the average change from baseline on the MWT at final visit.

The percentages of patients who showed any degree of improvement on the CGI-C in the two clinical trials are shown in Table 2 below.

Similar statistically significant treatment-related improvements were seen on other measures of impairment in narcolepsy, including a patient assessed level of daytime sleepiness on the ESS ($p<0.001$ for each dose in comparison to placebo).

Although PROVIGIL tended to be numerically superior to placebo on several of the other outcome measures, there were no consistent statistically significant differences between drug and placebo on these measures.

Nighttime sleep measured with polysomnography was not affected by the use of PROVIGIL.

The effectiveness of modafinil in long-term use (greater than 9 weeks) has not been systematically evaluated in placebo-controlled trials. The physician who elects to prescribe PROVIGIL tablets for an extended time in patients with narcolepsy should periodically re-evaluate long-term usefulness for the individual patient.

Obstructive Sleep Apnea/Hypopnea Syndrome (OSAHS)

The effectiveness of PROVIGIL in reducing the excessive sleepiness associated with OSAHS was established in two clinical trials. In both studies, patients were enrolled who met the International Classification of Sleep Disorders (ICSD) criteria for OSAHS (which are also consistent with the American Psychiatric Association DSM-IV criteria). These criteria include either, 1) excessive sleepiness or insomnia, plus frequent episodes of impaired breathing during sleep, and associated features such as loud snoring, morning headaches and dry mouth upon awakening; or 2) excessive sleepiness or insomnia and polysomnography demonstrating one of the following: more than five obstructive apneas, each greater than 10 seconds in duration, per hour of sleep and one or more of the following: frequent arousals from sleep associated with the apneas, bradytachycardia, and arterial oxygen desaturation in association with the apneas. In addition, for entry into these studies, all patients were required to have excessive sleepiness as demonstrated by a score ≥10 on the Epworth Sleepiness Scale, despite treatment with continuous positive airway pressure (CPAP). Evidence that CPAP was effective in reducing episodes of apnea/hypopnea was required along with documentation of CPAP use.

In the first study, a 12-week multicenter placebo-controlled trial, a total of 327 patients were randomized to receive PROVIGIL 200mg/day, PROVIGIL 400mg/day, or matching placebo. The majority of patients (80%) were fully compliant with CPAP, defined as CPAP use >4 hours/night on >70% nights. The remainder were partially CPAP compliant, defined as CPAP use <4 hours/night on >30% nights. CPAP use continued throughout the study. The primary measures of effectiveness were 1) sleep latency, as assessed by the Maintenance of Wakefulness Test (MWT) and 2) the change in the patient's overall disease status, as measured by the Clinical Global Impression of Change (CGI-C) at week 12 or the final visit. (See **CLINICAL TRIALS**, Narcolepsy section above for a description of these tests.)

Patients treated with PROVIGIL showed a statistically significant improvement in the ability to remain awake compared to placebo-treated patients as measured by the MWT ($p<0.001$) at endpoint [Table 1]. PROVIGIL-treated patients also showed a statistically significant improvement in clinical condition as rated by the CGI-C scale ($p<0.001$) [Table 2]. The two doses of PROVIGIL performed similarly.

In the second study, a 4-week multicenter placebo-controlled trial, 157 patients were randomized to either PROVIGIL 400 mg/day or placebo. Documentation of regular CPAP use (at least 4 hours/night on 70% of nights) was required for all patients.

The primary outcome measure was the change from baseline on the ESS at week 4 or final visit. The baseline ESS scores for the PROVIGIL and placebo groups were 14.2 and 14.4, respectively. At week 4, the ESS was reduced by 4.6 in the PROVIGIL group and by 2.0 in the placebo group, a difference that was statistically significant ($p<0.0001$).

Nighttime sleep measured with polysomnography was not affected by the use of PROVIGIL.

The effectiveness of modafinil in long-term use (greater than 12 weeks) has not been systematically evaluated in placebo-controlled trials. The physician who elects to prescribe PROVIGIL tablets for an extended time in patients with OSAHS should periodically reevaluate long-term usefulness for the individual patient.

Shift Work Sleep Disorder (SWSD)

The effectiveness of PROVIGIL for the excessive sleepiness associated with SWSD was demonstrated in a 12-week placebo-controlled clinical trial. A total of 209 patients with chronic SWSD were randomized to receive PROVIGIL 200mg/day or placebo. All patients met the International Classification of Sleep Disorders (ICSD-10) criteria for chronic SWSD (which are consistent with the American Psychiatric Association DSM-IV criteria for Circadian Rhythm Sleep Disorder: Shift Work Type). These criteria include 1) either: a) a primary complaint of excessive sleepiness or insomnia which is temporally associated with a work period (usually night work) that occurs during the habitual sleep phase, or b) polysomnography and the MSLT demonstrate loss of a normal sleep-wake pattern (i.e., disturbed chronobiological rhythmicity); and 2) no other medical or mental disorder accounts for the symptoms, and 3) the symptoms do not meet criteria for any other sleep disorder producing insomnia or excessive sleepiness (e.g., time zone change [jet lag] syndrome).

It should be noted that not all patients with a complaint of sleepiness who are also engaged in shift work meet the criteria for the diagnosis of SWSD. In the clinical trial, only patients who were symptomatic for at least 3 months were enrolled.

Enrolled patients were also required to work a minimum of 5 night shifts per month, have excessive sleepiness at the time of their night shifts (MSLT score < 6 minutes), and have daytime insomnia documented by a daytime polysomnogram (PSG).

The primary measures of effectiveness were 1) sleep latency, as assessed by the Multiple Sleep Latency Test (MSLT) performed during a simulated night shift at week 12 or the final visit and 2) the change in the patient's overall disease status, as measured by the Clinical Global Impression of Change (CGI-C) at week 12 or the final visit. Patients treated with PROVIGIL showed a statistically significant prolongation in the time to sleep onset compared to placebo-treated patients, as measured by the nighttime MSLT [Table 1] ($p<0.05$). Improvement on the CGI-C was also observed to be statistically significant ($p<0.001$).

Daytime sleep measured with polysomnography was not affected by the use of PROVIGIL.

The effectiveness of modafinil in long-term use (greater than 12 weeks) has not been systematically evaluated in placebo-controlled trials. The physician who elects to prescribe PROVIGIL for an extended time in patients with SWSD should periodically reevaluate long-term usefulness for the individual patient.

[See table 1 above]

Table 2. Clinical Global Impression of Change (CGI-C) (Percent of Patients Who Improved at Final Visit)

Disorder	PROVIGIL 200 mg*	PROVIGIL 400 mg*	Placebo
Narcolepsy I	64%	72%	37%
Narcolepsy II	58%	60%	38%
OSAHS	61%	68%	37%
SWSD	74%	—	36%

*Significantly different than placebo for all trials ($p<0.01$)

INDICATIONS AND USAGE

PROVIGIL is indicated to improve wakefulness in patients with excessive sleepiness associated with narcolepsy, obstructive sleep apnea/hypopnea syndrome, and shift work sleep disorder.

In OSAHS, PROVIGIL is indicated as an adjunct to standard treatment(s) for the underlying obstruction. If continuous positive airway pressure (CPAP) is the treatment of choice for a patient, a maximal effort to treat with CPAP for an adequate period of time should be made prior to initiating PROVIGIL. If PROVIGIL is used adjunctively with CPAP, the encouragement of and periodic assessment of CPAP compliance is necessary.

In all cases, careful attention to the diagnosis and treatment of the underlying sleep disorder(s) is of utmost importance. Prescribers should be aware that some patients may have more than one sleep disorder contributing to their excessive sleepiness.

CONTRAINDICATIONS

PROVIGIL is contraindicated in patients with known hypersensitivity to modafinil or its inactive ingredients.

WARNINGS

Patients with abnormal levels of sleepiness who take PROVIGIL should be advised that their level of wakefulness may not return to normal. Patients with excessive sleepiness, including those taking PROVIGIL, should be frequently reassessed for their degree of sleepiness and, if appropriate, advised to avoid driving or any other potentially dangerous activity. Prescribers should also be aware that patients may not acknowledge sleepiness or drowsiness until directly questioned about drowsiness or sleepiness during specific activities.

PRECAUTIONS

Diagnosis of Sleep Disorders

PROVIGIL should be used only in patients who have had a complete evaluation of their excessive sleepiness, and in whom a diagnosis of either narcolepsy, OSAHS, and/or SWSD has been made in accordance with ICSD or DSM diagnostic criteria (See **CLINICAL TRIALS** Section). Such an evaluation usually consists of a complete history and physical examination, and it may be supplemented with testing in a laboratory setting. Some patients may have more than one sleep disorder contributing to their excessive sleepiness (e.g., OSAHS and SWSD coincident in the same patient).

CPAP Use in Patients with OSAHS

In OSAHS, PROVIGIL is indicated as an adjunct to standard treatment(s) for the underlying obstruction. If continuous positive airway pressure (CPAP) is the treatment of choice for a patient, a maximal effort to treat with CPAP for an adequate period of time should be made prior to initiating PROVIGIL. If PROVIGIL is used adjunctively with CPAP, the encouragement of and periodic assessment of CPAP compliance is necessary.

General

Although modafinil has not been shown to produce functional impairment, any drug affecting the CNS may alter judgment, thinking or motor skills. Patients should be cautioned about operating an automobile or other hazardous machinery until they are reasonably certain that PROVIGIL therapy will not adversely affect their ability to engage in such activities.

Patients Using Contraceptives

The effectiveness of steroidal contraceptives may be reduced when used with PROVIGIL tablets and for one month after discontinuation of therapy (See **Drug Interactions**). Alternative or concomitant methods of contraception are recommended for patients treated with PROVIGIL tablets, and for one month after discontinuation of PROVIGIL.

Cardiovascular System

In clinical studies of PROVIGIL, signs and symptoms including chest pain, palpitations, dyspnea and transient ischemic T-wave changes on ECG were observed in three subjects in association with mitral valve prolapse or left ventricular hypertrophy. It is recommended that PROVIGIL tablets not be used in patients with a history of left ventricular hypertrophy or in patients with mitral valve prolapse who have experienced the mitral valve prolapse syndrome when previously receiving CNS stimulants. Such signs may include but are not limited to ischemic ECG changes, chest pain, or arrhythmia.

Modafinil has not been evaluated or used to any appreciable extent in patients with a recent history of myocardial infarction or unstable angina, and such patients should be treated with caution.

Continued on next page

Provigil—Cont.

Blood pressure monitoring in short-term (<3 months) controlled trials showed no clinically significant changes in mean systolic and diastolic blood pressure in patients receiving PROVIGIL as compared to placebo. However, a retrospective analysis of the use of antihypertensive medication in these studies showed that a greater proportion of patients on PROVIGIL required new or increased use of antihypertensive medications (2.4%) compared to patients on placebo (0.7%). The differential use was slightly larger when only studies in OSAHS were included, with 3.4% of patients on PROVIGIL and 1.1% of patients on placebo requiring such alterations in the use of antihypertensive medication. Increased monitoring of blood pressure may be appropriate in patients on PROVIGIL.

Central Nervous System

There have been reports of psychotic episodes associated with PROVIGIL use. One healthy male volunteer developed ideas of reference, paranoid delusions, and auditory hallucinations in association with multiple daily 600 mg doses of PROVIGIL and sleep deprivation. There was no evidence of psychosis 36 hours after drug discontinuation. Caution should be exercised when PROVIGIL is given to patients with a history of psychosis.

Patients with Severe Renal Impairment

In patients with severe renal impairment (mean creatinine clearance = 16.6 mL/min), a 200 mg single dose of modafinil did not lead to increased exposure to modafinil but resulted in much higher exposure to the inactive metabolite, modafinil acid, than is seen in subjects with normal renal function. There is little information available about the safety of such levels of this metabolite (See **CLINICAL PHARMACOLOGY**).

Patients with Severe Hepatic Impairment

In patients with severe hepatic impairment, with or without cirrhosis (See **CLINICAL PHARMACOLOGY**), PROVIGIL should be administered at a reduced dose as the clearance of modafinil was decreased compared to that in normal subjects (See **DOSAGE AND ADMINISTRATION**).

Elderly Patients

To the extent that elderly patients may have diminished renal and/or hepatic function, dosage reductions should be considered (See **DOSAGE AND ADMINISTRATION**).

Information for Patients

Physicians are advised to discuss the following issues with patients for whom they prescribe PROVIGIL.

PROVIGIL is indicated for patients who have abnormal levels of sleepiness. PROVIGIL has been shown to improve, but not eliminate this abnormal tendency to fall asleep. Therefore, patients should not alter their previous behavior with regard to potentially dangerous activities (e.g., driving, operating machinery) or other activities requiring appropriate levels of wakefulness, until and unless treatment with PROVIGIL has been shown to produce levels of wakefulness that permit such activities. Patients should be advised that PROVIGIL is not a replacement for sleep.

Patients should be informed that it may be critical that they continue to take their previously prescribed treatments (e.g., patients with OSAHS receiving CPAP should continue to do so).

Patients should be informed of the availability of a patient information leaflet, and they should be instructed to read the leaflet prior to taking PROVIGIL. See Patient Information at the end of this labeling for the text of the leaflet provided for patients.

Pregnancy

Patients should be advised to notify their physician if they become pregnant or intend to become pregnant during therapy. Patients should be cautioned regarding the potential increased risk of pregnancy when using steroidal contraceptives (including depot or implantable contraceptives) with PROVIGIL and for one month after discontinuation of therapy (See *Impairment of Fertility* and **Pregnancy**).

Nursing

Patients should be advised to notify their physician if they are breast feeding an infant.

Concomitant Medication

Patients should be advised to inform their physician if they are taking, or plan to take, any prescription or over-the-counter drugs, because of the potential for interactions between PROVIGIL and other drugs.

Alcohol

Patients should be advised that the use of PROVIGIL in combination with alcohol has not been studied. Patients should be advised that it is prudent to avoid alcohol while taking PROVIGIL.

Allergic Reactions

Patients should be advised to notify their physician if they develop a rash, hives, or a related allergic phenomenon.

Drug Interactions

CNS Active Drugs

Methylphenidate - In a single-dose study in healthy volunteers, simultaneous administration of modafinil (200 mg) with methylphenidate (40 mg) did not cause any significant alterations in the pharmacokinetics of either drug. However, the absorption of PROVIGIL may be delayed by approximately one hour when coadministered with methylphenidate.

Dextroamphetamine - In a single dose study in healthy volunteers, simultaneous administration of modafinil (200 mg) with dextroamphetamine (10 mg) did not cause any significant alterations in the pharmacokinetics of either drug. However, the absorption of PROVIGIL may be delayed by approximately one hour when coadministered with dextroamphetamine.

Clomipramine - The coadministration of a single dose of clomipramine (50 mg) on the first of three days of treatment with modafinil (200 mg/day) in healthy volunteers did not show an effect on the pharmacokinetics of either drug. However, one incident of increased levels of clomipramine and its active metabolite desmethylclomipramine has been reported in a patient with narcolepsy during treatment with modafinil.

Triazolam - In the drug interaction study between PROVIGIL and ethinyl estradiol (EE_2), on the same days as those for the plasma sampling for EE_2 pharmacokinetics, a single dose of triazolam (0.125 mg) was also administered. Mean C_{max} and $AUC_{0-\infty}$ of triazolam were decreased by 42% and 59%, respectively, and its elimination half-life was decreased by approximately an hour after the modafinil treatment.

Monoamine Oxidase (MAO) Inhibitors - Interaction studies with monoamine oxidase inhibitors have not been performed. Therefore, caution should be used when concomitantly administering MAO inhibitors and modafinil.

Other Drugs

Warfarin - There were no significant changes in the pharmacokinetic profiles of R- and S-warfarin in healthy subjects given a single dose of racemic warfarin (5 mg) following chronic administration of modafinil (200 mg/day for 7 days followed by 400 mg/day for 27 days) relative to the profiles in subjects given placebo. However, more frequent monitoring of prothrombin times/INR is advisable whenever PROVIGIL is coadministered with warfarin (See **CLINICAL PHARMACOLOGY, Pharmacokinetics**, Drug-Drug Interactions).

Ethinyl Estradiol - Administration of modafinil to female volunteers once daily at 200 mg/day for 7 days followed by 400 mg/day for 21 days resulted in a mean 11% decrease in C_{max} and 18% decrease in AUC_{0-24} of ethinyl estradiol (EE_2; 0.035 mg; administered orally with norgestimate). There was no apparent change in the elimination rate of ethinyl estradiol.

Cyclosporine - One case of an interaction between modafinil and cyclosporine, a substrate of CYP3A4, has been reported in a 41 year old woman who had undergone an organ transplant. After one month of administration of 200 mg/day of modafinil, cyclosporine blood levels were decreased by 50%. The interaction was postulated to be due to the increased metabolism of cyclosporine, since no other factor expected to affect the disposition of the drug had changed. Dosage adjustment for cyclosporine may be needed.

Potential Interactions with Drugs That Inhibit, Induce, or are Metabolized by Cytochrome P-450 Isoenzymes and Other Hepatic Enzymes

In *in vitro* studies using primary human hepatocyte cultures, modafinil was shown to slightly induce CYP1A2, CYP2B6 and CYP3A4 in a concentration-dependent manner. Although induction results based on *in vitro* experiments are not necessarily predictive of response *in vivo*, caution needs to be exercised when PROVIGIL is coadministered with drugs that depend on these three enzymes for their clearance. Specifically, lower blood levels of such drugs could result (See *Other Drugs*, Cyclosporine above).

The exposure of human hepatocytes to modafinil *in vitro* produced an apparent concentration-related suppression of expression of CYP2C9 activity suggesting that there is a potential for a metabolic interaction between modafinil and the substrates of this enzyme (e.g., S-warfarin and phenytoin). In a subsequent clinical study in healthy volunteers, chronic modafinil treatment did not show a significant effect on the single-dose pharmacokinetics of warfarin when compared to placebo (See **PRECAUTIONS, Drug Interactions**, Warfarin).

In vitro studies using human liver microsomes showed that modafinil reversibly inhibited CYP2C19 at pharmacologically relevant concentrations of modafinil. CYP2C19 is also reversibly inhibited, with similar potency, by a circulating metabolite, modafinil sulfone. Although the maximum plasma concentrations of modafinil sulfone are much lower than those of parent modafinil, the combined effect of both compounds could produce sustained partial inhibition of the enzyme. Drugs that are largely eliminated via CYP2C19 metabolism, such as diazepam, propranolol, phenytoin (also via CYP2C9) or S-mephenytoin may have prolonged elimination upon coadministration with PROVIGIL and may require dosage reduction and monitoring for toxicity.

Tricyclic antidepressants - CYP2C19 also provides an ancillary pathway for the metabolism of certain tricyclic antidepressants (e.g., clomipramine and desipramine) that are primarily metabolized by CYP2D6. In tricyclic-treated patients deficient in CYP2D6 (i.e., those who are poor metabolizers of debrisoquine; 7–10% of the Caucasian population; similar or lower in other populations), the amount of metabolism by CYP2C19 may be substantially increased. PROVIGIL may cause elevation of the levels of the tricyclics in this subset of patients. Physicians should be aware that a reduction in the dose of tricyclic agents might be needed in these patients.

In addition, due to the partial involvement of CYP3A4 in the metabolic elimination of modafinil, coadministration of potent inducers of CYP3A4 (e.g., carbamazepine, phenobarbital, rifampin) or inhibitors of CYP3A4 (e.g., ketoconazole, itraconazole) could alter the plasma levels of modafinil.

Carcinogenesis, Mutagenesis, Impairment of Fertility

Carcinogenesis

Carcinogenicity studies were conducted in which modafinil was administered in the diet to mice for 78 weeks and to rats for 104 weeks at doses of 6, 30 and 60 mg/kg/day. The highest dose studied represents 1.5 times (mouse) or 3 times (rat) greater than the recommended human daily dose of 200 mg on a mg/m^2 basis. There was no evidence of tumorigenesis associated with modafinil administration in these studies, but because the mouse study used an inadequate high dose that was not representative of a maximum tolerated dose, the carcinogenic potential of modafinil has not been fully evaluated.

Mutagenesis

There was no evidence of mutagenic or clastogenic potential of modafinil in a series of assays. It was not mutagenic in the *in vitro* Ames bacterial reverse mutation test, the *in vitro* mouse lymphoma/TK locus assay in the presence or absence of metabolic activation; and it was not clastogenic in the *in vitro* human lymphocyte chromosomal aberration assay in the presence or absence of metabolic activation, or in two *in vivo* mouse bone marrow micronucleus assays. Modafinil did not increase unscheduled DNA synthesis in rat hepatocytes. In a cell transformation assay in BALB/3T3 mouse embryo cells, modafinil did not cause an increase in the frequency of transformed foci in the presence or absence of metabolic activation.

Impairment of Fertility

Oral administration of modafinil to male and female rats had no effects on fertility when administered prior to and throughout mating, and continued in females through day 7 of gestation, at doses up to 480 mg/kg/day (23 times the recommended human dose of 200 mg/day on a mg/m^2 basis).

Pregnancy

Pregnancy Category C: Modafinil administered orally to pregnant rats throughout the period of organogenesis caused, in the absence of maternal toxicity, an increase in resorptions and an increased incidence of hydronephrosis and skeletal variations in the offspring at a dose of 200 mg/kg/day (10 times the recommended human dose of 200 mg/day on a mg/m^2 basis) but not at 100 mg/kg/day. However, in a subsequent study of up to 480 mg/kg/day (23 times the recommended human dose on a mg/m^2 basis), which included maternally toxic doses, no adverse effects on embryofetal development were seen.

Modafinil administered orally to pregnant rabbits throughout the period of organogenesis at doses up to 100 mg/kg/day (10 times the recommended human dose on a mg/m^2 basis) had no effects on embryofetal development.

However, in a subsequent study in pregnant rabbits, increased resorptions, and increased alterations in fetuses from a single litter (open eye lids, fused digits, rotated limbs), were observed at 180 mg/kg/day (17 times the recommended human dose on a mg/m^2 basis), a dose that was also maternally toxic.

Modafinil administered orally to rats throughout gestation and lactation at doses up to 200 mg/kg/day (5 times the recommended human dose on a mg/m^2 basis), had no effects on the postnatal development of the offspring.

There are no adequate and well-controlled studies in pregnant women. Modafinil should be used during pregnancy only if the potential benefit justifies the potential risk to the fetus.

Labor and Delivery

The effect of modafinil on labor and delivery in humans has not been systematically investigated. Seven normal births occurred in patients who had received modafinil during pregnancy. One patient gave birth 3 weeks earlier than the expected range of delivery dates (estimated using ultrasound) to a healthy male infant. One woman with a history of spontaneous abortions suffered a spontaneous abortion while being treated with modafinil.

Nursing Mothers

It is not known whether modafinil or its metabolites are excreted in human milk. Because many drugs are excreted in human milk, caution should be exercised when PROVIGIL tablets are administered to a nursing woman.

PEDIATRIC USE

Safety and effectiveness in individuals below 16 years of age have not been established. Leukopenia has been reported in pediatric patients taking PROVIGIL.

GERIATRIC USE

Safety and effectiveness in individuals above 65 years of age have not been established. Experience in a limited number of patients who were greater than 65 years of age in clinical trials showed an incidence of adverse experiences similar to other age groups.

ADVERSE REACTIONS

Modafinil has been evaluated for safety in over 3500 patients, of whom more than 2000 patients with excessive sleepiness associated with primary disorders of sleep and wakefulness were given at least one dose of modafinil. In clinical trials, modafinil has been found to be generally well tolerated and most adverse experiences were mild to moderate.

The most commonly observed adverse events (≥5%) associated with the use of PROVIGIL more frequently than placebo-treated patients in the placebo-controlled clinical studies in primary disorders of sleep and wakefulness were headache, nausea, nervousness, rhinitis, diarrhea, back pain, anxiety, insomnia, dizziness, and dyspepsia. The adverse event profile was similar across these studies.

In the placebo-controlled clinical trials, 74 of the 934 patients (8%) who received PROVIGIL discontinued due to an adverse experience compared to 3% of patients that received placebo. The most frequent reasons for discontinuation that occurred at a higher rate for PROVIGIL than placebo patients were headache (2%), nausea, anxiety, dizziness, insomnia, chest pain and nervousness (each <1%). In a Canadian clinical trial, a 35 year old obese narcoleptic male with a prior history of syncopal episodes experienced a 9-second episode of asystole after 27 days of modafinil treatment (300 mg/day in divided doses).

Incidence in Controlled Trials

The following table (Table 3) presents the adverse experiences that occurred at a rate of 1% or more and were more frequent in patients treated with PROVIGIL than in placebo patients in the principal, placebo-controlled clinical trials.

The prescriber should be aware that the figures provided below cannot be used to predict the frequency of adverse experiences in the course of usual medical practice, where patient characteristics and other factors may differ from those occurring during clinical studies. Similarly, the cited frequencies cannot be directly compared with figures obtained from other clinical investigations involving different treatments, uses, or investigators. Review of these frequencies, however, provides prescribers with a basis to estimate the relative contribution of drug and non-drug factors to the incidence of adverse events in the population studied.

[See table 3 at right]

Dose Dependency of Adverse Events

In the placebo-controlled clinical trials which compared doses of 200, 300, and 400 mg/day of PROVIGIL and placebo, the only adverse events that were clearly dose related were headache and anxiety.

Vital Sign Changes

While there was no consistent change in mean values of heart rate or systolic and diastolic blood pressure, the requirement for antihypertensive medication was slightly greater in patients on PROVIGIL compared to placebo (See **PRECAUTIONS**).

Weight Changes

There were no clinically significant differences in body weight change in patients treated with PROVIGIL compared to placebo-treated patients in the placebo-controlled clinical trials.

Laboratory Changes

Clinical chemistry, hematology, and urinalysis parameters were monitored in Phase 1, 2, and 3 studies. In these studies, mean plasma levels of gamma glutamyltransferase (GGT) and alkaline phosphatase (AP) were found to be higher following administration of PROVIGIL, but not placebo. Few subjects, however, had GGT or AP elevations outside of the normal range. Shifts to higher, but not clinically significantly abnormal, GGT and AP values appeared to increase with time in the population treated with PROVIGIL in the Phase 3 clinical trials. No differences were apparent in alanine aminotransferase, aspartate aminotransferase, total protein, albumin, or total bilirubin.

ECG Changes

No treatment-emergent pattern of ECG abnormalities was found in placebo-controlled clinical trials following administration of PROVIGIL.

Postmarketing Reports

In addition to the adverse events observed during clinical trials, the following adverse events have been identified during post-approval use of PROVIGIL in clinical practice. Because these adverse events are reported voluntarily from a population of uncertain size, reliable estimates of their frequency cannot be made.

Hematologic: agranulocytosis

Central Nervous System: symptoms of psychosis, symptoms of mania

Hypersensitivity: urticaria (hives), angioedema

DRUG ABUSE AND DEPENDENCE

Controlled Substance Class

Modafinil (PROVIGIL) is listed in Schedule IV of the Controlled Substances Act.

Abuse Potential and Dependence

In addition to its wakefulness-promoting effect and increased locomotor activity in animals, in humans, PROVIGIL produces psychoactive and euphoric effects, alterations in mood, perception, thinking and feelings typical of other CNS stimulants. In *in vitro* binding studies, modafinil binds to the dopamine reuptake site and causes an increase in extracellular dopamine, but no increase in dopamine release. Modafinil is reinforcing, as evidenced by its self-administration in monkeys previously trained to self-administer cocaine. In some studies, modafinil was also partially discriminated as stimulant-like. Physicians should follow patients closely, especially those with a history of drug and/or stimulant (e.g., methylphenidate, amphetamine, or cocaine) abuse. Patients should be observed for signs of misuse or abuse (e.g., incrementation of doses or drug-seeking behavior).

The abuse potential of modafinil (200, 400, and 800 mg) was assessed relative to methylphenidate (45 and 90 mg) in an inpatient study in individuals experienced with drugs of abuse. Results from this clinical study demonstrated that modafinil produced psychoactive and euphoric effects and feelings consistent with other scheduled CNS stimulants (methylphenidate).

Withdrawal

The effects of modafinil withdrawal were monitored following 9 weeks of modafinil use in one US Phase 3 controlled clinical trial. No specific symptoms of withdrawal were observed during 14 days of observation, although sleepiness returned in narcoleptic patients.

Table 3. Incidence Of Treatment-Emergent Adverse Experiences In Parallel-Group, Placebo-Controlled Clinical Trials[1] In Narcolepsy, OSAHS, and SWSD With PROVIGIL (200 mg, 300 mg and 400 mg)*

Body System	Preferred Term	Modafinil (n = 934)	Placebo (n = 567)
Body as a Whole	Headache	34%	23%
	Back pain	6%	5%
	Flu Syndrome	4%	3%
	Chest Pain	3%	1%
	Chills	1%	0%
	Neck Rigidity	1%	0%
Cardiovascular	Hypertension	3%	1%
	Tachycardia	2%	1%
	Palpitation	2%	1%
	Vasodilatation	2%	0%
Digestive	Nausea	11%	3%
	Diarrhea	6%	5%
	Dyspepsia	5%	4%
	Dry Mouth	4%	2%
	Anorexia	4%	1%
	Constipation	2%	1%
	Abnormal liver function[2]	2%	1%
	Flatulence	1%	0%
	Mouth Ulceration	1%	0%
	Thirst	1%	0%
Hemic/Lymphatic	Eosinophilia	1%	0%
Metabolic/Nutritional	Edema	1%	0%
Nervous	Nervousness	7%	3%
	Insomnia	5%	1%
	Anxiety	5%	1%
	Dizziness	5%	4%
	Depression	2%	1%
	Paresthesia	2%	0%
	Somnolence	2%	1%
	Hypertonia	1%	0%
	Dyskinesia[3]	1%	0%
	Hyperkinesia	1%	0%
	Agitation	1%	0%
	Confusion	1%	0%
	Tremor	1%	0%
	Emotional Lability	1%	0%
	Vertigo	1%	0%
Respiratory	Rhinitis	7%	6%
	Pharyngitis	4%	2%
	Lung Disorder	2%	1%
	Epistaxis	1%	0%
	Asthma	1%	0%
Skin/Appendages	Sweating	1%	0%
	Herpes Simplex	1%	0%
Special Senses	Amblyopia	1%	0%
	Abnormal Vision	1%	0%
	Taste Perversion	1%	0%
	Eye Pain	1%	0%
Urogenital	Urine Abnormality	1%	0%
	Hematuria	1%	0%
	Pyuria	1%	0%

* Six double-blind, placebo controlled clinical studies in narcolepsy, OSAHS, and SWSD.

[1] Events reported by at least 1% of patients treated with PROVIGIL that were more frequent than in the placebo group are included; incidence is rounded to the nearest 1%. The adverse experience terminology is coded using a standard modified COSTART Dictionary.

Events for which the PROVIGIL incidence was at least 1%, but equal to or less than placebo are not listed in the table. These events included the following: infection, pain, accidental injury, abdominal pain, hypothermia, allergic reaction, asthenia, fever, viral infection, neck pain, migraine, abnormal electrocardiogram, hypotension, tooth disorder, vomiting, periodontal abscess, increased appetite, ecchymosis, hyperglycemia, peripheral edema, weight loss, weight gain, myalgia, leg cramps, arthritis, cataplexy, thinking abnormality, sleep disorder, increased cough, sinusitis, dyspnea, bronchitis, rash, conjunctivitis, ear pain, dysmenorrhea[4], urinary tract infection.

[2] Elevated liver enzymes.

[3] Oro-facial dyskinesias.

[4] Incidence adjusted for gender.

OVERDOSAGE

Human Experience

In clinical trials, a total of 151 protocol-specified doses ranging from 1000 to 1600 mg/day (5 to 8 times the recommended daily dose of 200 mg) have been administered to 32 subjects, including 13 subjects who received doses of 1000 or 1200 mg/day for 7 to 21 consecutive days. In addition, several intentional acute overdoses occurred; the two largest being 4500 mg and 4000 mg taken by two subjects participating in foreign depression studies. None of these study subjects experienced any unexpected or life-threatening effects. Adverse experiences that were reported at these doses included excitation or agitation, insomnia, and slight or moderate elevations in hemodynamic parameters. Other observed high-dose effects in clinical studies have included anxiety, irritability, aggressiveness, confusion, nervousness, tremor, palpitations, sleep disturbances, nausea, diarrhea and decreased prothrombin time.

From post-marketing experience, there have been no reports of fatal overdoses involving modafinil alone (doses up to 12 grams). Overdoses involving multiple drugs, including modafinil, have resulted in fatal outcomes. Symptoms most often accompanying modafinil overdose, alone or in combination with other drugs have included: insomnia; central nervous system symptoms such as restlessness, disorientation, confusion, excitation and hallucination; digestive changes such as nausea and diarrhea; and cardiovascular changes such as tachycardia, bradycardia, hypertension and chest pain.

Cases of accidental ingestion/overdose have been reported in children as young as 11 months of age. The highest reported accidental ingestion on a mg/kg basis occurred in a three-year-old boy who ingested 800-1000 mg (50-63 mg/kg) of modafinil. The child remained stable. The symptoms associated with overdose in children were similar to those observed in adults.

Overdose Management

No specific antidote to the toxic effects of modafinil overdose has been identified to date. Such overdoses should be managed with primarily supportive care, including cardiovascular monitoring. If there are no contraindications, induced emesis or gastric lavage should be considered. There are no data to suggest the utility of dialysis or urinary acidification

Continued on next page

Provigil—Cont.

or alkalinization in enhancing drug elimination. The physician should consider contacting a poison-control center on the treatment of any overdose.

DOSAGE AND ADMINISTRATION

The recommended dose of PROVIGIL is 200 mg given once a day.

For patients with narcolepsy and OSAHS, PROVIGIL should be taken as a single dose in the morning.

For patients with SWSD, PROVIGIL should be taken approximately 1 hour prior to the start of their work shift.

Doses up to 400 mg/day, given as a single dose, have been well tolerated, but there is no consistent evidence that this dose confers additional benefit beyond that of the 200 mg dose (See **CLINICAL PHARMACOLOGY** and **CLINICAL TRIALS**).

Dosage adjustment should be considered for concomitant medications that are substrates for CYP3A4, such as triazolam and cyclosporine (See **PRECAUTIONS, Drug Interactions**).

Drugs that are largely eliminated via CYP2C19 metabolism, such as diazepam, propranolol, phenytoin (also via CYP2C9) or S-mephenytoin may have prolonged elimination upon coadministration with PROVIGIL and may require dosage reduction and monitoring for toxicity.

In patients with severe hepatic impairment, the dose of PROVIGIL should be reduced to one-half of that recommended for patients with normal hepatic function (See **CLINICAL PHARMACOLOGY** and **PRECAUTIONS**).

There is inadequate information to determine safety and efficacy of dosing in patients with severe renal impairment (See **CLINICAL PHARMACOLOGY** and **PRECAUTIONS**).

In elderly patients, elimination of PROVIGIL and its metabolites may be reduced as a consequence of aging. Therefore, consideration should be given to the use of lower doses in this population (See **CLINICAL PHARMACOLOGY** and **PRECAUTIONS**).

HOW SUPPLIED

PROVIGIL® (modafinil) Tablets

100 mg Each capsule-shaped, white, uncoated tablet is debossed with "PROVIGIL" on one side and "100 MG" on the other.

NDC 63459-101-01 - Bottles of 100

200 mg Each capsule-shaped, white, scored, uncoated tablet is debossed with "PROVIGIL" on one side and "200 MG" on the other.

NDC 63459-201-01 - Bottles of 100

Store at 20°-25° C (68°-77° F).

Manufactured for: **Cephalon, Inc.**
West Chester, PA 19380

U.S. Patent Nos. RE37,516 / 6,462,089

February 2004

PROV-006

PATIENT INFORMATION

PROVIGIL® (pro-vij-el) Tablets [C-IV]

Generic name: modafinil

Read the Patient Information that comes with PROVIGIL before you start taking it and each time you get a refill. There may be new information. This leaflet does not take the place of talking with your doctor about your condition or treatment.

What is the most important information I should know about PROVIGIL?

PROVIGIL may help treat the excessive sleepiness caused by certain sleep disorders, but it may not stop all your sleepiness. Regardless of how improved you may feel, do not change your daily habits until your doctor tells you it is okay. Discuss your level of sleepiness with your doctor at each visit. People with sleep disorders should always be careful about doing things that could be dangerous, including driving a car.

What is PROVIGIL?

PROVIGIL is a medicine to treat unusually sleepy people who have one of the following diagnosed sleep disorders:

- narcolepsy
- obstructive sleep apnea/hypopnea syndrome (OSAHS). PROVIGIL is used along with other medical treatments for OSAHS.
- shift work sleep disorder (SWSD)

You should be diagnosed with one of these sleep disorders before taking PROVIGIL, as sleepiness can be a symptom of other medical conditions that need to be treated.

PROVIGIL will not cure the above sleep disorders. PROVIGIL may help the sleepiness caused by these conditions, but it may not stop all your sleepiness. PROVIGIL is not meant to be used in place of getting enough sleep. You should follow your doctor's advice about good sleep habits and using other treatments.

PROVIGIL is a controlled substance [C-IV]. This means that PROVIGIL may be a target for people who abuse medicines or street drugs. Keep your PROVIGIL in a safe place. Giving away PROVIGIL is against the law.

Who should not take PROVIGIL?

Do not take PROVIGIL if you are allergic to any of its ingredients. The active ingredient is modafinil. See the end of this leaflet for a complete list of ingredients.

It is not known if PROVIGIL is right for children under the age of 16. Low levels of white blood cells (cells that fight infections) have happened in some children who have taken PROVIGIL.

Before starting PROVIGIL tell your doctor

- about all your medical conditions, including if you:
  - are pregnant, are planning to become pregnant, or are breastfeeding. It is not known if PROVIGIL may harm your unborn baby, or if PROVIGIL passes into your milk and if it can harm your baby.
  - have high blood pressure or heart problems.
  - have liver or kidney problems.
  - have abused medicines called "stimulants" or street drugs.
  - have or had a mental problem called psychosis.
- about all the medicines you take, including prescription and non-prescription medicines, vitamins, and herbal supplements. PROVIGIL and many other medicines can interact with each other causing side effects. PROVIGIL may affect the way other medicines work, and other medicines may affect how PROVIGIL works. Keep a list of all the medicines you take. Your doctor or pharmacist will tell you if it is safe to take PROVIGIL and other medicines together. Do not take other medicines with PROVIGIL unless your doctor has told you it is okay.

PROVIGIL can affect hormonal birth control methods (contraceptives). Women who use hormonal contraceptives such as birth control pills, shots, implants, intrauterine devices (IUDs), or patches, may have a higher chance for getting pregnant while taking PROVIGIL, and for one month after stopping PROVIGIL. Talk to your doctor about birth control methods that are right for you while using PROVIGIL.

How should I take PROVIGIL?

- Take PROVIGIL exactly as prescribed by your doctor. Your doctor will prescribe the dose of PROVIGIL that is right for you. Do not change your dose of PROVIGIL without talking to your doctor. Do not take more PROVIGIL than prescribed.
- Your doctor will tell you the right time of day to take PROVIGIL. Patients with narcolepsy or OSAHS usually take one dose of PROVIGIL every day in the morning. PROVIGIL may help you stay awake during the day but it should not affect nighttime sleep. Patients with SWSD usually take PROVIGIL about 1 hour before their work shift. Do not change the time of day you take PROVIGIL unless your have talked to your doctor.
- You can take PROVIGIL with or without food.
- If you take more than your prescribed dose, or take PROVIGIL too late in your waking day, you may find it harder to go to sleep. Call your doctor if you have any concerns.

What should I avoid while taking PROVIGIL?

- People with sleep disorders should always be careful about doing things that could be dangerous, including driving a car. Discuss your level of sleepiness with your doctor at each visit. Do not change your daily habits until your doctor tells you it is okay.
- Do not take other medicines including prescription and non-prescription medicines, vitamins or herbal supplements unless your doctor has told you it is okay.
- You should avoid drinking alcohol.

What are the possible side effects of PROVIGIL?

The most common side effects of PROVIGIL are headache, nausea, nervousness, stuffy nose, diarrhea, back pain, anxiety, trouble sleeping, dizziness, and upset stomach.

PROVIGIL may cause the following infrequent serious side effects. Call your doctor or get emergency help if you have any of these or any other serious side effects while taking PROVIGIL:

- chest pain.
- mental problems.
- allergic reactions, such as a rash, hives or other allergic reaction.

Some effects of PROVIGIL on the brain are similar to other medications called "stimulants". If you have a history of drug and/or stimulant use or abuse you should discuss this with your doctor before starting PROVIGIL.

Tell your doctor if you get any side effects while taking PROVIGIL.

These are not all the side effects of PROVIGIL. For more information, ask your doctor or pharmacist.

How should I store PROVIGIL?

- Store PROVIGIL at room temperature, 68° to 77° F (20° to 25° C).
- Store PROVIGIL in a safe place.
- Keep PROVIGIL and all medicines out of the reach of children.

General information about PROVIGIL

Medicines are sometimes prescribed for conditions that are not listed in patient information leaflets. Do not use PROVIGIL for a condition for which it was not prescribed. This medication is for your use only. Do not share this medication with others.

This leaflet summarizes the most important information about PROVIGIL. If you would like more information, talk with your doctor. You can ask your doctor or pharmacist for information about PROVIGIL that is written for health professionals. For more information, please call 1-800-896-5855, or go to www.provigil.com.

What are the ingredients in PROVIGIL?

Active Ingredient: modafinil

Inactive Ingredients: lactose, microcrystalline cellulose, pregelatinized starch, croscarmellose sodium, povidone, and magnesium stearate.

Rx Only

February 2004

Cephalon, Inc. West Chester, PA 19380.

This Patient Information Leaflet has been approved by the U.S. Food and Drug Administration.

Daiichi Pharmaceutical Corp.

11 PHILIPS PARKWAY
MONTVALE, NJ 07645

Direct Inquiries to:
Ph: (877) 324-4244 (877-DAIICHI)
Fax: (888) 727-5666

For Medical Emergencies and Product Information Contact:
Medical Services Department
Ph: (888) 727-2500
Fax: (888) 272-7979

FLOXIN® OTIC ℞

[flox-in]

(ofloxacin otic solution 0.3%)

Prescribing information for this product, which appears on pages 1184–1185 of the 2004 PDR, has been completely revised as follows. Please write "See Supplement A" next to the product heading.

DESCRIPTION

FLOXIN® Otic (ofloxacin otic solution) 0.3% is a sterile aqueous anti-infective (anti-bacterial) solution for otic use. Chemically, ofloxacin has three condensed 6-membered rings made up of a fluorinated carboxyquinolone with a benzoxazine ring. The chemical name of ofloxacin is (±)-9-fluoro-2,3-dihydro-3-methyl-10-(4-methyl-1-piperazinyl)-7-oxo-7H-pyrido [1,2,3-de]-1,4-benzoxazine-6-carboxylic acid. The empirical formula of ofloxacin is $C_{18}H_{20}FN_3O_4$ and its molecular weight is 361.38. The structural formula is:

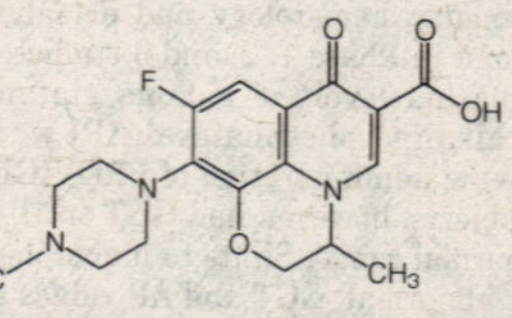

FLOXIN® Otic contains 0.3% (3mg/ml) ofloxacin with benzalkonium chloride (0.0025%), sodium chloride (0.9%), and water for injection. Hydrochloric acid and sodium hydroxide are added to adjust the pH to 6.5 ± 0.5.

CLINICAL PHARMACOLOGY

Pharmacokinetics: Drug concentrations in serum (in subjects with tympanostomy tubes and perforated tympanic membranes), in otorrhea, and in mucosa of the middle ear (in subjects with perforated tympanic membranes) were determined following otic administration of ofloxacin solution. In two single-dose studies, mean ofloxacin serum concentrations were low in adult patients with tympanostomy tubes, with and without otorrhea, after otic administration of a 0.3% solution (4.1 ng/ml (n=3) and 5.4 ng/ml (n=5), respectively). In adults with perforated tympanic membranes, the maximum serum drug level of ofloxacin detected was 10 ng/ml after administration of a 0.3% solution. Ofloxacin was detectable in the middle ear mucosa of some adult subjects with perforated tympanic membranes (11 of 16 subjects). The variability of ofloxacin concentration in middle ear mucosa was high. The concentrations ranged from 1.2 to 602 µg/g after otic administration of a 0.3% solution. Ofloxacin was present in high concentrations in otorrhea (389–2850 µg/g, n=13) 30 minutes after otic administration of a 0.3% solution in subjects with chronic suppurative otitis media and perforated tympanic membranes. However, the measurement of ofloxacin in the otorrhea does not necessarily reflect the exposure of the middle ear to ofloxacin.

Microbiology: Ofloxacin has *in vitro* activity against a wide range of gram-negative and gram-positive microorganisms. Ofloxacin exerts its antibacterial activity by inhibiting DNA gyrase, a bacterial topoisomerase. DNA gyrase is an essential enzyme which controls DNA topology and assists in DNA replication, repair, deactivation, and transcription. Cross-resistance has been observed between ofloxacin and other fluoroquinolones. There is generally no cross-resistance between ofloxacin and other classes of antibacterial agents such as beta-lactams or aminoglycosides.

Ofloxacin has been shown to be active against most isolates of the following microorganisms, both *in vitro* and clinically in otic infections as described in the **INDICATIONS AND USAGE** section.

Aerobic and facultative gram-positive microorganisms:

Staphylococcus aureus
Streptococcus pneumoniae

Aerobic and facultative gram-negative microorganisms:

Escherichia coli
Haemophilus influenzae
Moraxella catarrhalis
Proteus mirabilis
Pseudomonas aeruginosa

INDICATIONS AND USAGE

FLOXIN® Otic (ofloxacin otic solution) 0.3% is indicated for the treatment of infections caused by susceptible isolates of the designated microorganisms in the specific conditions listed below:

Otitis Externa in adults and pediatric patients, 6 months and older, due to *Escherichia coli, Pseudomonas aeruginosa, and Staphylococcus aureus.*

Chronic Suppurative Otitis Media in patients 12 years and older with perforated tympanic membranes due to *Proteus mirabilis, Pseudomonas aeruginosa,* and *Staphylococcus aureus.*

Acute Otitis Media in pediatric patients one year and older with tympanostomy tubes due to *Haemophilus influenzae, Moraxella catarrhalis, Pseudomonas aeruginosa Staphylococcus aureus,* and *Streptococcus pneumoniae.*

CONTRAINDICATIONS

FLOXIN® Otic (ofloxacin otic solution) 0.3% is contraindicated in patients with a history of hypersensitivity to ofloxacin, to other quinolones, or to any of the components in this medication.

WARNINGS

NOT FOR OPHTHALMIC USE.
NOT FOR INJECTION.

Serious and occasionally fatal hypersensitivity (anaphylactic) reactions, some following the first dose, have been reported in patients receiving systemic quinolones, including ofloxacin. Some reactions were accompanied by cardiovascular collapse, loss of consciousness, angioedema (including laryngeal, pharyngeal or facial edema), airway obstruction, dyspnea, urticaria, and itching. If an allergic reaction to ofloxacin is suspected, stop the drug. Serious acute hypersensitivity reactions may require immediate emergency treatment. Oxygen and airway management, including intubation, should be administered as clinically indicated.

PRECAUTIONS

General: As with other anti-infective preparations, prolonged use may result in over-growth of nonsusceptible organisms, including fungi. If the infection is not improved after one week, cultures should be obtained to guide further treatment. If otorrhea persists after a full course of therapy, or if two or more episodes of otorrhea occur within six months, further evaluation is recommended to exclude an underlying condition such as cholesteatoma, foreign body, or a tumor.

The systemic administration of quinolones, including ofloxacin at doses much higher than given or absorbed by the otic route, has led to lesions or erosions of the cartilage in weight-bearing joints and other signs of arthropathy in immature animals of various species.

Young growing guinea pigs dosed in the middle ear with 0.3% ofloxacin otic solution showed no systemic effects, lesions or erosions of the cartilage in weight-bearing joints, or other signs of arthropathy. No drug-related structural or functional changes of the cochlea and no lesions in the ossicles were noted in the guinea pig following otic administration of 0.3% ofloxacin for one month.

No signs of local irritation were found when 0.3% ofloxacin was applied topically in the rabbit eye. Ofloxacin was also shown to lack dermal sensitizing potential in the guinea pig maximization study.

Information for Patients: Avoid contaminating the applicator tip with material from the fingers or other sources. This precaution is necessary if the sterility of the drops is to be preserved. Systemic quinolones, including ofloxacin, have been associated with hypersensitivity reactions, even following a single dose. Discontinue use immediately and contact your physician at the first sign of a rash or allergic reaction.

Otitis Externa

Prior to administration of FLOXIN® Otic, the solution should be warmed by holding the bottle in the hand for one or two minutes to avoid dizziness which may result from the instillation of a cold solution. The patient should lie with the affected ear upward, and then the drops should be instilled. This position should be maintained for five minutes to facilitate penetration of the drops into the ear canal. Repeat, if necessary, for the opposite ear (see **DOSAGE AND ADMINISTRATION**).

Acute Otitis Media and Chronic Suppurative Otitis Media

Prior to administration of FLOXIN® Otic, the solution should be warmed by holding the bottle in the hand for one or two minutes to avoid dizziness which may result from the instillation of a cold solution. The patient should lie with the affected ear upward, and then the drops should be instilled. The tragus should then be pumped 4 times by pushing inward to facilitate penetration of the drops into the middle ear. This position should be maintained for five minutes. Repeat, if necessary, for the opposite ear (see **DOSAGE AND ADMINISTRATION**).

Drug Interactions: Specific drug interaction studies have not been conducted with FLOXIN® Otic.

Carcinogenesis, Mutagenesis, Impairment of Fertility

Long-term studies to determine the carcinogenic potential of ofloxacin have not been conducted. Ofloxacin was not mutagenic in the Ames test, the sister chromatid exchange assay (Chinese hamster and human cell lines), the unscheduled DNA synthesis (UDS) assay using human fibroblasts, the dominant lethal assay, or the mouse micronucleus assay. Ofloxacin was positive in the rat hepatocyte UDS assay, and in the mouse lymphoma assay. In rats, ofloxacin did not affect male or female reproductive performance at oral doses up to 360 mg/kg/day. This would be over 1000 times the maximum recommended clinical dose, based upon body surface area, assuming total absorption of ofloxacin from the ear of a patient treated with FLOXIN® Otic twice per day.

Adverse Event	Incidence Rate		
	Studies 002/003† BID (N=229)	Studies 016/017† QD (N=310)	Study 020† QD (N=489)
Application Site Reaction	3%	16.8%	0.6%
Pruritus	4%	1.2%	1.0%
Earache	1%	0.6%	0.8%
Dizziness	1%	0.0%	0.6%
Headache	0%	0.3%	0.2%
Vertigo	1%	0.0%	0.0%

† Studies 002/003 (BID) and 016/017 (QD) were active-controlled and comparative. Study 020 (QD) was open and non-comparative.

Pregnancy

Teratogenic effects: Pregnancy Category C. Ofloxacin has been shown to have an embryocidal effect in rats at a dose of 810 mg/kg/day and in rabbits at 160 mg/kg/day.

These dosages resulted in decreased fetal body weights and increased fetal mortality in rats and rabbits, respectively. Minor fetal skeletal variations were reported in rats receiving doses of 810 mg/kg/day. Ofloxacin has not been shown to be teratogenic at doses as high as 810 mg/kg/day and 160 mg/kg/day when administered to pregnant rats and rabbits, respectively.

Ofloxacin has not been shown to have any adverse effects on the developing embryo or fetus at doses relevant to the amount of ofloxacin that will be delivered ototopically at the recommended clinical doses.

Nonteratogenic Effects: Additional studies in the rat demonstrated that doses up to 360 mg/kg/day during late gestation had no adverse effects on late fetal development, labor, delivery, lactation, neonatal viability, or growth of the newborn. There are, however, no adequate and well-controlled studies in pregnant women. FLOXIN® Otic should be used during pregnancy only if the potential benefit justifies the potential risk to the fetus.

Nursing Mothers: In nursing women, a single 200 mg oral dose resulted in concentrations of ofloxacin in milk which were similar to those found in plasma. It is not known whether ofloxacin is excreted in human milk following topical otic administration. Because of the potential for serious adverse reactions from ofloxacin in nursing infants, a decision should be made whether to discontinue nursing or to discontinue the drug, taking into account the importance of the drug to the mother.

Pediatric Use: Safety and efficacy have been demonstrated in pediatric patients of the following ages for the listed indications:

- six months and older: otitis externa with intact tympanic membranes
- one year and older: acute otitis media with tympanostomy tubes
- twelve years and older: chronic suppurative otitis media with perforated tympanic membranes.

Safety and efficacy in pediatric patients below these ages have not been established.

Although no data are available on patients less than age 6 months, there are no known safety concerns or differences in the disease process in this population that will preclude use of this product.

No changes in hearing function occurred in 30 pediatric subjects treated with ofloxacin otic and tested for audiometric parameters.

Although quinolones, including ofloxacin, have been shown to cause arthropathy in immature animals after systemic administration, young growing guinea pigs dosed in the middle ear with 0.3% ofloxacin otic solution for one month showed no systemic effects, quinolone-induced lesions, erosions of the cartilage in weight-bearing joints, or other signs of arthropathy.

ADVERSE REACTIONS

Subjects with Otitis Externa

In the phase III clinical trials performed in support of once-daily dosing, 799 subjects with otitis externa and intact tympanic membranes were treated with ofloxacin otic solution. The studies, which served as the basis for approval, were 020 (pediatric, adolescents and adults), 016 (adolescents and adults) and 017 (pediatric). The following treatment-related adverse events occurred in two or more of the subjects.

[See table above]

An unexpected increase incidence of application site reaction was seen in studies 016/017 and was similar for both ofloxacin and the active control drug (neomycin-polymyxin B sulfate-hydrocortisone). This finding is believed to be the result of specific questioning of the subjects regarding the incidence of application site reactions.

In once daily dosing studies, there were also single reports of nausea, seborrhea, loss of hearing, tinnitus, otitis externa, otitis media, tremor, hypertension and fungal infection.

In twice daily dosing studies, the following treatment related adverse events were each reported in a single subject: dermatitis, eczema, erythematous rash, follicular rash, hypoaesthesia, tinnitus, dyspepsia, hot flushes, flushing and otorrhagia.

Subjects with Acute Otitis Media with Tympanostomy Tubes (AOM TT) and Subjects with Chronic Suppurative Otitis Media (CSOM) with Perforated Tympanic Membranes

In phase III clinical trials which formed the basis for approval, the following treatment-related adverse events occurred in 1% or more of the 656 subjects with non-intact tympanic membranes in AOM TT or CSOM treated twice-daily with ofloxacin otic solution:

Adverse Event	Incidence (N=656)
Taste Perversion	7%
Earache	1%
Pruritus	1%
Paraesthesia	1%
Rash	1%
Dizziness	1%

Other treatment-related adverse reactions reported in subjects with non-intact tympanic membranes included: diarrhea (0.6%), nausea (0.3%), vomiting (0.3%), dry mouth (0.5%), headache (0.3%), vertigo (0.5%), otorrhagia (0.6%), tinnitus (0.3%), fever (0.3%). The following treatment-related adverse events were each reported in a single subject: application site reaction, otitis externa, urticaria, abdominal pain, dysaesthesia, hyperkinesia, halitosis, inflammation, pain, insomnia, coughing, pharyngitis, rhinitis, sinusitis, and tachycardia.

Post-marketing Adverse Events

Cases of uncommon transient neuropsychiatric disturbances have been included in spontaneous post-marketing reports. A causal relationship with ofloxacin otic solution 0.3% is unknown.

DOSAGE AND ADMINISTRATION

Otitis Externa: The recommended dosage regimen for the treatment of otitis externa is:

For pediatric patients (from 6 months to 13 years old): Five drops (0.25 ml, 0.75 mg ofloxacin) instilled into the affected ear once daily for seven days.

For patients 13 years and older: Ten drops (0.5 ml, 1.5 mg ofloxacin) instilled into the affected ear once daily for seven days.

The solution should be warmed by holding the bottle in the hand for one or two minutes to avoid dizziness which may result from the instillation of a cold solution. The patient should lie with the affected ear upward, and then the drops should be instilled. This position should be maintained for five minutes to facilitate penetration of the drops into the ear canal. Repeat, if necessary, for the opposite ear.

Acute Otitis Media in pediatric patients with tympanostomy tubes: The recommended dosage regimen for the treatment of acute otitis media in pediatric patients (from 1 to 12 years old) with tympanostomy tubes is:

Five drops (0.25 ml, 0.75 mg ofloxacin) instilled into the affected ear twice daily for ten days. The solution should be warmed by holding the bottle in the hand for one or two minutes to avoid dizziness that may result from the instillation of a cold solution. The patient should lie with the affected ear upward, and then the drops should be instilled. The tragus should then be pumped 4 times by pushing inward to facilitate penetration of the drops into the middle ear. This position should be maintained for five minutes. Repeat, if necessary, for the opposite ear.

Chronic Suppurative Otitis Media with perforated tympanic membranes: The recommended dosage regimen for the treatment of chronic suppurative otitis media with perforated tympanic membranes in patients 12 years and older is:

Ten drops (0.5 ml, 1.5 mg ofloxacin) instilled into the affected ear twice daily for fourteen days. The solution should be warmed by holding the bottle in the hand for one or two minutes to avoid dizziness that may result from the instillation of a cold solution. The patient should lie with the affected ear upward, before instilling the drops. The tragus should then be pumped 4 times by pushing inward to facilitate penetration into the middle ear. This position should be maintained for five minutes. Repeat, if necessary, for the opposite ear.

HOW SUPPLIED

FLOXIN® Otic (ofloxacin otic solution) 0.3% is supplied in plastic dropper bottles containing 5 ml and 10 ml. The NDC codes are:

63395-101-05 FLOXIN® Otic 5ml

Continued on next page

Floxin—Cont.

63395-101-10 FLOXIN® Otic 10 ml
Store at 15-25° C (59-77° F).
Rx Only
Daiichi Pharmaceutical Corporation
Montvale, NJ 07645
Revised (November 7th, 2003)

Duramed Pharmaceuticals, Inc.
2 QUAKER RD.
POMONA, NY 10970

Direct Inquiries to:
877-405-0369

CENESTIN® ℞
[*sĕ'nĕ"stin*]
(synthetic conjugated estrogens, A)
Tablets
℞ only

Prescribing information for this product, which appears on pages 1204–1208 of the 2004 PDR, has been completely revised as follows. Please write "See Supplement A" next to the product heading.

ESTROGENS INCREASE THE RISK OF ENDOMETRIAL CANCER

Close clinical surveillance of all women taking estrogens is important. Adequate diagnostic measures, including endometrial sampling when indicated, should be undertaken to rule out malignancy in all cases of undiagnosed persistent or recurring abnormal vaginal bleeding. There is no evidence that the use of "natural" estrogens results in a different endometrial risk profile than synthetic estrogens at equivalent estrogen doses. (See **WARNINGS, Malignant neoplasms,** *Endometrial cancer.*)

CARDIOVASCULAR AND OTHER RISKS

Estrogens with and without progestins should not be used for the prevention of cardiovascular disease. (See **WARNINGS, Cardiovascular disorders.**)

The Women's Health Initiative (WHI) study reported increased risks of myocardial infarction, stroke, invasive breast cancer, pulmonary emboli, and deep vein thrombosis in postmenopausal women (50 to 79 years of age) during 5 years of treatment with oral conjugated equine estrogens (CE 0.625 mg) combined with medroxyprogesterone acetate (MPA 2.5 mg) relative to placebo. (See **CLINICAL PHARMACOLOGY, Clinical Studies.**)

Other doses of oral conjugated estrogens with medroxyprogesterone, and other combinations and dosage forms of estrogens and progestins were not studied in the WHI clinical trials and, in the absence of comparable data, these risks should be assumed to be similar. Because of these risks, estrogens with or without progestins should be prescribed at the lowest effective doses and for the shortest duration consistent with treatment goals and risks for the individual woman.

DESCRIPTION

Synthetic conjugated estrogens, A tablets contain a blend of nine (9) synthetic estrogenic substances. The estrogenic substances are sodium estrone sulfate, sodium equilin sulfate, sodium 17α-dihydroequilin sulfate, sodium 17α-estradiol sulfate, sodium 17β-dihydroequilin sulfate, sodium 17α-dihydroequilenin sulfate, sodium 17β-dihydroequilenin sulfate, sodium equilenin sulfate and sodium 17β-estradiol sulfate.

The structural formulae for these estrogens are:

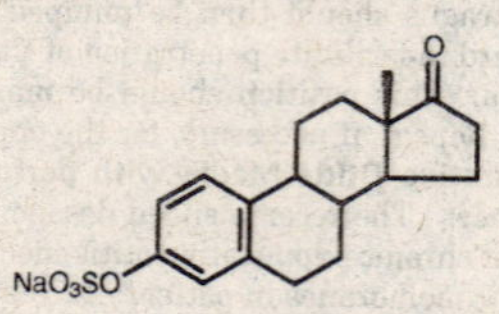

$C_{18}H_{21}NaO_5S$
372.42
Sodium Estrone Sulfate

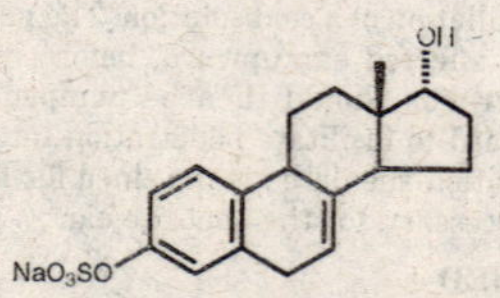

$C_{18}H_{21}NaO_5S$
372.42
Sodium 17α-Dihydroequilin Sulfate

[See first chemical structure at top of next column]
[See second chemical structure at top of next column]

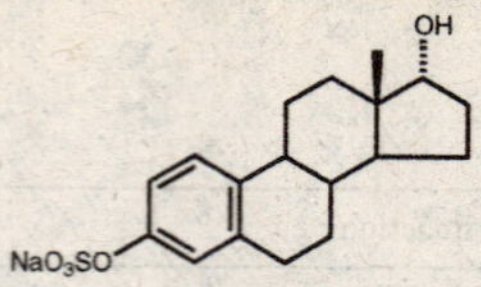

$C_{18}H_{23}NaO_5S$
374.44
Sodium 17α-Estradiol Sulfate

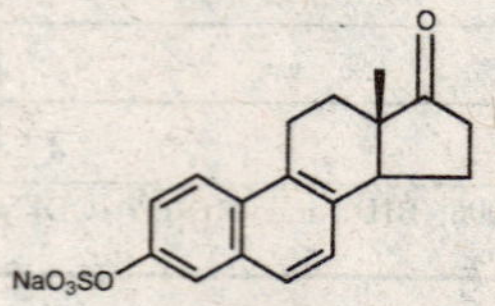

$C_{18}H_{17}NaO_5S$
368.39
Sodium Equilenin Sulfate

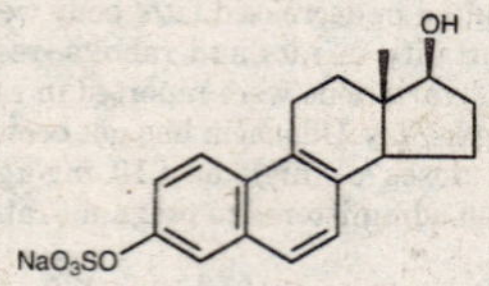

$C_{18}H_{19}NaO_5S$
370.41
Sodium 17β-Dihydroequilenin Sulfate

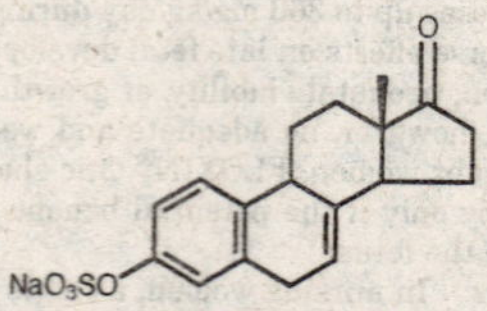

$C_{18}H_{19}NaO_5S$
370.41
Sodium Equilin Sulfate

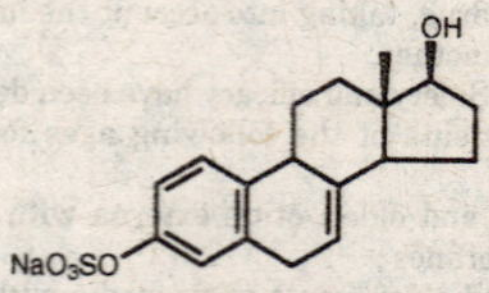

$C_{18}H_{21}NaO_5S$
372.42
Sodium 17β-Dihydroequilin Sulfate

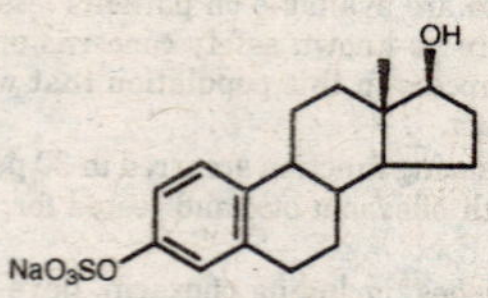

$C_{18}H_{23}NaO_5S$
374.44
Sodium 17β-Estradiol Sulfate

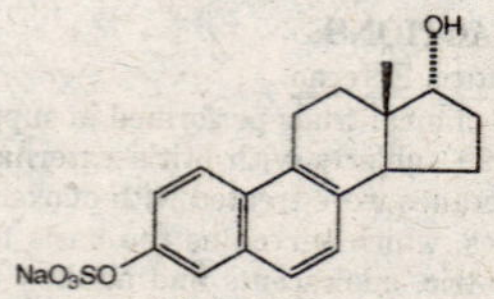

$C_{18}H_{19}NaO_5S$
370.41
Sodium 17α-Dihydroequilenin Sulfate

Tablets for oral administration, are available in 0.3 mg, 0.45 mg, 0.625 mg, 0.9 mg and 1.25 mg strengths of synthetic conjugated estrogens, A. Tablets also contain the following inactive ingredients: ethylcellulose, hypromellose, lactose monohydrate, magnesium stearate, polyethylene glycol, polysorbate 80, pregelatinized starch, titanium dioxide, and triethyl citrate.
-0.3 mg tablets also contain FD&C Blue No. 2 aluminum lake and D&C Yellow No. 10 aluminum lake.
-0.45 mg tablets also contain FD&C Yellow No. 6/Sunset Yellow FCF lake.
-0.625 mg tablets also contain FD&C Red No. 40 aluminum lake.
-0.9 mg tablets do not contain additional color additives.
-1.25 mg tablets also contain FD&C Blue No. 2 aluminum lake.

CLINICAL PHARMACOLOGY

Endogenous estrogens are largely responsible for the development and maintenance of the female reproductive system and secondary sexual characteristics. Although circulating estrogens exist in a dynamic equilibrium of metabolic interconversions, estradiol is the principal intracellular human estrogen and is substantially more potent than its metabolites, estrone and estriol at the receptor level.

The primary source of estrogen in normally cycling adult women is the ovarian follicle, which secretes 70 to 500 mcg of estradiol daily, depending on the phase of the menstrual cycle. After menopause, most endogenous estrogen is produced by conversion of androstenedione, secreted by the adrenal cortex, to estrone by peripheral tissues. Thus, estrone and the sulfate-conjugated form, estrone sulfate, are the most abundant circulating estrogens in postmenopausal women.

Estrogens act through binding to nuclear receptors in estrogen-responsive tissues. To date, two estrogen receptors have been identified. These vary in proportion from tissue to tissue.

Circulating estrogens modulate the pituitary secretion of the gonadotropins, luteinizing hormone (LH) and follicle stimulating hormone (FSH) through a negative feedback mechanism. Estrogens act to reduce the elevated levels of these hormones seen in postmenopausal women.

Pharmacokinetics

Absorption

Synthetic conjugated estrogens, A are soluble in water and are well absorbed from the gastrointestinal tract after release from the drug formulation. The Cenestin tablet releases the synthetic conjugated estrogens, A slowly over a period of several hours. The effect of food on the bioavailability of synthetic conjugated estrogens, A from Cenestin has not been studied.

[See table 1 at top of next page]

Figure 1

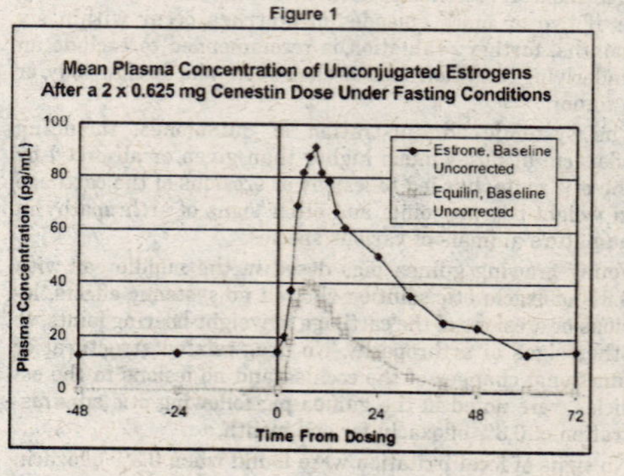

Distribution

The distribution of exogenous estrogens is similar to that of endogenous estrogens. Estrogens are widely distributed in the body and are generally found in higher concentrations in the sex hormone target organs. Estrogens circulate in the blood largely bound to sex hormone binding globulin (SHBG) and albumin.

Metabolism

Exogenous estrogens are metabolized in the same manner as endogenous estrogens. Circulating estrogens exist in a dynamic equilibrium of metabolic interconversions. These transformations take place mainly in the liver. Estradiol is converted reversibly to estrone, and both can be converted to estriol, which is the major urinary metabolite. Estrogens also undergo enterohepatic recirculation via sulfate and glucuronide conjugation in the liver, biliary secretion of conjugates into the intestine, and hydrolysis in the gut followed by reabsorption. In postmenopausal women a significant portion of the circulating estrogens exist as sulfate conjugates, especially estrone sulfate, which serves as a circulating reservoir for the formation of more active estrogens.

Excretion

Estradiol, estrone, and estriol are excreted in the urine along with glucuronide and sulfate conjugates.

Special Populations

Cenestin was investigated in postmenopausal women. No pharmacokinetic studies were conducted in special populations, including patients with renal or hepatic impairment.

Drug Interactions

In vitro and *in vivo* studies have shown that estrogens are metabolized partially by cytochrome P450 3A4 (CYP3A4). Therefore, inducers and inhibitors of CYP3A4 may affect estrogen drug metabolism. Inducers of CYP3A4 such as St. John's Wort preparations (Hypericum perforatum), phenobarbital, carbamazepine, and rifampin may reduce plasma concentrations of estrogens, possibly resulting in a decrease in therapeutic effects and/or changes in the uterine bleeding profile. Inhibitors of CYP3A4 such as erythromycin, clarithromycin, ketoconazole, itraconazole, ritonavir and grapefruit juice may increase plasma concentrations of estrogens and may result in side effects.

Clinical Studies

Effects on vasomotor symptoms

A randomized, placebo-controlled multicenter clinical study was conducted evaluating the effectiveness of Cenestin for the treatment of moderate to severe vasomotor symptoms in 120 postmenopausal women between 38 and 66 years of age (68% were Caucasian). Patients were randomized to receive

Table 1
PHARMACOKINETIC PARAMETERS FOR UNCONJUGATED AND CONJUGATED ESTROGENS IN HEALTHY POSTMENOPAUSAL WOMEN UNDER FASTING CONDITIONS
Pharmacokinetic Parameters of Unconjugated Estrogens Following a Dose of 2 × 0.625 mg Cenestin

Drug	C_{max} (pg/mL) CV%	t_{max} (h) CV%	AUC_{0-72h} (pg•hr/mL) CV%
Baseline-corrected estrone	84.5 (41.7)	8.25 (35.6)	1749 (43.8)
Equilin	45.6 (47.3)	7.78 (28.8)	723 (67.9)

Pharmacokinetic Parameters of Conjugated Estrogens Following a Dose of 2 × 0.625 mg Cenestin

Drug	C_{max} (ng/mL) CV%	t_{max} (h) CV%	$t_{½}$ (h) CV%	AUC_{0-72h} (ng•hr/mL) CV%
Baseline-corrected estrone	4.43 (40.4)	7.7 (30.3)	10.6 (25.4)	69.89 (39.2)
Equilin	3.27 (43.5)	5.8 (31.1)	9.7 (23.0)	46.46 (47.5)

either placebo or 0.625 mg Cenestin daily for 12 weeks. Dose titration was allowed after one week of treatment. The starting dose was either doubled (2 × 0.625 mg Cenestin or placebo taken daily) or reduced (0.3 mg Cenestin or placebo taken daily), if necessary. Efficacy was assessed at 4 and 12 weeks of treatment. By week 12, 10% of the study participants remained on a single 0.625 mg Cenestin tablet daily while 77% required two (0.625 mg) tablets daily. The results in Table 2 indicate that compared to placebo, Cenestin produced a reduction in moderate to severe vasomotor symptoms at weeks 4 and 12.

A second randomized, placebo-controlled multicenter clinical study was conducted evaluating the effectiveness of 0.45 mg Cenestin tablets, for the treatment of moderate to severe vasomotor symptoms in 104 menopausal women between 52 and 74 years of age (76% were Caucasian). Patients were randomized to receive either placebo or 0.45 mg Cenestin daily for 12 weeks. Efficacy was assessed at 4 and 12 weeks of treatment. The mean change in the number of moderate to severe hot flushes per week shown in Table 3 indicate that compared to placebo, 0.45 mg Cenestin produced a reduction in moderate to severe vasomotor symptoms at weeks 4 and 12. A corresponding reduction in the severity of hot flushes was demonstrated at weeks 5 and 12.

Table 2
Clinical Response[a]
Mean Change in the Number of Moderate to Severe Hot Flushes Per Week, 0.625 mg and 2 × 0.625 mg Cenestin, ITT Population

	Cenestin[b] 0.625 mg and 2 × 0.625 mg (n=70)	Placebo (n=47)
Baseline		
Mean # (SD)	96.8 (42.6)	94.1 (33.9)
Week 4		
Mean # (SD)	28.7 (28.8)	45.7 (36.8)
Mean Change from Baseline (SD)	-68.1 (43.9)	-48.4 (46.2)
P-value vs. Placebo	p=.022	
Week 12		
Mean # (SD)	16.5 (25.7)	37.8 (38.7)
Mean Change from Baseline (SD)	-80.3 (50.3)	-56.3 (48.0)
P-value vs. Placebo	p=.010	

Mean = Arithmetic Mean, SD = Standard Deviation
[a]Intent-to-treat population = 117
[b]: Combined results for 0.625 mg and 0.625 mg Cenestin tablets.

Table 3
Clinical Response*
Mean Change in the Number of Moderate to Severe Hot Flushes Per Week, 0.45 mg Cenestin, ITT Population

	Cenestin 0.45 mg (n=53)	Placebo (n=51)
Baseline		
Mean # (SD)	95.9 (37.0)	95.9 (41.6)
Week 4		
Mean # (SD)	45.7 (45.9)	59.4 (46.2)
Mean Change from Baseline (SD)	-50.3 (35.4)	-36.5 (42.9)
P-value vs. Placebo	p=.014	
Week 12		
Mean # (SD)	26.1 (43.0)	50.5 (48.4)
Mean Change from Baseline (SD)	-69.9 (38.1)	-45.4 (44.7)
P-value vs. Placebo	p<.001	

Mean = Arithmetic Mean, SD = Standard Deviation
*Intent-to-treat population = 104

Effects on vulvar and vaginal atrophy
The effects of 0.3 mg Cenestin on moderate to severe symptoms of vulvar and vaginal atrophy were confirmed in a 16-week, randomized, placebo-controlled, multicenter clinical study in 72 postmenopausal women between 30 and 77 years of age (53% were Caucasian). Patients were randomized to receive either placebo or 0.3 mg Cenestin daily for 16 weeks. Efficacy was assessed at weeks 12 and 16 for vaginal wall cytology and week 16 for vaginal pH. Results for percent of superficial cells from a maturation index of the vaginal mucosa are shown in Figure 2. Mean vaginal pH decreased from a baseline of 6.20 to 5.14 for Cenestin and increased to 6.15 from a baseline of 6.03 for placebo.

Figure 2
Summary of % Superficial Cells Results in Patients Following 16 Weeks of Treatment with Cenestin 0.3 mg
Mean +/- SE

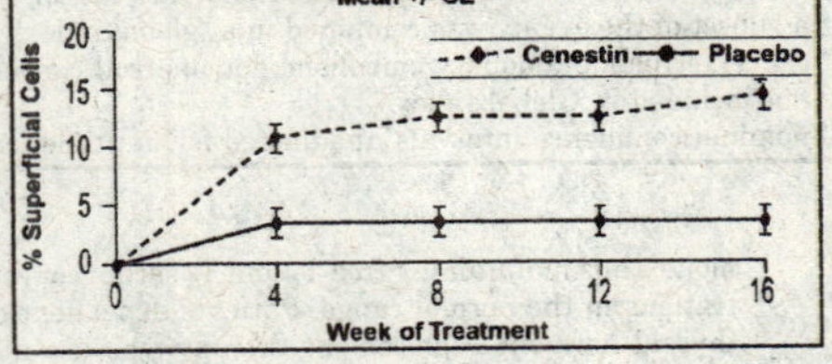

Women's Health Initiative Studies.
The Women's Health Initiative (WHI) enrolled a total of 27,000 predominantly healthy postmenopausal women to assess the risks and benefits of either the use of oral 0.625 mg conjugated equine estrogens (CE) per day alone or the use of oral 0.625 mg conjugated estrogens plus 2.5 mg medroxyprogesterone acetate (MPA) per day compared to placebo in prevention of certain chronic diseases. The primary endpoint was the incidence of coronary heart disease (CHD) (nonfatal myocardial infarction and CHD death), with invasive breast cancer as the primary adverse outcome studied. A "global index" included the earliest occurrence of CHD, invasive breast cancer, stroke, pulmonary embolism (PE), endometrial cancer, colorectal cancer, hip fracture, or death due to other cause. The study did not evaluate the effects of CE or CE/MPA on menopausal symptoms.

The CE-only substudy is continuing and results have not been reported. The CE/MPA substudy was stopped early because, according to the predefined stopping rule, the increased risk of breast cancer and cardiovascular events exceeded the specified benefits included in the "global index." Results of the CE/MPA substudy, which included 16,608 women (average age of 63 years range 50 to 79; 83.9% White, 6.5% Black, 5.5% Hispanic), after an average follow-up of 5.2 years are presented in Table 4 below:

[See table 4 at top of next page]

For those outcomes included in the "global index," absolute excess risks per 10,000 women-years in the group treated with CE/MPA were 7 more CHD events, 8 more strokes, 8 more PEs, and 8 more invasive breast cancers, while absolute risk reductions per 10,000 women-years were 6 fewer colorectal cancers and 5 fewer hip fractures. The absolute excess risk of events included in the "global index" was 19 per 10,000 women-years. There was no difference between the groups in terms of all-cause mortality. (See **BOXED WARNINGS, WARNINGS,** and **PRECAUTIONS.**)

INDICATIONS AND USAGE

Cenestin therapy is indicated for the:

1. Treatment of moderate-to-severe vasomotor symptoms associated with the menopause.
   - 0.45 mg Cenestin
   - 0.625 mg Cenestin
   - 0.9 mg Cenestin
   - 1.25 mg Cenestin
2. Treatment of moderate to severe symptoms of vulvar and vaginal atrophy associated with the menopause. When prescribing solely for the treatment of symptoms of vulvar and vaginal atrophy, topical vaginal products should be considered.
   - 0.3 mg Cenestin

CONTRAINDICATIONS

Cenestin should not be used in individuals with any of the following conditions:

1. Undiagnosed abnormal genital bleeding.
2. Known, suspected, or history of cancer of the breast.
3. Known or suspected estrogen-dependent neoplasia.
4. Active deep vein thrombosis, pulmonary embolism or a history of these conditions.
5. Active or recent (e.g., within the past year) arterial thromboembolic disease (e.g., stroke, myocardial infarction).
6. Liver dysfunction or disease.
7. Cenestin therapy should not be used in patients with known hypersensitivity to its ingredients.
8. Known or suspected pregnancy. There is no indication for Cenestin in pregnancy. There appears to be little or no increased risk of birth defects in children born to women who have used estrogens and progestins from oral contraceptives inadvertently during early pregnancy. (See **PRECAUTIONS.**)

WARNINGS

See **BOXED WARNINGS**.

1. Cardiovascular disorders.
Estrogen and estrogen/progestin therapy have been associated with an increased risk of cardiovascular events such as myocardial infarction and stroke, as well as venous thrombosis and pulmonary embolism (venous thromboembolism or VTE). Should any of these occur or be suspected, estrogens should be discontinued immediately.

Risk factors for arterial vascular disease (e.g., hypertension, diabetes mellitus, tobacco use, hypercholesterolemia, and obesity) and/or venous thromboembolism (e.g., personal history or family history of VTE, obesity, and systemic lupus erythematosus) should be managed appropriately.

a. Coronary heart disease and stroke. In the Women's Health Initiative (WHI) study, an increase in the number of myocardial infarctions and strokes has been observed in women receiving CE compared to placebo. These observations are preliminary, and the study is continuing. (See **CLINICAL PHARMACOLOGY, Clinical Studies.**)

In the CE/MPA substudy of WHI, an increased risk of coronary heart disease (CHD) events (defined as non-fatal myocardial infarction and CHD death) was observed in women receiving CE/MPA compared to women receiving placebo (37 vs 30 per 10,000 women-years). The increase in risk was observed in year one and persisted.

In the same substudy of WHI, an increased risk of stroke was observed in women receiving CE/MPA compared to women receiving placebo (29 vs 21 per 10,000 women-years). The increase in risk was observed after the first year and persisted.

In postmenopausal women with documented heart disease (n = 2,763, average age 66.7 years) a controlled clinical trial of secondary prevention of cardiovascular disease (Heart and Estrogen/Progestin Replacement Study; HERS) treatment with CE/MPA (0.625 mg/2.5 mg per day) demonstrated no cardiovascular benefit. During an average follow-up of 4.1 years, treatment with CE/MPA did not reduce the overall rate of CHD events in postmenopausal women with established coronary heart disease. There were more CHD events in the CE/MPA-treated group than in the placebo group in year 1, but not during the subsequent years. Two thousand three hundred and twenty one women from the original HERS trial agreed to participate in an open label extension of HERS, HERS II. Average follow-up in HERS II was an additional 2.7 years, for a total of 6.8 years overall. Rates of CHD events were comparable among women in the CE/MPA group and the placebo group in HERS, HERS II, and overall.

Large doses of estrogen (5 mg conjugated estrogens per day), comparable to those used to treat cancer of the prostate and breast, have been shown in a large prospective clinical trial in men to increase the risks of nonfatal myocardial infarction, pulmonary embolism, and thrombophlebitis.

b. Venous thromboembolism (VTE). In the Women's Health Initiative (WHI) study, an increase in VTE has been observed in women receiving CE compared to placebo. These observations are preliminary, and the study is continuing. (See **CLINICAL PHARMACOLOGY, Clinical Studies.**)

In the CE/MPA substudy of WHI, a 2-fold greater rate of VTE, including deep venous thrombosis and pulmonary embolism, was observed in women receiving CE/MPA compared to women receiving placebo. The rate of VTE was 34 per 10,000 women-years in the CE/MPA group compared to 16 per 10,000 women-years in the placebo group. The increase in VTE risk was observed during the first year and persisted.

If feasible, estrogens should be discontinued at least 4 to 6 weeks before surgery of the type associated with an increased risk of thromboembolism, or during periods of prolonged immobilization.

2. Malignant neoplasms.
a. Endometrial cancer. The use of unopposed estrogens in women with intact uteri has been associated with an increased risk of endometrial cancer. The reported endometrial cancer risk among unopposed estrogen users is about 2- to 12-fold greater than in non-users, and appears dependent on duration of treatment and on estrogen dose. Most studies show no significant increased risk associated with use of estrogens for less than one year. The greatest risk appears associated with prolonged use, with increased risks of 15- to 24-fold for five to ten years or more and this risk has been shown to persist for at least 8 to 15 years after estrogen therapy is discontinued.

Clinical surveillance of all women taking estrogen/progestin combinations is important. Adequate diagnostic measures, including endometrial sampling when indicated, should be

Continued on next page

Cenestin—Cont.

undertaken to rule out malignancy in all cases of undiagnosed persistent or recurring abnormal vaginal bleeding. There is no evidence that the use of natural estrogens results in a different endometrial risk profile than synthetic estrogens of equivalent estrogen dose. Adding a progestin to estrogen therapy has been shown to reduce the risk of endometrial hyperplasia, which may be a precursor to endometrial cancer.

b. Breast cancer. Estrogen and estrogen/progestin therapy in postmenopausal women has been associated with an increased risk of breast cancer. In the CE/MPA substudy of the Women's Health Initiative (WHI) study, a 26% increase of invasive breast cancer (38 vs 30 per 10,000 women-years) after an average of 5.2 years of treatment was observed in women receiving CE/MPA compared to women receiving placebo. The increased risk of breast cancer became apparent after 4 years on CE/MPA. The women reporting prior postmenopausal use of estrogen and/or estrogen with progestin had a higher relative risk for breast cancer associated with CE/MPA than those who had never used these hormones. (See **CLINICAL PHARMACOLOGY, Clinical Studies.**)

In the WHI, no increased risk of breast cancer in CE-treated women compared to placebo was reported after an average of 5.2 years of therapy. These data are preliminary and that substudy of WHI is continuing.

Epidemiologic studies have reported an increased risk of breast cancer in association with increasing duration of postmenopausal treatment with estrogens with or without a progestin. This association was reanalyzed in original data from 51 studies that involved various doses and types of estrogens, with and without progestins. In the reanalysis, an increased risk of having breast cancer diagnosed became apparent after about 5 years of continued treatment, and subsided after treatment had been discontinued for 5 years or longer. Some later studies have suggested that postmenopausal treatment with estrogen and progestin increases the risk of breast cancer more than treatment with estrogen alone.

A postmenopausal woman without a uterus who requires estrogen should receive estrogen-alone therapy, and should not be exposed unnecessarily to progestins. All postmenopausal women should receive yearly breast exams by a healthcare provider and perform monthly self-examinations. In addition, mammography examinations should be scheduled based on patient age and risk factors.

3. Gallbladder disease

A 2 to 4-fold increase in the risk of gallbladder disease requiring surgery in postmenopausal women receiving estrogens has been reported.

4. Hypercalcemia

Estrogen administration may lead to severe hypercalcemia in patients with breast cancer and bone metastases. If hypercalcemia occurs, use of the drug should be stopped and appropriate measures taken to reduce the serum calcium level.

5. Visual abnormalities

Retinal vascular thrombosis has been reported in patients receiving estrogens. Discontinue medication pending examination if there is sudden partial or complete loss of vision, or a sudden onset of proptosis, diplopia, or migraine. If examination reveals papilledema or renal vascular lesions, estrogens should be permanently discontinued.

Table 4
Relative and Absolute Risk Seen in the Estrogen/Progestin Substudy of the WHI[a]

Event[c]	Relative Risk Conjugated Equine Estrogens/ Medroxyprogesterone Acetate vs Placebo at 5.2 years (95% CI*)	Placebo n = 8102	CEE/MPA n = 8506
		Absolute Risk per 10,000 Person-years	
CHD events	1.29 (1.02-1.63)	30	37
Non-fatal MI	*1.32 (1.02-1.72)*	*23*	*30*
CHD death	*1.18 (0.70-1.97)*	*6*	*7*
Invasive breast cancer[b]	1.26 (1.00-1.59)	30	38
Stroke	1.41 (1.07-1.85)	21	29
Pulmonary embolism	2.13 (1.39-3.25)	8	16
Colorectal cancer	0.63 (0.43-0.92)	16	10
Endometrial cancer	0.83 (0.47-1.47)	6	5
Hip fracture	0.66 (0.45-0.98)	15	10
Death due to causes other than the events above	0.92 (0.74-1.14)	40	37
Global index[c]	1.15 (1.03-1.28)	151	170
Deep vein thrombosis[d]	2.07 (1.49-2.87)	13	26
Vertebral fractures[d]	0.66 (0.44-0.98)	15	9
Other osteoporotic fractures[d]	0.77 (0.69-0.86)	170	131

[a] adapted from JAMA, 2002; 288:321-333.
[b] Includes metastatic and non-metastatic breast cancer with the exception of in situ breast cancer.
[c] a subset of the events was combined in a "global index," defined as the earliest occurrence of CHD events, invasive breast cancer, stroke, pulmonary embolism, endometrial cancer, colorectal cancer, hip fracture, or death due to other causes.
[d] not included in Global Index.
* nominal confidence intervals unadjusted for multiple looks and multiple comparisons.

PRECAUTIONS

A. General

1. ***Addition of a progestin when a woman has not had a hysterectomy.*** Studies of the addition of a progestin for 10 or more days of a cycle of estrogen administration, or daily with estrogen in a continuous regimen, have reported a lowered incidence of endometrial hyperplasia than would be induced by estrogen treatment alone. Endometrial hyperplasia may be a precursor to endometrial cancer. There are, however, possible risks that may be associated with the use of progestins in estrogen replacement regimens. These include:
   a. A possible increased risk of breast cancer.
   b. Adverse effects on lipoprotein metabolism (e.g., lowering HDL, raising LDL).
   c. Impairment of glucose tolerance.
2. ***Elevated blood pressure.*** In a small number of case reports, substantial increases in blood pressure have been attributed to idiosyncratic reactions to estrogens. In a large, randomized, placebo controlled clinical trial, a generalized effect of estrogen therapy on blood pressure was not seen. Blood pressure should be monitored at regular intervals with estrogen use.
3. ***Hypertriglyceridemia.*** In patients with pre-existing hypertriglyceridemia, estrogen therapy may be associated with elevations of plasma triglycerides leading to pancreatitis and other complications.
4. ***Impaired liver function and past history of cholestatic jaundice.*** Estrogens may be poorly metabolized in patients with impaired liver function. For patients with a history of cholestatic jaundice associated with past estrogen use or with pregnancy, caution should be exercised and in the case of recurrence, medication should be discontinued.
5. ***Hypothyroidism.*** Estrogen administration leads to increased thyroid-binding globulin (TBG) levels. Patients with normal thyroid function can compensate for the increased TBG by making more thyroid hormone, thus maintaining free T_4 and T_3 serum concentrations in the normal range. Patients dependent on thyroid hormone replacement therapy who are also receiving estrogens may require increased doses of their thyroid replacement therapy. These patients should have their thyroid function monitored in order to maintain their free thyroid hormone levels in an acceptable range.
6. ***Fluid retention.*** Because estrogens may cause some degree of fluid retention, patients with conditions that might be influenced by this factor, such as a cardiac or renal dysfunction, warrant careful observation when estrogens are prescribed.
7. ***Hypocalcemia.*** Estrogens should be used with caution in individuals with severe hypocalcemia.
8. ***Ovarian cancer.*** Use of estrogen-only products, in particular for ten or more years, has been associated with an increased risk of ovarian cancer in some epidemiological studies. Other studies did not show a significant association. Data are insufficient to determine whether there is an increased risk with estrogen/progestin combination therapy in postmenopausal women.
9. ***Exacerbation of endometriosis.*** Endometriosis may be exacerbated with administration of estrogen therapy. A few cases of malignant transformation of residual endometrial implants have been reported in women treated post-hysterectomy with estrogen alone therapy. For patients known to have residual endometriosis post-hysterectomy, the addition of progestin should be considered.
10. ***Exacerbation of other conditions.*** Estrogens may cause an exacerbation of asthma, diabetes mellitus, epilepsy, migraine, porphyria, systemic lupus erythematosus, and hepatic hemangiomas and should be used with caution in women with these conditions.

B. Patient Information

Physicians are advised to discuss the PATIENT INFORMATION leaflet with patients for whom they prescribe Cenestin.

C. Laboratory Tests

Estrogen administration should be initiated at the lowest dose for the approved indication and then guided by clinical response, rather than by serum hormone levels (e.g., estradiol, FSH).

D. Drug/Laboratory Test Interactions

1. Accelerated prothrombin time, partial thromboplastin time, and platelet aggregation time; increased platelet count; increased factors II, VII antigen, VIII antigen, VIII coagulant activity, IX, X, XII, VII-X complex, II-VII-X complex, and beta-thromboglobulin; decreased levels of anti-factor Xa and antithrombin III, decreased antithrombin III activity; increased levels of fibrinogen and fibrinogen activity; increased plasminogen antigen and activity.
2. Increased thyroid-binding globulin (TBG) levels leading to increased circulating total thyroid hormone levels, as measured by protein-bound iodine (PBI), T_4 levels (by column or by radioimmunoassay) or T_3 levels by radioimmunoassay. T_3 resin uptake is decreased, reflecting the elevated TBG. Free T_4 and free T_3 concentrations are unaltered. Patients on thyroid replacement therapy may require higher doses of thyroid hormone.
3. Other binding proteins may be elevated in serum (i.e., corticosteroid binding globulin (CBG), sex hormone-binding globulin (SHBG)) leading to increased total circulating corticosteroids and sex steroids, respectively. Free hormone concentrations may be decreased. Other plasma proteins may be increased (angiotensinogen/renin substrate, alpha-1-antitrypsin, ceruloplasmin).
4. Increased plasma HDL and HDL_2 cholesterol subfraction concentrations, reduced LDL cholesterol concentration, increased triglyceride levels.
5. Impaired glucose tolerance.
6. Reduced response to metyrapone test.

E. Carcinogenesis, Mutagenesis, Impairment of Fertility

Long-term continuous administration of estrogen, with and without progestin, in women, with and without a uterus, has shown an increased risk of endometrial cancer, breast cancer, and ovarian cancer. (See **BOXED WARNINGS, WARNINGS** and **PRECAUTIONS.**)

Long-term continuous administration of natural and synthetic estrogens in certain animal species increases the frequency of carcinomas of the breast, uterus, cervix, vagina, testis, and liver.

F. Pregnancy

Cenestin should not be used in pregnancy. (See **CONTRAINDICATIONS.**)

G. Nursing Mothers

Estrogen administration to nursing mothers has been shown to decrease the quantity and quality of the milk. Detectable amounts of estrogens have been identified in the milk of mothers receiving this drug. Caution should be exercised when Cenestin is administered to a nursing woman.

H. Pediatric Use

Cenestin is not indicated in children.

I. Geriatric Use

There have not been sufficient numbers of geriatric patients involved in studies utilizing Cenestin to determine whether those over 65 years of age differ from younger subjects in their response to Cenestin.

ADVERSE REACTIONS

See **BOXED WARNINGS, WARNINGS** and **PRECAUTIONS.**

Because clinical trials are conducted under widely varying conditions, adverse reaction rates observed in the clinical trials of a drug cannot be directly compared to rates in the clinical trials of another drug and may not reflect the rates observed in practice. The adverse reaction information from clinical trials does, however, provide a basis for identifying the adverse events that appear to be related to drug use and for approximating rates.

In a 12-week clinical trial that included 72 women treated with 0.625 mg and 2 x 0.625 mg Cenestin and 48 women treated with placebo, adverse events that occurred at a rate of ≥ 5% are summarized in Table 5.

[See table 5 at top of next page]

In a second 12-week clinical trial that included 52 women treated with 0.45 mg Cenestin and 51 women treated with placebo, adverse events that occurred at a rate of >5% are summarized in Table 6

Table 5
Number (%) of Patients with Adverse Events With ≥5% Occurrence Rate By Body System and Treatment Group

Body System Adverse Event	Cenestin* 0.625 mg and 2 × 0.625 mg n (%)	Placebo n (%)	Total n (%)
Number of Patients Who Received Medication	72 (100)	48 (100)	120 (100)
Number of Patients With Adverse Events	68 (94)	43 (90)	111 (93)
Number of Patients Without Any Adverse Events	4 (6)	5 (10)	9 (8)
Body As A Whole			
Abdominal Pain	20 (28)	11 (23)	31 (26)
Asthenia	24 (33)	20 (42)	44 (37)
Back Pain	10 (14)	6 (13)	16 (13)
Fever	1 (1)	3 (6)	4 (3)
Headache	49 (68)	32 (67)	81 (68)
Infection	10 (14)	5 (10)	15 (13)
Pain	8 (11)	9 (19)	17 (14)
Cardiovascular System			
Palpitation	15 (21)	13 (27)	28 (23)
Digestive System			
Constipation	4 (6)	2 (4)	6 (5)
Diarrhea	4 (6)	0 (0)	4 (3)
Dyspepsia	7 (10)	3 (6)	10 (8)
Flatulence	21 (29)	14 (29)	35 (29)
Nausea	13 (18)	9 (19)	22 (18)
Vomiting	5 (7)	1 (2)	6 (5)
Metabolic and Nutritional			
Peripheral Edema	7 (10)	6 (13)	13 (11)
Musculoskeletal System			
Arthralgia	18 (25)	13 (27)	31 (26)
Myalgia	20 (28)	15 (31)	35 (29)
Nervous System			
Depression	20 (28)	18 (38)	38 (32)
Dizziness	8 (11)	5 (10)	13 (11)
Hypertonia	4 (6)	0 (0)	4 (3)
Insomnia	30 (42)	23 (48)	53 (44)
Leg Cramps	7 (10)	3 (6)	10 (8)
Nervousness	20 (28)	20 (42)	40 (33)
Paresthesia	24 (33)	15 (31)	39 (33)
Vertigo	12 (17)	12 (25)	24 (20)
Respiratory System			
Cough Increased	4 (6)	1 (2)	5 (4)
Pharyngitis	6 (8)	4 (8)	10 (8)
Rhinitis	6 (8)	7 (15)	13 (11)
Skin and Appendages			
Rash	3 (4)	3 (6)	6 (5)
Urogenital System			
Breast Pain	21 (29)	7 (15)	28 (23)
Dysmenorrhea	4 (6)	3 (6)	7 (6)
Metrorrhagia	10 (14)	3 (6)	13 (11)

*Combined results for 0.625 mg and 2 × 0.625 mg Cenestin Tablets

Table 6
Number (%) of Patients with a ≥5% Occurrence Rate By Body System and Treatment Group

Body System and Term	Cenestin 0.45 mg	Control	p-value
Any Adverse Event %	40 (75.5%)	39 (76.5%)	1.0000
Body As A Whole	20 (37.7%)	24 (47.1%)	0.4275
Asthenia	6 (11.3%)	7 (13.7%)	0.7731
Headache	6 (11.3%)	8 (15.7%)	0.5748
Infection	1 (1.9%)	6 (11.8%)	0.0576
Pain	6 (11.3%)	1 (2.0%)	0.1128
Pain abdominal	5 (9.4%)	3 (5.9%)	0.7159
Cardiovascular	5 (9.4%)	10 (19.6%)	0.1695
Palpitations	3 (5.7%)	3 (5.9%)	1.0000
Vasodilations	2 (3.8%)	4 (7.8%)	0.4324
Digestive	8 (15.1%)	7 (13.7%)	1.0000
Nausea	5 (9.4%)	2 (3.9%)	0.4374
Metabolic and Nutritional	5 (9.4%)	3 (5.9%)	0.7159
Weight increase	3 (5.7%)	2 (3.9%)	1.0000
Musculoskeletal	5 (9.4%)	6 (11.8%)	0.7582
Arthralgia	5 (9.4%)	5 (9.8%)	1.0000
Myalgia	2 (3.8%)	6 (11.8%)	0.1566
Neurological	15 (28.3%)	19 (37.3%)	0.4044
Anxiety	3 (5.7%)	1 (2.0%)	0.6179
Depression	2 (3.8%)	7 (13.7%)	0.0895
Insomnia	3 (5.7%)	5 (9.8%)	0.4839
Nervousness	2 (3.8%)	7 (13.7%)	0.0895
Paresthesia	4 (7.5%)	3 (5.9%)	1.0000
Vertigo	3 (5.7%)	3 (5.9%)	1.0000
Respiratory	10 (18.9%)	6 (11.8%)	0.4173
Upper Respiratory Tract Infection	7 (13.2%)	1 (2.0%)	0.0603
Rhinitis	3 (5.7%)	2 (3.9%)	1.0000
Pharyngitis	1 (1.9%)	3 (5.9%)	0.3581
Urogenital	19 (35.8%)	7 (13.7%)	0.0124
Endometrial thickening	10 (18.9%)	4 (7.8%)	0.1503
Vaginitis	4 (7.5%)	1 (2.0%)	0.3632

P-value by Fisher's Exact (2-tail) Test
If a subject experiences the same event more than once, the first occurrence is tabulated.

[See table 6 above]
The following additional adverse reactions have been reported with estrogen and/or progestin therapy:

1. Genitourinary system.
Changes in vaginal bleeding pattern and abnormal withdrawal bleeding or flow; breakthrough bleeding; spotting; dysmenorrhea, increase in size of uterine leiomyomata; vaginitis, including vaginal candidiasis; change in amount of cervical secretion; changes in cervical ectropion; ovarian cancer; endometrial hyperplasia; endometrial cancer.

2. Breasts.
Tenderness, enlargement, pain, nipple discharge, galactorrhea; fibrocystic breast changes; breast cancer.

3. Cardiovascular.
Deep and superficial venous thrombosis; pulmonary embolism; thrombophlebitis; myocardial infarction; stroke; increase in blood pressure.

4. Gastrointestinal.
Nausea, vomiting; abdominal cramps, bloating; cholestatic jaundice; increased incidence of gallbladder disease; pancreatitis, enlargement of hepatic hemangiomas.

5. Skin.
Chloasma or melasma, which may persist when drug is discontinued; erythema multiforme; erythema nodosum; hemorrhagic eruption; loss of scalp hair; hirsutism; pruritus, rash.

6. Eyes.
Retinal vascular thrombosis; intolerance to contact lenses.

7. Central nervous system.
Headache; migraine; dizziness; mental depression; chorea; nervousness; mood disturbances; irritability; exacerbation of epilepsy.

8. Miscellaneous.
Increase or decrease in weight; reduced carbohydrate tolerance; aggravation of porphyria; edema; arthalgias; leg cramps; changes in libido; anaphylactoid/anaphylactic reactions including urticaria and angioedema; hypocalcemia; exacerbation of asthma; increased triglycerides.

OVERDOSAGE

Serious ill effects have not been reported following acute ingestion of large doses of estrogen containing drug products by young children. Overdosage of estrogen may cause nausea and vomiting, and withdrawal bleeding may occur in females.

DOSAGE AND ADMINISTRATION

When estrogen is prescribed for a postmenopausal woman with a uterus, progestin should also be initiated to reduce the risk of endometrial cancer. A woman without a uterus does not need progestin. Use of estrogen, alone or in combination with a progestin, should be with the lowest effective dose and for the shortest duration consistent with treatment goals and risks for the individual woman. Patients should be reevaluated periodically as clinically appropriate (e.g., 3-month to 6-month intervals) to determine if treatment is still necessary (see **BOXED WARNINGS** and **WARNINGS**). For women who have a uterus, adequate diagnostic measures, such as endometrial sampling, when indicated, should be undertaken to rule out malignancy in cases of undiagnosed persistent or recurring abnormal vaginal bleeding.

1. For treatment of moderate to severe vasomotor symptoms associated with the menopause.
   - Cenestin 0.45 mg
   - Cenestin 0.625 mg
   - Cenestin 0.9 mg
   - Cenestin 1.25 mg

   Patients should be started at Cenestin 0.45 mg daily. Subsequent dosage adjustment may be made based upon the individual patient response.This dose should be periodically reassessed by the healthcare provider. The lowest effective dose of Cenestin for the treatment of moderate to severe vasomotor symptoms has not been determined.
2. For treatment of moderate to severe symptoms of vulvar and vaginal atrophy associated with the menopause. When prescribing solely for the treatment of symptoms of vulvar and vaginal atrophy, topical vaginal products should be considered.
   - Cenestin 0.3 mg daily

HOW SUPPLIED

Cenestin (synthetic conjugated estrogens, A) Tablets are available as:

0.3 mg: Round, green, film-coated, and are debossed with letters, **dp**, and number, 41.
Available in bottles of:

30	NDC 51285-441-30
100	NDC 51285-441-02
1000	NDC 51285-441-05

0.45 mg: Round, orange, film-coated, and are debossed with letters, **dp**, and number, 46.
Available in bottles of:

30	NDC 51285-446-30
100	NDC 51285-446-02
1000	NDC 51285-446-05

0.625 mg: Round, red, film-coated, and are debossed with letters, **dp**, and number, 42.
Available in bottles of:

30	NDC 51285-442-30
100	NDC 51285-442-02
1000	NDC 51285-442-05

0.9 mg: Round, white, film-coated, and are debossed with letters, **dp**, and number, 43.
Available in bottles of:

30	NDC 51285-443-30
100	NDC 51285-443-02
1000	NDC 51285-443-05

1.25 mg: Round, blue, film-coated, and are debossed with letters, **dp**, and number, 44.
Available in bottles of:

30	NDC 51285-444-30
100	NDC 51285-444-02
1000	NDC 51285-444-05

Store at 20-25°C (68-77°F); excursions are permitted to 15-30°C (59-86°F) [See USP Controlled Room Temperature].
Dispense in tight container.
Dispense in child-resistant packaging.
Pharmacist: Include one "Information for the patient" leaflet with each package dispensed.

PATIENT INFORMATION

Revised FEBRUARY 2004
Cenestin®
(synthetic conjugated estrogens, A) Tablets

Continued on next page

Cenestin—Cont.

Read this PATIENT INFORMATION before you start taking Cenestin and read what you get each time you refill Cenestin. There may be new information. This information does not take the place of talking to your healthcare provider about your medical condition or your treatment.

What is the most important information I should know about Cenestin (synthetic estrogen mixture)?

- Estrogens increase the chances of getting cancer of the uterus.

Report any unusual vaginal bleeding right away while you are taking estrogens. Vaginal bleeding after menopause may be a warning sign of cancer of the uterus (womb). Your healthcare provider should check any unusual vaginal bleeding to find out the cause.

- Do not use estrogens with or without progestins to prevent heart disease, heart attacks, or strokes.

Using estrogens with or without progestins may increase your chances of getting heart attack, strokes, breast cancer, and blood clots. You and your healthcare provider should talk regularly about whether you still need treatment with Cenestin.

What is Cenestin?
Cenestin is a medicine that contains a mixture of synthetic estrogens made from a plant source.

What is Cenestin used for?
Cenestin is used after menopause to:

- **reduce moderate or severe hot flashes.**
Estrogens are hormones made by a woman's ovaries. The ovaries normally stop making estrogens when a woman is between 45 to 55 years old. This drop in body estrogen levels causes the "change of life" or menopause (the end of monthly menstrual periods). Sometimes, both ovaries are removed during an operation before natural menopause takes place. The sudden drop in estrogen levels causes "surgical menopause."
When estrogen levels begin dropping, some women develop very uncomfortable symptoms, such as feelings of warmth in the face, neck, and chest, or sudden strong feelings of heat and sweating ("hot flashes" or "hot flushes"). In some women, the symptoms are mild, and they will not need estrogens. In other women, symptoms can be more severe.You and your healthcare provider should talk regularly about whether you still need treatment with Cenestin.
- **treat moderate to severe dryness, itching, and burning in and around the vagina.** You and your healthcare provider should talk regularly about whether you still need treatment with Cenestin to control these problems. If you use Cenestin only to treat your dryness, itching, and burning in and around your vagina, talk with your healthcare provider about whether a topical vaginal product would be better for you.

Who Should Not Take Cenestin?
Do not start taking Cenestin if you:

- **have unusual vaginal bleeding.**
- **currently have or have had certain cancers.** Estrogens may increase the risk of certain types of cancers, including cancer of the breast or uterus. If you have or had cancer, talk with your healthcare provider about whether you should take Cenestin.
- **had a stroke or heart attack in the past year.**
- **currently have or have had blood clots.**
- **currently have or have had liver problems.**
- **are allergic to Cenestin or any of its ingredients.** See the end of this leaflet for a list of ingredients in Cenestin.
- **think you may be pregnant.**

TELL YOUR HEALTHCARE PROVIDER:

- **if you are breastfeeding.** The synthetic estrogen hormones in Cenestin can pass into your milk.
- **about all of your medical problems.** Your healthcare provider may need to check you more carefully if you have certain conditions, such as asthma (wheezing), epilepsy (seizures), migraine, endometriosis, lupus, or problems with your heart, liver, thyroid, kidneys, or have high calcium levels in your blood.
- **about all the medicines you take,** including prescription and nonprescription medicines, vitamins, and herbal supplements. Some medicines may affect how Cenestin works. Cenestin may also affect how your other medicines work.
- **if you are going to have surgery or will be on bed rest.** You may need to stop taking estrogens.

How Should I Take Cenestin?
Take one Cenestin tablet each day at about the same time. If you miss a dose, take it as soon as possible. If it is almost time for your next dose, skip the missed dose and go back to your normal schedule. Do not take 2 doses at the same time. Start at the lowest dose and talk to your healthcare provider about how well that dose is working for you. Estrogens should be used only as long as needed. You and your healthcare provider should talk regularly (for example every 3 to 6 months) about whether you still need treatment with Cenestin.

What are the possible risks and side effects of estrogens?
Less common but serious side effects include:

- Breast cancer
- Cancer of the uterus
- Stroke
- Heart attack
- Blood clots
- Gallbladder disease
- Ovarian cancer

These are some of the warning signs of serious side effects:

- Breast lumps
- Unusual vaginal bleeding
- Dizziness and faintness
- Changes in speech
- Severe headaches
- Chest pain
- Shortness of breath
- Pains in your legs
- Changes in vision
- Vomiting

Call your healthcare provider right away if you get any of these warning signs, or any other unusual symptom that concerns you.

Common side effects include:

- Headache
- Breast pain
- Irregular vaginal bleeding or spotting
- Stomach/abdominal cramps, bloating
- Nausea and vomiting
- Hair loss

Other side effects include:

- High blood pressure
- Liver problems
- High blood sugar
- Fluid retention
- Enlargement of benign tumors of the uterus ("fibroids")
- Vaginal yeast infection

These are not all the possible side effects of Cenestin. For more information, ask your healthcare provider or pharmacist.

What can I do to lower my chances of getting a serious side effect with Cenestin?

- Talk with your healthcare provider regularly about whether you should continue taking Cenestin.
- If you have a uterus, talk to your healthcare provider about whether the addition of a progestin is right for you.
- See your healthcare provider right away if you get vaginal bleeding while taking Cenestin.
- Have a breast exam and mammogram (breast X-ray) every year unless your healthcare provider tells you something else. If members of your family have had breast cancer or if you have ever had breast lumps or an abnormal mammogram, you may need to have breast exams more often.
- If you have high blood pressure, high cholesterol (fat in the blood), diabetes, are overweight, or if you use tobacco, you may have higher chances for getting heart disease. Ask your healthcare provider for ways to lower your chances for getting heart disease.

General information about safe and effective use of Cenestin.
Medicines are sometimes prescribed for conditions that are not mentioned in patient information leaflets. Do not take Cenestin for conditions for which it was not prescribed. Do not give Cenestin to other people, even if they have the same symptoms you have. It may harm them.

Keep Cenestin out of the reach of children.
This leaflet provides a summary of the most important information about Cenestin. If you would like more information, talk with your healthcare provider or pharmacist. You can ask for information about Cenestin that is written for health professionals. You can get more information by calling the toll free number 877-405-0369.

What are the ingredients in Cenestin?
Tablets for oral administration, are available in 0.3 mg, 0.45 mg, 0.625 mg, 0.9 mg and 1.25 mg strengths of synthetic conjugated estrogens, A. Tablets also contain the following inactive ingredients: ethylcellulose, hypromellose, lactose monohydrate, magnesium stearate, polyethylene glycol, polysorbate 80, pregelatinized starch, titanium dioxide, and triethyl citrate.
-0.3 mg tablets also contain FD&C Blue No. 2 aluminum lake and D&C Yellow No. 10 aluminum lake.
-0.45 mg tablets also contain FD&C Yellow No. 6/Sunset Yellow FCF lake.
-0.625 mg tablets also contain FD&C Red No. 40 aluminum lake.
-0.9 mg tablets do not contain any additional color additives.
-1.25 mg tablets also contain FD&C Blue No. 2 aluminum lake.

Manufactured By:
Duramed Pharmaceuticals, Inc.
Subsidiary of Barr Pharmaceuticals, Inc.
Pomona, New York 10970
Revised FEBRUARY 2004
BR - 41, 46, 42, 43, 44

To keep your **PDR** up to date throughout the year, note these revisions on the corresponding pages of the annual volume. Simply write **"See Supplement A"** next to the product heading.

Forest Pharmaceuticals, Inc.

(Subsidiary of Forest Laboratories, Inc.)
13600 SHORELINE DRIVE
ST. LOUIS, MO 63045

Direct Inquiries to:
Professional Affairs Department
13600 Shoreline Drive
St. Louis, MO 63045
(800) 678-1605

AEROBID® ℞
AEROBID®-M
[*aər-ō-bĭd*]
(flunisolide)
Inhaler System
For oral inhalation only
℞ only

Prescribing information for this product, which appears on pages 1289–1291 of the 2004 PDR, has been completely revised as follows. Please write "See Supplement A" next to the product heading.

DESCRIPTION

Flunisolide, the active component of **AEROBID** Inhaler System, is an anti-inflammatory steroid having the chemical name 6α-fluoro-11β, 16α, 17, 21-tetrahydroxypregna-1, 4-diene-3, 20-dione cyclic-16, 17-acetal with acetone.
It has the following structure:

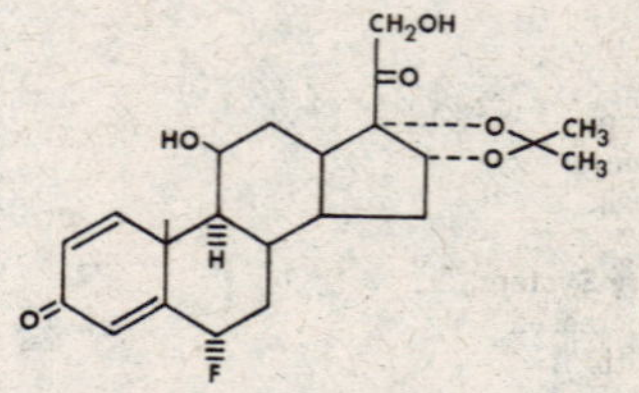

Flunisolide is a white to creamy white crystalline powder with a molecular weight of 434.49. It is soluble in acetone, sparingly soluble in chloroform, slightly soluble in methanol, and practically insoluble in water. It has a melting point of about 245°C.
AEROBID Inhaler is delivered in a metered-dose aerosol system containing a microcrystalline suspension of flunisolide as the hemihydrate in propellants (trichloromonofluoromethane, dichlorodifluoromethane and dichlorotetrafluoroethane) with sorbitan trioleate as a dispersing agent. **AEROBID-M** also contains menthol as a flavoring agent. Each activation delivers approximately 250 mcg of flunisolide to the patient. One **AEROBID** Inhaler System is designed to deliver at least 100 metered inhalations.

CLINICAL PHARMACOLOGY

Flunisolide has demonstrated marked anti-inflammatory and anti-allergic activity in classical test systems. It is a corticosteroid that is several hundred times more potent in animal anti-inflammatory assays than the cortisol standard. The molar dose of each activation of flunisolide in this preparation is approximately 2.5 to 7 times that of comparable inhaled corticosteroid products marketed for the same indication. The dose of flunisolide delivered per activation in this preparation is 10 times that per activation of Nasalide® (flunisolide) nasal solution. Clinical studies have shown therapeutic activity on bronchial mucosa with minimal evidence of systemic activity at recommended doses.
After oral inhalation of 1 mg flunisolide, total systemic availability was 40%. The flunisolide that is swallowed is rapidly and extensively converted to the 6β-OH metabolite and to water-soluble conjugates during the first pass through the liver. This offers a metabolic explanation for the low systemic activity of oral flunisolide itself since the metabolite has the low corticosteroid potency (on the order of the cortisol standard). The inhaled flunisolide absorbed through the bronchial tree is converted to the same metabolites. Repeated inhalation of 2.0 mg of flunisolide per day (the maximum recommended dose) for 14 days did not show accumulation of the drug in plasma. The plasma half-life of flunisolide is approximately 1.8 hours.
The following observations relevant to systemic absorption were made in clinical studies. In one uncontrolled study a statistically significant decrease in responsiveness to metyrapone was noted in 15 adult steroid-independent patients treated with 2.0 mg of flunisolide per day (the maximum recommended dose) for 3 months. A small but statistically significant drop in eosinophils from 11.5% to 7.4% of total circulating leucocytes was noted in another study in children who were not taking oral corticosteroids simultaneously. A 5% incidence of menstrual disturbances was reported during open studies, in which there were no control groups for comparison.
Aerosol administration of flunisolide 2.0 mg twice daily for one week to 6 healthy male subjects revealed neither suppression of adrenal function as measured by early morning cortisol levels nor impairment of HPA axis function as determined by insulin hypoglycemia tests.
Controlled clinical studies have included over 500 patients with asthma, among them 150 children age 6 and over.

More than 120 patients have been treated in open trials for two years or more. No significant adrenal suppression attributed to flunisolide was seen in these studies.
Significant decreases of systemic steroid dosages have been possible in flunisolide-treated patients. Recommended doses of flunisolide appear to be the therapeutic equivalent of an average of 10 mg/day of oral prednisone. Asthma patients have had further symptomatic improvement with flunisolide treatment even while reducing concomitant medication.

INDICATIONS AND USAGE

AEROBID (flunisolide) Inhaler is indicated in the maintenance treatment of asthma as prophylactic therapy. **AEROBID** is also indicated for asthma patients who require systemic corticosteroid administration, where adding **AEROBID** may reduce or eliminate the need for the systemic corticosteroids.
AEROBID Inhaler is NOT indicated for the relief of acute bronchospasm.

CONTRAINDICATIONS

AEROBID (flunisolide) Inhaler is contraindicated in the primary treatment of status asthmaticus or other acute episodes of asthma where intensive measures are required.
Hypersensitivity to any of the ingredients of this preparation contraindicates its use.

WARNINGS

Particular care is needed in patients who are transferred from systemically active corticosteroids to **AEROBID** Inhaler because deaths due to adrenal insufficiency have occurred in asthmatic patients during and after transfer from systemic corticosteroids to aerosol corticosteroids. After withdrawal from systemic corticosteroids, a number of months are required for recovery of hypothalamic-pituitary-adrenal (HPA) function. During this period of HPA suppression, patients may exhibit signs and symptoms of adrenal insufficiency when exposed to trauma, surgery or infections, particularly gastroenteritis. Although **AEROBID** Inhaler may provide control of asthmatic symptoms during these episodes, it does NOT provide the systemic steroid that is necessary for coping with these emergencies. During periods of stress or a severe asthmatic attack, patients who have been withdrawn from systemic corticosteroids should be instructed to resume systemic steroids (in large doses) immediately and to contact their physician for further instruction. These patients should also be instructed to carry a warning card indicating that they may need supplementary systemic steroids during periods of stress or a severe asthma attack. To assess the risk of adrenal insufficiency in emergency situations, routine tests of adrenal cortical function, including measurement of early morning resting cortisol levels, should be performed periodically in all patients. An early morning resting cortisol level may be accepted as normal if it falls at or near the normal mean level.
Localized infections with *Candida albicans* or *Aspergillus niger* have occurred in the mouth and pharynx and occasionally in the larynx. Positive cultures for oral *Candida* may be present in up to 34% of patients. Although the frequency of clinically apparent infection is considerably lower, these infections may require treatment with appropriate antifungal therapy or discontinuance of treatment with **AEROBID** Inhaler.
AEROBID Inhaler is not to be regarded as a bronchodilator and is not indicated for relief of bronchospasm.
Patients should be instructed to contact their physician immediately when episodes of asthma that are not responsive to bronchodilators occur during the course of treatment. During such episodes, patients may require therapy with systemic corticosteroids. Theoretically, the use of inhaled corticosteroids with alternate day prednisone systemic treatment should be accompanied by more HPA suppression than a therapeutically equivalent regimen of either alone.
Transfer of patients from systemic steroid therapy to **AEROBID** Inhaler may unmask allergic conditions previously suppressed by the systemic steroid therapy, e.g. rhinitis, conjunctivitis, and eczema.
Persons who are on drugs which suppress the immune system are more susceptible to infections than healthy individuals. Chicken pox and measles, for example, can have a more serious or even fatal course in non-immune children or adults on corticosteroids. In such children or adults who have not had these diseases, particular care should be taken to avoid exposure. How the dose, route and duration of corticosteroid administration affects the risk of developing a disseminated infection is not known. The contribution of the underlying disease and/or prior corticosteroid treatment to the risk is also not known. If exposed to chicken pox, prophylaxis with varicella zoster immune globulin (VZIG) may be indicated. If exposed to measles, prophylaxis with pooled intramuscular immunoglobulin (IG) may be indicated. (See the respective package inserts for complete VZIG and IG prescribing information.) If chicken pox develops, treatment with antiviral agents may be considered.

PRECAUTIONS

General: Because of the relatively high molar dose of flunisolide per activation in this preparation, and because of the evidence suggesting higher levels of systemic absorption with flunisolide than with other comparable inhaled corticosteroids (see CLINICAL PHARMACOLOGY section), patients treated with **AEROBID** (flunisolide) should be observed carefully for any evidence of systemic corticosteroid effect, including suppression of bone growth in children. Particular care should be taken in observing patients postoperatively or during periods of stress for evidence of a decrease in adrenal function. During withdrawal from oral steroids, some patients may experience symptoms of systemically active steroid withdrawal, e.g. joint and/or muscular pain, lassitude and depression, despite maintenance or even improvement of respiratory function. (See DOSAGE AND ADMINISTRATION for details.)
In responsive patients, flunisolide may permit control of asthmatic symptoms without suppression of HPA function. Since flunisolide is absorbed into the circulation and can be systemically active, the beneficial effects of **AEROBID** Inhaler in minimizing or preventing HPA dysfunction may be expected only when recommended dosages are not exceeded. The long-term local and systemic effects of **AEROBID** (flunisolide) in human subjects are still not fully known. In particular, the effects resulting from chronic use of **AEROBID** on developmental or immunologic processes in the mouth, pharynx, trachea, and lung are unknown.
Inhaled corticosteroids should be used with caution, if at all, in patients with active or quiescent tuberculosis infection of the respiratory tract; untreated systemic fungal, bacterial, parasitic or viral infections; or ocular herpes simplex.
Pulmonary infiltrates with eosinophilia may occur in patients on **AEROBID** Inhaler therapy. Although it is possible that in some patients this state may become manifest because of systemic steroid withdrawal when inhalational steroids are administered, a causative role for the drug and/or its vehicle cannot be ruled out.

Information for Patients:
Since the relief from **AEROBID** Inhaler depends on its regular use and on proper inhalation technique, patients must be instructed to take inhalations at regular intervals. They should also be instructed in the correct method of use. (See Patient Instruction Leaflet.)
Patients whose systemic corticosteroids have been reduced or withdrawn should be instructed to carry a warning card indicating they may need supplemental systemic steroids during periods of stress or a severe asthmatic attack that is not responsive to bronchodilators.
Persons who are on immunosuppressant doses of corticosteroids should be warned to avoid exposure to chicken pox or measles. Patients should also be advised that if they are exposed, medical advice should be sought without delay.
An illustrated leaflet of patient instructions for proper use accompanies each **AEROBID** Inhaler System.
CONTENTS UNDER PRESSURE
Do not puncture. Do not use or store near heat or open flame. Exposure to temperatures above 120°F (49°C) may cause container to explode. Never throw container into fire or incinerator. Keep out of reach of children.
Carcinogenesis: Long-term studies were conducted in mice and rats using oral administration to evaluate the carcinogenic potential of the drug. There was an increase in the incidence of pulmonary adenomas in mice, but not in rats. Female rats receiving the highest oral dose had an increased incidence of mammary adenocarcinoma compared to control rats. An increased incidence of this tumor type has been reported for other corticosteroids.
Impairment of Fertility: Female rats receiving high doses of flunisolide (200 mcg/kg/day) showed some evidence of impaired fertility. Reproductive performance in the low- (8 mcg/kg/day) and mid-dose (40 mcg/kg/day) groups was comparable to controls.
Pregnancy: Pregnancy Category C. As with other corticosteroids, flunisolide has been shown to be teratogenic in rabbits and rats at doses of 40 and 200 mcg/kg/day respectively. It was also fetotoxic in these animal reproductive studies. There are no adequate and well-controlled studies in pregnant women. Flunisolide should be used during pregnancy only if the potential benefit justifies the potential risk to the fetus.
Nursing Mothers: It is not known whether this drug is excreted in human milk. Because other corticosteroids are excreted in human milk, caution should be exercised when flunisolide is administered to nursing women.
Pediatric Use: Safety and effectiveness have not been established in children below the age of 6. Oral corticoids have been shown to cause growth suppression in children and adolescents, particularly with higher doses over extended periods. If a child or adolescent on any corticoid appears to have growth suppression, the possibility that they are particularly sensitive to this effect of steroids should be considered.

ADVERSE REACTIONS

Adverse events reported in controlled clinical trials and long-term open studies in 514 patients treated with **AEROBID** (flunisolide) are described below. Of those patients, 463 were treated for 3 months or longer, 407 for 6 months or longer, 287 for 1 year or longer, and 122 for 2 years or longer.
Musculoskeletal reactions were reported in 35% of steroid-dependent patients in whom the dose of oral steroid was being tapered. This is a well-known effect of steroid withdrawal.

Incidence 10% or greater:
Gastrointestinal: diarrhea (10%), nausea and/or vomiting (25%), upset stomach (10%)
General: flu (10%)
Mouth and Throat: sore throat (20%)
Nervous System: headache (25%)
Respiratory: cold symptoms (15%), nasal congestion (15%), upper respiratory infection (25%)
Special Senses: unpleasant taste (10%)

Incidence 3-9%
Cardiovascular: palpitations
Gastrointestinal: abdominal pain, heartburn
General: chest pain, decreased appetite, edema, fever
Mouth and Throat: *Candida* infection
Nervous System: dizziness, irritability, nervousness, shakiness
Reproductive: menstrual disturbances
Respiratory: chest congestion, cough*, hoarseness, rhinitis, runny nose, sinus congestion, sinus drainage, sinus infection, sinusitis, sneezing, sputum, wheezing*
Skin: eczema, itching (pruritus), rash
Special Senses: ear infection, loss of smell or taste

Incidence 1-3%
General: chills, increased appetite and weight gain, malaise, peripheral edema, sweating, weakness
Cardiovascular: hypertension, tachycardia
Gastrointestinal: constipation, dyspepsia, gas
Hemic/Lymph: capillary fragility, enlarged lymph nodes
Mouth and Throat: dry throat, glossitis, mouth irritation, pharyngitis, phlegm, throat irritation
Nervous System: anxiety, depression, faintness, fatigue, hyperactivity, hypoactivity, insomnia, moodiness, numbness, vertigo
Respiratory: bronchitis, chest tightness*, dyspnea, epistaxis, head stuffiness, laryngitis, nasal irritation, pleurisy, pneumonia, sinus discomfort
Skin: acne, hives or urticaria
Special Senses: blurred vision, earache, eye discomfort, eye infection

Incidence less than 1%, judged by investigators as possibly or probably drug related: abdominal fullness, shortness of breath.

*The incidences as shown of cough, wheezing, and chest tightness were judged by investigators to be possibly or probably drug related. In placebo-controlled trials, the *overall* incidences of these adverse events (regardless of investigators' judgement of drug relationship) were similar for drug and placebo-treated groups. They may be related to the vehicle or delivery system.

DOSAGE AND ADMINISTRATION

The **AEROBID** (flunisolide) Inhaler System is for oral inhalation only.
Adults: The recommended starting dose is 2 inhalations twice daily, morning and evening, for a total daily dose of 1 mg. The maximum daily dose should not exceed 4 inhalations twice a day for a total daily dose of 2 mg. When the drug is used chronically at 2 mg/day, patients should be monitored periodically for effects on the hypothalamic-pituitary-adrenal (HPA) axis.
Pediatric Patients: For children and adolescents 6-15 years of age, two inhalations may be administered twice daily for a total daily dose of 1 mg. Higher doses have not been studied. Insufficient information is available to warrant use in children under age 6. With chronic use, pediatric patients should be monitored for growth as well as for effects on the HPA axis.
Rinsing the mouth after inhalation is advised.
Different considerations must be given to the following groups of patients in order to obtain the full therapeutic benefit of **AEROBID** (flunisolide) Inhaler.

Patients Not Receiving Systemic Corticosteroids:
Patients who require maintenance therapy of their asthma may benefit from treatment with **AEROBID** at the doses recommended above. In patients who respond to **AEROBID**, improvement in pulmonary function is usually apparent within one to four weeks after the start of therapy. Once the desired effect is achieved, consideration should be given to tapering to the lowest effective dose.

Patients Maintained on Systemic Corticosteroids:
Clinical studies have shown that **AEROBID** may be effective in the management of asthmatics dependent or maintained on systemic corticosteroids and may permit replacement or significant reduction in the dosage of systemic corticosteroids.
The patient's asthma should be reasonably stable before treatment with **AEROBID** is started. Initially, **AEROBID** should be used concurrently with the patient's usual maintenance dose of systemic corticosteroid. After approximately one week, gradual withdrawal of the systemic corticosteroid is started by reducing the daily or alternate daily dose. Reductions may be made after an interval of one or two weeks, depending on the response of the patient. A slow rate of withdrawal is strongly recommended. Generally, these decrements should not exceed 2.5 mg of prednisone or its equivalent. During withdrawal, some patients may experience symptoms of systemic corticosteroid withdrawal; e.g. joint and/or muscular pain, lassitude and depression, despite maintenance or even improvement in pulmonary function. Such patients should be encouraged to continue with the inhaler but should be monitored for objective signs of adrenal insufficiency. If evidence of adrenal insufficiency occurs, the systemic corticosteroid doses should be increased temporarily and thereafter withdrawal should continue more slowly. During periods of stress or a severe asthma attack, transfer patients may require supplementary treatment with systemic corticosteroids.

HOW SUPPLIED

AEROBID (flunisolide) Inhaler Systems are available in canisters of 100 metered inhalations.
NDC 0456-0672-99 **AEROBID**
NDC 0456-0670-99 **AEROBID-M**

Continued on next page

Aerobid—Cont.

"Note: The indented statement below is required by the Federal government's Clean Air Act for all products containing or manufactured with chlorofluorocarbons (CFC's)."

WARNING: Contains trichloromonofluoromethane, dichlorodifluoromethane and dichlorotetrafluoroethane, substances which harm public health and environment by destroying ozone in the upper atmosphere.

"A notice similar to the above WARNING has been placed in the information for the patient of this product pursuant to EPA regulations."

mfd for Revised 3/02
FOREST PHARMACEUTICALS, INC.
St. Louis, MO 63045
mfd by
3M Pharmaceuticals
St. Paul, MN 624200

How to use your
AEROBID®
AEROBID®-M
(flunisolide)
Inhaler System
DIRECTIONS FOR USE:

Before using your new **AEROBID** Inhaler System, it is important that you read over the following simple instructions and familiarize yourself with the inhaler and its metal cartridge.

As your doctor has probably told you, the **AEROBID** Inhaler System must be used for a few days before it begins working, and then should be used regularly to help reduce the frequency and severity of your asthma attacks. It is not a bronchodilator and will not provide relief during an actual asthmatic attack, but it can cut down the number of bad attacks if used regularly every day.

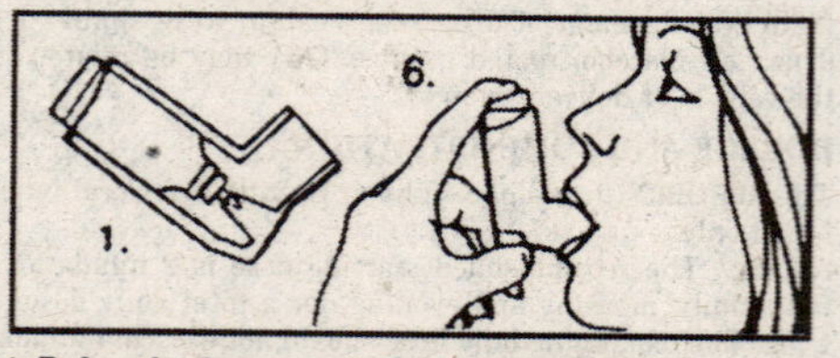

1. Before the first use, place the **AEROBID** metal cartridge inside the plastic container as shown.
2. Shake the inhaler system before each inhalation.
3. Before each use, remove dustcap and inspect mouthpiece for foreign objects.
4. Replace dustcap after each use.
5. Breathe out as completely as possible.
6. Hold the inhaler system upright and put plastic mouthpiece in your mouth as shown, being sure to close your lips tightly around the mouthpiece.
7. Breathe in slowly through your mouth. At the same time firmly press down on the metal cartridge with your index finger.
8. Hold your breath as long as you can.
9. While holding your breath, stop pressing on the cartridge and remove mouthpiece from your mouth.
10. If your doctor has prescribed two or more inhalations at each use, wait a minute to allow pressure to build up again in the metal canister, then repeat steps two through nine (2–9). Be sure to shake the inhaler system *again* before each inhalation.
11. After the prescribed number of inhalations, rinse out your mouth thoroughly with water.
12. Clean the inhaler system every few days. To do so, remove the metal cartridge, then rinse the plastic inhaler and cap with briskly running warm water. Dry thoroughly. Replace the cartridge and cap.

NOTE: If your mouth becomes sore or develops a rash, be sure to mention this to your doctor, but do not stop using your inhaler system unless he tells you.

WARNING: The contents of the metal cartridge are under pressure. Do not puncture. Do not use or store near heat or open flame. Exposure to temperature above 120°F (49°C) may cause cartridge to explode. Never throw cartridge into fire or incinerator. Use by children should always be supervised by an adult.

mfd by
3M Pharmaceuticals, Inc.
St. Paul, MN
For:
FOREST PHARMACEUTICALS, INC.
SUBSIDIARY OF FOREST LABORATORIES, INC.
ST. LOUIS, MISSOURI 63045

CELEXA™ ℞

[*sĕ-lĕk-să*]
(citalopram hydrobromide)
Tablets/Oral Solution
Rx Only

Prescribing information for this product, which appears on pages 1292–1296 of the 2004 PDR, has been completely revised as follows. Please write "See Supplement A" next to the product heading.

DESCRIPTION

Celexa™ (citalopram HBr) is an orally administered selective serotonin reuptake inhibitor (SSRI) with a chemical structure unrelated to that of other SSRIs or of tricyclic, tetracyclic, or other available antidepressant agents. Citalopram HBr is a racemic bicyclic phthalane derivative designated (±)-1-(3-dimethylaminopropyl)-1-(4-fluorophenyl)-1,3-dihydroisobenzofuran-5-carbonitrile, HBr with the following structural formula:

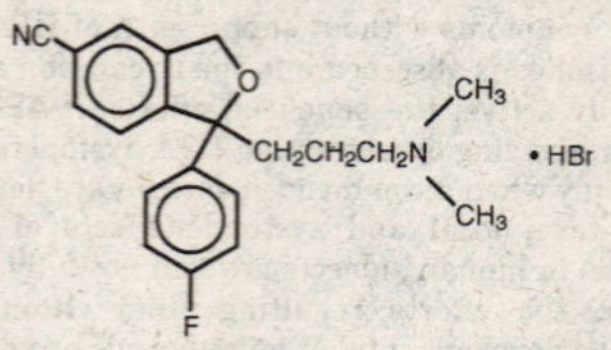

The molecular formula is $C_{20}H_{22}BrFN_2O$ and its molecular weight is 405.35.

Citalopram HBr occurs as a fine white to off-white powder. Citalopram HBr is sparingly soluble in water and soluble in ethanol.

Celexa (citalopram hydrobromide) is available as tablets or as an oral solution.

Celexa 10 mg tablets are film-coated, oval tablets containing citalopram HBr in strengths equivalent to 10 mg citalopram base. Celexa 20 mg and 40 mg tablets are film-coated, oval, scored tablets containing citalopram HBr in strengths equivalent to 20 mg or 40 mg citalopram base. The tablets also contain the following inactive ingredients: copolyvidone, corn starch, crosscarmellose sodium, glycerin, lactose monohydrate, magnesium stearate, hypromellose, microcrystalline cellulose, polyethylene glycol, and titanium dioxide. Iron oxides are used as coloring agents in the beige (10 mg) and pink (20 mg) tablets.

Celexa oral solution contains citalopram HBr equivalent to 2 mg/mL citalopram base. It also contains the following inactive ingredients: sorbitol, purified water, propylene glycol, methylparaben, natural peppermint flavor, and propylparaben.

CLINICAL PHARMACOLOGY

Pharmacodynamics

The mechanism of action of citalopram HBr as an antidepressant is presumed to be linked to potentiation of serotonergic activity in the central nervous system resulting from its inhibition of CNS neuronal reuptake of serotonin (5-HT). *In vitro* and *in vivo* studies in animals suggest that citalopram is a highly selective serotonin reuptake inhibitor (SSRI) with minimal effects on norepinephrine (NE) and dopamine (DA) neuronal reuptake. Tolerance to the inhibition of 5-HT uptake is not induced by long-term (14-day) treatment of rats with citalopram. Citalopram is a racemic mixture (50/50), and the inhibition of 5-HT reuptake by citalopram is primarily due to the (S)-enantiomer.

Citalopram has no or very low affinity for $5\text{-}HT_{1A}$, $5\text{-}HT_{2A}$, dopamine D_1 and D_2, α_1-, α_2-, and β-adrenergic, histamine H_1, gamma aminobutyric acid (GABA), muscarinic cholinergic, and benzodiazepine receptors. Antagonism of muscarinic, histaminergic, and adrenergic receptors has been hypothesized to be associated with various anticholinergic, sedative, and cardiovascular effects of other psychotropic drugs.

Pharmacokinetics

The single- and multiple-dose pharmacokinetics of citalopram are linear and dose-proportional in a dose range of 10–60 mg/day. Biotransformation of citalopram is mainly hepatic, with a mean terminal half-life of about 35 hours. With once daily dosing, steady state plasma concentrations are achieved within approximately one week. At steady state, the extent of accumulation of citalopram in plasma, based on the half-life, is expected to be 2.5 times the plasma concentrations observed after a single dose. The tablet and oral solution dosage forms of citalopram HBr are bioequivalent.

Absorption and Distribution

Following a single oral dose (40 mg tablet) of citalopram, peak blood levels occur at about 4 hours. The absolute bioavailability of citalopram was about 80% relative to an intravenous dose, and absorption is not affected by food. The volume of distribution of citalopram is about 12 L/kg and the binding of citalopram (CT), demethylcitalopram (DCT) and didemethylcitalopram (DDCT) to human plasma proteins is about 80%.

Metabolism and Elimination

Following intravenous administrations of citalopram, the fraction of drug recovered in the urine as citalopram and DCT was about 10% and 5%, respectively. The systemic clearance of citalopram was 330 mL/min, with approximately 20% of that due to renal clearance.

Citalopram is metabolized to demethylcitalopram (DCT), didemethylcitalopram (DDCT), citalopram-N-oxide, and a deaminated propionic acid derivative. In humans, unchanged citalopram is the predominant compound in plasma. At steady state, the concentrations of citalopram's metabolites, DCT and DDCT, in plasma are approximately one-half and one-tenth, respectively, that of the parent drug. *In vitro* studies show that citalopram is at least 8 times more potent than its metabolites in the inhibition of serotonin reuptake, suggesting that the metabolites evaluated do not likely contribute significantly to the antidepressant actions of citalopram.

In vitro studies using human liver microsomes indicated that CYP3A4 and CYP2C19 are the primary isozymes involved in the N-demethylation of citalopram.

Population Subgroups

Age—Citalopram pharmacokinetics in subjects ≥60 years of age were compared to younger subjects in two normal volunteer studies. In a single-dose study, citalopram AUC and half-life were increased in the elderly subjects by 30% and 50%, respectively, whereas in a multiple-dose study they were increased by 23% and 30%, respectively. 20 mg is the recommended dose for most elderly patients (see Dosage and Administration).

Gender—In three pharmacokinetic studies (total N=32), citalopram AUC in women was one and a half to two times that in men. This difference was not observed in five other pharmacokinetic studies (total N=114). In clinical studies, no differences in steady state serum citalopram levels were seen between men (N=237) and women (N=388). There were no gender differences in the pharmacokinetics of DCT and DDCT. No adjustment of dosage on the basis of gender is recommended.

Reduced hepatic function—Citalopram oral clearance was reduced by 37% and half-life was doubled in patients with reduced hepatic function compared to normal subjects. 20 mg is the recommended dose for most hepatically impaired patients (see Dosage and Administration).

Reduced renal function—In patients with mild to moderate renal function impairment, oral clearance of citalopram was reduced by 17% compared to normal subjects. No adjustment of dosage for such patients is recommended. No information is available about the pharmacokinetics of citalopram in patients with severely reduced renal function (creatinine clearance < 20 mL/min).

Drug-Drug Interactions

In vitro enzyme inhibition data did not reveal an inhibitory effect of citalopram on CYP3A4, -2C9, or -2E1, but did suggest that it is a weak inhibitor of CYP1A2, -2D6, and -2C19. Citalopram would be expected to have little inhibitory effect on *in vivo* metabolism mediated by these cytochromes. However, *in vivo* data to address this question are limited.

Since CYP3A4 and 2C19 are the primary enzymes involved in the metabolism of citalopram, it is expected that potent inhibitors of 3A4 (e.g., ketoconazole, itraconazole, and macrolide antibiotics) and potent inhibitors of CYP2C19 (e.g., omeprazole) might decrease the clearance of citalopram. However, coadministration of citalopram and the potent 3A4 inhibitor ketoconazole did not significantly affect the pharmacokinetics of citalopram. Because citalopram is metabolized by multiple enzyme systems, inhibition of a single enzyme may not appreciably decrease citalopram clearance. Citalopram steady state levels were not significantly different in poor metabolizers and extensive 2D6 metabolizers after multiple-dose administration of Celexa, suggesting that coadministration, with Celexa, of a drug that inhibits CYP2D6, is unlikely to have clinically significant effects on citalopram metabolism. See Drug Interactions under Precautions for more detailed information on available drug interaction data.

Clinical Efficacy Trials

The efficacy of Celexa as a treatment for depression was established in two placebo-controlled studies (of 4 to 6 weeks in duration) in adult outpatients (ages 18–66) meeting DSM-III or DSM-III-R criteria for major depression. Study 1, a 6-week trial in which patients received fixed Celexa doses of 10, 20, 40, and 60 mg/day, showed that Celexa at doses of 40 and 60 mg/day was effective as measured by the Hamilton Depression Rating Scale (HAMD) total score, the HAMD depressed mood item (Item 1), the Montgomery Asberg Depression Rating Scale, and the Clinical Global Impression (CGI) Severity scale. This study showed no clear effect of the 10 and 20 mg/day doses, and the 60 mg/day dose was not more effective than the 40 mg/day dose. In study 2, a 4-week, placebo-controlled trial in depressed patients, of whom 85% met criteria for melancholia, the initial dose was 20 mg/day, followed by titration to the maximum tolerated dose or a maximum dose of 80 mg/day. Patients treated with Celexa showed significantly greater improvement than placebo patients on the HAMD total score, HAMD item 1, and the CGI Severity score. In three additional placebo-controlled depression trials, the difference in response to treatment between patients receiving Celexa and patients receiving placebo was not statistically significant, possibly due to high spontaneous response rate, smaller sample size, or, in the case of one study, too low a dose.

In two long-term studies, depressed patients who had responded to Celexa during an initial 6 or 8 weeks of acute treatment (fixed doses of 20 or 40 mg/day in one study and flexible doses of 20–60 mg/day in the second study) were randomized to continuation of Celexa or to placebo. In both studies, patients receiving continued Celexa treatment experienced significantly lower relapse rates over the subsequent 6 months compared to those receiving placebo. In the fixed-dose study, the decreased rate of depression relapse was similar in patients receiving 20 or 40 mg/day of Celexa.

Analyses of the relationship between treatment outcome and age, gender, and race did not suggest any differential responsiveness on the basis of these patient characteristics.

Comparison of Clinical Trial Results

Highly variable results have been seen in the clinical development of all antidepressant drugs. Furthermore, in those circumstances when the drugs have not been studied in the same controlled clinical trial(s), comparisons among the results of studies evaluating the effectiveness of different antidepressant drug products are inherently unreliable. Because conditions of testing (e.g., patient samples, investigators, doses of the treatments administered and compared, outcome measures, etc.) vary among trials, it is virtually impossible to distinguish a difference in drug effect from a difference due to one of the confounding factors just enumerated.

INDICATIONS AND USAGE

Celexa (citalopram HBr) is indicated for the treatment of depression. The efficacy of Celexa in the treatment of depression was established in 4-6 week, controlled trials of outpatients whose diagnosis corresponded most closely to the DSM-III and DSM-III-R category of major depressive disorder (see Clinical Pharmacology).

A major depressive episode (DSM-IV) implies a prominent and relatively persistent (nearly every day for at least 2 weeks) depressed or dysphoric mood that usually interferes with daily functioning, and includes at least five of the following nine symptoms: depressed mood, loss of interest in usual activities, significant change in weight and/or appetite, insomnia or hypersomnia, psychomotor agitation or retardation, increased fatigue, feelings of guilt or worthlessness, slowed thinking or impaired concentration, a suicide attempt or suicidal ideation.

The antidepressant action of Celexa in hospitalized depressed patients has not been adequately studied.

The efficacy of Celexa in maintaining an antidepressant response for up to 24 weeks following 6 to 8 weeks of acute treatment was demonstrated in two placebo-controlled trials (see Clinical Pharmacology). Nevertheless, the physician who elects to use Celexa for extended periods should periodically re-evaluate the long-term usefulness of the drug for the individual patient.

CONTRAINDICATIONS

Concomitant use in patients taking monoamine oxidase inhibitors (MAOIs) is contraindicated (see Warnings).

Celexa is contraindicated in patients with a hypersensitivity to citalopram or any of the inactive ingredients in Celexa.

WARNINGS

Potential for Interaction with Monoamine Oxidase Inhibitors

In patients receiving serotonin reuptake inhibitor drugs in combination with a monoamine oxidase inhibitor (MAOI), there have been reports of serious, sometimes fatal, reactions including hyperthermia, rigidity, myoclonus, autonomic instability with possible rapid fluctuations of vital signs, and mental status changes that include extreme agitation progressing to delirium and coma. These reactions have also been reported in patients who have recently discontinued SSRI treatment and have been started on a MAOI. Some cases presented with features resembling neuroleptic malignant syndrome. Furthermore, limited animal data on the effects of combined use of SSRIs and MAOIs suggest that these drugs may act synergistically to elevate blood pressure and evoke behavioral excitation. Therefore, it is recommended that Celexa should not be used in combination with a MAOI, or within 14 days of discontinuing treatment with a MAOI. Similarly, at least 14 days should be allowed after stopping Celexa before starting a MAOI.

PRECAUTIONS

General

Discontinuation of Treatment with Celexa

During marketing of Celexa and other SSRIs and SNRIs (serotonin and norepinephrine reuptake inhibitors), there have been spontaneous reports of adverse events occurring upon discontinuation of these drugs, particularly when abrupt, including the following: dysphoric mood, irritability, agitation, dizziness, sensory disturbances (e.g., paresthesias such as electric shock sensations), anxiety, confusion, headache, lethargy, emotional lability, insomnia, and hypomania. While these events are generally self-limiting, there have been reports of serious discontinuation symptoms.

Patients should be monitored for these symptoms when discontinuing treatment with Celexa. A gradual reduction in the dose rather than abrupt cessation is recommended whenever possible. If intolerable symptoms occur following a decrease in the dose or upon discontinuation of treatment, then resuming the previously prescribed dose may be considered. Subsequently, the physician may continue decreasing the dose but at a more gradual rate (see DOSAGE AND ADMINISTRATION).

Abnormal Bleeding

Published case reports have documented the occurrence of bleeding episodes in patients treated with psychotropic drugs that interfere with serotonin reuptake. Subsequent epidemiological studies, both of the case-control and cohort design, have demonstrated an association between use of psychotropic drugs that interfere with serotonin reuptake and the occurrence of upper gastrointestinal bleeding. In two studies, concurrent use of a nonsteroidal anti-inflammatory drug (NSAID) or aspirin potentiated the risk of bleeding (see DRUG INTERACTIONS). Although these studies focused on upper gastrointestinal bleeding, there is reason to believe that bleeding at other sites may be similarly potentiated. Patients should be cautioned regarding the risk of bleeding associated with the concomitant use of Celexa with NSAIDs, aspirin, or other drugs that affect coagulation.

Hyponatremia

Several cases of hyponatremia and SIADH (syndrome of inappropriate antidiuretic hormone secretion) have been reported in association with Celexa treatment. All patients with these events have recovered with discontinuation of Celexa and/or medical intervention.

Activation of Mania/Hypomania

In placebo-controlled trials of Celexa, some of which included patients with bipolar disorder, activation of mania/hypomania was reported in 0.2% of 1063 patients treated with Celexa and in none of the 446 patients treated with placebo. Activation of mania/hypomania has also been reported in a small proportion of patients with major affective disorders treated with other marketed antidepressants. As with all antidepressants, Celexa should be used cautiously in patients with a history of mania.

Seizures

Although anticonvulsant effects of citalopram have been observed in animal studies, Celexa has not been systematically evaluated in patients with a seizure disorder. These patients were excluded from clinical studies during the product's premarketing testing. In clinical trials of Celexa, seizures occurred in 0.3% of patients treated with Celexa (a rate of one patient per 98 years of exposure) and 0.5% of patients treated with placebo (a rate of one patient per 50 years of exposure). Like other antidepressants, Celexa should be introduced with care in patients with a history of seizure disorder.

Suicide

The possibility of a suicide attempt is inherent in depression and may persist until significant remission occurs. Close supervision of high-risk patients should accompany initial drug therapy. Prescriptions for Celexa should be written for the smallest quantity of tablets consistent with good patient management, in order to reduce the risk of overdose.

Interference with Cognitive and Motor Performance

In studies in normal volunteers, Celexa in doses of 40 mg/day did not produce impairment of intellectual function or psychomotor performance. Because any psychoactive drug may impair judgement, thinking, or motor skills, however, patients should be cautioned about operating hazardous machinery, including automobiles, until they are reasonably certain that Celexa therapy does not affect their ability to engage in such activities.

Use in Patients with Concomitant Illness

Clinical experience with Celexa in patients with certain concomitant systemic illnesses is limited. Caution is advisable in using Celexa in patients with diseases or conditions that produce altered metabolism or hemodynamic responses.

Celexa has not been systematically evaluated in patients with a recent history of myocardial infarction or unstable heart disease. Patients with these diagnoses were generally excluded from clinical studies during the product's premarketing testing. However, the electrocardiograms of 1116 patients who received Celexa in clinical trials were evaluated and the data indicate that Celexa is not associated with the development of clinically significant ECG abnormalities.

In subjects with hepatic impairment, citalopram clearance was decreased and plasma concentrations were increased. The use of Celexa in hepatically impaired patients should be approached with caution and a lower maximum dosage is recommended (see Dosage and Administration).

Because citalopram is extensively metabolized, excretion of unchanged drug in urine is a minor route of elimination. Until adequate numbers of patients with severe renal impairment have been evaluated during chronic treatment with Celexa, however, it should be used with caution in such patients (see Dosage and Administration).

Information for Patients

Physicians are advised to discuss the following issues with patients for whom they prescribe Celexa.

Although in controlled studies Celexa has not been shown to impair psychomotor performance, any psychoactive drug may impair judgment, thinking, or motor skills, so patients should be cautioned about operating hazardous machinery, including automobiles, until they are reasonably certain that Celexa therapy does not affect their ability to engage in such activities.

Patients should be told that, although Celexa has not been shown in experiments with normal subjects to increase the mental and motor skill impairments caused by alcohol, the concomitant use of Celexa and alcohol in depressed patients is not advised.

Patients should be advised to inform their physician if they are taking, or plan to take, any prescription or over-the-counter drugs, as there is a potential for interactions.

Patients should be cautioned about the concomitant use of Celexa and NSAIDs, aspirin, or other drugs that affect coagulation since the combined use of psychotropic drugs that interfere with serotonin reuptake and these agents has been associated with an increased risk of bleeding.

Patients should be advised to notify their physician if they become pregnant or intend to become pregnant during therapy.

Patients should be advised to notify their physician if they are breastfeeding an infant.

While patients may notice improvement with Celexa therapy in 1 to 4 weeks, they should be advised to continue therapy as directed.

Laboratory Tests

There are no specific laboratory tests recommended.

Drug Interactions

CNS Drugs—Given the primary CNS effects of citalopram, caution should be used when it is taken in combination with other centrally acting drugs.

Alcohol—Although citalopram did not potentiate the cognitive and motor effects of alcohol in a clinical trial, as with other psychotropic medications, the use of alcohol by depressed patients taking Celexa is not recommended.

Monoamine Oxidase Inhibitors (MAOIs)—See Contraindications and Warnings.

Drugs That Interfere With Hemostasis (NSAIDs, Aspirin, Warfarin, etc.)

Serotonin release by platelets plays an important role in hemostasis. Epidemiological studies of the case-control and cohort design that have demonstrated an association between use of psychotropic drugs that interfere with serotonin reuptake and the occurrence of upper gastrointestinal bleeding have also shown that concurrent use of an NSAID or aspirin potentiated the risk of bleeding. Thus, patients should be cautioned about the use of such drugs concurrently with Celexa.

Cimetidine—In subjects who had received 21 days of 40 mg/day Celexa, combined administration of 400 mg/day cimetidine for 8 days resulted in an increase in citalopram AUC and C_{max} of 43% and 39%, respectively. The clinical significance of these findings is unknown.

Digoxin—In subjects who had received 21 days of 40 mg/day Celexa, combined administration of Celexa and digoxin (single dose of 1 mg) did not significantly affect the pharmacokinetics of either citalopram or digoxin.

Lithium—Coadministration of Celexa (40 mg/day for 10 days) and lithium (30 mmol/day for 5 days) had no significant effect on the pharmacokinetics of citalopram or lithium. Nevertheless, plasma lithium levels should be monitored with appropriate adjustment to the lithium dose in accordance with standard clinical practice. Because lithium may enhance the serotonergic effects of citalopram, caution should be exercised when Celexa and lithium are coadministered.

Theophylline—Combined administration of Celexa (40 mg/day for 21 days) and the CYP1A2 substrate theophylline (single dose of 300 mg) did not affect the pharmacokinetics of theophylline. The effect of theophylline on the pharmacokinetics of citalopram was not evaluated.

Sumatriptan—There have been rare postmarketing reports describing patients with weakness, hyperreflexia, and incoordination following the use of a selective serotonin reuptake inhibitor (SSRI) and sumatriptan. If concomitant treatment with sumatriptan and an SSRI (e.g., fluoxetine, fluvoxamine, paroxetine, sertraline, citalopram) is clinically warranted, appropriate observation of the patient is advised.

Warfarin—Administration of 40 mg/day Celexa for 21 days did not affect the pharmacokinetics of warfarin, a CYP3A4 substrate. Prothrombin time was increased by 5%, the clinical significance of which is unknown.

Carbamazepine—Combined administration of Celexa (40 mg/day for 14 days) and carbamazepine (titrated to 400 mg/day for 35 days) did not significantly affect the pharmacokinetics of carbamazepine, a CYP3A4 substrate. Although trough citalopram plasma levels were unaffected, given the enzyme-inducing properties of carbamazepine, the possibility that carbamazepine might increase the clearance of citalopram should be considered if the two drugs are coadministered.

Triazolam—Combined administration of Celexa (titrated to 40 mg/day for 28 days) and the CYP3A4 substrate triazolam (single dose of 0.25 mg) did not significantly affect the pharmacokinetics of either citalopram or triazolam.

Ketoconazole—Combined administration of Celexa (40 mg) and ketoconazole (200 mg) decreased the C_{max} and AUC of ketoconazole by 21% and 10%, respectively, and did not significantly affect the pharmacokinetics of citalopram.

CYP3A4 and 2C19 Inhibitors—*In vitro* studies indicated that CYP3A4 and 2C19 are the primary enzymes involved in the metabolism of citalopram. However, coadministration of citalopram (40 mg) and ketoconazole (200 mg), a potent inhibitor of CYP3A4, did not significantly affect the pharmacokinetics of citalopram. Because citalopram is metabolized by multiple enzyme systems, inhibition of a single enzyme may not appreciably decrease citalopram clearance.

Metoprolol—Administration of 40 mg/day Celexa for 22 days resulted in a two-fold increase in the plasma levels of the beta-adrenergic blocker metoprolol. Increased metoprolol plasma levels have been associated with decreased cardioselectivity. Coadministration of Celexa and metoprolol had no clinically significant effects on blood pressure or heart rate.

Imipramine and Other Tricyclic Antidepressants (TCAs)—*In vitro* studies suggest that citalopram is a relatively weak inhibitor of CYP2D6. Coadministration of Celexa (40 mg/day for 10 days) with the tricyclic antidepressant imipramine (single dose of 100 mg), a substrate for CYP2D6, did not significantly affect the plasma concentrations of imipramine or citalopram. However, the concentration of the imipramine metabolite desipramine was increased by approximately 50%. The clinical significance of the desipramine change is unknown. Nevertheless, caution is indicated in the coadministration of TCA's with Celexa.

Electroconvulsive Therapy (ECT)—There are no clinical studies of the combined use of electroconvulsive therapy (ECT) and Celexa.

Carcinogenesis, Mutagenesis, Impairment of Fertility

Carcinogenesis

Citalopram was administered in the diet to NMRI/BOM strain mice and COBS WI strain rats for 18 and 24 months, respectively. There was no evidence for carcinogenicity of citalopram in mice receiving up to 240 mg/kg/day, which is equivalent to 20 times the maximum recommended human daily dose (MRHD) of 60 mg on a surface area (mg/m^2) ba-

Continued on next page

Celexa—Cont.

sis. There was an increased incidence of small intestine carcinoma in rats receiving 8 or 24 mg/kg/day, doses which are approximately 1.3 and 4 times the MRHD, respectively, on a mg/m² basis. A no-effect dose for this finding was not established. The relevance of these findings to humans is unknown.

Mutagenesis

Citalopram was mutagenic in the *in vitro* bacterial reverse mutation assay (Ames test) in 2 of 5 bacterial strains (Salmonella TA98 and TA1537) in the absence of metabolic activation. It was clastogenic in the *in vitro* Chinese hamster lung cell assay for chromosomal aberrations in the presence and absence of metabolic activation. Citalopram was not mutagenic in the *in vitro* mammalian forward gene mutation assay (HPRT) in mouse lymphoma cells or in a coupled *in vitro/in vivo* unscheduled DNA synthesis (UDS) assay in rat liver. It was not clastogenic in the *in vitro* chromosomal aberration assay in human lymphocytes or in two *in vivo* mouse micronucleus assays.

Impairment of Fertility

When citalopram was administered orally to male and female rats prior to and throughout mating and gestation at doses of 16/24 (males/females), 32, 48, and 72 mg/kg/day, mating was decreased at all doses, and fertility was decreased at doses ≥ 32 mg/kg/day, approximately 5 times the maximum recommended human dose (MRHD) of 60 mg/day on a body surface area (mg/m²) basis. Gestation duration was increased at 48 mg/kg/day, approximately 8 times the MRHD.

Pregnancy

Pregnancy Category C

In animal reproduction studies, citalopram has been shown to have adverse effects on embryo/fetal and postnatal development, including teratogenic effects, when administered at doses greater than human therapeutic doses.

In two rat embryo/fetal development studies, oral administration of citalopram (32, 56, or 112 mg/kg/day) to pregnant animals during the period of organogenesis resulted in decreased embryo/fetal growth and survival and an increased incidence of fetal abnormalities (including cardiovascular and skeletal defects) at the high dose, which is approximately 18 times the maximum recommended human dose (MRHD) of 60 mg/day on a body surface area (mg/m²) basis. This dose was also associated with maternal toxicity (clinical signs, decreased BW gain). The developmental, no-effect dose of 56 mg/kg/day is approximately 9 times the MRHD on a mg/m² basis. In a rabbit study, no adverse effects on embryo/fetal development were observed at doses of up to 16 mg/kg/day, or approximately 5 times the MRHD on a mg/m² basis. Thus, teratogenic effects were observed at a maternally toxic dose in the rat and were not observed in the rabbit.

When female rats were treated with citalopram (4.8, 12.8, or 32 mg/kg/day) from late gestation through weaning, increased offspring mortality during the first 4 days after birth and persistent offspring growth retardation were observed at the highest dose, which is approximately 5 times the MRHD on a mg/m² basis. The no-effect dose of 12.8 mg/kg/day is approximately 2 times the MRHD on a mg/m² basis. Similar effects on offspring mortality and growth were seen when dams were treated throughout gestation and early lactation at doses ≥ 24 mg/kg/day, approximately 4 times the MRHD on a mg/m² basis. A no-effect dose was not determined in that study. There are no adequate and well-controlled studies in pregnant women; therefore, citalopram should be used during pregnancy only if the potential benefit justifies the potential risk to the fetus.

Pregnancy-Nonteratogenic Effects

Neonates exposed to Celexa and other SSRIs or SNRIs, late in the third trimester, have developed complications requiring prolonged hospitalization, respiratory support, and tube feeding. Such complications can arise immediately upon delivery. Reported clinical findings have included respiratory distress, cyanosis, apnea, seizures, temperature instability, feeding difficulty, vomiting, hypoglycemia, hypotonia, hypertonia, hyperreflexia, tremor, jitteriness, irritability, and constant crying. These features are consistent with either a direct toxic effect of SSRIs and SNRIs or, possibly, a drug discontinuation syndrome. It should be noted that, in some cases, the clinical picture is consistent with serotonin syndrome (see WARNINGS).

When treating a pregnant woman with Celexa during the third trimester, the physician should carefully consider the potential risks and benefits of treatment (see DOSAGE AND ADMINISTRATION).

Labor and Delivery

The effect of Celexa on labor and delivery in humans is unknown.

Nursing Mothers

As has been found to occur with many other drugs, citalopram is excreted in human breast milk. There have been two reports of infants experiencing excessive somnolence, decreased feeding, and weight loss in association with breastfeeding from a citalopram-treated mother; in one case, the infant was reported to recover completely upon discontinuation of citalopram by its mother and in the second case, no follow up information was available. The decision whether to continue or discontinue either nursing or Celexa therapy should take into account the risks of citalopram exposure for the infant and the benefits of Celexa treatment for the mother.

Pediatric Use

Safety and effectiveness in pediatric patients have not been established.

Geriatric Use

Of 4422 patients in clinical studies of Celexa, 1357 were 60 and over, 1034 were 65 and over, and 457 were 75 and over. No overall differences in safety or effectiveness were observed between these subjects and younger subjects, and other reported clinical experience has not identified differences in responses between the elderly and younger patients, but greater sensitivity of some older individuals cannot be ruled out. Most elderly patients treated with Celexa in clinical trials received daily doses between 20 and 40 mg (see Dosage and Administration).

In two pharmacokinetic studies, citalopram AUC was increased by 23% and 30%, respectively, in elderly subjects as compared to younger subjects, and its half-life was increased by 30% and 50%, respectively (see Clinical Pharmacology).

20 mg/day is the recommended dose for most elderly patients (see Dosage and Administration).

ADVERSE REACTIONS

The premarketing development program for Celexa included citalopram exposures in patients and/or normal subjects from 3 different groups of studies: 429 normal subjects in clinical pharmacology/pharmacokinetic studies; 4422 exposures from patients in controlled and uncontrolled clinical trials, corresponding to approximately 1370 patient-exposure years. There were, in addition, over 19,000 exposures from mostly open-label, European postmarketing studies. The conditions and duration of treatment with Celexa varied greatly and included (in overlapping categories) open-label and double-blind studies, inpatient and outpatient studies, fixed-dose and dose-titration studies, and short-term and long-term exposure. Adverse reactions were assessed by collecting adverse events, results of physical examinations, vital signs, weights, laboratory analyses, ECGs, and results of ophthalmologic examinations.

Adverse events during exposure were obtained primarily by general inquiry and recorded by clinical investigators using terminology of their own choosing. Consequently, it is not possible to provide a meaningful estimate of the proportion of individuals experiencing adverse events without first grouping similar types of events into a smaller number of standardized event categories. In the tables and tabulations that follow, standard World Health Organization (WHO) terminology has been used to classify reported adverse events.

The stated frequencies of adverse events represent the proportion of individuals who experienced, at least once, a treatment-emergent adverse event of the type listed. An event was considered treatment-emergent if it occurred for the first time or worsened while receiving therapy following baseline evaluation.

Adverse Findings Observed in Short-Term, Placebo-Controlled Trials

Adverse Events Associated with Discontinuation of Treatment

Among 1063 depressed patients who received Celexa at doses ranging from 10 to 80 mg/day in placebo-controlled trials of up to 6 weeks in duration, 16% discontinued treatment due to an adverse event, as compared to 8% of 446 patients receiving placebo. The adverse events associated with discontinuation and considered drug-related (i.e., associated with discontinuation in at least 1% of Celexa-treated patients at a rate at least twice that of placebo) are shown in TABLE 1. It should be noted that one patient can report more than one reason for discontinuation and be counted more than once in this table.

TABLE 1
Adverse Events Associated with Discontinuation of Treatment in Short-Term, Placebo-Controlled, Depression Trials

Body System/Adverse Event	Percentage of Patients Discontinuing Due to Adverse Event Citalopram (N=1063)	Placebo (N=446)
General		
Asthenia	1%	<1%
Gastrointestinal Disorders		
Nausea	4%	0%
Dry Mouth	1%	<1%
Vomiting	1%	0%
Central and Peripheral Nervous System Disorders		
Dizziness	2%	<1%
Psychiatric Disorders		
Insomnia	3%	1%
Somnolence	2%	1%
Agitation	1%	<1%

Adverse Events Occurring at an Incidence of 2% or More Among Celexa-Treated Patients

Table 2 enumerates the incidence, rounded to the nearest percent, of treatment-emergent adverse events that occurred among 1063 depressed patients who received Celexa at doses ranging from 10 to 80 mg/day in placebo-controlled trials of up to 6 weeks in duration. Events included are those occurring in 2% or more of patients treated with Celexa and for which the incidence in patients treated with Celexa was greater than the incidence in placebo-treated patients.

The prescriber should be aware that these figures cannot be used to predict the incidence of adverse events in the course of usual medical practice where patient characteristics and other factors differ from those which prevailed in the clinical trials. Similarly, the cited frequencies cannot be compared with figures obtained from other clinical investigations involving different treatments, uses, and investigators. The cited figures, however, do provide the prescribing physician with some basis for estimating the relative contribution of drug and non-drug factors to the adverse event incidence rate in the population studied.

The only commonly observed adverse event that occurred in Celexa patients with an incidence of 5% or greater and at least twice the incidence in placebo patients was ejaculation disorder (primarily ejaculatory delay) in male patients (see TABLE 2).

TABLE 2
Treatment-Emergent Adverse Events: Incidence in Placebo-Controlled Clinical Trials*

Body System/Adverse Event	(Percentage of Patients Reporting Event) Celexa (N=1063)	Placebo (N=446)
Autonomic Nervous System Disorders		
Dry Mouth	20%	14%
Sweating Increased	11%	9%
Central & Peripheral Nervous System Disorders		
Tremor	8%	6%
Gastrointestinal Disorders		
Nausea	21%	14%
Diarrhea	8%	5%
Dyspepsia	5%	4%
Vomiting	4%	3%
Abdominal Pain	3%	2%
General		
Fatigue	5%	3%
Fever	2%	<1%
Musculoskeletal System Disorders		
Arthralgia	2%	1%
Myalgia	2%	1%
Psychiatric Disorders		
Somnolence	18%	10%
Insomnia	15%	14%
Anxiety	4%	3%
Anorexia	4%	2%
Agitation	3%	1%
Dysmenorrhea[1]	3%	2%
Libido Decreased	2%	<1%
Yawning	2%	<1%
Respiratory System Disorders		
Upper Respiratory Tract Infection	5%	4%
Rhinitis	5%	3%
Sinusitis	3%	<1%
Urogenital		
Ejaculation Disorder[2,3]	6%	1%
Impotence[3]	3%	<1%

*Events reported by at least 2% of patients treated with Celexa are reported, except for the following events which had an incidence on placebo ≥ Celexa: headache, asthenia, dizziness, constipation, palpitation, vision abnormal, sleep disorder, nervousness, pharyngitis, micturition disorder, back pain.

[1]Denominator used was for females only (N=638 Celexa; N=252 placebo).

[2]Primarily ejaculatory delay.

[3]Denominator used was for males only (N=425 Celexa; N=194 placebo).

Dose Dependency of Adverse Events

The potential relationship between the dose of Celexa administered and the incidence of adverse events was examined in a fixed-dose study in depressed patients receiving placebo or Celexa 10, 20, 40, and 60 mg. Jonckheere's trend test revealed a positive dose response ($p<0.05$) for the following adverse events: fatigue, impotence, insomnia, sweating increased, somnolence, and yawning.

Male and Female Sexual Dysfunction with SSRIs

Although changes in sexual desire, sexual performance, and sexual satisfaction often occur as manifestations of a psychiatric disorder, they may also be a consequence of pharmacologic treatment. In particular, some evidence suggests that selective serotonin reuptake inhibitors (SSRIs) can cause such untoward sexual experiences.

Reliable estimates of the incidence and severity of untoward experiences involving sexual desire, performance, and satisfaction are difficult to obtain, however, in part because patients and physicians may be reluctant to discuss them. Accordingly, estimates of the incidence of untoward sexual experience and performance cited in product labeling, are likely to underestimate their actual incidence.

The table below displays the incidence of sexual side effects reported by at least 2% of patients taking Celexa in a pool of placebo-controlled clinical trials in patients with depression.

Treatment	Celexa (425 males)	Placebo (194 males)
Abnormal Ejaculation (mostly ejaculatory delay)	6.1% (males only)	1% (males only)
Libido Decreased	3.8% (males only)	<1% (males only)
Impotence	2.8% (males only)	<1% (males only)

In female depressed patients receiving Celexa, the reported incidence of decreased libido and anorgasmia was 1.3% (n=638 females) and 1.1% (n=252 females), respectively.
There are no adequately designed studies examining sexual dysfunction with citalopram treatment.
Priapism has been reported with all SSRIs.
While it is difficult to know the precise risk of sexual dysfunction associated with the use of SSRIs, physicians should routinely inquire about such possible side effects.

Vital Sign Changes
Celexa and placebo groups were compared with respect to (1) mean change from baseline in vital signs (pulse, systolic blood pressure, and diastolic blood pressure) and (2) the incidence of patients meeting criteria for potentially clinically significant changes from baseline in these variables. These analyses did not reveal any clinically important changes in vital signs associated with Celexa treatment. In addition, a comparison of supine and standing vital sign measures for Celexa and placebo treatments indicated that Celexa treatment is not associated with orthostatic changes.

Weight Changes
Patients treated with Celexa in controlled trials experienced a weight loss of about 0.5 kg compared to no change for placebo patients.

Laboratory Changes
Celexa and placebo groups were compared with respect to (1) mean change from baseline in various serum chemistry, hematology, and urinalysis variables, and (2) the incidence of patients meeting criteria for potentially clinically significant changes from baseline in these variables. These analyses revealed no clinically important changes in laboratory test parameters associated with Celexa treatment.

ECG Changes
Electrocardiograms from Celexa (N=802) and placebo (N=241) groups were compared with respect to (1) mean change from baseline in various ECG parameters, and (2) the incidence of patients meeting criteria for potentially clinically significant changes from baseline in these variables. The only statistically significant drug-placebo difference observed was a decrease in heart rate for Celexa of 1.7 bpm compared to no change in heart rate for placebo. There were no observed differences in QT or other ECG intervals.

Other Events Observed During the Premarketing Evaluation of Celexa (citalopram HBr)
Following is a list of WHO terms that reflect treatment-emergent adverse events, as defined in the introduction to the ADVERSE REACTIONS section, reported by patients treated with Celexa at multiple doses in a range of 10 to 80 mg/day during any phase of a trial within the premarketing database of 4422 patients. All reported events are included except those already listed in Table 2 or elsewhere in labeling, those events for which a drug cause was remote, those event terms which were so general as to be uninformative, and those occurring in only one patient. It is important to emphasize that, although the events reported occurred during treatment with Celexa, they were not necessarily caused by it.
Events are further categorized by body system and listed in order of decreasing frequency according to the following definitions: frequent adverse events are those occurring on one or more occasions in at least 1/100 patients; infrequent adverse events are those occurring in less than 1/100 patients but at least 1/1000 patients; rare events are those occurring in fewer than 1/1000 patients.
Cardiovascular—*Frequent*: tachycardia, postural hypotension, hypotension. *Infrequent*: hypertension, bradycardia, edema (extremities), angina pectoris, extrasystoles, cardiac failure, flushing, myocardial infarction, cerebrovascular accident, myocardial ischemia. *Rare*: transient ischemic attack, phlebitis, atrial fibrillation, cardiac arrest, bundle branch block.
Central and Peripheral Nervous System Disorders—*Frequent*: paresthesia, migraine. *Infrequent*: hyperkinesia, vertigo, hypertonia, extrapyramidal disorder, leg cramps, involuntary muscle contractions, hypokinesia, neuralgia, dystonia, abnormal gait, hypesthesia, ataxia. *Rare*: abnormal coordination, hyperesthesia, ptosis, stupor.
Endocrine Disorders—*Rare*: hypothyroidism, goiter, gynecomastia.
Gastrointestinal Disorders—*Frequent*: saliva increased, flatulence. *Infrequent*: gastritis, gastroenteritis, stomatitis, eructation, hemorrhoids, dysphagia, teeth grinding, gingivitis, esophagitis. *Rare*: colitis, gastric ulcer, cholecystitis, cholelithiasis, duodenal ulcer, gastroesophageal reflux, glossitis, jaundice, diverticulitis, rectal hemorrhage, hiccups.
General—*Infrequent*: hot flushes, rigors, alcohol intolerance, syncope, influenza-like symptoms. *Rare*: hayfever.
Hemic and Lymphatic Disorders—*Infrequent*: purpura, anemia, epistaxis, leukocytosis, leucopenia, lymphadenopathy. *Rare*: pulmonary embolism, granulocytopenia, lymphocytosis, lymphopenia, hypochromic anemia, coagulation disorder, gingival bleeding.
Metabolic and Nutritional Disorders—*Frequent*: decreased weight, increased weight. *Infrequent*: increased hepatic enzymes, thirst, dry eyes, increased alkaline phosphatase, abnormal glucose tolerance. *Rare*: bilirubinemia, hypokalemia, obesity, hypoglycemia, hepatitis, dehydration.
Musculoskeletal System Disorders—*Infrequent*: arthritis, muscle weakness, skeletal pain. *Rare*: bursitis, osteoporosis.
Psychiatric Disorders—*Frequent*: impaired concentration, amnesia, apathy, depression, increased appetite, aggravated depression, suicide attempt, confusion. *Infrequent*: increased libido, aggressive reaction, paroniria, drug dependence, depersonalization, hallucination, euphoria, psychotic depression, delusion, paranoid reaction, emotional lability, panic reaction, psychosis. *Rare*: catatonic reaction, melancholia.
Reproductive Disorders/Female*—*Frequent*: amenorrhea. *Infrequent*: galactorrhea, breast pain, breast enlargement, vaginal hemorrhage.
*% based on female subjects only: 2955
Respiratory System Disorders—*Frequent*: coughing. *Infrequent*: bronchitis, dyspnea, pneumonia. *Rare*: asthma, laryngitis, bronchospasm, pneumonitis, sputum increased.
Skin and Appendages Disorders—*Frequent*: rash, pruritus. *Infrequent*: photosensitivity reaction, urticaria, acne, skin discoloration, eczema, alopecia, dermatitis, skin dry, psoriasis. *Rare*: hypertrichosis, decreased sweating, melanosis, keratitis, cellulitis, pruritus ani.
Special Senses—*Frequent*: accommodation abnormal, taste perversion. *Infrequent*: tinnitus, conjunctivitis, eye pain. *Rare*: mydriasis, photophobia, diplopia, abnormal lacrimation, cataract, taste loss.
Urinary System Disorders—*Frequent*: polyuria. *Infrequent*: micturition frequency, urinary incontinence, urinary retention, dysuria. *Rare*: facial edema, hematuria, oliguria, pyelonephritis, renal calculus, renal pain.
Other Events Observed During the Postmarketing Evaluation of Celexa (citalopram HBr)
It is estimated that over 30 million patients have been treated with Celexa since market introduction. Although no causal relationship to Celexa treatment has been found, the following adverse events have been reported to be temporally associated with Celexa treatment, and have not been described elsewhere in labeling: acute renal failure, akathisia, allergic reaction, anaphylaxis, angioedema, choreoathetosis, chest pain, delirium, dyskinesia, ecchymosis, epidermal necrolysis, erythema multiforme, gastrointestinal hemorrhage, grand mal convulsions, hemolytic anemia, hepatic necrosis, myoclonus, neuroleptic malignant syndrome, nystagmus, pancreatitis, priapism, prolactinemia, prothrombin decreased, QT prolonged, rhabdomyolysis, serotonin syndrome, spontaneous abortion, thrombocytopenia, thrombosis, ventricular arrhythmia, Torsades de pointes, and withdrawal syndrome.

DRUG ABUSE AND DEPENDENCE
Controlled Substance Class
Celexa (citalopram HBr) is not a controlled substance.
Physical and Psychological Dependence
Animal studies suggest that the abuse liability of Celexa is low. Celexa has not been systematically studied in humans for its potential for abuse, tolerance, or physical dependence. The premarketing clinical experience with Celexa did not reveal any drug-seeking behavior. However, these observations were not systematic and it is not possible to predict, on the basis of this limited experience, the extent to which a CNS-active drug will be misused, diverted, and/or abused once marketed. Consequently, physicians should carefully evaluate Celexa patients for history of drug abuse and follow such patients closely, observing them for signs of misuse or abuse (e.g., development of tolerance, incrementations of dose, drug-seeking behavior).

OVERDOSAGE
Human Experience
Although there were no reports of fatal citalopram overdose in clinical trials involving overdoses of up to 2000 mg, postmarketing reports of drug overdoses involving citalopram have included 12 fatalities, 10 in combination with other drugs and/or alcohol and 2 with citalopram alone (3920 mg and 2800 mg), as well as non-fatal overdoses of up to 6000 mg. Symptoms most often accompanying citalopram overdose, alone or in combination with other drugs and/or alcohol, included dizziness, sweating, nausea, vomiting, tremor, somnolence, and sinus tachycardia. In more rare cases, observed symptoms included amnesia, confusion, coma, convulsions, hyperventilation, cyanosis, rhabdomyolysis, and ECG changes (including QTc prolongation, nodal rhythm, ventricular arrhythmia, and one possible case of Torsades de pointes).
Management of Overdose
Establish and maintain an airway to ensure adequate ventilation and oxygenation. Gastric evacuation by lavage and use of activated charcoal should be considered. Careful observation and cardiac and vital sign monitoring are recommended, along with general symptomatic and supportive care. Due to the large volume of distribution of citalopram, forced diuresis, dialysis, hemoperfusion, and exchange transfusion are unlikely to be of benefit. There are no specific antidotes for Celexa.
In managing overdosage, consider the possibility of multiple-drug involvement. The physician should consider contacting a poison control center for additional information on the treatment of any overdose.

DOSAGE AND ADMINISTRATION
Initial Treatment
Celexa (citalopram HBr) should be administered at an initial dose of 20 mg once daily, generally with an increase to a dose of 40 mg/day. Dose increases should usually occur in increments of 20 mg at intervals of no less than one week. Although certain patients may require a dose of 60 mg/day, the only study pertinent to dose response for effectiveness did not demonstrate an advantage for the 60 mg/day dose over the 40 mg/day dose; doses above 40 mg are therefore not ordinarily recommended.
Celexa should be administered once daily, in the morning or evening, with or without food.
Special Populations
20 mg/day is the recommended dose for most elderly patients and patients with hepatic impairment, with titration to 40 mg/day only for nonresponding patients.
No dosage adjustment is necessary for patients with mild or moderate renal impairment. Celexa should be used with caution in patients with severe renal impairment.
Treatment of Pregnant Women During the Third Trimester
Neonates exposed to Celexa and other SSRIs or SNRIs, late in the third trimester, have developed complications requiring prolonged hospitalization, respiratory support, and tube feeding (see PRECAUTIONS). When treating pregnant women with Celexa during the third trimester, the physician should carefully consider the potential risks and benefits of treatment. The physician may consider tapering Celexa in the third trimester.
Maintenance Treatment
It is generally agreed that acute episodes of depression require several months or longer of sustained pharmacologic therapy. Systematic evaluation of Celexa in two studies has shown that its antidepressant efficacy is maintained for periods of up to 24 weeks following 6 or 8 weeks of initial treatment (32 weeks total). In one study, patients were assigned randomly to placebo or to the same dose of Celexa (20–60 mg/day) during maintenance treatment as they had received during the acute stabilization phase, while in the other study, patients were assigned randomly to continuation of Celexa 20 or 40 mg/day, or placebo, for maintenance treatment. In the latter study, the rates of relapse to depression were similar for the two dose groups (see Clinical Trials under Clinical Pharmacology). Based on these limited data, it is not known whether the dose of citalopram needed to maintain euthymia is identical to the dose needed to induce remission. If adverse reactions are bothersome, a decrease in dose to 20 mg/day can be considered.
Discontinuation of Treatment with Celexa
Symptoms associated with discontinuation of Celexa and other SSRIs and SNRIs have been reported (see PRECAUTIONS). Patients should be monitored for these symptoms when discontinuing treatment. A gradual reduction in the dose rather than abrupt cessation is recommended whenever possible. If intolerable symptoms occur following a decrease in the dose or upon discontinuation of treatment, then resuming the previously prescribed dose may be considered. Subsequently, the physician may continue decreasing the dose but at a more gradual rate.
Switching Patients To or From a Monoamine Oxidase Inhibitor
At least 14 days should elapse between discontinuation of a MAOI and initiation of Celexa therapy. Similarly, at least 14 days should be allowed after stopping Celexa before starting a MAOI (see Contraindications and Warnings).

HOW SUPPLIED
Tablets:

10 mg	Bottle of 100	NDC # 0456-4010-01

Beige, oval, film-coated.
Imprint on one side with "FP". Imprint on the other side with "10 mg".

20 mg	Bottle of 100	NDC # 0456-4020-01
	10 × 10 Unit Dose	NDC # 0456-4020-63

Pink, oval, scored film-coated.
Imprint on scored side with "F" on the left side and "P" on the right side.
Imprint on the non-scored side with "20 mg".

40 mg	Bottle of 100	NDC # 0456-4040-01
	10 × 10 Unit Dose	NDC # 0456-4040-63

White, oval, scored film-coated.
Imprint on scored side with "F" on the left side and "P" on the right side.
Imprint on the non-scored side with "40 mg".
Oral Solution:
10 mg/5 mL, peppermint flavor (240 mL) NDC 0456-4130-08
Store at 25°C (77°F); excursions permitted to 15-30°C (59-86°F).

ANIMAL TOXICOLOGY
Retinal Changes in Rats
Pathologic changes (degeneration/atrophy) were observed in the retinas of albino rats in the 2-year carcinogenicity study with citalopram. There was an increase in both incidence and severity of retinal pathology in both male and female rats receiving 80 mg/kg/day (13 times the maximum recommended daily human dose of 60 mg on a mg/m^2 basis). Similar findings were not present in rats receiving 24 mg/kg/day for two years, in mice treated for 18 months at doses up to 240 mg/kg/day, or in dogs treated for one year at doses up to 20 mg/kg/day (4, 20, and 10 times, respectively, the maximum recommended daily human dose on a mg/m^2 basis).

Continued on next page

Celexa—Cont.

Additional studies to investigate the mechanism for this pathology have not been performed, and the potential significance of this effect in humans has not been established.

Cardiovascular Changes in Dogs

In a one-year toxicology study, 5 of 10 beagle dogs receiving oral doses of 8 mg/kg/day (4 times the maximum recommended daily human dose of 60 mg on a mg/m^2 basis) died suddenly between weeks 17 and 31 following initiation of treatment. Although appropriate data from that study are not available to directly compare plasma levels of citalopram (CT) and its metabolites, demethylcitalopram (DCT) and didemethylcitalopram (DDCT), to levels that have been achieved in humans, pharmacokinetic data indicate that the relative dog-to-human exposure was greater for the metabolites than for citalopram. Sudden deaths were not observed in rats at doses up to 120 mg/kg/day, which produced plasma levels of CT, DCT, and DDCT similar to those observed in dogs at doses of 8 mg/kg/day. A subsequent intravenous dosing study demonstrated that in beagle dogs, DDCT caused QT prolongation, a known risk factor for the observed outcome in dogs. This effect occurred in dogs at doses producing peak DDCT plasma levels of 810 to 3250 nM (39–155 times the mean steady state DDCT plasma level measured at the maximum recommended human daily dose of 60 mg). In dogs, peak DDCT plasma concentrations are approximately equal to peak CT plasma concentrations, whereas in humans, steady state DDCT plasma concentrations are less than 10% of steady state CT plasma concentrations. Assays of DDCT plasma concentrations in 2020 citalopram-treated individuals demonstrated that DDCT levels rarely exceeded 70 nM; the highest measured level of DDCT in human overdose was 138 nM. While DDCT is ordinarily present in humans at lower levels than in dogs, it is unknown whether there are individuals who may achieve higher DDCT levels. The possibility that DCT, a principal metabolite in humans, may prolong the QT interval in the dog has not been directly examined because DCT is rapidly converted to DDCT in that species.

Forest Pharmaceuticals, Inc.
Subsidiary of Forest Laboratories, Inc.
St. Louis, MO 63045 USA
Licensed from H. Lundbeck A/S
Rev. 1/04

MG #13940(15)

INFASURF® ℞
[in'fă-surf]
(calfactant)
Intratracheal Suspension
Sterile Suspension for Intratracheal Use Only
Rx Only

Prescribing information for this product, which appears on pages 1299–1300 of the 2004 PDR, has been completely revised as follows. Please write "See Supplement A" next to the product heading.

DESCRIPTION

Infasurf® (calfactant) Intratracheal Suspension is a sterile, non-pyrogenic lung surfactant intended for intratracheal instillation only. It is an extract of natural surfactant from calf lungs which includes phospholipids, neutral lipids, and hydrophobic surfactant-associated proteins B and C (SP-B and SP-C). It contains no preservatives.

Infasurf is an off-white suspension of calfactant in 0.9% aqueous sodium chloride solution. It has a pH of 5.0–6.2 (target pH 5.7). Each milliliter of Infasurf contains 35 mg total phospholipids (including 26 mg phosphatidylcholine of which 16 mg is disaturated phosphatidylcholine) and 0.65 mg proteins including 0.26 mg of SP-B.

CLINICAL PHARMACOLOGY

Endogenous lung surfactant is essential for effective ventilation because it modifies alveolar surface tension thereby stabilizing the alveoli. Lung surfactant deficiency is the cause of Respiratory Distress Syndrome (RDS) in premature infants. Infasurf restores surfactant activity to the lungs of these infants.

Activity: Infasurf adsorbs rapidly to the surface of the air: liquid interface and modifies surface tension similarly to natural lung surfactant. A minimum surface tension of ≤3 mN/m is produced *in vitro* by Infasurf as measured on a pulsating bubble surfactometer. *Ex vivo,* Infasurf restores the pressure volume mechanics and compliance of surfactant-deficient rat lungs. *In vivo,* Infasurf improves lung compliance, respiratory gas exchange, and survival in preterm lambs with profound surfactant deficiency.

Animal Metabolism: Infasurf is administered directly to the lung lumen surface, its site of action. No human studies of absorption, biotransformation, or excretion of Infasurf have been performed. The administration of Infasurf with radiolabeled phospholipids into the lungs of adult rabbits results in the persistence of 50% of radioactivity in the lung alveolar lining and 25% of radioactivity in the lung tissue 24 hours later. Less than 5% of the radioactivity is found in other organs. In premature lambs with lethal surfactant deficiency, less than 30% of instilled Infasurf is present in the lung lining after 24 hours.

Clinical Studies: The efficacy of Infasurf was demonstrated in two multiple-dose controlled clinical trials involving approximately 2,000 infants treated with Infasurf (approximately 100 mg phospholipid/kg) or Exosurf Neonatal®. In addition, two controlled trials of Infasurf versus Survanta®, and four uncontrolled trials were conducted that involved approximately 15,500 patients treated with Infasurf.

Infasurf versus Exosurf Neonatal®

Treatment Trial

A total of 1,126 infants ≤72 hours of age with RDS who required endotracheal intubation and had an a/A $PO_2 < 0.22$ were enrolled into a multiple-dose, randomized, double-blind treatment trial comparing Infasurf (3mL/kg) and Exosurf Neonatal® (5mL/kg). Patients were given an initial dose and one repeat dose 12 hours later if intubation was still required. The dose was instilled in two aliquots through a side port adapter into the proximal end of the endotracheal tube. Each aliquot was given in small bursts over 20-30 inspiratory cycles. After each aliquot was instilled, the infant was positioned with either the right or the left side dependent. Results for efficacy parameters evaluated at 28 days or to discharge for all treated patients from this treatment trial are shown in Table 1.

Table 1 - Infasurf vs Exosurf Neonatal®
Treatment Trial

Efficacy Parameter	Infasurf (N=570) %	Exosurf Neonatal® (N=556) %	p-Value
Incidence of air leaks[a]	11	22	≤0.001
Death due to RDS	4	4	0.95
Any death to 28 days	8	10	0.21
Any death before discharge	9	12	0.07
BPD[b]	5	6	0.41
Crossover to other surfactant[c]	4	4	1

[a] Pneumothorax and/or pulmonary interstitial emphysema.
[b] BPD is bronchopulmonary dysplasia, diagnosed by positive X-ray and oxygen dependence at 28 days.
[c] Protocol permitted use of comparator surfactant in patients who failed to respond to therapy with the initial randomized surfactant if the infant was < 96 hours of age, had received a full course of the randomized surfactant, and had an a/A PO_2 ratio < 0.10

Prophylaxis Trial

A total of 853 infants <29 weeks gestation were enrolled into a multiple-dose, randomized, double-blind prophylaxis trial comparing Infasurf (3mL/kg) and Exosurf Neonatal® (5mL/kg). The initial dose was administered within 30 minutes of birth. Repeat doses were administered at 12 and 24 hours if the patient remained intubated. Each dose was administered divided in 2 equal aliquots, and given through a side port adapter into the proximal end of the endotracheal tube. Each aliquot was given in small bursts over 20-30 inspiratory cycles. After each aliquot was instilled, the infant was positioned with either the right or the left side dependent. Results for efficacy parameters evaluated to day 28 or to discharge for all treated patients from this prophylaxis trial are shown in Table 2.

Table 2 - Infasurf vs Exosurf Neonatal®
Prophylaxis Trial

Efficacy Parameter	Infasurf (N=431) %	Exosurf Neonatal® (N=422) %	p-Value
Incidence of RDS	15	47	≤0.001
Incidence of air leaks[a]	10	15	0.01
Death due to RDS	2	5	≤0.01
Any death to 28 days	12	16	0.10
Any death before discharge	18	19	0.56
BPD[b]	16	17	0.60
Crossover to other surfactant[c]	0.2	3	≤0.001

[a] Pneumothorax and/or pulmonary interstitial emphysema.
[b] BPD is bronchopulmonary dysplasia, diagnosed by positive X-ray and oxygen dependence at 28 days.
[c] Protocol permitted use of comparator surfactant in patients who failed to respond to therapy with the initial randomized surfactant if the infant was < 72 hours of age, had received a full course of the randomized surfactant, and had an a/A PO_2 ratio < 0.10

Infasurf versus Survanta®

Treatment Trial

A total of 662 infants with RDS who required endotracheal intubation and had an a/A PO_2 <0.22 were enrolled into a multiple-dose, randomized, double-blind treatment trial comparing Infasurf (4mL/kg of a formulation that contained 25 mg of phospholipids/mL rather than the 35 mg/mL in the marketed formulation) and Survanta® (4mL/kg). Repeat doses were allowed ≥6 hours following the previous treatment (for up to three doses before 96 hours of age) if the patient required ≥30% oxygen. The surfactant was given through a 5 French feeding catheter inserted into the endotracheal tube. The total dose was instilled in four equal aliquots with the catheter removed between each of the instillations and mechanical ventilation resumed for 0.5 to 2 minutes. Each of the aliquots was administered with the patient in one of four different positions (prone, supine, right, and left lateral) to facilitate even distribution of the surfactant. Results for the major efficacy parameters evaluated at 28 days or to discharge (incidence of air leaks, death due to respiratory causes or to any cause, BPD, or treatment failure) for all treated patients from this treatment trial were not significantly different between Infasurf and Survanta®.

Prophylaxis Trial

A total of 457 infants ≤30 weeks gestation and <1251 grams birth weight were enrolled into a multiple-dose, randomized, double-blind trial comparing Infasurf (4mL/kg of a formulation that contained 25 mg of phospholipids/mL rather than the 35 mg/mL in the marketed formulation) and Survanta® (4mL/kg). The initial dose was administered within 15 minutes of birth and repeat doses were allowed ≥6 hours following the previous treatment (for up to three doses before 96 hours of age) if the patient required ≥30% oxygen. The surfactant was given through a 5 French feeding catheter inserted into the endotracheal tube. The total dose was instilled in four equal aliquots with the catheter removed between each of the instillations and mechanical ventilation resumed for 0.5 to 2 minutes. Each of the aliquots was administered with the patient in one of four different positions (prone, supine, right, and left lateral).

Results for efficacy endpoints evaluated at 28 days or to discharge for all treated patients from this prophylaxis trial showed an increase in mortality from any cause at 28 days (p=0.03) and in death due to respiratory causes (p=0.005) in Infasurf-treated infants. For evaluable patients (patients who met the protocol-defined entry criteria), mortality from any cause and mortality due to respiratory causes were also higher in the Infasurf group (p = 0.07 and 0.03, respectively). However, these observations have not been replicated in other adequate and well-controlled trials and their relevance to the intended population is unknown. All other efficacy outcomes (incidence of RDS, air leaks, BPD, and treatment failure) were not significantly different between Infasurf and Survanta® when analyzed for all treated patients and for evaluable patients.

Acute Clinical Effects: As with other surfactants, marked improvements in oxygenation and lung compliance may occur shortly after the administration of Infasurf. All controlled clinical trials with Infasurf demonstrated significant improvements in fraction of inspired oxygen (F_iO_2) and mean airway pressure (MAP) during the first 24 to 48 hours following initiation of Infasurf therapy.

INDICATIONS AND USAGE

Infasurf is indicated for the prevention of Respiratory Distress Syndrome (RDS) in premature infants at high risk for RDS and for the treatment ("rescue") of premature infants who develop RDS. Infasurf decreases the incidence of RDS, mortality due to RDS, and air leaks associated with RDS.

Prophylaxis

Prophylaxis therapy at birth with Infasurf is indicated for premature infants <29 weeks of gestational age at significant risk for RDS. Infasurf prophylaxis should be administered as soon as possible, preferably within 30 minutes after birth.

Treatment

Infasurf therapy is indicated for infants ≤72 hours of age with RDS (confirmed by clinical and radiologic findings) and requiring endotracheal intubation.

WARNINGS

Infasurf is intended for intratracheal use only.

THE ADMINISTRATION OF EXOGENOUS SURFACTANTS, INCLUDING INFASURF, OFTEN RAPIDLY IMPROVES OXYGENATION AND LUNG COMPLIANCE. Following administration of Infasurf, patients should be carefully monitored so that oxygen therapy and ventilatory support can be modified in response to changes in respiratory status.

Infasurf therapy is not a substitute for neonatal intensive care. Optimal care of premature infants at risk for RDS and newborn infants with RDS who need endotracheal intubation requires an acute care unit organized, staffed, equipped, and experienced with intubation, ventilator management, and general care of these patients.

TRANSIENT EPISODES OF REFLUX OF INFASURF INTO THE ENDOTRACHEAL TUBE, CYANOSIS, BRADYCARDIA, OR AIRWAY OBSTRUCTION HAVE OCCURRED DURING THE DOSING PROCEDURES. These events require stopping Infasurf administration and taking appropriate measures to alleviate the condition. After the patient is stable, dosing can proceed with appropriate monitoring.

PRECAUTIONS

When repeat dosing was given at fixed 12-hour intervals in the Infasurf vs. Exosurf Neonatal® trials, transient episodes of cyanosis, bradycardia, reflux of surfactant into the endotracheal tube, and airway obstruction were observed more frequently among infants in the Infasurf-treated group.

An increased proportion of patients with both intraventricular hemorrhage (IVH) and periventricular leukomalacia (PVL) was observed in Infasurf-treated infants in the Infasurf-Exosurf Neonatal® controlled trials. These observations were not associated with increased mortality.

No data are available on the use of Infasurf in conjunction with experimental therapies of RDS, e.g., high-frequency ventilation.

Table 3 - Common Complications of Prematurity and RDS in Controlled Trials

Complication	Infasurf (N=1001) %	Exosurf Neonatal® (N=978) %	Infasurf (N=553) %	Survanta® (N=566) %
Apnea	61	61	76	76
Patent ductus arteriosus	47	48	45	48
Intracranial hemorrhage	29	31	36	36
Severe intracranial hemorrhage[a]	12	10	9	7
IVH and PVL[b]	7	3	5	5
Sepsis	20	22	28	27
Pulmonary air leaks	12	22	15	15
Pulmonary interstitial emphysema	7	17	10	10
Pulmonary hemorrhage	7	7	7	6
Necrotizing enterocolitis	5	5	17	18

[a] Grade III and IV by the method of Papile.
[b] Patients with both intraventricular hemorrhage and periventricular leukomalacia.

Data from controlled trials on the efficacy of Infasurf are limited to doses of approximately 100 mg phospholipid/kg body weight and up to a total of 4 doses.

Carcinogenesis, Mutagenesis, Impairment of Fertility

Carcinogenesis studies and animal reproduction studies have not been performed with Infasurf. A single mutagenicity study (Ames assay) was negative.

ADVERSE REACTIONS

The most common adverse reactions associated with Infasurf dosing procedures in the controlled trials were cyanosis (65%), airway obstruction (39%), bradycardia (34%), reflux of surfactant into the endotracheal tube (21%), requirement for manual ventilation (16%), and reintubation (3%). These events were generally transient and not associated with serious complications or death.

The incidence of common complications of prematurity and RDS in the four controlled Infasurf trials are presented in Table 3. Prophylaxis and treatment study results for each surfactant are combined.

[See table 3 above]

Follow-up Evaluations

Two-year follow-up data of neurodevelopmental outcomes in 415 infants enrolled in 5 centers that participated in the Infasurf vs. Exosurf Neonatal® controlled trials demonstrated significant developmental delays in equal percentages of Infasurf and Exosurf Neonatal® patients.

OVERDOSAGE

There have been no reports of overdosage with Infasurf. While there are no known adverse effects of excess lung surfactant, overdosage would result in overloading the lungs with an isotonic solution. Ventilation should be supported until clearance of the liquid is accomplished.

DOSAGE AND ADMINISTRATION

FOR INTRATRACHEAL ADMINISTRATION ONLY

Infasurf should be administered under the supervision of clinicians experienced in the acute care of newborn infants with respiratory failure who require intubation.

Rapid and substantial increases in blood oxygenation and improved lung compliance often follow Infasurf instillation. Close clinical monitoring and surveillance following administration may be needed to adjust oxygen therapy and ventilator pressures appropriately.

Dosage

Each dose of Infasurf is 3 mL/kg body weight at birth. Infasurf has been administered every 12 hours for a total of up to 3 doses.

Directions for Use

Infasurf is a suspension which settles during storage. Gentle swirling or agitation of the vial is often necessary for redispersion. DO NOT SHAKE. Visible flecks in the suspension and foaming at the surface are normal for Infasurf.

Infasurf should be stored at refrigerated temperature 2° to 8°C (36° to 46°F). THE 3mL VIAL MUST BE STORED UPRIGHT. Date and time need to be recorded on the carton when Infasurf is removed from the refrigerator. Warming of Infasurf before administration is not necessary.

Unopened, unused vials of Infasurf that have warmed to room temperature can be returned to refrigerated storage within 24 hours for future use. **Infasurf should not be removed from the refrigerator for more than 24 hours. Infasurf should not be returned to the refrigerator more than once.** Repeated warming to room temperature should be avoided. Each single-use vial should be entered only once and the vial with any unused material should be discarded after the initial entry.

INFASURF DOES NOT REQUIRE RECONSTITUTION. DO NOT DILUTE OR SONICATE.

Dosing Procedures

General

Infasurf should only be administered intratracheally through an endotracheal tube. The dose of Infasurf is 3 mL/kg birth weight. The dose is drawn into a syringe from the single-use vial using a 20-gauge or larger needle with care taken to avoid excessive foaming. Administration is made by instillation of the Infasurf suspension into the endotracheal tube.

Administration for Treatment of RDS

Initial Dose

Infasurf should be administered intratracheally through a side-port adapter into the endotracheal tube. Two attendants, one to instill the Infasurf, the other to monitor the patient and assist in positioning, facilitate the dosing. The dose (3 mL/kg) should be administered in two aliquots of 1.5 mL/kg each. After each aliquot is instilled, the infant should be positioned with either the right or the left side dependent. Administration is made while ventilation is continued over 20–30 breaths for each aliquot, with small bursts timed only during the inspiratory cycles. A pause followed by evaluation of the respiratory status and repositioning should separate the two aliquots.

Repeat Doses

Repeat doses of 3 mL/kg of birth weight, up to a total of 3 doses 12 hours apart, have been given in the Infasurf controlled clinical trials if the patient was still intubated.

In the Infasurf vs. Survanta® trials, Infasurf was administered through a 5 French feeding catheter inserted into the endotracheal tube. The total dose was instilled in four equal aliquots with the catheter removed between each of the instillations and mechanical ventilation resumed for 0.5 to 2 minutes. Each of the aliquots was administered with the patient in one of four different positions (prone, supine, right, and left lateral) to facilitate even distribution of the surfactant. Repeat doses were administered as early as 6 hours after the previous dose for a total of up to 4 doses if the infant was still intubated and required at least 30% inspired oxygen to maintain a $P_aO_2 \leq 80$ torr.

Administration for Prophylaxis of RDS at Birth

The amount of a prophylaxis dose of Infasurf should be based on the infant's birth weight. Administration of Infasurf should be given as soon as possible after birth. Usually the immediate care and stabilization of the premature infant born with hypoxemia and/or bradycardia should precede Infasurf prophylaxis.

The dosing procedures are described under Administration for Treatment of RDS.

Dosing Precautions

During administration of Infasurf liquid suspension into the airway, infants often experience bradycardia, reflux of Infasurf into the endotracheal tube, airway obstruction, cyanosis, dislodgement of the endotracheal tube, or hypoventilation. If any of these events occur, the administration should be interrupted and the infant's condition should be stabilized using appropriate interventions before the administration of Infasurf is resumed. Endotracheal suctioning or reintubation is sometimes needed when there are signs of airway obstruction during the administration of the surfactant.

HOW SUPPLIED

Infasurf (calfactant) Intratracheal Suspension is supplied sterile in single-use, rubber-stoppered glass vials containing 3 mL (NDC 0456-4600-03) and 6 mL (NDC 0456-4600-06) off-white suspension.

Store Infasurf (calfactant) Intratracheal Suspension at refrigerated temperature 2° to 8°C (36° to 46°F) and protect from light. **THE 3mL VIAL MUST BE STORED UPRIGHT.** Vials are for single use only. After opening, discard unused drug.

Rx only

Manufactured for:
FOREST PHARMACEUTICALS, INC.
Subsidiary of Forest Laboratories, Inc.
St. Louis, MO 63045
by:
ONY, Inc.
Amherst, NY 14228
RMC 235 Rev. 06/03

LEVOTHROID® ℞
[lēv'o-throid"]
(levothyroxine sodium tablets, USP)
Rx Only

Prescribing information for this product, which appears on pages 1300–1302 of the 2004 PDR, has been completely revised as follows. Please write "See Supplement A" next to the product heading.

DESCRIPTION

LEVOTHROID® (levothyroxine sodium tablets, USP) contains synthetic crystalline L-3,3',5,5'-tetraiodothyronine sodium salt [levothyroxine (T_4) sodium]. Synthetic T_4 is identical to that produced in the human thyroid gland. Levothyroxine (T_4) sodium has an empirical formula of $C_{15}H_{10}I_4N\ NaO_4 \times H_2O$, molecular weight of 798.86 g/mol (anhydrous), and structural formula as shown:

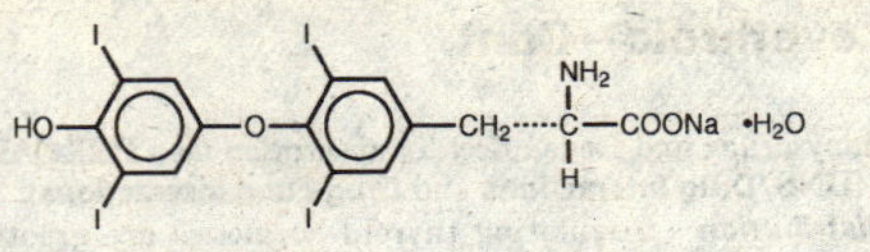

Inactive Ingredients: Microcrystalline cellulose, calcium phosphate dibasic, povidone and magnesium stearate. The following are the coloring additives per tablet strength.

Strength (mcg)	Color Additive(s)
25	FD&C Yellow No. 6 Aluminum Lake
50	None
75	FD&C Blue No. 2 Aluminum Lake, FD&C Red No. 40 Aluminum Lake
88	FD&C Yellow No. 6 Aluminum Lake, FD&C Blue No. 1 Aluminum Lake, D&C Yellow No. 10 Aluminum Lake
100	FD&C Yellow No. 6 Aluminum Lake, D&C Yellow No. 10 Aluminum Lake
112	D&C Red No. 27 Aluminum Lake, D&C Red No. 30 Aluminum Lake
125	FD&C Blue No. 1 Aluminum Lake, FD&C Red No. 40 Aluminum Lake, FD&C Yellow No. 6 Aluminum Lake
150	FD&C Blue No. 2 Aluminum Lake
175	FD&C Blue No. 1 Aluminum Lake, D&C Red No. 30 Aluminum Lake, D&C Red No. 27 Aluminum Lake
200	FD&C Red No. 40 Aluminum Lake
300	FD&C Yellow No. 6 Aluminum Lake, FD&C Blue No.1 Aluminum Lake, D&C Yellow No. 10 Aluminum Lake

CLINICAL PHARMACOLOGY

Thyroid hormone synthesis and secretion is regulated by the hypothalamic-pituitary-thyroid axis. Thyrotropin-releasing hormone (TRH) released from the hypothalamus stimulates secretion of thyrotropin-stimulating hormone, TSH, from the anterior pituitary. TSH, in turn, is the physiologic stimulus for the synthesis and secretion of thyroid hormones, L-thyroxine (T_4) and L-triiodothyronine (T_3), by the thyroid gland. Circulating serum T_3 and T_4 levels exert a feedback effect on both TRH and TSH secretion. When serum T_3 and T_4 levels increase, TRH and TSH secretion decrease. When thyroid hormone levels decrease, TRH and TSH secretion increase. The mechanisms by which thyroid hormones exert their physiologic actions are not completely understood, but it is thought that their principal effects are exerted through control of DNA transcription and protein synthesis. T_3 and T_4 diffuse into the cell nucleus and bind to thyroid receptor proteins attached to DNA. This hormone nuclear receptor complex activates gene transcription and synthesis of messenger RNA and cytoplasmic proteins.

Thyroid hormones regulate multiple metabolic processes and play an essential role in normal growth and development, and normal maturation of the central nervous system and bone. The metabolic actions of thyroid hormones include augmentation of cellular respiration and thermogenesis, as well as metabolism of proteins, carbohydrates and lipids. The protein anabolic effects of thyroid hormones are essential to normal growth and development.

The physiological actions of thyroid hormones are produced predominantly by T_3, the majority of which (approximately 80%) is derived from T_4 by deiodination in peripheral tissues.

Levothyroxine, at doses individualized according to patient response, is effective as replacement or supplemental therapy in hypothyroidism of any etiology, except transient hypothyroidism during the recovery phase of subacute thyroiditis.

Levothyroxine is also effective in the suppression of pituitary TSH secretion in the treatment or prevention of various types of euthyroid goiters, including thyroid nodules, Hashimoto's thyroiditis, multinodular goiter and, as adjunctive therapy in the management of thyrotropin-dependent well-differentiated thyroid cancer (see **INDICATIONS AND USAGE, PRECAUTIONS, DOSAGE AND ADMINISTRATION**).

PHARMACOKINETICS

Absorption - Absorption of orally administered T_4 from the gastrointestinal (GI) tract ranges from 40% to 80%. The majority of the levothyroxine dose is absorbed from the jejunum and upper ileum. The relative bioavailability of LEVOTHROID® tablets, compared to an equal nominal dose of oral levothyroxine sodium solution, is approximately 94%. T_4 absorption is increased by fasting, and decreased in malabsorption syndromes and by certain foods such as soybean infant formula. Dietary fiber decreases bioavailability of T_4. Absorption may also decrease with age. In addition,

Continued on next page

Levothroid—Cont.

many drugs and foods affect T_4 absorption (see **PRECAUTIONS, Drug Interactions and Drug-Food Interactions**).

Distribution - Circulating thyroid hormones are greater than 99% bound to plasma proteins, including thyroxine-binding globulin (TBG), thyroxine-binding prealbumin (TBPA), and albumin (TBA), whose capacities and affinities vary for each hormone. The higher affinity of both TBG and TBPA for T_4 partially explains the higher serum levels, slower metabolic clearance, and longer half-life of T_4 compared to T_3. Protein-bound thyroid hormones exist in reverse equilibrium with small amounts of free hormone. Only unbound hormone is metabolically active. Many drugs and physiologic conditions affect the binding of thyroid hormones to serum proteins (see **PRECAUTIONS, Drug Interactions** and **Drug-Laboratory Test Interactions**). Thyroid hormones do not readily cross the placental barrier (see **PRECAUTIONS, Pregnancy**).

Metabolism - T_4 is slowly eliminated (see **Table 1**). The major pathway of thyroid hormone metabolism is through sequential deiodination. Approximately eighty-percent of circulating T_3 is derived from peripheral T_4 by monodeiodination. The liver is the major site of degradation for both T_4 and T_3, with T_4 deiodination also occurring at a number of additional sites, including the kidney and other tissues. Approximately 80% of the daily dose of T_4 is deiodinated to yield equal amounts of T_3 and reverse T_3 (rT_3). T_3 and rT_3 are further deiodinated to diiodothyronine. Thyroid hormones are also metabolized via conjugation with glucuronides and sulfates and excreted directly into the bile and gut where they undergo enterohepatic recirculation.

Elimination - Thyroid hormones are primarily eliminated by the kidneys. A portion of the conjugated hormone reaches the colon unchanged and is eliminated in the feces. Approximately 20% of T_4 is eliminated in the stool. Urinary excretion of T_4 decreases with age.

Table 1: Pharmacokinetic Parameters of Thyroid Hormones in Euthyroid Patients

Hormone	Ratio in Thyroglobulin	Biologic Potency	$t_{1/2}$ (days)	Protein Binding (%)[2]
Levothyroxine (T_4)	10-20	1	6-7[1]	99.96
Liothyronine (T_3)	1	4	≤2	99.5

[1] 3 to 4 days in hyperthyroidism, 9 to 10 days in hypothyroidism; [2] Includes TBG, TBPA, and TBA

INDICATIONS AND USAGE

Levothyroxine sodium is used for the following indications:

Hypothyroidism - As replacement or supplemental therapy in congenital or acquired hypothyroidism of any etiology, except transient hypothyroidism during the recovery phase of subacute thyroiditis. Specific indications include: primary (thyroidal), secondary (pituitary), and tertiary (hypothalamic) hypothyroidism and subclinical hypothyroidism. Primary hypothyroidism may result from functional deficiency, primary atrophy, partial or total congenital absence of the thyroid gland, or from the effects of surgery, radiation, or drugs, with or without the presence of goiter.

Pituitary TSH Suppression - In the treatment or prevention of various types of euthyroid goiters (see **WARNINGS** and **PRECAUTIONS**), including thyroid nodules (see **WARNINGS** and **PRECAUTIONS**), subacute or chronic lymphocytic thyroiditis (Hashimoto's thyroiditis), multinodular goiter (see **WARNINGS** and **PRECAUTIONS**) and, as an adjunct to surgery and radioiodine therapy in the management of thyrotropin-dependent well-differentiated thyroid cancer.

CONTRAINDICATIONS

Levothyroxine is contraindicated in patients with untreated subclinical (suppressed serum TSH level with normal T_3 and T_4 levels) or overt thyrotoxicosis of any etiology and in patients with acute myocardial infarction. Levothyroxine is contraindicated in patients with uncorrected adrenal insufficiency since thyroid hormones may precipitate an acute adrenal crisis by increasing the metabolic clearance of glucocorticoids (see **PRECAUTIONS**). LEVOTHROID® is contraindicated in patients with hypersensitivity to any of the inactive ingredients in LEVOTHROID® tablets (see **DESCRIPTION, Inactive Ingredients**).

WARNINGS

WARNING: Thyroid hormones, including LEVOTHROID®, either alone or with other therapeutic agents, should not be used for the treatment of obesity or for weight loss. In euthyroid patients, doses within the range of daily hormonal requirements are ineffective for weight reduction. Larger doses may produce serious or even life threatening manifestations of toxicity, particularly when given in association with sympathomimetic amines such as those used for their anorectic effects.

Levothyroxine sodium should not be used in the treatment of male or female infertility unless this condition is associated with hypothyroidism.

In patients with nontoxic diffuse goiter or nodular thyroid disease, particularly the elderly or those with underlying cardiovascular disease, levothyroxine sodium therapy is contraindicated if the serum TSH level is already suppressed due to the risk of precipitating overt thyrotoxicosis (see **CONTRAINDICATIONS**). If the serum TSH level is not suppressed, LEVOTHROID® should be used with caution in conjunction with careful monitoring of thyroid function for evidence of hyperthyroidism and clinical monitoring for potential associated adverse cardiovascular signs and symptoms of hyperthyroidism.

PRECAUTIONS

General

Levothyroxine has a narrow therapeutic index. Regardless of the indication for use, careful dosage titration is necessary to avoid the consequences of over- or under-treatment. These consequences include, among others, effects on growth and development, cardiovascular function, bone metabolism, reproductive function, cognitive function, emotional state, gastrointestinal function, and on glucose and lipid metabolism. Many drugs interact with levothyroxine sodium, necessitating adjustments in dosing to maintain therapeutic response (see **Drug Interactions**).

Effects on bone mineral density - In women, long-term levothyroxine sodium therapy has been associated with in-

Table 2: Drug-Thyroidal Axis Interactions

Drugs that may reduce TSH secretion -the reduction is not sustained; therefore, hypothyroidism does not occur

Drug or Drug Class

Dopamine / Dopamine Agonists	Glucocorticoids	Octreotide

Effect - Use of these agents may result in a transient reduction in TSH secretion when administered at the following doses: Dopamine (≥1 μg/kg/min); Glucocorticoids (hydrocortisone ≥100 mg/day or equivalent); Octreotide (>100 μg/day).

Drugs that alter thyroid hormone secretion

Drugs that may decrease thyroid hormone secretion, which may result in hypothyroidism

Drug or Drug Class

Aminoglutethimide	Iodide	Methimazole
Amiodarone	(including iodine-containing	Propylthiouracil (PTU)
	Radiographic contrast agents)	Sulfonamides
	Lithium	Tolbutamide

Effect - Long-term lithium therapy can result in goiter in up to 50% of patients, and either subclinical or overt hypothyroidism, each in up to 20% of patients. The fetus, neonate, elderly and euthyroid patients with underlying thyroid disease (e.g., Hashimoto's thyroiditis or with Grave's disease previously treated with radioiodine or surgery) are among those individuals who are particularly susceptible to iodine-induced hypothyroidism. Oral cholecystographic agents and amiodarone are slowly excreted, producing more prolonged hypothyroidism than parenterally administered iodinated contrast agents. Long-term aminoglutethimide therapy may minimally decrease T_4 and T_3 levels and increase TSH, although all values remain within normal limits in most patients.

Drugs that may increase thyroid hormone secretion, which may result in hyperthyroidism

Drug or Drug Class

Amiodarone

Iodide (including iodine-containing Radiographic contrast agents)

Effect - Iodide and drugs that contain pharmacological amounts of iodide may cause hyperthyroidism in euthyroid patients with Grave's disease previously treated with antithyroid drugs or in euthyroid patients with thyroid autonomy (e.g., multinodular goiter or hyperfunctioning thyroid adenoma). Hyperthyroidism may develop over several weeks and may persist for several months after therapy discontinuation. Amiodarone may induce hyperthyroidism by causing thyroiditis.

Drugs that may decrease T_4 absorption, which may result in hypothyroidism

Drug or Drug Class

Antacids	Bile Acid Sequestrants	Cation Exchange Resins
- Aluminum & Magnesium Hydroxides	- Cholestyramine	- Kayexalate
	- Colestipol	Ferrous Sulfate
- Simethicone	Calcium Carbonate	Sucralfate

Effect - Concurrent use may reduce the efficacy of levothyroxine by binding and delaying or preventing absorption, potentially resulting in hypothyroidism. Calcium carbonate may form an insoluble chelate with levothyroxine, and ferrous sulfate likely forms a ferric-thyroxine complex. Administer levothyroxine at least 4 hours apart from these agents.

Drugs that may alter T_4 and T_3 serum transport - but FT_4 concentration remains normal; and, therefore, the patient remains euthyroid

Drugs that may increase serum TBG concentration

Clofibrate	Estrogens (oral)	Mitotane
Estrogen-containing oral contraceptives	Heroin/Methadone	Tamoxifen
	5-Flourouracil	

Drugs that may decrease serum TBG concentration

Androgens / Anabolic Steroids	Glucocorticoids
Asparaginase	Slow-Release Nicotinic Acid

Drugs that may cause protein-binding site displacement

Drug or Drug Class

Furosemide (> 80 mg IV)	Non Steroidal Anti-Inflammatory Drugs
Heparin	- Fenamates
Hydantoins	- Phenylbutazone
	Salicylates (>2 g/day)

Effect - Administration of these agents with levothyroxine results in an initial transient increase in FT_4. Continued administration results in a decrease in serum T_4 and normal FT_4 and TSH concentrations and, therefore, patients are clinically euthyroid. Salicylates inhibit binding of T_4 and T_3 to TBG and transthyretin. An initial increase in serum FT_4 is followed by return of FT_4 to normal levels with sustained therapeutic serum salicylate concentrations, although total-T_4 levels may decrease by as much as 30%.

Drugs that may alter T_4 and T_3 metabolism

Drugs that may increase hepatic metabolism, which may result in hypothyroidism

Drug or Drug Class

Carbamazepine	Hydantoins	Phenobarbital	Rifampin

Effect - Stimulation of hepatic microsomal drug-metabolizing enzyme activity may cause increased hepatic degradation of levothyroxine, resulting in increased levothyroxine requirements. Phenytoin and carbamazepine reduce serum protein binding of levothyroxine, and total- and free-T_4 may be reduced by 20% to 40%, but most patients have normal serum TSH levels and are clinically euthyroid.

(Table continued on next page)

Table 2 *(cont.)*: Drug-Thyroidal Axis Interactions

Drugs that may decrease T_4 5′-deiodinase activity

Drug or Drug Class
Amiodarone
Beta-adrenergic antagonists
- (e.g., Propranolol > 160 mg/day)
Glucocorticoids
- (e.g., Dexamethasone ≥4 mg/day)
- Propylthiouracil (PTU)

Effect - Administration of these enzyme inhibitors decreases the peripheral conversion of T_4 to T_3, leading to decreased T_3 levels. However, serum T_4 levels are usually normal but may occasionally be slightly increased. In patients treated with large doses of propranolol (> 160 mg/day), T_3 and T_4 levels change slightly, TSH levels remain normal, and patients are clinically euthyroid. It should be noted that actions of particular beta-adrenergic antagonists may be impaired when the hypothyroid patient is converted to the euthyroid state. Short-term administration of large doses of glucocorticoids may decrease serum T_3 concentrations by 30% with minimal change in serum T_4 levels. However, long-term glucocorticoid therapy may result in slightly decreased T_3 and T_4levels due to decreased TBG production (see above).

Miscellaneous

Drug or Drug Class
Anticoagulants (oral)
- Coumarin Derivatives
- Indandione Derivatives

Effect - Thyroid hormones appear to increase the catabolism of vitamin K-dependent clotting factors, thereby increasing the anticoagulant activity of oral anticoagulants. Concomitant use of these agents impairs the compensatory increases in clotting factor synthesis. Prothrombin time should be carefully monitored in patients taking levothyroxine and oral anticoagulants and the dose of anticoagulant therapy adjusted accordingly.

Drug or Drug Class
Antidepressants
- Tricyclics (e.g., Amitriptyline)
- Tetracyclics (e.g., Maprotiline)
- Selective Serotonin Reuptake Inhibitors (SSRIs; e.g., Sertraline)

Effect - Concurrent use of tri/tetracyclic antidepressants and levothyroxine may increase the therapeutic and toxic effects of both drugs, possibly due to increased receptor sensitivity to catecholamines. Toxic effects may include increased risk of cardiac arrhythmias and CNS stimulation; onset of action of tricyclics may be accelerated. Administration of sertraline in patients stabilized on levothyroxine may result in increased levothyroxine requirements.

Drug or Drug Class
Antidiabetic Agents
- Biguanides
- Meglitinides
- Thiazolidinediones
- Sulfonylureas
- Insulin

Effect - Addition of levothyroxine to antidiabetic or insulin therapy may result in increased antidiabetic agent or insulin requirements. Careful monitoring of diabetic control is recommended, especially when thyroid therapy is started, changed, or discontinued.

Drug or Drug Class
Cardiac Glycosides

Effect - Serum digitalis glycoside levels may be reduced in hyperthyroidism or when the hypothyroid patient is converted to the euthyroid state. Therapeutic effect of digitalis glycosides may be reduced.

Drug or Drug Class
Cytokines
- Interferon-α
- Interleukin-2

Effect - Therapy with interferon-α has been associated with the development of antithyroid microsomal antibodies in 20% of patients and some have transient hypothyroidism, hyperthyroidism, or both. Patients who have antithyroid antibodies before treatment are at higher risk for thyroid dysfunction during treatment. Interleukin-2 has been associated with transient painless thyroiditis in 20% of patients. Interferon-β and -γ have not been reported to cause thyroid dysfunction.

Drug or Drug Class
Growth Hormones
- Somatrem
- Somatropin

Effect - Excessive use of thyroid hormones with growth hormones may accelerate epiphyseal closure. However, untreated hypothyroidism may interfere with growth response to growth hormone.

Drug or Drug Class
Ketamine

Effect - Concurrent use may produce marked hypertension and tachycardia; cautious administration to patients receiving thyroid hormone therapy is recommended.

Drug or Drug Class
Methylxanthine Bronchodilators
- (e.g., Theophylline)

Effect - Decreased theophylline clearance may occur in hypothyroid patients; clearance returns to normal when the euthyroid state is achieved.

Drug or Drug Class
Radiographic Agents

Effect - Thyroid hormones may reduce the uptake of ^{123}I, ^{131}I, and ^{99m}Tc.

Drug or Drug Class
Sympathomimetics

Effect - Concurrent use may increase the effects of sympathomimetics or thyroid hormone. Thyroid hormones may increase the risk of coronary insufficiency when sympathomimetic agents are administered to patients with coronary artery disease.

Drug or Drug Class

Chloral Hydrate	Metoclopramide	Perphenazine
Diazepam	6-Mercaptopurine	Resorcinol (excessive topical use)
Ethionamide	Nitroprusside	Thiazide Diuretics
Lovastatin	Para-aminosalicylate sodium	

Effect - These agents have been associated with thyroid hormone and / or TSH level alterations by various mechanisms.

creased bone resorption, thereby decreasing bone mineral density, especially in post-menopausal women on greater than replacement doses or in women who are receiving suppressive doses of levothyroxine sodium. The increased bone resorption may be associated with increased serum levels and urinary excretion of calcium and phosphorous, elevations in bone alkaline phosphatase and suppressed serum parathyroid hormone levels. Therefore, it is recommended that patients receiving levothyroxine sodium be given the minimum dose necessary to achieve the desired clinical and biochemical response.

Patients with underlying cardiovascular disease - Exercise caution when administering levothyroxine to patients with cardiovascular disorders and to the elderly in whom there is an increased risk of occult cardiac disease. In these patients, levothyroxine therapy should be initiated at lower doses than those recommended in younger individuals or in patients without cardiac disease (see **WARNINGS; PRECAUTIONS, Geriatric Use;** and **DOSAGE AND ADMINISTRATION**). If cardiac symptoms develop or worsen, the levothyroxine dose should be reduced or withheld for one week and then cautiously restarted at a lower dose. Overtreatment with levothyroxine sodium may have adverse cardiovascular effects such as an increase in heart rate, cardiac wall thickness, and cardiac contractility and may precipitate angina or arrhythmias. Patients with coronary artery disease who are receiving levothyroxine therapy should be monitored closely during surgical procedures, since the possibility of precipitating cardiac arrhythmias may be greater in those treated with levothyroxine. Concomitant administration of levothyroxine and sympathomimetic agents to patients with coronary artery disease may precipitate coronary insufficiency.

Patients with nontoxic diffuse goiter or nodular thyroid disease - Exercise caution when administering levothyroxine to patients with nontoxic diffuse goiter or nodular thyroid disease in order to prevent precipitation of thyrotoxicosis (see **WARNINGS**). If the serum TSH is already suppressed, levothyroxine sodium should not be administered (see **CONTRAINDICATIONS**).

Associated endocrine disorders

Hypothalamic/pituitary hormone deficiencies - In patients with secondary or tertiary hypothyroidism, additional hypothalamic/pituitary hormone deficiencies should be considered, and, if diagnosed, treated (see **PRECAUTIONS, Autoimmune polyglandular syndrome** for adrenal insufficiency).

Autoimmune polyglandular syndrome - Occasionally, chronic autoimmune thyroiditis may occur in association with other autoimmune disorders such as adrenal insufficiency, pernicious anemia, and insulin-dependent diabetes mellitus. Patients with concomitant adrenal insufficiency should be treated with replacement glucocorticoids prior to initiation of treatment with levothyroxine sodium. Failure to do so may precipitate an acute adrenal crisis when thyroid hormone therapy is initiated, due to increased metabolic clearance of glucocorticoids by thyroid hormone. Patients with diabetes mellitus may require upward adjustments of their antidiabetic therapeutic regimens when treated with levothyroxine (see **PRECAUTIONS, Drug Interactions**).

Other associated medical conditions

Infants with congenital hypothyroidism appear to be at increased risk for other congenital anomalies, with cardiovascular anomalies (pulmonary stenosis, atrial septal defect, and ventricular septal defect) being the most common association.

Information for Patients

Patients should be informed of the following information to aid in the safe and effective use of LEVOTHROID®:

1. Notify your physician if you are allergic to any foods or medicines, are pregnant or intend to become pregnant, are breast-feeding or are taking any other medications, including prescription and over-the-counter preparations.
2. Notify your physician of any other medical conditions you may have, particularly heart disease, diabetes, clotting disorders, and adrenal or pituitary gland problems. Your dose of medications used to control these other conditions may need to be adjusted while you are taking LEVOTHROID®. If you have diabetes, monitor your blood and/or urinary glucose levels as directed by your physician and immediately report any changes to your physician. If you are taking anticoagulants (blood thinners), your clotting status should be checked frequently.
3. Use LEVOTHROID® only as prescribed by your physician. Do not discontinue or change the amount you take or how often you take it, unless directed to do so by your physician.
4. The levothyroxine in LEVOTHROID® is intended to replace a hormone that is normally produced by your thyroid gland. Generally, replacement therapy is to be taken for life, except in cases of transient hypothyroidism, which is usually associated with an inflammation of the thyroid gland (thyroiditis).
5. Take LEVOTHROID® as a single dose, preferably on an empty stomach, one-half to one hour before breakfast. Levothyroxine absorption is increased on an empty stomach.
6. It may take several weeks before you notice an improvement in your symptoms.
7. Notify your physician if you experience any of the following symptoms: rapid or irregular heartbeat, chest pain, shortness of breath, leg cramps, headache, nervousness, irritability, sleeplessness, tremors, change in appetite, weight gain or loss, vomiting, diarrhea, excessive sweating, heat intolerance, fever, changes in menstrual periods, hives or skin rash, or any other unusual medical event.
8. Notify your physician if you become pregnant while taking LEVOTHROID®. It is likely that your dose of LEVOTHROID® will need to be increased while you are pregnant
9. Notify your physician or dentist that you are taking LEVOTHROID® prior to any surgery.
10. Partial hair loss may occur rarely during the first few months of LEVOTHROID® therapy, but this is usually temporary.
11. LEVOTHROID® should not be used as a primary or adjunctive therapy in a weight control program.
12. Keep LEVOTHROID® out of the reach of children. Store LEVOTHROID® away from heat, moisture, and light.

Laboratory Tests

General

The diagnosis of hypothyroidism is confirmed by measuring TSH levels using a sensitive assay (second generation assay sensitivity ≤0.1 mIU/L or third generation assay sensitivity ≤0.01 mIU/L) and measurement of free-T_4.

The adequacy of therapy is determined by periodic assessment of appropriate laboratory tests and clinical evaluation. The choice of laboratory tests depends on various factors including the etiology of the underlying thyroid disease, the presence of concomitant medical conditions, including pregnancy, and the use of concomitant medications (see **PRECAUTIONS, Drug Interactions** and **Drug-Laboratory Test Interactions**). Persistent clinical and laboratory evidence of hypothyroidism despite an apparent adequate replacement dose of LEVOTHROID® may be evidence of inadequate absorption, poor compliance, drug interactions, or decreased T_4 potency of the drug product.

Adults

In adult patients with primary (thyroidal) hypothyroidism, serum TSH levels (using a sensitive assay) alone may be used to monitor therapy. The frequency of TSH monitoring during levothyroxine dose titration depends on the clinical

Continued on next page

Levothroid—Cont.

situation but it is generally recommended at 6-8 week intervals until normalization. For patients who have recently initiated levothyroxine therapy and whose serum TSH has normalized or in patients who have had their dosage or brand of levothyroxine changed, the serum TSH concentration should be measured after 8-12 weeks. When the optimum replacement dose has been attained, clinical (physical examination) and biochemical monitoring may be performed every 6-12 months, depending on the clinical situation, and whenever there is a change in the patient's status. It is recommended that a physical examination and a serum TSH measurement be performed at least annually in patients receiving LEVOTHROID® (see **WARNINGS, PRECAUTIONS,** and **DOSAGE AND ADMINISTRATION**).

Pediatrics

In patients with congenital hypothyroidism, the adequacy of replacement therapy should be assessed by measuring both serum TSH (using a sensitive assay) and total- or free-T_4. During the first three years of life, the serum total- or free-T_4 should be maintained at all times in the upper half of the normal range. While the aim of therapy is to also normalize the serum TSH level, this is not always possible in a small percentage of patients, particularly in the first few months of therapy. TSH may not normalize due to a resetting of the pituitary-thyroid feedback threshold as a result of *in utero* hypothyroidism. Failure of the serum T_4 to increase into the upper half of the normal range within 2 weeks of initiation of LEVOTHROID® therapy and/or of the serum TSH to decrease below 20mU/L within 4 weeks should alert the physician to the possibility that the child is not receiving adequate therapy. Careful inquiry should then be made regarding compliance, dose of medication administered, and method of administration prior to raising the dose of LEVOTHROID®.

The recommended frequency of monitoring of TSH and total- or free-T_4 in children is as follows: at 2 and 4 weeks after the initiation of treatment; every 1-2 months during the first year of life; every 2-3 months between 1 and 3 years of age; and every 3 to 12 months thereafter until growth is completed. More frequent intervals of monitoring may be necessary if poor compliance is suspected or abnormal values are obtained. It is recommended that TSH and T_4 levels, and a physical examination, if indicated, be performed 2 weeks after any change in LEVOTHROID® dosage. Routine clinical examination, including assessment of mental and physical growth and development, and bone maturation, should be performed at regular intervals (see **PRECAUTIONS, Pediatric Use** and **DOSAGE AND ADMINISTRATION**).

Secondary (pituitary) and tertiary (hypothalamic) hypothyroidism

Adequacy of therapy should be assessed by measuring serum free-T_4 levels, which should be maintained in the upper half of the normal range in these patients.

Drug Interactions

Many drugs affect thyroid hormone pharmacokinetics and metabolism (e.g., absorption, synthesis, secretion, catabolism, protein binding, and target tissue response) and may alter the therapeutic response to LEVOTHROID®. In addition, thyroid hormones and thyroid status have varied effects on the pharmacokinetics and actions of other drugs. A listing of drug-thyroidal axis interactions is contained in Table 2.

The list of drug-thyroidal axis interactions in Table 2 may not be comprehensive due to the introduction of new drugs that interact with the thyroidal axis or the discovery of previously unknown interactions. The prescriber should be aware of this fact and should consult appropriate reference sources (e.g., package inserts of newly approved drugs, medical literature) for additional information if a drug-drug interaction with levothyroxine is suspected.

[See table 2 on pages 174 and 175]

Oral anticoagulants - Levothyroxine increases the response to oral anticoagulant therapy. Therefore, a decrease in the dose of anticoagulant may be warranted with correction of the hypothyroid state or when the LEVOTHROID® dose is increased. Prothrombin time should be closely monitored to permit appropriate and timely dosage adjustments (see **Table 2**).

Digitalis glycosides - The therapeutic effects of digitalis glycosides may be reduced by levothyroxine. Serum digitalis glycoside levels may be decreased when a hypothyroid patient becomes euthyroid, necessitating an increase in the dose of digitalis glycosides (see **Table 2**).

Drug-Food Interactions - Consumption of certain foods may affect levothyroxine absorption thereby necessitating adjustments in dosing. Soybean flour (infant formula), cotton seed meal, walnuts, and dietary fiber may bind and decrease the absorption of levothyroxine sodium from the GI tract.

Drug-Laboratory Test Interactions - Changes in TBG concentration must be considered when interpreting T_4 and T_3 values, which necessitates measurement and evaluation of unbound (free) hormone and/or determination of the free-T_4 index (FT_4I). Pregnancy, infectious hepatitis, estrogens, estrogen-containing oral contraceptives, and acute intermittent porphyria increase TBG concentrations. Decreases in TBG concentrations are observed in nephrosis, severe hypoproteinemia, severe liver disease, acromegaly, and after androgen or corticosteroid therapy (see also **Table 2**). Familial hyper- or hypo-thyroxine binding globulinemias have been described, with the incidence of TBG deficiency approximating 1 in 9000.

Carcinogenesis, Mutagenesis, and Impairment of Fertility - Animal studies have not been performed to evaluate the carcinogenic potential, mutagenic potential or effects on fertility of levothyroxine. The synthetic T_4 in LEVOTHROID® is identical to that produced naturally by the human thyroid gland. Although there has been a reported association between prolonged thyroid hormone therapy and breast cancer, this has not been confirmed. Patients receiving LEVOTHROID® for appropriate clinical indications should be titrated to the lowest effective replacement dose.

Pregnancy - Category A - Studies in women taking levothyroxine sodium during pregnancy have not shown an increased risk of congenital abnormalities. Therefore, the possibility of fetal harm appears remote. LEVOTHROID® should not be discontinued during pregnancy and hypothyroidism diagnosed during pregnancy should be promptly treated.

Hypothyroidism during pregnancy is associated with a higher rate of complications, including spontaneous abortion, pre-eclampsia, stillbirth and premature delivery. Maternal hypothyroidism may have an adverse effect on fetal and childhood growth and development. During pregnancy, serum T_4 levels may decrease and serum TSH levels increase to values outside the normal range. Since elevations in serum TSH may occur as early as 4 weeks gestation, pregnant women taking LEVOTHROID® should have their TSH measured during each trimester. An elevated serum TSH level should be corrected by an increase in the dose of LEVOTHROID®. Since postpartum TSH levels are similar to preconception values, the LEVOTHROID® dosage should return to the pre-pregnancy dose immediately after delivery. A serum TSH level should be obtained 6-8 weeks postpartum.

Thyroid hormones cross the placental barrier to some extent as evidenced by levels in cord blood of athyreotic fetuses being approximately one-third maternal levels. Transfer of thyroid hormone from the mother to the fetus, however, may not be adequate to prevent *in utero* hypothyroidism.

Nursing Mothers - Although thyroid hormones are excreted only minimally in human milk, caution should be exercised when LEVOTHROID® is administered to a nursing woman. However, adequate replacement doses of levothyroxine are generally needed to maintain normal lactation.

Pediatric Use

General

The goal of treatment in pediatric patients with hypothyroidism is to achieve and maintain normal intellectual and physical growth and development.

The initial dose of levothyroxine varies with age and body weight (see **DOSAGE AND ADMINISTRATION, Table 3**). Dosing adjustments are based on an assessment of the individual patient's clinical and laboratory parameters (see **PRECAUTIONS, Laboratory Tests**).

In children in whom a diagnosis of permanent hypothyroidism has not been established, it is recommended that levothyroxine administration be discontinued for a 30-day trial period, but only after the child is at least 3 years of age. Serum T_4 and TSH levels should then be obtained. If the T_4 is low and the TSH high, the diagnosis of permanent hypothyroidism is established, and levothyroxine therapy should be reinstituted. If the T_4 and TSH levels are normal, euthyroidism may be assumed and, therefore, the hypothyroidism can be considered to have been transient. In this instance, however, the physician should carefully monitor the child and repeat the thyroid function tests if any signs or symptoms of hypothyroidism develop. In this setting, the clinician should have a high index of suspicion of relapse. If the results of the levothyroxine withdrawal test are inconclusive, careful follow-up and subsequent testing will be necessary.

Since some more severely affected children may become clinically hypothyroid when treatment is discontinued for 30 days, an alternate approach is to reduce the replacement dose of levothyroxine by half during the 30-day trial period. If, after 30 days, the serum TSH is elevated above 20 mU/L, the diagnosis of permanent hypothyroidism is confirmed, and full replacement therapy should be resumed. However, if the serum TSH has not risen to greater than 20 mU/L, levothyroxine treatment should be discontinued for another 30-day trial period followed by repeat serum T_4 and TSH testing.

The presence of concomitant medical conditions should be considered in certain clinical circumstances and, if present, appropriately treated (see **PRECAUTIONS**).

Congenital Hypothyroidism (see **PRECAUTIONS, Laboratory Tests** and **DOSAGE AND ADMINISTRATION**)

Rapid restoration of normal serum T_4 concentrations is essential for preventing the adverse effects of congenital hypothyroidism on intellectual development as well as on overall physical growth and maturation. Therefore, LEVOTHROID® therapy should be initiated immediately upon diagnosis and is generally continued for life.

During the first 2 weeks of LEVOTHROID® therapy, infants should be closely monitored for cardiac overload, arrhythmias, and aspiration from avid suckling.

The patient should be monitored closely to avoid undertreatment or overtreatment. Undertreatment may have deleterious effects on intellectual development and linear growth. Overtreatment has been associated with craniosynostosis in infants, and may adversely affect the tempo of brain maturation and accelerate the bone age with resultant premature closure of the epiphyses and compromised adult stature.

Acquired Hypothyroidism in Pediatric Patients

The patient should be monitored closely to avoid undertreatment and overtreatment. Undertreatment may result in poor school performance due to impaired concentration and slowed mentation and in reduced adult height. Overtreatment may accelerate the bone age and result in premature epiphyseal closure and compromised adult stature.

Treated children may manifest a period of catch-up growth, which may be adequate in some cases to normalize adult height. In children with severe or prolonged hypothyroidism, catch-up growth may not be adequate to normalize adult height.

Geriatric Use

Because of the increased prevalence of cardiovascular disease among the elderly, levothyroxine therapy should not be initiated at the full replacement dose (see **WARNINGS, PRECAUTIONS,** and **DOSAGE AND ADMINISTRATION**).

ADVERSE REACTIONS

Adverse reactions associated with levothyroxine therapy are primarily those of hyperthyroidism due to therapeutic overdosage (see **PRECAUTIONS** and **OVERDOSAGE**). They include the following:

General: fatigue, increased appetite, weight loss, heat intolerance, fever, excessive sweating;

Central nervous system: headache, hyperactivity, nervousness, anxiety, irritability, emotional lability, insomnia;

Musculoskeletal: tremors, muscle weakness;

Cardiovascular: palpitations, tachycardia, arrhythmias, increased pulse and blood pressure, heart failure, angina, myocardial infarction, cardiac arrest;

Respiratory: dyspnea;

Gastrointestinal: diarrhea, vomiting, abdominal cramps and elevations in liver function tests;

Dermatologic: hair loss, flushing;

Endocrine: decreased bone mineral density;

Reproductive: menstrual irregularities, impaired fertility.

Pseudotumor cerebri and slipped capital femoral epiphysis have been reported in children receiving levothyroxine therapy. Overtreatment may result in craniosynostosis in infants and premature closure of the epiphyses in children with resultant compromised adult height.

Seizures have been reported rarely with the institution of levothyroxine therapy.

Inadequate levothyroxine dosage will produce or fail to ameliorate the signs and symptoms of hypothyroidism.

Hypersensitivity reactions to inactive ingredients have occurred in patients treated with thyroid hormone products. These include urticaria, pruritus, skin rash, flushing, angioedema, various GI symptoms (abdominal pain, nausea, vomiting and diarrhea), fever, arthralgia, serum sickness and wheezing. Hypersensitivity to levothyroxine itself is not known to occur.

OVERDOSAGE

The signs and symptoms of overdosage are those of hyperthyroidism (see **PRECAUTIONS** and **ADVERSE REACTIONS**). In addition, confusion and disorientation may occur. Cerebral embolism, shock, coma, and death have been reported. Seizures have occurred in a child ingesting 18 mg of levothyroxine. Symptoms may not necessarily be evident or may not appear until several days after ingestion of levothyroxine sodium.

Treatment of Overdosage

Levothyroxine sodium should be reduced in dose or temporarily discontinued if signs or symptoms of overdosage occur.

Acute Massive Overdosage - This may be a life-threatening emergency, therefore, symptomatic and supportive therapy should be instituted immediately. If not contraindicated (e.g., by seizures, coma, or loss of the gag reflex), the stomach should be emptied by emesis or gastric lavage to decrease gastrointestinal absorption. Activated charcoal or cholestyramine may also be used to decrease absorption. Central and peripheral increased sympathetic activity may be treated by administering β-receptor antagonists, e.g., propranolol, provided there are no medical contraindications to their use. Provide respiratory support as needed; control congestive heart failure and arrhythmia; control fever, hypoglycemia, and fluid loss as necessary. Large doses of antithyroid drugs (e.g., methimazole or propylthiouracil) followed in one to two hours by large doses of iodine may be given to inhibit synthesis and release of thyroid hormones. Glucocorticoids may be given to inhibit the conversion of T_4 to T_3. Plasmapheresis, charcoal hemoperfusion and exchange transfusion have been reserved for cases in which continued clinical deterioration occurs despite conventional therapy. Because T_4 is highly protein bound, very little drug will be removed by dialysis.

DOSAGE AND ADMINISTRATION

General Principles

The goal of replacement therapy is to achieve and maintain a clinical and biochemical euthyroid state. The goal of suppressive therapy is to inhibit growth and/or function of abnormal thyroid tissue. The dose of LEVOTHROID® that is adequate to achieve these goals depends on a variety of factors including the patient's age, body weight, cardiovascular status, concomitant medical conditions, including pregnancy, concomitant medications, and the specific nature of the condition being treated (see **WARNINGS** and **PRECAUTIONS**). Hence, the following recommendations serve only as dosing guidelines. Dosing must be individualized and adjustments made based on periodic assessment of the patient's clinical response and laboratory parameters (see **PRECAUTIONS, Laboratory Tests**).

LEVOTHROID® is administered as a single daily dose, preferably one-half to one hour before breakfast. LEVOTHROID® should be taken at least 4 hours apart from drugs that are known to interfere with its absorption (see **PRECAUTIONS, Drug Interactions**).

Due to the long half-life of levothyroxine, the peak therapeutic effect at a given dose of levothyroxine sodium may not be attained for 4-6 weeks.

Caution should be exercised when administering LEVOTHROID® to patients with underlying cardiovascular disease, to the elderly, and to those with concomitant adrenal insufficiency (see **PRECAUTIONS**).

Specific Patient Populations

Hypothyroidism in Adults and in Children in Whom Growth and Puberty are Complete (see **WARNINGS** and **PRECAUTIONS, Laboratory Tests**)

Therapy may begin at full replacement doses in otherwise healthy individuals less than 50 years old and in those older than 50 years who have been recently treated for hyperthyroidism or who have been hypothyroid for only a short time (such as a few months). The average full replacement dose of levothyroxine sodium is approximately 1.7 mcg/kg/day (e.g., **100-125 mcg/day** for a 70 kg adult). Older patients may require less than 1 mcg/kg/day. Levothyroxine sodium doses greater than 200 mcg/day are seldom required. An inadequate response to daily doses ≥300 mcg/day is rare and may indicate poor compliance, malabsorption, and/or drug interactions.

For most patients older than 50 years or for patients under 50 years of age with underlying cardiac disease, an initial starting dose of **25-50 mcg/day** of levothyroxine sodium is recommended, with gradual increments in dose at 6-8 week intervals, as needed. The recommended starting dose of levothyroxine sodium in elderly patients with cardiac disease is **12.5-25 mcg/day**, with gradual dose increments at 4-6 week intervals. The levothyroxine sodium dose is generally adjusted in 12.5-25 mcg increments until the patient with primary hypothyroidism is clinically euthyroid and the serum TSH has normalized.

In patients with severe hypothyroidism, the recommended initial levothyroxine sodium dose is **12.5-25 mcg/day** with increases of 25 mcg/day every 2-4 weeks, accompanied by clinical and laboratory assessment, until the TSH level is normalized.

In patients with secondary (pituitary) or tertiary (hypothalamic) hypothyroidism, the levothyroxine sodium dose should be titrated until the patient is clinically euthyroid and the serum free-T_4 level is restored to the upper half of the normal range.

Pediatric Dosage - Congenital or Acquired Hypothyroidism (see **PRECAUTIONS, Laboratory Tests**)

General Principles

In general, levothyroxine therapy should be instituted at full replacement doses as soon as possible. Delays in diagnosis and institution of therapy may have deleterious effects on the child's intellectual and physical growth and development.

Undertreatment and overtreatment should be avoided (see **PRECAUTIONS, Pediatric Use**). LEVOTHROID® may be administered to infants and children who cannot swallow intact tablets by crushing the tablet and suspending the freshly crushed tablet in a small amount (5-10 mL or 1-2 teaspoons) of water. This suspension can be administered by spoon or dropper. **DO NOT STORE THE SUSPENSION.** Foods that decrease absorption of levothyroxine, such as soybean infant formula, should not be used for administering levothyroxine sodium tablets (see **PRECAUTIONS, Drug-Food Interactions**).

Newborns

The recommended starting dose of levothyroxine sodium in newborn infants is **10-15 mcg/kg/day**. A lower starting dose (e.g., 25 mcg/day) should be considered in infants at risk for cardiac failure, and the dose should be increased in 4-6 weeks as needed based on clinical and laboratory response to treatment. In infants with very low (<5 mcg/dL) or undetectable serum T_4 concentrations, the recommended initial starting dose is **50 mcg/day** of levothyroxine sodium.

Infants and Children

Levothyroxine therapy is usually initiated at full replacement doses, with the recommended dose per body weight decreasing with age (see **Table 3**). However, in children with chronic or severe hypothyroidism, an initial dose of **25 mcg/day** of levothyroxine sodium is recommended with increments of 25 mcg every 2-4 weeks until the desired effect is achieved.

Hyperactivity in an older child can be minimized if the starting dose is one-fourth of the recommended full replacement dose, and the dose is then increased on a weekly basis by an amount equal to one-fourth the full-recommended replacement dose until the full recommended replacement dose is reached.

Table 3: Levothyroxine Sodium Dosing Guidelines for Pediatric Hypothyroidism

AGE	Daily Dose Per Kg Body Weight[a]
0-3 months	10-15 mcg/kg/day
3-6 months	8-10 mcg/kg/day
6-12 months	6-8 mcg/kg/day
1-5 years	5-6 mcg/kg/day
6-12 years	4-5 mcg/kg/day
>12 years but growth and puberty incomplete	2-3 mcg/kg/day
Growth and puberty complete	1.7 mcg/kg/day

[a] The dose should be adjusted based on clinical response and laboratory parameters (see **PRECAUTIONS, Laboratory Tests** and **Pediatric Use**).

Pregnancy - Pregnancy may increase levothyroxine requirements (see **Pregnancy**).

Subclinical Hypothyroidism - If this condition is treated, a lower levothyroxine sodium dose (e.g., **1 mcg/kg/day**) than that used for full replacement may be adequate to normalize the serum TSH level. Patients who are not treated should be monitored yearly for changes in clinical status and thyroid laboratory parameters.

TSH Suppression in Well-differentiated Thyroid Cancer and Thyroid Nodules-The target level for TSH suppression in these conditions has not been established with controlled studies. In addition, the efficacy of TSH suppression for benign nodular disease is controversial. Therefore, the dose of LEVOTHROID® used for TSH suppression should be individualized based on the specific disease and the patient being treated.

In the treatment of well-differentiated (papillary and follicular) thyroid cancer, levothyroxine is used as an adjunct to surgery and radioiodine therapy. Generally, TSH is suppressed to <0.1 mU/L, and this usually requires a levothyroxine sodium dose of **greater than 2 mcg/kg/day**. However, in patients with high-risk tumors, the target level for TSH suppression may be <0.01 mU/L.

In the treatment of benign nodules and nontoxic multinodular goiter, TSH is generally suppressed to a higher target (e.g., 0.1 to either 0.5 or 1.0 mU/L) than that used for the treatment of thyroid cancer. Levothyroxine sodium is contraindicated if the serum TSH is already suppressed due to the risk of precipitating overt thyrotoxicosis (see **CONTRAINDICATIONS, WARNINGS** and **PRECAUTIONS**).

Myxedema Coma - Myxedema coma is a life-threatening emergency characterized by poor circulation and hypometabolism, and may result in unpredictable absorption of levothyroxine sodium from the gastrointestinal tract. Therefore, oral thyroid hormone drug products are not recommended to treat this condition. Thyroid hormone drug products formulated for intravenous administration should be administered.

HOW SUPPLIED

LEVOTHROID® (levothyroxine sodium tablets, USP) are caplet-shaped, color-coded, potency marked tablets and are supplied as follows:

Strength (mcg)	Color	NDC # for bottles of 100	NDC # for bottles of 1000
25	Orange	NDC 0456-1320-01	NDC 0456-1320-00
50	White	NDC 0456-1321-01	NDC 0456-1321-00
75	Violet	NDC 0456-1322-01	NDC 0456-1322-00
88	Mint Green	NDC 0456-1329-01	NDC 0456-1329-00
100	Yellow	NDC 0456-1323-01	NDC 0456-1323-00
112	Rose	NDC 0456-1330-01	NDC 0456-1330-00
125	Brown	NDC 0456-1324-01	NDC 0456-1324-00
150	Blue	NDC 0456-1325-01	NDC 0456-1325-00
175	Lilac	NDC 0456-1326-01	NDC 0456-1326-00
200	Pink	NDC 0456-1327-01	NDC 0456-1327-00
300	Green	NDC 0456-1328-01	NDC 0456-1328-00

STORAGE CONDITIONS

Store at 25°C (77°F) with excursions permitted to 15-30°C (59°-86°F).

Protect from moisture and light.

Manufactured for:

Forest Pharmaceuticals, Inc.
Subsidiary of Forest Laboratories, Inc.
St. Louis, Missouri, 63045

by:

Lloyd Pharmaceutical
Division of Lloyd, Inc.
Shenandoah, IA 51601

9/03 MG #19006

LEXAPRO™ ℞

[*lĕks'ă-prō*]

(escitalopram oxalate)
TABLETS/ORAL SOLUTION
Rx Only

Prescribing information for this product, which appears on pages 1302–1306 of the 2004 PDR, has been completely revised as follows. Please write "See Supplement A" next to the product heading.

DESCRIPTION

LEXAPRO™ (escitalopram oxalate) is an orally administered selective serotonin reuptake inhibitor (SSRI). Escitalopram is the pure S-enantiomer (single isomer) of the racemic bicyclic phthalane derivative citalopram. Escitalopram oxalate is designated S-(+)-1-[3-(dimethyl-amino)propyl]-1-(*p*-fluorophenyl)-5-phthalancarbonitrile oxalate with the following structural formula:

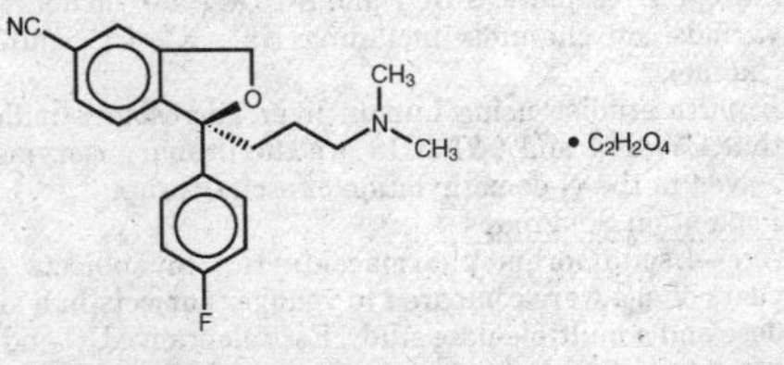

The molecular formula is $C_{20}H_{21}FN_2O$ • $C_2H_2O_4$ and the molecular weight is 414.40.

Escitalopram oxalate occurs as a fine white to slightly yellow powder and is freely soluble in methanol and dimethyl sulfoxide (DMSO), soluble in isotonic saline solution, sparingly soluble in water and ethanol, slightly soluble in ethyl acetate, and insoluble in heptane.

LEXAPRO (escitalopram oxalate) is available as tablets or as an oral solution.

LEXAPRO tablets are film coated, round tablets containing escitalopram oxalate in strengths equivalent to 5 mg, 10 mg and 20 mg escitalopram base. The 10 and 20 mg tablets are scored. The tablets also contain the following inactive ingredients: talc, croscarmellose sodium, microcrystalline cellulose/colloidal silicon dioxide, and magnesium stearate. The film coating contains hypromellose, titanium dioxide, and polyethylene glycol.

LEXAPRO oral solution contains escitalopram oxalate equivalent to 1 mg/mL escitalopram base. It also contains the following inactive ingredients: sorbitol, purified water, citric acid, sodium citrate, malic acid, glycerin, propylene glycol, methylparaben, propylparaben, and natural peppermint flavor.

CLINICAL PHARMACOLOGY

Pharmacodynamics

The mechanism of antidepressant action of escitalopram, the S-enantiomer of racemic citalopram, is presumed to be linked to potentiation of serotonergic activity in the central nervous system resulting from its inhibition of CNS neuronal reuptake of serotonin (5-HT). *In vitro* and *in vivo* studies in animals suggest that escitalopram is a highly selective serotonin reuptake inhibitor (SSRI) with minimal effects on norepinephrine and dopamine neuronal reuptake. Escitalopram is at least 100 fold more potent than the R-enantiomer with respect to inhibition of 5-HT reuptake and inhibition of 5-HT neuronal firing rate. Tolerance to a model of antidepressant effect in rats was not induced by long-term (up to 5 weeks) treatment with escitalopram. Escitalopram has no or very low affinity for serotonergic ($5\text{-}HT_{1-7}$) or other receptors including alpha- and beta-adrenergic, dopamine (D_{1-5}), histamine (H_{1-3}), muscarinic (M_{1-5}), and benzodiazepine receptors. Escitalopram also does not bind to or has low affinity for various ion channels including Na^+, K^+, Cl^- and Ca^{++} channels. Antagonism of muscarinic, histaminergic, and adrenergic receptors has been hypothesized to be associated with various anticholinergic, sedative, and cardiovascular side effects of other psychotropic drugs.

Pharmacokinetics

The single- and multiple-dose pharmacokinetics of escitalopram are linear and dose-proportional in a dose range of 10 to 30 mg/day. Biotransformation of escitalopram is mainly hepatic, with a mean terminal half-life of about 27-32 hours. With once daily dosing, steady state plasma concentrations are achieved within approximately one week. At steady state, the extent of accumulation of escitalopram in plasma in young healthy subjects was 2.2-2.5 times the plasma concentrations observed after a single dose. The tablet and the oral solution dosage forms of escitalopram oxalate are bioequivalent.

Absorption and Distribution

Following a single oral dose (20 mg tablet or solution) of escitalopram, peak blood levels occur at about 5 hours. Absorption of escitalopram is not affected by food.

Continued on next page

Lexapro—Cont.

The absolute bioavailability of citalopram is about 80% relative to an intravenous dose, and the volume of distribution of citalopram is about 12 L/kg. Data specific on escitalopram are unavailable.
The binding of escitalopram to human plasma proteins is approximately 56%.

Metabolism and Elimination

Following oral administrations of escitalopram, the fraction of drug recovered in the urine as escitalopram and S-demethylcitalopram (S-DCT) is about 8% and 10%, respectively. The oral clearance of escitalopram is 600 mL/min, with approximately 7% of that due to renal clearance.
Escitalopram is metabolized to S-DCT and S-didemethylcitalopram (S-DDCT). In humans, unchanged escitalopram is the predominant compound in plasma. At steady state, the concentration of the escitalopram metabolite S-DCT in plasma is approximately one-third that of escitalopram. The level of S-DDCT was not detectable in most subjects. *In vitro* studies show that escitalopram is at least 7 and 27 times more potent than S-DCT and S-DDCT, respectively, in the inhibition of serotonin reuptake, suggesting that the metabolites of escitalopram do not contribute significantly to the antidepressant actions of escitalopram. S-DCT and S-DDCT also have no or very low affinity for serotonergic ($5\text{-}HT_{1-7}$) or other receptors including alpha- and beta- adrenergic, dopamine (D_{1-5}), histamine (H_{1-3}), muscarinic (M_{1-5}), and benzodiazepine receptors. S-DCT and S-DDCT also do not bind to various ion channels including Na^+, K^+, Cl^- and Ca^{++} channels.
In vitro studies using human liver microsomes indicated that CYP3A4 and CYP2C19 are the primary isozymes involved in the N-demethylation of escitalopram.

Population Subgroups

Age—Escitalopram pharmacokinetics in subjects ≥ 65 years of age were compared to younger subjects in a single-dose and a multiple-dose study. Escitalopram AUC and half-life were increased by approximately 50% in elderly subjects, and C_{max} was unchanged. 10 mg is the recommended dose for elderly patients (see Dosage and Administration).
Gender—In a multiple-dose study of escitalopram (10 mg/day for 3 weeks) in 18 male (9 elderly and 9 young) and 18 female (9 elderly and 9 young) subjects, there were no differences in AUC, C_{max}, and half-life between the male and female subjects. No adjustment of dosage on the basis of gender is needed.
Reduced hepatic function—Citalopram oral clearance was reduced by 37% and half-life was doubled in patients with reduced hepatic function compared to normal subjects. 10 mg is the recommended dose of escitalopram for most hepatically impaired patients (see Dosage and Administration).
Reduced renal function—In patients with mild to moderate renal function impairment, oral clearance of citalopram was reduced by 17% compared to normal subjects. No adjustment of dosage for such patients is recommended. No information is available about the pharmacokinetics of escitalopram in patients with severely reduced renal function (creatinine clearance < 20 mL/min).

Drug-Drug Interactions

In vitro enzyme inhibition data did not reveal an inhibitory effect of escitalopram on CYP3A4, -1A2, -2C9, -2C19, and -2E1. Based on *in vitro* data, escitalopram would be expected to have little inhibitory effect on *in vivo* metabolism mediated by these cytochromes. While *in vivo* data to address this question are limited, results from drug interaction studies suggest that escitalopram, at a dose of 20 mg, has no 3A4 inhibitory effect and a modest 2D6 inhibitory effect. See Drug Interactions under Precautions for more detailed information on available drug interaction data.

Clinical Efficacy Trials

Major Depressive Disorder

The efficacy of LEXAPRO as a treatment for major depressive disorder was established in three, 8-week, placebo-controlled studies conducted in outpatients between 18 and 65 years of age who met DSM-IV criteria for major depressive disorder. The primary outcome in all three studies was change from baseline to endpoint in the Montgomery Asberg Depression Rating Scale (MADRS).
A fixed-dose study compared 10 mg/day LEXAPRO and 20 mg/day LEXAPRO to placebo and 40 mg/day citalopram. The 10 mg/day and 20 mg/day LEXAPRO treatment groups showed significantly greater mean improvement compared to placebo on the MADRS. The 10 mg and 20 mg LEXAPRO groups were similar on this outcome measure.
In a second fixed-dose study of 10 mg/day LEXAPRO and placebo, the 10 mg/day LEXAPRO treatment group showed significantly greater mean improvement compared to placebo on the MADRS.
In a flexible-dose study, comparing LEXAPRO, titrated between 10 and 20 mg/day, to placebo and citalopram, titrated between 20 and 40 mg/day, the LEXAPRO treatment group showed significantly greater mean improvement compared to placebo on the MADRS.
Analyses of the relationship between treatment outcome and age, gender, and race did not suggest any differential responsiveness on the basis of these patient characteristics.
In a longer-term trial, 274 patients meeting (DSM-IV) criteria for major depressive disorder, who had responded during an initial 8-week, open-label treatment phase with LEXAPRO 10 or 20 mg/day, were randomized to continuation of LEXAPRO at their same dose, or to placebo, for up to 36 weeks of observation for relapse. Response during the open label phase was defined by having a decrease of the MADRS total score to ≤ 12. Relapse during the double-blind phase was defined as an increase of the MADRS total score to ≥ 22, or discontinuation due to insufficient clinical response. Patients receiving continued LEXAPRO experienced a significantly longer time to relapse over the subsequent 36 weeks compared to those receiving placebo.

Generalized Anxiety Disorder

The efficacy of LEXAPRO in the treatment of Generalized Anxiety Disorder (GAD) was demonstrated in three, 8-week, multicenter, flexible-dose, placebo-controlled studies that compared LEXAPRO 10-20 mg/day to placebo in outpatients between 18 and 80 years of age who met DSM-IV criteria for GAD. In all three studies, LEXAPRO showed significantly greater mean improvement compared to placebo on the Hamilton Anxiety Scale (HAM-A).
There were too few patients in differing ethnic and age groups to adequately assess whether or not LEXAPRO has differential effects in these groups. There was no difference in response to LEXAPRO between men and women.

INDICATIONS AND USAGE

Major Depressive Disorder

LEXAPRO (escitalopram) is indicated for the treatment of major depressive disorder.
The efficacy of LEXAPRO in the treatment of major depressive disorder was established in three, 8-week, placebo-controlled trials of outpatients whose diagnoses corresponded most closely to the DSM-IV category of major depressive disorder (see Clinical Pharmacology).
A major depressive episode (DSM-IV) implies a prominent and relatively persistent (nearly every day for at least 2 weeks) depressed or dysphoric mood that usually interferes with daily functioning, and includes at least five of the following nine symptoms: depressed mood, loss of interest in usual activities, significant change in weight and/or appetite, insomnia or hypersomnia, psychomotor agitation or retardation, increased fatigue, feelings of guilt or worthlessness, slowed thinking or impaired concentration, a suicide attempt or suicidal ideation.
The efficacy of LEXAPRO in hospitalized patients with major depressive disorders has not been adequately studied.
The efficacy of LEXAPRO in maintaining a response, in patients with major depressive disorder who responded during an 8-week, acute-treatment phase while taking LEXAPRO and were then observed for relapse during a period of up to 36 weeks, was demonstrated in a placebo-controlled trial (see Clinical Efficacy Trials, under Clinical Pharmacology). Nevertheless, the physician who elects to use LEXAPRO for extended periods should periodically re-evaluate the long-term usefulness of the drug for the individual patient (see Dosage and Administration).

Generalized Anxiety Disorder

LEXAPRO is indicated for the treatment of Generalized Anxiety Disorder (GAD).
The efficacy of LEXAPRO was established in three, 8-week, placebo-controlled trials in patients with GAD (see Clinical Pharmacology).
Generalized Anxiety Disorder (DSM-IV) is characterized by excessive anxiety and worry (apprehensive expectation) that is persistent for at least 6 months and which the person finds difficult to control. It must be associated with at least 3 of the following symptoms: restlessness or feeling keyed up or on edge, being easily fatigued, difficulty concentrating or mind going blank, irritability, muscle tension, and sleep disturbance.
The efficacy of LEXAPRO in the long-term treatment of GAD, that is, for more than 8 weeks, has not been systematically evaluated in controlled trials. The physician who elects to use LEXAPRO for extended periods should periodically re-evaluate the long-term usefulness of the drug for the individual patient.

CONTRAINDICATIONS

Concomitant use in patients taking monoamine oxidase inhibitors (MAOIs) is contraindicated (see Warnings).
LEXAPRO is contraindicated in patients with a hypersensitivity to escitalopram or citalopram or any of the inactive ingredients in LEXAPRO.

WARNINGS

Potential for Interaction with Monoamine Oxidase Inhibitors

In patients receiving serotonin reuptake inhibitor drugs in combination with a monoamine oxidase inhibitor (MAOI), there have been reports of serious, sometimes fatal, reactions including hyperthermia, rigidity, myoclonus, autonomic instability with possible rapid fluctuations of vital signs, and mental status changes that include extreme agitation progressing to delirium and coma. These reactions have also been reported in patients who have recently discontinued SSRI treatment and have been started on a MAOI. Some cases presented with features resembling neuroleptic malignant syndrome. Furthermore, limited animal data on the effects of combined use of SSRIs and MAOIs suggest that these drugs may act synergistically to elevate blood pressure and evoke behavioral excitation. Therefore, it is recommended that LEXAPRO should not be used in combination with a MAOI, or within 14 days of discontinuing treatment with a MAOI. Similarly, at least 14 days should be allowed after stopping LEXAPRO before starting a MAOI.
Serotonin syndrome has been reported in two patients who were concomitantly receiving linezolid, an antibiotic which is a reversible non-selective MAOI.

PRECAUTIONS

General

Discontinuation of Treatment with LEXAPRO

During marketing of Lexapro and other SSRIs and SNRIs (Serotonin and Norepinephrine Reuptake Inhibitors), there have been spontaneous reports of adverse events occurring upon discontinuation of these drugs, particularly when abrupt, including the following: dysphoric mood, irritability, agitation, dizziness, sensory disturbances (e.g., paresthesias such as electric shock sensations), anxiety, confusion, headache, lethargy, emotional lability, insomnia, and hypomania. While these events are generally self-limiting, there have been reports of serious discontinuation symptoms.
Patients should be monitored for these symptoms when discontinuing treatment with LEXAPRO. A gradual reduction in the dose rather than abrupt cessation is recommended whenever possible. If intolerable symptoms occur following a decrease in the dose or upon discontinuation of treatment, then resuming the previously prescribed dose may be considered. Subsequently, the physician may continue decreasing the dose but at a more gradual rate (see DOSAGE AND ADMINISTRATION).

Abnormal Bleeding

Published case reports have documented the occurrence of bleeding episodes in patients treated with psychotropic drugs that interfere with serotonin reuptake. Subsequent epidemiological studies, both of the case-control and cohort design, have demonstrated an association between use of psychotropic drugs that interfere with serotonin reuptake and the occurrence of upper gastrointestinal bleeding. In two studies, concurrent use of a nonsteroidal anti-inflammatory drug (NSAID) or aspirin potentiated the risk of bleeding (see DRUG INTERACTIONS). Although these studies focused on upper gastrointestinal bleeding, there is reason to believe that bleeding at other sites may be similarly potentiated. Patients should be cautioned regarding the risk of bleeding associated with the concomitant use of LEXAPRO with NSAIDs, aspirin, or other drugs that affect coagulation.

Hyponatremia

One case of hyponatremia has been reported in association with LEXAPRO treatment. Several cases of hyponatremia or SIADH (syndrome of inappropriate antidiuretic hormone secretion) have been reported in association with racemic citalopram. All patients with these events have recovered with discontinuation of escitalopram or citalopram and/or medical intervention. Hyponatremia and SIADH have also been reported in association with other marketed drugs effective in the treatment of major depressive disorder.

Activation of Mania/Hypomania

In placebo-controlled trials of LEXAPRO in major depressive disorder, activation of mania/hypomania was reported in one (0.1%) of 715 patients treated with LEXAPRO and in none of the 592 patients treated with placebo. One additional case of hypomania has been reported in association with LEXAPRO treatment. Activation of mania/hypomania has also been reported in a small proportion of patients with major affective disorders treated with racemic citalopram and other marketed drugs effective in the treatment of major depressive disorder. As with all drugs effective in the treatment of major depressive disorder, LEXAPRO should be used cautiously in patients with a history of mania.

Seizures

Although anticonvulsant effects of racemic citalopram have been observed in animal studies, LEXAPRO has not been systematically evaluated in patients with a seizure disorder. These patients were excluded from clinical studies during the product's premarketing testing. In clinical trials of LEXAPRO, cases of convulsion have been reported in association with LEXAPRO treatment. Like other drugs effective in the treatment of major depressive disorder, LEXAPRO should be introduced with care in patients with a history of seizure disorder.

Suicide

The possibility of a suicide attempt is inherent in major depressive disorder and may persist until significant remission occurs. Close supervision of high-risk patients should accompany initial drug therapy. As with all drugs effective in the treatment of major depressive disorder, prescriptions for LEXAPRO should be written for the smallest quantity of tablets consistent with good patient management, in order to reduce the risk of overdose.

Interference with Cognitive and Motor Performance

In a study in normal volunteers, LEXAPRO 10 mg/day did not produce impairment of intellectual function or psychomotor performance. Because any psychoactive drug may impair judgment, thinking, or motor skills, however, patients should be cautioned about operating hazardous machinery, including automobiles, until they are reasonably certain that LEXAPRO therapy does not affect their ability to engage in such activities.

Use in Patients with Concomitant Illness

Clinical experience with LEXAPRO in patients with certain concomitant systemic illnesses is limited. Caution is advisable in using LEXAPRO in patients with diseases or conditions that produce altered metabolism or hemodynamic responses.
LEXAPRO has not been systematically evaluated in patients with a recent history of myocardial infarction or unstable heart disease. Patients with these diagnoses were generally excluded from clinical studies during the product's premarketing testing.
In subjects with hepatic impairment, clearance of racemic citalopram was decreased and plasma concentrations were

increased. The recommended dose of LEXAPRO in hepatically impaired patients is 10 mg/day (see Dosage and Administration).
Because escitalopram is extensively metabolized, excretion of unchanged drug in urine is a minor route of elimination. Until adequate numbers of patients with severe renal impairment have been evaluated during chronic treatment with LEXAPRO, however, it should be used with caution in such patients (see Dosage and Administration).

Information for Patients

Physicians are advised to discuss the following issues with patients for whom they prescribe LEXAPRO.
In a study in normal volunteers, LEXAPRO 10 mg/day did not impair psychomotor performance. The effect of LEXAPRO on psychomotor coordination, judgment, or thinking has not been systematically examined in controlled studies. Because psychoactive drugs may impair judgment, thinking, or motor skills, patients should be cautioned about operating hazardous machinery, including automobiles, until they are reasonably certain that LEXAPRO therapy does not affect their ability to engage in such activities.
Patients should be told that, although LEXAPRO has not been shown in experiments with normal subjects to increase the mental and motor skill impairments caused by alcohol, the concomitant use of LEXAPRO and alcohol in depressed patients is not advised.
Patients should be made aware that escitalopram is the active isomer of Celexa (citalopram hydrobromide) and that the two medications should not be taken concomitantly.
Patients should be advised to inform their physician if they are taking, or plan to take, any prescription or over-the-counter drugs, as there is a potential for interactions.
Patients should be cautioned about the concomitant use of LEXAPRO and NSAIDs, aspirin, or other drugs that affect coagulation since the combined use of psychotropic drugs that interfere with serotonin reuptake and these agents has been associated with an increased risk of bleeding.
Patients should be advised to notify their physician if they become pregnant or intend to become pregnant during therapy.
Patients should be advised to notify their physician if they are breast feeding an infant.
While patients may notice improvement with LEXAPRO therapy in 1 to 4 weeks, they should be advised to continue therapy as directed.

Laboratory Tests

There are no specific laboratory tests recommended.

Concomitant Administration with Racemic Citalopram

Citalopram—Since escitalopram is the active isomer of racemic citalopram (Celexa), the two agents should not be coadministered.

Drug Interactions

CNS Drugs—Given the primary CNS effects of escitalopram, caution should be used when it is taken in combination with other centrally acting drugs.
Alcohol—Although LEXAPRO did not potentiate the cognitive and motor effects of alcohol in a clinical trial, as with other psychotropic medications, the use of alcohol by patients taking LEXAPRO is not recommended.
Monoamine Oxidase Inhibitors (MAOIs)—See Contraindications and Warnings.

Drugs That Interfere With Hemostasis (NSAIDs, Aspirin, Warfarin, etc.)

Serotonin release by platelets plays an important role in hemostasis. Epidemiological studies of the case-control and cohort design that have demonstrated an association between use of psychotropic drugs that interfere with serotonin reuptake and the occurrence of upper gastrointestinal bleeding have also shown that concurrent use of an NSAID or aspirin potentiated the risk of bleeding. Thus, patients should be cautioned about the use of such drugs concurrently with LEXAPRO.
Cimetidine—In subjects who had received 21 days of 40 mg/day racemic citalopram, combined administration of 400 mg/day cimetidine for 8 days resulted in an increase in citalopram AUC and C_{max} of 43% and 39%, respectively. The clinical significance of these findings is unknown.
Digoxin—In subjects who had received 21 days of 40 mg/day racemic citalopram, combined administration of citalopram and digoxin (single dose of 1 mg) did not significantly affect the pharmacokinetics of either citalopram or digoxin.
Lithium—Coadministration of racemic citalopram (40 mg/day for 10 days) and lithium (30 mmol/day for 5 days) had no significant effect on the pharmacokinetics of citalopram or lithium. Nevertheless, plasma lithium levels should be monitored with appropriate adjustment to the lithium dose in accordance with standard clinical practice. Because lithium may enhance the serotonergic effects of escitalopram, caution should be exercised when LEXAPRO and lithium are coadministered.
Sumatriptan—There have been rare postmarketing reports describing patients with weakness, hyperreflexia, and incoordination following the use of a selective serotonin reuptake inhibitor (SSRI) and sumatriptan. If concomitant treatment with sumatriptan and an SSRI (e.g., fluoxetine, fluvoxamine, paroxetine, sertraline, citalopram, escitalopram) is clinically warranted, appropriate observation of the patient is advised.
Theophylline—Combined administration of racemic citalopram (40 mg/day for 21 days) and the CYP1A2 substrate theophylline (single dose of 300 mg) did not affect the pharmacokinetics of theophylline. The effect of theophylline on the pharmacokinetics of citalopram was not evaluated.
Warfarin—Administration of 40 mg/day racemic citalopram for 21 days did not affect the pharmacokinetics of warfarin, a CYP3A4 substrate. Prothrombin time was increased by 5%, the clinical significance of which is unknown.
Carbamazepine—Combined administration of racemic citalopram (40 mg/day for 14 days) and carbamazepine (titrated to 400 mg/day for 35 days) did not significantly affect the pharmacokinetics of carbamazepine, a CYP3A4 substrate. Although trough citalopram plasma levels were unaffected, given the enzyme-inducing properties of carbamazepine, the possibility that carbamazepine might increase the clearance of escitalopram should be considered if the two drugs are coadministered.
Triazolam—Combined administration of racemic citalopram (titrated to 40 mg/day for 28 days) and the CYP3A4 substrate triazolam (single dose of 0.25 mg) did not significantly affect the pharmacokinetics of either citalopram or triazolam.
Ketoconazole—Combined administration of racemic citalopram (40 mg) and ketoconazole (200 mg) decreased the C_{max} and AUC of ketoconazole by 21% and 10%, respectively, and did not significantly affect the pharmacokinetics of citalopram.
Ritonavir—Combined administration of a single dose of ritonavir (600 mg), both a CYP3A4 substrate and a potent inhibitor of CYP3A4, and escitalopram (20 mg) did not affect the pharmacokinetics of either ritonavir or escitalopram.
CYP3A4 and -2C19 Inhibitors—*In vitro* studies indicated that CYP3A4 and -2C19 are the primary enzymes involved in the metabolism of escitalopram. However, coadministration of escitalopram (20 mg) and ritonavir (600 mg), a potent inhibitor of CYP3A4, did not significantly affect the pharmacokinetics of escitalopram. Because escitalopram is metabolized by multiple enzyme systems, inhibition of a single enzyme may not appreciably decrease escitalopram clearance.
Drugs Metabolized by Cytochrome P4502D6—*In vitro* studies did not reveal an inhibitory effect of escitalopram on CYP2D6. In addition, steady state levels of racemic citalopram were not significantly different in poor metabolizers and extensive CYP2D6 metabolizers after multiple-dose administration of citalopram, suggesting that coadministration, with escitalopram, of a drug that inhibits CYP2D6, is unlikely to have clinically significant effects on escitalopram metabolism. However, there are limited *in vivo* data suggesting a modest CYP2D6 inhibitory effect for escitalopram, i.e., coadministration of escitalopram (20 mg/day for 21 days) with the tricyclic antidepressant desipramine (single dose of 50 mg), a substrate for CYP2D6, resulted in a 40% increase in C_{max} and a 100% increase in AUC of desipramine. The clinical significance of this finding is unknown. Nevertheless, caution is indicated in the coadministration of escitalopram and drugs metabolized by CYP2D6.
Metoprolol—Administration of 20 mg/day LEXAPRO for 21 days in healthy volunteers resulted in a 50% increase in C_{max} and 82% increase in AUC of the beta-adrenergic blocker metoprolol (given in a single dose of 100 mg). Increased metoprolol plasma levels have been associated with decreased cardioselectivity. Coadministration of LEXAPRO and metoprolol had no clinically significant effects on blood pressure or heart rate.
Electroconvulsive Therapy (ECT)—There are no clinical studies of the combined use of ECT and escitalopram.

Carcinogenesis, Mutagenesis, Impairment of Fertility

Carcinogenesis

Racemic citalopram was administered in the diet to NMRI/BOM strain mice and COBS WI strain rats for 18 and 24 months, respectively. There was no evidence for carcinogenicity of racemic citalopram in mice receiving up to 240 mg/kg/day. There was an increased incidence of small intestine carcinoma in rats receiving 8 or 24 mg/kg/day racemic citalopram. A no-effect dose for this finding was not established. The relevance of these findings to humans is unknown.

Mutagenesis

Racemic citalopram was mutagenic in the *in vitro* bacterial reverse mutation assay (Ames test) in 2 of 5 bacterial strains (Salmonella TA98 and TA1537) in the absence of metabolic activation. It was clastogenic in the *in vitro* Chinese hamster lung cell assay for chromosomal aberrations in the presence and absence of metabolic activation. Racemic citalopram was not mutagenic in the *in vitro* mammalian forward gene mutation assay (HPRT) in mouse lymphoma cells or in a coupled *in vitro*/*in vivo* unscheduled DNA synthesis (UDS) assay in rat liver. It was not clastogenic in the *in vitro* chromosomal aberration assay in human lymphocytes or in two *in vivo* mouse micronucleus assays.

Impairment of Fertility

When racemic citalopram was administered orally to 16 male and 24 female rats prior to and throughout mating and gestation at doses of 32, 48, and 72 mg/kg/day, mating was decreased at all doses, and fertility was decreased at doses ≥ 32 mg/kg/day. Gestation duration was increased at 48 mg/kg/day.

Pregnancy

Pregnancy Category C

In a rat embryo/fetal development study, oral administration of escitalopram (56, 112, or 150 mg/kg/day) to pregnant animals during the period of organogenesis resulted in decreased fetal body weight and associated delays in ossification at the two higher doses (approximately ≥ 56 times the maximum recommended human dose [MRHD] of 20 mg/day on a body surface area [mg/m^2] basis). Maternal toxicity (clinical signs and decreased body weight gain and food consumption), mild at 56 mg/kg/day, was present at all dose levels. The developmental no-effect dose of 56 mg/kg/day is approximately 28 times the MRHD on a mg/m^2 basis. No teratogenicity was observed at any of the doses tested (as high as 75 times the MRHD on a mg/m^2 basis).
When female rats were treated with escitalopram (6, 12, 24, or 48 mg/kg/day) during pregnancy and through weaning, slightly increased offspring mortality and growth retardation were noted at 48 mg/kg/day which is approximately 24 times the MRHD on a mg/m2 basis. Slight maternal toxicity (clinical signs and decreased body weight gain and food consumption) was seen at this dose. Slightly increased offspring mortality was seen at 24 mg/kg/day. The no-effect dose was 12 mg/kg/day which is approximately 6 times the MRHD on a mg/m^2 basis.
In animal reproduction studies, racemic citalopram has been shown to have adverse effects on embryo/fetal and postnatal development, including teratogenic effects, when administered at doses greater than human therapeutic doses.
In two rat embryo/fetal development studies, oral administration of racemic citalopram (32, 56, or 112 mg/kg/day) to pregnant animals during the period of organogenesis resulted in decreased embryo/fetal growth and survival and an increased incidence of fetal abnormalities (including cardiovascular and skeletal defects) at the high dose. This dose was also associated with maternal toxicity (clinical signs, decreased BW gain). The developmental no-effect dose was 56 mg/kg/day. In a rabbit study, no adverse effects on embryo/fetal development were observed at doses of racemic citalopram of up to 16 mg/kg/day. Thus, teratogenic effects of racemic citalopram were observed at a maternally toxic dose in the rat and were not observed in the rabbit.
When female rats were treated with racemic citalopram (4.8, 12.8, or 32 mg/kg/day) from late gestation through weaning, increased offspring mortality during the first 4 days after birth and persistent offspring growth retardation were observed at the highest dose. The no-effect dose was 12.8 mg/kg/day. Similar effects on offspring mortality and growth were seen when dams were treated throughout gestation and early lactation at doses ≥ 24 mg/kg/day. A no-effect dose was not determined in that study.
There are no adequate and well-controlled studies in pregnant women; therefore, escitalopram should be used during pregnancy only if the potential benefit justifies the potential risk to the fetus.

Pregnancy-Nonteratogenic Effects

Neonates exposed to LEXAPRO and other SSRIs or SNRIs, late in the third trimester, have developed complications requiring prolonged hospitalization, respiratory support, and tube feeding. Such complications can arise immediately upon delivery. Reported clinical findings have included respiratory distress, cyanosis, apnea, seizures, temperature instability, feeding difficulty, vomiting, hypoglycemia, hypotonia, hypertonia, hyperreflexia, tremor, jitteriness, irritability, and constant crying. These features are consistent with either a direct toxic effect of SSRIs and SNRIs or, possibly, a drug discontinuation syndrome. It should be noted that, in some cases, the clinical picture is consistent with serotonin syndrome (see WARNINGS).
When treating a pregnant woman with LEXAPRO during the third trimester, the physician should carefully consider the potential risks and benefits of treatment (see DOSAGE AND ADMINISTRATION).

Labor and Delivery

The effect of LEXAPRO on labor and delivery in humans is unknown.

Nursing Mothers

Racemic citalopram, like many other drugs, is excreted in human breast milk. There have been two reports of infants experiencing excessive somnolence, decreased feeding, and weight loss in association with breast feeding from a citalopram-treated mother; in one case, the infant was reported to recover completely upon discontinuation of citalopram by its mother and, in the second case, no follow up information was available. The decision whether to continue or discontinue either nursing or LEXAPRO therapy should take into account the risks of citalopram exposure for the infant and the benefits of LEXAPRO treatment for the mother.

Pediatric Use

Safety and effectiveness in pediatric patients have not been established.

Geriatric Use

Approximately 6% of the 1144 patients receiving escitalopram in controlled trials of LEXAPRO in major depressive disorder and GAD were 60 years of age or older; elderly patients in these trials received daily doses of LEXAPRO between 10 and 20 mg. The number of elderly patients in these trials was insufficient to adequately assess for possible differential efficacy and safety measures on the basis of age. Nevertheless, greater sensitivity of some elderly individuals to effects of LEXAPRO cannot be ruled out.
In two pharmacokinetic studies, escitalopram half-life was increased by approximately 50% in elderly subjects as compared to young subjects and C_{max} was unchanged (see Clinical Pharmacology). 10 mg/day is the recommended dose for elderly patients (see Dosage and Administration).
Of 4422 patients in clinical studies of racemic citalopram, 1357 were 60 and over, 1034 were 65 and over, and 457 were 75 and over. No overall differences in safety or effectiveness

Continued on next page

Lexapro—Cont.

were observed between these subjects and younger subjects, and other reported clinical experience has not identified differences in responses between the elderly and younger patients, but again, greater sensitivity of some elderly individuals cannot be ruled out.

ADVERSE REACTIONS

Adverse event information for LEXAPRO was collected from 715 patients with major depressive disorder who were exposed to escitalopram and from 592 patients who were exposed to placebo in double-blind, placebo-controlled trials. An additional 284 patients with major depressive disorder were newly exposed to escitalopram in open-label trials. The adverse event information for LEXAPRO in patients with GAD was collected from 429 patients exposed to escitalopram and from 427 patients exposed to placebo in double-blind, placebo-controlled trials.

Adverse events during exposure were obtained primarily by general inquiry and recorded by clinical investigators using terminology of their own choosing. Consequently, it is not possible to provide a meaningful estimate of the proportion of individuals experiencing adverse events without first grouping similar types of events into a smaller number of standardized event categories. In the tables and tabulations that follow, standard World Health Organization (WHO) terminology has been used to classify reported adverse events.

The stated frequencies of adverse events represent the proportion of individuals who experienced, at least once, a treatment-emergent adverse event of the type listed. An event was considered treatment-emergent if it occurred for the first time or worsened while receiving therapy following baseline evaluation.

Adverse Events Associated with Discontinuation of Treatment

Major Depressive Disorder

Among the 715 depressed patients who received LEXAPRO in placebo-controlled trials, 6% discontinued treatment due to an adverse event, as compared to 2% of 592 patients receiving placebo. In two fixed-dose studies, the rate of discontinuation for adverse events in patients receiving 10 mg/day LEXAPRO was not significantly different from the rate of discontinuation for adverse events in patients receiving placebo. The rate of discontinuation for adverse events in patients assigned to a fixed dose of 20 mg/day LEXAPRO was 10%, which was significantly different from the rate of discontinuation for adverse events in patients receiving 10 mg/day LEXAPRO (4%) and placebo (3%). Adverse events that were associated with the discontinuation of at least 1% of patients treated with LEXAPRO, and for which the rate was at least twice that of placebo, were nausea (2%) and ejaculation disorder (2% of male patients).

Generalized Anxiety Disorder

Among the 429 GAD patients who received LEXAPRO 10-20 mg/day in placebo-controlled trials, 8% discontinued treatment due to an adverse event, as compared to 4% of 427 patients receiving placebo. Adverse events that were associated with the discontinuation of at least 1% of patients treated with LEXAPRO, and for which the rate was at least twice the placebo rate, were nausea (2%), insomnia (1%), and fatigue (1%).

Incidence of Adverse Events in Placebo-Controlled Clinical Trials

Major Depressive Disorder

Table 1 enumerates the incidence, rounded to the nearest percent, of treatment emergent adverse events that occurred among 715 depressed patients who received LEXAPRO at doses ranging from 10 to 20 mg/day in placebo-controlled trials. Events included are those occurring in 2% or more of patients treated with LEXAPRO and for which the incidence in patients treated with LEXAPRO was greater than the incidence in placebo-treated patients.

The prescriber should be aware that these figures can not be used to predict the incidence of adverse events in the course of usual medical practice where patient characteristics and other factors differ from those which prevailed in the clinical trials. Similarly, the cited frequencies cannot be compared with figures obtained from other clinical investigations involving different treatments, uses, and investigators. The cited figures, however, do provide the prescribing physician with some basis for estimating the relative contribution of drug and non-drug factors to the adverse event incidence rate in the population studied.

The most commonly observed adverse events in LEXAPRO patients (incidence of approximately 5% or greater and approximately twice the incidence in placebo patients) were insomnia, ejaculation disorder (primarily ejaculatory delay), nausea, sweating increased, fatigue, and somnolence (see TABLE 1).

TABLE 1
Treatment-Emergent Adverse Events: Incidence in Placebo-Controlled Clinical Trials for Major Depressive Disorder*

Body System/ Adverse Event	(Percentage of Patients Reporting Event) LEXAPRO (N=715)	Placebo (N=592)
Autonomic Nervous System Disorders		
Dry Mouth	6%	5%
Sweating Increased	5%	2%
Central & Peripheral Nervous System Disorders		
Dizziness	5%	3%
Gastrointestinal Disorders		
Nausea	15%	7%
Diarrhea	8%	5%
Constipation	3%	1%
Indigestion	3%	1%
Abdominal Pain	2%	1%
General		
Influenza-like Symptoms	5%	4%
Fatigue	5%	2%
Psychiatric Disorders		
Insomnia	9%	4%
Somnolence	6%	2%
Appetitie Decreased	3%	1%
Libido Decreased	3%	1%
Respiratory System Disorders		
Rhinitis	5%	4%
Sinusitis	3%	2%
Urogenital		
Ejaculation Disorder[1,2]	9%	<1%
Impotence[2]	3%	<1%
Anorgasmia[3]	2%	<1%

*Events reported by at least 2% of patients treated with LEXAPRO are reported, except for the following events which had an incidence on placebo ≥ LEXAPRO: headache, upper respiratory tract infection, back pain, pharyngitis, inflicted injury, anxiety.

[1]Primarily ejaculatory delay.

[2]Denominator used was for males only (N=225 LEXAPRO; N=188 placebo).

[3]Denominator used was for females only (N=490 LEXAPRO; N=404 placebo).

Generalized Anxiety Disorder

Table 2 enumerates the incidence, rounded to the nearest percent of treatment-emergent adverse events that occurred among 429 GAD patients who received LEXAPRO 10 to 20 mg/day in placebo-controlled trials. Events included are those occurring in 2% or more of patients treated with LEXAPRO and for which the incidence in patients treated with LEXAPRO was greater than the incidence in placebo-treated patients.

The most commonly observed adverse events in LEXAPRO patients (incidence of approximately 5% or greater and approximately twice the incidence in placebo patients) were nausea, ejaculation disorder (primarily ejaculatory delay), insomnia, fatigue, decreased libido, and anorgasmia (see TABLE 2).

TABLE 2
Treatment-Emergent Adverse Events: Incidence in Placebo-Controlled Clinical Trials for Generalized Anxiety Disorder*

Body System/ Adverse Event	(Percentage of Patients Reporting Event) LEXAPRO (N=429)	Placebo (N=427)
Autonomic Nervous System Disorders		
Dry Mouth	9%	5%
Sweating Increased	4%	1%
Central & Peripheral Nervous System Disorders		
Headache	24%	17%
Paresthesia	2%	1%
Gastrointestinal Disorders		
Nausea	18%	8%
Diarrhea	8%	6%
Constipation	5%	4%
Indigestion	3%	2%
Vomiting	3%	1%
Abdominal Pain	2%	1%
Flatulence	2%	1%
Toothache	2%	0%
General		
Fatigue	8%	2%
Influenza-like Symptoms	5%	4%
Musculoskeletal		
Neck/Shoulder Pain	3%	1%
Psychiatric Disorders		
Somnolence	13%	7%
Insomnia	12%	6%
Libido Decreased	7%	2%
Dreaming Abnormal	3%	2%
Appetitie Decreased	3%	1%
Lethargy	3%	1%
Yawning	2%	1%
Urogenital		
Ejaculation Disorder[1,2]	14%	2%
Anorgasmia[3]	6%	<1%
Menstrual Disorder	2%	1%

*Events reported by at least 2% of patients treated with LEXAPRO are reported, except for the following events which had an incidence on placebo ≥ LEXAPRO: inflicted injury, dizziness, back pain, upper respiratory tract infection, rhinitis, pharyngitis.

[1]Primarily ejaculatory delay.

[2]Denominator used was for males only (N=182 LEXAPRO; N=195 placebo).

[3]Denominator used was for females only (N=247 LEXAPRO; N=232 placebo).

Dose Dependency of Adverse Events

The potential dose dependency of common adverse events (defined as an incidence rate of ≥5% in either the 10 mg or 20 mg LEXAPRO groups) was examined on the basis of the combined incidence of adverse events in two fixed-dose trials. The overall incidence rates of adverse events in 10 mg LEXAPRO-treated patients (66%) was similar to that of the placebo-treated patients (61%), while the incidence rate in 20 mg/day LEXAPRO-treated patients was greater (86%). Table 3 shows common adverse events that occurred in the 20 mg/day LEXAPRO group with an incidence that was approximately twice that of the 10 mg/day LEXAPRO group and approximately twice that of the placebo group.

TABLE 3
Incidence of Common Adverse Events* in Patients With Major Depressive Disorder Receiving Placebo, 10 mg/day LEXAPRO, or 20 mg/day LEXAPRO

Adverse Event	Placebo (N=311)	10 mg/day LEXAPRO (N=310)	20 mg/day LEXAPRO (N=125)
Insomnia	4%	7%	14%
Diarrhea	5%	6%	14%
Dry Mouth	3%	4%	9%
Somnolence	1%	4%	9%
Dizziness	2%	4%	7%
Sweating Increased	<1%	3%	8%
Constipation	1%	3%	6%
Fatigue	2%	2%	6%
Indigestion	1%	2%	6%

*Adverse events with an incidence rate of at least 5% in either of the LEXAPRO groups and with an incidence rate in the 20 mg/day LEXAPRO group that was approximately twice that of the 10 mg/day LEXAPRO group and the placebo group.

Male and Female Sexual Dysfunction with SSRIs

Although changes in sexual desire, sexual performance, and sexual satisfaction often occur as manifestations of a psychiatric disorder, they may also be a consequence of pharmacologic treatment. In particular, some evidence suggests that selective serotonin reuptake inhibitors (SSRIs) can cause such untoward sexual experiences.

Reliable estimates of the incidence and severity of untoward experiences involving sexual desire, performance and satisfaction are difficult to obtain, however, in part because patients and physicians may be reluctant to discuss them. Accordingly, estimates of the incidence of untoward sexual experience and performance cited in product labeling are likely to underestimate their actual incidence.

Table 4 shows the incidence rates of sexual side effects in patients with major depressive disorder and GAD in placebo-controlled trials.

TABLE 4
Incidence of Sexual Side Effects in Placebo-Controlled Clinical Trials

Adverse Event	LEXAPRO	Placebo
	In Males Only	
	(N=407)	(N=383)
Ejaculation Disorder (primarily ejaculatory delay)	12%	<1%
Libido Decreased	6%	2%
Impotence	2%	<1%
	In Females Only	
	(N=737)	(N=636)
Libido Decreased	3%	<1%
Anorgasmia	3%	<1%

There are no adequately designed studies examining sexual dysfunction with escitalopram treatment.

Priapism has been reported with all SSRIs.

While it is difficult to know the precise risk of sexual dysfunction associated with the use of SSRIs, physicians should routinely inquire about such possible side effects.

Vital Sign Changes

LEXAPRO and placebo groups were compared with respect to (1) mean change from baseline in vital signs (pulse, systolic blood pressure, and diastolic blood pressure) and (2) the incidence of patients meeting criteria for potentially clinically significant changes from baseline in these variables. These analyses did not reveal any clinically important changes in vital signs associated with LEXAPRO treatment. In addition, a comparison of supine and standing vital sign measures in subjects receiving LEXAPRO indicated that LEXAPRO treatment is not associated with orthostatic changes.

Weight Changes

Patients treated with LEXAPRO in controlled trials did not differ from placebo-treated patients with regard to clinically important change in body weight.

Laboratory Changes

LEXAPRO and placebo groups were compared with respect to (1) mean change from baseline in various serum chemistry, hematology, and urinalysis variables and (2) the incidence of patients meeting criteria for potentially clinically significant changes from baseline in these variables. These analyses revealed no clinically important changes in laboratory test parameters associated with LEXAPRO treatment.

ECG Changes

Electrocardiograms from LEXAPRO (N=625), racemic citalopram (N=351), and placebo (N=527) groups were compared with respect to (1) mean change from baseline in various ECG parameters and (2) the incidence of patients meeting criteria for potentially clinically significant changes from baseline in these variables. These analyses revealed (1) a decrease in heart rate of 2.2 bpm for LEXAPRO and 2.7 bpm for racemic citalopram, compared to an increase of 0.3 bpm for placebo and (2) an increase in QTc interval of 3.9 msec for LEXAPRO and 3.7 msec for racemic citalopram, compared to 0.5 msec for placebo. Neither LEXAPRO nor racemic citalopram were associated with the development of clinically significant ECG abnormalities.

Other Events Observed During the Premarketing Evaluation of LEXAPRO

Following is a list of WHO terms that reflect treatment-emergent adverse events, as defined in the introduction to the ADVERSE REACTIONS section, reported by the 1428 patients treated with LEXAPRO for periods of up to one year in double-blind or open-label clinical trials during its premarketing evaluation. All reported events are included except those already listed in Tables 1 & 2, those occurring in only one patient, event terms that are so general as to be uninformative, and those that are unlikely to be drug related. It is important to emphasize that, although the events reported occurred during treatment with LEXAPRO, they were not necessarily caused by it.

Events are further categorized by body system and listed in order of decreasing frequency according to the following definitions: frequent adverse events are those occurring on one or more occasions in at least 1/100 patients; infrequent adverse events are those occurring in less than 1/100 patients but at least 1/1000 patients.

Cardiovascular—*Frequent:* palpitation, hypertension. *Infrequent:* bradycardia, tachycardia, ECG abnormal, flushing, varicose vein.

Central and Peripheral Nervous System Disorders—*Frequent:* light-headed feeling, migraine. *Infrequent:* tremor, vertigo, restless legs, shaking, twitching, dysequilibrium, tics, carpal tunnel syndrome, muscle contractions involuntary, sluggishness, coordination abnormal, faintness, hyperreflexia, muscular tone increased.

Gastrointestinal Disorders—*Frequent:* heartburn, abdominal cramp, gastroenteritis. *Infrequent:* gastroesophageal reflux, bloating, abdominal discomfort, dyspepsia, increased stool frequency, belching, gastritis, hemorrhoids, gagging, polyposis gastric, swallowing difficult.

General—*Frequent:* allergy, pain in limb, fever, hot flushes, chest pain. *Infrequent:* edema of extremities, chills, tightness of chest, leg pain, asthenia, syncope, malaise, anaphylaxis, fall.

Hemic and Lymphatic Disorders—*Infrequent:* bruise, anemia, nosebleed, hematoma, lymphadenopathy cervical.

Metabolic and Nutritional Disorders—*Frequent:* increased weight. *Infrequent:* decreased weight, hyperglycemia, thirst, bilirubin increased, hepatic enzymes increased, gout, hypercholesterolemia.

Musculoskeletal System Disorders—*Frequent:* arthralgia, myalgia. *Infrequent:* jaw stiffness, muscle cramp, muscle stiffness, arthritis, muscle weakness, back discomfort, arthropathy, jaw pain, joint stiffness.

Psychiatric Disorders—*Frequent:* appetite increased, lethargy, irritability, concentration impaired. *Infrequent:* jitteriness, panic reaction, agitation, apathy, forgetfulness, depression aggravated, nervousness, restlessness aggravated, suicide attempt, amnesia, anxiety attack, bruxism, carbohydrate craving, confusion, depersonalization, disorientation, emotional lability, feeling unreal, tremulousness nervous, crying abnormal, depression, excitability, auditory hallucination, suicidal tendency.

Reproductive Disorders/Female*—*Frequent:* menstrual cramps, menstrual disorder. *Infrequent:* menorrhagia, breast neoplasm, pelvic inflammation, premenstrual syndrome, spotting between menses.

*% based on female subjects only: N= 905

Respiratory System Disorders—*Frequent:* bronchitis, sinus congestion, coughing, nasal congestion, sinus headache. *Infrequent:* asthma, breath shortness, laryngitis, pneumonia, tracheitis.

Skin and Appendages Disorders—*Frequent:* rash. *Infrequent:* pruritus, acne, alopecia, eczema, dermatitis, dry skin, folliculitis, lipoma, furunculosis, dry lips, skin nodule.

Special Senses—*Frequent:* vision blurred, tinnitus. *Infrequent:* taste alteration, earache, conjunctivitis, vision abnormal, dry eyes, eye irritation, visual disturbance, eye infection, pupils dilated, metallic taste.

Urinary System Disorders—*Frequent:* urinary frequency, urinary tract infection. *Infrequent:* urinary urgency, kidney stone, dysuria, blood in urine.

Events Reported Subsequent to the Marketing of Racemic Citalopram

Although no causal relationship to racemic citalopram treatment has been found, the following adverse events have been reported to be temporally associated with racemic citalopram treatment and were not observed during the premarketing evaluation of citalopram: acute renal failure, akathisia, allergic reaction, anaphylaxis, angioedema, choreoathetosis, delirium, dyskinesia, ecchymosis, epidermal necrolysis, erythema multiforme, gastrointestinal hemorrhage, grand mal convulsions, hemolytic anemia, hepatic necrosis, myoclonus, neuroleptic malignant syndrome, nystagmus, pancreatitis, priapism, prolactinemia, prothrombin decreased, QT prolonged, rhabdomyolysis, serotonin syndrome, spontaneous abortion, thrombocytopenia, thrombosis, Torsades de pointes, ventricular arrhythmia, and withdrawal syndrome.

DRUG ABUSE AND DEPENDENCE

Controlled Substance Class

LEXAPRO is not a controlled substance.

Physical and Psychological Dependence

Animal studies suggest that the abuse liability of racemic citalopram is low. LEXAPRO has not been systematically studied in humans for its potential for abuse, tolerance, or physical dependence. The premarketing clinical experience with LEXAPRO did not reveal any drug-seeking behavior. However, these observations were not systematic and it is not possible to predict on the basis of this limited experience the extent to which a CNS-active drug will be misused, diverted, and/or abused once marketed. Consequently, physicians should carefully evaluate LEXAPRO patients for history of drug abuse and follow such patients closely, observing them for signs of misuse or abuse (e.g., development of tolerance, incrementations of dose, drug-seeking behavior).

OVERDOSAGE

Human Experience

There have been five reports of LEXAPRO overdose involving doses of up to 600 mg. All five patients recovered and no symptoms associated with the overdoses were reported. In clinical trials of racemic citalopram, there were no reports of fatal citalopram overdose involving overdoses of up to 2000 mg. During the postmarketing evaluation of citalopram, like other SSRIs, a fatal outcome in a patient who has taken an overdose of citalopram has been rarely reported.

Postmarketing reports of drug overdoses involving citalopram have included 12 fatalities, 10 in combination with other drugs and/or alcohol and 2 with citalopram alone (3920 mg and 2800 mg), as well as non-fatal overdoses of up to 6000 mg. Symptoms most often accompanying citalopram overdose, alone or in combination with other drugs and/or alcohol, included dizziness, sweating, nausea, vomiting, tremor, somnolence, sinus tachycardia, and convulsions. In more rare cases, observed symptoms included amnesia, confusion, coma, hyperventilation, cyanosis, rhabdomyolysis, and ECG changes (including QTc prolongation, nodal rhythm, ventricular arrhythmia, and one possible case of Torsades de pointes).

Management of Overdose

Establish and maintain an airway to ensure adequate ventilation and oxygenation. Gastric evacuation by lavage and use of activated charcoal should be considered. Careful observation and cardiac and vital sign monitoring are recommended, along with general symptomatic and supportive care. Due to the large volume of distribution of escitalopram, forced diuresis, dialysis, hemoperfusion, and exchange transfusion are unlikely to be of benefit. There are no specific antidotes for LEXAPRO.

In managing overdosage, consider the possibility of multiple-drug involvement. The physician should consider contacting a poison control center for additional information on the treatment of any overdose.

DOSAGE AND ADMINISTRATION

Major Depressive Disorder

Initial Treatment

The recommended dose of LEXAPRO is 10 mg once daily. A fixed dose trial of LEXAPRO demonstrated the effectiveness of both 10 mg and 20 mg of LEXAPRO, but failed to demonstrate a greater benefit of 20 mg over 10 mg (see Clinical Efficacy Trials under Clinical Pharmacology). If the dose is increased to 20 mg, this should occur after a minimum of one week.

LEXAPRO should be administered once daily, in the morning or evening, with or without food.

Special Populations

10 mg/day is the recommended dose for most elderly patients and patients with hepatic impairment.

No dosage adjustment is necessary for patients with mild or moderate renal impairment. LEXAPRO should be used with caution in patients with severe renal impairment.

Treatment of Pregnant Women During the Third Trimester

Neonates exposed to LEXAPRO and other SSRIs or SNRIs, late in the third trimester, have developed complications requiring prolonged hospitalization, respiratory support, and tube feeding (see PRECAUTIONS). When treating pregnant women with LEXAPRO during the third trimester, the physician should carefully consider the potential risks and benefits of treatment. The physician may consider tapering LEXAPRO in the third trimester.

Maintenance Treatment

It is generally agreed that acute episodes of major depressive disorder require several months or longer of sustained pharmacological therapy beyond response to the acute episode. Systematic evaluation of continuing LEXAPRO 10 or 20 mg/day for periods of up to 36 weeks in patients with major depressive disorder who responded while taking LEXAPRO during an 8-week, acute-treatment phase demonstrated a benefit of such maintenance treatment (see Clinical Efficacy Trials, under Clinical Pharmacology). Nevertheless, patients should be periodically reassessed to determine the need for maintenance treatment.

Generalized Anxiety Disorder

Initial Treatment

The recommended starting dose of LEXAPRO is 10 mg once daily. If the dose is increased to 20 mg, this should occur after a minimum of one week. LEXAPRO should be administered once daily, in the morning or evening, with or without food.

Maintenance Treatment

Generalized anxiety disorder is recognized as a chronic condition. The efficacy of LEXAPRO in the treatment of GAD beyond 8 weeks has not been systematically studied. The physician who elects to use LEXAPRO for extended periods should periodically reevaluate the long-term usefulness of the drug for the individual patient.

Discontinuation of Treatment with LEXAPRO

Symptoms associated with discontinuation of LEXAPRO and other SSRIs and SNRIs, have been reported (see PRECAUTIONS). Patients should be monitored for these symptoms when discontinuing treatment. A gradual reduction in the dose rather than abrupt cessation is recommended whenever possible. If intolerable symptoms occur following a decrease in the dose or upon discontinuation of treatment, then resuming the previously prescribed dose may be considered. Subsequently, the physician may continue decreasing the dose but at a more gradual rate.

Switching Patients To or From a Monoamine Oxidase Inhibitor

At least 14 days should elapse between discontinuation of a MAOI and initiation of LEXAPRO therapy. Similarly, at least 14 days should be allowed after stopping LEXAPRO before starting a MAOI (see Contraindications and Warnings).

HOW SUPPLIED

5 mg Tablets:

Bottle of 100	NDC # 0456-2005-01

White to off-white, round, non-scored, film-coated. Imprint "FL" on one side of the tablet and "5" on the other side.

10 mg Tablets:

Bottle of 100	NDC # 0456-2010-01
10 x 10 Unit Dose	NDC # 0456-2010-63

White to off-white, round, scored, film-coated. Imprint on scored side with "F" on the left side and "L" on the right side.

Imprint on the non-scored side with "10".

20 mg Tablets:

Bottle of 100	NDC # 0456-2020-01
10 x 10 Unit Dose	NDC # 0456-2020-63

White to off-white, round, scored, film-coated. Imprint on scored side with "F" on the left side and "L" on the right side.

Imprint on the non-scored side with "20".

Oral Solution:

5 mg/5 mL, peppermint flavor (240 mL) NDC # 0456-2101-08

Store at 25°C (77°F); excursions permitted to 15-30°C (59-86°F).

ANIMAL TOXICOLOGY

Retinal Changes in Rats

Pathologic changes (degeneration/atrophy) were observed in the retinas of albino rats in the 2-year carcinogenicity study with racemic citalopram. There was an increase in both incidence and severity of retinal pathology in both male and female rats receiving 80 mg/kg/day. Similar findings were not present in rats receiving 24 mg/kg/day of racemic citalopram for two years, in mice receiving up to 240 mg/kg/day of racemic citalopram for 18 months, or in dogs receiving up to 20 mg/kg/day of racemic citalopram for one year. Additional studies to investigate the mechanism for this pathology have not been performed, and the potential significance of this effect in humans has not been established.

Cardiovascular Changes in Dogs

In a one year toxicology study, 5 of 10 beagle dogs receiving oral racemic citalopram doses of 8 mg/kg/day died suddenly between weeks 17 and 31 following initiation of treatment. Sudden deaths were not observed in rats at doses of racemic citalopram up to 120 mg/kg/day, which produced plasma levels of citalopram and its metabolites demethylcitalopram and didemethylcitalopram (DDCT) similar to those observed in dogs at 8 mg/kg/day. A subsequent intravenous dosing study demonstrated that in beagle dogs, racemic DDCT caused QT prolongation, a known risk factor for the observed outcome in dogs.

Forest Pharmaceuticals, Inc.
Subsidiary of Forest Laboratories, Inc.
St. Louis, MO 63045 USA
Licensed from H. Lundbeck A/S
Rev. 12/03

MG #17541(04)

GlaxoSmithKline
FIVE MOORE DRIVE
RESEARCH TRIANGLE PARK, NC 27709

For Medical Emergencies, Medical Information for Healthcare Professionals, and Consumer Inquiries, Contact:
1-888-825-5249
www.druginfo.gsk.com

ADVAIR DISKUS® 100/50 ℞
[ad'vair disk'us]
(fluticasone propionate 100 mcg and salmeterol* 50 mcg inhalation powder)
ADVAIR DISKUS® 250/50 ℞
(fluticasone propionate 250 mcg and salmeterol* 50 mcg inhalation powder)
ADVAIR DISKUS® 500/50 ℞
(fluticasone propionate 500 mcg and salmeterol* 50 mcg inhalation powder)
***As salmeterol xinafoate salt 72.5 mcg, equivalent to salmeterol base 50 mcg**
FOR ORAL INHALATION ONLY

Prescribing information for this product, which appears on pages 1406–1412 of the 2004 PDR, has been completely revised as follows. Please write "See Supplement A" next to the product heading.

WARNING: Data from a large placebo-controlled US study that compared the safety of salmeterol (SEREVENT® Inhalation Aerosol) or placebo added to usual asthma therapy showed a small but significant increase in asthma-related deaths in patients receiving salmeterol (13 deaths out of 13,174 patients treated for 28 weeks) versus those on placebo (4 of 13,179). Subgroup analyses suggest the risk may be greater in African American patients compared to Caucasians (see WARNINGS).

DESCRIPTION

ADVAIR DISKUS 100/50, ADVAIR DISKUS 250/50, and ADVAIR DISKUS 500/50 are combinations of fluticasone propionate and salmeterol xinafoate.

One active component of ADVAIR DISKUS is fluticasone propionate, a corticosteroid having the chemical name *S*-(fluoromethyl) 6α,9-difluoro-11β,17-dihydroxy-16α-methyl-3-oxoandrosta-1,4-diene-17β-carbothioate, 17-propionate. Fluticasone propionate is a white to off-white powder with a molecular weight of 500.6, and the empirical formula is $C_{25}H_{31}F_3O_5S$. It is practically insoluble in water, freely soluble in dimethyl sulfoxide and dimethylformamide, and slightly soluble in methanol and 95% ethanol.

The other active component of ADVAIR DISKUS is salmeterol xinafoate, a beta$_2$-adrenergic bronchodilator. Salmeterol xinafoate is the racemic form of the 1-hydroxy-2-naphthoic acid salt of salmeterol. The chemical name of salmeterol xinafoate is 4-hydroxy-α^1-[[[6-(4-phenylbutoxy) hexyl]amino]methyl]-1,3-benzenedimethanol, 1-hydroxy-2-naphthalenecarboxylate.

Salmeterol xinafoate is a white to off-white powder with a molecular weight of 603.8, and the empirical formula is $C_{25}H_{37}NO_4 \bullet C_{11}H_8O_3$. It is freely soluble in methanol; slightly soluble in ethanol, chloroform, and isopropanol; and sparingly soluble in water.

ADVAIR DISKUS 100/50, ADVAIR DISKUS 250/50, and ADVAIR DISKUS 500/50 are specially designed plastic devices containing a double-foil blister strip of a powder formulation of fluticasone propionate and salmeterol xinafoate intended for oral inhalation only. Each blister on the double-foil strip within the device contains 100, 250, or 500 mcg of microfine fluticasone propionate and 72.5 mcg of microfine salmeterol xinafoate salt, equivalent to 50 mcg of salmeterol base, in 12.5 mg of formulation containing lactose (which contains milk proteins). Each blister contains 1 complete dose of both medications. After a blister containing medication is opened by activating the device, the medication is dispersed into the airstream created by the patient inhaling through the mouthpiece.

Under standardized in vitro test conditions, ADVAIR DISKUS delivers 93, 233, and 465 mcg of fluticasone propionate and 45 mcg of salmeterol base per blister from ADVAIR DISKUS 100/50, 250/50, and 500/50, respectively, when tested at a flow rate of 60 L/min for 2 seconds. In adult patients with obstructive lung disease and severely compromised lung function (mean forced expiratory volume in 1 second [FEV$_1$] 20% to 30% of predicted), mean peak inspiratory flow (PIF) through a DISKUS® inhalation device was 82.4 L/min (range, 46.1 to 115.3 L/min).

Inhalation profiles for adolescent (N = 13, aged 12 to 17 years) and adult (N = 17, aged 18 to 50 years) patients with asthma inhaling maximally through the DISKUS device show mean PIF of 122.2 L/min (range, 81.6 to 152.1 L/min). The actual amount of drug delivered to the lung will depend on patient factors, such as inspiratory flow profile.

CLINICAL PHARMACOLOGY

Mechanism of Action: ***ADVAIR DISKUS:*** Since ADVAIR DISKUS contains both fluticasone propionate and salmeterol, the mechanisms of action described below for the individual components apply to ADVAIR DISKUS. These drugs represent 2 classes of medications (a synthetic corticosteroid and a selective, long-acting beta-adrenergic receptor agonist) that have different effects on clinical and physiological indices.

Fluticasone Propionate: Fluticasone propionate is a synthetic trifluorinated corticosteroid with potent anti-inflammatory activity. In vitro assays using human lung cytosol preparations have established fluticasone propionate as a human glucocorticoid receptor agonist with an affinity 18 times greater than dexamethasone, almost twice that of beclomethasone-17-monopropionate (BMP), the active metabolite of beclomethasone dipropionate, and over 3 times that of budesonide. Data from the McKenzie vasoconstrictor assay in man are consistent with these results.

Inflammation is an important component in the pathogenesis of asthma. Corticosteroids have been shown to inhibit multiple cell types (e.g., mast cells, eosinophils, basophils, lymphocytes, macrophages, and neutrophils) and mediator production or secretion (e.g., histamine, eicosanoids, leukotrienes, and cytokines) involved in the asthmatic response. These anti-inflammatory actions of corticosteroids contribute to their efficacy in asthma.

Inflammation is also a component in the pathogenesis of COPD. In contrast to asthma, however, the predominant inflammatory cells in COPD include neutrophils, CD8+ T-lymphocytes, and macrophages. The effects of corticosteroids in the treatment of COPD are not well defined and inhaled corticosteroids and fluticasone propionate when used apart from ADVAIR DISKUS are not indicated for the treatment of COPD.

Salmeterol Xinafoate: Salmeterol is a long-acting beta$_2$-adrenergic agonist. In vitro studies and in vivo pharmacologic studies demonstrate that salmeterol is selective for beta$_2$-adrenoceptors compared with isoproterenol, which has approximately equal agonist activity on beta$_1$- and beta$_2$-adrenoceptors. In vitro studies show salmeterol to be at least 50 times more selective for beta$_2$-adrenoceptors than albuterol. Although beta$_2$-adrenoceptors are the predominant adrenergic receptors in bronchial smooth muscle and beta$_1$-adrenoceptors are the predominant receptors in the heart, there are also beta$_2$-adrenoceptors in the human heart comprising 10% to 50% of the total beta-adrenoceptors. The precise function of these receptors has not been established, but they raise the possibility that even highly selective beta$_2$-agonists may have cardiac effects.

The pharmacologic effects of beta$_2$-adrenoceptor agonist drugs, including salmeterol, are at least in part attributable to stimulation of intracellular adenyl cyclase, the enzyme that catalyzes the conversion of adenosine triphosphate (ATP) to cyclic-3',5'-adenosine monophosphate (cyclic AMP). Increased cyclic AMP levels cause relaxation of bronchial smooth muscle and inhibition of release of mediators of immediate hypersensitivity from cells, especially from mast cells.

In vitro tests show that salmeterol is a potent and long-lasting inhibitor of the release of mast cell mediators, such as histamine, leukotrienes, and prostaglandin D_2, from human lung. Salmeterol inhibits histamine-induced plasma protein extravasation and inhibits platelet-activating factor-induced eosinophil accumulation in the lungs of guinea pigs when administered by the inhaled route. In humans, single doses of salmeterol administered via inhalation aerosol attenuate allergen-induced bronchial hyper-responsiveness.

Pharmacokinetics: ***ADVAIR DISKUS:*** Following administration of ADVAIR DISKUS to healthy subjects, peak plasma concentrations of fluticasone propionate were achieved in 1 to 2 hours and those of salmeterol were achieved in about 5 minutes.

In a single-dose crossover study, a higher than recommended dose of ADVAIR DISKUS was administered to 14 healthy subjects. Two (2) inhalations of the following treatments were administered: ADVAIR DISKUS 500/50, fluticasone propionate powder 500 mcg and salmeterol powder 50 mcg given concurrently, and fluticasone propionate powder 500 mcg alone. Mean peak plasma concentrations of fluticasone propionate averaged 107, 94, and 120 pg/mL, respectively, and of salmeterol averaged 200 and 150 pg/mL, respectively, indicating no significant changes in systemic exposures of fluticasone propionate and salmeterol.

In a repeat-dose study, the highest recommended dose of ADVAIR DISKUS was administered to 45 patients with asthma. One (1) inhalation twice daily of the following treatments was administered: ADVAIR DISKUS 500/50, fluticasone propionate powder 500 mcg and salmeterol powder 50 mcg given concurrently, or fluticasone propionate powder 500 mcg alone. Mean peak steady-state plasma concentrations of fluticasone propionate averaged 57, 73, and 70 pg/mL, respectively, indicating no significant changes in systemic exposure of fluticasone propionate. No plasma concentrations of salmeterol were measured in this repeat-dose study.

No significant changes in excretion of fluticasone propionate or salmeterol were observed. The terminal half-life of fluticasone propionate averaged 5.33 to 7.65 hours when ADVAIR DISKUS was administered, which is similar to that reported when fluticasone propionate was given concurrently with salmeterol or when fluticasone propionate was given alone (average, 5.30 to 6.91 hours). No terminal half-life of salmeterol was reported upon administration of ADVAIR DISKUS or salmeterol given concurrently with fluticasone propionate.

Special Populations: Formal pharmacokinetic studies using ADVAIR DISKUS have not been conducted to examine gender differences or in special populations, such as elderly patients or patients with hepatic or renal impairment.

Drug Interactions: In the repeat- and single-dose studies, there was no evidence of significant drug interaction in systemic exposure between fluticasone propionate and salmeterol when given as ADVAIR DISKUS.

Fluticasone Propionate: Absorption: Fluticasone propionate acts locally in the lung; therefore, plasma levels do not predict therapeutic effect. Studies using oral dosing of labeled and unlabeled drug have demonstrated that the oral systemic bioavailability of fluticasone propionate is negligible (<1%), primarily due to incomplete absorption and presystemic metabolism in the gut and liver. In contrast, the majority of the fluticasone propionate delivered to the lung is systemically absorbed. The systemic bioavailability of fluticasone propionate from the DISKUS device in healthy volunteers averages 18%.

Peak steady-state fluticasone propionate plasma concentrations in adult patients with asthma (N = 11) ranged from undetectable to 266 pg/mL after a 500-mcg twice-daily dose of fluticasone propionate inhalation powder using the DISKUS device. The mean fluticasone propionate plasma concentration was 110 pg/mL.

Peak steady-state fluticasone propionate plasma concentrations in subjects with COPD averaged 53 pg/mL (range, 19.3 to 159.3 pg/mL) after treatment with 250 mcg twice daily (N = 30) via the DISKUS device.

Distribution: Following intravenous administration, the initial disposition phase for fluticasone propionate was rapid and consistent with its high lipid solubility and tissue binding. The volume of distribution averaged 4.2 L/kg.

The percentage of fluticasone propionate bound to human plasma proteins averages 91%. Fluticasone propionate is weakly and reversibly bound to erythrocytes and is not significantly bound to human transcortin.

Metabolism: The total clearance of fluticasone propionate is high (average, 1,093 mL/min), with renal clearance accounting for less than 0.02% of the total. The only circulating metabolite detected in man is the 17β-carboxylic acid derivative of fluticasone propionate, which is formed through the cytochrome P450 3A4 pathway. This metabolite had less affinity (approximately 1/2,000) than the parent drug for the glucocorticoid receptor of human lung cytosol in vitro and negligible pharmacological activity in animal studies. Other metabolites detected in vitro using cultured human hepatoma cells have not been detected in man.

Elimination: Following intravenous dosing, fluticasone propionate showed polyexponential kinetics and had a terminal elimination half-life of approximately 7.8 hours. Less than 5% of a radiolabeled oral dose was excreted in the urine as metabolites, with the remainder excreted in the feces as parent drug and metabolites.

Special Populations: Hepatic Impairment: Since fluticasone propionate is predominantly cleared by hepatic metabolism, impairment of liver function may lead to accumulation of fluticasone propionate in plasma. Therefore, patients with hepatic disease should be closely monitored.

Gender: Full pharmacokinetic profiles were obtained from 9 female and 16 male patients with asthma given fluticasone propionate inhalation powder 500 mcg twice daily using the DISKUS device and from 14 female and 43 male patients with COPD given 250 or 500 mcg twice daily. No overall differences in fluticasone propionate pharmacokinetics were observed.

Age: No relationship between fluticasone propionate systemic exposure and age was observed in 57 patients with COPD (aged 40 to 82 years) given 250 or 500 mcg twice daily.

Other: Formal pharmacokinetic studies using fluticasone propionate have not been conducted in other special populations.

Drug Interactions: Fluticasone propionate is a substrate of cytochrome P450 3A4. Coadministration of fluticasone propionate and the highly potent cytochrome P450 3A4 inhibitor ritonavir is not recommended based upon a multiple-dose, crossover drug interaction study in 18 healthy subjects. Fluticasone propionate aqueous nasal spray (200 mcg once daily) was coadministered for 7 days with ritonavir (100 mg twice daily). Plasma fluticasone propionate concentrations following fluticasone propionate aqueous nasal spray alone were undetectable (<10 pg/mL) in most subjects, and when concentrations were detectable peak levels (C_{max} averaged 11.9 pg/mL [range, 10.8 to 14.1 pg/mL] and $AUC_{(0-\tau)}$ averaged 8.43 pg•hr/mL [range, 4.2 to 18.8 pg•hr/mL]). Fluticasone propionate C_{max} and $AUC_{(0-\tau)}$ increased to 318 pg/mL (range, 110 to 648 pg/mL) and 3,102.6 pg•hr/mL (range, 1,207.1 to 5,662.0 pg•hr/mL), respectively, after coadministration of ritonavir with fluticasone propionate aqueous nasal spray. This significant increase in plasma fluticasone propionate exposure resulted in a significant decrease (86%) in plasma cortisol area under the plasma concentration versus time curve (AUC).

Caution should be exercised when other potent cytochrome P450 3A4 inhibitors are coadministered with fluticasone propionate. In a drug interaction study, coadministration of orally inhaled fluticasone propionate (1,000 mcg) and ketoconazole (200 mg once daily) resulted in increased plasma fluticasone propionate exposure and reduced plasma cortisol AUC, but had no effect on urinary excretion of cortisol.

In another multiple-dose drug interaction study, coadministration of orally inhaled fluticasone propionate (500 mcg twice daily) and erythromycin (333 mg 3 times daily) did not affect fluticasone propionate pharmacokinetics.

Salmeterol Xinafoate: Salmeterol xinafoate, an ionic salt, dissociates in solution so that the salmeterol and 1-hydroxy-2-naphthoic acid (xinafoate) moieties are absorbed, distributed, metabolized, and eliminated independently. Salmeterol acts locally in the lung; therefore, plasma levels do not predict therapeutic effect.

Absorption: Because of the small therapeutic dose, systemic levels of salmeterol are low or undetectable after inhalation of recommended doses (50 mcg of salmeterol inhalation powder twice daily). Following chronic administration of an inhaled dose of 50 mcg of salmeterol inhalation powder twice daily, salmeterol was detected in plasma within 5 to 45 minutes in 7 patients with asthma; plasma concentrations were very low, with mean peak concentrations of 167 pg/mL at 20 minutes and no accumulation with repeated doses.

Distribution: The percentage of salmeterol bound to human plasma proteins averages 96% in vitro over the concentration range of 8 to 7,722 ng of salmeterol base per milliliter, much higher concentrations than those achieved following therapeutic doses of salmeterol.

Metabolism: Salmeterol base is extensively metabolized by hydroxylation, with subsequent elimination predominantly in the feces. No significant amount of unchanged salmeterol base was detected in either urine or feces.

Elimination: In 2 healthy subjects who received 1 mg of radiolabeled salmeterol (as salmeterol xinafoate) orally, approximately 25% and 60% of the radiolabeled salmeterol was eliminated in urine and feces, respectively, over a period of 7 days. The terminal elimination half-life was about 5.5 hours (1 volunteer only).

The xinafoate moiety has no apparent pharmacologic activity. The xinafoate moiety is highly protein bound (>99%) and has a long elimination half-life of 11 days.

Special Populations: Hepatic Impairment: Since salmeterol is predominantly cleared by hepatic metabolism, impairment of liver function may lead to accumulation of salmeterol in plasma. Therefore, patients with hepatic disease should be closely monitored.

Other: Formal pharmacokinetic studies using salmeterol base have not been conducted in other special populations.

Pharmacodynamics: ***ADVAIR DISKUS:*** Since systemic pharmacodynamic effects of salmeterol are not normally seen at the therapeutic dose, higher doses were used to produce measurable effects. Four studies were conducted in healthy subjects: (1) a single-dose crossover study using 2 inhalations of ADVAIR DISKUS 500/50, fluticasone propionate powder 500 mcg and salmeterol powder 50 mcg given concurrently, or fluticasone propionate powder 500 mcg given alone, (2) a cumulative dose study using 50 to 400 mcg of salmeterol powder given alone or as ADVAIR DISKUS 500/50, (3) a repeat-dose study for 11 days using 2 inhalations twice daily of ADVAIR DISKUS 250/50, fluticasone propionate powder 250 mcg, or salmeterol powder 50 mcg, and (4) a single-dose study using 5 inhalations of ADVAIR DISKUS 100/50, fluticasone propionate powder 100 mcg alone, or placebo. In these studies no significant differences were observed in the pharmacodynamic effects of salmeterol (pulse rate, blood pressure, QTc interval, potassium, and glucose) whether the salmeterol was given as ADVAIR DISKUS, concurrently with fluticasone propionate from separate inhalers, or as salmeterol alone. The systemic pharmacodynamic effects of salmeterol were not altered by the presence of fluticasone propionate in ADVAIR DISKUS. The potential effect of salmeterol on the effects of fluticasone propionate on the hypothalamic-pituitary-adrenal (HPA) axis was also evaluated in these studies. No significant differences across treatments were observed in 24-hour urinary cortisol excretion and, where measured, 24-hour plasma cortisol AUC. The systemic pharmacodynamic effects of fluticasone propionate were not altered by the presence of salmeterol in ADVAIR DISKUS in healthy subjects.

Asthma: In clinical studies with ADVAIR DISKUS in patients with asthma, no significant differences were observed in the systemic pharmacodynamic effects of salmeterol (pulse rate, blood pressure, QTc interval, potassium, and glucose) whether the salmeterol was given alone or as ADVAIR DISKUS. In 72 adolescent and adult patients with asthma given either ADVAIR DISKUS 100/50 or ADVAIR DISKUS 250/50, continuous 24-hour electrocardiographic monitoring was performed after the first dose and after 12 weeks of therapy, and no clinically significant dysrhythmias were noted.

In a 28-week study in patients with asthma, ADVAIR DISKUS 500/50 twice daily was compared with the concurrent use of salmeterol powder 50 mcg plus fluticasone propionate powder 500 mcg from separate inhalers or fluticasone propionate powder 500 mcg alone. No significant differences across treatments were observed in plasma cortisol AUC after 12 weeks of dosing or in 24-hour urinary cortisol excretion after 12 and 28 weeks.

In a 12-week study in patients with asthma, ADVAIR DISKUS 250/50 twice daily was compared with fluticasone propionate powder 250 mcg alone, salmeterol powder 50 mcg alone, and placebo. For most patients, the ability to increase cortisol production in response to stress, as assessed by 30-minute cosyntropin stimulation, remained intact with ADVAIR DISKUS. One patient (3%) who received ADVAIR DISKUS 250/50 had an abnormal response (peak serum cortisol <18 mcg/dL) after dosing, compared with 2 patients (6%) who received placebo, 2 patients (6%) who received fluticasone propionate 250 mcg, and no patients who received salmeterol.

Table 1. Percent of Patients Withdrawn Due to Worsening Asthma in Patients Previously Treated With Either Inhaled Corticosteroids or Salmeterol (Study 1)

ADVAIR DISKUS 100/50 (N = 87)	Fluticasone Propionate 100 mcg (N = 85)	Salmeterol 50 mcg (N = 86)	Placebo (N = 77)
3%	11%	35%	49%)

Chronic Obstructive Pulmonary Disease: In clinical studies with ADVAIR DISKUS in patients with COPD associated with chronic bronchitis, no significant differences were seen in pulse rate, blood pressure, potassium, and glucose between ADVAIR DISKUS, the individual components of ADVAIR DISKUS, and placebo. In a study of ADVAIR DISKUS 250/50, 8 subjects (2 [1.1%] in the group given ADVAIR DISKUS 250/50, 1 [0.5%] in the fluticasone propionate 250 mcg group, 3 [1.7%] in the salmeterol group, and 2 [1.1%] in the placebo group) had QTc intervals >470 msec at least 1 time during the treatment period. Five (5) of these 8 subjects had a prolonged QTc interval at baseline.

In a 24-week study, 130 patients with COPD associated with chronic bronchitis received continuous 24-hour electrocardiographic monitoring prior to the first dose and after 4 weeks of twice-daily treatment with either ADVAIR DISKUS 500/50, fluticasone propionate powder 500 mcg, salmeterol powder 50 mcg, or placebo. No significant differences in ventricular or supraventricular arrhythmias and heart rate were observed among the groups treated with ADVAIR DISKUS 500/50, the individual components, or placebo. One (1) subject in the fluticasone propionate group experienced atrial flutter/atrial fibrillation, and 1 subject in the group given ADVAIR DISKUS 500/50 experienced heart block. There were 3 cases of nonsustained ventricular tachycardia (1 each in the placebo, salmeterol, and fluticasone propionate 500 mcg treatment groups).

Short-cosyntropin stimulation testing was performed both at Day 1 and Endpoint in 101 patients with COPD receiving twice-daily ADVAIR DISKUS 250/50, fluticasone propionate powder 250 mcg, salmeterol powder 50 mcg, or placebo. For most patients, the ability to increase cortisol production in response to stress, as assessed by short cosyntropin stimulation, remained intact with ADVAIR DISKUS 250/50. One (1) patient (3%) who received ADVAIR DISKUS 250/50 had an abnormal stimulated cortisol response (peak cortisol <14.5 mcg/dL assessed by high-performance liquid chromatography) after dosing, compared with 2 patients (9%) who received fluticasone propionate 250 mcg, 2 patients (7%) who received salmeterol 50 mcg, and 1 patient (4%) who received placebo following 24 weeks of treatment or early discontinuation from study.

Fluticasone Propionate: Asthma: In clinical trials with fluticasone propionate inhalation powder using doses up to and including 250 mcg twice daily, occasional abnormal short cosyntropin tests (peak serum cortisol <18 mcg/dL) assessed by radioimmunoassay) were noted both in patients receiving fluticasone propionate and in patients receiving placebo. The incidence of abnormal tests at 500 mcg twice daily was greater than placebo. In a 2-year study carried out with the DISKHALER® inhalation device in 64 patients with mild, persistent asthma (mean FEV_1 91% of predicted) randomized to fluticasone propionate 500 mcg twice daily or placebo, no patient receiving fluticasone propionate had an abnormal response to 6-hour cosyntropin infusion (peak serum cortisol <18 mcg/dL). With a peak cortisol threshold of <35 mcg/dL, 1 patient receiving fluticasone propionate (4%) had an abnormal response at 1 year; repeat testing at 18 months and 2 years was normal. Another patient receiving fluticasone propionate (5%) had an abnormal response at 2 years. No patient on placebo had an abnormal response at 1 or 2 years.

Chronic Obstructive Pulmonary Disease: In a 24-week study, the steady-state fluticasone propionate pharmacokinetics and serum cortisol levels were described in a subset of patients with COPD associated with chronic bronchitis (N = 86) randomized to twice-daily fluticasone propionate inhalation powder via the DISKUS 500 mcg, fluticasone propionate inhalation powder 250 mcg, or placebo. Serial serum cortisol concentrations were measured across a 12-hour dosing interval following at least 4 weeks of dosing. Serum cortisol concentrations following 250 and 500 mcg twice-daily dosing were 10% and 21% lower than placebo, indicating a dose-dependent increase in systemic exposure to fluticasone propionate.

Salmeterol Xinafoate: Inhaled salmeterol, like other beta-adrenergic agonist drugs, can produce dose-related cardiovascular effects and effects on blood glucose and/or serum potassium (see PRECAUTIONS: General). The cardiovascular effects (heart rate, blood pressure) associated with salmeterol occur with similar frequency, and are of similar type and severity, as those noted following albuterol administration.

Asthma: The effects of rising doses of salmeterol and standard inhaled doses of albuterol were studied in volunteers and in patients with asthma. Salmeterol doses up to 84 mcg administered as inhalation aerosol resulted in heart rate increases of 3 to 16 beats/min, about the same as albuterol dosed at 180 mcg by inhalation aerosol (4 to 10 beats/min). Adolescent and adult patients receiving 50-mcg doses of salmeterol inhalation powder (N = 60) underwent continuous electrocardiographic monitoring during two 12-hour periods after the first dose and after 1 month of therapy, and no clinically significant dysrhythmias were noted.

Chronic Obstructive Pulmonary Disease: In 24-week clinical studies in patients with COPD associated with chronic bronchitis, the incidence of clinically significant electrocardiogram (ECG) abnormalities (myocardial ischemia, ventricular hypertrophy, clinically significant conduction abnormalities, clinically significant arrhythmias) was lower for patients who received salmeterol (1%, 9 of 688 patients who received either salmeterol 50 mcg or ADVAIR DISKUS) compared with placebo (3%, 10 of 370 subjects).

No significant differences with salmeterol 50 mcg alone or in combination with fluticasone propionate as ADVAIR DISKUS 500/50 was observed on pulse rate and systolic and diastolic blood pressure in a subset of patients with COPD who underwent 12-hour serial vital sign measurements after the first dose (N = 183) and after 12 weeks of therapy (N = 149). Median changes from baseline in pulse rate and systolic and diastolic blood pressure were similar to those seen with placebo (see ADVERSE REACTIONS: Chronic Obstructive Pulmonary Disease Associated With Chronic Bronchitis).

Studies in laboratory animals (minipigs, rodents, and dogs) have demonstrated the occurrence of cardiac arrhythmias and sudden death (with histologic evidence of myocardial necrosis) when beta-agonists and methylxanthines are administered concurrently. The clinical significance of these findings is unknown.

CLINICAL TRIALS

Asthma: In clinical trials comparing ADVAIR DISKUS with the individual components, improvements in most efficacy endpoints were greater with ADVAIR DISKUS than with the use of either fluticasone propionate or salmeterol alone. In addition, clinical trials showed similar results between ADVAIR DISKUS and the concurrent use of fluticasone propionate plus salmeterol at corresponding doses from separate inhalers.

Studies Comparing ADVAIR DISKUS to Fluticasone Propionate Alone or Salmeterol Alone: Three (3) double-blind, parallel-group clinical trials were conducted with ADVAIR DISKUS in 1,208 adolescent and adult patients (≥12 years, baseline FEV_1 63% to 72% of predicted normal) with asthma that was not optimally controlled on their current therapy. All treatments were inhalation powders, given as 1 inhalation from the DISKUS device twice daily, and other maintenance therapies were discontinued.

Study 1: Clinical Trial With ADVAIR DISKUS 100/50: This placebo-controlled, 12-week, US study compared ADVAIR DISKUS 100/50 with its individual components, fluticasone propionate 100 mcg and salmeterol 50 mcg. The study was stratified according to baseline asthma maintenance therapy; patients were using either inhaled corticosteroids (N = 250) (daily doses of beclomethasone dipropionate 252 to 420 mcg; flunisolide 1,000 mcg; fluticasone propionate inhalation aerosol 176 mcg; or triamcinolone acetonide 600 to 1,000 mcg) or salmeterol (N = 106). Baseline FEV_1 measurements were similar across treatments: ADVAIR DISKUS 100/50, 2.17 L; fluticasone propionate 100 mcg, 2.11 L; salmeterol, 2.13 L; and placebo, 2.15 L.

Predefined withdrawal criteria for lack of efficacy, an indicator of worsening asthma, were utilized for this placebo-controlled study. Worsening asthma was defined as a clinically important decrease in FEV_1 or peak expiratory flow (PEF), increase in use of VENTOLIN® (albuterol, USP) Inhalation Aerosol, increase in night awakenings due to asthma, emergency intervention or hospitalization due to asthma, or requirement for asthma medication not allowed by the protocol. As shown in Table 1, statistically significantly fewer patients receiving ADVAIR DISKUS 100/50 were withdrawn due to worsening asthma compared with fluticasone propionate, salmeterol, and placebo.

[See table 1 above]

The FEV_1 results are displayed in Figure 1. Because this trial used predetermined criteria for worsening asthma, which caused more patients in the placebo group to be withdrawn, FEV_1 results at Endpoint (last available FEV_1 result) are also provided. Patients receiving ADVAIR DISKUS 100/50 had significantly greater improvements in FEV_1 (0.51 L, 25%) compared with fluticasone propionate 100 mcg (0.28 L, 15%), salmeterol (0.11 L, 5%), and placebo (0.01 L, 1%). These improvements in FEV_1 with ADVAIR DISKUS were achieved regardless of baseline asthma maintenance therapy (inhaled corticosteroids or salmeterol).

[See figure at top of next column]

The effect of ADVAIR DISKUS 100/50 on morning and evening PEF endpoints is shown in Table 2.

[See table 2 at bottom of next page]

The subjective impact of asthma on patients' perception of health was evaluated through use of an instrument called the Asthma Quality of Life Questionnaire (AQLQ) (based on a 7-point scale where 1 = maximum impairment and 7 = none). Patients receiving ADVAIR DISKUS 100/50 had clinically meaningful improvements in overall asthma-specific

Continued on next page

Advair Diskus—Cont.

Figure 1. Mean Percent Change From Baseline in FEV₁ in Patients With Asthma Previously Treated With Either Inhaled Corticosteroids or Salmeterol (Study 1)

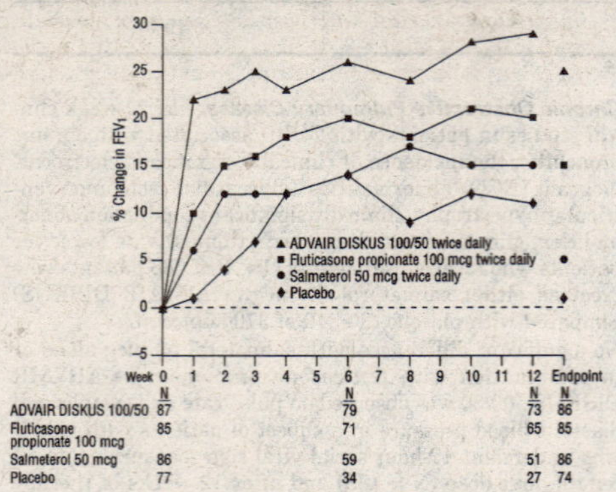

quality of life as defined by a difference between groups of ≥0.5 points in change from baseline AQLQ scores (difference in AQLQ score of 1.25 compared to placebo).

Study 2: Clinical Trial With ADVAIR DISKUS 250/50: This placebo-controlled, 12-week, US study compared ADVAIR DISKUS 250/50 with its individual components, fluticasone propionate 250 mcg and salmeterol 50 mcg in 349 patients with asthma using inhaled corticosteroids (daily doses of beclomethasone dipropionate 462 to 672 mcg; flunisolide 1,250 to 2,000 mcg; fluticasone propionate inhalation aerosol 440 mcg; or triamcinolone acetonide 1,100 to 1,600 mcg). Baseline FEV_1 measurements were similar across treatments: ADVAIR DISKUS 250/50, 2.23 L; fluticasone propionate 250 mcg, 2.12 L; salmeterol, 2.20 L; and placebo, 2.19 L.

Efficacy results in this study were similar to those observed in Study 1. Patients receiving ADVAIR DISKUS 250/50 had significantly greater improvements in FEV_1 (0.48 L, 23%) compared with fluticasone propionate 250 mcg (0.25 L, 13%), salmeterol (0.05 L, 4%), and placebo (decrease of 0.11 L, decrease of 5%). Statistically significantly fewer patients receiving ADVAIR DISKUS 250/50 were withdrawn from this study for worsening asthma (4%) compared with fluticasone propionate (22%), salmeterol (38%), and placebo (62%). In addition, ADVAIR DISKUS 250/50 was superior to fluticasone propionate, salmeterol, and placebo for improvements in morning and evening PEF. Patients receiving ADVAIR DISKUS 250/50 also had clinically meaningful improvements in overall asthma-specific quality of life as described in Study 1 (difference in AQLQ score of 1.29 compared to placebo).

Study 3: Clinical Trial With ADVAIR DISKUS 500/50: This 28-week, non-US study compared ADVAIR DISKUS 500/50 with fluticasone propionate 500 mcg alone and concurrent therapy (salmeterol 50 mcg plus fluticasone propionate 500 mcg administered from separate inhalers) twice daily in 503 patients with asthma using inhaled corticosteroids (daily doses of beclomethasone dipropionate 1,260 to 1,680 mcg; budesonide 1,500 to 2,000 mcg; flunisolide 1,500 to 2,000 mcg; or fluticasone propionate inhalation aerosol 660 to 880 mcg [750 to 1,000 mcg inhalation powder]). The primary efficacy parameter, morning PEF, was collected daily for the first 12 weeks of the study. The primary purpose of weeks 13 to 28 was to collect safety data.

Baseline PEF measurements were similar across treatments: ADVAIR DISKUS 500/50, 359 L/min; fluticasone propionate 500 mcg, 351 L/min; and concurrent therapy, 345 L/min. As shown in Figure 2, morning PEF improved significantly with ADVAIR DISKUS 500/50 compared with fluticasone propionate 500 mcg over the 12-week treatment period. Improvements in morning PEF observed with ADVAIR DISKUS 500/50 were similar to improvements observed with concurrent therapy.

[See figure at top of next column]

Onset of Action and Progression of Improvement in Asthma Control: The onset of action and progression of improvement in asthma control were evaluated in the 2 placebo-controlled US trials. Following the first dose, the median time to onset of clinically significant bronchodilatation (≥15% improvement in FEV_1) in most patients was seen within 30 to 60 minutes. Maximum improvement in FEV_1 generally occurred within 3 hours, and clinically significant

Figure 2. Mean Percent Change From Baseline in Morning Peak Expiratory Flow in Patients With Asthma Previously Treated With Inhaled Corticosteroids (Study 3)

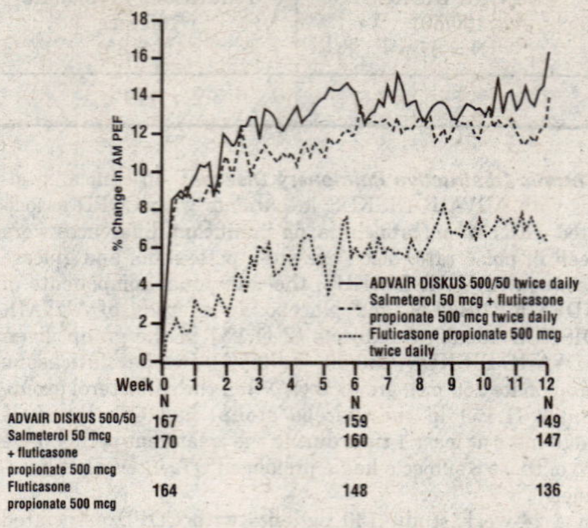

improvement was maintained for 12 hours (see Figure 3). Following the initial dose, predose FEV_1 relative to Day 1 baseline improved markedly over the first week of treatment and continued to improve over the 12 weeks of treatment in both studies.

No diminution in the 12-hour bronchodilator effect was observed with either ADVAIR DISKUS 100/50 (Figures 3 and 4) or ADVAIR DISKUS 250/50 as assessed by FEV_1 following 12 weeks of therapy.

Figure 3. Percent Change in Serial 12-hour FEV₁ in Patients With Asthma Previously Using Either Inhaled Corticosteroids or Salmeterol (Study 1)

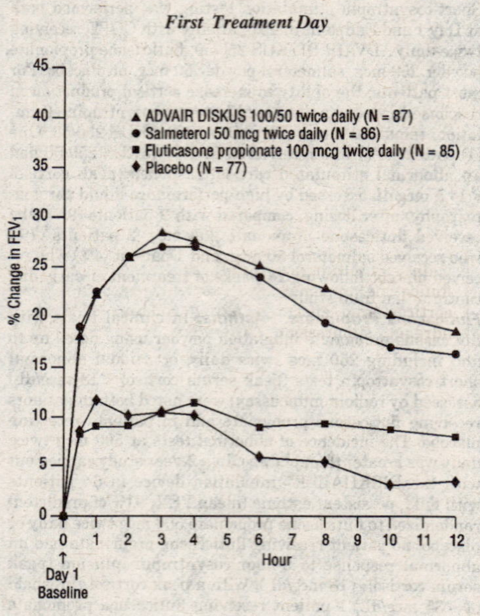

[See figure 4 at top of next column]

Reduction in asthma symptoms, use of rescue VENTOLIN Inhalation Aerosol, and improvement in morning and evening PEF also occurred within the first day of treatment with ADVAIR DISKUS, and continued to improve over the 12 weeks of therapy in both studies.

Chronic Obstructive Pulmonary Disease Associated With Chronic Bronchitis: In a clinical trial evaluating twice-daily treatment with ADVAIR DISKUS 250/50 in patients with COPD associated with chronic bronchitis, improvements in lung function (as defined by predose and postdose FEV_1) were significantly greater with ADVAIR DISKUS than with fluticasone propionate 250 mcg, salmeterol 50 mcg, or placebo. The study was a randomized, double-blind, parallel-group, 24-week trial. All patients had a history of cough productive of sputum that was not attributable to another disease process on most days for at least 3 months of the year for at least 2 years. Study treatments were inhalation powders given as 1 inhalation from the

Figure 4. Percent Change in Serial 12-hour FEV₁ in Patients With Asthma Previously Using Either Inhaled Corticosteroids or Salmeterol (Study 1)

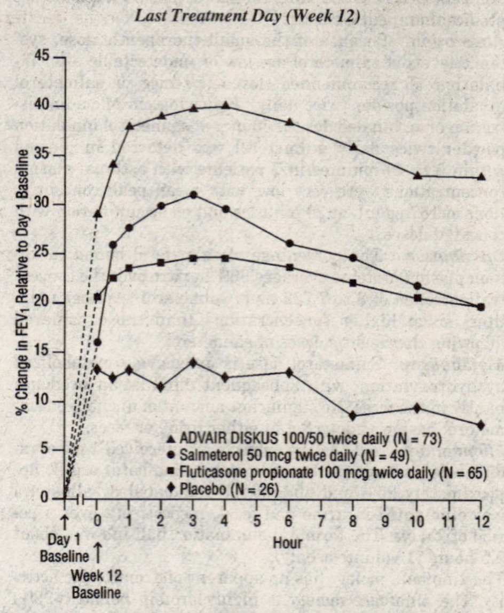

DISKUS device twice daily. Maintenance COPD therapies were discontinued, with the exception of theophylline.

Figures 5 and 6 display predose and 2-hour postdose FEV_1 results. To account for patient withdrawals during the study, FEV_1 at Endpoint (last evaluable FEV_1) was evaluated. Patients receiving ADVAIR DISKUS 250/50 had significantly greater improvements in predose FEV_1 at Endpoint (165 mL, 17%) compared with salmeterol 50 mcg (91 mL, 9%) and placebo (1 mL, 1%), demonstrating the contribution of fluticasone propionate to the improvement in lung function with ADVAIR DISKUS (Figure 5). Patients receiving ADVAIR DISKUS 250/50 had significantly greater improvements in postdose FEV_1 at Endpoint (281 mL, 27%) compared with fluticasone propionate 250 mcg (147 mL, 14%) and placebo (58 mL, 6%), demonstrating the contribution of salmeterol to the improvement in lung function with ADVAIR DISKUS (Figure 6).

A similar degree of improvement in lung function was also observed with ADVAIR DISKUS 500/50 twice daily.

Figure 5. Predose FEV₁: Mean Percent Change From Baseline in Patients With COPD Associated With Chronic Bronchitis

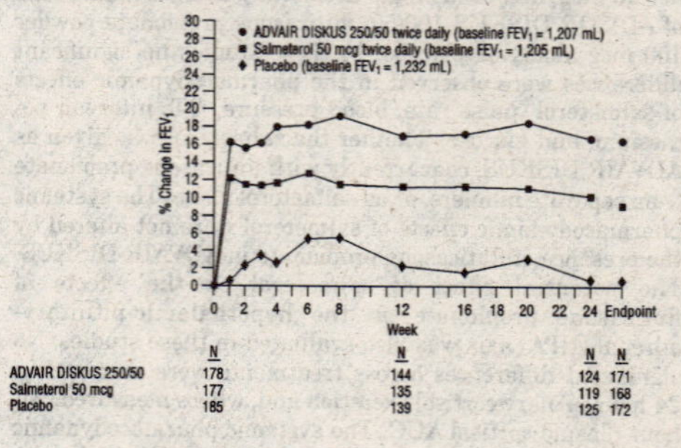

Figure 6. Two-Hour Postdose FEV₁: Mean Percent Changes From Baseline Over Time in Patients With COPD Associated With Chronic Bronchitis

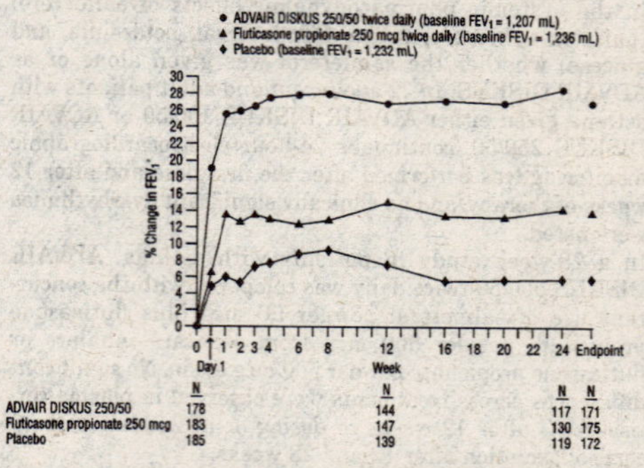

Patients treated with ADVAIR DISKUS 250/50 or ADVAIR DISKUS 500/50 did not have a significant reduction in chronic bronchitis symptoms (as measured by the Chronic Bronchitis Symptom Questionnaire) or in COPD exacerbations compared to patients treated with placebo over the 24 weeks of therapy. The improvement in lung function with ADVAIR DISKUS 500/50 was similar to the improvement seen with ADVAIR DISKUS 250/50. Since there is evidence of more systemic exposure to fluticasone propionate from this higher dose and no documented advantage for efficacy, ADVAIR DISKUS 500/50 is not recommended for use in COPD.

Table 2. Peak Expiratory Flow Results for Patients With Asthma Previously Treated With Either Inhaled Corticosteroids or Salmeterol (Study 1)

Efficacy Variable*	ADVAIR DISKUS 100/50 (N = 87)	Fluticasone Propionate 100 mcg (N = 85)	Salmeterol 50 mcg (N = 86)	Placebo (N = 77)
AM PEF (L/min)				
Baseline	393	374	369	382
Change from baseline	53	17	−2	−24
PM PEF (L/min)				
Baseline	418	390	396	398
Change from baseline	35	18	−7	−13

*Change from baseline = change from baseline at Endpoint (last available data).

The benefit of treatment of patients with COPD associated with chronic bronchitis with ADVAIR DISKUS 250/50 for periods longer than 6 months has not been evaluated.

INDICATIONS AND USAGE

Asthma: ADVAIR DISKUS is indicated for the long-term, twice-daily, maintenance treatment of asthma in patients 12 years of age and older.

ADVAIR DISKUS is NOT indicated for the relief of acute bronchospasm.

Chronic Obstructive Pulmonary Disease Associated With Chronic Bronchitis: ADVAIR DISKUS 250/50 is indicated for the twice-daily maintenance treatment of airflow obstruction in patients with COPD associated with chronic bronchitis.

ADVAIR DISKUS 250/50 mcg twice daily is the only approved dosage for the treatment of COPD associated with chronic bronchitis. Higher doses, including ADVAIR DISKUS 500/50, are not recommended (see DOSAGE AND ADMINISTRATION: Chronic Obstructive Pulmonary Disease Associated With Chronic Bronchitis).

The benefit of treating patients with COPD associated with chronic bronchitis with ADVAIR DISKUS 250/50 for periods longer than 6 months has not been evaluated. Patients who are treated with ADVAIR DISKUS 250/50 for COPD associated with chronic bronchitis for periods longer than 6 months should be reevaluated periodically to assess the continuing benefits and potential risks of treatment.

ADVAIR DISKUS is NOT indicated for the relief of acute bronchospasm.

CONTRAINDICATIONS

ADVAIR DISKUS is contraindicated in the primary treatment of status asthmaticus or other acute episodes of asthma or COPD where intensive measures are required.

Hypersensitivity to any of the ingredients of these preparations contraindicates their use (see DESCRIPTION and ADVERSE REACTIONS Observed During Clinical Practice: *Non-Site Specific*).

WARNINGS

DATA FROM A LARGE PLACEBO-CONTROLLED SAFETY STUDY THAT WAS STOPPED EARLY SUGGEST THAT SALMETEROL, A COMPONENT OF ADVAIR DISKUS, MAY BE ASSOCIATED WITH RARE SERIOUS ASTHMA EPISODES OR ASTHMA-RELATED DEATHS. The Salmeterol Multi-center Asthma Research Trial (SMART) enrolled long-acting beta$_2$-agonist-naive patients with asthma to assess the safety of salmeterol (SEREVENT Inhalation Aerosol) 42 mcg twice daily over 28 weeks compared to placebo, when added to usual asthma therapy. The primary endpoint was the combined number of respiratory-related deaths or respiratory-related life-threatening experiences (intubation and mechanical ventilation). Other endpoints included combined asthma-related deaths or life-threatening experiences and asthma-related deaths.

A planned interim analysis was conducted when approximately half of the intended number of patients had been enrolled (N = 26,353). The analysis showed no significant difference for the primary endpoint for the total population. However, a higher number of asthma-related deaths or life-threatening experiences (36 vs. 23) and a higher number of asthma-related deaths (13 vs. 4) occurred in the patients treated with SEREVENT Inhalation Aerosol. Post hoc subgroup analyses revealed no significant increase in respiratory- or asthma-related episodes, including deaths, in Caucasian patients. In African Americans, the study showed a small, though statistically significantly greater, number of primary events (20 vs. 7), asthma-related deaths or life-threatening experiences (19 vs. 4), and asthma-related deaths (8 vs. 1) in patients taking SEREVENT Inhalation Aerosol compared to those taking placebo. Even though SMART did not reach predetermined stopping criteria for the total population, the study was stopped due to the findings in African American patients and difficulties in enrollment. The data from the SMART study are not adequate to determine whether concurrent use of inhaled corticosteroids, such as fluticasone propionate, a component of ADVAIR DISKUS, provides protection from this risk. Therefore, it is not known whether the findings seen with SEREVENT Inhalation Aerosol would apply to ADVAIR DISKUS.

Findings similar to the SMART study findings were reported in a prior 16-week clinical study performed in the United Kingdom, the Salmeterol Nationwide Surveillance (SNS) study. In the SNS study, the incidence of asthma-related death was numerically, though not statistically, greater in patients with asthma treated with salmeterol (42 mcg twice daily) versus albuterol (180 mcg 4 times daily) added to usual asthma therapy.

Given the similar basic mechanisms of action of beta$_2$-agonists, it is possible that the findings seen in the SMART study may be consistent with a class effect.

1. **ADVAIR DISKUS SHOULD NOT BE USED FOR TRANSFERRING PATIENTS FROM SYSTEMIC CORTICOSTEROID THERAPY.** Particular care is needed for patients who have been transferred from systemically active corticosteroids to inhaled corticosteroids because deaths due to adrenal insufficiency have occurred in patients with asthma during and after transfer from systemic corticosteroids to less systemically available inhaled corticosteroids. After withdrawal from systemic corticosteroids, a number of months are required for recovery of HPA function.

Patients who have been previously maintained on 20 mg or more per day of prednisone (or its equivalent) may be most susceptible, particularly when their systemic corticosteroids have been almost completely withdrawn. During this period of HPA suppression, patients may exhibit signs and symptoms of adrenal insufficiency when exposed to trauma, surgery, or infection (particularly gastroenteritis) or other conditions associated with severe electrolyte loss. Although inhaled corticosteroids may provide control of asthma symptoms during these episodes, in recommended doses they supply less than normal physiological amounts of glucocorticoid systemically and do NOT provide the mineralocorticoid activity that is necessary for coping with these emergencies.

During periods of stress or a severe asthma attack, patients who have been withdrawn from systemic corticosteroids should be instructed to resume oral corticosteroids (in large doses) immediately and to contact their physicians for further instruction. These patients should also be instructed to carry a warning card indicating that they may need supplementary systemic corticosteroids during periods of stress or a severe asthma attack.

2. **ADVAIR DISKUS SHOULD NOT BE INITIATED IN PATIENTS DURING RAPIDLY DETERIORATING OR POTENTIALLY LIFE-THREATENING EPISODES OF ASTHMA. Serious acute respiratory events, including fatalities, have been reported both in the United States and worldwide when salmeterol, a component of ADVAIR DISKUS, has been initiated in patients with significantly worsening or acutely deteriorating asthma.** In most cases, these have occurred in patients with severe asthma (e.g., patients with a history of corticosteroid dependence, low pulmonary function, intubation, mechanical ventilation, frequent hospitalizations, or previous life-threatening acute asthma exacerbations) and/or in some patients in whom asthma has been acutely deteriorating (e.g., unresponsive to usual medications; increasing need for inhaled, short-acting beta$_2$-agonists; increasing need for systemic corticosteroids; significant increase in symptoms; recent emergency room visits; sudden or progressive deterioration in pulmonary function). However, they have occurred in a few patients with less severe asthma as well. It was not possible from these reports to determine whether salmeterol contributed to these events or simply failed to relieve the deteriorating asthma.

3. **Drug Interaction With Ritonavir:** A drug interaction study in healthy subjects has shown that ritonavir (a highly potent cytochrome P450 3A4 inhibitor) can significantly increase plasma fluticasone propionate exposure, resulting in significantly reduced serum cortisol concentrations (see CLINICAL PHARMACOLOGY: Pharmacokinetics: *Fluticasone Propionate: Drug Interactions* and PRECAUTIONS: Drug Interactions: *Inhibitors of Cytochrome P450*). During postmarketing use, there have been reports of clinically significant drug interactions in patients receiving fluticasone propionate and ritonavir, resulting in systemic corticosteroid effects including Cushing syndrome and adrenal suppression. Therefore, coadministration of fluticasone propionate and ritonavir is not recommended unless the potential benefit to the patient outweighs the risk of systemic corticosteroid side effects.

4. Do Not Use ADVAIR DISKUS to Treat Acute Symptoms: An inhaled, short-acting beta$_2$-agonist, not ADVAIR DISKUS, should be used to relieve acute symptoms of shortness of breath. When prescribing ADVAIR DISKUS, the physician must also provide the patient with an inhaled, short-acting beta$_2$-agonist (e.g., albuterol) for treatment of shortness of breath that occurs acutely, despite regular twice-daily (morning and evening) use of ADVAIR DISKUS. When beginning treatment with ADVAIR DISKUS, patients who have been taking oral or inhaled, short-acting beta$_2$-agonists on a regular basis (e.g., 4 times a day) should be instructed to discontinue the regular use of these drugs. For patients on ADVAIR DISKUS, inhaled, short-acting beta$_2$-agonists should only be used for symptomatic relief of acute symptoms of shortness of breath (see PRECAUTIONS: Information for Patients).

5. Watch for Increasing Use of Inhaled, Short-Acting Beta$_2$-Agonists, Which Is a Marker of Deteriorating Asthma: Asthma may deteriorate acutely over a period of hours or chronically over several days or longer. If the patient's inhaled, short-acting beta$_2$-agonist becomes less effective, the patient needs more inhalations than usual, or the patient develops a significant decrease in lung function, this may be a marker of destabilization of the disease. In this setting, the patient requires immediate reevaluation with reassessment of the treatment regimen, giving special consideration to the possible need for replacing the current strength of ADVAIR DISKUS with a higher strength, adding additional inhaled corticosteroid, or initiating systemic corticosteroids. Patients should not use more than 1 inhalation twice daily (morning and evening) of ADVAIR DISKUS.

6. Do Not Use an Inhaled, Long-Acting Beta$_2$-Agonist in Conjunction With ADVAIR DISKUS: Patients who are receiving ADVAIR DISKUS twice daily should not use additional salmeterol or other inhaled, long-acting beta$_2$-agonists (e.g., formoterol) for prevention of exercise-induced bronchospasm (EIB) or the maintenance treatment of asthma or the maintenance treatment of bronchospasm associated with COPD. Additional benefit would not be gained from using supplemental salmeterol or formoterol for prevention of EIB since ADVAIR DISKUS already contains an inhaled, long-acting beta$_2$-agonist.

7. Do Not Exceed Recommended Dosage: ADVAIR DISKUS should not be used more often or at higher doses than recommended. Fatalities have been reported in association with excessive use of inhaled sympathomimetic drugs. Large doses of inhaled or oral salmeterol (12 to 20 times the recommended dose) have been associated with clinically significant prolongation of the QTc interval, which has the potential for producing ventricular arrhythmias.

8. Paradoxical Bronchospasm: As with other inhaled asthma and COPD medications, ADVAIR DISKUS can produce paradoxical bronchospasm, which may be life threatening. If paradoxical bronchospasm occurs following dosing with ADVAIR DISKUS, it should be treated immediately with an inhaled, short-acting bronchodilator, ADVAIR DISKUS should be discontinued immediately, and alternative therapy should be instituted.

9. Immediate Hypersensitivity Reactions: Immediate hypersensitivity reactions may occur after administration of ADVAIR DISKUS, as demonstrated by cases of urticaria, angioedema, rash, and bronchospasm.

10. Upper Airway Symptoms: Symptoms of laryngeal spasm, irritation, or swelling, such as stridor and choking, have been reported in patients receiving fluticasone propionate and salmeterol, components of ADVAIR DISKUS.

11. Cardiovascular Disorders: ADVAIR DISKUS, like all products containing sympathomimetic amines, should be used with caution in patients with cardiovascular disorders, especially coronary insufficiency, cardiac arrhythmias, and hypertension. Salmeterol, a component of ADVAIR DISKUS, can produce a clinically significant cardiovascular effect in some patients as measured by pulse rate, blood pressure, and/or symptoms. Although such effects are uncommon after administration of salmeterol at recommended doses, if they occur, the drug may need to be discontinued. In addition, beta-agonists have been reported to produce ECG changes, such as flattening of the T wave, prolongation of the QTc interval, and ST segment depression. The clinical significance of these findings is unknown.

12. Discontinuation of Systemic Corticosteroids: Transfer of patients from systemic corticosteroid therapy to ADVAIR DISKUS may unmask conditions previously suppressed by the systemic corticosteroid therapy, e.g., rhinitis, conjunctivitis, eczema, arthritis, and eosinophilic conditions.

13. Immunosuppression: Persons who are using drugs that suppress the immune system are more susceptible to infections than healthy individuals. Chickenpox and measles, for example, can have a more serious or even fatal course in susceptible children or adults using corticosteroids. In such children or adults who have not had these diseases or been properly immunized, particular care should be taken to avoid exposure. How the dose, route, and duration of corticosteroid administration affect the risk of developing a disseminated infection is not known. The contribution of the underlying disease and/or prior corticosteroid treatment to the risk is also not known. If exposed to chickenpox, prophylaxis with varicella zoster immune globulin (VZIG) may be indicated. If exposed to measles, prophylaxis with pooled intramuscular immunoglobulin (IG) may be indicated. (See the respective package inserts for complete VZIG and IG prescribing information.) If chickenpox develops, treatment with antiviral agents may be considered.

PRECAUTIONS

General: ***Cardiovascular Effects:*** Cardiovascular and central nervous system effects seen with all sympathomimetic drugs (e.g., increased blood pressure, heart rate, excitement) can occur after use of salmeterol, a component of ADVAIR DISKUS, and may require discontinuation of ADVAIR DISKUS. ADVAIR DISKUS, like all medications containing sympathomimetic amines, should be used with caution in patients with cardiovascular disorders, especially coronary insufficiency, cardiac arrhythmias, and hypertension; in patients with convulsive disorders or thyrotoxicosis; and in patients who are unusually responsive to sympathomimetic amines.

As has been described with other beta-adrenergic agonist bronchodilators, clinically significant changes in ECGs have been seen infrequently in individual patients in controlled clinical studies with ADVAIR DISKUS and salmeterol. Clinically significant changes in systolic and/or diastolic blood pressure and pulse rate have been seen infrequently in individual patients in controlled clinical studies with salmeterol, a component of ADVAIR DISKUS.

Metabolic and Other Effects: Long-term use of orally inhaled corticosteroids may affect normal bone metabolism, resulting in a loss of bone mineral density (BMD). A 2-year study of 160 patients (females 18 to 40 and males 18 to 50 years of age) with asthma receiving chlorofluorocarbon-propelled fluticasone propionate inhalation aerosol 88 or 440 mcg twice daily demonstrated no statistically significant changes in BMD at any time point (24, 52, 76, and 104 weeks of double-blind treatment) as assessed by dual-energy x-ray absorptiometry at lumbar region L1 through L4. Long-term treatment effects of fluticasone propionate on BMD in the COPD population have not been studied.

In patients with major risk factors for decreased bone mineral content, such as tobacco use, advanced age, sedentary lifestyle, poor nutrition, family history of osteoporosis, or chronic use of drugs that can reduce bone mass (e.g., anticonvulsants and corticosteroids), ADVAIR DISKUS may pose an additional risk. Since patients with COPD often have multiple risk factors for reduced BMD, assessment of BMD is recommended, including prior to instituting ADVAIR DISKUS 250/50 and periodically thereafter. If significant reductions in BMD are seen and ADVAIR DISKUS 250/50 is still considered medically important for that pa-

Continued on next page

Advair Diskus—Cont.

tient's COPD therapy, use of medication to treat or prevent osteoporosis should be strongly considered. ADVAIR DISKUS 250/50 mcg twice daily is the only approved dosage for the treatment of COPD associated with chronic bronchitis, and higher doses, including ADVAIR DISKUS 500/50, are not recommended.

Glaucoma, increased intraocular pressure, and cataracts have been reported in patients with asthma and COPD following the long-term administration of inhaled corticosteroids, including fluticasone propionate, a component of ADVAIR DISKUS; therefore, regular eye examinations should be considered.

Lower respiratory tract infections, including pneumonia, have been reported following the inhaled administration of corticosteroids, including fluticasone propionate and ADVAIR DISKUS.

Doses of the related $beta_2$-adrenoceptor agonist albuterol, when administered intravenously, have been reported to aggravate preexisting diabetes mellitus and ketoacidosis. Beta-adrenergic agonist medications may produce significant hypokalemia in some patients, possibly through intracellular shunting, which has the potential to produce adverse cardiovascular effects. The decrease in serum potassium is usually transient, not requiring supplementation.

Clinically significant changes in blood glucose and/or serum potassium were seen infrequently during clinical studies with ADVAIR DISKUS at recommended doses.

During withdrawal from oral corticosteroids, some patients may experience symptoms of systemically active corticosteroid withdrawal, e.g., joint and/or muscular pain, lassitude, and depression, despite maintenance or even improvement of respiratory function.

Fluticasone propionate, a component of ADVAIR DISKUS, will often help control asthma symptoms with less suppression of HPA function than therapeutically equivalent oral doses of prednisone. Since fluticasone propionate is absorbed into the circulation and can be systemically active at higher doses, the beneficial effects of ADVAIR DISKUS in minimizing HPA dysfunction may be expected only when recommended dosages are not exceeded and individual patients are titrated to the lowest effective dose. A relationship between plasma levels of fluticasone propionate and inhibitory effects on stimulated cortisol production has been shown after 4 weeks of treatment with fluticasone propionate inhalation aerosol. Since individual sensitivity to effects on cortisol production exists, physicians should consider this information when prescribing ADVAIR DISKUS.

Because of the possibility of systemic absorption of inhaled corticosteroids, patients treated with ADVAIR DISKUS should be observed carefully for any evidence of systemic corticosteroid effects. Particular care should be taken in observing patients postoperatively or during periods of stress for evidence of inadequate adrenal response.

It is possible that systemic corticosteroid effects such as hypercorticism and adrenal suppression (including adrenal crisis) may appear in a small number of patients, particularly when fluticasone propionate is administered at higher than recommended doses over prolonged periods of time. If such effects occur, the dosage of ADVAIR DISKUS should be reduced slowly, consistent with accepted procedures for reducing systemic corticosteroids and for management of asthma symptoms.

Orally inhaled corticosteroids may cause a reduction in growth velocity when administered to pediatric patients (see PRECAUTIONS: Pediatric Use). Patients should be maintained on the lowest strength of ADVAIR DISKUS that effectively controls their asthma.

The long-term effects of ADVAIR DISKUS in human subjects are not fully known. In particular, the effects resulting from chronic use of fluticasone propionate on developmental or immunologic processes in the mouth, pharynx, trachea, and lung are unknown. Some patients have received inhaled fluticasone propionate on a continuous basis for periods of 3 years or longer. In clinical studies in patients with asthma treated for 2 years with inhaled fluticasone propionate, no apparent differences in the type or severity of adverse reactions were observed after long- versus short-term treatment.

In clinical studies with ADVAIR DISKUS, the development of localized infections of the pharynx with *Candida albicans* has occurred. When such an infection develops, it should be treated with appropriate local or systemic (i.e., oral antifungal) therapy while remaining on treatment with ADVAIR DISKUS, but at times therapy with ADVAIR DISKUS may need to be interrupted.

Inhaled corticosteroids should be used with caution, if at all, in patients with active or quiescent tuberculosis infections of the respiratory tract; untreated systemic fungal, bacterial, viral, or parasitic infections; or ocular herpes simplex.

Eosinophilic Conditions: In rare cases, patients on inhaled fluticasone propionate, a component of ADVAIR DISKUS, may present with systemic eosinophilic conditions, with some patients presenting with clinical features of vasculitis consistent with Churg-Strauss syndrome, a condition that is often treated with systemic corticosteroid therapy. These events usually, but not always, have been associated with the reduction and/or withdrawal of oral corticosteroid therapy following the introduction of fluticasone propionate. Cases of serious eosinophilic conditions have also been reported with other inhaled corticosteroids in this clinical setting. Physicians should be alert to eosinophilia, vasculitic rash, worsening pulmonary symptoms, cardiac complications, and/or neuropathy presenting in their patients. A causal relationship between fluticasone propionate and these underlying conditions has not been established (see ADVERSE REACTIONS: Observed During Clinical Practice: *Eosinophilic Conditions*).

Chronic Obstructive Pulmonary Disease: ADVAIR DISKUS 250/50 twice daily is the only dosage recommended for the treatment of airflow obstruction in patients with COPD associated with chronic bronchitis. Higher doses, including ADVAIR DISKUS 500/50, are not recommended, as no additional improvement in lung function (defined by predose and postdose FEV_1) was observed in clinical trials and higher doses of corticosteroids increase the risk of systemic effects.

The benefit of treatment of patients with COPD associated with chronic bronchitis with ADVAIR DISKUS 250/50 for periods longer than 6 months has not been evaluated. Patients who are treated with ADVAIR DISKUS 250/50 for COPD associated with chronic bronchitis for periods longer than 6 months should be reevaluated periodically to assess the continuing benefits and potential risks of treatment.

Information for Patients: Patients being treated with ADVAIR DISKUS should receive the following information and instructions. This information is intended to aid them in the safe and effective use of this medication. It is not a disclosure of all possible adverse or intended effects.

It is important that patients understand how to use the DISKUS inhalation device appropriately and how it should be used in relation to other asthma or COPD medications they are taking. Patients should be given the following information:

1. Patients should use ADVAIR DISKUS at regular intervals as directed. Results of clinical trials indicate significant improvement may occur within the first 30 minutes of taking the first dose; however, the full benefit may not be achieved until treatment has been administered for 1 week or longer. The patient should not use more than the prescribed dosage but should contact the physician if symptoms do not improve or if the condition worsens.
2. Most patients are able to taste or feel a dose delivered from ADVAIR DISKUS. However, whether or not patients are able to sense delivery of a dose, you should instruct them not to exceed the recommended dose of 1 inhalation each morning and evening, approximately 12 hours apart. You should instruct them to contact you or the pharmacist if they have questions.
3. The bronchodilation from a single dose of ADVAIR DISKUS may last up to 12 hours or longer. The recommended dosage (1 inhalation twice daily, morning and evening) should not be exceeded. Patients who are receiving ADVAIR DISKUS twice daily should not use salmeterol or other inhaled, long-acting $beta_2$-agonists (e.g., formoterol) for prevention of EIB or maintenance treatment of asthma or the maintenance treatment of bronchospasm in COPD.
4. ADVAIR DISKUS is not meant to relieve acute asthma symptoms and extra doses should not be used for that purpose. Acute symptoms should be treated with an inhaled, short-acting $beta_2$-agonist such as albuterol (the physician should provide the patient with such medication and instruct the patient in how it should be used). ADVAIR DISKUS is not meant to relieve acute asthma symptoms or exacerbations of COPD.
5. Patients should not stop therapy with ADVAIR DISKUS without physician/provider guidance since symptoms may recur after discontinuation.
6. The physician should be notified immediately if any of the following situations occur, which may be a sign of seriously worsening asthma:
   - decreasing effectiveness of inhaled, short-acting $beta_2$-agonists;
   - need for more inhalations than usual of inhaled, short-acting $beta_2$-agonists;
   - significant decrease in lung function as outlined by the physician.
7. Patients should be cautioned regarding common adverse effects associated with $beta_2$-agonists, such as palpitations, chest pain, rapid heart rate, tremor, or nervousness.
8. Patients who are at an increased risk for decreased BMD should be advised that the use of corticosteroids may pose an additional risk and should be told to monitor and, where appropriate, seek treatment for this condition.
9. Long-term use of inhaled corticosteroids, including fluticasone propionate, a component of ADVAIR DISKUS, may increase the risk of some eye problems (cataracts or glaucoma). Regular eye examinations should be considered.
10. When patients are prescribed ADVAIR DISKUS, other medications for asthma and COPD should be used only as directed by their physicians.
11. ADVAIR DISKUS should not be used with a spacer device.
12. Patients who are pregnant or nursing should contact their physicians about the use of ADVAIR DISKUS.
13. Effective and safe use of ADVAIR DISKUS includes an understanding of the way that it should be used:
    - Never exhale into the DISKUS.
    - Never attempt to take the DISKUS apart.
    - Always activate and use the DISKUS in a level, horizontal position.
    - After inhalation, rinse the mouth with water without swallowing.
    - Never wash the mouthpiece or any part of the DISKUS. KEEP IT DRY.
    - Always keep the DISKUS in a dry place.
    - Discard **1 month** after removal from the moisture-protective foil overwrap pouch or after all blisters have been used (when the dose indicator reads "0"), whichever comes first.
14. Patients should be warned to avoid exposure to chickenpox or measles and, if they are exposed, to consult their physicians without delay.
15. For the proper use of ADVAIR DISKUS and to attain maximum improvement, the patient should read and carefully follow the Patient's Instructions for Use accompanying the product.

Drug Interactions: ADVAIR DISKUS has been used concomitantly with other drugs, including short-acting $beta_2$-agonists, methylxanthines, and intranasal corticosteroids, commonly used in patients with asthma or COPD, without adverse drug reactions. No formal drug interaction studies have been performed with ADVAIR DISKUS.

Short-Acting $Beta_2$-Agonists: In clinical trials with patients with asthma, the mean daily need for albuterol by 166 patients using ADVAIR DISKUS was approximately 1.3 inhalations/day, and ranged from 0 to 9 inhalations/day. Five percent (5%) of patients using ADVAIR DISKUS in these trials averaged 6 or more inhalations per day over the course of the 12-week trials. No increase in frequency of cardiovascular adverse reactions was observed among patients who averaged 6 or more inhalations per day.

In a COPD clinical trial, the mean daily need for albuterol for patients using ADVAIR DISKUS 250/50 was 4.1 inhalations/day. Twenty-six percent (26%) of patients using ADVAIR DISKUS 250/50 averaged 6 or more inhalations per day over the course of the 24-week trial. No increase in frequency of cardiovascular adverse reactions was observed among patients who averaged 6 or more inhalations of albuterol per day.

Methylxanthines: The concurrent use of intravenously or orally administered methylxanthines (e.g., aminophylline, theophylline) by patients receiving ADVAIR DISKUS has not been completely evaluated. In clinical trials with patients with asthma, 39 patients receiving ADVAIR DISKUS 100/50, 250/50, or 500/50 twice daily concurrently with a theophylline product had adverse event rates similar to those in 304 patients receiving ADVAIR DISKUS without theophylline. Similar results were observed in patients receiving salmeterol 50 mcg plus fluticasone propionate 500 mcg twice daily concurrently with a theophylline product (N = 39) or without theophylline (N = 132).

In a COPD clinical trial, 17 patients receiving ADVAIR DISKUS 250/50 twice daily concurrently with a theophylline product had adverse event rates similar to those in 161 patients receiving ADVAIR DISKUS without theophylline. Based on the available data, the concomitant administration of methylxanthines with ADVAIR DISKUS did not alter the observed adverse event profile.

Fluticasone Propionate Nasal Spray: In patients taking ADVAIR DISKUS in clinical trials, no difference in the profile of adverse events or HPA axis effects was noted between patients taking FLONASE® (fluticasone propionate) Nasal Spray, 50 mcg concurrently (N = 46) and those who were not (N = 130).

Monoamine Oxidase Inhibitors and Tricyclic Antidepressants: ADVAIR DISKUS should be administered with extreme caution to patients being treated with monoamine oxidase inhibitors or tricyclic antidepressants, or within 2 weeks of discontinuation of such agents, because the action of salmeterol, a component of ADVAIR DISKUS, on the vascular system may be potentiated by these agents.

Beta-Adrenergic Receptor Blocking Agents: Beta-blockers not only block the pulmonary effect of beta-agonists, such as salmeterol, a component of ADVAIR DISKUS, but may produce severe bronchospasm in patients with asthma. Therefore, patients with asthma should not normally be treated with beta-blockers. However, under certain circumstances, there may be no acceptable alternatives to the use of beta-adrenergic blocking agents in patients with asthma. In this setting, cardioselective beta-blockers could be considered, although they should be administered with caution.

Diuretics: The ECG changes and/or hypokalemia that may result from the administration of nonpotassium-sparing diuretics (such as loop or thiazide diuretics) can be acutely worsened by beta-agonists, especially when the recommended dose of the beta-agonist is exceeded. Although the clinical significance of these effects is not known, caution is advised in the coadministration of beta-agonists with nonpotassium-sparing diuretics.

Inhibitors of Cytochrome P450: Fluticasone propionate is a substrate of cytochrome P450 3A4. A drug interaction study with fluticasone propionate aqueous nasal spray in healthy subjects has shown that ritonavir (a highly potent cytochrome P450 3A4 inhibitor) can significantly increase plasma fluticasone propionate exposure, resulting in significantly reduced serum cortisol concentrations (see CLINICAL PHARMACOLOGY: Pharmacokinetics: *Fluticasone Propionate: Drug Interactions*). During postmarketing use, there have been reports of clinically significant drug interactions in patients receiving fluticasone propionate and ritonavir, resulting in systemic corticosteroid effects including Cushing syndrome and adrenal suppression. Therefore, coadministration of fluticasone propionate and ritonavir is not recommended unless the potential benefit to the patient

outweighs the risk of systemic corticosteroid side effects.
In a placebo-controlled, crossover study in 8 healthy volunteers, coadministration of a single dose of orally inhaled fluticasone propionate (1,000 mcg) with multiple doses of ketoconazole (200 mg) to steady state resulted in increased plasma fluticasone propionate exposure, a reduction in plasma cortisol AUC, and no effect on urinary excretion of cortisol. This interaction may be due to an inhibition of cytochrome P450 3A4 by ketoconazole, which is also the route of metabolism of fluticasone propionate. Caution should be exercised when ADVAIR DISKUS is coadministered with ketoconazole and other known potent cytochrome P450 3A4 inhibitors.

Carcinogenesis, Mutagenesis, Impairment of Fertility: ***Fluticasone Propionate:*** Fluticasone propionate demonstrated no tumorigenic potential in mice at oral doses up to 1,000 mcg/kg (approximately 4 times the maximum recommended daily inhalation dose in adults on a mcg/m^2 basis) for 78 weeks or in rats at inhalation doses up to 57 mcg/kg (less than the maximum recommended daily inhalation dose in adults on a mcg/m^2 basis) for 104 weeks.
Fluticasone propionate did not induce gene mutation in prokaryotic or eukaryotic cells in vitro. No significant clastogenic effect was seen in cultured human peripheral lymphocytes in vitro or in the mouse micronucleus test.
No evidence of impairment of fertility was observed in reproductive studies conducted in male and female rats at subcutaneous doses up to 50 mcg/kg (less than the maximum recommended daily inhalation dose in adults on a mcg/m^2 basis). Prostate weight was significantly reduced at a subcutaneous dose of 50 mcg/kg.
Salmeterol: In an 18-month carcinogenicity study in CD-mice, salmeterol at oral doses of 1.4 mg/kg and above (approximately 20 times the maximum recommended daily inhalation dose in adults based on comparison of the plasma area under the curves [AUCs]) caused a dose-related increase in the incidence of smooth muscle hyperplasia, cystic glandular hyperplasia, leiomyomas of the uterus, and cysts in the ovaries. The incidence of leiomyosarcomas was not statistically significant. No tumors were seen at 0.2 mg/kg (approximately 3 times the maximum recommended daily inhalation doses in adults based on comparison of the AUCs).
In a 24-month oral and inhalation carcinogenicity study in Sprague Dawley rats, salmeterol caused a dose-related increase in the incidence of mesovarian leiomyomas and ovarian cysts at doses of 0.68 mg/kg and above (approximately 60 times the maximum recommended daily inhalation dose in adults on a mg/m^2 basis). No tumors were seen at 0.21 mg/kg (approximately 20 times the maximum recommended daily inhalation dose in adults on a mg/m^2 basis). These findings in rodents are similar to those reported previously for other beta-adrenergic agonist drugs. The relevance of these findings to human use is unknown.
Salmeterol produced no detectable or reproducible increases in microbial and mammalian gene mutation in vitro. No clastogenic activity occurred in vitro in human lymphocytes or in vivo in a rat micronucleus test. No effects on fertility were identified in male and female rats treated with salmeterol at oral doses up to 2 mg/kg (approximately 180 times the maximum recommended daily inhalation dose in adults on a mg/m^2 basis).

Pregnancy: ***Teratogenic Effects: ADVAIR DISKUS:*** Pregnancy Category C. From the reproduction toxicity studies in mice and rats, no evidence of enhanced toxicity was seen using combinations of fluticasone propionate and salmeterol compared to toxicity data from the components administered separately. In mice combining 150 mcg/kg subcutaneously of fluticasone propionate (less than the maximum recommended daily inhalation dose in adults on a mcg/m^2 basis) with 10 mg/kg orally of salmeterol (approximately 450 times the maximum recommended daily inhalation dose in adults on a mg/m^2 basis) was teratogenic. Cleft palate, fetal death, increased implantation loss and delayed ossification were seen. These observations are characteristic of glucocorticoids. No developmental toxicity was observed at combination doses up to 40 mcg/kg subcutaneously of fluticasone propionate (less than the maximum recommended daily inhalation dose in adults on a mcg/m^2 basis) and up to 1.4 mg/kg orally of salmeterol (approximately 65 times the maximum recommended daily inhalation dose in adults on a mg/m^2 basis). In rats, no teratogenicity was observed at combination doses up to 30 mcg/kg subcutaneously of fluticasone propionate (less than the maximum recommended daily inhalation dose in adults on a mcg/m^2 basis) and up to 1 mg/kg of salmeterol (approximately 90 times the maximum recommended daily inhalation dose in adults on a mg/m^2 basis). Combining 100 mcg/kg subcutaneously of fluticasone propionate (less than the maximum recommended daily inhalation dose in adults on a mcg/m^2 basis) with 10 mg/kg orally of salmeterol (approximately 900 times the maximum recommended daily inhalation dose in adults on a mg/m^2 basis) produced maternal toxicity, decreased placental weight, decreased fetal weight, umbilical hernia, delayed ossification, and changes in the occipital bone. There are no adequate and well-controlled studies with ADVAIR DISKUS in pregnant women. ADVAIR DISKUS should be used during pregnancy only if the potential benefit justifies the potential risk to the fetus.
Fluticasone Propionate: Pregnancy Category C. Subcutaneous studies in the mouse and rat at 45 and 100 mcg/kg (less than or equivalent to the maximum recommended daily inhalation dose in adults on a mcg/m^2 basis), respectively, revealed fetal toxicity characteristic of potent corticosteroid compounds, including embryonic growth retardation, omphalocele, cleft palate, and retarded cranial ossification.
In the rabbit, fetal weight reduction and cleft palate were observed at a subcutaneous dose of 4 mcg/kg (less than the maximum recommended daily inhalation dose in adults on a mcg/m^2 basis). However, no teratogenic effects were reported at oral doses up to 300 mcg/kg (approximately 5 times the maximum recommended daily inhalation dose in adults on a mcg/m^2 basis) of fluticasone propionate. No fluticasone propionate was detected in the plasma in this study, consistent with the established low bioavailability following oral administration (see CLINICAL PHARMACOLOGY: Pharmacokinetics: *Fluticasone Propionate: Absorption*).
Fluticasone propionate crossed the placenta following administration of a subcutaneous dose of 100 mcg/kg to mice (less than the maximum recommended daily inhalation dose in adults on a mcg/m^2 basis) administration of a subcutaneous or an oral dose of 100 mcg/kg to rats (approximately equivalent to the maximum recommended daily inhalation dose in adults on a mcg/m^2 basis) and an oral dose of 300 mcg/kg administered to rabbits (approximately 5 times the maximum recommended daily inhalation dose in adults on a mcg/m^2 basis).
There are no adequate and well-controlled studies in pregnant women. Fluticasone propionate should be used during pregnancy only if the potential benefit justifies the potential risk to the fetus.
Experience with oral corticosteroids since their introduction in pharmacologic, as opposed to physiologic, doses suggests that rodents are more prone to teratogenic effects from corticosteroids than humans. In addition, because there is a natural increase in corticosteroid production during pregnancy, most women will require a lower exogenous corticosteroid dose and many will not need corticosteroid treatment during pregnancy.
Salmeterol: Pregnancy Category C. No teratogenic effects occurred in rats at oral doses up to 2 mg/kg (approximately 180 times the maximum recommended daily inhalation dose in adults on a mg/m^2 basis). In pregnant Dutch rabbits administered oral doses of 1 mg/kg and above (approximately 50 times the maximum recommended daily inhalation dose in adults based on comparison of the AUCs), salmeterol exhibited fetal toxic effects characteristically resulting from beta-adrenoceptor stimulation. These included precocious eyelid openings, cleft palate, sternebral fusion, limb and paw flexures, and delayed ossification of the frontal cranial bones. No significant effects occurred at an oral dose of 0.6 mg/kg (approximately 20 times the maximum recommended daily inhalation dose in adults based on comparison of the AUCs).
New Zealand White rabbits were less sensitive since only delayed ossification of the frontal bones was seen at an oral dose of 10 mg/kg (approximately 1,800 times the maximum recommended daily inhalation dose in adults on a mg/m^2 basis). Extensive use of other beta-agonists has provided no evidence that these class effects in animals are relevant to their use in humans. There are no adequate and well-controlled studies with salmeterol in pregnant women. Salmeterol should be used during pregnancy only if the potential benefit justifies the potential risk to the fetus.
Salmeterol xinafoate crossed the placenta following oral administration of 10 mg/kg to mice and rats (approximately 450 and 900 times, respectively, the maximum recommended daily inhalation dose in adults on a mg/m^2 basis).

Use in Labor and Delivery: There are no well-controlled human studies that have investigated effects of ADVAIR DISKUS on preterm labor or labor at term. Because of the potential for beta-agonist interference with uterine contractility, use of ADVAIR DISKUS during labor should be restricted to those patients in whom the benefits clearly outweigh the risks.

Nursing Mothers: Plasma levels of salmeterol, a component of ADVAIR DISKUS, after inhaled therapeutic doses are very low. In rats, salmeterol xinafoate is excreted in the milk. There are no data from controlled trials on the use of salmeterol by nursing mothers. It is not known whether fluticasone propionate, a component of ADVAIR DISKUS, is excreted in human breast milk. However, other corticosteroids have been detected in human milk. Subcutaneous administration to lactating rats of 10 mcg/kg tritiated fluticasone propionate (less than the maximum recommended daily inhalation dose in adults on a mcg/m^2 basis) resulted in measurable radioactivity in milk.
Since there are no data from controlled trials on the use of ADVAIR DISKUS by nursing mothers, a decision should be made whether to discontinue nursing or to discontinue ADVAIR DISKUS, taking into account the importance of ADVAIR DISKUS to the mother.
Caution should be exercised when ADVAIR DISKUS is administered to a nursing woman.

Pediatric Use: The safety and effectiveness of ADVAIR DISKUS in children with asthma under 12 years of age have not been established. In one 12-week study, 257 patients 4 to 11 years inadequately controlled using inhaled corticosteroids were randomized to ADVAIR DISKUS 100/50 or concurrent therapy with fluticasone propionate inhalation powder 100 mcg plus salmeterol inhalation powder 50 mcg twice daily. The pattern of adverse events reported in patients 4 to 11 years of age was similar to that seen in patients 12 years of age and older treated with ADVAIR DISKUS.
Controlled clinical studies have shown that orally inhaled corticosteroids may cause a reduction in growth velocity in pediatric patients. This effect has been observed in the absence of laboratory evidence of HPA axis suppression, suggesting that growth velocity is a more sensitive indicator of systemic corticosteroid exposure in pediatric patients than some commonly used tests of HPA axis function. The long-term effects of this reduction in growth velocity associated with orally inhaled corticosteroids, including the impact on final adult height, are unknown. The potential for "catch-up" growth following discontinuation of treatment with orally inhaled corticosteroids has not been adequately studied.
Inhaled corticosteroids, including fluticasone propionate, a component of ADVAIR DISKUS, may cause a reduction in growth velocity in children and adolescents (see PRECAUTIONS: General: *Metabolic and Other Effects*). The growth of pediatric patients receiving orally inhaled corticosteroids, including ADVAIR DISKUS, should be monitored. If a child or adolescent on any corticosteroid appears to have growth suppression, the possibility that he/she is particularly sensitive to this effect of corticosteroids should be considered. The potential growth effects of prolonged treatment should be weighed against the clinical benefits obtained. To minimize the systemic effects of orally inhaled corticosteroids, including ADVAIR DISKUS, each patient should be titrated to the lowest strength that effectively controls his/her asthma (see DOSAGE AND ADMINISTRATION: Asthma).

Geriatric Use: Of the total number of patients in clinical studies of ADVAIR DISKUS for asthma, 44 were 65 years of age or older and 3 were 75 years of age or older. Of the total number of patients in a clinical study of ADVAIR DISKUS 250/50 for COPD, 85 were 65 years of age or older and 31 were 75 years of age or older. For both diseases, no overall differences in safety were observed between these patients and younger patients, and other reported clinical experience, including studies of the individual components, has not identified differences in responses between the elderly and younger patients, but greater sensitivity of some older individuals cannot be ruled out. As with other products containing beta$_2$-agonists, special caution should be observed when using ADVAIR DISKUS in geriatric patients who have concomitant cardiovascular disease that could be adversely affected by beta$_2$-agonists. Based on available data for ADVAIR DISKUS or its active components, no adjustment of dosage of ADVAIR DISKUS in geriatric patients is warranted.

ADVERSE REACTIONS

Asthma: The incidence of common adverse events in Table 3 is based upon 2 placebo-controlled, 12-week, US clinical studies (Studies 1 and 2). A total of 705 adolescent and adult patients (349 females and 356 males) previously treated with salmeterol or inhaled corticosteroids were treated twice daily with ADVAIR DISKUS (100/50- or 250/50-mcg doses), fluticasone propionate inhalation powder (100- or 250-mcg doses), salmeterol inhalation powder 50 mcg, or placebo.
[See table 3 at top of next page]
Table 3 includes all events (whether considered drug-related or nondrug-related by the investigator) that occurred at a rate of 3% or greater in either of the groups receiving ADVAIR DISKUS and were more common than in the placebo group. In considering these data, differences in average duration of exposure should be taken into account.
Rare cases of immediate and delayed hypersensitivity reactions, including rash and other rare events of angioedema and bronchospasm, have been reported.
These adverse reactions were mostly mild to moderate in severity.
Other adverse events that occurred in the groups receiving ADVAIR DISKUS in these studies with an incidence of 1% to 3% and that occurred at a greater incidence than with placebo were:
Blood and Lymphatic: Lymphatic signs and symptoms.
Cardiovascular: Palpitations.
Drug Interaction, Overdose, and Trauma: Muscle injuries, fractures, wounds and lacerations, contusions and hematomas, burns.
Ear, Nose, and Throat: Rhinorrhea/post-nasal drip; ear, nose, and throat infections; ear signs and symptoms; nasal signs and symptoms; nasal sinus disorders; rhinitis; sneezing; nasal irritation; blood in nasal mucosa.
Eye: Keratitis and conjunctivitis, viral eye infections, eye redness.
Gastrointestinal: Dental discomfort and pain, gastrointestinal signs and symptoms, gastrointestinal infections, gastroenteritis, gastrointestinal disorders, oral ulcerations, oral erythema and rashes, constipation, appendicitis, oral discomfort and pain.
Hepatobiliary Tract and Pancreas: Abnormal liver function tests.
Lower Respiratory: Lower respiratory signs and symptoms, pneumonia, lower respiratory infections.
Musculoskeletal: Arthralgia and articular rheumatism; muscle stiffness, tightness, and rigidity; bone and cartilage disorders.
Neurology: Sleep disorders, tremors, hypnagogic effects, compressed nerve syndromes.
Non-Site Specific: Allergies and allergic reactions, congestion, viral infections, pain, chest symptoms, fluid retention, bacterial infections, wheeze and hives, unusual taste.
Skin: Viral skin infections, urticaria, skin flakiness and acquired ichthyosis, disorders of sweat and sebum, sweating.
The incidence of common adverse events reported in Study 3, a 28-week, non-US clinical study of 503 patients previ-

Continued on next page

Advair Diskus—Cont.

ously treated with inhaled corticosteroids who were treated twice daily with ADVAIR DISKUS 500/50, fluticasone propionate inhalation powder 500 mcg and salmeterol inhalation powder 50 mcg used concurrently, or fluticasone propionate inhalation powder 500 mcg was similar to the incidences reported in Table 3.

Chronic Obstructive Pulmonary Disease Associated With Chronic Bronchitis: The incidence of common adverse events in Table 4 is based upon 1 placebo-controlled, 24-week, US clinical trial in patients with COPD associated with chronic bronchitis. A total of 723 adult patients (266 females and 457 males) were treated twice daily with ADVAIR DISKUS 250/50, fluticasone propionate inhalation powder 250 mcg, salmeterol inhalation powder 50 mcg, or placebo.

[See table 4 at right]

Table 4 includes all events (whether considered drug-related or nondrug-related by the investigator) that occurred at a rate of 3% or greater in the group receiving ADVAIR DISKUS 250/50 and were more common than in the placebo group.

These adverse reactions were mostly mild to moderate in severity.

Other adverse events that occurred in the groups receiving ADVAIR DISKUS 250/50 with an incidence of 1% to 3% and that occurred at a greater incidence than with placebo were:

Cardiovascular: Syncope.

Drug Interaction, Overdose, and Trauma: Postoperative complications.

Ear, Nose, and Throat: Ear, nose, and throat infections; ear signs and symptoms; laryngitis; nasal congestion/blockage; nasal sinus disorders; pharyngitis/throat infection.

Endocrine and Metabolic: Hypothyroidism.

Eye: Dry eyes, eye infections.

Gastrointestinal: Constipation, gastrointestinal signs and symptoms, oral lesions.

Hepatobiliary Tract and Pancreas: Abnormal liver function tests.

Lower Respiratory: Breathing disorders, lower respiratory signs and symptoms.

Non-Site Specific: Bacterial infections, candidiasis unspecified site, edema and swelling, nonspecific conditions, viral infections.

Psychiatry: Situational disorders.

Observed During Clinical Practice: In addition to adverse events reported from clinical trials, the following events have been identified during worldwide use of any formulation of ADVAIR, fluticasone propionate, and/or salmeterol regardless of indication. Because they are reported voluntarily from a population of unknown size, estimates of frequency cannot be made. These events have been chosen for inclusion due to either their seriousness, frequency of reporting, or causal connection to ADVAIR DISKUS, fluticasone propionate, and/or salmeterol or a combination of these factors.

In extensive US and worldwide postmarketing experience with salmeterol, a component of ADVAIR DISKUS, serious exacerbations of asthma, including some that have been fatal, have been reported. In most cases, these have occurred in patients with severe asthma and/or in some patients in whom asthma has been acutely deteriorating (see WARNINGS no. 2), but they have also occurred in a few patients with less severe asthma. It was not possible from these reports to determine whether salmeterol contributed to these events or simply failed to relieve the deteriorating asthma.

Cardiovascular: Arrhythmias (including atrial fibrillation, extrasystoles, supraventricular tachycardia), ventricular tachycardia.

Ear, Nose, and Throat: Aphonia, earache, facial and oropharyngeal edema, paranasal sinus pain, throat soreness.

Endocrine and Metabolic: Cushing syndrome, Cushingoid features, growth velocity reduction in children/adolescents, hypercorticism, hyperglycemia, weight gain, osteoporosis.

Eye: Cataracts, glaucoma.

Gastrointestinal: Abdominal pain, dyspepsia, xerostomia.

Musculoskeletal: Back pain, cramps, muscle spasm, myositis.

Neurology: Paresthesia, restlessness.

Non-Site Specific: Immediate and delayed hypersensitivity reaction (including very rare anaphylactic reaction), pallor. Very rare anaphylactic reaction in patients with severe milk protein allergy.

Psychiatry: Agitation, aggression, depression.

Respiratory: Chest congestion; chest tightness; dyspnea; immediate bronchospasm; influenza; paradoxical bronchospasm; tracheitis; wheezing; reports of upper respiratory symptoms of laryngeal spasm, irritation, or swelling such as stridor or choking.

Skin: Contact dermatitis, contusions, ecchymoses, photodermatitis.

Urogenital: Dysmenorrhea, irregular menstrual cycle, pelvic inflammatory disease, vaginal candidiasis, vaginitis, vulvovaginitis.

Eosinophilic Conditions: In rare cases, patients on inhaled fluticasone propionate, a component of ADVAIR DISKUS, may present with systemic eosinophilic conditions, with some patients presenting with clinical features of vasculitis consistent with Churg-Strauss syndrome, a condition that is often treated with systemic corticosteroid therapy. These events usually, but not always, have been associated with the reduction and/or withdrawal of oral corticosteroid therapy following the introduction of fluticasone propionate. Cases of serious eosinophilic conditions have also been reported with other inhaled corticosteroids in this clinical setting. While ADVAIR DISKUS should not be used for transferring patients from systemic corticosteroid therapy, physicians should be alert to eosinophilia, vasculitic rash, worsening pulmonary symptoms, cardiac complications, and/or neuropathy presenting in their patients. A causal relationship between fluticasone propionate and these underlying conditions has not been established (see PRECAUTIONS: General: *Eosinophilic Conditions*).

Table 3. Overall Adverse Effects With ≥3% Incidence in US Controlled Clinical Trials With ADVAIR DISKUS in Patients With Asthma

Adverse Event	ADVAIR DISKUS 100/50 (N = 92) %	ADVAIR DISKUS 250/50 (N = 84) %	Fluticasone Propionate 100 mcg (N = 90) %	Fluticasone Propionate 250 mcg (N = 84) %	Salmeterol 50 mcg (N = 180) %	Placebo (N = 175) %
Ear, nose, and throat						
Upper respiratory tract infection	27	21	29	25	19	14
Pharyngitis	13	10	7	12	8	6
Upper respiratory inflammation	7	6	7	8	8	5
Sinusitis	4	5	6	1	3	4
Hoarseness/dysphonia	5	2	2	4	<1	<1
Oral candidiasis	1	4	2	2	0	0
Lower respiratory						
Viral respiratory infections	4	4	4	10	6	3
Bronchitis	2	8	1	2	2	2
Cough	3	6	0	0	3	2
Neurology						
Headaches	12	13	14	8	10	7
Gastrointestinal						
Nausea & vomiting	4	6	3	4	1	1
Gastrointestinal discomfort & pain	4	1	0	2	1	1
Diarrhea	4	2	2	2	1	1
Viral gastrointestinal infections	3	0	3	1	2	2
Non-site specific						
Candidiasis unspecified site	3	0	1	4	0	1
Musculoskeletal						
Musculoskeletal pain	4	2	1	5	3	3
Average duration of exposure (days)	77.3	78.7	72.4	70.1	60.1	42.3

Table 4. Overall Adverse Events With ≥3% Incidence With ADVAIR DISKUS 250/50 in Patients With Chronic Obstructive Pulmonary Disease Associated With Chronic Bronchitis

Adverse Event	ADVAIR DISKUS 250/50 (N = 178) %	Fluticasone Propionate 250 mcg (N = 183) %	Salmeterol 50 mcg (N = 177) %	Placebo (N = 185) %
Ear, nose, and throat				
Candidiasis mouth/throat	10	6	3	1
Throat irritation	8	5	4	7
Hoarseness/dysphonia	5	3	≤1	0
Sinusitis	3	8	5	3
Lower respiratory				
Viral respiratory infections	6	4	3	3
Neurology				
Headaches	16	11	10	12
Dizziness	4	≤1	3	2
Non-site specific				
Fever	4	3	0	3
Malaise & fatigue	3	2	2	3
Musculoskeletal				
Musculoskeletal pain	9	8	12	9
Muscle cramps & spasms	3	3	1	1
Average duration of exposure (days)	141.3	138.5	136.1	131.6

Table 5. Recommended Dosages of ADVAIR DISKUS for Patients With Asthma Taking Inhaled Corticosteroids

Current **Daily Dose** of Inhaled Corticosteroid		Recommended Strength and Dosing Schedule of ADVAIR DISKUS
Beclomethasone dipropionate	≤420 mcg 462–840 mcg	100/50 twice daily 250/50 twice daily
Budesonide	≤400 mcg 800–1,200 mcg 1,600 mcg*	100/50 twice daily 250/50 twice daily 500/50 twice daily
Flunisolide	≤1,000 mcg 1,250–2,000 mcg	100/50 twice daily 250/50 twice daily
Fluticasone propionate inhalation aerosol	≤176 mcg 440 mcg 660–880 mcg*	100/50 twice daily 250/50 twice daily 500/50 twice daily
Fluticasone propionate inhalation powder	≤200 mcg 500 mcg 1,000 mcg*	100/50 twice daily 250/50 twice daily 500/50 twice daily
Triamcinolone acetonide	≤1,000 mcg 1,100–1,600 mcg	100/50 twice daily 250/50 twice daily

* ADVAIR DISKUS should not be used for transferring patients from systemic corticosteroid therapy.

OVERDOSAGE

ADVAIR DISKUS: No deaths occurred in rats given combinations of salmeterol and fluticasone propionate at acute inhalation doses of 3.6 and 1.9 mg/kg, respectively (approximately 320 and 15 times the maximum recommended daily inhalation dose in adults on a mg/m^2 basis).

Fluticasone Propionate: Chronic overdosage with fluticasone propionate may result in signs/symptoms of hypercorticism (see PRECAUTIONS: General: *Metabolic and Other Effects*). Inhalation by healthy volunteers of a single dose of 4,000 mcg of fluticasone propionate inhalation powder or single doses of 1,760 or 3,520 mcg of fluticasone propionate inhalation aerosol was well tolerated. Fluticasone propionate given by inhalation aerosol at doses of 1,320 mcg twice daily for 7 to 15 days to healthy human volunteers was also well tolerated. Repeat oral doses up to 80 mg daily for 10 days in healthy volunteers and repeat oral doses up to 20 mg daily for 42 days in patients were well tolerated. Adverse reactions were of mild or moderate severity, and incidences were similar in active and placebo treatment groups. The oral and subcutaneous median lethal doses in mice and rats were >1,000 mg/kg (>4,300 and >8,700 times, respectively, the maximum recommended daily inhalation dose in adults on a mg/m^2 basis).

Salmeterol: The expected signs and symptoms with overdosage of salmeterol are those of excessive beta-adrenergic stimulation and/or occurrence or exaggeration of any of the signs and symptoms listed under ADVERSE REACTIONS, e.g., seizures, angina, hypertension or hypotension, tachycardia with rates up to 200 beats/min, arrhythmias, nervousness, headache, tremor, muscle cramps, dry mouth, palpitation, nausea, dizziness, fatigue, malaise, and insomnia. Overdosage with salmeterol may be expected to result in exaggeration of the pharmacologic adverse effects associated with beta-adrenoceptor agonists, including tachycardia and/or arrhythmia, tremor, headache, and muscle cramps. Overdosage with salmeterol can lead to clinically significant prolongation of the QTc interval, which can produce ventricular arrhythmias. Other signs of overdosage may include hypokalemia and hyperglycemia.

As with all sympathomimetic medications, cardiac arrest and even death may be associated with abuse of salmeterol. Treatment consists of discontinuation of salmeterol together with appropriate symptomatic therapy. The judicious use of a cardioselective beta-receptor blocker may be considered, bearing in mind that such medication can produce bronchospasm. There is insufficient evidence to determine if dialysis is beneficial for overdosage of salmeterol. Cardiac monitoring is recommended in cases of overdosage.

No deaths were seen in rats given salmeterol at an inhalation dose of 2.9 mg/kg (approximately 250 times the maximum recommended daily inhalation dose in adults on a mg/m^2 basis) and in dogs at an inhalation dose of 0.7 mg/kg (approximately 190 times the maximum recommended daily inhalation dose in adults on a mg/m^2 basis). By the oral route, no deaths occurred in mice at 150 mg/kg (approximately 6,500 times the maximum recommended daily inhalation dose in adults on a mg/m^2 basis) and in rats at 1,000 mg/kg (approximately 86,000 times the maximum recommended daily inhalation dose in adults on a mg/m^2 basis).

DOSAGE AND ADMINISTRATION

ADVAIR DISKUS should be administered by the orally inhaled route only (see Patient's Instructions for Use).

Asthma: ADVAIR DISKUS is available in 3 strengths, ADVAIR DISKUS 100/50, ADVAIR DISKUS 250/50, and ADVAIR DISKUS 500/50, containing 100, 250, and 500 mcg of fluticasone propionate, respectively, and 50 mcg of salmeterol per inhalation.

For patients 12 years of age and older, the dosage is 1 inhalation twice daily (morning and evening, approximately 12 hours apart).

The recommended starting dosages for ADVAIR DISKUS are based upon patients' current asthma therapy.

- For patients who are not currently on an inhaled corticosteroid, whose disease severity warrants treatment with 2 maintenance therapies, including patients on non-corticosteroid maintenance therapy, the recommended starting dosage is ADVAIR DISKUS 100/50 twice daily.
- For patients on an inhaled corticosteroid, Table 5 provides the recommended starting dosage. The maximum recommended dosage is ADVAIR DISKUS 500/50 twice daily.

For all patients it is desirable to titrate to the lowest effective strength after adequate asthma stability is achieved.

[See table 5 on previous page]

ADVAIR DISKUS should be administered twice daily every day. More frequent administration (more than twice daily) or a higher number of inhalations (more than 1 inhalation twice daily) of the prescribed strength of ADVAIR DISKUS is not recommended as some patients are more likely to experience adverse effects with higher doses of salmeterol. The safety and efficacy of ADVAIR DISKUS when administered in excess of recommended doses have not been established.

If symptoms arise in the period between doses, an inhaled, short-acting beta$_2$-agonist should be taken for immediate relief.

Patients who are receiving ADVAIR DISKUS twice daily should not use additional salmeterol or other inhaled, long-acting beta$_2$-agonists (e.g., formoterol) for prevention of EIB, or for any other reason.

Improvement in asthma control following inhaled administration of ADVAIR DISKUS can occur within 30 minutes of beginning treatment, although maximum benefit may not be achieved for 1 week or longer after starting treatment. Individual patients will experience a variable time to onset and degree of symptom relief.

For patients who do not respond adequately to the starting dosage after 2 weeks of therapy, replacing the current strength of ADVAIR DISKUS with a higher strength may provide additional improvement in asthma control.

If a previously effective dosage regimen of ADVAIR DISKUS fails to provide adequate improvement in asthma control, the therapeutic regimen should be reevaluated and additional therapeutic options, e.g., replacing the current strength of ADVAIR DISKUS with a higher strength, adding additional inhaled corticosteroid, or initiating oral corticosteroids, should be considered.

Chronic Obstructive Pulmonary Disease Associated With Chronic Bronchitis: The dosage for adults is 1 inhalation (250/50 mcg) twice daily (morning and evening, approximately 12 hours apart).

ADVAIR DISKUS 250/50 mcg twice daily is the only approved dosage for the treatment of COPD associated with chronic bronchitis. Higher doses, including ADVAIR DISKUS 500/50, are not recommended, as no additional improvement in lung function was observed in clinical trials and higher doses of corticosteroids increase the risk of systemic effects.

If shortness of breath occurs in the period between doses, an inhaled, short-acting beta$_2$-agonist should be taken for immediate relief.

Patients who are receiving ADVAIR DISKUS twice daily should not use additional salmeterol or other inhaled, long-acting beta$_2$-agonists (e.g., formoterol) for the maintenance treatment of COPD or for any other reason.

Geriatric Use: In studies where geriatric patients (65 years of age or older, see PRECAUTIONS: Geriatric Use) have been treated with ADVAIR DISKUS, efficacy and safety did not differ from that in younger patients. Based on available data for ADVAIR DISKUS and its active components, no dosage adjustment is recommended.

Directions for Use: Illustrated Patient's Instructions for Use accompany each package of ADVAIR DISKUS.

HOW SUPPLIED

ADVAIR DISKUS 100/50 is supplied as a disposable, purple device containing 60 blisters. The DISKUS inhalation device is packaged within a purple, plastic-coated, moisture-protective foil pouch (NDC 0173-0695-00). ADVAIR DISKUS 100/50 is also supplied in an institutional pack of 1 purple, disposable DISKUS inhalation device containing 28 blisters. The DISKUS inhalation device is packaged within a purple, plastic-coated, moisture-protective foil pouch (NDC 0173-0695-02).

ADVAIR DISKUS 250/50 is supplied as a disposable, purple device containing 60 blisters. The DISKUS inhalation device is packaged within a purple, plastic-coated, moisture-protective foil pouch (NDC 0173-0696-00). ADVAIR DISKUS 250/50 is also supplied in an institutional pack of 1 purple, disposable DISKUS inhalation device containing 28 blisters. The DISKUS inhalation device is packaged within a purple, plastic-coated, moisture-protective foil pouch (NDC 0173-0696-02).

ADVAIR DISKUS 500/50 is supplied as a disposable, purple device containing 60 blisters. The DISKUS inhalation device is packaged within a purple, plastic-coated, moisture-protective foil pouch (NDC 0173-0697-00). ADVAIR DISKUS 500/50 is also supplied in an institutional pack of 1 purple, disposable DISKUS inhalation device containing 28 blisters. The DISKUS inhalation device is packaged within a purple, plastic-coated, moisture-protective foil pouch (NDC 0173-0697-02).

Store at controlled room temperature (see USP), 20° to 25°C (68° to 77°F) in a dry place away from direct heat or sunlight. Keep out of reach of children. The DISKUS inhalation device is not reusable. The device should be discarded 1 month after removal from the moisture-protective foil overwrap pouch or after all blisters have been used (when the dose indicator reads "0"), whichever comes first. Do not attempt to take the device apart.

GlaxoSmithKline, Research Triangle Park, NC 27709

November 2003/RL-2053

Table 9. Selected Clinical Adverse Events of All Grades Reported in >5% of Adult Patients

	PROAB3001 Therapy-Naive Patients		PROAB3006 NRTI-Experienced Patients	
Adverse Event	AGENERASE*/ Lamivudine/ Zidovudine (n = 113)	Lamivudine/ Zidovudine (n = 109)	AGENERASE*/ NRTI (n = 245)	Indinavir/ NRTI (n = 241)
Digestive				
Nausea	74%	50%	43%	35%
Vomiting	34%	17%	24%	20%
Diarrhea or loose stools	39%	35%	60%	41%
Taste disorders	10%	6%	2%	8%
Skin				
Rash	27%	6%	20%	15%
Nervous				
Paresthesia, oral/perioral	26%	6%	31%	2%
Paresthesia, peripheral	10%	4%	14%	10%
Psychiatric				
Depressive or mood disorders	16%	4%	9%	13%

*AGENERASE Capsules.

Table 10. Selected Clinical Adverse Events of All Grades Reported in Adult Patients in Open-Label Clinical Trials of AGENERASE Capsules in Combination with Ritonavir Capsules

Adverse Event	AGENERASE 1,200 mg plus Ritonavir 200 mg q.d.* (n = 101)	AGENERASE 600 mg plus Ritonavir 100 mg b.i.d.† (n = 239)
Nausea	31%	23%
Diarrhea/loose stools	30%	28%
Headache	16%	12%
Abdominal symptoms	14%	14%
Vomiting	11%	9%
Rash	10%	9%
Paresthesias	9%	11%
Fatigue	7%	14%
Depressive & mood disorders	4%	9%

*Data from 2 open-label studies in treatment-naive patients also receiving abacavir/lamivudine.

†Data from 3 open-label studies in treatment-naive and treatment-experienced patients receiving combination antiretroviral therapy.

AGENERASE® ℞

[*a-jin'ə-rās*]

(amprenavir)

Oral Solution

Prescribing information for this product, which appears on pages 1417–1422 of the 2004 PDR, has been revised as follows. Please write "See Supplement A" next to the product heading.

The ADVERSE REACTIONS *section was revised to:*

In clinical studies, adverse events leading to amprenavir discontinuation occurred primarily during the first 12 weeks of therapy, and were mostly due to gastrointestinal events (nausea, vomiting, diarrhea, and abdominal pain/discomfort), which were mild to moderate in severity.

Skin rash occurred in 22% of patients treated with amprenavir in studies PROAB3001 and PROAB3006. Rashes

Continued on next page

Agenerase—Cont.

were usually maculopapular and of mild or moderate intensity, some with pruritus. Rashes had a median onset of 11 days after amprenavir initiation and a median duration of 10 days. Skin rashes led to amprenavir discontinuation in approximately 3% of patients. In some patients with mild or moderate rash, amprenavir dosing was often continued without interruption; if interrupted, reintroduction of amprenavir generally did not result in rash recurrence.

Severe or life-threatening rash (Grade 3 or 4), including cases of Stevens-Johnson syndrome, occurred in approximately 1% of recipients of AGENERASE (see WARNINGS). Amprenavir therapy should be discontinued for severe or life-threatening rashes and for moderate rashes accompanied by systemic symptoms.

[See table 9 at top of previous page]

Among amprenavir-treated patients in Phase 3 studies, 2 patients developed de novo diabetes mellitus, 1 patient developed a dorsocervical fat enlargement (buffalo hump), and 9 patients developed fat redistribution.

In studies PROAB3001 and PROAB3006, no increased frequency of Grade 3 or 4 AST, ALT, amylase, or bilirubin elevations was seen compared to controls.

Pediatric Patients: An adverse event profile similar to that seen in adults was seen in pediatric patients.

Concomitant Therapy with Ritonavir: Tables 10 and 11 present adverse clinical events and laboratory abnormalities observed in subjects who received AGENERASE plus ritonavir. Since the trials were small, open-label, of varying duration, and often included different patient populations, direct comparisons to the frequency of events with AGENERASE Capsules alone (see Table 9) cannot be made.

[See table 10 at top of previous page]
[See table 11 below]

GlaxoSmithKline, Research Triangle Park, NC 27709
Licensed from Vertex Pharmaceuticals Incorporated
Cambridge, MA 02139

AGENERASE is a registered trademark of the GlaxoSmithKline group of companies.

February 2004/RL-2071

AMOXIL® ℞

[*ə-mäx'il*]

(amoxicillin capsules, tablets, chewable tablets, and powder for oral suspension)

Prescribing information for this product, which appears on pages 1427–1431 of the 2004 PDR, has been revised as follows. Please write "See Supplement A" next to the product heading.

The following subsection was added to ADVERSE REACTIONS:

Renal: Crystalluria has also been reported.

The following sentence was added to the second paragraph in OVERDOSAGE:

Crystalluria has also been reported after amoxicillin overdosage.

GlaxoSmithKline, Research Triangle Park, NC 27709

November 2003/AM:L25

ARGATROBAN ℞

[*är-ga' trō-ban*]

Injection

Prescribing information for this product, which appears on pages 1431–1435 of the 2004 PDR, has been revised as follows. Please write "See Supplement A" next to the product heading.

In ADVERSE REACTIONS, *the following subsection was revised to:*

Adverse Events Reported in Other Populations: The following safety information is based on a total of 1,127 individuals who were treated with Argatroban in clinical pharmacology studies (n = 211) or for various clinical indications (n = 916).

Intracranial Bleeding: Intracranial bleeding only occurred in patients with acute myocardial infarction who were started on both Argatroban and thrombolytic therapy with streptokinase. The overall frequency of this potentially life-threatening complication among patients receiving both Argatroban and thrombolytic therapy (streptokinase or tissue plasminogen activator) was 1% (8 out of 810 patients). Intracranial bleeding was not observed in 317 subjects or patients who did not receive concomitant thrombolysis (see PRECAUTIONS, Drug Interactions).

Intracranial bleeding was also observed in a prospective, placebo-controlled study of Argatroban in patients who had onset of acute stroke within 12 hours of study entry. Symptomatic intracranial hemorrhage was reported in 5 of 117 patients (4.3%) who received Argatroban and in none of the 54 patients who received placebo. Asymptomatic intracranial hemorrhage occurred in 5 (4.3%) and 2 (3.7%) of the patients, respectively.

In DOSAGE AND ADMINISTRATION, *the following subsections were revised to:*

Heparin-Induced Thrombocytopenia (HIT/HITTS): ***Dosage Adjustment:*** After the initial dose of Argatroban, the dose can be adjusted as clinically indicated (not to exceed 10 mcg/kg/min), until the steady-state aPTT is 1.5 to 3 times the initial baseline value (not to exceed 100 seconds) (see CLINICAL STUDIES for mean values of aPTT obtained after initial doses of Argatroban). Argatroban therapy should be continued until platelet counts have recovered substantially (i.e., >100 × 10^9/L or to pre-HIT/-HITTS baseline value).

Percutaneous Coronary Interventions (PCI) in HIT/HITTS Patients: ***Continued Anticoagulation after PCI:*** If a patient requires anticoagulation after the procedure, Argatroban may be continued, but at a lower infusion dose [see DOSAGE AND ADMINISTRATION, Heparin-Induced Thrombocytopenia (HIT/HITTS)]. If the patient has HIT or HITTS, Argatroban therapy should be continued until platelet counts have recovered substantially (i.e., >100 × 10^9/L or to pre-HIT/HITTS baseline value).

The following section was revised to:

CONVERSION TO ORAL ANTICOAGULANT THERAPY

Initiating Oral Anticoagulant Therapy: Once the decision is made to initiate oral anticoagulant therapy, recognize the potential for combined effects on INR with co-administration of Argatroban and warfarin. (See CLINICAL PHARMACOLOGY, Effect on INR.) Continue to monitor Argatroban using aPTT. Oral anticoagulation therapy (warfarin) should be initiated only after substantial recovery of platelet counts (e.g., >100 × 10^9/L or to pre-HIT/-HITTS baseline value). A loading dose of warfarin should not be used. Initiate therapy using the expected daily dose of warfarin. To avoid prothrombotic effects and to ensure continuous anticoagulation when initiating warfarin, it is recommended to overlap Argatroban and warfarin therapy for 4 or 5 days (see warfarin prescribing information).

Co-Administration of Warfarin and Argatroban at Doses Up to 2 mcg/kg/min: Use of Argatroban with warfarin results in prolongation of INR beyond that produced by warfarin alone. To avoid prothrombotic effects and to ensure continuous anticoagulation when initiating warfarin, it is recommended to continue co-administration for at least 4 or 5 days before discontinuing Argatroban. The previously established relationship between INR and bleeding risk is altered. The combination of Argatroban and warfarin does not cause further reduction in the vitamin K–dependent factor Xa activity than that which is seen with warfarin alone. The relationship between INR obtained on combined therapy and INR obtained on warfarin alone is dependent on both the dose of Argatroban and the thromboplastin reagent used. The INR value on warfarin alone (INR_W) can be calculated from the INR value on combination Argatroban and warfarin therapy (see CLINICAL PHARMACOLOGY, Figure 2 explanation and PRECAUTIONS, Drug Interactions).

Manufactured by Abbott Laboratories, North Chicago, IL 60064

Distributed by GlaxoSmithKline, Research Triangle Park, NC 27709

for Encysive Pharmaceuticals Inc. Bellaire, TX 77401

November 2003/AR:L5

AUGMENTIN® ℞

[*äg-mint' in*]

(amoxicillin/clavulanate potassium)

Powder for Oral Suspension and Chewable Tablets

Prescribing information for this product, which appears on pages 1435–1438 of the 2004 PDR, has been revised as follows. Please write "See Supplement A" next to the product heading.

The following paragraph was added before the DESCRIPTION *section:*

To reduce the development of drug-resistant bacteria and maintain the effectiveness of AUGMENTIN (amoxicillin/clavulanate potassium) and other antibacterial drugs, AUGMENTIN should be used only to treat or prevent infections that are proven or strongly suspected to be caused by bacteria.

The last 2 paragraphs of INDICATIONS AND USAGE *were revised to:*

To reduce the development of drug-resistant bacteria and maintain the effectiveness of AUGMENTIN and other antibacterial drugs, AUGMENTIN should be used only to treat or prevent infections that are proven or strongly suspected to be caused by susceptible bacteria. When culture and susceptibility information are available, they should be considered in selecting or modifying antibacterial therapy. In the absence of such data, local epidemiology and susceptibility patterns may contribute to the empiric selection of therapy.

Bacteriological studies, to determine the causative organisms and their susceptibility to AUGMENTIN, should be performed together with any indicated surgical procedures.

In PRECAUTIONS: General, *the following paragraph was added:*

Prescribing AUGMENTIN in the absence of a proven or strongly suspected bacterial infection or a prophylactic indication is unlikely to provide benefit to the patient and increases the risk of the development of drug-resistant bacteria.

PRECAUTIONS: Information for the Patient *was revised to:*

AUGMENTIN may be taken every 8 hours or every 12 hours, depending on the strength of the product prescribed. Each dose should be taken with a meal or snack to reduce the possibility of gastrointestinal upset. Many antibiotics can cause diarrhea. If diarrhea is severe or lasts more than 2 or 3 days, call your doctor.

Keep suspension refrigerated. Shake well before using. When dosing a child with the suspension (liquid) of AUGMENTIN, use a dosing spoon or medicine dropper. Be sure to rinse the spoon or dropper after each use. Bottles of suspension of AUGMENTIN may contain more liquid than required. Follow your doctor's instructions about the amount to use and the days of treatment your child requires. Discard any unused medicine.

Patients should be counseled that antibacterial drugs including AUGMENTIN, should only be used to treat bacterial infections. They do not treat viral infections (e.g., the common cold). When AUGMENTIN is prescribed to treat a bacterial infection, patients should be told that although it is common to feel better early in the course of therapy, the medication should be taken exactly as directed. Skipping doses or not completing the full course of therapy may: (1) decrease the effectiveness of the immediate treatment, and (2) increase the likelihood that bacteria will develop resistance and will not be treatable by AUGMENTIN or other antibacterial drugs in the future.

The following subsections were revised in ADVERSE REACTIONS:

Renal: Interstitial nephritis and hematuria have been reported rarely. Crystalluria has also been reported.

Miscellaneous: Tooth discoloration (brown, yellow, or gray staining) has been rarely reported. Most reports occurred in pediatric patients. Discoloration was reduced or eliminated with brushing or dental cleaning in most cases.

The following sentence was added to the third paragraph in OVERDOSAGE:

Crystalluria has also been reported after amoxicillin overdosage.

GlaxoSmithKline, Research Triangle Park, NC 27709

January 2004/AG:PL14

AUGMENTIN® ℞

[*äg-mint' in*]

amoxicillin/clavulanate potassium

Tablets

Prescribing information for this product, which appears on pages 1438–1441 of the 2004 PDR, has been revised as follows. Please write "See Supplement A" next to the product heading.

The following paragraph was added before the DESCRIPTION *section:*

To reduce the development of drug-resistant bacteria and maintain the effectiveness of AUGMENTIN (amoxicillin/clavulanate potassium) and other antibacterial drugs, AUGMENTIN should be used only to treat or prevent infections that are proven or strongly suspected to be caused by bacteria.

The last 2 paragraphs of INDICATIONS AND USAGE *were revised to:*

To reduce the development of drug-resistant bacteria and maintain the effectiveness of AUGMENTIN and other antibacterial drugs, AUGMENTIN should be used only to treat or prevent infections that are proven or strongly suspected to be caused by susceptible bacteria. When culture and susceptibility information are available, they should be considered in selecting or modifying antibacterial therapy. In the absence of such data, local epidemiology and susceptibility patterns may contribute to the empiric selection of therapy.

Bacteriological studies, to determine the causative organisms and their susceptibility to AUGMENTIN, should be performed together with any indicated surgical procedures.

Table 11. Grade 3/4 Laboratory Abnormalities Reported in ≥2% of Adult Patients in Open-Label Clinical Trials of AGENERASE Capsules in Combination with Ritonavir

Laboratory Abnormality (non-fasting specimens)	AGENERASE 1,200 mg plus Ritonavir 200 mg q.d.* (n = 101)	AGENERASE 600 mg plus Ritonavir 100 mg b.i.d.† (n = 239)
Hypertriglyceridemia (>750 mg/dL)	8%	13%
Hyperglycemia (>251 mg/dL)	2%	3%
AST (>5 x ULN)	3%	5%
ALT (>5 x ULN)	4%	4%
Amylase (>2 x ULN)	4%	3%

*Data from 2 open-label studies in treatment-naive patients also receiving abacavir/lamivudine.
† Data from 3 open-label studies in treatment-naive and treatment-experienced patients receiving combination antiretroviral therapy.

In PRECAUTIONS: General, *the following paragraph was added:*
Prescribing AUGMENTIN in the absence of a proven or strongly suspected bacterial infection or a prophylactic indication is unlikely to provide benefit to the patient and increases the risk of the development of drug-resistant bacteria.
The following subsection was added to PRECAUTIONS:
Information for Patients: Patients should be counseled that antibacterial drugs including AUGMENTIN, should only be used to treat bacterial infections. They do not treat viral infections (e.g., the common cold). When AUGMENTIN is prescribed to treat a bacterial infection, patients should be told that although it is common to feel better early in the course of therapy, the medication should be taken exactly as directed. Skipping doses or not completing the full course of therapy may: (1) decrease the effectiveness of the immediate treatment, and (2) increase the likelihood that bacteria will develop resistance and will not be treatable by AUGMENTIN or other antibacterial drugs in the future.
The following subsection was revised in ADVERSE REACTIONS:
Renal: Interstitial nephritis and hematuria have been reported rarely. Crystalluria has also been reported.
The following subsection was added to ADVERSE REACTIONS:
Miscellaneous: Tooth discoloration (brown, yellow, or gray staining) has been rarely reported. Most reports occurred in pediatric patients. Discoloration was reduced or eliminated with brushing or dental cleaning in most cases.
The following sentence was added to the third paragraph in OVERDOSAGE:
Crystalluria has also been reported after amoxicillin overdosage.
GlaxoSmithKline, Research Triangle Park, NC 27709

January 2004/AG:AL12

AUGMENTIN ES-600® ℞

[*äg-mint' in*]
amoxicillin/clavulanate potassium

Prescribing information for this product, which appears on pages 1441–1444 of the 2004 PDR, has been revised as follows. Please write "See Supplement A" next to the product heading.
The following paragraph was added before the DESCRIPTION *section:*
To reduce the development of drug-resistant bacteria and maintain the effectiveness of AUGMENTIN ES-600 (amoxicillin/clavulanate potassium) and other antibacterial drugs, AUGMENTIN ES-600 should be used only to treat or prevent infections that are proven or strongly suspected to be caused by bacteria.
The last paragraph of INDICATIONS AND USAGE *was revised to:*
To reduce the development of drug-resistant bacteria and maintain the effectiveness of AUGMENTIN ES-600 and other antibacterial drugs, AUGMENTIN ES-600 should be used only to treat or prevent infections that are proven or strongly suspected to be caused by susceptible bacteria. When culture and susceptibility information are available, they should be considered in selecting or modifying antibacterial therapy. In the absence of such data, local epidemiology and susceptibility patterns may contribute to the empiric selection of therapy when there is reason to believe the infection may involve both *S. pneumoniae* (penicillin MIC ≤2 mcg/mL) and the β-lactamase–producing organisms listed above. Once the results are known, therapy should be adjusted appropriately.
In PRECAUTIONS: General, *the following paragraph was added:*
Prescribing AUGMENTIN ES-600 in the absence of a proven or strongly suspected bacterial infection or a prophylactic indication is unlikely to provide benefit to the patient and increases the risk of the development of drug-resistant bacteria.
PRECAUTIONS: Information for the Patient *was revised to:*
AUGMENTIN ES-600 should be taken every 12 hours with a meal or snack to reduce the possibility of gastrointestinal upset. If diarrhea develops and is severe or lasts more than 2 or 3 days, call your doctor.
Keep suspension refrigerated. Shake well before using. When dosing a child with the suspension (liquid) of AUGMENTIN ES-600, use a dosing spoon or medicine dropper. Be sure to rinse the spoon or dropper after each use. Bottles of suspension of AUGMENTIN ES-600 may contain more liquid than required. Follow your doctor's instructions about the amount to use and the days of treatment your child requires. Discard any unused medicine.
Patients should be counseled that antibacterial drugs including AUGMENTIN ES-600, should only be used to treat bacterial infections. They do not treat viral infections (e.g., the common cold). When AUGMENTIN ES-600 is prescribed to treat a bacterial infection, patients should be told that although it is common to feel better early in the course of therapy, the medication should be taken exactly as directed. Skipping doses or not completing the full course of therapy may: (1) decrease the effectiveness of the immediate treatment, and (2) increase the likelihood that bacteria will develop resistance and will not be treatable by AUGMENTIN ES-600 or other antibacterial drugs in the future.
The following subsections were revised in ADVERSE REACTIONS:
Renal: Interstitial nephritis and hematuria have been reported rarely. Crystalluria has also been reported.
Miscellaneous: Tooth discoloration (brown, yellow, or gray staining) has been rarely reported. Most reports occurred in pediatric patients. Discoloration was reduced or eliminated with brushing or dental cleaning in most cases.
The following sentence was added to the third paragraph in OVERDOSAGE:
Crystalluria has also been reported after amoxicillin overdosage.
GlaxoSmithKline, Research Triangle Park, NC 27709

January 2004/AE:L8

AUGMENTIN XR™ ℞

[*äg-mint' in*]
(amoxicillin/clavulanate potassium)
Extended Release Tablets

Prescribing information for this product, which appears on pages 1444–1447 of the 2004 PDR, has been revised as follows. Please write "See Supplement A" next to the product heading.
The following paragraph was added before the DESCRIPTION *section:*
To reduce the development of drug-resistant bacteria and maintain the effectiveness of AUGMENTIN XR (amoxicillin/clavulanate potassium) and other antibacterial drugs, AUGMENTIN XR should be used only to treat or prevent infections that are proven or strongly suspected to be caused by bacteria.
The following paragraph was added to INDICATIONS AND USAGE:
To reduce the development of drug-resistant bacteria and maintain the effectiveness of AUGMENTIN XR and other antibacterial drugs, AUGMENTIN XR should be used only to treat or prevent infections that are proven or strongly suspected to be caused by susceptible bacteria. When culture and susceptibility information are available, they should be considered in selecting or modifying antibacterial therapy. In the absence of such data, local epidemiology and susceptibility patterns may contribute to the empiric selection of therapy.
In PRECAUTIONS: General, *the following paragraph was added:*
Prescribing AUGMENTIN XR in the absence of a proven or strongly suspected bacterial infection or a prophylactic indication is unlikely to provide benefit to the patient and increases the risk of the development of drug-resistant bacteria.
PRECAUTIONS: Information for Patients *was revised to:*
AUGMENTIN XR should be taken every 12 hours with a meal or snack to reduce the possibility of gastrointestinal upset. If diarrhea develops and is severe or lasts more than 2 or 3 days, call your doctor.
Patients should be counseled that antibacterial drugs, including AUGMENTIN XR, should only be used to treat bacterial infections. They do not treat viral infections (e.g., the common cold). When AUGMENTIN XR is prescribed to treat a bacterial infection, patients should be told that although it is common to feel better early in the course of therapy, the medication should be taken exactly as directed. Skipping doses or not completing the full course of therapy may: (1) decrease the effectiveness of the immediate treatment, and (2) increase the likelihood that bacteria will develop resistance and will not be treatable by AUGMENTIN XR or other antibacterial drugs in the future. Discard any unused medicine.
In ADVERSE REACTIONS, *the following changes were made to adverse reactions reported for ampicillin-class antibiotics:*
Renal: Interstitial nephritis and hematuria have been reported rarely. Crystalluria has also been reported.
Miscellaneous: Tooth discoloration (brown, yellow, or gray staining) has been rarely reported. Most reports occurred in pediatric patients. Discoloration was reduced or eliminated with brushing or dental cleaning in most cases.
The last paragraph of OVERDOSAGE *was revised to:*
Interstitial nephritis resulting in oliguric renal failure has been reported in a small number of patients after overdosage with amoxicillin. Crystalluria has also been reported after amoxicillin overdosage. Renal impairment appears to be reversible with cessation of drug administration. High blood levels may occur more readily in patients with impaired renal function because of decreased renal clearance of both amoxicillin and clavulanate. Both amoxicillin and clavulanate are removed from the circulation by hemodialysis (see DOSAGE AND ADMINISTRATION).
HOW SUPPLIED *was revised to:*
Each white, oval film-coated bilayer scored tablet, debossed with AUGMENTIN XR, contains amoxicillin trihydrate and amoxicillin sodium equivalent to a total of 1,000 mg of amoxicillin and clavulanate potassium equivalent to 62.5 mg of clavulanic acid.
NDC 0029-6096-48 Bottles of 28 (7 day XR pack)
NDC 0029-6096-60 Bottles of 40 (10 day XR pack)
GlaxoSmithKline, Research Triangle Park, NC 27709

January 2004/AX:L5

AVANDAMET™ ℞

[*ə-van' də-met*]
(rosiglitazone maleate and metformin hydrochloride)
Tablets

Prescribing information for this product, which appears on pages 1447–1452 of the 2004 PDR, has been revised as follows. Please write "See Supplement A" next to the product heading.
In DESCRIPTION, *the following paragraph was revised to:*
AVANDAMET is available for oral administration as tablets containing rosiglitazone maleate and metformin hydrochloride equivalent to: 1 mg rosiglitazone with 500 mg metformin hydrochloride (1 mg/500 mg), 2 mg rosiglitazone with 500 mg metformin hydrochloride (2 mg/500 mg), 4 mg rosiglitazone with 500 mg metformin hydrochloride (4 mg/500 mg), 2 mg rosiglitazone with 1000 mg metformin hydrochloride (2 mg/1000 mg), and 4 mg rosiglitazone with 1000 mg metformin hydrochloride (4 mg/1000 mg). In addition, each tablet contains the following inactive ingredients: Hypromellose 2910, lactose monohydrate, magnesium stearate, microcrystalline cellulose, polyethylene glycol 400, povidone 29–32, sodium starch glycolate, titanium dioxide, and 1 or more of the following: Red and yellow iron oxides.
In WARNINGS, *the following subsection was revised to:*
Rosiglitazone maleate
Cardiac Failure and Other Cardiac Effects: Rosiglitazone, like other thiazolidinediones, alone or in combination with other antidiabetic agents, can cause fluid retention, which may exacerbate or lead to heart failure. Patients should be observed for signs and symptoms of heart failure. AVANDAMET should be discontinued if any deterioration in cardiac status occurs. Patients with New York Heart Association (NYHA) Class 3 and 4 cardiac status were not studied during the clinical trials with rosiglitazone maleate. In patients requiring pharmacologic treatment for congestive heart failure, AVANDAMET should not be used (see CONTRAINDICATIONS).
In combination with insulin, thiazolidinediones may increase the risk of other cardiovascular adverse events. In three 26-week trials in patients with type 2 diabetes, 216 received 4 mg of rosiglitazone plus insulin, 322 received 8 mg of rosiglitazone plus insulin, and 338 received insulin alone. These trials included patients with long-standing diabetes and a high prevalence of pre-existing medical conditions, including peripheral neuropathy, retinopathy, ischemic heart disease, vascular disease, and congestive heart failure. In these clinical studies, an increased incidence of edema, cardiac failure, and other cardiovascular adverse events was seen in patients on rosiglitazone and insulin combination therapy compared to insulin and placebo. Patients who experienced cardiovascular events were on average older and had a longer duration of diabetes. These cardiovascular events were noted at both the 4 mg and 8 mg daily doses of rosiglitazone. In this population, however, it was not possible to determine specific risk factors that could be used to identify all patients at risk of heart failure and other cardiovascular events on combination therapy. Three of 10 patients who developed cardiac failure on combination therapy during the double-blind part of the fixed-dose studies had no known prior evidence of congestive heart failure, or pre-existing cardiac condition.
In a double-blind study in type 2 diabetes patients with chronic renal failure (112 received 4 mg or 8 mg of rosiglitazone plus insulin and 108 received insulin alone), there was no difference in cardiovascular adverse events with rosiglitazone in combination with insulin compared to insulin alone.
Patients treated with combination AVANDAMET and insulin should be monitored for cardiovascular adverse events. The combination therapy should be discontinued in patients who do not respond as manifested by a reduction in HbA1c or insulin dose after 4 to 5 months of therapy or who develop any significant adverse events. (See ADVERSE REACTIONS.) There are no studies that have evaluated the safety or effectiveness of AVANDAMET in combination with insulin. The use of AVANDAMET in combination with insulin is not indicated.
In DOSAGE AND ADMINISTRATION, *the following table was revised to:*

Table 1. AVANDAMET Starting Dose

PRIOR THERAPY	Usual AVANDAMET Starting Dose	
Total daily dose	Tablet strength	Number of tablets
Metformin HCl*		
1,000 mg/day	2 mg/500 mg	1 tablet twice a day
2,000 mg/day	2 mg/1,000 mg	1 tablet twice a day
Rosiglitazone		
4 mg/day	2 mg/500 mg	1 tablet twice a day
8 mg/day	4 mg/500 mg	1 tablet twice a day

*For patients on doses of metformin HCl between 1,000 and 2,000 mg/day, initiation of AVANDAMET requires individualization of therapy.

The following new tablet strengths and packs were added to HOW SUPPLIED:
2 mg/1,000 mg – yellow, film-coated oval tablet, debossed with gsk on one side and 2/1000 on the other.

Continued on next page

Avandamet—Cont.

4 mg/1,000 mg – pink, film-coated oval tablet, debossed with gsk on one side and 4/1000 on the other.
2 mg/1,000 mg bottles of 60: NDC 0007-3163-18
2 mg/1,000 mg bottles of 100: NDC 0007-3163-20
4 mg/1,000 mg bottles of 60: NDC 0007-3164-18
4 mg/1,000 mg bottles of 100: NDC 0007-3164-20
GlaxoSmithKline, Research Triangle Park, NC 27709

November 2003/AT:L3

CEFTIN® Tablets ℞
[*sĕf' tin*]
(cefuroxime axetil tablets)
CEFTIN® for Oral Suspension ℞
(cefuroxime axetil powder for oral suspension)

Prescribing information for this product, which appears on pages 1463–1467 of the 2004 PDR, has been revised as follows. Please write "See Supplement A" next to the product heading.

The following paragraph was added before the DESCRIPTION *section:*

To reduce the development of drug-resistant bacteria and maintain the effectiveness of CEFTIN and other antibacterial drugs, CEFTIN should be used only to treat or prevent infections that are proven or strongly suspected to be caused by bacteria.

In DESCRIPTION, *the following sentence was revised to:*

CEFTIN for Oral Suspension contains the inactive ingredients acesulfame potassium, aspartame, povidone K30, stearic acid, sucrose, tutti-frutti flavoring, and xanthan gum.

In INDICATIONS AND USAGE, *the last paragraph was deleted and the following paragraph was added:*

To reduce the development of drug-resistant bacteria and maintain the effectiveness of CEFTIN and other antibacterial drugs, CEFTIN should be used only to treat or prevent infections that are proven or strongly suspected to be caused by susceptible bacteria. When culture and susceptibility information are available, they should be considered in selecting or modifying antibacterial therapy. In the absence of such data, local epidemiology and susceptibility patterns may contribute to the empiric selection of therapy.

In PRECAUTIONS: General, *the following paragraph was added:*

Prescribing CEFTIN in the absence of a proven or strongly suspected bacterial infection or a prophylactic indication is unlikely to provide benefit to the patient and increases the risk of the development of drug-resistant bacteria.

The following paragraph was added to PRECAUTIONS: Information for Patients/Caregivers (Pediatric): *Phenylketonurics subsection:*

3. Patients should be counseled that antibacterial drugs, including CEFTIN, should only be used to treat bacterial infections. They do not treat viral infections (e.g., the common cold). When CEFTIN is prescribed to treat a bacterial infection, patients should be told that although it is common to feel better early in the course of therapy, the medication should be taken exactly as directed. Skipping doses or not completing the full course of therapy may: (1) decrease the effectiveness of the immediate treatment, and (2) increase the likelihood that bacteria will develop resistance and will not be treatable by CEFTIN or other antibacterial drugs in the future.

The last paragraph in DOSAGE AND ADMINISTRATION *was revised to:*

NOTE: SHAKE THE ORAL SUSPENSION WELL BEFORE EACH USE. Replace cap securely after each opening. Store the reconstituted suspension between 2° and 8°C (36° and 46°F) (in a refrigerator). DISCARD AFTER 10 DAYS.

HOW SUPPLIED *was revised to add the following new packs:*

CEFTIN Tablets, 250 mg:
Unit Dose Packs of 100 NDC 0173-0387-01
CEFTIN Tablets, 500 mg:
Unit Dose Packs of 50 NDC 0173-0394-01

The NDC numbers of the CEFTIN for Oral Suspension packs were revised to:

125 mg/5 mL:	100-mL Suspension	NDC 0173-0740-00
250 mg/5 mL:	50-mL Suspension	NDC 0173-0741-10
	100-mL Suspension	NDC 0173-0741-00

The storage conditions for CEFTIN for Oral Suspension were revised to:

Before reconstitution, store dry powder between 2° and 30°C (36° and 86°F).

After reconstitution, store suspension between 2° and 8°C (36° and 46°F), in a refrigerator. DISCARD AFTER 10 DAYS.

GlaxoSmithKline, Research Triangle Park, NC 27709

October 2003/RL-2046

COREG® ℞
[*kor' eg*]
(carvedilol)
Tablets

Prescribing information for this product, which appears on pages 1472–1477 of the 2004 PDR, has been revised as follows. Please write "See Supplement A" next to the product heading.

The WARNINGS: Hepatic Injury *subsection was deleted.*

The PRECAUTIONS: Geriatric Use *subsection was revised to:*

Of the 765 patients with congestive heart failure randomized to COREG in US clinical trials, 31% (235) were 65 years of age or older, and 7.3% (56) were 75 years of age or older. Of the 1,156 patients randomized to COREG in a long-term, placebo-controlled trial in severe heart failure, 47% (547) were 65 years of age or older, and 15% (174) were 75 years of age or older. Of 3,025 patients receiving COREG in congestive heart failure trials worldwide, 42% were 65 years of age or older.

Of the 975 myocardial infarction patients randomized to COREG in the CAPRICORN trial, 48% (468) were 65 years of age or older, and 11% (111) were 75 years of age or older.

Of the 2,065 hypertensive patients in US clinical trials of efficacy or safety who were treated with COREG, 21% (436) were 65 years of age or older. Of 3,722 patients receiving COREG in hypertension clinical trials conducted worldwide, 24% were 65 years of age or older.

With the exception of dizziness in hypertensive patients (incidence 8.8% in the elderly vs. 6% in younger patients), no overall differences in the safety or effectiveness (See Figures 2 and 4.) were observed between the older subjects and younger subjects in each of these populations. Similarly, other reported clinical experience has not identified differences in responses between the elderly and younger subjects, but greater sensitivity of some older individuals cannot be ruled out.

The ADVERSE REACTIONS *subsection was revised to:*

COREG has been evaluated for safety in patients with congestive heart failure (mild, moderate, and severe heart failure), in patients with left ventricular dysfunction following myocardial infarction and in hypertensive patients. The observed adverse event profile was consistent with the pharmacology of the drug and the health status of the patients in the clinical trials. Adverse events reported for each of these patient populations are provided below. Excluded are adverse events considered too general to be informative, and those not reasonably associated with the use of the drug because they were associated with the condition being treated or are very common in the treated population. Rates of adverse events were generally similar across demographic subsets (men and women, elderly and non-elderly, blacks and non-blacks).

Congestive Heart Failure: COREG has been evaluated for safety in congestive heart failure in more than 3,000 patients worldwide of whom more than 2,100 participated in placebo-controlled clinical trials. Approximately 60% of the total treated population received COREG for at least 6 months and 30% received COREG for at least 12 months. Both in US clinical trials in mild-to-moderate heart failure that compared COREG in daily doses up to 100 mg (n = 765) to placebo (n = 437), and in a multinational clinical trial in severe heart failure (COPERNICUS) that compared COREG in daily doses up to 50 mg (n = 1,156) with placebo (n = 1,133), discontinuation rates for adverse experiences were similar in carvedilol and placebo patients. In these databases, the only cause of discontinuation >1%, and occurring more often on carvedilol was dizziness (1.3% on carvedilol, 0.6% on placebo in the COPERNICUS trial).

Table 2 shows adverse events reported in patients with mild-to-moderate heart failure enrolled in US placebo-controlled clinical trials, and with severe heart failure enrolled in the COPERNICUS trial. Shown are adverse events that occurred more frequently in drug-treated patients than pla-

Table 2. Adverse Events (% Occurrence) Occurring More Frequently with COREG Than With Placebo in Patients With Mild-to-Moderate Heart Failure Enrolled in US Heart Failure Trials or in Patients With Severe Heart Failure in the COPERNICUS Trial (Incidence >3% in Patients Treated with Carvedilol, Regardless of Causality)

	Mild-to-Moderate HF		Severe Heart Failure	
	COREG	Placebo	COREG	Placebo
	(n = 765)	(n = 437)	(n = 1,156)	(n = 1,133)
Body as a Whole				
Asthenia	7	7	11	9
Fatigue	24	22	—	—
Digoxin level increased	5	4	2	1
Edema generalized	5	3	6	5
Edema dependent	4	2	—	—
Cardiovascular				
Bradycardia	9	1	10	3
Hypotension	9	3	14	8
Syncope	3	3	8	5
Angina Pectoris	2	3	6	4
Central Nervous System				
Dizziness	32	19	24	17
Headache	8	7	5	3
Gastrointestinal				
Diarrhea	12	6	5	3
Nausea	9	5	4	3
Vomiting	6	4	1	2
Metabolic				
Hyperglycemia	12	8	5	3
Weight increase	10	7	12	11
BUN increased	6	5	—	—
NPN increased	6	5	—	—
Hypercholesterolemia	4	3	1	1
Edema peripheral	2	1	7	6
Musculoskeletal				
Arthralgia	6	5	1	1
Respiratory				
Cough Increased	8	9	5	4
Rales	4	4	4	2
Vision				
Vision abnormal	5	2	—	—

cebo-treated patients with an incidence of >3% in patients treated with carvedilol regardless of causality. Median study medication exposure was 6.3 months for both carvedilol and placebo patients in the trials of mild-to-moderate heart failure, and 10.4 months in the trial of severe heart failure patients.
[See table 2 at top of previous page]
Cardiac failure and dyspnea were also reported in these studies, but the rates were equal or greater in patients who received placebo.
The following adverse events were reported with a frequency of >1% but ≤3% and more frequently with COREG in either the US placebo-controlled trials in patients with mild-to-moderate heart failure, or in patients with severe heart failure in the COPERNICUS trial.

Incidence >1% to ≤3%

Body as a Whole: Allergy, malaise, hypovolemia, fever, leg edema.
Cardiovascular: Fluid overload, postural hypotension, aggravated angina pectoris, AV block, palpitation, hypertension.
Central and Peripheral Nervous System: Hypesthesia, vertigo, paresthesia.
Gastrointestinal: Melena, periodontitis.
Liver and Biliary System: SGPT increased, SGOT increased.
Metabolic and Nutritional: Hyperuricemia, hypoglycemia, hyponatremia, increased alkaline phosphatase, glycosuria, hypervolemia, diabetes mellitus, GGT increased, weight loss, hyperkalemia, creatinine increased.
Musculoskeletal: Muscle cramps.
Platelet, Bleeding and Clotting: Prothrombin decreased, purpura, thrombocytopenia.
Psychiatric: Somnolence.
Reproductive, male: Impotence.
Special Senses: Blurred vision.
Urinary System: Renal insufficiency, albuminuria, hematuria.
Left Ventricular Dysfunction Following Myocardial Infarction: COREG has been evaluated for safety in survivors of an acute myocardial infarction with left ventricular dysfunction in the CAPRICORN trial which involved 969 patients who received COREG and 980 who received placebo. Approximately 75% of the patients received COREG for at least 6 months and 53% received COREG for at least 12 months. Patients were treated for an average of 12.9 months and 12.8 months with COREG and placebo, respectively.
The most common adverse events reported with COREG in the CAPRICORN trial were consistent with the profile of the drug in the US heart failure trials and the COPERNICUS trial. The only additional adverse events reported in CAPRICORN in >3% of the patients and more commonly on carvedilol were dyspnea, anemia, and lung edema. The following adverse events were reported with a frequency of >1% but ≤3% and more frequently with COREG: flu syndrome, cerebrovascular accident, peripheral vascular disorder, hypotonia, depression, gastrointestinal pain, arthritis and gout. The overall rates of discontinuations due to adverse events were similar in both groups of patients. In this database, the only cause of discontinuation >1%, and occurring more often on carvedilol was hypotension (1.5% on carvedilol, 0.2% on placebo).
Hypertension: COREG has been evaluated for safety in hypertension in more than 2,193 patients in US clinical trials and in 2,976 patients in international clinical trials. Approximately 36% of the total treated population received COREG for at least 6 months. In general, COREG was well tolerated at doses up to 50 mg daily. Most adverse events reported during COREG therapy were of mild to moderate severity. In US controlled clinical trials directly comparing COREG monotherapy in doses up to 50 mg (n = 1,142) to placebo (n = 462), 4.9% of COREG patients discontinued for adverse events vs. 5.2% of placebo patients. Although there was no overall difference in discontinuation rates, discontinuations were more common in the carvedilol group for postural hypotension (1% vs. 0). The overall incidence of adverse events in US placebo-controlled trials was found to increase with increasing dose of COREG. For individual adverse events this could only be distinguished for dizziness, which increased in frequency from 2% to 5% as total daily dose increased from 6.25 mg to 50 mg.
Table 3 shows adverse events in US placebo-controlled clinical trials for hypertension that occurred with an incidence of >1% regardless of causality, and that were more frequent in drug-treated patients than placebo-treated patients.

Table 3. Adverse Events in US Placebo-Controlled Hypertension Trials Incidence ≥1%, Regardless of Causality

	Adverse Reactions	
	COREG (n = 1,142) % occurrence	Placebo (n = 462) % occurrence
Cardiovascular		
Bradycardia	2	—
Postural hypotension	2	—
Peripheral Edema	1	—
Central Nervous System		
Dizziness	6	5
Insomnia	2	1
Gastrointestinal		
Diarrhea	2	1
Hematologic		
Thrombocytopenia	1	—
Metabolic		
Hypertriglyceridemia	1	—

Dyspnea and fatigue were also reported in these studies, but the rates were equal or greater in patients who received placebo.
The following adverse events not described above were reported as possibly or probably related to COREG in worldwide open or controlled trials with COREG in patients with hypertension or congestive heart failure.

Incidence >0.1% to ≤1%

Cardiovascular: Peripheral ischemia, tachycardia.
Central and Peripheral Nervous System: Hypokinesia.
Gastrointestinal: Bilirubinemia, increased hepatic enzymes (0.2% of hypertension patients and 0.4% of congestive heart failure patients were discontinued from therapy because of increases in hepatic enzymes; see Laboratory Abnormalities).
Psychiatric: Nervousness, sleep disorder, aggravated depression, impaired concentration, abnormal thinking, paroniria, emotional lability.
Respiratory System: Asthma (see CONTRAINDICATIONS).
Reproductive: Male: decreased libido.
Skin and Appendages: Pruritus, rash erythematous, rash maculopapular, rash psoriaform, photosensitivity reaction.
Special Senses: Tinnitus.
Urinary System: Micturition frequency increased.
Autonomic Nervous System: Dry mouth, sweating increased.
Metabolic and Nutritional: Hypokalemia, hypertriglyceridemia.
Hematologic: Anemia, leukopenia.
The following events were reported in ≤0.1% of patients and are potentially important: complete AV block, bundle branch block, myocardial ischemia, cerebrovascular disorder, convulsions, migraine, neuralgia, paresis, anaphylactoid reaction, alopecia, exfoliative dermatitis, amnesia, GI hemorrhage, bronchospasm, pulmonary edema, decreased hearing, respiratory alkalosis, increased BUN, decreased HDL, pancytopenia, and atypical lymphocytes.
Laboratory Abnormalities: Reversible elevations in serum transaminases (ALT or AST) have been observed during treatment with COREG. Rates of transaminase elevations (2- to 3-times the upper limit of normal) observed during controlled clinical trials have generally been similar between patients treated with COREG and those treated with placebo. However, transaminase elevations, confirmed by rechallenge, have been observed with COREG. In a long-term, placebo-controlled trial in severe heart failure, patients treated with COREG had lower values for hepatic transaminases than patients treated with placebo, possibly because COREG-induced improvements in cardiac function led to less hepatic congestion and/or improved hepatic blood flow.
COREG therapy has not been associated with clinically significant changes in serum potassium, total triglycerides, total cholesterol, HDL cholesterol, uric acid, blood urea nitrogen, or creatinine. No clinically relevant changes were noted in fasting serum glucose in hypertensive patients; fasting serum glucose was not evaluated in the congestive heart failure clinical trials.
Postmarketing Experience: The following adverse reaction has been reported in postmarketing experience: Reports of aplastic anemia have been rare and received only when carvedilol was administered concomitantly with other medications associated with the event.
GlaxoSmithKline, Research Triangle Park, NC 27709

October 2003/CO:L8

ENGERIX-B® ℞

[in' jə-rix]
[Hepatitis B Vaccine (Recombinant)]

Prescribing information for this product, which appears on pages 1486–1488 of the 2004 PDR, has been revised as follows. Please write "See Supplement A" next to the product heading.
CONTRAINDICATIONS *was revised to:*
Hypersensitivity to any component of the vaccine, including yeast, is a contraindication (see DESCRIPTION). This vaccine is contraindicated in patients with previous hypersensitivity to any hepatitis B-containing vaccine.
The following paragraph was added to WARNINGS:
The vial stopper is latex-free. The tip cap and the rubber plunger of the needleless prefilled syringes contain dry natural latex rubber that may cause allergic reactions in latex sensitive individuals.
Manufactured by GlaxoSmithKline Biologicals
Rixensart, Belgium, US License No. 1617
Distributed by GlaxoSmithKline, Research Triangle Park, NC 27709

August 2003/EB:L34

EPIVIR® TABLETS ℞

[ĕp' ə-vir]
(lamivudine tablets)

EPIVIR® ORAL SOLUTION ℞

(lamivudine oral solution)

Prescribing information for this product, which appears on pages 1489–1493 of the 2004 PDR, has been revised as follows. Please write "See Supplement A" next to the product heading.
The following paragraph was added to PRECAUTIONS: Information for Patients:
Diabetic patients should be advised that each 15-mL dose of EPIVIR Oral Solution contains 3 grams of sucrose.
The following paragraph was added to PRECAUTIONS: Drug Interactions:
Lamivudine is predominantly eliminated in the urine by active organic cationic secretion. The possibility of interactions with other drugs administered concurrently should be considered, particularly when their main route of elimination is active renal secretion via the organic cationic transport system (e.g., trimethoprim).
The following sentence was added to the end of OVERDOSAGE:
If overdose occurs, the patient should be monitored, and standard supportive treatment applied as required.
In HOW SUPPLIED, *the following sentence was revised to:*
EPIVIR Tablets, 150 mg, are white, modified diamond-shaped, film-coated tablets engraved with "GX CJ7" on one side and plain on the reverse side.
GlaxoSmithKline, Research Triangle Park, NC 27709
Manufactured under agreement from
Shire Pharmaceuticals Group plc, Basingstoke, UK

September 2003/RL-2035

EPIVIR-HBV® ℞

[ĕp' ə-vir]
(lamivudine)
Tablets

EPIVIR-HBV® ℞

(lamivudine)
Oral Solution

Prescribing information for this product, which appears on pages 1493–1496 of the 2004 PDR, has been revised as follows. Please write "See Supplement A" next to the product heading.
The following paragraph was added to PRECAUTIONS: Information for Patients:
Diabetic patients should be advised that each 20-mL dose of EPIVIR-HBV Oral Solution contains 4 grams of sucrose.
The following paragraph was added to PRECAUTIONS: Drug Interactions:
Lamivudine is predominantly eliminated in the urine by active organic cationic secretion. The possibility of interactions with other drugs administered concurrently should be considered, particularly when their main route of elimination is active renal secretion via the organic cationic transport system (e.g., trimethoprim).
The PRECAUTIONS: Nursing Mothers *subsection was revised to:*
A study in lactating rats administered 45 mg/kg of lamivudine showed that lamivudine concentrations in milk were slightly greater than those in plasma. Lamivudine is also excreted in human milk. Samples of breast milk obtained from 20 mothers receiving lamivudine monotherapy (300 mg twice daily) or combination therapy (150 mg lamivudine twice daily and 300 mg zidovudine twice daily) had measurable concentrations of lamivudine.
Because of the potential for serious adverse reactions in nursing infants, **mothers should be instructed not to breastfeed if they are receiving lamivudine.**
In ADVERSE REACTIONS: Lamivudine in Patients with HIV, *the following sentence was revised to:*
Pancreatitis was observed in 9 of the 2,613 adult patients (<0.5%) who received EPIVIR in controlled clinical trials.
In ADVERSE REACTIONS: Observed During Clinical Practice, *the following paragraph was revised to:*
Hemic and Lymphatic: Anemia (including pure red cell aplasia progressing on therapy), lymphadenopathy, splenomegaly.
The following sentence was added to the end of OVERDOSAGE:
If overdose occurs, the patient should be monitored, and standard supportive treatment applied as required.
GlaxoSmithKline, Research Triangle Park, NC 27709
Manufactured under agreement from Shire Pharmaceuticals Group plc
Basingstoke, UK

September 2003/RL-2034

ESKALITH® ℞
[*es'ka-lith*]
(lithium carbonate)
Capsules, 300 mg
ESKALITH CR® ℞
(lithium carbonate)
Controlled-Release
Tablets, 450 mg

Prescribing information for this product, which appears on pages 1496–1498 of the 2004 PDR, has been revised as follows. Please write "See Supplement A" next to the product heading.
In PRECAUTIONS: Drug Interactions, *the 4th paragraph was revised to:*
There is evidence that angiotensin-converting enzyme inhibitors, such as enalapril and captopril, and angiotensin II receptor antagonists, such as losartan, may substantially increase steady-state plasma lithium levels, sometimes resulting in lithium toxicity. When such combinations are used, lithium dosage may need to be decreased, and plasma lithium levels should be measured more often.
HOW SUPPLIED *was revised to:*
ESKALITH Capsules 300 mg are gray and yellow capsules imprinted with "ESKALITH" and "SB" on one side of each half of the capsule, in bottles of 100 (NDC 0007-4007-20).
ESKALITH CR Tablets 450 mg are round, yellow, biconvex, controlled-release tablets, debossed with "SKF" and "J10" on one side and scored on the other side, in bottles of 100 (NDC 0007-4010-20).
Manufactured by Cardinal Health, Winchester, KY 40391 for GlaxoSmithKline, Research Triangle Park, NC 27709

September 2003/EL:L50

FLONASE® ℞
[*flō' nāz*]
(fluticasone propionate)
Nasal Spray, 50 mcg

For Intranasal Use Only.
SHAKE GENTLY BEFORE USE.

Prescribing information for this product, which appears on pages 1502–1504 of the 2004 PDR, has been revised as follows. Please write "See Supplement A" next to the product heading.
The CLINICAL PHARMACOLOGY: Drug Interactions *subsection was revised to:*
Fluticasone propionate is a substrate of cytochrome P450 3A4. Coadministration of fluticasone propionate and the highly potent cytochrome P450 3A4 inhibitor ritonavir is not recommended based upon a multiple-dose, crossover drug interaction study in 18 healthy subjects. Fluticasone propionate aqueous nasal spray (200 mcg once daily) was coadministered for 7 days with three P450 3A4 inhibitors: ritonavir (100 mg twice daily), ketoconazole (200 mg once daily), and erythromycin (500 mg twice daily). Coadministration with ritonavir resulted in a significant increase in plasma fluticasone propionate exposure and a significant decrease (86%) in plasma cortisol area under the plasma concentration versus time curve (AUC). Coadministration with ketoconazole resulted in a slight increase in fluticasone propionate exposure and a 7% reduction in the area under the plasma cortisol AUC. Coadministration with erythromycin did not affect fluticasone propionate pharmacokinetics; there was a 2% reduction in the plasma cortisol AUC.
Caution should be exercised when potent cytochrome P450 3A4 inhibitors (e.g., ketoconazole) are coadministered with fluticasone propionate.
The following paragraph was added to WARNINGS:
A drug interaction study in healthy subjects has shown that ritonavir (a highly potent cytochrome P450 3A4 inhibitor) can significantly increase plasma fluticasone propionate exposure, resulting in significantly reduced serum cortisol concentrations (see CLINICAL PHARMACOLOGY: Drug Interactions and PRECAUTIONS: Drug Interactions). During postmarketing use, there have been reports of clinically significant drug interactions in patients receiving fluticasone propionate and ritonavir, resulting in systemic corticosteroid effects including Cushing syndrome and adrenal suppression. Therefore, coadministration of fluticasone propionate and ritonavir is not recommended unless the potential benefit to the patient outweighs the risk of systemic corticosteroid side effects.
The PRECAUTIONS: Drug Interactions *subsection was revised to:*
Fluticasone propionate is a substrate of cytochrome P450 3A4. A drug interaction study with fluticasone propionate aqueous nasal spray in healthy subjects has shown that ritonavir (a highly potent cytochrome P450 3A4 inhibitor) can significantly increase plasma fluticasone propionate exposure, resulting in significantly reduced serum cortisol concentrations (see CLINICAL PHARMACOLOGY: Drug Interactions). During postmarketing use, there have been reports of clinically significant drug interactions in patients receiving fluticasone propionate and ritonavir, resulting in systemic corticosteroid effects including Cushing syndrome and adrenal suppression. Therefore, coadministration of fluticasone propionate and ritonavir is not recommended unless the potential benefit to the patient outweighs the risk of systemic corticosteroid side effects.
In a placebo-controlled, crossover study in 8 healthy volunteers, coadministration of a single dose of orally inhaled fluticasone propionate (1,000 mcg; 5 times the maximum daily intranasal dose) with multiple doses of ketoconazole (200 mg) to steady state resulted in increased plasma fluticasone propionate exposure, a reduction in plasma cortisol AUC, and no effect on urinary excretion of cortisol. Caution should be exercised when FLONASE Nasal Spray is coadministered with ketoconazole and other known potent cytochrome P450 3A4 inhibitors.
GlaxoSmithKline, Research Triangle Park, NC 27709

July 2003/RL-2019

FLOVENT® 44 mcg ℞
[*flō' vent*]
(fluticasone propionate, 44 mcg)
Inhalation Aerosol

FLOVENT® 110 mcg ℞
(fluticasone propionate, 110 mcg)
Inhalation Aerosol

FLOVENT® 220 mcg ℞
(fluticasone propionate, 220 mcg)
Inhalation Aerosol

For Oral Inhalation Only

Prescribing information for this product, which appears on pages 1504–1507 of the 2004 PDR, has been revised as follows. Please write "See Supplement A" next to the product heading.
The CLINICAL PHARMACOLOGY: Drug Interactions *subsection was revised to:*
Fluticasone propionate is a substrate of cytochrome P450 3A4. Coadministration of fluticasone propionate and the highly potent cytochrome P450 3A4 inhibitor ritonavir is not recommended based upon a multiple-dose, crossover drug interaction study in 18 healthy subjects. Fluticasone propionate aqueous nasal spray (200 mcg once daily) was coadministered for 7 days with ritonavir (100 mg twice daily). This resulted in a significant increase in plasma fluticasone propionate exposure and a significant decrease (86%) in plasma cortisol area under the plasma concentration versus time curve (AUC).
Caution should be exercised when other potent cytochrome P450 3A4 inhibitors are coadministered with fluticasone propionate. In a drug interaction study, coadministration of orally inhaled fluticasone propionate (1,000 mcg) and ketoconazole (200 mg once daily) resulted in increased plasma fluticasone propionate exposure and reduced plasma cortisol AUC, but had no effect on urinary excretion of cortisol. In another multiple-dose drug interaction study, coadministration of orally inhaled fluticasone propionate (500 mcg twice daily) and erythromycin (333 mg 3 times daily) did not affect fluticasone propionate pharmacokinetics.
The following paragraph was added to WARNINGS:
A drug interaction study in healthy subjects has shown that ritonavir (a highly potent cytochrome P450 3A4 inhibitor) can significantly increase plasma fluticasone propionate exposure, resulting in significantly reduced serum cortisol concentrations (see CLINICAL PHARMACOLOGY: Drug Interactions and PRECAUTIONS: Drug Interactions). During postmarketing use, there have been reports of clinically significant drug interactions in patients receiving fluticasone propionate and ritonavir, resulting in systemic corticosteroid effects including Cushing syndrome and adrenal suppression. Therefore, coadministration of fluticasone propionate and ritonavir is not recommended unless the potential benefit to the patient outweighs the risk of systemic corticosteroid side effects.
The PRECAUTIONS: Drug Interactions *subsection was revised to:*
Fluticasone propionate is a substrate of cytochrome P450 3A4. A drug interaction study with fluticasone propionate aqueous nasal spray in healthy subjects has shown that ritonavir (a highly potent cytochrome P450 3A4 inhibitor) can significantly increase plasma fluticasone propionate exposure, resulting in significantly reduced serum cortisol concentrations (see CLINICAL PHARMACOLOGY: Drug Interactions). During postmarketing use, there have been reports of clinically significant drug interactions in patients receiving fluticasone propionate and ritonavir, resulting in systemic corticosteroid effects including Cushing syndrome and adrenal suppression. Therefore, coadministration of fluticasone propionate and ritonavir is not recommended unless the potential benefit to the patient outweighs the risk of systemic corticosteroid side effects.
In a placebo-controlled, crossover study in 8 healthy volunteers, coadministration of a single dose of orally inhaled fluticasone propionate (1,000 mcg) with multiple doses of ketoconazole (200 mg) to steady state resulted in increased mean plasma fluticasone propionate exposure, a reduction in plasma cortisol AUC, and no effect on urinary excretion of cortisol. Caution should be exercised when FLOVENT Inhalation Aerosol is coadministered with ketoconazole and other known potent cytochrome P450 3A4 inhibitors.
In ADVERSE REACTIONS: Observed During Clinical Practice, *the following paragraph was revised to:*
Skin: Contusions, cutaneous hypersensitivity reactions, ecchymoses, and pruritus.
GlaxoSmithKline, Research Triangle Park, NC 27709

July 2003/RL-2022

FLOVENT® ROTADISK® 50 mcg ℞
[*flō' vent*]
(fluticasone propionate inhalation powder, 50 mcg)
FLOVENT® ROTADISK® 100 mcg ℞
(fluticasone propionate inhalation powder, 100 mcg)
FLOVENT® ROTADISK® 250 mcg ℞
(fluticasone propionate inhalation powder, 250 mcg)

For Oral Inhalation Only
For Use With the DISKHALER® Inhalation Device

Prescribing information for this product, which appears on pages 1507–1510 of the 2004 PDR, has been revised as follows. Please write "See Supplement A" next to the product heading.
The CLINICAL PHARMACOLOGY: Drug Interactions *subsection was revised to:*
Fluticasone propionate is a substrate of cytochrome P450 3A4. Coadministration of fluticasone propionate and the highly potent cytochrome P450 3A4 inhibitor ritonavir is not recommended based upon a multiple-dose, crossover drug interaction study in 18 healthy subjects. Fluticasone propionate aqueous nasal spray (200 mcg once daily) was coadministered for 7 days with ritonavir (100 mg twice daily). This resulted in a significant increase in plasma fluticasone propionate exposure and a significant decrease (86%) in plasma cortisol area under the plasma concentration versus time curve (AUC).
Caution should be exercised when other potent cytochrome P450 3A4 inhibitors are coadministered with fluticasone propionate. In a drug interaction study, coadministration of orally inhaled fluticasone propionate (1,000 mcg) and ketoconazole (200 mg once daily) resulted in increased plasma fluticasone propionate exposure and reduced plasma cortisol AUC, but had no effect on urinary excretion of cortisol. In another multiple-dose drug interaction study, coadministration of orally inhaled fluticasone propionate (500 mcg twice daily) and erythromycin (333 mg 3 times daily) did not affect fluticasone propionate pharmacokinetics.
The following paragraph was added to WARNINGS:
A drug interaction study in healthy subjects has shown that ritonavir (a highly potent cytochrome P450 3A4 inhibitor) can significantly increase plasma fluticasone propionate exposure, resulting in significantly reduced serum cortisol concentrations (see CLINICAL PHARMACOLOGY: Drug Interactions and PRECAUTIONS: Drug Interactions). During postmarketing use, there have been reports of clinically significant drug interactions in patients receiving fluticasone propionate and ritonavir, resulting in systemic corticosteroid effects including Cushing syndrome and adrenal suppression. Therefore, coadministration of fluticasone propionate and ritonavir is not recommended unless the potential benefit to the patient outweighs the risk of systemic corticosteroid side effects.
The PRECAUTIONS: Drug Interactions *subsection was revised to:*
Fluticasone propionate is a substrate of cytochrome P450 3A4. A drug interaction study with fluticasone propionate aqueous nasal spray in healthy subjects has shown that ritonavir (a highly potent cytochrome P450 3A4 inhibitor) can significantly increase plasma fluticasone propionate exposure, resulting in significantly reduced serum cortisol concentrations (see CLINICAL PHARMACOLOGY: Drug Interactions). During postmarketing use, there have been reports of clinically significant drug interactions in patients receiving fluticasone propionate and ritonavir, resulting in systemic corticosteroid effects including Cushing syndrome and adrenal suppression. Therefore, coadministration of fluticasone propionate and ritonavir is not recommended unless the potential benefit to the patient outweighs the risk of systemic corticosteroid side effects.
In a placebo-controlled, crossover study in 8 healthy volunteers, coadministration of a single dose of orally inhaled fluticasone propionate (1,000 mcg) with multiple doses of ketoconazole (200 mg) to steady state resulted in increased plasma fluticasone propionate exposure, a reduction in plasma cortisol AUC, and no effect on urinary excretion of cortisol. Caution should be exercised when FLOVENT ROTADISK is coadministered with ketoconazole and other known potent cytochrome P450 3A4 inhibitors.
GlaxoSmithKline, Research Triangle Park, NC 27709

July 2003/RL-2023

FORTAZ® ℞
[*for' taz*]
(ceftazidime for injection)
FORTAZ® ℞
(ceftazidime injection)
For Intravenous or Intramuscular Use

Prescribing information for this product, which appears on pages 1510–1513 of the 2004 PDR, has been revised as follows. Please write "See Supplement A" next to the product heading.
The following paragraph was added before the DESCRIPTION *section:*
To reduce the development of drug-resistant bacteria and maintain the effectiveness of FORTAZ and other antibacte-

rial drugs, FORTAZ should be used only to treat or prevent infections that are proven or strongly suspected to be caused by bacteria.
The following paragraph was added to INDICATIONS AND USAGE:
To reduce the development of drug-resistant bacteria and maintain the effectiveness of FORTAZ and other antibacterial drugs, FORTAZ should be used only to treat or prevent infections that are proven or strongly suspected to be caused by susceptible bacteria. When culture and susceptibility information are available, they should be considered in selecting or modifying antibacterial therapy. In the absence of such data, local epidemiology and susceptibility patterns may contribute to the empiric selection of therapy.
The following paragraph was added to the PRECAUTIONS: General *subsection:*
Prescribing FORTAZ in the absence of a proven or strongly suspected bacterial infection or a prophylactic indication is unlikely to provide benefit to the patient and increases the risk of the development of drug-resistant bacteria.
The following subsection was added after PRECAUTIONS: General:
Information for Patients: Patients should be counseled that antibacterial drugs, including FORTAZ, should only be used to treat bacterial infections. They do not treat viral infections (e.g., the common cold). When FORTAZ is prescribed to treat a bacterial infection, patients should be told that although it is common to feel better early in the course of therapy, the medication should be taken exactly as directed. Skipping doses or not completing the full course of therapy may: (1) decrease the effectiveness of the immediate treatment, and (2) increase the likelihood that bacteria will develop resistance and will not be treatable by FORTAZ or other antibacterial drugs in the future.
FORTAZ® (ceftazidime for injection):
GlaxoSmithKline, Research Triangle Park, NC 27709
FORTAZ® (ceftazidime injection):
Manufactured for GlaxoSmithKline
Research Triangle Park, NC 27709
by Baxter Healthcare Corporation, Deerfield, IL 60015
October 2003/RL-2043

HAVRIX® ℞
[hav' rix]
(Hepatitis A Vaccine, Inactivated)

Prescribing information for this product, which appears on pages 1513–1515 of the 2004 PDR, has been revised as follows. Please write "See Supplement A" next to the product heading.
The following sentence was added to the end of DESCRIPTION:
Neomycin sulfate, an aminoglycoside antibiotic, is included in the cell growth media; only trace amounts (not more than 40 ng/mL) remain following purification.
The CONTRAINDICATIONS *section was revised to:*
Hypersensitivity to any component of the vaccine, including neomycin, is a contraindication (see DESCRIPTION). This vaccine is contraindicated in patients with previous hypersensitivity to any hepatitis A-containing vaccine.
The first 2 paragraphs of WARNINGS *were revised to:*
There have been rare reports of anaphylaxis/anaphylactoid reactions following commercial use of the vaccine.
The vial stopper is latex-free. The tip cap and the rubber plunger of the needleless prefilled syringes contain dry natural latex rubber that may cause allergic reactions in latex sensitive individuals.
Manufactured by GlaxoSmithKline Biologicals, Rixensart, Belgium, US License No. 1617
Distributed by GlaxoSmithKline
Research Triangle Park, NC 27709

August 2003/HA:L17

HYCAMTIN® ℞
[hī-kam' tin]
(topotecan hydrochloride)
For Injection
FOR INTRAVENOUS USE

Prescribing information for this product, which appears on pages 1516–1519 of the 2004 PDR, has been revised as follows. Please write "See Supplement A" next to the product heading.
The following subsection was added to PRECAUTIONS:
Geriatric Use: Of the 879 patients with metastatic ovarian cancer or small cell lung cancer in clinical studies of HYCAMTIN, 32% (n = 281) were 65 years of age and older, while 3.8% (n = 33) were 75 years of age and older. No overall differences in effectiveness or safety were observed between these patients and younger adult patients. Other reported clinical experience has not identified differences in responses between the elderly and younger adult patients, but greater sensitivity of some older individuals cannot be ruled out.
There were no apparent differences in the pharmacokinetics of topotecan in elderly patients, once the age-related decrease in renal function was considered (see CLINICAL PHARMACOLOGY).
This drug is known to be substantially excreted by the kidney, and the risk of toxic reactions to this drug may be greater in patients with impaired renal function. Because elderly patients are more likely to have decreased renal function, care should be taken in dose selection, and it may be useful to monitor renal function (see DOSAGE AND ADMINISTRATION).
GlaxoSmithKline, Research Triangle Park, NC 27709

July 2003/HY:L15

IMITREX® ℞
[ĭm'ĭ-trĕx]
(sumatriptan succinate)
Tablets

Prescribing information for this product, which appears on pages 1528–1532 of the 2004 PDR, has been revised as follows. Please write "See Supplement A" next to the product heading.
In DESCRIPTION, *the ingredients statements were revised to:*
Each tablet also contains the inactive ingredients croscarmellose sodium, dibasic calcium phosphate, magnesium stearate, microcrystalline cellulose, and sodium bicarbonate. Each 100-mg tablet also contains hypromellose, iron oxide, titanium dioxide, and triacetin.
The second paragraph of CLINICAL PHARMACOLOGY: Pharmacokinetics *was revised to:*
A food effect study involving administration of IMITREX Tablets 100 mg to healthy volunteers under fasting conditions and with a high-fat meal indicated that the C_{max} and AUC were increased by 15% and 12%, respectively, when administered in the fed state.
The HOW SUPPLIED *section was revised to:*
IMITREX Tablets, 25, 50, and 100 mg of sumatriptan (base) as the succinate.
IMITREX Tablets, 25 mg are white, triangular-shaped, film-coated tablets debossed with "I" on one side and "25" on the other in blister packs of 9 tablets (NDC 0173-0735-00).
IMITREX Tablets, 50 mg are white, triangular-shaped, film-coated tablets debossed with "IMITREX 50" on one side and a chevron shape (^) on the other in blister packs of 9 tablets (NDC 0173-0736-01).
IMITREX Tablets, 100 mg, are pink, triangular-shaped, film-coated tablets debossed with "IMITREX 100" on one side and a chevron shape (^) on the other in blister packs of 9 tablets (NDC 0173-0737-01).
Store between 36° and 86°F (2° and 30°C).
GlaxoSmithKline, Research Triangle Park, NC 27709

August 2003/RL-2026

LAMICTAL® ℞
[la-mĭk' tal]
(lamotrigine)
Tablets

LAMICTAL® ℞
(lamotrigine)
Chewable Dispersible Tablets

Prescribing information for this product, which appears on pages 1537–1545 of the 2004 PDR, has been revised as follows. Please write "See Supplement A" next to the product heading.
The CLINICAL PHARMACOLOGY: Pharmacokinetics and Drug Metabolism: *Gender subsection was revised to:*
The clearance of lamotrigine is not affected by gender. However, during dose escalation of LAMICTAL in one clinical trial in patients with epilepsy on a stable dose of valproate (n = 77), mean trough lamotrigine concentrations, unadjusted for weight, were 24% to 45% higher (0.3 to 1.7 mcg/mL) in females than in males.
The INDICATIONS AND USAGE: Epilepsy: *Monotherapy Use subsection was revised to:*
LAMICTAL is indicated for conversion to monotherapy in adults with partial seizures who are receiving treatment with a single EIAED or valproate.
Safety and effectiveness of LAMICTAL have not been established (1) as initial monotherapy, (2) for conversion to monotherapy from non–enzyme-inducing AEDs except valproate, or (3) for simultaneous conversion to monotherapy from 2 or more concomitant AEDs (see DOSAGE AND ADMINISTRATION).
Safety and effectiveness in patients below the age of 16 other than those with partial seizures and the generalized seizures of Lennox-Gastaut syndrome have not been established (see BOX WARNING).
The PRECAUTIONS: Drug Interactions: *Effects of Other Drugs on the Pharmacokinetics of Lamotrigine subsection was revised to:*
(see Table 3).
Valproate Added to LAMICTAL: The addition of valproate increases lamotrigine steady-state concentrations in normal volunteers by slightly more than 2-fold. In one study, maximal inhibition of lamotrigine clearance was reached at valproate doses between 250 mg/day and 500 mg/day and did not increase as the valproate dose was further increased.
The DOSAGE AND ADMINISTRATION: Epilepsy: *Monotherapy Use subsection was revised to:*
LAMICTAL is indicated for conversion to monotherapy in adults with partial seizures who are receiving treatment with a single EIAED (e.g., carbamazepine, phenytoin, phenobarbital, etc.) or valproate.
Safety and effectiveness of LAMICTAL have not been established (1) as initial monotherapy, (2) for conversion to monotherapy from non–enzyme-inducing AEDs except valproate, or (3) for simultaneous conversion to monotherapy from 2 or more concomitant AEDs.
Safety and effectiveness in pediatric patients below the age of 16 years other than those with partial seizures and the generalized seizures of Lennox-Gastaut syndrome have not been established (see BOX WARNING).
Epilepsy:
Conversion From Adjunctive Therapy With a Single Enzyme-Inducing Antiepileptic Drug or Valproate to Monotherapy With LAMICTAL in Patients ≥16 Years of Age With Epilepsy: The goal of the transition regimen is to effect the conversion to monotherapy with LAMICTAL under conditions that ensure adequate seizure control while mitigating the risk of serious rash associated with the rapid titration of LAMICTAL.
The recommended maintenance dose of LAMICTAL as monotherapy is 500 mg/day given in 2 divided doses.
To avoid an increased risk of rash, the recommended initial dose and subsequent dose escalations of LAMICTAL should not be exceeded (see BOX WARNING).
Conversion From Adjunctive Therapy With a Single Enzyme-Inducing Antiepileptic Drug to Monotherapy With LAMICTAL: After achieving a dose of 500 mg/day of LAMICTAL according to the guidelines in Table 12, the concomitant EIAED should be withdrawn by 20% decrements each week over a 4-week period. The regimen for the withdrawal of the concomitant EIAED is based on experience gained in the controlled monotherapy clinical trial.
Conversion from Adjunctive Therapy With Valproate to Monotherapy With LAMICTAL: The conversion regimen involves 4 steps. First, achieve a dose of 200 mg/day of LAMICTAL according to the guidelines in Table 11. Second, while keeping the LAMICTAL dose at 200 mg/day, valproate should be gradually decreased to a dose of 500 mg/day by decrements no greater than 500 mg/day per week. This dosage regimen is then maintained for 1 week. Third, LAMICTAL should then be increased to 300 mg/day while valproate is simultaneously decreased to 250 mg/day. This regimen should be maintained for 1 week. Fourth, valproate should then be discontinued completely and LAMICTAL increased by 100 mg/day every week until the recommended monotherapy dose of 500 mg/day is reached (see Table 13).

Table 13. Conversion from Adjunctive Therapy With Valproate to Monotherapy With LAMICTAL in Patients ≥16 Years of Age.

	LAMICTAL	Valproate
Step 1	Achieve a dose of 200 mg/day according to guidelines in Table 11 (if not already on 200 mg/day).	Maintain previous stable dose.
Step 2	Maintain at 200 mg/day.	Decrease to 500 mg/day by decrements no greater than 500 mg/day per week and then maintain the dose of 500 mg/day for 1 week.
Step 3	Increase to 300 mg/day and maintain for 1 week.	Simultaneously decrease to 250 mg/day and maintain for 1 week.
Step 4	Increase by 100 mg/day every week to achieve maintenance dose of 500 mg/day.	Discontinue.

Conversion from Adjunctive Therapy With Antiepileptic Drugs Other Than Enzyme-Inducing Antiepileptic Drugs and Valproate to Monotherapy With LAMICTAL: The effect of AEDs other than EIAEDs and valproate on the metabolism of LAMICTAL is not currently known. Therefore, no specific dosing guidelines can be provided for conversion to monotherapy with LAMICTAL.
Manufactured for GlaxoSmithKline
Research Triangle Park, NC 27709
by DSM Pharmaceuticals, Inc., Greenville, NC 27834
or GlaxoSmithKline, Research Triangle Park, NC 27709

January 2004/RL-2060

LEUKERAN® ℞
[lū' kŭh-răn]
(chlorambucil)
Tablets

Prescribing information for this product, which appears on pages 1562–1563 of the 2004 PDR, has been revised as follows. Please write "See Supplement A" next to the product heading.
The follow subsection was added to PRECAUTIONS:
Geriatric Use: Clinical studies of chlorambucil did not include sufficient numbers of subjects aged 65 and over to determine whether they respond differently from younger sub-

Continued on next page

Leukeran—Cont.

jects. Other reported clinical experience has not identified differences in responses between the elderly and younger patients. In general, dose selection for an elderly patient should be cautious, usually starting at the low end of the dosing range, reflecting the greater frequency of decreased hepatic, renal, or cardiac function, and of concomitant disease or other drug therapy.

GlaxoSmithKline, Research Triangle Park, NC 27709

November 2003/RL-2054

LOTRONEX® ℞

[lō' trə-nĕx]

(alosetron hydrochloride)

Tablets

Prescribing information for this product, which appears on pages 1563–1567 of the 2004 PDR, has been revised as follows. Please write "See Supplement A" next to the product heading.

The second paragraph of DESCRIPTION *was revised to:*

LOTRONEX Tablets are supplied for oral administration as 0.5 mg (white) and 1 mg (blue) tablets. The 0.5 mg tablet contains 0.562 mg alosetron HCl equivalent to 0.5 mg alosetron and the 1 mg tablet contains 1.124 mg alosetron HCl equivalent to 1 mg of alosetron. Each tablet also contains the inactive ingredients: lactose (anhydrous), magnesium stearate, microcrystalline cellulose, and pregelatinized starch. The white film-coat for the 0.5 mg tablet contains hypromellose, titanium dioxide, and triacetin. The blue film-coat for the 1 mg tablet contains hypromellose, titanium dioxide, triacetin, and indigo carmine.

The following paragraph was added to HOW SUPPLIED:

LOTRONEX Tablets, 0.5 mg (0.562 mg alosetron HCl equivalent to 0.5 mg alosetron) are white, oval, film-coated tablets debossed with GX EX1 on one face. Bottles of 30 (NDC 0173-0738-00) with child-resistant closures.

The storage conditions were revised to:

Store at 25°C (77°F); excursions permitted to 15–30°C (59–86°F) [see USP Controlled Room Temperature]. Protect from light and moisture.

The following section of the Medication Guide was revised to:

How should I take LOTRONEX?

- Take LOTRONEX exactly as your doctor prescribes it. You can take LOTRONEX with or without food.
- Begin with no more than 1 mg a day for 4 weeks to see how LOTRONEX affects you. Although the effect of 1 mg once a day on IBS symptoms has not been studied in clinical trials, you and your doctor may decide that you should keep taking this dose if it adequately controls your IBS symptoms and you have not become constipated or had ischemic colitis while taking LOTRONEX.
- If you miss a dose of LOTRONEX, just skip that dose. Do **not** take 2 doses the next time. Wait until the next time you are supposed to take it and then take your normal dose.
- If you try 1 mg once a day for 4 weeks and it does not control your symptoms, does not make you constipated, and does not give you ischemic colitis, tell your doctor. Your doctor may increase your dose up to 1 mg twice a day, the dose that was used in clinical trials.

If 1 mg twice a day does not work after 4 weeks, LOTRONEX is not likely to help you and you should stop using it and call your doctor.

Stop taking LOTRONEX and call your doctor right away if you get constipated or have any signs of low blood flow to parts of your intestines (ischemic colitis) such as new or worse abdominal pain, or blood in your diarrhea or stools.

The following paragraph in the Medication Guide was revised to:

Inactive Ingredients: lactose (anhydrous), magnesium stearate, microcrystalline cellulose, and pregelatinized starch. The white film-coat for the 0.5 mg tablet contains hypromellose, titanium dioxide, and triacetin. The blue film-coat for the 1 mg tablet contains hypromellose, titanium dioxide, triacetin, and indigo carmine.

GlaxoSmithKline, Research Triangle Park, NC 27709

December 2003/RL-1188

MALARONE® ℞

[mal' ə-rōn]

(atovaquone and proguanil hydrochloride)

Tablets

MALARONE® ℞

(atovaquone and proguanil hydrochloride)

Pediatric Tablets

Prescribing information for this product, which appears on pages 1567–1570 of the 2004 PDR, has been revised as follows. Please write "See Supplement A" next to the product heading.

The CLINICAL PHARMACOLOGY: Pharmacokinetics: *Distribution subsection was revised to:*

Atovaquone is highly protein bound (>99%) over the concentration range of 1 to 90 mcg/mL. A population pharmacokinetic analysis demonstrated that the apparent volume of distribution of atovaquone (V/F) in adult and pediatric patients after oral administration is approximately 8.8 L/kg.

Proguanil is 75% protein bound. A population pharmacokinetic analysis demonstrated that the apparent V/F of proguanil in adult and pediatric patients >15 years of age with body weights from 31 to 110 kg ranged from 1,617 to 2,502 L. In pediatric patients ≤15 years of age with body weights from 11 to 56 kg, the V/F of proguanil ranged from 462 to 966 L.

In human plasma, the binding of atovaquone and proguanil was unaffected by the presence of the other.

The CLINICAL PHARMACOLOGY: Pharmacokinetics: *Elimination subsection was revised to:*

The elimination half-life of atovaquone is about 2 to 3 days in adult patients.

The elimination half-life of proguanil is 12 to 21 hours in both adult patients and pediatric patients, but may be longer in individuals who are slow metabolizers.

A population pharmacokinetic analysis in adult and pediatric patients showed that the apparent clearance (CL/F) of both atovaquone and proguanil are related to the body weight. The values CL/F for both atovaquone and proguanil in subjects with body weights ≥11 kg are shown in Table 1. [See table 1 above]

Table 1. Apparent Clearance for Atovaquone and Proguanil in Patients as a Function of Body Weight

Body Weight	Atovaquone N	Atovaquone CL/F (L/hr) Mean ± SD* (range)	Proguanil N	Proguanil CL/F (L/hr) Mean ± SD* (range)
11–20 kg	159	1.34 ± 0.63 (0.52–4.26)	146	29.5 ± 6.5 (10.3–48.3)
21–30 kg	117	1.87 ± 0.81 (0.52–5.38)	113	40.0 ± 7.5 (15.9–62.7)
31–40 kg	95	2.76 ± 2.07 (0.97–12.5)	91	49.5 ± 8.30 (25.8–71.5)
>40 kg	368	6.61 ± 3.92 (1.32–20.3)	282	67.9 ± 19.9 (14.0–145)

*SD = standard deviation

The pharmacokinetics of atovaquone and proguanil in patients with body weight below 11 kg have not been adequately characterized.

The CLINICAL PHARMACOLOGY: Special Populations: *Pediatrics subsection was revised to:*

The pharmacokinetics of proguanil and cycloguanil are similar in adult patients and pediatric patients. However, the elimination half-life of atovaquone is shorter in pediatric patients (1 to 2 days) than in adult patients (2 to 3 days). In clinical trials, plasma trough levels of atovaquone and proguanil in pediatric patients weighing 5 to 40 kg were within the range observed in adults after dosing by body weight.

The PRECAUTIONS: Pediatric Use *subsection was revised to:*

Treatment of Malaria: The efficacy and safety of MALARONE for the treatment of malaria have been established in controlled studies involving pediatric patients weighing 5 kg or more (see CLINICAL STUDIES). Safety and effectiveness have not been established in pediatric patients who weigh less than 5 kg.

Prophylaxis of Malaria: The efficacy and safety of MALARONE have been established for the prophylaxis of malaria in controlled studies involving pediatric patients weighing 11 kg or more (see CLINICAL STUDIES). Safety and effectiveness have not been established in pediatric patients who weigh less than 11 kg.

ADVERSE REACTIONS *was revised to:*

Because MALARONE contains atovaquone and proguanil hydrochloride, the type and severity of adverse reactions associated with each of the compounds may be expected. The higher treatment doses of MALARONE were less well tolerated than the lower prophylactic doses.

Among adults who received MALARONE for treatment of malaria, attributable adverse experiences that occurred in ≥5% of patients were abdominal pain (17%), nausea (12%), vomiting (12%), headache (10%), diarrhea (8%), asthenia (8%), anorexia (5%), and dizziness (5%). Treatment was discontinued prematurely due to an adverse experience in 4 of 436 adults treated with MALARONE.

Among pediatric patients (weighing 11 to 40 kg) who received MALARONE for the treatment of malaria, attributable adverse experiences that occurred in ≥5% of patients were vomiting (10%) and pruritus (6%). Vomiting occurred in 43 of 319 (13%) pediatric patients who did not have symptomatic malaria but were given treatment doses of MALARONE for 3 days in a clinical trial. The design of this clinical trial required that any patient who vomited be withdrawn from the trial. Among pediatric patients with symptomatic malaria treated with MALARONE, treatment was discontinued prematurely due to an adverse experience in 1 of 116 (0.9%).

In a study of 100 pediatric patients (5 to <11 kg body weight) who received MALARONE for the treatment of uncomplicated *P. falciparum* malaria, only diarrhea (6%) occurred in ≥5% of patients as an adverse experience attributable to MALARONE. In 3 patients (3%), treatment was discontinued prematurely due to an adverse experience.

Abnormalities in laboratory tests reported in clinical trials were limited to elevations of transaminases in malaria pa-

Table 3. Adverse Experiences in Placebo-Controlled Clinical Trials of MALARONE for Prophylaxis of Malaria

Percent of Subjects With Adverse Experiences (Percent of Subjects With Adverse Experiences Attributable to Therapy)

Adverse Experience	Adults: Placebo n = 206	Adults: MALARONE* n = 206	Adults: MALARONE† n = 381	Children and Adolescents: Placebo n = 140	Children and Adolescents: MALARONE n = 125
Headache	27 (7)	22 (3)	17 (5)	21 (14)	19 (14)
Fever	13 (1)	5 (0)	3 (0)	11 (<1)	6 (0)
Myalgia	11 (0)	12 (0)	7 (0)	0 (0)	0 (0)
Abdominal pain	10 (5)	9 (4)	6 (3)	29 (29)	33 (31)
Cough	8 (<1)	6 (<1)	4 (1)	9 (0)	9 (0)
Diarrhea	8 (3)	6 (2)	4 (1)	3 (1)	2 (0)
Upper respiratory infection	7 (0)	8 (0)	5 (0)	0 (0)	<1 (0)
Dyspepsia	5 (4)	3 (2)	2 (1)	0 (0)	0 (0)
Back pain	4 (0)	8 (0)	4 (0)	0 (0)	0 (0)
Gastritis	3 (2)	3 (3)	2 (2)	0 (0)	0 (0)
Vomiting	2 (<1)	1 (<1)	<1 (<1)	6 (6)	7 (7)
Flu syndrome	1 (0)	2 (0)	4 (0)	6 (0)	9 (0)
Any adverse experience	65 (32)	54 (17)	49 (17)	62 (41)	60 (42)

* Subjects receiving the recommended dose of atovaquone and proguanil hydrochloride in placebo-controlled trials.

† Subjects receiving the recommended dose of atovaquone and proguanil hydrochloride in any trial.

Table 4. Adverse Experiences in Active-Controlled Clinical Trials of MALARONE for Prophylaxis of Malaria

Adverse Experience	Percent of Subjects With Adverse Experiences* (Percent of Subjects With Adverse Experiences Attributable to Therapy)							
	Study 1				Study 2			
	MALARONE n = 493		Mefloquine n = 483		MALARONE n = 511		Chloroquine plus Proguanil n = 511	
Diarrhea	38	(8)	36	(7)	34	(5)	39	(7)
Nausea	14	(3)	20	(8)	11	(2)	18	(7)
Abdominal pain	17	(5)	16	(5)	14	(3)	22	(6)
Headache	12	(4)	17	(7)	12	(4)	14	(4)
Dreams	7	(7)	16	(14)	6	(4)	7	(3)
Insomnia	5	(3)	16	(13)	4	(2)	5	(2)
Fever	9	(<1)	11	(1)	8	(<1)	8	(<1)
Dizziness	5	(2)	14	(9)	7	(3)	8	(4)
Vomiting	8	(1)	10	(2)	8	(0)	14	(2)
Oral ulcers	9	(6)	6	(4)	5	(4)	7	(5)
Pruritus	4	(2)	5	(2)	3	(1)	2	(<1)
Visual difficulties	2	(2)	5	(3)	3	(2)	3	(2)
Depression	<1	(<1)	5	(4)	<1	(<1)	1	(<1)
Anxiety	1	(<1)	5	(4)	<1	(<1)	1	(<1)
Any adverse experience	64	(30)	69	(42)	58	(22)	66	(28)
Any neuropsychiatric event	20	(14)	37	(29)	16	(10)	20	(10)
Any GI event	49	(16)	50	(19)	43	(12)	54	(20)

*Adverse experiences that started while receiving active study drug.

Table 6. Dosage for Treatment of Acute Malaria in Pediatric Patients

Weight (kg)	Atovaquone/ Proguanil HCl Total Daily Dose	Dosage Regimen
5–8	125 mg/50 mg	2 MALARONE Pediatric Tablets daily for 3 consecutive days
9–10	187.5 mg/75 mg	3 MALARONE Pediatric Tablets daily for 3 consecutive days
11–20	250 mg/100 mg	1 MALARONE Tablet (adult strength) daily for 3 consecutive days
21–30	500 mg/200 mg	2 MALARONE Tablets (adult strength) as a single dose daily for 3 consecutive days
31–40	750 mg/300 mg	3 MALARONE Tablets (adult strength) as a single dose daily for 3 consecutive days
>40	1 g/400 mg	4 MALARONE Tablets (adult strength) as a single dose daily for 3 consecutive days

tients being treated with MALARONE. The frequency of these abnormalities varied substantially across studies of treatment and were not observed in the randomized portions of the prophylaxis trials.

In one phase III trial of malaria treatment in Thai adults, early elevations of ALT and AST were observed to occur more frequently in patients treated with MALARONE compared to patients treated with an active control drug. Rates for patients who had normal baseline levels of these clinical laboratory parameters were: Day 7: ALT 26.7% vs. 15.6%; AST 16.9% vs. 8.6%. By day 14 of this 28-day study, the frequency of transaminase elevations equalized across the 2 groups.

In this and other studies in which transaminase elevations occurred, they were noted to persist for up to 4 weeks following treatment with MALARONE for malaria. None were associated with untoward clinical events.

Among subjects who received MALARONE for prophylaxis of malaria in placebo-controlled trials, adverse experiences occurred in similar proportions of subjects receiving MALARONE or placebo (Table 3). The most commonly reported adverse experiences possibly attributable to MALARONE or placebo were headache and abdominal pain. Prophylaxis with MALARONE was discontinued prematurely due to a treatment-related adverse experience in 3 of 381 adults and 0 of 125 pediatric patients.

[See table 3 at top of previous page]

In an additional placebo-controlled study of malaria prophylaxis with MALARONE involving 330 pediatric patients in a malaria-endemic area (see CLINICAL STUDIES), the safety profile of MALARONE was consistent with that described above. The most common treatment-emergent adverse events with MALARONE were abdominal pain (13%), headache (13%), and cough (10%). Abdominal pain (13% vs. 8%) and vomiting (5% vs. 3%) were reported more often with MALARONE than with placebo, while fever (5% vs. 12%) and diarrhea (1% vs. 5%) were more common with placebo. No patient withdrew from the study due to an adverse experience with MALARONE. No routine laboratory data were obtained during this study.

Among subjects who received MALARONE for prophylaxis of malaria in clinical trials with an active comparator, adverse experiences occurred in a similar or lower proportion of subjects receiving MALARONE than an active comparator (Table 4). The mean durations of dosing and the periods for which the adverse experiences are summarized in Table 3, were 28 days (Study 1) and 26 days (Study 2) for MALARONE, 53 days for mefloquine, and 49 days for chloroquine plus proguanil (reflecting the different recommended dosing regimens). Fewer neuropsychiatric adverse experiences occurred in subjects who received MALARONE than mefloquine. Fewer gastrointestinal adverse experiences occurred in subjects receiving MALARONE than chloroquine/proguanil. Compared with active comparator drugs, subjects receiving MALARONE had fewer adverse experiences overall that were attributed to prophylactic therapy (Table 4). Prophylaxis with MALARONE was discontinued prematurely due to a treatment-related adverse experience in 7 of 1,004 travelers.

[See table 4 above]

In a third active-controlled study, MALARONE (n = 110) was compared with chloroquine/proguanil (n = 111) for the prophylaxis of malaria in 221 nonimmune pediatric patients (see CLINICAL STUDIES). The mean duration of exposure was 23 days for MALARONE, 46 days for chloroquine, and 43 days for proguanil, reflecting the different recommended dosage regimens for these products. Fewer patients treated with MALARONE reported abdominal pain (2% vs. 7%) or nausea (<1% vs. 7%) than children who received chloroquine/proguanil. Oral ulceration (2% vs. 2%), vivid dreams (2% vs. <1%), and blurred vision (0% vs. 2%) occurred in similar proportions of patients receiving either MALARONE or chloroquine/proguanil, respectively. Two patients discontinued prophylaxis with chloroquine/proguanil due to adverse events, while none of those receiving MALARONE discontinued due to adverse events.

Post-Marketing Adverse Reactions: In addition to adverse events reported from clinical trials, the following events have been identified during world-wide post-approval use of MALARONE. Because they are reported voluntarily from a population of unknown size, estimates of frequency cannot be made. These events have been chosen for inclusion due to a combination of their seriousness, frequency of reporting, or potential causal connection to MALARONE.

Skin: Cutaneous reactions ranging from rash, photosensitivity, and urticaria to rare cases of erythema multiforme. In addition, one case of Stevens-Johnson syndrome has been reported.

OVERDOSAGE

There is limited information regarding overdosage from the administration of MALARONE.

There is no known antidote for atovaquone, and it is currently unknown if atovaquone is dialyzable. The median lethal dose is higher than the maximum oral dose tested in mice and rats (1,825 mg/kg/day). Overdoses up to 31,500 mg of atovaquone have been reported. In one such patient who also took an unspecified dose of dapsone, methemoglobinemia occurred. Rash has also been reported after overdose.

Overdoses of proguanil hydrochloride as large as 1,500 mg have been followed by complete recovery, and doses as high as 700 mg twice daily have been taken for over 2 weeks without serious toxicity. Adverse experiences occasionally associated with proguanil hydrochloride doses of 100 to 200 mg/day, such as epigastric discomfort and vomiting, would be likely to occur with overdose. There are also reports of reversible hair loss and scaling of the skin on the palms and/or soles, reversible aphthous ulceration, and hematologic side effects.

The following subsection was revised in DOSAGE AND ADMINISTRATION:

Treatment of Acute Malaria: ***Pediatric Patients:*** The dosage for treatment of acute malaria in pediatric patients is based upon body weight (Table 6).

[See table 6 at left]

MALARONE Tablets may be crushed and mixed with condensed milk just prior to administration for children who may have difficulty swallowing tablets.

GlaxoSmithKline, Research Triangle Park, NC 27709

December 2003/RL-2057

MYLERAN® ℞

[*mī′ lə-răn*]

(busulfan)

2-mg Scored Tablets

Prescribing information for this product, which appears on pages 1574–1576 of the 2004 PDR, has been revised as follows. Please write "See Supplement A" next to the product heading.

The following subsection was added to PRECAUTIONS:

Geriatric Use:

Clinical studies of busulfan did not include sufficient numbers of subjects aged 65 and over to determine whether they respond differently from younger subjects. Other reported clinical experience has not identified differences in responses between the elderly and younger patients. In general, dose selection for an elderly patient should be cautious, usually starting at the low end of the dosing range, reflecting the greater frequency of decreased hepatic, renal, or cardiac function, and of concomitant disease or other drug therapy.

Manufactured by DSM Pharmaceuticals, Inc.
Greenville, NC 27834
for GlaxoSmithKline, Research Triangle Park, NC 27709

January 2004/RL-2064

PAXIL® ℞

[*pax′il*]

(paroxetine hydrochloride)

Tablets and Oral Suspension

Prescribing information for this product, which appears on pages 1583–1589 of the 2004 PDR, has been revised as follows. Please write "See Supplement A" next to the product heading.

The DRUG ABUSE AND DEPENDENCE *section was revised to:*

Controlled Substance Class: PAXIL is not a controlled substance.

Physical and Psychologic Dependence: PAXIL has not been systematically studied in animals or humans for its potential for abuse, tolerance or physical dependence. While the clinical trials did not reveal any tendency for any drug-seeking behavior, these observations were not systematic and it is not possible to predict on the basis of this limited experience the extent to which a CNS-active drug will be

Continued on next page

Paxil—Cont.

misused, diverted, and/or abused once marketed. Consequently, patients should be evaluated carefully for history of drug abuse, and such patients should be observed closely for signs of misuse or abuse of PAXIL (e.g., development of tolerance, incrementations of dose, drug-seeking behavior).
GlaxoSmithKline, Research Triangle Park, NC 27709

October 2003/PX: L28

PAXIL CR™ ℞

[*păx'il*]
(paroxetine hydrochloride)
Controlled-Release Tablets

Prescribing information for this product, which appears on pages 1590–1594 of the 2004 PDR, has been completely revised as follows. Please write "See Supplement A" next to the product heading.

DESCRIPTION

PAXIL CR (paroxetine hydrochloride) is an orally administered psychotropic drug with a chemical structure unrelated to other selective serotonin reuptake inhibitors or to tricyclic, tetracyclic, or other available antidepressant or antipanic agents. It is the hydrochloride salt of a phenylpiperidine compound identified chemically as (-)-*trans*-4*R*-(4'-fluorophenyl)-3*S*-[(3',4'-methylenedioxyphenoxy) methyl] piperidine hydrochloride hemihydrate and has the empirical formula of $C_{19}H_{20}FNO_3 \bullet HCl \bullet 1/2H_2O$. The molecular weight is 374.8 (329.4 as free base). The structural formula of paroxetine hydrochloride is:

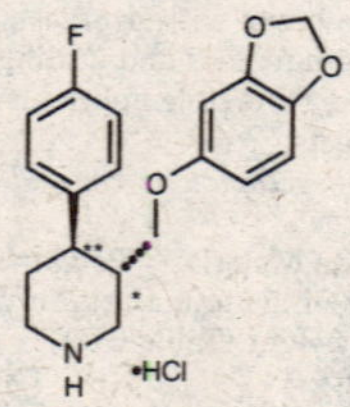

Paroxetine hydrochloride is an odorless, off-white powder, having a melting point range of 120° to 138°C and a solubility of 5.4 mg/mL in water.

Each enteric, film-coated, controlled-release tablet contains paroxetine hydrochloride equivalent to paroxetine as follows: 12.5 mg–yellow, 25 mg–pink, 37.5 mg–blue. One layer of the tablet consists of a degradable barrier layer and the other contains the active material in a hydrophilic matrix. Inactive ingredients consist of hypromellose, polyvinylpyrrolidone, lactose monohydrate, magnesium stearate, colloidal silicon dioxide, glyceryl behenate, methacrylic acid copolymer type C, sodium lauryl sulfate, polysorbate 80, talc, triethyl citrate, and 1 or more of the following colorants: Yellow ferric oxide, red ferric oxide, D&C Red No. 30, D&C Yellow No. 6, D&C Yellow No. 10, FD&C Blue No. 2.

CLINICAL PHARMACOLOGY

Pharmacodynamics: The efficacy of paroxetine in the treatment of major depressive disorder, panic disorder, social anxiety disorder, and premenstrual dysphoric disorder (PMDD) is presumed to be linked to potentiation of serotonergic activity in the central nervous system resulting from inhibition of neuronal reuptake of serotonin (5-hydroxytryptamine, 5-HT). Studies at clinically relevant doses in humans have demonstrated that paroxetine blocks the uptake of serotonin into human platelets. In vitro studies in animals also suggest that paroxetine is a potent and highly selective inhibitor of neuronal serotonin reuptake and has only very weak effects on norepinephrine and dopamine neuronal reuptake. In vitro radioligand binding studies indicate that paroxetine has little affinity for muscarinic, alpha$_1$-, alpha$_2$-, beta-adrenergic-, dopamine (D_2)-, 5-HT$_1$-, 5-HT$_2$-, and histamine (H_1)-receptors; antagonism of muscarinic, histaminergic, and alpha$_1$-adrenergic receptors has been associated with various anticholinergic, sedative, and cardiovascular effects for other psychotropic drugs.

Because the relative potencies of paroxetine's major metabolites are at most 1/50 of the parent compound, they are essentially inactive.

Pharmacokinetics: Tablets of PAXIL CR contain a degradable polymeric matrix (GEOMATRIX™) designed to control the dissolution rate of paroxetine over a period of approximately 4 to 5 hours. In addition to controlling the rate of drug release in vivo, an enteric coat delays the start of drug release until tablets of PAXIL CR have left the stomach.

Paroxetine hydrochloride is completely absorbed after oral dosing of a solution of the hydrochloride salt. In a study in which normal male and female subjects (n = 23) received single oral doses of PAXIL CR at 4 dosage strengths (12.5 mg, 25 mg, 37.5 mg, and 50 mg), paroxetine C_{max} and $AUC_{0\text{-}inf}$ increased disproportionately with dose (as seen also with immediate-release formulations). Mean C_{max} and $AUC_{0\text{-}inf}$ values at these doses were 2.0, 5.5, 9.0, and 12.5 ng/mL, and 121, 261, 338, and 540 ng•hr./mL, respectively. T_{max} was observed typically between 6 and 10 hours post-dose, reflecting a reduction in absorption rate compared with immediate-release formulations. The mean elimination half-life of paroxetine was 15 to 20 hours throughout this range of single doses of PAXIL CR. The bioavailability of 25 mg PAXIL CR is not affected by food.

During repeated administration of PAXIL CR (25 mg once daily), steady state was reached within 2 weeks (i.e., comparable to immediate-release formulations). In a repeat-dose study in which normal male and female subjects (n = 23) received PAXIL CR (25 mg daily), mean steady state C_{max}, C_{min}, and $AUC_{0\text{-}24}$ values were 30 ng/mL, 20 ng/mL, and 550 ng•hr./mL, respectively.

Based on studies using immediate-release formulations, steady-state drug exposure based on $AUC_{0\text{-}24}$ was several-fold greater than would have been predicted from single-dose data. The excess accumulation is a consequence of the fact that 1 of the enzymes that metabolizes paroxetine is readily saturable.

In steady-state dose proportionality studies involving elderly and nonelderly patients, at doses of the immediate-release formulation of 20 mg to 40 mg daily for the elderly and 20 mg to 50 mg daily for the nonelderly, some nonlinearity was observed in both populations, again reflecting a saturable metabolic pathway. In comparison to C_{min} values after 20 mg daily, values after 40 mg daily were only about 2 to 3 times greater than doubled.

Paroxetine is extensively metabolized after oral administration. The principal metabolites are polar and conjugated products of oxidation and methylation, which are readily cleared. Conjugates with glucuronic acid and sulfate predominate, and major metabolites have been isolated and identified. Data indicate that the metabolites have no more than 1/50 the potency of the parent compound at inhibiting serotonin uptake. The metabolism of paroxetine is accomplished in part by cytochrome $P_{450}IID_6$. Saturation of this enzyme at clinical doses appears to account for the nonlinearity of paroxetine kinetics with increasing dose and increasing duration of treatment. The role of this enzyme in paroxetine metabolism also suggests potential drug-drug interactions (see PRECAUTIONS).

Approximately 64% of a 30-mg oral solution dose of paroxetine was excreted in the urine with 2% as the parent compound and 62% as metabolites over a 10-day post-dosing period. About 36% was excreted in the feces (probably via the bile), mostly as metabolites and less than 1% as the parent compound over the 10-day post-dosing period.

Distribution: Paroxetine distributes throughout the body, including the CNS, with only 1% remaining in the plasma.

Protein Binding: Approximately 95% and 93% of paroxetine is bound to plasma protein at 100 ng/mL and 400 ng/mL, respectively. Under clinical conditions, paroxetine concentrations would normally be less than 400 ng/mL. Paroxetine does not alter the in vitro protein binding of phenytoin or warfarin.

Renal and Liver Disease: Increased plasma concentrations of paroxetine occur in subjects with renal and hepatic impairment. The mean plasma concentrations in patients with creatinine clearance below 30 mL/min. was approximately 4 times greater than seen in normal volunteers. Patients with creatinine clearance of 30 to 60 mL/min. and patients with hepatic functional impairment had about a 2-fold increase in plasma concentrations (AUC, C_{max}).

The initial dosage should therefore be reduced in patients with severe renal or hepatic impairment, and upward titration, if necessary, should be at increased intervals (see DOSAGE AND ADMINISTRATION).

Elderly Patients: In a multiple-dose study in the elderly at daily doses of 20, 30, and 40 mg of the immediate-release formulation, C_{min} concentrations were about 70% to 80% greater than the respective C_{min} concentrations in nonelderly subjects. Therefore the initial dosage in the elderly should be reduced (see DOSAGE AND ADMINISTRATION).

Clinical Trials

Major Depressive Disorder: The efficacy of PAXIL CR controlled-release tablets as a treatment for major depressive disorder has been established in two 12-week, flexible-dose, placebo-controlled studies of patients with DSM-IV Major Depressive Disorder. One study included patients in the age range 18 to 65 years, and a second study included elderly patients, ranging in age from 60 to 88. In both studies, PAXIL CR was shown to be significantly more effective than placebo in treating major depressive disorder as measured by the following: Hamilton Depression Rating Scale (HDRS), the Hamilton depressed mood item, and the Clinical Global Impression (CGI)–Severity of Illness score.

A study of outpatients with major depressive disorder who had responded to immediate-release paroxetine tablets (HDRS total score <8) during an initial 8-week open-treatment phase and were then randomized to continuation on immediate-release paroxetine tablets or placebo for 1 year demonstrated a significantly lower relapse rate for patients taking immediate-release paroxetine tablets (15%) compared to those on placebo (39%). Effectiveness was similar for male and female patients.

Panic Disorder: The effectiveness of PAXIL CR in the treatment of panic disorder was evaluated in three 10-week, multicenter, flexible-dose studies (Studies 1, 2, and 3) comparing paroxetine controlled-release (12.5 to 75 mg daily) to placebo in adult outpatients who had panic disorder (DSM-IV), with or without agoraphobia. These trials were assessed on the basis of their outcomes on 3 variables: (1) the proportions of patients free of full panic attacks at endpoint; (2) change from baseline to endpoint in the median number of full panic attacks; and (3) change from baseline to endpoint in the median Clinical Global Impression Severity score. For Studies 1 and 2, PAXIL CR was consistently superior to placebo on 2 of these 3 variables. Study 3 failed to consistently demonstrate a significant difference between PAXIL CR and placebo on any of these variables.

For all 3 studies, the mean dose of PAXIL CR for completers at endpoint was approximately 50 mg/day. Subgroup analyses did not indicate that there were any differences in treatment outcomes as a function of age or gender.

Long-term maintenance effects of the immediate-release formulation of paroxetine in panic disorder were demonstrated in an extension study. Patients who were responders during a 10-week double-blind phase with immediate-release paroxetine and during a 3-month double-blind extension phase were randomized to either immediate-release paroxetine or placebo in a 3-month double-blind relapse prevention phase. Patients randomized to paroxetine were significantly less likely to relapse than comparably treated patients who were randomized to placebo.

Social Anxiety Disorder: The efficacy of PAXIL CR as a treatment for social anxiety disorder has been established, in part, on the basis of extrapolation from the established effectiveness of the immediate-release formulation of paroxetine. In addition, the effectiveness of PAXIL CR in the treatment of social anxiety disorder was demonstrated in a 12-week, multicenter, double-blind, flexible-dose, placebo-controlled study of adult outpatients with a primary diagnosis of social anxiety disorder (DSM-IV). In the study, the effectiveness of PAXIL CR (12.5 to 37.5 mg daily) compared to placebo was evaluated on the basis of (1) change from baseline in the Liebowitz Social Anxiety Scale (LSAS) total score and (2) the proportion of responders who scored 1 or 2 (very much improved or much improved) on the Clinical Global Impression (CGI) Global Improvement score.

PAXIL CR demonstrated statistically significant superiority over placebo on both the LSAS total score and the CGI Improvement responder criterion. For patients who completed the trial, 64% of patients treated with PAXIL CR compared to 34.7% of patients treated with placebo were CGI Improvement responders.

Subgroup analyses did not indicate that there were any differences in treatment outcomes as a function of gender. Subgroup analyses of studies utilizing the immediate-release formulation of paroxetine generally did not indicate differences in treatment outcomes as a function of age, race, or gender.

Premenstrual Dysphoric Disorder: The effectiveness of PAXIL CR for the treatment of PMDD utilizing a continuous dosing regimen has been established in 2 placebo-controlled trials. Patients in these trials met DSM-IV criteria for PMDD. In a pool of 1,030 patients, treated with daily doses of PAXIL CR 12.5 or 25 mg/day, or placebo the mean duration of the PMDD symptoms was approximately 11 ± 7 years. Patients on systemic hormonal contraceptives were excluded from these trials. Therefore, the efficacy of PAXIL CR in combination with systemic (including oral) hormonal contraceptives for the continuous daily treatment of PMDD is unknown. In both positive studies, patients (N = 672) were treated with 12.5 mg/day or 25 mg/day of PAXIL CR or placebo continuously throughout the menstrual cycle for a period of 3 menstrual cycles. The VAS-Total score is a patient-rated instrument that mirrors the diagnostic criteria of PMDD as identified in the DSM-IV, and includes assessments for mood, physical symptoms, and other symptoms. 12.5 mg/day and 25 mg/day of PAXIL CR were significantly more effective than placebo as measured by change from baseline to the endpoint on the luteal phase VAS-Total score.

In a third study employing intermittent dosing, patients (N = 366) were treated for the 2 weeks prior to the onset of menses (luteal phase dosing, also known as intermittent dosing) with 12.5 mg/day or 25 mg/day of PAXIL CR or placebo for a period of 3 months. 12.5 mg/day and 25 mg/day of PAXIL CR, as luteal phase dosing, was significantly more effective than placebo as measured by change from baseline luteal phase VAS total score.

There is insufficient information to determine the effect of race or age on outcome in these studies.

INDICATIONS AND USAGE

Major Depressive Disorder: PAXIL CR is indicated for the treatment of major depressive disorder.

The efficacy of PAXIL CR in the treatment of a major depressive episode was established in two 12-week controlled trials of outpatients whose diagnoses corresponded to the DSM-IV category of major depressive disorder (see CLINICAL PHARMACOLOGY—Clinical Trials).

A major depressive episode (DSM-IV) implies a prominent and relatively persistent (nearly every day for at least 2 weeks) depressed mood or loss of interest or pleasure in nearly all activities, representing a change from previous functioning, and includes the presence of at least 5 of the following 9 symptoms during the same 2-week period: Depressed mood, markedly diminished interest or pleasure in usual activities, significant change in weight and/or appetite, insomnia or hypersomnia, psychomotor agitation or retardation, increased fatigue, feelings of guilt or worthlessness, slowed thinking or impaired concentration, a suicide attempt, or suicidal ideation.

The antidepressant action of paroxetine in hospitalized depressed patients has not been adequately studied.

PAXIL CR has not been systematically evaluated beyond 12 weeks in controlled clinical trials; however, the effectiveness of immediate-release paroxetine hydrochloride in maintaining a response in major depressive disorder for up to 1 year has been demonstrated in a placebo-controlled trial (see CLINICAL PHARMACOLOGY—Clinical Trials). The physician who elects to use PAXIL CR for extended periods should periodically re-evaluate the long-term usefulness of the drug for the individual patient.

Panic Disorder: PAXIL CR is indicated for the treatment of panic disorder, with or without agoraphobia, as defined in DSM-IV. Panic disorder is characterized by the occurrence of unexpected panic attacks and associated concern about having additional attacks, worry about the implications or consequences of the attacks, and/or a significant change in behavior related to the attacks.

The efficacy of PAXIL CR controlled-release tablets was established in two 10-week trials in panic disorder patients whose diagnoses corresponded to the DSM-IV category of panic disorder (see CLINICAL PHARMACOLOGY—Clinical Trials).

Panic disorder (DSM-IV) is characterized by recurrent unexpected panic attacks, i.e., a discrete period of intense fear or discomfort in which 4 (or more) of the following symptoms develop abruptly and reach a peak within 10 minutes: (1) palpitations, pounding heart, or accelerated heart rate; (2) sweating; (3) trembling or shaking; (4) sensations of shortness of breath or smothering; (5) feeling of choking; (6) chest pain or discomfort; (7) nausea or abdominal distress; (8) feeling dizzy, unsteady, lightheaded, or faint; (9) derealization (feelings of unreality) or depersonalization (being detached from oneself); (10) fear of losing control; (11) fear of dying; (12) paresthesias (numbness or tingling sensations); (13) chills or hot flushes.

Long-term maintenance of efficacy with the immediate-release formulation of paroxetine was demonstrated in a 3-month relapse prevention trial. In this trial, patients with panic disorder assigned to immediate-release paroxetine demonstrated a lower relapse rate compared to patients on placebo (see CLINICAL PHARMACOLOGY—Clinical Trials). Nevertheless, the physician who prescribes PAXIL CR for extended periods should periodically re-evaluate the long-term usefulness of the drug for the individual patient.

Social Anxiety Disorder: PAXIL CR is indicated for the treatment of social anxiety disorder, also known as social phobia, as defined in DSM-IV (300.23). Social anxiety disorder is characterized by a marked and persistent fear of 1 or more social or performance situations in which the person is exposed to unfamiliar people or to possible scrutiny by others. Exposure to the feared situation almost invariably provokes anxiety, which may approach the intensity of a panic attack. The feared situations are avoided or endured with intense anxiety or distress. The avoidance, anxious anticipation, or distress in the feared situation(s) interferes significantly with the person's normal routine, occupational or academic functioning, or social activities or relationships, or there is marked distress about having the phobias. Lesser degrees of performance anxiety or shyness generally do not require psychopharmacological treatment.

The efficacy of PAXIL CR as a treatment for social anxiety disorder has been established, in part, on the basis of extrapolation from the established effectiveness of the immediate-release formulation of paroxetine. In addition, the efficacy of PAXIL CR was established in a 12-week trial, in adult outpatients with social anxiety disorder (DSM-IV). PAXIL CR has not been studied in children or adolescents with social phobia (see CLINICAL PHARMACOLOGY—Clinical Trials).

The effectiveness of PAXIL CR in long-term treatment of social anxiety disorder, i.e., for more than 12 weeks, has not been systematically evaluated in adequate and well-controlled trials. Therefore, the physician who elects to prescribe PAXIL CR for extended periods should periodically re-evaluate the long-term usefulness of the drug for the individual patient (see DOSAGE AND ADMINISTRATION).

Premenstrual Dysphoric Disorder: PAXIL CR is indicated for the treatment of PMDD.

The efficacy of PAXIL CR in the treatment of PMDD has been established in 3 placebo-controlled trials (see CLINICAL PHARMACOLOGY—Clinical Trials).

The essential features of PMDD, according to DSM-IV, include markedly depressed mood, anxiety or tension, affective lability, and persistent anger or irritability. Other features include decreased interest in usual activities, difficulty concentrating, lack of energy, change in appetite or sleep, and feeling out of control. Physical symptoms associated with PMDD include breast tenderness, headache, joint and muscle pain, bloating, and weight gain. These symptoms occur regularly during the luteal phase and remit within a few days following the onset of menses; the disturbance markedly interferes with work or school or with usual social activities and relationships with others. In making the diagnosis, care should be taken to rule out other cyclical mood disorders that may be exacerbated by treatment with an antidepressant.

The effectiveness of PAXIL CR in long-term use, that is, for more than 3 menstrual cycles, has not been systematically evaluated in controlled trials. Therefore, the physician who elects to use PAXIL CR for extended periods should periodically re-evaluate the long-term usefulness of the drug for the individual patient.

CONTRAINDICATIONS

Concomitant use in patients taking either monoamine oxidase inhibitors (MAOIs) or thioridazine is contraindicated (see WARNINGS and PRECAUTIONS).

PAXIL CR is contraindicated in patients with a hypersensitivity to paroxetine or to any of the inactive ingredients in PAXIL CR.

WARNINGS

Potential for Interaction With Monoamine Oxidase Inhibitors: In patients receiving another serotonin reuptake inhibitor drug in combination with an MAOI, there have been reports of serious, sometimes fatal, reactions including hyperthermia, rigidity, myoclonus, autonomic instability with possible rapid fluctuations of vital signs, and mental status changes that include extreme agitation progressing to delirium and coma. These reactions have also been reported in patients who have recently discontinued that drug and have been started on an MAOI. Some cases presented with features resembling neuroleptic malignant syndrome. While there are no human data showing such an interaction with paroxetine hydrochloride, limited animal data on the effects of combined use of paroxetine and MAOIs suggest that these drugs may act synergistically to elevate blood pressure and evoke behavioral excitation. Therefore, it is recommended that PAXIL CR not be used in combination with an MAOI, or within 14 days of discontinuing treatment with an MAOI. At least 2 weeks should be allowed after stopping PAXIL CR before starting an MAOI.

Potential Interaction With Thioridazine: Thioridazine administration alone produces prolongation of the QTc interval, which is associated with serious ventricular arrhythmias, such as torsade de pointes–type arrhythmias, and sudden death. This effect appears to be dose related.

An in vivo study suggests that drugs which inhibit $P_{450}IID_6$, such as paroxetine, will elevate plasma levels of thioridazine. Therefore, it is recommended that paroxetine not be used in combination with thioridazine (see CONTRAINDICATIONS and PRECAUTIONS).

PRECAUTIONS

General: ***Activation of Mania/Hypomania:*** During premarketing testing of immediate-release paroxetine hydrochloride, hypomania or mania occurred in approximately 1.0% of paroxetine-treated unipolar patients compared to 1.1% of active-control and 0.3% of placebo-treated unipolar patients. In a subset of patients classified as bipolar, the rate of manic episodes was 2.2% for immediate-release paroxetine and 11.6% for the combined active-control groups. Among 1,627 patients with major depressive disorder, panic disorder, social anxiety disorder, or PMDD treated with PAXIL CR in controlled clinical studies, there were no reports of mania or hypomania. As with all drugs effective in the treatment of major depressive disorder, PAXIL CR should be used cautiously in patients with a history of mania.

Seizures: During premarketing testing of immediate-release paroxetine hydrochloride, seizures occurred in 0.1% of paroxetine-treated patients, a rate similar to that associated with other drugs effective in the treatment of major depressive disorder. Among 1,627 patients who received PAXIL CR in controlled clinical trials in major depressive disorder, panic disorder, social anxiety disorder, or PMDD, 1 patient (0.1%) experienced a seizure. PAXIL CR should be used cautiously in patients with a history of seizures. It should be discontinued in any patient who develops seizures.

Suicide: The possibility of a suicide attempt is inherent in major depressive disorder and may persist until significant remission occurs. Close supervision of high-risk patients should accompany initial drug therapy. Prescriptions for PAXIL CR should be written for the smallest quantity of tablets consistent with good patient management, in order to reduce the risk of overdose.

Because of well-established comorbidity between major depressive disorder and other psychiatric disorders, the same precautions observed when treating patients with major depressive disorder should be observed when treating patients with other psychiatric disorders.

Discontinuation of Treatment With PAXIL CR: Adverse events while discontinuing therapy with PAXIL CR were not systematically evaluated in most clinical trials; however, in recent placebo-controlled clinical trials utilizing daily doses of PAXIL CR up to 37.5 mg/day, spontaneously reported adverse events while discontinuing therapy with PAXIL CR were evaluated. Patients receiving 37.5 mg/day underwent an incremental decrease in the daily dose by 12.5 mg/day to a dose of 25 mg/day for 1 week before treatment was stopped. For patients receiving 25 mg/day or 12.5 mg/day, treatment was stopped without an incremental decrease in dose. With this regimen in those studies, the following adverse events were reported for PAXIL CR, at an incidence of 2% or greater for PAXIL CR and were at least twice that reported for placebo: Dizziness, nausea, nervousness, and additional symptoms described by the investigator as associated with tapering or discontinuing PAXIL CR (e.g., emotional lability, headache, agitation, electric shock sensations, fatigue, and sleep disturbances). These events were reported as serious in 0.3% of patients who discontinued therapy with PAXIL CR.

During marketing of PAXIL CR and other SSRIs and SNRIs (serotonin and norepinephrine reuptake inhibitors), there have been spontaneous reports of adverse events occurring upon discontinuation of these drugs, (particularly when abrupt), including the following: Dysphoric mood, irritability, agitation, dizziness, sensory disturbances (e.g., paresthesias such as electric shock sensations), anxiety, confusion, headache, lethargy, emotional lability, insomnia, and hypomania. While these events are generally self-limiting, there have been reports of serious discontinuation symptoms.

Patients should be monitored for these symptoms when discontinuing treatment with PAXIL CR. A gradual reduction in the dose rather than abrupt cessation is recommended whenever possible. If intolerable symptoms occur following a decrease in the dose or upon discontinuation of treatment, then resuming the previously prescribed dose may be considered. Subsequently, the physician may continue decreasing the dose but at a more gradual rate (see DOSAGE AND ADMINISTRATION).

Hyponatremia: Several cases of hyponatremia have been reported with immediate-release paroxetine hydrochloride. The hyponatremia appeared to be reversible when paroxetine was discontinued. The majority of these occurrences have been in elderly individuals, some in patients taking diuretics or who were otherwise volume depleted.

Abnormal Bleeding: Published case reports have documented the occurrence of bleeding episodes in patients treated with psychotropic drugs that interfere with serotonin reuptake. Subsequent epidemiological studies, both of the case-control and cohort design, have demonstrated an association between use of psychotropic drugs that interfere with serotonin reuptake and the occurrence of upper gastrointestinal bleeding. In 2 studies, concurrent use of a nonsteroidal anti-inflammatory drug (NSAID) or aspirin potentiated the risk of bleeding (see Drug Interactions). Although these studies focused on upper gastrointestinal bleeding, there is reason to believe that bleeding at other sites may be similarly potentiated. Patients should be cautioned regarding the risk of bleeding associated with the concomitant use of paroxetine with NSAIDs, aspirin, or other drugs that affect coagulation.

Use in Patients With Concomitant Illness: Clinical experience with immediate-release paroxetine hydrochloride in patients with certain concomitant systemic illness is limited. Caution is advisable in using PAXIL CR in patients with diseases or conditions that could affect metabolism or hemodynamic responses.

As with other SSRIs, mydriasis has been infrequently reported in premarketing studies with paroxetine hydrochloride. A few cases of acute angle closure glaucoma associated with therapy with immediate-release paroxetine have been reported in the literature. As mydriasis can cause acute angle closure in patients with narrow angle glaucoma, caution should be used when PAXIL CR is prescribed for patients with narrow angle glaucoma.

PAXIL CR or the immediate-release formulation has not been evaluated or used to any appreciable extent in patients with a recent history of myocardial infarction or unstable heart disease. Patients with these diagnoses were excluded from clinical studies during premarket testing. Evaluation of electrocardiograms of 682 patients who received immediate-release paroxetine hydrochloride in double-blind, placebo-controlled trials, however, did not indicate that paroxetine is associated with the development of significant ECG abnormalities. Similarly, paroxetine hydrochloride does not cause any clinically important changes in heart rate or blood pressure.

Increased plasma concentrations of paroxetine occur in patients with severe renal impairment (creatinine clearance <30 mL/min.) or severe hepatic impairment. A lower starting dose should be used in such patients (see DOSAGE AND ADMINISTRATION).

Information for Patients: Physicians are advised to discuss the following issues with patients for whom they prescribe PAXIL CR:

PAXIL CR should not be chewed or crushed, and should be swallowed whole.

Drugs That Interfere With Hemostasis (NSAIDs, Aspirin, Warfarin, etc.): Patients should be cautioned about the concomitant use of paroxetine and NSAIDs, aspirin, or other drugs that affect coagulation since the combined use of psychotropic drugs that interfere with serotonin reuptake and these agents has been associated with an increased risk of bleeding.

Interference With Cognitive and Motor Performance: Any psychoactive drug may impair judgment, thinking, or motor skills. Although in controlled studies immediate-release paroxetine hydrochloride has not been shown to impair psychomotor performance, patients should be cautioned about operating hazardous machinery, including automobiles, until they are reasonably certain that therapy with PAXIL CR does not affect their ability to engage in such activities.

Completing Course of Therapy: While patients may notice improvement with use of PAXIL CR in 1 to 4 weeks, they should be advised to continue therapy as directed.

Concomitant Medications: Patients should be advised to inform their physician if they are taking, or plan to take, any prescription or over-the-counter drugs, since there is a potential for interactions.

Alcohol: Although immediate-release paroxetine hydrochloride has not been shown to increase the impairment of mental and motor skills caused by alcohol, patients should be advised to avoid alcohol while taking PAXIL CR.

Pregnancy: Patients should be advised to notify their physician if they become pregnant or intend to become pregnant during therapy.

Nursing: Patients should be advised to notify their physician if they are breast-feeding an infant (see PRECAUTIONS—Nursing Mothers).

Laboratory Tests: There are no specific laboratory tests recommended.

Drug Interactions: ***Tryptophan:*** As with other serotonin reuptake inhibitors, an interaction between paroxetine and tryptophan may occur when they are coadministered. Adverse experiences, consisting primarily of headache, nausea, sweating, and dizziness, have been reported when tryptophan was administered to patients taking immediate-release paroxetine. Consequently, concomitant use of PAXIL CR with tryptophan is not recommended.

Monoamine Oxidase Inhibitors: See CONTRAINDICATIONS and WARNINGS.

Continued on next page

Paxil CR—Cont.

Thioridazine: See CONTRAINDICATIONS and WARNINGS.

Warfarin: Preliminary data suggest that there may be a pharmacodynamic interaction (that causes an increased bleeding diathesis in the face of unaltered prothrombin time) between paroxetine and warfarin. Since there is little clinical experience, the concomitant administration of PAXIL CR and warfarin should be undertaken with caution (see Drugs That Interfere With Hemostasis).

Sumatriptan: There have been rare postmarketing reports describing patients with weakness, hyperreflexia, and incoordination following the use of an SSRI and sumatriptan. If concomitant treatment with sumatriptan and an SSRI (e.g., fluoxetine, fluvoxamine, paroxetine, sertraline) is clinically warranted, appropriate observation of the patient is advised.

Drugs Affecting Hepatic Metabolism: The metabolism and pharmacokinetics of paroxetine may be affected by the induction or inhibition of drug-metabolizing enzymes.

Cimetidine: Cimetidine inhibits many cytochrome P_{450} (oxidative) enzymes. In a study where immediate-release paroxetine (30 mg once daily) was dosed orally for 4 weeks, steady-state plasma concentrations of paroxetine were increased by approximately 50% during coadministration with oral cimetidine (300 mg three times daily) for the final week. Therefore, when these drugs are administered concurrently, dosage adjustment of PAXIL CR after the starting dose should be guided by clinical effect. The effect of paroxetine on cimetidine's pharmacokinetics was not studied.

Phenobarbital: Phenobarbital induces many cytochrome P_{450} (oxidative) enzymes. When a single oral 30-mg dose of immediate-release paroxetine was administered at phenobarbital steady state (100 mg once daily for 14 days), paroxetine AUC and $T_{½}$ were reduced (by an average of 25% and 38%, respectively) compared to paroxetine administered alone. The effect of paroxetine on phenobarbital pharmacokinetics was not studied. Since paroxetine exhibits nonlinear pharmacokinetics, the results of this study may not address the case where the 2 drugs are both being chronically dosed. No initial dosage adjustment with PAXIL CR is considered necessary when coadministered with phenobarbital; any subsequent adjustment should be guided by clinical effect.

Phenytoin: When a single oral 30-mg dose of immediate-release paroxetine was administered at phenytoin steady state (300 mg once daily for 14 days), paroxetine AUC and $T_{½}$ were reduced (by an average of 50% and 35%, respectively) compared to immediate-release paroxetine administered alone. In a separate study, when a single oral 300-mg dose of phenytoin was administered at paroxetine steady state (30 mg once daily for 14 days), phenytoin AUC was slightly reduced (12% on average) compared to phenytoin administered alone. Since both drugs exhibit nonlinear pharmacokinetics, the above studies may not address the case where the 2 drugs are both being chronically dosed. No initial dosage adjustments are considered necessary when PAXIL CR is coadministered with phenytoin; any subsequent adjustments should be guided by clinical effect (see ADVERSE REACTIONS—Postmarketing Reports).

Drugs Metabolized by Cytochrome $P_{450}IID_6$: Many drugs, including most drugs effective in the treatment of major depressive disorder (paroxetine, other SSRIs, and many tricyclics), are metabolized by the cytochrome P_{450} isozyme $P_{450}IID_6$. Like other agents that are metabolized by $P_{450}IID_6$, paroxetine may significantly inhibit the activity of this isozyme. In most patients (>90%), this $P_{450}IID_6$ isozyme is saturated early during paroxetine dosing. In 1 study, daily dosing of immediate-release paroxetine (20 mg once daily) under steady-state conditions increased single-dose desipramine (100 mg) C_{max}, AUC, and $T_{½}$ by an average of approximately 2-, 5-, and 3-fold, respectively. Concomitant use of PAXIL CR with other drugs metabolized by cytochrome $P_{450}IID_6$ has not been formally studied but may require lower doses than usually prescribed for either PAXIL CR or the other drug.

Therefore, coadministration of PAXIL CR with other drugs that are metabolized by this isozyme, including certain drugs effective in the treatment of major depressive disorder (e.g., nortriptyline, amitriptyline, imipramine, desipramine, and fluoxetine), phenothiazines, risperidone, and Type 1C antiarrhythmics (e.g., propafenone, flecainide, and encainide), or that inhibit this enzyme (e.g., quinidine), should be approached with caution.

However, due to the risk of serious ventricular arrhythmias and sudden death potentially associated with elevated plasma levels of thioridazine, paroxetine and thioridazine should not be coadministered (see CONTRAINDICATIONS and WARNINGS).

At steady state, when the $P_{450}IID_6$ pathway is essentially saturated, paroxetine clearance is governed by alternative P_{450} isozymes that, unlike $P_{450}IID_6$, show no evidence of saturation (see PRECAUTIONS—Tricyclic Antidepressants).

Drugs Metabolized by Cytochrome $P_{450}IIIA_4$: An in vivo interaction study involving the coadministration under steady-state conditions of paroxetine and terfenadine, a substrate for $P_{450}IIIA_4$, revealed no effect of paroxetine on terfenadine pharmacokinetics. In addition, in vitro studies have shown ketoconazole, a potent inhibitor of $P_{450}IIIA_4$ activity, to be at least 100 times more potent than paroxetine as an inhibitor of the metabolism of several substrates for this enzyme, including terfenadine, astemizole, cisapride, triazolam, and cyclosporine. Based on the assumption that the relationship between paroxetine's in vitro K_i and its lack of effect on terfenadine's in vivo clearance predicts its effect on other $IIIA_4$ substrates, paroxetine's extent of inhibition of $IIIA_4$ activity is not likely to be of clinical significance.

	PAXIL CR 25 mg (n = 348)	PAXIL CR 12.5 mg (n = 333)	Placebo (n = 349)
TOTAL	15%	9.9%	6.3%
Nausea*	6.0%	2.4%	0.9%
Asthenia	4.9%	3.0%	1.4%
Somnolence*	4.3%	1.8%	0.3%
Insomnia	2.3%	1.5%	0.0%
Concentration Impaired*	2.0%	0.6%	0.3%
Dry mouth*	2.0%	0.6%	0.3%
Dizziness*	1.7%	0.6%	0.6%
Decreased Appetite*	1.4%	0.6%	0.0%
Sweating*	1.4%	0.0%	0.3%
Tremor*	1.4%	0.3%	0.0%
Yawn*	1.1%	0.0%	0.0%
Diarrhea	0.9%	1.2%	0.0%

*Events considered to be dose dependent are defined as events having an incidence rate with 25 mg of PAXIL CR that was at least twice that with 12.5 mg of PAXIL CR (as well as the placebo group).

Table 1. Treatment-Emergent Adverse Events Occurring in ≥1% of Patients Treated With PAXIL CR in a Pool of 2 Studies in Major Depressive Disorder[1,2]

Body System/Adverse Event	% Reporting Event	
	PAXIL CR (n = 212)	Placebo (n = 211)
Body as a Whole		
Headache	27%	20%
Asthenia	14%	9%
Infection[3]	8%	5%
Abdominal Pain	7%	4%
Back Pain	5%	3%
Trauma[4]	5%	1%
Pain[5]	3%	1%
Allergic Reaction[6]	2%	1%
Cardiovascular System		
Tachycardia	1%	0%
Vasodilatation[7]	2%	0%
Digestive System		
Nausea	22%	10%
Diarrhea	18%	7%
Dry Mouth	15%	8%
Constipation	10%	4%
Flatulence	6%	4%
Decreased Appetite	4%	2%
Vomiting	2%	1%
Nervous System		
Somnolence	22%	8%
Insomnia	17%	9%
Dizziness	14%	4%
Libido Decreased	7%	3%
Tremor	7%	1%
Hypertonia	3%	1%
Paresthesia	3%	1%
Agitation	2%	1%
Confusion	1%	0%
Respiratory System		
Yawn	5%	0%
Rhinitis	4%	1%
Cough Increased	2%	1%
Bronchitis	1%	0%
Skin and Appendages		
Sweating	6%	2%
Photosensitivity	2%	0%
Special Senses		
Abnormal Vision[8]	5%	1%
Taste Perversion	2%	0%
Urogenital System		
Abnormal Ejaculation[9,10]	26%	1%
Female Genital Disorder[9,11]	10%	<1%
Impotence[9]	5%	3%
Urinary Tract Infection	3%	1%
Menstrual Disorder[9]	2%	<1%
Vaginitis[9]	2%	0%

1. Adverse events for which the PAXIL CR reporting incidence was less than or equal to the placebo incidence are not included. These events are: Abnormal dreams, anxiety, arthralgia, depersonalization, dysmenorrhea, dyspepsia, hyperkinesia, increased appetite, myalgia, nervousness, pharyngitis, purpura, rash, respiratory disorder, sinusitis, urinary frequency, and weight gain.
2. <1% means greater than zero and less than 1%.
3. Mostly flu.
4. A wide variety of injuries with no obvious pattern.
5. Pain in a variety of locations with no obvious pattern.
6. Most frequently seasonal allergic symptoms.
7. Usually flushing.
8. Mostly blurred vision.
9. Based on the number of males or females.
10. Mostly anorgasmia or delayed ejaculation.
11. Mostly anorgasmia or delayed orgasm.

Tricyclic Antidepressants (TCAs): Caution is indicated in the coadministration of TCAs with PAXIL CR, because paroxetine may inhibit TCA metabolism. Plasma TCA concentrations may need to be monitored, and the dose of TCA may need to be reduced, if a TCA is coadministered with

PAXIL CR (see PRECAUTIONS—Drugs Metabolized by Cytochrome $P_{450}IID_6$).

Drugs Highly Bound to Plasma Protein: Because paroxetine is highly bound to plasma protein, administration of PAXIL CR to a patient taking another drug that is highly protein bound may cause increased free concentrations of the other drug, potentially resulting in adverse events. Conversely, adverse effects could result from displacement of paroxetine by other highly bound drugs.

Drugs That Interfere With Hemostasis (NSAIDs, Aspirin, Warfarin, etc.): Serotonin release by platelets plays an important role in hemostasis. Epidemiological studies of the case-control and cohort design that have demonstrated an association between use of psychotropic drugs that interfere with serotonin reuptake and the occurrence of upper gastrointestinal bleeding have also shown that concurrent use of an NSAID or aspirin potentiated the risk of bleeding. Thus, patients should be cautioned about the use of such drugs concurrently with paroxetine.

Alcohol: Although paroxetine does not increase the impairment of mental and motor skills caused by alcohol, patients should be advised to avoid alcohol while taking PAXIL CR.

Lithium: A multiple-dose study with immediate-release paroxetine hydrochloride has shown that there is no pharmacokinetic interaction between paroxetine and lithium carbonate. However, since there is little clinical experience, the concurrent administration of PAXIL CR and lithium should be undertaken with caution.

Digoxin: The steady-state pharmacokinetics of paroxetine was not altered when administered with digoxin at steady state. Mean digoxin AUC at steady state decreased by 15% in the presence of paroxetine. Since there is little clinical experience, the concurrent administration of PAXIL CR and digoxin should be undertaken with caution.

Diazepam: Under steady-state conditions, diazepam does not appear to affect paroxetine kinetics. The effects of paroxetine on diazepam were not evaluated.

Procyclidine: Daily oral dosing of immediate-release paroxetine (30 mg once daily) increased steady-state AUC_{0-24}, C_{max}, and C_{min} values of procyclidine (5 mg oral once daily) by 35%, 37%, and 67%, respectively, compared to procyclidine alone at steady state. If anticholinergic effects are seen, the dose of procyclidine should be reduced.

Beta-Blockers: In a study where propranolol (80 mg twice daily) was dosed orally for 18 days, the established steady-state plasma concentrations of propranolol were unaltered during coadministration with immediate-release paroxetine (30 mg once daily) for the final 10 days. The effects of propranolol on paroxetine have not been evaluated (see ADVERSE REACTIONS—Postmarketing Reports).

Theophylline: Reports of elevated theophylline levels associated with immediate-release paroxetine treatment have been reported. While this interaction has not been formally studied, it is recommended that theophylline levels be monitored when these drugs are concurrently administered.

Electroconvulsive Therapy (ECT): There are no clinical studies of the combined use of ECT and PAXIL CR.

Carcinogenesis, Mutagenesis, Impairment of Fertility:

Carcinogenesis: Two-year carcinogenicity studies were conducted in rodents given paroxetine in the diet at 1, 5, and 25 mg/kg/day (mice) and 1, 5, and 20 mg/kg/day (rats). These doses are up to approximately 2 (mouse) and 3 (rat) times the maximum recommended human dose (MRHD) on a mg/m^2 basis. There was a significantly greater number of male rats in the high-dose group with reticulum cell sarcomas (1/100, 0/50, 0/50, and 4/50 for control, low-, middle-, and high-dose groups, respectively) and a significantly increased linear trend across dose groups for the occurrence of lymphoreticular tumors in male rats. Female rats were not affected. Although there was a dose-related increase in the number of tumors in mice, there was no drug-related increase in the number of mice with tumors. The relevance of these findings to humans is unknown.

Mutagenesis: Paroxetine produced no genotoxic effects in a battery of 5 in vitro and 2 in vivo assays that included the following: Bacterial mutation assay, mouse lymphoma mutation assay, unscheduled DNA synthesis assay, and tests for cytogenetic aberrations in vivo in mouse bone marrow and in vitro in human lymphocytes and in a dominant lethal test in rats.

Impairment of Fertility: A reduced pregnancy rate was found in reproduction studies in rats at a dose of paroxetine of 15 mg/kg/day, which is approximately twice the MRHD on a mg/m^2 basis. Irreversible lesions occurred in the reproductive tract of male rats after dosing in toxicity studies for 2 to 52 weeks. These lesions consisted of vacuolation of epididymal tubular epithelium at 50 mg/kg/day and atrophic changes in the seminiferous tubules of the testes with arrested spermatogenesis at 25 mg/kg/day (approximately 8 and 4 times the MRHD on a mg/m^2 basis).

Pregnancy: Pregnancy Category C. Reproduction studies were performed at doses up to 50 mg/kg/day in rats and 6 mg/kg/day in rabbits administered during organogenesis. These doses are approximately 8 (rat) and 2 (rabbit) times the MRHD on an mg/m^2 basis. These studies have revealed no evidence of teratogenic effects. However, in rats, there was an increase in pup deaths during the first 4 days of lactation when dosing occurred during the last trimester of gestation and continued throughout lactation. This effect occurred at a dose of 1 mg/kg/day or approximately one-sixth of the MRHD on an mg/m^2 basis. The no-effect dose for rat pup mortality was not determined. The cause of these deaths is not known. There are no adequate and well-controlled studies in pregnant women. This drug should be

Table 2. Treatment-Emergent Adverse Events Occurring in ≥5% of Patients Treated With PAXIL CR in a Study of Elderly Patients With Major Depressive Disorder[1,2]

Body System/Adverse Event	% Reporting Event	
	PAXIL CR (n = 104)	Placebo (n = 109)
Body as a Whole		
Headache	17%	13%
Asthenia	15%	14%
Trauma	8%	5%
Infection	6%	2%
Digestive System		
Dry Mouth	18%	7%
Diarrhea	15%	9%
Constipation	13%	5%
Dyspepsia	13%	10%
Decreased Appetite	12%	5%
Flatulence	8%	7%
Nervous System		
Somnolence	21%	12%
Insomnia	10%	8%
Dizziness	9%	5%
Libido Decreased	8%	<1%
Tremor	7%	0%
Skin and Appendages		
Sweating	10%	<1%
Urogenital System		
Abnormal Ejaculation[3,4]	17%	3%
Impotence[3]	9%	3%

1. Adverse events for which the PAXIL CR reporting incidence was less than or equal to the placebo incidence are not included. These events are nausea and respiratory disorder.
2. <1% means greater than zero and less than 1%.
3. Based on the number of males.
4. Mostly anorgasmia or delayed ejaculation.

used during pregnancy only if the potential benefit justifies the potential risk to the fetus.

Nonteratogenic Effects: Neonates exposed to PAXIL CR and other SSRIs or SNRIs, late in the third trimester have developed complications requiring prolonged hospitalization, respiratory support, and tube feeding. Such complications can arise immediately upon delivery. Reported clinical findings have included respiratory distress, cyanosis, apnea, seizures, temperature instability, feeding difficulty, vomiting, hypoglycemia, hypotonia, hypertonia, hyperreflexia, tremor, jitteriness, irritability, and constant crying. These features are consistent with either a direct toxic effect of SSRIs and SNRIs or, possibly, a drug discontinuation syndrome. It should be noted that, in some cases, the clinical picture is consistent with serotonin syndrome (see WARNINGS—Potential for Interaction With Monoamine Oxidase Inhibitors). When treating a pregnant woman with paroxetine during the third trimester, the physician should carefully consider the potential risks and benefits of treatment (see DOSAGE AND ADMINISTRATION).

Labor and Delivery: The effect of paroxetine on labor and delivery in humans is unknown.

Nursing Mothers: Like many other drugs, paroxetine is secreted in human milk, and caution should be exercised when PAXIL CR is administered to a nursing woman.

Pediatric Use: Safety and effectiveness in the pediatric population have not been established.

Geriatric Use: In worldwide premarketing clinical trials with immediate-release paroxetine hydrochloride, 17% of paroxetine-treated patients (approximately 700) were 65 years or older. Pharmacokinetic studies revealed a decreased clearance in the elderly, and a lower starting dose is recommended; there were, however, no overall differences in the adverse event profile between elderly and younger patients, and effectiveness was similar in younger and older patients (see CLINICAL PHARMACOLOGY and DOSAGE AND ADMINISTRATION).

In a controlled study focusing specifically on elderly patients with major depressive disorder, PAXIL CR was demonstrated to be safe and effective in the treatment of elderly patients (>60 years) with major depressive disorder. (See CLINICAL PHARMACOLOGY—Clinical Trials and ADVERSE REACTIONS—Table 2.)

ADVERSE REACTIONS

The information included under the "Adverse Findings Observed in Short-Term, Placebo-Controlled Trials With PAXIL CR" subsection of ADVERSE REACTIONS is based on data from 11 placebo-controlled clinical trials. Three of these studies were conducted in patients with major depressive disorder, 3 studies were done in patients with panic disorder, 1 study was conducted in patients with social anxiety disorder, and 4 studies were done in female patients with PMDD. Two of the studies in major depressive disorder, which enrolled patients in the age range 18 to 65 years, are pooled. Information from a third study of major depressive disorder, which focused on elderly patients (60 to 88 years), is presented separately as is the information from the panic disorder studies and the information from the PMDD studies. Information on additional adverse events associated with PAXIL CR and the immediate-release formulation of paroxetine hydrochloride is included in a separate subsection (see Other Events).

Adverse Findings Observed in Short-Term, Placebo-Controlled Trials With PAXIL CR:

Adverse Events Associated With Discontinuation of Treatment: ***Major Depressive Disorder:*** Ten percent (21/212) of patients treated with PAXIL CR discontinued treatment due to an adverse event in a pool of 2 studies of patients with major depressive disorder. The most common events (≥1%) associated with discontinuation and considered to be drug related (i.e., those events associated with dropout at a rate approximately twice or greater for PAXIL CR compared to placebo) included the following:

	PAXIL CR (n = 212)	Placebo (n = 211)
Nausea	3.7%	0.5%
Asthenia	1.9%	0.5%
Dizziness	1.4%	0.0%
Somnolence	1.4%	0.0%

In a placebo-controlled study of elderly patients with major depressive disorder, 13% (13/104) of patients treated with PAXIL CR discontinued due to an adverse event. Events meeting the above criteria included the following:

	PAXIL CR (n = 104)	Placebo (n = 109)
Nausea	2.9%	0.0%
Headache	1.9%	0.9%
Depression	1.9%	0.0%
LFT's abnormal	1.9%	0.0%

Panic Disorder: Eleven percent (50/444) of patients treated with PAXIL CR in panic disorder studies discontinued treatment due to an adverse event. Events meeting the above criteria included the following:

	PAXIL CR (n = 444)	Placebo (n = 445)
Nausea	2.9%	0.4%
Insomnia	1.8%	0.0%
Headache	1.4%	0.2%
Asthenia	1.1%	0.0%

Social Anxiety Disorder: Three percent (5/186) of patients treated with PAXIL CR in the social anxiety disorder study discontinued treatment due to an adverse event. Events meeting the above criteria included the following:

	PAXIL CR (n = 186)	Placebo (n = 184)
Nausea	2.2%	0.5%
Headache	1.6%	0.5%
Diarrhea	1.1%	0.5%

Premenstrual Dysphoric Disorder: Spontaneously reported adverse events were monitored in studies of both continuous and intermittent dosing of PAXIL CR in the treatment of PMDD. Generally, there were few differences in the adverse event profiles of the 2 dosing regimens. Thirteen percent (88/681) of patients treated with PAXIL CR in PMDD studies of continuous dosing discontinued treatment due to an adverse event.

The most common events (≥1%) associated with discontinuation in either group treated with PAXIL CR with an inci-

Continued on next page

Paxil CR—Cont.

dence rate that is at least twice that of placebo in PMDD trials that employed a continuous dosing regimen are shown in the following table. This table also shows those events that were dose dependent (indicated with an asterisk) as defined as events having an incidence rate with 25 mg of PAXIL CR that was at least twice that with 12.5 mg of PAXIL CR (as well as the placebo group).

[See first table at top of page 200]

Commonly Observed Adverse Events: ***Major Depressive Disorder:*** The most commonly observed adverse events associated with the use of PAXIL CR in a pool of 2 trials (incidence of 5.0% or greater and incidence for PAXIL CR at least twice that for placebo, derived from Table 1) were: Abnormal ejaculation, abnormal vision, constipation, decreased libido, diarrhea, dizziness, female genital disorders, nausea, somnolence, sweating, trauma, tremor, and yawning.

Using the same criteria, the adverse events associated with the use of PAXIL CR in a study of elderly patients with major depressive disorder were: Abnormal ejaculation, constipation, decreased appetite, dry mouth, impotence, infection, libido decreased, sweating, and tremor.

Panic Disorder: In the pool of panic disorder studies, the adverse events meeting these criteria were: Abnormal ejaculation, somnolence, impotence, libido decreased, tremor, sweating, and female genital disorders (generally anorgasmia or difficulty achieving orgasm).

Social Anxiety Disorder: In the social anxiety disorder study, the adverse events meeting these criteria were: Nausea, asthenia, abnormal ejaculation, sweating, somnolence, impotence, insomnia, and libido decreased.

Premenstrual Dysphoric Disorder: The most commonly observed adverse events associated with the use of PAXIL CR either during continuous dosing or luteal phase dosing (incidence of 5% or greater and incidence for PAXIL CR at least twice that for placebo, derived from Table 5) were: Nausea, asthenia, libido decreased, somnolence, insomnia, female genital disorders, sweating, dizziness, diarrhea, and constipation.

In the luteal phase dosing PMDD trial, which employed dosing of 12.5 mg/day or 25 mg/day of PAXIL CR limited to the 2 weeks prior to the onset of menses over 3 consecutive menstrual cycles, adverse events were evaluated during the first 14 days of each off-drug phase. When the 3 off-drug phases were combined, the following adverse events were reported at an incidence of 2% or greater for PAXIL CR and were at least twice the rate of that reported for placebo: Infection (5.3% versus 2.5%), depression (2.8% versus 0.8%), insomnia (2.4% versus 0.8%), sinusitis (2.4% versus 0%), and asthenia (2.0% versus 0.8%).

Incidence in Controlled Clinical Trials: Table 1 enumerates adverse events that occurred at an incidence of 1% or more among patients treated with PAXIL CR, aged 18 to 65, who participated in 2 short-term (12-week) placebo-controlled trials in major depressive disorder in which patients were dosed in a range of 25 mg to 62.5 mg/day. Table 2 enumerates adverse events reported at an incidence of 5% or greater among elderly patients (ages 60 to 88) treated with PAXIL CR who participated in a short-term (12-week) placebo-controlled trial in major depressive disorder in which patients were dosed in a range of 12.5 mg to 50 mg/day. Table 3 enumerates adverse events reported at an incidence of 1% or greater among patients (19 to 72 years) treated with PAXIL CR who participated in short-term (10-week) placebo-controlled trials in panic disorder in which patients were dosed in a range of 12.5 mg to 75 mg/day. Table 4 enumerates adverse events reported at an incidence of 1% or greater among adult patients treated with PAXIL CR who participated in a short-term (12-week), double-blind, placebo-controlled trial in social anxiety disorder in which patients were dosed in a range of 12.5 to 37.5 mg/day. Table 5 enumerates adverse events that occurred at an incidence of 1% or more among patients treated with PAXIL CR who participated in three, 12-week, placebo-controlled trials in PMDD in which patients were dosed at 12.5 mg/day or 25 mg/day and in one 12-week placebo-controlled trial in which patients were dosed for 2 weeks prior to the onset of menses (luteal phase dosing) at 12.5 mg/day or 25 mg/day. Reported adverse events were classified using a standard COSTART-based Dictionary terminology.

The prescriber should be aware that these figures cannot be used to predict the incidence of side effects in the course of usual medical practice where patient characteristics and other factors differ from those that prevailed in the clinical trials. Similarly, the cited frequencies cannot be compared with figures obtained from other clinical investigations involving different treatments, uses, and investigators. The cited figures, however, do provide the prescribing physician with some basis for estimating the relative contribution of drug and nondrug factors to the side effect incidence rate in the population studied.

[See table 1 at top of page 200]
[See table 2 at top of previous page]
[See table 3 above]
[See table 4 at top of next page]
[See table 5 at top of page 204]

Dose Dependency of Adverse Events: The following table shows results in PMDD trials of common adverse events, defined as events with an incidence of ≥1% with 25 mg of PAXIL CR that was at least twice that with 12.5 mg of PAXIL CR and with placebo.

Table 3. Treatment-Emergent Adverse Events Occurring in ≥1% of Patients Treated With PAXIL CR in a Pool of 3 Panic Disorder Studies[1,2]

Body System/Adverse Event	% Reporting Event	
	PAXIL CR (n = 444)	Placebo (n = 445)
Body as a Whole		
Asthenia	15%	10%
Abdominal Pain	6%	4%
Trauma[3]	5%	4%
Cardiovascular System		
Vasodilation[4]	3%	2%
Digestive System		
Nausea	23%	17%
Dry Mouth	13%	9%
Diarrhea	12%	9%
Constipation	9%	6%
Decreased Appetite	8%	6%
Metabolic/Nutritional Disorder		
Weight Loss	1%	0%
Musculoskeletal System		
Myalgia	5%	3%
Nervous System		
Insomnia	20%	11%
Somnolence	20%	9%
Libido Decreased	9%	4%
Nervousness	8%	7%
Tremor	8%	2%
Anxiety	5%	4%
Agitation	3%	2%
Hypertonia[5]	2%	<1%
Myoclonus	2%	<1%
Respiratory System		
Sinusitis	8%	5%
Yawn	3%	0%
Skin and Appendages		
Sweating	7%	2%
Special Senses		
Abnormal Vision[6]	3%	<1%
Urogenital System		
Abnormal Ejaculation[7,8]	27%	3%
Impotence[7]	10%	1%
Female Genital Disorder[9,10]	7%	1%
Urinary Frequency	2%	<1%
Urination Impaired	2%	<1%
Vaginitis[9]	1%	<1%

1. Adverse events for which the reporting rate for PAXIL CR was less than or equal to the placebo rate are not included. These events are: Abnormal dreams, allergic reaction, back pain, bronchitis, chest pain, concentration impaired, confusion, cough increased, depression, dizziness, dysmenorrhea, dyspepsia, fever, flatulence, headache, increased appetite, infection, menstrual disorder, migraine, pain, paresthesia, pharyngitis, respiratory disorder, rhinitis, tachycardia, taste perversion, thinking abnormal, urinary tract infection, and vomiting.
2. <1% means greater than zero and less than 1%.
3. Various physical injuries.
4. Mostly flushing.
5. Mostly muscle tightness or stiffness.
6. Mostly blurred vision.
7. Based on the number of male patients.
8. Mostly anorgasmia or delayed ejaculation.
9. Based on the number of female patients.
10. Mostly anorgasmia or difficulty achieving orgasm.

Incidence of Common Adverse Events in Placebo, 12.5 mg and 25 mg of PAXIL CR in a Pool of 3 Fixed-Dose PMDD Trials

Common Adverse Event	PAXIL CR 25 mg (n = 348)	PAXIL CR 12.5 mg (n = 333)	Placebo (n = 349)
Sweating	8.9%	4.2%	0.9%
Tremor	6.0%	1.5%	0.3%
Concentration Impaired	4.3%	1.5%	0.6%
Yawn	3.2%	0.9%	0.3%
Paresthesia	1.4%	0.3%	0.3%
Hyperkinesia	1.1%	0.3%	0.0%
Vaginitis	1.1%	0.3%	0.3%

A comparison of adverse event rates in a fixed-dose study comparing immediate-release paroxetine with placebo in the treatment of major depressive disorder revealed a clear dose dependency for some of the more common adverse events associated with the use of immediate-release paroxetine.

Male and Female Sexual Dysfunction With SSRIs: Although changes in sexual desire, sexual performance, and sexual satisfaction often occur as manifestations of a psychiatric disorder, they may also be a consequence of pharmacologic treatment. In particular, some evidence suggests that SSRIs can cause such untoward sexual experiences.

Reliable estimates of the incidence and severity of untoward experiences involving sexual desire, performance, and satisfaction are difficult to obtain; however, in part because patients and physicians may be reluctant to discuss them. Accordingly, estimates of the incidence of untoward sexual experience and performance cited in product labeling, are likely to underestimate their actual incidence.

The percentage of patients reporting symptoms of sexual dysfunction in the pool of 2 placebo-controlled trials in nonelderly patients with major depressive disorder, in the pool of 3 placebo-controlled trials in patients with panic disorder, in the placebo-controlled trial in patients with social anxiety disorder, and in the intermittent dosing and the pool of 3 placebo-controlled continuous dosing trials in female patients with PMDD are as follows:

[See second table on page 204]

There are no adequate, controlled studies examining sexual dysfunction with paroxetine treatment.

Paroxetine treatment has been associated with several cases of priapism. In those cases with a known outcome, patients recovered without sequelae.

While it is difficult to know the precise risk of sexual dysfunction associated with the use of SSRIs, physicians should routinely inquire about such possible side effects.

Weight and Vital Sign Changes: Significant weight loss may be an undesirable result of treatment with paroxetine for some patients but, on average, patients in controlled trials with PAXIL CR or the immediate-release formulation, had minimal weight loss (about 1 pound). No significant changes in vital signs (systolic and diastolic blood pressure, pulse, and temperature) were observed in patients treated with PAXIL CR, or immediate-release paroxetine hydrochloride, in controlled clinical trials.

ECG Changes: In an analysis of ECGs obtained in 682 patients treated with immediate-release paroxetine and 415 patients treated with placebo in controlled clinical trials, no clinically significant changes were seen in the ECGs of either group.

Table 4. Treatment-Emergent Adverse Effects Occurring in ≥1% of Patients Treated With PAXIL CR in a Social Anxiety Disorder Study[1,2]

Body System/Adverse Event	% Reporting Event PAXIL CR (n = 186)	Placebo (n = 184)
Body as a Whole		
Headache	23%	17%
Asthenia	18%	7%
Abdominal Pain	5%	4%
Back Pain	4%	1%
Trauma[3]	3%	<1%
Allergic Reaction[4]	2%	<1%
Chest Pain	1%	<1%
Cardiovascular System		
Hypertension	2%	0%
Migraine	2%	1%
Tachycardia	2%	1%
Digestive System		
Nausea	22%	6%
Diarrhea	9%	8%
Constipation	5%	2%
Dry Mouth	3%	2%
Dyspepsia	2%	<1%
Decreased Appetite	1%	<1%
Tooth Disorder	1%	0%
Metabolic/Nutritional Disorders		
Weight Gain	3%	1%
Weight Loss	1%	0%
Nervous System		
Insomnia	9%	4%
Somnolence	9%	4%
Libido Decreased	8%	1%
Dizziness	7%	4%
Tremor	4%	2%
Anxiety	2%	1%
Concentration Impaired	2%	0%
Depression	2%	1%
Myoclonus	1%	<1%
Paresthesia	1%	<1%
Respiratory System		
Yawn	2%	0%
Skin and Appendages		
Sweating	14%	3%
Eczema	1%	0%
Special Senses		
Abnormal Vision[5]	2%	0%
Abnormality of Accommodation	2%	0%
Urogenital System		
Abnormal Ejaculation[6,7]	15%	1%
Impotence[6]	9%	0%
Female Genital Disorders[8,9]	3%	0%

1. Adverse events for which the reporting rate for PAXIL CR was less than or equal to the placebo rate are not included. These events are: Dysmenorrhea, flatulence, gastroenteritis, hypertonia, infection, pain, pharyngitis, rash, respiratory disorder, rhinitis, and vomiting.
2. <1% means greater than zero and less than 1%.
3. Various physical injuries.
4. Most frequently seasonal allergic symptoms.
5. Mostly blurred vision.
6. Based on the number of male patients.
7. Mostly anorgasmia or delayed ejaculation.
8. Based on the number of female patients.
9. Mostly anorgasmia or difficulty achieving orgasm.

Liver Function Tests: In a pool of 2 placebo-controlled clinical trials, patients treated with PAXIL CR or placebo exhibited abnormal values on liver function tests at comparable rates. In particular, the controlled-release paroxetine-versus-placebo comparisons for alkaline phosphatase, SGOT, SGPT, and bilirubin revealed no differences in the percentage of patients with marked abnormalities.

In a study of elderly patients with major depressive disorder, 3 of 104 patients treated with PAXIL CR and none of 109 placebo patients experienced liver transaminase elevations of potential clinical concern.

Two of the patients treated with PAXIL CR dropped out of the study due to abnormal liver function tests; the third patient experienced normalization of transaminase levels with continued treatment. Also, in the pool of 3 studies of patients with panic disorder, 4 of 444 patients treated with PAXIL CR and none of 445 placebo patients experienced liver transaminase elevations of potential clinical concern. Elevations in all 4 patients decreased substantially after discontinuation of PAXIL CR. The clinical significance of these findings is unknown.

In placebo-controlled clinical trials with the immediate-release formulation of paroxetine, patients exhibited abnormal values on liver function tests at no greater rate than that seen in placebo-treated patients.

Other Events Observed During the Clinical Development of Paroxetine: The following adverse events were reported during the clinical development of PAXIL CR and/or the clinical development of the immediate-release formulation of paroxetine.

Adverse events for which frequencies are provided below occurred in clinical trials with the controlled-release formulation of paroxetine. During its premarketing assessment in major depressive disorder, panic disorder, social anxiety disorder, and PMDD multiple doses of PAXIL CR were administered to 1,627 patients in phase 3 double-blind, controlled, outpatient studies. Untoward events associated with this exposure were recorded by clinical investigators using terminology of their own choosing. Consequently, it is not possible to provide a meaningful estimate of the proportion of individuals experiencing adverse events without first grouping similar types of untoward events into a smaller number of standardized event categories.

In the tabulations that follow, reported adverse events were classified using a COSTART-based dictionary. The frequencies presented, therefore, represent the proportion of the 1,627 patients exposed to PAXIL CR who experienced an event of the type cited on at least 1 occasion while receiving PAXIL CR. All reported events are included except those already listed in Tables 1 through 5 and those events where a drug cause was remote. If the COSTART term for an event was so general as to be uninformative, it was deleted or, when possible, replaced with a more informative term. It is important to emphasize that although the events reported occurred during treatment with paroxetine, they were not necessarily caused by it.

Events are further categorized by body system and listed in order of decreasing frequency according to the following definitions: Frequent adverse events are those occurring on 1 or more occasions in at least 1/100 patients (only those not already listed in the tabulated results from placebo-controlled trials appear in this listing); infrequent adverse events are those occurring in 1/100 to 1/1,000 patients; rare events are those occurring in fewer than 1/1,000 patients.

Adverse events for which frequencies are not provided occurred during the premarketing assessment of immediate-release paroxetine in phase 2 and 3 studies of major depressive disorder, obsessive compulsive disorder, panic disorder, social anxiety disorder, generalized anxiety disorder, and posttraumatic stress disorder. The conditions and duration of exposure to immediate-release paroxetine varied greatly and included (in overlapping categories) open and double-blind studies, uncontrolled and controlled studies, inpatient and outpatient studies, and fixed-dose and titration studies. Only those events not previously listed for controlled-release paroxetine are included. The extent to which these events may be associated with PAXIL CR is unknown.

Events are listed alphabetically within the respective body system. Events of major clinical importance are also described in the PRECAUTIONS section.

Body as a Whole: Infrequent were chills, face edema, fever, flu syndrome, malaise; rare were abscess, anaphylactoid reaction, anticholinergic syndrome, hypothermia; also observed were adrenergic syndrome, neck rigidity, sepsis.

Cardiovascular System: Infrequent were angina pectoris, bradycardia, hematoma, hypertension, hypotension, palpitation, postural hypotension, supraventricular tachycardia, syncope; rare were bundle branch block; also observed were arrhythmia nodal, atrial fibrillation, cerebrovascular accident, congestive heart failure, low cardiac output, myocardial infarct, myocardial ischemia, pallor, phlebitis, pulmonary embolus, supraventricular extrasystoles, thrombophlebitis, thrombosis, vascular headache, ventricular extrasystoles.

Digestive System: Infrequent were bruxism, dysphagia, eructation, gastritis, gastroenteritis, gastroesophageal reflux, gingivitis, hemorrhoids, liver function test abnormal, melena, pancreatitis, rectal hemorrhage, toothache, ulcerative stomatitis; rare were colitis, glossitis, gum hyperplasia, hepatosplenomegaly, increased salivation, intestinal obstruction, peptic ulcer, stomach ulcer, throat tightness; also observed were aphthous stomatitis, bloody diarrhea, bulimia, cardiospasm, cholelithiasis, duodenitis, enteritis, esophagitis, fecal impactions, fecal incontinence, gum hemorrhage, hematemesis, hepatitis, ileitis, ileus, jaundice, mouth ulceration, salivary gland enlargement, sialadenitis, stomatitis, tongue discoloration, tongue edema.

Endocrine System: Infrequent were ovarian cyst, testes pain; rare were diabetes mellitus, hyperthyroidism; also observed were goiter, hypothyroidism, thyroiditis.

Hemic and Lymphatic System: Infrequent were anemia, eosinophilia, hypochromic anemia, leukocytosis, leukopenia, lymphadenopathy, purpura; rare were thrombocytopenia; also observed were anisocytosis, basophilia, bleeding time increased, lymphedema, lymphocytosis, lymphopenia, microcytic anemia, monocytosis, normocytic anemia, thrombocythemia.

Metabolic and Nutritional Disorders: Infrequent were generalized edema, hyperglycemia, hypokalemia, peripheral edema, SGOT increased, SGPT increased, thirst; rare were bilirubinemia, dehydration, hyperkalemia, obesity; also observed were alkaline phosphatase increased, BUN increased, creatinine phosphokinase increased, gamma globulins increased, gout, hypercalcemia, hypercholesteremia, hyperphosphatemia, hypocalcemia, hypoglycemia, hyponatremia, ketosis, lactic dehydrogenase increased, non-protein nitrogen (NPN) increased.

Musculoskeletal System: Infrequent were arthritis, bursitis, tendonitis; rare were myasthenia, myopathy, myositis; also observed were generalized spasm, osteoporosis, tenosynovitis, tetany.

Nervous System: Frequent were depression; infrequent were amnesia, convulsion, depersonalization, dystonia, emotional lability, hallucinations, hyperkinesia, hypesthesia, hypokinesia, incoordination, libido increased, neuralgia, neuropathy, nystagmus, paralysis, vertigo; rare were ataxia, coma, diplopia, dyskinesia, hostility, paranoid reaction, torticollis, withdrawal syndrome; also observed were abnormal gait, akathisia, akinesia, aphasia, choreoathetosis, circumoral paresthesia, delirium, delusions, dysarthria, euphoria, extrapyramidal syndrome, fasciculations, grand mal convulsion, hyperalgesia, irritability, manic reaction, manic-depressive reaction, meningitis, myelitis, peripheral neuritis, psychosis, psychotic depression, reflexes decreased, reflexes increased, stupor, trismus.

Respiratory System: Frequent were pharyngitis; infrequent were asthma, dyspnea, epistaxis, laryngitis, pneumonia; rare were stridor; also observed were dysphonia, emphysema, hemoptysis, hiccups, hyperventilation, lung fibrosis, pulmonary edema, respiratory flu, sputum increased.

Skin and Appendages: Frequent were rash; infrequent were acne, alopecia, dry skin, eczema, pruritus, urticaria; rare were exfoliative dermatitis, furunculosis, pustular rash, seborrhea; also observed were angioedema, ecchymosis, erythema multiforme, erythema nodosum, hirsutism, maculopapular rash, skin discoloration, skin hypertrophy, skin ulcer, sweating decreased, vesiculobullous rash.

Special Senses: Infrequent were conjunctivitis, earache, keratoconjunctivitis, mydriasis, photophobia, retinal hemorrhage, tinnitus; rare were blepharitis, visual field defect;

Continued on next page

Paxil CR—Cont.

also observed were amblyopia, anisocoria, blurred vision, cataract, conjunctival edema, corneal ulcer, deafness, exophthalmos, glaucoma, hyperacusis, night blindness, parosmia, ptosis, taste loss.

Urogenital System: Frequent were dysmenorrhea*; infrequent were albuminuria, amenorrhea*, breast pain*, cystitis, dysuria, prostatitis*, urinary retention; rare were breast enlargement*, breast neoplasm*, female lactation, hematuria, kidney calculus, metrorrhagia*, nephritis, nocturia, pregnancy and puerperal disorders*, salpingitis, urinary incontinence, uterine fibroids enlarged*; also observed were breast atrophy, ejaculatory disturbance, endometrial disorder, epididymitis, fibrocystic breast, leukorrhea, mastitis, oliguria, polyuria, pyuria, urethritis, urinary casts, urinary urgency, urolith, uterine spasm, vaginal hemorrhage.

*Based on the number of men and women as appropriate.

Postmarketing Reports: Voluntary reports of adverse events in patients taking immediate-release paroxetine hydrochloride that have been received since market introduction and not listed above that may have no causal relationship with the drug include acute pancreatitis, elevated liver function tests (the most severe cases were deaths due to liver necrosis, and grossly elevated transaminases associated with severe liver dysfunction), Guillain-Barré syndrome, toxic epidermal necrolysis, priapism, syndrome of inappropriate ADH secretion, symptoms suggestive of prolactinemia and galactorrhea, neuroleptic malignant syndrome–like events; extrapyramidal symptoms which have included akathisia, bradykinesia, cogwheel rigidity, dystonia, hypertonia, oculogyric crisis which has been associated with concomitant use of pimozide; tremor and trismus; serotonin syndrome, associated in some cases with concomitant use of serotonergic drugs and with drugs which may have impaired paroxetine metabolism (symptoms have included agitation, confusion, diaphoresis, hallucinations, hyperreflexia, myoclonus, shivering, tachycardia, and tremor); status epilepticus, acute renal failure, pulmonary hypertension, allergic alveolitis, anaphylaxis, eclampsia, laryngismus, optic neuritis, porphyria, ventricular fibrillation, ventricular tachycardia (including torsade de pointes), thrombocytopenia, hemolytic anemia, events related to impaired hematopoiesis (including aplastic anemia, pancytopenia, bone marrow aplasia, and agranulocytosis), and vasculitic syndromes (such as Henoch-Schönlein purpura). There has been a case report of an elevated phenytoin level after 4 weeks of immediate-release paroxetine and phenytoin coadministration. There has been a case report of severe hypotension when immediate-release paroxetine was added to chronic metoprolol treatment.

DRUG ABUSE AND DEPENDENCE

Controlled Substance Class: PAXIL CR is not a controlled substance.

Physical and Psychologic Dependence: PAXIL CR has not been systematically studied in animals or humans for its potential for abuse, tolerance or physical dependence. While the clinical trials did not reveal any tendency for any drug-seeking behavior, these observations were not systematic and it is not possible to predict on the basis of this limited experience the extent to which a CNS-active drug will be misused, diverted, and/or abused once marketed. Consequently, patients should be evaluated carefully for history of drug abuse, and such patients should be observed closely for signs of misuse or abuse of PAXIL CR (e.g., development of tolerance, incrementations of dose, drug-seeking behavior).

OVERDOSAGE

Human Experience: Since the introduction of immediate-release paroxetine hydrochloride in the United States, 342 spontaneous cases of deliberate or accidental overdosage during paroxetine treatment have been reported worldwide (circa 1999). These include overdoses with paroxetine alone and in combination with other substances. Of these, 48 cases were fatal and of the fatalities, 17 appeared to involve paroxetine alone. Eight fatal cases that documented the amount of paroxetine ingested were generally confounded by the ingestion of other drugs or alcohol or the presence of significant comorbid conditions. Of 145 non-fatal cases with known outcome, most recovered without sequelae. The largest known ingestion involved 2,000 mg of paroxetine (33 times the maximum recommended daily dose) in a patient who recovered.

Commonly reported adverse events associated with paroxetine overdosage include somnolence, coma, nausea, tremor, tachycardia, confusion, vomiting, and dizziness. Other notable signs and symptoms observed with overdoses involving paroxetine (alone or with other substances) include mydriasis, convulsions (including status epilepticus), ventricular dysrhythmias (including torsade de pointes), hypertension, aggressive reactions, syncope, hypotension, stupor, bradycardia, dystonia, rhabdomyolysis, symptoms of hepatic dysfunction (including hepatic failure, hepatic necrosis, jaundice, hepatitis, and hepatic steatosis), serotonin syndrome, manic reactions, myoclonus, acute renal failure, and urinary retention.

Overdosage Management: Treatment should consist of those general measures employed in the management of overdosage with any drugs effective in the treatment of major depressive disorder.

Ensure an adequate airway, oxygenation, and ventilation. Monitor cardiac rhythm and vital signs. General supportive and symptomatic measures are also recommended. Induction of emesis is not recommended. Gastric lavage with a large-bore orogastric tube with appropriate airway protection, if needed, may be indicated if performed soon after ingestion, or in symptomatic patients.

Activated charcoal should be administered. Due to the large volume of distribution of this drug, forced diuresis, dialysis, hemoperfusion, and exchange transfusion are unlikely to be of benefit. No specific antidotes for paroxetine are known.

A specific caution involves patients taking or recently having taken paroxetine who might ingest excessive quantities of a tricyclic antidepressant. In such a case, accumulation of the parent tricyclic and an active metabolite may increase the possibility of clinically significant sequelae and extend the time needed for close medical observation (see PRECAUTIONS—Drugs Metabolized by Cytochrome $P_{450}IID_6$). In managing overdosage, consider the possibility of multiple-drug involvement. The physician should consider contacting a poison control center for additional information on the treatment of any overdose. Telephone numbers for certified poison control centers are listed in the *Physicians' Desk Reference* (PDR).

Table 5. Treatment-Emergent Adverse Events Occurring in ≥1% of Patients Treated With PAXIL CR in a Pool of 3 Premenstrual Dysphoric Disorder Studies with Continuous Dosing or in 1 Premenstrual Dysphoric Disorder Study with Luteal Phase Dosing[1,2,3]

	% Reporting Event			
	Continuous Dosing		Luteal Phase Dosing	
Body System/Adverse Event	PAXIL CR (n = 681)	Placebo (n = 349)	PAXIL CR (n = 246)	Placebo (n = 120)
Body as a Whole				
Asthenia	17%	6%	15%	4%
Headache	15%	12%	—	—
Infection	6%	4%	—	—
Abdominal Pain	—	—	3%	0%
Cardiovascular System				
Migraine	1%	<1%	—	—
Digestive System				
Nausea	17%	7%	18%	2%
Diarrhea	6%	2%	6%	0%
Constipation	5%	1%	2%	<1%
Dry Mouth	4%	2%	2%	<1%
Increased Appetite	3%	<1%	—	—
Decreased Appetite	2%	<1%	2%	0%
Dyspepsia	2%	1%	2%	2%
Gingivitis	—	—	1%	0%
Metabolic and Nutritional Disorders				
Generalized Edema	—	—	1%	<1%
Weight Gain	—	—	1%	<1%
Musculoskeletal System				
Arthralgia	2%	1%	—	—
Nervous System				
Libido Decreased	12%	5%	9%	6%
Somnolence	9%	2%	3%	<1%
Insomnia	8%	2%	7%	3%
Dizziness	7%	3%	6%	3%
Tremor	4%	<1%	5%	0%
Concentration Impaired	3%	<1%	1%	0%
Nervousness	2%	<1%	3%	2%
Anxiety	2%	1%	—	—
Lack of Emotion	2%	<1%	—	—
Depression	—	—	2%	<1%
Vertigo	—	—	2%	<1%
Abnormal Dreams	1%	<1%	—	—
Amnesia	—	—	1%	0%
Respiratory System				
Sinusitis	—	—	4%	2%
Yawn	2%	<1%	—	—
Bronchitis	—	—	2%	0%
Cough Increased	1%	<1%	—	—
Skin and Appendages				
Sweating	7%	<1%	6%	<1%
Special Senses				
Abnormal Vision	—	—	1%	0%
Urogenital System				
Female Genital Disorders[4]	8%	1%	2%	0%
Menorrhagia	1%	<1%	—	—
Vaginal Moniliasis	1%	<1%	—	—
Menstrual Disorder	—	—	1%	0%

1. Adverse events for which the reporting rate of PAXIL CR was less than or equal to the placebo rate are not included. These events for continuous dosing are: Abdominal pain, back pain, pain, trauma, weight gain, myalgia, pharyngitis, respiratory disorder, rhinitis, sinusitis, pruritis, dysmenorrhea, menstrual disorder, urinary tract infection, and vomiting. The events for luteal phase dosing are: Allergic reaction, back pain, headache, infection, pain, trauma, myalgia, anxiety, pharyngitis, respiratory disorder, cystitis, and dysmenorrhea.
2. <1% means greater than zero and less than 1%.
3. The luteal phase and continuous dosing PMDD trials were not designed for making direct comparisons between the 2 dosing regimens. Therefore, a comparison between the 2 dosing regimens of the PMDD trials of incidence rates shown in Table 5 should be avoided.
4. Mostly anorgasmia or difficulty achieving orgasm.

	Major Depressive Disorder		Panic Disorder		Social Anxiety Disorder		PMDD Continuous Dosing		PMDD Luteal Phase Dosing	
	PAXIL CR	Placebo	PAXIL CR	Placebo	PAXIL CR	Placebo	PAXIL CR	Placebo	PAXIL CR	Placebo
n (males)	**78**	**78**	**162**	**194**	**88**	**97**	**n/a**	**n/a**	**n/a**	**n/a**
Decreased Libido	10%	5%	9%	6%	13%	1%	n/a	n/a	n/a	n/a
Ejaculatory Disturbance	26%	1%	27%	3%	15%	1%	n/a	n/a	n/a	n/a
Impotence	5%	3%	10%	1%	9%	0%	n/a	n/a	n/a	n/a
n (females)	**134**	**133**	**282**	**251**	**98**	**87**	**681**	**349**	**246**	**120**
Decreased Libido	4%	2%	8%	2%	4%	1%	12%	5%	9%	6%
Orgasmic Disturbance	10%	<1%	7%	1%	3%	0%	8%	1%	2%	0%

DOSAGE AND ADMINISTRATION

Major Depressive Disorder: ***Usual Initial Dosage:*** PAXIL CR should be administered as a single daily dose, usually in the morning, with or without food. The recommended initial dose is 25 mg/day. Patients were dosed in a range of 25 mg to 62.5 mg/day in the clinical trials demonstrating the effectiveness of PAXIL CR in the treatment of major depressive disorder. As with all drugs effective in the treatment of major depressive disorder, the full effect may be delayed. Some patients not responding to a 25-mg dose may benefit from dose increases, in 12.5-mg/day increments, up to a maximum of 62.5 mg/day. Dose changes should occur at intervals of at least 1 week.

Patients should be cautioned that PAXIL CR should not be chewed or crushed, and should be swallowed whole.

Maintenance Therapy: There is no body of evidence available to answer the question of how long the patient treated with PAXIL CR should remain on it. It is generally agreed that acute episodes of major depressive disorder require several months or longer of sustained pharmacologic therapy. Whether the dose of an antidepressant needed to induce remission is identical to the dose needed to maintain and/or sustain euthymia is unknown.

Systematic evaluation of the efficacy of immediate-release paroxetine hydrochloride has shown that efficacy is maintained for periods of up to 1 year with doses that averaged about 30 mg, which corresponds to a 37.5-mg dose of PAXIL CR, based on relative bioavailability considerations (see CLINICAL PHARMACOLOGY—Pharmacokinetics).

Panic Disorder: ***Usual Initial Dosage:*** PAXIL CR should be administered as a single daily dose, usually in the morning. Patients should be started on 12.5 mg/day. Dose changes should occur in 12.5-mg/day increments and at intervals of at least 1 week. Patients were dosed in a range of 12.5 to 75 mg/day in the clinical trials demonstrating the effectiveness of PAXIL CR. The maximum dosage should not exceed 75 mg/day.

Patients should be cautioned that PAXIL CR should not be chewed or crushed, and should be swallowed whole.

Maintenance Therapy: Long-term maintenance of efficacy with the immediate-release formulation of paroxetine was demonstrated in a 3-month relapse prevention trial. In this trial, patients with panic disorder assigned to immediate-release paroxetine demonstrated a lower relapse rate compared to patients on placebo. Panic disorder is a chronic condition, and it is reasonable to consider continuation for a responding patient. Dosage adjustments should be made to maintain the patient on the lowest effective dosage, and patients should be periodically reassessed to determine the need for continued treatment.

Social Anxiety Disorder: ***Usual Initial Dosage:*** PAXIL CR should be administered as a single daily dose, usually in the morning, with or without food. The recommended initial dose is 12.5 mg/day. Patients were dosed in a range of 12.5 mg to 37.5 mg/day in the clinical trial demonstrating the effectiveness of PAXIL CR in the treatment of social anxiety disorder. If the dose is increased, this should occur at intervals of at least 1 week, in increments of 12.5 mg/day, up to a maximum of 37.5 mg/day.

Patients should be cautioned that PAXIL CR should not be chewed or crushed, and should be swallowed whole.

Maintenance Therapy: There is no body of evidence available to answer the question of how long the patient treated with PAXIL CR should remain on it. Although the efficacy of PAXIL CR beyond 12 weeks of dosing has not been demonstrated in controlled clinical trials, social anxiety disorder is recognized as a chronic condition, and it is reasonable to consider continuation of treatment for a responding patient. Dosage adjustments should be made to maintain the patient on the lowest effective dosage, and patients should be periodically reassessed to determine the need for continued treatment.

Premenstrual Dysphoric Disorder: ***Usual Initial Dosage:*** PAXIL CR should be administered as a single daily dose, usually in the morning, with or without food. PAXIL CR may be administered either daily throughout the menstrual cycle or limited to the luteal phase of the menstrual cycle, depending on physician assessment. The recommended initial dose is 12.5 mg/day. In clinical trials, both 12.5 mg/day and 25 mg/day were shown to be effective. Dose changes should occur at intervals of at least 1 week.

Patients should be cautioned that PAXIL CR should not be chewed or crushed, and should be swallowed whole.

Maintenance/Continuation Therapy: The effectiveness of PAXIL CR for a period exceeding 3 menstrual cycles has not been systematically evaluated in controlled trials. However, women commonly report that symptoms worsen with age until relieved by the onset of menopause. Therefore, it is reasonable to consider continuation of a responding patient. Patients should be periodically reassessed to determine the need for continued treatment.

Special Populations: ***Treatment of Pregnant Women During the Third Trimester:*** Neonates exposed to PAXIL CR and other SSRIs or SNRIs, late in the third trimester have developed complications requiring prolonged hospitalization, respiratory support, and tube feeding (see PRECAUTIONS). When treating pregnant women with paroxetine during the third trimester, the physician should carefully consider the potential risks and benefits of treatment. The physician may consider tapering paroxetine in the third trimester.

Dosage for Elderly or Debilitated Patients, and Patients With Severe Renal or Hepatic Impairment: The recommended initial dose of PAXIL CR is 12.5 mg/day for elderly patients, debilitated patients, and/or patients with severe renal or hepatic impairment. Increases may be made if indicated. Dosage should not exceed 50 mg/day.

Switching Patients to or From a Monoamine Oxidase Inhibitor: At least 14 days should elapse between discontinuation of an MAOI and initiation of therapy with PAXIL CR. Similarly, at least 14 days should be allowed after stopping PAXIL CR before starting an MAOI.

Discontinuation of Treatment With PAXIL CR: Symptoms associated with discontinuation of immediate-release paroxetine hydrochloride or PAXIL CR have been reported (see PRECAUTIONS). Patients should be monitored for these symptoms when discontinuing treatment, regardless of the indication for which PAXIL CR is being prescribed. A gradual reduction in the dose rather than abrupt cessation is recommended whenever possible. If intolerable symptoms occur following a decrease in the dose or upon discontinuation of treatment, then resuming the previously prescribed dose may be considered. Subsequently, the physician may continue decreasing the dose but at a more gradual rate.

HOW SUPPLIED

PAXIL CR is supplied as an enteric film-coated, controlled-release, round tablet, as follows:

12.5-mg yellow tablets, engraved with Paxil CR and 12.5
NDC 0029-3206-13 Bottles of 30
NDC 0029-3206-20 Bottles of 100
25-mg pink tablets, engraved with Paxil CR and 25
NDC 0029-3207-13 Bottles of 30
NDC 0029-3207-20 Bottles of 100
NDC 0029-3207-21 SUP 100s (intended for institutional use only)
37.5-mg blue tablets, engraved with Paxil CR and 37.5
NDC 0029-3208-13 Bottles of 30

Store at or below 25°C (77°F) [see USP].

PAXIL CR is a trademark of GlaxoSmithKline.
GEOMATRIX is a trademark of Jago Pharma, Muttenz, Switzerland.

GlaxoSmithKline
GlaxoSmithKline
Research Triangle Park, NC 27709

March 2004 PC:L9

RELENZA® ℞

[ra-lin' za]
(zanamivir for inhalation)
For Oral Inhalation Only
For Use with the DISKHALER® Inhalation Device

Prescribing information for this product, which appears on pages 1602–1604 of the 2004 PDR, has been revised as follows. Please write "See Supplement A" next to the product heading.

The following paragraph was added to INDICATIONS AND USAGE:

RELENZA is not recommended for treatment of patients with underlying airways disease (such as asthma or chronic obstructive pulmonary disease) (see WARNINGS and PRECAUTIONS).

GlaxoSmithKline, Research Triangle Park, NC 27709

April 2003/RL-2000

TABLOID® brand Thioguanine ℞

[tab' loid]
40-mg Scored Tablets

Prescribing information for this product, which appears on pages 1624–1626 of the 2004 PDR, has been revised as follows. Please write "See Supplement A" next to the product heading.

The third paragraph of WARNINGS *was revised to:*

There are individuals with an inherited deficiency of the enzyme thiopurine methyltransferase (TPMT) who may be unusually sensitive to the myelosuppressive effects of thioguanine and prone to developing rapid bone marrow suppression following the initiation of treatment. Substantial dosage reductions may be required to avoid the development of life-threatening bone marrow suppression in these patients. Prescribers should be aware that some laboratories offer testing for TPMT deficiency. Since bone marrow suppression may be associated with factors other than TPMT deficiency, TPMT testing may not identify all patients at risk for severe toxicity. Therefore, close monitoring of clinical and hematologic parameters is important. Bone marrow suppression could be exacerbated by coadministration with drugs that inhibit TPMT, such as olsalazine, mesalazine, or sulphasalazine.

The following sentence was added to the beginning of the PRECAUTIONS: Laboratory Tests *subsection:*

Prescribers should be aware that some laboratories offer testing for TPMT deficiency (see WARNINGS).

The following paragraph was added to DOSAGE AND ADMINISTRATION:

There are individuals with an inherited deficiency of the enzyme thiopurine methyltransferase (TPMT) who may be unusually sensitive to the myelosuppressive effects of thioguanine and prone to developing rapid bone marrow suppression following the initiation of treatment. Substantial dosage reductions may be required to avoid the development of life-threatening bone marrow suppression in these patients (see WARNINGS). Prescribers should be aware that some laboratories offer testing for TPMT deficiency.

Manufactured by DSM Pharmaceuticals, Inc.
Greenville, NC 27834
for GlaxoSmithKline, Research Triangle Park, NC 27709

January 2004/RL-2063

TIMENTIN® ℞

[tī-měn'tin]
brand of sterile ticarcillin disodium
and clavulanate potassium
for Intravenous Administration

Prescribing information for this product, which appears on pages 1632–1635 of the 2004 PDR, has been revised as follows. Please write "See Supplement A" next to the product heading.

The following paragraph was added before the DESCRIPTION *section:*

To reduce the development of drug-resistant bacteria and maintain the effectiveness of TIMENTIN (ticarcillin disodium and clavulanate potassium) and other antibacterial drugs, TIMENTIN should be used only to treat or prevent infections that are proven or strongly suspected to be caused by bacteria.

In INDICATIONS AND USAGE, *the following first 2 paragraphs were revised and the 3rd paragraph was added:*

Due to its broad spectrum of bactericidal activity against gram-positive and gram-negative bacteria, TIMENTIN is particularly useful for the treatment of mixed infections and for presumptive therapy prior to the identification of the causative organisms. TIMENTIN has been shown to be effective as single drug therapy in the treatment of some serious infections where normally combination antibiotic therapy might be employed.

Based on the in vitro synergism between ticarcillin/clavulanic acid and aminoglycosides against certain strains of *P. aeruginosa*, combined therapy has been successful, especially in patients with impaired host defenses. Both drugs should be used in full therapeutic doses.

To reduce the development of drug-resistant bacteria and maintain the effectiveness of TIMENTIN and other antibacterial drugs, TIMENTIN should be used only to treat or prevent infections that are proven or strongly suspected to be caused by susceptible bacteria. When culture and susceptibility information are available, they should be considered in selecting or modifying antibacterial therapy. In the absence of such data, local epidemiology and susceptibility patterns may contribute to the empiric selection of therapy.

In PRECAUTIONS: General, *the following paragraph was added:*

Prescribing TIMENTIN in the absence of a proven or strongly suspected bacterial infection or a prophylactic indication is unlikely to provide benefit to the patient and increases the risk of the development of drug-resistant bacteria.

In PRECAUTIONS, *the following subsection was added:*

Information for Patients: Patients should be counseled that antibacterial drugs, including TIMENTIN, should only be used to treat bacterial infections. They do not treat viral infections (e.g., the common cold). When TIMENTIN is prescribed to treat a bacterial infection, patients should be told that although it is common to feel better early in the course of therapy, the medication should be taken exactly as directed. Skipping doses or not completing the full course of therapy may: (1) decrease the effectiveness of the immediate treatment, and (2) increase the likelihood that bacteria will develop resistance and will not be treatable by TIMENTIN or other antibacterial drugs in the future.

In DOSAGE AND ADMINISTRATION, *all references to piggyback bottles were deleted.*

GlaxoSmithKline, Research Triangle Park, NC 27709

October 2003/TI:L131V

TIMENTIN® ℞

[tī-měn'tin]
sterile ticarcillin disodium
and clavulanate potassium
for Intravenous Administration
ADD-Vantage® ANTIBIOTIC VIAL

Prescribing information for this product, which appears on pages 1635–1639 of the 2004 PDR, has been revised as follows. Please write "See Supplement A" next to the product heading.

The following paragraph was added before the DESCRIPTION *section:*

To reduce the development of drug-resistant bacteria and maintain the effectiveness of TIMENTIN (ticarcillin disodium and clavulanate potassium) and other antibacterial drugs, TIMENTIN should be used only to treat or prevent infections that are proven or strongly suspected to be caused by bacteria.

In INDICATIONS AND USAGE, *the following first 2 paragraphs were revised and the 3rd paragraph was added:*

Due to its broad spectrum of bactericidal activity against gram-positive and gram-negative bacteria, TIMENTIN is particularly useful for the treatment of mixed infections and for presumptive therapy prior to the identification of the causative organisms. TIMENTIN has been shown to be ef-

Continued on next page

Timentin ADD-Vantage—Cont.

fective as single drug therapy in the treatment of some serious infections where normally combination antibiotic therapy might be employed.

Based on the in vitro synergism between ticarcillin/clavulanic acid and aminoglycosides against certain strains of *P. aeruginosa*, combined therapy has been successful, especially in patients with impaired host defenses. Both drugs should be used in full therapeutic doses.

To reduce the development of drug-resistant bacteria and maintain the effectiveness of TIMENTIN and other antibacterial drugs, TIMENTIN should be used only to treat or prevent infections that are proven or strongly suspected to be caused by susceptible bacteria. When culture and susceptibility information are available, they should be considered in selecting or modifying antibacterial therapy. In the absence of such data, local epidemiology and susceptibility patterns may contribute to the empiric selection of therapy.

In PRECAUTIONS: General, *the following paragraph was added:*

Prescribing TIMENTIN in the absence of a proven or strongly suspected bacterial infection or a prophylactic indication is unlikely to provide benefit to the patient and increases the risk of the development of drug-resistant bacteria.

In PRECAUTIONS: *the following subsection was added:*

Information for Patients: Patients should be counseled that antibacterial drugs, including TIMENTIN, should only be used to treat bacterial infections. They do not treat viral infections (e.g., the common cold). When TIMENTIN is prescribed to treat a bacterial infection, patients should be told that although it is common to feel better early in the course of therapy, the medication should be taken exactly as directed. Skipping doses or not completing the full course of therapy may: (1) decrease the effectiveness of the immediate treatment, and (2) increase the likelihood that bacteria will develop resistance and will not be treatable by TIMENTIN or other antibacterial drugs in the future.

GlaxoSmithKline, Research Triangle Park, NC 27709

October 2003/TI:L12AV

TIMENTIN® ℞

[*tī-mĕn' tin*]

brand of ticarcillin disodium and clavulanate potassium INJECTION

Galaxy® (PL 2040) Plastic Container (Product Package)

Prescribing information for this product, which appears on pages 1639–1642 of the 2004 PDR, has been revised as follows. Please write "See Supplement A" next to the product heading.

The following paragraph was added before the DESCRIPTION *section:*

To reduce the development of drug-resistant bacteria and maintain the effectiveness of TIMENTIN (ticarcillin disodium and clavulanate potassium) and other antibacterial drugs, TIMENTIN should be used only to treat or prevent infections that are proven or strongly suspected to be caused by bacteria.

In INDICATIONS AND USAGE, *the following first 2 paragraphs were revised and the 3rd paragraph was added:*

Due to its broad spectrum of bactericidal activity against gram-positive and gram-negative bacteria, TIMENTIN is particularly useful for the treatment of mixed infections and for presumptive therapy prior to the identification of the causative organisms. TIMENTIN has been shown to be effective as single drug therapy in the treatment of some serious infections where normally combination antibiotic therapy might be employed.

Based on the in vitro synergism between ticarcillin/clavulanic acid and aminoglycosides against certain strains of *P. aeruginosa*, combined therapy has been successful, especially in patients with impaired host defenses. Both drugs should be used in full therapeutic doses.

To reduce the development of drug-resistant bacteria and maintain the effectiveness of TIMENTIN and other antibacterial drugs, TIMENTIN should be used only to treat or prevent infections that are proven or strongly suspected to be caused by susceptible bacteria. When culture and susceptibility information are available, they should be considered in selecting or modifying antibacterial therapy. In the absence of such data, local epidemiology and susceptibility patterns may contribute to the empiric selection of therapy.

In PRECAUTIONS: General, *the following paragraph was added:*

Prescribing TIMENTIN in the absence of a proven or strongly suspected bacterial infection or a prophylactic indication is unlikely to provide benefit to the patient and increases the risk of the development of drug-resistant bacteria.

In PRECAUTIONS, *the following subsection was added:*

Information for Patients: Patients should be counseled that antibacterial drugs, including TIMENTIN, should only be used to treat bacterial infections. They do not treat viral infections (e.g., the common cold). When TIMENTIN is prescribed to treat a bacterial infection, patients should be told that although it is common to feel better early in the course of therapy, the medication should be taken exactly as directed. Skipping doses or not completing the full course of therapy may: (1) decrease the effectiveness of the immediate treatment, and (2) increase the likelihood that bacteria will develop resistance and will not be treatable by TIMENTIN or other antibacterial drugs in the future.

GlaxoSmithKline, Research Triangle Park, NC 27709

November 2003/TI:L15G

TIMENTIN® ℞

[*tī-mĕn'tin*]

brand of sterile ticarcillin disodium and clavulanate potassium for Intravenous Administration

PHARMACY BULK PACKAGE NOT FOR DIRECT INFUSION

RECONSTITUTED STOCK SOLUTION MUST BE TRANSFERRED AND FURTHER DILUTED FOR IV INFUSION.

Prescribing information for this product, which appears on pages 1642–1645 of the 2004 PDR, has been revised as follows. Please write "See Supplement A" next to the product heading.

The following paragraph was added before the DESCRIPTION *section:*

To reduce the development of drug-resistant bacteria and maintain the effectiveness of TIMENTIN (ticarcillin disodium and clavulanate potassium) and other antibacterial drugs, TIMENTIN should be used only to treat or prevent infections that are proven or strongly suspected to be caused by bacteria.

In INDICATIONS AND USAGE, *the following first 2 paragraphs were revised and the 3rd paragraph was added:*

Due to its broad spectrum of bactericidal activity against gram-positive and gram-negative bacteria, TIMENTIN is particularly useful for the treatment of mixed infections and for presumptive therapy prior to the identification of the causative organisms. TIMENTIN has been shown to be effective as single drug therapy in the treatment of some serious infections where normally combination antibiotic therapy might be employed.

Based on the in vitro synergism between ticarcillin/clavulanic acid and aminoglycosides against certain strains of *P. aeruginosa*, combined therapy has been successful, especially in patients with impaired host defenses. Both drugs should be used in full therapeutic doses.

To reduce the development of drug-resistant bacteria and maintain the effectiveness of TIMENTIN and other antibacterial drugs, TIMENTIN should be used only to treat or prevent infections that are proven or strongly suspected to be caused by susceptible bacteria. When culture and susceptibility information are available, they should be considered in selecting or modifying antibacterial therapy. In the absence of such data, local epidemiology and susceptibility patterns may contribute to the empiric selection of therapy.

In PRECAUTIONS: General, *the following paragraph was added:*

Prescribing TIMENTIN in the absence of a proven or strongly suspected bacterial infection or a prophylactic indication is unlikely to provide benefit to the patient and increases the risk of the development of drug-resistant bacteria.

In PRECAUTIONS, *the following subsection was added:*

Information for Patients: Patients should be counseled that antibacterial drugs, including TIMENTIN, should only be used to treat bacterial infections. They do not treat viral infections (e.g., the common cold). When TIMENTIN is prescribed to treat a bacterial infection, patients should be told that although it is common to feel better early in the course of therapy, the medication should be taken exactly as directed. Skipping doses or not completing the full course of therapy may: (1) decrease the effectiveness of the immediate treatment, and (2) increase the likelihood that bacteria will develop resistance and will not be treatable by TIMENTIN or other antibacterial drugs in the future.

GlaxoSmithKline, Research Triangle Park, NC 27709

October 2003/TI:L13PB

TWINRIX® ℞

[*twin' rix*]

[Hepatitis A Inactivated & Hepatitis B (Recombinant) Vaccine]

Prescribing information for this product, which appears on pages 1650–1653 of the 2004 PDR, has been revised as follows. Please write "See Supplement A" next to the product heading.

The CONTRAINDICATIONS *section was revised to:*

Hypersensitivity to any component of the vaccine, including yeast and neomycin, is a contraindication (see DESCRIPTION). This vaccine is contraindicated in patients with previous hypersensitivity to TWINRIX or monovalent hepatitis A or hepatitis B vaccines.

The following paragraph was added to WARNINGS:

The vial stopper is latex-free. The tip cap and the rubber plunger of the needleless prefilled syringes contain dry natural latex rubber that may cause allergic reactions in latex sensitive individuals.

The following subsection was added to PRECAUTIONS:

Carcinogenesis, Mutagenesis, Impairment of Fertility: TWINRIX has not been evaluated for its carcinogenic potential, mutagenic potential, or potential for impairment of fertility.

Manufactured by GlaxoSmithKline
Rixensart, Belgium, US License No. 1617

August 2003/TW:L5

ZINACEF® ℞

[*zin'a-sef*]

(cefuroxime for injection)

ZINACEF® ℞

(cefuroxime injection)

Prescribing information for this product, which appears on pages 1673–1676 of the 2004 PDR, has been revised as follows. Please write "See Supplement A" next to the product heading.

The following paragraph was added before the DESCRIPTION *section:*

To reduce the development of drug-resistant bacteria and maintain the effectiveness of ZINACEF and other antibacterial drugs, ZINACEF should be used only to treat or prevent infections that are proven or strongly suspected to be caused by bacteria.

The following section of INDICATIONS AND USAGE *was revised to:*

Clinical microbiological studies in skin and skin-structure infections frequently reveal the growth of susceptible strains of both aerobic and anaerobic organisms. ZINACEF has been used successfully in these mixed infections in which several organisms have been isolated.

In certain cases of confirmed or suspected gram-positive or gram-negative sepsis or in patients with other serious infections in which the causative organism has not been identified, ZINACEF may be used concomitantly with an aminoglycoside (see PRECAUTIONS). The recommended doses of both antibiotics may be given depending on the severity of the infection and the patient's condition.

To reduce the development of drug-resistant bacteria and maintain the effectiveness of ZINACEF and other antibacterial drugs, ZINACEF should be used only to treat or prevent infections that are proven or strongly suspected to be caused by susceptible bacteria. When culture and susceptibility information are available, they should be considered in selecting or modifying antibacterial therapy. In the absence of such data, local epidemiology and susceptibility patterns may contribute to the empiric selection of therapy.

In PRECAUTIONS: General, *the following paragraph was added:*

Prescribing ZINACEF in the absence of a proven or strongly suspected bacterial infection or a prophylactic indication is unlikely to provide benefit to the patient and increases the risk of the development of drug-resistant bacteria.

The following subsection was added to PRECAUTIONS:

Information for Patients: Patients should be counseled that antibacterial drugs, including ZINACEF, should only be used to treat bacterial infections. They do not treat viral infections (e.g., the common cold). When ZINACEF is prescribed to treat a bacterial infection, patients should be told that although it is common to feel better early in the course of therapy, the medication should be taken exactly as directed. Skipping doses or not completing the full course of therapy may: (1) decrease the effectiveness of the immediate treatment, and (2) increase the likelihood that bacteria will develop resistance and will not be treatable by ZINACEF or other antibacterial drugs in the future.

ZINACEF® (cefuroxime for injection):
GlaxoSmithKline, Research Triangle Park, NC 27709
ZINACEF® (cefuroxime injection):
Manufactured for GlaxoSmithKline
Research Triangle Park, NC 27709
by Baxter Healthcare Corporation, Deerfield, IL 60015
ZINACEF is a registered trademark of GlaxoSmithKline.
October 2003/RL-2045

ZOVIRAX® ℞

[*zō-vī'rax*]

(acyclovir)
Capsules

ZOVIRAX® ℞

(acyclovir)
Tablets

ZOVIRAX® ℞

(acyclovir)
Suspension

Prescribing information for this product, which appears on pages 1683–1685 of the 2004 PDR, has been revised as follows. Please write "See Supplement A" next to the product heading.

"Dysarthria" was added to ADVERSE REACTIONS: Observed During Clinical Practice: *Nervous:*

GlaxoSmithKline, Research Triangle Park, NC 27709

November 2003/RL-2049

ZOVIRAX® ℞

[*zō-vī ′rax*]

(acyclovir sodium)

for Injection

FOR INTRAVENOUS INFUSION ONLY

Prescribing information for this product, which appears on pages 1685–1687 of the 2004 PDR, has been revised as follows. Please write "See Supplement A" next to the product heading.

The following events were added to ADVERSE REACTIONS: Observed During Clinical Practice:

General: ... fatigue, ...

Digestive: Abdominal pain, ...

Nervous: ...dysarthria, ...

Manufactured by DSM Pharmaceuticals, Inc.
Greenville, NC 27834
for GlaxoSmithKline, Research Triangle Park, NC 27709

November 2003/RL-2050

Janssen Pharmaceutica Products, L.P.

1125 TRENTON-HARBOURTON ROAD
P.O. BOX 200
TITUSVILLE, NJ 08560-0200

For Medical Information Monday through Friday 9 am-5 pm EST Contact:
(800) JANSSEN
FAX: (609) 730-3138
After Hours and Weekends:
(800) JANSSEN

RISPERDAL® ℞

[*rĭs-pər-dăl*]

(risperidone)

Tablets/Oral Solution

RISPERDAL® M-TAB™

(risperidone)

Orally Disintegrating Tablets

Prescribing information for this product, which appears on pages 1764–1768 of the 2004 PDR, has been revised as follows. Please write "See Supplement A" next to the product heading.

DESCRIPTION

RISPERDAL® (risperidone) is a psychotropic agent belonging to the chemical class of benzisoxazole derivatives. The chemical designation is 3-[2-[4-(6-fluoro-1,2-benzisoxazol-3-yl)-1-piperidinyl]ethyl]-6,7,8,9-tetrahydro-2-methyl-4H-pyrido[1,2-a]pyrimidin-4-one. Its molecular formula is $C_{23}H_{27}FN_4O_2$ and its molecular weight is 410.49. The structural formula is:

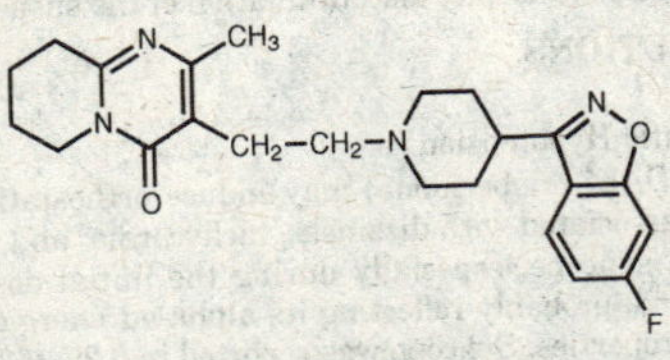

Risperidone is a white to slightly beige powder. It is practically insoluble in water, freely soluble in methylene chloride, and soluble in methanol and 0.1 N HCl.

RISPERDAL® tablets are available in 0.25 mg (dark yellow), 0.5 mg (red-brown), 1 mg (white), 2 mg (orange), 3 mg (yellow), and 4 mg (green) strengths. Inactive ingredients are colloidal silicon dioxide, hypromellose, lactose, magnesium stearate, microcrystalline cellulose, propylene glycol, sodium lauryl sulfate, and starch (corn). Tablets of 0.25, 0.5, 2, 3, and 4 mg also contain talc and titanium dioxide. The 0.25 mg tablets contain yellow iron oxide; the 0.5 mg tablets contain red iron oxide; the 2 mg tablets contain FD&C Yellow No. 6 Aluminum Lake; the 3 mg and 4 mg tablets contain D&C Yellow No. 10; the 4 mg tablets contain FD&C Blue No. 2 Aluminum Lake.

RISPERDAL® is also available as a 1 mg/mL oral solution. The inactive ingredients for this solution are tartaric acid, benzoic acid, sodium hydroxide, and purified water.

RISPERDAL® M-TAB™ Orally Disintegrating Tablets are available in 0.5 mg, 1 mg, and 2 mg strengths and are light coral in color.

RISPERDAL® M-TAB™ Orally Disintegrating Tablets contain the following inactive ingredients: Amberlite® resin, gelatin, mannitol, glycine, simethicone, carbomer, sodium hydroxide, aspartame, red ferric oxide, and peppermint oil.

CLINICAL PHARMACOLOGY

Pharmacodynamics

The mechanism of action of RISPERDAL® (risperidone), as with other drugs used to treat schizophrenia, is unknown. However, it has been proposed that the drug's therapeutic activity in schizophrenia is mediated through a combination of dopamine Type 2 (D_2) and serotonin Type 2 ($5HT_2$) receptor antagonism. Antagonism at receptors other than D_2 and $5HT_2$ may explain some of the other effects of RISPERDAL®.

RISPERDAL® is a selective monoaminergic antagonist with high affinity (Ki of 0.12 to 7.3 nM) for the serotonin Type 2 ($5HT_2$), dopamine Type 2 (D_2), α_1 and α_2 adrenergic, and H_1 histaminergic receptors. RISPERDAL® acts as an antagonist at other receptors, but with lower potency. RISPERDAL® has low to moderate affinity (Ki of 47 to 253 nM) for the serotonin $5HT_{1C}$, $5HT_{1D}$, and $5HT_{1A}$ receptors, weak affinity (Ki of 620 to 800 nM) for the dopamine D_1 and haloperidol-sensitive sigma site, and no affinity (when tested at concentrations $>10^{-5}$ M) for cholinergic muscarinic or β_1 and β_2 adrenergic receptors.

Pharmacokinetics

Absorption

Risperidone is well absorbed. The absolute oral bioavailability of risperidone is 70% (CV=25%). The relative oral bioavailability of risperidone from a tablet is 94% (CV=10%) when compared to a solution.

Pharmacokinetic studies showed that RISPERDAL® M-TAB™ Orally Disintegrating Tablets and RISPERDAL® Oral Solution are bioequivalent to RISPERDAL® Tablets.

Plasma concentrations of risperidone, its major metabolite, 9-hydroxyrisperidone, and risperidone plus 9-hydroxyrisperidone are dose proportional over the dosing range of 1 to 16 mg daily (0.5 to 8 mg BID). Following oral administration of solution or tablet, mean peak plasma concentrations of risperidone occurred at about 1 hour. Peak concentrations of 9-hydroxyrisperidone occurred at about 3 hours in extensive metabolizers, and 17 hours in poor metabolizers. Steady-state concentrations of risperidone are reached in 1 day in extensive metabolizers and would be expected to reach steady-state in about 5 days in poor metabolizers. Steady-state concentrations of 9-hydroxyrisperidone are reached in 5–6 days (measured in extensive metabolizers).

Food Effect

Food does not affect either the rate or extent of absorption of risperidone. Thus, risperidone can be given with or without meals.

Distribution

Risperidone is rapidly distributed. The volume of distribution is 1–2 L/kg. In plasma, risperidone is bound to albumin and α_1-acid glycoprotein. The plasma protein binding of risperidone is 90%, and that of its major metabolite, 9-hydroxyrisperidone, is 77%. Neither risperidone nor 9-hydroxyrisperidone displaces each other from plasma binding sites. High therapeutic concentrations of sulfamethazine (100 mcg/mL), warfarin (10 mcg/mL), and carbamazepine (10 mcg/mL) caused only a slight increase in the free fraction of risperidone at 10 ng/mL and 9-hydroxyrisperidone at 50 ng/mL, changes of unknown clinical significance.

Metabolism

Risperidone is extensively metabolized in the liver. The main metabolic pathway is through hydroxylation of risperidone to 9-hydroxyrisperidone by the enzyme, CYP 2D6. A minor metabolic pathway is through *N*-dealkylation. The main metabolite, 9-hydroxyrisperidone, has similar pharmacological activity as risperidone. Consequently, the clinical effect of the drug (e.g., the active moiety) results from the combined concentrations of risperidone plus 9-hydroxyrisperidone.

CYP 2D6, also called debrisoquin hydroxylase, is the enzyme responsible for metabolism of many neuroleptics, antidepressants, antiarrhythmics, and other drugs. CYP 2D6 is subject to genetic polymorphism (about 6%–8% of Caucasians, and a very low percentage of Asians, have little or no activity and are "poor metabolizers") and to inhibition by a variety of substrates and some non-substrates, notably quinidine. Extensive CYP 2D6 metabolizers convert risperidone rapidly into 9-hydroxyrisperidone, whereas poor CYP 2D6 metabolizers convert it much more slowly. Although extensive metabolizers have lower risperidone and higher 9-hydroxyrisperidone concentrations than poor metabolizers, the pharmacokinetics of the active moiety, after single and multiple doses, are similar in extensive and poor metabolizers.

Risperidone could be subject to two kinds of drug-drug interactions (see PRECAUTIONS—Drug Interactions). First, inhibitors of CYP 2D6 interfere with conversion of risperidone to 9-hydroxyrisperidone. This occurs with quinidine, giving essentially all recipients a risperidone pharmacokinetic profile typical of poor metabolizers. The therapeutic benefits and adverse effects of risperidone in patients receiving quinidine have not been evaluated, but observations in a modest number (n ≅ 70) of poor metabolizers given risperidone do not suggest important differences between poor and extensive metabolizers. Second, co-administration of known enzyme inducers (e.g., phenytoin, rifampin, and phenobarbital) with risperidone may cause a decrease in the combined plasma concentrations of risperidone and 9-hydroxyrisperidone. It would also be possible for risperidone to interfere with metabolism of other drugs metabolized by CYP 2D6. Relatively weak binding of risperidone to the enzyme suggests this is unlikely.

In a drug interaction study in schizophrenic patients, 11 subjects received risperidone titrated to 6 mg/day for 3 weeks, followed by concurrent administration of carbamazepine for an additional 3 weeks. During co-administration, the plasma concentrations of risperidone and its pharmacologically active metabolite, 9-hydroxyrisperidone, were decreased by about 50%. Plasma concentrations of carbamazepine did not appear to be affected. Co-administration of other known enzyme inducers (e.g., phenytoin, rifampin, and phenobarbital) with risperidone may cause similar decreases in the combined plasma concentrations of risperidone and 9-hydroxyrisperidone, which could lead to decreased efficacy of risperidone treatment (see PRECAUTIONS – Drug Interactions and DOSAGE AND ADMINISTRATION – Co-Administration of RISPERDAL® with Certain Other Medications).

Fluoxetine (20 mg QD) and paroxetine (20 mg QD) have been shown to increase the plasma concentration of risperidone 2.5–2.8 fold and 3–9 fold respectively. Fluoxetine did not affect the plasma concentration of 9-hydroxyrisperidone. Paroxetine lowered the concentration of 9-hydroxyrisperidone an average of 13% (see PRECAUTIONS – Drug Interactions and DOSAGE AND ADMINISTRATION – Co-Administration of RISPERDAL® with Certain Other Medications).

Repeated oral doses of risperidone (3 mg BID) did not affect the exposure (AUC) or peak plasma concentrations (C_{max}) of lithium (n=13) (see PRECAUTIONS – Drug Interactions).

Repeated oral doses of risperidone (4 mg QD) did not affect the pre-dose or average plasma concentrations and exposure (AUC) of valproate (1000 mg/day in three divided doses) compared to placebo (n=21). However, there was a 20% increase in valproate peak plasma concentration (C_{max}) after concomitant administration of risperidone (see PRECAUTIONS – Drug Interactions).

There were no significant interactions between risperidone (1 mg QD) and erythromycin (500 mg QID) (see PRECAUTIONS – Drug Interactions).

Excretion

Risperidone and its metabolites are eliminated via the urine and, to a much lesser extent, via the feces. As illustrated by a mass balance study of a single 1 mg oral dose of ^{14}C-risperidone administered as solution to three healthy male volunteers, total recovery of radioactivity at 1 week was 84%, including 70% in the urine and 14% in the feces.

The apparent half-life of risperidone was 3 hours (CV=30%) in extensive metabolizers and 20 hours (CV=40%) in poor metabolizers. The apparent half-life of 9-hydroxyrisperidone was about 21 hours (CV=20%) in extensive metabolizers and 30 hours (CV=25%) in poor metabolizers. The pharmacokinetics of the active moiety, after single and multiple doses, were similar in extensive and poor metabolizers, with an overall mean elimination half-life of about 20 hours.

Special Populations

Renal Impairment

In patients with moderate to severe renal disease, clearance of the sum of risperidone and its active metabolite decreased by 60% compared to young healthy subjects. RISPERDAL® doses should be reduced in patients with renal disease (see PRECAUTIONS and DOSAGE AND ADMINISTRATION).

Hepatic Impairment

While the pharmacokinetics of risperidone in subjects with liver disease were comparable to those in young healthy subjects, the mean free fraction of risperidone in plasma was increased by about 35% because of the diminished concentration of both albumin and α_1-acid glycoprotein. RISPERDAL® doses should be reduced in patients with liver disease (see PRECAUTIONS and DOSAGE AND ADMINISTRATION).

Elderly

In healthy elderly subjects, renal clearance of both risperidone and 9-hydroxyrisperidone was decreased, and elimination half-lives were prolonged compared to young healthy subjects. Dosing should be modified accordingly in the elderly patients (see DOSAGE AND ADMINISTRATION).

Race and Gender Effects

No specific pharmacokinetic study was conducted to investigate race and gender effects, but a population pharmacokinetic analysis did not identify important differences in the disposition of risperidone due to gender (whether corrected for body weight or not) or race.

Clinical Trials

Schizophrenia

Short-Term Efficacy

The efficacy of RISPERDAL® in the treatment of schizophrenia was established in four short-term (4- to 8-week) controlled trials of psychotic inpatients who met DSM-III-R criteria for schizophrenia.

Several instruments were used for assessing psychiatric signs and symptoms in these studies, among them the Brief Psychiatric Rating Scale (BPRS), a multi-item inventory of general psychopathology traditionally used to evaluate the effects of drug treatment in schizophrenia. The BPRS psychosis cluster (conceptual disorganization, hallucinatory behavior, suspiciousness, and unusual thought content) is considered a particularly useful subset for assessing actively psychotic schizophrenic patients. A second traditional assessment, the Clinical Global Impression (CGI), reflects the impression of a skilled observer, fully familiar with the manifestations of schizophrenia, about the overall clinical state of the patient. In addition, the Positive and Negative Syndrome Scale (PANSS) and the Scale for Assessing Negative Symptoms (SANS) were employed.

The results of the trials follow:

(1) In a 6-week, placebo-controlled trial (n=160) involving titration of RISPERDAL® in doses up to 10 mg/day (BID schedule), RISPERDAL® was generally superior to placebo on the BPRS total score, on the BPRS psychosis cluster, and marginally superior to placebo on the SANS.

(2) In an 8-week, placebo-controlled trial (n=513) involving

Continued on next page

Risperdal—Cont.

4 fixed doses of RISPERDAL® (2, 6, 10, and 16 mg/day, on a BID schedule), all 4 RISPERDAL® groups were generally superior to placebo on the BPRS total score, BPRS psychosis cluster, and CGI severity score; the 3 highest RISPERDAL® dose groups were generally superior to placebo on the PANSS negative subscale. The most consistently positive responses on all measures were seen for the 6 mg dose group, and there was no suggestion of increased benefit from larger doses.

(3) In an 8-week, dose comparison trial (n=1356) involving 5 fixed doses of RISPERDAL® (1, 4, 8, 12, and 16 mg/day, on a BID schedule), the four highest RISPERDAL® dose groups were generally superior to the 1 mg RISPERDAL® dose group on BPRS total score, BPRS psychosis cluster, and CGI severity score. None of the dose groups were superior to the 1 mg group on the PANSS negative subscale. The most consistently positive responses were seen for the 4 mg dose group.

(4) In a 4-week, placebo-controlled dose comparison trial (n=246) involving 2 fixed doses of RISPERDAL® (4 and 8 mg/day on a QD schedule), both RISPERDAL® dose groups were generally superior to placebo on several PANSS measures, including a response measure (> 20% reduction in PANSS total score), PANSS total score, and the BPRS psychosis cluster (derived from PANSS). The results were generally stronger for the 8 mg than for the 4 mg dose group.

Long-Term Efficacy

In a longer-term trial, 365 adult outpatients predominantly meeting DSM-IV criteria for schizophrenia and who had been clinically stable for at least 4 weeks on an antipsychotic medication were randomized to RISPERDAL® (2–8 mg/day) or to an active comparator, for 1 to 2 years of observation for relapse. Patients receiving RISPERDAL® experienced a significantly longer time to relapse over this time period compared to those receiving the active comparator.

Bipolar Mania

Monotherapy

The efficacy of RISPERDAL® in the treatment of acute manic or mixed episodes was established in 2 short-term (3-week) placebo-controlled trials in patients who met the DSM-IV criteria for Bipolar I Disorder with manic or mixed episodes. These trials included patients with or without psychotic features.

The primary rating instrument used for assessing manic symptoms in these trials was the Young Mania Rating Scale (Y-MRS), an 11-item clinician-rated scale traditionally used to assess the degree of manic symptomatology (irritability, disruptive/aggressive behavior, sleep, elevated mood, speech, increased activity, sexual interest, language/thought disorder, thought content, appearance, and insight) in a range from 0 (no manic features) to 60 (maximum score). The primary outcome in these trials was change from baseline in the Y-MRS total score. The results of the trials follow:

(1) In one 3-week placebo-controlled trial (n=246), limited to patients with manic episodes, which involved a dose range of RISPERDAL® 1–6 mg/day, once daily, starting at 3 mg/day (mean modal dose was 4.1 mg/day), RISPERDAL® was superior to placebo in the reduction of Y-MRS total score.

(2) In another 3-week placebo-controlled trial (n=286), which involved a dose range of 1–6 mg/day, once daily, starting at 3 mg/day (mean modal dose was 5.6 mg/day), RISPERDAL® was superior to placebo in the reduction of Y-MRS total score.

Combination Therapy

The efficacy of risperidone with concomitant lithium or valproate in the treatment of acute manic or mixed episodes was established in one controlled trial in patients who met the DSM-IV criteria for Bipolar I Disorder. This trial included patients with or without psychotic features and with or without a rapid-cycling course.

(1) In this 3-week placebo-controlled combination trial, 148 in- or outpatients on lithium or valproate therapy with inadequately controlled manic or mixed symptoms were randomized to receive RISPERDAL®, placebo, or an active comparator, in combination with their original therapy. RISPERDAL®, in a dose range of 1–6 mg/day, once daily, starting at 2 mg/day (mean modal dose of 3.8 mg/day), combined with lithium or valproate (in a therapeutic range of 0.6 mEq/L to 1.4 mEq/L or 50 mcg/mL to 120 mcg/mL, respectively) was superior to lithium or valproate alone in the reduction of Y-MRS total score.

(2) In a second 3-week placebo-controlled combination trial, 142 in- or outpatients on lithium, valproate, or carbamazepine therapy with inadequately controlled manic or mixed symptoms were randomized to receive RISPERDAL® or placebo, in combination with their original therapy. RISPERDAL®, in a dose range of 1-6 mg/day, once daily, starting at 2 mg/day (mean modal dose of 3.7 mg/day), combined with lithium, valproate, or carbamazepine (in therapeutic ranges of 0.6 mEq/L to 1.4 mEq/L for lithium, 50 mcg/mL to 125 mcg/mL for valproate, or 4–12 mcg/mL for carbamazepine, respectively) was not superior to lithium, valproate, or carbamazepine alone in the reduction of Y-MRS total score. A possible explanation for the failure of this trial was induction of risperidone and 9-hydroxyrisperidone clearance by carbamazepine, leading to subtherapeutic levels of risperidone and 9-hydroxyrisperidone.

INDICATIONS AND USAGE

Schizophrenia

RISPERDAL® (risperidone) is indicated for the treatment of schizophrenia.

The efficacy of RISPERDAL® in schizophrenia was established in short-term (6- to 8-weeks) controlled trials of schizophrenic inpatients (see CLINICAL PHARMACOLOGY).

The efficacy of RISPERDAL® in delaying relapse was demonstrated in schizophrenic patients who had been clinically stable for at least 4 weeks before initiation of treatment with RISPERDAL® or an active comparator and who were then observed for relapse during a period of 1 to 2 years (see CLINICAL PHARMACOLOGY – Clinical Trials). Nevertheless, the physician who elects to use RISPERDAL® for extended periods should periodically re-evaluate the long-term usefulness of the drug for the individual patient (see DOSAGE AND ADMINISTRATION).

Bipolar Mania

Monotherapy

RISPERDAL® is indicated for the short-term treatment of acute manic or mixed episodes associated with Bipolar I Disorder.

The efficacy of RISPERDAL® was established in two placebo-controlled trials (3-week) with patients meeting DSM-IV criteria for Bipolar I Disorder who currently displayed an acute manic or mixed episode with or without psychotic features (see CLINICAL PHARMACOLOGY).

Combination Therapy

The combination of RISPERDAL® with lithium or valproate is indicated for the short-term treatment of acute manic or mixed episodes associated with Bipolar I Disorder.

The efficacy of RISPERDAL® in combination with lithium or valproate was established in one placebo-controlled (3-week) trial with patients meeting DSM-IV criteria for Bipolar I Disorder who currently displayed an acute manic or mixed episode with or without psychotic features (see CLINICAL PHARMACOLOGY).

The effectiveness of RISPERDAL® for longer-term use, that is, for more than 3 weeks of treatment of an acute episode, and for prophylactic use in mania, has not been systematically evaluated in controlled clinical trials. Therefore, physicians who elect to use RISPERDAL® for extended periods should periodically re-evaluate the long-term risks and benefits of the drug for the individual patient (see DOSAGE AND ADMINISTRATION).

CONTRAINDICATIONS

RISPERDAL® (risperidone) is contraindicated in patients with a known hypersensitivity to the product.

WARNINGS

Neuroleptic Malignant Syndrome (NMS)

A potentially fatal symptom complex sometimes referred to as Neuroleptic Malignant Syndrome (NMS) has been reported in association with antipsychotic drugs. Clinical manifestations of NMS are hyperpyrexia, muscle rigidity, altered mental status, and evidence of autonomic instability (irregular pulse or blood pressure, tachycardia, diaphoresis, and cardiac dysrhythmia). Additional signs may include elevated creatinine phosphokinase, myoglobinuria (rhabdomyolysis), and acute renal failure.

The diagnostic evaluation of patients with this syndrome is complicated. In arriving at a diagnosis, it is important to identify cases in which the clinical presentation includes both serious medical illness (e.g., pneumonia, systemic infection, etc.) and untreated or inadequately treated extrapyramidal signs and symptoms (EPS). Other important considerations in the differential diagnosis include central anticholinergic toxicity, heat stroke, drug fever, and primary central nervous system pathology.

The management of NMS should include: (1) immediate discontinuation of antipsychotic drugs and other drugs not essential to concurrent therapy; (2) intensive symptomatic treatment and medical monitoring; and (3) treatment of any concomitant serious medical problems for which specific treatments are available. There is no general agreement about specific pharmacological treatment regimens for uncomplicated NMS.

If a patient requires antipsychotic drug treatment after recovery from NMS, the potential reintroduction of drug therapy should be carefully considered. The patient should be carefully monitored, since recurrences of NMS have been reported.

Tardive Dyskinesia

A syndrome of potentially irreversible, involuntary, dyskinetic movements may develop in patients treated with antipsychotic drugs. Although the prevalence of the syndrome appears to be highest among the elderly, especially elderly women, it is impossible to rely upon prevalence estimates to predict, at the inception of antipsychotic treatment, which patients are likely to develop the syndrome. Whether antipsychotic drug products differ in their potential to cause tardive dyskinesia is unknown.

The risk of developing tardive dyskinesia and the likelihood that it will become irreversible are believed to increase as the duration of treatment and the total cumulative dose of antipsychotic drugs administered to the patient increase. However, the syndrome can develop, although much less commonly, after relatively brief treatment periods at low doses.

There is no known treatment for established cases of tardive dyskinesia, although the syndrome may remit, partially or completely, if antipsychotic treatment is withdrawn. Antipsychotic treatment, itself, however, may suppress (or partially suppress) the signs and symptoms of the syndrome and thereby may possibly mask the underlying process. The effect that symptomatic suppression has upon the long-term course of the syndrome is unknown.

Given these considerations, RISPERDAL® (risperidone) should be prescribed in a manner that is most likely to minimize the occurrence of tardive dyskinesia. Chronic antipsychotic treatment should generally be reserved for patients who suffer from a chronic illness that (1) is known to respond to antipsychotic drugs, and (2) for whom alternative, equally effective, but potentially less harmful treatments are not available or appropriate. In patients who do require chronic treatment, the smallest dose and the shortest duration of treatment producing a satisfactory clinical response should be sought. The need for continued treatment should be reassessed periodically.

If signs and symptoms of tardive dyskinesia appear in a patient treated on RISPERDAL®, drug discontinuation should be considered. However, some patients may require treatment with RISPERDAL® despite the presence of the syndrome.

Cerebrovascular Adverse Events, Including Stroke, in Elderly Patients With Dementia

Cerebrovascular adverse events (e.g., stroke, transient ischemic attack), including fatalities, were reported in patients (mean age 85 years; range 73–97) in trials of risperidone in elderly patients with dementia-related psychosis. In placebo-controlled trials, there was a significantly higher incidence of cerebrovascular adverse events in patients treated with risperidone compared to patients treated with placebo. RISPERDAL® is not approved for the treatment of patients with dementia-related psychosis.

Hyperglycemia and Diabetes Mellitus

Hyperglycemia, in some cases extreme and associated with ketoacidosis or hyperosmolar coma or death, has been reported in patients treated with atypical antipsychotics including RISPERDAL®. Assessment of the relationship between atypical antipsychotic use and glucose abnormalities is complicated by the possibility of an increased background risk of diabetes mellitus in patients with schizophrenia and the increasing incidence of diabetes mellitus in the general population. Given these confounders, the relationship between atypical antipsychotic use and hyperglycemia-related adverse events is not completely understood. However, epidemiological studies suggest an increased risk of treatment-emergent hyperglycemia-related adverse events in patients treated with the atypical antipsychotics. Precise risk estimates for hyperglycemia-related adverse events in patients treated with atypical antipsychotics are not available.

Patients with an established diagnosis of diabetes mellitus who are started on atypical antipsychotics should be monitored regularly for worsening of glucose control. Patients with risk factors for diabetes mellitus (e.g., obesity, family history of diabetes) who are starting treatment with atypical antipsychotics should undergo fasting blood glucose testing at the beginning of treatment and periodically during treatment. Any patient treated with atypical antipsychotics should be monitored for symptoms of hyperglycemia including polydipsia, polyuria, polyphagia, and weakness. Patients who develop symptoms of hyperglycemia during treatment with atypical antipsychotics should undergo fasting blood glucose testing. In some cases, hyperglycemia has resolved when the atypical antipsychotic was discontinued; however, some patients required continuation of anti-diabetic treatment despite discontinuation of the suspect drug.

PRECAUTIONS

General

Orthostatic Hypotension

RISPERDAL® (risperidone) may induce orthostatic hypotension associated with dizziness, tachycardia, and in some patients, syncope, especially during the initial dose-titration period, probably reflecting its alpha-adrenergic antagonistic properties. Syncope was reported in 0.2% (6/2607) of RISPERDAL®-treated patients in Phase 2 and 3 studies. The risk of orthostatic hypotension and syncope may be minimized by limiting the initial dose to 2 mg total (either QD or 1 mg BID) in normal adults and 0.5 mg BID in the elderly and patients with renal or hepatic impairment (see DOSAGE AND ADMINISTRATION). Monitoring of orthostatic vital signs should be considered in patients for whom this is of concern. A dose reduction should be considered if hypotension occurs. RISPERDAL® should be used with particular caution in patients with known cardiovascular disease (history of myocardial infarction or ischemia, heart failure, or conduction abnormalities), cerebrovascular disease, and conditions which would predispose patients to hypotension, e.g., dehydration and hypovolemia. Clinically significant hypotension has been observed with concomitant use of RISPERDAL® and antihypertensive medication.

Seizures

During premarketing testing, seizures occurred in 0.3% (9/2607) of RISPERDAL®-treated patients, two in association with hyponatremia. RISPERDAL® should be used cautiously in patients with a history of seizures.

Dysphagia

Esophageal dysmotility and aspiration have been associated with antipsychotic drug use. Aspiration pneumonia is a common cause of morbidity and mortality in patients with advanced Alzheimer's dementia. RISPERDAL® and other antipsychotic drugs should be used cautiously in patients at risk for aspiration pneumonia.

Hyperprolactinemia

As with other drugs that antagonize dopamine D_2 receptors, risperidone elevates prolactin levels and the elevation persists during chronic administration. Tissue culture experiments indicate that approximately one-third of human breast cancers are prolactin dependent *in vitro*, a factor of potential importance if the prescription of these drugs is contemplated in a patient with previously detected breast cancer. Although disturbances such as galactorrhea, amenorrhea, gynecomastia, and impotence have been reported with prolactin-elevating compounds, the clinical significance of elevated serum prolactin levels is unknown for most patients. As is common with compounds which increase prolactin release, an increase in pituitary gland, mammary gland, and pancreatic islet cell hyperplasia and/or neoplasia was observed in the risperidone carcinogenicity studies conducted in mice and rats (see PRECAUTIONS – Carcinogenesis, Mutagenesis, Impairment of Fertility). However, neither clinical studies nor epidemiologic studies conducted to date have shown an association between chronic administration of this class of drugs and tumorigenesis in humans; the available evidence is considered too limited to be conclusive at this time.

Potential for Cognitive and Motor Impairment

Somnolence was a commonly reported adverse event associated with RISPERDAL® treatment, especially when ascertained by direct questioning of patients. This adverse event is dose-related, and in a study utilizing a checklist to detect adverse events, 41% of the high-dose patients (RISPERDAL® 16 mg/day) reported somnolence compared to 16% of placebo patients. Direct questioning is more sensitive for detecting adverse events than spontaneous reporting, by which 8% of RISPERDAL® 16 mg/day patients and 1% of placebo patients reported somnolence as an adverse event. Since RISPERDAL® has the potential to impair judgment, thinking, or motor skills, patients should be cautioned about operating hazardous machinery, including automobiles, until they are reasonably certain that RISPERDAL® therapy does not affect them adversely.

Priapism

Rare cases of priapism have been reported. While the relationship of the events to RISPERDAL® use has not been established, other drugs with alpha-adrenergic blocking effects have been reported to induce priapism, and it is possible that RISPERDAL® may share this capacity. Severe priapism may require surgical intervention.

Thrombotic Thrombocytopenic Purpura (TTP)

A single case of TTP was reported in a 28 year-old female patient receiving RISPERDAL® in a large, open premarketing experience (approximately 1300 patients). She experienced jaundice, fever, and bruising, but eventually recovered after receiving plasmapheresis. The relationship to RISPERDAL® therapy is unknown.

Antiemetic Effect

Risperidone has an antiemetic effect in animals; this effect may also occur in humans, and may mask signs and symptoms of overdosage with certain drugs or of conditions such as intestinal obstruction, Reye's syndrome, and brain tumor.

Body Temperature Regulation

Disruption of body temperature regulation has been attributed to antipsychotic agents. Both hyperthermia and hypothermia have been reported in association with oral RISPERDAL® use. Caution is advised when prescribing for patients who will be exposed to temperature extremes.

Suicide

The possibility of a suicide attempt is inherent in schizophrenia, and close supervision of high-risk patients should accompany drug therapy. Prescriptions for RISPERDAL® should be written for the smallest quantity of tablets, consistent with good patient management, in order to reduce the risk of overdose.

Use in Patients With Concomitant Illness

Clinical experience with RISPERDAL® in patients with certain concomitant systemic illnesses is limited. Caution is advisable in using RISPERDAL® in patients with diseases or conditions that could affect metabolism or hemodynamic responses.

RISPERDAL® has not been evaluated or used to any appreciable extent in patients with a recent history of myocardial infarction or unstable heart disease. Patients with these diagnoses were excluded from clinical studies during the product's premarket testing.

Increased plasma concentrations of risperidone and 9-hydroxyrisperidone occur in patients with severe renal impairment (creatinine clearance <30 mL/min/1.73 m²), and an increase in the free fraction of risperidone is seen in patients with severe hepatic impairment. A lower starting dose should be used in such patients (see DOSAGE AND ADMINISTRATION).

Information for Patients

Physicians are advised to discuss the following issues with patients for whom they prescribe RISPERDAL®:

Orthostatic Hypotension

Patients should be advised of the risk of orthostatic hypotension, especially during the period of initial dose titration.

Interference With Cognitive and Motor Performance

Since RISPERDAL® has the potential to impair judgment, thinking, or motor skills, patients should be cautioned about operating hazardous machinery, including automobiles, until they are reasonably certain that RISPERDAL® therapy does not affect them adversely.

Pregnancy

Patients should be advised to notify their physician if they become pregnant or intend to become pregnant during therapy.

Nursing

Patients should be advised not to breast-feed an infant if they are taking RISPERDAL®.

Tumor Type	Species	Sex	Multiples of Maximum Human Dose in mg/m² (mg/kg): Lowest Effect Level	Highest No-Effect Level
Pituitary adenomas	mouse	female	0.75 (9.4)	0.2 (2.4)
Endocrine pancreas adenomas	rat	male	1.5 (9.4)	0.4 (2.4)
Mammary gland adenocarcinomas	mouse	female	0.2 (2.4)	none
	rat	female	0.4 (2.4)	none
	rat	male	6.0 (37.5)	1.5 (9.4)
Mammary gland neoplasms, Total	rat	male	1.5 (9.4)	0.4 (2.4)

Concomitant Medication

Patients should be advised to inform their physicians if they are taking, or plan to take, any prescription or over-the-counter drugs, since there is a potential for interactions.

Alcohol

Patients should be advised to avoid alcohol while taking RISPERDAL®.

Phenylketonurics

Phenylalanine is a component of aspartame. Each 2 mg RISPERDAL® M-TAB™ Orally Disintegrating Tablet contains 0.56 mg phenylalanine; each 1 mg RISPERDAL® M-TAB™ Orally Disintegrating Tablet contains 0.28 mg phenylalanine; and each 0.5 mg RISPERDAL® M-TAB™ Orally Disintegrating Tablet contains 0.14 mg phenylalanine.

Laboratory Tests

No specific laboratory tests are recommended.

Drug Interactions

The interactions of RISPERDAL® and other drugs have not been systematically evaluated. Given the primary CNS effects of risperidone, caution should be used when RISPERDAL® is taken in combination with other centrally acting drugs and alcohol.

Because of its potential for inducing hypotension, RISPERDAL® may enhance the hypotensive effects of other therapeutic agents with this potential.

RISPERDAL® may antagonize the effects of levodopa and dopamine agonists.

Amytriptyline does not affect the pharmacokinetics of risperidone or the active antipsychotic fraction. Cimetidine and ranitidine increased the bioavailability of risperidone, but only marginally increased the plasma concentration of the active antipsychotic fraction.

Chronic administration of clozapine with risperidone may decrease the clearance of risperidone.

Carbamazepine and Other Enzyme Inducers

In a drug interaction study in schizophrenic patients, 11 subjects received risperidone titrated to 6 mg/day for 3 weeks, followed by concurrent administration of carbamazepine for an additional 3 weeks. During co-administration, the plasma concentrations of risperidone and its pharmacologically active metabolite, 9-hydroxyrisperidone, were decreased by about 50%. Plasma concentrations of carbamazepine did not appear to be affected. The dose of risperidone may need to be titrated accordingly for patients receiving carbamazepine, particularly during initiation or discontinuation of carbamazepine therapy. Co-administration of other known enzyme inducers (e.g., phenytoin, rifampin, and phenobarbital) with risperidone may cause similar decreases in the combined plasma concentrations of risperidone and 9-hydroxyrisperidone, which could lead to decreased efficacy of risperidone treatment.

Fluoxetine and Paroxetine

Fluoxetine (20 mg QD) and paroxetine (20 mg QD) have been shown to increase the plasma concentration of risperidone 2.5–2.8 fold and 3-9 fold respectively. Fluoxetine did not affect the plasma concentration of 9-hydroxyrisperidone. Paroxetine lowered the concentration of 9-hydroxyrisperidone an average of 13%. When either concomitant fluoxetine or paroxetine is initiated or discontinued, the physician should re-evaluate the dosing of RISPERDAL®. The effects of discontinuation of concomitant fluoxetine or paroxetine therapy on the pharmacokinetics of risperidone and 9-hydroxyrisperidone have not been studied.

Lithium

Repeated oral doses of risperidone (3 mg BID) did not affect the exposure (AUC) or peak plasma concentrations (C_{max}) of lithium (n=13).

Valproate

Repeated oral doses of risperidone (4 mg QD) did not affect the pre-dose or average plasma concentrations and exposure (AUC) of valproate (1000 mg/day in three divided doses) compared to placebo (n=21). However, there was a 20% increase in valproate peak plasma concentration (C_{max}) after concomitant administration of risperidone.

Digoxin

RISPERDAL® (0.25 mg BID) did not show a clinically relevant effect on the pharmacokinetics of digoxin.

Drugs That Inhibit CYP 2D6 and Other CYP Isozymes

Risperidone is metabolized to 9-hydroxyrisperidone by CYP 2D6, an enzyme that is polymorphic in the population and that can be inhibited by a variety of psychotropic and other drugs (see CLINICAL PHARMACOLOGY). Drug interactions that reduce the metabolism of risperidone to 9-hydroxyrisperidone would increase the plasma concentrations of risperidone and lower the concentrations of 9-hydroxyrisperidone. Analysis of clinical studies involving a modest number of poor metabolizers (n≅70) does not suggest that poor and extensive metabolizers have different rates of adverse effects. No comparison of effectiveness in the two groups has been made.

In vitro studies showed that drugs metabolized by other CYP isozymes, including 1A1, 1A2, 2C9, 2C19, and 3A4, are only weak inhibitors of risperidone metabolism.

There were no significant interactions between risperidone and erythromycin (see CLINICAL PHARMACOLOGY).

Drugs Metabolized by CYP 2D6

In vitro studies indicate that risperidone is a relatively weak inhibitor of CYP 2D6. Therefore, RISPERDAL® is not expected to substantially inhibit the clearance of drugs that are metabolized by this enzymatic pathway. In drug interaction studies, risperidone did not significantly affect the pharmacokinetics of donepezil and galantamine, which are metabolized by CYP 2D6.

Carcinogenesis, Mutagenesis, Impairment of Fertility

Carcinogenesis

Carcinogenicity studies were conducted in Swiss albino mice and Wistar rats. Risperidone was administered in the diet at doses of 0.63, 2.5, and 10 mg/kg for 18 months to mice and for 25 months to rats. These doses are equivalent to 2.4, 9.4, and 37.5 times the maximum recommended human dose (MRHD) (16 mg/day) on a mg/kg basis or 0.2, 0.75, and 3 times the MRHD (mice) or 0.4, 1.5, and 6 times the MRHD (rats) on a mg/m² basis. A maximum tolerated dose was not achieved in male mice. There were statistically significant increases in pituitary gland adenomas, endocrine pancreas adenomas, and mammary gland adenocarcinomas. The following table summarizes the multiples of the human dose on a mg/m² (mg/kg) basis at which these tumors occurred.

[See table above]

Antipsychotic drugs have been shown to chronically elevate prolactin levels in rodents. Serum prolactin levels were not measured during the risperidone carcinogenicity studies; however, measurements during subchronic toxicity studies showed that risperidone elevated serum prolactin levels 5–6 fold in mice and rats at the same doses used in the carcinogenicity studies. An increase in mammary, pituitary, and endocrine pancreas neoplasms has been found in rodents after chronic administration of other antipsychotic drugs and is considered to be prolactin-mediated. The relevance for human risk of the findings of prolactin-mediated endocrine tumors in rodents is unknown (see PRECAUTIONS, General—Hyperprolactinemia).

Mutagenesis

No evidence of mutagenic potential for risperidone was found in the Ames reverse mutation test, mouse lymphoma assay, in vitro rat hepatocyte DNA-repair assay, in vivo micronucleus test in mice, the sex-linked recessive lethal test in Drosophila, or the chromosomal aberration test in human lymphocytes or Chinese hamster cells.

Impairment of Fertility

Risperidone (0.16 to 5 mg/kg) was shown to impair mating, but not fertility, in Wistar rats in three reproductive studies (two Segment I and a multigenerational study) at doses 0.1 to 3 times the maximum recommended human dose (MRHD) on a mg/m² basis. The effect appeared to be in females, since impaired mating behavior was not noted in the Segment I study in which males only were treated. In a subchronic study in Beagle dogs in which risperidone was administered at doses of 0.31 to 5 mg/kg, sperm motility and concentration were decreased at doses 0.6 to 10 times the MRHD on a mg/m² basis. Dose-related decreases were also noted in serum testosterone at the same doses. Serum testosterone and sperm parameters partially recovered, but remained decreased after treatment was discontinued. No no-effect doses were noted in either rat or dog.

Pregnancy

Pregnancy Category C

The teratogenic potential of risperidone was studied in three Segment II studies in Sprague-Dawley and Wistar rats (0.63–10 mg/kg or 0.4 to 6 times the maximum recommended human dose [MRHD] on a mg/m² basis) and in one Segment II study in New Zealand rabbits (0.31–5 mg/kg or 0.4 to 6 times the MRHD on a mg/m² basis). The incidence of malformations was not increased compared to control in offspring of rats or rabbits given 0.4 to 6 times the MRHD on a mg/m² basis. In three reproductive studies in rats (two Segment III and a multigenerational study), there was an

Continued on next page

Risperdal—Cont.

increase in pup deaths during the first 4 days of lactation at doses of 0.16–5 mg/kg or 0.1 to 3 times the MRHD on a mg/m² basis. It is not known whether these deaths were due to a direct effect on the fetuses or pups or to effects on the dams.

There was no no-effect dose for increased rat pup mortality. In one Segment III study, there was an increase in stillborn rat pups at a dose of 2.5 mg/kg or 1.5 times the MRHD on a mg/m² basis. In a cross-fostering study in Wistar rats, toxic effects on the fetus or pups, as evidenced by a decrease in the number of live pups and an increase in the number of dead pups at birth (Day 0), and a decrease in birth weight in pups of drug-treated dams were observed. In addition, there was an increase in deaths by Day 1 among pups of drug-treated dams, regardless of whether or not the pups were cross-fostered. Risperidone also appeared to impair maternal behavior in that pup body weight gain and survival (from Day 1 to 4 of lactation) were reduced in pups born to control but reared by drug-treated dams. These effects were all noted at the one dose of risperidone tested, i.e., 5 mg/kg or 3 times the MRHD on a mg/m² basis.

Placental transfer of risperidone occurs in rat pups. There are no adequate and well-controlled studies in pregnant women. However, there was one report of a case of agenesis of the corpus callosum in an infant exposed to risperidone *in utero*. The causal relationship to RISPERDAL® therapy is unknown.

RISPERDAL® should be used during pregnancy only if the potential benefit justifies the potential risk to the fetus.

Labor and Delivery

The effect of RISPERDAL® on labor and delivery in humans is unknown.

Nursing Mothers

In animal studies, risperidone and 9-hydroxyrisperidone are excreted in milk. Risperidone and 9-hydroxyrisperidone are also excreted in human breast milk. Therefore, women receiving risperidone should not breast-feed.

Pediatric Use

Safety and effectiveness in children have not been established.

Geriatric Use

Clinical studies of RISPERDAL® did not include sufficient numbers of patients aged 65 and over to determine whether or not they respond differently than younger patients. Other reported clinical experience has not identified differences in responses between elderly and younger patients. In general, a lower starting dose is recommended for an elderly patient, reflecting a decreased pharmacokinetic clearance in the elderly, as well as a greater frequency of decreased hepatic, renal, or cardiac function, and of concomitant disease or other drug therapy (see CLINICAL PHARMACOLOGY and DOSAGE AND ADMINISTRATION). While elderly patients exhibit a greater tendency to orthostatic hypotension, its risk in the elderly may be minimized by limiting the initial dose to 0.5 mg BID followed by careful titration (see PRECAUTIONS). Monitoring of orthostatic vital signs should be considered in patients for whom this is of concern.

This drug is substantially excreted by the kidneys, and the risk of toxic reactions to this drug may be greater in patients with impaired renal function. Because elderly patients are more likely to have decreased renal function, care should be taken in dose selection, and it may be useful to monitor renal function (see DOSAGE AND ADMINISTRATION).

ADVERSE REACTIONS

The following findings are based on the short-term, placebo-controlled, North American, premarketing trials for schizophrenia and acute bipolar mania. In patients with Bipolar I Disorder, treatment-emergent adverse events are presented separately for risperidone as monotherapy and as adjunctive therapy to mood stabilizers.

Certain portions of the discussion below relating to objective or numeric safety parameters, namely dose-dependent adverse events, vital sign changes, weight gain, laboratory changes, and ECG changes are derived from studies in patients with schizophrenia. However, this information is also generally applicable to bipolar mania.

Associated With Discontinuation of Treatment

Schizophrenia

Approximately 9% (244/2607) of RISPERDAL® (risperidone)-treated patients in Phase 2 and 3 studies discontinued treatment due to an adverse event, compared with about 7% on placebo and 10% on active control drugs. The more common events (≥0.3%) associated with discontinuation and considered to be possibly or probably drug-related included:

Adverse Event	RISPERDAL®	Placebo
Extrapyramidal symptoms	2.1%	0%
Dizziness	0.7%	0%
Hyperkinesia	0.6%	0%
Somnolence	0.5%	0%
Nausea	0.3%	0%

Suicide attempt was associated with discontinuation in 1.2% of RISPERDAL®-treated patients compared to 0.6% of placebo patients, but, given the almost 40-fold greater exposure time in RISPERDAL® compared to placebo patients, it is unlikely that suicide attempt is a RISPERDAL®-related adverse event (see PRECAUTIONS). Discontinuation for extrapyramidal symptoms was 0% in placebo patients, but 3.8% in active-control patients in the Phase 2 and 3 trials.

Bipolar Mania

In the US placebo-controlled trial with risperidone as monotherapy, approximately 8% (10/134) of RISPERDAL®-treated patients discontinued treatment due to an adverse event, compared with approximately 6% (7/125) of placebo-treated patients. The adverse events associated with discontinuation and considered to be possibly, probably, or very likely drug-related included paroniria, somnolence, dizziness, extrapyramidal disorder, and muscle contractions involuntary. Each of these events occurred in one RISPERDAL®-treated patient (0.7%) and in no placebo-treated patients (0%).

In the US placebo-controlled trial with risperidone as adjunctive therapy to mood stabilizers, there was no overall difference in the incidence of discontinuation due to adverse events (4% for RISPERDAL® vs. 4% for placebo).

Incidence in Controlled Trials

Commonly Observed Adverse Events in Controlled Clinical Trials

Schizophrenia

In two 6- to 8-week placebo-controlled trials, spontaneously-reported, treatment-emergent adverse events with an incidence of 5% or greater in at least one of the RISPERDAL® groups and at least twice that of placebo were anxiety, somnolence, extra-pyramidal symptoms, dizziness, constipation, nausea, dyspepsia, rhinitis, rash, and tachycardia.

Adverse events were also elicited in one of these two trials (i.e., in the fixed-dose trial comparing RISPERDAL® at doses of 2, 6, 10, and 16 mg/day with placebo) utilizing a checklist for detecting adverse events, a method that is more sensitive than spontaneous reporting. By this method, the following additional common and drug-related adverse events occurred at an incidence of at least 5% and twice the rate of placebo: increased dream activity, increased duration of sleep, accommodation disturbances, reduced salivation, micturition disturbances, diarrhea, weight gain, menorrhagia, diminished sexual desire, erectile dysfunction, ejaculatory dysfunction, and orgastic dysfunction.

Bipolar Mania

In the US placebo-controlled trial with risperidone as monotherapy, the most commonly observed adverse events associated with the use of RISPERDAL® (incidence of 5% or greater and at least twice that of placebo) were somnolence, dystonia, akathisia, dyspepsia, nausea, parkinsonism, vision abnormal, and saliva increased. In the US placebo-controlled trial with risperidone as adjunctive therapy to mood stabilizers, the most commonly observed adverse events associated with the use of RISPERDAL® were somnolence, dizziness, parkinsonism, saliva increased, akathisia, abdominal pain, and urinary incontinence.

Adverse Events Occurring at an Incidence of 1% or More Among RISPERDAL®-Treated Patients - Schizophrenia

The table that follows enumerates adverse events that occurred at an incidence of 1% or more, and were more frequent among RISPERDAL®-treated patients treated at doses of ≤ 10 mg/day than among placebo-treated patients in the pooled results of two 6- to 8-week controlled trials. Patients received RISPERDAL® doses of 2, 6, 10, or 16 mg/day in the dose comparison trial, or up to a maximum dose of 10 mg/day in the titration study. This table shows the percentage of patients in each dose group (≤ 10 mg/day or 16 mg/day) who spontaneously reported at least one episode of an event at some time during their treatment. Patients given doses of 2, 6, or 10 mg did not differ materially in these rates. Reported adverse events were classified using the World Health Organization preferred terms.

The prescriber should be aware that these figures cannot be used to predict the incidence of side effects in the course of usual medical practice where patient characteristics and other factors differ from those which prevailed in this clinical trial. Similarly, the cited frequencies cannot be compared with figures obtained from other clinical investigations involving different treatments, uses, and investigators. The cited figures, however, do provide the prescribing physician with some basis for estimating the relative contribution of drug and non-drug factors to the side effect incidence rate in the population studied.

Table 1. Incidence of Treatment-Emergent Adverse Events in 6- to 8-Week Controlled Clinical Trials[1]

Body System/ Preferred Term	RISPERDAL® ≤10 mg/day (N=324)	RISPERDAL® 16 mg/day (N=77)	Placebo (N=142)
Psychiatric			
Insomnia	26%	23%	19%
Agitation	22%	26%	20%
Anxiety	12%	20%	9%
Somnolence	3%	8%	1%
Aggressive reaction	1%	3%	1%
Central & peripheral nervous system			
Extrapyramidal symptoms[2]	17%	34%	16%
Headache	14%	12%	12%
Dizziness	4%	7%	1%
Gastrointestinal			
Constipation	7%	13%	3%
Nausea	6%	4%	3%
Dyspepsia	5%	10%	4%
Vomiting	5%	7%	4%
Abdominal pain	4%	1%	0%
Saliva increased	2%	0%	1%
Toothache	2%	0%	0%
Respiratory system			
Rhinitis	10%	8%	4%
Coughing	3%	3%	1%
Sinusitis	2%	1%	1%
Pharyngitis	2%	3%	0%
Dyspnea	1%	0%	0%
Body as a whole-general			
Back pain	2%	0%	1%
Chest pain	2%	3%	1%
Fever	2%	3%	0%
Dermatological			
Rash	2%	5%	1%
Dry skin	2%	4%	0%
Seborrhea	1%	0%	0%
Infections			
Upper respiratory	3%	3%	1%
Visual			
Abnormal vision	2%	1%	1%
Musculo-Skeletal			
Arthralgia	2%	3%	0%
Cardiovascular			
Tachycardia	3%	5%	0%

[1] Events reported by at least 1% of patients treated with RISPERDAL® ≤ 10 mg/day are included, and are rounded to the nearest %. Comparative rates for RISPERDAL® 16 mg/day and placebo are provided as well. Events for which the RISPERDAL® incidence (in both dose groups) was equal to or less than placebo are not listed in the table, but included the following: nervousness, injury, and fungal infection.

[2] Includes tremor, dystonia, hypokinesia, hypertonia, hyperkinesia, oculogyric crisis, ataxia, abnormal gait, involuntary muscle contractions, hyporeflexia, akathisia, and extrapyramidal disorders. Although the incidence of 'extrapyramidal symptoms' does not appear to differ for the '10 mg/day' group and placebo, the data for individual dose groups in fixed dose trials do suggest a dose/response relationship (see ADVERSE REACTIONS – Dose Dependency of Adverse Events).

Adverse Events Occurring at an Incidence of 2% or More Among RISPERDAL®-Treated Patients - Bipolar Mania

Tables 2 and 3 display adverse events that occurred at an incidence of 2% or more, and were more frequent among patients treated with flexible doses of RISPERDAL® (1–6 mg daily as monotherapy and as adjunctive therapy to mood stabilizers, respectively) than among patients treated with placebo. Reported adverse events were classified using the World Health Organization preferred terms.

Table 2. Incidence of Treatment-Emergent Adverse Events in a 3-Week, Placebo-Controlled Trial - Monotherapy in Bipolar Mania[1]

Body System/ Preferred Term	RISPERDAL® (N=134)	Placebo (N=125)
Central & peripheral nervous system		
Dystonia	18%	6%
Akathisia	16%	6%
Dizziness	11%	9%
Parkinsonism	6%	3%
Hypoaesthesia	2%	1%
Psychiatric		
Somnolence	28%	7%
Agitation	8%	6%
Manic reaction	8%	6%
Anxiety	4%	2%
Concentration impaired	2%	1%
Gastrointestinal system		
Dyspepsia	11%	6%
Nausea	11%	2%
Saliva increased	5%	1%
Mouth dry	3%	2%
Body as a whole - general		
Pain	5%	3%
Fatigue	4%	2%
Injury	2%	0%
Respiratory system		
Sinusitis	4%	1%
Rhinitis	3%	2%
Coughing	2%	2%
Skin and appendages		
Acne	2%	0%
Pruritus	2%	1%
Musculo-Skeletal		
Myalgia	5%	2%
Skeletal pain	2%	1%
Metabolic and nutritional		
Weight increase	2%	0%
Vision disorders		
Vision abnormal	6%	2%
Cardiovascular, general		
Hypertension	3%	1%
Hypotension	2%	0%
Heart rate and rhythm		
Tachycardia	3%	2%

[1] Events reported by at least 2% of patients treated with RISPERDAL® are included and are rounded to the nearest %. Events reported by at least 2% of patients treated with RISPERDAL® that were less than the incidence reported by patients treated with placebo are not listed in the table, but included the following: headache, tremor, insomnia,

constipation, back pain, upper respiratory tract infection, pharyngitis, and arthralgia.

Table 3. Incidence of Treatment-Emergent Adverse Events in a 3-Week, Placebo-Controlled Trial - Adjunctive in Bipolar Mania[1]

Body System/ Preferred Term	RISPERDAL® + Mood Stabilizer (N=152)	Placebo + Mood Stabilizer (N=51)
Gastrointestinal system		
Saliva increased	10%	0%
Diarrhea	8%	4%
Abdominal pain	6%	0%
Constipation	6%	4%
Mouth dry	6%	4%
Tooth ache	4%	0%
Tooth disorder	4%	0%
Central & peripheral nervous sytem		
Dizziness	14%	2%
Parkinsonism	14%	4%
Akathisia	8%	0%
Dystonia	6%	4%
Psychiatric		
Somnolence	25%	12%
Anxiety	6%	4%
Confusion	4%	0%
Respiratory system		
Rhinitis	8%	4%
Pharyngitis	6%	4%
Coughing	4%	0%
Body as a whole - general		
Asthenia	4%	2%
Urinary system		
Urinary incontinence	6%	2%
Heart rate and rhythm		
Tachycardia	4%	2%
Metabolic and nutritional		
Weight increase	4%	2%
Skin and appendages		
Rash	4%	2%

[1] Events reported by at least 2% of patients treated with RISPERDAL® are included and are rounded to the nearest %. Events reported by at least 2% of patients treated with RISPERDAL® that were less than the incidence reported by patients treated with placebo are not listed in the table, but included the following: dyspepsia, nausea, vomiting, headache, tremor, insomnia, chest pain, fatigue, pain, skeletal pain, hypertension, and vision abnormal.

Dose Dependency of Adverse Events

Extrapyramidal Symptoms

Data from two fixed-dose trials provided evidence of dose-relatedness for extrapyramidal symptoms associated with risperidone treatment.

Two methods were used to measure extrapyramidal symptoms (EPS) in an 8-week trial comparing 4 fixed doses of risperidone (2, 6, 10, and 16 mg/day), including (1) a parkinsonism score (mean change from baseline) from the Extrapyramidal Symptom Rating Scale, and (2) incidence of spontaneous complaints of EPS:

Dose Groups	Placebo	Ris 2	Ris 6	Ris 10	Ris 16
Parkinsonism	1.2	0.9	1.8	2.4	2.6
EPS Incidence	13%	13%	16%	20%	31%

Similar methods were used to measure extrapyramidal symptoms (EPS) in an 8-week trial comparing 5 fixed doses of risperidone (1, 4, 8, 12, and 16 mg/day):

Dose Groups	Ris 1	Ris 4	Ris 8	Ris 12	Ris 16
Parkinsonism	0.6	1.7	2.4	2.9	4.1
EPS Incidence	7%	12%	18%	18%	21%

Other Adverse Events

Adverse event data elicited by a checklist for side effects from a large study comparing 5 fixed doses of RISPERDAL® (1, 4, 8, 12, and 16 mg/day) were explored for dose-relatedness of adverse events. A Cochran-Armitage Test for trend in these data revealed a positive trend ($p<0.05$) for the following adverse events: sleepiness, increased duration of sleep, accommodation disturbances, orthostatic dizziness, palpitations, weight gain, erectile dysfunction, ejaculatory dysfunction, orgastic dysfunction, asthenia/lassitude/increased fatigability, and increased pigmentation.

Vital Sign Changes

RISPERDAL® is associated with orthostatic hypotension and tachycardia (see PRECAUTIONS).

Weight Changes

The proportions of RISPERDAL® and placebo-treated patients meeting a weight gain criterion of ≥7% of body weight were compared in a pool of 6- to 8-week, placebo-controlled trials, revealing a statistically significantly greater incidence of weight gain for RISPERDAL® (18%) compared to placebo (9%).

Laboratory Changes

A between-group comparison for 6- to 8-week placebo-controlled trials revealed no statistically significant RISPERDAL®/placebo differences in the proportions of patients experiencing potentially important changes in routine serum chemistry, hematology, or urinalysis parameters. Similarly, there were no RISPERDAL®/placebo differences in the incidence of discontinuations for changes in serum chemistry, hematology, or urinalysis. However, RISPERDAL® administration was associated with increases in serum prolactin (see PRECAUTIONS).

ECG Changes

Between-group comparisons for pooled placebo-controlled trials revealed no statistically significant differences between risperidone and placebo in mean changes from baseline in ECG parameters, including QT, QTc, and PR intervals, and heart rate. When all RISPERDAL® doses were pooled from randomized controlled trials in several indications, there was a mean increase in heart rate of 1 beat per minute compared to no change for placebo patients. In short-term schizophrenia trials, higher doses of risperidone (8–16 mg/day) were associated with a higher mean increase in heart rate compared to placebo (4–6 beats per minute).

Other Events Observed During the Premarketing Evaluation of RISPERDAL®

During its premarketing assessment, multiple doses of RISPERDAL® were administered to 2607 patients in Phase 2 and 3 studies. The conditions and duration of exposure to RISPERDAL® varied greatly, and included (in overlapping categories) open-label and double-blind studies, uncontrolled and controlled studies, inpatient and outpatient studies, fixed-dose and titration studies, and short-term or longer-term exposure. In most studies, untoward events associated with this exposure were obtained by spontaneous report and recorded by clinical investigators using terminology of their own choosing. Consequently, it is not possible to provide a meaningful estimate of the proportion of individuals experiencing adverse events without first grouping similar types of untoward events into a smaller number of standardized event categories. In two large studies, adverse events were also elicited utilizing the UKU (direct questioning) side effect rating scale, and these events were not further categorized using standard terminology. (Note: These events are marked with an asterisk in the listings that follow.)

In the listings that follow, spontaneously reported adverse events were classified using World Health Organization (WHO) preferred terms. The frequencies presented, therefore, represent the proportion of the 2607 patients exposed to multiple doses of RISPERDAL® who experienced an event of the type cited on at least one occasion while receiving RISPERDAL®. All reported events are included, except those already listed in Table 1, those events for which a drug cause was remote, and those event terms which were so general as to be uninformative. It is important to emphasize that, although the events reported occurred during treatment with RISPERDAL®, they were not necessarily caused by it.

Events are further categorized by body system and listed in order of decreasing frequency according to the following definitions: frequent adverse events are those occurring in at least 1/100 patients (only those not already listed in the tabulated results from placebo-controlled trials appear in this listing); infrequent adverse events are those occurring in 1/100 to 1/1000 patients; rare events are those occurring in fewer than 1/1000 patients.

Psychiatric Disorders

Frequent: increased dream activity*, diminished sexual desire*, nervousness. *Infrequent*: impaired concentration, depression, apathy, catatonic reaction, euphoria, increased libido, amnesia. *Rare*: emotional lability, nightmares, delirium, withdrawal syndrome, yawning.

Central and Peripheral Nervous System Disorders

Frequent: increased sleep duration*. *Infrequent*: dysarthria, vertigo, stupor, paraesthesia, confusion. *Rare*: aphasia, cholinergic syndrome, hypoesthesia, tongue paralysis, leg cramps, torticollis, hypotonia, coma, migraine, hyperreflexia, choreoathetosis.

Gastrointestinal Disorders

Frequent: anorexia, reduced salivation*. *Infrequent*: flatulence, diarrhea, increased appetite, stomatitis, melena, dysphagia, hemorrhoids, gastritis. *Rare*: fecal incontinence, eructation, gastroesophageal reflux, gastroenteritis, esophagitis, tongue discoloration, cholelithiasis, tongue edema, diverticulitis, gingivitis, discolored feces, GI hemorrhage, hematemesis.

Body as a Whole/General Disorders

Frequent: fatigue. *Infrequent*: edema, rigors, malaise, influenza-like symptoms. *Rare*: pallor, enlarged abdomen, allergic reaction, ascites, sarcoidosis, flushing.

Respiratory System Disorders

Infrequent: hyperventilation, bronchospasm, pneumonia, stridor. *Rare*: asthma, increased sputum, aspiration.

Skin and Appendage Disorders

Frequent: increased pigmentation*, photosensitivity*. *Infrequent*: increased sweating, acne, decreased sweating, alopecia, hyperkeratosis, pruritus, skin exfoliation. *Rare*: bullous eruption, skin ulceration, aggravated psoriasis, furunculosis, verruca, dermatitis lichenoid, hypertrichosis, genital pruritus, urticaria.

Cardiovascular Disorders

Infrequent: palpitation, hypertension, hypotension, AV block, myocardial infarction. *Rare*: ventricular tachycardia, angina pectoris, premature atrial contractions, T wave inversions, ventricular extrasystoles, ST depression, myocarditis.

Vision Disorders

Infrequent: abnormal accommodation, xerophthalmia. *Rare*: diplopia, eye pain, blepharitis, photopsia, photophobia, abnormal lacrimation.

Metabolic and Nutritional Disorders

Infrequent: hyponatremia, weight increase, creatinine phosphokinase increase, thirst, weight decrease, diabetes mellitus. *Rare*: decreased serum iron, cachexia, dehydration, hypokalemia, hypoproteinemia, hyperphosphatemia, hypertriglyceridemia, hyperuricemia, hypoglycemia.

Urinary System Disorders

Frequent: polyuria/polydipsia*. *Infrequent*: urinary incontinence, hematuria, dysuria. *Rare*: urinary retention, cystitis, renal insufficiency.

Musculo-Skeletal System Disorders

Infrequent: myalgia. *Rare*: arthrosis, synostosis, bursitis, arthritis, skeletal pain.

Reproductive Disorders, Female

Frequent: menorrhagia*, orgastic dysfunction*, dry vagina*. *Infrequent*: nonpuerperal lactation, amenorrhea, female breast pain, leukorrhea, mastitis, dysmenorrhea, female perineal pain, intermenstrual bleeding, vaginal hemorrhage.

Liver and Biliary System Disorders

Infrequent: increased SGOT, increased SGPT. *Rare*: hepatic failure, cholestatic hepatitis, cholecystitis, cholelithiasis, hepatitis, hepatocellular damage.

Platelet, Bleeding, and Clotting Disorders

Infrequent: epistaxis, purpura. *Rare*: hemorrhage, superficial phlebitis, thrombophlebitis, thrombocytopenia.

Hearing and Vestibular Disorders

Rare: tinnitus, hyperacusis, decreased hearing.

Red Blood Cell Disorders

Infrequent: anemia, hypochromic anemia. *Rare*: normocytic anemia.

Reproductive Disorders, Male

Frequent: erectile dysfunction*. *Infrequent*: ejaculation failure.

White Cell and Resistance Disorders

Rare: leukocytosis, lymphadenopathy, leucopenia, Pelger-Huet anomaly.

Endocrine Disorders

Rare: gynecomastia, male breast pain, antidiuretic hormone disorder.

Special Senses

Rare: bitter taste.

* Incidence based on elicited reports.

Postintroduction Reports

Adverse events reported since market introduction which were temporally (but not necessarily causally) related to RISPERDAL® therapy, include the following: anaphylactic reaction, angioedema, apnea, atrial fibrillation, cerebrovascular disorder, including cerebrovascular accident, hyperglycemia, diabetes mellitus aggravated, including diabetic ketoacidosis, intestinal obstruction, jaundice, mania, pancreatitis, Parkinson's disease aggravated, pulmonary embolism. There have been rare reports of sudden death and/or cardiopulmonary arrest in patients receiving RISPERDAL®. A causal relationship with RISPERDAL® has not been established. It is important to note that sudden and unexpected death may occur in psychotic patients whether they remain untreated or whether they are treated with other antipsychotic drugs.

DRUG ABUSE AND DEPENDENCE

Controlled Substance Class

RISPERDAL® (risperidone) is not a controlled substance.

Physical and Psychological Dependence

RISPERDAL® has not been systematically studied in animals or humans for its potential for abuse, tolerance, or physical dependence. While the clinical trials did not reveal any tendency for any drug-seeking behavior, these observations were not systematic and it is not possible to predict on the basis of this limited experience the extent to which a CNS-active drug will be misused, diverted, and/or abused once marketed. Consequently, patients should be evaluated carefully for a history of drug abuse, and such patients should be observed closely for signs of RISPERDAL® misuse or abuse (e.g., development of tolerance, increases in dose, drug-seeking behavior).

OVERDOSAGE

Human Experience

Premarketing experience included eight reports of acute RISPERDAL® (risperidone) overdosage with estimated doses ranging from 20 to 300 mg and no fatalities. In general, reported signs and symptoms were those resulting from an exaggeration of the drug's known pharmacological effects, i.e., drowsiness and sedation, tachycardia and hypotension, and extrapyramidal symptoms. One case, involving an estimated overdose of 240 mg, was associated with hyponatremia, hypokalemia, prolonged QT, and widened QRS. Another case, involving an estimated overdose of 36 mg, was associated with a seizure.

Postmarketing experience includes reports of acute RISPERDAL® overdosage, with estimated doses of up to 360 mg. In general, the most frequently reported signs and symptoms are those resulting from an exaggeration of the drug's known pharmacological effects, i.e., drowsiness, sedation, tachycardia, hypotension, and extrapyramidal symptoms. Other adverse events reported since market introduction which were temporally (but not necessarily causally) related to RISPERDAL® overdose, include torsade de

Continued on next page

Risperdal—Cont.

pointes, prolonged QT interval, convulsions, cardiopulmonary arrest, and rare fatality associated with multiple drug overdose.

Management of Overdosage

In case of acute overdosage, establish and maintain an airway and ensure adequate oxygenation and ventilation. Gastric lavage (after intubation, if patient is unconscious) and administration of activated charcoal together with a laxative should be considered. Because of the rapid disintegration of RISPERDAL® M-TAB™ Orally Disintegrating Tablets, pill fragments may not appear in gastric contents obtained with lavage.

The possibility of obtundation, seizures, or dystonic reaction of the head and neck following overdose may create a risk of aspiration with induced emesis. Cardiovascular monitoring should commence immediately and should include continuous electrocardiographic monitoring to detect possible arrhythmias. If antiarrhythmic therapy is administered, disopyramide, procainamide, and quinidine carry a theoretical hazard of QT-prolonging effects that might be additive to those of risperidone. Similarly, it is reasonable to expect that the alpha-blocking properties of bretylium might be additive to those of risperidone, resulting in problematic hypotension.

There is no specific antidote to RISPERDAL®. Therefore, appropriate supportive measures should be instituted. The possibility of multiple drug involvement should be considered. Hypotension and circulatory collapse should be treated with appropriate measures, such as intravenous fluids and/or sympathomimetic agents (epinephrine and dopamine should not be used, since beta stimulation may worsen hypotension in the setting of risperidone-induced alpha blockade). In cases of severe extrapyramidal symptoms, anticholinergic medication should be administered. Close medical supervision and monitoring should continue until the patient recovers.

DOSAGE AND ADMINISTRATION

Schizophrenia

Usual Initial Dose

RISPERDAL® (risperidone) can be administered on either a BID or a QD schedule. In early clinical trials, RISPERDAL® was generally administered at 1 mg BID initially, with increases in increments of 1 mg BID on the second and third day, as tolerated, to a target dose of 3 mg BID by the third day. Subsequent controlled trials have indicated that total daily risperidone doses of up to 8 mg on a QD regimen are also safe and effective. However, regardless of which regimen is employed, in some patients a slower titration may be medically appropriate. Further dosage adjustments, if indicated, should generally occur at intervals of not less than 1 week, since steady state for the active metabolite would not be achieved for approximately 1 week in the typical patient. When dosage adjustments are necessary, small dose increments/decrements of 1–2 mg are recommended.

Efficacy in schizophrenia was demonstrated in a dose range of 4 to 16 mg/day in the clinical trials supporting effectiveness of RISPERDAL®; however, maximal effect was generally seen in a range of 4 to 8 mg/day. Doses above 6 mg/day for BID dosing were not demonstrated to be more efficacious than lower doses, were associated with more extrapyramidal symptoms and other adverse effects, and are not generally recommended. In a single study supporting QD dosing, the efficacy results were generally stronger for 8 mg than for 4 mg. The safety of doses above 16 mg/day has not been evaluated in clinical trials.

Maintenance Therapy

While there is no body of evidence available to answer the question of how long the schizophrenic patient treated with RISPERDAL® should remain on it, the effectiveness of RISPERDAL® 2 mg/day to 8 mg/day at delaying relapse was demonstrated in a controlled trial in patients who had been clinically stable for at least 4 weeks and were then followed for a period of 1 to 2 years. In this trial, RISPERDAL® was administered on a QD schedule, at 1 mg QD initially, with increases to 2 mg QD on the second day, and to a target dose of 4 mg QD on the third day (see CLINICAL PHARMACOLOGY – Clinical Trials). Nevertheless, patients should be periodically reassessed to determine the need for maintenance treatment with an appropriate dose.

Reinitiation of Treatment in Patients Previously Discontinued

Although there are no data to specifically address reinitiation of treatment, it is recommended that when restarting patients who have had an interval off RISPERDAL®, the initial titration schedule should be followed.

Switching From Other Antipsychotics

There are no systematically collected data to specifically address switching schizophrenic patients from other antipsychotics to RISPERDAL®, or concerning concomitant administration with other antipsychotics. While immediate discontinuation of the previous antipsychotic treatment may be acceptable for some schizophrenic patients, more gradual discontinuation may be most appropriate for others. In all cases, the period of overlapping antipsychotic administration should be minimized. When switching schizophrenic patients from depot antipsychotics, if medically appropriate, initiate RISPERDAL® therapy in place of the next scheduled injection. The need for continuing existing EPS medication should be re-evaluated periodically.

Bipolar Mania

Usual Dose

Risperidone should be administered on a once daily schedule, starting with 2 mg to 3 mg per day. Dosage adjustments, if indicated, should occur at intervals of not less than 24 hours and in dosage increments/decrements of 1 mg per day, as studied in the short-term, placebo-controlled trials. In these trials, short-term (3 week) anti-manic efficacy was demonstrated in a flexible dosage range of 1-6 mg per day (see CLINICAL PHARMACOLOGY – Clinical Trials). RISPERDAL® doses higher than 6 mg per day were not studied.

Maintenance Therapy

There is no body of evidence available from controlled trials to guide a clinician in the longer-term management of a patient who improves during treatment of an acute manic episode with risperidone. While it is generally agreed that pharmacological treatment beyond an acute response in mania is desirable, both for maintenance of the initial response and for prevention of new manic episodes, there are no systematically obtained data to support the use of risperidone in such longer-term treatment (i.e., beyond 3 weeks).

Pediatric Use

Safety and effectiveness of RISPERDAL® in pediatric patients with schizophrenia or acute mania associated with Bipolar I Disorder have not been established.

Dosage in Special Populations

The recommended initial dose is 0.5 mg BID in patients who are elderly or debilitated, patients with severe renal or hepatic impairment, and patients either predisposed to hypotension or for whom hypotension would pose a risk. Dosage increases in these patients should be in increments of no more than 0.5 mg BID. Increases to dosages above 1.5 mg BID should generally occur at intervals of at least 1 week. In some patients, slower titration may be medically appropriate.

Elderly or debilitated patients, and patients with renal impairment, may have less ability to eliminate RISPERDAL® than normal adults. Patients with impaired hepatic function may have increases in the free fraction of risperidone, possibly resulting in an enhanced effect (see CLINICAL PHARMACOLOGY). Patients with a predisposition to hypotensive reactions or for whom such reactions would pose a particular risk likewise need to be titrated cautiously and carefully monitored (see PRECAUTIONS). If a once-a-day dosing regimen in the elderly or debilitated patient is being considered, it is recommended that the patient be titrated on a twice-a-day regimen for 2–3 days at the target dose. Subsequent switches to a once-a-day dosing regimen can be done thereafter.

Co-Administration of RISPERDAL® with Certain Other Medications

Co-administration of carbamazepine and other enzyme inducers (e.g., phenytoin, rifampin, phenobarbital) with risperidone would be expected to cause decreases in the plasma concentrations of active moiety (the sum of risperidone and 9-hydroxyrisperidone), which could lead to decreased efficacy of risperidone treatment. The dose of risperidone needs to be titrated accordingly for patients receiving these enzyme inducers, especially during initiation or discontinuation of therapy with these inducers (see CLINICAL PHARMACOLOGY and PRECAUTIONS).

Fluoxetine and paroxetine have been shown to increase the plasma concentration of risperidone 2.5–2.8 fold and 3–9 fold respectively. Fluoxetine did not affect the plasma concentration of 9-hydroxyrisperidone. Paroxetine lowered the concentration of 9-hydroxyrisperidone an average of 13%. The dose of risperidone needs to be titrated accordingly when fluoxetine or paroxetine is co-administered (see CLINICAL PHARMACOLOGY and PRECAUTIONS).

Directions for Use of RISPERDAL® M-TAB™ Orally Disintegrating Tablets

RISPERDAL® M-TAB™ Orally Disintegrating Tablets are supplied in blister packs of 4 tablet units each.

Tablet Accessing

Do not open the blister until ready to administer. For single tablet removal, separate one of the four blister units by tearing apart at the perforations. Bend the corner where indicated. Peel back foil to expose the tablet. DO NOT push the tablet through the foil because this could damage the tablet.

Tablet Administration

Using dry hands, remove the tablet from the blister unit and immediately place the entire RISPERDAL® M-TAB™ Orally Disintegrating Tablet on the tongue. The RISPERDAL® M-TAB™ Orally Disintegrating Tablet should be consumed immediately, as the tablet cannot be stored once removed from the blister unit. RISPERDAL® M-TAB™ Orally Disintegrating Tablets disintegrate in the mouth within seconds and can be swallowed subsequently with or without liquid. Patients should not attempt to split or to chew the tablet.

HOW SUPPLIED

RISPERDAL® (risperidone) tablets are imprinted "JANSSEN", and either "Ris" and the strength "0.25", "0.5", or "R" and the strength "1", "2", "3", or "4".

0.25 mg dark yellow tablet: bottles of 60 NDC 50458-301-04, bottles of 500 NDC 50458-301-50, hospital unit dose packs of 100 NDC 50458-301-01.

0.5 mg red-brown tablet: bottles of 60 NDC 50458-302-06, bottles of 500 NDC 50458-302-50, hospital unit dose packs of 100 NDC 50458-302-01.

1 mg white tablet: bottles of 60 NDC 50458-300-06, blister pack of 100 NDC 50458-300-01, bottles of 500 NDC 50458-300-50.

2 mg orange tablet: bottles of 60 NDC 50458-320-06, blister pack of 100 NDC 50458-320-01, bottles of 500 NDC 50458-320-50.

3 mg yellow tablet: bottles of 60 NDC 50458-330-06, blister pack of 100 NDC 50458-330-01, bottles of 500 NDC 50458-330-50.

4 mg green tablet: bottles of 60 NDC 50458-350-06, blister pack of 100 NDC 50458-350-01.

RISPERDAL® (risperidone) 1 mg/mL oral solution (NDC 50458-305-03) is supplied in 30 mL bottles with a calibrated (in milligrams and milliliters) pipette. The minimum calibrated volume is 0.25 mL, while the maximum calibrated volume is 3 mL.

Tests indicate that RISPERDAL® (risperidone) oral solution is compatible in the following beverages: water, coffee, orange juice, and low-fat milk; it is NOT compatible with either cola or tea, however.

RISPERDAL® M-TAB™ (risperidone) Orally Disintegrating Tablets are etched on one side with "R0.5", "R1", and "R2", respectively, and are packaged in blister packs of 4 (2 × 2) tablets.

0.5 mg light coral, round, biconvex tablets: 7 blister packages per box, NDC 50458-395-28, long-term care packaging of 30 tablets NDC 50458-395-30.

1 mg light coral, square, biconvex tablets: 7 blister packages per box, NDC 50458-315-28, long-term care packaging of 30 tablets NDC 50458-315-30.

2 mg light coral, round, biconvex tablets: 7 blister packages per box, NDC 50458-325-28.

Storage and Handling

RISPERDAL® tablets should be stored at controlled room temperature 15°–25°C (59°–77°F). Protect from light and moisture.

Keep out of reach of children.

RISPERDAL® 1 mg/mL oral solution should be stored at controlled room temperature 15°–25°C (59°–77°F). Protect from light and freezing.

Keep out of reach of children.

RISPERDAL® M-TAB™ Orally Disintegrating Tablets should be stored at controlled room temperature 15°–25°C (59°–77°F).

Keep out of reach of children.

7503226

US Patent 4,804,663

December 2003

RISPERDAL® tablets are manufactured by:
JOLLC, Gurabo, Puerto Rico or
Janssen-Cilag, SpA, Latina, Italy
RISPERDAL® oral solution is manufactured by:
Janssen Pharmaceutica N.V.
Beerse, Belgium
RISPERDAL® M-TAB™ Orally Disintegrating Tablets are manufactured by:
JOLLC, Gurabo, Puerto Rico
RISPERDAL® tablets, RISPERDAL® M-TAB™ Orally Disintegrating Tablets, and oral solution are distributed by:
Janssen Pharmaceutica Products, L.P.
Titusville, NJ 08560
JANSSEN
PHARMACEUTICA PRODUCTS, L.P.

SPORANOX® CAPSULES ℞

itraconazole

Prescribing information for this product, which appears on pages 1768–1772 of the 2004 PDR, has been completely revised as follows. Please write "See Supplement A" next to the product heading.

Congestive Heart Failure

SPORANOX® (itraconazole) Capsules should not be administered for the treatment of onychomycosis in patients with evidence of ventricular dysfunction such as congestive heart failure (CHF) or a history of CHF. If signs or symptoms of congestive heart failure occur during administration of SPORANOX® Capsules, discontinue administration. When itraconazole was administered intravenously to dogs and healthy human volunteers, negative inotropic effects were seen. (See CLINICAL PHARMACOLOGY: Special Populations, CONTRAINDICATIONS, WARNINGS, PRECAUTIONS: Drug Interactions and ADVERSE REACTIONS: Post-marketing Experience for more information.)

Drug Interactions: Coadministration of cisapride, pimozide, quinidine, dofetilide, or levacetylmethadol (levomethadyl) with SPORANOX® (itraconazole) Capsules, Injection or Oral Solution is contraindicated. SPORANOX®, a potent cytochrome P450 3A4 isoenzyme system (CYP3A4) inhibitor, may increase plasma concentrations of drugs metabolized by this pathway. Serious cardiovascular events, including QT prolongation, torsades de pointes, ventricular tachycardia, cardiac arrest, and/or sudden death have occurred in patients using cisapride, pimozide, levacetylmethadol (levomethadyl), or quinidine concomitantly with SPORANOX® and/or other CYP3A4 inhibitors. See CONTRAINDICATIONS, WARNINGS, and PRECAUTIONS: Drug Interactions for more information.

DESCRIPTION

SPORANOX® is the brand name for itraconazole, a synthetic triazole antifungal agent. Itraconazole is a 1:1:1:1 racemic mixture of four diastereomers (two enantiomeric pairs), each possessing three chiral centers. It may be represented by the following structural formula and nomenclature:

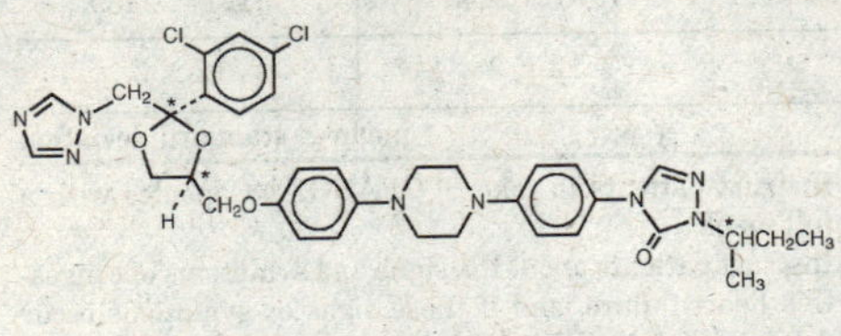

(±)-1-[(R*)-sec-butyl]-4-[p-[4-[p-[[(2R*,4S*)-2-(2,4-dichlorophenyl)-2-(1H-1,2,4-triazol-1-ylmethyl)-1,3-dioxolan-4-yl]methoxy] phenyl]-1-piperazinyl]phenyl]-Δ^2-1,2,4-triazolin-5-one mixture with (±)-1-[(R*)-sec-butyl]-4-[p-[4-[p-[[(2S*,4R*)-2-(2,4-dichlorophenyl)-2-(1H-1,2,4-triazol-1-ylmethyl)-1,3-dioxolan-4-yl]methoxy]phenyl]-1-piperazinyl] phenyl]-Δ^2-1,2,4-triazolin-5-one

or

(±)-1-[(RS)-sec-butyl]-4-[p-[4-[p-[[(2R,4S)-2-(2,4-dichlorophenyl)-2-(1H-1,2,4-triazol-1-ylmethyl)-1,3-dioxolan-4-yl] methoxy] phenyl]-1-piperazinyl]phenyl]-Δ^2-1,2,4-triazolin-5-one

Itraconazole has a molecular formula of $C_{35}H_{38}Cl_2N_8O_4$ and a molecular weight of 705.64. It is a white to slightly yellowish powder. It is insoluble in water, very slightly soluble in alcohols, and freely soluble in dichloromethane. It has a pKa of 3.70 (based on extrapolation of values obtained from methanolic solutions) and a log (n-octanol/water) partition coefficient of 5.66 at pH 8.1.

SPORANOX® Capsules contain 100 mg of itraconazole coated on sugar spheres. Inactive ingredients are gelatin, hypromellose, polyethylene glycol (PEG) 20,000, starch, sucrose, titanium dioxide, FD&C Blue No. 1, FD&C Blue No. 2, D&C Red No. 22 and D&C Red No. 28.

CLINICAL PHARMACOLOGY

Pharmacokinetics and Metabolism: NOTE: The plasma concentrations reported below were measured by high-performance liquid chromatography (HPLC) specific for itraconazole. When itraconazole in plasma is measured by a bioassay, values reported are approximately 3.3 times higher than those obtained by HPLC due to the presence of the bioactive metabolite, hydroxyitraconazole. (See MICROBIOLOGY.)

The pharmacokinetics of itraconazole after intravenous administration and its absolute oral bioavailability from an oral solution were studied in a randomized crossover study in 6 healthy male volunteers. The observed absolute oral bioavailability of itraconazole was 55%.

The oral bioavailability of itraconazole is maximal when SPORANOX® (itraconazole) Capsules are taken with a full meal. The pharmacokinetics of itraconazole were studied in 6 healthy male volunteers who received, in a crossover design, single 100-mg doses of itraconazole as a polyethylene glycol capsule, with or without a full meal. The same 6 volunteers also received 50 mg or 200 mg with a full meal in a crossover design. In this study, only itraconazole plasma concentrations were measured. The respective pharmacokinetic parameters for itraconazole are presented in the table below:

[See table below]

Doubling the SPORANOX® dose results in approximately a three-fold increase in the itraconazole plasma concentrations.

Values given in the table below represent data from a crossover pharmacokinetics study in which 27 healthy male volunteers each took a single 200-mg dose of SPORANOX® Capsules with or without a full meal:

[See table at top of next page]

Absorption of itraconazole under fasted conditions in individuals with relative or absolute achlorhydria, such as patients with AIDS or volunteers taking gastric acid secretion suppressors (e.g., H_2 receptor antagonists), was increased when SPORANOX® Capsules were administered with a cola beverage. Eighteen men with AIDS received single 200-mg doses of SPORANOX® Capsules under fasted conditions with 8 ounces of water or 8 ounces of a cola beverage in a crossover design. The absorption of itraconazole was increased when SPORANOX® Capsules were coadministered with a cola beverage, with AUC_{0-24} and C_{max} increasing 75% ± 121% and 95% ± 128%, respectively.

Thirty healthy men received single 200-mg doses of SPORANOX® Capsules under fasted conditions either 1) with water; 2) with water, after ranitidine 150 mg b.i.d. for 3 days; or 3) with cola, after ranitidine 150 mg b.i.d. for 3 days. When SPORANOX® Capsules were administered after ranitidine pretreatment, itraconazole was absorbed to a lesser extent than when SPORANOX® Capsules were administered alone, with decreases in AUC_{0-24} and C_{max} of 39% ± 37% and 42% ± 39%, respectively. When SPORANOX® Capsules were administered with cola after ranitidine pretreatment, itraconazole absorption was comparable to that observed when SPORANOX® Capsules were administered alone. (See PRECAUTIONS: Drug Interactions.)

Steady-state concentrations were reached within 15 days following oral doses of 50 mg to 400 mg daily. Values given in the table below are data at steady-state from a pharmacokinetics study in which 27 healthy male volunteers took 200-mg SPORANOX® Capsules b.i.d.(with a full meal) for 15 days:

	50 mg (fed)	100 mg (fed)	100 mg (fasted)	200 mg (fed)
C_{max} (ng/mL)	45 ± 16*	132 ± 67	38 ± 20	289 ± 100
T_{max} (hours)	3.2 ± 1.3	4.0 ± 1.1	3.3 ± 1.0	4.7 ± 1.4
$AUC_{0-\infty}$ (ng•h/mL)	567 ± 264	1899 ± 838	722 ± 289	5211 ± 2116

* mean ± standard deviation

	Itraconazole	Hydroxyitraconazole
C_{max} (ng/mL)	2282 ± 514*	3488 ± 742
C_{min} (ng/mL)	1855 ± 535	3349 ± 761
T_{max} (hours)	4.6 ± 1.8	3.4 ± 3.4
AUC_{0-12h} (ng•h/mL)	22569 ± 5375	38572 ± 8450
$t_{½}$ (hours)	64 ± 32	56 ± 24

* mean ± standard deviation

The plasma protein binding of itraconazole is 99.8% and that of hydroxyitraconazole is 99.5%. Following intravenous administration, the volume of distribution of itraconazole averaged 796 ± 185 liters.

Itraconazole is metabolized predominately by the cytochrome P450 3A4 isoenzyme system (CYP3A4), resulting in the formation of several metabolites, including hydroxyitraconazole, the major metabolite. Results of a pharmacokinetics study suggest that itraconazole may undergo saturable metabolism with multiple dosing. Fecal excretion of the parent drug varies between 3–18% of the dose. Renal excretion of the parent drug is less than 0.03% of the dose. About 40% of the dose is excreted as inactive metabolites in the urine. No single excreted metabolite represents more than 5% of a dose. Itraconazole total plasma clearance averaged 381 ± 95 mL/minute following intravenous administration. (See CONTRAINDICATIONS and PRECAUTIONS: Drug Interactions for more information.)

Special Populations:

Renal Insufficiency: A pharmacokinetic study using a single 200-mg dose of itraconazole (four 50-mg capsules) was conducted in three groups of patients with renal impairment (uremia: n=7; hemodialysis: n=7; and continuous ambulatory peritoneal dialysis: n=5). In uremic subjects with a mean creatinine clearance of 13 mL/min. x 1.73 m², the bioavailability was slightly reduced compared with normal population parameters. This study did not demonstrate any significant effect of hemodialysis or continuous ambulatory peritoneal dialysis on the pharmacokinetics of itraconazole (T_{max}, C_{max}, and AUC_{0-8}). Plasma concentration-versus-time profiles showed wide intersubject variation in all three groups.

Hepatic Insufficiency: A pharmacokinetic study using a single 100-mg dose of itraconazole (one 100-mg capsule) was conducted in 6 healthy and 12 cirrhotic subjects. No statistically significant differences in AUC were seen between these two groups. A statistically significant reduction in mean C_{max} (47%) and a twofold increase in the elimination half-life (37 ± 17 hours) of itraconazole were noted in cirrhotic subjects compared with healthy subjects. Patients with impaired hepatic function should be carefully monitored when taking itraconazole. The prolonged elimination half-life of itraconazole observed in cirrhotic patients should be considered when deciding to initiate therapy with other medications metabolized by CYP3A4. (See BOX WARNING, CONTRAINDICATIONS, and PRECAUTIONS: Drug Interactions.)

Decreased Cardiac Contractility: When itraconazole was administered intravenously to anesthetized dogs, a dose-related negative inotropic effect was documented. In a healthy volunteer study of SPORANOX® Injection (intravenous infusion), transient, asymptomatic decreases in left ventricular ejection fraction were observed using gated SPECT imaging; these resolved before the next infusion, 12 hours later. If signs or symptoms of congestive heart failure appear during administration of SPORANOX® Capsules, SPORANOX® should be discontinued. (See CONTRAINDICATIONS, WARNINGS, PRECAUTIONS: Drug Interactions and ADVERSE REACTIONS: Post-marketing Experience for more information.)

MICROBIOLOGY

Mechanism of Action: In vitro studies have demonstrated that itraconazole inhibits the cytochrome P450-dependent synthesis of ergosterol, which is a vital component of fungal cell membranes.

Activity In Vitro and In Vivo: Itraconazole exhibits in vitro activity against *Blastomyces dermatitidis, Histoplasma capsulatum, Histoplasma duboisii, Aspergillus flavus, Aspergillus fumigatus, Candida albicans,* and *Cryptococcus neoformans.* Itraconazole also exhibits varying in vitro activity against *Sporothrix schenckii, Trichophyton species, Candida krusei,* and other *Candida* species. The bioactive metabolite, hydroxyitraconazole, has not been evaluated against *Histoplasma capsulatum* and *Blastomyces dermatitidis.* Correlation between minimum inhibitory concentration (MIC) results in vitro and clinical outcome has yet to be established for azole antifungal agents.

Itraconazole administered orally was active in a variety of animal models of fungal infection using standard laboratory strains of fungi. Fungistatic activity has been demonstrated against disseminated fungal infections caused by *Blastomyces dermatitidis, Histoplasma duboisii, Aspergillus fumigatus, Coccidioides immitis, Cryptococcus neoformans, Paracoccidioides brasiliensis, Sporothrix schenckii, Trichophyton rubrum,* and *Trichophyton mentagrophytes.*

Itraconazole administered at 2.5 mg/kg and 5 mg/kg via the oral and parenteral routes increased survival rates and sterilized organ systems in normal and immunosuppressed guinea pigs with disseminated *Aspergillus fumigatus* infections. Oral itraconazole administered daily at 40 mg/kg and 80 mg/kg increased survival rates in normal rabbits with disseminated disease and in immunosuppressed rats with pulmonary *Aspergillus fumigatus* infection, respectively. Itraconazole has demonstrated antifungal activity in a variety of animal models infected with *Candida albicans* and other *Candida* species.

Resistance: Isolates from several fungal species with decreased susceptibility to itraconazole have been isolated in vitro and from patients receiving prolonged therapy.

Several in vitro studies have reported that some fungal clinical isolates, including *Candida* species, with reduced susceptibility to one azole antifungal agent may also be less susceptible to other azole derivatives. The finding of cross-resistance is dependent on a number of factors, including the species evaluated, its clinical history, the particular azole compounds compared, and the type of susceptibility test that is performed. The relevance of these in vitro susceptibility data to clinical outcome remains to be elucidated.

Studies (both in vitro and in vivo) suggest that the activity of amphotericin B may be suppressed by prior azole antifungal therapy. As with other azoles, itraconazole inhibits the ^{14}C-demethylation step in the synthesis of ergosterol, a cell wall component of fungi. Ergosterol is the active site for amphotericin B. In one study the antifungal activity of amphotericin B against *Aspergillus fumigatus* infections in mice was inhibited by ketoconazole therapy. The clinical significance of test results obtained in this study is unknown.

INDICATIONS AND USAGE

SPORANOX® (itraconazole) Capsules are indicated for the treatment of the following fungal infections in immunocompromised and non-immunocompromised patients:

1. Blastomycosis, pulmonary and extrapulmonary
2. Histoplasmosis, including chronic cavitary pulmonary disease and disseminated, non-meningeal histoplasmosis, and
3. Aspergillosis, pulmonary and extrapulmonary, in patients who are intolerant of or who are refractory to amphotericin B therapy.

Specimens for fungal cultures and other relevant laboratory studies (wet mount, histopathology, serology) should be obtained before therapy to isolate and identify causative organisms. Therapy may be instituted before the results of the cultures and other laboratory studies are known; however, once these results become available, antiinfective therapy should be adjusted accordingly.

SPORANOX® Capsules are also indicated for the treatment of the following fungal infections in non-immunocompromised patients:

1. Onychomycosis of the toenail, with or without fingernail involvement, due to dermatophytes (tinea unguium), and
2. Onychomycosis of the fingernail due to dermatophytes (tinea unguium).

Prior to initiating treatment, appropriate nail specimens for laboratory testing (KOH preparation, fungal culture, or nail biopsy) should be obtained to confirm the diagnosis of onychomycosis.

(See CLINICAL PHARMACOLOGY: Special Populations, CONTRAINDICATIONS, WARNINGS, and ADVERSE REACTIONS: Post-marketing Experience for more information.)

Description of Clinical Studies:

Blastomycosis: Analyses were conducted on data from two open-label, non-concurrently controlled studies (N=73 combined) in patients with normal or abnormal immune status. The median dose was 200 mg/day. A response for most signs and symptoms was observed within the first 2 weeks, and all signs and symptoms cleared between 3 and 6 months. Results of these two studies demonstrated substantial evidence of the effectiveness of itraconazole for the treatment of blastomycosis compared with the natural history of untreated cases.

Histoplasmosis: Analyses were conducted on data from two open-label, non-concurrently controlled studies (N=34 combined) in patients with normal or abnormal immune status (not including HIV-infected patients). The median dose was 200 mg/day. A response for most signs and symptoms was observed within the first 2 weeks, and all signs and symptoms cleared between 3 and 12 months. Results of these two studies demonstrated substantial evidence of the

Continued on next page

Sporanox Capsules—Cont.

effectiveness of itraconazole for the treatment of histoplasmosis, compared with the natural history of untreated cases.

Histoplasmosis in HIV-infected patients: Data from a small number of HIV-infected patients suggested that the response rate of histoplasmosis in HIV-infected patients is similar to that of non-HIV-infected patients. The clinical course of histoplasmosis in HIV-infected patients is more severe and usually requires maintenance therapy to prevent relapse.

Aspergillosis: Analyses were conducted on data from an open-label, "single-patient-use" protocol designed to make itraconazole available in the U.S. for patients who either failed or were intolerant of amphotericin B therapy (N=190). The findings were corroborated by two smaller open-label studies (N=31 combined) in the same patient population. Most adult patients were treated with a daily dose of 200 to 400 mg, with a median duration of 3 months. Results of these studies demonstrated substantial evidence of effectiveness of itraconazole as a second-line therapy for the treatment of aspergillosis compared with the natural history of the disease in patients who either failed or were intolerant of amphotericin B therapy.

Onychomycosis of the toenail: Analyses were conducted on data from three double-blind, placebo-controlled studies (N=214 total; 110 given SPORANOX® Capsules) in which patients with onychomycosis of the toenails received 200 mg of SPORANOX® Capsules once daily for 12 consecutive weeks. Results of these studies demonstrated mycologic cure, defined as simultaneous occurrence of negative KOH plus negative culture, in 54% of patients. Thirty-five percent (35%) of patients were considered an overall success (mycologic cure plus clear or minimal nail involvement with significantly decreased signs) and 14% of patients demonstrated mycologic cure plus clinical cure (clearance of all signs, with or without residual nail deformity). The mean time to overall success was approximately 10 months. Twenty-one percent (21%) of the overall success group had a relapse (worsening of the global score or conversion of KOH or culture from negative to positive).

Onychomycosis of the fingernail: Analyses were conducted on data from a double-blind, placebo-controlled study (N=73 total; 37 given SPORANOX® Capsules) in which patients with onychomycosis of the fingernails received a 1-week course (pulse) of 200 mg of SPORANOX® Capsules b.i.d., followed by a 3-week period without SPORANOX®, which was followed by a second 1-week pulse of 200 mg of SPORANOX® Capsules b.i.d. Results demonstrated mycologic cure in 61% of patients. Fifty-six percent (56%) of patients were considered an overall success and 47% of patients demonstrated mycologic cure plus clinical cure. The mean time to overall success was approximately 5 months. None of the patients who achieved overall success relapsed.

CONTRAINDICATIONS

Congestive Heart Failure: SPORANOX® (itraconazole) Capsules should not be administered for the treatment of onychomycosis in patients with evidence of ventricular dysfunction such as congestive heart failure (CHF) or a history of CHF. (See CLINICAL PHARMACOLOGY: Special Populations, WARNINGS, PRECAUTIONS: Drug Interactions-Calcium Channel Blockers, and ADVERSE REACTIONS: Post-marketing Experience.)

Drug Interactions: Concomitant administration of SPORANOX® (itraconazole) Capsules, Injection, or Oral Solution and certain drugs metabolized by the cytochrome P450 3A4 isoenzyme system (CYP3A4) may result in increased plasma concentrations of those drugs, leading to potentially serious and/or life-threatening adverse events. Cisapride, oral midazolam, pimozide, quinidine, dofetilide, triazolam and levacetylmethadol (levomethadyl) are contraindicated with SPORANOX®. HMG CoA-reductase inhibitors metabolized by CYP3A4, such as lovastatin and simvastatin, are also contraindicated with SPORANOX®. Ergot alkaloids metabolized by CYP3A4 such as dihydroergotamine, ergometrine (ergonovine), ergotamine and methylergometrine (methylergonovine) are contraindicated with SPORANOX®. (See BOX WARNING, and PRECAUTIONS: Drug Interactions.)

SPORANOX® should not be administered for the treatment of onychomycosis to pregnant patients or to women contemplating pregnancy.

SPORANOX® is contraindicated for patients who have shown hypersensitivity to itraconazole or its excipients. There is no information regarding cross-hypersensitivity between itraconazole and other azole antifungal agents. Caution should be used when prescribing SPORANOX® to patients with hypersensitivity to other azoles.

WARNINGS

SPORANOX® (itraconazole) Capsules and SPORANOX® Oral Solution should not be used interchangeably. This is because drug exposure is greater with the Oral Solution than with the Capsules when the same dose of drug is given. In addition, the topical effects of mucosal exposure may be different between the two formulations. Only the Oral Solution has been demonstrated effective for oral and/or esophageal candidiasis.

Hepatic Effects: SPORANOX® has been associated with rare cases of serious hepatotoxicity, including liver failure and death. Some of these cases had neither pre-existing liver disease nor a serious underlying medical condition, and some of these cases developed within the first week of treatment. If clinical signs or symptoms develop that are consistent with liver disease, treatment should be discontinued and liver function testing performed. Continued SPORANOX® use or reinstitution of treatment with SPORANOX® is strongly discouraged unless there is a serious or life threatening situation where the expected benefit exceeds the risk. (See PRECAUTIONS: Information for Patients and ADVERSE REACTIONS.)

	Itraconazole		Hydroxyitraconazole	
	Fed	Fasted	Fed	Fasted
C_{max} (ng/mL)	239 ± 85*	140 ± 65	397 ± 103	286 ± 101
T_{max} (hours)	4.5 ± 1.1	3.9 ± 1.0	5.1 ± 1.6	4.5 ± 1.1
$AUC_{0-\infty}$ (ng•h/mL)	3423 ± 1154	2094 ± 905	7978 ± 2648	5191 ± 2489
$t_{1/2}$ (hours)	21 ± 5	21 ± 7	12 ± 3	12 ± 3

* mean ± standard deviation

Cardiac Dysrhythmias: Life-threatening cardiac dysrhythmias and/or sudden death have occurred in patients using cisapride, pimozide, levacetylmethadol (levomethadyl), or quinidine concomitantly with SPORANOX® and/or other CYP3A4 inhibitors. Concomitant administration of these drugs with SPORANOX® is contraindicated. (See BOX WARNING, CONTRAINDICATIONS, and PRECAUTIONS: Drug Interactions.)

Cardiac Disease: SPORANOX® Capsules should not be administered for the treatment of onychomycosis in patients with evidence of ventricular dysfunction such as congestive heart failure (CHF) or a history of CHF. SPORANOX® Capsules should not be used for other indications in patients with evidence of ventricular dysfunction unless the benefit clearly outweighs the risk.

For patients with risk factors for congestive heart failure, physicians should carefully review the risks and benefits of SPORANOX® therapy. These risk factors include cardiac disease such as ischemic and valvular disease; significant pulmonary disease such as chronic obstructive pulmonary disease; and renal failure and other edematous disorders. Such patients should be informed of the signs and symptoms of CHF, should be treated with caution, and should be monitored for signs and symptoms of CHF during treatment. If signs or symptoms of CHF appear during administration of SPORANOX® Capsules, discontinue administration.

When itraconazole was administered intravenously to anesthetized dogs, a dose-related negative inotropic effect was documented. In a healthy volunteer study of SPORANOX® Injection (intravenous infusion), transient, asymptomatic decreases in left ventricular ejection fraction were observed using gated SPECT imaging; these resolved before the next infusion, 12 hours later.

Cases of CHF, peripheral edema, and pulmonary edema have been reported in the post-marketing period among patients being treated for onychomycosis and/or systemic fungal infections. (See CLINICAL PHARMACOLOGY: Special Populations, CONTRAINDICATIONS, PRECAUTIONS: Drug Interactions, and ADVERSE REACTIONS: Post-marketing Experience for more information.)

PRECAUTIONS

General: Rare cases of serious hepatotoxicity have been observed with SPORANOX® treatment, including some cases within the first week. In patients with elevated or abnormal liver enzymes or active liver disease, or who have experienced liver toxicity with other drugs, treatment with SPORANOX® is strongly discouraged unless there is a serious or life threatening situation where the expected benefit exceeds the risk. Liver function monitoring should be done in patients with pre-existing hepatic function abnormalities or those who have experienced liver toxicity with other medications and should be considered in all patients receiving SPORANOX®. Treatment should be stopped immediately and liver function testing should be conducted in patients who develop signs and symptoms suggestive of liver dysfunction.

If neuropathy occurs that may be attributable to SPORANOX® Capsules, the treatment should be discontinued.

SPORANOX® (itraconazole) Capsules should be administered after a full meal. (See CLINICAL PHARMACOLOGY: Pharmacokinetics and Metabolism.)

Under fasted conditions, itraconazole absorption was decreased in the presence of decreased gastric acidity. The absorption of itraconazole may be decreased with the concomitant administration of antacids or gastric acid secretion suppressors. Studies conducted under fasted conditions demonstrated that administration with 8 ounces of a cola beverage resulted in increased absorption of itraconazole in AIDS patients with relative or absolute achlorhydria. This increase relative to the effects of a full meal is unknown. (See CLINICAL PHARMACOLOGY: Pharmacokinetics and Metabolism.)

Information for Patients:

- The topical effects of mucosal exposure may be different between the SPORANOX® Capsules and Oral Solution. Only the Oral Solution has been demonstrated effective for oral and/or esophageal candidiasis. SPORANOX® Capsules should not be used interchangeably with SPORANOX® Oral Solution.
- Instruct patients to take SPORANOX® Capsules with a full meal.
- Instruct patients about the signs and symptoms of congestive heart failure, and if these signs or symptoms occur during SPORANOX® administration, they should discontinue SPORANOX® and contact their healthcare provider immediately.
- Instruct patients to stop SPORANOX® treatment immediately and contact their healthcare provider if any signs and symptoms suggestive of liver dysfunction develop. Such signs and symptoms may include unusual fatigue, anorexia, nausea and/or vomiting, jaundice, dark urine, or pale stools.
- Instruct patients to contact their physician before taking any concomitant medications with itraconazole to ensure there are no potential drug interactions.

Drug Interactions: Itraconazole and its major metabolite, hydroxyitraconazole, are inhibitors of CYP3A4. Therefore, the following drug interactions may occur (See Table 1 below and the following drug class subheadings that follow):

1. SPORANOX® may decrease the elimination of drugs metabolized by CYP3A4, resulting in increased plasma concentrations of these drugs when they are administered with SPORANOX®. These elevated plasma concentrations may increase or prolong both therapeutic and adverse effects of these drugs. Whenever possible, plasma concentrations of these drugs should be monitored, and dosage adjustments made after concomitant SPORANOX® therapy is initiated. When appropriate, clinical monitoring for signs or symptoms of increased or prolonged pharmacologic effects is advised. Upon discontinuation, depending on the dose and duration of treatment, itraconazole plasma concentrations decline gradually (especially in patients with hepatic cirrhosis or in those receiving CYP3A4 inhibitors). This is particularly important when initiating therapy with drugs whose metabolism is affected by itraconazole.
2. Inducers of CYP3A4 may decrease the plasma concentrations of itraconazole. SPORANOX® may not be effective in patients concomitantly taking SPORANOX® and one of these drugs. Therefore, administration of these drugs with SPORANOX® is not recommended.
3. Other inhibitors of CYP3A4 may increase the plasma concentrations of itraconazole. Patients who must take SPORANOX® concomitantly with one of these drugs should be monitored closely for signs or symptoms of increased or prolonged pharmacologic effects of SPORANOX®.

Table 1. Selected Drugs that are predicted to alter the plasma concentration of itraconazole or have their plasma concentration altered by SPORANOX®[1]

Drug plasma concentration increased by itraconazole	
Antiarrhythmics	digoxin, dofetilide,[2] quinidine[2], disopyramide
Anticonvulsants	carbamazepine
Antimycobacterials	rifabutin
Antineoplastics	busulfan, docetaxel, vinca alkaloids
Antipsychotics	pimozide[2]
Benzodiazepines	alprazolam, diazepam, midazolam,[2,3] triazolam[2]
Calcium Channel Blockers	dihydropyridines, verapamil
Gastrointestinal Motility Agents	cisapride[2]
HMG CoA-Reductase Inhibitors	atorvastatin, cerivastatin, lovastatin,[2] simvastatin[2]
Immunosuppressants	cyclosporine, tacrolimus, sirolimus
Oral Hypoglycemics	oral hypoglycemics
Protease Inhibitors	indinavir, ritonavir, saquinavir
Other	levacetylmethadol (levomethadyl), ergot alkaloids, halofantrine, alfentanil, buspirone, methylprednisolone, budesonide, dexamethasone, trimetrexate, warfarin, cilostazol, eletriptan

Decrease plasma concentration of itraconazole

Anticonvulsants	carbamazepine, phenobarbital, phenytoin
Antimycobacterials	isoniazid, rifabutin, rifampin
Gastric Acid Suppressors/ Neutralizers	antacids, H_2-receptor antagonists, proton pump inhibitors
Non-nucleoside Reverse Transcriptase Inhibitors	nevirapine

Increase plasma concentration of itraconazole

Macrolide Antibiotics	clarithromycin, erythromycin
Protease Inhibitors	indinavir, ritonavir

[1] This list is not all-inclusive.
[2] Contraindicated with SPORANOX® based on clinical and/or pharmacokinetics studies. (See WARNINGS and below.)
[3] For information on parenterally administered midazolam, see the Benzodiazepine paragraph below.

Antiarrhythmics: The class IA antiarrhythmic quinidine and class III antiarrhythmic dofetilide are known to prolong the QT interval. Coadministration of quinidine or dofetilide with SPORANOX® may increase plasma concentrations of quinidine or dofetilide which could result in serious cardiovascular events. Therefore, concomitant administration of SPORANOX® and quinidine or dofetilide is contraindicated. (See BOX WARNING, CONTRAINDICATIONS, and WARNINGS.)

The class IA antiarrhythmic disopyramide has the potential to increase the QT interval at high plasma concentrations. Caution is advised when SPORANOX® and disopyramide are administered concomitantly.

Concomitant administration of digoxin and SPORANOX® has led to increased plasma concentrations of digoxin.

Anticonvulsants: Reduced plasma concentrations of itraconazole were reported when SPORANOX® was administered concomitantly with phenytoin. Carbamazepine, phenobarbital, and phenytoin are all inducers of CYP3A4. Although interactions with carbamazepine and phenobarbital have not been studied, concomitant administration of SPORANOX® and these drugs would be expected to result in decreased plasma concentrations of itraconazole. In addition, in vivo studies have demonstrated an increase in plasma carbamazepine concentrations in subjects concomitantly receiving ketoconazole. Although there are no data regarding the effect of itraconazole on carbamazepine metabolism, because of the similarities between ketoconazole and itraconazole, concomitant administration of SPORANOX® and carbamazepine may inhibit the metabolism of carbamazepine.

Antimycobacterials: Drug interaction studies have demonstrated that plasma concentrations of azole antifungal agents and their metabolites, including itraconazole and hydroxyitraconazole, were significantly decreased when these agents were given concomitantly with rifabutin or rifampin. In vivo data suggest that rifabutin is metabolized in part by CYP3A4. SPORANOX® may inhibit the metabolism of rifabutin. Although no formal study data are available for isoniazid, similar effects should be anticipated. Therefore, the efficacy of SPORANOX® could be substantially reduced if given concomitantly with one of these agents. Coadministration is not recommended.

Antineoplastics: SPORANOX® may inhibit the metabolism of busulfan, docetaxel, and vinca alkaloids.

Antipsychotics: Pimozide is known to prolong the QT interval and is partially metabolized by CYP3A4. Coadministration of pimozide with SPORANOX® could result in serious cardiovascular events. Therefore, concomitant administration of SPORANOX® and pimozide is contraindicated. (See BOX WARNING, CONTRAINDICATIONS, and WARNINGS.)

Benzodiazepines: Concomitant administration of SPORANOX® and alprazolam, diazepam, oral midazolam, or triazolam could lead to increased plasma concentrations of these benzodiazepines. Increased plasma concentrations could potentiate and prolong hypnotic and sedative effects. Concomitant administration of SPORANOX® and oral midazolam or triazolam is contraindicated. (See CONTRAINDICATIONS and WARNINGS.) If midazolam is administered parenterally, special precaution and patient monitoring is required since the sedative effect may be prolonged.

Calcium Channel Blockers: Edema has been reported in patients concomitantly receiving SPORANOX® and dihydropyridine calcium channel blockers. Appropriate dosage adjustment may be necessary.

Calcium channel blockers can have a negative inotropic effect which may be additive to those of itraconazole; itraconazole can inhibit the metabolism of calcium channel blockers such as dihydropyridines (e.g., nifedipine and felodipine) and verapamil. Therefore, caution should be used when co-administering itraconazole and calcium channel blockers. (See CLINICAL PHARMACOLOGY: Special Populations, CONTRAINDICATIONS, WARNINGS, and ADVERSE REACTIONS: Post-marketing Experience for more information).

Gastric Acid Suppressors/Neutralizers: Reduced plasma concentrations of itraconazole were reported when SPORANOX® Capsules were administered concomitantly with H_2-receptor antagonists. Studies have shown that absorption of itraconazole is impaired when gastric acid production is decreased. Therefore, SPORANOX® should be administered with a cola beverage if the patient has achlorhydria or is taking H_2-receptor antagonists or other gastric acid suppressors. Antacids should be administered at least 1 hour before or 2 hours after administration of SPORANOX® Capsules. In a clinical study, when SPORANOX® Capsules were administered with omeprazole (a proton pump inhibitor), the bioavailability of itraconazole was significantly reduced.

Gastrointestinal Motility Agents: Coadministration of SPORANOX® with cisapride can elevate plasma cisapride concentrations which could result in serious cardiovascular events. Therefore, concomitant administration of SPORANOX® with cisapride is contraindicated. (See BOX WARNING, CONTRAINDICATIONS, and WARNINGS.)

HMG CoA-Reductase Inhibitors: Human pharmacokinetic data suggest that SPORANOX® inhibits the metabolism of atorvastatin, cerivastatin, lovastatin, and simvastatin, which may increase the risk of skeletal muscle toxicity, including rhabdomyolysis. Concomitant administration of SPORANOX® with HMG CoA-reductase inhibitors, such as lovastatin and simvastatin, is contraindicated. (See CONTRAINDICATIONS and WARNINGS.)

Immunosuppressants: Concomitant administration of SPORANOX® and cyclosporine or tacrolimus has led to increased plasma concentrations of these immunosuppressants. Concomitant administration of SPORANOX® and sirolimus could increase plasma concentrations of sirolimus.

Macrolide Antibiotics: Erythromycin and clarithromycin are known inhibitors of CYP3A4 (See Table 1) and may increase plasma concentrations of itraconazole. In a small pharmacokinetic study involving HIV infected patients, clarithromycin was shown to increase plasma concentrations of itraconazole. Similarly, following administration of 1 gram of erythromycin ethyl succinate and 200 mg itraconazole as single doses, the mean C_{max} and $AUC_{0-\infty}$ of itraconazole increased by 44% (90% CI: 119-175%) and 36% (90% CI: 108-171%), respectively.

Non-nucleoside Reverse Transcriptase Inhibitors: Nevirapine is an inducer of CYP3A4. In vivo studies have shown that nevirapine induces the metabolism of ketoconazole, significantly reducing the bioavailability of ketoconazole. Studies involving nevirapine and itraconazole have not been conducted. However, because of the similarities between ketoconazole and itraconazole, concomitant administration of SPORANOX® and nevirapine is not recommended.

In a clinical study, when 8 HIV-infected subjects were treated concomitantly with SPORANOX® Capsules 100 mg twice daily and the nucleoside reverse transcriptase inhibitor zidovudine 8 ± 0.4 mg/kg/day, the pharmacokinetics of zidovudine were not affected. Other nucleoside reverse transcriptase inhibitors have not been studied.

Oral Hypoglycemic Agents: Severe hypoglycemia has been reported in patients concomitantly receiving azole antifungal agents and oral hypoglycemic agents. Blood glucose concentrations should be carefully monitored when SPORANOX® and oral hypoglycemic agents are coadministered.

Polyenes: Prior treatment with itraconazole, like other azoles, may reduce or inhibit the activity of polyenes such as amphotericin B. However, the clinical significance of this drug effect has not been clearly defined.

Protease Inhibitors: Concomitant administration of SPORANOX® and protease inhibitors metabolized by CYP3A4, such as indinavir, ritonavir, and saquinavir, may increase plasma concentrations of these protease inhibitors. In addition, concomitant administration of SPORANOX® and indinavir and ritonavir (but not saquinavir) may increase plasma concentrations of itraconazole. Caution is advised when SPORANOX® and protease inhibitors must be given concomitantly.

Other:

- Levacetylmethadol (levomethadyl) is known to prolong the QT interval and is metabolized by CYP3A4. Coadministration of levacetylmethadol with SPORANOX® could result in serious cardiovascular events. Therefore, concomitant administration of SPORANOX® and levacetylmethadol is contraindicated.
- Elevated concentrations of ergot alkaloids can cause ergotism, ie. a risk for vasospasm potentially leading to cerebral ischemia and/or ischemia of the extremities. Concomitant administration of ergot alkaloids such as dihydroergotamine, ergometrine (ergonovine), ergotamine and methylergometrine (methylergonovine) with SPORANOX® is contraindicated.
- Halofantrine has the potential to prolong the QT interval at high plasma concentrations. Caution is advised when SPORANOX® and halofantrine are administered concomitantly.
- In vitro data suggest that alfentanil is metabolized by CYP3A4. Administration with SPORANOX® may increase plasma concentrations of alfentanil.
- Human pharmacokinetic data suggest that concomitant administration of SPORANOX® and buspirone results in significant increases in plasma concentrations of buspirone.
- SPORANOX® may inhibit the metabolism of certain glucocorticosteroids such as budesonide, dexamethasone and methylprednisolone.
- In vitro data suggest that trimetrexate is extensively metabolized by CYP3A4. In vitro animal models have demonstrated that ketoconazole potently inhibits the metabolism of trimetrexate. Although there are no data regarding the effect of itraconazole on trimetrexate metabolism, because of the similarities between ketoconazole and itraconazole, concomitant administration of SPORANOX® and trimetrexate may inhibit the metabolism of trimetrexate.
- SPORANOX® enhances the anticoagulant effect of coumarin-like drugs, such as warfarin.
- Cilostazol and eletriptan are CYP3A4 metabolized drugs that should be used with caution when co-administered with SPORANOX®.

Carcinogenesis, Mutagenesis, and Impairment of Fertility: Itraconazole showed no evidence of carcinogenicity potential in mice treated orally for 23 months at dosage levels up to 80 mg/kg/day (approximately 10x the maximum recommended human dose [MRHD]). Male rats treated with 25 mg/kg/day (3.1× MRHD) had a slightly increased incidence of soft tissue sarcoma. These sarcomas may have been a consequence of hypercholesterolemia, which is a response of rats, but not dogs or humans, to chronic itraconazole administration. Female rats treated with 50 mg/kg/day (6.25× MRHD) had an increased incidence of squamous cell carcinoma of the lung (2/50) as compared to the untreated group. Although the occurrence of squamous cell carcinoma in the lung is extremely uncommon in untreated rats, the increase in this study was not statistically significant.

Itraconazole produced no mutagenic effects when assayed in DNA repair test (unscheduled DNA synthesis) in primary rat hepatocytes, in Ames tests with *Salmonella typhimurium* (6 strains) and *Escherichia coli*, in the mouse lymphoma gene mutation tests, in a sex-linked recessive lethal mutation (*Drosophila melanogaster*) test, in chromosome aberration tests in human lymphocytes, in a cell transformation test with C3H/10T½ C18 mouse embryo fibroblasts cells, in a dominant lethal mutation test in male and female mice, and in micronucleus tests in mice and rats.

Itraconazole did not affect the fertility of male or female rats treated orally with dosage levels of up to 40 mg/kg/day (5× MRHD), even though parental toxicity was present at this dosage level. More severe signs of parental toxicity, including death, were present in the next higher dosage level, 160 mg/kg/day (20× MRHD).

Pregnancy: Teratogenic effects. Pregnancy Category C: Itraconazole was found to cause a dose-related increase in maternal toxicity, embryotoxicity, and teratogenicity in rats at dosage levels of approximately 40–160 mg/kg/day (5–20× MRHD), and in mice at dosage levels of approximately 80 mg/kg/day (10× MRHD). In rats, the teratogenicity consisted of major skeletal defects; in mice, it consisted of encephaloceles and/or macroglossia.

There are no studies in pregnant women. SPORANOX® should be used for the treatment of systemic fungal infections in pregnancy only if the benefit outweighs the potential risk. SPORANOX® should not be administered for the treatment of onychomycosis to pregnant patients or to women contemplating pregnancy. SPORANOX® should not be administered to women of childbearing potential for the treatment of onychomycosis unless they are using effective measures to prevent pregnancy and they begin therapy on the second or third day following the onset of menses. Effective contraception should be continued throughout SPORANOX® therapy and for 2 months following the end of treatment.

During post-marketing experience, cases of congenital abnormalities have been reported. (See ADVERSE REACTIONS, Post-marketing Experience.)

Nursing Mothers: Itraconazole is excreted in human milk; therefore, the expected benefits of SPORANOX® therapy for the mother should be weighed against the potential risk from exposure of itraconazole to the infant. The U.S. Public Health Service Centers for Disease Control and Prevention advises HIV-infected women not to breast-feed to avoid potential transmission of HIV to uninfected infants.

Pediatric Use: The efficacy and safety of SPORANOX® have not been established in pediatric patients. No pharmacokinetic data on SPORANOX® Capsules are available in children. A small number of patients ages 3 to 16 years have been treated with 100 mg/day of itraconazole capsules for systemic fungal infections, and no serious unexpected adverse events have been reported. SPORANOX® Oral Solution (5 mg/kg/day) has been administered to pediatric patients (N=26; ages 6 months to 12 years) for 2 weeks and no serious unexpected adverse events were reported.

The long-term effects of itraconazole on bone growth in children are unknown. In three toxicology studies using rats, itraconazole induced bone defects at dosage levels as low as 20 mg/kg/day (2.5× MRHD). The induced defects included reduced bone plate activity, thinning of the zona compacta of the large bones, and increased bone fragility. At a dosage level of 80 mg/kg/day (10× MRHD) over 1 year or 160 mg/kg/day (20× MRHD) for 6 months, itraconazole induced small tooth pulp with hypocellular appearance in some rats. No such bone toxicity has been reported in adult patients.

HIV-Infected Patients: Because hypochlorhydria has been reported in HIV-infected individuals, the absorption of itraconazole in these patients may be decreased.

ADVERSE REACTIONS

SPORANOX® has been associated with rare cases of serious hepatotoxicity, including liver failure and death. Some

Continued on next page

Sporanox Capsules—Cont.

of these cases had neither pre-existing liver disease nor a serious underlying medical condition. If clinical signs or symptoms develop that are consistent with liver disease, treatment should be discontinued and liver function testing performed. The risks and benefits of SPORANOX® use should be reassessed. (See WARNINGS: Hepatic Effects and PRECAUTIONS: General and Information for Patients.)

Adverse Events in the Treatment of Systemic Fungal Infections

Adverse event data were derived from 602 patients treated for systemic fungal disease in U.S. clinical trials who were immunocompromised or receiving multiple concomitant medications. Treatment was discontinued in 10.5% of patients due to adverse events. The median duration before discontinuation of therapy was 81 days (range: 2 to 776 days). The table lists adverse events reported by at least 1% of patients.

Clinical Trials of Systemic Fungal Infections: Adverse Events Occurring with an Incidence of Greater than or Equal to 1%

Body System/Adverse Event	Incidence (%) (N=602)
Gastrointestinal	
Nausea	11
Vomiting	5
Diarrhea	3
Abdominal Pain	2
Anorexia	1
Body as a Whole	
Edema	4
Fatigue	3
Fever	3
Malaise	1
Skin and Appendages	
Rash*	9
Pruritus	3
Central/Peripheral Nervous System	
Headache	4
Dizziness	2
Psychiatric	
Libido Decreased	1
Somnolence	1
Cardiovascular	
Hypertension	3
Metabolic/Nutritional	
Hypokalemia	2
Urinary System	
Albuminuria	1
Liver and Biliary System	
Hepatic Function Abnormal	3
Reproductive System, Male	
Impotence	1

*Rash tends to occur more frequently in immunocompromised patients receiving immunosuppressive medications.

Adverse events infrequently reported in all studies included constipation, gastritis, depression, insomnia, tinnitus, menstrual disorder, adrenal insufficiency, gynecomastia, and male breast pain.

Adverse Events Reported in Toenail Onychomycosis Clinical Trials

Patients in these trials were on a continuous dosing regimen of 200 mg once daily for 12 consecutive weeks.

The following adverse events led to temporary or permanent discontinuation of therapy.

Clinical Trials of Onychomycosis of the Toenail: Adverse Events Leading to Temporary or Permanent Discontinuation of Therapy

Adverse Event	Incidence (%) Itraconazole (N=112)
Elevated Liver Enzymes (greater than twice the upper limit of normal)	4
Gastrointestinal Disorders	4
Rash	3
Hypertension	2
Orthostatic Hypotension	1
Headache	1
Malaise	1
Myalgia	1
Vasculitis	1
Vertigo	1

The following adverse events occurred with an incidence of greater than or equal to 1% (N=112): headache: 10%; rhinitis: 9%; upper respiratory tract infection: 8%; sinusitis, injury: 7%; diarrhea, dyspepsia, flatulence, abdominal pain, dizziness, rash: 4%; cystitis, urinary tract infection, liver function abnormality, myalgia, nausea: 3%; appetite increased, constipation, gastritis, gastroenteritis, pharyngitis, asthenia, fever, pain, tremor, herpes zoster, abnormal dreaming: 2%.

Adverse Events Reported in Fingernail Onychomycosis Clinical Trials

Patients in these trials were on a pulse regimen consisting of two 1-week treatment periods of 200 mg twice daily, separated by a 3-week period without drug.

The following adverse events led to temporary or permanent discontinuation of therapy.

Clinical Trials of Onychomycosis of the Fingernail: Adverse Events Leading to Temporary or Permanent Discontinuation of Therapy

Adverse Event	Incidence (%) Itraconazole (N=37)
Rash/Pruritus	3
Hypertriglyceridemia	3

The following adverse events occurred with an incidence of greater than or equal to 1% (N=37): headache: 8%; pruritus, nausea, rhinitis: 5%; rash, bursitis, anxiety, depression, constipation, abdominal pain, dyspepsia, ulcerative stomatitis, gingivitis, hypertriglyceridemia, sinusitis, fatigue, malaise, pain, injury: 3%.

Post-marketing Experience

Worldwide post-marketing experiences with the use of SPORANOX® include adverse events of gastrointestinal origin, such as dyspepsia, nausea, vomiting, diarrhea, abdominal pain and constipation. Other reported adverse events include peripheral edema, congestive heart failure and pulmonary edema, headache, dizziness, peripheral neuropathy, menstrual disorders, reversible increases in hepatic enzymes, hepatitis, liver failure, hypokalemia, hypertriglyceridemia, alopecia, allergic reactions (such as pruritus, rash, urticaria, angioedema, anaphylaxis), Stevens-Johnson syndrome, anaphylactic, anaphylactoid and allergic reactions, photosensitivity and neutropenia. There is limited information on the use of SPORANOX® during pregnancy. Cases of congenital abnormalities including skeletal, genitourinary tract, cardiovascular and ophthalmic malformations as well as chromosomal and multiple malformations have been reported during post-marketing experience. A causal relationship with SPORANOX® has not been established. (See CLINICAL PHARMACOLOGY: Special Populations, CONTRAINDICATIONS, WARNINGS, and PRECAUTIONS: Drug Interactions for more information).

OVERDOSAGE

Itraconazole is not removed by dialysis. In the event of accidental overdosage, supportive measures, including gastric lavage with sodium bicarbonate, should be employed.

Limited data exist on the outcomes of patients ingesting high doses of itraconazole. In patients taking either 1000 mg of SPORANOX® (itraconazole) Oral Solution or up to 3000 mg of SPORANOX® (itraconazole) Capsules, the adverse event profile was similar to that observed at recommended doses.

DOSAGE AND ADMINISTRATION

SPORANOX® (itraconazole) Capsules should be taken with a full meal to ensure maximal absorption.

SPORANOX® Capsules is a different preparation than SPORANOX® Oral Solution and should not be used interchangeably.

Treatment of Blastomycosis and Histoplasmosis: The recommended dose is 200 mg once daily (2 capsules). If there is no obvious improvement, or there is evidence of progressive fungal disease, the dose should be increased in 100-mg increments to a maximum of 400 mg daily. Doses above 200 mg/day should be given in two divided doses.

Treatment of Aspergillosis: A daily dose of 200 to 400 mg is recommended.

Treatment in Life-Threatening Situations: In life-threatening situations, a loading dose should be used whether given as oral capsules or intravenously.

- IV Injection: the recommended intravenous dose is 200 mg b.i.d. for four consecutive doses, followed by 200 mg once daily thereafter. Each intravenous dose should be infused over 1 hour. The safety and efficacy of SPORANOX® Injection administered for greater than 14 days is not known. See complete prescribing information for SPORANOX® (itraconazole) Injection.
- Capsules: although clinical studies did not provide for a loading dose, it is recommended, based on pharmacokinetic data, that a loading dose of 200 mg (2 capsules) three times daily (600 mg/day) be given for the first 3 days of treatment.

Treatment should be continued for a minimum of three months and until clinical parameters and laboratory tests indicate that the active fungal infection has subsided. An inadequate period of treatment may lead to recurrence of active infection.

SPORANOX® Capsules and SPORANOX® Oral Solution should not be used interchangeably. Only the oral solution has been demonstrated effective for oral and/or esophageal candidiasis.

Treatment of Onychomycosis: Toenails with or without fingernail involvement: The recommended dose is 200 mg (2 capsules) once daily for 12 consecutive weeks.

Treatment of Onychomycosis: Fingernails only: The recommended dosing regimen is 2 treatment pulses, each consisting of 200 mg (2 capsules) b.i.d. (400 mg/day) for 1 week. The pulses are separated by a 3-week period without SPORANOX®.

HOW SUPPLIED

SPORANOX® (itraconazole) Capsules are available containing 100 mg of itraconazole, with a blue opaque cap and pink transparent body, imprinted with "JANSSEN" and "SPORANOX 100." The capsules are supplied in unit-dose blister packs of 3 × 10 capsules (NDC 50458-290-01), bottles of 30 capsules (NDC 50458-290-04) and in the PulsePak® containing 7 blister packs × 4 capsules each (NDC 50458-290-28).

Store at controlled room temperature 15°-25°C (59°-77°F). Protect from light and moisture.

Keep out of reach of children.

 7501622

U.S. Patent Nos. 4,267,179; 5,633,015

Revised January 2004

Distributed by:
JANSSEN PHARMACEUTICA PRODUCTS, L.P.
Titusville, New Jersey 08560, USA

Capsule contents manufactured by:
JANSSEN PHARMACEUTICA N.V.
Beerse, Belgium

SPORANOX IV® ℞

itraconazole

Prescribing information for this product, which appears on page(s) 1772–1776 of the 2004 PDR, has been completely revised as follows. Please write "See Supplement A" next to the product heading.

Congestive Heart Failure: When itraconazole was administered intravenously to dogs and healthy human volunteers, negative inotropic effects were seen. If signs or symptoms of congestive heart failure occur during administration of SPORANOX® (itraconazole) Injection, continued SPORANOX® use should be reassessed. (See CLINICAL PHARMACOLOGY: Special Populations, CONTRAINDICATIONS, WARNINGS, PRECAUTIONS: Drug Interactions and ADVERSE REACTIONS: Post-marketing Experience for more information.)

Drug Interactions: Coadministration of cisapride, pimozide, quinidine, dofetilide, or levacetylmethadol (levomethadyl) with SPORANOX® (itraconazole) Capsules, Injection or Oral Solution is contraindicated. SPORANOX®, a potent cytochrome P450 3A4 isoenzyme system (CYP3A4) inhibitor, may increase plasma concentrations of drugs metabolized by this pathway. Serious cardiovascular events, including QT prolongation, torsades de pointes, ventricular tachycardia, cardiac arrest, and/or sudden death have occurred in patients using cisapride, pimozide, levacetylmethadol (levomethadyl), or quinidine concomitantly with SPORANOX® and/or other CYP3A4 inhibitors. (See CONTRAINDICATIONS, WARNINGS, and PRECAUTIONS: Drug Interactions for more information.)

DESCRIPTION

For intravenous infusion (NOT FOR IV BOLUS INJECTION)

SPORANOX® is the brand name for itraconazole, a synthetic triazole antifungal agent. Itraconazole is a 1:1:1:1 racemic mixture of four diastereomers (two enantiomeric pairs), each possessing three chiral centers. It may be represented by the following structural formula and nomenclature:

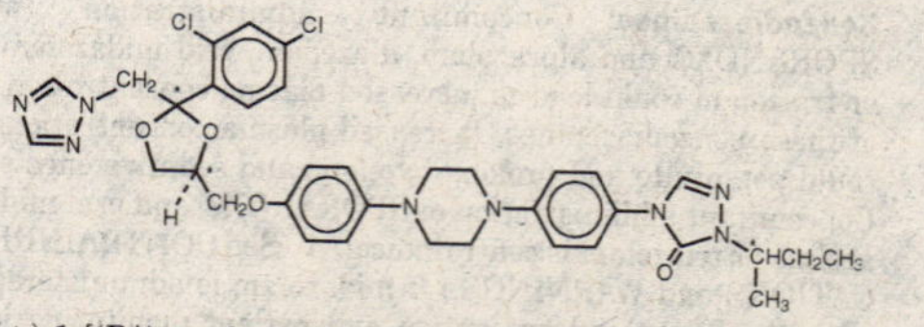

(±)-1-[(R*)-sec-butyl]-4-[p-[4-[p-[[(2R*,4S*)-2-(2,4-dichlorophenyl)-2-(1H-1,2,4-triazol-1-ylmethyl)-1,3-dioxolan-4-yl]methoxy]phenyl]-1-piperazinyl]phenyl]-Δ^2-1,2,4-triazolin-5-one mixture with (±)-1-[(R*)-sec-butyl]-4-[p-[4-[p-[[(2S*,4R*)-2-(2,4-dichlorophenyl)-2-(1H-1,2,4-triazol-1-ylmethyl)-1,3-dioxolan-4-yl]methoxy] phenyl]-1-piperazinyl]phenyl]-Δ^2-1,2,4-triazolin-5-one.

or

(±)-1-[(RS)-sec-butyl]-4-[p-[4-[p-[[(2R,4S)-2-(2,4-dichlorophenyl)-2-(1H-1,2,4-triazol-1-ylmethyl)-1,3-dioxolan-4-yl]methoxy]phenyl]-1-piperazinyl]phenyl]-Δ^2-1,2,4-triazolin-5-one.

Itraconazole has a molecular formula of $C_{35}H_{38}Cl_2N_8O_4$ and a molecular weight of 705.64. It is a white to slightly yellowish powder. It is insoluble in water, very slightly soluble in alcohols, and freely soluble in dichloromethane. It has a pKa of 3.70 (based on extrapolation of values obtained from methanolic solutions) and a log (n-octanol/water) partition coefficient of 5.66 at pH 8.1.

SPORANOX® (itraconazole) Injection is a sterile pyrogen-free clear, colorless to slightly yellow solution for intravenous infusion. Each mL contains 10 mg of itraconazole, solubilized by hydroxypropyl-cyclodextrin (400 mg) as a molecular inclusion complex, with 3.8 µL hydrochloric acid, 25 µL propylene glycol, and sodium hydroxide for pH adjustment to 4.5, in water for injection. SPORANOX® Injection is packaged in 25 mL colorless glass ampules, containing 250 mg of itraconazole, contents of which are diluted in 50 mL 0.9% Sodium Chloride Injection, USP (Normal Saline) prior to infusion. When properly administered, contents of one ampule will supply 200 mg of itraconazole.

CLINICAL PHARMACOLOGY

Pharmacokinetics and Metabolism: NOTE: The plasma concentrations reported below were measured by high-performance liquid chromatography (HPLC) specific for itraconazole. When itraconazole in plasma is measured by a bioassay, values reported may be higher than those obtained by HPLC due to the presence of the bioactive metabolite, hydroxyitraconazole. (See MICROBIOLOGY.)

The pharmacokinetics of SPORANOX® (itraconazole) Injection (200 mg b.i.d. for two days, then 200 mg q.d. for five days) followed by oral dosing of SPORANOX® Capsules were studied in patients with advanced HIV infection. Steady-state plasma concentrations were reached after the fourth dose for itraconazole and by the seventh dose for hydroxyitraconazole. Steady-state plasma concentrations were maintained by administration of SPORANOX® Capsules, 200 mg b.i.d. Pharmacokinetic parameters for itraconazole and hydroxyitraconazole are presented in the table below:

[See first table above]

The estimated mean ±SD half-life at steady-state of itraconazole after intravenous infusion was 35.4 ± 29.4 hours. In previous studies, the mean elimination half-life for itraconazole at steady-state after daily oral administration of 100 to 400 mg was 30-40 hours. Approximately 93-101% of hydroxypropyl-β-cyclodextrin was excreted unchanged in the urine within 12 hours after dosing.

The plasma protein binding of itraconazole is 99.8% and that of hydroxyitraconazole is 99.5%. Following intravenous administration, the volume of distribution of itraconazole averaged 796 ± 185 L.

Itraconazole is metabolized predominately by the cytochrome P450 3A4 isoenzyme system (CYP3A4), resulting in the formation of several metabolites, including hydroxyitraconazole, the major metabolite. Results of a pharmacokinetics study suggest that itraconazole may undergo saturable metabolism with multiple dosing. Fecal excretion of the parent drug varies between 3-18% of the dose. Renal excretion of the parent drug is less than 0.03% of the dose. About 40% of the dose is excreted as inactive metabolites in the urine. No single excreted metabolite represents more than 5% of a dose. Itraconazole total plasma clearance averaged 381 ± 95 mL/min following intravenous administration. Approximately 80–90% of hydroxypropyl-β-cyclodextrin is eliminated through the kidneys. (See CONTRAINDICATIONS and PRECAUTIONS: Drug Interactions for more information.)

Special Populations

Renal Insufficiency: Plasma concentrations of itraconazole in patients with mild to moderate renal insufficiency were comparable to those obtained in healthy subjects. The majority of the 8-gram dose of hydroxypropyl-β-cyclodextrin was eliminated in the urine during the 120-hour collection period in normal subjects and in patients with mild to severe renal insufficiency. Following a single intravenous dose of 200 mg to subjects with severe renal impairment (creatinine clearance ≤ 19 mL/minute), clearance of hydroxypropyl-β-cyclodextrin was reduced six-fold compared with subjects with normal renal function. SPORANOX® Injection should not be used in patients with creatinine clearance < 30 mL/min.

In patients with mild to moderate renal impairment, SPORANOX® Injection should be used with caution. Serum creatinine levels should be closely monitored and, if renal toxicity is suspected, consideration should be given to changing to SPORANOX® Capsules.

Hepatic Insufficiency: Patients with impaired hepatic function should be carefully monitored when taking itraconazole. The prolonged elimination half-life of itraconazole observed in a clinical trial with itraconazole capsules in cirrhotic patients should be considered when deciding to initiate therapy with other medications metabolized by CYP3A4. (See BOX WARNING, CONTRAINDICATIONS, and PRECAUTIONS: Drug Interactions.)

Decreased Cardiac Contractility: When itraconazole was administered intravenously to anesthetized dogs, a dose-related negative inotropic effect was documented. In a healthy volunteer study of SPORANOX® Injection (intravenous infusion), transient, asymptomatic decreases in left ventricular ejection fraction were observed using gated SPECT imaging; these resolved before the next infusion, 12 hours later. If signs or symptoms of congestive heart failure appear during administration of SPORANOX® Injection, monitor carefully and consider other treatment alternatives which may include discontinuation of SPORANOX® Injection administration. (See WARNINGS, PRECAUTIONS: Drug Interactions and ADVERSE REACTIONS: Post-marketing Experience for more information.)

Parameter	Injection Day 7 n=29		Capsules, 200 mg b.i.d. Day 36 n=12	
	itraconazole	hydroxyitraconazole	itraconazole	hydroxyitraconazole
C_{max} (ng/mL)	2856 ± 866*	1906 ± 612	2010 ± 1420	2614 ± 1703
t_{max} (hr)	1.08 ± 0.14	8.53 ± 6.36	3.92 ± 1.83	5.92 ± 6.14
$AUC_{0\text{-}12h}$ (ng•h/mL)	—	—	18768 ± 13933	28516 ± 19149
$AUC_{0\text{-}24h}$ (ng•h/mL)	30605 ± 8961	42445 ± 13282	—	—

*mean ± standard deviation

Overview of Efficacy (Intent-to-Treat Population)

Efficacy Parameters	SPORANOX® N=179 (%)	Amphotericin B N=181 (%)
Success	84 (47%)	68 (38%)
Unevaluable*	24 (13%)	44 (24%)
Failure	71 (40%)	69 (38%)
Reason for Failure		
Intolerance after > 3 days of antifungal medication	12	37
Persistent fever	20	7
Change in antifungal medication due to fever	13	1
Emergent fungal infection	10	9
Documented bacterial or viral infection	7	8
Insufficient response	6	5
Deterioration of signs and symptoms	2	0
Death after > 3 days antifungal medication	1	2
Resolution of fever	131 (73%)	127 (70%)
Survival	161 (90%)	156 (86%)

* Treatment duration ≤ 3 days (including patients who died within 3 days, withdrew because of adverse events or were deemed ineligible due to a confirmed pre-treatment infection).

MICROBIOLOGY

Mechanism of Action: In vitro studies have demonstrated that itraconazole inhibits the cytochrome P450-dependent synthesis of ergosterol, which is a vital component of fungal cell membranes.

Activity In Vitro and In Vivo: Itraconazole exhibits in vitro activity against *Blastomyces dermatitidis, Histoplasma capsulatum, Histoplasma duboisii, Aspergillus flavus, Aspergillus fumigatus, Candida albicans,* and *Cryptococcus neoformans.* Itraconazole also exhibits varying in vitro activity against *Sporothrix schenckii, Trichophyton* species, *Candida krusei*, and other *Candida* species. The bioactive metabolite, hydroxyitraconazole, has not been evaluated against *Histoplasma capsulatum* and *Blastomyces dermatitidis.* Correlation between minimum inhibitory concentration (MIC) results in vitro and clinical outcome has yet to be established for azole antifungal agents.

Itraconazole administered orally was active in a variety of animal models of fungal infection using standard laboratory strains of fungi. Fungistatic activity has been demonstrated against disseminated fungal infections caused by *Blastomyces dermatitidis, Histoplasma duboisii, Aspergillus fumigatus, Coccidioides immitis, Cryptococcus neoformans, Paracoccidioides brasiliensis, Sporothrix schenckii, Trichophyton rubrum,* and *Trichophyton mentagrophytes.*

Itraconazole administered at 2.5 mg/kg and 5 mg/kg via the oral and parenteral routes increased survival rates and sterilized organ systems in normal and immunosuppressed guinea pigs with disseminated *Aspergillus fumigatus* infections. Oral itraconazole administered daily at 40 mg/kg and 80 mg/kg increased survival rates in normal rabbits with disseminated disease and in immunosuppressed rats with pulmonary *Aspergillus fumigatus* infection, respectively. Itraconazole has demonstrated antifungal activity in a variety of animal models infected with *Candida albicans* and other *Candida* species.

Resistance: Isolates from several fungal species with decreased susceptibility to itraconazole have been isolated in vitro and from patients receiving prolonged therapy.

Several in vitro studies have reported that some fungal clinical isolates, including *Candida* species, with reduced susceptibility to one azole antifungal agent may also be less susceptible to other azole derivatives. The finding of cross-resistance is dependent on a number of factors, including the species evaluated, its clinical history, the particular azole compounds compared, and the type of susceptibility test that is performed. The relevance of these in vitro susceptibility data to clinical outcome remains to be elucidated. Studies (both in vitro and in vivo) suggest that the activity of amphotericin B may be suppressed by prior azole antifungal therapy. As with other azoles, itraconazole inhibits the ^{14}C-demethylation step in the synthesis of ergosterol, a cell wall component of fungi. Ergosterol is the active site for amphotericin B. In one study the anti-fungal activity of amphotericin B against *Aspergillus fumigatus* infections in mice was inhibited by ketoconazole therapy. The clinical significance of test results obtained in this study is unknown.

CLINICAL STUDIES

Empiric Therapy in Febrile Neutropenic Patients: An open randomized trial compared the efficacy and safety of itraconazole (intravenous followed by oral solution) with amphotericin B for empiric therapy in 384 febrile, neutropenic patients with hematologic malignancies who had suspected fungal infections. Patients received either itraconazole (injection, 200 mg b.i.d. for 2 days followed by 200 mg once daily for up to 14 days, followed by oral solution, 200 mg b.i.d.) or amphotericin B (total daily dose of 0.7-1.0 mg/kg body weight). The longest treatment duration was 28 days. An outcome assignment of "success" required (a) patient survival with resolution of fever and neutropenia within 28 days of treatment, (b) absence of emergent fungal infections, (c) no discontinuation of therapy due to toxicity or lack of efficacy, and (d) treatment for three or more days. The success rate using an intent-to-treat analysis was 47% for the itraconazole group and 38% for the amphotericin B arm.

[See second table above]

INDICATIONS AND USAGE

SPORANOX® (itraconazole) Injection/Oral Solution is indicated for empiric therapy of febrile neutropenic patients with suspected fungal infections. (NOTE: In a comparative trial, the overall response rate for itraconazole-treated subjects was higher than for amphotericin B-treated subjects. However, compared to amphotericin B-treated subjects, a larger number of itraconazole-treated subjects discontinued treatment due to persistent fever and a change in antifun-

Continued on next page

Sporanox IV—Cont.

gal medication due to fever. Whereas, a larger number of amphotericin B-treated subjects discontinued due to drug intolerance. (See CLINICAL STUDIES section.)

SPORANOX® (itraconazole) Injection is also indicated for the treatment of the following fungal infections in immunocompromised and non-immunocompromised patients:

1. Blastomycosis, pulmonary and extrapulmonary;
2. Histoplasmosis, including chronic cavitary pulmonary disease and disseminated, non-meningeal histoplasmosis; and
3. Aspergillosis, pulmonary and extrapulmonary, in patients who are intolerant of or who are refractory to amphotericin B therapy.

Specimens for fungal cultures and other relevant laboratory studies (wet mount, histopathology, serology) should be obtained prior to therapy to isolate and identify causative organisms. Therapy may be instituted before the results of the cultures and other laboratory studies are known; however, once these results become available, anti-infective therapy should be adjusted accordingly.

(See CLINICAL PHARMACOLOGY: Special Populations, WARNINGS, and ADVERSE REACTIONS: Post-marketing Experience for more information).

CONTRAINDICATIONS

Drug Interactions: Concomitant administration of SPORANOX® (itraconazole) Capsules, Injection, or Oral Solution and certain drugs metabolized by the cytochrome P450 3A4 isoenzyme system (CYP3A4) may result in increased plasma concentrations of those drugs, leading to potentially serious and/or life-threatening adverse events. Cisapride, oral midazolam, pimozide, quinidine, dofetilide, triazolam and levacetylmethadol (levomethadyl) are contraindicated with SPORANOX®. HMG CoA-reductase inhibitors metabolized by CYP3A4, such as lovastatin and simvastatin, are also contraindicated with SPORANOX®. Ergot alkaloids metabolized by CYP3A4 such as dihydroergotamine, ergometrine (ergonovine), ergotamine and methylergometrine (methylergonovine) are contraindicated with SPORANOX®. (See BOX WARNING, and PRECAUTIONS: Drug Interactions.)

SPORANOX® is contraindicated for patients who have shown hypersensitivity to itraconazole or its excipients. There is no information regarding cross-hypersensitivity between itraconazole and other azole antifungal agents. Caution should be used when prescribing SPORANOX® to patients with hypersensitivity to other azoles.

WARNINGS

SPORANOX® (itraconazole) Injection contains the excipient hydroxypropyl-β-cyclodextrin which produced pancreatic adenocarcinomas in a rat carcinogenicity study. These findings were not observed in a similar mouse carcinogenicity study. The clinical relevance of these findings is unknown. (See PRECAUTIONS: Carcinogenesis, Mutagenesis, and Impairment of Fertility.)

Hepatic Effects: SPORANOX® has been associated with rare cases of serious hepatotoxicity, including liver failure and death. Some of these cases had neither pre-existing liver disease nor a serious underlying medical condition, and some of these cases developed within the first week of treatment. If clinical signs or symptoms develop that are consistent with liver disease, treatment should be discontinued and liver function testing performed. Continued SPORANOX® use or reinstitution of treatment with SPORANOX® is strongly discouraged unless there is a serious or life threatening situation where the expected benefit exceeds the risk. (See PRECAUTIONS: Information for Patients and ADVERSE REACTIONS.)

Cardiac Dysrhythmias: Life-threatening cardiac dysrhythmias and/or sudden death have occurred in patients using cisapride, pimozide, levacetylmethadol (levomethadyl), or quinidine concomitantly with SPORANOX® and/or other CYP3A4 inhibitors. Concomitant administration of these drugs with SPORANOX® is contraindicated. (See BOX WARNING, CONTRAINDICATIONS, and PRECAUTIONS: Drug Interactions.)

Cardiac Disease: SPORANOX® Injection should not be used in patients with evidence of ventricular dysfunction unless the benefit clearly outweighs the risk. For patients with risk factors for congestive heart failure, physicians should carefully review the risks and benefits of SPORANOX® therapy. These risk factors include cardiac disease such as ischemic and valvular disease; significant pulmonary disease such as chronic obstructive pulmonary disease; and renal failure and other edematous disorders. Such patients should be informed of the signs and symptoms of CHF, should be treated with caution, and should be monitored for signs and symptoms of CHF during treatment. If signs or symptoms of CHF appear during administration of SPORANOX® Injection, monitor carefully and consider other treatment alternatives which may include discontinuation of SPORANOX® Injection administration.

When itraconazole was administered intravenously to anesthetized dogs, a dose-related negative inotropic effect was documented. In a healthy volunteer study of SPORANOX® Injection (intravenous infusion), transient, asymptomatic decreases in left ventricular ejection fraction were observed using gated SPECT imaging; these resolved before the next infusion, 12 hours later.

Cases of CHF, peripheral edema, and pulmonary edema have been reported in the post-marketing period among patients being treated for onychomycosis and/or systemic fungal infections. (See CLINICAL PHARMACOLOGY: Special Populations, PRECAUTIONS: Drug Interactions, and ADVERSE REACTIONS: Post-marketing Experience for more information.)

Table 1. Selected Drugs that are predicted to alter the plasma concentration of itraconazole or have their plasma concentration altered by SPORANOX®[1]

Drug plasma concentration increased by itraconazole	
Antiarrhythmics	digoxin, dofetilide[2], quinidine disopyramide
Anticonvulsants	carbamazepine
Antimycobacterials	rifabutin
Antineoplastics	busulfan, docetaxel, vinca alkaloids
Antipsychotics	pimozide[2]
Benzodiazepines	alprazolam, diazepam, midazolam,[2,3] triazolam[2]
Calcium Channel Blockers	dihydropyridines, verapamil
Gastrointestinal Motility Agents	cisapride[2]
HMG CoA-Reductase Inhibitors	atorvastatin, cerivastatin, lovastatin,[2] simvastatin[2]
Immunosuppressants	cyclosporine, tacrolimus, sirolimus
Oral Hypoglycemics	oral hypoglycemics
Protease Inhibitors	indinavir, ritonavir, saquinavir
Other	levacetylmethadol (levomethadyl), ergot alkaloids, halofantrine, alfentanil, buspirone, methylprednisolone, budesonide, dexamethasone trimetrexate, warfarin, cilostazol, eletripan
Decrease plasma concentration of itraconazole	
Anticonvulsants	carbamazepine, phenobarbital, phenytoin
Antimycobacterials	isoniazid, rifabutin, rifampin
Reverse Transcriptase Inhibitors	nevirapine
Increase plasma concentration of itraconazole	
Macrolide Antibiotics	clarithromycin, erythromycin
Protease Inhibitors	indinavir, ritonavir

[1] This list is not all-inclusive.
[2] Contraindicated with SPORANOX® based on clinical and/or pharmacokinetics studies. (See WARNINGS and below.)
[3] For information on parenterally administered midazolam, see the Benzodiazepine paragraph below.

PRECAUTIONS

General: Rare cases of serious hepatotoxicity have been observed with SPORANOX® treatment, including some cases within the first week. In patients with elevated or abnormal liver enzymes or active liver disease, or who have experienced liver toxicity with other drugs, treatment with SPORANOX® is strongly discouraged unless there is a serious or life threatening situation where the expected benefit exceeds the risk. Liver function monitoring should be done in patients with pre-existing hepatic function abnormalities or those who have experienced liver toxicity with other medications and should be considered in all patients receiving SPORANOX®. Treatment should be stopped immediately and liver function testing should be conducted in patients who develop signs and symptoms suggestive of liver dysfunction.

If neuropathy occurs that may be attributable to SPORANOX® Injection, the treatment should be discontinued.

As severe renal impairment prolongs the elimination rate of hydroxypropyl-β-cyclodextrin, SPORANOX® (itraconazole) Injection should not be used in patients with severe renal dysfunction (creatinine clearance < 30 mL/min). (See CLINICAL PHARMACOLOGY: Special Populations.)

Information for Patients: SPORANOX® Injection contains the excipient hydroxypropyl-β-cyclodextrin which produced pancreatic adenocarcinomas in a rat carcinogenicity study. These findings were not observed in a similar mouse carcinogenicity study. The clinical relevance of these findings is unknown. (See PRECAUTIONS: Carcinogenesis, Mutagenesis, and Impairment of Fertility.)

Drug Interactions: Itraconazole and its major metabolite, hydroxyitraconazole, are inhibitors of CYP3A4. Therefore, the following drug interactions may occur (See Table 1 below and the following drug class subheadings that follow):

1. SPORANOX® may decrease the elimination of drugs metabolized by CYP3A4, resulting in increased plasma concentrations of these drugs when they are administered with SPORANOX®. These elevated plasma concentrations may increase or prolong both therapeutic and adverse effects of these drugs. Whenever possible, plasma concentrations of these drugs should be monitored, and dosage adjustments made after concomitant SPORANOX® therapy is initiated. When appropriate, clinical monitoring for signs or symptoms of increased or prolonged pharmacologic effects is advised. Upon discontinuation, depending on the dose and duration of treatment, itraconazole plasma concentrations decline gradually (especially in patients with hepatic cirrhosis or in those receiving CYP3A4 inhibitors). This is particularly important when initiating therapy with drugs whose metabolism is affected by itraconazole.
2. Inducers of CYP3A4 may decrease the plasma concentrations of itraconazole. SPORANOX® may not be effective in patients concomitantly taking SPORANOX® and one of these drugs. Therefore, administration of these drugs with SPORANOX® is not recommended.
3. Other inhibitors of CYP3A4 may increase the plasma concentrations of itraconazole. Patients who must take SPORANOX® concomitantly with one of these drugs should be monitored closely for signs or symptoms of increased or prolonged pharmacologic effects of SPORANOX®.

[See table 1 above]

Antiarrhythmics: The class IA antiarrhythmic quinidine and class III antiarrhythmic dofetilide are known to prolong the QT interval. Coadministration of quinidine or dofetilide with SPORANOX® may increase plasma concentrations of quinidine or dofetilide which could result in serious cardiovascular events. Therefore, concomitant administration of SPORANOX® and quinidine or dofetilide is contraindicated. (See BOX WARNING, CONTRAINDICATIONS, and WARNINGS.)

The class IA antiarrhythmic disopyramide has the potential to increase the QT interval at high plasma concentrations. Caution is advised when SPORANOX® and disopyramide are administered concomitantly.

Concomitant administration of digoxin and SPORANOX® has led to increased plasma concentrations of digoxin.

Anticonvulsants: Reduced plasma concentrations of itraconazole were reported when SPORANOX® was administered concomitantly with phenytoin. Carbamazepine, phenobarbital, and phenytoin are all inducers of CYP3A4. Although interactions with carbamazepine and phenobarbital have not been studied, concomitant administration of SPORANOX® and these drugs would be expected to result in decreased plasma concentrations of itraconazole. In addition, in vivo studies have demonstrated an increase in plasma carbamazepine concentrations in subjects concomitantly receiving ketoconazole. Although there are no data regarding the effect of itraconazole on carbamazepine metabolism, because of the similarities between ketoconazole and itraconazole, concomitant administration of SPORANOX® and carbamazepine may inhibit the metabolism of carbamazepine.

Antimycobacterials: Drug interaction studies have demonstrated that plasma concentrations of azole antifungal agents and their metabolites, including itraconazole and hydroxyitraconazole, were significantly decreased when these agents were given concomitantly with rifabutin or rifampin. In vivo data suggest that rifabutin is metabolized in part by CYP3A4. SPORANOX® may inhibit the metabolism of rifabutin. Although no formal study data are available for isoniazid, similar effects should be anticipated. Therefore, the efficacy of SPORANOX® could be substantially reduced if given concomitantly with one of these agents. Coadministration is not recommended.

Antineoplastics: SPORANOX® may inhibit the metabolism of busulfan, docetaxel, and vinca alkaloids.

Antipsychotics: Pimozide is known to prolong the QT interval and is partially metabolized by CYP3A4. Coadministration of pimozide with SPORANOX® could result in serious cardiovascular events. Therefore, concomitant administration of SPORANOX® and pimozide is contraindicated. (See BOX WARNING, CONTRAINDICATIONS, and WARNINGS.)

Benzodiazepines: Concomitant administration of SPORANOX® and alprazolam, diazepam, oral midazolam, or triazolam could lead to increased plasma concentrations of these benzodiazepines. Increased plasma concentrations could potentiate and prolong hypnotic and sedative effects. Concomitant administration of SPORANOX® and oral midazolam or triazolam is contraindicated. (See CONTRAINDICATIONS and WARNINGS.) If midazolam is administered parenterally, special precaution and patient monitoring is required since the sedative effect may be prolonged.

Calcium Channel Blockers: Edema has been reported in patients concomitantly receiving SPORANOX® and dihydropyridine calcium channel blockers. Appropriate dosage adjustment may be necessary.

Calcium channel blockers can have a negative inotropic effect which may be additive to those of itraconazole; itraconazole can inhibit the metabolism of calcium channel blockers such as dihydropyridines (e.g., nifedipine and felodipine) and verapamil. Therefore, caution should be used when co-administering itraconazole and calcium channel blockers. (See CLINICAL PHARMACOLOGY: Special Populations, WARNINGS, and ADVERSE REACTIONS: Post-marketing Experience for more information.)

Gastrointestinal Motility Agents: Coadministration of SPORANOX® with cisapride can elevate plasma cisapride concentrations which could result in serious cardiovascular events. Therefore, concomitant administration of SPORANOX® with cisapride is contraindicated. (See BOX WARNING, CONTRAINDICATIONS, and WARNINGS.)

HMG CoA-Reductase Inhibitors: Human pharmacokinetic data suggest that SPORANOX® inhibits the metabolism of atorvastatin, cerivastatin, lovastatin, and simvastatin, which may increase the risk of skeletal muscle toxicity, including rhabdomyolysis. Concomitant administration of SPORANOX® with HMG CoA-reductase inhibitors, such as lovastatin and simvastatin, is contraindicated. (See CONTRAINDICATIONS, and WARNINGS.)

Immunosuppressants: Concomitant administration of SPORANOX® and cyclosporine or tacrolimus has led to increased plasma concentrations of these immunosuppressants. Concomitant administration of SPORANOX® and sirolimus could increase plasma concentrations of sirolimus.

Macrolide Antibiotics: Erythromycin and clarithromycin are known inhibitors of CYP3A4 (See Table 1) and may increase plasma concentrations of itraconazole. In a small pharmacokinetic study involving HIV infected patients, clarithromycin was shown to increase plasma concentrations of itraconazole. Similarly, following administration of 1 gram of erythromycin ethyl succinate and 200 mg itraconazole as single doses, the mean C_{max} and $AUC_{0-\infty}$ of itraconazole increased by 44% (90% CI: 119-175%) and 36% (90% CI: 108-171%), respectively.

Oral Hypoglycemic Agents: Severe hypoglycemia has been reported in patients concomitantly receiving azole antifungal agents and oral hypoglycemic agents. Blood glucose concentrations should be carefully monitored when SPORANOX® and oral hypoglycemic agents are coadministered.

Polyenes: Prior treatment with itraconazole, like other azoles, may reduce or inhibit the activity of polyenes such as amphotericin B. However, the clinical significance of this drug effect has not been clearly defined.

Protease Inhibitors: Concomitant administration of SPORANOX® and protease inhibitors metabolized by CYP3A4, such as indinavir, ritonavir, and saquinavir, may increase plasma concentrations of these protease inhibitors. In addition, concomitant administration of SPORANOX® and indinavir and ritonavir (but not saquinavir) may increase plasma concentrations of itraconazole. Caution is advised when SPORANOX® and protease inhibitors must be given concomitantly.

Reverse Transcriptase Inhibitors: Nevirapine is an inducer of CYP3A4. In vivo studies have shown that nevirapine induces the metabolism of ketoconazole, significantly reducing the bioavailability of ketoconazole. Studies involving nevirapine and itraconazole have not been conducted. However, because of the similarities between ketoconazole and itraconazole, concomitant administration of SPORANOX® and nevirapine is not recommended. In a clinical study, when 8 HIV-infected subjects were treated concomitantly with SPORANOX® Capsules 100 mg twice daily and the nucleoside reverse transcriptase inhibitor zidovudine 8 ± 0.4 mg/kg/day, the pharmacokinetics of zidovudine were not affected. Other nucleoside reverse transcriptase inhibitors have not been studied.

Other:

- Levacetylmethadol (levomethadyl) is known to prolong the QT interval and is metabolized by CYP3A4. Coadministration of levacetylmethadol with SPORANOX® could result in serious cardiovascular events. Therefore, concomitant administration of SPORANOX® and levacetylmethadol is contraindicated.
- Elevated concentrations of ergot alkaloids can cause ergotism, ie. a risk for vasospasm potentially leading to cerebral ischemia and/or ischemia of the extremities. Concomitant administration of ergot alkaloids such as dihydroergotamine, ergometrine (ergonovine), ergotamine and methylergometrine (methylergonovine) with SPORANOX® is contraindicated.
- Halofantrine has the potential to prolong the QT interval at high plasma concentrations. Caution is advised when SPORANOX® and halofantrine are administered concomitantly.
- In vitro data suggest that alfentanil is metabolized by CYP3A4. Administration with SPORANOX® may increase plasma concentrations of alfentanil.
- Human pharmacokinetic data suggest that concomitant administration of SPORANOX® and buspirone results in significant increases in plasma concentrations of buspirone.
- SPORANOX® may inhibit the metabolism of certain glucocorticosteroids such as budesonide, dexamethasone and methylprednisolone.
- In vitro data suggest that trimetrexate is extensively metabolized by CYP3A4. In vitro animal models have demonstrated that ketoconazole potently inhibits the metabolism of trimetrexate. Although there are no data regarding the effect of itraconazole on trimetrexate metabolism, because of the similarities between ketoconazole and itraconazole, concomitant administration of SPORANOX® and trimetrexate may inhibit the metabolism of trimetrexate.
- Cilostazol and eletriptan are CYP3A4 metabolized drugs that should be used with caution when co-administered with SPORANOX®.
- SPORANOX® enhances the anticoagulant effect of coumarin-like drugs, such as warfarin.

Table 2. Summary of Possibly or Definitely Drug-Related Adverse Events Reported by ≥2% of Subjects

Adverse Event	Total SPORANOX® Injection (N=360) %	Comparative Studies		
		SPORANOX® Injection (N=234) %	Intravenous Fluconazole (N=32) %	Intravenous Amphotericin B (N=202) %
Gastrointestinal system disorders				
Nausea	8	9	0	15
Diarrhea	6	6	3	9
Vomiting	4	6	0	10
Abdominal pain	2	2	0	3
Constipation	0	1	3	0
Metabolic and nutritional disorders				
Hypokalemia	5	8	0	29
Alkaline phosphatase increased	1	2	3	2
Serum creatinine increased	2	2	3	26
Hypomagnesemia	1	1	0	5
Blood urea nitrogen increased	0	1	0	7
Fluid overload	0	0	0	3
Hypocalcemia	0	0	0	3
Liver and biliary system disorders				
Bilirubinemia	4	6	9	3
SGPT/ALT increased	2	3	3	1
Hepatic function abnormal	1	2	0	2
Jaundice	1	2	0	0
SGOT/AST increased	1	2	0	0
Body as a whole – General disorders				
Pain	1	2	0	0
Rigors	0	0	0	34
Fever	0	0	0	6
Skin and appendages disorders				
Rash	3	3	3	3
Sweating increased	1	2	0	0
Respiratory system disorder				
Dyspnea	0	0	0	3
Central and peripheral nervous system disorders				
Dizziness	1	2	0	1
Headache	2	2	0	3
Urinary system disorders				
Renal function abnormal	1	1	0	11
Application site disorder				
Application site reaction	4	0	0	0
Cardiovascular disorders, general				
Hypotension	0	0	0	3
Hypertension	0	0	0	2
Heart rate and rhythm disorders				
Tachycardia	0	1	0	3
Vascular (extracardiac) disorders				
Vein disorder	3	0	0	0

Carcinogenesis, Mutagenesis and Impairment of Fertility: Itraconazole showed no evidence of carcinogenicity potential in mice treated orally for 23 months at dosage levels up to 80 mg/kg/day (approximately 10× the maximum recommended human dose [MRHD]). Male rats treated with 25 mg/kg/day (3.1× MRHD) had a slightly increased incidence of soft tissue sarcoma. These sarcomas may have been a consequence of hypercholesterolemia, which is a response of rats, but not dogs or humans, to chronic itraconazole administration. Female rats treated with 50 mg/kg/day (6.25× MRHD) had an increased incidence of squamous cell carcinoma of the lung (2/50) as compared to the untreated group. Although the occurrence of squamous cell carcinoma in the lung is extremely uncommon in untreated rats, the increase in this study was not statistically significant.

Hydroxypropyl-β-cyclodextrin (HP-β-CD), the solubilizing excipient used in SPORANOX® Injection and Oral Solution, was found to produce pancreatic exocrine hyperplasia and neoplasia when administered orally to rats at doses of 500, 2000 or 5000 mg/kg/day for 25 months. Adenocarcinomas of the exocrine pancreas produced in the treated animals were not seen in the untreated group and are not reported in the historical controls. Development of these tumors may be related to a mitogenic action of cholecystokinin. This finding was not observed in the mouse carcinogenicity study at doses of 500, 2000 or 5000 mg/kg/day for 22-23 months; however, the clinical relevance of these findings is unknown. Based on body surface area comparisons, the expo-

Continued on next page

Sporanox IV—Cont.

sure to humans of HP-β-CD at the recommended clinical dose of SPORANOX® Oral Solution, is approximately equivalent to 1.7 times the exposure at the lowest dose in the rat study. The relevance of the findings with orally administered HP-β-CD to potential carcinogenic effects for SPORANOX® Injection is uncertain.

Itraconazole produced no mutagenic effects when assayed in a DNA repair test (unscheduled DNA synthesis) in primary rat hepatocytes, in Ames tests with *Salmonella typhimurium* (6 strains) and *Escherichia coli*, in the mouse lymphoma gene mutation tests, in a sex-linked recessive lethal mutation (*Drosophila melanogaster*) test, in chromosome aberration tests in human lymphocytes, in a cell transformation test with C3H/10T½ C18 mouse embryo fibroblasts cells, in a dominant lethal mutation test in male and female mice, and in micronucleus tests in mice and rats.

Itraconazole did not affect the fertility of male or female rats treated orally with dosage levels of up to 40 mg/kg/day (5× MRHD), even though parental toxicity was present at this dosage level. More severe signs of parental toxicity, including death, were present in the next higher dosage level, 160 mg/kg/day (20× MRHD).

Pregnancy: Teratogenic Effects. Pregnancy Category C: Itraconazole was found to cause a dose-related increase in maternal toxicity, embryotoxicity, and teratogenicity in rats at dosage levels of approximately 40-160 mg/kg/day (5-20× MRHD), and in mice at dosage levels of approximately 80 mg/kg/day (10× MRHD). In rats, the teratogenicity consisted of major skeletal defects; in mice, it consisted of encephaloceles and/or macroglossia.

There are no studies in pregnant women. SPORANOX® should be used for the treatment of systemic fungal infections in pregnancy only if the benefit outweighs the potential risk.

During post-marketing experience, cases of congenital abnormalities have been reported. (See ADVERSE REACTIONS, Post-marketing Experience.)

Nursing Mothers: Itraconazole is excreted in human milk; therefore, the expected benefits of SPORANOX® therapy for the mother should be weighed against the potential risk from exposure of itraconazole to the infant. The U.S. Public Health Service Centers for Disease Control and Prevention advises HIV-infected women not to breast-feed to avoid potential transmission of HIV to uninfected infants.

Pediatric Use: The efficacy and safety of SPORANOX® have not been established in pediatric patients. No pharmacokinetic data on SPORANOX® Capsules or Injection are available in children. A small number of patients ages 3 to 16 years have been treated with 100 mg/day of itraconazole capsules for systemic fungal infections, and no serious unexpected adverse effects have been reported. SPORANOX® Oral Solution (5 mg/kg/day) has been administered to pediatric patients (N=26, ages 6 months to 12 years) for 2 weeks and no serious unexpected adverse events were reported.

The long-term effects of itraconazole on bone growth in children are unknown. In three toxicology studies using rats, itraconazole induced bone defects at dosage levels as low as 20 mg/kg/day (2.5× MRHD). The induced defects included reduced bone plate activity, thinning of the zona compacta of the large bones, and increased bone fragility. At a dosage level of 80 mg/kg/day (10× MRHD) over 1 year or 160 mg/kg/day (20× MRHD) for 6 months, itraconazole induced small tooth pulp with hypocellular appearance in some rats. No such bone toxicity has been reported in adult patients.

Geriatric Use: Clinical studies of SPORANOX® Injection did not include sufficient numbers of subjects aged 65 and over to determine whether they respond differently from younger subjects. Other reported clinical experience has not identified differences in responses between the elderly and younger patients. In general, dose selection for an elderly patient should be cautious, reflecting the greater frequency of decreased hepatic, renal, or cardiac function, and of concomitant disease or other drug therapy.

ADVERSE REACTIONS

SPORANOX® has been associated with rare cases of serious hepatotoxicity, including liver failure and death. Some of these cases had neither pre-existing liver disease nor a serious underlying medical condition. If clinical signs or symptoms develop that are consistent with liver disease, treatment should be discontinued and liver function testing performed. The risks and benefits of SPORANOX® use should be reassessed. (See WARNINGS: Hepatic Effects and PRECAUTIONS: General and Information for Patients.)

Adverse Events Reported in Trials in Patients with SPORANOX® Injection

Adverse events considered at least possibly drug related are shown in Table 2 and are based on the experience of 360 patients treated with SPORANOX® Injection in four pharmacokinetic, one uncontrolled and four active controlled studies where the control was amphotericin B or fluconazole. Nearly all patients were neutropenic or were otherwise immunocompromised and were treated empirically for febrile episodes, for documented systemic fungal infections, or in trials to determine pharmacokinetics. The dose of SPORANOX® Injection was 200 mg twice daily for the first two days followed by a single daily dose of 200 mg for the remainder of the intravenous treatment period. The majority of patients received between 7 and 14 days of SPORANOX® Injection.

[See table 2 at top of previous page]

The following adverse events occurred in less than 2% of patients in clinical trials of SPORANOX® Injection: LDH increased, edema, albuminuria, hyperglycemia, and hepatitis.

Post-marketing Experience

Worldwide post-marketing experiences with the use of SPORANOX® include adverse events of gastrointestinal origin, such as dyspepsia, nausea, vomiting, diarrhea, abdominal pain and constipation. Other reported adverse events include peripheral edema, congestive heart failure and pulmonary edema, headache, dizziness, peripheral neuropathy, menstrual disorders, reversible increases in hepatic enzymes, hepatitis, liver failure, hypokalemia, hypertriglyceridemia, alopecia, allergic reactions (such as pruritus, rash, urticaria, angioedema, anaphylaxis), Stevens-Johnson syndrome, anaphylactic, anaphylactoid and allergic reactions, photosensitivity and neutropenia. There is limited information on the use of SPORANOX® during pregnancy. Cases of congenital abnormalities including skeletal, genitourinary tract, cardiovascular and ophthalmic malformations as well as chromosomal and multiple malformations have been reported during post-marketing experience. A causal relationship with SPORANOX® has not been established. (See CLINICAL PHARMACOLOGY: Special Populations, CONTRAINDICATIONS, WARNINGS, and PRECAUTIONS: Drug Interactions for more information.)

OVERDOSAGE

Itraconazole is not removed by dialysis.

There are limited data on the outcomes of patients ingesting high doses of itraconazole. In patients taking either 1000 mg of SPORANOX® (itraconazole) Oral Solution or up to 3000 mg of SPORANOX® Capsules, or b.i.d. dosing for four days with SPORANOX® Injection, the adverse event profile was similar to that observed at recommended doses.

DOSAGE AND ADMINISTRATION

Use only the components [SPORANOX® (itraconazole) Injection ampule, 0.9% Sodium Chloride Injection, USP (Normal Saline) bag and filtered infusion set] provided in the kit: **DO NOT SUBSTITUTE.**

SPORANOX® Injection should not be diluted with 5% Dextrose Injection, USP, or with Lactated Ringer's Injection, USP, alone or in combination with any other diluent. The compatibility of SPORANOX® Injection with diluents other than 0.9% Sodium Chloride Injection, USP (Normal Saline) is not known. **NOT FOR IV BOLUS INJECTION.**

NOTE: After reconstitution, the diluted SPORANOX® Injection may be stored refrigerated (2-8°C) or at room temperature (15-25°C) for up to 48 hours, when protected from direct light. During administration, exposure to normal room light is acceptable.

NOTE: Use only a dedicated infusion line for administration of SPORANOX® Injection. Do not introduce concomitant medication in the same bag nor through the same line as SPORANOX® Injection. Other medications may be administered after flushing the line/catheter with 0.9% Sodium Chloride Injection, USP, as described below, and removing and replacing the entire infusion line. Alternatively, utilize another lumen, in the case of a multi-lumen catheter. Correct preparation and administration of SPORANOX® Injection are necessary to ensure maximal efficacy and safety. A precise mixing ratio is required in order to obtain a stable admixture. It is critical to maintain a 3.33 mg/mL itraconazole:diluent ratio. Failure to maintain this concentration will lead to the formation of a precipitate.

Add the full contents (25 mL) of the SPORANOX® Injection ampule into the infusion bag provided, which contains 50 mL of 0.9% Sodium Chloride Injection, USP (Normal Saline). Mix gently after the solution is completely transferred. Withdraw and discard 15 mL of the solution before administering to the patient. Using a flow control device, infuse 60 mL of the dilute solution (3.33 mg/mL = 200 mg itraconazole, pH apx. 4.8) intravenously over 60 minutes, using an extension line and the infusion set provided. After administration, flush the infusion set with 15-20 mL of 0.9% Sodium Chloride Injection, USP, over 30 seconds-15 minutes, via the two-way stopcock. Do not use Bacteriostatic Sodium Chloride Injection, USP. The compatibility of SPORANOX® Injection with flush solutions other than 0.9% Sodium Chloride Injection, USP (Normal Saline) is not known. Discard the entire infusion line.

Parenteral drug products should be inspected visually for particulate matter and discoloration prior to administration, whenever solution and container permit.

Empiric Therapy in Febrile, Neutropenic Patients with Suspected Fungal Infections (ETFN): The recommended dose of SPORANOX® Injection is 200 mg b.i.d. for four doses, followed by 200 mg once daily for up to 14 days. Each intravenous dose should be infused over 1 hour. Treatment should be continued with SPORANOX® Oral Solution 200 mg (20 mL) b.i.d. until resolution of clinically significant neutropenia. The safety and efficacy of SPORANOX® use exceeding 28 days in ETFN is not known.

Treatment of Blastomycosis, Histoplasmosis and Aspergillosis: The recommended intravenous dose is 200 mg b.i.d. for four doses, followed by 200 mg q.d. Each intravenous dose should be infused over 1 hour.

For the treatment of blastomycosis, histoplasmosis and aspergillosis, SPORANOX® can be given as oral capsules or intravenously. The safety and efficacy of SPORANOX® Injection administered for greater than 14 days is not known. Total itraconazole therapy (SPORANOX® Injection followed by SPORANOX® Capsules) should be continued for a minimum of 3 months and until clinical parameters and laboratory tests indicate that the active fungal infection has subsided. An inadequate period of treatment may lead to recurrence of active infection.

SPORANOX® Injection should not be used in patients with creatinine clearance <30 mL/min.

HOW SUPPLIED

SPORANOX® (itraconazole) Injection for intravenous infusion is supplied as a kit (NDC 50458-298-01), containing one 25 mL colorless glass ampule of itraconazole 10 mg/mL sterile, pyrogen-free solution (NDC 50458-297-10), one 50 mL bag (100 mL capacity) of 0.9% Sodium Chloride Injection, USP (Normal Saline) and one filtered infusion set.

Store at or below 25°C (77°F). Protect from light and freezing.

SPORANOX®
(ITRACONAZOLE)
INJECTION

Manufactured by:
Abbott Laboratories, Inc.
North Chicago, IL 60064
631-10-938-7
Distributed by:
Ortho Biotech Products, L.P.
Raritan, NJ 08869
ORTHO BIOTECH
U.S. Patent 4,727,064
58-7309-R7
Revised January 2004

SPORANOX® ℞
(itraconazole)
ORAL SOLUTION

Prescribing information for this product, which appears on pages 1776–1781 of the 2004 PDR, has been completely revised as follows. Please write "See Supplement A" next to the product heading.

Congestive Heart Failure: When itraconazole was administered intravenously to dogs and healthy human volunteers, negative inotropic effects were seen. If signs or symptoms of congestive heart failure occur during administration of SPORANOX® (itraconazole) Oral Solution, continued SPORANOX® use should be reassessed. (See CLINICAL PHARMACOLOGY: Special Populations, CONTRAINDICATIONS, WARNINGS, PRECAUTIONS: Drug Interactions and ADVERSE REACTIONS: Post-marketing Experience for more information.)

Drug Interactions: Coadministration of cisapride, pimozide, quinidine, dofetilide, or levacetylmethadol (levomethadyl) with SPORANOX® (itraconazole) Capsules, Injection or Oral Solution is contraindicated. SPORANOX®, a potent cytochrome P450 3A4 isoenzyme system (CYP3A4) inhibitor, may increase plasma concentrations of drugs metabolized by this pathway. Serious cardiovascular events, including QT prolongation, torsades de pointes, ventricular tachycardia, cardiac arrest, and/or sudden death have occurred in patients using cisapride, pimozide, levacetylmethadol (levomethadyl), or quinidine concomitantly with SPORANOX® and/or other CYP3A4 inhibitors. (See CONTRAINDICATIONS, WARNINGS, and PRECAUTIONS: Drug Interactions for more information.)

DESCRIPTION

SPORANOX® is the brand name for itraconazole, a synthetic triazole antifungal agent. Itraconazole is a 1:1:1:1 racemic mixture of four diastereomers (two enantiomeric pairs), each possessing three chiral centers. It may be represented by the following structural formula and nomenclature:

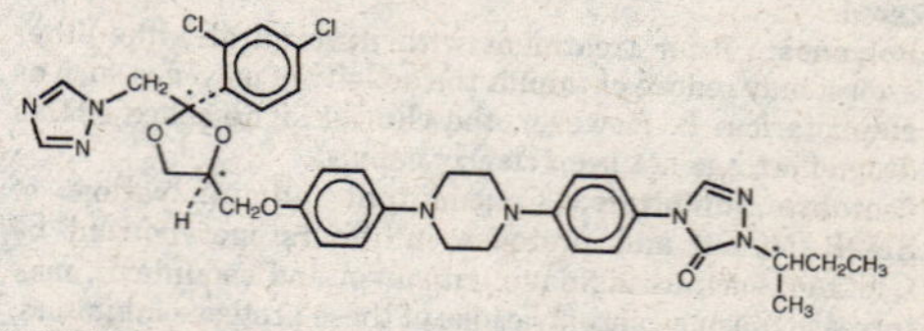

(±)-1-[(R*)-sec-butyl]-4-[p-[4-[p-[[(2R*,4S*)-2-(2,4-dichlorophenyl)-2-(1H-1,2,4-triazol-1-ylmethyl)-1,3-dioxolan-4-yl] methoxy]phenyl]-1-piperazinyl] phenyl]-Δ^2-1,2,4-triazolin-5-one mixture with (±)-1-[(R*)-sec-butyl]-4-[p-[4-[p-[[(2S*, 4R*)-2-(2,4-dichlorophenyl)-2-(1H-1,2,4-triazol-1-ylmethyl)-1,3-dioxolan-4-yl]methoxy]phenyl]-1-piperazinyl]phenyl]-Δ^2-1,2,4-triazolin-5-one

or

(±)-1-[(RS)-sec-butyl]-4-[p-[4-[p-[[(2R,4S)-2-(2,4-dichlorophenyl)-2-(1H-1,2,4-triazol-1-ylmethyl)-1,3-dioxolan-4-yl] methoxy]phenyl]-1-piperazinyl] phenyl]-Δ^2-1,2,4-triazolin-5-one.

Itraconazole has a molecular formula of $C_{35}H_{38}Cl_2N_8O_4$ and a molecular weight of 705.64. It is a white to slightly yellowish powder. It is insoluble in water, very slightly soluble in alcohols, and freely soluble in dichloromethane. It has a pKa of 3.70 (based on extrapolation of values obtained from methanolic solutions) and a log (n-octanol/water) partition coefficient of 5.66 at pH 8.1.

SPORANOX® (itraconazole) Oral Solution contains 10 mg of itraconazole per mL, solubilized by hydroxypropyl-β-cyclodextrin (400 mg/mL) as a molecular inclusion complex. SPORANOX® Oral Solution is clear and yellowish in color with a target pH of 2. Other ingredients are hydrochloric acid, propylene glycol, purified water, sodium hydroxide, sodium saccharin, sorbitol, cherry flavor 1, cherry flavor 2 and caramel flavor.

CLINICAL PHARMACOLOGY

Pharmacokinetics and Metabolism: NOTE: The plasma concentrations reported below were measured by high-performance liquid chromatography (HPLC) specific for itraconazole. When itraconazole in plasma is measured by a bioassay, values reported may be higher than those obtained by HPLC due to the presence of the bioactive metabolite, hydroxyitraconazole. (See MICROBIOLOGY.)

The absolute bioavailability of itraconazole administered as a non-marketed solution formulation under fed conditions was 55% in 6 healthy male volunteers. However, the bioavailability of SPORANOX® (itraconazole) Oral Solution is increased under fasted conditions reaching higher maximum plasma concentrations (C_{max}) in a shorter period of time. In 27 healthy male volunteers, the steady-state area under the plasma concentration versus time curve (AUC_{0-24h}) of itraconazole (SPORANOX® Oral Solution, 200 mg daily for 15 days) under fasted conditions was 131 ± 30% of that obtained under fed conditions. Therefore, unlike SPORANOX® Capsules, it is recommended that SPORANOX® Oral Solution be administered without food. Presented in the table below are the steady-state (Day 15) pharmacokinetic parameters for itraconazole and hydroxyitraconazole (SPORANOX® Oral Solution) under fasted and fed conditions:

[See first table at right]

The bioavailability of SPORANOX® Oral Solution relative to SPORANOX® Capsules was studied in 30 healthy male volunteers who received 200 mg of itraconazole as the oral solution and capsules under fed conditions. The $AUC_{0-\infty}$ from SPORANOX® Oral Solution was 149 ± 68% of that obtained from SPORANOX® Capsules; a similar increase was observed for hydroxyitraconazole. In addition, a cross study comparison of itraconazole and hydroxyitraconazole pharmacokinetics following the administration of single 200 mg doses of SPORANOX® Oral Solution (under fasted conditions) or SPORANOX® Capsules (under fed conditions) indicates that when these two formulations are administered under conditions which optimize their systemic absorption, the bioavailability of the solution relative to capsules is expected to be increased further. Therefore, it is recommended that SPORANOX® Oral Solution and SPORANOX® Capsules not be used interchangeably. The following table contains pharmacokinetic parameters for itraconazole and hydroxyitraconazole following single 200 mg doses of SPORANOX® Oral Solution (n=27) or SPORANOX® Capsules (n=30) administered to healthy male volunteers under fasted and fed conditions, respectively:

[See second table at right]

The plasma protein binding of itraconazole is 99.8% and that of hydroxyitraconazole is 99.5%. Following intravenous administration, the volume of distribution of itraconazole averaged 796 ± 185 L.

Itraconazole is metabolized predominately by the cytochrome P450 3A4 isoenzyme system (CYP3A4), resulting in the formation of several metabolites, including hydroxyitraconazole, the major metabolite. Results of a pharmacokinetics study suggest that itraconazole may undergo saturable metabolism with multiple dosing. Fecal excretion of the parent drug varies between 3-18% of the dose. Renal excretion of the parent drug is less than 0.03% of the dose. About 40% of the dose is excreted as inactive metabolites in the urine. No single excreted metabolite represents more than 5% of a dose. Itraconazole total plasma clearance averaged 381 ± 95 mL/minute following intravenous administration. (See CONTRAINDICATIONS and PRECAUTIONS: Drug Interactions for more information.)

Special Populations:

Pediatrics: The pharmacokinetics of SPORANOX® Oral Solution were studied in 26 pediatric patients requiring systemic antifungal therapy. Patients were stratified by age: 6 months to 2 years (n=8), 2 to 5 years (n=7) and 5 to 12 years (n=11), and received itraconazole oral solution 5 mg/kg once daily for 14 days. Pharmacokinetic parameters at steady-state (Day 14) were not significantly different among the age strata and are summarized in the table below for all 26 patients:

	Itraconazole	Hydroxyitraconazole
C_{max} (ng/mL)	582.5 ± 382.4*	692.4 ± 355.0
C_{min} (ng/mL)	187.5 ± 161.4	403.8 ± 336.1
AUC_{0-24h} (ng·h/mL)	7706.7 ± 5245.2	13356.4 ± 8942.4
$t_{1/2}$ (hours)	35.8 ± 35.6	17.7 ± 13.0

*mean ± standard deviation

Renal Insufficiency: A pharmacokinetic study using a single 200-mg dose of itraconazole (four 50-mg capsules) was conducted in three groups of patients with renal impairment (uremia: n=7; hemodialysis: n=7; and continuous ambulatory peritoneal dialysis: n=5). In uremic subjects with a mean creatinine clearance of 13 mL/min. × 1.73 m², the bioavailability was slightly reduced compared with normal

	Itraconazole		Hydroxyitraconazole	
	Fasted	Fed	Fasted	Fed
C_{max} (ng/mL)	1963 ± 601*	1435 ± 477	2055 ± 487	1781 ± 397
T_{max} (hours)	2.5 ± 0.8	4.4 ± 0.7	5.3 ± 4.3	4.3 ± 1.2
AUC_{0-24h} (ng·h/mL)	29271 ± 10285	22815 ± 7098	45184 ± 10981	38823 ± 8907
$t_{1/2}$ (hours)	39.7 ± 13	37.4 ± 13	27.3 ± 13	26.1 ± 10

*mean ± standard deviation

	Itraconazole		Hydroxyitraconazole	
	Oral Solution fasted	Capsules fed	Oral Solution fasted	Capsules fed
C_{max} (ng/mL)	544 ± 213*	302 ± 119	622 ± 116	504 ± 132
T_{max} (hours)	2.2 ± 0.8	5 ± 0.8	3.5 ± 1.2	5 ± 1
AUC_{0-24h} (ng·h/mL)	4505 ± 1670	2682 ± 1084	9552 ± 1835	7293 ± 2144

*mean ± standard deviation

population parameters. This study did not demonstrate any significant effect of hemodialysis or continuous ambulatory peritoneal dialysis on the pharmacokinetics of itraconazole (T_{max}, C_{max}, and AUC_{0-8}). Plasma concentration-versus-time profiles showed wide intersubject variation in all three groups.

Hepatic Insufficiency: Patients with impaired hepatic function should be carefully monitored when taking itraconazole. The prolonged elimination half-life of itraconazole observed in cirrhotic patients should be considered when deciding to initiate therapy with other medications metabolized by CYP3A4. (See BOX WARNING, CONTRAINDICATIONS, and PRECAUTIONS: Drug Interactions.)

Decreased Cardiac Contractility: When itraconazole was administered intravenously to anesthetized dogs, a dose-related negative inotropic effect was documented. In a healthy volunteer study of SPORANOX® Injection (intravenous infusion), transient, asymptomatic decreases in left ventricular ejection fraction were observed using gated SPECT imaging; these resolved before the next infusion, 12 hours later. If signs or symptoms of congestive heart failure appear during administration of SPORANOX® Oral Solution, monitor carefully and consider other treatment alternatives which may include discontinuation of SPORANOX® Oral Solution administration. (See WARNINGS, PRECAUTIONS: Drug Interactions and ADVERSE REACTIONS: Post-marketing Experience for more information.)

Cystic Fibrosis: Seventeen cystic fibrosis patients, ages 7 to 28 years old, were administered itraconazole oral solution 2.5 mg/kg bid for 14 days in a pharmacokinetic study. Sixteen patients completed the study. Steady state trough concentrations >250ng/mL were achieved in 6 out of 11 patients ≥16 years of age but in none of the 5 patients <16 years of age. Large variability was observed in the pharmacokinetic data (%CV for trough concentrations = 98% and 70% for ≥16 and <16 years, respectively; %CV for AUC = 75% and 58% for ≥16 and <16 years, respectively). If a patient with cystic fibrosis does not respond to SPORANOX® Oral Solution, consideration should be given to switching to alternative therapy.

MICROBIOLOGY

Mechanism of Action: In vitro studies have demonstrated that itraconazole inhibits the cytochrome P450-dependent synthesis of ergosterol, which is a vital component of fungal cell membranes.

Activity In Vitro and In Vivo: Itraconazole exhibits in vitro activity against *Blastomyces dermatitidis, Histoplasma capsulatum, Histoplasma duboisii, Aspergillus flavus, Aspergillus fumigatus, Candida albicans,* and *Cryptococcus neoformans.* Itraconazole also exhibits varying in vitro activity against *Sporothrix schenckii, Trichophyton* species, *Candida krusei,* and other *Candida* species. The bioactive metabolite, hydroxyitraconazole, has not been evaluated against *Histoplasma capsulatum* and *Blastomyces dermatitidis.* Correlation between minimum inhibitory concentration (MIC) results in vitro and clinical outcome has yet to be established for azole antifungal agents.

Itraconazole administered orally was active in a variety of animal models of fungal infection using standard laboratory strains of fungi. Fungistatic activity has been demonstrated against disseminated fungal infections caused by *Blastomyces dermatitidis, Histoplasma duboisii, Aspergillus fumigatus, Coccidioides immitis, Cryptococcus neoformans, Paracoccidioides brasiliensis, Sporothrix schenckii, Trichophyton rubrum,* and *Trichophyton mentagrophytes.*

Itraconazole administered at 2.5 mg/kg and 5 mg/kg via the oral and parenteral routes increased survival rates and sterilized organ systems in normal and immunosuppressed guinea pigs with disseminated *Aspergillus fumigatus* infections. Oral itraconazole administered daily at 40 mg/kg and 80 mg/kg increased survival rates in normal rabbits with disseminated disease and in immunosuppressed rats with pulmonary *Aspergillus fumigatus* infection, respectively. Itraconazole has demonstrated antifungal activity in a variety of animal models infected with *Candida albicans* and other *Candida* species.

Resistance: Isolates from several fungal species with decreased susceptibility to itraconazole have been isolated in vitro and from patients receiving prolonged therapy.

Several in vitro studies have reported that some fungal clinical isolates, including *Candida* species, with reduced susceptibility to one azole antifungal agent may also be less susceptible to other azole derivatives. The finding of cross-resistance is dependent on a number of factors, including the species evaluated, its clinical history, the particular azole compounds compared, and the type of susceptibility test that is performed. The relevance of these in vitro susceptibility data to clinical outcome remains to be elucidated.

Studies (both in vitro and in vivo) suggest that the activity of amphotericin B may be suppressed by prior azole antifungal therapy. As with other azoles, itraconazole inhibits the ^{14}C-demethylation step in the synthesis of ergosterol, a cell wall component of fungi. Ergosterol is the active site for amphotericin B. In one study the antifungal activity of amphotericin B against *Aspergillus fumigatus* infections in mice was inhibited by ketoconazole therapy. The clinical significance of test results obtained in this study is unknown.

CLINICAL STUDIES

Empiric Therapy in Febrile Neutropenic Patients: An open randomized trial compared the efficacy and safety of itraconazole (intravenous followed by oral solution) with amphotericin B for empiric therapy in 384 febrile, neutropenic patients with hematologic malignancies who had suspected fungal infections. Patients received either itraconazole (injection, 200 mg b.i.d. for 2 days followed by 200 mg once daily for up to 14 days, followed by oral solution, 200 mg b.i.d.) or amphotericin B (total daily dose of 0.7-1.0 mg/kg body weight). The longest treatment duration was 28 days. An outcome assignment of "success" required (a) patient survival with resolution of fever and neutropenia within 28 days of treatment, (b) absence of emergent fungal infections, (c) no discontinuation of therapy due to toxicity or lack of efficacy, and (d) treatment for three or more days. The success rate using an intent-to-treat analysis was 47% for the itraconazole group and 38% for the amphotericin B arm.

[See first table at top of next page]

Oropharyngeal Candidiasis: Two randomized, controlled studies for the treatment of oropharyngeal candidiasis have been conducted (total n=344). In one trial, clinical response to either 7 or 14 days of itraconazole oral solution, 200 mg/day, was similar to fluconazole tablets and averaged 84% across all arms. Clinical response in this study was defined as cured or improved (only minimal signs and symptoms with no visible lesions). Approximately 5% of subjects were lost to follow-up before any evaluations could be performed. Response to 14 days therapy of itraconazole oral solution was associated with a lower relapse rate than 7 days of itraconazole therapy. In another trial, the clinical response rate (defined as cured or improved) for itraconazole oral solution was similar to clotrimazole troches and averaged approximately 71% across both arms, with approximately 3% of subjects lost to follow-up before any evaluations could be performed. Ninety-two percent of the patients in these studies were HIV seropositive.

In an uncontrolled, open-label study of selected patients clinically unresponsive to fluconazole tablets (n=74, all patients HIV seropositive), patients were treated with itraconazole oral solution 100 mg b.i.d. (Clinically unresponsive to fluconazole in this study was defined as having received a dose of fluconazole tablets at least 200 mg/day for a minimum of 14 days.) Treatment duration was 14-28 days based on response. Approximately 55% of patients had complete resolution of oral lesions. Of patients who responded and then entered a follow-up phase (n=22), all relapsed

Continued on next page

Sporanox Oral Solution—Cont.

within 1 month (median 14 days) when treatment was discontinued. Although baseline endoscopies had not been performed, several patients in this study developed symptoms of esophageal candidiasis while receiving therapy with itraconazole oral solution. Itraconazole oral solution has not been directly compared to other agents in a controlled trial of similar patients.

Esophageal Candidiasis: A double-blind randomized study (n=119, 111 of whom were HIV seropositive) compared itraconazole oral solution (100 mg/day) to fluconazole tablets (100 mg/day). The dose of each was increased to 200 mg/day for patients not responding initially. Treatment continued for 2 weeks following resolution of symptoms, for a total duration of treatment of 3-8 weeks. Clinical response (a global assessment of cured or improved) was not significantly different between the two study arms, and averaged approximately 86% with 8% lost to follow-up. Six of 53 (11%) itraconazole-treated patients and 12/57 (21%) fluconazole-treated patients were escalated to the 200 mg dose in this trial. Of the subgroup of patients who responded and entered a follow-up phase (n=88), approximately 23% relapsed across both arms within 4 weeks.

INDICATIONS AND USAGE

SPORANOX® (itraconazole) Injection/Oral Solution is indicated for empiric therapy of febrile neutropenic patients with suspected fungal infections. (NOTE: In a comparative trial, the overall response rate for itraconazole-treated subjects was higher than for amphotericin B-treated subjects. However, compared to amphotericin B-treated subjects, a larger number of itraconazole-treated subjects discontinued treatment due to persistent fever and a change in antifungal medication due to fever. Whereas, a larger number of amphotericin B-treated subjects discontinued due to drug intolerance. (See CLINICAL STUDIES section.)

SPORANOX® (itraconazole) Oral Solution is also indicated for the treatment of oropharyngeal and esophageal candidiasis.

(See CLINICAL PHARMACOLOGY: Special Populations, WARNINGS, and ADVERSE REACTIONS: Post-marketing Experience for more information.)

CONTRAINDICATIONS

Drug Interactions: Concomitant administration of SPORANOX® (itraconazole) Capsules, Injection, or Oral Solution and certain drugs metabolized by the cytochrome P450 3A4 isoenzyme system (CYP3A4) may result in increased plasma concentrations of those drugs, leading to potentially serious and/or life-threatening adverse events. Cisapride, oral midazolam, pimozide, quinidine, dofetilide, triazolam and levacetylmethadol (levomethadyl) are contraindicated with SPORANOX®. HMG CoA-reductase inhibitors metabolized by CYP3A4, such as lovastatin and simvastatin, are also contraindicated with SPORANOX®. Ergot alkaloids metabolized by CYP3A4 such as dihydroergotamine, ergometrine (ergonovine), ergotamine and methylergometrine (methylergonovine) are contraindicated with SPORANOX®. (See BOX WARNING, and PRECAUTIONS: Drug Interactions.)

SPORANOX® is contraindicated for patients who have shown hypersensitivity to itraconazole or its excipients. There is no information regarding cross-hypersensitivity between itraconazole and other azole antifungal agents. Caution should be used when prescribing SPORANOX® to patients with hypersensitivity to other azoles.

WARNINGS

SPORANOX® (itraconazole) Oral Solution and SPORANOX® Capsules should not be used interchangeably. Only SPORANOX® Oral Solution has been demonstrated effective for oral and/or esophageal candidiasis. SPORANOX® Oral Solution contains the excipient hydroxypropyl-β-cyclodextrin which produced pancreatic adenocarcinomas in a rat carcinogenicity study. These findings were not observed in a similar mouse carcinogenicity study. The clinical relevance of these findings is unknown. (See Carcinogenesis, Mutagenesis, and Impairment of Fertility.)

Hepatic Effects: SPORANOX® has been associated with rare cases of serious hepatotoxicity, including liver failure and death. Some of these cases had neither pre-existing liver disease nor a serious underlying medical condition and some of these cases developed within the first week of treatment. If clinical signs or symptoms develop that are consistent with liver disease, treatment should be discontinued and liver function testing performed. Continued SPORANOX® use or reinstitution of treatment with SPORANOX® is strongly discouraged unless there is a serious or life threatening situation where the expected benefit exceeds the risk. (See PRECAUTIONS: Information for Patients and ADVERSE REACTIONS.)

Cardiac Dysrhythmias: Life-threatening cardiac dysrhythmias and/or sudden death have occurred in patients using cisapride, pimozide, levacetylmethadol (levomethadyl), or quinidine concomitantly with SPORANOX® and/or other CYP3A4 inhibitors. Concomitant administration of these drugs with SPORANOX® is contraindicated. (See BOX WARNING, CONTRAINDICATIONS, and PRECAUTIONS: Drug Interactions.)

Cardiac Disease: SPORANOX® Oral Solution should not be used in patients with evidence of ventricular dysfunction unless the benefit clearly outweighs the risk. For patients with risk factors for congestive heart failure, physicians should carefully review the risks and benefits of SPORANOX® therapy. These risk factors include cardiac

Overview of Efficacy
(Intent-to-Treat Population)

Efficacy Parameters	SPORANOX® N=179 (%)	Amphotericin B N=181 (%)
Success	84 (47%)	68 (38%)
Unevaluable*	24 (13%)	44 (24%)
Failure	71 (40%)	69 (38%)
Reason for Failure		
Intolerance after > 3 days of antifungal medication	12	37
Persistent fever	20	7
Change in antifungal medication due to fever	13	1
Emergent fungal infection	10	9
Documented bacterial or viral infection	7	8
Insufficient response	6	5
Deterioration of signs and symptoms	2	0
Death after > 3 days antifungal medication	1	2
Resolution of fever	131 (73%)	127 (70%)
Survival	161 (90%)	156 (86%)

*Treatment duration ≤ 3 days (including patients who died within 3 days, withdrew because of adverse events or were deemed ineligible due to a confirmed pre-treatment infection).

Table 1. Selected Drugs that are predicted to alter the plasma concentration of itraconazole or have their plasma concentration altered by SPORANOX®[1]

Drug plasma concentration increased by itraconazole	
Antiarrhythmics	digoxin, dofetilide[2], quinidine[2], disopyramide
Anticoagulants	Warfarin
Anticonvulsants	Carbamazepine
Antimycobacterials	Rifabutin
Antineoplastics	busulfan, docetaxel, vinca alkaloids
Antipsychotics	pimozide[2],
Benzodiazepines	alprazolam, diazepam, midazolam,[2,3] triazolam[2]
Calcium Channel Blockers	dihydropyridines, verapamil
Gastrointestinal Motility Agents	cisapride[2]
HMG CoA-Reductase Inhibitors	atorvastatin, cerivastatin, lovastatin,[2] simvastatin[2]
Immunosuppressants	cyclosporine, tacrolimus, sirolimus
Oral Hypoglycemics	oral hypoglycemics
Protease Inhibitors	indinavir, ritonavir, saquinavir
Other	levacetylmethadol, (levomethadyl), ergot alkaloids, halofantrine, alfentanil, buspirone, methylprednisolone, budesonide, dexamethasone, trimetrexate, warfarin, cilostazol, eletriptan
Decrease plasma concentration of itraconazole	
Anticonvulsants	carbamazepine, phenobarbital, phenytoin
Antimycobacterials	isoniazid, rifabutin, rifampin
Gastric Acid Suppressors/Neutralizers	antacids, H_2-receptor antagonists, proton pump inhibitors
Reverse Transcriptase Inhibitors	Nevirapine
Increase plasma concentration of itraconazole	
Macrolide Antibiotics	clarithromycin, erythromycin
Protease Inhibitors	indinavir, ritonavir

[1]This list is not all-inclusive.
[2]Contraindicated with SPORANOX® based on clinical and/or pharmacokinetics studies. (See WARNINGS and below.)
[3]For information on parenterally administered midazolam, see the Benzodiazepine paragraph below.

disease such as ischemic and valvular disease; significant pulmonary disease such as chronic obstructive pulmonary disease; and renal failure and other edematous disorders. Such patients should be informed of the signs and symptoms of CHF, should be treated with caution, and should be monitored for signs and symptoms of CHF during treatment. If signs or symptoms of CHF appear during administration of SPORANOX® Oral Solution, monitor carefully and consider other treatment alternatives which may include discontinuation of SPORANOX® Oral Solution administration.

When itraconazole was administered intravenously to anesthetized dogs, a dose-related negative inotropic effect was documented. In a healthy volunteer study of SPORANOX® Injection (intravenous infusion), transient, asymptomatic decreases in left ventricular ejection fraction were observed using gated SPECT imaging; these resolved before the next infusion, 12 hours later.

Cases of CHF, peripheral edema, and pulmonary edema have been reported in the post-marketing period among patients being treated for onychomycosis and/or systemic fungal infections. (See CLINICAL PHARMACOLOGY: Special Populations, PRECAUTIONS: Drug Interactions, and ADVERSE REACTIONS: Post-marketing Experience for more information.)

Cystic Fibrosis: If a patient with cystic fibrosis does not respond to SPORANOX® Oral Solution, consideration should be given to switching to alternative therapy (see CLINICAL PHARMACOLOGY/Special Populations).

Treatment of Severely Neutropenic Patients: SPORANOX® Oral Solution as treatment for oropharyngeal and/or esophageal candidiasis was not investigated in severely neutropenic patients. Due to its pharmacokinetic properties, SPORANOX® Oral Solution is not recommended for initiation of treatment in patients at immediate risk of systemic candidiasis.

PRECAUTIONS

General: Rare cases of serious hepatotoxicity have been observed with SPORANOX® treatment, including some cases within the first week. In patients with elevated or abnormal liver enzymes or active liver disease, or who have experienced liver toxicity with other drugs, treatment with SPORANOX® is strongly discouraged unless there is a serious or life threatening situation where the expected benefit exceeds the risk. Liver function monitoring should be done in patients with pre-existing hepatic function abnormalities or those who have experienced liver toxicity with other medications and should be considered in all patients receiving SPORANOX®. Treatment should be stopped immediately and liver function testing should be conducted in patients who develop signs and symptoms suggestive of liver dysfunction.

If neuropathy occurs that may be attributable to SPORANOX® Oral Solution, the treatment should be discontinued.

Information for Patients:

- Only SPORANOX® Oral Solution has been demonstrated effective for oral and/or esophageal candidiasis. SPORANOX® Oral Solution contains the excipient hydroxypropyl-β-cyclodextrin which produced pancreatic adenocarcinomas in a rat carcinogenicity study. These findings were not observed in a similar mouse carcinogenicity study. The clinical relevance of these findings is unknown. (See Carcinogenesis, Mutagenesis, and Impairment of Fertility.)
- Taking SPORANOX® Oral Solution under fasted conditions improves the systemic availability of itraconazole. Instruct patients to take SPORANOX® Oral Solution without food, if possible.
- SPORANOX® Oral Solution should not be used interchangeably with SPORANOX® Capsules.
- Instruct patients about the signs and symptoms of congestive heart failure, and if these signs or symptoms occur during SPORANOX® administration, they should discontinue SPORANOX® and contact their healthcare provider immediately.
- Instruct patients to stop SPORANOX® treatment immediately and contact their healthcare provider if any signs and symptoms suggestive of liver dysfunction develop. Such signs and symptoms may include unusual fatigue, anorexia, nausea and/or vomiting, jaundice, dark urine or pale stools.
- Instruct patients to contact their physician before taking any concomitant medications with itraconazole to ensure there are no potential drug interactions.

Drug Interactions: Itraconazole and its major metabolite, hydroxyitraconazole, are inhibitors of CYP3A4. Therefore, the following drug interactions may occur (See Table 1 below and the following drug class subheadings that follow):

1. SPORANOX® may decrease the elimination of drugs metabolized by CYP3A4, resulting in increased plasma concentrations of these drugs when they are administered with SPORANOX®. These elevated plasma concentrations may increase or prolong both therapeutic and adverse effects of these drugs. Whenever possible, plasma concentrations of these drugs should be monitored, and dosage adjustments made after concomitant SPORANOX® therapy is initiated. When appropriate, clinical monitoring for signs or symptoms of increased or prolonged pharmacologic effects is advised. Upon discontinuation, depending on the dose and duration of treatment, itraconazole plasma concentrations decline gradually (especially in patients with hepatic cirrhosis or in those receiving CYP3A4 inhibitors). This is particularly important when initiating therapy with drugs whose metabolism is affected by itraconazole.
2. Inducers of CYP3A4 may decrease the plasma concentrations of itraconazole. SPORANOX® may not be effective in patients concomitantly taking SPORANOX® and one of these drugs. Therefore, administration of these drugs with SPORANOX® is not recommended.
3. Other inhibitors of CYP3A4 may increase the plasma concentrations of itraconazole. Patients who must take SPORANOX® concomitantly with one of these drugs should be monitored closely for signs or symptoms of increased or prolonged pharmacologic effects of SPORANOX®.

[See table 1 at top of previous page]

Antiarrhythmics: The class IA antiarrhythmic quinidine and class III antiarrhythmic dofetilide are known to prolong the QT interval. Coadministration of quinidine or dofetilide with SPORANOX® may increase plasma concentrations of quinidine or dofetilide which could result in serious cardiovascular events. Therefore, concomitant administration of SPORANOX® and quinidine or dofetilide is contraindicated. (See BOX WARNING, CONTRAINDICATIONS, and WARNINGS.)

The class IA antiarrhythmic disopyramide has the potential to increase the QT interval at high plasma concentrations. Caution is advised when SPORANOX® and disopyramide are administered concomitantly.

Concomitant administration of digoxin and SPORANOX® has led to increased plasma concentrations of digoxin.

Anticoagulants: SPORANOX® enhances the anticoagulant effect of coumarin-like drugs, such as warfarin.

Table 2: Summary of possibly or definitely drug-related adverse events reported in ≥ 2% of subjects (Empiric Therapy Trial in Febrile Neutropenic Patients)

Adverse Event	SPORANOX® (N=192) %	Amphotericin B (N=192) %
Gastrointestinal system disorders		
Nausea	11	15
Diarrhea	10	9
Vomiting	7	10
Abdominal pain	3	3
Metabolic and nutritional disorders		
Hypokalemia	9	28
Serum creatinine increased	3	25
LDH increased	2	0
Alkaline phosphatase increased	2	2
Hypomagnesemia	2	4
Blood urea nitrogen increased	1	6
Fluid overload	1	3
Hypocalcemia	1	2
Liver and biliary system disorders		
Bilirubinemia	6	3
Hepatic function abnormal	3	2
SGPT/ALT increased	3	1
Jaundice	2	1
SGOT/AST increased	2	1
Skin and appendage disorders		
Rash	5	3
Sweating increased	2	1
CNS and peripheral nervous system		
Headache	2	2
Body as a whole		
Edema	2	2
Rigors	1	34
Fever	0	7
Respiratory system disorder		
Dyspnea	1	3
Urinary system disorder		
Renal function abnormal	1	12
Cardiovascular disorders, general		
Hypotension	1	3
Hypertension	0	2
Heart rate and rhythm disorders		
Tachycardia	1	3

Anticonvulsants: Reduced plasma concentrations of itraconazole were reported when SPORANOX® was administered concomitantly with phenytoin. Carbamazepine, phenobarbital, and phenytoin are all inducers of CYP3A4. Although interactions with carbamazepine and phenobarbital have not been studied, concomitant administration of SPORANOX® and these drugs would be expected to result in decreased plasma concentrations of itraconazole. In addition, in vivo studies have demonstrated an increase in plasma carbamazepine concentrations in subjects concomitantly receiving ketoconazole. Although there are no data regarding the effect of itraconazole on carbamazepine metabolism, because of the similarities between ketoconazole and itraconazole, concomitant administration of SPORANOX® and carbamazepine may inhibit the metabolism of carbamazepine.

Antimycobacterials: Drug interaction studies have demonstrated that plasma concentrations of azole antifungal agents and their metabolites, including itraconazole and hydroxyitraconazole, were significantly decreased when these agents were given concomitantly with rifabutin or rifampin. In vivo data suggest that rifabutin is metabolized in part by CYP3A4. SPORANOX® may inhibit the metabolism of rifabutin. Although no formal study data are available for isoniazid, similar effects should be anticipated. Therefore, the efficacy of SPORANOX® could be substantially reduced if given concomitantly with one of these agents. Coadministration is not recommended.

Antineoplastics: SPORANOX® may inhibit the metabolism of busulfan, docetaxel, and vinca alkaloids.

Antipsychotics: Pimozide is known to prolong the QT interval and is partially metabolized by CYP3A4. Coadministration of pimozide with SPORANOX® could result in serious cardiovascular events. Therefore, concomitant administration of SPORANOX® and pimozide is contraindicated. (See BOX WARNING, CONTRAINDICATIONS, and WARNINGS.)

Benzodiazepines: Concomitant administration of SPORANOX® and alprazolam, diazepam, oral midazolam, or triazolam could lead to increased plasma concentrations of these benzodiazepines. Increased plasma concentrations could potentiate and prolong hypnotic and sedative effects. Concomitant administration of SPORANOX® and oral midazolam or triazolam is contraindicated. (See CONTRAINDICATIONS and WARNINGS.) If midazolam is administered parenterally, special precaution and patient monitoring is required since the sedative effect may be prolonged.

Calcium Channel Blockers: Edema has been reported in patients concomitantly receiving SPORANOX® and dihy-

Continued on next page

Sporanox Oral Solution—Cont.

dropyridine calcium channel blockers. Appropriate dosage adjustment may be necessary.

Calcium channel blockers can have a negative inotropic effect which may be additive to those of itraconazole; itraconazole can inhibit the metabolism of calcium channel blockers such as dihydropyridines (e.g., nifedipine and felodipine) and verapamil. Therefore, caution should be used when co-administering itraconazole and calcium channel blockers. (See CLINICAL PHARMACOLOGY: Special Populations, WARNINGS, and ADVERSE REACTIONS: Post-marketing Experience for more information.)

Gastric Acid Suppressors/Neutralizers: Reduced plasma concentrations of itraconazole were reported when SPORANOX® Capsules were administered concomitantly with H_2-receptor antagonists. Studies have shown that absorption of itraconazole is impaired when gastric acid production is decreased. Therefore, SPORANOX® should be administered with a cola beverage if the patient has achlorhydria or is taking H_2-receptor antagonists or other gastric acid suppressors. Antacids should be administered at least 1 hour before or 2 hours after administration of SPORANOX® Capsules. In a clinical study, when SPORANOX® Capsules were administered with omeprazole (a proton pump inhibitor), the bioavailability of itraconazole was significantly reduced. However, as itraconazole is already dissolved in SPORANOX® Oral Solution, the effect of H_2 antagonists is expected to be substantially less than with the capsules. Nevertheless, caution is advised when the two drugs are co-administered.

Gastrointestinal Motility Agents: Coadministration of SPORANOX® with cisapride can elevate plasma cisapride concentrations which could result in serious cardiovascular events. Therefore, concomitant administration of SPORANOX® with cisapride is contraindicated. (See BOX WARNING, CONTRAINDICATIONS, and WARNINGS.)

HMG CoA-Reductase Inhibitors: Human pharmacokinetic data suggest that SPORANOX® inhibits the metabolism of atorvastatin, cerivastatin, lovastatin, and simvastatin, which may increase the risk of skeletal muscle toxicity, including rhabdomyolysis. Concomitant administration of SPORANOX® with HMG CoA-reductase inhibitors, such as lovastatin or simvastatin is contraindicated. (See CONTRAINDICATIONS and WARNINGS.)

Immunosuppressants: Concomitant administration of SPORANOX® and cyclosporine or tacrolimus has led to increased plasma concentrations of these immunosuppressants. Concomitant administration of SPORANOX® and sirolimus could increase plasma concentrations of sirolimus.

Macrolide Antibiotics: Erythromycin and clarithromycin are known inhibitors of CYP3A4 (See Table 1) and may increase plasma concentrations of itraconazole. In a small pharmacokinetic study involving HIV infected patients, clarithromycin was shown to increase plasma concentrations of itraconazole. Similarly, following administration of 1 gram of erythromycin ethyl succinate and 200 mg itraconazole as single doses, the mean C_{max} and $AUC_{0-\infty}$ of itraconazole increased by 44% (90% CI: 119-175%) and 36% (90% CI: 108-171%), respectively.

Oral Hypoglycemic Agents: Severe hypoglycemia has been reported in patients concomitantly receiving azole antifungal agents and oral hypoglycemic agents. Blood glucose concentrations should be carefully monitored when SPORANOX® and oral hypoglycemic agents are coadministered.

Polyenes: Prior treatment with itraconazole, like other azoles, may reduce or inhibit the activity of polyenes such as amphotericin B. However, the clinical significance of this drug effect has not been clearly defined.

Protease Inhibitors: Concomitant administration of SPORANOX® and protease inhibitors metabolized by CYP3A4, such as indinavir, ritonavir, and saquinavir, may increase plasma concentrations of these protease inhibitors. In addition, concomitant administration of SPORANOX® and indinavir and ritonavir (but not saquinavir) may increase plasma concentrations of itraconazole. Caution is advised when SPORANOX® and protease inhibitors must be given concomitantly.

Reverse Transcriptase Inhibitors: Nevirapine is an inducer of CYP3A4. In vivo studies have shown that nevirapine induces the metabolism of ketoconazole, significantly reducing the bioavailability of ketoconazole. Studies involving nevirapine and itraconazole have not been conducted. However, because of the similarities between ketoconazole and itraconazole, concomitant administration of SPORANOX® and nevirapine is not recommended. In a clinical study, when 8 HIV-infected subjects were treated concomitantly with SPORANOX® Capsules 100 mg twice daily and the nucleoside reverse transcriptase inhibitor zidovudine 8 ± 0.4 mg/kg/day, the pharmacokinetics of zidovudine were not affected. Other nucleoside reverse transcriptase inhibitors have not been studied.

Other:

- Levacetylmethadol (levomethadyl) is known to prolong the QT interval and is metabolized by CYP3A4. Co-administration of levacetylmethadol with SPORANOX® could result in serious cardiovascular events. Therefore, concomitant administration of SPORANOX® and levacetylmethadol is contraindicated.
- Elevated concentrations of ergot alkaloids can cause ergotism, ie. a risk for vasospasm potentially leading to cerebral ischemia and/or ischemia of the extremities. Concomitant administration of ergot alkaloids such as dihydroergotamine, ergometrine (ergonovine), ergotamine and methylergometrine (methylergonovine) with SPORANOX® is contraindicated.
- Halofantrine has the potential to prolong the QT interval at high plasma concentrations. Caution is advised when SPORANOX® and halofantrine are administered concomitantly.
- In vitro data suggest that alfentanil is metabolized by CYP3A4. Administration with SPORANOX® may increase plasma concentrations of alfentanil.
- Human pharmacokinetic data suggest that concomitant administration of SPORANOX® and buspirone results in significant increases in plasma concentrations of buspirone.
- SPORANOX® may inhibit the metabolism of certain glucocorticosteroids such as budesonide, dexamethasone and methylprednisolone.
- In vitro data suggest that trimetrexate is extensively metabolized by CYP3A4. In vitro animal models have demonstrated that ketoconazole potently inhibits the metabolism of trimetrexate. Although there are no data regarding the effect of itraconazole on trimetrexate metabolism, because of the similarities between ketoconazole and itraconazole, concomitant administration of SPORANOX® and trimetrexate may inhibit the metabolism of trimetrexate.
- Cilostazol and eletriptan are CYP3A4 metabolized drugs that should be used with caution when co-administered with SPORANOX®.

Table 3: Summary of Adverse Events Reported by ≥2% of SPORANOX® Treated Patients in U.S. Clinical Trials (Total)

Body System/Adverse Event	Itraconazole		Clotrimazole (n=125**)%	(n=81***)%
	All Total (n=350*)%	Fluconazole controlled studies (n=272)%		
Gastrointestinal disorders				
Nausea	11	10	11	5
Diarrhea	11	10	10	4
Vomiting	7	6	8	1
Abdominal pain	6	4	7	7
Constipation	2	2	1	0
Body as a whole				
Fever	7	6	8	5
Chest pain	3	3	2	0
Pain	2	2	4	0
Fatigue	2	1	2	0
Respiratory disorders				
Coughing	4	4	10	0
Dyspnea	2	3	5	1
Pneumonia	2	2	0	0
Sinusitis	2	2	4	0
Sputum increased	2	3	3	1
Skin and appendages disorders				
Rash	4	5	4	6
Increased sweating	3	4	6	1
Skin disorder, unspecified	2	2	2	1
Central/peripheral nervous system				
Headache	4	4	6	6
Dizziness	2	2	4	1
Resistance mechanism disorders				
Pneumocystis carinii infection	2	2	2	0
Psychiatric disorders				
Depression	2	1	0	1

* Of the 350 patients, 209 were treated for oropharyngeal candidiasis in controlled studies, 63 were treated for esophageal candidiasis in controlled studies and 78 were treated for oropharyngeal candidiasis in an open study.

** Of the 125 patients, 62 were treated for oropharyngeal candidiasis and 63 were treated for esophageal candidiasis.

*** All 81 patients were treated for oropharyngeal candidiasis.

Carcinogenesis, Mutagenesis, and Impairment of Fertility: Itraconazole showed no evidence of carcinogenicity potential in mice treated orally for 23 months at dosage levels up to 80 mg/kg/day (approximately 10x the maximum recommended human dose [MRHD]). Male rats treated with 25 mg/kg/day (3.1× MRHD) had a slightly increased incidence of soft tissue sarcoma. These sarcomas may have been a consequence of hypercholesterolemia, which is a response of rats, but not dogs or humans, to chronic itraconazole administration. Female rats treated with 50 mg/kg/day (6.25× MRHD) had an increased incidence of squamous cell carcinoma of the lung (2/50) as compared to the untreated group. Although the occurrence of squamous cell carcinoma in the lung is extremely uncommon in untreated rats, the increase in this study was not statistically significant.

Hydroxypropyl-β-cyclodextrin (HP-β-CD), the solubilizing excipient used in SPORANOX® Oral Solution, was found to produce pancreatic exocrine hyperplasia and neoplasia when administered orally to rats at doses of 500, 2000 or 5000 mg/kg/day for 25 months. Adenocarcinomas of the exocrine pancreas produced in the treated animals were not seen in the untreated group and are not reported in the historical controls. Development of these tumors may be related to a mitogenic action of cholecystokinin. This finding was not observed in the mouse carcinogenicity study at doses of 500, 2000 or 5000 mg/kg/day for 22-23 months; however, the clinical relevance of these findings is unknown. Based on body surface area comparisons, the exposure to humans of HP-β-CD at the recommended clinical dose of SPORANOX® Oral Solution, is approximately equivalent to 1.7 times the exposure at the lowest dose in the rat study.

Itraconazole produced no mutagenic effects when assayed in a DNA repair test (unscheduled DNA synthesis) in primary rat hepatocytes, in Ames tests with *Salmonella typhimurium* (6 strains) and *Escherichia coli*, in the mouse lymphoma gene mutation tests, in a sex-linked recessive lethal mutation (*Drosophila melanogaster*) test, in chromosome aberration tests in human lymphocytes, in a cell transformation test with C3H/10T½ C18 mouse embryo fibroblasts cells, in a dominant lethal mutation test in male and female mice, and in micronucleus tests in mice and rats.

Itraconazole did not affect the fertility of male or female rats treated orally with dosage levels of up to 40 mg/kg/day (5× MRHD), even though parental toxicity was present at this dosage level. More severe signs of parental toxicity, including death, were present in the next higher dosage level, 160 mg/kg/day (20× MRHD).

Pregnancy: Teratogenic Effects. Pregnancy Category C: Itraconazole was found to cause a dose-related increase in maternal toxicity, embryotoxicity, and teratogenicity in rats at dosage levels of approximately 40-160 mg/kg/day (5-20× MRHD), and in mice at dosage levels of approximately 80 mg/kg/day (10× MRHD). In rats, the teratogenicity consisted of major skeletal defects; in mice, it consisted of encephaloceles and/or macroglossia.

There are no studies in pregnant women. SPORANOX® should be used in pregnancy only if the benefit outweighs the potential risk.

During post-marketing experience, cases of congenital abnormalities have been reported. (See ADVERSE REACTIONS, Post-marketing Experience.)

Nursing Mothers: Itraconazole is excreted in human milk; therefore, the expected benefits of SPORANOX® therapy for the mother should be weighed against the potential risk from exposure of itraconazole to the infant. The U.S. Public Health Service Centers for Disease Control and Prevention advises HIV-infected women not to breast-feed to avoid potential transmission of HIV to uninfected infants.

Pediatric Use: The efficacy and safety of SPORANOX® have not been established in pediatric patients. A pharmacokinetic study was conducted with SPORANOX® Oral Solution in 26 pediatric patients, ages 6 months to 12 years, requiring systemic antifungal treatment. Itraconazole was dosed at 5 mg/kg once daily for two weeks and no serious unexpected adverse events were reported. (See CLINICAL PHARMACOLOGY.)

The long-term effects of itraconazole on bone growth in children are unknown. In three toxicology studies using rats, itraconazole induced bone defects at dosage levels as low as 20 mg/kg/day (2.5× MRHD). The induced defects included reduced bone plate activity, thinning of the zona compacta of the large bones, and increased bone fragility. At a dosage level of 80 mg/kg/day (10× MRHD) over 1 year or 160 mg/kg/day (20× MRHD) for 6 months, itraconazole induced small tooth pulp with hypocellular appearance in some rats. No such bone toxicity has been reported in adult patients.

ADVERSE REACTIONS

SPORANOX® has been associated with rare cases of serious hepatotoxicity, including liver failure and death. Some of these cases had neither pre-existing liver disease nor a serious underlying medical condition. If clinical signs or symptoms develop that are consistent with liver disease, treatment should be discontinued and liver function testing performed. The risks and benefits of SPORANOX® use should be reassessed. (See WARNINGS: Hepatic Effects and PRECAUTIONS: General and Information for Patients.)

Adverse Events Reported in Empiric Therapy in Febrile Neutropenic (ETFN) Patients

Adverse events considered at least possibly drug related in a clinical trial of empiric therapy in 384 febrile, neutropenic patients (192 treated with SPORANOX® and 192 with amphotericin B) with suspected fungal infections are listed in Table 2 below. Patients received a regimen of SPORANOX® Injection followed by SPORANOX® Oral Solution. The dose of SPORANOX® Injection was 200 mg twice daily for the first two days followed by a single daily dose of 200 mg for the remainder of the intravenous treatment period. The majority of patients received between 7 and 14 days of SPORANOX® Injection. The dose of SPORANOX® Oral Solution was 200 mg (20 mL) b.i.d. for the remainder of therapy.

[See table 2 at top of page 223]

The following additional adverse events considered at least possibly related occurred in between 1 and 2% of patients who received SPORANOX® Injection and Oral Solution: constipation, hypophosphatemia, gamma-GT increased, erythematous rash, pruritus, dizziness, tremor, and pulmonary infiltration.

Adverse Events Reported in Oropharyngeal or Esophageal Candidiasis Trials

U.S. adverse experience data are derived from 350 immunocompromised patients (332 HIV seropositive/AIDS) treated for oropharyngeal or esophageal candidiasis. Table 3 below lists adverse events reported by at least 2% of patients treated with SPORANOX® Oral Solution in U.S. clinical trials. Data on patients receiving comparator agents in these trials are included for comparison.

[See table 3 at top of previous pag]

Adverse events reported by less than 2% of patients in U.S. clinical trials with SPORANOX® included: adrenal insufficiency, asthenia, back pain, dehydration, dyspepsia, dysphagia, flatulence, gynecomastia, hematuria, hemorrhoids, hot flushes, implantation complication, infection unspecified, injury, insomnia, male breast pain, myalgia, pharyngitis, pruritus, rhinitis, rigors, stomatitis ulcerative, taste perversion, tinnitus, upper respiratory tract infection, vision abnormal, and weight decrease. Edema, hypokalemia and menstrual disorders have been reported in clinical trials with itraconazole capsules.

Post-marketing Experience

Worldwide post-marketing experiences with the use of SPORANOX® include adverse events of gastrointestinal origin, such as dyspepsia, nausea, vomiting, diarrhea, abdominal pain and constipation. Other reported adverse events include peripheral edema, congestive heart failure and pulmonary edema, headache, dizziness, peripheral neuropathy, menstrual disorders, reversible increases in hepatic enzymes, hepatitis, liver failure, hypokalemia, hypertriglyceridemia, alopecia, allergic reactions (such as pruritus, rash, urticaria, angioedema, anaphylaxis), Stevens-Johnson syndrome, anaphylactic, anaphylactoid and allergic reactions, photosensitivity and neutropenia. There is limited information on the use of SPORANOX® during pregnancy. Cases of congenital abnormalities including skeletal, genitourinary tract, cardiovascular and ophthalmic malformations as well as chromosomal and multiple malformations have been reported during post-marketing experience. A causal relationship with SPORANOX® has not been established. (See CLINICAL PHARMACOLOGY: Special Populations, CONTRAINDICATIONS, WARNINGS, and PRECAUTIONS: Drug Interactions for more information.)

OVERDOSAGE

Itraconazole is not removed by dialysis. In the event of accidental overdosage, supportive measures, including gastric lavage with sodium bicarbonate, should be employed.

There are limited data on the outcomes of patients ingesting high doses of itraconazole. In patients taking either 1000 mg of SPORANOX® (itraconazole) Oral Solution or up to 3000 mg of SPORANOX® Capsules, the adverse event profile was similar to that observed at recommended doses.

DOSAGE AND ADMINISTRATION

Empiric Therapy in Febrile, Neutropenic Patients with Suspected Fungal Infections (ETFN): The recommended dose of SPORANOX® Injection is 200 mg b.i.d. for four doses, followed by 200 mg once daily for up to 14 days. Each intravenous dose should be infused over 1 hour. Treatment should be continued with SPORANOX® Oral Solution 200 mg (20 mL) b.i.d. until resolution of clinically significant neutropenia. The safety and efficacy of SPORANOX® use exceeding 28 days in ETFN is not known.

SPORANOX® Oral Solution is a different preparation than SPORANOX® Capsules and should not be used interchangeably.

Treatment of Oropharyngeal and Esophageal Candidiasis: The solution should be vigorously swished in the mouth (10 mL at a time) for several seconds and swallowed.

The recommended dosage of SPORANOX® (itraconazole) Oral Solution for oropharyngeal candidiasis is 200 mg (20 mL) daily for 1 to 2 weeks. Clinical signs and symptoms of oropharyngeal candidiasis generally resolve within several days.

For patients with oropharyngeal candidiasis unresponsive/refractory to treatment with fluconazole tablets, the recommended dose is 100 mg (10 mL) b.i.d. For patients responding to therapy, clinical response will be seen in 2 to 4 weeks. Patients may be expected to relapse shortly after discontinuing therapy. Limited data on the safety of long-term use (>6 months) of SPORANOX® Oral Solution are available at this time.

The recommended dosage of SPORANOX® Oral Solution for esophageal candidiasis is 100 mg (10 mL) daily for a minimum treatment of three weeks. Treatment should continue for 2 weeks following resolution of symptoms. Doses up to 200 mg (20 mL) per day may be used based on medical judgement of the patient's response to therapy.

SPORANOX® Oral Solution and SPORANOX® Capsules should not be used interchangeably. Patients should be instructed to take SPORANOX® Oral Solution without food, if possible. Only SPORANOX® Oral Solution has been demonstrated effective for oral and/or esophageal candidiasis.

HOW SUPPLIED

SPORANOX® (itraconazole) Oral Solution is available in 150 mL amber glass bottles (NDC 50458-295-15) containing 10 mg of itraconazole per mL.

Store at or below 25°C (77°F). Do not freeze.

Keep out of reach of children.

U.S. Patent No. 4,267,179; 5,707,975; 4,727,064

Revised January 2004 631-10-939-6

© Janssen 2003

Manufactured by:
Janssen Pharmaceutica N.V.
Beerse, Belgium
Distributed by:
Ortho Biotech Products, L.P.
Raritan, NJ 08869
ORTHO BIOTECH

Jones Pharma Incorporated

(a wholly owned subsidiary of King Pharmaceuticals, Inc.)
1945 CRAIG ROAD
ST LOUIS, MO 63146

Contact information in the Manufacturers' Index, which appears on page 8 of the 2004 PDR, has been completely revised as follows. Please write "See Supplement A" next to the heading.

Direct Inquiries to:
Customer Service:
800-776-3637
Fax:
423-989-6279

To report an Adverse Drug Experience:
(800) 546-4905
Fax: (423) 990-0519

MedPointe Pharmaceuticals
MedPointe Healthcare Inc.

SOMERSET, NJ 08873

For Medical Information, Contact:
Generally:
Medical Information
800-526-3840
After Hours and Weekend Emergencies:
800-526-3840

MedPointe Pharmaceuticals
MedPointe Healthcare Inc.
Sales and Ordering
Somerset, NJ 08873

ZOMIG® ℞
[zō'mig]
(zolmitriptan)
TABLETS
ZOMIG-ZMT®
(zolmitriptan)
Orally Disintegrating Tablets

Prescribing information for this product, which appears on pages 707–710 of the 2004 PDR, has been completely revised as follows. Please write "See Supplement A" next to the product heading.

DESCRIPTION

ZOMIG® (zolmitriptan) Tablets and ZOMIG-ZMT® (zolmitriptan) Orally Disintegrating Tablets contain zolmitriptan, which is a selective 5 hydroxytryptamine 1B/1D (5-$HT_{1B/1D}$) receptor agonist. Zolmitriptan is chemically designated as (S)-4-[[3-[2-(dimethylamino)ethyl]-1H-indol-5-yl]methyl]-2-oxazolidinone and has the following chemical structure:

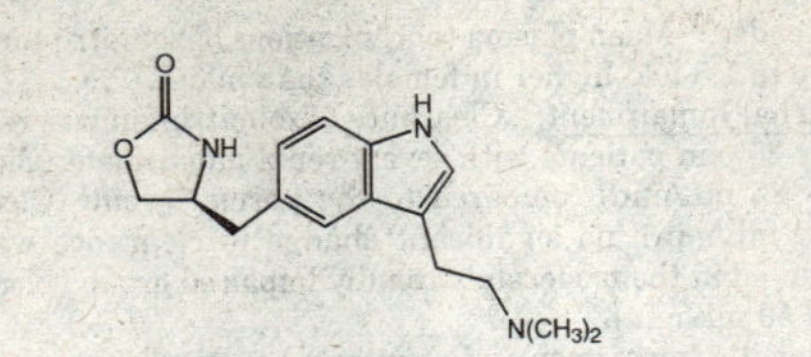

The empirical formula is $C_{16}H_{21}N_3O_2$, representing a molecular weight of 287.36. Zolmitriptan is a white to almost white powder that is readily soluble in water. ZOMIG Tablets are available as 2.5 mg (yellow) and 5 mg (pink) film coated tablets for oral administration. The film coated tablets contain anhydrous lactose NF, microcrystalline cellulose NF, sodium starch glycolate NF, magnesium stearate NF, hydroxypropyl methylcellulose USP, titanium dioxide USP, polyethylene glycol 400 NF, yellow iron oxide NF (2.5 mg tablet), red iron oxide NF (5 mg tablet), and polyethylene glycol 8000 NF.

ZOMIG-ZMT® Orally Disintegrating Tablets are available as 2.5 mg and 5.0 mg white uncoated tablets for oral administration. The orally disintegrating tablets contain mannitol USP, microcrystalline cellulose NF, crospovidone NF, aspartame NF, sodium bicarbonate USP, citric acid anhydrous USP, colloidal silicon dioxide NF, magnesium stearate NF and orange flavor SN 027512.

CLINICAL PHARMACOLOGY

Mechanism of Action

Zolmitriptan binds with high affinity to human recombinant 5-HT_{1D} and 5-HT_{1B} receptors. Zolmitriptan exhibits modest affinity for 5-HT_{1A} receptors, but has no significant affinity (as measured by radioligand binding assays) or pharmacological activity at 5-HT_2, 5-HT_3, 5-HT_4, alpha$_1$-, alpha$_2$, or beta$_1$-adrenergic; H_1, H_2, histaminic; muscarinic; dopamine$_1$, or dopamine$_2$ receptors. The N-desmethyl metabolite also has high affinity for 5-$HT_{1B/1D}$ and modest affinity for 5-HT_{1A} receptors.

Current theories proposed to explain the etiology of migraine headache suggest that symptoms are due to local cranial vasodilatation and/or to the release of sensory neuropeptides (vasoactive intestinal peptide, substance P and calcitonin gene-related peptide) through nerve endings in the trigeminal system. The therapeutic activity of zolmitriptan for the treatment of migraine headache can most likely be attributed to the agonist effects at the 5-$HT_{1B/1D}$ receptors on intracranial blood vessels (including the arterio-venous anastomoses) and sensory nerves of the trigeminal system which result in cranial vessel constriction and inhibition of pro-inflammatory neuropeptide release.

Clinical Pharmacokinetics and Bioavailability

Absorption

Zolmitriptan is well absorbed after oral administration for both the conventional tablets and the orally disintegrating tablets. Zolmitriptan displays linear kinetics over the dose range of 2.5 to 50 mg.

The AUC and C_{max} of zolmitriptan are similar following administration of ZOMIG Tablets and ZOMIG-ZMT Orally Disintegrating Tablets, but the T_{max} is somewhat later with ZOMIG-ZMT, with a median T_{max} of 3 hours for the orally disintegrating tablet compared with 1.5 hours for the conventional tablet. The AUC, C_{max}, and T_{max} for the active N-desmethyl metabolite are similar for the two formulations.

During a moderate to severe migraine attack, mean AUC_{0-4} and C_{max} for zolmitriptan, dosed as a conventional tablet, were decreased by 40% and 25%, respectively, and mean T_{max} was delayed by one-half hour compared to the same patients during a migraine free period.

Food has no significant effect on the bioavailability of zolmitriptan. No accumulation occurred on multiple dosing.

Distribution:

Mean absolute bioavailability is approximately 40%. The mean apparent volume of distribution is 7.0 L/kg. Plasma protein binding of zolmitriptan is 25% over the concentration range of 10–1000ng/mL.

Metabolism:

Zolmitriptan is converted to an active N-desmethyl metabolite such that the metabolite concentrations are about two-thirds that of zolmitriptan. Because the $5HT_{1B/1D}$ potency of the metabolite is 2 to 6 times that of the parent, the metabolite may contribute a substantial portion of the overall effect after zolmitriptan administration.

Elimination:

Total radioactivity recovered in urine and feces was 65% and 30% of the administered dose, respectively. About 8% of the dose was recovered in the urine as unchanged zolmitriptan. Indole acetic acid metabolite accounted for 31% of the dose, followed by N-oxide (7%) and N-desmethyl (4%) metabolites. The indole acetic acid and N-oxide metabolites are inactive.

Mean total plasma clearance is 31.5mL/min/kg, of which one-sixth is renal clearance. The renal clearance is greater than the glomerular filtration rate suggesting renal tubular secretion.

Special Populations:

Age: Zolmitriptan pharmacokinetics in healthy elderly non-migraineur volunteers (age 65–76 yrs) were similar to

Continued on next page

Zomig—Cont.

those in younger non-migraineur volunteers (age 18–39 yrs).

Gender: Mean plasma concentrations of zolmitriptan were up to 1.5-fold higher in females than males.

Renal Impairment: Clearance of zolmitriptan was reduced by 25% in patients with severe renal impairment (Clcr ≥ 5 ≤ 25 mL/min) compared to the normal group (Clcr > = 70 mL/min); no significant change in clearance was observed in the moderately renally impaired group (Clcr ≥ 26 ≤ 50 mL/min).

Hepatic Impairment: In severely hepatically impaired patients, the mean C_{max}, T_{max}, and $AUC_{0-\infty}$ of zolmitriptan were increased 1.5, 2 (2 vs 4 hr), and 3-fold, respectively, compared to normals. Seven out of 27 patients experienced 20 to 80 mm Hg elevations in systolic and/or diastolic blood pressure after a 10 mg dose. Zolmitriptan should be administered with caution in subjects with liver disease, generally using doses less than 2.5 mg (see WARNINGS and PRECAUTIONS).

Hypertensive Patients: No differences in the pharmacokinetics of zolmitriptan or its effects on blood pressure were seen in mild to moderate hypertensive volunteers compared to normotensive controls.

Race: Retrospective analysis of pharmacokinetic data between Japanese and Caucasians revealed no significant differences.

Drug Interactions

All drug interaction studies were performed in healthy volunteers using a single 10 mg dose of zolmitriptan and a single dose of the other drug except where otherwise noted.

Fluoxetine: The pharmacokinetics of zolmitriptan, as well as its effect on blood pressure, were unaffected by 4 weeks of pretreatment with oral fluoxetine (20 mg/day).

MAO Inhibitors: Following one week of administration of 150 mg bid moclobemide, a specific MAO-A inhibitor, there was an increase of about 25% in both C_{max} and AUC for zolmitriptan and a 3-fold increase in the C_{max} and AUC of the active N-desmethyl metabolite of zolmitriptan (see CONTRAINDICATIONS and PRECAUTIONS).

Selegiline, a selective MAO-B inhibitor, at a dose of 10 mg/day for 1 week, had no effect on the pharmacokinetics of zolmitriptan and its metabolite.

Propranolol: C_{max} and AUC of zolmitriptan increased 1.5-fold after one week of dosing with propranolol (160 mg/day). C_{max} and AUC of the N-desmethyl metabolite were reduced by 30% and 15%, respectively. There were no interactive effects on blood pressure or pulse rate following administration of propranolol with zolmitriptan.

Acetaminophen: A single 1 g dose of acetaminophen does not alter the pharmacokinetics of zolmitriptan and its N-desmethyl metabolite. However, zolmitriptan delayed the T_{max} of acetaminophen by one hour.

Metoclopramide: A single 10 mg dose of metoclopramide had no effect on the pharmacokinetics of zolmitriptan or its metabolites.

Oral Contraceptives: Retrospective analysis of pharmacokinetic data across studies indicated that mean plasma concentrations of zolmitriptan were generally higher in females taking oral contraceptives compared to those not taking oral contraceptives. Mean C_{max} and AUC of zolmitriptan were found to be higher by 30% and 50%, respectively, and T_{max} was delayed by one-half hour in females taking oral contraceptives. The effect of zolmitriptan on the pharmacokinetics of oral contraceptives has not been studied.

Cimetidine: Following the administration of cimetidine, the half-life and AUC of a 5 mg dose of zolmitriptan and its active metabolite were approximately doubled (see PRECAUTIONS).

Clinical Studies

The efficacy of ZOMIG Tablets in the acute treatment of migraine headaches was demonstrated in five randomized, double-blind, placebo controlled studies, of which 2 utilized the 1 mg dose, 2 utilized the 2.5 mg dose and 4 utilized the 5 mg dose; all studies used the marketed formulation. In study 1, patients treated their headaches in a clinic setting. In the other studies, patients treated their headaches as outpatients. In study 4, patients who had previously used sumatriptan were excluded, whereas in the other studies no such exclusion was applied. Patients enrolled in these five studies were predominantly female (82%) and Caucasian (97%) with a mean age of 40 years (range 12–65). Patients were instructed to treat a moderate to severe headache. Headache response, defined as a reduction in headache severity from moderate or severe pain to mild or no pain, was assessed at 1, 2, and, in most studies, 4 hours after dosing. Associated symptoms such as nausea, photophobia, and phonophobia were also assessed. Maintenance of response was assessed for up to 24 hours postdose. A second dose of ZOMIG Tablets or other medication was allowed 2 to 24 hours after the initial treatment for persistent and recurrent headache. The frequency and time to use of these additional treatments were also recorded. In all studies, the effect of zolmitriptan was compared to placebo in the treatment of a single migraine attack.

In all five studies, the percentage of patients achieving headache response 2 hours after treatment was significantly greater among patients receiving ZOMIG Tablets at all doses (except for the 1 mg dose in the smallest study) compared to those who received placebo. In the two studies that evaluated the 1 mg dose, there was a statistically significant greater percentage of patients with headache response at 2 hours in the higher dose groups (2.5 and/or 5 mg) compared to the 1 mg dose group. There were no statistically significant differences between the 2.5 and 5 mg dose groups (or of doses up to 20 mg) for the primary end point of headache response at 2 hours in any study. The results of these controlled clinical studies are summarized in Table 1.

Comparisons of drug performance based upon results obtained in different clinical trials are never reliable. Because studies are conducted at different times, with different samples of patients, by different investigators, employing different criteria and/or different interpretations of the same criteria, under different conditions (dose, dosing regimen, etc.), quantitative estimates of treatment response and the timing of response may be expected to vary considerably from study to study.

Table 1:
Percentage of Patients with Headache Response (Mild or no Headache) 2 Hours Following Treatment (n=number of patients randomized)

	Placebo	ZOMIG 1.0 mg	ZOMIG 2.5 mg	ZOMIG 5 mg
Study 1[a]	16% (n=19)	27% (n=22)	NA	60%*# (n=20)
Study 2	19% (n=88)	NA	NA	66%* (n=179)
Study 3	34% (n=121)	50%* (n=140)	65%*# (n=260)	67%*# (n=245)
Study 4[b]	44% (n=55)	NA	NA	59%* (n=491)
Study 5	36% (n=92)	NA NA	62%* (n=178)	NA

* p<0.05 in comparison with placebo.
\# p<0.05 in comparison with 1 mg.
a This was the only study in which patients treated the headache in a clinic setting.
b This was the only study where patients were excluded who had previously used sumatriptan.
NA - not applicable

The estimated probability of achieving an initial headache response by 4 hours following treatment is depicted in Figure 1.

Figure 1: Estimated Probability of achieving initial headache response within 4 hours*

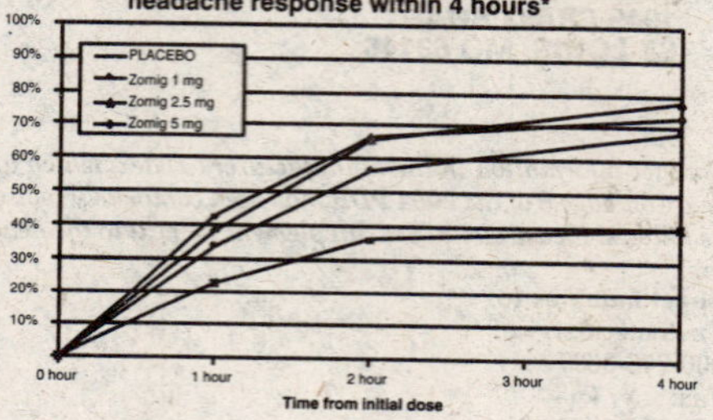

*Figure 1 shows the Kaplan-Meier plot of the probability over time of obtaining headache response (no or mild pain) following treatment with zolmitriptan. The averages displayed are based on pooled data from 3 placebo-controlled, outpatient trials providing evidence of efficacy (Trials 2, 3 and 5). Patients not achieving headache response or taking additional treatment prior to 4 hours were censored to 4 hours.

For patients with migraine associated photophobia, phonophobia, and nausea at baseline, there was a decreased incidence of these symptoms following administration of ZOMIG as compared to placebo.

Two to 24 hours following the initial dose of study treatment, patients were allowed to use additional treatment for pain relief in the form of a second dose of study treatment or other medication. The estimated probability of patients taking a second dose or other medication for migraine over the 24 hours following the initial dose of study treatment is summarized in Figure 2.

[See figure 2 at top of next column]

The efficacy of ZOMIG was unaffected by presence of aura; duration of headache prior to treatment; relationship to menses; gender, age, or weight of the patient; pretreatment nausea, or concomitant use of common migraine prophylactic drugs.

ZOMIG-ZMT Orally Disintegrating Tablets

The efficacy of ZOMIG-ZMT 2.5 mg was demonstrated in a randomized, placebo-controlled trial that was similar in design to the trials of ZOMIG Tablets. Patients were instructed to treat a moderate to severe headache. Of the 471 patients treated in the study, 87% were female and 97% were Caucasian, with a mean age of 41 years (range 18–62). At 2 hours post-dosing response rates in patients treated with ZOMIG-ZMT 2.5 mg were 63% compared to 22% in the placebo group. The difference was statistically significant. The estimated probability of achieving an initial headache response by 2 hours following treatment with ZOMIG-ZMT Tablets is depicted in Figure 3.

[See figure 3 at top of next column]

Figure 2: The Estimated Probability Of Patients Taking A Second Dose Or Other Medication For Migraines Over The 24 Hours Following The Initial Dose Of Study Treatment*

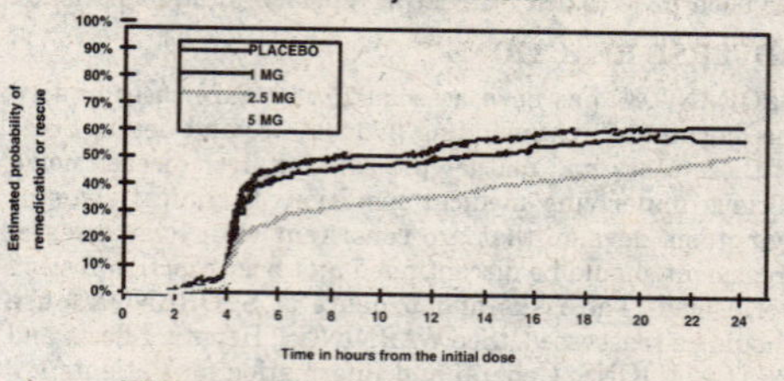

*This Kaplan-Meier plot is based on data obtained in 3 placebo controlled clinical trials (Study 2, 3 and 5). Patients not using additional treatments were censored at 24 hours. The plot includes both patients who had headache response at 2 hours and those who had no response to the initial dose. It should be noted that the protocols did not allow remedication within 2 hours postdose.

Figure 3: Estimated Probability of Achieving Initial Headache Response by 2 Hours

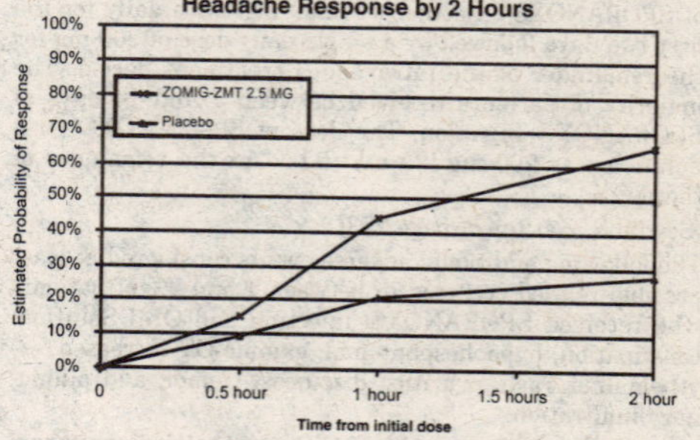

Figure 3 shows the Kaplan-Meier plot of the probability over time of obtaining headache response (no or mild pain) following treatment with ZOMIG-ZMT Tablets or placebo. Patients taking additional treatment or not achieving headache response prior to 2 hours were censored at 2 hours.

For patients with migraine-associated photophobia, phonophobia and nausea at baseline, there was a decreased incidence of these symptoms following administration of ZOMIG-ZMT as compared to placebo.

Two to 24 hours following the initial dose of study treatment, patients were allowed to use additional treatment in the form of a second dose of study treatment or other medication. The estimated probability of patients taking a second dose or other medication for migraine over the 24 hours following the initial dose of study treatment is summarized in Figure 4.

Figure 4: The Estimated Probability of Patients Taking a Second Dose or Other Medication for Migraines Over the 24 Hours Following The Initial Dose of Study Treatment

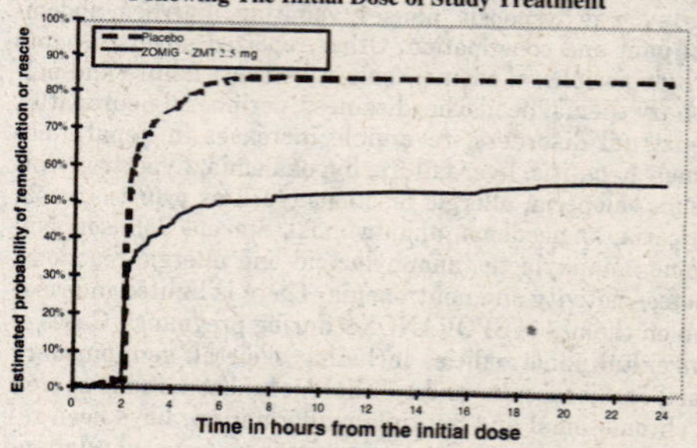

In this Kaplan-Meier plot, patients not using additional treatments were censored at 24 hours. The plot includes both patients who had headache response at 2 hours and those who had no response to the initial dose. Remedication was allowed 2 hours post-dose, and unlike the conventional tablet, remedication prior to 4 hours was not discouraged.

INDICATIONS AND USAGE

ZOMIG is indicated for the acute treatment of migraine with or without aura in adults.

ZOMIG is not intended for the prophylactic therapy of migraine or for use in the management of hemiplegic or basilar migraine (see CONTRAINDICATIONS). Safety and effectiveness of ZOMIG have not been established for cluster headache, which is present in an older, predominantly male population.

CONTRAINDICATIONS

ZOMIG should not be given to patients with ischemic heart disease (angina pectoris, history of myocardial infarction, or documented silent ischemia) or to patients who have symptoms or findings consistent with ischemic heart disease, coronary artery vasospasm, including Prinzmetal's variant angina, or other significant underlying cardiovascular disease (see WARNINGS).

Because ZOMIG may increase blood pressure, it should not be given to patients with uncontrolled hypertension (see WARNINGS).

ZOMIG should not be used within 24 hours of treatment with another 5-HT1 agonist, or an ergotamine-containing or ergot-type medication like dihydroergotamine or methysergide.

ZOMIG should not be administered to patients with hemiplegic or basilar migraine.

Concurrent administration of MAO-A inhibitors or use of zolmitriptan within 2 weeks of discontinuation of MAO-A inhibitor therapy is contraindicated (see CLINICAL PHARMACOLOGY: Drug Interactions and PRECAUTIONS: Drug Interactions).

ZOMIG is contraindicated in patients who are hypersensitive to zolmitriptan or any of its inactive ingredients.

WARNINGS

ZOMIG should only be used where a clear diagnosis of migraine has been established.

Risk of Myocardial Ischemia and/or Infarction and Other Adverse Cardiac Events: ZOMIG should not be given to patients with documented ischemic or vasospastic coronary artery disease (see CONTRAINDICATIONS). It is strongly recommended that zolmitriptan not be given to patients in whom unrecognized coronary artery disease (CAD) is predicted by the presence of risk factors (e.g., hypertension, hypercholesterolemia, smoker, obesity, diabetes, strong family history of CAD, female with surgical or physiological menopause, or male over 40 years of age) unless a cardiovascular evaluation provides satisfactory clinical evidence that the patient is reasonably free of coronary artery and ischemic myocardial disease or other significant underlying cardiovascular disease. The sensitivity of cardiac diagnostic procedures to detect cardiovascular disease or predisposition to coronary artery vasospasm is modest, at best. If, during the cardiovascular evaluation, the patient's medical history, electrocardiographic or other investigations reveal findings indicative of, or consistent with, coronary artery vasospasm or myocardial ischemia, zolmitriptan should not be administered (see CONTRAINDICATIONS). For patients with risk factors predictive of CAD, who are determined to have a satisfactory cardiovascular evaluation, it is strongly recommended that administration of the first dose of zolmitriptan take place in the setting of a physician's office or similar medically staffed and equipped facility unless the patient has previously received zolmitriptan. Because cardiac ischemia can occur in the absence of clinical symptoms, consideration should be given to obtaining on the first occasion of use an electrocardiogram (ECG) during the interval immediately following ZOMIG, in these patients with risk factors.

It is recommended that patients who are intermittent long-term users of ZOMIG and who have or acquire risk factors predictive of CAD, as described above, undergo periodic interval cardiovascular evaluation as they continue to use ZOMIG.

The systematic approach described above is intended to reduce the likelihood that patients with unrecognized cardiovascular disease will be inadvertently exposed to zolmitriptan.

Cardiac Events and Fatalities:

Serious adverse cardiac events, including acute myocardial infarction, have been reported within a few hours following administration of zolmitriptan. Life-threatening disturbances of cardiac rhythm, and death have been reported within a few hours following the administration of other $5\text{-}HT_1$ agonists. Considering the extent of use of $5\text{-}HT_1$ agonists in patients with migraine, the incidence of these events is extremely low.

ZOMIG can cause coronary vasospasm; at least one of these events occurred in a patient with no cardiac disease history and with documented absence of coronary artery disease. Because of the close proximity of the events to ZOMIG use, a causal relationship cannot be excluded. In the cases where there has been known underlying coronary artery disease, the relationship is uncertain.

Patients with symptomatic Wolff-Parkinson-White syndrome or arrhythmias associated with other cardiac accessory conduction pathway disorders should not receive ZOMIG.

Premarketing experience with zolmitriptan:

Among the more than 2,500 patients with migraine who participated in premarketing controlled clinical trials of ZOMIG Tablets, no deaths or serious cardiac events were reported.

Postmarketing experience with zolmitriptan:

Serious cardiovascular events have been reported in association with the use of ZOMIG Tablets, and in very rare cases, these events have occurred in the absence of known cardiovascular disease. The uncontrolled nature of postmarketing surveillance, however, makes it impossible to determine definitively the proportion of the reported cases that were actually caused by zolmitriptan or to reliably assess causation in individual cases.

Cerebrovascular Events and Fatalities with $5\text{-}HT_1$ agonists:

Cerebral hemorrhage, subarachnoid hemorrhage, stroke, and other cerebrovascular events have been reported in patients treated with $5\text{-}HT_1$ agonists; and some have resulted in fatalities. In a number of cases, it appears possible that the cerebrovascular events were primary, the agonist having been administered in the incorrect belief that the symptoms experienced were a consequence of migraine, when they were not. It should be noted that patients with migraine may be at increased risk of certain cerebrovascular events (eg, stroke, hemorrhage, transient ischemic attack).

Other Vasospasm-Related Events:

$5\text{-}HT_1$ agonists may cause vasospastic reactions other than coronary artery vasospasm such as peripheral and gastrointestinal vascular ischemia. As with other serotonin $5HT_1$ agonists, very rare gastrointestinal ischemic events including ischemic colitis and gastrointestinal infarction or necrosis have been reported with ZOMIG Tablets; these may present as bloody diarrhea or abdominal pain.

Increase in Blood Pressure:

As with other $5\text{-}HT_1$ agonists, significant elevations in systemic blood pressure have been reported on rare occasions with ZOMIG Tablet use, in patients with and without a history of hypertension; very rarely these increases in blood pressure have been associated with significant clinical events. Zolmitriptan is contraindicated in patients with uncontrolled hypertension. In volunteers, an increase of 1 and 5 mm Hg in the systolic and diastolic blood pressure, respectively, was seen at 5 mg. In the headache trials, vital signs were measured only in the small inpatient study and no effect on blood pressure was seen. In a study of patients with moderate to severe liver disease, 7 of 27 experienced 20 to 80 mm Hg elevations in systolic and/or diastolic blood pressure after a dose of 10 mg of zolmitriptan (see CONTRAINDICATIONS).

An 18% increase in mean pulmonary artery pressure was seen following dosing with another $5\text{-}HT_1$ agonist in a study evaluating subjects undergoing cardiac catheterization.

PRECAUTIONS

General

As with other $5\text{-}HT_{1B/1D}$ agonists, sensations of tightness, pain, pressure, and heaviness have been reported after treatment with ZOMIG Tablets in the precordium, throat, neck, and jaw. Because zolmitriptan may cause coronary artery vasospasm, patients who experience signs or symptoms suggestive of angina following dosing should be evaluated for the presence of CAD or a predisposition to Prinzmetal's variant angina before receiving additional doses of medication, and should be monitored electrocardiographically if dosing is resumed and similar symptoms recur. Similarly, patients who experience other symptoms or signs suggestive of decreased arterial flow, such as ischemic bowel syndrome or Raynaud's syndrome following the use of any $5\text{-}HT_1$ agonist are candidates for further evaluation. (see WARNINGS).

Zolmitriptan should also be administered with caution to patients with diseases that may alter the absorption, metabolism, or excretion of drugs, such as impaired hepatic function (see CLINICAL PHARMACOLOGY).

For a given attack, if a patient does not respond to the first dose of zolmitriptan, the diagnosis of migraine headache should be reconsidered before administration of a second dose.

Binding to Melanin-Containing Tissues:

When pigmented rats were given a single oral dose of 10 mg/kg of radiolabeled zolmitriptan, the radioactivity in the eye after 7 days, the latest time point examined, was still 75% of the value measured after 4 hours. This suggests that zolmitriptan and/or its metabolites may bind to the melanin of the eye. Because there could be accumulation in melanin rich tissues over time, this raises the possibility that zolmitriptan could cause toxicity in these tissues after extended use. However, no effects on the retina related to treatment with zolmitriptan were noted in any of the toxicity studies. Although no systematic monitoring of ophthalmologic function was undertaken in clinical trials, and no specific recommendations for ophthalmologic monitoring are offered, prescribers should be aware of the possibility of long-term ophthalmologic effects.

Phenylketonurics:

Phenylketonuric patients should be informed that ZOMIG-ZMT contain phenylalanine (a component of aspartame). Each 2.5 mg orally disintegrating tablet contains 2.81 mg phenylalanine. Each 5 mg orally disintegrating tablet contains 5.62 mg phenylalanine.

Information for Patients:

See PATIENT INFORMATION at the end of this labeling for the text of the separate leaflet provided for patients.

ZOMIG-ZMT Orally Disintegrating Tablets:

The orally disintegrating tablet is packaged in a blister. Patients should be instructed not to remove the tablet from the blister until just prior to dosing. The blister pack should then be peeled open, and the orally disintegrating tablet placed on the tongue, where it will dissolve and be swallowed with the saliva.

Laboratory Tests:

No monitoring of specific laboratory tests is recommended.

Drug Interactions:

Ergot-containing drugs have been reported to cause prolonged vasospastic reactions. Because there is a theoretical basis that these effects may be additive, use of ergotamine-containing or ergot-type medications (like dihydroergotamine or methysergide) and zolmitriptan within 24 hours of each other should be avoided (see CONTRAINDICATIONS).

MAO-A inhibitors increase the systemic exposure of zolmitriptan. Therefore, the use of zolmitriptan in patients receiving MAO-A inhibitors is contraindicated (see CLINICAL PHARMACOLOGY and CONTRAINDICATIONS).

Concomitant use of other $5\text{-}HT_{1B/1D}$ agonists within 24 hours of ZOMIG treatment is not recommended. (see CONTRAINDICATIONS).

Following administration of cimetidine, the half-life and AUC of zolmitriptan and its active metabolites were approximately doubled (see CLINICAL PHARMACOLOGY).

Selective serotonin reuptake inhibitors (SSRIs) (eg, fluoxetine, fluvoxamine, paroxetine, sertraline) have been reported, rarely, to cause weakness, hyperreflexia, and incoordination when coadministered with $5\text{-}HT_1$ agonists. If concomitant treatment with zolmitriptan and an SSRI is clinically warranted, appropriate observation of the patient is advised.

Drug/Laboratory Test Interactions:

Zolmitriptan is not known to interfere with commonly employed clinical laboratory tests.

Carcinogenesis, Mutagenesis, Impairment of Fertility:

Carcinogenicity studies by oral gavage were carried out in mice and rats at doses up to 400 mg/kg/day. Mice were dosed for 85 weeks (males) and 92 weeks (females). The exposure (plasma AUC of parent drug) at the highest dose level was approximately 800 times that seen in humans after a single 10 mg dose (the maximum recommended total daily dose). There was no effect of zolmitriptan on tumor incidence. Control, low dose, and middle dose rats were dosed for 104–105 weeks; the high dose group was sacrificed after 101 weeks (males) and 86 weeks (females) due to excess mortality. Aside from an increase in the incidence of thyroid follicular cell hyperplasia and thyroid follicular cell adenomas seen in male rats receiving 400 mg/kg/day, an exposure approximately 3000 times that seen in humans after dosing with 10 mg, no tumors were noted.

Mutagenesis:

Zolmitriptan was mutagenic in an Ames test, in 2 of 5 strains of *S. typhimurium* tested, in the presence of, but not in the absence of, metabolic activation. It was not mutagenic in an *in vitro* mammalian gene cell mutation (CHO/HGPRT) assay. Zolmitriptan was clastogenic in an *in vitro* human lymphocyte assay both in the absence of and the presence of metabolic activation; it was not clastogenic in an *in vivo* mouse micronucleus assay. It was also not genotoxic in an unscheduled DNA synthesis study.

Impairment of Fertility:

Studies of male and female rats administered zolmitriptan prior to and during mating and up to implantation have shown no impairment of fertility at doses up to 400 mg/kg/day. Exposure at this dose was approximately 3000 times exposure at the maximum recommended human dose of 10 mg/day.

Pregnancy

Pregnancy Category C

There are no adequate and well controlled studies in pregnant women; therefore, zolmitriptan should be used during pregnancy only if the potential benefit justifies the potential risk to the fetus.

In reproductive toxicity studies in rats and rabbits, oral administration of zolmitriptan to pregnant animals was associated with embryolethality and fetal abnormalities. When pregnant rats were administered oral zolmitriptan during the period of organogenesis at doses of 100, 400, and 1200 mg/kg/day, there was a dose-related increase in embryolethality which became statistically significant at the high dose. The maternal plasma exposures at these doses were approximately 280, 1100, and 5000 times the exposure in humans receiving the maximum recommended total daily dose of 10 mg. The high dose was maternally toxic, as evidenced by a decreased maternal body weight gain during gestation. In a similar study in rabbits, embryolethality was increased at the maternally toxic doses of 10 and 30 mg/kg/day (maternal plasma exposures equivalent to 11 and 42 times exposure in humans receiving the maximum recommended total daily dose of 10 mg), and increased incidences of fetal malformations (fused sternebrae, rib anomalies) and variations (major blood vessel variations, irregular ossification pattern of ribs) were observed at 30 mg/kg/day. Three mg/kg/day was a no effect dose (equivalent to human exposure at a dose of 10 mg). When female rats were given zolmitriptan during gestation, parturition, and lactation, an increased incidence of hydronephrosis was found in the offspring at the maternally toxic dose of 400 mg/kg/day (1100 times human exposure).

Nursing Mothers

It is not known whether zolmitriptan is excreted in human milk. Because many drugs are excreted in human milk, caution should be exercised when zolmitriptan is administered to a nursing woman. Lactating rats dosed with zolmitriptan had milk levels equivalent to maternal plasma levels at 1 hour and 4 times higher than plasma levels at 4 hours

Pediatric Use

Safety and effectiveness of ZOMIG in pediatric patients have not been established therefore, ZOMIG is not recommended for use in patients under 18 years of age.

Postmarketing experience with other triptans includes a limited number of reports that describe pediatric patients who have experienced clinically serious adverse events that are similar in nature to those reported rarely in adults.

Geriatric Use

Although the pharmacokinetic disposition of the drug in the elderly is similar to that seen in younger adults, there is no information about the safety and effectiveness of zolmitriptan in this population because patients over age 65 were excluded from the controlled clinical trials. (see CLINICAL PHARMACOLOGY: Special Populations)

ADVERSE REACTIONS

Serious cardiac events, including myocardial infarction, have occurred following the use of ZOMIG Tablets. These

Continued on next page

Zomig—Cont.

events are extremely rare and most have been reported in patients with risk factors predictive of CAD. Events reported, in association with drugs of this class, have included coronary artery vasospasm, transient myocardial ischemia, myocardial infarction, ventricular tachycardia, and ventricular fibrillation (see CONTRAINDICATIONS, WARNINGS, and PRECAUTIONS).

Incidence in Controlled Clinical Trials:

Among 2,633 patients treated with ZOMIG Tablets in the active and placebo controlled trials, no patients withdrew for reasons related to adverse events, but as patients treated a single headache in these trials, the opportunity for discontinuation was limited. In a long-term, open label study where patients were allowed to treat multiple migraine attacks for up to 1 year, 8% (167 out of 2,058) withdrew from the trial because of adverse experience. The most common events were paresthesia, asthenia, nausea, dizziness, pain, chest or neck tightness or heaviness, somnolence, and warm sensation.

Table 2 lists the adverse events that occurred in ≥ 2% of the 2,074 patients in any one of the ZOMIG 1 mg, ZOMIG 2.5 mg or ZOMIG 5 mg Tablets dose groups of the controlled clinical trials. Only events that were more frequent in a ZOMIG Tablets group compared to the placebo groups are included. The events cited reflect experience gained under closely monitored conditions of clinical trials in a highly selected patient population. In actual clinical practice or in other clinical trials, these frequency estimates may not apply, as the conditions of use, reporting behavior, and the kinds of patients treated may differ.

Several of the adverse events appear dose related, notably paresthesia, sensation of heaviness or tightness in chest, neck, jaw, and throat, dizziness, somnolence, and possibly asthenia and nausea.

[See table 2 below]

ZOMIG is generally well tolerated. Across all doses, most adverse reactions were mild and transient and did not lead to long-lasting effects. The incidence of adverse events in controlled clinical trials was not affected by gender, weight, or age of the patients; use of prophylactic medications; or presence of aura. There were insufficient data to assess the impact of race on the incidence of adverse events.

Other Events:

In the paragraphs that follow, the frequencies of less commonly reported adverse clinical events are presented. Because the reports include events observed in open and uncontrolled studies, the role of ZOMIG in their causation cannot be reliably determined. Furthermore, variability associated with adverse event reporting, the terminology used to describe adverse events, etc., limit the value of the quantitative frequency estimates provided. Event frequencies are calculated as the number of patients who used ZOMIG Tablets (n=4,027) and reported an event divided by the total number of patients exposed to ZOMIG Tablets. All reported events are included except those already listed in the previous table, those too general to be informative, and those not reasonably associated with the use of the drug. Events are further classified within body system categories and enumerated in order of decreasing frequency using the following definitions: infrequent adverse events are those occurring in 1/100 to 1/1,000 patients and rare adverse events are those occurring in fewer than 1/1,000 patients.

Atypical sensation: Infrequent was hyperesthesia.

General: Infrequent were allergy reaction, chills, facial edema, fever, malaise, and photosensitivity.

Cardiovascular: Infrequent were arrhythmias, hypertension, and syncope. Rare were bradycardia, extrasystoles, postural hypotension, QT prolongation, tachycardia, and thrombophlebitis.

Digestive: Infrequent were increased appetite, tongue edema, esophagitis, gastroenteritis, liver function abnormality, and thirst. Rare were anorexia, constipation, gastritis, hematemesis, pancreatitis, melena, and ulcer.

Hemic: Infrequent was ecchymosis. Rare were cyanosis, thrombocytopenia, eosinophilia, and leukopenia.

Metabolic: Infrequent was edema. Rare were hyperglycemia and alkaline phosphatase increased.

Musculoskeletal: Infrequent were back pain, leg cramps, and tenosynovitis. Rare were arthritis, asthenia, tetany, and twitching.

Neurological: Infrequent were agitation, anxiety, depression, emotional lability, and insomnia; Rare were akathisia, amnesia, apathy, ataxia, dystonia, euphoria, hallucinations, cerebral ischemia, hyperkinesia, hypotonia, hypertonia, and irritability.

Respiratory: Infrequent were bronchitis, bronchospasm, epistaxis, hiccup, laryngitis, and yawn. Rare were apnea and voice alteration.

Skin: Infrequent were pruritus, rash, and urticaria.

Special Senses: Infrequent were dry eye, eye pain, hyperacusis, ear pain, parosmia, and tinnitus. Rare were diplopia and lacrimation.

Urogenital: Infrequent were hematuria, cystitis, polyuria, urinary frequency, urinary urgency. Rare were miscarriage and dysmenorrhea.

The adverse experiences profile seen with ZOMIG-ZMT Tablets was similar to that seen with ZOMIG Tablets.

Postmarketing Experience with ZOMIG Tablets:

The following section enumerates potentially important adverse events that have occurred in clinical practice and which have been reported spontaneously to various surveillance systems. The events enumerated represent reports arising from both domestic and non-domestic use of oral zolmitriptan. The events enumerated include all except those already listed in the ADVERSE REACTIONS section above or those too general to be informative. Because the reports cite events reported spontaneously from worldwide postmarketing experience, frequency of events and the role of zolmitriptan in their causation cannot be reliably determined.

Cardiovascular

Coronary artery vasospasm; transient myocardial ischemia, angina pectoris, and myocardial infarction.

Digestive

Very rare gastrointestinal ischemic events including splenic infarction, ischemic colitis and gastrointestinal infarction or necrosis have been reported; these may present as bloody diarrhea or abdominal pain. (See WARNINGS.)

Neurological: As with other acute migraine treatments including other $5HT_1$ agonists, there have been rare reports of headache.

General

As with other $5\text{-}HT_{1B/1D}$ agonists, there have been very rare reports of anaphylaxis or anaphylactoid reactions in patients receiving ZOMIG. There have been rare reports of hypersensitivity reactions, including angioedema.

DRUG ABUSE AND DEPENDENCE

The abuse potential of ZOMIG has not been assessed in clinical trials.

OVERDOSAGE

There is no experience with clinical overdose. Volunteers receiving single 50 mg oral doses of zolmitriptan commonly experienced sedation.

The elimination half-life of ZOMIG is 3 hours (see CLINICAL PHARMACOLOGY), and therefore monitoring of patients after overdose with ZOMIG should continue for at least 15 hours or while symptoms or signs persist.

There is no specific antidote to zolmitriptan. In cases of severe intoxication, intensive care procedures are recommended, including establishing and maintaining a patent airway, ensuring adequate oxygenation and ventilation, and monitoring and support of the cardiovascular system.

It is unknown what effect hemodialysis or peritoneal dialysis has on the plasma concentrations of zolmitriptan.

DOSAGE AND ADMINISTRATION

ZOMIG Tablets

In controlled clinical trials, single doses of 1, 2.5 and 5 mg of ZOMIG Tablets were effective for the acute treatment of migraines in adults. A greater proportion of patients had headache response following a 2.5 or 5 mg dose than following a 1 mg dose (see Table 1). In the only direct comparison of 2.5 and 5 mg, there was little added benefit from the larger dose but side effects are generally increased at 5 mg (see Table 2). Patients should, therefore, be started on 2.5 mg or lower. A dose lower than 2.5 mg can be achieved by manually breaking the scored 2.5 mg tablet in half.

If the headache returns, the dose may be repeated after 2 hours, not to exceed 10 mg within a 24 hour period. Controlled trials have not adequately established the effectiveness of a second dose if the initial dose is ineffective.

The safety of treating an average of more than three headaches in a 30-day period has not been established.

ZOMIG-ZMT Orally Disintegrating Tablets

In a controlled clinical trial, a single dose of 2.5 mg of ZOMIG-ZMT Tablets was effective for the acute treatment of migraines in adults.

If the headache returns, the dose may be repeated after 2 hours, not to exceed 10 mg within a 24 hour period. Controlled trials have not adequately established the effectiveness of a second dose if the initial dose is ineffective.

The safety of treating an average of more than three headaches in a 30-day period has not been established.

Administration with liquid is not necessary. The orally disintegrating tablet is packaged in a blister. Patients should be instructed not to remove the tablet from the blister until just prior to dosing. The blister pack should then be peeled open, and the orally disintegrating tablet placed on the tongue, where it will dissolve and be swallowed with the saliva. It is not recommended to break the orally disintegrating tablet.

Hepatic Impairment

Patients with moderate to severe hepatic impairment have decreased clearance of zolmitriptan and significant elevation in blood pressure was observed in some patients. Use of a low dose with blood pressure monitoring is recommended (see CLINICAL PHARMACOLOGY AND WARNINGS).

HOW SUPPLIED

2.5 mg Tablets - Yellow, biconvex, round film-coated, scored tablets containing 2.5 mg of zolmitriptan identified with "ZOMIG" and "2.5" debossed on one side are supplied in cartons containing a blister pack of 6 tablets (NDC 0310-0210-20).

2.5 mg Orally Disintegrating Tablets - White, flat faced, uncoated, bevelled tablet containing 2.5 mg of zolmitriptan identified with a debossed "Z" on one side are supplied in cartons containing a blister pack of 6 tablets (NDC 0310-209-20).

5 mg Tablets - Pink, biconvex, film-coated tablets containing 5 mg of zolmitriptan identified with "ZOMIG" and "5" debossed on one side are supplied in cartons containing a blister pack of 3 tablets (NDC 0310-0211-25).

5 mg Orally Disintegrating Tablets - White, flat faced, round, uncoated, bevelled tablet containing 5.0 mg of zolmitriptan identified with a debossed "Z" and "5" on one side and plain on the other are supplied in cartons containing a blister pack of 3 tablets (NDC 0310-0213-21).

Storage:

Store both ZOMIG Tablets and ZOMIG-ZMT Tablets at controlled room temperature, 20–25°C (68–77°F) [see USP]. Protect from light and moisture.

ZOMIG®
(zolmitriptan)
TABLETS
ZOMIG-ZMT®
(zolmitriptan)
ORALLY DISINTEGRATING TABLETS

PATIENT INFORMATION

The following wording is contained in a separate leaflet provided for patients.

ZOMIG® (zolmitriptan) Tablets
ZOMIG-ZMT® (zolmitriptan) Orally Disintegrating Tablets
Patient Information about ZOMIG (Zo-mig) for Migraines
Generic Name: zolmitriptan (zol-mi-trip-tan)

Information for the Consumer on ZOMIG (zolmitriptan) Tablets

Please read this leaflet carefully before you administer ZOMIG Tablets. This provides a summary of the information available on your medicine. Please do not throw away this leaflet until you have finished your medicine. You may need to read this leaflet again. This leaflet does not contain all the information on ZOMIG Tablets. For further information or advice, ask your doctor or pharmacist.

Information About Your Medicine

The name of your medicine is ZOMIG Tablets. It can be obtained only by prescription from your doctor. The decision to use ZOMIG Tablets is one that you and your doctor should make jointly, taking into account your individual prefer-

Table 2:
Adverse Experience Incidence in Five Placebo-Controlled Migraine Clinical Trials:
Events Reported By ≥ 2% Patients Treated With ZOMIG Tablets

Adverse Event Type	Placebo (n=401)	ZOMIG 1 mg (n=163)	ZOMIG 2.5 mg (n=498)	ZOMIG 5 mg (n=1012)
ATYPICAL SENSATIONS	**6%**	**12%**	**12%**	**18%**
Hypesthesia	1%	1%	1%	2%
Paresthesia (all types)	2%	5%	7%	9%
Sensation warm/cold	4%	6%	5%	7%
PAIN AND PRESSURE SENSATIONS	**7%**	**13%**	**14%**	**22%**
Chest - pain/tightness/pressure and/or heaviness	1%	2%	3%	4%
Neck/throat/jaw - pain/tightness/pressure	3%	4%	7%	10%
Heaviness other than chest or neck	1%	1%	2%	5%
Pain – location specified	1%	2%	2%	3%
Other – Pressure/tightness/heaviness	0%	2%	2%	2%
DIGESTIVE	**8%**	**11%**	**16%**	**14%**
Dry mouth	2%	5%	3%	3%
Dyspepsia	1%	3%	2%	1%
Dysphagia	0%	0%	0%	2%
Nausea	4%	4%	9%	6%
NEUROLOGICAL	**10%**	**11%**	**17%**	**21%**
Dizziness	4%	6%	8%	10%
Somnolence	3%	5%	6%	8%
Vertigo	0%	0%	0%	2%
OTHER				
Asthenia	3%	5%	3%	9%
Palpitations	1%	0%	<1%	2%
Myalgia	<1%	1%	1%	2%
Myasthenia	<1%	0%	1%	2%
Sweating	1%	0%	2%	3%

ences and medical circumstances. If you have risk factors for heart disease (such as high blood pressure, high cholesterol, obesity, diabetes, smoking, strong family history of heart disease, or you are postmenopausal or a male over the age of 40), you should tell your doctor, who should evaluate you for heart disease in order to determine if ZOMIG Tablets are appropriate for you.

1. The Purpose of Your Medicine: ZOMIG Tablets are intended to relieve your migraine, but not to prevent or reduce the number of attacks you experience. Use ZOMIG Tablets only to treat an actual migraine attack.

2. Important Questions to Consider Before Using ZOMIG Tablets: If the answer to any of the following questions is **YES** or if you do not know the answer, then you must discuss it with your doctor before you use ZOMIG Tablets.

- Do you have any chest pain, heart disease, shortness of breath, or irregular heartbeats? Have you had a heart attack?
- Do you have risk factors for heart disease (such as high blood pressure, high cholesterol, obesity, diabetes, smoking, strong family history of heart disease, or you are postmenopausal or a male over the age of 40)?
- Do you have high blood pressure?
- Are you pregnant? Do you think you might be pregnant? Are you trying to become pregnant? Are you not using adequate contraception? Are you breast feeding an infant?
- If you are taking ZOMIG-ZMT®, are you sensitive to phenylalanine (a component of the artificial sweetener aspartame)?
- Have you ever had to stop taking this or any other medication because of an allergy or other problems?
- Are you taking any other migraine medications, including 5-HT_1 agonists (triptans) or migraine medications containing ergotamine, dihydroergotamine, or methysergide?
- Are you taking any medication for depression (monoamine oxidase inhibitors or selective serotonin reuptake inhibitors [SSRIs])?
- Are you taking cimetidine for gastrointestinal symptoms?
- Have you had, or do you have, any disease of the liver or kidney?
- Have you had, or do you have, epilepsy or seizures?
- Is this headache different from your usual migraine attacks?

Remember, if you answered **YES** to any of the above questions, then you must discuss it with your doctor.

3. The Use of ZOMIG Tablets During Pregnancy: Do not use ZOMIG Tablets if you are pregnant, think you might be pregnant, are trying to become pregnant, or are not using adequate contraception unless you have discussed this with your doctor.

4. How to Use ZOMIG Tablets and ZOMIG-ZMT Orally Disintegrating Tablets: Adults should be started on a 2.5 mg dose or lower administered by mouth. A dose lower than 2.5 mg can be achieved by manually breaking the conventional film-coated, scored 2.5 mg tablet in half. It is not recommended to break the ZOMIG-ZMT Tablet. If your headache comes back after your initial dose, a second dose may be administered anytime after 2 hours of administering the dose. For any attack where you have no response to the first dose, do not take a second dose without first consulting with your doctor. Do not administer more than a total of 10 mg of ZOMIG in any 24-hour period. Discard any unused tablets or its portion that have been removed from the blister packaging. Do not take ZOMIG with any other drug in the same class (triptans) within 24 hours or within 24 hours of taking ergotamine-type medications such as ergotamine, dihydroergotamine or methysergide to treat your migraine.

Additionally for ZOMIG-ZMT Tablets, the blister pack should be peeled open and the orally disintegrating tablet placed on the tongue, where it will dissolve and be swallowed with the saliva.

5. Side Effects to Watch for: Some patients experience pain or tightness in the chest or throat, including muscle aches and pains, when using ZOMIG. If this happens to you, then discuss it with your doctor before using any more ZOMIG. If the chest pain is severe or does not go away, call your doctor immediately. As with other drugs in this class (triptans), there have been very rare reports of heart attack occurring in patients with and without risk factors for heart and blood vessel disease.

- Some people experience; alterations of heart rate; temporary increase in blood pressure; sudden and severe stomach pain.
- Shortness of breath; wheeziness; heart throbbing; swelling of eyelids, face, or lips; or a skin rash, skin lumps, or hives happens rarely. If it happens to you, then tell your doctor immediately. Do not take any more ZOMIG unless your doctor tells you to do so.
- Some people may have feelings of dry mouth, tingling, heat, heaviness, or pressure after treatment with ZOMIG. A few people may feel drowsy, dizzy, tired, or sick. Tell your doctor immediately if you have symptoms that you do not understand.

6. What to Do if an Overdose Is Taken: If you have taken more medication than you have been told, contact either your doctor, hospital emergency department, or nearest poison control center immediately. This medicine was prescribed for your particular condition and should not be used by others or for any other condition.

7. Storing Your Medicine: Keep your medicine in a safe place where children cannot reach it. It may be harmful to children. Store your medication away from light and moisture, and at a controlled room temperature. If your medication has expired (the expiration date is printed on the treatment pack), throw it away as instructed. If your doctor decides to stop your treatment, do not keep any leftover medicine unless your doctor tells you to. Throw away your medicine as instructed. Be sure that discarded tablets are out of the reach of children.

ZOMIG® (zolmitriptan) Tablets
Manufactured for:
AstraZeneca Pharmaceuticals LP
Wilmington, Delaware 19850
By: IPR Pharmaceuticals, Inc.
Carolina, Puerto Rico 00984-1967

ZOMIG-ZMT® (zolmitriptan) Orally Disintegrating Tablets
Manufactured for:
AstraZeneca Pharmaceuticals LP
Wilmington, Delaware 19850
By: CIMA Labs, Inc.
Eden Prairie, Minnesota 55344
Rev 08/03
SIC 64195-01

Merck & Co., Inc.
WEST POINT, PA 19486

For Medical Information Contact:
Generally:
Product and service information:
Call the Merck National Service Center, 8:00 AM to 7:00 PM (ET), Monday through Friday:
(800) NSC-MERCK
(800) 672-6372
FAX: (800) MERCK-68
FAX: (800) 637-2568

Adverse Drug Experiences:
Call the Merck National Service Center, 8:00 AM to 7:00 PM (ET), Monday through Friday:
(800) NSC-MERCK
(800) 672-6372

In Emergencies:
24-hour emergency information for healthcare professionals:
(800) NSC-MERCK
(800) 672-6372

Sales and Ordering:
For product orders and direct account inquiries only, call the Order Management Center,
8:00 AM to 7:00 PM (ET), Monday through Friday:
(800) MERCK RX
(800) 637-2579

EMEND® CAPSULES ℞
[ē′mĕnd]
(aprepitant)

Prescribing information for this product, which appears on pages 1980–1984 of the 2004 PDR, has been revised as follows. Please write "See Supplement A" next to the product heading.

In the **CLINICAL PHARMACOLOGY** section, under *Clinical Studies, Multiple-Cycle Extension*, in the first sentence, delete the numeral 6.

In the **ADVERSE REACTIONS** section, in Table 4, change "Creatine" to "Creatinine."

Revisions based on 9565001, issued May 2003.

FOSAMAX® ℞
(alendronate sodium)
Tablets and Oral Solution

Prescribing information for this product, which appears on pages 1986–1992 of the 2004 PDR, has been revised as follows. Please write "See Supplement A" next to the product heading.

In the **DESCRIPTION** section, after the last paragraph ending "contain carnauba wax." add the following new paragraph:

"Each bottle of the oral solution contains 91.35 mg of alendronate monosodium salt trihydrate, which is the molar equivalent to 70 mg of free acid. Each bottle also contains the following inactive ingredients: sodium citrate dihydrate and citric acid anhydrous as buffering agents, sodium saccharin, artificial raspberry flavor, and purified water. Added as preservatives are sodium propylparaben 0.0225% and sodium butylparaben 0.0075%."

In the **CLINICAL PHARMACOLOGY** section, under *Pharmacokinetics, Absorption*, after the end of the first paragraph ending with "before breakfast." add the following new paragraph:

"FOSAMAX 70 mg oral solution and FOSAMAX 70 mg tablet are equally bioavailable."

In the **CONTRAINDICATIONS** section, after the second bullet ending with "at least 30 minutes" insert the following new bullet:

"• Patients at increased risk of aspiration should not receive FOSAMAX oral solution."

In the **WARNINGS** section, in the first sentence of the third paragraph, delete the words "a full glass (6-8 oz)" and add "the recommended amount"

In the **PRECAUTIONS** section, under *Information for Patients, Dosing Instructions*, in the first sentence, delete the words "each tablet is swallowed" and replace with "it is taken".

In the second paragraph, the first sentence should be changed to the following 3 sentences: "To facilitate delivery to the stomach and thus reduce the potential for esophageal irritation patients should be instructed to swallow each tablet of FOSAMAX with a full glass of water (6–8 oz). To facilitate gastric emptying patients should drink at least 2 oz (a quarter of a cup) of water after taking FOSAMAX oral solution. Patients should be instructed not to lie down for at least 30 minutes and until after their first food of the day."

In the **PRECAUTIONS** section, under *Information for Patients, Dosing Instructions*, in the first sentence of the third paragraph beginning "Patients should be" replace the word "tablet" with "dose". In the second sentence, replace the word "tablets" with "doses" and then again replace "tablet" with "dose".

In the **ADVERSE REACTIONS** section, under *Post-Marketing Experience* and *Body as a Whole:*, delete the second sentence and replace with: "Transient symptoms of myalgia, malaise and rarely, fever have been reported with FOSAMAX, typically in association with initiation of treatment."

In the **DOSAGE AND ADMINISTRATION** section, delete the first sentence of the second paragraph. The first 4 sentences should now read, " FOSAMAX should only be taken upon arising for the day. To facilitate delivery to the stomach and thus reduce the potential for esophageal irritation, a FOSAMAX tablet should be swallowed with a full glass of water (6–8 oz). To facilitate gastric emptying FOSAMAX oral solution should be followed by at least 2 oz (a quarter of a cup) of water. Patients should not lie down for at least 30 minutes and until after their first food of the day."

In the **DOSAGE AND ADMINISTRATION** section, under the subheading *Treatment of osteoporosis in postmenopausal women* (see INDICATIONS AND USAGE), add the following bullet after "one 70 mg tablet once weekly or": "• one bottle of 70 mg oral solution once weekly". On the next line, add "or" directly under the previous "or". In the second sentence of the next section under the subheading *Treatment to increase bone mass in men with osteoporosis*, in the second sentence after the word "tablet" add the following: "or one bottle of 70 mg oral solution".

At the end of the **HOW SUPPLIED** section, add the following on a new line:

"No. 3833 — Oral Solution FOSAMAX, 70 mg, is a clear, colorless solution with a raspberry flavor and is supplied as follows:

NDC 0006-3833-34 unit-of-use cartons of 4 single-dose bottles containing 75 mL each."

In the **HOW SUPPLIED** section, under *Storage*, insert the following subhead, *"FOSAMAX Tablets:"*. At the end of the next sentence, add the following subhead and text:

"FOSAMAX Oral Solution:
Store at 25°C (77°F), excursions permitted to 15–30°C (59–86°F). [See USP Controlled Room Temperature.] Do not freeze."

Revisions based on 7957023, issued September 2003.

In the Patient Information about FOSAMAX Once Daily, in the **What are the possible side effects of FOSAMAX?** section, in the third paragraph that begins "Bone, muscle" add the following sentence at the end of the second sentence that ends "eye pain have occurred." "Rarely, severe skin reactions have occurred."

Revisions based on 7969413, issued April 2003.

In the Patient Information about FOSAMAX Once Weekly, in the **How should I take once weekly FOSAMAX?** section, under item 1, delete second sentence and add the following sentence: **"Every week, take one dose of FOSAMAX (one tablet or one entire bottle of solution) on your chosen day."**

In the **How should I take once weekly FOSAMAX?** section, under item 2, first sentence, delete words beginning with "swallow" to "Not juice". Replace with the following: "**take your FOSAMAX with plain water only as follows:**

• TABLETS: Swallow one tablet with a full glass (6–8 oz) of plain water.

• ORAL SOLUTION: Drink one entire bottle of solution followed by at least 2 ounces (a quarter of a cup) of plain water.

Do not take FOSAMAX with:
Mineral water
Coffee or tea
Juice

In the **How should I take once weekly FOSAMAX?** section, under item 3, first sentence, replace the word "swallowing" with "taking" and delete "tablet". In the second sentence, delete "the FOSAMAX tablet" and replace with "FOSAMAX". In the same section, under item 4, first sentence, replace the word "swallowing" with "taking" and delete "tablet".

In the same section, under item 7, delete the text and replace with the following: "If you miss a dose, take only one

Continued on next page

Information on the Merck & Co., Inc., products listed on these pages is from the full prescribing information in use April 1, 2004.

Fosamax—Cont.

dose of FOSAMAX on the morning after you remember. *Do not take two doses on the same day.* Return to taking one dose once a week, as originally scheduled on your chosen day."

In the **What is FOSAMAX?** section, insert the following new paragraph after the second bullet: "FOSAMAX tablets are for treatment and prevention, and FOSAMAX oral solution is for treatment of osteoporosis."

In the **Who should not take FOSAMAX?** section after the second bullet, add the following new bullet:

• Difficulty swallowing liquids should not take FOSAMAX oral solution

In the **What are the possible side effects of FOSAMAX?** section, first paragraph, third sentence, delete "a full glass" and replace with "the recommended amount".

In the **What are the possible side effects of FOSAMAX?** section, in the third paragraph that begins "Bone, muscle" add the following sentence at the end of the second one that ends "have occurred."

"Rarely, severe skin reactions have occurred." Continue with next sentence that begins "Allergic reactions".

Revisions based on 9364104, issued April 2003; and 9364105, issued September 2003.

HYZAAR® 50-12.5 ℞

[*hīz-är*]

(losartan potassium-hydrochlorothiazide tablets)

HYZAAR® 100-25 ℞

(losartan potassium-hydrochlorothiazide tablets)

Prescribing information for this product, which appears on pages 1997–2000 of the 2004 PDR, has been revised as follows. Please write "See Supplement A" next to the product heading.

In the **CLINICAL PHARMACOLOGY** section under *Renal Insufficiency:* replace the existing paragraph with the following paragraphs:

"*Losartan:* Following oral administration, plasma concentrations and AUCs of losartan and its active metabolite are increased by 50-90% in patients with mild (creatinine clearance of 50 to 74 mL/min) or moderate (creatinine clearance 30 to 49 mL/min) renal insufficiency. In this study, renal clearance was reduced by 55-85% for both losartan and its active metabolite in patients with mild or moderate renal insufficiency. Neither losartan nor its active metabolite can be removed by hemodialysis."

"*Hydrochlorothiazide:* Following oral administration, the AUC for hydrochlorothiazide is increased by 70 and 700% for patients with mild and moderate renal insufficiency, respectively. In this study, renal clearance of hydrochlorothiazide decreased by 45 and 85% in patients with mild and moderate renal impairment, respectively."

"The usual regimens of therapy with HYZAAR may be followed as long as the patient's creatinine clearance is >30 mL/min. In patients with more severe renal impairment, loop diuretics are preferred to thiazides, so HYZAAR is not recommended. (See DOSAGE AND ADMINISTRATION.)"

In the **CLINICAL PHARMACOLOGY** section under *Drug Interaction/Losartan Potassium* after the second sentence in the first paragraph replace the remaining part of the paragraph with the following:

"There is no pharmacokinetic interaction between losartan and hydrochlorothiazide. Coadministration of losartan and cimetidine led to an increase of about 18% in AUC of losartan but did not affect the pharmacokinetics of its active metabolite. Coadministration of losartan and phenobarbital led to a reduction of about 20% in the AUC of losartan and that of its active metabolite. A somewhat greater interaction (approximately 40% reduction in the AUC of active metabolite and approximately 30% reduction in the AUC of losartan) has been reported with rifampin. Fluconazole, an inhibitor of cytochrome P450 2C9, decreased the AUC of the active metabolite by approximately 40%, but increased the AUC of losartan by approximately 70% following multiple doses. Conversion of losartan to its active metabolite after intravenous administration is not affected by ketoconazole, an inhibitor of P450 3A4. The AUC of active metabolite following oral losartan was not affected by erythromycin, another inhibitor of P450 3A4, but the AUC of losartan was increased by 30%."

In the **CLINICAL PHARMACOLOGY** section after *Losartan Potassium-Hydrochlorothiazide* paragraph ending with "...Black and non-Black patients." add the following subhead: *Severe Hypertension (Sitting Diastolic Blood Pressure [SiDBP] •110 mmHg*

Under that header insert the following paragraphs:

"The safety and efficacy of HYZAAR as initial therapy for severe hypertension (defined as a mean SiDBP •110 mmHg confirmed on 2 separate occasions off all antihypertensive therapy) was studied in a 6-week double-blind, randomized, multicenter study. Patients were randomized to either losartan and hydrochlorothiazide (50-12.5 mg, once daily) or to losartan (50 mg, once daily) and followed for blood pressure response. Patients were titrated at 2-week intervals if their SiDBP did not reach goal (<90 mmHg). Patients on combination therapy were titrated from losartan 50 mg/hydrochlorothiazide 12.5 mg to losartan 50 mg/hydrochlorothiazide 12.5 mg (sham titration to maintain the blind) to losartan 100 mg/hydrochlorothiazide 25 mg. Patients on monotherapy were titrated from losartan 50 mg to losartan 100 mg to losartan 150 mg, as needed. The primary endpoint was a comparison at 4 weeks of patients who achieved goal diastolic blood pressure (trough SiDBP <90 mmHg)."

"The study enrolled 585 patients, including 264 (45%) females, 124 (21%) blacks, and 21 (4%) •65 years of age. The mean blood pressure at baseline for the total population was 171/113 mmHg. The mean age was 53 years. After 4 weeks of therapy, the mean SiDBP was 3.1 mmHg lower and the mean SiSBP was 5.6 mmHg lower in the group treated with HYZAAR. As a result, a greater proportion of the patients on HYZAAR reached the target diastolic blood pressure (17.6% for HYZAAR, 9.4% for losartan; p=0.006). Similar trends were seen when the patients were grouped according to gender, race or age (<, • 65)."

"After 6 weeks of therapy, more patients who received the combination regimen reached target diastolic blood pressure than those who received the monotherapy regimen (29.8% versus 12.5%)."

"During the study period, there were no reported cases of syncope in either treatment group. There were 2 (0.6%) and 0 (0.0%) cases of hypotension reported in the group treated with HYZAAR and the group treated with losartan, respectively. The overall pattern of adverse events reported for patients treated with HYZAAR as initial therapy was similar to the adverse event profile for patients treated with losartan as initial therapy. For information on the specific adverse events observed during the study period, see ADVERSE REACTIONS, *Severe Hypertension*."

In the **INDICATIONS AND USAGE** section, replace the entire paragraph with the following: "HYZAAR is indicated for the treatment of hypertension. This fixed dose combination is not indicated for initial therapy of hypertension, except when the hypertension is severe enough that the value of achieving prompt blood pressure control exceeds the risk of initiating combination therapy in these patients (see CLINICAL PHARMACOLOGY, *Pharmacodynamics and Clinical Effects*, and DOSAGE AND ADMINISTRATION).

In the **PRECAUTIONS** section, under *Drug Interactions/Losartan Potassium* replace the entire first paragraph with the following:

"No significant drug-drug pharmacokinetic interactions have been found in interaction studies with hydrochlorothiazide, digoxin, warfarin, cimetidine and phenobarbital. Rifampin, an inducer of drug metabolism, decreased the concentrations of losartan and its active metabolite. (See CLINICAL PHARMACOLOGY, *Drug Interactions*.) In humans, two inhibitors of P450 3A4 have been studied. Ketoconazole did not affect the conversion of losartan to the active metabolite after intravenous administration of losartan, and erythromycin had no clinically significant effect after oral administration. Fluconazole, an inhibitor of P450 2C9, decreased active metabolite concentration and increased losartan concentration. The pharmacodynamic consequences of concomitant use of losartan and inhibitors of P450 2C9 have not been examined. Subjects who do not metabolize losartan to active metabolite have been shown to have a specific, rare defect in cytochrome P450 2C9. These data suggest that the conversion of losartan to its active metabolite is mediated primarily by P450 2C9 and not P450 3A4."

In the **PRECAUTIONS** section, replace *Use in the Elderly* with *Geriatric Use*.

Delete the first paragraph under *Use in the Elderly* beginning with "Of the total number...."

Add the following paragraphs under *Geriatric Use*:

"Clinical studies of HYZAAR did not include sufficient numbers of subjects aged 65 and over to determine whether they respond differently from younger subjects. Other reported clinical experience has not identified differences in responses between the elderly and younger patients. In general, dose selection for an elderly patient should be cautious, usually starting at the low end of the dosing range, reflecting the greater frequency of decreased hepatic, renal, or cardiac function, and of concomitant disease or other drug therapy."

"Hydrochlorothiazide is known to be substantially excreted by the kidney, and the risk of toxic reactions to this drug may be greater in patients with impaired renal function (see CLINICAL PHARMACOLOGY, *Special Populations*)."

In the **ADVERSE REACTIONS** section after the sentence beginning with "Cases of cough,...losartan in post-marketing experience." Add subhead *Severe Hypertension:* In a clinical study in patients with severe hypertension (SiDBP •110 mmHg), the overall pattern of adverse events reported through six weeks of follow-up was similar in patients treated with HYZAAR as initial therapy and in patients treated with losartan as initial therapy. There were no reported cases of syncope in either treatment group. There were 2 (0.6%) and 0 (0.0%) cases of hypotension reported in the group treated with HYZAAR and the group treated with losartan, respectively. There were 3 (0.8%) and 2 (1.2%) cases of increased serum creatinine (>0.5 mg/dL) in the group treated with HYZAAR and the group treated with losartan, respectively, during the same time period. (See CLINICAL PHARMACOLOGY, *Pharmacodynamics and Clinical Effects, Severe Hypertension*.)

Under **DOSAGE AND ADMINISTRATION** add the following subhead above the first paragraph:

Hypertension

In the **DOSAGE AND ADMINISTRATION** section after **Patients with Hepatic Impairment**: paragraph add the following subhead:

Severe Hypertension

Add the following paragraph under the subhead:

"The starting dose of HYZAAR for initial treatment of severe hypertension is one tablet of HYZAAR 50-12.5 once daily (see CLINICAL PHARMACOLOGY, *Pharmacodynamics and Clinical Effects*). For patients who do not respond adequately to HYZAAR 50-12.5 after 2 to 4 weeks of therapy, the dosage may be increased to one tablet of HYZAAR 100-25 once daily. The maximum dose is one tablet of HYZAAR 100-25 once daily. HYZAAR is not recommended as initial therapy in patients with hepatic impairment (see WARNINGS, *Impaired Hepatic Function*) because the appropriate 25 mg starting dose of losartan cannot be given. It is also not recommended for use as initial therapy in patients with intravascular volume depletion (e.g., patients treated with diuretics, see WARNINGS, *Hypotension—Volume-Depleted Patients*)."

Revision based on and 9573622, issued September 2003.

INDOCIN® IV ℞

[*in-dō-sĭn*]

(Indomethacin for Injection)

Prescribing information for this product, which appears on pages 2003–2005 of the 2004 PDR, has been revised as follows. Please write "See Supplement A" next to the product heading.

In the second line of the title, in the parentheses, change "Sodium Trihydrate)" to "for Injection)."

In the **DESCRIPTION** section, in the first sentence of the first paragraph, in the parentheses, change "Sodium Trihydrate)" to "for Injection)," and at the end of the same sentence, change "sodium trihydrate" to "for injection". In the second sentence of the first paragraph, change "sodium trihydrate" to "for injection."

Also in the **DESCRIPTION** section, in the first sentence of the second paragraph, change "sodium trihydrate" to "for injection."

In the **ADVERSE REACTIONS** section, in the second paragraph, change "sodium trihydrate" to "for injection."

Also in the **ADVERSE REACTIONS** section, in the first sentence of the last paragraph, change "(see section **ADDITIONAL ADVERSE REACTIONS–ADULTS**)." to "(see package circular for Capsules INDOCIN (Indomethacin) for additional information concerning adverse reactions and other cautionary statements)."

In the **HOW SUPPLIED** section, in the first paragraph, change "sodium trihydrate" to "for injection"

Delete the **ADDITIONAL ADVERSE REACTIONS–ADULTS** section.

Revisions based on 9408719, issued January 2003.

INVANZ® ℞

[*ĭn-vănz*]

(ertapenem for injection)

For Intravenous or Intramuscular Use

Prescribing information for this product, which appears on pages 2005–2009 of the 2004 PDR, has been revised as follows. Please write "See Supplement A" alongside product heading.

After the main heading, add the following paragraph: "To reduce the development of drug-resistant bacteria and maintain the effectiveness of INVANZ and other antibacterial drugs, INVANZ should be used only to treat or prevent infections that are proven or strongly suspected to be caused by bacteria."

At the end of the INDICATIONS AND USAGE section, add the following paragraph: "To reduce the development of drug-resistant bacteria and maintain the effectiveness of INVANZ and other antibacterial drugs, INVANZ should be used only to treat or prevent infections that are proven or strongly suspected to be caused by susceptible bacteria. When culture and susceptibility information are available, they should be considered in selecting or modifying antibacterial therapy. In the absence of such data, local epidemiology and susceptibility patterns may contribute to the empiric selection of therapy."

In the PRECAUTIONS section, under *General*, after the second paragraph, add the following paragraph: "Prescribing INVANZ in the absence of a proven or strongly suspected bacterial infection or a prophylactic indication is unlikely to provide benefit to the patient and increases the risk of the development of drug-resistant bacteria."

In the PRECAUTIONS section, before *Laboratory Tests*, add the following: "*Information for patients* Patients should be counseled that antibacterial drugs including INVANZ should only be used to treat bacterial infections. They do not treat viral infections (e.g., the common cold). When INVANZ is prescribed to treat a bacterial infection, patients should be told that although it is common to feel better early in the course of therapy, the medication should be taken exactly as directed. Skipping doses or not completing the full course of therapy may (1) decrease the effectiveness of the immediate treatment and (2) increase the likelihood that bacteria will develop resistance and will not be treatable by INVANZ or other antibacterial drugs in the future."

In the ADVERSE REACTIONS section, before *Adverse Laboratory Changes*, add the following: "*Post-Marketing Experience*: The following post-marketing adverse experiences have been reported: *Immune System*: anaphylaxis including anaphylactoid reactions (very rare) *Nervous System & Psychiatric*: hallucinations (very rare)"

Revisions based on 9500001, issued June 2003, and 9500002, issued August 2003.

MEFOXIN® ℞
[*mĕ-fŏk-sĭn*]
cefoxitin for injection

Prescribing information for this product, which appears on pages 2017–2020 of the 2004 PDR, has been revised as follows. Please write "See Supplement A" next to the product heading.

Place the following paragraph below the MEFOXIN brand name and generic name:

To reduce the development of drug-resistant bacteria and maintain the effectiveness of MEFOXIN* and other antibacterial drugs, MEFOXIN should be used only to treat or prevent infections that are proven or strongly suspected to be caused by bacteria.

In the **INDICATIONS AND USAGE** section, under the *Prevention* subhead, add the following text after the first two paragraphs:

To reduce the development of drug-resistant bacteria and maintain the effectiveness of MEFOXIN and other antibacterial drugs, MEFOXIN should be used only to treat or prevent infections that are proven or strongly suspected to be caused by susceptible bacteria. When culture and susceptibility information are available, they should be considered in selecting or modifying antibacterial therapy. In the absence of such data, local epidemiology and susceptibility patterns may contribute to the empiric selection of therapy.

In the **PRECAUTIONS** section, beneath the *General* subhead, and before the subhead *Laboratory Tests*, add the following text:

Prescribing MEFOXIN in the absence of a proven or strongly suspected bacterial infection or a prophylactic indication is unlikely to provide benefit to the patient and increases the risk of the development of drug-resistant bacteria.

Information for Patients

Patients should be counseled that antibacterial drugs including MEFOXIN should only be used to treat bacterial infections. They do not treat viral infections (e.g., the common cold). When MEFOXIN is prescribed to treat a bacterial infection, patients should be told that although it is common to feel better early in the course of therapy, the medication should be taken exactly as directed. Skipping doses or not completing the full course of therapy may (1) decrease the effectiveness of the immediate treatment and (2) increase the likelihood that bacteria will develop resistance and will not be treatable by MEFOXIN or other antibacterial drugs in the future.

After **REFERENCES** section, change code and issue date to:

7882341 Issued August 2003

MEFOXIN® PREMIXED INTRAVENOUS SOLUTION ℞
[*mĕ-fŏk-sĭn*]
(cefoxitin injection)

Prescribing information for this product, which appears on pages 2020–2022 of the 2004 PDR, has been revised as follows. Please write "See Supplement A" next to the product heading.

Place the following paragraph right below the MEFOXIN brand name and generic name:

To reduce the development of drug-resistant bacteria and maintain the effectiveness of MEFOXIN* and other antibacterial drugs, MEFOXIN should be used only to treat or prevent infections that are proven or strongly suspected to be caused by bacteria.

In the **INDICATIONS AND USAGE** section, under the *Prevention* subhead, add the following text after the first two paragraphs:

To reduce the development of drug-resistant bacteria and maintain the effectiveness of MEFOXIN and other antibacterial drugs, MEFOXIN should be used only to treat or prevent infections that are proven or strongly suspected to be caused by susceptible bacteria. When culture and susceptibility information are available, they should be considered in selecting or modifying antibacterial therapy. In the absence of such data, local epidemiology and susceptibility patterns may contribute to the empiric selection of therapy.

In the **PRECAUTIONS** section, beneath the *General* subhead, and before the subhead *Laboratory Tests*, add the following text:

Prescribing MEFOXIN in the absence of a proven or strongly suspected bacterial infection or a prophylactic indication is unlikely to provide benefit to the patient and increases the risk of the development of drug-resistant bacteria.

Information for Patients

Patients should be counseled that antibacterial drugs including MEFOXIN should only be used to treat bacterial infections. They do not treat viral infections (e.g., the common cold). When MEFOXIN is prescribed to treat a bacterial infection, patients should be told that although it is common to feel better early in the course of therapy, the medication should be taken exactly as directed. Skipping doses or not completing the full course of therapy may (1) decrease the effectiveness of the immediate treatment and (2) increase the likelihood that bacteria will develop resistance and will not be treatable by MEFOXIN or other antibacterial drugs in the future.

REFERENCES section, change the code number and issue date to

7948525 Issued August 2003

MINTEZOL® CHEWABLE TABLETS AND SUSPENSION ℞
[*mĭn-tĕ-zŏl*]
(Thiabendazole)

Prescribing information for this product, which appears on pages 2031–2032 of the 2004 PDR, has been revised as follows. Please write "See Supplement A" next to the product heading.

In the **PRECAUTIONS** section, after the last paragraph, add the subhead "*Geriatric Use*" under that, as a new paragraph, add:

"Clinical studies of MINTEZOL did not include sufficient numbers of subjects aged 65 and over to determine whether they respond differently from younger subjects. Other reported clinical experience has not identified differences in responses between the elderly and younger patients. In general, dose selection for an elderly patient should be cautious, usually starting at the low end of the dosing range, reflecting the greater frequency of decreased hepatic, renal, or cardiac function, and of concomitant disease or other drug therapy."

After that paragraph, add as a new paragraph, "This drug is metabolized almost completely by the liver, and the metabolites are known to be substantially excreted by the kidney, therefore the risk of toxicity may be greater in patients with impaired renal function. Because elderly patients are more likely to have decreased renal function, care should be taken in dose selection, and it may be useful to monitor renal function."

Revision based on 7930815, issued June 2003.

NOROXIN® ℞
[*nōr-ŏk-sĭn*]
(NORFLOXACIN)
TABLETS

Prescribing information for this product, which appears on pages 2039–2042 of the 2004 PDR, has been completely revised as follows. Please write "See Supplement A" next to the product heading.

To reduce the development of drug-resistant bacteria and maintain the effectiveness of NOROXIN† and other antibacterial drugs, NOROXIN should be used only to treat or prevent infections that are proven or strongly suspected to be caused by bacteria.

DESCRIPTION

NOROXIN (Norfloxacin) is a synthetic, broad-spectrum antibacterial agent for oral administration. Norfloxacin, a fluoroquinolone, is 1-ethyl-6-fluoro-1,4-dihydro-4-oxo-7-(1-piperazinyl)-3-quinolinecarboxylic acid. Its empirical formula is $C_{16}H_{18}FN_3O_3$ and the structural formula is:

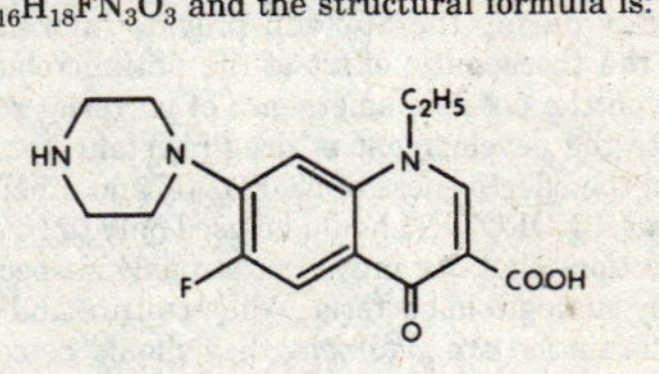

Norfloxacin is a white to pale yellow crystalline powder with a molecular weight of 319.34 and a melting point of about 221°C. It is freely soluble in glacial acetic acid, and very slightly soluble in ethanol, methanol and water.

NOROXIN is available in 400-mg tablets. Each tablet contains the following inactive ingredients: cellulose, croscarmellose sodium, hydroxypropyl cellulose, hydroxypropyl methylcellulose, iron oxide, magnesium stearate, and titanium dioxide.

Norfloxacin, a fluoroquinolone, differs from non-fluorinated quinolones by having a fluorine atom at the 6 position and a piperazine moiety at the 7 position.

† Registered trademark of MERCK & CO., Inc.

CLINICAL PHARMACOLOGY

In fasting healthy volunteers, at least 30-40% of an oral dose of NOROXIN is absorbed. Absorption is rapid following single doses of 200 mg, 400 mg and 800 mg. At the respective doses, mean peak serum and plasma concentrations of 0.8, 1.5 and 2.4 μg/mL are attained approximately one hour after dosing. The presence of food and/or dairy products may decrease absorption. The effective half-life of norfloxacin in serum and plasma is 3-4 hours. Steady-state concentrations of norfloxacin will be attained within two days of dosing.

In healthy elderly volunteers (65-75 years of age with normal renal function for their age), norfloxacin is eliminated more slowly because of their slightly decreased renal function. Following a single 400-mg dose of norfloxacin, the mean (± SD) AUC and C_{max} of 9.8 (2.83) μg•hr/mL and 2.02 (0.77) μg/mL, respectively, were observed in healthy elderly volunteers. The extent of systemic exposure was slightly higher than that seen in younger adults (AUC 6.4 μg•hr/mL and C_{max} 1.5 μg/mL). Drug absorption appears unaffected. However, the effective half-life of norfloxacin in these elderly subjects is 4 hours.

There is no information on accumulation of norfloxacin with repeated administration in elderly patients. However, no dosage adjustment is required based on age alone. In elderly patients with reduced renal function, the dosage should be adjusted as for other patients with renal impairment (see DOSAGE AND ADMINISTRATION, *Renal Impairment*).

The disposition of norfloxacin in patients with creatinine clearance rates greater than 30 mL/min/1.73 m^2 is similar to that in healthy volunteers. In patients with creatinine clearance rates equal to or less than 30 mL/min/1.73 m^2, the renal elimination of norfloxacin decreases so that the effective serum half-life is 6.5 hours. In these patients, alteration of dosage is necessary (see DOSAGE AND ADMINISTRATION). Drug absorption appears unaffected by decreasing renal function.

Norfloxacin is eliminated through metabolism, biliary excretion, and renal excretion. After a single 400-mg dose of NOROXIN, mean antimicrobial activities equivalent to 278, 773, and 82 μg of norfloxacin/g of feces were obtained at 12, 24, and 48 hours, respectively. Renal excretion occurs by both glomerular filtration and tubular secretion as evidenced by the high rate of renal clearance (approximately 275 mL/min). Within 24 hours of drug administration, 26 to 32% of the administered dose is recovered in the urine as norfloxacin with an additional 5-8% being recovered in the urine as six active metabolites of lesser antimicrobial potency. Only a small percentage (less than 1%) of the dose is recovered thereafter. Fecal recovery accounts for another 30% of the administered dose. In elderly subjects (average creatinine clearance 91 mL/min/1.73 m^2) approximately 22% of the administered dose was recovered in urine and renal clearance averaged 154 mL/min.

Two to three hours after a single 400-mg dose, urinary concentrations of 200 μg/mL or more are attained in the urine. In healthy volunteers, mean urinary concentrations of norfloxacin remain above 30 μg/mL for at least 12 hours following a 400-mg dose. The urinary pH may affect the solubility of norfloxacin. Norfloxacin is least soluble at urinary pH of 7.5 with greater solubility occurring at pHs above and below this value. The serum protein binding of norfloxacin is between 10 and 15%.

The following are mean concentrations of norfloxacin in various fluids and tissues measured 1 to 4 hours post-dose after two 400-mg doses, unless otherwise indicated:

Renal Parenchyma	7.3 μg/g
Prostate	2.5 μg/g
Seminal Fluid	2.7 μg/mL
Testicle	1.6 μg/g
Uterus/Cervix	3.0 μg/g
Vagina	4.3 μg/g
Fallopian Tube	1.9 μg/g
Bile	6.9 μg/mL (after two 200-mg doses)

Microbiology

Norfloxacin has *in vitro* activity against a broad range of gram-positive and gram-negative aerobic bacteria. The fluorine atom at the 6 position provides increased potency against gram-negative organisms, and the piperazine moiety at the 7 position is responsible for antipseudomonal activity.

Norfloxacin inhibits bacterial deoxyribonucleic acid synthesis and is bactericidal. At the molecular level, three specific events are attributed to norfloxacin in *E. coli* cells:

1) inhibition of the ATP-dependent DNA supercoiling reaction catalyzed by DNA gyrase,
2) inhibition of the relaxation of supercoiled DNA,
3) promotion of double-stranded DNA breakage.

Resistance to norfloxacin due to spontaneous mutation *in vitro* is a rare occurrence (range: 10^{-9} to 10^{-12} cells). Resistant organisms have emerged during therapy with norfloxacin in less than 1% of patients treated. Organisms in which development of resistance is greatest are the following:

Pseudomonas aeruginosa
Klebsiella pneumoniae
Acinetobacter spp.
Enterococcus spp.

For this reason, when there is a lack of satisfactory clinical response, repeat culture and susceptibility testing should be done. Nalidixic acid-resistant organisms are generally susceptible to norfloxacin *in vitro*; however, these organisms may have higher minimum inhibitory concentrations (MIC's) to norfloxacin than nalidixic acid-susceptible strains. There is generally no cross-resistance between norfloxacin and other classes of antibacterial agents. Therefore, norfloxacin may demonstrate activity against indicated organisms resistant to some other antimicrobial agents including the aminoglycosides, penicillins, cephalosporins, tetracyclines, macrolides, and sulfonamides, including com-

Continued on next page

Information on the Merck & Co., Inc., products listed on these pages is from the full prescribing information in use April 1, 2004.

Noroxin—Cont.

binations of sulfamethoxazole and trimethoprim. Antagonism has been demonstrated *in vitro* between norfloxacin and nitrofurantoin.

Norfloxacin has been shown to be active against most strains of the following microorganisms both *in vitro* and in clinical infections as described in the **INDICATIONS AND USAGE** section.

Gram-positive aerobes:

Enterococcus faecalis
Staphylococcus aureus
Staphylococcus epidermidis
Staphylococcus saprophyticus
Streptococcus agalactiae

Gram-negative aerobes:

Citrobacter freundii
Enterobacter aerogenes
Enterobacter cloacae
Escherichia coli
Klebsiella pneumoniae
Neisseria gonorrhoeae
Proteus mirabilis
Proteus vulgaris
Pseudomonas aeruginosa
Serratia marcescens

The following *in vitro* data are available, **but their clinical significance is unknown.**

Norfloxacin exhibits *in vitro* minimal inhibitory concentrations (MIC's) of ≤4 μg/mL against most (≥90%) strains of the following microorganisms; however, the safety and effectiveness of norfloxacin in treating clinical infections due to these microorganisms have not been established in adequate and well-controlled clinical trials.

Gram-negative aerobes:

Citrobacter diversus
Edwardsiella tarda
Enterobacter agglomerans
Haemophilus ducreyi
Klebsiella oxytoca
Morganella morganii
Providencia alcalifaciens
Providencia rettgeri
Providencia stuartii
Pseudomonas fluorescens
Pseudomonas stutzeri

Other:

Ureaplasma urealyticum

NOROXIN is not generally active against obligate anaerobes.

Norfloxacin has not been shown to be active against *Treponema pallidum*. (See WARNINGS.)

Susceptibility Tests

Dilution Techniques:

Quantitative methods are used to determine antimicrobial minimal inhibitory concentrations (MIC's). These MIC's provide estimates of the susceptibility of bacteria to antimicrobial compounds. The MIC's should be determined using a standardized procedure. Standardized procedures are based on a dilution method[1] (broth, agar, or microdilution) or equivalent with standardized inoculum concentrations and standardized concentrations of norfloxacin powder. The MIC values should be interpreted according to the following criteria*:

MIC (μg/mL)	Interpretation
≤4	Susceptible (S)
8	Intermediate (I)
≥16	Resistant (R)

A report of "Susceptible" indicates that the pathogen is likely to be inhibited if the antimicrobial compound in the blood reaches the concentrations usually achievable. A report of "Intermediate" indicates that the result should be considered equivocal, and, if the microorganism is not fully susceptible to alternative, clinically feasible drugs, the test should be repeated. This category implies possible clinical applicability in body sites where the drug is physiologically concentrated or in situations where high dosage of drug can be used. This category also provides a buffer zone which prevents small uncontrolled technical factors from causing major discrepancies in interpretation. A report of "Resistant" indicates that the pathogen is not likely to be inhibited if the antimicrobial compound in the blood reaches the concentrations usually achievable; other therapy should be selected.

Standardized susceptibility test procedures require the use of laboratory control microorganisms to control the technical aspects of the laboratory procedures. Standard norfloxacin powder should provide the following MIC values:

Organism	MIC range (μg/mL)
E. coli ATCC 25922	0.03-0.12
E. faecalis ATCC 29212	2-8
P. aeruginosa ATCC 27853	1-4
S. aureus ATCC 29213	0.5-2

Diffusion Techniques:

Quantitative methods that require measurement of zone diameters also provide reproducible estimates of the susceptibility of bacteria to antimicrobial compounds. One such standardized procedure[2] requires the use of standardized inoculum concentrations. This procedure uses paper disks impregnated with 10-μg norfloxacin to test the susceptibility of microorganisms to norfloxacin. Reports from the laboratory providing results of the standard single-disk susceptibility test with a 10-μg norfloxacin disk should be interpreted according to the following criteria*:

Zone diameter (mm)	Interpretation
≥17	Susceptible (S)
13-16	Intermediate (I)
≤12	Resistant (R)

Interpretation should be as stated above for results using dilution techniques. Interpretation involves correlation of the diameter obtained in the disk test with the MIC for norfloxacin.

As with standard dilution techniques, diffusion methods require the use of laboratory control microorganisms that are used to control the technical aspects of the laboratory procedures. For the diffusion techniques, the 10-μg norfloxacin disk should provide the following zone diameters in these laboratory test quality control strains:

Organism	Zone Diameter (mm)
E. coli ATCC 25922	28-35
P. aeruginosa ATCC 27853	22-29
S. aureus ATCC 25923	17-28

*These interpretative criteria apply only to isolates from urinary tract infections. There are no established norfloxacin interpretive criteria for *Neisseria gonorrhoeae* or organisms isolated from other infection sites.

INDICATIONS AND USAGE

NOROXIN is indicated for the treatment of adults with the following infections caused by susceptible strains of the designated microorganisms:

Urinary tract infections:

Uncomplicated urinary tract infections (including cystitis) due to *Enterococcus faecalis, Escherichia coli, Klebsiella pneumoniae, Proteus mirabilis, Pseudomonas aeruginosa, Staphylococcus epidermidis, Staphylococcus saprophyticus, Citrobacter freundii***, *Enterobacter aerogenes***, *Enterobacter cloacae***, *Proteus vulgaris***, *Staphylococcus aureus***, or *Streptococcus agalactiae***.

Complicated urinary tract infections due to *Enterococcus faecalis, Escherichia coli, Klebsiella pneumoniae, Proteus mirabilis, Pseudomonas aeruginosa*, or *Serratia marcescens***.

Sexually transmitted diseases (see WARNINGS):

Uncomplicated urethral and cervical gonorrhea due to *Neisseria gonorrhoeae*.

Prostatitis:

Prostatitis due to *Escherichia coli*.

(See DOSAGE AND ADMINISTRATION for appropriate dosing instructions.)

Penicillinase production should have no effect on norfloxacin activity.

Appropriate culture and susceptibility tests should be performed before treatment in order to isolate and identify organisms causing the infection and to determine their susceptibility to norfloxacin. Therapy with norfloxacin may be initiated before results of these tests are known; once results become available, appropriate therapy should be given. Repeat culture and susceptibility testing performed periodically during therapy will provide information not only on the therapeutic effect of the antimicrobial agents but also on the possible emergence of bacterial resistance.

To reduce the development of drug-resistant bacteria and maintain the effectiveness of NOROXIN and other antibacterial drugs, NOROXIN should be used only to treat or prevent infections that are proven or strongly suspected to be caused by susceptible bacteria. When culture and susceptibility information are available, they should be considered in selecting or modifying antibacterial therapy. In the absence of such data, local epidemiology and susceptibility patterns may contribute to the empiric selection of therapy.

**Efficacy for this organism in this organ system was studied in fewer than 10 infections.

CONTRAINDICATIONS

NOROXIN (norfloxacin) is contraindicated in persons with a history of hypersensitivity, tendinitis, or tendon rupture associated with the use of norfloxacin or any member of the quinolone group of antimicrobial agents.

WARNINGS

Safety in Children, Adolescents, Nursing mothers, and during Pregnancy: THE SAFETY AND EFFICACY OF ORAL NORFLOXACIN IN PEDIATRIC PATIENTS, ADOLESCENTS (UNDER THE AGE OF 18), PREGNANT WOMEN, AND NURSING MOTHERS HAVE NOT BEEN ESTABLISHED. (See PRECAUTIONS, *Pediatric Use, Pregnancy*, and *Nursing Mothers* subsections.) The oral administration of single doses of norfloxacin, 6 times*** the recommended human clinical dose (on a mg/kg basis), caused lameness in immature dogs. Histologic examination of the weight-bearing joints of these dogs revealed permanent lesions of the cartilage. Other quinolones also produced erosions of the cartilage in weight-bearing joints and other signs of arthropathy in immature animals of various species. (See ANIMAL PHARMACOLOGY.)

QT interval prolongation/torsades de pointes: QT interval prolongation and episodes of torsades de pointes have been reported in patients receiving quinolones, including norfloxacin. This drug should be avoided in patients with known prolongation of the QT interval, patients with uncorrected hypokalemia, and patients receiving class IA (quinidine, procainamide), or class III (amiodarone, sotalol) antiarrhythmic agents.

Seizures: Convulsions have been reported in patients receiving norfloxacin. Convulsions, increased intracranial pressure, and toxic psychoses have been reported in patients receiving drugs in this class. Quinolones may also cause central nervous system (CNS) stimulation which may lead to tremors, restlessness, lightheadedness, confusion, and hallucinations. If these reactions occur in patients receiving norfloxacin, the drug should be discontinued and appropriate measures instituted.

The effects of norfloxacin on brain function or on the electrical activity of the brain have not been tested. Therefore, until more information becomes available, norfloxacin, like all other quinolones, should be used with caution in patients with known or suspected CNS disorders, such as severe cerebral arteriosclerosis, epilepsy, and other factors which predispose to seizures. (See ADVERSE REACTIONS.)

Hypersensitivity/anaphylaxis: Serious and occasionally fatal hypersensitivity (anaphylactoid or anaphylactic) reactions, some following the first dose, have been reported in patients receiving quinolone therapy. Some reactions were accompanied by cardiovascular collapse, loss of consciousness, tingling, pharyngeal or facial edema, dyspnea, urticaria and itching. Only a few patients had a history of hypersensitivity reactions. If an allergic reaction to norfloxacin occurs, discontinue the drug. Serious acute hypersensitivity reactions may require immediate emergency treatment with epinephrine. Oxygen, intravenous fluids, antihistamines, corticosteroids, pressor amines, and airway management, including intubation, should be administered as indicated.

***Pseudomembranous colitis:* Pseudomembranous colitis has been reported with nearly all antibacterial agents, including norfloxacin, and may range in severity from mild to life-threatening. Therefore, it is important to consider this diagnosis in patients who present with diarrhea subsequent to the administration of antibacterial agents.**

Treatment with antibacterial agents alters the normal flora of the colon and may permit overgrowth of clostridia. Studies indicate that a toxin produced by *Clostridium difficile* is one primary cause of "antibiotic-associated colitis".

After the diagnosis of pseudomembranous colitis has been established, therapeutic measures should be initiated. Mild cases of pseudomembranous colitis usually respond to drug discontinuation alone. In moderate to severe cases, consideration should be given to management with fluids and electrolytes, protein supplementation, and treatment with an antibacterial drug clinically effective against *C. difficile* colitis.

Peripheral neuropathy: Sensory or sensorimotor axonal polyneuropathy affecting small (pain, burning, tingling) and/or large (numbness, vibration) axons has been reported in patients receiving quinolones, including norfloxacin. Post-marketing surveillance reports indicate that these neuropathies can have a rapid onset after the initiation of fluoroquinolone use and can be rapidly progressive and in some cases can be irreversible. NOROXIN should be discontinued if the patient experiences symptoms of neuropathy including pain, burning, tingling, numbness, and/or vibration in order to prevent the development of an irreversible condition.

Tendon rupture: Ruptures of the shoulder, hand, or Achilles tendons that required surgical repair or resulted in prolonged disability have been reported in patients receiving quinolones, including norfloxacin. Post-marketing surveillance reports indicate that this risk may be increased in patients receiving concomitant corticosteroids, especially in the elderly. Norfloxacin should be discontinued if the patient experiences pain, inflammation, or rupture of a tendon. Patients should rest and refrain from exercise until the diagnosis of tendinitis or tendon rupture has been confidently excluded. Tendon rupture can occur during or after therapy with quinolones, including norfloxacin.

*Syphilis treatment: Norfloxacin has **not** been shown to be effective in the treatment of syphilis.* Antimicrobial agents used in high doses for short periods of time to treat gonorrhea may mask or delay the symptoms of incubating syphilis. All patients with gonorrhea should have a serologic test for syphilis at the time of diagnosis. Patients treated with norfloxacin should have a follow-up serologic test for syphilis after three months.

***Based on a patient weight of 50 kg.

PRECAUTIONS

General

Needle-shaped crystals were found in the urine of some volunteers who received either placebo, 800 mg norfloxacin, or 1600 mg norfloxacin (at or twice the recommended daily dose, respectively) while participating in a double-blind, crossover study comparing single doses of norfloxacin with placebo. While crystalluria is not expected to occur under usual conditions with a dosage regimen of 400 mg b.i.d., as a precaution, the daily recommended dosage should not be exceeded and the patient should drink sufficient fluids to ensure a proper state of hydration and adequate urinary output.

Alteration in dosage regimen is necessary for patients with impaired renal function (see DOSAGE AND ADMINISTRATION).

Moderate to severe phototoxicity reactions have been observed in patients who are exposed to excessive sunlight while receiving some members of this drug class. Excessive sunlight should be avoided. Therapy should be discontinued if phototoxicity occurs.

Rarely, hemolytic reactions have been reported in patients with latent or actual defects in glucose-6-phosphate dehydrogenase activity who take quinolone antibacterial agents, including norfloxacin. (See ADVERSE REACTIONS.)

Quinolones, including norfloxacin, may exacerbate the signs of myasthenia gravis and lead to life-threatening weakness of the respiratory muscles. Caution should be exercised when using quinolones, including NOROXIN, in patients with myasthenia gravis (see ADVERSE REACTIONS).

Prescribing NOROXIN in the absence of a proven or strongly suspected bacterial infection or a prophylactic indication is unlikely to provide benefit to the patient and increases the risk of the development of drug-resistant bacteria.

Information for Patients

Patients should be advised:

— that norfloxacin may cause changes in the electrocardiogram (QTc interval prolongation).

— that norfloxacin should be avoided in patients receiving class IA (e.g., quinidine, procainamide) or class III (e.g., amiodarone, sotalol) antiarrhythmic agents.

— that norfloxacin should be used with caution in subjects receiving drugs that affect the QTc interval such as cisapride, erythromycin, antipsychotics, and tricyclic antidepressants.

— to inform their physicians of any personal or family history of QTc prolongation or proarrhythmic conditions such as hypokalemia, bradycardia or recent myocardial ischemia.

— that peripheral neuropathies have been associated with norfloxacin use. If symptoms of peripheral neuropathy including pain, burning, tingling, numbness, and/or vibration develop, they should discontinue treatment and contact their physicians.

— to drink fluids liberally.

— that norfloxacin should be taken at least one hour before or at least two hours after a meal or ingestion of milk and/or other dairy products.

— that multivitamins or other products containing iron or zinc, antacids or Videx®‡ (Didanosine), chewable/buffered tablets or the pediatric powder for oral solution, should not be taken within the two-hour period before or within the two-hour period after taking norfloxacin. (See PRECAUTIONS, *Drug Interactions*.)

— that norfloxacin can cause dizziness and lightheadedness and, therefore, patients should know how they react to norfloxacin before they operate an automobile or machinery or engage in activities requiring mental alertness and coordination.

— to discontinue treatment and inform their physician if they experience pain, inflammation, or rupture of a tendon, and to rest and refrain from exercise until the diagnosis of tendinitis or tendon rupture has been confidently excluded.

— that norfloxacin may be associated with hypersensitivity reactions, even following the first dose, and to discontinue the drug at the first sign of a skin rash or other allergic reaction.

— to avoid undue exposure to excessive sunlight while receiving norfloxacin and to discontinue therapy if phototoxicity occurs.

— that some quinolones may increase the effects of theophylline and/or caffeine. (See PRECAUTIONS, *Drug Interactions*.)

— that convulsions have been reported in patients taking quinolones, including norfloxacin, and to notify their physician before taking this drug if there is a history of this condition.

‡Registered trademark of Bristol-Myers Squibb Company

Patients should be counseled that antibacterial drugs including NOROXIN should only be used to treat bacterial infections. They do not treat viral infections (e.g., the common cold). When NOROXIN is prescribed to treat a bacterial infection, patients should be told that although it is common to feel better early in the course of therapy, the medication should be taken exactly as directed. Skipping doses or not completing the full course of therapy may (1) decrease the effectiveness of the immediate treatment and (2) increase the likelihood that bacteria will develop resistance and will not be treatable by NOROXIN or other antibacterial drugs in the future.

Laboratory Tests

As with any potent antibacterial agent, periodic assessment of organ system functions, including renal, hepatic, and hematopoietic, is advisable during prolonged therapy.

Drug Interactions

Elevated plasma levels of theophylline have been reported with concomitant quinolone use. There have been reports of theophylline-related side effects in patients on concomitant therapy with norfloxacin and theophylline. Therefore, monitoring of theophylline plasma levels should be considered and dosage of theophylline adjusted as required.

Elevated serum levels of cyclosporine have been reported with concomitant use of cyclosporine with norfloxacin. Therefore, cyclosporine serum levels should be monitored and appropriate cyclosporine dosage adjustments made when these drugs are used concomitantly.

Quinolones, including norfloxacin, may enhance the effects of oral anticoagulants, including warfarin or its derivatives or similar agents. When these products are administered concomitantly, prothrombin time or other suitable coagulation tests should be closely monitored.

The concomitant administration of quinolones including norfloxacin with glyburide (a sulfonylurea agent) has, on rare occasions, resulted in severe hypoglycemia. Therefore, monitoring of blood glucose is recommended when these agents are co-administered.

Diminished urinary excretion of norfloxacin has been reported during the concomitant administration of probenecid and norfloxacin.

The concomitant use of nitrofurantoin is not recommended since nitrofurantoin may antagonize the antibacterial effect of NOROXIN in the urinary tract.

Multivitamins, or other products containing iron or zinc, antacids or sucralfate should not be administered concomitantly with, or within 2 hours of, the administration of norfloxacin, because they may interfere with absorption resulting in lower serum and urine levels of norfloxacin.

Videx® (Didanosine) chewable/buffered tablets or the pediatric powder for oral solution should not be administered concomitantly with, or within 2 hours of, the administration of norfloxacin, because these products may interfere with absorption resulting in lower serum and urine levels of norfloxacin.

Some quinolones have also been shown to interfere with the metabolism of caffeine. This may lead to reduced clearance of caffeine and a prolongation of its plasma half-life.

Carcinogenesis, Mutagenesis, Impairment of Fertility

No increase in neoplastic changes was observed with norfloxacin as compared to controls in a study in rats, lasting up to 96 weeks at doses 8-9 times*** the usual human dose (on a mg/kg basis).

Norfloxacin was tested for mutagenic activity in a number of *in vivo* and *in vitro* tests. Norfloxacin had no mutagenic effect in the dominant lethal test in mice and did not cause chromosomal aberrations in hamsters or rats at doses 30-60 times*** the usual human dose (on a mg/kg basis). Norfloxacin had no mutagenic activity *in vitro* in the Ames microbial mutagen test, Chinese hamster fibroblasts and V-79 mammalian cell assay. Although norfloxacin was weakly positive in the Rec-assay for DNA repair, all other mutagenic assays were negative including a more sensitive test (V-79).

Norfloxacin did not adversely affect the fertility of male and female mice at oral doses up to 30 times*** the usual human dose (on a mg/kg basis).

Pregnancy

Teratogenic Effects. Pregnancy Category C. Norfloxacin has been shown to produce embryonic loss in monkeys when given in doses 10 times*** the maximum daily total human dose (on a mg/kg basis). At this dose, peak plasma levels obtained in monkeys were approximately 2 times those obtained in humans. There has been no evidence of a teratogenic effect in any of the animal species tested (rat, rabbit, mouse, monkey) at 6-50 times*** the maximum daily human dose (on a mg/kg basis). There are, however, no adequate and well-controlled studies in pregnant women. Norfloxacin should be used during pregnancy only if the potential benefit justifies the potential risk to the fetus.

Nursing Mothers

It is not known whether norfloxacin is excreted in human milk.

When a 200-mg dose of NOROXIN was administered to nursing mothers, norfloxacin was not detected in human milk. However, because the dose studied was low, because other drugs in this class are secreted in human milk, and because of the potential for serious adverse reactions from norfloxacin in nursing infants, a decision should be made to discontinue nursing or to discontinue the drug, taking into account the importance of the drug to the mother.

Pediatric Use

The safety and effectiveness of oral norfloxacin in pediatric patients and adolescents below the age of 18 years have not been established. Norfloxacin causes arthropathy in juvenile animals of several animal species. (See WARNINGS and ANIMAL PHARMACOLOGY.)

Geriatric Use

Of the 340 subjects in one large clinical study of NOROXIN for treatment of urinary tract infections, 103 patients were 65 and older, 77 of whom were 70 and older; no overall differences in safety and effectiveness were evident between these subjects and younger subjects. In clinical practice, no difference in the type of reported adverse experiences have been observed between the elderly and younger patients except for a possible increased risk of tendon rupture in elderly patients receiving concomitant corticosteroids (see WARNINGS). In addition, increased risk for other adverse experiences in some older individuals cannot be ruled out (see ADVERSE REACTIONS).

This drug is known to be substantially excreted by the kidney, and the risk of toxic reactions to this drug may be greater in patients with impaired renal function. Because elderly patients are more likely to have decreased renal function, care should be taken in dose selection, and it may be useful to monitor renal function (see DOSAGE AND ADMINISTRATION).

A pharmacokinetic study of NOROXIN in elderly volunteers (65 to 75 years of age with normal renal function for their age) was carried out (see CLINICAL PHARMACOLOGY).

ADVERSE REACTIONS

Single-Dose Studies

In clinical trials involving 82 healthy subjects and 228 patients with gonorrhea, treated with a single dose of norfloxacin, 6.5% reported drug-related adverse experiences. However, the following incidence figures were calculated without reference to drug relationship.

The most common adverse experiences (>1.0%) were: dizziness (2.6%), nausea (2.6%), headache (2.0%), and abdominal cramping (1.6%).

Additional reactions (0.3%-1.0%) were: anorexia, diarrhea, hyperhidrosis, asthenia, anal/rectal pain, constipation, dyspepsia, flatulence, tingling of the fingers, and vomiting.

Laboratory adverse changes considered drug-related were reported in 4.5% of patients/subjects. These laboratory changes were: increased AST (SGOT) (1.6%), decreased WBC (1.3%), decreased platelet count (1.0%), increased urine protein (1.0%), decreased hematocrit and hemoglobin (0.6%), and increased eosinophils (0.6%).

Multiple-Dose Studies

In clinical trials involving 52 healthy subjects and 1980 patients with urinary tract infections or prostatitis treated with multiple doses of norfloxacin, 3.6% reported drug-related adverse experiences. However, the incidence figures below were calculated without reference to drug relationship.

The most common adverse experiences (>1.0%) were: nausea (4.2%), headache (2.8%), dizziness (1.7%), and asthenia (1.3%).

Additional reactions (0.3%-1.0%) were: abdominal pain, back pain, constipation, diarrhea, dry mouth, dyspepsia/heartburn, fever, flatulence, hyperhidrosis, loose stools, pruritus, rash, somnolence, and vomiting.

Less frequent reactions (0.1%-0.2%) included: abdominal swelling, allergies, anorexia, anxiety, bitter taste, blurred vision, bursitis, chest pain, chills, depression, dysmenorrhea, edema, erythema, foot or hand swelling, insomnia, mouth ulcer, myocardial infarction, palpitation, pruritus ani, renal colic, sleep disturbances, and urticaria.

Abnormal laboratory values observed in these patients/subjects were: eosinophilia (1.5%), elevation of ALT (SGPT) (1.4%), decreased WBC and/or neutrophil count (1.4%), elevation of AST (SGOT) (1.4%), and increased alkaline phosphatase (1.1%). Those occurring less frequently included increased BUN, increased LDH, increased serum creatinine, decreased hematocrit, and glycosuria.

Post Marketing

The most frequently reported adverse reaction in post-marketing experience is rash.

CNS effects characterized as generalized seizures, myoclonus and tremors have been reported with NOROXIN (see WARNINGS). Visual disturbances have been reported with drugs in this class.

The following additional adverse reactions have been reported since the drug was marketed:

Hypersensitivity Reactions

Hypersensitivity reactions have been reported including anaphylactoid reactions, angioedema, dyspnea, vasculitis, urticaria, arthritis, arthralgia and myalgia (see WARNINGS).

Skin

Toxic epidermal necrolysis, Stevens-Johnson syndrome and erythema multiforme, exfoliative dermatitis, photosensitivity.

Gastrointestinal

Pseudomembranous colitis, hepatitis, jaundice including cholestatic jaundice and elevated liver function tests, pancreatitis (rare), stomatitis. The onset of pseudomembranous colitis symptoms may occur during or after antibacterial treatment (see WARNINGS).

Cardiovascular

On rare occasions, prolonged QTc interval and ventricular arrhythmia (including torsades de pointes).

Renal

Interstitial nephritis, renal failure.

Nervous System/Psychiatric

Peripheral neuropathy, Guillain-Barré syndrome, ataxia, paresthesia; psychic disturbances including psychotic reactions and confusion.

Musculoskeletal

Tendinitis, tendon rupture; exacerbation of myasthenia gravis (see PRECAUTIONS); elevated creatine kinase (CK).

Hematologic

Neutropenia; leukopenia; agranulocytosis; hemolytic anemia, sometimes associated with glucose-6-phosphate dehydrogenase deficiency; thrombocytopenia.

Special Senses

Hearing loss, tinnitus, diplopia, dysgeusia.

Other adverse events reported with quinolones include: agranulocytosis, albuminuria, candiduria, crystalluria, cylindruria, dysphagia, elevation of blood glucose, elevation of serum cholesterol, elevation of serum potassium, elevation of serum triglycerides, hematuria, hepatic necrosis, symptomatic hypoglycemia, nystagmus, postural hypotension, prolongation of prothrombin time, and vaginal candidiasis.

OVERDOSAGE

No significant lethality was observed in male and female mice and rats at single oral doses up to 4 g/kg.

In the event of acute overdosage, the stomach should be emptied by inducing vomiting or by gastric lavage, and the patient carefully observed and given symptomatic and supportive treatment. Adequate hydration must be maintained.

Continued on next page

Information on the Merck & Co., Inc., products listed on these pages is from the full prescribing information in use April 1, 2004.

Noroxin—Cont.

DOSAGE AND ADMINISTRATION

Tablets NOROXIN should be taken at least one hour before or at least two hours after a meal or ingestion of milk and/or other dairy products. Multivitamins, other products containing iron or zinc, antacids containing magnesium and aluminum, sucralfate, or Videx® (Didanosine), chewable/buffered tablets or the pediatric powder for oral solution, should not be taken within 2 hours of administration of norfloxacin.

Tablets NOROXIN should be taken with a glass of water. Patients receiving NOROXIN should be well hydrated (see PRECAUTIONS).

Normal Renal Function

The recommended daily dose of NOROXIN is as described in the following chart:

[See table below]

Renal Impairment

NOROXIN may be used for the treatment of urinary tract infections in patients with renal insufficiency. In patients with a creatinine clearance rate of 30 mL/min/1.73 m^2 or less, the recommended dosage is one 400-mg tablet once daily for the duration given above. At this dosage, the urinary concentration exceeds the MICs for most urinary pathogens susceptible to norfloxacin, even when the creatinine clearance is less than 10 mL/min/1.73 m^2.

When only the serum creatinine level is available, the following formula (based on sex, weight, and age of the patient) may be used to convert this value into creatinine clearance. The serum creatinine should represent a steady state of renal function.

$$\text{Males: } \frac{(\text{weight in kg}) \times (140 - \text{age})}{(72) \times \text{serum creatinine (mg/100 mL)}}$$

$$\text{Females: } (0.85) \times (\text{above value})$$

Elderly

Elderly patients being treated for urinary tract infections who have a creatinine clearance of greater than 30 mL/min/1.73 m^2 should receive the dosages recommended under *Normal Renal Function*.

Elderly patients being treated for urinary tract infections who have a creatinine clearance of 30 mL/min/1.73 m^2 or less should receive 400 mg once daily as recommended under *Renal Impairment*.

HOW SUPPLIED

No. 3522 — Tablets NOROXIN 400 mg are dark pink, oval shaped, film-coated tablets, coded MSD 705 on one side and NOROXIN on the other. They are supplied as follows:

NDC 0006-0705-68 bottles of 100

NDC 0006-0705-20 unit of use bottles of 20

NDC 0006-0705-28 unit dose packages of 100.

Storage

Store at 25°C (77°F); excursions permitted to 15-30°C (59-86°F) [see USP Controlled Room Temperature]. Keep container tightly closed.

ANIMAL PHARMACOLOGY

Norfloxacin and related drugs have been shown to cause arthropathy in immature animals of most species tested (see WARNINGS).

Crystalluria has occurred in laboratory animals tested with norfloxacin. In dogs, needle-shaped drug crystals were seen in the urine at doses of 50 mg/kg/day. In rats, crystals were reported following doses of 200 mg/kg/day.

Embryo lethality and slight maternotoxicity (vomiting and anorexia) were observed in cynomolgus monkeys at doses of 150 mg/kg/day or higher.

Ocular toxicity, seen with some related drugs, was not observed in any norfloxacin-treated animals.

REFERENCES

1. National Committee for Clinical Laboratory Standards, Methods for dilution antimicrobial susceptibility tests for bacteria that grow aerobically - 3rd ed., Approved Standard NCCLS Document M7-A3, Vol. 13, No. 25, NCCLS, Villanova, PA, 1993.
2. National Committee for Clinical Laboratory Standards, Performance standards for antimicrobial disk susceptibility tests - 5th ed., Approved Standard NCCLS Document M2-A5, Vol. 13, No. 24, NCCLS, Villanova, PA, 1993.

MERCK & CO., INC., Whitehouse Station, NJ 08889, USA

Revisions based on 7898531, issued November 2003, 7898532, issued November 2003, and 7898533, issued November 2003.

Infection	Description	Unit Dose	Frequency	Duration	Daily Dose
Urinary Tract	Uncomplicated UTI's (cystitis) due to *E. coli*, *K. pneumoniae*, or *P. mirabilis*	400 mg	q12h	3 days	800 mg
	Uncomplicated UTI's due to other indicated organisms	400 mg	q12h	7-10 days	800 mg
	Complicated UTI's	400 mg	q12h	10-21 days	800 mg
Sexually Transmitted Diseases	Uncomplicated Gonorrhea	800 mg	single dose	1 day	800 mg
Prostatitis	Acute or Chronic	400 mg	q12h	28 days	800 mg

PNEUMOVAX® 23 ℞

[*new-mō-văks*]

(Pneumococcal Vaccine Polyvalent)

Prescribing information for this product, which appears on pages 2051–2053 of the 2004 PDR, has been revised as follows. Please write "See Supplement A" next to the product heading.

In the **ADVERSE REACTIONS** section, replace all text beginning with "The following adverse experiences have been reported with PNEUMOVAX 23" and ending with "Fever ≤102°F." with the following:

"The following adverse experiences have been reported with PNEUMOVAX 23 in clinical trials and/or post-marketing experience:

Local reactions at injection site including soreness, warmth, erythema, swelling and induration.‡ Very rarely, cellulitis-like reactions were reported. These cellulitis-like reactions, reported in post-marketing experience, show short onset time from vaccine administration and were transient in nature.

Fever ≤102°F.‡"

‡ Most common adverse experiences reported in clinical trials."

In the **ADVERSE REACTIONS** section, under *Body as a Whole*, before "Asthenia", add "Cellulitis".

Revisions based on 7999820, issued July 2003.

PRIMAXIN® I.M. ℞

(Imipenem and Cilastatin for Injectable Suspension)

Prescribing information for this product, which appears on pages 2053–2055 of the 2004 PDR, has been revised as follows. Please write "See Supplement A" next to the product heading.

At the beginning, after the brand name and the generic, add the following paragraph:

"To reduce the development of drug-resistant bacteria and maintain the effectiveness of PRIMAXIN I.M.† and other antibacterial drugs, PRIMAXIN I.M. should be used only to treat or prevent infections that are proven or strongly suspected to be caused by bacteria."

In the **INDICATIONS AND USAGE** section, at the end, add the following paragraph:

"To reduce the development of drug-resistant bacteria and maintain the effectiveness of PRIMAXIN I.M. and other antibacterial drugs, PRIMAXIN I.M. should be used only to treat or prevent infections that are proven or strongly suspected to be caused by susceptible bacteria. When culture and susceptibility information are available, they should be considered in selecting or modifying antibacterial therapy. In the absence of such data, local epidemiology and susceptibility patterns may contribute to the empiric selection of therapy."

In the **PRECAUTIONS** section, under *General*, after the second paragraph, add the following paragraph:

"Prescribing PRIMAXIN I.M. in the absence of a proven or strongly suspected bacterial infection or a prophylactic indication is unlikely to provide benefit to the patient and increases the risk of the development of drug-resistant bacteria."

After the *General* subsection, add the following subsection:

"*Information for Patients*

Patients should be counseled that antibacterial drugs including PRIMAXIN I.M. should only be used to treat bacterial infections. They do not treat viral infections (e.g., the common cold). When PRIMAXIN I.M. is prescribed to treat a bacterial infection, patients should be told that although it is common to feel better early in the course of therapy, the medication should be taken exactly as directed. Skipping doses or not completing the full course of therapy may (1) decrease the effectiveness of the immediate treatment and (2) increase the likelihood that bacteria will develop resistance and will not be treatable by PRIMAXIN I.M. or other antibacterial drugs in the future."

Also in the **PRECAUTIONS** section, under *Carcinogenesis, Mutagenesis, Impairment of Fertility*, in the second paragraph, replace the first sentence with "Reproductive tests in male and female rats were performed with imipenem-cilastatin sodium at intravenous doses up to 80 mg/kg/day and at a subcutaneous dose of 320 mg/kg/day, 2.1 times*** the maximum recommended daily human dose of the intramuscular formulation (on a mg/m^2 body surface area basis)." Replace the corresponding footnote with "*** Based on patient body surface area of 1.6 m^2 (weight of 60 kg)." In addition, delete the last sentence of the paragraph.

Also in the **PRECAUTIONS** section, under *Pregnancy: Teratogenic Effects*, replace the first two paragraphs with the following:

"*Pregnancy Category C:* Teratology studies with cilastatin sodium at doses of 30, 100, and 300 mg/kg/day administered intravenously to rabbits and 40, 200, and 1000 mg/kg/day administered subcutaneously to rats, up to approximately 3.9 and 6.5 times*** the maximum recommended daily human dose (on a mg/m^2 body surface area basis) of the intramuscular formulation of PRIMAXIN (25 mg/kg/day) in the two species, respectively, showed no evidence of adverse effects on the fetus. No evidence of teratogenicity was observed in rabbits given imipenem at intravenous doses of 15, 30, or 60 mg/kg/day and rats given imipenem at intravenous doses of 225, 450, or 900 mg/kg/day, up to approximately 0.8 and 5.8 times*** the maximum recommended daily human dose (on a mg/m^2 body surface area basis) in the two species, respectively.

Teratology studies with imipenem-cilastatin sodium at intravenous doses of 20 and 80 and a subcutaneous dose of 320 mg/kg/day, approximately equal to (mice) and up to 2.1 times*** (rats) the maximum recommended daily intramuscular human dose (on a mg/m^2 body surface area basis) in pregnant rodents during the period of major organogenesis, revealed no evidence of teratogenicity."

In the third paragraph, in the first sentence, after "pregnant rabbits", add "subcutaneously".

In the fourth paragraph, in the third sentence, replace "3 times*** the maximum daily recommended human dose" with "1.3 times*** the maximum recommended daily human dose".

After the fourth paragraph, add the following paragraph:

"No adverse effects on the fetus or on lactation were observed when imipenem-cilastatin sodium was administered subcutaneously to rats late in gestation at dosages up to 320 mg/kg/day, 2.1 times the maximum recommended daily human dose (on a mg/m^2 body surface area basis)."

At the end, replace "7632909 Issued November 2001" with "7632911 Issued August 2003".

PRIMAXIN® I.V. ℞

[*prī-măk-sĭn*]

(Imipenem and Cilastatin for Injection)

Prescribing information for this product, which appears on pages 2055–2059 of the 2004 PDR, has been revised as follows. Please write "See Supplement A" next to the product heading.

At the beginning, after the brand name and the generic, add the following paragraph:

"To reduce the development of drug-resistant bacteria and maintain the effectiveness of PRIMAXIN I.V.† and other antibacterial drugs, PRIMAXIN I.V. should be used only to treat or prevent infections that are proven or strongly suspected to be caused by bacteria."

In the **INDICATIONS AND USAGE** section, at the end, add the following paragraph:

"To reduce the development of drug-resistant bacteria and maintain the effectiveness of PRIMAXIN I.V. and other antibacterial drugs, PRIMAXIN I.V. should be used only to treat or prevent infections that are proven or strongly suspected to be caused by susceptible bacteria. When culture and susceptibility information are available, they should be considered in selecting or modifying antibacterial therapy. In the absence of such data, local epidemiology and susceptibility patterns may contribute to the empiric selection of therapy."

In the **PRECAUTIONS** section, under *General*, at the end, add the following paragraph:

"Prescribing PRIMAXIN I.V. in the absence of a proven or strongly suspected bacterial infection or a prophylactic indication is unlikely to provide benefit to the patient and increases the risk of the development of drug-resistant bacteria."

After the *General* subsection, add the following subsection:

"*Information for Patients*

Patients should be counseled that antibacterial drugs including PRIMAXIN I.V. should only be used to treat bacterial infections. They do not treat viral infections (e.g., the common cold). When PRIMAXIN I.V. is prescribed to treat a bacterial infection, patients should be told that although it is common to feel better early in the course of therapy, the medication should be taken exactly as directed. Skipping doses or not completing the full course of therapy may (1) decrease the effectiveness of the immediate treatment and (2) increase the likelihood that bacteria will develop resistance and will not be treatable by PRIMAXIN I.V. or other antibacterial drugs in the future."

In the **PRECAUTIONS** section, under *Carcinogenesis, Mutagenesis, Impairment of Fertility*, in the second paragraph, replace the first sentence with "Reproductive tests in male and female rats were performed with imipenem-cilastatin sodium at intravenous doses up to 80 mg/kg/day and at a subcutaneous dose of 320 mg/kg/day, approximately equal to the highest recommended human dose of the intravenous formulation (on a mg/m^2 body surface area basis)." Also, delete the last sentence of the paragraph.

In the **PRECAUTIONS** section, under *Pregnancy: Teratogenic Effects*, replace the first two paragraphs with the following:

"*Pregnancy Category C:* Teratology studies with cilastatin sodium at doses of 30, 100, and 300 mg/kg/day administered intravenously to rabbits and 40, 200, and 1000 mg/kg/day administered subcutaneously to rats, up to approximately 1.9 and 3.2 times†† the maximum recommended daily human dose (on a mg/m^2 body surface area basis) of the intravenous formulation of imipenem-cilastatin sodium (50 mg/kg/day) in the two species, respectively, showed no evidence of adverse effect on the fetus. No evidence of teratogenicity was observed in rabbits given imipenem at intravenous doses of 15, 30 or 60 mg/kg/day and rats given imipenem at intravenous doses of 225, 450, or 900 mg/kg/day, up to approximately 0.4 and 2.9 times†† the maximum recommended daily human dose (on a mg/m^2 body surface area basis) in the two species, respectively.
Teratology studies with imipenem-cilastatin sodium at intravenous doses of 20 and 80, and a subcutaneous dose of 320 mg/kg/day, up to 0.5 times†† (mice) to approximately equal to (rats) the highest recommended daily intravenous human dose (on a mg/m^2 body surface area basis) in pregnant rodents during the period of major organogenesis, revealed no evidence of teratogenicity."
In addition, replace the corresponding footnote with "†† Based on patient body surface area of 1.6 m^2 (weight of 60 kg)."
Also under *Pregnancy: Teratogenic Effects*, in the third paragraph, in the first sentence, after "when administered", add "subcutaneously" and after "higher" add "(1000-4000 mg/day),".
In the fourth paragraph, in the third sentence, replace "2 times††" with "0.6 times††".
Before the last paragraph, add the following paragraph:
"No adverse effects on the fetus or on lactation were observed when imipenem-cilastatin sodium was administered subcutaneously to rats late in gestation at dosages up to 320 mg/kg/day, approximately equal to the highest recommended human dose (on a mg/m^2 body surface area basis)."
At the end, after the **REFERENCES** section, replace "7882126 Issued November 2001" with "7882128 Issued August 2003".

PRINIVIL® ℞

[*prĭn-ĭ-vĭl*]
lisinopril

Prescribing information for this product, which appears on pages 2059–2063 of the 2004 PDR, has been revised as follows. Please write "See Supplement A" next to the product heading.
In the **CLINICAL PHARMACOLOGY** section, under *Pharmacokinetics and Metabolism*, in the first paragraph, at the beginning of the first sentence, add "*Adult Patients:*".
After the sixth paragraph, as a new paragraph, add the following: "*Pediatric Patients:* The pharmacokinetics of lisinopril were studied in 29 pediatric hypertensive patients between 6 years and 16 years with glomerular filtration rate >30 mL/min/1.73 m^2. After doses of 0.1 to 0.2 mg/kg, steady state peak plasma concentrations of lisinopril occurred within 6 hours and the extent of absorption based on urinary recovery was about 28%. These values are similar to those obtained previously in adults. The typical value of lisinopril oral clearance (systemic clearance/absolute bioavailability) in a child weighing 30 kg is 10 L/h, which increases in proportion to renal function."
In the **CLINICAL PHARMACOLOGY** section, under *Pharmacodynamics and Clinical Effects*, after *Hypertension*, insert "*Adult Patients:*" before Administration.
In the **CLINICAL PHARMACOLOGY** section, under *Pharmacodynamics and Clinical Effects*, after the eighth paragraph, as a new paragraph, insert the following: "*Pediatric Patients:* In a clinical study involving 115 hypertensive pediatric patients 6 to 16 years of age, patients who weighed <50 kg received either 0.625, 2.5, or 20 mg of lisinopril daily and patients who weighed ≥50 kg received either 1.25, 5, or 40 mg of lisinopril daily. At the end of 2 weeks, lisinopril administered once daily lowered trough blood pressure in a dose-dependent manner with consistent antihypertensive efficacy demonstrated at doses >1.25 mg (0.02 mg/kg). This effect was confirmed in a withdrawal phase, where the diastolic pressure rose by about 9 mmHg more in patients randomized to placebo than it did in patients who were randomized to remain on the middle and high doses of lisinopril. The dose-dependent antihypertensive effect of lisinopril was consistent across several demographic subgroups: age, Tanner stage, gender, race. In this study, lisinopril was generally well-tolerated." After this paragraph, as a new paragraph, insert the following: "In the above pediatric studies, lisinopril was given either as tablets or in a suspension for those children and infants who were unable to swallow tablets or who required a lower dose than is available in tablet form (see DOSAGE AND ADMINISTRATION, *Preparation of Suspension*)."
In the **CLINICAL PHARMACOLOGY** section, under *Pharmacodynamics and Clinical Effects*, in the tenth paragraph, after 12-week clinical studies insert "using doses of PRINIVIL up to 20 mg".
In the **INDICATIONS AND USAGE** section, under *Acute Myocardial Infarction*, at the end of the third paragraph, after compared to non-blacks insert "(see WARNINGS, *Anaphylactoid and Possibly Related Reactions, Angioedema*)".
In the **WARNINGS** section, under ***Anaphylactoid and Possibly Related Reactions***, at the beginning of the second paragraph before ***Angioedema:***, add "***Head and Neck***". In the second paragraph, after the second sentence, insert the following sentence: "ACE inhibitors have been associated with a higher rate of angioedema in Black than in non-Black patients." After the third paragraph, insert the following as a new paragraph: "***Intestinal Angioedema:*** Intestinal angioedema has been reported in patients treated with ACE inhibitors. These patients presented with abdominal pain (with or without nausea or vomiting); in some cases there was no prior history of facial angioedema and C-1 esterase levels were normal. The angioedema was diagnosed by procedures including abdominal CT scan or ultrasound, or at surgery, and symptoms resolved after stopping the ACE inhibitor. Intestinal angioedema should be included in the differential diagnosis of patients on ACE inhibitors presenting with abdominal pain." In the fifth paragraph, after *Anaphylactoid reactions during membrane exposure:*, replace the first sentence with the following: "Sudden and potentially life-threatening anaphylactoid reactions have been reported in some patients dialyzed with high-flux membranes (e.g., AN69®) and treated concomitantly with an ACE inhibitor. In such patients, dialysis must be stopped immediately, and aggressive therapy for anaphylactoid reactions be initiated. Symptoms have not been relieved by antihistamines in these situations. In these patients, consideration should be given to using a different type of dialysis membrane or a different class of antihypertensive agent."
In the **WARNINGS** section, replace the subheading "*Neutropenia/Agranulocytosis*" with "*Leukopenia/Neutropenia/Agranulocytosis*". In the first paragraph after this subheading, in the third sentence, replace "neutropenia" with "leukopenia/neutropenia".
In the **PRECAUTIONS** section, under *Information for Patients*, in the fifth paragraph, before the first sentence, replace "*Neutropenia:*" with *Leukopenia/Neutropenia:* and in the first sentence replace "neutropenia" with "leukopenia/neutropenia".
In the **PRECAUTIONS** section, under *Drug Interactions*, after the third paragraph, as a new paragraph, insert the following: "In a study in 36 patients with mild to moderate hypertension where the antihypertensive effects of PRINIVIL alone were compared to PRINIVIL given concomitantly with indomethacin, the use of indomethacin was associated with a reduced antihypertensive effect, although the difference between the two regimens was not significant."
In the **PRECAUTIONS** section, under *Nursing Mothers*, in the third sentence, after discontinue insert "nursing or discontinue".
In the **PRECAUTIONS** section, under *Pediatric Use*, replace the text with the following: "Antihypertensive effects of PRINIVIL have been established in hypertensive pediatric patients aged 6 to 16 years." As a new paragraph, add: "There are no data on the effect of PRINIVIL on blood pressure in pediatric patients under the age of 6 or in pediatric patients with glomerular filtration rate <30 mL/min/1.73 m^2 (see CLINICAL PHARMACOLOGY, *Pharmacokinetics and Metabolism* and *Pharmacodynamics and Clinical Effects*, and DOSAGE AND ADMINISTRATION)."
In the **ADVERSE REACTIONS** section, under *ACUTE MYOCARDIAL INFARCTION*, in the eighth paragraph, after bone marrow depression, insert "hemolytic anemia," and replace "neutropenia" with "leukopenia/neutropenia".
In the **ADVERSE REACTIONS** section, under *ACUTE MYOCARDIAL INFARCTION*, in the seventeenth paragraph, after *Miscellaneous:* replace the text with the following: "A symptom complex has been reported which may include a positive ANA, an elevated erythrocyte sedimentation rate, arthralgia/arthritis, myalgia, fever, vasculitis, eosinophilia and leukocytosis. Rash, photosensitivity or other dermatological manifestations may occur alone or in combination with these symptoms." In the eighteenth paragraph, after PRINIVIL insert "(0.1%)". After the third sentence, insert "In rare cases, intestinal angioedema has been reported with angiotensin converting enzyme inhibitors including lisinopril." After the twenty-first paragraph, insert the following: "*Pediatric Patients:* No relevant differences between the adverse experience profile for pediatric patients and that previously reported for adult patients were identified."
In the **DOSAGE AND ADMINISTRATION** section, under *Heart Failure*, in the first sentence, before digitalis insert "(usually)". After the *Use in Elderly* subsection, insert the following subsections: As a subheading, insert "*Pediatric Hypertensive Patients ≥ 6 years of age*". As a new paragraph, insert "The usual recommended starting dose is 0.07 mg/kg once daily (up to 5 mg total). Dosage should be adjusted according to blood pressure response. Doses above 0.61 mg/kg (or in excess of 40 mg) have not been studied in pediatric patients. (See CLINICAL PHARMACOLOGY, *Pharmacokinetics and Metabolism* and *Pharmacodynamics and Clinical Effects*.)" As a new paragraph, insert "PRINIVIL is not recommended in pediatric patients <6 years or in pediatric patients with glomerular filtration rate <30 mL/min/1.73 m^2 (see CLINICAL PHARMACOLOGY, *Pharmacokinetics and Metabolism, Pharmacodynamics and Clinical Effects* and PRECAUTIONS)." As a subheading, insert "*Preparation of Suspension (for 200 mL of a 1.0 mg/mL suspension)*". As a new paragraph, insert "Add 10 mL of Purified Water USP to a polyethylene terephthalate (PET) bottle containing ten 20-mg tablets of PRINIVIL and shake for at least one minute. Add 30 mL of Bicitra®** diluent and 160 mL of Ora-Sweet SF™*** to the concentrate in the PET bottle and gently shake for several seconds to disperse the ingredients. The suspension should be stored at or below 25°C (77°F) and can be stored for up to four weeks. Shake the suspension before each use." As a footnote, insert "** Registered trademark of Alza Corporation *** Trademark of Paddock Laboratories, Inc."
In the **HOW SUPPLIED** section, delete the following lines:
"**NDC** 0006-0015-28 unit dose packages of 100"
"**NDC** 0006-0015-31 unit of use bottles of 30"
"**NDC** 0006-0019-28 unit dose packages of 100"
"**NDC** 0006-0019-58 unit of use bottles of 100"
"**NDC** 0006-0019-94 unit of use bottles of 90"
"**NDC** 0006-0019-72 carton of 25 UNIBLISTER™ cards of 31 tablets each."
"**NDC** 0006-0106-28 unit dose packages of 100"
"**NDC** 0006-0106-31 unit of use bottles of 30"
"**NDC** 0006-0106-58 unit of use bottles of 100"
"**NDC** 0006-0106-94 unit of use bottles of 90"
"**NDC** 0006-0106-72 carton of 25 UNIBLISTER™ cards of 31 tablets each."
"**NDC** 0006-0207-28 unit dose packages of 100"
"**NDC** 0006-0207-31 unit of use bottles of 30"
"**NDC** 0006-0207-58 unit of use bottles of 100"
"**NDC** 0006-0207-94 unit of use bottles of 90"
"**NDC** 0006-0207-72 carton of 25 UNIBLISTER™ cards of 31 tablets each."
Revisions based on 7825248 and 7825249, issued April 2003.

PRINZIDE® ℞

[*prĭn-zīd*]
lisinopril-hydrochlorothiazide

Prescribing information for this product, which appears on pages 2063–2067 of the 2004 PDR, has been revised as follows. Please write "See Supplement A" next to the product heading.
In the **WARNINGS** section, under subheading ***Anaphylactoid and Possibly Related Reactions:***, in the second paragraph, at the beginning of the subheading ***Angioedema:***, add "***Head and Neck***". After the third paragraph, add the following paragraph: "***Intestinal Angioedema:*** Intestinal angioedema has been reported in patients treated with ACE inhibitors. These patients presented with abdominal pain (with or without nausea or vomiting); in some cases there was no prior history of facial angioedema and C-1 esterase levels were normal. The angioedema was diagnosed by procedures including abdominal CT scan or ultrasound, or at surgery, and symptoms resolved after stopping the ACE inhibitor. Intestinal angioedema should be included in the differential diagnosis of patients on ACE inhibitors presenting with abdominal pain."
In the **PRECAUTIONS** section, after the last paragraph, add the subheading "*Geriatric Use*". Under that, as a new paragraph, add the following: "Clinical studies of PRINZIDE did not include sufficient numbers of subjects aged 65 and over to determine whether they respond differently from younger subjects. Other reported clinical experience has not identified differences in responses between the elderly and younger patients. In general, dose selection for an elderly patient should be cautious, usually starting at the low end of the dosing range, reflecting the greater frequency of decreased hepatic, renal, or cardiac function, and of concomitant disease or other drug therapy. In a multiple dose pharmacokinetic study in elderly versus young hypertensive patients using the lisinopril/hydrochlorothiazide combination, area under the plasma concentration time curve (AUC) increased approximately 120% for lisinopril and approximately 80% for hydrochlorothiazide in older patients." Under that, as a new paragraph, add the following: "This drug is known to be substantially excreted by the kidney, and the risk of toxic reactions to this drug may be greater in patients with impaired renal function. Because elderly patients are more likely to have decreased renal function, care should be taken in dose selection. Evaluation of the hypertensive patient should always include assessment of renal function. (See DOSAGE AND ADMINISTRATION.)"
In the **ADVERSE REACTIONS** section, in the sixth paragraph, before "(See WARNINGS.)", insert the following sentence: "In rare cases, intestinal angioedema has been reported with angiotensin converting enzyme inhibitors including lisinopril."
In the **DOSAGE AND ADMINISTRATION** section, delete the last paragraph.
Revision based on 7836335 and 7836336, issued April 2003.

PROPECIA® TABLETS ℞

[*prō-pē-sha*]
(finasteride)

Prescribing information for this product, which appears on pages 2067-2070 of the 2004 PDR, has been revised as follows. Please write "See Supplement A" next to the product heading.
In the **PRECAUTIONS** section, under *Information for Patients*, after the first paragraph, insert the following:

Continued on next page

Information on the Merck & Co., Inc., products listed on these pages is from the full prescribing information in use April 1, 2004.

Propecia—Cont.

Physicians should instruct their patients to promptly report any changes in their breasts such as lumps, pain or nipple discharge. Breast changes including breast enlargement, tenderness and neoplasm have been reported (see **ADVERSE REACTIONS**).

In the **ADVERSE REACTIONS** section, at the end, add the following:

The relationship between long-term use of finasteride and male breast neoplasia is currently unknown. During a 4- to 6-year placebo- and comparator-controlled study that enrolled 3047 men, there were 4 cases of breast cancer in men treated with PROSCAR but no cases in men not treated with PROSCAR. In another 4-year, placebo-controlled study that enrolled 3040 men, there were 2 cases of breast cancer in placebo-treated men, but no cases were reported in men treated with PROSCAR.

In a 7-year placebo-controlled trial that enrolled 18,882 healthy men, 9060 had prostate needle biopsy data available for analysis. In the PROSCAR group, 280 (6.4%) men had prostate cancer with Gleason scores of 7–10 detected on needle biopsy vs. 237 (5.1%) men in the placebo group. Of the total cases of prostate cancer diagnosed in this study, approximately 98% were classified as intracapsular (stage T1 or T2). The clinical significance of these findings is unknown.

Revisions based on 9328503, issued October 2003, and 9328504, issued October 2003.

In the "Patient Information," under **What are the possible side effects of PROPECIA?**, at the end of the second paragraph, add the following:

You should promptly report to your doctor any changes in your breasts such as lumps, pain or nipple discharge. Tell your doctor promptly about these or any other unusual side effects.

Also under **What are the possible side effects of PROPECIA?**, delete the third paragraph.

Revisions based on 9329303, issued October 2003.

PROSCAR® TABLETS ℞

[*prō' skär*]

(Finasteride)

Prescribing information for this product, which appears on pages 2070-2073 of the 2004 PDR, has been revised as follows. Please write "See Supplement A" next to the product heading.

In the **PRECAUTIONS** section, under *Effects on PSA and Prostate Cancer Detection*, in the first paragraph, replace the third and fourth sentences with the following:

"In these BPH studies, PROSCAR did not appear to alter the rate of prostate cancer detection, and the overall incidence of prostate cancer was not significantly different in patients treated with PROSCAR or placebo."

Also in the **PRECAUTIONS** section, under *Information for Patients*, after the second paragraph, add the following paragraph:

"Physicians should instruct their patients to promptly report any changes in their breasts such as lumps, pain or nipple discharge. Breast changes including breast enlargement, tenderness and neoplasm have been reported (see **ADVERSE REACTIONS**)."

In the **ADVERSE REACTIONS** section, in the *Phase III Studies and 5-Year Open Extensions* subsection, replace the second paragraph with the following:

Long-Term Data

"There is no evidence of increased adverse experiences with increased duration of treatment with PROSCAR. New reports of drug-related sexual adverse experiences decreased with duration of therapy.

"The relationship between long-term use of finasteride and male breast neoplasia is currently unknown. During a 4- to 6-year placebo- and comparator-controlled study that enrolled 3047 men, there were 4 cases of breast cancer in men treated with finasteride but no cases in men not treated with finasteride. During the 4-year, placebo-controlled PLESS study that enrolled 3040 men, there were 2 cases of breast cancer in placebo-treated men, but no cases were reported in men treated with finasteride.

"In a 7-year placebo-controlled trial that enrolled 18,882 healthy men, 9060 had prostate needle biopsy data available for analysis. In the PROSCAR group, 280 (6.4%) men had prostate cancer with Gleason scores of 7–10 detected on needle biopsy vs. 237 (5.1%) men in the placebo group. Of the total cases of prostate cancer diagnosed in this study, approximately 98% were classified as intracapsular (stage T1 or T2). The clinical significance of these findings is unknown."

Post-Marketing Experience

Revisions based on 9556705, issued July 2003, and 9556706, issued August 2003.

In the **Patient Information**, under **What you need to know while taking PROSCAR**, in the paragraph that begins "In addition, some men", replace "swelling" with "enlargement" and add the following after the first sentence in that paragraph:

"You should promptly report to your doctor any changes in your breasts such as lumps, pain or nipple discharge."

Revisions based on 7819308, issued July 2003.

RECOMBIVAX HB® ℞

[*rē-kŏm-bī-văks*]

(Hepatitis B Vaccine [recombinant])

Prescribing information for this product, which appears on pages 2073-2076 of the 2004 PDR, has been revised as follows. Please write "See Supplement A" next to the product heading.

In the **DESCRIPTION** section, in the seventh paragraph, replace "**Pediatric/Adolescent Formulation (With and Without Preservative)**" with "**Pediatric/Adolescent Formulation (Without Preservative)**"; in the eighth paragraph, replace "**Adult Formulation (With and Without Preservative)**" with "**Adult Formulation (Without Preservative)**"; and in the ninth paragraph, replace "**Dialysis Formulation (With and Without Preservative)**" with "**Dialysis Formulation (Without Preservative)**".

In the **DESCRIPTION** section, in the tenth paragraph, delete the first sentence: "Formulations that contain a preservative include thimerosal, a mercury derivative, at 1:20,000 or 50 mcg/mL."

In the **DOSAGE AND ADMINISTRATION** section, replace the second, third, and fourth paragraphs with the following: *"RECOMBIVAX HB Hepatitis B Vaccine (Recombinant) DIALYSIS FORMULATION [(40 mcg/mL) (WITHOUT PRESERVATIVE)] IS INTENDED ONLY FOR ADULT PREDIALYSIS/DIALYSIS PATIENTS.*

RECOMBIVAX HB Hepatitis B Vaccine (Recombinant) PEDIATRIC/ADOLESCENT (WITHOUT PRESERVATIVE) and ADULT FORMULATIONS (WITHOUT PRESERVATIVE) ARE NOT INTENDED FOR USE IN PREDIALYSIS/DIALYSIS PATIENTS."

In the **DOSAGE AND ADMINISTRATION** section, in Table 1, delete superscript double asterisk from column heading "Dose/Regimen**". In column 2, replace "10 mcg" with "10 mcg**" in the Dose/Regimen information for the Adolescents group and the Adults group.

In the** footnote for Table 1, delete "(see text regarding use of the formulations without preservative)".

In the **DOSAGE AND ADMINISTRATION** section, replace the fourth paragraph after Table 1 with the following: "*For All Formulations:* Since none of the formulations contain a preservative, once the single-dose vial has been penetrated, the withdrawn vaccine should be used promptly, and the vial must be discarded." In the fifth paragraph after Table 1, delete the heading "*For All Formulations With and Without Preservative:*". In the seventh paragraph after Table 1, delete the heading "*For Vials With and Without Preservative:*".

In the **HOW SUPPLIED** section, under PEDIATRIC/ADOLESCENT FORMULATION (PRESERVATIVE-FREE), delete the supply numbers and respective descriptions for numbers 4982, 4983, and 4994. Also delete the PEDIATRIC/ADOLESCENT FORMULATION section, which contains the supply numbers and respective descriptions for numbers 4769, 4876, 4849, and 4969. Delete the ADULT FORMULATION section, which contains the supply numbers and descriptions for numbers 4775, 4773, 4872, 4873, and 4848. Also delete the DIALYSIS FORMULATION section, which contains the supply number and description for number 4776.

Revisions based on 7994325, issued August 2002, and 7994326, issued June 2003.

STROMECTOL® TABLETS ℞

[*strō'mĕk-tōl*]

(Ivermectin)

Prescribing information for this product, which appears on pages 2081–2083 of the 2004 PDR, has been revised as follows. Please write "See Supplement A" next to the product heading.

In the **PRECAUTIONS** section, under *General*, in the second sentence of the second paragraph, replace "standing" with "standing/walking."

In the **ADVERSE REACTIONS** section, under *Onchocerciasis*, in the first sentence of the fifth paragraph, replace "orthostatic hypotension) and worsening of bronchial asthma" with "orthostatic hypotension), worsening of bronchial asthma, and toxic epidermal necrolysis."

Revisions based on 9032306, issued October 2003.

TIMOLIDE® TABLETS ℞

[*tĭm-ō-līd*]

timolol maleate-hydrochlorothiazide

Prescribing information for this product, which appears on pages 2084–2087 of the 2004 PDR, has been revised as follows. Please write "See Supplement A" alongside product heading.

In the **PRECAUTIONS** section, under *Geriatric Use*, in the second paragraph, replace the first sentence with the following: "Both timolol and hydrochlorothiazide are known to be substantially excreted by the kidney, and the risk of toxic reactions to these drugs may be greater in patients with impaired renal function."

"Revisions based on 7928435, Issued October 2003."

VIOXX® ℞

[*vī-ŏks*]

(rofecoxib tablets and oral suspension)

Prescribing information for this product, which appears on pages 2108–2113 of the 2004 PDR, has been revised as follows. Please write "See Supplement A" next to the product heading.

In the CLINICAL PHARMACOLOGY section, under *Hepatic Insufficiency*, after the second sentence, add "Since patients with hepatic insufficiency are prone to fluid retention and hemodynamic compromise, the maximum recommended chronic dose of VIOXX for patients with moderate hepatic insufficiency is 12.5 mg daily. (See PRECAUTIONS, *Hepatic Effects* and DOSAGE AND ADMINISTRATION, *Hepatic Insufficiency*.)"

In the CLINICAL STUDIES section, under *Upper Endoscopy in Patients with Osteoarthritis and Rheumatoid Arthritis*, after the fourth paragraph, add this new paragraph: "A similarly designed 12-week endoscopy study was conducted in OA patients treated with low-dose enteric coated aspirin 81 mg daily, low-dose enteric coated aspirin 81 mg plus VIOXX 25 mg daily, ibuprofen 2400 mg daily, or placebo. There was no difference in the cumulative incidence of endoscopic gastroduodenal ulcers in patients taking low-dose aspirin plus VIOXX 25 mg as compared to those taking ibuprofen 2400 mg daily alone. Patients taking low-dose aspirin plus ibuprofen were not studied. (See PRECAUTIONS, *Drug Interactions, Aspirin*.)"

In the PRECAUTIONS section, under *Hepatic Effects*, in the second paragraph, after the first sentence, add "The maximum recommended chronic daily dose in patients with moderate hepatic insufficiency is 12.5 mg daily." In the second paragraph, replace *Pharmacokinetics*, with "CLINICAL PHARMACOLOGY," and after *Special Populations*, add "and DOSAGE AND ADMINISTRATION, *Hepatic Insufficiency*

In the PRECAUTIONS section, under *Laboratory Tests, Aspirin:*, after the first sentence, add "In a 12-week endoscopy study conducted in OA patients there was no difference in the cumulative incidence of endoscopic gastroduodenal ulcers in patients taking low-dose (81 mg) enteric coated aspirin plus VIOXX 25 mg daily, as compared to those taking ibuprofen 2400 mg daily alone. Patients taking low-dose aspirin plus ibuprofen were not studied. (See CLINICAL STUDIES, *Special Studies, Upper Endoscopy in Patients with Osteoarthritis and Rheumatoid Arthritis*.)" The next sentence begins a new paragraph.

In the DOSAGE AND ADMINISTRATION section, under *Hepatic Insufficiency*, between Cmax, and patients, add "in". Replace "should be treated with the lowest possible dose" with "the maximum recommended chronic daily dose is 12.5 mg." Replace "see" with "See". Add the sentence, "The efficacy of 12.5 mg in rheumatoid arthritis patients with moderate hepatic insufficiency has not been studied."

Revisions based on 9556413, issued August 2003.

In the Patient Information, under "**Can I take VIOXX with other medicines?**", in the second paragraph, after the first sentence, add "If you take both aspirin and VIOXX, you may have a greater chance of serious stomach problems than if you take VIOXX alone." In the second sentence, replace "this purpose" with "prevention of heart attack or stroke".

In the Patient Information, under "**What are the possible side effects of VIOXX?**", in the second paragraph, after "confusion," add "constipation,".

Revisions based on 9183910, issued August 2003, and 9183911, issued September 2003.

ZOCOR® Tablets ℞

[*zō'kōr*]

(simvastatin)

Prescribing information for this product, which appears on pages 2113–2118 of the 2004 PDR, has been revised as follows. Please write "See Supplement A" next to the product heading.

In the **WARNINGS** section, under *Myopathy/Rhabdomyolysis*, under Other drugs:, delete the first paragraph and add two new paragraphs:

"**Gemfibrozil particularly with higher doses of simvastatin** (see below; PRECAUTIONS, *Drug Interactions, Interactions with lipid-lowering drugs that can cause myopathy when given alone*; DOSAGE AND ADMINISTRATION).

Other lipid-lowering drugs (other fibrates or ≥1 g/day of niacin) that can cause myopathy when given alone (see below; PRECAUTIONS, *Drug Interactions, Interactions with lipid-lowering drugs that can cause myopathy when given alone*."

In the **WARNINGS** section, under ***Myopathy/Rhabdomyolysis***, under Other drugs:, in the paragraph beginning "**Other drugs: Amiodarone or verapamil with higher doses of simvastatin**" delete "**Other drugs:**". After **Amiodarone or verapamil with higher doses of simvastatin** (see" insert the word "below".

In the **WARNINGS** section, under ***Myopathy/Rhabdomyolysis***, under **Consequently:**, replace existing point "**2.**" with the following two new points.

"**2. The dose of simvastatin should not exceed 10 mg daily in patients receiving concomitant medication with gemfibrozil. The combined use of simvastatin with gemfibrozil should be avoided, unless the benefits are likely to outweigh the increased risks of this drug combination.** Caution should be used when prescribing other lipid-lowering drugs (other fibrates or lipid-lowering doses (≥1 g/day) of niacin) with simvastatin, as these agents can cause myopathy when given alone. **The benefit of further alterations in lipid levels by the combined use of simvastatin with fibrates or niacin should be carefully weighed against the potential risks of these combinations.** Addition of fibrates or niacin to simvastatin typically provides little additional reduction in LDL-C, but further reductions of TG and further increases in HDL-C may be obtained.

3. The dose of simvastatin should not exceed 10 mg daily in patients receiving concomitant medication with cyclosporine. The benefits of the use of simvastatin in patients receiving cyclosporine should be carefully weighed against the risks of this combination."

Renumber subsequent points in appropriate sequential order, so "**3.**" becomes "**4.**", "**4.**" becomes "**5.**", and **5.**" becomes "**6.**"

In the **PRECAUTIONS** section, under *Interactions with lipid-lowering drugs that can cause myopathy when given alone,* replace all text beginning with "The risk of myopathy is also increased by the following lipid-lowering drugs that are not potent CYP3A4 inhibitors, but which can cause myopathy when given alone." up to and including "**Niacin (nicotinic acid) (≥1 g/day)**" with the following:

"**See WARNINGS, *Myopathy/Rhabdomyolysis.***

The risk of myopathy is increased by gemfibrozil **(see DOSAGE AND ADMINISTRATION)** and to a lesser extent by other fibrates and niacin (nicotinic acid) (≥1 g/day)."

In the **ADVERSE REACTIONS** section, under *Concomitant Lipid-Lowering Therapy,* in the third sentence, delete ", other fibrates or lipid-lowering doses (≥1 g/day) of niacin".

In the **OVERDOSAGE** section, replace the existing second paragraph with the following new paragraph:

"A few cases of overdosage with ZOCOR have been reported; the maximum dose taken was 3.6 g. All patients recovered without sequelae. Until further experience is obtained, no specific treatment of overdosage with ZOCOR can be recommended."

In the **DOSAGE AND ADMINISTRATION** section, in the last sentence of the second paragraph, delete "fibrates or niacin" and add "or gemfibrozil".

In the **DOSAGE AND ADMINISTRATION** section, under *Concomitant Lipid-Lowering Therapy,* in the second sentence, delete "other fibrates or lipid-lowering doses (≥1 g/day) of niacin,".

Revisions based on 9556644 and 9556645, issued September 2003.

Monarch Pharmaceuticals

A wholly owned subsidiary of King Pharmaceuticals, Inc.
501 FIFTH STREET
BRISTOL, TN 37620

Contact information in the Manufacturers' Index, which appears on page 10 of the 2004 PDR, has been completely revised as follows. Please write "See Supplement A" next to the product heading.

Direct Inquiries to:
Customer Service:
800-776-3637
Fax:
423-989-6279
To report an Adverse Drug Experience:
(800) 546-4905
Fax: (423) 990-0519

Ortho-McNeil Pharmaceutical

RARITAN, NJ 08869-0602

www.ortho-mcneil.com
For Medical Information Contact:
(800) 682-6532
In Emergencies:
(908) 218-7325
For Patient Education Materials Contact:
877-323-2200
For Customer Service (Sales and Ordering):
800-631-5273

LEVAQUIN® ℞
[*lĕv-ă-kwĭn*]
(levofloxacin) Tablets
LEVAQUIN®
(levofloxacin) Injection
LEVAQUIN®
(levofloxacin in 5% dextrose) Injection

Prescribing information for this product, which appears on pages 2445–2452 of the 2004 PDR, has been revised as follows. Please write "See Supplement A" next to the product heading.

UPDATED DOSAGE AND ADMINISTRATION SECTION

The DOSAGE AND ADMINISTRATION section has been revised as follows:

Patients with Normal Renal Function

Infection*	Unit Dose	Freq.	Duration**	Daily Dose
Comm. Acquired Pneumonia	500 mg	q24h	7-14 days	500 mg
Comm. Acquired Pneumonia	750 mg***	q24h	5 days	750 mg
Nosocomial Pneumonia	750 mg	q24h	7-14 days	750 mg
Complicated SSSI	750 mg	q24h	7-14 days	750 mg
Acute Bacterial Exacerbation of Chronic Bronchitis	500 mg	q24h	7 days	500 mg
Acute Maxillary Sinusitis	500 mg	q24h	10-14 days	500 mg
Uncomplicated SSSI	500 mg	q24h	7-10 days	500 mg
Chronic Bacterial Prostatitis	500 mg	q24h	28 days	500 mg
Complicated UTI	250 mg	q24h	10 days	250 mg
Acute pyelonephritis	250 mg	q24h	10 days	250 mg
Uncomplicated UTI	250 mg	q24h	3 days	250 mg

* **DUE TO THE DESIGNATED PATHOGENS** (See **INDICATIONS AND USAGE.**)
** Sequential therapy (intravenous to oral) may be instituted at the discretion of the physician.
*** Efficacy of this alternative regimen has only been documented for infections caused by penicillin-susceptible *Streptococcus pneumoniae, Haemophilius influenzae, Haemophilus parainfluenzae, Mycoplasma pneumoniae* and *Chlamydia pneumoniae.*

Patients with Impaired Renal Function

Renal Status	Initial Dose	Subsequent Dose
Acute Bacterial Exacerbation of Chronic Bronchitis/Comm. Acquired Pneumonia/Acute Maxillary Sinusitis/ Uncomplicated SSSI/Chronic Bacterial Prostatitis		
CL_{CR} from 50 to 80 mL/min	No dosage adjustment required	
CL_{CR} from 20 to 49 mL/min	500 mg	250 mg q24h
CL_{CR} from 10 to 19 mL/min	500 mg	250 mg q48h
Hemodialysis	500 mg	250 mg q48h
CAPD	500 mg	250 mg q48h
Complicated SSSI/Nosocomial Pneumonia/Comm. Acquired Pneumonia		
CL_{CR} from 50 to 80 mL/min	No dosage adjustment required	
CL_{CR} from 20 to 49 mL/min	750 mg	750 mg q48h
CL_{CR} from 10 to 19 mL/min	750 mg	500 mg q48h
Hemodialysis	750 mg	500 mg q48h
CAPD	750 mg	500 mg q48h
Complicated UTI/Acute Pyelonephritis		
CL_{CR} ≥20 mL/min	No dosage adjustment required	
CL_{CR} from 10 to 19 mL/min	250 mg	250 mg q48h
Uncomplicated UTI	No dosage adjustment required	

CL_{CR}=creatinine clearances
CAPD=chronic ambulatory peritoneal dialysis

DOSAGE AND ADMINISTRATION

LEVAQUIN Injection should only be administered by intravenous infusion. It is not for intramuscular, intrathecal, intraperitoneal, or subcutaneous administration.

CAUTION: RAPID OR BOLUS INTRAVENOUS INFUSION MUST BE AVOIDED. Levofloxacin Injection should be infused intravenously slowly over a period of not less than 60 or 90 minutes, depending on the dosage. (See **PRECAUTIONS.**)

Single-use vials require dilution prior to administration. (See **PREPARATION FOR ADMINISTRATION.**)

The usual dose of LEVAQUIN Tablets or Injection is 250 mg or 500 mg administered orally or by slow infusion over 60 minutes every 24 hours or 750 mg administered orally or by slow infusion over 90 minutes every 24 hours, as indicated by infection and described in the following dosing chart. These recommendations apply to patients with normal renal function (i.e., creatinine clearance > 80 mL/min). For patients with altered renal function see the **Patients with Impaired Renal Function** subsection. Oral doses should be administered at least two hours before or two hours after antacids containing magnesium, aluminum, as well as sucralfate, metal cations such as iron, and multivitamin preparations with zinc or Videx® (didanosine), chewable/buffered tablets or the pediatric powder for oral solution.

[See first table above]
[See second table above]

When only the serum creatinine is known, the following formula may be used to estimate creatinine clearance.

$$\text{Men: Creatinine Clearance (mL/min)} = \frac{\text{Weight (kg)} \times (140 - \text{age})}{72 \times \text{serum creatinine (mg/dL)}}$$

Women: 0.85 × the value calculated for men.

The serum creatinine should represent a steady state of renal function.

Preparation of Levofloxacin Injection for Administration

LEVAQUIN Injection in Single-Use Vials: LEVAQUIN Injection is supplied in single-use vials containing a concentrated levofloxacin solution with the equivalent of 500 mg (20 mL vial) and 750 mg (30 mL vial) of levofloxacin in Water for Injection, USP. The 20 mL and 30 mL vials each contain 25 mg of levofloxacin/mL. **THESE LEVAQUIN INJECTION SINGLE-USE VIALS MUST BE FURTHER DILUTED WITH AN APPROPRIATE SOLUTION PRIOR TO INTRAVENOUS ADMINISTRATION.** (See **COMPATIBLE INTRAVENOUS SOLUTIONS.**) The concentration of the resulting diluted solution should be 5 mg/mL prior to administration. This intravenous drug product should be inspected visually for particulate matter prior to administration. Samples containing visible particles should be discarded.

Since no preservative or bacteriostatic agent is present in this product, aseptic technique must be used in preparation of the final intravenous solution. **Since the vials are for single-use only, any unused portion remaining in the vial should be discarded. When used to prepare two 250 mg doses from the 20 mL vial containing 500 mg of levofloxacin, the full content of the vial should be withdrawn at once using a single-entry procedure, and a second dose should be prepared and stored for subsequent use.** (See **Stability of LEVAQUIN Injection Following Dilution.**)

Since only limited data are available on the compatibility of levofloxacin intravenous injection with other intravenous substances, **additives or other medications should not be added to LEVAQUIN Injection in single-use vials or infused simultaneously through the same intravenous line.** If the same intravenous line is used for sequential infusion of several different drugs, the line should be flushed before and after infusion of LEVAQUIN Injection with an infusion solution compatible with LEVAQUIN Injection and with any other drug(s) administered via this common line.

Prepare the desired dosage of levofloxacin according to the following chart:

[See first table at top of next page]

For example, to prepare a 500 mg dose using the 20 mL vial (25 mg/mL), withdraw 20 mL and dilute with a compatible intravenous solution to a total volume of 100 mL.

Compatible Intravenous Solutions: Any of the following intravenous solutions may be used to prepare a 5 mg/mL levofloxacin solution with the approximate pH values:

Intravenous Fluids	Final pH of LEVAQUIN Solution
0.9% Sodium Chloride Injection, USP	4.71
5% Dextrose Injection, USP	4.58
5% Dextrose/0.9% NaCl Injection	4.62
5% Dextrose in Lactated Ringers	4.92
Plasma-Lyte® 56/5% Dextrose Injection	5.03
5% Dextrose, 0.45% Sodium Chloride, and 0.15% Potassium Chloride Injection	4.61
Sodium Lactate Injection (M/6)	5.54

LEVAQUIN Injection Premix in Single-Use Flexible Containers: LEVAQUIN Injection is also supplied in flexible containers containing a premixed, ready-to-use levofloxacin solution in D_5W for single-use. The fill volume is either 50 or 100 mL for the 100 mL flexible container or 150 mL for the 150 mL container. **NO FURTHER DILUTION OF THESE PREPARATIONS ARE NECESSARY. Consequently each 50 mL, 100 mL, and 150 mL premix flexible container already contains a dilute solution with the equivalent of 250 mg, 500 mg, and 750 mg of levofloxacin, respectively (5 mg/mL) in 5% Dextrose (D_5W).**

This parenteral drug product should be inspected visually for particulate matter prior to administration. Samples containing visible particles should be discarded.

Continued on next page

Levaquin—Cont.

Since the premix flexible containers are for single-use only, any unused portion should be discarded.

Since only limited data are available on the compatibility of levofloxacin intravenous injection with other intravenous substances, **additives or other medications should not be added to LEVAQUIN Injection in flexible containers or infused simultaneously through the same intravenous line.** If the same intravenous line is used for sequential infusion of several different drugs, the line should be flushed before and after infusion of LEVAQUIN Injection with an infusion solution compatible with LEVAQUIN Injection and with any other drug(s) administered via this common line.

Instructions for the Use of LEVAQUIN Injection Premix in Flexible Containers

To open:

1. Tear outer wrap at the notch and remove solution container.
2. Check the container for minute leaks by squeezing the inner bag firmly. If leaks are found, or if the seal is not intact, discard the solution, as the sterility may be compromised.
3. Do not use if the solution is cloudy or a precipitate is present.
4. Use sterile equipment.
5. **WARNING: Do not use flexible containers in series connections.** Such use could result in air embolism due to residual air being drawn from the primary container before administration of the fluid from the secondary container is complete.

Preparation for administration:

1. Close flow control clamp of administration set.
2. Remove cover from port at bottom of container.
3. Insert piercing pin of administration set into port with a twisting motion until the pin is firmly seated. **NOTE: See full directions on administration set carton.**
4. Suspend container from hanger.
5. Squeeze and release drip chamber to establish proper fluid level in chamber during infusion of LEVAQUIN Injection in Premix Flexible Containers.
6. Open flow control clamp to expel air from set. Close clamp.
7. Regulate rate of administration with flow control clamp.

Stability of LEVAQUIN Injection as Supplied

When stored under recommended conditions, LEVAQUIN Injection, as supplied in 20 mL and 30 mL vials, or 100 mL and 150 mL flexible containers, is stable through the expiration date printed on the label.

Stability of LEVAQUIN Injection Following Dilution

LEVAQUIN Injection, when diluted in a compatible intravenous fluid to a concentration of 5 mg/mL, is stable for 72 hours when stored at or below 25°C (77°F) and for 14 days when stored under refrigeration at 5°C (41°F) in plastic intravenous containers. Solutions that are diluted in a compatible intravenous solution and frozen in glass bottles or plastic intravenous containers are stable for 6 months when stored at -20°C (-4°F). **THAW FROZEN SOLUTIONS AT ROOM TEMPERATURE 25°C (77°F) OR IN A REFRIGERATOR 8°C (46°F). DO NOT FORCE THAW BY MICROWAVE IRRADIATION OR WATER BATH IMMERSION. DO NOT REFREEZE AFTER INITIAL THAWING.**

Desired Dosage Strength	From Appropriate Vial, Withdraw Volume	Volume of Diluent	Infusion Time
250 mg	10 mL (20 mL Vial)	40 mL	60 min
500 mg	20 mL (20 mL Vial)	80 mL	60 min
750 mg	30 mL (30 mL Vial)	120 mL	90 min

CLINICAL STUDIES

Nosocomial Pneumonia

Adult patients with clinically and radiologically documented nosocomial pneumonia were enrolled in a multicenter, randomized, open-label study comparing intravenous levofloxacin (750 mg once daily) followed by oral levofloxacin (750 mg once daily) for a total of 7-15 days to intravenous imipenem/cilastatin (500-1000 mg q6-8 hours daily) followed by oral ciprofloxacin (750 mg q12 hours daily) for a total of 7-15 days. Levofloxacin-treated patients received an average of 7 days of intravenous therapy (range: 1-16 days); comparator-treated patients received an average of 8 days of intravenous therapy (range: 1-19 days).

Overall, in the clinically and microbiologically evaluable population, adjunctive therapy was empirically initiated at study entry in 56 of 93 (60.2%) patients in the levofloxacin arm and 53 of 94 (56.4%) patients in the comparator arm. The average duration of adjunctive therapy was 7 days in the levofloxacin arm and 7 days in the comparator. In clinically and microbiologically evaluable patients with documented Pseudomonas aeruginosa infection, 15 of 17 (88.2%) received ceftazidime (N=11) or piperacillin/tazobactam (N=4) in the levofloxacin arm and 16 of 17 (94.1%) received an aminoglycoside in the comparator arm. Overall, in clinically and microbiologically evaluable patients, vancomycin was added to the treatment regimen of 37 of 93 (39.8%) patients in the levofloxacin arm and 28 of 94 (29.8%) patients in the comparator arm for suspected methicillin-resistant *S. aureus* infection.

Clinical success rates in clinically and microbiologically evaluable patients at the posttherapy visit (primary study endpoint assessed on day 3-15 after completing therapy) were for levofloxacin and 60.6% for comparator. The 95% CI for the difference of response rates (levofloxacin minus comparator) was [-17.2, 12.0]. The microbiological eradication rates at the posttherapy visit were 66.7% for levofloxacin and 60.6% for comparator. The 95% CI for the difference of eradication rates (levofloxacin minus comparator) was [-8.3, 20.3]. Clinical success and microbiological eradication rates by pathogen were as follows:

[See second table above]

Pathogen	N	Levofloxacin No. (%) of Patients Microbiologic/Clinical Outcomes		N	Imipenem/Cilastatin No. (%) of Patients Microbiologic/Clinical Outcomes	
MSSA[a]	21	14 (66.7)/	13 (61.9)	19	13 (68.4)/	15 (78.9)
P. aeruginosa[b]	17	10 (58.8)/	11 (64.7)	17	5 (29.4)/	7 (41.2)
S. marcescens	11	9 (81.8)/	7 (63.6)	7	2 (28.6)/	3 (42.9)
E. coli	12	10 (83.3)/	7 (58.3)	11	7 (63.6)/	8 (72.7)
K. pneumoniae[c]	11	9 (81.8)/	5 (45.5)	7	6 (85.7)/	3 (42.9)
H. influenzae	16	13 (81.3)/	10 (62.5)	15	14 (93.3)	11 (73.3)
S. pneumoniae	4	3 (75.0)/	3 (75.0)	7	5 (71.4)/	4 (57.1)

[a]Methicillin-susceptible *S. aureus*
[b]See above text for use of combination therapy.
[c]The observed differences in rates for the clinical and microbiological outcomes may reflect other factors that were not accounted for in the study.

Pathogen	Levofloxacin (N=136) N	Levofloxacin (N=136) Eradication	Ciprofloxacin (N=125) N	Ciprofloxacin (N=125) Eradication
E. coli	15	14 (93.3%)	11	9 (81.8%)
E. faecalis	54	39 (72.2%)	44	33 (75.0%)
**S. epidermidis*	11	9 (81.8%)	14	11 (78.6%)

*Eradication rates shown are for patients who had a sole pathogen only; mixed cultures were excluded.

Community-Acquired Bacterial Pneumonia
7 to 14 Day Treatment Regimen

Adult inpatients and outpatients with a diagnosis of community-acquired bacterial pneumonia were evaluated in two pivotal clinical studies. In the first study, 590 patients were enrolled in a prospective, multi-center, unblinded randomized trial comparing levofloxacin 500 mg once daily orally or intravenously for 7 to 14 days to ceftriaxone 1 to 2 grams intravenously once or in equally divided doses twice daily followed by cefuroxime axetil 500 mg orally twice daily for a total of 7 to 14 days. Patients assigned to treatment with the control regimen were allowed to receive erythromycin (or doxycycline if intolerant of erythromycin) if an infection due to atypical pathogens was suspected or proven. Clinical and microbiologic evaluations were performed during treatment, 5 to 7 days posttherapy, and 3 to 4 weeks posttherapy. Clinical success (cure plus improvement) with levofloxacin at 5 to 7 days posttherapy, the primary efficacy variable in this study, was superior (95%) to the control group (83%). The 95% CI for the difference of response rates (levofloxacin minus comparator) was [-6, 19]. In the second study, 264 patients were enrolled in a prospective, multi-center, non-comparative trial of 500 mg levofloxacin administered orally or intravenously once daily for 7 to 14 days. Clinical success for clinically evaluable patients was 93%. For both studies, the clinical success rate in patients with atypical pneumonia due to *Chlamydia pneumoniae, Mycoplasma pneumoniae*, and *Legionella pneumophila* were 96%, 96%, and 70%, respectively.

Microbiologic eradication rates across both studies were as follows:

Pathogen	No. Pathogens	Microbiologic Eradication Rate (%)
H. influenzae	55	98
S. pneumoniae	83	95
S. aureus	17	88
M. catarrhalis	18	94
H. parainfluenzae	19	95
K. pneumoniae	10	100.0

Additional studies were initiated to evaluate the utility of LEVAQUIN in community-acquired pneumonia due to *S. pneumoniae*, with particular interest in penicillin-resistant strains (MIC value for penicillin ≥2 μg/mL). In addition to the studies previously discussed, inpatients and outpatients with mild to severe community-acquired pneumonia were evaluated in six additional clinical studies; one double-blind study, two open label randomized studies, and three open label non-comparative studies. The total number of clinically evaluable patients with *S. pneumoniae* across all 8 studies was 250 for levofloxacin and 41 for comparators. The clinical success rate (cured or improved) among the 250 levofloxacin-treated patients with *S. pneumoniae* was 245/250 (98%). The clinical success rate among the 41 comparator-treated patients with *S. pneumoniae* was 39/41 (95%). Across these 8 studies, 18 levofloxacin-treated and 4 non-quinolone comparator-treated patients with community-acquired pneumonia due to penicillin-resistant *S. pneumoniae* (MIC value for penicillin ≥2 μg/mL) were identified. Of the 18 levofloxacin-treated patients, 15 were evaluable following the completion of therapy. Fifteen out of the 15 evaluable levofloxacin-treated patients with community-acquired pneumonia due to penicillin-resistant *S. pneumoniae* achieved clinical success (cure or improvement). Of these 15 patients, 6 were bacteremic and 5 were classified as having severe disease. Of the 4 comparator-treated patients with community-acquired pneumonia due to penicillin-resistant *S. pneumoniae*, 3 were evaluable for clinical efficacy. Three out of the 3 evaluable comparator-treated patients achieved clinical success. All three of the comparator-treated patients were bacteremic and had disease classified as severe.

Community-Acquired Bacterial Pneumonia
5-Day Treatment Regimen

To evaluate the safety and efficacy of higher dose and shorter course of levofloxacin, 528 outpatient and hospitalized adults with clinically and radiologically determined mild to severe community-acquired pneumonia were evaluated in a double-blind, randomized, prospective, multicenter study comparing levofloxacin 750 mg, i.v. or p.o., q.d. for five days or levofloxacin 500 mg i.v. or p.o., q.d. for 10 days.

Clinical success rates (cure plus improvement) in the clinically evaluable population were 90.9% in the levofloxacin 750mg group and 91.1% in the levofloxacin 500 mg group. The 95% CI for the difference of response rates (levofloxacin 750 minus levofloxacin 500) was [-5.9, 5.4]. In the clinically evaluable population (31-38 days after enrollment) pneumonia was observed in 7 out of 151 patients in the levofloxacin 750 mg group and 2 out of 147 patients in the levofloxacin 500 mg group. Given the small numbers observed, the significance of this finding can not be determined statistically. The microbiological efficacy of the 5-day regimen was documented for infections listed in the table below.

	Eradication rate
Penicillin susceptible *S. pneumoniae*	19/20
Haemophilus influenzae	12/12
Haemophilus parainfluenzae	10/10
Mycoplasma pneumoniae	26/27
Chlamydia pneumoniae	13/15

Complicated Skin and Skin Infections

Three hundred ninety-nine patients were enrolled in an open-label, randomized, comparative study for complicated skin and skin structure infections. The patients were randomized to receive either levofloxacin 750 mg QD (IV followed by oral), or an approved comparator for a median of 10 ± 4.7 days. As is expected in complicated skin and skin structure infections, surgical procedures were performed in the levofloxacin and comparator groups. Surgery (incision and drainage or debridement) was performed on 45% of the levofloxacin treated patients and 44% of the comparator treated patients, either shortly before or during antibiotic treatment and formed an integral part of therapy for this indication.

Among those who could be evaluated clinically 2-5 days after completion of study drug, overall success rates (improved or cured) were 116/138 (84.1%) for patients treated with levofloxacin and 106/132 (80.3%) for patients treated with the comparator.

Success rates varied with the type of diagnosis ranging from 68% in patients with infected ulcers to 90% in patients with infected wounds and abscesses. These rates were equivalent to those seen with comparator drugs.

Chronic Bacterial Prostatitis

Adult patients with a clinical diagnosis of prostatitis and microbiological culture results from urine sample collected after prostatic massage (VB3) or expressed prostatic secretion (EPS) specimens obtained via the Meares-Stamey procedure were enrolled in a multicenter, randomized, double-blind study comparing oral levofloxacin 500 mg, once daily for a total of 28 days to oral ciprofloxacin 500 mg, twice daily for a total of 28 days. The primary efficacy endpoint was microbiologic efficacy in microbiologically evaluable patients. A total of 136 and 125 microbiologically evaluable patients were enrolled in the levofloxacin and ciprofloxacin groups, respectively. The microbiologic eradication rate by patient infection at 5-18 days after completion of therapy was 75.0%

in the levofloxacin group and 76.8% in the ciprofloxacin group (95% CI [-12.58, 8.98] for levofloxacin minus ciprofloxacin). The overall eradication rates for pathogens of interest are presented below:

[See third table at top of previous page]

Eradication rates for *S. epidermidis* when found with other co-pathogens are consistent with rates seen in pure isolates. Clinical success (cure + improvement with no need for further antibiotic therapy) rates in microbiologically evaluable population 5-18 days after completion of therapy were 75.0% for levofloxacin-treated patients and 72.8% for ciprofloxacin-treated patients (95% CI [-8.87, 13.27] for levofloxacin minus ciprofloxacin). Clinical long-term success (24-45 days after completion of therapy) rates were 66.7% for the levofloxacin-treated patients and 76.9% for the ciprofloxacin-treated patients (95% CI [-23.40, 2.89] for levofloxacin minus ciprofloxacin).

 Revised February 2004 7518209

TOPAMAX® ℞
[*tō-pā-māks*]
(topiramate)
Tablets

TOPAMAX® ℞
(topiramate capsules)
Sprinkle Capsules

Prescribing information for this product, which appears on pages 2484–2490 of the 2004 PDR, has been revised as follows. Please write "See Supplement A" next to the product heading.

UPDATED WARNINGS SECTION

Metabolic Acidosis

Hyperchloremic, non-anion gap, metabolic acidosis (i.e., decreased serum bicarbonate below the normal reference range in the absence of chronic respiratory alkalosis) is associated with topiramate treatment. This metabolic acidosis is caused by renal bicarbonate loss due to the inhibitory effect of topiramate on carbonic anhydrase. Such electrolyte imbalance has been observed with the use of topiramate in placebo-controlled clinical trials and in the post-marketing period. Generally, topiramate-induced metabolic acidosis occurs early in treatment although cases can occur at any time during treatment. Bicarbonate decrements are usually mild-moderate (average decrease of 4 mEq/L at daily doses of 400 mg in adults and at approximately 6 mg/kg/day in pediatric patients); rarely, patients can experience severe decrements to values below 10 mEq/L. Conditions or therapies that predispose to acidosis (such as renal disease, severe respiratory disorders, status epilepticus, diarrhea, surgery, ketogenic diet, or drugs) may be additive to the bicarbonate lowering effects of topiramate.

In adults, the incidence of persistent treatment-emergent decreases in serum bicarbonate (levels of <20 mEq/L at two consecutive visits or at the final visit) in controlled clinical trials for adjunctive treatment of epilepsy was 32% for 400 mg/day, and 1% for placebo. Metabolic acidosis has been observed at doses as low as 50 mg/day. The incidence of a markedly abnormally low serum bicarbonate (i.e., absolute value <17 mEq/L and >5 mEq/L decrease from pretreatment) in these trials was 3% for 400 mg/day, and 0% for placebo. Serum bicarbonate levels have not been systematically evaluated at daily doses greater than 400 mg/day.

In pediatric patients (<16 years of age), the incidence of persistent treatment-emergent decreases in serum bicarbonate in placebo-controlled trials for adjunctive treatment of Lennox-Gastaut syndrome or refractory partial onset seizures was 67% for TOPAMAX (at approximately 6 mg/kg/day), and 10% for placebo. The incidence of a markedly abnormally low serum bicarbonate (i.e., absolute value <17 mEq/L and >5 mEq/L decrease from pretreatment) in these trials was 11% for TOPAMAX and 0% for placebo. Cases of moderately severe metabolic acidosis have been reported in patients as young as 5 months old, especially at daily doses above 5 mg/kg/day.

Although not approved for the prophylaxis of migraine, the incidence of persistent treatment-emergent decreases in serum bicarbonate in placebo-controlled trials for adults for prophylaxis of migraine was 44% for 200 mg/day, 39% for 100 mg/day, 23% for 50 mg/day, and 7% for placebo. The incidence of a markedly abnormally low serum bicarbonate (i.e., absolute value <17 mEq/L and >5 mEq/L decrease from pretreatment) in these trials was 11% for 200 mg/day, 9% for 100 mg/day, 2% for 50 mg/day, and <1% for placebo.

Some manifestations of acute or chronic metabolic acidosis may include hyperventilation, nonspecific symptoms such as fatigue and anorexia, or more severe sequelae including cardiac arrhythmias or stupor. Chronic, untreated metabolic acidosis may increase the risk for neprolithiasis or nephrocalcinosis, and may also result in osteomalacia (referred to as rickets in pediatric patients) and/or osteoporosis with an increased risk for fractures. Chronic metabolic acidosis in pediatric patients may also reduce growth rates. A reduction in growth rate may eventually decrease the maximal height achieved. The effect of topiramate on growth and bone-related sequelae has not been systematically investigated.

Measurement of baseline and periodic serum bicarbonate during topiramate treatment is recommended. If metabolic acidosis develops and persists, consideration should be given to reducing the dose or discontinuing topiramate (using dose tapering). If the decision is made to continue patients on topiramate in the face of persistent acidosis, alkali treatment should be considered.

Acute Myopia and Secondary Angle Closure Glaucoma

A syndrome consisting of acute myopia associated with secondary angle closure glaucoma has been reported in patients receiving TOPAMAX®. Symptoms include acute onset of decreased visual acuity and/or ocular pain. Opthalmologic findings can include myopia, anterior chamber shallowing, ocular hyperemia (redness) and increased intraocular pressure. Mydriasis may or may not be present. This syndrome may be associated with supraciliary effusion resulting in anterior displacement of the lens and iris, with secondary angle closure glaucoma. Symptoms typically occur within 1 month of initiating TOPAMAX® therapy. In contrast to primary narrow angle glaucoma, which is rare under 40 years of age, secondary angle closure glaucoma associated with topiramate has been reported in pediatric patients as well as adults. The primary treatment to reverse symptoms is discontinuation of TOPAMAX® as rapidly as possible, according to the judgement of the treating physician. Other measures, in conjunction with discontinuation of TOPAMAX®, may be helpful.

Elevated intraocular pressure of any etiology, if left untreated, can lead to serious sequelae including permanent vision loss.

Oligohidrosis and Hyperthermia

Oligohidrosis (decreased sweating), infrequently resulting in hospitalization, has been reported in association with TOPAMAX® use. Decreased sweating and an elevation in body temperature above normal characterized these cases. Some of the cases were reported after exposure to elevated environmental temperatures.

The majority of the reports have been in children. Patients, especially pediatric patients, treated with TOPAMAX® should be monitored closely for evidence of decreased sweating and increased body temperature, especially in hot weather. Caution should be used when TOPAMAX® is prescribed with other drugs that predispose patients to heat-related disorders; these drugs include, but are not limited to, other carbonic anhydrase inhibitors and drugs with anticholinergic activity.

Withdrawal of AEDs

Antiepileptic drugs, including TOPAMAX®, should be withdrawn gradually to minimize the potential of increased seizure frequency.

Cognitive/Neuropsychiatric Adverse Events

Adults

Adverse events most often associated with the use of TOPAMAX® were central nervous system related. In adults, the most significant of these can be classified into two general categories: 1) psychomotor slowing, difficulty with concentration, and speech or language problems, in particular, word-finding difficulties and 2) somnolence or fatigue. Additional nonspecific CNS effects occasionally observed with topiramate as add-on therapy include dizziness or imbalance, confusion, memory problems, and exacerbation of mood disturbances (e.g., irritability and depression). Reports of psychomotor slowing, speech and language problems, and difficulty with concentration and attention were common in adults. Although in some cases these events were mild to moderate, they at times led to withdrawal from treatment. The incidence of psychomotor slowing is only marginally dose-related, but both language problems and difficulty with concentration or attention clearly increased in frequency with increasing dosage in the five double-blind trials [see **ADVERSE REACTIONS, Table 6** in full Prescribing Information].

Somnolence and fatigue were the most frequently reported adverse events during clinical trials with TOPAMAX®. These events were generally mild to moderate and occurred early in therapy. While the incidence of somnolence does not appear to be dose-related, that of fatigue increases at dosages above 400 mg/day.

Pediatric Patients

In double-blind clinical studies, the incidences of cognitive/neuropsychiatric adverse events in pediatric patients were generally lower than previously observed in adults.These events included psychomotor slowing, difficulty with concentration/attention, speech disorders/related speech problems and language problems. The most frequently reported neuropsychiatric events in this population were somnolence and fatigue. No patients discontinued treatment due to adverse events in double-blind trials.

Sudden Unexplained Death in Epilepsy (SUDEP)

During the course of premarketing development of TOPAMAX® (topiramate) Tablets, 10 sudden and unexplained deaths were recorded among a cohort of treated patients (2,796 subject years of exposure). This represents an incidence of 0.0035 deaths per patient year. Although this rate exceeds that expected in a healthy population matched for age and sex, it is within the range of estimates for the incidence of sudden unexplained deaths in patients with epilepsy not receiving TOPAMAX® (ranging from 0.0005 for the general population of patients with epilepsy, to 0.003 for a clinical trial population similar to that in the TOPAMAX® program, to 0.005 for patients with refractory epilepsy).

OMP DIVISION
ORTHO-McNEIL PHARMACEUTICAL, INC.
Raritan, NJ 08869

 Revision Date December 2003 7517109

Parkedale Pharmaceuticals

(a wholly owned subsidiary of King Pharmaceuticals, Inc.)
870 PARKDALE ROAD
ROCHESTER, MI 48307

Contact information in the Manufacturers' Index, which appears on page 13 of the 2004 PDR, has been completely revised as follows. Please write "See Supplement A" next to the product heading.

Direct Inquiries to:
Customer Service:
800-776-3637
Fax:
423-989-6279
To report an Adverse Drug Experience:
(800) 546-4905
Fax: (423) 990-0519

Parke-Davis

A Division of Warner-Lambert Company LLC
A Pfizer Company
235 E 42ND ST
NEW YORK, NY 10017-5755

For Medical Information Contact:
(800) 438-1985
24 hours a day, 7 days a week
Distribution:
1855 Shelby Oaks Drive North
Memphis, TN 38134
(901) 387-5200
Customer Service:
(800) 533-4535
EXPORT INQUIRIES:
Pfizer International Inc.
(212) 733-2323

ACCUPRIL® ℞
[*ă'kew-prĭl*]
(Quinapril Hydrochloride Tablets)

Prescribing information for this product, which appears on pages 2516–2519 of the 2004 PDR, has been completely revised as follows. Please write "See Supplement A" next to the product heading.

USE IN PREGNANCY
When used in pregnancy during the second and third trimesters, ACE inhibitors can cause injury and even death to the developing fetus. When pregnancy is detected, ACCUPRIL should be discontinued as soon as possible. See WARNINGS, Fetal/Neonatal Morbidity and Mortality.

DESCRIPTION

ACCUPRIL® (quinapril hydrochloride) is the hydrochloride salt of quinapril, the ethyl ester of a non-sulfhydryl, angiotensin-converting enzyme (ACE) inhibitor, quinaprilat.

Quinapril hydrochloride is chemically described as [3S-[2[R*(R*)], 3R*]]-2-[2-[[1-(ethoxycarbonyl)-3-phenylpropyl] amino]-1-oxopropyl]-1,2,3,4-tetrahydro-3-isoquinolinecarboxylic acid, monohydrochloride. Its empirical formula is $C_{25}H_{30}N_2O_5$ •HCl and its structural formula is:

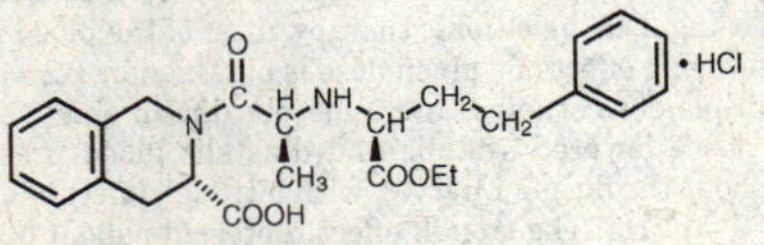

M.W.=474.98

Quinapril hydrochloride is a white to off-white amorphous powder that is freely soluble in aqueous solvents.

ACCUPRIL tablets contain 5 mg, 10 mg, 20 mg, or 40 mg of quinapril for oral administration. Each tablet also contains candelilla wax, crospovidone, gelatin, lactose, magnesium carbonate, magnesium stearate, synthetic red iron oxide, and titanium dioxide.

CLINICAL PHARMACOLOGY

Mechanism of Action: Quinapril is deesterified to the principal metabolite, quinaprilat, which is an inhibitor of ACE activity in human subjects and animals. ACE is a peptidyl dipeptidase that catalyzes the conversion of angiotensin I to the vasoconstrictor, angiotensin II. The effect of quinapril in hypertension and in congestive heart failure (CHF) appears to result primarily from the inhibition of circulating and tissue ACE activity, thereby reducing angiotensin II formation. Quinapril inhibits the elevation in blood pressure caused by intravenously administered angiotensin I, but has no effect on the pressor response to angio-

Continued on next page

Accupril—Cont.

tensin II, norepinephrine or epinephrine. Angiotensin II also stimulates the secretion of aldosterone from the adrenal cortex, thereby facilitating renal sodium and fluid reabsorption. Reduced aldosterone secretion by quinapril may result in a small increase in serum potassium. In controlled hypertension trials, treatment with ACCUPRIL alone resulted in mean increases in potassium of 0.07 mmol/L (see PRECAUTIONS). Removal of angiotensin II negative feedback on renin secretion leads to increased plasma renin activity (PRA).

While the principal mechanism of antihypertensive effect is thought to be through the renin-angiotensin-aldosterone system, quinapril exerts antihypertensive actions even in patients with low renin hypertension. ACCUPRIL was an effective antihypertensive in all races studied, although it was somewhat less effective in blacks (usually a predominantly low renin group) than in nonblacks. ACE is identical to kininase II, an enzyme that degrades bradykinin, a potent peptide vasodilator; whether increased levels of bradykinin play a role in the therapeutic effect of quinapril remains to be elucidated.

Pharmacokinetics and Metabolism: Following oral administration, peak plasma quinapril concentrations are observed within one hour. Based on recovery of quinapril and its metabolites in urine, the extent of absorption is at least 60%. The rate and extent of quinapril absorption are diminished moderately (approximately 25-30%) when ACCUPRIL tablets are administered during a high-fat meal. Following absorption, quinapril is deesterified to its major active metabolite, quinaprilat (about 38% of oral dose), and to other minor inactive metabolites. Following multiple oral dosing of ACCUPRIL, there is an effective accumulation half-life of quinaprilat of approximately 3 hours, and peak plasma quinaprilat concentrations are observed approximately 2 hours post-dose. Quinaprilat is eliminated primarily by renal excretion, up to 96% of an IV dose, and has an elimination half-life in plasma of approximately 2 hours and a prolonged terminal phase with a half-life of 25 hours. The pharmacokinetics of quinapril and quinaprilat are linear over a single-dose range of 5-80 mg doses and 40-160 mg in multiple daily doses. Approximately 97% of either quinapril or quinaprilat circulating in plasma is bound to proteins.

In patients with renal insufficiency, the elimination half-life of quinaprilat increases as creatinine clearance decreases. There is a linear correlation between plasma quinaprilat clearance and creatinine clearance. In patients with end-stage renal disease, chronic hemodialysis or continuous ambulatory peritoneal dialysis has little effect on the elimination of quinapril and quinaprilat. Elimination of quinaprilat may be reduced in elderly patients (≥65 years) and in those with heart failure; this reduction is attributable to decrease in renal function (see DOSAGE AND ADMINISTRATION). Quinaprilat concentrations are reduced in patients with alcoholic cirrhosis due to impaired deesterification of quinapril. Studies in rats indicate that quinapril and its metabolites do not cross the blood-brain barrier.

Pharmacodynamics and Clinical Effects

Hypertension: Single doses of 20 mg of ACCUPRIL provide over 80% inhibition of plasma ACE for 24 hours. Inhibition of the pressor response to angiotensin I is shorter-lived, with a 20 mg dose giving 75% inhibition for about 4 hours, 50% inhibition for about 8 hours, and 20% inhibition at 24 hours. With chronic dosing, however, there is substantial inhibition of angiotensin II levels at 24 hours by doses of 20-80 mg.

Administration of 10 to 80 mg of ACCUPRIL to patients with mild to severe hypertension results in a reduction of sitting and standing blood pressure to about the same extent with minimal effect on heart rate. Symptomatic postural hypotension is infrequent although it can occur in patients who are salt- and/or volume-depleted (see WARNINGS). Antihypertensive activity commences within 1 hour with peak effects usually achieved by 2 to 4 hours after dosing. During chronic therapy, most of the blood pressure lowering effect of a given dose is obtained in 1-2 weeks. In multiple-dose studies, 10-80 mg per day in single or divided doses lowered systolic and diastolic blood pressure throughout the dosing interval, with a trough effect of about 5-11/3-7 mm Hg. The trough effect represents about 50% of the peak effect. While the dose-response relationship is relatively flat, doses of 40-80 mg were somewhat more effective at trough than 10-20 mg, and twice daily dosing tended to give a somewhat lower trough blood pressure than once daily dosing with the same total dose. The antihypertensive effect of ACCUPRIL continues during long-term therapy, with no evidence of loss of effectiveness.

Hemodynamic assessments in patients with hypertension indicate that blood pressure reduction produced by quinapril is accompanied by a reduction in total peripheral resistance and renal vascular resistance with little or no change in heart rate, cardiac index, renal blood flow, glomerular filtration rate, or filtration fraction.

Use of ACCUPRIL with a thiazide diuretic gives a blood-pressure lowering effect greater than that seen with either agent alone.

In patients with hypertension, ACCUPRIL 10-40 mg was similar in effectiveness to captopril, enalapril, propranolol, and thiazide diuretics.

Therapeutic effects appear to be the same for elderly (≥65 years of age) and younger adult patients given the same daily dosages, with no increase in adverse events in elderly patients.

Heart Failure: In a placebo-controlled trial involving patients with congestive heart failure treated with digitalis and diuretics, parenteral quinaprilat, the active metabolite of quinapril, reduced pulmonary capillary wedge pressure and systemic vascular resistance and increased cardiac output/index. Similar favorable hemodynamic effects were seen with oral quinapril in baseline-controlled trials, and such effects appeared to be maintained during chronic oral quinapril therapy. Quinapril reduced renal hepatic vascular resistance and increased renal and hepatic blood flow with glomerular filtration rate remaining unchanged.

A significant dose response relationship for improvement in maximal exercise tolerance has been observed with ACCUPRIL therapy. Beneficial effects on the severity of heart failure as measured by New York Heart Association (NYHA) classification and Quality of Life and on symptoms of dyspnea, fatigue, and edema were evident after 6 months in a double-blind, placebo-controlled study. Favorable effects were maintained for up to two years of open label therapy. The effects of quinapril on long-term mortality in heart failure have not been evaluated.

INDICATIONS AND USAGE

Hypertension

ACCUPRIL is indicated for the treatment of hypertension. It may be used alone or in combination with thiazide diuretics.

Heart Failure

ACCUPRIL is indicated in the management of heart failure as adjunctive therapy when added to conventional therapy including diuretics and/or digitalis.

In using ACCUPRIL, consideration should be given to the fact that another angiotensin-converting enzyme inhibitor, captopril, has caused agranulocytosis, particularly in patients with renal impairment or collagen vascular disease. Available data are insufficient to show that ACCUPRIL does not have a similar risk (see WARNINGS).

Angioedema in black patients: Black patients receiving ACE inhibitor monotherapy have been reported to have a higher incidence of angioedema compared to non-blacks. It should also be noted that in controlled clinical trials ACE inhibitors have an effect on blood pressure that is less in black patients than in non-blacks.

CONTRAINDICATIONS

ACCUPRIL is contraindicated in patients who are hypersensitive to this product and in patients with a history of angioedema related to previous treatment with an ACE inhibitor.

WARNINGS

Anaphylactoid and Possibly Related Reactions

Presumably because angiotensin-converting inhibitors affect the metabolism of eicosanoids and polypeptides, including endogenous bradykinin, patients receiving ACE inhibitors (including **ACCUPRIL**) may be subject to a variety of adverse reactions, some of them serious.

Head and Neck Angioedema: Angioedema of the face, extremities, lips, tongue, glottis, and larynx has been reported in patients treated with ACE inhibitors and has been seen in 0.1% of patients receiving ACCUPRIL.

In two similarly sized U.S. postmarketing trials that, combined, enrolled over 3,000 black patients and over 19,000 non-blacks, angioedema was reported in 0.30% and 0.55% of blacks (in study 1 and 2 respectively) and 0.39% and 0.17% of non-blacks.

Angioedema associated with laryngeal edema can be fatal. If laryngeal stridor or angioedema of the face, tongue, or glottis occurs, treatment with ACCUPRIL should be discontinued immediately, the patient treated in accordance with accepted medical care, and carefully observed until the swelling disappears. In instances where swelling is confined to the face and lips, the condition generally resolves without treatment; antihistamines may be useful in relieving symptoms. **Where there is involvement of the tongue, glottis, or larynx likely to cause airway obstruction, emergency therapy including, but not limited to, subcutaneous epinephrine solution 1:1000 (0.3 to 0.5 mL) should be promptly administered** (see ADVERSE REACTIONS).

Intestinal Angioedema: Intestinal angioedema has been reported in patients treated with ACE inhibitors. These patients presented with abdominal pain (with or without nausea or vomiting); in some cases there was no prior history of facial angioedema and C-1 esterase levels were normal. The angioedema was diagnosed by procedures including abdominal CT scan or ultrasound, or at surgery, and symptoms resolved after stopping the ACE inhibitor. Intestinal angioedema should be included in the differential diagnosis of patients on ACE inhibitors presenting with abdominal pain.

Patients with a history of angioedema: Patients with a history of angioedema unrelated to ACE inhibitor therapy may be at increased risk of angioedema while receiving an ACE inhibitor (see also CONTRAINDICATIONS).

Anaphylactoid reactions during desensitization: Two patients undergoing desensitizing treatment with hymenoptera venom while receiving ACE inhibitors sustained life-threatening anaphylactoid reactions. In the same patients, these reactions were avoided when ACE inhibitors were temporarily withheld, but they reappeared upon inadvertent rechallenge.

Anaphylactoid reactions during membrane exposure: Anaphylactoid reactions have been reported in patients dialyzed with high-flux membranes and treated concomitantly with an ACE inhibitor. Anaphylactoid reactions have also been reported in patients undergoing low-density lipoprotein apheresis with dextran sulfate absorption.

Hepatic Failure: Rarely, ACE inhibitors have been associated with a syndrome that starts with cholestatic jaundice and progresses to fulminant hepatic necrosis and (sometimes) death. The mechanism of this syndrome is not understood. Patients receiving ACE inhibitors who develop jaundice or marked elevations of hepatic enzymes should discontinue the ACE inhibitor and receive appropriate medical follow-up.

Hypotension: Excessive hypotension is rare in patients with uncomplicated hypertension treated with ACCUPRIL alone. Patients with heart failure given ACCUPRIL commonly have some reduction in blood pressure, but discontinuation of therapy because of continuing symptomatic hypotension usually is not necessary when dosing instructions are followed. Caution should be observed when initiating therapy in patients with heart failure (see DOSAGE AND ADMINISTRATION). In controlled studies, syncope was observed in 0.4% of patients (N=3203); this incidence was similar to that observed for captopril (1%) and enalapril (0.8%).

Patients at risk of excessive hypotension, sometimes associated with oliguria and/or progressive azotemia, and rarely with acute renal failure and/or death, include patients with the following conditions or characteristics: heart failure, hyponatremia, high dose diuretic therapy, recent intensive diuresis or increase in diuretic dose, renal dialysis, or severe volume and/or salt depletion of any etiology. It may be advisable to eliminate the diuretic (except in patients with heart failure), reduce the diuretic dose or cautiously increase salt intake (except in patients with heart failure) before initiating therapy with ACCUPRIL in patients at risk for excessive hypotension who are able to tolerate such adjustments.

In patients at risk of excessive hypotension, therapy with ACCUPRIL should be started under close medical supervision. Such patients should be followed closely for the first two weeks of treatment and whenever the dose of ACCUPRIL and/or diuretic is increased. Similar considerations may apply to patients with ischemic heart or cerebrovascular disease in whom an excessive fall in blood pressure could result in a myocardial infarction or a cerebrovascular accident.

If excessive hypotension occurs, the patient should be placed in the supine position and, if necessary, receive an intravenous infusion of normal saline. A transient hypotensive response is not a contraindication to further doses of ACCUPRIL, which usually can be given without difficulty once the blood pressure has stabilized. If symptomatic hypotension develops, a dose reduction or discontinuation of ACCUPRIL or concomitant diuretic may be necessary.

Neutropenia/Agranulocytosis: Another ACE inhibitor, captopril, has been shown to cause agranulocytosis and bone marrow depression rarely in patients with uncomplicated hypertension, but more frequently in patients with renal impairment, especially if they also have a collagen vascular disease, such as systemic lupus erythematosus or scleroderma. Agranulocytosis did occur during ACCUPRIL treatment in one patient with a history of neutropenia during previous captopril therapy. Available data from clinical trials of ACCUPRIL are insufficient to show that, in patients without prior reactions to other ACE inhibitors, ACCUPRIL does not cause agranulocytosis at similar rates. As with other ACE inhibitors, periodic monitoring of white blood cell counts in patients with collagen vascular disease and/or renal disease should be considered.

Fetal/Neonatal Morbidity and Mortality: ACE inhibitors can cause fetal and neonatal morbidity and death when administered to pregnant women. Several dozen cases have been reported in the world literature. When pregnancy is detected, ACE inhibitors should be discontinued as soon as possible.

The use of ACE inhibitors during the second and third trimesters of pregnancy has been associated with fetal and neonatal injury, including hypotension, neonatal skull hypoplasia, anuria, reversible or irreversible renal failure, and death. Oligohydramnios has also been reported, presumably resulting from decreased fetal renal function; oligohydramnios in this setting has been associated with fetal limb contractures, craniofacial deformation, and hypoplastic lung development. Prematurity, intrauterine growth retardation, and patent ductus arteriosus have also been reported, although it is not clear whether these occurrences were due to the ACE inhibitor exposure.

These adverse effects do not appear to have resulted from intrauterine ACE inhibitor exposure that has been limited to the first trimester. Mothers whose embryos and fetuses are exposed to ACE inhibitors only during the first trimester should be so informed. Nonetheless, when patients become pregnant, physicians should make every effort to discontinue the use of ACCUPRIL as soon as possible.

Rarely (probably less often than once in every thousand pregnancies), no alternative to ACE inhibitors will be found. In these rare cases, the mothers should be apprised of the potential hazards to their fetuses, and serial ultrasound examinations should be performed to assess the intraamniotic environment.

If oligohydramnios is observed, ACCUPRIL should be discontinued unless it is considered life-saving for the mother. Contraction stress testing (CST), a non-stress test (NST), or biophysical profiling (BPP) may be appropriate, depending upon the week of pregnancy. Patients and physicians should be aware, however, that oligohydramnios may not appear until after the fetus has sustained irreversible injury.

Infants with histories of *in utero* exposure to ACE inhibitors should be closely observed for hypotension, oliguria, and hyperkalemia. If oliguria occurs, attention should be directed toward support of blood pressure and renal perfusion. Exchange transfusion or dialysis may be required as a means of reversing hypotension and/or substituting for disordered renal function. Removal of ACCUPRIL, which crosses the placenta, from the neonatal circulation is not significantly accelerated by these means.

No teratogenic effects of ACCUPRIL were seen in studies of pregnant rats and rabbits. On a mg/kg basis, the doses used were up to 180 times (in rats) and one time (in rabbits) the maximum recommended human dose.

PRECAUTIONS

General

Impaired renal function: As a consequence of inhibiting the renin-angiotensin-aldosterone system, changes in renal function may be anticipated in susceptible individuals. In patients with severe heart failure whose renal function may depend on the activity of the renin-angiotensin-aldosterone system, treatment with ACE inhibitors, including ACCUPRIL, may be associated with oliguria and/or progressive azotemia and rarely acute renal failure and/or death.

In clinical studies in hypertensive patients with unilateral or bilateral renal artery stenosis, increases in blood urea nitrogen and serum creatinine have been observed in some patients following ACE inhibitor therapy. These increases were almost always reversible upon discontinuation of the ACE inhibitor and/or diuretic therapy. In such patients, renal function should be monitored during the first few weeks of therapy.

Some patients with hypertension or heart failure with no apparent preexisting renal vascular disease have developed increases in blood urea and serum creatinine, usually minor and transient, especially when ACCUPRIL has been given concomitantly with a diuretic. This is more likely to occur in patients with preexisting renal impairment. Dosage reduction and/or discontinuation of any diuretic and/or ACCUPRIL may be required.

Evaluation of patients with hypertension or heart failure should always include assessment of renal function (see DOSAGE AND ADMINISTRATION).

Hyperkalemia and potassium-sparing diuretics: In clinical trials, hyperkalemia (serum potassium ≥5.8 mmol/L) occurred in approximately 2% of patients receiving ACCUPRIL. In most cases, elevated serum potassium levels were isolated values which resolved despite continued therapy. Less than 0.1% of patients discontinued therapy due to hyperkalemia. Risk factors for the development of hyperkalemia include renal insufficiency, diabetes mellitus, and the concomitant use of potassium-sparing diuretics, potassium supplements, and/or potassium-containing salt substitutes, which should be used cautiously, if at all, with ACCUPRIL (see PRECAUTIONS, Drug Interactions).

Cough: Presumably due to the inhibition of the degradation of endogenous bradykinin, persistent non-productive cough has been reported with all ACE inhibitors, always resolving after discontinuation of therapy. ACE inhibitor-induced cough should be considered in the differential diagnosis of cough.

Surgery/anesthesia: In patients undergoing major surgery or during anesthesia with agents that produce hypotension, ACCUPRIL will block angiotensin II formation secondary to compensatory renin release. If hypotension occurs and is considered to be due to this mechanism, it can be corrected by volume expansion.

Information for Patients

Pregnancy: Female patients of childbearing age should be told about the consequences of second- and third-trimester exposure to ACE inhibitors, and they should also be told that these consequences do not appear to have resulted from intrauterine ACE-inhibitor exposure that has been limited to the first trimester. These patients should be asked to report pregnancies to their physicians as soon as possible.

Angioedema: Angioedema, including laryngeal edema can occur with treatment with ACE inhibitors, especially following the first dose. Patients should be so advised and told to report immediately any signs or symptoms suggesting angioedema (swelling of face, extremities, eyes, lips, tongue, difficulty in swallowing or breathing) and to stop taking the drug until they have consulted with their physician (see WARNINGS).

Symptomatic hypotension: Patients should be cautioned that lightheadedness can occur, especially during the first few days of ACCUPRIL therapy, and that it should be reported to a physician. If actual syncope occurs, patients should be told to not take the drug until they have consulted with their physician (see WARNINGS).

All patients should be cautioned that inadequate fluid intake or excessive perspiration, diarrhea, or vomiting can lead to an excessive fall in blood pressure because of reduction in fluid volume, with the same consequences of lightheadedness and possible syncope.

Patients planning to undergo any surgery and/or anesthesia should be told to inform their physician that they are taking an ACE inhibitor.

Hyperkalemia: Patients should be told not to use potassium supplements or salt substitutes containing potassium without consulting their physician (see PRECAUTIONS).

Neutropenia: Patients should be told to report promptly any indication of infection (eg, sore throat, fever) which could be a sign of neutropenia.

NOTE: As with many other drugs, certain advice to patients being treated with ACCUPRIL is warranted. This information is intended to aid in the safe and effective use of this medication. It is not a disclosure of all possible adverse or intended effects.

Drug Interactions

Concomitant diuretic therapy: As with other ACE inhibitors, patients on diuretics, especially those on recently instituted diuretic therapy, may occasionally experience an excessive reduction of blood pressure after initiation of therapy with ACCUPRIL. The possibility of hypotensive effects with ACCUPRIL may be minimized by either discontinuing the diuretic or cautiously increasing salt intake prior to initiation of treatment with ACCUPRIL. If it is not possible to discontinue the diuretic, the starting dose of quinapril should be reduced (see DOSAGE AND ADMINISTRATION).

Agents increasing serum potassium: Quinapril can attenuate potassium loss caused by thiazide diuretics and increase serum potassium when used alone. If concomitant therapy of ACCUPRIL with potassium-sparing diuretics (eg, spironolactone, triamterene, or amiloride), potassium supplements, or potassium-containing salt substitutes is indicated, they should be used with caution along with appropriate monitoring of serum potassium (see PRECAUTIONS).

Tetracycline and other drugs that interact with magnesium: Simultaneous administration of tetracycline with ACCUPRIL reduced the absorption of tetracycline by approximately 28% to 37%, possibly due to the high magnesium content in ACCUPRIL tablets. This interaction should be considered if coprescribing ACCUPRIL and tetracycline or other drugs that interact with magnesium.

Lithium: Increased serum lithium levels and symptoms of lithium toxicity have been reported in patients receiving concomitant lithium and ACE inhibitor therapy. These drugs should be coadministered with caution and frequent monitoring of serum lithium levels is recommended. If a diuretic is also used, it may increase the risk of lithium toxicity.

Other agents: Drug interaction studies of ACCUPRIL with other agents showed:

- Multiple dose therapy with propranolol or cimetidine has no effect on the pharmacokinetics of single doses of ACCUPRIL.
- The anticoagulant effect of a single dose of warfarin (measured by prothrombin time) was not significantly changed by quinapril coadministration twice-daily.
- ACCUPRIL treatment did not affect the pharmacokinetics of digoxin.
- No pharmacokinetic interaction was observed when single doses of ACCUPRIL and hydrochlorothiazide were administered concomitantly.
- Co-administration of multiple 10 mg doses of atorvastatin with 80 mg of ACCUPRIL resulted in no significant change in the steady-state pharmacokinetic parameters of atorvastatin.

Carcinogenesis, Mutagenesis, Impairment of Fertility

Quinapril hydrochloride was not carcinogenic in mice or rats when given in doses up to 75 or 100 mg/kg/day (50 to 60 times the maximum human daily dose, respectively, on an mg/kg basis and 3.8 to 10 times the maximum human daily dose when based on an mg/m^2 basis) for 104 weeks. Female rats given the highest dose level had an increased incidence of mesenteric lymph node hemangiomas and skin/subcutaneous lipomas. Neither quinapril nor quinaprilat were mutagenic in the Ames bacterial assay with or without metabolic activation. Quinapril was also negative in the following genetic toxicology studies: *in vitro* mammalian cell point mutation, sister chromatid exchange in cultured mammalian cells, micronucleus test with mice, *in vitro* chromosome aberration with V79 cultured lung cells, and in an *in vivo* cytogenetic study with rat bone marrow. There were no adverse effects on fertility or reproduction in rats at doses up to 100 mg/kg/day (60 and 10 times the maximum daily human dose when based on mg/kg and mg/m^2, respectively).

Pregnancy

Pregnancy Categories C (first trimester) and D (second and third trimesters): See WARNINGS, Fetal/Neonatal Morbidity and Mortality.

Nursing Mothers

Because ACCUPRIL is secreted in human milk, caution should be exercised when this drug is administered to a nursing woman.

Pediatric Use

The safety and effectiveness of ACCUPRIL in pediatric patients have not been established.

Geriatric Use

Clinical studies of ACCUPRIL did not include sufficient numbers of subjects aged 65 and over to determine whether they respond differently from younger subjects. Other reported clinical experience has not identified differences in responses between the elderly and younger patients. In general, dose selection for an elderly patient should be cautious, usually starting at the low end of the dosing range, reflecting the greater frequency of decreased hepatic, renal or cardiac function, and of concomitant disease or other drug therapy.

This drug is known to be substantially excreted by the kidney, and the risk of toxic reactions to this drug may be greater in patients with impaired renal function. Because elderly patients are more likely to have decreased renal function, care should be taken in dose selection, and it may be useful to monitor renal function.

Elderly patients exhibited increased area under the plasma concentration time curve and peak levels for quinaprilat compared to values observed in younger patients; this appeared to relate to decreased renal function rather than to age itself.

ADVERSE REACTIONS

Hypertension

ACCUPRIL has been evaluated for safety in 4960 subjects and patients. Of these, 3203 patients, including 655 elderly patients, participated in controlled clinical trials. ACCUPRIL has been evaluated for long-term safety in over 1400 patients treated for 1 year or more.

Adverse experiences were usually mild and transient.

In placebo-controlled trials, discontinuation of therapy because of adverse events was required in 4.7% of patients with hypertension.

Adverse experiences probably or possibly related to therapy or of unknown relationship to therapy occurring in 1% or more of the 1563 patients in placebo-controlled hypertension trials who were treated with ACCUPRIL are shown below.

Adverse Events in Placebo-Controlled Trials

	Accupril (N=1563) Incidence (Discontinuance)	Placebo (N=579) Incidence (Discontinuance)
Headache	5.6 (0.7)	10.9 (0.7)
Dizziness	3.9 (0.8)	2.6 (0.2)
Fatigue	2.6 (0.3)	1.0
Coughing	2.0 (0.5)	0.0
Nausea and/or Vomiting	1.4 (0.3)	1.9 (0.2)
Abdominal Pain	1.0 (0.2)	0.7

Heart Failure

ACCUPRIL has been evaluated for safety in 1222 ACCUPRIL treated patients. Of these, 632 patients participated in controlled clinical trials. In placebo-controlled trials, discontinuation of therapy because of adverse events was required in 6.8% of patients with congestive heart failure.

Adverse experiences probably or possibly related or of unknown relationship to therapy occurring in 1% or more of the 585 patients in placebo-controlled congestive heart failure trials who were treated with ACCUPRIL are shown below.

	Accupril (N=585) Incidence (Discontinuance)	Placebo (N=295) Incidence (Discontinuance)
Dizziness	7.7 (0.7)	5.1 (1.0)
Coughing	4.3 (0.3)	1.4
Fatigue	2.6 (0.2)	1.4
Nausea and/or Vomiting	2.4 (0.2)	0.7
Chest Pain	2.4	1.0
Hypotension	2.9 (0.5)	1.0
Dyspnea	1.9 (0.2)	2.0
Diarrhea	1.7	1.0
Headache	1.7	1.0 (0.3)
Myalgia	1.5	2.0
Rash	1.4 (0.2)	1.0
Back Pain	1.2	0.3

See PRECAUTIONS, Cough.

Hypertension and/or Heart Failure

Clinical adverse experiences probably, possibly, or definitely related, or of uncertain relationship to therapy occurring in 0.5% to 1.0% (except as noted) of the patients with CHF or hypertension treated with ACCUPRIL (with or without concomitant diuretic) in controlled or uncontrolled trials (N=4847) and less frequent, clinically significant events seen in clinical trials or post-marketing experience (the rarer events are in italics) include (listed by body system):

General: back pain, malaise, viral infections, *anaphylactoid reaction.*

Cardiovascular: palpitation, vasodilation, tachycardia, *heart failure, hyperkalemia, myocardial infarction, cerebrovascular accident, hypertensive crisis, angina pectoris, orthostatic hypotension, cardiac rhythm disturbances, cardiogenic shock*

Hematology: *hemolytic anemia*

Gastrointestinal: flatulence, dry mouth or throat, constipation, *gastrointestinal hemorrhage, pancreatitis, abnormal liver function tests, dyspepsia*

Nervous/Psychiatric: somnolence, vertigo, syncope, nervousness, depression, insomnia, paresthesia

Integumentary: alopecia, increased sweating, pemphigus, pruritus, *exfoliative dermatitis, photosensitivity reaction, dermatopolymyositis*

Urogenital: urinary tract infection, impotence, *acute renal failure, worsening renal failure*

Respiratory: *eosinophilic pneumonitis*

Other: amblyopia, edema, arthralgia, pharyngitis, *agranulocytosis, hepatitis, thrombocytopenia*

Fetal/Neonatal Morbidity and Mortality

See WARNINGS, Fetal/Neonatal Morbidity and Mortality.

Continued on next page

Accupril—Cont.

Angioedema
Angioedema has been reported in patients receiving ACCUPRIL (0.1%). Angioedema associated with laryngeal edema may be fatal. If angioedema of the face, extremities, lips, tongue, glottis, and/or larynx occurs, treatment with ACCUPRIL should be discontinued and appropriate therapy instituted immediately. (See WARNINGS.)

Clinical Laboratory Test Findings
Hematology: (See WARNINGS)
Hyperkalemia: (See PRECAUTIONS)
Creatinine and Blood Urea Nitrogen: Increases (>1.25 times the upper limit of normal) in serum creatinine and blood urea nitrogen were observed in 2% and 2%, respectively, of all patients treated with ACCUPRIL alone. Increases are more likely to occur in patients receiving concomitant diuretic therapy than in those on ACCUPRIL alone. These increases often remit on continued therapy. In controlled studies of heart failure, increases in blood urea nitrogen and serum creatinine were observed in 11% and 8%, respectively, of patients treated with ACCUPRIL; most often these patients were receiving diuretics with or without digitalis.

OVERDOSAGE

Doses of 1440 to 4280 mg/kg of quinapril cause significant lethality in mice and rats.
No specific information is available on the treatment of overdosage with quinapril. The most likely clinical manifestation would be symptoms attributable to severe hypotension.
Laboratory determinations of serum levels of quinapril and its metabolites are not widely available, and such determinations have, in any event, no established role in the management of quinapril overdose.
No data are available to suggest physiological maneuvers (eg, maneuvers to change pH of the urine) that might accelerate elimination of quinapril and its metabolites.
Hemodialysis and peritoneal dialysis have little effect on the elimination of quinapril and quinaprilat. Angiotensin II could presumably serve as a specific antagonist-antidote in the setting of quinapril overdose, but angiotensin II is essentially unavailable outside of scattered research facilities. Because the hypotensive effect of quinapril is achieved through vasodilation and effective hypovolemia, it is reasonable to treat quinapril overdose by infusion of normal saline solution.

DOSAGE AND ADMINISTRATION

Hypertension
Monotherapy: The recommended initial dosage of ACCUPRIL in patients not on diuretics is 10 or 20 mg once daily. Dosage should be adjusted according to blood pressure response measured at peak (2-6 hours after dosing) and trough (predosing). Generally, dosage adjustments should be made at intervals of at least 2 weeks. Most patients have required dosages of 20, 40, or 80 mg/day, given as a single dose or in two equally divided doses. In some patients treated once daily, the antihypertensive effect may diminish toward the end of the dosing interval. In such patients an increase in dosage or twice daily administration may be warranted. In general, doses of 40-80 mg and divided doses give a somewhat greater effect at the end of the dosing interval.
Concomitant Diuretics: If blood pressure is not adequately controlled with ACCUPRIL monotherapy, a diuretic may be added. In patients who are currently being treated with a diuretic, symptomatic hypotension occasionally can occur following the initial dose of ACCUPRIL. To reduce the likelihood of hypotension, the diuretic should, if possible, be discontinued 2 to 3 days prior to beginning therapy with ACCUPRIL (see WARNINGS). Then, if blood pressure is not controlled with ACCUPRIL alone, diuretic therapy should be resumed.
If the diuretic cannot be discontinued, an initial dose of 5 mg ACCUPRIL should be used with careful medical supervision for several hours and until blood pressure has stabilized.
The dosage should subsequently be titrated (as described above) to the optimal response (see WARNINGS, PRECAUTIONS, and Drug Interactions).
Renal Impairment: Kinetic data indicate that the apparent elimination half-life of quinaprilat increases as creatinine clearance decreases. Recommended starting doses, based on clinical and pharmacokinetic data from patients with renal impairment, are as follows:

Creatinine Clearance	Maximum Recommended Initial Dose
>60 mL/min	10 mg
30-60 mL/min	5 mg
10-30 mL/min	2.5 mg
<10 mL/min	Insufficient data for dosage recommendation

Patients should subsequently have their dosage titrated (as described above) to the optimal response.
Elderly (≥65 years): The recommended initial dosage of ACCUPRIL in elderly patients is 10 mg given once daily followed by titration (as described above) to the optimal response.

Heart Failure
ACCUPRIL is indicated as adjunctive therapy when added to conventional therapy including diuretics and/or digitalis. The recommended starting dose is 5 mg twice daily. This dose may improve symptoms of heart failure, but increases in exercise duration have generally required higher doses. Therefore, if the initial dosage of ACCUPRIL is well tolerated, patients should then be titrated at weekly intervals until an effective dose, usually 20 to 40 mg daily given in two equally divided doses, is reached or undesirable hypotension, orthostasis, or azotemia (see WARNINGS) prohibit reaching this dose.
Following the initial dose of ACCUPRIL, the patient should be observed under medical supervision for at least two hours for the presence of hypotension or orthostatis and, if present, until blood pressure stabilizes. The appearance of hypotension, orthostatis, or azotemia early in dose titration should not preclude further careful dose titration. Consideration should be given to reducing the dose of concomitant diuretics.

DOSE ADJUSTMENTS IN PATIENTS WITH HEART FAILURE AND RENAL IMPAIRMENT OR HYPONATREMIA
Pharmacokinetic data indicate that quinapril elimination is dependent on level of renal function. In patients with heart failure and renal impairment, the recommended initial dose of ACCUPRIL is 5 mg in patients with a creatinine clearance above 30 mL/min and 2.5 mg in patients with a creatinine clearance of 10 to 30 mL/min. There is insufficient data for dosage recommendation in patients with a creatinine clearance less than 10 mL/min (see DOSAGE AND ADMINISTRATION, Heart Failure WARNINGS, and PRECAUTIONS, Drug Interactions).
If the initial dose is well tolerated, ACCUPRIL may be administered the following day as a twice daily regimen. In the absence of excessive hypotension or significant deterioration of renal function, the dose may be increased at weekly intervals based on clinical and hemodynamic response.

HOW SUPPLIED

ACCUPRIL tablets are supplied as follows:
5-mg tablets: brown, film-coated, elliptical scored tablets, coded "PD 527" on one side and "5" on the other.
N0071-0527-23 bottles of 90 tablets
N0071-0527-40 10 × 10 unit dose blisters
10-mg tablets: brown, film-coated, triangular tablets, coded "PD 530" on one side and "10" on the other.
N0071-0530-23 bottles of 90 tablets
N0071-0530-40 10 × 10 unit dose blisters
20-mg tablets: brown, film-coated, round tablets, coded "PD 532" on one side and "20" on the other.
N0071-0532-23 bottles of 90 tablets
N0071-0532-40 10 × 10 unit dose blisters
40-mg tablets: brown, film-coated, elliptical tablets, coded "PD 535" on one side and "40" on the other.
N0071-0535-23 bottles of 90 tablets
Dispense in well-closed containers as defined in the USP.
Storage: Store at controlled room temperature 15°-30°C (59°-86°F).
Protect from light.
Rx only

Revised February 2003
Manufactured by:
Pfizer Pharmaceuticals, Ltd.
Vega Baja, PR 00694
Distributed by:
Parke-Davis
Division of Pfizer Inc, NY, NY 10017
69-5825-00-2

ACCURETIC™ ℞

[ā' kew-rĕ' tĭk]
(quinapril HCl/hydrochlorothiazide) Tablets

Prescribing information for this product, which appears on pages 2519–2522 of the 2004 PDR, has been completely revised as follows. Please write "See Supplement A" next to the product heading.

USE IN PREGNANCY
When used in pregnancy during the second and third trimesters, ACE inhibitors can cause injury and even death to the developing fetus. When pregnancy is detected, ACCURETIC should be discontinued as soon as possible. See **WARNINGS: Fetal/Neonatal Morbidity and Mortality.**

DESCRIPTION

ACCURETIC is a fixed-combination tablet that combines an angiotensin-converting enzyme (ACE) inhibitor, quinapril hydrochloride, and a thiazide diuretic, hydrochlorothiazide.
Quinapril hydrochloride is chemically described as [3S-[2[R*(R*)], 3R*]]-2-[2-[[1-(ethoxycarbonyl)-3-phenylpropyl] amino]-1-oxopropyl]-1,2,3,4-tetrahydro-3-isoquinolinecarboxylic acid, monohydrochloride. Its empirical formula is $C_{25}H_{30}N_2O_5$•HCl and its structural formula is:
[See chemical structure at top of next column]
Quinapril hydrochloride is a white to off-white amorphous powder that is freely soluble in aqueous solvents.
Hydrochlorothiazide is chemically described as: 6-Chloro-3,4-dihydro-2H-1,2,4-benzothiadiazine-7-sulfonamide 1,1-

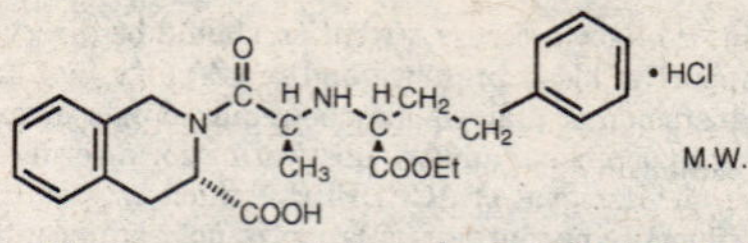

M.W. = 474.98

dioxide. Its empirical formula is $C_7H_8ClN_3O_4S_2$ and its structural formula is:

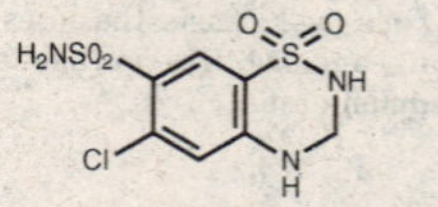

M.W. = 297.72

Hydrochlorothiazide is a white to off-white, crystalline powder which is slightly soluble in water but freely soluble in sodium hydroxide solution.
ACCURETIC is available for oral use as fixed combination tablets in three strengths of quinapril with hydrochlorothiazide: 10 mg with 12.5 mg (ACCURETIC 10/12.5), 20 mg with 12.5 mg (ACCURETIC 20/12.5), and 20 mg with 25 mg (ACCURETIC 20/25). Inactive ingredients: candelilla wax, crospovidone, hydroxypropyl cellulose, hypromellose, iron oxide red, iron oxide yellow, lactose, magnesium carbonate, magnesium stearate, polyethylene glycol, povidone, and titanium dioxide.

CLINICAL PHARMACOLOGY

Mechanism of Action: The principal metabolite of quinapril, quinaprilat, is an inhibitor of ACE activity in human subjects and animals. ACE is peptidyl dipeptidase that catalyzes the conversion of angiotensin I to the vasoconstrictor, angiotensin II. The effect of quinapril in hypertension appears to result primarily from the inhibition of circulating and tissue ACE activity, thereby reducing angiotensin II formation. Quinapril inhibits the elevation in blood pressure caused by intravenously administered angiotensin I, but has no effect on the pressor response to angiotensin II, norepinephrine, or epinephrine. Angiotensin II also stimulates the secretion of aldosterone from the adrenal cortex, thereby facilitating renal sodium and fluid reabsorption. Reduced aldosterone secretion by quinapril may result in a small increase in serum potassium. In controlled hypertension trials, treatment with quinapril alone resulted in mean increases in potassium of 0.07 mmol/L (see **PRECAUTIONS**). Removal of angiotensin II negative feedback on renin secretion leads to increased plasma renin activity (PRA).
While the principal mechanism of antihypertensive effect is thought to be through the renin-angiotensin-aldosterone system, quinapril exerts antihypertensive actions even in patients with low renin hypertension. Quinapril was an effective antihypertensive in all races studied, although it was somewhat less effective in blacks (usually a predominantly low renin group) than in non-blacks. ACE is identical to kininase II, an enzyme that degrades bradykinin, a potent peptide vasodilator; whether increased levels of bradykinin play a role in the therapeutic effect of quinapril remains to be elucidated.
Hydrochlorothiazide is a thiazide diuretic. Thiazides affect the renal tubular mechanisms of electrolyte reabsorption, directly increasing excretion of sodium and chloride in approximately equivalent amounts. Indirectly, the diuretic action of hydrochlorothiazide reduces plasma volume, with consequent increases in plasma renin activity, increases in aldosterone secretion, increases in urinary potassium loss, and decreases in serum potassium. The renin-aldosterone link is mediated by angiotensin, so coadministration of an ACE inhibitor tends to reverse the potassium loss associated with these diuretics.
The mechanism of the antihypertensive effect of thiazides is unknown.
Pharmacokinetics and Metabolism: The rate and extent of absorption of quinapril and hydrochlorothiazide from ACCURETIC tablets are not different, respectively, from the rate and extent of absorption of quinapril and hydrochlorothiazide from immediate-release monotherapy formulations, either administered concurrently or separately. Following oral administration of Accupril (quinapril monotherapy) tablets, peak plasma quinapril concentrations are observed within 1 hour. Based on recovery of quinapril and its metabolites in urine, the extent of absorption is at least 60%. The absorption of hydrochlorothiazide is somewhat slower (1 to 2.5 hours) and more complete (50% to 80%).
The rate of quinapril absorption was reduced by 14% when ACCURETIC tablets were administered with a high-fat meal as compared to fasting, while the extent of absorption was not affected. The rate of hydrochlorothiazide absorption was reduced by 12% when ACCURETIC tablets were administered with a high-fat meal, while the extent of absorption was not significantly affected. Therefore, ACCURETIC may be administered without regard to food.
Following absorption, quinapril is deesterified to its major active metabolite, quinaprilat (about 38% of oral dose), and to other minor inactive metabolites. Following multiple oral dosing of quinapril, there is an effective accumulation half-life of quinaprilat of approximately 3 hours, and peak plasma quinaprilat concentrations are observed approximately 2 hours postdose. Approximately 97% of either quinapril or quinaprilat circulating in plasma is bound to proteins. Hydrochlorothiazide is not metabolized. Its apparent volume of distribution is 3.6 to 7.8 L/kg, consistent with measured plasma protein binding of 67.9%. The drug also accumulates in red blood cells, so that whole blood levels are 1.6 to 1.8 times those measured in plasma.

Some placental passage occurred when quinapril was administered to pregnant rats. Studies in rats indicate that quinapril and its metabolites do not cross the blood-brain barrier. Hydrochlorothiazide crosses the placenta freely but not the blood-brain barrier.

Quinaprilat is eliminated primarily by renal excretion, up to 96% of an IV dose, and has an elimination half-life in plasma of approximately 2 hours and a prolonged terminal phase with a half-life of 25 hours. Hydrochlorothiazide is excreted unchanged by the kidney. When plasma levels have been followed for at least 24 hours, the plasma half-life has been observed to vary between 4 to 15 hours. At least 61% of the oral dose is eliminated unchanged within 24 hours.

In patients with renal insufficiency, the elimination half-life of quinaprilat increases as creatinine clearance decreases. There is a linear correlation between plasma quinaprilat clearance and creatinine clearance. In patients with end-stage renal disease, chronic hemodialysis or continuous ambulatory peritoneal dialysis have little effect on the elimination of quinapril and quinaprilat. Elimination of quinaprilat is reduced in elderly patients (≥65 years) and in those with heart failure; this reduction is attributable to decrease in renal function (see **DOSAGE AND ADMINISTRATION**). Quinaprilat concentrations are reduced in patients with alcoholic cirrhosis due to impaired deesterification of quinapril. In a study of patients with impaired renal function (mean creatinine clearance of 19 mL/min), the half-life of hydrochlorothiazide elimination was lengthened to 21 hours.

The pharmacokinetics of quinapril and quinaprilat are linear over a single-dose range of 5- to 80-mg doses and 40- to 160-mg in multiple daily doses.

Pharmacodynamics and Clinical Effects: Single doses of 20 mg of quinapril provide over 80% inhibition of plasma ACE for 24 hours. Inhibition of the pressor response to angiotensin I is shorter-lived, with a 20-mg dose giving 75% inhibition for about 4 hours, 50% inhibition for about 8 hours, and 20% inhibition at 24 hours. With chronic dosing, however, there is substantial inhibition of angiotensin II levels at 24 hours by doses of 20 to 80 mg.

Administration of 10 to 80 mg of quinapril to patients with mild to severe hypertension results in a reduction of sitting and standing blood pressure to about the same extent with minimal effect on heart rate. Symptomatic postural hypotension is infrequent, although it can occur in patients who are salt- and/or volume-depleted (see **WARNINGS**).

Antihypertensive activity commences within 1 hour with peak effects usually achieved by 2 to 4 hours after dosing. During chronic therapy, most of the blood pressure lowering effect of a given dose is obtained in 1 to 2 weeks. In multiple-dose studies, 10 to 80 mg per day in single or divided doses lowered systolic and diastolic blood pressure throughout the dosing interval, with a trough effect of about 5 to 11/3 to 7 mm Hg. The trough effect represents about 50% of the peak effect.

While the dose-response relationship is relatively flat, doses of 40 to 80 mg were somewhat more effective at trough than 10 to 20 mg, and twice-daily dosing tended to give a somewhat lower trough blood pressure than once-daily dosing with the same total dose. The antihypertensive effect of quinapril continues during long-term therapy, with no evidence of loss of effectiveness.

Hemodynamic assessments in patients with hypertension indicate that blood pressure reduction produced by quinapril is accompanied by a reduction in total peripheral resistance and renal vascular resistance with little or no change in heart rate, cardiac index, renal blood flow, glomerular filtration rate, or filtration fraction.

Therapeutic effects of quinapril appear to be the same for elderly (≥65 years of age) and younger adult patients given the same daily dosages, with no increase in adverse events in elderly patients. In patients with hypertension, quinapril 10 to 40 mg was similar in effectiveness to captopril, enalapril, propranolol, and thiazide diuretics.

After oral administration of hydrochlorothiazide, diuresis begins within 2 hours, peaks in about 4 hours, and lasts about 6 to 12 hours. Use of quinapril with a thiazide diuretic gives blood pressure lowering effect greater than that seen with either agent alone. In clinical trials of quinapril/hydrochlorothiazide using quinapril doses of 2.5 to 40 mg and hydrochlorothiazide doses of 6.25 to 25 mg, the antihypertensive effects were sustained for at least 24 hours, and increased with increasing dose of either component. Although quinapril monotherapy is somewhat less effective in blacks than in non-blacks, the efficacy of combination therapy appears to be independent of race. By blocking the renin-angiotensin-aldosterone axis, administration of quinapril tends to reduce the potassium loss associated with the diuretic. In clinical trials of ACCURETIC, the average change in serum potassium was near zero when 2.5 to 40 mg of quinapril was combined with hydrochlorothiazide 6.25 mg, and the average subject who received 10 to 20/12.5 to 25 mg experienced a milder reduction in serum potassium than that experienced by the average subject receiving the same dose of hydrochlorothiazide monotherapy.

INDICATIONS AND USAGE

ACCURETIC is indicated for the treatment of hypertension. This fixed combination is not indicated for the initial therapy of hypertension (see **DOSAGE AND ADMINISTRATION**).

In using ACCURETIC, consideration should be given to the fact that another angiotensin-converting enzyme inhibitor, captopril, has caused agranulocytosis, particularly in patients with renal impairment or collagen-vascular disease. Available data are insufficient to show that quinapril does not have a similar risk (see **WARNINGS: Neutropenia/Agranulocytosis**).

Angioedema in Black Patients: Black patients receiving ACE inhibitor monotherapy have been reported to have a higher incidence of angioedema compared to non-blacks. It should also be noted that in controlled clinical trials, ACE inhibitors have an effect on blood pressure that is less in black patients than in non-blacks.

CONTRAINDICATIONS

ACCURETIC is contraindicated in patients who are hypersensitive to quinapril or hydrochlorothiazide and in patients with a history of angioedema related to previous treatment with an ACE inhibitor.

Because of the hydrochlorothiazide components, this product is contraindicated in patients with anuria or hypersensitivity to other sulfonamide-derived drugs.

WARNINGS

Anaphylactoid and Possibly Related Reactions: Presumably because angiotensin converting inhibitors affect the metabolism of eicosanoids and polypeptides, including endogenous bradykinin, patients receiving ACE inhibitors (including quinapril) may be subject to a variety of adverse reactions, some of them serious.

Head and Neck Angioedema: Angioedema of the face, extremities, lips, tongue, glottis, and larynx has been reported in patients treated with ACE inhibitors and has been seen in 0.1% of patients receiving quinapril. In two similarly sized US postmarketing quinapril trials that, combined, enrolled over 3,000 black patients and over 19,000 non-blacks, angioedema was reported in 0.30% and 0.55% of blacks (in Study 1 and 2, respectively) and 0.39% and 0.17% of non-blacks. Angioedema associated with laryngeal edema can be fatal. If laryngeal stridor or angioedema of the face, tongue, or glottis occurs, treatment with ACCURETIC should be discontinued immediately, the patient treated in accordance with accepted medical care, and carefully observed until the swelling disappears. In instances where swelling is confined to the face and lips, the condition generally resolves without treatment; antihistamines may be useful in relieving symptoms. **Where there is involvement of the tongue, glottis, or larynx likely to cause airway obstruction, emergency therapy including, but not limited to, subcutaneous epinephrine solution 1:1000 (0.3 to 0.5 mL) should be promptly administered** (see **PRECAUTIONS** and **ADVERSE REACTIONS**).

Intestinal Angioedema: Intestinal angioedema has been reported in patients treated with ACE inhibitors. These patients presented with abdominal pain (with or without nausea or vomiting); in some cases there was no prior history of facial angioedema and C-1 esterase levels were normal. The angioedema was diagnosed by procedures including abdominal CT scan or ultrasound, or at surgery, and symptoms resolved after stopping the ACE inhibitor. Intestinal angioedema should be included in the differential diagnosis of patients on ACE inhibitors presenting with abdominal pain.

Patients With a History of Angioedema: Patients with a history of angioedema unrelated to ACE inhibitor therapy may be at increased risk of angioedema while receiving an ACE inhibitor (see also **CONTRAINDICATIONS**).

Anaphylactoid Reactions During Desensitization: Two patients undergoing desensitizing treatment with Hymenoptera venom while receiving ACE inhibitors sustained life-threatening anaphylactoid reactions. In the same patients, these reactions were avoided when ACE inhibitors were temporarily withheld, but they reappeared upon inadvertent challenge.

Anaphylactoid Reactions During Membrane Exposure: Anaphylactoid reactions have been reported in patients dialyzed with high-flux membranes and treated concomitantly with an ACE inhibitor. Anaphylactoid reactions have also been reported in patients undergoing low-density lipoprotein apheresis with dextran sulfate absorption.

Hepatic Failure: Rarely, ACE inhibitors have been associated with a syndrome that starts with cholestatic jaundice and progresses to fulminant hepatic necrosis and (sometimes) death. The mechanism of this syndrome is not understood. Patients receiving ACE inhibitors who develop jaundice or marked elevations of hepatic enzymes should discontinue the ACE inhibitor and receive appropriate medical follow-up.

Hypotension: ACCURETIC can cause symptomatic hypotension, probably not more frequently than either monotherapy. It was reported in 1.2% of 1,571 patients receiving ACCURETIC during clinical trials. Like other ACE inhibitors, quinapril has been only rarely associated with hypotension in uncomplicated hypertensive patients.

Symptomatic hypotension sometimes associated with oliguria and/or progressive azotemia, and rarely acute renal failure and/or death, include patients with the following conditions or characteristics: heart failure, hyponatremia, high dose diuretic therapy, recent intensive diuresis or increase in diuretic dose, renal dialysis or severe volume and/or salt depletion of any etiology. Volume and/or salt depletion should be corrected before initiating therapy with ACCURETIC.

ACCURETIC should be used cautiously in patients receiving concomitant therapy with other antihypertensives. The thiazide component of ACCURETIC may potentiate the action of other antihypertensive drugs, especially ganglionic or peripheral adrenergic-blocking drugs. The antihypertensive effects of the thiazide component may also be enhanced in the postsympathectomy patients.

In patients at risk of excessive hypotension, therapy with ACCURETIC should be started under close medical supervision. Such patients should be followed closely for the first 2 weeks of treatment and whenever the dosage of quinapril or diuretic is increased. Similar considerations may apply to patients with ischemic heart or cerebrovascular disease in whom an excessive fall in blood pressure could result in myocardial infarction or cerebrovascular accident.

If excessive hypotension occurs, the patient should be placed in a supine position and, if necessary, treated with intravenous infusion of normal saline. ACCURETIC treatment usually can be continued following restoration of blood pressure and volume. If symptomatic hypotension develops, a dose reduction or discontinuation of ACCURETIC may be necessary.

Impaired Renal Function: ACCURETIC should be used with caution in patients with severe renal disease. Thiazides may precipitate azotemia in such patients, and the effects of repeated dosing may be cumulative.

When the renin-angiotensin-aldosterone system is inhibited by quinapril, changes in renal function may be anticipated in susceptible individuals. In patients with severe congestive heart failure, whose renal function may depend on the activity of the renin-angiotensin-aldosterone system, treatment with angiotensin-converting enzyme inhibitors (including quinapril) may be associated with oliguria and/or progressive azotemia and (rarely) with acute renal failure and/or death.

In clinical studies in hypertensive patients with unilateral renal artery stenosis, treatment with ACE inhibitors was associated with increases in blood urea nitrogen and serum creatinine; these increases were reversible upon discontinuation of ACE inhibitor, concomitant diuretic, or both. When such patients are treated with ACCURETIC, renal function should be monitored during the first few weeks of therapy.

Some quinapril-treated hypertensive patients with no apparent preexisting renal vascular diseases have developed increases in blood urea nitrogen and serum creatinine, usually minor and transient, especially when quinapril has been given concomitantly with a diuretic. This is more likely to occur in patients with pre-existing renal impairment. Dosage reduction of ACCURETIC may be required. **Evaluation of the hypertensive patients should also include assessment of the renal function.** (see **DOSAGE AND ADMINISTRATION**).

Neutropenia/Agranulocytosis: Another ACE inhibitor, captopril, has been shown to cause agranulocytosis and bone marrow depression rarely in patients with uncomplicated hypertension, but more frequently in patients with renal impairment, especially if they also have a collagen vascular disease, such as systemic lupus erythematosus or scleroderma. Agranulocytosis did occur during quinapril treatment in one patient with a history of neutropenia during previous captopril therapy. Available data from clinical trials of quinapril are insufficient to show that, in patients without prior reactions to other ACE inhibitors, quinapril does not cause agranulocytosis at similar rates. As with other ACE inhibitors, periodic monitoring of white blood cell counts in patients with collagen vascular disease and/or renal disease should be considered.

Fetal/Neonatal Morbidity and Mortality: ACE inhibitors can cause fetal and neonatal morbidity and death when administered to pregnant women. Several dozen cases have been reported in the world literature. When pregnancy is detected, ACCURETIC should be discontinued as soon as possible.

The use of ACE inhibitors during the second and third trimesters of pregnancy has been associated with fetal and neonatal injury, including hypotension, neonatal skull hypoplasia, anuria, reversible or irreversible renal failure, and death. Oligohydramnios has also been reported, presumably resulting from decreased fetal renal function; oligohydramnios in this setting has been associated with fetal limb contractures, craniofacial deformation, and hypoplastic lung development. Prematurity, intrauterine growth retardation, and patent ductus arteriosus have also been reported, although it is not clear whether these occurrences were due to the ACE inhibitor exposure.

These adverse effects do not appear to have resulted from intrauterine ACE inhibitor exposure that has been limited to the first trimester. Mothers whose embryos and fetuses are exposed to ACE inhibitors only during the first trimester should be so informed. Nonetheless, when patients become pregnant, physicians should make every effort to discontinue the use of quinapril as soon as possible.

Rarely (probably less often than once in every thousand pregnancies), no alternative ACE inhibitors will be found. In these rare cases, the mothers should be apprised of the potential hazards to their fetuses, and serial ultrasound examinations should be performed to assess the intraamniotic environment.

If oligohydramnios is observed, quinapril should be discontinued unless it is considered life-saving for the mother. Contraction stress testing (CST), a nonstress test (NST), or biophysical profiling (BPP) may be appropriate, depending upon the week of pregnancy. Patients and physicians should be aware, however, that oligohydramnios may not appear until after the fetus has sustained irreversible injury.

Infants with histories of *in utero* exposure to ACE inhibitors should be closely observed for hypotension, oliguria, and hyperkalemia. If oliguria occurs, attention should be directed toward support of blood pressure and renal perfusion. Ex-

Continued on next page

Accuretic—Cont.

change transfusion or peritoneal dialysis may be required as a means of reversing hypotension and/or substituting for disordered renal function. Removal of quinapril, which crosses the placenta, from the neonatal circulation is not significantly accelerated by these means.

Intrauterine exposure to thiazide diuretics is associated with fetal or neonatal jaundice, thrombocytopenia, and possibly other adverse reactions that occurred in adults.

No teratogenic effects of quinapril were seen in studies of pregnant rats and rabbits. On a mg/kg basis, the doses used were up to 180 times (in rats) and one time (in rabbits) the maximum recommended human dose. No teratogenic effects of ACCURETIC were seen in studies of pregnant rats and rabbits. On a mg/kg (quinapril/hydrochlorothiazide) basis, the doses used were up to 188/94 times (in rats) and 0.6/0.3 times (in rabbits) the maximum recommended human dose.

Impaired Hepatic Function: ACCURETIC should be used with caution in patients with impaired hepatic function or progressive liver disease, since minor alterations of fluid and electrolyte balance may precipitate hepatic coma. Also, since the metabolism of quinapril to quinaprilat is normally dependent upon hepatic esterases, patients with impaired liver function could develop markedly elevated plasma levels of quinapril. No normal pharmacokinetic studies have been carried out in hypertensive patients with impaired liver function.

Systemic Lupus Erythematosus: Thiazide diuretics have been reported to cause exacerbation or activation of systemic lupus erythematosus.

PRECAUTIONS

General

Derangements of Serum Electrolytes: In clinical trials, hyperkalemia (serum potassium ≥5.8 mmol/L) occurred in approximately 2% of patients receiving quinapril. In most cases, elevated serum potassium levels were isolated values which resolved despite continued therapy. Less than 0.1% of patients discontinued therapy due to hyperkalemia. Risk factors for the development of hyperkalemia include renal insufficiency, diabetes mellitus, and the concomitant use of potassium-sparing diuretics, potassium supplements, and/or potassium-containing salt substitutes.

Treatment with thiazide diuretics has been associated with hypokalemia, hyponatremia, and hypochloremic alkalosis. These disturbances have sometimes been manifest as one or more of dryness of mouth, thirst, weakness, lethargy, drowsiness, restlessness, muscle pains or cramps, muscular fatigue, hypotension, oliguria, tachycardia, nausea, and vomiting. Hypokalemia can also sensitize or exaggerate the response of the heart to the toxic effects of digitalis. The risk of hypokalemia is greatest in patients with cirrhosis of the liver, in patients experiencing a brisk diuresis, in patients who are receiving inadequate oral intake of electrolytes, and in patients receiving concomitant therapy with corticosteroids or ACTH.

The opposite effects of quinapril and hydrochlorothiazide on serum potassium will approximately balance each other in many patients, so that no net effect upon serum potassium will be seen. In other patients, one or the other effect may be dominant. Initial and periodic determinations of serum electrolytes to detect possible electrolyte imbalance should be performed at appropriate intervals.

Chloride deficits secondary to thiazide therapy are generally mild and require specific treatment only under extraordinary circumstances (eg, in liver disease or renal disease). Dilutional hyponatremia may occur in edematous patients in hot weather; appropriate therapy is water restriction rather than administration of salt, except in rare instances when the hyponatremia is life threatening. In actual salt depletion, appropriate replacement is the therapy of choice.

Calcium excretion is decreased by thiazides. In a few patients on prolonged thiazide therapy, pathological changes in the parathyroid gland have been observed, with hypercalcemia and hypophosphatemia. More serious complications of hyperparathyroidism (renal lithiasis, bone resorption, and peptic ulceration) have not been seen.

Thiazides increase the urinary excretion of magnesium, and hypomagnesemia may result.

Other Metabolic Disturbances: Thiazide diuretics tend to reduce glucose tolerance and to raise serum levels of cholesterol, triglycerides, and uric acid. These effects are usually minor, but frank gout or overt diabetes may be precipitated in susceptible patients.

Cough: Presumably due to the inhibition of the degradation of endogenous bradykinin, persistent nonproductive cough has been reported with all ACE inhibitors, resolving after discontinuation of therapy. ACE inhibitor-induced cough should be considered in the differential diagnosis of cough.

Surgery/Anesthesia: In patients undergoing surgery or during anesthesia with agents that produce hypotension, quinapril will block the angiotensin II formation that could otherwise occur secondary to compensatory renin release. Hypotension that occurs as a result of this mechanism can be corrected by volume expansion.

Information for Patients

Angioedema: Angioedema, including laryngeal edema, can occur with treatment with ACE inhibitors, especially following the first dose. Patients receiving ACCURETIC should be told to report immediately any signs or symptoms suggesting angioedema (swelling of face, eyes, lips, or tongue, or difficulty in breathing) and to take no more drug until after consulting with the prescribing physician.

Pregnancy: Female patients of childbearing age should be told about the consequences of second- and third-trimester exposure to ACE inhibitors, and they should also be told that these consequences do not appear to have resulted from intrauterine ACE-inhibitor exposure that has been limited to the first trimester. These patients should be asked to report pregnancies to their physicians as soon as possible.

Symptomatic Hypotension: A patient receiving ACCURETIC should be cautioned that lightheadedness can occur, especially during the first days of therapy, and that it should be reported to the prescribing physician. The patient should be told that if syncope occurs, ACCURETIC should be discontinued until the physician has been consulted.

All patients should be cautioned that inadequate fluid intake, excessive perspiration, diarrhea, or vomiting can lead to an excessive fall in blood pressure because of reduction in fluid volume, with the same consequences of lightheadedness and possible syncope.

Patients planning to undergo major surgery and/ or general or spinal anesthesia should be told to inform their physicians that they are taking an ACE inhibitor.

Hyperkalemia: A patient receiving ACCURETIC should be told not to use potassium supplements or salt substitutes containing potassium without consulting the prescribing physician.

Neutropenia: Patients should be told to promptly report any indication of infection (eg, sore throat, fever) which could be a sign of neutropenia.

NOTE: As with many other drugs, certain advice to patients being treated with quinapril is warranted. This information is intended to aid in the safe and effective use of this medication. It is not a disclosure of all possible adverse or intended effects.

Laboratory Tests

The hydrochlorothiazide component of ACCURETIC may decrease serum PBI levels without signs of thyroid disturbance.

Therapy with ACCURETIC should be interrupted for a few days before carrying out tests of parathyroid function.

Drug Interactions

Potassium Supplements and Potassium-Sparing Diuretics: As noted above ("Derangements of Serum Electrolytes"), the net effect of ACCURETIC may be to elevate a patient's serum potassium, to reduce it, or to leave it unchanged. Potassium-sparing diuretics (spironolactone, amiloride, triamterene, and others) or potassium supplements can increase the risk of hyperkalemia. If concomitant use of such agents is indicated, they should be given with caution, and the patient's serum potassium should be monitored frequently.

Lithium: Increased serum lithium levels and symptoms of lithium toxicity have been reported in patients receiving ACE inhibitors during therapy with lithium. Because renal clearance of lithium is reduced by thiazides, the risk of lithium toxicity is presumably raised further when, as in therapy with ACCURETIC, a thiazide diuretic is coadministered with the ACE inhibitor. ACCURETIC and lithium should be coadministered with caution, and frequent monitoring of serum lithium levels is recommended.

Tetracycline and Other Drugs That Interact with Magnesium: Simultaneous administration of tetracycline with quinapril reduced the absorption of tetracycline by approximately 28% to 37%, possibly due to the high magnesium content in quinapril tablets. This interaction should be considered if coprescribing quinapril and tetracycline or other drugs that interact with magnesium.

Other Agents:

Drug interaction studies of quinapril and other agents showed:

- Multiple dose therapy with propranolol or cimetidine has no effect on the pharmacokinetics of single doses of quinapril.
- The anticoagulant effect of a single dose of warfarin (measured by prothrombin time) was not significantly changed by quinapril coadministration twice daily.
- Quinapril treatment did not affect the pharmacokinetics of digoxin.
- No pharmacokinetic interaction was observed when single doses of quinapril and hydrochlorothiazide were administered concomitantly.

When administered concurrently, the following drugs may interact with thiazide diuretics.

- Alcohol, Barbiturates, or Narcotics—potentiation of orthostatic hypotension may occur.
- Antidiabetic Drugs (oral hypoglycemic agents and insulin)—dosage adjustments of the antidiabetic drug may be required.
- Cholestyramine and Colestipol Resin—absorption of hydrochlorothiazide is impaired in the presence of anionic exchange resins. Single doses of either cholestyramine or colestipol resins bind the hydrochlorothiazide and reduce its absorption from the gastrointestinal tract by up to 85% and 43%, respectively.
- Corticosteroids, ACTH—intensified electrolyte depletion, particularly hypokalemia.
- Pressor Amines (eg, norepinephrine)—possible decreased response to pressor amines, but not sufficient to preclude their therapeutic use.
- Skeletal Muscle Relaxants, Nondepolarizing (eg, tubocurarine)—possible increased responsiveness to the muscle relaxant.
- Nonsteroidal Antiinflammatory Drugs—the diuretic, natriuretic, and antihypertensive effects of thiazide diuretics may be reduced by concurrent administration of nonsteroidal antiinflammatory agents.

Carcinogenesis, Mutagenesis, Impairment of Fertility

Carcinogenicity, mutagenicity, and fertility studies have not been conducted in animals with ACCURETIC.

Quinapril hydrochloride was not carcinogenic in mice or rats when given in doses up to 75 or 100 mg/kg/day (50 or 60 times the maximum human daily dose, respectively, on a mg/kg basis and 3.8 or 10 times the maximum human daily dose on a mg/m^2 basis) for 104 weeks. Female rats given the highest dose level had an increased incidence of mesenteric lymph node hemangiomas and skin/subcutaneous lipomas. Neither quinapril nor quinaprilat were mutagenic in the Ames bacterial assay with or without metabolic activation. Quinapril was also negative in the following genetic toxicology studies: *in vitro* mammalian cell point mutation, sister chromatid exchange in cultured mammalian cells, micronucleus test with mice, *in vitro* chromosome aberration with V79 cultured lung cells, and in an *in vivo* cytogenetic study with rat bone marrow. There were no adverse effects on fertility or reproduction in rats at doses up to 100 mg/kg/day (60 and 10 times the maximum daily human dose when based on mg/kg and mg/m^2, respectively).

Under the auspices of the National Toxicology Program, rats and mice received hydrochlorothiazide in their feed for 2 years, at doses up to 600 mg/kg/day in mice and up to 100 mg/kg/day in rats. These studies uncovered no evidence of a carcinogenic potential of hydrochlorothiazide in rats or female mice, but there was "equivocal" evidence of hepatocarcinogenicity in male mice. Hydrochlorothiazide was not genotoxic in *in vitro* assays using strains TA 98, TA 100, TA 1535, TA 1537, and TA 1538 of *Salmonella typhimurium* (the Ames test); in the Chinese hamster ovary (CHO) test for chromosomal aberrations; or *in vivo* assays using mouse germinal cell chromosomes, Chinese hamster bone marrow chromosomes, and the *Drosophila* sex-linked recessive lethal trait gene. Positive test results were obtained in the *in vitro* CHO sister chromatid exchange (clastogenicity) test and in the mouse lymphoma cell (mutagenicity) assays, using concentrations of hydrochlorothiazide of 43 to 1300 µg/mL. Positive test results were also obtained in the *Aspergillus nidulans* nondisjunction assay, using an unspecified concentration of hydrochlorothiazide.

Hydrochlorothiazide had no adverse effects on the fertility of mice and rats of either sex in studies wherein these species were exposed, via their diets, to doses of up to 100 and 4 mg/kg/day, respectively, prior to mating and throughout gestation.

Pregnancy

Pregnancy Categories C (first trimester) and D (second and third trimesters): See WARNINGS: Fetal/Neonatal Morbidity and Mortality.

Nursing Mothers

Because quinapril and hydrochlorothiazide are secreted in human milk, caution should be exercised when ACCURETIC is administered to a nursing woman.

Because of the potential for serious adverse reactions in nursing infants from hydrochlorothiazide and the unknown effects of quinapril in infants, a decision should be made whether to discontinue nursing or to discontinue ACCURETIC, taking into account the importance of the drug to the mother.

Geriatric Use

Clinical studies of quinapril HCl/hydrochlorothiazide did not include sufficient numbers of subjects aged 65 and over to determine whether they respond differently from younger subjects. Other reported clinical experience has not identified differences in responses between the elderly and younger patients. In general, dose selection for an elderly patient should be cautious, usually starting at the low end of the dosing range, reflecting the greater frequency of decreased hepatic, renal, or cardiac function, and of concomitant disease or other drug therapy.

Pediatric Use

Safety and effectiveness of ACCURETIC in children have not been established.

ADVERSE REACTIONS

ACCURETIC has been evaluated for safety in 1571 patients in controlled and uncontrolled studies. Of these, 498 were given quinapril plus hydrochlorothiazide for at least 1 year, with 153 patients extending combination therapy for over 2 years. In clinical trials with ACCURETIC, no adverse experience specific to the combination has been observed.

Adverse experiences that have occurred have been limited to those that have been previously reported with quinapril or hydrochlorothiazide.

Adverse experiences were usually mild and transient, and there was no relationship between side effects and age, sex, race, or duration of therapy. Discontinuation of therapy because of adverse effects was required in 2.1% in patients in controlled studies. The most common reasons for discontinuation of therapy with ACCURETIC were cough (1.0%; see **PRECAUTIONS**) and headache (0.7%).

Adverse experiences probably or possibly related to therapy or of unknown relationship to therapy occurring in 1% or more of the 943 patients treated with quinapril plus hydrochlorothiazide in controlled trials are shown below.

[See first table at top of next page]

Clinical adverse experiences probably, possibly, or definitely related or of uncertain relationship to therapy occurring in ≥0.5% to <1.0% (except as noted) of the patients treated with quinapril/HCTZ in controlled and uncontrolled trials (N=1571) and less frequent, clinically significant events seen in clinical trials or postmarketing experience (the rarer events are in italics) include (listed by body system):

[See second table at top of next page]

	Percent of Patients in Controlled Trials	
	Quinapril/HCTZ N = 943	Placebo N = 100
Headache	6.7	30.0
Dizziness	4.8	4.0
Coughing	3.2	2.0
Fatigue	2.9	3.0
Myalgia	2.4	5.0
Viral Infection	1.9	4.0
Rhinitis	2.0	3.0
Nausea and/or Vomiting	1.8	6.0
Abdominal Pain	1.7	4.0
Back Pain	1.5	2.0
Diarrhea	1.4	1.0
Upper Respiratory Infection	1.3	4.0
Insomnia	1.2	2.0
Somnolence	1.2	0.0
Bronchitis	1.2	1.0
Dyspepsia	1.2	2.0
Asthenia	1.1	1.0
Pharyngitis	1.1	2.0
Vasodilatation	1.0	1.0
Vertigo	1.0	2.0
Chest Pain	1.0	2.0

BODY AS A WHOLE:	Asthenia, Malaise
CARDIOVASCULAR:	Palpitation, Tachycardia, *Heart Failure, Hyperkalemia, Myocardial Infarction, Cerebrovascular Accident, Hypertensive Crisis, Angina Pectoris, Orthostatic Hypotension, Cardiac Rhythm Disturbance*
GASTROINTESTINAL:	Mouth or Throat Dry, *Gastrointestinal Hemorrhage, Pancreatitis, Abnormal Liver Function Tests*
NERVOUS/PSYCHIATRIC:	Nervousness, Vertigo, *Paresthesia*
RESPIRATORY:	Sinusitis, Dyspnea
INTEGUMENTARY:	Pruritus, Sweating Increased, *Erythema Multiforme, Exfoliative Dermatitis, Photosensitivity Reaction, Alopecia, Pemphigus*
UROGENITAL SYSTEM:	*Acute Renal Failure, Impotence*
OTHER:	*Agranulocytosis, Thrombocytopenia, Arthralgia*
Angioedema:	Angioedema has been reported in 0.1% of patients receiving quinapril (0.1%) (see **WARNINGS**).
Fetal/Neonatal Morbidity and Mortality:	See **WARNINGS:** Fetal/Neonatal Morbidity and Mortality

BODY AS A WHOLE:	Weakness.
CARDIOVASCULAR:	Orthostatic hypotension (may be potentiated by alcohol, barbiturates, or narcotics).
DIGESTIVE:	Pancreatitis, jaundice (intrahepatic cholestatic), sialadenitis, vomiting, diarrhea, cramping, nausea, gastric irritation, constipation, and anorexia.
NEUROLOGIC:	Vertigo, lightheadedness, transient blurred vision, headache, paresthesia, xanthopsia, weakness, and restlessness.
MUSCULOSKELETAL:	Muscle spasm.
HEMATOLOGIC:	Aplastic anemia, agranulocytosis, leukopenia, thrombocytopenia, and hemolytic anemia.
RENAL:	Renal failure, renal dysfunction, interstitial nephritis (see **WARNINGS**).
METABOLIC:	Hyperglycemia, glycosuria, and hyperuricemia.
HYPERSENSITIVITY:	Necrotizing angiitis, Stevens-Johnson syndrome, respiratory distress (including pneumonitis and pulmonary edema), purpura, urticaria, rash, and photosensitivity.

Postmarketing Experience
The following serious nonfatal adverse events, regardless of their relationship to quinapril and HCTZ combination tablets, have been reported during extensive postmarketing experience:
BODY AS A WHOLE: Shock, accidental injury, neoplasm, cellulitis, ascites, generalized edema, hernia and anaphylactoid reaction.
CARDIOVASCULAR SYSTEM: Bradycardia, cor pulmonale, vasculitis, and deep thrombosis.
DIGESTIVE SYSTEM: Gastrointestinal carcinoma, cholestatic jaundice, hepatitis, esophagitis, vomiting, and diarrhea.
HEMIC SYSTEM: Anemia.
METABOLIC AND NUTRITIONAL DISORDERS: Weight loss.
MUSCULOSKELETAL SYSTEM: Myopathy, myositis, and arthritis.
NERVOUS SYSTEM: Paralysis, hemiplegia, speech disorder, abnormal gait, meningism, and amnesia.
RESPIRATORY SYSTEM: Pneumonia, asthma, respiratory infiltration, and lung disorder.
SKIN AND APPENDAGES: Urticaria, macropapular rash, and petechiases.
SPECIAL SENSES: Abnormal vision.
UROGENITAL SYSTEM: Kidney function abnormal, albuminuria, pyuria, hematuria, and nephrosis.
Quinapril monotherapy has been evaluated for safety in 4960 patients. In clinical trials adverse events which occurred with quinapril were also seen with ACCURETIC. In addition, the following were reported for quinapril at an incidence >0.5%: depression, back pain, constipation, syncope, and amblyopia.
Hydrochlorothiazide has been extensively prescribed for many years, but there has not been enough systematic collection of data to support an estimate of the frequency of the observed adverse reactions. Within organ-system groups, the reported reactions are listed here in decreasing order of severity, without regard to frequency.
[See third table above]

Clinical Laboratory Test Findings
Serum Electrolytes: See **PRECAUTIONS**.
Creatinine, Blood Urea Nitrogen: Increases (>1.25 times the upper limit of normal) in serum creatinine and blood urea nitrogen were observed in 3% and 4%, respectively, of patients treated with ACCURETIC. Most increases were minor and reversible, which can occur in patients with essential hypertension but most frequently in patients with renal artery stenosis (see **PRECAUTIONS**).
PBI and Tests of Parathyroid Function: See **PRECAUTIONS**.
Hematology: See **WARNINGS**.
Other (causal relationships unknown): Other clinically important changes in standard laboratory tests were rarely associated with ACCURETIC administration. Elevations in uric acid, glucose, magnesium, cholesterol, triglyceride, and calcium (see **PRECAUTIONS**) have been reported.

OVERDOSAGE

No specific information is available on the treatment of overdosage with ACCURETIC or quinapril monotherapy; treatment should be symptomatic and supportive. Therapy with ACCURETIC should be discontinued, and the patient should be observed. Dehydration, electrolyte imbalance, and hypotension should be treated by established procedures.
The oral median lethal dose of quinapril/hydrochlorothiazide in combination ranges from 1063/664 to 4640/2896 mg/kg in mice and rats. Doses of 1440 to 4280 mg/kg of quinapril cause significant lethality in mice and rats. In single-dose studies of hydrochlorothiazide, most rats survived doses up to 2.75 g/kg.
Data from human overdoses of ACE inhibitors are scanty; the most likely manifestation of human quinapril overdosage is hypotension. In human hydrochlorothiazide overdose, the most common signs and symptoms observed have been those of dehydration and electrolyte depletion (hypokalemia, hypochloremia, hyponatremia). If digitalis has also been administered, hypokalemia may accentuate cardiac arrhythmias.
Laboratory determinations of serum levels of quinapril and its metabolites are not widely available, and such determinations have, in any event, no established role in the management of quinapril overdose.
No data are available to suggest physiological maneuvers (eg, maneuvers to change the pH of the urine) that might accelerate elimination of quinapril and its metabolites. Hemodialysis and peritoneal dialysis have little effect on the elimination of quinapril and quinaprilat.
Angiotensin II could presumably serve as a specific antagonist-antidote in the setting of quinapril overdose, but angiotensin II is essentially unavailable outside of scattered research facilities. Because the hypotensive effect of quinapril is achieved through vasodilation and effective hypovolemia, it is reasonable to treat quinapril overdose by infusion of normal saline solution.

DOSAGE AND ADMINISTRATION

As individual monotherapy, quinapril is an effective treatment of hypertension in once-daily doses of 10 to 80 mg and hydrochlorothiazide is effective in doses of 12.5 to 50 mg. In clinical trials of quinapril/hydrochlorothiazide combination therapy using quinapril doses of 2.5 to 40 mg and hydrochlorothiazide doses of 6.25 to 25 mg, the antihypertensive effects increased with increasing dose of either component.
The side effects (see **WARNINGS**) of quinapril are generally rare and apparently independent of dose; those of hydrochlorothiazide are a mixture of dose-dependent phenomena (primarily hypokalemia) and dose-independent phenomena (eg, pancreatitis), the former much more common than the latter. Therapy with any combination of quinapril and hydrochlorothiazide will be associated with both sets of dose-independent side effects, but regimens that combine low doses of hydrochlorothiazide with quinapril produce minimal effects on serum potassium. In clinical trials of ACCURETIC, the average change in serum potassium was near zero in subjects who received HCTZ 6.25 mg in the combination, and the average subject who received 10 to 40/12.5 to 25 mg experienced a milder reduction in serum potassium than that experienced by the average subject receiving the same dose of hydrochlorothiazide monotherapy.
To minimize dose-independent side effects, it is usually appropriate to begin combination therapy only after a patient has failed to achieve the desired effect with monotherapy.

Therapy Guided by Clinical Effect
Patients whose blood pressures are not adequately controlled with quinapril monotherapy may instead be given ACCURETIC 10/12.5 or 20/12.5. Further increases of either or both components could depend on clinical response. The hydrochlorothiazide dose should generally not be increased until 2 to 3 weeks have elapsed. Patients whose blood pressures are adequately controlled with 25 mg of daily hydrochlorothiazide, but who experience significant potassium loss with this regimen, may achieve blood pressure control with less electrolyte disturbance if they are switched to ACCURETIC 10/12.5 or 20/12.5.

Replacement Therapy
For convenience, patients who are adequately treated with 20 mg of quinapril and 25 mg of hydrochlorothiazide and experience no significant electrolyte disturbances may instead wish to receive ACCURETIC 20/25.

Use in Renal Impairment
Regimens of therapy with ACCURETIC need not take account of renal function as long as the patient's creatinine clearance is >30 mL/min/1.73 m^2 (serum creatinine roughly ≤3 mg/dL or 265 µmol/L). In patients with more severe renal impairment, loop diuretics are preferred to thiazides. Therefore, ACCURETIC is not recommended for use in these patients.

HOW SUPPLIED

ACCURETIC is available in tablets of three different strengths:
10/12.5 tablets: pink, scored elliptical, biconvex, film-coated tablets coded "PD 222" on one side. Each tablet contains 10 mg of quinapril and 12.5 mg of hydrochlorothiazide.
N0071-0222-23: 90 tablet bottles
20/12.5 tablets: pink, scored triangular, film-coated tablets coded "PD 220" on one side. Each tablet contains 20 mg of quinapril and 12.5 mg of hydrochlorothiazide.
N0071-0220-23: 90 tablet bottles
20/25 tablets: pink, round, biconvex, film-coated tablets coded "PD 223" on one side. Each tablet contains 20 mg of quinapril and 25 mg of hydrochlorothiazide.
N0071-0223-23: 90 tablet bottles
Dispense in tight containers as defined in the USP.
Store at Controlled Room Temperature 20°-25°C (68°-77°F) [see USP].
Rx only.
69-5822-00-2
Manufactured by:
Pfizer Pharmaceuticals, Ltd
Vega Baja, PR 00694
MADE IN GERMANY
Distributed by:
PARKE-DAVIS
Division of Pfizer Inc
NY, NY 10017

Revised August 2003

KAPSEALS®
DILANTIN® ℞
[*dī-lăn-tĭn*]
(Extended Phenytoin Sodium Capsules, USP)

Prescribing information for this product, which appears on pages 2526–2528 of the 2004 PDR, has been completely revised as follows. Please write "See Supplement A" next to the product heading.

DESCRIPTION

Phenytoin sodium is an antiepileptic drug. Phenytoin sodium is related to the barbiturates in chemical structure, but has a five-membered ring. The chemical name is sodium

Continued on next page

Dilantin Kapseals—Cont.

5,5-diphenyl-2, 4-imidazolidinedione, having the following structural formula:

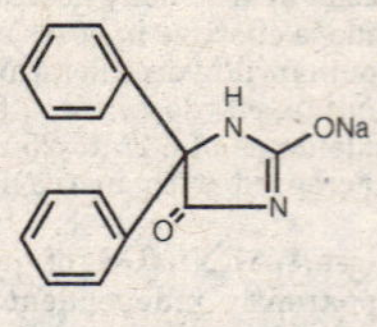

Each Dilantin—*Extended Phenytoin Sodium Capsule,* USP—contains 30 mg or 100 mg phenytoin sodium, USP. Also contains lactose, NF; confectioner's sugar, NF; talc, USP; and magnesium stearate, NF. The capsule shell and band contain colloidal silicon dioxide, NF; FD&C red No. 3; gelatin, NF; glyceryl monooleate; sodium lauryl sulfate, NF. The Dilantin 30-mg capsule shell and band also contain citric acid, USP; FD&C blue No. 1; sodium benzoate, NF; titanium dioxide, USP. The Dilantin 100-mg capsule shell and band also contain FD&C yellow No. 6; purified water, USP; polyethylene glycol 200. Product *in vivo* performance is characterized by a slow and extended rate of absorption with peak blood concentrations expected in 4 to 12 hours as contrasted to *Prompt Phenytoin Sodium Capsules,* USP with a rapid rate of absorption with peak blood concentration expected in 1½ to 3 hours.

CLINICAL PHARMACOLOGY

Phenytoin is an antiepileptic drug which can be used in the treatment of epilepsy. The primary site of action appears to be the *motor cortex* where spread of seizure activity is inhibited. Possibly by promoting sodium efflux from neurons, phenytoin tends to *stabilize* the threshold against hyperexcitability caused by excessive stimulation or environmental changes capable of reducing membrane sodium gradient. This includes the reduction of posttetanic potentiation at synapses. Loss of posttetanic potentiation prevents cortical seizure foci from detonating adjacent cortical areas. Phenytoin reduces the maximal activity of brain stem centers responsible for the tonic phase of tonic-clonic (grand mal) seizures.

The plasma half-life in man after oral administration of phenytoin averages 22 hours, with a range of 7 to 42 hours. Steady-state therapeutic levels are achieved at least 7 to 10 days (5–7 half-lives) after initiation of therapy with recommended doses of 300 mg/day.

When serum level determinations are necessary, they should be obtained at least 5–7 half-lives after treatment initiation, dosage change, or addition or subtraction of another drug to the regimen so that equilibrium or steady-state will have been achieved. Trough levels provide information about clinically effective serum level range and confirm patient compliance and are obtained just prior to the patient's next scheduled dose. Peak levels indicate an individual's threshold for emergence of dose-related side effects and are obtained at the time of expected peak concentration. For Dilantin Kapseals peak serum levels occur 4 to 12 hours after administration.

Optimum control without clinical signs of toxicity occurs more often with serum levels between 10 and 20 mcg/mL, although some mild cases of tonic-clonic (grand mal) epilepsy may be controlled with lower serum levels of phenytoin.

In most patients maintained at a steady dosage, stable phenytoin serum levels are achieved. There may be wide interpatient variability in phenytoin serum levels with equivalent dosages. Patients with unusually low levels may be noncompliant or hypermetabolizers of phenytoin. Unusually high levels result from liver disease, congenital enzyme deficiency, or drug interactions which result in metabolic interference. The patient with large variations in phenytoin plasma levels, despite standard doses, presents a difficult clinical problem. Serum level determinations in such patients may be particularly helpful. As phenytoin is highly protein bound, free phenytoin levels may be altered in patients whose protein binding characteristics differ from normal.

Most of the drug is excreted in the bile as inactive metabolites which are then reabsorbed from the intestinal tract and excreted in the urine. Urinary excretion of phenytoin and its metabolites occurs partly with glomerular filtration but more importantly by tubular secretion. Because phenytoin is hydroxylated in the liver by an enzyme system which is saturable at high plasma levels, small incremental doses may increase the half-life and produce very substantial increases in serum levels, when these are in the upper range. The steady-state level may be disproportionately increased, with resultant intoxication, from an increase in dosage of 10% or more.

INDICATIONS AND USAGE

Dilantin is indicated for the control of generalized tonic-clonic (grand mal) and complex partial (psychomotor, temporal lobe) seizures and prevention and treatment of seizures occurring during or following neurosurgery.

Phenytoin serum level determinations may be necessary for optimal dosage adjustments (see DOSAGE AND ADMINISTRATION and CLINICAL PHARMACOLOGY sections).

CONTRAINDICATIONS

Phenytoin is contraindicated in those patients who are hypersensitive to phenytoin or other hydantoins.

WARNINGS

Abrupt withdrawal of phenytoin in epileptic patients may precipitate status epilepticus. When, in the judgment of the clinician, the need for dosage reduction, discontinuation, or substitution of alternative antiepileptic medication arises, this should be done gradually. However, in the event of an allergic or hypersensitivity reaction, rapid substitution of alternative therapy may be necessary. In this case, alternative therapy should be an antiepileptic drug not belonging to the hydantoin chemical class.

There have been a number of reports suggesting a relationship between phenytoin and the development of lymphadenopathy (local or generalized) including benign lymph node hyperplasia, pseudolymphoma, lymphoma, and Hodgkin's disease. Although a cause and effect relationship has not been established, the occurrence of lymphadenopathy indicates the need to differentiate such a condition from other types of lymph node pathology. Lymph node involvement may occur with or without symptoms and signs resembling serum sickness, eg, fever, rash, and liver involvement.

In all cases of lymphadenopathy, follow-up observation for an extended period is indicated and every effort should be made to achieve seizure control using alternative antiepileptic drugs.

Acute alcoholic intake may increase phenytoin serum levels, while chronic alcohol use may decrease serum levels.

In view of isolated reports associating phenytoin with exacerbation of porphyria, caution should be exercised in using this medication in patients suffering from this disease.

Usage In Pregnancy:

Clinical:

A. *Risks to Mother.* An increase in seizure frequency may occur during pregnancy because of altered phenytoin pharmacokinetics. Periodic measurement of plasma phenytoin concentrations may be valuable in the management of pregnant women as a guide to appropriate adjustment of dosage (see PRECAUTIONS, Laboratory Tests). However, postpartum restoration of the original dosage will probably be indicated.

B. *Risks to the Fetus.* If this drug is used during pregnancy, or if the patient becomes pregnant while taking the drug, the patient should be apprised of the potential harm to the fetus.

Prenatal exposure to phenytoin may increase the risks for congenital malformations and other adverse developmental outcomes. Increased frequencies of major malformations (such as orofacial clefts and cardiac defects), minor anomalies (dysmorphic facial features, nail and digit hypoplasia), growth abnormalities (including microcephaly), and mental deficiency have been reported among children born to epileptic women who took phenytoin alone or in combination with other antiepileptic drugs during pregnancy. There have also been several reported cases of malignancies, including neuroblastoma, in children whose mothers received phenytoin during pregnancy. The overall incidence of malformations for children of epileptic women treated with antiepileptic drugs (phenytoin and/or others) during pregnancy is about 10%, or two- to three-fold that in the general population. However, the relative contributions of antiepileptic drugs and other factors associated with epilepsy to this increased risk are uncertain and in most cases it has not been possible to attribute specific developmental abnormalities to particular antiepileptic drugs.

Patients should consult with their physicians to weigh the risks and benefits of phenytoin during pregnancy.

C. *Postpartum Period.* A potentially life-threatening bleeding disorder related to decreased levels of vitamin K-dependent clotting factors may occur in newborns exposed to phenytoin *in utero.* This drug-induced condition can be prevented with vitamin K administration to the mother before delivery and to the neonate after birth.

Preclinical:

Increased resorption and malformation rates have been reported following administration of phenytoin doses of 75 mg/kg or higher (approximately 120% of the maximum human loading dose or higher on a mg/m^2 basis) to pregnant rabbits.

PRECAUTIONS

General:

The liver is the chief site of biotransformation of phenytoin; patients with impaired liver function, elderly patients, or those who are gravely ill may show early signs of toxicity.

A small percentage of individuals who have been treated with phenytoin have been shown to metabolize the drug slowly. Slow metabolism may be due to limited enzyme availability and lack of induction; it appears to be genetically determined.

Phenytoin should be discontinued if a skin rash appears (see WARNINGS section regarding drug discontinuation). If the rash is exfoliative, purpuric, or bullous or if lupus erythematosus, Stevens-Johnson syndrome, or toxic epidermal necrolysis is suspected, use of this drug should not be resumed and alternative therapy should be considered. (See ADVERSE REACTIONS section.) If the rash is of a milder type (measles-like or scarlatiniform), therapy may be resumed after the rash has completely disappeared. If the rash recurs upon reinstitution of therapy, further phenytoin medication is contraindicated.

Phenytoin and other hydantoins are contraindicated in patients who have experienced phenytoin hypersensitivity (see CONTRAINDICATIONS). Additionally, caution should be exercised if using structurally similar compounds (eg, barbiturates, succinimides, oxazolidinediones, and other related compounds) in these same patients.

Hyperglycemia, resulting from the drug's inhibitory effects on insulin release, has been reported. Phenytoin may also raise the serum glucose level in diabetic patients.

Osteomalacia has been associated with phenytoin therapy and is considered to be due to phenytoin's interference with vitamin D metabolism.

Phenytoin is not indicated for seizures due to hypoglycemic or other metabolic causes. Appropriate diagnostic procedures should be performed as indicated.

Phenytoin is not effective for absence (petit mal) seizures. If tonic-clonic (grand mal) and absence (petit mal) seizures are present, combined drug therapy is needed.

Serum levels of phenytoin sustained above the optimal range may produce confusional states referred to as "delirium," "psychosis," or "encephalopathy," or rarely irreversible cerebellar dysfunction. Accordingly, at the first sign of acute toxicity, plasma levels are recommended. Dose reduction of phenytoin therapy is indicated if plasma levels are excessive; if symptoms persist, termination is recommended. (See WARNINGS section.)

Information for Patients:

Patients taking phenytoin should be advised of the importance of adhering strictly to the prescribed dosage regimen, and of informing the physician of any clinical condition in which it is not possible to take the drug orally as prescribed, eg, surgery, etc.

Patients should also be cautioned on the use of other drugs or alcoholic beverages without first seeking the physician's advice.

Patients should be instructed to call their physician if skin rash develops.

The importance of good dental hygiene should be stressed in order to minimize the development of gingival hyperplasia and its complications.

Do not use capsules which are discolored.

Laboratory Tests:

Phenytoin serum level determinations may be necessary to achieve optimal dosage adjustments.

Drug Interactions:

There are many drugs which may increase or decrease phenytoin levels or which phenytoin may affect. Serum level determinations for phenytoin are especially helpful when possible drug interactions are suspected. The most commonly occurring drug interactions are listed below:

1. Drugs which may increase phenytoin serum levels include: acute alcohol intake, amiodarone, chloramphenicol, chlordiazepoxide, cimetidine, diazepam, dicumarol, disulfiram, estrogens, ethosuximide, fluoxetine, H2-antagonists, halothane, isoniazid, methylphenidate, phenothiazines, phenylbutazone, salicylates, succinimides, sulfonamides, ticlopidine, tolbutamide, trazodone.
2. Drugs which may decrease phenytoin levels include: carbamazepine, chronic alcohol abuse, reserpine, and sucralfate. Moban® brand of molindone hydrochloride contains calcium ions which interfere with the absorption of phenytoin. Ingestion times of phenytoin and antacid preparations containing calcium should be staggered in patients with low serum phenytoin levels to prevent absorption problems.
3. Drugs which may either increase or decrease phenytoin serum levels include: phenobarbital, sodium valproate, and valproic acid. Similarly, the effect of phenytoin on phenobarbital, valproic acid, and sodium valproate serum levels is unpredictable.
4. Although not a true drug interaction, tricyclic antidepressants may precipitate seizures in susceptible patients and phenytoin dosage may need to be adjusted.
5. Drugs whose efficacy is impaired by phenytoin include: corticosteroids, coumarin anticoagulants, digitoxin, doxycycline, estrogens, furosemide, oral contraceptives, paroxetine, quinidine, rifampin, theophylline, vitamin D.

Drug Enteral Feeding/Nutritional Preparations Interaction:

Literature reports suggest that patients who have received enteral feeding preparations and/or related nutritional supplements have lower than expected phenytoin plasma levels. It is therefore suggested that phenytoin not be administered concomitantly with an enteral feeding preparation. More frequent serum phenytoin level monitoring may be necessary in these patients.

Drug/Laboratory Test Interactions:

Phenytoin may decrease serum concentrations of T4. It may also produce lower than normal values for dexamethasone or metyrapone tests. Phenytoin may cause increased serum levels of glucose, alkaline phosphatase, and gamma glutamyl transpeptidase (GGT).

Care should be taken when using immunoanalytical methods to measure plasma phenytoin concentrations.

Carcinogenesis:

See WARNINGS section for information on carcinogenesis.

Pregnancy:

Pregnancy Category D; See WARNINGS section.

Nursing Mothers:

Infant breast-feeding is not recommended for women taking this drug because phenytoin appears to be secreted in low concentrations in human milk.

Pediatric Use: See DOSAGE AND ADMINISTRATION section.

ADVERSE REACTIONS

Central Nervous System: The most common manifestations encountered with phenytoin therapy are referable to this system and are usually dose-related. These include nystagmus, ataxia, slurred speech, decreased coordination, and

mental confusion. Dizziness, insomnia, transient nervousness, motor twitchings, and headaches have also been observed. There have also been rare reports of phenytoin induced dyskinesias, including chorea, dystonia, tremor, and asterixis, similar to those induced by phenothiazine and other neuroleptic drugs.
A predominantly sensory peripheral polyneuropathy has been observed in patients receiving long-term phenytoin therapy.
Gastrointestinal System: Nausea, vomiting, constipation, toxic hepatitis, and liver damage.
Integumentary System: Dermatological manifestations sometimes accompanied by fever have included scarlatiniform or morbilliform rashes. A morbilliform rash (measles-like) is the most common; other types of dermatitis are seen more rarely. Other more serious forms which may be fatal have included bullous, exfoliative or purpuric dermatitis, lupus erythematosus, Stevens-Johnson syndrome, and toxic epidermal necrolysis (see PRECAUTIONS section).
Hemopoietic System: Hemopoietic complications, some fatal, have occasionally been reported in association with administration of phenytoin. These have included thrombocytopenia, leukopenia, granulocytopenia, agranulocytosis, and pancytopenia with or without bone marrow suppression. While macrocytosis and megaloblastic anemia have occurred, these conditions usually respond to folic acid therapy. Lymphadenopathy including benign lymph node hyperplasia, pseudolymphoma, lymphoma, and Hodgkin's disease have been reported (see WARNINGS section).
Connective Tissue System: Coarsening of the facial features, enlargement of the lips, gingival hyperplasia, hypertrichosis, and Peyronie's disease.
Immunologic: Hypersensitivity syndrome (which may include, but is not limited to, symptoms such as arthralgias, eosinophilia, fever, liver dysfunction, lymphadenopathy, or rash), systemic lupus erythematosus, periarteritis nodosa and immunoglobulin abnormalities.

OVERDOSAGE

The lethal dose in pediatric patients is not known. The lethal dose in adults is estimated to be 2 to 5 grams. The initial symptoms are nystagmus, ataxia, and dysarthria. Other signs are tremor, hyperreflexia, lethargy, slurred speech, nausea, vomiting. The patient may become comatose and hypotensive. Death is due to respiratory and circulatory depression.
There are marked variations among individuals with respect to phenytoin plasma levels where toxicity may occur. Nystagmus, on lateral gaze, usually appears at 20 mcg/mL, ataxia at 30 mcg/mL; dysarthria and lethargy appear when the plasma concentration is over 40 mcg/mL, but as high a concentration as 50 mcg/mL has been reported without evidence of toxicity. As much as 25 times the therapeutic dose has been taken to result in a serum concentration over 100 mcg/mL with complete recovery.
Treatment:
Treatment is nonspecific since there is no known antidote. The adequacy of the respiratory and circulatory systems should be carefully observed and appropriate supportive measures employed. Hemodialysis can be considered since phenytoin is not completely bound to plasma proteins. Total exchange transfusion has been used in the treatment of severe intoxication in pediatric patients.
In acute overdosage, the possibility of other CNS depressants, including alcohol, should be borne in mind.

DOSAGE AND ADMINISTRATION

Serum concentrations should be monitored in changing from Extended Phenytoin Sodium Capsules, USP (Dilantin) to Prompt Phenytoin Sodium Capsules, USP, and from the sodium salt to the free acid form.
Dilantin® Kapseals® is formulated with the sodium salt of phenytoin. The free acid form of phenytoin is used in Dilantin-125 Suspension and Dilantin Infatabs. Because there is approximately an 8% increase in drug content with the free acid form over that of the sodium salt, dosage adjustments and serum level monitoring may be necessary when switching from a product formulated with the free acid to a product formulated with the sodium salt and vice versa.
General:
Dosage should be individualized to provide maximum benefit. In some cases, serum blood level determinations may be necessary for optimal dosage adjustments—the clinically effective serum level is usually 10-20 mcg/mL. With recommended dosage, a period of seven to ten days may be required to achieve steady-state blood levels with phenytoin and changes in dosage (increase or decrease) should not be carried out at intervals shorter than seven to ten days.
Adult Dosage:
Divided daily dosage:
Patients who have received no previous treatment may be started on one 100-mg Dilantin (Extended Phenytoin Sodium Capsule) three times daily and the dosage then adjusted to suit individual requirements. For most adults, the satisfactory maintenance dosage will be one capsule three to four times a day. An increase up to two capsules three times a day may be made, if necessary.
Once-a-day dosage:
In adults, if seizure control is established with divided doses of three 100-mg Dilantin capsules daily, once-a-day dosage with 300 mg of extended phenytoin sodium capsules may be considered. Studies comparing divided doses of 300 mg with a single daily dose of this quantity indicated absorption, peak plasma levels, biologic half-life, difference between peak and minimum values, and urinary recovery were equivalent. Once-a-day dosage offers a convenience to the individual patient or to nursing personnel for institutionalized patients and is intended to be used only for patients requiring this amount of drug daily. A major problem in motivating noncompliant patients may also be lessened when the patient can take this drug once a day. However, patients should be cautioned not to miss a dose, inadvertently.
Only extended phenytoin sodium capsules are recommended for once-a-day dosing. Inherent differences in dissolution characteristics and resultant absorption rates of phenytoin due to different manufacturing procedures and/or dosage forms preclude such recommendation for other phenytoin products. When a change in the dosage form or brand is prescribed, careful monitoring of phenytoin serum levels should be carried out.
Loading dose:
Some authorities have advocated use of an oral loading dose of phenytoin in adults who require rapid steady-state serum levels and where intravenous administration is not desirable. This dosing regimen should be reserved for patients in a clinic or hospital setting where phenytoin serum levels can be closely monitored. Patients with a history of renal or liver disease should not receive the oral loading regimen.
Initially, one gram of phenytoin capsules is divided into three doses (400 mg, 300 mg, 300 mg) and administered at two-hour intervals. Normal maintenance dosage is then instituted 24 hours after the loading dose, with frequent serum level determinations.
Pediatric Dosage:
Initially, 5 mg/kg/day in two or three equally divided doses, with subsequent dosage individualized to a maximum of 300 mg daily. A recommended daily maintenance dosage is usually 4 to 8 mg/kg. Children over 6 years old and adolescents may require the minimum adult dose (300 mg/day).

HOW SUPPLIED

Kapseal, transparent #3 capsule with an orange band—imprinted Dilantin 100 mg:
100's (NDC 0071-0362-24)
1,000's (NDC 0071-0362-32)
Unit Dose 100's (NDC 0071-0362-40)
Kapseal 365, transparent #4 capsule with a pink band—Dilantin 30 mg:
100's (NDC 0071-0365-24)
Store at controlled room temperature. Preserve in tight, light-resistant containers. Protect from moisture.
Rx only

Revised February 2003
Distributed by:
Pfizer Parke-Davis
Division of Pfizer Inc, NY, NY 10017
70-5965-00-3

INFATABS®
DILANTIN® ℞
[*dī-lăn' tĭn" ĭn' fă-tăbs"*]
(Phenytoin Tablets, USP)
NOT FOR ONCE A DAY DOSING

Prescribing information for this product, which appears on pages 2528–2529 of the 2004 PDR, has been completely revised as follows. Please write "See Supplement A" next to the product heading.

DESCRIPTION

Dilantin is an antiepileptic drug.
Dilantin (phenytoin) is related to the barbiturates in chemical structure, but has a five-membered ring. The chemical name is 5,5-diphenyl-2,4-imidazolidinedione, having the following structural formula:

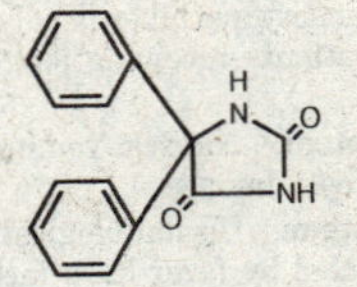

Each Dilantin Infatab, for oral administration, contains 50 mg phenytoin, USP. Also contains: D&C yellow No. 10, Al lake; FD&C yellow No. 6, Al lake; flavor; saccharin sodium, USP; sucrose, NF; talc, USP; and other ingredients.

CLINICAL PHARMACOLOGY

Phenytoin is an antiepileptic drug which can be useful in the treatment of epilepsy. The primary site of action appears to be the motor cortex where spread of seizure activity is inhibited. Possibly by promoting sodium efflux from neurons, phenytoin tends to stabilize the threshold against hyperexcitability caused by excessive stimulation or environmental changes capable of reducing membrane sodium gradient. This includes the reduction of posttetanic potentiation at synapses. Loss of posttetanic potentiation prevents cortical seizure foci from detonating adjacent cortical areas. Phenytoin reduces the maximal activity of brain stem centers responsible for the tonic phase of tonic-clonic (grand mal) seizures.
Clinical studies using Dilantin Infatabs have shown an average plasma half-life of 14 hours with a range of 7 to 29 hours. Steady-state therapeutic levels are achieved at least 7 to 10 days (5-7 half-lives) after initiation of therapy with recommended doses of 300 mg/day.
When serum level determinations are necessary, they should be obtained at least 5-7 half-lives after treatment initiation, dosage change, or addition or subtraction of another drug to the regimen so that equilibrium or steady-state will have been achieved. Trough levels provide information about clinically effective serum level range and confirm patient compliance and are obtained just prior to the patient's next scheduled dose. Peak levels indicate an individual's threshold for emergence of dose-related side effects and are obtained at the time of expected peak concentration. For Dilantin Infatabs peak levels occur 1½-3 hours after administration.
Optimum control without clinical signs of toxicity occurs more often with serum levels between 10 and 20 mcg/mL, although some mild cases of tonic-clonic (grand mal) epilepsy may be controlled with lower serum levels of phenytoin.
In most patients maintained at a steady dosage, stable phenytoin serum levels are achieved. There may be wide interpatient variability in phenytoin serum levels with equivalent dosages. Patients with unusually low levels may be noncompliant or hypermetabolizers of phenytoin. Unusually high levels result from liver disease, congenital enzyme deficiency, or drug interactions which result in metabolic interference. The patient with large variations in phenytoin plasma levels, despite standard doses, presents a difficult clinical problem. Serum level determinations in such patients may be particularly helpful. As phenytoin is highly protein bound, free phenytoin levels may be altered in patients whose protein binding characteristics differ from normal.
Most of the drug is excreted in the bile as inactive metabolites which are then reabsorbed from the intestinal tract and excreted in the urine. Urinary excretion of phenytoin and its metabolites occurs partly with glomerular filtration but, more importantly, by tubular secretion. Because phenytoin is hydroxylated in the liver by an enzyme system which is saturable at high plasma levels, small incremental doses may increase the half-life and produce very substantial increases in serum levels, when these are in the upper range. The steady-state level may be disproportionately increased, with resultant intoxication, from an increase in dosage of 10% or more.
Clinical studies show that chewed and unchewed Dilantin Infatabs are bioequivalent, yield approximately equivalent plasma levels, and are more rapidly absorbed than 100-mg Dilantin Kapseals®.

INDICATIONS AND USAGE

Dilantin Infatabs (Phenytoin Tablets, USP) are indicated for the control of generalized tonic-clonic (grand mal) and complex partial (psychomotor, temporal lobe) seizures and prevention and treatment of seizures occurring during or following neurosurgery. Phenytoin serum level determinations may be necessary for optimal dosage adjustments (see DOSAGE AND ADMINISTRATION and CLINICAL PHARMACOLOGY sections).

CONTRAINDICATIONS

Phenytoin is contraindicated in those patients who are hypersensitive to phenytoin or other hydantoins.

WARNINGS

Abrupt withdrawal of phenytoin in epileptic patients may precipitate status epilepticus. When, in the judgment of the clinician, the need for dosage reduction, discontinuation, or substitution of alternative antiepileptic medication arises, this should be done gradually. However, in the event of an allergic or hypersensitivity reaction, rapid substitution of alternative therapy may be necessary. In this case, alternative therapy should be an antiepileptic drug not belonging to the hydantoin chemical class.
There have been a number of reports suggesting a relationship between phenytoin and the development of lymphadenopathy (local or generalized) including benign lymph node hyperplasia, pseudolymphoma, lymphoma, and Hodgkin's disease. Although a cause and effect relationship has not been established, the occurrence of lymphadenopathy indicates the need to differentiate such a condition from other types of lymph node pathology. Lymph node involvement may occur with or without symptoms and signs resembling serum sickness, eg, fever, rash, and liver involvement. In all cases of lymphadenopathy, follow-up observation for an extended period is indicated and every effort should be made to achieve seizure control using alternative antiepileptic drugs.
Acute alcoholic intake may increase phenytoin serum levels while chronic alcoholic use may decrease serum levels.
In view of isolated reports associating phenytoin with exacerbation of porphyria, caution should be exercised in using this medication in patients suffering from this disease.
Usage in Pregnancy
Clinical:
A. *Risks to Mother.* An increase in seizure frequency may occur during pregnancy because of altered phenytoin pharmacokinetics. Periodic measurement of plasma phenytoin concentrations may be valuable in the management of pregnant women as a guide to appropriate adjustment of dosage (see PRECAUTIONS, Laboratory Tests). However, postpartum restoration of the original dosage will probably be indicated.
B. *Risks to the Fetus.* If this drug is used during pregnancy,

Continued on next page

Dilantin Infatabs—Cont.

or if the patient becomes pregnant while taking the drug, the patient should be apprised of the potential harm to the fetus.

Prenatal exposure to phenytoin may increase the risks for congenital malformations and other adverse developmental outcomes. Increased frequencies of major malformations (such as orofacial clefts and cardiac defects), minor anomalies (dysmorphic facial features, nail and digit hypoplasia), growth abnormalities (including microcephaly), and mental deficiency have been reported among children born to epileptic women who took phenytoin alone or in combination with other antiepileptic drugs during pregnancy. There have also been several reported cases of malignancies, including neuroblastoma, in children whose mothers received phenytoin during pregnancy. The overall incidence of malformations for children of epileptic women treated with antiepileptic drugs (phenytoin and/or others) during pregnancy is about 10%, or two- to three-fold that in the general population. However, the relative contributions of antiepileptic drugs and other factors associated with epilepsy to this increased risk are uncertain and in most cases it has not been possible to attribute specific developmental abnormalities to particular antiepileptic drugs.

Patients should consult with their physicians to weigh the risks and benefits of phenytoin during pregnancy.

C. *Postpartum Period.* A potentially life-threatening bleeding disorder related to decreased levels of vitamin K-dependent clotting factors may occur in newborns exposed to phenytoin *in utero*. This drug-induced condition can be prevented with vitamin K administration to the mother before delivery and to the neonate after birth.

Preclinical:

Increased resorption and malformation rates have been reported following administration of phenytoin doses of 75 mg/kg or higher (approximately 120% of the maximum human loading dose or higher on a mg/m^2 basis) to pregnant rabbits.

PRECAUTIONS

General

The liver is the chief site of biotransformation of phenytoin; patients with impaired liver function, elderly patients, or those who are gravely ill may show early signs of toxicity.

A small percentage of individuals who have been treated with phenytoin have been shown to metabolize the drug slowly. Slow metabolism may be due to limited enzyme availability and lack of induction; it appears to be genetically determined.

Phenytoin should be discontinued if a skin rash appears (see WARNINGS section regarding drug discontinuation). If the rash is exfoliative, purpuric, or bullous or if lupus erythematosus, Stevens-Johnson syndrome, or toxic epidermal necrolysis is suspected, use of this drug should not be resumed and alternative therapy should be considered. (See ADVERSE REACTIONS.) If the rash is of a milder type (measles-like or scarlatiniform), therapy may be resumed after the rash has completely disappeared. If the rash recurs upon reinstitution of therapy, further phenytoin medication is contraindicated.

Phenytoin and other hydantoins are contraindicated in patients who have experienced phenytoin hypersensitivity (see CONTRAINDICATIONS). Additionally, caution should be exercised if using structurally similar (eg, barbiturates, succinimides, oxazolidinediones, and other related compounds) in these same patients.

Hyperglycemia, resulting from the drug's inhibitory effects on insulin release, has been reported. Phenytoin may also raise the serum glucose level in diabetic patients.

Osteomalacia has been associated with phenytoin therapy and is considered to be due to phenytoin's interference with vitamin D metabolism.

Phenytoin is not indicated for seizures due to hypoglycemic or other metabolic causes. Appropriate diagnostic procedures should be performed as indicated.

Phenytoin is not effective for absence (petit mal) seizures. If tonic-clonic (grand mal) and absence (petit mal) seizures are present, combined drug therapy is needed.

Serum levels of phenytoin sustained above the optimal range may produce confusional states referred to as "delirium," "psychosis," or "encephalopathy," or rarely irreversible cerebellar dysfunction. Accordingly, at the first sign of acute toxicity, plasma levels are recommended. Dose reduction of phenytoin therapy is indicated if plasma levels are excessive; if symptoms persist, termination is recommended. (See WARNINGS section.)

Information for Patients

Patients taking phenytoin should be advised of the importance of adhering strictly to the prescribed dosage regimen, and of informing the physician of any clinical condition in which it is not possible to take the drug orally as prescribed, eg, surgery, etc.

Patients should also be cautioned on the use of other drugs or alcoholic beverages without first seeking the physician's advice.

Patients should be instructed to call their physician if skin rash develops.

The importance of good dental hygiene should be stressed in order to minimize the development of gingival hyperplasia and its complications.

Laboratory Tests

Phenytoin serum level determinations may be necessary to achieve optimal dosage adjustments.

Drug Interactions

There are many drugs which may increase or decrease phenytoin levels or which phenytoin may affect. Serum level determinations for phenytoin are especially helpful when possible drug interactions are suspected. The most commonly occurring drug interactions are listed below:

1. Drugs which may increase phenytoin serum levels include: acute alcohol intake, amiodarone, chloramphenicol, chlordiazepoxide, cimetidine, diazepam, dicumarol, disulfiram, estrogens, ethosuximide, fluoxetine, H_2-antagonists, halothane, isoniazid, methylphenidate, phenothiazines, phenylbutazone, salicylates, succinimides, sulfonamides, ticlopidine, tolbutamide, trazodone.
2. Drugs which may decrease phenytoin serum levels include: carbamazepine, chronic alcohol abuse, reserpine, and sucralfate. Moban® brand of Molindone Hydrochloride contains calcium ions which interfere with the absorption of phenytoin. Ingestion times of phenytoin and antacid preparations containing calcium should be staggered in patients with low serum phenytoin levels to prevent absorption problems.
3. Drugs which may either increase or decrease phenytoin serum levels include: phenobarbital, sodium valproate, and valproic acid. Similarly, the effect of phenytoin on phenobarbital, valproic acid, and sodium valproate serum levels is unpredictable.
4. Although not a true drug interaction, tricyclic antidepressants may precipitate seizures in susceptible patients and phenytoin dosage may need to be adjusted.
5. Drugs whose efficacy is impaired by phenytoin include: corticosteroids, coumarin anticoagulants, digitoxin, doxycycline, estrogens, furosemide, oral contraceptives, paroxetine, quinidine, rifampin, theophylline, vitamin D.

Drug Enteral Feeding/Nutritional Preparations Interaction:
Literature reports suggest that patients who have received enteral feeding preparations and/or related nutritional supplements have lower than expected phenytoin plasma levels. It is therefore suggested that phenytoin not be administered concomitantly with an enteral feeding preparation. More frequent serum phenytoin levels monitoring may be necessary in these patients.

Drug/Laboratory Test Interactions

Phenytoin may decrease serum concentrations of T4. It may also produce lower than normal values for dexamethasone or metyrapone tests. Phenytoin may cause increased serum levels of glucose, alkaline phosphatase, and gamma glutamyl transpeptidase (GGT).

Care should be taken when using immunoanalytical methods to measure plasma phenytoin concentrations.

Carcinogenesis

See WARNINGS section for information on carcinogenesis.

Pregnancy

Pregnancy Category D: See WARNINGS section.

Nursing Mothers

Infant breast-feeding is not recommended for women taking this drug because phenytoin appears to be secreted in low concentrations in human milk.

Pediatric Use: See DOSAGE AND ADMINISTRATION section.

ADVERSE REACTIONS

Central Nervous System: The most common manifestations encountered with phenytoin therapy are referable to this system and are usually dose-related. These include nystagmus, ataxia, slurred speech, decreased coordination, and mental confusion. Dizziness, insomnia, transient nervousness, motor twitchings, and headache have also been observed.

There have also been rare reports of phenytoin induced dyskinesias, including chorea, dystonia, tremor and asterixis, similar to those induced by phenothiazine and other neuroleptic drugs.

A predominantly sensory peripheral polyneuropathy has been observed in patients receiving long-term phenytoin therapy.

Gastrointestinal System: Nausea, vomiting, constipation, toxic hepatitis and liver damage.

Integumentary System: Dermatological manifestations sometimes accompanied by fever have included scarlatiniform or morbilliform rashes. A morbilliform rash (measles-like) is the most common; other types of dermatitis are seen more rarely. Other more serious forms which may be fatal have included bullous, exfoliative or purpuric dermatitis, lupus erythematosus, Stevens-Johnson syndrome, and toxic epidermal necrolysis (see PRECAUTIONS section).

Hemopoietic System: Hemopoietic complications, some fatal, have occasionally been reported in association with administration of phenytoin. These have included thrombocytopenia, leukopenia, granulocytopenia, agranulocytosis, and pancytopenia with or without bone marrow suppression. While macrocytosis and megaloblastic anemia have occurred, these conditions usually respond to folic acid therapy. Lymphadenopathy including benign lymph node hyperplasia, pseudolymphoma, lymphoma, and Hodgkin's disease have been reported (see WARNINGS section).

Connective Tissue System: Coarsening of the facial features, enlargement of the lips, gingival hyperplasia, hypertrichosis, and Peyronie's disease.

Immunologic: Hypersensitivity syndrome (which may include, but is not limited to, symptoms such as arthralgias, eosinophilia, fever, liver dysfunction, lymphadenopathy, or rash), systemic lupus erythematosus, periarteritis nodosa and immunoglobulin abnormalities.

OVERDOSAGE

The lethal dose in pediatric patients is not known. The lethal dose in adults is estimated to be 2 to 5 grams. The initial symptoms are nystagmus, ataxia, and dysarthria. Other signs are tremor, hyperreflexia, lethargy, slurred speech, nausea, vomiting. The patient may become comatose and hypotensive. Death is due to respiratory and circulatory depression.

There are marked variations among individuals with respect to phenytoin plasma levels where toxicity may occur. Nystagmus on lateral gaze usually appears at 20 mcg/mL, ataxia at 30 mcg/mL, dysarthria and lethargy appear when the plasma concentration is over 40 mcg/mL, but as high a concentration as 50 mcg/mL has been reported without evidence of toxicity. As much as 25 times the therapeutic dose has been taken to result in a serum concentration over 100 mcg/mL with complete recovery.

Treatment

Treatment is nonspecific since there is no known antidote. The adequacy of the respiratory and circulatory systems should be carefully observed and appropriate supportive measures employed.

Hemodialysis can be considered since phenytoin is not completely bound to plasma proteins. Total exchange transfusion has been used in the treatment of severe intoxication in pediatric patients.

In acute overdosage the possibility of other CNS depressants, including alcohol, should be borne in mind.

DOSAGE AND ADMINISTRATION

When given in equal doses, Dilantin Infatabs yield higher plasma levels than Dilantin Kapseals®. For this reason serum concentrations should be monitored and care should be taken when switching a patient from the sodium salt to the free acid form.

Dilantin® Kapseals® is formulated with the sodium salt of phenytoin. The free acid form of phenytoin is used in Dilantin-125 Suspensions and Dilantin Infatabs. Because there is approximately an 8% increase in drug content with the free acid form over that of the sodium salt, dosage adjustments and serum level monitoring may be necessary when switching from a product formulated with the free acid to a product formulated with the sodium salt and vice versa.

General

Not for once a day dosing.

Dosage should be individualized to provide maximum benefit. In some cases, serum blood level determinations may be necessary for optimal dosage adjustments—the clinically effective serum level is usually 10-20 mcg/mL. With recommended dosage, a period of seven to ten days may be required to achieve steady-state blood levels with phenytoin and changes in dosage (increase or decrease) should not be carried out at intervals shorter than seven to ten days.

Dilantin Infatabs can be either chewed thoroughly before being swallowed or swallowed whole.

Adult Dosage

Patients who have received no previous treatment may be started on two Infatabs three times daily, and the dose is then adjusted to suit individual requirements. For most adults, the satisfactory maintenance dosage will be six to eight Infatabs daily; an increase to twelve Infatabs daily may be made, if necessary.

Pediatric Dosage

Initially, 5 mg/kg/day in two or three equally divided doses, with subsequent dosage individualized to a maximum 300 mg daily. A recommended daily maintenance dosage is usually 4 to 8 mg/kg. Children over 6 years old and adolescents may require the minimum adult dose (300 mg/day). If the daily dosage cannot be divided equally, the larger dose should be given before retiring.

HOW SUPPLIED

Dilantin Infatabs are supplied as:

N 0071-0007-24—Bottle of 100.

Store at a room temperature below 30°C (86°F).

N 0071-0007-40—Unit dose (10/10's).

Store at controlled room temperature 15°-30°C (59°-86°F).

Protect from moisture.

Each tablet contains 50 mg phenytoin in a yellow triangular scored chewable tablet.

Rx only

Revised February 2003

Manufactured by:

Pfizer Pharmaceuticals, Ltd.

Vega Baja, PR 00694

Distributed by:

Pfizer Parke-Davis

Division of Pfizer Inc, NY, NY 10017

69-5830-00-2

LIPITOR® ℞

[*lĭ'pĭ-tōr*]

(Atorvastatin Calcium)

Tablets

Prescribing information for this product, which appears on pages 2543–2546 of the 2004 PDR, has been completely revised as follows. Please write "See Supplement A" next to the product heading.

DESCRIPTION

Lipitor® (atorvastatin calcium) is a synthetic lipid-lowering agent. Atorvastatin is an inhibitor of 3-hydroxy-3-methylglutaryl-coenzyme A (HMG-CoA) reductase. This enzyme catalyzes the conversion of HMG-CoA to mevalonate, an early and rate-limiting step in cholesterol biosynthesis.
Atorvastatin calcium is [R-(R*, R*)]-2-(4-fluorophenyl)-β, δ-dihydroxy-5-(1-methylethyl)-3-phenyl-4-[(phenylamino)-carbonyl]-1H-pyrrole-1-heptanoic acid, calcium salt (2:1) trihydrate. The empirical formula of atorvastatin calcium is $(C_{33}H_{34}FN_2O_5)_2Ca \cdot 3H_2O$ and its molecular weight is 1209.42. Its structural formula is:

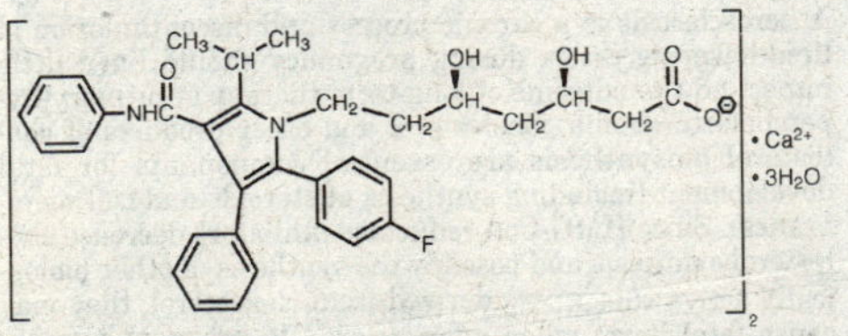

Atorvastatin calcium is a white to off-white crystalline powder that is insoluble in aqueous solutions of pH 4 and below. Atorvastatin calcium is very slightly soluble in distilled water, pH 7.4 phosphate buffer, and acetonitrile, slightly soluble in ethanol, and freely soluble in methanol.
Lipitor tablets for oral administration contain 10, 20, 40 or 80 mg atorvastatin and the following inactive ingredients: calcium carbonate, USP; candelilla wax, FCC; croscarmellose sodium, NF; hydroxypropyl cellulose, NF; lactose monohydrate, NF; magnesium stearate, NF; microcrystalline cellulose, NF; Opadry White YS-1-7040 (hypromellose, polyethylene glycol, talc, titanium dioxide); polysorbate 80, NF; simethicone emulsion.

CLINICAL PHARMACOLOGY

Mechanism of Action

Atorvastatin is a selective, competitive inhibitor of HMG-CoA reductase, the rate-limiting enzyme that converts 3-hydroxy-3-methylglutaryl-coenzyme A to mevalonate, a precursor of sterols, including cholesterol. Cholesterol and triglycerides circulate in the bloodstream as part of lipoprotein complexes. With ultracentrifugation, these complexes separate into HDL (high-density lipoprotein), IDL (intermediate-density lipoprotein), LDL (low-density lipoprotein), and VLDL (very-low-density lipoprotein) fractions. Triglycerides (TG) and cholesterol in the liver are incorporated into VLDL and released into the plasma for delivery to peripheral tissues. LDL is formed from VLDL and is catabolized primarily through the high-affinity LDL receptor. Clinical and pathologic studies show that elevated plasma levels of total cholesterol (total-C), LDL-cholesterol (LDL-C), and apolipoprotein B (apo B) promote human atherosclerosis and are risk factors for developing cardiovascular disease, while increased levels of HDL-C are associated with a decreased cardiovascular risk.
In animal models, Lipitor lowers plasma cholesterol and lipoprotein levels by inhibiting HMG-CoA reductase and cholesterol synthesis in the liver and by increasing the number of hepatic LDL receptors on the cell-surface to enhance uptake and catabolism of LDL; Lipitor also reduces LDL production and the number of LDL particles. Lipitor reduces LDL-C in some patients with homozygous familial hypercholesterolemia (FH), a population that rarely responds to other lipid-lowering medication(s).
A variety of clinical studies have demonstrated that elevated levels of total-C, LDL-C, and apo B (a membrane complex for LDL-C) promote human atherosclerosis. Similarly, decreased levels of HDL-C (and its transport complex, apo A) are associated with the development of atherosclerosis. Epidemiologic investigations have established that cardiovascular morbidity and mortality vary directly with the level of total-C and LDL-C, and inversely with the level of HDL-C.
Lipitor reduces total-C, LDL-C, and apo B in patients with homozygous and heterozygous FH, nonfamilial forms of hypercholesterolemia, and mixed dyslipidemia. Lipitor also reduces VLDL-C and TG and produces variable increases in HDL-C and apolipoprotein A-1. Lipitor reduces total-C, LDL-C, VLDL-C, apo B, TG, and non-HDL-C, and increases HDL-C in patients with isolated hypertriglyceridemia. Lipitor reduces intermediate density lipoprotein cholesterol (IDL-C) in patients with dysbetalipoproteinemia. The effect of Lipitor on cardiovascular morbidity and mortality has not been determined.
Like LDL, cholesterol-enriched triglyceride-rich lipoproteins, including VLDL, intermediate density lipoprotein (IDL), and remnants, can also promote atherosclerosis. Elevated plasma triglycerides are frequently found in a triad with low HDL-C levels and small LDL particles, as well as in association with non-lipid metabolic risk factors for coronary heart disease. As such, total plasma TG has not consistently been shown to be an independent risk factor for CHD. Furthermore, the independent effect of raising HDL or lowering TG on the risk of coronary and cardiovascular morbidity and mortality has not been determined.

Pharmacodynamics

Atorvastatin as well as some of its metabolites are pharmacologically active in humans. The liver is the primary site of action and the principal site of cholesterol synthesis and LDL clearance. Drug dosage rather than systemic drug concentration correlates better with LDL-C reduction. Individualization of drug dosage should be based on therapeutic response (see DOSAGE AND ADMINISTRATION).

TABLE 1. Dose-Response in Patients With Primary Hypercholesterolemia (Adjusted Mean % Change From Baseline)[a]

Dose	N	TC	LDL-C	Apo B	TG	HDL-C	Non-HDL-C/ HDL-C
Placebo	21	4	4	3	10	-3	7
10	22	-29	-39	-32	-19	6	-34
20	20	-33	-43	-35	-26	9	-41
40	21	-37	-50	-42	-29	6	-45
80	23	-45	-60	-50	-37	5	-53

[a]Results are pooled from 2 dose-response studies.

TABLE 2. Mean Percent Change From Baseline at End Point (Double-Blind, Randomized, Active-Controlled Trials)

Treatment (Daily Dose)	N	Total-C	LDL-C	Apo B	TG	HDL-C	Non-HDL-C/ HDL-C
Study 1							
Atorvastatin 10 mg	707	-27[a]	-36[a]	-28[a]	-17[a]	+7	-37[a]
Lovastatin 20 mg	191	-19	-27	-20	-6	+7	-28
95% CI for Diff[1]		-9.2, -6.5	-10.7, -7.1	-10.0, -6.5	-15.2, -7.1	-1.7, 2.0	-11.1, -7.1
Study 2							
Atorvastatin 10 mg	222	-25[b]	-35[b]	-27[b]	-17[b]	+6	-36[b]
Pravastatin 20 mg	77	-17	-23	-17	-9	+8	-28
95% CI for Diff[1]		-10.8, -6.1	-14.5, -8.2	-13.4, -7.4	-14.1, -0.7	-4.9, 1.6	-11.5, -4.1
Study 3							
Atorvastatin 10 mg	132	-29[c]	-37[c]	-34[c]	-23[c]	+7	-39[c]
Simvastatin 10 mg	45	-24	-30	-30	-15	+7	-33
95% CI for Diff[1]		-8.7, -2.7	-10.1, -2.6	-8.0, -1.1	-15.1, -0.7	-4.3, 3.9	-9.6, -1.9

[1] A negative value for the 95% CI for the difference between treatments favors atorvastatin for all except HDL-C, for which a positive value favors atorvastatin. If the range does not include 0, this indicates a statistically significant difference.
[a] Significantly different from lovastatin, ANCOVA, $p \leq 0.05$
[b] Significantly different from pravastatin, ANCOVA, $p \leq 0.05$
[c] Significantly different from simvastatin, ANCOVA, $p \leq 0.05$

Pharmacokinetics and Drug Metabolism

Absorption: Atorvastatin is rapidly absorbed after oral administration; maximum plasma concentrations occur within 1 to 2 hours. Extent of absorption increases in proportion to atorvastatin dose. The absolute bioavailability of atorvastatin (parent drug) is approximately 14% and the systemic availability of HMG-CoA reductase inhibitory activity is approximately 30%. The low systemic availability is attributed to presystemic clearance in gastrointestinal mucosa and/or hepatic first-pass metabolism. Although food decreases the rate and extent of drug absorption by approximately 25% and 9%, respectively, as assessed by Cmax and AUC, LDL-C reduction is similar whether atorvastatin is given with or without food. Plasma atorvastatin concentrations are lower (approximately 30% for Cmax and AUC) following evening drug administration compared with morning. However, LDL-C reduction is the same regardless of the time of day of drug administration (see DOSAGE AND ADMINISTRATION).
Distribution: Mean volume of distribution of atorvastatin is approximately 381 liters. Atorvastatin is ≥98% bound to plasma proteins. A blood/plasma ratio of approximately 0.25 indicates poor drug penetration into red blood cells. Based on observations in rats, atorvastatin is likely to be secreted in human milk (see CONTRAINDICATIONS, Pregnancy and Lactation, and PRECAUTIONS, Nursing Mothers).
Metabolism: Atorvastatin is extensively metabolized to ortho- and parahydroxylated derivatives and various beta-oxidation products. *In vitro* inhibition of HMG-CoA reductase by ortho- and parahydroxylated metabolites is equivalent to that of atorvastatin. Approximately 70% of circulating inhibitory activity for HMG-CoA reductase is attributed to active metabolites. *In vitro* studies suggest the importance of atorvastatin metabolism by cytochrome P450 3A4, consistent with increased plasma concentrations of atorvastatin in humans following coadministration with erythromycin, a known inhibitor of this isozyme (see PRECAUTIONS, Drug Interactions). In animals, the ortho-hydroxy metabolite undergoes further glucuronidation.
Excretion: Atorvastatin and its metabolites are eliminated primarily in bile following hepatic and/or extra-hepatic metabolism; however, the drug does not appear to undergo enterohepatic recirculation. Mean plasma elimination half-life of atorvastatin in humans is approximately 14 hours, but the half-life of inhibitory activity for HMG-CoA reductase is 20 to 30 hours due to the contribution of active metabolites. Less than 2% of a dose of atorvastatin is recovered in urine following oral administration.

Special Populations

Geriatric: Plasma concentrations of atorvastatin are higher (approximately 40% for Cmax and 30% for AUC) in healthy elderly subjects (age ≥65 years) than in young adults. Clinical data suggest a greater degree of LDL-lowering at any dose of drug in the elderly patient population compared to younger adults (see PRECAUTIONS section; Geriatric Use subsection).
Pediatric: Pharmacokinetic data in the pediatric population are not available.
Gender: Plasma concentrations of atorvastatin in women differ from those in men (approximately 20% higher for Cmax and 10% lower for AUC); however, there is no clinically significant difference in LDL-C reduction with Lipitor between men and women.
Renal Insufficiency: Renal disease has no influence on the plasma concentrations or LDL-C reduction of atorvastatin; thus, dose adjustment in patients with renal dysfunction is not necessary (see DOSAGE AND ADMINISTRATION).
Hemodialysis: While studies have not been conducted in patients with end-stage renal disease, hemodialysis is not expected to significantly enhance clearance of atorvastatin since the drug is extensively bound to plasma proteins.
Hepatic Insufficiency: In patients with chronic alcoholic liver disease, plasma concentrations of atorvastatin are markedly increased. Cmax and AUC are each 4-fold greater in patients with Childs-Pugh A disease. Cmax and AUC are approximately 16-fold and 11-fold increased, respectively, in patients with Childs-Pugh B disease (see CONTRAINDICATIONS).

Clinical Studies

Hypercholesterolemia (Heterozygous Familial and Nonfamilial) and Mixed Dyslipidemia (*Fredrickson* Types IIa and IIb)

Lipitor reduces total-C, LDL-C, VLDL-C, apo B, and TG, and increases HDL-C in patients with hypercholesterolemia and mixed dyslipidemia. Therapeutic response is seen within 2 weeks, and maximum response is usually achieved within 4 weeks and maintained during chronic therapy.
Lipitor is effective in a wide variety of patient populations with hypercholesterolemia, with and without hypertriglyceridemia, in men and women, and in the elderly. Experience in pediatric patients has been limited to patients with homozygous FH. In two multicenter, placebo-controlled, dose-response studies in patients with hypercholesterolemia, Lipitor given as a single dose over 6 weeks significantly reduced total-C, LDL-C, apo B, and TG (Pooled results are provided in Table 1).
[See table 1 above]
In patients with *Fredrickson* Types IIa and IIb hyperlipoproteinemia pooled from 24 controlled trials, the median (25th and 75th percentile) percent changes from baseline in HDL-C for atorvastatin 10, 20, 40, and 80 mg were 6.4 (-1.4, 14), 8.7(0, 17), 7.8(0, 16), and 5.1 (-2.7, 15), respectively. Additionally, analysis of the pooled data demonstrated consistent and significant decreases in total-C, LDL-C, TG, total-C/HDL-C, and LDL-C/HDL-C.
In three multicenter, double-blind studies in patients with hypercholesterolemia, Lipitor was compared to other HMG-CoA reductase inhibitors. After randomization, patients were treated for 16 weeks with either Lipitor 10 mg per day or a fixed dose of the comparative agent (Table 2).
[See table 2 above]
The impact on clinical outcomes of the differences in lipid-altering effects between treatments shown in Table 2 is not known. Table 2 does not contain data comparing the effects of atorvastatin 10 mg and higher doses of lovastatin, pravastatin, and simvastatin. The drugs compared in the studies summarized in the table are not necessarily interchangeable.

Hypertriglyceridemia (*Fredrickson* Type IV)

The response to Lipitor in 64 patients with isolated hypertriglyceridemia treated across several clinical trials is shown in the table below. For the atorvastatin-treated patients, median (min, max) baseline TG level was 565 (267-1502).

Continued on next page

Lipitor—Cont.

[See table 3 below]

Dysbetalipoproteinemia (*Fredrickson* Type III)

The results of an open-label crossover study of 16 patients (genotypes: 14 apo E2/E2 and 2 apo E3/E2) with dysbetalipoproteinemia (*Fredrickson* Type III) are shown in the table below.

[See table 4 below]

Homozygous Familial Hypercholesterolemia

In a study without a concurrent control group, 29 patients ages 6 to 37 years with homozygous FH received maximum daily doses of 20 to 80 mg of Lipitor. The mean LDL-C reduction in this study was 18%. Twenty-five patients with a reduction in LDL-C had a mean response of 20% (range of 7% to 53%, median of 24%); the remaining 4 patients had 7% to 24% increases in LDL-C. Five of the 29 patients had absent LDL-receptor function. Of these, 2 patients also had a portacaval shunt and had no significant reduction in LDL-C. The remaining 3 receptor-negative patients had a mean LDL-C reduction of 22%.

Heterozygous Familial Hypercholesterolemia in Pediatric Patients

In a double-blind, placebo-controlled study followed by an open-label phase, 187 boys and postmenarchal girls 10-17 years of age (mean age 14.1 years) with heterozygous familial hypercholesterolemia (FH) or severe hypercholesterolemia were randomized to Lipitor (n=140) or placebo (n=47) for 26 weeks and then all received Lipitor for 26 weeks. Inclusion in the study required 1) a baseline LDL-C level ≥ 190 mg/dL or 2) a baseline LDL-C ≥ 160 mg/dL and positive family history of FH or documented premature cardiovascular disease in a first- or second-degree relative. The mean baseline LDL-C value was 218.6 mg/dL (range: 138.5-385.0 mg/dL) in the Lipitor group compared to 230.0 mg/dL (range: 160.0-324.5 mg/dL) in the placebo group. The dosage of Lipitor (once daily) was 10 mg for the first 4 weeks and up-titrated to 20 mg if the LDL-C level was > 130 mg/dL. The number of Lipitor-treated patients who required up-titration to 20 mg after Week 4 during the double-blind phase was 80 (57.1%).

Lipitor significantly decreased plasma levels of total-C, LDL-C, triglycerides, and apolipoprotein B during the 26 week double-blind phase (see Table 5).

[See table 5 below]

The mean achieved LDL-C value was 130.7 mg/dL (range: 70.0-242.0 mg/dL) in the Lipitor group compared to 228.5 mg/dL (range: 152.0-385.0 mg/dL) in the placebo group during the 26 week double-blind phase.

The safety and efficacy of doses above 20 mg have not been studied in controlled trials in children. The long-term efficacy of Lipitor therapy in childhood to reduce morbidity and mortality in adulthood has not been established.

INDICATIONS AND USAGE

Lipitor is indicated:

1. as an adjunct to diet to reduce elevated total-C, LDL-C, apo B, and TG levels and to increase HDL-C in patients with primary hypercholesterolemia (heterozygous familial and nonfamilial) and mixed dyslipidemia (*Fredrickson* Types IIa and IIb);
2. as an adjunct to diet for the treatment of patients with elevated serum TG levels (*Fredrickson* Type IV);
3. for the treatment of patients with primary dysbetalipoproteinemia (*Fredrickson* Type III) who do not respond adequately to diet;
4. to reduce total-C and LDL-C in patients with homozygous familial hypercholesterolemia as an adjunct to other lipid-lowering treatments (eg, LDL apheresis) or if such treatments are unavailable;
5. as an adjunct to diet to reduce total-C, LDL-C, and apo B levels in boys and postmenarchal girls, 10 to 17 years of age, with heterozygous familial hypercholesterolemia if after an adequate trial of diet therapy the following findings are present:
   a. LDL-C remains ≥ 190 mg/dL or
   b. LDL-C remains ≥ 160 mg/dL and:
      - there is a positive family history of premature cardiovascular disease or
      - two or more other CVD risk factors are present in the pediatric patient

Therapy with lipid-altering agents should be a component of multiple-risk-factor intervention in individuals at increased risk for atherosclerotic vascular disease due to hypercholesterolemia. Lipid-altering agents should be used in addition to a diet restricted in saturated fat and cholesterol only when the response to diet and other nonpharmacological measures has been inadequate (see *National Cholesterol Education Program (NCEP) Guidelines*, summarized in Table 6).

[See table 6 at top of next page]

After the LDL-C goal has been achieved, if the TG is still ≥200 mg/dL, non HDL-C (total-C minus HDL-C) becomes a secondary target of therapy. Non-HDL-C goals are set 30 mg/dL higher than LDL-C goals for each risk category.

Prior to initiating therapy with Lipitor, secondary causes for hypercholesterolemia (eg, poorly controlled diabetes mellitus, hypothyroidism, nephrotic syndrome, dysproteinemias, obstructive liver disease, other drug therapy, and alcoholism) should be excluded, and a lipid profile performed to measure total-C, LDL-C, HDL-C, and TG. For patients with TG <400 mg/dL (<4.5 mmol/L), LDL-C can be estimated using the following equation: LDL-C = total-C - (0.20 × [TG] + HDL-C). For TG levels >400 mg/dL (>4.5 mmol/L), this equation is less accurate and LDL-C concentrations should be determined by ultracentrifugation.

Lipitor has not been studied in conditions where the major lipoprotein abnormality is elevation of chylomicrons (*Fredrickson* Types I and V).

The NCEP classification of cholesterol levels in pediatric patients with a familial history of hypercholesterolemia or premature cardiovascular disease is summarized below:

Category	Total-C (mg/dL)	LDL-C (mg/dL)
Acceptable	<170	<110
Borderline	170-199	110-129
High	≥200	≥130

CONTRAINDICATIONS

Active liver disease or unexplained persistent elevations of serum transaminases.

Hypersensitivity to any component of this medication.

Pregnancy and Lactation

Atherosclerosis is a chronic process and discontinuation of lipid-lowering drugs during pregnancy should have little impact on the outcome of long-term therapy of primary hypercholesterolemia. Cholesterol and other products of cholesterol biosynthesis are essential components for fetal development (including synthesis of steroids and cell membranes). Since HMG-CoA reductase inhibitors decrease cholesterol synthesis and possibly the synthesis of other biologically active substances derived from cholesterol, they may cause fetal harm when administered to pregnant women. Therefore, HMG-CoA reductase inhibitors are contraindicated during pregnancy and in nursing mothers. ATORVASTATIN SHOULD BE ADMINISTERED TO WOMEN OF CHILDBEARING AGE ONLY WHEN SUCH PATIENTS ARE HIGHLY UNLIKELY TO CONCEIVE AND HAVE BEEN INFORMED OF THE POTENTIAL HAZARDS. If the patient becomes pregnant while taking this drug, therapy should be discontinued and the patient apprised of the potential hazard to the fetus.

WARNINGS

Liver Dysfunction

HMG-CoA reductase inhibitors, like some other lipid-lowering therapies, have been associated with biochemical abnormalities of liver function. **Persistent elevations (>3 times the upper limit of normal [ULN] occurring on 2 or more occasions) in serum transaminases occurred in 0.7% of patients who received atorvastatin in clinical trials. The incidence of these abnormalities was 0.2%, 0.2%, 0.6%, and 2.3% for 10, 20, 40, and 80 mg, respectively.**

One patient in clinical trials developed jaundice. Increases in liver function tests (LFT) in other patients were not associated with jaundice or other clinical signs or symptoms. Upon dose reduction, drug interruption, or discontinuation, transaminase levels returned to or near pretreatment levels without sequelae. Eighteen of 30 patients with persistent LFT elevations continued treatment with a reduced dose of atorvastatin.

It is recommended that liver function tests be performed prior to and at 12 weeks following both the initiation of therapy and any elevation of dose, and periodically (eg, semiannually) thereafter. Liver enzyme changes generally occur in the first 3 months of treatment with atorvastatin. Patients who develop increased transaminase levels should be monitored until the abnormalities resolve. Should an increase in ALT or AST of >3 times ULN persist, reduction of dose or withdrawal of atorvastatin is recommended.

Atorvastatin should be used with caution in patients who consume substantial quantities of alcohol and/or have a history of liver disease. Active liver disease or unexplained persistent transaminase elevations are contraindications to the use of atorvastatin (see CONTRAINDICATIONS).

Skeletal Muscle

Rare cases of rhabdomyolysis with acute renal failure secondary to myoglobinuria have been reported with atorvastatin and with other drugs in this class.

Uncomplicated myalgia has been reported in atorvastatin-treated patients (see ADVERSE REACTIONS). Myopathy, defined as muscle aches or muscle weakness in conjunction with increases in creatine phosphokinase (CPK) values >10 times ULN, should be considered in any patient with diffuse myalgias, muscle tenderness or weakness, and/or marked elevation of CPK. Patients should be advised to report promptly unexplained muscle pain, tenderness or weakness, particularly if accompanied by malaise or fever. Atorvastatin therapy should be discontinued if markedly elevated CPK levels occur or myopathy is diagnosed or suspected.

The risk of myopathy during treatment with drugs in this class is increased with concurrent administration of cyclosporine, fibric acid derivatives, erythromycin, niacin, or azole antifungals. Physicians considering combined therapy with atorvastatin and fibric acid derivatives, erythromycin, immunosuppressive drugs, azole antifungals, or lipid-lowering doses of niacin should carefully weigh the potential benefits and risks and should carefully monitor patients for any signs or symptoms of muscle pain, tenderness, or weakness, particularly during the initial months of therapy and during any periods of upward dosage titration of either drug. Periodic creatine phosphokinase (CPK) determinations may be considered in such situations, but there is no assurance that such monitoring will prevent the occurrence of severe myopathy.

Atorvastatin therapy should be temporarily withheld or discontinued in any patient with an acute, serious condition suggestive of a myopathy or having a risk factor predisposing to the development of renal failure secondary to rhabdomyolysis (eg, severe acute infection, hypotension, major surgery, trauma, severe metabolic, endocrine and electrolyte disorders, and uncontrolled seizures).

PRECAUTIONS

General

Before instituting therapy with atorvastatin, an attempt should be made to control hypercholesterolemia with appro-

TABLE 3. Combined Patients With Isolated Elevated TG: Median (min, max) Percent Changes From Baseline

	Placebo (N=12)	Atorvastatin 10 mg (N=37)	Atorvastatin 20 mg (N=13)	Atorvastatin 80 mg (N=14)
Triglycerides	-12.4 (-36.6, 82.7)	-41.0 (-76.2, 49.4)	-38.7 (-62.7, 29.5)	-51.8 (-82.8, 41.3)
Total-C	-2.3 (-15.5, 24.4)	-28.2 (-44.9, -6.8)	-34.9 (-49.6, -15.2)	-44.4 (-63.5, -3.8)
LDL-C	3.6 (-31.3, 31.6)	-26.5 (-57.7, 9.8)	-30.4 (-53.9, 0.3)	-40.5 (-60.6, -13.8)
HDL-C	3.8 (-18.6, 13.4)	13.8 (-9.7, 61.5)	11.0 (-3.2, 25.2)	7.5 (-10.8, 37.2)
VLDL-C	-1.0 (-31.9, 53.2)	-48.8 (-85.8, 57.3)	-44.6 (-62.2, -10.8)	-62.0 (-88.2, 37.6)
non-HDL-C	-2.8 (-17.6, 30.0)	-33.0 (-52.1, -13.3)	-42.7 (-53.7, -17.4)	-51.5 (-72.9, -4.3)

TABLE 4. Open-Label Crossover Study of 16 Patients With Dysbetalipoproteinemia (*Fredrickson* Type III)

	Median (min, max) at Baseline (mg/dL)	Median % Change (min, max)	
		Atorvastatin 10 mg	Atorvastatin 80 mg
Total-C	442 (225, 1320)	-37 (-85, 17)	-58 (-90, -31)
Triglycerides	678 (273, 5990)	-39 (-92, -8)	-53 (-95, -30)
IDL-C + VLDL-C	215 (111, 613)	-32 (-76, 9)	-63 (-90, -8)
non-HDL-C	411 (218, 1272)	-43 (-87, -19)	-64 (-92, -36)

TABLE 5
Lipid-altering Effects of Lipitor in Adolescent Boys and Girls with Heterozygous Familial Hypercholesterolemia or Severe Hypercholesterolemia
(Mean Percent Change from Baseline at Endpoint in Intention-to-Treat Population)

DOSAGE	N	Total-C	LDL-C	HDL-C	TG	Apolipoprotein B
Placebo	47	-1.5	-0.4	-1.9	1.0	0.7
Lipitor	140	-31.4	-39.6	2.8	-12.0	-34.0

TABLE 6. NCEP Treatment Guidelines: LDL-C Goals and Cutpoints for Therapeutic Lifestyle Changes and Drug Therapy in Different Risk Categories

Risk Category	LDL Goal (mg/dL)	LDL Level at Which to Initiate Therapeutic Lifestyle Changes (mg/dL)	LDL Level at Which to Consider Drug Therapy (mg/dL)
CHD[a] or CHD risk equivalents (10-year risk >20%)	<100	≥100	≥130 (100-129: drug optional)[b]
2+ Risk Factors (10-year risk ≤20%)	<130	≥130	10-year risk 10%-20%: ≥130 10-year risk <10%: ≥160
0-1 Risk factor[c]	<160	≥160	≥190 (160-189: LDL-lowering drug optional)

[a] CHD, coronary heart disease
[b] Some authorities recommend use of LDL-lowering drugs in this category if an LDL-C level of <100 mg/dL cannot be achieved by therapeutic lifestyle changes. Others prefer use of drugs that primarily modify triglycerides and HDL-C, e.g., nicotinic acid or fibrate. Clinical judgement also may call for deferring drug therapy in this subcategory.
[c] Almost all people with 0-1 risk factor have 10-year risk <10%; thus, 10-year risk assessment in people with 0-1 risk factor is not necessary.

TABLE 7. Adverse Events in Placebo-Controlled Studies (% of Patients)

BODY SYSTEM/ Adverse Event	Placebo N = 270	Atorvastatin 10 mg N = 863	Atorvastatin 20 mg N = 36	Atorvastatin 40 mg N = 79	Atorvastatin 80 mg N = 94
BODY AS A WHOLE					
Infection	10.0	10.3	2.8	10.1	7.4
Headache	7.0	5.4	16.7	2.5	6.4
Accidental Injury	3.7	4.2	0.0	1.3	3.2
Flu Syndrome	1.9	2.2	0.0	2.5	3.2
Abdominal Pain	0.7	2.8	0.0	3.8	2.1
Back Pain	3.0	2.8	0.0	3.8	1.1
Allergic Reaction	2.6	0.9	2.8	1.3	0.0
Asthenia	1.9	2.2	0.0	3.8	0.0
DIGESTIVE SYSTEM					
Constipation	1.8	2.1	0.0	2.5	1.1
Diarrhea	1.5	2.7	0.0	3.8	5.3
Dyspepsia	4.1	2.3	2.8	1.3	2.1
Flatulence	3.3	2.1	2.8	1.3	1.1
RESPIRATORY SYSTEM					
Sinusitis	2.6	2.8	0.0	2.5	6.4
Pharyngitis	1.5	2.5	0.0	1.3	2.1
SKIN AND APPENDAGES					
Rash	0.7	3.9	2.8	3.8	1.1
MUSCULOSKELETAL SYSTEM					
Arthralgia	1.5	2.0	0.0	5.1	0.0
Myalgia	1.1	3.2	5.6	1.3	0.0

priate diet, exercise, and weight reduction in obese patients, and to treat other underlying medical problems (see INDICATIONS AND USAGE).

Information for Patients

Patients should be advised to report promptly unexplained muscle pain, tenderness, or weakness, particularly if accompanied by malaise or fever.

Drug Interactions

The risk of myopathy during treatment with drugs of this class is increased with concurrent administration of cyclosporine, fibric acid derivatives, niacin (nicotinic acid), erythromycin, azole antifungals (see WARNINGS, Skeletal Muscle).

Antacid: When atorvastatin and Maalox® TC suspension were coadministered, plasma concentrations of atorvastatin decreased approximately 35%. However, LDL-C reduction was not altered.

Antipyrine: Because atorvastatin does not affect the pharmacokinetics of antipyrine, interactions with other drugs metabolized via the same cytochrome isozymes are not expected.

Colestipol: Plasma concentrations of atorvastatin decreased approximately 25% when colestipol and atorvastatin were coadministered. However, LDL-C reduction was greater when atorvastatin and colestipol were coadministered than when either drug was given alone.

Cimetidine: Atorvastatin plasma concentrations and LDL-C reduction were not altered by coadministration of cimetidine.

Digoxin: When multiple doses of atorvastatin and digoxin were coadministered, steady-state plasma digoxin concentrations increased by approximately 20%. Patients taking digoxin should be monitored appropriately.

Erythromycin: In healthy individuals, plasma concentrations of atorvastatin increased approximately 40% with coadministration of atorvastatin and erythromycin, a known inhibitor of cytochrome P450 3A4 (see WARNINGS, Skeletal Muscle).

Oral Contraceptives: Coadministration of atorvastatin and an oral contraceptive increased AUC values for norethindrone and ethinyl estradiol by approximately 30% and 20%. These increases should be considered when selecting an oral contraceptive for a woman taking atorvastatin.

Warfarin: Atorvastatin had no clinically significant effect on prothrombin time when administered to patients receiving chronic warfarin treatment.

Endocrine Function

HMG-CoA reductase inhibitors interfere with cholesterol synthesis and theoretically might blunt adrenal and/or gonadal steroid production. Clinical studies have shown that atorvastatin does not reduce basal plasma cortisol concentration or impair adrenal reserve. The effects of HMG-CoA reductase inhibitors on male fertility have not been studied in adequate numbers of patients. The effects, if any, on the pituitary-gonadal axis in premenopausal women are unknown. Caution should be exercised if an HMG-CoA reductase inhibitor is administered concomitantly with drugs that may decrease the levels or activity of endogenous steroid hormones, such as ketoconazole, spironolactone, and cimetidine.

CNS Toxicity

Brain hemorrhage was seen in a female dog treated for 3 months at 120 mg/kg/day. Brain hemorrhage and optic nerve vacuolation were seen in another female dog that was sacrificed in moribund condition after 11 weeks of escalating doses up to 280 mg/kg/day. The 120 mg/kg dose resulted in a systemic exposure approximately 16 times the human plasma area-under-the-curve (AUC, 0-24 hours) based on the maximum human dose of 80 mg/day. A single tonic convulsion was seen in each of 2 male dogs (one treated at 10 mg/kg/day and one at 120 mg/kg/day) in a 2-year study. No CNS lesions have been observed in mice after chronic treatment for up to 2 years at doses up to 400 mg/kg/day or in rats at doses up to 100 mg/kg/day. These doses were 6 to 11 times (mouse) and 8 to 16 times (rat) the human AUC (0-24) based on the maximum recommended human dose of 80 mg/day.

CNS vascular lesions, characterized by perivascular hemorrhages, edema, and mononuclear cell infiltration of perivascular spaces, have been observed in dogs treated with other members of this class. A chemically similar drug in this class produced optic nerve degeneration (Wallerian degeneration of retinogeniculate fibers) in clinically normal dogs in a dose-dependent fashion at a dose that produced plasma drug levels about 30 times higher than the mean drug level in humans taking the highest recommended dose.

Carcinogenesis, Mutagenesis, Impairment of Fertility

In a 2-year carcinogenicity study in rats at dose levels of 10, 30, and 100 mg/kg/day, 2 rare tumors were found in muscle in high-dose females: in one, there was a rhabdomyosarcoma and, in another, there was a fibrosarcoma. This dose represents a plasma AUC (0-24) value of approximately 16 times the mean human plasma drug exposure after an 80 mg oral dose.

A 2-year carcinogenicity study in mice given 100, 200, or 400 mg/kg/day resulted in a significant increase in liver adenomas in high-dose males and liver carcinomas in high-dose females. These findings occurred at plasma AUC (0-24) values of approximately 6 times the mean human plasma drug exposure after an 80 mg oral dose.

In vitro, atorvastatin was not mutagenic or clastogenic in the following tests with and without metabolic activation: the Ames test with *Salmonella typhimurium* and *Escherichia coli*, the HGPRT forward mutation assay in Chinese hamster lung cells, and the chromosomal aberration assay in Chinese hamster lung cells. Atorvastatin was negative in the *in vivo* mouse micronucleus test.

Studies in rats performed at doses up to 175 mg/kg (15 times the human exposure) produced no changes in fertility. There was aplasia and aspermia in the epididymis of 2 of 10 rats treated with 100 mg/kg/day of atorvastatin for 3 months (16 times the human AUC at the 80 mg dose); testis weights were significantly lower at 30 and 100 mg/kg and epididymal weight was lower at 100 mg/kg. Male rats given 100 mg/kg/day for 11 weeks prior to mating had decreased sperm motility, spermatid head concentration, and increased abnormal sperm. Atorvastatin caused no adverse effects on semen parameters, or reproductive organ histopathology in dogs given doses of 10, 40, or 120 mg/kg for two years.

Pregnancy

Pregnancy Category X

See CONTRAINDICATIONS

Safety in pregnant women has not been established. Atorvastatin crosses the rat placenta and reaches a level in fetal liver equivalent to that of maternal plasma. Atorvastatin was not teratogenic in rats at doses up to 300 mg/kg/day or in rabbits at doses up to 100 mg/kg/day. These doses resulted in multiples of about 30 times (rat) or 20 times (rabbit) the human exposure based on surface area (mg/m^2).

In a study in rats given 20, 100, or 225 mg/kg/day, from gestation day 7 through to lactation day 21 (weaning), there was decreased pup survival at birth, neonate, weaning, and maturity in pups of mothers dosed with 225 mg/kg/day. Body weight was decreased on days 4 and 21 in pups of mothers dosed at 100 mg/kg/day; pup body weight was decreased at birth and at days 4, 21, and 91 at 225 mg/kg/day. Pup development was delayed (rotorod performance at 100 mg/kg/day and acoustic startle at 225 mg/kg/day; pinnae detachment and eye opening at 225 mg/kg/day). These doses correspond to 6 times (100 mg/kg) and 22 times (225 mg/kg) the human AUC at 80 mg/day. Rare reports of congenital anomalies have been received following intrauterine exposure to HMG-CoA reductase inhibitors. There has been one report of severe congenital bony deformity, tracheo-esophageal fistula, and anal atresia (VATER association) in a baby born to a woman who took lovastatin with dextroamphetamine sulfate during the first trimester of pregnancy. Lipitor should be administered to women of child-bearing potential only when such patients are highly unlikely to conceive and have been informed of the potential hazards. If the woman becomes pregnant while taking Lipitor, it should be discontinued and the patient advised again as to the potential hazards to the fetus.

Nursing Mothers

Nursing rat pups had plasma and liver drug levels of 50% and 40%, respectively, of that in their mother's milk. Because of the potential for adverse reactions in nursing infants, women taking Lipitor should not breast-feed (see CONTRAINDICATIONS).

Pediatric Use

Safety and effectiveness in patients 10-17 years of age with heterozygous familial hypercholesterolemia have been evaluated in a controlled clinical trial of 6 months duration in adolescent boys and postmenarchal girls. Patients treated with Lipitor had an adverse experience profile generally similar to that of patients treated with placebo, the most common adverse experiences observed in both groups, regardless of causality assessment, were infections. **Doses greater than 20 mg have not been studied in this patient population.** In this limited controlled study, there was no detectable effect on growth or sexual maturation in boys or on menstrual cycle length in girls (see CLINICAL PHARMACOLOGY, Clinical Studies section; ADVERSE REACTIONS, Pediatric Patients (ages 10-17 years); and DOSAGE AND ADMINISTRATION Heterozygous Familial Hypercholesterolemia in Pediatric Patients (10-17 years of age). Adolescent females should be counseled on appropriate contraceptive methods while on Lipitor therapy (see CONTRAINDICATIONS and PRECAUTIONS Pregnancy). **Lipitor has not been studied in controlled clinical trials involving pre-pubertal patients or patients younger than 10 years of age.**

Clinical efficacy with doses up to 80 mg/day for 1 year have been evaluated in an uncontrolled study of patients with homozygous FH including 8 pediatric patients (see CLINICAL PHARMACOLOGY, Clinical Studies: Homozygous Familial Hypercholesterolemia).

Geriatric Use

The safety and efficacy of atorvastatin (10-80 mg) in the geriatric population (≥65 years of age) was evaluated in the ACCESS study. In this 54-week open-label trial 1,958 patients initiated therapy with atorvastatin 10 mg. Of these, 835 were elderly (≥65 years) and 1,123 were non-elderly. The mean change in LDL-C from baseline after 6 weeks of treatment with atorvastatin 10 mg was –38.2% in the elderly patients versus –34.6% in the non-elderly group.

The rates of discontinuation due to adverse events were similar between the two age groups. There were no differences in clinically relevant laboratory abnormalities between the age groups.

Continued on next page

Lipitor—Cont.

ADVERSE REACTIONS

Lipitor is generally well-tolerated. Adverse reactions have usually been mild and transient. In controlled clinical studies of 2502 patients, <2% of patients were discontinued due to adverse experiences attributable to atorvastatin. The most frequent adverse events thought to be related to atorvastatin were constipation, flatulence, dyspepsia, and abdominal pain.

Clinical Adverse Experiences

Adverse experiences reported in ≥2% of patients in placebo-controlled clinical studies of atorvastatin, regardless of causality assessment, are shown in Table 7.

[See table 7 at top of previous page]

The following adverse events were reported, regardless of causality assessment in patients treated with atorvastatin in clinical trials. The events in italics occurred in ≥2% of patients and the events in plain type occurred in <2% of patients.

Body as a Whole: *Chest pain*, face edema, fever, neck rigidity, malaise, photosensitivity reaction, generalized edema.

Digestive System: *Nausea*, gastroenteritis, liver function tests abnormal, colitis, vomiting, gastritis, dry mouth, rectal hemorrhage, esophagitis, eructation, glossitis, mouth ulceration, anorexia, increased appetite, stomatitis, biliary pain, cheilitis, duodenal ulcer, dysphagia, enteritis, melena, gum hemorrhage, stomach ulcer, tenesmus, ulcerative stomatitis, hepatitis, pancreatitis, cholestatic jaundice.

Respiratory System: *Bronchitis*, *rhinitis*, pneumonia, dyspnea, asthma, epistaxis.

Nervous System: *Insomnia*, *dizziness*, paresthesia, somnolence, amnesia, abnormal dreams, libido decreased, emotional lability, incoordination, peripheral neuropathy, torticollis, facial paralysis, hyperkinesia, depression, hypesthesia, hypertonia.

Musculoskeletal System: *Arthritis*, leg cramps, bursitis, tenosynovitis, myasthenia, tendinous contracture, myositis.

Skin and Appendages: Pruritus, contact dermatitis, alopecia, dry skin, sweating, acne, urticaria, eczema, seborrhea, skin ulcer.

Urogenital System: *Urinary tract infection*, urinary frequency, cystitis, hematuria, impotence, dysuria, kidney calculus, nocturia, epididymitis, fibrocystic breast, vaginal hemorrhage, albuminuria, breast enlargement, metrorrhagia, nephritis, urinary incontinence, urinary retention, urinary urgency, abnormal ejaculation, uterine hemorrhage.

Special Senses: Amblyopia, tinnitus, dry eyes, refraction disorder, eye hemorrhage, deafness, glaucoma, parosmia, taste loss, taste perversion.

Cardiovascular System: Palpitation, vasodilatation, syncope, migraine, postural hypotension, phlebitis, arrhythmia, angina pectoris, hypertension.

Metabolic and Nutritional Disorders: *Peripheral edema*, hyperglycemia, creatine phosphokinase increased, gout, weight gain, hypoglycemia.

Hemic and Lymphatic System: Ecchymosis, anemia, lymphadenopathy, thrombocytopenia, petechia.

Postintroduction Reports

Adverse events associated with Lipitor therapy reported since market introduction, that are not listed above, regardless of causality assessment, include the following: anaphylaxis, angioneurotic edema, bullous rashes (including erythema multiforme, Stevens-Johnson syndrome, and toxic epidermal necrolysis), and rhabdomyolysis.

Pediatric Patients (ages 10-17 years)

In a 26-week controlled study in boys and postmenarchal girls (n=140), the safety and tolerability profile of Lipitor 10 to 20 mg daily was generally similar to that of placebo (see CLINICAL PHARMACOLOGY, Clinical Studies, section and PRECAUTIONS, Pediatric Use).

OVERDOSAGE

There is no specific treatment for atorvastatin overdosage. In the event of an overdose, the patient should be treated symptomatically, and supportive measures instituted as required. Due to extensive drug binding to plasma proteins, hemodialysis is not expected to significantly enhance atorvastatin clearance.

DOSAGE AND ADMINISTRATION

The patient should be placed on a standard cholesterol-lowering diet before receiving Lipitor and should continue on this diet during treatment with Lipitor.

Hypercholesterolemia (Heterozygous Familial and Nonfamilial) and Mixed Dyslipidemia (*Fredrickson* Types IIa and IIb)

The recommended starting dose of Lipitor is 10 or 20 mg once daily. Patients who require a large reduction in LDL-C (more than 45%) may be started at 40 mg once daily. The dosage range of Lipitor is 10 to 80 mg once daily. Lipitor can be administered as a single dose at any time of the day, with or without food. The starting dose and maintenance doses of Lipitor should be individualized according to patient characteristics such as goal of therapy and response (see *NCEP Guidelines* summarized in Table 5). After initiation and/or upon titration of Lipitor, lipid levels should be analyzed within 2 to 4 weeks and dosage adjusted accordingly.

Since the goal of treatment is to lower LDL-C, the NCEP recommends that LDL-C levels be used to initiate and assess treatment response. Only if LDL-C levels are not available, should total-C be used to monitor therapy.

Heterozygous Familial Hypercholesterolemia in Pediatric Patients (10-17 years of age)

The recommended starting dose of Lipitor is 10 mg/day; the maximum recommended dose is 20 mg/day (doses greater than 20 mg have not been studied in this patient population). Doses should be individualized according to the recommended goal of therapy (see NCEP Pediatric Panel Guidelines[1], CLINICAL PHARMACOLOGY, and INDICATIONS AND USAGE). Adjustments should be made at intervals of 4 weeks or more.

[1] National Cholesterol Education Program (NCEP): Highlights of the Report of the Expert Panel on Blood Cholesterol Levels in Children Adolescents, *Pediatrics*. 89(3):495-501. 1992.

Homozygous Familial Hypercholesterolemia

The dosage of Lipitor in patients with homozygous FH is 10 to 80 mg daily. Lipitor should be used as an adjunct to other lipid-lowering treatments (eg, LDL apheresis) in these patients or if such treatments are unavailable.

Concomitant Therapy

Atorvastatin may be used in combination with a bile acid binding resin for additive effect. The combination of HMG-CoA reductase inhibitors and fibrates should generally be avoided (see WARNINGS, Skeletal Muscle, and PRECAUTIONS, Drug Interactions for other drug-drug interactions).

Dosage in Patients With Renal Insufficiency

Renal disease does not affect the plasma concentrations nor LDL-C reduction of atorvastatin; thus, dosage adjustment in patients with renal dysfunction is not necessary (see CLINICAL PHARMACOLOGY, Pharmacokinetics).

HOW SUPPLIED

Lipitor is supplied as white, elliptical, film-coated tablets of atorvastatin calcium containing 10, 20, 40 and 80 mg atorvastatin.

10 mg tablets: coded "PD 155" on one side and "10" on the other.
NDC 0071-0155-23 bottles of 90
NDC 0071-0155-34 bottles of 5000
NDC 0071-0155-40 10 × 10 unit dose blisters

20 mg tablets: coded "PD 156" on one side and "20" on the other.
NDC 0071-0156-23 bottles of 90
NDC 0071-0156-40 10 × 10 unit dose blisters
NDC 0071-0156-94 bottles of 5000

40 mg tablets: coded "PD 157" on one side and "40" on the other.
NDC 0071-0157-23 bottles of 90
NDC 0071-0157-73 bottles of 500

80 mg tablets: coded "PD 158" on one side and "80" on the other.
NDC 0071-0158-23 bottles of 90
NDC 0071-0158-73 bottles of 500

Storage

Store at controlled room temperature 20-25°C (68-77°F) [see USP].

Rx Only

Manufactured by:
Pfizer Ireland Pharmaceuticals
Dublin, Ireland
Distributed by:
Pfizer Parke-Davis
Division of Pfizer Inc, NY, NY 10017
69-5884-00-4 Revised August 2003

LOPID®

[lō'pĭd]

(Gemfibrozil Tablets, USP) ℞

Prescribing information for this product, which appears on pages 2554–2557 of the 2004 PDR, has been completely revised as follows. Please write "See Supplement A" next to the product heading.

DESCRIPTION

LOPID® (gemfibrozil tablets, USP) is a lipid regulating agent. It is available as tablets for oral administration. Each tablet contains 600 mg gemfibrozil. Each also contains calcium stearate, NF; candelilla wax, FCC; microcrystalline cellulose, NF; hydroxypropyl cellulose, NF; hypromellose, USP; methylparaben, NF; Opaspray white; polyethylene glycol, NF; polysorbate 80, NF; propylparaben, NF; colloidal silicon dioxide, NF; pregelatinized starch, NF. The chemical name is 5-(2,5-dimethylphenoxy)-2,2-dimethylpentanoic acid, with the following structural formula:

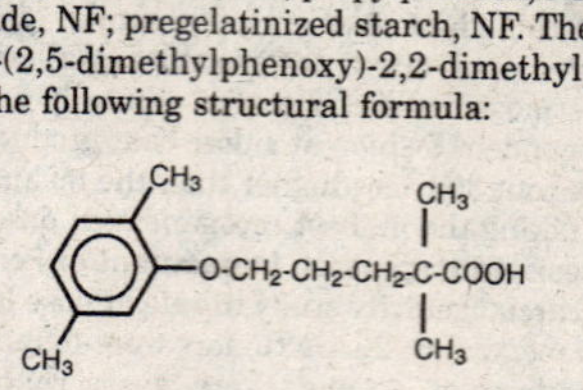

The empirical formula is $C_{15}H_{22}O_3$ and the molecular weight is 250.35; the solubility in water and acid is 0.0019% and in dilute base it is greater than 1%. The melting point is 58° -61° C. Gemfibrozil is a white solid which is stable under ordinary conditions.

CLINICAL PHARMACOLOGY

LOPID (gemfibrozil tablets, USP) is a lipid regulating agent which decreases serum triglycerides and very low density lipoprotein (VLDL) cholesterol, and increases high density lipoprotein (HDL) cholesterol. While modest decreases in total and low density lipoprotein (LDL) cholesterol may be observed with LOPID therapy, treatment of patients with elevated triglycerides due to Type IV hyperlipoproteinemia often results in a rise in LDL-cholesterol. LDL-cholesterol levels in Type IIb patients with elevations of both serum LDL-cholesterol and triglycerides are, in general, minimally affected by LOPID treatment; however, LOPID usually raises HDL-cholesterol significantly in this group. LOPID increases levels of high density lipoprotein (HDL) subfractions HDL_2 and HDL_3, as well as apolipoproteins AI and AII. Epidemiological studies have shown that both low HDL-cholesterol and high LDL-cholesterol are independent risk factors for coronary heart disease.

In the primary prevention component of the Helsinki Heart Study (refs. 1,2), in which 4081 male patients between the ages of 40 and 55 were studied in a randomized, double-blind, placebo-controlled fashion, LOPID therapy was associated with significant reductions in total plasma triglycerides and a significant increase in high density lipoprotein cholesterol. Moderate reductions in total plasma cholesterol and low density lipoprotein cholesterol were observed for the LOPID treatment group as a whole, but the lipid response was heterogeneous, especially among different Fredrickson types. The study involved subjects with serum non-HDL-cholesterol of over 200 mg/dL and no previous history of coronary heart disease. Over the five-year study period, the LOPID group experienced a 1.4% absolute (34% relative) reduction in the rate of serious coronary events (sudden cardiac deaths plus fatal and nonfatal myocardial infarctions) compared to placebo, p=0.04 (see Table I). There was a 37% relative reduction in the rate of nonfatal myocardial infarction compared to placebo, equivalent to a treatment-related difference of 13.1 events per thousand persons. Deaths from any cause during the double-blind portion of the study totaled 44 (2.2%) in the LOPID randomization group and 43 (2.1%) in the placebo group.

[See table I on next page]

Among Fredrickson types, during the 5-year double-blind portion of the primary prevention component of the Helsinki Heart Study, the greatest reduction in the incidence of serious coronary events occurred in Type IIb patients who had elevations of both LDL-cholesterol and total plasma triglycerides. This subgroup of Type IIb gemfibrozil group patients had a lower mean HDL-cholesterol level at baseline than the Type IIa subgroup that had elevations of LDL-cholesterol and normal plasma triglycerides. The mean increase in HDL-cholesterol among the Type IIb patients in this study was 12.6% compared to placebo. The mean change in LDL-cholesterol among Type IIb patients was –4.1% with LOPID compared to a rise of 3.9% in the placebo subgroup. The Type IIb subjects in the Helsinki Heart Study had 26 fewer coronary events per thousand persons over five years in the gemfibrozil group compared to placebo. The difference in coronary events was substantially greater between LOPID and placebo for that subgroup of patients with the triad of LDL-cholesterol >175 mg/dL (>4.5 mmol), triglycerides >200 mg/dL (>2.2 mmol), and HDL-cholesterol <35 mg/dL (<0.90 mmol) (see Table I).

Further information is available from a 3.5 year (8.5 year cumulative) follow-up of all subjects who had participated in the Helsinki Heart Study. At the completion of the Helsinki Heart Study, subjects could choose to start, stop, or continue to receive LOPID; without knowledge of their own lipid values or double-blind treatment, 60% of patients originally randomized to placebo began therapy with LOPID and 60% of patients originally randomized to LOPID continued medication. After approximately 6.5 years following randomization, all patients were informed of their original treatment group and lipid values during the five years of the double-blind treatment. After further elective changes in LOPID treatment status, 61% of patients in the group originally randomized to LOPID were taking drug; in the group originally randomized to placebo, 65% were taking LOPID. The event rate per 1000 occurring during the open-label follow-up period is detailed in Table II.

[See table II at bottom of next page]

Cumulative mortality through 8.5 years showed a 20% relative excess of deaths in the group originally randomized to LOPID versus the originally randomized placebo group and a 20% relative decrease in cardiac events in the group originally randomized to LOPID versus the originally randomized placebo group (see Table III). This analysis of the originally randomized "intent-to-treat" population neglects the possible complicating effects of treatment switching during the open-label phase. Adjustment of hazard ratios taking into account open-label treatment status from years 6.5 to 8.5 could change the reported hazard ratios for mortality toward unity.

[See table III at bottom of next page]

It is not clear to what extent the findings of the primary prevention component of the Helsinki Heart Study can be extrapolated to other segments of the dyslipidemic population not studied (such as women, younger or older males, or those with lipid abnormalities limited solely to HDL-cholesterol) or to other lipid-altering drugs.

The secondary prevention component of the Helsinki Heart Study was conducted over five years in parallel and at the same centers in Finland in 628 middle-aged males excluded from the primary prevention component of the Helsinki Heart Study because of a history of angina, myocardial infarction or unexplained ECG changes (ref. 3). The primary efficacy endpoint of the study was cardiac events (the sum of fatal and non-fatal myocardial infarctions and sudden cardiac deaths). The hazard ratio (LOPID:placebo) for cardiac events was 1.47 (95% confidence limits 0.88-2.48, p=0.14). Of the 35 patients in the LOPID group who experienced cardiac events, 12 patients suffered events after discontinuation from the study. Of the 24 patients in the placebo group with cardiac events, 4 patients suffered events after discontinuation from the study. There were 17 cardiac deaths in the LOPID group and 8 in the placebo group (hazard ratio 2.18; 95% confidence limits 0.94-5.05, p=0.06). Ten of these deaths in the LOPID group and 3 in the placebo group occurred after discontinuation from therapy. In this study of patients with known or suspected coronary heart disease, no benefit from LOPID treatment was observed in reducing cardiac events or cardiac deaths. Thus, LOPID has shown benefit only in selected dyslipidemic patients without suspected or established coronary heart disease. Even in patients with coronary heart disease and the triad of elevated LDL-cholesterol, elevated triglycerides, plus low HDL-cholesterol, the possible effect of LOPID on coronary events has not been adequately studied.

No efficacy in the patients with established coronary heart disease was observed during the Coronary Drug Project with the chemically and pharmacologically related drug, clofibrate. The Coronary Drug Project was a 6-year randomized, double-blind study involving 1000 clofibrate, 1000 nicotinic acid, and 3000 placebo patients with known coronary heart disease. A clinically and statistically significant reduction in myocardial infarctions was seen in the concurrent nicotinic acid group compared to placebo; no reduction was seen with clofibrate.

The mechanism of action of gemfibrozil has not been definitely established. In man, LOPID has been shown to inhibit peripheral lipolysis and to decrease the hepatic extraction of free fatty acids, thus reducing hepatic triglyceride production. LOPID inhibits synthesis and increases clearance of VLDL carrier apolipoprotein B, leading to a decrease in VLDL production.

Animal studies suggest that gemfibrozil may, in addition to elevating HDL-cholesterol, reduce incorporation of long-chain fatty acids into newly formed triglycerides, accelerate turnover and removal of cholesterol from the liver, and increase excretion of cholesterol in the feces. LOPID is well absorbed from the gastrointestinal tract after oral administration. Peak plasma levels occur in 1 to 2 hours with a plasma half-life of 1.5 hours following multiple doses.

Gemfibrozil is completely absorbed after oral administration of LOPID tablets, reaching peak plasma concentrations 1 to 2 hours after dosing. Gemfibrozil pharmacokinetics are affected by the timing of meals relative to time of dosing. In one study (ref. 4), both the rate and extent of absorption of the drug were significantly increased when administered 0.5 hour before meals. Average AUC was reduced by 14-44% when LOPID was administered after meals compared to 0.5 hour before meals. In a subsequent study (ref. 4), rate of absorption of LOPID was maximum when administered 0.5 hour before meals with the Cmax 50-60% greater than when given either with meals or fasting. In this study, there were no significant effects on AUC of timing of dose relative to meals (see DOSAGE AND ADMINISTRATION).

LOPID mainly undergoes oxidation of a ring methyl group to successively form a hydroxymethyl and a carboxyl metabolite. Approximately seventy percent of the administered human dose is excreted in the urine, mostly as the glucuronide conjugate, with less than 2% excreted as unchanged gemfibrozil. Six percent of the dose is accounted for in the feces. Gemfibrozil is highly bound to plasma proteins and there is potential for displacement interactions with other drugs (see PRECAUTIONS).

INDICATIONS AND USAGE

LOPID (gemfibrozil tablets, USP) is indicated as adjunctive therapy to diet for:

1. Treatment of adult patients with very high elevations of serum triglyceride levels (Types IV and V hyperlipidemia) who present a risk of pancreatitis and who do not respond adequately to a determined dietary effort to control them. Patients who present such risk typically have serum triglycerides over 2000 mg/dL and have elevations of VLDL-cholesterol as well as fasting chylomicrons (Type V hyperlipidemia). Subjects who consistently have total serum or plasma triglycerides below 1000 mg/dL are unlikely to present a risk of pancreatitis. LOPID therapy may be considered for those subjects with triglyceride elevations between 1000 and 2000 mg/dL who have a history of pancreatitis or of recurrent abdominal pain typical of pancreatitis. It is recognized that some Type IV patients with triglycerides under 1000 mg/dL may, through dietary or alcoholic indiscretion, convert to a Type V pattern with massive triglyceride elevations accompanying fasting chylomicronemia, but the influence of LOPID therapy on the risk of pancreatitis in such situations has not been adequately studied. Drug therapy is not indicated for patients with Type I hyperlipoproteinemia, who have elevations of chylomicrons and plasma triglycerides, but who have normal levels of very low density lipoprotein (VLDL). Inspection of plasma refrigerated for 14 hours is helpful in distinguishing Types I, IV, and V hyperlipoproteinemia (ref. 5).
2. Reducing the risk of developing coronary heart disease **only** in Type IIb patients without history of or symptoms of existing coronary heart disease who have had an inadequate response to weight loss, dietary therapy, exercise, and other pharmacologic agents (such as bile acid sequestrants and nicotinic acid, known to reduce LDL- and raise HDL-cholesterol) **and** who have the following triad of lipid abnormalities: low HDL-cholesterol levels in addition to elevated LDL-cholesterol and elevated triglycerides (see WARNINGS, PRECAUTIONS, and CLINICAL PHARMACOLOGY). The National Cholesterol Education Program has defined a serum HDL-cholesterol value that is consistently below 35 mg/dL as constituting an independent risk factor for coronary heart disease (ref. 6). Patients with significantly elevated triglycerides should be closely observed when treated with gemfibrozil. In some patients with high triglyceride levels, treatment with gemfibrozil is associated with a significant increase in LDL-cholesterol. BECAUSE OF POTENTIAL TOXICITY SUCH AS MALIGNANCY, GALLBLADDER DISEASE, ABDOMINAL PAIN LEADING TO APPENDECTOMY AND OTHER ABDOMINAL SURGERIES, AN INCREASED INCIDENCE IN NON-CORONARY MORTALITY, AND THE 44% RELATIVE INCREASE DURING THE TRIAL PERIOD IN AGE-ADJUSTED ALL-CAUSE MORTALITY SEEN WITH THE CHEMICALLY AND PHARMACOLOGICALLY RELATED DRUG, CLOFIBRATE, THE POTENTIAL BENEFIT OF GEMFIBROZIL IN TREATING TYPE IIA PATIENTS WITH ELEVATIONS OF LDL-CHOLESTEROL ONLY IS NOT LIKELY TO OUTWEIGH THE RISKS. LOPID IS ALSO NOT INDICATED FOR THE TREATMENT OF PATIENTS WITH LOW HDL-CHOLESTEROL AS THEIR ONLY LIPID ABNORMALITY.

In a subgroup analysis of patients in the Helsinki Heart Study with above-median HDL-cholesterol values at baseline (greater than 46.4 mg/dL), the incidence of serious coronary events was similar for gemfibrozil and placebo subgroups (see Table I).

The initial treatment for dyslipidemia is dietary therapy specific for the type of lipoprotein abnormality. Excess body weight and excess alcohol intake may be important factors in hypertriglyceridemia and should be managed prior to any drug therapy. Physical exercise can be an important ancillary measure, and has been associated with rises in HDL-cholesterol. Diseases contributory to hyperlipidemia such as hypothyroidism or diabetes mellitus should be looked for and adequately treated. Estrogen therapy is sometimes associated with massive rises in plasma triglycerides, especially in subjects with familial hypertriglyceridemia. In such cases, discontinuation of estrogen therapy may obviate the need for specific drug therapy of hypertriglyceridemia. The use of drugs should be considered only when reasonable attempts have been made to obtain satisfactory results with nondrug methods. If the decision is made to use drugs, the patient should be instructed that this does not reduce the importance of adhering to diet.

CONTRAINDICATIONS

1. Combination therapy of LOPID with cerivastatin due to the increased risk of myopathy and rhabdomyolysis (see WARNINGS).

2. Hepatic or severe renal dysfunction, including primary biliary cirrhosis.

3. Preexisting gallbladder disease (see WARNINGS).

4. Hypersensitivity to gemfibrozil.

WARNINGS

1. Because of chemical, pharmacological, and clinical similarities between gemfibrozil and clofibrate, the adverse findings with clofibrate in two large clinical studies may also apply to gemfibrozil. In the first of those studies, the Coronary Drug Project, 1000 subjects with previous myocardial infarction were treated for five years with clofibrate. There was no difference in mortality between the clofibrate-treated subjects and 3000 placebo-treated subjects, but twice as many clofibrate-treated subjects developed cholelithiasis and cholecystitis requiring surgery. In the other study, conducted by the World Health Organization (WHO), 5000 subjects without known coronary heart disease were treated with clofibrate for five years and followed one year beyond. There was a statistically significant, 44%, higher age-adjusted total mortality in the clofibrate-treated than in a comparable placebo-treated control group during the trial period. The excess mortality was due to a 33% increase in non-cardiovascular causes, including malignancy, post-cholecystectomy complications, and pancreatitis. The higher risk of clofibrate-treated subjects for gallbladder disease was confirmed.

Because of the more limited size of the Helsinki Heart Study, the observed difference in mortality from any cause between the LOPID and placebo group is not statistically significantly different from the 29% excess mortality reported in the clofibrate group in the separate WHO study at the nine year follow-up (see CLINICAL PHARMACOLOGY). Noncoronary heart disease related mortality showed an excess in the group originally randomized to LOPID primarily due to cancer deaths observed during the open-label extension.

During the five year primary prevention component of the Helsinki Heart Study, mortality from any cause was 44

Table I

Reduction in CHD Rates (events per 1000 patients) by Baseline Lipids[1] in the Helsinki Heart Study, Years 0-5[2]

	All Patients			LDL-C>175; HDL-C>46.4			LDL-C>175; TG>177			LDL-C>175; TG>200; HDL-C<35		
	P	L	Dif[3]	P	L	Dif	P	L	Dif	P	L	Dif
Incidence of Events[4]	41	27	14	32	29	3	71	44	27	149	64	85

[1]lipid values in mg/dL at baseline

[2]P = placebo group; L = LOPID group

[3]difference in rates between placebo and LOPID groups

[4]fatal and nonfatal myocardial infarctions plus sudden cardiac deaths (events per 1000 patients over 5 years)

Table II

Cardiac Events and All-Cause Mortality (events per 1000 patients) Occurring During the 3.5 Year Open-Label Follow-up to the Helsinki Heart Study[1]

Group:	PDrop N=215	PN N=494	PL N=1283	LDrop N=221	LN N=574	LL N=1207
Cardiac Events	38.8	22.9	22.5	37.2	28.3	25.4
All-Cause Mortality	41.9	22.3	15.6	72.3	19.2	24.9

[1]The six open-label groups are designated first by the original randomization (P = placebo, L = LOPID) and then by the drug taken in the follow-up period (N = Attend clinic but took no drug, L = LOPID, Drop = No attendance at clinic during open-label).

Table III

Cardiac Events, Cardiac Deaths, Non-Cardiac Deaths and All-Cause Mortality in the Helsinki Heart Study, Years 0-8.5[1]

Event	LOPID at Study Start	Placebo at Study Start	LOPID:Placebo Hazard Ratio[2]	CI Hazard Ratio[3]
Cardiac Events[4]	110	131	0.80	0.62-1.03
Cardiac Deaths	36	38	0.98	0.63-1.54
Non-Cardiac Deaths	65	45	1.40	0.95-2.05
All-Cause Mortality	101	83	1.20	0.90-1.61

[1]Intention-to-Treat Analysis of originally randomized patients neglecting the open-label treatment switches and exposure to study conditions.

[2]Hazard ration for risk event in the group originally randomized to LOPID compared to the group originally randomized to placebo neglecting open-label treatment switch and exposure to study condition.

[3]95% confidence intervals of LOPID:placebo group hazard ratio

[4]Fatal and non-fatal myocardial infarctions plus sudden cardiac deaths over the 8.5 year period.

Continued on next page

Lopid—Cont.

(2.2%) in the LOPID group and 43 (2.1%) in the placebo group; including the 3.5 year follow-up period since the trial was completed, cumulative mortality from any cause was 101 (4.9%) in the LOPID group and 83 (4.1%) in the group originally randomized to placebo (hazard ratio 1:20 in favor of placebo). Because of the more limited size of the Helsinki Heart Study, the observed difference in mortality from any cause between the LOPID and placebo groups at Year-5 or at Year-8.5 is not statistically significantly different from the 29% excess mortality reported in the clofibrate group in the separate WHO study at the nine year follow-up. Noncoronary heart disease related mortality showed an excess in the group originally randomized to LOPID at the 8.5 year follow-up (65 LOPID versus 45 placebo noncoronary deaths).

The incidence of cancer (excluding basal cell carcinoma) discovered during the trial and in the 3.5 years after the trial was completed was 51 (2.5%) in both originally randomized groups. In addition, there were 16 basal cell carcinomas in the group originally randomized to LOPID and 9 in the group randomized to placebo (p=0.22). There were 30 (1.5%) deaths attributed to cancer in the group originally randomized to LOPID and 18 (0.9%) in the group originally randomized to placebo (p=0.11). Adverse outcomes, including coronary events, were higher in gemfibrozil patients in a corresponding study in men with a history of known or suspected coronary heart disease in the secondary prevention component of the Helsinki Heart Study. (See CLINICAL PHARMACOLOGY.)

A comparative carcinogenicity study was also done in rats comparing three drugs in this class: fenofibrate (10 and 60 mg/kg; 0.3 and 1.6 times the human dose), clofibrate (400 mg/kg; 1.6 times the human dose), and gemfibrozil (250 mg/kg; 1.7 times the human dose). Pancreatic acinar adenomas were increased in males and females on fenofibrate; hepatocellular carcinoma and pancreatic acinar adenomas were increased in males and hepatic neoplastic nodules in females treated with clofibrate; hepatic neoplastic nodules were increased in males and females treated with clofibrate; hepatic neoplastic nodules were increased in males and females treated with gemfibrozil while testicular interstitial cell (Leydig cell) tumors were increased in males on all three drugs.

2. A gallstone prevalence substudy of 450 Helsinki Heart Study participants showed a trend toward a greater prevalence of gallstones during the study within the LOPID treatment group (7.5% vs 4.9% for the placebo group, a 55% excess for the gemfibrozil group). A trend toward a greater incidence of gallbladder surgery was observed for the LOPID group (17 vs 11 subjects, a 54% excess). This result did not differ statistically from the increased incidence of cholecystectomy observed in the WHO study in the group treated with clofibrate. Both clofibrate and gemfibrozil may increase cholesterol excretion into the bile leading to cholelithiasis. If cholelithiasis is suspected, gallbladder studies are indicated. LOPID therapy should be discontinued if gallstones are found. Cases of cholelithiasis have been reported with gemfibrozil therapy (ref. 7).

3. Since a reduction of mortality from coronary heart disease has not been demonstrated and because liver and interstitial cell testicular tumors were increased in rats, LOPID should be administered only to those patients described in the INDICATIONS AND USAGE section. If a significant serum lipid response is not obtained, LOPID should be discontinued.

4. Concomitant Anticoagulants–Caution should be exercised when anticoagulants are given in conjunction with LOPID. The dosage of the anticoagulant should be reduced to maintain the prothrombin time at the desired level to prevent bleeding complications. Frequent prothrombin determinations are advisable until it has been definitely determined that the prothrombin level has stabilized.

5. Concomitant therapy with LOPID and an HMG-CoA reductase inhibitor is associated with an increased risk of skeletal muscle toxicity manifested as rhabdomyolysis, markedly elevated creatine kinase (CPK) levels and myoglobinuria, leading in a high proportion of cases to acute renal failure and death. **Because of an observed marked increased risk of myopathy and rhabdomyolysis, the specific combination of LOPID and cerivastatin is absolutely contraindicated (see CONTRAINDICATIONS).** IN PATIENTS WHO HAVE HAD AN UNSATISFACTORY LIPID RESPONSE TO EITHER DRUG ALONE, THE BENEFIT OF COMBINED THERAPY WITH LOPID AND HMG-CoA REDUCTASE INHIBITORS OTHER THAN CERIVASTATIN DOES NOT OUTWEIGH THE RISKS OF SEVERE MYOPATHY, RHABDOMYOLYSIS, AND ACUTE RENAL FAILURE (refs. 8, 9, 10, 11) (see Drug Interactions). The use of fibrates alone, including LOPID, may occasionally be associated with myositis. Patients receiving LOPID and complaining of muscle pain, tenderness or weakness should have prompt medical evaluation for myositis, including serum creatine–kinase level determination. If myositis is suspected or diagnosed, LOPID therapy should be withdrawn.

6. Cataracts–Subcapsular bilateral cataracts occurred in 10%, and unilateral in 6.3%, of male rats treated with gemfibrozil at 10 times the human dose.

PRECAUTIONS

1. **Initial Therapy**—Laboratory studies should be done to ascertain that the lipid levels are consistently abnormal. Before instituting LOPID therapy, every attempt should be made to control serum lipids with appropriate diet, exercise, weight loss in obese patients, and control of any medical problems such as diabetes mellitus and hypothyroidism that are contributing to the lipid abnormalities.

2. **Continued Therapy**—Periodic determination of serum lipids should be obtained, and the drug withdrawn if lipid response is inadequate after three months of therapy.

3. **Drug Interactions**—(A) **HMG-CoA reductase inhibitors:** The risk of myopathy and rhabdomyolysis is increased with combined gemfibrozil and HMG-CoA reductase inhibitor therapy (see CONTRAINDICATIONS). Myopathy or rhabdomyolysis with or without acute renal failure have been reported as early as three weeks after initiation of combined therapy or after several months (refs. 8, 9, 10, 11). (See WARNINGS.) There is no assurance that periodic monitoring of creatine kinase will prevent the occurrence of severe myopathy and kidney damage.

(B) **Anticoagulants:** CAUTION SHOULD BE EXERCISED WHEN ANTICOAGULANTS ARE GIVEN IN CONJUNCTION WITH LOPID. THE DOSAGE OF THE ANTICOAGULANT SHOULD BE REDUCED TO MAINTAIN THE PROTHROMBIN TIME AT THE DESIRED LEVEL TO PREVENT BLEEDING COMPLICATIONS. FREQUENT PROTHROMBIN DETERMINATIONS ARE ADVISABLE UNTIL IT HAS BEEN DEFINITELY DETERMINED THAT THE PROTHROMBIN LEVEL HAS STABILIZED.

4. **Carcinogenesis, Mutagenesis, Impairment of Fertility**—Long-term studies have been conducted in rats at 0.2 and 1.3 times the human exposure (based on AUC). The incidence of benign liver nodules and liver carcinomas was significantly increased in high dose male rats. The incidence of liver carcinomas increased also in low dose males, but this increase was not statistically significant (p=0.1). Male rats had a dose-related and statistically significant increase of benign Leydig cell tumors. The higher dose female rats had a significant increase in the combined incidence of benign and malignant liver neoplasms.

Long-term studies have been conducted in mice at 0.1 and 0.7 times the human exposure (based on AUC). There were no statistically significant differences from controls in the incidence of liver tumors, but the doses tested were lower than those shown to be carcinogenic with other fibrates.

Electron microscopy studies have demonstrated a florid hepatic peroxisome proliferation following LOPID administration to the male rat. An adequate study to test for peroxisome proliferation has not been done in humans but changes in peroxisome morphology have been observed. Peroxisome proliferation has been shown to occur in humans with either of two other drugs of the fibrate class when liver biopsies were compared before and after treatment in the same individual.

Administration of approximately 2 times the human dose (based on surface area) to male rats for 10 weeks resulted in a dose-related decrease of fertility. Subsequent studies demonstrated that this effect was reversed after a drug-free period of about eight weeks, and it was not transmitted to the offspring.

5. **Pregnancy Category C**—LOPID has been shown to produce adverse effects in rats and rabbits at doses between 0.5 and 3 times the human dose (based on surface area). There are no adequate and well-controlled studies in pregnant women. LOPID should be used during pregnancy only if the potential benefit justifies the potential risk to the fetus.

Administration of LOPID to female rats at 2 times the human dose (based on surface area) before and throughout gestation caused a dose-related decrease in conception rate and, an increase in stillborns and a slight reduction in pup weight during lactation. There were also dose-related increased skeletal variations. Anophthalmia occurred, but rarely.

Administration of 0.6 and 2 times the human dose (based on surface area) of LOPID to female rats from gestation day 15 through weaning caused dose-related decreases in birth weight and suppressions of pup growth during lactation.

Administration of 1 and 3 times the human dose (based on surface area) of LOPID to female rabbits during organogenesis caused a dose-related decrease in litter size and, at the high dose, an increased incidence of parietal bone variations.

6. **Nursing Mothers**—It is not known whether this drug is excreted in human milk. Because many drugs are excreted in human milk and because of the potential for tumorigenicity shown for LOPID in animal studies, a decision should be made whether to discontinue nursing or to discontinue the drug, taking into account the importance of the drug to the mother.

7. **Hematologic Changes**—Mild hemoglobin, hematocrit and white blood cell decreases have been observed in occasional patients following initiation of LOPID therapy. However, these levels stabilize during long-term administration. Rarely, severe anemia, leukopenia, thrombocytopenia, and bone marrow hypoplasia have been reported. Therefore, periodic blood counts are recommended during the first 12 months of LOPID administration.

8. **Liver Function**—Abnormal liver function tests have been observed occasionally during LOPID administration, including elevations of AST (SGOT), ALT (SGPT), LDH, bilirubin, and alkaline phosphatase. These are usually reversible when LOPID is discontinued. Therefore, periodic liver function studies are recommended and LOPID therapy should be terminated if abnormalities persist.

9. **Kidney Function**—There have been reports of worsening renal insufficiency upon the addition of LOPID therapy in individuals with baseline plasma creatinine >2.0 mg/dL. In such patients, the use of alternative therapy should be considered against the risks and benefits of a lower dose of LOPID.

10. **Pediatric Use**—Safety and efficacy in pediatric patients have not been established.

ADVERSE REACTIONS

In the double-blind controlled phase of the primary prevention component of the Helsinki Heart Study, 2046 patients received LOPID for up to five years. In that study, the following adverse reactions were statistically more frequent in subjects in the LOPID group:

	LOPID (N = 2046)	PLACEBO (N = 2035)
	Frequency in percent of subjects	
Gastrointestinal reactions	34.2	23.8
Dyspepsia	19.6	11.9

	CAUSAL RELATIONSHIP PROBABLE	CAUSAL RELATIONSHIP NOT ESTABLISHED
General:		weight loss
Cardiac:		extrasystoles
Gastrointestinal:	cholestatic jaundice	pancreatitis hepatoma colitis
Central Nervous System:	dizziness somnolence paresthesia peripheral neuritis decreased libido depression headache	confusion convulsions syncope
Eye:	blurred vision	retinal edema
Genitourinary:	impotence	decreased male fertility renal dysfunction
Musculoskeletal:	myopathy myasthenia myalgia painful extremities arthralgia synovitis rhabdomyolysis (see WARNINGS and Drug Interactions under PRECAUTIONS)	
Clinical Laboratory:	increased creatine phosphokinase increased bilirubin increased liver transaminases (AST [SGOT], ALT [SGPT]) increased alkaline phosphatase	positive antinuclear antibody
Hematopoietic:	anemia leukopenia bone marrow hypoplasia eosinophilia	thrombocytopenia
Immunologic:	angioedema laryngeal edema urticaria	anaphylaxis Lupus-like syndrome vasculitis
Integumentary:	exfoliative dermatitis rash dermatitis pruritus	alopecia photosensitivity

Abdominal pain	9.8	5.6
Acute appendicitis (histologically confirmed in most cases where data were available)	1.2	0.6
Atrial fibrillation	0.7	0.1
Adverse events reported by more than 1% of subjects, but without a significant difference between groups:		
Diarrhea	7.2	6.5
Fatigue	3.8	3.5
Nausea/Vomiting	2.5	2.1
Eczema	1.9	1.2
Rash	1.7	1.3
Vertigo	1.5	1.3
Constipation	1.4	1.3
Headache	1.2	1.1

Gallbladder surgery was performed in 0.9% of LOPID and 0.5% of placebo subjects in the primary prevention component, a 64% excess, which is not statistically different from the excess of gallbladder surgery observed in the clofibrate compared to the placebo group of the WHO study. Gallbladder surgery was also performed more frequently in the LOPID group compared to placebo (1.9% vs 0.3%, p=0.07) in the secondary prevention component. A statistically significant increase in appendectomy in the gemfibrozil group was seen also in the secondary prevention component (6 on gemfibrozil vs 0 on placebo, p=0.014).

Nervous system and special senses adverse reactions were more common in the LOPID group. These included hypesthesia, paresthesias, and taste perversion. Other adverse reactions that were more common among LOPID treatment group subjects but where a causal relationship was not established include cataracts, peripheral vascular disease, and intracerebral hemorrhage.

From other studies it seems probable that LOPID is causally related to the occurrence of MUSCULOSKELETAL SYMPTOMS (see WARNINGS), and to ABNORMAL LIVER FUNCTION TESTS and HEMATOLOGIC CHANGES (see PRECAUTIONS).

Reports of viral and bacterial infections (common cold, cough, urinary tract infections) were more common in gemfibrozil treated patients in other controlled clinical trials of 805 patients. Additional adverse reactions that have been reported for gemfibrozil are listed below by system. These are categorized according to whether a causal relationship to treatment with LOPID is probable or not established:

[See table at top of previous page]

Additional adverse reactions that have been reported include cholecystitis and cholelithiasis (ref. 12) (see WARNINGS).

DOSAGE AND ADMINISTRATION

The recommended dose for adults is 1200 mg administered in two divided doses 30 minutes before the morning and evening meal (see CLINICAL PHARMACOLOGY).

OVERDOSAGE

There have been reported cases of overdosage with LOPID. In one case, a 7-year-old child recovered after ingesting up to 9 grams of LOPID. Symptoms reported with overdosage were abdominal cramps, abnormal liver function tests, diarrhea, increased CPK, joint and muscle pain, nausea and vomiting. Symptomatic supportive measures should be taken, should an overdose occur.

HOW SUPPLIED

LOPID (Tablet 737), white, elliptical, film-coated, scored tablets, each containing 600 mg gemfibrozil, are available as follows:

N 0071-0737-20: Bottles of 60

N 0071-0737-30: Bottles of 500

Parcode® No. 737

Store at controlled room temperature 20°–25°C (68°–77°F) [see USP]. Protect from light and humidity.

REFERENCES

1. Frick MH, Elo O, Haapa K, et al: Helsinki Heart Study: Primary prevention trial with gemfibrozil in middle-aged men with dyslipidemia. *N Engl J Med* 1987; 317:1237-1245.
2. Manninen V, Elo O, Frick MH, et al: Lipid alterations and decline in the incidence of coronary heart disease in the Helsinki Heart Study. *JAMA* 1988; 260:641-651.
3. Frick MH, Heinonen OP, et al: Efficacy of gemfibrozil in dyslipidemic subjects with suspected heart disease. An ancillary study in the Helsinki Heart Study frame population. *Annals of Medicine* 1993; 25:41-45.
4. Data on file. Parke-Davis; Morris Plains, NJ.
5. Nikkila EA: Familial lipoprotein lipase deficiency and related disorders of chylomicron metabolism. In Stanbury JB et al. (eds.): *The Metabolic Basis of Inherited Disease*, 5th ed., McGraw-Hill, 1983, Chap. 30, pp. 622-642.
6. Report of the National Cholesterol Education Program Expert Panel on Detection, Evaluation, and Treatment of High Blood Cholesterol. *Arch Int Med* 1988;148:36-69.
7. Data on file. Pfizer; NY, NY.
8. Pierce LR, Wysowski DK, Gross TP. Myopathy and rhabdomyolysis associated with lovastatin/gemfibrozil combination therapy. *JAMA* 1990;264:71-75.
9. Bermingham RP, Whitsitt TB, Smart ML et al. Rhabdomyolysis in a patient receiving the combination of cerivastatin and gemfibrozil. Am J Health-Syst Pharm 2000;57:461-464.
10. Duell PB, Connor WE, Illingworth DR. Rhabdomyolysis after taking atorvastatin with gemfibrozil. Am J Cardiol 1998;81:368-369.
11. Tal A, Rajeshawari M, Isley W. Rhabdomyolysis associated with simvastatin/gemfibrozil therapy. South Med J 1997;90:546-547.
12. Data on file. Pfizer; NY, NY.

℞ only

Revised August 2003

Manufactured by:

Pfizer Pharmaceuticals, Ltd.

Vega Baja, PR 00694

Distributed by:

PARKE-DAVIS

Division of Pfizer Inc, NY, NY 10017

69-5829-00-3

NARDIL® ℞

[*när-dĭl*]

(Phenelzine Sulfate Tablets, USP)

Prescribing information for this product, which appears on pages 2557–2559 of the 2004 PDR, has been completely revised as follows. Please write "See Supplement A" next to the product heading.

DESCRIPTION

NARDIL® (phenelzine sulfate) is a potent inhibitor of monoamine oxidase (MAO). Phenelzine sulfate is a hydrazine derivative. It has a molecular weight of 234.27 and is chemically described as $C_8H_{12}N_2 \bullet H_2SO_4$. Its chemical structure is shown below:

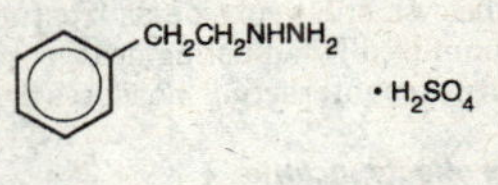

Molecular weight: 234.27

Each NARDIL film-coated tablet for oral administration contains phenelzine sulfate equivalent to 15 mg of phenelzine base and the following inactive ingredients: mannitol, USP; croscarmellose sodium, NF; povidone, USP; edetate disodium, USP; magnesium stearate, NF; isopropyl alcohol, USP; purified water, USP; opadry orange Y30-13242A; simethicone emulsion, USP.

CLINICAL PHARMACOLOGY

Monoamine oxidase is a complex enzyme system, widely distributed throughout the body. Drugs that inhibit monoamine oxidase in the laboratory are associated with a number of clinical effects. Thus, it is unknown whether MAO inhibition per se, other pharmacologic actions, or an interaction of both is responsible for the clinical effects observed. Therefore, the physician should become familiar with all the effects produced by drugs of this class.

INDICATIONS AND USAGE

NARDIL has been found to be effective in depressed patients clinically characterized as "atypical," "nonendogenous," or "neurotic." These patients often have mixed anxiety and depression and phobic or hypochondriacal features. There is less conclusive evidence of its usefulness with severely depressed patients with endogenous features.

NARDIL should rarely be the first antidepressant drug used. Rather, it is more suitable for use with patients who have failed to respond to the drugs more commonly used for these conditions.

CONTRAINDICATIONS

NARDIL should not be used in patients who are hypersensitive to the drug or its ingredients, with pheochromocytoma, congestive heart failure, a history of liver disease, or abnormal liver function tests.

The potentiation of sympathomimetic substances and related compounds by MAO inhibitors may result in hypertensive crises (see WARNINGS). Therefore, patients being treated with NARDIL should not take sympathomimetic drugs (including amphetamines, cocaine, methylphenidate, dopamine, epinephrine, and norepinephrine) or related compounds (including methyldopa, L-dopa, L-tryptophan, L-tyrosine, and phenylalanine). Hypertensive crises during NARDIL therapy may also be caused by the ingestion of foods with a high concentration of tyramine or dopamine. Therefore, patients being treated with NARDIL should avoid high protein food that has undergone protein breakdown by aging, fermentation, pickling, smoking, or bacterial contamination. Patients should also avoid cheeses (especially aged varieties), pickled herring, beer, wine, liver, yeast extract (including brewer's yeast in large quantities), dry sausage (including Genoa salami, hard salami, pepperoni, and Lebanon bologna), pods of broad beans (fava beans), and yogurt. Excessive amounts of caffeine and chocolate may also cause hypertensive reactions.

NARDIL should not be used in combination with dextromethorphan or with CNS depressants such as alcohol and certain narcotics. Excitation, seizures, delirium, hyperpyrexia, circulatory collapse, coma, and death have been reported in patients receiving MAOI therapy who have been given a single dose of meperidine. NARDIL should not be administered together with or in rapid succession to other MAO inhibitors because HYPERTENSIVE CRISES and convulsive seizures, fever, marked sweating, excitation, delirium, tremor, coma, and circulatory collapse may occur.

A List of MAO Inhibitors by Generic Name Follows:

pargyline hydrochloride
pargyline hydrochloride
  and methylclothiazide
furazolidone
isocarboxazid
procarbazine
tranylcypromine

NARDIL should also not be used in combination with buspirone HCl, since several cases of elevated blood pressure have been reported in patients taking MAO inhibitors who were then given buspirone HCl. At least 10 days should elapse between the discontinuation of NARDIL and the institution of another antidepressant or buspirone HCl, or the discontinuation of another MAO inhibitor and the institution of NARDIL.

There have been reports of serious reactions (including hyperthermia, rigidity, myoclonic movements and death) when serotoninergic drugs (e.g., dexfenfluramine, fluoxetine, fluvoxamine, paroxetine, sertraline, citalopram, venlafaxine) have been combined with an MAO inhibitor. Therefore, the concomitant use of NARDIL with serotoninergic agents is contraindicated (see PRECAUTIONS-Drug Interactions). Allow at least five weeks between discontinuation of fluoxetine and initiation of NARDIL and at least 10 days between discontinuation of NARDIL and initiation of fluoxetine, or other serotoninergic agents. Before initiating NARDIL after using other serotoninergic agents, a sufficient amount of time must be allowed for clearance of the serotoninergic agent and its active metabolites.

The combination of MAO inhibitors and tryptophan has been reported to cause behavioral and neurologic syndromes including disorientation, confusion, amnesia, delirium, agitation, hypomanic signs, ataxia, myoclonus, hyperreflexia, shivering, ocular oscillations, and Babinski signs.

The concurrent administration of an MAO inhibitor and bupropion hydrochloride (Wellbutrin®) is contraindicated. At least 14 days should elapse between discontinuation of an MAO inhibitor and initiation of treatment with bupropion hydrochloride.

Patients taking NARDIL should not undergo elective surgery requiring general anesthesia. Also, they should not be given cocaine or local anesthesia containing sympathomimetic vasoconstrictors. The possible combined hypotensive effects of NARDIL and spinal anesthesia should be kept in mind. NARDIL should be discontinued at least 10 days prior to elective surgery.

MAO inhibitors, including NARDIL, are contraindicated in patients receiving guanethidine.

WARNINGS

The most serious reactions to NARDIL involve changes in blood pressure.

Hypertensive Crises: The most important reaction associated with NARDIL administration is the occurrence of hypertensive crises, which have sometimes been fatal.

These crises are characterized by some or all of the following symptoms: occipital headache which may radiate frontally, palpitation, neck stiffness or soreness, nausea, vomiting, sweating (sometimes with fever and sometimes with cold, clammy skin), dilated pupils, and photophobia. Either tachycardia or bradycardia may be present and can be associated with constricting chest pain.

NOTE: Intracranial bleeding has been reported in association with the increase in blood pressure.

Blood pressure should be observed frequently to detect evidence of any pressor response in all patients receiving NARDIL. Therapy should be discontinued immediately upon the occurrence of palpitation or frequent headaches during therapy.

Recommended treatment in hypertensive crisis: If a hypertensive crisis occurs, NARDIL should be discontinued immediately and therapy to lower blood pressure should be instituted immediately. On the basis of present evidence, phentolamine is recommended. (The dosage reported for phentolamine is 5 mg intravenously.) Care should be taken to administer this drug slowly in order to avoid producing an excessive hypotensive effect. Fever should be managed by means of external cooling.

Warning to the Patient: All patients should be warned that the following foods, beverages, and medications must be avoided while taking NARDIL, and for two weeks after discontinuing use.

Foods and Beverages To Avoid

Meat and Fish
- Pickled herring
- Liver
- Dry sausage (including Genoa salami, hard salami, pepperoni, and Lebanon bologna)

Vegetables
- Broad bean pods (fava bean pods)
- Sauerkraut

Dairy Products
- Cheese (cottage cheese and cream cheese are allowed)
- Yogurt

Beverages
- Beer and wine
- Alcohol-free and reduced-alcohol beer and wine products

Miscellaneous
- Yeast extract (including brewer's yeast in large quantities)
- Meat extract
- Excessive amounts of chocolate and caffeine

Continued on next page

Nardil—Cont.

Also, any spoiled or improperly refrigerated, handled, or stored protein-rich foods such as meats, fish, and dairy products, including foods that may have undergone protein changes by aging, pickling, fermentation, or smoking to improve flavor should be avoided.

OTC Medications To Avoid

Cold and cough preparations (including those containing dextromethorphan)
Nasal decongestants (tablets, drops, or spray)
Hay-fever medications
Sinus medications
Asthma inhalant medications
Antiappetite medicines
Weight-reducing preparations
"Pep" pills
L-tryptophan containing preparations

Also, certain prescription drugs should be avoided. Therefore, patients under the care of another physician or dentist should inform him/her that they are taking NARDIL.

Patients should be warned that the use of the above foods, beverages, or medications may cause a reaction characterized by headache and other serious symptoms due to a rise in blood pressure, with the exception of dextromethorphan which may cause reactions similar to those seen with meperidine. Also, there has been a report of an interaction between NARDIL and dextromethorphan (ingested as a lozenge) causing drowsiness and bizarre behavior.

Patients should be instructed to report promptly the occurrence of headache or other unusual symptoms.

Concomitant Use with Dibenzazepine Derivative Drugs

If the decision is made to administer NARDIL concurrently with other antidepressant drugs, or within less than 10 days after discontinuation of antidepressant therapy, the patient should be cautioned by the physician regarding the possibility of adverse drug interaction.

A List of Dibenzazepine Derivative Drugs by Generic Name Follows:

nortriptyline hydrochloride
amitriptyline hydrochloride
perphenazine andamitriptyline hydrochloride
clomipramine hydrochloride
desipramine hydrochloride
imipramine hydrochloride
doxepin
carbamazepine
cyclobenzaprine HCl
amoxapine
maprotiline HCl
trimipramine maleate
protriptyline HCl
mirtazapine

NARDIL should be used with caution in combination with antihypertensive drugs, including thiazide diuretics and β-blockers, since exaggerated hypotensive effects may result.

Use in Pregnancy: The safe use of NARDIL during pregnancy or lactation has not been established. The potential benefit of this drug, if used during pregnancy, lactation, or in women of childbearing age, should be weighed against the possible hazard to the mother or fetus.

Doses of NARDIL in pregnant mice well exceeding the maximum recommended human dose have caused a significant decrease in the number of viable offspring per mouse. In addition, the growth of young dogs and rats has been retarded by doses exceeding the maximum human dose.

Use in Pediatric Patients: NARDIL is not recommended for pediatric patients under 16 years of age, since there are no controlled studies of safety in this age group. NARDIL, as with other hydrazine derivatives, has been reported to induce pulmonary and vascular tumors in an uncontrolled lifetime study in mice.

PRECAUTIONS

In depressed patients, the possibility of suicide should always be considered and adequate precautions taken. It is recommended that careful observations of patients undergoing NARDIL treatment be maintained until control of depression is achieved. If necessary, additional measures (ECT, hospitalization, etc) should be instituted.

All patients undergoing treatment with NARDIL should be closely followed for symptoms of postural hypotension. Hypotensive side effects have occurred in hypertensive as well as normotensive and hypotensive patients. Blood pressure usually returns to pretreatment levels rapidly when the drug is discontinued or the dosage is reduced.

Because the effect of NARDIL on the convulsive threshold may be variable, adequate precautions should be taken when treating epileptic patients.

Of the more severe side effects that have been reported with any consistency, hypomania has been the most common. This reaction has been largely limited to patients in whom disorders characterized by hyperkinetic symptoms coexist with, but are obscured by, depressive affect; hypomania usually appeared as depression improved. If agitation is present, it may be increased with NARDIL. Hypomania and agitation have also been reported at higher than recommended doses or following long-term therapy.

NARDIL may cause excessive stimulation in schizophrenic patients; in manic-depressive states it may result in a swing from a depressive to a manic phase.

MAO inhibitors, including NARDIL, potentiate hexobarbital hypnosis in animals. Therefore, barbiturates should be given at a reduced dose with NARDIL.

MAO inhibitors inhibit the destruction of serotonin and norepinephrine, which are believed to be released from tissue stores by rauwolfia alkaloids. Accordingly, caution should be exercised when rauwolfia is used concomitantly with an MAO inhibitor, including NARDIL.

There is conflicting evidence as to whether or not MAO inhibitors affect glucose metabolism or potentiate hypoglycemic agents. This should be kept in mind if NARDIL is administered to diabetics.

Drug Interactions

In patients receiving nonselective monoamine oxidase (MAO) inhibitors in combination with serotoninergic agents (e.g., dexfenfluramine, fluoxetine, fluvoxamine, paroxetine, sertraline, citalopram, venlafaxine) there have been reports of serious, sometimes fatal, reactions. Because NARDIL is a monoamine oxidase (MAO) inhibitor, NARDIL should not be used concomitantly with a serotoninergic agent (See CONTRAINDICATIONS).

Geriatric Use

Clinical studies of NARDIL did not include sufficient numbers of subjects aged 65 and over to determine whether they respond differently from younger subjects. Other reported clinical experience has not identified differences in responses between the elderly and younger patients. In general, dose selection for an elderly patient should be cautious, usually starting at the low end of the dosing range, reflecting the greater frequency of decreased hepatic, renal, or cardiac function, and of concomitant disease or other drug therapy.

ADVERSE REACTIONS

NARDIL is a potent inhibitor of monoamine oxidase. Because this enzyme is widely distributed throughout the body, diverse pharmacologic effects can be expected to occur. When they occur, such effects tend to be mild or moderate in severity (see below), often subside as treatment continues, and can be minimized by adjusting dosage; rarely is it necessary to institute counteracting measures or to discontinue NARDIL.

Common side effects include:

Nervous System—Dizziness, headache, drowsiness, sleep disturbances (including insomnia and hypersomnia), fatigue, weakness, tremors, twitching, myoclonic movements, hyperreflexia.

Gastrointestinal—Constipation, dry mouth, gastrointestinal disturbances, elevated serum transaminases (without accompanying signs and symptoms).

Metabolic—Weight gain.

Cardiovascular—Postural hypotension, edema.

Genitourinary—Sexual disturbances, eg, anorgasmia and ejaculatory disturbances and impotence.

Less common mild to moderate side effects (some of which have been reported in a single patient or by a single physician) include:

Nervous System—Jitteriness, palilalia, euphoria, nystagmus, paresthesias.

Genitourinary—Urinary retention.

Metabolic—Hypernatremia.

Dermatologic—Pruritus, skin rash, sweating.

Special Senses—Blurred vision, glaucoma.

Although reported less frequently, and sometimes only once, additional severe side effects include:

Nervous System—Ataxia, shock-like coma, toxic delirium, manic reaction, convulsions, acute anxiety reaction, precipitation of schizophrenia, transient respiratory and cardiovascular depression following ECT.

Gastrointestinal—To date, fatal progressive necrotizing hepatocellular damage has been reported in very few patients. Reversible jaundice.

Hematologic—Leukopenia.

Immunologic—Lupus-like syndrome

Metabolic—Hypermetabolic syndrome (which may include, but is not limited to, hyperpyrexia, tachycardia, tachypnea, muscular rigidity, elevated CK levels, metabolic acidosis, hypoxia, coma and may resemble an overdose).

Respiratory—Edema of the glottis.

General—Fever associated with increased muscle tone.

Withdrawal may be associated with nausea, vomiting, and malaise.

An uncommon withdrawal syndrome following abrupt withdrawal of NARDIL has been infrequently reported. Signs and symptoms of this syndrome generally commence 24 to 72 hours after drug discontinuation and may range from vivid nightmares with agitation to frank psychosis and convulsions. This syndrome generally responds to reinstitution of low-dose NARDIL therapy followed by cautious downward titration and discontinuation.

DOSAGE AND ADMINISTRATION

Initial dose: The usual starting dose of NARDIL is one tablet (15 mg) three times a day.

Early phase treatment: Dosage should be increased to at least 60 mg per day at a fairly rapid pace consistent with patient tolerance. It may be necessary to increase dosage up to 90 mg per day to obtain sufficient MAO inhibition. Many patients do not show a clinical response until treatment at 60 mg has been continued for at least 4 weeks.

Maintenance dose: After maximum benefit from NARDIL is achieved, dosage should be reduced slowly over several weeks. Maintenance dose may be as low as one tablet, 15 mg, a day or every other day, and should be continued for as long as is required.

OVERDOSAGE

Note—For management of *hypertensive crises* see WARNINGS section.

Accidental or intentional overdosage may be more common in patients who are depressed. It should be remembered that multiple drugs and/or alcohol may have been ingested. Depending on the amount of overdosage with NARDIL, a varying and mixed clinical picture may develop, including signs and symptoms of central nervous system and cardiovascular stimulation and/or depression. Signs and symptoms may be absent or minimal during the initial 12-hour period following ingestion and may develop slowly thereafter, reaching a maximum in 24-48 hours. Death has been reported following overdosage. Therefore, immediate hospitalization, with continuous patient observation and monitoring throughout this period, is essential.

Signs and symptoms of overdosage may include, alone or in combination, any of the following: drowsiness, dizziness, faintness, irritability, hyperactivity, agitation, severe headache, hallucinations, trismus, opisthotonus, rigidity, convulsions, and coma; rapid and irregular pulse, hypertension, hypotension, and vascular collapse; precordial pain, respiratory depression and failure, hyperpyrexia, diaphoresis, and cool, clammy skin.

Treatment

Intensive symptomatic and supportive treatment may be required. Induction of emesis or gastric lavage with instillation of charcoal slurry may be helpful in early poisoning, provided the airway has been protected against aspiration. Signs and symptoms of central nervous system stimulation, including convulsions, should be treated with diazepam, given slowly intravenously. Phenothiazine derivatives and central nervous system stimulants should be avoided. Hypotension and vascular collapse should be treated with intravenous fluids and, if necessary, blood pressure titration with an intravenous infusion of dilute pressor agent. It should be noted that adrenergic agents may produce a markedly increased pressor response.

Respiration should be supported by appropriate measures, including management of the airway, use of supplemental oxygen, and mechanical ventilatory assistance, as required. Body temperature should be monitored closely. Intensive management of hyperpyrexia may be required. Maintenance of fluid and electrolyte balance is essential.

There are no data on the lethal dose in man. The pathophysiologic effects of massive overdosage may persist for several days, since the drug acts by inhibiting physiologic enzyme systems. With symptomatic and supportive measures, recovery from *mild* overdosage may be expected within 3 to 4 days.

Hemodialysis, peritoneal dialysis, and charcoal hemoperfusion may be of value in massive overdosage, but sufficient data are not available to recommend their routine use in these cases.

Toxic blood levels of phenelzine have not been established, and assay methods are not practical for clinical or toxicological use.

HOW SUPPLIED

Each NARDIL tablet is orange, biconvex, film-coated, and engraved with "P-D 270" and contains phenelzine sulfate equivalent to 15 mg of phenelzine base.
NDC 0071-0350-24. Bottle of 100

Storage:
Store between 15° - 30°C (59° - 86°F).

Rx only

Revised May 2003
Distributed by:
Pfizer
Parke-Davis
Div of Pfizer Inc, NY, NY 10017 ©2003, Warner-Lambert Co.
69-5985-00-3

NEURONTIN® ℞
(gabapentin) Capsules

NEURONTIN®
(gabapentin) Tablets

NEURONTIN®
(gabapentin) Oral Solution

Prescribing information for this product, which appears on pages 2559–2564 of the 2004 PDR, has been completely revised as follows. Please write "See Supplement A" next to the product heading.

DESCRIPTION

Neurontin® (gabapentin) Capsules, Neurontin® (gabapentin) Tablets, and Neurontin® (gabapentin) Oral Solution are supplied as imprinted hard shell capsules containing 100 mg, 300 mg, and 400 mg of gabapentin, elliptical film-coated tablets containing 600 mg and 800 mg of gabapentin or an oral solution containing 250 mg/5 mL of gabapentin.

The inactive ingredients for the capsules are lactose, cornstarch, and talc. The 100 mg capsule shell contains gelatin and titanium dioxide. The 300 mg capsule shell contains gelatin, titanium dioxide, and yellow iron oxide. The 400 mg capsule shell contains gelatin, red iron oxide, titanium dioxide, and yellow iron oxide. The imprinting ink contains FD&C Blue No. 2 and titanium dioxide.

The inactive ingredients for the tablets are poloxamer 407, copolyvidonum, cornstarch, magnesium stearate, hydroxypropyl cellulose, talc, candelilla wax and purified water.

The inactive ingredients for the oral solution are glycerin, xylitol, purified water and artificial cool strawberry anise flavor.

Gabapentin is described as 1-(aminomethyl)cyclohexaneacetic acid with a molecular formula of $C_9H_{17}NO_2$ and a molecular weight of 171.24. The structural formula of gabapentin is:

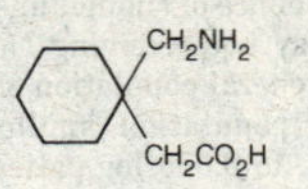

Gabapentin is a white to off-white crystalline solid with a pK_{a1} of 3.7 and a pK_{a2} of 10.7. It is freely soluble in water and both basic and acidic aqueous solutions. The log of the partition coefficient (n-octanol/0.05M phosphate buffer) at pH 7.4 is –1.25.

CLINICAL PHARMACOLOGY

Mechanism of Action

The mechanism by which gabapentin exerts its analgesic action is unknown, but in animal models of analgesia, gabapentin prevents allodynia (pain-related behavior in response to a normally innocuous stimulus) and hyperalgesia (exaggerated response to painful stimuli). In particular, gabapentin prevents pain-related responses in several models of neuropathic pain in rats or mice (e.g. spinal nerve ligation models, streptozocin-induced diabetes model, spinal cord injury model, acute herpes zoster infection model). Gabapentin also decreases pain-related responses after peripheral inflammation (carrageenan footpad test, late phase of formalin test). Gabapentin did not alter immediate pain-related behaviors (rat tail flick test, formalin footpad acute phase, acetic acid abdominal constriction test, footpad heat irradiation test). The relevance of these models to human pain is not known.

The mechanism by which gabapentin exerts its anticonvulsant action is unknown, but in animal test systems designed to detect anticonvulsant activity, gabapentin prevents seizures as do other marketed anticonvulsants. Gabapentin exhibits antiseizure activity in mice and rats in both the maximal electroshock and pentylenetetrazole seizure models and other preclinical models (e.g., strains with genetic epilepsy, etc.). The relevance of these models to human epilepsy is not known.

Gabapentin is structurally related to the neurotransmitter GABA (gamma-aminobutyric acid) but it does not modify $GABA_A$ or $GABA_B$ radioligand binding, it is not converted metabolically into GABA or a GABA agonist, and it is not an inhibitor of GABA uptake or degradation. Gabapentin was tested in radioligand binding assays at concentrations up to 100 μM and did not exhibit affinity for a number of other common receptor sites, including benzodiazepine, glutamate, N-methyl-D-aspartate (NMDA), quisqualate, kainate, strychnine-insensitive or strychnine-sensitive glycine, alpha 1, alpha 2, or beta adrenergic, adenosine A1 or A2, cholinergic muscarinic or nicotinic, dopamine D1 or D2, histamine H1, serotonin S1 or S2, opiate mu, delta or kappa, cannabinoid 1, voltage-sensitive calcium channel sites labeled with nitrendipine or diltiazem, or at voltage-sensitive sodium channel sites labeled with batrachotoxinin A 20-alpha-benzoate. Furthermore, gabapentin did not alter the cellular uptake of dopamine, noradrenaline, or serotonin.

In vitro studies with radiolabeled gabapentin have revealed a gabapentin binding site in areas of rat brain including neocortex and hippocampus. A high-affinity binding protein in animal brain tissue has been identified as an auxiliary subunit of voltage-activated calcium channels. However, functional correlates of gabapentin binding, if any, remain to be elucidated.

Pharmacokinetics and Drug Metabolism

All pharmacological actions following gabapentin administration are due to the activity of the parent compound; gabapentin is not appreciably metabolized in humans.

Oral Bioavailability: Gabapentin bioavailability is not dose proportional; i.e., as dose is increased, bioavailability decreases. Bioavailability of gabapentin is approximately 60%, 47%, 34%, 33%, and 27% following 900, 1200, 2400, 3600, and 4800 mg/day given in 3 divided doses, respectively. Food has only a slight effect on the rate and extent of absorption of gabapentin (14% increase in AUC and C_{max}).

Distribution: Less than 3% of gabapentin circulates bound to plasma protein. The apparent volume of distribution of gabapentin after 150 mg intravenous administration is 58±6 L (Mean±SD). In patients with epilepsy, steady-state predose (C_{min}) concentrations of gabapentin in cerebrospinal fluid were approximately 20% of the corresponding plasma concentrations.

Elimination: Gabapentin is eliminated from the systemic circulation by renal excretion as unchanged drug. Gabapentin is not appreciably metabolized in humans.

Gabapentin elimination half-life is 5 to 7 hours and is unaltered by dose or following multiple dosing. Gabapentin elimination rate constant, plasma clearance, and renal clearance are directly proportional to creatinine clearance (see Special Populations: Patients With Renal Insufficiency, below). In elderly patients, and in patients with impaired renal function, gabapentin plasma clearance is reduced. Gabapentin can be removed from plasma by hemodialysis.

Dosage adjustment in patients with compromised renal function or undergoing hemodialysis is recommended (see DOSAGE AND ADMINISTRATION, Table 5).

Special Populations: *Adult Patients With Renal Insufficiency:* Subjects (N=60) with renal insufficiency (mean creatinine clearance ranging from 13-114 mL/min) were administered single 400 mg oral doses of gabapentin. The mean gabapentin half-life ranged from about 6.5 hours (patients with creatinine clearance >60 mL/min) to 52 hours (creatinine clearance <30 mL/min) and gabapentin renal clearance from about 90 mL/min (>60 mL/min group) to about 10 mL/min (<30 mL/min). Mean plasma clearance (CL/F) decreased from approximately 190 mL/min to 20 mL/min.

Dosage adjustment in adult patients with compromised renal function is necessary (see DOSAGE AND ADMINISTRATION). Pediatric patients with renal insufficiency have not been studied.

Hemodialysis: In a study in anuric adult subjects (N=11), the apparent elimination half-life of gabapentin on nondialysis days was about 132 hours; during dialysis the apparent half-life of gabapentin was reduced to 3.8 hours. Hemodialysis thus has a significant effect on gabapentin elimination in anuric subjects.

Dosage adjustment in patients undergoing hemodialysis is necessary (see DOSAGE AND ADMINISTRATION).

Hepatic Disease: Because gabapentin is not metabolized, no study was performed in patients with hepatic impairment.

Age: The effect of age was studied in subjects 20-80 years of age. Apparent oral clearance (CL/F) of gabapentin decreased as age increased, from about 225 mL/min in those under 30 years of age to about 125 mL/min in those over 70 years of age. Renal clearance (CLr) and CLr adjusted for body surface area also declined with age; however, the decline in the renal clearance of gabapentin with age can largely be explained by the decline in renal function. Reduction of gabapentin dose may be required in patients who have age related compromised renal function. (See PRECAUTIONS, Geriatric Use, and DOSAGE AND ADMINISTRATION.)

Pediatric: Gabapentin pharmacokinetics were determined in 48 pediatric subjects between the ages of 1 month and 12 years following a dose of approximately 10 mg/kg. Peak plasma concentrations were similar across the entire age group and occurred 2 to 3 hours postdose. In general, pediatric subjects between 1 month and <5 years of age achieved approximately 30% lower exposure (AUC) than that observed in those 5 years of age and older. Accordingly, oral clearance normalized per body weight was higher in the younger children. Apparent oral clearance of gabapentin was directly proportional to creatinine clearance. Gabapentin elimination half-life averaged 4.7 hours and was similar across the age groups studied.

A population pharmacokinetic analysis was performed in 253 pediatric subjects between 1 month and 13 years of age. Patients received 10 to 65 mg/kg/day given TID. Apparent oral clearance (CL/F) was directly proportional to creatinine clearance and this relationship was similar following a single dose and at steady state. Higher oral clearance values were observed in children <5 years of age compared to those observed in children 5 years of age and older, when normalized per body weight. The clearance was highly variable in infants <1 year of age. The normalized CL/F values observed in pediatric patients 5 years of age and older were consistent with values observed in adults after a single dose. The oral volume of distribution normalized per body weight was constant across the age range.

These pharmacokinetic data indicate that the effective daily dose in pediatric patients with epilepsy ages 3 and 4 years should be 40 mg/kg/day to achieve average plasma concentrations similar to those achieved in patients 5 years of age and older receiving gabapentin at 30 mg/kg/day (see DOSAGE AND ADMINISTRATION).

Gender: Although no formal study has been conducted to compare the pharmacokinetics of gabapentin in men and women, it appears that the pharmacokinetic parameters for males and females are similar and there are no significant gender differences.

Race: Pharmacokinetic differences due to race have not been studied. Because gabapentin is primarily renally excreted and there are no important racial differences in creatinine clearance, pharmacokinetic differences due to race are not expected.

Clinical Studies

Postherpetic Neuralgia

Neurontin® was evaluated for the management of postherpetic neuralgia (PHN) in 2 randomized, double-blind, placebo-controlled, multicenter studies; N=563 patients in the intent-to-treat (ITT) population (Table 1). Patients were enrolled if they continued to have pain for more than 3 months after healing of the herpes zoster skin rash.

[See table 1 above]

TABLE 1. Controlled PHN Studies: Duration, Dosages, and Number of Patients

Study	Study Duration	Gabapentin (mg/day)[a] Target Dose	Patients Receiving Gabapentin	Patients Receiving Placebo
1	8 weeks	3600	113	116
2	7 weeks	1800, 2400	223	111
		Total	336	227

[a] Given in 3 divided doses (TID)

Each study included a 1-week baseline during which patients were screened for eligibility and a 7- or 8-week double-blind phase (3 or 4 weeks of titration and 4 weeks of fixed dose). Patients initiated treatment with titration to a maximum of 900 mg/day gabapentin over 3 days. Dosages were then to be titrated in 600 to 1200 mg/day increments at 3- to 7-day intervals to target dose over 3 to 4 weeks. In Study 1, patients were continued on lower doses if not able to achieve the target dose. During baseline and treatment, patients recorded their pain in a daily diary using an 11-point numeric pain rating scale ranging from 0 (no pain) to 10 (worst possible pain). A mean pain score during baseline of at least 4 was required for randomization (baseline mean pain score for Studies 1 and 2 combined was 6.4). Analyses were conducted using the ITT population (all randomized patients who received at least one dose of study medication). Both studies showed significant differences from placebo at all doses tested.

A significant reduction in weekly mean pain scores was seen by Week 1 in both studies, and significant differences were maintained to the end of treatment. Comparable treatment effects were observed in all active treatment arms. Pharmacokinetic/pharmacodynamic modeling provided confirmatory evidence of efficacy across all doses. Figures 1 and 2 show these changes for Studies 1 and 2.

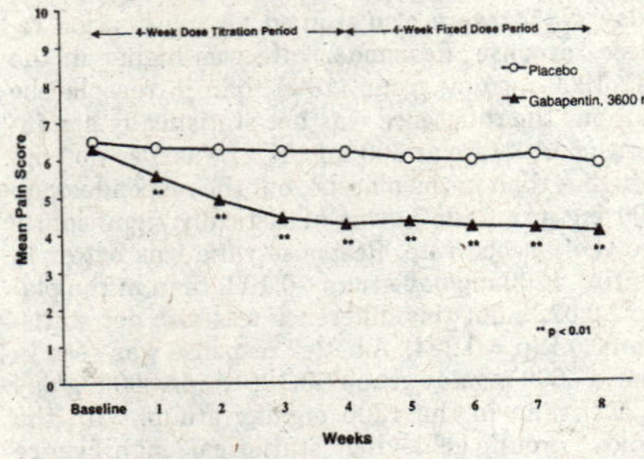

Figure 1. Weekly Mean Pain Scores (Observed Cases in ITT Population): Study 1

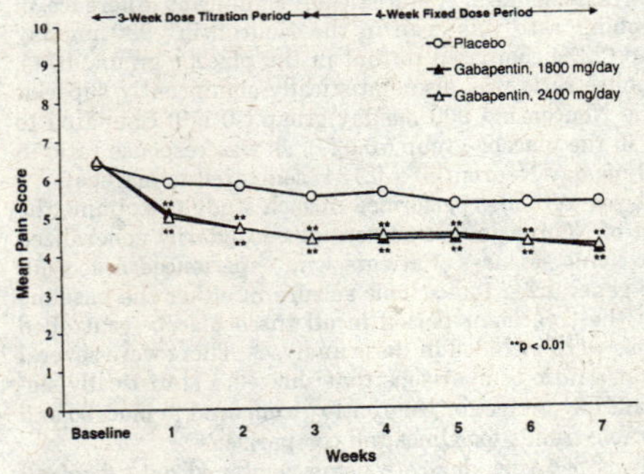

Figure 2. Weekly Mean Pain Scores (Observed Cases in ITT Population): Study 2

The proportion of responders (those patients reporting at least 50% improvement in endpoint pain score compared with baseline) was calculated for each study (Figure 3).

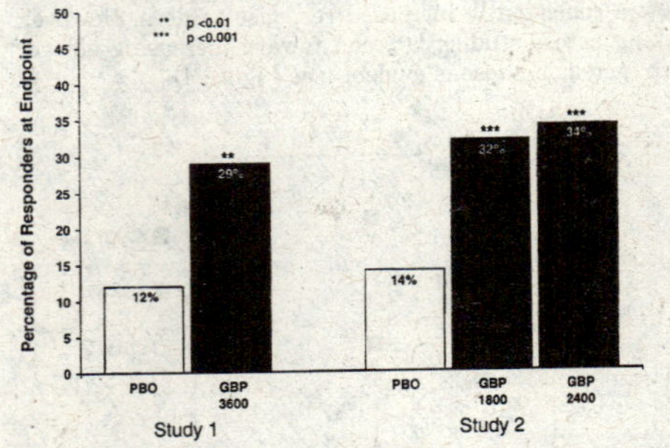

Figure 3. Proportion of Responders (patients with ≥50% reduction in pain score) at Endpoint: Controlled PHN Studies

Epilepsy

The effectiveness of Neurontin® as adjunctive therapy (added to other antiepileptic drugs) was established in multicenter placebo-controlled, double-blind, parallel-group clinical trials in adult and pediatric patients (3 years and older) with refractory partial seizures.

Evidence of effectiveness was obtained in three trials conducted in 705 patients (age 12 years and above) and one trial conducted in 247 pediatric patients (3 to 12 years of age). The patients enrolled had a history of at least 4 partial seizures per month in spite of receiving one or more antiep-

Continued on next page

Neurontin—Cont.

ileptic drugs at therapeutic levels and were observed on their established antiepileptic drug regimen during a 12-week baseline period (6 weeks in the study of pediatric patients). In patients continuing to have at least 2 (or 4 in some studies) seizures per month, Neurontin® or placebo was then added on to the existing therapy during a 12-week treatment period. Effectiveness was assessed primarily on the basis of the percent of patients with a 50% or greater reduction in seizure frequency from baseline to treatment (the "responder rate") and a derived measure called response ratio, a measure of change defined as (T - B)/(T + B), where B is the patient's baseline seizure frequency and T is the patient's seizure frequency during treatment. Response ratio is distributed within the range -1 to +1. A zero value indicates no change while complete elimination of seizures would give a value of -1; increased seizure rates would give positive values. A response ratio of -0.33 corresponds to a 50% reduction in seizure frequency. The results given below are for all partial seizures in the intent-to-treat (all patients who received any doses of treatment) population in each study, unless otherwise indicated.

One study compared Neurontin® 1200 mg/day divided TID with placebo. Responder rate was 23% (14/61) in the Neurontin® group and 9% (6/66) in the placebo group; the difference between groups was statistically significant. Response ratio was also better in the Neurontin® group (-0.199) than in the placebo group (-0.044), a difference that also achieved statistical significance.

A second study compared primarily 1200 mg/day divided TID Neurontin® (N=101) with placebo (N=98). Additional smaller Neurontin® dosage groups (600 mg/day, N=53; 1800 mg/day, N=54) were also studied for information regarding dose response. Responder rate was higher in the Neurontin® 1200 mg/day group (16%) than in the placebo group (8%), but the difference was not statistically significant. The responder rate at 600 mg (17%) was also not significantly higher than in the placebo, but the responder rate in the 1800 mg group (26%) was statistically significantly superior to the placebo rate. Response ratio was better in the Neurontin® 1200 mg/day group (-0.103) than in the placebo group (-0.022); but this difference was also not statistically significant (p = 0.224). A better response was seen in the Neurontin® 600 mg/day group (-0.105) and 1800 mg/day group (-0.222) than in the 1200 mg/day group, with the 1800 mg/day group achieving statistical significance compared to the placebo group.

A third study compared Neurontin® 900 mg/day divided TID (N=111) and placebo (N=109). An additional Neurontin® 1200 mg/day dosage group (N=52) provided dose-response data. A statistically significant difference in responder rate was seen in the Neurontin® 900 mg/day group (22%) compared to that in the placebo group (10%). Response ratio was also statistically significantly superior in the Neurontin® 900 mg/day group (-0.119) compared to that in the placebo group (-0.027), as was response ratio in 1200 mg/day Neurontin® (-0.184) compared to placebo.

Analyses were also performed in each study to examine the effect of Neurontin® on preventing secondarily generalized tonic-clonic seizures. Patients who experienced a secondarily generalized tonic-clonic seizure in either the baseline or in the treatment period in all three placebo-controlled studies were included in these analyses. There were several response ratio comparisons that showed a statistically significant advantage for Neurontin® compared to placebo and favorable trends for almost all comparisons.

Analysis of responder rate using combined data from all three studies and all doses (N=162, Neurontin®; N=89, placebo) also showed a significant advantage for Neurontin® over placebo in reducing the frequency of secondarily generalized tonic-clonic seizures.

In two of the three controlled studies, more than one dose of Neurontin® was used. Within each study the results did not show a consistently increased response to dose. However, looking across studies, a trend toward increasing efficacy with increasing dose is evident (see Figure 4).

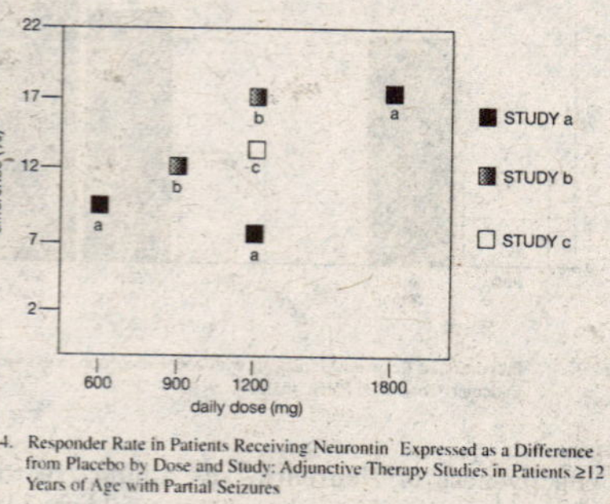

FIGURE 4. Responder Rate in Patients Receiving Neurontin® Expressed as a Difference from Placebo by Dose and Study: Adjunctive Therapy Studies in Patients ≥12 Years of Age with Partial Seizures

In the figure, treatment effect magnitude, measured on the Y axis in terms of the difference in the proportion of gabapentin and placebo assigned patients attaining a 50% or greater reduction in seizure frequency from baseline, is plotted against the daily dose of gabapentin administered (X axis).

Although no formal analysis by gender has been performed, estimates of response (Response Ratio) derived from clinical trials (398 men, 307 women) indicate no important gender differences exist. There was no consistent pattern indicating that age had any effect on the response to Neurontin®. There were insufficient numbers of patients of races other than Caucasian to permit a comparison of efficacy among racial groups.

A fourth study in pediatric patients age 3 to 12 years compared 25 – 35 mg/kg/day Neurontin® (N=118) with placebo (N=127). For all partial seizures in the intent-to-treat population, the response ratio was statistically significantly better for the Neurontin® group (-0.146) than for the placebo group (-0.079). For the same population, the responder rate for Neurontin® (21%) was not significantly different from placebo (18%).

A study in pediatric patients age 1 month to 3 years compared 40 mg/kg/day Neurontin® (N=38) with placebo (N=38) in patients who were receiving at least one marketed antiepileptic drug and had at least one partial seizure during the screening period (within 2 weeks prior to baseline). Patients had up to 48 hours of baseline and up to 72 hours of double-blind video EEG monitoring to record and count the occurrence of seizures. There were no statistically significant differences between treatments in either the response ratio or responder rate.

INDICATIONS AND USAGE

Postherpetic Neuralgia

Neurontin® (gabapentin) is indicated for the management of postherpetic neuralgia in adults.

Epilepsy

Neurontin® (gabapentin) is indicated as adjunctive therapy in the treatment of partial seizures with and without secondary generalization in patients over 12 years of age with epilepsy. Neurontin is also indicated as adjunctive therapy in the treatment of partial seizures in pediatric patients age 3 – 12 years.

CONTRAINDICATIONS

Neurontin® is contraindicated in patients who have demonstrated hypersensitivity to the drug or its ingredients.

WARNINGS

Neuropsychiatric Adverse Events—Pediatric Patients 3-12 years of age

Gabapentin use in pediatric patients with epilepsy 3–12 years of age is associated with the occurrence of central nervous system related adverse events. The most significant of these can be classified into the following categories: 1) emotional lability (primarily behavioral problems), 2) hostility, including aggressive behaviors, 3) thought disorder, including concentration problems and change in school performance, and 4) hyperkinesia (primarily restlessness and hyperactivity). Among the gabapentin-treated patients, most of the events were mild to moderate in intensity.

In controlled trials in pediatric patients 3–12 years of age the incidence of these adverse events was: emotional lability 6% (gabapentin-treated patients) vs 1.3% (placebo-treated patients); hostility 5.2% vs 1.3%; hyperkinesia 4.7% vs 2.9%; and thought disorder 1.7% vs 0%. One of these events, a report of hostility, was considered serious. Discontinuation of gabapentin treatment occurred in 1.3% of patients reporting emotional lability and hyperkinesia and 0.9% of gabapentin-treated patients reporting hostility and thought disorder. One placebo-treated patient (0.4%) withdrew due to emotional lability.

Withdrawal Precipitated Seizure, Status Epilepticus

Antiepileptic drugs should not be abruptly discontinued because of the possibility of increasing seizure frequency.

In the placebo-controlled studies in patients >12 years of age, the incidence of status epilepticus in patients receiving Neurontin® was 0.6% (3 of 543) versus 0.5% in patients receiving placebo (2 of 378). Among the 2074 patients >12 years of age treated with Neurontin® across all studies (controlled and uncontrolled) 31 (1.5%) had status epilepticus. Of these, 14 patients had no prior history of status epilepticus either before treatment or while on other medications. Because adequate historical data are not available, it is impossible to say whether or not treatment with Neurontin® is associated with a higher or lower rate of status epilepticus than would be expected to occur in a similar population not treated with Neurontin®.

Tumorigenic Potential

In standard preclinical *in vivo* lifetime carcinogenicity studies, an unexpectedly high incidence of pancreatic acinar adenocarcinomas was identified in male, but not female, rats. (See PRECAUTIONS: Carcinogenesis, Mutagenesis, Impairment of Fertility.) The clinical significance of this finding is unknown. Clinical experience during gabapentin's premarketing development provides no direct means to assess its potential for inducing tumors in humans.

In clinical studies in adjunctive therapy in epilepsy comprising 2085 patient-years of exposure in patients >12 years of age, new tumors were reported in 10 patients (2 breast, 3 brain, 2 lung, 1 adrenal, 1 non-Hodgkin's lymphoma, 1 endometrial carcinoma *in situ*), and preexisting tumors worsened in 11 patients (9 brain, 1 breast, 1 prostate) during or up to 2 years following discontinuation of Neurontin®. Without knowledge of the background incidence and recurrence in a similar population not treated with Neurontin®, it is impossible to know whether the incidence seen in this cohort is or is not affected by treatment.

Sudden and Unexplained Death in Patients With Epilepsy

During the course of premarketing development of Neurontin® 8 sudden and unexplained deaths were recorded among a cohort of 2203 patients treated (2103 patient-years of exposure).

Some of these could represent seizure-related deaths in which the seizure was not observed, e.g., at night. This represents an incidence of 0.0038 deaths per patient-year. Although this rate exceeds that expected in a healthy population matched for age and sex, it is within the range of estimates for the incidence of sudden unexplained deaths in patients with epilepsy not receiving Neurontin® (ranging from 0.0005 for the general population of epileptics to 0.003 for a clinical trial population similar to that in the Neurontin® program, to 0.005 for patients with refractory epilepsy). Consequently, whether these figures are reassuring or raise further concern depends on comparability of the populations reported upon to the Neurontin® cohort and the accuracy of the estimates provided.

PRECAUTIONS

Information for Patients

Patients should be instructed to take Neurontin® only as prescribed.

Patients should be advised that Neurontin® may cause dizziness, somnolence and other symptoms and signs of CNS depression. Accordingly, they should be advised neither to drive a car nor to operate other complex machinery until they have gained sufficient experience on Neurontin® to gauge whether or not it affects their mental and/or motor performance adversely.

Patients who require concomitant treatment with morphine may experience increases in gabapentin concentrations. Patients should be carefully observed for signs of CNS depression, such as somnolence, and the dose of Neurontin® or morphine should be reduced appropriately (see Drug Interactions).

Laboratory Tests

Clinical trials data do not indicate that routine monitoring of clinical laboratory parameters is necessary for the safe use of Neurontin®. The value of monitoring gabapentin blood concentrations has not been established. Neurontin® may be used in combination with other antiepileptic drugs without concern for alteration of the blood concentrations of gabapentin or of other antiepileptic drugs.

Drug Interactions

In vitro studies were conducted to investigate the potential of gabapentin to inhibit the major cytochrome P450 enzymes (CYP1A2, CYP2A6, CYP2C9, CYP2C19, CYP2D6, CYP2E1, and CYP3A4) that mediate drug and xenobiotic metabolism using isoform selective marker substrates and human liver microsomal preparations. Only at the highest concentration tested (171 μg/mL; 1 mM) was a slight degree of inhibition (14%-30%) of isoform CYP2A6 observed. No inhibition of any of the other isoforms tested was observed at gabapentin concentrations up to 171 μg/mL (approximately 15 times the C_{max} at 3600 mg/day).

Gabapentin is not appreciably metabolized nor does it interfere with the metabolism of commonly coadministered antiepileptic drugs.

The drug interaction data described in this section were obtained from studies involving healthy adults and adult patients with epilepsy.

Phenytoin: In a single (400 mg) and multiple dose (400 mg TID) study of Neurontin® in epileptic patients (N=8) maintained on phenytoin monotherapy for at least 2 months, gabapentin had no effect on the steady-state trough plasma concentrations of phenytoin and phenytoin had no effect on gabapentin pharmacokinetics.

Carbamazepine: Steady-state trough plasma carbamazepine and carbamazepine 10, 11 epoxide concentrations were not affected by concomitant gabapentin (400 mg TID; N=12) administration. Likewise, gabapentin pharmacokinetics were unaltered by carbamazepine administration.

Valproic Acid: The mean steady-state trough serum valproic acid concentrations prior to and during concomitant gabapentin administration (400 mg TID; N=17) were not different and neither were gabapentin pharmacokinetic parameters affected by valproic acid.

Phenobarbital: Estimates of steady-state pharmacokinetic parameters for phenobarbital or gabapentin (300 mg TID; N=12) are identical whether the drugs are administered alone or together.

Naproxen: Coadministration (N=18) of naproxen sodium capsules (250 mg) with Neurontin® (125 mg) appears to increase the amount of gabapentin absorbed by 12% to 15%. Gabapentin had no effect on naproxen pharmacokinetic parameters. These doses are lower than the therapeutic doses for both drugs. The magnitude of interaction within the recommended dose ranges of either drug is not known.

Hydrocodone: Coadministration of Neurontin® (125 to 500 mg; N=48) decreases hydrocodone (10 mg; N=50) C_{max} and AUC values in a dose-dependent manner relative to administration of hydrocodone alone; C_{max} and AUC values are 3% to 4% lower, respectively, after administration of 125 mg Neurontin® and 21% to 22% lower, respectively, after administration of 500 mg Neurontin®. The mechanism for this interaction is unknown. Hydrocodone increases gabapentin AUC values by 14%. The magnitude of interaction at other doses is not known.

Morphine: A literature article reported that when a 60-mg controlled-release morphine capsule was administered 2 hours prior to a 600-mg Neurontin® capsule (N=12), mean gabapentin AUC increased by 44% compared to gabapentin administered without morphine (see PRECAUTIONS). Morphine pharmacokinetic parameter values were not affected by administration of Neurontin® 2 hours after morphine. The magnitude of interaction at other doses is not known.

Cimetidine: In the presence of cimetidine at 300 mg QID (N=12) the mean apparent oral clearance of gabapentin fell by 14% and creatinine clearance fell by 10%. Thus cimetidine appeared to alter the renal excretion of both gabapentin and creatinine, an endogenous marker of renal function. This small decrease in excretion of gabapentin by cimetidine is not expected to be of clinical importance. The effect of gabapentin on cimetidine was not evaluated.

Oral Contraceptive: Based on AUC and half-life, multiple-dose pharmacokinetic profiles of norethindrone and ethinyl estradiol following administration of tablets containing 2.5 mg of norethindrone acetate and 50 mcg of ethinyl estradiol were similar with and without coadministration of gabapentin (400 mg TID; N=13). The Cmax of norethindrone was 13% higher when it was coadministered with gabapentin; this interaction is not expected to be of clinical importance.

Antacid (Maalox®): Maalox reduced the bioavailability of gabapentin (N=16) by about 20%. This decrease in bioavailability was about 5% when gabapentin was administered 2 hours after Maalox. It is recommended that gabapentin be taken at least 2 hours following Maalox administration.

Effect of Probenecid: Probenecid is a blocker of renal tubular secretion. Gabapentin pharmacokinetic parameters without and with probenecid were comparable. This indicates that gabapentin does not undergo renal tubular secretion by the pathway that is blocked by probenecid.

Drug/Laboratory Tests Interactions

Because false positive readings were reported with the Ames N-Multistix SG® dipstick test for urinary protein when gabapentin was added to other antiepileptic drugs, the more specific sulfosalicylic acid precipitation procedure is recommended to determine the presence of urine protein.

Carcinogenesis, Mutagenesis, Impairment of Fertility

Gabapentin was given in the diet to mice at 200, 600, and 2000 mg/kg/day and to rats at 250, 1000, and 2000 mg/kg/day for 2 years. A statistically significant increase in the incidence of pancreatic acinar cell adenomas and carcinomas was found in male rats receiving the high dose; the no-effect dose for the occurrence of carcinomas was 1000 mg/kg/day. Peak plasma concentrations of gabapentin in rats receiving the high dose of 2000 mg/kg were 10 times higher than plasma concentrations in humans receiving 3600 mg per day, and in rats receiving 1000 mg/kg/day peak plasma concentrations were 6.5 times higher than in humans receiving 3600 mg/day. The pancreatic acinar cell carcinomas did not affect survival, did not metastasize and were not locally invasive. The relevance of this finding to carcinogenic risk in humans is unclear.

Studies designed to investigate the mechanism of gabapentin-induced pancreatic carcinogenesis in rats indicate that gabapentin stimulates DNA synthesis in rat pancreatic acinar cells *in vitro* and, thus, may be acting as a tumor promoter by enhancing mitogenic activity. It is not known whether gabapentin has the ability to increase cell proliferation in other cell types or in other species, including humans.

Gabapentin did not demonstrate mutagenic or genotoxic potential in three *in vitro* and four *in vivo* assays. It was negative in the Ames test and the *in vitro* HGPRT forward mutation assay in Chinese hamster lung cells; it did not produce significant increases in chromosomal aberrations in the *in vitro* Chinese hamster lung cell assay; it was negative in the *in vivo* chromosomal aberration assay and in the *in vivo* micronucleus test in Chinese hamster bone marrow; it was negative in the *in vivo* mouse micronucleus assay; and it did not induce unscheduled DNA synthesis in hepatocytes from rats given gabapentin.

No adverse effects on fertility or reproduction were observed in rats at doses up to 2000 mg/kg (approximately 5 times the maximum recommended human dose on a mg/m^2 basis).

Pregnancy

Pregnancy Category C: Gabapentin has been shown to be fetotoxic in rodents, causing delayed ossification of several bones in the skull, vertebrae, forelimbs, and hindlimbs. These effects occurred when pregnant mice received oral doses of 1000 or 3000 mg/kg/day during the period of organogenesis, or approximately 1 to 4 times the maximum dose of 3600 mg/day given to epileptic patients on a mg/m^2 basis. The no-effect level was 500 mg/kg/day or approximately ½ of the human dose on a mg/m^2 basis.

When rats were dosed prior to and during mating, and throughout gestation, pups from all dose groups (500, 1000 and 2000 mg/kg/day) were affected. These doses are equivalent to less than approximately 1 to 5 times the maximum human dose on a mg/m^2 basis. There was an increased incidence of hydroureter and/or hydronephrosis in rats in a study of fertility and general reproductive performance at 2000 mg/kg/day with no effect at 1000 mg/kg/day, in a teratology study at 1500 mg/kg/day with no effect at 300 mg/kg/day, and in a perinatal and postnatal study at all doses studied (500, 1000 and 2000 mg/kg/day). The doses at which the effects occurred are approximately 1 to 5 times the maximum human dose of 3600 mg/day on a mg/m^2 basis; the no-effect doses were approximately 3 times (Fertility and General Reproductive Performance study) and approximately equal to (Teratogenicity study) the maximum human dose on a mg/m^2 basis. Other than hydroureter and hydronephrosis, the etiologies of which are unclear, the incidence of malformations was not increased compared to controls in offspring of mice, rats, or rabbits given doses up to 50 times (mice), 30 times (rats), and 25 times (rabbits) the human daily dose on a mg/kg basis, or 4 times (mice), 5 times (rats), or 8 times (rabbits) the human daily dose on a mg/m^2 basis.

In a teratology study in rabbits, an increased incidence of postimplantation fetal loss occurred in dams exposed to 60, 300, and 1500 mg/kg/day, or less than approximately ¼ to 8 times the maximum human dose on a mg/m^2 basis. There are no adequate and well-controlled studies in pregnant women. This drug should be used during pregnancy only if the potential benefit justifies the potential risk to the fetus.

Use in Nursing Mothers

Gabapentin is secreted into human milk following oral administration. A nursed infant could be exposed to a maximum dose of approximately 1 mg/kg/day of gabapentin. Because the effect on the nursing infant is unknown, Neurontin® should be used in women who are nursing only if the benefits clearly outweigh the risks.

Pediatric Use

Safety and effectiveness of Neurontin® (gabapentin) in the management of postherpetic neuralgia in pediatric patients have not been established.

Effectiveness as adjunctive therapy in the treatment of partial seizures in pediatric patients below the age of 3 years has not been established (see CLINICAL PHARMACOLOGY, Clinical Studies).

Geriatric Use

The total number of patients treated with Neurontin® in controlled clinical trials in patients with postherpetic neuralgia was 336, of which 102 (30%) were 65 to 74 years of age, and 168 (50%) were 75 years of age and older. There was a larger treatment effect in patients 75 years of age and older compared with younger patients who received the same dosage. Since gabapentin is almost exclusively eliminated by renal excretion, the larger treatment effect observed in patients ≥75 years may be a consequence of increased gabapentin exposure for a given dose that results from an age-related decrease in renal function. However, other factors cannot be excluded. The types and incidence of adverse events were similar across age groups except for peripheral edema and ataxia, which tended to increase in incidence with age.

Clinical studies of Neurontin® in epilepsy did not include sufficient numbers of subjects aged 65 and over to determine whether they responded differently from younger subjects. Other reported clinical experience has not identified differences in responses between the elderly and younger patients. In general, dose selection for an elderly patient should be cautious, usually starting at the low end of the dosing range, reflecting the greater frequency of decreased hepatic, renal, or cardiac function, and of concomitant disease or other drug therapy.

This drug is known to be substantially excreted by the kidney, and the risk of toxic reactions to this drug may be greater in patients with impaired renal function. Because elderly patients are more likely to have decreased renal function, care should be taken in dose selection, and dose should be adjusted based on creatinine clearance values in these patients (see CLINICAL PHARMACOLOGY, ADVERSE REACTIONS, and DOSAGE AND ADMINISTRATION sections).

ADVERSE REACTIONS

Postherpetic Neuralgia

The most commonly observed adverse events associated with the use of Neurontin® in adults, not seen at an equivalent frequency among placebo-treated patients, were dizziness, somnolence, and peripheral edema.

In the 2 controlled studies in postherpetic neuralgia, 16% of the 336 patients who received Neurontin® and 9% of the 227 patients who received placebo discontinued treatment because of an adverse event. The adverse events that most frequently led to withdrawal in Neurontin®-treated patients were dizziness, somnolence, and nausea.

Incidence in Controlled Clinical Trials

Table 2 lists treatment-emergent signs and symptoms that occurred in at least 1% of Neurontin®-treated patients with postherpetic neuralgia participating in placebo-controlled trials and that were numerically more frequent in the Neurontin® group than in the placebo group. Adverse events were usually mild to moderate in intensity.

TABLE 2. Treatment-Emergent Adverse Event Incidence in Controlled Trials in Postherpetic Neuralgia (Events in at least 1% of Neurontin®-Treated Patients and Numerically More Frequent Than in the Placebo Group)

Body System/ Preferred Term	Neurontin® N=336 %	Placebo N=227 %
Body as a Whole		
Asthenia	5.7	4.8
Infection	5.1	3.5
Headache	3.3	3.1
Accidental injury	3.3	1.3
Abdominal pain	2.7	2.6
Digestive System		
Diarrhea	5.7	3.1
Dry mouth	4.8	1.3
Constipation	3.9	1.8
Nausea	3.9	3.1
Vomiting	3.3	1.8
Flatulence	2.1	1.8
Metabolic and Nutritional Disorders		
Peripheral edema	8.3	2.2
Weight gain	1.8	0.0
Hyperglycemia	1.2	0.4
Nervous System		
Dizziness	28.0	7.5
Somnolence	21.4	5.3
Ataxia	3.3	0.0
Thinking abnormal	2.7	0.0
Abnormal gait	1.5	0.0
Incoordination	1.5	0.0
Amnesia	1.2	0.9
Hypesthesia	1.2	0.9
Respiratory System		
Pharyngitis	1.2	0.4
Skin and Appendages		
Rash	1.2	0.9
Special Senses		
Amblyopia[a]	2.7	0.9
Conjuctivitis	1.2	0.0
Diplopia	1.2	0.0
Otitis media	1.2	0.0

[a] Reported as blurred vision

Other events in more than 1% of patients but equally or more frequent in the placebo group included pain, tremor, neuralgia, back pain, dyspepsia, dyspnea, and flu syndrome.

There were no clinically important differences between men and women in the types and incidence of adverse events. Because there were few patients whose race was reported as other than white, there are insufficient data to support a statement regarding the distribution of adverse events by race.

Epilepsy

The most commonly observed adverse events associated with the use of Neurontin® in combination with other antiepileptic drugs in patients >12 years of age, not seen at an equivalent frequency among placebo-treated patients, were somnolence, dizziness, ataxia, fatigue, and nystagmus. The most commonly observed adverse events reported with the use of Neurontin® in combination with other antiepileptic drugs in pediatric patients 3 to 12 years of age, not seen at an equal frequency among placebo-treated patients, were viral infection, fever, nausea and/or vomiting, somnolence, and hostility (see WARNINGS, Neuropsychiatric Adverse Events).

Approximately 7% of the 2074 patients >12 years of age and approximately 7% of the 449 pediatric patients 3 to 12 years of age who received Neurontin® in premarketing clinical trials discontinued treatment because of an adverse event. The adverse events most commonly associated with withdrawal in patients >12 years of age were somnolence (1.2%), ataxia (0.8%), fatigue (0.6%), nausea and/or vomiting (0.6%), and dizziness (0.6%). The adverse events most commonly associated with withdrawal in pediatric patients were emotional lability (1.6%), hostility (1.3%), and hyperkinesia (1.1%).

Incidence in Controlled Clinical Trials

Table 3 lists treatment-emergent signs and symptoms that occurred in at least 1% of Neurontin®-treated patients >12 years of age with epilepsy participating in placebo-controlled trials and were numerically more common in the Neurontin® group. In these studies, either Neurontin® or placebo was added to the patient's current antiepileptic drug therapy. Adverse events were usually mild to moderate in intensity.

The prescriber should be aware that these figures, obtained when Neurontin® was added to concurrent antiepileptic drug therapy, cannot be used to predict the frequency of adverse events in the course of usual medical practice where patient characteristics and other factors may differ from those prevailing during clinical studies. Similarly, the cited frequencies cannot be directly compared with figures obtained from other clinical investigations involving different treatments, uses, or investigators. An inspection of these frequencies, however, does provide the prescribing physician with one basis to estimate the relative contribution of drug and nondrug factors to the adverse event incidences in the population studied.

TABLE 3. Treatment-Emergent Adverse Event Incidence in Controlled Add-On Trials In Patients >12 years of age (Events in at least 1% of Neurontin® patients and numerically more frequent than in the placebo group)

Body System/ Adverse Event	Neurontin®[a] N=543 %	Placebo[a] N=378 %
Body As A Whole		
Fatigue	11.0	5.0
Weight Increase	2.9	1.6
Back Pain	1.8	0.5
Peripheral Edema	1.7	0.5
Cardiovascular		
Vasodilatation	1.1	0.3
Digestive System		
Dyspepsia	2.2	0.5
Mouth or Throat Dry	1.7	0.5
Constipation	1.5	0.8
Dental Abnormalities	1.5	0.3
Increased Appetite	1.1	0.8
Hematologic and Lymphatic Systems		
Leukopenia	1.1	0.5
Musculoskeletal System		
Myalgia	2.0	1.9
Fracture	1.1	0.8

Continued on next page

Neurontin—Cont.

Nervous System		
Somnolence	19.3	8.7
Dizziness	17.1	6.9
Ataxia	12.5	5.6
Nystagmus	8.3	4.0
Tremor	6.8	3.2
Nervousness	2.4	1.9
Dysarthria	2.4	0.5
Amnesia	2.2	0.0
Depression	1.8	1.1
Thinking Abnormal	1.7	1.3
Twitching	1.3	0.5
Coordination Abnormal	1.1	0.3
Respiratory System		
Rhinitis	4.1	3.7
Pharyngitis	2.8	1.6
Coughing	1.8	1.3
Skin and Appendages		
Abrasion	1.3	0.0
Pruritus	1.3	0.5
Urogenital System		
Impotence	1.5	1.1
Special Senses		
Diplopia	5.9	1.9
Amblyopia[b]	4.2	1.1
Laboratory Deviations		
WBC Decreased	1.1	0.5

[a] Plus background antiepileptic drug therapy
[b] Amblyopia was often described as blurred vision.

Other events in more than 1% of patients >12 years of age but equally or more frequent in the placebo group included: headache, viral infection, fever, nausea and/or vomiting, abdominal pain, diarrhea, convulsions, confusion, insomnia, emotional lability, rash, acne.

Among the treatment-emergent adverse events occurring at an incidence of at least 10% of Neurontin®-treated patients, somnolence and ataxia appeared to exhibit a positive dose-response relationship.

The overall incidence of adverse events and the types of adverse events seen were similar among men and women treated with Neurontin®. The incidence of adverse events increased slightly with increasing age in patients treated with either Neurontin® or placebo. Because only 3% of patients (28/921) in placebo-controlled studies were identified as nonwhite (black or other), there are insufficient data to support a statement regarding the distribution of adverse events by race.

Table 4 lists treatment-emergent signs and symptoms that occurred in at least 2% of Neurontin®-treated patients age 3 to 12 years of age with epilepsy participating in placebo-controlled trials and were numerically more common in the Neurontin® group. Adverse events were usually mild to moderate in intensity.

TABLE 4. Treatment-Emergent Adverse Event Incidence in Pediatric Patients Age 3 to 12 Years in a Controlled Add-On Trial (Events in at least 2% of Neurontin® patients and numerically more frequent than in the placebo group)

Body System/ Adverse Event	Neurontin®[a] N=119 %	Placebo[a] N=128 %
Body As A Whole		
Viral Infection	10.9	3.1
Fever	10.1	3.1
Weight Increase	3.4	0.8
Fatigue	3.4	1.6
Digestive System		
Nausea and/or Vomiting	8.4	7.0
Nervous System		
Somnolence	8.4	4.7
Hostility	7.6	2.3
Emotional Lability	4.2	1.6
Dizziness	2.5	1.6
Hyperkinesia	2.5	0.8
Respiratory System		
Bronchitis	3.4	0.8
Respiratory Infection	2.5	0.8

[a] Plus background antiepileptic drug therapy

Other events in more than 2% of pediatric patients 3 to 12 years of age but equally or more frequent in the placebo group included: pharyngitis, upper respiratory infection, headache, rhinitis, convulsions, diarrhea, anorexia, coughing, and otitis media.

Other Adverse Events Observed During All Clinical Trials Clinical Trials in Adults and Adolescents (Except Clinical Trials in Neuropathic Pain)

Neurontin® has been administered to 2074 patients >12 years of age during all adjunctive therapy clinical trials (except clinical trials in patients with neuropathic pain), only some of which were placebo-controlled. During these trials, all adverse events were recorded by the clinical investigators using terminology of their own choosing. To provide a meaningful estimate of the proportion of individuals having adverse events, similar types of events were grouped into a smaller number of standardized categories using modified COSTART dictionary terminology. These categories are used in the listing below. The frequencies presented represent the proportion of the 2074 patients >12 years of age exposed to Neurontin® who experienced an event of the type cited on at least one occasion while receiving Neurontin®. All reported events are included except those already listed in Table 3, those too general to be informative, and those not reasonably associated with the use of the drug.

Events are further classified within body system categories and enumerated in order of decreasing frequency using the following definitions: frequent adverse events are defined as those occurring in at least 1/100 patients; infrequent adverse events are those occurring in 1/100 to 1/1000 patients; rare events are those occurring in fewer than 1/1000 patients.

Body As A Whole: *Frequent:* asthenia, malaise, face edema; *Infrequent:* allergy, generalized edema, weight decrease, chill; *Rare:* strange feelings, lassitude, alcohol intolerance, hangover effect.

Cardiovascular System: *Frequent:* hypertension; *Infrequent:* hypotension, angina pectoris, peripheral vascular disorder, palpitation, tachycardia, migraine, murmur; *Rare:* atrial fibrillation, heart failure, thrombophlebitis, deep thrombophlebitis, myocardial infarction, cerebrovascular accident, pulmonary thrombosis, ventricular extrasystoles, bradycardia, premature atrial contraction, pericardial rub, heart block, pulmonary embolus, hyperlipidemia, hypercholesterolemia, pericardial effusion, pericarditis.

Digestive System: *Frequent:* anorexia, flatulence, gingivitis; *Infrequent:* glossitis, gum hemorrhage, thirst, stomatitis, increased salivation, gastroenteritis, hemorrhoids, bloody stools, fecal incontinence, hepatomegaly; *Rare:* dysphagia, eructation, pancreatitis, peptic ulcer, colitis, blisters in mouth, tooth discolor, perlèche, salivary gland enlarged, lip hemorrhage, esophagitis, hiatal hernia, hematemesis, proctitis, irritable bowel syndrome, rectal hemorrhage, esophageal spasm.

Endocrine System: *Rare:* hyperthyroid, hypothyroid, goiter, hypoestrogen, ovarian failure, epididymitis, swollen testicle, cushingoid appearance.

Hematologic and Lymphatic System: *Frequent:* purpura most often described as bruises resulting from physical trauma; *Infrequent:* anemia, thrombocytopenia, lymphadenopathy; *Rare:* WBC count increased, lymphocytosis, non-Hodgkin's lymphoma, bleeding time increased.

Musculoskeletal System: *Frequent:* arthralgia; *Infrequent:* tendinitis, arthritis, joint stiffness, joint swelling, positive Romberg test; *Rare:* costochondritis, osteoporosis, bursitis, contracture.

Nervous System: *Frequent:* vertigo, hyperkinesia, paresthesia, decreased or absent reflexes, increased reflexes, anxiety, hostility; *Infrequent:* CNS tumors, syncope, dreaming abnormal, aphasia, hypesthesia, intracranial hemorrhage, hypotonia, dysesthesia, paresis, dystonia, hemiplegia, facial paralysis, stupor, cerebellar dysfunction, positive Babinski sign, decreased position sense, subdural hematoma, apathy, hallucination, decrease or loss of libido, agitation, paranoia, depersonalization, euphoria, feeling high, doped-up sensation, suicidal, psychosis; *Rare:* choreoathetosis, orofacial dyskinesia, encephalopathy, nerve palsy, personality disorder, increased libido, subdued temperament, apraxia, fine motor control disorder, meningismus, local myoclonus, hyperesthesia, hypokinesia, mania, neurosis, hysteria, antisocial reaction, suicide gesture.

Respiratory System: *Frequent:* pneumonia; *Infrequent:* epistaxis, dyspnea, apnea; *Rare:* mucositis, aspiration pneumonia, hyperventilation, hiccup, laryngitis, nasal obstruction, snoring, bronchospasm, hypoventilation, lung edema.

Dermatological: *Infrequent:* alopecia, eczema, dry skin, increased sweating, urticaria, hirsutism, seborrhea, cyst, herpes simplex; *Rare:* herpes zoster, skin discolor, skin papules, photosensitive reaction, leg ulcer, scalp seborrhea, psoriasis, desquamation, maceration, skin nodules, subcutaneous nodule, melanosis, skin necrosis, local swelling.

Urogenital System: *Infrequent:* hematuria, dysuria, urination frequency, cystitis, urinary retention, urinary incontinence, vaginal hemorrhage, amenorrhea, dysmenorrhea, menorrhagia, breast cancer, unable to climax, ejaculation abnormal; *Rare:* kidney pain, leukorrhea, pruritus genital, renal stone, acute renal failure, anuria, glycosuria, nephrosis, nocturia, pyuria, urination urgency, vaginal pain, breast pain, testicle pain.

Special Senses: *Frequent:* abnormal vision; *Infrequent:* cataract, conjunctivitis, eyes dry, eye pain, visual field defect, photophobia, bilateral or unilateral ptosis, eye hemorrhage, hordeolum, hearing loss, earache, tinnitus, inner ear infection, otitis, taste loss, unusual taste, eye twitching, ear fullness; *Rare:* eye itching, abnormal accommodation, perforated ear drum, sensitivity to noise, eye focusing problem, watery eyes, retinopathy, glaucoma, iritis, corneal disorders, lacrimal dysfunction, degenerative eye changes, blindness, retinal degeneration, miosis, chorioretinitis, strabismus, eustachian tube dysfunction, labyrinthitis, otitis externa, odd smell.

Clinical trials in Pediatric Patients With Epilepsy

Adverse events occurring during epilepsy clinical trials in 449 pediatric patients 3 to 12 years of age treated with gabapentin that were not reported in adjunctive trials in adults are:

Body as a Whole: dehydration, infectious mononucleosis
Digestive System: hepatitis
Hemic and Lymphatic System: coagulation defect
Nervous System: aura disappeared, occipital neuralgia
Psychobiologic Function: sleepwalking
Respiratory System: pseudocroup, hoarseness

Clinical Trials in Adults With Neuropathic Pain of Various Etiologies

Safety information was obtained in 1173 patients during double-blind and open-label clinical trials including neuropathic pain conditions for which efficacy has not been demonstrated. Adverse events reported by investigators were grouped into standardized categories using modified COSTART IV terminology. Listed below are all reported events except those already listed in Table 2 and those not reasonably associated with the use of the drug.

Events are further classified within body system categories and enumerated in order of decreasing frequency using the following definitions: frequent adverse events are defined as those occurring in at least 1/100 patients; infrequent adverse events are those occurring in 1/100 to 1/1000 patients; rare events are those occurring in fewer than 1/1000 patients.

Body as a Whole: *Infrequent:* chest pain, cellulitis, malaise, neck pain, face edema, allergic reaction, abscess, chills, chills and fever, mucous membrane disorder; *Rare:* body odor, cyst, fever, hernia, abnormal BUN value, lump in neck, pelvic pain, sepsis, viral infection.

Cardiovascular System: *Infrequent:* hypertension, syncope, palpitation, migraine, hypotension, peripheral vascular disorder, cardiovascular disorder, cerebrovascular accident, congestive heart failure, myocardial infarction, vasodilatation; *Rare:* angina pectoris, heart failure, increased capillary fragility, phlebitis, thrombophlebitis, varicose vein.

Digestive System: *Infrequent:* gastroenteritis, increased appetite, gastrointestinal disorder, oral moniliasis, gastritis, tongue disorder, thirst, tooth disorder, abnormal stools, anorexia, liver function tests abnormal, periodontal abscess; *Rare:* cholecystitis, cholelithiasis, duodenal ulcer, fecal incontinence, gamma glutamyl transpeptidase increased, gingivitis, intestinal obstruction, intestinal ulcer, melena, mouth ulceration, rectal disorder, rectal hemorrhage, stomatitis.

Endocrine System: *Infrequent:* diabetes mellitus.

Hemic and Lymphatic System: *Infrequent:* ecchymosis, anemia; *Rare:* lymphadenopathy, lymphoma-like reaction, prothrombin decreased.

Metabolic and Nutritional: *Infrequent:* edema, gout, hypoglycemia, weight loss; *Rare:* alkaline phosphatase increased, diabetic ketoacidosis, lactic dehydrogenase increased.

Musculoskeletal: *Infrequent:* arthritis, arthralgia, myalgia, arthrosis, leg cramps, myasthenia; *Rare:* shin bone pain, joint disorder, tendon disorder.

Nervous System: *Frequent:* confusion, depression; *Infrequent:* vertigo, nervousness, paresthesia, insomnia, neuropathy, libido decreased, anxiety, depersonalization, reflexes decreased, speech disorder, abnormal dreams, dysarthria, emotional lability, nystagmus, stupor, circumoral paresthesia, euphoria, hyperesthesia, hypokinesia; *Rare:* agitation, hypertonia, libido increased, movement disorder, myoclonus, vestibular disorder.

Respiratory System: *Infrequent:* cough increased, bronchitis, rhinitis, sinusitis, pneumonia, asthma, lung disorder, epistaxis; *Rare:* hemoptysis, voice alteration.

Skin and Appendages: *Infrequent:* pruritus, skin ulcer, dry skin, herpes zoster, skin disorder, fungal dermatitis, furunculosis, herpes simplex, psoriasis, sweating, urticaria, vesiculobullous rash; *Rare:* acne, hair disorder, maculopapular rash, nail disorder, skin carcinoma, skin discoloration, skin hypertrophy.

Special Senses: *Infrequent:* abnormal vision, ear pain, eye disorder, taste perversion, deafness; *Rare:* conjunctival hyperemia, diabetic retinopathy, eye pain, fundi with microhemorrhage, retinal vein thrombosis, taste loss.

Urogenital System: *Infrequent:* urinary tract infection, dysuria, impotence, urinary incontinence, vaginal moniliasis, breast pain, menstrual disorder, polyuria, urinary retention; *Rare:* cystitis, ejaculation abnormal, swollen penis, gynecomastia, nocturia, pyelonephritis, swollen scrotum, urinary frequency, urinary urgency, urine abnormality.

Postmarketing and Other Experience

In addition to the adverse experiences reported during clinical testing of Neurontin®, the following adverse experiences have been reported in patients receiving marketed Neurontin®. These adverse experiences have not been listed above and data are insufficient to support an estimate of their incidence or to establish causation. The listing is alphabetized: angioedema, blood glucose fluctuation, erythema multiforme, elevated liver function tests, fever, hyponatremia, jaundice, movement disorder such as dyskinesia, Stevens-Johnson syndrome.

Adverse events following the abrupt discontinuation of gabapentin have also been reported. The most frequently reported events were anxiety, insomnia, nausea, pain and sweating.

DRUG ABUSE AND DEPENDENCE

The abuse and dependence potential of Neurontin® has not been evaluated in human studies.

OVERDOSAGE

A lethal dose of gabapentin was not identified in mice and rats receiving single oral doses as high as 8000 mg/kg. Signs of acute toxicity in animals included ataxia, labored breathing, ptosis, sedation, hypoactivity, or excitation.

Acute oral overdoses of Neurontin® up to 49 grams have been reported. In these cases, double vision, slurred speech, drowsiness, lethargy and diarrhea were observed. All patients recovered with supportive care.

TABLE 5. Neurontin® Dosage Based on Renal Function

Renal Function Creatinine Clearance (mL/min)	Total Daily Dose Range (mg/day)	Dose Regimen (mg)				
≥60	900-3600	300 TID	400 TID	600 TID	800 TID	1200 TID
>30-59	400-1400	200 BID	300 BID	400 BID	500 BID	700 BID
>15-29	200-700	200 QD	300 QD	400 QD	500 QD	700 QD
15[a]	100-300	100 QD	125 QD	150 QD	200 QD	300 QD
		Post-Hemodialysis Supplemental Dose (mg)[b]				
Hemodialysis		125[b]	150[b]	200[b]	250[b]	350[b]

[a] For patients with creatinine clearance <15 mL/min, reduce daily dose in proportion to creatinine clearance (e.g., patients with a creatinine clearance of 7.5 mL/min should receive one-half the daily dose that patients with a creatinine clearance of 15 mL/min receive).

[b] Patients on hemodialysis should receive maintenance doses based on estimates of creatinine clearance as indicated in the upper portion of the table and a supplemental post-hemodialysis dose administered after each 4 hours of hemodialysis as indicated in the lower portion of the table.

Gabapentin can be removed by hemodialysis. Although hemodialysis has not been performed in the few overdose cases reported, it may be indicated by the patient's clinical state or in patients with significant renal impairment.

DOSAGE AND ADMINISTRATION

Neurontin® is given orally with or without food.

If Neurontin® dose is reduced, discontinued or substituted with an alternative medication, this should be done gradually over a minimum of 1 week.

Postherpetic Neuralgia

In adults with postherpetic neuralgia, Neurontin® therapy may be initiated as a single 300-mg dose on Day 1, 600 mg/day on Day 2 (divided BID), and 900 mg/day on Day 3 (divided TID). The dose can subsequently be titrated up as needed for pain relief to a daily dose of 1800 mg (divided TID). In clinical studies, efficacy was demonstrated over a range of doses from 1800 mg/day to 3600 mg/day with comparable effects across the dose range. Additional benefit of using doses greater than 1800 mg/day was not demonstrated.

Epilepsy

Neurontin® is recommended for add-on therapy in patients 3 years of age and older. Effectiveness in pediatric patients below the age of 3 years has not been established.

Patients >12 years of age: The effective dose of Neurontin® is 900 to 1800 mg/day and given in divided doses (three times a day) using 300 or 400 mg capsules, or 600 or 800 mg tablets. The starting dose is 300 mg three times a day. If necessary, the dose may be increased using 300 or 400 mg capsules, or 600 or 800 mg tablets three times a day up to 1800 mg/day. Dosages up to 2400 mg/day have been well tolerated in long-term clinical studies. Doses of 3600 mg/day have also been administered to a small number of patients for a relatively short duration, and have been well tolerated. The maximum time between doses in the TID schedule should not exceed 12 hours.

Pediatric Patients Age 3–12 years: The starting dose should range from 10-15 mg/kg/day in 3 divided doses, and the effective dose reached by upward titration over a period of approximately 3 days. The effective dose of Neurontin® in patients 5 years of age and older is 25–35 mg/kg/day and given in divided doses (three times a day). The effective dose in pediatric patients ages 3 and 4 years is 40 mg/kg/day and given in divided doses (three times a day) (see CLINICAL PHARMACOLOGY, Pediatrics.) Neurontin® may be administered as the oral solution, capsule, or tablet, or using combinations of these formulations. Dosages up to 50 mg/kg/day have been well-tolerated in a long-term clinical study. The maximum time interval between doses should not exceed 12 hours.

It is not necessary to monitor gabapentin plasma concentrations to optimize Neurontin® therapy. Further, because there are no significant pharmacokinetic interactions among Neurontin® and other commonly used antiepileptic drugs, the addition of Neurontin® does not alter the plasma levels of these drugs appreciably.

If Neurontin® is discontinued and/or an alternate anticonvulsant medication is added to the therapy, this should be done gradually over a minimum of 1 week.

Dosage in Renal Impairment

Creatinine clearance is difficult to measure in outpatients. In patients with stable renal function, creatinine clearance (C_{Cr}) can be reasonably well estimated using the equation of Cockcroft and Gault:

for females $C_{Cr}=(0.85)(140\text{-age})(\text{weight})/[(72)(S_{Cr})]$

for males $C_{Cr}=(140\text{-age})(\text{weight})/[(72)(S_{Cr})]$

where age is in years, weight is in kilograms and S_{Cr} is serum creatinine in mg/dL.

Dosage adjustment in patients ≥12 years of age with compromised renal function or undergoing hemodialysis is recommended as follows (see dosing recommendations above for effective doses in each indication).

[See table 5 above]

The use of Neurontin® in patients <12 years of age with compromised renal function has not been studied.

Dosage in Elderly

Because elderly patients are more likely to have decreased renal function, care should be taken in dose selection, and dose should be adjusted based on creatinine clearance values in these patients.

HOW SUPPLIED

Neurontin® (gabapentin) capsules, tablets and oral solution are supplied as follows:

100 mg capsules;
White hard gelatin capsules printed with "PD" on one side and "Neurontin®/100 mg" on the other; available in:
Bottles of 100: N 0071-0803-24
Unit dose 50's: N 0071-0803-40

300 mg capsules;
Yellow hard gelatin capsules printed with "PD" on one side and "Neurontin®/300 mg" on the other; available in:
Bottles of 100: N 0071-0805-24
Unit dose 50's: N 0071-0805-40

400 mg capsules;
Orange hard gelatin capsules printed with "PD" on one side and "Neurontin®/400 mg" on the other; available in:
Bottles of 100: N 0071-0806-24
Unit dose 50's: N 0071-0806-40

600 mg tablets;
White elliptical film-coated scored tablets debossed with "NT" and "16" on one side; available in:
Bottles of 100: N 0071-0513-24

800 mg tablets;
White elliptical film-coated scored tablets debossed with "NT" and "26" on one side; available in:
Bottles of 100: N 0071-0401-24

250 mg/5 mL oral solution;
Clear colorless to slightly yellow solution; each 5 mL of oral solution contains 250 mg of gabapentin; available in:
Bottles containing 470 mL: N0071-2012-23

Storage (Capsules)

Store at 25°C (77°F); excursions permitted to 15° - 30°C (59° - 86°F) [see USP Controlled Room Temperature].

Storage (Tablets)

Store at 25°C (77°F); excursions permitted to 15° - 30°C (59° - 86°F) [see USP Controlled Room Temperature].

Storage (Oral Solution)

Store refrigerated, 2°-8°C (36°-46°F)

Rx only

Revised September 2003

Capsules and Tablets:
Manufactured by:
Pfizer Pharmaceuticals, Ltd.
Vega Baja, PR 00694

Oral Solution:
Manufactured for:
Pfizer Pharmaceuticals, Ltd.
Vega Baja, PR 00694

Distributed by:
Parke-Davis
Division of Pfizer Inc, NY, NY 10017

75-5800-00-4

Pfizer Inc.
235 EAST 42ND STREET
NEW YORK, NY 10017–5755

For Medical Information Contact:
(800) 438-1985
24 hours a day, 7 days a week

Pfizer Labs and Roerig Division:
For Medical Information Contact:
24 hours a day, seven days a week:
(800) 438-1985

Distribution:
1855 Shelby Oaks Drive North
Memphis, TN 38134
(901) 387-5200
Customer Service:
(800) 533-4535
EXPORT INQUIRIES:
Pfizer International Inc.
(212) 573-2323

ARICEPT® ℞

[ă'rĭ-sĕpt]

(Donepezil Hydrochloride Tablets)

Prescribing information for this product, which appears on pages 2570–2573 of the 2004 PDR, has been completely revised as follows. Please write "See Supplement A" next to the product heading.

DESCRIPTION

ARICEPT® (donepezil hydrochloride) is a reversible inhibitor of the enzyme acetylcholinesterase, known chemically as (±)-2,3-dihydro-5,6-dimethoxy-2-[[1-(phenylmethyl)-4-piperidinyl]methyl]-1*H*-inden-1-one hydrochloride. Donepezil hydrochloride is commonly referred to in the pharmacological literature as E2020. It has an empirical formula of $C_{24}H_{29}NO_3HCl$ and a molecular weight of 415.96. Donepezil hydrochloride is a white crystalline powder and is freely soluble in chloroform, soluble in water and in glacial acetic acid, slightly soluble in ethanol and in acetonitrile and practically insoluble in ethyl acetate and in n-hexane.

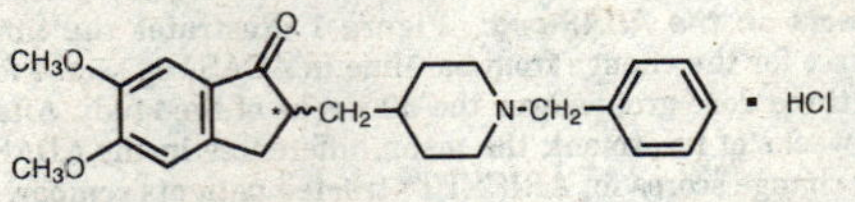

ARICEPT® is available for oral administration in film-coated tablets containing 5 or 10 mg of donepezil hydrochloride. Inactive ingredients are lactose monohydrate, corn starch, microcrystalline cellulose, hydroxypropyl cellulose, and magnesium stearate. The film coating contains talc, polyethylene glycol, hypromellose and titanium dioxide. Additionally, the 10 mg tablet contains yellow iron oxide (synthetic) as a coloring agent.

CLINICAL PHARMACOLOGY

Current theories on the pathogenesis of the cognitive signs and symptoms of Alzheimer's Disease attribute some of them to a deficiency of cholinergic neurotransmission.

Donepezil hydrochloride is postulated to exert its therapeutic effect by enhancing cholinergic function. This is accomplished by increasing the concentration of acetylcholine through reversible inhibition of its hydrolysis by acetylcholinesterase. If this proposed mechanism of action is correct, donepezil's effect may lessen as the disease process advances and fewer cholinergic neurons remain functionally intact. There is no evidence that donepezil alters the course of the underlying dementing process.

Clinical Trial Data

The effectiveness of ARICEPT® as a treatment for Alzheimer's Disease is demonstrated by the results of two randomized, double-blind, placebo-controlled clinical investigations in patients with Alzheimer's Disease (diagnosed by NINCDS and DSM III-R criteria, Mini-Mental State Examination ≥ 10 and ≤ 26 and Clinical Dementia Rating of 1 or 2). The mean age of patients participating in ARICEPT® trials was 73 years with a range of 50 to 94. Approximately 62% of patients were women and 38% were men. The racial distribution was white 95%, black 3% and other races 2%.

Study Outcome Measures: In each study, the effectiveness of treatment with ARICEPT® was evaluated using a dual outcome assessment strategy.

The ability of ARICEPT® to improve cognitive performance was assessed with the cognitive subscale of the Alzheimer's Disease Assessment Scale (ADAS-cog), a multi-item instrument that has been extensively validated in longitudinal cohorts of Alzheimer's Disease patients. The ADAS-cog examines selected aspects of cognitive performance including elements of memory, orientation, attention, reasoning, language and praxis. The ADAS-cog scoring range is from 0 to 70, with higher scores indicating greater cognitive impairment. Elderly normal adults may score as low as 0 or 1, but it is not unusual for non-demented adults to score slightly higher.

The patients recruited as participants in each study had mean scores on the Alzheimer's Disease Assessment Scale (ADAS-cog) of approximately 26 units, with a range from 4 to 61. Experience gained in longitudinal studies of ambulatory patients with mild to moderate Alzheimer's Disease suggest that they gain 6 to 12 units a year on the ADAS-cog. However, lesser degrees of change are seen in patients with very mild or very advanced disease because the ADAS-cog is not uniformly sensitive to change over the course of the disease. The annualized rate of decline in the placebo patients participating in ARICEPT® trials was approximately 2 to 4 units per year.

The ability of ARICEPT® to produce an overall clinical effect was assessed using a Clinician's Interview Based Impression of Change that required the use of caregiver information, the CIBIC plus. The CIBIC plus is not a single instrument and is not a standardized instrument like the ADAS-cog. Clinical trials for investigational drugs have used a variety of CIBIC formats, each different in terms of depth and structure.

As such, results from a CIBIC plus reflect clinical experience from the trial or trials in which it was used and cannot be compared directly with the results of CIBIC plus evaluations from other clinical trials. The CIBIC plus used in ARICEPT® trials was a semi-structured instrument that was intended to examine four major areas of patient function: General, Cognitive, Behavioral and Activities of Daily Living. It represents the assessment of a skilled clinician based upon his/her observations at an interview with the

Continued on next page

Aricept—Cont.

patient, in combination with information supplied by a caregiver familiar with the behavior of the patient over the interval rated. The CIBIC plus is scored as a seven point categorical rating, ranging from a score of 1, indicating "markedly improved," to a score of 4, indicating "no change" to a score of 7, indicating "markedly worse." The CIBIC plus has not been systematically compared directly to assessments not using information from caregivers (CIBIC) or other global methods.

Thirty-Week Study

In a study of 30 weeks duration, 473 patients were randomized to receive single daily doses of placebo, 5 mg/day or 10 mg/day of ARICEPT®. The 30-week study was divided into a 24-week double-blind active treatment phase followed by a 6-week single-blind placebo washout period. The study was designed to compare 5 mg/day or 10 mg/day fixed doses of ARICEPT® to placebo. However, to reduce the likelihood of cholinergic effects, the 10 mg/day treatment was started following an initial 7-day treatment with 5 mg/day doses.

Effects on the ADAS-cog: Figure 1 illustrates the time course for the change from baseline in ADAS-cog scores for all three dose groups over the 30 weeks of the study. After 24 weeks of treatment, the mean differences in the ADAS-cog change scores for ARICEPT® treated patients compared to the patients on placebo were 2.8 and 3.1 units for the 5 mg/day and 10 mg/day treatments, respectively. These differences were statistically significant. While the treatment effect size may appear to be slightly greater for the 10 mg/day treatment, there was no statistically significant difference between the two active treatments.

Following 6 weeks of placebo washout, scores on the ADAS-cog for both the ARICEPT® treatment groups were indistinguishable from those patients who had received only placebo for 30 weeks. This suggests that the beneficial effects of ARICEPT® abate over 6 weeks following discontinuation of treatment and do not represent a change in the underlying disease. There was no evidence of a rebound effect 6 weeks after abrupt discontinuation of therapy.

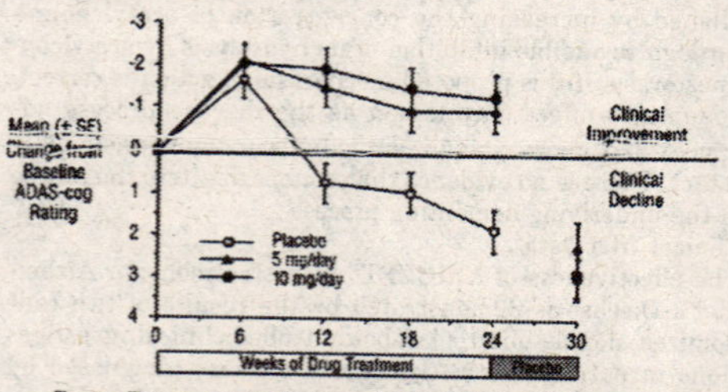

Figure 1. Time-course of the Change from Baseline in ADAS-cog Score for Patients Completing 24 Weeks of Treatment.

Figure 2 illustrates the cumulative percentages of patients from each of the three treatment groups who had attained the measure of improvement in ADAS-cog score shown on the X axis. Three change scores, (7-point and 4-point reductions from baseline or no change in score) have been identified for illustrative purposes and the percent of patients in each group achieving that result is shown in the inset table. The curves demonstrate that both patients assigned to placebo and ARICEPT® have a wide range of responses, but that the active treatment groups are more likely to show the greater improvements. A curve for an effective treatment would be shifted to the left of the curve for placebo, while an ineffective or deleterious treatment would be superimposed upon or shifted to the right of the curve for placebo, respectively.

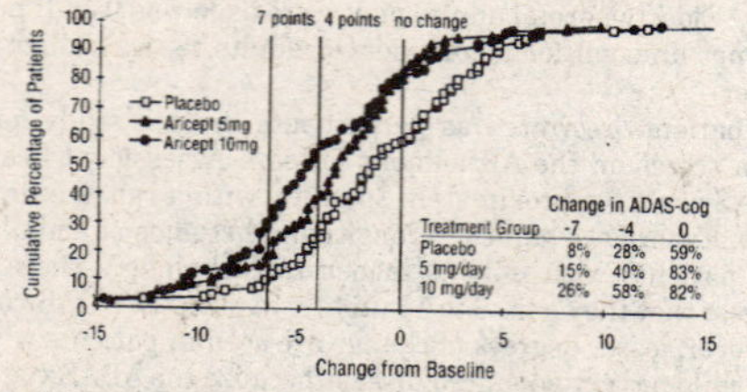

Figure 2. Cumulative Percentage of Patients Completing 24 Weeks of Double-blind Treatment with Specified Changes from Baseline ADAS-cog Scores. The Percentages of Randomized Patients who Completed the Study were: Placebo 80%, 5 mg/day 85% and 10 mg/day 68%.

Effects on the CIBIC plus: Figure 3 is a histogram of the frequency distribution of CIBIC plus scores attained by patients assigned to each of the three treatment groups who completed 24 weeks of treatment. The mean drug-placebo differences for these groups of patients were 0.35 units and 0.39 units for 5 mg/day and 10 mg/day of ARICEPT®, respectively. These differences were statistically significant. There was no statistically significant difference between the two active treatments.

[See figure 3 at top of next column]

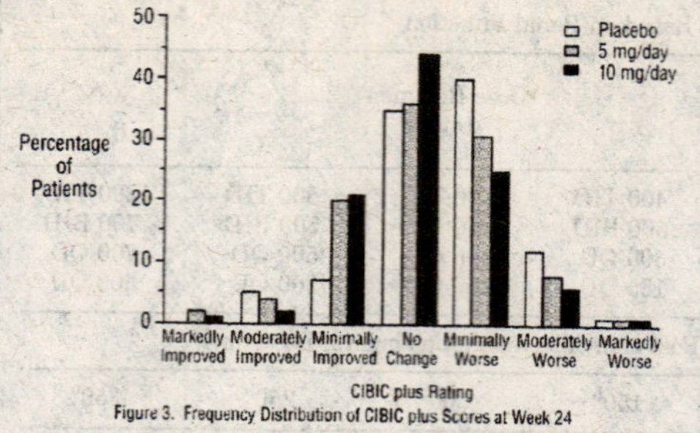

Figure 3. Frequency Distribution of CIBIC plus Scores at Week 24

Fifteen-Week Study

In a study of 15 weeks duration, patients were randomized to receive single daily doses of placebo or either 5 mg/day or 10 mg/day of ARICEPT® for 12 weeks, followed by a 3-week placebo washout period. As in the 30-week study, to avoid acute cholinergic effects, the 10 mg/day treatment followed an initial 7-day treatment with 5 mg/day doses.

Effects on the ADAS-Cog: Figure 4 illustrates the time course of the change from baseline in ADAS-cog scores for all three dose groups over the 15 weeks of the study. After 12 weeks of treatment, the differences in mean ADAS-cog change scores for the ARICEPT® treated patients compared to the patients on placebo were 2.7 and 3.0 units each, for the 5 and 10 mg/day ARICEPT® treatment groups respectively. These differences were statistically significant. The effect size for the 10 mg/day group may appear to be slightly larger than that for 5 mg/day. However, the differences between active treatments were not statistically significant.

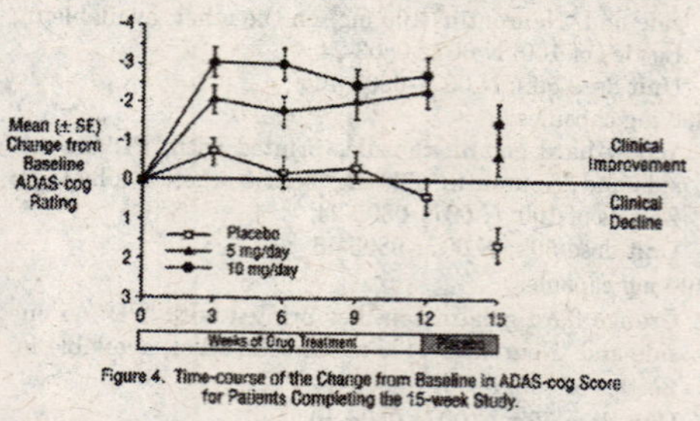

Figure 4. Time-course of the Change from Baseline in ADAS-cog Score for Patients Completing the 15-week Study.

Following 3 weeks of placebo washout, scores on the ADAS-cog for both the ARICEPT® treatment groups increased, indicating that discontinuation of ARICEPT® resulted in a loss of its treatment effect. The duration of this placebo washout period was not sufficient to characterize the rate of loss of the treatment effect, but, the 30-week study (see above) demonstrated that treatment effects associated with the use of ARICEPT® abate within 6 weeks of treatment discontinuation.

Figure 5 illustrates the cumulative percentages of patients from each of the three treatment groups who attained the measure of improvement in ADAS-cog score shown on the X axis. The same three change scores, (7-point and 4-point reductions from baseline or no change in score) as selected for the 30-week study have been used for this illustration. The percentages of patients achieving those results are shown in the inset table.

As observed in the 30-week study, the curves demonstrate that patients assigned to either placebo or to ARICEPT® have a wide range of responses, but that the ARICEPT® treated patients are more likely to show the greater improvements in cognitive performance.

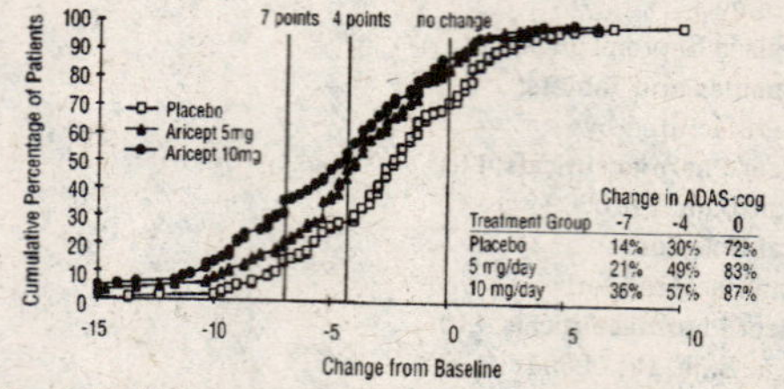

Figure 5. Cumulative Percentage of Patients with Specified Changes from Baseline ADAS-cog Scores. The Percentages of Randomized Patients Within Each Treatment Group Who Completed the Study Were: Placebo 93%, 5 mg/day 90% and 10 mg/day 82%.

Effects on the CIBIC plus: Figure 6 is a histogram of the frequency distribution of CIBIC plus scores attained by patients assigned to each of the three treatment groups who completed 12 weeks of treatment. The differences in mean scores for ARICEPT® treated patients compared to the patients on placebo at Week 12 were 0.36 and 0.38 units for the 5 mg/day and 10 mg/day treatment groups, respectively. These differences were statistically significant.

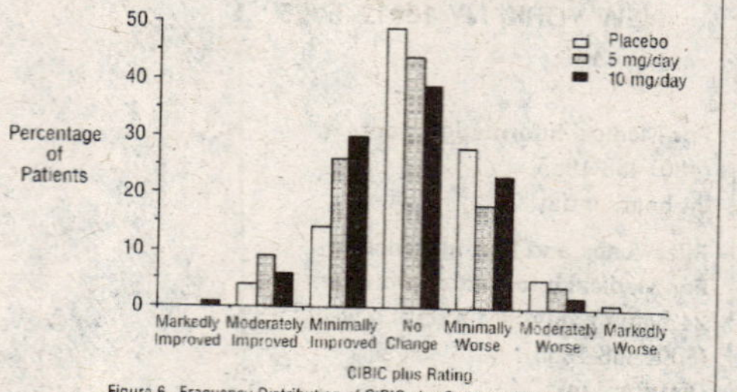

Figure 6. Frequency Distribution of CIBIC plus Scores at Week 12

In both studies, patient age, sex and race were not found to predict the clinical outcome of ARICEPT® treatment.

Clinical Pharmacokinetics

Donepezil is well absorbed with a relative oral bioavailability of 100% and reaches peak plasma concentrations in 3 to 4 hours. Pharmacokinetics are linear over a dose range of 1-10 mg given once daily. Neither food nor time of administration (morning vs. evening dose) influences the rate or extent of absorption. The elimination half life of donepezil is about 70 hours and the mean apparent plasma clearance (Cl/F) is 0.13 L/hr/kg. Following multiple dose administration, donepezil accumulates in plasma by 4-7 fold and steady state is reached within 15 days. The steady state volume of distribution is 12 L/kg. Donepezil is approximately 96% bound to human plasma proteins, mainly to albumins (about 75%) and $alpha_1$ - acid glycoprotein (about 21%) over the concentration range of 2–1000 ng/mL.

Donepezil is both excreted in the urine intact and extensively metabolized to four major metabolites, two of which are known to be active, and a number of minor metabolites, not all of which have been identified. Donepezil is metabolized by CYP 450 isoenzymes 2D6 and 3A4 and undergoes glucuronidation. Following administration of ^{14}C-labeled donepezil, plasma radioactivity, expressed as a percent of the administered dose, was present primarily as intact donepezil (53%) and as 6-O-desmethyl donepezil (11%), which has been reported to inhibit AChE to the same extent as donepezil *in vitro* and was found in plasma at concentrations equal to about 20% of donepezil. Approximately 57% and 15% of the total radioactivity was recovered in urine and feces, respectively, over a period of 10 days, while 28% remained unrecovered, with about 17% of the donepezil dose recovered in the urine as unchanged drug.

Special Populations:

Hepatic Disease: In a study of 10 patients with stable alcoholic cirrhosis, the clearance of ARICEPT® was decreased by 20% relative to 10 healthy age and sex matched subjects.

Renal Disease: In a study of 4 patients with moderate to severe renal impairment (Cl_{Cr} < 22 mL/min/1.73 m^2) the clearance of ARICEPT® did not differ from 4 age and sex matched healthy subjects.

Age: No formal pharmacokinetic study was conducted to examine age related differences in the pharmacokinetics of ARICEPT®. However, mean plasma ARICEPT® concentrations measured during therapeutic drug monitoring of elderly patients with Alzheimer's Disease are comparable to those observed in young healthy volunteers.

Gender and Race: No specific pharmacokinetic study was conducted to investigate the effects of gender and race on the disposition of ARICEPT®. However, retrospective pharmacokinetic analysis indicates that gender and race (Japanese and Caucasians) did not affect the clearance of ARICEPT®.

Drug-Drug Interactions

Drugs Highly Bound to Plasma Proteins: Drug displacement studies have been performed *in vitro* between this highly bound drug (96%) and other drugs such as furosemide, digoxin, and warfarin. ARICEPT® at concentrations of 0.3–10 µg/mL did not affect the binding of furosemide (5 µg/mL), digoxin (2 ng/mL), and warfarin (3 µg/mL) to human albumin. Similarly, the binding of ARICEPT® to human albumin was not affected by furosemide, digoxin and warfarin.

Effect of ARICEPT® on the Metabolism of Other Drugs: No *in vivo* clinical trials have investigated the effect of ARICEPT® on the clearance of drugs metabolized by CYP 3A4 (e.g. cisapride, terfenadine) or by CYP 2D6 (e.g. imipramine). However, *in vitro* studies show a low rate of binding to these enzymes (mean K_i about 50–130 µM), that, given the therapeutic plasma concentrations of donepezil (164 nM), indicates little likelihood of interference.

Whether ARICEPT® has any potential for enzyme induction is not known.

Formal pharmacokinetic studies evaluated the potential of ARICEPT® for interaction with theophylline, cimetidine, warfarin and digoxin. No significant effects on the pharmacokinetics of these drugs were observed.

Effect of Other Drugs on the Metabolism of ARICEPT®: Ketoconazole and quinidine, inhibitors of CYP450, 3A4 and 2D6, respectively, inhibit donepezil metabolism *in vitro*. Whether there is a clinical effect of these inhibitors is not known. Inducers of CYP 2D6 and CYP 3A4 (e.g., phenytoin, carbamazepine, dexamethasone, rifampin, and phenobarbital) could increase the rate of elimination of ARICEPT®. Formal pharmacokinetic studies demonstrated that the metabolism of ARICEPT® is not significantly affected by concurrent administration of digoxin or cimetidine.

INDICATIONS AND USAGE

ARICEPT® is indicated for the treatment of mild to moderate dementia of the Alzheimer's type.

CONTRAINDICATIONS

ARICEPT® is contraindicated in patients with known hypersensitivity to donepezil hydrochloride or to piperidine derivatives.

WARNINGS

Anesthesia: ARICEPT®, as a cholinesterase inhibitor, is likely to exaggerate succinylcholine-type muscle relaxation during anesthesia.

Cardiovascular Conditions: Because of their pharmacological action, cholinesterase inhibitors may have vagotonic effects on the sinoatrial and atrioventricular nodes. This effect may manifest as bradycardia or heart block in patients both with and without known underlying cardiac conduction abnormalities. Syncopal episodes have been reported in association with the use of ARICEPT®.

Gastrointestinal Conditions: Through their primary action, cholinesterase inhibitors may be expected to increase gastric acid secretion due to increased cholinergic activity. Therefore, patients should be monitored closely for symptoms of active or occult gastrointestinal bleeding, especially those at increased risk for developing ulcers, e.g., those with a history of ulcer disease or those receiving concurrent nonsteroidal anti-inflammatory drugs (NSAIDS). Clinical studies of ARICEPT® have shown no increase, relative to placebo, in the incidence of either peptic ulcer disease or gastrointestinal bleeding.

ARICEPT®, as a predictable consequence of its pharmacological properties, has been shown to produce diarrhea, nausea and vomiting. These effects, when they occur, appear more frequently with the 10 mg/day dose than with the 5 mg/day dose. In most cases, these effects have been mild and transient, sometimes lasting one to three weeks, and have resolved during continued use of ARICEPT®.

Genitourinary: Although not observed in clinical trials of ARICEPT®, cholinomimetics may cause bladder outflow obstruction.

Neurological Conditions: Seizures: Cholinomimetics are believed to have some potential to cause generalized convulsions. However, seizure activity also may be a manifestation of Alzheimer's Disease.

Pulmonary Conditions: Because of their cholinomimetic actions, cholinesterase inhibitors should be prescribed with care to patients with a history of asthma or obstructive pulmonary disease.

PRECAUTIONS

Drug-Drug Interactions (see Clinical Pharmacology: Clinical Pharmacokinetics: Drug-drug Interactions)

Effect of ARICEPT® on the Metabolism of Other Drugs: No *in vivo* clinical trials have investigated the effect of ARICEPT® on the clearance of drugs metabolized by CYP 3A4 (e.g. cisapride, terfenadine) or by CYP 2D6 (e.g. imipramine). However, *in vitro* studies show a low rate of binding to these enzymes (mean K_i about 50–130 μM), that, given the therapeutic plasma concentrations of donepezil (164 nM), indicates little likelihood of interference.

Whether ARICEPT® has any potential for enzyme induction is not known.

Effect of Other Drugs on the Metabolism of ARICEPT®: Ketoconazole and quinidine, inhibitors of CYP450, 3A4 and 2D6, respectively, inhibit donepezil metabolism *in vitro*. Whether there is a clinical effect of these inhibitors is not known. Inducers of CYP 2D6 and CYP 3A4 (e.g., phenytoin, carbamazepine, dexamethasone, rifampin, and phenobarbital) could increase the rate of elimination of ARICEPT®.

Use with Anticholinergics: Because of their mechanism of action, cholinesterase inhibitors have the potential to interfere with the activity of anticholinergic medications.

Use with Cholinomimetics and Other Cholinesterase Inhibitors: A synergistic effect may be expected when cholinesterase inhibitors are given concurrently with succinylcholine, similar neuromuscular blocking agents or cholinergic agonists such as bethanechol.

Carcinogenesis, Mutagenesis, Impairment of Fertility

Carcinogenicity studies of donepezil have not been completed.

Donepezil was not mutagenic in the Ames reverse mutation assay in bacteria. In the chromosome aberration test in cultures of Chinese hamster lung (CHL) cells, some clastogenic effects were observed. Donepezil was not clastogenic in the *in vivo* mouse micronucleus test.

Donepezil had no effect on fertility in rats at doses up to 10 mg/kg/day (approximately 8 times the maximum recommended human dose on a mg/m² basis).

Pregnancy

Pregnancy Category C: Teratology studies conducted in pregnant rats at doses up to 16 mg/kg/day (approximately 13 times the maximum recommended human dose on a mg/m² basis) and in pregnant rabbits at doses up to 10 mg/kg/day (approximately 16 times the maximum recommended human dose on a mg/m² basis) did not disclose any evidence for a teratogenic potential of donepezil. However, in a study in which pregnant rats were given up to 10 mg/kg/day (approximately 8 times the maximum recommended human dose on a mg/m² basis) from day 17 of gestation through day 20 postpartum, there was a slight increase in still births and a slight decrease in pup survival through day 4 postpartum at this dose; the next lower dose tested was 3 mg/kg/day. There are no adequate or well-controlled studies in pregnant women. ARICEPT® should be used during pregnancy only if the potential benefit justifies the potential risk to the fetus.

Nursing Mothers

It is not known whether donepezil is excreted in human breast milk. ARICEPT® has no indication for use in nursing mothers.

Pediatric Use

There are no adequate and well-controlled trials to document the safety and efficacy of ARICEPT® in any illness occurring in children.

ADVERSE REACTIONS

Adverse Events Leading to Discontinuation

The rates of discontinuation from controlled clinical trials of ARICEPT® due to adverse events for the ARICEPT® 5 mg/day treatment groups were comparable to those of placebo-treatment groups at approximately 5%. The rate of discontinuation of patients who received 7-day escalations from 5 mg/day to 10 mg/day, was higher at 13%.

The most common adverse events leading to discontinuation, defined as those occurring in at least 2% of patients and at twice the incidence seen in placebo patients, are shown in Table 1.

Table 1. Most Frequent Adverse Events Leading to Withdrawal from Controlled Clinical Trials by Dose Group

Dose Group	Placebo	5 mg/day ARICEPT®	10 mg/day ARICEPT®
Patients Randomized	355	350	315
Event/% Discontinuing			
Nausea	1%	1%	3%
Diarrhea	0%	<1%	3%
Vomiting	<1%	<1%	2%

Most Frequent Adverse Clinical Events Seen in Association with the Use of ARICEPT®

The most common adverse events, defined as those occurring at a frequency of at least 5% in patients receiving 10 mg/day and twice the placebo rate, are largely predicted by ARICEPT®'s cholinomimetic effects. These include nausea, diarrhea, insomnia, vomiting, muscle cramp, fatigue and anorexia. These adverse events were often of mild intensity and transient, resolving during continued ARICEPT® treatment without the need for dose modification.

There is evidence to suggest that the frequency of these common adverse events may be affected by the rate of titration. An open-label study was conducted with 269 patients who received placebo in the 15 and 30-week studies. These patients were titrated to a dose of 10 mg/day over a 6-week period. The rates of common adverse events were lower than those seen in patients titrated to 10 mg/day over one week in the controlled clinical trials and were comparable to those seen in patients on 5 mg/day.

See Table 2 for a comparison of the most common adverse events following one and six week titration regimens.

[See table 2 below]

Table 2. Comparison of rates of adverse events in patients titrated to 10 mg/day over 1 and 6 weeks

	No titration		One week titration	Six week titration
Adverse Event	Placebo (n=315)	5 mg/day (n=311)	10 mg/day (n=315)	10 mg/day (n=269)
Nausea	6%	5%	19%	6%
Diarrhea	5%	8%	15%	9%
Insomnia	6%	6%	14%	6%
Fatigue	3%	4%	8%	3%
Vomiting	3%	3%	8%	5%
Muscle cramps	2%	6%	8%	3%
Anorexia	2%	3%	7%	3%

Adverse Events Reported in Controlled Trials

The events cited reflect experience gained under closely monitored conditions of clinical trials in a highly selected patient population. In actual clinical practice or in other clinical trials, these frequency estimates may not apply, as the conditions of use, reporting behavior, and the kinds of patients treated may differ. Table 3 lists treatment emergent signs and symptoms that were reported in at least 2% of patients in placebo-controlled trials who received ARICEPT® and for which the rate of occurrence was greater for ARICEPT® assigned than placebo assigned patients. In general, adverse events occurred more frequently in female patients and with advancing age.

Table 3. Adverse Events Reported in Controlled Clinical Trials in at Least 2% of Patients Receiving ARICEPT® and at a Higher Frequency than Placebo-treated Patients

Body System/ Adverse Event	Placebo (n=355)	ARICEPT® (n=747)
Percent of Patients with any Adverse Event	72	74
Body as a Whole		
Headache	9	10
Pain, various locations	8	9
Accident	6	7
Fatigue	3	5
Cardiovascular System		
Syncope	1	2
Digestive System		
Nausea	6	11
Diarrhea	5	10
Vomiting	3	5
Anorexia	2	4
Hemic and Lymphatic System		
Ecchymosis	3	4
Metabolic and Nutritional Systems		
Weight Decrease	1	3
Musculoskeletal System		
Muscle Cramps	2	6
Arthritis	1	2
Nervous System		
Insomnia	6	9
Dizziness	6	8
Depression	<1	3
Abnormal Dreams	0	3
Somnolence	<1	2
Urogenital System		
Frequent Urination	1	2

Other Adverse Events Observed During Clinical Trials

ARICEPT® has been administered to over 1700 individuals during clinical trials worldwide. Approximately 1200 of these patients have been treated for at least 3 months and more than 1000 patients have been treated for at least 6 months. Controlled and uncontrolled trials in the United States included approximately 900 patients. In regards to the highest dose of 10 mg/day, this population includes 650 patients treated for 3 months, 475 patients treated for 6 months and 116 patients treated for over 1 year. The range of patient exposure is from 1 to 1214 days.

Treatment emergent signs and symptoms that occurred during 3 controlled clinical trials and two open-label trials in the United States were recorded as adverse events by the clinical investigators using terminology of their own choosing. To provide an overall estimate of the proportion of individuals having similar types of events, the events were grouped into a smaller number of standardized categories using a modified COSTART dictionary and event frequencies were calculated across all studies. These categories are used in the listing below. The frequencies represent the proportion of 900 patients from these trials who experienced that event while receiving ARICEPT®. All adverse events occurring at least twice are included, except for those already listed in Tables 2 or 3, COSTART terms too general to be informative, or events less likely to be drug caused. Events are classified by body system and listed using the following definitions: *frequent adverse events* - those occurring in at least 1/100 patients; *infrequent adverse events* - those occurring in 1/100 to 1/1000 patients. These adverse events are not necessarily related to ARICEPT® treatment and in most cases were observed at a similar frequency in placebo-treated patients in the controlled studies. No important additional adverse events were seen in studies conducted outside the United States.

Body as a Whole: *Frequent:* influenza, chest pain, toothache; *Infrequent:* fever, edema face, periorbital edema, hernia hiatal, abscess, cellulitis, chills, generalized coldness, head fullness, listlessness.

Continued on next page

Aricept—Cont.

Cardiovascular System: *Frequent:* hypertension, vasodilation, atrial fibrillation, hot flashes, hypotension; *Infrequent:* angina pectoris, postural hypotension, myocardial infarction, AV block (first degree), congestive heart failure, arteritis, bradycardia, peripheral vascular disease, supraventricular tachycardia, deep vein thrombosis.

Digestive System: *Frequent:* fecal incontinence, gastrointestinal bleeding, bloating, epigastric pain; *Infrequent:* eructation, gingivitis, increased appetite, flatulence, periodontal abscess, cholelithiasis, diverticulitis, drooling, dry mouth, fever sore, gastritis, irritable colon, tongue edema, epigastric distress, gastroenteritis, increased transaminases, hemorrhoids, ileus, increased thirst, jaundice, melena, polydipsia, duodenal ulcer, stomach ulcer.

Endocrine System: *Infrequent:* diabetes mellitus, goiter.

Hemic and Lymphatic System: *Infrequent:* anemia, thrombocythemia, thrombocytopenia, eosinophilia, erythrocytopenia.

Metabolic and Nutritional Disorders: *Frequent:* dehydration; *Infrequent:* gout, hypokalemia, increased creatine kinase, hyperglycemia, weight increase, increased lactate dehydrogenase.

Musculoskeletal System: *Frequent:* bone fracture; *Infrequent:* muscle weakness, muscle fasciculation.

Nervous System: *Frequent:* delusions, tremor, irritability, paresthesia, aggression, vertigo, ataxia, increased libido, restlessness, abnormal crying, nervousness, aphasia; *Infrequent:* cerebrovascular accident, intracranial hemorrhage, transient ischemic attack, emotional lability, neuralgia, coldness (localized), muscle spasm, dysphoria, gait abnormality, hypertonia, hypokinesia, neurodermatitis, numbness (localized), paranoia, dysarthria, dysphasia, hostility, decreased libido, melancholia, emotional withdrawal, nystagmus, pacing.

Respiratory System: *Frequent:* dyspnea, sore throat, bronchitis; *Infrequent:* epistaxis, post nasal drip, pneumonia, hyperventilation, pulmonary congestion, wheezing, hypoxia, pharyngitis, pleurisy, pulmonary collapse, sleep apnea, snoring.

Skin and Appendages: *Frequent:* pruritus, diaphoresis, urticaria; *Infrequent:* dermatitis, erythema, skin discoloration, hyperkeratosis, alopecia, fungal dermatitis, herpes zoster, hirsutism, skin striae, night sweats, skin ulcer.

Special Senses: *Frequent:* cataract, eye irritation, vision blurred; *Infrequent:* dry eyes, glaucoma, earache, tinnitus, blepharitis, decreased hearing, retinal hemorrhage, otitis externa, otitis media, bad taste, conjunctival hemorrhage, ear buzzing, motion sickness, spots before eyes.

Urogenital System: *Frequent:* urinary incontinence, nocturia; *Infrequent:* dysuria, hematuria, urinary urgency, metrorrhagia, cystitis, enuresis, prostate hypertrophy, pyelonephritis, inability to empty bladder, breast fibroadenosis, fibrocystic breast, mastitis, pyuria, renal failure, vaginitis.

Postintroduction Reports

Voluntary reports of adverse events temporally associated with ARICEPT® that have been received since market introduction that are not listed above, and that there is inadequate data to determine the causal relationship with the drug include the following: abdominal pain, agitation, cholecystitis, confusion, convulsions, hallucinations, heart block (all types), hemolytic anemia, hepatitis, hyponatremia, neuroleptic malignant syndrome, pancreatitis, and rash.

OVERDOSAGE

Because strategies for the management of overdose are continually evolving, it is advisable to contact a Poison Control Center to determine the latest recommendations for the management of an overdose of any drug.

As in any case of overdose, general supportive measures should be utilized. Overdosage with cholinesterase inhibitors can result in cholinergic crisis characterized by severe nausea, vomiting, salivation, sweating, bradycardia, hypotension, respiratory depression, collapse and convulsions. Increasing muscle weakness is a possibility and may result in death if respiratory muscles are involved. Tertiary anticholinergics such as atropine may be used as an antidote for ARICEPT® overdosage. Intravenous atropine sulfate titrated to effect is recommended: an initial dose of 1.0 to 2.0 mg IV with subsequent doses based upon clinical response. Atypical responses in blood pressure and heart rate have been reported with other cholinomimetics when coadministered with quaternary anticholinergics such as glycopyrrolate. It is not known whether ARICEPT® and/or its metabolites can be removed by dialysis (hemodialysis, peritoneal dialysis, or hemofiltration).

Dose-related signs of toxicity in animals included reduced spontaneous movement, prone position, staggering gait, lacrimation, clonic convulsions, depressed respiration, salivation, miosis, tremors, fasciculation and lower body surface temperature.

DOSAGE AND ADMINISTRATION

The dosages of ARICEPT® shown to be effective in controlled clinical trials are 5 mg and 10 mg administered once per day.

The higher dose of 10 mg did not provide a statistically significantly greater clinical benefit than 5 mg. There is a suggestion, however, based upon order of group mean scores and dose trend analyses of data from these clinical trials, that a daily dose of 10 mg of ARICEPT® might provide additional benefit for some patients. Accordingly, whether or not to employ a dose of 10 mg is a matter of prescriber and patient preference.

Evidence from the controlled trials indicates that the 10 mg dose, with a one week titration, is likely to be associated with a higher incidence of cholinergic adverse events than the 5 mg dose. In open label trials using a 6 week titration, the frequency of these same adverse events was similar between the 5 mg and 10 mg dose groups. Therefore, because steady state is not achieved for 15 days and because the incidence of untoward effects may be influenced by the rate of dose escalation, treatment with a dose of 10 mg should not be contemplated until patients have been on a daily dose of 5 mg for 4 to 6 weeks.

ARICEPT® should be taken in the evening, just prior to retiring. ARICEPT® can be taken with or without food.

HOW SUPPLIED

ARICEPT® is supplied as film-coated, round tablets containing either 5 mg or 10 mg of donepezil hydrochloride.

The 5 mg tablets are white. The strength, in mg (5), is debossed on one side and ARICEPT is debossed on the other side.

The 10 mg tablets are yellow. The strength, in mg (10), is debossed on one side and ARICEPT is debossed on the other side.

5 mg (White)	Bottles of 30 (NDC# 62856-245-30)
	Bottles of 90 (NDC# 62856-245-90)
	Unit Dose Blister Package 100 (10×10) (NDC# 62856-245-41)
10 mg (Yellow)	Bottles of 30 (NDC# 62856-246-30)
	Bottles of 90 (NDC# 62856-246-90)
	Unit Dose Blister Package 100 (10×10) (NDC# 62856-246-41)

Storage: Store at controlled room temperature, 15°C to 30°C (59°F to 86°F).

℞ only

ARICEPT® is a registered trademark of Eisai Co., Ltd.

Manufactured and Marketed by Eisai Inc., Teaneck, NJ 07666

Marketed by
Pfizer Inc, New York, NY 10017

200305
Revised October 2003

BEXTRA® ℞
[*bĕks'trā*]
valdecoxib tablets

Prescribing information for this product, which appears on pages 2573–2577 of the 2004 PDR, has been completely revised as follows. Please write "See Supplement A" next to the product heading.

DESCRIPTION

Valdecoxib is chemically designated as 4-(5-methyl-3-phenyl-4-isoxazolyl) benzenesulfonamide and is a diaryl substituted isoxazole. It has the following chemical structure:

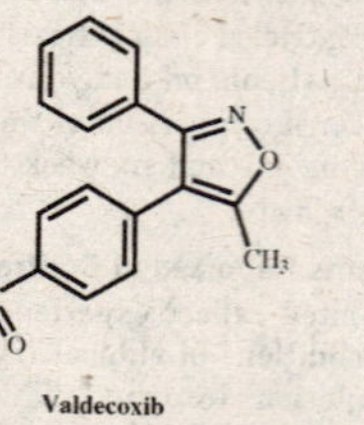

Valdecoxib

The empirical formula for valdecoxib is $C_{16}H_{14}N_2O_3S$, and the molecular weight is 314.36. Valdecoxib is a white crystalline powder that is relatively insoluble in water (10 µg/mL) at 25°C and pH 7.0, soluble in methanol and ethanol, and freely soluble in organic solvents and alkaline (pH=12) aqueous solutions.

BEXTRA Tablets for oral administration contain either 10 mg or 20 mg of valdecoxib. Inactive ingredients include lactose monohydrate, microcrystalline cellulose, pregelatinized starch, croscarmellose sodium, magnesium stearate, hypromellose, polyethylene glycol, polysorbate 80, and titanium dioxide.

CLINICAL PHARMACOLOGY

Mechanism of Action

Valdecoxib is a nonsteroidal anti-inflammatory drug (NSAID) that exhibits anti-inflammatory, analgesic and antipyretic properties in animal models. The mechanism of action is believed to be due to inhibition of prostaglandin synthesis primarily through inhibition of cyclooxygenase-2 (COX-2). At therapeutic plasma concentrations in humans valdecoxib does not inhibit cyclooxygenase-1 (COX-1).

Pharmacokinetics

Absorption

Valdecoxib achieves maximal plasma concentrations in approximately 3 hours. The absolute bioavailability of valdecoxib is 83% following oral administration of BEXTRA compared to intravenous infusion of valdecoxib.

Dose proportionality was demonstrated after single doses (1-400 mg) of valdecoxib. With multiple doses (up to 100 mg/day for 14 days), valdecoxib exposure as measured by the AUC, increases in a more than proportional manner at doses above 10 mg BID. Steady state plasma concentrations of valdecoxib are achieved by day 4.

The steady state pharmacokinetic parameters of valdecoxib in healthy male subjects are shown in Table 1.

Table 1
Mean (SD) Steady State Pharmacokinetic Parameters

Steady State Pharmacokinetic Parameters after Valdecoxib 10 mg Once Daily for 14 Days	Healthy Male Subjects (n=8, 20 to 42 yr.)
$AUC_{(0-24hr)}$ (hr·ng/mL)	1479.0 (291.9)
C_{max} (ng/mL)	161.1 (48.1)
T_{max} (hr)	2.25 (0.71)
C_{min} (ng/mL)	21.9 (7.68)
Elimination Half-life (hr)	8.11 (1.32)

No clinically significant age or gender differences were seen in pharmacokinetic parameters that would require dosage adjustments.

Effect of Food and Antacid

BEXTRA can be taken with or without food. Food had no significant effect on either the peak plasma concentration (C_{max}) or extent of absorption (AUC) of valdecoxib when BEXTRA was taken with a high fat meal. The time to peak plasma concentration (T_{max}), however, was delayed by 1-2 hours. Administration of BEXTRA with antacid (aluminum/magnesium hydroxide) had no significant effect on either the rate or extent of absorption of valdecoxib.

Distribution

Plasma protein binding for valdecoxib is about 98% over the concentration range (21-2384 ng/mL). Steady state apparent volume of distribution (Vss/F) of valdecoxib is approximately 86 L after oral administration. Valdecoxib and its active metabolite preferentially partition into erythrocytes with a blood to plasma concentration ratio of about 2.5:1. This ratio remains approximately constant with time and therapeutic blood concentrations.

Metabolism

In humans, valdecoxib undergoes extensive hepatic metabolism involving both P450 isoenzymes (3A4 and 2C9) and non-P450 dependent pathways (i.e., glucuronidation). Concomitant administration of BEXTRA with known CYP 3A4 and 2C9 inhibitors (e.g., fluconazole and ketoconazole) can result in increased plasma exposure of valdecoxib (see PRECAUTIONS — Drug Interactions).

One active metabolite of valdecoxib has been identified in human plasma at approximately 10% the concentration of valdecoxib. This metabolite, which is a less potent COX-2 specific inhibitor than the parent, also undergoes extensive metabolism and constitutes less than 2% of the valdecoxib dose excreted in the urine and feces. Due to its low concentration in the systemic circulation, it is not likely to contribute significantly to the efficacy profile of BEXTRA.

Excretion

Valdecoxib is eliminated predominantly via hepatic metabolism with less than 5% of the dose excreted unchanged in the urine and feces. About 70% of the dose is excreted in the urine as metabolites, and about 20% as valdecoxib N-glucuronide. The apparent oral clearance (CL/F) of valdecoxib is about 6 L/hr. The mean elimination half-life ($T_{1/2}$) ranges from 8-11 hours, and increases with age.

Special Populations

Geriatric

In elderly subjects (> 65 years), weight-adjusted steady state plasma concentrations ($AUC_{(0-12hr)}$) are about 30% higher than in young subjects. No dose adjustment is needed based on age.

Pediatric

BEXTRA has not been investigated in pediatric patients below 18 years of age.

Race

Pharmacokinetic differences due to race have not been identified in clinical and pharmacokinetic studies conducted to date.

Hepatic Insufficiency

Valdecoxib plasma concentrations are significantly increased (130%) in patients with moderate (Child-Pugh Class B) hepatic impairment. In clinical trials, doses of BEXTRA above those recommended have been associated with fluid retention. Hence, treatment with BEXTRA should be initiated with caution in patients with mild to moderate hepatic impairment and fluid retention. The use of BEXTRA in patients with severe hepatic impairment (Child-Pugh Class C) is not recommended.

Renal Insufficiency

The pharmacokinetics of valdecoxib have been studied in patients with varying degrees of renal impairment. Because renal elimination of valdecoxib is not important to its disposition, no clinically significant changes in valdecoxib clearance were found even in patients with severe renal impairment or in patients undergoing renal dialysis. In patients undergoing hemodialysis the plasma clearance (CL/F) of valdecoxib was similar to the CL/F found in healthy elderly subjects (CL/F about 6 to 7 L/hr.) with normal renal function (based on creatinine clearance).

NSAIDs have been associated with worsening renal function and use in advanced renal disease is not recommended (see PRECAUTIONS – Renal Effects).

Drug Interactions

Also see **PRECAUTIONS — Drug Interactions.**

General

Valdecoxib undergoes both P450 (CYP) dependent and non-P450 dependent (glucuronidation) metabolism. In vitro studies indicate that valdecoxib is not a significant inhibitor of CYP 1A2, 3A4, or 2D6 and is only a weak inhibitor of CYP 2C9 and 2C19 at therapeutic concentrations. The P450-mediated metabolic pathway of valdecoxib predominantly

Figure 1
Incidence of Endoscopically Observed Gastroduodenal Ulcers in OA Patients

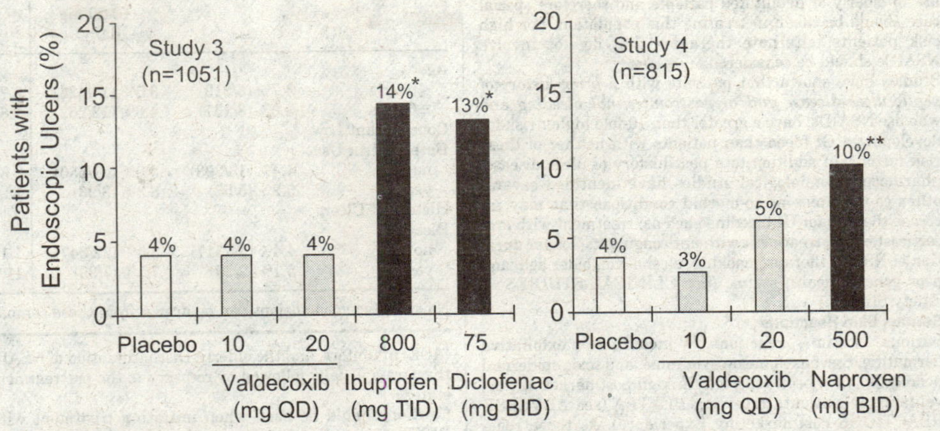

* Significantly different vs placebo and both valdecoxib treatment groups; p<0.05
** Significantly different vs placebo and valdecoxib 10 mg; p<0.05

Figure 2
Incidence of Endoscopic Gastroduodenal Ulcers and Renal Events in the High-dose Safety Study

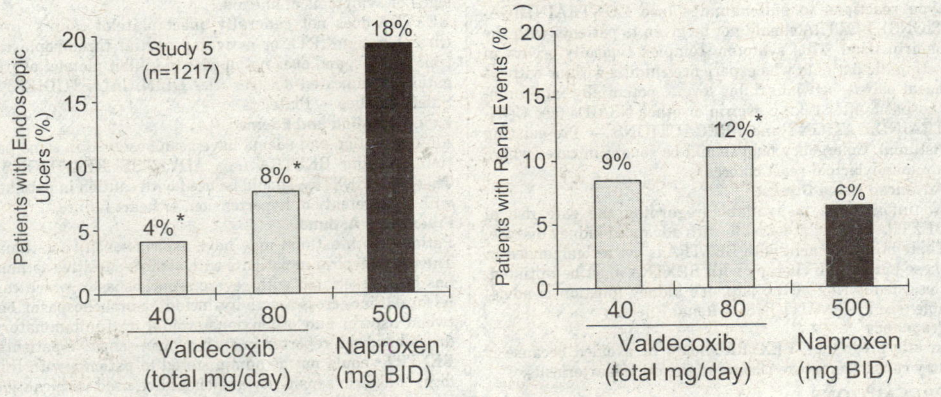

* Significantly different vs naproxen, p<0.05

involves the 3A4 and 2C9 isozymes. Using prototype inhibitors and substrates of these isozymes, the following results were obtained. Coadministration of a known inhibitor of CYP 2C9/3A4 (fluconazole) and a CYP 3A4 (ketoconazole) inhibitor enhanced the total plasma exposure (AUC) of valdecoxib. Coadministration of valdecoxib with warfarin caused a small, but statistically significant increase in plasma exposures of R-warfarin and S-warfarin, and also in the pharmacodynamic effects (International Normalized Ratio - INR) of warfarin. (See PRECAUTIONS — Drug Interactions.)

Coadministration of valdecoxib, or its injectable prodrug, with substrates of CYP 2C9 (propofol) and CYP 3A4 (midazolam, alfentanil, fentanyl) did not inhibit the metabolism of either substrate.

Coadministration of valdecoxib with a CYP 3A4 substrate (glyburide) or a CYP 2D6 substrate (dextromethorphan) did not result in clinically important inhibition in the metabolism of these agents.

CLINICAL STUDIES

The efficacy and clinical utility of BEXTRA Tablets have been demonstrated in osteoarthritis (OA), rheumatoid arthritis (RA) and in the treatment of primary dysmenorrhea.

Osteoarthritis

BEXTRA was evaluated for treatment of the signs and symptoms of osteoarthritis of the knee or hip, in five double-blind, randomized, controlled trials in which 3918 patients were treated for 3 to 6 months. BEXTRA was shown to be superior to placebo in improvement in three domains of OA symptoms: (1) the WOMAC (Western Ontario and McMaster Universities) osteoarthritis index, a composite of pain, stiffness and functional measures in OA, (2) the overall patient assessment of pain, and (3) the overall patient global assessment. The two 3-month pivotal trials in OA generally showed changes statistically significantly different from placebo, and comparable to the naproxen control, in measures of these domains for the 10 mg/day dose. No additional benefit was seen with a valdecoxib 20-mg daily dose.

Rheumatoid Arthritis

BEXTRA demonstrated significant reduction compared to placebo in the signs and symptoms of RA, as measured by the ACR (American College of Rheumatology) 20 improvement, a composite defined as both improvement of 20% in the number of tender and number of swollen joints, and a 20% improvement in three of the following five: patient global, physician global, patient pain, patient function assessment, and C-reactive protein (CRP). BEXTRA was evaluated for treatment of the signs and symptoms of rheumatoid arthritis in four double-blind, randomized, controlled studies in which 3444 patients were treated for 3 to 6 months. The two 3-month pivotal trials compared valdecoxib to naproxen and placebo. The results for the ACR20 responses in these trials are shown below (Table 2). Trials of BEXTRA in rheumatoid arthritis allowed concomitant use of corticosteroids and/or disease-modifying antirheumatic drugs (DMARDs), such as methotrexate, gold salts, and hydroxychloroquine. No additional benefit was seen with a valdecoxib 20-mg daily dose.

Table 2
ACR20 Response Rate (%) in Rheumatoid Arthritis

	Study 1		Study 2	
BEXTRA 10 mg/day	49%**	(103/209)	46%**	(103/226)
BEXTRA 20 mg/day	48%**	(102/212)	47%*	(103/219)
Naproxen 500 mg BID	44%*	(100/225)	53%**	(115/219)
Placebo	32%	(70/222)	32%	(71/220)

* p<0.01; ** p<0.001 compared to placebo

Primary Dysmenorrhea

BEXTRA was compared to naproxen sodium 550 mg in two placebo-controlled studies of women with moderate to severe primary dysmenorrhea. The onset of analgesia was within 60 minutes for BEXTRA 20 mg. The onset, magnitude, and duration of analgesic effect with BEXTRA 20 mg were comparable to naproxen sodium 550 mg.

Safety Studies

Gastrointestinal (GI) Endoscopy Studies with Therapeutic Doses: Scheduled upper GI endoscopic evaluations were performed with BEXTRA at doses of 10 and 20 mg daily in over 800 OA patients who were enrolled into two randomized 3-month studies using active comparators and placebo controls (Study 3 and Study 4). These studies enrolled patients free of endoscopic ulcers at baseline and compared rates of endoscopic ulcers, defined as any gastroduodenal ulcer seen endoscopically provided it was of "unequivocal depth" and at least 3 mm in diameter.

In both studies, BEXTRA 10 mg daily was associated with a statistically significant lower incidence of endoscopic gastroduodenal ulcers over the study period compared to the active comparators. Figure 1 summarizes the incidence of gastroduodenal ulcers in Studies 3 and 4 for the placebo, valdecoxib, and active control arms.

[See figure 1 above]

Safety Study with Supratherapeutic Doses: Scheduled upper GI endoscopic evaluations were performed in a randomized 6-month study of 1217 patients with OA and RA comparing valdecoxib 20 mg BID (40 mg daily) and 40 mg BID (80 mg daily) (4 to 8 times the recommended therapeutic dose) to naproxen 500 mg BID (Study 5). This study also formally assessed renal events as a primary outcome with supratherapeutic doses of BEXTRA. The renal endpoint was defined as any of the following: new/increase in edema, new/increase in congestive heart failure, increase in blood pressure (BP; >20 mm Hg systolic, >10 mm Hg diastolic), new/increase in BP treatment, new/increase in diuretic therapy, creatinine increase over 30% (or >1.2 mg/dL if baseline <0.9 mg/dL), BUN increase over 200% or >50 mg/dL, 24-hr urinary protein increase to >500 mg (if baseline 0-150 mg or >750 if baseline 151-300 or >1000 if baseline 301-500), serum potassium increase to >6 mEq/L, or serum sodium decrease to <130 mEq/L.

Figure 2 summarizes the incidence rates of gastroduodenal ulcers and renal events that were seen in Study 5. BEXTRA 40 mg daily and 80 mg daily were associated with a statistically significant lower incidence of endoscopic gastroduodenal ulcers over the study period compared to naproxen. The incidence of renal events was significantly different between the BEXTRA 80 mg daily group and naproxen. The clinical relevance of renal events observed with supratherapeutic doses (4 to 8 times the recommended therapeutic dose) of BEXTRA is not known (see PRECAUTIONS – Renal Effects).

[See figure 2 above]

Renal Safety at the Therapeutic Chronic Dose: The renal effects of valdecoxib compared with placebo and conventional NSAIDs were also assessed by prospectively designed pooled analyses of renal events data (see definition above — Supratherapeutic Doses) from five placebo- and active-controlled 12-week arthritis trials that included 995 OA or RA patients given valdecoxib 10 mg daily. The incidence of renal events observed in this analysis with valdecoxib 10 mg daily (3%), ibuprofen 800 mg TID (7%), naproxen 500 mg BID (2%) and diclofenac 75 mg BID (4%) were significantly higher than placebo-treated patients (1%). In all treatment groups, the majority of renal events were either due to the occurrence of edema or worsening BP.

Gastrointestinal Ulcers in High-Risk Patients: Subset analyses were performed of patients with risk factors (age, concomitant low-dose aspirin use, history of prior ulcer disease) enrolled in four upper GI endoscopic studies. Table 3 summarizes the trends seen.

[See table 3 at top of next page]

The correlation between findings of endoscopic studies, and the incidence of clinically significant serious upper GI events has not been established.

Platelets: In four clinical studies with young and elderly (≥65 years) subjects, single and multiple doses up to 7 days of BEXTRA 10 to 40 mg BID had no effect on platelet aggregation.

INDICATIONS AND USAGE

BEXTRA Tablets are indicated:

- For relief of the signs and symptoms of osteoarthritis and adult rheumatoid arthritis.
- For the treatment of primary dysmenorrhea.

CONTRAINDICATIONS

BEXTRA should not be given to patients who have demonstrated allergic-type reactions to sulfonamides. BEXTRA Tablets are contraindicated in patients with known hypersensitivity to valdecoxib. BEXTRA should not be given to patients who have experienced asthma, urticaria, or allergic-type reactions after taking aspirin or NSAIDs. Severe, rarely fatal, anaphylactic-like reactions to NSAIDs are possible in such patients (see WARNINGS — Anaphylactoid Reactions, and PRECAUTIONS — Preexisting Asthma).

WARNINGS

Gastrointestinal (GI) Effects — Risk of GI Ulceration, Bleeding, and Perforation

Serious gastrointestinal toxicity such as bleeding, ulceration and perforation of the stomach, small intestine or large intestine can occur at any time with or without warning symptoms in patients treated with nonsteroidal anti-inflammatory drugs (NSAIDs). Minor gastrointestinal problems such as dyspepsia are common and may also occur at any time during NSAID therapy. Therefore, physicians and patients should remain alert for ulceration and bleeding even in the absence of previous GI tract symptoms. Patients should be informed about the signs and symptoms of serious GI toxicity and the steps to take if they occur. The utility of periodic laboratory monitoring has not been demonstrated, nor has it been adequately assessed. Only one in five patients who develop a serious upper GI adverse event on NSAID therapy is symptomatic. It has been demonstrated that upper GI ulcers, gross bleeding or perforation caused by NSAIDs appear to occur in approximately 1% of patients treated for 3 to 6 months and 2-4% of patients treated for one year. These trends continue, thus increasing the likelihood of developing a serious GI event at some time during the course of therapy. However, even short-term therapy is not without risk.

Continued on next page

Bextra—Cont.

NSAIDs should be prescribed with extreme caution in patients with a prior history of ulcer disease or gastrointestinal bleeding. Most spontaneous reports of fatal GI events are in elderly or debilitated patients and therefore special care should be taken in treating this population. For high risk patients, alternate therapies that do not involve NSAIDs should be considered.

Studies have shown that patients with a *prior history of peptic ulcer disease and/or gastrointestinal bleeding* and who use NSAIDs, have a greater than 10-fold higher risk for developing a GI bleed than patients with neither of these risk factors. In addition to a past history of ulcer disease, pharmacoepidemiological studies have identified several other co-therapies or co-morbid conditions that may increase the risk for GI bleeding such as: treatment with oral corticosteroids, treatment with anticoagulants, longer duration of NSAID therapy, smoking, alcoholism, older age, and poor general health status. (See CLINICAL STUDIES — Safety Studies.)

Serious Skin Reactions

Serious skin reactions, including exfoliative dermatitis, Stevens-Johnson syndrome, and toxic epidermal necrolysis, have been reported through postmarketing surveillance in patients receiving BEXTRA (see ADVERSE REACTIONS-Postmarketing Experience). As these reactions can be life-threatening, BEXTRA should be discontinued at the first appearance of skin rash or any other sign of hypersensitivity.

Anaphylactoid Reactions

In postmarketing experience, cases of hypersensitivity reactions (anaphylactic reactions and angioedema) have been reported in patients receiving BEXTRA (see ADVERSE REACTIONS-Postmarketing Experience). These cases have occurred in patients with and without a history of allergic-type reactions to sulfonamides (see CONTRAINDICATIONS). BEXTRA should not be given to patients with the aspirin triad. This symptom complex typically occurs in asthmatic patients who experience rhinitis with or without nasal polyps, or who exhibit severe, potentially fatal bronchospasm after taking aspirin or other NSAIDs (see CONTRAINDICATIONS and PRECAUTIONS — Pre-existing Asthma). Emergency help should be sought in cases where an anaphylactoid reaction occurs.

Advanced Renal Disease

No information is available regarding the safe use of BEXTRA Tablets in patients with advanced kidney disease. Therefore, treatment with BEXTRA is not recommended in these patients. If therapy with BEXTRA must be initiated, close monitoring of the patient's kidney function is advisable (see PRECAUTIONS — Renal Effects).

Pregnancy

In late pregnancy, BEXTRA should be avoided because it may cause premature closure of the ductus arteriosus.

PRECAUTIONS

General

BEXTRA Tablets cannot be expected to substitute for corticosteroids or to treat corticosteroid insufficiency. Abrupt discontinuation of corticosteroids may lead to exacerbation of corticosteroid-responsive illness. Patients on prolonged corticosteroid therapy should have their therapy tapered slowly if a decision is made to discontinue corticosteroids.

The pharmacological activity of valdecoxib in reducing fever and inflammation may diminish the utility of these diagnostic signs in detecting complications of presumed noninfectious, painful conditions.

Hepatic Effects

Borderline elevations of one or more liver tests may occur in up to 15% of patients taking NSAIDs. Notable elevations of ALT or AST (approximately three or more times the upper limit of normal) have been reported in approximately 1% of patients in clinical trials with NSAIDs. These laboratory abnormalities may progress, may remain unchanged, or may remain transient with continuing therapy. Rare cases of severe hepatic reactions, including jaundice and fatal fulminant hepatitis, liver necrosis and hepatic failure (some with fatal outcome) have been reported with NSAIDs. In controlled clinical trials of valdecoxib, the incidence of borderline (defined as 1.2- to 3.0-fold) elevations of liver tests was 8.0% for valdecoxib and 8.4% for placebo, while approximately 0.3% of patients taking valdecoxib, and 0.2% of patients taking placebo, had notable (defined as greater than 3-fold) elevations of ALT or AST.

A patient with symptoms and/or signs suggesting liver dysfunction, or in whom an abnormal liver test has occurred, should be monitored carefully for evidence of the development of a more severe hepatic reaction while on therapy with BEXTRA. If clinical signs and symptoms consistent with liver disease develop, or if systemic manifestations occur (e.g., eosinophilia, rash), BEXTRA should be discontinued.

Renal Effects

Long-term administration of NSAIDs has resulted in renal papillary necrosis and other renal injury. Renal toxicity has also been seen in patients in whom renal prostaglandins have a compensatory role in the maintenance of renal perfusion. In these patients, administration of a nonsteroidal anti-inflammatory drug may cause a dose-dependent reduction in prostaglandin formation and, secondarily, in renal blood flow, which may precipitate overt renal decompensation. Patients at greatest risk of this reaction are those with impaired renal function, heart failure, liver dysfunction, those taking diuretics and Angiotensin Converting Enzyme

Table 3
Incidence of Endoscopic Gastroduodenal Ulcers
in Patients With and Without Selected Risk Factors

Risk Factor	Placebo-controlled Studies Placebo	Valdecoxib (10-20 mg daily)	Valdecoxib (10-80 mg daily)	Active-controlled Studies Ibuprofen 800 mg TID	Naproxen 500 mg BID	Diclofenac 75 mg BID
Age						
<65 yrs	3.7% (8/219)	3.5% (17/484)	3.7% (48/1306)	8.2% (9/110)	12.8% (51/397)	13.2% (34/258)
≥65 yrs	5.8% (8/137)	4.6% (12/262)	7.6% (43/568)	21.6% (16/74)	22.0% (33/150)	18.2% (25/137)
Concomitant Low Dose Aspirin Use						
no	4.4% (13/298)	3.2% (21/650)	3.8% (64/1671)	9.8% (15/153)	16.0% (75/468)	12.8% (45/351)
yes	5.2% (3/58)	8.3% (8/96)	13.3% (27/203)	32.3% (10/31)	11.4% (9/79)	31.8% (14/44)
History of Ulcer Disease						
no	4.4% (14/317)	3.4% (22/647)	4.1% (68/1666)	13.8% (22/160)	13.3% (63/475)	14.7% (52/354)
yes	5.1% (2/39)	7.1% (7/99)	11.1% (23/208)	12.5% (3/24)	29.2% (21/72)	17.1% (7/41)

No statistical conclusions can be drawn from these comparisons.

(ACE) inhibitors, and the elderly. Discontinuation of NSAID therapy is usually followed by recovery to the pretreatment state.

Caution should be used when initiating treatment with BEXTRA in patients with considerable dehydration. It is advisable to rehydrate patients first and then start therapy with BEXTRA. Caution is also recommended in patients with preexisting kidney disease. (See WARNINGS — Advanced Renal Disease.)

Hematological Effects

Anemia is sometimes seen in patients receiving BEXTRA. Patients on long-term treatment with BEXTRA should have their hemoglobin or hematocrit checked if they exhibit any signs or symptoms of anemia.

BEXTRA does not generally affect platelet counts, prothrombin time (PT), or activated partial thromboplastin time (APTT), and does not appear to inhibit platelet aggregation at indicated dosages (See CLINICAL STUDIES — Safety Studies — Platelets).

Fluid Retention and Edema

Fluid retention and edema have been observed in some patients taking BEXTRA (see ADVERSE REACTIONS). Therefore, BEXTRA should be used with caution in patients with fluid retention, hypertension, or heart failure.

Preexisting Asthma

Patients with asthma may have aspirin-sensitive asthma. The use of aspirin in patients with aspirin-sensitive asthma has been associated with severe bronchospasm, which can be fatal. Since cross reactivity, including bronchospasm, between aspirin and other nonsteroidal anti-inflammatory drugs has been reported in such aspirin-sensitive patients, BEXTRA should not be administered to patients with this form of aspirin sensitivity and should be used with caution in patients with preexisting asthma.

Information for Patients

BEXTRA can cause GI discomfort and, rarely, more serious GI side effects, which may result in hospitalization and even fatal outcomes. Although serious GI tract ulcerations and bleeding can occur without warning symptoms, patients should be alert for the signs and symptoms of ulcerations and bleeding, and should ask for medical advice when observing any indicative sign or symptoms. Patients should be apprised of the importance of this follow-up (see WARNINGS — Gastrointestinal (GI) Effects — Risk of GI Ulceration, Bleeding, and Perforation).

Patients should report to their physicians, signs or symptoms of gastrointestinal ulceration or bleeding, skin rash, weight gain, or edema.

Patients should be informed of the warning signs and symptoms of hepatotoxicity (e.g., nausea, fatigue, lethargy, pruritus, jaundice, right upper quadrant tenderness, and flu-like symptoms). If these occur, patients should be instructed to stop therapy and seek immediate medical attention.

Patients should also be instructed to seek immediate emergency help in the case of an anaphylactoid reaction (see WARNINGS — Anaphylactoid Reactions).

In late pregnancy, BEXTRA should be avoided because it may cause premature closure of the ductus arteriosus.

Laboratory Tests

Because serious GI tract ulcerations and bleeding can occur without warning symptoms, physicians should monitor for signs and symptoms of GI bleeding.

Drug Interactions

The drug interaction studies with valdecoxib were performed both with valdecoxib and a rapidly hydrolyzed intravenous prodrug form. The results from trials using the intravenous prodrug are reported in this section as they relate to the role of valdecoxib in drug interactions.

General: In humans, valdecoxib metabolism is predominantly mediated via CYP 3A4 and 2C9 with glucuronidation being a further (20%) route of metabolism. In vitro studies indicate that valdecoxib is a moderate inhibitor of CYP 2C19 (IC50 = 6 μ/mL), and a weak inhibitor of both 3A4 (IC50 = 44 μ/mL) and 2C9 (IC50 = 13 μ/mL). In view of the limitations of in vitro studies and the high valdecoxib IC50 values, the potential for such metabolic inhibitory effects in vivo at therapeutic doses of valdecoxib is low.

Aspirin: Concomitant administration of aspirin with valdecoxib may result in an increased risk of GI ulceration and complications compared to valdecoxib alone. Because of its lack of anti-platelet effect valdecoxib is not a substitute for aspirin for cardiovascular prophylaxis.

In a parallel group drug interaction study comparing the intravenous prodrug form of valdecoxib at 40 mg BID (n=10) vs placebo (n=9), valdecoxib had no effect on in vitro aspirin-mediated inhibition of arachidonate- or collagen-stimulated platelet aggregation.

Methotrexate: Valdecoxib 10 mg BID did not show a significant effect on the plasma exposure or renal clearance of methotrexate.

ACE-inhibitors: Reports suggest that NSAIDs may diminish the antihypertensive effect of ACE-inhibitors. This interaction should be given consideration in patients taking BEXTRA concomitantly with ACE-inhibitors.

Furosemide: Clinical studies, as well as post-marketing observations, have shown that NSAIDs can reduce the natriuretic effect of furosemide and thiazides in some patients. This response has been attributed to inhibition of renal prostaglandin synthesis.

Anticonvulsants: Anticonvulsant drug interaction studies with valdecoxib have not been conducted. As with other drugs, routine monitoring should be performed when therapy with BEXTRA is either initiated or discontinued in patients on anticonvulsant therapy.

Dextromethorphan: Dextromethorphan is primarily metabolized by CYP 2D6 and to a lesser extent by 3A4. Coadministration with valdecoxib (40 mg BID for 7 days) resulted in a significant increase in dextromethorphan plasma levels suggesting that, at these doses, valdecoxib is a weak inhibitor of 2D6. Dextromethorphan plasma concentrations in the presence of high doses of valdecoxib were almost 5-fold lower than those seen in CYP 2D6 poor metabolizers.

Lithium: Valdecoxib 40 mg BID for 7 days produced significant decreases in lithium serum clearance (25%) and renal clearance (30%) with a 34% higher serum exposure compared to lithium alone. Lithium serum concentrations should be monitored closely when initiating or changing therapy with BEXTRA in patients receiving lithium. Lithium carbonate (450 mg BID for 7 days) had no effect on valdecoxib pharmacokinetics.

Warfarin: The effect of valdecoxib on the anticoagulant effect of warfarin (1 - 8 mg/day) was studied in healthy subjects by coadministration of BEXTRA 40 mg BID for 7 days. Valdecoxib caused a statistically significant increase in plasma exposures of R-warfarin and S-warfarin (12% and 15%, respectively), and in the pharmacodynamic effects (prothrombin time, measured as INR) of warfarin. While mean INR values were only slightly increased with coadministration of valdecoxib, the day-to-day variability in individual INR values was increased. Anticoagulant therapy should be monitored, particularly during the first few weeks, after initiating therapy with BEXTRA in patients receiving warfarin or similar agents.

Fluconazole and Ketoconazole: Ketoconazole and fluconazole are predominantly CYP 3A4 and 2C9 inhibitors, respectively. Concomitant single dose administration of valdecoxib 20 mg with multiple doses of ketoconazole and fluconazole produced a significant increase in exposure of valdecoxib. Plasma exposure (AUC) to valdecoxib was increased 62% when coadministered with fluconazole and 38% when coadministered with ketoconazole.

Glyburide: Glyburide is a CYP 3A4 substrate. Coadministration of valdecoxib (10 mg BID for 7 days) with glyburide (5 mg QD or 10 mg BID) did not affect the pharmacokinetics (exposure) of glyburide.

Carcinogenesis, Mutagenesis, Impairment of Fertility

Valdecoxib was not carcinogenic in rats given oral doses up to 7.5 mg/kg/day for males and 1.5 mg/kg/day for females (equivalent to approximately 2- to 6-fold human exposure at 20 mg QD as measured by the $AUC_{(0-24hr)}$) or in mice given oral doses up to 25 mg/kg/day for males and 50 mg/kg/day for females (equivalent to approximately 0.6- to 2.4-fold human exposure at 20 mg QD as measured by the $AUC_{(0-24hr)}$) for two years.

Valdecoxib was not mutagenic in an Ames test or a mutation assay in Chinese hamster ovary (CHO) cells, nor was it clastogenic in a chromosome aberration assay in CHO cells or in an *in vivo* micronucleus test in rat bone marrow.

Valdecoxib did not impair male rat fertility at oral doses up to 9.0 mg/kg/day (equivalent to approximately 3- to 6-fold human exposure at 20 mg QD as measured by the $AUC_{(0-24hr)}$). In female rats, a decrease in ovulation with increased pre- and post-implantation loss resulted in decreased live embryos/fetuses at doses ≥2 mg/kg/day (equivalent to approximately 2-fold human exposure at 20 mg QD as measured by the $AUC_{(0-24hr)}$ for valdecoxib). The effects on female fertility were reversible. This effect is expected with inhibition of prostaglandin synthesis and is not the result of irreversible alteration of female reproductive function.

Pregnancy

Teratogenic Effects: Pregnancy Category C.

The incidence of fetuses with skeletal anomalies such as semi-bipartite thoracic vertebra centra and fused sternebrae was slightly higher in rabbits at an oral dose of 40 mg/kg/day (equivalent to approximately 72-fold human exposures at 20 mg QD as measured by the $AUC_{(0-24hr)}$) throughout organogenesis. Valdecoxib was not teratogenic in rabbits up to an oral dose of 10 mg/kg/day (equivalent to approximately 8-fold human exposures at 20 mg QD as measured by the $AUC_{(0-24hr)}$).

Valdecoxib was not teratogenic in rats up to an oral dose of 10 mg/kg/day (equivalent to approximately 19-fold human exposure at 20 mg QD as measured by the $AUC_{(0-24hr)}$). There are no studies in pregnant women. However, valdecoxib crosses the placenta in rats and rabbits. BEXTRA should be used during pregnancy only if the potential benefit justifies the potential risk to the fetus.

Non-Teratogenic Effects: Valdecoxib caused increased pre- and post-implantation loss with reduced live fetuses at oral doses ≥10 mg/kg/day (equivalent to approximately 19-fold human exposure at 20 mg QD as measured by the $AUC_{(0-24hr)}$) in rats and an oral dose of 40 mg/kg/day (equivalent to approximately 72-fold human exposure at 20 mg QD as measured by the $AUC_{(0-24hr)}$) in rabbits throughout organogenesis. In addition, reduced neonatal survival and decreased neonatal body weight when rats were treated with valdecoxib at oral doses ≥6 mg/kg/day (equivalent to approximately 7-fold human exposure at 20 mg QD as measured by the $AUC_{(0-24hr)}$) throughout organogenesis and lactation period. No studies have been conducted to evaluate the effect of valdecoxib on the closure of the ductus arteriosus in humans. Therefore, as with other drugs known to inhibit prostaglandin synthesis, use of BEXTRA during the third trimester of pregnancy should be avoided.

Labor and Delivery

Valdecoxib produced no evidence of delayed labor or parturition at oral doses up to 10 mg/kg/day in rats (equivalent to approximately 19-fold human exposure at 20 mg QD as measured by the $AUC_{(0-24hr)}$). The effects of BEXTRA on labor and delivery in pregnant women are unknown.

Nursing Mothers

Valdecoxib and its active metabolite are excreted in the milk of lactating rats. It is not known whether this drug is excreted in human milk. Because many drugs are excreted in human milk, and because of the potential for adverse reactions in nursing infants from BEXTRA, a decision should be made whether to discontinue nursing or to discontinue the drug, taking into account the importance of the drug to the mother and the importance of nursing to the infant.

Pediatric Use

Safety and effectiveness of BEXTRA in pediatric patients below the age of 18 years have not been evaluated.

Geriatric Use

Of the patients who received BEXTRA in arthritis clinical trials of three months duration, or greater, approximately 2100 were 65 years of age or older, including 570 patients who were 75 years or older. No overall differences in effectiveness were observed between these patients and younger patients.

ADVERSE REACTIONS

Of the patients treated with BEXTRA Tablets in controlled arthritis trials, 2665 were patients with OA, and 2684 were patients with RA. More than 4000 patients have received a chronic total daily dose of BEXTRA 10 mg or more. More than 2800 patients have received BEXTRA 10 mg/day, or more, for at least 6 months and 988 of these have received BEXTRA for at least 1 year.

Osteoarthritis and Rheumatoid Arthritis

Table 4 lists all adverse events, regardless of causality, that occurred in ≥2.0% of patients receiving BEXTRA 10 and 20 mg/day in studies of three months or longer from 7 controlled studies conducted in patients with OA or RA that included a placebo and/or a positive control group.

[See table 4 above]

In these placebo- and active-controlled clinical trials, the discontinuation rate due to adverse events was 7.5% for arthritis patients receiving valdecoxib 10 mg daily, 7.9% for arthritis patients receiving valdecoxib 20 mg daily and 6.0% for patients receiving placebo.

In the seven controlled OA and RA studies, the following adverse events occurred in 0.1 - 1.9% of patients treated with BEXTRA 10 – 20 mg daily, regardless of causality.

Application site disorders: Cellulitis, dermatitis contact

Cardiovascular: Aggravated hypertension, aneurysm, angina pectoris, arrhythmia, cardiomyopathy, congestive heart failure, coronary artery disorder, heart murmur, hypotension

Central, peripheral nervous system: Cerebrovascular disorder, hypertonia, hypoesthesia, migraine, neuralgia, neuropathy, paresthesia, tremor, twitching, vertigo

Endocrine: Goiter

Female reproductive: Amenorrhea, dysmenorrhea, leukorrhea, mastitis, menstrual disorder, menorrhagia, menstrual bloating, vaginal hemorrhage

Gastrointestinal: Abnormal stools, constipation, diverticulosis, dry mouth, duodenal ulcer, duodenitis, eructation, esophagitis, fecal incontinence, gastric ulcer, gastritis, gastroenteritis, gastroesophageal reflux, hematemesis, hematochezia, hemorrhoids, hemorrhoids bleeding, hiatal hernia, melena, stomatitis, stool frequency increased, tenesmus, tooth disorder, vomiting

Table 4
Adverse Events with Incidence ≥ 2.0% in Valdecoxib Treatment Groups:
Controlled Arthritis Trials of Three Months or Longer

				(Total Daily Dose)		
		Valdecoxib		Diclofenac	Ibuprofen	Naproxen
Adverse Event	**Placebo**	**10 mg**	**20 mg**	**150 mg**	**2400 mg**	**1000 mg**
Number Treated	973	1214	1358	711	207	766
Autonomic Nervous System Disorders						
Hypertension	0.6	1.6	2.1	2.5	2.4	1.7
Body as a Whole						
Back pain	1.6	1.6	2.7	2.8	1.4	1.0
Edema peripheral	0.7	2.4	3.0	3.2	2.9	2.1
Influenza-like symptoms	2.2	2.0	2.2	3.1	2.9	2.0
Injury accidental	2.8	4.0	3.7	3.9	3.9	3.0
Central and Peripheral Nervous System Disorders						
Dizziness	2.1	2.6	2.7	4.2	3.4	2.7
Headache	7.1	4.8	8.5	6.6	4.3	5.5
Gastrointestinal System Disorders						
Abdominal fullness	2.0	2.1	1.9	3.0	2.9	2.5
Abdominal pain	6.3	7.0	8.2	17.0	8.2	10.1
Diarrhea	4.2	5.4	6.0	10.8	3.9	4.7
Dyspepsia	6.3	7.9	8.7	13.4	15.0	12.9
Flatulence	4.1	2.9	3.5	3.1	7.7	5.4
Nausea	5.9	7.0	6.3	8.4	7.7	8.7
Musculoskeletal System Disorders						
Myalgia	1.6	2.0	1.9	2.4	2.4	1.4
Respiratory System Disorders						
Sinusitis	2.2	2.6	1.8	1.1	3.4	3.4
Upper respiratory tract infection	6.0	6.7	5.7	6.3	4.3	6.4
Skin and Appendages Disorders						
Rash	1.0	1.4	2.1	1.5	0.5	1.4

General: Allergy aggravated, allergic reaction, asthenia, chest pain, chills, cyst NOS, edema generalized, face edema, fatigue, fever, hot flushes, halitosis, malaise, pain, periorbital swelling, peripheral pain

Hearing and vestibular: Ear abnormality, earache, tinnitus

Heart rate and rhythm: Bradycardia, palpitation, tachycardia

Hemic: Anemia

Liver and biliary system: Hepatic function abnormal, hepatitis, ALT increased, AST increased

Male reproductive: Impotence, prostatic disorder

Metabolic and nutritional: Alkaline phosphatase increased, BUN increased, CPK increased, creatinine increased, diabetes mellitus, glycosuria, gout, hypercholesterolemia, hyperglycemia, hyperkalemia, hyperlipemia, hyperuricemia, hypocalcemia, hypokalemia, LDH increased, thirst increased, weight decrease, weight increase, xerophthalmia

Musculoskeletal: Arthralgia, fracture accidental, neck stiffness, osteoporosis, synovitis, tendonitis

Neoplasm: Breast neoplasm, lipoma, malignant ovarian cyst

Platelets (bleeding or clotting): Ecchymosis, epistaxis, hematoma NOS, thrombocytopenia

Psychiatric: Anorexia, anxiety, appetite increased, confusion, depression, depression aggravated, insomnia, nervousness, morbid dreaming, somnolence

Resistance mechanism disorders: Herpes simplex, herpes zoster, infection fungal, infection soft tissue, infection viral, moniliasis, moniliasis genital, otitis media

Respiratory: Abnormal breath sounds, bronchitis, bronchospasm, coughing, dyspnea, emphysema, laryngitis, pneumonia, pharyngitis, pleurisy, rhinitis

Skin and appendages: Acne, alopecia, dermatitis, dermatitis fungal, eczema, photosensitivity allergic reaction, pruritus, rash erythematous, rash maculopapular, rash psoriaform, skin dry, skin hypertrophy, skin ulceration, sweating increased, urticaria

Special senses: Taste perversion

Urinary system: Albuminuria, cystitis, dysuria, hematuria, micturition frequency increased, pyuria, urinary incontinence, urinary tract infection

Vascular: Claudication intermittent, hemangioma acquired, varicose vein

Vision: Blurred vision, cataract, conjunctival hemorrhage, conjunctivitis, eye pain, keratitis, vision abnormal

White cell and RES disorders: Eosinophilia, leukopenia, leukocytosis, lymphadenopathy, lymphangitis, lymphopenia

Other serious adverse events that were reported rarely (estimated <0.1%) in clinical trials, regardless of causality, in patients taking BEXTRA:

Autonomic nervous system disorders: Hypertensive encephalopathy, vasospasm

Cardiovascular: Abnormal ECG, aortic stenosis, åtrial fibrillation, carotid stenosis, coronary thrombosis, heart block, heart valve disorders, mitral insufficiency, myocardial infarction, myocardial ischemia, pericarditis, syncope, thrombophlebitis, unstable angina, ventricular fibrillation

Central, peripheral nervous system: Convulsions

Endocrine: Hyperparathyroidism

Female reproductive: Cervical dysplasia

Gastrointestinal: Appendicitis, colitis with bleeding, dysphagia, esophageal perforation, gastrointestinal bleeding, ileus, intestinal obstruction, peritonitis

Hemic: Lymphoma-like disorder, pancytopenia

Liver and biliary system: Cholelithiasis

Metabolic: Dehydration

Musculoskeletal: Pathological fracture, osteomyelitis

Neoplasm: Benign brain neoplasm, bladder carcinoma, carcinoma, gastric carcinoma, prostate carcinoma, pulmonary carcinoma

Platelets (bleeding or clotting): Embolism, pulmonary embolism, thrombosis

Psychiatric: Manic reaction, psychosis

Renal: Acute renal failure

Resistance mechanism disorders: Sepsis

Respiratory: Apnea, pleural effusion, pulmonary edema, pulmonary fibrosis, pulmonary infarction, pulmonary hemorrhage, respiratory insufficiency

Skin: Basal cell carcinoma, malignant melanoma

Urinary system: Pyelonephritis, renal calculus

Vision: Retinal detachment

Postmarketing Eperience

The following reactions have been identified during postmarketing use of BEXTRA. These reactions have been chosen for inclusion either due to their seriousness, reporting frequency, possible causal relationship to BEXTRA, or a combination of these factors. Because these reactions were reported voluntarily from a population of uncertain size, it is not possible to reliably estimate their frequency or establish a causal relationship to drug exposure.

General: Hypersensitivity reactions (including anaphylactic reactions and angioedema)

Skin and appendages: Erythema multiforme, exfoliative dermatitis, Stevens-Johnson syndrome, toxic epidermal necrolysis

OVERDOSAGE

Symptoms following acute NSAID overdoses are usually limited to lethargy, drowsiness, nausea, vomiting, and epigastric pain, which are generally reversible with supportive care. Gastrointestinal bleeding can occur. Hypertension, acute renal failure, respiratory depression and coma may occur, but are rare.

Anaphylactoid reactions have been reported with therapeutic ingestion of NSAIDs, and may occur following an overdose.

Patients should be managed by symptomatic and supportive care following an NSAID overdose. There are no specific antidotes. Hemodialysis removed only about 2% of administered valdecoxib from the systemic circulation of 8 patients with end-stage renal disease and, based on its degree of plasma protein binding (>98%), dialysis is unlikely to be useful in overdose. Forced diuresis, alkalinization of urine, or hemoperfusion also may not be useful due to high protein binding.

DOSAGE AND ADMINISTRATION

Osteoarthritis and Adult Rheumatoid Arthritis

The recommended dose of BEXTRA Tablets for the relief of the signs and symptoms of arthritis is 10 mg once daily.

Primary Dysmenorrhea

The recommended dose of BEXTRA Tablets for treatment of primary dysmenorrhea is 20 mg twice daily, as needed.

HOW SUPPLIED

BEXTRA Tablets 10 mg are white, film-coated, and capsule-shaped, debossed "10" on one side with a four pointed star shape on the other, supplied as:

NDC Number	Size
0025-1975-31	Bottle of 100
0025-1975-51	Bottle of 500
0025-1975-34	Carton of 100 unit dose

BEXTRA Tablets 20 mg are white, film-coated, and capsule-shaped, debossed "20" on one side with a four pointed star shape on the other, supplied as:

Continued on next page

Bextra—Cont.

NDC Number	Size
0025-1980-31	Bottle of 100
0025-1980-51	Bottle of 500
0025-1980-34	Carton of 100 unit dose

Store at 25°C (77°F); excursions permitted to 15-30°C (59-86°F) [See USP Controlled Room Temperature].
Rx only
Revised: July 2003
Manufactured for:
G.D. Searle LLC
A subsidiary of Pharmacia Corporation
Chicago, IL 60680, USA
Pfizer Inc
New York, NY 10017, USA
by: Searle Ltd.
Caguas, PR 00725
818 763 003 P04001-2 / PS4001-2

CELEBREX® ℞
[*sĕ-lĕ-brĕks*]
celecoxib capsules

Prescribing information for this product, which appears on pages 2585–2589 of the 2004 PDR, has been completely revised as follows. Please write "See Supplement A" next to the product heading.

DESCRIPTION

CELEBREX (celecoxib) is chemically designated as 4-[5-(4-methylphenyl)-3-(trifluoromethyl)-1H-pyrazol-1-yl] benzenesulfonamide and is a diaryl-substituted pyrazole. It has the following chemical structure:

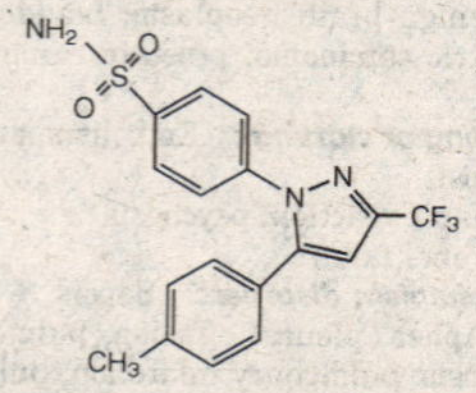

The empirical formula for celecoxib is $C_{17}H_{14}F_3N_3O_2S$, and the molecular weight is 381.38.
CELEBREX oral capsules contain either 100 mg, 200 mg or 400 mg of celecoxib.
The inactive ingredients in CELEBREX capsules include: croscarmellose sodium, edible inks, gelatin, lactose monohydrate, magnesium stearate, povidone, sodium lauryl sulfate and titanium dioxide.

CLINICAL PHARMACOLOGY

Mechanism of Action: CELEBREX is a nonsteroidal anti-inflammatory drug that exhibits anti-inflammatory, analgesic, and antipyretic activities in animal models. The mechanism of action of CELEBREX is believed to be due to inhibition of prostaglandin synthesis, primarily via inhibition of cyclooxygenase-2 (COX-2), and at therapeutic concentrations in humans, CELEBREX does not inhibit the cyclooxygenase-1 (COX-1) isoenzyme. In animal colon tumor models, celecoxib reduced the incidence and multiplicity of tumors.

Pharmacokinetics:

Absorption

Peak plasma levels of celecoxib occur approximately 3 hrs after an oral dose. Under fasting conditions, both peak plasma levels (C_{max}) and area under the curve (AUC) are roughly dose proportional up to 200 mg BID; at higher doses there are less than proportional increases in C_{max} and AUC (see Food Effects). Absolute bioavailability studies have not been conducted. With multiple dosing, steady state conditions are reached on or before day 5.
The pharmacokinetic parameters of celecoxib in a group of healthy subjects are shown in Table 1.
[See table 1 below]

Food Effects

When CELEBREX capsules were taken with a high fat meal, peak plasma levels were delayed for about 1 to 2 hours with an increase in total absorption (AUC) of 10% to 20%. Under fasting conditions, at doses above 200 mg, there is less than a proportional increase in C_{max} and AUC, which is thought to be due to the low solubility of the drug in aqueous media.
Coadministration of CELEBREX with an aluminum- and magnesium-containing antacid resulted in a reduction in plasma celecoxib concentrations with a decrease of 37% in C_{max} and 10% in AUC. CELEBREX, at doses up to 200 mg BID can be administered without regard to timing of meals. Higher doses (400 mg BID) should be administered with food to improve absorption.

Distribution

In healthy subjects, celecoxib is highly protein bound (~97%) within the clinical dose range. *In vitro* studies indicate that celecoxib binds primarily to albumin and, to a lesser extent, α_1-acid glycoprotein. The apparent volume of distribution at steady state (V_{ss}/F) is approximately 400 L, suggesting extensive distribution into the tissues. Celecoxib is not preferentially bound to red blood cells.

Metabolism

Celecoxib metabolism is primarily mediated via cytochrome P450 2C9. Three metabolites, a primary alcohol, the corresponding carboxylic acid and its glucuronide conjugate, have been identified in human plasma. These metabolites are inactive as COX-1 or COX-2 inhibitors. Patients who are known or suspected to be P450 2C9 poor metabolizers based on a previous history should be administered celecoxib with caution as they may have abnormally high plasma levels due to reduced metabolic clearance.

Excretion

Celecoxib is eliminated predominantly by hepatic metabolism with little (<3%) unchanged drug recovered in the urine and feces. Following a single oral dose of radiolabeled drug, approximately 57% of the dose was excreted in the feces and 27% was excreted into the urine. The primary metabolite in both urine and feces was the carboxylic acid metabolite (73% of dose) with low amounts of the glucuronide also appearing in the urine. It appears that the low solubility of the drug prolongs the absorption process making terminal half-life ($t_{1/2}$) determinations more variable. The effective half-life is approximately 11 hours under fasted conditions. The apparent plasma clearance (CL/F) is about 500 mL/min.

Special Populations

Geriatric: At steady state, elderly subjects (over 65 years old) had a 40% higher C_{max} and a 50% higher AUC compared to the young subjects. In elderly females, celecoxib C_{max} and AUC are higher than those for elderly males, but these increases are predominantly due to lower body weight in elderly females. Dose adjustment in the elderly is not generally necessary. However, for patients of less than 50 kg in body weight, initiate therapy at the lowest recommended dose.

Pediatric: CELEBREX capsules have not been investigated in pediatric patients below 18 years of age.

Race: Meta-analysis of pharmacokinetic studies has suggested an approximately 40% higher AUC of celecoxib in Blacks compared to Caucasians. The cause and clinical significance of this finding is unknown.

Hepatic Insufficiency: A pharmacokinetic study in subjects with mild (Child-Pugh Class A) and moderate (Child-Pugh Class B) hepatic impairment has shown that steady-state celecoxib AUC is increased about 40% and 180%, respectively, above that seen in healthy control subjects. Therefore, the daily recommended dose of CELEBREX capsules should be reduced by approximately 50% in patients with moderate (Child-Pugh Class B) hepatic impairment. Patients with severe hepatic impairment (Child-Pugh Class C) have not been studied. The use of CELEBREX in patients with severe hepatic impairment is not recommended.

Renal Insufficiency: In a cross-study comparison, celecoxib AUC was approximately 40% lower in patients with chronic renal insufficiency (GFR 35-60 mL/min) than that seen in subjects with normal renal function. No significant relationship was found between GFR and celecoxib clearance. Patients with severe renal insufficiency have not been studied. Similar to other NSAIDs, CELEBREX is not recommended in patients with severe renal insufficiency (see WARNINGS – Advanced Renal Disease).

Drug Interactions

Also see **PRECAUTIONS – Drug Interactions.**

General: Significant interactions may occur when celecoxib is administered together with drugs that inhibit P450 2C9. *In vitro* studies indicate that celecoxib is not an inhibitor of cytochrome P450 2C9, 2C19 or 3A4.
Clinical studies with celecoxib have identified potentially significant interactions with fluconazole and lithium. Experience with nonsteroidal anti-inflammatory drugs (NSAIDs) suggests the potential for interactions with furosemide and ACE inhibitors. The effects of celecoxib on the pharmacokinetics and/or pharmacodynamics of glyburide, ketoconazole, methotrexate, phenytoin, and tolbutamide have been studied *in vivo* and clinically important interactions have not been found.

CLINICAL STUDIES

Osteoarthritis (OA): CELEBREX has demonstrated significant reduction in joint pain compared to placebo. CELEBREX was evaluated for treatment of the signs and the symptoms of OA of the knee and hip in approximately 4,200 patients in placebo- and active-controlled clinical trials of up to 12 weeks duration. In patients with OA, treatment with CELEBREX 100 mg BID or 200 mg QD resulted in improvement in WOMAC (Western Ontario and McMaster Universities) osteoarthritis index, a composite of pain, stiffness, and functional measures in OA. In three 12-week studies of pain accompanying OA flare, CELEBREX doses of 100 mg BID and 200 mg BID provided significant reduction of pain within 24-48 hours of initiation of dosing. At doses of 100 mg BID or 200 mg BID the effectiveness of CELEBREX was shown to be similar to that of naproxen 500 mg BID. Doses of 200 mg BID provided no additional benefit above that seen with 100 mg BID. A total daily dose of 200 mg has been shown to be equally effective whether administered as 100 mg BID or 200 mg QD.

Rheumatoid Arthritis (RA): CELEBREX has demonstrated significant reduction in joint tenderness/pain and joint swelling compared to placebo. CELEBREX was evaluated for treatment of the signs and symptoms of RA in approximately 2,100 patients in placebo- and active-controlled clinical trials of up to 24 weeks in duration. CELEBREX was shown to be superior to placebo in these studies, using the ACR20 Responder Index, a composite of clinical, laboratory, and functional measures in RA. CELEBREX doses of 100 mg BID and 200 mg BID were similar in effectiveness and both were comparable to naproxen 500 mg BID.
Although CELEBREX 100 mg BID and 200 mg BID provided similar overall effectiveness, some patients derived additional benefit from the 200 mg BID dose. Doses of 400 mg BID provided no additional benefit above that seen with 100-200 mg BID.

Analgesia, including primary dysmenorrhea: In acute analgesic models of post-oral surgery pain, post-orthopedic surgical pain, and primary dysmenorrhea, CELEBREX relieved pain that was rated by patients as moderate to severe. Single doses (see DOSAGE AND ADMINISTRATION) of CELEBREX provided pain relief within 60 minutes.

Familial Adenomatous Polyposis (FAP): CELEBREX was evaluated to reduce the number of adenomatous colorectal polyps. A randomized double-blind placebo-controlled study was conducted in 83 patients with FAP. The study population included 58 patients with a prior subtotal or total colectomy and 25 patients with an intact colon. Thirteen patients had the attenuated FAP phenotype.
One area in the rectum and up to four areas in the colon were identified at baseline for specific follow-up, and polyps were counted at baseline and following six months of treatment. The mean reduction in the number of colorectal polyps was 28% for CELEBREX 400 mg BID, 12% for CELEBREX 100 mg BID and 5% for placebo. The reduction in polyps observed with CELEBREX 400 mg BID was statistically superior to placebo at the six-month timepoint (p=0.003). (See Figure 1.)

Figure 1
Percent Change from Baseline in Number of Colorectal Polyps (FAP Patients)

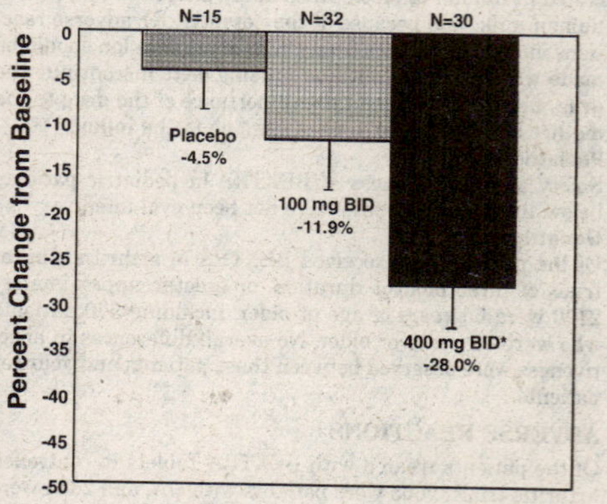

*p=0.003 versus placebo

Special Studies

Endoscopic Studies: Scheduled upper GI endoscopic evaluations were performed in over 4,500 arthritis patients who were enrolled in five controlled randomized 12-24 week trials using active comparators, two of which also included placebo controls. There was no consistent relationship between the incidence of gastroduodenal ulcers and the dose of CELEBREX over the range studied.
Table 2 summarizes the incidence of endoscopic ulcers in two 12-week studies that enrolled patients in whom baseline endoscopies revealed no ulcers.

Table 2
Incidence of Gastroduodenal Ulcers from Endoscopic Studies in OA and RA Patients

	3 Month Studies	
	Study 1 (n = 1108)	Study 2 (n = 1049)
Placebo	2.3% (5/217)	2.0% (4/200)
Celebrex 50 mg BID	3.4% (8/233)	—
Celebrex 100 mg BID	3.1% (7/227)	4.0% (9/223)
Celebrex 200 mg BID	5.9% (13/221)	2.7% (6/219)
Celebrex 400 mg BID	—	4.1% (8/197)
Naproxen 500 mg BID	16.2% (34/210)*	17.6% (37/210)*

*p≤0.05 vs all other treatments

Table 3 summarizes data from two 12-week studies that enrolled patients in whom baseline endoscopies revealed no ulcers. Patients underwent interval endoscopies every 4 weeks to give information on ulcer risk over time.

Table 1
Summary of Single Dose (200 mg) Disposition Kinetics of Celecoxib in Healthy Subjects[1]

Mean (%CV) PK Parameter Values				
C_{max}, ng/mL	T_{max}, hr	Effective $t_{1/2}$, hr	V_{ss}/F, L	CL/F, L/hr
705 (38)	2.8 (37)	11.2 (31)	429 (34)	27.7 (28)

[1]Subjects under fasting conditions (n=36, 19-52 yrs.)

Table 3
Incidence of Gastroduodenal Ulcers from 3-Month Serial Endoscopy Studies in OA and RA Patients

	Week 4	Week 8	Week 12	Final
Study 3 (n=523)				
Celebrex 200 mg BID	4.0% (10/252)*	2.2% (5/227)*	1.5% (3/196)*	7.5% (20/266)*
Naproxen 500 mg BID	19.0% (47/247)	14.2% (26/182)	9.9% (14/141)	34.6% (89/257)
Study 4 (n=1062)				
Celebrex 200 mg BID	3.9% (13/337)†	2.4% (7/296)†	1.8% (5/274)†	7.0% (25/356)†
Diclofenac 75 mg BID	5.1% (18/350)	3.3% (10/306)	2.9% (8/278)	9.7% (36/372)
Ibuprofen 800 mg TID	13.0% (42/323)	6.2% (15/241)	9.6% (21/219)	23.3% (78/334)

*p ≤0.05 Celebrex vs. naproxen based on interval and cumulative analyses
†p ≤0.05 Celebrex vs. ibuprofen based on interval and cumulative analyses

[See table 3 above]
One randomized and double-blind 6-month study in 430 RA patients was conducted in which an endoscopic examination was performed at 6 months. The incidence of endoscopic ulcers in patients taking Celebrex 200 mg BID was 4% vs 15% for patients taking diclofenac SR 75 mg BID (p<0.001).
In 4 of the 5 endoscopic studies, approximately 11% of patients (440/4,000) were taking aspirin (≤325 mg/day). In the Celebrex groups, the endoscopic ulcer rate appeared to be higher in aspirin users than in non-users. However, the increased rate of ulcers in these aspirin users was less than the endoscopic ulcer rates observed in the active comparator groups, with or without aspirin.
The correlation between findings of endoscopic studies, and the relative incidence of clinically significant serious upper GI events has not been established. Serious clinically significant upper GI bleeding has been observed in patients receiving Celebrex in controlled and open-labeled trials, albeit infrequently (see *Use with Aspirin* and WARNINGS — Gastrointestinal (GI) Effects).
Use with Aspirin: The Celecoxib Long-Term Arthritis Safety Study (CLASS) was a prospective long-term safety outcome study conducted postmarketing in approximately 5,800 OA patients and 2,200 RA patients. Patients received Celebrex 400 mg BID (4-fold and 2-fold the recommended OA and RA doses, respectively, and the approved dose for FAP), ibuprofen 800 mg TID or diclofenac 75 mg BID (common therapeutic doses). Median exposures for Celebrex (n = 3,987) and diclofenac (n = 1,996) were 9 months while ibuprofen (n = 1,985) was 6 months. The Kaplan-Meier cumulative rates at 9 months are provided for all analyses. The primary endpoint of this outcome study was the incidence of *complicated ulcers* (gastrointestinal bleeding, perforation or obstruction). Patients were allowed to take concomitant low-dose (≤ 325 mg/day) aspirin (ASA) for cardiovascular prophylaxis (ASA subgroups: Celebrex, n = 882; diclofenac, n = 445; ibuprofen, n = 412). Differences in the incidence of *complicated ulcers* between Celebrex and the combined group of ibuprofen and diclofenac were not statistically significant. Those patients on Celebrex and concomitant low-dose ASA experienced 4-fold higher rates of *complicated ulcers* compared to those not on ASA (see WARNINGS — Gastrointestinal (GI) Effects). The results for Celebrex are displayed in Table 4. For *complicated and symptomatic ulcer* rates, see WARNINGS — Gastrointestinal (GI) Effects – Risk of GI Ulceration, Bleeding, and Perforation.

Table 4
Effects of Co-Administration of Low-Dose Aspirin on *Complicated Ulcer* Rates with Celebrex 400 mg BID (Kaplan-Meier Rates at 9 months [%])

	Non-Aspirin Users n=3105	Aspirin Users n=882
Complicated Ulcers	0.32	1.12

Platelets: In clinical trials, Celebrex at single doses up to 800 mg and multiple doses of 600 mg BID for up to 7 days duration (higher than recommended therapeutic doses) had no effect on platelet aggregation and bleeding time. Comparators (naproxen 500 mg BID, ibuprofen 800 mg TID, diclofenac 75 mg BID) significantly reduced platelet aggregation and prolonged bleeding time.
Because of its lack of platelet effects, Celebrex is not a substitute for aspirin for cardiovascular prophylaxis.

INDICATIONS AND USAGE
Celebrex is indicated:
1) For relief of the signs and symptoms of osteoarthritis.
2) For relief of the signs and symptoms of rheumatoid arthritis in adults.
3) For the management of acute pain in adults (see CLINICAL STUDIES).
4) For the treatment of primary dysmenorrhea.
5) To reduce the number of adenomatous colorectal polyps in familial adenomatous polyposis (FAP), as an adjunct to usual care (e.g., endoscopic surveillance, surgery). It is not known whether there is a clinical benefit from a reduction in the number of colorectal polyps in FAP patients. It is also not known whether the effects of Celebrex treatment will persist after Celebrex is discontinued. The efficacy and safety of Celebrex treatment in patients with FAP beyond six months have not been studied (see CLINICAL STUDIES, WARNINGS and PRECAUTIONS sections).

CONTRAINDICATIONS
Celebrex is contraindicated in patients with known hypersensitivity to celecoxib.
Celebrex should not be given to patients who have demonstrated allergic-type reactions to sulfonamides.
Celebrex should not be given to patients who have experienced asthma, urticaria, or allergic-type reactions after taking aspirin or other NSAIDs. Severe, rarely fatal, anaphylactic-like reactions to NSAIDs have been reported in such patients (see WARNINGS — Anaphylactoid Reactions, and PRECAUTIONS — Preexisting Asthma).

WARNINGS
Gastrointestinal (GI) Effects—Risk of GI Ulceration, Bleeding, and Perforation
Serious gastrointestinal toxicity such as bleeding, ulceration, and perforation of the stomach, small intestine or large intestine, can occur at any time, with or without warning symptoms, in patients treated with nonsteroidal anti-inflammatory drugs (NSAIDs). Minor upper gastrointestinal problems, such as dyspepsia, are common and may also occur at any time during NSAID therapy. Therefore, physicians and patients should remain alert for ulceration and bleeding, even in the absence of previous GI tract symptoms (see PRECAUTIONS – Hematological Effects). Patients should be informed about the signs and/or symptoms of serious GI toxicity and the steps to take if they occur. The utility of periodic laboratory monitoring has not been demonstrated, nor has it been adequately assessed. Only one in five patients who develop a serious upper GI adverse event on NSAID therapy is symptomatic. It has been demonstrated that upper GI ulcers, gross bleeding or perforation, caused by NSAIDs, appear to occur in approximately 1% of patients treated for 3-6 months, and in about 2-4% of patients treated for one year. These trends continue thus, increasing the likelihood of developing a serious GI event at some time during the course of therapy. However, even short-term therapy is not without risk.
NSAIDs should be prescribed with extreme caution in patients with a prior history of ulcer disease or gastrointestinal bleeding. Most spontaneous reports of fatal GI events are in elderly or debilitated patients and therefore special care should be taken in treating this population. **To minimize the potential risk for an adverse GI event, the lowest effective dose should be used for the shortest possible duration.** For high risk patients, alternate therapies that do not involve NSAIDs should be considered.
Studies have shown that patients with a *prior history of peptic ulcer disease and/or gastrointestinal bleeding* and who use NSAIDs, have a greater than 10-fold higher risk for developing a GI bleed than patients with neither of these risk factors. In addition to a past history of ulcer disease, pharmacoepidemiological studies have identified several other co-therapies or co-morbid conditions that may increase the risk for GI bleeding such as: treatment with oral corticosteroids, treatment with anticoagulants, longer duration of NSAID therapy, smoking, alcoholism, older age, and poor general health status.
CLASS Study: The estimated cumulative rates at 9 months of *complicated and symptomatic ulcers* (an adverse event similar but not identical to the "upper GI ulcers, gross bleeding or perforation" described in the preceding paragraphs) for patients treated with Celebrex 400 mg BID (see Special Studies – *Use with Aspirin*) are described in Table 5. Table 5 also displays results for patients less than or greater than or equal to the age of 65 years. The differences in rates between Celebrex alone and Celebrex with ASA groups may be due to the higher risk for GI events in ASA users.

Table 5
***Complicated and Symptomatic Ulcer* Rates in Patients Taking Celebrex 400 mg BID (Kaplan-Meier Rates at 9 months [%]) Based on Risk Factors**

	Complicated and Symptomatic Ulcer Rates
All Patients	
Celebrex alone (n=3105)	0.78
Celebrex with ASA (n=882)	2.19
Patients <65 Years	
Celebrex alone (n=2025)	0.47
Celebrex with ASA (n=403)	1.26
Patients ≥65 Years	
Celebrex alone (n=1080)	1.40
Celebrex with ASA (n=479)	3.06

In a small number of patients with a history of ulcer disease, the *complicated and symptomatic ulcer* rates in patients taking Celebrex alone or Celebrex with ASA were, respectively, 2.56% (n=243) and 6.85% (n=91) at 48 weeks. These results are to be expected in patients with a prior history of ulcer disease (see WARNINGS – Gastrointestinal (GI) Effects – Risk of GI Ulceration, Bleeding, and Perforation).
Anaphylactoid Reactions
As with NSAIDs in general, anaphylactoid reactions have occurred in patients without known prior exposure to Celebrex. In post-marketing experience, rare cases of anaphylactic reactions and angioedema have been reported in patients receiving Celebrex. Celebrex should not be given to patients with the aspirin triad. This symptom complex typically occurs in asthmatic patients who experience rhinitis with or without nasal polyps, or who exhibit severe, potentially fatal bronchospasm after taking aspirin or other NSAIDs (see CONTRAINDICATIONS and PRECAUTIONS — Preexisting Asthma). Emergency help should be sought in cases where an anaphylactoid reaction occurs.
Advanced Renal Disease
No information is available from controlled clinical studies regarding the use of Celebrex in patients with advanced kidney disease. Therefore, treatment with Celebrex is not recommended in these patients with advanced kidney disease. If Celebrex therapy must be initiated, close monitoring of the patient's kidney function is advisable (see PRECAUTIONS — Renal Effects).
Pregnancy
In late pregnancy Celebrex should be avoided because it may cause premature closure of the ductus arteriosus (see PRECAUTIONS – Pregnancy).
Familial Adenomatous Polyposis (FAP): Treatment with Celebrex in FAP has not been shown to reduce the risk of gastrointestinal cancer or the need for prophylactic colectomy or other FAP-related surgeries. Therefore, the usual care of FAP patients should not be altered because of the concurrent administration of Celebrex. In particular, the frequency of routine endoscopic surveillance should not be decreased and prophylactic colectomy or other FAP-related surgeries should not be delayed.

PRECAUTIONS
General: Celebrex cannot be expected to substitute for corticosteroids or to treat corticosteroid insufficiency. Abrupt discontinuation of corticosteroids may lead to exacerbation of corticosteroid-responsive illness. Patients on prolonged corticosteroid therapy should have their therapy tapered slowly if a decision is made to discontinue corticosteroids.
The pharmacological activity of Celebrex in reducing inflammation, and possibly fever, may diminish the utility of these diagnostic signs in detecting infectious complications of presumed noninfectious, painful conditions.
Hepatic Effects: Borderline elevations of one or more liver associated enzymes may occur in up to 15% of patients taking NSAIDs, and notable elevations of ALT or AST (approximately 3 or more times the upper limit of normal) have been reported in approximately 1% of patients in clinical trials with NSAIDs. These laboratory abnormalities may progress, may remain unchanged, or may be transient with continuing therapy. Rare cases of severe hepatic reactions, including jaundice and fatal fulminant hepatitis, liver necrosis and hepatic failure (some with fatal outcome) have been reported with NSAIDs, including Celebrex (see ADVERSE REACTIONS – post-marketing experience). In controlled clinical trials of Celebrex, the incidence of borderline elevations (greater than or equal to 1.2 times and less than 3 times the upper limit of normal) of liver associated enzymes was 6% for Celebrex and 5% for placebo, and approximately 0.2% of patients taking Celebrex and 0.3% of patients taking placebo had notable elevations of ALT and AST.
A patient with symptoms and/or signs suggesting liver dysfunction, or in whom an abnormal liver test has occurred, should be monitored carefully for evidence of the development of a more severe hepatic reaction while on therapy with Celebrex. If clinical signs and symptoms consistent with liver disease develop, or if systemic manifestations occur (e.g., eosinophilia, rash, etc.), Celebrex should be discontinued.
Renal Effects: Long-term administration of NSAIDs has resulted in renal papillary necrosis and other renal injury. Renal toxicity has also been seen in patients in whom renal prostaglandins have a compensatory role in the maintenance of renal perfusion. In these patients, administration of a nonsteroidal anti-inflammatory drug may cause a dose-dependent reduction in prostaglandin formation and, secondarily, in renal blood flow, which may precipitate overt renal decompensation. Patients at greatest risk of this reaction are those with impaired renal function, heart failure, liver dysfunction, those taking diuretics and ACE inhibitors, and the elderly. Discontinuation of NSAID therapy is usually followed by recovery to the pretreatment state. Clinical trials with Celebrex have shown renal effects similar to those observed with comparator NSAIDs.

Continued on next page

Celebrex—Cont.

Caution should be used when initiating treatment with Celebrex in patients with considerable dehydration. It is advisable to rehydrate patients first and then start therapy with Celebrex. Caution is also recommended in patients with preexisting kidney disease (see WARNINGS—Advanced Renal Disease).

Hematological Effects: Anemia is sometimes seen in patients receiving Celebrex. In controlled clinical trials the incidence of anemia was 0.6% with Celebrex and 0.4% with placebo. Patients on long-term treatment with Celebrex should have their hemoglobin or hematocrit checked if they exhibit any signs or symptoms of anemia or blood loss. Celebrex does not generally affect platelet counts, prothrombin time (PT), or partial thromboplastin time (PTT), and does not inhibit platelet aggregation at indicated dosages (see CLINICAL STUDIES—Special Studies—Platelets).

Fluid Retention, Edema, and Hypertension: Fluid retention and edema have been observed in some patients taking Celebrex (see ADVERSE REACTIONS). In the CLASS study (see Special Studies – *Use with Aspirin*), the Kaplan-Meier cumulative rates at 9 months of peripheral edema in patients on Celebrex 400 mg BID (4-fold and 2-fold the recommended OA and RA doses, respectively, and the approved dose for FAP), ibuprofen 800 mg TID and diclofenac 75 mg BID were 4.5%, 6.9% and 4.7%, respectively. The rates of hypertension in the Celebrex, ibuprofen and diclofenac treated patients were 2.4%, 4.2% and 2.5%, respectively. As with other NSAIDs, Celebrex should be used with caution in patients with fluid retention, hypertension, or heart failure.

Preexisting Asthma: Patients with asthma may have aspirin-sensitive asthma. The use of aspirin in patients with aspirin-sensitive asthma has been associated with severe bronchospasm which can be fatal. Since cross reactivity, including bronchospasm, between aspirin and other nonsteroidal anti-inflammatory drugs has been reported in such aspirin-sensitive patients, Celebrex should not be administered to patients with this form of aspirin sensitivity and should be used with caution in patients with preexisting asthma.

Information for Patients: Celebrex can cause discomfort and, rarely, more serious side effects, such as gastrointestinal bleeding, which may result in hospitalization and even fatal outcomes. Although serious GI tract ulcerations and bleeding can occur without warning symptoms, patients should be alert for the signs and symptoms of ulcerations and bleeding, and should ask for medical advice when observing any indicative signs or symptoms. Patients should be apprised of the importance of this follow-up (see WARNINGS — Gastrointestinal (GI) Effects – Risk of Gastrointestinal Ulceration, Bleeding, and Perforation).

Patients should promptly report signs or symptoms of gastrointestinal ulceration or bleeding, skin rash, unexplained weight gain, or edema to their physicians.

Patients should be informed of the warning signs and symptoms of hepatotoxicity (e.g., nausea, fatigue, lethargy, pruritus, jaundice, right upper quadrant tenderness, and "flu-like" symptoms). If these occur, patients should be instructed to stop therapy and seek immediate medical therapy.

Patients should also be instructed to seek immediate emergency help in the case of an anaphylactoid reaction (see WARNINGS).

In late pregnancy Celebrex should be avoided because it may cause premature closure of the ductus arteriosus.

Patients with familial adenomatous polyposis (FAP) should be informed that Celebrex has not been shown to reduce colorectal, duodenal or other FAP-related cancers, or the need for endoscopic surveillance, prophylactic or other FAP-related surgery. Therefore, all patients with FAP should be instructed to continue their usual care while receiving Celebrex.

Laboratory Tests: Because serious GI tract ulcerations and bleeding can occur without warning symptoms, physicians should monitor for signs or symptoms of GI bleeding. In controlled clinical trials, elevated BUN occurred more frequently in patients receiving Celebrex compared with patients on placebo. This laboratory abnormality was also seen in patients who received comparator NSAIDs in these studies. The clinical significance of this abnormality has not been established.

Drug Interactions

General: Celecoxib metabolism is predominantly mediated via cytochrome P450 2C9 in the liver. Co-administration of celecoxib with drugs that are known to inhibit 2C9 should be done with caution.

In vitro studies indicate that celecoxib, although not a substrate, is an inhibitor of cytochrome P450 2D6. Therefore, there is a potential for an *in vivo* drug interaction with drugs that are metabolized by P450 2D6.

ACE-inhibitors: Reports suggest that NSAIDs may diminish the antihypertensive effect of Angiotensin Converting Enzyme (ACE) inhibitors. This interaction should be given consideration in patients taking Celebrex concomitantly with ACE-inhibitors.

Furosemide: Clinical studies, as well as post marketing observations, have shown that NSAIDs can reduce the natriuretic effect of furosemide and thiazides in some patients. This response has been attributed to inhibition of renal prostaglandin synthesis.

Aspirin: Celebrex can be used with low-dose aspirin. However, concomitant administration of aspirin with Celebrex increases the rate of GI ulceration or other complications, compared to use of Celebrex alone (see CLINICAL STUDIES — Special Studies — *Use with Aspirin* and WARNINGS – Gastrointestinal (GI) Effects – Risk of GI Ulceration, Bleeding, and Perforation – CLASS Study).

Because of its lack of platelet effects, Celebrex is not a substitute for aspirin for cardiovascular prophylaxis.

Fluconazole: Concomitant administration of fluconazole at 200 mg QD resulted in a two-fold increase in celecoxib plasma concentration. This increase is due to the inhibition of celecoxib metabolism via P450 2C9 by fluconazole (see Pharmacokinetics — Metabolism). Celebrex should be introduced at the lowest recommended dose in patients receiving fluconazole.

Lithium: In a study conducted in healthy subjects, mean steady-state lithium plasma levels increased approximately 17% in subjects receiving lithium 450 mg BID with Celebrex 200 mg BID as compared to subjects receiving lithium alone. Patients on lithium treatment should be closely monitored when Celebrex is introduced or withdrawn.

Methotrexate: In an interaction study of rheumatoid arthritis patients taking methotrexate, Celebrex did not have a significant effect on the pharmacokinetics of methotrexate.

Warfarin: Anticoagulant activity should be monitored, particularly in the first few days, after initiating or changing Celebrex therapy in patients receiving warfarin or similar agents, since these patients are at an increased risk of bleeding complications. The effect of celecoxib on the anticoagulant effect of warfarin was studied in a group of healthy subjects receiving daily doses of 2-5 mg of warfarin. In these subjects, celecoxib did not alter the anticoagulant effect of warfarin as determined by prothrombin time. However, in post-marketing experience, bleeding events have been reported, predominantly in the elderly, in association with increases in prothrombin time in patients receiving Celebrex concurrently with warfarin.

Carcinogenesis, mutagenesis, impairment of fertility: Celecoxib was not carcinogenic in rats given oral doses up to 200 mg/kg for males and 10 mg/kg for females (approximately 2- to 4-fold the human exposure as measured by the AUC_{0-24} at 200 mg BID) or in mice given oral doses up to 25 mg/kg for males and 50 mg/kg for females (approximately equal to human exposure as measured by the AUC_{0-24} at 200 mg BID) for two years.

Celecoxib was not mutagenic in an Ames test and a mutation assay in Chinese hamster ovary (CHO) cells, nor clastogenic in a chromosome aberration assay in CHO cells and an *in vivo* micronucleus test in rat bone marrow.

Celecoxib did not impair male and female fertility in rats at oral doses up to 600 mg/kg/day (approximately 11-fold human exposure at 200 mg BID based on the AUC_{0-24}).

Pregnancy

Teratogenic effects: Pregnancy Category C. Celecoxib at oral doses ≥150 mg/kg/day (approximately 2-fold human exposure at 200 mg BID as measured by AUC_{0-24}), caused an increased incidence of ventricular septal defects, a rare event, and fetal alterations, such as ribs fused, sternebrae fused and sternebrae misshapen when rabbits were treated throughout organogenesis. A dose-dependent increase in diaphragmatic hernias was observed when rats were given celecoxib at oral doses ≥30 mg/kg/day (approximately 6-fold human exposure based on the AUC_{0-24} at 200 mg BID) throughout organogenesis. There are no studies in pregnant women. Celebrex should be used during pregnancy only if the potential benefit justifies the potential risk to the fetus.

Nonteratogenic effects: Celecoxib produced pre-implantation and post-implantation losses and reduced embryo/fetal survival in rats at oral dosages ≥50 mg/kg/day (approximately 6-fold human exposure based on the AUC_{0-24} at 200 mg BID). These changes are expected with inhibition of prostaglandin synthesis and are not the result of permanent alteration of female reproductive function, nor are they expected at clinical exposures. No studies have been conducted to evaluate the effect of celecoxib on the closure of the ductus arteriosus in humans. Therefore, use of Celebrex during the third trimester of pregnancy should be avoided.

Labor and delivery: Celecoxib produced no evidence of delayed labor or parturition at oral doses up to 100 mg/kg in rats (approximately 7-fold human exposure as measured by the AUC_{0-24} at 200 mg BID). The effects of Celebrex on labor and delivery in pregnant women are unknown.

Nursing mothers: Celecoxib is excreted in the milk of lactating rats at concentrations similar to those in plasma. Limited data from one subject indicate that celecoxib is also excreted in human milk. Because many drugs are excreted in human milk and because of the potential for serious adverse reactions in nursing infants from Celebrex, a decision should be made whether to discontinue nursing or to discontinue the drug, taking into account the importance of the drug to the mother.

Pediatric Use

Safety and effectiveness in pediatric patients below the age of 18 years have not been evaluated.

Geriatric Use

Of the total number of patients who received Celebrex in clinical trials, more than 3,300 were 65-74 years of age, while approximately 1,300 additional patients were 75 years and over. No substantial differences in effectiveness were observed between these subjects and younger subjects. In clinical studies comparing renal function as measured by the GFR, BUN and creatinine, and platelet function as measured by bleeding time and platelet aggregation, the results were not different between elderly and young volunteers. However, as with other NSAIDs, including those that selectively inhibit COX-2, there have been more spontaneous post-marketing reports of fatal GI events and acute renal failure in the elderly than in younger patients (see WARNINGS – Gastrointestinal (GI) Effects – Risk of GI Ulceration, Bleeding, and Perforation).

ADVERSE REACTIONS

Of the Celebrex treated patients in the premarketing controlled clinical trials, approximately 4,250 were patients with OA, approximately 2,100 were patients with RA, and approximately 1,050 were patients with post-surgical pain. More than 8,500 patients have received a total daily dose of Celebrex of 200 mg (100 mg BID or 200 mg QD) or more, including more than 400 treated at 800 mg (400 mg BID). Approximately 3,900 patients have received Celebrex at these doses for 6 months or more; approximately 2,300 of these have received it for 1 year or more and 124 of these have received it for 2 years or more.

Adverse events from Celebrex premarketing controlled arthritis trials: Table 6 lists all adverse events, regardless of causality, occurring in ≥2% of patients receiving Celebrex from 12 controlled studies conducted in patients with OA or RA that included a placebo and/or a positive control group.

[See table at left]

Table 6
Adverse Events Occurring in ≥2% of Celebrex Patients From Celebrex Premarketing Controlled Arthritis Trials

	Celebrex (100-200 mg BID or 200 mg QD) (n=4146)	Placebo (n=1864)	Naproxen 500 mg BID (n=1366)	Diclofenac 75 mg BID (n=387)	Ibuprofen 800 mg TID (n=345)
Gastrointestinal					
Abdominal Pain	4.1%	2.8%	7.7%	9.0%	9.0%
Diarrhea	5.6%	3.8%	5.3%	9.3%	5.8%
Dyspepsia	8.8%	6.2%	12.2%	10.9%	12.8%
Flatulence	2.2%	1.0%	3.6%	4.1%	3.5%
Nausea	3.5%	4.2%	6.0%	3.4%	6.7%
Body as a whole					
Back Pain	2.8%	3.6%	2.2%	2.6%	0.9%
Peripheral edema	2.1%	1.1%	2.1%	1.0%	3.5%
Injury-accidental	2.9%	2.3%	3.0%	2.6%	3.2%
Central and peripheral nervous system					
Dizziness	2.0%	1.7%	2.6%	1.3%	2.3%
Headache	15.8%	20.2%	14.5%	15.5%	15.4%
Psychiatric					
Insomnia	2.3%	2.3%	2.9%	1.3%	1.4%
Respiratory					
Pharyngitis	2.3%	1.1%	1.7%	1.6%	2.6%
Rhinitis	2.0%	1.3%	2.4%	2.3%	0.6%
Sinusitis	5.0%	4.3%	4.0%	5.4%	5.8%
Upper respiratory tract infection	8.1%	6.7%	9.9%	9.8%	9.9%
Skin					
Rash	2.2%	2.1%	2.1%	1.3%	1.2%

In placebo- or active-controlled clinical trials, the discontinuation rate due to adverse events was 7.1% for patients receiving Celebrex and 6.1% for patients receiving placebo. Among the most common reasons for discontinuation due to adverse events in the Celebrex treatment groups were dyspepsia and abdominal pain (cited as reasons for discontinuation in 0.8% and 0.7% of Celebrex patients, respectively). Among patients receiving placebo, 0.6% discontinued due to dyspepsia and 0.6% withdrew due to abdominal pain.

The following adverse events occurred in 0.1-1.9% of patients regardless of causality.

[See first table at top of next page]

Other serious adverse reactions which occur rarely (estimated <0.1%), regardless of causality: The following seri-

CELEBREX (100-200 mg BID or 200 mg QD)	
Gastrointestinal:	Constipation, diverticulitis, dysphagia, eructation, esophagitis, gastritis, gastroenteritis, gastroesophageal reflux, hemorrhoids, hiatal hernia, melena, dry mouth, stomatitis, tenesmus, tooth disorder, vomiting
Cardiovascular:	Aggravated hypertension, angina pectoris, coronary artery disorder, myocardial infarction
General:	Allergy aggravated, allergic reaction, asthenia, chest pain, cyst NOS, edema generalized, face edema, fatigue, fever, hot flushes, influenza-like symptoms, pain, peripheral pain
Resistance mechanism disorders:	Herpes simplex, herpes zoster, infection bacterial, infection fungal, infection soft tissue, infection viral, moniliasis, moniliasis genital, otitis media
Central, peripheral nervous system:	Leg cramps, hypertonia, hypoesthesia, migraine, neuralgia, neuropathy, paresthesia, vertigo
Female reproductive:	Breast fibroadenosis, breast neoplasm, breast pain, dysmenorrhea, menstrual disorder, vaginal hemorrhage, vaginitis
Male reproductive:	Prostatic disorder
Hearing and vestibular:	Deafness, ear abnormality, earache, tinnitus
Heart rate and rhythm:	Palpitation, tachycardia
Liver and biliary system:	Hepatic function abnormal, SGOT increased, SGPT increased
Metabolic and nutritional:	BUN increased, CPK increased, diabetes mellitus, hypercholesterolemia, hyperglycemia, hypokalemia, NPN increase, creatinine increased, alkaline phosphatase increased, weight increase
Musculoskeletal:	Arthralgia, arthrosis, bone disorder, fracture accidental, myalgia, neck stiffness, synovitis, tendinitis
Platelets (bleeding or clotting):	Ecchymosis, epistaxis, thrombocythemia
Psychiatric:	Anorexia, anxiety, appetite increased, depression, nervousness, somnolence
Hemic:	Anemia
Respiratory:	Bronchitis, bronchospasm, bronchospasm aggravated, coughing, dyspnea, laryngitis, pneumonia
Skin and appendages:	Alopecia, dermatitis, nail disorder, photosensitivity reaction, pruritus, rash erythematous, rash maculopapular, skin disorder, skin dry, sweating increased, urticaria
Application site disorders:	Cellulitis, dermatitis contact, injection site reaction, skin nodule
Special senses:	Taste perversion
Urinary system:	Albuminuria, cystitis, dysuria, hematuria, micturition frequency, renal calculus, urinary incontinence, urinary tract infection
Vision:	Blurred vision, cataract, conjunctivitis, eye pain, glaucoma

Cardiovascular:	Syncope, congestive heart failure, ventricular fibrillation, pulmonary embolism, cerebrovascular accident, peripheral gangrene, thrombophlebitis, *vasculitis*
Gastrointestinal:	Intestinal obstruction, intestinal perforation, gastrointestinal bleeding, colitis with bleeding, esophageal perforation, pancreatitis, ileus
Liver and biliary system:	Cholelithiasis, *hepatitis, jaundice, liver failure*
Hemic and lymphatic:	Thrombocytopenia, *agranulocytosis, aplastic anemia, pancytopenia, leukopenia*
Metabolic:	*Hypoglycemia, hyponatremia*
Nervous system:	*Aseptic meningitis*, ataxia, suicide
Renal:	Acute renal failure, *interstitial nephritis*
Skin:	*Erythema multiforme, exfoliative dermatitis, Stevens-Johnson syndrome, toxic epidermal necrolysis*
General:	Sepsis, sudden death, *anaphylactoid reaction, angioedema*

ous adverse events have occurred rarely in patients taking CELEBREX. Cases reported only in the post-marketing experience are indicated in italics.

[See second table above]

Safety Data from CLASS Study:

Hematological Events:

During this study (see Special Studies – *Use with Aspirin*), the incidence of clinically significant decreases in hemoglobin (>2 g/dL) confirmed by repeat testing was lower in patients on CELEBREX 400 mg BID (4-fold and 2-fold the recommended OA and RA doses, respectively, and the approved dose for FAP) compared to patients on either diclofenac 75 mg BID or ibuprofen 800 mg TID: 0.5%, 1.3% and 1.9%, respectively. The lower incidence of events with CELEBREX was maintained with or without ASA use (see CLINICAL STUDIES – Special Studies – Platelets).

Withdrawals/Serious Adverse Events:

Kaplan-Meier cumulative rates at 9 months for withdrawals due to adverse events for CELEBREX, diclofenac and ibuprofen were 24%, 29%, and 26%, respectively. Rates for serious adverse events (i.e. those causing hospitalization or felt to be life threatening or otherwise medically significant) regardless of causality were not different across treatment groups, respectively, 8%, 7%, and 8%.

Based on Kaplan-Meier cumulative rates for investigator-reported serious cardiovascular thromboembolic adverse events*, there were no differences between the CELEBREX, diclofenac, or ibuprofen treatment groups. The rates in all patients at 9 months for CELEBREX, diclofenac, and ibuprofen were 1.2%, 1.4%, and 1.1%, respectively. The rates for non-ASA users in each of the three treatment groups were less than 1%. The rates for myocardial infarction in each of the three non-ASA treatment groups were less than 0.2%.

*includes myocardial infarction, pulmonary embolism, deep venous thrombosis, unstable angina, transient ischemic attacks or ischemic cerebrovascular accidents.

Adverse events from analgesia and dysmenorrhea studies: Approximately 1,700 patients were treated with CELEBREX in analgesia and dysmenorrhea studies. All patients in post-oral surgery pain studies received a single dose of study medication. Doses up to 600 mg/day of CELEBREX were studied in primary dysmenorrhea and post-orthopedic surgery pain studies. The types of adverse events in the analgesia and dysmenorrhea studies were similar to those reported in arthritis studies. The only additional adverse event reported was post-dental extraction alveolar osteitis (dry socket) in the post-oral surgery pain studies.

Adverse events from the controlled trial in familial adenomatous polyposis: The adverse event profile reported for the 83 patients with familial adenomatous polyposis enrolled in the randomized, controlled clinical trial was similar to that reported for patients in the arthritis controlled trials. Intestinal anastomotic ulceration was the only new adverse event reported in the FAP trial, regardless of causality, and was observed in 3 of 58 patients (one at 100 mg BID, and two at 400 mg BID) who had prior intestinal surgery.

OVERDOSAGE

No overdoses of CELEBREX were reported during clinical trials. Doses up to 2400 mg/day for up to 10 days in 12 patients did not result in serious toxicity. Symptoms following acute NSAID overdoses are usually limited to lethargy, drowsiness, nausea, vomiting, and epigastric pain, which are generally reversible with supportive care. Gastrointestinal bleeding can occur. Hypertension, acute renal failure, respiratory depression and coma may occur, but are rare. Anaphylactoid reactions have been reported with therapeutic ingestion of NSAIDs, and may occur following an overdose. Patients should be managed by symptomatic and supportive care following an NSAID overdose. There are no specific antidotes. No information is available regarding the removal of celecoxib by hemodialysis, but based on its high degree of plasma protein binding (>97%) dialysis is unlikely to be useful in overdose. Emesis and/or activated charcoal (60 to 100 g in adults, 1 to 2 g/kg in children) and/or osmotic cathartic may be indicated in patients seen within 4 hours of ingestion with symptoms or following a large overdose. Forced diuresis, alkalinization of urine, hemodialysis, or hemoperfusion may not be useful due to high protein binding.

DOSAGE AND ADMINISTRATION

For osteoarthritis and rheumatoid arthritis, the lowest dose of CELEBREX should be sought for each patient. These doses can be given without regard to timing of meals.

Osteoarthritis: For relief of the signs and symptoms of osteoarthritis the recommended oral dose is 200 mg per day administered as a single dose or as 100 mg twice per day.

Rheumatoid arthritis: For relief of the signs and symptoms of rheumatoid arthritis the recommended oral dose is 100 to 200 mg twice per day.

Management of Acute Pain and Treatment of Primary Dysmenorrhea: The recommended dose of CELEBREX is 400 mg initially, followed by an additional 200 mg dose if needed on the first day. On subsequent days, the recommended dose is 200 mg twice daily as needed.

Familial adenomatous polyposis (FAP): Usual medical care for FAP patients should be continued while on CELEBREX. To reduce the number of adenomatous colorectal polyps in patients with FAP, the recommended oral dose is 400 mg twice per day to be taken with food.

Special Populations

Hepatic insufficiency: The daily recommended dose of CELEBREX capsules in patients with moderate hepatic impairment (Child-Pugh Class B) should be reduced by approximately 50% (see CLINICAL PHARMACOLOGY – Special Populations).

HOW SUPPLIED

CELEBREX 100-mg capsules are white, reverse printed white on blue band of body and cap with markings of 7767 on the cap and 100 on the body, supplied as:

NDC Number	Size
0025-1520-31	bottle of 100
0025-1520-51	bottle of 500
0025-1520-34	carton of 100 unit dose

CELEBREX 200-mg capsules are white, with reverse printed white on gold band with markings of 7767 on the cap and 200 on the body, supplied as:

NDC Number	Size
0025-1525-31	bottle of 100
0025-1525-51	bottle of 500
0025-1525-34	carton of 100 unit dose

CELEBREX 400-mg capsules are white, with reverse printed white on green band with markings of 7767 on the cap and 400 on the body, supplied as:

NDC Number	Size
0025-1530-02	bottle of 60
0025-1530-01	carton of 100 unit dose

Store at 25°C (77°F); excursions permitted to 15-30°C (59-86°F) [see USP Controlled Room Temperature].

Rx only Revised: January 2004

Manufactured for: *G.D. Searle LLC*
A subsidiary of Pharmacia Corporation
Chicago, IL 60680, USA
Pfizer Inc
New York, NY 10017, USA

by: *Searle Ltd.*
Caguas, PR 00725

PHARMACIA Pfizer

CELEBREX®
celecoxib capsules
819 059 006 PS4025-7

DIFLUCAN® ℞

[*dī-flew-kăn*]

(Fluconazole Tablets)
(Fluconazole Injection - for intravenous infusion only)
(Fluconazole for Oral Suspension)

Prescribing information for this product, which appears on pages 2590–2594 of the 2004 PDR, has been completely revised as follows. Please write "See Supplement A" next to the product heading.

DESCRIPTION

DIFLUCAN® (fluconazole), the first of a new subclass of synthetic triazole antifungal agents, is available as tablets for oral administration, as a powder for oral suspension and as a sterile solution for intravenous use in glass and in Viaflex® Plus plastic containers.

Fluconazole is designated chemically as 2,4-difluoro-α,α[1]-bis(1H-1,2,4-triazol-1-ylmethyl) benzyl alcohol with an empirical formula of $C_{13}H_{12}F_2N_6O$ and molecular weight 306.3. The structural formula is:

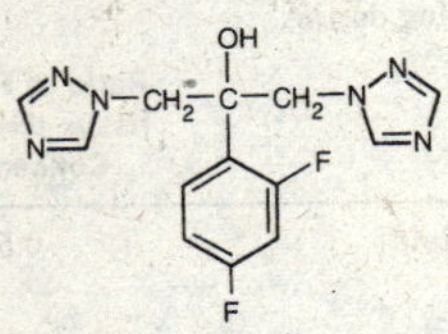

Fluconazole is a white crystalline solid which is slightly soluble in water and saline.

DIFLUCAN tablets contain 50, 100, 150, or 200 mg of fluconazole and the following inactive ingredients: microcrystalline cellulose, dibasic calcium phosphate anhydrous, povidone, croscarmellose sodium, FD&C Red No. 40 aluminum lake dye, and magnesium stearate.

DIFLUCAN for oral suspension contains 350 mg or 1400 mg of fluconazole and the following inactive ingredients: sucrose, sodium citrate dihydrate, citric acid anhydrous, sodium benzoate, titanium dioxide, colloidal silicon dioxide, xanthan gum and natural orange flavor. After reconstitution with 24 mL of distilled water or Purified Water (USP), each mL of reconstituted suspension contains 10 mg or 40 mg of fluconazole.

DIFLUCAN injection is an iso-osmotic, sterile, nonpyrogenic solution of fluconazole in a sodium chloride or dextrose diluent. Each mL contains 2 mg of fluconazole and 9 mg of sodium chloride or 56 mg of dextrose, hydrous. The pH ranges from 4.0 to 8.0 in the sodium chloride diluent and from 3.5 to 6.5 in the dextrose diluent. Injection volumes of 100 mL and 200 mL are packaged in glass and in Viaflex® Plus plastic containers.

The Viaflex® Plus plastic container is fabricated from a specially formulated polyvinyl chloride (PL 146® Plastic) (Viaflex and PL 146 are registered trademarks of Baxter International, Inc.). The amount of water that can permeate from inside the container into the overwrap is insufficient to affect the solution significantly. Solutions in contact with the plastic container can leach out certain of its chemical components in very small amounts within the expiration pe-

Continued on next page

Diflucan—Cont.

riod, e.g., di-2-ethylhexylphthalate (DEHP), up to 5 parts per million. However, the suitability of the plastic has been confirmed in tests in animals according to USP biological tests for plastic containers as well as by tissue culture toxicity studies.

CLINICAL PHARMACOLOGY

Mode of Action

Fluconazole is a highly selective inhibitor of fungal cytochrome P-450 sterol C-14 alpha-demethylation. Mammalian cell demethylation is much less sensitive to fluconazole inhibition. The subsequent loss of normal sterols correlates with the accumulation of 14 alpha-methyl sterols in fungi and may be responsible for the fungistatic activity of fluconazole.

Pharmacokinetics and Metabolism

The pharmacokinetic properties of fluconazole are similar following administration by the intravenous or oral routes. In normal volunteers, the bioavailability of orally administered fluconazole is over 90% compared with intravenous administration. Bioequivalence was established between the 100 mg tablet and both suspension strengths when administered as a single 200 mg dose.

Peak plasma concentrations (Cmax) in fasted normal volunteers occur between 1 and 2 hours with a terminal plasma elimination half-life of approximately 30 hours (range: 20-50 hours) after oral administration.

In fasted normal volunteers, administration of a single oral 400 mg dose of DIFLUCAN (fluconazole) leads to a mean Cmax of 6.72 µg/mL (range: 4.12 to 8.08 µg/mL) and after single oral doses of 50-400 mg, fluconazole plasma concentrations and AUC (area under the plasma concentration-time curve) are dose proportional.

Administration of a single oral 150 mg tablet of DIFLUCAN (fluconazole) to ten lactating women resulted in a mean Cmax of 2.61 µg/mL (range: 1.57 to 3.65 µg/mL).

Steady-state concentrations are reached within 5-10 days following oral doses of 50-400 mg given once daily. Administration of a loading dose (on day 1) of twice the usual daily dose results in plasma concentrations close to steady-state by the second day. The apparent volume of distribution of fluconazole approximates that of total body water. Plasma protein binding is low (11-12%). Following either single- or multiple-oral doses for up to 14 days, fluconazole penetrates into all body fluids studied (see table below). In normal volunteers, saliva concentrations of fluconazole were equal to or slightly greater than plasma concentrations regardless of dose, route, or duration of dosing. In patients with bronchiectasis, sputum concentrations of fluconazole following a single 150 mg oral dose were equal to plasma concentrations at both 4 and 24 hours post dose. In patients with fungal meningitis, fluconazole concentrations in the CSF are approximately 80% of the corresponding plasma concentrations.

A single oral 150 mg dose of fluconazole administered to 27 patients penetrated into vaginal tissue, resulting in tissue: plasma ratios ranging from 0.94 to 1.14 over the first 48 hours following dosing.

A single oral 150 mg dose of fluconazole administered to 14 patients penetrated into vaginal fluid, resulting in fluid: plasma ratios ranging from 0.36 to 0.71 over the first 72 hours following dosing.

Tissue or Fluid	Ratio of Fluconazole Tissue (Fluid)/Plasma Concentration*
Cerebrospinal fluid†	0.5-0.9
Saliva	1
Sputum	1
Blister fluid	1
Urine	10
Normal skin	10
Nails	1
Blister skin	2
Vaginal tissue	1
Vaginal fluid	0.4-0.7

*Relative to concurrent concentrations in plasma in subjects with normal renal function.
†Independent of degree of meningeal inflammation.

In normal volunteers, fluconazole is cleared primarily by renal excretion, with approximately 80% of the dose appearing in the urine as unchanged drug. About 11% of the dose is excreted in the urine as metabolites.

The pharmacokinetics of fluconazole are markedly affected by reduction in renal function. There is an inverse relationship between the elimination half-life and creatinine clearance. The dose of DIFLUCAN may need to be reduced in patients with impaired renal function. (See **DOSAGE AND ADMINISTRATION.**) A 3-hour hemodialysis session decreases plasma concentrations by approximately 50%.

In normal volunteers, DIFLUCAN administration (doses ranging from 200 mg to 400 mg once daily for up to 14 days) was associated with small and inconsistent effects on testosterone concentrations, endogenous corticosteroid concentrations, and the ACTH-stimulated cortisol response.

Pharmacokinetics in Children

In children, the following pharmacokinetic data {Mean(%cv)} have been reported:

[See table below]

Clearance corrected for body weight was not affected by age in these studies. Mean body clearance in adults is reported to be 0.23 (17%) mL/min/kg.

In premature newborns (gestational age 26 to 29 weeks), the mean (%cv) clearance within 36 hours of birth was 0.180 (35%, N=7) mL/min/kg, which increased with time to a mean of 0.218 (31%, N=9) mL/min/kg six days later and 0.333 (56%, N=4) mL/min/kg 12 days later. Similarly, the half-life was 73.6 hours, which decreased with time to a mean of 53.2 hours six days later and 46.6 hours 12 days later.

Drug Interaction Studies

Oral contraceptives: Oral contraceptives were administered as a single dose both before and after the oral administration of DIFLUCAN 50 mg once daily for 10 days in 10 healthy women. There was no significant difference in ethinyl estradiol or levonorgestrel AUC after the administration of 50 mg of DIFLUCAN. The mean increase in ethinyl estradiol AUC was 6% (range: –47 to 108%) and levonorgestrel AUC increased 17% (range: –33 to 141%).

In a second study, twenty-five normal females received daily doses of both 200 mg DIFLUCAN tablets or placebo for two, ten-day periods. The treatment cycles were one month apart with all subjects receiving DIFLUCAN during one cycle and placebo during the other. The order of study treatment was random. Single doses of an oral contraceptive tablet containing levonorgestrel and ethinyl estradiol were administered on the final treatment day (day 10) of both cycles. Following administration of 200 mg of DIFLUCAN, the mean percentage increase of AUC for levonorgestrel compared to placebo was 25% (range: -12 to 82%) and the mean percentage increase for ethinyl estradiol compared to placebo was 38% (range: -11 to 101%). Both of these increases were statistically significantly different from placebo.

Cimetidine: DIFLUCAN 100 mg was administered as a single oral dose alone and two hours after a single dose of cimetidine 400 mg to six healthy male volunteers. After the administration of cimetidine, there was a significant decrease in fluconazole AUC and Cmax. There was a mean ± SD decrease in fluconazole AUC of 13% ± 11% (range: –3.4 to –31%) and Cmax decreased 19% ± 14% (range: –5 to –40%). However, the administration of cimetidine 600 mg to 900 mg intravenously over a four-hour period (from one hour before to 3 hours after a single oral dose of DIFLUCAN 200 mg) did not affect the bioavailability or pharmacokinetics of fluconazole in 24 healthy male volunteers.

Antacid: Administration of Maalox® (20 mL) to 14 normal male volunteers immediately prior to a single dose of DIFLUCAN 100 mg had no effect on the absorption or elimination of fluconazole.

Hydrochlorothiazide: Concomitant oral administration of 100 mg DIFLUCAN and 50 mg hydrochlorothiazide for 10 days in 13 normal volunteers resulted in a significant increase in fluconazole AUC and Cmax compared to DIFLUCAN given alone. There was a mean ± SD increase in fluconazole AUC and Cmax of 45% ± 31% (range: 19 to 114%) and 43% ± 31% (range: 19 to 122%), respectively. These changes are attributed to a mean ± SD reduction in renal clearance of 30% ± 12% (range: –10 to –50%).

Rifampin: Administration of a single oral 200 mg dose of DIFLUCAN after 15 days of rifampin administered as 600 mg daily in eight healthy male volunteers resulted in a significant decrease in fluconazole AUC and a significant increase in apparent oral clearance of fluconazole. There was a mean ± SD reduction in fluconazole AUC of 23% ± 9% (range: –13 to –42%). Apparent oral clearance of fluconazole increased 32% ± 17% (range: 16 to 72%). Fluconazole half-life decreased from 33.4 ± 4.4 hours to 26.8 ± 3.9 hours. (See **PRECAUTIONS.**)

Warfarin: There was a significant increase in prothrombin time response (area under the prothrombin time-time curve) following a single dose of warfarin (15 mg) administered to 13 normal male volunteers following oral DIFLUCAN 200 mg administered daily for 14 days as compared to the administration of warfarin alone. There was a mean ± SD increase in the prothrombin time response (area under the prothrombin time-time curve) of 7% ± 4% (range: –2 to 13%). (See **PRECAUTIONS.**) Mean is based on data from 12 subjects as one of 13 subjects experienced a 2-fold increase in his prothrombin time response.

Phenytoin: Phenytoin AUC was determined after 4 days of phenytoin dosing (200 mg daily, orally for 3 days followed by 250 mg intravenously for one dose) both with and without the administration of fluconazole (oral DIFLUCAN 200 mg daily for 16 days) in 10 normal male volunteers. There was a significant increase in phenytoin AUC. The mean ± SD increase in phenytoin AUC was 88% ± 68% (range: 16 to 247%). The absolute magnitude of this interaction is unknown because of the intrinsically nonlinear disposition of phenytoin. (See **PRECAUTIONS.**)

Cyclosporine: Cyclosporine AUC and Cmax were determined before and after the administration of fluconazole 200 mg daily for 14 days in eight renal transplant patients who had been on cyclosporine therapy for at least 6 months and on a stable cyclosporine dose for at least 6 weeks. There was a significant increase in cyclosporine AUC, Cmax, Cmin (24-hour concentration), and a significant reduction in apparent oral clearance following the administration of fluconazole. The mean ± SD increase in AUC was 92% ± 43% (range: 18 to 147%). The Cmax increased 60% ± 48% (range: –5 to 133%). The Cmin increased 157% ± 96% (range: 33 to 360%). The apparent oral clearance decreased 45% ± 15% (range: –15 to –60%). (See **PRECAUTIONS.**)

Zidovudine: Plasma zidovudine concentrations were determined on two occasions (before and following fluconazole 200 mg daily for 15 days) in 13 volunteers with AIDS or ARC who were on a stable zidovudine dose for at least two weeks. There was a significant increase in zidovudine AUC following the administration of fluconazole. The mean ± SD increase in AUC was 20% ± 32% (range: –27 to 104%). The metabolite, GZDV, to parent drug ratio significantly decreased after the administration of fluconazole, from 7.6 ± 3.6 to 5.7 ± 2.2.

Theophylline: The pharmacokinetics of theophylline were determined from a single intravenous dose of aminophylline (6 mg/kg) before and after the oral administration of fluconazole 200 mg daily for 14 days in 16 normal male volunteers. There were significant increases in theophylline AUC, Cmax, and half-life with a corresponding decrease in clearance. The mean ± SD theophylline AUC increased 21% ± 16% (range: –5 to 48%). The Cmax increased 13% ± 17% (range: –13 to 40%). Theophylline clearance decreased 16% ± 11% (range: –32 to 5%). The half-life of theophylline increased from 6.6 ± 1.7 hours to 7.9 ± 1.5 hours. (See **PRECAUTIONS.**)

Terfenadine: Six healthy volunteers received terfenadine 60 mg BID for 15 days. Fluconazole 200 mg was administered daily from days 9 through 15. Fluconazole did not affect terfenadine plasma concentrations. Terfenadine acid metabolite AUC increased 36% ± 36% (range: 7 to 102%) from day 8 to day 15 with the concomitant administration of fluconazole. There was no change in cardiac repolarization as measured by Holter QTc intervals. Another study at a 400-mg and 800-mg daily dose of fluconazole demonstrated that DIFLUCAN taken in doses of 400 mg per day or greater significantly increases plasma levels of terfenadine when taken concomitantly. (See **CONTRAINDICATIONS** and **PRECAUTIONS.**)

Oral hypoglycemics: The effects of fluconazole on the pharmacokinetics of the sulfonylurea oral hypoglycemic agents tolbutamide, glipizide, and glyburide were evaluated in three placebo-controlled studies in normal volunteers. All subjects received the sulfonylurea alone as a single dose and again as a single dose following the administration of DIFLUCAN 100 mg daily for 7 days. In these three studies 22/46 (47.8%) of DIFLUCAN treated patients and 9/22 (40.1%) of placebo treated patients experienced symptoms consistent with hypoglycemia. (See **PRECAUTIONS.**)

Tolbutamide: In 13 normal male volunteers, there was significant increase in tolbutamide (500 mg single dose) AUC and Cmax following the administration of fluconazole. There was a mean ± SD increase in tolbutamide AUC of 26% ± 9% (range: 12 to 39%). Tolbutamide Cmax increased 11% ± 9% (range: –6 to 27%). (See **PRECAUTIONS.**)

Glipizide: The AUC and Cmax of glipizide (2.5 mg single dose) were significantly increased following the administration of fluconazole in 13 normal male volunteers. There was a mean ± SD increase in AUC of 49% ± 13% (range: 27 to 73%) and an increase in Cmax of 19% ± 23% (range: –11 to 79%). (See **PRECAUTIONS.**)

Glyburide: The AUC and Cmax of glyburide (5 mg single dose) were significantly increased following the administration of fluconazole in 20 normal male volunteers. There was a mean ± SD increase in AUC of 44% ± 29% (range: –13 to 115%) and Cmax increased 19% ± 19% (range: –23 to 62%). Five subjects required oral glucose following the ingestion of glyburide after 7 days of fluconazole administration. (See **PRECAUTIONS.**)

Rifabutin: There have been published reports that an interaction exists when fluconazole is administered concomitantly with rifabutin, leading to increased serum levels of rifabutin. (See **PRECAUTIONS.**)

Tacrolimus: There have been published reports that an interaction exists when fluconazole is administered concomi-

Age Studied	Dose (mg/kg)	Clearance (mL/min/kg)	Half-life (Hours)	Cmax (µg/mL)	Vdss (L/kg)
9 Months-13 years	Single-Oral 2 mg/kg	0.40 (38%) N=14	25.0	2.9 (22%) N=16	—
9 Months-13 years	Single-Oral 8 mg/kg	0.51 (60%) N=15	19.5	9.8 (20%) N=15	—
5-15 years	Multiple IV 2 mg/kg	0.49 (40%) N=4	17.4	5.5 (25%) N=5	0.722 (36%) N=4
5-15 years	Multiple IV 4 mg/kg	0.59 (64%) N=5	15.2	11.4 (44%) N=6	0.729 (33%) N=5
5-15 years	Multiple IV 8 mg/kg	0.66 (31%) N=7	17.6	14.1 (22%) N=8	1.069 (37%) N=7

tantly with tacrolimus, leading to increased serum levels of tacrolimus. (See **PRECAUTIONS**.)

Cisapride: A preliminary report from a placebo-controlled, randomized multiple-dose study in subjects given fluconazole 200 mg daily and cisapride 20 mg four times daily starting after 7 days of fluconazole dosing found that fluconazole significantly increased the AUC and Cmax of cisapride both after single (AUC 102% and Cmax 92% increases) and multiple (AUC 192% and Cmax 153% increases) dosing of cisapride. Fluconazole significantly increased the QTc interval in subjects receiving cisapride 20 mg four times daily for 5 days. (See **CONTRAINDICATIONS** and **PRECAUTIONS**.)

Microbiology

Fluconazole exhibits *in vitro* activity against *Cryptococcus neoformans* and *Candida* spp. Fungistatic activity has also been demonstrated in normal and immunocompromised animal models for systemic and intracranial fungal infections due to *Cryptococcus neoformans* and for systemic infections due to *Candida albicans*.

In common with other azole antifungal agents, most fungi show a higher apparent sensitivity to fluconazole *in vivo* than *in vitro*. Fluconazole administered orally and/or intravenously was active in a variety of animal models of fungal infection using standard laboratory strains of fungi. Activity has been demonstrated against fungal infections caused by *Aspergillus flavus* and *Aspergillus fumigatus* in normal mice. Fluconazole has also been shown to be active in animal models of endemic mycoses, including one model of *Blastomyces dermatitidis* pulmonary infections in normal mice; one model of *Coccidioides immitis* intracranial infections in normal mice; and several models of *Histoplasma capsulatum* pulmonary infection in normal and immunosuppressed mice. The clinical significance of results obtained in these studies is unknown.

Oral fluconazole has been shown to be active in an animal model of vaginal candidiasis.

Concurrent administration of fluconazole and amphotericin B in infected normal and immunosuppressed mice showed the following results: a small additive antifungal effect in systemic infection with *C. albicans*, no interaction in intracranial infection with *Cr. neoformans*, and antagonism of the two drugs in systemic infection with *Asp. fumigatus*. The clinical significance of results obtained in these studies is unknown.

There have been reports of cases of superinfection with *Candida* species other than *C. albicans*, which are often inherently not susceptible to DIFLUCAN (e.g., *Candida krusei*). Such cases may require alternative antifungal therapy.

INDICATIONS AND USAGE

DIFLUCAN (fluconazole) is indicated for the treatment of:

1. Vaginal candidiasis (vaginal yeast infections due to *Candida*).
2. Oropharyngeal and esophageal candidiasis. In open noncomparative studies of relatively small numbers of patients, DIFLUCAN was also effective for the treatment of *Candida* urinary tract infections, peritonitis, and systemic *Candida* infections including candidemia, disseminated candidiasis, and pneumonia.
3. Cryptococcal meningitis. Before prescribing DIFLUCAN (fluconazole) for AIDS patients with cryptococcal meningitis, please see **CLINICAL STUDIES** section. Studies comparing DIFLUCAN to amphotericin B in non-HIV infected patients have not been conducted.

Prophylaxis. DIFLUCAN is also indicated to decrease the incidence of candidiasis in patients undergoing bone marrow transplantation who receive cytotoxic chemotherapy and/or radiation therapy.

Specimens for fungal culture and other relevant laboratory studies (serology, histopathology) should be obtained prior to therapy to isolate and identify causative organisms. Therapy may be instituted before the results of the cultures and other laboratory studies are known; however, once these results become available, anti-infective therapy should be adjusted accordingly.

CLINICAL STUDIES

Cryptococcal meningitis: In a multicenter study comparing DIFLUCAN (200 mg/day) to amphotericin B (0.3 mg/kg/day) for treatment of cryptococcal meningitis in patients with AIDS, a multivariate analysis revealed three pretreatment factors that predicted death during the course of therapy: abnormal mental status, cerebrospinal fluid cryptococcal antigen titer greater than 1:1024, and cerebrospinal fluid white blood cell count of less than 20 cells/mm^3. Mortality among high risk patients was 33% and 40% for amphotericin B and DIFLUCAN patients, respectively (p=0.58), with overall deaths 14% (9 of 63 subjects) and 18% (24 of 131 subjects) for the 2 arms of the study (p=0.48). Optimal doses and regimens for patients with acute cryptococcal meningitis and at high risk for treatment failure remain to be determined. (Saag, *et al.* N Engl J Med 1992; 326:83-9.)

Vaginal candidiasis: Two adequate and well-controlled studies were conducted in the U.S. using the 150 mg tablet. In both, the results of the fluconazole regimen were comparable to the control regimen (clotrimazole or miconazole intravaginally for 7 days) both clinically and statistically at the one month post-treatment evaluation.

The therapeutic cure rate, defined as a complete resolution of signs and symptoms of vaginal candidiasis (clinical cure), along with a negative KOH examination and negative culture for *Candida* (microbiologic eradication), was 55% in both the fluconazole group and the vaginal products group.

	Fluconazole PO 150 mg tablet	Vaginal Product qhs × 7 days
Enrolled	448	422
Evaluable at Late Follow-Up	347 (77%)	327 (77%)
Clinical cure	239/347 (69%)	235/327 (72%)
Mycologic erad.	213/347 (61%)	196/327 (60%)
Therapeutic cure	190/347 (55%)	179/327 (55%)

[See table above]

Approximately three-fourths of the enrolled patients had acute vaginitis (<4 episodes/12 months) and achieved 80% clinical cure, 67% mycologic eradication and 59% therapeutic cure when treated with a 150 mg DIFLUCAN tablet administered orally. These rates were comparable to control products. The remaining one-fourth of enrolled patients had recurrent vaginitis (≥4 episodes/12 months) and achieved 57% clinical cure, 47% mycologic eradication and 40% therapeutic cure. The numbers are too small to make meaningful clinical or statistical comparisons with vaginal products in the treatment of patients with recurrent vaginitis.

Substantially more gastrointestinal events were reported in the fluconazole group compared to the vaginal product group. Most of the events were mild to moderate. Because fluconazole was given as a single dose, no discontinuations occurred.

[See table at top of next page]

Pediatric Studies

Oropharyngeal candidiasis: An open-label, comparative study of the efficacy and safety of DIFLUCAN (2-3 mg/kg/day) and oral nystatin (400,000 I.U. 4 times daily) in immunocompromised children with oropharyngeal candidiasis was conducted. Clinical and mycological response rates were higher in the children treated with fluconazole.

Clinical cure at the end of treatment was reported for 86% of fluconazole treated patients compared to 46% of nystatin treated patients. Mycologically, 76% of fluconazole treated patients had the infecting organism eradicated compared to 11% for nystatin treated patients.

	Fluconazole	Nystatin
Enrolled	96	90
Clinical Cure	76/88 (86%)	36/78 (46%)
Mycological eradication*	55/72 (76%)	6/54 (11%)

*Subjects without follow-up cultures for any reason were considered nonevaluable for mycological response.

The proportion of patients with clinical relapse 2 weeks after the end of treatment was 14% for subjects receiving DIFLUCAN and 16% for subjects receiving nystatin. At 4 weeks after the end of treatment the percentages of patients with clinical relapse were 22% for DIFLUCAN and 23% for nystatin.

CONTRAINDICATIONS

DIFLUCAN (fluconazole) is contraindicated in patients who have shown hypersensitivity to fluconazole or to any of its excipients. There is no information regarding cross-hypersensitivity between fluconazole and other azole antifungal agents. Caution should be used in prescribing DIFLUCAN to patients with hypersensitivity to other azoles. Coadministration of terfenadine is contraindicated in patients receiving DIFLUCAN (fluconazole) at multiple doses of 400 mg or higher based upon results of a multiple dose interaction study. Coadministration of cisapride is contraindicated in patients receiving DIFLUCAN (fluconazole). (See **CLINICAL PHARMACOLOGY: Drug Interaction Studies** and **PRECAUTIONS**.)

WARNINGS

(1) Hepatic injury: DIFLUCAN has been associated with rare cases of serious hepatic toxicity, including fatalities primarily in patients with serious underlying medical conditions. In cases of DIFLUCAN-associated hepatotoxicity, no obvious relationship to total daily dose, duration of therapy, sex or age of the patient has been observed.

DIFLUCAN hepatotoxicity has usually, but not always, been reversible on discontinuation of therapy. Patients who develop abnormal liver function tests during DIFLUCAN therapy should be monitored for the development of more severe hepatic injury. DIFLUCAN should be discontinued if clinical signs and symptoms consistent with liver disease develop that may be attributable to DIFLUCAN.

(2) Anaphylaxis: In rare cases, anaphylaxis has been reported.

(3) Dermatologic: Patients have rarely developed exfoliative skin disorders during treatment with DIFLUCAN. In patients with serious underlying diseases (predominantly AIDS and malignancy), these have rarely resulted in a fatal outcome. Patients who develop rashes during treatment with DIFLUCAN should be monitored closely and the drug discontinued if lesions progress.

PRECAUTIONS

General

Some azoles, including fluconazole, have been associated with prolongation of the QT interval on the electrocardiogram. During post-marketing surveillance, there have been very rare cases of QT prolongation and torsade de pointes in patients taking fluconazole. These reports included seriously ill patients with multiple confounding risk factors, such as structural heart disease, electrolyte abnormalities and concomitant medications that may have been contributory.

Fluconazole should be administered with caution to patients with these potentially proarrhythmic conditions.

Single Dose

The convenience and efficacy of the single dose oral tablet of fluconazole regimen for the treatment of vaginal yeast infections should be weighed against the acceptability of a higher incidence of drug related adverse events with DIFLUCAN (26%) versus intravaginal agents (16%) in U.S. comparative clinical studies. (See **ADVERSE REACTIONS** and **CLINICAL STUDIES**.)

Drug Interactions: (See **CLINICAL PHARMACOLOGY: Drug Interaction Studies** and **CONTRAINDICATIONS**.) Clinically or potentially significant drug interactions between DIFLUCAN and the following agents/classes have been observed. These are described in greater detail below:

- Oral hypoglycemics
- Coumarin-type anticoagulants
- Phenytoin
- Cyclosporine
- Rifampin
- Theophylline
- Terfenadine
- Cisapride
- Astemizole
- Rifabutin
- Tacrolimus

Oral hypoglycemics: Clinically significant hypoglycemia may be precipitated by the use of DIFLUCAN with oral hypoglycemic agents; one fatality has been reported from hypoglycemia in association with combined DIFLUCAN and glyburide use. DIFLUCAN reduces the metabolism of tolbutamide, glyburide, and glipizide and increases the plasma concentration of these agents. When DIFLUCAN is used concomitantly with these or other sulfonylurea oral hypoglycemic agents, blood glucose concentrations should be carefully monitored and the dose of the sulfonylurea should be adjusted as necessary. (See **CLINICAL PHARMACOLOGY: Drug Interaction Studies.**)

Coumarin-type anticoagulants: Prothrombin time may be increased in patients receiving concomitant DIFLUCAN and coumarin-type anticoagulants. Careful monitoring of prothrombin time in patients receiving DIFLUCAN and coumarin-type anticoagulants is recommended. (See **CLINICAL PHARMACOLOGY: Drug Interaction Studies.**)

Phenytoin: DIFLUCAN increases the plasma concentrations of phenytoin. Careful monitoring of phenytoin concentrations in patients receiving DIFLUCAN and phenytoin is recommended. (See **CLINICAL PHARMACOLOGY: Drug Interaction Studies.**)

Cyclosporine: DIFLUCAN may significantly increase cyclosporine levels in renal transplant patients with or without renal impairment. Careful monitoring of cyclosporine concentrations and serum creatinine is recommended in patients receiving DIFLUCAN and cyclosporine. (See **CLINICAL PHARMACOLOGY: Drug Interaction Studies.**)

Rifampin: Rifampin enhances the metabolism of concurrently administered DIFLUCAN. Depending on clinical circumstances, consideration should be given to increasing the dose of DIFLUCAN when it is administered with rifampin. (See **CLINICAL PHARMACOLOGY: Drug Interaction Studies.**)

Theophylline: DIFLUCAN increases the serum concentrations of theophylline. Careful monitoring of serum theophylline concentrations in patients receiving DIFLUCAN and theophylline is recommended. (See **CLINICAL PHARMACOLOGY: Drug Interaction Studies.**)

Terfenadine: Because of the occurrence of serious cardiac dysrhythmias secondary to prolongation of the QTc interval in patients receiving azole antifungals in conjunction with terfenadine, interaction studies have been performed. One study at a 200-mg daily dose of fluconazole failed to demonstrate a prolongation in QTc interval. Another study at a 400-mg and 800-mg daily dose of fluconazole demonstrated that DIFLUCAN taken in doses of 400 mg per day or greater significantly increases plasma levels of terfenadine when taken concomitantly. The combined use of fluconazole at doses of 400 mg or greater with terfenadine is contraindicated. (See **CONTRAINDICATIONS** and **CLINICAL PHARMACOLOGY: Drug Interaction Studies.**) The coadministration of fluconazole at doses lower than 400 mg/day with terfenadine should be carefully monitored.

Cisapride: There have been reports of cardiac events, including torsade de pointes in patients to whom fluconazole and cisapride were coadministered. The combined use of fluconazole with cisapride is contraindicated. (See **CONTRAINDICATIONS** and **CLINICAL PHARMACOLOGY: Drug Interaction Studies.**)

Astemizole: The use of fluconazole in patients concurrently taking astemizole or other drugs metabolized by the cytochrome P450 system may be associated with elevations in serum levels of these drugs. In the absence of definitive information, caution should be used when coadministering fluconazole. Patients should be carefully monitored.

Rifabutin: There have been reports of uveitis in patients to whom fluconazole and rifabutin were coadministered. Patients receiving rifabutin and fluconazole concomitantly should be carefully monitored. (See **CLINICAL PHARMACOLOGY: Drug Interaction Studies.**)

Continued on next page

Diflucan—Cont.

Tacrolimus: There have been reports of nephrotoxicity in patients to whom fluconazole and tacrolimus were coadministered. Patients receiving tacrolimus and fluconazole concomitantly should be carefully monitored. (See **CLINICAL PHARMACOLOGY: Drug Interaction Studies.**)

Fluconazole tablets coadministered with ethinyl estradiol- and levonorgestrel-containing oral contraceptives produced an overall mean increase in ethinyl estradiol and levonorgestrel levels; however, in some patients there were decreases up to 47% and 33% of ethinyl estradiol and levonorgestrel levels. (See **CLINICAL PHARMACOLOGY: Drug Interaction Studies.**) The data presently available indicate that the decreases in some individual ethinyl estradiol and levonorgestrel AUC values with fluconazole treatment are likely the result of random variation. While there is evidence that fluconazole can inhibit the metabolism of ethinyl estradiol and levonorgestrel, there is no evidence that fluconazole is a net inducer of ethinyl estradiol or levonorgestrel metabolism. The clinical significance of these effects is presently unknown.

Physicians should be aware that interaction studies with medications other than those listed in the **CLINICAL PHARMACOLOGY** section have not been conducted, but such interactions may occur.

Carcinogenesis, Mutagenesis and Impairment of Fertility

Fluconazole showed no evidence of carcinogenic potential in mice and rats treated orally for 24 months at doses of 2.5, 5 or 10 mg/kg/day (approximately 2-7× the recommended human dose). Male rats treated with 5 and 10 mg/kg/day had an increased incidence of hepatocellular adenomas.

Fluconazole, with or without metabolic activation, was negative in tests for mutagenicity in 4 strains of *S. typhimurium*, and in the mouse lymphoma L5178Y system. Cytogenetic studies *in vivo* (murine bone marrow cells, following oral administration of fluconazole) and *in vitro* (human lymphocytes exposed to fluconazole at 1000 µg/mL) showed no evidence of chromosomal mutations.

Fluconazole did not affect the fertility of male or female rats treated orally with daily doses of 5, 10 or 20 mg/kg or with parenteral doses of 5, 25 or 75 mg/kg, although the onset of parturition was slightly delayed at 20 mg/kg PO. In an intravenous perinatal study in rats at 5, 20 and 40 mg/kg, dystocia and prolongation of parturition were observed in a few dams at 20 mg/kg (approximately 5-15× the recommended human dose) and 40 mg/kg, but not at 5 mg/kg. The disturbances in parturition were reflected by a slight increase in the number of still-born pups and decrease of neonatal survival at these dose levels. The effects on parturition in rats are consistent with the species specific estrogen-lowering property produced by high doses of fluconazole. Such a hormone change has not been observed in women treated with fluconazole. (See **CLINICAL PHARMACOLOGY.**)

Pregnancy

Teratogenic Effects. Pregnancy Category C: Fluconazole was administered orally to pregnant rabbits during organogenesis in two studies, at 5, 10 and 20 mg/kg and at 5, 25, and 75 mg/kg, respectively. Maternal weight gain was impaired at all dose levels, and abortions occurred at 75 mg/kg (approximately 20-60× the recommended human dose); no adverse fetal effects were detected. In several studies in which pregnant rats were treated orally with fluconazole during organogenesis, maternal weight gain was impaired and placental weights were increased at 25 mg/kg. There were no fetal effects at 5 or 10 mg/kg; increases in fetal anatomical variants (supernumerary ribs, renal pelvis dilation) and delays in ossification were observed at 25 and 50 mg/kg and higher doses. At doses ranging from 80 mg/kg (approximately 20-60× the recommended human dose) to 320 mg/kg embryolethality in rats was increased and fetal abnormalities included wavy ribs, cleft palate and abnormal cranio-facial ossification. These effects are consistent with the inhibition of estrogen synthesis in rats and may be a result of known effects of lowered estrogen on pregnancy, organogenesis and parturition.

There are no adequate and well controlled studies in pregnant women. There have been reports of multiple congenital abnormalities in infants whose mothers were being treated for 3 or more months with high dose (400-800 mg/day) fluconazole therapy for coccidioidomycosis (an unindicated use). The relationship between fluconazole use and these events is unclear. DIFLUCAN should be used in pregnancy only if the potential benefit justifies the possible risk to the fetus.

Nursing Mothers

Fluconazole is secreted in human milk at concentrations similar to plasma. Therefore, the use of DIFLUCAN in nursing mothers is not recommended.

Pediatric Use

An open-label, randomized, controlled trial has shown DIFLUCAN to be effective in the treatment of oropharyngeal candidiasis in children 6 months to 13 years of age. (See **CLINICAL STUDIES.**)

The use of DIFLUCAN in children with cryptococcal meningitis, *Candida* esophagitis, or systemic *Candida* infections is supported by the efficacy shown for these indications in adults and by the results from several small noncomparative pediatric clinical studies. In addition, pharmacokinetic studies in children (see **CLINICAL PHARMACOLOGY**) have established a dose proportionality between children and adults. (See **DOSAGE AND ADMINISTRATION.**)

Parameter	Fluconazole PO	Vaginal Products
Evaluable patients	448	422
With any adverse event	141 (31%)	112 (27%)
Nervous System	90 (20%)	69 (16%)
Gastrointestinal	73 (16%)	18 (4%)
With drug-related event	117 (26%)	67 (16%)
Nervous System	61 (14%)	29 (7%)
Headache	58 (13%)	28 (7%)
Gastrointestinal	68 (15%)	13 (3%)
Abdominal pain	25 (6%)	7 (2%)
Nausea	30 (7%)	3 (1%)
Diarrhea	12 (3%)	2 (<1%)
Application site event	0 (0%)	19 (5%)
Taste Perversion	6 (1%)	0 (0%)

In a noncomparative study of children with serious systemic fungal infections, most of which were candidemia, the effectiveness of DIFLUCAN was similar to that reported for the treatment of candidemia in adults. Of 17 subjects with culture-confirmed candidemia, 11 of 14 (79%) with baseline symptoms (3 were asymptomatic) had a clinical cure; 13/15 (87%) of evaluable patients had a mycologic cure at the end of treatment but two of these patients relapsed at 10 and 18 days, respectively, following cessation of therapy.

The efficacy of DIFLUCAN for the suppression of cryptococcal meningitis was successful in 4 of 5 children treated in a compassionate-use study of fluconazole for the treatment of life-threatening or serious mycosis. There is no information regarding the efficacy of fluconazole for primary treatment of cryptococcal meningitis in children.

The safety profile of DIFLUCAN in children has been studied in 577 children ages 1 day to 17 years who received doses ranging from 1 to 15 mg/kg/day for 1 to 1,616 days. (See **ADVERSE REACTIONS.**)

Efficacy of DIFLUCAN has not been established in infants less than 6 months of age. (See **CLINICAL PHARMACOLOGY.**) A small number of patients (29) ranging in age from 1 day to 6 months have been treated safely with DIFLUCAN.

ADVERSE REACTIONS

In Patients Receiving a Single Dose for Vaginal Candidiasis:

During comparative clinical studies conducted in the United States, 448 patients with vaginal candidiasis were treated with DIFLUCAN, 150 mg single dose. The overall incidence of side effects possibly related to DIFLUCAN was 26%. In 422 patients receiving active comparative agents, the incidence was 16%. The most common treatment-related adverse events reported in the patients who received 150 mg single dose fluconazole for vaginitis were headache (13%), nausea (7%), and abdominal pain (6%). Other side effects reported with an incidence equal to or greater than 1% included diarrhea (3%), dyspepsia (1%), dizziness (1%), and taste perversion (1%). Most of the reported side effects were mild to moderate in severity. Rarely, angioedema and anaphylactic reaction have been reported in marketing experience.

In Patients Receiving Multiple Doses for Other Infections:

Sixteen percent of over 4000 patients treated with DIFLUCAN (fluconazole) in clinical trials of 7 days or more experienced adverse events. Treatment was discontinued in 1.5% of patients due to adverse clinical events and in 1.3% of patients due to laboratory test abnormalities.

Clinical adverse events were reported more frequently in HIV infected patients (21%) than in non-HIV infected patients (13%); however, the patterns in HIV infected and non-HIV infected patients were similar. The proportions of patients discontinuing therapy due to clinical adverse events were similar in the two groups (1.5%).

The following treatment-related clinical adverse events occurred at an incidence of 1% or greater in 4048 patients receiving DIFLUCAN for 7 or more days in clinical trials: nausea 3.7%, headache 1.9%, skin rash 1.8%, vomiting 1.7%, abdominal pain 1.7%, and diarrhea 1.5%.

The following adverse events have occurred under conditions where a causal association is probable:

Hepatobiliary: In combined clinical trials and marketing experience, there have been rare cases of serious hepatic reactions during treatment with DIFLUCAN. (See **WARNINGS.**) The spectrum of these hepatic reactions has ranged from mild transient elevations in transaminases to clinical hepatitis, cholestasis and fulminant hepatic failure, including fatalities. Instances of fatal hepatic reactions were noted to occur primarily in patients with serious underlying medical conditions (predominantly AIDS or malignancy) and often while taking multiple concomitant medications. Transient hepatic reactions, including hepatitis and jaundice, have occurred among patients with no other identifiable risk factors. In each of these cases, liver function returned to baseline on discontinuation of DIFLUCAN.

In two comparative trials evaluating the efficacy of DIFLUCAN for the suppression of relapse of cryptococcal meningitis, a statistically significant increase was observed in median AST (SGOT) levels from a baseline value of 30 IU/L to 41 IU/L in one trial and 34 IU/L to 66 IU/L in the other. The overall rate of serum transaminase elevations of more than 8 times the upper limit of normal was approximately 1% in fluconazole-treated patients in clinical trials. These elevations occurred in patients with severe underlying disease, predominantly AIDS or malignancies, most of whom were receiving multiple concomitant medications, including many known to be hepatotoxic. The incidence of abnormally elevated serum transaminases was greater in patients taking DIFLUCAN concomitantly with one or more of the following medications: rifampin, phenytoin, isoniazid, valproic acid, or oral sulfonylurea hypoglycemic agents.

Immunologic: In rare cases, anaphylaxis has been reported.

The following adverse events have occurred under conditions where a causal association is uncertain:

Cardiovascular: QT prolongation, torsade de pointes. (See **PRECAUTIONS.**)

Central Nervous System: Seizures.

Dermatologic: Exfoliative skin disorders including Stevens-Johnson syndrome and toxic epidermal necrolysis (see **WARNINGS**), alopecia.

Hematopoietic and Lymphatic: Leukopenia, including neutropenia and agranulocytosis, thrombocytopenia.

Metabolic: Hypercholesterolemia, hypertriglyceridemia, hypokalemia.

Adverse Reactions in Children:

In Phase II/III clinical trials conducted in the United States and in Europe, 577 pediatric patients, ages 1 day to 17 years were treated with DIFLUCAN at doses up to 15 mg/kg/day for up to 1,616 days. Thirteen percent of children experienced treatment related adverse events. The most commonly reported events were vomiting (5%), abdominal pain (3%), nausea (2%), and diarrhea (2%). Treatment was discontinued in 2.3% of patients due to adverse clinical events and in 1.4% of patients due to laboratory test abnormalities. The majority of treatment-related laboratory abnormalities were elevations of transaminases or alkaline phosphatase.

Percentage of Patients With Treatment-Related Side Effects

	Fluconazole (N=577)	Comparative Agents (N=451)
With any side effect	13.0	9.3
Vomiting	5.4	5.1
Abdominal pain	2.8	1.6
Nausea	2.3	1.6
Diarrhea	2.1	2.2

OVERDOSAGE

There has been one reported case of overdosage with DIFLUCAN (fluconazole). A 42-year-old patient infected with human immunodeficiency virus developed hallucinations and exhibited paranoid behavior after reportedly ingesting 8200 mg of DIFLUCAN. The patient was admitted to the hospital, and his condition resolved within 48 hours.

In the event of overdose, symptomatic treatment (with supportive measures and gastric lavage if clinically indicated) should be instituted.

Fluconazole is largely excreted in urine. A three-hour hemodialysis session decreases plasma levels by approximately 50%.

In mice and rats receiving very high doses of fluconazole, clinical effects in both species included decreased motility and respiration, ptosis, lacrimation, salivation, urinary incontinence, loss of righting reflex and cyanosis; death was sometimes preceded by clonic convulsions.

DOSAGE AND ADMINISTRATION

Dosage and Administration in Adults:

Single Dose

Vaginal candidiasis: The recommended dosage of DIFLUCAN for vaginal candidiasis is 150 mg as a single oral dose.

Multiple Dose

SINCE ORAL ABSORPTION IS RAPID AND ALMOST COMPLETE, THE DAILY DOSE OF DIFLUCAN (FLUCONAZOLE) IS THE SAME FOR ORAL (TABLETS AND SUSPENSION) AND INTRAVENOUS ADMINISTRATION. In general, a loading dose of twice the daily dose is recommended on the first day of therapy to result in plasma concentrations close to steady-state by the second day of therapy.

The daily dose of DIFLUCAN for the treatment of infections other than vaginal candidiasis should be based on the infecting organism and the patient's response to therapy. Treatment should be continued until clinical parameters or laboratory tests indicate that active fungal infection has subsided. An inadequate period of treatment may lead to recurrence of active infection. Patients with AIDS and cryptococcal meningitis or recurrent oropharyngeal candidiasis usually require maintenance therapy to prevent relapse.

Oropharyngeal candidiasis: The recommended dosage of DIFLUCAN for oropharyngeal candidiasis is 200 mg on the first day, followed by 100 mg once daily. Clinical evidence of oropharyngeal candidiasis generally resolves within several days, but treatment should be continued for at least 2 weeks to decrease the likelihood of relapse.

Esophageal candidiasis: The recommended dosage of DIFLUCAN for esophageal candidiasis is 200 mg on the first day, followed by 100 mg once daily. Doses up to 400 mg/day may be used, based on medical judgment of the patient's response to therapy. Patients with esophageal candidiasis should be treated for a minimum of three weeks and for at least two weeks following resolution of symptoms.

Systemic Candida infections: For systemic *Candida* infections including candidemia, disseminated candidiasis, and pneumonia, optimal therapeutic dosage and duration of therapy have not been established. In open, noncomparative studies of small numbers of patients, doses of up to 400 mg daily have been used.

Urinary tract infections and peritonitis: For the treatment of *Candida* urinary tract infections and peritonitis, daily doses of 50-200 mg have been used in open, noncomparative studies of small numbers of patients.

Cryptococcal meningitis: The recommended dosage for treatment of acute cryptococcal meningitis is 400 mg on the first day, followed by 200 mg once daily. A dosage of 400 mg once daily may be used, based on medical judgment of the patient's response to therapy. The recommended duration of treatment for initial therapy of cryptococcal meningitis is 10-12 weeks after the cerebrospinal fluid becomes culture negative. The recommended dosage of DIFLUCAN for suppression of relapse of cryptococcal meningitis in patients with AIDS is 200 mg once daily.

Prophylaxis in patients undergoing bone marrow transplantation: The recommended DIFLUCAN daily dosage for the prevention of candidiasis of patients undergoing bone marrow transplantation is 400 mg, once daily. Patients who are anticipated to have severe granulocytopenia (less than 500 neutrophils per cu mm) should start DIFLUCAN prophylaxis several days before the anticipated onset of neutropenia, and continue for 7 days after the neutrophil count rises above 1000 cells per cu mm.

Dosage and Administration in Children:

The following dose equivalency scheme should generally provide equivalent exposure in pediatric and adult patients:

Pediatric Patients	Adults
3 mg/kg	100 mg
6 mg/kg	200 mg
12* mg/kg	400 mg

*Some older children may have clearances similar to that of adults. Absolute doses exceeding 600 mg/day are not recommended.

Experience with DIFLUCAN in neonates is limited to pharmacokinetic studies in premature newborns. (See **CLINICAL PHARMACOLOGY.**) Based on the prolonged half-life seen in premature newborns (gestational age 26 to 29 weeks), these children, in the first two weeks of life, should receive the same dosage (mg/kg) as in older children, but administered every 72 hours. After the first two weeks, these children should be dosed once daily. No information regarding DIFLUCAN pharmacokinetics in full-term newborns is available.

Oropharyngeal candidiasis: The recommended dosage of DIFLUCAN for oropharyngeal candidiasis in children is 6 mg/kg on the first day, followed by 3 mg/kg once daily. Treatment should be administered for at least 2 weeks to decrease the likelihood of relapse.

Esophageal candidiasis: For the treatment of esophageal candidiasis, the recommended dosage of DIFLUCAN in children is 6 mg/kg on the first day, followed by 3 mg/kg once daily. Doses up to 12 mg/kg/day may be used based on medical judgment of the patient's response to therapy. Patients with esophageal candidiasis should be treated for a minimum of three weeks and for at least 2 weeks following the resolution of symptoms.

Systemic Candida infections: For the treatment of candidemia and disseminated *Candida* infections, daily doses of 6-12 mg/kg/day have been used in an open, noncomparative study of a small number of children.

Cryptococcal meningitis: For the treatment of acute cryptococcal meningitis, the recommended dosage is 12 mg/kg on the first day, followed by 6 mg/kg once daily. A dosage of 12 mg/kg once daily may be used, based on medical judgment of the patient's response to therapy. The recommended duration of treatment for initial therapy of cryptococcal meningitis is 10-12 weeks after the cerebrospinal fluid becomes culture negative. For suppression of relapse of cryptococcal meningitis in children with AIDS, the recommended dose of DIFLUCAN is 6 mg/kg once daily.

Dosage In Patients With Impaired Renal Function:

Fluconazole is cleared primarily by renal excretion as unchanged drug. There is no need to adjust single dose therapy for vaginal candidiasis because of impaired renal function. In patients with impaired renal function who will receive multiple doses of DIFLUCAN, an initial loading dose of 50 to 400 mg should be given. After the loading dose, the daily dose (according to indication) should be based on the following table:

Creatinine Clearance (mL/min)	Percent of Recommended Dose
>50	100%
≤50 (no dialysis)	50%
Regular dialysis	100% after each dialysis

These are suggested dose adjustments based on pharmacokinetics following administration of multiple doses. Further adjustment may be needed depending upon clinical condition.

When serum creatinine is the only measure of renal function available, the following formula (based on sex, weight, and age of the patient) should be used to estimate the creatinine clearance in adults:

Males: $\dfrac{\text{Weight (kg)} \times (140\text{-age})}{72 \times \text{serum creatinine (mg/100 mL)}}$

Females: $0.85 \times$ above value

Although the pharmacokinetics of fluconazole has not been studied in children with renal insufficiency, dosage reduction in children with renal insufficiency should parallel that recommended for adults. The following formula may be used to estimate creatinine clearance in children:

$$K \times \frac{\text{linear length or height (cm)}}{\text{serum creatinine (mg/100 mL)}}$$

(Where K=0.55 for children older than 1 year and 0.45 for infants.)

Administration

DIFLUCAN may be administered either orally or by intravenous infusion. DIFLUCAN injection has been used safely for up to fourteen days of intravenous therapy. The intravenous infusion of DIFLUCAN should be administered at a maximum rate of approximately 200 mg/hour, given as a continuous infusion.

DIFLUCAN injections in glass and Viaflex® Plus plastic containers are intended only for intravenous administration using sterile equipment.

Parenteral drug products should be inspected visually for particulate matter and discoloration prior to administration whenever solution and container permit.

Do not use if the solution is cloudy or precipitated or if the seal is not intact.

Directions for Mixing the Oral Suspension

Prepare a suspension at time of dispensing as follows: tap bottle until all the powder flows freely. To reconstitute, add 24 mL of distilled water or Purified Water (USP) to fluconazole bottle and shake vigorously to suspend powder. Each bottle will deliver 35 mL of suspension. The concentrations of the reconstituted suspensions are as follows:

Fluconazole Content per Bottle	Concentration of Reconstituted Suspension
350 mg	10 mg/mL
1400 mg	40 mg/mL

Note: Shake oral suspension well before using. Store reconstituted suspension between 86°F (30°C) and 41°F (5°C) and discard unused portion after 2 weeks. Protect from freezing.

Directions for IV Use of DIFLUCAN in Viaflex® Plus Plastic Containers

Do not remove unit from overwrap until ready for use. The overwrap is a moisture barrier. The inner bag maintains the sterility of the product.

CAUTION: Do not use plastic containers in series connections. Such use could result in air embolism due to residual air being drawn from the primary container before administration of the fluid from the secondary container is completed.

To Open

Tear overwrap down side at slit and remove solution container. Some opacity of the plastic due to moisture absorption during the sterilization process may be observed. This is normal and does not affect the solution quality or safety. The opacity will diminish gradually. After removing overwrap, check for minute leaks by squeezing inner bag firmly. If leaks are found, discard solution as sterility may be impaired.

DO NOT ADD SUPPLEMENTARY MEDICATION.

Preparation for Administration:

1. Suspend container from eyelet support.
2. Remove plastic protector from outlet port at bottom of container.
3. Attach administration set. Refer to complete directions accompanying set.

HOW SUPPLIED

DIFLUCAN® Tablets: Pink trapezoidal tablets containing 50, 100 or 200 mg of fluconazole are packaged in bottles or unit dose blisters. The 150 mg fluconazole tablets are pink and oval shaped, packaged in a single dose unit blister.

DIFLUCAN® Tablets are supplied as follows:

DIFLUCAN® 50 mg Tablets: Engraved with "DIFLUCAN" and "50" on the front and "ROERIG" on the back.
NDC 0049-3410-30 Bottles of 30

DIFLUCAN® 100 mg Tablets: Engraved with "DIFLUCAN" and "100" on the front and "ROERIG" on the back.
NDC 0049-3420-30 Bottles of 30
NDC 0049-3420-41 Unit dose package of 100

DIFLUCAN® 150 mg Tablets: Engraved with "DIFLUCAN" and "150" on the front and "ROERIG" on the back.
NDC 0049-3500-79 Unit dose package of 1

DIFLUCAN® 200 mg Tablets: Engraved with "DIFLUCAN" and "200" on the front and "ROERIG" on the back.
NDC 0049-3430-30 Bottles of 30
NDC 0049-3430-41 Unit dose package of 100

Storage: Store tablets below 86°F (30°C).

DIFLUCAN® for Oral Suspension: DIFLUCAN® for oral suspension is supplied as an orange-flavored powder to provide 35 mL per bottle as follows:
NDC 0049-3440-19 Fluconazole 350 mg per bottle
NDC 0049-3450-19 Fluconazole 1400 mg per bottle

Storage: Store dry powder below 86°F (30°C). Store reconstituted suspension between 86°F (30°C) and 41°F (5°C) and discard unused portion after 2 weeks. Protect from freezing.

DIFLUCAN® Injections: DIFLUCAN® injections for intravenous infusion administration are formulated as sterile iso-osmotic solutions containing 2 mg/mL of fluconazole. They are supplied in glass bottles or in Viaflex® Plus plastic containers containing volumes of 100 mL or 200 mL affording doses of 200 mg and 400 mg of fluconazole, respectively. DIFLUCAN® injections in Viaflex® Plus plastic containers are available in both sodium chloride and dextrose diluents.

DIFLUCAN® Injections in Glass Bottles:
NDC 0049-3371-26 Fluconazole in Sodium Chloride Diluent 200 mg/100 mL × 6
NDC 0049-3372-26 Fluconazole in Sodium Chloride Diluent 400 mg/200 mL × 6

Storage: Store between 86°F (30°C) and 41°F (5°C). Protect from freezing.

DIFLUCAN® Injections in Viaflex® Plus Plastic Containers:
NDC 0049-3435-26 Fluconazole in Sodium Chloride Diluent 200 mg/100 mL × 6
NDC 0049-3436-26 Fluconazole in Sodium Chloride Diluent 400 mg/200 mL × 6
NDC 0049-3437-26 Fluconazole in Dextrose Diluent 200 mg/100 mL × 6
NDC 0049-3438-26 Fluconazole in Dextrose Diluent 400 mg/200 mL × 6

Storage: Store between 77°F (25°C) and 41°F (5°C). Brief exposure up to 104°F (40°C) does not adversely affect the product. Protect from freezing.

Rx only

Pfizer Roerig
Division of Pfizer Inc, NY, NY 10017
70-4526-00-8 Revised June 2003

GEOCILLIN® ℞
[*gē'ō-sil-ĭn*]
(carbenicillin indanyl sodium)
TABLETS
For Oral Use

Prescribing information for this product, which appears on pages 2596–2597 of the 2004 PDR, has been completely revised as follows. Please write "See Supplement A" next to the product heading.

To reduce the development of drug-resistant bacteria and maintain the effectiveness of Geocillin® and other antibacterial drugs, Geocillin should be used only to treat or prevent infections that are proven or strongly suspected to be caused by bacteria.

DESCRIPTION

Geocillin, a semisynthetic penicillin, is the sodium salt of the indanyl ester of Geopen® (carbenicillin disodium). The chemical name is: 1-(5-Indanyl)-N-(2-carboxy-3,3-dimethyl-7-oxo-4-thia-1-azabicyclo[3.2.0] hept-6-yl)-2-phenylmalonamate monosodium salt.

The structural formula is:

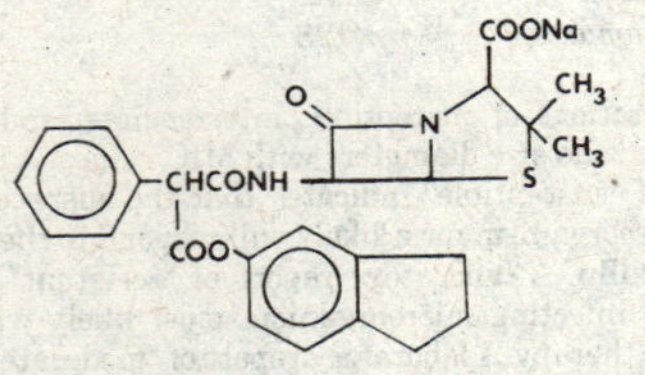

The empirical formula is: $C_{26}H_{25}N_2NaO_6S$ and mol. wt. is 516.55.

Geocillin tablets are yellow, capsule-shaped and film-coated, made of a white crystalline solid. Carbenicillin is freely soluble in water. Each Geocillin tablet contains 382 mg of carbenicillin, 118 mg of indanyl sodium ester. Each Geocillin tablet contains 23 mg of sodium.

Inert ingredients are: glycine; magnesium stearate and sodium lauryl sulfate. May also include the following: hydroxypropyl cellulose; hypromellose; opaspray (which may include Blue 2 Lake, Yellow 6 Lake, Yellow 10 Lake, and other inert ingredients); opadry light yellow (which may contain D&C Yellow 10 Lake, FD&C Yellow 6 Lake and other inert ingredients); opadry clear (which may contain other inert ingredients).

CLINICAL PHARMACOLOGY

Free carbenicillin is the predominant pharmacologically active fraction of Geocillin. Carbenicillin exerts its antibacterial activity by interference with final cell wall synthesis of susceptible bacteria.

Geocillin is acid stable, and rapidly absorbed from the small intestine following oral administration. It provides relatively low plasma concentrations of antibiotic and is primarily excreted in the urine. After absorption, Geocillin is rapidly converted to carbenicillin by hydrolysis of the ester linkage. Following ingestion of a single 500 mg tablet of Geocillin, a peak carbenicillin plasma concentration of approximately 6.5 mcg/ml is reached in 1 hour. About 30% of this dose is excreted in the urine unchanged within 12 hours, with another 6% excreted over the next 12 hours.

In a multiple dose study utilizing volunteers with normal renal function, the following mean urine and serum levels of carbenicillin were achieved:

[See table at top of next page]

Microbiology

The antibacterial activity of Geocillin is due to its rapid conversion to carbenicillin by hydrolysis after absorption.

Continued on next page

Geocillin—Cont.

Though Geocillin provides substantial *in vitro* activity against a variety of both gram-positive and gram-negative microorganisms, the most important aspect of its profile is in its antipseudomonal and antiproteal activity. Because of the high urine levels obtained following administration, Geocillin has demonstrated clinical efficacy in urinary infections due to susceptible strains of:

Escherichia coli
Proteus mirabilis
Proteus vulgaris
Morganella morganii (formerly *Proteus morganii*)
Pseudomonas species
Providencia rettgeri (formerly *Proteus rettgeri*)
Enterobacter species
Enterococci *(S. faecalis)*

In addition, *in vitro* data, not substantiated by clinical studies, indicate the following pathogens to be usually susceptible to Geocillin:

Staphylococcus species (nonpenicillinase producing)
Streptococcus species

Resistance

Most *Klebsiella* species are usually resistant to the action of Geocillin. Some strains of *Pseudomonas* species have developed resistance to carbenicillin.

Susceptibility Testing

Geopen (carbenicillin disodium) Susceptibility Powder or 100 µg Geopen Susceptibility Discs may be used to determine microbial susceptibility to Geocillin using one of the following standard methods recommended by the National Committee for Clinical Laboratory Standards:

M2-A3, "Performance Standards for Antimicrobial Disk Susceptibility Tests"
M7-A, "Methods for Dilution Antimicrobial Susceptibility Tests for Bacteria that Grow Aerobically"
M11-A, "Reference Agar Dilution Procedure for Antimicrobial Susceptibility Testing of Anaerobic Bacteria"
M17-P, "Alternative Methods for Antimicrobial Susceptibility Testing of Anaerobic Bacteria"

Tests should be interpreted by the following criteria:

Organisms	Disk Diffusion Zone diameter (mm) Suscept.	Intermed.	Resist.
Enterobacter	≥23	18-22	≤17
Pseudomonas sp.	≥17	14-16	≤13

Organisms	Dilution MIC (µg/ml) Suscept.	Moderately Suscept.	Resist.
Enterobacter	≤16	32	≥64
Pseudomonas sp.	≤128	—	≥156

Interpretations of susceptible, intermediate, and resistant correlate zone size diameters with MIC values. A laboratory report of "susceptible" indicates that the suspected causative microorganism most likely will respond to therapy with carbenicillin. A laboratory report of "resistant" indicates that the infecting microorganism most likely will not respond to therapy. A laboratory report of "moderately susceptible" indicates that the microorganism is most likely susceptible if a high dosage of carbenicillin is used, or if the infection is such that high levels of carbenicillin may be attained as in urine. A report of "intermediate" using the disk diffusion method may be considered an equivocal result, and dilution tests may be indicated.

INDICATIONS AND USAGE

Geocillin (carbenicillin indanyl sodium) is indicated in the treatment of acute and chronic infections of the upper and lower urinary tract and in asymptomatic bacteriuria due to susceptible strains of the following organisms:

Escherichia coli
Proteus mirabilis
Morganella morganii (formerly *Proteus morganii*)
Providencia rettgeri (formerly *Proteus rettgeri*)
Proteus vulgaris
Pseudomonas
Enterobacter
Enterococci

Geocillin is also indicated in the treatment of prostatitis due to susceptible strains of the following organisms:

Escherichia coli
Enterococcus *(S. faecalis)*
Proteus mirabilis
Enterobacter sp.

WHEN HIGH AND RAPID BLOOD AND URINE LEVELS OF ANTIBIOTIC ARE INDICATED, THERAPY WITH GEOPEN (CARBENICILLIN DISODIUM) SHOULD BE INITIATED BY PARENTERAL ADMINISTRATION FOLLOWED, AT THE PHYSICIAN'S DISCRETION, BY ORAL THERAPY.

NOTE: Susceptibility testing should be performed prior to and during the course of therapy to detect the possible emergence of resistant organisms which may develop.

To reduce the development of drug-resistant bacteria and maintain effectiveness of Geocillin and other antibacterial drugs, Geocillin should be used only to treat or prevent infections that are proven or strongly suspected to be caused by susceptible bacteria. When culture and susceptibility information are available, they should be considered in selecting or modifying antibacterial therapy. In the absence of such data, local epidemiology and susceptibility patterns may contribute to the empiric selection of therapy.

DRUG	DOSE	Mean Urine Concentration of Carbenicillin mcg/ml Hours After Initial Dose 0-3	3-6	6-24
Geocillin	1 tablet q.6 hr	1130	352	292
Geocillin	2 tablets q.6 hr	1428	789	809

Mean serum concentrations of carbenicillin in this study for these dosages are:

DRUG	DOSE	Mean Serum Concentration mcg/ml Hours After Initial Dose ½	1	2	4	6	24	25	26	28
Geocillin	1 tablet q.6 hr	5.1	6.5	3.2	1.9	0.0	0.4	8.8	5.4	0.4
Geocillin	2 tablets q.6 hr	6.1	9.6	7.9	2.6	0.4	0.8	13.2	12.8	3.8

CONTRAINDICATIONS

Geocillin is ordinarily contraindicated in patients who have a known penicillin allergy.

WARNINGS

Serious and occasionally fatal hypersensitivity (anaphylactic) reactions have been reported in patients on oral penicillin therapy. Although anaphylaxis is more frequent following parenteral therapy, it has occurred in patients on oral penicillins. These reactions are more apt to occur in individuals with a history of penicillin hypersensitivity and/or a history of sensitivity to multiple allergens.

There have been reports of individuals with a history of penicillin hypersensitivity who have experienced severe hypersensitivity reactions when treated with a cephalosporin, and vice versa. Before initiating therapy with a penicillin, careful inquiry should be made concerning previous hypersensitivity reactions to penicillins, cephalosporins, or other allergens. If an allergic reaction occurs, the drug should be discontinued and the appropriate therapy instituted.

SERIOUS ANAPHYLACTOID REACTIONS REQUIRE IMMEDIATE EMERGENCY TREATMENT WITH EPINEPHRINE. OXYGEN, INTRAVENOUS STEROIDS AND AIRWAY MANAGEMENT, INCLUDING INTUBATION, SHOULD ALSO BE ADMINISTERED AS INDICATED.

PRECAUTIONS

General: As with any penicillin preparation, an allergic response, including anaphylaxis, may occur particularly in a hypersensitive individual.

Long term use of Geocillin may result in the overgrowth of nonsusceptible organisms. If superinfection occurs during therapy, appropriate measures should be taken.

Since carbenicillin is primarily excreted by the kidney, patients with severe renal impairment (creatinine clearance of less than 10 ml/min) will not achieve therapeutic urine levels of carbenicillin.

In patients with creatinine clearance of 10-20 ml/min it may be necessary to adjust dosage to prevent accumulation of drug.

Prescribing Geocillin in the absence of proven or strongly suspected bacterial infection or a prophylactic indication is unlikely to provide benefit to the patient and increases the risk of the development of drug-resistant bacteria.

Information for Patients: Patients should be counseled that antibacterial drugs including Geocillin should only be used to treat bacterial infections. They do not treat viral infections (e.g., the common cold). When Geocillin is prescribed to treat a bacterial infection, patients should be told that although it is common to feel better early in the course of therapy, the medication should be taken exactly as directed. Skipping doses or not completing the full course of therapy may (1) decrease the effectiveness of the immediate treatment and (2) increase the likelihood that bacteria will develop resistance and will not be treatable by Geocillin or other antibacterial drugs in the future.

Laboratory Tests: As with other penicillins, periodic assessment of organ system function including renal, hepatic, and hematopoietic systems is recommended during prolonged therapy.

Drug Interactions: Geocillin (carbenicillin indanyl sodium) blood levels may be increased and prolonged by concurrent administration of probenecid.

Carcinogenesis, Mutagenesis, Impairment of Fertility: There are no long-term animal or human studies to evaluate carcinogenic potential. Rats fed 250-1000 mg/kg/day for 18 months developed mild liver pathology (e.g., bile duct hyperplasia) at all dose levels, but there was no evidence of drug-related neoplasia. Geocillin administered at daily doses ranging to 1000 mg/kg had no apparent effect on the fertility or reproductive performance of rats.

Pregnancy Category B: Reproduction studies have been performed at dose levels of 1000 or 500 mg/kg in rats, 200 mg/kg in mice, and at 500 mg/kg in monkeys with no harm to fetus due to Geocillin. There are, however, no adequate and well controlled studies in pregnant women. Because animal reproduction studies are not always predictive of human response, this drug should be used during pregnancy only if clearly needed.

Labor and Delivery: It is not known whether the use of Geocillin in humans during labor or delivery has immediate or delayed adverse effects on the fetus, prolongs the duration of labor, or increases the likelihood that forceps delivery or other obstetrical intervention or resuscitation of the newborn will be necessary.

Nursing Mothers: Carbenicillin class antibiotics are excreted in milk although the amounts excreted are unknown; therefore, caution should be exercised if administered to a nursing woman.

Pediatric Use: Since only limited clinical data is available to date in children, the safety of Geocillin administration in this age group has not yet been established.

ADVERSE REACTIONS

The following adverse reactions have been reported as possibly related to Geocillin administration in controlled studies which include 344 patients receiving Geocillin.

Gastrointestinal: The most frequent adverse reactions associated with Geocillin therapy are related to the gastrointestinal tract. Nausea, bad taste, diarrhea, vomiting, flatulence, and glossitis were reported. Abdominal cramps, dry mouth, furry tongue, rectal bleeding, anorexia, and unspecified epigastric distress were rarely reported.

Dermatologic: Hypersensitivity reactions such as skin rash, urticaria, and less frequently pruritus.

Hematologic: As with other penicillins, anemia, thrombocytopenia, leukopenia, neutropenia, and eosinophilia have infrequently been observed. The clinical significance of these abnormalities is not known.

Miscellaneous: Other reactions rarely reported were hyperthermia, headache, itchy eyes, vaginitis, and loose stools.

Abnormalities of Hepatic Function Tests: Mild SGOT elevations have been observed following Geocillin administration.

OVERDOSAGE

Geocillin is generally nontoxic. Geocillin when taken in excessive amounts may produce mild gastrointestinal irritation. The drug is rapidly excreted in the urine and symptoms are transitory. The usual symptoms of anaphylaxis may occur in hypersensitive individuals.

Carbenicillin blood levels achievable with Geocillin are very low, and toxic reactions as a function of overdosage should not occur systematically. The oral LD_{50} in mice is 3,600 mg/kg, in rats 2,000 mg/kg, and in dogs is in excess of 500 mg/kg. The lethal human dose is not known.

Although never reported, the possibility of accumulation of indanyl should be considered when large amounts of Geocillin are ingested. Free indole, which is a phenol derivative, may be potentially toxic. In general 8-15 grams of phenol, and presumably a similar amount of indole, are required orally before toxicity (peripheral vascular collapse) may occur. The metabolic by-products of indole are nontoxic. In patients with hepatic failure it may be possible for unmetabolized indole to accumulate.

The metabolic by-products of Geocillin, indanyl sulfate and glucuronide, as well as free carbenicillin, are dialyzable.

DOSAGE AND ADMINISTRATION

Geocillin is available as a coated tablet to be administered orally.

Usual Adult Dose

URINARY TRACT INFECTIONS	
Escherichia coli, Proteus species, and *Enterobacter*	1-2 tablets 4 times daily
Pseudomonas and *Enterococcus*	2 tablets 4 times daily
PROSTATITIS	
Escherichia coli, Proteus mirabilis, Enterobacter and *Enterococcus*	2 tablets 4 times daily

HOW SUPPLIED

Geocillin® is available as film-coated tablets in bottles of 100's (NDC 0049-1430-66). Each tablet contains carbenicillin indanyl sodium equivalent to 382 mg of carbenicillin.

℞ only

Pfizer Roerig
Division of Pfizer Inc, NY, NY 10017
69-1970-00-4 Revised September 2003

GEODON® ℞
[gē-ō-dōn]
(ziprasidone HCl)
GEODON® for Injection
(ziprasidone mesylate)
FOR IM USE ONLY

Prescribing information for this product, which appears on pages 2597–2603 of the 2004 PDR, has been completely revised as follows. Please write "See Supplement A" next to the product heading.

DESCRIPTION

GEODON® is available as GEODON Capsules (ziprasidone hydrochloride) for oral administration and as GEODON for Injection (ziprasidone mesylate) for intramuscular injection. Ziprasidone is an antipsychotic agent that is chemically unrelated to phenothiazine or butyrophenone antipsychotic agents. It has a molecular weight of 412.94 (free base), with the following chemical name: 5-[2-[4-(1,2-benzisothiazol-3-yl)-1-piperazinyl]ethyl]-6-chloro-1,3-dihydro-2*H*-indol-2-one. The empirical formula of $C_{21}H_{21}ClN_4OS$ (free base of ziprasidone) represents the following structural formula:

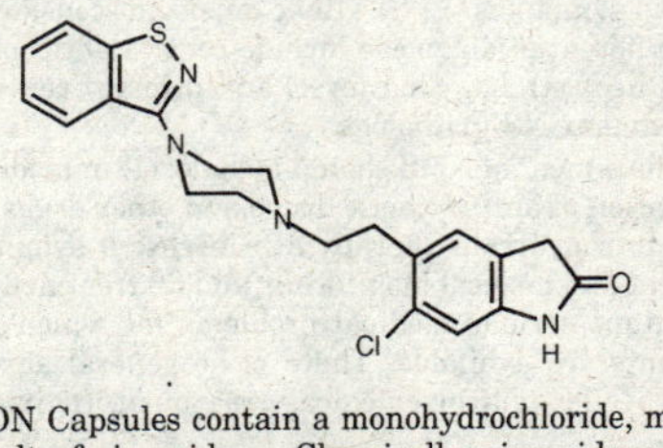

GEODON Capsules contain a monohydrochloride, monohydrate salt of ziprasidone. Chemically, ziprasidone hydrochloride monohydrate is 5-[2-[4-(1,2-benzisothiazol-3-yl)-1-piperazinyl]ethyl]-6-chloro-1,3-dihydro-2*H*-indol-2-one, monohydrochloride, monohydrate. The empirical formula is $C_{21}H_{21}ClN_4OS \cdot HCl \cdot H_2O$ and its molecular weight is 467.42. Ziprasidone hydrochloride monohydrate is a white to slightly pink powder.

GEODON Capsules are supplied for oral administration in 20 mg (blue/white), 40 mg (blue/blue), 60 mg (white/white), and 80 mg (blue/white) capsules. GEODON Capsules contain ziprasidone hydrochloride monohydrate, lactose, pregelatinized starch, and magnesium stearate.

GEODON for Injection contains a lyophilized form of ziprasidone mesylate trihydrate. Chemically, ziprasidone mesylate trihydrate is 5-[2-[4-(1,2-benzisothiazol-3-yl)-1-piperazinyl]ethyl]-6-chloro-1,3-dihydro-2*H*-indol-2-one, methanesulfonate, trihydrate. The empirical formula is $C_{21}H_{21}ClN_4OS \cdot CH_3SO_3H \cdot 3H_2O$ and its molecular weight is 563.09.

GEODON for Injection is available in a single dose vial as ziprasidone mesylate (20 mg ziprasidone/mL when reconstituted according to label instructions - see **Preparation for Administration**) for intramuscular administration. Each mL of ziprasidone mesylate for injection (when reconstituted) contains 20 mg of ziprasidone and 4.7 mg of methanesulfonic acid solubilized by 294 mg of sulfobutylether β-cyclodextrin sodium (SBECD).

CLINICAL PHARMACOLOGY

Pharmacodynamics

Ziprasidone exhibited high *in vitro* binding affinity for the dopamine D_2 and D_3, the serotonin $5HT_{2A}$, $5HT_{2C}$, $5HT_{1A}$, $5HT_{1D}$, and α_1-adrenergic receptors (K_i s of 4.8, 7.2, 0.4, 1.3, 3.4, 2, and 10 nM, respectively), and moderate affinity for the histamine H_1 receptor (K_i=47 nM). Ziprasidone functioned as an antagonist at the D_2, $5HT_{2A}$, and $5HT_{1D}$ receptors, and as an agonist at the $5HT_{1A}$ receptor. Ziprasidone inhibited synaptic reuptake of serotonin and norepinephrine. No appreciable affinity was exhibited for other receptor/binding sites tested, including the cholinergic muscarinic receptor (IC_{50} >1 μM).

The mechanism of action of ziprasidone, as with other drugs having efficacy in schizophrenia, is unknown. However, it has been proposed that this drug's efficacy in schizophrenia is mediated through a combination of dopamine type 2 (D_2) and serotonin type 2 ($5HT_2$) antagonism. Antagonism at receptors other than dopamine and $5HT_2$ with similar receptor affinities may explain some of the other therapeutic and side effects of ziprasidone.

Ziprasidone's antagonism of histamine H_1 receptors may explain the somnolence observed with this drug.

Ziprasidone's antagonism of α_1-adrenergic receptors may explain the orthostatic hypotension observed with this drug.

Oral Pharmacokinetics

Ziprasidone's activity is primarily due to the parent drug. The multiple-dose pharmacokinetics of ziprasidone are dose-proportional within the proposed clinical dose range, and ziprasidone accumulation is predictable with multiple dosing. Elimination of ziprasidone is mainly via hepatic metabolism with a mean terminal half-life of about 7 hours within the proposed clinical dose range. Steady-state concentrations are achieved within one to three days of dosing. The mean apparent systemic clearance is 7.5 mL/min/kg. Ziprasidone is unlikely to interfere with the metabolism of drugs metabolized by cytochrome P450 enzymes.

Absorption: Ziprasidone is well absorbed after oral administration, reaching peak plasma concentrations in 6 to 8 hours. The absolute bioavailability of a 20 mg dose under fed conditions is approximately 60%. The absorption of ziprasidone is increased up to two-fold in the presence of food.

Distribution: Ziprasidone has a mean apparent volume of distribution of 1.5 L/kg. It is greater than 99% bound to plasma proteins, binding primarily to albumin and α_1-acid glycoprotein. The *in vitro* plasma protein binding of ziprasidone was not altered by warfarin or propranolol, two highly protein-bound drugs, nor did ziprasidone alter the binding of these drugs in human plasma. Thus, the potential for drug interactions with ziprasidone due to displacement is minimal.

Metabolism and Elimination: Ziprasidone is extensively metabolized after oral administration with only a small amount excreted in the urine (<1%) or feces (<4%) as unchanged drug. Ziprasidone is primarily cleared via three metabolic routes to yield four major circulating metabolites, benzisothiazole (BITP) sulphoxide, BITP-sulphone, ziprasidone sulphoxide, and S-methyl-dihydroziprasidone. Approximately 20% of the dose is excreted in the urine, with approximately 66% being eliminated in the feces. Unchanged ziprasidone represents about 44% of total drug-related material in serum. *In vitro* studies using human liver subcellular fractions indicate that S-methyl-dihydroziprasidone is generated in two steps. The data indicate that the reduction reaction is mediated by aldehyde oxidase and the subsequent methylation is mediated by thiol methyltransferase. *In vitro* studies using human liver microsomes and recombinant enzymes indicate that CYP3A4 is the major CYP contributing to the oxidative metabolism of ziprasidone. CYP1A2 may contribute to a much lesser extent. Based on *in vivo* abundance of excretory metabolites, less than one-third of ziprasidone metabolic clearance is mediated by cytochrome P450 catalyzed oxidation and approximately two-thirds via reduction by aldehyde oxidase. There are no known clinically relevant inhibitors or inducers of aldehyde oxidase.

Intramuscular Pharmacokinetics

Systemic Bioavailability: The bioavailability of ziprasidone administered intramuscularly is 100%. After intramuscular administration of single doses, peak serum concentrations typically occur at approximately 60 minutes post-dose or earlier and the mean half-life ($T_{½}$) ranges from two to five hours. Exposure increases in a dose-related manner and following three days of intramuscular dosing, little accumulation is observed.

Metabolism and Elimination: Although the metabolism and elimination of IM ziprasidone have not been systematically evaluated, the intramuscular route of administration would not be expected to alter the metabolic pathways.

Special Populations

Age and Gender Effects—In a multiple-dose (8 days of treatment) study involving 32 subjects, there was no difference in the pharmacokinetics of ziprasidone between men and women or between elderly (>65 years) and young (18 to 45 years) subjects. Additionally, population pharmacokinetic evaluation of patients in controlled trials has revealed no evidence of clinically significant age or gender-related differences in the pharmacokinetics of ziprasidone. Dosage modifications for age or gender are, therefore, not recommended.

Ziprasidone intramuscular has not been systematically evaluated in elderly patients (65 years and over).

Race—No specific pharmacokinetic study was conducted to investigate the effects of race. Population pharmacokinetic evaluation has revealed no evidence of clinically significant race-related differences in the pharmacokinetics of ziprasidone. Dosage modifications for race are, therefore, not recommended.

Smoking—Based on *in vitro* studies utilizing human liver enzymes, ziprasidone is not a substrate for CYP1A2; smoking should therefore not have an effect on the pharmacokinetics of ziprasidone. Consistent with these *in vitro* results, population pharmacokinetic evaluation has not revealed any significant pharmacokinetic differences between smokers and nonsmokers.

Renal Impairment—Because ziprasidone is highly metabolized, with less than 1% of the drug excreted unchanged, renal impairment alone is unlikely to have a major impact on the pharmacokinetics of ziprasidone. The pharmacokinetics of ziprasidone following 8 days of 20 mg BID dosing were similar among subjects with varying degrees of renal impairment (n=27), and subjects with normal renal function, indicating that dosage adjustment based upon the degree of renal impairment is not required. Ziprasidone is not removed by hemodialysis.

Hepatic Impairment—As ziprasidone is cleared substantially by the liver, the presence of hepatic impairment would be expected to increase the AUC of ziprasidone; a multiple-dose study at 20 mg BID for 5 days in subjects (n=13) with clinically significant (Childs-Pugh Class A and B) cirrhosis revealed an increase in AUC_{0-12} of 13% and 34% in Childs-Pugh Class A and B, respectively, compared to a matched control group (n=14). A half-life of 7.1 hours was observed in subjects with cirrhosis compared to 4.8 hours in the control group.

Intramuscular ziprasidone has not been systematically evaluated in elderly patients or in patients with hepatic or renal impairment. As the cyclodextrin excipient is cleared by renal filtration, ziprasidone intramuscular should be administered with caution to patients with impaired renal function.

Drug-Drug Interactions

An *in vitro* enzyme inhibition study utilizing human liver microsomes showed that ziprasidone had little inhibitory effect on CYP1A2, CYP2C9, CYP2C19, CYP2D6 and CYP3A4, and thus would not likely interfere with the metabolism of drugs primarily metabolized by these enzymes. *In vivo* studies have revealed no effect of ziprasidone on the pharmacokinetics of dextromethorphan, estrogen, progesterone, or lithium (see **Drug Interactions** under **PRECAUTIONS**).

In vivo studies have revealed an approximately 35% decrease in ziprasidone AUC by concomitantly administered carbamazepine, an approximately 35-40% increase in ziprasidone AUC by concomitantly administered ketoconazole, but no effect on ziprasidone's pharmacokinetics by cimetidine or antacid (see **Drug Interactions** under **PRECAUTIONS**).

Clinical Trials

The efficacy of oral ziprasidone in the treatment of schizophrenia was evaluated in 5 placebo-controlled studies, 4 short-term (4- and 6-week) trials and one long-term (52-week) trial. All trials were in inpatients, most of whom met DSM III-R criteria for schizophrenia. Each study included 2 to 3 fixed doses of ziprasidone as well as placebo. Four of the 5 trials were able to distinguish ziprasidone from placebo; one short-term study did not. Although a single fixed-dose haloperidol arm was included as a comparative treatment in one of the three short-term trials, this single study was inadequate to provide a reliable and valid comparison of ziprasidone and haloperidol.

Several instruments were used for assessing psychiatric signs and symptoms in these studies. The Brief Psychiatric Rating Scale (BPRS) and the Positive and Negative Syndrome Scale (PANSS) are both multi-item inventories of general psychopathology usually used to evaluate the effects of drug treatment in schizophrenia. The BPRS psychosis cluster (conceptual disorganization, hallucinatory behavior, suspiciousness, and unusual thought content) is considered a particularly useful subset for assessing actively psychotic schizophrenic patients. A second widely used assessment, the Clinical Global Impression (CGI), reflects the impression of a skilled observer, fully familiar with the manifestations of schizophrenia, about the overall clinical state of the patient. In addition, the Scale for Assessing Negative Symptoms (SANS) was employed for assessing negative symptoms in one trial.

The results of the oral ziprasidone trials follow:

(1) In a 4-week, placebo-controlled trial (n=139) comparing 2 fixed doses of ziprasidone (20 and 60 mg BID) with placebo, only the 60 mg BID dose was superior to placebo on the BPRS total score and the CGI severity score. This higher dose group was not superior to placebo on the BPRS psychosis cluster or on the SANS.

(2) In a 6-week, placebo-controlled trial (n=302) comparing 2 fixed doses of ziprasidone (40 and 80 mg BID) with placebo, both dose groups were superior to placebo on the BPRS total score, the BPRS psychosis cluster, the CGI severity score and the PANSS total and negative subscale scores. Although 80 mg BID had a numerically greater effect than 40 mg BID, the difference was not statistically significant.

(3) In a 6-week, placebo-controlled trial (n=419) comparing 3 fixed doses of ziprasidone (20, 60, and 100 mg BID) with placebo, all three dose groups were superior to placebo on the PANSS total score, the BPRS total score, the BPRS psychosis cluster, and the CGI severity score. Only the 100 mg BID dose group was superior to placebo on the PANSS negative subscale score. There was no clear evidence for a dose-response relationship within the 20 mg BID to 100 mg BID dose range.

(4) In a 4-week, placebo-controlled trial (n=200) comparing 3 fixed doses of ziprasidone (5, 20, and 40 mg BID), none of the dose groups was statistically superior to placebo on any outcome of interest.

(5) A study was conducted in chronic, symptomatically stable schizophrenic inpatients (n=294) randomized to 3 fixed doses of ziprasidone (20, 40, or 80 mg BID) or placebo and followed for 52 weeks. Patients were observed for "impending psychotic relapse," defined as CGI-improvement score of ≥6 (much worse or very much worse) and/or scores ≥6 (moderately severe) on the hostility or uncooperativeness items of the PANSS on two consecutive days. Ziprasidone was significantly superior to placebo in both time to relapse and rate of relapse, with no significant difference between the different dose groups.

There were insufficient data to examine population subsets based on age and race. Examination of population subsets based on gender did not reveal any differential responsiveness.

The efficacy of intramuscular ziprasidone in the management of agitated schizophrenic patients was established in two short-term, double-blind trials of schizophrenic subjects who were considered by the investigators to be "acutely agitated" and in need of IM antipsychotic medication. In addition, patients were required to have a score of 3 or more on at least 3 of the following items of the PANSS: anxiety, tension, hostility and excitement. Efficacy was evaluated by analysis of the area under the curve (AUC) of the Behavioural Activity Rating Scale (BARS) and Clinical Global Impression (CGI) severity rating. The BARS is a seven point scale with scores ranging from 1 (difficult or unable to rouse) to 7 (violent, requires restraint). Patients' scores on the BARS at baseline were mostly 5 (signs of overt activity [physical or verbal], calms down with instructions) and as determined by investigators, exhibited a degree of agitation that warranted intramuscular therapy. There were few patients with a rating higher than 5 on the BARS, as the most severely agitated patients were generally unable to provide informed consent for participation in pre-marketing clinical trials.

Continued on next page

Geodon—Cont.

Both studies compared higher doses of ziprasidone intramuscular with a 2 mg control dose. In one study, the higher dose was 20 mg, which could be given up to 4 times in the 24 hours of the study, at interdose intervals of no less than 4 hours. In the other study, the higher dose was 10 mg, which could be given up to 4 times in the 24 hours of the study, at interdose intervals of no less than 2 hours.

The results of the intramuscular ziprasidone trials follow:
(1) In a one-day, double-blind, randomized trial (n=79) involving doses of ziprasidone intramuscular of 20 mg or 2 mg, up to QID, ziprasidone intramuscular 20 mg was statistically superior to ziprasidone intramuscular 2 mg, as assessed by AUC of the BARS at 0 to 4 hours, and by CGI severity at 4 hours and study endpoint.
(2) In another one-day, double-blind, randomized trial (n=117) involving doses of ziprasidone intramuscular of 10 mg or 2 mg, up to QID, ziprasidone intramuscular 10 mg was statistically superior to ziprasidone intramuscular 2 mg, as assessed by AUC of the BARS at 0 to 2 hours, but not by CGI severity.

INDICATIONS AND USAGE

Ziprasidone is indicated for the treatment of schizophrenia. When deciding among the alternative treatments available for this condition, the prescriber should consider the finding of ziprasidone's greater capacity to prolong the QT/QTc interval compared to several other antipsychotic drugs (see **WARNINGS**). Prolongation of the QTc interval is associated in some other drugs with the ability to cause torsade de pointes-type arrhythmia, a potentially fatal polymorphic ventricular tachycardia, and sudden death. In many cases this would lead to the conclusion that other drugs should be tried first. Whether ziprasidone will cause torsade de pointes or increase the rate of sudden death is not yet known (see **WARNINGS**).

The efficacy of oral ziprasidone was established in short-term (4- and 6-week) controlled trials of schizophrenic inpatients (see **CLINICAL PHARMACOLOGY**).

In a placebo-controlled trial involving the follow-up for up to 52 weeks of stable schizophrenic inpatients, GEODON was demonstrated to delay the time to and rate of relapse. The physician who elects to use GEODON for extended periods should periodically re-evaluate the long-term usefulness of the drug for the individual patient.

Ziprasidone intramuscular is indicated for the treatment of acute agitation in schizophrenic patients for whom treatment with ziprasidone is appropriate and who need intramuscular antipsychotic medication for rapid control of the agitation. "Psychomotor agitation" is defined in DSM-IV as "excessive motor activity associated with a feeling of inner tension." Schizophrenic patients experiencing agitation often manifest behaviors that interfere with their diagnosis and care, e.g., threatening behaviors, escalating or urgently distressing behavior, or self-exhausting behavior, leading clinicians to the use of intramuscular antipsychotic medications to achieve immediate control of the agitation. The efficacy of intramuscular ziprasidone for acute agitation in schizophrenia was established in single-day controlled trials of schizophrenic inpatients (see **CLINICAL PHARMACOLOGY**). Since there is no experience regarding the safety of administering ziprasidone intramuscular to schizophrenic patients already taking oral ziprasidone, the practice of co-administration is not recommended.

CONTRAINDICATIONS

QT Prolongation

Because of ziprasidone's dose-related prolongation of the QT interval and the known association of fatal arrhythmias with QT prolongation by some other drugs, ziprasidone is contraindicated in patients with a known history of QT prolongation (including congenital long QT syndrome), with recent acute myocardial infarction, or with uncompensated heart failure (see **WARNINGS**).

Pharmacokinetic/pharmacodynamic studies between ziprasidone and other drugs that prolong the QT interval have not been performed. An additive effect of ziprasidone and other drugs that prolong the QT interval cannot be excluded. Therefore, ziprasidone should not be given with dofetilide, sotalol, quinidine, other Class Ia and III anti-arrhythmics, mesoridazine, thioridazine, chlorpromazine, droperidol, pimozide, sparfloxacin, gatifloxacin, moxifloxacin, halofantrine, mefloquine, pentamidine, arsenic trioxide, levomethadyl acetate, dolasetron mesylate, probucol or tacrolimus. Ziprasidone is also contraindicated with drugs that have demonstrated QT prolongation as one of their pharmacodynamic effects and have this effect described in the full prescribing information as a contraindication or a boxed or bolded warning (see **WARNINGS**).

Hypersensitivity

Ziprasidone is contraindicated in individuals with a known hypersensitivity to the product.

WARNINGS

QT Prolongation and Risk of Sudden Death

Ziprasidone use should be avoided in combination with other drugs that are known to prolong the QTc interval (see CONTRAINDICATIONS, and see Drug Interactions under PRECAUTIONS). Additionally, clinicians should be alert to the identification of other drugs that have been consistently observed to prolong the QTc interval. Such drugs should not be prescribed with ziprasidone. Ziprasidone should also be avoided in patients with congenital long QT syndrome and in patients with a history of cardiac arrhythmias (see CONTRAINDICATIONS).

A study directly comparing the QT/QTc prolonging effect of oral ziprasidone with several other drugs effective in the treatment of schizophrenia was conducted in patient volunteers. In the first phase of the trial, ECGs were obtained at the time of maximum plasma concentration when the drug was administered alone. In the second phase of the trial, ECGs were obtained at the time of maximum plasma concentration while the drug was co-administered with an inhibitor of the CYP4503A4 metabolism of the drug.

In the first phase of the study, the mean change in QTc from baseline was calculated for each drug, using a sample-based correction that removes the effect of heart rate on the QT interval. The mean increase in QTc from baseline for ziprasidone ranged from approximately 9 to 14 msec greater than for four of the comparator drugs (risperidone, olanzapine, quetiapine, and haloperidol), but was approximately 14 msec less than the prolongation observed for thioridazine.

In the second phase of the study, the effect of ziprasidone on QTc length was not augmented by the presence of a metabolic inhibitor (ketoconazole 200 mg BID).

In placebo-controlled trials, oral ziprasidone increased the QTc interval compared to placebo by approximately 10 msec at the highest recommended daily dose of 160 mg. In clinical trials with oral ziprasidone, the electrocardiograms of 2/2988 (0.06%) patients who received GEODON and 1/440 (0.23%) patients who received placebo revealed QTc intervals exceeding the potentially clinically relevant threshold of 500 msec. In the ziprasidone-treated patients, neither case suggested a role of ziprasidone. One patient had a history of prolonged QTc and a screening measurement of 489 msec; QTc was 503 msec during ziprasidone treatment. The other patient had a QTc of 391 msec at the end of treatment with ziprasidone and upon switching to thioridazine experienced QTc measurements of 518 and 593 msec.

Some drugs that prolong the QT/QTc interval have been associated with the occurrence of torsade de pointes and with sudden unexplained death. The relationship of QT prolongation to torsade de pointes is clearest for larger increases (20 msec and greater) but it is possible that smaller QT/QTc prolongations may also increase risk, or increase it in susceptible individuals, such as those with hypokalemia, hypomagnesemia, or genetic predisposition. Although torsade de pointes has not been observed in association with the use of ziprasidone at recommended doses in premarketing studies, experience is too limited to rule out an increased risk.

A study evaluating the QT/QTc prolonging effect of intramuscular ziprasidone, with intramuscular haloperidol as a control, was conducted in patient volunteers. In the trial, ECGs were obtained at the time of maximum plasma concentration following two injections of ziprasidone (20 mg then 30 mg) or haloperidol (7.5 mg then 10 mg) given four hours apart. Note that a 30 mg dose of intramuscular ziprasidone is 50% higher than the recommended therapeutic dose. The mean change in QTc from baseline was calculated for each drug, using a sample-based correction that removes the effect of heart rate on the QT interval. The mean increase in QTc from baseline for ziprasidone was 4.6 msec following the first injection and 12.8 msec following the second injection. The mean increase in QTc from baseline for haloperidol was 6.0 msec following the first injection and 14.7 msec following the second injection. In this study, no patients had a QTc interval exceeding 500 msec.

As with other antipsychotic drugs and placebo, sudden unexplained deaths have been reported in patients taking ziprasidone at recommended doses. The premarketing experience for ziprasidone did not reveal an excess risk of mortality for ziprasidone compared to other antipsychotic drugs or placebo, but the extent of exposure was limited, especially for the drugs used as active controls and placebo. Nevertheless, ziprasidone's larger prolongation of QTc length compared to several other antipsychotic drugs raises the possibility that the risk of sudden death may be greater for ziprasidone than for other available drugs for treating schizophrenia. This possibility needs to be considered in deciding among alternative drug products (see INDICATIONS AND USAGE).

Certain circumstances may increase the risk of the occurrence of torsade de pointes and/or sudden death in association with the use of drugs that prolong the QTc interval, including (1) bradycardia; (2) hypokalemia or hypomagnesemia; (3) concomitant use of other drugs that prolong the QTc interval; and (4) presence of congenital prolongation of the QT interval.

It is recommended that patients being considered for ziprasidone treatment who are at risk for significant electrolyte disturbances, hypokalemia in particular, have baseline serum potassium and magnesium measurements. Hypokalemia (and/or hypomagnesemia) may increase the risk of QT prolongation and arrhythmia. Hypokalemia may result from diuretic therapy, diarrhea, and other causes. Patients with low serum potassium and/or magnesium should be repleted with those electrolytes before proceeding with treatment. It is essential to periodically monitor serum electrolytes in patients for whom diuretic therapy is introduced during ziprasidone treatment. Persistently prolonged QTc intervals may also increase the risk of further prolongation and arrhythmia, but it is not clear that routine screening ECG measures are effective in detecting such patients. Rather, ziprasidone should be avoided in patients with histories of significant cardiovascular illness, e.g., QT prolongation, recent acute myocardial infarction, uncompensated heart failure, or cardiac arrhythmia. Ziprasidone should be discontinued in patients who are found to have persistent QTc measurements >500 msec.

For patients taking ziprasidone who experience symptoms that could indicate the occurrence of torsade de pointes, e.g., dizziness, palpitations, or syncope, the prescriber should initiate further evaluation, e.g., Holter monitoring may be useful.

Neuroleptic Malignant Syndrome (NMS)

A potentially fatal symptom complex sometimes referred to as Neuroleptic Malignant Syndrome (NMS) has been reported in association with administration of antipsychotic drugs. Clinical manifestations of NMS are hyperpyrexia, muscle rigidity, altered mental status and evidence of autonomic instability (irregular pulse or blood pressure, tachycardia, diaphoresis, and cardiac dysrhythmia). Additional signs may include elevated creatinine phosphokinase, myoglobinuria (rhabdomyolysis), and acute renal failure.

The diagnostic evaluation of patients with this syndrome is complicated. In arriving at a diagnosis, it is important to exclude cases where the clinical presentation includes both serious medical illness (e.g., pneumonia, systemic infection, etc.) and untreated or inadequately treated extrapyramidal signs and symptoms (EPS). Other important considerations in the differential diagnosis include central anticholinergic toxicity, heat stroke, drug fever, and primary central nervous system (CNS) pathology.

The management of NMS should include: (1) immediate discontinuation of antipsychotic drugs and other drugs not essential to concurrent therapy; (2) intensive symptomatic treatment and medical monitoring; and (3) treatment of any concomitant serious medical problems for which specific treatments are available. There is no general agreement about specific pharmacological treatment regimens for NMS.

If a patient requires antipsychotic drug treatment after recovery from NMS, the potential reintroduction of drug therapy should be carefully considered. The patient should be carefully monitored, since recurrences of NMS have been reported.

Tardive Dyskinesia

A syndrome of potentially irreversible, involuntary, dyskinetic movements may develop in patients undergoing treatment with antipsychotic drugs. Although the prevalence of the syndrome appears to be highest among the elderly, especially elderly women, it is impossible to rely upon prevalence estimates to predict, at the inception of antipsychotic treatment, which patients are likely to develop the syndrome. Whether antipsychotic drug products differ in their potential to cause tardive dyskinesia is unknown.

The risk of developing tardive dyskinesia and the likelihood that it will become irreversible are believed to increase as the duration of treatment and the total cumulative dose of antipsychotic drugs administered to the patient increase. However, the syndrome can develop, although much less commonly, after relatively brief treatment periods at low doses.

There is no known treatment for established cases of tardive dyskinesia, although the syndrome may remit, partially or completely, if antipsychotic treatment is withdrawn. Antipsychotic treatment itself, however, may suppress (or partially suppress) the signs and symptoms of the syndrome and thereby may possibly mask the underlying process. The effect that symptomatic suppression has upon the long-term course of the syndrome is unknown.

Given these considerations, ziprasidone should be prescribed in a manner that is most likely to minimize the occurrence of tardive dyskinesia. Chronic antipsychotic treatment should generally be reserved for patients who suffer from a chronic illness that (1) is known to respond to antipsychotic drugs, and (2) for whom alternative, equally effective, but potentially less harmful treatments are not available or appropriate. In patients who do require chronic treatment, the smallest dose and the shortest duration of treatment producing a satisfactory clinical response should be sought. The need for continued treatment should be reassessed periodically.

If signs and symptoms of tardive dyskinesia appear in a patient on ziprasidone, drug discontinuation should be considered. However, some patients may require treatment with ziprasidone despite the presence of the syndrome.

PRECAUTIONS

General

Rash—In premarketing trials with ziprasidone, about 5% of patients developed rash and/or urticaria, with discontinuation of treatment in about one-sixth of these cases. The occurrence of rash was related to dose of ziprasidone, although the finding might also be explained by the longer exposure time in the higher dose patients. Several patients with rash had signs and symptoms of associated systemic illness, e.g., elevated WBCs. Most patients improved promptly with adjunctive treatment with antihistamines or steroids and/or upon discontinuation of ziprasidone, and all patients experiencing these events were reported to recover completely. Upon appearance of rash for which an alternative etiology cannot be identified, ziprasidone should be discontinued.

Orthostatic Hypotension—Ziprasidone may induce orthostatic hypotension associated with dizziness, tachycardia, and, in some patients, syncope, especially during the initial dose-titration period, probably reflecting its α_1-adrenergic antagonist properties. Syncope was reported in 0.6% of the patients treated with ziprasidone.

Ziprasidone should be used with particular caution in patients with known cardiovascular disease (history of myocardial infarction or ischemic heart disease, heart failure or conduction abnormalities), cerebrovascular disease or conditions which would predispose patients to hypotension (dehydration, hypovolemia, and treatment with antihypertensive medications).

Seizures—During clinical trials, seizures occurred in 0.4% of patients treated with ziprasidone. There were confounding factors that may have contributed to the occurrence of seizures in many of these cases. As with other antipsychotic drugs, ziprasidone should be used cautiously in patients with a history of seizures or with conditions that potentially lower the seizure threshold, e.g., Alzheimer's dementia. Conditions that lower the seizure threshold may be more prevalent in a population of 65 years or older.

Hyperprolactinemia—As with other drugs that antagonize dopamine D_2 receptors, ziprasidone elevates prolactin levels in humans. Increased prolactin levels were also observed in animal studies with this compound, and were associated with an increase in mammary gland neoplasia in mice; a similar effect was not observed in rats (see **Carcinogenesis**). Tissue culture experiments indicate that approximately one-third of human breast cancers are prolactin-dependent *in vitro*, a factor of potential importance if the prescription of these drugs is contemplated in a patient with previously detected breast cancer. Although disturbances such as galactorrhea, amenorrhea, gynecomastia, and impotence have been reported with prolactin-elevating compounds, the clinical significance of elevated serum prolactin levels is unknown for most patients. Neither clinical studies nor epidemiologic studies conducted to date have shown an association between chronic administration of this class of drugs and tumorigenesis in humans; the available evidence is considered too limited to be conclusive at this time.

Potential for Cognitive and Motor Impairment—Somnolence was a commonly reported adverse event in patients treated with ziprasidone. In the 4- and 6-week placebo-controlled trials, somnolence was reported in 14% of patients on ziprasidone compared to 7% of placebo patients. Somnolence led to discontinuation in 0.3% of patients in short-term clinical trials. Since ziprasidone has the potential to impair judgment, thinking, or motor skills, patients should be cautioned about performing activities requiring mental alertness, such as operating a motor vehicle (including automobiles) or operating hazardous machinery until they are reasonably certain that ziprasidone therapy does not affect them adversely.

Priapism—One case of priapism was reported in the premarketing database. While the relationship of the event to ziprasidone use has not been established, other drugs with alpha-adrenergic blocking effects have been reported to induce priapism, and it is possible that ziprasidone may share this capacity. Severe priapism may require surgical intervention.

Body Temperature Regulation—Although not reported with ziprasidone in premarketing trials, disruption of the body's ability to reduce core body temperature has been attributed to antipsychotic agents. Appropriate care is advised when prescribing ziprasidone for patients who will be experiencing conditions which may contribute to an elevation in core body temperature, e.g., exercising strenuously, exposure to extreme heat, receiving concomitant medication with anticholinergic activity, or being subject to dehydration.

Dysphagia—Esophageal dysmotility and aspiration have been associated with antipsychotic drug use. Aspiration pneumonia is a common cause of morbidity and mortality in elderly patients, in particular those with advanced Alzheimer's dementia. Ziprasidone and other antipsychotic drugs should be used cautiously in patients at risk for aspiration pneumonia.

Suicide—The possibility of a suicide attempt is inherent in psychotic illness and close supervision of high-risk patients should accompany drug therapy. Prescriptions for ziprasidone should be written for the smallest quantity of capsules consistent with good patient management in order to reduce the risk of overdose.

Use in Patients with Concomitant Illness—Clinical experience with ziprasidone in patients with certain concomitant systemic illnesses (see **Renal Impairment** and **Hepatic Impairment** under **CLINICAL PHARMACOLOGY, Special Populations**) is limited.

Ziprasidone has not been evaluated or used to any appreciable extent in patients with a recent history of myocardial infarction or unstable heart disease. Patients with these diagnoses were excluded from premarketing clinical studies. Because of the risk of QTc prolongation and orthostatic hypotension with ziprasidone, caution should be observed in cardiac patients (see **QTc Prolongation** under **WARNINGS** and **Orthostatic Hypotension** under **PRECAUTIONS**).

Information for Patients

Please refer to the patient package insert. To assure safe and effective use of GEODON, the information and instructions provided in the patient information should be discussed with patients.

Laboratory Tests

Patients being considered for ziprasidone treatment that are at risk of significant electrolyte disturbances should have baseline serum potassium and magnesium measurements. Low serum potassium and magnesium should be repleted before proceeding with treatment. Patients who are started on diuretics during ziprasidone therapy need periodic monitoring of serum potassium and magnesium. Ziprasidone should be discontinued in patients who are found to have persistent QTc measurements >500 msec (see **WARNINGS**).

Drug Interactions

Drug-drug interactions can be pharmacodynamic (combined pharmacologic effects) or pharmacokinetic (alteration of plasma levels). The risks of using ziprasidone in combination with other drugs have been evaluated as described below. All interactions studies have been conducted with oral ziprasidone. Based upon the pharmacodynamic and pharmacokinetic profile of ziprasidone, possible interactions could be anticipated:

Pharmacodynamic Interactions

(1) Ziprasidone should not be used with any drug that prolongs the QT interval (see **CONTRAINDICATIONS**).

(2) Given the primary CNS effects of ziprasidone, caution should be used when it is taken in combination with other centrally acting drugs.

(3) Because of its potential for inducing hypotension, ziprasidone may enhance the effects of certain antihypertensive agents.

(4) Ziprasidone may antagonize the effects of levodopa and dopamine agonists.

Pharmacokinetic Interactions

The Effect of Other Drugs on Ziprasidone

Carbamazepine—Carbamazepine is an inducer of CYP3A4; administration of 200 mg BID for 21 days resulted in a decrease of approximately 35% in the AUC of ziprasidone. This effect may be greater when higher doses of carbamazepine are administered.

Ketoconazole—Ketoconazole, a potent inhibitor of CYP3A4, at a dose of 400 mg QD for 5 days, increased the AUC and Cmax of ziprasidone by about 35-40%. Other inhibitors of CYP3A4 would be expected to have similar effects.

Cimetidine—Cimetidine at a dose of 800 mg QD for 2 days did not affect ziprasidone pharmacokinetics.

Antacid—The coadministration of 30 mL of Maalox® with ziprasidone did not affect the pharmacokinetics of ziprasidone.

In addition, population pharmacokinetic analysis of schizophrenic patients enrolled in controlled clinical trials has not revealed evidence of any clinically significant pharmacokinetic interactions with benztropine, propranolol, or lorazepam.

Effect of Ziprasidone on Other Drugs

In vitro studies revealed little potential for ziprasidone to interfere with the metabolism of drugs cleared primarily by CYP1A2, CYP2C9, CYP2C19, CYP2D6, and CYP3A4, and little potential for drug interactions with ziprasidone due to displacement (see **CLINICAL PHARMACOLOGY, Pharmacokinetics**).

Lithium—Ziprasidone at a dose of 40 mg BID administered concomitantly with lithium at a dose of 450 mg BID for 7 days did not affect the steady-state level or renal clearance of lithium.

Oral Contraceptives—Ziprasidone at a dose of 20 mg BID did not affect the pharmacokinetics of concomitantly administered oral contraceptives, ethinyl estradiol (0.03 mg) and levonorgestrel (0.15 mg).

Dextromethorphan—Consistent with *in vitro* results, a study in normal healthy volunteers showed that ziprasidone did not alter the metabolism of dextromethorphan, a CYP2D6 model substrate, to its major metabolite, dextrorphan. There was no statistically significant change in the urinary dextromethorphan/dextrorphan ratio.

Carcinogenesis, Mutagenesis, Impairment of Fertility

Carcinogenesis—Lifetime carcinogenicity studies were conducted with ziprasidone in Long Evans rats and CD-1 mice. Ziprasidone was administered for 24 months in the diet at doses of 2, 6, or 12 mg/kg/day to rats, and 50, 100, or 200 mg/kg/day to mice (0.1 to 0.6 and 1 to 5 times the maximum recommended human dose [MRHD] of 200 mg/day on a mg/m² basis, respectively). In the rat study, there was no evidence of an increased incidence of tumors compared to controls. In male mice, there was no increase in incidence of tumors relative to controls. In female mice, there were dose-related increases in the incidences of pituitary gland adenoma and carcinoma, and mammary gland adenocarcinoma at all doses tested (50 to 200 mg/kg/day or 1 to 5 times the MRHD on a mg/m² basis). Proliferative changes in the pituitary and mammary glands of rodents have been observed following chronic administration of other antipsychotic agents and are considered to be prolactin-mediated. Increases in serum prolactin were observed in a 1-month dietary study in female, but not male, mice at 100 and 200 mg/kg/day (or 2.5 and 5 times the MRHD on a mg/m² basis). Ziprasidone had no effect on serum prolactin in rats in a 5-week dietary study at the doses that were used in the carcinogenicity study. The relevance for human risk of the findings of prolactin-mediated endocrine tumors in rodents is unknown (see **Hyperprolactinemia** under **PRECAUTIONS, General**).

Mutagenesis—Ziprasidone was tested in the Ames bacterial mutation assay, the *in vitro* mammalian cell gene mutation mouse lymphoma assay, the *in vitro* chromosomal aberration assay in human lymphocytes, and the *in vivo* chromosomal aberration assay in mouse bone marrow. There was a reproducible mutagenic response in the Ames assay in one strain of *S. typhimurium* in the absence of metabolic activation. Positive results were obtained in both the *in vitro* mammalian cell gene mutation assay and the *in vitro* chromosomal aberration assay in human lymphocytes.

Impairment of Fertility—Ziprasidone was shown to increase time to copulation in Sprague-Dawley rats in two fertility and early embryonic development studies at doses of 10 to 160 mg/kg/day (0.5 to 8 times the MRHD of 200 mg/day on a mg/m² basis). Fertility rate was reduced at 160 mg/kg/day (8 times the MRHD on a mg/m² basis). There was no effect on fertility at 40 mg/kg/day (2 times the MRHD on a mg/m² basis). The effect on fertility appeared to be in the female since fertility was not impaired when males given 160 mg/kg/day (8 times the MRHD on a mg/m² basis) were mated with untreated females. In a 6-month study in male rats given 200 mg/kg/day (10 times the MRHD on a mg/m² basis) there were no treatment-related findings observed in the testes.

Pregnancy - Pregnancy Category C—In animal studies ziprasidone demonstrated developmental toxicity, including possible teratogenic effects at doses similar to human therapeutic doses. When ziprasidone was administered to pregnant rabbits during the period of organogenesis, an increased incidence of fetal structural abnormalities (ventricular septal defects and other cardiovascular malformations and kidney alterations) was observed at a dose of 30 mg/kg/day (3 times the MRHD of 200 mg/day on a mg/m² basis). There was no evidence to suggest that these developmental effects were secondary to maternal toxicity. The developmental no-effect dose was 10 mg/kg/day (equivalent to the MRHD on a mg/m² basis). In rats, embryofetal toxicity (decreased fetal weights, delayed skeletal ossification) was observed following administration of 10 to 160 mg/kg/day (0.5 to 8 times the MRHD on a mg/m² basis) during organogenesis or throughout gestation, but there was no evidence of teratogenicity. Doses of 40 and 160 mg/kg/day (2 and 8 times the MRHD on a mg/m² basis) were associated with maternal toxicity. The developmental no-effect dose was 5 mg/kg/day (0.2 times the MRHD on a mg/m² basis).

There was an increase in the number of pups born dead and a decrease in postnatal survival through the first 4 days of lactation among the offspring of female rats treated during gestation and lactation with doses of 10 mg/kg/day (0.5 times the MRHD on a mg/m² basis) or greater. Offspring developmental delays and neurobehavioral functional impairment were observed at doses of 5 mg/kg/day (0.2 times the MRHD on a mg/m² basis) or greater. A no-effect level was not established for these effects.

There are no adequate and well-controlled studies in pregnant women. Ziprasidone should be used during pregnancy only if the potential benefit justifies the potential risk to the fetus.

Labor and Delivery—The effect of ziprasidone on labor and delivery in humans is unknown.

Nursing Mothers—It is not known whether, and if so in what amount, ziprasidone or its metabolites are excreted in human milk. It is recommended that women receiving ziprasidone should not breast feed.

Pediatric Use—The safety and effectiveness of ziprasidone in pediatric patients have not been established.

Geriatric Use—Of the approximately 4500 patients treated with ziprasidone in clinical studies, 2.4% (109) were 65 years of age or over. In general, there was no indication of any different tolerability of ziprasidone or for reduced clearance of ziprasidone in the elderly compared to younger adults. Nevertheless, the presence of multiple factors that might increase the pharmacodynamic response to ziprasidone, or cause poorer tolerance or orthostasis, should lead to consideration of a lower starting dose, slower titration, and careful monitoring during the initial dosing period for some elderly patients.

ADVERSE REACTIONS

The premarketing development program for oral ziprasidone included over 5400 patients and/or normal subjects exposed to one or more doses of ziprasidone. Of these 5400 subjects, over 4500 were patients who participated in multiple-dose effectiveness trials, and their experience corresponded to approximately 1733 patient years. The conditions and duration of treatment with ziprasidone included open-label and double-blind studies, inpatient and outpatient studies, and short-term and longer-term exposure. The premarketing development program for intramuscular ziprasidone included 570 patients and/or normal subjects who received one or more injections of ziprasidone. Over 325 of these subjects participated in trials involving the administration of multiple doses.

Adverse events during exposure were obtained by collecting voluntarily reported adverse experiences, as well as results of physical examinations, vital signs, weights, laboratory analyses, ECGs, and results of ophthalmologic examinations. Adverse experiences were recorded by clinical investigators using terminology of their own choosing. Consequently, it is not possible to provide a meaningful estimate of the proportion of individuals experiencing adverse events without first grouping similar types of events into a smaller number of standardized event categories. In the tables and tabulations that follow, standard COSTART dictionary terminology has been used to classify reported adverse events.

The stated frequencies of adverse events represent the proportion of individuals who experienced, at least once, a treatment-emergent adverse event of the type listed. An event was considered treatment emergent if it occurred for the first time or worsened while receiving therapy following baseline evaluation.

Adverse Findings Observed in Short-Term, Placebo-Controlled Trials with Oral Ziprasidone

The following findings are based on a pool of two 6-week, and two 4-week placebo-controlled trials in which ziprasidone was administered in doses ranging from 10 to 200 mg/day.

Continued on next page

Geodon—Cont.

Adverse Events Associated with Discontinuation of Treatment in Short-Term, Placebo-Controlled Trials of Oral Ziprasidone
Approximately 4.1% (29/702) of ziprasidone-treated patients in short-term, placebo-controlled studies discontinued treatment due to an adverse event, compared with about 2.2% (6/273) on placebo. The most common event associated with dropout was rash, including 7 dropouts for rash among ziprasidone patients (1%) compared to no placebo patients (see **PRECAUTIONS**).

Adverse Events Occurring at an Incidence of 1% or More Among Ziprasidone-Treated Patients in Short-Term, Oral, Placebo-Controlled Trials
Table 1 enumerates the incidence, rounded to the nearest percent, of treatment-emergent adverse events that occurred during acute therapy (up to 6 weeks) in predominantly schizophrenic patients, including only those events that occurred in 1% or more of patients treated with ziprasidone and for which the incidence in patients treated with ziprasidone was greater than the incidence in placebo-treated patients.

The prescriber should be aware that these figures cannot be used to predict the incidence of side effects in the course of usual medical practice where patient characteristics and other factors differ from those which prevailed in the clinical trials. Similarly, the cited frequencies cannot be compared with figures obtained from other clinical investigations involving different treatments, uses, and investigators. The cited figures, however, do provide the prescribing physician with some basis for estimating the relative contribution of drug and non-drug factors to the side effect incidence rate in the population studied.

In these studies, the most commonly observed adverse events associated with the use of ziprasidone (incidence of 5% or greater) and observed at a rate on ziprasidone at least twice that of placebo were somnolence (14%), extrapyramidal syndrome (5%), and respiratory disorder (8%).

Table 1. Treatment-Emergent Adverse Event Incidence In Short-Term Oral Placebo-Controlled Trials

Body System/Adverse Event	Percentage of Patients Reporting Event Ziprasidone (N=702)	Placebo (N=273)
Body as a Whole		
Asthenia	5	3
Accidental Injury	4	2
Cardiovascular		
Tachycardia	2	1
Postural Hypotension	1	0
Digestive		
Nausea	10	7
Constipation	9	8
Dyspepsia	8	7
Diarrhea	5	4
Dry Mouth	4	2
Anorexia	2	1
Musculoskeletal		
Myalgia	1	0
Nervous		
Somnolence	14	7
Akathisia	8	7
Dizziness	8	6
Extrapyramidal Syndrome	5	1
Dystonia	4	2
Hypertonia	3	2
Respiratory		
Respiratory Disorder*	8	3
Rhinitis	4	2
Cough Increased	3	1
Skin and Appendages		
Rash	4	3
Fungal Dermatitis	2	1
Special Senses		
Abnormal Vision	3	2

*Cold symptoms and upper respiratory infection account for >90% of investigator terms pointing to "respiratory disorder".

Explorations for interactions on the basis of gender did not reveal any clinically meaningful differences in the adverse event occurrence on the basis of this demographic factor.

Dose Dependency of Adverse Events in Short-Term, Placebo-Controlled Trials
An analysis for dose response in this 4-study pool revealed an apparent relation of adverse event to dose for the following events: asthenia, postural hypotension, anorexia, dry mouth, increased salivation, arthralgia, anxiety, dizziness, dystonia, hypertonia, somnolence, tremor, rhinitis, rash, and abnormal vision.

Extrapyramidal Symptoms (EPS)—The incidence of reported EPS for ziprasidone-treated patients in the short-term, placebo-controlled trials was 5% vs. 1% for placebo. Objectively collected data from those trials on the Simpson Angus Rating Scale (for EPS) and the Barnes Akathisia Scale (for akathisia) did not generally show a difference between ziprasidone and placebo.

Vital Sign Changes—Ziprasidone is associated with orthostatic hypotension (see **PRECAUTIONS**).

Weight Gain—The proportions of patients meeting a weight gain criterion of ≥7% of body weight were compared in a pool of four 4- and 6- week placebo-controlled clinical trials, revealing a statistically significantly greater incidence of weight gain for ziprasidone (10%) compared to placebo (4%). A median weight gain of 0.5 kg was observed in ziprasidone patients compared to no median weight change in placebo patients. In this set of clinical trials, weight gain was reported as an adverse event in 0.4% and 0.4% of ziprasidone and placebo patients, respectively. During long-term therapy with ziprasidone, a categorization of patients at baseline on the basis of body mass index (BMI) revealed the greatest mean weight gain and highest incidence of clinically significant weight gain (>7% of body weight) in patients with low BMI (<23) compared to normal (23-27) or overweight patients (>27). There was a mean weight gain of 1.4 kg for those patients with a "low" baseline BMI, no mean change for patients with a "normal" BMI, and a 1.3 kg mean weight loss for patients who entered the program with a "high" BMI.

ECG Changes—Ziprasidone is associated with an increase in the QTc interval (see **WARNINGS**). Ziprasidone was associated with a mean increase in heart rate of 1.4 beats per minute compared to a 0.2 beats per minute decrease among placebo patients.

Other Adverse Events Observed During the Premarketing Evaluation of Oral Ziprasidone
Following is a list of COSTART terms that reflect treatment-emergent adverse events as defined in the introduction to the **ADVERSE REACTIONS** section reported by patients treated with ziprasidone at multiple doses >4 mg/day within the database of 3834 patients. All reported events are included except those already listed in Table 1 or elsewhere in labeling, those event terms that were so general as to be uninformative, events reported only once and that did not have a substantial probability of being acutely life-threatening, events that are part of the illness being treated or are otherwise common as background events, and events considered unlikely to be drug-related. It is important to emphasize that, although the events reported occurred during treatment with ziprasidone, they were not necessarily caused by it.

Events are further categorized by body system and listed in order of decreasing frequency according to the following definitions: frequent adverse events are those occurring in at least 1/100 patients (only those not already listed in the tabulated results from placebo-controlled trials appear in this listing); infrequent adverse events are those occurring in 1/100 to 1/1000 patients; rare events are those occurring in fewer than 1/1000 patients.

Body as a Whole: *Frequent:* abdominal pain, flu syndrome, fever, accidental fall, face edema, chills, photosensitivity reaction, flank pain, hypothermia, motor vehicle accident.

Cardiovascular System: *Frequent:* hypertension; *Infrequent:* bradycardia, angina pectoris, atrial fibrillation; *Rare:* first degree AV block, bundle branch block, phlebitis, pulmonary embolus, cardiomegaly, cerebral infarct, cerebrovascular accident, deep thrombophlebitis, myocarditis, thrombophlebitis.

Digestive System: *Frequent:* vomiting; *Infrequent:* rectal hemorrhage, dysphagia, tongue edema; *Rare:* gum hemorrhage, jaundice, fecal impaction, gamma glutamyl transpeptidase increased, hematemesis, cholestatic jaundice, hepatitis, hepatomegaly, leukoplakia of mouth, fatty liver deposit, melena.

Endocrine: *Rare:* hypothyroidism, hyperthyroidism, thyroiditis.

Hemic and Lymphatic System: *Infrequent:* anemia, ecchymosis, leukocytosis, leukopenia, eosinophilia, lymphadenopathy; *Rare:* thrombocytopenia, hypochromic anemia, lymphocytosis, monocytosis, basophilia, lymphedema, polycythemia, thrombocythemia.

Metabolic and Nutritional Disorders: *Infrequent:* thirst, transaminase increased, peripheral edema, hyperglycemia, creatine phosphokinase increased, alkaline phosphatase increased, hypercholesteremia, dehydration, lactic dehydrogenase increased, albuminuria, hypokalemia; *Rare:* BUN increased, creatinine increased, hyperlipemia, hypocholesteremia, hyperkalemia, hypochloremia, hypoglycemia, hyponatremia, hypoproteinemia, glucose tolerance decreased, gout, hyperchloremia, hyperuricemia, hypocalcemia, hypoglycemic reaction, hypomagnesemia, ketosis, respiratory alkalosis.

Musculoskeletal System: *Infrequent:* tenosynovitis; *Rare:* myopathy.

Nervous System: *Frequent:* agitation, tremor, dyskinesia, hostility, paresthesia, confusion, vertigo, hypokinesia, hyperkinesia, abnormal gait, oculogyric crisis, hypesthesia, ataxia, amnesia, cogwheel rigidity, delirium, hypotonia, akinesia, dysarthria, withdrawal syndrome, buccoglossal syndrome, choreoathetosis, diplopia, incoordination, neuropathy; *Rare:* myoclonus, nystagmus, torticollis, circumoral paresthesia, opisthotonos, reflexes increased, trismus.

Respiratory System: *Frequent:* dyspnea; *Infrequent:* pneumonia, epistaxis; *Rare:* hemoptysis, laryngismus.

Skin and Appendages: *Infrequent:* maculopapular rash, urticaria, alopecia, eczema, exfoliative dermatitis, contact dermatitis, vesiculobullous rash.

Special Senses: *Infrequent:* conjunctivitis, dry eyes, tinnitus, blepharitis, cataract, photophobia; *Rare:* eye hemorrhage, visual field defect, keratitis, keratoconjunctivitis.

Urogenital System: *Infrequent:* impotence, abnormal ejaculation, amenorrhea, hematuria, menorrhagia, female lactation, polyuria, urinary retention, metrorrhagia, male sexual dysfunction, anorgasmia, glycosuria; *Rare:* gynecomastia, vaginal hemorrhage, nocturia, oliguria, female sexual dysfunction, uterine hemorrhage.

Adverse Findings Observed in Trials of Intramuscular Ziprasidone

Adverse Events Occurring at an Incidence of 1% or More Among Ziprasidone-Treated Patients in Short-Term Trials of Intramuscular Ziprasidone
Table 2 enumerates the incidence, rounded to the nearest percent, of treatment-emergent adverse events that occurred during acute therapy with intramuscular ziprasidone in 1% or more of patients.

In these studies, the most commonly observed adverse events associated with the use of intramuscular ziprasidone (incidence of 5% or greater) and observed at a rate on intramuscular ziprasidone (in the higher dose groups) at least twice that of the lowest intramuscular ziprasidone group were headache (13%), nausea (12%), and somnolence (20%).
[See table 2 on next page]

DRUG ABUSE AND DEPENDENCE

Controlled Substance Class—Ziprasidone is not a controlled substance.

Physical and Psychological Dependence—Ziprasidone has not been systematically studied, in animals or humans, for its potential for abuse, tolerance, or physical dependence. While the clinical trials did not reveal any tendency for drug-seeking behavior, these observations were not systematic and it is not possible to predict on the basis of this limited experience the extent to which ziprasidone will be misused, diverted, and/or abused once marketed. Consequently, patients should be evaluated carefully for a history of drug abuse, and such patients should be observed closely for signs of ziprasidone misuse or abuse (e.g., development of tolerance, increases in dose, drug-seeking behavior).

OVERDOSAGE

Human Experience—In premarketing trials involving more than 5400 patients and/or normal subjects, accidental or intentional overdosage of oral ziprasidone was documented in 10 patients. All of these patients survived without sequelae. In the patient taking the largest confirmed amount, 3240 mg, the only symptoms reported were minimal sedation, slurring of speech, and transitory hypertension (200/95).

Management of Overdosage—In case of acute overdosage, establish and maintain an airway and ensure adequate oxygenation and ventilation. Intravenous access should be established, and gastric lavage (after intubation, if patient is unconscious) and administration of activated charcoal together with a laxative should be considered. The possibility of obtundation, seizure, or dystonic reaction of the head and neck following overdose may create a risk of aspiration with induced emesis.

Cardiovascular monitoring should commence immediately and should include continuous electrocardiographic monitoring to detect possible arrhythmias. If antiarrhythmic therapy is administered, disopyramide, procainamide, and quinidine carry a theoretical hazard of additive QT-prolonging effects that might be additive to those of ziprasidone.

Hypotension and circulatory collapse should be treated with appropriate measures such as intravenous fluids. If sympathomimetic agents are used for vascular support, epinephrine and dopamine should not be used, since beta stimulation combined with α_1 antagonism associated with ziprasidone may worsen hypotension. Similarly, it is reasonable to expect that the alpha-adrenergic-blocking properties of bretylium might be additive to those of ziprasidone, resulting in problematic hypotension.

In cases of severe extrapyramidal symptoms, anticholinergic medication should be administered. There is no specific antidote to ziprasidone, and it is not dialyzable. The possibility of multiple drug involvement should be considered. Close medical supervision and monitoring should continue until the patient recovers.

DOSAGE AND ADMINISTRATION

When deciding among the alternative treatments available for schizophrenia, the prescriber should consider the finding of ziprasidone's greater capacity to prolong the QT/QTc interval compared to several other antipsychotic drugs (see **WARNINGS**).

Initial Treatment

GEODON® Capsules should be administered at an initial daily dose of 20 mg BID with food. In some patients, daily dosage may subsequently be adjusted on the basis of individual clinical status up to 80 mg BID. Dosage adjustments, if indicated, should generally occur at intervals of not less than 2 days, as steady-state is achieved within 1 to 3 days. In order to ensure use of the lowest effective dose, ordinarily patients should be observed for improvement for several weeks before upward dosage adjustment.

Efficacy in schizophrenia was demonstrated in a dose range of 20 to 100 mg BID in short-term, placebo-controlled clinical trials. There were trends toward dose response within the range of 20 to 80 mg BID, but results were not consistent. An increase to a dose greater than 80 mg BID is not generally recommended. The safety of doses above 100 mg BID has not been systematically evaluated in clinical trials.

TABLE 2. Treatment-Emergent Adverse Event Incidence In Short-Term Fixed-Dose Intramuscular Trials

Body System/Adverse Event	Percentage of Patients Reporting Event		
	Ziprasidone 2 mg (N=92)	Ziprasidone 10 mg (N=63)	Ziprasidone 20 mg (N=41)
Body as a Whole			
Headache	3	13	5
Injection Site Pain	9	8	7
Asthenia	2	0	0
Abdominal Pain	0	2	0
Flu Syndrome	1	0	0
Back Pain	1	0	0
Cardiovascular			
Postural Hypotension	0	0	5
Hypertension	2	0	0
Bradycardia	0	0	2
Vasodilation	1	0	0
Digestive			
Nausea	4	8	12
Rectal Hemorrhage	0	0	2
Diarrhea	3	3	0
Vomiting	0	3	0
Dyspepsia	1	3	2
Anorexia	0	2	0
Constipation	0	0	2
Tooth Disorder	1	0	0
Dry Mouth	1	0	0
Nervous			
Dizziness	3	3	10
Anxiety	2	0	0
Insomnia	3	0	0
Somnolence	8	8	20
Akathisia	0	2	0
Agitation	2	2	0
Extrapyramidal Syndrome	2	0	0
Hypertonia	1	0	0
Cogwheel Rigidity	1	0	0
Paresthesia	0	2	0
Personality Disorder	0	2	0
Psychosis	1	0	0
Speech Disorder	0	2	0
Respiratory			
Rhinitis	1	0	0
Skin and Appendages			
Furunculosis	0	2	0
Sweating	0	0	2
Urogenital			
Dysmenorrhea	0	2	0
Priapism	1	0	0

Maintenance Treatment

While there is no body of evidence available to answer the question of how long a patient treated with ziprasidone should remain on it, systematic evaluation of ziprasidone has shown that its efficacy in schizophrenia is maintained for periods of up to 52 weeks at a dose of 20 to 80 mg BID (see **CLINICAL PHARMACOLOGY**). No additional benefit was demonstrated for doses above 20 mg BID. Patients should be periodically reassessed to determine the need for maintenance treatment.

Intramuscular Administration

The recommended dose is 10 to 20 mg administered as required up to a maximum dose of 40 mg per day. Doses of 10 mg may be administered every two hours; doses of 20 mg may be administered every four hours up to a maximum of 40 mg/day. Intramuscular administration of ziprasidone for more than three consecutive days has not been studied.

If long-term therapy is indicated, oral ziprasidone hydrochloride capsules should replace the intramuscular administration as soon as possible.

Since there is no experience regarding the safety of administering ziprasidone intramuscular to schizophrenic patients already taking oral ziprasidone, the practice of co-administration is not recommended.

Dosing in Special Populations

Oral: Dosage adjustments are generally not required on the basis of age, gender, race, or renal or hepatic impairment.

Intramuscular: Ziprasidone intramuscular has not been systematically evaluated in elderly patients or in patients with hepatic or renal impairment. As the cyclodextrin excipient is cleared by renal filtration, ziprasidone intramuscular should be administered with caution to patients with impaired renal function. Dosing adjustments are not required on the basis of gender or race.

Preparation for Administration

GEODON® for Injection (ziprasidone mesylate) should only be administered by intramuscular injection. Single-dose vials require reconstitution prior to administration; any unused portion should be discarded.

Add 1.2 mL of Sterile Water for Injection to the vial and shake vigorously until all the drug is dissolved. Each mL of reconstituted solution contains 20 mg ziprasidone. To administer a 10 mg dose, draw up 0.5 mL of the reconstituted solution. To administer a 20 mg dose, draw up 1.0 mL of the reconstituted solution. Since no preservative or bacteriostatic agent is present in this product, aseptic technique must be used in preparation of the final solution. This medicinal product must not be mixed with other medicinal products or solvents other than Sterile Water for Injection. Parenteral drug products should be inspected visually for particulate matter and discoloration prior to administration, whenever solution and container permit.

HOW SUPPLIED

GEODON® Capsules are differentiated by capsule color/size and are imprinted in black ink with "Pfizer" and a unique number. GEODON Capsules are supplied for oral administration in 20 mg (blue/white), 40 mg (blue/blue), 60 mg (white/white), and 80 mg (blue/white) capsules. They are supplied in the following strengths and package configurations:

GEODON® Capsules

Package Configuration	Capsule Strength (mg)	NDC Code	Imprint
Bottles of 60	20	NDC-0049-3960-60	396
Bottles of 60	40	NDC-0049-3970-60	397
Bottles of 60	60	NDC-0049-3980-60	398
Bottles of 60	80	NDC-0049-3990-60	399
Unit dose/80	20	NDC-0049-3960-41	396
Unit dose/80	40	NDC-0049-3970-41	397
Unit dose/80	60	NDC-0049-3980-41	398
Unit dose/80	80	NDC-0049-3990-41	399

Storage and Handling—GEODON® Capsules should be stored at controlled room temperature, 15°-30°C (59°-86°F). GEODON® for Injection is available in a single dose vial as ziprasidone mesylate (20 mg ziprasidone/mL when reconstituted according to label instructions—see **Preparation for Administration**) for intramuscular administration. Each mL of ziprasidone mesylate for injection (when reconstituted) affords a colorless to pale pink solution that contains 20 mg of ziprasidone and 4.7 mg of methanesulfonic acid solubilized by 294 mg of sulfobutylether β-cyclodextrin sodium (SBECD).

GEODON® for Injection

Package	Concentration	NDC Code
Single Use Vials	20 mg/mL	NDC-0049-3920-83

Continued on next page

Geodon—Cont.

Storage and Handling—GEODON® for Injection should be stored at controlled room temperature, 15°-30°C (59°-86°F) in dry form. Protect from light. Following reconstitution, GEODON for Injection can be stored, when protected from light, for up to 24 hours at 15°-30°C (59°-86°F) or up to 7 days refrigerated, 2°-8°C (36°-46°F).

Rx only

Distributed by
Pfizer Roerig
Division of Pfizer Inc, NY, NY 10017
69-5770-00-5 Revised December 2003

LIPITOR® ℞

[*lĭ'pĭ-tōr*]
(Atorvastatin Calcium)
Tablets

Prescribing information for this product, which appears on pages 2606–2610 of the 2004 PDR, has been completely revised as follows. Please write "See Supplement A" next to the product heading.

DESCRIPTION

Lipitor® (atorvastatin calcium) is a synthetic lipid-lowering agent. Atorvastatin is an inhibitor of 3-hydroxy-3-methylglutaryl-coenzyme A (HMG-CoA) reductase. This enzyme catalyzes the conversion of HMG-CoA to mevalonate, an early and rate-limiting step in cholesterol biosynthesis.

Atorvastatin calcium is [R-(R*, R*)]-2-(4-fluorophenyl)-β, δ-dihydroxy-5-(1-methylethyl)-3-phenyl-4-[(phenylamino)-carbonyl]-1H-pyrrole-1-heptanoic acid, calcium salt (2:1) trihydrate. The empirical formula of atorvastatin calcium is $(C_{33}H_{34}FN_2O_5)_2Ca \cdot 3H_2O$ and its molecular weight is 1209.42. Its structural formula is:

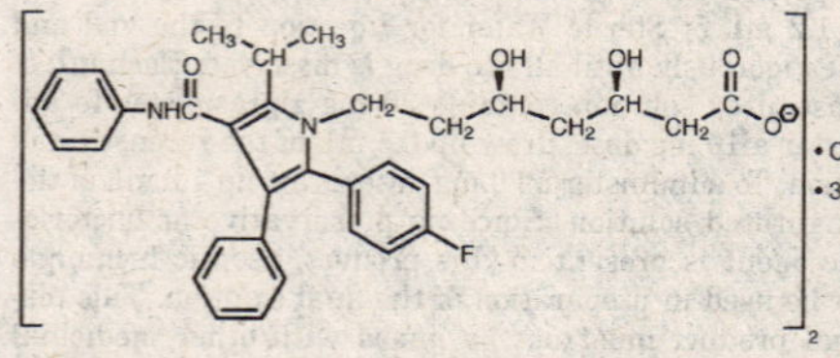

Atorvastatin calcium is a white to off-white crystalline powder that is insoluble in aqueous solutions of pH 4 and below. Atorvastatin calcium is very slightly soluble in distilled water, pH 7.4 phosphate buffer, and acetonitrile, slightly soluble in ethanol, and freely soluble in methanol.

Lipitor tablets for oral administration contain 10, 20, 40 or 80 mg atorvastatin and the following inactive ingredients: calcium carbonate, USP; candelilla wax, FCC; croscarmellose sodium, NF; hydroxypropyl cellulose, NF; lactose monohydrate, NF; magnesium stearate, NF; microcrystalline cellulose, NF; Opadry White YS-1-7040 (hypromellose, polyethylene glycol, talc, titanium dioxide); polysorbate 80, NF; simethicone emulsion.

CLINICAL PHARMACOLOGY

Mechanism of Action

Atorvastatin is a selective, competitive inhibitor of HMG-CoA reductase, the rate-limiting enzyme that converts 3-hydroxy-3-methylglutaryl-coenzyme A to mevalonate, a precursor of sterols, including cholesterol. Cholesterol and triglycerides circulate in the bloodstream as part of lipoprotein complexes. With ultracentrifugation, these complexes separate into HDL (high-density lipoprotein), IDL (intermediate-density lipoprotein), LDL (low-density lipoprotein), and VLDL (very-low-density lipoprotein) fractions. Triglycerides (TG) and cholesterol in the liver are incorporated into VLDL and released into the plasma for delivery to peripheral tissues. LDL is formed from VLDL and is catabolized primarily through the high-affinity LDL receptor. Clinical and pathologic studies show that elevated plasma levels of total cholesterol (total-C), LDL-cholesterol (LDL-C), and apolipoprotein B (apo B) promote human atherosclerosis and are risk factors for developing cardiovascular disease, while increased levels of HDL-C are associated with a decreased cardiovascular risk.

In animal models, Lipitor lowers plasma cholesterol and lipoprotein levels by inhibiting HMG-CoA reductase and cholesterol synthesis in the liver and by increasing the number of hepatic LDL receptors on the cell-surface to enhance uptake and catabolism of LDL; Lipitor also reduces LDL production and the number of LDL particles. Lipitor reduces LDL-C in some patients with homozygous familial hypercholesterolemia (FH), a population that rarely responds to other lipid-lowering medication(s).

A variety of clinical studies have demonstrated that elevated levels of total-C, LDL-C, and apo B (a membrane complex for LDL-C) promote human atherosclerosis. Similarly, decreased levels of HDL-C (and its transport complex, apo A) are associated with the development of atherosclerosis. Epidemiologic investigations have established that cardiovascular morbidity and mortality vary directly with the level of total-C and LDL-C, and inversely with the level of HDL-C.

Lipitor reduces total-C, LDL-C, and apo B in patients with homozygous and heterozygous FH, nonfamilial forms of hypercholesterolemia, and mixed dyslipidemia. Lipitor also reduces VLDL-C and TG and produces variable increases in HDL-C and apolipoprotein A-1. Lipitor reduces total-C, LDL-C, VLDL-C, apo B, TG, and non-HDL-C, and increases HDL-C in patients with isolated hypertriglyceridemia. Lipitor reduces intermediate density lipoprotein cholesterol (IDL-C) in patients with dysbetalipoproteinemia. The effect of Lipitor on cardiovascular morbidity and mortality has not been determined.

Like LDL, cholesterol-enriched triglyceride-rich lipoproteins, including VLDL, intermediate density lipoprotein (IDL), and remnants, can also promote atherosclerosis. Elevated plasma triglycerides are frequently found in a triad with low HDL-C levels and small LDL particles, as well as in association with non-lipid metabolic risk factors for coronary heart disease. As such, total plasma TG has not consistently been shown to be an independent risk factor for CHD. Furthermore, the independent effect of raising HDL or lowering TG on the risk of coronary and cardiovascular morbidity and mortality has not been determined.

Pharmacodynamics

Atorvastatin as well as some of its metabolites are pharmacologically active in humans. The liver is the primary site of action and the principal site of cholesterol synthesis and LDL clearance. Drug dosage rather than systemic drug concentration correlates better with LDL-C reduction. Individualization of drug dosage should be based on therapeutic response (see DOSAGE AND ADMINISTRATION).

Pharmacokinetics and Drug Metabolism

Absorption: Atorvastatin is rapidly absorbed after oral administration; maximum plasma concentrations occur within 1 to 2 hours. Extent of absorption increases in proportion to atorvastatin dose. The absolute bioavailability of atorvastatin (parent drug) is approximately 14% and the systemic availability of HMG-CoA reductase inhibitory activity is approximately 30%. The low systemic availability is attributed to presystemic clearance in gastrointestinal mucosa and/or hepatic first-pass metabolism. Although food decreases the rate and extent of drug absorption by approximately 25% and 9%, respectively, as assessed by Cmax and AUC, LDL-C reduction is similar whether atorvastatin is given with or without food. Plasma atorvastatin concentrations are lower (approximately 30% for Cmax and AUC) following evening drug administration compared with morning. However, LDL-C reduction is the same regardless of the time of day of drug administration (see DOSAGE AND ADMINISTRATION).

Distribution: Mean volume of distribution of atorvastatin is approximately 381 liters. Atorvastatin is ≥98% bound to plasma proteins. A blood/plasma ratio of approximately 0.25 indicates poor drug penetration into red blood cells. Based on observations in rats, atorvastatin is likely to be secreted in human milk (see CONTRAINDICATIONS, Pregnancy and Lactation, and PRECAUTIONS, Nursing Mothers).

Metabolism: Atorvastatin is extensively metabolized to ortho- and parahydroxylated derivatives and various beta-oxidation products. *In vitro* inhibition of HMG-CoA reductase by ortho- and parahydroxylated metabolites is equivalent to that of atorvastatin. Approximately 70% of circulating inhibitory activity for HMG-CoA reductase is attributed to active metabolites. *In vitro* studies suggest the importance of atorvastatin metabolism by cytochrome P450 3A4, consistent with increased plasma concentrations of atorvastatin in humans following coadministration with erythromycin, a known inhibitor of this isozyme (see PRECAUTIONS, Drug Interactions). In animals, the ortho-hydroxy metabolite undergoes further glucuronidation.

Excretion: Atorvastatin and its metabolites are eliminated primarily in bile following hepatic and/or extra-hepatic metabolism; however, the drug does not appear to undergo enterohepatic recirculation. Mean plasma elimination half-life of atorvastatin in humans is approximately 14 hours, but the half-life of inhibitory activity for HMG-CoA reductase is 20 to 30 hours due to the contribution of active metabolites. Less than 2% of a dose of atorvastatin is recovered in urine following oral administration.

Special Populations

Geriatric: Plasma concentrations of atorvastatin are higher (approximately 40% for Cmax and 30% for AUC) in healthy elderly subjects (age ≥65 years) than in young adults. Clinical data suggest a greater degree of LDL-lowering at any dose of drug in the elderly patient population compared to younger adults (see PRECAUTIONS section; Geriatric Use subsection).

Pediatric: Pharmacokinetic data in the pediatric population are not available.

Gender: Plasma concentrations of atorvastatin in women differ from those in men (approximately 20% higher for Cmax and 10% lower for AUC); however, there is no clinically significant difference in LDL-C reduction with Lipitor between men and women.

Renal Insufficiency: Renal disease has no influence on the plasma concentrations or LDL-C reduction of atorvastatin; thus, dose adjustment in patients with renal dysfunction is not necessary (see DOSAGE AND ADMINISTRATION).

Hemodialysis: While studies have not been conducted in patients with end-stage renal disease, hemodialysis is not expected to significantly enhance clearance of atorvastatin since the drug is extensively bound to plasma proteins.

Hepatic Insufficiency: In patients with chronic alcoholic liver disease, plasma concentrations of atorvastatin are markedly increased. Cmax and AUC are each 4-fold greater in patients with Childs-Pugh A disease. Cmax and AUC are approximately 16-fold and 11-fold increased, respectively, in patients with Childs-Pugh B disease (see CONTRAINDICATIONS).

Clinical Studies

Hypercholesterolemia (Heterozygous Familial and Nonfamilial) and Mixed Dyslipidemia (*Fredrickson* Types IIa and IIb)

Lipitor reduces total-C, LDL-C, VLDL-C, apo B, and TG, and increases HDL-C in patients with hypercholesterolemia and mixed dyslipidemia. Therapeutic response is seen within 2 weeks, and maximum response is usually achieved within 4 weeks and maintained during chronic therapy.

Lipitor is effective in a wide variety of patient populations with hypercholesterolemia, with and without hypertriglyceridemia, in men and women, and in the elderly. Experience in pediatric patients has been limited to patients with homozygous FH. In two multicenter, placebo-controlled, dose-response studies in patients with hypercholesterolemia, Lipitor given as a single dose over 6 weeks significantly reduced total-C, LDL-C, apo B, and TG (Pooled results are provided in Table 1).

[See table 1 below]

In patients with *Fredrickson* Types IIa and IIb hyperlipoproteinemia pooled from 24 controlled trials, the median (25th and 75th percentile) percent changes from baseline in HDL-C for atorvastatin 10, 20, 40, and 80 mg were 6.4 (-1.4, 14), 8.7(0, 17), 7.8(0, 16), and 5.1 (-2.7, 15), respectively. Additionally, analysis of the pooled data demonstrated consistent and significant decreases in total-C, LDL-C, TG, total-C/HDL-C, and LDL-C/HDL-C.

In three multicenter, double-blind studies in patients with hypercholesterolemia, Lipitor was compared to other HMG-CoA reductase inhibitors. After randomization, patients were treated for 16 weeks with either Lipitor 10 mg per day or a fixed dose of the comparative agent (Table 2).

[See table 2 at top of next page]

The impact on clinical outcomes of the differences in lipid-altering effects between treatments shown in Table 2 is not known. Table 2 does not contain data comparing the effects of atorvastatin 10 mg and higher doses of lovastatin, pravastatin, and simvastatin. The drugs compared in the studies summarized in the table are not necessarily interchangeable.

Hypertriglyceridemia (*Fredrickson* Type IV)

The response to Lipitor in 64 patients with isolated hypertriglyceridemia treated across several clinical trials is shown in the table below. For the atorvastatin-treated patients, median (min, max) baseline TG level was 565 (267-1502).

[See table 3 at top of next page]

Dysbetalipoproteinemia (*Fredrickson* Type III)

The results of an open-label crossover study of 16 patients (genotypes: 14 apo E2/E2 and 2 apo E3/E2) with dysbetalipoproteinemia (*Fredrickson* Type III) are shown in the table below.

[See table 4 on next page]

Homozygous Familial Hypercholesterolemia

In a study without a concurrent control group, 29 patients ages 6 to 37 years with homozygous FH received maximum daily doses of 20 to 80 mg of Lipitor. The mean LDL-C reduction in this study was 18%. Twenty-five patients with a reduction in LDL-C had a mean response of 20% (range of 7% to 53%, median of 24%); the remaining 4 patients had 7% to 24% increases in LDL-C. Five of the 29 patients had absent LDL-receptor function. Of these, 2 patients also had a portacaval shunt and had no significant reduction in LDL-C. The remaining 3 receptor-negative patients had a mean LDL-C reduction of 22%.

Heterozygous Familial Hypercholesterolemia in Pediatric Patients

In a double-blind, placebo-controlled study followed by an open-label phase, 187 boys and postmenarchal girls 10-17 years of age (mean age 14.1 years) with heterozygous familial hypercholesterolemia (FH) or severe hypercholesterolemia were randomized to Lipitor (n=140) or placebo (n=47) for 26 weeks and then all received Lipitor for 26 weeks. Inclusion in the study required 1) a baseline LDL-C level ≥ 190 mg/dL or 2) a baseline LDL-C ≥ 160 mg/dL and positive family history of FH or documented premature cardiovascular disease in a first- or second-degree relative. The mean baseline LDL-C value was 218.6 mg/dL (range: 138.5-

TABLE 1. Dose-Response in Patients With Primary Hypercholesterolemia (Adjusted Mean % Change From Baseline)[a]

Dose	N	TC	LDL-C	Apo B	TG	HDL-C	Non-HDL-C/ HDL-C
Placebo	21	4	4	3	10	-3	7
10	22	-29	-39	-32	-19	6	-34
20	20	-33	-43	-35	-26	9	-41
40	21	-37	-50	-42	-29	6	-45
80	23	-45	-60	-50	-37	5	-53

[a]Results are pooled from 2 dose-response studies.

TABLE 2. Mean Percent Change From Baseline at End Point (Double-Blind, Randomized, Active-Controlled Trials)

Treatment (Daily Dose)	N	Total-C	LDL-C	Apo B	TG	HDL-C	Non-HDL-C/ HDL-C
Study 1							
Atorvastatin 10 mg	707	-27[a]	-36[a]	-28[a]	-17[a]	+7	-37[a]
Lovastatin 20 mg	191	-19	-27	-20	-6	+7	-28
95% CI for Diff[1]		-9.2, -6.5	-10.7, -7.1	-10.0, -6.5	-15.2, -7.1	-1.7, 2.0	-11.1, -7.1
Study 2							
Atorvastatin 10 mg	222	-25[b]	-35[b]	-27[b]	-17[b]	+6	-36[b]
Pravastatin 20 mg	77	-17	-23	-17	-9	+8	-28
95% CI for Diff[1]		-10.8, -6.1	-14.5, -8.2	-13.4, -7.4	-14.1, -0.7	-4.9, 1.6	-11.5, -4.1
Study 3							
Atorvastatin 10 mg	132	-29[c]	-37[c]	-34[c]	-23[c]	+7	-39[c]
Simvastatin 10 mg	45	-24	-30	-30	-15	+7	-33
95% CI for Diff[1]		-8.7, -2.7	-10.1, -2.6	-8.0, -1.1	-15.1, -0.7	-4.3, 3.9	-9.6, -1.9

[1] A negative value for the 95% CI for the difference between treatments favors atorvastatin for all except HDL-C, for which a positive value favors atorvastatin. If the range does not include 0, this indicates a statistically significant difference.
[a] Significantly different from lovastatin, ANCOVA, p ≤0.05
[b] Significantly different from pravastatin, ANCOVA, p ≤0.05
[c] Significantly different from simvastatin, ANCOVA, p ≤0.05

TABLE 3. Combined Patients With Isolated Elevated TG: Median (min, max) Percent Changes From Baseline

	Placebo (N=12)	Atorvastatin 10 mg (N=37)	Atorvastatin 20 mg (N=13)	Atorvastatin 80 mg (N=14)
Triglycerides	-12.4 (-36.6, 82.7)	-41.0 (-76.2, 49.4)	-38.7 (-62.7, 29.5)	-51.8 (-82.8, 41.3)
Total-C	-2.3 (-15.5, 24.4)	-28.2 (-44.9, -6.8)	-34.9 (-49.6, -15.2)	-44.4 (-63.5, -3.8)
LDL-C	3.6 (-31.3, 31.6)	-26.5 (-57.7, 9.8)	-30.4 (-53.9, 0.3)	-40.5 (-60.6, -13.8)
HDL-C	3.8 (-18.6, 13.4)	13.8 (-9.7, 61.5)	11.0 (-3.2, 25.2)	7.5 (-10.8, 37.2)
VLDL-C	-1.0 (-31.9, 53.2)	-48.8 (-85.8, 57.3)	-44.6 (-62.2, -10.8)	-62.0 (-88.2, 37.6)
non-HDL-C	-2.8 (-17.6, 30.0)	-33.0 (-52.1, -13.3)	-42.7 (-53.7, -17.4)	-51.5 (-72.9, -4.3)

TABLE 4. Open-Label Crossover Study of 16 Patients With Dysbetalipoproteinemia (*Fredrickson* Type III)

		Median % Change (min, max)	
	Median (min, max) at Baseline (mg/dL)	Atorvastatin 10 mg	Atorvastatin 80 mg
Total-C	442 (225, 1320)	-37 (-85, 17)	-58 (-90, -31)
Triglycerides	678 (273, 5990)	-39 (-92, -8)	-53 (-95, -30)
IDL-C + VLDL-C	215 (111, 613)	-32 (-76, 9)	-63 (-90, -8)
non-HDL-C	411 (218, 1272)	-43 (-87, -19)	-64 (-92, -36)

TABLE 5
Lipid-altering Effects of Lipitor in Adolescent Boys and Girls with Heterozygous Familial Hypercholesterolemia or Severe Hypercholesterolemia
(Mean Percent Change from Baseline at Endpoint in Intention-to-Treat Population)

DOSAGE	N	Total-C	LDL-C	HDL-C	TG	Apolipoprotein B
Placebo	47	-1.5	-0.4	-1.9	1.0	0.7
Lipitor	140	-31.4	-39.6	2.8	-12.0	-34.0

385.0 mg/dL) in the Lipitor group compared to 230.0 mg/dL (range: 160.0-324.5 mg/dL) in the placebo group. The dosage of Lipitor (once daily) was 10 mg for the first 4 weeks and up-titrated to 20 mg if the LDL-C level was > 130 mg/dL. The number of Lipitor-treated patients who required up-titration to 20 mg after Week 4 during the double-blind phase was 80 (57.1%).

Lipitor significantly decreased plasma levels of total-C, LDL-C, triglycerides, and apolipoprotein B during the 26 week double-blind phase (see Table 5).

[See table 5 above]

The mean achieved LDL-C value was 130.7 mg/dL (range: 70.0-242.0 mg/dL) in the Lipitor group compared to 228.5 mg/dL (range: 152.0-385.0 mg/dL) in the placebo group during the 26 week double-blind phase.

The safety and efficacy of doses above 20 mg have not been studied in controlled trials in children. The long-term efficacy of Lipitor therapy in childhood to reduce morbidity and mortality in adulthood has not been established.

INDICATIONS AND USAGE

Lipitor is indicated:

1. as an adjunct to diet to reduce elevated total-C, LDL-C, apo B, and TG levels and to increase HDL-C in patients with primary hypercholesterolemia (heterozygous familial and nonfamilial) and mixed dyslipidemia (*Fredrickson* Types IIa and IIb);
2. as an adjunct to diet for the treatment of patients with elevated serum TG levels (*Fredrickson* Type IV);
3. for the treatment of patients with primary dysbetalipoproteinemia (*Fredrickson* Type III) who do not respond adequately to diet;
4. to reduce total-C and LDL-C in patients with homozygous familial hypercholesterolemia as an adjunct to other lipid-lowering treatments (eg, LDL apheresis) or if such treatments are unavailable;
5. as an adjunct to diet to reduce total-C, LDL-C, and apo B levels in boys and postmenarchal girls, 10 to 17 years of age, with heterozygous familial hypercholesterolemia if after an adequate trial of diet therapy the following findings are present:
   a. LDL-C remains ≥ 190 mg/dL or
   b. LDL-C remains ≥ 160 mg/dL and:
      - there is a positive family history of premature cardiovascular disease or
      - two or more other CVD risk factors are present in the pediatric patient

Therapy with lipid-altering agents should be a component of multiple-risk-factor intervention in individuals at increased risk for atherosclerotic vascular disease due to hypercholesterolemia. Lipid-altering agents should be used in addition to a diet restricted in saturated fat and cholesterol only when the response to diet and other nonpharmacological measures has been inadequate (see *National Cholesterol Education Program (NCEP) Guidelines*, summarized in Table 6).

[See table 6 at top of next page]

After the LDL-C goal has been achieved, if the TG is still ≥200 mg/dL, non HDL-C (total-C minus HDL-C) becomes a secondary target of therapy. Non-HDL-C goals are set 30 mg/dL higher than LDL-C goals for each risk category.

Prior to initiating therapy with Lipitor, secondary causes for hypercholesterolemia (eg, poorly controlled diabetes mellitus, hypothyroidism, nephrotic syndrome, dysproteinemias, obstructive liver disease, other drug therapy, and alcoholism) should be excluded, and a lipid profile performed to measure total-C, LDL-C, HDL-C, and TG. For patients with TG <400 mg/dL (<4.5 mmol/L), LDL-C can be estimated using the following equation: LDL-C = total-C - (0.20 × [TG] + HDL-C). For TG levels >400 mg/dL (>4.5 mmol/L), this equation is less accurate and LDL-C concentrations should be determined by ultracentrifugation.

Lipitor has not been studied in conditions where the major lipoprotein abnormality is elevation of chylomicrons (*Fredrickson* Types I and V).

The NCEP classification of cholesterol levels in pediatric patients with a familial history of hypercholesterolemia or premature cardiovascular disease is summarized below:

Category	Total-C (mg/dL)	LDL-C (mg/dL)
Acceptable	<170	<110
Borderline	170-199	110-129
High	≥200	≥130

CONTRAINDICATIONS

Active liver disease or unexplained persistent elevations of serum transaminases.

Hypersensitivity to any component of this medication.

Pregnancy and Lactation

Atherosclerosis is a chronic process and discontinuation of lipid-lowering drugs during pregnancy should have little impact on the outcome of long-term therapy of primary hypercholesterolemia. Cholesterol and other products of cholesterol biosynthesis are essential components for fetal development (including synthesis of steroids and cell membranes). Since HMG-CoA reductase inhibitors decrease cholesterol synthesis and possibly the synthesis of other biologically active substances derived from cholesterol, they may cause fetal harm when administered to pregnant women. Therefore, HMG-CoA reductase inhibitors are contraindicated during pregnancy and in nursing mothers. ATORVASTATIN SHOULD BE ADMINISTERED TO WOMEN OF CHILDBEARING AGE ONLY WHEN SUCH PATIENTS ARE HIGHLY UNLIKELY TO CONCEIVE AND HAVE BEEN INFORMED OF THE POTENTIAL HAZARDS. If the patient becomes pregnant while taking this drug, therapy should be discontinued and the patient apprised of the potential hazard to the fetus.

WARNINGS

Liver Dysfunction

HMG-CoA reductase inhibitors, like some other lipid-lowering therapies, have been associated with biochemical abnormalities of liver function. **Persistent elevations (>3 times the upper limit of normal [ULN] occurring on 2 or more occasions) in serum transaminases occurred in 0.7% of patients who received atorvastatin in clinical trials. The incidence of these abnormalities was 0.2%, 0.2%, 0.6%, and 2.3% for 10, 20, 40, and 80 mg, respectively.**

One patient in clinical trials developed jaundice. Increases in liver function tests (LFT) in other patients were not associated with jaundice or other clinical signs or symptoms. Upon dose reduction, drug interruption, or discontinuation, transaminase levels returned to or near pretreatment levels without sequelae. Eighteen of 30 patients with persistent LFT elevations continued treatment with a reduced dose of atorvastatin.

It is recommended that liver function tests be performed prior to and at 12 weeks following both the initiation of therapy and any elevation of dose, and periodically (eg, semiannually) thereafter. Liver enzyme changes generally occur in the first 3 months of treatment with atorvastatin. Patients who develop increased transaminase levels should be monitored until the abnormalities resolve. Should an increase in ALT or AST of >3 times ULN persist, reduction of dose or withdrawal of atorvastatin is recommended.

Atorvastatin should be used with caution in patients who consume substantial quantities of alcohol and/or have a history of liver disease. Active liver disease or unexplained persistent transaminase elevations are contraindications to the use of atorvastatin (see CONTRAINDICATIONS).

Skeletal Muscle

Rare cases of rhabdomyolysis with acute renal failure secondary to myoglobinuria have been reported with atorvastatin and with other drugs in this class.

Uncomplicated myalgia has been reported in atorvastatin-treated patients (see ADVERSE REACTIONS). Myopathy, defined as muscle aches or muscle weakness in conjunction with increases in creatine phosphokinase (CPK) values >10 times ULN, should be considered in any patient with diffuse myalgias, muscle tenderness or weakness, and/or marked elevation of CPK. Patients should be advised to report promptly unexplained muscle pain, tenderness or weakness, particularly if accompanied by malaise or fever. Atorvastatin therapy should be discontinued if markedly elevated CPK levels occur or myopathy is diagnosed or suspected.

The risk of myopathy during treatment with drugs in this class is increased with concurrent administration of cyclosporine, fibric acid derivatives, erythromycin, niacin, or azole antifungals. Physicians considering combined therapy with atorvastatin and fibric acid derivatives, erythromycin, immunosuppressive drugs, azole antifungals, or lipid-lowering doses of niacin should carefully weigh the potential ben-

Continued on next page

Lipitor—Cont.

efits and risks and should carefully monitor patients for any signs or symptoms of muscle pain, tenderness, or weakness, particularly during the initial months of therapy and during any periods of upward dosage titration of either drug. Periodic creatine phosphokinase (CPK) determinations may be considered in such situations, but there is no assurance that such monitoring will prevent the occurrence of severe myopathy.

Atorvastatin therapy should be temporarily withheld or discontinued in any patient with an acute, serious condition suggestive of a myopathy or having a risk factor predisposing to the development of renal failure secondary to rhabdomyolysis (eg, severe acute infection, hypotension, major surgery, trauma, severe metabolic, endocrine and electrolyte disorders, and uncontrolled seizures).

PRECAUTIONS

General

Before instituting therapy with atorvastatin, an attempt should be made to control hypercholesterolemia with appropriate diet, exercise, and weight reduction in obese patients, and to treat other underlying medical problems (see INDICATIONS AND USAGE).

Information for Patients

Patients should be advised to report promptly unexplained muscle pain, tenderness, or weakness, particularly if accompanied by malaise or fever.

Drug Interactions

The risk of myopathy during treatment with drugs of this class is increased with concurrent administration of cyclosporine, fibric acid derivatives, niacin (nicotinic acid), erythromycin, azole antifungals (see WARNINGS, Skeletal Muscle).

Antacid: When atorvastatin and Maalox® TC suspension were coadministered, plasma concentrations of atorvastatin decreased approximately 35%. However, LDL-C reduction was not altered.

Antipyrine: Because atorvastatin does not affect the pharmacokinetics of antipyrine, interactions with other drugs metabolized via the same cytochrome isozymes are not expected.

Colestipol: Plasma concentrations of atorvastatin decreased approximately 25% when colestipol and atorvastatin were coadministered. However, LDL-C reduction was greater when atorvastatin and colestipol were coadministered than when either drug was given alone.

Cimetidine: Atorvastatin plasma concentrations and LDL-C reduction were not altered by coadministration of cimetidine.

Digoxin: When multiple doses of atorvastatin and digoxin were coadministered, steady-state plasma digoxin concentrations increased by approximately 20%. Patients taking digoxin should be monitored appropriately.

Erythromycin: In healthy individuals, plasma concentrations of atorvastatin increased approximately 40% with coadministration of atorvastatin and erythromycin, a known inhibitor of cytochrome P450 3A4 (see WARNINGS, Skeletal Muscle).

Oral Contraceptives: Coadministration of atorvastatin and an oral contraceptive increased AUC values for norethindrone and ethinyl estradiol by approximately 30% and 20%. These increases should be considered when selecting an oral contraceptive for a woman taking atorvastatin.

Warfarin: Atorvastatin had no clinically significant effect on prothrombin time when administered to patients receiving chronic warfarin treatment.

Endocrine Function

HMG-CoA reductase inhibitors interfere with cholesterol synthesis and theoretically might blunt adrenal and/or gonadal steroid production. Clinical studies have shown that atorvastatin does not reduce basal plasma cortisol concentration or impair adrenal reserve. The effects of HMG-CoA reductase inhibitors on male fertility have not been studied in adequate numbers of patients. The effects, if any, on the pituitary-gonadal axis in premenopausal women are unknown. Caution should be exercised if an HMG-CoA reductase inhibitor is administered concomitantly with drugs that may decrease the levels or activity of endogenous steroid hormones, such as ketoconazole, spironolactone, and cimetidine.

CNS Toxicity

Brain hemorrhage was seen in a female dog treated for 3 months at 120 mg/kg/day. Brain hemorrhage and optic nerve vacuolation were seen in another female dog that was sacrificed in moribund condition after 11 weeks of escalating doses up to 280 mg/kg/day. The 120 mg/kg dose resulted in a systemic exposure approximately 16 times the human plasma area-under-the-curve (AUC, 0-24 hours) based on the maximum human dose of 80 mg/day. A single tonic convulsion was seen in each of 2 male dogs (one treated at 10 mg/kg/day and one at 120 mg/kg/day) in a 2-year study. No CNS lesions have been observed in mice after chronic treatment for up to 2 years at doses up to 400 mg/kg/day or in rats at doses up to 100 mg/kg/day. These doses were 6 to 11 times (mouse) and 8 to 16 times (rat) the human AUC (0-24) based on the maximum recommended human dose of 80 mg/day.

CNS vascular lesions, characterized by perivascular hemorrhages, edema, and mononuclear cell infiltration of perivascular spaces, have been observed in dogs treated with other members of this class. A chemically similar drug in this class produced optic nerve degeneration (Wallerian degeneration of retinogeniculate fibers) in clinically normal dogs

TABLE 6. NCEP Treatment Guidelines: LDL-C Goals and Cutpoints for Therapeutic Lifestyle Changes and Drug Therapy in Different Risk Categories

Risk Category	LDL Goal (mg/dL)	LDL Level at Which to Initiate Therapeutic Lifestyle Changes (mg/dL)	LDL Level at Which to Consider Drug Therapy (mg/dL)
CHD[a] or CHD risk equivalents (10-year risk >20%)	<100	≥100	≥130 (100-129: drug optional)[b]
2+ Risk Factors (10-year risk ≤20%)	<130	≥130	10-year risk 10%-20%: ≥130 10-year risk <10%: ≥160
0-1 Risk factor[c]	<160	≥160	≥190 (160-189: LDL-lowering drug optional)

[a] CHD, coronary heart disease

[b] Some authorities recommend use of LDL-lowering drugs in this category if an LDL-C level of <100 mg/dL cannot be achieved by therapeutic lifestyle changes. Others prefer use of drugs that primarily modify triglycerides and HDL-C, e.g., nicotinic acid or fibrate. Clinical judgement also may call for deferring drug therapy in this subcategory.

[c] Almost all people with 0-1 risk factor have 10-year risk <10%; thus, 10-year risk assessment in people with 0-1 risk factor is not necessary.

in a dose-dependent fashion at a dose that produced plasma drug levels about 30 times higher than the mean drug level in humans taking the highest recommended dose.

Carcinogenesis, Mutagenesis, Impairment of Fertility

In a 2-year carcinogenicity study in rats at dose levels of 10, 30, and 100 mg/kg/day, 2 rare tumors were found in muscle in high-dose females: in one, there was a rhabdomyosarcoma and, in another, there was a fibrosarcoma. This dose represents a plasma AUC (0-24) value of approximately 16 times the mean human plasma drug exposure after an 80 mg oral dose.

A 2-year carcinogenicity study in mice given 100, 200, or 400 mg/kg/day resulted in a significant increase in liver adenomas in high-dose males and liver carcinomas in high-dose females. These findings occurred at plasma AUC (0-24) values of approximately 6 times the mean human plasma drug exposure after an 80 mg oral dose.

In vitro, atorvastatin was not mutagenic or clastogenic in the following tests with and without metabolic activation: the Ames test with *Salmonella typhimurium* and *Escherichia coli*, the HGPRT forward mutation assay in Chinese hamster lung cells, and the chromosomal aberration assay in Chinese hamster lung cells. Atorvastatin was negative in the *in vivo* mouse micronucleus test.

Studies in rats performed at doses up to 175 mg/kg (15 times the human exposure) produced no changes in fertility. There was aplasia and aspermia in the epididymis of 2 of 10 rats treated with 100 mg/kg/day of atorvastatin for 3 months (16 times the human AUC at the 80 mg dose); testis weights were significantly lower at 30 and 100 mg/kg and epididymal weight was lower at 100 mg/kg. Male rats given 100 mg/kg/day for 11 weeks prior to mating had decreased sperm motility, spermatid head concentration, and increased abnormal sperm. Atorvastatin caused no adverse effects on semen parameters, or reproductive organ histopathology in dogs given doses of 10, 40, or 120 mg/kg for two years.

Pregnancy

Pregnancy Category X

See CONTRAINDICATIONS

Safety in pregnant women has not been established. Atorvastatin crosses the rat placenta and reaches a level in fetal liver equivalent to that of maternal plasma. Atorvastatin was not teratogenic in rats at doses up to 300 mg/kg/day or in rabbits at doses up to 100 mg/kg/day. These doses resulted in multiples of about 30 times (rat) or 20 times (rabbit) the human exposure based on surface area (mg/m^2).

In a study in rats given 20, 100, or 225 mg/kg/day, from gestation day 7 through to lactation day 21 (weaning), there was decreased pup survival at birth, neonate, weaning, and maturity in pups of mothers dosed with 225 mg/kg/day. Body weight was decreased on days 4 and 21 in pups of mothers dosed at 100 mg/kg/day; pup body weight was decreased at birth and at days 4, 21, and 91 at 225 mg/kg/day. Pup development was delayed (rotorod performance at 100 mg/kg/day and acoustic startle at 225 mg/kg/day; pinnae detachment and eye opening at 225 mg/kg/day). These doses correspond to 6 times (100 mg/kg) and 22 times (225 mg/kg) the human AUC at 80 mg/day. Rare reports of congenital anomalies have been received following intrauterine exposure to HMG-CoA reductase inhibitors. There has been one report of severe congenital bony deformity, tracheo-esophageal fistula, and anal atresia (VATER association) in a baby born to a woman who took lovastatin with dextroamphetamine sulfate during the first trimester of pregnancy. Lipitor should be administered to women of child-bearing potential only when such patients are highly unlikely to conceive and have been informed of the potential hazards. If the woman becomes pregnant while taking Lipitor, it should be discontinued and the patient advised again as to the potential hazards to the fetus.

Nursing Mothers

Nursing rat pups had plasma and liver drug levels of 50% and 40%, respectively, of that in their mother's milk. Because of the potential for adverse reactions in nursing infants, women taking Lipitor should not breast-feed (see CONTRAINDICATIONS).

Pediatric Use

Safety and effectiveness in patients 10-17 years of age with heterozygous familial hypercholesterolemia have been evaluated in a controlled clinical trial of 6 months duration in adolescent boys and postmenarchal girls. Patients treated with Lipitor had an adverse experience profile generally similar to that of patients treated with placebo, the most common adverse experiences observed in both groups, regardless of causality assessment, were infections. **Doses greater than 20 mg have not been studied in this patient population.** In this limited controlled study, there was no detectable effect on growth or sexual maturation in boys or on menstrual cycle length in girls (see CLINICAL PHARMACOLOGY, Clinical Studies section; ADVERSE REACTIONS, Pediatric Patients (ages 10-17 years); and DOSAGE AND ADMINISTRATION Heterozygous Familial Hypercholesterolemia in Pediatric Patients (10-17 years of age). Adolescent females should be counseled on appropriate contraceptive methods while on Lipitor therapy (see CONTRAINDICATIONS and PRECAUTIONS Pregnancy). **Lipitor has not been studied in controlled clinical trials involving pre-pubertal patients or patients younger than 10 years of age.**

Clinical efficacy with doses up to 80 mg/day for 1 year have been evaluated in an uncontrolled study of patients with homozygous FH including 8 pediatric patients (see CLINICAL PHARMACOLOGY, Clinical Studies: Homozygous Familial Hypercholesterolemia).

Geriatric Use

The safety and efficacy of atorvastatin (10-80 mg) in the geriatric population (≥65 years of age) was evaluated in the ACCESS study. In this 54-week open-label trial 1,958 patients initiated therapy with atorvastatin 10 mg. Of these, 835 were elderly (≥65 years) and 1,123 were non-elderly. The mean change in LDL-C from baseline after 6 weeks of treatment with atorvastatin 10 mg was –38.2% in the elderly patients versus –34.6% in the non-elderly group.

The rates of discontinuation due to adverse events were similar between the two age groups. There were no differences in clinically relevant laboratory abnormalities between the age groups.

ADVERSE REACTIONS

Lipitor is generally well-tolerated. Adverse reactions have usually been mild and transient. In controlled clinical studies of 2502 patients, <2% of patients were discontinued due to adverse experiences attributable to atorvastatin. The most frequent adverse events thought to be related to atorvastatin were constipation, flatulence, dyspepsia, and abdominal pain.

Clinical Adverse Experiences

Adverse experiences reported in ≥2% of patients in placebo-controlled clinical studies of atorvastatin, regardless of causality assessment, are shown in Table 7.

[See table at top of next page]

The following adverse events were reported, regardless of causality assessment in patients treated with atorvastatin in clinical trials. The events in italics occurred in ≥2% of patients and the events in plain type occurred in <2% of patients.

Body as a Whole: *Chest pain*, face edema, fever, neck rigidity, malaise, photosensitivity reaction, generalized edema.

Digestive System: *Nausea*, gastroenteritis, liver function tests abnormal, colitis, vomiting, gastritis, dry mouth, rectal hemorrhage, esophagitis, eructation, glossitis, mouth ulceration, anorexia, increased appetite, stomatitis, biliary pain, cheilitis, duodenal ulcer, dysphagia, enteritis, melena, gum hemorrhage, stomach ulcer, tenesmus, ulcerative stomatitis, hepatitis, pancreatitis, cholestatic jaundice.

Respiratory System: *Bronchitis*, *rhinitis*, pneumonia, dyspnea, asthma, epistaxis.

Nervous System: *Insomnia*, *dizziness*, paresthesia, somnolence, amnesia, abnormal dreams, libido decreased, emotional lability, incoordination, peripheral neuropathy, torticollis, facial paralysis, hyperkinesia, depression, hypesthesia, hypertonia.

Musculoskeletal System: *Arthritis*, leg cramps, bursitis, tenosynovitis, myasthenia, tendinous contracture, myositis.

Skin and Appendages: Pruritus, contact dermatitis, alopecia, dry skin, sweating, acne, urticaria, eczema, seborrhea, skin ulcer.

Urogenital System: *Urinary tract infection*, urinary frequency, cystitis, hematuria, impotence, dysuria, kidney cal-

TABLE 7. Adverse Events in Placebo-Controlled Studies (% of Patients)

BODY SYSTEM/ Adverse Event	Placebo N = 270	Atorvastatin 10 mg N = 863	Atorvastatin 20 mg N = 36	Atorvastatin 40 mg N = 79	Atorvastatin 80 mg N = 94
BODY AS A WHOLE					
Infection	10.0	10.3	2.8	10.1	7.4
Headache	7.0	5.4	16.7	2.5	6.4
Accidental Injury	3.7	4.2	0.0	1.3	3.2
Flu Syndrome	1.9	2.2	0.0	2.5	3.2
Abdominal Pain	0.7	2.8	0.0	3.8	2.1
Back Pain	3.0	2.8	0.0	3.8	1.1
Allergic Reaction	2.6	0.9	2.8	1.3	0.0
Asthenia	1.9	2.2	0.0	3.8	0.0
DIGESTIVE SYSTEM					
Constipation	1.8	2.1	0.0	2.5	1.1
Diarrhea	1.5	2.7	0.0	3.8	5.3
Dyspepsia	4.1	2.3	2.8	1.3	2.1
Flatulence	3.3	2.1	2.8	1.3	1.1
RESPIRATORY SYSTEM					
Sinusitis	2.6	2.8	0.0	2.5	6.4
Pharyngitis	1.5	2.5	0.0	1.3	2.1
SKIN AND APPENDAGES					
Rash	0.7	3.9	2.8	3.8	1.1
MUSCULOSKELETAL SYSTEM					
Arthralgia	1.5	2.0	0.0	5.1	0.0
Myalgia	1.1	3.2	5.6	1.3	0.0

culus, nocturia, epididymitis, fibrocystic breast, vaginal hemorrhage, albuminuria, breast enlargement, metrorrhagia, nephritis, urinary incontinence, urinary retention, urinary urgency, abnormal ejaculation, uterine hemorrhage.

Special Senses: Amblyopia, tinnitus, dry eyes, refraction disorder, eye hemorrhage, deafness, glaucoma, parosmia, taste loss, taste perversion.

Cardiovascular System: Palpitation, vasodilatation, syncope, migraine, postural hypotension, phlebitis, arrhythmia, angina pectoris, hypertension.

Metabolic and Nutritional Disorders: *Peripheral edema*, hyperglycemia, creatine phosphokinase increased, gout, weight gain, hypoglycemia.

Hemic and Lymphatic System: Ecchymosis, anemia, lymphadenopathy, thrombocytopenia, petechia.

Postintroduction Reports

Adverse events associated with Lipitor therapy reported since market introduction, that are not listed above, regardless of causality assessment, include the following: anaphylaxis, angioneurotic edema, bullous rashes (including erythema multiforme, Stevens-Johnson syndrome, and toxic epidermal necrolysis), and rhabdomyolysis.

Pediatric Patients (ages 10-17 years)

In a 26-week controlled study in boys and postmenarchal girls (n=140), the safety and tolerability profile of Lipitor 10 to 20 mg daily was generally similar to that of placebo (see CLINICAL PHARMACOLOGY, Clinical Studies, section and PRECAUTIONS, Pediatric Use).

OVERDOSAGE

There is no specific treatment for atorvastatin overdosage. In the event of an overdose, the patient should be treated symptomatically, and supportive measures instituted as required. Due to extensive drug binding to plasma proteins, hemodialysis is not expected to significantly enhance atorvastatin clearance.

DOSAGE AND ADMINISTRATION

The patient should be placed on a standard cholesterol-lowering diet before receiving Lipitor and should continue on this diet during treatment with Lipitor.

Hypercholesterolemia (Heterozygous Familial and Nonfamilial) and Mixed Dyslipidemia (*Fredrickson* Types IIa and IIb)

The recommended starting dose of Lipitor is 10 or 20 mg once daily. Patients who require a large reduction in LDL-C (more than 45%) may be started at 40 mg once daily. The dosage range of Lipitor is 10 to 80 mg once daily. Lipitor can be administered as a single dose at any time of the day, with or without food. The starting dose and maintenance doses of Lipitor should be individualized according to patient characteristics such as goal of therapy and response (see *NCEP Guidelines* summarized in Table 5). After initiation and/or upon titration of Lipitor, lipid levels should be analyzed within 2 to 4 weeks and dosage adjusted accordingly.

Since the goal of treatment is to lower LDL-C, the NCEP recommends that LDL-C levels be used to initiate and assess treatment response. Only if LDL-C levels are not available, should total-C be used to monitor therapy.

Heterozygous Familial Hypercholesterolemia in Pediatric Patients (10-17 years of age)

The recommended starting dose of Lipitor is 10 mg/day; the maximum recommended dose is 20 mg/day (doses greater than 20 mg have not been studied in this patient population). Doses should be individualized according to the recommended goal of therapy (see NCEP Pediatric Panel Guidelines[1], CLINICAL PHARMACOLOGY, and INDICATIONS AND USAGE). Adjustments should be made at intervals of 4 weeks or more.

[1] National Cholesterol Education Program (NCEP): Highlights of the Report of the Expert Panel on Blood Cholesterol Levels in Children Adolescents, *Pediatrics*. 89(3):495-501. 1992.

Homozygous Familial Hypercholesterolemia

The dosage of Lipitor in patients with homozygous FH is 10 to 80 mg daily. Lipitor should be used as an adjunct to other lipid-lowering treatments (eg, LDL apheresis) in these patients or if such treatments are unavailable.

Concomitant Therapy

Atorvastatin may be used in combination with a bile acid binding resin for additive effect. The combination of HMG-CoA reductase inhibitors and fibrates should generally be avoided (see WARNINGS, Skeletal Muscle, and PRECAUTIONS, Drug Interactions for other drug-drug interactions).

Dosage in Patients With Renal Insufficiency

Renal disease does not affect the plasma concentrations nor LDL-C reduction of atorvastatin; thus, dosage adjustment in patients with renal dysfunction is not necessary (see CLINICAL PHARMACOLOGY, Pharmacokinetics).

HOW SUPPLIED

Lipitor is supplied as white, elliptical, film-coated tablets of atorvastatin calcium containing 10, 20, 40 and 80 mg atorvastatin.

10 mg tablets: coded "PD 155" on one side and "10" on the other.

NDC 0071-0155-23 bottles of 90
NDC 0071-0155-34 bottles of 5000
NDC 0071-0155-40 10 × 10 unit dose blisters

20 mg tablets: coded "PD 156" on one side and "20" on the other.

NDC 0071-0156-23 bottles of 90
NDC 0071-0156-40 10 × 10 unit dose blisters
NDC 0071-0156-94 bottles of 5000

40 mg tablets: coded "PD 157" on one side and "40" on the other.

NDC 0071-0157-23 bottles of 90
NDC 0071-0157-73 bottles of 500

80 mg tablets: coded "PD 158" on one side and "80" on the other.

NDC 0071-0158-23 bottles of 90
NDC 0071-0158-73 bottles of 500

Storage

Store at controlled room temperature 20-25°C (68-77°F) [see USP].

Rx Only

Manufactured by:
Pfizer Ireland Pharmaceuticals
Dublin, Ireland
Distributed by:
Pfizer Parke-Davis
Division of Pfizer Inc, NY, NY 10017
69-5884-00-4 Revised August 2003

NORVASC® ℞

[*nor'vask*]
(amlodipine besylate)
Tablets

Prescribing information for this product, which appears on pages 2615–2617 of the 2004 PDR, has been completely revised as follows. Please write "See Supplement A" next to the product heading.

DESCRIPTION

NORVASC® is the besylate salt of amlodipine, a long-acting calcium channel blocker.

NORVASC is chemically described as (R.S.) 3-ethyl-5-methyl-2-(2-aminoethoxymethyl)-4-(2-chlorophenyl)-1,4-dihydro-6-methyl-3,5-pyridinedicarboxylate benzenesulphonate. Its empirical formula is $C_{20}H_{25}ClN_2O_5 \cdot C_6H_6O_3S$, and its structural formula is:

[See chemical structure at top of next column]

Amlodipine besylate is a white crystalline powder with a molecular weight of 567.1. It is slightly soluble in water and sparingly soluble in ethanol. NORVASC (amlodipine besylate) tablets are formulated as white tablets equivalent to 2.5, 5 and 10 mg of amlodipine for oral administration. In addition to the active ingredient, amlodipine besylate, each

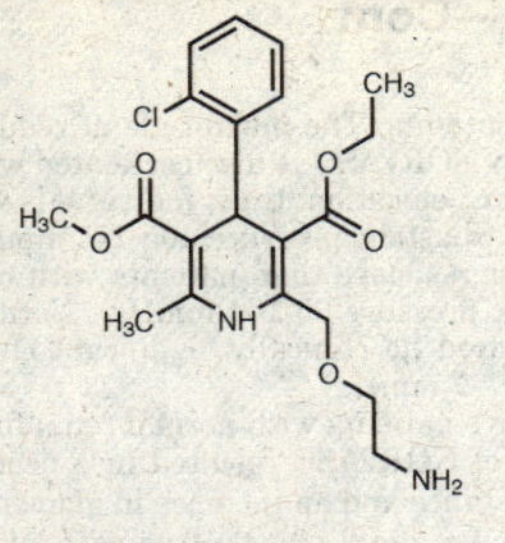

$C_6H_6O_3S$

tablet contains the following inactive ingredients: microcrystalline cellulose, dibasic calcium phosphate anhydrous, sodium starch glycolate, and magnesium stearate.

CLINICAL PHARMACOLOGY

Mechanism of Action: NORVASC is a dihydropyridine calcium antagonist (calcium ion antagonist or slow-channel blocker) that inhibits the transmembrane influx of calcium ions into vascular smooth muscle and cardiac muscle. Experimental data suggest that NORVASC binds to both dihydropyridine and nondihydropyridine binding sites. The contractile processes of cardiac muscle and vascular smooth muscle are dependent upon the movement of extracellular calcium ions into these cells through specific ion channels. NORVASC inhibits calcium ion influx across cell membranes selectively, with a greater effect on vascular smooth muscle cells than on cardiac muscle cells. Negative inotropic effects can be detected *in vitro* but such effects have not been seen in intact animals at therapeutic doses. Serum calcium concentration is not affected by NORVASC. Within the physiologic pH range, NORVASC is an ionized compound (pKa=8.6), and its kinetic interaction with the calcium channel receptor is characterized by a gradual rate of association and dissociation with the receptor binding site, resulting in a gradual onset of effect.

NORVASC is a peripheral arterial vasodilator that acts directly on vascular smooth muscle to cause a reduction in peripheral vascular resistance and reduction in blood pressure.

The precise mechanisms by which NORVASC relieves angina have not been fully delineated, but are thought to include the following:

Exertional Angina: In patients with exertional angina, NORVASC reduces the total peripheral resistance (afterload) against which the heart works and reduces the rate pressure product, and thus myocardial oxygen demand, at any given level of exercise.

Vasospastic Angina: NORVASC has been demonstrated to block constriction and restore blood flow in coronary arteries and arterioles in response to calcium, potassium epinephrine, serotonin, and thromboxane A_2 analog in experimental animal models and in human coronary vessels *in vitro*. This inhibition of coronary spasm is responsible for the effectiveness of NORVASC in vasospastic (Prinzmetal's or variant) angina.

Pharmacokinetics and Metabolism: After oral administration of therapeutic doses of NORVASC, absorption produces peak plasma concentrations between 6 and 12 hours. Absolute bioavailability has been estimated to be between 64 and 90%. The bioavailability of NORVASC is not altered by the presence of food.

NORVASC is extensively (about 90%) converted to inactive metabolites via hepatic metabolism with 10% of the parent compound and 60% of the metabolites excreted in the urine. *Ex vivo* studies have shown that approximately 93% of the circulating drug is bound to plasma proteins in hypertensive patients. Elimination from the plasma is biphasic with a terminal elimination half-life of about 30-50 hours. Steady-state plasma levels of NORVASC are reached after 7 to 8 days of consecutive daily dosing.

The pharmacokinetics of NORVASC are not significantly influenced by renal impairment. Patients with renal failure may therefore receive the usual initial dose.

Elderly patients and patients with hepatic insufficiency have decreased clearance of amlodipine with a resulting increase in AUC of approximately 40-60%, and a lower initial dose may be required. A similar increase in AUC was observed in patients with moderate to severe heart failure.

Pediatric Patients: Sixty-two hypertensive patients aged greater than 6 years received doses of NORVASC between 1.25 mg and 20 mg. Weight-adjusted clearance and volume of distribution were similar to values in adults.

Pharmacodynamics: *Hemodynamics* Following administration of therapeutic doses to patients with hypertension, NORVASC produces vasodilation resulting in a reduction of supine and standing blood pressures. These decreases in blood pressure are not accompanied by a significant change in heart rate or plasma catecholamine levels with chronic dosing. Although the acute intravenous administration of amlodipine decreases arterial blood pressure and increases heart rate in hemodynamic studies of patients with chronic stable angina, chronic administration of oral amlodipine in clinical trials did not lead to clinically significant changes in heart rate or blood pressures in normotensive patients with angina.

With chronic once daily oral administration, antihypertensive effectiveness is maintained for at least 24 hours. Plasma concentrations correlate with effect in both young

Continued on next page

Norvasc—Cont.

and elderly patients. The magnitude of reduction in blood pressure with NORVASC is also correlated with the height of pretreatment elevation; thus, individuals with moderate hypertension (diastolic pressure 105-114 mmHg) had about a 50% greater response than patients with mild hypertension (diastolic pressure 90-104 mmHg). Normotensive subjects experienced no clinically significant change in blood pressures (+1/–2 mmHg).

In hypertensive patients with normal renal function, therapeutic doses of NORVASC resulted in a decrease in renal vascular resistance and an increase in glomerular filtration rate and effective renal plasma flow without change in filtration fraction or proteinuria.

As with other calcium channel blockers, hemodynamic measurements of cardiac function at rest and during exercise (or pacing) in patients with normal ventricular function treated with NORVASC have generally demonstrated a small increase in cardiac index without significant influence on dP/dt or on left ventricular end diastolic pressure or volume. In hemodynamic studies, NORVASC has not been associated with a negative inotropic effect when administered in the therapeutic dose range to intact animals and man, even when co-administered with beta-blockers to man. Similar findings, however, have been observed in normals or well-compensated patients with heart failure with agents possessing significant negative inotropic effects.

Studies in Patients with Congestive Heart Failure: NORVASC has been compared to placebo in four 8-12 week studies of patients with NYHA class II/III heart failure, involving a total of 697 patients. In these studies, there was no evidence of worsened heart failure based on measures of exercise tolerance, NYHA classification, symptoms, or LVEF. In a long-term (follow-up at least 6 months, mean 13.8 months) placebo-controlled mortality/morbidity study of NORVASC 5-10 mg in 1153 patients with NYHA classes III (n=931) or IV (n=222) heart failure on stable doses of diuretics, digoxin, and ACE inhibitors, NORVASC had no effect on the primary endpoint of the study which was the combined endpoint of all-cause mortality and cardiac morbidity (as defined by life-threatening arrhythmia, acute myocardial infarction, or hospitalization for worsened heart failure), or on NYHA classification, or symptoms of heart failure. Total combined all-cause mortality and cardiac morbidity events were 222/571 (39%) for patients on NORVASC and 246/583 (42%) for patients on placebo; the cardiac morbid events represented about 25% of the endpoints in the study.

Another study (PRAISE-2) randomized patients with NYHA class III (80%) or IV (20%) heart failure without clinical symptoms or objective evidence of underlying ischemic disease, on stable doses of ACE inhibitor (99%), digitalis (99%) and diuretics (99%), to placebo (n=827) or NORVASC (n=827) and followed them for a mean of 33 months. There was no statistically significant difference between NORVASC and placebo in the primary endpoint of all cause mortality (95% confidence limits from 8% reduction to 29% increase on NORVASC). With NORVASC there were more reports of pulmonary edema.

Electrophysiologic Effects: NORVASC does not change sinoatrial nodal function or atrioventricular conduction in intact animals or man. In patients with chronic stable angina, intravenous administration of 10 mg did not significantly alter A-H and H-V conduction and sinus node recovery time after pacing. Similar results were obtained in patients receiving NORVASC and concomitant beta blockers. In clinical studies in which NORVASC was administered in combination with beta-blockers to patients with either hypertension or angina, no adverse effects on electrocardiographic parameters were observed. In clinical trials with angina patients alone, NORVASC therapy did not alter electrocardiographic intervals or produce higher degrees of AV blocks.

Effects in Hypertension

Adult Patients: The antihypertensive efficacy of NORVASC has been demonstrated in a total of 15 double-blind, placebo-controlled, randomized studies involving 800 patients on NORVASC and 538 on placebo. Once daily administration produced statistically significant placebo-corrected reductions in supine and standing blood pressures at 24 hours postdose, averaging about 12/6 mmHg in the standing position and 13/7 mmHg in the supine position in patients with mild to moderate hypertension. Maintenance of the blood pressure effect over the 24-hour dosing interval was observed, with little difference in peak and trough effect. Tolerance was not demonstrated in patients studied for up to 1 year. The 3 parallel, fixed dose, dose response studies showed that the reduction in supine and standing blood pressures was dose-related within the recommended dosing range. Effects on diastolic pressure were similar in young and older patients. The effect on systolic pressure was greater in older patients, perhaps because of greater baseline systolic pressure. Effects were similar in black patients and in white patients.

Pediatric Patients: Two hundred sixty-eight hypertensive patients aged 6 to 17 years were randomized first to NORVASC 2.5 or 5 mg once daily for 4 weeks and then randomized again to the same dose or to placebo for another 4 weeks. Patients receiving 5 mg at the end of 8 weeks had lower blood pressure than those secondarily randomized to placebo. The magnitude of the treatment effect is difficult to interpret, but it is probably less than 5 mmHg systolic on the 5 mg dose. Adverse events were similar to those seen in adults.

Effects in Chronic Stable Angina: The effectiveness of 5-10 mg/day of NORVASC in exercise-induced angina has been evaluated in 8 placebo-controlled, double-blind clinical trials of up to 6 weeks duration involving 1038 patients (684 NORVASC, 354 placebo) with chronic stable angina. In 5 of the 8 studies significant increases in exercise time (bicycle or treadmill) were seen with the 10 mg dose. Increases in symptom-limited exercise time averaged 12.8% (63 sec) for NORVASC 10 mg, and averaged 7.9% (38 sec) for NORVASC 5 mg. NORVASC 10 mg also increased time to 1 mm ST segment deviation in several studies and decreased angina attack rate. The sustained efficacy of NORVASC in angina patients has been demonstrated over long-term dosing. In patients with angina there were no clinically significant reductions in blood pressures (4/1 mmHg) or changes in heart rate (+0.3 bpm).

Effects in Vasospastic Angina: In a double-blind, placebo-controlled clinical trial of 4 weeks duration in 50 patients, NORVASC therapy decreased attacks by approximately 4/week compared with a placebo decrease of approximately 1/week ($p<0.01$). Two of 23 NORVASC and 7 of 27 placebo patients discontinued from the study due to lack of clinical improvement.

INDICATIONS AND USAGE

1. Hypertension

NORVASC is indicated for the treatment of hypertension. It may be used alone or in combination with other antihypertensive agents.

2. Chronic Stable Angina

NORVASC is indicated for the treatment of chronic stable angina. NORVASC may be used alone or in combination with other antianginal agents.

3. Vasospastic Angina (Prinzmetal's or Variant Angina)

NORVASC is indicated for the treatment of confirmed or suspected vasospastic angina. NORVASC may be used as monotherapy or in combination with other antianginal drugs.

CONTRAINDICATIONS

NORVASC is contraindicated in patients with known sensitivity to amlodipine.

WARNINGS

Increased Angina and/or Myocardial Infarction: Rarely, patients, particularly those with severe obstructive coronary artery disease, have developed documented increased frequency, duration and/or severity of angina or acute myocardial infarction on starting calcium channel blocker therapy or at the time of dosage increase. The mechanism of this effect has not been elucidated.

PRECAUTIONS

General: Since the vasodilation induced by NORVASC is gradual in onset, acute hypotension has rarely been reported after oral administration of NORVASC. Nonetheless, caution should be exercised when administering NORVASC as with any other peripheral vasodilator particularly in patients with severe aortic stenosis.

Use in Patients with Congestive Heart Failure: In general, calcium channel blockers should be used with caution in patients with heart failure. NORVASC (5-10 mg per day) has been studied in a placebo-controlled trial of 1153 patients with NYHA Class III or IV heart failure (see CLINICAL PHARMACOLOGY) on stable doses of ACE inhibitor, digoxin, and diuretics. Follow-up was at least 6 months, with a mean of about 14 months. There was no overall adverse effect on survival or cardiac morbidity (as defined by life-threatening arrhythmia, acute myocardial infarction, or hospitalization for worsened heart failure). NORVASC has been compared to placebo in four 8-12 week studies of patients with NYHA class II/III heart failure, involving a total of 697 patients. In these studies, there was no evidence of worsened heart failure based on measures of exercise tolerance, NYHA classification, symptoms, or LVEF.

Beta-Blocker Withdrawal: NORVASC is not a beta-blocker and therefore gives no protection against the dangers of abrupt beta-blocker withdrawal; any such withdrawal should be by gradual reduction of the dose of beta-blocker.

Patients with Hepatic Failure: Since NORVASC is extensively metabolized by the liver and the plasma elimination half-life (t 1/2) is 56 hours in patients with impaired hepatic function, caution should be exercised when administering NORVASC to patients with severe hepatic impairment.

Drug Interactions: *In vitro* data in human plasma indicate that NORVASC has no effect on the protein binding of drugs tested (digoxin, phenytoin, warfarin, and indomethacin).

Special Studies: Effect of other agents on NORVASC.

CIMETIDINE: Co-administration of NORVASC with cimetidine did not alter the pharmacokinetics of NORVASC.

GRAPEFRUIT JUICE: Co-administration of 240 mL of grapefruit juice with a single oral dose of amlodipine 10 mg in 20 healthy volunteers had no significant effect on the pharmacokinetics of amlodipine.

MAALOX (antacid): Co-administration of the antacid Maalox with a single dose of NORVASC had no significant effect on the pharmacokinetics of NORVASC.

SILDENAFIL: A single 100 mg dose of sildenafil (Viagra®) in subjects with essential hypertension had no effect on the pharmacokinetic parameters of NORVASC. When NORVASC and sildenafil were used in combination, each agent independently exerted its own blood pressure lowering effect.

Special Studies: Effect of NORVASC on other agents.

ATORVASTATIN: Co-administration of multiple 10 mg doses of NORVASC with 80 mg of atorvastatin resulted in no significant change in the steady state pharmacokinetic parameters of atorvastatin.

DIGOXIN: Co-administration of NORVASC with digoxin did not change serum digoxin levels or digoxin renal clearance in normal volunteers.

ETHANOL (alcohol): Single and multiple 10 mg doses of NORVASC had no significant effect on the pharmacokinetics of ethanol.

WARFARIN: Co-administration of NORVASC with warfarin did not change the warfarin prothrombin response time.

In clinical trials, NORVASC has been safely administered with thiazide diuretics, beta-blockers, angiotensin-converting enzyme inhibitors, long-acting nitrates, sublingual nitroglycerin, digoxin, warfarin, non-steroidal anti-inflammatory drugs, antibiotics, and oral hypoglycemic drugs.

Drug/Laboratory Test Interactions: None known.

Carcinogenesis, Mutagenesis, Impairment of Fertility: Rats and mice treated with amlodipine in the diet for two years, at concentrations calculated to provide daily dosage levels of 0.5, 1.25, and 2.5 mg/kg/day showed no evidence of carcinogenicity. The highest dose (for mice, similar to, and for rats twice* the maximum recommended clinical dose of 10 mg on a mg/m^2 basis) was close to the maximum tolerated dose for mice but not for rats.

Mutagenicity studies revealed no drug related effects at either the gene or chromosome levels.

There was no effect on the fertility of rats treated with amlodipine (males for 64 days and females 14 days prior to mating) at doses up to 10 mg/kg/day (8 times* the maximum recommended human dose of 10 mg on a mg/m^2 basis).

Pregnancy Category C: No evidence of teratogenicity or other embryo/fetal toxicity was found when pregnant rats or rabbits were treated orally with up to 10 mg/kg amlodipine (respectively 8 times* and 23 times* the maximum recommended human dose of 10 mg on a mg/m^2 basis) during their respective periods of major organogenesis. However, litter size was significantly decreased (by about 50%) and the number of intrauterine deaths was significantly increased (about 5-fold) in rats administered 10 mg/kg amlodipine for 14 days before mating and throughout mating and gestation. Amlodipine has been shown to prolong both the gestation period and the duration of labor in rats at this dose. There are no adequate and well-controlled studies in pregnant women. Amlodipine should be used during pregnancy only if the potential benefit justifies the potential risk to the fetus.

*Based on patient weight of 50 kg.

Nursing Mothers: It is not known whether amlodipine is excreted in human milk. In the absence of this information, it is recommended that nursing be discontinued while NORVASC is administered.

Pediatric Use: The effect of NORVASC on blood pressure in patients less than 6 years of age is not known.

Geriatric Use: Clinical studies of NORVASC did not include sufficient numbers of subjects aged 65 and over to determine whether they respond differently from younger subjects. Other reported clinical experience has not identified differences in responses between the elderly and younger patients. In general, dose selection for an elderly patient should be cautious, usually starting at the low end of the dosing range, reflecting the greater frequency of decreased hepatic, renal, or cardiac function, and of concomitant disease or other drug therapy. Elderly patients have decreased clearance of amlodipine with a resulting increase of AUC of approximately 40-60%, and a lower initial dose may be required (see **DOSAGE AND ADMINISTRATION**).

ADVERSE REACTIONS

NORVASC has been evaluated for safety in more than 11,000 patients in U.S. and foreign clinical trials. In general, treatment with NORVASC was well-tolerated at doses up to 10 mg daily. Most adverse reactions reported during therapy with NORVASC were of mild or moderate severity. In controlled clinical trials directly comparing NORVASC (N=1730) in doses up to 10 mg to placebo (N=1250), discontinuation of NORVASC due to adverse reactions was required in only about 1.5% of patients and was not significantly different from placebo (about 1%). The most common side effects are headache and edema. The incidence (%) of side effects which occurred in a dose related manner are as follows:

Adverse Event	2.5 mg N=275	5.0 mg N=296	10.0 mg N=268	Placebo N=520
Edema	1.8	3.0	10.8	0.6
Dizziness	1.1	3.4	3.4	1.5
Flushing	0.7	1.4	2.6	0.0
Palpitation	0.7	1.4	4.5	0.6

Other adverse experiences which were not clearly dose related but which were reported with an incidence greater than 1.0% in placebo-controlled clinical trials include the following:

Placebo-Controlled Studies

	NORVASC (%) (N=1730)	PLACEBO (%) (N=1250)
Headache	7.3	7.8
Fatigue	4.5	2.8
Nausea	2.9	1.9
Abdominal Pain	1.6	0.3
Somnolence	1.4	0.6

For several adverse experiences that appear to be drug and dose related, there was a greater incidence in women than men associated with amlodipine treatment as shown in the following table:

ADR	NORVASC M=% (N=1218)	NORVASC F=% (N=512)	PLACEBO M=% (N=914)	PLACEBO F=% (N=336)
Edema	5.6	14.6	1.4	5.1
Flushing	1.5	4.5	0.3	0.9
Palpitations	1.4	3.3	0.9	0.9
Somnolence	1.3	1.6	0.8	0.3

The following events occurred in ≤1% but >0.1% of patients in controlled clinical trials or under conditions of open trials or marketing experience where a causal relationship is uncertain; they are listed to alert the physician to a possible relationship:

Cardiovascular: arrhythmia (including ventricular tachycardia and atrial fibrillation), bradycardia, chest pain, hypotension, peripheral ischemia, syncope, tachycardia, postural dizziness, postural hypotension, vasculitis.

Central and Peripheral Nervous System: hypoesthesia, neuropathy peripheral, paresthesia, tremor, vertigo.

Gastrointestinal: anorexia, constipation, dyspepsia,** dysphagia, diarrhea, flatulence, pancreatitis, vomiting, gingival hyperplasia.

General: allergic reaction, asthenia,** back pain, hot flushes, malaise, pain, rigors, weight gain, weight decrease.

Musculoskeletal System: arthralgia, arthrosis, muscle cramps,** myalgia.

Psychiatric: sexual dysfunction (male** and female), insomnia, nervousness, depression, abnormal dreams, anxiety, depersonalization.

Respiratory System: dyspnea,** epistaxis.

Skin and Appendages: angioedema, erythema multiforme, pruritus,** rash,** rash erythematous, rash maculopapular.

**These events occurred in less than 1% in placebo-controlled trials, but the incidence of these side effects was between 1% and 2% in all multiple dose studies.

Special Senses: abnormal vision, conjunctivitis, diplopia, eye pain, tinnitus.

Urinary System: micturition frequency, micturition disorder, nocturia.

Autonomic Nervous System: dry mouth, sweating increased.

Metabolic and Nutritional: hyperglycemia, thirst.

Hemopoietic: leukopenia, purpura, thrombocytopenia.

The following events occurred in ≤0.1% of patients: cardiac failure, pulse irregularity, extrasystoles, skin discoloration, urticaria, skin dryness, alopecia, dermatitis, muscle weakness, twitching, ataxia, hypertonia, migraine, cold and clammy skin, apathy, agitation, amnesia, gastritis, increased appetite, loose stools, coughing, rhinitis, dysuria, polyuria, parosmia, taste perversion, abnormal visual accommodation, and xerophthalmia.

Other reactions occurred sporadically and cannot be distinguished from medications or concurrent disease states such as myocardial infarction and angina.

NORVASC therapy has not been associated with clinically significant changes in routine laboratory tests. No clinically relevant changes were noted in serum potassium, serum glucose, total triglycerides, total cholesterol, HDL cholesterol, uric acid, blood urea nitrogen, or creatinine.

The following postmarketing event has been reported infrequently where a causal relationship is uncertain: gynecomastia. In postmarketing experience, jaundice and hepatic enzyme elevations (mostly consistent with cholestasis or hepatitis) in some cases severe enough to require hospitalization have been reported in association with use of amlodipine.

NORVASC has been used safely in patients with chronic obstructive pulmonary disease, well-compensated congestive heart failure, peripheral vascular disease, diabetes mellitus, and abnormal lipid profiles.

OVERDOSAGE

Single oral doses of 40 mg/kg and 100 mg/kg in mice and rats, respectively, caused deaths. A single oral dose of 4 mg/kg or higher in dogs caused a marked peripheral vasodilation and hypotension.

Overdosage might be expected to cause excessive peripheral vasodilation with marked hypotension and possibly a reflex tachycardia. In humans, experience with intentional overdosage of NORVASC is limited. Reports of intentional overdosage include a patient who ingested 250 mg and was asymptomatic and was not hospitalized; another (120 mg) was hospitalized, underwent gastric lavage and remained normotensive; the third (105 mg) was hospitalized and had hypotension (90/50 mmHg) which normalized following plasma expansion. A patient who took 70 mg amlodipine and an unknown quantity of benzodiazepine in a suicide attempt developed shock which was refractory to treatment and died the following day with abnormally high benzodiazepine plasma concentration. A case of accidental drug overdose has been documented in a 19-month-old male who ingested 30 mg amlodipine (about 2 mg/kg). During the emergency room presentation, vital signs were stable with no evidence of hypotension, but a heart rate of 180 bpm. Ipecac was administered 3.5 hours after ingestion and on subsequent observation (overnight) no sequelae were noted.

If massive overdose should occur, active cardiac and respiratory monitoring should be instituted. Frequent blood pressure measurements are essential. Should hypotension occur, cardiovascular support including elevation of the extremities and the judicious administration of fluids should be initiated. If hypotension remains unresponsive to these conservative measures, administration of vasopressors (such as phenylephrine) should be considered with attention to circulating volume and urine output. Intravenous calcium gluconate may help to reverse the effects of calcium entry blockade. As NORVASC is highly protein bound, hemodialysis is not likely to be of benefit.

DOSAGE AND ADMINISTRATION

Adults: The usual initial antihypertensive oral dose of NORVASC is 5 mg once daily with a maximum dose of 10 mg once daily. Small, fragile, or elderly individuals, or patients with hepatic insufficiency may be started on 2.5 mg once daily and this dose may be used when adding NORVASC to other antihypertensive therapy.

Dosage should be adjusted according to each patient's need. In general, titration should proceed over 7 to 14 days so that the physician can fully assess the patient's response to each dose level. Titration may proceed more rapidly, however, if clinically warranted, provided the patient is assessed frequently.

The recommended dose for chronic stable or vasospastic angina is 5-10 mg, with the lower dose suggested in the elderly and in patients with hepatic insufficiency. Most patients will require 10 mg for adequate effect. See ADVERSE REACTIONS section for information related to dosage and side effects.

Children: The effective antihypertensive oral dose in pediatric patients ages 6-17 years is 2.5 mg to 5 mg once daily. Doses in excess of 5 mg daily have not been studied in pediatric patients. See **CLINICAL PHARMACOLOGY.**

Co-administration with Other Antihypertensive and/or Antianginal Drugs: NORVASC has been safely administered with thiazides, ACE inhibitors, beta-blockers, long-acting nitrates, and/or sublingual nitroglycerin.

HOW SUPPLIED

NORVASC®—2.5 mg Tablets (amlodipine besylate equivalent to 2.5 mg of amlodipine per tablet) are supplied as white, diamond, flat-faced, beveled edged engraved with "NORVASC" on one side and "2.5" on the other side and supplied as follows:

NDC 0069-1520-68	Bottle of 90

NORVASC®—5 mg Tablets (amlodipine besylate equivalent to 5 mg of amlodipine per tablet) are white, elongated octagon, flat-faced, beveled edged engraved with both "NORVASC" and "5" on one side and plain on the other side and supplied as follows:

NDC 0069-1530-68	Bottle of 90
NDC 0069-1530-41	Unit Dose package of 100
NDC 0069-1530-72	Bottle of 300

NORVASC®—10 mg Tablets (amlodipine besylate equivalent to 10 mg of amlodipine per tablet) are white, round, flat-faced, beveled edged engraved with both "NORVASC" and "10" on one side and plain on the other side and supplied as follows:

NDC 0069-1540-68	Bottle of 90
NDC 0069-1540-41	Unit Dose package of 100

Store bottles at controlled room temperature, 59° to 86°F (15° to 30°C) and dispense in tight, light-resistant containers (USP).

Rx only

Pfizer Labs
Division of Pfizer Inc, NY, NY 10017
70-4782-00-1
Revised June 2003

Buffered PFIZERPEN® ℞

[*fizər pĕn*]
(penicillin G potassium)
for Injection

Prescribing information for this product, which appears on pages 2617–2618 of the 2004 PDR, has been completely revised as follows. Please write "See Supplement A" next to the product heading.

To reduce the development of drug-resistant bacteria and maintain the effectiveness of Pfizerpen® and other antibacterial drugs, Pfizerpen should be used only to treat or prevent infections that are proven or strongly suspected to be caused by bacteria.

DESCRIPTION

Buffered Pfizerpen (penicillin G potassium) for Injection is a sterile, pyrogen-free powder for reconstitution. Buffered Pfizerpen for Injection is an antibacterial agent for intramuscular, continuous intravenous drip, intrapleural or other local infusion, and intrathecal administration.

Each million units contains approximately 6.8 milligrams of sodium (0.3 mEq) and 65.6 milligrams of potassium (1.68 mEq).

Chemically, Pfizerpen is monopotassium 3,3-dimethyl-7-oxo-6-(2-phenylacetamido)-4-thia-1-azabicyclo (3.2.0) heptane-2-carboxylate. It has a molecular weight of 372.48 and the following chemical structure:

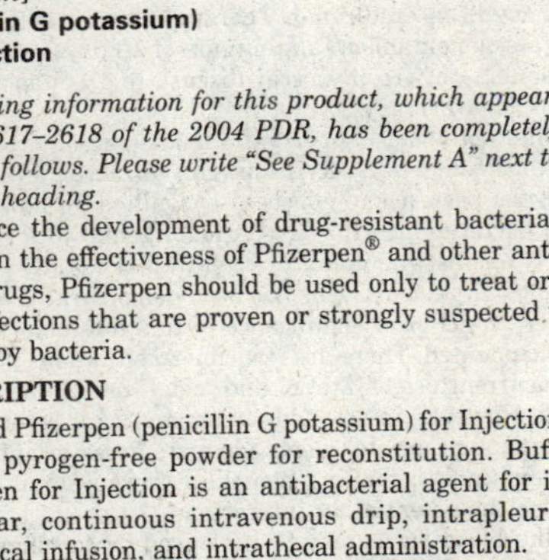

Formula
$C_{16}H_{17}KN_2O_4S$

Penicillin G potassium is a colorless or white crystal, or a white crystalline powder which is odorless, or practically so, and moderately hygroscopic. Penicillin G potassium is very soluble in water. The pH of the reconstituted product is between 6.0–8.5.

CLINICAL PHARMACOLOGY

Aqueous penicillin G is rapidly absorbed following both intramuscular and subcutaneous injection. Initial blood levels following parenteral administration are high but transient. Penicillins bind to serum proteins, mainly albumin. Therapeutic levels of the penicillins are easily achieved under normal circumstances in extracellular fluid and most other body tissues. Penicillins are distributed in varying degrees into pleural, pericardial, peritoneal, ascitic, synovial, and interstitial fluids. Penicillins are excreted in breast milk. Penetration into the cerebrospinal fluid, eyes, and prostate is poor. Penicillins are rapidly excreted in the urine by glomerular filtration and active tubular secretion, primarily as unchanged drug. Approximately 60 percent of the total dose of 300,000 units is excreted in the urine within this 5-hour period. For this reason, high and frequent doses are required to maintain the elevated serum levels desirable in treating certain severe infections in individuals with normal kidney function. In neonates and young infants, and in individuals with impaired kidney function, excretion is considerably delayed.

Microbiology

Penicillin G exerts a bactericidal action against penicillin-susceptible microorganisms during the stage of active multiplication. It acts through the inhibition of biosynthesis of cell wall mucopeptide rendering the cell wall osmotically unstable. It is not active against the penicillinase-producing bacteria, which include many strains of staphylococci. While *in vitro* studies have demonstrated the susceptibility of most strains of the following organisms, clinical efficacy for infections other than those included in the INDICATIONS AND USAGE section has not been documented. Penicillin G exerts high *in vitro* activity against staphylococci (except penicillinase-producing strains), streptococci (groups A, C, G, H, L, and M), and pneumococci. Other organisms susceptible to penicillin G are *N. gonorrhoeae, Corynebacterium diphtheriae, Bacillus anthracis,* Clostridia, *Actinomyces bovis, Streptobacillus moniliformis, Listeria monocytogenes* and Leptospira. *Treponema pallidum* is extremely sensitive to the bactericidal action of penicillin G. Some species of gram-negative bacilli are sensitive to moderate to high concentrations of the drug obtained with intravenous administration. These include most strains of *Escherichia coli;* all strains of *Proteus mirabilis,* Salmonella and Shigella; and some strains of *Aerobacter aerogenes* and *Alcaligenes faecalis.*

Penicillin acts synergistically with gentamicin or tobramycin against many strains of enterococci.

Susceptibility Testing: Penicillin G Susceptibility Powder or 10 units Penicillin G Susceptibility Discs may be used to determine microbial susceptibility to penicillin G using one of the following standard methods recommended by the National Committee for Laboratory Standards:

M2-A3, "Performance Standards for Antimicrobial Disk Susceptibility Tests"
M7-A, "Methods for Dilution Antimicrobial Susceptibility Tests for Bacteria that Grow Aerobically"
M11-A, "Reference Agar Dilution Procedure for Antimicrobial Susceptibility Testing of Anaerobic Bacteria"
M17-P, "Alternative Methods for Antimicrobial Susceptibility Testing of Anaerobic Bacteria"

Tests should be interpreted by the following criteria:
[See first table at top of next page]
[See second table at top of next page]

Interpretations of susceptible, intermediate, and resistant correlate zone size diameters with MIC values. A laboratory report of "susceptible" indicates that the suspected causative microorganism most likely will respond to therapy with penicillin G. A laboratory report of "resistant" indicates that the infecting microorganism most likely will not respond to therapy. A laboratory report of "moderately susceptible" indicates that the microorganism is most likely susceptible if a high dosage of penicillin G is used, or if the infection is such that high levels of penicillin G may be attained, as in urine. A report of "intermediate" using the disk diffusion method may be considered an equivocal result, and dilution tests may be indicated.

Control organisms are recommended for susceptibility testing. Each time the test is performed the following organisms should be included. The range for zones of inhibition is shown below:

Control Organism	Zone of Inhibition Range
Staphylococcus aureus (ATCC 25923)	27-35

INDICATIONS AND USAGE

Aqueous penicillin G (parenteral) is indicated in the therapy of severe infections caused by penicillin G-susceptible microorganisms when rapid and high penicillin levels are required in the conditions listed below. Therapy should be guided by bacteriological studies (including susceptibility tests) and by clinical response.

The following infections will usually respond to adequate dosage of aqueous penicillin G (parenteral):

Streptococcal infections.

NOTE: Streptococci in groups A, C, H, G, L, and M are very sensitive to penicillin G. Some group D organisms are sensitive to the high serum levels obtained with aqueous penicillin G.

Continued on next page

Pfizerpen—Cont.

Aqueous penicillin G (parenteral) is the penicillin dosage form of choice for bacteremia, empyema, severe pneumonia, pericarditis, endocarditis, meningitis, and other severe infections caused by sensitive strains of the gram-positive species listed above.

Pneumococcal infections.
Staphylococcal infections–penicillin G sensitive.
Other infections:
Anthrax.
Actinomycosis.
Clostridial infections (including tetanus).
Diphtheria (to prevent carrier state).
Erysipeloid (*Erysipelothrix insidiosa*) endocarditis.
Fusospirochetal infections—severe infections of the oropharynx (Vincent's), lower respiratory tract and genital area due to *Fusobacterium fusiformisans* spirochetes.
Gram-negative bacillary infections (bacteremias)–(*E. coli, A. aerogenes, A. faecalis,* Salmonella, Shigella and *P. mirabilis*).
Listeria infections (*Listeria monocytogenes*).
Meningitis and endocarditis.
Pasteurella infections (*Pasteurella multocida*).
Bacteremia and meningitis.
Rat-bite fever (*Spirillum minus* or *Streptobacillus moniliformis*).
Gonorrheal endocarditis and arthritis (*N. gonorrhoeae*).
Syphilis (*T. pallidum*) including congenital syphilis.
Meningococcic meningitis.

Although no controlled clinical efficacy studies have been conducted, aqueous crystalline penicillin G for injection and penicillin G procaine suspension have been suggested by the American Heart Association and the American Dental Association for use as part of a combined parenteral-oral regimen for prophylaxis against bacterial endocarditis in patients with congenital heart disease or rheumatic, or other acquired valvular heart disease when they undergo dental procedures and surgical procedures of the upper respiratory tract.[1] Since it may happen that *alpha* hemolytic streptococci relatively resistant to penicillin may be found when patients are receiving continuous oral penicillin for secondary prevention of rheumatic fever, prophylactic agents other than penicillin may be chosen for these patients and prescribed in addition to their continuous rheumatic fever prophylactic regimen.

NOTE: When selecting antibiotics for the prevention of bacterial endocarditis, the physician or dentist should read the full joint statement of the American Heart Association and the American Dental Association.[1]

To reduce the development of drug-resistant bacteria and maintain effectiveness of Pfizerpen and other antibacterial drugs, Pfizerpen should be used only to treat or prevent infections that are proven or strongly suspected to be caused by susceptible bacteria. When culture and susceptibility information are available, they should be considered in selecting or modifying antibacterial therapy. In the absence of such data, local epidemiology and susceptibility patterns may contribute to the empiric selection of therapy.

CONTRAINDICATIONS

A history of a previous hypersensitivity reaction to any penicillin is a contraindication.

WARNINGS

Serious and occasionally fatal hypersensitivity (anaphylactoid) reactions have been reported in patients on penicillin therapy. These reactions are more likely to occur in individuals with a history of penicillin hypersensitivity and/or a history of sensitivity to multiple allergens. There have been reports of individuals with a history of penicillin hypersensitivity who have experienced severe reactions when treated with cephalosporins. Before initiating therapy with any penicillin, careful inquiry should be made concerning previous hypersensitivity reactions to penicillin, cephalosporins, or other allergens. If an allergic reaction occurs, the drug should be discontinued and the appropriate therapy instituted. Serious anaphylactoid reactions require immediate emergency treatment with epinephrine. Oxygen, intravenous steroids, and airway management including intubation, should also be administered as indicated.

PRECAUTIONS

General: Penicillin should be used with caution in individuals with histories of significant allergies and/or asthma.

Prescribing Pfizerpen in the absence of proven or strongly suspected bacterial infection or a prophylactic indication is unlikely to provide benefit to the patient and increases the risk of the development of drug-resistant bacteria.

Information for Patients: Patients should be counseled that antibacterial drugs including Pfizerpen should only be used to treat bacterial infections. They do not treat viral infections (e.g., the common cold). When Pfizerpen is prescribed to treat a bacterial infection, patients should be told that although it is common to feel better early in the course of therapy, the medication should be taken exactly as directed. Skipping doses or not completing the full course of therapy may (1) decrease the effectiveness of the immediate treatment and (2) increase the likelihood that bacteria will develop resistance and will not be treatable by Pfizerpen or other antibacterial drugs in the future.

Intramuscular Therapy: Care should be taken to avoid intravenous or accidental intraarterial administration, or injection into or near major peripheral nerves or blood vessels, since such injections may produce neurovascular damage.

Zone Diameter, nearest whole mm	Susceptible	Moderately Susceptible	Resistant
Staphylococci	≥29	—	≤28
N. gonorrhoeae	≥20	—	≤19
Enterococci	—	≥15	≤14
Non-enterococcal streptococci and *L. monocytogenes*	≥28	20-27	≤19

Approximate MIC Correlates	Susceptible	Resistant
Staphylococci	≤0.1 μg/mL	β-lactamase
N. gonorrhoeae	≤0.1 μg/mL	β-lactamase
Enterococci	—	≥16 μg/mL
Non-enterococcal streptococci and *L. monocytogenes*	≤0.12 μg/mL	≥ 4 μg/mL

Particular care should be taken with IV administration because of the possibility of thrombophlebitis.

In streptococcal infections, therapy must be sufficient to eliminate the organism (10 days minimum), otherwise the sequelae of streptococcal disease may occur. Cultures should be taken following the completion of treatment to determine whether streptococci have been eradicated.

The use of antibiotics may result in overgrowth of nonsusceptible organisms. Constant observation of the patient is essential. If new infections due to bacteria or fungi appear during therapy, the drug should be discontinued and appropriate measures taken. Whenever allergic reactions occur, penicillin should be withdrawn unless, in the opinion of the physician, the condition being treated is life threatening and amenable only to penicillin therapy.

Aqueous penicillin G by the intravenous route in high doses (above 10 million units) should be administered slowly because of the adverse effects of electrolyte imbalance from either the potassium or sodium content of the penicillin. Penicillin G potassium contains 1.7 mEq potassium and 0.3 mEq sodium per million units. The patient's renal, cardiac, and vascular status should be evaluated and if impairment of function is suspected or known to exist a reduction in the total dosage should be considered. Frequent evaluation of electrolyte balance, renal and hematopoietic function is recommended during therapy when high doses of intravenous aqueous penicillin G are used.

Laboratory Tests: In prolonged therapy with penicillin, periodic evaluation of the renal, hepatic, and hematopoietic systems is recommended for organ system dysfunction. This is particularly important in prematures, neonates and other infants, and when high doses are used.

Positive Coomb's tests have been reported after large intravenous doses.

Monitor serum potassium and implement corrective measures when necessary.

When treating gonococcal infections in which primary and secondary syphilis are suspected, proper diagnostic procedures, including dark field examinations, should be done before receiving penicillin and monthly serological tests made for at least four months. All cases of penicillin treated syphilis should receive clinical and serological examinations every six months for two to three years.

In suspected staphylococcal infections, proper laboratory studies, including susceptibility tests, should be performed.

In streptococcal infections, cultures should be taken following completion of treatment to determine whether streptococci have been eradicated. Therapy must be sufficient to eliminate the organism (a minimum of 10 days), otherwise the sequelae of streptococcal disease (e.g., endocarditis, rheumatic fever) may occur.

Drug Interactions: Concurrent administration of bacteriostatic antibiotics (e.g., erythromycin, tetracycline) may diminish the bactericidal effects of penicillins by slowing the rate of bacterial growth. Bactericidal agents work most effectively against the immature cell wall of rapidly proliferating microorganisms. This has been demonstrated *in vitro;* however, the clinical significance of this interaction is not well documented. There are few clinical situations in which the concurrent use of "static" and "cidal" antibiotics are indicated. However, in selected circumstances in which such therapy is appropriate, using adequate doses of antibacterial agents and beginning penicillin therapy first, should minimize the potential for interaction.

Penicillin blood levels may be prolonged by concurrent administration of probenecid which blocks the renal tubular secretion of penicillins.

Displacement of penicillin from plasma protein binding sites will elevate the level of free penicillin in the serum.

Carcinogenesis, Mutagenesis, Impairment of Fertility: No information on long-term studies are available on the carcinogenesis, mutagenesis, or the impairment of fertility with the use of penicillins.

Pregnancy Category B–*Teratogenic Effects:* Reproduction studies performed in the mouse, rat, and rabbit have revealed no evidence of impaired fertility or harm to the fetus due to penicillin G. Human experience with the penicillins during pregnancy has not shown any positive evidence of adverse effects on the fetus. There are, however, no adequate and well controlled studies in pregnant women showing conclusively that harmful effects of these drugs on the fetus can be excluded. Because animal reproduction studies are not always predictive of human response, this drug should be used during pregnancy only if clearly needed.

Nursing Mothers: Penicillins are excreted in human milk. Caution should be exercised when penicillin G is administered to a nursing woman.

Pediatric Use: Penicillins are excreted largely unchanged by the kidney. Because of incompletely developed renal function in infants, the rate of elimination will be slow. Use caution in administering to newborns and evaluate organ system function frequently.

ADVERSE REACTIONS

Penicillin is a substance of low toxicity but does have a significant index of sensitization. The following hypersensitivity reactions have been reported: skin rashes ranging from maculopapular eruptions to exfoliative dermatitis; urticaria; and reactions resembling serum sickness, including chills, fever, edema, arthralgia and prostration. Severe and occasionally fatal anaphylaxis has occurred (see WARNINGS).

Hemolytic anemia, leucopenia, thrombocytopenia, nephropathy, and neuropathy are rarely observed adverse reactions and are usually associated with high intravenous dosage.

Patients given continuous intravenous therapy with penicillin G potassium in high dosage (10 million to 100 million units daily) may suffer severe or even fatal potassium poisoning, particularly if renal insufficiency is present. Hyperreflexia, convulsions, and coma may be indicative of this syndrome.

Cardiac arrhythmias and cardiac arrest may also occur. (High dosage of penicillin G sodium may result in congestive heart failure due to high sodium intake.)

The Jarisch-Herxheimer reaction has been reported in patients treated for syphilis.

OVERDOSAGE

Neurological adverse reactions, including convulsions, may occur with the attainment of high CSF levels of beta-lactams. In case of overdosage, discontinue medication, treat symptomatically, and institute supportive measures as required.

Penicillin G potassium is hemodialyzable.

DOSAGE AND ADMINISTRATION

Severe infections due to Susceptible Strains of Streptococci, Pneumococci, and Staphylococci–bacteremia, pneumonia, endocarditis, pericarditis, empyema, meningitis, and other severe infections–a minimum of 5 million units daily.

Syphilis–Aqueous penicillin G may be used in the treatment of acquired and congenital syphilis, but because of the necessity of frequent dosage, hospitalization is recommended. Dosage and duration of therapy will be determined by age of patient and stage of the disease.

Gonorrheal endocarditis–a minimum of 5 million units daily.

Meningococcic meningitis–1-2 million units intramuscularly every 2 hours, or continuous IV drip of 20-30 million units/day.

Actinomycosis–1-6 million units/day for cervicofacial cases; 10–20 million units/day for thoracic and abdominal disease.

Clostridial infections–20 million units/day; penicillin is adjunctive therapy to antitoxin.

Fusospirochetal infections–severe infections of oropharynx, lower respiratory tract, and genital area–5-10 million units/day.

Rat-bite fever (Spirillum minus or *Streptobacillus moniliformis)*–12-15 million units/day for 3-4 weeks.

Listeria infections (Listeria monocytogenes)
Neonates–500,000 to 1 million units/day.
Adults with meningitis–15-20 million units/day for 2 weeks.
Adults with endocarditis–15-20 million units/day for 4 weeks.

Pasteurella infections (Pasteurella multocida)
Bacteremia and meningitis–4-6 million units/day for 2 weeks.

Erysipeloid (Erysipelothrix insidiosa)
Endocarditis–2-20 million units/day for 4-6 weeks.

Gram-negative bacillary infections (E. coli, Enterobacter aerogenes, A. faecalis, Salmonella, Shigella and *Proteus mirabilis)*
Bacteremia–20-80 million units/day.

Diphtheria (carrier state)–300,000–400,000 units of penicillin/day in divided doses for 10-12 days.

Approx. Desired Concentration (units/mL)	Approx. Volume (mL) 1,000,000 units	Solvent for Vial of 5,000,000 units	Infusion Only 20,000,000 units
50,000	20.0	—	—
100,000	10.0	—	—
250,000	4.0	18.2	75.0
500,000	1.8	8.2	33.0
750,000	—	4.8	—
1,000,000	—	3.2	11.5

Anthrax–A minimum of 5 million units of penicillin/day in divided doses until cure is effected.

For prophylaxis against bacterial endocarditis[1] in patients with congenital heart disease or rheumatic or other acquired valvular heart disease, when undergoing dental procedures or surgical procedures of the upper respiratory tract, use a combined parenteral-oral regimen. One million units of aqueous crystalline penicillin G (30,000 units/kg in children) intramuscularly, mixed with 600,000 units procaine penicillin G (600,000 units for children) should be given one-half to one hour before the procedure. Oral penicillin V (phenoxymethyl penicillin), 500 mg for adults or 250 mg for children less than 60 lb, should be given every 6 hours for 8 doses. Doses for children should not exceed recommendations for adults for a single dose or for a 24 hour period.

Reconstitution

The following table shows the amount of solvent required for solution of various concentrations:

[See table above]

When the required volume of solvent is greater than the capacity of the vial, the penicillin can be dissolved by first injecting only a portion of the solvent into the vial, then withdrawing the resultant solution and combining it with the remainder of the solvent in a larger sterile container.

Buffered Pfizerpen (penicillin G potassium) for Injection is highly water soluble. It may be dissolved in small amounts of Water for Injection, or Sterile Isotonic Sodium Chloride Solution for Parenteral Use. All solutions should be stored in a refrigerator. When refrigerated, penicillin solutions may be stored for seven days without significant loss of potency.

Buffered Pfizerpen for Injection may be given intramuscularly or by continuous intravenous drip for dosages of 500,000, 1,000,000, or 5,000,000 units. It is also suitable for intrapleural, intraarticular, and other local instillations.

THE 20,000,000 UNIT DOSAGE MAY BE ADMINISTERED BY INTRAVENOUS INFUSION ONLY.

(1) Intramuscular Injection: Keep total volume of injection small. The intramuscular route is the preferred route of administration. Solutions containing up to 100,000 units of penicillin per mL of diluent may be used with a minimum of discomfort. Greater concentration of penicillin G per mL is physically possible and may be employed where therapy demands. When large dosages are required, it may be advisable to administer aqueous solutions of penicillin by means of continuous intravenous drip.

(2) Continuous Intravenous Drip: Determine the volume of fluid and rate of its administration required by the patient in a 24 hour period in the usual manner for fluid therapy, and add the appropriate daily dosage of penicillin to this fluid. For example, if an adult patient requires 2 liters of fluid in 24 hours and a daily dosage of 10 million units of penicillin, add 5 million units to 1 liter and adjust the rate of flow so the liter will be infused in 12 hours.

(3) Intrapleural or Other Local Infusion: If fluid is aspirated, give infusion in a volume equal to ¼ or ½ the amount of fluid aspirated, otherwise, prepare as for intramuscular injection.

(4) Intrathecal Use: The intrathecal use of penicillin in meningitis must be highly individualized. It should be employed only with full consideration of the possible irritating effects of penicillin when used by this route. The preferred route of therapy in bacterial meningitides is intravenous, supplemented by intramuscular injection.

Parenteral drug products should be inspected visually for particulate matter and discoloration prior to administration, whenever solution and container permit.

Sterile solution may be left in refrigerator for one week without significant loss of potency.

HOW SUPPLIED

Buffered Pfizerpen® (penicillin G potassium) for Injection is available in vials containing respectively 5,000,000 units × 10's (NDC 0049-0520-83) and 20,000,000 units 1's (NDC 0049-0530-28); buffered with sodium citrate and citric acid to an optimum pH.

Each million units contains approximately 6.8 milligrams of sodium (0.3 mEq) and 65.6 milligrams of potassium (1.68 mEq).

Store the dry powder below 86°F (30°C).

Reference

1. American Heart Association, 1977. Prevention of bacterial endocarditis. Circulation. **56**:139A–143A.

Rx only

Pfizer Roerig

Division of Pfizer Inc, NY, NY 10017

70-4209-44-7 Revised September 2003

PROCARDIA XL® ℞

[*pro-car' dē-ă*]

(nifedipine)

Extended Release Tablets

For Oral Use

Prescribing information for this product, which appears on pages 2621–2623 of the 2004 PDR, has been completely revised as follows. Please write "See Supplement A" next to the product heading.

DESCRIPTION

Nifedipine is a drug belonging to a class of pharmacological agents known as the calcium channel blockers. Nifedipine is 3,5-pyridinedicarboxylic acid, 1,4-dihydro-2,6-dimethyl-4-(2-nitrophenyl)-, dimethyl ester, $C_{17}H_{18}N_2O_6$, and has the structural formula:

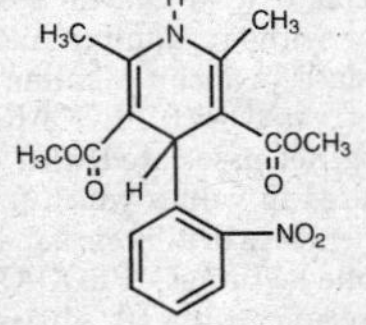

Nifedipine is a yellow crystalline substance, practically insoluble in water but soluble in ethanol. It has a molecular weight of 346.3. PROCARDIA XL is a registered trademark for Nifedipine GITS. Nifedipine GITS (Gastrointestinal Therapeutic System) Tablet is formulated as a once-a-day controlled-release tablet for oral administration designed to deliver 30, 60, or 90 mg of nifedipine.

Inert ingredients in the formulations are: cellulose acetate; hydroxypropyl cellulose; hypromellose; magnesium stearate; polyethylene glycol; polyethylene oxide; red ferric oxide; sodium chloride; titanium dioxide.

System Components and Performance

PROCARDIA XL® Extended Release Tablet is similar in appearance to a conventional tablet. It consists, however, of a semipermeable membrane surrounding an osmotically active drug core. The core itself is divided into two layers: an "active" layer containing the drug, and a "push" layer containing pharmacologically inert (but osmotically active) components. As water from the gastrointestinal tract enters the tablet, pressure increases in the osmotic layer and "pushes" against the drug layer, releasing drug through the precision laser-drilled tablet orifice in the active layer.

PROCARDIA XL Extended Release Tablet is designed to provide nifedipine at an approximately constant rate over 24 hours. This controlled rate of drug delivery into the gastrointestinal lumen is independent of pH or gastrointestinal motility. PROCARDIA XL depends for its action on the existence of an osmotic gradient between the contents of the bi-layer core and fluid in the GI tract. Drug delivery is essentially constant as long as the osmotic gradient remains constant, and then gradually falls to zero. Upon swallowing, the biologically inert components of the tablet remain intact during GI transit and are eliminated in the feces as an insoluble shell.

CLINICAL PHARMACOLOGY

Nifedipine is a calcium ion influx inhibitor (slow-channel blocker or calcium ion antagonist) and inhibits the transmembrane influx of calcium ions into cardiac muscle and smooth muscle. The contractile processes of cardiac muscle and vascular smooth muscle are dependent upon the movement of extracellular calcium ions into these cells through specific ion channels. Nifedipine selectively inhibits calcium ion influx across the cell membrane of cardiac muscle and vascular smooth muscle without altering serum calcium concentrations.

Mechanism of Action

A) Angina

The precise mechanisms by which inhibition of calcium influx relieves angina has not been fully determined, but includes at least the following two mechanisms:

1) Relaxation and Prevention of Coronary Artery Spasm

Nifedipine dilates the main coronary arteries and coronary arterioles, both in normal and ischemic regions, and is a potent inhibitor of coronary artery spasm, whether spontaneous or ergonovine-induced. This property increases myocardial oxygen delivery in patients with coronary artery spasm, and is responsible for the effectiveness of nifedipine in vasospastic (Prinzmetal's or variant) angina. Whether this effect plays any role in classical angina is not clear, but studies of exercise tolerance have not shown an increase in the maximum exercise rate-pressure product, a widely accepted measure of oxygen utilization. This suggests that, in general, relief of spasm or dilation of coronary arteries is not an important factor in classical angina.

2) Reduction of Oxygen Utilization

Nifedipine regularly reduces arterial pressure at rest and at a given level of exercise by dilating peripheral arterioles and reducing the total peripheral vascular resistance (afterload) against which the heart works. This unloading of the heart reduces myocardial energy consumption and oxygen requirements, and probably accounts for the effectiveness of nifedipine in chronic stable angina.

B) Hypertension

The mechanism by which nifedipine reduces arterial blood pressure involves peripheral arterial vasodilatation and the resulting reduction in peripheral vascular resistance. The increased peripheral vascular resistance that is an underlying cause of hypertension results from an increase in active tension in the vascular smooth muscle. Studies have demonstrated that the increase in active tension reflects an increase in cytosolic free calcium.

Nifedipine is a peripheral arterial vasodilator which acts directly on vascular smooth muscle. The binding of nifedipine to voltage-dependent and possibly receptor-operated channels in vascular smooth muscle results in an inhibition of calcium influx through these channels. Stores of intracellular calcium in vascular smooth muscle are limited and thus dependent upon the influx of extracellular calcium for contraction to occur. The reduction in calcium influx by nifedipine causes arterial vasodilation and decreased peripheral vascular resistance which results in reduced arterial blood pressure.

Pharmacokinetics and Metabolism

Nifedipine is completely absorbed after oral administration. Plasma drug concentrations rise at a gradual, controlled rate after a PROCARDIA XL Extended Release Tablet dose and reach a plateau at approximately six hours after the first dose. For subsequent doses, relatively constant plasma concentrations at this plateau are maintained with minimal fluctuations over the 24-hour dosing interval. About a four-fold higher fluctuation index (ratio of peak to trough plasma concentration) was observed with the conventional immediate-release Procardia® capsule at t.i.d. dosing than with once daily PROCARDIA XL Extended Release Tablet. At steady-state the bioavailability of the PROCARDIA XL Extended Release Tablet is 86% relative to Procardia capsules. Administration of the PROCARDIA XL Extended Release Tablet in the presence of food slightly alters the early rate of drug absorption, but does not influence the extent of drug bioavailability. Markedly reduced GI retention time over prolonged periods (i.e., short bowel syndrome), however, may influence the pharmacokinetic profile of the drug which could potentially result in lower plasma concentrations. Pharmacokinetics of PROCARDIA XL Extended Release Tablets are linear over the dose range of 30 to 180 mg in that plasma drug concentrations are proportional to dose administered. There was no evidence of dose dumping either in the presence or absence of food for over 150 subjects in pharmacokinetic studies.

Nifedipine is extensively metabolized to highly water-soluble, inactive metabolites accounting for 60 to 80% of the dose excreted in the urine. The elimination half-life of nifedipine is approximately two hours. Only traces (less than 0.1% of the dose) of unchanged form can be detected in the urine. The remainder is excreted in the feces in metabolized form, most likely as a result of biliary excretion. Thus, the pharmacokinetics of nifedipine are not significantly influenced by the degree of renal impairment. Patients in hemodialysis or chronic ambulatory peritoneal dialysis have not reported significantly altered pharmacokinetics of nifedipine. Since hepatic biotransformation is the predominant route for the disposition of nifedipine, the pharmacokinetics may be altered in patients with chronic liver disease. Patients with hepatic impairment (liver cirrhosis) have a longer disposition half-life and higher bioavailability of nifedipine than healthy volunteers. The degree of serum protein binding of nifedipine is high (92-98%). Protein binding may be greatly reduced in patients with renal or hepatic impairment.

Hemodynamics

Like other slow-channel blockers, nifedipine exerts a negative inotropic effect on isolated myocardial tissue. This is rarely, if ever, seen in intact animals or man, probably because of reflex responses to its vasodilating effects. In man, nifedipine decreases peripheral vascular resistance which leads to a fall in systolic and diastolic pressures, usually minimal in normotensive volunteers (less than 5-10 mm Hg systolic), but sometimes larger. With PROCARDIA XL Extended Release Tablets, these decreases in blood pressure are not accompanied by any significant change in heart rate. Hemodynamic studies in patients with normal ventricular function have generally found a small increase in cardiac index without major effects on ejection fraction, left ventricular end diastolic pressure (LVEDP) or volume (LVEDV). In patients with impaired ventricular function, most acute studies have shown some increase in ejection fraction and reduction in left ventricular filling pressure.

Electrophysiologic Effects

Although, like other members of its class, nifedipine causes a slight depression of sinoatrial node function and atrioventricular conduction in isolated myocardial preparations, such effects have not been seen in studies in intact animals or in man. In formal electrophysiologic studies, predominantly in patients with normal conduction systems, nifedipine has had no tendency to prolong atrioventricular conduction or sinus node recovery time, or to slow sinus rate.

INDICATIONS AND USAGE

I. Vasospastic Angina

Continued on next page

Procardia XL—Cont.

PROCARDIA XL is indicated for the management of vasospastic angina confirmed by any of the following criteria: 1) classical pattern of angina at rest accompanied by ST segment elevation, 2) angina or coronary artery spasm provoked by ergonovine, or 3) angiographically demonstrated coronary artery spasm. In those patients who have had angiography, the presence of significant fixed obstructive disease is not incompatible with the diagnosis of vasospastic angina, provided that the above criteria are satisfied. PROCARDIA XL may also be used where the clinical presentation suggests a possible vasospastic component but where vasospasm has not been confirmed, e.g., where pain has a variable threshold on exertion or in unstable angina where electrocardiographic findings are compatible with intermittent vasospasm, or when angina is refractory to nitrates and/or adequate doses of beta blockers.

II. Chronic Stable Angina
(Classical Effort-Associated Angina)

PROCARDIA XL is indicated for the management of chronic stable angina (effort-associated angina) without evidence of vasospasm in patients who remain symptomatic despite adequate doses of beta blockers and/or organic nitrates or who cannot tolerate those agents.

In chronic stable angina (effort-associated angina) nifedipine has been effective in controlled trials of up to eight weeks duration in reducing angina frequency and increasing exercise tolerance, but confirmation of sustained effectiveness and evaluation of long-term safety in these patients is incomplete.

Controlled studies in small numbers of patients suggest concomitant use of nifedipine and beta-blocking agents may be beneficial in patients with chronic stable angina, but available information is not sufficient to predict with confidence the effects of concurrent treatment, especially in patients with compromised left ventricular function or cardiac conduction abnormalities. When introducing such concomitant therapy, care must be taken to monitor blood pressure closely since severe hypotension can occur from the combined effects of the drugs. (See WARNINGS.)

III. Hypertension

PROCARDIA XL is indicated for the treatment of hypertension. It may be used alone or in combination with other antihypertensive agents.

CONTRAINDICATIONS

Known hypersensitivity reaction to nifedipine.

WARNINGS

Excessive Hypotension

Although in most angina patients the hypotensive effect of nifedipine is modest and well tolerated, occasional patients have had excessive and poorly tolerated hypotension. These responses have usually occurred during initial titration or at the time of subsequent upward dosage adjustment, and may be more likely in patients on concomitant beta blockers.

Severe hypotension and/or increased fluid volume requirements have been reported in patients receiving nifedipine together with a beta-blocking agent who underwent coronary artery bypass surgery using high dose fentanyl anesthesia. The interaction with high dose fentanyl appears to be due to the combination of nifedipine and a beta blocker, but the possibility that it may occur with nifedipine alone, with low doses of fentanyl, in other surgical procedures, or with other narcotic analgesics cannot be ruled out. In nifedipine-treated patients where surgery using high dose fentanyl anesthesia is contemplated, the physician should be aware of these potential problems and if the patient's condition permits, sufficient time (at least 36 hours) should be allowed for nifedipine to be washed out of the body prior to surgery.

The following information should be taken into account in those patients who are being treated for hypertension as well as angina:

Increased Angina and/or Myocardial Infarction

Rarely, patients, particularly those who have severe obstructive coronary artery disease, have developed well documented increased frequency, duration and/or severity of angina or acute myocardial infarction on starting nifedipine or at the time of dosage increase. The mechanism of this effect is not established.

Beta Blocker Withdrawal

It is important to taper beta blockers if possible, rather than stopping them abruptly before beginning nifedipine. Patients recently withdrawn from beta blockers may develop a withdrawal syndrome with increased angina, probably related to increased sensitivity to catecholamines. Initiation of nifedipine treatment will not prevent this occurrence and on occasion has been reported to increase it.

Congestive Heart Failure

Rarely, patients, usually receiving a beta blocker, have developed heart failure after beginning nifedipine. Patients with tight aortic stenosis may be at greater risk for such an event, as the unloading effect of nifedipine would be expected to be of less benefit to those patients, owing to their fixed impedance to flow across the aortic valve.

PRECAUTIONS

General—Hypotension: Because nifedipine decreases peripheral vascular resistance, careful monitoring of blood pressure during the initial administration and titration of nifedipine is suggested. Close observation is especially recommended for patients already taking medications that are known to lower blood pressure. (See WARNINGS.)

Peripheral Edema: Mild to moderate peripheral edema occurs in a dose dependent manner with an incidence ranging from approximately 10% to about 30% at the highest dose studied (180 mg). It is a localized phenomenon thought to be associated with vasodilation of dependent arterioles and small blood vessels and not due to left ventricular dysfunction or generalized fluid retention. With patients whose angina or hypertension is complicated by congestive heart failure, care should be taken to differentiate this peripheral edema from the effects of increasing left ventricular dysfunction.

Other: As with any other non-deformable material, caution should be used when administering PROCARDIA XL in patients with preexisting severe gastrointestinal narrowing (pathologic or iatrogenic). There have been rare reports of obstructive symptoms in patients with known strictures in association with the ingestion of PROCARDIA XL.

Information for Patients: PROCARDIA XL Extended Release Tablets should be swallowed whole. Do not chew, divide or crush tablets. Do not be concerned if you occasionally notice in your stool something that looks like a tablet. In PROCARDIA XL, the medication is contained within a nonabsorbable shell that has been specially designed to slowly release the drug for your body to absorb. When this process is completed, the empty tablet is eliminated from your body.

Laboratory Tests: Rare, usually transient, but occasionally significant elevations of enzymes such as alkaline phosphatase, CPK, LDH, SGOT and SGPT have been noted. The relationship to nifedipine therapy is uncertain in most cases, but probable in some. These laboratory abnormalities have rarely been associated with clinical symptoms; however, cholestasis with or without jaundice has been reported. A small (5.4%) increase in mean alkaline phosphatase was noted in patients treated with PROCARDIA XL. This was an isolated finding not associated with clinical symptoms and it rarely resulted in values which fell outside the normal range. Rare instances of allergic hepatitis have been reported. In controlled studies, PROCARDIA XL did not adversely affect serum uric acid, glucose, or cholesterol. Serum potassium was unchanged in patients receiving PROCARDIA XL in the absence of concomitant diuretic therapy, and slightly decreased in patients receiving concomitant diuretics.

Nifedipine, like other calcium channel blockers, decreases platelet aggregation *in vitro*. Limited clinical studies have demonstrated a moderate but statistically significant decrease in platelet aggregation and an increase in bleeding time in some nifedipine patients. This is thought to be a function of inhibition of calcium transport across the platelet membrane. No clinical significance for these findings has been demonstrated.

Positive direct Coombs test with/without hemolytic anemia has been reported but a causal relationship between nifedipine administration and positivity of this laboratory test, including hemolysis, could not be determined.

Although nifedipine has been used safely in patients with renal dysfunction and has been reported to exert a beneficial effect, in certain cases, rare, reversible elevations in BUN and serum creatinine have been reported in patients with pre-existing chronic renal insufficiency. The relationship to nifedipine therapy is uncertain in most cases but probable in some.

Drug Interactions: Beta-adrenergic blocking agents: (See INDICATIONS AND USAGE and WARNINGS.) Experience in over 1400 patients with Procardia capsules in a noncomparative clinical trial has shown that concomitant administration of nifedipine and beta-blocking agents is usually well tolerated, but there have been occasional literature reports suggesting that the combination may increase the likelihood of congestive heart failure, severe hypotension, or exacerbation of angina.

Long-acting Nitrates: Nifedipine may be safely co-administered with nitrates, but there have been no controlled studies to evaluate the antianginal effectiveness of this combination.

Digitalis: Administration of nifedipine with digoxin increased digoxin levels in nine of twelve normal volunteers. The average increase was 45%. Another investigator found no increase in digoxin levels in thirteen patients with coronary artery disease. In an uncontrolled study of over two hundred patients with congestive heart failure during which digoxin blood levels were not measured, digitalis toxicity was not observed. Since there have been isolated reports of patients with elevated digoxin levels, it is recommended that digoxin levels be monitored when initiating, adjusting, and discontinuing nifedipine to avoid possible over- or under-digitalization.

Coumarin Anticoagulants: There have been rare reports of increased prothrombin time in patients taking coumarin anticoagulants to whom nifedipine was administered. However, the relationship to nifedipine therapy is uncertain.

Cimetidine: A study in six healthy volunteers has shown a significant increase in peak nifedipine plasma levels (80%) and area-under-the-curve (74%), after a one week course of cimetidine at 1000 mg per day and nifedipine at 40 mg per day. Ranitidine produced smaller, non-significant increases. The effect may be mediated by the known inhibition of cimetidine on hepatic cytochrome P-450, the enzyme system probably responsible for the first-pass metabolism of nifedipine. If nifedipine therapy is initiated in a patient currently receiving cimetidine, cautious titration is advised.

Carcinogenesis, Mutagenesis, Impairment of Fertility: Nifedipine was administered orally to rats for two years and was not shown to be carcinogenic. When given to rats prior to mating, nifedipine caused reduced fertility at a dose approximately 30 times the maximum recommended human dose. There is a literature report of reversible reduction in the ability of human sperm obtained from a limited number of infertile men taking recommended doses of nifedipine to bind to and fertilize an ovum *in vitro*. *In vivo* mutagenicity studies were negative.

Pregnancy: Pregnancy Category C: Nifedipine has been shown to produce teratogenic findings in rats and rabbits, including digital anomalies similar to those reported for phenytoin. Digital anomalies have been reported to occur with other members of the dihydropyridine class and are possibly a result of compromised uterine blood flow. Nifedipine administration was associated with a variety of embryotoxic, placentotoxic, and fetotoxic effects, including stunted fetuses (rats, mice, rabbits), rib deformities (mice), cleft palate (mice), small placentas and underdeveloped chorionic villi (monkeys), embryonic and fetal deaths (rats, mice, rabbits), and prolonged pregnancy/decreased neonatal survival (rats; not evaluated in other species). On a mg/kg basis, all of the doses associated with the teratogenic embryotoxic or fetotoxic effects in animals were higher (3.5 to 42 times) than the maximum recommended human dose of 120 mg/day. On a mg/m^2 basis, some doses were higher and some were lower than the maximum recommended human dose but all are within an order of magnitude of it. The doses associated with placentotoxic effects in monkeys were equivalent to or lower than the maximum recommended human dose on a mg/m^2 basis.

There are no adequate and well-controlled studies in pregnant women. PROCARDIA XL Extended Release Tablets should be used during pregnancy only if the potential benefit justifies the potential risk to the fetus.

Pediatric Use: Safety and effectiveness in pediatric patients have not been established.

ADVERSE EXPERIENCES

Over 1000 patients from both controlled and open trials with PROCARDIA XL Extended Release Tablets in hypertension and angina were included in the evaluation of adverse experiences. All side effects reported during PROCARDIA XL Extended Release Tablet therapy were tabulated independent of their causal relation to medication. The most common side effect reported with PROCARDIA XL was edema which was dose related and ranged in frequency from approximately 10% to about 30% at the highest dose studied (180 mg). Other common adverse experiences reported in placebo-controlled trials include:

Adverse Effect	PROCARDIA XL (%) (N=707)	Placebo (%) (N=266)
Headache	15.8	9.8
Fatigue	5.9	4.1
Dizziness	4.1	4.5
Constipation	3.3	2.3
Nausea	3.3	1.9

Of these, only edema and headache were more common in PROCARDIA XL patients than placebo patients.

The following adverse reactions occurred with an incidence of less than 3.0%. With the exception of leg cramps, the incidence of these side effects was similar to that of placebo alone.

Body as a Whole/Systemic: asthenia, flushing, pain
Cardiovascular: palpitations
Central Nervous System: insomnia, nervousness, paresthesia, somnolence
Dermatologic: pruritus, rash
Gastrointestinal: abdominal pain, diarrhea, dry mouth, dyspepsia, flatulence
Musculoskeletal: arthralgia, leg cramps
Respiratory: chest pain (nonspecific), dyspnea
Urogenital: impotence, polyuria

Other adverse reactions were reported sporadically with an incidence of 1.0% or less. These include:

Body as a Whole/Systemic: face edema, fever, hot flashes, malaise, periorbital edema, rigors
Cardiovascular: arrhythmia, hypotension, increased angina, tachycardia, syncope
Central Nervous System: anxiety, ataxia, decreased libido, depression, hypertonia, hypoesthesia, migraine, paroniria, tremor, vertigo
Dermatologic: alopecia, increased sweating, urticaria, purpura
Gastrointestinal: eructation, gastroesophageal reflux, gum hyperplasia, melena, vomiting, weight increase
Musculoskeletal: back pain, gout, myalgias
Respiratory: coughing, epistaxis, upper respiratory tract infection, respiratory disorder, sinusitis
Special Senses: abnormal lacrimation, abnormal vision, taste perversion, tinnitus
Urogenital/Reproductive: breast pain, dysuria, hematuria, nocturia

Adverse experiences which occurred in less than 1 in 1000 patients cannot be distinguished from concurrent disease states or medications.

The following adverse experiences, reported in less than 1% of patients, occurred under conditions (e.g., open trials, marketing experience) where a causal relationship is uncertain: gastrointestinal irritation, gastrointestinal bleeding, gynecomastia.

In multiple-dose U.S. and foreign controlled studies with nifedipine capsules in which adverse reactions were reported spontaneously, adverse effects were frequent but generally not serious and rarely required discontinuation of therapy or dosage adjustment. Most were expected consequences of the vasodilator effects of nifedipine.

Adverse Effect	PROCARDIA CAPSULES (%) (N=226)	Placebo (%) (N=235)
Dizziness, lightheadedness, giddiness	27	15
Flushing, heat sensation	25	8
Headache	23	20
Weakness	12	10
Nausea, heartburn	11	8
Muscle cramps, tremor	8	3
Peripheral edema	7	1
Nervousness, mood changes	7	4
Palpitation	7	5
Dyspnea, cough, wheezing	6	3
Nasal congestion, sore throat	6	8

There is also a large uncontrolled experience in over 2100 patients in the United States. Most of the patients had vasospastic or resistant angina pectoris, and about half had concomitant treatment with beta-adrenergic blocking agents. The relatively common adverse events were similar in nature to those seen with PROCARDIA XL.

In addition, more serious adverse events were observed, not readily distinguishable from the natural history of the disease in these patients. It remains possible, however, that some or many of these events were drug related. Myocardial infarction occurred in about 4% of patients and congestive heart failure or pulmonary edema in about 2%. Ventricular arrhythmias or conduction disturbances each occurred in fewer than 0.5% of patients.

In a subgroup of over 1000 patients receiving PROCARDIA with concomitant beta blocker therapy, the pattern and incidence of adverse experiences was not different from that of the entire group of PROCARDIA (nifedipine) treated patients. (See PRECAUTIONS.)

In a subgroup of approximately 250 patients with a diagnosis of congestive heart failure as well as angina, dizziness or lightheadedness, peripheral edema, headache or flushing each occurred in one in eight patients. Hypotension occurred in about one in 20 patients. Syncope occurred in approximately one patient in 250. Myocardial infarction or symptoms of congestive heart failure each occurred in about one patient in 15. Atrial or ventricular dysrhythmias each occurred in about one patient in 150.

In post-marketing experience, there have been rare reports of exfoliative dermatitis caused by nifedipine. There have been rare reports of exfoliative or bullous skin adverse events (such as erythema multiforme, Stevens-Johnson Syndrome, and toxic epidermal necrolysis) and photosensitivity reactions.

OVERDOSAGE

Experience with nifedipine overdosage is limited. Generally, overdosage with nifedipine leading to pronounced hypotension calls for active cardiovascular support including monitoring of cardiovascular and respiratory function, elevation of extremities, judicious use of calcium infusion, pressor agents and fluids. Clearance of nifedipine would be expected to be prolonged in patients with impaired liver function. Since nifedipine is highly protein-bound, dialysis is not likely to be of any benefit.

There has been one reported case of massive overdosage with PROCARDIA XL Extended Release Tablets. The main effects of ingestion of approximately 4800 mg of PROCARDIA XL in a young man attempting suicide as a result of cocaine-induced depression was initial dizziness, palpitations, flushing, and nervousness. Within several hours of ingestion, nausea, vomiting, and generalized edema developed. No significant hypotension was apparent at presentation, 18 hours post-ingestion. Electrolyte abnormalities consisted of a mild, transient elevation of serum creatinine, and modest elevations of LDH and CPK, but normal SGOT. Vital signs remained stable, no electrocardiographic abnormalities were noted and renal function returned to normal within 24 to 48 hours with routine supportive measures alone. No prolonged sequelae were observed.

The effect of a single 900 mg ingestion of Procardia capsules in a depressed anginal patient also on tricyclic antidepressants was loss of consciousness within 30 minutes of ingestion, and profound hypotension, which responded to calcium infusion, pressor agents, and fluid replacement. A variety of ECG abnormalities were seen in this patient with a history of bundle branch block, including sinus bradycardia and varying degrees of AV block. These dictated the prophylactic placement of a temporary ventricular pacemaker, but otherwise resolved spontaneously. Significant hyperglycemia was seen initially in this patient, but plasma glucose levels rapidly normalized without further treatment.

A young hypertensive patient with advanced renal failure ingested 280 mg of Procardia capsules at one time, with resulting marked hypotension responding to calcium infusion and fluids. No AV conduction abnormalities, arrhythmias, or pronounced changes in heart rate were noted, nor was there any further deterioration in renal function.

DOSAGE AND ADMINISTRATION

Dosage must be adjusted according to each patient's needs. Therapy for either hypertension or angina should be initiated with 30 or 60 mg once daily. PROCARDIA XL Extended Release Tablets should be swallowed whole and should not be bitten or divided. In general, titration should proceed over a 7-14 day period so that the physician can fully assess the response to each dose level and monitor blood pressure before proceeding to higher doses. Since steady-state plasma levels are achieved on the second day of dosing, if symptoms so warrant, titration may proceed more rapidly provided the patient is assessed frequently. Titration to doses above 120 mg are not recommended.

Angina patients controlled on Procardia capsules alone or in combination with other antianginal medications may be safely switched to PROCARDIA XL Extended Release Tablets at the nearest equivalent total daily dose (e.g., 30 mg t.i.d. of Procardia capsules may be changed to 90 mg once daily of PROCARDIA XL Extended Release Tablets). Subsequent titration to higher or lower doses may be necessary and should be initiated as clinically warranted. Experience with doses greater than 90 mg in patients with angina is limited. Therefore, doses greater than 90 mg should be used with caution and only when clinically warranted.

No "rebound effect" has been observed upon discontinuation of PROCARDIA XL Extended Release Tablets. However, if discontinuation of nifedipine is necessary, sound clinical practice suggests that the dosage should be decreased gradually with close physician supervision.

Care should be taken when dispensing PROCARDIA XL to assure that the extended release dosage form has been prescribed.

Co-Administration with Other Antianginal Drugs

Sublingual nitroglycerin may be taken as required for the control of acute manifestations of angina, particularly during nifedipine titration. See PRECAUTIONS, Drug Interactions, for information on co-administration of nifedipine with beta blockers or long-acting nitrates.

HOW SUPPLIED

PROCARDIA XL® Extended Release Tablets are supplied as 30 mg, 60 mg and 90 mg round, biconvex, rose-pink, film-coated tablets in:

Bottles of 100:	30 mg	(NDC 0069-2650-66)
		(NDC 59012-265-66)
	60 mg	(NDC 0069-2660-66)
		(NDC 59012-266-66)
	90 mg	(NDC 0069-2670-66)
		(NDC 59012-267-66)
Bottles of 300:	30 mg	(NDC 0069-2650-72)
		(NDC 59012-265-72)
	60 mg	(NDC 0069-2660-72)
		(NDC 59012-266-72)
Bottles of 5000:	30 mg	(NDC 0069-2650-94)
		(NDC 59012-265-94)
	60 mg	(NDC 0069-2660-94)
		(NDC 59012-266-94)
Unit dose packages of 100:	30 mg	(NDC 0069-2650-41)
		(NDC 59012-265-41)
	60 mg	(NDC 0069-2660-41)
		(NDC 59012-266-41)
	90 mg	(NDC 0069-2670-41)
		(NDC 59012-267-41)

Store below 86°F (30°C).
Protect from moisture and humidity.
Rx only

Pfizer Labs
Division of Pfizer Inc, NY, NY 10017
69-4467-00-8 Revised August 2003

RESCRIPTOR® ℞

[*rē-skrĭp'tōr*]
brand of delavirdine mesylate tablets

Prescribing information for this product, which appears on pages 2630–2636 of the 2004 PDR, has been completely revised as follows. Please write "See Supplement A" next to the product heading.

DESCRIPTION

RESCRIPTOR Tablets contain delavirdine mesylate, a synthetic non-nucleoside reverse transcriptase inhibitor of the human immunodeficiency virus type 1 (HIV-1). The chemical name of delavirdine mesylate is piperazine, 1-[3-[(1-methyl-ethyl)amino]-2-pyridinyl]-4-[[5-[(methylsulfonyl)-amino]-1H-indol-2-yl]carbonyl]-, monomethanesulfonate. Its molecular formula is $C_{22}H_{28}N_6O_3S \bullet CH_4O_3S$, and its molecular weight is 552.68. The structural formula is:

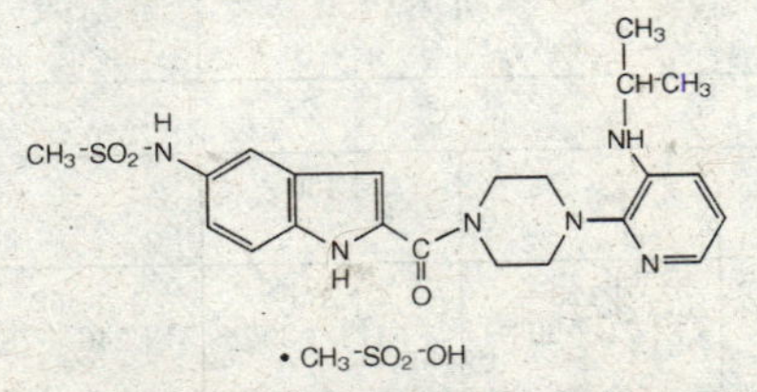

Delavirdine mesylate is an odorless white-to-tan crystalline powder. The aqueous solubility of delavirdine free base at 23° C is 2942 μg/mL at pH 1.0, 295 μg/mL at pH 2.0, and 0.81 μg/mL at pH 7.4.

Each RESCRIPTOR Tablet, for oral administration, contains 100 or 200 mg of delavirdine mesylate (henceforth referred to as delavirdine). Inactive ingredients consist of lactose, microcrystalline cellulose, croscarmellose sodium, magnesium stearate, colloidal silicon dioxide, and carnauba wax. In addition, the 100-mg tablet contains Opadry White YS-1-7000-E and the 200-mg tablet contains hypromellose, Opadry White YS-1-18202-A and Pharmaceutical Ink Black.

MICROBIOLOGY

Mechanism of Action: Delavirdine is a non-nucleoside reverse transcriptase inhibitor (NNRTI) of HIV-1. Delavirdine binds directly to reverse transcriptase (RT) and blocks RNA-dependent and DNA-dependent DNA polymerase activities. Delavirdine does not compete with template: primer or deoxynucleoside triphosphates. HIV-2 RT and human cellular DNA polymerases α, γ, or δ are not inhibited by delavirdine. In addition, HIV-1 group O, a group of highly divergent strains that are uncommon in North America, may not be inhibited by delavirdine.

In Vitro HIV-1 Susceptibility: *In vitro* anti–HIV-1 activity of delavirdine was assessed by infecting cell lines of lymphoblastic and monocytic origin and peripheral blood lymphocytes with laboratory and clinical isolates of HIV-1. IC_{50} and IC_{90} values (50% and 90% inhibitory concentrations) for laboratory isolates (N=5) ranged from 0.005 to 0.030 μM and 0.04 to 0.10 μM, respectively. Mean IC_{50} of clinical isolates (N=74) was 0.038 μM (range 0.001 to 0.69 μM); 73 of 74 clinical isolates had an $IC_{50} \leq 0.18$ μM. The IC_{90} of 24 of these clinical isolates ranged from 0.05 to 0.10 μM. In drug combination studies of delavirdine with zidovudine, didanosine, zalcitabine, lamivudine, interferon-α, and protease inhibitors, additive to synergistic anti–HIV-1 activity was observed in cell culture. The relationship between the *in vitro* susceptibility of HIV-1 RT inhibitors and the inhibition of HIV replication in humans has not been established.

Drug Resistance: Phenotypic analyses of isolates from patients treated with RESCRIPTOR as monotherapy showed a 50-fold to 500-fold reduced susceptibility in 14 of 15 patients by week 8 of therapy. Genotypic analysis of HIV-1 isolates from patients receiving RESCRIPTOR plus zidovudine combination therapy (N=79) showed resistance conferring mutations in all isolates by week 24 of therapy. In RESCRIPTOR treated patients the mutations in RT occurred predominantly at amino acid positions 103 and less frequently at positions 181 and 236. In a separate study, an average of 86-fold increase in the zidovudine susceptibility of patient isolates (N=24) was observed after 24-weeks of RESCRIPTOR and zidovudine combination therapy. The clinical relevance of the phenotypic and the genotypic changes associated with RESCRIPTOR therapy has not been established.

Cross-resistance: RESCRIPTOR may confer cross-resistance to other non-nucleoside RT inhibitors when used alone or in combination. Mutations at positions 103 and/or 181 have been found in resistant virus during treatment with RESCRIPTOR and other non-nucleoside RT inhibitors. These mutations have been associated with cross-resistance among non-nucleoside RT inhibitors *in vitro*.

CLINICAL PHARMACOLOGY

Pharmacokinetics

Absorption and Bioavailability: Delavirdine is rapidly absorbed following oral administration, with peak plasma concentrations occurring at approximately one hour. Following administration of delavirdine 400 mg tid (n=67, HIV-1–infected patients), the mean ± SD steady-state peak plasma concentration (C_{max}) was 35 ± 20 μM (range 2 to 100 μM), systemic exposure (AUC) was 180 ± 100 μM • hr (range 5 to 515 μM • hr) and trough concentration (C_{min}) was 15 ± 10 μM (range 0.1 to 45 μM). The single-dose bioavailability of delavirdine tablets relative to an oral solution was 85 ± 25% (n=16, non-HIV–infected subjects). The single-dose bioavailability of delavirdine tablets (100 mg strength) was increased by approximately 20% when a slurry of drug was prepared by allowing delavirdine tablets to disintegrate in water before administration (n=16, non-HIV–infected subjects). The bioavailability of the 200 mg strength delavirdine tablets has not been evaluated when administered as a slurry, because they are not readily dispersed in water (see DOSAGE AND ADMINISTRATION).

Delavirdine may be administered with or without food. In a multiple-dose, crossover study, delavirdine was administered every eight hours with food or every eight hours, one hour before or two hours after a meal (n=13, HIV-1–infected patients). Patients remained on their typical diet throughout the study; meal content was not standardized. When multiple doses of delavirdine were administered with food, geometric mean C_{max} was reduced by approximately 25%, but AUC and C_{min} were not altered.

Distribution: Delavirdine is extensively bound (approximately 98%) to plasma proteins, primarily albumin. The percentage of delavirdine that is protein bound is constant over a delavirdine concentration range of 0.5 to 196 μM. In five HIV-1–infected patients whose total daily dose of delavirdine ranged from 600 to 1200 mg, cerebrospinal fluid concentrations of delavirdine averaged 0.4% ± 0.07% of the corresponding plasma delavirdine concentrations; this represents about 20% of the fraction not bound to plasma proteins. Steady-state delavirdine concentrations in saliva (n=5, HIV-1–infected patients who received delavirdine 400 mg tid) and semen (n=5 healthy volunteers who received delavirdine 300 mg tid) were about 6% and 2%, respectively, of the corresponding plasma delavirdine concentrations collected at the end of a dosing interval.

Metabolism and Elimination: Delavirdine is extensively converted to several inactive metabolites. Delavirdine is primarily metabolized by cytochrome P450 3A (CYP3A), but *in vitro* data suggest that delavirdine may also be metabolized by CYP2D6. The major metabolic pathways for delavirdine are N-desalkylation and pyridine hydroxylation. Delavirdine exhibits nonlinear steady-state elimination

Continued on next page

Rescriptor—Cont.

pharmacokinetics, with apparent oral clearance decreasing by about 22-fold as the total daily dose of delavirdine increases from 60 to 1200 mg/day. In a study of ^{14}C-delavirdine in six healthy volunteers who received multiple doses of delavirdine tablets 300 mg tid, approximately 44% of the radiolabeled dose was recovered in feces, and approximately 51% of the dose was excreted in urine. Less than 5% of the dose was recovered unchanged in urine. The parent plasma half-life of delavirdine increases with dose; mean half-life following 400 mg tid is 5.8 hours, with a range of 2 to 11 hours.

In vitro and *in vivo* studies have shown that delavirdine reduces CYP3A activity and inhibits its own metabolism. *In vitro* studies have also shown that delavirdine reduces CYP2C9, CYP2D6, and CYP2C19 activity. Inhibition of hepatic CYP3A activity by delavirdine is reversible within 1 week after discontinuation of drug.

Special Populations

Hepatic or Renal Impairment: The pharmacokinetics of delavirdine in patients with hepatic or renal impairment have not been investigated (see PRECAUTIONS).

Age: The pharmacokinetics of delavirdine have not been adequately studied in patients <16 years or >65 years of age.

Gender: Data from population pharmacokinetics suggest that the plasma concentrations of delavirdine tend to be higher in females than in males. However, this difference is not considered to be clinically significant.

Race: No significant differences in the mean trough delavirdine concentrations were observed between different racial or ethnic groups.

Drug Interactions (see also PRECAUTIONS: Drug Interactions)

Specific drug interaction studies were performed with delavirdine and a number of drugs. Table 1 summarizes the effects of delavirdine on the geometric mean AUC, C_{max} and C_{min} of coadministered drugs. Table 2 shows the effects of coadministered drugs on the geometric mean AUC, C_{max} and C_{min} of delavirdine.

For information regarding clinical recommendations, see **CONTRAINDICATIONS, WARNINGS, and PRECAUTIONS: Drug Interactions.**

[See table 1 below]
[See table 2 at top of next page]

INDICATIONS AND USAGE

RESCRIPTOR Tablets are indicated for the treatment of HIV-1 infection in combination with at least 2 other active antiretroviral agents when therapy is warranted.

The following should be considered before initiating therapy with RESCRIPTOR in treatment-naive patients. There are insufficient data directly comparing RESCRIPTOR-containing antiretroviral regimens with currently preferred 3-drug regimens for initial treatment of HIV. In studies comparing regimens consisting of 2 NRTIs (currently considered suboptimal) to RESCRIPTOR plus 2 NRTIs, the proportion of patients receiving the RESCRIPTOR regimen who achieved and sustained an HIV-1 RNA level <400 copies/mL over one year of therapy was relatively low (see DESCRIPTION OF CLINICAL STUDIES).

Resistant virus emerges rapidly when RESCRIPTOR is administered as monotherapy. Therefore, RESCRIPTOR should always be administered in combination with other antiretroviral agents.

DESCRIPTION OF CLINICAL STUDIES

For clinical Studies 21 Part II and 13C described below, efficacy was evaluated by the percentage of patients with a plasma HIV RNA level <400 copies/mL through Week 52 as measured by the Roche Amplicor® HIV-1 Monitor (standard assay). An intent-to-treat analysis was performed where only subjects who achieved confirmed suppression and sustained it through Week 52 are regarded as responders. All other subjects (including never suppressed, discontinued, and those who rebounded after initial suppression of < 400 copies/mL) are considered failures at Week 52. Results of an interim analysis of efficacy conducted for studies 21 Part II and 13C by independent Data and Safety Monitoring Boards (DSMBs) revealed that the triple therapy arms in both studies produced significantly greater antiviral benefit than the dual therapy arms, and early termination of the studies was recommended.

Study 21 Part II: Study 21 Part II was a double-blind, randomized, placebo-controlled trial comparing treatment with RESCRIPTOR (DLV; 400 mg tid), zidovudine (ZDV; 200 mg tid), and lamivudine (3TC; 150 mg bid) versus RESCRIPTOR (400 mg tid) and zidovudine (200 mg tid) versus zidovudine (200 mg tid) and lamivudine (150 mg bid) in 373 HIV-1–infected patients (mean age 35 years [range 17 to 67], 87% male and 60% Caucasian) who were antiretroviral treatment naive (84%) or had limited nucleoside experience (16%). Mean baseline CD_4 cell count was 359 cells/mm^3 and mean baseline plasma HIV RNA was 4.4 log_{10} copies/mL.

Results showed that the mean increase from baseline in CD_4 count at 52 weeks was 111 cells/mL for RESCRIPTOR + ZDV + 3TC, 27 cells/mL for RESCRIPTOR + ZDV, and 74 cells/mL for ZDV + 3TC.

The results of the intent-to-treat analysis of the percentage of patients with a plasma HIV RNA level <400 copies/mL are presented in Figure 1. HIV-1 RNA status and reasons for discontinuation of randomized treatment at 52 weeks are summarized in Table 3. Subjects who were never suppressed before discontinuation were placed in the discontinuation category.

[See figure at top of next column]

Figure 1
Percentage of Patients with HIV RNA Below 400 copies/mL
Standard PCR Assay
Protocol 21 Part 2
Intent-to-Treat Analysis

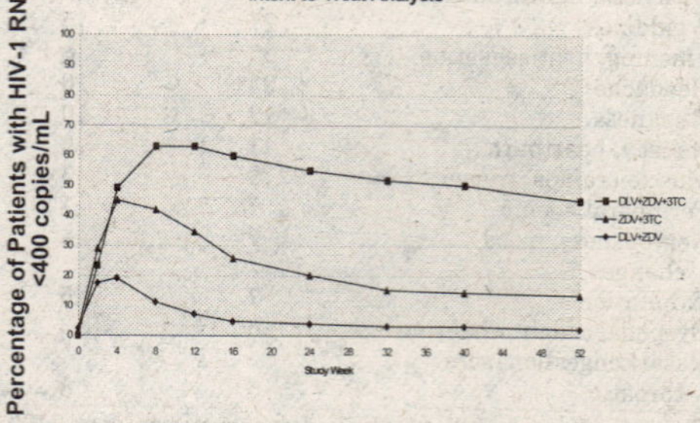

[See table 3 on next page]

Study 13C: Study 13C was a double-blind, randomized, placebo-controlled trial comparing treatment with RESCRIPTOR (400 mg tid), zidovudine (200 mg tid or 300 bid) and either didanosine (ddI; 200 mg bid), zalcitabine (ddC; 0.75 mg tid) or lamivudine (150 mg bid) versus zidovudine (200 mg tid or 300 mg bid) and either didanosine (200 mg bid), zalcitabine (0.75 mg tid) or lamivudine (150 mg bid) in 345 HIV-1–infected patients (mean age 35.8 years [range 18 to 72], 66% male and 63% Caucasian) who were antiretroviral treatment naive (63%) or had limited antiretroviral experience (37%). Mean baseline CD_4 cell count was 210 cells/mm^3 and mean baseline plasma HIV RNA was 4.9 log_{10} copies/mL.

Results showed that the mean increase from baseline in CD_4 count at 54 weeks was 102 cells/mL for RESCRIPTOR + ZDV + ddI or ddC or 3TC and 56 cells/mL for ZDV + ddI or ddC or 3TC.

Figure 2
Percentage of Patients with HIV RNA Below 400 copies/mL
Standard PCR Assay
Protocol 13C
Intent-to-Treat Analysis

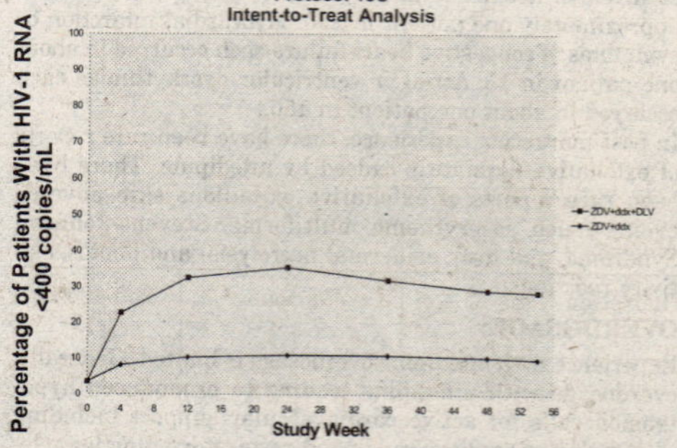

The results of the intent-to-treat analysis of the percentage of patients with a plasma HIV RNA level <400 copies/mL are presented in Figure 2. HIV-1 RNA status and reasons for discontinuation of randomized treatment at 54 weeks are summarized in Table 4. Subjects who were never suppressed before discontinuation were placed in the discontinuation category.

Table 4. Outcomes of Randomized Treatment Through Week 54 for Protocol 13C

Outcome	ZDV + ddx† (N = 173) %	ZDV + ddx + DLV (N = 172) %
HIV RNA <400 copies/mL*	10	29
HIV RNA ≥400 copies/mL§,‡	69	42
Discontinued due to adverse events§	7	12
Discontinued due to other reasons§ǁ	14	17

* Corresponds to rates at Week 54 in proportion curve
† ddx = ddI or ddC or 3TC
‡ Virologic failures at or before Week 54
§ Considered to be treatment failure in the analysis
ǁ Includes discontinuations due to consent withdrawn, loss to follow-up, protocol violations, non-compliance, pregnancy, never treated, and other reasons

Results from several smaller supportive studies evaluating the use of RESCRIPTOR in treatment-naive patients suggest that it may have activity when used in combination with protease inhibitors and NRTIs in 3- or 4-drug combinations.

CONTRAINDICATIONS

RESCRIPTOR Tablets are contraindicated in patients with known hypersensitivity to any of its ingredients. Coadministration of RESCRIPTOR is contraindicated with drugs that are highly dependent on CYP3A for clearance and for which elevated plasma concentrations are associated with serious and/or life-threatening events. These drugs are listed in Table 5. **Also, see PRECAUTIONS, Table 6, Drugs That Should Not Be Coadministered With RESCRIPTOR.**

Table 1. Pharmacokinetic Parameters for Coadministered Drugs in the Presence of Delavirdine.

Coadministered Drug	Dose of Coadministered Drug	Dose of RESCRIPTOR	n	% Change in Pharmacokinetic Parameters of Coadministered Drug (90% CI)		
				C_{max}	AUC	C_{min}
HIV-Protease Inhibitors						
Indinavir	400 mg tid × 7 days	400 mg tid × 7 days	28	↓36* (↓52-↓14)	↔*	↑118* (↑16-↑312)
	600 mg tid × 7 days	400 mg tid × 7 days	28	↔	↑53* (↑7-↑120)	↑298* (↑104-↑678)
Nelfinavir†	750 mg tid × 14 days	400 mg tid × 7 days	12	↑88 (↑66-↑113)	↑107 (↑83-↑135)	↑136 (↑103-↑175)
Saquinavir	Soft gel capsule 1000 mg tid × 28 days	400 mg tid × 28 days	20	↑98‡ (↑4-↑277)	↑121‡ (↑14-↑340)	↑199‡ (↑37-↑553)
Nucleoside Reverse Transcriptase Inhibitors						
Didanosine (buffered tablets)	125 or 250 mg bid × 28 days	400 mg tid × 28 days	9	↓20§ (↓44-↑15)	↓21§ (↓40-↑5)	–
Zidovudine	200 mg tid for >38 days	100 mg qid to 400 mg tid for 8-10 days	34	↔	↔	–
Anti-infective Agents						
Clarithromycin	500 mg bid × 15 days	300 mg tid × 30 days	6	–	↑100	–
Rifabutin	300 mg qd for 15-99 days	400-1000 mg tid for 45-129 days	5	↑128 (↑71-↑203)	↑230 (↑119-↑396)	↑452 (↑246-↑781)

↑ Indicates increase
↓ Indicates decrease
↔ Indicates no significant change
* Relative to indinavir 800 mg tid without RESCRIPTOR
† Plasma concentrations of the nelfinavir active metabolite (nelfinavir hydroxy-t-butylamide) were significantly reduced by delavirdine, which is more than compensated for by increased nelfinavir concentration
‡ Saquinavir soft gel capsule 1000 mg tid plus RESCRIPTOR 400 mg tid relative to saquinavir soft gel capsule 1200 mg tid without RESCRIPTOR
§ RESCRIPTOR taken with didanosine (buffered tablets) relative to doses of RESCRIPTOR and didanosine (buffered tablets) separated by at least 1 hr
– Indicates no data available

Table 2. Pharmacokinetic Parameters for Delavirdine in the Presence of Coadministered Drugs

Coadministered Drug	Dose of Coadministered Drug	Dose of RESCRIPTOR	n	% Change in Delavirdine Pharmacokinetic Parameters (90% CI)		
				C_{max}	AUC	C_{min}
HIV-Protease Inhibitors						
Indinavir	400 or 600 mg tid × 7 days	400 mg tid × 7 days	81	No apparent changes based on a comparison to historical data		
Nelfinavir	750 mg tid × 7 days	400 mg tid × 14 days	7	↓27 (↓49-↑4)	↓31 (↓57-↑10)	↓33 (↓70-↑49)
Saquinavir	Soft gel capsule 1000 mg tid × 28 days	400 mg tid for 7-28 days	23	No apparent changes based on a comparison to historical data		
Nucleoside Reverse Transcriptase Inhibitors						
Didanosine (buffered tablets)	125 or 200 mg bid × 28 days	400 mg tid × 28 days	9	↓32* (↓48-↓11)	↓19* (↓37-↑6)	↔*
Zidovudine	200 mg tid for ≥ 7 days	400 mg tid for 7-14 days	42	No apparent changes based on a comparison to historical data		
Anti-infective Agents						
Clarithromycin	500 mg bid × 15 days	300 mg tid × 30 days	6	↔	↔	↔
Fluconazole	400 mg qd × 15 days	300 mg tid × 30 days	8	↔	↔	↔
Ketoconazole	Various	200-400 mg tid	26	–	–	↑50[†]
Rifabutin	300 mg qd × 14 days	400 mg tid × 28 days	7	↓72 (↓61-↓80)	↓82 (↓74-↓88)	↓94 (↓90-↓96)
Rifampin	600 mg qd × 15 days	400 mg tid × 30 days	7	↓90 (↓94-↓83)	↓97 (↓98-↓95)	↓100
Sulfamethoxazole or Trimethoprim & Sulfamethoxazole	Various	200-400 mg tid	311	–	–	↔[†]
Other						
Antacid (Maalox® TC)	20 mL	300 mg single dose	12	↓52 (↓68-↓29)	↓44 (↓58-↓27)	–
Fluoxetine	Various	200-400 mg tid	36	–	–	↑50[†]
Phenytoin, Phenobarbital, Carbamazepine	Various	300-400 mg tid	8	–	–	↓90[†]

↑ Indicates increase
↓ Indicates decrease
↔ Indicates no significant change
* RESCRIPTOR taken with didanosine (buffered tablets) relative to doses of RESCRIPTOR and didanosine (buffered tablets) separated by at least 1 hr
† Population pharmacokinetic data from efficacy studies
– Indicates no data available

Table 3: Outcomes of Randomized Treatment Through Week 52 for Protocol 21 Part 2

Outcome	ZDV + 3TC (N = 124) %	DLV + ZDV (N = 125) %	DLV + ZDV + 3TC (N = 124) %
HIV RNA <400 copies/mL*	14	2	45
HIV RNA ≥400 copies/mL[†,‡]	64	52	31
Discontinued due to adverse events[‡]	8	13	10
Discontinued due to other reasons[‡,§]	14	33	14

*Corresponds to rates at Week 52 in proportion curve
† Virologic failures at or before Week 52
‡ Considered to be treatment failure in the analysis
§ Includes discontinuations due to consent withdrawn, loss to follow-up, protocol violations, non-compliance, pregnancy, never treated, and other reasons

Table 5. Drugs That Are Contraindicated With RESCRIPTOR

Drug Class	Drugs Within Class That Are Contraindicated With RESCRIPTOR
Antihistamines	Astemizole, terfenadine
Ergot derivatives	Dihydroergotamine, ergonovine, ergotamine, methylergonovine
GI motility agent	Cisapride
Neuroleptic	Pimozide
Sedative/hypnotics	Alprazolam, midazolam, triazolam

WARNINGS

ALERT: Find out about medicines that should NOT be taken with RESCRIPTOR. This statement is included on the product's bottle label.

Drug Interactions

Because delavirdine may inhibit the metabolism of many different drugs (eg, antiarrhythmics, calcium channel blockers, sedative hypnotics, and others), **serious and/or life threatening drug interactions could result from inappropriate coadministration of some drugs with delavirdine.** In addition, some drugs may markedly reduce delavirdine plasma concentrations, resulting in suboptimal antiviral activity and subsequent emergence of drug resistance. All prescribers should become familiar with the following tables in this package insert: **Table 5, Drugs That Are Contraindicated With RESCRIPTOR; Table 6, Drugs That Should Not Be Coadministered With RESCRIPTOR; and Table 7, Established and Other Potentially Significant Drug Interactions: Alteration in Dose or Regimen May Be Recommended Based on Drug Interaction Studies or Predicted Interaction.** Additional details on drug interactions can be found in Tables 1 and 2 under the **CLINICAL PHARMACOLOGY** section.

Concomitant use of lovastatin or simvastatin with RESCRIPTOR is not recommended. Caution should be exercised if RESCRIPTOR is used concurrently with other HMG-CoA reductase inhibitors that are also metabolized by the CYP3A4 pathway (eg, atorvastatin or cerivastatin). The risk of myopathy including rhabdomyolysis may be increased when RESCRIPTOR is used in combination with these drugs.

Particular caution should be used when prescribing sildenafil in patients receiving RESCRIPTOR. Coadministration of sildenafil with RESCRIPTOR is expected to substantially increase sildenafil concentrations and may result in an increase in sildenafil-associated adverse events, including hypotension, visual changes, and priapism (see **PRECAUTIONS, Drug Interactions** and **Information for Patients**, and the complete prescribing information for sildenafil).

Concomitant use of St. John's wort (hypericum perforatum) or St. John's wort containing products and RESCRIPTOR is not recommended. Coadministration of St. John's wort with non-nucleoside reverse transcriptase inhibitors (NNRTIs), including RESCRIPTOR, is expected to substantially decrease NNRTI concentrations and may result in sub-optimal levels of RESCRIPTOR and lead to loss of virologic response and possible resistance to RESCRIPTOR or to the class of NNRTIs.

PRECAUTIONS

General: Delavirdine is metabolized primarily by the liver. Therefore, caution should be exercised when administering RESCRIPTOR Tablets to patients with impaired hepatic function.

Resistance/Cross-Resistance: Non-nucleoside reverse transcriptase inhibitors, when used alone or in combination, may confer cross-resistance to other non-nucleoside reverse transcriptase inhibitors.

Fat Redistribution: Redistribution/accumulation of body fat including central obesity, dorsocervical fat enlargement (buffalo hump), peripheral wasting, facial wasting, breast enlargement, and "cushingoid appearance" have been observed in patients receiving antiretroviral therapy. The mechanism and long-term consequences of these events are currently unknown. A causal relationship has not been established.

Skin Rash: Severe rash, including rare cases of erythema multiforme and Stevens-Johnson syndrome, has been reported in patients receiving RESCRIPTOR. Erythema multiforme and Stevens-Johnson syndrome were rarely seen in clinical trials and resolved after withdrawal of RESCRIPTOR. Any patient experiencing severe rash or rash accompanied by symptoms such as fever, blistering, oral lesions, conjunctivitis, swelling, and muscle or joint aches should discontinue RESCRIPTOR and consult a physician. Two cases of Stevens-Johnson syndrome have been reported through postmarketing surveillance out of a total of 339 surveillance reports.

In Studies 21 Part II and 13C (see **DESCRIPTION OF CLINICAL STUDIES**), rash (including maculopapular rash) was reported in more patients who were treated with RESCRIPTOR 400 mg tid (35% and 32%, respectively) than in those who were not treated with RESCRIPTOR (21% and 16%, respectively). The highest intensity of rash reported in these studies was severe (grade 3), which was observed in approximately 4% of patients treated with RESCRIPTOR in each study and in none of the patients who were not treated with RESCRIPTOR. Also in Studies 21 Part II and 13C, discontinuations due to rash were reported in more patients who received RESCRIPTOR 400 mg tid (3% and 4%, respectively) than in those who did not receive RESCRIPTOR (0% and 1%, respectively).

In most cases, the duration of the rash was less than two weeks and did not require dose reduction or discontinuation of RESCRIPTOR. Most patients were able to resume therapy after rechallenge with RESCRIPTOR following a treatment interruption due to rash. The distribution of the rash was mainly on the upper body and proximal arms, with decreasing intensity of the lesions on the neck and face, and progressively less on the rest of the trunk and limbs. Occurrence of a delavirdine-associated rash after one month is uncommon. Symptomatic relief has been obtained using diphenhydramine hydrochloride, hydroxyzine hydrochloride, and/or topical corticosteroids.

Information for Patients: A statement to patients and healthcare providers is included on the product's bottle label: **ALERT: Find out about medicines that should NOT be taken with RESCRIPTOR.** A patient package insert (PPI) for RESCRIPTOR is available for patient information.

Patients should be informed that RESCRIPTOR is not a cure for HIV-1 infection and that they may continue to acquire illnesses associated with HIV-1 infection, including opportunistic infections. Treatment with RESCRIPTOR has

Continued on next page

Rescriptor—Cont.

not been shown to reduce the incidence or frequency of such illnesses, and patients should be advised to remain under the care of a physician when using RESCRIPTOR.

Patients should be advised that the use of RESCRIPTOR has not been shown to reduce the risk of transmission of HIV-1.

Patients should be instructed that the major toxicity of RESCRIPTOR is rash and should be advised to promptly notify their physician should rash occur. The majority of rashes associated with RESCRIPTOR occur within 1 to 3 weeks after initiating treatment with RESCRIPTOR. The rash normally resolves in 3 to 14 days and may be treated symptomatically while therapy with RESCRIPTOR is continued. Any patient experiencing severe rash or rash accompanied by symptoms such as fever, blistering, oral lesions, conjunctivitis, swelling, and muscle or joint aches should discontinue medication and consult a physician.

Patients should be informed that redistribution or accumulation of body fat may occur in patients receiving antiretroviral therapy and that the cause and long-term health effects of these conditions are not known at this time.

Patients should be informed to take RESCRIPTOR every day as prescribed. Patients should not alter the dose of RESCRIPTOR without consulting their doctor. If a dose is missed, patients should take the next dose as soon as possible. However, if a dose is skipped, the patient should not double the next dose.

Patients with achlorhydria should take RESCRIPTOR with an acidic beverage (e.g., orange or cranberry juice). However, the effect of an acidic beverage on the absorption of delavirdine in patients with achlorhydria has not been investigated.

Patients taking both RESCRIPTOR and antacids should be advised to take them at least 1 hour apart.

Because RESCRIPTOR may interact with certain drugs, patients should be advised to report to their doctor the use of any prescription, nonprescription medication or herbal products, particularly St. John's wort.

Patients receiving sildenafil and RESCRIPTOR should be advised that they may be at an increased risk of sildenafil-associated adverse events, including hypotension, visual changes, and prolonged penile erection, and should promptly report any symptoms to their doctor.

Drug Interactions (see also CONTRAINDICATIONS, WARNINGS, and CLINICAL PHARMACOLOGY: Drug Interactions)

Delavirdine is an inhibitor of CYP3A isoform and other CYP isoforms to a lesser extent including CYP2C9, CYP2D6, and CYP2C19. Coadministration of RESCRIPTOR and drugs primarily metabolized by CYP3A (e.g., HMG-CoA reductase inhibitors, and sildenafil) may result in increased plasma concentrations of the coadministered drug that could increase or prolong both its therapeutic or adverse effects.

Delavirdine is metabolized primarily by CYP3A, but *in vitro* data suggest that delavirdine may also be metabolized by CYP2D6. Coadministration of RESCRIPTOR and drugs that induce CYP3A, such as rifampin, may decrease delavirdine plasma concentrations and reduce its therapeutic effect. Coadministration of RESCRIPTOR and drugs that inhibit CYP3A may increase delavirdine plasma concentrations. **(See Table 6, Drugs That Should Not Be Coadministered With RESCRIPTOR, and Table 7, Established and Other Potentially Significant Drug Interactions: Alteration in Dose or Regimen May Be Recommended Based on Drug Interaction Studies or Predicted Interaction.)**

[See table 6 above]

[See table 7 at right]

Carcinogenesis, Mutagenesis and Impairment of Fertility: Delavirdine was negative in a battery of genetic toxicology tests which included an Ames assay, an *in vitro* rat hepatocyte unscheduled DNA synthesis assay, an *in vitro* chromosome aberration assay in human peripheral lymphocytes, an *in vitro* mutation assay in Chinese hamster ovary cells, and an *in vivo* micronucleus test in mice.

Lifetime carcinogenicity studies were conducted in rats at doses of 10, 32 and 100 mg/kg/day and in mice at doses of 62.5, 250 and 500 mg/kg/day for males and 62.5, 125 and 250 mg/kg/day for females. In rats, delavirdine was noncarcinogenic at maximally tolerated doses that produced exposures (AUC) up to 12 (male rats) and 9 (female rats) times human exposure at the recommended clinical dose. In mice, delavirdine produced significant increases in the incidence of hepatocellular adenoma/adenocarcinoma in both males and females, hepatocellular adenoma in females, and mesenchymal urinary bladder tumors in males. The systemic drug exposures (AUC) in female mice were 0.5- to 3-fold and in male mice 0.2- to 4-fold of those in humans at the recommended clinical dose. Given the lack of genotoxic activity of delavirdine, the relevance of urinary bladder and hepatocellular neoplasm in delavirdine-treated mice to humans is not known.

Delavirdine at doses of 20, 100, and 200 mg/kg/day did not cause impairment of fertility in rats when males were treated for 70 days and females were treated for 14 days prior to mating.

Pregnancy: Pregnancy Category C: Delavirdine has been shown to be teratogenic in rats. Delavirdine caused ventricular septal defects in rats at doses of 50, 100, and 200 mg/kg/day when administered during the period of organogenesis. The lowest dose of delavirdine that caused malformations produced systemic exposures in pregnant rats equal to or lower than the expected human exposure to RESCRIPTOR (C_{min} 15 µM) at the recommended dose. Exposure in rats approximately 5-fold higher than the expected human exposure resulted in marked maternal toxicity, embryotoxicity, fetal developmental delay, and reduced pup survival. Additionally, reduced pup survival on postpartum day 0 occurred at an exposure (mean C_{min}) approximately equal to the expected human exposure. Delavirdine was excreted in the milk of lactating rats at a concentration three to five times that of rat plasma.

Delavirdine at doses of 200 and 400 mg/kg/day administered during the period of organogenesis caused maternal toxicity, embryotoxicity and abortions in rabbits. The lowest dose of delavirdine that resulted in these toxic effects produced systemic exposures in pregnant rabbits approximately 6-fold higher than the expected human exposure to RESCRIPTOR (C_{min} 15 µM) at the recommended dose. The no-observed-adverse-effect dose in the pregnant rabbit was 100 mg/kg/day. Various malformations were observed at this dose, but the incidence of such malformations was not statistically significantly different from those observed in the control group. Systemic exposures in pregnant rabbits at a dose of 100 mg/kg/day were lower than those expected in humans at the recommended clinical dose. Malformations

Table 6. Drugs That Should Not Be Coadministered With RESCRIPTOR

Drug Class: Drug Name	Clinical Comment
Anticonvulsant agents: phenytoin, phenobarbital, carbamazepine	May lead to loss of virologic response and possible resistance to RESCRIPTOR or to the class of non-nucleoside reverse transcriptase inhibitors.
Antihistamines: astemizole, terfenadine	CONTRAINDICATED due to potential for serious and/or life-threatening reactions such as cardiac arrhythmias.
Antimycobacterials: rifabutin,* rifampin*	May lead to loss of virologic response and possible resistance to RESCRIPTOR or to the class of non-nucleoside reverse transcriptase inhibitors or other coadministered antiviral agents.
Ergot Derivatives: dihydroergotamine, ergonovine, ergotamine, methylergonovine	CONTRAINDICATED due to potential for serious and/or life-threatening reactions such as acute ergot toxicity characterized by peripheral vasospasm and ischemia of the extremities and other tissues.
GI motility agent: cisapride	CONTRAINDICATED due to potential for serious and/or life-threatening reactions such as cardiac arrhythmias.
Herbal Products: St. John's wort (hypericum perforatum)	May lead to loss of virologic response and possible resistance to RESCRIPTOR or to the class of non-nucleoside reverse transcriptase inhibitors.
HMG-CoA reductase inhibitors: lovastatin, simvastatin	Potential for serious reactions such as risk of myopathy including rhabdomyolysis.
Neuroleptic: pimozide	CONTRAINDICATED due to potential for serious and/or life-threatening reactions such as cardiac arrhythmias.
Sedative/hypnotics: alprazolam, midazolam, triazolam	CONTRAINDICATED due to potential for serious and/or life-threatening reactions such as prolonged or increased sedation or respiratory depression.

*See **CLINICAL PHARMACOLOGY** for magnitude of interaction, Tables 1 and 2.

Table 7. Established and Other Potentially Significant Drug Interactions: Alteration in Dose or Regimen May Be Recommended Based on Drug Interaction Studies or Predicted Interaction

Concomitant Drug Class: Drug Name	Effect on Concentration of Delavirdine or Concomitant Drug	Clinical Comment
HIV-Antiviral Agents		
Amprenavir	↑ Amprenavir	Appropriate doses of this combination, with respect to safety, efficacy and pharmacokinetics, have not been established.
Didanosine*	↓ Delavirdine ↓ Didanosine	Administration of didanosine (buffered tablets) and RESCRIPTOR should be separated by at least one hour.
Indinavir*	↑ Indinavir	A dose reduction of indinavir to 600 mg tid should be considered when RESCRIPTOR and indinavir are coadministered.
Lopinavir/Ritonavir	↑ Lopinavir ↑ Ritonavir	Appropriate doses of this combination, with respect to safety, efficacy and pharmacokinetics, have not been established.
Nelfinavir*	↑ Nelfinavir ↓ Delavirdine	Appropriate doses of this combination, with respect to safety, efficacy and pharmacokinetics, have not been established. (See **CLINICAL PHARMACOLOGY:** Tables 1 and 2.)
Ritonavir	↑ Ritonavir	Appropriate doses of this combination, with respect to safety, efficacy and pharmacokinetics, have not been established.
Saquinavir*	↑ Saquinavir	A dose reduction of saquinavir (soft gelatin capsules) may be considered when RESCRIPTOR and saquinavir are coadministered. (See **CLINICAL PHARMACOLOGY:** Table 1.) Appropriate doses with respect to safety, efficacy and pharmacokinetics, have not been established.
Other Agents		
Acid blockers: antacids*	↓ Delavirdine	Doses of an antacid and RESCRIPTOR should be separated by at least one hour, because the absorption of delavirdine is reduced when coadministered with antacids.
H_2Receptor antagonists: cimetidine, famotidine, nizatidine, ranitidine Proton pump inhibitors: omeprazole, lansoprazole		These agents increase gastric pH and may reduce the absorption of delavirdine. Although the effect of these drugs on delavirdine absorption has not been evaluated, chronic use of these drugs with RESCRIPTOR is not recommended.

(Table continued on next page)

Table 7 *(cont)*. Established and Other Potentially Significant Drug Interactions: Alteration in Dose or Regimen May Be Recommended Based on Drug Interaction Studies or Predicted Interaction

Concomitant Drug Class: Drug Name	Effect on Concentration of Delavirdine or Concomitant Drug	Clinical Comment
Other Agents (continued)		
Amphetamines	↑ Amphetamines	Use with caution.
Antiarrhythmics: bepridil	↑ Antiarrhythmics	Use with caution. Increased bepridil exposure may be associated with life-threatening reactions such as cardiac arrythmias.
Amiodarone, lidocaine (systemic), quinidine, flecainide, propafenone		Caution is warranted and therapeutic concentration monitoring is recommended, if available, for antiarrhythmics when coadministered with RESCRIPTOR.
Anticoagulant: warfarin	↑ Warfarin	It is recommended that INR (international normalized ratio) be monitored.
Anti-infective: clarithromycin*	↑ Clarithromycin	When coadministered with RESCRIPTOR, clarithromycin should be adjusted in patients with impaired renal function: • For patients with CL_{CR} 30 to 60 mL/min the dose of clarithromycin should be reduced by 50%. • For patients with CL_{CR} <30 mL/min the dose of clarithromycin should be reduced by 75%.
Dihydropyridine calcium channel blockers: amlodipine, diltiazem, felodipine, isradipine, nifedipine, nicardipine, nimodipine, nisoldipine, verapamil	↑ Dihydropyridine calcium channel blockers	Caution is warranted and clinical monitoring of patients is recommended.
Corticosteroid: dexamethasone	↓ Delavirdine	Use with caution. RESCRIPTOR may be less effective due to decreased delavirdine plasma concentrations in patients taking these agents concomitantly.
Erectile dysfunction agents: sildenafil	↑ Sildenafil	Sildenafil should not exceed a maximum single dose of 25 mg in a 48 hour period.
HMG-CoA reductase inhibitors: atorvastatin, cerivastatin, fluvastatin	↑ Atorvastatin ↑ Cerivastatin ↑ Fluvastatin	Use lowest possible dose of atorvastatin or cerivastatin, or fluvastatin with careful monitoring, or consider other HMG-CoA reductase inhibitors such as pravastatin in combination with RESCRIPTOR.
Immunosuppressants: cyclosporine, tacrolimus, rapamycin	↑ Immunosuppressants	Therapeutic concentration monitoring is recommended for immunosuppressant agents when coadministered with RESCRIPTOR.
Narcotic analgesic: methadone	↑ Methadone	Dosage of methadone may need to be decreased when coadministered with RESCRIPTOR.
Oral contraceptives: ethinyl estradiol	↑ Ethinyl estradiol	Concentrations of ethinyl estradiol may increase. However, the clinical significance is unknown.

↑ Indicates increase
↓ Indicates decrease
*See **CLINICAL PHARMACOLOGY** for magnitude of interaction, Tables 1 and 2.

Table 8. Percent of Patients With Treatment-Emergent Rash in Pivotal Trials (Studies 21 Part II and 13C)*

Percent of Patients with:	Description of Rash Grade†	RESCRIPTOR 400 mg TID (N = 412)	Control Group Patients (N = 295)
Grade 1 Rash	Erythema, pruritus	69 (16.7%)	35 (11.9%)
Grade 2 Rash	Diffuse maculopapular rash, dry desquamation	59 (14.3%)	17 (5.8%)
Grade 3 Rash	Vesiculation, moist desquamation, ulceration	18 (4.4%)	0 (0.0%)
Grade 4 Rash	Erythema multiforme, Stevens-Johnson syndrome, toxic epideral necrolysis, necrosis requiring surgery, exfoliative dermatitis	0 (0.0%)	0 (0.0%)
Rash of any Grade		146 (35.4%)	52 (17.6%)
Treatment discontinuation as a result of rash		13 (3.2%)	1 (0.3%)

*Includes events reported regardless of causality
† ACTG Toxicity Grading System; includes events reported as "rash", "maculopapular rash", and "urticaria".

were not apparent at 200 and 400 mg/kg/day; however, only a limited number of fetuses were available for examination as a result of maternal and embryo death.

No adequate and well-controlled studies in pregnant women have been conducted. RESCRIPTOR should be used during pregnancy only if the potential benefit justifies the potential risk to the fetus. Of 9 pregnancies reported in premarketing clinical studies and postmarketing experience, a total of 10 infants were born (including 1 set of twins). Eight of the infants were born healthy. One infant was born HIV-positive but was otherwise healthy and with no congenital abnormalities detected, and 1 infant was born prematurely (34 to 35 weeks) with a small muscular ventricular septal defect that spontaneously resolved. The patient received approximately six weeks of treatment with delavirdine and zidovudine early in the course of the pregnancy.

Antiretroviral Pregnancy Registry: To monitor maternal-fetal outcomes of pregnant women exposed to RESCRIPTOR and other antiretroviral agents, an Antiretroviral Pregnancy Registry has been established. Physicians are encouraged to register patients by calling (800) 258-4263.

Nursing Mothers: The Centers for Disease Control and Prevention recommend that HIV-infected mothers not breast-feed their infants to avoid risking postnatal transmission of HIV. Because of both the potential for HIV transmission and any possible adverse reactions in nursing infants, **mothers should be instructed not to breast-feed if they are receiving RESCRIPTOR.**

Pediatric Use: Safety and effectiveness of delavirdine in combination with other antiretroviral agents have not been established in HIV-1–infected individuals younger than 16 years of age.

Geriatric Use: Clinical studies of RESCRIPTOR did not include sufficient numbers of subjects aged 65 and over to determine whether they respond differently from younger subjects. In general, caution should be taken when dosing RESCRIPTOR in elderly patients due to the greater frequency of decreased hepatic, renal or cardiac function and of concomitant disease or other drug therapy.

ADVERSE REACTIONS

The safety of RESCRIPTOR Tablets alone and in combination with other therapies has been studied in approximately 6,000 patients receiving RESCRIPTOR. The majority of adverse events were of mild or moderate (ie, ACTG grade 1 or 2) intensity. The most frequently reported drug-related adverse event (ie, events considered by the investigator to be related to the blinded study medication, or events with an unknown or missing causal relationship to the blinded medication) among patients receiving RESCRIPTOR was skin rash (see **Table 8** and **PRECAUTIONS: Skin Rash**).

[See table 8 at left]

Adverse events of moderate to severe intensity reported by at least 5% of evaluable patients in any treatment group in the pivotal trials, which includes patients receiving RESCRIPTOR in combination with zidovudine and/or lamivudine in Study 21 Part II for up to 98 weeks and in combination with zidovudine and either lamivudine, didanosine, or zalcitabine in Study 13C for up to 72 weeks are summarized in Table 9.

[See table 9 on next page]

Other adverse events that occurred in patients receiving RESCRIPTOR (in combination treatment) in all phase II and III studies, and considered possibly related to treatment, and of at least ACTG grade 2 in intensity are listed below by body system.

Body as a Whole: Abdominal cramps, abdominal distention, abdominal pain (localized), abscess, allergic reaction, chills, edema (generalized or localized), epidermal cyst, fever, infection, infection viral, lip edema, malaise, Mycobacterium tuberculosis infection, neck rigidity, sebaceous cyst, and redistribution/accumulation of body fat (see **PRECAUTIONS, Fat Redistribution**).

Cardiovascular System: Abnormal cardiac rate and rhythm, cardiac insufficiency, cardiomyopathy, hypertension, migraine, pallor, peripheral vascular disorder, and postural hypotension.

Digestive System: Anorexia, bloody stool, colitis, constipation, decreased appetite, diarrhea (*Clostridium difficile*), diverticulitis, dry mouth, dyspepsia, dysphagia, enteritis at all levels, eructation, fecal incontinence, flatulence, gagging, gastroenteritis, gastroesophageal reflux, gastrointestinal bleeding, gastrointestinal disorder, gingivitis, gum hemorrhage, hepatomegaly, increased appetite, increased saliva, increased thirst, jaundice, mouth or tongue inflammation or ulcers, nonspecific hepatitis, oral/enteric moniliasis, pancreatitis, rectal disorder, sialadenitis, tooth abscess, and toothache.

Hemic and Lymphatic System: Adenopathy, bruising, eosinophilia, granulocytosis, leukopenia, pancytopenia, purpura, spleen disorder, thrombocytopenia, and prolonged prothrombin time.

Metabolic and Nutritional Disorders: Alcohol intolerance, amylase increased, bilirubinemia, hyperglycemia, hyperkalemia, hypertriglyceridemia, hyperuricemia, hypocalcemia, hyponatremia, hypophosphatemia, increased AST (SGOT), increased gamma glutamyl transpeptidase, increased lipase, increased serum alkaline phosphatase, increased serum creatinine, and weight increase or decrease.

Musculoskeletal System: Arthralgia or arthritis of single and multiple joints, bone disorder, bone pain, myalgia, tendon disorder, tenosynovitis, tetany, and vertigo.

Nervous System: Abnormal coordination, agitation, amnesia, change in dreams, cognitive impairment, confusion, decreased libido, disorientation, dizziness, emotional lability, euphoria, hallucination, hyperesthesia, hyperreflexia, hypertonia, hypesthesia, impaired concentration, manic symptoms, muscle cramp, nervousness, neuropathy, nystagmus, paralysis, paranoid symptoms, restlessness, sleep cycle disorder, somnolence, tingling, tremor, vertigo, and weakness.

Respiratory System: Chest congestion, dyspnea, epistaxis, hiccups, laryngismus, pneumonia, and rhinitis.

Skin and Appendages: Angioedema, dermal leukocytoclastic vasculitis, dermatitis, desquamation, diaphoresis, discolored skin, dry skin, erythema, erythema multiforme, folliculitis, fungal dermatitis, hair loss, herpes zoster or simplex, nail disorder, petechiae, non-application site pruritus, seborrhea, skin hypertrophy, skin disorder, skin nodule, Stevens-Johnson syndrome, urticaria, vesiculobullous rash, and wart.

Continued on next page

Rescriptor—Cont.

Special Senses: Blepharitis, blurred vision, conjunctivitis, diplopia, dry eyes, ear pain, parosmia, otitis media, photophobia, taste perversion, and tinnitus.
Urogenital System: Amenorrhea, breast enlargement, calculi of the kidney, chromaturia, epididymitis, hematuria, hemospermia, impaired urination, impotence, kidney pain, metrorrhagia, nocturia, polyuria, proteinuria, testicular pain, urinary tract infection, and vaginal moniliasis.
Postmarketing Experience: Adverse event terms reported from postmarketing surveillance that were not reported in the phase II and III trials are presented below.
Digestive System: Hepatic failure.
Hemic and Lymphatic System: Hemolytic anemia.
Musculoskeletal System: Rhabdomyolysis.
Urogenital System: Acute kidney failure.
Laboratory Abnormalities: Marked laboratory abnormalities observed in at least 2% of patients during Studies 21 Part II and 13C are summarized in Table 10. Marked laboratory abnormalities are defined as any Grade 3 or 4 abnormality found in patients at any time during study.
[See table 10 on next page]

Table 9. Treatment-Emergent Events, Regardless of Causality, of Moderate-to-Severe or Life-Threatening Intensity Reported by at Least 5% of Evaluable* Patients in any Treatment Group

	Study 21 Part II			Study 13C	
Adverse Events	ZDV + 3TC (N = 123)	400 mg tid RESCRIPTOR + ZDV (N = 123)	400 mg tid RESCRIPTOR + ZDV + 3TC (N = 119)	ZDV + ddI, ddC, or 3TC (N = 172)	400 mg tid RESCRIPTOR + ZDV + ddI, ddC, or 3TC (N = 170)
	% of pts. (N)	% of pts. (N)	% of pts. (N)	% of pts. (N)	% of pts. (N)
Body as a Whole					
Abdominal pain, generalized	2.4 (3)	3.3 (4)	5.0 (6)	1.7 (3)	2.4 (4)
Asthenia/fatigue	16.3 (20)	15.4 (19)	16.0 (19)	8.1 (14)	5.3 (9)
Fever	2.4 (3)	1.6 (2)	3.4 (4)	6.4 (11)	7.1 (12)
Flu syndrome	4.9 (6)	7.3 (9)	5.0 (6)	5.2 (9)	2.4 (4)
Headache	14.6 (18)	12.2 (15)	16.8 (20)	12.8 (22)	11.2 (19)
Localized pain	4.9 (6)	5.7 (7)	5.0 (6)	2.9 (5)	1.8 (3)
Digestive					
Diarrhea	8.1 (10)	2.4 (3)	4.2 (5)	8.1 (14)	5.9 (10)
Nausea	17.1 (21)	20.3 (25)	16.8 (20)	9.3 (16)	14.7 (25)
Vomiting	8.9 (11)	4.9 (6)	2.5 (3)	4.1 (7)	6.5 (11)
Nervous					
Anxiety	1.6 (2)	2.4 (3)	6.7 (8)	4.1 (7)	3.5 (6)
Depressive symptoms	6.5 (8)	4.9 (6)	12.6 (15)	3.5 (6)	5.9 (10)
Insomnia	4.9 (6)	4.9 (6)	5.0 (6)	2.9 (5)	1.2 (2)
Respiratory					
Bronchitis	4.1 (5)	6.5 (8)	6.7 (8)	3.5 (6)	3.5 (6)
Cough	9.8 (12)	4.1 (5)	5.0 (6)	5.2 (9)	3.5 (6)
Pharyngitis	6.5 (8)	1.6 (2)	5.0 (6)	4.1 (7)	3.5 (6)
Sinusitis	8.9 (11)	7.3 (9)	5.0 (6)	2.3 (4)	1.2 (2)
Upper respiratory infection	11.4 (14)	6.5 (8)	7.6 (9)	8.7 (15)	4.7 (8)
Skin					
Rashes	3.3 (4)	19.5 (24)	13.4 (16)	7.6 (13)	18.8 (32)

*Evaluable patients in Study 21 Part II were those who received at least 1 dose of study medication and returned for at least 1 clinic study visit. Evaluable patients in Study 13C were those who received at least 1 dose of study medication.

OVERDOSAGE

Human experience of acute overdose with RESCRIPTOR is limited.
Management of Overdosage: Treatment of overdosage with RESCRIPTOR should consist of general supportive measures, including monitoring of vital signs and observation of the patient's clinical status. There is no specific antidote for overdosage with RESCRIPTOR. If indicated, elimination of unabsorbed drug should be achieved by emesis or gastric lavage. Since delavirdine is extensively metabolized by the liver and is highly protein bound, dialysis is unlikely to result in significant removal of the drug.

DOSAGE AND ADMINISTRATION

The recommended dosage for RESCRIPTOR Tablets is 400 mg (four 100-mg or two 200-mg tablets) three times daily. RESCRIPTOR should be used in combination with other antiretroviral therapy. The complete prescribing information for other antiretroviral agents should be consulted for information on dosage and administration.
The 100-mg RESCRIPTOR Tablets may be dispersed in water prior to consumption. To prepare a dispersion, add four 100-mg RESCRIPTOR Tablets to at least 3 ounces of water, allow to stand for a few minutes, and then stir until a uniform dispersion occurs (see **CLINICAL PHARMACOLOGY: Pharmacokinetics: Absorption and Bioavailability**). The dispersion should be consumed promptly. The glass should be rinsed with water and the rinse swallowed to insure the entire dose is consumed. **The 200-mg tablets should be taken as intact tablets, because they are not readily dispersed in water.** Note: The 200-mg tablets are approximately one third smaller in size than the 100-mg tablets.
RESCRIPTOR Tablets may be administered with or without food (see **CLINICAL PHARMACOLOGY: Pharmacokinetics-Absorption and Bioavailability**). Patients with achlorhydria should take RESCRIPTOR with an acidic beverage (e.g., orange or cranberry juice). However, the effect of an acidic beverage on the absorption of delavirdine in patients with achlorhydria has not been investigated.
Patients taking both RESCRIPTOR and antacids should be advised to take them at least one hour apart.

HOW SUPPLIED

RESCRIPTOR Tablets are available as follows:
100 mg: white, capsule-shaped tablets marked with "U 3761".
Bottles of 360 tablets NDC 63010-020-36
200 mg: white, capsule-shaped tablets marked with "RESCRIPTOR 200 mg".
Bottles of 180 tablets NDC 63010-021-18
Store at controlled room temperature 20° to 25°C (68° to 77°F) [see USP]. Keep container tightly closed. Protect from high humidity.
Rx only

ANIMAL TOXICOLOGY

Toxicities among various organs and organ systems in rats, mice, rabbits, dogs, and monkeys were observed following the administration of delavirdine. Necrotizing vasculitis was the most significant toxicity that occurred in dogs when mean nadir serum concentrations of delavirdine were at least 7-fold higher than the expected human exposure to RESCRIPTOR (C_{min} 15 μM) at the recommended dose. Vasculitis in dogs was not reversible during a 2.5-month recovery period; however, partial resolution of the vascular lesion characterized by reduced inflammation, diminished necrosis, and intimal thickening occurred during this period. Other major target organs included the gastrointestinal tract, endocrine organs, liver, kidneys, bone marrow, lymphoid tissue, lung, and reproductive organs.
Agouron Pharmaceuticals, Inc.
La Jolla, CA 92037, USA
RESCRIPTOR is a registered trademark of Pharmacia & Upjohn Company.
L416-0001 Rev. 08/11/03

SINEQUAN® ℞
[sĭn 'a-kwŏn]
(doxepin HCl)
Capsules
Oral Concentrate

Prescribing information for this product, which appears on pages 2636–2637 of the 2004 PDR, has been completely revised as follows. Please write "See Supplement A" next to the product heading.

DESCRIPTION

SINEQUAN® (doxepin hydrochloride) is one of a class of psychotherapeutic agents known as dibenzoxepin tricyclic compounds. The molecular formula of the compound is $C_{19}H_{21}NO \cdot HCl$ having a molecular weight of 316. It is a white crystalline solid readily soluble in water, lower alcohols and chloroform.
Inert ingredients for the capsule formulations are: hard gelatin capsules (which may contain Blue 1, Red 3, Red 40, Yellow 10, and other inert ingredients); magnesium stearate; sodium lauryl sulfate; starch.
Inert ingredients for the oral concentrate formulation are: glycerin; methylparaben; peppermint oil; propylparaben; water.

CHEMISTRY
SINEQUAN (doxepin HCl) is a dibenzoxepin derivative and is the first of a family of tricyclic psychotherapeutic agents. Specifically, it is an isomeric mixture of:
1-Propanamine, 3-dibenz[*b,e*]oxepin-11 (6*H*)ylidene-*N,N*-dimethyl-, hydrochloride.

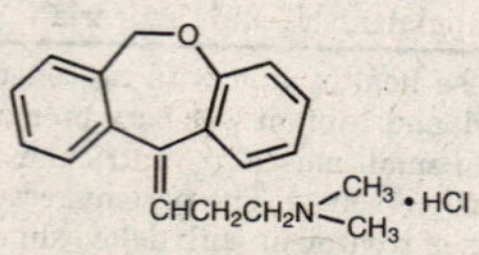

SINEQUAN (doxepin HCl)

ACTIONS

The mechanism of action of SINEQUAN (doxepin HCl) is not definitely known. It is not a central nervous system stimulant nor a monoamine oxidase inhibitor. The current hypothesis is that the clinical effects are due, at least in part, to influences on the adrenergic activity at the synapses so that deactivation of norepinephrine by reuptake into the nerve terminals is prevented. Animal studies suggest that doxepin HCl does not appreciably antagonize the antihypertensive action of guanethidine. In animal studies anticholinergic, antiserotonin and antihistamine effects on smooth muscle have been demonstrated. At higher than usual clinical doses, norepinephrine response was potentiated in animals. This effect was not demonstrated in humans.
At clinical dosages up to 150 mg per day, SINEQUAN can be given to man concomitantly with guanethidine and related compounds without blocking the antihypertensive effect. At dosages above 150 mg per day blocking of the antihypertensive effect of these compounds has been reported.
SINEQUAN is virtually devoid of euphoria as a side effect. Characteristic of this type of compound, SINEQUAN has not been demonstrated to produce the physical tolerance or psychological dependence associated with addictive compounds.

INDICATIONS

SINEQUAN is recommended for the treatment of:
1. Psychoneurotic patients with depression and/or anxiety.
2. Depression and/or anxiety associated with alcoholism (not to be taken concomitantly with alcohol).
3. Depression and/or anxiety associated with organic disease (the possibility of drug interaction should be considered if the patient is receiving other drugs concomitantly).
4. Psychotic depressive disorders with associated anxiety including involutional depression and manic-depressive disorders.

The target symptoms of psychoneurosis that respond particularly well to SINEQUAN include anxiety, tension, depression, somatic symptoms and concerns, sleep disturbances, guilt, lack of energy, fear, apprehension and worry.
Clinical experience has shown that SINEQUAN is safe and well tolerated even in the elderly patient. Owing to lack of clinical experience in the pediatric population, SINEQUAN is not recommended for use in children under 12 years of age.

Table 10. Marked Laboratory Abnormalities Reported by ≥2% of Patients

Adverse Events	Toxicity Limit	Study 21 Part II			Study 13C	
		ZDV + 3TC N = 123	400 mg tid RESCRIPTOR + ZDV N = 123	400 mg tid RESCRIPTOR + ZDV + 3TC N = 119	ZDV + ddI, ddC, or 3TC N = 172	400 mg tid RESCRIPTOR + ZDV + ddI, ddC, or 3TC N = 170
		% pts.	% pts.	% pts.	% pts.	% pts.
Hematology						
Hemoglobin	<7 mg/dL	4.1	2.5	0.9	1.7	2.9
Neutrophils	<750/mm^3	5.7	4.9	3.4	10.4	7.6
Prothrombin time (PT)	>1.5 × ULN	0	0	1.7	2.9	2.4
Activated partial thromboplastin (APTT)	>2.33 × ULN	0	0.8	0	5.8	2.4
Chemistry						
Alanine aminotransferase (ALT/SGPT)	>5 × ULN	2.5	4.1	5.1	3.5	4.1
Amylase	>2 × ULN	0.8	2.5	2.6	3.5	2.9
Aspartate aminotransferase (AST/SGOT)	>5 × ULN	1.6	2.5	3.4	3.5	2.3
Bilirubin	>2.5 × ULN	0.8	2.5	1.7	1.2	0
Gamma glutamyl transferase (GGT)	>5 × ULN	N/A	N/A	N/A	4.1	1.8
Glucose (hypo-/hyperglycemia)	<40 mg/dL >250 mg/dL	4.1	0.8	1.7	1.2	0.0

N/A = not applicable because no predose values were obtained for patients

CONTRAINDICATIONS

SINEQUAN is contraindicated in individuals who have shown hypersensitivity to the drug. Possibility of cross sensitivity with other dibenzoxepines should be kept in mind. SINEQUAN is contraindicated in patients with glaucoma or a tendency to urinary retention. These disorders should be ruled out, particularly in older patients.

WARNINGS

The once-a-day dosage regimen of SINEQUAN in patients with intercurrent illness or patients taking other medications should be carefully adjusted. This is especially important in patients receiving other medications with anticholinergic effects.

Usage in Geriatrics: The use of SINEQUAN on a once-a-day dosage regimen in geriatric patients should be adjusted carefully based on the patient's condition (see PRECAUTIONS—Geriatric Use).

Usage in Pregnancy: Reproduction studies have been performed in rats, rabbits, monkeys and dogs and there was no evidence of harm to the animal fetus. The relevance to humans is not known. Since there is no experience in pregnant women who have received this drug, safety in pregnancy has not been established. There has been a report of apnea and drowsiness occurring in a nursing infant whose mother was taking SINEQUAN.

Usage in Children: The use of SINEQUAN in children under 12 years of age is not recommended because safe conditions for its use have not been established.

PRECAUTIONS

Drug Interactions: *Drugs Metabolized by P450 2D6:* The biochemical activity of the drug metabolizing isozyme cytochrome P450 2D6 (debrisoquin hydroxylase) is reduced in a subset of the Caucasian population (about 7-10% of Caucasians are so-called "poor metabolizers"); reliable estimates of the prevalence of reduced P450 2D6 isozyme activity among Asian, African and other populations are not yet available. Poor metabolizers have higher than expected plasma concentrations of tricyclic antidepressants (TCAs) when given usual doses. Depending on the fraction of drug metabolized by P450 2D6, the increase in plasma concentration may be small, or quite large (8-fold increase in plasma AUC of the TCA).

In addition, certain drugs inhibit the activity of this isozyme and make normal metabolizers resemble poor metabolizers. An individual who is stable on a given dose of TCA may become abruptly toxic when given one of these inhibiting drugs as concomitant therapy. The drugs that inhibit cytochrome P450 2D6 include some that are not metabolized by the enzyme (quinidine; cimetidine) and many that are substrates for P450 2D6 (many other antidepressants, phenothiazines, and the Type 1C antiarrhythmics propafenone and flecainide). While all the selective serotonin reuptake inhibitors (SSRIs), e.g., citalopram, escitalopram, fluoxetine, sertraline, and paroxetine, inhibit P450 2D6, they may vary in the extent of inhibition. The extent to which SSRI-TCA interactions may pose clinical problems will depend on the degree of inhibition and the pharmacokinetics of the SSRI involved. Nevertheless, caution is indicated in the coadministration of TCAs with any of the SSRIs and also in switching from one class to the other. Of particular importance, sufficient time must elapse before initiating TCA treatment in a patient being withdrawn from fluoxetine, given the long half-life of the parent and active metabolite (at least 5 weeks may be necessary).

Concomitant use of tricyclic antidepressants with drugs that can inhibit cytochrome P450 2D6 may require lower doses than usually prescribed for either the tricyclic antidepressant or the other drug. Furthermore, whenever one of these other drugs is withdrawn from co-therapy, an increased dose of tricyclic antidepressant may be required. It is desirable to monitor TCA plasma levels whenever a TCA is going to be co-administered with another drug known to be an inhibitor of P450 2D6.

Doxepin is primarily metabolized by CYP2D6 (with CYP1A2 & CYP3A4 as minor pathways). Inhibitors or substrates of CYP2D6 (i.e., quinidine, selective serotonin reuptake inhibitors [SSRIs]) may increase the plasma concentration of doxepin when administered concomitantly. The extent of interaction depends on the variability of effect on CYP2D6. The clinical significance of this interaction with doxepin has not been systematically evaluated.

MAO Inhibitors: Serious side effects and even death have been reported following the concomitant use of certain drugs with MAO inhibitors. Therefore, MAO inhibitors should be discontinued at least two weeks prior to the cautious initiation of therapy with SINEQUAN. The exact length of time may vary and is dependent upon the particular MAO inhibitor being used, the length of time it has been administered, and the dosage involved.

Cimetidine: Cimetidine has been reported to produce clinically significant fluctuations in steady-state serum concentrations of various tricyclic antidepressants. Serious anticholinergic symptoms (i.e., severe dry mouth, urinary retention and blurred vision) have been associated with elevations in the serum levels of tricyclic antidepressant when cimetidine therapy is initiated. Additionally, higher than expected tricyclic antidepressant levels have been observed when they are begun in patients already taking cimetidine. In patients who have been reported to be well controlled on tricyclic antidepressants receiving concurrent cimetidine therapy, discontinuation of cimetidine has been reported to decrease established steady-state serum tricyclic antidepressant levels and compromise their therapeutic effects.

Alcohol: It should be borne in mind that alcohol ingestion may increase the danger inherent in any intentional or unintentional SINEQUAN overdosage. This is especially important in patients who may use alcohol excessively.

Tolazamide: A case of severe hypoglycemia has been reported in a type II diabetic patient maintained on tolazamide (1 gm/day) 11 days after the addition of doxepin (75 mg/day).

Drowsiness: Since drowsiness may occur with the use of this drug, patients should be warned of the possibility and cautioned against driving a car or operating dangerous machinery while taking the drug. Patients should also be cautioned that their response to alcohol may be potentiated.

Sedating drugs may cause confusion and oversedation in the elderly; elderly patients generally should be started on low doses of SINEQUAN and observed closely. (See PRECAUTIONS—Geriatric Use.)

Suicide: Since suicide is an inherent risk in any depressed patient and may remain so until significant improvement has occurred, patients should be closely supervised during the early course of therapy. Prescriptions should be written for the smallest feasible amount.

Psychosis: Should increased symptoms of psychosis or shift to manic symptomatology occur, it may be necessary to reduce dosage or add a major tranquilizer to the dosage regimen.

Geriatric Use: A determination has not been made whether controlled clinical studies of SINEQUAN included sufficient numbers of subjects aged 65 and over to define a difference in response from younger subjects. Other reported clinical experience has not identified differences in responses between the elderly and younger patients. In general, dose selection for an elderly patient should be cautious, usually starting at the low end of the dosing range, reflecting the greater frequency of decreased hepatic, renal or cardiac function, and of concomitant disease or other drug therapy.

The extent of renal excretion of SINEQUAN has not been determined. Because elderly patients are more likely to have decreased renal function, care should be taken in dose selections.

Sedating drugs may cause confusion and oversedation in the elderly; elderly patients generally should be started on low doses of SINEQUAN and observed closely. (See WARNINGS.)

ADVERSE REACTIONS

NOTE: Some of the adverse reactions noted below have not been specifically reported with SINEQUAN use. However, due to the close pharmacological similarities among the tricyclics, the reactions should be considered when prescribing SINEQUAN (doxepin HCl).

Anticholinergic Effects: Dry mouth, blurred vision, constipation, and urinary retention have been reported. If they do not subside with continued therapy, or become severe, it may be necessary to reduce the dosage.

Central Nervous System Effects: Drowsiness is the most commonly noticed side effect. This tends to disappear as therapy is continued. Other infrequently reported CNS side effects are confusion, disorientation, hallucinations, numbness, paresthesias, ataxia, extrapyramidal symptoms, seizures, tardive dyskinesia, and tremor.

Cardiovascular: Cardiovascular effects including hypotension, hypertension, and tachycardia have been reported occasionally.

Allergic: Skin rash, edema, photosensitization, and pruritus have occasionally occurred.

Hematologic: Eosinophilia has been reported in a few patients. There have been occasional reports of bone marrow depression manifesting as agranulocytosis, leukopenia, thrombocytopenia, and purpura.

Gastrointestinal: Nausea, vomiting, indigestion, taste disturbances, diarrhea, anorexia, and aphthous stomatitis have been reported. (See Anticholinergic Effects.)

Endocrine: Raised or lowered libido, testicular swelling, gynecomastia in males, enlargement of breasts and galactorrhea in the female, raising or lowering of blood sugar levels, and syndrome of inappropriate antidiuretic hormone secretion have been reported with tricyclic administration.

Other: Dizziness, tinnitus, weight gain, sweating, chills, fatigue, weakness, flushing, jaundice, alopecia, headache, exacerbation of asthma, and hyperpyrexia (in association with chlorpromazine) have been occasionally observed as adverse effects.

Withdrawal Symptoms: The possibility of development of withdrawal symptoms upon abrupt cessation of treatment after prolonged SINEQUAN administration should be borne in mind. These are not indicative of addiction and gradual withdrawal of medication should not cause these symptoms.

DOSAGE AND ADMINISTRATION

For most patients with illness of mild to moderate severity, a starting daily dose of 75 mg is recommended. Dosage may subsequently be increased or decreased at appropriate intervals and according to individual response. The usual optimum dose range is 75 mg/day to 150 mg/day.

In more severely ill patients higher doses may be required with subsequent gradual increase to 300 mg/day if necessary. Additional therapeutic effect is rarely to be obtained by exceeding a dose of 300 mg/day.

In patients with very mild symptomatology or emotional symptoms accompanying organic disease, lower doses may suffice. Some of these patients have been controlled on doses as low as 25-50 mg/day.

The total daily dosage of SINEQUAN may be given on a divided or once-a-day dosage schedule. If the once-a-day schedule is employed, the maximum recommended dose is 150 mg/day. This dose may be given at bedtime. **The 150 mg capsule strength is intended for maintenance therapy only and is not recommended for initiation of treatment.**

Anti-anxiety effect is apparent before the antidepressant effect. Optimal antidepressant effect may not be evident for two to three weeks.

OVERDOSAGE

Deaths may occur from overdosage with this class of drugs. Multiple drug ingestion (including alcohol) is common in de-

Continued on next page

Sinequan—Cont.

liberate tricyclic antidepressant overdose. As the management is complex and changing, it is recommended that the physician contact a poison control center for current information on treatment. Signs and symptoms of toxicity develop rapidly after tricyclic antidepressant overdose; therefore, hospital monitoring is required as soon as possible.

Manifestations: Critical manifestations of overdose include: cardiac dysrhythmias, severe hypotension, convulsions, and CNS depression, including coma. Changes in the electrocardiogram, particularly in QRS axis or width, are clinically significant indicators of tricyclic antidepressant toxicity.

Other signs of overdose may include: confusion, disturbed concentration, transient visual hallucinations, dilated pupils, agitation, hyperactive reflexes, stupor, drowsiness, muscle rigidity, vomiting, hypothermia, hyperpyrexia, or any of the symptoms listed under ADVERSE REACTIONS. Deaths have been reported involving overdoses of doxepin.

General Recommendations:

General: Obtain an ECG and immediately initiate cardiac monitoring. Protect the patient's airway, establish an intravenous line and initiate gastric decontamination. A minimum of six hours of observation with cardiac monitoring and observation for signs of CNS or respiratory depression, hypotension, cardiac dysrhythmias and/or conduction blocks, and seizures is strongly advised. If signs of toxicity occur at any time during this period, extended monitoring is recommended. There are case reports of patients succumbing to fatal dysrhythmias late after overdose; these patients had clinical evidence of significant poisoning prior to death and most received inadequate gastrointestinal decontamination. Monitoring of plasma drug levels should not guide management of the patient.

Gastrointestinal Decontamination: All patients suspected of tricyclic antidepressant overdose should receive gastrointestinal decontamination. This should include large volume gastric lavage followed by activated charcoal. If consciousness is impaired, the airway should be secured prior to lavage. Emesis is contraindicated.

Cardiovascular: A maximal limb-lead QRS duration of ≥0.10 seconds may be the best indication of the severity of the overdose. Intravenous sodium bicarbonate should be used to maintain the serum pH in the range of 7.45 to 7.55. If the pH response is inadequate, hyperventilation may also be used. Concomitant use of hyperventilation and sodium bicarbonate should be done with extreme caution, with frequent pH monitoring. A pH >7.60 or a pCO_2 <20 mm Hg is undesirable. Dysrhythmias unresponsive to sodium bicarbonate therapy/hyperventilation may respond to lidocaine, bretylium or phenytoin. Type 1A and 1C antiarrhythmics are generally contraindicated (e.g., quinidine, disopyramide, and procainamide).

In rare instances, hemoperfusion may be beneficial in acute refractory cardiovascular instability in patients with acute toxicity. However, hemodialysis, peritoneal dialysis, exchange transfusions, and forced diuresis generally have been reported as ineffective in tricyclic antidepressant poisoning.

CNS: In patients with CNS depression, early intubation is advised because of the potential for abrupt deterioration. Seizures should be controlled with benzodiazepines, or if these are ineffective, other anticonvulsants (e.g., phenobarbital, phenytoin). Physostigmine is not recommended except to treat life-threatening symptoms that have been unresponsive to other therapies, and then only in consultation with a poison control center.

Psychiatric Follow-up: Since overdosage is often deliberate, patients may attempt suicide by other means during the recovery phase. Psychiatric referral may be appropriate.

Pediatric Management: The principles of management of child and adult overdosages are similar. It is strongly recommended that the physician contact the local poison control center for specific pediatric treatment.

HOW SUPPLIED

SINEQUAN® is available as capsules containing doxepin HCl equivalent to:

10 mg—100's (NDC 0049-5340-66)
25 mg—100's (NDC 0049-5350-66)
50 mg—100's (NDC 0049-5360-66)
75 mg—100's (NDC 0049-5390-66)
100 mg—100's (NDC 0049-5380-66)
150 mg—50's (NDC 0049-5370-50)

SINEQUAN® Oral Concentrate is available in 120 mL bottles (NDC 0049-5100-47) with an accompanying dropper calibrated at 5 mg, 10 mg, 15 mg, 20 mg, and 25 mg. Each mL contains doxepin HCl equivalent to 10 mg doxepin. Just prior to administration, SINEQUAN® Oral Concentrate should be diluted with approximately 120 mL of water, whole or skimmed milk, or orange, grapefruit, tomato, prune or pineapple juice. SINEQUAN® Oral Concentrate is not physically compatible with a number of carbonated beverages. For those patients requiring antidepressant therapy who are on methadone maintenance, SINEQUAN® Oral Concentrate and methadone syrup can be mixed together with Gatorade®, lemonade, orange juice, sugar water, Tang®, or water; but not with grape juice. Preparation and storage of bulk dilutions is not recommended.

Rx only

Distributed by:
Roerig
Division of Pfizer Inc, NY, NY 10017

69-2135-00-2 Revised October 2003

UNASYN® ℞

[*ew-nā-sĭn*]
(ampicillin sodium/sulbactam sodium)

Prescribing information for this product, which appears on pages 2651–2654 of the 2004 PDR, has been completely revised as follows. Please write "See Supplement A" next to the product heading.

To reduce the development of drug-resistant bacteria and maintain the effectiveness of UNASYN® and other antibacterial drugs, UNASYN should be used only to treat or prevent infections that are proven or strongly suspected to be caused by bacteria.

DESCRIPTION

UNASYN is an injectable antibacterial combination consisting of the semisynthetic antibiotic ampicillin sodium and the beta-lactamase inhibitor sulbactam sodium for intravenous and intramuscular administration.

Ampicillin sodium is derived from the penicillin nucleus, 6-aminopenicillanic acid. Chemically, it is monosodium (2S, 5R, 6R)-6-[(R)-2-amino-2-phenylacetamido]-3,3-dimethyl-7-oxo-4-thia-1-azabicyclo[3.2.0]heptane-2-carboxylate and has a molecular weight of 371.39. Its chemical formula is $C_{16}H_{18}N_3NaO_4S$. The structural formula is:

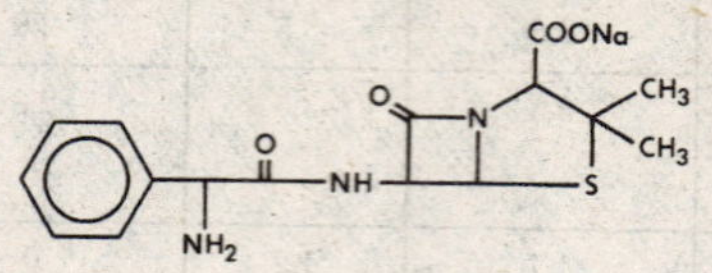

Sulbactam sodium is a derivative of the basic penicillin nucleus. Chemically, sulbactam sodium is sodium penicillinate sulfone; sodium (2S, 5R)-3,3-dimethyl-7-oxo-4-thia- 1-azabicyclo [3.2.0] heptane-2-carboxylate 4,4-dioxide. Its chemical formula is $C_8H_{10}NNaO_5S$ with a molecular weight of 255.22. The structural formula is:

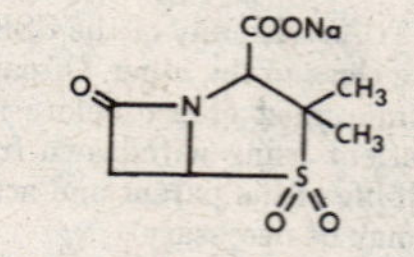

UNASYN, ampicillin sodium/sulbactam sodium parenteral combination, is available as a white to off-white dry powder for reconstitution. UNASYN dry powder is freely soluble in aqueous diluents to yield pale yellow to yellow solutions containing ampicillin sodium and sulbactam sodium equivalent to 250 mg ampicillin per mL and 125 mg sulbactam per mL. The pH of the solutions is between 8.0 and 10.0.

Dilute solutions (up to 30 mg ampicillin and 15 mg sulbactam per mL) are essentially colorless to pale yellow. The pH of dilute solutions remains the same.

1.5 g of UNASYN (1 g ampicillin as the sodium salt plus 0.5 g sulbactam as the sodium salt) parenteral contains approximately 115 mg (5 mEq) of sodium.

3 g of UNASYN (2 g ampicillin as the sodium salt plus 1 g sulbactam as the sodium salt) parenteral contains approximately 230 mg (10 mEq) of sodium.

CLINICAL PHARMACOLOGY

General: Immediately after completion of a 15-minute intravenous infusion of UNASYN, peak serum concentrations of ampicillin and sulbactam are attained. Ampicillin serum levels are similar to those produced by the administration of equivalent amounts of ampicillin alone. Peak ampicillin serum levels ranging from 109 to 150 mcg/mL are attained after administration of 2000 mg of ampicillin plus 1000 mg sulbactam and 40 to 71 mcg/mL after administration of 1000 mg ampicillin plus 500 mg sulbactam. The corresponding mean peak serum levels for sulbactam range from 48 to 88 mcg/mL and 21 to 40 mcg/mL, respectively. After an intramuscular injection of 1000 mg ampicillin plus 500 mg sulbactam, peak ampicillin serum levels ranging from 8 to 37 mcg/mL and peak sulbactam serum levels ranging from 6 to 24 mcg/mL are attained.

The mean serum half-life of both drugs is approximately 1 hour in healthy volunteers.

Approximately 75 to 85% of both ampicillin and sulbactam are excreted unchanged in the urine during the first 8 hours after administration of UNASYN to individuals with normal renal function. Somewhat higher and more prolonged serum levels of ampicillin and sulbactam can be achieved with the concurrent administration of probenecid.

In patients with impaired renal function the elimination kinetics of ampicillin and sulbactam are similarly affected, hence the ratio of one to the other will remain constant whatever the renal function. The dose of UNASYN in such patients should be administered less frequently in accordance with the usual practice for ampicillin (see DOSAGE and ADMINISTRATION).

Ampicillin has been found to be approximately 28% reversibly bound to human serum protein and sulbactam approximately 38% reversibly bound.

The following average levels of ampicillin and sulbactam were measured in the tissues and fluids listed:

TABLE A
Concentration of UNASYN in Various Body Tissues and Fluids

Fluid or Tissue	Dose (grams) Ampicillin/ Sulbactam	Concentration (mcg/mL or mcg/g) Ampicillin/ Sulbactam
Peritoneal Fluid	0.5/0.5 IV	7/14
Blister Fluid (Cantharides)	0.5/0.5 IV	8/20
Tissue Fluid	1/0.5 IV	8/4
Intestinal Mucosa	0.5/0.5 IV	11/18
Appendix	2/1 IV	3/40

Penetration of both ampicillin and sulbactam into cerebrospinal fluid in the presence of inflamed meninges has been demonstrated after IV administration of UNASYN.

The pharmacokinetics of ampicillin and sulbactam in pediatric patients receiving UNASYN are similar to those observed in adults. Immediately after a 15-minute infusion of 50 to 75 mg UNASYN/kg body weight, peak serum and plasma concentrations of 82 to 446 mcg ampicillin/mL and 44 to 203 mcg sulbactam/mL were obtained. Mean half-life values were approximately 1 hour.

MICROBIOLOGY

Ampicillin is similar to benzyl penicillin in its bactericidal action against susceptible organisms during the stage of active multiplication. It acts through the inhibition of cell wall mucopeptide biosynthesis. Ampicillin has a broad spectrum of bactericidal activity against many gram-positive and gram-negative aerobic and anaerobic bacteria. (Ampicillin is, however, degraded by beta-lactamases and therefore the spectrum of activity does not normally include organisms which produce these enzymes.)

A wide range of beta-lactamases found in microorganisms resistant to penicillins and cephalosporins have been shown in biochemical studies with cell free bacterial systems to be irreversibly inhibited by sulbactam. Although sulbactam alone possesses little useful antibacterial activity except against the *Neisseriaceae*, whole organism studies have shown that sulbactam restores ampicillin activity against beta-lactamase producing strains. In particular, sulbactam has good inhibitory activity against the clinically important plasmid mediated beta-lactamases most frequently responsible for transferred drug resistance. Sulbactam has no effect on the activity of ampicillin against ampicillin susceptible strains.

The presence of sulbactam in the UNASYN formulation effectively extends the antibiotic spectrum of ampicillin to include many bacteria normally resistant to it and to other beta-lactam antibiotics. Thus, UNASYN possesses the properties of a broad-spectrum antibiotic and a beta-lactamase inhibitor.

While *in vitro* studies have demonstrated the susceptibility of most strains of the following organisms, clinical efficacy for infections other than those included in the indications section has not been documented.

Gram-Positive Bacteria: *Staphylococcus aureus* (beta-lactamase and non-beta-lactamase producing), *Staphylococcus epidermidis* (beta-lactamase and non-beta-lactamase producing), *Staphylococcus saprophyticus* (beta-lactamase and non-beta-lactamase producing), *Streptococcus faecalis*† (Enterococcus), *Streptococcus pneumoniae*† (formerly *D. pneumoniae*), *Streptococcus pyogenes*†, *Streptococcus viridans*†.

Gram-Negative Bacteria: *Hemophilus influenzae* (beta-lactamase and non-beta-lactamase producing), *Moraxella (Branhamella) catarrhalis* (beta-lactamase and non-beta-lactamase producing), *Escherichia coli* (beta-lactamase and non-beta-lactamase producing), *Klebsiella* species (all known strains are beta-lactamase producing), *Proteus mirabilis* (beta-lactamase and non-beta-lactamase producing), *Proteus vulgaris, Providencia rettgeri, Providencia stuartii, Morganella morganii*, and *Neisseria gonorrhoeae* (beta-lactamase and non-beta-lactamase producing).

Anaerobes: *Clostridium* species†, *Peptococcus* species†, *Peptostreptococcus* species, *Bacteroides* species, including *B. fragilis*.

†These are not beta-lactamase producing strains and, therefore, are susceptible to ampicillin alone.

Susceptibility Testing

Diffusion Technique: For the Kirby-Bauer method of susceptibility testing, a 20 mcg (10 mcg ampicillin + 10 mcg sulbactam) diffusion disk should be used. The method is one outlined in the NCCLS publication M2-A4.[1] With this procedure, a report from the laboratory of "Susceptible" indicates that the infecting organism is likely to respond to UNASYN therapy and a report of "Resistant" indicates that the infecting organism is not likely to respond to therapy. An "Intermediate" susceptibility report suggests that the infecting organism would be susceptible to UNASYN if a higher dosage is used or if the infection is confined to tissues or fluids (e.g., urine) in which high antibiotic levels are attained.

Dilution Techniques: Broth or agar dilution methods may be used to determine the minimal inhibitory concentration (MIC) value for susceptibility of bacterial isolates to ampicillin/sulbactam. The method used is one outlined in the NCCLS publication M7-A2.[2] Tubes should be inoculated to contain 10^5 to 10^6 organisms/mL or plates "spotted" with 10^4 organisms.

The recommended dilution method employs a constant ampicillin/sulbactam ratio of 2:1 in all tubes with increasing

concentrations of ampicillin. MIC's are reported in terms of ampicillin concentration in the presence of sulbactam at a constant 2 parts ampicillin to 1 part sulbactam.
[See table above]

Recommended ampicillin/sulbactam, Susceptibility Ranges[1,2,3]

	Resistant	Intermediate	Susceptible
Gram(-) and Staphylococcus			
Bauer/Kirby Zone Sizes	≤11 mm	12-13 mm	≥14 mm
MIC (mcg of ampicillin/mL)	≥32	16	≤ 8
Hemophilus influenzae			
Bauer/Kirby Zone Sizes	≤19	—	≥20
MIC (mcg of ampicillin/mL)	≥ 4	—	≤ 2

[1] The non-beta-lactamase producing organisms which are normally susceptible to ampicillin, such as *Streptococci*, will have similar zone sizes as for ampicillin disks.
[2] *Staphylococci* resistant to methicillin, oxacillin, or nafcillin must be considered resistant to UNASYN.
[3] The quality control cultures should have the following assigned daily ranges for ampicillin/sulbactam:

		Disks	Mode MIC (mcg/mL ampicillin/ mcg/mL sulbactam)
E. coli	(ATCC 25922)	20-24 mm	2/1
S. aureus	(ATCC 25923)	29-37 mm	0.12/0.06
E. coli	(ATCC 35218)	13-19 mm	8/4

INDICATIONS AND USAGE

UNASYN is indicated for the treatment of infections due to susceptible strains of the designated microorganisms in the conditions listed below.

Skin and Skin Structure Infections caused by beta-lactamase producing strains of *Staphylococcus aureus, Escherichia coli,* Klebsiella* spp.* (including *K. pneumoniae*), Proteus mirabilis,* Bacteroides fragilis,* Enterobacter* spp.,* and *Acinetobacter calcoaceticus.**

NOTE: For information on use in pediatric patients see PRECAUTIONS–Pediatric Use and CLINICAL STUDIES sections.

Intra-Abdominal Infections caused by beta-lactamase producing strains of *Escherichia coli, Klebsiella* spp. (including *K. pneumoniae*), Bacteroides* spp. (including *B. fragilis*), and *Enterobacter* spp.*

Gynecological Infections caused by beta-lactamase producing strains of *Escherichia coli,** and *Bacteroides* spp.* (including *B. fragilis**).

*Efficacy for this organism in this organ system was studied in fewer than 10 infections.

While UNASYN is indicated only for the conditions listed above, infections caused by ampicillin-susceptible organisms are also amenable to treatment with UNASYN due to its ampicillin content. Therefore, mixed infections caused by ampicillin-susceptible organisms and beta-lactamase producing organisms susceptible to UNASYN should not require the addition of another antibiotic.

Appropriate culture and susceptibility tests should be performed before treatment in order to isolate and identify the organisms causing infection and to determine their susceptibility to UNASYN.

Therapy may be instituted prior to obtaining the results from bacteriological and susceptibility studies, when there is reason to believe the infection may involve any of the beta-lactamase producing organisms listed above in the indicated organ systems. Once the results are known, therapy should be adjusted if appropriate.

To reduce the development of drug-resistant bacteria and maintain effectiveness of UNASYN and other antibacterial drugs, UNASYN should be used only to treat or prevent infections that are proven or strongly suspected to be caused by susceptible bacteria. When culture and susceptibility information are available, they should be considered in selecting or modifying antibacterial therapy. In the absence of such data, local epidemiology and susceptibility patterns may contribute to the empiric selection of therapy.

CONTRAINDICATIONS

The use of UNASYN is contraindicated in individuals with a history of hypersensitivity reactions to any of the penicillins.

WARNINGS

SERIOUS AND OCCASIONALLY FATAL HYPERSENSITIVITY (ANAPHYLACTIC) REACTIONS HAVE BEEN REPORTED IN PATIENTS ON PENICILLIN THERAPY. THESE REACTIONS ARE MORE APT TO OCCUR IN INDIVIDUALS WITH A HISTORY OF PENICILLIN HYPERSENSITIVITY AND/OR HYPERSENSITIVITY REACTIONS TO MULTIPLE ALLERGENS. THERE HAVE BEEN REPORTS OF INDIVIDUALS WITH A HISTORY OF PENICILLIN HYPERSENSITIVITY WHO HAVE EXPERIENCED SEVERE REACTIONS WHEN TREATED WITH CEPHALOSPORINS. BEFORE THERAPY WITH A PENICILLIN, CAREFUL INQUIRY SHOULD BE MADE CONCERNING PREVIOUS HYPERSENSITIVITY REACTIONS TO PENICILLINS, CEPHALOSPORINS, AND OTHER ALLERGENS. IF AN ALLERGIC REACTION OCCURS, UNASYN SHOULD BE DISCONTINUED AND THE APPROPRIATE THERAPY INSTITUTED.

SERIOUS ANAPHYLACTOID REACTIONS REQUIRE IMMEDIATE EMERGENCY TREATMENT WITH EPINEPHRINE. OXYGEN, INTRAVENOUS STEROIDS, AND AIRWAY MANAGEMENT, INCLUDING INTUBATION, SHOULD ALSO BE ADMINISTERED AS INDICATED.

Pseudomembranous colitis has been reported with nearly all antibacterial agents, including UNASYN, and has ranged in severity from mild to life-threatening. Therefore, it is important to consider this diagnosis in patients who present with diarrhea subsequent to the administration of antibacterial agents.

Treatment with antibacterial agents alters the normal flora of the colon and may permit overgrowth of clostridia. Studies indicate that toxin produced by *Clostridium difficile* is one primary cause of "antibiotic-associated colitis."

Mild cases of pseudomembranous colitis usually respond to drug discontinuation alone. In moderate to severe cases, consideration should be given to management with fluids and electrolytes, protein supplementation and treatment with an antibacterial drug clinically effective against *C. difficile* colitis.

PRECAUTIONS

General: A high percentage of patients with mononucleosis who receive ampicillin develop a skin rash. Thus, ampicillin class antibiotics should not be administered to patients with mononucleosis. In patients treated with UNASYN the possibility of superinfections with mycotic or bacterial pathogens should be kept in mind during therapy. If superinfections occur (usually involving *Pseudomonas* or *Candida*), the drug should be discontinued and/or appropriate therapy instituted.

Prescribing UNASYN in the absence of proven or strongly suspected bacterial infection or a prophylactic indication is unlikely to provide benefit to the patient and increases the risk of the development of drug-resistant bacteria.

Information for Patients: Patients should be counseled that antibacterial drugs including UNASYN should only be used to treat bacterial infections. They do not treat viral infections (e.g., the common cold). When UNASYN is prescribed to treat a bacterial infection, patients should be told that although it is common to feel better early in the course of therapy, the medication should be taken exactly as directed. Skipping doses or not completing the full course of therapy may (1) decrease the effectiveness of the immediate treatment and (2) increase the likelihood that bacteria will develop resistance and will not be treatable by UNASYN or other antibacterial drugs in the future.

Drug Interactions: Probenecid decreases the renal tubular secretion of ampicillin and sulbactam. Concurrent use of probenecid with UNASYN may result in increased and prolonged blood levels of ampicillin and sulbactam. The concurrent administration of allopurinol and ampicillin increases substantially the incidence of rashes in patients receiving both drugs as compared to patients receiving ampicillin alone. It is not known whether this potentiation of ampicillin rashes is due to allopurinol or the hyperuricemia present in these patients. There are no data with UNASYN and allopurinol administered concurrently. UNASYN and aminoglycosides should not be reconstituted together due to the *in vitro* inactivation of aminoglycosides by the ampicillin component of UNASYN.

Drug/Laboratory Test Interactions: Administration of UNASYN will result in high urine concentration of ampicillin. High urine concentrations of ampicillin may result in false positive reactions when testing for the presence of glucose in urine using Clinitest™, Benedict's Solution or Fehling's Solution. It is recommended that glucose tests based on enzymatic glucose oxidase reactions (such as Clinistix™ or Testape™) be used. Following administration of ampicillin to pregnant women, a transient decrease in plasma concentration of total conjugated estriol, estriol-glucuronide, conjugated estrone and estradiol has been noted. This effect may also occur with UNASYN.

Carcinogenesis, Mutagenesis, Impairment of Fertility: Long-term studies in animals have not been performed to evaluate carcinogenic or mutagenic potential.

Pregnancy

Pregnancy Category B: Reproduction studies have been performed in mice, rats, and rabbits at doses up to ten (10) times the human dose and have revealed no evidence of impaired fertility or harm to the fetus due to UNASYN. There are, however, no adequate and well controlled studies in pregnant women. Because animal reproduction studies are not always predictive of human response, this drug should be used during pregnancy only if clearly needed. (See–Drug/Laboratory Test Interactions.)

Labor and Delivery: Studies in guinea pigs have shown that intravenous administration of ampicillin decreased the uterine tone, frequency of contractions, height of contractions, and duration of contractions. However, it is not known whether the use of UNASYN in humans during labor or delivery has immediate or delayed adverse effects on the fetus, prolongs the duration of labor, or increases the likelihood that forceps delivery or other obstetrical intervention or resuscitation of the newborn will be necessary.

Nursing Mothers: Low concentrations of ampicillin and sulbactam are excreted in the milk; therefore, caution should be exercised when UNASYN is administered to a nursing woman.

Pediatric Use: The safety and effectiveness of UNASYN have been established for pediatric patients one year of age and older for skin and skin structure infections as approved in adults. Use of UNASYN in pediatric patients is supported by evidence from adequate and well-controlled studies in adults with additional data from pediatric pharmacokinetic studies, a controlled clinical trial conducted in pediatric patients and post-marketing adverse events surveillance. (See **CLINICAL PHARMACOLOGY, INDICATIONS AND USAGE, ADVERSE REACTIONS, DOSAGE AND ADMINISTRATION**, and **CLINICAL STUDIES** sections.)

The safety and effectiveness of UNASYN have not been established for pediatric patients for intra-abdominal infections.

ADVERSE REACTIONS

Adult Patients: UNASYN is generally well tolerated. The following adverse reactions have been reported.

Local Adverse Reactions

Pain at IM injection site – 16%
Pain at IV injection site – 3%
Thrombophlebitis – 3%

Systemic Adverse Reactions

The most frequently reported adverse reactions were diarrhea in 3% of the patients and rash in less than 2% of the patients.

Additional systemic reactions reported in less than 1% of the patients were: itching, nausea, vomiting, candidiasis, fatigue, malaise, headache, chest pain, flatulence, abdominal distension, glossitis, urine retention, dysuria, edema, facial swelling, erythema, chills, tightness in throat, substernal pain, epistaxis and mucosal bleeding.

Pediatric Patients: Available safety data for pediatric patients treated with UNASYN demonstrate a similar adverse events profile to those observed in adult patients. Additionally, atypical lymphocytosis has been observed in one pediatric patient receiving UNASYN.

Adverse Laboratory Changes

Adverse laboratory changes without regard to drug relationship that were reported during clinical trials were:

Hepatic: Increased AST (SGOT), ALT (SGPT), alkaline phosphatase, and LDH.

Hematologic: Decreased hemoglobin, hematocrit, RBC, WBC, neutrophils, lymphocytes, platelets and increased lymphocytes, monocytes, basophils, eosinophils, and platelets.

Blood Chemistry: Decreased serum albumin and total proteins.

Renal: Increased BUN and creatinine.

Urinalysis: Presence of RBC's and hyaline casts in urine.

The following adverse reactions have been reported with ampicillin-class antibiotics and can also occur with UNASYN.

Gastrointestinal: Gastritis, stomatitis, black "hairy" tongue and enterocolitis. Onset of pseudomembranous colitis symptoms may occur during or after antibiotic treatment. (See WARNINGS.)

Hypersensitivity Reactions: Urticaria, erythema multiforme, and an occasional case of exfoliative dermatitis have been reported. These reactions may be controlled with antihistamines and, if necessary, systemic corticosteroids. Whenever such reactions occur, the drug should be discontinued, unless the opinion of the physician dictates otherwise. Serious and occasional fatal hypersensitivity (anaphylactic) reactions can occur with a penicillin. (See WARNINGS.)

Hematologic: In addition to the adverse laboratory changes listed above for UNASYN, agranulocytosis has been reported during therapy with penicillins. All of these reactions are usually reversible on discontinuation of therapy and are believed to be hypersensitivity phenomena. Some individuals have developed positive direct Coombs Tests during treatment with UNASYN, as with other beta-lactam antibiotics.

OVERDOSAGE

Neurological adverse reactions, including convulsions, may occur with the attainment of high CSF levels of beta-lactams. Ampicillin may be removed from circulation by hemodialysis. The molecular weight, degree of protein binding and pharmacokinetics profile of sulbactam suggest that this compound may also be removed by hemodialysis.

CLINICAL STUDIES

Skin and Skin Structure Infections in Pediatric Patients: Data from a controlled clinical trial conducted in pediatric patients provided evidence supporting the safety and efficacy of UNASYN for the treatment of skin and skin structure infections. Of 99 pediatric patients evaluable for clinical efficacy, 60 patients received a regimen containing intravenous UNASYN, and 39 patients received a regimen containing intravenous cefuroxime. This trial demonstrated

Continued on next page

Unasyn—Cont.

similar outcomes (assessed at an appropriate interval after discontinuation of all antimicrobial therapy) for UNASYN- and cefuroxime-treated patients:

Therapeutic Regimen	Clinical Success	Clinical Failure
UNASYN	51/60 (85%)	9/60 (15%)
Cefuroxime	34/39 (87%)	5/39 (13%)

Most patients received a course of oral antimicrobials following initial treatment with intravenous administration of parenteral antimicrobials. The study protocol required that the following three criteria be met prior to transition from intravenous to oral antimicrobial therapy: 1) receipt of a minimum of 72 hours of intravenous therapy; 2) no documented fever for prior 24 hours; and 3) improvement or resolution of the signs and symptoms of infection.
The choice of oral antimicrobial agent used in this trial was determined by susceptibility testing of the original pathogen, if isolated, to oral agents available. The course of oral antimicrobial therapy should not routinely exceed 14 days.

DOSAGE AND ADMINISTRATION

UNASYN may be administered by either the IV or the IM routes.
For IV administration, the dose can be given by slow intravenous injection over at least 10-15 minutes or can also be delivered, in greater dilutions with 50-100 mL of a compatible diluent as an intravenous infusion over 15-30 minutes.
UNASYN may be administered by deep intramuscular injection. (See Preparation for Intramuscular Injection.)
The recommended adult dosage of UNASYN is 1.5 g (1 g ampicillin as the sodium salt plus 0.5 g sulbactam as the sodium salt) to 3 g (2 g ampicillin as the sodium salt plus 1 g sulbactam as the sodium salt) every six hours. This 1.5 to 3 g range represents the total of ampicillin content plus the sulbactam content of UNASYN, and corresponds to a range of 1 g ampicillin/0.5 g sulbactam to 2 g ampicillin/1 g sulbactam. The total dose of sulbactam should not exceed 4 grams per day.

Pediatric Patients 1 Year of Age or Older: The recommended daily dose of UNASYN in pediatric patients is 300 mg per kg of body weight administered via intravenous infusion in equally divided doses every 6 hours. This 300 mg/kg/day dosage represents the total ampicillin content plus the sulbactam content of UNASYN, and corresponds to 200 mg ampicillin/100 mg sulbactam per kg per day. The safety and efficacy of UNASYN administered via intramuscular injection in pediatric patients have not been established. Pediatric patients weighing 40 kg or more should be dosed according to adult recommendations, and the total dose of sulbactam should not exceed 4 grams per day. The course of intravenous therapy should not routinely exceed 14 days. In clinical trials, most children received a course of oral antimicrobials following initial treatment with intravenous UNASYN. (See **CLINICAL STUDIES** section.)

Impaired Renal Function

In patients with impairment of renal function the elimination kinetics of ampicillin and sulbactam are similarly affected, hence the ratio of one to the other will remain constant whatever the renal function. The dose of UNASYN in such patients should be administered less frequently in accordance with the usual practice for ampicillin and according to the following recommendations:

UNASYN Dosage Guide For Patients With Renal Impairment

Creatinine Clearance (mL/min/1.73m²)	Ampicillin/ Sulbactam Half-Life (Hours)	Recommended UNASYN Dosage
≥30	1	1.5-3.0 g q 6h-q 8h
15-29	5	1.5-3.0 g q 12h
5-14	9	1.5-3.0 g q 24h

When only serum creatinine is available, the following formula (based on sex, weight, and age of the patient) may be used to convert this value into creatinine clearance. The serum creatinine should represent a steady state of renal function.

Males $\dfrac{\text{weight (kg)} \times (140 - \text{age})}{72 \times \text{serum creatinine}}$

Females $0.85 \times$ above value

COMPATIBILITY, RECONSTITUTION AND STABILITY

UNASYN sterile powder is to be stored at or below 30°C (86°F) prior to reconstitution.
When concomitant therapy with aminoglycosides is indicated, UNASYN and aminoglycosides should be reconstituted and administered separately, due to the *in vitro* inactivation of aminoglycosides by any of the aminopenicillins.

DIRECTIONS FOR USE

General Dissolution Procedures: UNASYN sterile powder for intravenous and intramuscular use may be reconstituted with any of the compatible diluents described in this insert. Solutions should be allowed to stand after dissolution to allow any foaming to dissipate in order to permit visual inspection for complete solubilization.

Preparation for Intravenous Use

1.5 g and 3.0 g Bottles: UNASYN sterile powder in piggyback units may be reconstituted directly to the desired concentrations using any of the following parenteral diluents. Reconstitution of UNASYN, at the specified concentrations, with these diluents provide stable solutions for the time periods indicated in the following table: (After the indicated time periods, any unused portions of solutions should be discarded.)
[See table below]
If piggyback bottles are unavailable, standard vials of UNASYN sterile powder may be used. Initially, the vials may be reconstituted with Sterile Water for Injection to yield solutions containing 375 mg UNASYN per mL (250 mg ampicillin/125 mg sulbactam per mL). An appropriate volume should then be immediately diluted with a suitable parenteral diluent to yield solutions containing 3 to 45 mg UNASYN per mL (2 to 30 mg ampicillin/1 to 15 mg sulbactam/per mL).
1.5 g ADD-Vantage® Vials: UNASYN in the ADD-Vantage® system is intended as a single dose for intravenous administration after dilution with the ADD-Vantage® Flexible Diluent Container containing 50 mL, 100 mL or 250 mL of 0.9% Sodium Chloride Injection, USP.
3 g ADD-Vantage® Vials: UNASYN in the ADD-Vantage® system is intended as a single dose for intravenous administration after dilution with the ADD-Vantage® Flexible Diluent Container containing 100 mL or 250 mL of 0.9% Sodium Chloride Injection, USP.
UNASYN in the ADD-Vantage® system is to be reconstituted with 0.9% Sodium Chloride Injection, USP only. See INSTRUCTIONS FOR USE OF THE ADD-Vantage® VIAL. Reconstitution of UNASYN, at the specified concentration, with 0.9% Sodium Chloride Injection, USP provides stable solutions for the time period indicated below:

Diluent	Maximum Concentration (mg/mL) UNASYN (Ampicillin/ Sulbactam)	Use Period
0.9% Sodium Chloride Injection	30 (20/10)	8 hrs @ 25°C

In 0.9% Sodium Chloride Injection, USP

The final diluted solution of UNASYN should be completely administered *within 8 hours* in order to assure proper potency.

Preparation for Intramuscular Injection

1.5 g and 3.0 g Standard Vials: Vials for intramuscular use may be reconstituted with Sterile Water for Injection USP, 0.5% Lidocaine Hydrochloride Injection USP or 2% Lidocaine Hydrochloride Injection USP. Consult the following table for recommended volumes to be added to obtain solutions containing 375 mg UNASYN per mL (250 mg ampicillin/125 mg sulbactam per mL). Note: *Use only freshly prepared solutions and administer within one hour after preparation.*

UNASYN Vial Size	Volume of Diluent to be Added	Withdrawal Volume*
1.5 g	3.2 mL	4.0 mL
3.0 g	6.4 mL	8.0 mL

*There is sufficient excess present to allow withdrawal and administration of the stated volumes.

Animal Pharmacology: While reversible glycogenosis was observed in laboratory animals, this phenomenon was dose- and time-dependent and is not expected to develop at the therapeutic doses and corresponding plasma levels attained during the relatively short periods of combined ampicillin/sulbactam therapy in man.

HOW SUPPLIED

UNASYN® (ampicillin sodium/sulbactam sodium) is supplied as a sterile off-white dry powder in glass vials and piggyback bottles. The following packages are available:
Vials containing 1.5 g (NDC 0049-0013-83) equivalent of UNASYN (1 g ampicillin as the sodium salt plus 0.5 g sulbactam as the sodium salt)
Vials containing 3 g (NDC 0049-0014-83) equivalent of UNASYN (2 g ampicillin as the sodium salt plus 1 g sulbactam as the sodium salt)
Bottles containing 1.5 g (NDC 0049-0022-83) equivalent of UNASYN (1 g ampicillin as the sodium salt plus 0.5 g sulbactam as the sodium salt)
Bottles containing 3 g (NDC 0049-0023-83) equivalent of UNASYN (2 g ampicillin as the sodium salt plus 1 g sulbactam as the sodium salt)
Pharmacy Bulk Package containing 15 g (NDC 0049-0024-28) equivalent of UNASYN (10 g ampicillin as the sodium salt plus 5 g sulbactam as the sodium salt)
ADD-Vantage® vials containing 1.5 g (NDC 0049-0031-83) equivalent of UNASYN (1 g ampicillin as the sodium salt plus 0.5 g sulbactam as the sodium salt) are distributed by Pfizer Inc.
ADD-Vantage® vials containing 3 g (NDC 0049-0032-83) equivalent of UNASYN (2 g ampicillin as the sodium salt plus 1 g sulbactam as the sodium salt) are distributed by Pfizer Inc.
The 1.5 g UNASYN ADD-Vantage® vials are only to be used with Abbott Laboratories' ADD-Vantage® Flexible Diluent Container containing 0.9% Sodium Chloride Injection, USP, 50 mL, 100 mL, or 250 mL sizes.
The 3 g UNASYN ADD-Vantage® vials are only to be used with Abbott Laboratories' ADD-Vantage® Flexible Diluent Container containing 0.9% Sodium Chloride Injection, USP, 100 mL or 250 mL sizes.

INSTRUCTIONS FOR USE OF THE ADD-Vantage® VIAL

To Open Diluent Container: Peel overwrap from the corner and remove container. Some opacity of the plastic due to moisture absorption during the sterilization process may be observed. This is normal and does not affect the solution quality or safety. The opacity will diminish gradually.

To Assemble Vial and Flexible Diluent Container: (Use Aseptic Technique)

1. Remove the protective covers from the top of the vial and the vial port on the diluent container as follows:
a. To remove the breakaway vial cap, swing the pull ring over the top of the vial and pull down far enough to start the opening (see Figure 1), pull the ring approximately half way around the cap and then pull straight up to remove the cap (see Figure 2).
NOTE: Do not access vial with syringe.

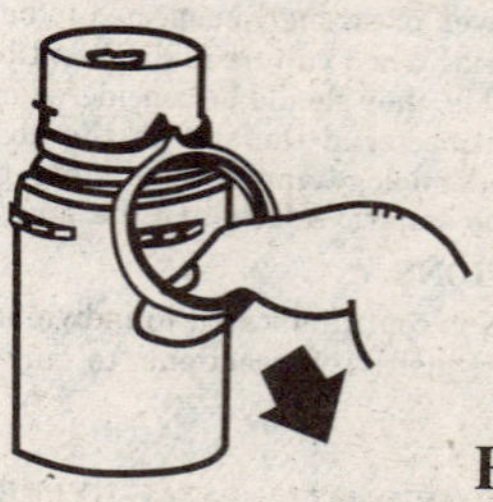

Fig. 1

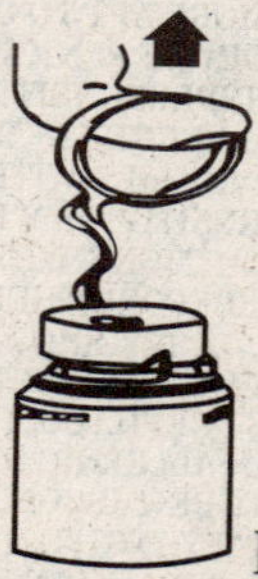

Fig. 2

b. To remove the vial port cover, grasp the tab on the pull ring, pull up to break the three tie strings, then pull back to remove the cover. (See Figure 3.)
2. Screw the vial into the vial port until it will go no further. THE VIAL MUST BE SCREWED IN TIGHTLY TO ASSURE A SEAL. This occurs approximately 1/2 turn (180°) after the first audible click. (See Figure 4.) The clicking sound does not assure a seal, the vial must be turned as far as it will go.
NOTE: Once vial is sealed, do not attempt to remove. (See Figure 4.)
3. Recheck the vial to assure that it is tight by trying to turn it further in the direction of assembly.
4. Label appropriately.
[See figure at top of next column]
[See figure at top of next column]

To Prepare Admixture

1. Squeeze the bottom of the diluent container gently to inflate the portion of the container surrounding the end of the drug vial.

Diluent	Maximum Concentration (mg/mL) UNASYN (Ampicillin/Sulbactam)	Use Periods
Sterile Water for Injection	45 (30/15)	8 hrs @ 25°C
	45 (30/15)	48 hrs @ 4°C
	30 (20/10)	72 hrs @ 4°C
0.9% Sodium Chloride Injection	45 (30/15)	8 hrs @ 25°C
	45 (30/15)	48 hrs @ 4°C
	30 (20/10)	72 hrs @ 4°C
5% Dextrose Injection	30 (20/10)	2 hrs @ 25°C
	30 (20/10)	4 hrs @ 4°C
	3 (2/1)	4 hrs @ 25°C
Lactated Ringer's Injection	45 (30/15)	8 hrs @ 25°C
	45 (30/15)	24 hrs @ 4°C
M/6 Sodium Lactate Injection	45 (30/15)	8 hrs @ 25°C
	45 (30/15)	8 hrs @ 4°C
5% Dextrose in 0.45% Saline	3 (2/1)	4 hrs @ 25°C
	15 (10/5)	4 hrs @ 4°C
10% Invert Sugar	3 (2/1)	4 hrs @ 25°C
	30 (20/10)	3 hrs @ 4°C

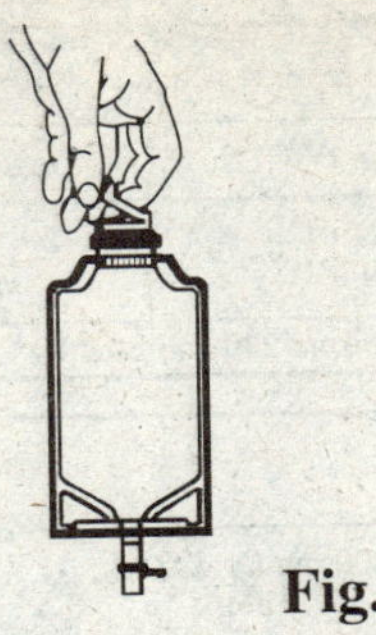

Fig. 3

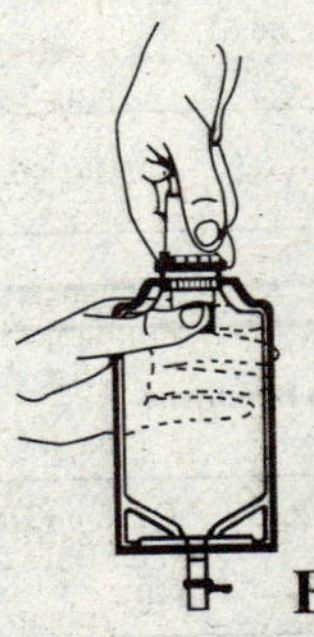

Fig. 4

2. With the other hand, push the drug vial down into the container telescoping the walls of the container. Grasp the inner cap of the vial through the walls of the container. (See Figure 5.)
3. Pull the inner cap from the drug vial. (See Figure 6.) Verify that the rubber stopper has been pulled out, allowing the drug and diluent to mix.
4. Mix container contents thoroughly and use within the specified time.

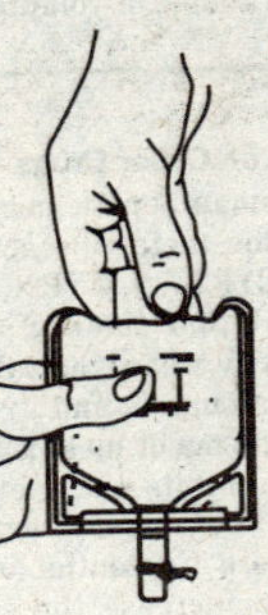

Fig. 5

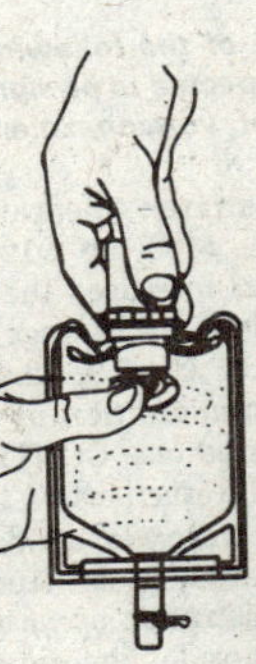

Fig. 6

REFERENCES

1. National Committee for Clinical Laboratory Standards, *Performance Standards for Antimicrobial Disk Susceptibility Tests*–Fourth Edition. Approved Standard NCCLS Document M2-A4, Vol. 10, No. 7 NCCLS, Villanova, PA, April 1990.
2. National Committee for Clinical Laboratory Standards, *Methods for Dilution Antimicrobial Susceptibility Tests for Bacteria that Grow Aerobically*, Second Edition. Approved Standard NCCLS Document M7-A2, Vol. 10, No. 8 NCCLS, Villanova, PA, April 1990.

Rx only

Pfizer Roerig
Division of Pfizer Inc, NY, NY 10017
70-4361-44-4 Revised September 2003

VFEND® I.V. ℞
[*vee'fənd*]
(voriconazole) for Injection
VFEND® Tablets ℞
(voriconazole)
VFEND® for Oral Suspension ℞
(voriconazole)

Prescribing information for this product, which appears on pages 2654–2662 of the 2004 PDR, has been completely revised as follows. Please write "See Supplement A" next to the product heading.

DESCRIPTION

VFEND® (voriconazole), a triazole antifungal agent, is available as a lyophilized powder for solution for intravenous infusion, film-coated tablets for oral administration, and as a powder for oral suspension. The structural formula is:

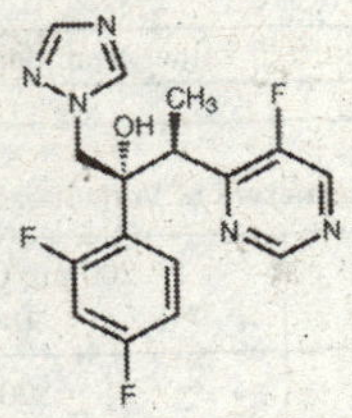

Voriconazole is designated chemically as (2R, 3S)-2-(2,4-difluorophenyl)-3-(5-fluoro-4-pyrimidinyl)-1-(1*H* -1,2,4-triazol-1-yl)-2-butanol with an empirical formula of $C_{16}H_{14}F_3N_5O$ and a molecular weight of 349.3.

Voriconazole drug substance is a white to light-colored powder.

VFEND I.V. is a white lyophilized powder containing nominally 200 mg voriconazole and 3200 mg sulfobutyl ether beta-cyclodextrin sodium in a 30 mL Type I clear glass vial.

VFEND I.V. is intended for administration by intravenous infusion. It is a single dose, unpreserved product. Vials containing 200 mg lyophilized voriconazole are intended for reconstitution with Water for Injection to produce a solution containing 10 mg/mL VFEND and 160 mg/mL of sulfobutyl ether beta-cyclodextrin sodium. The resultant solution is further diluted prior to administration as an intravenous infusion (see DOSAGE AND ADMINISTRATION).

VFEND Tablets contain 50 mg or 200 mg of voriconazole. The inactive ingredients include lactose monohydrate, pregelatinized starch, croscarmellose sodium, povidone, magnesium stearate and a coating containing hypromellose, titanium dioxide, lactose monohydrate and triacetin.

VFEND for Oral Suspension is a white to off-white powder providing a white to off-white orange-flavored suspension when reconstituted. Bottles containing 45 g powder for oral suspension are intended for reconstitution with water to produce a suspension containing 40 mg/mL voriconazole. The inactive ingredients include colloidal silicon dioxide, titanium dioxide, xanthan gum, sodium citrate dihydrate, sodium benzoate, anhydrous citric acid, natural orange flavor, and sucrose.

CLINICAL PHARMACOLOGY

Pharmacokinetics

General Pharmacokinetic Characteristics

The pharmacokinetics of voriconazole have been characterized in healthy subjects, special populations and patients. The pharmacokinetics of voriconazole are non-linear due to saturation of its metabolism. The interindividual variability of voriconazole pharmacokinetics is high. Greater than proportional increase in exposure is observed with increasing dose. It is estimated that, on average, increasing the oral dose in healthy subjects from 200 mg Q12h to 300 mg Q12h leads to a 2.5-fold increase in exposure (AUC_τ) while increasing the intravenous dose from 3 mg/kg Q12h to 4 mg/kg Q12h produces a 2.3-fold increase in exposure (Table 1).

[See table 1 at top of next page]

During oral administration of 200 mg or 300 mg twice daily for 14 days in patients at risk of aspergillosis (mainly patients with malignant neoplasms of lymphatic or hematopoietic tissue), the observed pharmacokinetic characteristics were similar to those observed in healthy subjects (Table 2).

[See table 2 at top of next page]

Sparse plasma sampling for pharmacokinetics was conducted in the therapeutic studies in patients aged 12-18 years. In 11 adolescent patients who received a mean voriconazole maintenance dose of 4 mg/kg IV, the median of the calculated mean plasma concentrations was 1.60 µg/mL (inter-quartile range 0.28 to 2.73 µg/mL). In 17 adolescent patients for whom mean plasma concentrations were calculated following a mean oral maintenance dose of 200 mg Q12h, the median of the calculated mean plasma concentrations was 1.16 µg/mL (inter-quartile range 0.85 to 2.14 µg/mL).

When the recommended intravenous or oral loading dose regimens are administered to healthy subjects, peak plasma concentrations close to steady state are achieved within the first 24 hours of dosing. Without the loading dose, accumulation occurs during twice-daily multiple dosing with steady-state peak plasma voriconazole concentrations being achieved by day 6 in the majority of subjects (Table 3).

[See table 3 at top of next page]

Steady state trough plasma concentrations with voriconazole are achieved after approximately 5 days of oral or intravenous dosing without a loading dose regimen. However, when an intravenous loading dose regimen is used, steady state trough plasma concentrations are achieved within one day.

Absorption

The pharmacokinetic properties of voriconazole are similar following administration by the intravenous and oral routes. Based on a population pharmacokinetic analysis of pooled data in healthy subjects (N=207), the oral bioavailability of voriconazole is estimated to be 96% (CV 13%). Bioequivalence was established between the 200 mg tablet and the 40 mg/mL oral suspension when administered as a 400 mg Q12h loading dose followed by a 200 mg Q12h maintenance dose.

Maximum plasma concentrations (C_{max}) are achieved 1-2 hours after dosing. When multiple doses of voriconazole are administered with high fat meals, the mean C_{max} and AUC_τ are reduced by 34% and 24%, respectively when administered as a tablet and by 58% and 37% respectively when administered as the oral suspension (see DOSAGE AND ADMINISTRATION).

In healthy subjects, the absorption of voriconazole is not affected by coadministration of oral ranitidine, cimetidine, or omeprazole, drugs that are known to increase gastric pH.

Distribution

The volume of distribution at steady state for voriconazole is estimated to be 4.6 L/kg, suggesting extensive distribution into tissues. Plasma protein binding is estimated to be 58% and was shown to be independent of plasma concentrations achieved following single and multiple oral doses of 200 mg or 300 mg (approximate range: 0.9-15 µg/mL). Varying degrees of hepatic and renal insufficiency do not affect the protein binding of voriconazole.

Metabolism

In vitro studies showed that voriconazole is metabolized by the human hepatic cytochrome P450 enzymes, CYP2C19, CYP2C9 and CYP3A4 (see CLINICAL PHARMACOLOGY - Drug Interactions).

In vivo studies indicated that CYP2C19 is significantly involved in the metabolism of voriconazole. This enzyme exhibits genetic polymorphism. For example, 15-20% of Asian populations may be expected to be poor metabolizers. For Caucasians and Blacks, the prevalence of poor metabolizers is 3-5%. Studies conducted in Caucasian and Japanese healthy subjects have shown that poor metabolizers have, on average, 4-fold higher voriconazole exposure (AUC_τ) than their homozygous extensive metabolizer counterparts. Subjects who are heterozygous extensive metabolizers have, on average, 2-fold higher voriconazole exposure than their homozygous extensive metabolizer counterparts.

The major metabolite of voriconazole is the N-oxide, which accounts for 72% of the circulating radiolabelled metabolites in plasma. Since this metabolite has minimal antifungal activity, it does not contribute to the overall efficacy of voriconazole.

Excretion

Voriconazole is eliminated via hepatic metabolism with less than 2% of the dose excreted unchanged in the urine. After administration of a single radiolabelled dose of either oral or IV voriconazole, preceded by multiple oral or IV dosing, approximately 80% to 83% of the radioactivity is recovered in the urine. The majority (>94%) of the total radioactivity is excreted in the first 96 hours after both oral and intravenous dosing.

As a result of non-linear pharmacokinetics, the terminal half-life of voriconazole is dose dependent and therefore not useful in predicting the accumulation or elimination of voriconazole.

Pharmacokinetic-Pharmacodynamic Relationships

Clinical Efficacy and Safety

In ten clinical trials, the median values for the average and maximum voriconazole plasma concentrations in individual patients across these studies (N=1121) was 2.51 µg/mL (inter-quartile range 1.21 to 4.44 µg/mL) and 3.79 µg/mL (inter-quartile range 2.06 to 6.31 µg/mL), respectively. A pharmacokinetic-pharmacodynamic analysis of patient data from 6 of these 10 clinical trials (N=280) could not detect a positive association between mean, maximum or minimum plasma voriconazole concentration and efficacy. However, PK/PD analyses of the data from all 10 clinical trials identified positive associations between plasma voriconazole concentrations and rate of both liver function test abnormalities and visual disturbances (see ADVERSE REACTIONS).

Electrocardiogram

A placebo-controlled, randomized, crossover study to evaluate the effect on the QT interval of healthy male and female volunteers was conducted with three single oral doses of voriconazole and ketoconazole. Serial ECGs and plasma samples were obtained at specified intervals over a 24-hour post dose observation period. The placebo-adjusted mean maximum increases in QTc from baseline after 800, 1200 and 1600 mg of voriconazole and after ketoconazole 800 mg were all <10 msec. Females exhibited a greater increase in QTc than males, although all mean changes were <10 msec. Age was not found to affect the magnitude of increase in QTc. No subject in any group had an increase in QTc of ≥60 msec from baseline. No subject experienced an interval exceeding the potentially clinically relevant threshold of 500 msec. However, the QT effect of voriconazole combined with drugs known to prolong the QT interval is unknown. (See CONTRAINDICATIONS, PRECAUTIONS-Drug Interactions).

Pharmacokinetics in Special Populations

Gender

In a multiple oral dose study, the mean C_{max} and AUC_τ for healthy young females were 83% and 113% higher, respectively, than in healthy young males (18-45 years), after tablet dosing. In the same study, no significant differences in the mean C_{max} and AUC_τ were observed between healthy elderly males and healthy elderly females (≥65 years). In a similar study, after dosing with the oral suspension, the mean AUC for healthy young females was 45% higher than in healthy young males whereas the mean C_{max} was comparable between genders. The steady state trough

Continued on next page

Vfend—Cont.

voriconazole concentrations (C_{min}) seen in females were 100% and 91% higher than in males receiving the tablet and the oral suspension, respectively.

In the clinical program, no dosage adjustment was made on the basis of gender. The safety profile and plasma concentrations observed in male and female subjects were similar. Therefore, no dosage adjustment based on gender is necessary.

Geriatric

In an oral multiple dose study the mean C_{max} and AUC_{τ} in healthy elderly males (≥ 65 years) were 61% and 86% higher, respectively, than in young males (18-45 years). No significant differences in the mean C_{max} and AUC_{τ} were observed between healthy elderly females (≥ 65 years) and healthy young females (18-45 years).

In the clinical program, no dosage adjustment was made on the basis of age. An analysis of pharmacokinetic data obtained from 552 patients from 10 voriconazole clinical trials showed that the median voriconazole plasma concentrations in the elderly patients (>65 years) were approximately 80% to 90% higher than those in the younger patients (≤65 years) after either IV or oral administration. However, the safety profile of voriconazole in young and elderly subjects was similar and, therefore, no dosage adjustment is necessary for the elderly.

Pediatric

A population pharmacokinetic analysis was conducted on pooled data from 35 immunocompromised pediatric patients aged 2 to <12 years old who were included in two pharmacokinetic studies of intravenous voriconazole (single dose and multiple dose). Twenty-four of these patients received multiple intravenous maintenance doses of 3 mg/kg and 4 mg/kg. A comparison of the pediatric and adult population pharmacokinetic data revealed that the predicted average steady state plasma concentrations were similar at the maintenance dose of 4 mg/kg every 12 hours in children and 3 mg/kg every 12 hours in adults (medians of 1.19 μg/mL and 1.16 μg/mL in children and adults, respectively). (See PRECAUTIONS, Pediatric Use.)

Hepatic Insufficiency

After a single oral dose (200 mg) of voriconazole in 8 patients with mild (Child-Pugh Class A) and 4 patients with moderate (Child-Pugh Class B) hepatic insufficiency, the mean systemic exposure (AUC) was 3.2-fold higher than in age and weight matched controls with normal hepatic function. There was no difference in mean peak plasma concentrations (C_{max}) between the groups. When only the patients with mild (Child-Pugh Class A) hepatic insufficiency were compared to controls, there was still a 2.3-fold increase in the mean AUC in the group with hepatic insufficiency compared to controls.

In an oral multiple dose study, AUC_{τ} was similar in six subjects with moderate hepatic impairment (Child-Pugh Class B) given a lower maintenance dose of 100 mg twice daily compared to six subjects with normal hepatic function given the standard 200 mg twice daily maintenance dose. The mean peak plasma concentrations (C_{max}) were 20% lower in the hepatically impaired group.

It is recommended that the standard loading dose regimens be used but that the maintenance dose be halved in patients with mild to moderate hepatic cirrhosis (Child-Pugh Class A and B) receiving voriconazole. No pharmacokinetic data are available for patients with severe hepatic cirrhosis (Child-Pugh Class C) (see DOSAGE AND ADMINISTRATION).

Renal Insufficiency

In a single oral dose (200 mg) study in 24 subjects with normal renal function and mild to severe renal impairment, systemic exposure (AUC) and peak plasma concentration (C_{max}) of voriconazole were not significantly affected by renal impairment. Therefore, no adjustment is necessary for oral dosing in patients with mild to severe renal impairment.

In a multiple dose study of IV voriconazole (6 mg/kg IV loading dose × 2, then 3 mg/kg IV × 5.5 days) in 7 patients with moderate renal dysfunction (creatinine clearance 30-50 mL/min), the systemic exposure (AUC) and peak plasma concentrations (C_{max}) were not significantly different from those in 6 volunteers with normal renal function.

However, in patients with moderate renal dysfunction (creatinine clearance 30-50 mL/min), accumulation of the intravenous vehicle, SBECD, occurs. The mean systemic exposure (AUC) and peak plasma concentrations (C_{max}) of SBECD were increased by 4-fold and almost 50%, respectively, in the moderately impaired group compared to the normal control group.

Intravenous voriconazole should be avoided in patients with moderate or severe renal impairment (creatinine clearance <50 mL/min), unless an assessment of the benefit/risk to the patient justifies the use of intravenous voriconazole (see DOSAGE AND ADMINISTRATION - Dosage Adjustment).

A pharmacokinetic study in subjects with renal failure undergoing hemodialysis showed that voriconazole is dialyzed with clearance of 121 mL/min. The intravenous vehicle, SBECD, is hemodialyzed with clearance of 55 mL/min. A 4-hour hemodialysis session does not remove a sufficient amount of voriconazole to warrant dose adjustment.

Drug Interactions

Effects of Other Drugs on Voriconazole

Voriconazole is metabolized by the human hepatic cytochrome P450 enzymes CYP2C19, CYP2C9, and CYP3A4. Results of *in vitro* metabolism studies indicate that the affinity of voriconazole is highest for CYP2C19, followed by CYP2C9, and is appreciably lower for CYP3A4. Inhibitors or inducers of these three enzymes may increase or decrease voriconazole systemic exposure (plasma concentrations), respectively.

Table 1
Population Pharmacokinetic Parameters of Voriconazole in Volunteers

	200 mg Oral Q12h	300 mg Oral Q12h	3 mg/kg IV Q12h	4 mg/kg IV Q12h
AUC_{τ}* (μg•h/mL) (CV%)	19.86 (94%)	50.32 (74%)	21.81 (100%)	50.40 (83%)

*Mean AUC_{τ} are predicted values from population pharmacokinetic analysis of data from 236 volunteers

Table 2
Pharmacokinetic Parameters of Voriconazole in Patients at Risk for Aspergillosis

	200 mg Oral Q12h (n=9)	300 mg Oral Q12h (n=9)
AUC_{τ}* (μg•h/mL) (CV%)	20.31 (69%)	36.51 (45%)
C_{max}* (μg/mL) (CV%)	3.00 (51%)	4.66 (35%)

*Geometric mean values on Day 14 of multiple dosing in 2 cohorts of patients

Table 3
Pharmacokinetic Parameters of Voriconazole from Loading Dose and Maintenance Dose Regimens (Individual Studies in Volunteers)

	400 mg Q12h on Day 1, 200 mg Q12h on Days 2 to 10 (n=17)		6 mg/kg IV** Q12h on Day 1, 3 mg/kg IV Q12h on Days 2 to 10 (n=9)	
	Day 1, 1st dose	Day 10	Day 1, 1st dose	Day 10
AUC_{τ}* (μg•h/mL) (CV%)	9.31 (38%)	11.13 (103%)	13.22 (22%)	13.25 (58%)
C_{max} (μg/mL) (CV%)	2.30 (19%)	2.08 (62%)	4.70 (22%)	3.06 (31%)

*AUC_{τ} values are calculated over dosing interval of 12 hours
Pharmacokinetic parameters for loading and maintenance doses summarized for same cohort of volunteers
**IV infusion over 60 minutes

The systemic exposure to voriconazole is significantly reduced or is expected to be reduced by the concomitant administration of the following agents and their use is contraindicated:

***Rifampin* (potent CYP450 inducer):** Rifampin (600 mg once daily) decreased the steady state C_{max} and AUC_{τ} of voriconazole (200 mg Q12h × 7 days) by an average of 93% and 96%, respectively, in healthy subjects. Doubling the dose of voriconazole to 400 mg Q12h does not restore adequate exposure to voriconazole during coadministration with rifampin.

Coadministration of voriconazole and rifampin is contraindicated (see CONTRAINDICATIONS, PRECAUTIONS - Drug Interactions).

***Ritonavir* (potent CYP450 inducer; CYP3A4 inhibitor and substrate):** Ritonavir (400 mg Q12h for 9 days) decreased the steady state C_{max} and AUC_{τ} of oral voriconazole (400 mg Q12h for 1 day, then 200 mg Q12h for 8 days) by an average of 66% and 82%, respectively, in healthy subjects. The effect of ritonavir (100 mg Q12h as used to inhibit CYP3A and increase concentrations of other antiretroviral drugs) on voriconazole concentrations has not been studied. Repeat oral administration of voriconazole (400 mg Q12h for 1 day, then 200 mg Q12h for 8 days) did not have a significant effect on steady state C_{max} and AUC_{τ} of ritonavir following repeat dose administration (400 mg Q12h for 9 days) in healthy subjects. **Coadministration of voriconazole and ritonavir (400 mg Q12h) is contraindicated** (see CONTRAINDICATIONS, PRECAUTIONS - Drug Interactions).

***Carbamazepine and long acting barbiturates* (potent CYP450 inducers):** Although not studied *in vitro* or *in vivo*, carbamazepine and long acting barbiturates (e.g. phenobarbital, mephobarbital) are likely to significantly decrease plasma voriconazole concentrations. **Coadministration of voriconazole with carbamazepine or long acting barbiturates is contraindicated** (see CONTRAINDICATIONS, PRECAUTIONS - Drug Interactions).

Minor or no significant pharmacokinetic interactions that do not require dosage adjustment:

***Cimetidine* (non-specific CYP450 inhibitor and increases gastric pH):** Cimetidine (400 mg Q12h × 8 days) increased voriconazole steady state C_{max} and AUC_{τ} by an average of 18% (90% CI: 6%, 32%) and 23% (90% CI: 13%, 33%), respectively, following oral doses of 200 mg Q12h × 7 days to healthy subjects.

***Ranitidine* (increases gastric pH):** Ranitidine (150 mg Q12h) had no significant effect on voriconazole C_{max} and AUC_{τ} following oral doses of 200 mg Q12h × 7 days to healthy subjects.

Macrolide antibiotics: Co-administration of **erythromycin** (CYP3A4 inhibitor;1g Q12h for 7 days) or **azithromycin** (500 mg qd for 3 days) with voriconazole 200 mg Q12h for 14 days had no significant effect on voriconazole steady state C_{max} and AUC_{τ} in healthy subjects. The effects of voriconazole on the pharmacokinetics of either erythromycin or azithromycin are not known.

Effects of Voriconazole on Other Drugs

In vitro studies with human hepatic microsomes show that voriconazole inhibits the metabolic activity of the cytochrome P450 enzymes CYP2C19, CYP2C9, and CYP3A4. In these studies, the inhibition potency of voriconazole for CYP3A4 metabolic activity was significantly less than that of two other azoles, ketoconazole and itraconazole. *In vitro* studies also show that the major metabolite of voriconazole, voriconazole N-oxide, inhibits the metabolic activity of CYP2C9 and CYP3A4 to a greater extent than that of CYP2C19. Therefore, there is potential for voriconazole and its major metabolite to increase the systemic exposure (plasma concentrations) of other drugs metabolized by these CYP450 enzymes.

The systemic exposure of the following drugs is significantly increased or is expected to be significantly increased by coadministration of voriconazole and their use is contraindicated:

***Sirolimus* (CYP3A4 substrate):** Repeat dose administration of oral voriconazole (400 mg Q12h for 1 day, then 200 mg Q12h for 8 days) increased the C_{max} and AUC of sirolimus (2 mg single dose) an average of 7-fold (90% CI: 5.7, 7.5) and 11-fold (90% CI: 9.9, 12.6), respectively, in healthy subjects. **Coadministration of voriconazole and sirolimus is contraindicated** (see CONTRAINDICATIONS, PRECAUTIONS - Drug Interactions).

***Terfenadine, astemizole, cisapride, pimozide and quinidine* (CYP3A4 substrates):** Although not studied *in vitro* or *in vivo*, concomitant administration of voriconazole with terfenadine, astemizole, cisapride, pimozide or quinidine may result in inhibition of the metabolism of these drugs. Increased plasma concentrations of these drugs can lead to QT prolongation and rare occurrences of *torsade de pointes*. **Coadministration of voriconazole and terfenadine, astemizole, cisapride, pimozide and quinidine is contraindicated** (see CONTRAINDICATIONS, PRECAUTIONS - Drug Interactions).

Ergot alkaloids: Although not studied *in vitro* or *in vivo*, voriconazole may increase the plasma concentration of ergot alkaloids (ergotamine and dihydroergotamine) and lead to ergotism. **Coadministration of voriconazole with ergot alkaloids is contraindicated** (see CONTRAINDICATIONS, PRECAUTIONS - Drug Interactions).

Coadministration of voriconazole with the following agents results in increased exposure or is expected to result in increased exposure to these drugs. Therefore, careful monitoring and/or dosage adjustment of these drugs is needed:

***Cyclosporine* (CYP3A4 substrate):** In stable renal transplant recipients receiving chronic cyclosporine therapy, concomitant administration of oral voriconazole (200 mg Q12h for 8 days) increased cyclosporine C_{max} and AUC_{τ} an average of 1.1 times (90% CI: 0.9, 1.41) and 1.7 times (90% CI: 1.5, 2.0), respectively, as compared to when cyclosporine was administered without voriconazole. When initiating therapy with voriconazole in patients already receiving cyclosporine, it is recommended that the cyclosporine dose be reduced to one-half of the original dose and followed with frequent monitoring of the cyclosporine blood levels. Increased cyclosporine levels have been associated with nephrotoxicity.

When voriconazole is discontinued, cyclosporine levels should be frequently monitored and the dose increased as necessary (see PRECAUTIONS - Drug Interactions).

***Tacrolimus* (CYP3A4 substrate):** Repeat oral dose administration of voriconazole (400 mg Q12h × 1 day then 200 mg Q12h × 6 days) increased tacrolimus (0.1 mg/kg single dose) C_{max} and AUC_τ in healthy subjects by an average of 2-fold (90% CI: 1.9, 2.5) and 3-fold (90% CI: 2.7, 3.8), respectively. When initiating therapy with voriconazole in patients already receiving tacrolimus, it is recommended that the tacrolimus dose be reduced to one-third of the original dose and followed with frequent monitoring of the tacrolimus blood levels. Increased tacrolimus levels have been associated with nephrotoxicity. When voriconazole is discontinued, tacrolimus levels should be carefully monitored and the dose increased as necessary (see PRECAUTIONS - Drug Interactions).

***Warfarin* (CYP2C9 substrate):** Coadministration of voriconazole (300 mg Q12h × 12 days) with warfarin (30 mg single dose) significantly increased maximum prothrombin time by approximately 2-times that of placebo in healthy subjects. Close monitoring of prothrombin time or other suitable anti-coagulation tests is recommended if warfarin and voriconazole are coadministered and the warfarin dose adjusted accordingly (see PRECAUTIONS - Drug Interactions).

***Oral Coumarin Anticoagulants* (CYP2C9, CYP3A4 substrates):** Although not studied *in vitro* or *in vivo*, voriconazole may increase the plasma concentrations of coumarin anticoagulants and therefore may cause an increase in prothrombin time. If patients receiving coumarin preparations are treated simultaneously with voriconazole, the prothrombin time or other suitable anti-coagulation tests should be monitored at close intervals and the dosage of anticoagulants adjusted accordingly (see PRECAUTIONS - Drug Interactions).

***Statins* (CYP3A4 substrates):** Although not studied clinically, voriconazole has been shown to inhibit lovastatin metabolism *in vitro* (human liver microsomes). Therefore, voriconazole is likely to increase the plasma concentrations of statins that are metabolized by CYP3A4. It is recommended that dose adjustment of the statin be considered during coadministration. Increased statin concentrations in plasma have been associated with rhabdomyolysis (see PRECAUTIONS - Drug Interactions).

***Benzodiazepines* (CYP3A4 substrates):** Although not studied clinically, voriconazole has been shown to inhibit midazolam metabolism *in vitro* (human liver microsomes). Therefore, voriconazole is likely to increase the plasma concentrations of benzodiazepines that are metabolized by CYP3A4 (e.g., midazolam, triazolam, and alprazolam) and lead to a prolonged sedative effect. It is recommended that dose adjustment of the benzodiazepine be considered during coadministration (see PRECAUTIONS - Drug Interactions).

***Calcium Channel Blockers* (CYP3A4 substrates):** Although not studied clinically, voriconazole has been shown to inhibit felodipine metabolism *in vitro* (human liver microsomes). Therefore, voriconazole may increase the plasma concentrations of calcium channel blockers that are metabolized by CYP3A4. Frequent monitoring for adverse events and toxicity related to calcium channel blockers is recommended during coadministration. Dose adjustment of the calcium channel blocker may be needed (see PRECAUTIONS - Drug Interactions).

***Sulfonylureas* (CYP2C9 substrates):** Although not studied *in vitro* or *in vivo*, voriconazole may increase plasma concentrations of sulfonylureas (e.g., tolbutamide, glipizide, and glyburide) and therefore cause hypoglycemia. Frequent monitoring of blood glucose and appropriate adjustment (i.e., reduction) of the sulfonylurea dosage is recommended during coadministration (see PRECAUTIONS - Drug Interactions).

***Vinca Alkaloids* (CYP3A4 substrates):** Although not studied *in vitro* or *in vivo*, voriconazole may increase the plasma concentrations of the vinca alkaloids (e.g., vincristine and vinblastine) and lead to neurotoxicity. Therefore, it is recommended that dose adjustment of the vinca alkaloid be considered.

No significant pharmacokinetic interactions were observed when voriconazole was coadministered with the following agents. Therefore, no dosage adjustment for these agents is recommended:

***Prednisolone* (CYP3A4 substrate):** Voriconazole (200 mg Q12h × 30 days) increased C_{max} and AUC of prednisolone (60 mg single dose) by an average of 11% and 34%, respectively, in healthy subjects.

***Digoxin* (P-glycoprotein mediated transport):** Voriconazole (200 mg Q12h × 12 days) had no significant effect on steady state C_{max} and AUC_τ of digoxin (0.25 mg once daily for 10 days) in healthy subjects.

***Mycophenolic acid* (UDP-glucuronyl transferase substrate):** Voriconazole (200 mg Q12h × 5 days) had no significant effect on the C_{max} and AUC_τ of mycophenolic acid and its major metabolite, mycophenolic acid glucuronide after administration of a 1 g single oral dose of mycophenolate mofetil.

Two-Way Interactions

Concomitant use of the following agents with voriconazole is contraindicated:

***Efavirenz, a non-nucleoside reverse transcriptase inhibitor* (CYP450 inducer; CYP3A4 inhibitor and substrate):** Steady state efavirenz (400 mg PO QD) decreased the steady state C_{max} and AUC_τ of voriconazole (400 mg PO Q12h 1 day, then 200 mg PO Q12h for 8 days) by an average of 61% and 77%, respectively, in healthy subjects. Voriconazole at steady state (400 mg PO Q12h for 1 day, then 200 mg Q12h for 8 days) increased the steady state C_{max} and AUC_τ of efavirenz (400 mg PO QD for 9 days) by an average of 38% and 44%, respectively, in healthy subjects. **Coadministration of voriconazole and efavirenz is contraindicated** (see CONTRAINDICATIONS, PRECAUTIONS – Drug Interactions).

***Rifabutin* (potent CYP450 inducer):** Rifabutin (300 mg once daily) decreased the C_{max} and AUC_τ of voriconazole at 200 mg twice daily by an average of 67% (90% CI: 58%, 73%) and 79% (90% CI: 71%, 84%), respectively, in healthy subjects. During coadministration with rifabutin (300 mg once daily), the steady state C_{max} and AUC_τ of voriconazole following an increased dose of 400 mg twice daily were on average approximately 2-times higher, compared with voriconazole alone at 200 mg twice daily. Coadministration of voriconazole at 400 mg twice daily with rifabutin 300 mg twice daily increased the C_{max} and AUC_τ of rifabutin by an average of 3-times (90% CI: 2.2, 4.0) and 4-times (90% CI: 3.5, 5.4), respectively, compared to rifabutin given alone. **Coadministration of voriconazole and rifabutin is contraindicated.**

Significant drug interactions that may require dosage adjustment, frequent monitoring of drug levels and/or frequent monitoring of drug-related adverse events/toxicity:

***Phenytoin* (CYP2C9 substrate and potent CYP450 inducer):** Repeat dose administration of phenytoin (300 mg once daily) decreased the steady state C_{max} and AUC_τ of orally administered voriconazole (200 mg Q12h × 14 days) by an average of 50% and 70%, respectively, in healthy subjects. Administration of a higher voriconazole dose (400 mg Q12h × 7 days) with phenytoin (300 mg once daily) resulted in comparable steady state voriconazole C_{max} and AUC_τ estimates as compared to when voriconazole was given at 200 mg Q12h without phenytoin.

Phenytoin may be coadministered with voriconazole if the maintenance dose of voriconazole is increased from 4 mg/kg to 5 mg/kg intravenously every 12 hours or from 200 mg to 400 mg orally, every 12 hours (100 mg to 200 mg orally, every 12 hours in patients less than 40 kg) (see DOSAGE AND ADMINISTRATION).

Repeat dose administration of voriconazole (400 mg Q12h × 10 days) increased the steady state C_{max} and AUC_τ of phenytoin (300 mg once daily) by an average of 70% and 80%, respectively, in healthy subjects. The increase in phenytoin C_{max} and AUC when coadministered with voriconazole may be expected to be as high as 2-times the C_{max} and AUC estimates when phenytoin is given without voriconazole. Therefore, frequent monitoring of plasma phenytoin concentrations and phenytoin-related adverse effects is recommended when phenytoin is coadministered with voriconazole (see PRECAUTIONS - Drug Interactions).

***Omeprazole* (CYP2C19 inhibitor; CYP2C19 and CYP3A4 substrate):** Coadministration of omeprazole (40 mg once daily × 10 days) with oral voriconazole (400 mg Q12h × 1 day, then 200 mg Q12h × 9 days) increased the steady state C_{max} and AUC_τ of voriconazole by an average of 15% (90% CI: 5%, 25%) and 40% (90% CI: 29%, 55%), respectively, in healthy subjects. No dosage adjustment of voriconazole is recommended.

Coadministration of voriconazole (400 mg Q12h × 1 day, then 200 mg × 6 days) with omeprazole (40 mg once daily × 7 days) to healthy subjects significantly increased the steady state C_{max} and AUC_τ of omeprazole an average of 2-times (90% CI: 1.8, 2.6) and 4-times (90% CI: 3.3, 4.4), respectively, as compared to when omeprazole is given without voriconazole. When initiating voriconazole in patients already receiving omeprazole doses of 40 mg or greater, it is recommended that the omeprazole dose be reduced by one-half (see PRECAUTIONS - Drug Interactions).

The metabolism of other proton pump inhibitors that are CYP2C19 substrates may also be inhibited by voriconazole and may result in increased plasma concentrations of these drugs.

No significant pharmacokinetic interaction was seen and no dosage adjustment of these drugs is recommended:

***Indinavir* (CYP3A4 inhibitor and substrate):** Repeat dose administration of indinavir (800 mg TID for 10 days) had no significant effect on voriconazole C_{max} and AUC following repeat dose administration (200 mg Q12h for 17 days) in healthy subjects.

Repeat dose administration of voriconazole (200 mg Q12h for 7 days) did not have a significant effect on steady state C_{max} and AUC_τ of indinavir following repeat dose administration (800 mg TID for 7 days) in healthy subjects.

Other Two-Way Interactions Expected to be Significant Based on *In Vitro* Findings:

***Other HIV Protease Inhibitors* (CYP3A4 substrates and inhibitors):** *In vitro* studies (human liver microsomes) suggest that voriconazole may inhibit the metabolism of HIV protease inhibitors (e.g. saquinavir, amprenavir and nelfinavir). *In vitro* studies (human liver microsomes) also show that the metabolism of voriconazole may be inhibited by HIV protease inhibitors (e.g., saquinavir and amprenavir). Patients should be frequently monitored for drug toxicity during the coadministration of voriconazole and HIV protease inhibitors (see PRECAUTIONS - Drug Interactions).

***Other Non-Nucleoside Reverse Transcriptase Inhibitors (NNRTI)* (CYP3A4 substrates, inhibitors or CYP450 inducers):** *In vitro* studies (human liver microsomes) show that the metabolism of voriconazole may be inhibited by an NNRTI (e.g., delavirdine). Although not studied *in vitro* or *in vivo*, the metabolism of voriconazole may be induced by an NNRTI, such as nevirapine. *In vitro* studies (human liver microsomes) show that voriconazole may also inhibit the metabolism of an NNRTI (e.g., delavirdine). Patients should be frequently monitored for drug toxicity during the coadministration of voriconazole and an NNRTI (see PRECAUTIONS - Drug Interactions).

MICROBIOLOGY

Mechanism of Action

Voriconazole is a triazole antifungal agent. The primary mode of action of voriconazole is the inhibition of fungal cytochrome P-450-mediated 14 alpha-lanosterol demethylation, an essential step in fungal ergosterol biosynthesis. The accumulation of 14 alpha-methyl sterols correlates with the subsequent loss of ergosterol in the fungal cell wall and may be responsible for the antifungal activity of voriconazole. Voriconazole has been shown to be more selective for fungal cytochrome P-450 enzymes than for various mammalian cytochrome P-450 enzyme systems.

Activity *In Vitro* and *In Vivo*

Voriconazole has demonstrated *in vitro* activity against *Aspergillus* species (*A. fumigatus, A. flavus, A. niger* and *A. terreus*), *Candida* species (*C. albicans, C. glabrata* and *C. krusei*), *Scedosporium apiospermum* and *Fusarium* spp., including *Fusarium solani*. (see INDICATIONS AND USAGE, CLINICAL STUDIES).

In vitro susceptibility testing was performed according to the National Committee for Clinical Laboratory Standards (NCCLS) methods (M38-P for moulds and M27-A for yeasts). Voriconazole breakpoints have not been established for any fungi. The relationship between clinical outcome and *in vitro* susceptibility results remains to be elucidated.

Voriconazole was active in normal and/or immunocompromised guinea pigs with systemic and/or pulmonary infections due to *A. fumigatus* (including an isolate with reduced susceptibility to itraconazole) or *Candida* species *[C.albicans* (including an isolate with reduced susceptibility to fluconazole), *C. krusei and C. glabrata]* in which the endpoints were prolonged survival of infected animals and/or reduction of mycological burden from target organs. In one experiment, voriconazole exhibited activity against *Scedosporium apiospermum* infections in immune competent guinea pigs.

Drug Resistance

Voriconazole drug resistance development has not been adequately studied *in vitro* against *Candida, Aspergillus, Scedosporium* and *Fusarium* species. The frequency of drug resistance development for the various fungi for which this drug is indicated is not known.

Fungal isolates exhibiting reduced susceptibility to fluconazole or itraconazole may also show reduced susceptibility to voriconazole, suggesting cross-resistance can occur among these azoles. The relevance of cross-resistance and clinical outcome has not been fully characterized. Clinical cases where azole cross-resistance is demonstrated may require alternative antifungal therapy.

INDICATIONS AND USAGE

VFEND is indicated for use in the treatment of the following fungal infections:

Invasive aspergillosis. In clinical trials, the majority of isolates recovered were *Aspergillus fumigatus*. There was a small number of cases of culture-proven disease due to species of *Aspergillus* other than *A. fumigatus* (see CLINICAL STUDIES, MICROBIOLOGY).

Esophageal candidiasis. (see CLINICAL STUDIES, MICROBIOLOGY).

Serious fungal infections caused by *Scedosporium apiospermum* (asexual form of *Pseudallescheria boydii*) and *Fusarium* spp. including *Fusarium solani*, in patients intolerant of, or refractory to, other therapy. (see CLINICAL STUDIES, MICROBIOLOGY).

Specimens for fungal culture and other relevant laboratory studies (including histopathology) should be obtained prior to therapy to isolate and identify causative organism(s). Therapy may be instituted before the results of the cultures and other laboratory studies are known. However, once these results become available, antifungal therapy should be adjusted accordingly.

CLINICAL STUDIES

Voriconazole, administered orally or parenterally, has been evaluated as primary or salvage therapy in 520 patients aged 12 years and older with infections caused by *Aspergillus* spp., *Fusarium* spp., and *Scedosporium* spp.

Invasive Aspergillosis

Voriconazole was studied in patients for primary therapy of invasive aspergillosis (randomized, controlled study 307/602), for primary and salvage therapy of aspergillosis (non-comparative study 304) and for treatment of patients with invasive aspergillosis who were refractory to, or intolerant of, other antifungal therapy (non-comparative study 309/604).

Study 307/602

The efficacy of voriconazole compared to amphotericin B in the primary treatment of acute invasive aspergillosis was demonstrated in 277 patients treated for 12 weeks in Study 307/602. The majority of study patients had underlying hematologic malignancies, including bone marrow transplantation. The study also included patients with solid organ transplantation, solid tumors, and AIDS. The patients were mainly treated for definite or probable invasive aspergillosis of the lungs. Other aspergillosis infections included disseminated disease, CNS infections and sinus infections. Diagnosis of definite or probable invasive aspergillosis was made according to criteria modified from those established by the

Continued on next page

Vfend—Cont.

National Institute of Allergy and Infectious Diseases Mycoses Study Group/European Organisation for Research and Treatment of Cancer (NIAID MSG/EORTC).

Voriconazole was administered intravenously with a loading dose of 6 mg/kg every 12 hours for the first 24 hours followed by a maintenance dose of 4 mg/kg every 12 hours for a minimum of seven days. Therapy could then be switched to the oral formulation at a dose of 200 mg Q12h. Median duration of IV voriconazole therapy was 10 days (range 2-90 days). After IV voriconazole therapy, the median duration of PO voriconazole therapy was 76 days (range 2-232 days).

Patients in the comparator group received conventional amphotericin B as a slow infusion at a daily dose of 1.0-1.5 mg/kg/day. Median duration of IV amphotericin therapy was 12 days (range 1-85 days). Treatment was then continued with other licensed antifungal therapy (OLAT), including itraconazole and lipid amphotericin B formulations. Although initial therapy with conventional amphotericin B was to be continued for at least two weeks, actual duration of therapy was at the discretion of the investigator. Patients who discontinued initial randomized therapy due to toxicity or lack of efficacy were eligible to continue in the study with OLAT treatment.

A satisfactory global response at 12 weeks (complete or partial resolution of all attributable symptoms, signs, radiographic/bronchoscopic abnormalities present at baseline) was seen in 53% of voriconazole treated patients compared to 32% of amphotericin B treated patients (Table 4). A benefit of voriconazole compared to amphotericin B on patient survival at Day 84 was seen with a 71% survival rate on voriconazole compared to 58% on amphotericin B (Table 4). Table 4 also summarizes the response (success) based on mycological confirmation and species.

[See table 4 at right]

Study 304

The results of this comparative trial (Study 307/602) confirmed the results of an earlier trial in the primary and salvage treatment of patients with acute invasive aspergillosis (Study 304). In this earlier study, an overall success rate of 52% (26/50) was seen in patients treated with voriconazole for primary therapy. Success was seen in 17/29 (59%) with *Aspergillus fumigatus* infections and 3/6 (50%) patients with infections due to non-*fumigatus* species [*A. flavus* (1/1); *A. nidulans* (0/2); *A. niger* (2/2); *A. terreus* (0/1)]. Success in patients who received voriconazole as salvage therapy is presented in Table 5.

Study 309/604

Additional data regarding response rates in patients who were refractory to, or intolerant of, other antifungal agents are also provided in Table 5. Overall mycological eradication for culture-documented infections due to *fumigatus* and non-*fumigatus* species of *Aspergillus* was 36/82 (44%) and 12/30 (40%), respectively, in voriconazole treated patients. Patients had various underlying diseases and species other than *A. fumigatus* contributed to mixed infections in some cases.

For patients who were infected with a single pathogen and were refractory to, or intolerant of, other antifungal agents, the satisfactory response rates for voriconazole in studies 304 and 309/604 are presented in Table 5.

Table 5 Combined Response Data in Salvage Patients with Single Aspergillus Species (Studies 304 and 309/604)

	Success n/N
A. fumigatus	43/97 (44%)
A. flavus	5/12
A. nidulans	1/3
A. niger	4/5
A. terreus	3/8
A. versicolor	0/1

Nineteen patients had more than one species of *Aspergillus* isolated. Success was seen in 4/17 (24%) of these patients.

Esophageal Candidiasis

The efficacy of oral voriconazole 200 mg bid compared to oral fluconazole 200 mg od in the primary treatment of esophageal candidiasis was demonstrated in Study 150-305, a double-blind, double-dummy, study in immunocompromised patients with endoscopically-proven esophageal candidiasis. Patients were treated for a median of 15 days (range 1 to 49 days). Outcome was assessed by repeat endoscopy at end of treatment (EOT). A successful response was defined as a normal endoscopy at EOT or at least a 1 grade improvement over baseline endoscopic score. For patients in the Intent To Treat (ITT) population with only a baseline endoscopy, a successful response was defined as symptomatic cure or improvement at EOT compared to baseline. Voriconazole and fluconazole (200 mg od) showed comparable efficacy rates against esophageal candidiasis, as presented in Table 6.

[See table 6 above]

Microbiologic success rates by *Candida* species are presented in Table 7.

[See table 7 above]

Table 4
Overall Efficacy and Success by Species in the Primary Treatment of Acute Invasive Aspergillosis Study 307/602

	Voriconazole	Ampho B[c]	Stratified Difference (95% CI)[d]
	n/N (%)	n/N (%)	
Efficacy as Primary Therapy			
Satisfactory Global Response[a]	76/144 (53)	42/133 (32)	21.8% (10.5%, 33.0%) p<0.0001
Survival at Day 84[b]	102/144 (71)	77/133 (58)	13.1% (2.1%, 24.2%)
Success by Species			
	Success n/N (%)		
Overall success	76/144 (53)	42/133 (32)	
Mycologically confirmed[e]	37/84 (44)	16/67 (24)	
Aspergillus spp.[f]			
A. fumigatus	28/63 (44)	12/47 (26)	
A. flavus	3/6	4/9	
A. terreus	2/3	0/3	
A. niger	1/4	0/9	
A. nidulans	1/1	0/0	

[a] Assessed by independent Data Review Committee (DRC)
[b] Proportion of subjects alive
[c] Amphotericin B followed by other licensed antifungal therapy
[d] Difference and corresponding 95% confidence interval are stratified by protocol
[e] Not all mycologically confirmed specimens were speciated
[f] Some patients had more than one species isolated at baseline

Table 6
Success Rates in Patients Treated for Esophageal Candidiasis

Population	Voriconazole	Fluconazole	Difference % (95% CI)[a]
PP[b]	113/115 (98.2%)	134/141 (95.0%)	3.2 (-1.1, 7.5)
ITT[c]	175/200 (87.5%)	171/191 (89.5%)	-2.0 (-8.3, 4.3)

[a] Confidence Interval for the difference (Voriconazole – Fluconazole) in success rates.
[b] PP (Per Protocol) patients had confirmation of *Candida* esophagitis by endoscopy, received at least 12 days of treatment, and had a repeat endoscopy at EOT (end of treatment).
[c] ITT (Intent to Treat) patients without endoscopy or clinical assessment at EOT were treated as failures.

Table 7
Clinical and mycological outcome by baseline pathogen in patients with esophageal candidiasis (Study 150-305).

Pathogen[a]	Voriconazole		Fluconazole	
	Favorable endoscopic response[b]	**Mycological eradication[b]**	**Favorable endoscopic response[b]**	**Mycological eradication[b]**
	Success/Total (%)	Eradication/Total (%)	Success/Total (%)	Eradication/Total (%)
C. albicans	134/140 (96%)	90/107 (84%)	147/156 (94%)	91/115 (79%)
C. glabrata	8/8 (100%)	4/7 (57%)	4/4 (100%)	1/4 (25%)
C. krusei	1/1	1/1	2/2 (100%)	0/0

[a] Some patients had more than one species isolated at baseline
[b] Patients with endoscopic and/or mycological assessment at end of therapy

Other Serious Fungal Pathogens

In pooled analyses of patients, voriconazole was shown to be effective against the following additional fungal pathogens:

Scedosporium apiospermum - Successful response to voriconazole therapy was seen in 15 of 24 patients (63%). Three of these patients relapsed within 4 weeks, including 1 patient with pulmonary, skin and eye infections, 1 patient with cerebral disease, and 1 patient with skin infection. Ten patients had evidence of cerebral disease and 6 of these had a successful outcome (1 relapse). In addition, a successful response was seen in one of three patients with mixed organism infections.

Fusarium spp. - Nine of 21 (43%) patients were successfully treated with voriconazole. Of these nine patients, three had eye infections, one had an eye and blood infection, one had a skin infection, one had a blood infection alone, two had sinus infections, and one had disseminated infection (pulmonary, skin, hepatosplenic). Three of these patients (one with disseminated disease, one with an eye infection and one with a blood infection) had *Fusarium solani* and were complete successes. Two of these patients relapsed, one with a sinus infection and profound neutropenia and one post surgical patient with blood and eye infections.

CONTRAINDICATIONS

VFEND is contraindicated in patients with known hypersensitivity to voriconazole or its excipients. There is no information regarding cross-sensitivity between VFEND (voriconazole) and other azole antifungal agents. Caution should be used when prescribing VFEND to patients with hypersensitivity to other azoles.

Coadministration of the CYP3A4 substrates, terfenadine, astemizole, cisapride, pimozide or quinidine with VFEND are contraindicated since increased plasma concentrations of these drugs can lead to QT prolongation and rare occurrences of *torsade de pointes* (see CLINICAL PHARMACOLOGY - Drug Interactions, PRECAUTIONS - Drug Interactions).

Coadministration of VFEND with sirolimus is contraindicated because VFEND significantly increases sirolimus concentrations in healthy subjects (see CLINICAL PHARMACOLOGY - Drug Interactions, PRECAUTIONS - Drug Interactions).

Coadministration of VFEND with rifampin, carbamazepine and long-acting barbiturates is contraindicated since these drugs are likely to decrease plasma voriconazole concentrations significantly (see CLINICAL PHARMACOLOGY - Drug Interactions, PRECAUTIONS - Drug Interactions).

Coadministration of VFEND with ritonavir (400 mg Q12h) is contraindicated because ritonavir (400 mg Q12h) significantly decreases plasma voriconazole concentrations in healthy subjects. The effect of ritonavir (100 mg Q12h as used to inhibit CYP3A and increase concentrations of other antiretroviral drugs) on voriconazole concentrations has not been studied (see CLINICAL PHARMACOLOGY - Drug Interactions, PRECAUTIONS - Drug Interactions).

Coadministration of VFEND with efavirenz is contraindicated because efavirenz significantly decreases voriconazole plasma concentrations while VFEND also significantly increases efavirenz plasma concentrations (see CLINICAL PHARMACOLOGY - Drug Interactions, PRECAUTIONS - Drug Interactions).

Coadministration of VFEND with rifabutin is contraindicated since VFEND significantly increases rifabutin plasma concentrations and rifabutin also significantly decreases voriconazole plasma concentrations (see CLINICAL PHARMACOLOGY - Drug Interactions, PRECAUTIONS - Drug Interactions).

Coadministration of VFEND with ergot alkaloids (ergotamine and dihydroergotamine) is contraindicated because VFEND may increase the plasma concentration of ergot alkaloids, which may lead to ergotism.

WARNINGS

VISUAL DISTURBANCES: The effect of VFEND on visual function is not known if treatment continues beyond 28 days. If treatment continues beyond 28 days, visual function including visual acuity, visual field and color perception should be monitored **(see PRECAUTIONS – Information for Patients and ADVERSE EVENTS – Visual Disturbances).**

HEPATIC TOXICITY: In clinical trials, there have been uncommon cases of serious hepatic reactions during treatment with VFEND (including clinical hepatitis, cholestasis and fulminant hepatic failure, including fatalities). Instances of hepatic reactions were noted to occur primarily in patients with serious underlying medical conditions (predominantly hematological malignancy). Hepatic reactions, including hepatitis and jaundice, have occurred among patients with no other identifiable risk factors. Liver dysfunction has usually been reversible on discontinuation of therapy **(see PRECAUTIONS – Laboratory Tests and ADVERSE EVENTS – Clinical Laboratory Values).**

Monitoring of hepatic function: Liver function tests should be evaluated at the start of and during the course of VFEND therapy. Patients who develop abnormal liver function tests during VFEND therapy should be monitored for the development of more severe hepatic injury. Patient management should include laboratory evaluation of hepatic function (particularly liver function tests and bilirubin). Discontinuation of VFEND must be considered if clinical signs and symptoms consistent with liver disease develop that may be attributable to VFEND (see PRECAUTIONS - Laboratory Tests, DOSAGE AND ADMINISTRATION - Dosage Adjustment, ADVERSE EVENTS - Clinical Laboratory Tests).

Pregnancy Category D: Voriconazole can cause fetal harm when administered to a pregnant woman.

Voriconazole was teratogenic in rats (cleft palates, hydronephrosis/hydroureter) from 10 mg/kg (0.3 times the recommended maintenance dose (RMD) on a mg/m^2 basis) and embryotoxic in rabbits at 100 mg/kg (6 times the RMD). Other effects in rats included reduced ossification of sacral and caudal vertebrae, skull, pubic and hyoid bone, super numerary ribs, anomalies of the sternebrae and dilatation of the ureter/renal pelvis. Plasma estradiol in pregnant rats was reduced at all dose levels. Voriconazole treatment in rats produced increased gestational length and dystocia, which were associated with increased perinatal pup mortality at the 10 mg/kg dose. The effects seen in rabbits were an increased embryomortality, reduced fetal weight and increased incidences of skeletal variations, cervical ribs and extra sternebral ossification sites.

If this drug is used during pregnancy, or if the patient becomes pregnant while taking this drug, the patient should be apprised of the potential hazard to the fetus.

Galactose intolerance: VFEND tablets contain lactose and should not be given to patients with rare hereditary problems of galactose intolerance, Lapp lactase deficiency or glucose-galactose malabsorption.

PRECAUTIONS

General

(See WARNINGS, DOSAGE AND ADMINISTRATION)

Some azoles, including voriconazole, have been associated with prolongation of the QT interval on the electrocardiogram. During clinical development and post-marketing surveillance, there have been rare cases of torsade de pointes in patients taking voriconazole. These reports involved seriously ill patients with multiple confounding risk factors, such as history of cardiotoxic chemotherapy, cardiomyopathy, hypokalemia and concomitant medications that may have been contributory.

Voriconazole should be administered with caution to patients with these potentially proarrhythmic conditions.

Rigorous attempts to correct potassium, magnesium and calcium should be made before starting voriconazole (see CLINICAL PHARMACOLOGY - Pharmacokinetic-pharmacodynamic Relationships - Electrocardiogram).

Infusion Related Reactions

During infusion of the intravenous formulation of voriconazole in healthy subjects, anaphylactoid-type reactions, including flushing, fever, sweating, tachycardia, chest tightness, dyspnea, faintness, nausea, pruritus and rash, have occurred uncommonly. Symptoms appeared immediately upon initiating the infusion. Consideration should be given to stopping the infusion should these reactions occur.

Information for Patients

Patients should be advised:

Table 8 Effect of Other Drugs on Voriconazole Pharmacokinetics

Drug/Drug Class (Mechanism of Interaction by the Drug)	Voriconazole Plasma Exposure (C_{max} and AUC, after 200 mg Q12h)	Recommendations for Voriconazole Dosage Adjustment/Comments
Rifampin*, Efavirenz** and Rifabutin* (CYP450 Induction)	Significantly Reduced	**Contraindicated**
Ritonavir (400mg Q12h HIV Protease Inhibitor)** (CYP450 Induction)	Significantly Reduced	**Contraindicated** The effect of ritonavir (100 mg Q12h as used to inhibit CYP3A and increase concentrations of other antiretroviral drugs) on voriconazole concentrations has not been studied.
Carbamazepine (CYP450 Induction)	Not Studied *In Vivo* or *In Vitro*, but Likely to Result in Significant Reduction	**Contraindicated**
Long Acting Barbiturates (CYP450 Induction)	Not Studied *In Vivo* or *In Vitro*, but Likely to Result in Significant Reduction	**Contraindicated**
Phenytoin* (CYP450 Induction)	Significantly Reduced	Increase voriconazole maintenance dose from 4 mg/kg to 5 mg/kg IV every 12 hrs or from 200 mg to 400 mg orally every 12 hrs (100 mg to 200 mg orally every 12 hrs in patients weighing less than 40 kg)
Other HIV Protease Inhibitors (CYP3A4 Inhibition)	*In Vivo* Studies Showed No Significant Effects of Indinavir on Voriconazole Exposure *In Vitro* Studies Demonstrate Potential for Inhibition of Voriconazole Metabolism (Increased Plasma Exposure)	No dosage adjustment in the voriconazole dosage needed when coadministered with indinavir Frequent monitoring for adverse events and toxicity related to voriconazole when coadministered with other HIV protease inhibitors
Other NNRTIs*** (CYP3A4 Inhibition or CYP450 Induction)	*In Vitro* Studies Demonstrate Potential for Inhibition of Voriconazole Metabolism (Increased Plasma Exposure) Not Studied *In Vitro* or *In Vivo*, but Metabolism of Voriconazole May also be Induced (Decreased Plasma Exposure)	Frequent monitoring for adverse events and toxicity related to voriconazole Careful assessment of voriconazole effectiveness

*Results based on *in vivo* clinical studies generally following repeat oral dosing with 200 mg Q12h voriconazole to healthy subjects

**Results based on *in vivo* clinical study following repeat oral dosing with 400 mg Q12h for 1 day, then 200 mg Q12h for 8 days voriconazole to healthy subjects

***Non-Nucleoside Reverse Transcriptase Inhibitors

- that VFEND Tablets or Oral Suspension should be taken at least one hour before, or one hour following, a meal.
- **that they should not drive at night while taking VFEND. VFEND may cause changes to vision, including blurring and/or photophobia.**
- **that they should avoid potentially hazardous tasks, such as driving or operating machinery if they perceive any change in vision.**
- that strong, direct sunlight should be avoided during VFEND therapy.
- that VFEND for Oral Suspension contains sucrose and is not recommended for patients with rare hereditary problems of fructose intolerance, sucrase-isomaltase deficiency or glucose-galactose malabsorption.

Laboratory Tests

Electrolyte disturbances such as hypokalemia, hypomagnesemia and hypocalcemia should be corrected prior to initiation of VFEND therapy.

Patient management should include laboratory evaluation of renal (particularly serum creatinine) and hepatic function (particularly liver function tests and bilirubin).

Drug Interactions

Tables 8 and 9 provide a summary of significant drug interactions with voriconazole that either have been studied *in vivo* (clinically) or that may be expected to occur based on results of *in vitro* metabolism studies with human liver microsomes. For more details, see CLINICAL PHARMACOLOGY - Drug Interactions.

[See table 8 above]

[See table 9 on pages 306 and 307]

Patients with Hepatic Insufficiency

It is recommended that the standard loading dose regimens be used but that the maintenance dose be halved in patients with mild to moderate hepatic cirrhosis (Child-Pugh Class A and B) receiving VFEND (see CLINICAL PHARMACOLOGY - Hepatic Insufficiency, DOSAGE AND ADMINISTRATION - Hepatic Insufficiency).

VFEND has not been studied in patients with severe cirrhosis (Child-Pugh Class C). VFEND has been associated with elevations in liver function tests and clinical signs of liver damage, such as jaundice, and should only be used in patients with severe hepatic insufficiency if the benefit outweighs the potential risk. Patients with hepatic insufficiency must be carefully monitored for drug toxicity.

Patients with Renal Insufficiency

In patients with moderate to severe renal dysfunction (creatinine clearance <50 mL/min), accumulation of the intravenous vehicle, SBECD, occurs. Oral voriconazole should be administered to these patients, unless an assessment of the benefit/risk to the patient justifies the use of intravenous voriconazole. Serum creatinine levels should be closely monitored in these patients, and if increases occur, consideration should be given to changing to oral voriconazole therapy (see CLINICAL PHARMACOLOGY - Renal Insufficiency, DOSAGE AND ADMINISTRATION - Renal Insufficiency).

Renal Adverse Events

Acute renal failure has been observed in severely ill patients undergoing treatment with VFEND. Patients being treated with voriconazole are likely to be treated concomitantly with nephrotoxic medications and have concurrent conditions that may result in decreased renal function.

Monitoring of Renal Function

Patients should be monitored for the development of abnormal renal function. This should include laboratory evaluation, particularly serum creatinine.

Dermatological Reactions

Patients have rarely developed serious cutaneous reactions, such as Stevens-Johnson syndrome, during treatment with VFEND. If patients develop a rash, they should be monitored closely and consideration given to discontinuation of VFEND. VFEND has been infrequently associated with photosensitivity skin reaction, especially during long-term therapy. It is recommended that patients avoid strong, direct sunlight during VFEND therapy.

Carcinogenesis, Mutagenesis, Impairment of Fertility

Two-year carcinogenicity studies were conducted in rats and mice. Rats were given oral doses of 6, 18 or 50 mg/kg voriconazole, or 0.2, 0.6, or 1.6 times the recommended maintenance dose (RMD) on a mg/m^2 basis. Hepatocellular adenomas were detected in females at 50 mg/kg and hepatocellular carcinomas were found in males at 6 and 50 mg/kg. Mice were given oral doses of 10, 30 or 100 mg/kg voriconazole, or 0.1, 0.4, or 1.4 times the RMD on a mg/m^2 basis. In mice, hepatocellular adenomas were detected in males and females and hepatocellular carcinomas were detected in males at 1.4 times the RMD of voriconazole.

Voriconazole demonstrated clastogenic activity (mostly chromosome breaks) in human lymphocyte cultures *in vitro*. Voriconazole was not genotoxic in the Ames assay, CHO assay, the mouse micronucleus assay or the DNA repair test (Unscheduled DNA Synthesis assay).

Voriconazole produced a reduction in the pregnancy rates of rats dosed at 50 mg/kg, or 1.6 times the RMD. This was statistically significant only in the preliminary study and not in a larger fertility study.

Teratogenic Effects

Pregnancy category D. See WARNINGS

Women of Childbearing Potential

Women of childbearing potential should use effective contraception during treatment.

Nursing Mothers

The excretion of voriconazole in breast milk has not been investigated. VFEND should not be used by nursing mothers unless the benefit clearly outweighs the risk.

Continued on next page

Vfend—Cont.

Pediatric Use
Safety and effectiveness in pediatric patients below the age of 12 years have not been established.
A total of 22 patients aged 12-18 years with invasive aspergillosis were included in the therapeutic studies. Twelve out of 22 (55%) patients had successful response after treatment with a maintenance dose of voriconazole 4 mg/kg Q12h.
Sparse plasma sampling for pharmacokinetics in adolescents was conducted in the therapeutic studies (see CLINICAL PHARMACOLOGY - Pharmacokinetics, General Pharmacokinetic Characteristics).
Geriatric Use
In multiple dose therapeutic trials of voriconazole, 9.2% of patients were ≥ 65 years of age and 1.8% of patients were ≥ 75 years of age. In a study in healthy volunteers, the systemic exposure (AUC) and peak plasma concentrations (C_{max}) were increased in elderly males compared to young males. Pharmacokinetic data obtained from 552 patients from 10 voriconazole therapeutic trials showed that voriconazole plasma concentrations in the elderly patients were approximately 80% to 90% higher than those in younger patients after either IV or oral administration. However, the overall safety profile of the elderly patients was similar to that of the young so no dosage adjustment is recommended (see CLINICAL PHARMACOLOGY - Pharmacokinetics in Special Populations).

ADVERSE REACTIONS
Overview
The most frequently reported adverse events (all causalities) in the therapeutic trials were visual disturbances, fever, rash, vomiting, nausea, diarrhea, headache, sepsis, peripheral edema, abdominal pain, and respiratory disorder. The treatment-related adverse events which most often led to discontinuation of voriconazole therapy were elevated liver function tests, rash, and visual disturbances (see hepatic toxicity under WARNINGS and discussion of Clinical Laboratory Values and dermatological and visual adverse events below).
Discussion of Adverse Reactions
The data described in the table below reflect exposure to voriconazole in 1493 patients in the therapeutic studies. This represents a heterogeneous population, including immunocompromised patients, e.g., patients with hematological malignancy or HIV and non-neutropenic patients. This subgroup does not include healthy volunteers and patients treated in the compassionate use and non-therapeutic studies. This patient population was 62% male, had a mean age of 45.1 years (range 12-90, including 49 patients aged 12-18 years), and was 81% white and 9% black. Five hundred sixty-one patients had a duration of voriconazole therapy of greater than 12 weeks, with 136 patients receiving voriconazole for over six months. Table 10 includes all adverse events which were reported in therapeutic studies at an incidence of ≥1% as well as events of concern which occurred at an incidence of <1% during voriconazole therapy.
In study 307/602, 381 patients (196 on voriconazole, 185 on amphotericin B) were treated to compare voriconazole to amphotericin B followed by other licensed antifungal therapy in the primary treatment of patients with acute invasive aspergillosis. Study 305 evaluated the effects of oral voriconazole (200 patients) and oral fluconazole (191 patients) in the treatment of esophageal candidiasis. Laboratory test abnormalities for these studies are discussed under Clinical Laboratory Values below.
[See table 10 on pages 307 and 308]
VISUAL DISTURBANCES: Voriconazole treatment-related visual disturbances are common. In clinical trials, approximately 30% of patients experienced altered/enhanced visual perception, blurred vision, color vision change and/or photophobia. The visual disturbances were generally mild and rarely resulted in discontinuation. Visual disturbances may be associated with higher plasma concentrations and/or doses.
The mechanism of action of the visual disturbance is unknown, although the site of action is most likely to be within the retina. In a study in healthy volunteers investigating the effect of 28-day treatment with voriconazole on retinal function, voriconazole caused a decrease in the electroretinogram (ERG) waveform amplitude, a decrease in the visual field, and an alteration in color perception. The ERG measures electrical currents in the retina. The effects were noted early in administration of voriconazole and continued through the course of study drug dosing. Fourteen days after end of dosing, ERG, visual fields and color perception returned to normal (see WARNINGS, PRECAUTIONS – Information For Patients).
Dermatological Reactions: Dermatological reactions were common in the patients treated with voriconazole. The mechanism underlying these dermatologic adverse events remains unknown. In clinical trials, rashes considered related to therapy were reported by 6% (86/1493) of voriconazole-treated patients. The majority of rashes were of mild to moderate severity. Cases of photosensitivity reactions appear to be more likely to occur with long-term treatment. Patients have rarely developed serious cutaneous reactions, including Stevens-Johnson syndrome, toxic epidermal necrolysis and erythema multiforme during treatment with VFEND. If patients develop a rash, they should be monitored closely and consideration given to dis-

Table 9 Effect of Voriconazole on Pharmacokinetics of Other Drugs

Drug/Drug Class (Mechanism of Interaction by Voriconazole)	Drug Plasma Exposure (C_{max} and AUC_τ)	Recommendations for Drug Dosage Adjustment/Comments
Sirolimus* (CYP3A4 Inhibition)	Significantly Increased	**Contraindicated**
Rifabutin* and Efavirenz** (CYP3A4 Inhibition)	Significantly Increased	**Contraindicated**
Ritonavir (400 mg Q12h HIV Protease Inhibitor)** (CYP3A4 Inhibition)	No significant effect of voriconazole on ritonavir C_{max} or AUC_τ	**Contraindicated** because of significant reduction of voriconazole C_{max} and AUC_τ
Terfenadine, Astemizole, Cisapride, Pimozide, Quinidine (CYP3A4 Inhibition)	Not Studied *In Vivo* or *In Vitro*, but Drug Plasma Exposure Likely to be Increased	**Contraindicated** because of potential for QT prolongation and rare occurrence of *torsade de pointes*
Ergot Alkaloids (CYP450 Inhibition)	Not Studied *In Vivo* or *In Vitro*, but Drug Plasma Exposure Likely to be Increased	**Contraindicated**
Cyclosporine* (CYP3A4 Inhibition)	AUC_τ Significantly Increased; No Significant Effect on C_{max}	When initiating therapy with VFEND in patients already receiving cyclosporine, reduce the cyclosporine dose to one-half of the starting dose and follow with frequent monitoring of cyclosporine blood levels. Increased cyclosporine levels have been associated with nephrotoxicity. When VFEND is discontinued, cyclosporine concentrations must be frequently monitored and the dose increased as necessary.
Tacrolimus* (CYP3A4 Inhibition)	Significantly Increased	When initiating therapy with VFEND in patients already receiving tacrolimus, reduce the tacrolimus dose to one-third of the starting dose and follow with frequent monitoring of tacrolimus blood levels. Increased tacrolimus levels have been associated with nephrotoxicity. When VFEND is discontinued, tacrolimus concentrations must be frequently monitored and the dose increased as necessary.
Phenytoin* (CYP2C9 Inhibition)	Significantly Increased	Frequent monitoring of phenytoin plasma concentrations and frequent monitoring of adverse effects related to phenytoin.
Warfarin* (CYP2C9 Inhibition)	Prothrombin Time Significantly Increased	Monitor PT or other suitable anticoagulation tests. Adjustment of warfarin dosage may be needed.
Omeprazole* (CYP2C19/3A4 Inhibition)	Significantly Increased	When initiating therapy with VFEND in patients already receiving omeprazole doses of 40 mg or greater, reduce the omeprazole dose by one-half. The metabolism of other proton pump inhibitors that are CYP2C19 substrates may also be inhibited by voriconazole and may result in increased plasma concentrations of other proton pump inhibitors.
Other HIV Protease Inhibitors (CYP3A4 Inhibition)	*In Vivo* Studies showed No Significant Effects on Indinavir Exposure *In Vitro* Studies Demonstrate Potential for Voriconazole to Inhibit Metabolism (Increased Plasma Exposure)	No dosage adjustment for indinavir when coadministered with VFEND Frequent monitoring for adverse events and toxicity related to other HIV protease inhibitors
Other NNRTIs*** (CYP3A4 Inhibition)	*In Vitro* Studies Demonstrate Potential for Voriconazole to Inhibit Metabolism (Increased Plasma Exposure)	Frequent monitoring for adverse events and toxicity related to NNRTI
Benzodiazepines (CYP3A4 Inhibition)	*In Vitro* Studies Demonstrate Potential for Voriconazole to Inhibit Metabolism (Increased Plasma Exposure)	Frequent monitoring for adverse events and toxicity (i.e., prolonged sedation) related to benzodiazepines metabolized by CYP3A4 (e.g., midazolam, triazolam, alprazolam). Adjustment of benzodiazepine dosage may be needed.
HMG-CoA Reductase Inhibitors (Statins) (CYP3A4 Inhibition)	*In Vitro* Studies Demonstrate Potential for Voriconazole to Inhibit Metabolism (Increased Plasma Exposure)	Frequent monitoring for adverse events and toxicity related to statins. Increased statin concentrations in plasma have been associated with rhabdomyolysis. Adjustment of the statin dosage may be needed.
Dihydropyridine Calcium Channel Blockers (CYP3A4 Inhibition)	*In Vitro* Studies Demonstrate Potential for Voriconazole to Inhibit Metabolism (Increased Plasma Exposure)	Frequent monitoring for adverse events and toxicity related to calcium channel blockers. Adjustment of calcium channel blocker dosage may be needed.
Sulfonylurea Oral Hypoglycemics (CYP2C9 Inhibition)	Not Studied *In Vivo* or *In Vitro*, but Drug Plasma Exposure Likely to be Increased	Frequent monitoring of blood glucose and for signs and symptoms of hypoglycemia. Adjustment of oral hypoglycemic drug dosage may be needed.

(Table continued on next page)

Table 9 (cont.) Effect of Voriconazole on Pharmacokinetics of Other Drugs

Drug/Drug Class (Mechanism of Interaction by Voriconazole)	Drug Plasma Exposure (C_{max} and AUC_τ)	Recommendations for Drug Dosage Adjustment/Comments
Vinca Alkaloids (CYP3A4 Inhibition)	Not Studied *In Vivo* or *In Vitro*, but Drug Plasma Exposure Likely to be Increased	Frequent monitoring for adverse events and toxicity (i.e., neurotoxicity) related to vinca alkaloids. Adjustment of vinca alkaloid dosage may be needed.

*Results based on *in vivo* clinical studies generally following repeat oral dosing with 200 mg BID voriconazole to healthy subjects
**Results based on *in vivo* clinical study following repeat oral doing with 400 mg Q12h for 1 day, then 200 mg Q12h for 8 days voriconazole to healthy subjects
***Non-Nucleoside Reverse Transcriptase Inhibitors

Table 10
Treatment Emergent Adverse Events
Rate ≥ 1% or Adverse Events of Concern in All Therapeutic Studies
Possibly Related to Therapy or Causality Unknown

	All Therapeutic Studies	Protocol 305 (oral therapy)		Protocol 307/602 (IV/oral therapy)	
	Voriconazole N = 1493	Voriconazole N = 200	Fluconazole N = 191	Voriconazole N = 196	Ampho B** N = 185
	N (%)	N (%)	N (%)	N (%)	N (%)
Special Senses*					
Abnormal vision	307 (20.6)	31 (15.5)	8 (4.2)	55 (28.1)	1 (0.5)
Photophobia	36 (2.4)	5 (2.5)	2 (1.0)	7 (3.6)	0
Chromatopsia	20 (1.3)	2 (1.0)	0	2 (1.0)	0
Eye hemorrhage	3 (0.2)	0	0	0	0
Body as a Whole					
Fever	93 (6.2)	0	0	7 (3.6)	25 (13.5)
Chills	61 (4.1)	1 (0.5)	0	0	36 (19.5)
Headache	48 (3.2)	0	1 (0.5)	7 (3.6)	8 (4.3)
Abdominal pain	25 (1.7)	0	0	5 (2.6)	6 (3.2)
Chest pain	13 (0.9)	0	0	4 (2.0)	2 (1.1)
Cardiovascular System					
Tachycardia	37 (2.5)	0	0	5 (2.6)	5 (2.7)
Hypertension	29 (1.9)	0	0	1 (0.5)	2 (1.1)
Hypotension	26 (1.7)	1 (0.5)	0	1 (0.5)	3 (1.6)
Vasodilatation	23 (1.5)	0	0	2 (1.0)	2 (1.1)
Digestive System					
Nausea	88 (5.9)	2 (1.0)	3 (1.6)	14 (7.1)	29 (15.7)
Vomiting	71 (4.8)	2 (1.0)	1 (0.5)	11 (5.6)	18 (9.7)
Liver function tests abnormal	41 (2.7)	6 (3.0)	2 (1.0)	9 (4.6)	4 (2.2)
Diarrhea	16 (1.1)	0	0	3 (1.5)	6 (3.2)
Cholestatic jaundice	16 (1.1)	3 (1.5)	0	4 (2.0)	0
Dry mouth	15 (1.0)	0	1 (0.5)	3 (1.5)	0
Jaundice	3 (0.2)	1 (0.5)	0	0	0
Hemic and Lymphatic System					
Thrombocytopenia	7 (0.5)	0	1 (0.5)	2 (1.0)	2 (1.1)
Anemia	2 (0.1)	0	0	0	5 (2.7)
Leukopenia	4 (0.3)	0	0	1 (0.5)	0
Pancytopenia	1 (0.1)	0	0	0	0
Metabolic and Nutritional Systems					
Alkaline phosphatase increased	54 (3.6)	10 (5.0)	3 (1.6)	6 (3.1)	4 (2.2)
Hepatic enzymes increased	28 (1.9)	3 (1.5)	0	7 (3.6)	5 (2.7)
SGOT increased	28 (1.9)	8 (4.0)	2 (1.0)	1 (0.5)	0
SGPT increased	27 (1.8)	6 (3.0)	2 (1.0)	3 (1.5)	1 (0.5)
Hypokalemia	24 (1.6)	0	0	1 (0.5)	36 (19.5)
Peripheral edema	16 (1.1)	1 (0.5)	0	7 (3.6)	9 (4.9)
Hypomagnesemia	16 (1.1)	0	0	2 (1.0)	10 (5.4)

(Table continued on next page)

continuation of VFEND. It is recommended that patients avoid strong, direct sunlight during VFEND therapy.

Less Common Adverse Events

The following adverse events occurred in <1% of all voriconazole-treated patients, including healthy volunteers and patients treated under compassionate use protocols (total N = 2090). This listing includes events where a causal relationship to voriconazole cannot be ruled out or those which may help the physician in managing the risks to the patients. The list does not include events included in Table 10 above and does not include every event reported in the voriconazole clinical program.

Body as a Whole: abdomen enlarged, allergic reaction, anaphylactoid reaction (see PRECAUTIONS), ascites, asthenia, back pain, cellulitis, edema, face edema, flank pain, flu syndrome, graft versus host reaction, granuloma, infection, bacterial infection, fungal infection, injection site pain, injection site infection/inflammation, mucous membrane disorder, multi-organ failure, pain, pelvic pain, peritonitis, sepsis, substernal chest pain

Cardiovascular: atrial arrhythmia, atrial fibrillation, AV block complete, bigeminy, bradycardia, bundle branch block, cardiomegaly, cardiomyopathy, cerebral hemorrhage, cerebral ischemia, cerebrovascular accident, congestive heart failure, deep thrombophlebitis, endocarditis, extrasystoles, heart arrest, myocardial infarction, nodal arrhythmia, palpitation, phlebitis, postural hypotension, pulmonary embolus, QT interval prolonged, supraventricular tachycardia, syncope, thrombophlebitis, vasodilatation, ventricular arrhythmia, ventricular fibrillation, ventricular tachycardia (including *torsade de pointes*)

Digestive: anorexia, cheilitis, cholecystitis, cholelithiasis, constipation, duodenal ulcer perforation, duodenitis, dyspepsia, dysphagia, esophageal ulcer, esophagitis, flatulence, gastroenteritis, gastrointestinal hemorrhage, GGT/LDH elevated, gingivitis, glossitis, gum hemorrhage, gum hyperplasia, hematemesis, hepatic coma, hepatic failure, hepatitis, intestinal perforation, intestinal ulcer, enlarged liver, melena, mouth ulceration, pancreatitis, parotid gland enlargement, periodontitis, proctitis, pseudomembranous colitis, rectal disorder, rectal hemorrhage, stomach ulcer, stomatitis, tongue edema

Endocrine: adrenal cortex insufficiency, diabetes insipidus, hyperthyroidism, hypothyroidism

Hemic and Lymphatic: agranulocytosis, anemia (macrocytic, megaloblastic, microcytic, normocytic), aplastic anemia, hemolytic anemia, bleeding time increased, cyanosis, DIC, ecchymosis, eosinophilia, hypervolemia, lymphadenopathy, lymphangitis, marrow depression, petechia, purpura, enlarged spleen, thrombotic thrombocytopenic purpura

Metabolic and Nutritional: albuminuria, BUN increased, creatine phosphokinase increased, edema, glucose tolerance decreased, hypercalcemia, hypercholesteremia, hyperglycemia, hyperkalemia, hypermagnesemia, hypernatremia, hyperuricemia, hypocalcemia, hypoglycemia, hyponatremia, hypophosphatemia, uremia

Musculoskeletal: arthralgia, arthritis, bone necrosis, bone pain, leg cramps, myalgia, myasthenia, myopathy, osteomalacia, osteoporosis

Nervous System: abnormal dreams, acute brain syndrome, agitation, akathisia, amnesia, anxiety, ataxia, brain edema, coma, confusion, convulsion, delirium, dementia, depersonalization, depression, diplopia, encephalitis, encephalopathy, euphoria, Extrapyramidal Syndrome, grand mal convulsion, Guillain-Barré syndrome, hypertonia, hypesthesia, insomnia, intracranial hypertension, libido decreased, neuralgia, neuropathy, nystagmus, oculogyric crisis, paresthesia, psychosis, somnolence, suicidal ideation, tremor, vertigo

Respiratory System: cough increased, dyspnea, epistaxis, hemoptysis, hypoxia, lung edema, pharyngitis, pleural effusion, pneumonia, respiratory disorder, respiratory distress syndrome, respiratory tract infection, rhinitis, sinusitis, voice alteration

Skin and Appendages: alopecia, angioedema, contact dermatitis, discoid lupus erythematosis, eczema, erythema multiforme, exfoliative dermatitis, fixed drug eruption, furunculosis, herpes simplex, melanosis, photosensitivity skin reaction, psoriasis, skin discoloration, skin disorder, skin dry, Stevens-Johnson syndrome, sweating, toxic epidermal necrolysis, urticaria

Special Senses: abnormality of accommodation, blepharitis, color blindness, conjunctivitis, corneal opacity, deafness, ear pain, eye pain, dry eyes, keratitis, keratoconjunctivitis, mydriasis, night blindness, optic atrophy, optic neuritis, otitis externa, papilledema, retinal hemorrhage, retinitis, scleritis, taste loss, taste perversion, tinnitus, uveitis, visual field defect

Urogenital: anuria, blighted ovum, creatinine clearance decreased, dysmenorrhea, dysuria, epididymitis, glycosuria, hemorrhagic cystitis, hematuria, hydronephrosis, impotence, kidney pain, kidney tubular necrosis, metrorrhagia, nephritis, nephrosis, oliguria, scrotal edema, urinary incontinence, urinary retention, urinary tract infection, uterine hemorrhage, vaginal hemorrhage

Clinical Laboratory Values

The overall incidence of clinically significant transaminase abnormalities in the voriconazole clinical program was 13.4% (200/1493) of patients treated with voriconazole. Increased incidence of liver function test abnormalities may be associated with higher plasma concentrations and/or doses. The majority of abnormal liver function tests either

Continued on next page

Vfend—Cont.

resolved during treatment without dose adjustment or following dose adjustment, including discontinuation of therapy.

Voriconazole has been infrequently associated with cases of serious hepatic toxicity including cases of jaundice and rare cases of hepatitis and hepatic failure leading to death. Most of these patients had other serious underlying conditions.

Liver function tests should be evaluated at the start of and during the course of VFEND therapy. Patients who develop abnormal liver function tests during VFEND therapy should be monitored for the development of more severe hepatic injury. Patient management should include laboratory evaluation of hepatic function (particularly liver function tests and bilirubin). Discontinuation of VFEND must be considered if clinical signs and symptoms consistent with liver disease develop that may be attributable to VFEND (see WARNINGS and PRECAUTIONS - Laboratory Tests).

Acute renal failure has been observed in severely ill patients undergoing treatment with VFEND. Patients being treated with voriconazole are likely to be treated concomitantly with nephrotoxic medications and have concurrent conditions that may result in decreased renal function. It is recommended that patients are monitored for the development of abnormal renal function. This should include laboratory evaluation, particularly serum creatinine.

Tables 11 and 12 show the number of patients with hypokalemia and clinically significant changes in renal and liver function tests in two randomized, comparative multicenter studies. In study 305, patients were randomized to either oral voriconazole or oral fluconazole to evaluate an indication other than invasive aspergillosis in immunocompromised patients. In study 307/602, patients with definite or probable invasive aspergillosis were randomized to either voriconazole or amphotericin B therapy.

[See table 11 below]

[See table 12 at top of next page]

OVERDOSE

In clinical trials, there were three cases of accidental overdose. All occurred in pediatric patients who received up to five times the recommended intravenous dose of voriconazole. A single adverse event of photophobia of 10 minutes duration was reported.

There is no known antidote to voriconazole.

Voriconazole is hemodialyzed with clearance of 121 mL/min. The intravenous vehicle, SBECD, is hemodialyzed with clearance of 55 mL/min. In an overdose, hemodialysis may assist in the removal of voriconazole and SBECD from the body.

The minimum lethal oral dose in mice and rats was 300 mg/kg (equivalent to 4 and 7 times the recommended maintenance dose (RMD), based on body surface area). At this dose, clinical signs observed in both mice and rats included salivation, mydriasis, titubation (loss of balance while moving), depressed behavior, prostration, partially closed eyes, and dyspnea. Other signs in mice were convulsions, corneal opacification and swollen abdomen.

DOSAGE AND ADMINISTRATION

Administration

VFEND Tablets or Oral Suspension should be taken at least one hour before, or one hour following, a meal.

VFEND I.V. for Injection requires reconstitution to 10 mg/mL and subsequent dilution to 5 mg/mL or less prior to administration as an infusion, at a maximum rate of 3 mg/kg per hour over 1-2 hours (see Intravenous Administration).

NOT FOR IV BOLUS INJECTION

Electrolyte disturbances such as hypokalemia, hypomagnesemia and hypocalcemia should be corrected prior to initiation of VFEND therapy (see PRECAUTIONS).

Use In Adults

Invasive aspergillosis and serious fungal infections due to *Fusarium* spp. and *Scedosporium apiospermum*:

For the treatment of adults with invasive aspergillosis and infections due to *Fusarium* spp. and *Scedosporium apiospermum*, therapy must be initiated with the specified loading dose regimen of intravenous VFEND to achieve plasma concentrations on Day 1 that are close to steady state. On the basis of high oral bioavailability, switching between intravenous and oral administration is appropriate when clinically indicated (see CLINICAL PHARMACOLOGY). Once the patient can tolerate medication given by mouth, the oral tablet form or oral suspension form of VFEND may be utilized.

The recommended dosing regimen of VFEND is as follows:

Loading Dose Regimen	6 mg/kg IV every 12 hours (for the first 24 hours)	
Maintenance Dose	IV	Oral*
	4 mg/kg every 12 hours	200 mg every 12 hours

*Patients who weigh 40 kg or more should receive an oral maintenace dose of 200 mg VFEND every 12 hours. Adult patients who weigh less than 40 kg should receive an oral maintenance dose of 100 mg every 12 hours.

Dosage Adjustment

If patient response is inadequate, the oral maintenance dose may be increased from 200 mg every 12 hours to 300 mg every 12 hours. For adult patients weighing less than 40 kg, the oral maintenance dose may be increased from 100 mg every 12 hours to 150 mg every 12 hours.

If patients are unable to tolerate treatment, reduce the intravenous maintenance dose to 3 mg/kg every 12 hours and the oral maintenance dose by 50 mg steps to a minimum of 200 mg every 12 hours (or to 100 mg every 12 hours for adult patients weighing less than 40 kg).

Phenytoin may be coadministered with VFEND if the intravenous maintenance dose of VFEND is increased to 5 mg/kg every 12 hours, or the oral maintenance dose is increased from 200 mg to 400 mg every 12 hours (100 mg to 200 mg every 12 hours in adult patients weighing less than 40 kg) (see CLINICAL PHARMACOLOGY, PRECAUTIONS - Drug Interactions).

Duration of therapy should be based on the severity of the patient's underlying disease, recovery from immunosuppression, and clinical response.

Esophageal Candidiasis:

The recommended dosing regimen is an oral dose of 200 mg every 12 hours for patients who weigh 40 kg or more. Adult patients who weigh less than 40 kg should receive an oral dose of 100 mg every 12 hours. Patients should be treated for a minimum of 14 days and for at least 7 days following resolution of symptoms.

Use in Geriatric Patients

No dose adjustment is necessary for geriatric patients.

Use in Patients with Hepatic Insufficiency

In the clinical program, patients were included who had baseline liver function tests (ALT, AST) up to 5 times the upper limit of normal. No dose adjustment is necessary in patients with this degree of abnormal liver function, but continued monitoring of liver function tests for further elevations is recommended (see WARNINGS).

It is recommended that the standard loading dose regimens be used but that the maintenance dose be halved in patients with mild to moderate hepatic cirrhosis (Child-Pugh Class A and B).

VFEND has not been studied in patients with severe hepatic cirrhosis (Child-Pugh Class C) or in patients with chronic hepatitis B or chronic hepatitis C disease. VFEND has been associated with elevations in liver function tests and clinical signs of liver damage, such as jaundice, and should only be used in patients with severe hepatic insufficiency if the benefit outweighs the potential risk. Patients with hepatic insufficiency must be carefully monitored for drug toxicity.

Use in Patients with Renal Insufficiency

The pharmacokinetics of orally administered VFEND are not significantly affected by renal insufficiency. Therefore, no adjustment is necessary for oral dosing in patients with mild to severe renal impairment (see CLINICAL PHARMACOLOGY - Special Populations).

In patients with moderate or severe renal insufficiency (creatinine clearance <50 mL/min), accumulation of the intravenous vehicle, SBECD, occurs. Oral voriconazole should be administered to these patients, unless an assessment of the benefit/risk to the patient justifies the use of intravenous voriconazole. Serum creatinine levels should be closely monitored in these patients, and, if increases occur, consideration should be given to changing to oral voriconazole therapy (see DOSAGE and ADMINISTRATION).

Voriconazole is hemodialyzed with clearance of 121 mL/min. The intravenous vehicle, SBECD, is hemodialyzed with clearance of 55 mL/min. A 4-hour hemodialysis session does not remove a sufficient amount of voriconazole to warrant dose adjustment.

Intravenous Administration

VFEND I.V. For Injection:

Reconstitution

The powder is reconstituted with 19 mL of Water For Injection to obtain an extractable volume of 20 mL of clear concentrate containing 10 mg/mL of voriconazole. It is recommended that a standard 20 mL (non-automated) syringe be used to ensure that the exact amount (19.0 mL) of water for injection is dispensed. Discard the vial if a vacuum does not pull the diluent into the vial. Shake the vial until all the powder is dissolved.

Dilution

VFEND must be infused over 1-2 hours, at a concentration of 5 mg/mL or less. Therefore, the required volume of the 10 mg/mL VFEND concentrate should be further diluted as follows (appropriate diluents listed below):

Table 10 *(cont.)*
Treatment Emergent Adverse Events
Rate ≥ 1% or Adverse Events of Concern in All Therapeutic Studies
Possibly Related to Therapy or Causality Unknown

	All Therapeutic Studies	Protocol 305 (oral therapy)		Protocol 307/602 (IV/oral therapy)	
	Voriconazole N = 1493	Voriconazole N = 200	Fluconazole N = 191	Voriconazole N = 196	Ampho B** N = 185
	N (%)	N (%)	N (%)	N (%)	N (%)
Hypomagnesemia	16 (1.1)	0	0	2 (1.0)	10 (5.4)
Bilirubinemia	12 (0.8)	1 (0.5)	0	1 (0.5)	3 (1.6)
Creatinine increased	4 (0.3)	1 (0.5)	0	0	59 (31.9)
Nervous System					
Hallucinations	37 (2.5)	0	0	10 (5.1)	1 (0.5)
Dizziness	20 (1.3)	0	2 (1.0)	5 (2.6)	0
Skin and Appendages					
Rash	86 (5.8)	3 (1.5)	1 (0.5)	13 (6.6)	7 (3.8)
Pruritus	16 (1.1)	0	0	2 (1.0)	2 (1.1)
Maculopapular rash	17 (1.1)	3 (1.5)	0	1 (0.5)	0
Urogenital					
Kidney function abnormal	8 (0.5)	1 (0.5)	1 (0.5)	4 (2.0)	40 (21.6)
Acute kidney failure	7 (0.5)	0	0	0	11 (5.9)

* See WARNINGS – Visual Disturbances, PRECAUTIONS – Information For Patients
**Amphotericin B followed by other licensed antifungal therapy

Table 11
PROTOCOL 305
Clinically Significant Laboratory Test Abnormalities

	Criteria*	VORICONAZOLE	FLUCONAZOLE
		n/N (%)	n/N (%)
T. Bilirubin	>1.5× ULN	8/185 (4.3)	7/186 (3.8)
AST	>3.0× ULN	38/187 (20.3)	15/186 (8.1)
ALT	>3.0× ULN	20/187 (10.7)	12/186 (6.5)
Alk phos	>3.0× ULN	19/187 (10.2)	14/186 (7.5)

* Without regard to baseline value
n number of patients with a clinically significant abnormality while on study therapy
N total number of patients with at least one observation of the given lab test while on study therapy
ULN upper limit of normal

Table 12
PROTOCOL 307/602
Clinically Significant Laboratory Test Abnormalities

	Criteria*	VORICONAZOLE	AMPHOTERICIN B**
		n/N (%)	n/N (%)
T. Bilirubin	>1.5× ULN	35/180 (19.4)	46/173 (26.6)
AST	>3.0× ULN	21/180 (11.7)	18/174 (10.3)
ALT	>3.0× ULN	34/180 (18.9)	40/173 (23.1)
Alk phos	>3.0× ULN	29/181 (16.0)	38/173 (22.0)
Creatinine	>1.3× ULN	39/182 (21.4)	102/177 (57.6)
Potassium	<0.9× LLN	30/181 (16.6)	70/178 (39.3)

* Without regard to baseline value
** Amphotericin B followed by other licensed antifungal therapy
n number of patients with a clinically significant abnormality while on study therapy
N total number of patients with at least one observation of the given lab test while on study therapy
ULN upper limit of normal
LLN lower limit of normal

Table 13 Required Volumes of 10 mg/mL VFEND Concentrate

Body Weight (kg)	Volume of VFEND Concentrate (10 mg/mL) required for:		
	3 mg/kg dose (number of vials)	4 mg/kg dose (number of vials)	6 mg/kg dose (number of vials)
30	9.0 mL (1)	12 mL (1)	18 mL (1)
35	10.5 mL (1)	14 mL (1)	21 mL (2)
40	12.0 mL (1)	16 mL (1)	24 mL (2)
45	13.5 mL (1)	18 mL (1)	27 mL (2)
50	15.0 mL (1)	20 mL (1)	30 mL (2)
55	16.5 mL (1)	22 mL (2)	33 mL (2)
60	18.0 mL (1)	24 mL (2)	36 mL (2)
65	19.5 mL (1)	26 mL (2)	39 mL (2)
70	21.0 mL (2)	28 mL (2)	42 mL (3)
75	22.5 mL (2)	30 mL (2)	45 mL (3)
80	24.0 mL (2)	32 mL (2)	48 mL (3)
85	25.5 mL (2)	34 mL (2)	51 mL (3)
90	27.0 mL (2)	36 mL (2)	54 mL (3)
95	28.5 mL (2)	38 mL (2)	57 mL (3)
100	30.0 mL (2)	40 mL (2)	60 mL (3)

1. Calculate the volume of 10 mg/mL VFEND concentrate required based on the patient's weight (see Table 13).
2. In order to allow the required volume of VFEND concentrate to be added, withdraw and discard at least an equal volume of diluent from the infusion bag or bottle to be used. The volume of diluent remaining in the bag or bottle should be such that when the 10 mg/mL VFEND concentrate is added, the final concentration is not less than 0.5 mg/mL nor greater than 5 mg/mL.
3. Using a suitable size syringe and aseptic technique, withdraw the required volume of VFEND concentrate from the appropriate number of vials and add to the infusion bag or bottle. DISCARD PARTIALLY USED VIALS.

The final VFEND solution must be infused over 1-2 hours at a maximum rate of 3 mg/kg per hour.
[See table 13 above]
VFEND I.V. for Injection is a single dose unpreserved sterile lyophile. Therefore, from a microbiological point of view, once reconstituted, the product should be used immediately. If not used immediately, in-use storage times and conditions prior to use are the responsibility of the user and should not be longer than 24 hours at 2° to 8°C (37° to 46°F). This medicinal product is for single use only and any unused solution should be discarded. Only clear solutions without particles should be used.
The reconstituted solution can be diluted with:
9 mg/mL (0.9%) Sodium Chloride USP
Lactated Ringers USP
5% Dextrose and Lactated Ringers USP
5% Dextrose and 0.45% Sodium Chloride, USP
5% Dextrose USP
5% Dextrose and 20 mEq Potassium Chloride, USP
0.45% Sodium Chloride USP
5% Dextrose and 0.9% Sodium Chloride, USP
The compatibility of VFEND I.V. with diluents other than those described above is unknown (see Incompatibilities below).
Parenteral drug products should be inspected visually for particulate matter and discoloration prior to administration, whenever solution and container permit.
Incompatibilities:
VFEND I.V. must not be infused into the same line or cannula concomitantly with other drug infusions, including parenteral nutrition, e.g., Aminofusin 10% Plus. Aminofusin 10% Plus is physically incompatible, with an increase in subvisible particulate matter after 24 hours storage at 4°C. Infusions of blood products must not occur simultaneously with VFEND I.V.
Infusions of total parenteral nutrition can occur simultaneously with VFEND I.V.
VFEND I.V. must not be diluted with 4.2% Sodium Bicarbonate Infusion. The mildly alkaline nature of this diluent caused slight degradation of VFEND after 24 hours storage at room temperature. Although refrigerated storage is recommended following reconstitution, use of this diluent is not recommended as a precautionary measure. Compatibility with other concentrations is unknown.

VFEND for Oral Suspension
Reconstitution
Tap the bottle to release the powder. Add 46 mL of water to the bottle. Shake the closed bottle vigorously for about 1 minute. Remove child-resistant cap and push bottle adaptor into the neck of the bottle. Replace the cap. Write the date of expiration of the reconstituted suspension on the bottle label (the shelf-life of the reconstituted suspension is 14 days at controlled room temperature 15-30°C (59-86°F)).
Instructions for use
Shake the closed bottle of reconstituted suspension for approximately 10 seconds before each use. The reconstituted oral suspension should only be administered using the oral dispenser supplied with each pack.
Incompatibilities
VFEND for Oral Suspension and the 40 mg/mL reconstituted oral suspension should not be mixed with any other medication or additional flavoring agent. It is not intended that the suspension be further diluted with water or other vehicles.

HOW SUPPLIED
Powder for Solution for Injection
VFEND I.V. for Injection is supplied in a single use vial as a sterile lyophilized powder equivalent to 200 mg VFEND and 3200 mg sulfobutyl ether beta-cyclodextrin sodium (SBECD).
Individually packaged vials of 200 mg VFEND I.V.
(NDC 0049-3190-28)
Tablets
VFEND 50 mg tablets - white, film-coated, round, debossed with "Pfizer" on one side and "VOR50" on the reverse.
Bottles of 30 (NDC 0049-3170-30)
VFEND 200 mg tablets – white, film-coated, capsule shaped, debossed with "Pfizer" on one side and "VOR200" on the reverse.
Bottles of 30 (NDC 0049-3180-30)
Powder for Oral Suspension
VFEND for Oral Suspension is supplied in 100 mL high density polyethylene (HDPE) bottles. Each bottle contains 45 g of powder for oral suspension. Following reconstitution, the volume of the suspension is 75 mL, providing a usable volume of 70 mL (40 mg voriconazole/mL). A 5 mL oral dispenser and a press-in bottle adaptor are also provided.
(NDC 0049-3160-44)

STORAGE
VFEND I.V. for injection unreconstituted-vials should be stored at 15° - 30°C (59° - 86°F) [see USP Controlled Room Temperature]. VFEND is a single dose unpreserved sterile lyophile. From a microbiological point of view, following reconstitution of the lyophile with Water for Injection, the reconstituted solution should be used immediately. If not used immediately, in-use storage times and conditions prior to use are the responsibility of the user and should not be longer than 24 hours at 2° to 8°C (36° to 46°F). Chemical and physical in-use stability has been demonstrated for 24 hours at 2° to 8°C (36° to 46°F). This medicinal product is for single use only and any unused solution should be discarded. Only clear solutions without particles should be used (see DOSAGE AND ADMINISTRATION - Intravenous Administration).
VFEND Tablets should be stored at 15° - 30°C (59° - 86 ° F) [see USP Controlled Room Temperature].
VFEND Powder for Oral Suspension should be stored at 2 - 8°C (36 - 46°F) (in a refrigerator) before reconstitution. The shelf-life of the powder for oral suspension is 18 months. The reconstituted suspension should be stored at 15 - 30°C (59 - 86°F) [see USP Controlled Room Temperature]. Do not refrigerate or freeze. Keep the container tightly closed. The shelf-life of the reconstituted suspension is 14 days. Any remaining suspension should be discarded 14 days after reconstitution.

REFERENCES
1. National Committee for Clinical Laboratory Standards. Reference method for broth dilution antifungal susceptibility testing of conidium-forming filamentous fungi. Approved Standard M38-P. National Committee for Clinical Laboratory Standards, Villanova, Pa.
2. National Committee for Clinical Laboratory Standards. Reference method for broth dilution antifungal susceptibility testing of yeasts. Approved Standard M27-A. National Committee for Clinical Laboratory Standards, Villanova, Pa.

Rx only

Distributed by
Pfizer Roerig
Division of Pfizer Inc, NY, NY 10017
69-5906-00-4 Revised December 2003

VIAGRA® ℞
[*vī-ă-grə*]
(sildenafil citrate)
Tablets

Prescribing information for this product, which appears on pages 2662–2665 of the 2004 PDR, has been completely revised as follows. Please write "See Supplement A" next to the product heading.

DESCRIPTION
VIAGRA®, an oral therapy for erectile dysfunction, is the citrate salt of sildenafil, a selective inhibitor of cyclic guanosine monophosphate (cGMP)-specific phosphodiesterase type 5 (PDE5).
Sildenafil citrate is designated chemically as 1-[[3-(6,7-dihydro-1-methyl-7-oxo-3-propyl-1*H*-pyrazolo[4,3-*d*]pyrimidin-5-yl)-4-ethoxyphenyl]sulfonyl]-4-methylpiperazine citrate and has the following structural formula:

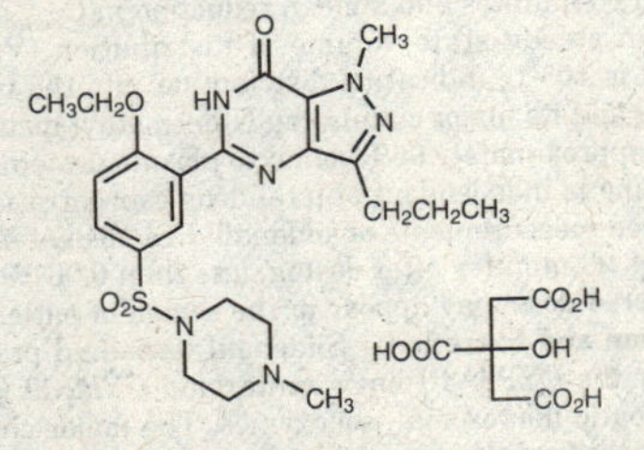

Sildenafil citrate is a white to off-white crystalline powder with a solubility of 3.5 mg/mL in water and a molecular weight of 666.7. VIAGRA (sildenafil citrate) is formulated as blue, film-coated rounded-diamond-shaped tablets equivalent to 25 mg, 50 mg and 100 mg of sildenafil for oral administration. In addition to the active ingredient, sildenafil

Continued on next page

Viagra—Cont.

citrate, each tablet contains the following inactive ingredients: microcrystalline cellulose, anhydrous dibasic calcium phosphate, croscarmellose sodium, magnesium stearate, hypromellose, titanium dioxide, lactose, triacetin, and FD & C Blue #2 aluminum lake.

CLINICAL PHARMACOLOGY

Mechanism of Action

The physiologic mechanism of erection of the penis involves release of nitric oxide (NO) in the corpus cavernosum during sexual stimulation. NO then activates the enzyme guanylate cyclase, which results in increased levels of cyclic guanosine monophosphate (cGMP), producing smooth muscle relaxation in the corpus cavernosum and allowing inflow of blood. Sildenafil has no direct relaxant effect on isolated human corpus cavernosum, but enhances the effect of nitric oxide (NO) by inhibiting phosphodiesterase type 5 (PDE5), which is responsible for degradation of cGMP in the corpus cavernosum. When sexual stimulation causes local release of NO, inhibition of PDE5 by sildenafil causes increased levels of cGMP in the corpus cavernosum, resulting in smooth muscle relaxation and inflow of blood to the corpus cavernosum. Sildenafil at recommended doses has no effect in the absence of sexual stimulation.

Studies *in vitro* have shown that sildenafil is selective for PDE5. Its effect is more potent on PDE5 than on other known phosphodiesterases (10-fold for PDE6, >80-fold for PDE1, >700-fold for PDE2, PDE3, PDE4, PDE7, PDE8, PDE9, PDE10, and PDE11). The approximately 4,000-fold selectivity for PDE5 versus PDE3 is important because PDE3 is involved in control of cardiac contractility. Sildenafil is only about 10-fold as potent for PDE5 compared to PDE6, an enzyme found in the retina which is involved in the phototransduction pathway of the retina. This lower selectivity is thought to be the basis for abnormalities related to color vision observed with higher doses or plasma levels (see **Pharmacodynamics**).

In addition to human corpus cavernosum smooth muscle, PDE5 is also found in lower concentrations in other tissues including platelets, vascular and visceral smooth muscle, and skeletal muscle. The inhibition of PDE5 in these tissues by sildenafil may be the basis for the enhanced platelet antiaggregatory activity of nitric oxide observed *in vitro*, an inhibition of platelet thrombus formation *in vivo* and peripheral arterial-venous dilatation *in vivo*.

Pharmacokinetics and Metabolism

VIAGRA is rapidly absorbed after oral administration, with absolute bioavailability of about 40%. Its pharmacokinetics are dose-proportional over the recommended dose range. It is eliminated predominantly by hepatic metabolism (mainly cytochrome P450 3A4) and is converted to an active metabolite with properties similar to the parent, sildenafil. The concomitant use of potent cytochrome P450 3A4 inhibitors (e.g., erythromycin, ketoconazole, itraconazole) as well as the nonspecific CYP inhibitor, cimetidine, is associated with increased plasma levels of sildenafil (see **DOSAGE AND ADMINISTRATION**). Both sildenafil and the metabolite have terminal half lives of about 4 hours.

Mean sildenafil plasma concentrations measured after the administration of a single oral dose of 100 mg to healthy male volunteers is depicted below:

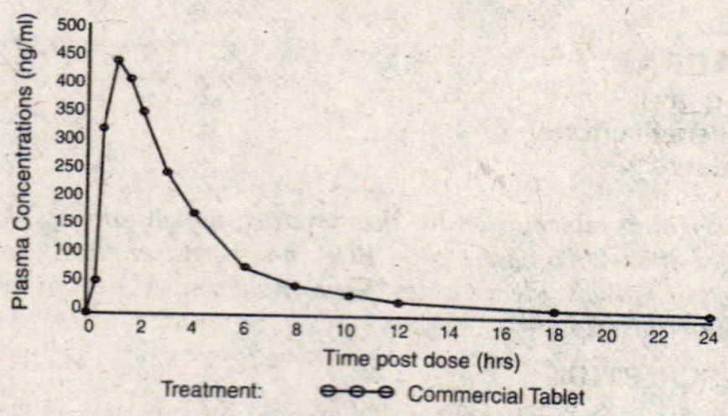

Figure 1: Mean Sildenafil Plasma Concentrations in Healthy Male Volunteers.

Absorption and Distribution: VIAGRA is rapidly absorbed. Maximum observed plasma concentrations are reached within 30 to 120 minutes (median 60 minutes) of oral dosing in the fasted state. When VIAGRA is taken with a high fat meal, the rate of absorption is reduced, with a mean delay in T_{max} of 60 minutes and a mean reduction in C_{max} of 29%. The mean steady state volume of distribution (Vss) for sildenafil is 105 L, indicating distribution into the tissues. Sildenafil and its major circulating N-desmethyl metabolite are both approximately 96% bound to plasma proteins. Protein binding is independent of total drug concentrations.

Based upon measurements of sildenafil in semen of healthy volunteers 90 minutes after dosing, less than 0.001% of the administered dose may appear in the semen of patients.

Metabolism and Excretion: Sildenafil is cleared predominantly by the CYP3A4 (major route) and CYP2C9 (minor route) hepatic microsomal isoenzymes. The major circulating metabolite results from N-desmethylation of sildenafil, and is itself further metabolized. This metabolite has a PDE selectivity profile similar to sildenafil and an *in vitro* potency for PDE5 approximately 50% of the parent drug. Plasma concentrations of this metabolite are approximately 40% of those seen for sildenafil, so that the metabolite accounts for about 20% of sildenafil's pharmacologic effects.

After either oral or intravenous administration, sildenafil is excreted as metabolites predominantly in the feces (approximately 80% of administered oral dose) and to a lesser extent in the urine (approximately 13% of the administered oral dose). Similar values for pharmacokinetic parameters were seen in normal volunteers and in the patient population, using a population pharmacokinetic approach.

Pharmacokinetics in Special Populations

Geriatrics: Healthy elderly volunteers (65 years or over) had a reduced clearance of sildenafil, with free plasma concentrations approximately 40% greater than those seen in healthy younger volunteers (18–45 years).

Renal Insufficiency: In volunteers with mild (CLcr=50-80 mL/min) and moderate (CLcr=30-49 mL/min) renal impairment, the pharmacokinetics of a single oral dose of VIAGRA (50 mg) were not altered. In volunteers with severe (CLcr=<30 mL/min) renal impairment, sildenafil clearance was reduced, resulting in approximately doubling of AUC and C_{max} compared to age-matched volunteers with no renal impairment.

Hepatic Insufficiency: In volunteers with hepatic cirrhosis (Child-Pugh A and B), sildenafil clearance was reduced, resulting in increases in AUC (84%) and C_{max} (47%) compared to age-matched volunteers with no hepatic impairment.

Therefore, age >65, hepatic impairment and severe renal impairment are associated with increased plasma levels of sildenafil. A starting oral dose of 25 mg should be considered in those patients (see **DOSAGE AND ADMINISTRATION**).

Pharmacodynamics

Effects of VIAGRA on Erectile Response: In eight double-blind, placebo-controlled crossover studies of patients with either organic or psychogenic erectile dysfunction, sexual stimulation resulted in improved erections, as assessed by an objective measurement of hardness and duration of erections (RigiScan®), after VIAGRA administration compared with placebo. Most studies assessed the efficacy of VIAGRA approximately 60 minutes post dose. The erectile response, as assessed by RigiScan®, generally increased with increasing sildenafil dose and plasma concentration. The time course of effect was examined in one study, showing an effect for up to 4 hours but the response was diminished compared to 2 hours.

Effects of VIAGRA on Blood Pressure: Single oral doses of sildenafil (100 mg) administered to healthy volunteers produced decreases in supine blood pressure (mean maximum decrease in systolic/diastolic blood pressure of 8.4/5.5 mmHg). The decrease in blood pressure was most notable approximately 1–2 hours after dosing, and was not different than placebo at 8 hours. Similar effects on blood pressure were noted with 25 mg, 50 mg and 100 mg of VIAGRA, therefore the effects are not related to dose or plasma levels within this dosage range. Larger effects were recorded among patients receiving concomitant nitrates (see **CONTRAINDICATIONS**).

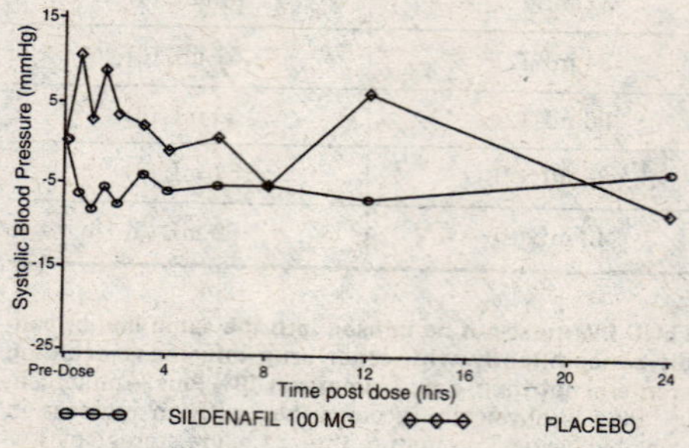

Figure 2: Mean Change from Baseline in Sitting Systolic Blood Pressure, Healthy Volunteers.

Effects of VIAGRA on Cardiac Parameters: Single oral doses of sildenafil up to 100 mg produced no clinically relevant changes in the ECGs of normal male volunteers.

Studies have produced relevant data on the effects of VIAGRA on cardiac output. In one small, open-label, uncontrolled, pilot study, eight patients with stable ischemic heart disease underwent Swan-Ganz catheterization. A total dose of 40 mg sildenafil was administered by four intravenous infusions.

The results from this pilot study are shown in Table 1; the mean resting systolic and diastolic blood pressures decreased by 7% and 10% compared to baseline in these patients. Mean resting values for right atrial pressure, pulmonary artery pressure, pulmonary artery occluded pressure and cardiac output decreased by 28%, 28%, 20% and 7% respectively. Even though this total dosage produced plasma sildenafil concentrations which were approximately 2 to 5 times higher than the mean maximum plasma concentrations following a single oral dose of 100 mg in healthy male volunteers, the hemodynamic response to exercise was preserved in these patients.

[See table 1 below]

In a double-blind study, 144 patients with erectile dysfunction and chronic stable angina limited by exercise, not receiving chronic oral nitrates, were randomized to a single dose of placebo or VIAGRA 100 mg 1 hour prior to exercise testing. The primary endpoint was time to limiting angina in the evaluable cohort. The mean times (adjusted for baseline) to onset of limiting angina were 423.6 and 403.7 seconds for sildenafil (N=70) and placebo, respectively. These results demonstrated that the effect of VIAGRA on the primary endpoint was statistically non-inferior to placebo.

Effects of VIAGRA on Vision: At single oral doses of 100 mg and 200 mg, transient dose-related impairment of color discrimination (blue/green) was detected using the Farnsworth-Munsell 100-hue test, with peak effects near the time of peak plasma levels. This finding is consistent with the inhibition of PDE6, which is involved in phototransduction in the retina. An evaluation of visual function at doses up to twice the maximum recommended dose revealed no effects of VIAGRA on visual acuity, intraocular pressure, or pupillometry.

Clinical Studies

In clinical studies, VIAGRA was assessed for its effect on the ability of men with erectile dysfunction (ED) to engage in sexual activity and in many cases specifically on the ability to achieve and maintain an erection sufficient for satisfactory sexual activity. VIAGRA was evaluated primarily at doses of 25 mg, 50 mg and 100 mg in 21 randomized, double-blind, placebo-controlled trials of up to 6 months in duration, using a variety of study designs (fixed dose, titration, parallel, crossover). VIAGRA was administered to more than 3,000 patients aged 19 to 87 years, with ED of various etiologies (organic, psychogenic, mixed) with a mean duration of 5 years. VIAGRA demonstrated statistically significant improvement compared to placebo in all 21 studies. The studies that established benefit demonstrated improvements in success rates for sexual intercourse compared with placebo.

The effectiveness of VIAGRA was evaluated in most studies using several assessment instruments. The primary measure in the principal studies was a sexual function questionnaire (the International Index of Erectile Function - IIEF) administered during a 4-week treatment-free run-in period, at baseline, at follow-up visits, and at the end of double-blind, placebo-controlled, at-home treatment. Two of the questions from the IIEF served as primary study endpoints; categorical responses were elicited to questions about (1) the ability to achieve erections sufficient for sexual intercourse and (2) the maintenance of erections after penetration. The patient addressed both questions at the final visit for the last 4 weeks of the study. The possible categorical responses to these questions were (0) no attempted intercourse, (1) never or almost never, (2) a few times, (3) sometimes, (4) most times, and (5) almost always or always. Also collected as part of the IIEF was information about other aspects of sexual function, including information on erectile function, orgasm, desire, satisfaction with intercourse, and overall sexual satisfaction. Sexual function data were also recorded by patients in a daily diary. In addition, patients were asked a global efficacy question and an optional partner questionnaire was administered.

The effect on one of the major end points, maintenance of erections after penetration, is shown in Figure 3, for the pooled results of 5 fixed-dose, dose-response studies of greater than one month duration, showing response according to baseline function. Results with all doses have been pooled, but scores showed greater improvement at the 50 and 100 mg doses than at 25 mg. The pattern of responses was similar for the other principal question, the ability to achieve an erection sufficient for intercourse. The titration studies, in which most patients received 100 mg, showed similar results. Figure 3 shows that regardless of the base-

TABLE 1. HEMODYNAMIC DATA IN PATIENTS WITH STABLE ISCHEMIC HEART DISEASE AFTER IV ADMINISTRATION OF 40 MG SILDENAFIL

Means ± SD	At rest				After 4 minutes of exercise			
	n	Baseline (B2)	n	Sildenafil (D1)	n	Baseline	n	Sildenafil
PAOP (mmHg)	8	8.1 ± 5.1	8	6.5 ± 4.3	8	36.0 ± 13.7	8	27.8 ± 15.3
Mean PAP (mmHg)	8	16.7 ± 4	8	12.1 ± 3.9	8	39.4 ± 12.9	8	31.7 ± 13.2
Mean RAP (mmHg)	7	5.7 ± 3.7	8	4.1 ± 3.7	–	–	–	–
Systolic SAP (mmHg)	8	150.4 ± 12.4	8	140.6 ± 16.5	8	199.5 ± 37.4	8	187.8 ± 30.0
Diastolic SAP (mmHg)	8	73.6 ± 7.8	8	65.9 ± 10	8	84.6 ± 9.7	8	79.5 ± 9.4
Cardiac output (L/min)	8	5.6 ± 0.9	8	5.2 ± 1.1	8	11.5 ± 2.4	8	10.2 ± 3.5
Heart rate (bpm)	8	67 ± 11.1	8	66.9 ± 12	8	101.9 ± 11.6	8	99.0 ± 20.4

line levels of function, subsequent function in patients treated with VIAGRA was better than that seen in patients treated with placebo. At the same time, on-treatment function was better in treated patients who were less impaired at baseline.

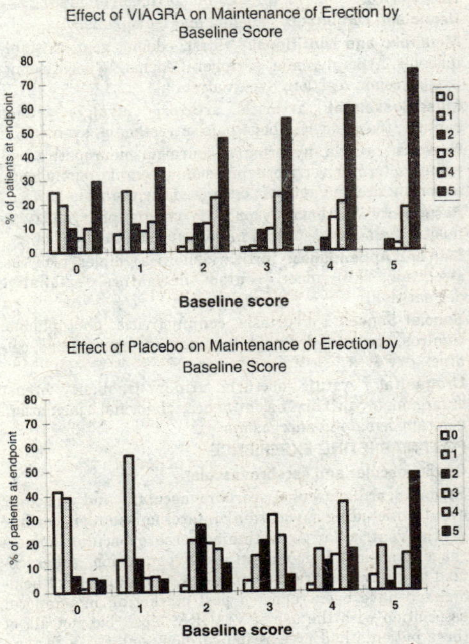

Figure 3. Effect of VIAGRA and Placebo on Maintenance of Erection by Baseline Score.

The frequency of patients reporting improvement of erections in response to a global question in four of the randomized, double-blind, parallel, placebo-controlled fixed dose studies (1797 patients) of 12 to 24 weeks duration is shown in Figure 4. These patients had erectile dysfunction at baseline that was characterized by median categorical scores of 2 (a few times) on principal IIEF questions. Erectile dysfunction was attributed to organic (58%; generally not characterized, but including diabetes and excluding spinal cord injury), psychogenic (17%), or mixed (24%) etiologies. Sixty-three percent, 74%, and 82% of the patients on 25 mg, 50 mg and 100 mg of VIAGRA, respectively, reported an improvement in their erections, compared to 24% on placebo. In the titration studies (n=644) (with most patients eventually receiving 100 mg), results were similar.

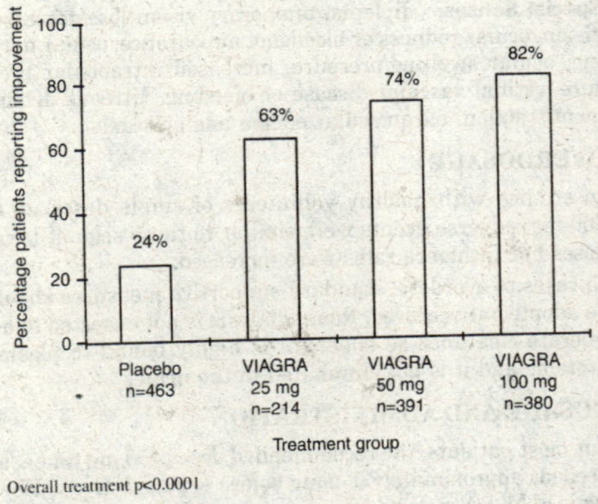

Figure 4. Percentage of Patients Reporting an Improvement in Erections.

The patients in studies had varying degrees of ED. One-third to one-half of the subjects in these studies reported successful intercourse at least once during a 4-week, treatment-free run-in period.

In many of the studies, of both fixed dose and titration designs, daily diaries were kept by patients. In these studies, involving about 1600 patients, analyses of patient diaries showed no effect of VIAGRA on rates of attempted intercourse (about 2 per week), but there was clear treatment-related improvement in sexual function: per patient weekly success rates averaged 1.3 on 50–100 mg of VIAGRA vs 0.4 on placebo; similarly, group mean success rates (total successes divided by total attempts) were about 66% on VIAGRA vs about 20% on placebo.

During 3 to 6 months of double-blind treatment or longer-term (1 year), open-label studies, few patients withdrew from active treatment for any reason, including lack of effectiveness. At the end of the long-term study, 88% of patients reported that VIAGRA improved their erections.

Men with untreated ED had relatively low baseline scores for all aspects of sexual function measured (again using a 5-point scale) in the IIEF. VIAGRA improved these aspects of sexual function: frequency, firmness and maintenance of erections; frequency of orgasm; frequency and level of desire; frequency, satisfaction and enjoyment of intercourse; and overall relationship satisfaction.

One randomized, double-blind, flexible-dose, placebo-controlled study included only patients with erectile dysfunction attributed to complications of diabetes mellitus (n=268). As in the other titration studies, patients were started on 50 mg and allowed to adjust the dose up to 100 mg or down to 25 mg of VIAGRA; all patients, however, were receiving 50 mg or 100 mg at the end of the study. There were highly statistically significant improvements on the two principal IIEF questions (frequency of successful penetration during sexual activity and maintenance of erections after penetration) on VIAGRA compared to placebo. On a global improvement question, 57% of VIAGRA patients reported improved erections versus 10% on placebo. Diary data indicated that on VIAGRA, 48% of intercourse attempts were successful versus 12% on placebo.

One randomized, double-blind, placebo-controlled, crossover, flexible-dose (up to 100 mg) study of patients with erectile dysfunction resulting from spinal cord injury (n=178) was conducted. The changes from baseline in scoring on the two end point questions (frequency of successful penetration during sexual activity and maintenance of erections after penetration) were highly statistically significantly in favor of VIAGRA. On a global improvement question, 83% of patients reported improved erections on VIAGRA versus 12% on placebo. Diary data indicated that on VIAGRA, 59% of attempts at sexual intercourse were successful compared to 13% on placebo.

Across all trials, VIAGRA improved the erections of 43% of radical prostatectomy patients compared to 15% on placebo.

Subgroup analyses of responses to a global improvement question in patients with psychogenic etiology in two fixed-dose studies (total n=179) and two titration studies (total n=149) showed 84% of VIAGRA patients reported improvement in erections compared with 26% of placebo. The changes from baseline in scoring on the two end point questions (frequency of successful penetration during sexual activity and maintenance of erections after penetration) were highly statistically significantly in favor of VIAGRA. Diary data in two of the studies (n=178) showed rates of successful intercourse per attempt of 70% for VIAGRA and 29% for placebo.

A review of population subgroups demonstrated efficacy regardless of baseline severity, etiology, race and age. VIAGRA was effective in a broad range of ED patients, including those with a history of coronary artery disease, hypertension, other cardiac disease, peripheral vascular disease, diabetes mellitus, depression, coronary artery bypass graft (CABG), radical prostatectomy, transurethral resection of the prostate (TURP) and spinal cord injury, and in patients taking antidepressants/antipsychotics and antihypertensives/diuretics.

Analysis of the safety database showed no apparent difference in the side effect profile in patients taking VIAGRA with and without antihypertensive medication. This analysis was performed retrospectively, and was not powered to detect any pre-specified difference in adverse reactions.

INDICATION AND USAGE

VIAGRA is indicated for the treatment of erectile dysfunction.

CONTRAINDICATIONS

Consistent with its known effects on the nitric oxide/cGMP pathway (see **CLINICAL PHARMACOLOGY**), VIAGRA was shown to potentiate the hypotensive effects of nitrates, and its administration to patients who are using organic nitrates, either regularly and/or intermittently, in any form is therefore contraindicated.

After patients have taken VIAGRA, it is unknown when nitrates, if necessary, can be safely administered. Based on the pharmacokinetic profile of a single 100 mg oral dose given to healthy normal volunteers, the plasma levels of sildenafil at 24 hours post dose are approximately 2 ng/mL (compared to peak plasma levels of approximately 440 ng/mL) (see **CLINICAL PHARMACOLOGY: Pharmacokinetics and Metabolism**). In the following patients: age >65, hepatic impairment (e.g., cirrhosis), severe renal impairment (e.g., creatinine clearance <30 mL/min), and concomitant use of potent cytochrome P450 3A4 inhibitors (erythromycin), plasma levels of sildenafil at 24 hours post dose have been found to be 3 to 8 times higher than those seen in healthy volunteers. Although plasma levels of sildenafil at 24 hours post dose are much lower than at peak concentration, it is unknown whether nitrates can be safely coadministered at this time point.

VIAGRA is contraindicated in patients with a known hypersensitivity to any component of the tablet.

WARNINGS

There is a potential for cardiac risk of sexual activity in patients with preexisting cardiovascular disease. Therefore, treatments for erectile dysfunction, including VIAGRA, should not be generally used in men for whom sexual activity is inadvisable because of their underlying cardiovascular status.

VIAGRA has systemic vasodilatory properties that resulted in transient decreases in supine blood pressure in healthy volunteers (mean maximum decrease of 8.4/5.5 mmHg), (see **CLINICAL PHARMACOLOGY: Pharmacodynamics**). While this normally would be expected to be of little consequence in most patients, prior to prescribing VIAGRA, physicians should carefully consider whether their patients with underlying cardiovascular disease could be affected adversely by such vasodilatory effects, especially in combination with sexual activity.

Patients with the following underlying conditions can be particularly sensitive to the actions of vasodilators including VIAGRA – those with left ventricular outflow obstruction (e.g. aortic stenosis, idiopathic hypertrophic subaortic stenosis) and those with severely impaired autonomic control of blood pressure.

There is no controlled clinical data on the safety or efficacy of VIAGRA in the following groups; if prescribed, this should be done with caution.

- Patients who have suffered a myocardial infarction, stroke, or life-threatening arrhythmia within the last 6 months;
- Patients with resting hypotension (BP <90/50) or hypertension (BP >170/110);
- Patients with cardiac failure or coronary artery disease causing unstable angina;
- Patients with retinitis pigmentosa (a minority of these patients have genetic disorders of retinal phosphodiesterases).

Prolonged erection greater than 4 hours and priapism (painful erections greater than 6 hours in duration) have been reported infrequently since market approval of VIAGRA. In the event of an erection that persists longer than 4 hours, the patient should seek immediate medical assistance. If priapism is not treated immediately, penile tissue damage and permanent loss of potency could result.

The concomitant administration of the protease inhibitor ritonavir substantially increases serum concentrations of sildenafil (**11-fold increase in AUC**). If VIAGRA is prescribed to patients taking ritonavir, caution should be used. Data from subjects exposed to high systemic levels of sildenafil are limited. Visual disturbances occurred more commonly at higher levels of sildenafil exposure. Decreased blood pressure, syncope, and prolonged erection were reported in some healthy volunteers exposed to high doses of sildenafil (200–800 mg). To decrease the chance of adverse events in patients taking ritonavir, a decrease in sildenafil dosage is recommended (see **Drug Interactions, ADVERSE REACTIONS** and **DOSAGE AND ADMINISTRATION**).

PRECAUTIONS

General

The evaluation of erectile dysfunction should include a determination of potential underlying causes and the identification of appropriate treatment following a complete medical assessment.

Before prescribing VIAGRA, it is important to note the following:

Patients on multiple antihypertensive medications were included in the pivotal clinical trials for VIAGRA. In a separate drug interaction study, when amlodipine, 5 mg or 10 mg, and VIAGRA, 100 mg were orally administered concomitantly to hypertensive patients mean additional blood pressure reduction of 8 mmHg systolic and 7 mmHg diastolic were noted (see **Drug Interactions**).

When the alpha blocker doxazosin (4 mg) and VIAGRA (25 mg) were administered simultaneously to patients with benign prostatic hyperplasia (BPH), mean additional reductions of supine blood pressure of 7 mmHg systolic and 7 mmHg diastolic were observed. When higher doses of VIAGRA and doxazosin (4 mg) were administered simultaneously, there were infrequent reports of patients who experienced symptomatic postural hypotension within 1 to 4 hours of dosing. Simultaneous administration of VIAGRA to patients taking alpha-blocker therapy may lead to symptomatic hypotension in some patients. Therefore, VIAGRA doses above 25 mg should not be taken within 4 hours of taking an alpha-blocker.

The safety of VIAGRA is unknown in patients with bleeding disorders and patients with active peptic ulceration.

VIAGRA should be used with caution in patients with anatomical deformation of the penis (such as angulation, cavernosal fibrosis or Peyronie's disease), or in patients who have conditions which may predispose them to priapism (such as sickle cell anemia, multiple myeloma, or leukemia).

The safety and efficacy of combinations of VIAGRA with other treatments for erectile dysfunction have not been studied. Therefore, the use of such combinations is not recommended.

In humans, VIAGRA has no effect on bleeding time when taken alone or with aspirin. *In vitro* studies with human platelets indicate that sildenafil potentiates the antiaggregatory effect of sodium nitroprusside (a nitric oxide donor). The combination of heparin and VIAGRA had an additive effect on bleeding time in the anesthetized rabbit, but this interaction has not been studied in humans.

Information for Patients

Physicians should discuss with patients the contraindication of VIAGRA with regular and/or intermittent use of organic nitrates.

Physicians should discuss with patients the potential cardiac risk of sexual activity in patients with preexisting cardiovascular risk factors. Patients who experience symptoms (e.g., angina pectoris, dizziness, nausea) upon initiation of sexual activity should be advised to refrain from further activity and should discuss the episode with their physician.

Physicians should warn patients that prolonged erections greater than 4 hours and priapism (painful erections greater than 6 hours in duration) have been reported infrequently since market approval of VIAGRA. In the event of an erection that persists longer than 4 hours, the patient

Continued on next page

Viagra—Cont.

should seek immediate medical assistance. If priapism is not treated immediately, penile tissue damage and permanent loss of potency may result.

Physicians should advise patients that simultaneous administration of VIAGRA doses above 25 mg and an alpha-blocker may lead to symptomatic hypotension in some patients. Therefore, VIAGRA doses above 25 mg should not be taken within four hours of taking an alpha-blocker.

The use of VIAGRA offers no protection against sexually transmitted diseases. Counseling of patients about the protective measures necessary to guard against sexually transmitted diseases, including the Human Immunodeficiency Virus (HIV), may be considered.

Drug Interactions

Effects of Other Drugs on VIAGRA

***In vitro* studies:** Sildenafil metabolism is principally mediated by the cytochrome P450 (CYP) isoforms 3A4 (major route) and 2C9 (minor route). Therefore, inhibitors of these isoenzymes may reduce sildenafil clearance.

***In vivo* studies:** Cimetidine (800 mg), a nonspecific CYP inhibitor, caused a 56% increase in plasma sildenafil concentrations when coadministered with VIAGRA (50 mg) to healthy volunteers.

When a single 100 mg dose of VIAGRA was administered with erythromycin, a specific CYP3A4 inhibitor, at steady state (500 mg bid for 5 days), there was a 182% increase in sildenafil systemic exposure (AUC). In addition, in a study performed in healthy male volunteers, coadministration of the HIV protease inhibitor saquinavir, also a CYP3A4 inhibitor, at steady state (1200 mg tid) with VIAGRA (100 mg single dose) resulted in a 140% increase in sildenafil C_{max} and a 210% increase in sildenafil AUC. VIAGRA had no effect on saquinavir pharmacokinetics. Stronger CYP3A4 inhibitors such as ketoconazole or itraconazole would be expected to have still greater effects, and population data from patients in clinical trials did indicate a reduction in sildenafil clearance when it was coadministered with CYP3A4 inhibitors (such as ketoconazole, erythromycin, or cimetidine) (see **DOSAGE AND ADMINISTRATION**).

In another study in healthy male volunteers, coadministration with the HIV protease inhibitor ritonavir, which is a highly potent P450 inhibitor, at steady state (500 mg bid) with VIAGRA (100 mg single dose) resulted in a 300% (4-fold) increase in sildenafil C_{max} and a 1000% (11-fold) increase in sildenafil plasma AUC. At 24 hours the plasma levels of sildenafil were still approximately 200 ng/mL, compared to approximately 5 ng/mL when sildenafil was dosed alone. This is consistent with ritonavir's marked effects on a broad range of P450 substrates. VIAGRA had no effect on ritonavir pharmacokinetics (see **DOSAGE AND ADMINISTRATION**).

Although the interaction between other protease inhibitors and sildenafil has not been studied, their concomitant use is expected to increase sildenafil levels.

It can be expected that concomitant administration of CYP3A4 inducers, such as rifampin, will decrease plasma levels of sildenafil.

Single doses of antacid (magnesium hydroxide/aluminum hydroxide) did not affect the bioavailability of VIAGRA.

Pharmacokinetic data from patients in clinical trials showed no effect on sildenafil pharmacokinetics of CYP2C9 inhibitors (such as tolbutamide, warfarin), CYP2D6 inhibitors (such as selective serotonin reuptake inhibitors, tricyclic antidepressants), thiazide and related diuretics, ACE inhibitors, and calcium channel blockers. The AUC of the active metabolite, N-desmethyl sildenafil, was increased 62% by loop and potassium-sparing diuretics and 102% by nonspecific beta-blockers. These effects on the metabolite are not expected to be of clinical consequence.

Effects of VIAGRA on Other Drugs

***In vitro* studies:** Sildenafil is a weak inhibitor of the cytochrome P450 isoforms 1A2, 2C9, 2C19, 2D6, 2E1 and 3A4 (IC50 >150 µM). Given sildenafil peak plasma concentrations of approximately 1 µM after recommended doses, it is unlikely that VIAGRA will alter the clearance of substrates of these isoenzymes.

***In vivo* studies:** When VIAGRA 100 mg oral was coadministered with amlodipine, 5 mg or 10 mg oral, to hypertensive patients, the mean additional reduction on supine blood pressure was 8 mmHg systolic and 7 mmHg diastolic.

No significant interactions were shown with tolbutamide (250 mg) or warfarin (40 mg), both of which are metabolized by CYP2C9.

VIAGRA (50 mg) did not potentiate the increase in bleeding time caused by aspirin (150 mg).

VIAGRA (50 mg) did not potentiate the hypotensive effect of alcohol in healthy volunteers with mean maximum blood alcohol levels of 0.08%.

In a study of healthy male volunteers, sildenafil (100 mg) did not affect the steady state pharmacokinetics of the HIV protease inhibitors, saquinavir and ritonavir, both of which are CYP3A4 substrates.

Carcinogenesis, Mutagenesis, Impairment of Fertility

Sildenafil was not carcinogenic when administered to rats for 24 months at a dose resulting in total systemic drug exposure (AUCs) for unbound sildenafil and its major metabolite of 29- and 42-times, for male and female rats, respectively, the exposures observed in human males given the Maximum Recommended Human Dose (MRHD) of 100 mg. Sildenafil was not carcinogenic when administered to mice for 18–21 months at dosages up to the Maximum Tolerated Dose (MTD) of 10 mg/kg/day, approximately 0.6 times the MRHD on a mg/m² basis.

Sildenafil was negative in *in vitro* bacterial and Chinese hamster ovary cell assays to detect mutagenicity, and *in vitro* human lymphocytes and *in vivo* mouse micronucleus assays to detect clastogenicity.

There was no impairment of fertility in rats given sildenafil up to 60 mg/kg/day for 36 days to females and 102 days to males, a dose producing an AUC value of more than 25 times the human male AUC.

There was no effect on sperm motility or morphology after single 100 mg oral doses of VIAGRA in healthy volunteers.

Pregnancy, Nursing Mothers and Pediatric Use

VIAGRA is not indicated for use in newborns, children, or women.

Pregnancy Category B. No evidence of teratogenicity, embryotoxicity or fetotoxicity was observed in rats and rabbits which received up to 200 mg/kg/day during organogenesis. These doses represent, respectively, about 20 and 40 times the MRHD on a mg/m² basis in a 50 kg subject. In the rat pre- and postnatal development study, the no observed adverse effect dose was 30 mg/kg/day given for 36 days. In the nonpregnant rat the AUC at this dose was about 20 times human AUC. There are no adequate and well-controlled studies of sildenafil in pregnant women.

Geriatric Use: Healthy elderly volunteers (65 years or over) had a reduced clearance of sildenafil (see **CLINICAL PHARMACOLOGY: Pharmacokinetics in Special Populations**). Since higher plasma levels may increase both the efficacy and incidence of adverse events, a starting dose of 25 mg should be considered (see **DOSAGE AND ADMINISTRATION**).

ADVERSE REACTIONS

PRE-MARKETING EXPERIENCE:

VIAGRA was administered to over 3700 patients (aged 19–87 years) during clinical trials worldwide. Over 550 patients were treated for longer than one year.

In placebo-controlled clinical studies, the discontinuation rate due to adverse events for VIAGRA (2.5%) was not significantly different from placebo (2.3%). The adverse events were generally transient and mild to moderate in nature.

In trials of all designs, adverse events reported by patients receiving VIAGRA were generally similar. In fixed-dose studies, the incidence of some adverse events increased with dose. The nature of the adverse events in flexible-dose studies, which more closely reflect the recommended dosage regimen, was similar to that for fixed-dose studies.

When VIAGRA was taken as recommended (on an as-needed basis) in flexible-dose, placebo-controlled clinical trials, the following adverse events were reported:

TABLE 2. ADVERSE EVENTS REPORTED BY ≥2% OF PATIENTS TREATED WITH VIAGRA AND MORE FREQUENT ON DRUG THAN PLACEBO IN PRN FLEXIBLE-DOSE PHASE II/III STUDIES

Adverse Event	Percentage of Patients Reporting Event	
	VIAGRA N=734	PLACEBO N=725
Headache	16%	4%
Flushing	10%	1%
Dyspepsia	7%	2%
Nasal Congestion	4%	2%
Urinary Tract Infection	3%	2%
Abnormal Vision†	3%	0%
Diarrhea	3%	1%
Dizziness	2%	1%
Rash	2%	1%

† Abnormal Vision: Mild and transient, predominantly color tinge to vision, but also increased sensitivity to light or blurred vision. In these studies, only one patient discontinued due to abnormal vision.

Other adverse reactions occurred at a rate of >2%, but equally common on placebo: respiratory tract infection, back pain, flu syndrome, and arthralgia.

In fixed-dose studies, dyspepsia (17%) and abnormal vision (11%) were more common at 100 mg than at lower doses. At doses above the recommended dose range, adverse events were similar to those detailed above but generally were reported more frequently.

The following events occurred in <2% of patients in controlled clinical trials; a causal relationship to VIAGRA is uncertain. Reported events include those with a plausible relation to drug use; omitted are minor events and reports too imprecise to be meaningful:

Body as a whole: face edema, photosensitivity reaction, shock, asthenia, pain, chills, accidental fall, abdominal pain, allergic reaction, chest pain, accidental injury.

Cardiovascular: angina pectoris, AV block, migraine, syncope, tachycardia, palpitation, hypotension, postural hypotension, myocardial ischemia, cerebral thrombosis, cardiac arrest, heart failure, abnormal electrocardiogram, cardiomyopathy.

Digestive: vomiting, glossitis, colitis, dysphagia, gastritis, gastroenteritis, esophagitis, stomatitis, dry mouth, liver function tests abnormal, rectal hemorrhage, gingivitis.

Hemic and Lymphatic: anemia and leukopenia.

Metabolic and Nutritional: thirst, edema, gout, unstable diabetes, hyperglycemia, peripheral edema, hyperuricemia, hypoglycemic reaction, hypernatremia.

Musculoskeletal: arthritis, arthrosis, myalgia, tendon rupture, tenosynovitis, bone pain, myasthenia, synovitis.

Nervous: ataxia, hypertonia, neuralgia, neuropathy, paresthesia, tremor, vertigo, depression, insomnia, somnolence, abnormal dreams, reflexes decreased, hypesthesia.

Respiratory: asthma, dyspnea, laryngitis, pharyngitis, sinusitis, bronchitis, sputum increased, cough increased.

Skin and Appendages: urticaria, herpes simplex, pruritus, sweating, skin ulcer, contact dermatitis, exfoliative dermatitis.

Special Senses: mydriasis, conjunctivitis, photophobia, tinnitus, eye pain, deafness, ear pain, eye hemorrhage, cataract, dry eyes.

Urogenital: cystitis, nocturia, urinary frequency, breast enlargement, urinary incontinence, abnormal ejaculation, genital edema and anorgasmia.

POST-MARKETING EXPERIENCE:

Cardiovascular and cerebrovascular

Serious cardiovascular, cerebrovascular, and vascular events, including myocardial infarction, sudden cardiac death, ventricular arrhythmia, cerebrovascular hemorrhage, transient ischemic attack, hypertension, subarachnoid and intracerebral hemorrhages, and pulmonary hemorrhage have been reported post-marketing in temporal association with the use of VIAGRA. Most, but not all, of these patients had preexisting cardiovascular risk factors. Many of these events were reported to occur during or shortly after sexual activity, and a few were reported to occur shortly after the use of VIAGRA without sexual activity. Others were reported to have occurred hours to days after the use of VIAGRA and sexual activity. It is not possible to determine whether these events are related directly to VIAGRA, to sexual activity, to the patient's underlying cardiovascular disease, to a combination of these factors, or to other factors (see **WARNINGS** for further important cardiovascular information).

Other events

Other events reported post-marketing to have been observed in temporal association with VIAGRA and not listed in the pre-marketing adverse reactions section above include:

Nervous: seizure and anxiety.

Urogenital: prolonged erection, priapism (see **WARNINGS**) and hematuria.

Special Senses: diplopia, temporary vision loss/decreased vision, ocular redness or bloodshot appearance, ocular burning, ocular swelling/pressure, increased intraocular pressure, retinal vascular disease or bleeding, vitreous detachment/traction, paramacular edema and epistaxis.

OVERDOSAGE

In studies with healthy volunteers of single doses up to 800 mg, adverse events were similar to those seen at lower doses but incidence rates were increased.

In cases of overdose, standard supportive measures should be adopted as required. Renal dialysis is not expected to accelerate clearance as sildenafil is highly bound to plasma proteins and it is not eliminated in the urine.

DOSAGE AND ADMINISTRATION

For most patients, the recommended dose is 50 mg taken, as needed, approximately 1 hour before sexual activity. However, VIAGRA may be taken anywhere from 4 hours to 0.5 hour before sexual activity. Based on effectiveness and toleration, the dose may be increased to a maximum recommended dose of 100 mg or decreased to 25 mg. The maximum recommended dosing frequency is once per day.

The following factors are associated with increased plasma levels of sildenafil: age >65 (40% increase in AUC), hepatic impairment (e.g., cirrhosis, 80%), severe renal impairment (creatinine clearance <30 mL/min, 100%), and concomitant use of potent cytochrome P450 3A4 inhibitors [ketoconazole, itraconazole, erythromycin (182%), saquinavir (210%)]. Since higher plasma levels may increase both the efficacy and incidence of adverse events, a starting dose of 25 mg should be considered in these patients.

Ritonavir greatly increased the systemic level of sildenafil in a study of healthy, non-HIV infected volunteers (11-fold increase in AUC, see **Drug Interactions**.) Based on these pharmacokinetic data, it is recommended not to exceed a maximum single dose of 25 mg of VIAGRA in a 48 hour period.

	25 mg	50 mg	100 mg
Obverse	VGR25	VGR50	VGR100
Reverse	PFIZER	PFIZER	PFIZER
Bottle of 30	NDC-0069-4200-30	NDC-0069-4210-30	NDC-0069-4220-30
Bottle of 100	N/A	NDC-0069-4210-66	NDC-0069-4220-66

VIAGRA was shown to potentiate the hypotensive effects of nitrates and its administration in patients who use nitric oxide donors or nitrates in any form is therefore contraindicated.
Simultaneous administration of VIAGRA doses above 25 mg and an alpha-blocker may lead to symptomatic hypotension in some patients. Doses of 50 mg or 100 mg of VIAGRA should not be taken within 4 hours of alpha-blocker administration. A 25 mg dose of VIAGRA may be taken at any time.

HOW SUPPLIED

VIAGRA® (sildenafil citrate) is supplied as blue, film-coated, rounded-diamond-shaped tablets containing sildenafil citrate equivalent to the nominally indicated amount of sildenafil as follows:
[See table at bottom of previous page]
Recommended Storage: Store at 25°C (77°F); excursions permitted to 15-30°C (59-86°F) [see USP Controlled Room Temperature].
Rx only

Distributed by
Pfizer Labs
Division of Pfizer Inc, NY, NY 10017
69-5485-00-9 Revised August 2003

VIBRAMYCIN® ℞

[*vī-bra-mī-sĭn*]
Hyclate
(doxycycline hyclate)
CAPSULES
Monohydrate
(doxycycline monohydrate)
for ORAL SUSPENSION
Calcium
(doxycycline calcium)
oral suspension
SYRUP
VIBRA-TABS®
(doxycycline hyclate)
FILM COATED TABLETS

Prescribing information for this product, which appears on pages 2665–2668 of the 2004 PDR, has been completely revised as follows. Please write "See Supplement A" next to the product heading.
To reduce the development of drug-resistant bacteria and maintain the effectiveness of Vibramycin® and other antibacterial drugs, Vibramycin should be used only to treat or prevent infections that are proven or strongly suspected to be caused by bacteria.

DESCRIPTION

Vibramycin® is a broad-spectrum antibiotic synthetically derived from oxytetracycline, and is available as Vibramycin Monohydrate (doxycycline monohydrate); Vibramycin Hyclate and Vibra-Tabs (doxycycline hydrochloride hemiethanolate hemihydrate); and Vibramycin Calcium (doxycycline calcium) for oral administration.
The structural formula of doxycycline monohydrate is

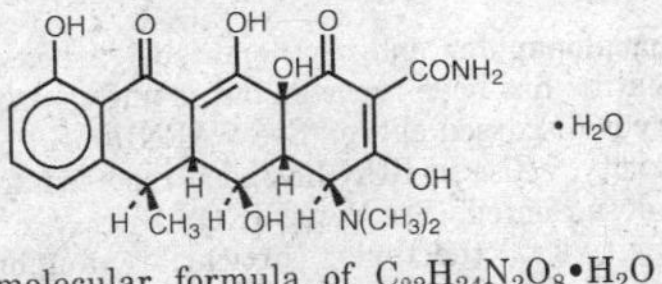

with a molecular formula of $C_{22}H_{24}N_2O_8 \bullet H_2O$ and a molecular weight of 462.46. The chemical designation for doxycycline is 4-(Dimethylamino)-1, 4, 4a, 5, 5a, 6, 11, 12a-octahydro-3, 5, 10, 12, 12a-pentahydroxy-6-methyl-1, 11-dioxo-2-naphthacenecarboxamide monohydrate. The molecular formula for doxycycline hydrochloride hemiethanolate hemihydrate is $(C_{22}H_{24}N_2O_8 \bullet HCl)_2 \bullet C_2H_6O \bullet H_2O$ and the molecular weight is 1025.89. Doxycycline is a light-yellow crystalline powder. Doxycycline hyclate is soluble in water, while doxycycline monohydrate is very slightly soluble in water.
Doxycycline has a high degree of lipoid solubility and a low affinity for calcium binding. It is highly stable in normal human serum. Doxycycline will not degrade into an epianhydro form.
Inert ingredients in the syrup formulation are: apple flavor; butylparaben; calcium chloride; carmine; glycerin; hydrochloric acid; magnesium aluminum silicate; povidone; propylene glycol; propylparaben; raspberry flavor; simethicone emulsion; sodium hydroxide; sodium metabisulfite; sorbitol solution; water.
Inert ingredients in the capsule formulations are: hard gelatin capsules (which may contain Blue 1 and other inert ingredients); magnesium stearate; microcrystalline cellulose; sodium lauryl sulfate.
Inert ingredients for the oral suspension formulation are: carboxymethylcellulose sodium; Blue 1; methylparaben; microcrystalline cellulose; propylparaben; raspberry flavor; Red 28; simethicone emulsion; sucrose.
Inert ingredients for the tablet formulation are: ethylcellulose; hypromellose; magnesium stearate; microcrystalline cellulose; propylene glycol; sodium lauryl sulfate; talc; titanium dioxide; Yellow 6 Lake.

CLINICAL PHARMACOLOGY

Tetracyclines are readily absorbed and are bound to plasma proteins in varying degree. They are concentrated by the liver in the bile, and excreted in the urine and feces at high concentrations and in a biologically active form. Doxycycline is virtually completely absorbed after oral administration. Following a 200 mg dose, normal adult volunteers averaged peak serum levels of 2.6 mcg/mL of doxycycline at 2 hours decreasing to 1.45 mcg/mL at 24 hours. Excretion of doxycycline by the kidney is about 40%/72 hours in individuals with normal function (creatinine clearance about 75 mL/min.). This percentage excretion may fall as low as 1-5%/72 hours in individuals with severe renal insufficiency (creatinine clearance below 10 mL/min.). Studies have shown no significant difference in serum half-life of doxycycline (range 18-22 hours) in individuals with normal and severely impaired renal function.
Hemodialysis does not alter serum half-life.
Results of animal studies indicate that tetracyclines cross the placenta and are found in fetal tissues.

Microbiology
The tetracyclines are primarily bacteriostatic and are thought to exert their antimicrobial effect by the inhibition of protein synthesis. The tetracyclines, including doxycycline, have a similar antimicrobial spectrum of activity against a wide range of gram-positive and gram-negative organisms. Cross-resistance of these organisms to tetracyclines is common.

Gram-Negative Bacteria
Neisseria gonorrhoeae
Calymmatobacterium granulomatis
Haemophilus ducreyi
Haemophilus influenzae
Yersinia pestis (formerly *Pasteurella pestis*)
Francisella tularensis (formerly *Pasteurella tularensis*)
Vibrio cholerae (formerly *Vibrio comma*)
Bartonella bacilliformis
Brucella species
Because many strains of the following groups of gram-negative microorganisms have been shown to be resistant to tetracyclines, culture and susceptibility testing are recommended:
Escherichia coli
Klebsiella species
Enterobacter aerogenes
Shigella species
Acinetobacter species (formerly *Mima* species and *Herellea* species)
Bacteroides species

Gram-Positive Bacteria
Because many strains of the following groups of gram-positive microorganisms have been shown to be resistant to tetracycline, culture and susceptibility testing are recommended. Up to 44 percent of strains of *Streptococcus pyogenes* and 74 percent of *Streptococcus faecalis* have been found to be resistant to tetracycline drugs. Therefore, tetracycline should not be used for streptococcal disease unless the organism has been demonstrated to be susceptible.
Streptococcus pyogenes
Streptococcus pneumoniae
Enterococcus group (*Streptococcus faecalis* and *Streptococcus faecium*)
Alpha-hemolytic streptococci (viridans group)

Other Microorganisms
Rickettsiae
Chlamydia psittaci
Chlamydia trachomatis
Mycoplasma pneumoniae
Ureaplasma urealyticum
Borrelia recurrentis
Treponema pallidum
Treponema pertenue
Clostridium species
Fusobacterium fusiforme
Actinomyces species
Bacillus anthracis
Propionibacterium acnes
Entamoeba species
Balantidium coli
Plasmodium falciparum
Doxycycline has been found to be active against the asexual erythrocytic forms of *Plasmodium falciparum* but not against the gametocytes of *P. falciparum*. The precise mechanism of action of the drug is not known.

Susceptibility tests: Diffusion techniques: Quantitative methods that require measurement of zone diameters give the most precise estimate of the susceptibility of bacteria to antimicrobial agents. One such standard procedure[1] which has been recommended for use with disks to test susceptibility of organisms to doxycycline uses the 30-mcg tetracycline-class disk or the 30-mcg doxycycline disk. Interpretation involves the correlation of the diameter obtained in the disk test with the minimum inhibitory concentration (MIC) for tetracycline or doxycycline, respectively.
Reports from the laboratory giving results of the standard single-disk susceptibility test with a 30-mcg tetracycline-class disk or the 30-mcg doxycycline disk should be interpreted according to the following criteria:

Zone Diameter (mm)		Interpretation
tetracycline	doxycycline	
≥19	≥16	Susceptible
15-18	13-15	Intermediate
≤14	≤12	Resistant

A report of "Susceptible" indicates that the pathogen is likely to be inhibited by generally achievable blood levels. A report of "Intermediate" suggests that the organism would be susceptible if a high dosage is used or if the infection is confined to tissues and fluids in which high antimicrobial levels are attained. A report of "Resistant" indicates that achievable concentrations are unlikely to be inhibitory, and other therapy should be selected.
Standardized procedures require the use of laboratory control organisms. The 30-mcg tetracycline-class disk or the 30-mcg doxycycline disk should give the following zone diameters:

Organism	Zone Diameter (mm)	
	tetracycline	doxycycline
E. coli ATCC 25922	18-25	18-24
S. aureus ATCC 25923	19-28	23-29

Dilution techniques: Use a standardized dilution method[2] (broth, agar, microdilution) or equivalent with tetracycline powder. The MIC values obtained should be interpreted according to the following criteria:

MIC (mcg/mL)	Interpretation
≤4	Susceptible
8	Intermediate
≥16	Resistant

As with standard diffusion techniques, dilution methods require the use of laboratory control organisms. Standard tetracycline powder should provide the following MIC values:

Organism	MIC (mcg/mL)
E. coli ATCC 25922	1.0-4.0
S. aureus ATCC 29213	0.25-1.0
E. faecalis ATCC 29212	8-32
P. aeruginosa ATCC 27853	8-32

INDICATIONS AND USAGE

To reduce the development of drug-resistant bacteria and maintain effectiveness of Vibramycin and other antibacterial drugs, Vibramycin should be used only to treat or prevent infections that are proven or strongly suspected to be caused by susceptible bacteria. When culture and susceptibility information are available, they should be considered in selecting or modifying antibacterial therapy. In the absence of such data, local epidemiology and susceptibility patterns may contribute to the empiric selection of therapy.

Treatment:
Doxycycline is indicated for the treatment of the following infections:
Rocky Mountain spotted fever, typhus fever and the typhus group, Q fever, rickettsialpox, and tick fevers caused by Rickettsiae.
Respiratory tract infections caused by *Mycoplasma pneumoniae*.
Lymphogranuloma venereum caused by *Chlamydia trachomatis*.
Psittacosis (ornithosis) caused by *Chlamydia psittaci*.
Trachoma caused by *Chlamydia trachomatis*, although the infectious agent is not always eliminated as judged by immunofluorescence.
Inclusion conjunctivitis caused by *Chlamydia trachomatis*.
Uncomplicated urethral, endocervical or rectal infections in adults caused by *Chlamydia trachomatis*.
Nongonococcal urethritis caused by *Ureaplasma urealyticum*.
Relapsing fever due to *Borrelia recurrentis*.
Doxycycline is also indicated for the treatment of infections caused by the following gram-negative microorganisms:
Chancroid caused by *Haemophilus ducreyi*.
Plague due to *Yersinia pestis* (formerly *Pasteurella pestis*).
Tularemia due to *Francisella tularensis* (formerly *Pasteurella tularensis*).
Cholera caused by *Vibrio cholerae* (formerly *Vibrio comma*).
Campylobacter fetus infections caused by *Campylobacter fetus* (formerly *Vibrio fetus*).
Brucellosis due to *Brucella* species (in conjunction with streptomycin).
Bartonellosis due to *Bartonella bacilliformis*.
Granuloma inguinale caused by *Calymmatobacterium granulomatis*.
Because many strains of the following groups of microorganisms have been shown to be resistant to doxycycline, culture and susceptibility testing are recommended.
Doxycycline is indicated for treatment of infections caused by the following gram-negative microorganisms, when bacteriologic testing indicates appropriate susceptibility to the drug:
Escherichia coli.
Enterobacter aerogenes (formerly *Aerobacter aerogenes*).
Shigella species.
Acinetobacter species (formerly *Mima* species and *Herellea* species).
Respiratory tract infections caused by *Haemophilus influenzae*.
Respiratory tract and urinary tract infections caused by *Klebsiella* species.
Doxycycline is indicated for treatment of infections caused by the following gram-positive microorganisms when bacteriologic testing indicates appropriate susceptibility to the drug:
Upper respiratory infections caused by *Streptococcus pneumoniae* (formerly *Diplococcus pneumoniae*).

Continued on next page

Vibramycin—Cont.

Anthrax due to *Bacillus anthracis*, including inhalational anthrax (post-exposure): to reduce the incidence or progression of disease following exposure to aerosolized *Bacillus anthracis*.

When penicillin is contraindicated, doxycycline is an alternative drug in the treatment of the following infections:

Uncomplicated gonorrhea caused by *Neisseria gonorrhoeae*.
Syphilis caused by *Treponema pallidum*.
Yaws caused by *Treponema pertenue*.
Listeriosis due to *Listeria monocytogenes*.
Vincent's infection caused by *Fusobacterium fusiforme*.
Actinomycosis caused by *Actinomyces israelii*.
Infections caused by *Clostridium* species.

In acute intestinal amebiasis, doxycycline may be a useful adjunct to amebicides.

In severe acne, doxycycline may be useful adjunctive therapy.

Prophylaxis:

Doxycycline is indicated for the prophylaxis of malaria due to *Plasmodium falciparum* in short-term travelers (<4 months) to areas with chloroquine and/or pyrimethamine-sulfadoxine resistant strains. See DOSAGE AND ADMINISTRATION section and Information for Patients subsection of the PRECAUTIONS section.

CONTRAINDICATIONS

This drug is contraindicated in persons who have shown hypersensitivity to any of the tetracyclines.

WARNINGS

THE USE OF DRUGS OF THE TETRACYCLINE CLASS DURING TOOTH DEVELOPMENT (LAST HALF OF PREGNANCY, INFANCY AND CHILDHOOD TO THE AGE OF 8 YEARS) MAY CAUSE PERMANENT DISCOLORATION OF THE TEETH (YELLOW-GRAY-BROWN). This adverse reaction is more common during long-term use of the drugs, but it has been observed following repeated short-term courses. Enamel hypoplasia has also been reported. TETRACYCLINE DRUGS, THEREFORE, SHOULD NOT BE USED IN THIS AGE GROUP, EXCEPT FOR ANTHRAX, INCLUDING INHALATIONAL ANTHRAX (POST-EXPOSURE), UNLESS OTHER DRUGS ARE NOT LIKELY TO BE EFFECTIVE OR ARE CONTRAINDICATED.

Pseudomembranous colitis has been reported with nearly all antibacterial agents, including doxycycline, and may range in severity from mild to life-threatening. Therefore, it is important to consider this diagnosis in patients who present with diarrhea subsequent to the administration of antibacterial agents.

Treatment with antibacterial agents alters the normal flora of the colon and may permit overgrowth of clostridia. Studies indicate that a toxin produced by *Clostridium difficile* is a primary cause of "antibiotic-associated colitis."

After the diagnosis of pseudomembranous colitis has been established, therapeutic measures should be initiated. Mild cases of pseudomembranous colitis usually respond to discontinuation of the drug alone. In moderate to severe cases, consideration should be given to management with fluids and electrolytes, protein supplementation and treatment with an antibacterial drug clinically effective against *Clostridium difficile* colitis.

All tetracyclines form a stable calcium complex in any bone-forming tissue. A decrease in fibula growth rate has been observed in prematures given oral tetracycline in doses of 25 mg/kg every 6 hours. This reaction was shown to be reversible when the drug was discontinued.

Results of animal studies indicate that tetracyclines cross the placenta, are found in fetal tissues, and can have toxic effects on the developing fetus (often related to retardation of skeletal development). Evidence of embryotoxicity has also been noted in animals treated early in pregnancy. If any tetracycline is used during pregnancy or if the patient becomes pregnant while taking this drug, the patient should be apprised of the potential hazard to the fetus.

The antianabolic action of the tetracyclines may cause an increase in BUN. Studies to date indicate that this does not occur with the use of doxycycline in patients with impaired renal function.

Photosensitivity manifested by an exaggerated sunburn reaction has been observed in some individuals taking tetracyclines. Patients apt to be exposed to direct sunlight or ultraviolet light should be advised that this reaction can occur with tetracycline drugs, and treatment should be discontinued at the first evidence of skin erythema.

Vibramycin Syrup contains sodium metabisulfite, a sulfite that may cause allergic-type reactions, including anaphylactic symptoms and life-threatening or less severe asthmatic episodes in certain susceptible people. The overall prevalence of sulfite sensitivity in the general population is unknown and probably low. Sulfite sensitivity is seen more frequently in asthmatic than in non-asthmatic people.

PRECAUTIONS

General

As with other antibiotic preparations, use of this drug may result in overgrowth of nonsusceptible organisms, including fungi. If superinfection occurs, the antibiotic should be discontinued and appropriate therapy instituted.

Bulging fontanels in infants and benign intracranial hypertension in adults have been reported in individuals receiving tetracyclines. These conditions disappeared when the drug was discontinued.

Incision and drainage or other surgical procedures should be performed in conjunction with antibiotic therapy, when indicated.

Doxycycline offers substantial but not complete suppression of the asexual blood stages of *Plasmodium* strains.

Doxycycline does not suppress *P. falciparum's* sexual blood stage gametocytes. Subjects completing this prophylactic regimen may still transmit the infection to mosquitoes outside endemic areas.

Prescribing Vibramycin in the absence of proven or strongly suspected bacterial infection or a prophylactic indication is unlikely to provide benefit to the patient and increases the risk of the development of drug-resistant bacteria.

Information for Patients

Patients taking doxycycline for malaria prophylaxis should be advised:

— that no present-day antimalarial agent, including doxycycline, guarantees protection against malaria.
— to avoid being bitten by mosquitoes by using personal protective measures that help avoid contact with mosquitoes, especially from dusk to dawn (e.g., staying in well-screened areas, using mosquito nets, covering the body with clothing, and using an effective insect repellent).
— that doxycycline prophylaxis:
  — should begin 1-2 days before travel to the malarious area,
  — should be continued daily while in the malarious area and after leaving the malarious area,
  — should be continued for 4 further weeks to avoid development of malaria after returning from an endemic area,
  — should not exceed 4 months.

All patients taking doxycycline should be advised:

— to avoid excessive sunlight or artificial ultraviolet light while receiving doxycycline and to discontinue therapy if phototoxicity (e.g., skin eruption, etc.) occurs. Sunscreen or sunblock should be considered (See WARNINGS.)
— to drink fluids liberally along with doxycycline to reduce the risk of esophageal irritation and ulceration. (See ADVERSE REACTIONS.)
— that the absorption of tetracyclines is reduced when taken with foods, especially those which contain calcium. However, the absorption of doxycycline is not markedly influenced by simultaneous ingestion of food or milk. (See DRUG INTERACTIONS.)
— that the absorption of tetracyclines is reduced when taking bismuth subsalicylate (See DRUG INTERACTIONS.)
— that the use of doxycycline might increase the incidence of vaginal candidiasis.

Patients should be counseled that antibacterial drugs including Vibramycin should only be used to treat bacterial infections. They do not treat viral infections (e.g., the common cold). When Vibramycin is prescribed to treat a bacterial infection, patients should be told that although it is common to feel better early in the course of therapy, the medication should be taken exactly as directed. Skipping doses or not completing the full course of therapy may (1) decrease the effectiveness of the immediate treatment and (2) increase the likelihood that bacteria will develop resistance and will not be treatable by Vibramycin or other antibacterial drugs in the future.

Laboratory Tests

In venereal disease, when co-existent syphilis is suspected, dark field examinations should be done before treatment is started and the blood serology repeated monthly for at least 4 months.

In long-term therapy, periodic laboratory evaluation of organ systems, including hematopoietic, renal, and hepatic studies, should be performed.

Drug Interactions

Because tetracyclines have been shown to depress plasma prothrombin activity, patients who are on anticoagulant therapy may require downward adjustment of their anticoagulant dosage.

Since bacteriostatic drugs may interfere with the bactericidal action of penicillin, it is advisable to avoid giving tetracyclines in conjunction with penicillin.

Absorption of tetracyclines is impaired by antacids containing aluminum, calcium, or magnesium, and iron-containing preparations.

Absorption of tetracyclines is impaired by bismuth subsalicylate.

Barbiturates, carbamazepine, and phenytoin decrease the half-life of doxycycline.

The concurrent use of tetracycline and Penthrane® (methoxyflurane) has been reported to result in fatal renal toxicity.

Concurrent use of tetracycline may render oral contraceptives less effective.

Drug/Laboratory Test Interactions

False elevations of urinary catecholamine levels may occur due to interference with the fluorescence test.

Carcinogenesis, Mutagenesis, Impairment of Fertility

Long-term studies in animals to evaluate carcinogenic potential of doxycycline have not been conducted. However, there has been evidence of oncogenic activity in rats in studies with the related antibiotics, oxytetracycline (adrenal and pituitary tumors), and minocycline (thyroid tumors).

Likewise, although mutagenicity studies of doxycycline have not been conducted, positive results in *in vitro* mammalian cell assays have been reported for related antibiotics (tetracycline, oxytetracycline).

Doxycycline administered orally at dosage levels as high as 250 mg/kg/day had no apparent effect on the fertility of female rats. Effect on male fertility has not been studied.

Pregnancy: Teratogenic Effects. Pregnancy Category D: There are no adequate and well-controlled studies on the use of doxycycline in pregnant women. The vast majority of reported experience with doxycycline during human pregnancy is short-term, first trimester exposure. There are no human data available to assess the effects of long-term therapy of doxycycline in pregnant women such as that proposed for treatment of anthrax exposure. An expert review of published data on experiences with doxycycline use during pregnancy by TERIS – the Teratogen Information System – concluded that therapeutic doses during pregnancy are unlikely to pose a substantial teratogenic risk (the quantity and quality of data were assessed as limited to fair), but the data are insufficient to state that there is no risk[a]. A case-control study (18,515 mothers of infants with congenital anomalies and 32,804 mothers of infants with no congenital anomalies) shows a weak but marginally statistically significant association with total malformations and use of doxycycline anytime during pregnancy. Sixty-three (0.19%) of the controls and fifty-six (0.30%) of the cases were treated with doxycycline. This association was not seen when the analysis was confined to maternal treatment during the period of organogenesis (i.e., in the second and third months of gestation) with the exception of a marginal relationship with neural tube defect based on only two exposed cases[b].

A small prospective study of 81 pregnancies describes 43 pregnant women treated for 10 days with doxycycline during early first trimester. All mothers reported their exposed infants were normal at 1 year of age[c].

Nonteratogenic effects: (See WARNINGS).

Labor and Delivery

The effect of tetracyclines on labor and delivery is unknown.

Nursing Mothers

Tetracyclines are excreted in human milk; however, the extent of absorption of tetracyclines, including doxycycline, by the breastfed infant is not known. Short-term use by lactating women is not necessarily contraindicated; however, the effects of prolonged exposure to doxycycline in breast milk are unknown[d]. Because of the potential for serious adverse reactions in nursing infants from doxycycline, a decision should be made whether to discontinue nursing or to discontinue the drug, taking into account the importance of the drug to the mother. (See WARNINGS.)

Pediatric Use

See WARNINGS and DOSAGE AND ADMINISTRATION.

ADVERSE REACTIONS

Due to oral doxycycline's virtually complete absorption, side effects of the lower bowel, particularly diarrhea, have been infrequent. The following adverse reactions have been observed in patients receiving tetracyclines:

Gastrointestinal: anorexia, nausea, vomiting, diarrhea, glossitis, dysphagia, enterocolitis, and inflammatory lesions (with monilial overgrowth) in the anogenital region. Hepatotoxicity has been reported rarely. These reactions have been caused by both the oral and parenteral administration of tetracyclines. Rare instances of esophagitis and esophageal ulcerations have been reported in patients receiving capsule and tablet forms of the drugs in the tetracycline class. Most of these patients took medications immediately before going to bed. (See DOSAGE AND ADMINISTRATION.)

Skin: maculopapular and erythematous rashes. Exfoliative dermatitis has been reported but is uncommon. Photosensitivity is discussed above. (See WARNINGS.)

Renal toxicity: Rise in BUN has been reported and is apparently dose related. (See WARNINGS.)

Hypersensitivity reactions: urticaria, angioneurotic edema, anaphylaxis, anaphylactoid purpura, serum sickness, pericarditis, and exacerbation of systemic lupus erythematosus.

Blood: Hemolytic anemia, thrombocytopenia, neutropenia, and eosinophilia have been reported.

Other: bulging fontanels in infants and intracranial hypertension in adults. (See PRECAUTIONS – General.)

When given over prolonged periods, tetracyclines have been reported to produce brown-black microscopic discoloration of the thyroid gland. No abnormalities of thyroid function studies are known to occur.

OVERDOSAGE

In case of overdosage, discontinue medication, treat symptomatically and institute supportive measures. Dialysis does not alter serum half-life and thus would not be of benefit in treating cases of overdosage.

DOSAGE AND ADMINISTRATION

THE USUAL DOSAGE AND FREQUENCY OF ADMINISTRATION OF DOXYCYCLINE DIFFERS FROM THAT OF THE OTHER TETRACYCLINES. EXCEEDING THE RECOMMENDED DOSAGE MAY RESULT IN AN INCREASED INCIDENCE OF SIDE EFFECTS. Adults: The usual dose of oral doxycycline is 200 mg on the first day of treatment (administered 100 mg every 12 hours) followed by a maintenance dose of 100 mg/day. The maintenance dose may be administered as a single dose or as 50 mg every 12 hours.

In the management of more severe infections (particularly chronic infections of the urinary tract), 100 mg every 12 hours is recommended.

For children above eight years of age: The recommended dosage schedule for children weighing 100 pounds or less is 2 mg/lb of body weight divided into two doses on the first day of treatment, followed by 1 mg/lb of body weight given as a single daily dose or divided into two doses, on subsequent days. For more severe infections up to 2 mg/lb of body weight may be used. For children over 100 lb the usual adult dose should be used.

The therapeutic antibacterial serum activity will usually persist for 24 hours following recommended dosage.

When used in streptococcal infections, therapy should be continued for 10 days.

Administration of adequate amounts of fluid along with capsule and tablet forms of drugs in the tetracycline class is recommended to wash down the drugs and reduce the risk of esophageal irritation and ulceration. (See ADVERSE REACTIONS.)

If gastric irritation occurs, it is recommended that doxycycline be given with food or milk. The absorption of doxycycline is not markedly influenced by simultaneous ingestion of food or milk.

Studies to date have indicated that administration of doxycycline at the usual recommended doses does not lead to excessive accumulation of the antibiotic in patients with renal impairment.

Uncomplicated gonococcal infections in adults (except anorectal infections in men): 100 mg, by mouth, twice a day for 7 days. As an alternate single visit dose, administer 300 mg stat followed in one hour by a second 300 mg dose. The dose may be administered with food, including milk or carbonated beverage, as required.

Uncomplicated urethral, endocervical, or rectal infection in adults caused by *Chlamydia trachomatis:* 100 mg by mouth twice a day for 7 days.

Nongonococcal urethritis (NGU) caused by *C. trachomatis* or *U. urealyticum:* 100 mg by mouth twice a day for 7 days.

Syphilis – early: Patients who are allergic to penicillin should be treated with doxycycline 100 mg by mouth twice a day for 2 weeks.

Syphilis of more than one year's duration: Patients who are allergic to penicillin should be treated with doxycycline 100 mg by mouth twice a day for 4 weeks.

Acute epididymo-orchitis caused by *N. gonorrhoeae:* 100 mg, by mouth, twice a day for at least 10 days.

Acute epididymo-orchitis caused by *C. trachomatis:* 100 mg, by mouth, twice a day for at least 10 days.

For prophylaxis of malaria: For adults, the recommended dose is 100 mg daily. For children over 8 years of age, the recommended dose is 2 mg/kg given once daily up to the adult dose. Prophylaxis should begin 1-2 days before travel to the malarious area. Prophylaxis should be continued daily during travel in the malarious area and for 4 weeks after the traveler leaves the malarious area.

Inhalational anthrax (post-exposure):

ADULTS: 100 mg of doxycycline, by mouth, twice a day for 60 days.

CHILDREN: weighing less than 100 lb (45 kg); 1 mg/lb (2.2 mg/kg) of body weight, by mouth, twice a day for 60 days. Children weighing 100 lb or more should receive the adult dose.

HOW SUPPLIED

Vibramycin® Hyclate (doxycycline hyclate) is available in capsules containing doxycycline hyclate equivalent to:

<u>50 mg doxycycline</u>
bottles of 50 (NDC 0069-0940-50)

The capsules are white and light blue and are imprinted with "VIBRA" on one half and "PFIZER 094" on the other half.

<u>100 mg doxycycline</u>
bottles of 50 (NDC 0069-0950-50)

The capsules are light blue and are imprinted with "VIBRA" on one half and "PFIZER 095" on the other half.

Vibra-Tabs® (doxycycline hyclate) is available in salmon colored film-coated tablets containing doxycycline hyclate equivalent to:

<u>100 mg doxycycline</u>
bottles of 50 (NDC 0069-0990-50)

The tablets are imprinted on one side with "VIBRA-TABS" and "PFIZER 099" on the other side.

Vibramycin® Calcium Syrup (doxycycline calcium) oral suspension is available as a raspberry-apple flavored oral suspension. Each teaspoonful (5 mL) contains doxycycline calcium equivalent to 50 mg of doxycycline: 1 pint (473 mL) bottles (NDC 0069-0971-93).

Vibramycin® Monohydrate (doxycycline monohydrate) for Oral Suspension is available as a raspberry-flavored, dry powder for oral suspension. When reconstituted, each teaspoonful (5 mL) contains doxycycline monohydrate equivalent to 25 mg of doxycycline: 2 oz (60 mL) bottles (NDC 0069-0970-65).

All products are to be stored below 86°F (30°C) and dispensed in tight, light-resistant containers (USP).

ANIMAL PHARMACOLOGY AND ANIMAL TOXICOLOGY

Hyperpigmentation of the thyroid has been produced by members of the tetracycline class in the following species: in rats by oxytetracycline, doxycycline, tetracycline PO_4, and methacycline; in minipigs by doxycycline, minocycline, tetracycline PO_4, and methacycline; in dogs by doxycycline and minocycline; in monkeys by minocycline.

Minocycline, tetracycline PO_4, methacycline, doxycycline, tetracycline base, oxytetracycline HCl, and tetracycline HCl were goitrogenic in rats fed a low iodine diet. This goitrogenic effect was accompanied by high radioactive iodine uptake. Administration of minocycline also produced a large goiter with high radioiodine uptake in rats fed a relatively high iodine diet.

Treatment of various animal species with this class of drugs has also resulted in the induction of thyroid hyperplasia in the following: in rats and dogs (minocycline); in chickens (chlortetracycline); and in rats and mice (oxytetracycline). Adrenal gland hyperplasia has been observed in goats and rats treated with oxytetracycline.

REFERENCES

1. National Committee for Clinical Laboratory Standards, *Performance Standards for Antimicrobial Disk Susceptibility Tests*, Fourth Edition. Approved Standard NCCLS Document M2-A4, Vol. 10, No. 7 NCCLS, Villanova, PA, April 1990.

2. National Committee for Clinical Laboratory Standards, *Methods for Dilution Antimicrobial Susceptibility Tests for Bacteria that Grow Aerobically*, Second Edition. Approved Standard NCCLS Document M7-A2, Vol. 10, No. 8 NCCLS, Villanova, PA, April 1990.

3. [a]Friedman JM and Polifka JE. *Teratogenic Effects of Drugs. A Resource for Clinicians (TERIS).* Baltimore, MD: The Johns Hopkins University Press, 2000: 149–195.

[b]Cziezel AE and Rockenbauer M. Teratogenic study of doxycycline. *Obstet Gynecol* 1997; 89: 524–528.

[c]Horne HW Jr and Kundsin RB. The role of mycoplasma among 81 consecutive pregnancies: a prospective study. *Int J Fertil* 1980; 25: 315–317.

[d]Hale T. *Medications and Mothers Milk.* 9th edition. Amarillo, TX: Pharmasoft Publishing, 2000: 225–226.

Rx only

Pfizer Labs
Division of Pfizer Inc, NY, NY 10017
69-1680-32-9 Revised September 2003

VIRACEPT® ℞

[*vī-ră-cept*]
(nelfinavir mesylate)
TABLETS and ORAL POWDER

Prescribing information for this product, which appears on pages 2669–2675 of the 2004 PDR, has been completely revised as follows. Please write "See Supplement A" next to the product heading.

DESCRIPTION

VIRACEPT® (nelfinavir mesylate) is an inhibitor of the human immunodeficiency virus (HIV) protease. VIRACEPT Tablets are available for oral administration as a light blue, capsule-shaped tablet with a clear film coating in 250 mg strength (as nelfinavir free base) and as a white oval tablet with a clear film coating in 625 mg strength (as nelfinavir free base). Each tablet contains the following common inactive ingredients: calcium silicate, crospovidone, magnesium stearate, hypromellose, and triacetin. In addition, the 250 mg tablet contains FD&C blue #2 powder and the 625 mg tablet contains colloidal silicon dioxide. VIRACEPT Oral Powder is available for oral administration in a 50 mg/g strength (as nelfinavir free base) in bottles. The oral powder also contains the following inactive ingredients: microcrystalline cellulose, maltodextrin, dibasic potassium phosphate, crospovidone, hypromellose, aspartame, sucrose palmitate, and natural and artificial flavor. The chemical name for nelfinavir mesylate is [3*S*-[2(2*S**, 3*S**), 3α,4aβ,8aβ]]-*N*-(1,1-dimethylethyl)decahydro-2-[2-hydroxy-3-[(3-hydroxy-2-methylbenzoyl)amino]-4-(phenylthio)butyl]-3-isoquinoline carboxamide mono-methanesulfonate (salt) and the molecular weight is 663.90 (567.79 as the free base). Nelfinavir mesylate has the following structural formula:

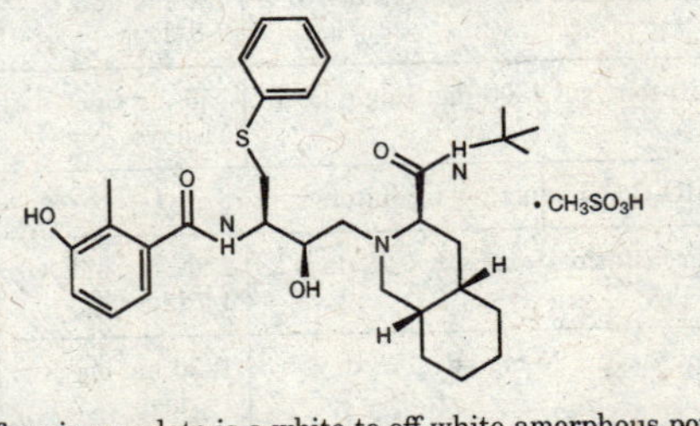

Nelfinavir mesylate is a white to off-white amorphous powder, slightly soluble in water at pH ≤4 and freely soluble in methanol, ethanol, 2-propanol and propylene glycol.

MICROBIOLOGY

Mechanism of Action: Nelfinavir is an inhibitor of the HIV-1 protease. Inhibition of the viral protease prevents cleavage of the *gag* and *gag-pol* polyprotein resulting in the production of immature, non-infectious virus.

Antiviral Activity In Vitro: The antiviral activity of nelfinavir *in vitro* has been demonstrated in both acute and/or chronic HIV infections in lymphoblastoid cell lines, peripheral blood lymphocytes and monocytes/macrophages. Nelfinavir was found to be active against several laboratory strains and clinical isolates of HIV-1 and the HIV-2 strain ROD. The EC_{95} (95% effective concentration) of nelfinavir ranged from 7 to 196 nM. Drug combination studies with protease inhibitors showed nelfinavir had antagonistic interactions with indinavir, additive interactions with ritonavir or saquinavir and synergistic interactions with amprenavir and lopinavir. Minimal to no cellular cytotoxicity was observed with any of these protease inhibitors alone or in combination with nelfinavir. In combination with reverse transcriptase inhibitors, nelfinavir demonstrated additive (didanosine or stavudine) to synergistic (abacavir, delavirdine, efavirenz, lamivudine, nevirapine, tenofovir, zalcitabine or zidovudine) antiviral activity *in vitro* without enhanced cytotoxicity.

Drug Resistance: HIV-1 isolates with reduced susceptibility to nelfinavir have been selected *in vitro.* HIV isolates from selected patients treated with nelfinavir alone or in combination with reverse transcriptase inhibitors were monitored for phenotypic (n=19) and genotypic (n=195, 157 of which were evaluable) changes in clinical trials over a period of 2 to 82 weeks. One or more viral protease mutations at amino acid positions 30, 35, 36, 46, 71, 77 and 88 were detected in the HIV-1 of >10% of patients with evaluable isolates. The overall incidence of the D30N mutation in the viral protease of evaluable isolates (n=157) from patients receiving nelfinavir monotherapy or nelfinavir in combination with zidovudine and lamivudine or stavudine was 54.8%. The overall incidence of other mutations associated with primary protease inhibitor resistance was 9.6% for the L90M substitution whereas substitutions at 48, 82, or 84 were not observed. Of the 19 clinical isolates for which both phenotypic and genotypic analyses were performed, 9 showed reduced susceptibility (5- to 93-fold) to nelfinavir *in vitro.* All 9 patient isolates possessed one or more mutations in the viral protease gene. Amino acid position 30 appeared to be the most frequent mutation site.

Cross-resistance: Non-clinical Studies—Patient-derived recombinant HIV isolates containing the D30N mutation (n=4) and demonstrating high-level (>10-fold) NFV-resistance remained susceptible (<2.5-fold resistance) to amprenavir, indinavir, lopinavir, and saquinavir, *in vitro.* Patient-derived recombinant HIV isolates containing the L90M mutation (n=8) demonstrated moderate to high-level resistance to NFV and had varying levels of susceptibility to amprenavir, indinavir, lopinavir, and saquinavir, *in vitro.* Most patient-derived recombinant isolates with phenotypic and genotypic evidence of reduced susceptibility (>2.5-fold) to amprenavir, indinavir, lopinavir, and/or saquinavir demonstrated high-level cross-resistance to nelfinavir, *in vitro.* Mutations associated with resistance to other PIs (e.g. G48V, V82A/F/T, I84V, L90M) appeared to confer high-level cross-resistance to NFV. Following ritonavir therapy 6 of 7 clinical isolates with decreased ritonavir susceptibility (8- to 113-fold) *in vitro* compared to baseline also exhibited decreased susceptibility to nelfinavir *in vitro* (5- to 40-fold). Cross-resistance between nelfinavir and reverse transcriptase inhibitors is unlikely because different enzyme targets are involved. Clinical isolates (n=5) with decreased susceptibility to lamivudine, nevirapine or zidovudine remain fully susceptible to nelfinavir *in vitro.*

Clinical Studies—There have been no controlled or comparative studies evaluating the virologic response to subsequent protease inhibitor-containing regimens in patients who have demonstrated loss of virologic response to a nelfinavir-containing regimen. However, virologic response was evaluated in a single-arm prospective study of 26 patients with extensive prior antiretroviral experience with reverse transcriptase inhibitors (mean 2.9) who had received VIRACEPT for a mean duration of 59.7 weeks and were switched to a ritonavir (400 mg BID)/saquinavir hardgel (400 mg BID) containing regimen after a prolonged period of VIRACEPT failure (median 48 weeks). Sequence analysis of HIV-1 isolates prior to switch demonstrated a D30N or an L90M substitution in 18 and 6 patients, respectively. Subjects remained on therapy for a mean of 48 weeks (range 40 to 56 weeks) where 17 of 26 (65%) subjects and 13 of 26 (50%) subjects were treatment responders with HIV RNA below the assay limit of detection (<500 HIV RNA copies/mL, Chiron bDNA) at 24 and 48 weeks, respectively.

CLINICAL PHARMACOLOGY

Pharmacokinetics

The pharmacokinetic properties of nelfinavir were evaluated in healthy volunteers and HIV-infected patients; no substantial differences were observed between the two groups.

Absorption: Pharmacokinetic parameters of nelfinavir (area under the plasma concentration-time curve during a 24-hour period at steady-state [AUC_{24}], peak plasma concentrations [C_{max}], morning and evening trough concentrations [C_{trough}]) from a pharmacokinetic study in HIV-positive patients after multiple dosing with 1250 mg (five 250 mg tablets) twice daily (BID) for 28 days (10 patients) and 750 mg (three 250 mg tablets) three times daily (TID) for 28 days (11 patients) are summarized in Table 1.

Table 1
Summary of a Pharmacokinetic Study in HIV-positive Patients with Multiple Dosing of 1250 mg BID for 28 days and 750 mg TID for 28 days

Regimen	AUC_{24} mg.h/L	C_{max} mg/L	C_{trough} Morning mg/L	C_{trough} Afternoon or Evening mg/L
1250 mg BID	52.8 ± 15.7	4.0 ± 0.8	2.2 ± 1.3	0.7 ± 0.4
750 mg TID	43.6 ± 17.8	3.0 ± 1.6	1.4 ± 0.6	1.0 ± 0.5

data are mean ± SD

Continued on next page

Viracept—Cont.

The difference between morning and afternoon or evening trough concentrations for the TID and BID regimens was also observed in healthy volunteers who were dosed at precisely 8- or 12-hour intervals.

In healthy volunteers receiving a single 1250 mg dose, the 625 mg tablet was not bioequivalent to the 250 mg tablet formulation. Under fasted conditions (n=27), the AUC and C_{max} were 34% and 24% higher, respectively, for the 625 mg tablets. In a relative bioavailability assessment under fed conditions (n=28), the AUC was 24% higher for the 625 mg tablet; the C_{max} was comparable for both formulations. (See ADVERSE REACTIONS).

In healthy volunteers receiving a single 750 mg dose under fed conditions, nelfinavir concentrations were similar following administration of the 250 mg tablet and oral powder.

Effect of Food on Oral Absorption: Food increases nelfinavir exposure and decreases nelfinavir pharmacokinetic variability relative to the fasted state. Healthy volunteers received a single dose of 1250 mg of VIRACEPT 250 mg tablets (5 tablets) under fasted or fed conditions (three different meals). Results from the study are summarized in Table 2.

Table 2
Changes in AUC, C_{max} and T_{max} for Nelfinavir in Fed State Relative to Fasted State Following 1250 mg VIRACEPT (5 × 250 mg tablets)

Number of Kcal	% Fat	Number of subjects	AUC fold increase	C_{max} fold increase	Increase in T_{max} (hr)
125	20	n=21	2.2	2.0	1.00
500	20	n=22	3.1	2.3	2.00
1000	50	n=23	5.2	3.3	2.00

A food effect study has not been conducted with the 625 mg tablet. However, based on a cross-study comparison (n=26 fed vs. n=26 fasted) following single dose administration of nelfinavir 1250 mg, the magnitude of the food effect for the 625 mg nelfinavir tablet appears comparable to that of the 250 mg tablets. VIRACEPT should be taken with a meal.

Distribution: The apparent volume of distribution following oral administration of nelfinavir was 2–7 L/kg. Nelfinavir in serum is extensively protein-bound (>98%).

Metabolism: Unchanged nelfinavir comprised 82-86% of the total plasma radioactivity after a single oral 750 mg dose of ^{14}C-nelfinavir. *In vitro*, multiple cytochrome P-450 enzymes including CYP3A and CYP2C19 are responsible for metabolism of nelfinavir. One major and several minor oxidative metabolites were found in plasma. The major oxidative metabolite has *in vitro* antiviral activity comparable to the parent drug.

Elimination: The terminal half-life in plasma was typically 3.5 to 5 hours. The majority (87%) of an oral 750 mg dose containing ^{14}C-nelfinavir was recovered in the feces; fecal radioactivity consisted of numerous oxidative metabolites (78%) and unchanged nelfinavir (22%). Only 1-2% of the dose was recovered in urine, of which unchanged nelfinavir was the major component.

Special Populations

Hepatic Insufficiency: The multi-dose pharmacokinetics of nelfinavir have not been studied in HIV-positive patients with hepatic insufficiency.

Renal Insufficiency: The pharmacokinetics of nelfinavir have not been studied in patients with renal insufficiency; however, less than 2% of nelfinavir is excreted in the urine, so the impact of renal impairment on nelfinavir elimination should be minimal.

Gender and Race: No significant pharmacokinetic differences have been detected between males and females. Pharmacokinetic differences due to race have not been evaluated.

Pediatrics: The pharmacokinetics of nelfinavir have been investigated in 5 studies in pediatric patients from birth to 13 years of age either receiving VIRACEPT three times or twice daily. The dosing regimens and associated AUC_{24} values are summarized in Table 3.

Table 3
Summary of Steady-state AUC_{24} of Nelfinavir in Pediatric Studies

Protocol No.	Dosing Regimen[1]	N[2]	Age	AUC_{24} (mg.hr/L) Arithmetic mean ± SD
AG1343-524	20 (19-28) mg/kg TID	14	2-13 years	56.1 ± 29.8
PACTG-725	55 (48-60) mg/kg BID	6	3-11 years	101.8 ± 56.1
PENTA 7	40 (34-43) mg/kg TID	4	2-9 months	33.8 ± 8.9
PENTA 7	75 (55-83) mg/kg BID	12	2-9 months	37.2 ± 19.2
PACTG-353	40 (14-56) mg/kg BID	10	6 weeks 1 week	44.1 ± 27.4 45.8 ± 32.1

[1] Protocol specified dose (actual dose range)
[2] N: number of subjects with evaluable pharmacokinetic results
C_{trough} values are not presented in the table because they are not available for all studies

Pharmacokinetic data are also available for 86 patients (age 2 to 12 years) who received VIRACEPT 25-35 mg/kg TID in Study AG1343-556. The pharmacokinetic data from Study AG1343-556 were more variable than data from other studies conducted in the pediatric population; the 95% confidence interval for AUC_{24} was 9 to 121 mg.hr/L.

Overall, use of VIRACEPT in the pediatric population is associated with highly variable drug exposure. The high variability may be due to inconsistent food intake in pediatric patients. (See PRECAUTIONS Pediatric Use; DOSAGE AND ADMINISTRATION.)

Geriatric Patients: The pharmacokinetics of nelfinavir have not been studied in patients over 65 years of age.

Drug Interactions (also see CONTRAINDICATIONS, WARNINGS, PRECAUTIONS: Drug Interactions)

CYP3A and CYP2C19 appear to be the predominant enzymes that metabolize nelfinavir in humans. The potential ability of nelfinavir to inhibit the major human cytochrome P450 enzymes (CYP3A, CYP2C19, CYP2D6, CYP2C9, CYP1A2 and CYP2E1) has been investigated *in vitro*. Only CYP3A was inhibited at concentrations in the therapeutic range. Specific drug interaction studies were performed

Table 4: Drug Interactions:
Changes in Pharmacokinetic Parameters for Coadministered Drug in the Presence of VIRACEPT

Coadministered Drug	Nelfinavir Dose	N	% Change of Coadministered Drug Pharmacokinetic Parameters[1] (90% CI) AUC	C_{max}	C_{min}
HIV-Protease Inhibitors					
Indinavir 800 mg Single Dose	750 mg q8h × 7 days	6	↑51% (↑29- ↑77%)	↓10% (↓28- ↑13%)	NA
Ritonavir 500 mg Single Dose	750 mg q8h × 5 doses	10	↔	↔	NA
Saquinavir 1200 mg Single Dose[2]	750 mg tid × 4 days	14	↑392% (↑291- ↑521%)	↑179% (↑117- ↑259%)	NA
Amprenavir 800 mg tid × 14 days	750 mg tid × 14 days	6	↔	↓14% (↓38- ↑20%)	↑189% (↑52- ↑448%)
Nucleoside Reverse Transcriptase Inhibitors					
Lamivudine 150 mg Single Dose	750 mg q8h × 7-10 days	11	↑10% (↑2- ↑18%)	↑31% (↑9- ↑56%)	NA
Stavudine 30-40 mg bid × 56 days	750 mg tid × 56 days	8	See footnote[3]		
Zidovudine 200 mg Single Dose	750 mg q8h × 7-10 days	11	↓35% (↓29- ↓40%)	↓31% (↓13- ↓46%)	NA
Non-Nucleoside Reverse Transcriptase Inhibitors					
Efavirenz 600 mg qd × 7 days	750 mg q8h × 7 days	10	↓12% (↓31- ↑12%)	↓12% (↓29- ↑8%)	↓22% (↓54- ↑32%)
Nevirapine 200 mg qd × 14 days[3] Followed by 200 mg bid × 14 days	750 mg tid × 36 days	23	See footnote[3]		
Delavirdine 400 mg q8h × 14 days	750 mg q8h × 7 days	7	↓31% (↓57- ↑10%)	↓27% (↓49- ↑4%)	↓33% (↓70 - ↑49%)
Anti-infective Agents					
Rifabutin 150 mg qd × 8 days[4]	750 mg q8h × 7-8 days[5]	12	↑83% (↑72- ↑96%)	↑19% (↑11- ↑28%)	↑177% (↑144- ↑215%)
Rifabutin 300 mg qd × 8 days	750 mg q8h × 7-8 days	10	↑207% (↑161- ↑263%)	↑146% (↑118- ↑178%)	↑305% (↑245- ↑375%)
Azithromycin 1200 mg Single Dose	750 mg tid × 11 days	12	↑112% (↑80- ↑150%)	↑136% (↑77- ↑215%)	NA
HMG-CoA Reductase Inhibitors					
Atorvastatin 10 mg qd × 28 days	1250 mg bid × 14 days	15	↑74% (↑41- ↑116%)	↑122% (↑68- ↑193%)	↑39% (↓21- ↑145%)
Simvastatin 20 mg qd × 28 days	1250 mg bid × 14 days	16	↑505% (↑393 - ↑643%)	↑517% (↑367 - ↑715%)	ND
Other Agents					
Ethinyl estradiol 35 μg qd × 15 days	750 mg q8h × 7 days	12	↓47% (↓42 - ↓52%)	↓28% (↓16 - ↓37%)	↓62% (↓57 - ↓67%)
Norethindrone 0.4 mg qd × 15 days	750 mg q8h × 7 days	12	↓18% (↓13 - ↓23%)	↔	↓46% (↓38- ↓53%)
Methadone 80 mg +/−21 mg qd[6] >1 month	1250 mg bid × 8 days	13	↓47% (↓42 - ↓51%)	↓46% (↓42 - ↓49%)	↓53% (↓49 - ↓57%)
Phenytoin 300 mg qd × 14 days[7]	1250 mg bid × 7 days	12	↓29% (↓17 - ↓39%)	↓21% (↓12- ↓29%)	↓39% (↓27- ↓49%)

NA: Not relevent for single-dose treatment; ND: Cannot be determined
[1] ↑ Indicates increase ↓ Indicates decrease ↔ Indicates no change (geometric mean exposure increased or decreased <10%)
[2]Using the soft-gelatin capsule formulation of saquinavir 1200 mg
[3]Based on non-definitive cross-study comparison, drug plasma concentrations appeared to be unaffected by coadministration
[4]Rifabutin 150 mg qd changes are relative to Rifabutin 300 mg qd × 8 days without coadministration with nelfinavir
[5]Comparable changes in rifabutin concentrations were observed with VIRACEPT 1250 mg q12h × 7 days
[6]Changes are reported for total plasma methadone; changes for the individual R-enantiomer and S-enantiomer were similar
[7]Phenytoin exposure measures are reported for total phenytoin exposure. The effect of nelfinavir on unbound phenytoin was similar

Table 5: Drug Interactions:
Changes in Pharmacokinetic Parameters for Nelfinavir in the Presence of the Coadministered Drug

Coadministered Drug	Nelfinavir Dose	N	% Change of Nelfinavir Pharmacokinetic Parameters[1] (90% CI)		
			AUC	C_{max}	C_{min}
HIV-Protease Inhibitors					
Indinavir 800 mg q8h × 7 days	750 mg Single Dose	6	↑83% (↑42-↑137%)	↑31% (↑16-↑48%)	NA
Ritonavir 500 mg q12h × 3 doses	750 mg Single Dose	10	↑152% (↑96-↑224%)	↑44% (↑28-↑63%)	NA
Saquinavir 1200 mg tid × 4 days[2]	750 mg Single Dose	14	↑18% (↑7-↑30%)	↔	NA
Amprenavir 800 mg tid × 14 days	750 mg tid × 14 days	6	See footnote[3]		
Nucleoside Reverse Transcriptase Inhibitors					
Didanosine 200 mg Single Dose	750 mg Single Dose	9	↔	↔	NA
Zidovudine 200 mg + Lamivudine 150 mg Single Dose	750 mg q8h × 7-10 days	11	↔	↔	↔
Non-Nucleoside Reverse Transcriptase Inhibitors					
Efavirenz 600 mg qd × 7 days	750 mg q8h × 7 days	7	↑20% (↑8-↑34%)	↑21% (↑10-↑33%)	↔
Nevirapine 200 mg qd × 14 days Followed by 200 mg bid × 14 days	750 mg tid × 36 days	23	↔	↔	↓32% (↓50 - ↑5%)
Delavirdine 400 mg q8h × 7 days	750 mg q8h × 14 days	12	↑107% (↑83-↑135%)	↑88% (↑66-↑113%)	↑136% (↑103-↑175%)
Anti-infective Agents					
Ketoconazole 400 mg qd × 7 days	500 mg q8h × 5-6 days	12	↑35% (↑24-↑46%)	↑25% (↑11-↑40%)	↑14% (↓23-↑69%)
Rifabutin 150 mg qd × 8 days	750 mg q8h × 7-8 days	11	↓23% (↓14-↓31%)	↓18% (↓8-↓27%)	↓25% (↓8-↓39%)
	1250 mg q12h × 7-8 days	11	↔	↔	↓15% (↓43-↑27%)
Rifabutin 300 mg qd × 8 days	750 mg q8h × 7-8 days	10	↓32% (↓15-↓46%)	↓24% (↓10-↓36%)	↓53% (↓15-↓73%)
Rifampin 600 mg qd × 7 days	750 mg q8h × 5-6 days	12	↓83% (↓79-↓86%)	↓76% (↓69-↓82%)	↓92% (↓86-↓95%)
Azithromycin 1200 mg Single Dose	750 mg tid × 9 days	12	↓15% (↓7-↓22%)	↓10% (↓19-↑1%)	↓29% (↓19-↓38%)
HMG-CoA Reductase Inhibitors					
Atorvastatin 10 mg qd × 28 days	1250 mg bid × 14 days	15	See footnote[3]		
Simvastatin 20 mg qd × 28 days	1250 mg bid × 14 days	16	See footnote[3]		
Other Agents					
Methadone 80 mg +/−21 mg qd >1 month	1250 mg bid × 8 days	13	See footnote[3]		
Phenytoin 300 mg qd × 7 days	1250 mg bid × 14 days	15	↔	↔	↓18% (↓45-↑23%)

NA: Not relevent for single-dose treatment
[1] ↑ Indicates increase ↓ Indicates decrease ↔ Indicates no change (geometric mean exposure increased or decreased <10%)
[2]Using the soft-gelatin capsule formulation of saquinavir 1200 mg
[3]Based on non-definitive cross-study comparison, nelfinavir plasma concentrations appeared to be unaffected by co-administration

with nelfinavir and a number of drugs. Table 4 summarizes the effects of nelfinavir on the geometric mean AUC, C_{max} and C_{min} of coadministered drugs. Table 5 shows the effects of coadministered drugs on the geometric mean AUC, C_{max} and C_{min} of nelfinavir.

[See table 4 on previous page]

[See table 5 above]

For information regarding clinical recommendations see CONTRAINDICATIONS, WARNINGS, PRECAUTIONS: Drug Interactions.

INDICATIONS AND USAGE

VIRACEPT in combination with other antiretroviral agents is indicated for the treatment of HIV infection.

Description of Studies

In the clinical studies described below, efficacy was evaluated by the percent of patients with plasma HIV RNA < 400 copies/mL (Studies 511 and 542) or < 500 copies/mL (Study ACTG 364), using the Roche RT-PCR (Amplicor) HIV-1 Monitor or < 50 copies/mL, using the Roche HIV-1 Ultrasensitive assay (Study Avanti 3). In the analysis presented in each figure, patients who terminated the study early for any reason, switched therapy due to inadequate efficacy or who had a missing HIV-RNA measurement that was either preceded or followed by a measurement above the limit of assay quantification were considered to have HIV-RNA above 400 copies/mL, above 500 copies/mL, or above 50 copies/mL at subsequent time points, depending on the assay that was used.

a. Studies in Antiretroviral Treatment Naïve Patients

Study 511: VIRACEPT + zidovudine + lamivudine versus zidovudine + lamivudine

Study 511 was a double-blind, randomized, placebo controlled trial comparing treatment with zidovudine (ZDV; 200 mg TID) and lamivudine (3TC; 150 mg BID) plus 2 doses of VIRACEPT (750 mg and 500 mg TID) to zidovudine (200 mg TID) and lamivudine (150 mg BID) alone in 297 antiretroviral naive HIV-1 infected patients (median age 35 years [range 21 to 63], 89% male and 78% Caucasian). Mean baseline CD4 cell count was 288 cells/mm³ and mean baseline plasma HIV RNA was 5.21 $\log_{10}$ copies/mL (160,394 copies/mL). The percent of patients with plasma HIV RNA < 400 copies/mL and mean changes in CD4 cell count are summarized in Figures 1 and 2, respectively.

[See figure 1 at top of next column]

[See figure 2 at top of next column]

Study 542: VIRACEPT BID + stavudine + lamivudine compared to VIRACEPT TID + stavudine + lamivudine

Study 542 is an ongoing, randomized, open-label trial comparing the HIV RNA suppression achieved by VIRACEPT

Figure 1
Study 511: Percentage of Patients With HIV RNA Below 400 Copies/mL

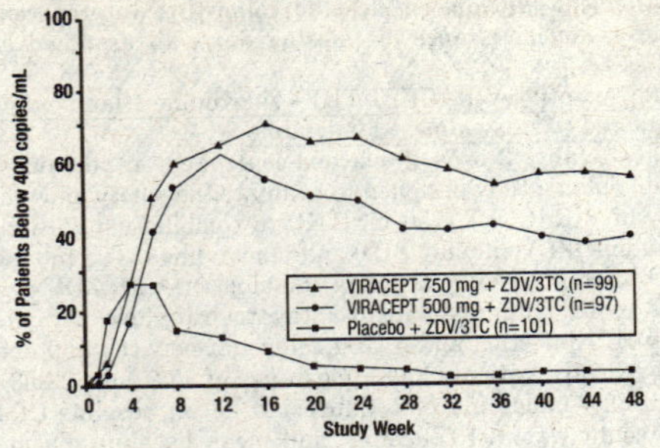

Figure 2
Study 511: Mean Change From Baseline in CD_4 Cell Counts

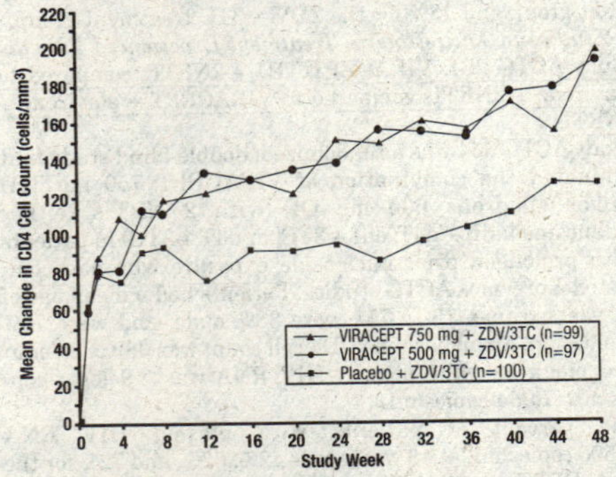

1250 mg BID versus VIRACEPT 750 mg TID in patients also receiving stavudine (d4T; 30-40 mg BID) and lamivudine (3TC; 150 mg BID). Patients had a median age of 36 years (range 18 to 83), were 84% male, and were 91% Caucasian. Patients had received less than 6 months of therapy with nucleoside transcriptase inhibitors and were naïve to protease inhibitors. Mean baseline CD4 cell count was 296 cells/mm³ and mean baseline plasma HIV RNA was 5.0 $\log_{10}$ copies/mL (100,706 copies/mL).

Results showed that there was no significant difference in mean CD4 cell count among treatment groups; the mean increases from baseline for the BID and TID arms were 150 cells/mm³ at 24 weeks and approximately 200 cells/mm³ at 48 weeks.

The percent of patients with HIV RNA < 400 copies/mL is summarized in Figure 3. The outcomes of patients through 48 weeks of treatment are summarized in Table 6.

Figure 3
Study 542: Percentage of Patients With HIV RNA Below 400 Copies/mL

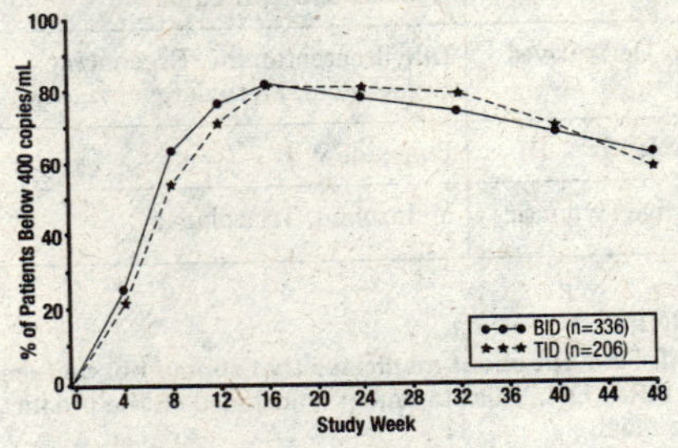

Table 6
Outcomes of Randomized Treatment Through 48 Weeks

Outcome	VIRACEPT 1250 mg BID Regimen	VIRACEPT 750 mg TID Regimen
Number of patients evaluable*	323	192
HIV RNA <400 copies/mL	198 (61%)	111 (58%)
HIV RNA ≥400 copies/mL	46 (14%)	22 (11%)
Discontinued due to VIRICEPT toxicity**	9 (3%)	2 (1%)
Discontinued due to other antiretroviral agents' toxicity**	3 (1%)	3 (2%)
Others***	67 (21%)	54 (28%)

*Twelve patients in the BID arm and fourteen patients in the TID arm have not yet reached 48 weeks of therapy.
**These rates only reflect dose-limiting toxicities that were counted as the initial reason for treatment failure in the anlysis (see ADVERSE REACTIONS for a description of the safety profile of these regimens).

Continued on next page

Viracept—Cont.

***Consent withdrawn, lost to follow-up, intercurrent illness, noncompliance or missing data; all assumed as failures.

Study Avanti 3: VIRACEPT TID + zidovudine + lamivudine compared to zidovudine + lamivudine

Study Avanti 3 was a placebo-controlled, randomized, double-blind study designed to evaluate the safety and efficacy of VIRACEPT (750 mg TID) in combination with zidovudine (ZDV; 300 mg BID) and lamivudine (3TC; 150 mg BID) (n=53) versus placebo in combination with ZDV and 3TC (n=52) administered to antiretroviral-naive patients with HIV infection and a CD4 cell count between 150 and 500 cells/μL. Patients had a mean age of 35 (range 22-59), were 89% male, and 88% Caucasian. Mean baseline CD4 cell count was 304 cells/mm^3 and mean baseline plasma HIV RNA was 4.8 $\log_{10}$ copies/mL (57,887 copies/mL). The percent of patients with plasma HIV RNA < 50 copies/mL at 52 weeks was 54% for the VIRACEPT + ZDV + 3TC treatment group and 13% for the ZDV + 3TC treatment group.

b. Studies in Antiretroviral Treatment Experienced Patients

Study ACTG 364: VIRACEPT TID + 2NRTIs compared to efavirenz + 2NRTIs compared to VIRACEPT + efavirenz + 2NRTIs

Study ACTG 364 was a randomized, double-blind study that evaluated the combination of VIRACEPT 750 mg TID and/or efavirenz 600 mg QD with 2 NRTIs (either didanosine [ddI] + d4T, ddI + 3TC, or d4T + 3TC) in patients with prolonged prior nucleoside exposure who had completed 2 previous ACTG studies. Patients had a mean age of 41 years (range 18 to 75), were 88% male, and were 74% Caucasian. Mean baseline CD4 cell count was 389 cells/mm^3 and mean baseline plasma HIV RNA was 3.9 $\log_{10}$ copies/mL (7,954 copies/mL).

The percent of patients with plasma HIV RNA < 500 copies/mL at 48 weeks was 42%, 62%, and 72% for the VIRACEPT (n=66), EFV (n=65), and VIRACEPT + EFV (n=64) treatment groups, respectively. The 4-drug combination of VIRACEPT + EFV + 2 NRTIs was more effective in suppressing plasma HIV RNA in these patients than either 3-drug regimen.

CONTRAINDICATIONS

VIRACEPT is contraindicated in patients with clinically significant hypersensitivity to any of its components.

Coadministration of VIRACEPT is contraindicated with drugs that are highly dependent on CYP3A for clearance and for which elevated plasma concentrations are associated with serious and/or life-threatening events. These drugs are listed in Table 7.

Table 7
Drugs That Are Contraindicated With VIRACEPT

Drug Class	Drugs Within Class That Are Contraindicated With VIRACEPT
Antiarrhythmics	Amiodarone, Quinidine
Ergot Derivatives	Dihydroergotamine, Ergonovine, Ergotamine, Methylergonovine
Neuroleptic	Pimoxide
Sedative/Hypnotics	Midazolam, Triazolam

WARNINGS

ALERT: Find out about medicines that should not be taken with VIRACEPT. This statement is included on the product's bottle label.

Drug Interactions (also see PRECAUTIONS)

Nelfinavir is an inhibitor of the CYP3A enzyme. Coadministration of VIRACEPT and drugs primarily metabolized by CYP3A may result in increased plasma concentrations of the other drug that could increase or prolong its therapeutic and adverse effects. Caution should be exercised when inhibitors of CYP3A, including VIRACEPT, are coadministered with drugs that are metabolized by CYP3A and that prolong the QT interval. (See ADVERSE REACTIONS; Post-Marketing Experience). Nelfinavir is metabolized by CYP3A and CYP2C19. Coadministration of VIRACEPT and drugs that induce CYP3A or CYP2C19 may decrease nelfinavir plasma concentrations and reduce its therapeutic effect. Coadministration of VIRACEPT and drugs that inhibit CYP3A or CYP2C19 may increase nelfinavir plasma concentrations. (Also see **PRECAUTIONS: Table 8: Drugs That Should Not Be Coadministered With VIRACEPT - Table 9: Established and Other Potentially Significant Drug Interactions With VIRACEPT.**)

Concomitant use of VIRACEPT with lovastatin or simvastatin is not recommended. Caution should be exercised if HIV protease inhibitors, including VIRACEPT, are used concurrently with other HMG-CoA reductase inhibitors that are also metabolized by the CYP3A pathway (e.g., atorvastatin). (Also see **Tables 4 and 5: Drug Interactions**). The risk of myopathy including rhabdomyolysis may be increased when protease inhibitors, including VIRACEPT, are used in combination with these drugs.

Particular caution should be used when prescribing sildenafil in patients receiving protease inhibitors, including VIRACEPT. Coadministration of a protease inhibitor with sildenafil is expected to substantially increase sildenafil concentrations and may result in an increase in sildenafil-associated adverse events, including hypotension, visual changes, and priapism. (See PRECAUTIONS, Drug Interactions and Information for Patients, and the complete prescribing information for sildenafil.)

Concomitant use of St. John's wort (hypericum perforatum) or St. John's wort containing products and VIRACEPT is not recommended. Coadministration of St. John's wort with protease inhibitors, including VIRACEPT, is expected to substantially decrease protease inhibitor concentrations and may result in sub-optimal levels of VIRACEPT and lead to loss of virologic response and possible resistance to VIRACEPT or to the class of protease inhibitors.

Patients with Phenylketonuria

Patients with Phenylketonuria: VIRACEPT Oral Powder contains 11.2 mg phenylalanine per gram of powder.

Diabetes mellitus/Hyperglycemia

New onset diabetes mellitus, exacerbation of pre-existing diabetes mellitus and hyperglycemia have been reported during post-marketing surveillance in HIV-infected patients receiving protease inhibitor therapy. Some patients required either initiation or dose adjustments of insulin or oral hypoglycemic agents for treatment of these events. In some cases diabetic ketoacidosis has occurred. In those patients who discontinued protease inhibitor therapy, hyperglycemia persisted in some cases. Because these events have been reported voluntarily during clinical practice, estimates of frequency cannot be made and a causal relationship between protease inhibitor therapy and these events has not been established.

PRECAUTIONS

General

Nelfinavir is principally metabolized by the liver. Therefore, caution should be exercised when administering this drug to patients with hepatic impairment.

Resistance/Cross Resistance

HIV cross-resistance between protease inhibitors has been observed. (See MICROBIOLOGY.)

Hemophilia

There have been reports of increased bleeding, including spontaneous skin hematomas and hemarthrosis, in patients with hemophilia type A and B treated with protease inhibitors. In some patients, additional factor VIII was given. In more than half of the reported cases, treatment with protease inhibitors was continued or reintroduced. A causal relationship has not been established.

Fat Redistribution

Redistribution/accumulation of body fat including central obesity, dorsocervical fat enlargement (buffalo hump), peripheral wasting, facial wasting, breast enlargement, and "cushingoid appearance" have been observed in patients receiving antiretroviral therapy. The mechanism and long-term consequences of these events are currently unknown. A causal relationship has not been established.

Information For Patients

"A statement to patients and health care providers is included on the product's bottle label: **ALERT: Find out about medicines that should NOT be taken with VIRACEPT.** A Patient Package Insert (PPI) for VIRACEPT is available for patient information."

For optimal absorption, patients should be advised to take VIRACEPT with food (see CLINICAL PHARMACOLOGY: Pharmacokinetics and DOSAGE AND ADMINISTRATION).

Patients should be informed that VIRACEPT is not a cure for HIV infection and that they may continue to acquire illnesses associated with advanced HIV infection, including opportunistic infections.

Patients should be told that there is currently no data demonstrating that VIRACEPT therapy can reduce the risk of transmitting HIV to others through sexual contact or blood contamination.

Patients should be told that sustained decreases in plasma HIV RNA have been associated with a reduced risk of progression to AIDS and death. Patients should be advised to take VIRACEPT and other concomitant antiretroviral therapy every day as prescribed. Patients should not alter the dose or discontinue therapy without consulting with their doctor. If a dose of VIRACEPT is missed, patients should take the dose as soon as possible and then return to their normal schedule. However, if a dose is skipped, the patient should not double the next dose.

Patients should be informed that VIRACEPT Tablets are film-coated and that this film-coating is intended to make the tablets easier to swallow.

The most frequent adverse event associated with VIRACEPT is diarrhea, which can usually be controlled with non-prescription drugs, such as loperamide, which slow gastrointestinal motility.

Patients should be informed that redistribution or accumulation of body fat may occur in patients receiving antiretroviral therapy and that the cause and long term health effects of these conditions are not known at this time.

VIRACEPT may interact with some drugs, therefore, patients should be advised to report to their doctor the use of any other prescription, non-prescription medication or herbal products, particularly St. John's wort.

Patients receiving oral contraceptives should be instructed that alternate or additional contraceptive measures should be used during therapy with VIRACEPT.

Patients receiving sildenafil and nelfinavir should be advised that they may be at an increased risk of sildenafil-associated adverse events including hypotension, visual changes, and prolonged penile erection, and should promptly report any symptoms to their doctor.

Drug Interactions (Also see CONTRAINDICATIONS, WARNINGS, CLINICAL PHARMACOLOGY: Drug Interactions)

Nelfinavir is an inhibitor of CYP3A. Coadministration of VIRACEPT and drugs primarily metabolized by CYP3A (e.g., dihydropyridine calcium channel blockers, HMG-CoA reductase inhibitors, immunosuppressants and sildenafil) may result in increased plasma concentrations of the other drug that could increase or prolong both its therapeutic and adverse effects. (See Tables 8 and 9). Nelfinavir is metabolized by CYP3A and CYP2C19. Coadministration of VIRACEPT and drugs that induce CYP3A or CYP2C19, such as rifampin, may decrease nelfinavir plasma concentrations and reduce its therapeutic effect. Coadministration of VIRACEPT and drugs that inhibit CYP3A or CYP2C19 may increase nelfinavir plasma concentrations.

Drug interaction studies reveal no clinically significant drug interactions between nelfinavir and didanosine, lamivudine, stavudine, zidovudine, efavirenz, nevirapine, or ketoconazole and no dose adjustments are needed. In the case of didanosine, it is recommended that didanosine be administered on an empty stomach; therefore, nelfinavir should be administered with food one hour after or more than 2 hours before didanosine.

Based on known metabolic profiles, clinically significant drug interactions are not expected between VIRACEPT and dapsone, trimethoprim/sulfamethoxazole, or itraconazole.

Table 8
Drugs That Should Not Be Coadministered With VIRACEPT

Drug Class: Drug Name	Clinical Comment
Antiarrhythmics: amiodarone, quinidine	CONTRAINDICATED due to potential for serious and/or life threatening reactions such as cardiac arrhythmias.
Antimycobacterial: rifampin	May lead to loss of virologic response and possible resistance to VIRACEPT or other coadministered antiretroviral agents.
Ergot Derivatives: dihydroergotamine, ergonovine, ergotamine, methylergonovine	CONTRAINDICATED due to potential for serious and/or life threatening reactions such as acute ergot toxicity characterized by peripheral vasospasm and ischemia of the extremities and other tissues.
Herbal Products: St. John's wort (hypericum perforatum)	May lead to loss of virologic response and possible resistance to VIRACEPT or other coadministered antiretroviral agents.
HMG-CoA Reductase Inhibitors: lovastatin, simvastatin	Potential for serious reactions such as risk of myopathy including rhabdomyolysis.
Neuroleptic: pimozide	CONTRAINDICATED due to potential for serious and/or life threatening reactions such as cardiac arrhythmias.
Sedative/Hypnotics: midazolam, triazolam	CONTRAINDICTED due to potential for serious and/or life threatening reactions such as prolonged or increased sedation or respiratory depression.

[See table 9 on next page]

Carcinogenesis, Mutagenesis, Impairment of Fertility

Long-term carcinogenicity studies in rats have been conducted with nelfinavir at doses of 0, 100, 300, and 1000 mg/kg/day via oral gavage. Thyroid follicular cell adenomas and carcinomas were increased in male rats at 300 mg/kg/day and higher and in female rats at 1000 mg/kg/day. The systemic exposures (C_{max}) at 300 and 1000 mg/kg/day were 1- to 3-fold, respectively, of those measured in humans at the recommended therapeutic dose (750 mg TID or 1250 mg BID). The mechanism of nelfinavir-induced tumorogenesis in rats is unknown. However, nelfinavir showed no evidence of mutagenic or clastogenic activity in a battery of *in vitro* and *in vivo* genetic toxicology assays. These studies included bacterial mutation assays in *S. typhimurium* and *E. coli*, a mouse lymphoma tyrosine kinase assay, a chromosomal aberration assay in human lymphocytes, and an *in vivo* mouse bone marrow micronucleus assay. Given the lack of genotoxic activity of nelfinavir, the relevance to humans of neoplasms in nelfinavir-treated rats is not known.

Nelfinavir produced no effects on either male or female mating and fertility or embryo survival in rats at systemic exposures comparable to the human therapeutic exposure.

Pregnancy—Pregnancy Category B

There were no effects on fetal development or maternal toxicity when nelfinavir was administered to pregnant rats at systemic exposures (AUC) comparable to human exposure. Administration of nelfinavir to pregnant rabbits resulted in no fetal development effects up to a dose at which a slight decrease in maternal body weight was observed; however, even at the highest dose evaluated, systemic exposure in rabbits was significantly lower than human exposure. Additional studies in rats indicated that exposure to nelfinavir in females from mid-pregnancy through lactation had no effect on the survival, growth, and development of the offspring to weaning. Subsequent reproductive performance of these offspring was also not affected by maternal exposure to nelfinavir. However, there are no adequate and well-controlled studies in pregnant women taking VIRACEPT. Because animal reproduction studies are not always predictive of human response, VIRACEPT should be used during pregnancy only if clearly needed.

Antiretroviral Pregnancy Registry: (APR): To monitor maternal-fetal outcomes of pregnant women exposed to VIRACEPT and other antiretroviral agents, an Antiretroviral Pregnancy Registry has been established. Physicians are encouraged to register patients by calling (800) 258-4263.

Nursing Mothers

The Centers for Disease Control and Prevention recommends that HIV-infected mothers not breast-feed their infants to avoid risking postnatal transmission of HIV. Studies in lactating rats have demonstrated that nelfinavir is excreted in milk. Because of both the potential for HIV transmission and the potential for serious adverse reactions in nursing infants, **mothers should be instructed not to breast-feed if they are receiving VIRACEPT.**

Pediatric Use

The safety and effectiveness of VIRACEPT have been established in patients from 2 to 13 years of age. The use of VIRACEPT in these age groups is supported by evidence from adequate and well-controlled studies of VIRACEPT in adults and pharmacokinetic studies and studies supporting activity in pediatric patients. In patients less than 2 years of age, VIRACEPT was found to be safe at the doses studied, but a reliably effective dose could not be established (see CLINICAL PHARMACOLOGY: Special Populations, ADVERSE REACTIONS: Pediatric Population, and DOSAGE AND ADMINISTRATION: Pediatric Patients).

The following issues should be considered when initiating VIRACEPT in pediatric patients:

- In pediatric patients ≥ 2 years of age receiving VIRACEPT as part of triple combination antiretroviral therapy in randomized studies, the proportion of patients achieving a HIV RNA level <400 copies/mL through 48 weeks ranged from 26% to 42%.
- Response rates in children <2 years of age appeared to be poorer than those in patients ≥ 2 years of age in some studies.
- Highly variable drug exposure remains a significant problem in the use of VIRACEPT in pediatric patients. Unpredictable drug exposure may be exacerbated in pediatric patients because of increased clearance compared to adults and difficulties with compliance and adequate food intake with dosing. Pharmacokinetic results from the pediatric studies are reported in Table 3 (see Clinical Pharmacology, Special Populations).

Study 556 was a randomized, double-blind, placebo-controlled trial with VIRACEPT or placebo coadministered with ZDV and ddI in 141 HIV-positive children who had received minimal antiretroviral therapy. The mean age of the children was 3.9 years. 94 (67%) children were between 2-12 years, and 47 (33%) were < 2 years of age. The mean baseline HIV RNA value was 5.0 log for all patients and the mean CD4 cell count was 886 cells/mm^3 for all patients. The efficacy of VIRACEPT measured by HIV RNA <400 at 48 weeks in children ≥ 2 years of age was 26% compared to 2% of placebo patients (p=0.0008). In the children < 2 years of age, only 1 of 27 and 2 of 20 maintained an undetectable HIV RNA level at 48 weeks for placebo and VIRACEPT patients respectively.

PACTG 377 was an open-label study that randomized 181 HIV treatment-experienced pediatric patients to receive: d4T+NVP+RTV, d4T+3TC+NFV, or d4T+3TC+NVP+NFV with NFV given on a TID schedule. The median age was 5.9 years and 46% were male. At baseline the median HIV RNA was 4.4 log and median CD4 cell count was 690 cells/mm^3. Substudy PACTG 725 evaluated d4T+3TC+NFV with NFV given on a BID schedule. The proportion of patients with detectable viral load at baseline achieving HIV RNA <400 copies/mL at 48 weeks was: 41% for d4T+NVP+RTV, 42% for d4T+3TC+NFV, 30% for d4T+NVP+NFV, and 52% for d4T+3TC+NVP+NFV. No significant clinical differences were identified between patients receiving VIRACEPT in BID or TID schedules.

VIRACEPT has been evaluated in 2 studies of young infants. The PENTA 7 study was an open-label study to evaluate the toxicity, tolerability, pharmacokinetics, and activity of NFV+d4T+ddI in 20 HIV-infected infants less than 12 weeks of age. PACTG 353 evaluated the pharmacokinetics and safety of VIRACEPT in infants born to HIV-infected women receiving NFV as part of combination therapy during pregnancy.

Geriatric Use

Clinical studies of VIRACEPT did not include sufficient numbers of subjects aged 65 and over to determine whether they respond differently from younger subjects.

ADVERSE REACTIONS

The safety of VIRACEPT was studied in over 5000 patients who received drug either alone or in combination with nucleoside analogues. The majority of adverse events were of mild intensity. The most frequently reported adverse event among patients receiving VIRACEPT was diarrhea, which was generally of mild to moderate intensity. The frequency of nelfinavir-associated diarrhea may be increased in patients receiving the 625 mg tablet because of the increased bioavailability of this formulation.

Drug-related clinical adverse experiences of moderate or severe intensity in ≥ 2% of patients treated with VIRACEPT coadministered with d4T and 3TC (Study 542) for up to 48 weeks or with ZDV plus 3TC (Study 511) for up to 24 weeks are presented in Table 10.

[See table 10 on next page]

Adverse events occurring in less than 2% of patients receiving VIRACEPT in all phase II/III clinical trials and considered at least possibly related or of unknown relationship to treatment and of at least moderate severity are listed below.

Body as a Whole: abdominal pain, accidental injury, allergic reaction, asthenia, back pain, fever, headache, malaise, pain, and redistribution/accumulation of body fat (see PRECAUTIONS, Fat Redistribution).

Digestive System: anorexia, dyspepsia, epigastric pain, gastrointestinal bleeding, hepatitis, mouth ulceration, pancreatitis and vomiting.

Hemic/Lymphatic System: anemia, leukopenia and thrombocytopenia.

Metabolic/Nutritional System: increases in alkaline phosphatase, amylase, creatine phosphokinase, lactic dehydrogenase, SGOT, SGPT and gamma glutamyl transpeptidase; hyperlipemia, hyperuricemia, hyperglycemia, hypoglycemia, dehydration, and liver function tests abnormal.

Musculoskeletal System: arthralgia, arthritis, cramps, myalgia, myasthenia and myopathy.

Nervous System: anxiety, depression, dizziness, emotional lability, hyperkinesia, insomnia, migraine, paresthesia, seizures, sleep disorder, somnolence and suicide ideation.

Respiratory System: dyspnea, pharyngitis, rhinitis, and sinusitis.

Skin/Appendages: dermatitis, folliculitis, fungal dermatitis, maculopapular rash, pruritus, sweating, and urticaria.

Special Senses: acute iritis and eye disorder.

Urogenital System: kidney calculus, sexual dysfunction and urine abnormality.

Post-Marketing Experience

The following additional adverse experiences have been reported from postmarketing surveillance as at least possibly related or of unknown relationship to VIRACEPT:

Body as a Whole: hypersensitivity reactions (including bronchospasm, moderate to severe rash, fever and edema)

Cardiovascular System: QTc prolongation, torsades de pointes

Digestive System: jaundice

Metabolic/Nutritional System: bilirubinemia, metabolic acidosis

Laboratory Abnormalities

The percentage of patients with marked laboratory abnormalities in Studies 542 and 511 are presented in Table 11. Marked laboratory abnormalities are defined as a Grade 3

Continued on next page

Table 9
Established and Other Potentially Significant Drug Interactions:
Alteration in Dose or Regimen May Be Recommended Based on Drug Interaction Studies
(see CLINICAL PHARMACOLOGY, for Magnitude of Interaction, Tables 4 and 5)

Concomitant Drug Class: Drug Name	Effect on Concentration	Clinical Comment
HIV-Antiviral Agents		
Protease Inhibitors: indinavir ritonavir saquinavir	 ↑ nelfinavir ↑ indinavir ↑ nelfinavir ↑ saquinavir	Appropriate doses for these combinations, with respect to safety and efficacy, have not been established.
Non-nucleoside Reverse Transcriptase Inhibitors, delavirdine nevirapine	 ↑ nelfinavir ↓ delavirdine ↓ nelfinavir (C_{min})	Appropriate doses for these combinations, with respect to safety and efficacy, have not been established.
Nucleoside Reverse Transcriptase Inhibitor: didanosine		It is recommended that didanosine be administered on an empty stomach; therefore, didanosine should be given one hour before or two hours after VIRACEPT (given with food).
Other Agents		
Anti-Convulsants: carbamazepine phenobarbital	↓ nelfinavir	May decrease nelfinavir plasma concentrations. VIRACEPT may not be effective due to decreased nelfinavir plasma concentrations in patients taking these agents concomitantly.
Anti-Convulsant: phenytoin	↓ phenytoin	Phenytoin plasma/serum concentrations should be monitored; phenytoin dose may require adjustment to compensate for altered phenytoin concentration.
Anti-Mycobacterial: rifabutin	↑ rifabutin ↓ nelfinavir (750 mg TID) ↔nelfinavir (1250 mg BID)	It is recommended that the dose of rifabutin be reduced to one-half the usual dose when administered with VIRACEPT; 1250 mg BID is the preferred dose of VIRACEPT when coadministered with rifabutin.
Erectile Dysfunction Agent: sildenafil	↑ sildenafil	Sildenafil should not exceed a maximum single dose of 25 mg in a 48 hour period.
HMG-CoA Reductase Inhibitor: atorvastatin	↑ atorvastatin	Use lowest possible dose of atorvastatin with careful monitoring, or consider other HMG-CoA reductase inhibitors such as pravastatin or fluvastatin in combination with VIRACEPT.
Immuno-suppressants: cyclosporine tacrolimus sirolimus	↑ immuno-suppressants	Plasma concentrations may be increased by VIRACEPT.
Narcotic Analgesia: methadone	↓ methadone	Dosage of methadone may need to be increased when coadministered with VIRACEPT.
Oral Contraceptive: ethinyl estradiol	↓ ethinyl estradiol	Alternative or additional contraceptive measures should be used when oral contraceptives and VIRACEPT are coadministered.
Macrolide Antibiotic: azithromycin	↑ azithromycin	Dose adjustment of azithromycin is not recommended, but close monitoring for known side effects such as liver enzyme abnormalities and hearing impairment is warranted.

Viracept—Cont.

or 4 abnormality in a patient with a normal baseline value or a Grade 4 abnormality in a patient with a Grade 1 abnormality at baseline.
[See table 11 below]

Pediatric Population

VIRACEPT has been studied in approximately 400 pediatric patients in clinical trials from birth to 13 years of age. The adverse event profile seen during pediatric clinical trials was similar to that for adults.

The most commonly reported drug-related, treatment-emergent adverse events reported in the pediatric studies included: diarrhea, leukopenia/neutropenia, rash, anorexia and abdominal pain. Diarrhea, regardless of assigned relationship to study drug, was reported in 39% to 47% of pediatric patients receiving VIRACEPT in 2 of the larger treatment trials. Leukopenia/neutropenia was the laboratory abnormality most commonly reported as a significant event across the pediatric studies.

OVERDOSAGE

Human experience of acute overdose with VIRACEPT is limited. There is no specific antidote for overdose with VIRACEPT. If indicated, elimination of unabsorbed drug should be achieved by emesis or gastric lavage. Administration of activated charcoal may also be used to aid removal of unabsorbed drug. Since nelfinavir is highly protein bound, dialysis is unlikely to significantly remove drug from blood.

DOSAGE AND ADMINISTRATION

Adults: The recommended dose is 1250 mg (five 250 mg tablets or two 625 mg tablets) twice daily or 750 mg (three 250 mg tablets) three times daily. VIRACEPT should be taken with a meal. Patients unable to swallow the 250 or 625 mg tablets may dissolve the tablets in a small amount of water. Once dissolved, patients should mix the cloudy liquid well, and consume it immediately. The glass should be rinsed with water and the rinse swallowed to ensure the entire dose is consumed.

Pediatric Patients (2-13 years): In children 2 years of age and older, the recommended oral dose of VIRACEPT oral powder or 250 mg tablets is 45 to 55 mg/kg twice daily or 25 to 35 mg/kg three times daily. All doses should be taken **with a meal.** Doses higher than the adult maximum dose of 2500 mg per day have not been studied in children. For children unable to take tablets, VIRACEPT Oral Powder may be administered. The oral powder may be mixed with a small amount of water, milk, formula, soy formula, soy milk or dietary supplements; once mixed, the entire contents must be consumed in order to obtain the full dose. If the mixture is not consumed immediately, it must be stored under refrigeration, but storage must not exceed 6 hours. Acidic food or juice (e.g., orange juice, apple juice or apple sauce) are not recommended to be used in combination with VIRACEPT, because the combination may result in a bitter taste. VIRACEPT Oral Powder should not be reconstituted with water in its original container.

The healthcare provider should assess appropriate formulation and dosage for each patient. Crushed 250 mg tablets can be used in lieu of powder. Tables 12 and 13 provide dosing guidelines for VIRACEPT tablets and powder based on age and body weight.

Table 10
Percentage of Patients with Treatment-Emergent[1] Adverse Events of Moderate or Severe Intensity Reported in ≥ 2% of Patients

	Study 511 24 weeks			Study 542 48 weeks	
Adverse Events	Placebo + ZDV/3TC (n=101)	500 mg TID VIRACEPT + ZDV/3TC (n=97)	750 mg TID VIRACEPT + ZDV/3TC (n=100)	1250 mg BID VIRACEPT + d4T/3TC (n=344)	750 mg TID VIRACEPT + d4T/3TC (n=210)
Digestive System					
Diarrhea	3%	14%	20%	20%	15%
Nausea	4%	3%	7%	3%	3%
Flatulence	0	5%	2%	1%	1%
Skin/Appendages					
Rash	1%	1%	3%	2%	1%

[1] Includes those adverse events at least possibly related to study drug or of unknown relationship and excludes concurrent HIV conditions

Table 11
Percentage of Patients by Treatment Group With Marked Laboratory Abnormalities[1] in > 2% of Patients

	Study 511			Study 542	
	Placebo + ZDV/3TC (n=101)	500 mg TID VIRACEPT + ZDV/3TC (n=97)	750 mg TID VIRACEPT + ZDV/3TC (n=100)	1250 mg BID VIRACEPT + d4T/3TC (n=344)	750 mg TID VIRACEPT + d4T/3TC (n=210)
Hematology					
Hemoglobin	6%	3%	2%	0	0
Neutrophils	4%	3%	5%	2%	1%
Lymphocytes	1%	6%	1%	1%	0
Chemistry					
ALT (SGPT)	6%	1%	1%	2%	1%
AST (SGOT)	4%	1%	0	2%	1%
Creatine Kinase	7%	2%	2%	NA	NA

[1] Marked laboratory abnormalities are defined as a shift from Grade 0 at baseline to at least Grade 3 or from Grade 1 to Grade 4

Table 13
Dosing Table for Children ≥2 years of age (powder)

Body Weight		Twice Daily (BID) 45–55 mg/kg		Three Times Daily (TID) 25–35 mg/kg	
Kg.	Lbs.	Scoops of powder (50 mg/1 g)	Teaspoons[1] of Powder	Scoops of powder (50 mg/1 g)	Teaspoons[1] of Powder
9.0 to < 10.5	20 to < 23	10	2½	6	1½
10.5 to < 12	23 to < 26.5	11	2¾	7	1¾
12 to < 14	26.5 to < 31	13	3¼	8	2
14 to < 16	31 to < 35	15	3¾	9	2¼
16 to < 18	35 to < 39.5	Not recommended[2]	Not recommended[2]	10	2½
18 to < 23	39.5 to < 50.5	Not recommended[2]	Not recommended[2]	12	3
≥23	≥50.5	Not recommended[2]	Not recommended[2]	15	3¾

[1] If a teaspoon is used to measure VIRACEPT oral powder, 1 level teaspoon contains 200 mg of VIRACEPT (4 level scoops equals 1 level teaspoon)
[2] Use VIRACEPT 250 mg tablet

Table 12
Dosing Table for Children ≥ 2 years of age (tablets)

Body Weight		Twice Daily (BID) 45–55 mg/kg ≥2 years	Three Times Daily (TID) 25–35 mg/kg ≥2 years
Kg.	Lbs.	# of tablets (250 mg)	# of tablets (250 mg)
10–12	22–26.4	2	1
13–18	28.6–39.6	3	2
19–20	41.8–44	4	2
≥21	≥46.2	4–5[1]	3[2]

[1] For BID dosing, the maximum dose per day is 5 tablets BID
[2] For TID dosing, the maximum dose per day is 3 tablets TID

[See table 13 at left]

HOW SUPPLIED

VIRACEPT (nelfinavir mesylate) 250 mg: Light blue, capsule-shaped tablets with a clear film coating engraved with "VIRACEPT" on one side and "250 mg" on the other.
Bottles of 300, 250 mg tablets .... NDC 63010-010-30
VIRACEPT (nelfinavir mesylate) 625 mg: White oval tablet with a clear film coating engraved with "V" on one side and "625" on the other.
Bottles of 120, 625 mg tablets .... NDC 63010-027-70
VIRACEPT (nelfinavir mesylate) Oral Powder is available as a 50 mg/g off-white powder containing 50 mg (as nelfinavir free base) in each level scoopful (1 gram).
Multiple use bottles of 144 grams of powder with scoop .... NDC 63010-011-90
VIRACEPT TABLETS AND ORAL POWDER SHOULD BE STORED AT 15° TO 30°C (59° TO 86°F).
Keep container tightly closed. Dispense in original container.
RX only
VIRACEPT and Agouron are registered trademarks of Agouron Pharmaceuticals, Inc.

69-6003-00-8 Revised April 2004

ZITHROMAX®

℞

[*zĭth-rō-măks*]
(azithromycin tablets)
and
(azithromycin for oral suspension)

Prescribing information for this product, which appears on pages 2675–2682 of the 2004 PDR, has been completely revised as follows. Please write "See Supplement A" next to the product heading.

To reduce the development of drug-resistant bacteria and maintain the effectiveness of ZITHROMAX® (azithromycin) and other bacterial drugs, ZITHROMAX (azithromycin) should be used only to treat or prevent infections that are proven or strongly suspected to be caused by bacteria.

DESCRIPTION

ZITHROMAX (azithromycin tablets and azithromycin for oral suspension) contain the active ingredient azithromycin, an azalide, a subclass of macrolide antibiotics, for oral administration. Azithromycin has the chemical name (*2R,3S,4R,5R,8R, 10R,11R,12S,13S,14R*)- 13-[(2,6-dideoxy-3-*C*-methyl-3-*O*-methyl-α-*L*-*ribo*-hexopyranosyl)oxy]-2-ethyl-3,4,10-trihydroxy-3,5,6,8,10,12,14-heptamethyl-11-[[3,4,6-trideoxy-3-(dimethylamino)-β-*D*-*xylo*-hexopyranosyl]oxy]-1-oxa-6-azacyclopentadecan-15-one. Azithromycin is derived from erythromycin; however, it differs chemically from erythromycin in that a methyl-substituted nitrogen atom is incorporated into the lactone ring. Its molecular formula is $C_{38}H_{72}N_2O_{12}$, and its molecular weight is 749.00. Azithromycin has the following structural formula:
[See chemical structure at top of next column]

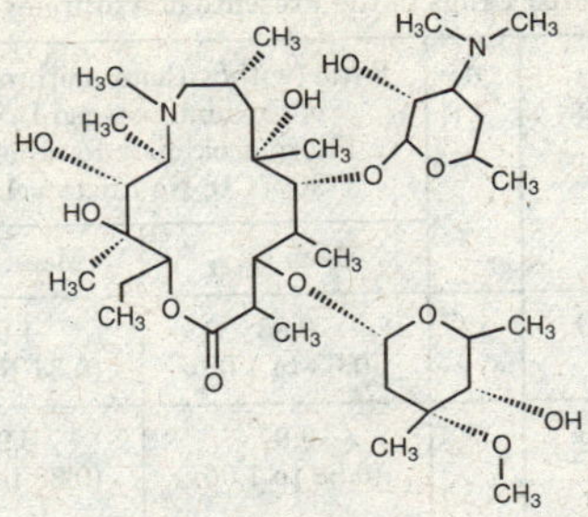

Azithromycin, as the dihydrate, is a white crystalline powder with a molecular formula of $C_{38}H_{72}N_2O_{12}\bullet 2H_2O$ and a molecular weight of 785.0.

ZITHROMAX is supplied for oral administration as film-coated, modified capsular shaped tablets containing azithromycin dihydrate equivalent to either 250 mg or 500 mg azithromycin and the following inactive ingredients: dibasic calcium phosphate anhydrous, pregelatinized starch, sodium croscarmellose, magnesium stearate, sodium lauryl sulfate, hypromellose, lactose, titanium dioxide, triacetin and D&C Red #30 aluminum lake.

ZITHROMAX for oral suspension is supplied in bottles containing azithromycin dihydrate powder equivalent to 300 mg, 600 mg, 900 mg, or 1200 mg azithromycin per bottle and the following inactive ingredients: sucrose; sodium phosphate, tribasic, anhydrous; hydroxypropyl cellulose; xanthan gum; FD&C Red #40; and spray dried artificial cherry, creme de vanilla and banana flavors. After constitution, each 5 mL of suspension contains 100 mg or 200 mg of azithromycin.

CLINICAL PHARMACOLOGY

Pharmacokinetics

Following oral administration of a single 500 mg dose (two 250 mg tablets) to 36 fasted healthy male volunteers, the mean (SD) pharmacokinetic parameters were AUC_{0-72} = 4.3 (1.2) μg•h/mL; C_{max} = 0.5 (0.2) μg/mL; T_{max} = 2.2 (0.9) hours.

With a regimen of 500 mg (two 250 mg capsules*) on day 1, followed by 250 mg daily (one 250 mg capsule) on days 2 through 5, the pharmacokinetic parameters of azithromycin in plasma in healthy young adults (18-40 years of age) are portrayed in the chart below. C_{min} and C_{max} remained essentially unchanged from day 2 through day 5 of therapy.

Pharmacokinetic Parameters (Mean)	Total n=12 Day 1	Day 5
C_{max} (μg/mL)	0.41	0.24
T_{max} (h)	2.5	3.2
AUC_{0-24} (μg•h/mL)	2.6	2.1
C_{min} (μg/mL)	0.05	0.05
Urinary Excret. (% dose)	4.5	6.5

*Azithromycin 250 mg tablets are bioequivalent to 250 mg capsules in the fasted state. Azithromycin 250 mg capsules are no longer commercially available.

In a two-way crossover study, 12 adult healthy volunteers (6 males, 6 females) received 1,500 mg of azithromycin administered in single daily doses over either 5 days (two 250 mg tablets on day 1, followed by one 250 mg tablet on days 2-5) or 3 days (500 mg per day for days 1-3). Due to limited serum samples on day 2 (3-day regimen) and days 2-4 (5-day regimen), the serum concentration-time profile of each subject was fit to a 3-compartment model and the $AUC_{0-\infty}$ for the fitted concentration profile was comparable between the 5-day and 3-day regimens.

[See first table above]

Median azithromycin exposure (AUC_{0-288}) in mononuclear (MN) and polymorphonuclear (PMN) leukocytes following either the 5-day or 3-day regimen was more than a 1000-fold and 800-fold greater than in serum, respectively. Administration of the same total dose with either the 5-day or 3-day regimen may be expected to provide comparable concentrations of azithromycin within MN and PMN leukocytes.

Two azithromycin 250 mg tablets are bioequivalent to a single 500 mg tablet.

Absorption

The absolute bioavailability of azithromycin 250 mg capsules is 38%.

In a two-way crossover study in which 12 healthy subjects received a single 500 mg dose of azithromycin (two 250 mg tablets) with or without a high fat meal, food was shown to increase C_{max} by 23% but had no effect on AUC.

When azithromycin suspension was administered with food to 28 adult healthy male subjects, C_{max} increased by 56% and AUC was unchanged.

The AUC of azithromycin was unaffected by co-administration of an antacid containing aluminum and magnesium hydroxide with azithromycin capsules; however, the C_{max} was reduced by 24%. Administration of cimetidine (800 mg) two hours prior to azithromycin had no effect on azithromycin absorption.

Distribution

The serum protein binding of azithromycin is variable in the concentration range approximating human exposure, decreasing from 51% at 0.02 μg/mL to 7% at 2 μg/mL.

Following oral administration, azithromycin is widely distributed throughout the body with an apparent steady-state

Pharmackoinetic Parameter [mean (SD)]	3-Day Regimen Day 1	Day 3	5-Day Regimen Day 1	Day 5
C_{max} (serum, μg/mL)	0.44 (0.22)	0.54 (0.25)	0.43 (0.20)	0.24 (0.06)
Serum $AUC_{0-\infty}$ (μg•hr/mL)	17.4 (6.2)*		14.9 (3.1)*	
Serum $T_{½}$	71.8 hr		68.9 hr	

*Total AUC for the entire 3-day and 5-day regimens

AZITHROMYCIN CONCENTRATIONS FOLLOWING A 500 mg DOSE (TWO 250 mg CAPSULES) IN ADULTS[1]

TISSUE OR FLUID	TIME AFTER DOSE (h)	TISSUE OR FLUID CONCENTRATION (μg/g or μg/mL)	CORRESPONSING PLASMA OR SERUM LEVEL (μg/mL)	TISSUE (FLUID) PLASMA (SERUM) RATIO
SKIN	72-96	0.4	0.012	35
LUNG	72-96	4.0	0.012	>100
SPUTUM*	2-4	1.0	0.64	2
SPUTUM**	10-12	2.9	0.1	30
TONSIL***	9-18	4.5	0.03	>100
TONSIL***	180	0.9	0.006	>100
CERVIX****	19	2.8	0.04	70

[1] Azithromycin tissue concentrations were originally determined using 250 mg capsules.
* Sample was obtained 2–4 hours after the first dose.
** Sample was obtained 10–12 hours after the first dose.
*** Dosing regimen of two doses of 250 mg each, separated by 12 hours.
**** Sample was obtained 19 hours after a single 500 mg dose.

volume of distribution of 31.1 L/kg. Greater azithromycin concentrations in tissues than in plasma or serum were observed. High tissue concentrations should not be interpreted to be quantitatively related to clinical efficacy. The antimicrobial activity of azithromycin is pH related and appears to be reduced with decreasing pH. However, the extensive distribution of drug to tissues may be relevant to clinical activity.

Selected tissue (or fluid) concentration and tissue (or fluid) to plasma/serum concentration ratios are shown in the following table:

[See second table above]

The extensive tissue distribution was confirmed by examination of additional tissues and fluids (bone, ejaculum, prostate, ovary, uterus, salpinx, stomach, liver, and gallbladder). As there are no data from adequate and well-controlled studies of azithromycin treatment of infections in these additional body sites, the clinical importance of these tissue concentration data is unknown.

Following a regimen of 500 mg on the first day and 250 mg daily for 4 days, only very low concentrations were noted in cerebrospinal fluid (less than 0.01 μg/mL) in the presence of non-inflamed meninges.

Metabolism

In vitro and *in vivo* studies to assess the metabolism of azithromycin have not been performed.

Elimination

Plasma concentrations of azithromycin following single 500 mg oral and i.v. doses declined in a polyphasic pattern with a mean apparent plasma clearance of 630 mL/min and terminal elimination half-life of 68 hours. The prolonged terminal half-life is thought to be due to extensive uptake and subsequent release of drug from tissues.

Biliary excretion of azithromycin, predominantly as unchanged drug, is a major route of elimination. Over the course of a week, approximately 6% of the administered dose appears as unchanged drug in urine.

Special Populations

Renal Insufficiency

Azithromycin pharmacokinetics were investigated in 42 adults (21 to 85 years of age) with varying degrees of renal impairment. Following the oral administration of a single 1,000 mg dose of azithromycin, mean C_{max} and AUC_{0-120} increased by 5.1% and 4.2%, respectively in subjects with mild to moderate renal impairment (GFR 10 to 80 mL/min) compared to subjects with normal renal function (GFR >80 mL/min). The mean C_{max} and AUC_{0-120} increased 61% and 35%, respectively in subjects with severe renal impairment (GFR <10 mL/min) compared to subjects with normal renal function (GFR >80 mL/min). (See **DOSAGE AND ADMINISTRATION**.)

Hepatic Insufficiency

The pharmacokinetics of azithromycin in subjects with hepatic impairment have not been established.

Gender

There are no significant differences in the disposition of azithromycin between male and female subjects. No dosage adjustment is recommended based on gender.

Geriatric Patients

When studied in healthy elderly subjects aged 65 to 85 years, the pharmacokinetic parameters of azithromycin in elderly men were similar to those in young adults; however, in elderly women, although higher peak concentrations (increased by 30 to 50%) were observed, no significant accumulation occurred.

Pediatric Patients

In two clinical studies, azithromycin for oral suspension was dosed at 10 mg/kg on day 1, followed by 5 mg/kg on days 2 through 5 to two groups of pediatric patients (aged 1-5 years and 5-15 years, respectively). The mean pharmacokinetic parameters on day 5 were C_{max}=0.216 μg/mL, T_{max}=1.9 hours, and AUC_{0-24}=1.822 μg•hr/mL for the 1- to 5-year-old group and were C_{max}=0.383 μg/mL, T_{max}=2.4 hours, and AUC_{0-24}=3.109 μg•hr/mL for the 5- to 15-year-old group.

Two clinical studies were conducted in 68 pediatric patients aged 3-16 years to determine the pharmacokinetics and safety of azithromycin for oral suspension. Azithromycin was administered following a low-fat breakfast.

The first study consisted of 35 pediatric patients treated with 20 mg/kg/day (maximum daily dose 500 mg) for 3 days of whom 34 patients were evaluated for pharmacokinetics.

In the second study, 33 pediatric patients received doses of 12 mg/kg/day (maximum daily dose 500 mg) for 5 days of whom 31 patients were evaluated for pharmacokinetics.

In both studies, azithromycin concentrations were determined over a 24 hour period following the last daily dose. Patients weighing above 25.0 kg in the 3-day study or 41.7 kg in the 5-day study received the maximum adult daily dose of 500 mg. Eleven patients (weighing 25.0 kg or less) in the first study and 17 patients (weighing 41.7 kg or less) in the second study received a total dose of 60 mg/kg. The following table shows pharmacokinetic data in the subset of pediatric patients who received a total dose of 60 mg/kg.

Pharmacokinetic Parameter [mean (SD)]	3-Day Regimen (20 mg/kg × 3 days)	5-Day Regimen (12 mg/kg × 5 days)
n	11	17
C_{max} (μg/mL)	1.1 (0.4)	0.5 (0.4)
T_{max} (hr)	2.7 (1.9)	2.2 (0.8)
AUC_{0-24} (μg•hr/mL)	7.9 (2.9)	3.9 (1.9)

The similarity of the overall exposure ($AUC_{0-\infty}$) between the 3-day and 5-day regimens in pediatric patients is unknown. Single dose pharmacokinetics in pediatric patients given doses of 30 mg/kg have not been studied. (See **DOSAGE AND ADMINISTRATION**.)

Drug-Drug Interactions

Drug interaction studies were performed with azithromycin and other drugs likely to be co-administered. The effects of co-administration of azithromycin on the pharmacokinetics of other drugs are shown in Table 1 and the effect of other drugs on the pharmacokinetics of azithromycin are shown in Table 2.

Co-administration of azithromycin at therapeutic doses had a modest effect on the pharmacokinetics of the drugs listed in Table 1. No dosage adjustment of drugs listed in Table 1 is recommended when co-administered with azithromycin.

Co-administration of azithromycin with efavirenz or fluconazole had a modest effect on the pharmacokinetics of azithromycin. Nelfinavir significantly increased the C_{max} and AUC of azithromycin. No dosage adjustment of azithromycin is recommended when administered with drugs listed in Table 2. (See **PRECAUTIONS - Drug Interactions.**)

[See table 1 at top of next page]

Mean rifabutin concentrations one-half day after the last dose of rifabutin were 60 ng/mL when co-administered with azithromycin and 71 ng/mL when co-administered with placebo.

[See table 2 on next page]

Microbiology: Azithromycin acts by binding to the 50S ribosomal subunit of susceptible microorganisms and, thus,

Continued on next page

Zithromax Tabs/O.S.—Cont.

interfering with microbial protein synthesis. Nucleic acid synthesis is not affected.

Azithromycin concentrates in phagocytes and fibroblasts as demonstrated by *in vitro* incubation techniques. Using such methodology, the ratio of intracellular to extracellular concentration was >30 after one hour incubation. *In vivo* studies suggest that concentration in phagocytes may contribute to drug distribution to inflamed tissues.

Azithromycin has been shown to be active against most isolates of the following microorganisms, both *in vitro* and in clinical infections as described in the **INDICATIONS AND USAGE** section.

Aerobic and facultative gram-positive microorganisms

Staphylococcus aureus
Streptococcus agalactiae
Streptococcus pneumoniae
Streptococcus pyogenes

NOTE: Azithromycin demonstrates cross-resistance with erythromycin-resistant gram-positive strains. Most strains of *Enterococcus faecalis* and methicillin-resistant staphylococci are resistant to azithromycin.

Aerobic and facultative gram-negative microorganisms

Haemophilus ducreyi
Haemophilus influenzae
Moraxella catarrhalis
Neisseria gonorrhoeae

"Other" microorganisms

Chlamydia pneumoniae
Chlamydia trachomatis
Mycoplasma pneumoniae

Beta-lactamase production should have no effect on azithromycin activity.

The following *in vitro* data are available, **but their clinical significance is unknown.**

At least 90% of the following microorganisms exhibit an *in vitro* minimum inhibitory concentration (MIC) less than or equal to the susceptible breakpoints for azithromycin. However, the safety and effectiveness of azithromycin in treating clinical infections due to these microorganisms have not been established in adequate and well-controlled trials.

Aerobic and facultative gram-positive microorganisms

Streptococci (Groups C, F, G)
Viridans group streptococci

Aerobic and facultative gram-negative microorganisms

Bordetella pertussis
Legionella pneumophila

Anaerobic microorganisms

Peptostreptococcus species
Prevotella bivia

"Other" microorganisms

Ureaplasma urealyticum

Susceptibility Testing Methods:

When available, the results of *in vitro* susceptibility test results for antimicrobial drugs used in resident hospitals should be provided to the physician as periodic reports which describe the susceptibility profile of nosocomial and community-acquired pathogens. These reports may differ from susceptibility data obtained from outpatient use, but could aid the physician in selecting the most effective antimicrobial.

Dilution techniques:

Quantitative methods are used to determine antimicrobial minimum inhibitory concentrations (MICs). These MICs provide estimates of the susceptibility of bacteria to antimicrobial compounds. The MICs should be determined using a standardized procedure. Standardized procedures are based on a dilution method[1,3] (broth or agar) or equivalent with standardized inoculum concentrations and standardized concentrations of azithromycin powder. The MIC values should be interpreted according to criteria provided in Table 1.

Diffusion techniques:

Quantitative methods that require measurement of zone diameters also provide reproducible estimates of the susceptibility of bacteria to antimicrobial compounds. One such standardized procedure[2,3] requires the use of standardized inoculum concentrations. This procedure uses paper disks impregnated with 15-µg azithromycin to test the susceptibility of microorganisms to azithromycin. The disk diffusion interpretive criteria are provided in Table 1.

[See table 1 at top of next page]

No interpretive criteria have been established for testing *Neisseria gonorrhoeae*. This species is not usually tested.

A report of "susceptible" indicates that the pathogen is likely to be inhibited if the antimicrobial compound reaches the concentrations usually achievable. A report of "intermediate" indicates that the result should be considered equivocal, and, if the microorganism is not fully susceptible to alternative, clinically feasible drugs, the test should be repeated. This category implies possible clinical applicability in body sites where the drug is physiologically concentrated or in situations where high dosage of drug can be used. This category also provides a buffer zone which prevents small uncontrolled technical factors from causing major discrepancies in interpretation. A report of "resistant" indicates that the pathogen is not likely to be inhibited if the antimicrobial compound reaches the concentrations usually achievable; other therapy should be selected.

QUALITY CONTROL:

Standardized susceptibility test procedures require the use of quality control microorganisms to control the technical aspects of the test procedures. Standard azithromycin powder should provide the following range of values noted in Table 2. Quality control microorganisms are specific strains of organisms with intrinsic biological properties. QC strains are very stable strains which will give a standard and repeatable susceptibility pattern. The specific strains used for microbiological quality control are not clinically significant.

Table 1. Drug Interactions: Pharmacokinetic Parameters for Co-administered Drugs in the Presence of Azithromycin

Co-administered Drug	Dose of Co-administered Drug	Dose of Azithromycin	n	Ratio (with/without azithromycin) of Co-administered Drug Pharmacokinetic Parameters (90% CI); No Effect = 1.00	
				Mean C_{max}	Mean AUC
Atrovastatin	10 mg/day × 8 days	500 mg/day PO on days 6-8	12	0.83 (0.63 to 1.08)	1.01 (0.81 to 1.25)
Carbamazepine	200 mg/day × 2 days, then 200 mg BID × 18 days	500 mg/day PO for days 16-18	7	0.97 (0.88 to 1.06)	0.96 (0.88 to 1.06)
Cetirizine	20 mg/day × 11 days	500 mg PO on day 7, then 250 mg day on days 8-11	14	1.03 (0.93 to 1.14)	1.02 (0.92 to 1.13)
Didanosine	200 mg PO BID × 21 days	1,200 mg/day PO on days 8-21	6	1.44 (0.85 to 2.43)	1.14 (0.83 to 1.57)
Efavirenz	400 mg/day × 7 days	600 mg PO on day 7	14	1.04*	0.95*
Fluconazole	200 mg PO single dose	1,200 mg PO single dose	18	1.04 (0.98 to 1.11)	1.01 (0.97 to 1.05)
Indinavir	800 mg TID × 5 days	1,200 mg PO on day 5	18	0.96 (0.86 to 1.08)	0.90 (0.81 to 1.00)
Midazolam	15 mg PO on day 3	500 mg/day PO × 3 days	12	1.27 (0.89 to 1.81)	1.26 (1.01 to 1.56)
Nelfinavir	750 mg TID × 11 days	1,200 mg PO on day 9	14	0.90 (0.81 to 1.01)	0.85 (0.78 to 0.93)
Rifabutin	300 mg/day × 10 days	500 mg PO on day 1, then 250 mg/day on days 2-10	6	See footnote below	NA
Sildenafil	100 mg on days 1 and 4	500 mg/day PO × 3 days	12	1.16 (0.86 to 1.57)	0.92 (0.75 to 1.12)
Theophylline	4 mg/kg IV on days 1, 11, 25	500 mg PO on day 7, 250 mg/ day on days 8-11	10	1.19 (1.02 to 1.40)	1.02 (0.86 to 1.22)
Theophylline	300 mg PO BID × 15 days	500 mg PO on day 6, then 250 mg/day on days 7-10	8	1.09 (0.92 to 1.29)	1.08 (0.89 to 1.31)
Triazolam	0.125 mg on day 2	500 mg PO on day 1, then 250 mg/day on day 2	12	1.06*	1.02*
Trimethoprim/Sulfamethoxazole	160 mg/800 mg/day PO × 7 days	1,200 mg PO on day 7	12	0.85 (0.75 to 0.97)/ 0.90 (0.78 to 1.03)	0.87 (0.80 to 0.95)/ 0.96 (0.88 to 1.03)
Zidovudine	500 mg/day PO × 21 days	600 mg/day PO × 14 days	5	1.12 (0.42 to 3.02)	0.94 (0.52 to 1.70)
Zidovudine	500 mg/day PO × 21 days	1,200 mg/day PO × 14 days	4	1.31 (0.43 to 3.97)	1.30 (0.69 to 2.43)

NA - Not Available
* - 90% Confidence interval not reported

Table 2. Drug Interactions: Pharmacokinetic Parameters for Azithromycin in the Presence of Co-administered Drugs (See **PRECAUTIONS—Drug Interactions.**)

Co-administered Drug	Dose of Co-administered Drug	Dose of Azithromycin	n	Ratio (with/without co-administered drug) of Azithromycin Pharmacokinetic Parameters (90% CI); No Effect = 1.00	
				Mean C_{max}	Mean AUC
Efavirenz	400 mg/day × 7 days	600 mg PO on day 7	14	1.22 (1.04 to 1.42)	0.92*
Fluconazole	200 mg PO single dose	1,200 mg PO single dose	18	0.82 (0.66 to 1.02)	1.07 (0.94 to 1.22)
Nelfinavir	750 mg TID × 11 days	1,200 mg PO on day 9	14	2.36 (1.77 to 3.15)	2.12 (1.80 to 2.50)
Rifabutin	300 mg/day × 10 days	500 mg PO on day 1, then 250 mg/ day on days 2-10	6	See footnote below	NA

NA – Not available
* - 90% Confidence interval not reported
Mean azithromycin concentrations one day after the last dose were 53 ng/mL when coadministered with 300 mg daily rifabutin and 49 ng/mL when coadministered with placebo.

Table 1. Susceptibility Interpretive Criteria for Azithromycin
Susceptibility Test Result Interpretive Criteria

Pathogen	Minimum Inhibitory Concentrations (μg/mL)			Disk Diffusion (zone diameters in mm)		
	S	I	R[a]	S	I	R[a]
Haemophilus spp.	≤ 4	—	—	≥ 12	—	—
Staphylococcus aureus	≤ 2	4	≥ 8	≥ 18	14-17	≤ 13
Streptococci including *S. pneumoniae*[b]	≤ 0.5	1	≥ 2	≥ 18	14-17	≤ 13

[a]The current absence of data on resistant strains precludes defining any category other than "susceptible." If strains yield MIC results other than susceptible, they should be submitted to a reference laboratory for further testing.
[b]Susceptibility of streptococci including *S. pneumoniae* to azithromycin and other macrolides can be predicted by testing erythromycin.

Table 2. Acceptable Quality Control Ranges for Azithromycin

QC Strain	Minimum Inhibitory Concentrations (μg/mL)	Disk Diffusion (zone diameters in mm)
Haemophilus influenzae ATCC 49247	1.0-4.0	13-21
Staphylococcus aureus ATCC 29213	0.5-2.0	
Staphylococcus aureus ATCC 25923		21-26
Streptococcus pneumoniae ATCC 49619	0.06-0.25	19-25

[See table 2 above]

INDICATIONS AND USAGE

ZITHROMAX (azithromycin) is indicated for the treatment of patients with mild to moderate infections (pneumonia: see **WARNINGS**) caused by susceptible strains of the designated microorganisms in the specific conditions listed below. As recommended dosages, durations of therapy and applicable patient populations vary among these infections, please see **DOSAGE AND ADMINISTRATION** for specific dosing recommendations.

Adults:

Acute bacterial exacerbations of chronic obstructive pulmonary disease due to *Haemophilus influenzae, Moraxella catarrhalis* or *Streptococcus pneumoniae.*

Acute bacterial sinusitis due to *Haemophilus influenzae, Moraxella catarrhalis* or *Streptococcus pneumoniae.*

Community-**acquired pneumonia** due to *Chlamydia pneumoniae, Haemophilus influenzae, Mycoplasma pneumoniae* or *Streptococcus pneumoniae* in patients appropriate for oral therapy.

NOTE: Azithromycin should not be used in patients with pneumonia who are judged to be inappropriate for oral therapy because of moderate to severe illness or risk factors such as any of the following:

patients with cystic fibrosis,
patients with nosocomially acquired infections,
patients with known or suspected bacteremia,
patients requiring hospitalization,
elderly or debilitated patients, or
patients with significant underlying health problems that may compromise their ability to respond to their illness (including immunodeficiency or functional asplenia).

Pharyngitis/tonsillitis caused by *Streptococcus pyogenes* as an alternative to first-line therapy in individuals who cannot use first-line therapy.

NOTE: Penicillin by the intramuscular route is the usual drug of choice in the treatment of *Streptococcus pyogenes* infection and the prophylaxis of rheumatic fever. ZITHROMAX is often effective in the eradication of susceptible strains of *Streptococcus pyogenes* from the nasopharynx. Because some strains are resistant to ZITHROMAX, susceptibility tests should be performed when patients are treated with ZITHROMAX. Data establishing efficacy of azithromycin in subsequent prevention of rheumatic fever are not available.

Uncomplicated skin and skin structure infections due to *Staphylococcus aureus, Streptococcus pyogenes*, or *Streptococcus agalactiae.* Abscesses usually require surgical drainage.

Urethritis and cervicitis due to *Chlamydia trachomatis* or *Neisseria gonorrhoeae.*

Genital ulcer disease in men due to *Haemophilus ducreyi* (chancroid). Due to the small number of women included in clinical trials, the efficacy of azithromycin in the treatment of chancroid in women has not been established.

ZITHROMAX, at the recommended dose, should not be relied upon to treat syphilis. Antimicrobial agents used in high doses for short periods of time to treat non-gonococcal urethritis may mask or delay the symptoms of incubating syphilis. All patients with sexually-transmitted urethritis or cervicitis should have a serologic test for syphilis and appropriate cultures for gonorrhea performed at the time of diagnosis. Appropriate antimicrobial therapy and follow-up tests for these diseases should be initiated if infection is confirmed.

Appropriate culture and susceptibility tests should be performed before treatment to determine the causative organism and its susceptibility to azithromycin. Therapy with ZITHROMAX may be initiated before results of these tests are known; once the results become available, antimicrobial therapy should be adjusted accordingly.

To reduce the development of drug-resistant bacteria and maintain the effectiveness of ZITHROMAX (azithromycin) and other antibacterial drugs, ZITHROMAX (azithromycin) should be used only to treat or prevent infections that are proven or strongly suspected to be caused by susceptible bacteria. When culture and susceptibility information are available, they should be considered in selecting or modifying antibacterial therapy. In the absence of such data, local epidemiology and susceptibility patterns may contribute to the empiric selection of therapy.

Pediatric Patients: (See **PRECAUTIONS—Pediatric Use** and **CLINICAL STUDIES IN PEDIATRIC PATIENTS.**)

Acute otitis media caused by *Haemophilus influenzae, Moraxella catarrhalis* or *Streptococcus pneumoniae.* (For specific dosage recommendation, see **DOSAGE AND ADMINISTRATION.**)

Community-acquired pneumonia due to *Chlamydia pneumoniae, Haemophilus influenzae, Mycoplasma pneumoniae* or *Streptococcus pneumoniae* in patients appropriate for oral therapy. (For specific dosage recommendation, see **DOSAGE AND ADMINISTRATION.**)

NOTE: Azithromycin should not be used in pediatric patients with pneumonia who are judged to be inappropriate for oral therapy because of moderate to severe illness or risk factors such as any of the following:

patients with cystic fibrosis,
patients with nosocomially acquired infections,
patients with known or suspected bacteremia,
patients requiring hospitalization, or
patients with significant underlying health problems that may compromise their ability to respond to their illness (including immunodeficiency or functional asplenia).

Pharyngitis/tonsillitis caused by *Streptococcus pyogenes* as an alternative to first-line therapy in individuals who cannot use first-line therapy. (For specific dosage recommendation, see **DOSAGE AND ADMINISTRATION.**)

NOTE: Penicillin by the intramuscular route is the usual drug of choice in the treatment of *Streptococcus pyogenes* infection and the prophylaxis of rheumatic fever. ZITHROMAX is often effective in the eradication of susceptible strains of *Streptococcus pyogenes* from the nasopharynx. Because some strains are resistant to ZITHROMAX, susceptibility tests should be performed when patients are treated with ZITHROMAX. Data establishing efficacy of azithromycin in subsequent prevention of rheumatic fever are not available.

Appropriate culture and susceptibility tests should be performed before treatment to determine the causative organism and its susceptibility to azithromycin. Therapy with ZITHROMAX may be initiated before results of these tests are known; once the results become available, antimicrobial therapy should be adjusted accordingly.

CONTRAINDICATIONS

ZITHROMAX is contraindicated in patients with known hypersensitivity to azithromycin, erythromycin or any macrolide antibiotic.

WARNINGS

Serious allergic reactions, including angioedema, anaphylaxis, and dermatologic reactions including Stevens Johnson Syndrome and toxic epidermal necrolysis have been reported rarely in patients on azithromycin therapy. Although rare, fatalities have been reported. (See **CONTRAINDICATIONS.**) Despite initially successful symptomatic treatment of the allergic symptoms, when symptomatic therapy was discontinued, the allergic symptoms **recurred soon thereafter in some patients without further azithromycin exposure.** These patients required prolonged periods of observation and symptomatic treatment. The relationship of these episodes to the long tissue half-life of azithromycin and subsequent prolonged exposure to antigen is unknown at present.

If an allergic reaction occurs, the drug should be discontinued and appropriate therapy should be instituted. Physicians should be aware that reappearance of the allergic symptoms may occur when symptomatic therapy is discontinued.

In the treatment of pneumonia, azithromycin has only been shown to be safe and effective in the treatment of community-acquired pneumonia due to *Chlamydia pneumoniae, Haemophilus influenzae, Mycoplasma pneumoniae* or *Streptococcus pneumoniae* in patients appropriate for oral therapy. Azithromycin should not be used in patients with pneumonia who are judged to be inappropriate for oral therapy because of moderate to severe illness or risk factors such as any of the following: patients with cystic fibrosis, patients with nosocomially acquired infections, patients with known or suspected bacteremia, patients requiring hospitalization, elderly or debilitated patients, or patients with significant underlying health problems that may compromise their ability to respond to their illness (including immunodeficiency or functional asplenia).

Pseudomembranous colitis has been reported with nearly all antibacterial agents and may range in severity from mild to life-threatening. Therefore, it is important to consider this diagnosis in patients who present with diarrhea subsequent to the administration of antibacterial agents.

Treatment with antibacterial agents alters the normal flora of the colon and may permit overgrowth of clostridia. Studies indicate that a toxin produced by *Clostridium difficile* is a primary cause of "antibiotic-associated colitis."

After the diagnosis of pseudomembranous colitis has been established, therapeutic measures should be initiated. Mild cases of pseudomembranous colitis usually respond to discontinuation of the drug alone. In moderate to severe cases, consideration should be given to management with fluids and electrolytes, protein supplementation, and treatment with an antibacterial drug clinically effective against *Clostridium difficile* colitis.

PRECAUTIONS

General: Because azithromycin is principally eliminated via the liver, caution should be exercised when azithromycin is administered to patients with impaired hepatic function. Due to the limited data in subjects with GFR <10 mL/min, caution should be exercised when prescribing azithromycin in these patients. (See **CLINICAL PHARMACOLOGY – Special Populations – Renal Insufficiency.**)

Prolonged cardiac repolarization and QT interval, imparting a risk of developing cardiac arrhythmia and *torsades de pointes*, have been seen in treatment with other macrolides. A similar effect with azithromycin cannot be completely ruled out in patients at increased risk for prolonged cardiac repolarization.

Prescribing ZITHROMAX (azithromycin) in the absence of a proven or strongly suspected bacterial infection or a prophylactic indication is unlikely to provide benefit to the patient and increases the risk of the development of drug-resistant bacteria.

Information for Patients:

ZITHROMAX tablets and oral suspension can be taken with or without food.

Patients should also be cautioned not to take aluminum- and magnesium-containing antacids and azithromycin simultaneously.

The patient should be directed to discontinue azithromycin immediately and contact a physician if any signs of an allergic reaction occur.

Patients should be counseled that antibacterial drugs including ZITHROMAX (azithromycin) should only be used to treat bacterial infections. They do not treat viral infections (e.g., the common cold). When ZITHROMAX (azithromycin) is prescribed to treat a bacterial infection, patients should be told that although it is common to feel better early in the course of the therapy, the medication should be taken exactly as directed. Skipping doses or not completing the full course of therapy may (1) decrease the effectiveness of the immediate treatment and (2) increase the likelihood that bacteria will develop resistance and will not be treatable by ZITHROMAX (azithromycin) or other antibacterial drugs in the future.

Drug Interactions:

Co-administration of nelfinavir at steady-state with a single oral dose of azithromycin resulted in increased azithromycin serum concentrations. Although a dose adjustment of azithromycin is not recommended when administered in combination with nelfinavir, close monitoring for known side effects of azithromycin, such as liver enzyme abnormalities and hearing impairment, is warranted. (See **ADVERSE REACTIONS.**)

Azithromycin did not affect the prothrombin time response to a single dose of warfarin. However, prudent medical practice dictates careful monitoring of prothrombin time in all patients treated with azithromycin and warfarin concomitantly. Concurrent use of macrolides and warfarin in clinical practice has been associated with increased anticoagulant effects.

Drug interaction studies were performed with azithromycin and other drugs likely to be co-administered. (See **CLINICAL PHARMACOLOGY—Drug-Drug Interactions.**) When used in therapeutic doses, azithromycin had a modest effect on the pharmacokinetics of atorvastatin, carbamazepine, cetirizine, didanosine, efavirenz, fluconazole, indinavir, midazolam, rifabutin, sildenafil, theophylline (intravenous and oral), triazolam, trimethoprim/sulfamethoxazole or zidovudine. Co-administration with efavirenz, or fluconazole had a modest effect on the pharmacokinetics of azithromycin. No dosage adjustment of either drug is recommended when azithromycin is coadministered with any of the above agents.

Continued on next page

Zithromax Tabs/O.S.—Cont.

Interactions with the drugs listed below have not been reported in clinical trials with azithromycin; however, no specific drug interaction studies have been performed to evaluate potential drug-drug interaction. Nonetheless, they have been observed with macrolide products. Until further data are developed regarding drug interactions when azithromycin and these drugs are used concomitantly, careful monitoring of patients is advised:

Digoxin–elevated digoxin concentrations.

Ergotamine or dihydroergotamine–acute ergot toxicity characterized by severe peripheral vasospasm and dysesthesia.

Terfenadine, cyclosporine, hexobarbital and phenytoin concentrations.

Laboratory Test Interactions: There are no reported laboratory test interactions.

Carcinogenesis, Mutagenesis, Impairment of Fertility: Long-term studies in animals have not been performed to evaluate carcinogenic potential. Azithromycin has shown no mutagenic potential in standard laboratory tests: mouse lymphoma assay, human lymphocyte clastogenic assay, and mouse bone marrow clastogenic assay. No evidence of impaired fertility due to azithromycin was found.

Pregnancy: Teratogenic Effects. Pregnancy Category B: Reproduction studies have been performed in rats and mice at doses up to moderately maternally toxic dose concentrations (i.e., 200 mg/kg/day). These doses, based on a mg/m^2 basis, are estimated to be 4 and 2 times, respectively, the human daily dose of 500 mg. In the animal studies, no evidence of harm to the fetus due to azithromycin was found. There are, however, no adequate and well-controlled studies in pregnant women. Because animal reproduction studies are not always predictive of human response, azithromycin should be used during pregnancy only if clearly needed.

Nursing Mothers: It is not known whether azithromycin is excreted in human milk. Because many drugs are excreted in human milk, caution should be exercised when azithromycin is administered to a nursing woman.

Pediatric Use: (See **CLINICAL PHARMACOLOGY, INDICATIONS AND USAGE,** and **DOSAGE AND ADMINISTRATION.**)

Acute Otitis Media (total dosage regimen: 30 mg/kg, see **DOSAGE AND ADMINISTRATION**): Safety and effectiveness in the treatment of pediatric patients with otitis media under 6 months of age have not been established.

Acute Bacterial Sinusitis (dosage regimen: 10 mg/kg on Days 1-3): Safety and effectiveness in the treatment of pediatric patients with acute bacterial sinusitis under 6 months of age have not been established. Use of Zithromax® for the treatment of acute bacterial sinusitis pediatric patients (6 months of age or greater) is supported by adequate and well-controlled studies in adults, similar pathophysiology of acute sinusitis in adults and pediatric patients, and studies of acute otitis media in pediatric patients.

Community-Acquired Pneumonia (dosage regimen: 10 mg/kg on Day 1 followed by 5 mg/kg on Days 2-5): Safety and effectiveness in the treatment of pediatric patients with community-acquired pneumonia under 6 months of age have not been established. Safety and effectiveness for pneumonia due to *Chlamydia pneumoniae* and *Mycoplasma pneumoniae* were documented in pediatric clinical trials. Safety and effectiveness for pneumonia due to *Haemophilus influenzae* and *Streptococcus pneumoniae* were not documented bacteriologically in the pediatric clinical trial due to difficulty in obtaining specimens. Use of azithromycin for these two microorganisms is supported, however, by evidence from adequate and well-controlled studies in adults.

Pharyngitis/Tonsillitis (dosage regimen: 12 mg/kg on Days 1-5): Safety and effectiveness in the treatment of pediatric patients with pharyngitis/tonsillitis under 2 years of age have not been established.

Studies evaluating the use of repeated courses of therapy have not been conducted. (See **CLINICAL PHARMACOLOGY and ANIMAL TOXICOLOGY.**)

Geriatric Use: Pharmacokinetic parameters in older volunteers (65–85 years old) were similar to those in younger volunteers (18–40 years old) for the 5-day therapeutic regimen. Dosage adjustment does not appear to be necessary for older patients with normal renal and hepatic function receiving treatment with this dosage regimen. (See **CLINICAL PHARMACOLOGY.**)

In multiple-dose clinical trials of oral azithromycin, 9% of patients were at least 65 years of age (458/4949) and 3% of patients (144/4949) were at least 75 years of age. No overall differences in safety or effectiveness were observed between these subjects and younger subjects, and other reported clinical experience has not identified differences in response between the elderly and younger patients, but greater sensitivity of some older individuals cannot be ruled out.

ZITHROMAX 250 mg tablets contain 0.9 mg of sodium per tablet.

ZITHROMAX 500 mg tablets contain 1.8 mg of sodium per tablet.

ZITHROMAX for oral suspension 100 mg/5 mL contains 3.7 mg of sodium per 5 mL of constituted solution.

ZITHROMAX for oral suspension 200 mg/5 mL contains 7.4 mg of sodium per 5 mL of constituted solution.

ADVERSE REACTIONS

In clinical trials, most of the reported side effects were mild to moderate in severity and were reversible upon discontinuation of the drug. Potentially serious side effects of angioedema and cholestatic jaundice were reported rarely. Approximately 0.7% of the patients (adults and pediatric patients) from the 5-day multiple-dose clinical trials discontinued ZITHROMAX (azithromycin) therapy because of treatment-related side effects. In adults given 500 mg/day for 3 days, the discontinuation rate due to treatment-related side effects was 0.6%. In clinical trials in pediatric patients given 30 mg/kg, either as a single dose or over 3 days, discontinuation from the trials due to treatment-related side effects was approximately 1%. (See **DOSAGE AND ADMINISTRATION.**) Most of the side effects leading to discontinuation were related to the gastrointestinal tract, e.g., nausea, vomiting, diarrhea, or abdominal pain. (See **CLINICAL STUDIES IN PEDIATRIC PATIENTS.**)

Clinical:

Adults:

Multiple-dose regimens: Overall, the most common treatment-related side effects in adult patients receiving multiple-dose regimens of ZITHROMAX were related to the gastrointestinal system with diarrhea/loose stools (4-5%), nausea (3%) and abdominal pain (2-3%) being the most frequently reported.

No other treatment-related side effects occurred in patients on the multiple-dose regimens of ZITHROMAX with a frequency greater than 1%. Side effects that occurred with a frequency of 1% or less included the following:

Cardiovascular: Palpitations, chest pain.

Gastrointestinal: Dyspepsia, flatulence, vomiting, melena and cholestatic jaundice.

Genitourinary: Monilia, vaginitis and nephritis.

Nervous System: Dizziness, headache, vertigo and somnolence.

General: Fatigue.

Allergic: Rash, pruritus, photosensitivity and angioedema.

Single 1-gram dose regimen: Overall, the most common side effects in patients receiving a single-dose regimen of 1 gram of ZITHROMAX were related to the gastrointestinal system and were more frequently reported than in patients receiving the multiple-dose regimen.

Side effects that occurred in patients on the single one-gram dosing regimen of ZITHROMAX with a frequency of 1% or greater included diarrhea/loose stools (7%), nausea (5%), abdominal pain (5%), vomiting (2%), dyspepsia (1%) and vaginitis (1%).

Single 2-gram dose regimen: Overall, the most common side effects in patients receiving a single 2-gram dose of ZITHROMAX were related to the gastrointestinal system. Side effects that occurred in patients in this study with a frequency of 1% or greater included nausea (18%), diarrhea/loose stools (14%), vomiting (7%), abdominal pain (7%), vaginitis (2%), dyspepsia (1%) and dizziness (1%). The majority of these complaints were mild in nature.

Pediatric Patients:

Single and Multiple-dose regimens: The types of side effects in pediatric patients were comparable to those seen in adults, with different incidence rates for the dosage regimens recommended in pediatric patients.

Acute Otitis Media: For the recommended total dosage regimen of 30 mg/kg, the most frequent side effects (≥ 1%) attributed to treatment were diarrhea, abdominal pain, vomiting, nausea and rash. (See **DOSAGE AND ADMINISTRATION** and **CLINICAL STUDIES IN PEDIATRIC PATIENTS.**)

The incidence, based on dosing regimen, is described in the table below:

[See table below]

Community-Acquired Pneumonia: For the recommended dosage regimen of 10 mg/kg on Day 1 followed by 5 mg/kg on Days 2-5, the most frequent side effects attributed to treatment were diarrhea/loose stools, abdominal pain, vomiting, nausea and rash.

The incidence is described in the table below:

[See first table at top of next page]

Pharyngitis/tonsillitis: For the recommended dosage regimen of 12 mg/kg on Days 1–5, the most frequent side effects attributed to treatment were diarrhea, vomiting, abdominal pain, nausea and headache.

The incidence is described in the table below:

[See second table at top of next page]

With any of the treatment regimens, no other treatment-related side effects occurred in pediatric patients treated with ZITHROMAX with a frequency greater than 1%. Side effects that occurred with a frequency of 1% or less included the following:

Cardiovascular: Chest pain.

Gastrointestinal: Dyspepsia, constipation, anorexia, enteritis, flatulence, gastritis, jaundice, loose stools and oral moniliasis.

Hematologic and Lymphatic: Anemia and leukopenia.

Nervous System: Headache (otitis media dosage), hyperkinesia, dizziness, agitation, nervousness and insomnia.

Dosage Regimen	Diarrhea, %	Abdominal Pain, %	Vomiting, %	Nausea, %	Rash, %
1-day	4.3%	1.4%	4.9%	1.0%	1.0%
3-day	2.6%	1.7%	2.3%	0.4%	0.6%
5-day	1.8%	1.2%	1.1%	0.5%	0.4%

General: Fever, face edema, fatigue, fungal infection, malaise and pain.

Allergic: Rash and allergic reaction.

Respiratory: Cough increased, pharyngitis, pleural effusion and rhinitis.

Skin and Appendages: Eczema, fungal dermatitis, pruritus, sweating, urticaria and vesiculobullous rash.

Special Senses: Conjunctivitis.

Post-Marketing Experience:

Adverse events reported with azithromycin during the post-marketing period in adult and/or pediatric patients for which a causal relationship may not be established include:

Allergic: Arthralgia, edema, urticaria and angioedema.

Cardiovascular: Arrhythmias including ventricular tachycardia and hypotension. There have been rare reports of QT prolongation and *torsades de pointes.*

Gastrointestinal: Anorexia, constipation, dyspepsia, flatulence, vomiting/diarrhea rarely resulting in dehydration, pseudomembranous colitis, pancreatitis, oral candidiasis and rare reports of tongue discoloration.

General: Asthenia, paresthesia, fatigue, malaise and anaphylaxis (rarely fatal).

Genitourinary: Interstitial nephritis and acute renal failure and vaginitis.

Hematopoietic: Thrombocytopenia.

Liver/Biliary: Abnormal liver function including hepatitis and cholestatic jaundice, as well as rare cases of hepatic necrosis and hepatic failure, some of which have resulted in death.

Nervous System: Convulsions, dizziness/vertigo, headache, somnolence, hyperactivity, nervousness, agitation and syncope.

Psychiatric: Aggressive reaction and anxiety.

Skin/Appendages: Pruritus, rarely serious skin reactions including erythema multiforme, Stevens Johnson Syndrome and toxic epidermal necrolysis.

Special Senses: Hearing disturbances including hearing loss, deafness and/or tinnitus and rare reports of taste perversion.

Laboratory Abnormalities:

Adults:

Clinically significant abnormalities (irrespective of drug relationship) occurring during the clinical trials were reported as follows: with an incidence of greater than 1%: decreased hemoglobin, hematocrit, lymphocytes, neutrophils and blood glucose; elevated serum creatine phosphokinase, potassium, ALT, GGT, AST, BUN, creatinine, blood glucose, platelet count, lymphocytes, neutrophils and eosinophils; with an incidence of less than 1%: leukopenia, neutropenia, decreased sodium, potassium, platelet count, elevated monocytes, basophils, bicarbonate, serum alkaline phosphatase, bilirubin, LDH and phosphate. The majority of subjects with elevated serum creatinine also had abnormal values at baseline.

When follow-up was provided, changes in laboratory tests appeared to be reversible.

In multiple-dose clinical trials involving more than 5000 patients, four patients discontinued therapy because of treatment-related liver enzyme abnormalities and one because of a renal function abnormality.

Pediatric Patients:

One, Three and Five Day Regimens

Laboratory data collected from comparative clinical trials employing two 3-day regimens (30 mg/kg or 60 mg/kg in divided doses over 3 days), or two 5-day regimens (30 mg/kg or 60 mg/kg in divided doses over 5 days) were similar for regimens of azithromycin and all comparators combined, with most clinically significant laboratory abnormalities occurring at incidences of 1-5%. Laboratory data for patients receiving 30 mg/kg as a single dose were collected in one single center trial. In that trial, an absolute neutrophil count between 500-1500 cells/mm^3 was observed in 10/64 patients receiving 30 mg/kg as a single dose, 9/62 patients receiving 30 mg/kg given over 3 days, and 8/63 comparator patients. No patient had an absolute neutrophil count <500 cells/mm^3. (See **DOSAGE AND ADMINISTRATION.**)

In multiple-dose clinical trials involving approximately 4700 pediatric patients, no patients discontinued therapy because of treatment-related laboratory abnormalities.

DOSAGE AND ADMINISTRATION

(See **INDICATIONS AND USAGE** and **CLINICAL PHARMACOLOGY**

Adults:

[See third table on next page]

ZITHROMAX® tablets can be taken with or without food.

Renal Insufficiency:

No dosage adjustment is recommended for subjects with renal impairment (GFR ≤80 mL/min). The mean AUC_{0-120} was similar in subjects with GFR 10-80 mL/min compared to subjects with normal renal function, whereas it increased 35% in subjects with GFR <10 mL/min compared to subjects with normal renal function. Caution should be exercised when azithromycin is administered to subjects with severe renal impairment. (See **CLINICAL PHARMACOLOGY, Special Populations, Renal Insufficiency.**)

Hepatic Insufficiency:

The pharmacokinetics of azithromycin in subjects with hepatic impairment have not been established. No dose adjustment recommendations can be made in patients with impaired hepatic function (See **CLINICAL PHARMACOLOGY, Special Populations, Hepatic Insufficiency.**)

No dosage adjustment is recommended based on age or gender. (See **CLINICAL PHARMACOLOGY, Special Populations.**)

Dosage Regimen	Diarrhea/Loose stools, %	Abdominal Pain, %	Vomiting, %	Nausea, %	Rash, %
5-day	5.8%	1.9%	1.9%	1.9%	1.6%

Dosage Regimen	Diarrhea, %	Abdominal Pain, %	Vomiting, %	Nausea, %	Rash, %	Headache, %
5-day	5.4%	3.4%	5.6%	1.8%	0.7%	1.1%

Infection*	Recommended Dose/Duration of Therapy
Community-acquired pneumonia (mild severity) Pharyngitis/tonsillitis (second line therapy) Skin/skin structure (uncomplicated)	500 mg as a single dose on Day 1, followed by 250 mg once daily on Days 2 through 5.
Acute bacterial exacerbations of chronic obstructive pulmonary disease (mild to moderate)	500 mg QD × 3 days OR 500 mg as a single dose on Day 1, followed by 250 mg once daily on Days 2 through 5.
Acute bacterial sinusitis	500 mg QD × 3 days
Genital ulcer disease (chancroid)	One single 1 gram dose
Non-gonococcal urethritis and cervicitis	One single 1 gram dose
Gonococcal urethritis and cervicitis	One single 2 gram dose

*DUE TO THE INDICATED ORGANISMS (See **INDICATIONS AND USAGE.**)

PEDIATRIC DOSAGE GUIDELINES FOR OTITIS MEDIA, ACUTE BACTERIAL SINUSITIS AND COMMUNITY-ACQUIRED PNEUMONIA
(Age 6 months and above, see PRECAUTIONS—Pediatric Use.)
Based on Body Weight

OTITIS MEDIA AND COMMUNITY-ACQUIRED PNEUMONIA: (5-Day Regimen)*

Dosing Calculated on 10 mg/kg/day Day 1 and 5 mg/kg/day Days 2 to 5.

Weight		100 mg/5 mL		200 mg/5 mL		Total mL per Treatment Course	Total mg per Treatment Course
Kg	Lbs.	Day 1	Days 2–5	Day 1	Days 2–5		
5	11	2.5 mL (½ tsp)	1.25 mL (¼ tsp)			7.5 mL	150 mg
10	22	5 mL (1 tsp)	2.5 mL (½ tsp)			15 mL	300 mg
20	44			5 mL (1 tsp)	2.5 mL (½ tsp)	15 mL	600 mg
30	66			7.5 mL (1½ tsp)	3.75 mL (¾ tsp)	22.5 mL	900 mg
40	88			10 mL (2 tsp)	5 mL (1 tsp)	30 mL	1200 mg
50 and above	110 and above			12.5 mL (2½ tsp)	6.25 mL (1¼ tsp)	37.5 mL	1500 mg

*Effectiveness of the 3-day or 1-day regimen in pediatric patients with community-acquired pneumonia has not been established.

Pediatric Patients:
ZITHROMAX for oral suspension can be taken with or without food.

Acute Otitis Media: The recommended dose of ZITHROMAX for oral suspension for the treatment of pediatric patients with acute otitis media is 30 mg/kg given as a single dose or 10 mg/kg once daily for 3 days or 10 mg/kg as a single dose on the first day followed by 5 mg/kg/day on Days 2 through 5. (See chart below.)

Acute Bacterial Sinusitis: The recommended dose of ZITHROMAX® for oral suspension for the treatment of pediatric patients with acute bacterial sinusitis is 10 mg/kg once daily for 3 days. (See chart below.)

Community-Acquired Pneumonia: The recommended dose of ZITHROMAX for oral suspension for the treatment of pediatric patients with community-acquired pneumonia is 10 mg/kg as a single dose on the first day followed by 5 mg/kg on Days 2 through 5. (See chart below.)

[See fourth table above]
[See first table at top of next page]
[See second table at top of next page]

The safety of re-dosing azithromycin in pediatric patients who vomit after receiving 30 mg/kg as a single dose has not been established. In clinical studies involving 487 patients with acute otitis media given a single 30 mg/kg dose of azithromycin, eight patients who vomited within 30 minutes of dosing were re-dosed at the same total dose.

Pharyngitis/Tonsillitis: The recommended dose of ZITHROMAX for children with pharyngitis/tonsillitis is 12 mg/kg once daily for 5 days. (See chart below.)

[See third table on next page]

Constituting instructions for ZITHROMAX Oral Suspension, 300, 600, 900, 1200 mg bottles. The table below indicates the volume of water to be used for constitution:

[See fourth table on next page]

Shake well before each use. Oversized bottle provides shake space. Keep tightly closed.

After mixing, store suspension at 5° to 30°C (41° to 86°F) and use within 10 days. Discard after full dosing is completed.

HOW SUPPLIED

ZITHROMAX 250 mg tablets are supplied as pink modified capsular shaped, engraved, film-coated tablets containing azithromycin dihydrate equivalent to 250 mg of azithromycin. ZITHROMAX 250 mg tablets are engraved with "PFIZER" on one side and "306" on the other. These are packaged in bottles and blister cards of 6 tablets (Z-PAKS®) as follows:

Bottles of 30	NDC 0069-3060-30
Boxes of 3 (Z-PAKS® of 6)	NDC 0069-3060-75
Unit Dose package of 50	NDC 0069-3060-86

ZITHROMAX 500 mg tablets are supplied as pink modified capsular shaped, engraved, film-coated tablets containing azithromycin dihydrate equivalent to 500 mg of azithromycin. ZITHROMAX 500 mg tablets are engraved with "Pfizer" on one side and "ZTM500" on the other. These are packaged in bottles and blister cards of 3 tablets (TRI-PAKS™) as follows:

Bottles of 30	NDC 0069-3070-30
Boxes of 3 (TRI-PAKS™ of 3 tablets)	NDC 0069-3070-75
Unit Dose package of 50	NDC 0069-3070-86

ZITHROMAX tablets should be stored between 15° to 30°C (59° to 86°F).

ZITHROMAX for oral suspension after constitution contains a flavored suspension. ZITHROMAX® for oral suspension is supplied to provide 100 mg/5 mL or 200 mg/5 mL suspension in bottles as follows:

Azithromycin contents per bottle	NDC
300 mg	0069-3110-19
600 mg	0069-3120-19
900 mg	0069-3130-19
1200 mg	0069-3140-19

See **DOSAGE AND ADMINISTRATION** for constitution instructions with each bottle type.

Storage: Store dry powder below 30°C (86°F). Store constituted suspension between 5° to 30°C (41° to 86°F) and discard when full dosing is completed.

CLINICAL STUDIES (See INDICATIONS AND USAGE and Pediatric Use.)

Pediatric Patients

From the perspective of evaluating pediatric clinical trials, Days 11-14 were considered on-therapy evaluations because of the extended half-life of azithromycin. Day 11-14 data are provided for clinical guidance. Day 24-32 evaluations were considered the primary test of cure endpoint.

Acute Otitis Media

Safety and efficacy using azithromycin 30 mg/kg given over 5 days

Protocol 1

In a double-blind, controlled clinical study of acute otitis media performed in the United States, azithromycin (10 mg/kg on Day 1 followed by 5 mg/kg on Days 2-5) was compared to amoxicillin/clavulanate potassium (4:1). For the 553 patients who were evaluated for clinical efficacy, the clinical success rate (i.e., cure plus improvement) at the Day 11 visit was 88% for azithromycin and 88% for the control agent. For the 521 patients who were evaluated at the Day 30 visit, the clinical success rate was 73% for azithromycin and 71% for the control agent.

In the safety analysis of the above study, the incidence of treatment-related adverse events, primarily gastrointestinal, in all patients treated was 9% with azithromycin and 31% with the control agent. The most common side effects were diarrhea/loose stools (4% azithromycin vs. 20% control), vomiting (2% azithromycin vs. 7% control), and abdominal pain (2% azithromycin vs. 5% control).

Protocol 2

In a non-comparative clinical and microbiologic trial performed in the United States, where significant rates of beta-lactamase producing organisms (35%) were found, 131 patients were evaluable for clinical efficacy. The combined clinical success rate (i.e., cure and improvement) at the Day 11 visit was 84% for azithromycin. For the 122 patients who were evaluated at the Day 30 visit, the clinical success rate was 70% for azithromycin.

Microbiologic determinations were made at the pre-treatment visit. Microbiology was not reassessed at later visits. The following presumptive bacterial/clinical cure outcomes (i.e., clinical success) were obtained from the evaluable group:

Presumed Bacteriologic Eradication

	Day 11 Azithromycin	Day 30 Azithromycin
S. pneumoniae	61/74 (82%)	40/56 (71%)
H. influenzae	43/54 (80%)	30/47 (64%)
M. catarrhalis	28/35 (80%)	19/26 (73%)
S. pyogenes	11/11 (100%)	7/7
Overall	177/217 (82%)	97/137 (73%)

In the safety analysis of this study, the incidence of treatment-related adverse events, primarily gastrointestinal, in all patients treated was 9%. The most common side effect was diarrhea (4%).

Protocol 3

In another controlled comparative clinical and microbiologic study of otitis media performed in the United States, azithromycin was compared to amoxicillin/clavulanate potassium (4:1). This study utilized two of the same investigators as Protocol 2 (above), and these two investigators enrolled 90% of the patients in Protocol 3. For this reason, Protocol 3 was not considered to be an independent study. Significant rates of beta-lactamase producing organisms (20%) were found. Ninety-two (92) patients were evaluable for clinical and microbiologic efficacy. The combined clinical success rate (i.e., cure and improvement) of those patients with a baseline pathogen at the Day 11 visit was 88% for azithromycin vs. 100% for control; at the Day 30 visit, the clinical success rate was 82% for azithromycin vs. 80% for control.

Microbiologic determinations were made at the pre-treatment visit. Microbiology was not reassessed at later visits. At the Day 11 and Day 30 visits, the following presumptive bacterial/clinical cure outcomes (i.e., clinical success) were obtained from the evaluable group:

[See fifth table on next page]

In the safety analysis of the above study, the incidence of treatment-related adverse events, primarily gastrointestinal, in all patients treated was 4% with azithromycin and 31% with the control agent. The most common side effect was diarrhea/loose stools (2% azithromycin vs. 29% control).

Safety and efficacy using azithromycin 30 mg/kg given over 3 days

Protocol 4

In a double-blind, controlled, randomized clinical study of acute otitis media in pediatric patients from 6 months to 12 years of age, azithromycin (10 mg/kg per day for 3 days) was compared to amoxicillin/clavulanate potassium (7:1) in divided doses q12h for 10 days. Each patient received active drug and placebo matched for the comparator.

For the 366 patients who were evaluated for clinical efficacy at the Day 12 visit, the clinical success rate (i.e., cure plus improvement) was 83% for azithromycin and 88% for the control agent. For the 362 patients who were evaluated at the Day 24–28 visit, the clinical success rate was 74% for azithromycin and 69% for the control agent.

In the safety analysis of the above study, the incidence of treatment-related adverse events, primarily gastrointestinal, in all patients treated was 10.6% with azithromycin and 20.0% with the control agent. The most common side

Continued on next page

Zithromax Tabs/O.S.—Cont.

effects were diarrhea/loose stools (5.9% azithromycin vs. 14.6% control), vomiting (2.1% azithromycin vs. 1.1% control), and rash (0.0% azithromycin vs. 4.3% control).

Safety and efficacy using azithromycin 30 mg/kg given as a single dose

Protocol 5

A double blind, controlled, randomized trial was performed at nine clinical centers. Pediatric patients from 6 months to 12 years of age were randomized 1:1 to treatment with either azithromycin (given at 30 mg/kg as a single dose on Day 1) or amoxicillin/clavulanate potassium (7:1), divided q12h for 10 days. Each child received active drug, and placebo matched for the comparator.

Clinical response (Cure, Improvement, Failure) was evaluated at End of Therapy (Day 12–16) and Test of Cure (Day 28–32). Safety was evaluated throughout the trial for all treated subjects. For the 321 subjects who were evaluated at End of Treatment, the clinical success rate (cure plus improvement) was 87% for azithromycin, and 88% for the comparator. For the 305 subjects who were evaluated at Test of Cure, the clinical success rate was 75% for both azithromycin and the comparator.

In the safety analysis, the incidence of treatment-related adverse events, primarily gastrointestinal, was 16.8% with azithromycin, and 22.5% with the comparator. The most common side effects were diarrhea (6.4% with azithromycin vs. 12.7% with the comparator), vomiting (4% with each agent), rash (1.7% with azithromycin vs. 5.2% with the comparator) and nausea (1.7% with azithromycin vs. 1.2% with the comparator).

Protocol 6

In a non-comparative clinical and microbiological trial, 248 patients from 6 months to 12 years of age with documented acute otitis media were dosed with a single oral dose of azithromycin (30 mg/kg on Day 1).

For the 240 patients who were evaluable for clinical modified Intent-to-Treat (MITT) analysis, the clinical success rate (i.e., cure plus improvement) at Day 10 was 89% and for the 242 patients evaluable at Day 24–28, the clinical success rate (cure) was 85%.

Presumed Bacteriologic Eradication

	Day 10	Day 24-28
S. pneumoniae	70/76 (92%)	67/76 (88%)
H. influenzae	30/42 (71%)	28/44 (64%)
M. catarrhalis	10/10 (100%)	10/10 (100%)
Overall	110/128 (86%)	105/130 (81%)

In the safety analysis of this study, the incidence of treatment-related adverse events, primarily gastrointestinal, in all the subjects treated was 12.1%. The most common side effects were vomiting (5.6%), diarrhea (3.2%), and abdominal pain (1.6%).

Pharyngitis/Tonsillitis

In three double-blind controlled studies, conducted in the United States, azithromycin (12 mg/kg once a day for 5 days) was compared to penicillin V (250 mg three times a day for 10 days) in the treatment of pharyngitis due to documented Group A β-hemolytic streptococci (GABHS or *S. pyogenes*). Azithromycin was clinically and microbiologically statistically superior to penicillin at Day 14 and Day 30 with the following clinical success (i.e., cure and improvement) and bacteriologic efficacy rates (for the combined evaluable patient with documented GABHS):

[See table at top of next page]

Approximately 1% of azithromycin-susceptible *S. pyogenes* isolates were resistant to azithromycin following therapy.

The incidence of treatment-related adverse events, primarily gastrointestinal, in all patients treated was 18% on azithromycin and 13% on penicillin. The most common side effects were diarrhea/loose stools (6% azithromycin vs. 2% penicillin), vomiting (6% azithromycin vs. 4% penicillin), and abdominal pain (3% azithromycin vs. 1% penicillin).

Adult Patients

Acute Bacterial Exacerbations of Chronic Obstructive Pulmonary Disease

In a randomized, double-blind controlled clinical trial of acute exacerbation of chronic bronchitis (AECB), azithromycin (500 mg once daily for 3 days) was compared with clarithromycin (500 mg twice daily for 10 days). The primary endpoint of this trial was the clinical cure rate at Day 21–24. For the 304 patients analyzed in the modified intent to treat analysis at the Day 21–24 visit, the clinical cure rate for 3 days of azithromycin was 85% (125/147) compared to 82% (129/157) for 10 days of clarithromycin.

The following outcomes were the clinical cure rates at the Day 21–24 visit for the bacteriologically evaluable patients by pathogen:

Pathogen	Azithromycin (3 Days)	Clarithromycin (10 Days)
S. pneumoniae	29/32 (91%)	21/27 (78%)
H. influenzae	12/14 (86%)	14/16 (88%)
M. catarrhalis	11/12 (92%)	12/15 (80%)

In the safety analysis of this study, the incidence of treatment-related adverse events, primarily gastrointestinal, were comparable between treatment arms (25% with azithromycin and 29% with clarithromycin). The most common side effects were diarrhea, nausea and abdominal pain with comparable incidence rates for each symptom of 5-9% between the two treatment arms. (See **ADVERSE REACTIONS**.)

OTITIS MEDIA AND ACUTE BACTERIAL SINUSITIS: (3-Day Regimen)*

Dosing Calculated on 10 mg/kg/day

Weight		100 mg/5 mL	200 mg/5 mL	Total mL per Treatment Course	Total mg per Treatment Course
Kg	Lbs.	Day 1–3	Day 1–3		
5	11	2.5 mL (½ tsp)		7.5 mL	150 mg
10	22	5 mL (1 tsp)		15 mL	300 mg
20	44		5 mL (1 tsp)	15 mL	600 mg
30	66		7.5 mL (1½ tsp)	22.5 mL	900 mg
40	88		10 mL (2 tsp)	30 mL	1200 mg
50 and above	110 and above		12.5 mL (2½ tsp)	37.5 mL	1500 mg

*Effectiveness of the 5-day or 1-day regimen in pediatric patients with acute bacterial sinusitis has not been established.

OTITIS MEDIA: (1-Day Regimen)

Dosing Calculated on 30 mg/kg as a single dose

Weight		200 mg/5 mL	Total mL per Treatment Course	Total mg per Treatment Course
Kg	Lbs.	Day 1		
5	11	3.75 mL (¾ tsp)	3.75 mL	150 mg
10	22	7.5 mL (1½ tsp)	7.5 mL	300 mg
20	44	15 mL (3 tsp)	15 mL	600 mg
30	66	22.5 mL (4½ tsp)	22.5 mL	900 mg
40	88	30 mL (6 tsp)	30 mL	1200 mg
50 and above	110 and above	37.5 mL (7½ tsp)	37.5 mL	1500 mg

PEDIATRIC DOSAGE GUIDELINES FOR PHARYNGITIS/TONSILLITIS
(Age 2 years and above, see PRECAUTIONS—Pediatric Use.)
Based on Body Weight

PHARYNGITIS/TONSILLITIS: (5-Day Regimen)

Dosing Calculated on 12 mg/kg/day for 5 days.

Weight		200 mg/5 mL	Total mL per Treatment Course	Total mg per Treatment Course
Kg	Lbs.	Day 1–5		
8	18	2.5 mL (½ tsp)	12.5 mL	500 mg
17	37	5 mL (1 tsp)	25 mL	1000 mg
25	55	7.5 mL (1½ tsp)	37.5 mL	1500 mg
33	73	10 mL (2 tsp)	50 mL	2000 mg
40	88	12.5 mL (2½ tsp)	62.5 mL	2500 mg

Amount of water to be added	Total volume after constitution (azithromycin content)	Azithromycin concentration after constitution
9 mL (300 mg)	15 mL (300 mg)	100 mg/5 mL
9 mL (600 mg)	15 mL (600 mg)	200 mg/5 mL
12 mL (900 mg)	22.5 mL (900 mg)	200 mg/5 mL
15 mL (1200 mg)	30 mL (1200 mg)	200 mg/5 mL

Presumed Bacteriologic Eradication

	Day 11		Day 30	
	Azithromycin	Control	Azithromycin	Control
S. pneumoniae	25/29 (86%)	26/26 (100%)	22/28 (79%)	18/22 (82%)
H. influenzae	9/11 (82%)	9/9	8/10 (80%)	6/8
M. catarrhalis	7/7	5/5	5/5	2/3
S. pyogenes	2/2	5/5	2/2	4/4
Overall	43/49 (88%)	45/45 (100%)	37/45 (82%)	30/37 (81%)

Acute Bacterial Sinusitis

In a randomized, double blind, double-dummy controlled clinical trial of acute bacterial sinusitis, azithromycin (500 mg once daily for 3 days) was compared with amoxicillin/clavulanate (500/125 mg tid for 10 days). Clinical response assessments were made at Day 10 and Day 28. The primary endpoint of this trial was prospectively defined as the clinical cure rate at Day 28. For the 594 patients analyzed in the modified intent to treat analysis at the Day 10 visit, the clinical cure rate for 3 days azithromycin was 88% (268/303) compared to 85% (248/291) for 10 days of amoxicillin/clavulanate. For the 586 patients analyzed in the modified intent to treat analysis at the Day 28 visit, the clinical cure rate for 3 days of azithromycin was 71.5% (213/

Three U.S. Streptococcal Pharyngitis Studies
Azithromycin vs. Penicillin V
EFFICACY RESULTS

	Day 14	Day 30
Bacteriologic Eradication:		
Azithromycin	323/340 (95%)	255/330 (77%)
Penicillin V	242/332 (73%)	206/325 (63%)
Clinical Success (Cure plus improvement):		
Azithromycin	336/343 (98%)	310/330 (94%)
Penicillin V	284/338 (84%)	241/325 (74%)

298) compared to 71.5% (206/288), with a 97.5% confidence interval of –8.4 to 8.3, for 10 days of amoxicillin/clavulanate. In the safety analysis of this study, the overall incidence of treatment-related adverse events, primarily gastrointestinal, was lower in the azithromycin treatment arm (31%) than in the amoxicillin/clavulanate arm (51%). The most common side effects were diarrhea (17% in the azithromycin arm vs. 32% in the amoxicillin/clavulanate arm), and nausea (7% in the azithromycin arm vs. 12% in the amoxicillin/clavulanate arm). (See **ADVERSE REACTIONS**).

In an open label, noncomparative study requiring baseline transantral sinus punctures the following outcomes were the clinical success rates at the Day 7 and Day 28 visits for the modified intent to treat patients administered 500 mg of azithromycin once daily for 3 days with the following pathogens:

Pathogen	**Azithromycin (500 mg per day for 3 Days)**	
	Day 7	***Day 28***
S. pneumoniae	23/26 (88%)	21/25 (84%)
H. influenzae	28/32 (87%)	24/32 (75%)
M. catarrhalis	14/15 (93%)	13/15 (87%)

The overall incidence of treatment-related adverse events in the noncomparative study was 21% in modified intent to treat patients treated with azithromycin at 500 mg once daily for 3 days with the most common side effects being diarrhea (9%), abdominal pain (4%) and nausea (3%). (See **ADVERSE REACTIONS**).

ANIMAL TOXICOLOGY

Phospholipidosis (intracellular phospholipid accumulation) has been observed in some tissues of mice, rats, and dogs given multiple doses of azithromycin. It has been demonstrated in numerous organ systems (e.g., eye, dorsal root ganglia, liver, gallbladder, kidney, spleen, and pancreas) in dogs treated with azithromycin at doses which, expressed on the basis of mg/m^2, are approximately equal to the recommended adult human dose, and in rats treated at doses approximately one-sixth of the recommended adult human dose. This effect has been shown to be reversible after cessation of azithromycin treatment. Phospholipidosis has been observed to a similar extent in the tissues of neonatal rats and dogs given daily doses of azithromycin ranging from 10 days to 30 days. Based on the pharmacokinetic data, phospholipidosis has been seen in the rat (30 mg/kg dose) at observed C_{max} value of 1.3 µg/mL (six times greater than the observed C_{max} of 0.216 µg/mL at the pediatric dose of 10 mg/kg). Similarly, it has been shown in the dog (10 mg/kg dose) at observed C_{max} value of 1.5 µg/mL (seven times greater than the observed same C_{max} and drug dose in the studied pediatric population). On a mg/m^2 basis, 30 mg/kg dose in the neonatal rat (135 mg/m^2) and 10 mg/kg dose in the neonatal dog (79 mg/m^2) are approximately 0.5 and 0.3 times, respectively, the recommended dose in the pediatric patients with an average body weight of 25 kg. Phospholipidosis, similar to that seen in the adult animals, is reversible after cessation of azithromycin treatment. The significance of these findings for animals and for humans is unknown.

REFERENCES:

1. National Committee for Clinical Laboratory Standards, *Methods for Dilution Antimicrobial Susceptibility Tests for Bacteria That Grow Aerobically* – Fifth Edition. Approved Standard NCCLS Document M7-A5, Vol. 20, No. 2 (ISBN 1-56238-394-9). NCCLS, 940 West Valley Road, Suite 1400, Wayne, PA 19087-1898, January 2000.
2. National Committee for Clinical Laboratory Standards, *Performance Standards for Antimicrobial Disk Susceptibility Tests* – Seventh Edition. Approved Standard NCCLS Document M2-A7, Vol. 20, No. 1 (ISBN 1-56238-393-0). NCCLS, 940 West Valley Road, Suite 1400, Wayne, PA 19087-1898, January 2000.
3. National Committee for Clinical Laboratory Standards. *Performance Standards for Antimicrobial Susceptibility Testing* – Eleventh Informational Supplement. NCCLS Document M100-S11, Vol. 21, No. 1 (ISBN 1-56238-426-0). NCCLS, 940 West Valley Road, Suite 1400, Wayne, PA 19087-1898, January 2001.

Rx only

Licensed from Pliva

Distributed by:
Pfizer Labs
Division of Pfizer Inc, NY, NY 10017
70-5179-00-4 Revised January 2004

ZITHROMAX® ℞
[*zĭth'rō-măks*]
(azithromycin capsules)
(azithromycin tablets)
and (azithromycin for oral suspension)

Prescribing information for this product, which appears on pages 2682–2687of the 2004 PDR, has been completely revised as follows. Please write "See Supplement A" next to the product heading.

To reduce the development of drug-resistant bacteria and maintain the effectiveness of Zithromax® (azithromycin) and other antibacterial drugs, Zithromax (azithromycin) should be used only to treat or prevent infections that are proven or strongly suspected to be caused by bacteria.

DESCRIPTION

ZITHROMAX® (azithromycin capsules, azithromycin tablets and azithromycin for oral suspension) contain the active ingredient azithromycin, an azalide, a subclass of macrolide antibiotics, for oral administration. Azithromycin has the chemical name (*2R,3S,4R,5R,8R,10R,11R,12S,13S,14R*)-13-[(2,6-dideoxy-3-*C*-methyl-3-*O*-methyl-α-*L*-*ribo*-hexopyranosyl)oxy]-2-ethyl-3,4,10-trihydroxy-3,5,6,8,10,12,14-heptamethyl-11-[[3,4,6-trideoxy-3-(dimethylamino)-β-*D*-*xylo*-hexopyranosyl]oxy]-1-oxa-6-azacyclopentadecan-15-one. Azithromycin is derived from erythromycin; however, it differs chemically from erythromycin in that a methyl-substituted nitrogen atom is incorporated into the lactone ring. Its molecular formula is $C_{38}H_{72}N_2O_{12}$, and its molecular weight is 749.0. Azithromycin has the following structural formula: Azithromycin, as the dihydrate, is a white crystalline pow-

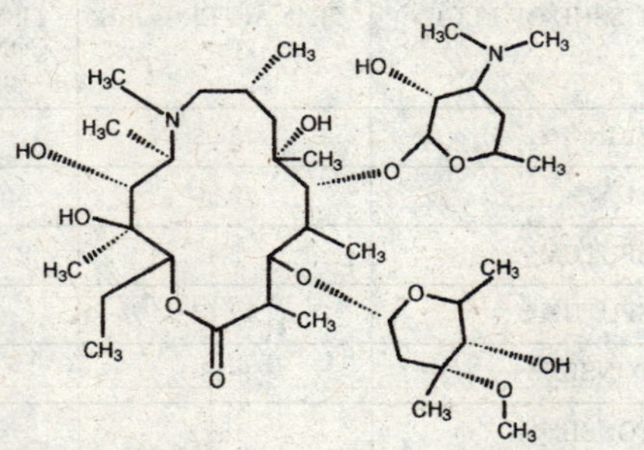

der with a molecular formula of $C_{38}H_{72}N_2O_{12} \bullet 2H_2O$ and a molecular weight of 785.0.

ZITHROMAX® capsules contain azithromycin dihydrate equivalent to 250 mg of azithromycin. The capsules are supplied in red opaque hard-gelatin capsules (containing FD&C Red #40). They also contain the following inactive ingredients: anhydrous lactose, corn starch, magnesium stearate, and sodium lauryl sulfate.

ZITHROMAX® tablets contain azithromycin dihydrate equivalent to 600 mg azithromycin. The tablets are supplied as white, modified oval-shaped, film-coated tablets. They also contain the following inactive ingredients: dibasic calcium phosphate anhydrous, pregelatinized starch, sodium croscarmellose, magnesium stearate, sodium lauryl sulfate and an aqueous film coat consisting of hypromellose, titanium dioxide, lactose and triacetin.

ZITHROMAX® for oral suspension is supplied in a single dose packet containing azithromycin dihydrate equivalent to 1 g azithromycin. It also contains the following inactive ingredients: colloidal silicon dioxide, sodium phosphate tribasic, anhydrous; spray dried artificial banana flavor, spray dried artificial cherry flavor, and sucrose.

CLINICAL PHARMACOLOGY

Pharmacokinetics: Following oral administration, azithromycin is rapidly absorbed and widely distributed throughout the body. Rapid distribution of azithromycin into tissues and high concentration within cells result in significantly higher azithromycin concentrations in tissues than in plasma or serum. The 1 g single dose packet is bioequivalent to four 250 mg capsules.

The pharmacokinetic parameters of azithromycin in plasma after dosing as per labeled recommendations in healthy young adults and asymptomatic HIV-seropositive adults (age 18-40 years old) are portrayed in the following chart:

[See first table at top of next page]

In these studies (500 mg Day 1, 250 mg Days 2–5), there was no significant difference in the disposition of azithromycin between male and female subjects. Plasma concentrations of azithromycin following single 500 mg oral and i.v. doses declined in a polyphasic pattern resulting in an average terminal half-life of 68 hours. With a regimen of 500 mg on Day 1 and 250 mg/day on Days 2–5, C_{min} and C_{max} remained essentially unchanged from Day 2 through Day 5 of therapy. However, without a loading dose, azithromycin C_{min} levels required 5 to 7 days to reach steady-state.

In asymptomatic HIV-seropositive adult subjects receiving 600-mg ZITHROMAX® tablets once daily for 22 days, steady state azithromycin serum levels were achieved by Day 15 of dosing.

When azithromycin capsules were administered with food, the rate of absorption (C_{max}) of azithromycin was reduced by 52% and the extent of absorption (AUC) by 43%.

When the oral suspension of azithromycin was administered with food, the C_{max} increased by 46% and the AUC by 14%.

The absolute bioavailability of two 600 mg tablets was 34% (CV=56%). Administration of two 600 mg tablets with food increased C_{max} by 31% (CV=43%) while the extent of absorption (AUC) was unchanged (mean ratio of AUCs=1.00; CV=55%).

The AUC of azithromycin in 250 mg capsules was unaffected by coadministration of an antacid containing aluminum and magnesium hydroxide with ZITHROMAX® (azithromycin); however, the C_{max} was reduced by 24%. Administration of cimetidine (800 mg) two hours prior to azithromycin had no effect on azithromycin absorption.

When studied in healthy elderly subjects from age 65 to 85 years, the pharmacokinetic parameters of azithromycin (500 mg Day 1, 250 mg Days 2-5) in elderly men were similar to those in young adults; however, in elderly women, although higher peak concentrations (increased by 30 to 50%) were observed, no significant accumulation occurred.

The high values in adults for apparent steady-state volume of distribution (31.1 L/kg) and plasma clearance (630 mL/min) suggest that the prolonged half-life is due to extensive uptake and subsequent release of drug from tissues. Selected tissue (or fluid) concentration and tissue (or fluid) to plasma/serum concentration ratios are shown in the following table:

[See second table on next page]

The extensive tissue distribution was confirmed by examination of additional tissues and fluids (bone, ejaculum, prostate, ovary, uterus, salpinx, stomach, liver, and gallbladder). As there are no data from adequate and well-controlled studies of azithromycin treatment of infections in these additional body sites, the clinical significance of these tissue concentration data is unknown.

Following a regimen of 500 mg on the first day and 250 mg daily for 4 days, only very low concentrations were noted in cerebrospinal fluid (less than 0.01 µg/mL) in the presence of non-inflamed meninges.

Following oral administration of a single 1200 mg dose (two 600 mg tablets), the mean maximum concentration in peripheral leukocytes was 140 µg/mL. Concentrations remained above 32 µg/mL for approximately 60 hr. The mean half-lives for 6 males and 6 females were 34 hr and 57 hr, respectively. Leukocyte to plasma C_{max} ratios for males and females were 258 (±77%) and 175 (±60%), respectively, and the AUC ratios were 804 (±31%) and 541 (±28%), respectively. The clinical relevance of these findings is unknown.

Following oral administration of multiple daily doses of 600 mg (1 tablet/day) to asymptomatic HIV-seropositive adults, mean maximum concentration in peripheral leukocytes was 252 µg/mL (±49%). Trough concentrations in peripheral leukocytes at steady-state averaged 146 µg/mL (±33%). The mean leukocyte to serum C_{max} ratio was 456 (±38%) and the mean leukocyte to serum AUC ratio was 816 (±31%). The clinical relevance of these findings is unknown.

The serum protein binding of azithromycin is variable in the concentration range approximating human exposure, decreasing from 51% at 0.02 µg/mL to 7% at 2 µg/mL. Biliary excretion of azithromycin, predominantly as unchanged drug, is a major route of elimination. Over the course of a week, approximately 6% of the administered dose appears as unchanged drug in urine.

There are no pharmacokinetic data available from studies in hepatically- or renally-impaired individuals.

The effect of azithromycin on the plasma levels or pharmacokinetics of theophylline administered in multiple doses adequate to reach therapeutic steady-state plasma levels is not known. (See PRECAUTIONS.)

Mechanism of Action: Azithromycin acts by binding to the 50S ribosomal subunit of susceptible microorganisms and, thus, interfering with microbial protein synthesis. Nucleic acid synthesis is not affected.

Azithromycin concentrates in phagocytes and fibroblasts as demonstrated by *in vitro* incubation techniques. Using such methodology, the ratio of intracellular to extracellular concentration was >30 after one hour incubation. *In vivo* studies suggest that concentration in phagocytes may contribute to drug distribution to inflamed tissues.

Microbiology:

Azithromycin has been shown to be active against most strains of the following microorganisms, both *in vitro* and in clinical infections as described in the INDICATIONS AND USAGE section.

Aerobic Gram-Positive Microorganisms

Staphylococcus aureus
Streptococcus agalactiae
Streptococcus pneumoniae
Streptococcus pyogenes

NOTE: Azithromycin demonstrates cross-resistance with erythromycin-resistant gram-positive strains. Most strains of *Enterococcus faecalis* and methicillin-resistant staphylococci are resistant to azithromycin.

Aerobic Gram-Negative Microorganisms

Haemophilus influenzae
Moraxella catarrhalis

"Other" Microorganisms

Chlamydia trachomatis

Beta-lactamase production should have no effect on azithromycin activity.

Continued on next page

Zithromax Caps/Tabs/O.S.—Cont.

Azithromycin has been shown to be active *in vitro* and in the prevention and treatment of disease caused by the following microorganisms:

Mycobacteria

Mycobacterium avium complex (MAC) consisting of:
Mycobacterium avium
Mycobacterium intracellulare.

The following *in vitro* data are available, *but their clinical significance is unknown.*

Azithromycin exhibits *in vitro* minimal inhibitory concentrations (MICs) of 2.0 μg/mL or less against most (≥90%) strains of the following microorganisms; however, the safety and effectiveness of azithromycin in treating clinical infections due to these microorganisms have not been established in adequate and well-controlled trials.

Aerobic Gram-Positive Microorganisms

Streptococci (Groups C, F, G)
Viridans group streptococci

Aerobic Gram-Negative Microorganisms

Bordetella pertussis
Campylobacter jejuni
Haemophilus ducreyi
Legionella pneumophila

Anaerobic Microorganisms

Bacteroides bivius
Clostridium perfringens
Peptostreptococcus species

"Other" Microorganisms

Borrelia burgdorferi
Mycoplasma pneumoniae
Treponema pallidum
Ureaplasma urealyticum

Susceptibility Testing of Bacteria Excluding Mycobacteria

The *in vitro* potency of azithromycin is markedly affected by the pH of the microbiological growth medium during incubation. Incubation in a 10% CO_2 atmosphere will result in lowering of media pH (7.2 to 6.6) within 18 hours and in an apparent reduction of the *in vitro* potency of azithromycin. Thus, the initial pH of the growth medium should be 7.2-7.4, and the CO_2 content of the incubation atmosphere should be as low as practical.

Azithromycin can be solubilized for *in vitro* susceptibility testing by dissolving in a minimum amount of 95% ethanol and diluting to working concentration with water.

Dilution Techniques:

Quantitative methods are used to determine minimal inhibitory concentrations that provide reproducible estimates of the susceptibility of bacteria to antimicrobial compounds. One such standardized procedure uses a standardized dilution method[1] (broth, agar or microdilution) or equivalent with azithromycin powder. The MIC values should be interpreted according to the following criteria:

MIC (μg/mL)	Interpretation
≤ 2	Susceptible (S)
4	Intermediate (I)
≥ 8	Resistant (R)

A report of "Susceptible" indicates that the pathogen is likely to respond to monotherapy with azithromycin. A report of "Intermediate" indicates that the result should be considered equivocal, and, if the microorganism is not fully susceptible to alternative, clinically feasible drugs, the test should be repeated. This category also provides a buffer zone which prevents small uncontrolled technical factors from causing major discrepancies in interpretation. A report of "Resistant" indicates that usually achievable drug concentrations are unlikely to be inhibitory and that other therapy should be selected.

Measurement of MIC or MBC and achieved antimicrobial compound concentrations may be appropriate to guide therapy in some infections. (See CLINICAL PHARMACOLOGY section for further information on drug concentrations achieved in infected body sites and other pharmacokinetic properties of this antimicrobial drug product.)

Standardized susceptibility test procedures require the use of laboratory control microorganisms. Standard azithromycin powder should provide the following MIC values:

Microorganism	MIC (μg/mL)
Escherichia coli ATCC 25922	2.0-8.0
Enterococcus faecalis ATCC 29212	1.0-4.0
Staphylococcus aureus ATCC 29213	0.25-1.0

Diffusion Techniques:

Quantitative methods that require measurement of zone diameters also provide reproducible estimates of the susceptibility of bacteria to antimicrobial compounds. One such standardized procedure[2] that has been recommended for use with disks to test the susceptibility of microorganisms to azithromycin uses the 15-μg azithromycin disk. Interpretation involves the correlation of the diameter obtained in the disk test with the minimal inhibitory concentration (MIC) for azithromycin.

Reports from the laboratory providing results of the standard single-disk susceptibility test with a 15 μg azithromycin disk should be interpreted according to the following criteria:

Zone Diameter (mm)	Interpretation
≥ 18	(S) Susceptible
14–17	(I) Intermediate
≤ 13	(R) Resistant

MEAN (CV%) PK PARAMETER

DOSE/DOSAGE FORM (serum, except as indicated)	Subjects	Day No.	C_{max} (μg/mL)	T_{max} (hr)	C_{24} (μg/mL)	ACU (μg•hr/mL)	$T_{½}$ (hr)	Urinary Excretion (% of dose)
500 mg/250 mg capsule	12	Day 1	0.41	2.5	0.05	2.6[a]	—	4.5
and 250 mg on Days 2-5	12	Day 5	0.24	3.2	0.05	2.1[a]	—	6.5
1200 mg/600 mg tablets	12	Day 1	0.66	2.5	0.074	6.8[b]	40	—
%CV			(62%)	(79%)	(49%)	(64%)	(33%)	
600 mg tablet/day	7	1	0.33	2.0	0.039	2.4[a]		
%CV			25%	(50%)	(36%)	(19%)		
	7	22	0.55	2.1	0.14	5.8[a]	84.5	—
%CV			(18%)	(52%)	(26%)	(25%)		—
600 mg tablet/day (leukocytes)	7	22	252	10.9	146	4763[a]	82.8	—
%CV			(49%)	(28%)	(33%)	(42%)	—	—

[a]AUC_{0-24}; [b]0–last.

AZITHROMYCIN CONCENTRATIONS FOLLOWING TWO 250 mg (500 mg) CAPSULES IN ADULTS

TISSUE OR FLUID	TIME AFTER DOSE (h)	TISSUE OR FLUID CONCENTRATION (μg/g or μg/mL)[1]	CORRESPONDING PLASMA OR SERUM LEVEL (μg/mL)	TISSUE (FLUID) PLASMA (SERUM) RATIO[1]
SKIN	72-96	0.4	0.012	35
LUNG	72-96	4.0	0.012	>100
SPUTUM*	2-4	1.0	0.64	2
SPUTUM**	10-12	2.9	0.1	30
TONSIL***	9-18	4.5	0.03	>100
TONSIL***	180	0.9	0.006	>100
CERVIX****	19	2.8	0.04	70

[1] High tissue concentrations should not be interpreted to be quantitatively related to clinical efficacy. The antimicrobial activity of azithromycin is pH related. Azithromycin is concentrated in cell lysosomes which have a low intraorganelle pH, at which the drug's activity is reduced. However, the extensive distribution of drug to tissues may be relevant to clinical activity.

* Sample was obtained 2-4 hours after the first dose

** Sample was obtained 10-12 hours after the first dose.

*** Dosing regimen of 2 doses of 250 mg each, separated by 12 hours.

**** Sample was obtained 19 hours after a single 500 mg dose.

Interpretation should be as stated above for results using dilution techniques.

As with standardized dilution techniques, diffusion methods require the use of laboratory control microorganisms. The 15-μg azithromycin disk should provide the following zone diameters in these laboratory test quality control strains:

Microorganism	Zone Diameter (mm)
Staphylococcus aureus ATCC 25923	21-26

***In Vitro* Activity of Azithromycin Against Mycobacteria.**

Azithromycin has demonstrated *in vitro* activity against *Mycobacterium avium* complex (MAC) organisms. While gene probe techniques may be used to distinguish between *M. avium* and *M. intracellulare*, many studies only reported results on *M. avium* complex (MAC) isolates. Azithromycin has also been shown to be active against phagocytized *M. avium* complex (MAC) organisms in mouse and human macrophage cell cultures as well as in the beige mouse infection model.

Various *in vitro* methodologies employing broth or solid media at different pHs, with and without oleic acid-albumin dextrose-catalase (OADC), have been used to determine azithromycin MIC values for *Mycobacterium avium* complex strains. In general, azithromycin MIC values decreased 4 to 8 fold as the pH of Middlebrook 7H11 agar media increased from 6.6 to 7.4. At pH 7.4, azithromycin MIC values determined with Mueller-Hinton agar were 4 fold higher than that observed with Middlebrook 7H12 media at the same pH. Utilization of oleic acid-albumin-dextrose-catalase (OADC) in these assays has been shown to further alter MIC values. The relationship between azithromycin and clarithromycin MIC values has not been established. In general, azithromycin MIC values were observed to be 2 to 32 fold higher than clarithromycin independent of the susceptibility method employed.

The ability to correlate MIC values and plasma drug levels is difficult as azithromycin concentrates in macrophages and tissues. (See CLINICAL PHARMACOLOGY)

Drug Resistance:

Complete cross-resistance between azithromycin and clarithromycin has been observed with *Mycobacterium avium* complex (MAC) isolates. In most isolates, a single point mutation at a position that is homologous to the *Escherichia coli* positions 2058 or 2059 on the 23S rRNA gene is the mechanism producing this cross-resistance pattern.[3,4] *Mycobacterium avium* complex (MAC) isolates exhibiting cross-resistance show an increase in azithromycin MICs to ≥128 μg/mL with clarithromycin MICs increasing to ≥32 μg/mL. These MIC values were determined employing the radiometric broth dilution susceptibility testing method with Middlebrook 7H12 medium. The clinical significance of azithromycin and clarithromycin cross-resistance is not fully understood at this time but preclinical data suggest that reduced activity to both agents will occur after *M. avium* complex strains produce the 23S rRNA mutation.

Susceptibility testing for *Mycobacterium avium* complex (MAC):

The disk diffusion techniques and dilution methods for susceptibility testing against Gram-positive and Gram-negative bacteria should not be used for determining azithromycin MIC values against mycobacteria. *In vitro* susceptibility testing methods and diagnostic products currently available for determining minimal inhibitory concentration (MIC) values against *Mycobacterium avium* complex (MAC) organisms have not been standardized or validated. Azithromycin MIC values will vary depending on the susceptibility testing method employed, composition and pH of media and the utilization of nutritional supplements. Breakpoints to determine whether clinical isolates of *M. avium* or *M. intracellulare* are susceptible or resistant to azithromycin have not been established.

The clinical relevance of azithromycin *in vitro* susceptibility test results for other mycobacterial species, including *Mycobacterium tuberculosis*, using any susceptibility testing method has not been determined.

INDICATIONS AND USAGE

ZITHROMAX® (azithromycin) is indicated for the treatment of patients with mild to moderate infections (pneumonia: see WARNINGS) caused by susceptible strains of the designated microorganisms in the specific conditions listed below.

Lower Respiratory Tract:

Acute bacterial exacerbations of chronic obstructive pulmonary disease due to *Haemophilus influenzae, Moraxella catarrhalis*, or *Streptococcus pneumoniae*.

Community-acquired pneumonia of mild severity due to *Streptococcus pneumoniae* or *Haemophilus influenzae* in patients appropriate for outpatient oral therapy.

NOTE: Azithromycin should not be used in patients with pneumonia who are judged to be inappropriate for outpatient oral therapy because of moderate to severe illness or risk factors such as any of the following:

patients with nosocomially acquired infections,
patients with known or suspected bacteremia,
patients requiring hospitalization,
elderly or debilitated patients, or
patients with significant underlying health problems that may compromise their ability to respond to their illness (including immunodeficiency or functional asplenia).

Upper Respiratory Tract:
Streptococcal pharyngitis/tonsillitis–As an alternative to first line therapy of acute pharyngitis/tonsillitis due to *Streptococcus pyogenes* occurring in individuals who cannot use first line therapy.

NOTE: Penicillin is the usual drug of choice in the treatment of *Streptococcus pyogenes* infection and the prophylaxis of rheumatic fever. ZITHROMAX® is often effective in the eradication of susceptible strains of *Streptococcus pyogenes* from the nasopharynx. Data establishing efficacy of azithromycin in subsequent prevention of rheumatic fever are not available.

Skin and Skin Structure
Uncomplicated skin and skin structure infections due to *Staphylococcus aureus, Streptococcus pyogenes,* or *Streptococcus agalactiae.* Abscesses usually require surgical drainage.

Sexually Transmitted Diseases
Non-gonococcal urethritis and cervicitis due to *Chlamydia trachomatis.*

ZITHROMAX®, at the recommended dose, should not be relied upon to treat gonorrhea or syphilis. Antimicrobial agents used in high doses for short periods of time to treat non-gonococcal urethritis may mask or delay the symptoms of incubating gonorrhea or syphilis. All patients with sexually-transmitted urethritis or cervicitis should have a serologic test for syphilis and appropriate cultures for gonorrhea performed at the time of diagnosis. Appropriate antimicrobial therapy and follow-up tests for these diseases should be initiated if infection is confirmed.

Appropriate culture and susceptibility tests should be performed before treatment to determine the causative organism and its susceptibility to azithromycin. Therapy with ZITHROMAX® may be initiated before results of these tests are known; once the results become available, antimicrobial therapy should be adjusted accordingly.

To reduce the development of drug-resistant bacteria and maintain the effectiveness of Zithromax (azithromycin) and other antibacterial drugs, Zithromax (azithromycin) should be used only to treat or prevent infections that are proven or strongly suspected to be caused by susceptible bacteria. When culture and susceptibility information are available, they should be considered in selecting or modifying antibacterial therapy. In the absence of such data, local epidemiology and susceptibility patterns may contribute to the empiric selection of therapy.

Mycobacterial Infections

Prophylaxis of Disseminated *Mycobacterium avium* complex (MAC) Disease
ZITHROMAX®, taken alone or in combination with rifabutin at its approved dose, is indicated for the prevention of disseminated *Mycobacterium avium* complex (MAC) disease in persons with advanced HIV infection. (See DOSAGE AND ADMINISTRATION, CLINICAL STUDIES)

Treatment of Disseminated *Mycobacterium avium* complex (MAC) Disease
ZITHROMAX®, taken in combination with ethambutol, is indicated for the treatment of disseminated MAC infections in persons with advanced HIV infection. (See DOSAGE AND ADMINISTRATION, CLINICAL STUDIES)

CONTRAINDICATIONS

ZITHROMAX® is contraindicated in patients with known hypersensitivity to azithromycin, erythromycin, or any macrolide antibiotic.

WARNINGS

Rare serious allergic reactions, including angioedema and anaphylaxis, have been reported rarely in patients on azithromycin therapy. (See **CONTRAINDICATIONS.**) Despite initially successful symptomatic treatment of the allergic symptoms, when symptomatic therapy was discontinued, the allergic symptoms **recurred soon thereafter in some patients without further azithromycin exposure.** These patients required prolonged periods of observation and symptomatic treatment. The relationship of these episodes to the long tissue half-life of azithromycin and subsequent prolonged exposure to antigen is unknown at present.

If an allergic reaction occurs, the drug should be discontinued and appropriate therapy should be instituted. Physicians should be aware that reappearance of the allergic symptoms may occur when symptomatic therapy is discontinued.

In the treatment of pneumonia, azithromycin has only been shown to be safe and effective in the treatment of community-acquired pneumonia of mild severity due to *Streptococcus pneumoniae* or *Haemophilus influenzae* in patients appropriate for outpatient oral therapy. Azithromycin should not be used in patients with pneumonia who are judged to be inappropriate for outpatient oral therapy because of moderate to severe illness or risk factors such as any of the following: patients with nosocomially acquired infections, patients with known or suspected bacteremia, patients requiring hospitalization, elderly or debilitated patients, or patients with significant underlying health problems that may compromise their ability to respond to their illness (including immunodeficiency or functional asplenia).

Pseudomembranous colitis has been reported with nearly all antibacterial agents and may range in severity from mild to life-threatening. Therefore, it is important to consider this diagnosis in patients who present with diarrhea subsequent to the administration of antibacterial agents.

Treatment with antibacterial agents alters the normal flora of the colon and may permit overgrowth of clostridia. Studies indicate that a toxin produced by *Clostridium difficile* is a primary cause of "antibiotic-associated colitis."

After the diagnosis of pseudomembranous colitis has been established, therapeutic measures should be initiated. Mild cases of pseudomembranous colitis usually respond to discontinuation of the drug alone. In moderate to severe cases, consideration should be given to management with fluids and electrolytes, protein supplementation, and treatment with an antibacterial drug clinically effective against *Clostridium difficile* colitis.

PRECAUTIONS

General: Because azithromycin is principally eliminated via the liver, caution should be exercised when azithromycin is administered to patients with impaired hepatic function. There are no data regarding azithromycin usage in patients with renal impairment; thus, caution should be exercised when prescribing azithromycin in these patients.

Prolonged cardiac repolarization and QT interval, imparting a risk of developing cardiac arrhythmia and *torsades de pointes*, have been seen in treatment with other macrolides. A similar effect with azithromycin cannot be completely ruled out in patients at increased risk for prolonged cardiac repolarization.

Prescribing Zithromax (azithromycin) in the absence of a proven or strongly suspected bacterial infection or a prophylactic indication is unlikely to provide benefit to the patient and increases the risk of the development of drug-resistant bacteria.

Information for Patients:
Patients should be cautioned to take ZITHROMAX® capsules at least one hour prior to a meal or at least two hours after a meal. Azithromycin capsules should not be taken with food.

ZITHROMAX® tablets may be taken with or without food. However, increased tolerability has been observed when tablets are taken with food.

ZITHROMAX® for oral suspension in single 1 g packets can be taken with or without food after constitution.

Patients should also be cautioned not to take aluminum- and magnesium-containing antacids and azithromycin simultaneously.

The patient should be directed to discontinue azithromycin immediately and contact a physician if any signs of an allergic reaction occur.

Patients should be counseled that antibacterial drugs including Zithromax (azithromycin) should only be used to treat bacterial infections. They do not treat viral infections (e.g., the common cold). When Zithromax (azithromycin) is prescribed to treat bacterial infection, patients should be told that although it is common to feel better early in the course of therapy, the medication should be taken exactly as directed. Skipping doses or not completing the full course of therapy may (1) decrease the effectiveness of the immediate treatment and (2) increase the likelihood that bacteria will develop resistance and will not be treatable by Zithromax (azithromycin) or other antibacterial drugs in the future.

Drug Interactions: Aluminum- and magnesium-containing antacids reduce the peak serum levels (rate) but not the AUC (extent) of azithromycin (500 mg) absorption.

Administration of cimetidine (800 mg) two hours prior to azithromycin had no effect on azithromycin (500 mg) absorption.

A single oral dose of 1200 mg azithromycin (2 x 600 mg ZITHROMAX® tablets) did not alter the pharmacokinetics of a single 800 mg oral dose of fluconazole in healthy adult subjects.

Total exposure (AUC) and half-life of azithromycin following the single oral tablet dose of 1200 mg were unchanged and the reduction in Cmax was not significant (mean decrease of 18%) by coadministration with 800 mg fluconazole.

A single oral dose of 1200 mg azithromycin (2 x 600 mg ZITHROMAX® tablets) had no significant effect on the pharmacokinetics of indinavir (800 mg indinavir tid for 5 days) in healthy adult subjects.

Coadministration of a single oral dose of 1200 mg azithromycin (2 x 600 mg ZITHROMAX® tablets) with steady-state nelfinavir (750 mg tid) to healthy adult subjects produced a decrease of approximately 15% in mean AUC_{0-8} of nelfinavir and its M8 metabolite. Mean Cmax of nelfinavir and its M8 metabolite were not significantly affected. No dosage adjustment of nelfinavir is required when nelfinavir is coadministered with azithromycin.

Coadministration of nelfinavir (750 mg tid) at steady state with a single oral dose of 1200 mg azithromycin increased the mean $AUC_{0-\infty}$ of azithromycin by approximately a factor of 2-times (range of up to 4 times) of that when azithromycin was given alone. The mean Cmax of azithromycin was also increased by approximately a factor of 2-times (range of up to 5 times) of that when azithromycin was given alone. Dose adjustment of azithromycin is not recommended. However, when administered in conjunction with nelfinavir, close monitoring for known side effects of azithromycin, such as liver enzyme abnormalities and hearing impairment, is warranted. (See ADVERSE REACTIONS.)

Following administration of trimethoprim/sulfamethoxazole DS (160 mg/800 mg) for 7 days to healthy adult subjects, coadministration of 1200 mg azithromycin (2 x 600 mg ZITHROMAX® tablets) on the 7th day had no significant effects on peak concentrations (C_{max}), total exposure (AUC), and the urinary excretion of either trimethoprim or sulfamethoxazole.

Coadministration of trimethoprim/sulfamethoxazole DS for 7 days had no significant effect on the peak concentration (C_{max}) and total exposure (AUC) of azithromycin following administration of the single 1200 mg tablet dose to healthy adult subjects.

Administration of a 600 mg single oral dose of azithromycin had no effect on the pharmacokinetics of efavirenz given at 400 mg doses for 7 days to healthy adult subjects.

Efavirenz, when administered at a dose of 400 mg for seven days produced a 22% increase in the C_{max} of azithromycin administered as a 600 mg single oral dose, while the AUC of azithromycin was not affected.

Azithromycin (500 mg Day 1, 250 mg Days 2-5) did not affect the plasma levels or pharmacokinetics of theophylline administered as a single intravenous dose. The effect of azithromycin on the plasma levels or pharmacokinetics of theophylline administered in multiple doses resulting in therapeutic steady-state levels of theophylline is not known. However, concurrent use of macrolides and theophylline has been associated with increases in the serum concentrations of theophylline. Therefore, until further data are available, prudent medical practice dictates careful monitoring of plasma theophylline levels in patients receiving azithromycin and theophylline concomitantly.

Azithromycin (500 mg Day 1, 250 mg Days 2-5) did not affect the prothrombin time response to a single dose of warfarin. However, prudent medical practice dictates careful monitoring of prothrombin time in all patients treated with azithromycin and warfarin concomitantly. Concurrent use of macrolides and warfarin in clinical practice has been associated with increased anticoagulant effects.

Dose adjustments are not indicated when azithromycin and zidovudine are coadministered. When zidovudine (100 mg q3h x5) was coadministered with daily azithromycin (600 mg, n=5 or 1200 mg, n=7), mean C_{max}, AUC and Clr increased by 26% (CV 54%), 10% (CV 26%) and 38% (CV 114%), respectively. The mean AUC of phosphorylated zidovudine increased by 75% (CV 95%), while zidovudine glucuronide C_{max} and AUC increased by less than 10%. In another study, addition of 1 gram azithromycin per week to a regimen of 10 mg/kg daily zidovudine resulted in 25% (CV 70%) and 13% (CV 37%) increases in zidovudine C_{max} and AUC, respectively. Zidovudine glucuronide mean C_{max} and AUC increased by 16% (CV 61%) and 8.0% (CV 32%), respectively.

Doses of 1200 mg/day azithromycin for 14 days in 6 subjects increased C_{max} of concurrently administered didanosine (200 mg *q*.12h) by 44% (54% CV) and AUC by 14% (23% CV). However, none of these changes were significantly different from those produced in a parallel placebo control group of subjects.

Preliminary data suggest that coadministration of azithromycin and rifabutin did not markedly affect the mean serum concentrations of either drug. Administration of 250 mg azithromycin daily for 10 days (500 mg on the first day) produced mean concentrations of azithromycin 1 day after the last dose of 53 ng/mL when coadministered with 300 mg daily rifabutin and 49 mg/mL when coadministered with placebo. Mean concentrations 5 days after the last dose were 23 ng/mL and 21 ng/mL in the two groups of subjects. Administration of 300 mg rifabutin for 10 days produced mean concentrations of rifabutin one half day after the last dose of 60 mg/ml when coadministered with daily 250 mg azithromycin and 71 ng/mL when coadministered with placebo. Mean concentrations 5 days after the last dose were 8.1 ng/mL and 9.2 ng/mL in the two groups of subjects.

The following drug interactions have not been reported in clinical trials with azithromycin; however, no specific drug interaction studies have been performed to evaluate potential drug-drug interaction. Nonetheless, they have been observed with macrolide products. Until further data are developed regarding drug interactions when azithromycin and these drugs are used concomitantly, careful monitoring of patients is advised:

Digoxin–elevated digoxin levels.

Ergotamine or dihydroergotamine–acute ergot toxicity characterized by severe peripheral vasospasm and dysesthesia.

Triazolam–decrease the clearance of triazolam and thus may increase the pharmacologic effect of triazolam.

Drugs metabolized by the cytochrome P^{450} system–elevations of serum carbamazepine, cyclosporine, hexobarbital, and phenytoin levels.

Laboratory Test Interactions: There are no reported laboratory test interactions.

Carcinogenesis, Mutagenesis, Impairment of Fertility: Long-term studies in animals have not been performed to evaluate carcinogenic potential. Azithromycin has shown no mutagenic potential in standard laboratory tests: mouse lymphoma assay, human lymphocyte clastogenic assay, and mouse bone marrow clastogenic assay.

Continued on next page

Zithromax Caps/Tabs/O.S.—Cont.

Pregnancy: Teratogenic Effects. Pregnancy Category B: Reproduction studies have been performed in rats and mice at doses up to moderately maternally toxic dose levels (i.e., 200 mg/kg/day). These doses, based on a mg/m^2 basis, are estimated to be 4 and 2 times, respectively, the human daily dose of 500 mg.

With regard to the MAC treatment dose of 600 mg daily, on a mg/m^2/day basis, the doses in rats and mice are approximately 3.3 and 1.7 times the human dose, respectively.

With regard to the MAC prophylaxis dose of 1200 mg weekly, on a mg/m^2/day basis, the doses in rats and mice are approximately 2 and 1 times the human dose, respectively.

No evidence of impaired fertility or harm to the fetus due to azithromycin was found. There are, however, no adequate and well-controlled studies in pregnant women. Because animal reproduction studies are not always predictive of human response, azithromycin should be used during pregnancy only if clearly needed.

Nursing Mothers: It is not known whether azithromycin is excreted in human milk. Because many drugs are excreted in human milk, caution should be exercised when azithromycin is administered to a nursing woman.

Pediatric Use:

In controlled clinical studies, azithromycin has been administered to pediatric patients ranging in age from 6 months to 12 years. For information regarding the use of ZITHROMAX (azithromycin for oral suspension) in the treatment of pediatric patients, please refer to the INDICATIONS AND USAGE and DOSAGE AND ADMINISTRATION sections of the prescribing information for ZITHROMAX (azithromycin for oral suspension) 100 mg/5 mL and 200 mg/5 mL bottles.

Safety in HIV-Infected Pediatric Patients: Safety and efficacy of azithromycin for the prevention or treatment of MAC in HIV-infected children have not been established. Safety data are available for 72 children 5 months to 18 years of age (mean 7 years) who received azithromycin for treatment of opportunistic infections. The mean duration of therapy was 242 days (range 3–2004 days) at doses of <1 to 52 mg/kg/day (mean 12 mg/kg/day). Adverse events were similar to those observed in the adult population, most of which involved the gastrointestinal tract. Treatment related reversible hearing impairment in children was observed in 4 subjects (5.6%). Two (2.8%) children prematurely discontinued treatment due to side effects: one due to back pain and one due to abdominal pain, hot and cold flushes, dizziness, headache, and numbness. A third child discontinued due to a laboratory abnormality (eosinophilia). The protocols upon which these data are based specified a daily dose of 10–20 mg/kg/day (oral and/or i.v.) of azithromycin.

Geriatric Use: Pharmacokinetic parameters in older volunteers (65–85 years old) were similar to those in younger volunteers (18–40 years old) for the 5-day therapeutic regimen. Dosage adjustment does not appear to be necessary for older patients with normal renal and hepatic function receiving treatment with this dosage regimen. (See CLINICAL PHARMACOLOGY.)

In multiple-dose clinical trials of oral azithromycin, 9% of patients were at least 65 years of age (458/4949) and 3% of patients (144/4949) were at least 75 years of age. No overall differences in safety or effectiveness were observed between these subjects and younger subjects, and other reported clinical experience has not identified differences in responses between the elderly and younger patients, but greater sensitivity of some older individuals cannot be ruled out.

ZITHROMAX® 600 mg tablets contain 2.1 mg of sodium per tablet. ZITHROMAX® for oral suspension 1 gram single-dose packets contain 37.0 mg of sodium per packet.

Geriatric Patients with Opportunistic Infections, Including *Mycobacterium avium* complex (MAC) Disease: Safety data are available for 30 patients (65–94 years old) treated with azithromycin at doses >300 mg/day for a mean of 207 days. These patients were treated for a variety of opportunistic infections, including MAC. The side effect profile was generally similar to that seen in younger patients, except for a higher incidence of side effects relating to the gastrointestinal system and to reversible impairment of hearing. (See DOSAGE AND ADMINISTRATION.)

ADVERSE REACTIONS

In clinical trials, most of the reported side effects were mild to moderate in severity and were reversible upon discontinuation of the drug. Approximately 0.7% of the patients from the multiple-dose clinical trials discontinued ZITHROMAX® (azithromycin) therapy because of treatment-related side effects. Most of the side effects leading to discontinuation were related to the gastrointestinal tract, e.g., nausea, vomiting, diarrhea, or abdominal pain. Rarely but potentially serious side effects were angioedema and cholestatic jaundice.

Clinical:

Multiple-dose regimen:

Overall, the most common side effects in adult patients receiving a multiple-dose regimen of ZITHROMAX® were related to the gastrointestinal system with diarrhea/loose stools (5%), nausea (3%), and abdominal pain (3%) being the most frequently reported.

No other side effects occurred in patients on the multiple-dose regimen of ZITHROMAX® with a frequency greater than 1%. Side effects that occurred with a frequency of 1% or less included the following:

Cardiovascular: Palpitations, chest pain.

Gastrointestinal: Dyspepsia, flatulence, vomiting, melena, and cholestatic jaundice.

Genitourinary: Monilia, vaginitis, and nephritis.

Nervous System: Dizziness, headache, vertigo, and somnolence.

General: Fatigue.

Allergic: Rash, photosensitivity, and angioedema.

Chronic therapy with 1200 mg weekly regimen: The nature of side effects seen with the 1200 mg weekly dosing regimen for the prevention of *Mycobacterium avium* infection in severely immunocompromised HIV-infected patients were similar to those seen with short term dosing regimens. (See CLINICAL STUDIES.)

Chronic therapy with 600 mg daily regimen combined with ethambutol: The nature of side effects seen with the 600 mg daily dosing regimen for the treatment of *Mycobacterium avium* complex infection in severely immunocompromised HIV-infected patients were similar to those seen with short term dosing regimens. Five percent of patients experienced reversible hearing impairment in the pivotal clinical trial for the treatment of disseminated MAC in patients with AIDS. Hearing impairment has been reported with macrolide antibiotics, especially at higher doses. Other treatment related side effects occurring in >5% of subjects and seen at any time during a median of 87.5 days of therapy include: abdominal pain (14%), nausea (14%), vomiting (13%), diarrhea (12%), flatulence (5%), headache (5%) and abnormal vision (5%). Discontinuations from treatment due to laboratory abnormalities or side effects considered related to study drug occurred in 8/88 (9.1%) of subjects.

Single 1-gram dose regimen: Overall, the most common side effects in patients receiving a single-dose regimen of 1 gram of ZITHROMAX® were related to the gastrointestinal system and were more frequently reported than in patients receiving the multiple-dose regimen.

Side effects that occurred in patients on the single one-gram dosing regimen of ZITHROMAX® with a frequency of 1% or greater included diarrhea/loose stools (7%), nausea (5%), abdominal pain (5%), vomiting (2%), dyspepsia (1%), and vaginitis (1%).

Post-Marketing Experience:

Adverse events reported with azithromycin during the post-marketing period in adult and/or pediatric patients for which a causal relationship may not be established include:

Allergic: Arthralgia, edema, urticaria, angioedema.

Cardiovascular: Arrhythmias including ventricular tachycardia, hypotension. There have been rare reports of QT prolongation and *torsades de pointes*.

Gastrointestinal: Anorexia, constipation, dyspepsia, flatulence, vomiting/diarrhea rarely resulting in dehydration, pseudomembranous colitis, pancreatitis, oral candidiasis and rare reports of tongue discoloration.

General: Asthenia, paresthesia, fatigue, malaise and anaphylaxis (rarely fatal).

Genitourinary: Interstitial nephritis and acute renal failure, vaginitis.

Hematopoietic: Thrombocytopenia.

Liver/Biliary: Abnormal liver function including hepatitis and cholestatic jaundice, as well as rare cases of hepatic necrosis and hepatic failure, some of which have resulted in death.

Nervous System: Convulsions, dizziness/vertigo, headache, somnolence, hyperactivity, nervousness, agitation and syncope.

Psychiatric: Aggressive reaction and anxiety.

Skin/Appendages: Pruritus, rarely serious skin reactions including erythema multiforme, Stevens Johnson Syndrome, and toxic epidermal necrolysis.

Special Senses: Hearing disturbances including hearing loss, deafness, and/or tinnitus, rare reports of taste perversion.

Laboratory Abnormalities:

Significant abnormalities (irrespective of drug relationship) occurring during the clinical trials were reported as follows:

With an incidence of 1-2%, elevated serum creatine phosphokinase, potassium, ALT (SGPT), GGT, and AST (SGOT).

With an incidence of less than 1%, leukopenia, neutropenia, decreased platelet count, elevated serum alkaline phosphatase, bilirubin, BUN, creatinine, blood glucose, LDH, and phosphate.

When follow-up was provided, changes in laboratory tests appeared to be reversible.

In multiple-dose clinical trials involving more than 3000 patients, 3 patients discontinued therapy because of treatment-related liver enzyme abnormalities and 1 because of a renal function abnormality.

In a phase I drug interaction study performed in normal volunteers, 1 of 6 subjects given the combination of azithromycin and rifabutin, 1 of 7 given rifabutin alone and 0 of 6 given azithromycin alone developed a clinically significant neutropenia (<500 cells/mm^3).

Laboratory abnormalities seen in clinical trials for the prevention of disseminated *Mycobacterium avium* disease in severely immunocompromised HIV-infected patients are presented in the CLINICAL STUDIES section.

Chronic therapy (median duration: 87.5 days, range: 1-229 days) that resulted in laboratory abnormalities in >5% subjects with normal baseline values in the pivotal trial for treatment of disseminated MAC in severely immunocompromised HIV infected patients treated with azithromycin 600 mg daily in combination with ethambutol include: a reduction in absolute neutrophils to <50% of the lower limit of normal (10/52, 19%) and an increase to five times the upper limit of normal in alkaline phosphatase (3/35, 9%). These findings in subjects with normal baseline values are similar when compared to all subjects for analyses of neutrophil reductions (22/75 [29%]) and elevated alkaline phosphatase (16/80 [20%]). Causality of these laboratory abnormalities due to the use of study drug has not been established.

DOSAGE AND ADMINISTRATION

(See INDICATIONS AND USAGE.)

ZITHROMAX® capsules should be given at least 1 hour before or 2 hours after a meal. ZITHROMAX® capsules should not be mixed with or taken with food.

ZITHROMAX® for oral suspension (single dose 1 g packet) can be taken with or without food after constitution. Not for pediatric use. For pediatric suspension, please refer to the INDICATIONS AND USAGE and DOSAGE AND ADMINISTRATION sections of the prescribing information for ZITHROMAX (azithromycin for oral suspension) 100 mg/5 mL and 200 mg/5 mL bottles.

ZITHROMAX® tablets may be taken without regard to food. However, increased tolerability has been observed when tablets are taken with food.

The recommended dose of ZITHROMAX® for the treatment of individuals 16 years of age and older with mild to moderate acute bacterial exacerbations of chronic obstructive pulmonary disease, pneumonia, pharyngitis/tonsillitis (as second line therapy), and uncomplicated skin and skin structure infections due to the indicated organisms is: 500 mg as a single dose on the first day followed by 250 mg once daily on Days 2 through 5 for a total dose of 1.5 grams of ZITHROMAX®.

The recommended dose of ZITHROMAX® for the treatment of non-gonococcal urethritis and cervicitis due to *C. trachomatis* is: a single 1 gram (1000 mg) dose of ZITHROMAX®. This dose can be administered as four 250 mg capsules or as one single dose packet (1 g).

Prevention of Disseminated MAC Infections

The recommended dose of ZITHROMAX® for the prevention of disseminated *Mycobacterium avium* complex (MAC) disease is: 1200 mg taken once weekly. This dose of ZITHROMAX® may be combined with the approved dosage regimen of rifabutin.

Treatment of Disseminated MAC Infections

ZITHROMAX® should be taken at a daily dose of 600 mg, in combination with ethambutol at the recommended daily dose of 15 mg/kg. Other antimycobacterial drugs that have shown *in vitro* activity against MAC may be added to the regimen of azithromycin plus ethambutol at the discretion of the physician or health care provider.

DIRECTIONS FOR ADMINISTRATION OF ZITHROMAX® for oral suspension in the single dose packet (1 g): The entire contents of the packet should be mixed thoroughly with two ounces (approximately 60 mL) of water. Drink the entire contents immediately; add an additional two ounces of water, mix, and drink to assure complete consumption of dosage. **The single dose packet should not be used to administer doses other than 1000 mg of azithromycin. This packet not for pediatric use.**

HOW SUPPLIED

ZITHROMAX® capsules (imprinted with "Pfizer 305") are supplied in red opaque hard-gelatin capsules containing

Cumulative Incidence Rate, %: Placebo (n=89)

Month	MAC Free and Alive	MAC	Adverse Experience	Lost to Follow-up
6	69.7	13.5	6.7	10.1
12	47.2	19.1	15.7	18.0
18	37.1	22.5	18.0	22.5

Cumulative Incidence Rate, %: Azithromycin (n=85)

Month	MAC Free and Alive	MAC	Adverse Experience	Lost to Follow-up
6	84.7	3.5	9.4	2.4
12	63.5	8.2	16.5	11.8
18	44.7	11.8	25.9	17.6

Cumulative Incidence Rate, %: Rifabutin (n=223)

Month	MAC Free and Alive	MAC	Adverse Experience	Lost to Follow-up
6	83.4	7.2	8.1	1.3
12	60.1	15.2	16.1	8.5
18	40.8	21.5	24.2	13.5

Cumulative Incidence Rate, %: Azithromycin (n=223)

Month	MAC Free and Alive	MAC	Adverse Experience	Lost to Follow-up
6	85.2	3.6	5.8	5.4
12	65.5	7.6	16.1	10.8
18	45.3	12.1	23.8	18.8

Cumulative Incidence Rate, %: Azithromycin/Rifabutin Combination (n=218)

Month	MAC Free and Alive	MAC	Adverse Experience	Lost to Follow-up
6	89.4	1.8	5.5	3.2
12	71.6	2.8	15.1	10.6
18	49.1	6.4	29.4	15.1

INCIDENCE OF ONE OR MORE TREATMENT RELATED* ADVERSE EVENTS IN HIV INFECTED PATIENTS RECEIVING PROPHYLAXIS FOR DISSEMINATED MAC OVER APPROXIMATELY 1 YEAR**

	Study 155		Study 174		
	Placebo (N=91)	Azithromycin 1200 mg weekly (N=89)	Azithromycin 1200 mg weekly (N=233)	Rifabutin 300 mg daily (N=236)	Azithromycin + Rifabutin (N=224)
Mean Duration of Therapy (days)	303.8	402.9	315	296.1	344.4
Discontinuation of Therapy	2.3	8.2	13.5	15.9	22.7
Autonomic Nervous System					
Mouth Dry	0	0	0	3.0	2.7
Central Nervous System					
Dizziness	0	1.1	3.9	1.7	0.4
Headache	0	0	3.0	5.5	4.5
Gastrointestinal					
Diarrhea	15.4	52.8	50.2	19.1	50.9
Loose Stools	6.6	19.1	12.9	3.0	9.4
Abdominal Pain	6.6	27	32.2	12.3	31.7
Dyspepsia	1.1	9	4.7	1.7	1.8
Flatulence	4.4	9	10.7	5.1	5.8
Nausea	11	32.6	27.0	16.5	28.1
Vomiting	1.1	6.7	9.0	3.8	5.8
General					
Fever	1.1	0	2.1	4.2	4.9
Fatigue	0	2.2	3.9	2.1	3.1
Malaise	0	1.1	0.4	0	2.2
Musculoskeletal					
Arthralgia	0	0	3.0	4.2	7.1
Psychiatric					
Anorexia	1.1	0	2.1	2.1	3.1
Skin & Appendages					
Pruritus	3.3	0	3.9	3.4	7.6
Rash	3.2	3.4	8.1	9.4	11.1
Skin discoloration	0	0	0	2.1	2.2
Special Senses					
Tinnitus	4.4	3.4	0.9	1.3	0.9
Hearing Decreased	2.2	1.1	0.9	0.4	0
Uveitis	0	0	0.4	1.3	1.8
Taste Perversion	0	0	1.3	2.5	1.3

* Includes those events considered possibly or probably related to study drug
** >2% adverse event rates for any group (except uveitis).

Prophylaxis Against Disseminated MAC Abnormal Laboratory Values*

		Placebo		Azithromycin 1200 mg weekly		Rifabutin 300 mg daily		Azithromycin & Rifabutin	
Hemoglobin	<8 g/dl	1/51	2%	4/170	2%	4/114	4%	8/107	8%
Platelet Count	<50 × 10³/mm³	1/71	1%	4/260	2%	2/182	1%	6/181	3%
WBC Count	<1 × 10³/mm³	0/8	0%	2/70	3%	2/47	4%	0/43	0%
Neutrophils	<500/mm³	0/26	0%	4/106	4%	3/82	4%	2/78	3%
SGOT	>5 × ULN[a]	1/41	2%	8/158	5%	3/121	3%	6/114	5%
SGPT	>5 × ULN	0/49	0%	8/166	5%	3/130	2%	5/117	4%
Alk Phos	>5 × ULN	1/80	1%	4/247	2%	2/172	1%	3/164	2%

[a]=Upper Limit of Normal
*excludes subjects outside of the relevant normal range at baseline

azithromycin dihydrate equivalent to 250 mg of azithromycin. These are packaged in bottles and blister cards of 6 capsules (Z-PAKS®) as follows:

Bottles of 50 NDC 0069-3050-50
Boxes of 3 (Z-PAKS® of 6) NDC 0069-3050-34
Unit Dose package of 50 NDC 0069-3050-86

Store capsules below 30°C (86°F).

ZITHROMAX® 600 mg tablets (engraved on front with "PFIZER" and on back with "308") are supplied as white, modified oval-shaped, film-coated tablets containing azithromycin dihydrate equivalent to 600 mg azithromycin. These are packaged in bottles of 30 tablets. ZITHROMAX® tablets are supplied as follows:

Bottles of 30 NDC 0069-3080-30

Tablets should be stored at or below 30°C (86°F).

ZITHROMAX® for oral suspension is supplied in single dose packets containing azithromycin dihydrate equivalent to 1 gram of azithromycin as follows:

Boxes of 10 Single Dose Packets (1 g) NDC 0069-3051-07
Boxes of 3 Single Dose Packets (1 g) NDC 0069-3051-75

Store single dose packets between 5° and 30°C (41° and 86°F).

CLINICAL STUDIES IN PATIENTS WITH ADVANCED HIV INFECTION FOR THE PREVENTION AND TREATMENT OF DISEASE DUE TO DISSEMINATED *MYCOBACTERIUM AVIUM* COMPLEX (MAC)

(See INDICATIONS AND USAGE):

Prevention of Disseminated MAC Disease

Two randomized, double blind clinical trials were performed in patients with CD4 counts <100 cells/μL. The first study (155) compared azithromycin (1200 mg once weekly) to placebo and enrolled 182 patients with a mean CD4 count of 35 cells/μL. The second study (174) randomized 723 patients to either azithromycin (1200 mg once weekly), rifabutin (300 mg daily) or the combination of both. The mean CD4 count was 51 cells/μL. The primary endpoint in these studies was disseminated MAC disease. Other endpoints included the incidence of clinically significant MAC disease and discontinuations from therapy for drug-related side effects.

MAC bacteremia

In trial 155, 85 patients randomized to receive azithromycin and 89 patients randomized to receive placebo met study entrance criteria. Cumulative incidences at 6, 12 and 18 months of the possible outcomes are in the following table:

[See table at bottom of previous page]

The difference in the one year cumulative incidence rates of disseminated MAC disease (placebo–azithromycin) is 10.9%. This difference is statistically significant (p=0.037) with a 95% confidence interval for this difference of (0.8%, 20.9%). The comparable number of patients experiencing adverse events and the fewer number of patients lost to follow-up on azithromycin should be taken into account when interpreting the significance of this difference.

In trial 174, 223 patients randomized to receive rifabutin, 223 patients randomized to receive azithromycin, and 218 patients randomized to receive both rifabutin and azithromycin met study entrance criteria. Cumulative incidences at 6, 12 and 18 months of the possible outcomes are recorded in the following table:

[See first table at left]

Comparing the cumulative one year incidence rates, azithromycin monotherapy is at least as effective as rifabutin monotherapy. The difference (rifabutin–azithromycin) in the one year rates (7.6%) is statistically significant (p=0.022) with an adjusted 95% confidence interval (0.9%, 14.3%). Additionally, azithromycin/rifabutin combination therapy is more effective than rifabutin alone. The difference (rifabutin–azithromycin/rifabutin) in the cumulative one year incidence rates (12.5%) is statistically significant (p<0.001) with an adjusted 95% confidence interval of (6.6%, 18.4%). The comparable number of patients experiencing adverse events and the fewer number of patients lost to follow-up on rifabutin should be taken into account when interpreting the significance of this difference.

In Study 174, sensitivity testing[5] was performed on all available MAC isolates from subjects randomized to either azithromycin, rifabutin or the combination. The distribution of MIC values for azithromycin from susceptibility testing of the breakthrough isolates was similar between study arms. As the efficacy of azithromycin in the treatment of disseminated MAC has not been established, the clinical relevance of these *in vitro* MICs as an indicator of susceptibility or resistance is not known.

Clinically Significant Disseminated MAC Disease

In association with the decreased incidence of bacteremia, patients in the groups randomized to either azithromycin alone or azithromycin in combination with rifabutin showed reductions in the signs and symptoms of disseminated MAC disease, including fever or night sweats, weight loss and anemia.

Discontinuations From Therapy For Drug-Related Side Effects

In Study 155, discontinuations for drug-related toxicity occurred in 8.2% of subjects treated with azithromycin and 2.3% of those given placebo (p=0.121). In Study 174, more subjects discontinued from the combination of azithromycin and rifabutin (22.7%) than from azithromycin alone (13.5%; p=0.026) or rifabutin alone (15.9%; p=0.209).

Safety

As these patients with advanced HIV disease were taking multiple concomitant medications and experienced a variety of intercurrent illnesses, it was often difficult to attribute adverse events to study medication. Overall, the nature of side effects seen on the weekly dosage regimen of azithromycin over a period of approximately one year in patients with advanced HIV disease was similar to that previously reported for shorter course therapies.

[See second table at left]

Side effects related to the gastrointestinal tract were seen more frequently in patients receiving azithromycin than in those receiving placebo or rifabutin. In Study 174, 86% of diarrheal episodes were mild to moderate in nature with discontinuation of therapy for this reason occurring in only 9/233 (3.8%) of patients.

Changes in Laboratory Values

In these immunocompromised patients with advanced HIV infection, it was necessary to assess laboratory abnormalities developing on study with additional criteria if baseline values were outside the relevant normal range.

[See third table at left]

Continued on next page

Zithromax Caps/Tabs/O.S.—Cont.

Treatment of Disseminated MAC Disease

One randomized, double blind clinical trial (Study 189) was performed in patients with disseminated MAC. In this trial, 246 HIV infected patients with disseminated MAC received either azithromycin 250 mg qd (N=65), azithromycin 600 mg qd (N=91) or clarithromycin 500 mg bid (N=90), each administered with ethambutol 15 mg/kg qd, for 24 weeks. Patients were cultured and clinically assessed every 3 weeks through week 12 and monthly thereafter through week 24. After week 24, patients were switched to any open label therapy at the discretion of the investigator and followed every 3 months through the last follow up visit of the trial. Patients were followed from the baseline visit for a period of up to 3.7 years (median: 9 months). MAC isolates recovered during study treatment or post-treatment were obtained whenever possible.

The primary endpoint was sterilization by week 24. Sterilization was based on data from the central laboratory, and was defined as two consecutive observed negative blood cultures for MAC, independent of missing culture data between the two negative observations. Analyses were performed on all randomized patients who had a positive baseline culture for MAC.

The azithromycin 250 mg arm was discontinued after an interim analysis at 12 weeks showed a significantly lower clearance of bacteremia compared to clarithromycin 500 mg bid.

Efficacy results for the azithromycin 600 mg qd and clarithromycin 500 mg bid treatment regimens are described in the following table:

Response to therapy of patients taking ethambutol and either azithromycin 600 mg qd or clarithromycin 500 mg bid

	Azithromycin 600 mg qd	Clarithromycin 500 mg bid	**95.1% CI on difference
Patients with positive culture at baseline	68	57	
Week 24			
Two consecutive negative blood cultures*	31/68 (46%)	32/57 (56%)	[-28, 7]
Mortality	16/68 (24%)	15/57 (26%)	[-18, 13]

*Primary endpoint

**[95% confidence interval] on difference in rates (azithromycin-clarithromycin)

The primary endpoint, rate of sterilization of blood cultures (two consecutive negative cultures) at 24 weeks, was lower in the azithromycin 600 mg qd group than in the clarithromycin 500 mg bid group.

Sterilization by Baseline Colony Count

Within both treatment groups, the sterilization rates at week 24 decreased as the range of MAC cfu/mL increased.

	Azithromycin 600 mg (N=68)	Clarithromycin 500 mg bid (N=57)
Groups Stratified by MAC Colony Counts at Baseline	No. (%) Subjects in Stratified Group Sterile at Week 24	No. (%) Subjects in Stratified Group Sterile at Week 24
≤ 10 cfu/mL	10/15 (66.7%)	12/17 (70.6%)
11-100 cfu/mL	13/28 (46.4%)	13/19 (68.4%)
101-1,000 cfu/mL	7/19 (36.8%)	5/13 (38.5%)
1,001-10,000 cfu/mL	1/5 (20.0%)	1/5 (20%)
>10,000 cfu/mL	0/1 (0.0%)	1/3 (33.3%)

Susceptibility Pattern of MAC Isolates:

Susceptibility testing was performed on MAC isolates recovered at baseline, at the time of breakthrough on therapy or during post-therapy follow-up. The T100 radiometric broth method was employed to determine azithromycin and clarithromycin MIC values. Azithromycin MIC values ranged from <4 to >256 μg/mL and clarithromycin MICs ranged from <1 to >32 μg/mL. The individual MAC susceptibility results demonstrated that azithromycin MIC values could be 4 to 32 fold higher than clarithromycin MIC values. During study treatment and post-treatment follow up for up to 3.7 years (median: 9 months) in study 189, a total of 6/68 (9%) and 6/57 (11%) of the patients randomized to azithromycin 600 mg daily and clarithromycin 500 mg bid, respectively, developed MAC blood culture isolates that had a sharp increase in MIC values. All twelve MAC isolates had azithromycin MIC's ≥256 μg/mL and clarithromycin MIC's >32 μg/mL. These high MIC values suggest development of drug resistance. However, at this time, specific breakpoints for separating susceptible and resistant MAC isolates have not been established for either macrolide.

ANIMAL TOXICOLOGY

Phospholipidosis (intracellular phospholipid binding) has been observed in some tissues of mice, rats, and dogs given multiple doses of azithromycin. It has been demonstrated in numerous organ systems (e.g., eye, dorsal root ganglia, liver, gallbladder, kidney, spleen, and pancreas) in dogs administered doses which, based on pharmacokinetics, are as low as 2 times greater than the recommended adult human dose and in rats at doses comparable to the recommended adult human dose. This effect has been reversible after cessation of azithromycin treatment. The significance of these findings for humans is unknown.

REFERENCES

1. National Committee for Clinical Laboratory Standards. Methods for Dilution Antimicrobial Susceptibility Tests for Bacteria that Grow Aerobically–Third Edition. Approved Standard NCCLS Document M7-A3, Vol. 13, No. 25, NCCLS, Villanova, PA, December 1993.
2. National Committee for Clinical Laboratory Standards. Performance Standards for Antimicrobial Disk Susceptibility Tests–Fifth Edition. Approved Standard NCCLS Document M2-A5, Vol. 13, No. 24, NCCLS, Villanova, PA, December 1993.
3. Dunne MW, Foulds G, Retsema JA. Rationale for the use of azithromycin as *Mycobacterium avium* chemoprophylaxis. *American J Medicine* 1997; 102(5C):37-49.
4. Meier A, Kirshner P, Springer B, et al. Identification of mutations in 23S rRNA gene of clarithromycin-resistant *Mycobacterium intracellulare. Antimicrob Agents Chemother.* 1994;38:381-384.
5. Methodology per Inderlied CB, et al. Determination of *In Vitro* Susceptibility of *Mycobacterium avium* Complex Isolates to Antimicrobial Agents by Various Methods. *Antimicrob Agents Chemother* 1987; 31:1697-1702.

Rx only

Licensed from Pliva **©2003 PFIZER INC**
Distributed by:
Pfizer Labs
Division of Pfizer Inc, NY, NY 10017
69-4763-00-9 Revised October 2003

ZITHROMAX® ℞

[*zĭth-ro-măks*]
(azithromycin for injection)
For IV infusion only

Prescribing information for this product, which appears on pages 2687–2690 of the 2004 PDR, has been completely revised as follows. Please write "See Supplement A" next to the product heading.

To reduce the development of drug-resistant bacteria and maintain the effectiveness of ZITHROMAX® (azithromycin) and other bacterial drugs, ZITHROMAX (azithromycin) should be used only to treat or prevent infections that are proven or strongly suspected to be caused by bacteria.

DESCRIPTION

ZITHROMAX (azithromycin for injection) contains the active ingredient azithromycin, an azalide, a subclass of macrolide antibiotics, for intravenous injection. Azithromycin has the chemical name *(2R,3S,4R,5R,8R,10R,11R,12S,13S,14R)*-13-[(2,6-dideoxy-3-*C*-methyl-3-*O*-methyl-*α-L-ribo*-hexopyranosyl)oxy]-2-ethyl-3,4,10-trihydroxy-3,5,6,8,10,12,14-hepta-methyl-11-[[3,4,6-trideoxy-3-(dimethylamino)-*β-D-xylo*-hexopyranosyl]oxy]-1-oxa-6-azacyclopentadecan-15-one. Azithromycin is derived from erythromycin; however, it differs chemically from erythromycin in that a methyl-substituted nitrogen atom is incorporated into the lactone ring. Its molecular formula is $C_{38}H_{72}N_2O_{12}$, and its molecular weight is 749.00. Azithromycin has the following structural formula:

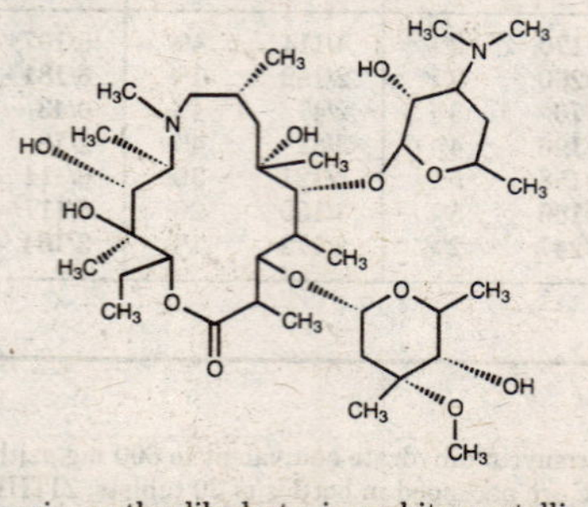

Azithromycin, as the dihydrate, is a white crystalline powder with a molecular formula of $C_{38}H_{72}N_2O_{12} \cdot 2H_2O$ and a molecular weight of 785.0.

ZITHROMAX (azithromycin for injection) consists of azithromycin dihydrate and the following inactive ingredients: citric acid and sodium hydroxide. ZITHROMAX (azithromycin for injection) is supplied in lyophilized form in a 10-mL vial equivalent to 500 mg of azithromycin for intravenous administration. Reconstitution, according to label directions, results in approximately 5 mL of ZITHROMAX for intravenous injection with each mL containing azithromycin dihydrate equivalent to 100 mg of azithromycin.

CLINICAL PHARMACOLOGY

Pharmacokinetics

In patients hospitalized with community-acquired pneumonia receiving single daily one-hour intravenous infusions for 2 to 5 days of 500 mg azithromycin at a concentration of 2 mg/mL, the mean C_{max} ± S.D. achieved was 3.63 ± 1.60 μg/mL, while the 24-hour trough level was 0.20 ± 0.15 μg/mL, and the AUC_{24} was 9.60 ± 4.80 μg•h/mL.

The mean C_{max}, 24-hour trough and AUC_{24} values were 1.14 ± 0.14 μg/mL, 0.18 ± 0.02 μg/mL, and 8.03 ±0.86 μg•h/mL, respectively, in normal volunteers receiving a 3-hour intravenous infusion of 500 mg azithromycin at a concentration of 1 mg/mL. Similar pharmacokinetic values were obtained in patients hospitalized with community-acquired pneumonia that received the same 3-hour dosage regimen for 2–5 days.

[See first table at bottom of next page]

The average CL_t and V_d values were 10.18 mL/min/kg and 33.3 L/kg, respectively, in 18 normal volunteers receiving 1000 to 4000-mg doses given as 1 mg/mL over 2 hours.

Comparison of the plasma pharmacokinetic parameters following the 1st and 5th daily doses of 500 mg intravenous azithromycin showed only an 8% increase in C_{max} but a 61% increase in AUC_{24} reflecting a threefold rise in C_{24} trough levels.

Following single oral doses of 500 mg azithromycin (two 250 mg capsules) to 12 healthy volunteers, C_{max}, trough level, and AUC_{24} were reported to be 0.41 μg/mL, 0.05 μg/mL, and 2.6 μg•h/mL, respectively. These oral values are approximately 38%, 83%, and 52% of the values observed following a single 500-mg I.V. 3-hour infusion (C_{max}: 1.08 μg/mL, trough: 0.06 μg/mL, and AUC^{24}: 5.0 μg•h/mL). Thus, plasma concentrations are higher following the intravenous regimen throughout the 24-hour interval. The pharmacokinetic parameters on day 5 of azithromycin 250-mg capsules following a 500-mg oral loading dose to healthy young adults (age 18-40 years old) were as follows: C_{max}: 0.24 μg/mL, AUC_{24}: 2.1 μg•h/mL. Azithromycin 250 mg capsules are no longer commercially available. Azithromycin 250 mg tablets are bioequivalent to 250 mg capsules in the fasting state.

Median azithromycin exposure (AUC_{0-288}) in mononuclear (MN) and polymorphonuclear (PMN) leukocytes following 1,500 mg of oral azithromycin, administered in single daily doses over either 5 days (two 250 mg tablets on day 1, followed by one 250 mg tablet on days 2-5) or 3 days (500 mg per day for days 1-3) to 12 healthy volunteers, was more than a 1000-fold and 800-fold greater than in serum, respectively.

Distribution:

The serum protein binding of azithromycin is variable in the concentration range approximating human exposure, decreasing from 51% at 0.02 μg/mL to 7% at 2 μg/mL.

Tissue concentrations have not been obtained following intravenous infusions of azithromycin. Selected tissue (or fluid) concentration and tissue (or fluid) to plasma/serum concentration ratios following oral administration of azithromycin are shown in the following table:

[See second table at bottom of next page]

Tissue levels were determined following a single oral dose of 500 mg azithromycin in 7 gynecological patients. Approximately 17 hours after dosing, azithromycin concentrations were 2.7 μg/g in ovarian tissue, 3.5 μg/g in uterine tissue, and 3.3 μg/g in salpinx. Following a regimen of 500 mg on the first day followed by 250 mg daily for 4 days, concentrations in the cerebrospinal fluid were less than 0.01 μg/mL in the presence of non-inflamed meninges.

Metabolism

In vitro and *in vivo* studies to assess the metabolism of azithromycin have not been performed.

Elimination

Plasma concentrations of azithromycin following single 500 mg oral and i.v. doses declined in a polyphasic pattern with a mean apparent plasma clearance of 630 mL/min and terminal elimination half-life of 68 hours. The prolonged terminal half-life is thought to be due to extensive uptake and subsequent release of drug from tissues.

In a multiple-dose study in 12 normal volunteers utilizing a 500-mg (1 mg/mL) one-hour intravenous-dosage regimen for five days, the amount of administered azithromycin dose excreted in urine in 24 hours was about 11% after the 1st dose and 14% after the 5th dose. These values are greater than the reported 6% excreted unchanged after oral administration of azithromycin. Biliary excretion is a major route of elimination for unchanged drug, following oral administration.

Special Populations

Renal Insufficiency

Azithromycin pharmacokinetics were investigated in 42 adults (21 to 85 years of age) with varying degrees of renal impairment. Following the oral administration of a single 1,000 mg dose of azithromycin, mean C_{max} and AUC_{0-120} increased by 5.1% and 4.2%, respectively in subjects with mild to moderate renal impairment (GFR 10 to 80 mL/min) compared to subjects with normal renal function (GFR >80 mL/min). The mean C_{max} and AUC_{0-120} increased 61% and 35%, respectively in subjects with severe renal impairment (GFR <10 mL/min) compared to subjects with normal renal function (GFR >80 mL/min). (See **DOSAGE AND ADMINISTRATION**.)

Hepatic Insufficiency
The pharmacokinetics of azithromycin in subjects with hepatic impairment have not been established.
Gender
There are no significant differences in the disposition of azithromycin between male and female subjects. No dosage adjustment is recommended based on gender.
Geriatric Patients
Pharmacokinetic studies with intravenous azithromycin have not been performed in older volunteers. Pharmacokinetics of azithromycin following oral administration in older volunteers (65-85 years old) were similar to those in younger volunteers (18-40 years old) for the 5-day therapeutic regimen.
Pediatric Patients
Pharmacokinetic studies with intravenous azithromycin have not been performed in children.
Drug-Drug Interactions
Drug interaction studies were performed with oral azithromycin and other drugs likely to be co-administered. The effects of co-administration of azithromycin on the pharmacokinetics of other drugs are shown in Table 1 and the effect of other drugs on the pharmacokinetics of azithromycin are shown in Table 2.
Co-administration of azithromycin at therapeutic doses had a modest effect on the pharmacokinetics of the drugs listed in Table 1. No dosage adjustment of drugs listed in Table 1 is recommended when co-administered with azithromycin.
Co-administration of azithromycin with efavirenz or fluconazole had a modest effect on the pharmacokinetics of azithromycin. Nelfinavir significantly increased the C_{max} and AUC of azithromycin. No dosage adjustment of azithromycin is recommended when administered with drugs listed in Table 2. (See **PRECAUTIONS - Drug Interactions.**)
[See table 1 at top of next page]
Mean rifabutin concentrations one-half day after the last dose rifabutin were 60 ng/mL when co-administered with azithromycin and 71 ng/mL when co-administered with placebo.
[See table 2 on next page]
Microbiology: Azithromycin acts by binding to the 50S ribosomal subunit of susceptible microorganisms and, thus, interfering with microbial protein synthesis. Nucleic acid synthesis is not affected.
Azithromycin concentrates in phagocytes and fibroblasts as demonstrated by *in vitro* incubation techniques. Using such methodology, the ratio of intracellular to extracellular concentration was >30 after one hour incubation. *In vivo* studies suggest that concentration in phagocytes may contribute to drug distribution to inflamed tissues.
Azithromycin has been shown to be active against most isolates of the following microorganisms, both *in vitro* and in clinical infections as described in the **INDICATIONS AND USAGE** section of the package insert for ZITHROMAX (azithromycin for injection).
Aerobic and facultative gram-positive microorganisms
Staphylococcus aureus
Streptococcus pneumoniae
NOTE: Azithromycin demonstrates cross-resistance with erythromycin-resistant gram-positive strains. Most strains of *Enterococcus faecalis* and methicillin-resistant staphylococci are resistant to azithromycin.
Aerobic and facultative gram-negative microorganisms
Haemophilus influenzae
Moraxella catarrhalis
Neisseria gonorrhoeae
"Other" microorganisms
Chlamydia pneumoniae
Chlamydia trachomatis
Legionella pneumophila
Mycoplasma hominis
Mycoplasma pneumoniae
Beta-lactamase production should have no effect on azithromycin activity.
Azithromycin has been shown to be active against most strains of the following microorganisms, both *in vitro* and in clinical infections as described in the **INDICATIONS AND USAGE** section of the package insert for ZITHROMAX (azithromycin tablets) and ZITHROMAX (azithromycin for oral suspension).
Aerobic and facultative gram-positive microorganisms
Staphylococcus aureus
Streptococcus agalactiae
Streptococcus pneumoniae
Streptococcus pyogenes
Aerobic and facultative gram-negative microorganisms
Haemophilus ducreyi
Haemophilus influenzae
Moraxella catarrhalis
Neisseria gonorrhoeae
"Other" microorganisms
Chlamydia pneumoniae
Chlamydia trachomatis
Mycoplasma pneumoniae
Beta-lactamase production should have no effect on azithromycin activity.
The following *in vitro* data are available, **but their clinical significance is unknown.**
At least 90% of the following microorganisms exhibit an *in vitro* minimum inhibitory concentration (MIC) less than or equal to the susceptible breakpoints for azithromycin. However, the safety and effectiveness of azithromycin in treating clinical infections due to these microorganisms have not been established in adequate and well-controlled clinical trials.
Aerobic and facultative gram-positive microorganisms
Streptococci (Groups C, F, G)
Viridans group streptococci
Aerobic and facultative gram-negative microorganisms
Bordetella pertussis
Anaerobic microorganisms
Peptostreptococcus species
Prevotella bivia
"Other" microorganisms
Ureaplasma urealyticum
Beta-lactamase production should have no effect on azithromycin activity.
Susceptibility Testing Methods:
When available, the results of *in vitro* susceptibility test results for antimicrobial drugs used in resident hospitals should be provided to the physician as periodic reports which describe the susceptibility profile nosocomial and community-acquired pathogens. These reports may differ from susceptibility data obtained from outpatient use, but could aid the physician in selecting the most effective antimicrobial.
Dilution techniques:
Quantitative methods are used to determine antimicrobial minimum inhibitory concentrations (MICs). These MICs provide estimates of the susceptibility of bacteria to antimicrobial compounds. The MICs should be determined using a standardized procedure. Standardized procedures are based on a dilution method[1,3] (broth or agar) or equivalent with standardized inoculum concentrations and standardized concentrations of azithromycin powder. The MIC values should be interpreted according to criteria provided in Table 1.
Diffusion techniques:
Quantitative methods that require measurement of zone diameters also provide reproducible estimates of the susceptibility of bacteria to antimicrobial compounds. One such standardized procedure[2,3] requires the use of standardized inoculum concentrations. This procedure uses paper disks impregnated with 15-μg azithromycin to test the susceptibility of microorganisms to azithromycin. The disk diffusion interpretive criteria are provided in Table 1.
[See table 1 at top of page 335]
No interpretive criteria have been established for testing *Neisseria gonorrhoeae*. This species is not usually tested.
A report of "susceptible" indicates that the pathogen is likely to be inhibited if the antimicrobial compound reaches the concentrations usually achievable. A report of "intermediate" indicates that the result should be considered equivocal, and, if the microorganism is not fully susceptible to alternative, clinically feasible drugs, the test should be repeated. This category implies possible clinical applicability in body sites where the drug is physiologically concentrated or in situations where high dosage of drug can be used. This category also provides a buffer zone which prevents small uncontrolled technical factors from causing major discrepancies in interpretation. A report of "resistant" indicates that the pathogen is not likely to be inhibited if the antimicrobial compound reaches the concentrations usually achievable; other therapy should be selected.
QUALITY CONTROL:
Standardized susceptibility test procedures require the use of quality control microorganisms to control the technical aspects of the test procedures. Standard azithromycin powder should provide the following range of values noted in Table 2. Quality control microorganisms are specific strains of organisms with intrinsic biological properties. QC strains are very stable strains which will give a standard and repeatable susceptibility pattern. The specific strains used for microbiological quality control are not clinically significant.

Table 2. Acceptable Quality Control Ranges for Azithromycin

QC Strain	Minimum Inhibitory Concentrations (μg/mL)	Disk Diffusion (zone diameters in mm)
Haemophilus influenzae ATCC 49247	1.0-4.0	13-21
Staphylococcus aureus ATCC 29213	0.5-2.0	
Staphylococcus aureus ATCC 25923		21-26
Streptococcus pneumoniae ATCC 49619	0.06-0.25	19-25

Plasma concentrations (μg/mL ± S.D.) after the last daily intravenous infusion of 500 mg azithromycin

Infusion Concentration, Duration	Time after starting the infusion (hr)								
	0.5	1	2	3	4	6	8	12	24
2 mg/mL, 1 hr[a]	2.98 ±1.12	3.63 ±1.73	0.60 ±0.31	0.40 ±0.23	0.33 ±0.16	0.26 ±0.14	0.27 ±0.15	0.20 ±0.12	0.20 ±0.15
1 mg/mL, 3 hr[b]	0.91 ±0.13	1.02 ±0.11	1.14 ±0.13	1.13 ±0.16	0.32 ±0.05	0.28 ±0.04	0.27 ±0.03	0.22 ±0.02	0.18 ±0.02

a = 500 mg (2 mg/mL) for 2-5 days in Community-acquired pneumonia patients.
b = 500 mg (1 mg/mL) for 5 days in healthy subjects.

AZITHROMYCIN CONCENTRATIONS FOLLOWING
A 500 mg DOSE (TWO 250 mg CAPSULES) IN ADULTS

TISSUE OR FLUID	TIME AFTER DOSE (h)	TISSUE OR FLUID CONCENTRATION (μg/g or μg/mL)[1]	CORRESPONDING PLASMA OR SERUM LEVEL (μg/mL)	TISSUE (FLUID) PLASMA (SERUM) RATIO[1]
SKIN	72-96	0.4	0.012	35
LUNG	72-96	4.0	0.012	>100
SPUTUM*	2-4	1.0	0.64	2
SPUTUM**	10-12	2.9	0.1	30
TONSIL***	9-18	4.5	0.03	>100
TONSIL***	180	0.9	0.006	>100
CERVIX****	19	2.8	0.04	70

[1]High tissue concentrations should not be interpreted to be quantitatively related to clinical efficacy. The antimicrobial activity of azithromycin is pH related and appears to be reduced with decreasing pH. However, the extensive distribution of drug to tissues may be relevant to clinical activity.
* Sample was obtained 2-4 hours after the first dose.
** Sample was obtained 10-12 hours after the first dose.
*** Dosing regimen of 2 doses of 250 mg each, separated by 12 hours.
**** Sample was obtained 19 hours after a single 500 mg dose.

INDICATIONS AND USAGE
ZITHROMAX (azithromycin for injection) is indicated for the treatment of patients with infections caused by susceptible strains of the designated microorganisms in the conditions listed below. As recommended dosages, durations of therapy, and applicable patient populations vary among these infections, please see **DOSAGE AND ADMINISTRATION** for dosing recommendations.
Community-acquired pneumonia due to *Chlamydia pneumoniae, Haemophilus influenzae, Legionella pneumophila, Moraxella catarrhalis, Mycoplasma pneumoniae, Staphylococcus aureus,* or *Streptococcus pneumoniae* in patients who require initial intravenous therapy.
Pelvic inflammatory disease due to *Chlamydia trachomatis, Neisseria gonorrhoeae,* or *Mycoplasma hominis* in patients who require initial intravenous therapy. If anaerobic microorganisms are suspected of contributing to the infection, an antimicrobial agent with anaerobic activity should be administered in combination with ZITHROMAX.
ZITHROMAX® (azithromycin for injection) should be followed by ZITHROMAX by the oral route as required. (See **DOSAGE AND ADMINISTRATION.**)
Appropriate culture and susceptibility tests should be performed before treatment to determine the causative microorganism and its susceptibility to azithromycin. Therapy with ZITHROMAX may be initiated before results of these tests are known; once the results become available, antimicrobial therapy should be adjusted accordingly.
To reduce the development of drug-resistant bacteria and maintain the effectiveness of ZITHROMAX (azithromycin) and other antibacterial drugs, ZITHROMAX (azithromycin) should be used only to treat or prevent infections that are proven or strongly suspected to be caused by susceptible bacteria. When culture and susceptibility information are available, they should be considered in selecting or modify-

Continued on next page

Zithromax IV—Cont.

ing antibacterial therapy. In the absence of such data, local epidemiology and susceptibility patterns may contribute to the empiric selection of therapy.

CONTRAINDICATIONS

ZITHROMAX is contraindicated in patients with known hypersensitivity to azithromycin, erythromycin, or any macrolide antibiotic.

WARNINGS

Serious allergic reactions, including angioedema, anaphylaxis, and dermatologic reactions including Stevens Johnson Syndrome and toxic epidermal necrolysis have been reported rarely in patients on azithromycin therapy. Although rare, fatalities have been reported. (See **CONTRAINDICATIONS.**) Despite initially successful symptomatic treatment of the allergic symptoms, when symptomatic therapy was discontinued, the allergic symptoms **recurred soon thereafter in some patients without further azithromycin exposure.** These patients required prolonged periods of observation and symptomatic treatment. The relationship of these episodes to the long tissue half-life of azithromycin and subsequent prolonged exposure to antigen is unknown at present.

If an allergic reaction occurs, the drug should be discontinued and appropriate therapy should be instituted. Physicians should be aware that reappearance of the allergic symptoms may occur when symptomatic therapy is discontinued.

Pseudomembranous colitis has been reported with nearly all antibacterial agents and may range in severity from mild to life-threatening. Therefore, it is important to consider this diagnosis in patients who present with diarrhea subsequent to the administration of antibacterial agents.

Treatment with antibacterial agents alters the normal flora of the colon and may permit overgrowth of clostridia. Studies indicate that a toxin produced by *Clostridium difficile* is a primary cause of "antibiotic-associated colitis."

After the diagnosis of pseudomembranous colitis has been established, therapeutic measures should be initiated. Mild cases of pseudomembranous colitis usually respond to discontinuation of the drug alone. In moderate to severe cases, consideration should be given to management with fluids and electrolytes, protein supplementation, and treatment with an antibacterial drug clinically effective against *Clostridium difficile* colitis.

PRECAUTIONS

General: Because azithromycin is principally eliminated via the liver, caution should be exercised when azithromycin is administered to patients with impaired hepatic function. Due to the limited data in subjects with GFR <10 mL/min, caution should be exercised when prescribing azithromycin in these patients. (See **CLINICAL PHARMACOLOGY - Special Populations - Renal Insufficiency.**)

ZITHROMAX (azithromycin for injection) should be reconstituted and diluted as directed and administered as an intravenous infusion over not less than 60 minutes. (See **DOSAGE AND ADMINISTRATION.**)

Local I.V. site reactions have been reported with the intravenous administration of azithromycin. The incidence and severity of these reactions were the same when 500 mg azithromycin were given over 1 hour (2 mg/mL as 250 mL infusion) or over 3 hours (1 mg/mL as 500 mL infusion). (See **ADVERSE REACTIONS.**) All volunteers who received infusate concentrations above 2.0 mg/mL experienced local I.V. site reactions and, therefore, higher concentrations should be avoided.

Prolonged cardiac repolarization and QT interval, imparting a risk of developing cardiac arrhythmia and *torsades de pointes*, have been seen in treatment with other macrolides. A similar effect with azithromycin cannot be completely ruled out in patients at increased risk for prolonged cardiac repolarization.

Prescribing ZITHROMAX (azithromycin) in the absence of a proven or strongly suspected bacterial infection or a prophylactic indication is unlikely to provide benefit to the patient and increases the risk of the development of drug-resistant bacteria.

Information for Patients:

Patients should be directed to discontinue azithromycin and contact a physician if any signs of an allergic reaction occur.

Patients should be counseled that antibacterial drugs including ZITHROMAX (azithromycin) should only be used to treat bacterial infections. They do not treat viral infections (e.g., the common cold). When ZITHROMAX (azithromycin) is prescribed to treat a bacterial infection, patients should be told that although it is common to feel better early in the course of the therapy, the medication should be taken exactly as directed. Skipping doses or not completing the full course of therapy may (1) decrease the effectiveness of the immediate treatment and (2) increase the likelihood that bacteria will develop resistance and will not be treatable by ZITHROMAX (azithromycin) or other antibacterial drugs in the future.

Drug Interactions: Co-administration of nelfinavir at steady-state with a single oral dose of azithromycin resulted in increased azithromycin serum concentrations. Although a dose adjustment of azithromycin is not recommended when administered in combination with nelfinavir, close monitoring for known side effects of azithromycin, such as liver enzyme abnormalities and hearing impairment, is warranted. (See **ADVERSE REACTIONS.**)

Azithromycin given by the oral route did not affect the prothrombin time response to a single dose of warfarin. However, prudent medical practice dictates careful monitoring of prothrombin time in all patients treated with azithromycin and warfarin concomitantly. Concurrent use of macrolides and warfarin in clinical practice has been associated with increased anticoagulant effects.

Drug interaction studies were performed with azithromycin and other drugs likely to be co-administered. (See CLINICAL PHARMACOLOGY-Drug-Drug Interactions.) When used in therapeutic doses, azithromycin had a modest effect on the pharmacokinetics of atorvastatin, carbamazepine, cetirizine, didanosine, efavirenz, fluconazole, indinavir, midazolam, rifabutin, sildenafil, theophylline (intravenous and oral), triazolam, trimethoprim/sulfamethoxazole or zidovudine. Co-administration with efavirenz or fluconazole had a

Table 1. Drug Interactions: Pharmacokinetic Parameters for Co-administered Drugs in the Presence of Azithromycin

Co-administered Drug	Dose of Co-administered Drug	Dose of Azithromycin	n	Ratio (with/without azithromycin) of Co-administered Drug Pharmacokinetic Parameters (90% CI); No Effect = 1.00	
				Mean C_{max}	Mean AUC
Atorvastatin	10 mg/day × 8 days	500 mg/day PO on days 6-8	12	0.83 (0.63 to 1.08)	1.01 (0.81 to 1.25)
Carbamazepine	200 mg/day × 2 days, then 200 mg BID × 18 days	500 mg/day PO for days 16-18	7	0.97 (0.88 to 1.06)	0.96 (0.88 to 1.06)
Cetirizine	20 mg/day × 11 days	500 mg PO on day 7, then 250 mg/day on days 8-11	14	1.03 (0.93 to 1.14)	1.02 (0.92 to 1.13)
Didanosine	200 mg PO BID × 21 days	1,200 mg/day PO on days 8-21	6	1.44 (0.85 to 2.43)	1.14 (0.83 to 1.57)
Efavirenz	400 mg/day × 7 days	600 mg PO on day 7	14	1.04*	0.95*
Fluconazole	200 mg PO single dose	1,200 mg PO single dose	18	1.04 (0.98 to 1.11)	1.01 (0.97 to 1.05)
Indinavir	800 mg TID × 5 days	1,200 mg PO on day 5	18	0.96 (0.86 to 1.08)	0.90 (0.81 to 1.00)
Midazolam	15 mg PO on day 3	500 mg/day PO × 3 days	12	1.27 (0.89 to 1.81)	1.26 (1.01 to 1.56)
Nelfinavir	750 mg TID × 11 days	1,200 mg PO on day 9	14	0.90 (0.81 to 1.01)	0.85 (0.78 to 0.93)
Rifabutin	300 mg/day × 10 days	500 mg PO on day 1, then 250 mg/day on days 2-10	6	See footnote below	NA
Sildenafil	100 mg on days 1 and 4	500 mg/day PO × 3 days	12	1.16 (0.86 to 1.57)	0.92 (0.75 to 1.12)
Theophylline	4 mg/kg IV on days 1, 11, 25	500 mg PO on day 7, 250 mg/day on days 8-11	10	1.19 (1.02 to 1.40)	1.02 (0.86 to 1.22)
Theophylline	300 mg PO BID × 15 days	500 mg PO on day 6, then 250 mg/day on days 7-10	8	1.09 (0.92 to 1.29)	1.08 (0.89 to 1.31)
Triazolam	0.125 mg on day 2	500 mg PO on day 1, then 250 mg/day on day 2	12	1.06*	1.02*
Trimethoprim/ Sulfamethoxazole	160 mg/800 mg/day PO × 7 days	1,200 mg PO on day 7	12	0.85 (0.75 to 0.97)/ 0.90 (0.78 to 1.03)	0.87 (0.80 to 0.95)/ 0.96 (0.88 to 1.03)
Zidovudine	500 mg/day PO × 21 days	600 mg/day PO × 14 days	5	1.12 (0.42 to 3.02)	0.94 (0.52 to 1.70)
Zidovudine	500 mg/day PO × 21 days	1,200 mg/day PO × 14 days	4	1.31 (0.43 to 3.97)	1.30 (0.69 to 2.43)

NA - Not Available
* - 90% Confidence interval not reported

Table 2. Drug Interactions: Pharmacokinetic Parameters for Azithromycin in the Presence of Co-administered Drugs (See **PRECAUTIONS - Drug Interactions.**)

Co-administered Drug	Dose of Co-administered Drug	Dose of Azithromycin	n	Ratio (with/without co-administered drug) of Azithromycin Pharmacokinetic Parameters (90% CI); No Effect = 1.00	
				Mean C_{max}	Mean AUC
Efavirenz	400 mg/day × 7 days	600 mg PO on day 7	14	1.22 (1.04 to 1.42)	0.92*
Fluconazole	200 mg PO single dose	1,200 mg PO single dose	18	0.82 (0.66 to 1.02)	1.07 (0.94 to 1.22)
Nelfinavir	750 mg TID × 11 days	1,200 mg PO on day 9	14	2.36 (1.77 to 3.15)	2.12 (1.80 to 2.50)
Rifabutin	300 mg/day × 10 days	500 mg PO on day 1, then 250 mg/day on days 2-10	6	See footnote below	NA

NA – Not available
* - 90% Confidence interval not reported
Mean azithromycin concentrations one day after the last dose were 53 ng/mL when coadministered with 300 mg daily rifabutin and 49 ng/mL when coadministered with placebo.

Table 1. Susceptibility Interpretive Criteria for Azithromycin Susceptibility Test Result Interpretive Criteria

Pathogen	Minimum Inhibitory Concentrations (μg/mL)			Disk Diffusion (zone diameters in mm)		
	S	I	R[a]	S	I	R[a]
Haemophilus spp.	≤ 4	--	--	≥ 12	--	--
Staphylococcus aureus	≤ 2	4	≥ 8	≥ 18	14-17	≤ 13
Streptococci including S. pneumoniae[b]	≤ 0.5	1	≥ 2	≥ 18	14-17	≤ 13

[a] The current absence of data on resistant strains precludes defining any category other than "susceptible". If strains yield MIC results other than susceptible, they should be submitted to a reference laboratory for further testing.

[b] Susceptibility of streptococci including *S. pneumoniae* to azithromycin and other macrolides can be predicted by testing erythromycin.

modest effect on the pharmacokinetics of azithromycin. No dosage adjustment of either drug is recommended when azithromycin is coadministered with any of these agents.

Interactions with the drugs listed below have not been reported in clinical trials with azithromycin; however, no specific drug interaction studies have been performed to evaluate potential drug-drug interaction. Nonetheless, they have been observed with macrolide products. Until further data are developed regarding drug interactions when azithromycin and these drugs are used concomitantly, careful monitoring of patients is advised:

Digoxin - elevated digoxin concentrations.

Ergotamine or dihydroergotamine - acute ergot toxicity characterized by severe peripheral vasospasm and dysesthesia.

Terfenadine, cyclosporine, hexobarbital and phenytoin - elevated concentrations.

Laboratory Test Interactions: There are no reported laboratory test interactions.

Carcinogenesis, Mutagenesis, Impairment of Fertility: Long-term studies in animals have not been performed to evaluate carcinogenic potential. Azithromycin has shown no mutagenic potential in standard laboratory tests: mouse lymphoma assay, human lymphocyte clastogenic assay, and mouse bone marrow clastogenic assay. No evidence of impaired fertility due to azithromycin was found.

Pregnancy: Teratogenic Effects. Pregnancy Category B: Reproduction studies have been performed in rats and mice at doses up to moderately maternally toxic dose concentrations (i.e., 200 mg/kg/day by the oral route). These doses, based on a mg/m^2 basis, are estimated to be 4 and 2 times, respectively, the human daily dose of 500 mg by the oral route. In the animal studies, no evidence of harm to the fetus due to azithromycin was found. There are, however, no adequate and well-controlled studies in pregnant women. Because animal reproduction studies are not always predictive of human response, azithromycin should be used during pregnancy only if clearly needed.

Nursing Mothers: It is not known whether azithromycin is excreted in human milk. Because many drugs are excreted in human milk, caution should be exercised when azithromycin is administered to a nursing woman.

Pediatric Use: Safety and effectiveness of azithromycin for injection in children or adolescents under 16 years have not been established. In controlled clinical studies, azithromycin has been administered to pediatric patients (age 6 months to 16 years) by the oral route. For information regarding the use of ZITHROMAX (azithromycin for oral suspension) in the treatment of pediatric patients, refer to the **INDICATIONS AND USAGE** and **DOSAGE AND ADMINISTRATION** sections of the prescribing information for ZITHROMAX (azithromycin for oral suspension) 100 mg/5 mL and 200 mg/5 mL bottles.

Geriatric Use: Pharmacokinetic studies with intravenous azithromycin have not been performed in older volunteers. Pharmacokinetics of azithromycin following oral administration in older volunteers (65-85 years old) were similar to those in younger volunteers (18-40 years old) for the 5-day therapeutic regimen.

In multiple-dose clinical trials of intravenous azithromycin in the treatment of community-acquired pneumonia, 45% of patients (188/414) were at least 65 years of age and 22% of patients (91/414) were at least 75 years of age. No overall differences in safety were observed between these subjects and younger subjects in terms of adverse events, laboratory abnormalities, and discontinuations. Similar decreases in clinical response were noted in azithromycin- and comparator-treated patients with increasing age.

ZITHROMAX (azithromycin for injection) contains 114 mg (4.96 mEq) of sodium per vial. At the usual recommended doses, patients would receive 114 mg (4.96 mEq) of sodium. The geriatric population may respond with a blunted natriuresis to salt loading. The total sodium content from dietary and non-dietary sources may be clinically important with regard to such diseases as congestive heart failure.

ADVERSE REACTIONS

In clinical trials of intravenous azithromycin for community-acquired pneumonia, in which 2-5 I.V. doses were given, most of the reported side effects were mild to moderate in severity and were reversible upon discontinuation of the drug. The majority of patients in these trials had one or more comorbid diseases and were receiving concomitant medications. Approximately 1.2% of the patients discontinued intravenous ZITHROMAX therapy, and a total of 2.4% discontinued azithromycin therapy by either the intravenous or oral route because of clinical or laboratory side effects.

In clinical trials conducted in patients with pelvic inflammatory disease, in which 1-2 I.V. doses were given, 2% of women who received monotherapy with azithromycin and 4% who received azithromycin plus metronidazole discontinued therapy due to clinical side effects.

Clinical side effects leading to discontinuations from these studies were most commonly gastrointestinal (abdominal pain, nausea, vomiting, diarrhea), and rashes; laboratory side effects leading to discontinuation were increases in transaminase levels and/or alkaline phosphatase levels.

Clinical:

Overall, the most common side effects associated with treatment in adult patients who received I.V./P.O. ZITHROMAX in studies of community-acquired pneumonia were related to the gastrointestinal system with diarrhea/loose stools (4.3%), nausea (3.9%), abdominal pain (2.7%), and vomiting (1.4%) being the most frequently reported. Approximately 12% of patients experienced a side effect related to the intravenous infusion; most common were pain at the injection site (6.5%) and local inflammation (3.1%).

The most common side effects associated with treatment in adult women who received I.V./P.O. ZITHROMAX® in studies of pelvic inflammatory disease were related to the gastrointestinal system. Diarrhea (8.5%) and nausea (6.6%) were most commonly reported, followed by vaginitis (2.8%), abdominal pain (1.9%), anorexia (1.9%), rash and pruritus (1.9%). When azithromycin was co-administered with metronidazole in these studies, a higher proportion of women experienced side effects of nausea (10.3%), abdominal pain (3.7%), vomiting (2.8%), application site reaction, stomatitis, dizziness, or dyspnea (all at 1.9%).

No other side effects occurred in patients on the multiple dose I.V./P.O. regimen of ZITHROMAX® in these studies with a frequency greater than 1%.

Side effects that occurred with a frequency of 1% or less included the following:

Gastrointestinal: dyspepsia, flatulence, mucositis, oral moniliasis, and gastritis

Nervous System: headache, somnolence

Allergic: bronchospasm

Special Senses: taste perversion

Post-Marketing Experience:

Adverse events reported with azithromycin during the post-marketing period in adult and/or pediatric patients for which a causal relationship may not be established include:

Allergic: Arthralgia, edema, urticaria and angioedema.

Cardiovascular: Arrhythmias including ventricular tachycardia and hypotension. There have been rare reports of QT prolongation and *torsades de pointes*.

Gastrointestinal: Anorexia, constipation, dyspepsia, flatulence, vomiting/diarrhea rarely resulting in dehydration, pseudomembranous colitis, pancreatitis, oral candidiasis and rare reports of tongue discoloration.

General: Asthenia, paresthesia, fatigue, malaise and anaphylaxis (rarely fatal).

Genitourinary: Interstitial nephritis and acute renal failure and vaginitis.

Hematopoietic: Thrombocytopenia.

Liver/Biliary: Abnormal liver function including hepatitis and cholestatic jaundice, as well as rare cases of hepatic necrosis and hepatic failure, some of which have resulted in death.

Nervous System: Convulsions, dizziness/vertigo, headache, somnolence, hyperactivity, nervousness, agitation and syncope.

Psychiatric: Aggressive reaction and anxiety.

Skin/Appendages: Pruritus, rarely serious skin reactions including erythema multiforme, Stevens-Johnson Syndrome and toxic epidermal necrolysis.

Special Senses: Hearing disturbances including hearing loss, deafness and/or tinnitus and rare reports of taste perversion.

Laboratory Abnormalities:

Significant abnormalities (irrespective of drug relationship) occurring during the clinical trials were reported as follows: with an incidence of 4-6%, elevated ALT (SGPT), AST (SGOT), creatinine

with an incidence of 1-3%, elevated LDH, bilirubin

with an incidence of less than 1%, leukopenia, neutropenia, decreased platelet count, and elevated serum alkaline phosphatase

When follow-up was provided, changes in laboratory tests appeared to be reversible.

In multiple-dose clinical trials involving more than 750 patients treated with ZITHROMAX (I.V./P.O.), less than 2% of patients discontinued azithromycin therapy because of treatment-related liver enzyme abnormalities.

DOSAGE AND ADMINISTRATION

(See INDICATIONS AND USAGE and CLINICAL PHARMACOLOGY.)

The recommended dose of ZITHROMAX (azithromycin for injection) for the treatment of adult patients with community-acquired pneumonia due to the indicated organisms is: 500 mg as a single daily dose by the intravenous route for at least two days. Intravenous therapy should be followed by azithromycin by the oral route at a single, daily dose of 500 mg, administered as two 250-mg tablets to complete a 7- to 10-day course of therapy. The timing of the switch to oral therapy should be done at the discretion of the physician and in accordance with clinical response.

The recommended dose of ZITHROMAX (azithromycin) for the treatment of adult patients with pelvic inflammatory disease due to the indicated organisms is: 500 mg as a single daily dose by the intravenous route for one or two days. Intravenous therapy should be followed by azithromycin by the oral route at a single, daily dose of 250 mg to complete a 7-day course of therapy. The timing of the switch to oral therapy should be done at the discretion of the physician and in accordance with clinical response. If anaerobic microorganisms are suspected of contributing to the infection, an antimicrobial agent with anaerobic activity should be administered in combination with ZITHROMAX.

Renal Insufficiency:

No dosage adjustment is recommended for subjects with renal impairment (GFR ≤ 80 mL/min). The mean AUC_{0-120} was similar in subjects with GFR 10-80 mL/min compared to subjects with normal renal function, whereas it increased 35% in subjects with GFR <10 mL/min compared to subjects with normal renal function. Caution should be exercised when azithromycin is administered to subjects with severe renal impairment. (See **CLINICAL PHARMACOLOGY, Special Populations, Renal Insufficiency.**)

Hepatic Insufficiency:

The pharmacokinetics of azithromycin in subjects with hepatic impairment have not been established. No dose adjustment recommendations can be made in patients with impaired hepatic function (See **CLINICAL PHARMACOLOGY, Special Populations, Hepatic Insufficiency.**)

No dosage adjustment is recommended based on age or gender. (See **CLINICAL PHARMACOLOGY, Special Populations.**)

The infusate concentration and rate of infusion for ZITHROMAX (azithromycin for injection) should be either 1 mg/mL over 3 hours or 2 mg/mL over 1 hour.

Preparation of the solution for intravenous administration is as follows:

Reconstitution

Prepare the initial solution of ZITHROMAX (azithromycin for injection) by adding 4.8 mL of Sterile Water For Injection to the 500 mg vial and shaking the vial until all of the drug is dissolved. Since ZITHROMAX (azithromycin for injection) is supplied under vacuum, it is recommended that a standard 5 mL (non-automated) syringe be used to ensure that the exact amount of 4.8 mL of Sterile Water is dispensed. Each mL of reconstituted solution contains 100 mg azithromycin. Reconstituted solution is stable for 24 hours when stored below 30°C or 86°F.

Parenteral drug products should be inspected visually for particulate matter prior to administration. If particulate matter is evident in reconstituted fluids, the drug solution should be discarded.

Dilute this solution further prior to administration as instructed below.

Dilution

To provide azithromycin over a concentration range of 1.0-2.0 mg/mL, transfer 5 mL of the 100 mg/mL azithromycin solution into the appropriate amount of any of the diluents listed below:

Normal Saline (0.9% sodium chloride)
1/2 Normal Saline (0.45% sodium chloride)
5% Dextrose in Water
Lactated Ringer's Solution
5% Dextrose in 1/2 Normal Saline (0.45% sodium chloride) with 20 mEq KCl
5% Dextrose in Lactated Ringer's Solution
5% Dextrose in 1/3 Normal Saline (0.3% sodium chloride)
5% Dextrose in 1/2 Normal Saline (0.45% sodium chloride)
Normosol®-M in 5% Dextrose
Normosol®-R in 5% Dextrose

When used with the Vial-Mate™ drug reconstitution device, please reference the Vial-Mate™ instructions for assembly and reconstitution.

Final Infusion Solution Concentration (mg/mL)	Amount of Diluent (mL)
1.0 mg/mL	500 mL
2.0 mg/mL	250 mL

It is recommended that a 500-mg dose of ZITHROMAX (azithromycin for injection), diluted as above, be infused over a period of not less than 60 minutes.

ZITHROMAX (azithromycin for injection) should not be given as a bolus or as an intramuscular injection.

Other intravenous substances, additives, or medications should not be added to ZITHROMAX (azithromycin for injection), or infused simultaneously through the same intravenous line.

Storage

When diluted according to the instructions (1.0 mg/mL to 2.0 mg/mL), ZITHROMAX (azithromycin for injection) is stable for 24 hours at or below room temperature (30°C or 86°F), or for 7 days if stored under refrigeration (5°C or 41°F).

Continued on next page

Zithromax IV—Cont.

HOW SUPPLIED

ZITHROMAX® (azithromycin for injection) is supplied in lyophilized form under a vacuum in a 10-mL vial equivalent to 500 mg of azithromycin for intravenous administration. Each vial also contains sodium hydroxide and 413.6 mg citric acid.

These are packaged as follows:

10 vials of 500 mg	NDC 0069-3150-83
10 vials of 500 mg with 1 Vial-Mate™ Adaptor each	NDC 0069-3150-14

CLINICAL STUDIES

Community-Acquired Pneumonia

In a controlled study of community-acquired pneumonia performed in the U.S., azithromycin (500 mg as a single daily dose by the intravenous route for 2–5 days, followed by 500 mg/day by the oral route to complete 7–10 days therapy) was compared to cefuroxime (2250 mg/day in three divided doses by the intravenous route for 2–5 days followed by 1000 mg/day in two divided doses by the oral route to complete 7–10 days therapy), with or without erythromycin. For the 291 patients who were evaluable for clinical efficacy, the clinical outcome rates, i.e., cure, improved, and success (cure + improved) among the 277 patients seen at 10–14 days post-therapy were as follows:

Clinical Outcome	Azithromycin	Comparator
Cure	46%	44%
Improved	32%	30%
Success (Cure + Improved)	78%	74%

In a separate, uncontrolled clinical and microbiological trial performed in the U.S., 94 patients with community-acquired pneumonia who received azithromycin in the same regimen were evaluable for clinical efficacy. The clinical outcome rates, i.e., cure, improved, and success (cure + improved) among the 84 patients seen at 10-14 days post-therapy were as follows:

Clinical Outcome	Azithromycin
Cure	60%
Improved	29%
Success (Cure + Improved)	89%

Microbiological determinations in both trials were made at the pre-treatment visit and, where applicable, were reassessed at later visits. Serological testing was done on baseline and final visit specimens. The following combined presumptive bacteriological eradication rates were obtained from the evaluable groups:

Combined Bacteriological Eradication Rates for Azithromycin:

(at last completed visit)	Azithromycin
S. pneumoniae	64/67 (96%)[a]
H. influenzae	41/43 (95%)
M. catarrhalis	9/10
S. aureus	9/10

[a] Nineteen of twenty-four patients (79%) with positive blood cultures for *S. pneumoniae* were cured (intent to treat analysis) with eradication of the pathogen.

The presumed bacteriological outcomes at 10-14 days post-therapy for patients treated with azithromycin with evidence (serology and/or culture) of atypical pathogens for both trials were as follows:

Evidence of Infection	Total	Cure	Improved	Cure + Improved
Mycoplasma pneumoniae	18	11 (61%)	5 (28%)	16 (89%)
Chlamydia pneumoniae	34	15 (44%)	13 (38%)	28 (82%)
Legionella pneumophila	16	5 (31%)	8 (50%)	13 (81%)

ANIMAL TOXICOLOGY

Phospholipidosis (intracellular phospholipid accumulation) has been observed in some tissues of mice, rats, and dogs given multiple doses of azithromycin. It has been demonstrated in numerous organ systems (e.g., eye, dorsal root ganglia, liver, gallbladder, kidney, spleen, and pancreas) in dogs treated with azithromycin at doses which, expressed on the basis of mg/m², are approximately equal to the recommended adult human dose, and in rats treated at doses approximately one-sixth of the recommended adult human dose. This effect has been shown to be reversible after cessation of azithromycin treatment. Phospholipidosis has been observed to a similar extent in the tissues of neonatal rats and dogs given daily doses of azithromycin ranging from 10 days to 30 days. Based on the pharmacokinetic data, phospholipidosis has been seen in the rat (30 mg/kg dose) at observed C_{max} value of 1.3 µg/mL (six times greater than the observed C_{max} of 0.216 µg/mL at the pediatric dose of 10 mg/kg). Similarly, it has been shown in the dog (10 mg/kg dose) at observed C_{max} value of 1.5 µg/mL (seven times greater than the observed same C_{max} and drug dose in the studied pediatric population). On a mg/m² basis, 30 mg/kg dose in the neonatal rat (135 mg/m²) and 10 mg/kg dose in the neonatal dog (79 mg/m²) are approximately 0.45 and 0.3 times, respectively, the recommended dose in the pediatric patients with an average body weight of 25 kg. Phospholipidosis, similar to that seen in the adult animals, is reversible after cessation of azithromycin treatment. The significance of these findings for animals and for humans is unknown.

REFERENCES

1. National Committee for Clinical Laboratory Standards, *Methods for Dilution Antimicrobial Susceptibility Tests for Bacteria That Grow Aerobically* – Fifth Edition. Approved Standard NCCLS Document M7-A5, Vol. 20, No. 2 (ISBN 1-56238-394-9). NCCLS, 940 West Valley Road, Suite 1400, Wayne, PA 19087-1898, January, 2000.
2. National Committee for Clinical Laboratory Standards, *Performance Standards for Antimicrobial Disk Susceptibility Tests* - Seventh Edition. Approved Standard NCCLS Document M2-A7, Vol. 20, No. 1 (ISBN 1-56238-393-0). NCCLS, 940 West Valley Road, Suite 1400, Wayne, PA 19087-1898, January, 2000.
3. National Committee for Clinical Laboratory Standards. *Performance Standards for Antimicrobial Susceptibility Testing* – Eleventh Informational Supplement. NCCLS Document M100-S11, Vol. 21, No. 1 (ISBN 1-56238-426-0). NCCLS, 940 West Valley Road, Suite 1400, Wayne, PA 19087-1898, January, 2001.

Rx only

Distributed by:

Pfizer Labs

Division of Pfizer Inc

NY, NY 10017

70-5191-00-8 Revised October 2003

ZOLOFT® ℞

[*zō-lŏft*]

(sertraline hydrochloride)

Tablets and Oral Concentrate

Prescribing information for this product, which appears on pages 2690-2696 of the 2004 PDR, has been completely revised as follows. Please write "See Supplement A" next to the product heading.

DESCRIPTION

ZOLOFT® (sertraline hydrochloride) is a selective serotonin reuptake inhibitor (SSRI) for oral administration. It has a molecular weight of 342.7. Sertraline hydrochloride has the following chemical name: (1S-cis)-4-(3,4-dichlorophenyl)-1,2,3,4-tetrahydro-N-methyl-1-naphthalenamine hydrochloride. The empirical formula $C_{17}H_{17}NCl_2 \bullet HCl$ is represented by the following structural formula:

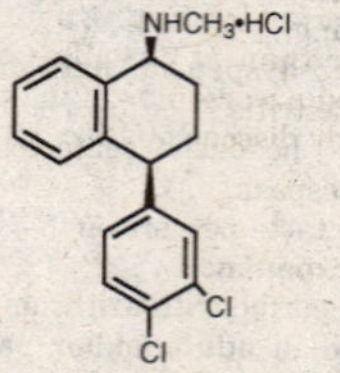

Sertraline hydrochloride is a white crystalline powder that is slightly soluble in water and isopropyl alcohol, and sparingly soluble in ethanol.

ZOLOFT is supplied for oral administration as scored tablets containing sertraline hydrochloride equivalent to 25, 50 and 100 mg of sertraline and the following inactive ingredients: dibasic calcium phosphate dihydrate, D & C Yellow #10 aluminum lake (in 25 mg tablet), FD & C Blue #1 aluminum lake (in 25 mg tablet), FD & C Red #40 aluminum lake (in 25 mg tablet), FD & C Blue #2 aluminum lake (in 50 mg tablet), hydroxypropyl cellulose, hypromellose, magnesium stearate, microcrystalline cellulose, polyethylene glycol, polysorbate 80, sodium starch glycolate, synthetic yellow iron oxide (in 100 mg tablet), and titanium dioxide.

ZOLOFT oral concentrate is available in a multidose 60 mL bottle. Each mL of solution contains sertraline hydrochloride equivalent to 20 mg of sertraline. The solution contains the following inactive ingredients: glycerin, alcohol (12%), menthol, butylated hydroxytoluene (BHT). The oral concentrate must be diluted prior to administration (see PRECAUTIONS, Information for Patients and DOSAGE AND ADMINISTRATION).

CLINICAL PHARMACOLOGY

Pharmacodynamics

The mechanism of action of sertraline is presumed to be linked to its inhibition of CNS neuronal uptake of serotonin (5HT). Studies at clinically relevant doses in man have demonstrated that sertraline blocks the uptake of serotonin into human platelets. *In vitro* studies in animals also suggest that sertraline is a potent and selective inhibitor of neuronal serotonin reuptake and has only very weak effects on norepinephrine and dopamine neuronal reuptake. *In vitro* studies have shown that sertraline has no significant affinity for adrenergic (alpha$_1$, alpha$_2$, beta), cholinergic, GABA, dopaminergic, histaminergic, serotonergic ($5HT_{1A}$, $5HT_{1B}$, $5HT_2$), or benzodiazepine receptors; antagonism of such receptors has been hypothesized to be associated with various anticholinergic, sedative, and cardiovascular effects for other psychotropic drugs. The chronic administration of sertraline was found in animals to downregulate brain norepinephrine receptors, as has been observed with other drugs effective in the treatment of major depressive disorder. Sertraline does not inhibit monoamine oxidase.

Pharmacokinetics

Systemic Bioavailability–In man, following oral once-daily dosing over the range of 50 to 200 mg for 14 days, mean peak plasma concentrations (Cmax) of sertraline occurred between 4.5 to 8.4 hours post-dosing. The average terminal elimination half-life of plasma sertraline is about 26 hours. Based on this pharmacokinetic parameter, steady-state sertraline plasma levels should be achieved after approximately one week of once-daily dosing. Linear dose-proportional pharmacokinetics were demonstrated in a single dose study in which the Cmax and area under the plasma concentration time curve (AUC) of sertraline were proportional to dose over a range of 50 to 200 mg. Consistent with the terminal elimination half-life, there is an approximately two-fold accumulation, compared to a single dose, of sertraline with repeated dosing over a 50 to 200 mg dose range. The single dose bioavailability of sertraline tablets is approximately equal to an equivalent dose of solution.

In a relative bioavailability study comparing the pharmacokinetics of 100 mg sertraline as the oral solution to a 100 mg sertraline tablet in 16 healthy adults, the solution to tablet ratio of geometric mean AUC and Cmax values were 114.8% and 120.6%, respectively. 90% confidence intervals (CI) were within the range of 80-125% with the exception of the upper 90% CI limit for Cmax which was 126.5%.

The effects of food on the bioavailability of the sertraline tablet and oral concentrate were studied in subjects administered a single dose with and without food. For the tablet, AUC was slightly increased when drug was administered with food but the Cmax was 25% greater, while the time to reach peak plasma concentration (Tmax) decreased from 8 hours post-dosing to 5.5 hours. For the oral concentrate, Tmax was slightly prolonged from 5.9 hours to 7.0 hours with food.

Metabolism–Sertraline undergoes extensive first pass metabolism. The principal initial pathway of metabolism for sertraline is N-demethylation. N-desmethylsertraline has a plasma terminal elimination half-life of 62 to 104 hours. Both *in vitro* biochemical and *in vivo* pharmacological testing have shown N-desmethylsertraline to be substantially less active than sertraline. Both sertraline and N-desmethylsertraline undergo oxidative deamination and subsequent reduction, hydroxylation, and glucuronide conjugation. In a study of radiolabeled sertraline involving two healthy male subjects, sertraline accounted for less than 5% of the plasma radioactivity. About 40-45% of the administered radioactivity was recovered in urine in 9 days. Unchanged sertraline was not detectable in the urine. For the same period, about 40-45% of the administered radioactivity was accounted for in feces, including 12-14% unchanged sertraline.

Desmethylsertraline exhibits time-related, dose dependent increases in AUC (0-24 hour), Cmax and Cmin, with about a 5-9 fold increase in these pharmacokinetic parameters between day 1 and day 14.

Protein Binding–*In vitro* protein binding studies performed with radiolabeled ^{3}H-sertraline showed that sertraline is highly bound to serum proteins (98%) in the range of 20 to 500 ng/mL. However, at up to 300 and 200 ng/mL concentrations, respectively, sertraline and N-desmethylsertraline did not alter the plasma protein binding of two other highly protein bound drugs, viz., warfarin and propranolol (see PRECAUTIONS).

Pediatric Pharmacokinetics–Sertraline pharmacokinetics were evaluated in a group of 61 pediatric patients (29 aged 6-12 years, 32 aged 13-17 years) with a DSM-III-R diagnosis of major depressive disorder or obsessive-compulsive disorder. Patients included both males (N=28) and females (N=33). During 42 days of chronic sertraline dosing, sertraline was titrated up to 200 mg/day and maintained at that dose for a minimum of 11 days. On the final day of sertraline 200 mg/day, the 6-12 year old group exhibited a mean sertraline AUC (0-24 hr) of 3107 ng-hr/mL, mean Cmax of 165 ng/mL, and mean half-life of 26.2 hr. The 13-17 year old group exhibited a mean sertraline AUC (0-24 hr) of 2296 ng-hr/mL, mean Cmax of 123 ng/mL, and mean half-life of 27.8 hr. Higher plasma levels in the 6-12 year old group were largely attributable to patients with lower body weights. No gender associated differences were observed. By comparison, a group of 22 separately studied adults between 18 and 45 years of age (11 male, 11 female) received 30 days of 200 mg/day sertraline and exhibited a mean sertraline AUC (0-24 hr) of 2570 ng-hr/mL, mean Cmax of 142 ng/mL, and mean half-life of 27.2 hr. Relative to the adults, both the 6-12 year olds and the 13-17 year olds showed about 22% lower AUC (0-24 hr) and Cmax values when plasma concentration was adjusted for weight. These data suggest that pediatric patients metabolize sertraline with slightly greater efficiency than adults. Nevertheless, lower doses may be advisable for pediatric patients given their lower body weights, especially in very young patients, in order to avoid excessive plasma levels (see DOSAGE AND ADMINISTRATION).

Age–Sertraline plasma clearance in a group of 16 (8 male, 8 female) elderly patients treated for 14 days at a dose of 100 mg/day was approximately 40% lower than in a similarly studied group of younger (25 to 32 y.o.) individuals. Steady-state, therefore, should be achieved after 2 to 3 weeks in older patients. The same study showed a decreased clearance of desmethylsertraline in older males, but not in older females.

Liver Disease–As might be predicted from its primary site of metabolism, liver impairment can affect the elimination of sertraline. In patients with chronic mild liver impairment (N=10, 8 patients with Child-Pugh scores of 5-6 and 2 patients with Child-Pugh scores of 7-8) who received 50 mg sertraline per day maintained for 21 days, sertraline clearance was reduced, resulting in approximately 3-fold greater exposure compared to age-matched volunteers with no hepatic impairment (N=10). The exposure to desmethylsertraline was approximately 2-fold greater compared to age-matched volunteers with no hepatic impairment. There were no significant differences in plasma protein binding observed between the two groups. The effects of sertraline in patients with moderate and severe hepatic impairment have not been studied. The results suggest that the use of sertraline in patients with liver disease must be approached with caution. If sertraline is administered to patients with liver impairment, a lower or less frequent dose should be used (see PRECAUTIONS and DOSAGE AND ADMINISTRATION).

Renal Disease–Sertraline is extensively metabolized and excretion of unchanged drug in urine is a minor route of elimination. In volunteers with mild to moderate (CLcr=30-60 mL/min), moderate to severe (CLcr=10-29 mL/min) or severe (receiving hemodialysis) renal impairment (N=10 each group), the pharmacokinetics and protein binding of 200 mg sertraline per day maintained for 21 days were not altered compared to age-matched volunteers (N=12) with no renal impairment. Thus sertraline multiple dose pharmacokinetics appear to be unaffected by renal impairment (see PRECAUTIONS).

Clinical Trials

Major Depressive Disorder–The efficacy of ZOLOFT as a treatment for major depressive disorder was established in two placebo-controlled studies in adult outpatients meeting DSM-III criteria for major depressive disorder. Study 1 was an 8-week study with flexible dosing of ZOLOFT in a range of 50 to 200 mg/day; the mean dose for completers was 145 mg/day. Study 2 was a 6-week fixed-dose study, including ZOLOFT doses of 50, 100, and 200 mg/day. Overall, these studies demonstrated ZOLOFT to be superior to placebo on the Hamilton Depression Rating Scale and the Clinical Global Impression Severity and Improvement scales. Study 2 was not readily interpretable regarding a dose response relationship for effectiveness.

Study 3 involved depressed outpatients who had responded by the end of an initial 8-week open treatment phase on ZOLOFT 50-200 mg/day. These patients (N=295) were randomized to continuation for 44 weeks on double-blind ZOLOFT 50-200 mg/day or placebo. A statistically significantly lower relapse rate was observed for patients taking ZOLOFT compared to those on placebo. The mean dose for completers was 70 mg/day.

Analyses for gender effects on outcome did not suggest any differential responsiveness on the basis of sex.

Obsessive-Compulsive Disorder (OCD)–The effectiveness of ZOLOFT in the treatment of OCD was demonstrated in three multicenter placebo-controlled studies of adult outpatients (Studies 1-3). Patients in all studies had moderate to severe OCD (DSM-III or DSM-III-R) with mean baseline ratings on the Yale–Brown Obsessive-Compulsive Scale (YBOCS) total score ranging from 23 to 25.

Study 1 was an 8-week study with flexible dosing of ZOLOFT in a range of 50 to 200 mg/day; the mean dose for completers was 186 mg/day. Patients receiving ZOLOFT experienced a mean reduction of approximately 4 points on the YBOCS total score which was significantly greater than the mean reduction of 2 points in placebo-treated patients.

Study 2 was a 12-week fixed-dose study, including ZOLOFT doses of 50, 100, and 200 mg/day. Patients receiving ZOLOFT doses of 50 and 200 mg/day experienced mean reductions of approximately 6 points on the YBOCS total score which were significantly greater than the approximately 3 point reduction in placebo-treated patients.

Study 3 was a 12-week study with flexible dosing of ZOLOFT in a range of 50 to 200 mg/day; the mean dose for completers was 185 mg/day. Patients receiving ZOLOFT experienced a mean reduction of approximately 7 points on the YBOCS total score which was significantly greater than the mean reduction of approximately 4 points in placebo-treated patients.

Analyses for age and gender effects on outcome did not suggest any differential responsiveness on the basis of age or sex.

The effectiveness of ZOLOFT for the treatment of OCD was also demonstrated in a 12-week, multicenter, placebo-controlled, parallel group study in a pediatric outpatient population (children and adolescents, ages 6-17). Patients receiving ZOLOFT in this study were initiated at doses of either 25 mg/day (children, ages 6-12) or 50 mg/day (adolescents, ages 13-17), and then titrated over the next four weeks to a maximum dose of 200 mg/day, as tolerated. The mean dose for completers was 178 mg/day. Dosing was once a day in the morning or evening. Patients in this study had moderate to severe OCD (DSM-III-R) with mean baseline ratings on the Children's Yale-Brown Obsessive-Compulsive Scale (CYBOCS) total score of 22. Patients receiving sertraline experienced a mean reduction of approximately 7 units on the CYBOCS total score which was significantly greater than the 3 unit reduction for placebo patients. Analyses for age and gender effects on outcome did not suggest any differential responsiveness on the basis of age or sex.

In a longer-term study, patients meeting DSM-III-R criteria for OCD who had responded during a 52-week single-blind trial on ZOLOFT 50-200 mg/day (n=224) were randomized to continuation of ZOLOFT or to substitution of placebo for up to 28 weeks of observation for discontinuation due to relapse or insufficient clinical response. Response during the single-blind phase was defined as a decrease in the YBOCS score of ≥ 25% compared to baseline and a CGI-I of 1 (very much improved), 2 (much improved) or 3 (minimally improved). Relapse during the double-blind phase was defined as the following conditions being met (on three consecutive visits for 1 and 2, and for visit 3 for condition 3): (1) YBOCS score increased by ≥ 5 points, to a minimum of 20, relative to baseline; (2) CGI-I increased by ≥ one point; and (3) worsening of the patient's condition in the investigator's judgment, to justify alternative treatment. Insufficient clinical response indicated a worsening of the patient's condition that resulted in study discontinuation, as assessed by the investigator. Patients receiving continued ZOLOFT treatment experienced a significantly lower rate of discontinuation due to relapse or insufficient clinical response over the subsequent 28 weeks compared to those receiving placebo. This pattern was demonstrated in male and female subjects.

Panic Disorder–The effectiveness of ZOLOFT in the treatment of panic disorder was demonstrated in three double-blind, placebo-controlled studies (Studies 1-3) of adult outpatients who had a primary diagnosis of panic disorder (DSM-III-R), with or without agoraphobia.

Studies 1 and 2 were 10-week flexible dose studies. ZOLOFT was initiated at 25 mg/day for the first week, and then patients were dosed in a range of 50-200 mg/day on the basis of clinical response and toleration. The mean ZOLOFT doses for completers to 10 weeks were 131 mg/day and 144 mg/day, respectively, for Studies 1 and 2. In these studies, ZOLOFT was shown to be significantly more effective than placebo on change from baseline in panic attack frequency and on the Clinical Global Impression Severity of Illness and Global Improvement scores. The difference between ZOLOFT and placebo in reduction from baseline in the number of full panic attacks was approximately 2 panic attacks per week in both studies.

Study 3 was a 12-week fixed-dose study, including ZOLOFT doses of 50, 100, and 200 mg/day. Patients receiving ZOLOFT experienced a significantly greater reduction in panic attack frequency than patients receiving placebo. Study 3 was not readily interpretable regarding a dose response relationship for effectiveness.

Subgroup analyses did not indicate that there were any differences in treatment outcomes as a function of age, race, or gender.

In a longer-term study, patients meeting DSM-III-R criteria for Panic Disorder who had responded during a 52-week open trial on ZOLOFT 50-200 mg/day (n=183) were randomized to continuation of ZOLOFT or to substitution of placebo for up to 28 weeks of observation for discontinuation due to relapse or insufficient clinical response. Response during the open phase was defined as a CGI-I score of 1 (very much improved) or 2 (much improved). Relapse during the double-blind phase was defined as the following conditions being met on three consecutive visits: (1) CGI-I ≥ 3; (2) meets DSM-III-R criteria for Panic Disorder; (3) number of panic attacks greater than at baseline. Insufficient clinical response indicated a worsening of the patient's condition that resulted in study discontinuation, as assessed by the investigator. Patients receiving continued ZOLOFT treatment experienced a significantly lower rate of discontinuation due to relapse or insufficient clinical response over the subsequent 28 weeks compared to those receiving placebo. This pattern was demonstrated in male and female subjects.

Posttraumatic Stress Disorder (PTSD)–The effectiveness of ZOLOFT in the treatment of PTSD was established in two multicenter placebo-controlled studies (Studies 1-2) of adult outpatients who met DSM-III-R criteria for PTSD. The mean duration of PTSD for these patients was 12 years (Studies 1 and 2 combined) and 44% of patients (169 of the 385 patients treated) had secondary depressive disorder.

Studies 1 and 2 were 12-week flexible dose studies. ZOLOFT was initiated at 25 mg/day for the first week, and patients were then dosed in the range of 50-200 mg/day on the basis of clinical response and toleration. The mean ZOLOFT dose for completers was 146 mg/day and 151 mg/day, respectively for Studies 1 and 2. Study outcome was assessed by the Clinician-Administered PTSD Scale Part 2 (CAPS) which is a multi-item instrument that measures the three PTSD diagnostic symptom clusters of reexperiencing/intrusion, avoidance/numbing, and hyperarousal as well as the patient-rated Impact of Event Scale (IES) which measures intrusion and avoidance symptoms. ZOLOFT was shown to be significantly more effective than placebo on change from baseline to endpoint on the CAPS, IES and on the Clinical Global Impressions (CGI) Severity of Illness and Global Improvement scores. In two additional placebo-controlled PTSD trials, the difference in response to treatment between patients receiving ZOLOFT and patients receiving placebo was not statistically significant. One of these additional studies was conducted in patients similar to those recruited for Studies 1 and 2, while the second additional study was conducted in predominantly male veterans.

As PTSD is a more common disorder in women than men, the majority (76%) of patients in these trials were women (152 and 139 women on sertraline and placebo versus 39 and 55 men on sertraline and placebo; Studies 1 and 2 combined). Post hoc exploratory analyses revealed a significant difference between ZOLOFT and placebo on the CAPS, IES and CGI in women, regardless of baseline diagnosis of comorbid major depressive disorder, but essentially no effect in the relatively smaller number of men in these studies. The clinical significance of this apparent gender interaction is unknown at this time. There was insufficient information to determine the effect of race or age on outcome.

In a longer-term study, patients meeting DSM-III-R criteria for PTSD who had responded during a 24-week open trial on ZOLOFT 50-200 mg/day (n=96) were randomized to continuation of ZOLOFT or to substitution of placebo for up to 28 weeks of observation for relapse. Response during the open phase was defined as a CGI-I of 1 (very much improved) or 2 (much improved), and a decrease in the CAPS-2 score of > 30% compared to baseline. Relapse during the double-blind phase was defined as the following conditions being met on two consecutive visits: (1) CGI-I ≥ 3; (2) CAPS-2 score increased by ≥ 30% and by ≥ 15 points relative to baseline; and (3) worsening of the patient's condition in the investigator's judgment. Patients receiving continued ZOLOFT treatment experienced significantly lower relapse rates over the subsequent 28 weeks compared to those receiving placebo. This pattern was demonstrated in male and female subjects.

Premenstrual Dysphoric Disorder (PMDD) – The effectiveness of ZOLOFT for the treatment of PMDD was established in two double-blind, parallel group, placebo-controlled flexible dose trials (Studies 1 and 2) conducted over 3 menstrual cycles. Patients in Study 1 met DSM-III-R criteria for Late Luteal Phase Dysphoric Disorder (LLPDD), the clinical entity now referred to as Premenstrual Dysphoric Disorder (PMDD) in DSM-IV. Patients in Study 2 met DSM-IV criteria for PMDD. Study 1 utilized daily dosing throughout the study, while Study 2 utilized luteal phase dosing for the 2 weeks prior to the onset of menses. The mean duration of PMDD symptoms for these patients was approximately 10.5 years in both studies. Patients on oral contraceptives were excluded from these trials; therefore, the efficacy of sertraline in combination with oral contraceptives for the treatment of PMDD is unknown.

Efficacy was assessed with the Daily Record of Severity of Problems (DRSP), a patient-rated instrument that mirrors the diagnostic criteria for PMDD as identified in the DSM-IV, and includes assessments for mood, physical symptoms, and other symptoms. Other efficacy assessments included the Hamilton Depression Rating Scale (HAMD-17), and the Clinical Global Impression Severity of Illness (CGI-S) and Improvement (CGI-I) scores.

In Study 1, involving n=251 randomized patients, ZOLOFT treatment was initiated at 50 mg/day and administered daily throughout the menstrual cycle. In subsequent cycles, patients were dosed in the range of 50-150 mg/day on the basis of clinical response and toleration. The mean dose for completers was 102 mg/day. ZOLOFT administered daily throughout the menstrual cycle was significantly more effective than placebo on change from baseline to endpoint on the DRSP total score, the HAMD-17 total score, and the CGI-S score, as well as the CGI-I score at endpoint.

In Study 2, involving n=281 randomized patients, ZOLOFT treatment was initiated at 50 mg/day in the late luteal phase (last 2 weeks) of each menstrual cycle and then discontinued at the onset of menses. In subsequent cycles, patients were dosed in the range of 50-100 mg/day in the luteal phase of each cycle, on the basis of clinical response and toleration. Patients who were titrated to 100 mg/day received 50 mg/day for the first 3 days of the cycle, then 100 mg/day for the remainder of the cycle. The mean ZOLOFT dose for completers was 74 mg/day. ZOLOFT administered in the late luteal phase of the menstrual cycle was significantly more effective than placebo on change from baseline to endpoint on the DRSP total score and the CGI-S score, as well as the CGI-I score at endpoint.

There was insufficient information to determine the effect of race or age on outcome in these studies.

Social Anxiety Disorder – The effectiveness of ZOLOFT in the treatment of social anxiety disorder (also known as social phobia) was established in two multicenter placebo-controlled studies (Study 1 and 2) of adult outpatients who met DSM-IV criteria for social anxiety disorder.

Study 1 was a 12-week, multicenter, flexible dose study comparing ZOLOFT (50-200 mg/day) to placebo, in which ZOLOFT was initiated at 25 mg/day for the first week. Study outcome was assessed by (a) the Liebowitz Social Anxiety Scale (LSAS), a 24-item clinician administered instrument that measures fear, anxiety and avoidance of social and performance situations, and by (b) the proportion of responders as defined by the Clinical Global Impression of Improvement (CGI-I) criterion of CGI-I ≤ 2 (very much or much improved). ZOLOFT was statistically significantly more effective than placebo as measured by the LSAS and the percentage of responders.

Study 2 was a 20-week, multicenter, flexible dose study that compared ZOLOFT (50-200 mg/day) to placebo. Study outcome was assessed by the (a) Duke Brief Social Phobia Scale (BSPS), a multi-item clinician-rated instrument that measures fear, avoidance and physiologic response to social or performance situations, (b) the Marks Fear Questionnaire Social Phobia Subscale (FQ-SPS), a 5-item patient-rated instrument that measures change in the severity of phobic avoidance and distress, and (c) the CGI-I responder criterion of ≤ 2. ZOLOFT was shown to be statistically significantly more effective than placebo as measured by the BSPS total score and fear, avoidance and physiologic factor scores, as well as the FQ-SPS total score, and to have significantly more responders than placebo as defined by the CGI-I.

Subgroup analyses did not suggest differences in treatment outcome on the basis of gender. There was insufficient information to determine the effect of race or age on outcome.

In a longer-term study, patients meeting DSM-IV criteria for social anxiety disorder who had responded while as-

Continued on next page

Zoloft—Cont.

signed to ZOLOFT (CGI-I of 1 or 2) during a 20-week placebo-controlled trial on ZOLOFT 50-200 mg/day were randomized to continuation of ZOLOFT or to substitution of placebo for up to 24 weeks of observation for relapse. Relapse was defined as ≥ 2 point increase in the Clinical Global Impression – Severity of Illness (CGI-S) score compared to baseline or study discontinuation due to lack of efficacy. Patients receiving ZOLOFT continuation treatment experienced a statistically significantly lower relapse rate over this 24-week study than patients randomized to placebo substitution.

INDICATIONS AND USAGE

Major Depressive Disorder–ZOLOFT® (sertraline hydrochloride) is indicated for the treatment of major depressive disorder.

The efficacy of ZOLOFT in the treatment of a major depressive episode was established in six to eight week controlled trials of outpatients whose diagnoses corresponded most closely to the DSM-III category of major depressive disorder (see Clinical Trials under CLINICAL PHARMACOLOGY).

A major depressive episode implies a prominent and relatively persistent depressed or dysphoric mood that usually interferes with daily functioning (nearly every day for at least 2 weeks); it should include at least 4 of the following 8 symptoms: change in appetite, change in sleep, psychomotor agitation or retardation, loss of interest in usual activities or decrease in sexual drive, increased fatigue, feelings of guilt or worthlessness, slowed thinking or impaired concentration, and a suicide attempt or suicidal ideation.

The antidepressant action of ZOLOFT in hospitalized depressed patients has not been adequately studied.

The efficacy of ZOLOFT in maintaining an antidepressant response for up to 44 weeks following 8 weeks of open-label acute treatment (52 weeks total) was demonstrated in a placebo-controlled trial. The usefulness of the drug in patients receiving ZOLOFT for extended periods should be re-evaluated periodically (see Clinical Trials under CLINICAL PHARMACOLOGY).

Obsessive-Compulsive Disorder–ZOLOFT is indicated for the treatment of obsessions and compulsions in patients with obsessive-compulsive disorder (OCD), as defined in the DSM-III-R; i.e., the obsessions or compulsions cause marked distress, are time-consuming, or significantly interfere with social or occupational functioning.

The efficacy of ZOLOFT was established in 12-week trials with obsessive-compulsive outpatients having diagnoses of obsessive-compulsive disorder as defined according to DSM-III or DSM-III-R criteria (see Clinical Trials under CLINICAL PHARMACOLOGY).

Obsessive-compulsive disorder is characterized by recurrent and persistent ideas, thoughts, impulses, or images (obsessions) that are ego-dystonic and/or repetitive, purposeful, and intentional behaviors (compulsions) that are recognized by the person as excessive or unreasonable.

The efficacy of ZOLOFT in maintaining a response, in patients with OCD who responded during a 52-week treatment phase while taking ZOLOFT and were then observed for relapse during a period of up to 28 weeks, was demonstrated in a placebo-controlled trial (see Clinical Trials under CLINICAL PHARMACOLOGY). Nevertheless, the physician who elects to use ZOLOFT for extended periods should periodically re-evaluate the long-term usefulness of the drug for the individual patient (see DOSAGE AND ADMINISTRATION).

Panic Disorder–ZOLOFT is indicated for the treatment of panic disorder, with or without agoraphobia, as defined in DSM-IV. Panic disorder is characterized by the occurrence of unexpected panic attacks and associated concern about having additional attacks, worry about the implications or consequences of the attacks, and/or a significant change in behavior related to the attacks.

The efficacy of ZOLOFT was established in three 10-12 week trials in panic disorder patients whose diagnoses corresponded to the DSM-III-R category of panic disorder (see Clinical Trials under CLINICAL PHARMACOLOGY).

Panic disorder (DSM-IV) is characterized by recurrent unexpected panic attacks, i.e., a discrete period of intense fear or discomfort in which four (or more) of the following symptoms develop abruptly and reach a peak within 10 minutes: (1) palpitations, pounding heart, or accelerated heart rate; (2) sweating; (3) trembling or shaking; (4) sensations of shortness of breath or smothering; (5) feeling of choking; (6) chest pain or discomfort; (7) nausea or abdominal distress; (8) feeling dizzy, unsteady, lightheaded, or faint; (9) derealization (feelings of unreality) or depersonalization (being detached from oneself); (10) fear of losing control; (11) fear of dying; (12) paresthesias (numbness or tingling sensations); (13) chills or hot flushes.

The efficacy of ZOLOFT in maintaining a response, in patients with panic disorder who responded during a 52-week treatment phase while taking ZOLOFT and were then observed for relapse during a period of up to 28 weeks, was demonstrated in a placebo-controlled trial (see Clinical Trials under CLINICAL PHARMACOLOGY). Nevertheless, the physician who elects to use ZOLOFT for extended periods should periodically re-evaluate the long-term usefulness of the drug for the individual patient (see DOSAGE AND ADMINISTRATION).

Posttraumatic Stress Disorder (PTSD)–ZOLOFT (sertraline hydrochloride) is indicated for the treatment of posttraumatic stress disorder.

The efficacy of ZOLOFT in the treatment of PTSD was established in two 12-week placebo-controlled trials of outpatients whose diagnosis met criteria for the DSM-III-R category of PTSD (see Clinical Trials under CLINICAL PHARMACOLOGY).

PTSD, as defined by DSM-III-R/IV, requires exposure to a traumatic event that involved actual or threatened death or serious injury, or threat to the physical integrity of self or others, and a response which involves intense fear, helplessness, or horror. Symptoms that occur as a result of exposure to the traumatic event include reexperiencing of the event in the form of intrusive thoughts, flashbacks or dreams, and intense psychological distress and physiological reactivity on exposure to cues to the event; avoidance of situations reminiscent of the traumatic event, inability to recall details of the event, and/or numbing of general responsiveness manifested as diminished interest in significant activities, estrangement from others, restricted range of affect, or sense of foreshortened future; and symptoms of autonomic arousal including hypervigilance, exaggerated startle response, sleep disturbance, impaired concentration, and irritability or outbursts of anger. A PTSD diagnosis requires that the symptoms are present for at least a month and that they cause clinically significant distress or impairment in social, occupational, or other important areas of functioning.

The efficacy of ZOLOFT in maintaining a response in patients with PTSD for up to 28 weeks following 24 weeks of open-label treatment was demonstrated in a placebo-controlled trial. Nevertheless, the physician who elects to use ZOLOFT for extended periods should periodically re-evaluate the long-term usefulness of the drug for the individual patient (see DOSAGE AND ADMINISTRATION).

Premenstrual Dysphoric Disorder (PMDD) – ZOLOFT is indicated for the treatment of premenstrual dysphoric disorder (PMDD).

The efficacy of ZOLOFT in the treatment of PMDD was established in 2 placebo-controlled trials of female outpatients treated for 3 menstrual cycles who met criteria for the DSM-III-R/IV category of PMDD (see Clinical Trials under CLINICAL PHARMACOLOGY).

The essential features of PMDD include markedly depressed mood, anxiety or tension, affective lability, and persistent anger or irritability. Other features include decreased interest in activities, difficulty concentrating, lack of energy, change in appetite or sleep, and feeling out of control. Physical symptoms associated with PMDD include breast tenderness, headache, joint and muscle pain, bloating and weight gain. These symptoms occur regularly during the luteal phase and remit within a few days following onset of menses; the disturbance markedly interferes with work or school or with usual social activities and relationships with others. In making the diagnosis, care should be taken to rule out other cyclical mood disorders that may be exacerbated by treatment with an antidepressant.

The effectiveness of ZOLOFT in long-term use, that is, for more than 3 menstrual cycles, has not been systematically evaluated in controlled trials. Therefore, the physician who elects to use ZOLOFT for extended periods should periodically re-evaluate the long-term usefulness of the drug for the individual patient (see DOSAGE AND ADMINISTRATION).

Social Anxiety Disorder – ZOLOFT (sertraline hydrochloride) is indicated for the treatment of social anxiety disorder, also known as social phobia.

The efficacy of ZOLOFT in the treatment of social anxiety disorder was established in two placebo-controlled trials of outpatients with a diagnosis of social anxiety disorder as defined by DSM-IV criteria (see Clinical Trials under CLINICAL PHARMACOLOGY).

Social anxiety disorder, as defined by DSM-IV, is characterized by marked and persistent fear of social or performance situations involving exposure to unfamiliar people or possible scrutiny by others and by fears of acting in a humiliating or embarrassing way. Exposure to the feared social situation almost always provokes anxiety and feared social or performance situations are avoided or else are endured with intense anxiety or distress. In addition, patients recognize that the fear is excessive or unreasonable and the avoidance and anticipatory anxiety of the feared situation is associated with functional impairment or marked distress.

The efficacy of ZOLOFT in maintaining a response in patients with social anxiety disorder for up to 24 weeks following 20 weeks of ZOLOFT treatment was demonstrated in a placebo-controlled trial. Physicians who prescribe ZOLOFT for extended periods should periodically re-evaluate the long-term usefulness of the drug for the individual patient (see Clinical Trials under CLINICAL PHARMACOLOGY).

CONTRAINDICATIONS

All Dosage Forms of ZOLOFT:

Concomitant use in patients taking monoamine oxidase inhibitors (MAOIs) is contraindicated (see WARNINGS). Concomitant use in patients taking pimozide is contraindicated (see PRECAUTIONS).

ZOLOFT is contraindicated in patients with a hypersensitivity to sertraline or any of the inactive ingredients in ZOLOFT.

Oral Concentrate:

ZOLOFT oral concentrate is contraindicated with ANTABUSE (disulfiram) due to the alcohol content of the concentrate.

WARNINGS

Cases of serious sometimes fatal reactions have been reported in patients receiving ZOLOFT® (sertraline hydrochloride), a selective serotonin reuptake inhibitor (SSRI), in combination with a monoamine oxidase inhibitor (MAOI). Symptoms of a drug interaction between an SSRI and an MAOI include: hyperthermia, rigidity, myoclonus, autonomic instability with possible rapid fluctuations of vital signs, mental status changes that include confusion, irritability, and extreme agitation progressing to delirium and coma. These reactions have also been reported in patients who have recently discontinued an SSRI and have been started on an MAOI. Some cases presented with features resembling neuroleptic malignant syndrome. Therefore, ZOLOFT should not be used in combination with an MAOI, or within 14 days of discontinuing treatment with an MAOI. Similarly, at least 14 days should be allowed after stopping ZOLOFT before starting an MAOI.

PRECAUTIONS

General

Activation of Mania/Hypomania–During premarketing testing, hypomania or mania occurred in approximately 0.4% of ZOLOFT® (sertraline hydrochloride) treated patients.

Weight Loss–Significant weight loss may be an undesirable result of treatment with sertraline for some patients, but on average, patients in controlled trials had minimal, 1 to 2 pound weight loss, versus smaller changes on placebo. Only rarely have sertraline patients been discontinued for weight loss.

Seizure–ZOLOFT has not been evaluated in patients with a seizure disorder. These patients were excluded from clinical studies during the product's premarket testing. No seizures were observed among approximately 3000 patients treated with ZOLOFT in the development program for major depressive disorder. However, 4 patients out of approximately 1800 (220<18 years of age) exposed during the development program for obsessive-compulsive disorder experienced seizures, representing a crude incidence of 0.2%. Three of these patients were adolescents, two with a seizure disorder and one with a family history of seizure disorder, none of whom were receiving anticonvulsant medication. Accordingly, ZOLOFT should be introduced with care in patients with a seizure disorder.

Suicide–The possibility of a suicide attempt is inherent in major depressive disorder and may persist until significant remission occurs. Close supervision of high risk patients should accompany initial drug therapy. Prescriptions for ZOLOFT should be written for the smallest quantity of tablets consistent with good patient management, in order to reduce the risk of overdose.

Because of the well-established comorbidity between OCD, panic disorder, PTSD, PMDD or social anxiety disorder and major depressive disorder, the same precautions observed when treating patients with major depressive disorder should be observed when treating patients with OCD, panic disorder, PTSD, PMDD or social anxiety disorder.

Weak Uricosuric Effect–ZOLOFT® (sertraline hydrochloride) is associated with a mean decrease in serum uric acid of approximately 7%. The clinical significance of this weak uricosuric effect is unknown.

Use in Patients with Concomitant Illness–Clinical experience with ZOLOFT in patients with certain concomitant systemic illness is limited. Caution is advisable in using ZOLOFT in patients with diseases or conditions that could affect metabolism or hemodynamic responses.

ZOLOFT has not been evaluated or used to any appreciable extent in patients with a recent history of myocardial infarction or unstable heart disease. Patients with these diagnoses were excluded from clinical studies during the product's premarket testing. However, the electrocardiograms of 774 patients who received ZOLOFT in double-blind trials were evaluated and the data indicate that ZOLOFT is not associated with the development of significant ECG abnormalities.

ZOLOFT is extensively metabolized by the liver. In patients with chronic mild liver impairment, sertraline clearance was reduced, resulting in increased AUC, Cmax and elimination half-life. The effects of sertraline in patients with moderate and severe hepatic impairment have not been studied. The use of sertraline in patients with liver disease must be approached with caution. If sertraline is administered to patients with liver impairment, a lower or less frequent dose should be used (see CLINICAL PHARMACOLOGY and DOSAGE AND ADMINISTRATION).

Since ZOLOFT is extensively metabolized, excretion of unchanged drug in urine is a minor route of elimination. A clinical study comparing sertraline pharmacokinetics in healthy volunteers to that in patients with renal impairment ranging from mild to severe (requiring dialysis) indicated that the pharmacokinetics and protein binding are unaffected by renal disease. Based on the pharmacokinetic results, there is no need for dosage adjustment in patients with renal impairment (see CLINICAL PHARMACOLOGY).

Interference with Cognitive and Motor Performance–In controlled studies, ZOLOFT did not cause sedation and did not interfere with psychomotor performance. (See **Information for Patients.**)

Hyponatremia–Several cases of hyponatremia have been reported and appeared to be reversible when ZOLOFT was discontinued. Some cases were possibly due to the syndrome of inappropriate antidiuretic hormone secretion. The majority of these occurrences have been in elderly individuals, some in patients taking diuretics or who were otherwise volume depleted.

Platelet Function–There have been rare reports of altered platelet function and/or abnormal results from laboratory studies in patients taking ZOLOFT. While there have been reports of abnormal bleeding or purpura in several patients taking ZOLOFT, it is unclear whether ZOLOFT had a causative role.

Information for Patients

Physicians are advised to discuss the following issues with patients for whom they prescribe ZOLOFT:

Patients should be told that although ZOLOFT has not been shown to impair the ability of normal subjects to perform tasks requiring complex motor and mental skills in laboratory experiments, drugs that act upon the central nervous system may affect some individuals adversely. Therefore, patients should be told that until they learn how they respond to ZOLOFT they should be careful doing activities when they need to be alert, such as driving a car or operating machinery.

Patients should be told that although ZOLOFT has not been shown in experiments with normal subjects to increase the mental and motor skill impairments caused by alcohol, the concomitant use of ZOLOFT and alcohol is not advised.

Patients should be told that while no adverse interaction of ZOLOFT with over-the-counter (OTC) drug products is known to occur, the potential for interaction exists. Thus, the use of any OTC product should be initiated cautiously according to the directions of use given for the OTC product.

Patients should be advised to notify their physician if they become pregnant or intend to become pregnant during therapy.

Patients should be advised to notify their physician if they are breast feeding an infant.

ZOLOFT oral concentrate is contraindicated with ANTABUSE (disulfiram) due to the alcohol content of the concentrate.

ZOLOFT Oral Concentrate contains 20 mg/mL of sertraline (as the hydrochloride) as the active ingredient and 12% alcohol. ZOLOFT Oral Concentrate must be diluted before use. Just before taking, use the dropper provided to remove the required amount of ZOLOFT Oral Concentrate and mix with 4 oz (1/2 cup) of water, ginger ale, lemon/lime soda, lemonade or orange juice ONLY. Do not mix ZOLOFT Oral Concentrate with anything other than the liquids listed. The dose should be taken immediately after mixing. Do not mix in advance. At times, a slight haze may appear after mixing; this is normal. Note that caution should be exercised for persons with latex sensitivity, as the dropper dispenser contains dry natural rubber.

Laboratory Tests

None.

Drug Interactions

Potential Effects of Coadministration of Drugs Highly Bound to Plasma Proteins–Because sertraline is tightly bound to plasma protein, the administration of ZOLOFT® (sertraline hydrochloride) to a patient taking another drug which is tightly bound to protein (e.g., warfarin, digitoxin) may cause a shift in plasma concentrations potentially resulting in an adverse effect. Conversely, adverse effects may result from displacement of protein bound ZOLOFT by other tightly bound drugs.

In a study comparing prothrombin time AUC (0-120 hr) following dosing with warfarin (0.75 mg/kg) before and after 21 days of dosing with either ZOLOFT (50-200 mg/day) or placebo, there was a mean increase in prothrombin time of 8% relative to baseline for ZOLOFT compared to a 1% decrease for placebo ($p<0.02$). The normalization of prothrombin time for the ZOLOFT group was delayed compared to the placebo group. The clinical significance of this change is unknown. Accordingly, prothrombin time should be carefully monitored when ZOLOFT therapy is initiated or stopped.

Cimetidine–In a study assessing disposition of ZOLOFT (100 mg) on the second of 8 days of cimetidine administration (800 mg daily), there were significant increases in ZOLOFT mean AUC (50%), Cmax (24%) and half-life (26%) compared to the placebo group. The clinical significance of these changes is unknown.

CNS Active Drugs–In a study comparing the disposition of intravenously administered diazepam before and after 21 days of dosing with either ZOLOFT (50 to 200 mg/day escalating dose) or placebo, there was a 32% decrease relative to baseline in diazepam clearance for the ZOLOFT group compared to a 19% decrease relative to baseline for the placebo group ($p<0.03$). There was a 23% increase in Tmax for desmethyldiazepam in the ZOLOFT group compared to a 20% decrease in the placebo group ($p<0.03$). The clinical significance of these changes is unknown.

In a placebo-controlled trial in normal volunteers, the administration of two doses of ZOLOFT did not significantly alter steady-state lithium levels or the renal clearance of lithium.

Nonetheless, at this time, it is recommended that plasma lithium levels be monitored following initiation of ZOLOFT therapy with appropriate adjustments to the lithium dose.

In a controlled study of a single dose (2 mg) of pimozide, 200 mg sertraline (q.d.) co-administration to steady state was associated with a mean increase in pimozide AUC and Cmax of about 40%, but was not associated with any changes in EKG. Since the highest recommended pimozide dose (10 mg) has not been evaluated in combination with sertraline, the effect on QT interval and PK parameters at doses higher than 2 mg at this time are not known. While the mechanism of this interaction is unknown, due to the narrow therapeutic index of pimozide and due to the interaction noted at a low dose of pimozide, concomitant administration of ZOLOFT and pimozide should be contraindicated (see CONTRAINDICATIONS).

The risk of using ZOLOFT in combination with other CNS active drugs has not been systematically evaluated. Consequently, caution is advised if the concomitant administration of ZOLOFT and such drugs is required.

There is limited controlled experience regarding the optimal timing of switching from other drugs effective in the treatment of major depressive disorder, obsessive-compulsive disorder, panic disorder, posttraumatic stress disorder, premenstrual dysphoric disorder and social anxiety disorder to ZOLOFT. Care and prudent medical judgment should be exercised when switching, particularly from long-acting agents. The duration of an appropriate washout period which should intervene before switching from one selective serotonin reuptake inhibitor (SSRI) to another has not been established.

Monoamine Oxidase Inhibitors–See CONTRAINDICATIONS and WARNINGS.

Drugs Metabolized by P450 3A4–In three separate *in vivo* interaction studies, sertraline was co- administered with cytochrome P450 3A4 substrates, terfenadine, carbamazepine, or cisapride under steady-state conditions. The results of these studies indicated that sertraline did not increase plasma concentrations of terfenadine, carbamazepine, or cisapride. These data indicate that sertraline's extent of inhibition of P450 3A4 activity is not likely to be of clinical significance. Results of the interaction study with cisapride indicate that sertraline 200 mg (q.d.) induces the metabolism of cisapride (cisapride AUC and Cmax were reduced by about 35%).

Drugs Metabolized by P450 2D6–Many drugs effective in the treatment of major depressive disorder, e.g., the SSRIs, including sertraline, and most tricyclic antidepressant drugs effective in the treatment of major depressive disorder inhibit the biochemical activity of the drug metabolizing isozyme cytochrome P450 2D6 (debrisoquin hydroxylase), and, thus, may increase the plasma concentrations of co-administered drugs that are metabolized by P450 2D6. The drugs for which this potential interaction is of greatest concern are those metabolized primarily by 2D6 and which have a narrow therapeutic index, e.g., the tricyclic antidepressant drugs effective in the treatment of major depressive disorder and the Type 1C antiarrhythmics propafenone and flecainide. The extent to which this interaction is an important clinical problem depends on the extent of the inhibition of P450 2D6 by the antidepressant and the therapeutic index of the co-administered drug. There is variability among the drugs effective in the treatment of major depressive disorder in the extent of clinically important 2D6 inhibition, and in fact sertraline at lower doses has a less prominent inhibitory effect on 2D6 than some others in the class. Nevertheless, even sertraline has the potential for clinically important 2D6 inhibition. Consequently, concomitant use of a drug metabolized by P450 2D6 with ZOLOFT may require lower doses than usually prescribed for the other drug. Furthermore, whenever ZOLOFT is withdrawn from co-therapy, an increased dose of the co-administered drug may be required (see Tricyclic Antidepressant Drugs Effective in the Treatment of Major Depressive Disorder under PRECAUTIONS).

Sumatriptan–There have been rare postmarketing reports describing patients with weakness, hyperreflexia, and incoordination following the use of a selective serotonin reuptake inhibitor (SSRI) and sumatriptan. If concomitant treatment with sumatriptan and an SSRI (e.g., citalopram, fluoxetine, fluvoxamine, paroxetine, sertraline) is clinically warranted, appropriate observation of the patient is advised.

Tricyclic Antidepressant Drugs Effective in the Treatment of Major Depressive Disorder (TCAs)–The extent to which SSRI–TCA interactions may pose clinical problems will depend on the degree of inhibition and the pharmacokinetics of the SSRI involved. Nevertheless, caution is indicated in the co-administration of TCAs with ZOLOFT, because sertraline may inhibit TCA metabolism. Plasma TCA concentrations may need to be monitored, and the dose of TCA may need to be reduced, if a TCA is co-administered with ZOLOFT (see Drugs Metabolized by P450 2D6 under PRECAUTIONS).

Hypoglycemic Drugs–In a placebo-controlled trial in normal volunteers, administration of ZOLOFT for 22 days (including 200 mg/day for the final 13 days) caused a statistically significant 16% decrease from baseline in the clearance of tolbutamide following an intravenous 1000 mg dose. ZOLOFT administration did not noticeably change either the plasma protein binding or the apparent volume of distribution of tolbutamide, suggesting that the decreased clearance was due to a change in the metabolism of the drug. The clinical significance of this decrease in tolbutamide clearance is unknown.

Atenolol–ZOLOFT (100 mg) when administered to 10 healthy male subjects had no effect on the beta-adrenergic blocking ability of atenolol.

Digoxin–In a placebo-controlled trial in normal volunteers, administration of ZOLOFT for 17 days (including 200 mg/day for the last 10 days) did not change serum digoxin levels or digoxin renal clearance.

Microsomal Enzyme Induction–Preclinical studies have shown ZOLOFT to induce hepatic microsomal enzymes. In clinical studies, ZOLOFT was shown to induce hepatic enzymes minimally as determined by a small (5%) but statistically significant decrease in antipyrine half-life following administration of 200 mg/day for 21 days. This small change in antipyrine half-life reflects a clinically insignificant change in hepatic metabolism.

Electroconvulsive Therapy–There are no clinical studies establishing the risks or benefits of the combined use of electroconvulsive therapy (ECT) and ZOLOFT.

Alcohol–Although ZOLOFT did not potentiate the cognitive and psychomotor effects of alcohol in experiments with normal subjects, the concomitant use of ZOLOFT and alcohol is not recommended.

Carcinogenesis–Lifetime carcinogenicity studies were carried out in CD-1 mice and Long-Evans rats at doses up to 40 mg/kg/day. These doses correspond to 1 times (mice) and 2 times (rats) the maximum recommended human dose (MRHD) on a mg/m^2 basis. There was a dose-related increase of liver adenomas in male mice receiving sertraline at 10-40 mg/kg (0.25-1.0 times the MRHD on a mg/m^2 basis). No increase was seen in female mice or in rats of either sex receiving the same treatments, nor was there an increase in hepatocellular carcinomas. Liver adenomas have a variable rate of spontaneous occurrence in the CD-1 mouse and are of unknown significance to humans. There was an increase in follicular adenomas of the thyroid in female rats receiving sertraline at 40 mg/kg (2 times the MRHD on a mg/m^2 basis); this was not accompanied by thyroid hyperplasia. While there was an increase in uterine adenocarcinomas in rats receiving sertraline at 10-40 mg/kg (0.5-2.0 times the MRHD on a mg/m^2 basis) compared to placebo controls, this effect was not clearly drug related.

Mutagenesis–Sertraline had no genotoxic effects, with or without metabolic activation, based on the following assays: bacterial mutation assay; mouse lymphoma mutation assay; and tests for cytogenetic aberrations *in vivo* in mouse bone marrow and *in vitro* in human lymphocytes.

Impairment of Fertility–A decrease in fertility was seen in one of two rat studies at a dose of 80 mg/kg (4 times the maximum recommended human dose on a mg/m^2 basis).

Pregnancy–Pregnancy Category C–Reproduction studies have been performed in rats and rabbits at doses up to 80 mg/kg/day and 40 mg/kg/day, respectively. These doses correspond to approximately 4 times the maximum recommended human dose (MRHD) on a mg/m^2 basis. There was no evidence of teratogenicity at any dose level. When pregnant rats and rabbits were given sertraline during the period of organogenesis, delayed ossification was observed in fetuses at doses of 10 mg/kg (0.5 times the MRHD on a mg/m^2 basis) in rats and 40 mg/kg (4 times the MRHD on a mg/m^2 basis) in rabbits. When female rats received sertraline during the last third of gestation and throughout lactation, there was an increase in the number of stillborn pups and in the number of pups dying during the first 4 days after birth. Pup body weights were also decreased during the first four days after birth. These effects occurred at a dose of 20 mg/kg (1 times the MRHD on a mg/m^2 basis). The no effect dose for rat pup mortality was 10 mg/kg (0.5 times the MRHD on a mg/m^2 basis). The decrease in pup survival was shown to be due to *in utero* exposure to sertraline. The clinical significance of these effects is unknown. There are no adequate and well-controlled studies in pregnant women. ZOLOFT® (sertraline hydrochloride) should be used during pregnancy only if the potential benefit justifies the potential risk to the fetus.

Labor and Delivery–The effect of ZOLOFT on labor and delivery in humans is unknown.

Nursing Mothers–It is not known whether, and if so in what amount, sertraline or its metabolites are excreted in human milk. Because many drugs are excreted in human milk, caution should be exercised when ZOLOFT is administered to a nursing woman.

Pediatric Use–The efficacy of ZOLOFT for the treatment of obsessive-compulsive disorder was demonstrated in a 12-week, multicenter, placebo-controlled study with 187 outpatients ages 6-17 (see Clinical Trials under CLINICAL PHARMACOLOGY). The efficacy of ZOLOFT in pediatric patients with major depressive disorder, panic disorder, PTSD, PMDD or social anxiety disorder has not been established.

The safety of ZOLOFT use in children and adolescents with OCD, ages 6-18, was evaluated in a 12-week, multicenter, placebo-controlled study with 187 outpatients, ages 6-17, and in a flexible dose, 52 week open extension study of 137 patients, ages 6-18, who had completed the initial 12-week, double-blind, placebo-controlled study. ZOLOFT was administered at doses of either 25 mg/day (children, ages 6-12) or 50 mg/day (adolescents, ages 13-18) and then titrated in weekly 25 mg/day or 50 mg/day increments, respectively, to a maximum dose of 200 mg/day based upon clinical response. The mean dose for completers was 157 mg/day. In the acute 12 week pediatric study and in the 52 week study, ZOLOFT had an adverse event profile generally similar to that observed in adults.

Sertraline pharmacokinetics were evaluated in 61 pediatric patients between 6 and 17 years of age with major depressive disorder or OCD and revealed similar drug exposures to those of adults when plasma concentration was adjusted for weight (see Pharmacokinetics under CLINICAL PHARMACOLOGY).

Approximately 600 patients with major depressive disorder or OCD between 6 and 17 years of age have received ZOLOFT in clinical trials, both controlled and uncontrolled. The adverse event profile observed in these patients was generally similar to that observed in adult studies with ZOLOFT (see ADVERSE REACTIONS). As with other

Continued on next page

Zoloft—Cont.

SSRIs, decreased appetite and weight loss have been observed in association with the use of ZOLOFT. In a pooled analysis of two 10-week, double-blind, placebo-controlled, flexible dose (50-200 mg) outpatient trials for major depressive disorder (n=373), there was a difference in weight change between sertraline and placebo of roughly 1 kilogram, for both children (ages 6-11) and adolescents (ages 12-17), in both cases representing a slight weight loss for sertraline compared to a slight gain for placebo. At baseline the mean weight for children was 39.0 kg for sertraline and 38.5 kg for placebo. At baseline the mean weight for adolescents was 61.4 kg for sertraline and 62.5 kg for placebo. There was a bigger difference between sertraline and placebo in the proportion of outliers for clinically important weight loss in children than in adolescents. For children, about 7% had a weight loss > 7% of body weight compared to none of the placebo patients; for adolescents, about 2% had a weight loss > 7% of body weight compared to about 1% of the placebo patients. A subset of these patients who completed the randomized controlled trials (sertraline n=99, placebo n=122) were continued into a 24-week, flexible-dose, open-label, extension study. A mean weight loss of approximately 0.5 kg was seen during the first eight weeks of treatment for subjects with first exposure to sertraline during the open-label extension study, similar to mean weight loss observed among sertralinetreated subjects during the first eight weeks of the randomized controlled trials. The subjects continuing in the open label study began gaining weight compared to baseline by week 12 of sertraline treatment. Those subjects who completed 34 weeks of sertraline treatment (10 weeks in a placebo controlled trial + 24 weeks open label, n=68) had weight gain that was similar to that expected using data from age-adjusted peers. Regular monitoring of weight and growth is recommended if treatment of a pediatric patient with an SSRI is to be continued long term. Safety and effectiveness in pediatric patients below the age of 6 have not been established.

The risks, if any, that may be associated with ZOLOFT's use beyond 1 year in children and adolescents with OCD or major depressive disorder have not been systematically assessed. The prescriber should be mindful that the evidence relied upon to conclude that sertraline is safe for use in children and adolescents derives from clinical studies that were 10 to 52 weeks in duration and from the extrapolation of experience gained with adult patients. In particular, there are no studies that directly evaluate the effects of long-term sertraline use on the growth, development, and maturation of children and adolescents. Although there is no affirmative finding to suggest that sertraline possesses a capacity to adversely affect growth, development or maturation, the absence of such findings is not compelling evidence of the absence of the potential of sertraline to have adverse effects in chronic use.

Geriatric Use–U.S. geriatric clinical studies of ZOLOFT in major depressive disorder included 663 ZOLOFT-treated subjects ≥ 65 years of age, of those, 180 were ≥ 75 years of age. No overall differences in the pattern of adverse reactions were observed in the geriatric clinical trial subjects relative to those reported in younger subjects (see ADVERSE REACTIONS), and other reported experience has not identified differences in safety patterns between the elderly and younger subjects. As with all medications, greater sensitivity of some older individuals cannot be ruled out. There were 947 subjects in placebo-controlled geriatric clinical studies of ZOLOFT in major depressive disorder. No overall differences in the pattern of efficacy were observed in the geriatric clinical trial subjects relative to those reported in younger subjects.

Other Adverse Events in Geriatric Patients. In 354 geriatric subjects treated with ZOLOFT in placebo-controlled trials, the overall profile of adverse events was generally similar to that shown in Tables 1 and 2. Urinary tract infection was the only adverse event not appearing in Tables 1 and 2 and reported at an incidence of at least 2% and at a rate greater than placebo in placebo-controlled trials.

As with other SSRIs, ZOLOFT has been associated with cases of clinically significant hyponatremia in elderly patients (see Hyponatremia under PRECAUTIONS).

ADVERSE REACTIONS

During its premarketing assessment, multiple doses of ZOLOFT were administered to over 4000 adult subjects as of February 18, 2000. The conditions and duration of exposure to ZOLOFT varied greatly, and included (in overlapping categories) clinical pharmacology studies, open and double-blind studies, uncontrolled and controlled studies, inpatient and outpatient studies, fixed-dose and titration studies, and studies for multiple indications, including major depressive disorder, OCD, panic disorder, PTSD, PMDD and social anxiety disorder.

Untoward events associated with this exposure were recorded by clinical investigators using terminology of their own choosing. Consequently, it is not possible to provide a meaningful estimate of the proportion of individuals experiencing adverse events without first grouping similar types of untoward events into a smaller number of standardized event categories.

In the tabulations that follow, a World Health Organization dictionary of terminology has been used to classify reported adverse events. The frequencies presented, therefore, represent the proportion of the over 4000 adult individuals exposed to multiple doses of ZOLOFT who experienced a treatment-emergent adverse event of the type cited on at least one occasion while receiving ZOLOFT. An event was considered treatment-emergent if it occurred for the first time or worsened while receiving therapy following baseline evaluation. It is important to emphasize that events reported during therapy were not necessarily caused by it.

TABLE 1
MOST COMMON TREATMENT-EMERGENT ADVERSE EVENTS: INCIDENCE IN PLACEBO-CONTROLLED CLINICAL TRIALS

	Percentage of Patients Reporting Event													
	Major Depressive Disorder/Other*		OCD		Panic Disorder		PTSD		PMDD Daily Dosing		PMDD Luteal Phase Dosing[2]		Social Anxiety Disorder	
Body System/ Adverse Event	ZOLOFT (N=861)	Placebo (N=853)	ZOLOFT (N=533)	Placebo (N=373)	ZOLOFT (N=430)	Placebo (N=275)	ZOLOFT (N=374)	Placebo (N=376)	ZOLOFT (N=121)	Placebo (N=122)	ZOLOFT (N=136)	Placebo (N=127)	ZOLOFT (N=344)	Placebo (N=268)
Autonomic Nervous System Disorders														
Ejaculation Failure[1]	7	<1	17	2	19	1	11	1	N/A	N/A	N/A	N/A	14	–
Mouth Dry	16	9	14	9	15	10	11	6	6	3	10	3	12	4
Sweating Increased	8	3	6	1	5	1	4	2	6	<1	3	0	11	2
Centr. & Periph. Nerv. System Disorders														
Somnolence	13	6	15	8	15	9	13	9	7	<1	2	0	9	6
Tremor	11	3	8	1	5	1	5	1	2	0	<1	<1	9	3
Dizziness	12	7	17	9	10	10	8	5	6	3	7	5	14	6
General														
Fatigue	11	8	14	10	11	6	10	5	16	7	10	<1	12	6
Pain	1	2	3	1	3	3	4	6	6	<1	3	2	1	3
Malaise	<1	1	1	1	7	14	10	10	9	5	7	5	8	3
Gastrointestinal Disorders														
Abdominal Pain	2	2	5	5	6	7	6	5	7	<1	3	3	5	5
Anorexia	3	2	11	2	7	2	8	2	3	2	5	0	6	3
Constipation	8	6	6	4	7	3	3	3	2	3	1	2	5	3
Diarrhea/Loose Stools	18	9	24	10	20	9	24	15	13	3	13	7	21	8
Dyspepsia	6	3	10	4	10	8	6	6	7	2	7	3	13	5
Nausea	26	12	30	11	29	18	21	11	23	9	13	3	22	8
Psychiatric Disorders														
Agitation	6	4	6	3	6	2	5	5	2	<1	1	0	4	2
Insomnia	16	9	28	12	25	18	20	11	17	11	12	10	25	10
Libido Decreased	1	<1	11	2	7	1	7	2	11	2	4	2	9	3

[1]Primarily ejaculatory delay. Denominator used was for male patients only (N=271 ZOLOFT major depressive disorder/other*; N=271 placebo major depressive disorder/other*; N=296 ZOLOFT OCD; N=219 placebo OCD; N=216 ZOLOFT panic disorder; N=134 placebo panic disorder; N=130 ZOLOFT PTSD; N=149 placebo PTSD; No male patients in PMDD studies; N=205 ZOLOFT social anxiety disorder; N=153 placebo social anxiety disorder).

*Major depressive disorder and other premarketing controlled trials.

[2]The luteal phase and daily dosing PMDD trials were not designed for making direct comparisons between the two dosing regimens. Therefore, a comparison between the two dosing regimens of the PMDD trials of incidence rates shown in Table 1 should be avoided.

The prescriber should be aware that the figures in the tables and tabulations cannot be used to predict the incidence of side effects in the course of usual medical practice where patient characteristics and other factors differ from those that prevailed in the clinical trials. Similarly, the cited frequencies cannot be compared with figures obtained from other clinical investigations involving different treatments, uses, and investigators. The cited figures, however, do provide the prescribing physician with some basis for estimating the relative contribution of drug and nondrug factors to the side effect incidence rate in the population studied.

Incidence in Placebo-Controlled Trials–Table 1 enumerates the most common treatment-emergent adverse events associated with the use of ZOLOFT (incidence of at least 5% for ZOLOFT and at least twice that for placebo within at least one of the indications) for the treatment of adult patients with major depressive disorder/other*, OCD, panic disorder, PTSD, PMDD and social anxiety disorder in placebo-controlled clinical trials. Most patients in major depressive disorder/other*, OCD, panic disorder, PTSD and social anxiety disorder studies received doses of 50 to 200 mg/day. Patients in the PMDD study with daily dosing throughout the menstrual cycle received doses of 50 to 150 mg/day, and in the PMDD study with dosing during the luteal phase of the menstrual cycle received doses of 50 to 100 mg/day. Table 2 enumerates treatment-emergent adverse events that occurred in 2% or more of adult patients treated with ZOLOFT and with incidence greater than placebo who participated in controlled clinical trials comparing ZOLOFT with placebo in the treatment of major depressive disorder/other*, OCD, panic disorder, PTSD, PMDD and social anxiety disorder. Table 2 provides combined data for the pool of studies that are provided separately by indication in Table 1.

[See table 1 at bottom of previous page]

TABLE 2
TREATMENT-EMERGENT ADVERSE EVENTS: INCIDENCE IN PLACEBO-CONTROLLED CLINICAL TRIALS
Percentage of Patients Reporting Event
Major Depressive Disorder/Other*, OCD, Panic Disorder, PTSD, PMDD and Social Anxiety Disorder combined

Body System/Adverse Event**	ZOLOFT (N=2799)	Placebo (N=2394)
Autonomic Nervous System Disorders		
Ejaculation Failure[(1)]	14	1
Mouth Dry	14	8
Sweating Increased	7	2
Centr. & Periph. Nerv. System Disorders		
Somnolence	13	7
Dizziness	12	7
Headache	25	23
Paresthesia	2	1
Tremor	8	2
Disorders of Skin and Appendages		
Rash	3	2
Gastrointestinal Disorders		
Anorexia	6	2
Constipation	6	4
Diarrhea/Loose Stools	20	10
Dyspepsia	8	4
Nausea	25	11
Vomiting	4	2
General		
Fatigue	12	7
Psychiatric Disorders		
Agitation	5	3
Anxiety	4	3
Insomnia	21	11
Libido Decreased	6	2
Nervousness	5	4
Special Senses		
Vision Abnormal	3	2

(1)Primarily ejaculatory delay. Denominator used was for male patients only (N=1118 ZOLOFT; N=926 placebo).
*Major depressive disorder and other premarketing controlled trials.
**Included are events reported by at least 2% of patients taking ZOLOFT except the following events, which had an incidence on placebo greater than or equal to ZOLOFT: abdominal pain, back pain, flatulence, malaise, pain, pharyngitis, respiratory disorder, upper respiratory tract infection.

TABLE 3
MOST COMMON ADVERSE EVENTS ASSOCIATED WITH DISCONTINUATION IN PLACEBO-CONTROLLED CLINICAL TRIALS

Adverse Event	Major Depressive Disorder/ Other*, OCD, Panic Disorder, PTSD, PMDD and Social Anxiety Disorder combined (N=2799)	Major Depressive Disorder/ Other* (N=861)	OCD (N=533)	Panic Disorder (N=430)	PTSD (N=374)	PMDD Daily Dosing (N=121)	PMDD Luteal Phase Dosing (N=136)	Social Anxiety Disorder (N=344)
Abdominal Pain	–	–	–	–	–	–	–	1%
Agitation	–	1%	–	2%	–	–	–	–
Anxiety	–	–	–	–	–	–	–	2%
Diarrhea/Loose Stools	2%	2%	2%	1%	–	2%	–	–
Dizziness	–	–	1%	–	–	–	–	–
Dry Mouth	–	1%	–	–	–	–	–	–
Dyspepsia	–	–	–	1%	–	–	–	–
Ejaculation Failure[(1)]	1%	1%	1%	2%	–	N/A	N/A	2%
Fatigue	–	–	–	–	–	–	–	2%
Headache	1%	2%	–	–	1%	–	–	2%
Hot Flushes	–	–	–	–	–	–	1%	–
Insomnia	2%	1%	3%	2%	–	–	1%	3%
Nausea	3%	4%	3%	3%	2%	2%	1%	2%
Nervousness	–	–	–	–	–	2%	–	–
Palpitation	–	–	–	–	–	–	1%	–
Somnolence	1%	1%	2%	2%	–	–	–	–
Tremor	–	2%	–	–	–	–	–	–

(1)Primarily ejaculatory delay. Denominator used was for male patients only (N=271 major depressive disorder/other*; N=296 OCD; N=216 panic disorder; N=130 PTSD; No male patients in PMDD studies; N=205 social anxiety disorder).
*Major depressive disorder and other premarketing controlled trials.

Associated with Discontinuation in Placebo-Controlled Clinical Trials

Table 3 lists the adverse events associated with discontinuation of ZOLOFT® (sertraline hydrochloride) treatment (incidence at least twice that for placebo and at least 1% for ZOLOFT in clinical trials) in major depressive disorder/other*, OCD, panic disorder, PTSD, PMDD and social anxiety disorder.

[See table 3 above]

Male and Female Sexual Dysfunction with SSRIs

Although changes in sexual desire, sexual performance and sexual satisfaction often occur as manifestations of a psychiatric disorder, they may also be a consequence of pharmacologic treatment. In particular, some evidence suggests that selective serotonin reuptake inhibitors (SSRIs) can cause such untoward sexual experiences. Reliable estimates of the incidence and severity of untoward experiences involving sexual desire, performance and satisfaction are difficult to obtain, however, in part because patients and physicians may be reluctant to discuss them. Accordingly, estimates of the incidence of untoward sexual experience and performance cited in product labeling, are likely to underestimate their actual incidence.

Table 4 below displays the incidence of sexual side effects reported by at least 2% of patients taking ZOLOFT in placebo-controlled trials.

TABLE 4

Adverse Event	ZOLOFT	Placebo
Ejaculation failure* (primarily delayed ejaculation)	14%	1%
Decreased libido**	6%	1%

* Denominator used was for male patients only (N=1118 ZOLOFT; N=926 placebo)
** Denominator used was for male and female patients (N=2799 ZOLOFT; N=2394 placebo)

There are no adequate and well-controlled studies examining sexual dysfunction with sertraline treatment.

Priapism has been reported with all SSRIs.

While it is difficult to know the precise risk of sexual dysfunction associated with the use of SSRIs, physicians should routinely inquire about such possible side effects.

Other Adverse Events in Pediatric Patients–In over 600 pediatric patients treated with ZOLOFT, the overall profile of adverse events was generally similar to that seen in adult studies. However, the following adverse events, from controlled trials, not appearing in Tables 1 and 2, were reported at an incidence of at least 2% and occurred at a rate of at least twice the placebo rate (N=281 patients treated with ZOLOFT): fever, hyperkinesia, urinary incontinence, aggressive reaction, sinusitis, epistaxis and purpura.

Other Events Observed During the Premarketing Evaluation of ZOLOFT® (sertraline hydrochloride)–Following is a list of treatment-emergent adverse events reported during premarketing assessment of ZOLOFT in clinical trials (over 4000 adult subjects) except those already listed in the previous tables or elsewhere in labeling.

In the tabulations that follow, a World Health Organization dictionary of terminology has been used to classify reported adverse events. The frequencies presented, therefore, represent the proportion of the over 4000 adult individuals exposed to multiple doses of ZOLOFT who experienced an event of the type cited on at least one occasion while receiving ZOLOFT. All events are included except those already listed in the previous tables or elsewhere in labeling and those reported in terms so general as to be uninformative and those for which a causal relationship to ZOLOFT treatment seemed remote. It is important to emphasize that although the events reported occurred during treatment with ZOLOFT, they were not necessarily caused by it. Events are further categorized by body system and listed in order of decreasing frequency according to the following definitions: frequent adverse events are those occurring on one or more occasions in at least 1/100 patients; infrequent adverse events are those occurring in 1/100 to 1/1000 patients; rare events are those occurring in fewer than 1/1000 patients. Events of major clinical importance are also described in the PRECAUTIONS section.

Autonomic Nervous System Disorders–*Frequent:* impotence; *Infrequent:* flushing, increased saliva, cold clammy skin, mydriasis; *Rare:* pallor, glaucoma, priapism, vasodilation.

Body as a Whole–General Disorders–*Rare:* allergic reaction, allergy.

Cardiovascular–*Frequent:* palpitations, chest pain; *Infrequent:* hypertension, tachycardia, postural dizziness, postural hypotension, periorbital edema, peripheral edema, hypotension, peripheral ischemia, syncope, edema, depen-

Continued on next page

Zoloft—Cont.

dent edema; *Rare:* precordial chest pain, substernal chest pain, aggravated hypertension, myocardial infarction, cerebrovascular disorder.

Central and Peripheral Nervous System Disorders–*Frequent:* hypertonia, hypoesthesia; *Infrequent:* twitching, confusion, hyperkinesia, vertigo, ataxia, migraine, abnormal coordination, hyperesthesia, leg cramps, abnormal gait, nystagmus, hypokinesia; *Rare:* dysphonia, coma, dyskinesia, hypotonia, ptosis, choreoathetosis, hyporeflexia.

Disorders of Skin and Appendages–*Infrequent:* pruritus, acne, urticaria, alopecia, dry skin, erythematous rash, photosensitivity reaction, maculopapular rash; *Rare:* follicular rash, eczema, dermatitis, contact dermatitis, bullous eruption, hypertrichosis, skin discoloration, pustular rash.

Endocrine Disorders–*Rare:* exophthalmos, gynecomastia.

Gastrointestinal Disorders–*Frequent:* appetite increased; *Infrequent:* dysphagia, tooth caries aggravated, eructation, esophagitis, gastroenteritis; *Rare:* melena, glossitis, gum hyperplasia, hiccup, stomatitis, tenesmus, colitis, diverticulitis, fecal incontinence, gastritis, rectum hemorrhage, hemorrhagic peptic ulcer, proctitis, ulcerative stomatitis, tongue edema, tongue ulceration.

General–*Frequent:* back pain, asthenia, malaise, weight increase; *Infrequent:* fever, rigors, generalized edema; *Rare:* face edema, aphthous stomatitis.

Hearing and Vestibular Disorders–*Rare:* hyperacusis, labyrinthine disorder.

Hematopoietic and Lymphatic–*Rare:* anemia, anterior chamber eye hemorrhage.

Liver and Biliary System Disorders–*Rare:* abnormal hepatic function.

Metabolic and Nutritional Disorders–*Infrequent:* thirst; *Rare:* hypoglycemia, hypoglycemia reaction.

Musculoskeletal System Disorders–*Frequent:* myalgia; *Infrequent:* arthralgia, dystonia, arthrosis, muscle cramps, muscle weakness.

Psychiatric Disorders–*Frequent:* yawning, other male sexual dysfunction, other female sexual dysfunction; *Infrequent:* depression, amnesia, paroniria, teeth-grinding, emotional lability, apathy, abnormal dreams, euphoria, paranoid reaction, hallucination, aggressive reaction, aggravated depression, delusions; *Rare:* withdrawal syndrome, suicide ideation, libido increased, somnambulism, illusion.

Reproductive–*Infrequent:* menstrual disorder, dysmenorrhea, intermenstrual bleeding, vaginal hemorrhage, amenorrhea, leukorrhea; *Rare:* female breast pain, menorrhagia, balanoposthitis, breast enlargement, atrophic vaginitis, acute female mastitis.

Respiratory System Disorders–*Frequent:* rhinitis; *Infrequent:* coughing, dyspnea, upper respiratory tract infection, epistaxis, bronchospasm, sinusitis; *Rare:* hyperventilation, bradypnea, stridor, apnea, bronchitis, hemoptysis, hypoventilation, laryngismus, laryngitis.

Special Senses–*Frequent:* tinnitus; *Infrequent:* conjunctivitis, earache, eye pain, abnormal accommodation; *Rare:* xerophthalmia, photophobia, diplopia, abnormal lacrimation, scotoma, visual field defect.

Urinary System Disorders–*Infrequent:* micturition frequency, polyuria, urinary retention, dysuria, nocturia, urinary incontinence; *Rare:* cystitis, oliguria, pyelonephritis, hematuria, renal pain, strangury.

Laboratory Tests–In man, asymptomatic elevations in serum transaminases (SGOT [or AST] and SGPT [or ALT]) have been reported infrequently (approximately 0.8%) in association with ZOLOFT® (sertraline hydrochloride) administration. These hepatic enzyme elevations usually occurred within the first 1 to 9 weeks of drug treatment and promptly diminished upon drug discontinuation.

ZOLOFT therapy was associated with small mean increases in total cholesterol (approximately 3%) and triglycerides (approximately 5%), and a small mean decrease in serum uric acid (approximately 7%) of no apparent clinical importance.

The safety profile observed with ZOLOFT treatment in patients with major depressive disorder, OCD, panic disorder, PTSD, PMDD and social anxiety disorder is similar.

Other Events Observed During the Postmarketing Evaluation of ZOLOFT–Reports of adverse events temporally associated with ZOLOFT that have been received since market introduction, that are not listed above and that may have no causal relationship with the drug, include the following: acute renal failure, anaphylactoid reaction, angioedema, blindness, optic neuritis, cataract, increased coagulation times, bradycardia, AV block, atrial arrhythmias, QT-interval prolongation, ventricular tachycardia (including torsade de pointes-type arrhythmias), hypothyroidism, agranulocytosis, aplastic anemia and pancytopenia, leukopenia, thrombocytopenia, lupus-like syndrome, serum sickness, hyperglycemia, galactorrhea, hyperprolactinemia, neuroleptic malignant syndrome-like events, extrapyramidal symptoms, oculogyric crisis, serotonin syndrome, psychosis, pulmonary hypertension, severe skin reactions, which potentially can be fatal, such as Stevens-Johnson syndrome, vasculitis, photosensitivity and other severe cutaneous disorders, rare reports of pancreatitis, and liver events—clinical features (which in the majority of cases appeared to be reversible with discontinuation of ZOLOFT) occurring in one or more patients include: elevated enzymes, increased bilirubin, hepatomegaly, hepatitis, jaundice, abdominal pain, vomiting, liver failure and death.

DRUG ABUSE AND DEPENDENCE

Controlled Substance Class–ZOLOFT® (sertraline hydrochloride) is not a controlled substance.

Physical and Psychological Dependence–In a placebo-controlled, double-blind, randomized study of the comparative abuse liability of ZOLOFT, alprazolam, and d-amphetamine in humans, ZOLOFT did not produce the positive subjective effects indicative of abuse potential, such as euphoria or drug liking, that were observed with the other two drugs. Premarketing clinical experience with ZOLOFT did not reveal any tendency for a withdrawal syndrome or any drug-seeking behavior. In animal studies ZOLOFT does not demonstrate stimulant or barbiturate-like (depressant) abuse potential. As with any CNS active drug, however, physicians should carefully evaluate patients for history of drug abuse and follow such patients closely, observing them for signs of ZOLOFT misuse or abuse (e.g., development of tolerance, incrementation of dose, drug-seeking behavior).

OVERDOSAGE

Human Experience–Of 1,027 cases of overdose involving sertraline hydrochloride worldwide, alone or with other drugs, there were 72 deaths (circa 1999).

Among 634 overdoses in which sertraline hydrochloride was the only drug ingested, 8 resulted in fatal outcome, 75 completely recovered, and 27 patients experienced sequelae after overdosage to include alopecia, decreased libido, diarrhea, ejaculation disorder, fatigue, insomnia, somnolence and serotonin syndrome. The remaining 524 cases had an unknown outcome. The most common signs and symptoms associated with non-fatal sertraline hydrochloride overdosage were somnolence, vomiting, tachycardia, nausea, dizziness, agitation and tremor.

The largest known ingestion was 13.5 grams in a patient who took sertraline hydrochloride alone and subsequently recovered. However, another patient who took 2.5 grams of sertraline hydrochloride alone experienced a fatal outcome. Other important adverse events reported with sertraline hydrochloride overdose (single or multiple drugs) include bradycardia, bundle branch block, coma, convulsions, delirium, hallucinations, hypertension, hypotension, manic reaction, pancreatitis, QT-interval prolongation, serotonin syndrome, stupor and syncope.

Overdose Management–Treatment should consist of those general measures employed in the management of overdosage with any antidepressant.

Ensure an adequate airway, oxygenation and ventilation. Monitor cardiac rhythm and vital signs. General supportive and symptomatic measures are also recommended. Induction of emesis is not recommended. Gastric lavage with a large-bore orogastric tube with appropriate airway protection, if needed, may be indicated if performed soon after ingestion, or in symptomatic patients.

Activated charcoal should be administered. Due to large volume of distribution of this drug, forced diuresis, dialysis, hemoperfusion and exchange transfusion are unlikely to be of benefit. No specific antidotes for sertraline are known.

In managing overdosage, consider the possibility of multiple drug involvement. The physician should consider contacting a poison control center on the treatment of any overdose. Telephone numbers for certified poison control centers are listed in the *Physicians' Desk Reference*® (PDR®).

DOSAGE AND ADMINISTRATION

Initial Treatment

Dosage for Adults

Major Depressive Disorder and Obsessive-Compulsive Disorder–ZOLOFT treatment should be administered at a dose of 50 mg once daily.

Panic Disorder, Posttraumatic Stress Disorder and Social Anxiety Disorder–ZOLOFT treatment should be initiated with a dose of 25 mg once daily. After one week, the dose should be increased to 50 mg once daily.

While a relationship between dose and effect has not been established for major depressive disorder, OCD, panic disorder, PTSD or social anxiety disorder, patients were dosed in a range of 50-200 mg/day in the clinical trials demonstrating the effectiveness of ZOLOFT for the treatment of these indications. Consequently, a dose of 50 mg, administered once daily, is recommended as the initial therapeutic dose. Patients not responding to a 50 mg dose may benefit from dose increases up to a maximum of 200 mg/day. Given the 24 hour elimination half-life of ZOLOFT, dose changes should not occur at intervals of less than 1 week.

Premenstrual Dysphoric Disorder–ZOLOFT treatment should be initiated with a dose of 50 mg/day, either daily throughout the menstrual cycle or limited to the luteal phase of the menstrual cycle, depending on physician assessment.

While a relationship between dose and effect has not been established for PMDD, patients were dosed in the range of 50-150 mg/day with dose increases at the onset of each new menstrual cycle (see Clinical Trials under CLINICAL PHARMACOLOGY). Patients not responding to a 50 mg/day dose may benefit from dose increases (at 50 mg increments/menstrual cycle) up to 150 mg/day when dosing daily throughout the menstrual cycle, or 100 mg/day when dosing during the luteal phase of the menstrual cycle. If a 100 mg/day dose has been established with luteal phase dosing, a 50 mg/day titration step for three days should be utilized at the beginning of each luteal phase dosing period.

ZOLOFT should be administered once daily, either in the morning or evening.

Dosage for Pediatric Population (Children and Adolescents)

Obsessive-Compulsive Disorder–ZOLOFT treatment should be initiated with a dose of 25 mg once daily in children (ages 6-12) and at a dose of 50 mg once daily in adolescents (ages 13-17).

While a relationship between dose and effect has not been established for OCD, patients were dosed in a range of 25-200 mg/day in the clinical trials demonstrating the effectiveness of ZOLOFT for pediatric patients (6-17 years) with OCD. Patients not responding to an initial dose of 25 or 50 mg/day may benefit from dose increases up to a maximum of 200 mg/day. For children with OCD, their generally lower body weights compared to adults should be taken into consideration in advancing the dose, in order to avoid excess dosing. Given the 24 hour elimination half-life of ZOLOFT, dose changes should not occur at intervals of less than 1 week.

ZOLOFT should be administered once daily, either in the morning or evening.

Dosage for Hepatically Impaired Patients

The use of sertraline in patients with liver disease should be approached with caution. The effects of sertraline in patients with moderate and severe hepatic impairment have not been studied. If sertraline is administered to patients with liver impairment, a lower or less frequent dose should be used (see CLINICAL PHARMACOLOGY and PRECAUTIONS).

Maintenance/Continuation/Extended Treatment

Major Depressive Disorder–It is generally agreed that acute episodes of major depressive disorder require several months or longer of sustained pharmacologic therapy beyond response to the acute episode. Systematic evaluation of ZOLOFT has demonstrated that its antidepressant efficacy is maintained for periods of up to 44 weeks following 8 weeks of initial treatment at a dose of 50-200 mg/day (mean dose of 70 mg/day) (see Clinical Trials under CLINICAL PHARMACOLOGY). It is not known whether the dose of ZOLOFT needed for maintenance treatment is identical to the dose needed to achieve an initial response. Patients should be periodically reassessed to determine the need for maintenance treatment.

Posttraumatic Stress Disorder–It is generally agreed that PTSD requires several months or longer of sustained pharmacological therapy beyond response to initial treatment. Systematic evaluation of ZOLOFT has demonstrated that its efficacy in PTSD is maintained for periods of up to 28 weeks following 24 weeks of treatment at a dose of 50-200 mg/day (see Clinical Trials under CLINICAL PHARMACOLOGY). It is not known whether the dose of ZOLOFT needed for maintenance treatment is identical to the dose needed to achieve an initial response. Patients should be periodically reassessed to determine the need for maintenance treatment.

Social Anxiety Disorder–Social anxiety disorder is a chronic condition that may require several months or longer of sustained pharmacological therapy beyond response to initial treatment. Systematic evaluation of ZOLOFT has demonstrated that its efficacy in social anxiety disorder is maintained for periods of up to 24 weeks following 20 weeks of treatment at a dose of 50-200 mg/day (see Clinical Trials under CLINICAL PHARMACOLOGY). Dosage adjustments should be made to maintain patients on the lowest effective dose and patients should be periodically reassessed to determine the need for long-term treatment.

Obsessive-Compulsive Disorder and Panic Disorder–It is generally agreed that OCD and Panic Disorder require several months or longer of sustained pharmacological therapy beyond response to initial treatment. Systematic evaluation of continuing ZOLOFT for periods of up to 28 weeks in patients with OCD and Panic Disorder who have responded while taking ZOLOFT during initial treatment phases of 24 to 52 weeks of treatment at a dose range of 50-200 mg/day has demonstrated a benefit of such maintenance treatment (see Clinical Trials under CLINICAL PHARMACOLOGY). It is not known whether the dose of ZOLOFT needed for maintenance treatment is identical to the dose needed to achieve an initial response. Nevertheless, patients should be periodically reassessed to determine the need for maintenance treatment.

Premenstrual Dysphoric Disorder–The effectiveness of ZOLOFT in long-term use, that is, for more than 3 menstrual cycles, has not been systematically evaluated in controlled trials. However, as women commonly report that symptoms worsen with age until relieved by the onset of menopause, it is reasonable to consider continuation of a responding patient. Dosage adjustments, which may include changes between dosage regimens (e.g., daily throughout the menstrual cycle versus during the luteal phase of the menstrual cycle), may be needed to maintain the patient on the lowest effective dosage and patients should be periodically reassessed to determine the need for continued treatment.

Switching Patients to or from a Monoamine Oxidase Inhibitor–At least 14 days should elapse between discontinuation of an MAOI and initiation of therapy with ZOLOFT. In addition, at least 14 days should be allowed after stopping ZOLOFT before starting an MAOI (see CONTRAINDICATIONS and WARNINGS).

ZOLOFT Oral Concentrate

ZOLOFT Oral Concentrate contains 20 mg/mL of sertraline (as the hydrochloride) as the active ingredient and 12% alcohol. ZOLOFT Oral Concentrate must be diluted before use. Just before taking, use the dropper provided to remove the required amount of ZOLOFT Oral Concentrate and mix with 4 oz (1/2 cup) of water, ginger ale, lemon/lime soda, lemonade or orange juice ONLY. Do not mix ZOLOFT Oral Concentrate with anything other than the liquids listed. The dose should be taken immediately after mixing. Do not mix in advance. At times, a slight haze may appear after mixing; this is normal. Note that caution should be exercised for patients with latex sensitivity, as the dropper dispenser contains dry natural rubber.

ZOLOFT Oral Concentrate is contraindicated with ANTABUSE (disulfiram) due to the alcohol content of the concentrate.

HOW SUPPLIED

ZOLOFT® (sertraline hydrochloride) capsular-shaped scored tablets, containing sertraline hydrochloride equivalent to 25, 50 and 100 mg of sertraline, are packaged in bottles.

ZOLOFT® 25 mg Tablets: light green film coated tablets engraved on one side with ZOLOFT and on the other side scored and engraved with 25 mg.

NDC 0049-4960-50	Bottles of 50

ZOLOFT® 50 mg Tablets: light blue film coated tablets engraved on one side with ZOLOFT and on the other side scored and engraved with 50 mg.

NDC 0049-4900-66	Bottles of 100
NDC 0049-4900-73	Bottles of 500
NDC 0049-4900-94	Bottles of 5000
NDC 0049-4900-41	Unit Dose Packages of 100

ZOLOFT® 100 mg Tablets: light yellow film coated tablets engraved on one side with ZOLOFT and on the other side scored and engraved with 100 mg.

NDC 0049-4910-66	Bottles of 100
NDC 0049-4910-73	Bottles of 500
NDC 0049-4910-94	Bottles of 5000
NDC 0049-4910-41	Unit Dose Packages of 100

Store at 25°C (77°F); excursions permitted to 15°-30°C (59°-86°F) [see USP Controlled Room Temperature].

ZOLOFT® Oral Concentrate: ZOLOFT Oral Concentrate is a clear, colorless solution with a menthol scent containing sertraline hydrochloride equivalent to 20 mg of sertraline per mL and 12% alcohol. It is supplied as a 60 mL bottle with an accompanying calibrated dropper.

NDC 0049-4940-23	Bottles of 60 mL

Store at 25°C (77°F); excursions permitted to 15°-30°C (59°-86°F) [see USP Controlled Room Temperature].

Rx only

Distributed by

Pfizer Roerig

Division of Pfizer Inc, NY, NY 10017

69-4721-00-7 Revised September 2003

Pharmacia & Upjohn

A DIVISION OF PFIZER
235 EAST 42ND ST
NEW YORK, NY 10017-5755

Direct Inquiries to:
212-733-2323

For Medical Information, Contact:
800-323-4204
24 hours a day, 7 days a week

AROMASIN® ℞

[ărŏ-mă-sĭn]

(exemestane tablets)

Prescribing information for this product, which appears on pages 2705–2707 of the 2004 PDR, has been completely revised as follows. Please write "See Supplement A" next to the product heading.

DESCRIPTION

AROMASIN® Tablets for oral administration contain 25 mg of exemestane, an irreversible, steroidal aromatase inactivator. Exemestane is chemically described as 6-methylenandrosta-1,4-diene-3,17-dione. Its molecular formula is $C_{20}H_{24}O_2$ and its structural formula is as follows:

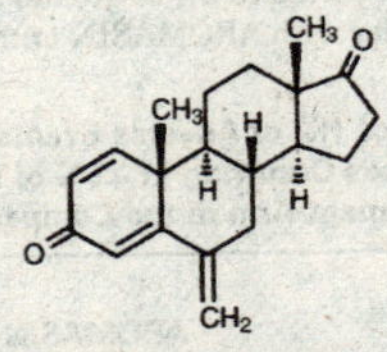

The active ingredient is a white to slightly yellow crystalline powder with a molecular weight of 296.41. Exemestane is freely soluble in N, N-dimethylformamide, soluble in methanol, and practically insoluble in water.

Each AROMASIN Tablet contains the following inactive ingredients: mannitol, crospovidone, polysorbate 80, hypromellose, colloidal silicon dioxide, microcrystalline cellulose, sodium starch glycolate, magnesium stearate, simethicone, polyethylene glycol 6000, sucrose, magnesium carbonate, titanium dioxide, methylparaben, and polyvinyl alcohol.

CLINICAL PHARMACOLOGY

Mechanism of Action

Breast cancer cell growth may be estrogen-dependent. Aromatase is the principal enzyme that converts androgens to estrogens both in pre- and postmenopausal women. While the main source of estrogen (primarily estradiol) is the ovary in premenopausal women, the principal source of circulating estrogens in postmenopausal women is from conversion of adrenal and ovarian androgens (androstenedione and testosterone) to estrogens (estrone and estradiol) by the aromatase enzyme in peripheral tissues. Estrogen deprivation through aromatase inhibition is an effective and selective treatment for some postmenopausal patients with hormone-dependent breast cancer.

Exemestane is an irreversible, steroidal aromatase inactivator, structurally related to the natural substrate androstenedione. It acts as a false substrate for the aromatase enzyme, and is processed to an intermediate that binds irreversibly to the active site of the enzyme causing its inactivation, an effect also known as "suicide inhibition." Exemestane significantly lowers circulating estrogen concentrations in postmenopausal women, but has no detectable effect on adrenal biosynthesis of corticosteroids or aldosterone. Exemestane has no effect on other enzymes involved in the steroidogenic pathway up to a concentration at least 600 times higher than that inhibiting the aromatase enzyme.

Pharmacokinetics

Following oral administration to healthy postmenopausal women, exemestane is rapidly absorbed. After maximum plasma concentration is reached, levels decline polyexponentially with a mean terminal half-life of about 24 hours. Exemestane is extensively distributed and is cleared from the systemic circulation primarily by metabolism. The pharmacokinetics of exemestane are dose proportional after single (10 to 200 mg) or repeated oral doses (0.5 to 50 mg). Following repeated daily doses of exemestane 25 mg, plasma concentrations of unchanged drug are similar to levels measured after a single dose.

Pharmacokinetic parameters in postmenopausal women with advanced breast cancer following single or repeated doses have been compared with those in healthy, postmenopausal women. Exemestane appeared to be more rapidly absorbed in the women with breast cancer than in the healthy women, with a mean t_{max} of 1.2 hours in the women with breast cancer and 2.9 hours in the healthy women. After repeated dosing, the average oral clearance in women with advanced breast cancer was 45% lower than the oral clearance in healthy postmenopausal women, with corresponding higher systemic exposure. Mean AUC values following repeated doses in women with breast cancer (75.4 ng•h/mL) were about twice those in healthy women (41.4 ng•h/mL).

Absorption: Following oral administration of radiolabeled exemestane, at least 42% of radioactivity was absorbed from the gastrointestinal tract. Exemestane plasma levels increased by approximately 40% after a high-fat breakfast.

Distribution: Exemestane is distributed extensively into tissues. Exemestane is 90% bound to plasma proteins and the fraction bound is independent of the total concentration. Albumin and α_1-acid glycoprotein both contribute to the binding. The distribution of exemestane and its metabolites into blood cells is negligible.

Metabolism and Excretion: Following administration of radiolabeled exemestane to healthy postmenopausal women, the cumulative amounts of radioactivity excreted in urine and feces were similar (42 ± 3% in urine and 42 ± 6% in feces over a 1-week collection period). The amount of drug excreted unchanged in urine was less than 1% of the dose. Exemestane is extensively metabolized, with levels of the unchanged drug in plasma accounting for less than 10% of the total radioactivity. The initial steps in the metabolism of exemestane are oxidation of the methylene group in position 6 and reduction of the 17-keto group with subsequent formation of many secondary metabolites. Each metabolite accounts only for a limited amount of drug-related material. The metabolites are inactive or inhibit aromatase with decreased potency compared with the parent drug. One metabolite may have androgenic activity (see Pharmacodynamics, Other Endocrine Effects). Studies using human liver preparations indicate that cytochrome P-450 3A4 (CYP 3A4) is the principal isoenzyme involved in the oxidation of exemestane.

Special Populations

Geriatric: Healthy postmenopausal women aged 43 to 68 years were studied in the pharmacokinetic trials. Age-related alterations in exemestane pharmacokinetics were not seen over this age range.

Gender: The pharmacokinetics of exemestane following administration of a single, 25-mg tablet to fasted healthy males (mean age 32 years) were similar to the pharmacokinetics of exemestane in fasted healthy postmenopausal women (mean age 55 years).

Race: The influence of race on exemestane pharmacokinetics has not been evaluated.

Hepatic Insufficiency: The pharmacokinetics of exemestane have been investigated in subjects with moderate or severe hepatic insufficiency (Childs-Pugh B or C). Following a single 25-mg oral dose, the AUC of exemestane was approximately 3 times higher than that observed in healthy volunteers (see PRECAUTIONS).

Renal Insufficiency: The AUC of exemestane after a single 25-mg dose was approximately 3 times higher in subjects with moderate or severe renal insufficiency (creatinine clearance <35 mL/min/1.73 m^2) compared with the AUC in healthy volunteers (see PRECAUTIONS

Pediatric: The pharmacokinetics of exemestane have not been studied in pediatric patients.

Drug-Drug Interactions

Exemestane is metabolized by cytochrome P-450 3A4 (CYP 3A4) and aldoketoreductases. It does not inhibit any of the major CYP isoenzymes, including CYP 1A2, 2C9, 2D6, 2E1, and 3A4. In a clinical pharmacokinetic study, ketoconazole showed no significant influence on the pharmacokinetics of exemestane. Although no other formal drug-drug interaction studies have been conducted, significant effects on exemestane clearance by CYP isoenzymes inhibitors appear unlikely. In a pharmacokinetic interaction study of 10 healthy postmenopausal volunteers pretreated with potent CYP 3A4 inducer rifampicin 600 mg daily for 14 days followed by a single dose of exemestane 25 mg, the mean plasma Cmax and AUC0 of exemestane were decreased by 41% and 54%, respectively (see PRECAUTIONS AND DOSAGE AND ADMINISTRATION).

Pharmacodynamics

Effect on Estrogens: Multiple doses of exemestane ranging from 0.5 to 600 mg/day were administered to postmenopausal women with advanced breast cancer. Plasma estrogen (estradiol, estrone, and estrone sulfate) suppression was seen starting at a 5-mg daily dose of exemestane, with a maximum suppression of at least 85% to 95% achieved at a 25-mg dose. Exemestane 25 mg daily reduced whole body aromatization (as measured by injecting radiolabeled androstenedione) by 98% in postmenopausal women with breast cancer. After a single dose of exemestane 25 mg, the maximal suppression of circulating estrogens occurred 2 to 3 days after dosing and persisted for 4 to 5 days.

Effect on Corticosteroids: In multiple-dose trials of doses up to 200 mg daily, exemestane selectivity was assessed by examining its effect on adrenal steroids. Exemestane did not affect cortisol or aldosterone secretion at baseline or in response to ACTH at any dose. Thus, no glucocorticoid or mineralocorticoid replacement therapy is necessary with exemestane treatment.

Other Endocrine Effects: Exemestane does not bind significantly to steroidal receptors, except for a slight affinity for the androgen receptor (0.28% relative to dihydrotestosterone). The binding affinity of its 17-dihydrometabolite for the androgen receptor, however, is 100-times that of the parent compound. Daily doses of exemestane up to 25 mg had no significant effect on circulating levels of testosterone, androstenedione, dehydroepiandrosterone sulfate, or 17-hydroxyprogesterone. Increases in testosterone and androstenedione levels have been observed at daily doses of 200 mg or more. A dose-dependent decrease in sex hormone binding globulin (SHBG) has been observed with daily exemestane doses of 2.5 mg or higher. Slight, nondose-dependent increases in serum luteinizing hormone (LH) and follicle-stimulating hormone (FSH) levels have been observed even at low doses as a consequence of feedback at the pituitary level.

CLINICAL STUDIES

Exemestane 25 mg administered once daily was evaluated in a randomized double-blind, multicenter, multinational comparative study and in two multicenter single-arm studies of postmenopausal women with advanced breast cancer who had disease progression after treatment with tamoxifen for metastatic disease or as adjuvant therapy. Some patients also have received prior cytotoxic therapy, either as adjuvant treatment or for metastatic disease.

The primary purpose of the three studies was evaluation of objective response rate (complete response [CR] and partial response [PR]). Time to tumor progression and overall survival were also assessed in the comparative trial. Response rates were assessed based on World Health Organization (WHO) criteria, and in the comparative study, were submitted to an external review committee that was blinded to patient treatment. In the comparative study, 769 patients were randomized to receive AROMASIN (exemestane tablets) 25 mg once daily (N = 366) or megestrol acetate 40 mg four times daily (N = 403). Demographics and baseline characteristics are presented in Table 1.

[See table 1 at top of next page]

The efficacy results from the comparative study are shown in Table 2. The objective response rates observed in the two treatment arms showed that AROMASIN was not different from megestrol acetate. Response rates for exemestane from the two single-arm trials were 23.4% and 28.1%.

[See table 2 on next page]

There were too few deaths occurring across treatment groups to draw conclusions on overall survival differences. The Kaplan-Meier curve for time to tumor progression in the comparative study is shown in Figure 1.

Figure 1. Time to Tumor Progression in the Comparative Study of Postmenopausal Women With Advanced Breast Cancer Whose Disease Had Progressed After Tamoxifen Therapy

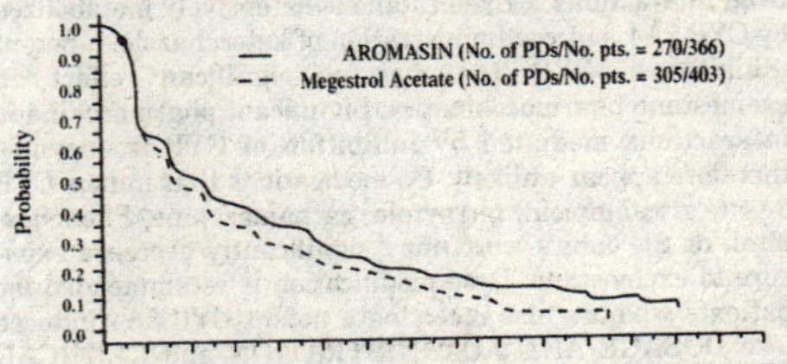

INDICATIONS AND USAGE

AROMASIN Tablets are indicated for the treatment of advanced breast cancer in postmenopausal women whose disease has progressed following tamoxifen therapy.

Continued on next page

Aromasin—Cont.

CONTRAINDICATIONS

AROMASIN Tablets are contraindicated in patients with a known hypersensitivity to the drug or to any of the excipients.

WARNINGS

AROMASIN Tablets may cause fetal harm when administered to a pregnant woman. Radioactivity related to ^{14}C-exemestane crossed the placenta of rats following oral administration of 1 mg/kg exemestane. The concentration of exemestane and its metabolites was approximately equivalent in maternal and fetal blood. When rats were administered exemestane from 14 days prior to mating until either days 15 or 20 of gestation, and resuming for the 21 days of lactation, an increase in placental weight was seen at 4 mg/kg/day (approximately 1.5 times the recommended human daily dose on a mg/m^2 basis). Prolonged gestation and abnormal or difficult labor was observed at doses equal to or greater than 20 mg/kg/day. Increased resorption, reduced number of live fetuses, decreased fetal weight, and retarded ossification were also observed at these doses. No malformations were noted when exemestane was administered to pregnant rats during the organogenesis period at doses up to 810 mg/kg/day (approximately 320 times the recommended human dose on a mg/m^2 basis). Daily doses of exemestane, given to rabbits during organogenesis caused a decrease in placental weight at 90 mg/kg/day (approximately 70 times the recommended human daily dose on a mg/m^2 basis). Abortions, an increase in resorptions, and a reduction in fetal body weight were seen at 270 mg/kg/day. There was no increase in the incidence of malformations in rabbits at doses up to 270 mg/kg/day (approximately 210 times the recommended human dose on a mg/m^2 basis).

There are no studies in pregnant women using AROMASIN. AROMASIN is indicated for postmenopausal women. If there is exposure to AROMASIN during pregnancy, the patient should be apprised of the potential hazard to the fetus and potential risk for loss of the pregnancy.

PRECAUTIONS

General. AROMASIN Tablets should not be administered to premenopausal women. AROMASIN should not be coadministered with estrogen-containing agents as these could interfere with its pharmacologic action.

Hepatic Insufficiency. The pharmacokinetics of exemestane have been investigated in subjects with moderate or severe hepatic insufficiency (Childs-Pugh B or C). Following a single 25-mg oral dose, the AUC of exemestane was approximately 3 times higher than that observed in healthy volunteers. The safety of chronic dosing in patients with moderate or severe hepatic impairment has not been studied. Based on experience with exemestane at repeated doses up to 200 mg daily that demonstrated a moderate increase in non-life threatening adverse events, dosage adjustment does not appear to be necessary.

Renal Insufficiency. The AUC of exemestane after a single 25-mg dose was approximately 3 times higher in subjects with moderate or severe renal insufficiency (creatinine clearance <35 mL/min/1.73 m^2) compared with the AUC in healthy volunteers. The safety of chronic dosing in patients with moderate or severe renal impairment has not been studied. Based on experience with exemestane at repeated doses up to 200 mg daily that demonstrated a moderate increase in non-life threatening adverse events, dosage adjustment does not appear to be necessary.

Laboratory Tests. Approximately 20% of patients receiving exemestane in clinical studies, experienced Common Toxicity Criteria (CTC) grade 3 or 4 lymphocytopenia. Of these patients, 89% had a pre-exisiting lower grade lymphopenia. Forty percent of patients either recovered or improved to a lesser severity while on treatment. Patients did not have a significant increase in viral infections, and no opportunistic infections were observed. Elevations of serum levels of AST, ALT, alkaline phosphatase and gamma glutamyl transferase > 5 times the upper value of the normal range (i.e., ≥ CTC grade 3) have been rarely reported but appear mostly attributable to the underlying presence of liver and/or bone metastases. In the comparative study, CTC grade 3 or 4 elevation of gamma glutamyl transferase without documented evidence of liver metastasis was reported in 2.7% of patients treated with AROMASIN and in 1.8% of patients treated with megestrol acetate.

Drug Interactions. Exemestane is extensively metabolized by CYP 3A4, but coadministration of ketoconazole, a potent inhibitor of CYP 3A4, has no significant effect on exemestane pharmacokinetics. Significant pharmacokinetic interactions mediated by inhibition of CYP isoenzymes therefore appear unlikely. Co-medications that induce CYP 3A4 (e.g. rifampicin, phenytoin, carbamazepine, Phenobarbital, or St. John's wort) may significantly decrease exposure to exemestane. Dose modification is recommended for patients who are also receiving a potent CYP 3A4 inducer (see DOSAGE AND ADMINISTRATION and CLINICAL PHARMACOLOGY).

Drug/Laboratory Tests Interactions. No clinically relevant changes in the results of clinical laboratory tests have been observed.

Carcinogenesis, Mutagenesis, Impairment of Fertility. Carcinogenicity studies have not been conducted with exemestane. Exemestane was not mutagenic in bacteria (Ames test) or mammalian cells (V79 Chinese hamster lung cells). Exemestane was clastogenic in human lymphocytes in vitro without metabolic activation but was not clastogenic in vivo (micronucleus assay in mouse bone marrow). Exemestane did not increase unscheduled DNA synthesis in rat hepatocytes.

Untreated female rats showed reduced fertility when mated to males treated with 500 mg/kg/day exemestane (approximately 200 times the recommended human dose on a mg/m^2 basis) for 63 days prior to and during cohabitation. Exemestane given to female rats 14 days prior to mating and through day 15 or 20 of gestation increased the placental weights at 4 mg/kg/day (approximately 1.5 times the human dose on a mg/m^2 basis). Exemestane showed no effects on female fertility parameters (e.g., ovarian function, mating behavior, conception rate) in rats given doses up to 20 mg/kg/day (approximately 8 times the human dose on a mg/m^2 basis), but mean litter size was decreased at this dose. In general toxicology studies, changes in the ovary, including hyperplasia, an increase in ovarian cysts and a decrease in corpora lutea were observed with variable frequency in mice, rats and dogs at doses that ranged from 3-20 times the human dose on a mg/m^2 basis.

Pregnancy. Pregnancy Category D. See WARNINGS.

Nursing Mothers. AROMASIN is only indicated in postmenopausal women. However, radioactivity related to exemestane appeared in rat milk within 15 minutes of oral administration of radiolabeled exemestane. Concentrations of exemestane and its metabolites were approximately equivalent in the milk and plasma of rats for 24 hours after a single oral dose of 1 mg/kg ^{14}C-exemestane. It is not known whether exemestane is excreted in human milk. Because many drugs are excreted in human milk, caution should be exercised if a nursing woman is inadvertently exposed to AROMASIN (see WARNINGS).

Pediatric Use. The safety and effectiveness of AROMASIN in pediatric patients have not been established.

Geriatric Use. The use of AROMASIN in geriatric patients does not require special precautions.

ADVERSE REACTIONS

A total of 1058 patients were treated with exemestane 25 mg once daily in the clinical trials program. Exemestane was generally well tolerated, and adverse events were usually mild to moderate. Only one death was considered possibly related to treatment with exemestane; an 80-year-old woman with known coronary artery disease had a myocardial infarction with multiple organ failure after 9 weeks on study treatment. In the clinical trials program, only 3% of the patients discontinued treatment with exemestane because of adverse events, mainly within the first 10 weeks of treatment; late discontinuations because of adverse events were uncommon (0.3%).

In the comparative study, adverse reactions were assessed for 358 patients treated with AROMASIN and 400 patients treated with megestrol acetate. Fewer patients receiving AROMASIN discontinued treatment because of adverse events than those treated with megestrol acetate (2% vs. 5%). Adverse events that were considered drug related or of indeterminate cause included hot flashes (13% vs. 5%), nausea (9% vs. 5%), fatigue (8% vs. 10%), increased sweating (4% vs. 8%), and increased appetite (3% vs. 6%). The proportion of patients experiencing an excessive weight gain (>10% of their baseline weight) was significantly higher with megestrol acetate than with AROMASIN (17% vs. 8%). Table 3 shows the adverse events of all CTC grades, regardless of causality, reported in 5% or greater of patients in the study treated either with AROMASIN or megestrol acetate.

Table 1. Demographics and Baseline Characteristics from the Comparative Study of Postmenopausal Women with Advanced Breast Cancer Whose Disease Had Progressed after Tamoxifen Therapy

Parameter	AROMASIN (N = 366)	Megestrol Acetate (N = 403)
Median Age (range)	65 (35-89)	65 (30-91)
ECOG Performance Status		
0	167 (46%)	187 (46%)
1	162 (44%)	172 (43%)
2	34 (9%)	42 (10%)
Receptor Status		
ER and/or PgR +	246 (67%)	274 (68%)
ER and PgR unknown	116 (32%)	128 (32%)
Responders to prior tamoxifen	68 (19%)	85 (21%)
NE for response to prior tamoxifen	46 (13%)	41 (10%)
Site of Metastasis		
Visceral ± other sites	207 (57%)	239 (59%)
Bone only	61 (17%)	73 (18%)
Soft tissue only	54 (15%)	51 (13%)
Bone & soft tissue	43 (12%)	38 (9%)
Measurable Disease	287 (78%)	314 (78%)
Prior Tamoxifen Therapy		
Adjuvant or Neoadjuvant	145 (40%)	152 (38%)
Advanced Disease, Outcome		
CR, PR or SD≥ 6 months	179 (49%)	210 (52%)
SD< 6 months, PD or NE	42 (12%)	41 (10%)
Prior Chemotherapy		
For advanced disease ± adjuvant	58 (16%)	67 (17%)
Adjuvant only	104 (28%)	108 (27%)
No chemotherapy	203 (56%)	226 (56%)

Table 2. Efficacy Results from the Comparative Study of Postmenopausal Women with Advanced Breast Cancer Whose Disease Had Progressed after Tamoxifen Therapy

Response Characteristics	AROMASIN (N=366)		Megestrol Acetate (N=403)
Objective Response Rate = CR+ PR (%)	15.0		12.4
Difference in Response Rate (AR-MA)		2.6	
95% C. I.		7.5, -2.3	
CR (%)	2.2		1.2
PR (%)	12.8		11.2
SD ≥ 24 Weeks (%)	21.3		21.1
Median Duration of Response (weeks)	76.1		71.0
Median TTP (weeks)	20.3		16.6
Hazard Ratio (AR-MA)		0.84	

Abbreviations: CR = complete response, PR = partial response, SD = stable disease (no change), TTP = time to tumor progression, C. I. = confidence interval, MA = megestrol acetate, AR = AROMASIN

Table 3. Incidence (%) of Adverse Events of all Grades* and Causes Occurring in ≥5% of Patients in Each Treatment Arm in the Comparative Study

Event	AROMASIN 25 mg once daily (N=358)	Megestrol Acetate 40 mg QID (N=400)
Autonomic Nervous		
Increased sweating	6	9
Body as a Whole		
Fatigue	22	29
Hot flashes	13	6
Pain	13	13
Influenza-like symptoms	6	5
Edema (includes edema, peripheral edema, leg edema)	7	6
Cardiovascular		
Hypertension	5	6
Nervous		
Depression	13	9
Insomnia	11	9

Anxiety	10	11
Dizziness	8	6
Headache	8	7
Gastrointestinal		
Nausea	18	12
Vomiting	7	4
Abdominal pain	6	11
Anorexia	6	5
Constipation	5	8
Diarrhea	4	5
Increased appetite	3	6
Respiratory		
Dyspnea	10	15
Coughing	6	7

* Graded according to Common Toxicity Criteria

Less frequent adverse events of any cause (from 2% to 5%) reported in the comparative study for patients receiving AROMASIN 25 mg once daily were fever, generalized weakness, paresthesia, pathological fracture, bronchitis, sinusitis, rash, itching, urinary tract infection, and lymphedema. Additional adverse events of any cause observed in the overall clinical trials program (N = 1058) in 5% or greater of patients treated with exemestane 25 mg once daily but not in the comparative study included pain at tumor sites (8%), asthenia (6%) and fever (5%). Adverse events of any cause reported in 2% to 5% of all patients treated with exemestane 25 mg in the overall clinical trials program but not in the comparative study included chest pain, hypoesthesia, confusion, dyspepsia, arthralgia, back pain, skeletal pain, infection, upper respiratory tract infection, pharyngitis, rhinitis, and alopecia.

OVERDOSAGE

Clinical trials have been conducted with exemestane given as a single dose to healthy female volunteers at doses as high as 800 mg and daily for 12 weeks to postmenopausal women with advanced breast cancer at doses as high as 600 mg. These dosages were well tolerated. There is no specific antidote to overdosage and treatment must be symptomatic. General supportive care, including frequent monitoring of vital signs and close observation of the patient, is indicated.

A male child (age unknown) accidentally ingested a 25-mg tablet of exemestane. The initial physical examination was normal, but blood tests performed 1 hour after ingestion indicated leucocytosis (WBC 25000/mm^3 with 90% neutrophils). Blood tests were repeated 4 days after the incident and were normal. No treatment was given.

In mice, mortality was observed after a single oral dose of exemestane of 3200 mg/kg, the lowest dose tested (about 640 times the recommended human dose on a mg/m^2 basis). In rats and dogs, mortality was observed after single oral doses of exemestane of 5000 mg/kg (about 2000 times the recommended human dose on a mg/m^2 basis) and of 3000 mg/kg (about 4000 times the recommended human dose on a mg/m^2 basis), respectively.

Convulsions were observed after single doses of exemestane of 400 mg/kg and 3000 mg/kg in mice and dogs (approximately 80 and 4000 times the recommended human dose on a mg/m^2 basis), respectively.

DOSAGE AND ADMINISTRATION

The recommended dose of AROMASIN Tablets is 25 mg once daily after a meal. Treatment with AROMASIN should continue until tumor progression is evident.

For patients receiving AROMASIN with a potent CYP 3A4 inducer such as rifampicin or phenytoin the recommended dose of AROMASIN is 50 mg once daily after a meal.

The safety of chronic dosing in patients with moderate or severe hepatic or renal impairment has not been studied. Based on experience with exemestane at repeated doses up to 200 mg daily that demonstrated a moderate increase in non-life threatening adverse events, dosage adjustment does not appear to be necessary (see CLINICAL PHARMACOLOGY, Special Populations and PRECAUTIONS).

HOW SUPPLIED

AROMASIN Tablets are round, biconvex, and off-white to slightly gray. Each tablet contains 25 mg of exemestane. The tablets are printed on one side with the number "7663" in black. AROMASIN is packaged in HDPE bottles with a child-resistant screw cap, supplied in packs of 30 tablets.

30-tablet HDPE bottle NDC 0009-7663-04

Store at 25°C (77°F); excursions permitted to 15°-30°C (59°-86°F) [see USP Controlled Room Temperature].

℞ only MADE IN ITALY

Manufactured for: Pharmacia & Upjohn Company
A subsidiary of Pharmacia Corporation
Kalamazoo, Michigan 49001, USA
By: Pharmacia Italia S.p.A.
Ascoli Piceno, Italy

Revised March 2004 420079800 817 885 003

BEXTRA® ℞

[bĕks'tră]

valdecoxib tablets

Prescribing information for this product, which appears on pages 2709–2713 of the 2004 PDR, has been completely revised as follows. Please write "See Supplement A" next to the product heading.

DESCRIPTION

Valdecoxib is chemically designated as 4-(5-methyl-3-phenyl-4-isoxazolyl) benzenesulfonamide and is a diaryl substituted isoxazole. It has the following chemical structure:

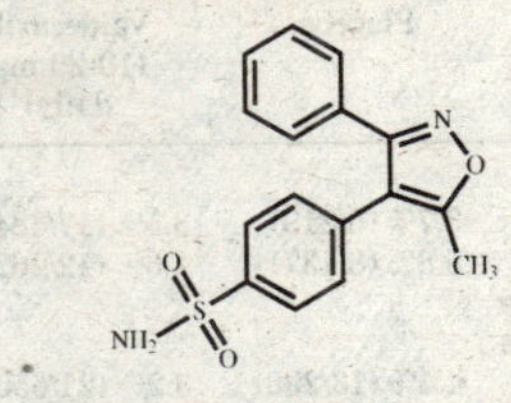

Valdecoxib

The empirical formula for valdecoxib is $C_{16}H_{14}N_2O_3S$, and the molecular weight is 314.36. Valdecoxib is a white crystalline powder that is relatively insoluble in water (10 µ/mL) at 25°C and pH 7.0, soluble in methanol and ethanol, and freely soluble in organic solvents and alkaline (pH=12) aqueous solutions.

BEXTRA Tablets for oral administration contain either 10 mg or 20 mg of valdecoxib. Inactive ingredients include lactose monohydrate, microcrystalline cellulose, pregelatinized starch, croscarmellose sodium, magnesium stearate, hypromellose, polyethylene glycol, polysorbate 80, and titanium dioxide.

CLINICAL PHARMACOLOGY

Mechanism of Action

Valdecoxib is a nonsteroidal anti-inflammatory drug (NSAID) that exhibits anti-inflammatory, analgesic and antipyretic properties in animal models. The mechanism of action is believed to be due to inhibition of prostaglandin synthesis primarily through inhibition of cyclooxygenase-2 (COX-2). At therapeutic plasma concentrations in humans valdecoxib does not inhibit cyclooxygenase-1 (COX-1).

Pharmacokinetics

Absorption

Valdecoxib achieves maximal plasma concentrations in approximately 3 hours. The absolute bioavailability of valdecoxib is 83% following oral administration of BEXTRA compared to intravenous infusion of valdecoxib.

Dose proportionality was demonstrated after single doses (1-400 mg) of valdecoxib. With multiple doses (up to 100 mg/day for 14 days), valdecoxib exposure as measured by the AUC, increases in a more than proportional manner at doses above 10 mg BID. Steady state plasma concentrations of valdecoxib are achieved by day 4.

The steady state pharmacokinetic parameters of valdecoxib in healthy male subjects are shown in Table 1.

Table 1

Mean (SD) Steady State Pharmacokinetic Parameters

Steady State Pharmacokinetic Parameters after Valdecoxib 10 mg Once Daily for 14 Days	Healthy Male Subjects (n=8, 20 to 42 yr.)
$AUC_{(0-24hr)}$ (hr·ng/mL)	1479.0 (291.9)
C_{max} (ng/mL)	161.1 (48.1)
T_{max} (hr)	2.25 (0.71)
C_{min} (ng/mL)	21.9 (7.68)
Elimination Half-life (hr)	8.11 (1.32)

No clinically significant age or gender differences were seen in pharmacokinetic parameters that would require dosage adjustments.

Effect of Food and Antacid

BEXTRA can be taken with or without food. Food had no significant effect on either the peak plasma concentration (C_{max}) or extent of absorption (AUC) of valdecoxib when BEXTRA was taken with a high fat meal. The time to peak plasma concentration (T_{max}), however, was delayed by 1-2 hours. Administration of BEXTRA with antacid (aluminum/magnesium hydroxide) had no significant effect on either the rate or extent of absorption of valdecoxib.

Distribution

Plasma protein binding for valdecoxib is about 98% over the concentration range (21-2384 ng/mL). Steady state apparent volume of distribution (Vss/F) of valdecoxib is approximately 86 L after oral administration. Valdecoxib and its active metabolite preferentially partition into erythrocytes with a blood to plasma concentration ratio of about 2.5:1. This ratio remains approximately constant with time and therapeutic blood concentrations.

Metabolism

In humans, valdecoxib undergoes extensive hepatic metabolism involving both P450 isoenzymes (3A4 and 2C9) and non-P450 dependent pathways (i.e., glucuronidation). Concomitant administration of BEXTRA with known CYP 3A4 and 2C9 inhibitors (e.g., fluconazole and ketoconazole) can result in increased plasma exposure of valdecoxib (see PRECAUTIONS — Drug Interactions).

One active metabolite of valdecoxib has been identified in human plasma at approximately 10% the concentration of valdecoxib. This metabolite, which is a less potent COX-2 specific inhibitor than the parent, also undergoes extensive metabolism and constitutes less than 2% of the valdecoxib dose excreted in the urine and feces. Due to its low concentration in the systemic circulation, it is not likely to contribute significantly to the efficacy profile of BEXTRA.

Excretion

Valdecoxib is eliminated predominantly via hepatic metabolism with less than 5% of the dose excreted unchanged in the urine and feces. About 70% of the dose is excreted in the urine as metabolites, and about 20% as valdecoxib N-glucuronide. The apparent oral clearance (CL/F) of valdecoxib is about 6 L/hr. The mean elimination half-life ($T_{1/2}$) ranges from 8-11 hours, and increases with age.

Special Populations

Geriatric

In elderly subjects (> 65 years), weight-adjusted steady state plasma concentrations ($AUC_{(0-12hr)}$) are about 30% higher than in young subjects. No dose adjustment is needed based on age.

Pediatric

BEXTRA has not been investigated in pediatric patients below 18 years of age.

Race

Pharmacokinetic differences due to race have not been identified in clinical and pharmacokinetic studies conducted to date.

Hepatic Insufficiency

Valdecoxib plasma concentrations are significantly increased (130%) in patients with moderate (Child-Pugh Class B) hepatic impairment. In clinical trials, doses of BEXTRA above those recommended have been associated with fluid retention. Hence, treatment with BEXTRA should be initiated with caution in patients with mild to moderate hepatic impairment and fluid retention. The use of BEXTRA in patients with severe hepatic impairment (Child-Pugh Class C) is not recommended.

Renal Insufficiency

The pharmacokinetics of valdecoxib have been studied in patients with varying degrees of renal impairment. Because renal elimination of valdecoxib is not important to its disposition, no clinically significant changes in valdecoxib clearance were found even in patients with severe renal impairment or in patients undergoing renal dialysis. In patients undergoing hemodialysis the plasma clearance (CL/F) of valdecoxib was similar to the CL/F found in healthy elderly subjects (CL/F about 6 to 7 L/hr.) with normal renal function (based on creatinine clearance).

NSAIDs have been associated with worsening renal function and use in advanced renal disease is not recommended (see PRECAUTIONS – Renal Effects).

Drug Interactions

Also see **PRECAUTIONS — Drug Interactions.**

General

Valdecoxib undergoes both P450 (CYP) dependent and non-P450 dependent (glucuronidation) metabolism. In vitro studies indicate that valdecoxib is not a significant inhibitor of CYP 1A2, 3A4, or 2D6 and is only a weak inhibitor of CYP 2C9 and 2C19 at therapeutic concentrations. The P450-mediated metabolic pathway of valdecoxib predominantly involves the 3A4 and 2C9 isozymes. Using prototype inhibitors and substrates of these isozymes, the following results were obtained. Coadministration of a known inhibitor of CYP 2C9/3A4 (fluconazole) and a CYP 3A4 (ketoconazole) inhibitor enhanced the total plasma exposure (AUC) of valdecoxib. Coadministration of valdecoxib with warfarin caused a small, but statistically significant increase in plasma exposures of R-warfarin and S-warfarin, and also in the pharmacodynamic effects (International Normalized Ratio - INR) of warfarin. (See PRECAUTIONS — Drug Interactions.)

Coadministration of valdecoxib, or its injectable prodrug, with substrates of CYP 2C9 (propofol) and CYP 3A4 (midazolam, alfentanil, fentanyl) did not inhibit the metabolism of either substrate.

Coadministration of valdecoxib with a CYP 3A4 substrate (glyburide) or a CYP 2D6 substrate (dextromethorphan) did not result in clinically important inhibition in the metabolism of these agents.

CLINICAL STUDIES

The efficacy and clinical utility of BEXTRA Tablets have been demonstrated in osteoarthritis (OA), rheumatoid arthritis (RA) and in the treatment of primary dysmenorrhea.

Osteoarthritis

BEXTRA was evaluated for treatment of the signs and symptoms of osteoarthritis of the knee or hip, in five double-blind, randomized, controlled trials in which 3918 patients were treated for 3 to 6 months. BEXTRA was shown to be superior to placebo in improvement in three domains of OA symptoms: (1) the WOMAC (Western Ontario and McMaster Universities) osteoarthritis index, a composite of pain, stiffness and functional measures in OA, (2) the overall patient assessment of pain, and (3) the overall patient global assessment. The two 3-month pivotal trials in OA generally showed changes statistically significantly different from placebo, and comparable to the naproxen control, in measures of these domains for the 10 mg/day dose. No additional benefit was seen with a valdecoxib 20-mg daily dose.

Rheumatoid Arthritis

BEXTRA demonstrated significant reduction compared to placebo in the signs and symptoms of RA, as measured by the ACR (American College of Rheumatology) 20 improvement, a composite defined as both improvement of 20% in the number of tender and number of swollen joints, and a 20% improvement in three of the following five: patient global, physician global, patient pain, patient function assessment, and C-reactive protein (CRP). BEXTRA was evaluated for treatment of the signs and symptoms of rheumatoid arthritis in four double-blind, randomized, controlled studies in which 3444 patients were treated for 3 to 6 months. The two 3-month pivotal trials compared

Continued on next page

Bextra—Cont.

valdecoxib to naproxen and placebo. The results for the ACR20 responses in these trials are shown below (Table 2). Trials of BEXTRA in rheumatoid arthritis allowed concomitant use of corticosteroids and/or disease-modifying antirheumatic drugs (DMARDs), such as methotrexate, gold salts, and hydroxychloroquine. No additional benefit was seen with a valdecoxib 20-mg daily dose.

Table 2
ACR20 Response Rate (%) in Rheumatoid Arthritis

	Study 1		Study 2	
BEXTRA 10 mg/day	49%**	(103/209)	46%**	(103/226)
BEXTRA 20 mg/day	48%**	(102/212)	47%*	(103/219)
Naproxen 500 mg BID	44%*	(100/225)	53%**	(115/219)
Placebo	32%	(70/222)	32%	(71/220)

* $p<0.01$; ** $p<0.001$ compared to placebo

Primary Dysmenorrhea
BEXTRA was compared to naproxen sodium 550 mg in two placebo-controlled studies of women with moderate to severe primary dysmenorrhea. The onset of analgesia was within 60 minutes for BEXTRA 20 mg. The onset, magnitude, and duration of analgesic effect with BEXTRA 20 mg were comparable to naproxen sodium 550 mg.

Safety Studies
Gastrointestinal (GI) Endoscopy Studies with Therapeutic Doses: Scheduled upper GI endoscopic evaluations were performed with BEXTRA at doses of 10 and 20 mg daily in over 800 OA patients who were enrolled into two randomized 3-month studies using active comparators and placebo controls (Study 3 and Study 4). These studies enrolled patients free of endoscopic ulcers at baseline and compared rates of endoscopic ulcers, defined as any gastroduodenal ulcer seen endoscopically provided it was of "unequivocal depth" and at least 3 mm in diameter.
In both studies, BEXTRA 10 mg daily was associated with a statistically significant lower incidence of endoscopic gastroduodenal ulcers over the study period compared to the active comparators. Figure 1 summarizes the incidence of gastroduodenal ulcers in Studies 3 and 4 for the placebo, valdecoxib, and active control arms.
[See figure 1 below]
Safety Study with Supratherapeutic Doses: Scheduled upper GI endoscopic evaluations were performed in a randomized 6-month study of 1217 patients with OA and RA comparing valdecoxib 20 mg BID (40 mg daily) and 40 mg BID (80 mg daily) (4 to 8 times the recommended therapeutic dose) to naproxen 500 mg BID (Study 5). This study also formally assessed renal events as a primary outcome with supratherapeutic doses of BEXTRA. The renal endpoint was defined as any of the following: new/increase in edema, new/increase in congestive heart failure, increase in blood pressure (BP; >20 mm Hg systolic, >10 mm Hg diastolic), new/increase in BP treatment, new/increase in diuretic therapy, creatinine increase over 30% (or >1.2 mg/dL if baseline <0.9 mg/dL), BUN increase over 200% or >50 mg/dL, 24-hr urinary protein increase to >500 mg (if baseline 0-150 mg or >750 if baseline 151-300 or >1000 if baseline 301-500), serum potassium increase to >6 mEq/L, or serum sodium decrease to <130 mEq/L.

Table 3
Incidence of Endoscopic Gastroduodenal Ulcers
in Patients With and Without Selected Risk Factors

Risk Factor	Placebo-controlled Studies: Placebo	Placebo-controlled Studies: Valdecoxib (10-20 mg daily)	Active-controlled Studies: Valdecoxib (10-80 mg daily)	Ibuprofen 800 mg TID	Naproxen 500 mg BID	Diclofenac 75 mg BID
Age						
<65 yrs	3.7% (8/219)	3.5% (17/484)	3.7% (48/1306)	8.2% (9/110)	12.8% (51/397)	13.2% (34/258)
≥65 yrs	5.8% (8/137)	4.6% (12/262)	7.6% (43/568)	21.6% (16/74)	22.0% (33/150)	18.2% (25/137)
Concomitant Low Dose Aspirin Use						
no	4.4% (13/298)	3.2% (21/650)	3.8% (64/1671)	9.8% (15/153)	16.0% (75/468)	12.8% (45/351)
yes	5.2% (3/58)	8.3% (8/96)	13.3% (27/203)	32.3% (10/31)	11.4% (9/79)	31.8% (14/44)
History of Ulcer Disease						
no	4.4% (14/317)	3.4% (22/647)	4.1% (68/1666)	13.8% (22/160)	13.3% (63/475)	14.7% (52/354)
yes	5.1% (2/39)	7.1% (7/99)	11.1% (23/208)	12.5% (3/24)	29.2% (21/72)	17.1% (7/41)

No statistical conclusions can be drawn from these comparisons.

Figure 1
Incidence of Endoscopically Observed
Gastroduodenal Ulcers in OA Patients

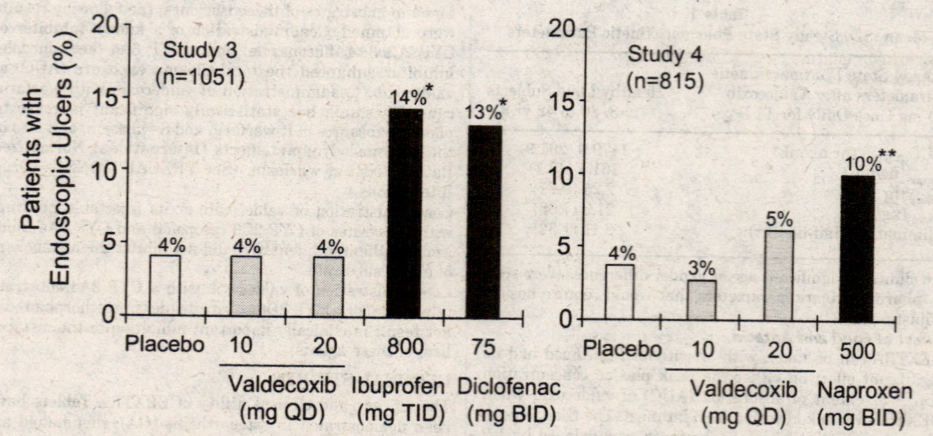

* Significantly different vs placebo and both valdecoxib treatment groups; p<0.05
** Significantly different vs placebo and valdecoxib 10 mg; p<0.05

Figure 2
Incidence of Endoscopic Gastroduodenal Ulcers and
Renal Events in the High-dose Safety Study

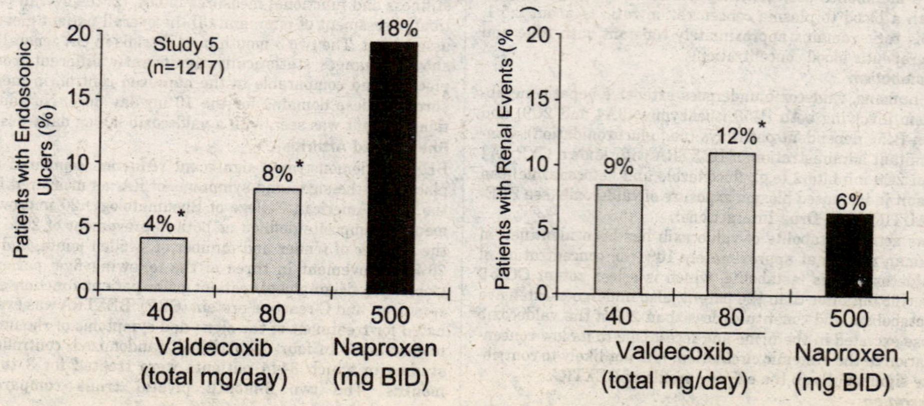

* Significantly different vs naproxen, p<0.05

Figure 2 summarizes the incidence rates of gastroduodenal ulcers and renal events that were seen in Study 5. BEXTRA 40 mg daily and 80 mg daily were associated with a statistically significant lower incidence of endoscopic gastroduodenal ulcers over the study period compared to naproxen. The incidence of renal events was significantly different between the BEXTRA 80 mg daily group and naproxen. The clinical relevance of renal events observed with supratherapeutic doses (4 to 8 times the recommended therapeutic dose) of BEXTRA is not known (see PRECAUTIONS – Renal Effects).
[See figure at left]
Renal Safety at the Therapeutic Chronic Dose: The renal effects of valdecoxib compared with placebo and conventional NSAIDs were also assessed by prospectively designed pooled analyses of renal events data (see definition above — Supratherapeutic Doses) from five placebo- and active-controlled 12-week arthritis trials that included 995 OA or RA patients given valdecoxib 10 mg daily. The incidence of renal events observed in this analysis with valdecoxib 10 mg daily (3%), ibuprofen 800 mg TID (7%), naproxen 500 mg BID (2%) and diclofenac 75 mg BID (4%) were significantly higher than placebo-treated patients (1%). In all treatment groups, the majority of renal events were either due to the occurrence of edema or worsening BP.
Gastrointestinal Ulcers in High-Risk Patients: Subset analyses were performed of patients with risk factors (age, concomitant low-dose aspirin use, history of prior ulcer disease) enrolled in four upper GI endoscopic studies. Table 3 summarizes the trends seen.
[See table 3 above]
The correlation between findings of endoscopic studies, and the incidence of clinically significant serious upper GI events has not been established.
Platelets: In four clinical studies with young and elderly (≥65 years) subjects, single and multiple doses up to 7 days of BEXTRA 10 to 40 mg BID had no effect on platelet aggregation.

INDICATIONS AND USAGE

BEXTRA Tablets are indicated:
- For relief of the signs and symptoms of osteoarthritis and adult rheumatoid arthritis.
- For the treatment of primary dysmenorrhea.

CONTRAINDICATIONS

BEXTRA should not be given to patients who have demonstrated allergic-type reactions to sulfonamides. BEXTRA Tablets are contraindicated in patients with known hypersensitivity to valdecoxib. BEXTRA should not be given to patients who have experienced asthma, urticaria, or allergic-type reactions after taking aspirin or NSAIDs. Severe, rarely fatal, anaphylactic-like reactions to NSAIDs are possible in such patients (see WARNINGS — Anaphylactoid Reactions, and PRECAUTIONS — Preexisting Asthma).

WARNINGS

Gastrointestinal (GI) Effects — Risk of GI Ulceration, Bleeding, and Perforation
Serious gastrointestinal toxicity such as bleeding, ulceration and perforation of the stomach, small intestine or large intestine can occur at any time with or without warning symptoms in patients treated with nonsteroidal anti-inflammatory drugs (NSAIDs). Minor gastrointestinal problems such as dyspepsia are common and may also occur at any time during NSAID therapy. Therefore, physicians and patients should remain alert for ulceration and bleeding even in the absence of previous GI tract symptoms. Patients should be informed about the signs and symptoms of serious GI toxicity and the steps to take if they occur. The utility of periodic laboratory monitoring has not been demonstrated, nor has it been adequately assessed. Only one in five patients who develop a serious upper GI adverse event on NSAID therapy is symptomatic. It has been demonstrated that upper GI ulcers, gross bleeding or perforation caused by NSAIDs appear to occur in approximately 1% of patients treated for 3 to 6 months and 2-4% of patients treated for one year. These trends continue, thus increasing the likelihood of developing a serious GI event at some time during the course of therapy. However, even short-term therapy is not without risk.

NSAIDs should be prescribed with extreme caution in patients with a prior history of ulcer disease or gastrointestinal bleeding. Most spontaneous reports of fatal GI events are in elderly or debilitated patients and therefore special care should be taken in treating this population. For high risk patients, alternate therapies that do not involve NSAIDs should be considered.

Studies have shown that patients with a *prior history of peptic ulcer disease and/or gastrointestinal bleeding* and who use NSAIDs, have a greater than 10-fold higher risk for developing a GI bleed than patients with neither of these risk factors. In addition to a past history of ulcer disease, pharmacoepidemiological studies have identified several other co-therapies or co-morbid conditions that may increase the risk for GI bleeding such as: treatment with oral corticosteroids, treatment with anticoagulants, longer duration of NSAID therapy, smoking, alcoholism, older age, and poor general health status. (See CLINICAL STUDIES — Safety Studies.)

Serious Skin Reactions

Serious skin reactions, including exfoliative dermatitis, Stevens-Johnson syndrome, and toxic epidermal necrolysis, have been reported through postmarketing surveillance in patients receiving BEXTRA (see ADVERSE REACTIONS-Postmarketing Experience). As these reactions can be life-threatening, BEXTRA should be discontinued at the first appearance of skin rash or any other sign of hypersensitivity.

Anaphylactoid Reactions

In postmarketing experience, cases of hypersensitivity reactions (anaphylactic reactions and angioedema) have been reported in patients receiving BEXTRA (see ADVERSE REACTIONS-Postmarketing Experience). These cases have occurred in patients with and without a history of allergic-type reactions to sulfonamides (see CONTRAINDICATIONS). BEXTRA should not be given to patients with the aspirin triad. This symptom complex typically occurs in asthmatic patients who experience rhinitis with or without nasal polyps, or who exhibit severe, potentially fatal bronchospasm after taking aspirin or other NSAIDs (see CONTRAINDICATIONS and PRECAUTIONS — Pre-existing Asthma). Emergency help should be sought in cases where an anaphylactoid reaction occurs.

Advanced Renal Disease

No information is available regarding the safe use of BEXTRA Tablets in patients with advanced kidney disease. Therefore, treatment with BEXTRA is not recommended in these patients. If therapy with BEXTRA must be initiated, close monitoring of the patient's kidney function is advisable (see PRECAUTIONS — Renal Effects).

Pregnancy

In late pregnancy, BEXTRA should be avoided because it may cause premature closure of the ductus arteriosus.

PRECAUTIONS

General

BEXTRA Tablets cannot be expected to substitute for corticosteroids or to treat corticosteroid insufficiency. Abrupt discontinuation of corticosteroids may lead to exacerbation of corticosteroid-responsive illness. Patients on prolonged corticosteroid therapy should have their therapy tapered slowly if a decision is made to discontinue corticosteroids.

The pharmacological activity of valdecoxib in reducing fever and inflammation may diminish the utility of these diagnostic signs in detecting complications of presumed noninfectious, painful conditions.

Hepatic Effects

Borderline elevations of one or more liver tests may occur in up to 15% of patients taking NSAIDs. Notable elevations of ALT or AST (approximately three or more times the upper limit of normal) have been reported in approximately 1% of patients in clinical trials with NSAIDs. These laboratory abnormalities may progress, may remain unchanged, or may remain transient with continuing therapy. Rare cases of severe hepatic reactions, including jaundice and fatal fulminant hepatitis, liver necrosis and hepatic failure (some with fatal outcome) have been reported with NSAIDs. In controlled clinical trials of valdecoxib, the incidence of borderline (defined as 1.2- to 3.0-fold) elevations of liver tests was 8.0% for valdecoxib and 8.4% for placebo, while approximately 0.3% of patients taking valdecoxib, and 0.2% of patients taking placebo, had notable (defined as greater than 3-fold) elevations of ALT or AST.

A patient with symptoms and/or signs suggesting liver dysfunction, or in whom an abnormal liver test has occurred, should be monitored carefully for evidence of the development of a more severe hepatic reaction while on therapy with BEXTRA. If clinical signs and symptoms consistent with liver disease develop, or if systemic manifestations occur (e.g., eosinophilia, rash), BEXTRA should be discontinued.

Renal Effects

Long-term administration of NSAIDs has resulted in renal papillary necrosis and other renal injury. Renal toxicity has also been seen in patients in whom renal prostaglandins have a compensatory role in the maintenance of renal perfusion. In these patients, administration of a nonsteroidal anti-inflammatory drug may cause a dose-dependent reduction in prostaglandin formation and, secondarily, in renal blood flow, which may precipitate overt renal decompensation. Patients at greatest risk of this reaction are those with impaired renal function, heart failure, liver dysfunction, those taking diuretics and Angiotensin Converting Enzyme (ACE) inhibitors, and the elderly. Discontinuation of NSAID therapy is usually followed by recovery to the pretreatment state.

Caution should be used when initiating treatment with BEXTRA in patients with considerable dehydration. It is advisable to rehydrate patients first and then start therapy with BEXTRA. Caution is also recommended in patients with preexisting kidney disease. (See WARNINGS — Advanced Renal Disease.)

Hematological Effects

Anemia is sometimes seen in patients receiving BEXTRA. Patients on long-term treatment with BEXTRA should have their hemoglobin or hematocrit checked if they exhibit any signs or symptoms of anemia.

BEXTRA does not generally affect platelet counts, prothrombin time (PT), or activated partial thromboplastin time (APTT), and does not appear to inhibit platelet aggregation at indicated dosages (See CLINICAL STUDIES — Safety Studies — Platelets).

Fluid Retention and Edema

Fluid retention and edema have been observed in some patients taking BEXTRA (see ADVERSE REACTIONS). Therefore, BEXTRA should be used with caution in patients with fluid retention, hypertension, or heart failure.

Preexisting Asthma

Patients with asthma may have aspirin-sensitive asthma. The use of aspirin in patients with aspirin-sensitive asthma has been associated with severe bronchospasm, which can be fatal. Since cross reactivity, including bronchospasm, between aspirin and other nonsteroidal anti-inflammatory drugs has been reported in such aspirin-sensitive patients, BEXTRA should not be administered to patients with this form of aspirin sensitivity and should be used with caution in patients with preexisting asthma.

Information for Patients

BEXTRA can cause GI discomfort and, rarely, more serious GI side effects, which may result in hospitalization and even fatal outcomes. Although serious GI tract ulcerations and bleeding can occur without warning symptoms, patients should be alert for the signs and symptoms of ulcerations and bleeding, and should ask for medical advice when observing any indicative sign or symptoms. Patients should be apprised of the importance of this follow-up (see WARNINGS — Gastrointestinal (GI) Effects — Risk of GI Ulceration, Bleeding, and Perforation).

Patients should report to their physicians, signs or symptoms of gastrointestinal ulceration or bleeding, skin rash, weight gain, or edema.

Patients should be informed of the warning signs and symptoms of hepatotoxicity (e.g., nausea, fatigue, lethargy, pruritus, jaundice, right upper quadrant tenderness, and flu-like symptoms). If these occur, patients should be instructed to stop therapy and seek immediate medical attention.

Patients should also be instructed to seek immediate emergency help in the case of an anaphylactoid reaction (see WARNINGS — Anaphylactoid Reactions).

In late pregnancy, BEXTRA should be avoided because it may cause premature closure of the ductus arteriosus.

Laboratory Tests

Because serious GI tract ulcerations and bleeding can occur without warning symptoms, physicians should monitor for signs and symptoms of GI bleeding.

Drug Interactions

The drug interaction studies with valdecoxib were performed both with valdecoxib and a rapidly hydrolyzed intravenous prodrug form. The results from trials using the intravenous prodrug are reported in this section as they relate to the role of valdecoxib in drug interactions.

General: In humans, valdecoxib metabolism is predominantly mediated via CYP 3A4 and 2C9 with glucuronidation being a further (20%) route of metabolism. In vitro studies indicate that valdecoxib is a moderate inhibitor of CYP 2C19 (IC50 = 6 μ/mL), and a weak inhibitor of both 3A4 (IC50 = 44 μ/mL) and 2C9 (IC50 = 13 μ/mL). In view of the limitations of in vitro studies and the high valdecoxib IC50 values, the potential for such metabolic inhibitory effects in vivo at therapeutic doses of valdecoxib is low.

Aspirin: Concomitant administration of aspirin with valdecoxib may result in an increased risk of GI ulceration and complications compared to valdecoxib alone. Because of its lack of anti-platelet effect valdecoxib is not a substitute for aspirin for cardiovascular prophylaxis.

In a parallel group drug interaction study comparing the intravenous prodrug form of valdecoxib at 40 mg BID (n=10) vs placebo (n=9), valdecoxib had no effect on in vitro aspirin-mediated inhibition of arachidonate- or collagen-stimulated platelet aggregation.

Methotrexate: Valdecoxib 10 mg BID did not show a significant effect on the plasma exposure or renal clearance of methotrexate.

ACE-inhibitors: Reports suggest that NSAIDs may diminish the antihypertensive effect of ACE-inhibitors. This interaction should be given consideration in patients taking BEXTRA concomitantly with ACE-inhibitors.

Furosemide: Clinical studies, as well as post-marketing observations, have shown that NSAIDs can reduce the natriuretic effect of furosemide and thiazides in some patients. This response has been attributed to inhibition of renal prostaglandin synthesis.

Anticonvulsants: Anticonvulsant drug interaction studies with valdecoxib have not been conducted. As with other drugs, routine monitoring should be performed when therapy with BEXTRA is either initiated or discontinued in patients on anticonvulsant therapy.

Dextromethorphan: Dextromethorphan is primarily metabolized by CYP 2D6 and to a lesser extent by 3A4. Coadministration with valdecoxib (40 mg BID for 7 days) resulted in a significant increase in dextromethorphan plasma levels suggesting that, at these doses, valdecoxib is a weak inhibitor of 2D6. Dextromethorphan plasma concentrations in the presence of high doses of valdecoxib were almost 5-fold lower than those seen in CYP 2D6 poor metabolizers.

Lithium: Valdecoxib 40 mg BID for 7 days produced significant decreases in lithium serum clearance (25%) and renal clearance (30%) with a 34% higher serum exposure compared to lithium alone. Lithium serum concentrations should be monitored closely when initiating or changing therapy with BEXTRA in patients receiving lithium. Lithium carbonate (450 mg BID for 7 days) had no effect on valdecoxib pharmacokinetics.

Warfarin: The effect of valdecoxib on the anticoagulant effect of warfarin (1 - 8 mg/day) was studied in healthy subjects by coadministration of BEXTRA 40 mg BID for 7 days. Valdecoxib caused a statistically significant increase in plasma exposures of R-warfarin and S-warfarin (12% and 15%, respectively), and in the pharmacodynamic effects (prothrombin time, measured as INR) of warfarin. While mean INR values were only slightly increased with coadministration of valdecoxib, the day-to-day variability in individual INR values was increased. Anticoagulant therapy should be monitored, particularly during the first few weeks, after initiating therapy with BEXTRA in patients receiving warfarin or similar agents.

Fluconazole and Ketoconazole: Ketoconazole and fluconazole are predominantly CYP 3A4 and 2C9 inhibitors, respectively. Concomitant single dose administration of valdecoxib 20 mg with multiple doses of ketoconazole and fluconazole produced a significant increase in exposure of valdecoxib. Plasma exposure (AUC) to valdecoxib was increased 62% when coadministered with fluconazole and 38% when coadministered with ketoconazole.

Glyburide: Glyburide is a CYP 3A4 substrate. Coadministration of valdecoxib (10 mg BID for 7 days) with glyburide (5 mg QD or 10 mg BID) did not affect the pharmacokinetics (exposure) of glyburide.

Carcinogenesis, Mutagenesis, Impairment of Fertility

Valdecoxib was not carcinogenic in rats given oral doses up to 7.5 mg/kg/day for males and 1.5 mg/kg/day for females (equivalent to approximately 2- to 6-fold human exposure at 20 mg QD as measured by the $AUC_{(0-24hr)}$) or in mice given oral doses up to 25 mg/kg/day for males and 50 mg/kg/day for females (equivalent to approximately 0.6- to 2.4-fold human exposure at 20 mg QD as measured by the $AUC_{(0-24hr)}$) for two years.

Valdecoxib was not mutagenic in an Ames test or a mutation assay in Chinese hamster ovary (CHO) cells, nor was it clastogenic in a chromosome aberration assay in CHO cells or in an *in vivo* micronucleus test in rat bone marrow.

Valdecoxib did not impair male rat fertility at oral doses up to 9.0 mg/kg/day (equivalent to approximately 3- to 6-fold human exposure at 20 mg QD as measured by the $AUC_{(0-24hr)}$). In female rats, a decrease in ovulation with increased pre- and post-implantation loss resulted in decreased live embryos/fetuses at doses ≥2 mg/kg/day (equivalent to approximately 2-fold human exposure at 20 mg QD as measured by the $AUC_{(0-24hr)}$ for valdecoxib). The effects on female fertility were reversible. This effect is expected with inhibition of prostaglandin synthesis and is not the result of irreversible alteration of female reproductive function.

Pregnancy

Teratogenic Effects: Pregnancy Category C.

The incidence of fetuses with skeletal anomalies such as semi-bipartite thoracic vertebra centra and fused sternebrae was slightly higher in rabbits at an oral dose of 40 mg/kg/day (equivalent to approximately 72-fold human exposures at 20 mg QD as measured by the $AUC_{(0-24hr)}$) throughout organogenesis. Valdecoxib was not teratogenic in rabbits up to an oral dose of 10 mg/kg/day (equivalent to approximately 8-fold human exposures at 20 mg QD as measured by the $AUC_{(0-24hr)}$).

Valdecoxib was not teratogenic in rats up to an oral dose of 10 mg/kg/day (equivalent to approximately 19-fold human exposure at 20 mg QD as measured by the $AUC_{(0-24hr)}$). There are no studies in pregnant women. However, valdecoxib crosses the placenta in rats and rabbits. BEXTRA should be used during pregnancy only if the potential benefit justifies the potential risk to the fetus.

Non-Teratogenic Effects: Valdecoxib caused increased pre- and post-implantation loss with reduced live fetuses at oral doses ≥10 mg/kg/day (equivalent to approximately 19-fold human exposure at 20 mg QD as measured by the $AUC_{(0-24hr)}$) in rats and an oral dose of 40 mg/kg/day (equivalent to approximately 72-fold human exposure at 20 mg QD as measured by the $AUC_{(0-24hr)}$) in rabbits throughout organogenesis. In addition, reduced neonatal survival and decreased neonatal body weight when rats were treated with valdecoxib at oral doses ≥6 mg/kg/day (equivalent to approximately 7-fold human exposure at 20 mg QD as measured by the $AUC_{(0-24hr)}$) throughout organogenesis and lactation period. No studies have been conducted to evaluate the effect of valdecoxib on the closure of the ductus arteriosus in humans. Therefore, as with other drugs known to inhibit prostaglandin synthesis, use of BEXTRA during the third trimester of pregnancy should be avoided.

Labor and Delivery

Valdecoxib produced no evidence of delayed labor or parturition at oral doses up to 10 mg/kg/day in rats (equivalent to approximately 19-fold human exposure at 20 mg QD as measured by the $AUC_{(0-24hr)}$). The effects of BEXTRA on labor and delivery in pregnant women are unknown.

Continued on next page

Bextra—Cont.

Nursing Mothers
Valdecoxib and its active metabolite are excreted in the milk of lactating rats. It is not known whether this drug is excreted in human milk. Because many drugs are excreted in human milk, and because of the potential for adverse reactions in nursing infants from BEXTRA, a decision should be made whether to discontinue nursing or to discontinue the drug, taking into account the importance of the drug to the mother and the importance of nursing to the infant.

Pediatric Use
Safety and effectiveness of BEXTRA in pediatric patients below the age of 18 years have not been evaluated.

Geriatric Use
Of the patients who received BEXTRA in arthritis clinical trials of three months duration, or greater, approximately 2100 were 65 years of age or older, including 570 patients who were 75 years or older. No overall differences in effectiveness were observed between these patients and younger patients.

ADVERSE REACTIONS

Of the patients treated with BEXTRA Tablets in controlled arthritis trials, 2665 were patients with OA, and 2684 were patients with RA. More than 4000 patients have received a chronic total daily dose of BEXTRA 10 mg or more. More than 2800 patients have received BEXTRA 10 mg/day, or more, for at least 6 months and 988 of these have received BEXTRA for at least 1 year.

Osteoarthritis and Rheumatoid Arthritis
Table 4 lists all adverse events, regardless of causality, that occurred in ≥2.0% of patients receiving BEXTRA 10 and 20 mg/day in studies of three months or longer from 7 controlled studies conducted in patients with OA or RA that included a placebo and/or a positive control group.
[See table 4 below]
In these placebo- and active-controlled clinical trials, the discontinuation rate due to adverse events was 7.5% for arthritis patients receiving valdecoxib 10 mg daily, 7.9% for arthritis patients receiving valdecoxib 20 mg daily and 6.0% for patients receiving placebo.
In the seven controlled OA and RA studies, the following adverse events occurred in 0.1 - 1.9% of patients treated with BEXTRA 10 – 20 mg daily, regardless of causality.
Application site disorders: Cellulitis, dermatitis contact
Cardiovascular: Aggravated hypertension, aneurysm, angina pectoris, arrhythmia, cardiomyopathy, congestive heart failure, coronary artery disorder, heart murmur, hypotension
Central, peripheral nervous system: Cerebrovascular disorder, hypertonia, hypoesthesia, migraine, neuralgia, neuropathy, paresthesia, tremor, twitching, vertigo
Endocrine: Goiter
Female reproductive: Amenorrhea, dysmenorrhea, leukorrhea, mastitis, menstrual disorder, menorrhagia, menstrual bloating, vaginal hemorrhage
Gastrointestinal: Abnormal stools, constipation, diverticulosis, dry mouth, duodenal ulcer, duodenitis, eructation, esophagitis, fecal incontinence, gastric ulcer, gastritis, gastroenteritis, gastroesophageal reflux, hematemesis, hematochezia, hemorrhoids, hemorrhoids bleeding, hiatal hernia, melena, stomatitis, stool frequency increased, tenesmus, tooth disorder, vomiting
General: Allergy aggravated, allergic reaction, asthenia, chest pain, chills, cyst NOS, edema generalized, face edema, fatigue, fever, hot flushes, halitosis, malaise, pain, periorbital swelling, peripheral pain
Hearing and vestibular: Ear abnormality, earache, tinnitus
Heart rate and rhythm: Bradycardia, palpitation, tachycardia
Hemic: Anemia
Liver and biliary system: Hepatic function abnormal, hepatitis, ALT increased, AST increased
Male reproductive: Impotence, prostatic disorder
Metabolic and nutritional: Alkaline phosphatase increased, BUN increased, CPK increased, creatinine increased, diabetes mellitus, glycosuria, gout, hypercholesterolemia, hyperglycemia, hyperkalemia, hyperlipemia, hyperuricemia, hypocalcemia, hypokalemia, LDH increased, thirst increased, weight decrease, weight increase, xerophthalmia
Musculoskeletal: Arthralgia, fracture accidental, neck stiffness, osteoporosis, synovitis, tendonitis
Neoplasm: Breast neoplasm, lipoma, malignant ovarian cyst
Platelets (bleeding or clotting): Ecchymosis, epistaxis, hematoma NOS, thrombocytopenia
Psychiatric: Anorexia, anxiety, appetite increased, confusion, depression, depression aggravated, insomnia, nervousness, morbid dreaming, somnolence
Resistance mechanism disorders: Herpes simplex, herpes zoster, infection fungal, infection soft tissue, infection viral, moniliasis, moniliasis genital, otitis media
Respiratory: Abnormal breath sounds, bronchitis, bronchospasm, coughing, dyspnea, emphysema, laryngitis, pneumonia, pharyngitis, pleurisy, rhinitis
Skin and appendages: Acne, alopecia, dermatitis, dermatitis fungal, eczema, photosensitivity allergic reaction, pruritus, rash erythematous, rash maculopapular, rash psoriaform, skin dry, skin hypertrophy, skin ulceration, sweating increased, urticaria
Special senses: Taste perversion
Urinary system: Albuminuria, cystitis, dysuria, hematuria, micturition frequency increased, pyuria, urinary incontinence, urinary tract infection
Vascular: Claudication intermittent, hemangioma acquired, varicose vein
Vision: Blurred vision, cataract, conjunctival hemorrhage, conjunctivitis, eye pain, keratitis, vision abnormal
White cell and RES disorders: Eosinophilia, leukopenia, leukocytosis, lymphadenopathy, lymphangitis, lymphopenia
Other serious adverse events that were reported rarely (estimated <0.1%) in clinical trials, regardless of causality, in patients taking BEXTRA:
Autonomic nervous system disorders: Hypertensive encephalopathy, vasospasm
Cardiovascular: Abnormal ECG, aortic stenosis, atrial fibrillation, carotid stenosis, coronary thrombosis, heart block, heart valve disorders, mitral insufficiency, myocardial infarction, myocardial ischemia, pericarditis, syncope, thrombophlebitis, unstable angina, ventricular fibrillation
Central, peripheral nervous system: Convulsions
Endocrine: Hyperparathyroidism
Female reproductive: Cervical dysplasia
Gastrointestinal: Appendicitis, colitis with bleeding, dysphagia, esophageal perforation, gastrointestinal bleeding, ileus, intestinal obstruction, peritonitis
Hemic: Lymphoma-like disorder, pancytopenia
Liver and biliary system: Cholelithiasis
Metabolic: Dehydration
Musculoskeletal: Pathological fracture, osteomyelitis
Neoplasm: Benign brain neoplasm, bladder carcinoma, carcinoma, gastric carcinoma, prostate carcinoma, pulmonary carcinoma
Platelets (bleeding or clotting): Embolism, pulmonary embolism, thrombosis
Psychiatric: Manic reaction, psychosis
Renal: Acute renal failure

Table 4
Adverse Events with Incidence ≥ 2.0% in Valdecoxib Treatment Groups:
Controlled Arthritis Trials of Three Months or Longer

		(Total Daily Dose)				
		Valdecoxib				
Adverse Event Number Treated	**Placebo** 973	**10 mg** 1214	**20 mg** 1358	**Diclofenac 150 mg** 711	**Ibuprofen 2400 mg** 207	**Naproxen 1000 mg** 766
Autonomic Nervous System Disorders						
Hypertension	0.6	1.6	2.1	2.5	2.4	1.7
Body as a Whole						
Back pain	1.6	1.6	2.7	2.8	1.4	1.0
Edema peripheral	0.7	2.4	3.0	3.2	2.9	2.1
Influenza-like symptoms	2.2	2.0	2.2	3.1	2.9	2.0
Injury accidental	2.8	4.0	3.7	3.9	3.9	3.0
Central and Peripheral Nervous System Disorders						
Dizziness	2.1	2.6	2.7	4.2	3.4	2.7
Headache	7.1	4.8	8.5	6.6	4.3	5.5
Gastrointestinal System Disorders						
Abdominal fullness	2.0	2.1	1.9	3.0	2.9	2.5
Abdominal pain	6.3	7.0	8.2	17.0	8.2	10.1
Diarrhea	4.2	5.4	6.0	10.8	3.9	4.7
Dyspepsia	6.3	7.9	8.7	13.4	15.0	12.9
Flatulence	4.1	2.9	3.5	3.1	7.7	5.4
Nausea	5.9	7.0	6.3	8.4	7.7	8.7
Musculoskeletal System Disorders						
Myalgia	1.6	2.0	1.9	2.4	2.4	1.4
Respiratory System Disorders						
Sinusitis	2.2	2.6	1.8	1.1	3.4	3.4
Upper respiratory tract infection	6.0	6.7	5.7	6.3	4.3	6.4
Skin and Appendages Disorders						
Rash	1.0	1.4	2.1	1.5	0.5	1.4

Resistance mechanism disorders: Sepsis
Respiratory: Apnea, pleural effusion, pulmonary edema, pulmonary fibrosis, pulmonary infarction, pulmonary hemorrhage, respiratory insufficiency
Skin: Basal cell carcinoma, malignant melanoma
Urinary system: Pyelonephritis, renal calculus
Vision: Retinal detachment

Postmarketing Eperience
The following reactions have been identified during postmarketing use of BEXTRA. These reactions have been chosen for inclusion either due to their seriousness, reporting frequency, possible causal relationship to BEXTRA, or a combination of these factors. Because these reactions were reported voluntarily from a population of uncertain size, it is not possible to reliably estimate their frequency or establish a causal relationship to drug exposure.
General: Hypersensitivity reactions (including anaphylactic reactions and angioedema)
Skin and appendages: Erythema multiforme, exfoliative dermatitis, Stevens-Johnson syndrome, toxic epidermal necrolysis

OVERDOSAGE

Symptoms following acute NSAID overdoses are usually limited to lethargy, drowsiness, nausea, vomiting, and epigastric pain, which are generally reversible with supportive care. Gastrointestinal bleeding can occur. Hypertension, acute renal failure, respiratory depression and coma may occur, but are rare.
Anaphylactoid reactions have been reported with therapeutic ingestion of NSAIDs, and may occur following an overdose.
Patients should be managed by symptomatic and supportive care following an NSAID overdose. There are no specific antidotes. Hemodialysis removed only about 2% of administered valdecoxib from the systemic circulation of 8 patients with end-stage renal disease and, based on its degree of plasma protein binding (>98%), dialysis is unlikely to be useful in overdose. Forced diuresis, alkalinization of urine, or hemoperfusion also may not be useful due to high protein binding.

DOSAGE AND ADMINISTRATION

Osteoarthritis and Adult Rheumatoid Arthritis
The recommended dose of BEXTRA Tablets for the relief of the signs and symptoms of arthritis is 10 mg once daily.

Primary Dysmenorrhea
The recommended dose of BEXTRA Tablets for treatment of primary dysmenorrhea is 20 mg twice daily, as needed.

HOW SUPPLIED

BEXTRA Tablets 10 mg are white, film-coated, and capsule-shaped, debossed "10" on one side with a four pointed star shape on the other, supplied as:

NDC Number	Size
0025-1975-31	Bottle of 100
0025-1975-51	Bottle of 500
0025-1975-34	Carton of 100 unit dose

BEXTRA Tablets 20 mg are white, film-coated, and capsule-shaped, debossed "20" on one side with a four pointed star shape on the other, supplied as:

NDC Number	Size
0025-1980-31	Bottle of 100
0025-1980-51	Bottle of 500
0025-1980-34	Carton of 100 unit dose

Store at 25°C (77°F); excursions permitted to 15-30°C (59-86°F) [See USP Controlled Room Temperature].
Rx only
Revised: July 2003
Manufactured for:
G.D. Searle LLC
A subsidiary of Pharmacia Corporation
Chicago, IL 60680, USA
Pfizer Inc
New York, NY 10017, USA
by: Searle Ltd.
Caguas, PR 00725
818 763 003 P04001-2 / PS4001-2

CAVERJECT® ℞
[kă-vər-jĕkt]
(alprostadil for injection)
For Intracavernosal Use

Prescribing information for this product, which appears on pages 2721–2724 of the 2004 PDR, has been completely revised as follows. Please write "See Supplement A" next to the product heading.

DESCRIPTION

CAVERJECT Sterile Powder contains alprostadil as the naturally occurring form of prostaglandin E_1 (PGE_1) and is designated chemically as (11α, 13E, 15S)-11,15-dihydroxy-9-oxoprost-13-en-1-oic acid. The molecular weight is 354.49. Alprostadil is a white to off-white crystalline powder with a melting point between 115° and 116°C. Its solubility at 35°C is 8000 micrograms per 100 milliliter double distilled water. CAVERJECT is available as a sterile freeze-dried powder for intracavernosal use in four sizes: 5, 10, 20 and 40 micrograms per vial—When reconstituted as directed with 1 milliliter of bacteriostatic water for injection or sterile water, both preserved with benzyl alcohol 0.945% w/v, gives 1.13 milliliters of reconstituted solution. Each milliliter of CAVERJECT contains 5.4, 10.5, 20.5 or 41.1 micrograms of alprostadil depending on vial strength, 172 milligrams of lactose, 47 micrograms of sodium citrate and 8.4 milligrams of benzyl alcohol. The deliverable amount of alprostadil is 5, 10, 20 or 40 micrograms per milliliter because approximately 0.4 microgram for the 5 microgram strength, 0.5 microgram for the 10 and 20 microgram strengths and 1.1 microgram for the 40 microgram strength is lost due to adsorption to the vial and syringe. When necessary, the pH of alprostadil for injection was adjusted with hydrochloric acid and/or sodium hydroxide before lyophilization.

The structural formula of alprostadil is represented below:

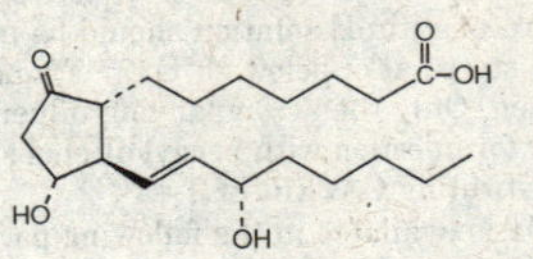

CLINICAL PHARMACOLOGY

Alprostadil has a wide variety of pharmacological actions; vasodilation and inhibition of platelet aggregation are among the most notable of these effects. In most animal species tested, alprostadil relaxed retractor penis and corpus cavernosum urethrae *in vitro*. Alprostadil also relaxed isolated preparations of human corpus cavernosum and spongiosum, as well as cavernous arterial segments contracted by either noradrenaline or $PGF_{2\alpha}$ *in vitro*. In pigtail monkeys *(Macaca nemestrina)*, alprostadil increased cavernous arterial blood flow *in vivo*. The degree and duration of cavernous smooth muscle relaxation in this animal model was dose-dependent.

Alprostadil induces erection by relaxation of trabecular smooth muscle and by dilation of cavernosal arteries. This leads to expansion of lacunar spaces and entrapment of blood by compressing the venules against the tunica albuginea, a process referred to as the corporal veno-occlusive mechanism.

Pharmacokinetics:

Absorption: For the treatment of erectile dysfunction, alprostadil is administered by injection into the corpora cavernosa. The absolute bioavailability of alprostadil has not been determined.

Distribution: Following intracavernosal injection of 20 micrograms alprostadil, mean peripheral plasma concentrations of alprostadil at 30 and 60 minutes after injection (89 and 102 picograms/milliliter, respectively) were not significantly greater than baseline levels of endogenous alprostadil (96 picograms/milliliter). Alprostadil is bound in plasma primarily to albumin (81% bound) and to a lesser extent α-globulin IV-4 fraction (55% bound). No significant binding to erythrocytes or white blood cells was observed.

Metabolism: Alprostadil is rapidly converted to compounds which are further metabolized prior to excretion. Following intravenous administration, approximately 80% of circulating alprostadil is metabolized in one pass through the lungs, primarily by *beta-* and *omega-*oxidation. Hence, any alprostadil entering the systemic circulation following intracavernosal injection is very rapidly metabolized. Following intracavernosal injection of 20 micrograms alprostadil, peripheral levels of the major circulating metabolite, 13,14-dihydro-15-oxo-PGE_1, increased to reach a peak 30 minutes after injection and returned to pre-dose levels by 60 minutes after injection.

Excretion: The metabolites of alprostadil are excreted primarily by the kidney, with almost 90% of an administered intravenous dose excreted in urine within 24 hours post-dose. The remainder of the dose is excreted in the feces. There is no evidence of tissue retention of alprostadil or its metabolites following intravenous administration.

Pharmacokinetics in Special Populations:

Geriatric: The potential effect of age on the pharmacokinetics of alprostadil has not been formally evaluated. In patients with acute respiratory distress syndrome (ARDS), the mean (± SD) pulmonary extraction of alprostadil was 72% ± 15% in 11 elderly patients aged 65 years or older (mean, 71 ± 6 years) and 65% ± 20% in 6 young patients aged 35 years or younger (mean, 28 ± 5 years).

Pediatric: Alprostadil plasma concentrations were measured in 10 neonates (gestational age of 34 weeks in 2 infants and 38 to 40 weeks in 8 infants) receiving steady-state intravenous infusions of alprostadil to treat underlying cardiac malformations. Infusion rates of alprostadil ranged from 5 to 50 (median, 45) nanograms/kilogram/minute, resulting in alprostadil plasma concentrations ranging between 22 and 530 (median, 56) picograms/milliliter. The wide range of alprostadil plasma concentrations in neonates reflects high variability in individual clearances of alprostadil in this patient population.

Gender: The potential influence of gender on the pharmacokinetics of alprostadil has not been formally studied in healthy subjects. Two studies determined the pulmonary extraction of alprostadil following intravascular administration in 23 patients with ARDS. The mean (± SD) pulmonary extraction was 66% ± 20% in 17 male patients and 69% ± 18% in 6 female patients, suggesting that the pharmacokinetics of alprostadil are not influenced by gender.

Race: The potential influence of race on the pharmacokinetics of alprostadil has not been formally evaluated.

Renal and Hepatic Insufficiency: The pharmacokinetics of alprostadil have not been formally examined in patients with renal or hepatic insufficiency.

Pulmonary Disease: The pulmonary extraction of alprostadil following intravascular administration was reduced by 15% (66 ± 3.2% vs 78 ± 2.4%) in patients with ARDS compared with a control group of patients with normal respiratory function who were undergoing cardiopulmonary bypass surgery. Pulmonary clearance was found to vary as a function of cardiac output and pulmonary intrinsic clearance in a group of 14 patients with ARDS or at risk of developing ARDS following trauma or sepsis. In this study, the extraction efficiency of alprostadil ranged from subnormal (11%) to normal (90%), with an overall mean of 67%.

Drug-Drug Interactions:

The potential for pharmacokinetic drug-drug interactions between alprostadil and other agents has not been formally studied.

INDICATION AND USAGE

CAVERJECT is indicated for the treatment of erectile dysfunction due to neurogenic, vasculogenic, psychogenic, or mixed etiology.

Intracavernosal CAVERJECT may be a useful adjunct to other diagnostic tests in the diagnosis of erectile dysfunction.

CONTRAINDICATIONS

CAVERJECT should not be used in patients who have a known hypersensitivity to the drug, in patients who have conditions that might predispose them to priapism, such as sickle cell anemia or trait, multiple myeloma, or leukemia, or in patients with anatomical deformation of the penis, such as angulation, cavernosal fibrosis, or Peyronie's disease. Patients with penile implants should not be treated with CAVERJECT.

CAVERJECT should not be used in women or children and is not for use in newborns.

CAVERJECT should not be used in men for whom sexual activity is inadvisable or contraindicated.

PRECAUTIONS

General Precautions: Prolonged erection (erection lasting 4 to 6 hours) and priapism (erection lasting over 6 hours) are known to occur following intracavernosal administration of vasoactive substances, including CAVERJECT. The patient should be instructed to immediately report to his physician or, if unavailable, to seek immediate medical assistance for any erection that persists for longer than 4 hours. Treatment of priapism should be according to established medical practice.

The overall incidence of penile fibrosis, including Peyronie's disease, reported in clinical studies with CAVERJECT was 3%. In one self-injection clinical study where duration of use was up to 18 months, the incidence of fibrosis was 7.8%. Regular follow-up of patients, with careful examination of the penis, is strongly recommended to detect signs of penile fibrosis. Treatment with CAVERJECT should be discontinued in patients who develop penile angulation, cavernosal fibrosis, or Peyronie's disease.

Patients on anticoagulants, such as warfarin or heparin, may have increased propensity for bleeding after intracavernosal injection.

Underlying treatable medical causes of erectile dysfunction should be diagnosed and treated prior to initiation of therapy with CAVERJECT.

The safety and efficacy of combinations of CAVERJECT and other vasoactive agents have not been systematically studied. Therefore, the use of such combinations is not recommended.

The patient should be instructed not to re-use or to share needles or syringes. As with all prescription medicines, the patient should not allow anyone else to use his medicine.

Information for the Patient:

To ensure safe and effective use of CAVERJECT, the patient should be thoroughly instructed and trained in the self-injection technique before he begins intracavernosal treatment with CAVERJECT at home. The desirable dose should be established in the physician's office. The instructions for preparation of the solution of CAVERJECT should be carefully followed. Vials with precipitates or discoloration should be discarded. The reconstituted vial is designed for one use only and should be discarded after withdrawal of proper volume of the solution. The content of the reconstituted vial should not be shaken. The needle must be properly discarded after use; it must not be re-used or shared with other persons. Patient instructions for administration are included in each package of CAVERJECT.

The dose of CAVERJECT that is established in the physician's office should not be changed by the patient without consulting the physician. The patient may expect an erection to occur within 5 to 20 minutes. A standard treatment goal is to produce an erection lasting no longer than 1 hour. Generally, CAVERJECT should be used no more than 3 times per week, with at least 24 hours between each use.

Patients should be aware of possible side effects of therapy with CAVERJECT; the most frequently occurring is penile pain after injection, usually mild to moderate in severity. A potentially serious adverse reaction with intracavernosal therapy is priapism. Accordingly, the patient should be instructed to contact the physician's office immediately or, if unavailable, to seek immediate medical assistance if an erection persists for longer than 4 hours.

The patient should report any penile pain that was not present before or that increased in intensity, as well as the occurrence of nodules or hard tissue in the penis to his physician as soon as possible. As with any intravenous injection, an infection is a possibility. Patients should be instructed to report to the physician any penile redness, swelling, tenderness or curvature of the erect penis. The patient must visit the physician's office for regular checkups for assessment of the therapeutic benefit and safety of treatment with CAVERJECT.

Note: Use of intracavernosal CAVERJECT offers no protection from the transmission of sexually transmitted diseases. Individuals who use CAVERJECT should be counseled about the protective measures that are necessary to guard against the spread of sexually transmitted diseases, including the human immunodeficiency virus (HIV).

The injection of CAVERJECT can induce a small amount of bleeding at the site of injection (see ADVERSE REACTIONS section—hematoma, ecchymosis, hemorrhage at the site of injection). In patients infected with blood-borne diseases, this could increase the risk of transmission of blood-borne diseases between partners.

In clinical trials, concomitant use of agents such as antihypertensive drugs, diuretics, antidiabetic agents (including insulin), or non-steroidal anti-inflammatory drugs had no effect on the efficacy or safety of CAVERJECT.

Carcinogenesis, Mutagenesis, and Impairment of Fertility:

Long-term carcinogenicity studies have not been conducted. Rat reproductive studies indicate that alprostadil at doses of up to 0.2 milligram/kilogram/day does not adversely affect or alter rat spermatogenesis, providing a 200-fold margin of safety compared with the usual human doses. The following battery of mutagenicity assays revealed no potential for mutagenesis: bacterial mutation (Ames), alkaline elution, rat micronucleus, sister chromatid exchange, CHO/HGPRT mammalian cell forward gene mutation, and unscheduled DNA synthesis (UDS).

A 1-year irritancy study was conducted in three groups of 5 male Cynomolgus monkeys injected intracavernosally twice weekly with either vehicle or 3 or 8.25 micrograms of alprostadil per injection. An additional two groups of 6 monkeys each were injected with vehicle or with 8.25 micrograms/injection twice weekly as described previously plus they received multiple doses during weeks 44, 48, and 52. Three monkeys from each group were retained for a 4-week recovery period. There was no evidence of drug-related penile irritancy or nonpenile tissue lesions, which could be directly related to alprostadil. The irritancy which was noted for control and treated monkeys was considered to be a result of the injection procedure itself, and any lesions noted were shown to be reversible. At the end of the 4-week recovery period, the histological changes in the penis had regressed.

Pregnancy, Nursing Mothers, and Pediatric Use:

CAVERJECT is not indicated for use in newborns, children, or women.

Geriatric Use

A total of 341 subjects included in clinical studies were 65 and over. No overall differences in safety and effectiveness were observed between these subjects and younger subjects, and the other reported clinical experience has not identified differences in responses between elderly and younger patients, but decreased sensitivity of some older individuals cannot be ruled out.

ADVERSE REACTIONS

Local Adverse Reactions: The following local adverse reaction information was derived from controlled and uncontrolled studies, including an uncontrolled 18-month safety study.

Local Adverse Reactions Reported by ≥ 1% of Patients Treated with CAVERJECT for up to 18 Months*

Event	CAVERJECT N = 1861
Penile pain	37%
Prolonged erection	4%
Penile fibrosis**	3%
Injection site hematoma	3%
Penis disorder***	3%
Injection site ecchymosis	2%
Penile rash	1%
Penile edema	1%

* Except for penile pain (2%), no significant local adverse reactions were reported by 294 patients who received 1 to 3 injections of placebo.

** See General Precautions.

*** Includes numbness, yeast infection, irritation, sensitivity, phimosis, pruritus, erythema, venous leak, penile skin tear, strange feeling of penis, discoloration of penile head, itch at tip of penis.

Penile Pain: Penile pain after intracavernosal administration of CAVERJECT was reported at least once by 37% of patients in clinical studies of up to 18 months in duration. In the majority of the cases, penile pain was rated mild or moderate in intensity. Three percent of patients discontinued treatment because of penile pain. The frequency of penile pain was 2% in 294 patients who received 1 to 3 injections of placebo.

Prolonged Erection/Priapism: In clinical trials, prolonged erection was defined as an erection that lasted for 4 to 6 hours; priapism was defined as erection that lasted 6 hours or longer. The frequency of prolonged erection after intracavernosal administration of CAVERJECT was 4%, while the frequency of priapism was 0.4%. In the majority of cases, spontaneous detumescence occurred. To minimize the chances of prolonged erection or priapism, CAVERJECT

Continued on next page

Caverject—Cont.

should be titrated slowly to the lowest effect dose (see DOSAGE AND ADMINISTRATION section). The patient must be instructed to immediately report to his physician or, if unavailable, to seek immediate medical assistance for any erection that persists for longer than 4 hours. If priapism is not treated immediately, penile tissue damage and permanent loss of potency may result.

Hematoma/Ecchymosis: The frequency of hematoma and ecchymosis was 3% and 2%, respectively. In most cases, hematoma/ecchymosis was judged to be a complication of a faulty injection technique. Accordingly, proper instruction of the patient in self-injection is of importance to minimize the potential of hematoma/ecchymosis (see DOSAGE AND ADMINISTRATION).

The following local adverse reactions were reported by fewer than 1% of patients after injection of CAVERJECT: balanitis, injection site hemorrhage, injection site inflammation, injection site itching, injection site swelling, injection site edema, urethral bleeding, penile warmth, numbness, yeast infection, irritation, sensitivity, phimosis, pruritus, erythema, venous leak, painful erection, and abnormal ejaculation.

Systemic Adverse Events: The following systemic adverse event information was derived from controlled and uncontrolled studies, including an uncontrolled 18-month safety study.

Systemic Adverse Events Reported by ≥ 1% of Patients Treated with CAVERJECT for up to 18 Months*

Body System/Reaction	CAVERJECT N = 1861
Cardiovascular System	
Hypertension	2%
Central Nervous System	
Headache	2%
Dizziness	1%
Musculoskeletal System	
Back pain	1%
Respiratory System	
Upper respiratory infection	4%
Flu syndrome	2%
Sinusitis	2%
Nasal congestion	1%
Cough	1%
Urogenital System	
Prostatic Disorder**	2%
Miscellaneous	
Localized pain***	2%
Trauma****	2%

* No significant adverse events were reported by 294 patients who received 1 to 3 injections of placebo.

** prostatitis, pain, hypertrophy, enlargement

*** pain in various anatomical structures other than injection site

**** injuries, fractures, abrasions, lacerations, dislocations

The following systemic events, which were reported for < 1% of patients in clinical studies, were judged by investigators to be possibly related to use of CAVERJECT: testicular pain, scrotal disorder, scrotal edema, hematuria, testicular disorder, impaired urination, urinary frequency, urinary urgency, pelvic pain, hypotension, vasodilation, peripheral vascular disorder, supraventricular extrasystoles, vasovagal reactions, hypesthesia, non-generalized weakness, diaphoresis, rash, non-application site pruritus, skin neoplasm, nausea, dry mouth, increased serum creatinine, leg cramps, and mydriasis.

Hemodynamic changes, manifested as decreases in blood pressure and increases in pulse rate, were observed during clinical studies, principally at doses above 20 micrograms and above 30 micrograms of alprostadil, respectively, and appeared to be dose-dependent. However, these changes were usually clinically unimportant; only three patients discontinued the treatment because of symptomatic hypotension.

CAVERJECT had no clinically important effect on serum or urine laboratory tests.

OVERDOSAGE

Overdosage was not observed in clinical trials with CAVERJECT. If intracavernous overdose of CAVERJECT occurs, the patient should be under medical supervision until any systemic effects have resolved and/or until penile detumescence has occurred. Symptomatic treatment of any systemic symptoms would be appropriate.

DOSAGE AND ADMINISTRATION

The dose of CAVERJECT should be individualized for each patient by careful titration under supervision by the physician. In clinical studies, patients were treated with CAVERJECT in doses ranging from 0.2 to 140 micrograms; however, since 99% of patients received doses of 60 micrograms or less, doses of greater than 60 micrograms are not recommended. In general, the lowest possible effective dose should always be employed. In clinical studies, over 80% of patients experienced an erection sufficient for sexual intercourse after intracavernosal injection of CAVERJECT. A 1/2-inch, 27- to 30-gauge needle is generally recommended.

Initial Titration in Physician's Office:

Erectile Dysfunction of Vasculogenic, Psychogenic, or Mixed Etiology. Dosage titration should be initiated at 2.5 micrograms of alprostadil. If there is a partial response, the dose may be increased by 2.5 micrograms to a dose of 5 micrograms and then in increments of 5 to 10 micrograms, depending upon erectile response, until the dose that produces an erection suitable for intercourse and not exceeding a duration of 1 hour is reached. If there is no response to the initial 2.5-microgram dose, the second dose may be increased to 7.5 micrograms, followed by increments of 5 to 10 micrograms. The patient must stay in the physician's office until complete detumescence occurs. If there is no response, then the next higher dose may be given within 1 hour. If there is a response, then there should be at least a 1-day interval before the next dose is given.

Erectile Dysfunction of Pure Neurogenic Etiology (Spinal Cord Injury). Dosage titration should be initiated at 1.25 micrograms of alprostadil. The dose may be increased by 1.25 micrograms to a dose of 2.5 micrograms, followed by an increment of 2.5 micrograms to a dose of 5 micrograms, and then in 5-microgram increments until the dose that produces an erection suitable for intercourse and not exceeding a duration of 1 hour is reached. The patient must stay in the physician's office until complete detumescence occurs. If there is no response, then the next higher dose may be given within 1 hour. If there is a response, then there should be at least a 1-day interval before the next dose is given.

The majority of patients (56%) in one clinical study involving 579 patients were titrated to doses of greater than 5 micrograms but less than or equal to 20 micrograms. The mean dose at the end of the titration phase was 17.8 micrograms of alprostadil.

Maintenance Therapy:

The first injections of CAVERJECT must be done at the physician's office by medically trained personnel. Self-injection therapy by the patient can be started only after the patient is properly instructed and well trained in the self-injection technique. The physician should make a careful assessment of the patient's skills and competence with this procedure. The intracavernosal injection must be done under sterile conditions. The site of injection is usually along the dorso-lateral aspect of the proximal third of the penis. Visible veins should be avoided. The side of the penis that is injected and the site of injection must be alternated; the injection site must be cleansed with an alcohol swab.

The dose of CAVERJECT that is selected for self-injection treatment should provide the patient with an erection that is satisfactory for sexual intercourse and that is maintained for no longer than 1 hour. If the duration of erection is longer than 1 hour, the dose of CAVERJECT should be reduced. Self-injection therapy for use at home should be initiated at the dose that was determined in the physician's office; however, dose adjustment, if required (up to 57% of patients in one clinical study), should be made only after consultation with the physician. The dose should be adjusted in accordance with the titration guidelines described above. The effectiveness of CAVERJECT for long-term use of up to 6 months has been documented in an uncontrolled, self-injection study. The mean dose of CAVERJECT at the end of 6 months was 20.7 micrograms in this study.

Careful and continuous follow-up of the patient while in the self-injection program must be exercised. This is especially true for the initial self-injections, since adjustments in the dose of CAVERJECT may be needed. The recommended frequency of injection is no more than 3 times weekly, with at least 24 hours between each dose. The reconstituted vial of CAVERJECT is intended for single use only and should be discarded after use. The user should be instructed in the proper disposal of the syringe, needle, and vial.

While on self-injection treatment, it is recommended that the patient visit the prescribing physician's office every 3 months. At that time, the efficacy and safety of the therapy should be assessed, and the dose of CAVERJECT should be adjusted, if needed.

CAVERJECT as an Adjunct to the Diagnosis of Erectile Dysfunction:

In the simplest diagnostic test for erectile dysfunction (pharmacologic testing), patients are monitored for the occurrence of an erection after an intracavernosal injection of CAVERJECT. Extensions of this testing are the use of CAVERJECT as an adjunct to laboratory investigations, such as duplex or Doppler imaging, ^{133}Xenon washout tests, radioisotope penogram, and penile arteriography, to allow visualization and assessment of penile vasculature. For any of these tests, a single dose of CAVERJECT that induces an erection with firm rigidity should be used.

General Procedure for Solution Preparation:

CAVERJECT is packaged in a 5-milliliter glass vial. Bacteriostatic water for injection or sterile water, both preserved with benzyl alcohol 0.945% w/v, must be used as the diluent for reconstitution. After reconstitution with 1 milliliter of diluent, the volume of the resulting solution is 1.13 milliliters. One milliliter of this solution will contain 5.4, 10.5, 20.5 or 41.1 micrograms of alprostadil depending on vial strength, 172 milligrams of lactose, 47 micrograms of sodium citrate and 8.4 milligrams of benzyl alcohol. The deliverable amount of alprostadil is 5, 10, 20 or 40 micrograms per milliliter because approximately 0.4 microgram for the 5 microgram strength, 0.5 microgram for the 10 and 20 microgram strengths and 1.1 microgram for the 40 microgram strength is lost due to adsorption to the vial and syringe. After reconstitution, the solution of CAVERJECT should be used within 24 hours when stored at or below 25°C (77°F) and not refrigerated or frozen. Parenteral drug products should be inspected visually for particulate matter and discoloration prior to administration whenever the solution and container permit.

HOW SUPPLIED

CAVERJECT is a dry lyophilized powder and is supplied in vials containing 6.15, 11.9, 23.2 or 46.4 micrograms of alprostadil for intracavernosal administration. Store the 5, 10 and 20 microgram strengths at or below 25°C (77°F). **Store the 40 microgram strength at 2° to 8°C (36° to 46°F) until dispensed. After dispensing, the CAVERJECT 40 microgram strength may be stored at or below 25°C (77°F) for 3 months or until expiration date, whichever occurs first.**

When reconstituted and used as directed, the deliverable amount of alprostadil is 5, 10, 20 or 40 micrograms, respectively. The reconstituted solution should be used within 24 hours when stored at or below 25°C (77°F) and not refrigerated or frozen. Only the accompanying diluent or bacteriostatic water for injection with benzyl alcohol should be used when reconstituting CAVERJECT.

CAVERJECT is available in the following package:

6–20 microgram vials with diluent syringes	NDC 0009-3701-01

An autoinjector **(PenInject 2.25™ AutoInjector)**, designed for use with the vials with diluent syringe package described above is available separately. A pamphlet containing instructions on loading, using, and maintaining the **PenInject 2.25 AutoInjector** is included with the device.

Other available packages:

6–5 microgram vials	NDC 0009-5131-02
6–10 microgram vials	NDC 0009-3778-05
6–20 microgram vials	NDC 0009-3701-05
6–40 microgram vials	NDC 0009-7686-04

PATIENT INSTRUCTIONS FOR Caverject®

alprostadil for injection

PRE-FILLED DILUENT

(bacteriostatic water for injection) SYRINGE

IMPOTENCE: CAUSES AND TREATMENTS

There are several causes of impotence, a condition known medically as erectile dysfunction. These include: medications that you may be taking for other conditions, impaired blood circulation in the penis, nerve damage, emotional problems, excessive smoking or alcohol use, use of street drugs, and hormonal imbalances. Often, impotence is due to more than one cause.

Treatments for impotence include: switching medications (if you are taking a medication that causes impotence), administration of hormones, penile injections, use of medical devices that produce an erection, surgical procedures to correct blood flow in the penis, penile implants, and psychological counseling. Your doctor has selected CAVERJECT for injection to treat your impotence. Your doctor can also discuss other available treatments. You should not stop taking any prescription medications, unless told to do so by your doctor.

USE OF CAVERJECT

CAVERJECT is injected into a specific area of the penis and should produce an erection in 5 to 20 minutes. The erection should last for about 1 hour. Generally, you should not use CAVERJECT more than 3 times a week, with at least 24 hours between uses.

Who Should Not Use CAVERJECT?

Men who have conditions that might result in long-lasting erections should not use CAVERJECT. Some of these conditions include: sickle cell anemia or trait, leukemia, and tumor of the bone marrow (multiple myeloma). Men with penile implants, or an abnormally formed penis, or who have been advised not to engage in sexual activity should not use CAVERJECT. CAVERJECT should not be used by women or children.

What Are The Risks Of Using CAVERJECT?

Erections that last more than 4 hours can cause serious and permanent damage. **Call your doctor or seek professional help immediately if you still have an erection 4 hours after injection.**

The most common side effect of CAVERJECT is mild to moderate pain after injection. About one-third of patients report this effect.

Call your doctor if you notice any redness, lumps, swelling, tenderness, or curving of the erect penis.

A small amount of bleeding at the injection site may occur. Tell your doctor if you have a condition or are taking a medicine that interferes with blood clotting.

NOTE: CAVERJECT offers no protection from the transmission of sexually transmitted diseases such as HIV (the virus that causes AIDS). Small amounts of bleeding at the injection site can increase the risk of transmission of blood-borne diseases between partners.

There is no approved injectable treatment using multiple drug components or "cocktails" for erectile dysfunction. Moreover, there are no data on the efficacy and safety of these combinations.

STORAGE

1. Unused packs of 5, 10 and 20 microgram vials of CAVERJECT may be stored at or below 25°C (77°F). **Unused packs of the 40 microgram vial may be stored at or below 25°C (77°F) for 3 months or until expiration date, whichever occurs first.** Do not freeze.
2. After reconstitution, the solution of CAVERJECT should be used within 24 hours when stored at or below 25°C (77°F) and not refrigerated or frozen.
3. During travel, care should be taken to avoid allowing the product to freeze or be stored at temperatures above 25°C (77°F). Therefore, do not store in checked luggage during air travel or leave in a closed automobile.

ADDITIONAL INFORMATION

There is a technical leaflet discussion of CAVERJECT written for health-care professionals that your pharmacist can let you read.

More information about erectile dysfunction and its treatment is available from the National Institutes of Health (Washington, DC), the American Foundation for Urological Diseases (Baltimore, MD), or the Impotence Institute of America (Washington, DC).

PREPARING AND INJECTING CAVERJECT

You must be properly instructed and trained in the injection technique by your doctor before using CAVERJECT.

Before using CAVERJECT, talk to your doctor about what to expect when using it, possible side effects, and what to do if side effects occur. Your dose has been selected for your individual needs. Do not change your dose without consulting your doctor. If you are not sure of the volume or dose to be used, talk to your doctor or pharmacist.

Follow these instructions exactly to prepare and inject a sterile dose of CAVERJECT. A dose may be administered manually as described in the "Inject Your Dose of Caverject" section below, or with the use of an autoinjector **(PenInject 2.25 AutoInjector)** which is available separately. If you choose to use the **PenInject 2.25 AutoInjector**, see the pamphlet provided with it for instructions on loading, using and maintaining this device.

If the needle is severely bent at any time, do not use it for injecting CAVERJECT and do not attempt to straighten it prior to injecting CAVERJECT. A severely bent and re-straightened needle may be predisposed to breakage. Needle breakage, with a portion of the needle remaining in the penis, has been reported and, in some cases, required hospitalization and surgical removal. If the needle is severely bent while preparing the injection, discard the syringe/needle and use a new self-injection system.

Use the needle/syringe, and vial **only once** then safely discard the supplies and any unused solution (see the "Disposal of Injection Materials" section of these instructions).

Supplies Needed

To prepare and inject CAVERJECT you will need a vial of CAVERJECT Sterile Powder, the pre-filled diluent syringe with attached needle, and two alcohol swabs (Figure A). All required materials are provided in the blue plastic case in which CAVERJECT is supplied.

The pre-filled syringe contains the diluent (bacteriostatic water for injection preserved with benzyl alcohol 0.945% w/v) you will use to dissolve the CAVERJECT Sterile Powder. You will use the same syringe to inject the solution of CAVERJECT into your penis.

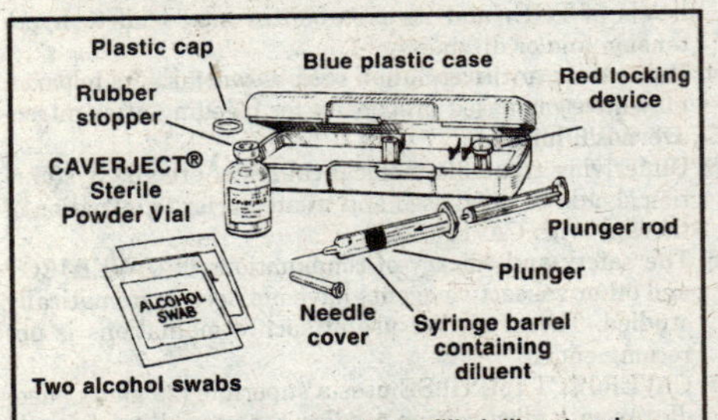

A. Self-injection system with pre-filled diluent syringe

CAVERJECT, with pre-filled diluent syringe, comes in 5, 10 or 20 microgram strengths. **MAKE SURE YOU HAVE THE RIGHT STRENGTH VIAL OF CAVERJECT.**

Prepare the Dose

1. Wash your hands thoroughly, and dry them with a clean towel.
2. Handle the syringe by the syringe barrel only. Do not touch the needle with your hands. Do not allow the needle to touch any surface.
3. Insert plunger rod into open end of syringe barrel. Gently screw threaded end of plunger rod into rubber stopper. Do not overtighten.
4. With the needle cover still in place, slowly push the plunger slightly forward toward the needle end of the syringe. Allow the plunger to slide back to its initial position. Repeat this procedure several times to spread the plunger stopper lubricant evenly.
5. Remove the plastic cap from the vial of CAVERJECT.
6. Wipe the rubber stopper on the vial of CAVERJECT with alcohol swab. Discard this alcohol swab.
7. Grasp the syringe barrel (not the plunger) and remove the needle cover. Do not discard the needle cover, you will need to use it again (see 14). Do not touch the exposed needle. Hold the syringe with the needle pointing up and push the plunger to the 1-cc (mL) mark on the syringe. This is to expel air and excess diluent.
8. Holding the syringe/needle in a straight line with the vial of CAVERJECT to avoid bending the needle, push the needle through the center of the vial's rubber stopper and push the syringe plunger all the way down to expel all the diluent into the vial. Proceed immediately to step 9.
9. Without removing the needle or touching the needle or stopper, **gently** swirl (do not shake) the vial until all the powder is dissolved in the diluent. Then turn the vial and needle/syringe upside down and **gently** swirl the vial to dissolve any powder in the neck of the vial. **DO NOT USE THE SOLUTION IF IT IS CLOUDY, COLORED OR CONTAINS PARTICLES.**
10. Keeping the needle in the vial, firmly hold the vial and syringe upside down in one hand (see Figure B).

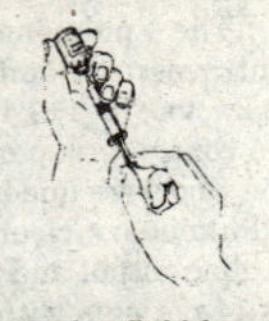

B. Removing fluid from the vial

11. Keeping the needle tip below the level of fluid, slowly pull back on the syringe plunger until all the fluid is removed from the vial.
12. If there are air bubbles, gently tap the syringe barrel until they float to the top of the solution (see Figure C). Holding the syringe upright, push the syringe plunger to the correct volume mark for the dose prescribed by your doctor. This will expel any air and excess solution into the vial.

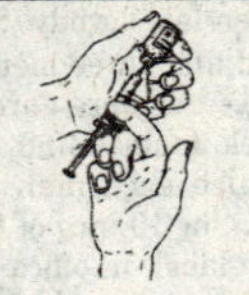

C. Tapping the syringe to release air bubbles

13. Grasp the syringe barrel (not the plunger) and pull the needle/syringe from the vial of CAVERJECT in a straight line to avoid bending the needle.
14. Place the needle cover over the needle and set the syringe down on a level surface.

Select Injection Site

1. CAVERJECT will be injected into a corpus cavernosum (spongy tissue) of the penis. One corpus cavernosum runs the length of the right side of the penis. Another corpus cavernosum runs the length of the left side of the penis (see Figures D and E).

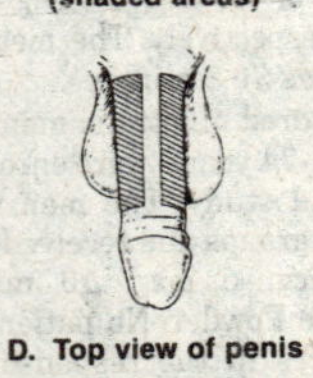

D. Top view of penis

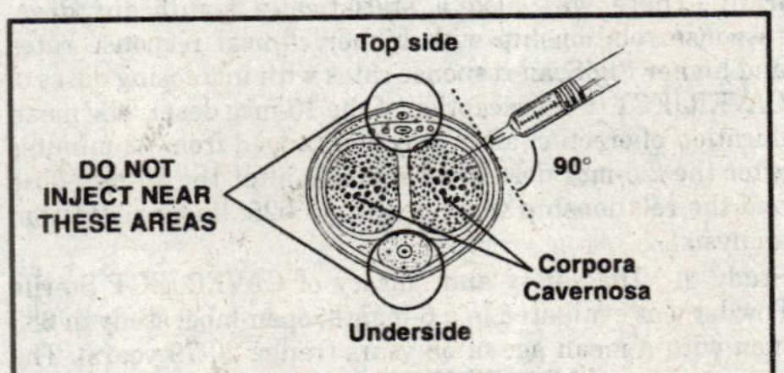

E. Cross-section of penis

2. Choose an injection site on one side of the shaft of the penis as shown in Figure D. AVOID VISIBLE BLOOD VESSELS.
3. WITH EACH USE OF CAVERJECT, ALTERNATE THE SIDE OF THE PENIS AND VARY THE SITE OF THE INJECTION.

Inject Your Dose of CAVERJECT

1. You should be sitting upright or slightly reclined when injecting CAVERJECT.
2. If your penis is not circumcised, pull the foreskin back. Holding the head of your penis with your thumb and forefinger, stretch it lengthwise along your thigh so that you can clearly see the selected injection site.
3. Clean the injection site with a new alcohol swab. Do not discard this swab, you will need to use it again (see step 7).
4. Remove the cover from the needle. Reposition the penis firmly against your thigh as in step 2 to keep it from moving during the injection.

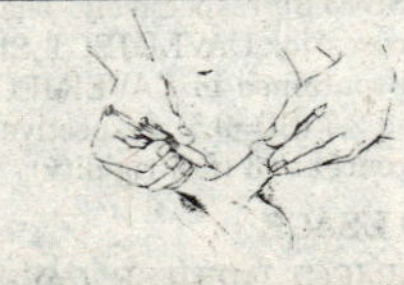

F. Inserting the needle into the injection site

5. Hold the syringe between your thumb and index finger (Figure F). Using a steady motion, push the needle straight into the selected site until the metal part of the needle is almost entirely in the penis.
6. Holding the syringe barrel between two fingers, move your thumb or finger to the top of the plunger and, with a steady motion, push down on the plunger so that the entire volume of CAVERJECT is slowly injected (Figure G). [See figure at top of next column]

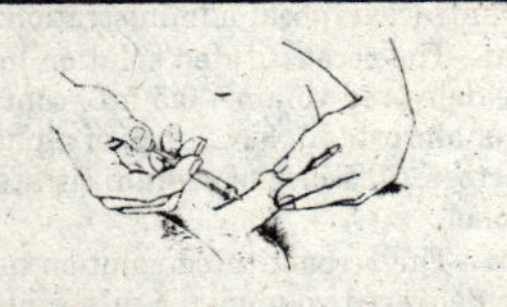

G. Injecting the contents of the syringe

7. Grasp the syringe barrel and pull the needle out of your penis. **APPLY PRESSURE TO THE INJECTION SITE WITH THE ALCOHOL SWAB FOR ABOUT 5 MINUTES OR UNTIL ANY BLEEDING STOPS.**

Disposal of Injection Materials

After use, dispose of all injection materials safely. Your pharmacist may be able to supply a disposal box especially for syringes. If not, the blue plastic case of CAVERJECT may be used as follows:

1. Place the used syringe and vial into the blue plastic case. Then remove the red plastic locking device. Close the case firmly so that it snaps shut (Figure H).

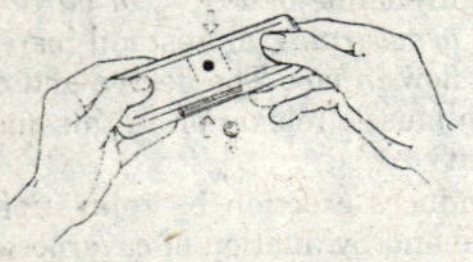

H. Closing the plastic case

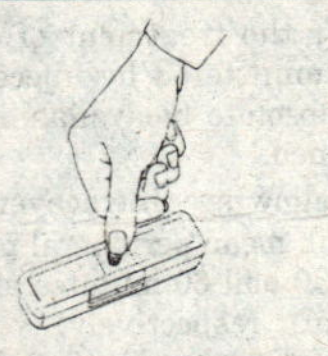

I. Locking the plastic case

2. Push the red locking device through the case label where a picture of a padlock appears and push down until completely inserted. (Figure I). **Once the locking device is in position, the case will be permanently closed.** The case can now be discarded safely. This case, which contains used supplies of CAVERJECT, is not suitable for recycling.
3. **Do not re-use or share needles or syringes. As with all prescription medicines, do not allow anyone else to use your medicine.**

℞ only

Pharmacia & Upjohn Company
A subsidiary of Pharmacia Corporation
Kalamazoo, MI 49001, USA
Revised October 2003 816 442 109 691800

CAVERJECT IMPULSE® ℞

[*kā-vər-jĕkt*]

Dual Chamber System
alprostadil for injection
For Intracavernosal Use

Prescribing information for this product, which appears on pages 2724–2727 of the 2004 PDR, has been completely revised as follows. Please write "See Supplement A" next to the product heading.

DESCRIPTION

CAVERJECT contains alprostadil as the naturally occurring form of prostaglandin E_1 (PGE_1) and is designated chemically as (11α,13E,15S)-11,15-dihydroxy-9-oxoprost-13-en-1-oic acid. The molecular weight is 354.49.

Alprostadil is a white to off-white crystalline powder with a melting point between 115° and 116°C. Its solubility at 35°C is 8000 micrograms (mcg) per 100 milliliter double distilled water.

The structural formula of alprostadil is represented below:

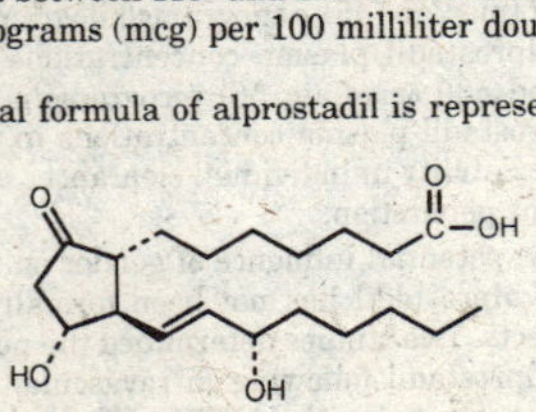

CAVERJECT IMPULSE is available as a disposable, single-dose, dual chamber syringe system. The system includes a glass cartridge which contains sterile, freeze-dried alprostadil in the front chamber and sterile bacteriostatic

Continued on next page

Caverject Impulse—Cont.

water for injection in the rear chamber. The alprostadil is reconstituted with the sterile bacteriostatic water just before injection. CAVERJECT IMPULSE is available in two strengths for intracavernosal administration:

10 microgram—The reconstituted solution has a volume of 0.64 mL. The delivered volume, 0.5 mL, contains 10 micrograms (mcg) of alprostadil, 324.7 mcg of alpha cyclodextrin, 45.4 mg of lactose, 23.5 mcg of sodium citrate, and 4.45 mg of benzyl alcohol.

20 microgram—The reconstituted solution has a volume of 0.64 mL. The delivered volume, 0.5 mL, contains 20 micrograms (mcg) of alprostadil, 649.3 mcg of alpha cyclodextrin, 45.4 mg of lactose, 23.5 mcg of sodium citrate, and 4.45 mg of benzyl alcohol.

When necessary, the pH of the alprostadil for injection was adjusted with hydrochloric acid and/or sodium hydroxide before lyophilization.

CLINICAL PHARMACOLOGY

Alprostadil has a wide variety of pharmacological actions; vasodilation and inhibition of platelet aggregation are among the most notable of these effects. In most animal species tested, alprostadil relaxed retractor penis and corpus cavernosum urethrae *in vitro*. Alprostadil also relaxed isolated preparations of human corpus cavernosum and spongiosum, as well as cavernous arterial segments contracted by either noradrenaline or PGF_{2a} *in vitro*. In pigtail monkeys (*Macaca nemestrina*), alprostadil increased cavernous arterial blood flow *in vivo* The degree and duration of cavernous smooth muscle relaxation in this animal model was dose-dependent.

Alprostadil induces erection by relaxation of trabecular smooth muscle and by dilation of cavernosal arteries. This leads to expansion of lacunar spaces and entrapment of blood by compressing the venules against the tunica albuginea, a process referred to as the corporal veno-occlusive mechanism.

Pharmacokinetics

Absorption: For the treatment of erectile dysfunction, alprostadil is administered by injection into the corpora cavernosa. The absolute bioavailability of alprostadil has not been determined.

Distribution: Following intracavernosal injection of 20 mcg alprostadil, mean peripheral plasma concentrations of alprostadil at 30 and 60 minutes after injection (89 and 102 picograms/mL, respectively) were not significantly greater than baseline levels of endogenous alprostadil (96 picograms/mL). Plasma levels of alprostadil were measured using a radioimmunoassay method. Alprostadil is bound in plasma primarily to albumin (81% bound) and to a lesser extent I-globulin IV-4 fraction (55% bound). No significant binding to erythrocytes or white blood cells was observed.

Metabolism: Alprostadil is rapidly converted to compounds, which are further metabolized prior to excretion. Following intravenous administration, approximately 80% of circulating alprostadil is metabolized in one pass through the lungs, primarily by beta- and omega-oxidation. Hence, any alprostadil entering the systemic circulation following intracavernosal injection is very rapidly metabolized. Following intracavernosal injection of 20 mcg alprostadil, peripheral levels of the major circulating metabolite, 13,14-dihydro-15-oxo-PGE_1, increased to reach a peak 30 minutes after injection and returned to pre-dose levels by 60 minutes after injection.

Excretion: The metabolites of alprostadil are excreted primarily by the kidney, with almost 90% of an administered intravenous dose excreted in urine within 24 hours post-dose. The remainder of the dose is excreted in the feces. There is no evidence of tissue retention of alprostadil or its metabolites following intravenous administration.

Pharmacokinetics in Special Populations

Geriatric: The potential effect of age on the pharmacokinetics of alprostadil has not been formally evaluated. In patients with acute respiratory distress syndrome (ARDS), the mean (± SD) pulmonary extraction of alprostadil was 72% ± 15% in 11 elderly patients aged 65 years or older (mean, 71 ± 6 years) and 65% ± 20% in 6 young patients aged 35 years or younger (mean, 28 ± 5 years).

Pediatric: Alprostadil plasma concentrations were measured in 10 neonates (gestational age of 34 weeks in 2 infants and 38 to 40 weeks in 8 infants) receiving steady-state intravenous infusions of alprostadil to treat underlying cardiac malformations. Infusion rates of alprostadil ranged from 5 to 50 (median, 45) nanograms/kilogram/minute, resulting in alprostadil plasma concentrations ranging between 22 and 530 (median, 56) picograms/mL. The wide range of alprostadil plasma concentrations in neonates reflects high variability in individual clearances of alprostadil in this patient population.

Gender: The potential influence of gender on the pharmacokinetics of alprostadil has not been formally studied in healthy subjects. Two studies determined the pulmonary extraction of alprostadil following intravascular administration in 23 patients with ARDS. The mean (± SD) pulmonary extraction was 66% ± 20% in 17 male patients and 69% ± 18% in 6 female patients, suggesting that the pharmacokinetics of alprostadil are not influenced by gender.

Race: The potential influence of race in the pharmacokinetics of alprostadil has not been formally evaluated.

Renal and Hepatic Insufficiency: The pharmacokinetics of alprostadil have not been formally studied in patients with renal or hepatic insufficiency.

Pulmonary Disease: The pulmonary extraction of alprostadil following intravascular administration was reduced by 15% (66 ± 3.2% vs. 78 ± 2.4%) in patients with ARDS compared with a control group of patients with normal respiratory function who were undergoing cardiopulmonary bypass surgery. Pulmonary clearance was found to vary as a function of cardiac output and pulmonary intrinsic clearance in a group of 14 patients with ARDS or at risk of developing ARDS following trauma or sepsis. In this study, the extraction efficiency of alprostadil ranged from subnormal (11%) to normal (90%), with an overall mean of 67%.

Drug-Drug Interactions: The potential for pharmacokinetic drug-drug interactions between alprostadil and other agents has not been formally studied.

CLINICAL STUDIES

The safety and efficacy of CAVERJECT Sterile Powder was investigated in men with a diagnosis of erectile dysfunction due to psychogenic, vasculogenic, neurogenic, and/or mixed etiology in two well-controlled studies (Study 1 and Study 2) and in one 6-month open-label study (Study 3).

Study 1: One hundred fifty-three men with a mean age of 53 years (range 23-69 years) were enrolled. The study had three phases: a 2.5 week double-blind, in-office randomized crossover phase in which each man received placebo or 2.5 mcg, 5 mcg, 7.5 mcg, or 10 mcg of CAVERJECT Sterile Powder; a 2 week open-label, in-office dose-titration phase to identify the optimum home-use dose (the latter dose was defined as a dose inducing an erection sufficient for penetration and lasting ≤ 60 minutes); and a 4-week open-label, self-injection phase. In the double-blind phase, each dose of CAVERJECT was significantly more effective than placebo by clinical evaluation ("full penile rigidity") and by RigiScan criteria (≥ 70% rigidity for at least 10 minutes); there was no response to placebo. The percentage of responders increased with increasing doses of CAVERJECT. The overall response in the dose-ranging phases was 76% (117/153) by clinical evaluation and 51% (78/152) by RigiScan criteria. The optimum dose for self-injection ranged from 1.25 to 65 mcg (median 20 mcg). Seventy-three percent of the injections in 102 men who self-injected CAVERJECT resulted in satisfactory intercourse. Seventy-five percent of the patients remained on the dose identified during the dose-ranging phase; 17% and 8% of the patients slightly decreased or increased the dose, respectively. The mean duration of erection per injection was 70.8 minutes.

Study 2: Two hundred ninety-six men with a mean age of 53.8 years (range 21-74 years) were enrolled in this parallel-design, double-blind study. The men were randomly assigned to one of five groups and received either a single dose of placebo, 2.5 mcg, 5 mcg, 10 mcg, or 20 mcg of CAVERJECT Sterile Powder. No patient responded to placebo. The differences in the response rates in both the clinical and the RigiScan evaluations between each of the doses of CAVERJECT and placebo were statistically significant. There was also a statistically significant dose-response relationship with higher clinical response rates and higher RigiScan response rates with increasing doses of CAVERJECT (with exception of the 10-mcg dose). The mean duration of erection after injection ranged from 12 minutes after the 2.5-mcg dose to 44 minutes after the 20-mcg dose and the relationship was linear (p = .025, linear regression analysis).

Study 3: The safety and efficacy of CAVERJECT Sterile Powder was evaluated in a 6-month, open-label study in 683 men with a mean age of 58 years (range 20-79 years). The optimum dose of CAVERJECT was established by titration in 89% of men (606/683). Four hundred seventy-one men (69%) completed the 6-month study. At the start of the study, the mean dose was 17.7 mcg of CAVERJECT and at the end of the study it was 20.7 mcg. Eighty-seven percent of the 13,762 injections of CAVERJECT, administered by self-injection by the men in the study, resulted in satisfactory sexual activity. The mean duration of erection was 67.5 minutes.

The formulation of alprostadil contained in CAVERJECT IMPULSE includes the inactive excipient alpha cyclodextrin. This formulation was compared with CAVERJECT Sterile Powder in 87 men in a single-blind, crossover study designed to evaluate efficacy and safety. The doses used by the patients in the study ranged from 2.5 mcg to 20 mcg and were the same for both formulations. The efficacy of the two formulations was shown to be comparable, as assessed by the 30-point erectile function (EF) domain score from the International Index of Erectile Function (IIEF) and by a physician-assessment score for erectile response. The mean EF domain scores for CAVERJECT Sterile Powder and the formulation contained in CAVERJECT IMPULSE were 26.6 (SD=5.3) and 27.6 (SD=3.8), respectively. The mean physician's assessment scores for CAVERJECT Sterile Powder and the formulation contained in CAVERJECT IMPULSE were 2.6 (SD=0.6) and 2.7 (SD=0.5), respectively, based on a scale of 0 (no tumescence) to 3 (full rigidity).

INDICATION AND USAGE

CAVERJECT (CAVERJECT IMPULSE, CAVERJECT Sterile Powder, and CAVERJECT Injection) is indicated for the treatment of erectile dysfunction due to neurogenic, vasculogenic, psychogenic, or mixed etiology.

Intracavernosal CAVERJECT is also indicated as an adjunct to other diagnostic tests in the diagnosis of erectile dysfunction.

CONTRAINDICATIONS

CAVERJECT should not be used in patients who have a known hypersensitivity to the drug, in patients who have conditions that might predispose them to priapism, such as sickle cell anemia or trait, multiple myeloma, or leukemia, or in patients with anatomical deformation of the penis, such as angulation, cavernosal fibrosis, or Peyronie's disease. Patients with penile implants should not be treated with CAVERJECT.

CAVERJECT is intended for use in adult men only.

CAVERJECT is not indicated for use in children or newborns.

CAVERJECT should not be used in men for whom sexual activity is inadvisable or contraindicated.

WARNINGS

Prolonged erection defined as erection lasting > 4 to ≤ 6 hours in duration occurred in 4% of 1,861 patients treated up to 18 months in studies of CAVERJECT Sterile Powder. The incidence of priapism (erections lasting > 6 hours in duration) was 0.4% with the same length of use. Pharmacologic intervention and/or aspiration of blood from the corpora cavernosum was performed in 2 of the 7 patients with priapism. To minimize the chances of prolonged erection or priapism, CAVERJECT should be titrated slowly to the lowest effective dose (see DOSAGE AND ADMINISTRATION). The patient must be instructed to immediately report to his prescribing physician, or, if unavailable, to seek immediate medical assistance for any erection that persists longer than 4 hours. If priapism is not treated immediately, penile tissue damage and permanent loss of potency may result.

PRECAUTIONS

General Precautions

1. CAVERJECT IMPULSE is designed for one use only. Following a single use, the injection device and any remaining solution should be properly discarded.
2. The overall incidence of penile fibrosis, including Peyronie's disease, reported in clinical studies with CAVERJECT Sterile Powder was 3%. In one self-injection clinical study where duration of use was up to 18 months, the incidence of fibrosis was 7.8%.
   Regular follow-up of patients, with careful examination of the penis, is strongly recommended to detect signs of penile fibrosis. Treatment with CAVERJECT should be discontinued in patients who develop penile angulation, cavernosal fibrosis, or Peyronie's disease.
3. Intracavernous injections of CAVERJECT can lead to increased peripheral blood levels of PGE_1 and its metabolites, especially in those patients with significant corpora cavernosa venous leakage. Increased peripheral blood levels of PGE_1 and its metabolites may lead to hypotension and/or dizziness.
4. Patients on anticoagulants, such as warfarin or heparin, may have increased propensity for bleeding after intracavernosal injection.
5. Underlying treatable medical causes of erectile dysfunction should be diagnosed and treated prior to initiation of therapy with CAVERJECT.
6. The safety and efficacy of combinations of CAVERJECT and other vasoactive agents have not been systematically studied. Therefore, the use of such combinations is not recommended.
7. CAVERJECT IMPULSE uses a superfine (29 gauge) needle. As with all superfine needles, the possibility of needle breakage exists. Careful instruction in proper patient handling and injection techniques may minimize the potential for needle breakage.
8. The patient should be instructed not to re-use or to share needles or syringes. As with all prescription medicines, the patient should not allow anyone else to use his medicine.

Information for the Patient:

To ensure safe and effective use of CAVERJECT, the patient should be thoroughly instructed and trained in the self-injection technique before he begins intracavernosal treatment with CAVERJECT at home. The desirable dose should be established in the physician's office.

Any reconstituted solution with precipitates or discoloration should be discarded. The CAVERJECT IMPULSE syringe system is designed for one use only and should be discarded after use. The device and the needle must be properly discarded after use. Needles must not be re-used or shared with other persons. Patient instructions for administration are included in each package of CAVERJECT IMPULSE.

The dose of CAVERJECT that is established in the physician's office should not be changed by the patient without consulting the physician. The patient may expect an erection to occur within 5 to 20 minutes. A standard treatment goal is to produce an erection lasting no longer than 1 hour. Generally, CAVERJECT should be used no more than 3 times per week, with at least 24 hours between each use.

Patients should be aware of possible side effects of therapy with CAVERJECT; the most frequently occurring is penile pain after injection, usually mild to moderate in severity. A potentially serious adverse reaction with intracavernosal therapy is priapism. Accordingly, the patient should be instructed to contact the physician's office immediately or, if unavailable, to seek immediate medical assistance if an erection persists for longer than 4 hours.

The patient should report any penile pain that was not present before or that increased in intensity, as well as the occurrence of nodules or hard tissue in the penis to his physician as soon as possible. As with any injection, an infection is a possibility. Patients should be instructed to report to the physician any penile redness, swelling, tenderness or curvature of the erect penis. The patient must visit the physician's office for regular checkups for assessment of the therapeutic benefit and safety of treatment with CAVERJECT.

Note: Use of intracavernosal CAVERJECT offers no protection from the transmission of sexually transmitted diseases. Individuals who use CAVERJECT should be counseled about the protective measures that are necessary to guard against the spread of sexually transmitted diseases, including the human immunodeficiency virus (HIV).

The injection of CAVERJECT can induce a small amount of bleeding at the site of injection (see ADVERSE REACTIONS section hematoma, ecchymosis, hemorrhage at the site of injection). In patients infected with blood-borne diseases, this could increase the risk of transmission of blood-borne diseases between partners.

In clinical trials, concomitant use of agents such as antihypertensive drugs, diuretics, antidiabetic agents (including insulin), or non-steroidal anti-inflammatory drugs had no effect on the efficacy or safety of CAVERJECT.

Carcinogenesis, Mutagenesis, and Impairment of Fertility: Long-term carcinogenicity studies have not been conducted. Rat reproductive studies indicate that alprostadil at doses of up to 0.2 mg/kg/day does not adversely affect or alter rat spermatogenesis, providing a 200-fold margin of safety compared with the usual human doses. The following battery of mutagenicity assays revealed no potential for mutagenesis: bacterial mutation (Ames), alkaline elution, rat micronucleus, sister chromatid exchange, CHO/HGPRT mammalian cell forward gene mutation, and unscheduled DNA synthesis (UDS).

A 1-year irritancy study was conducted in three groups of 5 male Cynomolgus monkeys injected intracavernosally twice weekly with either vehicle or 3 or 8.25 mcg of alprostadil/injection. An additional two groups of 6 monkeys each were injected with vehicle or with 8.25 mcg/injection twice weekly as described previously plus they received multiple doses during weeks 44, 48, and 52. Three monkeys from each group were retained for a 4-week recovery period. There was no evidence of drug-related penile irritancy or nonpenile tissue lesions, which could be directly related to alprostadil. The irritancy, which was noted for control and treated monkeys, was considered to be a result of the injection procedure itself, and any lesions noted were shown to be reversible. At the end of the 4-week recovery period, the histological changes in the penis had regressed.

Pregnancy, Nursing Mothers, and Pediatric Use:
CAVERJECT is not indicated for use in pediatric patients or women.

Geriatric Use:
A total of 341 subjects included in clinical studies were 65 and older. No overall differences in safety and effectiveness were observed between these subjects and younger subjects, and the other reported clinical experience has not identified differences in responses between elderly and younger patients, but decreased sensitivity of some older individuals cannot be ruled out.

ADVERSE REACTIONS

Local Adverse Reactions: The following local adverse reaction information was derived from controlled and uncontrolled studies of CAVERJECT Sterile Powder, including an uncontrolled 18-month safety study.

Local Adverse Reactions Reported by ≥ 1% of Patients Treated with CAVERJECT Sterile Powder for up to 18 Months*

Event	CAVERJECT N = 1861
Penile pain	37%
Prolonged erection	4%
Penile fibrosis**	3%
Injection site hematoma	3%
Penis disorder***	3%
Injection site ecchymosis	2%
Penile rash	1%
Penile edema	1%

* Except for penile pain (2%), no significant local adverse reactions were reported by 294 patients who received 1 to 3 injections of placebo.
** See General Precautions.
*** Includes numbness, yeast infection, irritation, sensitivity, phimosis, pruritus, erythema, venous leak, penile skin tear, strange feeling of penis, discoloration of penile head, itch at tip of penis.

Penile Pain: Penile pain after intracavernosal administration of CAVERJECT was reported at least once by 37% of patients in clinical studies of up to 18 months in duration. In the majority of the cases, penile pain was rated mild or moderate in intensity. Three percent of patients discontinued treatment because of penile pain. The frequency of penile pain was 2% in 294 patients who received 1 to 3 injections of placebo.

Prolonged Erection/Priapism: In clinical trials, prolonged erection was defined as an erection that lasted for 4 to 6 hours; priapism was defined as erection that lasted 6 hours or longer. The frequency of prolonged erection after intracavernosal administration of CAVERJECT was 4%, while the frequency of priapism was 0.4% (see WARNINGS).

Hematoma/Ecchymosis: The frequency of hematoma and ecchymosis was 3% and 2%, respectively. In most cases, hematoma/ecchymosis was judged to be a complication of a faulty injection technique. Accordingly, proper instruction of the patient in self-injection is of importance to minimize the potential of hematoma/ecchymosis (see DOSAGE AND ADMINISTRATION).

The following local adverse reactions were reported by fewer than 1% of patients after injection of CAVERJECT: balanitis, injection site hemorrhage, injection site inflammation, injection site itching, injection site swelling, injection site edema, urethral bleeding, penile warmth, numbness, yeast infection, irritation, sensitivity, phimosis, pruritus, erythema, venous leak, painful erection, and abnormal ejaculation.

Systemic Adverse Events: The following systemic adverse event information was derived from controlled and uncontrolled studies of CAVERJECT Sterile Powder, including an uncontrolled 18-month safety study.

Systemic Adverse Events Reported by ≥ 1% of Patients Treated with CAVERJECT Sterile Powder for up to 18 Months*

Body System/Reaction	CAVERJECT N = 1861
Cardiovascular System	
Hypertension	2%
Central Nervous System	
Headache	2%
Dizziness	1%
Musculoskeletal System	
Back pain	1%
Respiratory System	
Upper respiratory infection	4%
Flu syndrome	2%
Sinusitis	2%
Nasal congestion	1%
Cough	1%
Urogenital System	
Prostatic Disorder**	2%
Miscellaneous	
Localized pain***	2%
Trauma****	2%

* No significant adverse events were reported by 294 patients who received 1 to 3 injections of placebo.
** Prostatitis, pain, hypertrophy, enlargement
*** Pain in various anatomical structures other than injection site
**** Injuries, fractures, abrasions, lacerations, dislocations

The following systemic events, which were reported for < 1% of patients in clinical studies, were judged by investigators to be possibly related to use of CAVERJECT: testicular pain, scrotal disorder, scrotal edema, hematuria, testicular disorder, impaired urination, urinary frequency, urinary urgency, pelvic pain, hypotension, vasodilation, peripheral vascular disorder, supraventricular extrasystoles, vasovagal reactions, hypesthesia, non-generalized weakness, diaphoresis, rash, non-application site pruritus, skin neoplasm, nausea, dry mouth, increased serum creatinine, leg cramps, and mydriasis.

Hemodynamic changes, manifested as decreases in blood pressure and increases in pulse rate, were observed during clinical studies, principally at doses above 20 mcg and above 30 mcg of alprostadil, respectively, and appeared to be dose-dependent. However, these changes were usually clinically unimportant; only three patients discontinued the treatment because of symptomatic hypotension.

CAVERJECT had no clinically important effect on serum or urine laboratory tests.

The safety of CAVERJECT IMPULSE was evaluated in a study that compared the formulation of alprostadil for injection contained in CAVERJECT IMPULSE with the formulation contained in CAVERJECT Sterile Powder. The doses used by the 87 patients in this crossover study were the same for both formulations. The number and type of events reported for CAVERJECT IMPULSE were consistent between formulations in this study and in other controlled and uncontrolled studies with CAVERJECT Sterile Powder.

OVERDOSAGE

Overdosage was not observed in clinical trials with CAVERJECT. If intracavernous overdose of CAVERJECT occurs, the patient should be under medical supervision until any systemic effects have resolved and/or until penile detumescence has occurred. Symptomatic treatment of any systemic symptoms would be appropriate.

DOSAGE AND ADMINISTRATION

The dose of CAVERJECT should be individualized for each patient by careful titration under supervision by the physician. In clinical studies, patients were treated with CAVERJECT Sterile Powder in doses ranging from 0.2 to 140 mcg; however, since 99% of patients received doses of 60 mcg or less, doses of greater than 60 mcg are not recommended. In general, the lowest possible effective dose should always be employed. In clinical studies, over 80% of patients experienced an erection sufficient for sexual intercourse after intracavernosal injection of CAVERJECT.

Initial Titration in Physician's Office:

Erectile Dysfunction of Vasculogenic, Psychogenic, or Mixed Etiology. Dosage titration should be initiated at 2.5 mcg of alprostadil. The 10 mcg strength of CAVERJECT IMPULSE is designed to allow delivery of a 2.5 mcg dose of alprostadil (see General Procedure for Solution Preparation). If there is a partial response at 2.5 mcg, the dose may be increased by 2.5 mcg to a dose of 5 mcg within 1 hour. No more than 2 doses during initial titration should be given within a 24-hour period. If additional titration is required, doses in increments of 5 to 10 mcg may be given at least 24 hours apart until the dose that produces an erection suitable for intercourse and not exceeding a duration of 1 hour is reached. If there is no response to the initial 2.5-mcg dose, the second dose may be increased to 7.5 mcg within 1 hour. No more than 2 doses during initial titration should be given within a 24-hour period. If additional titration is required, doses in increments of 5 to 10 mcg may be given at least 24 hours apart. The patient must stay in the physician's office until complete detumescence occurs.

Erectile Dysfunction of Pure Neurogenic Etiology (Spinal Cord Injury). Dosage titration should be initiated at 1.25 mcg of alprostadil. Because CAVERJECT IMPULSE is designed to deliver doses of 2.5 mcg or greater (see General Procedure for Solution Preparation), CAVERJECT Sterile Powder or CAVERJECT Injection may be used for an initial dose of 1.25 mcg. The initial dose may be increased by 1.25 mcg to a dose of 2.5 mcg within 1 hour. No more than 2 doses during initial titration should be given within a 24-hour period. If additional titration is required, a dose of 5 mcg may be given during the next 24 hours. Thereafter, doses in increments of 5 mcg may be given at least 24 hours apart until the dose that produces an erection suitable for intercourse and not exceeding a duration of 1 hour is reached. The patient must stay in the physician's office until complete detumescence occurs.

The majority of patients (56%) in one clinical study involving 579 patients with erectile dysfunction of various etiologies were titrated to doses of greater than 5 mcg but less than or equal to 20 mcg. The mean dose at the end of the titration phase was 17.8 mcg of alprostadil.

Maintenance Therapy:

The first injections of CAVERJECT must be done at the physician's office by medically trained personnel. Self-injection therapy by the patient should be started only after the patient is properly instructed and well trained in the self-injection technique. The physician should make a careful assessment of the patient's skills and competence with this procedure. The intracavernosal injection must be done under sterile conditions. The site of injection is usually along the dorso-lateral aspect of the proximal third of the penis. Visible veins should be avoided. The side of the penis that is injected and the site of injection must be alternated; the injection site must be cleansed with an alcohol swab.

The dose of CAVERJECT that is selected for self-injection treatment should provide the patient with an erection that is satisfactory for sexual intercourse and that is maintained for no longer than 1 hour. If the duration of erection is longer than 1 hour, the dose of CAVERJECT should be reduced. Self-injection therapy for use at home should be initiated at the dose that was determined in the physician's office; however, dose adjustment, if required (up to 57% of patients in one clinical study), should be made only after consultation with the physician. The dose should be adjusted in accordance with the titration guidelines described above. The effectiveness of CAVERJECT for long-term use of up to 6 months has been documented in an uncontrolled, self-injection study. The mean dose of CAVERJECT Sterile Powder at the end of 6 months was 20.7 mcg in this study. CAVERJECT IMPULSE in the 10 mcg strength is designed to deliver a minimum dose of 2.5 mcg and a maximum dose of 10 mcg. CAVERJECT IMPULSE in the 20 mcg strength is designed to deliver a minimum dose of 5 mcg and a maximum dose of 20 mcg. The physician should determine the most suitable formulation of CAVERJECT for the individual patient (CAVERJECT IMPULSE, CAVERJECT Sterile Powder, or CAVERJECT Injection).

Careful and continuous follow-up of the patient while in the self-injection program must be exercised. This is especially true for the initial self-injections, since adjustments in the dose of CAVERJECT may be needed. The recommended frequency of injection is no more than 3 times weekly, with at least 24 hours between each dose. All formulations of CAVERJECT are intended for single use only and should be discarded after use. The user should be instructed in the proper disposal of the injection materials (e.g., device, needles).

While on self-injection treatment, it is recommended that the patient visit the prescribing physician's office every 3 months. At that time, the efficacy and safety of the therapy should be assessed, and the dose of CAVERJECT should be adjusted, if needed.

CAVERJECT as an Adjunct to the Diagnosis of Erectile Dysfunction:

In the simplest diagnostic test for erectile dysfunction (pharmacologic testing), patients are monitored for the occurrence of an erection after an intracavernosal injection of CAVERJECT. Extensions of this testing are the use of CAVERJECT as an adjunct to laboratory investigations, such as duplex or Doppler imaging, ^{133}Xenon washout tests, radioisotope penogram, and penile arteriography, to allow visualization and assessment of penile vasculature. For any of these tests, a single dose of CAVERJECT that induces an erection with firm rigidity should be used.

General Procedure for Solution Preparation:

CAVERJECT IMPULSE consists of a disposable, single-dose, dual-chamber syringe system. The system includes a glass cartridge, which contains sterile, freeze-dried alprostadil in the front chamber and sterile bacteriostatic water for injection in the rear chamber. Following proper reconstitution instructions, the 10 mcg strength syringe can deliver up to 0.5 mL of solution. Each 0.5 mL of solution

Continued on next page

Caverject Impulse—Cont.

contains 10 mcg of alprostadil, 324.7 mcg of alpha cyclodextrin, 45.4 mg of lactose, 23.5 mcg of sodium citrate, and 4.45 mg of benzyl alcohol. The delivery device can be set to deliver a solution volume of 0.125, 0.25, 0.375, or 0.50 mL to enable administration of 2.5, 5, 7.5, or 10 mcg of alprostadil. Following proper reconstitution instructions, the 20 mcg strength syringe can deliver up to 0.5 mL of solution. Each 0.5 mL of solution contains 20 mcg of alprostadil, 649.3 mcg of alpha cyclodextrin, 45.4 mg of lactose, 23.5 mcg of sodium citrate, and 4.45 mg of benzyl alcohol. The delivery device can be set to deliver a solution volume of 0.125, 0.25, 0.375, or 0.50 mL to enable administration of 5, 10, 15, or 20 mcg of alprostadil. After reconstitution, the solution of CAVERJECT should be used within 24 hours when stored at or below 25°C (77°F). Parenteral drug products should be inspected visually for particulate matter and discoloration prior to administration whenever the solution and container permit. The product should not be used if particulate matter or discoloration are present. Following a single use, the injection device and any remaining solution should be properly discarded.

Caution: CAVERJECT IMPULSE is for single use only. Do not use any remaining CAVERJECT solution.

HOW SUPPLIED

CAVERJECT IMPULSE is supplied as a disposable, single-dose, dual chamber syringe system. The system includes a glass cartridge, which contains sterile, freeze-dried alprostadil in the front chamber and sterile bacteriostatic water for reconstitution in the rear chamber. The syringes contain either 12.8 or 25.6 mcg of alprostadil to allow delivery of a maximum of 10 or 20 mcg/0.5mL. Store the unreconstituted product at 25°C (77°F); excursions permitted to 15° to 30°C (59° to 86°F) [see USP Controlled Room Temperature].

When reconstituted and used as directed, the deliverable amount for the 10 mcg strength is 10 mcg/0.5 mL or an increment of 10 mcg/0.5 mL, 2.5 mcg/0.125 mL, 5 mcg/0.25 mL, or 7.5 mcg/0.375 mL of alprostadil and the deliverable amount for the 20 microgram strength is 20 mcg/0.5 mL or an increment of 20 mcg/0.5 mL, 5 mcg/ 0.125 mL, 10 mcg/0.250 mL, or 15 mcg/0.375 mL of alprostadil. The reconstituted solution should be used within 24 hours when stored at or below 25°C (77°F).

CAVERJECT IMPULSE is supplied in a carton containing 2 blister trays. Each blister tray contains one dual chamber syringe system, one needle and 2 alcohol swabs. It is available in the following strengths:

10 mcg	NDC 0009-5181-01
20 mcg	NDC 0009-5182-01

CAVERJECT is also available as follows:

CAVERJECT Sterile Powder (alprostadil for injection) packaged in vials, 6 vials per carton

10 mcg	NDC 0009-3778-05
20 mcg	NDC 0009-3701-05
40 mcg	NDC 0009-7686-04

CAVERJECT Sterile Powder (alprostadil for injection) vials with diluent syringe, 6 syringe systems per carton

5 mcg	NDC 0009-7212-03
10 mcg	NDC 0009-3778-08
20 mcg	NDC 0009-3701-01

CAVERJECT Injection ([alprostadil injection] aqueous), 5 ampoules per carton

10 mcg (10 mcg/mL)	NDC 0009-7655-02
20 mcg (20 mcg/mL)	NDC 0009-7654-02
40 mcg (40 mcg/2mL)	NDC 0009-7650-02

℞ only

MADE IN SWEDEN

Manufactured for:
Pharmacia & Upjohn Company
A subsidiary of Pharmacia Corporation
Kalamazoo, MI 49001, USA
By:
Pharmacia AB
Stockholm, Sweden
September 2003
819 369 001
1-001-481

Patient Instructions For:
Caverject *impulse*®

Dual Chamber System
alprostadil for injection

Read this information carefully before using CAVERJECT [KAV-er-jeckt]. Read the information you get each time you renew your prescription, in case anything has changed. This is a summary and does not replace talking with your doctor when you start this medication and at check-ups. If you have any questions or concerns, talk to your doctor about them.

What is CAVERJECT?

CAVERJECT is a medicine to treat male impotence (erectile dysfunction). CAVERJECT is injected into a specific area of the penis and should produce an erection in 5 to 20 minutes. The erection should last for no longer than 1 hour.

CAVERJECT IMPULSE is for one use only and should be thrown away properly after a single use.

CAVERJECT does not protect you from sexually transmitted diseases (STDs), such as HIV (the virus that causes AIDS). In addition, small amounts of bleeding at the injection site can increase the risk of passing diseases carried by the blood, such as HIV.

What are the causes of and treatments for impotence?

There are several causes of impotence. These include medications that you may be taking for other conditions, poor blood circulation in the penis, nerve damage, emotional problems, too much smoking or alcohol use, use of street drugs, and hormonal problems. Often, impotence is due to more than one cause.

Treatments for impotence include switching medications if you are taking a medication that causes impotence, prescription medications, medical devices that produce an erection, surgical procedures to correct blood flow in the penis, penile implants, and psychological counseling.

You should not stop taking any prescription medications, unless told to do so by your doctor.

The use of other medical treatments for impotence in combination with CAVERJECT is not recommended. Discuss any concerns you may have about combination treatment with your doctor.

Who should not use CAVERJECT?

Do not use CAVERJECT if you have certain conditions that might cause long-lasting erections (lasting more than 4 hours). Long-lasting erections may cause penis damage. These conditions include:

- sickle cell anemia or trait
- leukemia
- tumor of the bone marrow (multiple myeloma)

Do not use CAVERJECT if you

- have a penile implant
- have an abnormally formed penis
- have other penis problems
- were told by your doctor not to have sex

Women and children should not use CAVERJECT.

How should I use CAVERJECT?

You will be treated with CAVERJECT in your doctor's office to find out what dose is best for you. After that, you can inject it yourself at home. Do not use it more than 3 times a week. There should be at least 24 hours between doses. See your doctor for regular check-ups to be sure CAVERJECT is not causing damage and that it is working as well as possible.

See the section "Instructions for Use" at the end of this leaflet for details about how to use CAVERJECT.

What are the possible side effects of CAVERJECT?

About 4 in 100 men who use CAVERJECT may get erections that last more than 4 hours. These can cause serious and permanent damage. **Call your doctor or seek professional help immediately if you still have an erection 4 hours after injection.**

The most common side effect of CAVERJECT is mild to moderate pain after injection. About one-third of patients report this effect.

You may get a small amount of bleeding at the injection site. This is more likely if you have a medical condition or are taking a medicine that interferes with blood clotting.

Call your doctor if you notice any redness, lumps, swelling, tenderness, or curving of the erect penis. Also, tell your doctor about any penis pain you did not have before or other penis problems you have.

There is a possibility of needle breakage with use of CAVERJECT IMPULSE. To best avoid breaking the needle, you should pay careful attention to your doctor's instructions and try to handle the device properly. If the needle breaks during injection and you are able to see and grasp the broken end, you should remove it and contact your doctor. If you cannot see or cannot grasp the broken end, you should promptly contact your doctor.

How should I store CAVERJECT IMPULSE?

1. Unmixed packages of CAVERJECT IMPULSE should be stored at room temperature. Temperatures between 59° to 86°F (15° to 30°C) are allowed. Avoid storing CAVERJECT IMPULSE at very high and very low temperatures.
2. During travel, do not let the medicine freeze or be stored at a temperature above 77°F (25°C). For example, do not store it in checked luggage during air travel or leave it in a closed automobile.
3. After mixing, CAVERJECT IMPULSE should be used within 24 hours. It should be kept at a temperature of 77°F or below during this storage time.

General advice about prescription medicines

Medicines are sometimes prescribed for purposes other than those listed in a Patient Information Leaflet. If you have any concerns about CAVERJECT, ask your doctor. Your doctor or pharmacist can give you information about CAVERJECT that was written for health care professionals. Do not use CAVERJECT for a condition for which it was not prescribed. Do not share CAVERJECT with other people.

You can get more information about impotence (erectile dysfunction) and its treatment from the National Institutes of Health (Washington, DC), the American Foundation for Urological Diseases (Baltimore, MD), or the Impotence Institute of America (Washington, DC).

INSTRUCTIONS FOR USE

Before you use CAVERJECT, your doctor must train you in how to prepare and give the injection properly.

Before using CAVERJECT, talk to your doctor about what to expect when using it, possible side effects, and what to do if side effects occur. Your dose has been selected for your individual needs. Do not change your dose without consulting your doctor. If you are not sure of the volume or dose to be used, talk to your doctor or pharmacist.

Follow these instructions exactly to prepare and inject a sterile (germ-free) dose of CAVERJECT.

Supplies Needed

CAVERJECT IMPULSE is packaged with a needle for injection (Figure A) and alcohol swab.

Figure A

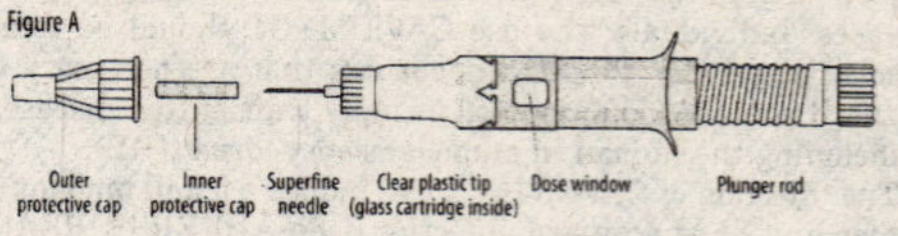

CAVERJECT IMPULSE is available in 10 and 20 mcg strengths.

MAKE SURE YOU HAVE THE RIGHT STRENGTH OF CAVERJECT IMPULSE.

Prepare the Dose

1. Wash your hands thoroughly and dry them with a clean towel.
2. Remove the device, needle, and alcohol swabs from the blistered tray.
3. Using one of the alcohol swabs, clean the rubber membrane at the tip of the syringe (Figure B).

Figure B

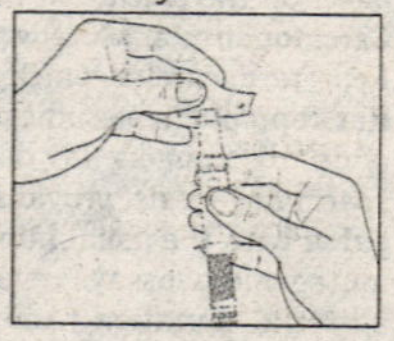

4. Peel the paper lid from the needle (Figure C).

Figure C

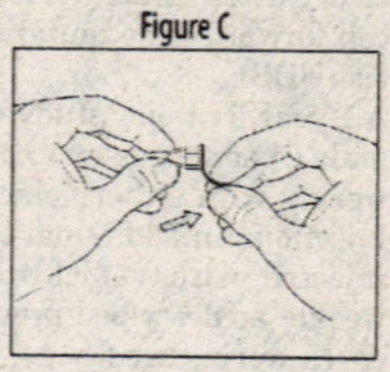

5. Attach the needle to the device by pressing the needle on to the tip of the device and turning clockwise until the needle is firmly in place. Remove the outer protective cap from the needle (Figure D).

Figure D

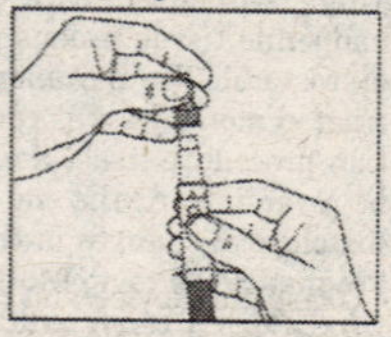

6. Hold the device with the needle pointing upward. The white plunger rod is in the extended position (Figure E).

Figure E

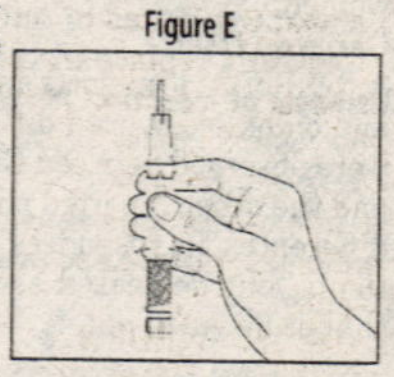

7. Turn the plunger rod slowly clockwise until it stops. This automatically mixes the alprostadil powder and the diluent. Turn the device upside down several times to make sure the solution is evenly mixed. The solution should be clear. Do not use it if it is cloudy or contains particles (Figure F).

Figure F

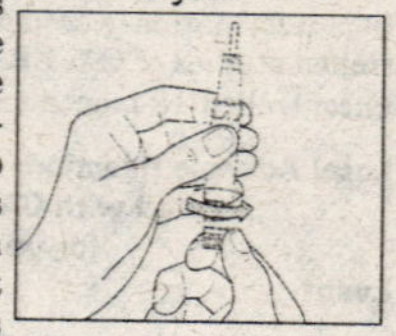

8. Hold the device with the needle upward and carefully remove the inner protective cap from the needle (Figure G).

Figure G

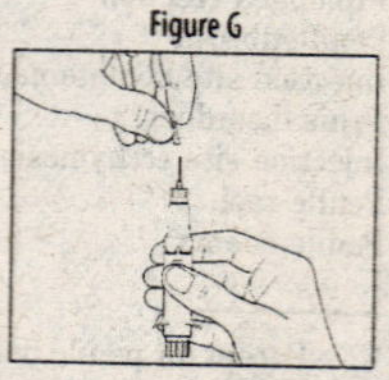

9. Keeping the device upright, press the plunger rod as far as it will go. A few drops will appear at the needlepoint and the solution will be free of bubbles although typically there may be some very small bubbles at the side of the glass cartridge (Figure H).

Figure H

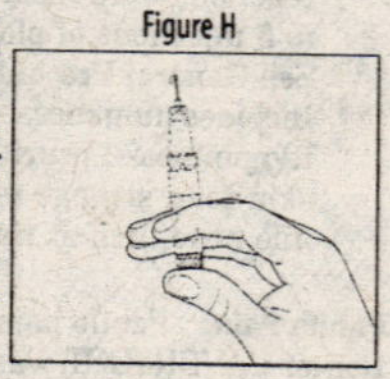

10. Turn the end of the plunger rod clockwise slowly to choose the dose your physician has determined is appropriate for you. The number that appears in the window shows the dose in micrograms. If the number is higher than your prescribed dose, continue to turn the plunger rod clockwise slowly until you reach the correct dose (Figure I).

Figure I

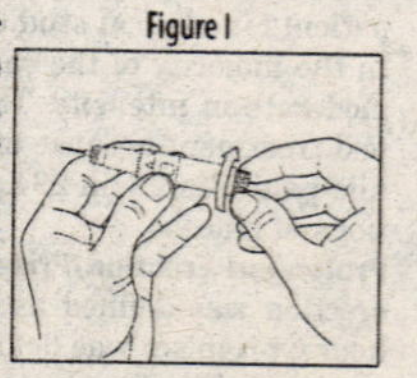

11. Set the device down on a level surface making sure the needle is not in contact with the surface.

Select Injection Site

1. CAVERJECT IMPULSE will be injected into a corpus cavernosum (spongy tissue) of the penis. One corpus cavernosum runs the length of the right side of the penis.

Another corpus cavernosum runs the length of the left side of the penis (see Figures J and K).

Figure J

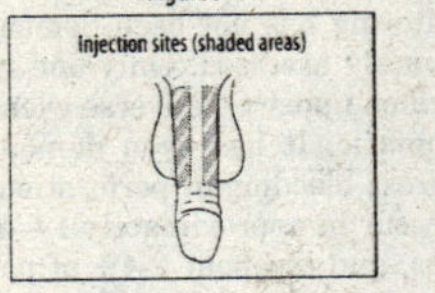

Figure K

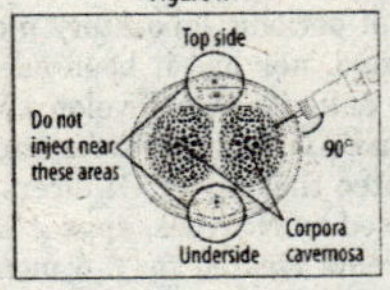

2. Choose an injection site on one side of the shaft of the penis as shown in Figure J. **Avoid visible veins.**
3. **With each use of CAVERJECT, alternate the side of the penis and vary the site of injection.**

Inject Your Dose of CAVERJECT

1. You should be sitting upright or slightly reclined when injecting CAVERJECT.
2. Holding the head of your penis with your thumb and forefinger, stretch your penis lengthwise along your thigh so that the skin is tight and you can clearly see the selected injection site.
3. Clean the injection site with a new alcohol swab. Do not discard this swab, you will need to use it again (see step 6).
4. Reposition the penis firmly against your thigh as in step 2 to keep it from moving during the injection.
5. Holding the device between your thumb and index finger, push the needle into the selected site through the skin and into the tissue as far as it will go. Push the plunger rod as far as it will go so the entire dose is injected (Figure L). If the injection solution does not flow easily, move the needle slightly and push as before. When using a dose less than the full capacity, a small amount of liquid will remain in the device.

Figure L

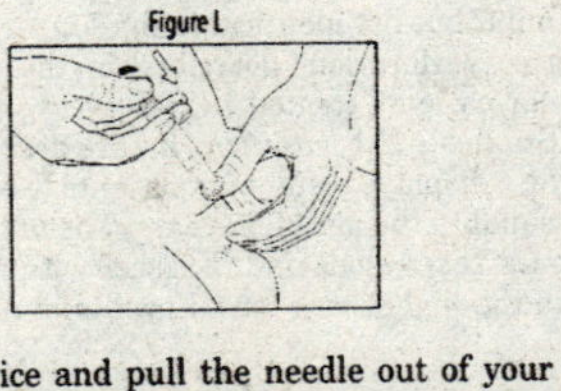

6. Grasp the device and pull the needle out of your penis. **Push on the injection site with the alcohol swab for about 5 minutes or until any bleeding stops.**
7. Carefully replace the outer protective cap on the needle.

Disposal of Injection Materials

After use, dispose of all injection materials safely. Your pharmacist may be able to supply a disposal box especially for disposable injection devices. **As with all prescription medicines, do not allow anyone else to use your medicine.**

℞ only
MADE IN SWEDEN
Manufactured for:
Pharmacia & Upjohn Company
A subsidiary of Pharmacia Corporation
Kalamazoo, MI 49001, USA
By:
Pharmacia AB
Stockholm, Sweden
September 2003
819 369 001
1-001-481

CELEBREX® ℞
[*sĕ-lĕ-brĕks*]
celecoxib capsules

Prescribing information for this product, which appears on pages 2727–2731 of the 2004 PDR, has been completely revised as follows. Please write "See Supplement A" next to the product heading.

DESCRIPTION

CELEBREX (celecoxib) is chemically designated as 4-[5-(4-methylphenyl)-3-(trifluoromethyl)-1H-pyrazol-1-yl] benzenesulfonamide and is a diaryl-substituted pyrazole. It has the following chemical structure:

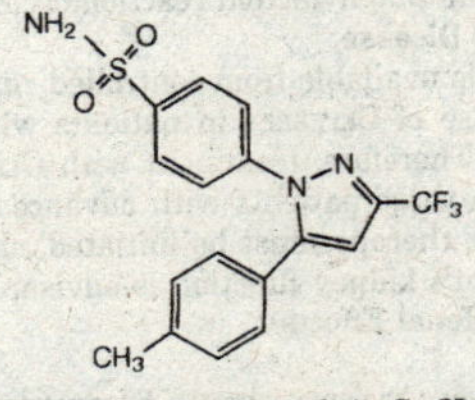

The empirical formula for celecoxib is $C_{17}H_{14}F_3N_3O_2S$, and the molecular weight is 381.38.

CELEBREX oral capsules contain either 100 mg, 200 mg or 400 mg of celecoxib.

The inactive ingredients in CELEBREX capsules include: croscarmellose sodium, edible inks, gelatin, lactose monohydrate, magnesium stearate, povidone, sodium lauryl sulfate and titanium dioxide.

CLINICAL PHARMACOLOGY

Mechanism of Action: CELEBREX is a nonsteroidal anti-inflammatory drug that exhibits anti-inflammatory, analgesic, and antipyretic activities in animal models. The mechanism of action of CELEBREX is believed to be due to inhibition of prostaglandin synthesis, primarily via inhibition of cyclooxygenase-2 (COX-2), and at therapeutic concentrations in humans, CELEBREX does not inhibit the cyclooxygenase-1 (COX-1) isoenzyme. In animal colon tumor models, celecoxib reduced the incidence and multiplicity of tumors.

Pharmacokinetics:

Absorption

Peak plasma levels of celecoxib occur approximately 3 hrs after an oral dose. Under fasting conditions, both peak plasma levels (C_{max}) and area under the curve (AUC) are roughly dose proportional up to 200 mg BID; at higher doses there are less than proportional increases in C_{max} and AUC (see Food Effects). Absolute bioavailability studies have not been conducted. With multiple dosing, steady state conditions are reached on or before day 5.

The pharmacokinetic parameters of celecoxib in a group of healthy subjects are shown in Table 1.

[See table 1 above]

Table 1
Summary of Single Dose (200 mg) Disposition Kinetics of Celecoxib in Healthy Subjects[1]

Mean (%CV) PK Parameter Values				
C_{max}, ng/mL	T_{max}, hr	Effective $t_{1/2}$, hr	V_{ss}/F, L	CL/F, L/hr
705 (38)	2.8 (37)	11.2 (31)	429 (34)	27.7 (28)

[1]Subjects under fasting conditions (n=36, 19-52 yrs.)

Food Effects

When CELEBREX capsules were taken with a high fat meal, peak plasma levels were delayed for about 1 to 2 hours with an increase in total absorption (AUC) of 10% to 20%. Under fasting conditions, at doses above 200 mg, there is less than a proportional increase in C_{max} and AUC, which is thought to be due to the low solubility of the drug in aqueous media. Coadministration of CELEBREX with an aluminum- and magnesium-containing antacid resulted in a reduction in plasma celecoxib concentrations with a decrease of 37% in C_{max} and 10% in AUC. CELEBREX, at doses up to 200 mg BID can be administered without regard to timing of meals. Higher doses (400 mg BID) should be administered with food to improve absorption.

Distribution

In healthy subjects, celecoxib is highly protein bound (~97%) within the clinical dose range. *In vitro* studies indicate that celecoxib binds primarily to albumin and, to a lesser extent, α_1-acid glycoprotein. The apparent volume of distribution at steady state (V_{ss}/F) is approximately 400 L, suggesting extensive distribution into the tissues. Celecoxib is not preferentially bound to red blood cells.

Metabolism

Celecoxib metabolism is primarily mediated via cytochrome P450 2C9. Three metabolites, a primary alcohol, the corresponding carboxylic acid and its glucuronide conjugate, have been identified in human plasma. These metabolites are inactive as COX-1 or COX-2 inhibitors. Patients who are known or suspected to be P450 2C9 poor metabolizers based on a previous history should be administered celecoxib with caution as they may have abnormally high plasma levels due to reduced metabolic clearance.

Excretion

Celecoxib is eliminated predominantly by hepatic metabolism with little (<3%) unchanged drug recovered in the urine and feces. Following a single oral dose of radiolabeled drug, approximately 57% of the dose was excreted in the feces and 27% was excreted into the urine. The primary metabolite in both urine and feces was the carboxylic acid metabolite (73% of dose) with low amounts of the glucuronide also appearing in the urine. It appears that the low solubility of the drug prolongs the absorption process making terminal half-life ($t_{1/2}$) determinations more variable. The effective half-life is approximately 11 hours under fasted conditions. The apparent plasma clearance (CL/F) is about 500 mL/min.

Special Populations

Geriatric: At steady state, elderly subjects (over 65 years old) had a 40% higher C_{max} and a 50% higher AUC compared to the young subjects. In elderly females, celecoxib C_{max} and AUC are higher than those for elderly males, but these increases are predominantly due to lower body weight in elderly females. Dose adjustment in the elderly is not generally necessary. However, for patients of less than 50 kg in body weight, initiate therapy at the lowest recommended dose.

Pediatric: CELEBREX capsules have not been investigated in pediatric patients below 18 years of age.

Race: Meta-analysis of pharmacokinetic studies has suggested an approximately 40% higher AUC of celecoxib in Blacks compared to Caucasians. The cause and clinical significance of this finding is unknown.

Hepatic Insufficiency: A pharmacokinetic study in subjects with mild (Child-Pugh Class A) and moderate (Child-Pugh Class B) hepatic impairment has shown that steady-state celecoxib AUC is increased about 40% and 180%, respectively, above that seen in healthy control subjects. Therefore, the daily recommended dose of CELEBREX capsules should be reduced by approximately 50% in patients with moderate (Child-Pugh Class B) hepatic impairment. Patients with severe hepatic impairment (Child-Pugh Class C) have not been studied. The use of CELEBREX in patients with severe hepatic impairment is not recommended.

Renal Insufficiency: In a cross-study comparison, celecoxib AUC was approximately 40% lower in patients with chronic renal insufficiency (GFR 35-60 mL/min) than that seen in subjects with normal renal function. No significant relationship was found between GFR and celecoxib clearance. Patients with severe renal insufficiency have not been studied. Similar to other NSAIDs, CELEBREX is not recommended in patients with severe renal insufficiency (see WARNINGS – Advanced Renal Disease).

Drug Interactions

Also see **PRECAUTIONS – Drug Interactions.**

General: Significant interactions may occur when celecoxib is administered together with drugs that inhibit P450 2C9. *In vitro* studies indicate that celecoxib is not an inhibitor of cytochrome P450 2C9, 2C19 or 3A4.

Clinical studies with celecoxib have identified potentially significant interactions with fluconazole and lithium. Experience with nonsteroidal anti-inflammatory drugs (NSAIDs) suggests the potential for interactions with furosemide and ACE inhibitors. The effects of celecoxib on the pharmacokinetics and/or pharmacodynamics of glyburide, ketoconazole, methotrexate, phenytoin, and tolbutamide have been studied *in vivo* and clinically important interactions have not been found.

CLINICAL STUDIES

Osteoarthritis (OA): CELEBREX has demonstrated significant reduction in joint pain compared to placebo. CELEBREX was evaluated for treatment of the signs and the symptoms of OA of the knee and hip in approximately 4,200 patients in placebo- and active-controlled clinical trials of up to 12 weeks duration. In patients with OA, treatment with CELEBREX 100 mg BID or 200 mg QD resulted in improvement in WOMAC (Western Ontario and McMaster Universities) osteoarthritis index, a composite of pain, stiffness, and functional measures in OA. In three 12-week studies of pain accompanying OA flare, CELEBREX doses of 100 mg BID and 200 mg BID provided significant reduction of pain within 24-48 hours of initiation of dosing. At doses of 100 mg BID or 200 mg BID the effectiveness of CELEBREX was shown to be similar to that of naproxen 500 mg BID. Doses of 200 mg BID provided no additional benefit above that seen with 100 mg BID. A total daily dose of 200 mg has been shown to be equally effective whether administered as 100 mg BID or 200 mg QD.

Rheumatoid Arthritis (RA): CELEBREX has demonstrated significant reduction in joint tenderness/pain and joint swelling compared to placebo. CELEBREX was evaluated for treatment of the signs and symptoms of RA in approximately 2,100 patients in placebo- and active-controlled clinical trials of up to 24 weeks in duration. CELEBREX was shown to be superior to placebo in these studies, using the ACR20 Responder Index, a composite of clinical, laboratory, and functional measures in RA. CELEBREX doses of 100 mg BID and 200 mg BID were similar in effectiveness and both were comparable to naproxen 500 mg BID.

Although CELEBREX 100 mg BID and 200 mg BID provided similar overall effectiveness, some patients derived additional benefit from the 200 mg BID dose. Doses of 400 mg BID provided no additional benefit above that seen with 100-200 mg BID.

Analgesia, including primary dysmenorrhea: In acute analgesic models of post-oral surgery pain, post-orthopedic surgical pain, and primary dysmenorrhea, CELEBREX relieved pain that was rated by patients as moderate to severe. Single doses (see DOSAGE AND ADMINISTRATION) of CELEBREX provided pain relief within 60 minutes.

Familial Adenomatous Polyposis (FAP): CELEBREX was evaluated to reduce the number of adenomatous colorectal polyps. A randomized double-blind placebo-controlled study was conducted in 83 patients with FAP. The study population included 58 patients with a prior subtotal or total colectomy and 25 patients with an intact colon. Thirteen patients had the attenuated FAP phenotype.

One area in the rectum and up to four areas in the colon were identified at baseline for specific follow-up, and polyps were counted at baseline and following six months of treatment. The mean reduction in the number of colorectal polyps was 28% for CELEBREX 400 mg BID, 12% for CELEBREX 100 mg BID and 5% for placebo. The reduction in polyps observed with CELEBREX 400 mg BID was statistically superior to placebo at the six-month timepoint (p=0.003). (See Figure 1.)

[See figure 1 at top of next column]

Special Studies

Endoscopic Studies: Scheduled upper GI endoscopic evaluations were performed in over 4,500 arthritis patients who were enrolled in five controlled randomized 12-24 week trials using active comparators, two of which also included placebo controls. There was no consistent relationship between the incidence of gastroduodenal ulcers and the dose of CELEBREX over the range studied.

Table 2 summarizes the incidence of endoscopic ulcers in two 12-week studies that enrolled patients in whom baseline endoscopies revealed no ulcers.

Continued on next page

Celebrex—Cont.

Figure 1
Percent Change from Baseline in Number of Colorectal Polyps (FAP Patients)

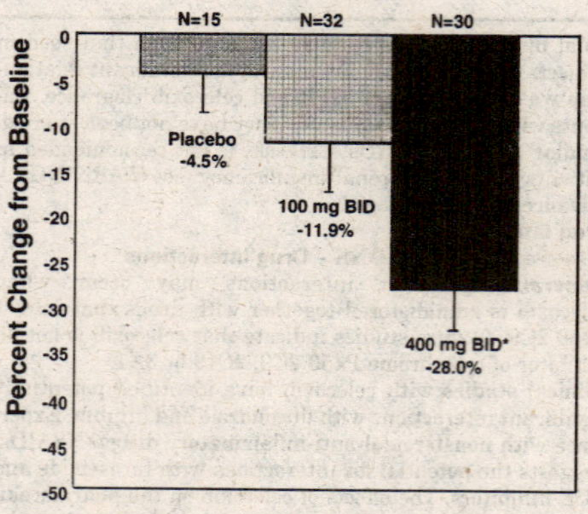

*p=0.003 versus placebo

Table 2
Incidence of Gastroduodenal Ulcers from Endoscopic Studies in OA and RA Patients

	3 Month Studies	
	Study 1 (n = 1108)	Study 2 (n = 1049)
Placebo	2.3% (5/217)	2.0% (4/200)
Celebrex 50 mg BID	3.4% (8/233)	—
Celebrex 100 mg BID	3.1% (7/227)	4.0% (9/223)
Celebrex 200 mg BID	5.9% (13/221)	2.7% (6/219)
Celebrex 400 mg BID	—	4.1% (8/197)
Naproxen 500 mg BID	16.2% (34/210)*	17.6% (37/210)*

*p≤0.05 vs all other treatments

Table 3 summarizes data from two 12-week studies that enrolled patients in whom baseline endoscopies revealed no ulcers. Patients underwent interval endoscopies every 4 weeks to give information on ulcer risk over time.
[See table 3 below]
One randomized and double-blind 6-month study in 430 RA patients was conducted in which an endoscopic examination was performed at 6 months. The incidence of endoscopic ulcers in patients taking CELEBREX 200 mg BID was 4% vs 15% for patients taking diclofenac SR 75 mg BID (p<0.001).
In 4 of the 5 endoscopic studies, approximately 11% of patients (440/4,000) were taking aspirin (≤325 mg/day). In the CELEBREX groups, the endoscopic ulcer rate appeared to be higher in aspirin users than in non-users. However, the increased rate of ulcers in these aspirin users was less than the endoscopic ulcer rates observed in the active comparator groups, with or without aspirin.
The correlation between findings of endoscopic studies, and the relative incidence of clinically significant serious upper GI events has not been established. Serious clinically significant upper GI bleeding has been observed in patients receiving CELEBREX in controlled and open-labeled trials, albeit infrequently (see *Use with Aspirin* and WARNINGS — Gastrointestinal (GI) Effects).
Use with Aspirin: The Celecoxib Long-Term Arthritis Safety Study (CLASS) was a prospective long-term safety outcome study conducted postmarketing in approximately 5,800 OA patients and 2,200 RA patients. Patients received CELEBREX 400 mg BID (4-fold and 2-fold the recommended OA and RA doses, respectively, and the approved dose for FAP), ibuprofen 800 mg TID or diclofenac 75 mg BID (common therapeutic doses). Median exposures for CELEBREX (n = 3,987) and diclofenac (n = 1,996) were 9 months while ibuprofen (n = 1,985) was 6 months. The Kaplan-Meier cumulative rates at 9 months are provided for all analyses. The primary endpoint of this outcome study was the incidence of *complicated ulcers* (gastrointestinal bleeding, perforation or obstruction). Patients were allowed to take concomitant low-dose (≤ 325 mg/day) aspirin (ASA) for cardiovascular prophylaxis (ASA subgroups: CELEBREX, n = 882; diclofenac, n = 445; ibuprofen, n = 412). Differences in the incidence of *complicated ulcers* between CELEBREX and the combined group of ibuprofen and diclofenac were not statistically significant. Those patients on CELEBREX and concomitant low-dose ASA experienced 4-fold higher rates of *complicated ulcers* compared to those not on ASA (see WARNINGS — Gastrointestinal (GI) Effects). The results for CELEBREX are displayed in Table 4. For *complicated and symptomatic ulcer* rates, see WARNINGS — Gastrointestinal (GI) Effects – Risk of GI Ulceration, Bleeding, and Perforation.

Table 4
Effects of Co-Administration of Low-Dose Aspirin on *Complicated Ulcer* Rates with CELEBREX 400 mg BID (Kaplan-Meier Rates at 9 months [%])

	Non-Aspirin Users n=3105	Aspirin Users n=882
Complicated Ulcers	0.32	1.12

Platelets: In clinical trials, CELEBREX at single doses up to 800 mg and multiple doses of 600 mg BID for up to 7 days duration (higher than recommended therapeutic doses) had no effect on platelet aggregation and bleeding time. Comparators (naproxen 500 mg BID, ibuprofen 800 mg TID, diclofenac 75 mg BID) significantly reduced platelet aggregation and prolonged bleeding time.
Because of its lack of platelet effects, CELEBREX is not a substitute for aspirin for cardiovascular prophylaxis.

INDICATIONS AND USAGE

CELEBREX is indicated:
1) For relief of the signs and symptoms of osteoarthritis.
2) For relief of the signs and symptoms of rheumatoid arthritis in adults.
3) For the management of acute pain in adults (see CLINICAL STUDIES).
4) For the treatment of primary dysmenorrhea.
5) To reduce the number of adenomatous colorectal polyps in familial adenomatous polyposis (FAP), as an adjunct to usual care (e.g., endoscopic surveillance, surgery). It is not known whether there is a clinical benefit from a reduction in the number of colorectal polyps in FAP patients. It is also not known whether the effects of CELEBREX treatment will persist after CELEBREX is discontinued. The efficacy and safety of CELEBREX treatment in patients with FAP beyond six months have not been studied (see CLINICAL STUDIES, WARNINGS and PRECAUTIONS sections).

CONTRAINDICATIONS

CELEBREX is contraindicated in patients with known hypersensitivity to celecoxib.
CELEBREX should not be given to patients who have demonstrated allergic-type reactions to sulfonamides.
CELEBREX should not be given to patients who have experienced asthma, urticaria, or allergic-type reactions after taking aspirin or other NSAIDs. Severe, rarely fatal, anaphylactic-like reactions to NSAIDs have been reported in such patients (see WARNINGS — Anaphylactoid Reactions, and PRECAUTIONS — Preexisting Asthma).

WARNINGS

Gastrointestinal (GI) Effects—Risk of GI Ulceration, Bleeding, and Perforation
Serious gastrointestinal toxicity such as bleeding, ulceration, and perforation of the stomach, small intestine or large intestine, can occur at any time, with or without warning symptoms, in patients treated with nonsteroidal anti-inflammatory drugs (NSAIDs). Minor upper gastrointestinal problems, such as dyspepsia, are common and may also occur at any time during NSAID therapy. Therefore, physicians and patients should remain alert for ulceration and bleeding, even in the absence of previous GI tract symptoms (see PRECAUTIONS – Hematological Effects). Patients should be informed about the signs and/or symptoms of serious GI toxicity and the steps to take if they occur. The utility of periodic laboratory monitoring has not been demonstrated, nor has it been adequately assessed. Only one in five patients who develop a serious upper GI adverse event on NSAID therapy is symptomatic. It has been demonstrated that upper GI ulcers, gross bleeding or perforation, caused by NSAIDs, appear to occur in approximately 1% of patients treated for 3-6 months, and in about 2-4% of patients treated for one year. These trends continue thus, increasing the likelihood of developing a serious GI event at some time during the course of therapy. However, even short-term therapy is not without risk.
NSAIDs should be prescribed with extreme caution in patients with a prior history of ulcer disease or gastrointestinal bleeding. Most spontaneous reports of fatal GI events are in elderly or debilitated patients and therefore special care should be taken in treating this population. **To minimize the potential risk for an adverse GI event, the lowest effective dose should be used for the shortest possible duration.** For high risk patients, alternate therapies that do not involve NSAIDs should be considered.
Studies have shown that patients with a *prior history of peptic ulcer disease and/or gastrointestinal bleeding* and who use NSAIDs, have a greater than 10-fold higher risk for developing a GI bleed than patients with neither of these risk factors. In addition to a past history of ulcer disease, pharmacoepidemiological studies have identified several other co-therapies or co-morbid conditions that may increase the risk for GI bleeding such as: treatment with oral corticosteroids, treatment with anticoagulants, longer duration of NSAID therapy, smoking, alcoholism, older age, and poor general health status.
CLASS Study: The estimated cumulative rates at 9 months of *complicated and symptomatic ulcers* (an adverse event similar but not identical to the "upper GI ulcers, gross bleeding or perforation" described in the preceding paragraphs) for patients treated with CELEBREX 400 mg BID (see Special Studies – *Use with Aspirin*) are described in Table 5. Table 5 also displays results for patients less than or greater than or equal to the age of 65 years. The differences in rates between CELEBREX alone and CELEBREX with ASA groups may be due to the higher risk for GI events in ASA users.

Table 5
***Complicated and Symptomatic Ulcer* Rates in Patients Taking CELEBREX 400 mg BID (Kaplan-Meier Rates at 9 months [%]) Based on Risk Factors**

	Complicated and Symptomatic Ulcer Rates
All Patients	
Celebrex alone (n=3105)	0.78
Celebrex with ASA (n=882)	2.19
Patients <65 Years	
Celebrex alone (n=2025)	0.47
Celebrex with ASA (n=403)	1.26
Patients ≥65 Years	
Celebrex alone (n=1080)	1.40
Celebrex with ASA (n=479)	3.06

In a small number of patients with a history of ulcer disease, the *complicated and symptomatic ulcer* rates in patients taking CELEBREX alone or CELEBREX with ASA were, respectively, 2.56% (n=243) and 6.85% (n=91) at 48 weeks. These results are to be expected in patients with a prior history of ulcer disease (see WARNINGS – Gastrointestinal (GI) Effects – Risk of GI Ulceration, Bleeding, and Perforation).

Anaphylactoid Reactions
As with NSAIDs in general, anaphylactoid reactions have occurred in patients without known prior exposure to CELEBREX. In post-marketing experience, rare cases of anaphylactic reactions and angioedema have been reported in patients receiving CELEBREX. CELEBREX should not be given to patients with the aspirin triad. This symptom complex typically occurs in asthmatic patients who experience rhinitis with or without nasal polyps, or who exhibit severe, potentially fatal bronchospasm after taking aspirin or other NSAIDs (see CONTRAINDICATIONS and PRECAUTIONS — Preexisting Asthma). Emergency help should be sought in cases where an anaphylactoid reaction occurs.

Advanced Renal Disease
No information is available from controlled clinical studies regarding the use of CELEBREX in patients with advanced kidney disease. Therefore, treatment with CELEBREX is not recommended in these patients with advanced kidney disease. If CELEBREX therapy must be initiated, close monitoring of the patient's kidney function is advisable (see PRECAUTIONS — Renal Effects).

Pregnancy
In late pregnancy CELEBREX should be avoided because it may cause premature closure of the ductus arteriosus (see PRECAUTIONS – Pregnancy).

Familial Adenomatous Polyposis (FAP): Treatment with CELEBREX in FAP has not been shown to reduce the risk of gastrointestinal cancer or the need for prophylactic colectomy or other FAP-related surgeries. Therefore, the usual care of FAP patients should not be altered because of the concurrent administration of CELEBREX. In particular, the frequency of routine endoscopic surveillance should not be decreased and prophylactic colectomy or other FAP-related surgeries should not be delayed.

Table 3
Incidence of Gastroduodenal Ulcers from 3-Month Serial Endoscopy Studies in OA and RA Patients

	Week 4	Week 8	Week 12	Final
Study 3 (n=523)				
Celebrex 200 mg BID	4.0% (10/252)*	2.2% (5/227)*	1.5% (3/196)*	7.5% (20/266)*
Naproxen 500 mg BID	19.0% (47/247)	14.2% (26/182)	9.9% (14/141)	34.6% (89/257)
Study 4 (n=1062)				
Celebrex 200 mg BID	3.9% (13/337)†	2.4% (7/296)†	1.8% (5/274)†	7.0% (25/356)†
Diclofenac 75 mg BID	5.1% (18/350)	3.3% (10/306)	2.9% (8/278)	9.7% (36/372)
Ibuprofen 800 mg TID	13.0% (42/323)	6.2% (15/241)	9.6% (21/219)	23.3% (78/334)

*p ≤0.05 Celebrex vs. naproxen based on interval and cumulative analyses
†p ≤0.05 Celebrex vs. ibuprofen based on interval and cumulative analyses

PRECAUTIONS

General: Celebrex cannot be expected to substitute for corticosteroids or to treat corticosteroid insufficiency. Abrupt discontinuation of corticosteroids may lead to exacerbation of corticosteroid-responsive illness. Patients on prolonged corticosteroid therapy should have their therapy tapered slowly if a decision is made to discontinue corticosteroids.

The pharmacological activity of Celebrex in reducing inflammation, and possibly fever, may diminish the utility of these diagnostic signs in detecting infectious complications of presumed noninfectious, painful conditions.

Hepatic Effects: Borderline elevations of one or more liver associated enzymes may occur in up to 15% of patients taking NSAIDs, and notable elevations of ALT or AST (approximately 3 or more times the upper limit of normal) have been reported in approximately 1% of patients in clinical trials with NSAIDs. These laboratory abnormalities may progress, may remain unchanged, or may be transient with continuing therapy. Rare cases of severe hepatic reactions, including jaundice and fatal fulminant hepatitis, liver necrosis and hepatic failure (some with fatal outcome) have been reported with NSAIDs, including Celebrex (see ADVERSE REACTIONS – post-marketing experience). In controlled clinical trials of Celebrex, the incidence of borderline elevations (greater than or equal to 1.2 times and less than 3 times the upper limit of normal) of liver associated enzymes was 6% for Celebrex and 5% for placebo, and approximately 0.2% of patients taking Celebrex and 0.3% of patients taking placebo had notable elevations of ALT and AST.

A patient with symptoms and/or signs suggesting liver dysfunction, or in whom an abnormal liver test has occurred, should be monitored carefully for evidence of the development of a more severe hepatic reaction while on therapy with Celebrex. If clinical signs and symptoms consistent with liver disease develop, or if systemic manifestations occur (e.g., eosinophilia, rash, etc.), Celebrex should be discontinued.

Renal Effects: Long-term administration of NSAIDs has resulted in renal papillary necrosis and other renal injury. Renal toxicity has also been seen in patients in whom renal prostaglandins have a compensatory role in the maintenance of renal perfusion. In these patients, administration of a nonsteroidal anti-inflammatory drug may cause a dose-dependent reduction in prostaglandin formation and, secondarily, in renal blood flow, which may precipitate overt renal decompensation. Patients at greatest risk of this reaction are those with impaired renal function, heart failure, liver dysfunction, those taking diuretics and ACE inhibitors, and the elderly. Discontinuation of NSAID therapy is usually followed by recovery to the pretreatment state. Clinical trials with Celebrex have shown renal effects similar to those observed with comparator NSAIDs.

Caution should be used when initiating treatment with Celebrex in patients with considerable dehydration. It is advisable to rehydrate patients first and then start therapy with Celebrex. Caution is also recommended in patients with preexisting kidney disease (see WARNINGS—Advanced Renal Disease).

Hematological Effects: Anemia is sometimes seen in patients receiving Celebrex. In controlled clinical trials the incidence of anemia was 0.6% with Celebrex and 0.4% with placebo. Patients on long-term treatment with Celebrex should have their hemoglobin or hematocrit checked if they exhibit any signs or symptoms of anemia or blood loss. Celebrex does not generally affect platelet counts, prothrombin time (PT), or partial thromboplastin time (PTT), and does not inhibit platelet aggregation at indicated dosages (see CLINICAL STUDIES—Special Studies—Platelets).

Fluid Retention, Edema, and Hypertension: Fluid retention and edema have been observed in some patients taking Celebrex (see ADVERSE REACTIONS). In the CLASS study (see Special Studies – *Use with Aspirin*), the Kaplan-Meier cumulative rates at 9 months of peripheral edema in patients on Celebrex 400 mg BID (4-fold and 2-fold the recommended OA and RA doses, respectively, and the approved dose for FAP), ibuprofen 800 mg TID and diclofenac 75 mg BID were 4.5%, 6.9% and 4.7%, respectively. The rates of hypertension in the Celebrex, ibuprofen and diclofenac treated patients were 2.4%, 4.2% and 2.5%, respectively. As with other NSAIDs, Celebrex should be used with caution in patients with fluid retention, hypertension, or heart failure.

Preexisting Asthma: Patients with asthma may have aspirin-sensitive asthma. The use of aspirin in patients with aspirin-sensitive asthma has been associated with severe bronchospasm which can be fatal. Since cross reactivity, including bronchospasm, between aspirin and other nonsteroidal anti-inflammatory drugs has been reported in such aspirin-sensitive patients, Celebrex should not be administered to patients with this form of aspirin sensitivity and should be used with caution in patients with preexisting asthma.

Information for Patients: Celebrex can cause discomfort and, rarely, more serious side effects, such as gastrointestinal bleeding, which may result in hospitalization and even fatal outcomes. Although serious GI tract ulcerations and bleeding can occur without warning symptoms, patients should be alert for the signs and symptoms of ulcerations and bleeding, and should ask for medical advice when observing any indicative signs or symptoms. Patients should be apprised of the importance of this follow-up (see WARNINGS — Gastrointestinal (GI) Effects – Risk of Gastrointestinal Ulceration, Bleeding, and Perforation).

Patients should promptly report signs or symptoms of gastrointestinal ulceration or bleeding, skin rash, unexplained weight gain, or edema to their physicians.

Patients should be informed of the warning signs and symptoms of hepatotoxicity (e.g., nausea, fatigue, lethargy, pruritus, jaundice, right upper quadrant tenderness, and "flu-like" symptoms). If these occur, patients should be instructed to stop therapy and seek immediate medical therapy.

Patients should also be instructed to seek immediate emergency help in the case of an anaphylactoid reaction (see WARNINGS).

In late pregnancy Celebrex should be avoided because it may cause premature closure of the ductus arteriosus.

Patients with familial adenomatous polyposis (FAP) should be informed that Celebrex has not been shown to reduce colorectal, duodenal or other FAP-related cancers, or the need for endoscopic surveillance, prophylactic or other FAP-related surgery. Therefore, all patients with FAP should be instructed to continue their usual care while receiving Celebrex.

Laboratory Tests: Because serious GI tract ulcerations and bleeding can occur without warning symptoms, physicians should monitor for signs or symptoms of GI bleeding. In controlled clinical trials, elevated BUN occurred more frequently in patients receiving Celebrex compared with patients on placebo. This laboratory abnormality was also seen in patients who received comparator NSAIDs in these studies. The clinical significance of this abnormality has not been established.

Drug Interactions

General: Celecoxib metabolism is predominantly mediated via cytochrome P450 2C9 in the liver. Co-administration of celecoxib with drugs that are known to inhibit 2C9 should be done with caution.

In vitro studies indicate that celecoxib, although not a substrate, is an inhibitor of cytochrome P450 2D6. Therefore, there is a potential for an *in vivo* drug interaction with drugs that are metabolized by P450 2D6.

ACE-inhibitors: Reports suggest that NSAIDs may diminish the antihypertensive effect of Angiotensin Converting Enzyme (ACE) inhibitors. This interaction should be given consideration in patients taking Celebrex concomitantly with ACE-inhibitors.

Furosemide: Clinical studies, as well as post marketing observations, have shown that NSAIDs can reduce the natriuretic effect of furosemide and thiazides in some patients. This response has been attributed to inhibition of renal prostaglandin synthesis.

Aspirin: Celebrex can be used with low-dose aspirin. However, concomitant administration of aspirin with Celebrex increases the rate of GI ulceration or other complications, compared to use of Celebrex alone (see CLINICAL STUDIES — Special Studies — *Use with Aspirin* and WARNINGS – Gastrointestinal (GI) Effects – Risk of GI Ulceration, Bleeding, and Perforation – CLASS Study).

Because of its lack of platelet effects, Celebrex is not a substitute for aspirin for cardiovascular prophylaxis.

Fluconazole: Concomitant administration of fluconazole at 200 mg QD resulted in a two-fold increase in celecoxib plasma concentration. This increase is due to the inhibition of celecoxib metabolism via P450 2C9 by fluconazole (see Pharmacokinetics — Metabolism). Celebrex should be introduced at the lowest recommended dose in patients receiving fluconazole.

Lithium: In a study conducted in healthy subjects, mean steady-state lithium plasma levels increased approximately 17% in subjects receiving lithium 450 mg BID with Celebrex 200 mg BID as compared to subjects receiving lithium alone. Patients on lithium treatment should be closely monitored when Celebrex is introduced or withdrawn.

Methotrexate: In an interaction study of rheumatoid arthritis patients taking methotrexate, Celebrex did not have a significant effect on the pharmacokinetics of methotrexate.

Warfarin: Anticoagulant activity should be monitored, particularly in the first few days, after initiating or changing Celebrex therapy in patients receiving warfarin or similar agents, since these patients are at an increased risk of bleeding complications. The effect of celecoxib on the anticoagulant effect of warfarin was studied in a group of healthy subjects receiving daily doses of 2-5 mg of warfarin. In these subjects, celecoxib did not alter the anticoagulant effect of warfarin as determined by prothrombin time. However, in post-marketing experience, bleeding events have been reported, predominantly in the elderly, in association with increases in prothrombin time in patients receiving Celebrex concurrently with warfarin.

Carcinogenesis, mutagenesis, impairment of fertility: Celecoxib was not carcinogenic in rats given oral doses up to 200 mg/kg for males and 10 mg/kg for females (approximately 2- to 4-fold the human exposure as measured by the AUC_{0-24} at 200 mg BID) or in mice given oral doses up to 25 mg/kg for males and 50 mg/kg for females (approximately equal to human exposure as measured by the AUC_{0-24} at 200 mg BID) for two years.

Celecoxib was not mutagenic in an Ames test and a mutation assay in Chinese hamster ovary (CHO) cells, nor clastogenic in a chromosome aberration assay in CHO cells and an *in vivo* micronucleus test in rat bone marrow.

Celecoxib did not impair male and female fertility in rats at oral doses up to 600 mg/kg/day (approximately 11-fold human exposure at 200 mg BID based on the AUC_{0-24}).

Pregnancy

Teratogenic effects: Pregnancy Category C. Celecoxib at oral doses ≥150 mg/kg/day (approximately 2-fold human exposure at 200 mg BID as measured by AUC_{0-24}), caused an increased incidence of ventricular septal defects, a rare event, and fetal alterations, such as ribs fused, sternebrae fused and sternebrae misshapen when rabbits were treated throughout organogenesis. A dose-dependent increase in diaphragmatic hernias was observed when rats were given celecoxib at oral doses ≥30 mg/kg/day (approximately 6-fold human exposure based on the AUC_{0-24} at 200 mg BID) throughout organogenesis. There are no studies in pregnant women. Celebrex should be used during pregnancy only if the potential benefit justifies the potential risk to the fetus.

Nonteratogenic effects: Celecoxib produced pre-implantation and post-implantation losses and reduced embryo/fetal survival in rats at oral dosages ≥50 mg/kg/day (approximately 6-fold human exposure based on the AUC_{0-24} at 200 mg BID). These changes are expected with inhibition of prostaglandin synthesis and are not the result of permanent alteration of female reproductive function, nor are they expected at clinical exposures. No studies have been conducted to evaluate the effect of celecoxib on the closure of the ductus arteriosus in humans. Therefore, use of Celebrex during the third trimester of pregnancy should be avoided.

Labor and delivery: Celecoxib produced no evidence of delayed labor or parturition at oral doses up to 100 mg/kg in rats (approximately 7-fold human exposure as measured by the AUC_{0-24} at 200 mg BID). The effects of Celebrex on labor and delivery in pregnant women are unknown.

Nursing mothers: Celecoxib is excreted in the milk of lactating rats at concentrations similar to those in plasma. Limited data from one subject indicate that celecoxib is also excreted in human milk. Because many drugs are excreted in human milk and because of the potential for serious adverse reactions in nursing infants from Celebrex, a decision should be made whether to discontinue nursing or to discontinue the drug, taking into account the importance of the drug to the mother.

Pediatric Use

Safety and effectiveness in pediatric patients below the age of 18 years have not been evaluated.

Geriatric Use

Of the total number of patients who received Celebrex in clinical trials, more than 3,300 were 65-74 years of age, while approximately 1,300 additional patients were 75 years and over. No substantial differences in effectiveness were observed between these subjects and younger subjects. In clinical studies comparing renal function as measured by the GFR, BUN and creatinine, and platelet function as measured by bleeding time and platelet aggregation, the results were not different between elderly and young volunteers. However, as with other NSAIDs, including those that selectively inhibit COX-2, there have been more spontaneous post-marketing reports of fatal GI events and acute renal failure in the elderly than in younger patients (see WARNINGS – Gastrointestinal (GI) Effects – Risk of GI Ulceration, Bleeding, and Perforation).

ADVERSE REACTIONS

Of the Celebrex treated patients in the premarketing controlled clinical trials, approximately 4,250 were patients with OA, approximately 2,100 were patients with RA, and approximately 1,050 were patients with post-surgical pain. More than 8,500 patients have received a total daily dose of Celebrex of 200 mg (100 mg BID or 200 mg QD) or more, including more than 400 treated at 800 mg (400 mg BID). Approximately 3,900 patients have received Celebrex at these doses for 6 months or more; approximately 2,300 of these have received it for 1 year or more and 124 of these have received it for 2 years or more.

Adverse events from Celebrex premarketing controlled arthritis trials: Table 6 lists all adverse events, regardless of causality, occurring in ≥2% of patients receiving Celebrex from 12 controlled studies conducted in patients with OA or RA that included a placebo and/or a positive control group.

[See table 6 on next page]

In placebo- or active-controlled clinical trials, the discontinuation rate due to adverse events was 7.1% for patients receiving Celebrex and 6.1% for patients receiving placebo. Among the most common reasons for discontinuation due to adverse events in the Celebrex treatment groups were dyspepsia and abdominal pain (cited as reasons for discontinuation in 0.8% and 0.7% of Celebrex patients, respectively). Among patients receiving placebo, 0.6% discontinued due to dyspepsia and 0.6% withdrew due to abdominal pain.

The following adverse events occurred in 0.1-1.9% of patients regardless of causality.

[See second table on next page]

Other serious adverse reactions which occur rarely (estimated <0.1%), regardless of causality: The following serious adverse events have occurred rarely in patients taking Celebrex. Cases reported only in the post-marketing experience are indicated in italics.

[See third table at bottom of next page]

Safety Data from CLASS Study:

Hematological Events:

During this study (see Special Studies – *Use with Aspirin*), the incidence of clinically significant decreases in hemoglobin (>2 g/dL) confirmed by repeat testing was lower in pa-

Continued on next page

Celebrex—Cont.

tients on Celebrex 400 mg BID (4-fold and 2-fold the recommended OA and RA doses, respectively, and the approved dose for FAP) compared to patients on either diclofenac 75 mg BID or ibuprofen 800 mg TID: 0.5%, 1.3% and 1.9%, respectively. The lower incidence of events with Celebrex was maintained with or without ASA use (see CLINICAL STUDIES – Special Studies – Platelets).

Withdrawals/Serious Adverse Events:
Kaplan-Meier cumulative rates at 9 months for withdrawals due to adverse events for Celebrex, diclofenac and ibuprofen were 24%, 29%, and 26%, respectively. Rates for serious adverse events (i.e. those causing hospitalization or felt to be life threatening or otherwise medically significant) regardless of causality were not different across treatment groups, respectively, 8%, 7%, and 8%.

Based on Kaplan-Meier cumulative rates for investigator-reported serious cardiovascular thromboembolic adverse events*, there were no differences between the Celebrex, diclofenac, or ibuprofen treatment groups. The rates in all patients at 9 months for Celebrex, diclofenac, and ibuprofen were 1.2%, 1.4%, and 1.1%, respectively. The rates for non-ASA users in each of the three treatment groups were less than 1%. The rates for myocardial infarction in each of the three non-ASA treatment groups were less than 0.2%.

*includes myocardial infarction, pulmonary embolism, deep venous thrombosis, unstable angina, transient ischemic attacks or ischemic cerebrovascular accidents.

Adverse events from analgesia and dysmenorrhea studies: Approximately 1,700 patients were treated with Celebrex in analgesia and dysmenorrhea studies. All patients in post-oral surgery pain studies received a single dose of study medication. Doses up to 600 mg/day of Celebrex were studied in primary dysmenorrhea and post-orthopedic surgery pain studies. The types of adverse events in the analgesia and dysmenorrhea studies were similar to those reported in arthritis studies. The only additional adverse event reported was post-dental extraction alveolar osteitis (dry socket) in the post-oral surgery pain studies.

Adverse events from the controlled trial in familial adenomatous polyposis: The adverse event profile reported for the 83 patients with familial adenomatous polyposis enrolled in the randomized, controlled clinical trial was similar to that reported for patients in the arthritis controlled trials. Intestinal anastomotic ulceration was the only new adverse event reported in the FAP trial, regardless of causality, and was observed in 3 of 58 patients (one at 100 mg BID, and two at 400 mg BID) who had prior intestinal surgery.

Table 6
Adverse Events Occurring in ≥2% of Celebrex Patients From Celebrex Premarketing Controlled Arthritis Trials

	Celebrex (100-200 mg BID or 200 mg QD) (n=4146)	Placebo (n=1864)	Naproxen 500 mg BID (n=1366)	Diclofenac 75 mg BID (n=387)	Ibuprofen 800 mg TID (n=345)
Gastrointestinal					
Abdominal Pain	4.1%	2.8%	7.7%	9.0%	9.0%
Diarrhea	5.6%	3.8%	5.3%	9.3%	5.8%
Dyspepsia	8.8%	6.2%	12.2%	10.9%	12.8%
Flatulence	2.2%	1.0%	3.6%	4.1%	3.5%
Nausea	3.5%	4.2%	6.0%	3.4%	6.7%
Body as a whole					
Back Pain	2.8%	3.6%	2.2%	2.6%	0.9%
Peripheral edema	2.1%	1.1%	2.1%	1.0%	3.5%
Injury-accidental	2.9%	2.3%	3.0%	2.6%	3.2%
Central and peripheral nervous system					
Dizziness	2.0%	1.7%	2.6%	1.3%	2.3%
Headache	15.8%	20.2%	14.5%	15.5%	15.4%
Psychiatric					
Insomnia	2.3%	2.3%	2.9%	1.3%	1.4%
Respiratory					
Pharyngitis	2.3%	1.1%	1.7%	1.6%	2.6%
Rhinitis	2.0%	1.3%	2.4%	2.3%	0.6%
Sinusitis	5.0%	4.3%	4.0%	5.4%	5.8%
Upper respiratory tract infection	8.1%	6.7%	9.9%	9.8%	9.9%
Skin					
Rash	2.2%	2.1%	2.1%	1.3%	1.2%

Celebrex (100-200 mg BID or 200 mg QD)	
Gastrointestinal:	Constipation, diverticulitis, dysphagia, eructation, esophagitis, gastritis, gastroenteritis, gastroesophageal reflux, hemorrhoids, hiatal hernia, melena, dry mouth, stomatitis, tenesmus, tooth disorder, vomiting
Cardiovascular:	Aggravated hypertension, angina pectoris, coronary artery disorder, myocardial infarction
General:	Allergy aggravated, allergic reaction, asthenia, chest pain, cyst NOS, edema generalized, face edema, fatigue, fever, hot flushes, influenza-like symptoms, pain, peripheral pain
Resistance mechanism disorders:	Herpes simplex, herpes zoster, infection bacterial, infection fungal, infection soft tissue, infection viral, moniliasis, moniliasis genital, otitis media
Central, peripheral nervous system:	Leg cramps, hypertonia, hypoesthesia, migraine, neuralgia, neuropathy, paresthesia, vertigo
Female reproductive:	Breast fibroadenosis, breast neoplasm, breast pain, dysmenorrhea, menstrual disorder, vaginal hemorrhage, vaginitis
Male reproductive:	Prostatic disorder
Hearing and vestibular:	Deafness, ear abnormality, earache, tinnitus
Heart rate and rhythm:	Palpitation, tachycardia
Liver and biliary system:	Hepatic function abnormal, SGOT increased, SGPT increased
Metabolic and nutritional:	BUN increased, CPK increased, diabetes mellitus, hypercholesterolemia, hyperglycemia, hypokalemia, NPN increase, creatinine increased, alkaline phosphatase increased, weight increase
Musculoskeletal:	Arthralgia, arthrosis, bone disorder, fracture accidental, myalgia, neck stiffness, synovitis, tendinitis
Platelets (bleeding or clotting):	Ecchymosis, epistaxis, thrombocythemia
Psychiatric:	Anorexia, anxiety, appetite increased, depression, nervousness, somnolence
Hemic:	Anemia
Respiratory:	Bronchitis, bronchospasm, bronchospasm aggravated, coughing, dyspnea, laryngitis, pneumonia
Skin and appendages:	Alopecia, dermatitis, nail disorder, photosensitivity reaction, pruritus, rash erythematous, rash maculopapular, skin disorder, skin dry, sweating increased, urticaria
Application site disorders:	Cellulitis, dermatitis contact, injection site reaction, skin nodule
Special senses:	Taste perversion
Urinary system:	Albuminuria, cystitis, dysuria, hematuria, micturition frequency, renal calculus, urinary incontinence, urinary tract infection
Vision:	Blurred vision, cataract, conjunctivitis, eye pain, glaucoma

Cardiovascular:	Syncope, congestive heart failure, ventricular fibrillation, pulmonary embolism, cerebrovascular accident, peripheral gangrene, thrombophlebitis, *vasculitis*
Gastrointestinal:	Intestinal obstruction, intestinal perforation, gastrointestinal bleeding, colitis with bleeding, esophageal perforation, pancreatitis, ileus
Liver and biliary system:	Cholelithiasis, *hepatitis, jaundice, liver failure*
Hemic and lymphatic:	Thrombocytopenia, *agranulocytosis, aplastic anemia, pancytopenia, leukopenia*
Metabolic:	*Hypoglycemia, hyponatremia*
Nervous system:	*Aseptic meningitis,* ataxia, suicide
Renal:	Acute renal failure, *interstitial nephritis*
Skin:	*Erythema multiforme, exfoliative dermatitis, Stevens-Johnson syndrome, toxic epidermal necrolysis*
General:	Sepsis, sudden death, *anaphylactoid reaction, angioedema*

OVERDOSAGE

No overdoses of Celebrex were reported during clinical trials. Doses up to 2400 mg/day for up to 10 days in 12 patients did not result in serious toxicity. Symptoms following acute NSAID overdoses are usually limited to lethargy, drowsiness, nausea, vomiting, and epigastric pain, which are generally reversible with supportive care. Gastrointestinal bleeding can occur. Hypertension, acute renal failure, respiratory depression and coma may occur, but are rare. Anaphylactoid reactions have been reported with therapeutic ingestion of NSAIDs, and may occur following an overdose. Patients should be managed by symptomatic and supportive care following an NSAID overdose. There are no specific antidotes. No information is available regarding the removal of celecoxib by hemodialysis, but based on its high degree of plasma protein binding (>97%) dialysis is unlikely to be useful in overdose. Emesis and/or activated charcoal (60 to 100 g in adults, 1 to 2 g/kg in children) and/or osmotic cathartic may be indicated in patients seen within 4 hours of ingestion with symptoms or following a large overdose. Forced diuresis, alkalinization of urine, hemodialysis, or hemoperfusion may not be useful due to high protein binding.

DOSAGE AND ADMINISTRATION

For osteoarthritis and rheumatoid arthritis, the lowest dose of Celebrex should be sought for each patient. These doses can be given without regard to timing of meals.

Osteoarthritis: For relief of the signs and symptoms of osteoarthritis the recommended oral dose is 200 mg per day administered as a single dose or as 100 mg twice per day.

Rheumatoid arthritis: For relief of the signs and symptoms of rheumatoid arthritis the recommended oral dose is 100 to 200 mg twice per day.

Management of Acute Pain and Treatment of Primary Dysmenorrhea: The recommended dose of Celebrex is 400 mg initially, followed by an additional 200 mg dose if needed on the first day. On subsequent days, the recommended dose is 200 mg twice daily as needed.

Familial adenomatous polyposis (FAP): Usual medical care for FAP patients should be continued while on Celebrex. To reduce the number of adenomatous colorectal polyps in patients with FAP, the recommended oral dose is 400 mg twice per day to be taken with food.

Special Populations

Hepatic insufficiency: The daily recommended dose of Celebrex capsules in patients with moderate hepatic impairment (Child-Pugh Class B) should be reduced by approximately 50% (see CLINICAL PHARMACOLOGY – Special Populations).

HOW SUPPLIED

Celebrex 100-mg capsules are white, reverse printed white on blue band of body and cap with markings of 7767 on the cap and 100 on the body, supplied as:

NDC Number	Size
0025-1520-31	bottle of 100
0025-1520-51	bottle of 500
0025-1520-34	carton of 100 unit dose

Celebrex 200-mg capsules are white, with reverse printed white on gold band with markings of 7767 on the cap and 200 on the body, supplied as:

NDC Number	Size
0025-1525-31	bottle of 100
0025-1525-51	bottle of 500
0025-1525-34	carton of 100 unit dose

Celebrex 400-mg capsules are white, with reverse printed white on green band with markings of 7767 on the cap and 400 on the body, supplied as:

NDC Number	Size
0025-1530-02	bottle of 60
0025-1530-01	carton of 100 unit dose

Store at 25°C (77°F); excursions permitted to 15-30°C (59-86°F) [see USP Controlled Room Temperature].

Rx only Revised: January 2004

Manufactured for: G.D. Searle LLC
A subsidiary of Pharmacia Corporation
Chicago, IL 60680, USA
Pfizer Inc
New York, NY 10017, USA
by: *Searle Ltd.*
Caguas, PR 00725

PHARMACIA Pfizer
Celebrex®
celecoxib capsules
819 059 006

PS4025-7

CLEOCIN HCL® ℞
[*klē-ō-sĭn*]
(clindamycin hydrochloride)
capsules, USP

Prescribing information for this product, which appears on pages 2731–2732 of the 2004 PDR, has been completely revised as follows. Please write "See Supplement A" next to the product heading.

To reduce the development of drug-resistant bacteria and maintain the effectiveness of CLEOCIN HCl and other antibacterial drugs, CLEOCIN HCl should be used only to treat or prevent infections that are proven or strongly suspected to be caused by bacteria.

WARNING

Pseudomembranous colitis has been reported with nearly all antibacterial agents, including clindamycin, and may range in severity from mild to life-threatening. Therefore, it is important to consider this diagnosis in patients who present with diarrhea subsequent to the administration of antibacterial agents.

Because clindamycin therapy has been associated with severe colitis which may end fatally, it should be reserved for serious infections where less toxic antimicrobial agents are inappropriate, as described in the **INDICATIONS AND USAGE** section. It should not be used in patients with nonbacterial infections such as most upper respiratory tract infections. Treatment with antibacterial agents alters the normal flora of the colon and may permit over-growth of clostridia. Studies indicate that a toxin produced by *Clostridium difficile* is one primary cause of "antibiotic-associated colitis".

After the diagnosis of pseudomembranous colitis has been established, therapeutic measures should be initiated. Mild cases of pseudomembranous colitis usually respond to drug discontinuation alone. In moderate to severe cases, consideration should be given to management with fluids and electrolytes, protein supplementation, and treatment with an antibacterial drug clinically effective against *C. difficile* colitis.

Diarrhea, colitis, and pseudomembranous colitis have been observed to begin up to several weeks following cessation of therapy with clindamycin.

DESCRIPTION

Clindamycin hydrochloride is the hydrated hydrochloride salt of clindamycin. Clindamycin is a semisynthetic antibiotic produced by a 7(S)-chloro-substitution of the 7(R)-hydroxyl group of the parent compound lincomycin.

CLEOCIN HCl Capsules contain clindamycin hydrochloride equivalent to 75 mg, 150 mg or 300 mg of clindamycin.

Inactive ingredients: **75 mg**—corn starch, FD&C blue no. 1, FD&C yellow no. 5, gelatin, lactose, magnesium stearate and talc; **150 mg**—corn starch, FD&C blue no. 1, FD&C yellow no. 5, gelatin, lactose, magnesium stearate, talc and titanium dioxide; **300 mg**—corn starch, FD&C blue no. 1, gelatin, lactose, magnesium stearate, talc and titanium dioxide.

The structural formula is represented below:

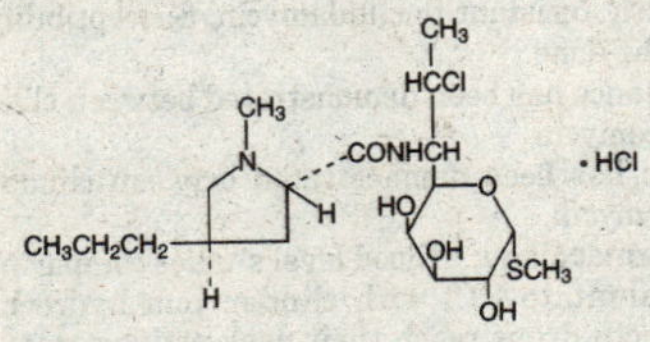

The chemical name for clindamycin hydrochloride is Methyl 7-chloro-6,7,8-trideoxy-6-(1-methyl-*trans*-4-propyl-L-2-pyrrolidinecarboxamido)-1-thio-L-*threo*-α-D-*galacto*-octopyranoside monohydrochloride.

CLINICAL PHARMACOLOGY

Microbiology: Clindamycin has been shown to have *in vitro* activity against isolates of the following organisms:

Aerobic gram-positive cocci, including:
- *Staphylococcus aureus*
- *Staphylococcus epidermidis*
- *(penicillinase and nonpenicillinase producing strains).* When tested by *in vitro* methods some staphylococcal strains originally resistant to erythromycin rapidly develop resistance to clindamycin.
- Streptococci (except *Streptococcus faecalis*)
- Pneumococci

Anaerobic gram-negative bacilli, including:
- Bacteroides species (including *Bacteroides fragilis* group and *Bacteroides melaninogenicus* group)
- Fusobacterium species

Anaerobic gram-positive nonsporeforming bacilli, including:
- Propionibacterium
- Eubacterium
- Actinomyces species

Anaerobic and microaerophilic gram-positive cocci, including:
- Peptococcus species
- Peptostreptococcus species
- Microaerophilic streptococci

Clostridia: Clostridia are more resistant than most anaerobes to clindamycin. Most *Clostridium perfringens* are susceptible, but other species, eg, *Clostridium sporogenes* and *Clostridium tertium* are frequently resistant to clindamycin. Susceptibility testing should be done.

Cross resistance has been demonstrated between clindamycin and lincomycin.

Antagonism has been demonstrated between clindamycin and erythromycin.

Human Pharmacology: Serum level studies with a 150 mg oral dose of clindamycin hydrochloride in 24 normal adult volunteers showed that clindamycin was rapidly absorbed after oral administration. An average peak serum level of 2.50 mcg/mL was reached in 45 minutes; serum levels averaged 1.51 mcg/mL at 3 hours and 0.70 mcg/mL at 6 hours. Absorption of an oral dose is virtually complete (90%), and the concomitant administration of food does not appreciably modify the serum concentrations; serum levels have been uniform and predictable from person to person and dose to dose. Serum level studies following multiple doses of CLEOCIN HCl for up to 14 days show no evidence of accumulation or altered metabolism of drug.

Serum half-life of clindamycin is increased slightly in patients with markedly reduced renal function. Hemodialysis and peritoneal dialysis are not effective in removing clindamycin from the serum.

Concentrations of clindamycin in the serum increased linearly with increased dose. Serum levels exceed the MIC (minimum inhibitory concentration) for most indicated organisms for at least six hours following administration of the usually recommended doses. Clindamycin is widely distributed in body fluids and tissues (including bones). The average biological half-life is 2.4 hours. Approximately 10% of the bioactivity is excreted in the urine and 3.6% in the feces; the remainder is excreted as bioinactive metabolites. Doses of up to 2 grams of clindamycin per day for 14 days have been well tolerated by healthy volunteers, except that the incidence of gastrointestinal side effects is greater with the higher doses.

No significant levels of clindamycin are attained in the cerebrospinal fluid, even in the presence of inflamed meninges. Pharmacokinetic studies in elderly volunteers (61–79 years) and younger adults (18–39 years) indicate that age alone does not alter clindamycin pharmacokinetics (clearance, elimination half-life, volume of distribution, and area under the serum concentration-time curve) after IV administration of clindamycin phosphate. After oral administration of clindamycin hydrochloride, elimination half-life is increased to approximately 4.0 hours (range 3.4–5.1 h) in the elderly compared to 3.2 hours (range 2.1–4.2 h) in younger adults. The extent of absorption, however, is not different between age groups and no dosage alteration is necessary for the elderly with normal hepatic function and normal (age-adjusted) renal function[1].

INDICATIONS AND USAGE

Clindamycin is indicated in the treatment of serious infections caused by susceptible anaerobic bacteria.

Clindamycin is also indicated in the treatment of serious infections due to susceptible strains of streptococci, pneumococci, and staphylococci. Its use should be reserved for penicillin-allergic patients or other patients for whom, in the judgment of the physician, a penicillin is inappropriate. Because of the risk of colitis, as described in the WARNING box, before selecting clindamycin the physician should consider the nature of the infection and the suitability of less toxic alternatives (eg, erythromycin).

Anaerobes: Serious respiratory tract infections such as empyema, anaerobic pneumonitis and lung abscess; serious skin and soft tissue infections; septicemia; intra-abdominal infections such as peritonitis and intra-abdominal abscess (typically resulting from anaerobic organisms resident in the normal gastrointestinal tract); infections of the female pelvis and genital tract such as endometritis, nongonococcal tuboovarian abscess, pelvic cellulitis and postsurgical vaginal cuff infection.

Streptococci: Serious respiratory tract infections; serious skin and soft tissue infections.

Staphylococci: Serious respiratory tract infections; serious skin and soft tissue infections.

Pneumococci: Serious respiratory tract infections.

Bacteriologic studies should be performed to determine the causative organisms and their susceptibility to clindamycin.

***In Vitro* Susceptibility Testing:** A standardized disk testing procedure* is recommended for determining susceptibility of aerobic bacteria to clindamycin. A description is contained in the CLEOCIN® Susceptibility Disk insert. Using this method, the laboratory can designate isolates as resistant, intermediate, or susceptible. Tube or agar dilution methods may be used for both anaerobic and aerobic bacteria. When the directions in the CLEOCIN® Susceptibility Powder insert are followed, an MIC of 1.6 mcg/mL may be considered susceptible; MICs of 1.6 to 4.8 mcg/mL may be considered intermediate and MICs greater than 4.8 mcg/mL may be considered resistant.

*Bauer AW, Kirby WMM, Sherris JC, et al: Antibiotic susceptibility testing by a standardized single disc method. *Am J Clin Pathol* **45**:493-496, 1966. Standardized disc susceptibility test. *Federal Register* **37**:20527-29, 1972.

CLEOCIN Susceptibility Disks 2 mcg. See package insert for use.

CLEOCIN Susceptibility Powder 20 mg. See package insert for use.

For anaerobic bacteria the minimal inhibitory concentration (MIC) of clindamycin can be determined by agar dilution and broth dilution (including microdilution) techniques. If MICs are not determined routinely, the disk broth method is recommended for routine use. THE KIRBY-BAUER DISK DIFFUSION METHOD AND ITS INTERPRETIVE STANDARDS ARE NOT RECOMMENDED FOR ANAEROBES.

To reduce the development of drug-resistant bacteria and maintain the effectiveness of CLEOCIN HCl and other antibacterial drugs, CLEOCIN HCl should be used only to treat or prevent infections that are proven or strongly suspected to be caused by susceptible bacteria. When culture and susceptibility information are available, they should be considered in selecting or modifying antibacterial therapy. In the absence of such data, local epidemiology and susceptibility patterns may contribute to the empiric selection of therapy.

CONTRAINDICATIONS

CLEOCIN HCl is contraindicated in individuals with a history of hypersensitivity to preparations containing clindamycin or lincomycin.

WARNINGS

See WARNING box.

Pseudomembranous colitis has been reported with nearly all antibacterial agents, including clindamycin, and may range in severity from mild to life-threatening. Therefore, it is important to consider this diagnosis in patients who present with diarrhea subsequent to the administration of antibacterial agents.

Treatment with antibacterial agents alters the normal flora of the colon and may permit overgrowth of clostridia. Studies indicate that a toxin produced by *Clostridium difficile* is one primary cause of "antibiotic-associated colitis".

After the diagnosis of pseudomembranous colitis has been established, therapeutic measures should be initiated. Mild cases of pseudomembranous colitis usually respond to drug discontinuation alone. In moderate to severe cases, consideration should be given to management with fluids and electrolytes, protein supplementation, and treatment with an antibacterial drug clinically effective against *C. difficile* colitis.

A careful inquiry should be made concerning previous sensitivities to drugs and other allergens.

Usage in Meningitis—Since clindamycin does not diffuse adequately into the cerebrospinal fluid, the drug should not be used in the treatment of meningitis.

PRECAUTIONS

General

Review of experience to date suggests that a subgroup of older patients with associated severe illness may tolerate diarrhea less well. When clindamycin is indicated in these patients, they should be carefully monitored for change in bowel frequency.

CLEOCIN HCl should be prescribed with caution in individuals with a history of gastrointestinal disease, particularly colitis.

CLEOCIN HCl should be prescribed with caution in atopic individuals.

Indicated surgical procedures should be performed in conjunction with antibiotic therapy.

The use of CLEOCIN HCl occasionally results in overgrowth of nonsusceptible organisms—particularly yeasts. Should superinfections occur, appropriate measures should be taken as indicated by the clinical situation.

Clindamycin dosage modification may not be necessary in patients with renal disease. In patients with moderate to severe liver disease, prolongation of clindamycin half-life has been found. However, it was postulated from studies that when given every eight hours, accumulation should rarely occur. Therefore, dosage modification in patients with liver disease may not be necessary. However, periodic liver enzyme determinations should be made when treating patients with severe liver disease.

The 75 mg and 150 mg capsules contain FD&C yellow no. 5 (tartrazine) which may cause allergic-type reactions (including bronchial asthma) in certain susceptible individuals. Although the overall incidence of FD&C yellow no. 5 (tartrazine) sensitivity in the general population is low, it is frequently seen in patients who also have aspirin hypersensitivity.

Prescribing CLEOCIN HCl in the absence of a proven or strongly suspected bacterial infection or a prophylactic indication is unlikely to provide benefit to the patient and increases the risk of the development of drug-resistant bacteria.

Information for Patients

Patients should be counseled that antibacterial drugs including CLEOCIN HCl should only be to treat bacterial infections. They do not treat viral infections (e.g., the common cold). When CLEOCIN HCl is prescribed to treat a bacterial infection, patients should be told that although it is common to feel better early in the course of therapy, the medication should be taken exactly as directed. Skipping doses or not completing the full course of therapy may (1) decrease the effectiveness of the immediate treatment and (2) increase the likelihood that bacteria will develop resistance and will not be treatable by CLEOCIN HCl or other antibacterial drugs in the future.

Continued on next page

Cleocin HCL—Cont.

Laboratory Tests
During prolonged therapy, periodic liver and kidney function tests and blood counts should be performed.
Drug Interactions
Clindamycin has been shown to have neuromuscular blocking properties that may enhance the action of other neuromuscular blocking agents. Therefore, it should be used with caution in patients receiving such agents.
Antagonism has been demonstrated between clindamycin and erythromycin *in vitro*. Because of possible clinical significance, these two drugs should not be administered concurrently.
Carcinogenesis, Mutagenesis, Impairment of Fertility
Long term studies in animals have not been performed with clindamycin to evaluate carcinogenic potential. Genotoxicity tests performed included a rat micronucleus test and an Ames Salmonella reversion test. Both tests were negative. Fertility studies in rats treated orally with up to 300 mg/kg/day (approximately 1.6 times the highest recommended adult human dose based on mg/m^2) revealed no effects on fertility or mating ability.
Pregnancy: Teratogenic effects
Pregnancy category B
Reproduction studies performed in rats and mice using oral doses of clindamycin up to 600 mg/kg/day (3.2 and 1.6 times the highest recommended adult human dose based on mg/m^2, respectively) or subcutaneous doses of clindamycin up to 250 mg/kg/day (1.3 and 0.7 times the highest recommended adult human dose based on mg/m^2, respectively) revealed no evidence of teratogenicity.
There are, however, no adequate and well-controlled studies in pregnant women. Because animal reproduction studies are not always predictive of the human response, this drug should be used during pregnancy only if clearly needed.
Nursing Mothers
Clindamycin has been reported to appear in breast milk in the range of 0.7 to 3.8 mcg/mL.
Pediatric Use
When CLEOCIN HCl is administered to the pediatric population (birth to 16 years), appropriate monitoring of organ system functions is desirable.
Geriatric Use
Clinical studies of clindamycin did not include sufficient numbers of patients age 65 and over to determine whether they respond differently from younger patients. However, other reported clinical experience indicates that antibiotic-associated colitis and diarrhea (due to *Clostridium difficile*) seen in association with most antibiotics occur more frequently in the elderly >60 years) and may be more severe. These patients should be carefully monitored for the development of diarrhea.
Pharmacokinetic studies with clindamycin have shown no clinically important differences between young and elderly subjects with normal hepatic function and normal (age-adjusted) renal function after oral or intravenous administration.

ADVERSE REACTIONS

The following reactions have been reported with the use of clindamycin.
Gastrointestinal: Abdominal pain, pseudomembranous colitis, esophagitis, nausea, vomiting and diarrhea (see **WARNING** box). The onset of pseudomembranous colitis symptoms may occur during or after antibacterial treatment (see **WARNINGS**).
Hypersensitivity Reactions: Generalized mild to moderate morbilliform-like (maculopapular) skin rashes are the most frequently reported adverse reactions. Vesiculobullous rashes, as well as urticaria, have been observed during drug therapy. Rare instances of erythema multiforme, some resembling Stevens-Johnson syndrome, and a few cases of anaphylactoid reactions have also been reported.
Skin and Mucous Membranes: Pruritus, vaginitis, and rare instances of exfoliative dermatitis have been reported. (See *Hypersensitivity Reactions.*)
Liver: Jaundice and abnormalities in liver function tests have been observed during clindamycin therapy.
Renal: Although no direct relationship of clindamycin to renal damage has been established, renal dysfunction as evidenced by azotemia, oliguria, and/or proteinuria has been observed in rare instances.
Hematopoietic: Transient neutropenia (leukopenia) and eosinophilia have been reported. Reports of agranulocytosis and thrombocytopenia have been made. No direct etiologic relationship to concurrent clindamycin therapy could be made in any of the foregoing.
Musculoskeletal: Rare instances of polyarthritis have been reported.

OVERDOSAGE

Significant mortality was observed in mice at an intravenous dose of 855 mg/kg and in rats at an oral or subcutaneous dose of approximately 2618 mg/kg. In the mice, convulsions and depression were observed.
Hemodialysis and peritoneal dialysis are not effective in removing clindamycin from the serum.

DOSAGE AND ADMINISTRATION

If significant diarrhea occurs during therapy, this antibiotic should be discontinued (see **WARNING** box).
Adults: *Serious infections*—150 to 300 mg every 6 hours. *More severe infections*—300 to 450 mg every 6 hours. **Pediatric Patients:** *Serious infections*—8 to 16 mg/kg/day (4 to 8 mg/lb/day) divided into three or four equal doses. *More severe infections*—16 to 20 mg/kg/day (8 to 10 mg/lb/day) divided into three or four equal doses.
To avoid the possibility of esophageal irritation, CLEOCIN HCl Capsules should be taken with a full glass of water.
Serious infections due to anaerobic bacteria are usually treated with CLEOCIN PHOSPHATE® Sterile Solution. However, in clinically appropriate circumstances, the physician may elect to initiate treatment or continue treatment with CLEOCIN HCI Capsules.
In cases of β-hemolytic streptococcal infections, treatment should continue for at least 10 days.

HOW SUPPLIED

CLEOCIN HCl Capsules are available in the following strengths, colors and sizes:

75 mg Green	
Bottles of 100	NDC 0009-0331-02
150 mg Light Blue and Green	
Bottles of 16	NDC 0009-0225-01
Bottles of 100	NDC 0009-0225-02
Unit dose package of 100	NDC 0009-0225-03
300 mg Light Blue	
Bottles of 16	NDC 0009-0395-13
Bottles of 100	NDC 0009-0395-14
Unit dose package of 100	NDC 0009-0395-02

Store at controlled room temperature 20° to 25° C (68° to 77° F) [see USP].

ANIMAL TOXICOLOGY

One year oral toxicity studies in Spartan Sprague-Dawley rats and beagle dogs at dose levels up to 300 mg/kg/day (approximately 1.6 and 5.4 times the highest recommended adult human dose based on mg/m^2, respectively) have shown clindamycin to be well tolerated. No appreciable difference in pathological findings has been observed between groups of animals treated with clindamycin and comparable control groups. Rats receiving clindamycin hydrochloride at 600 mg/kg/day (approximately 3.2 times the highest recommended adult human dose based on mg/m^2) for 6 months tolerated the drug well; however, dogs dosed at this level (approximately 10.8 times the highest recommended adult human dose based on mg/m^2) vomited, would not eat, and lost weight.
℞ only

REFERENCES

1. Smith RB, Phillips JP: Evaluation of CLEOCIN HCl and CLEOCIN Phosphate in an Aged Population. Upjohn TR 8147-82-9122-021, December 1982.

Made in Canada for
Pharmacia & Upjohn Company
A subsidiary of Pharmacia Corporation
Kalamazoo, MI 49001, USA
By Patheon YM, Inc.
Toronto, Ontario
M3B 1Y5
Canada
Revised September 2003 810 570 927
692851

CLEOCIN PEDIATRIC® ℞

[*klē-ō-sĭn*]
(clindamycin palmitate hydrochloride)
for oral solution, USP
Not for Injection

Prescribing information for this product, which appears on pages 2733–2734 of the 2004 PDR, has been completely revised as follows. Please write "See Supplement A" next to the product heading.

To reduce the development of drug-resistant bacteria and maintain the effectiveness of CLEOCIN PEDIATRIC and other antibacterial drugs, CLEOCIN PEDIATRIC should be used only to treat or prevent infections that are proven or strongly suspected to be caused by bacteria.

WARNING

Pseudomembranous colitis has been reported with nearly all antibacterial agents, including clindamycin, and may range in severity from mild to life-threatening. Therefore, it is important to consider this diagnosis in patients who present with diarrhea subsequent to the administration of antibacterial agents.
Because clindamycin therapy has been associated with severe colitis which may end fatally, it should be reserved for serious infections where less toxic antimicrobial agents are inappropriate, as described in the **INDICATIONS AND USAGE** section. It should not be used in patients with nonbacterial infections such as most upper respiratory tract infections. Treatment with antibacterial agents alters the normal flora of the colon and may permit overgrowth of clostridia. Studies indicate that a toxin produced by *Clostridium difficile* is one primary cause of "antibiotic-associated colitis".
After the diagnosis of pseudomembranous colitis has been established, therapeutic measures should be initiated. Mild cases of pseudomembranous colitis usually respond to drug discontinuation alone. In moderate to severe cases, consideration should be given to management with fluids and electrolytes, protein supplementation, and treatment with an antibacterial drug clinically effective against *C. difficile* colitis.
Diarrhea, colitis, and pseudomembranous colitis have been observed to begin up to several weeks following cessation of therapy with clindamycin.

DESCRIPTION

Clindamycin palmitate hydrochloride is a water soluble hydrochloride salt of the ester of clindamycin and palmitic acid. Clindamycin is a semisynthetic antibiotic produced by a 7(S)-chloro-substitution of the 7(R)-hydroxyl group of the parent compound lincomycin.
The structural formula is represented below:

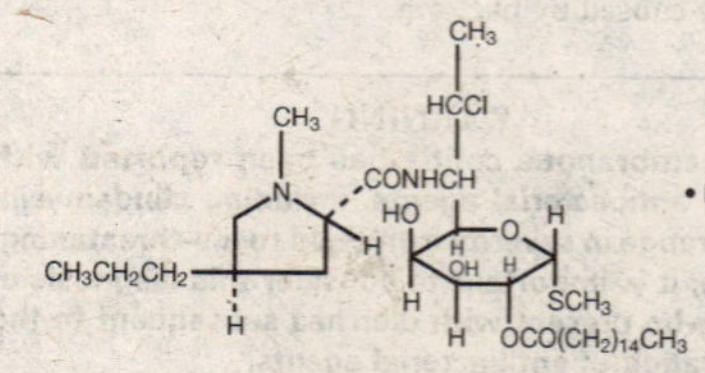

The chemical name for clindamycin palmitate hydrochloride is Methyl 7-chloro-6, 7, 8-trideoxy-6-(1-methyl-*trans*-4-propyl-L-2-pyrrolidinecarboxamido)-1-thio-L-*threo*-α-D-*galacto*-octopyranoside 2-palmitate monohydrochloride.
CLEOCIN PEDIATRIC Flavored Granules contain clindamycin palmitate hydrochloride for reconstitution. Each 5 mL contains the equivalent of 75 mg clindamycin. Inactive ingredients: artificial cherry flavor, dextrin, ethylparaben, pluronic F68, polymethylsiloxane, sucrose.

CLINICAL PHARMACOLOGY

Microbiology: Although clindamycin palmitate HCl is inactive *in vitro*, rapid *in vivo* hydrolysis converts this compound to the antibacterially active clindamycin.
Clindamycin has been shown to have *in vitro* activity against isolates of the following organisms:
Aerobic gram positive cocci, including:
Staphylococcus aureus / *Staphylococcus epidermidis* (penicillinase and non-penicillinase producing strains). When tested by *in vitro* methods some staphylococcal strains originally resistant to erythromycin rapidly develop resistance to clindamycin.
Streptococci (except *Streptococcus faecalis*)
Pneumococci
Anaerobic gram negative bacilli, including:
Bacteroides species (including *Bacteroides fragilis* group and *Bacteroides melaninogenicus* group)
Fusobacterium species
Anaerobic gram positive nonsporeforming bacilli, including:
Propionibacterium
Eubacterium
Actinomyces species
Anaerobic and microaerophilic gram positive cocci, including:
Peptococcus species
Peptostreptococcus species
Microaerophilic streptococci
Clostridia: Clostridia are more resistant than most anaerobes to clindamycin.
Most *Clostridium perfringens* are susceptible, but other species, eg, *Clostridium sporogenes* and *Clostridium tertium* are frequently resistant to clindamycin. Susceptibility testing should be done.
Cross resistance has been demonstrated between clindamycin and lincomycin.
Antagonism has been demonstrated between clindamycin and erythromycin.
Human Pharmacology: Blood level studies comparing clindamycin palmitate HCl with clindamycin hydrochloride show that both drugs reach their peak active serum levels at the same time, indicating a rapid hydrolysis of the palmitate to the clindamycin.
Clindamycin is widely distributed in body fluids and tissues (including bones). Approximately 10% of the biological activity is excreted in the urine. The average serum half-life after doses of CLEOCIN PEDIATRIC is approximately two hours in pediatric patients.
Serum half-life of clindamycin is increased slightly in patients with markedly reduced renal function. Hemodialysis and peritoneal dialysis are not effective in removing clindamycin from the serum.
Serum level studies with clindamycin palmitate HCl in normal pediatric patients weighing 50–100 lbs given 2, 3 or 4 mg/kg every 6 hours (8, 12 or 16 mg/kg/day) demonstrated mean peak clindamycin serum levels of 1.24, 2.25 and 2.44 mcg/mL respectively, one hour after the first dose. By the fifth dose, the 6-hour serum concentration had reached equilibrium. Peak serum concentrations after this time would be about 2.46, 2.98 and 3.79 mcg/mL with doses of 8, 12 and 16 mg/kg/day, respectively. Serum levels have been uniform and predictable from person to person and dose to dose. Multiple-dose studies in neonates and infants up to 6 months of age show that the drug does not accumulate in the serum and is excreted rapidly. Serum levels exceed the MICs for most indicated organisms for at least six hours following administration of the usually recommended doses of CLEOCIN PEDIATRIC in adults and pediatric patients.
No significant levels of clindamycin are attained in the cerebrospinal fluid, even in the presence of inflamed meninges.
Pharmacokinetic studies in elderly volunteers (61–79 years) and younger adults (18–39 years) indicate that age alone

does not alter clindamycin pharmacokinetics (clearance, elimination half-life, volume of distribution, and area under the serum concentration-time curve) after IV administration of clindamycin phosphate. After oral administration of clindamycin hydrochloride, elimination half-life is increased to approximately 4.0 hours (range 3.4–5.1 h) in the elderly compared to 3.2 hours (range 2.1–4.2 h) in younger adults; administration of clindamycin palmitate HCl resulted in a similar elimination half-life value of about 4.5 hours in elderly subjects. However, the extent of absorption is not different between age groups and no dosage alteration is necessary for the elderly with normal hepatic function and normal (age-adjusted) renal function[1].

INDICATIONS AND USAGE

CLEOCIN PEDIATRIC (clindamycin palmitate HCl) is indicated in the treatment of serious infections caused by susceptible anaerobic bacteria.

Clindamycin is also indicated in the treatment of serious infections due to susceptible strains of streptococci, pneumococci and staphylococci. Its use should be reserved for penicillin-allergic patients or other patients for whom, in the judgment of the physician, a penicillin is inappropriate. Because of the risk of colitis, as described in the WARNING box, before selecting clindamycin the physician should consider the nature of the infection and the suitability of less toxic alternatives (eg, erythromycin).

Anaerobes: Serious respiratory tract infections such as empyema, anaerobic pneumonitis and lung abscess; serious skin and soft tissue infections; septicemia; intra-abdominal infections such as peritonitis and intra-abdominal abscess (typically resulting from anaerobic organisms resident in the normal gastrointestinal tract); infections of the female pelvis and genital tract such as endometritis, nongonococcal tubo-ovarian abscess, pelvic cellulitis and postsurgical vaginal cuff infection.

Streptococci: Serious respiratory tract infections; serious skin and soft tissue infections.

Staphylococci: Serious respiratory tract infections; serious skin and soft tissue infections.

Pneumococci: Serious respiratory tract infections. Bacteriologic studies should be performed to determine the causative organisms and their susceptibility to clindamycin.

In Vitro Susceptibility Testing: A standardized disk testing procedure[2] is recommended for determining susceptibility of aerobic bacteria to clindamycin. A description is contained in the CLEOCIN® Susceptibility Disk (clindamycin) insert. Using this method, the laboratory can designate isolates as resistant, intermediate, or susceptible. Tube or agar dilution methods may be used for both anaerobic and aerobic bacteria. When the directions in the CLEOCIN® Susceptibility Powder insert are followed, an MIC (minimal inhibitory concentration) of 1.6 mcg/mL may be considered susceptible; MICs of 1.6 to 4.8 mcg/mL may be considered intermediate and MICs greater than 4.8 mcg/mL may be considered resistant.

CLEOCIN Susceptibility Disks 2 mcg. See package insert for use.

CLEOCIN Susceptibility Powder 20 mg. See package insert for use.

For anaerobic bacteria the minimal inhibitory concentration (MIC) of clindamycin can be determined by agar dilution and broth dilution (including microdilution) techniques. If MICs are not determined routinely, the disk broth method is recommended for routine use. THE KIRBY-BAUER DISK DIFFUSION METHOD AND ITS INTERPRETIVE STANDARDS ARE NOT RECOMMENDED FOR ANAEROBES.

To reduce the development of drug-resistant bacteria and maintain the effectiveness of CLEOCIN PEDIATRIC and other antibacterial drugs, CLEOCIN PEDIATRIC should be used only to treat or prevent infections that are proven or strongly suspected to be caused by susceptible bacteria. When culture and susceptibility information are available, they should be considered in selecting or modifying antibacterial therapy. In the absence of such data, local epidemiology and susceptibility patterns may contribute to the empiric selection of therapy.

CONTRAINDICATIONS

This drug is contraindicated in individuals with a history of hypersensitivity to preparations containing clindamycin or lincomycin.

WARNINGS

See WARNING box.

Pseudomembranous colitis has been reported with nearly all antibacterial agents, including clindamycin, and may range in severity from mild to life-threatening. Therefore, it is important to consider this diagnosis in patients who present with diarrhea subsequent to the administration of antibacterial agents.

Treatment with antibacterial agents alters the normal flora of the colon and may permit overgrowth of clostridia. Studies indicate that a toxin produced by *Clostridium difficile* is one primary cause of "antibiotic-associated colitis".

After the diagnosis of pseudomembranous colitis has been established, therapeutic measures should be initiated. Mild cases of pseudomembranous colitis usually respond to drug discontinuation alone. In moderate to severe cases, consideration should be given to management with fluids and electrolytes, protein supplementation, and treatment with an antibacterial drug clinically effective against *C. difficile* colitis.

A careful inquiry should be made concerning previous sensitivities to drugs and other allergens.

Usage in Meningitis: Since clindamycin does not diffuse adequately into the cerebrospinal fluid, the drug should not be used in the treatment of meningitis.

PRECAUTIONS

General

Review of experience to date suggests that a subgroup of older patients with associated severe illness may tolerate diarrhea less well. When clindamycin is indicated in these patients, they should be carefully monitored for change in bowel frequency.

CLEOCIN PEDIATRIC (clindamycin palmitate HCl) should be prescribed with caution in individuals with a history of gastrointestinal disease, particularly colitis.

CLEOCIN PEDIATRIC should be prescribed with caution in atopic individuals.

Indicated surgical procedures should be performed in conjunction with antibiotic therapy.

The use of CLEOCIN PEDIATRIC occasionally results in overgrowth of nonsusceptible organisms-particularly yeasts. Should superinfections occur, appropriate measures should be taken as indicated by the clinical situation.

Clindamycin dosage modification may not be necessary in patients with renal disease. In patients with moderate to severe liver disease, prolongation of clindamycin half-life has been found. However, it was postulated from studies that when given every eight hours, accumulation should rarely occur. Therefore, dosage modification in patients with liver disease may not be necessary. However, periodic liver enzyme determinations should be made when treating patients with severe liver disease.

Prescribing CLEOCIN PEDIATRIC in the absence of a proven or strongly suspected bacterial infection or a prophylactic indication is unlikely to provide benefit to the patient and increases the risk of the development of drug-resistant bacteria.

Information for Patients

Patients should be counseled that antibacterial drugs including CLEOCIN PEDIATRIC should only be used to treat bacterial infections. They do not treat viral infections (e.g., the common cold). When CLEOCIN PEDIATRIC is prescribed to treat a bacterial infection, patients should be told that although it is common to feel better early in the course of therapy, the medication should be taken exactly as directed. Skipping doses or not completing the full course of therapy may (1) decrease the effectiveness of the immediate treatment and (2) increase the likelihood that bacteria will develop resistance and will not be treatable by CLEOCIN PEDIATRIC or other antibacterial drugs in the future.

Laboratory Tests

During prolonged therapy, periodic liver and kidney function tests and blood counts should be performed.

Drug Interactions

Clindamycin has been shown to have neuromuscular blocking properties that may enhance the action of other neuromuscular blocking agents. Therefore, it should be used with caution in patients receiving such agents.

Antagonism has been demonstrated between clindamycin and erythromycin *in vitro*. Because of possible clinical significance, these two drugs should not be administered concurrently.

Carcinogenesis, Mutagenesis, Impairment of Fertility

Long term studies in animals have not been performed with clindamycin to evaluate carcinogenic potential. Genotoxicity tests performed included a rat micronucleus test and an Ames Salmonella reversion test. Both tests were negative. Fertility studies in rats treated orally with up to 300 mg/kg/day (approximately 1.6 times the highest recommended adult human oral dose based on mg/m^2) revealed no effects on fertility or mating ability.

Pregnancy: Teratogenic Effects

Pregnancy Category B

Reproduction studies performed in rats and mice using oral doses of clindamycin up to 600 mg/kg/day (3.2 and 1.6 times the highest recommended adult human oral dose based on mg/m^2, respectively) or subcutaneous doses of clindamycin up to 250 mg/kg/day (1.3 and 0.7 times the highest recommended adult human oral dose based on mg/m^2, respectively) revealed no evidence of teratogenicity.

There are, however, no adequate and well-controlled studies in pregnant women. Because animal reproduction studies are not always predictive of the human response, this drug should be used during pregnancy only if clearly needed.

Nursing Mothers

Clindamycin has been reported to appear in breast milk in the range of 0.7 to 3.8 mcg/mL.

Pediatric Use

When CLEOCIN HCl is administered to the pediatric population (birth to 16 years), appropriate monitoring of organ system functions is desirable.

Geriatric Use

Clinical studies of clindamycin did not include sufficient numbers of patients age 65 and over to determine whether they respond differently from younger patients. However, other reported clinical experience indicates that antibiotic-associated colitis and diarrhea (due to *Clostridium difficile*) seen in association with most antibiotics occur more frequently in the elderly (>60 years) and may be more severe. These patients should be carefully monitored for the development of diarrhea.

Pharmacokinetic studies with clindamycin have shown no clinically important differences between young subjects (18–39 years) and elderly subjects (61–79 years) with normal hepatic function and normal (age-adjusted) renal function after oral or intravenous administration.

ADVERSE REACTIONS

The following reactions have been reported with the use of clindamycin.

Gastrointestinal: Abdominal pain, pseudomembraneous colitis, esophagitis, nausea, vomiting and diarrhea (see **WARNING** box). The onset of pseudomembranous colitis symptoms may occur during or after antibacterial treatment (see **WARNINGS**).

Hypersensitivity Reactions: Generalized mild to moderate morbilliform-like (maculopapular) skin rashes are the most frequently reported adverse reactions. Vesiculobullous rashes, as well as urticaria, have been observed during drug therapy. Rare instances of erythema multiforme, some resembling Stevens-Johnson syndrome, and a few cases of anaphylactoid reactions have also been reported.

Skin and Mucous Membranes: Pruritus, vaginitis, and rare instances of exfoliative dermatitis have been reported. (See *Hypersensitivity Reactions*.)

Liver: Jaundice and abnormalities in liver function tests have been observed during clindamycin therapy.

Renal: Although no direct relationship of clindamycin to renal damage has been established, renal dysfunction as evidenced by azotemia, oliguria, and/or proteinuria has been observed in rare instances.

Hematopoietic: Transient neutropenia (leukopenia) and eosinophilia have been reported. Reports of agranulocytosis and thrombocytopenia have been made. No direct etiologic relationship to concurrent clindamycin therapy could be made in any of the foregoing.

Musculoskeletal: Rare instances of polyarthritis have been reported.

OVERDOSAGE

Significant mortality was observed in mice at an intravenous dose of 855 mg/kg and in rats at an oral or subcutaneous dose of approximately 2618 mg/kg. In the mice, convulsions and depression were observed. Hemodialysis and peritoneal dialysis are not effective in removing clindamycin from the serum.

DOSAGE AND ADMINISTRATION

If significant diarrhea occurs during therapy, this antibiotic should be discontinued (see **WARNING** box).

Concomitant administration of food does not adversely affect the absorption of clindamycin palmitate HCl contained in CLEOCIN PEDIATRIC Flavored Granules.

Serious infections: 8-12 mg/kg/day (4-6 mg/lb/day) divided into 3 or 4 equal doses.

Severe infections: 13-16 mg/kg/day (6.5-8 mg/lb/day) divided into 3 or 4 equal doses.

More severe infections: 17-25 mg/kg/day (8.5-12.5 mg/lb/day) divided into 3 or 4 equal doses.

In pediatric patients weighing 10 kg or less, ½ teaspoon (37.5 mg) three times a day should be considered the minimum recommended dose.

Serious infections due to anaerobic bacteria are usually treated with CLEOCIN PHOSPHATE® Sterile Solution. However, in clinically appropriate circumstances, the physician may elect to initiate treatment or continue treatment with CLEOCIN PEDIATRIC.

NOTE: In cases of ß-hemolytic streptococcal infections, treatment should be continued for at least 10 days.

Reconstitution Instructions: When reconstituted with water as follows, each 5 mL (teaspoon) of solution contains clindamycin palmitate HCl equivalent to 75 mg clindamycin.

Reconstitute bottles of 100 mL with **75 mL** of water. Add a large portion of the water and shake vigorously; add the remainder of the water and shake until the solution is uniform.

Storage Conditions: Store at controlled room temperature 20° to 25°C (68° to 77°F) [see USP].

Do **NOT** refrigerate the reconstituted solution; when chilled, the solution may thicken and be difficult to pour. The solution is stable for 2 weeks at room temperature.

HOW SUPPLIED

CLEOCIN PEDIATRIC Flavored Granules for oral solution is available in bottles of 100 mL (NDC 0009-0760-04).

When reconstituted as directed, each bottle yields a solution containing 75 mg of clindamycin per 5 mL.

ANIMAL TOXICOLOGY

One year oral toxicity studies in Spartan Sprague-Dawley rats and beagle dogs at dose levels up to 300 mg/kg/day (approximately 1.6 and 5.4 times the highest recommended adult human oral dose based on mg/m^2, respectively) have shown clindamycin to be well tolerated. No appreciable difference in pathological findings has been observed between groups of animals treated with clindamycin and comparable control groups. Rats receiving clindamycin hydrochloride at 600 mg/kg/day (approximately 3.2 times the highest recommended adult human oral dose based on mg/m^2) for 6 months tolerated the drug well; however, dogs dosed at this level (approximately 10.8 times the highest recommended adult human oral dose based on mg/m^2) vomited, would not eat, and lost weight.

℞ only

REFERENCES

1. Smith RB, Phillips JP: Evaluation of CLEOCIN HCl and CLEOCIN Phosphate in an Aged Population. Upjohn TR 8147-82-9122-021, December 1982.
2. Bauer AW, Kirby WMM, Sherris JC, Turck M: Antibiotic susceptibility testing by a standardized single disk

Continued on next page

Cleocin Pediatric—Cont.

method. *Am J. Clin. Path.*, **45**:493–496, 1966. Standardized Disk Susceptibility Test, *Federal Register,* **37**:20527–29, 1972.

Manufactured for
Pharmacia & Upjohn Company
A subsidiary of Pharmacia Corporation
Kalamazoo, Michigan 49001, USA
By
International Processing Corporation
Winchester, Kentucky 40391, USA
Revised September 2003

810 568 315
692167
0760-04

CLEOCIN PHOSPHATE® ℞
[*klē-ō-sĭn*]
(clindamycin injection, USP and clindamycin injection in 5% dextrose)
Sterile Solution is for Intramuscular and Intravenous Use
CLEOCIN PHOSPHATE in the ADD-Vantage™ Vial is For Intravenous Use Only

Prescribing information for this product, which appears on pages 2734–2736 of the 2004 PDR, has been completely revised as follows. Please write "See Supplement A" next to the product heading.

To reduce the development of drug-resistant bacteria and maintain the effectiveness of CLEOCIN PHOSPHATE and other antibacterial drugs, CLEOCIN PHOSPHATE should be used only to treat or prevent infections that are proven or strongly suspected to be caused by bacteria.

WARNING

Pseudomembranous colitis has been reported with nearly all antibacterial agents, including clindamycin, and may range in severity from mild to life-threatening. Therefore, it is important to consider this diagnosis in patients who present with diarrhea subsequent to the administration of antibacterial agents.

Because clindamycin therapy has been associated with severe colitis which may end fatally, it should be reserved for serious infections where less toxic antimicrobial agents are inappropriate, as described in the **INDICATIONS AND USAGE** section. It should not be used in patients with nonbacterial infections such as most upper respiratory tract infections. Treatment with antibacterial agents alters the normal flora of the colon and may permit overgrowth of clostridia. Studies indicate that a toxin produced by *Clostridium difficile* is one primary cause of "antibiotic-associated colitis".

After the diagnosis of pseudomembranous colitis has been established, therapeutic measures should be initiated. Mild cases of pseudomembranous colitis usually respond to drug discontinuation alone. In moderate to severe cases, consideration should be given to management with fluids and electrolytes, protein supplementation, and treatment with an antibacterial drug clinically effective against *C. difficile* colitis.

Diarrhea, colitis, and pseudomembranous colitis have been observed to begin up to several weeks following cessation of therapy with clindamycin.

DESCRIPTION

CLEOCIN PHOSPHATE Sterile Solution in vials contains clindamycin phosphate, a water soluble ester of clindamycin and phosphoric acid. Each mL contains the equivalent of 150 mg clindamycin, 0.5 mg disodium edetate and 9.45 mg benzyl alcohol added as preservative in each mL.

Clindamycin is a semisynthetic antibiotic produced by a 7(S)-chloro-substitution of the 7(R)-hydroxyl group of the parent compound lincomycin.

The chemical name of clindamycin phosphate is L-*threo*-α-D-*galacto*-Octopyranoside, methyl 7-chloro-6,7,8-trideoxy-6-[[(1-methyl-4-propyl-2-pyrrolidinyl) carbonyl] amino]-1-thio-, 2-(dihydrogen phosphate), (2*S*-*trans*)-.

The molecular formula is $C_{18}H_{34}ClN_2O_8PS$ and the molecular weight is 504.96.

The structural formula is represented below:

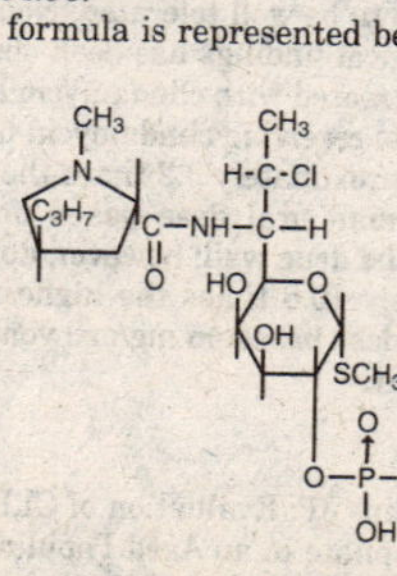

CLEOCIN PHOSPHATE in the ADD-Vantage Vial is intended for intravenous use only after further dilution with appropriate volume of ADD-Vantage diluent base solution.

CLEOCIN PHOSPHATE IV Solution in the Galaxy® plastic container for intravenous use is composed of clindamycin phosphate equivalent to 300, 600 and 900 mg of clindamycin premixed with 5% dextrose as a sterile solution. Disodium edetate has been added at a concentration of 0.04 mg/mL. The pH has been adjusted with sodium hydroxide and/or hydrochloric acid.

The plastic container is fabricated from a specially designed multilayer plastic, PL 2501. Solutions in contact with the plastic container can leach out certain of its chemical components in very small amounts within the expiration period. The suitability of the plastic has been confirmed in tests in animals according to the USP biological tests for plastic containers, as well as by tissue culture toxicity studies.

CLINICAL PHARMACOLOGY

Biologically inactive clindamycin phosphate is rapidly converted to active clindamycin.

By the end of short-term intravenous infusion, peak serum levels of active clindamycin are reached. Biologically inactive clindamycin phosphate disappears rapidly from the serum; the average elimination half-life is 6 minutes; however, the serum elimination half-life of active clindamycin is about 3 hours in adults and 2½ hours in pediatric patients.

After intramuscular injection of clindamycin phosphate, peak levels of active clindamycin are reached within 3 hours in adults and 1 hour in pediatric patients. Serum level curves may be constructed from IV peak serum levels as given in Table 1 by application of elimination half-lives listed above.

Serum levels of clindamycin can be maintained above the *in vitro* minimum inhibitory concentrations for most indicated organisms by administration of clindamycin phosphate every 8 to 12 hours in adults and every 6 to 8 hours in pediatric patients, or by continuous intravenous infusion. An equilibrium state is reached by the third dose.

The elimination half-life of clindamycin is increased slightly in patients with markedly reduced renal or hepatic function. Hemodialysis and peritoneal dialysis are not effective in removing clindamycin from the serum. Dosage schedules need not be modified in the presence of mild or moderate renal or hepatic disease.

No significant levels of clindamycin are attained in the cerebrospinal fluid even in the presence of inflamed meninges.

Pharmacokinetic studies in elderly volunteers (61-79 years) and younger adults (18-39 years) indicate that age alone does not alter clindamycin pharmacokinetics (clearance, elimination half-life, volume of distribution, and area under the serum concentration-time curve) after IV administration of clindamycin phosphate. After oral administration of clindamycin hydrochloride, elimination half-life is increased to approximately 4.0 hours (range 3.4–5.1 h) in the elderly compared to 3.2 hours (range 2.1–4.2 h) in younger adults. The extent of absorption, however, is not different between age groups and no dosage alteration is necessary for the elderly with normal hepatic function and normal (age-adjusted) renal function[1].

Serum assays for active clindamycin require an inhibitor to prevent *in vitro* hydrolysis of clindamycin phosphate.

Table 1. Average Peak and Trough Serum Concentrations of Active Clindamycin After Dosing with Clindamycin Phosphate

Dosage Regimen	Peak mcg/mL	Trough mcg/mL
Healthy Adult Males (Post equilibrium)		
600 mg IV in 30 min q6h	10.9	2.0
600 mg IV in 30 min q8h	10.8	1.1
900 mg IV in 30 min q8h	14.1	1.7
600 mg IM q12h*	9	
Pediatric Patients (first dose)*		
5–7 mg/kg IV in 1 hour	10	
5–7 mg/kg IM	8	
3–5 mg/kg IM	4	

*Data in this group from patients being treated for infection.

Microbiology: Although clindamycin phosphate is inactive *in vitro*, rapid *in vivo* hydrolysis converts this compound to the antibacterially active clindamycin.

Clindamycin has been shown to have *in vitro* activity against isolates of the following organisms:

Aerobic gram positive cocci, including:
- Staphylococcus aureus
- Staphylococcus epidermidis (penicillinase and non-penicillinase producing strains). When tested by *in vitro* methods, some staphylococcal strains originally resistant to erythromycin rapidly develop resistance to clindamycin.
- Streptococci (except *Enterococcus faecalis*)
- Pneumococci

Anaerobic gram negative bacilli, including:
- *Bacteroides* species (including *Bacteroides fragilis* group and *Bacteroides melaninogenicus* group)
- *Fusobacterium* species

Anaerobic gram positive nonsporeforming bacilli, including:
- *Propionibacterium*
- *Eubacterium*
- *Actinomyces* species

Anaerobic and *microaerophilic gram positive cocci*, including:
- *Peptococcus* species
- *Peptostreptococcus* species
- Microaerophilic streptococci

Clostridia: Clostridia are more resistant than most anaerobes to clindamycin. Most *Clostridium perfringens* are susceptible, but other species, e.g., *Clostridium sporogenes* and *Clostridium tertium* are frequently resistant to clindamycin. Susceptibility testing should be done.

Cross resistance has been demonstrated between clindamycin and lincomycin.

Antagonism has been demonstrated between clindamycin and erythromycin.

In vitro Susceptibility Testing:

Disk diffusion technique-Quantitative methods that require measurement of zone diameters give the most precise estimates of antibiotic susceptibility. One such procedure[2] has been recommended for use with disks to test susceptibility to clindamycin.

Reports from a laboratory using the standardized single-disk susceptibility test[1] with a 2 mcg clindamycin disk should be interpreted according to the following criteria:

Susceptible organisms produce zones of 17 mm or greater, indicating that the tested organism is likely to respond to therapy.

Organisms of intermediate susceptibility produce zones of 15–16 mm, indicating that the tested organism would be susceptible if a high dosage is used or if the infection is confined to tissues and fluids (e.g., urine), in which high antibiotic levels are attained.

Resistant organisms produce zones of 14 mm or less, indicating that other therapy should be selected.

Standardized procedures require the use of control organisms. The 2 mcg clindamycin disk should give a zone diameter between 24 and 30 mm for *S. aureus* ATCC 25923.

Dilution techniques—A bacterial isolate may be considered susceptible if the minimum inhibitory concentration (MIC) for clindamycin is not more than 1.6 mcg/mL. Organisms are considered moderately susceptible if the MIC is greater than 1.6 mcg/mL and less than or equal to 4.8 mcg/mL. Organisms are considered resistant if the MIC is greater than 4.8 mcg per mL.

The range of MICs for the control strains are as follows:
S. aureus ATCC 29213, 0.06 — 0.25 mcg/mL.
E. faecalis ATCC 29212, 4.0 — 16 mcg/mL.

For anaerobic bacteria the minimum inhibitory concentration (MIC) of clindamycin can be determined by agar dilution and broth dilution (including microdilution) techniques.[3] If MICs are not determined routinely, the disk broth method is recommended for routine use. THE KIRBY-BAUER DISK DIFFUSION METHOD AND ITS INTERPRETIVE STANDARDS ARE NOT RECOMMENDED FOR ANAEROBES.

INDICATIONS AND USAGE

CLEOCIN PHOSPHATE products are indicated in the treatment of serious infections caused by susceptible anaerobic bacteria.

CLEOCIN PHOSPHATE products are also indicated in the treatment of serious infections due to susceptible strains of streptococci, pneumococci, and staphylococci. Its use should be reserved for penicillin-allergic patients or other patients for whom, in the judgment of the physician, a penicillin is inappropriate. Because of the risk of antibiotic-associated pseudomembranous colitis, as described in the WARNING box, before selecting clindamycin the physician should consider the nature of the infection and the suitability of less toxic alternatives (e.g., erythromycin).

Bacteriologic studies should be performed to determine the causative organisms and their susceptibility to clindamycin.

Indicated surgical procedures should be performed in conjunction with antibiotic therapy.

CLEOCIN PHOSPHATE is indicated in the treatment of serious infections caused by susceptible strains of the designated organisms in the conditions listed below:

Lower respiratory tract infections including pneumonia, empyema, and lung abscess caused by anaerobes, *Streptococcus pneumoniae*, other streptococci (except *E. faecalis*), and *Staphylococcus aureus*.

Skin and skin structure infections caused by *Streptococcus pyogenes*, *Staphylococcus aureus*, and anaerobes.

Gynecological infections including endometritis, nongonococcal tubo-ovarian abscess, pelvic cellulitis, and postsurgical vaginal cuff infection caused by susceptible anaerobes.

Intra-abdominal infections including peritonitis and intra-abdominal abscess caused by susceptible anaerobic organisms.

Septicemia caused by *Staphylococcus aureus*, streptococci (except *Enterococcus faecalis*), and susceptible anaerobes.

Bone and joint infections including acute hematogenous osteomyelitis caused by *Staphylococcus aureus* and as adjunctive therapy in the surgical treatment of chronic bone and joint infections due to susceptible organisms.

To reduce the development of drug-resistant bacteria and maintain the effectiveness of CLEOCIN PHOSPHATE and other antibacterial drugs, CLEOCIN PHOSPHATE should be used only to treat or prevent infections that are proven or strongly suspected to be caused by susceptible bacteria. When culture and susceptibility information are available, they should be considered in selecting or modifying antibacterial therapy. In the absence of such data, local epidemiology and susceptibility patterns may contribute to the empiric selection of therapy.

CONTRAINDICATIONS

This drug is contraindicated in individuals with a history of hypersensitivity to preparations containing clindamycin or lincomycin.

WARNINGS

See **WARNING** box.

Pseudomembranous colitis has been reported with nearly all antibacterial agents, including clindamycin, and may range in severity from mild to life-threatening. Therefore, it is important to consider this diagnosis in patients who present with diarrhea subsequent to the administration of antibacterial agents.

Treatment with antibacterial agents alters the normal flora of the colon and may permit overgrowth of clostridia. Studies indicate that a toxin produced by *clostridium difficile* is one primary cause of "antibiotic-associated colitis".

After the diagnosis of pseudomembranous colitis has been established, therapeutic measures should be initiated. Mild cases of pseudomembranous colitis usually respond to drug discontinuation alone. In moderate to severe cases, consideration should be given to management with fluids and electrolytes, protein supplementation, and treatment with an antibacterial drug clinically effective against *C. difficile* colitis.

A careful inquiry should be made concerning previous sensitivities to drugs and other allergens.

This product contains benzyl alcohol as a preservative. Benzyl alcohol has been associated with a fatal "Gasping Syndrome" in premature infants. (See **PRECAUTIONS–Pediatric Use.**)

Usage in Meningitis—Since clindamycin does not diffuse adequately into the cerebrospinal fluid, the drug should not be used in the treatment of meningitis.

SERIOUS ANAPHYLACTOID REACTIONS REQUIRE IMMEDIATE EMERGENCY TREATMENT WITH EPINEPHRINE. OXYGEN AND INTRAVENOUS CORTICOSTEROIDS SHOULD ALSO BE ADMINISTERED AS INDICATED.

PRECAUTIONS

General

Review of experience to date suggests that a subgroup of older patients with associated severe illness may tolerate diarrhea less well. When clindamycin is indicated in these patients, they should be carefully monitored for change in bowel frequency.

CLEOCIN PHOSPHATE products should be prescribed with caution in individuals with a history of gastrointestinal disease, particularly colitis.

CLEOCIN PHOSPHATE should be prescribed with caution in atopic individuals.

Certain infections may require incision and drainage or other indicated surgical procedures in addition to antibiotic therapy.

The use of CLEOCIN PHOSPHATE may result in overgrowth of nonsusceptible organisms—particularly yeasts. Should superinfections occur, appropriate measures should be taken as indicated by the clinical situation.

CLEOCIN PHOSPHATE should not be injected intravenously undiluted as a bolus, but should be infused over at least 10–60 minutes as directed in the DOSAGE AND ADMINISTRATION section.

Clindamycin dosage modification may not be necessary in patients with renal disease. In patients with moderate to severe liver disease, prolongation of clindamycin half-life has been found. However, it was postulated from studies that when given every eight hours, accumulation should rarely occur. Therefore, dosage modification in patients with liver disease may not be necessary. However, periodic liver enzyme determinations should be made when treating patients with severe liver disease.

Prescribing CLEOCIN PHOSPHATE in the absence of a proven or strongly suspected bacterial infection or a prophylactic indication is unlikely to provide benefit to the patient and increases the risk of the development of drug-resistant bacteria.

Information for Patients

Patients should be counseled that antibacterial drugs including CLEOCIN PHOSPHATE should only be used to treat bacterial infections. They do not treat viral infections (e.g., the common cold). When CLEOCIN PHOSPHATE is prescribed to treat a bacterial infection, patients should be told that although it is common to feel better early in the course of therapy, the medication should be taken exactly as directed. Skipping doses or not completing the full course of therapy may (1) decrease the effectiveness of the immediate treatment and (2) increase the likelihood that bacteria will develop resistance and will not be treatable by CLEOCIN PHOSPHATE or other antibacterial drugs in the future.

Laboratory Tests

During prolonged therapy periodic liver and kidney function tests and blood counts should be performed.

Drug Interactions

Clindamycin has been shown to have neuromuscular blocking properties that may enhance the action of other neuromuscular blocking agents. Therefore, it should be used with caution in patients receiving such agents.

Antagonism has been demonstrated between clindamycin and erythromycin *in vitro*. Because of possible clinical significance, the two drugs should not be administered concurrently.

Carcinogenesis, Mutagenesis, Impairment of Fertility

Long term studies in animals have not been performed with clindamycin to evaluate carcinogenic potential. Genotoxicity tests performed included a rat micronucleus test and an Ames Salmonella reversion test. Both tests were negative.

Fertility studies in rats treated orally with up to 300 mg/kg/day (approximately 1.1 times the highest recommended adult human dose based on mg/m^2) revealed no effects on fertility or mating ability.

Pregnancy: Teratogenic effects

Pregnancy category B

Reproduction studies performed in rats and mice using oral doses of clindamycin up to 600 mg/kg/day (2.1 and 1.1 times the highest recommended adult human dose based on mg/m^2, respectively) or subcutaneous doses of clindamycin up to 250 mg/kg/day (0.9 and 0.5 times the highest recommended adult human dose based on mg/m^2, respectively) revealed no evidence of teratogenicity.

There are, however, no adequate and well-controlled studies in pregnant women. Because animal reproduction studies are not always predictive of the human response, this drug should be used during pregnancy only if clearly needed.

Nursing Mothers

Clindamycin has been reported to appear in breast milk in the range of 0.7 to 3.8 mcg/mL at dosages of 150 mg orally to 600 mg intravenously. Because of the potential for adverse reactions due to clindamycin in neonates (see **Pediatric Use**), the decision to discontinue the drug should be made, taking into account the importance of the drug to the mother.

Pediatric Use

When CLEOCIN PHOSPHATE Sterile Solution is administered to the pediatric population (birth to 16 years) appropriate monitoring of organ system functions is desirable.

Usage in Newborns and Infants

This product contains benzyl alcohol as a preservative. Benzyl alcohol has been associated with a fatal "Gasping Syndrome" in premature infants.

The potential for the toxic effect in the pediatric population from chemicals that may leach from the single dose premixed IV preparation in plastic has not been evaluated.

Geriatric Use

Clinical studies of clindamycin did not include sufficient numbers of patients age 65 and over to determine whether they respond differently from younger patients. However, other reported clinical experience indicates that antibiotic-associated colitis and diarrhea (due to *Clostridium difficile*) seen in association with most antibiotics occur more frequently in the elderly (>60 years) and may be more severe. These patients should be carefully monitored for the development of diarrhea.

Pharmacokinetic studies with clindamycin have shown no clinically important differences between young and elderly subjects with normal hepatic function and normal (age-adjusted) renal function after oral or intravenous administration.

ADVERSE REACTIONS

The following reactions have been reported with the use of clindamycin.

Gastrointestinal: Antibiotic-associated colitis (see **WARNINGS**), pseudomembranous colitis, abdominal pain, nausea, and vomiting. The onset of pseudomembranous colitis symptoms may occur during or after antibacterial treatment (see **WARNINGS**). An unpleasant or metallic taste occasionally has been reported after intravenous administration of the higher doses of clindamycin phosphate.

Hypersensitivity Reactions: Maculopapular rash and urticaria have been observed during drug therapy. Generalized mild to moderate morbilliform-like skin rashes are the most frequently reported of all adverse reactions. Rare instances of erythema multiforme, some resembling Stevens-Johnson syndrome, have been associated with clindamycin. A few cases of anaphylactoid reactions have been reported. If a hypersensitivity reaction occurs, the drug should be discontinued. The usual agents (epinephrine, corticosteroids, antihistamines) should be available for emergency treatment of serious reactions.

Skin and Mucous Membranes: Pruritus, vaginitis, and rare instances of exfoliative dermatitis have been reported (see *Hypersensitivity Reactions*).

Liver: Jaundice and abnormalities in liver function tests have been observed during clindamycin therapy.

Renal: Although no direct relationship of clindamycin to renal damage has been established, renal dysfunction as evidenced by azotemia, oliguria, and/or proteinuria has been observed in rare instances.

Hematopoietic: Transient neutropenia (leukopenia) and eosinophilia have been reported. Reports of agranulocytosis and thrombocytopenia have been made. No direct etiologic relationship to concurrent clindamycin therapy could be made in any of the foregoing.

Local Reactions: Pain, induration and sterile abscess have been reported after intramuscular injection and thrombophlebitis after intravenous infusion. Reactions can be minimized or avoided by giving deep intramuscular injections and avoiding prolonged use of indwelling intravenous catheters.

Musculoskeletal: Rare instances of polyarthritis have been reported.

Cardiovascular: Rare instances of cardiopulmonary arrest and hypotension have been reported following too rapid intravenous administration. (See **DOSAGE AND ADMINISTRATION** section.)

OVERDOSAGE

Significant mortality was observed in mice at an intravenous dose of 855 mg/kg and in rats at an oral or subcutaneous dose of approximately 2618 mg/kg. In the mice, convulsions and depression were observed.

Hemodialysis and peritoneal dialysis are not effective in removing clindamycin from the serum.

DOSAGE AND ADMINISTRATION

If diarrhea occurs during therapy, this antibiotic should be discontinued (see **WARNING** box).

Adults: Parenteral (IM or IV Administration): Serious infections due to aerobic gram-positive cocci and the more susceptible anaerobes (NOT generally including *Bacteroides fragilis, Peptococcus* species and *Clostridium* species other than *Clostridium perfringens*):

600–1200 mg/day in 2, 3 or 4 equal doses.

More severe infections, particularly those due to proven or suspected *Bacteroides fragilis, Peptococcus* species, or *Clostridium* species other than *Clostridium perfringens*:

1200–2700 mg/day in 2, 3 or 4 equal doses.

For more serious infections, these doses may have to be increased. In life-threatening situations due to either aerobes or anaerobes these doses may be increased. Doses of as much as 4800 mg daily have been given intravenously to adults. See **Dilution and Infusion Rates** section below.

Single intramuscular injections of greater than 600 mg are not recommended.

Alternatively, drug may be administered in the form of a single rapid infusion of the first dose followed by continuous IV infusion as follows:

To maintain serum clindamycin levels	Rapid infusion rate	Maintenance infusion rate
Above 4 mcg/mL	10 mg/min for 30 min	0.75 mg/min
Above 5 mcg/mL	15 mg/min for 30 min	1.00 mg/min
Above 6 mcg/mL	20 mg/min for 30 min	1.25 mg/min

Neonates (less than 1 month):

15 to 20 mg/kg/day in 3 to 4 equal doses. The lower dosage may be adequate for small prematures.

Pediatric patients 1 month of age to 16 years: Parenteral (IM or IV) administration: 20 to 40 mg/kg/day in 3 or 4 equal doses. The higher doses would be used for more severe infections. As an alternative to dosing on a body weight basis, pediatric patients may be dosed on the basis of square meters body surface: 350 mg/m^2/day for serious infections and 450 mg/m^2/day for more severe infections.

Parenteral therapy may be changed to oral CLEOCIN PEDIATRIC® Flavored Granules (clindamycin palmitate hydrochloride) or CLEOCIN HCl® Capsules (clindamycin hydrochloride) when the condition warrants and at the discretion of the physician.

In cases of β-hemolytic streptococcal infections, treatment should be continued for at least 10 days.

Dilution and Infusion Rates: Clindamycin phosphate must be diluted prior to IV administration. The concentration of clindamycin in diluent for infusion should not exceed 18 mg per mL. Infusion rates should not exceed 30 mg per minute. The usual infusion dilutions and rates are as follows:

Dose	Diluent	Time
300 mg	50 mL	10 min
600 mg	50 mL	20 min
900 mg	50-100 mL	30 min
1200 mg	100 mL	40 min

Administration of more than 1200 mg in a single 1-hour infusion is not recommended.

Parenteral drug products should be inspected visually for particulate matter and discoloration prior to administration, whenever solution and container permit.

Dilution and Compatibility: Physical and biological compatibility studies monitored for 24 hours at room temperature have demonstrated no inactivation or incompatibility with the use of CLEOCIN PHOSPHATE Sterile Solution (clindamycin phosphate) in IV solutions containing sodium chloride, glucose, calcium or potassium, and solutions containing vitamin B complex in concentrations usually used clinically. No incompatibility has been demonstrated with the antibiotics cephalothin, kanamycin, gentamicin, penicillin or carbenicillin.

The following drugs are physically incompatible with clindamycin phosphate: ampicillin sodium, phenytoin sodium, barbiturates, aminophylline, calcium gluconate, and magnesium sulfate.

The compatibility and duration of stability of drug admixtures will vary depending on concentration and other conditions. For current information regarding compatibilities of clindamycin phosphate under specific conditions, please contact the Medical and Drug Information Unit, Pharmacia & Upjohn Company.

Physico-Chemical Stability of diluted solutions of CLEOCIN PHOSPHATE

Room temperature: 6, 9 and 12 mg/mL (equivalent to clindamycin base) in dextrose injection 5%, sodium chloride injection 0.9%, or Lactated Ringers Injection in glass bottles or minibags, demonstrated physical and chemical stability for at least 16 days at 25°C. Also, 18 mg/mL (equivalent to clindamycin base) in dextrose injection 5%, in minibags, demonstrated physical and chemical stability for at least 16 days at 25°C.

Refrigeration: 6, 9 and 12 mg/mL (equivalent to clindamycin base) in dextrose injection 5%, sodium chloride injection

Continued on next page

Cleocin Phosphate—Cont.

0.9%, or Lactated Ringers Injection in glass bottles or minibags, demonstrated physical and chemical stability for at least 32 days at 4°C.
IMPORTANT: This chemical stability information in no way indicates that it would be acceptable practice to use this product well after the preparation time. Good professional practice suggests that compounded admixtures should be administered as soon after preparation as is feasible.
Frozen: 6, 9 and 12 mg/mL (equivalent to clindamycin base) in dextrose injection 5%, sodium chloride injection 0.9%, or Lactated Ringers Injection in minibags demonstrated physical and chemical stability for at least eight weeks at -10°C. Frozen solutions should be thawed at room temperature and not refrozen.

DIRECTIONS FOR DISPENSING

Pharmacy Bulk Package — Not for Direct Infusion
The Pharmacy Bulk Package is for use in a Pharmacy Admixture Service only under a laminar flow hood. Entry into the vial should be made with a small diameter sterile transfer set or other small diameter sterile dispensing device, and contents dispensed in aliquots using aseptic technique. Multiple entries with a needle and syringe are not recommended. AFTER ENTRY USE ENTIRE CONTENTS OF VIAL PROMPTLY. ANY UNUSED PORTION MUST BE DISCARDED WITHIN 24 HOURS AFTER INITIAL ENTRY.

DIRECTIONS FOR USE

CLEOCIN PHOSPHATE IV Solution in Galaxy Plastic Container

Premixed CLEOCIN PHOSPHATE IV Solution is for intravenous administration using sterile equipment. Check for minute leaks prior to use by squeezing bag firmly. If leaks are found, discard solution as sterility may be impaired. Do not add supplementary medication. Parenteral drug products should be inspected visually for particulate matter and discoloration prior to administration whenever solution and container permit. Do not use unless solution is clear and seal is intact.
Caution: Do not use plastic containers in series connections. Such use could result in air embolism due to residual air being drawn from the primary container before administration of the fluid from the secondary container is complete.

Preparation for Administration:
1. Suspend container from eyelet support.
2. Remove protector from outlet port at bottom of container.
3. Attach administration set. Refer to complete directions accompanying set.

Preparation of CLEOCIN PHOSPHATE in ADD-Vantage System—For IV Use Only. CLEOCIN PHOSPHATE 600 mg and 900 mg may be reconstituted in 50 mL or 100 mL, respectively, of Dextrose Injection 5% or Sodium Chloride Injection 0.9% in the ADD-diluent container. Refer to separate instructions for ADD-Vantage‡ System.

HOW SUPPLIED

Each mL of CLEOCIN PHOSPHATE Sterile Solution contains clindamycin phosphate equivalent to 150 mg clindamycin; 0.5 mg disodium edetate; 9.45 mg benzyl alcohol added as preservative. When necessary, pH is adjusted with sodium hydroxide and/or hydrochloric acid. CLEOCIN PHOSPHATE is available in the following packages:

25-2 mL vials	NDC 0009-0870-26
25-4 mL vials	NDC 0009-0775-26
25-6 mL vials	NDC 0009-0902-11
1-60 mL Pharmacy Bulk Package	NDC 0009-0728-05

CLEOCIN PHOSPHATE is supplied in ADD-Vantage vials as follows:

NDC	Vial Size	Total Clindamycin Phosphate/vial	Amount of Diluent
0009-3124-01	4 mL	600 mg	50 mL
0009-3447-01	6 mL	900 mg	100 mL

Store at controlled room temperature 20° to 25°C (68° to 77°F) [see USP].
CLEOCIN PHOSPHATE IV Solution in Galaxy plastic containers is a sterile solution of clindamycin phosphate with 5% dextrose. The single dose Galaxy plastic containers are available as follows:

24-300 mg/50 mL containers	NDC 0009-3381-01
24-600 mg/50 mL containers	NDC 0009-3375-01
24-900 mg/50 mL containers	NDC 0009-3382-01

Exposure of pharmaceutical products to heat should be minimized. It is recommended that Galaxy plastic containers be stored at room temperature (25°C). Avoid temperatures above 30°C.

ANIMAL TOXICOLOGY

One year oral toxicity studies in Spartan Sprague-Dawley rats and beagle dogs at dose levels up to 300 mg/kg/day (approximately 1.1 and 3.6 times the highest recommended adult human dose based on mg/m², respectively) have shown clindamycin to be well tolerated. No appreciable difference in pathological findings has been observed between groups of animals treated with clindamycin and comparable control groups. Rats receiving clindamycin hydrochloride at 600 mg/kg/day (approximately 2.1 times the highest recommended adult human dose based on mg/m²) for 6 months tolerated the drug well; however, dogs dosed at this level (approximately 7.2 times the highest recommended adult human dose based on mg/m²) vomited, would not eat, and lost weight.

℞ only
Pharmacia & Upjohn Company
A subsidiary of Pharmacia Corporation
Kalamazoo, MI 49001, USA
Revised September 2003 810 020 140
691273
0775-26

REFERENCES

1. Smith RB, Phillips JP: Evaluation of CLEOCIN HCl and CLEOCIN Phosphate in an Aged Population. Upjohn TR 8147-82-9122-021, December 1982.
2. Bauer AW, Kirby WMM, Sherris JC, Turck M; Antibiotic susceptibility testing by a standardized single disk method. *Am. J. Clin. Path.*, **45**:493–496, 1966. Standardized Disk Susceptibility Test, *Federal Register*, **37**:20527–29, 1972.
3. National Committee for Clinical Lab. Standards. Methods for Antimicrobial Susceptibility Testing of Anaerobic Bacteria—Second Edition; Tentative Standard. NCCLS publication M11-T2. Villanova, PA; NCCLS; 1988.

‡ADD-Vantage is a registered trademark of Abbott Laboratories.
CLEOCIN PHOSPHATE IV Solution in the Galaxy plastic containers is manufactured for Pharmacia & Upjohn Company by Baxter Healthcare Corporation, Deerfield, IL 60015.
Galaxy® is a registered trademark of Baxter International, Inc.

CLEOCIN® ℞
[*klē-ō-sĭn*]
(clindamycin phosphate vaginal cream, USP)

FOR INTRAVAGINAL USE ONLY
NOT FOR OPHTHALMIC, DERMAL, OR ORAL USE

Prescribing information for this product, which appears on pages 2736–2739 of the 2004 PDR, has been completely revised as follows. Please write "See Supplement A" next to the product heading.

DESCRIPTION

Clindamycin phosphate is a water soluble ester of the semi-synthetic antibiotic produced by a 7(S)-chloro-substitution of the 7(R)-hydroxyl group of the parent antibiotic lincomycin. The chemical name for clindamycin phosphate is methyl 7-chloro-6,7,8-trideoxy-6-(1-methyl-*trans*-4-propyl-L-2-pyrrolidinecarboxamido)-1-thio-L-*threo*-α-*D*-*galacto*-octopyranoside 2-(dihydrogen phosphate). It has a molecular weight of 504.96, and the molecular formula is $C_{18}H_{34}ClN_2O_8PS$. The structural formula is represented at right:

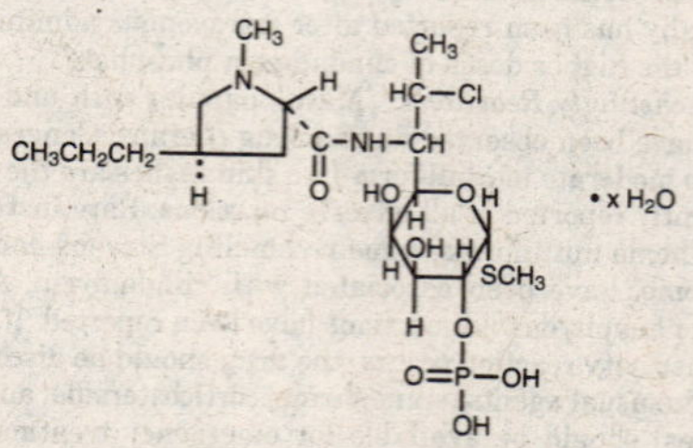

CLEOCIN Vaginal Cream 2%, is a semi-solid, white cream, which contains 2% clindamycin phosphate, USP, at a concentration equivalent to 20 mg clindamycin per gram. The pH of the cream is between 3.0 and 6.0. The cream also contains benzyl alcohol, cetostearyl alcohol, mixed fatty acid esters, mineral oil, polysorbate 60, propylene glycol, purified water, sorbitan monostearate, and stearic acid.
Each applicatorful of 5 grams of vaginal cream contains approximately 100 mg of clindamycin phosphate.

CLINICAL PHARMACOLOGY

Following a once a day intravaginal dose of 100 mg of clindamycin phosphate vaginal cream 2%, administered to 6 healthy female volunteers for 7 days, approximately 5% (range 0.6% to 11%) of the administered dose was absorbed systemically. The peak serum clindamycin concentration observed on the first day averaged 18 ng/mL (range 4 to 47 ng/mL) and on day 7 it averaged 25 ng/mL (range 6 to 61ng/mL). These peak concentrations were attained approximately 10 hours post-dosing (range 4-24 hours).
Following a once a day intravaginal dose of 100 mg of clindamycin phosphate vaginal cream 2%, administered for 7 consecutive days to 5 women with bacterial vaginosis, absorption was slower and less variable than that observed in healthy females. Approximately 5% (range 2% to 8%) of the dose was absorbed systemically. The peak serum clindamycin concentration observed on the first day averaged 13 ng/mL (range 6 to 34 ng/mL) and on day 7 it averaged 16 ng/mL (range 7 to 26 ng/mL). These peak concentrations were attained approximately 14 hours post-dosing (range 4-24 hours).
There was little or no systemic accumulation of clindamycin after repeated vaginal dosing of clindamycin phosphate vaginal cream 2%. The systemic half-life was 1.5 to 2.6 hours.

MICROBIOLOGY

Clindamycin inhibits bacterial protein synthesis at the level of the bacterial ribosome. The antibiotic binds preferentially to the 50S ribosomal subunit and affects the process of peptide chain initiation. Although clindamycin phosphate is inactive *in vitro*, rapid *in vivo* hydrolysis converts this compound to the antibacterially active clindamycin.
Culture and sensitivity testing of bacteria are not routinely performed to establish the diagnosis of bacterial vaginosis. (See INDICATIONS AND USAGE). Standard methodology for the susceptibility testing of the potential bacterial vaginosis pathogens, *Gardnerella vaginalis, Mobiluncus* spp., or *Mycoplasma hominis,* has not been defined. Nonetheless, clindamycin is an antimicrobial agent active *in vitro* against most strains of the following organisms that have been reported to be associated with bacterial vaginosis:
Bacteroides spp.
Gardnerella vaginalis
Mobiluncus spp.
Mycoplasma hominis
Peptostreptococcus spp.

INDICATIONS AND USAGE

CLEOCIN Vaginal Cream 2%, is indicated in the treatment of bacterial vaginosis (formerly referred to as *Haemophilus* vaginitis, *Gardnerella* vaginitis, nonspecific vaginitis, *Corynebacterium* vaginitis, or anaerobic vaginosis). CLEOCIN Vaginal Cream 2%, can be used to treat non-pregnant women and pregnant women during the second and third trimester. (See CLINICAL STUDIES.)

NOTE: For purposes of this indication, a clinical diagnosis of bacterial vaginosis is usually defined by the presence of a homogeneous vaginal discharge that (a) has a pH of greater than 4.5, (b) emits a "fishy" amine odor when mixed with a 10% KOH solution, and (c) contains clue cells on microscopic examination. Gram's stain results consistent with a diagnosis of bacterial vaginosis include (a) markedly reduced or absent *Lactobacillus* morphology, (b) predominance of *Gardnerella* morphotype, and (c) absent or few white blood cells.
Other pathogens commonly associated with vulvovaginitis, eg, *Trichomonas vaginalis, Chlamydia trachomatis, N. gonorrhoeae, Candida albicans,* and *Herpes simplex* virus should be ruled out.

CONTRAINDICATIONS

CLEOCIN Vaginal Cream 2%, is contraindicated in individuals with a history of hypersensitivity to clindamycin, lincomycin, or any of the components of this vaginal cream. CLEOCIN Vaginal Cream 2%, is also contraindicated in individuals with a history of regional enteritis, ulcerative colitis, or a history of "antibiotic-associated" colitis.

WARNINGS

Pseudomembranous colitis has been reported with nearly all antibacterial agents, including clindamycin, and may range in severity from mild to life-threatening. Orally and parenterally administered clindamycin has been associated with severe colitis which may end fatally. Diarrhea, bloody diarrhea, and colitis (including pseudomembranous colitis) have been reported with the use of orally and parenterally administered clindamycin, as well as with topical (dermal) formulations of clindamycin. Therefore, it is important to consider this diagnosis in patients who present with diarrhea subsequent to the administration of clindamycin, even when administered by the vaginal route, because approximately 5% of the clindamycin dose is systemically absorbed from the vagina.
Treatment with antibacterial agents alters the normal flora of the colon and may permit overgrowth of clostridia. Studies indicate that a toxin produced by *Clostridium difficile* is a primary cause of "antibiotic-associated" colitis.
After the diagnosis of pseudomembranous colitis has been established, therapeutic measures should be initiated. Mild cases of pseudomembranous colitis usually respond to discontinuation of the drug alone. In moderate to severe cases, consideration should be given to management with fluids and electrolytes, protein supplementation, and treatment with an antibacterial drug clinically effective against *Clostridium difficile* colitis.
Onset of pseudomembranous colitis symptoms may occur during or after antimicrobial treatment.

PRECAUTIONS

General

CLEOCIN Vaginal Cream 2%, contains ingredients that will cause burning and irritation of the eye. In the event of accidental contact with the eye, rinse the eye with copious amounts of cool tap water.
The use of CLEOCIN Vaginal Cream 2% may result in the overgrowth of nonsusceptible organisms in the vagina. In clinical studies involving 600 non-pregnant women who received treatment for 3 days, *Candida albicans* was detected, either symptomatically or by culture, in 8.8% of patients. In 9% of the patients, vaginitis was recorded. In clinical studies involving 1325 non-pregnant women who received treatment for 7 days, *Candida albicans* was detected, either symptomatically or by culture, in 10.5% of patients. Vaginitis was recorded in 10.7% of the patients. In 180 pregnant women who received treatment for 7 days, *Candida albicans* was detected, either symptomatically or by culture, in 13.3% of patients. In 7.2% of the patients, vaginitis was recorded. *Candida albicans,* as reported here, includes the terms: vaginal moniliasis and moniliasis (body as a whole).

Vaginitis includes the terms: vulvo-vaginal disorder, vulvovaginitis, vaginal discharge, trichomonal vaginitis, and vaginitis.

Information for the Patient:

The patient should be instructed not to engage in vaginal intercourse, or use other vaginal products (such as tampons or douches) during treatment with this product.

The patient should also be advised that this cream contains mineral oil that may weaken latex or rubber products such as condoms or vaginal contraceptive diaphragms. Therefore, use of such products within 72 hours following treatment with CLEOCIN Vaginal Cream 2%, is not recommended.

Drug Interactions

Clindamycin has been shown to have neuromuscular blocking properties that may enhance the action of other neuromuscular blocking agents. Therefore, it should be used with caution in patients receiving such agents.

Carcinogenesis, Mutagenesis, Impairment of Fertility

Long term studies in animals have not been performed with clindamycin to evaluate carcinogenic potential. Genotoxicity tests performed included a rat micronucleus test and an Ames test. Both tests were negative. Fertility studies in rats treated orally with up to 300 mg/kg/day (31 times the human exposure based on mg/m^2) revealed no effects on fertility or mating ability.

Pregnancy: Teratogenic effects

Pregnancy Category B

There are no adequate and well-controlled studies in pregnant women during the first trimester of pregnancy. This drug should be used during the first trimester of pregnancy only if clearly needed.

CLEOCIN Vaginal Cream 2% has been studied in pregnant women during the second trimester. In women treated for seven days, abnormal labor was reported in 1.1% of patients who received clindamycin vaginal cream 2% compared with 0.5% of patients who received placebo.

Reproduction studies have been performed in rats and mice using oral and parenteral doses of clindamycin up to 600 mg/kg/day (62 and 25 times, respectively, the maximum human exposure based on mg/m^2) and have revealed no evidence of harm to the fetus due to clindamycin. In one mouse strain, cleft palates were observed in treated fetuses; this outcome was not produced in other mouse strains or in other species and is, therefore, considered to be a strain specific effect.

See INDICATIONS AND USAGE; PRECAUTIONS, General; and ADVERSE REACTIONS.

Nursing Mothers

Clindamycin has been detected in human milk after oral or parenteral administration. It is not known if clindamycin is excreted in human milk following the use of vaginally administered clindamycin phosphate.

Because of the potential for serious adverse reactions in nursing infants from clindamycin phosphate, a decision should be made whether to discontinue nursing or to discontinue the drug, taking into account the importance of the drug to the mother.

Pediatric Use

Safety and effectiveness in pediatric patients have not been established.

Geriatric Use

Clinical studies for CLEOCIN Vaginal Cream 2% did not include sufficient numbers of subjects aged 65 and over to determine whether they respond differently from younger subjects. Other reported clinical experience has not identified differences in responses between the elderly and younger patients.

ADVERSE REACTIONS

Clinical trials

Non-pregnant Women: In clinical trials involving non-pregnant women, 1.8% of 600 patients who received treatment with CLEOCIN Vaginal Cream 2% for 3 days and 2.7% of 1325 patients who received treatment for 7 days discontinued therapy due to drug-related adverse events. Medical events judged to be related, probably related, possibly related, or of unknown relationship to vaginally administered clindamycin phosphate vaginal cream 2%, were reported for 20.7% of the patients receiving treatment for 3 days and 21.3% of the patients receiving treatment for 7 days. Events occurring in ≥1% of patients receiving clindamycin phosphate vaginal cream 2% are shown in Table 1.

TABLE 1 – Events Occurring in ≥1% of Non-pregnant Patients Receiving Clindamycin Phosphate Vaginal Cream 2%

Event	CLEOCIN Vaginal Cream	
	3 Day n=600	7 Day n=1325
Urogenital		
Vaginal moniliasis	7.7	10.4
Vulvovaginitis	6.0	4.4
Vulvovaginal disorder	3.2	5.3
Trichomonal vaginitis	0	1.3
Body as a Whole		
Moniliasis (body)	1.3	0.2

Other events occurring in < 1% of the clindamycin vaginal cream 2% groups include:

Urogenital system: vaginal discharge, metrorrhagia, urinary tract infection, endometriosis, menstrual disorder, vaginitis/vaginal infection, and vaginal pain.

Body as a whole: localized abdominal pain, generalized abdominal pain, abdominal cramps, halitosis, headache, bacterial infection, inflammatory swelling, allergic reaction, and fungal infection.

Digestive system: nausea, vomiting, constipation, dyspepsia, flatulence, diarrhea, and gastrointestinal disorder.

Endocrine system: hyperthyroidism.

Central nervous system: dizziness and vertigo.

Respiratory system: epistaxis.

Skin: pruritus (non-application site), moniliasis, rash, maculopapular rash, erythema, and urticaria.

Special senses: taste perversion.

Pregnant Women: In a clinical trial involving pregnant women during the second trimester, 1.7% of 180 patients who received treatment for 7 days discontinued therapy due to drug-related adverse events. Medical events judged to be related, probably related, possibly related, or of unknown relationship to vaginally administered clindamycin phosphate vaginal cream 2%, were reported for 22.8% of pregnant patients. Events occurring in ≥1% of patients receiving either clindamycin phosphate vaginal cream 2% or placebo are shown in Table 2.

TABLE 2 – Events Occurring in ≥ 1% of Pregnant Patients Receiving Clindamycin Phosphate Vaginal Cream 2% or Placebo

Event	CLEOCIN Vaginal Cream	Placebo
	7 DAY n=180	7 Day n=184
Urogenital		
Vaginal moniliasis	13.3	7.1
Vulvovaginal disorder	6.7	7.1
Abnormal labor	1.1	0.5
Body as a Whole		
Fungal infection	1.7	0
Skin		
Pruritus, non-application site	1.1	0

Other events occurring in <1% of the clindamycin vaginal cream 2% group include:

Urogenital system: dysuria, metrorrhagia, vaginal pain, and trichomonal vaginitis.

Body as a whole: upper respiratory infection.

Skin: pruritus (topical application site) and erythema.

Other clindamycin formulations:

Clindamycin vaginal cream affords minimal peak serum levels and systemic exposure (AUCs) of clindamycin compared to 100 mg oral clindamycin dosing. Although these lower levels of exposure are less likely to produce the common reactions seen with oral clindamycin, the possibility of these and other reactions cannot be excluded presently. Data from well-controlled trials directly comparing clindamycin administered orally to clindamycin administered vaginally are not available.

The following adverse reactions and altered laboratory tests have been reported with the **oral or parenteral** use of clindamycin:

Gastrointestinal: Abdominal pain, esophagitis, nausea, vomiting, and diarrhea. (See WARNINGS.)

Hematopoietic: Transient neutropenia (leukopenia), eosinophilia, agranulocytosis, and thrombocytopenia have been reported. No direct etiologic relationship to concurrent clindamycin therapy could be made in any of these reports.

Hypersensitivity Reactions: Maculopapular rash and urticaria have been observed during drug therapy. Generalized mild to moderate morbilliform-like skin rashes are the most frequently reported of all adverse reactions. Rare instances of erythema multiforme, some resembling Stevens-Johnson syndrome, have been associated with clindamycin. A few cases of anaphylactoid reactions have been reported. If a hypersensitivity reaction occurs, the drug should be discontinued.

Liver: Jaundice and abnormalities in liver function tests have been observed during clindamycin therapy.

Musculoskeletal: Rare instances of polyarthritis have been reported.

Renal: Although no direct relationship of clindamycin to renal damage has been established, renal dysfunction as evidenced by azotemia, oliguria, and/or proteinuria has been observed in rare instances.

OVERDOSAGE

Vaginally applied clindamycin phosphate vaginal cream 2% could be absorbed in sufficient amounts to produce systemic effects. (See WARNINGS.)

DOSAGE AND ADMINISTRATION

The recommended dose is one applicatorful of clindamycin phosphate vaginal cream 2%, (5 grams containing approximately 100 mg of clindamycin phosphate) intravaginally, preferably at bedtime, for 3 or 7 consecutive days in non-pregnant patients and for 7 consecutive days in pregnant patients. (See CLINICAL STUDIES.)

HOW SUPPLIED

CLEOCIN Vaginal Cream 2%, (clindamycin phosphate vaginal cream) is supplied as follows:

40 g tube
(with 7 disposable applicators) NDC 0009-3448-01

Store at controlled room temperature 20° to 25° C (68° to 77° F) [see USP]. Protect from freezing.

CLINICAL STUDIES

In two clinical studies involving 674 evaluable non-pregnant women with bacterial vaginosis comparing CLEOCIN Vaginal Cream 2% for 3 or 7 days, the clinical cure rates, determined at 1 month posttherapy, ranged from 72% to 81% for the 3-day treatment and 84% to 86% for the 7-day treatment.

	CLEOCIN 3 Day		CLEOCIN 7 Day	
US Study	94/131	72%	110/128	86%
European Study	161/199	81%	181/216	84%

In a clinical study involving 249 evaluable pregnant patients in the second and third trimester treated for 7 days, the clinical cure rate, determined at 1 month posttherapy, was 60% (77/129) in the clindamycin arm and 9% (11/120) for the vehicle arm. The determination of clinical cure was based on the absence of a "fishy" amine odor when the vaginal discharge was mixed with a 10% KOH solution and the absence of clue cells on microscopic examination.

℞ only

Pharmacia & Upjohn Company
A subsidiary of Pharmacia Corporation
Kalamazoo, Michigan 49001, USA

Revised August 2003 815 255 609
692910

DIRECTIONS FOR USE

Disposable plastic applicators are provided with this package. They are designed to allow proper vaginal administration of the cream.

Remove cap from cream tube. Screw a plastic applicator on the threaded end of the tube.

Rolling tube from the bottom, squeeze gently and force the medication into the applicator. The applicator is filled when the plunger reaches its predetermined stopping point.

Unscrew the applicator from the tube and replace the cap.

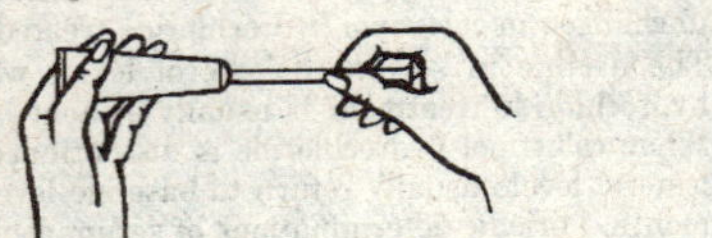

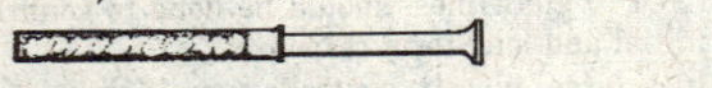

While lying on your back, firmly grasp the applicator barrel and insert into vagina as far as possible without causing discomfort.

Slowly push the plunger until it stops.

Carefully withdraw applicator from vagina, and discard applicator.

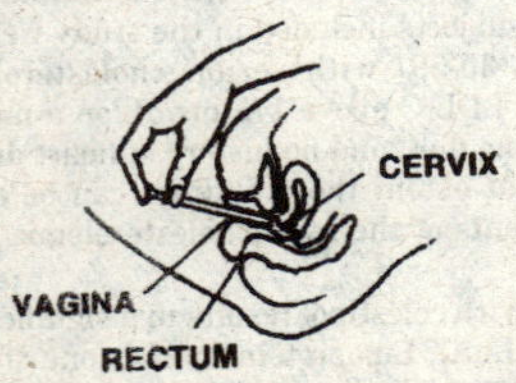

REMEMBER TO APPLY ONE APPLICATORFUL EACH NIGHT BEFORE BEDTIME, OR AS PRESCRIBED BY YOUR DOCTOR.

COLESTID® ℞

[kō'lĕs-tĭd]

(micronized colestipol hydrochloride tablets)

Prescribing information for this product, which appears on pages 2740–2742 of the 2004 PDR, has been completely revised as follows. Please write "See Supplement A" next to the product heading.

DESCRIPTION

The active ingredient in COLESTID Tablets is micronized colestipol hydrochloride, which is a lipid lowering agent for oral use. Colestipol is an insoluble, high molecular weight basic anion-exchange copolymer of diethylenetriamine and 1-chloro-2, 3-epoxypropane, with approximately 1 out of 5 amine nitrogens protonated (chloride form). It is a light yellow water-insoluble resin which is hygroscopic and swells when suspended in water or aqueous fluids.

Each COLESTID Tablet contains one gram of micronized colestipol hydrochloride. COLESTID Tablets are light yellow in color and are tasteless and odorless. Inactive ingre-

Continued on next page

Colestid—Cont.

dients: cellulose acetate phthalate, glyceryl triacetate, carnauba wax, hypromellose, magnesium stearate, povidone, silicon dioxide. COLESTID Tablets contain no calories.

CLINICAL PHARMACOLOGY

Cholesterol is the major, and probably the sole precursor of bile acids. During normal digestion, bile acids are secreted via the bile from the liver and gall bladder into the intestines. Bile acids emulsify the fat and lipid materials present in food, thus facilitating absorption. A major portion of the bile acids secreted is reabsorbed from the intestines and returned via the portal circulation to the liver, thus completing the enterohepatic cycle. Only very small amounts of bile acids are found in normal serum.

Colestipol hydrochloride binds bile acids in the intestine forming a complex that is excreted in the feces. This nonsystemic action results in a partial removal of the bile acids from the enterohepatic circulation, preventing their reabsorption. Since colestipol hydrochloride is an anion exchange resin, the chloride anions of the resin can be replaced by other anions, usually those with a greater affinity for the resin than the chloride ion.

Colestipol hydrochloride is hydrophilic, but it is virtually water insoluble (99.75%) and it is not hydrolyzed by digestive enzymes. The high molecular weight polymer in colestipol hydrochloride apparently is not absorbed. In humans, less than 0.17% of a single ^{14}C-labeled colestipol hydrochloride dose is excreted in the urine when given following 60 days of dosing of 20 grams of colestipol hydrochloride per day.

The increased fecal loss of bile acids due to colestipol hydrochloride administration leads to an increased oxidation of cholesterol to bile acids. This results in an increase in the number of low-density lipoprotein (LDL) receptors, increased hepatic uptake of LDL and a decrease in beta lipoprotein or LDL serum levels, and a decrease in serum cholesterol levels. Although colestipol hydrochloride produces an increase in the hepatic synthesis of cholesterol in man, serum cholesterol levels fall.

There is evidence to show that this fall in cholesterol is secondary to an increased rate of clearance of cholesterol-rich lipoproteins (beta or low-density lipoproteins) from the plasma. Serum triglyceride levels may increase or remain unchanged in colestipol hydrochloride treated patients.

The decline in serum cholesterol levels with colestipol hydrochloride treatment is usually evident by one month. When colestipol hydrochloride is discontinued, serum cholesterol levels usually return to baseline levels within one month. Periodic determinations of serum cholesterol levels as outlined in the National Cholesterol Education Program (NCEP) guidelines, should be done to confirm a favorable initial and long-term response.[1]

In a large, placebo-controlled, multiclinic study, the LRC-CPPT[2], hypercholesterolemic subjects treated with cholestyramine, a bile-acid sequestrant with a mechanism of action and an effect on serum cholesterol similar to that of colestipol hydrochloride, had reductions in total and LDL-C. Over the 7-year study period the cholestyramine group experienced a 19% reduction (relative to the incidence in the placebo group) in the combined rate of coronary heart disease (CHD) death plus nonfatal myocardial infarction (cumulative incidences of 7% cholestyramine and 8.6% placebo). The subjects included in the study were middle-aged men (aged 35-59) with serum cholesterol levels above 265 mg/dL, LDL-C above 175 mg/dL on a moderate cholesterol-lowering diet, and no history of heart disease. It is not clear to what extent these findings can be extrapolated to other segments of the hypercholesterolemic population not studied.

Treatment with colestipol results in a significant increase in lipoprotein LpAI. Lipoprotein LpAI is one of the two major lipoprotein particles within the high-density lipoprotein (HDL) density range[3], and has been shown in cell culture to promote cholesterol efflux or removal from cells[4]. Although the significance of this finding has not been established in clinical studies, the elevation of the lipoprotein LpAI particle within the HDL fraction is consistent with an antiatherogenic effect of colestipol hydrochloride, even though little change is observed in HDL cholesterol (HDL-C).

In patients with heterozygous familial hypercholesterolemia who have not obtained an optimal response to colestipol hydrochloride alone in maximal doses, the combination of colestipol hydrochloride and nicotinic acid has been shown to further lower serum cholesterol, triglyceride, and LDL-cholesterol (LDL-C) values. Simultaneously, HDL-C values increased significantly. In many such patients it is possible to normalize serum lipid values.[5-7]

Preliminary evidence suggests that the cholesterol-lowering effects of lovastatin and the bile acid sequestrant, colestipol hydrochloride, are additive.

The effect of intensive lipid-lowering therapy on coronary atherosclerosis has been assessed by arteriography in hyperlipidemic patients. In these randomized, controlled clinical trials, patients were treated for two to four years by either conventional measures (diet, placebo, or in some cases low-dose resin), or with intensive combination therapy using diet and COLESTID Granules plus either nicotinic acid or lovastatin. When compared to conventional measures, intensive lipid-lowering combination therapy significantly reduced the frequency of progression and increased the frequency of regression of coronary atherosclerotic lesions in patients with or at risk for coronary artery disease.[8-11]

INDICATIONS AND USAGE

Since no drug is innocuous, strict attention should be paid to the indications and contraindications, particularly when selecting drugs for chronic long-term use.

COLESTID Tablets are indicated as adjunctive therapy to diet for the reduction of elevated serum total and LDL-C in patients with primary hypercholesterolemia (elevated LDL-C) who do not respond adequately to diet. Generally, COLESTID Tablets have no clinically significant effect on serum triglycerides, but with their use, triglyceride levels may be raised in some patients.

Therapy with lipid-altering agents should be a component of multiple risk factor intervention in those individuals at significantly increased risk for atherosclerotic vascular disease due to hypercholesterolemia. Treatment should begin and continue with dietary therapy (see NCEP guidelines). A minimum of six months of intensive dietary therapy and counseling should be carried out prior to initiation of drug therapy. Shorter periods may be considered in patients with severe elevations of LDL-C or with definite CHD.

According to the NCEP guidelines, the goal of treatment is to lower LDL-C, and LDL-C is to be used to initiate and assess treatment response. Only if LDL-C levels are not available, should the Total-C be used to monitor therapy. The NCEP treatment guidelines are shown below.

		LDL-Cholesterol mg/dL (mmol/L)	
Definite Atherosclerotic Disease*	Two or More Other Risk Factors**	Initiation Level	Goal
No	No	≥190 (≥4.9)	<160 (<4.1)
No	Yes	≥160 (≥4.1)	<130 (<3.4)
Yes	Yes or No	≥130 (≥3.4)	≤100 (≤2.6)

*Coronary heart disease or peripheral vascular disease (including symptomatic carotid artery disease).

**Other risk factors for coronary heart disease (CHD) include: age (males: ≥45 years; female: ≥55 years or premature menopause without estrogen replacement therapy); family history of premature CHD; current cigarette smoking; hypertension; confirmed HDL-C <35 mg/dL (0.91 mmol/L); and diabetes mellitus. Subtract one risk factor if HDL-C is ≥60 mg/dL (1.6 mmol/L).

CONTRAINDICATIONS

COLESTID Tablets are contraindicated in those individuals who have shown hypersensitivity to any of their components.

PRECAUTIONS

Prior to initiating therapy with COLESTID Tablets, secondary causes of hypercholesterolemia (e.g., poorly controlled diabetes mellitus, hypothyroidism, nephrotic syndrome, dysproteinemias, obstructive liver disease, other drug therapy, alcoholism), should be excluded, and a lipid profile performed to assess total cholesterol, HDL-C, and triglycerides (TG). For individuals with TG less than 400 mg/dL (<4.5 mmol/L), LDL-C can be estimated using the following equation:

LDL-C = Total cholesterol – [(Triglycerides/5) + HDL-C]

For TG levels >400 mg/dL, this equation is less accurate and LDL-C concentrations should be determined by ultracentrifugation. In hypertriglyceridemic patients, LDL-C may be low or normal despite elevated Total-C. In such cases COLESTID Tablets may not be indicated.

Because it sequesters bile acids, colestipol hydrochloride may interfere with normal fat absorption and, thus, may reduce absorption of folic acid and fat soluble vitamins such as A, D, and K.

Chronic use of colestipol hydrochloride may be associated with an increased bleeding tendency due to hypoprothrombinemia from vitamin K deficiency. This will usually respond promptly to parenteral vitamin K_1 and recurrences can be prevented by oral administration of vitamin K_1.

Serum cholesterol and triglyceride levels should be determined periodically based on NCEP guidelines to confirm a favorable initial and adequate long-term response.

COLESTID Tablets may produce or severely worsen pre-existing constipation. The dosage should be increased gradually in patients to minimize the risk of developing fecal impaction. In patients with pre-existing constipation, the starting dose should be 2 grams once or twice a day. Increased fluid and fiber intake should be encouraged to alleviate constipation and a stool softener may occasionally be indicated. If the initial dose is well tolerated, the dose may be increased as needed by a further 2 to 4 grams/day (at monthly intervals) with periodic monitoring of serum lipoproteins. If constipation worsens or the desired therapeutic response is not achieved at 2 to 16 grams/day, combination therapy or alternate therapy should be considered. Particular effort should be made to avoid constipation in patients with symptomatic coronary artery disease. Constipation associated with COLESTID Tablets may aggravate hemorrhoids.

While there have been no reports of hypothyroidism induced in individuals with normal thyroid function, the theoretical possibility exists, particularly in patients with limited thyroid reserve.

Since colestipol hydrochloride is a chloride form of an anion exchange resin, there is a possibility that prolonged use may lead to the development of hyperchloremia acidosis.

Carcinogenesis, Mutagenesis and Impairment of Fertility

In studies conducted in rats in which cholestyramine resin (a bile acid sequestering agent similar to colestipol hydrochloride) was used as a tool to investigate the role of various intestinal factors, such as fat, bile salts, and microbial flora, in the development of intestinal tumors induced by potent carcinogens, the incidence of such tumors was observed to be greater in cholestyramine resin treated rats than in control rats.

The relevance of this laboratory observation from studies in rats with cholestyramine resin to the clinical use of COLESTID Tablets is not known. In the LRC-CPPT study referred to above, the total incidence of fatal and nonfatal neoplasms was similar in both treatment groups. When the many different categories of tumors are examined, various alimentary system cancers were somewhat more prevalent in the cholestyramine group. The small numbers and the multiple categories prevent conclusions from being drawn. Further follow-up of the LRC-CPPT participants by the sponsors of that study is planned for cause-specific mortality and cancer morbidity. When colestipol hydrochloride was administered in the diet to rats for 18 months, there was no evidence of any drug related intestinal tumor formation. In the Ames assay, colestipol hydrochloride was not mutagenic.

Use in Pregnancy

Since colestipol hydrochloride is essentially not absorbed systemically (less than 0.17% of the dose), it is not expected to cause fetal harm when administered during pregnancy in recommended dosages. There are no adequate and well-controlled studies in pregnant women, and the known interference with absorption of fat-soluble vitamins may be detrimental even in the presence of supplementation.

Nursing Mothers: Caution should be exercised when COLESTID Tablets are administered to a nursing mother. The possible lack of proper vitamin absorption described in the "Pregnancy" section may have an effect on nursing infants.

Pediatric Use

Safety and effectiveness in the pediatric population have not been established.

Information for Patients

COLESTID Tablets may be larger than pills you have taken before. If you have had swallowing problems or choking with food, liquids or other tablets or capsules in the past, you should discuss this with your doctor before taking COLESTID Tablets.

It is important that you take COLESTID Tablets correctly:

1. Always take one tablet at a time and swallow promptly.
2. Swallow each tablet whole. Do not cut, crush, or chew the tablets.
3. COLESTID Tablets must be taken with water or another liquid that you prefer. Swallowing the tablets will be easier if you drink plenty of liquid as you swallow each tablet.

Difficulty swallowing and temporary obstruction of the esophagus (the tube between your mouth and stomach) have been rarely reported in patients taking COLESTID Tablets. If a tablet does get stuck after you swallow it, you may notice pressure or discomfort. If this happens to you, you should contact your doctor. Do not take COLESTID Tablets again without your doctor's advice.

If you are taking other medications, you should take them at least one hour before or four hours after taking COLESTID Tablets.

DRUG INTERACTIONS

Since colestipol hydrochloride is an anion exchange resin, it may have a strong affinity for anions other than the bile acids. *In vitro* studies have indicated that colestipol hydrochloride binds a number of drugs. Therefore, COLESTID Tablets may delay or reduce the absorption of concomitant oral medication. The interval between the administration of COLESTID Tablets and any other medication should be as long as possible. Patients should take other drugs at least one hour before or four hours after COLESTID Tablets to avoid impeding their absorption.

Repeated doses of colestipol hydrochloride given prior to a single dose of propranolol in human trials have been reported to decrease propranolol absorption. However, in a follow-up study in normal subjects, single-dose administration of colestipol hydrochloride and propranolol and twice-a-day administration for 5 days of both agents did not affect the extent of propranolol absorption, but had a small yet statistically significant effect on its rate of absorption; the time to reach maximum concentration was delayed approximately 30 minutes. Effects on the absorption of other beta-blockers have not been determined. Therefore, patients on propranolol should be observed when COLESTID Tablets are either added or deleted from a therapeutic regimen.

Studies in humans show that the absorption of chlorothiazide as reflected in urinary excretion is markedly decreased even when administered one hour before colestipol hydrochloride. The absorption of tetracycline, furosemide, penicillin G, hydrochlorothiazide, and gemfibrozil was significantly decreased when given simultaneously with colestipol hydrochloride; these drugs were not tested to determine the effect of administration one hour before colestipol hydrochloride.

No depressant effect on blood levels in humans was noted when colestipol hydrochloride was administered with any of the following drugs: aspirin, clindamycin, clofibrate, methyldopa, nicotinic acid (niacin), tolbutamide, phenytoin or warfarin. Particular caution should be observed with dig-

italis preparations since there are conflicting results for the effect of colestipol hydrochloride on the availability of digoxin and digitoxin. The potential for binding of these drugs if given concomitantly is present. Discontinuing colestipol hydrochloride could pose a hazard to health if a potentially toxic drug that is significantly bound to the resin has been titrated to a maintenance level while the patient was taking colestipol hydrochloride.
Bile acid binding resins may also interfere with the absorption of oral phosphate supplements and hydrocortisone.

ADVERSE REACTIONS

Gastrointestinal
The most common adverse reactions are confined to the gastrointestinal tract. To achieve minimal GI disturbance with an optimal LDL-C lowering effect, a gradual increase of dosage starting with 2 grams, once or twice daily is recommended. Constipation is the major single complaint and at times is severe. Most instances of constipation are mild, transient, and controlled with standard treatment. Increased fluid intake and inclusion of additional dietary fiber should be the first step; a stool softener may be added if needed. Some patients require decreased dosage or discontinuation of therapy. Hemorrhoids may be aggravated.
Other, less frequent gastrointestinal complaints consist of abdominal discomfort (abdominal pain and cramping), intestinal gas (bloating and flatulence), indigestion and heartburn, diarrhea and loose stools, and nausea and vomiting. Bleeding hemorrhoids and blood in the stool have been infrequently reported. Peptic ulceration, cholecystitis, and cholelithiasis have been rarely reported in patients receiving colestipol hydrochloride granules, and are not necessarily drug related.
Difficulty swallowing and transient esophageal obstruction have been rarely reported in patients taking COLESTID Tablets.
Transient and modest elevations of aspartate aminotransferase (AST, SGOT), alanine aminotransferase (ALT, SGPT) and alkaline phosphatase were observed on one or more occasions in various patients treated with colestipol hydrochloride.
The following nongastrointestinal adverse reactions have been reported with generally equal frequency in patients receiving COLESTID Tablets, colestipol granules, or placebo in clinical studies:
Cardiovascular
Chest pain, angina, and tachycardia have been infrequently reported.
Hypersensitivity
Rash has been infrequently reported. Urticaria and dermatitis have been rarely noted in patients receiving colestipol hydrochloride granules.
Musculoskeletal
Musculoskeletal pain, aches and pains in the extremities, joint pain and arthritis, and backache have been reported.
Neurologic
Headache, migraine headache, and sinus headache have been reported. Other infrequently reported complaints include dizziness, light-headedness, and insomnia.
Miscellaneous
Anorexia, fatigue, weakness, shortness of breath, and swelling of the hands or feet, have been infrequently reported.

OVERDOSAGE

Overdosage of COLESTID Tablets has not been reported. Should overdosage occur, however, the chief potential harm would be obstruction of the gastrointestinal tract. The location of such potential obstruction, the degree of obstruction and the presence or absence of normal gut motility would determine treatment.

DOSAGE AND ADMINISTRATION

For adults, COLESTID Tablets are recommended in doses of 2 to 16 grams/day given once or in divided doses. The starting dose should be 2 grams once or twice daily. Dosage increases of 2 grams, once or twice daily should occur at 1- or 2-month intervals. Appropriate use of lipid profiles as per NCEP guidelines including LDL-C and triglycerides, is advised so that optimal but not excessive doses are used to obtain the desired therapeutic effect on LDL-C level. If the desired therapeutic effect is not obtained at a dose of 2 to 16 grams/day with good compliance and acceptable side effects, combined therapy or alternate treatment should be considered.
COLESTID Tablets must be taken one at a time and be promptly swallowed whole, using plenty of water or other appropriate liquid. Do not cut, crush, or chew the tablets. Patients should take other drugs at least one hour before or four hours after COLESTID Tablets to minimize possible interference with their absorption. (See DRUG INTERACTIONS.)

Before Administration of COLESTID Tablets

1. Define the type of hyperlipoproteinemia, as described in NCEP guidelines.
2. Institute a trial of diet and weight reduction.
3. Establish baseline serum total and LDL-C and triglyceride levels.

During Administration of COLESTID Tablets

1. The patient should be carefully monitored clinically, including serum cholesterol and triglyceride levels. Periodic determinations of serum cholesterol levels as outlined in the NCEP guidelines should be done to confirm a favorable initial and long-term response.
2. Failure of total or LDL-C to fall within the desired range should lead one to first examine dietary and drug compliance. If these are deemed acceptable, combined therapy or alternate treatment should be considered.
3. Significant rise in triglyceride level should be considered as indication for dose reduction, drug discontinuation, or combined or alternate therapy.

HOW SUPPLIED

COLESTID Tablets are yellow, elliptical, imprinted U, and are supplied as follows:

Bottles of 120	NDC 0009-0450-03
Bottles of 500	NDC 0009-0450-04

Each tablet contains 1 gram of colestipol hydrochloride.
Store at controlled room temperature 20° to 25°C (68° to 77°F) [see USP].

REFERENCES

1. Summary of the Second Report of the National Cholesterol Education Program (NCEP) Expert Panel on Detection, Evaluation, and Treatment of High Blood Cholesterol in Adults (Adult Treatment Panel II). *JAMA* 1993; 269(23):3015-3023.
2. Lipid Metabolism-Atherogenesis Branch, National Heart, Lung, and Blood Institute, Bethesda, MD: The Lipid Research Clinics Coronary Primary Prevention Trial Results. I. Reduction in Incidence of Coronary Heart Disease. *JAMA* 1984; 251:351-364.
3. Parra HJ, et al. Differential electroimmunoassay of human LpA-I lipoprotein particles on ready-to-use plates. *Clin. Chem.* 1990; 36(8):1431-1435.
4. Barbaras R, et al. Cholesterol efflux from cultured adipose cells is mediated by LpAI particles but not by LpAI:AII particles. *Biochem. Biophys. Res. Comm.* 1987; 142(1):63-69.
5. Kane JP, et al. Normalization of low-density-lipoprotein levels in heterozygous familial hypercholesterolemia with a combined drug regimen. *N Engl. J. Med.* 1981; 304:251-258.
6. Illingworth DR, et al. Colestipol plus nicotinic acid in treatment of heterozygous familial hypercholesterolemia. *Lancet* 1981; 1:296-298.
7. Kuo PT, et al. Familial type II hyperlipoproteinemia with coronary heart disease: Effect of diet-cholestipol-nicotinic acid treatment. *Chest* 1981; 79:286-291.
8. Blankenhorn DH, et al. Beneficial Effects of Combined Colestipol-Niacin Therapy on Coronary Atherosclerosis and Coronary Venous Bypass Grafts. *JAMA* 1987; 257(23):3233-3240.
9. Cashin-Hemphill L, et al. Beneficial Effects of Colestipol-Niacin on Coronary Atherosclerosis: A 4-Year Follow-up. *JAMA* 1990; 264:3013-3017.
10. Brown G. et al. Regression of Coronary Artery Disease as a Result of Intensive Lipid-Lowering Therapy in Men with High Levels of Apolipoprotein B. *N. Engl. J. Med.* 1990; 323:1289-1298.
11. Kane JP, et al. Regression of Coronary Atherosclerosis During Treatment of Familial Hypercholesterolemia with Combined Drug Regimens. *JAMA* 1990; 264:3007-3012.

℞ only
Manufactured for:
Pharmacia & Upjohn Company
A subsidiary of Pharmacia Corporation
Kalamazoo, MI 49001, USA
By:
International Processing Corporation
Winchester, KY 40391, USA
Revised July 2003 815 838 308
692851

DETROL® LA ℞

[*dĕ-trōl*]
(tolterodine tartrate extended release capsules)

Prescribing information for this product, which appears on pages 2751–2753 of the 2004 PDR, has been completely revised as follows. Please write "See Supplement A" next to the product heading.

DESCRIPTION

DETROL LA Capsules contain tolterodine tartrate. The active moiety, tolterodine, is a muscarinic receptor antagonist. The chemical name of tolterodine tartrate is (R)-N,N-diisopropyl-3-(2-hydroxy-5-methylphenyl)-3-phenylpropanamine L-hydrogen tartrate. The empirical formula of tolterodine tartrate is $C_{26}H_{37}NO_7$, and its molecular weight is 475.6. The structural formula of tolterodine tartrate is represented below.

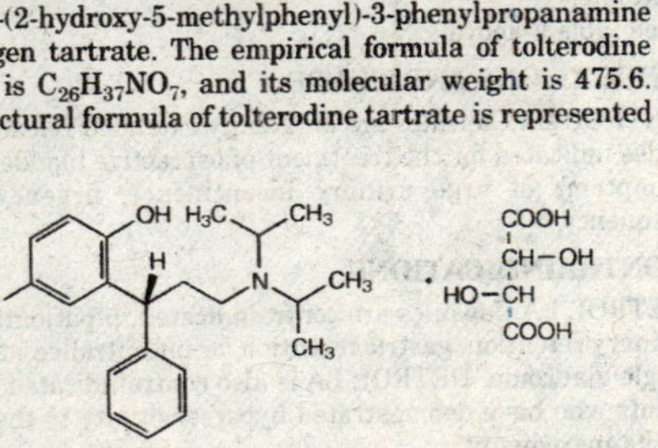

Tolterodine tartrate is a white, crystalline powder. The pKa value is 9.87 and the solubility in water is 12 mg/mL. It is soluble in methanol, slightly soluble in ethanol, and practically insoluble in toluene. The partition coefficient (Log D) between n-octanol and water is 1.83 at pH 7.3.
DETROL LA for oral administration contains 2 mg or 4 mg of tolterodine tartrate. Inactive ingredients are sucrose, starch, hypromellose, ethylcellulose, medium chain triglycerides, oleic acid, gelatin, and FD&C Blue #2. The 2-mg capsules also contain yellow iron oxide. Both capsule strengths are imprinted with a pharmaceutical grade printing ink that contains shellac glaze, titanium dioxide, propylene glycol, and simethicone.

CLINICAL PHARMACOLOGY

Tolterodine is a competitive muscarinic receptor antagonist. Both urinary bladder contraction and salivation are mediated via cholinergic muscarinic receptors.
After oral administration, tolterodine is metabolized in the liver, resulting in the formation of the 5-hydroxymethyl derivative, a major pharmacologically active metabolite. The 5-hydroxymethyl metabolite, which exhibits an antimuscarinic activity similar to that of tolterodine, contributes significantly to the therapeutic effect. Both tolterodine and the 5-hydroxymethyl metabolite exhibit a high specificity for muscarinic receptors, since both show negligible activity or affinity for other neurotransmitter receptors and other potential cellular targets, such as calcium channels.
Tolterodine has a pronounced effect on bladder function. Effects on urodynamic parameters before and 1 and 5 hours after a single 6.4-mg dose of tolterodine immediate release were determined in healthy volunteers. The main effects of tolterodine at 1 and 5 hours were an increase in residual urine, reflecting an incomplete emptying of the bladder, and a decrease in detrusor pressure. These findings are consistent with an antimuscarinic action on the lower urinary tract.

Pharmacokinetics

Absorption: In a study with ^{14}C-tolterodine solution in healthy volunteers who received a 5-mg oral dose, at least 77% of the radiolabeled dose was absorbed. C_{max} and area under the concentration-time curve (AUC) determined after dosage of tolterodine immediate release are dose-proportional over the range of 1 to 4 mg. Based on the sum of unbound serum concentrations of tolterodine and the 5-hydroxymethyl metabolite ("active moiety"), the AUC of tolterodine extended release 4 mg daily is equivalent to tolterodine immediate release 4 mg (2 mg bid). C_{max} and C_{min} levels of tolterodine extended release are about 75% and 150% of tolterodine immediate release, respectively. Maximum serum concentrations of tolterodine extended release are observed 2 to 6 hours after dose administration.
Effect of Food: There is no effect of food on the pharmacokinetics of tolterodine extended release.
Distribution: Tolterodine is highly bound to plasma proteins, primarily α_1-acid glycoprotein. Unbound concentrations of tolterodine average 3.7% ± 0.13% over the concentration range achieved in clinical studies. The 5-hydroxymethyl metabolite is not extensively protein bound, with unbound fraction concentrations averaging 36% ± 4.0%. The blood to serum ratio of tolterodine and the 5-hydroxymethyl metabolite averages 0.6 and 0.8, respectively, indicating that these compounds do not distribute extensively into erythrocytes. The volume of distribution of tolterodine following administration of a 1.28-mg intravenous dose is 113 ± 26.7 L.
Metabolism: Tolterodine is extensively metabolized by the liver following oral dosing. The primary metabolic route involves the oxidation of the 5-methyl group and is mediated by the cytochrome P450 2D6 (CYP2D6) and leads to the formation of a pharmacologically active 5-hydroxymethyl metabolite. Further metabolism leads to formation of the 5-carboxylic acid and *N*-dealkylated 5-carboxylic acid metabolites, which account for 51% ± 14% and 29% ± 6.3% of the metabolites recovered in the urine, respectively.
Variability in Metabolism: A subset (about 7%) of the Caucasian population is devoid of CYP2D6, the enzyme responsible for the formation of the 5-hydroxymethyl metabolite of tolterodine. The identified pathway of metabolism for these individuals ("poor metabolizers") is dealkylation via cytochrome P450 3A4 (CYP3A4) to *N*-dealkylated tolterodine. The remainder of the population is referred to as "extensive metabolizers." Pharmacokinetic studies revealed that tolterodine is metabolized at a slower rate in poor metabolizers than in extensive metabolizers; this results in significantly higher serum concentrations of tolterodine and in negligible concentrations of the 5-hydroxymethyl metabolite.
Excretion: Following administration of a 5-mg oral dose of ^{14}C-tolterodine solution to healthy volunteers, 77% of radioactivity was recovered in urine and 17% was recovered in feces in 7 days. Less than 1% (< 2.5% in poor metabolizers) of the dose was recovered as intact tolterodine, and 5% to 14% (<1% in poor metabolizers) was recovered as the active 5-hydroxymethyl metabolite.
A summary of mean (± standard deviation) pharmacokinetic parameters of tolterodine extended release and the 5-hydroxymethyl metabolite in extensive (EM) and poor (PM) metabolizers is provided in Table 1. These data were obtained following single and multiple doses of tolterodine extended release administered daily to 17 healthy male volunteers (13 EM, 4 PM).
[See table 1 at top of next page]

Pharmacokinetics in Special Populations

Age: In Phase 1, multiple-dose studies in which tolterodine immediate release 4 mg (2 mg bid) was administered, serum concentrations of tolterodine and of the 5-hydroxymethyl metabolite were similar in healthy elderly volunteers (aged 64 through 80 years) and healthy young volunteers (aged less than 40 years). In another Phase 1 study, elderly volunteers (aged 71 through 81 years) were given tolterodine immediate release 2 or 4 mg (1 or 2 mg bid). Mean serum concentrations of tolterodine and the

Continued on next page

Detrol LA—Cont.

5-hydroxymethyl metabolite in these elderly volunteers were approximately 20% and 50% higher, respectively, than reported in young healthy volunteers. However, no overall differences were observed in safety between older and younger patients on tolterodine in the Phase 3, 12-week, controlled clinical studies; therefore, no tolterodine dosage adjustment for elderly patients is recommended (see **PRECAUTIONS, Geriatric Use**).

Pediatric: The pharmacokinetics of tolterodine has not been established in pediatric patients.

Gender: The pharmacokinetics of tolterodine immediate release and the 5-hydroxymethyl metabolite are not influenced by gender. Mean C_{max} of tolterodine immediate release (1.6 µg/L in males versus 2.2 µg/L in females) and the active 5-hydroxymethyl metabolite (2.2 µg/L in males versus 2.5 µg/L in females) are similar in males and females who were administered tolterodine immediate release 2 mg. Mean AUC values of tolterodine (6.7 µg•h/L in males versus 7.8 µg•h/L in females) and the 5-hydroxymethyl metabolite (10 µg•h/L in males versus 11 µg•h/L in females) are also similar. The elimination half-life of tolterodine immediate release for both males and females is 2.4 hours, and the half-life of the 5-hydroxymethyl metabolite is 3.0 hours in females and 3.3 hours in males.

Race: Pharmacokinetic differences due to race have not been established.

Renal Insufficiency: Renal impairment can significantly alter the disposition of tolterodine immediate release and its metabolites. In a study conducted in patients with creatinine clearance between 10 and 30 mL/min, tolterodine immediate release and the 5-hydroxymethyl metabolite levels were approximately 2-3 fold higher in patients with renal impairment than in healthy volunteers. Exposure levels of other metabolites of tolterodine (eg, tolterodine acid, *N*-dealkylated tolterodine acid, *N*-dealkylated tolterodine and *N*-dealkylated hydroxy tolterodine) were significantly higher (10-30 fold) in renally impaired patients as compared to the healthy volunteers. The recommended dose for patients with significantly reduced renal function is tolterodine 2 mg daily (see **PRECAUTIONS, General**).

Hepatic Insufficiency: Liver impairment can significantly alter the disposition of tolterodine immediate release. In a study of tolterodine immediate release conducted in cirrhotic patients, the elimination half-life of tolterodine immediate release was longer in cirrhotic patients (mean, 7.8 hours) than in healthy, young, and elderly volunteers (mean, 2 to 4 hours). The clearance of orally administered tolterodine immediate release was substantially lower in cirrhotic patients (1.0 ± 1.7 L/h/kg) than in the healthy volunteers (5.7 ± 3.8 L/h/kg). The recommended dose for patients with significantly reduced hepatic function is tolterodine 2 mg daily (see **PRECAUTIONS, General**).

Drug-Drug Interactions

Fluoxetine: Fluoxetine is a selective serotonin reuptake inhibitor and a potent inhibitor of CYP2D6 activity. In a study to assess the effect of fluoxetine on the pharmacokinetics of tolterodine immediate release and its metabolites, it was observed that fluoxetine significantly inhibited the metabolism of tolterodine immediate release in extensive metabolizers, resulting in a 4.8-fold increase in tolterodine AUC. There was a 52% decrease in C_{max} and a 20% decrease in AUC of the 5-hydroxymethyl metabolite. Fluoxetine thus alters the pharmacokinetics in patients who would otherwise be extensive metabolizers of tolterodine immediate release to resemble the pharmacokinetic profile in poor metabolizers. The sums of unbound serum concentrations of tolterodine immediate release and the 5-hydroxymethyl metabolite are only 25% higher during the interaction. No dose adjustment is required when tolterodine and fluoxetine are coadministered.

Other Drugs Metabolized by Cytochrome P450 Isoenzymes: Tolterodine immediate release does not cause clinically significant interactions with other drugs metabolized by the major drug metabolizing CYP enzymes. In vivo drug-interaction data show that tolterodine immediate release does not result in clinically relevant inhibition of CYP1A2, 2D6, 2C9, 2C19, or 3A4 as evidenced by lack of influence on the marker drugs caffeine, debrisoquine, S-warfarin, and omeprazole. In vitro data show that tolterodine immediate release is a competitive inhibitor of CYP2D6 at high concentrations (Ki 1.05 µM), while tolterodine immediate release as well as the 5-hydroxymethyl metabolite are devoid of any significant inhibitory potential regarding the other isoenzymes.

CYP3A4 Inhibitors: The effect of a 200-mg daily dose of ketoconazole on the pharmacokinetics of tolterodine immediate release was studied in 8 healthy volunteers, all of whom were poor metabolizers (see **Pharmacokinetics**, Variability in Metabolism for discussion of poor metabolizers). In the presence of ketoconazole, the mean C_{max} and AUC of tolterodine increased by 2 and 2.5 fold, respectively. Based on these findings, other potent CYP3A4 inhibitors such as other azole antifungals (eg, itraconazole, miconazole) or macrolide antibiotics (eg, erythromycin, clarithromycin) or cyclosporine or vinblastine may also lead to increases of tolterodine plasma concentrations (see **PRECAUTIONS** and **DOSAGE AND ADMINISTRATION**).

Warfarin: In healthy volunteers, coadministration of tolterodine immediate release 4 mg (2 mg bid) for 7 days and a single dose of warfarin 25 mg on day 4 had no effect on prothrombin time, Factor VII suppression, or on the pharmacokinetics of warfarin.

Table 1. Summary of Mean (±SD) Pharmacokinetic Parameters of Tolterodine Extended Release and its Active Metabolite (5-hydroxymethyl metabolite) in Healthy Volunteers

	Tolterodine				5-hydroxymethyl metabolite			
	t_{max}† (h)	C_{max} (µg/L)	C_{avg} (µg/L)	t1/2 (h)	t_{max}† (h)	C_{max} (µg/L)	C_{avg} (µg/L)	t1/2 (h)
Single dose 4 mg* EM	4 (2 - 6)	1.3 (0.8)	0.8 (0.57)	8.4 (3.2)	4 (3 - 6)	1.6 (0.5)	1.0 (0.32)	8.8 (5.9)
Multiple dose 4 mg EM	4 (2 - 6)	3.4 (4.9)	1.7 (2.8)	6.9 (3.5)	4 (2 - 6)	2.7 (0.90)	1.4 (0.6)	9.9 (4.0)
PM	4 (3 - 6)	19 (16)	13 (11)	18 (16)	—‡	—	—	—

*Parameter dose-normalized from 8 to 4 mg for the single-dose data.
C_{max} = Maximum serum concentration; t_{max} = Time of occurrence of C_{max};
C_{avg} = Average serum concentration; t1/2 = Terminal elimination half-life.
†Data presented as median (range).
‡ = not applicable.

Table 2. 95% Confidence Intervals (CI) for the Difference between DETROL LA (4 mg daily) and Placebo for Mean Change at Week 12 from Baseline*

	DETROL LA (n=507)	Placebo (n=508) †	Treatment Difference, vs Placebo (95% CI)
Number of incontinence episodes/week			
Mean Baseline	22.1	23.3	−4.8‡
Mean Change from Baseline	−11.8 (SD 17.8)	−6.9 (SD 15.4)	(−6.9, −2.8)
Number of micturitions/day			
Mean Baseline	10.9	11.3	
Mean Change from Baseline	−1.8 (SD 3.4)	−1.2 (SD 2.9)	−0.6‡ (−1.0, −0.2)
Volume Voided per micturition (mL)			
Mean Baseline	141	136	
Mean Change from Baseline	34 (SD 51)	14 (SD 41)	20‡ (14, 26)

SD = Standard Deviation.
* Intent-to-treat analysis.
† 1 to 2 patients missing in placebo group for each efficacy parameter.
‡ The difference between DETROL LA and placebo was statistically significant.

Oral Contraceptives: Tolterodine immediate release 4 mg (2 mg bid) had no effect on the pharmacokinetics of an oral contraceptive (ethinyl estradiol 30 µg/levo-norgestrel 150 µg) as evidenced by the monitoring of ethinyl estradiol and levo-norgestrel over a 2-month period in healthy female volunteers.

Diuretics: Coadministration of tolterodine immediate release up to 8 mg (4 mg bid) for up to 12 weeks with diuretic agents, such as indapamide, hydrochlorothiazide, triamterene, bendroflumethiazide, chlorothiazide, methylchlorothiazide, or furosemide, did not cause any adverse electrocardiographic (ECG) effects.

CLINICAL STUDIES

DETROL LA Capsules 2 mg were evaluated in 29 patients in a Phase 2 dose-effect study. DETROL LA 4 mg was evaluated for the treatment of overactive bladder with symptoms of urge urinary incontinence and frequency in a randomized, placebo-controlled, multicenter, double-blind, Phase 3, 12-week study. A total of 507 patients received DETROL LA 4 mg once daily in the morning and 508 received placebo. The majority of patients were Caucasian (95%) and female (81%), with a mean age of 61 years (range, 20 to 93 years). In the study, 642 patients (42%) were 65 to 93 years of age. The study included patients known to be responsive to tolterodine immediate release and other anticholinergic medications, however, 47% of patients never received prior pharmacotherapy for overactive bladder. At study entry, 97% of patients had at least 5 urge incontinence episodes per week and 91% of patients had 8 or more micturitions per day. The primary efficacy endpoint was change in mean number of incontinence episodes per week at week 12 from baseline. Secondary efficacy endpoints included change in mean number of micturitions per day and mean volume voided per micturition at week 12 from baseline.

[See table 2 above]

INDICATIONS AND USAGE

DETROL LA Capsules are once daily extended release capsules indicated for the treatment of overactive bladder with symptoms of urge urinary incontinence, urgency, and frequency.

CONTRAINDICATIONS

DETROL LA Capsules are contraindicated in patients with urinary retention, gastric retention, or uncontrolled narrow-angle glaucoma. DETROL LA is also contraindicated in patients who have demonstrated hypersensitivity to the drug or its ingredients.

PRECAUTIONS

General

Risk of Urinary Retention and Gastric Retention: DETROL LA Capsules should be administered with caution to patients with clinically significant bladder outflow obstruction because of the risk of urinary retention and to patients with gastrointestinal obstructive disorders, such as pyloric stenosis, because of the risk of gastric retention (see **CONTRAINDICATIONS**).

Controlled Narrow-Angle Glaucoma: DETROL LA should be used with caution in patients being treated for narrow-angle glaucoma.

Reduced Hepatic and Renal Function: For patients with significantly reduced hepatic function or renal function, the recommended dose for DETROL LA is 2 mg daily (see **CLINICAL PHARMACOLOGY, Pharmacokinetics in Special Populations**).

Information for Patients

Patients should be informed that antimuscarinic agents such as DETROL LA may produce the following effects: blurred vision, dizziness, or drowsiness.

Drug Interactions

CYP3A4 Inhibitors: Ketoconazole, an inhibitor of the drug metabolizing enzyme CYP3A4, significantly increased plasma concentrations of tolterodine when coadministered to subjects who were poor metabolizers (see **CLINICAL PHARMACOLOGY,** Variability in Metabolism and **Drug-Drug Interactions**). For patients receiving ketoconazole or other potent CYP3A4 inhibitors such as other azole antifungals (eg, itraconazole, miconazole) or macrolide antibiotics (eg, erythromycin, clarithromycin) or cyclosporine or vinblastine, the recommended dose of DETROL LA is 2 mg daily.

Drug-Laboratory-Test Interactions

Interactions between tolterodine and laboratory tests have not been studied.

Carcinogenesis, Mutagenesis, Impairment of Fertility

Carcinogenicity studies with tolterodine immediate release were conducted in mice and rats. At the maximum tolerated dose in mice (30 mg/kg/day), female rats (20 mg/kg/day), and male rats (30 mg/kg/day), AUC values obtained for tolterodine were 355, 291, and 462 µg•h/L, respectively. In comparison, the human AUC value for a 2-mg dose administered twice daily is estimated at 34 µg•h/L. Thus, tolterodine exposure in the carcinogenicity studies was 9- to 14-fold higher than expected in humans. No increase in tumors was found in either mice or rats.

No mutagenic effects of tolterodine were detected in a battery of in vitro tests, including bacterial mutation assays (Ames test) in 4 strains of *Salmonella typhimurium* and in 2 strains of *Escherichia coli*, a gene mutation assay in L5178Y mouse lymphoma cells, and chromosomal aberration tests in human lymphocytes. Tolterodine was also negative in vivo in the bone marrow micronucleus test in the mouse.

In female mice treated for 2 weeks before mating and during gestation with 20 mg/kg/day (corresponding to AUC value of about 500 µg•h/L), neither effects on reproductive performance or fertility were seen. Based on AUC values, the systemic exposure was about 15-fold higher in animals than in humans. In male mice, a dose of 30 mg/kg/day did not induce any adverse effects on fertility.

Pregnancy

Pregnancy Category C. At oral doses of 20 mg/kg/day (approximately 14 times the human exposure), no anomalies or malformations were observed in mice. When given at doses of 30 to 40 mg/kg/day, tolterodine has been shown to be embryolethal and reduce fetal weight, and increase the incidence of fetal abnormalities (cleft palate, digital abnormalities, intra-abdominal hemorrhage, and various skeletal abnormalities, primarily reduced ossification) in mice. At these doses, the AUC values were about 20- to 25-fold

Table 3. Incidence* (%) of Adverse Events Exceeding Placebo Rate and Reported in ≥1% of Patients Treated with DETROL LA (4 mg daily) in a 12-week, Phase 3 Clinical Trial

Body System	Adverse Event	% DETROL LA n=505	% Placebo n=507
Autonomic Nervous	dry mouth	23	8
General	headache	6	4
	fatigue	2	1
Central/Peripheral Nervous	dizziness	2	1
Gastrointestinal	constipation	6	4
	abdominal pain	4	2
	dyspepsia	3	1
Vision	xerophthalmia	3	2
	vision abnormal	1	0
Psychiatric	somnolence	3	2
	anxiety	1	0
Respiratory	sinusitis	2	1
Urinary	dysuria	1	0

* in nearest integer.

Bottle of 30		Bottles of 500	
2 mg Capsules	NDC 0009-5190-01	2 mg Capsules	NDC 0009-5190-03
4 mg Capsules	NDC 0009-5191-01	4 mg Capsules	NDC 0009-5191-03
Bottles of 90		Unit Dose Blisters	
2 mg Capsules	NDC 0009-5190-02	2 mg Capsules	NDC 0009-5190-04
4 mg Capsules	NDC 0009-5191-02	4 mg Capsules	NDC 0009-5191-04

higher than in humans. Rabbits treated subcutaneously at a dose of 0.8 mg/kg/day achieved an AUC of 100 µg•h/L, which is about 3-fold higher than that resulting from the human dose. This dose did not result in any embryotoxicity or teratogenicity. There are no studies of tolterodine in pregnant women. Therefore, DETROL LA should be used during pregnancy only if the potential benefit for the mother justifies the potential risk to the fetus.

Nursing Mothers

Tolterodine immediate release is excreted into the milk in mice. Offspring of female mice treated with tolterodine 20 mg/kg/day during the lactation period had slightly reduced body-weight gain. The offspring regained the weight during the maturation phase. It is not known whether tolterodine is excreted in human milk; therefore, DETROL LA should not be administered during nursing. A decision should be made whether to discontinue nursing or to discontinue DETROL LA in nursing mothers.

Pediatric Use

The safety and effectiveness of tolterodine in pediatric patients has not been established.

Geriatric Use

No overall differences in safety were observed between the older and younger patients treated with tolterodine (see **CLINICAL PHARMACOLOGY, Pharmacokinetics in Special Populations**).

ADVERSE REACTIONS

The Phase 2 and 3 clinical trial program for DETROL LA Capsules included 1073 patients who were treated with DETROL LA (n=537) or placebo (n=536). The patients were treated with 2, 4, 6, or 8 mg/day for up to 15 months. Because clinical trials are conducted under widely varying conditions, adverse reaction rates observed in the clinical trials of a drug cannot be directly compared to rates in the clinical trials of another drug and may not reflect the rates observed in practice. The adverse reaction information from clinical trials does, however, provide a basis for identifying the adverse events that appear to be related to drug use and for approximating rates. The data described below reflect exposure to DETROL LA 4 mg once daily every morning in 505 patients and to placebo in 507 patients exposed for 12 weeks in the Phase 3, controlled clinical study.

Adverse events were reported in 52% (n=263) of patients receiving DETROL LA and in 49% (n=247) of patients receiving placebo. The most common adverse events reported by patients receiving DETROL LA were dry mouth, headache, constipation, and abdominal pain. Dry mouth was the most frequently reported adverse event for patients treated with DETROL LA occurring in 23.4% of patients treated with DETROL LA and 7.7% of placebo-treated patients. Dry mouth, constipation, abnormal vision (accommodation abnormalities), urinary retention, and dry eyes are expected side effects of antimuscarinic agents. A serious adverse event was reported by 1.4% (n=7) of patients receiving DETROL LA and by 3.6% (n=18) of patients receiving placebo.

The frequency of discontinuation due to adverse events was highest during the first 4 weeks of treatment. Similar percentages of patients treated with DETROL LA or placebo discontinued treatment due to adverse events. Treatment was discontinued due to adverse events and dry mouth was reported as an adverse event in 2.4% (n=12) of patients treated with DETROL LA and in 1.2% (n=6) of patients treated with placebo.

Table 3 lists the adverse events reported in 1% or more of patients treated with DETROL LA 4 mg once daily in the 12-week study. The adverse events were reported regardless of causality.

[See table 3 above]

Postmarketing Surveillance

The following events have been reported in association with tolterodine use in clinical practice: anaphylactoid reactions, including angioedema; tachycardia; palpitations; peripheral edema; and hallucinations. Because these spontaneously reported events are from the worldwide postmarketing experience, the frequency of events and the role of tolterodine in their causation cannot be reliably determined.

OVERDOSAGE

A 27-month-old child who ingested 5 to 7 tolterodine immediate release tablets 2 mg was treated with a suspension of activated charcoal and was hospitalized overnight with symptoms of dry mouth. The child fully recovered.

Management of Overdosage

Overdosage with DETROL LA Capsules can potentially result in severe central anticholinergic effects and should be treated accordingly.

ECG monitoring is recommended in the event of overdosage. In dogs, changes in the QT interval (slight prolongation of 10% to 20%) were observed at a suprapharmacologic dose of 4.5 mg/kg, which is about 68 times higher than the recommended human dose. In clinical trials of normal volunteers and patients, QT interval prolongation was not observed with tolterodine immediate release at doses up to 8 mg (4 mg bid) and higher doses were not evaluated.

DOSAGE AND ADMINISTRATION

The recommended dose of DETROL LA Capsules are 4 mg daily. DETROL LA should be taken once daily with liquids and swallowed whole. The dose may be lowered to 2 mg daily based on individual response and tolerability, however, limited efficacy data is available for DETROL LA 2 mg (see **CLINICAL STUDIES**).

For patients with significantly reduced hepatic or renal function or who are currently taking drugs that are potent inhibitors of CYP3A4, the recommended dose of DETROL LA is 2 mg daily (see **CLINICAL PHARMACOLOGY** and **PRECAUTIONS, Drug Interactions**).

HOW SUPPLIED

DETROL LA Capsules 2 mg are blue-green with symbol and 2 printed in white ink. DETROL LA Capsules 4 mg are blue with symbol and 4 printed in white ink. DETROL LA Capsules are supplied as follows:

[See second table above]

Store at 25°C (77°F); excursions permitted to 15-30°C (59-86°F) [see USP Controlled Room Temperature].

Protect from light.

℞ only

U.S. Patent No. 5,382,600

Manufactured for
Pharmacia & Upjohn Company
A subsidiary of Pharmacia Corporation
Kalamazoo, MI 49001, USA
By
International Processing Corporation
Winchester, Kentucky 40391, USA

Revised July 2003 818 229 006
692167
4688-76

ELLENCE® ℞

[ĕl-ĕns]

(epirubicin hydrochloride) injection

Prescribing information for this product, which appears on pages 2755–2759 of the 2004 PDR, has been completely revised as follows. Please write "See Supplement A" next to the product heading.

WARNING

1. Severe local tissue necrosis will occur if there is extravasation during administration (See PRECAUTIONS). Epirubicin must not be given by the intramuscular or subcutaneous route.
2. Myocardial toxicity, manifested in its most severe form by potentially fatal congestive heart failure (CHF), may occur either during therapy with epirubicin or months to years after termination of therapy. The probability of developing clinically evident CHF is estimated as approximately 0.9% at a cumulative dose of 550 mg/m², 1.6% at 700 mg/m², and 3.3% at 900 mg/m². In the adjuvant treatment of breast cancer, the maximum cumulative dose used in clinical trials was 720 mg/m². The risk of developing CHF increases rapidly with increasing total cumulative doses of epirubicin in excess of 900 mg/m²; this cumulative dose should only be exceeded with extreme caution. Active or dormant cardiovascular disease, prior or concomitant radiotherapy to the mediastinal/pericardial area, previous therapy with other anthracyclines or anthracenediones, or concomitant use of other cardiotoxic drugs may increase the risk of cardiac toxicity. Cardiac toxicity with ELLENCE may occur at lower cumulative doses whether or not cardiac risk factors are present.
3. Secondary acute myelogenous leukemia (AML) has been reported in patients with breast cancer treated with anthracyclines, including epirubicin. The occurrence of refractory secondary leukemia is more common when such drugs are given in combination with DNA-damaging antineoplastic agents, when patients have been heavily pretreated with cytotoxic drugs, or when doses of anthracyclines have been escalated. The cumulative risk of developing treatment-related AML, in 3844 patients with breast cancer who received adjuvant treatment with epirubicin-containing regimens, was estimated as 0.2% at 3 years and 0.8% at 5 years.
4. Dosage should be reduced in patients with impaired hepatic function (see DOSAGE AND ADMINISTRATION).
5. Severe myelosuppression may occur.
6. Epirubicin should be administered only under the supervision of a physician who is experienced in the use of cancer chemotherapeutic agents.

DESCRIPTION

ELLENCE Injection (epirubicin hydrochloride injection) is an anthracycline cytotoxic agent, intended for intravenous administration. ELLENCE is supplied as a sterile, clear, red solution and is available in polypropylene vials containing 50 and 200 mg of epirubicin hydrochloride as a preservative-free, ready-to-use solution. Each milliliter of solution contains 2 mg of epirubicin hydrochloride. Inactive ingredients include sodium chloride, USP, and water for injection, USP. The pH of the solution has been adjusted to 3.0 with hydrochloric acid, NF.

Epirubicin hydrochloride is the 4-epimer of doxorubicin and is a semi-synthetic derivative of daunorubicin. The chemical name is (8S- ***cis***)-10-[(3-amino-2,3,6-trideoxy-α-L- ***arabino***-hexopyranosyl)oxy]-7,8,9,10- tetrahydro-6,8,11-trihydroxy-8-(hydroxyacetyl)-1-methoxy-5,12-naphthacenedione hydrochloride. The active ingredient is a red-orange hygroscopic powder, with the empirical formula $C_{27}H_{29}NO_{11}$ HCl and a molecular weight of 579.95. The structural formula is as follows:

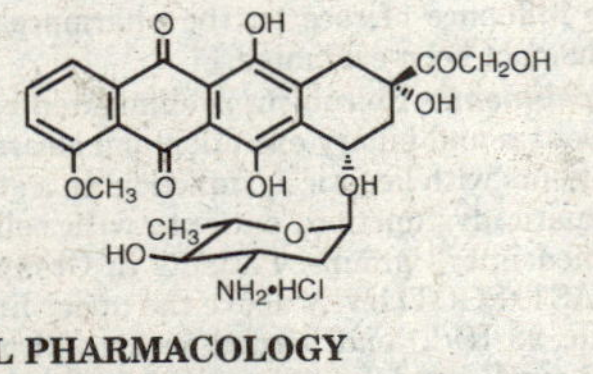

CLINICAL PHARMACOLOGY

Epirubicin is an anthracycline cytotoxic agent. Although it is known that anthracyclines can interfere with a number of biochemical and biological functions within eukaryotic cells, the precise mechanisms of epirubicin's cytotoxic and/or antiproliferative properties have not been completely elucidated.

Epirubicin forms a complex with DNA by intercalation of its planar rings between nucleotide base pairs, with consequent inhibition of nucleic acid (DNA and RNA) and protein synthesis. Such intercalation triggers DNA cleavage by

Continued on next page

Ellence—Cont.

topoisomerase II, resulting in cytocidal activity. Epirubicin also inhibits DNA helicase activity, preventing the enzymatic separation of double-stranded DNA and interfering with replication and transcription. Epirubicin is also involved in oxidation/reduction reactions by generating cytotoxic free radicals. The antiproliferative and cytotoxic activity of epirubicin is thought to result from these or other possible mechanisms.

Epirubicin is cytotoxic in vitro to a variety of established murine and human cell lines and primary cultures of human tumors. It is also active in vivo against a variety of murine tumors and human xenografts in athymic mice, including breast tumors.

Pharmacokinetics

Epirubicin pharmacokinetics are linear over the dose range of 60 to 150 mg/m^2 and plasma clearance is not affected by the duration of infusion or administration schedule. Pharmacokinetic parameters for epirubicin following 6- to 10-minute, single-dose intravenous infusions of epirubicin at doses of 60 to 150 mg/m^2 in patients with solid tumors are shown in Table 1. The plasma concentration declined in a triphasic manner with mean half-lives for the alpha, beta, and gamma phases of about 3 minutes, 2.5 hours, and 33 hours, respectively.

[See table 1 at right]

Distribution. Following intravenous administration, epirubicin is rapidly and widely distributed into the tissues. Binding of epirubicin to plasma proteins, predominantly albumin, is about 77% and is not affected by drug concentration. Epirubicin also appears to concentrate in red blood cells; whole blood concentrations are approximately twice those of plasma.

Metabolism. Epirubicin is extensively and rapidly metabolized by the liver and is also metabolized by other organs and cells, including red blood cells. Four main metabolic routes have been identified:

(1) reduction of the C-13 keto-group with the formation of the 13(S)-dihydro derivative, epirubicinol;

(2) conjugation of both the unchanged drug and epirubicinol with glucuronic acid; (3) loss of the amino sugar moiety through a hydrolytic process with the formation of the doxorubicin and doxorubicinol aglycones; and (4) loss of the amino sugar moiety through a redox process with the formation of the 7-deoxy-doxorubicin aglycone and 7-deoxydoxorubicinol aglycone. Epirubicinol has in vitro cytotoxic activity one-tenth that of epirubicin. As plasma levels of epirubicinol are lower than those of the unchanged drug, they are unlikely to reach in vivo concentrations sufficient for cytotoxicity. No significant activity or toxicity has been reported for the other metabolites.

Excretion. Epirubicin and its major metabolites are eliminated through biliary excretion and, to a lesser extent, by urinary excretion. Mass-balance data from 1 patient found about 60% of the total radioactive dose in feces (34%) and urine (27%). These data are consistent with those from 3 patients with extrahepatic obstruction and percutaneous drainage, in whom approximately 35% and 20% of the administered dose were recovered as epirubicin or its major metabolites in bile and urine, respectively, in the 4 days after treatment.

Pharmacokinetics in Special Populations

Age. A population analysis of plasma data from 36 cancer patients (13 males and 23 females, 20 to 73 years) showed that age affects plasma clearance of epirubicin in female patients. The predicted plasma clearance for a female patient of 70 years of age was about 35% lower than that for a female patient of 25 years of age. An insufficient number of males > 50 years of age were included in the study to draw conclusions about age-related alterations in clearance in males. Although a lower epirubicin starting dose does not appear necessary in elderly female patients, and was not used in clinical trials, particular care should be taken in monitoring toxicity when epirubicin is administered to female patients > 70 years of age. (See PRECAUTIONS).

Gender. In patients ≤ 50 years of age, mean clearance values in adult male and female patients were similar. The clearance of epirubicin is decreased in elderly women (see Pharmacokinetics in Special Populations - Age).

Pediatric. The pharmacokinetics of epirubicin in pediatric patients have not been evaluated.

Race. The influence of race on the pharmacokinetics of epirubicin has not been evaluated.

Hepatic Impairment. Epirubicin is eliminated by both hepatic metabolism and biliary excretion and clearance is reduced in patients with hepatic dysfunction. In a study of the effect of hepatic dysfunction, patients with solid tumors were classified into 3 groups. Patients in Group 1 (n=22) had serum AST (SGOT) levels above the upper limit of normal (median: 93 IU/L) and normal serum bilirubin levels (median: 0.5 mg/dL) and were given epirubicin doses of 12.5 to 90 mg/m^2. Patients in Group 2 had alterations in both serum AST (median: 175 IU/L) and bilirubin levels (median: 2.7 mg/dL) and were treated with an epirubicin dose of 25 mg/m^2 (n=8). Their pharmacokinetics were compared to those of patients with normal serum AST and bilirubin values, who received epirubicin doses of 12.5 to 120 mg/m^2. The median plasma clearance of epirubicin was decreased compared to patients with normal hepatic function by about 30% in patients in Group 1 and by 50% in patients in Group 2. Patients with more severe hepatic impairment have not been evaluated. (See WARNINGS and DOSAGE AND ADMINISTRATION.)

Table 1. Summary of Mean (±SD) Pharmacokinetic Parameters in Patients[1] with Solid Tumors Receiving Intravenous Epirubicin 60 to 150 mg/m^2

Dose[2] (mg/m^2)	C_{max}[3] (µg/mL)	AUC[4] (µg • h/mL)	t ½[5] (hours)	CL[6] (L/hour)	Vss[7] (L/kg)
60	5.7 ± 1.6	1.6 ± 0.2	35.3 ± 9	65 ± 8	21 ± 2
75	5.3 ± 1.5	1.7 ± 0.3	32.1 ± 5	83 ± 14	27 ± 11
120	9.0 ± 3.5	3.4 ± 0.7	33.7 ± 4	65 ± 13	23 ± 7
150	9.3 ± 2.9	4.2 ± 0.8	31.1 ± 6	69 ± 13	21 ± 7

[1] Advanced solid tumor cancers, primarily of the lung
[2] N=6 patients per dose level
[3] Plasma concentration at the end of 6 to 10 minute infusion
[4] Area under the plasma concentration curve
[5] Half-life of terminal phase
[6] Plasma clearance
[7] Steady state volume of distribution

Table 2. Treatment Regimens Used in Phase 3 Studies of Patients with Early Breast Cancer

	Treatment Groups	Agent	Regimen
MA-5[1] N=716	**CEF-120** (total, 6 cycles)[2] N=356	Cyclophosphamide	75 mg/m^2 PO, d 1-14, q 28 days
		ELLENCE	60 mg/m^2 IV, d 1 & 8, q 28 days
		Fluorouracil	500 mg/m^2 IV, d 1 & 8, q 28 days
	CMF (total, 6 cycles) N=360	Cyclophosphamide	100 mg/m^{2}PO, d 1-14, q 28 days
		Methotrexate	40 mg/m^2 IV, d 1 & 8, q 28 days
		Fluorouracil	600 mg/m^2 IV, d 1 & 8, q 28 days
GFEA-05[3] N=565	**FEC-100** (total, 6 cycles) N=276	Fluorouracil	500 mg/m^{2}IV, d 1, q 21 days
		ELLENCE	100 mg/m^2 IV, d 1, q 21 days
		Cyclophosphamide	500 mg/m^2 IV, d 1, q 21 days
	FEC-50 (total, 6 cycles) N=289	Fluorouracil	500 mg/m^{2}IV, d 1, q 21 days
		ELLENCE	50 mg/m^2 IV, d 1, q 21 days
		Cyclophosphamide	500 mg/m^2 IV, d 1, 21 days
	Tamoxifen 30 mg daily × 3 years, postmenopausal women, any receptor status		

[1] In women who underwent lumpectomy, breast irradiation was to be administered after completion of study chemotherapy.
[2] Patients also received prophylactic antibiotic therapy with trimethoprim-sulfamethoxazole or fluroquinolone for the duration of their chemotherapy.
[3] All women were to receive breast irradiation after the completion of chemotherapy.

Table 3. Efficacy Results from Phase 3 Studies of Patients with Early Breast Cancer*

	MA-5 Study		GFEA-05 Study	
	CEF-120 N=356	CMF N=360	FEC-100 N=276	FEC-50 N=289
RFS at 5 yrs (%)	62	53	65	52
Log-rank Test	(stratified p=0.013)		(p=0.007)	
OS at 5 yrs	77	70	76	65
Log-rank Test	(stratified p=0.043) (unstratified p=0.13)		(p=0.007)	

*Based on Kaplan-Meier estimates

Renal Impairment. No significant alterations in the pharmacokinetics of epirubicin or its major metabolite, epirubicinol, have been observed in patients with serum creatinine < 5 mg/dL. A 50% reduction in plasma clearance was reported in four patients with serum creatinine ≥ 5 mg/dL (see WARNINGS and DOSAGE AND ADMINISTRATION). Patients on dialysis have not been studied.

Drug-Drug Interactions

Taxanes. Coadministration of paclitaxel or docetaxel did not affect the pharmacokinetics of epirubicin when given immediately following the taxane.

Cimetidine. Coadministration of cimetidine (400 mg twice daily for 7 days starting 5 days before chemotherapy) increased the mean AUC of epirubicin (100 mg/m^2) by 50% and decreased its plasma clearance by 30% (see PRECAUTIONS).

Drugs metabolized by cytochrome P-450 enzymes. No systematic in vitro or in vivo evaluation has been performed to examine the potential for inhibition or induction by epirubicin of oxidative cytochrome P-450 isoenzymes.

CLINICAL STUDIES

Two randomized, open-label, multicenter studies evaluated the use of ELLENCE Injection 100 to 120 mg/m^2 in combination with cyclophosphamide and fluorouracil for the adjuvant treatment of patients with axiliary-node-positive breast cancer and no evidence of distant metastatic disease (Stage II or III). Study MA-5 evaluated 120 mg/m^2 of epirubicin per course in combination with cyclophosphamide and fluorouracil (CEF-120 regimen). This study randomized premenopausal and perimenopausal women with one or more positive lymph nodes to an epirubicin-containing CEF-120 regimen or to a CMF regimen. Study GFEA-05 evaluated the use of 100 mg/m^2 of epirubicin per course in combination with fluorouracil and cyclophosphamide (FEC-100). This study randomized pre- and postmenopausal women to the FEC-100 regimen or to a lower-dose FEC-50 regimen. In the GFEA-05 study, eligible patients were either required to have ≥ 4 nodes involved with tumor or, if only 1 to 3 nodes were positive, to have negative estrogen- and progesterone-receptors and a histologic tumor grade of 2 or 3. A total of 1281 women participated in these studies. Patients with T4 tumors were not eligible for either study. Table 2 shows the treatment regimens that the patients received.

[See table 2 above]

In the MA-5 trial, the median age of the study population was 45 years. Approximately 60% of patients had 1 to 3 involved nodes and approximately 40% had ≥ 4 nodes involved with tumor. In the GFEA-05 study, the median age was 51 years and approximately half of the patients were postmenopausal. About 17% of the study population had 1 to 3 positive nodes and 80% of patients had ≥ 4 involved lymph nodes. Demographic and tumor characteristics were well-balanced between treatment arms in each study.

The efficacy endpoints of relapse-free survival (RFS) and overall survival (OS) were analyzed using Kaplan-Meier methods in the intent-to-treat (ITT) patient populations in each study. Results for endpoints are described in terms of the outcomes at 5 years. In Study MA-5, epirubicin-containing combination therapy (CEF-120) showed significantly longer 5-year RFS than CMF (62% versus 53%; stratified log rank p=0.013). The overall reduction in risk of relapse was 24%. The 5-year OS was also greater for the epirubicin-containing CEF-120 regimen than for the CMF regimen (77% versus 70%; stratified log rank p=0.043; nonstratified log rank p=0.13). The overall relative reduction in the risk of death was 29%.

In Study GFEA-05, patients treated with the higher-dose epirubicin regimen (FEC-100) had a significantly longer 5-year RFS (65% versus 52%, log rank p=0.007) and OS (76% versus 65%, log rank p=0.007) than patients given the lower dose regimen (FEC-50). The overall reduction in risk of relapse was 32%. The relative reduction in the risk of death was 31%.

Although the trials were not powered for subset analyses, improvement in RFS and OS were observed both in patients with 1-3 nodes positive and in those with ≥ 4 nodes positive for tumor involvement when comparing the CEF-120 or FEC-100 groups with the control groups. In addition, in the

Figure 1. Relapse-Free Survival in Study MA-5

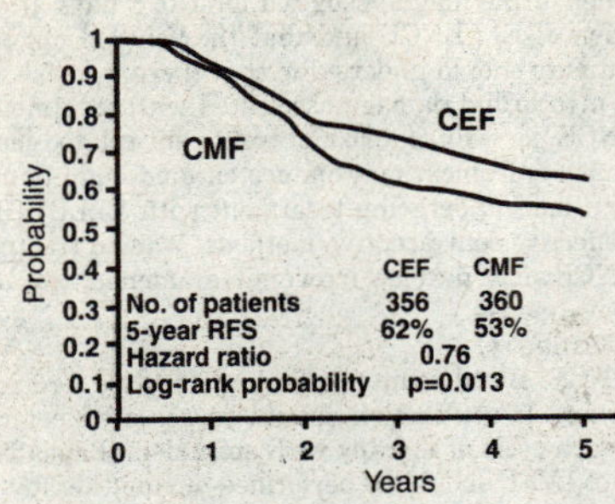

Figure 2. Overall Survival in Study MA-5

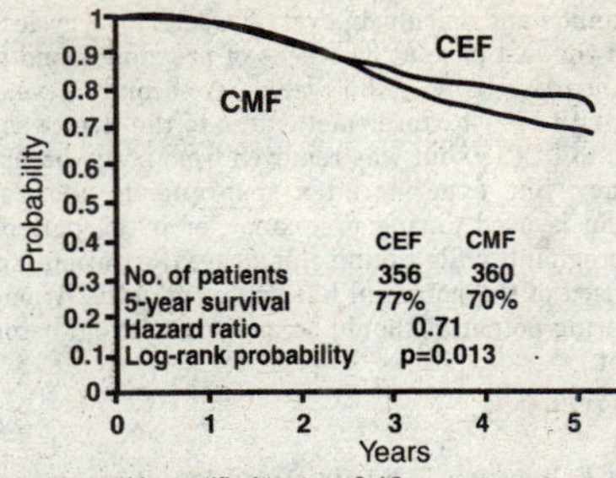

*Unstratified test, p=0.13

Figure 3. Relapse-Free Survival in Study GFEA-05

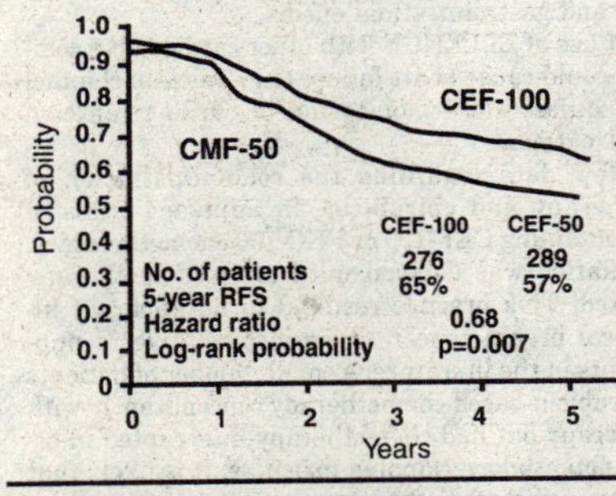

Figure 4. Overall Survival in Study GFEA-0

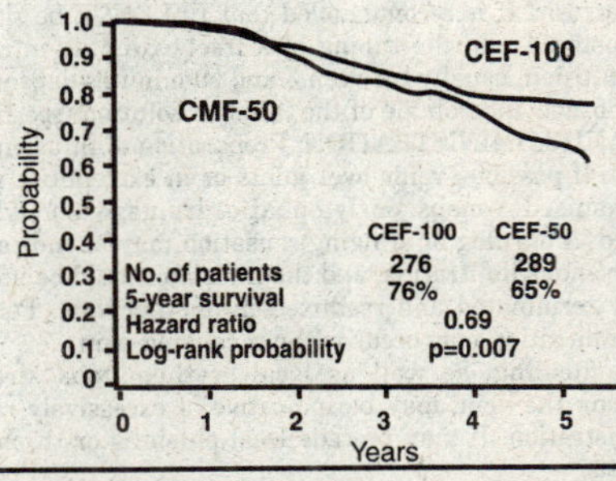

GFEA-05 study, similar improvements in RFS and OS were observed in both pre- and postmenopausal women treated with FEC-100 compared to FEC-50. Efficacy results for the two studies are shown in Table 3.

[See table 3 on previous page]

The Kaplan-Meier curves for RFS and OS from Study MA-5 are shown in Figures 1 and 2 and those for Study GFEA-05 are shown in Figures 3 and 4.

[See figures 1, 2, 3 & 4 above]

INDICATIONS AND USAGE

ELLENCE Injection is indicated as a component of adjuvant therapy in patients with evidence of axillary node tumor involvement following resection of primary breast cancer.

CONTRAINDICATIONS

Patients should not be treated with ELLENCE Injection if they have any of the following conditions: baseline neutrophil count < 1500 cells/mm^3; severe myocardial insufficiency, recent myocardial infarction, severe arrhythmias; previous treatment with anthracyclines up to the maximum cumulative dose; hypersensitivity to epirubicin, other anthracyclines, or anthracenediones; or severe hepatic dysfunction (see WARNINGS and DOSAGE AND ADMINISTRATION).

WARNINGS

ELLENCE Injection should be administered only under the supervision of qualified physicians experienced in the use of cytotoxic therapy. Before beginning treatment with epirubicin, patients should recover from acute toxicities (such as stomatitis, neutropenia, thrombocytopenia, and generalized infections) of prior cytotoxic treatment. Also, initial treatment with ELLENCE should be preceded by a careful baseline assessment of blood counts; serum levels of total bilirubin, AST, and creatinine; and cardiac function as measured by left ventricular ejection function (LVEF). Patients should be carefully monitored during treatment for possible clinical complications due to myelosuppression. Supportive care may be necessary for the treatment of severe neutropenia and severe infectious complications. Monitoring for potential cardiotoxicity is also important, especially with greater cumulative exposure to epirubicin.

Hematologic Toxicity. A dose-dependent, reversible leukopenia and/or neutropenia is the predominant manifestation of hematologic toxicity associated with epirubicin and represents the most common acute dose-limiting toxicity of this drug. In most cases, the white blood cell (WBC) nadir is reached 10 to 14 days from drug administration. Leukopenia/neutropenia is usually transient, with WBC and neutrophil counts generally returning to normal values by Day 21 after drug administration. As with other cytotoxic agents, ELLENCE at the recommended dose in combination with cyclophosphamide and fluorouracil can produce severe leukopenia and neutropenia. Severe thrombocytopenia and anemia may also occur. Clinical consequences of severe myelosuppression include fever, infection, septicemia, septic shock, hemorrhage, tissue hypoxia, symptomatic anemia, or death. If myelosuppressive complications occur, appropriate supportive measures (e.g., intravenous antibiotics, colony-stimulating factors, transfusions) may be required. Myelosuppression requires careful monitoring. Total and differential WBC, red blood cell (RBC), and platelet counts should be assessed before and during each cycle of therapy with ELLENCE.

Cardiac Function. Cardiotoxicity is a known risk of anthracycline treatment. Anthracycline-induced cardiac toxicity may be manifested by early (or acute) or late (delayed) events. Early cardiac toxicity of epirubicin consists mainly of sinus tachycardia and/or ECG abnormalities such as nonspecific ST-T wave changes, but tachyarrhythmias, including premature ventricular contractions and ventricular tachycardia, bradycardia, as well as atrioventricular and bundle-branch block have also been reported. These effects do not usually predict subsequent development of delayed cardiotoxicity, are rarely of clinical importance, and are generally not considered an indication for the suspension of epirubicin treatment. Delayed cardiac toxicity results from a characteristic cardiomyopathy that is manifested by reduced LVEF and/or signs and symptoms of congestive heart failure (CHF) such as tachycardia, dyspnea, pulmonary edema, dependent edema, hepatomegaly, ascites, pleural effusion, gallop rhythm. Life-theatening CHF is the most severe form of anthracycline-induced cardiomyopathy. This toxicity appears to be dependent on the cumulative dose of ELLENCE and represents the cumulative dose-limiting toxicity of the drug. If it occurs, delayed cardiotoxicity usually develops late in the course of therapy with ELLENCE or within 2 to 3 months after completion of treatment, but later events (several months to years after treatment termination) have been reported.

In a retrospective survey, including 9144 patients, mostly with solid tumors in advanced stages, the probability of developing CHF increased with increasing cumulative doses of ELLENCE (Figure 5). The estimated risk of epirubicin-treated patients developing clinically evident CHF was 0.9% at a cumulative dose of 550 mg/m^2, 1.6% at 700 mg/m^2, and 3.3% at 900 mg/m^2. The risk of developing CHF in the absence of other cardiac risk factors increased steeply after an epirubicin cumulative dose of 900 mg/m^2.

Figure 5. Risk of CHF in 9144 Patients Treated with Epirubicin

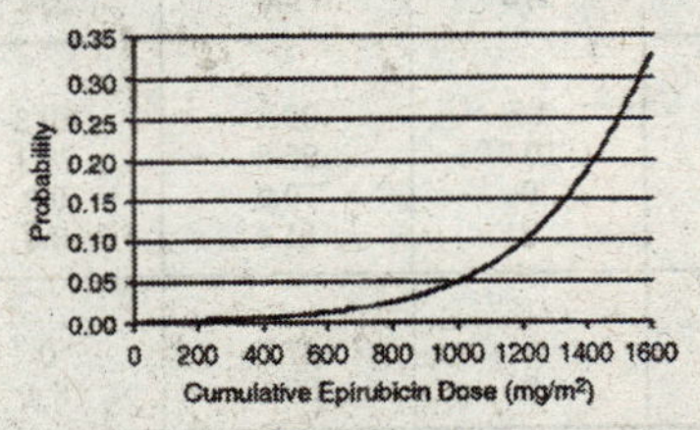

In another retrospective survey of 469 epirubicin-treated patients with metastatic or early breast cancer, the reported risk of CHF was comparable to that observed in the larger study of over 9000 patients.

Given the risk of cardiomyopathy, a cumulative dose of 900 mg/m^2 ELLENCE should be exceeded only with extreme caution. Risk factors (active or dormant cardiovascular disease, prior or concomitant radiotherapy to the mediastinal/pericardial area, previous therapy with other anthracyclines or anthracenediones, concomitant use of other drugs with the ability to suppress cardiac contractility) may increase the risk of cardiac toxicity. Although not formally tested, it is probable that the toxicity of epirubicin and other anthracyclines or anthracenediones is additive. Cardiac toxicity with ELLENCE may occur at lower cumulative doses whether or not cardiac risk factors are present. Although endomyocardial biopsy is recognized as the most sensitive diagnostic tool to detect anthracycline-induced cardiomyopathy, this invasive examination is not practically performed on a routine basis. Electrocardiogram (ECG) changes such as dysrhythmias, a reduction of the QRS voltage, or a prolongation beyond normal limits of the systolic time interval may be indicative of anthracycline-induced cardiomyopathy, but ECG is not a sensitive or specific method for following anthracycline-related cardiotoxicity. The risk of serious cardiac impairment may be decreased through regular monitoring of LVEF during the course of treatment with prompt discontinuation of ELLENCE at the first sign of impaired function. The preferred method for repeated assessment of cardiac function is evaluation of LVEF measured by multi-gated radionuclide angiography (MUGA) or echocardiography (ECHO). A baseline cardiac evaluation with an ECG and a MUGA scan or an ECHO is recommended, especially in patients with risk factors for increased cardiac toxicity. Repeated MUGA or ECHO determinations of LVEF should be performed, particularly with higher, cumulative anthracycline doses. The technique used for assessment should be consistent through follow-up. In patients with risk factors, particularly prior anthracycline or anthracenedione use, the monitoring of cardiac function must be particularly strict and the risk-benefit of continuing treatment with ELLENCE in patients with impaired cardiac function must be carefully evaluated.

Secondary Leukemia. The occurrence of secondary acute myelogenous leukemia, with or without a preleukemic phase, has been reported in patients treated with anthracyclines. Secondary leukemia is more common when such drugs are given in combination with DNA-damaging antineoplastic agents, when patients have been heavily pretreated with cytotoxic drugs, or when doses of the anthracyclines have been escalated. These leukemias can have a short 1- to 3- year latency period. An analysis of 3844 patients who received adjuvant treatment with epirubicin in controlled clinical trials, showed a cumulative risk of secondary acute myelogenous leukemia of about 0.2% (approximate 95% CI, 0.05-0.4) at 3 years and approximately 0.8% (approximate 95% CI, 0.3-1.2) at 5 years. ELLENCE is mutagenic, clastogenic, and carcinogenic in animals (see next section, Carcinogenesis, Mutagenesis and Impairment of Fertility).

Carcinogenesis, Mutagenesis & Impairment of Fertility. Treatment-related acute myelogenous leukemia has been reported in women treated with epirubicin-based adjuvant chemotherapy regimens (see above section, WARNINGS, Secondary Leukemia). Conventional long-term animal studies to evaluate the carcinogenic potential of epirubicin have not been conducted, but intravenous administration of a single 3.6 mg/kg epirubicin dose to female rats (about 0.2 times the maximum recommended human dose on a body surface area basis) approximately doubled the incidence of mammary tumors (primarily fibroadenomas) observed at 1 year. Administration of 0.5 mg/kg epirubicin intravenously to rats (about 0.025 times the maximum recommended human dose on a body surface area basis) every 3 weeks for ten doses increased the incidence of subcutaneous fibromas in males over an 18-month observation period. In addition, subcutaneous administration of 0.75 or 1.0 mg/kg/day (about 0.015 times the maximum recommended human dose on a body surface area basis) to newborn rats for 4 days on both the first and tenth day after birth for a total of eight doses increased the incidence of animals with tumors compared to controls during a 24-month observation period.

Epirubicin was mutagenic in vitro to bacteria (Ames test) either in the presence or absence of metabolic activation and to mammalian cells (HGPRT assay in V79 Chinese hamster lung fibroblasts) in the absence but not in the presence of metabolic activation. Epirubicin was clastogenic in vitro (chromosome aberrations in human lymphocytes) both in the presence and absence of metabolic activation and was also clastogenic in vivo (chromosome aberration in mouse bone marrow).

In fertility studies in rats, males were given epirubicin daily for 9 weeks and mated with females that were given epirubicin daily for 2 weeks prior to mating and through Day 7 of gestation. When 0.3 mg/kg/day (about 0.015 times the maximum recommended human single dose on a body surface area basis) was administered to both sexes, no pregnancies resulted. No effects on mating behavior or fertility were observed at 0.1 mg/kg/day, but male rats had atrophy of the testes and epididymis, and reduced spermatogenesis. The 0.1 mg/kg/day dose also caused embryolethality. An increased incidence of fetal growth retardation was observed in these studies at 0.03 mg/kg/day (about 0.0015 times the maximum recommended human single dose on a body surface area basis). Multiple daily doses of epirubicin to rabbits and dogs also caused atrophy of male reproductive organs. Single 20.5 and 12 mg/kg doses of intravenous epirubicin caused testicular atrophy in mice and rats, respectively (both approximately 0.5 times the maximum recommended human dose on a body surface area basis). A single dose of 16.7 mg/kg epirubicin caused uterine atrophy in rats.

Although experimental data are not available, ELLENCE could induce chromosomal damage in human spermatozoa due to its genotoxic potential. Men undergoing treatment with ELLENCE should use effective contraceptive methods. ELLENCE may cause irreversible amenorrhea (premature menopause) in premenopausal women.

Liver Function. The major route of elimination of epirubicin is the hepatobiliary system (see CLINICAL PHARMACOLOGY, Pharmacokinetics in Special Populations). Serum total bilirubin and AST levels should be evaluated before and during treatment with ELLENCE. Patients with elevated bilirubin or AST may experience slower clearance of drug with an increase in overall toxicity. Lower doses are recommended in these patients (see DOSAGE AND ADMINISTRATION). Patients with severe hepatic impairment have not been evaluated; therefore, epirubicin should not be used in this patient population.

Renal Function. Serum creatinine should be assessed before and during therapy. Dosage adjustment is necessary in

Continued on next page

Ellence—Cont.

patients with serum creatinine >5 mg/dL (see DOSAGE AND ADMINISTRATION). Patients undergoing dialysis have not been studied.

Tumor-Lysis Syndrome. As with other cytotoxic agents, ELLENCE may induce hyperuricemia as a consequence of the extensive purine catabolism that accompanies drug-induced rapid lysis of highly chemosensitive neoplastic cells (tumor lysis syndrome). Other metabolic abnormalities may also occur. While not generally a problem in patients with breast cancer, physicians should consider the potential for tumor-lysis syndrome in potentially susceptible patients and should consider monitoring serum uric acid, potassium, calcium, phosphate, and creatinine immediately after initial chemotherapy administration. Hydration, urine alkalinization, and prophylaxis with allopurinol to prevent hyperuricemia may minimize potential complications of tumor-lysis syndrome.

Pregnancy - Category D. ELLENCE may cause fetal harm when administered to a pregnant woman. Administration of 0.8 mg/kg/day intravenously of epirubicin to rats (about 0.04 times the maximum recommended single human dose on a body surface area basis) during Days 5 to 15 of gestation was embryotoxic (increased resorptions and post-implantation loss) and caused fetal growth retardation (decreased body weight), but was not teratogenic up to this dose. Administration of 2 mg/kg/day intravenously of epirubicin to rats (about 0.1 times the maximum recommended single human dose on a body surface area basis) on Days 9 and 10 of gestation was embryotoxic (increased late resorptions, post-implantation losses, and dead fetuses; and decreased live fetuses), retarded fetal growth (decreased body weight), and caused decreased placental weight. This dose was also teratogenic, causing numerous external (anal atresia, misshapen tail, abnormal genital tubercle), visceral (primarily gastrointestinal, urinary, and cardiovascular systems), and skeletal (deformed long bones and girdles, rib abnormalities, irregular spinal ossification) malformations. Administration of intravenous epirubicin to rabbits at doses up to 0.2 mg/kg/day (about 0.02 times the maximum recommended single human dose on a body surface area basis) during Days 6 to 18 of gestation was not embryotoxic or teratogenic, but a maternally toxic dose of 0.32 mg/kg/day increased abortions and delayed ossification. Administration of a maternally toxic intravenous dose of 1 mg/kg/day epirubicin to rabbits (about 0.1 times the maximum recommended single human dose on a body surface area basis) on Days 10 to 12 of gestation induced abortion, but no other signs of embryofetal toxicity or teratogenicity were observed. When doses up to 0.5 mg/kg/day epirubicin were administered to rat dams from Day 17 of gestation to Day 21 after delivery (about 0.025 times the maximum recommended single human dose on a body surface area basis), no permanent changes were observed in the development, functional activity, behavior, or reproductive performance of the offspring.

There are no adequate and well-controlled studies in pregnant women. Two pregnancies have been reported in women taking epirubicin. A 34-year-old woman, 28 weeks pregnant at her diagnosis of breast cancer, was treated with cyclophosphamide and epirubicin every 3 weeks for 3 cycles. She received the last dose at 34 weeks of pregnancy and delivered a healthy baby at 35 weeks. A second 34-year-old woman with breast cancer metastatic to the liver was randomized to FEC-50 but was removed from study because of pregnancy. She experienced a spontaneous abortion. If epirubicin is used during pregnancy, or if the patient becomes pregnant while taking this drug, the patient should be apprised of the potential hazard to the fetus. Women of childbearing potential should be advised to avoid becoming pregnant.

PRECAUTIONS

General

ELLENCE Injection is administered by intravenous infusion. Venous sclerosis may result from an injection into a small vessel or from repeated injections into the same vein. Extravasation of epirubicin during the infusion may cause local pain, severe tissue lesions (vesication, severe cellulitis) and necrosis. It is recommended that ELLENCE be slowly administered into the tubing of a freely running intravenous infusion, usually between 3 and 20 minutes depending upon dosage and volume of the infusion solution (see DOSAGE AND ADMINISTRATION, Preparation of Infusion Solution). If possible, veins over joints or in extremities with compromised venous or lymphatic drainage should be avoided. A burning or stinging sensation may be indicative of perivenous infiltration, and the infusion should be immediately terminated and restarted in another vein. Perivenous infiltration may occur without causing pain.

Facial flushing, as well as local erythematous streaking along the vein, may be indicative of excessively rapid administration. It may precede local phlebitis or thrombophlebitis.

Patients administered the 120-mg/m^2 regimen of ELLENCE as a component of combination chemotherapy should also receive prophylactic antibiotic therapy with trimethoprim-sulfamethoxazole (e.g., Septra®, Bactrim®) or a fluoroquinolone (see CLINICAL STUDIES, Early Breast Cancer, and DOSAGE AND ADMINISTRATION).

Epirubicin is emetigenic. Antiemetics may reduce nausea and vomiting; prophylactic use of antiemetics should be considered before administration of ELLENCE, particularly when given in conjunction with other emetigenic drugs.

As with other anthracyclines, administration of ELLENCE after previous radiation therapy may induce an inflammatory recall reaction at the site of the irradiation.

As with other cytotoxic agents, thrombophlebitis and thromboembolic phenomena, including pulmonary embolism (in some cases fatal) have been coincidentally reported with the use of epirubicin.

Information for Patients

Patients should be informed of the expected adverse effects of epirubicin, including gastrointestinal symptoms (nausea, vomiting, diarrhea, and stomatitis) and potential neutropenic complications. Patients should consult their physician if vomiting, dehydration, fever, evidence of infection, symptoms of CHF, or injection-site pain occurs following therapy with ELLENCE. Patients should be informed that they will almost certainly develop alopecia. Patients should be advised that their urine may appear red for 1 to 2 days after administration of ELLENCE and that they should not be alarmed. Patients should understand that there is a risk of irreversible myocardial damage associated with treatment with ELLENCE, as well as a risk of treatment-related leukemia. Because epirubicin may induce chromosomal damage in sperm, men undergoing treatment with ELLENCE should use effective contraceptive methods. Women treated with ELLENCE may develop irreversible amenorrhea, or premature menopause.

Laboratory Testing

See WARNINGS. Blood counts, including absolute neutrophil counts, and liver function should be assessed before and during each cycle of therapy with epirubicin. Repeated evaluations of LVEF should be performed during therapy.

Drug Interactions

ELLENCE when used in combination with other cytotoxic drugs may show on-treatment additive toxicity, especially hematologic and gastrointestinal effects.

Concomitant use of ELLENCE with other cardioactive compounds that could cause heart failure (e.g., calcium channel blockers), requires close monitoring of cardiac function throughout treatment.

There are few data regarding the coadministration of radiation therapy and epirubicin. In adjuvant trials of epirubicin-containing CEF-120 or FEC-100 chemotherapies, breast irradiation was delayed until after chemotherapy was completed. This practice resulted in no apparent increase in local breast cancer recurrence relative to published accounts in the literature. A small number of patients received epirubicin-based chemotherapy concomitantly with radiation therapy but had chemotherapy interrupted in order to avoid potential overlapping toxicities. It is likely that use of epirubicin with radiotherapy may sensitize tissues to the cytotoxic actions of irradiation. Administration of ELLENCE after previous radiation therapy may induce an inflammatory recall reaction at the site of the irradiation.

Epirubicin is extensively metabolized by the liver. Changes in hepatic function induced by concomitant therapies may affect epirubicin metabolism, pharmacokinetics, therapeutic efficacy, and/or toxicity.

Cimetidine increased the AUC of epirubicin by 50%. Cimetidine treatment should be stopped during treatment with ELLENCE (see CLINICAL PHARMACOLOGY).

Drug-Laboratory Test Interactions

There are no known interactions between ELLENCE and laboratory tests.

Carcinogenesis, Mutagenesis & Impairment of Fertility

See WARNINGS.

Pregnancy

Pregnancy Category D - see WARNINGS.

Nursing Mothers

Epirubicin was excreted into the milk of rats treated with 0.50 mg/kg/day of epirubicin during peri- and postnatal periods. It is not known whether epirubicin is excreted in human milk. Because many drugs, including other anthracyclines, are excreted in human milk and because of the potential for serious adverse reactions in nursing infants from epirubicin, mothers should discontinue nursing prior to taking this drug.

Geriatric Use

Although a lower starting dose of ELLENCE was not used in trials in elderly female patients, particular care should be taken in monitoring toxicity when ELLENCE is administered to female patients ≥ 70 years of age. (See CLINICAL PHARMACOLOGY, Pharmacokinetics in Special Populations).

Pediatric Use

The safety and effectiveness of epirubicin in pediatric patients have not been established in adequate and well-controlled clinical trials. Pediatric patients may be at greater risk for anthracycline-induced acute manifestations of cardiotoxicity and for chronic CHF.

ADVERSE REACTIONS

On-Study Events

Integrated safety data are available from two studies (Studies MA-5 and GFEA-05, see CLINICAL STUDIES) evaluating epirubicin-containing combination regimens in patients with early breast cancer. Of the 1260 patients treated in these studies, 620 patients received the higher-dose epirubicin regimen (FEC-100/CEF-120), 280 patients received the lower-dose epirubicin regimen (FEC-50), and 360 patients received CMF. Serotonin-specific antiemetic therapy and colony-stimulating factors were not used in these trials. Clinically relevant acute adverse events are summarized in Table 4.

[See table 4 at left]

Table 4. Clinically Relevant Acute Adverse Events in Patients with Early Breast Cancer

Event	% of Patients					
	FEC-100/CEF-120 (N = 620)		FEC-50 (N = 280)		CMF (N = 360)	
	Grades 1-4	Grades 3/4	Grades 1-4	Grades 3/4	Grades 1-4	Grades 3/4
Hematologic						
Leukopenia	80.3	58.6	49.6	1.5	98.1	60.3
Neutropenia	80.3	67.2	53.9	10.5	95.8	78.1
Anemia	72.2	5.8	12.9	0	70.9	0.9
Thrombocytopenia	48.8	5.4	4.6	0	51.4	3.6
Endocrine						
Amenorrhea	71.8	0	69.3	0	67.7	0
Hot flashes	38.9	4.0	5.4	0	69.1	6.4
Body as a Whole						
Lethargy	45.8	1.9	1.1	0	72.7	0.3
Fever	5.2	0	1.4	0	4.5	0
Gastrointestinal						
Nausea/vomiting	92.4	25.0	83.2	22.1	85.0	6.4
Mucositis	58.5	8.9	9.3	0	52.9	1.9
Diarrhea	24.8	0.8	7.1	0	50.7	2.8
Anorexia	2.9	0	1.8	0	5.8	0.3
Infection						
Infection	21.5	1.6	15.0	0	25.9	0.6
Febrile neutropenia	NA	6.1	0	0	NA	1.1
Ocular						
Conjunctivitis/keratitis	14.8	0	1.1	0	38.4	0
Skin						
Alopecia	95.5	56.6	69.6	19.3	84.4	6.7
Local toxicity	19.5	0.3	2.5	0.4	8.1	0
Rash/itch	8.9	0.3	1.4	0	14.2	0
Skin changes	4.7	0	0.7	0	7.2	0

FEC & CEF = cyclophosphamide + epirubicin + fluorouracil; CMF = cyclophosphamide + methotrexate + flurouracil
NA = not available

Grade 1 or 2 changes in transaminase levels were observed but were more frequently seen with CMF than with CEF.

Delayed Events

Table 5 describes the incidence of delayed adverse events in patients participating in the MA-5 and GFEA-05 trials.

[Set table 5 at top of next page]

Two cases of acute lymphoid leukemia (ALL) were also observed in patients receiving epirubicin. However, an association between anthracyclines such as epirubicin and ALL has not been clearly established.

Overview of Acute and Delayed Toxicities

Hematologic—See WARNINGS.

Gastrointestinal. A dose-dependent mucositis (mainly oral stomatitis, less often esophagitis) may occur in patients treated with epirubicin. Clinical manifestations of mucositis

Table 5. Long-Term Adverse Events in Patients with Early Breast Cancer

Event	% of Patients		
	FEC-100/CEF-120 (N=620)	FEC-50 (N=280)	CMF (N=360)
Cardiac toxicity			
Asymptomatic drops in LVEF	1.8	1.4	0.8
CHF	1.5	0.4	0.3
Leukemia			
AML	0.8	0	0.3

CEF-120:	Cyclophosphamide	75 mg/m^2 PO D 1-14
	ELLENCE	60 mg/m^2 IV D 1, 8
	5-Fluorouracil	500 mg/m^2 IV D 1, 8
	Repeated every 28 days for 6 cycles	
FEC-100:	5-Fluorouracil	500 mg/m^2
	ELLENCE	100 mg/m^2
	Cyclophosphamide	500 mg/m^2
	All drugs administered intravenously on Day 1 and repeated every 21 days for 6 cycles	

may include a pain or burning sensation, erythema, erosions, ulcerations, bleeding, or infections. Mucositis generally appears early after drug administration and, if severe, may progress over a few days to mucosal ulcerations; most patients recover from this adverse event by the third week of therapy. Hyperpigmentation of the oral mucosa may also occur.

Nausea, vomiting, and occasionally diarrhea and abdominal pain can also occur. Severe vomiting and diarrhea may produce dehydration. Antiemetics may reduce nausea and vomiting; prophylactic use of antiemetics should be considered before therapy (see PRECAUTIONS).

Cutaneous and Hypersensitivity Reactions. Alopecia occurs frequently, but is usually reversible, with hair regrowth occurring within 2 to 3 months from the termination of therapy. Flushes, skin and nail hyperpigmentation, photosensitivity, and hypersensitivity to irradiated skin (radiation-recall reaction) have been observed. Urticaria and anaphylaxis have been reported in patients treated with epirubicin; signs and symptoms of these reactions may vary from skin rash and pruritus to fever, chills, and shock.

Cardiovascular—See WARNINGS.

Secondary Leukemia—See WARNINGS

Injection-Site Reactions—See PRECAUTIONS.

OVERDOSAGE

A 36-year-old man with non-Hodgkin's lymphoma received a daily 95 mg/m^2 dose of ELLENCE Injection for 5 consecutive days. Five days later, he developed bone marrow aplasia, grade 4 mucositis, and gastrointestinal bleeding. No signs of acute cardiac toxicity were observed. He was treated with antibiotics, colony-stimulating factors, and antifungal agents, and recovered completely. A 63-year-old woman with breast cancer and liver metastasis received a single 320 mg/m^2 dose of ELLENCE. She was hospitalized with hyperthermia and developed multiple organ failure (respiratory and renal), with lactic acidosis, increased lactate dehydrogenase, and anuria. Death occurred within 24 hours after administration of ELLENCE. Additional instances of administration of doses higher than recommended have been reported at doses ranging from 150 to 250 mg/m^2. The observed adverse events in these patients were qualitatively similar to known toxicities of epirubicin. Most of the patients recovered with appropriate supportive care.

If an overdose occurs, supportive treatment (including antibiotic therapy, blood and platelet transfusions, colony-stimulating factors, and intensive care as needed) should be provided until the recovery of toxicities. Delayed CHF has been observed months after anthracycline administration. Patients must be observed carefully over time for signs of CHF and provided with appropriate supportive therapy.

DOSAGE AND ADMINISTRATION

ELLENCE Injection is administered to patients by intravenous infusion. ELLENCE is given in repeated 3- to 4-week cycles. The total dose of ELLENCE may be given on Day 1 of each cycle or divided equally and given on Days 1 and 8 of each cycle. The recommended dosages of ELLENCE are as follows:

Starting Doses

The recommended starting dose of ELLENCE is 100 to 120 mg/m^2. The following regimens were used in the trials supporting use of ELLENCE as a component of adjuvant therapy in patients with axillary-node positive breast cancer:

[See second table above]

Patients administered the 120-mg/m^2 regimen of ELLENCE also received prophylactic antibiotic therapy with trimethoprim-sulfamethoxazole (e.g., Septra®, Bactrim®) or a fluoroquinolone.

Bone Marrow Dysfunction. Consideration should be given to administration of lower starting doses (75-90 mg/m^2) for heavily pretreated patients, patients with pre-existing bone marrow depression, or in the presence of neoplastic bone marrow infiltration (see WARNINGS and PRECAUTIONS).

Hepatic Dysfunction. Definitive recommendations regarding use of ELLENCE in patients with hepatic dysfunction are not available because patients with hepatic abnormalities were excluded from participation in adjuvant trials of FEC-100/CEF-120 therapy. In patients with elevated serum AST or serum total bilirubin concentrations, the following dose reductions were recommended in clinical trials, although few patients experienced hepatic impairment:

- Bilirubin 1.2 to 3 mg/dL or AST 2 to 4 times upper limit of normal
  1/2 of recommended starting dose
- Bilirubin > 3 mg/dL or AST > 4 times upper limit of normal
  1/4 of recommended starting dose

Information regarding experience in patients with hepatic dysfunction is provided in CLINICAL PHARMACOLOGY, Pharmacokinetics In Special Populations.

Renal Dysfunction. While no specific dose recommendation can be made based on the limited available data in patients with renal impairment, lower doses should be considered in patients with severe renal impairment (serum creatinine > 5 mg/dL).

Dose Modifications

Dosage adjustments after the first treatment cycle should be made based on hematologic and nonhematologic toxicities. Patients experiencing during treatment cycle nadir platelet counts <50,000/mm^3, absolute neutrophil counts (ANC) <250/mm^3, neutropenic fever, or Grades 3/4 nonhematologic toxicity should have the Day 1 dose in subsequent cycles reduced to 75% of the Day 1 dose given in the current cycle. Day 1 chemotherapy in subsequent courses of treatment should be delayed until platelet counts are ≥100,000/mm^3, ANC ≥1500/mm^3, and nonhematologic toxicities have recovered to ≤ Grade 1.

For patients receiving a divided dose of ELLENCE (Day 1 and Day 8), the Day 8 dose should be 75% of Day 1 if platelet counts are 75,000-100,000/mm^3 and ANC is 1000 to 1499/mm^3. If Day 8 platelet counts are <75,000/mm^3, ANC <1000/mm^3, or Grade 3/4 nonhematologic toxicity has occurred, the Day 8 dose should be omitted.

Preparation & Administration Precautions

Parenteral drug products should be inspected visually for particulate matter and discoloration prior to administration, whenever solution and container permit. Procedures normally used for proper handling and disposal of anticancer drugs should be considered for use with ELLENCE. Several guidelines on this subject have been published.[1–8]

Protective measures. The following protective measures should be taken when handling ELLENCE:

- Personnel should be trained in appropriate techniques for reconstitution and handling.
- Pregnant staff should be excluded from working with this drug.
- Personnel handling ELLENCE should wear protective clothing: goggles, gowns and disposable gloves and masks.
- A designated area should be defined for syringe preparation (preferably under a laminar flow system), with the work surface protected by disposable, plastic-backed, absorbent paper.
- All items used for reconstitution, administration or cleaning (including gloves) should be placed in high-risk, waste-disposal bags for high temperature incineration.

Spillage or leakage should be treated with dilute sodium hypochlorite (1% available chlorine) solution, preferably by soaking, and then water. All contaminated and cleaning materials should be placed in high-risk, waste-disposal bags for incineration. Accidental contact with the skin or eyes should be treated immediately by copious lavage with water, or soap and water, or sodium bicarbonate solution. However, do not abrade the skin by using a scrub brush. Medical attention should be sought. Always wash hands after removing gloves.

Incompatibilities. Prolonged contact with any solution of an alkaline pH should be avoided as it will result in hydrolysis of the drug. ELLENCE should not be mixed with heparin or fluorouracil due to chemical incompatibility that may lead to precipitation.

ELLENCE can be used in combination with other antitumor agents, but it is not recommended that it be mixed with other drugs in the same syringe.

Preparation of Infusion Solution

ELLENCE is provided as a preservative-free, ready-to-use solution.

ELLENCE should be administered into the tubing of a freely flowing intravenous infusion (0.9% sodium chloride or 5% glucose solution). The usual infusion time ranges between 3 and 20 minutes depending upon dosage and volume of the infusion solution. This technique is intended to minimize the risk of thrombosis or perivenous extravasation, which could lead to severe cellulitis, vesication, or tissue necrosis. A direct push injection is not recommended due to the risk of extravasation, which may occur even in the presence of adequate blood return upon needle aspiration. Venous sclerosis may result from injection into small vessels or repeated injections into the same vein (see PRECAUTIONS). ELLENCE should be used within 24 hours of first penetration of the rubber stopper. Discard any unused solution.

HOW SUPPLIED

ELLENCE Injection is available in polypropylene single-use vials containing 2 mg epirubicin hydrochloride per mL as a sterile, preservative-free, ready-to-use solution in the following strengths:

50 mg/25 mL single-use vial NDC 0009-5091-01
200 mg/100 mL single-use vial NDC 0009-5093-01

Store refrigerated between 2°C and 8°C (36°F and 46°F). Do not freeze. Protect from light. Discard unused portion.

℞ only

US Patent No. 5,977,082

Manufactured for: Pharmacia & Upjohn Company, A subsidiary of Pharmacia Corporation, Kalamazoo, MI 49001 USA
By: Pharmacia (Perth) Pty Limited, Bentley WA 6102 Australia

April 2003 817 911 105
692532

REFERENCES

1. ONS Clinical Practice Committee. Cancer Chemotherapy Guidelines and Recommendations Practice. Pittsburgh, PA: Oncology Nursing Society; 1999: 32-41.
2. Recommendations for the Safe Handling of Parenteral Antineoplastic Drugs. Washington, DC: Division of Safety, Clinical Center Pharmacy Department and Cancer Nursing Services, National Institutes of Health; 1992 US Dept of Health and Human Services. Public Health Service Publication NIH 92-2621.
3. AMA Council on Scientific Affairs. Guidelines for Handling Parenteral Antineoplastics. JAMA 1985; 253(11):1590-1592.
4. National Study Commission on Cytotoxic Exposure - Recommendations for Handling of Cytotoxic Agents. 1987. Available from Louis P. Jeffrey, ScD., Chairman, National Study Commission on Cytotoxic Exposure, Massachusetts College of Pharmacy and Allied Health Sciences, 179 Longwood Avenue, Boston, MA 02115.
5. Clinical Oncology Society of Australia, Guidelines and Recommendations for Safe Handling of Antineoplastic Agents. Med J Australia 1983; 1:426-428.
6. Jones RB, Frank R, Mass T. Safe Handling of Chemotherapeutic Agents: A Report from the Mount Sinai Medical Center. CA-A Cancer J for Clin 1983; 33:258-263.
7. American Society of Hospital Pharmacists. ASHP Technical Assistance Bulletin on Handling Cytotoxic and Hazardous Drugs. Am J Hosp Pharm 1990; 47:1033-1049.
8. Controlling Occupational Exposure to Hazardous Drugs (OSHA Work-Practice Guidelines). Am J Health-Syst Pharm 1996; 53:1669-1685.

Jun 2003 PAM274AC

FRAGMIN® ℞

[*frăg-mĭn*]

dalteparin sodium injection

For *Subcutaneous* Use Only

Prescribing information for this product, which appears on pages 2762–2765 of the 2004 PDR, has been completely revised as follows. Please write "See Supplement A" next to the product heading.

SPINAL/EPIDURAL HEMATOMAS

When neuraxial anesthesia (epidural/spinal anesthesia) or spinal puncture is employed, patients anticoagulated or scheduled to be anticoagulated with low molecular weight heparins or heparinoids for prevention of thromboembolic complications are at risk of developing an epidural or spinal hematoma which can result in long-term or permanent paralysis.

The risk of these events is increased by the use of indwelling epidural catheters for administration of analgesia or by the concomitant use of drugs affecting hemostasis such as non steroidal anti-inflammatory drugs (NSAIDs), platelet inhibitors, or other anticoagulants. The risk also appears to be increased by traumatic or repeated epidural or spinal puncture.

Patients should be frequently monitored for signs and symptoms of neurological impairment. If neurological compromise is noted, urgent treatment is necessary.

The physician should consider the potential benefit versus risk before neuraxial intervention in patients anticoagulated or to be anticoagulated for thromboprophylaxis (also see **WARNINGS, Hemorrhage** and **PRECAUTIONS, Drug Interactions**).

DESCRIPTION

FRAGMIN Injection (dalteparin sodium injection) is a sterile, low molecular weight heparin. It is available in single-

Continued on next page

Fragmin—Cont.

dose, prefilled syringes preassembled with a needle guard device, and multiple-dose vials. With reference to the W.H.O. First International Low Molecular Weight Heparin Reference Standard, each syringe contains either 2500, 5000, 7500, or 10,000 anti-Factor Xa international units (IU), equivalent to 16, 32, 48, or 64 mg dalteparin sodium, respectively. Each vial contains either 10,000 or 25,000 anti-Factor Xa IU per 1 mL (equivalent to 64 or 160 mg dalteparin sodium, respectively), for a total of 95,000 anti-Factor Xa IU per vial.

Each prefilled syringe also contains Water for Injection and sodium chloride, when required, to maintain physiologic ionic strength. The prefilled syringes are preservative free. Each multiple-dose vial also contains Water for Injection and 14 mg of benzyl alcohol per mL as a preservative. The pH of both formulations is 5.0 to 7.5.

Dalteparin sodium is produced through controlled nitrous acid depolymerization of sodium heparin from porcine intestinal mucosa followed by a chromatographic purification process. It is composed of strongly acidic sulphated polysaccharide chains (oligosaccharide, containing 2,5-anhydro-D-mannitol residues as end groups) with an average molecular weight of 5000 and about 90% of the material within the range 2000-9000. The molecular weight distribution is:

< 3000 daltons	3.0-15.0%
3000 to 8000 daltons	65.0-78.0%
> 8000 daltons	14.0-26.0%

Structural Formula

[See chemical structure below]

CLINICAL PHARMACOLOGY

Dalteparin is a low molecular weight heparin with antithrombotic properties. It acts by enhancing the inhibition of Factor Xa and thrombin by antithrombin. In man, dalteparin potentiates preferentially the inhibition of coagulation Factor Xa, while only slightly affecting clotting time, e.g., activated partial thromboplastin time (APTT).

Pharmacodynamics:

Doses of FRAGMIN Injection of up to 10,000 anti-Factor Xa IU administered subcutaneously as a single dose or two 5000 IU doses 12 hours apart to healthy subjects do not produce a significant change in platelet aggregation, fibrinolysis, or global clotting tests such as prothrombin time (PT), thrombin time (TT) or APTT. Subcutaneous (s.c.) administration of doses of 5000 IU bid of FRAGMIN for seven consecutive days to patients undergoing abdominal surgery did not markedly affect APTT, Platelet Factor 4 (PF4), or lipoprotein lipase.

Pharmacokinetics:

Mean peak levels of plasma anti-Factor Xa activity following single s.c. doses of 2500, 5000 and 10,000 IU were 0.19 ± 0.04, 0.41 ± 0.07 and 0.82 ± 0.10 IU/mL, respectively, and were attained in about 4 hours in most subjects. Absolute bioavailability in healthy volunteers, measured as the anti-Factor Xa activity, was 87 ± 6%. Increasing the dose from 2500 to 10,000 IU resulted in an overall increase in anti-Factor Xa AUC that was greater than proportional by about one-third.

Peak anti-Factor Xa activity increased more or less linearly with dose over the same dose range. There appeared to be no appreciable accumulation of anti-Factor Xa activity with twice-daily dosing of 100 IU/kg s.c. for up to 7 days.

The volume of distribution for dalteparin anti-Factor Xa activity was 40 to 60 mL/kg. The mean plasma clearances of dalteparin anti-Factor Xa activity in normal volunteers following single intravenous bolus doses of 30 and 120 anti-Factor Xa IU/kg were 24.6 ± 5.4 and 15.6 ± 2.4 mL/hr/kg, respectively. The corresponding mean disposition half-lives are 1.47 ± 0.3 and 2.5 ± 0.3 hours.

Following intravenous doses of 40 and 60 IU/kg, mean terminal half-lives were 2.1 ± 0.3 and 2.3 ± 0.4 hours, respectively. Longer apparent terminal half-lives (3 to 5 hours) are observed following s.c. dosing, possibly due to delayed absorption. In patients with chronic renal insufficiency requiring hemodialysis, the mean terminal half-life of anti-Factor Xa activity following a single intravenous dose of 5000 IU FRAGMIN was 5.7 ± 2.0 hours, i.e. considerably longer than values observed in healthy volunteers, therefore, greater accumulation can be expected in these patients.

CLINICAL TRIALS

Prophylaxis of Ischemic Complications in Unstable Angina and Non-Q-Wave Myocardial Infarction:

In a double-blind, randomized, placebo-controlled clinical trial, patients who recently experienced unstable angina with EKG changes or non-Q-wave myocardial infarction (MI) were randomized to FRAGMIN Injection 120 IU/kg every 12 hours subcutaneously (s.c.) or placebo every 12 hours s.c. In this trial, unstable angina was defined to include only angina with EKG changes. All patients, except when contraindicated, were treated concurrently with aspirin (75 mg once daily) and beta blockers. Treatment was initiated within 72 hours of the event (the majority of patients received treatment within 24 hours) and continued for 5 to 8 days. A total of 1506 patients were enrolled and treated; 746 received FRAGMIN and 760 received placebo. The mean age of the study population was 68 years (range 40 to 90 years) and the majority of patients were white (99.7%) and male (63.9%). The combined incidence of the double endpoint of death or myocardial infarction was lower for FRAGMIN compared with placebo at 6 days after initiation of therapy. These results were observed in an analysis of all-randomized and all-treated patients. The combined incidence of death, MI, need for intravenous (i.v.) heparin or i.v. nitroglycerin, and revascularization was also lower for FRAGMIN than for placebo (see Table 1).

[See table 1 below]

In a second randomized, controlled trial designed to evaluate long-term treatment with FRAGMIN (days 6 to 45), data were also collected comparing 1-week (5 to 8 days) treatment of FRAGMIN 120 IU/kg every 12 hours s.c. with heparin at an APTT-adjusted dosage. All patients, except when contraindicated, were treated concurrently with aspirin (100 to 165 mg per day). Of the total enrolled study population of 1499 patients, 1482 patients were treated; 751 received FRAGMIN and 731 received heparin. The mean age of the study population was 64 years (range 25 to 92 years) and the majority of patients were white (96.0%) and male (64.2%). The incidence of the combined triple endpoint of death, myocardial infarction, or recurrent angina during this 1-week treatment period (5 to 8 days) was 9.3% for FRAGMIN and 7.6% for heparin (p=0.323).

Prophylaxis of Deep Vein Thrombosis in Patients Following Hip Replacement Surgery:

In an open-label randomized study, FRAGMIN 5000 IU administered once daily s.c. was compared with warfarin sodium, administered orally, in patients undergoing hip replacement surgery. Treatment with FRAGMIN was initiated with a 2500 IU dose s.c. within 2 hours before surgery, followed by a 2500 IU dose s.c. the evening of the day of surgery. Then, a dosing regimen of FRAGMIN 5000 IU s.c. once daily was initiated on the first postoperative day. The first dose of warfarin sodium was given the evening before surgery, then continued daily at a dose adjusted for INR 2.0 to 3.0. Treatment in both groups was then continued for 5 to 9 days postoperatively. Of the total enrolled study population of 580 patients, 553 were treated and 550 underwent surgery. Of those who underwent surgery, 271 received FRAGMIN and 279 received warfarin sodium. The mean age of the study population was 63 years (range 20 to 92 years) and the majority of patients were white (91.1%) and female (52.9%). The incidence of deep vein thrombosis (DVT), any vein, as determined by evaluable venography, was significantly lower for the group treated with FRAGMIN compared with patients treated with warfarin sodium (28/192 vs 49/190; p=0.006) [see Table 2].

[See table 2 at top of next page]

In a second single-center, double-blind study of patients undergoing hip replacement surgery, FRAGMIN 5000 IU once daily s.c. starting the evening before surgery, was compared with heparin 5000 U s.c. tid, starting the morning of surgery. Treatment in both groups was continued for up to 9 days postoperatively. Of the total enrolled study population of 140 patients, 139 were treated and 136 underwent surgery. Of those who underwent surgery, 67 received FRAGMIN and 69 received heparin. The mean age of the study population was 69 years (range 42 to 87 years) and the majority of patients were female (58.8%). In the intent-to-treat analysis, the incidence of proximal DVT was significantly lower for patients treated with FRAGMIN compared with patients treated with heparin (6/67 vs 18/69; p=0.012). Further, the incidence of pulmonary embolism detected by lung scan was also significantly lower in the group treated with FRAGMIN (9/67 vs 19/69; p=0.032).

A third multi-center, double-blind, randomized study evaluated a postoperative dosing regimen of FRAGMIN for thromboprophylaxis following total hip replacement surgery. Patients received either FRAGMIN or warfarin sodium, randomized into one of three treatment groups. One group of patients received the first dose of FRAGMIN 2500 IU s.c. within 2 hours before surgery, followed by another dose of FRAGMIN 2500 IU s.c. at least 4 hours (6.6 ± 2.3 hr) after surgery. Another group received the first dose of FRAGMIN 2500 IU s.c. at least 4 hours (6.6 ± 2.4 hr) after surgery. Then, **both** of these groups began a dosing regimen of FRAGMIN 5000 IU once daily s.c. on postoperative day 1. The third group of patients received warfarin sodium the evening of the day of surgery, then continued daily at a dose adjusted for INR 2.0 to 3.0. Treatment for all groups was continued for 4 to 8 days postoperatively, after which time all patients underwent bilateral venography.

In the total enrolled study population of 1501 patients, 1472 patients were treated; 496 received FRAGMIN (first dose before surgery), 487 received FRAGMIN (first dose after surgery) and 489 received warfarin sodium. The mean age of the study population was 63 years (range 18 to 91 years) and the majority of patients were white (94.4%) and female (51.8%).

Administration of the first dose of FRAGMIN after surgery was as effective in reducing the incidence of thromboembolic events as administration of the first dose of FRAGMIN before surgery (44/336 vs 37/338; p=0.448). Both dosing regimens of FRAGMIN were more effective than warfarin sodium in reducing the incidence of thromboembolic events following hip replacement surgery.

Prophylaxis of Deep Vein Thrombosis Following Abdominal Surgery in Patients at Risk for Thromboembolic Complications:

Abdominal surgery patients at risk include those who are over 40 years of age, obese, undergoing surgery under general anesthesia lasting longer than 30 minutes, or who have additional risk factors such as malignancy or a history of deep vein thrombosis or pulmonary embolism.

FRAGMIN administered once daily s.c. beginning prior to surgery and continuing for 5 to 10 days after surgery, was shown to reduce the risk of DVT in patients at risk for thromboembolic complications in two double-blind, randomized, controlled clinical trials performed in patients undergoing major abdominal surgery. In the first study, a total of 204 patients were enrolled and treated; 102 received FRAGMIN and 102 received placebo. The mean age of the study population was 64 years (range 40 to 98 years) and the majority of patients were female (54.9%). In the second study, a total of 391 patients were enrolled and treated; 195 received FRAGMIN and 196 received heparin. The mean age of the study population was 59 years (range 30 to 88 years) and the majority of patients were female (51.9%). As summarized in the following tables, FRAGMIN 2500 IU was superior to placebo and similar to heparin in reducing the risk of DVT (see Tables 3 and 4).

[See table 3 on next page]

[See table 4 on next page]

In a third double-blind, randomized study performed in patients undergoing major abdominal surgery with malignancy, FRAGMIN 5000 IU once daily was compared with FRAGMIN 2500 IU once daily. Treatment was continued for 6 to 8 days. A total of 1375 patients were enrolled and treated; 679 received FRAGMIN 5000 IU and 696 received 2500 IU. The mean age of the combined groups was 71 years (range 40 to 95 years). The majority of patients were female (51.0%). The study showed that FRAGMIN 5000 IU once daily was more effective than FRAGMIN 2500 IU once daily in reducing the risk of DVT in patients undergoing abdominal surgery with malignancy (see Table 5).

[See table 5 on next page]

Prophylaxis of Deep Vein Thrombosis in Medical Patients at Risk for Thromboembolic Complications Due to Severely Restricted Mobility During Acute Illness:

In a double-blind, multi-center, randomized, placebo-controlled clinical trial, general medical patients with severely restricted mobility who were at risk of venous thromboembolism were randomized to receive either FRAGMIN 5000 IU or placebo s.c. once daily during Days 1 to 14 of the study. The primary endpoint was evaluated at Day 21, and the follow-up period was up to Day 90. These patients had an acute medical condition requiring a projected hospital stay of at least 4 days, and were confined to bed during waking hours. The study included patients with congestive heart failure (NYHA Class III or IV), acute respiratory failure not requiring ventilatory support, and the following acute conditions with at least one risk factor occurring in > 1% of treated patients: acute infection (excluding septic shock), acute rheumatic disorder, acute lumbar or sciatic pain, vertebral compression, or acute arthritis of the lower extremities. Risk factors include > 75 years of age, cancer, previous DVT/PE, obesity and chronic venous insufficiency. A total of 3681 patients were enrolled and treated: 1848 received FRAGMIN and 1833 received placebo. The mean age

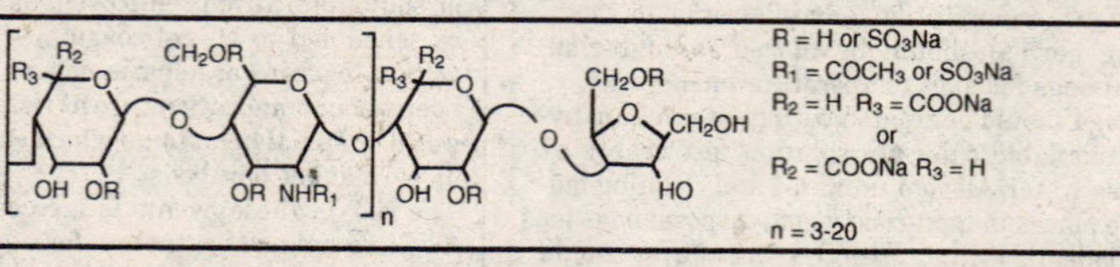

Table 1
Efficacy of FRAGMIN in the Prophylaxis of Ischemic Complications in Unstable Angina and Non-Q-Wave Myocardial Infarction

Indication	Dosing Regimen: FRAGMIN 120 IU/kg/12 hr s.c.	Placebo q 12 hr s.c.
All Treated Unstable Angina and Non-Q-Wave MI Patients	746	760
Primary Endpoints – 6 day timepoint Death, MI	13/741 (1.8%)[1]	36/757 (4.8%)
Secondary Endpoints – 6 day timepoint Death, MI, i.v. heparin, i.v. nitroglycerin, Revascularization	59/739 (8.0%)[1]	106/756 (14.0%)

[1] p-value = 0.001

Table 2
Efficacy of FRAGMIN in the Prophylaxis of Deep Vein Thrombosis Following Hip Replacement Surgery

Indication	Dosing Regimen	
	FRAGMIN 5000 IU qd[1] s.c.	Warfarin Sodium qd[2] oral
All Treated Hip Replacement Surgery Patients	271	279
Treatment Failures in Evaluable Patients DVT, Total	28/192 (14.6%)[3]	49/190 (25.8%)
Proximal DVT	10/192 (5.2%)[4]	16/190 (8.4%)
PE	2/271 (0.7%)	2/279 (0.7%)

[1] The daily dose on the day of surgery was divided: 2500 IU was given two hours before surgery and again in the evening of the day of surgery.
[2] Warfarin sodium dosage was adjusted to maintain a prothrombin time index of 1.4 to 1.5, corresponding to an International Normalized Ratio (INR) of approximately 2.5.
[3] p-value = 0.006
[4] p-value = 0.185

Table 3
Efficacy of FRAGMIN in the Prophylaxis of Deep Vein Thrombosis Following Abdominal Surgery

Indication	Dosing Regimen	
	FRAGMIN 2500 IU qd s.c.	Placebo qd s.c.
All Treated Abdominal Surgery Patients	102	102
Treatment Failures in Evaluable Patients Total Thromboembolic Events	4/91 (4.4%)[1]	16/91 (17.6%)
Proximal DVT	0	5/91 (5.5%)
Distal DVT	4/91 (4.4%)	11/91 (12.1%)
PE	0	2/91 (2.2%)[2]

[1] p-value = 0.008
[2] Both patients also had DVT, 1 proximal and 1 distal

Table 4
Efficacy of FRAGMIN in the Prophylaxis of Deep Vein Thrombosis Following Abdominal Surgery

Indication	Dosing Regimen	
	FRAGMIN 2500 IU qd s.c.	Heparin 5000 U bid s.c.
All Treated Abdominal Surgery Patients	195	196
Treatment Failures in Evaluable Patients Total Thromboembolic Events	7/178 (3.9%)[1]	7/174 (4.0%)
Proximal DVT	3/178 (1.7%)	4/174 (2.3%)
Distal DVT	3/178 (1.7%)	3/174 (1.7%)
PE	1/178 (0.6%)	0

[1] p-value = 0.74

Table 5
Efficacy of FRAGMIN in the Prophylaxis of Deep Vein Thrombosis Following Abdominal Surgery

Indication	Dosing Regimen	
	FRAGMIN 2500 IU qd s.c.	FRAGMIN 5000 IU qd s.c.
All Treated Abdominal Surgery Patients[1]	696	679
Treatment Failures in Evaluable Patients Total Thromboembolic Events	99/656 (15.1%)[2]	60/645 (9.3%)
Proximal DVT	18/657 (2.7%)	14/646 (2.2%)
Distal DVT	80/657 (12.2%)	41/646 (6.3%)
PE Fatal	1/674 (0.1%)	1/669 (0.1%)
Non-fatal	2	4

[1] Major abdominal surgery with malignancy
[2] p-value = 0.001

of the study population was 69 years (range 26 to 99 years), 92.1% were white and 51.9% were female. The primary efficacy endpoint was defined as at least one of the following within Days 1 to 21 of the study: asymptomatic DVT (diagnosed by compression ultrasound), a confirmed symptomatic DVT, a confirmed pulmonary embolism or sudden death.

When given at a dose of 5000 IU once a day s.c., FRAGMIN significantly reduced the incidence of thromboembolic events including verified DVT by Day 21 (see Table 6). The prophylactic effect was sustained through Day 90.

[See table 6 at bottom of next page]

INDICATIONS AND USAGE

FRAGMIN Injection is indicated for the prophylaxis of ischemic complications in unstable angina and non-Q-wave myocardial infarction, when concurrently administered with aspirin therapy (as described in CLINICAL TRIALS, Prophylaxis of Ischemic Complications in Unstable Angina and Non-Q-Wave Myocardial Infarction).

FRAGMIN is also indicated for the prophylaxis of deep vein thrombosis (DVT), which may lead to pulmonary embolism (PE):

- In patients undergoing hip replacement surgery;
- In patients undergoing abdominal surgery who are at risk for thromboembolic complications;
- In medical patients who are at risk for thromboembolic complications due to severely restricted mobility during acute illness.

CONTRAINDICATIONS

FRAGMIN Injection is contraindicated in patients with known hypersensitivity to the drug, active major bleeding, or thrombocytopenia associated with positive ***in vitro*** tests for anti-platelet antibody in the presence of FRAGMIN.

Patients undergoing regional anesthesia should not receive FRAGMIN for unstable angina or non-Q-wave myocardial infarction due to an increased risk of bleeding associated with the dosage of FRAGMIN recommended for unstable angina and non-Q-wave myocardial infarction.

Patients with known hypersensitivity to heparin or pork products should not be treated with FRAGMIN.

WARNINGS

FRAGMIN Injection is not intended for intramuscular administration.

FRAGMIN cannot be used interchangeably (unit for unit) with unfractionated heparin or other low molecular weight heparins.

FRAGMIN should be used with extreme caution in patients with history of heparin-induced thrombocytopenia.

Hemorrhage:

FRAGMIN, like other anticoagulants, should be used with extreme caution in patients who have an increased risk of hemorrhage, such as those with severe uncontrolled hypertension, bacterial endocarditis, congenital or acquired bleeding disorders, active ulceration and angiodysplastic gastrointestinal disease, hemorrhagic stroke, or shortly after brain, spinal or ophthalmological surgery.

Spinal or epidural hematomas can occur with the associated use of low molecular weight heparins or heparinoids and neuraxial (spinal/epidural) anesthesia or spinal puncture, which can result in long-term or permanent paralysis. The risk of these events is higher with the use of indwelling epidural catheters or concomitant use of additional drugs affecting hemostasis such as NSAIDs (see boxed WARNING and ADVERSE REACTIONS, Ongoing Safety Surveillance).

As with other anticoagulants, bleeding can occur at any site during therapy with FRAGMIN. An unexpected drop in hematocrit or blood pressure should lead to a search for a bleeding site.

Thrombocytopenia:

In clinical trials, thrombocytopenia with platelet counts of $< 100{,}000/mm^3$ and $< 50{,}000/mm^3$ occurred in $< 1\%$ and $< 1\%$, respectively. In clinical practice, rare cases of thrombocytopenia with thrombosis have also been observed.

Thrombocytopenia of any degree should be monitored closely. Heparin-induced thrombocytopenia can occur with the administration of FRAGMIN. The incidence of this complication is unknown at present.

Miscellaneous:

The multiple-dose vial of FRAGMIN contains benzyl alcohol as a preservative. Benzyl alcohol has been reported to be associated with a fatal "Gasping Syndrome" in premature infants. Because benzyl alcohol may cross the placenta, FRAGMIN preserved with benzyl alcohol should not be used in pregnant women (see **PRECAUTIONS, Pregnancy Category B, Nonteratogenic Effects**).

PRECAUTIONS

General:

FRAGMIN Injection should not be mixed with other injections or infusions unless specific compatibility data are available that support such mixing.

FRAGMIN should be used with caution in patients with bleeding diathesis, thrombocytopenia or platelet defects; severe liver or kidney insufficiency, hypertensive or diabetic retinopathy, and recent gastrointestinal bleeding.

If a thromboembolic event should occur despite dalteparin prophylaxis, FRAGMIN should be discontinued and appropriate therapy initiated.

Drug Interactions:

FRAGMIN should be used with care in patients receiving oral anticoagulants, platelet inhibitors, and thrombolytic agents because of increased risk of bleeding (see **PRECAUTIONS, Laboratory Tests**). Aspirin, unless contraindicated, is recommended in patients treated for unstable angina or non-Q-wave myocardial infarction (see **DOSAGE AND ADMINISTRATION**).

Laboratory Tests:

Periodic routine complete blood counts, including platelet count, and stool occult blood tests are recommended during the course of treatment with FRAGMIN. No special monitoring of blood clotting times (e.g., APTT) is needed.

When administered at recommended prophylaxis doses, routine coagulation tests such as Prothrombin Time (PT) and Activated Partial Thromboplastin Time (APTT) are relatively insensitive measures of FRAGMIN activity and, therefore, unsuitable for monitoring.

Drug/Laboratory Test Interactions:

Elevations of Serum Transaminases:

Asymptomatic increases in transaminase levels (SGOT/AST and SGPT/ALT) greater than three times the upper limit of normal of the laboratory reference range have been reported in 1.7 and 4.3%, respectively, of patients during treatment with FRAGMIN. Similar significant increases in transami-

Continued on next page

Fragmin—Cont.

nase levels have also been observed in patients treated with heparin and other low molecular weight heparins. Such elevations are fully reversible and are rarely associated with increases in bilirubin. Since transaminase determinations are important in the differential diagnosis of myocardial infarction, liver disease and pulmonary emboli, elevations that might be caused by drugs like FRAGMIN should be interpreted with caution.

Carcinogenicity, Mutagenesis, Impairment of Fertility:
Dalteparin sodium has not been tested for its carcinogenic potential in long-term animal studies. It was not mutagenic in the ***in vitro*** Ames Test, mouse lymphoma cell forward mutation test and human lymphocyte chromosomal aberration test and in the ***in vivo*** mouse micronucleus test. Dalteparin sodium at subcutaneous doses up to 1200 IU/kg (7080 IU/m^2) did not affect the fertility or reproductive performance of male and female rats.

Pregnancy: Pregnancy Category B.

Teratogenic Effects:
Reproduction studies with dalteparin sodium at intravenous doses up to 2400 IU/kg (14,160 IU/m^2) in pregnant rats and 4800 IU/kg (40,800 IU/m^2) in pregnant rabbits did not produce any evidence of impaired fertility or harm to the fetuses. There are, however, no adequate and well-controlled studies in pregnant women. Because animal reproduction studies are not always predictive of human response, this drug should be used during pregnancy only if clearly needed.

Nonteratogenic Effects:
Cases of "Gasping Syndrome" have occurred when large amounts of benzyl alcohol have been administered (99-404 mg/kg/day). The 9.5 mL multiple-dose vial of FRAGMIN contains 14 mg/mL of benzyl alcohol.

Nursing Mothers:
It is not known whether dalteparin sodium is excreted in human milk. Because many drugs are excreted in human milk, caution should be exercised when FRAGMIN is administered to a nursing mother.

Pediatric Use:
Safety and effectiveness in pediatric patients have not been established.

Geriatric Use:
Of the total number of patients in clinical studies of FRAGMIN, 5204 patients were 65 years of age or older and 2123 were 75 or older. No overall differences in effectiveness were observed between these subjects and younger subjects. Some studies suggest that the risk of bleeding increases with age. Postmarketing surveillance and literature reports have not revealed additional differences in the safety of FRAGMIN between elderly and younger patients. Careful attention to dosing intervals and concomitant medications (especially antiplatelet medications) is advised, particularly in geriatric patients with low body weight (< 45 kg) and those predisposed to decreased renal function (see also **CLINICAL PHARMACOLOGY** and **General** and **Drug Interactions** subsections of **PRECAUTIONS**).

ADVERSE REACTIONS

Hemorrhage:
The incidence of hemorrhagic complications during treatment with FRAGMIN Injection has been low. The most commonly reported side effect is hematoma at the injection site. The incidence of bleeding may increase with higher doses; however, in abdominal surgery patients with malignancy, no significant increase in bleeding was observed when comparing FRAGMIN 5000 IU to either FRAGMIN 2500 IU or low dose heparin.

In a trial comparing FRAGMIN 5000 IU once daily to FRAGMIN 2500 IU once daily in patients undergoing surgery for malignancy, the incidence of bleeding events was 4.6% and 3.6%, respectively (n.s.). In a trial comparing FRAGMIN 5000 IU once daily to heparin 5000 U twice daily, the incidence of bleeding events was 3.2% and 2.7%, respectively (n.s.) in the malignancy subgroup.

Unstable Angina and Non-Q-Wave Myocardial Infarction:
Table 7 summarizes major bleeding events that occurred with FRAGMIN, heparin, and placebo in clinical trials of unstable angina and non-Q-wave myocardial infarction.
[See table 7 at left]

Hip Replacement Surgery:
Table 8 summarizes: 1) all major bleeding events and, 2) other bleeding events possibly or probably related to treatment with FRAGMIN (preoperative dosing regimen), warfarin sodium, or heparin in two hip replacement surgery clinical trials.
[See table 8 at left]

Six of the patients treated with FRAGMIN experienced seven major bleeding events. Two of the events were wound hematoma (one requiring reoperation), three were bleeding from the operative site, one was intraoperative bleeding due to vessel damage, and one was gastrointestinal bleeding. None of the patients experienced retroperitoneal or intracranial hemorrhage nor died of bleeding complications.

In the third hip replacement surgery clinical trial, the incidence of major bleeding events was similar in all three treatment groups: 3.6% (18/496) for patients who started FRAGMIN before surgery; 2.5% (12/487) for patients who started FRAGMIN after surgery; and 3.1% (15/489) for patients treated with warfarin sodium.

Abdominal Surgery:
Table 9 summarizes bleeding events that occurred in clinical trials which studied FRAGMIN 2500 and 5000 IU administered once daily to abdominal surgery patients.
[See table 9 at top of next page]

Medical Patients with Severely Restricted Mobility During Acute Illness:
Table 10 summarizes major bleeding events that occurred in a clinical trial of medical patients with severely restricted mobility during acute illness.
[See table 10 at top of next page]

Three of the major bleeding events that occurred by Day 21 were fatal, all due to gastrointestinal hemorrhage (two patients in the group treated with FRAGMIN and one in the group receiving placebo). Two deaths occurred after Day 21: one patient in the placebo group died from a subarachnoid hemorrhage that started on Day 55, and one patient died on day 71 (two months after receiving the last dose of FRAGMIN) from a subdural hematoma.

Thrombocytopenia: See WARNINGS: Thrombocytopenia.

Other:

Allergic Reactions:
Allergic reactions (i.e., pruritus, rash, fever, injection site reaction, bulleous eruption) and skin necrosis have occurred rarely. A few cases of anaphylactoid reactions have been reported.

Local Reactions:
Pain at the injection site, the only non-bleeding event determined to be possibly or probably related to treatment with FRAGMIN and reported at a rate of at least 2% in the group treated with FRAGMIN, was reported in 4.5% of patients treated with FRAGMIN 5000 IU qd vs 11.8% of patients treated with heparin 5000 U bid in the abdominal surgery trials. In the hip replacement trials, pain at injection site was reported in 12% of patients treated with FRAGMIN 5000 IU qd vs 13% of patients treated with heparin 5000 U tid.

Ongoing Safety Surveillance:
Since first international market introduction in 1985, there have been nine reports of epidural or spinal hematoma formation with concurrent use of dalteparin sodium and spinal/epidural anesthesia or spinal puncture. Five of the nine patients had post-operative indwelling epidural catheters placed for analgesia or received additional drugs affecting hemostasis. The hematomas caused long-term or permanent paralysis (partial or complete) in seven of these cases. One patient experienced temporary paraplegia but made a full recovery, and one patient had no neurological deficit. Because these events were reported voluntarily from a population of unknown size, estimates of frequency cannot be made.

OVERDOSAGE

Symptoms/Treatment:
An excessive dosage of FRAGMIN Injection may lead to hemorrhagic complications. These may generally be stopped by the slow intravenous injection of protamine sulfate (1% solution), at a dose of 1 mg protamine for every 100 anti-Xa IU of FRAGMIN given. A second infusion of 0.5 mg protamine sulfate per 100 anti-Xa IU of FRAGMIN may be administered if the APTT measured 2 to 4 hours after the first infusion remains prolonged. Even with these additional doses of protamine, the APTT may remain more prolonged than would usually be found following administration of conventional heparin. In all cases, the anti-Factor Xa activity is never completely neutralized (maximum about 60 to 75%).

Table 6
Efficacy of FRAGMIN in the Prophylaxis of Deep Vein Thrombosis in Medical Patients with Severely Restricted Mobility During Acute Illness

Indication	Dosing Regimen	
	FRAGMIN 5000 IU qd s.c.	Placebo qd s.c.
All Treated Medical Patients During Acute Illness	1848	1833
Treatment failure in evaluable patients (Day 21)[1] DVT, PE, or sudden death	42/1518 (2.77%)[2]	73/1473 (4.96%)
Total thromboembolic events (Day 21)	37/1513 (2.45%)	70/1470 (4.76%)
Total DVT	32/1508 (2.12%)	64/1464 (4.37%)
Proximal DVT	29/1518 (1.91%)	60/1474 (4.07%)
Symptomatic VTE	10/1759 (0.57%)	17/1740 (0.98%)
PE	5/1759 (0.28%)	6/1740 (0.34%)
Sudden Death	5/1829 (0.27%)	3/1807 (0.17%)

[1] Defined as DVT (diagnosed by compression ultrasound at Day 21 + 3), confirmed symptomatic DVT, confirmed PE or sudden death.
[2] p-value = 0.0015

Table 7
Major Bleeding Events in Unstable Angina and Non-Q-Wave Myocardial Infarction

Indication	Dosing Regimen		
Unstable Angina and Non-Q-Wave MI	FRAGMIN 120 IU/kg/12 hr s.c.[1]	Heparin i.v. and s.c.[2]	Placebo q 12 hr s.c.
Major Bleeding Events[3,4]	15/1497 (1.0%)	7/731 (1.0%)	4/760 (0.5%)

[1] Treatment was administered for 5 to 8 days.
[2] Heparin i.v. infusion for at least 48 hours, APPT 1.5 to 2 times control, then 12,500 U s.c. every 12 hours for 5 to 8 days.
[3] Aspirin (75 to 165 mg per day) and beta blocker therapies were administered concurrently.
[4] Bleeding events were considered major if: 1) accompanied by a decrease in hemoglobin of ≥2 g/dL in connection with clinical symptoms; 2) a transfusion was required; 3) bleeding led to interruption of treatment or death; or 4) intracranial bleeding.

Table 8
Bleeding Events Following Hip Replacement Surgery

Indication	FRAGMIN vs Warfarin Sodium		FRAGMIN vs Heparin	
	Dosing Regimen		Dosing Regimen	
Hip Replacement Surgery	FRAGMIN 5000 IU qd s.c. (n=274[2])	Warfarin Sodium[1] oral (n=279)	FRAGMIN 5000 IU qd s.c. (n=69[4])	Heparin 5000 U tid s.c. (n=69)
Major Bleeding Events[3]	7/274 (2.6%)	1/279 (0.4%)	0	3/69 (4.3%)
Other Bleeding Events[5]				
Hematuria	8/274 (2.9%)	5/279 (1.8%)	0	0
Wound Hematoma	6/274 (2.2%)	0	0	0
Injection Site Hematoma	3/274 (1.1%)	NA	2/69 (2.9%)	7/69 (10.1%)

[1] Warfarin sodium dosage was adjusted to maintain a prothrombin time index of 1.4 to 1.5, corresponding to an International Normalized Ratio (INR) of approximately 2.5.
[2] Includes three treated patients who did not undergo a surgical procedure.
[3] A bleeding event was considered major if: 1) hemorrhage caused a significant clinical event, 2) it was associated with a hemoglobin decrease of ≥ 2 g/dL or transfusion of 2 or more units of blood products, 3) it resulted in reoperation due to bleeding, or 4) it involved retroperitoneal or intracranial hemorrhage.
[4] Includes two treated patients who did not undergo a surgical procedure.
[5] Occurred at a rate of at least 2% in the group treated with FRAGMIN 5000 IU once daily.

Table 9
Bleeding Events Following Abdominal Surgery

Indication	FRAGMIN vs Heparin				FRAGMIN vs Placebo		FRAGMIN vs FRAGMIN	
	Dosing Regimen				Dosing Regimen		Dosing Regimen	
Abdominal Surgery	**FRAGMIN** 2500 IU qd s.c.	**Heparin** 5000 U bid s.c.	**FRAGMIN** 5000 IU qd s.c.	**Heparin** 5000 U bid s.c.	**FRAGMIN** 2500 IU qd s.c.	**Placebo** qd s.c.	**FRAGMIN** 2500 IU qd s.c.	**FRAGMIN** 5000 IU qd s.c.
Postoperative Transfusions	26/459 (5.7%)	36/454 (7.9%)	81/508 (15.9%)	63/498 (12.7%)	14/182 (7.7%)	13/182 (7.1%)	89/1025 (8.7%)	125/1033 (12.1%)
Wound Hematoma	16/467 (3.4%)	18/467 (3.9%)	12/508 (2.4%)	6/498 (1.2%)	2/79 (2.5%)	2/77 (2.6%)	1/1030 (0.1%)	4/1039 (0.4%)
Reoperation Due to Bleeding	2/392 (0.5%)	3/392 (0.8%)	4/508 (0.8%)	2/498 (0.4%)	1/79 (1.3%)	1/78 (1.3%)	2/1030 (0.2%)	13/1038 (1.3%)
Injection Site Hematoma	1/466 (0.2%)	5/464 (1.1%)	36/506 (7.1%)	47/493 (9.5%)	8/172 (4.7%)	2/174 (1.1%)	36/1026 (3.5%)	57/1035 (5.5%)

Table 10
Bleeding Events in Medical Patients with Severely Restricted Mobility During Acute Illness

Indication	Dosing Regimen	
Medical Patients with Severely Restricted Mobility	**FRAGMIN** 5000 IU qd s.c.	**Placebo** qd s.c.
Major Bleeding Events[1] at Day 14	8/1848 (0.43%)	0/1833 (0%)
Major Bleeding Events[1] at Day 21	9/1848 (0.49%)	3/1833 (0.16%)

[1] A bleeding event was considered major if: 1) it was accompanied by a decrease in hemoglobin of ≥2 g/dL in connection with clinical symptoms; 2) intraocular, spinal/epidural, intracranial, or retroperitoneal bleeding; 3) required transfusion of ≥2 units of blood products; 4) required significant medical or surgical intervention; or 5) led to death.

Table 11
Volume of FRAGMIN to be Administered by Patient Weight, Based on 9.5 mL Vial (10,000 IU/mL)

Patient weight (lb)	< 110	110 to 131	132 to 153	154 to 175	176 to 197	≥ 198
Patient weight (kg)	< 50	50 to 59	60 to 69	70 to 79	80 to 89	≥ 90
Volume of FRAGMIN (mL)	0.55	0.65	0.75	0.90	1.00	1.00

Table 12
Dosing Options for Patients Undergoing Hip Replacement Surgery

Timing of First Dose of FRAGMIN	Dose of FRAGMIN to be Given Subcutaneously			
	10 to 14 Hours Before Surgery	Within 2 Hours Before Surgery	4 to 8 Hours After Surgery[1]	Postoperative Period[2]
Postoperative Start	—	—	2500 IU[3]	5000 IU qd
Preoperative Start - Day of Surgery	—	2500 IU	2500 IU[3]	5000 IU qd
Preoperative Start - Evening Before Surgery[4]	5000 IU	—	5000 IU	5000 IU qd

[1] Or later, if hemostasis has not been achieved.
[2] Up to 14 days of treatment was well tolerated in controlled clinical trials, where the usual duration of treatment was 5 to 10 days postoperatively.
[3] Allow a minimum of 6 hours between this dose and the dose to be given on Postoperative Day 1. Adjust the timing of the dose on Postoperative Day 1 accordingly.
[4] Allow approximately 24 hours between doses.

Particular care should be taken to avoid overdosage with protamine sulfate. Administration of protamine sulfate can cause severe hypotensive and anaphylactoid reactions. Because fatal reactions, often resembling anaphylaxis, have been reported with protamine sulfate, it should be given only when resuscitation techniques and treatment of anaphylactic shock are readily available. For additional information, consult the labeling of Protamine Sulfate Injection, USP, products. A single subcutaneous dose of 100,000 IU/kg of FRAGMIN to mice caused a mortality of 8% (1/12) whereas 50,000 IU/kg was a non-lethal dose. The observed sign was hematoma at the site of injection.

DOSAGE AND ADMINISTRATION

Unstable Angina and Non-Q-Wave Myocardial Infarction:
In patients with unstable angina or non-Q-wave myocardial infarction, the recommended dose of FRAGMIN Injection is 120 IU/kg of body weight, but not more than 10,000 IU, subcutaneously (s.c.) every 12 hours with concurrent oral aspirin (75 to 165 mg once daily) therapy. Treatment should be continued until the patient is clinically stabilized. The usual duration of administration is 5 to 8 days. Concurrent aspirin therapy is recommended except when contraindicated.
Table 11 lists the volume of FRAGMIN, based on the 9.5 mL multiple-dose vial (10,000 IU/mL), to be administered for a range of patient weights.
[See table 11 above]

Hip Replacement Surgery:
Table 12 presents the dosing options for patients undergoing hip replacement surgery. The usual duration of administration is 5 to 10 days after surgery; up to 14 days of treatment with FRAGMIN have been well tolerated in clinical trials.
[See table 12 above]

Abdominal Surgery:
In patients undergoing abdominal surgery with a risk of thromboembolic complications, the recommended dose of FRAGMIN is 2500 IU administered by s.c. injection once daily, starting 1 to 2 hours prior to surgery and repeated once daily postoperatively. The usual duration of administration is 5 to 10 days.
In patients undergoing abdominal surgery associated with a high risk of thromboembolic complications, such as malignant disorder, the recommended dose of FRAGMIN is 5000 IU s.c. the evening before surgery, then once daily postoperatively. The usual duration of administration is 5 to 10 days. Alternatively, in patients with malignancy, 2500 IU of FRAGMIN can be administered s.c. 1 to 2 hours before surgery followed by 2500 IU s.c. 12 hours later, and then 5000 IU once daily postoperatively. The usual duration of administration is 5 to 10 days.
Dosage adjustment and routine monitoring of coagulation parameters are not required if the dosage and administration recommendations specified above are followed.

Medical Patients with Severely Restricted Mobility During Acute Illness:
In medical patients with severely restricted mobility during acute illness, the recommended dose of FRAGMIN is 5000 IU administered by s.c. injection once daily. In clinical trials, the usual duration of administration was 12 to 14 days.

Administration:
FRAGMIN is administered by subcutaneous injection. It must not be administered by intramuscular injection.
Subcutaneous injection technique: Patients should be sitting or lying down and FRAGMIN administered by deep s.c. injection. FRAGMIN may be injected in a U-shape area around the navel, the upper outer side of the thigh or the upper outer quadrangle of the buttock. The injection site should be varied daily. When the area around the navel or the thigh is used, using the thumb and forefinger, you **must** lift up a fold of skin while giving the injection. The entire length of the needle should be inserted at a 45 to 90 degree angle.
Parenteral drug products should be inspected visually for particulate matter and discoloration prior to administration, whenever solution and container permit.
After first penetration of the rubber stopper, store the multiple-dose vials at room temperature for up to 2 weeks. Discard any unused solution after 2 weeks.
Instructions for using the prefilled single-dose syringes preassembled with needle guard devices:

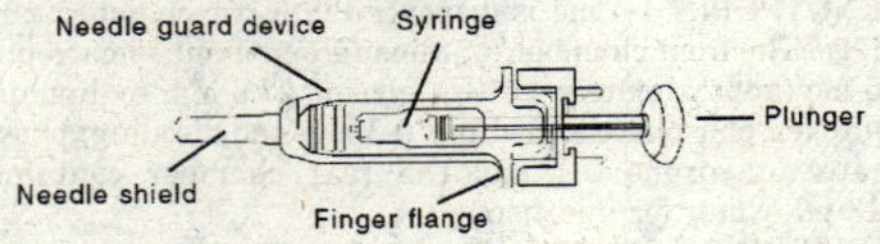

Fixed dose syringes: To ensure delivery of the full dose, do not expel the air bubble from the prefilled syringe before injection. Hold the syringe assembly by the open sides of the device. Remove the needle shield. Insert the needle into the injection area as instructed above. Depress the plunger of the syringe while holding the finger flange **until the entire dose has been given.** The needle guard will **not** be activated unless the **entire** dose has been given. Remove needle from the patient. Let go of the plunger and allow syringe to move up inside the device until the entire needle is guarded. Discard the syringe assembly in approved containers.
Graduated syringes: Hold the syringe assembly by the open sides of the device. Remove the needle shield. With the needle pointing up, prepare the syringe by expelling the air bubble and then continuing to push the plunger down to the desired dose or volume, discarding the extra solution in an appropriate manner. Insert the needle into the injection area as instructed above. Depress the plunger of the syringe while holding the finger flange **until the entire dose remaining in the syringe has been given.** The needle guard will **not** be activated unless the **entire** dose has been given. Remove needle from the patient. Let go of the plunger and allow syringe to move up inside the device until the entire needle is guarded. Discard the syringe assembly in approved containers.

HOW SUPPLIED

FRAGMIN Injection is available in the following strengths and package sizes:
0.2 mL single-dose prefilled syringe, affixed with a 27-gauge × 1/2 inch needle and preassembled with UltraSafe Passive™ Needle Guard* devices.
Package of 10:
2500 anti-Factor Xa IU NDC 0013-2406-91
5000 anti-Factor Xa IU NDC 0013-2426-91
0.3 mL single-dose prefilled syringe, affixed with a 27-gauge × 1/2 inch needle and preassembled with UltraSafe Passive™ Needle Guard* devices.
Package of 10:
7500 anti-Factor Xa IU NDC 0013-2426-01
1.0 mL single-dose graduated syringe, affixed with a 27-gauge × 1/2 inch needle and preassembled with UltraSafe Passive™ Needle Guard* devices.
Package of 10:
10,000 anti-Factor Xa IU NDC 0013-5190-01
3.8 mL multiple-dose vial:
25,000 anti-Factor Xa IU/mL NDC 0013-5191-01
(95,000 anti-Factor Xa IU/vial)
9.5 mL multiple-dose vial:
10,000 anti-Factor Xa IU/mL NDC 0013-2436-06
(95,000 anti-Factor Xa IU/vial)
Store at controlled room temperature 20° to 25°C (68° to 77°F) [see USP].
℞ only
U.S. Patent 4,303,651
*UltraSafe Passive™ Needle Guard is a trademark of Safety Syringes, Inc.
Manufactured for: Pharmacia & Upjohn Company
A subsidiary of Pharmacia Corporation
Kalamazoo, MI 49001, USA
By: Vetter Pharma-Fertigung
Ravensburg, Germany
(prefilled syringes)
Pharmacia N.V./S.A.
Puurs, Belgium
(multiple-dose vial)

Continued on next page

Fragmin—Cont.

818 312 111 Revised December 2003
R7065
SR7065

GENOTROPIN® ℞
[*gen-ō" trō-pĭn*]
(somatropin [rDNA origin]) for injection
In a Two-Chamber Cartridge

Prescribing information for this product, which appears on 2765–2768 of the 2004 PDR, has been completely revised as follows. Please write "See Supplement A" next to the product heading.

DESCRIPTION

GENOTROPIN Lyophilized Powder contains somatropin [rDNA origin], which is a polypeptide hormone of recombinant DNA origin. It has 191 amino acid residues and a molecular weight of 22,124 daltons. The amino acid sequence of the product is identical to that of human growth hormone of pituitary origin (somatropin). GENOTROPIN is synthesized in a strain of *Escherichia coli* that has been modified by the addition of the gene for human growth hormone.

GENOTROPIN is a sterile white lyophilized powder intended for subcutaneous injection.

GENOTROPIN 1.5 mg is dispensed in a two-chamber cartridge. The front chamber contains recombinant somatropin 1.5 mg (approximately 4.5 IU), glycine 27.6 mg, sodium dihydrogen phosphate anhydrous 0.3 mg, and disodium phosphate anhydrous 0.3 mg; the rear chamber contains 1.13 mL water for injection.

GENOTROPIN 5.8 mg is dispensed in a two-chamber cartridge. The front chamber contains recombinant somatropin 5.8 mg (approximately 17.4 IU), glycine 2.2 mg, mannitol 1.8 mg, sodium dihydrogen phosphate anhydrous 0.32 mg, and disodium phosphate anhydrous 0.31 mg; the rear chamber contains 0.3% m-Cresol (as a preservative) and mannitol 45 mg in 1.14 mL water for injection.

GENOTROPIN 13.8 mg is dispensed in a two-chamber cartridge. The front chamber contains recombinant somatropin 13.8 mg (approximately 41.4 IU), glycine 2.3 mg, mannitol 14.0 mg, sodium dihydrogen phosphate anhydrous 0.47 mg, and disodium phosphate anhydrous 0.46 mg; the rear chamber contains 0.3% m-Cresol (as a preservative) and mannitol 32 mg in 1.13 mL water for injection.

GENOTROPIN MINIQUICK® is dispensed as a single-use syringe device containing a two-chamber cartridge. GENOTROPIN MINIQUICK is available as individual doses of 0.2 mg to 2.0 mg in 0.2-mg increments. The front chamber contains recombinant somatropin 0.22 to 2.2 mg (approximately 0.66 to 6.6 IU), glycine 0.23 mg, mannitol 1.14 mg, sodium dihydrogen phosphate 0.05 mg, and disodium phosphate anhydrous 0.027 mg; the rear chamber contains mannitol 12.6 mg in water for injection 0.275 mL.

GENOTROPIN is a highly purified preparation. The reconstituted recombinant somatropin solution has an osmolality of approximately 300 mOsm/kg, and a pH of approximately 6.7. The concentration of the reconstituted solution varies by strength and presentation (see HOW SUPPLIED).

CLINICAL PHARMACOLOGY

In vitro, preclinical, and clinical tests have demonstrated that GENOTROPIN Lyophilized Powder is therapeutically equivalent to human growth hormone of pituitary origin and achieves similar pharmacokinetic profiles in normal adults. In pediatric patients who have growth hormone deficiency (GHD) or Prader-Willi syndrome (PWS), or who were born small for gestational age (SGA), treatment with GENOTROPIN stimulates linear growth. In patients with GHD or PWS, treatment with GENOTROPIN also normalizes concentrations of IGF-I (Insulin-like Growth Factor-I/Somatomedin C). In adults with GHD, treatment with GENOTROPIN results in reduced fat mass, increased lean body mass, metabolic alterations that include beneficial changes in lipid metabolism, and normalization of IGF-I concentrations.

In addition, the following actions have been demonstrated for GENOTROPIN and/or somatropin.

1. Tissue Growth

A. ***Skeletal Growth:*** GENOTROPIN stimulates skeletal growth in pediatric patients with GHD, PWS, or SGA. The measurable increase in body length after administration of GENOTROPIN results from an effect on the epiphyseal plates of long bones. Concentrations of IGF-I, which may play a role in skeletal growth, are generally low in the serum of pediatric patients with GHD, PWS, or SGA, but tend to increase during treatment with GENOTROPIN. Elevations in mean serum alkaline phosphatase concentration are also seen.

B. ***Cell Growth:*** It has been shown that there are fewer skeletal muscle cells in short-statured pediatric patients who lack endogenous growth hormone as compared with the normal pediatric population. Treatment with somatropin results in an increase in both the number and size of muscle cells.

2. Protein Metabolism

Linear growth is facilitated in part by increased cellular protein synthesis. Nitrogen retention, as demonstrated by decreased urinary nitrogen excretion and serum urea nitrogen, follows the initiation of therapy with GENOTROPIN.

3. Carbohydrate Metabolism

Pediatric patients with hypopituitarism sometimes experience fasting hypoglycemia that is improved by treatment with GENOTROPIN. Large doses of growth hormone may impair glucose tolerance.

4. Lipid Metabolism

In GHD patients, administration of somatropin has resulted in lipid mobilization, reduction in body fat stores, and increased plasma fatty acids.

5. Mineral Metabolism

Somatropin induces retention of sodium, potassium, and phosphorus. Serum concentrations of inorganic phosphate are increased in patients with GHD after therapy with GENOTROPIN. Serum calcium is not significantly altered by GENOTROPIN. Growth hormone could increase calciuria.

6. Body Composition

Adult GHD patients treated with GENOTROPIN at the recommended adult dose (see DOSAGE AND ADMINISTRATION) demonstrate a decrease in fat mass and an increase in lean body mass. When these alterations are coupled with the increase in total body water, the overall effect of GENOTROPIN is to modify body composition, an effect that is maintained with continued treatment.

PHARMACOKINETICS

Absorption

Following a 0.03 mg/kg subcutaneous (SC) injection in the thigh of 1.3 mg/mL GENOTROPIN to adult GHD patients, approximately 80% of the dose was systemically available as compared with that available following intravenous dosing. Results were comparable in both male and female patients. Similar bioavailability has been observed in healthy adult male subjects.

In healthy adult males, following an SC injection in the thigh of 0.03 mg/kg, the extent of absorption (AUC) of a concentration of 5.3 mg/mL GENOTROPIN was 35% greater than that for 1.3 mg/mL GENOTROPIN. The mean (± standard deviation) peak (C_{max}) serum levels were 23.0 (± 9.4) ng/mL and 17.4 (± 9.2) ng/mL, respectively.

In a similar study involving pediatric GHD patients, 5.3 mg/mL GENOTROPIN yielded a mean AUC that was 17% greater than that for 1.3 mg/mL GENOTROPIN. The mean C_{max} levels were 21.0 ng/mL and 16.3 ng/mL, respectively.

Adult GHD patients received two single SC doses of 0.03 mg/kg of GENOTROPIN at a concentration of 1.3 mg/mL, with a one- to four-week washout period between injections. Mean C_{max} levels were 12.4 ng/mL (first injection) and 12.2 ng/mL (second injection), achieved at approximately six hours after dosing.

There are no data on the bioequivalence between the 12-mg/mL formulation and either the 1.3-mg/mL or the 5.3-mg/mL formulations.

Distribution

The mean volume of distribution of GENOTROPIN following administration to GHD adults was estimated to be 1.3 (± 0.8) L/kg.

Metabolism

The metabolic fate of GENOTROPIN involves classical protein catabolism in both the liver and kidneys. In renal cells, at least a portion of the breakdown products are returned to the systemic circulation. The mean terminal half-life of intravenous GENOTROPIN in normal adults is 0.4 hours, whereas subcutaneously administered GENOTROPIN has a half-life of 3.0 hours in GHD adults. The observed difference is due to slow absorption from the subcutaneous injection site.

Excretion

The mean clearance of subcutaneously administered GENOTROPIN in 16 GHD adult patients was 0.3 (± 0.11) L/hrs/kg.

Special Populations

Pediatric: The pharmacokinetics of GENOTROPIN are similar in GHD pediatric and adult patients.

Gender: No gender studies have been performed in pediatric patients; however, in GHD adults, the absolute bioavailability of GENOTROPIN was similar in males and females.

Race: No studies have been conducted with GENOTROPIN to assess pharmacokinetic differences among races.

Renal or hepatic insufficiency: No studies have been conducted with GENOTROPIN in these patient populations.

[See table 1 below]

Table 1
Mean SC Pharmacokinetic Parameters in Adult GHD Patients

	Bioavailability (%) (N=15)	T_{max} (hours) (N=16)	CL/F (L/hr × kg) (N=16)	Vss/F (L/kg) (N=16)	$T_{1/2}$ (hours) (N=16)
Mean (± SD)	80.5 *	5.9 (± 1.65)	0.3 (± 0.11)	1.3 (± 0.80)	3.0 (± 1.44)
95% CI	70.5 – 92.1	5.0 – 6.7	0.2 – 0.4	0.9 – 1.8	2.2 – 3.7

T_{max} = time of maximum plasma concentration
CL/F = plasma clearance
Vss/F = volume of distribution
$T_{1/2}$ = terminal half-life
SD = standard deviation
CI = confidence interval

*The absolute bioavailability was estimated under the assumption that the log-transformed data follow a normal distribution. The mean and standard deviation of the log-transformed data were mean = 0.22 (± 0.241).

CLINICAL STUDIES

Adult Patients with Growth Hormone Deficiency (GHD)

GENOTROPIN Lyophilized Powder was compared with placebo in six randomized clinical trials involving a total of 172 adult GHD patients. These trials included a 6-month double-blind treatment period, during which 85 patients received GENOTROPIN and 87 patients received placebo, followed by an open-label treatment period in which participating patients received GENOTROPIN for up to a total of 24 months. GENOTROPIN was administered as a daily SC injection at a dose of 0.04 mg/kg/week for the first month of treatment and 0.08 mg/kg/week for subsequent months.

Beneficial changes in body composition were observed at the end of the 6-month treatment period for the patients receiving GENOTROPIN as compared with the placebo patients. Lean body mass, total body water, and lean/fat ratio increased while total body fat mass and waist circumference decreased. These effects on body composition were maintained when treatment was continued beyond 6 months. Bone mineral density declined after 6 months of treatment but returned to baseline values after 12 months of treatment.

Pediatric Patients with Prader-Willi Syndrome (PWS)

The safety and efficacy of GENOTROPIN in the treatment of pediatric patients with Prader-Willi syndrome (PWS) were evaluated in two randomized, open-label, controlled clinical trials. Patients received either GENOTROPIN or no treatment for the first year of the studies, while all patients received GENOTROPIN during the second year. GENOTROPIN was administered as a daily SC injection, and the dose was calculated for each patient every 3 months. In Study 1, the treatment group received GENOTROPIN at a dose of 0.24 mg/kg/week during the entire study. During the second year, the control group received GENOTROPIN at a dose of 0.48 mg/kg/week. In Study 2, the treatment group received GENOTROPIN at a dose of 0.36 mg/kg/week during the entire study. During the second year, the control group received GENOTROPIN at a dose of 0.36 mg/kg/week.

Patients who received GENOTROPIN showed significant increases in linear growth during the first year of study, compared with patients who received no treatment (see Table 2). Linear growth continued to increase in the second year, when both groups received treatment with GENOTROPIN.

[See table 2 at bottom of next page]

Changes in body composition were also observed in the patients receiving GENOTROPIN (see Table 3). These changes included a decrease in the amount of fat mass, and increases in the amount of lean body mass and the ratio of lean-to-fat tissue, while changes in body weight were similar to those seen in patients who received no treatment. Treatment with GENOTROPIN did not accelerate bone age, compared with patients who received no treatment.

[See table 3 at bottom of next page]

Pediatric Patients Born Small for Gestational Age (SGA) Who Fail to Manifest Catch-up Growth by Age 2

The safety and efficacy of GENOTROPIN in the treatment of children born small for gestational age (SGA) were evaluated in 4 randomized, open-label, controlled clinical trials. Patients (age range of 2 to 8 years) were observed for 12 months before being randomized to receive either GENOTROPIN (two doses per study, most often 0.24 and 0.48 mg/kg/week) as a daily SC injection or no treatment for the first 24 months of the studies. After 24 months in the studies, all patients received GENOTROPIN.

Patients who received any dose of GENOTROPIN showed significant increases in growth during the first 24 months of study, compared with patients who received no treatment (see Table 4). Children receiving 0.48 mg/kg/week demonstrated a significant improvement in height standard deviation score (SDS) compared with children treated with 0.24 mg/kg/week. Both of these doses resulted in a slower but constant increase in growth between months 24 to 72 (data not shown).

[See table 4 at bottom of next page]

INDICATIONS AND USAGE

GENOTROPIN Lyophilized Powder is indicated for:

- Long-term treatment of pediatric patients who have growth failure due to an inadequate secretion of endogenous growth hormone.
- Long-term treatment of pediatric patients who have growth failure due to Prader-Willi syndrome (PWS). The diagnosis of PWS should be confirmed by appropriate genetic testing (see CONTRAINDICATIONS).

- Long-term treatment of growth failure in children born small for gestational age (SGA) who fail to manifest catch-up growth by age 2.

Other causes of short stature in pediatric patients should be excluded.

- Long-term replacement therapy in adults with growth hormone deficiency (GHD) of either childhood- or adult-onset etiology. GHD should be confirmed by an appropriate growth hormone stimulation test.

CONTRAINDICATIONS

GENOTROPIN Lyophilized Powder should not be used when there is any evidence of neoplastic activity. Intracranial lesions must be inactive and antitumor therapy complete prior to the institution of therapy. GENOTROPIN should be discontinued if there is evidence of tumor growth. Growth hormone should not be used for growth promotion in pediatric patients with fused epiphyses.

Growth hormone should not be initiated to treat patients with acute critical illness due to complications following open heart or abdominal surgery, multiple accidental trauma, or to patients having acute respiratory failure. Two placebo-controlled clinical trials in non-growth hormone deficient adult patients (n=522) with these conditions revealed a significant increase in mortality (41.9% vs 19.3%) among somatropin treated patients (doses 5.3 to 8 mg/day) compared to those receiving placebo (see WARNINGS).

Growth hormone is contraindicated in patients with Prader-Willi syndrome who are severely obese or have severe respiratory impairment (see WARNINGS).

WARNINGS

The 5.8-mg and 13.8-mg presentations of GENOTROPIN Lyophilized Powder contain m-Cresol as a preservative. These products should not be used by patients with a known sensitivity to this preservative. The GENOTROPIN 1.5-mg and GENOTROPIN MINIQUICK presentations are preservative-free (see HOW SUPPLIED).

See CONTRAINDICATIONS for information on increased mortality in patients with acute critical illnesses in intensive care units due to complications following open heart or abdominal surgery, multiple accidental trauma, or with acute respiratory failure. The safety of continuing growth hormone treatment in patients receiving replacement doses for approved indications who concurrently develop these illnesses has not been established. Therefore, the potential benefit of treatment continuation with growth hormone in patients having acute critical illnesses should be weighed against the potential risk.

There have been reports of fatalities after initiating therapy with growth hormone in pediatric patients with Prader-Willi syndrome who had one or more of the following risk factors: severe obesity, history of upper airway obstruction or sleep apnea, or unidentified respiratory infection. Male patients with one or more of these factors may be at greater risk than females. Patients with Prader-Willi syndrome should be evaluated for signs of upper airway obstruction and sleep apnea before initiation of treatment with growth hormone. If during treatment with growth hormone patients show signs of upper airway obstruction (including onset of or increased snoring) and/or new onset sleep apnea, treatment should be interrupted. All patients with Prader-Willi syndrome treated with growth hormone should also have effective weight control and be monitored for signs of respiratory infections, which should be diagnosed as early as possible and treated aggressively (see CONTRAINDICATIONS).

PRECAUTIONS

General

Treatment with GENOTROPIN Lyophilized Powder, as with other growth hormone preparations, should be directed by physicians who are experienced in the diagnosis and management of patients with GHD or Prader-Willi syndrome (PWS), or those who were born small for gestational age (SGA).

Patients and caregivers who will administer GENOTROPIN in medically unsupervised situations should receive appropriate training and instruction on the proper use of GENOTROPIN from the physician or other suitably qualified health professional.

Patients with GHD secondary to an intracranial lesion should be examined frequently for progression or recurrence of the underlying disease process. Review of literature reports of pediatric use of somatropin replacement therapy reveals no relationship between this therapy and recurrence of central nervous system (CNS) tumors. In adults, it is unknown whether there is any relationship between somatropin treatment and CNS tumor recurrence.

Patients should be monitored carefully for any malignant transformation of skin lesions.

Caution should be used if growth hormone is administered to patients with diabetes mellitus, and insulin dosage may need to be adjusted. Patients with diabetes or glucose intolerance should be monitored closely during treatment with GENOTROPIN. Patients with risk factors for glucose intolerance, such as obesity (including obese patients with PWS) or a family history of Type II diabetes, should be monitored closely as well. Because growth hormone may induce a state of insulin resistance, patients should be observed for evidence of glucose intolerance.

In patients with hypopituitarism (multiple hormonal deficiencies) standard hormonal replacement therapy should be monitored closely when treatment with GENOTROPIN is instituted. Hypothyroidism may develop during treatment with GENOTROPIN, and inadequate treatment of hypothyroidism may prevent optimal response to GENOTROPIN. Therefore, patients should have periodic thyroid function tests and be treated with thyroid hormone when indicated.

Pediatric patients with endocrine disorders, including GHD, have a higher incidence of slipped capital femoral epiphyses. Any pediatric patient with the onset of a limp or complaints of hip or knee pain during growth hormone therapy should be evaluated.

Progression of scoliosis can occur in patients who experience rapid growth. Because growth hormone increases growth rate, patients with a history of scoliosis who are treated with growth hormone should be monitored for progression of scoliosis. However, growth hormone has not been shown to increase the incidence of scoliosis. Scoliosis is commonly seen in untreated patients with PWS. Physicians should be alert to this abnormality, which may manifest during growth hormone therapy.

Intracranial hypertension (IH) with papilledema, visual changes, headache, nausea and/or vomiting has been reported in a small number of patients treated with growth hormone products. Symptoms usually occurred within the first 8 weeks of the initiation of growth hormone therapy. In all reported cases, IH-associated signs and symptoms resolved after termination of therapy or a reduction of the growth hormone dose. Funduscopic examination of patients is recommended at the initiation, and periodically during the course of, growth hormone therapy. Patients with PWS may be at increased risk for development of IH.

Before continuing treatment as an adult, a post-pubertal GHD patient who received growth hormone replacement therapy in childhood should be reevaluated with proper testing as described in INDICATIONS AND USAGE. If continued treatment is appropriate, GENOTROPIN should be administered at the reduced dose level recommended for adult GHD patients.

Drug Interactions

Concomitant glucocorticoid treatment may inhibit the growth-promoting effect of growth hormone. Pediatric GHD patients with coexisting ACTH deficiency should have their glucocorticoid replacement dose carefully adjusted to avoid an inhibitory effect on growth (see also PRECAUTIONS - General). Limited published data indicate that growth hormone treatment increases cytochrome P450 (CP450) mediated antipyrine clearance in man. These data suggest that growth hormone administration may alter the clearance of compounds known to be metabolized by CP450 liver enzymes (e.g. corticosteroids, sex steroids, anticonvulsants, cyclosporine). Careful monitoring is advisable when growth hormone is administered in combination with other drugs known to be metabolized by CP450 liver enzymes.

Carcinogenesis, Mutagenesis, Impairment of Fertility

Carcinogenicity studies have not been conducted with rhGH. No potential mutagenicity of rhGH was revealed in a battery of tests including induction of gene mutations in bacteria (the Ames test), gene mutations in mammalian cells grown in vitro (mouse L5178Y cells), and chromosomal damage in intact animals (bone marrow cells in rats). See PREGNANCY section for effect on fertility.

Pregnancy: Pregnancy Category B

Reproduction studies carried out with GENOTROPIN at doses of 0.3, 1, and 3.3 mg/kg/day administered SC in the rat and 0.08, 0.3, and 1.3 mg/kg/day administered intramuscularly in the rabbit (highest doses approximately 24 times and 19 times the recommended human therapeutic levels, respectively, based on body surface area) resulted in decreased maternal body weight gains but were not teratogenic. In rats receiving SC doses during gametogenesis and up to 7 days of pregnancy, 3.3 mg/kg/day (approximately 24

Continued on next page

Table 2
Efficacy of GENOTROPIN in Pediatric Patients with Prader-Willi Syndrome (Mean ± SD)

	Study 1		Study 2	
	GENOTROPIN (0.24 mg/kg/week) n=15	Untreated Control n=12	GENOTROPIN (0.36 mg/kg/week) n=7	Untreated Control n=9
Linear growth (cm) Baseline height	112.7 ± 14.9	109.5 ± 12.0	120.3 ± 17.5	120.5 ± 11.2
Growth from months 0 to 12	11.6* ± 2.3	5.0 ± 1.2	10.7* ± 2.3	4.3 ± 1.5
Height Standard Deviation Score (SDS) for age Baseline SDS	-1.6 ± 1.3	-1.8 ± 1.5	-2.6 ± 1.7	-2.1 ± 1.4
SDS at 12 months	-0.5† ± 1.3	-1.9 ± 1.4	-1.4† ± 1.5	-2.2 ± 1.4

* $p \leq 0.001$
† $p \leq 0.002$ (when comparing SDS change at 12 months)

Table 3
Effect of GENOTROPIN on Body Composition in Pediatric Patients with Prader-Willi Syndrome (Mean ± SD)

	GENOTROPIN n=14	Untreated Control n=10
Fat mass (kg) Baseline	12.3 ± 6.8	9.4 ± 4.9
Change from months 0 to 12	-0.9* ± 2.2	2.3 ± 2.4
Lean body mass (kg) Baseline	15.6 ± 5.7	14.3 ± 4.0
Change from months 0 to 12	4.7* ± 1.9	0.7 ± 2.4
Lean body mass/Fat mass Baseline	1.4 ± 0.4	1.8 ± 0.8
Change from months 0 to 12	1.0* ± 1.4	-0.1 ± 0.6
Body weight (kg)† Baseline	27.2 ± 12.0	23.2 ± 7.0
Change from months 0 to 12	3.7‡ ± 2.0	3.5 ± 1.9

* $p < 0.005$
† n=15 for the group receiving GENOTROPIN; n=12 for the Control group
‡ n.s.

Table 4
Efficacy of GENOTROPIN in Children Born Small for Gestational Age (Mean ± SD)

	GENOTROPIN (0.24 mg/kg/week) n=76	GENOTROPIN (0.48 mg/kg/week) n=93	Untreated Control n=40
Height Standard Deviation Score (SDS) Baseline SDS	-3.2 ± 0.8	-3.4 ± 1.0	-3.1 ± 0.9
SDS at 24 months	-0.2 ± 0.8	-1.7 ± 1.0	-2.9 ± 0.9
Change in SDS from baseline to month 24	1.2* ± 0.5	1.7*† ± 0.6	0.1 ± 0.3

* p = 0.0001 vs Untreated Control group
† p = 0.0001 vs group treated with GENOTROPIN 0.24 mg/kg/week

Genotropin—Cont.

times human dose) produced anestrus or extended estrus cycles in females and fewer and less motile sperm in males. When given to pregnant female rats (days 1 to 7 of gestation) at 3.3 mg/kg/day a very slight increase in fetal deaths was observed. At 1 mg/kg/day (approximately seven times human dose) rats showed slightly extended estrus cycles, whereas at 0.3 mg/kg/day no effects were noted.

In perinatal and postnatal studies in rats, GENOTROPIN doses of 0.3, 1, and 3.3 mg/kg/day produced growth-promoting effects in the dams but not in the fetuses. Young rats at the highest dose showed increased weight gain during suckling but the effect was not apparent by 10 weeks of age. No adverse effects were observed on gestation, morphogenesis, parturition, lactation, postnatal development, or reproductive capacity of the offsprings due to GENOTROPIN. There are, however, no adequate and well-controlled studies in pregnant women. Because animal reproduction studies are not always predictive of human response, this drug should be used during pregnancy only if clearly needed.

Nursing Mothers

There have been no studies conducted with GENOTROPIN in nursing mothers. It is not known whether this drug is excreted in human milk. Because many drugs are excreted in human milk, caution should be exercised when GENOTROPIN is administered to a nursing woman.

Geriatric Use

The safety and effectiveness of GENOTROPIN in patients aged 65 and over has not been evaluated in clinical studies. Elderly patients may be more sensitive to the action of GENOTROPIN and may be more prone to develop adverse reactions.

ADVERSE REACTIONS

As with all protein drugs, a small number of patients may develop antibodies to the protein. Growth hormone antibody with binding lower than 2 mg/L has not been associated with growth attenuation. In some cases when binding capacity is > 2 mg/L, interference with growth response has been observed.

In 419 pediatric patients evaluated in clinical studies with GENOTROPIN Lyophilized Powder, 244 had been treated previously with GENOTROPIN or other growth hormone preparations and 175 had received no previous growth hormone therapy. Antibodies to growth hormone (anti-hGH antibodies) were present in six previously treated patients at baseline. Three of the six became negative for anti-hGH antibodies during 6 to 12 months of treatment with GENOTROPIN. Of the remaining 413 patients, eight (1.9%) developed detectable anti-hGH antibodies during treatment with GENOTROPIN; none had an antibody binding capacity > 2 mg/L. There was no evidence that the growth response to GENOTROPIN was affected in these antibody-positive patients.

Preparations of GENOTROPIN contain a small amount of periplasmic *Escherichia coli* peptides (PECP). Anti-PECP antibodies are found in a small number of patients treated with GENOTROPIN, but these appear to be of no clinical significance.

In clinical studies with GENOTROPIN in pediatric GHD patients, the following events were reported infrequently: injection site reactions, including pain or burning associated with the injection, fibrosis, nodules, rash, inflammation, pigmentation, or bleeding; lipoatrophy; headache; hematuria; hypothyroidism; and mild hyperglycemia.

Leukemia has been reported in a small number of pediatric patients who have been treated with growth hormone, including growth hormone of pituitary origin and recombinant somatropin. The relationship, if any, between leukemia and growth hormone therapy is uncertain.

In two clinical studies with GENOTROPIN in pediatric patients with Prader-Willi syndrome, the following drug-related events were reported: edema, aggressiveness, arthralgia, benign intracranial hypertension, hair loss, headache, and myalgia.

In clinical studies of 273 pediatric patients born small for gestational age treated with GENOTROPIN, the following clinically significant events were reported: mild transient hyperglycemia, one patient with benign intracranial hypertension, two patients with central precocious puberty, two patients with jaw prominence, and several patients with aggravation of pre-existing scoliosis, injection site reactions, and self-limited progression of pigmented nevi. Anti-hGH antibodies were not detected in any of the patients treated with GENOTROPIN.

In clinical trials with GENOTROPIN in 1,145 GHD adults, the majority of the adverse events consisted of mild to moderate symptoms of fluid retention, including peripheral swelling, arthralgia, pain and stiffness of the extremities, peripheral edema, myalgia, paresthesia, and hypoesthesia. These events were reported early during therapy, and tended to be transient and/or responsive to dosage reduction.

Table 5 displays the adverse events reported by 5% or more of adult GHD patients in clinical trials after various durations of treatment with GENOTROPIN. Also presented are the corresponding incidence rates of these adverse events in placebo patients during the 6-month double-blind portion of the clinical trials.

[See table 5 below]

In expanded post-trial extension studies, diabetes mellitus developed in 12 of 3,031 patients (0.4%) during treatment with GENOTROPIN. All 12 patients had predisposing factors, e.g., elevated glycated hemoglobin levels and/or marked obesity, prior to receiving GENOTROPIN. Of the 3,031 patients receiving GENOTROPIN, 61 (2%) developed symptoms of carpal tunnel syndrome, which lessened after dosage reduction or treatment interruption (52) or surgery (9). Other adverse events that have been reported include generalized edema and hypoesthesia.

OVERDOSAGE

There is little information on acute or chronic overdosage with GENOTROPIN Lyophilized Powder. Intravenously administered growth hormone has been shown to result in an acute decrease in plasma glucose. Subsequently, hyperglycemia was seen. It is thought that the same effect might occur on rare occasions with a high dosage of GENOTROPIN administered SC. Long-term overdosage may result in signs and symptoms of acromegaly consistent with overproduction of growth hormone.

DOSAGE AND ADMINISTRATION

The dosage of GENOTROPIN Lyophilized Powder must be adjusted for the individual patient. The weekly dose should be divided into 6 or 7 **subcutaneous** injections. GENOTROPIN may be given in the thigh, buttocks, or abdomen; the site of SC injections should be rotated daily to help prevent lipoatrophy.

Pediatric GHD Patients: Generally, a dose of 0.16 to 0.24 mg/kg body weight/week is recommended.

Pediatric PWS Patients: Generally, a dose of 0.24 mg/kg body weight/week is recommended.

Pediatric SGA Patients: Generally, a dose of 0.48 mg/kg body weight/week is recommended.

Adult GHD Patients: The recommended dosage at the start of therapy is not more than 0.04 mg/kg/week. The dose may be increased at 4- to 8-week intervals according to individual patient requirements to a maximum of 0.08 mg/kg/week, depending upon patient tolerance of treatment. Clinical response, side effects, and determination of age-adjusted serum IGF-I may be used as guidance in dose titration. This approach will tend to result in weight-adjusted doses that are larger for women compared with men and smaller for older and obese patients.

GENOTROPIN must not be injected intravenously.

GENOTROPIN is supplied in a two-chamber cartridge, with the lyophilized powder in the front chamber and a diluent in the rear chamber. A reconstitution device is used to mix the diluent and powder.

Follow the directions for reconstitution provided with each device. **Do not shake**; shaking may cause denaturation of the active ingredient.

Table 5
Adverse Events Reported by ≥ 5% of 1,145 Adult GHD Patients During Clinical Trials of GENOTROPIN and Placebo, Grouped by Duration of Treatment

Adverse Event	Double Blind Phase		Open Label Phase GENOTROPIN		
	Placebo 0-6 mo. n = 572 % Patients	GENOTROPIN 0-6 mo. n = 573 % Patients	6-12 mo. n = 504 % Patients	12-18 mo. n = 63 % Patients	18-24 mo. n = 60 % Patients
Swelling, peripheral	5.1	17.5*	5.6	0	1.7
Arthralgia	4.2	17.3*	6.9	6.3	3.3
Upper respiratory infection	14.5	15.5	13.1	15.9	13.3
Pain, extremities	5.9	14.7*	6.7	1.6	3.3
Edema, peripheral	2.6	10.8*	3.0	0	0
Paresthesia	1.9	9.6*	2.2	3.2	0
Headache	7.7	9.9	6.2	0	0
Stiffness of extremities	1.6	7.9*	2.4	1.6	0
Fatigue	3.8	5.8	4.6	6.3	1.7
Myalgia	1.6	4.9*	2.0	4.8	6.7
Back pain	4.4	2.8	3.4	4.8	5.0

* Increased significantly when compared to placebo, $P \leq .025$: Fisher's Exact Test (one-sided)
n = number of patients receiving treatment during the indicated period.
% = percentage of patients who reported the event during the indicated period.

All parenteral drug products should be inspected visually for particulate matter and discoloration prior to administration, whenever solution and container permit. If the solution is cloudy, the contents **MUST NOT** be injected.

Patients and caregivers who will administer GENOTROPIN in medically unsupervised situations should receive appropriate training and instruction on the proper use of GENOTROPIN from the physician or other suitably qualified health professional.

STABILITY AND STORAGE

Except as noted below, store GENOTROPIN Lyophilized Powder under refrigeration at 2° to 8°C (36° to 46°F). Do not freeze. Protect from light.

The 1.5-mg cartridge of GENOTROPIN contains a diluent with no preservative. After reconstitution, the cartridge may be stored under refrigeration for up to 24 hours. Use only once and discard any remaining solution.

The 5.8-mg and 13.8-mg cartridges of GENOTROPIN contain a diluent with a preservative. Thus, after reconstitution, they may be stored under refrigeration for up to 21 days.

The GENOTROPIN MINIQUICK Growth Hormone Delivery Device should be refrigerated prior to dispensing, but may be stored at or below 25°C (77°F) for up to three months after dispensing. The diluent has no preservative. After reconstitution, the GENOTROPIN MINIQUICK may be stored under refrigeration for up to 24 hours before use. The GENOTROPIN MINIQUICK should be used only once and then discarded.

HOW SUPPLIED

GENOTROPIN Lyophilized Powder is available in the following packages:

1.5-mg two-chamber cartridge (without preservative)
concentration of 1.3 mg/mL (approximately 4 IU/mL)
Pre-assembled in a GENOTROPIN INTRA-MIX® Growth Hormone Reconstitution Device and packaged with a pressure release needle
Package of 5 NDC 0013-2606-94

5.8-mg two-chamber cartridge (with preservative)
concentration of 5 mg/mL (approximately 15 IU/mL)
For use with the GENOTROPIN PEN® 5 Growth Hormone Delivery Device and/or the GENOTROPIN MIXER™ Growth Hormone Reconstitution Device
Package of 5 NDC 0013-2626-94
Package of 1 NDC 0013-2626-81
Pre-assembled in a GENOTROPIN INTRA-MIX Growth Hormone Reconstitution Device and packaged with a pressure release needle
Package of 5 NDC 0013-2616-94
Package of 1 NDC 0013-2616-81

13.8-mg two-chamber cartridge (with preservative)
concentration of 12 mg/mL (approximately 36 IU/mL)
For use with the GENOTROPIN PEN 12 Growth Hormone Delivery Device and/or the GENOTROPIN MIXER Growth Hormone Reconstitution Device
Package of 5 NDC 0013-2646-94
Package of 1 NDC 0013-2646-81

Manufactured by: Pharmacia AB
Stockholm, Sweden
or
Vetter Pharma-Fertigung GmbH & Co. KG
Langenargen, Germany

GENOTROPIN MINIQUICK Growth Hormone Delivery Device containing a two-chamber cartridge of GENOTROPIN (without preservative)

After reconstitution, each GENOTROPIN MINIQUICK delivers a fixed volume of 0.25 mL, regardless of strength. Available in the following strengths, each in a package of 7:

0.2 mg	NDC 0013-2649-02
0.4 mg	NDC 0013-2650-02
0.6 mg	NDC 0013-2651-02
0.8 mg	NDC 0013-2652-02
1.0 mg	NDC 0013-2653-02
1.2 mg	NDC 0013-2654-02
1.4 mg	NDC 0013-2655-02
1.6 mg	NDC 0013-2656-02
1.8 mg	NDC 0013-2657-02
2.0 mg	NDC 0013-2658-02

Please see accompanying directions for use of the reconstitution and/or delivery device.

Manufactured by: Pharmacia AB
Stockholm, Sweden

Rx only

Manufactured for: Pharmacia & Upjohn Company
A subsidiary of Pharmacia Corporation
Kalamazoo, MI 49001, USA

Revised February 2004
818 279 005

GLYSET® ℞

[*glī-sĕt*]
(miglitol tablets)

Prescribing information for this product, which appears on pages 2768–2771 of the 2004 PDR, has been completely revised as follows. Please write "See Supplement A" next to the product heading.

DESCRIPTION

GLYSET Tablets contain miglitol, an oral alpha-glucosidase inhibitor for use in the management of non-insulin-dependent diabetes mellitus (NIDDM). Miglitol is a desoxynojirimycin derivative, and is chemically known as 3,4,5-piperidinetriol, 1-(2-hydroxyethyl)-2-(hydroxymethyl)-, [2R-(2α,3β,4α,5β)]-. It is a white to pale-yellow powder with a molecular weight of 207.2. Miglitol is soluble in water and has a pK_a of 5.9. Its empirical formula is $C_8H_{17}NO_5$ and its chemical structure is as follows:

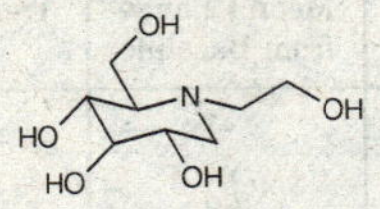

GLYSET is available as 25 mg, 50 mg and 100 mg tablets for oral use. The inactive ingredients are starch, microcrystalline cellulose, magnesium stearate, hypromellose, polyethylene glycol, titanium dioxide, and polysorbate 80.

CLINICAL PHARMACOLOGY

Miglitol is a desoxynojirimycin derivative that delays the digestion of ingested carbohydrates, thereby resulting in a smaller rise in blood glucose concentration following meals. As a consequence of plasma glucose reduction, GLYSET Tablets reduce levels of glycosylated hemoglobin in patients with Type II (non-insulin-dependent) diabetes mellitus. Systemic nonenzymatic protein glycosylation, as reflected by levels of glycosylated hemoglobin, is a function of average blood glucose concentration over time.

Mechanism of Action

In contrast to sulfonylureas, GLYSET does not enhance insulin secretion. The antihyperglycemic action of miglitol results from a reversible inhibition of membrane-bound intestinal α-glucoside hydrolase enzymes. Membrane-bound intestinal α-glucosidases hydrolyze oligosaccharides and disaccharides to glucose and other monosaccharides in the brush border of the small intestine. In diabetic patients, this enzyme inhibition results in delayed glucose absorption and lowering of postprandial hyperglycemia.

Because its mechanism of action is different, the effect of GLYSET to enhance glycemic control is additive to that of sulfonylureas when used in combination. In addition, GLYSET diminishes the insulinotropic and weight-increasing effects of sulfonylureas.

Miglitol has minor inhibitory activity against lactase and consequently, at the recommended doses, would not be expected to induce lactose intolerance.

Pharmacokinetics

Absorption: Absorption of miglitol is saturable at high doses: a dose of 25 mg is completely absorbed, whereas a dose of 100 mg is only 50% - 70% absorbed. For all doses, peak concentrations are reached in 2-3 hours. There is no evidence that systemic absorption of miglitol contributes to its therapeutic effect.

Distribution: The protein binding of miglitol is negligible (<4.0%). Miglitol has a volume of distribution of 0.18 L/kg, consistent with distribution primarily into the extracellular fluid.

Metabolism: Miglitol is not metabolized in man or in any animal species studied. No metabolites have been detected in plasma, urine, or feces, indicating a lack of either systemic or pre-systemic metabolism.

Excretion: Miglitol is eliminated by renal excretion as unchanged drug. Thus, following a 25-mg dose, over 95% of the dose is recovered in the urine within 24 hours. At higher doses, the cumulative recovery of drug from urine is somewhat lower due to the incomplete bioavailability. The elimination half-life of miglitol from plasma is approximately 2 hours.

Special Populations

Renal Impairment: Because miglitol is excreted primarily by the kidneys, accumulation of miglitol is expected in patients with renal impairment. Patients with creatinine clearance < 25 mL/min taking 25 mg 3 times daily exhibited a greater than two-fold increase in miglitol plasma levels as compared to subjects with creatinine clearance >60 mL/min. Dosage adjustment to correct the increased plasma concentrations is not feasible because miglitol acts locally. Little information is available on the safety of miglitol in patients with creatinine clearance <25 mL/min.

Hepatic impairment: Miglitol pharmacokinetics were not altered in cirrhotic patients relative to healthy control subjects. Since miglitol is not metabolized, no influence of hepatic function on the kinetics of miglitol is expected.

Gender: No significant difference in the pharmacokinetics of miglitol was observed between elderly men and women when body weight was taken into account.

Race: Several pharmacokinetic studies were conducted in Japanese volunteers, with results similar to those observed in Caucasians. A study comparing the pharmacodynamic response to a single 50-mg dose in Black and Caucasian healthy volunteers indicated similar glucose and insulin responses in both populations.

CLINICAL STUDIES

Clinical Experience in Non-Insulin-Dependent Diabetes Mellitus (NIDDM) Patients on Dietary Treatment Only

GLYSET Tablets were evaluated in two U.S. and three non-U.S. controlled, fixed-dose, monotherapy studies, in which 735 patients treated with GLYSET were evaluated for efficacy analyses (see Table 1).

In Study 1, a one-year study in which GLYSET was evaluated as monotherapy and also as combination therapy, there was a statistically significantly smaller increase in mean glycosylated hemoglobin (HbA1c) over time in the miglitol 50 mg 3 times daily monotherapy arm compared to placebo. Significant reductions in mean fasting and postprandial plasma glucose levels and in mean postprandial insulin levels were observed in patients treated with GLYSET compared with the placebo group.

Table 1
Results of Monotherapy Study with GLYSET

Study	Treatment	HbA1c (%) Mean Change from Baseline*	HbA1c (%) Treatment Effect**	1-hour Postprandial Glucose (mg/dL) Mean Change from Baseline	1-hour Postprandial Glucose (mg/dL) Treatment Effect**
1 (U.S.)	Placebo	+0.71	—	+24	—
	GLYSET 50 mg t.i.d.***	+0.13	-0.58†	-39	-63†
2 (U.S.)	Placebo	+0.47	—	+15	—
	GLYSET 50 mg t.i.d.	-0.22	-0.69†	-52	-67†
	GLYSET 100 mg t.i.d.	-0.28	-0.75†	-59	-74†
3 (non-U.S.)	Placebo	+0.18	—	+2	—
	GLYSET 25 mg t.i.d.	-0.08	-0.26	-33	-35†
	GLYSET 50 mg t.i.d.	-0.22	-0.40	-45	-47†
	GLYSET 100 mg t.i.d.	-0.63	-0.81†	-62	-64†
	GLYSET 200 mg t.i.d.‡	-0.84	-1.02†	-85	-87†
4 (non-U.S.)	Placebo	+0.01	—	+8	—
	GLYSET 50 mg t.i.d.	-0.35	-0.36†	-20	-28†
	GLYSET 100 mg t.i.d.	-0.57	-0.58†	-25	-33†
5 (non-U.S.)	Placebo	+0.32	—	+17	—
	GLYSET 100 mg t.i.d.	-0.43	-0.75†	-38	-55†

* Mean baseline ranged from 7.54 to 8.72% in these studies.
** The result of subtracting the placebo group average.
*** t.i.d. = 3 times daily
† p≤ 0.05
‡ Although results for the 200 mg 3 times daily are presented for completeness, the maximum recommended dosage of GLYSET is 100 mg 3 times daily.

In Study 2, a 14-week study, there was a significant decrease in HbA1c in patients receiving GLYSET 50 mg 3 times daily or 100 mg 3 times daily compared to placebo. In addition, there were significant reductions in postprandial plasma glucose and postprandial serum insulin levels compared to placebo.

Study 3 was a 6-month dose-ranging trial evaluating GLYSET at doses from 25 mg 3 times daily to 200 mg 3 times daily. GLYSET produced a greater reduction in HbA1c than placebo at all doses, although the effect was statistically significant only at the 100 mg 3 times daily and 200 mg 3 times daily doses. In addition, all doses of GLYSET produced significant reductions in postprandial plasma glucose and postprandial insulin levels compared to placebo.

Studies 4 and 5 were 6-month studies evaluating GLYSET at 50 and 100 mg 3 times daily, and 100 mg 3 times daily, respectively. As compared to placebo, GLYSET produced significant reductions in HbA1c, as well as a significant reduction in postprandial plasma glucose in both studies at the doses employed.

[See table 1 above]

Clinical Experience in NIDDM Patients Receiving Sulfonylureas

GLYSET was studied as adjunctive therapy to a background of maximal or near-maximal sulfonylurea (SFU) treatment in three large, double-blind, randomized studies (two U.S. and one non-U.S.) in which 471 patients treated with GLYSET were evaluated for efficacy (see Table 2).

Study 6 included patients under treatment with maximal doses of SFU at entry. At the end of this 14-week study, the mean treatment effects on glycosylated hemoglobin (HbA1c) were -0.82% and -0.74% for patients receiving GLYSET 50 mg 3 times daily plus SFU, and GLYSET 100 mg 3 times daily plus SFU, respectively.

Study 7 was a one-year study in which GLYSET at 25, 50 or 100 mg 3 times daily was added to a maximal dose of glyburide (10 mg twice daily). At the end of this study, the mean treatment effects on HbA1c of GLYSET when added to maximum glyburide therapy were -0.30%, -0.62%, and -0.73% with the 25, 50 and 100 mg 3 times daily dosages of GLYSET, respectively.

In Study 8, the addition of GLYSET 100 mg 3 times daily to a background of treatment with glyburide produced an additional mean treatment effect on HbA1c of -0.66%.

[See table 2 at top of next page]

Dose-Response

Results from controlled, fixed-dose studies of GLYSET as monotherapy or as combination treatment with a sulfonylurea were combined to derive a pooled estimate of the difference from placebo in the mean change from baseline in glycosylated hemoglobin (HbA1c) and postprandial plasma glucose as shown in Figures 1 and 2:

[See figure 1 at top of next column]
[See figure 2 at top of next column]

Because of its mechanism of action, the primary pharmacologic effect of miglitol is manifested as a reduction in postprandial plasma glucose, as shown previously in all of the major clinical trials. GLYSET was statistically significantly different from placebo at all doses in each of the individual studies with respect to effect on mean one-hour postprandial plasma glucose, and there is a dose response from 25 to 100 mg 3 times daily for this efficacy parameter.

Figure 1
HbA1c (%)
Mean Change From Baseline:
Treatment Effect
Pooled Results from Controlled Fixed-Dose Studies in Tables 1 and 2

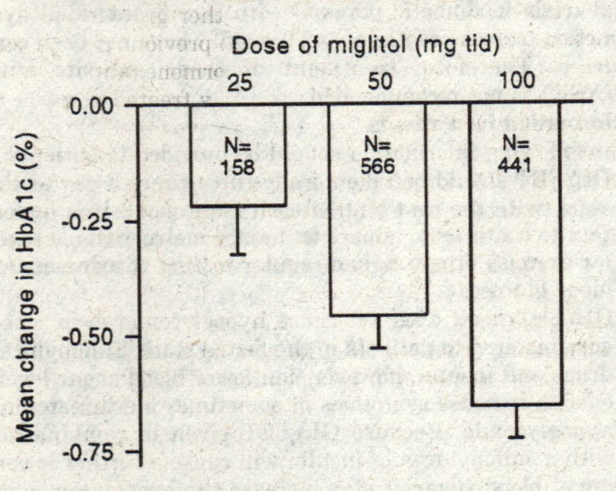

Figure 2
1-Hour Postprandial Plasma Glucose
Mean Change From Baseline:
Treatment Effect
Pooled Results from Controlled Fixed-Dose Studies in Tables 1 and 2

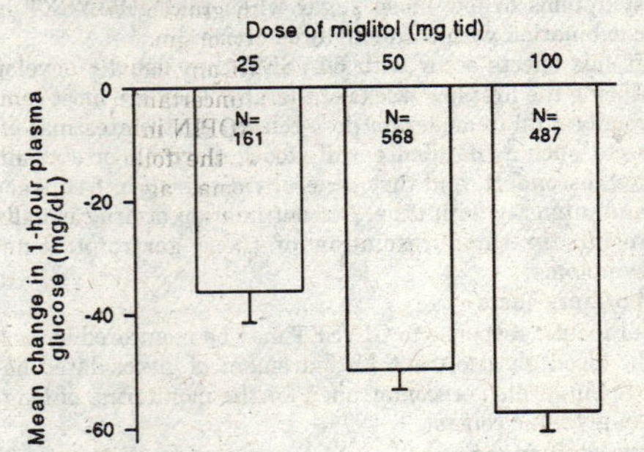

INDICATIONS AND USAGE

GLYSET Tablets, as monotherapy, are indicated as an adjunct to diet to improve glycemic control in patients with non-insulin-dependent diabetes mellitus (NIDDM) whose hyperglycemia cannot be managed with diet alone. GLYSET may also be used in combination with a sulfonylurea when diet plus either GLYSET or a sulfonylurea alone do not result in adequate glycemic control. The effect of GLYSET to enhance glycemic control is additive to that of sulfonylureas when used in combination, presumably because its mechanism of action is different.

In initiating treatment for NIDDM, diet should be emphasized as the primary form of treatment. Caloric restriction and weight loss are essential in the obese diabetic patient. Proper dietary management alone may be effective in controlling blood glucose and symptoms of hyperglycemia. The importance of regular physical activity when appropriate should also be stressed. If this treatment program fails to result in adequate glycemic control, the use of GLYSET

Continued on next page

Glyset—Cont.

should be considered. The use of GLYSET must be viewed by both the physician and patient as a treatment in addition to diet and not as a substitute for diet or as a convenient mechanism for avoiding dietary restraint.

CONTRAINDICATIONS

GLYSET Tablets are contraindicated in patients with:
- Diabetic ketoacidosis
- Inflammatory bowel disease, colonic ulceration, or partial intestinal obstruction, and in patients predisposed to intestinal obstruction
- Chronic intestinal diseases associated with marked disorders of digestion or absorption, or with conditions that may deteriorate as a result of increased gas formation in the intestine
- Hypersensitivity to the drug or any of its components.

PRECAUTIONS

General

Hypoglycemia: Because of its mechanism of action, GLYSET when administered alone should not cause hypoglycemia in the fasted or postprandial state. Sulfonylurea agents may cause hypoglycemia. Because GLYSET Tablets given in combination with a sulfonylurea will cause a further lowering of blood glucose, it may increase the hypoglycemic potential of the sulfonylurea, although this was not observed in clinical trials. Oral glucose (dextrose), whose absorption is not delayed by GLYSET, should be used instead of sucrose (cane sugar) in the treatment of mild-to-moderate hypoglycemia. Sucrose, whose hydrolysis to glucose and fructose is inhibited by GLYSET, is unsuitable for the rapid correction of hypoglycemia. Severe hypoglycemia may require the use of either intravenous glucose infusion or glucagon injection.

Loss of Control of Blood Glucose: When diabetic patients are exposed to stress such as fever, trauma, infection, or surgery, a temporary loss of control of blood glucose may occur. At such times, temporary insulin therapy may be necessary.

Renal Impairment: Plasma concentrations of GLYSET in renally impaired volunteers were proportionally increased relative to the degree of renal dysfunction. Long-term clinical trials in diabetic patients with significant renal dysfunction (serum creatinine >2.0 mg/dL) have not been conducted. Therefore, treatment of these patients with GLYSET is not recommended.

Information for Patients

The following information should be provided to patients:
- GLYSET should be taken orally three times a day at the start (with the first bite) of each main meal. It is important to continue to adhere to dietary instructions, a regular exercise program, and regular testing of urine and/or blood glucose.
- GLYSET itself does not cause hypoglycemia even when administered to patients in the fasted state. Sulfonylurea drugs and insulin, however, can lower blood sugar levels enough to cause symptoms or sometimes life-threatening hypoglycemia. Because GLYSET given in combination with a sulfonylurea or insulin will cause a further lowering of blood sugar, it may increase the hypoglycemic potential of these agents. The risk of hypoglycemia, its symptoms and treatment, and conditions that predispose to its development should be well understood by patients and responsible family members. Because GLYSET prevents the breakdown of table sugar, a source of glucose (dextrose, D-glucose) should be readily available to treat symptoms of low blood sugar when taking GLYSET in combination with a sulfonylurea or insulin.
- If side effects occur with GLYSET, they usually develop during the first few weeks of therapy. They are most commonly mild-to-moderate dose-related gastrointestinal effects, such as flatulence, soft stools, diarrhea, or abdominal discomfort, and they generally diminish in frequency and intensity with time. Discontinuation of drug usually results in rapid resolution of these gastrointestinal symptoms.

Laboratory Tests

Therapeutic response to GLYSET may be monitored by periodic blood glucose tests. Measurement of glycosylated hemoglobin levels is recommended for the monitoring of long-term glycemic control.

Drug Interactions

Several studies investigated the possible interaction between miglitol and glyburide. In six healthy volunteers given a single dose of 5-mg glyburide on a background of 6 days treatment with miglitol (50 mg 3 times daily for 4 days followed by 100 mg 3 times daily for 2 days) or placebo, the mean C_{max} and AUC values for glyburide were 17% and 25% lower, respectively, when glyburide was given with miglitol. In a study in diabetic patients in which the effects of adding miglitol 100 mg 3 times daily × 7 days or placebo to a background regimen of 3.5 mg glyburide daily were investigated, the mean AUC value for glyburide was 18% lower in the group treated with miglitol, although this difference was not statistically significant. Further information on a potential interaction with glyburide was obtained from one of the large U.S. clinical trials (Study 7) in which patients were dosed with either miglitol or placebo on a background of glyburide 10 mg twice daily. At the 6-month and 1-year clinic visits, patients taking concomitant miglitol 100 mg 3 times daily exhibited mean C_{max} values for glyburide that were 16% and 8% lower, respectively, compared to patients taking glyburide alone. However, these differences were not statistically significant. Thus, although there was a trend toward lower AUC and C_{max} values for glyburide when co-administered with GLYSET, no definitive statement regarding a potential interaction can be made based on the foregoing three studies.

Table 2
Results of Combination Therapy with GLYSET Plus Sulfonylurea (SFU)

Study	Treatment	HbA1c (%)		1-hour Postprandial Glucose (mg/dL)	
		Mean Change from Baseline*	Treatment Effect**	Mean Change from Baseline	Treatment Effect**
6 (U.S.)	Placebo + SFU	+0.33	—	-1	—
	GLYSET 50 mg t.i.d.*** + SFU	-0.49	-0.82†	-69	-68†
	GLYSET 100 mg t.i.d. + SFU	-0.41	-0.74†	-73	-72†
7 (U.S.)	Placebo + SFU	+1.01	—	48	—
	GLYSET 25 mg t.i.d. + SFU	+0.71	-0.30	-2	-50†
	GLYSET 50 mg t.i.d. + SFU	+0.39	-0.62†	-13	-61†
	GLYSET 100 mg t.i.d. + SFU	+0.28	-0.73†	-33	-81†
8 (non-U.S.)	Placebo + SFU	+0.16	—	+10	—
	GLYSET 100 mg t.i.d. + SFU	-0.50	-0.66†	-36	-46†

* Mean baseline ranged from 8.56 to 9.16% in these studies.
** The result of subtracting the placebo group average.
*** t.i.d. = 3 times daily
† $p \leq 0.05$

The effect of miglitol (100 mg 3 times daily × 7 days) on the pharmacokinetics of a single 1000-mg dose of metformin was investigated in healthy volunteers. Mean AUC and C_{max} values for metformin were 12% to 13% lower when the volunteers were given miglitol as compared with placebo, but this difference was not statistically significant.

In a healthy volunteer study, co-administration of either 50 mg or 100 mg miglitol 3 times daily together with digoxin reduced the average plasma concentrations of digoxin by 19% and 28%, respectively. However, in diabetic patients under treatment with digoxin, plasma digoxin concentrations were not altered by co-administration of miglitol 100 mg 3 times daily × 14 days.

Other healthy volunteer studies have demonstrated that miglitol may significantly reduce the bioavailability of ranitidine and propranolol by 60% and 40%, respectively. No effect of miglitol was observed on the pharmacokinetics or pharmacodynamics of either warfarin or nifedipine.

Intestinal adsorbents (e.g., charcoal) and digestive enzyme preparations containing carbohydrate-splitting enzymes (e.g., amylase, pancreatin) may reduce the effect of GLYSET and should not be taken concomitantly.

In 12 healthy males, concomitantly administered antacid did not influence the pharmacokinetics of miglitol.

Carcinogenesis, Mutagenesis, and Impairment of Fertility

Miglitol was administered to mice by the dietary route at doses as high as approximately 500 mg/kg body weight (corresponding to greater than 5 times the exposure in humans based on AUC) for 21 months. In a two-year rat study, miglitol was administered in the diet at exposures comparable to the maximum human exposures based on AUC. There was no evidence of carcinogenicity resulting from dietary treatment with miglitol.

In vitro, miglitol was found to be non-mutagenic in the bacterial mutagenesis (Ames) assay and the eukaryotic forward mutation assay (CHO/HGPRT). Miglitol did not have any clastogenic effects *in vivo* in the mouse micronucleus test. There were no heritable mutations detected in dominant lethal assay.

A combined male and female fertility study conducted in Wistar rats treated orally with miglitol at dose levels of 300 mg/kg body weight (approximately 8 times the maximum human exposure based on body surface area) produced no untoward effect on reproductive performance or capability to reproduce. In addition, survival, growth, development, and fertility of the offspring were not compromised.

Pregnancy

Teratogenic Effects: Pregnancy Category B. The safety of GLYSET in pregnant women has not been established. Developmental toxicology studies have been performed in rats at doses of 50, 150 and 450 mg/kg, corresponding to levels of approximately 1.5, 4, and 12 times the maximum recommended human exposure based on body surface area. In rabbits, doses of 10, 45, and 200 mg/kg corresponding to levels of approximately 0.5, 3, and 10 times the human exposure were examined. These studies revealed no evidence of fetal malformations attributable to miglitol. Doses of miglitol up to 4 and 3 times the human dose (based on body surface area), for rats and rabbits, respectively, did not reveal evidence of impaired fertility or harm to the fetus. The highest doses tested in these studies, 450 mg/kg in the rat and 200 mg/kg in the rabbit promoted maternal and/or fetal toxicity. Fetotoxicity was indicated by a slight but significant reduction in fetal weight in the rat study and slight reduction in fetal weight, delayed ossification of the fetal skeleton and increase in the percentage of non-viable fetuses in the rabbit study. In the peri-postnatal study in rats, the NOAEL (No Observed Adverse Effect Level) was 100 mg/kg (corresponding to approximately four times the exposure to humans, based on body surface area). An increase in stillborn progeny was noted at the high dose (300 mg/kg) in the rat peri-postnatal study, but not at the high dose (450 mg/kg) in the delivery segment of the rat developmental toxicity study. Otherwise, there was no adverse effect on survival, growth, development, behavior, or fertility in either the rat developmental toxicity or peri-postnatal studies. There are, however, no adequate and well-controlled studies in pregnant women. Because animal reproduction studies are not always predictive of human response, this drug should be used during pregnancy only if clearly needed.

Nursing Mothers

Miglitol has been shown to be excreted in human milk to a very small degree. Total excretion into milk accounted for 0.02% of a 100-mg maternal dose. The estimated exposure to a nursing infant is approximately 0.4% of the maternal dose. Although the levels of miglitol reached in human milk are exceedingly low, it is recommended that GLYSET not be administered to a nursing woman.

Pediatric Use

Safety and effectiveness of GLYSET in pediatric patients have not been established.

Geriatric Use

Of the total number of subjects in clinical studies of GLYSET in the United States, patients valid for safety analyses included 24% over 65, and 3% over 75. No overall differences in safety and effectiveness were observed between these subjects and younger subjects. The pharmacokinetics of miglitol were studied in elderly and young males (n=8 per group). At the dosage of 100 mg 3 times daily for 3 days, no differences between the two groups were found.

ADVERSE REACTIONS

Gastrointestinal: Gastrointestinal symptoms are the most common reactions to GLYSET Tablets. In U.S. placebo-controlled trials, the incidences of abdominal pain, diarrhea, and flatulence were 11.7%, 28.7%, and 41.5% respectively in 962 patients treated with GLYSET 25-100 mg 3 times daily, whereas the corresponding incidences were 4.7%, 10.0%, and 12.0% in 603 placebo-treated patients. The incidence of diarrhea and abdominal pain tended to diminish considerably with continued treatment.

Dermatologic: Skin rash was reported in 4.3% of patients treated with GLYSET compared to 2.4% of placebo-treated patients. Rashes were generally transient and most were assessed as unrelated to GLYSET by physician-investigators.

Abnormal Laboratory Findings: Low serum iron occurred more often in patients treated with GLYSET (9.2%) than in placebo-treated patients (4.2%) but did not persist in the majority of cases and was not associated with reductions in hemoglobin or changes in other hematologic indices.

OVERDOSAGE

Unlike sulfonylureas or insulin, an overdose of GLYSET Tablets will not result in hypoglycemia. An overdose may result in transient increases in flatulence, diarrhea, and abdominal discomfort. Because of the lack of extra-intestinal effects seen with GLYSET, no serious systemic reactions are expected in the event of an overdose.

DOSAGE AND ADMINISTRATION

There is no fixed dosage regimen for the management of diabetes mellitus with GLYSET Tablets or any other pharmacologic agent. Dosage of GLYSET must be individualized on the basis of both effectiveness and tolerance while not exceeding the maximum recommended dosage of 100 mg 3 times daily. GLYSET should be taken three times daily at the start (with the first bite) of each main meal. GLYSET should be started at 25 mg, and the dosage gradually increased as described below, both to reduce gastrointestinal adverse effects and to permit identification of the minimum dose required for adequate glycemic control of the patient. During treatment initiation and dose titration (see below), one-hour postprandial plasma glucose may be used to determine the therapeutic response to GLYSET and identify the minimum effective dose for the patient. Thereafter, glycosylated hemoglobin should be measured at intervals of approximately three months. The therapeutic goal should be to decrease both postprandial plasma glucose and glycosylated hemoglobin levels to normal or near normal by using the lowest effective dose of GLYSET, either as monotherapy or in combination with a sulfonylurea.

Initial Dosage: The recommended starting dosage of GLYSET is 25 mg, given orally three times daily at the start (with the first bite) of each main meal. However, some patients may benefit by starting at 25 mg once daily to minimize gastrointestinal adverse effects, and gradually increasing the frequency of administration to 3 times daily.

Maintenance Dosage: The usual maintenance dose of GLYSET is 50 mg 3 times daily, although some patients may benefit from increasing the dose to 100 mg 3 times daily. In order to allow adaptation to potential gastrointestinal adverse effects, it is recommended that GLYSET therapy be initiated at a dosage of 25 mg 3 times daily, the lowest effective dosage, and then gradually titrated upward to allow adaptation. After 4 - 8 weeks of the 25 mg 3 times daily regimen, the dosage should be increased to 50 mg 3 times daily for approximately three months, following which a glycosylated hemoglobin level should be measured to assess therapeutic response. If, at that time, the glycosylated hemoglobin level is not satisfactory, the dosage may be further increased to 100 mg 3 times daily, the maximum recommended dosage. Pooled data from controlled studies suggest a dose-response for both HbA1c and one-hour postprandial plasma glucose throughout the recommended dosage range. However, no single study has examined the effect on glycemic control of titrating patients' doses upwards within the same study. If no further reduction in postprandial glucose or glycosylated hemoglobin levels is observed with titration to 100 mg 3 times daily, consideration should be given to lowering the dose. Once an effective and tolerated dosage is established, it should be maintained.

Maximum Dosage: The maximum recommended dosage of GLYSET is 100 mg 3 times daily. In one clinical trial, 200 mg 3 times daily gave additional improved glycemic control but increased the incidence of the gastrointestinal symptoms described above.

Patients Receiving Sulfonylureas: Sulfonylurea agents may cause hypoglycemia. There was no increased incidence of hypoglycemia in patients who took GLYSET in combination with sulfonylurea agents compared to the incidence of hypoglycemia in patients receiving sulfonylureas alone in any clinical trial. However, GLYSET given in combination with a sulfonylurea will cause a further lowering of blood glucose and may increase the risk of hypoglycemia due to the additive effects of the two agents. If hypoglycemia occurs, appropriate adjustments in the dosage of these agents should be made.

HOW SUPPLIED

GLYSET Tablets are available as 25 mg, 50 mg, and 100 mg white, round, film-coated tablets. The tablets are debossed with the word "GLYSET" on one side and the strength on the other side, as indicated below.

Strength	NDC	Tablet Identification Front	Back
Bottles of 100:			
25 mg	0009-5012-01	GLYSET	25
50 mg	0009-5013-01	GLYSET	50
100 mg	0009-5014-01	GLYSET	100

Store at 25°C (77°F); excursions permitted to 15°-30°C (59°-86°F) [see USP Controlled Room Temperature].

℞ only

U.S. Patent No. 4,639,436

Manufactured for:
Pharmacia & Upjohn Company
A subsidiary of Pharmacia Corporation
Kalamazoo, MI 49001, USA
By:
Bayer Corporation
West Haven, CT 06516, USA

GLYSET is a registered trademark of Bayer Corporation used under license.

Revised July 2003

817 700 405
692460

VANTIN® ℞

[văn-tĭn]

Tables and Oral Suspension
(cefpodoxime proxetil tablets and cefpodoxime proxetil for oral suspension, USP)
For Oral Use Only

Prescribing information for this product, which appears on pages 2793–2797 of the 2004 PDR, has been completely revised as follows. Please write "See Supplement A" next to the product heading.

DESCRIPTION

Cefpodoxime proxetil is an orally administered, extended spectrum, semi-synthetic antibiotic of the cephalosporin class. The chemical name is (RS)-1(isopropoxycarbonyloxy) ethyl (+)-(6R,7R)-7-[2- (2-amino-4-thiazolyl)-2-{(Z)methoxyimino}acetamido]-3-methoxymethyl-8-oxo- 5-thia-1-azabicyclo [4.2.0] oct-2-ene-2-carboxylate.

Its empirical formula is $C_{21}H_{27}N_5O_9S_2$ and its structural formula is represented below:

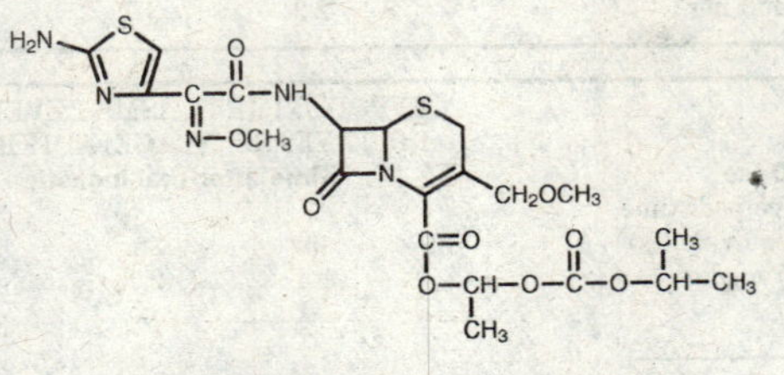

The molecular weight of cefpodoxime proxetil is 557,6.

Cefpodoxime proxetil is a prodrug; its active metabolite is cefpodoxime. All doses of cefpodoxime proxetil in this insert are expressed in terms of the active cefpodoxime moiety. The drug is supplied both as film-coated tablets and as flavored granules for oral suspension.

VANTIN Tablets contain cefpodoxime proxetil equivalent to 100 mg or 200 mg of cefpodoxime activity and the following inactive ingredients: carboxymethylcellulose calcium, carnauba wax, FD&C Yellow No. 6, hydroxypropylcellulose, hypromellose, lactose hydrous, magnesium stearate, propylene glycol, sodium lauryl sulfate and titanium dioxide. In addition, the 100 mg film-coated tablets contain D&C Yellow No. 10 and the 200 mg film-coated tablets contain FD&C Red No. 40.

Each 5 mL of VANTIN Oral Suspension contains cefpodoxime proxetil equivalent to 50 mg or 100 mg of cefpodoxime activity after constitution and the following inactive ingredients: artificial flavorings, butylated hydroxy anisole (BHA), carboxymethylcellulose sodium, microcrystalline cellulose, carrageenan, citric acid, colloidal silicon dioxide, croscarmellose sodium, hydroxypropylcellulose, lactose, maltodextrin, natural flavorings, propylene glycol alginate, sodium citrate, sodium benzoate, starch, sucrose, and vegetable oil.

CLINICAL PHARMACOLOGY

Absorption and Excretion:

Cefpodoxime proxetil is a prodrug that is absorbed from the gastrointestinal tract and de-esterified to its active metabolite, cefpodoxime. Following oral administration of 100 mg of cefpodoxime proxetil to fasting subjects, approximately 50% of the administered cefpodoxime dose was absorbed systemically. Over the recommended dosing range (100 to 400 mg), approximately 29 to 33% of the administered cefpodoxime dose was excreted unchanged in the urine in 12 hours. There is minimal metabolism of cefpodoxime *in vivo*.

Effects of Food:

The extent of absorption (mean AUC) and the mean peak plasma concentration increased when film-coated tablets were administered with food. Following a 200 mg tablet dose taken with food, the AUC was 21 to 33% higher than under fasting conditions, and the peak plasma concentration averaged 3.1 mcg/mL in fed subjects versus 2.6 mcg/mL in fasted subjects. Time to peak concentration was not significantly different between fed and fasted subjects.

When a 200 mg dose of the suspension was taken with food, the extent of absorption (mean AUC) and mean peak plasma concentration in fed subjects were not significantly different from fasted subjects, but the rate of absorption was slower with food (48% increase in T_{max}).

Pharmacokinetics of Cefpodoxime Proxetil Film-coated Tablets:

Over the recommended dosing range, (100 to 400 mg), the rate and extent of cefpodoxime absorption exhibited dose-dependency; dose-normalized C_{max} and AUC decreased by up to 32% with increasing dose. Over the recommended dosing range, the T_{max} was approximately 2 to 3 hours and the $T_{1/2}$ ranged from 2.09 to 2.84 hours. Mean C_{max} was 1.4 mcg/mL for the 100 mg dose, 2.3 mcg/mL for the 200 mg dose, and 3.9 mcg/mL for the 400 mg dose. In patients with normal renal function, neither accumulation nor significant changes in other pharmacokinetic parameters were noted following multiple oral doses of up to 400 mg Q 12 hours.

[See first table at top of next page]

Pharmacokinetics of Cefpodoxime Proxetil Suspension:

In adult subjects, a 100 mg dose of oral suspension produced an average peak cefpodoxime concentration of approximately 1.5 mcg/mL (range: 1.1 to 2.1 mcg/mL), which is equivalent to that reported following administration of the 100 mg tablet. Time to peak plasma concentration and area under the plasma concentration-time curve (AUC) for the oral suspension were also equivalent to those produced with film-coated tablets in adults following a 100 mg oral dose.

The pharmacokinetics of cefpodoxime were investigated in 29 patients aged 1 to 17 years. Each patient received a single, oral, 5 mg/kg dose of cefpodoxime oral suspension. Plasma and urine samples were collected for 12 hours after dosing. The plasma levels reported from this study are as follows:

[See second table at top of next page]

Distribution:

Protein binding of cefpodoxime ranges from 22 to 33% in serum and from 21 to 29% in plasma.

Skin Blister:

Following multiple-dose administration every 12 hours for 5 days of 200 mg or 400 mg cefpodoxime proxetil, the mean maximum cefpodoxime concentration in skin blister fluid averaged 1.6 and 2.8 mcg/mL, respectively. Skin blister fluid cefpodoxime levels at 12 hours after dosing averaged 0.2 and 0.4 mcg/mL for the 200 mg and 400 mg multiple-dose regimens, respectively.

Tonsil Tissue:

Following a single, oral 100 mg cefpodoxime proxetil film-coated tablet, the mean maximum cefpodoxime concentration in tonsil tissue averaged 0.24 mcg/g at 4 hours post-dosing and 0.09 mcg/g at 7 hours post-dosing. Equilibrium was achieved between plasma and tonsil tissue within 4 hours of dosing. No detection of cefpodoxime in tonsillar tissue was reported 12 hours after dosing. These results demonstrated that concentrations of cefpodoxime exceeded the MIC_{90} of *S. pyogenes* for at least 7 hours after dosing of 100 mg of cefpodoxime proxetil.

Lung Tissue:

Following a single, oral 200 mg cefpodoxime proxetil film-coated tablet, the mean maximum cefpodoxime concentration in lung tissue averaged 0.63 mcg/g at 3 hours post-dosing, 0.52 mcg/g at 6 hours post-dosing, and 0.19 mcg/g at 12 hours post-dosing. The results of this study indicated that cefpodoxime penetrated into lung tissue and produced sustained drug concentrations for at least 12 hours after dosing at levels that exceeded the MIC_{90} for *S. pneumoniae* and *H. influenzae*.

CSF:

Adequate data on CSF levels of cefpodoxime are not available.

Effects of Decreased Renal Function:

Elimination of cefpodoxime is reduced in patients with moderate to severe renal impairment (< 50mL/min creatinine clearance). (See **PRECAUTIONS** and **DOSAGE AND ADMINISTRATION**.) In subjects with mild impairment of renal function (50 to 80 mL/min creatinine clearance), the average plasma half-life of cefpodoxime was 3.5 hours. In subjects with moderate (30 to 49 mL/min creatinine clearance) or severe renal impairment (5 to 29 mL/min creatinine clearance), the half-life increased to 5.9 and 9.8 hours, respectively. Approximately 23% of the administered dose was cleared from the body during a standard 3-hour hemodialysis procedure.

Effect of Hepatic Impairment (cirrhosis):

Absorption was somewhat diminished and elimination unchanged in patients with cirrhosis. The mean cefpodoxime $T_{1/2}$ and renal clearance in cirrhotic patients were similar to those derived in studies of healthy subjects. Ascites did not appear to affect values in cirrhotic subjects. No dosage adjustment is recommended in this patient population.

Pharmacokinetics in Elderly Subjects:

Elderly subjects do not require dosage adjustments unless they have diminished renal function. (See **PRECAUTIONS**.) In healthy geriatric subjects, cefpodoxime half-life in plasma averaged 4.2 hours (vs 3.3 in younger subjects) and urinary recovery averaged 21% after a 400 mg dose was administered every 12 hours. Other pharmacokinetic parameters (C_{max}, AUC, and T_{max}) were unchanged relative to those observed in healthy young subjects.

Microbiology:

Cefpodoxime is active against a wide-spectrum of Gram-positive and Gram-negative bacteria.

Cefpodoxime is stable in the presence of beta-lactamase enzymes. As a result, many organisms resistant to penicillins and cephalosporins, due to their production of beta lactamase, may be susceptible to cefpodoxime. Cefpodoxime is inactivated by certain extended spectrum beta-lactamases. The bactericidal activity of cefpodoxime results from its inhibition of cell wall synthesis.

Cefpodoxime has been shown to be active against most strains of the following microorganisms, both *in vitro* and in clinical infections, as described in the **INDICATIONS AND USAGE** section.

Aerobic Gram-positive microorganisms:

Staphylococcus aureus (including penicillinase-producing strains)

NOTE: Cefpodoxime is inactive against methicillin-resistant staphylococci.

Staphylococcus saprophyticus

Streptococcus pneumoniae (excluding penicillin-resistant strains)

Streptococcus pyogenes

Aerobic Gram-negative microorganisms:

Escherichia coli

Klebsiella pneumoniae

Proteus mirabilis

Haemophilus influenzae (including beta-lactamase producing strains)

Moraxella (Branhamella) catarrhalis

Neisseria gonorrhoeae (including penicillinase-producing strains)

The following *in vitro* data are available, but their clinical significance is unknown. Cefpodoxime exhibits *in vitro* minimum inhibitory concentrations (MICs) of ≤ 2.0 mcg/mL against most (≥90%) of isolates of the following microorganisms. However, the safety and efficacy of cefpodoxime in treating clinical infections due to these microorganisms have not been established in adequate and well controlled clinical trials.

Aerobic Gram-positive microorganisms:

Streptococcus agalactiae

Streptococcus spp. (Groups C, F, G)

NOTE: Cefpodoxime is inactive against enterococci.

Continued on next page

Vantin—Cont.

Aerobic Gram-negative microorganisms:
Citrobacter diversus
Klebsiella oxytoca
Proteus vulgaris
Providencia rettgeri
Haemophilus parainfluenzae
NOTE: Cefpodoxime is inactive against most strains of Pseudomonas and Enterobacter.
Anaerobic Gram-positive microorganisms:
Peptostreptococcus magnus

SUSCEPTIBILITY TESTING

Dilution Techniques: Quantitative methods are used to determine antimicrobial inhibitory concentrations (MICs). These MICs provide estimates of the susceptibility of microorganisms to antimicrobial compounds. The MICs should be determined using a standardized procedure. Standardized procedures are based on dilution methods[1,2] (broth or agar) or equivalent using standardized inoculum concentrations, and standardized concentrations of cefpodoxime from a powder of known potency. The MIC values should be interpreted according to the following criteria:

For Susceptibility Testing of *Enterobacteriaceae* and *Staphylococcus* spp.

MIC (mcg/mL)	Interpretation
≤ 2.0	Susceptible (S)
4.0	Intermediate (I)
≥ 8.0	Resistant (R)

For Susceptibility Testing of *Haemophilus* spp.[a]

MIC (mcg/mL)	Interpretation[b]
≤ 2.0	Susceptible (S)

[a] The interpretive criteria for *Haemophilus* spp. is applicable only to broth microdilution susceptibility testing done with Haemophilus Test Medium (HTM) broth.[2]
[b] "Intermediate" and "Resistant" categories have not been determined.

For Susceptibility Testing of *Neisseria gonorrhoeae*.[c]

MIC (mcg/mL)	Interpretation[d]
≤ 0.5	Susceptible (S)

[c] The interpretive value for *N. gonorroheae* is applicable only to agar dilution susceptibility testing done with *Neisseria gonorrhoeae* susceptibility test medium.[2]
[d] "Intermediate" and "Resistant" categories have not been determined.

For Susceptibility Testing of Streptococcus pneumoniae.

MIC (mcg/mL)	Interpretation[e]
≤ 0.5	Susceptible (S)
1.0	Intermediate (I)
≥ 2.0	Resistant (R)

[e] The interpretive value for *S. pneumoniae* is applicable only to broth microdilution susceptibility testing done with cation-adjusted Mueller-Hinton broth with lysed horse blood (LHB) (2-5% v/v).[2]

For Susceptibility Testing of *Streptococcus* spp. other than *Streptococcus pneumoniae*.[f]
A streptococcal isolate that is susceptible to penicillin (MIC ≤ 0.12 mcg/mL) can be considered susceptible to cefpodoxime for approved indications, and need not be tested against cefpodoxime.

[f] The interpretive value for *Streptococcus* spp. is applicable only to broth microdilution susceptibility testing done with cation-adjusted Mueller-Hinton broth with lysed horse blood (LHB) (2-5% v/v).[2]

A report of "Susceptible" indicates that the pathogen is likely to be inhibited if the concentration of the antimicrobial compound in the blood reaches usually achievable levels. A report of "Intermediate" indicates that the results should be considered equivocal, and, if the microorganism is not fully susceptible to alternative, clinically feasible drugs, the test should be repeated. This category implies possible clinical applicability in body sites where the drug is physiologically concentrated or in situations where high dosage of drug can be used. This category also provides a buffer zone which prevents small technical factors from causing major discrepancies in interpretation. A report of "Resistant" indicates that the pathogen is not likely to be inhibited if the antimicrobial compound in the blood reaches the concentrations usually achievable; other therapy should be selected.

Quality Control
A standardized susceptibility test procedure requires the use of laboratory control organisms to control the technical aspects of the laboratory procedures. Standard cefpodoxime powder should provide the following MIC values with the indicated quality control strains:

Microorganism (ATCC®#)	MIC Range (mcg/mL)
Escherichia coli (25922)	0.25 - 1.0
Staphylococcus aureus (29213)	1.0 - 8.0
Haemophilus influenzae (49247)	0.25 - 1.0[g]
Neisseria gonorrhoeae (49226)	0.03 - 0.12[h]
Streptococcus pneumoniae(49619)[j]	0.03 - 0.12[i]

CEFPODOXIME PLASMA LEVELS (mcg/mL) IN FASTED ADULTS AFTER FILM-COATED TABLET ADMINISTRATION (Single Dose)

Dose (cefpodoxime equivalents)	Time after oral ingestion 1hr	2hr	3hr	4hr	6hr	8hr	12hr
100 mg	0.98	1.4	1.3	1.0	0.59	0.29	0.08
200 mg	1.5	2.2	2.2	1.8	1.2	0.62	0.18
400 mg	2.2	3.7	3.8	3.3	2.3	1.3	0.38

CEFPODOXIME PLASMA LEVELS (mcg/mL) IN FASTED PATIENTS (1 to 17 YEARS OF AGE) AFTER SUSPENSION ADMINISTRATION

Dose (cefpodoxime equivalents)	Time after oral ingestion 1hr	2hr	3hr	4hr	6hr	8hr	12hr
5 mg/kg[1]	1.4	2.1	2.1	1.7	0.90	0.40	0.090

[1] Dose did not exceed 200 mg.

[g] These quality control ranges are applicable to tests performed by a broth microdilution procedure using Haemophilus Test Medium (HTM).
[h] These quality control ranges are applicable to tests performed by agar dilution only using GC agar base with 1% defined growth supplement.
[i] These quality control ranges are applicable to tests performed by the broth microdilution method only using cation-adjusted Mueller-Hinton broth with 2 to 5% lysed horse blood.
[j] When susceptibility testing *Streptococcus pneumoniae* or *Streptococcus* spp. this quality control strain should be tested.

Diffusion Techniques: Quantitative methods that require measurement of zone diameters also provide reproducible estimates of the susceptibility of bacteria to antimicrobial compounds. One such standardized procedure[3] requires the use of standardized inoculum concentrations. This procedure uses paper disks impregnated with 10 mcg cefpodoxime to test the susceptibility of microorganisms to cefpodoxime. Reports from the laboratory providing results of the standard single-disk susceptibility test with a 10 mcg cefpodoxime disk should be interpreted according to the following criteria:

For Susceptibility Testing of *Enterobacteriaceae* and *Staphylococcus* spp.

Zone Diameter (mm)	Interpretation
≥ 21	Susceptible (S)
18-20	Intermediate (I)
≤ 17	Resistant (R)

For Susceptibility Testing of *Haemophilus* spp.[k]

Zone Diameter (mm)	Interpretation[l]
≥ 21	Susceptible (S)

[k] The zone diameter for *Haemophilus spp.* is applicable only to tests performed on Haemophilus Test Medium (HTM) agar incubated under 5% CO_2.[2]
[l] "Intermediate" and "Resistant" criteria have not been determined.

For Susceptibility Testing of *Neisseria gonorrhoeae*.[m]

Zone Diameter (mm)	Interpretation[n]
≥ 29	Susceptible (S)

[m] The zone diameter for *N. gonorrhoeae* is applicable only to tests performed on GC agar base and 1% defined growth supplement incubated under 5% CO_2.[2]
[n] "Intermediate" and "Resistant" categories have not been determined.

For Susceptibility Testing of *Streptococcus pneumoniae*.[o]
Isolates of pneumococci with oxacillin zone sizes of ≥20 mm are susceptible (MIC ≤ 0.06 mcg/mL) to penicillin and can be considered susceptible to cefpodoxime for approved indications, and cefpodoxime need not be tested.

[o] The zone diameter for *S. pneumoniae* is applicable only to tests performed on Mueller-Hinton agar with 5% sheep blood incubated in 5% CO_2.[2]

For Susceptibility Testing of *Streptococcus* spp. other than *Streptococcus pneumoniae*.[p]
A streptococcal isolate that is susceptible to penicillin (zone diameter ≥ 28 mm) can be considered susceptible to cefpodoxime for approved indications, and cefpodoxime need not be tested.

[p] The zone diameter for *Streptococcus* spp. is applicable only to tests performed on Mueller-Hinton agar with 5% sheep blood incubated in 5% CO_2.[2]

Quality Control
As with standardized dilution techniques, diffusion methods require the use of laboratory control microorganisms that are used to control the technical aspects of the laboratory procedures. For the diffusion technique, the 10 mcg cefpodoxime disk should provide the following zone diameters with the quality control strains listed below:

Microorganism (ATCC®#)	Zone Diameter Range (mm)
Escherichia coli (25922)	23-28
Staphylococcus aureus (25923)	19-25
Haemophilus influenzae (49247)	25-31[q]
Neisseria gonorrhoeae (49226)	35-43[r]
Streptococcus pneumoniae(49619)[t]	28-34[s]

[q] This zone diameter range is only applicable to tests performed on Haemophilus Test Medium (HTM) agar incubated in 5% CO_2.
[r] This zone diameter range is only applicable to tests performed on GC agar base and 1% defined growth supplement incubated in 5% CO_2.
[s] This zone diameter range is only applicable to tests performed on Mueller-Hinton agar supplemented with 5% defibrinated sheep blood, incubated in 5% CO_2.
[t] This organism is to be used for quality control testing for both *S. pneumoniae* and *Streptococcus* spp.
ATCC® is a registered trademark of the American Type Culture Collection.

INDICATIONS AND USAGE
Cefpodoxime proxetil is indicated for the treatment of patients with mild to moderate infections caused by susceptible strains of the designated microorganisms in the conditions listed below. **Recommended dosages, durations of therapy, and applicable patient populations vary among these infections. Please see DOSAGE AND ADMINISTRATION for specific recommendations.**

Acute otitis media caused by *Streptococcus pneumoniae*, (excluding penicillin-resistant strains), *Streptococcus pyogenes, Haemophilus influenzae* (including beta-lactamase-producing strains), or *Moraxella (Branhamella) catarrhalis* (including beta-lactamase producing strains).

Pharyngitis and/or tonsillitis caused by *Streptococcus pyogenes*.

NOTE: Only penicillin by the intramuscular route of administration has been shown to be effective in the prophylaxis of rheumatic fever. Cefpodoxime proxetil is generally effective in the eradication of streptococci from the oropharynx. However, data establishing the efficacy of cefpodoxime proxetil for the prophylaxis of subsequent rheumatic fever are not available.

Community-acquired pneumonia caused by *S. pneumoniae* or *H. influenzae* (including beta-lactamase-producing strains).

Acute bacterial exacerbation of chronic bronchitis caused by *S. pneumoniae, H. influenzae* (non-beta-lactamase-producing strains only), or *M. catarrhalis*. Data are insufficient at this time to establish efficacy in patients with acute bacterial exacerbations of chronic bronchitis caused by beta-lactamase-producing strains of *H. influenzae*.

Acute, uncomplicated urethral and cervical gonorrhea caused by *Neisseria gonorrhoeae* (including penicillinase-producing strains).

Acute, uncomplicated ano-rectal infections in women due to *Neisseria gonorrhoeae* (including penicillinase-producing strains).

NOTE: The efficacy of cefpodoxime in treating male patients with rectal infections caused by *N. gonorrhoeae* has not been established. Data do not support the use of cefpodoxime proxetil in the treatment of pharyngeal infections due to *N. gonorrhoeae* in men or women.

Uncomplicated skin and skin structure infections caused by *Staphylococcus aureus* (including penicillinase-producing strains) or *Streptococcus pyogenes*. Abscesses should be surgically drained as clinically indicated.

NOTE: In clinical trials, successful treatment of uncomplicated skin and skin structure infections was dose-related. The effective therapeutic dose for skin infections was higher than those used in other recommended indications. (See **DOSAGE AND ADMINISTRATION**.)

Acute maxillary sinusitis caused by *Haemophilus influenzae* (including beta-lactamase producing strains), *Streptococcus pneumoniae*, and *Moraxella catarrhalis*.

Uncomplicated urinary tract infections (cystitis) caused by *Escherichia coli, Klebsiella pneumoniae, Proteus mirabilis*, or *Staphylococcus saprophyticus*.

NOTE: In considering the use of cefpodoxime proxetil in the treatment of cystitis, cefpodoxime proxetil's lower bacterial eradication rates should be weighed against the increased eradication rates and different safety profiles of some other classes of approved agents. (See **CLINICAL STUDIES** section.)

Appropriate specimens for bacteriological examination should be obtained in order to isolate and identify causative organisms and to determine their susceptibility to cefpodoxime. Therapy may be instituted while awaiting the results of these studies. Once these results become available, antimicrobial therapy should be adjusted accordingly.

CONTRAINDICATIONS

Cefpodoxime proxetil is contraindicated in patients with a known allergy to cefpodoxime or to the cephalosporin group of antibiotics.

WARNINGS

BEFORE THERAPY WITH CEFPODOXIME PROXETIL IS INSTITUTED, CAREFUL INQUIRY SHOULD BE MADE TO DETERMINE WHETHER THE PATIENT HAS HAD PREVIOUS HYPERSENSITIVITY REACTIONS TO CEFPODOXIME, OTHER CEPHALOSPORINS, PENICILLINS, OR OTHER DRUGS. IF CEFPODOXIME IS TO BE ADMINISTERED TO PENICILLIN SENSITIVE PATIENTS, CAUTION SHOULD BE EXERCISED BECAUSE CROSS HYPERSENSITIVITY AMONG BETA-LACTAM ANTIBIOTICS HAS BEEN CLEARLY DOCUMENTED AND MAY OCCUR IN UP TO 10% OF PATIENTS WITH A HISTORY OF PENICILLIN ALLERGY. IF AN ALLERGIC REACTION TO CEFPODOXIME PROXETIL OCCURS, DISCONTINUE THE DRUG. SERIOUS ACUTE HYPERSENSITIVITY REACTIONS MAY REQUIRE TREATMENT WITH EPINEPHRINE AND OTHER EMERGENCY MEASURES, INCLUDING OXYGEN, INTRAVENOUS FLUIDS, INTRAVENOUS ANTIHISTAMINE, AND AIRWAY MANAGEMENT, AS CLINICALLY INDICATED. PSEUDOMEMBRANOUS COLITIS HAS BEEN REPORTED WITH NEARLY ALL ANTIBACTERIAL AGENTS, INCLUDING CEFPODOXIME, AND MAY RANGE IN SEVERITY FROM MILD TO LIFE-THREATENING. THEREFORE, IT IS IMPORTANT TO CONSIDER THIS DIAGNOSIS IN PATIENTS WHO PRESENT WITH DIARRHEA SUBSEQUENT TO THE ADMINISTRATION OF ANTIBACTERIAL AGENTS.

Extreme caution should be observed when using this product in patients at increased risk for antibiotic-induced, pseudomembranous colitis because of exposure to institutional settings, such as nursing homes or hospitals with endemic *C. difficile*.

Treatment with broad-spectrum antibiotics, including cefpodoxime proxetil, alters the normal flora of the colon and may permit overgrowth of clostridia. Studies indicate a toxin produced by *Clostridium difficile* is the primary cause of "antibiotic-associated colitis".

After the diagnosis of pseudomembranous colitis has been established, therapeutic measures should be initiated. Mild cases of pseudomembranous colitis usually respond to drug discontinuation alone. In moderate to severe cases, consideration should be given to management with fluids and electrolytes, protein supplementation, and treatment with an oral antibacterial drug effective against *C. difficile*.

A concerted effort to monitor for *C. difficile* in cefpodoxime-treated patients with diarrhea was undertaken because of an increased incidence of diarrhea associated with *C. difficile* in early trials in normal subjects. *C.difficile* organisms or toxin was reported in 10% of the cefpodoxime-treated adult patients with diarrhea; however, no specific diagnosis of pseudomembranous colitis was made in these patients.

In post-marketing experience outside the United States, reports of pseudomembranous colitis associated with the use of cefpodoxime proxetil have been received.

PRECAUTIONS

General:

In patients with transient or persistent reduction in urinary output due to renal insufficiency, the total daily dose of cefpodoxime proxetil should be reduced because high and prolonged serum antibiotic concentrations can occur in such individuals following usual doses. Cefpodoxime, like other cephalosporins, should be administered with caution to patients receiving concurrent treatment with potent diuretics. (See **DOSAGE AND ADMINISTRATION**.)

As with other antibiotics, prolonged use of cefpodoxime proxetil may result in overgrowth of non-susceptible organisms. Repeated evaluation of the patient's condition is essential. If superinfection occurs during therapy, appropriate measures should be taken.

Drug Interactions:

Antacids: Concomitant administration of high doses of antacids (sodium bicarbonate and aluminum hydroxide) or H_2 blockers reduces peak plasma levels by 24% to 42% and the extent of absorption by 27% to 32%, respectively. The rate of absorption is not altered by these concomitant medications. Oral anti-cholinergics (e.g., propantheline) delay peak plasma levels (47% increase in T_{max}), but do not affect the extent of absorption (AUC).

Probenecid: As with other beta-lactam antibiotics, renal excretion of cefpodoxime was inhibited by probenecid and resulted in an approximately 31% increase in AUC and 20% increase in peak cefpodoxime plasma levels.

Nephrotoxic drugs: Although nephrotoxicity has not been noted when cefpodoxime proxetil was given alone, close monitoring of renal function is advised when cefpodoxime proxetil is administered concomitantly with compounds of known nephrotoxic potential.

Drug/Laboratory Test Interactions:

Cephalosporins, including cefpodoxime proxetil, are known to occasionally induce a positive direct Coombs' test.

Carcinogenesis, Mutagenesis, Impairment of Fertility:

Long-term animal carcinogenesis studies of cefpodoxime proxetil have not been performed. Mutagenesis studies of cefpodoxime, including the Ames test both with and without metabolic activation, the chromosome aberration test, the unscheduled DNA synthesis assay, mitotic recombination and gene conversion, the forward gene mutation assay and the *in vivo* micronucleus test, were all negative. No untoward effects on fertility or reproduction were noted when 100 mg/kg/day or less (2 times the human dose based on mg/m^2) was administered orally to rats.

Pregnancy - Teratogenic Effects:

Pregnancy Category B

Cefpodoxime proxetil was neither teratogenic nor embryocidal when administered to rats during organogenesis at doses up to 100 mg/kg/day (2 times the human dose based on mg/m^2) or to rabbits at doses up to 30 mg/kg/day (1-2 times the human dose based on mg/m^2).

There are, however, no adequate and well-controlled studies of cefpodoxime proxetil use in pregnant women. Because animal reproduction studies are not always predictive of human response, this drug should be used during pregnancy only if clearly needed.

Labor and Delivery:

Cefpodoxime proxetil has not been studied for use during labor and delivery. Treatment should only be given if clearly needed.

Nursing Mothers:

Cefpodoxime is excreted in human milk. In a study of 3 lactating women, levels of cefpodoxime in human milk were 0%, 2% and 6% of concomitant serum levels at 4 hours following a 200 mg oral dose of cefpodoxime proxetil. At 6 hours post-dosing, levels were 0%, 9% and 16% of concomitant serum levels. Because of the potential for serious reactions in nursing infants, a decision should be made whether to discontinue nursing or to discontinue the drug, taking into account the importance of the drug to the mother.

Pediatric Use:

Safety and efficacy in infants less than 2 months of age have not been established.

Geriatric Use:

Of the 3338 patients in multiple-dose clinical studies of cefpodoxime proxetil film-coated tablets, 521 (16%) were 65 and over, while 214 (6%) were 75 and over. No overall differences in effectiveness or safety were observed between the elderly and younger patients. In healthy geriatric subjects with normal renal function, cefpodoxime half-life in plasma averaged 4.2 hours and urinary recovery averaged 21% after a 400 mg dose was given every 12 hours for 15 days. Other pharmacokinetic parameters were unchanged relative to those observed in healthy younger subjects.

Dose adjustment in elderly patients with normal renal function is not necessary.

ADVERSE REACTIONS

Clinical Trials:

Film-coated Tablets (Multiple dose):

In clinical trials using **multiple doses** of cefpodoxime proxetil film-coated tablets, 4696 patients were treated with the recommended dosages of cefpodoxime (100 to 400 mg Q 12 hours). There were no deaths or permanent disabilities thought related to drug toxicity. One-hundred twenty-nine (2.7%) patients discontinued medication due to adverse events thought possibly- or probably-related to drug toxicity. Ninety-three (52%) of the 178 patients who discontinued therapy (whether thought related to drug therapy or not) did so because of gastrointestinal disturbances, nausea, vomiting, or diarrhea. The percentage of cefpodoxime proxetil-treated patients who discontinued study drug because of adverse events was significantly greater at a dose of 800 mg daily than at a dose of 400 mg daily or at a dose of 200 mg daily. Adverse events thought possibly- or probably-related to cefpodoxime in multiple dose clinical trials (N=4696 cefpodoxime-treated patients) were:

Incidence Greater Than 1%:

Diarrhea	7.0%

Diarrhea or loose stools were dose related: decreasing from 10.4% of patients receiving 800 mg per day to 5.7% for those receiving 200 mg per day. Of patients with diarrhea, 10% had *C. difficile* organism or toxin in the stool. (See **WARNINGS**.)

Nausea	3.3%
Vaginal Fungal Infections	1.0%
Vulvovaginal Infections	1.3%
Abdominal Pain	1.2%
Headache	1.0%

Incidence Less Than 1%: By body system in decreasing order:

Clinical Studies

Adverse events thought possibly- or probably-related to cefpodoxime proxetil that occurred in **less than 1%** of patients (N=4696)

Body - fungal infections, abdominal distention, malaise, fatigue, asthenia, fever, chest pain, back pain, chills, generalized pain, abnormal microbiological tests, moniliasis, abscess, allergic reaction, facial edema, bacterial infections, parasitic infections, localized edema, localized pain.

Cardiovascular - congestive heart failure, migraine, palpitations, vasodilation, hematoma, hypertension, hypotension.

Digestive - vomiting, dyspepsia, dry mouth, flatulence, decreased appetite, constipation, oral moniliasis, anorexia, eructation, gastritis, mouth ulcers, gastrointestinal disorders, rectal disorders, tongue disorders, tooth disorders, increased thirst, oral lesions, tenesmus, dry throat, toothache.

Hemic and Lymphatic - anemia.

Metabolic and Nutritional - dehydration, gout, peripheral edema, weight increase.

Musculo-skeletal - myalgia.

Nervous - dizziness, insomnia, somnolence, anxiety, shakiness, nervousness, cerebral infarction, change in dreams, impaired concentration, confusion, nightmares, paresthesia, vertigo.

Respiratory - asthma, cough, epistaxis, rhinitis, wheezing, bronchitis, dyspnea, pleural effusion, pneumonia, sinusitis.

Skin - urticaria, rash, pruritus non-application site, diaphoresis, maculopapular rash, fungal dermatitis, desquamation, dry skin non-application site, hair loss, vesiculobullous rash, sunburn.

Special Senses - taste alterations, eye irritation, taste loss, tinnitus.

Urogenital - hematuria, urinary tract infections, metrorrhagia, dysuria, urinary frequency, nocturia, penile infection, proteinuria, vaginal pain.

Granules for Oral Suspension (Multiple dose):

In clinical trials using multiple doses of cefpodoxime proxetil granules for oral suspension, 2128 pediatric patients (93% of whom were less than 12 years of age) were treated with the recommended dosages of cefpodoxime (10 mg/kg/day Q 24 hours or divided Q 12 hours to a maximum equivalent adult dose). There were no deaths or permanent disabilities in any of the patients in these studies. Twenty-four patients (1.1%) discontinued medication due to adverse events thought possibly- or probably-related to study drug. Primarily, these discontinuations were for gastrointestinal disturbances, usually diarrhea, vomiting, or rashes.

Adverse events thought possibly- or probably-related, or of unknown relationship to cefpodoxime proxetil for oral suspension in multiple dose clinical trials (N=2128 patients treated with cefpodoxime) were:

Incidence Greater Than 1%:

Diarrhea	6.0%

The incidence of diarrhea in infants and toddlers (age 1 month to 2 years) was 12.8%

Diaper rash/Fungal skin rash	2.0% (includes moniliasis)

The incidence of diaper rash in infants and toddlers was 8.5%.

Other skin rashes	1.8%
Vomiting	2.3%

Incidence Less Than 1%:

Body: Localized abdominal pain, abdominal cramp, headache, monilia, generalized abdominal pain, asthenia, fever, fungal infection.

Digestive: Nausea, monilia, anorexia, dry mouth, stomatitis, pseudomembranous colitis.

Hemic & Lymphatic: Thrombocythemia, positive direct Coombs' test, eosinophilia, leukocytosis, leukopenia, prolonged partial thromboplastin time, thrombocytopenic purpura.

Metabolic & Nutritional: Increased SGPT.

Musculo-Skeletal: Myalgia.

Nervous: Hallucination, hyperkinesia, nervousness, somnolence.

Respiratory: Epistaxis, rhinitis.

Skin: Skin moniliasis, urticaria, fungal dermatitis, acne, exfoliative dermatitis, maculopapular rash.

Special Senses: Taste perversion.

Film-coated Tablets (Single dose):

In clinical trials using **a single dose** of cefpodoxime proxetil film-coated tablets, 509 patients were treated with the recommended dosage of cefpodoxime (200 mg). There were no deaths or permanent disabilities thought related to drug toxicity in these studies.

Adverse events thought possibly- or probably-related to cefpodoxime in single dose clinical trials conducted in the United States were:

Incidence Greater Than 1%:

Nausea	1.4%
Diarrhea	1.2%

Incidence Less Than 1%:

Central Nervous System: Dizziness, headache, syncope.

Dermatologic: Rash.

Genital: Vaginitis.

Gastrointestinal: Abdominal pain.

Psychiatric: Anxiety.

Laboratory Changes

Significant laboratory changes that have been reported in adult and pediatric patients in clinical trials of cefpodoxime proxetil, without regard to drug relationship, were:

Hepatic: Transient increases in AST (SGOT), ALT (SGPT), GGT, alkaline phosphatase, bilirubin, and LDH.

Hematologic: Eosinophilia, leukocytosis, lymphocytosis, granulocytosis, basophilia, monocytosis, thrombocytosis, decreased hemoglobin, decreased hematocrit, leukopenia, neutropenia, lymphocytopenia, thrombocytopenia, thrombocythemia, positive Coombs' test, and prolonged PT, and PTT.

Serum Chemistry: Hyperglycemia, hypoglycemia, hypoalbuminemia, hypoproteinemia, hyperkalemia, and hyponatremia.

Renal: Increases in BUN and creatinine.

Most of these abnormalities were transient and not clinically significant.

Post-marketing Experience:

The following serious adverse experiences have been reported: allergic reactions including Stevens-Johnson syndrome, toxic epidermal necrolysis, erythema multiforme

Continued on next page

Vantin—Cont.

and serum sickness-like reactions, pseudomembranous colitis, bloody diarrhea with abdominal pain, ulcerative colitis, rectorrhagia with hypotension, anaphylactic shock, acute liver injury, *in utero* exposure with miscarriage, purpuric nephritis, pulmonary infiltrate with eosinophilia, and eyelid dermatitis.

One death was attributed to pseudomembranous colitis and disseminated intravascular coagulation.

Cephalosporin Class Labeling:

In addition to the adverse reactions listed above which have been observed in patients treated with cefpodoxime proxetil, the following adverse reactions and altered laboratory tests have been reported for cephalosporin class antibiotics:

Adverse Reactions and Abnormal Laboratory Tests: Renal dysfunction, toxic nephropathy, hepatic dysfunction including cholestasis, aplastic anemia, hemolytic anemia, serum sickness-like reaction, hemorrhage, agranulocytosis, and pancytopenia.

Several cephalosporins have been implicated in triggering seizures, particularly in patients with renal impairment when the dosage was not reduced. (See **DOSAGE AND ADMINISTRATION** and **OVERDOSAGE**.) If seizures associated with drug therapy occur, the drug should be discontinued. Anticonvulsant therapy can be given if clinically indicated.

OVERDOSAGE

In acute rodent toxicity studies, a single 5 g/kg oral dose produced no adverse effects.

In the event of serious toxic reaction from overdosage, hemodialysis or peritoneal dialysis may aid in the removal of cefpodoxime from the body, particularly if renal function is compromised.

The toxic symptoms following an overdose of beta-lactam antibiotics may include nausea, vomiting, epigastric distress, and diarrhea.

DOSAGE AND ADMINISTRATION

(See INDICATIONS AND USAGE for indicated pathogens.)

FILM-COATED TABLETS:

VANTIN Tablets should be administered orally with food to enhance absorption. (See **CLINICAL PHARMACOLOGY**.)

The recommended dosages, durations of treatment, and applicable patient population are as described in the following chart:

[See first table below]

GRANULES FOR ORAL SUSPENSION:

VANTIN Oral Suspension may be given without regard to food. The recommended dosages, durations of treatment, and applicable patient populations are as described in the following chart:

[See second table below]

Patients with Renal Dysfunction:

For patients with severe renal impairment (< 30 mL/min creatinine clearance), the dosing intervals should be increased to Q 24 hours. In patients maintained on hemodialysis, the dose frequency should be 3 times/week after hemodialysis.

When only the serum creatinine level is available, the following formula (based on sex, weight, and age of the patient) may be used to estimate creatinine clearance (mL/min). For this estimate to be valid, the serum creatinine level should represent a steady state of renal function.

Males: $\frac{\text{Weight (kg)} \times (140 - \text{age})}{72 \times \text{serum creatinine (mg/100 mL)}}$ (mL/min)

Females: $0.85 \times$ above value (mL/min)

Patients with Cirrhosis:

Cefpodoxime pharmacokinetics in cirrhotic patients (with or without ascites) are similar to those in healthy subjects. Dose adjustment is not necessary in this population.

Preparation of Suspension:

[See third table below]

After mixing, the suspension should be stored in a refrigerator, 2° to 8°C (36° to 46°F). Shake well before using. Keep container tightly closed. The mixture may be used for 14 days. Discard unused portion after 14 days.

HOW SUPPLIED

VANTIN Tablets are available in the following strengths (cefpodoxime equivalent), colors, and sizes:

100 mg, (light orange, elliptical, debossed with U3617)

Bottles of 20	NDC 0009-3617-01
Bottles of 100	NDC 0009-3617-02
Unit dose packs of 100	NDC 0009-3617-03

200 mg, (coral red, elliptical, debossed with U3618)

Bottles of 20	NDC 0009-3618-01
Bottles of 100	NDC 0009-3618-02
Unit dose packs of 100	NDC 0009-3618-03

Store tablets at controlled room temperature 20° to 25°C (68° to 77°F) [see USP]. Replace cap securely after each opening. Protect unit dose packs from excessive moisture.

VANTIN Oral Suspension provides the equivalent of 50 mg or 100 mg cefpodoxime per 5 mL suspension (when constituted as directed) and is available in lemon creme flavor in the following sizes:

50 mg/5 mL

100-mL suspension	NDC 0009-3531-01
75-mL suspension	NDC 0009-3531-02
50-mL suspension	NDC 0009-3531-03

100 mg/5 mL

100-mL suspension	NDC 0009-3615-01
75-mL suspension	NDC 0009-3615-02
50-mL suspension	NDC 0009-3615-03

Store unsuspended granules at controlled room temperature 20° to 25°C (68° to 77°F) [see USP].

Directions for mixing are included on the label. After mixing, suspension should be stored in a refrigerator, 2° to 8°C (36° to 46°F). Shake well before using. Keep container tightly closed. The mixture may be used for 14 days. Discard unused portion after 14 days.

REFERENCES

1. NCCLS. Methods for dilution antimicrobial susceptibility tests for bacteria that grow aerobically - fourth edition; Approved standard. NCCLS document M7-A4 (ISBN 1-56238-309-4). NCCLS, 940 West Valley Rd., Suite 1400, Wayne, PA 19087-1898, 1997.
2. NCCLS. Performance standards for antimicrobial susceptibility testing; Eighth informational supplement. NCCLS document M100-S8 (ISBN 1-56238-337-x). NCCLS, 940 West Valley Rd., Suite 1400, Wayne, PA 19087-1898, 1998.
3. NCCLS. Performance standards for antimicrobial disk susceptibility tests - sixth edition; Approved standard. NCCLS document M2-A6 (ISBN 1-56238-306-6). NCCLS, 940 West Valley Rd., Suite 1400, Wayne, PA 19087-1898, 1997.

CLINICAL TRIALS

Cystitis

In two double-blind, 2:1 randomized, comparative trials performed in adults in the United States, cefpodoxime proxetil was compared to other beta-lactam antibiotics. In these studies, the following bacterial eradication rates were obtained at 5 to 9 days after therapy:

Pathogen	Cefpodoxime	Comparator
E. coli	200/243 (82%)	99/123 (80%)
Other pathogens	34/42 (81%)	23/28 (82%)
K. pneumoniae		
P. mirabilis		
S. saprophyticus		
TOTAL	234/285 (82%)	122/151 (81%)

In these studies, clinical cure rates and bacterial eradication rates for cefpodoxime proxetil were comparable to the comparator agents; however, the clinical cure rates and bacteriologic eradication rates were lower than those observed with some other classes of approved agents for cystitis.

Acute Otitis Media Studies

In controlled studies of acute otitis media performed in the United States, where significant rates of beta-lactamase-producing organisms were found, cefpodoxime proxetil was compared to cefixime. In these studies, using very strict evaluability criteria and microbiologic and clinical response criteria at the 4 to 21 day post-therapy follow-up, the following presumptive bacterial eradication/clinical success outcomes (cured and improved) were obtained.

Pathogen	Cefpodoxime Proxetil **5 mg/kg Q 12h × 5 d**	Cefixime
S. pneumoniae	88/122 (72%)	72/124 (58%)
H. influenzae	50/76 (66%)	61/81 (75%)
M. catarrhalis	22/39 (56%)	23/41 (56%)
S. pyogenes	20/25 (80%)	13/23 (57%)
Clinical succes rate	171/254 (67%)	165/258 (64%)

℞ only

U.S. Patent No. 4,668,783.

Adults and Adolescents (age 12 years and older):

Type of Infection	Total Daily Dose	Dose Frequency	Duration
Pharyngitis and/or tonsillitis	200 mg	100 mg Q 12 hours	5 to 10 days
Acute community-acquired pneumonia	400 mg	200 mg Q 12 hours	14 days
Acute bacterial exacerbations of chronic bronchitis	400 mg	200 mg Q 12 hours	10 days
Uncomplicated gonorrhea (men and women) and rectal gonococcal infections (women)	200 mg	single dose	
Skin and skin structure	800 mg	400 mg Q 12 hours	7 to 14 days
Acute maxillary sinusitis	400 mg	200 mg Q 12 hours	10 days
Uncomplicated urinary tract infection	200 mg	100 mg Q 12 hours	7 days

Adults and Adolescents (age 12 years and older):

Type of Infection	Total Daily Dose	Dose Frequency	Duration
Pharyngitis and/or tonsillitis	200 mg	100 mg Q 12 hours	5 to 10 days
Acute community-acquired pneumonia	400 mg	200 mg Q 12 hours	14 days
Uncomplicated gonorrhea (men and women) and rectal gonococcal infections (women)	200 mg	single dose	
Skin and skin structure	800 mg	400 mg Q 12 hours	7 to 14 days
Acute maxillary sinusitis	400 mg	200 mg Q 12 hours	10 days
Uncomplicated urinary tract infection	200 mg	100 mg Q 12 hours	7 days

Infants and Pediatric Patients (age 2 months through 12 years):

Type of Infection	Total Daily Dose	Dose Frequency	Duration
Acute otitis media	10 mg/kg/day (Max 400 mg/day)	5 mg/kg Q 12 h (Max 200 mg/dose)	5 days
Pharyngitis and/or tonsillitis	10 mg/kg/day (Max 200 mg/day)	5 mg/kg/dose Q 12 h (Max 100 mg/dose)	5 to 10 days
Acute maxillary sinusitis	10 mg/kg/day (Max 400 mg/kg/day)	5 mg/kg Q 12 hours (Max 200 mg/dose)	10 days

Constitution Directions For Oral Suspension

Constituted Volume	Final Concentration	Directions
50 mL	50 mg per 5 mL	Suspend in a total of 29 mL of distilled water. Method: First, shake the bottle to loosen granules. Then add the water in two approximately equal portions, shaking vigorously after each aliquot of water.
75 mL	50 mg per 5 mL	Suspend in a total of 44 mL of distilled water. Method: First, shake the bottle to loosen granules. Then add the water in two approximately equal portions, shaking vigorously after each aliquot of water.
100 mL	50 mg per 5 mL	Suspend in a total of 58 mL of distilled water. Method: First, shake the bottle to loosen granules. Then add the water in two approximately equal portions, shaking vigorously after each aliquot of water.
50 mL	100 mg per 5 mL	Suspend in a total of 29 mL of distilled water. Method: First, shake the bottle to loosen granules. Then add the water in two approximately equal portions, shaking vigorously after each aliquot of water.
75 mL	100 mg per 5 mL	Suspend in a total of 43 mL of distilled water. Method: First, shake the bottle to loosen granules. Then add the water in two approximately equal portions, shaking vigorously after each aliquot of water.
100 mL	100 mg per 5 mL	Suspend in a total of 57 mL of distilled water. Method: First, shake the bottle to loosen granules. Then add the water in two approximately equal portions, shaking vigorously after each aliquot of water.

Licensed from Sankyo Company, Ltd., Japan
Made by: Pharmacia N.V./S.A., Puurs - Belgium
For: Pharmacia & Upjohn Company, A subsidiary of Pharmacia Corporation, Kalamazoo, Michigan 49001, USA
Revised August 2003 815 267 317 5R6847

XALATAN® ℞
[*ză-lă-tăn*]
(latanoprost ophthalmic solution)
0.005% (50 µg/mL)

Prescribing information for this product, which appears on pages 2797–2798 of the 2004 PDR, has been completely revised as follows. Please write "See Supplement A" next to the product heading.

DESCRIPTION

Latanoprost is a prostaglandin $F_{2\alpha}$ analogue. Its chemical name is isopropyl - (Z)- 7 [(1R,2R,3R,5S) 3,5-dihydroxy-2-[(3R)-3-hydroxy-5-phenylpentyl] cyclopentyl] -5-heptenoate. Its molecular formula is $C_{26}H_{40}O_5$ and its chemical structure is:

M.W. 432.58

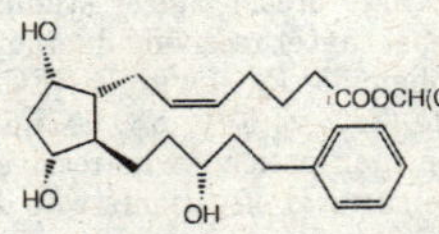

Latanoprost is a colorless to slightly yellow oil that is very soluble in acetonitrile and freely soluble in acetone, ethanol, ethyl acetate, isopropanol, methanol and octanol. It is practically insoluble in water.

XALATAN Sterile Ophthalmic Solution (latanoprost ophthalmic solution) is supplied as a sterile, isotonic, buffered aqueous solution of latanoprost with a pH of approximately 6.7 and an osmolality of approximately 267 mOsmol/kg. Each mL of XALATAN contains 50 micrograms of latanoprost. Benzalkonium chloride, 0.02% is added as a preservative. The inactive ingredients are: sodium chloride, sodium dihydrogen phosphate monohydrate, disodium hydrogen phosphate anhydrous and water for injection. One drop contains approximately 1.5 µg of latanoprost.

CLINICAL PHARMACOLOGY

Mechanism of Action

Latanoprost is a prostanoid selective FP receptor agonist that is believed to reduce the intraocular pressure (IOP) by increasing the outflow of aqueous humor. Studies in animals and man suggest that the main mechanism of action is increased uveoscleral outflow. Elevated IOP represents a major risk factor for glaucomatous field loss. The higher the level of IOP, the greater the likelihood of optic nerve damage and visual field loss.

Pharmacokinetics/Pharmacodynamics

Absorption: Latanoprost is absorbed through the cornea where the isopropyl ester prodrug is hydrolyzed to the acid form to become biologically active. Studies in man indicate that the peak concentration in the aqueous humor is reached about two hours after topical administration.

Distribution: The distribution volume in humans is 0.16 ± 0.02 L/kg. The acid of latanoprost can be measured in aqueous humor during the first 4 hours, and in plasma only during the first hour after local administration.

Metabolism: Latanoprost, an isopropyl ester prodrug, is hydrolyzed by esterases in the cornea to the biologically active acid. The active acid of latanoprost reaching the systemic circulation is primarily metabolized by the liver to the 1,2-dinor and 1,2,3,4-tetranor metabolites via fatty acid β-oxidation.

Excretion: The elimination of the acid of latanoprost from human plasma is rapid ($t_{1/2}$ =17 min) after both intravenous and topical administration. Systemic clearance is approximately 7 mL/min/kg. Following hepatic β-oxidation, the metabolites are mainly eliminated via the kidneys. Approximately 88% and 98% of the administered dose is recovered in the urine after topical and intravenous dosing, respectively.

Animal Studies

In monkeys, latanoprost has been shown to induce increased pigmentation of the iris. The mechanism of increased pigmentation seems to be stimulation of melanin production in melanocytes of the iris, with no proliferative changes observed. The change in iris color may be permanent.

Ocular administration of latanoprost at a dose of 6 µg/eye/day (4 times the daily human dose) to cynomolgus monkeys has also been shown to induce increased palpebral fissure. This effect was reversible upon discontinuation of the drug.

INDICATIONS AND USAGE

XALATAN Sterile Ophthalmic Solution is indicated for the reduction of elevated intraocular pressure in patients with open-angle glaucoma or ocular hypertension.

CLINICAL STUDIES

Patients with mean baseline intraocular pressure of 24 – 25 mmHg who were treated for 6 months in multi-center, randomized, controlled trials demonstrated 6 – 8 mmHg reductions in intraocular pressure. This IOP reduction with XALATAN Sterile Ophthalmic Solution 0.005% dosed once daily was equivalent to the effect of timolol 0.5% dosed twice daily.

A 3-year open-label, prospective safety study with a 2-year extension phase was conducted to evaluate the progression of increased iris pigmentation with continuous use of XALATAN once-daily as adjunctive therapy in 519 patients with open-angle glaucoma. The analysis was based on observed-cases population of the 380 patients who continued in the extension phase.

Results showed that the onset of noticeable increased iris pigmentation occurred within the first year of treatment for the majority of the patients who developed noticeable increased iris pigmentation. Patients continued to show signs of increasing iris pigmentation throughout the five years of the study. Observation of increased iris pigmentation did not affect the incidence, nature or severity of adverse events (other than increased iris pigmentation) recorded in the study. IOP reduction was similar regardless of the development of increased iris pigmentation during the study.

CONTRAINDICATIONS

Known hypersensitivity to latanoprost, benzalkonium chloride or any other ingredients in this product.

WARNINGS

XALATAN Sterile Ophthalmic Solution has been reported to cause changes to pigmented tissues. The most frequently reported changes have been increased pigmentation of the iris, periorbital tissue (eyelid) and eyelashes, and growth of eyelashes. Pigmentation is expected to increase as long as XALATAN is administered. After discontinuation of XALATAN, pigmentation of the iris is likely to be permanent while pigmentation of the periorbital tissue and eyelash changes have been reported to be reversible in some patients. Patients who receive treatment should be informed of the possibility of increased pigmentation. The effects of increased pigmentation beyond 5 years are not known.

PRECAUTIONS

General: XALATAN Sterile Ophthalmic Solution may gradually increase the pigmentation of the iris. The eye color change is due to increased melanin content in the stromal melanocytes of the iris rather than to an increase in the number of melanocytes. This change may not be noticeable for several months to years (see **WARNINGS**). Typically, the brown pigmentation around the pupil spreads concentrically towards the periphery of the iris and the entire iris or parts of the iris become more brownish. Neither nevi nor freckles of the iris appear to be affected by treatment. While treatment with XALATAN can be continued in patients who develop noticeably increased iris pigmentation, these patients should be examined regularly.

During clinical trials, the increase in brown iris pigment has not been shown to progress further upon discontinuation of treatment, but the resultant color change may be permanent.

Eyelid skin darkening, which may be reversible, has been reported in association with the use of XALATAN (see **WARNINGS**).

XALATAN may gradually change eyelashes and vellus hair in the treated eye; these changes include increased length, thickness, pigmentation, the number of lashes or hairs, and misdirected growth of eyelashes. Eyelash changes are usually reversible upon discontinuation of treatment.

XALATAN should be used with caution in patients with a history of intraocular inflammation (iritis/uveitis) and should generally not be used in patients with active intraocular inflammation.

Macular edema, including cystoid macular edema, has been reported during treatment with XALATAN. These reports have mainly occurred in aphakic patients, in pseudophakic patients with a torn posterior lens capsule, or in patients with known risk factors for macular edema. XALATAN should be used with caution in patients who do not have an intact posterior capsule or who have known risk factors for macular edema.

There is limited experience with XALATAN in the treatment of angle closure, inflammatory or neovascular glaucoma.

There have been reports of bacterial keratitis associated with the use of multiple-dose containers of topical ophthalmic products. These containers had been inadvertently contaminated by patients who, in most cases, had a concurrent corneal disease or a disruption of the ocular epithelial surface (see **PRECAUTIONS**, *Information for Patients*).

Contact lenses should be removed prior to the administration of XALATAN, and may be reinserted 15 minutes after administration (see **PRECAUTIONS**, *Information for Patients*).

Information for Patients (see **WARNINGS** and **PRECAUTIONS**): Patients should be advised about the potential for increased brown pigmentation of the iris, which may be permanent. Patients should also be informed about the possibility of eyelid skin darkening, which may be reversible after discontinuation of XALATAN.

Patients should also be informed of the possibility of eyelash and vellus hair changes in the treated eye during treatment with XALATAN. These changes may result in a disparity between eyes in length, thickness, pigmentation, number of eyelashes or vellus hairs, and/or direction of eyelash growth. Eyelash changes are usually reversible upon discontinuation of treatment.

Patients should be instructed to avoid allowing the tip of the dispensing container to contact the eye or surrounding structures because this could cause the tip to become contaminated by common bacteria known to cause ocular infections. Serious damage to the eye and subsequent loss of vision may result from using contaminated solutions.

Patients also should be advised that if they develop an intercurrent ocular condition (e.g., trauma, or infection) or have ocular surgery, they should immediately seek their physician's advice concerning the continued use of the multiple-dose container.

Patients should be advised that if they develop any ocular reactions, particularly conjunctivitis and lid reactions, they should immediately seek their physician's advice.

Patients should also be advised that XALATAN contains benzalkonium chloride, which may be absorbed by contact lenses. Contact lenses should be removed prior to administration of the solution. Lenses may be reinserted 15 minutes following administration of XALATAN.

If more than one topical ophthalmic drug is being used, the drugs should be administered at least five (5) minutes apart.

Drug Interactions: In vitro studies have shown that precipitation occurs when eye drops containing thimerosal are mixed with XALATAN. If such drugs are used they should be administered at least five (5) minutes apart.

Carcinogenesis, Mutagenesis, Impairment of Fertility: Latanoprost was not mutagenic in bacteria, in mouse lymphoma or in mouse micronucleus tests.

Chromosome aberrations were observed *in vitro* with human lymphocytes.

Latanoprost was not carcinogenic in either mice or rats when administered by oral gavage at doses of up to 170 µg/kg/day (approximately 2,800 times the recommended maximum human dose) for up to 20 and 24 months, respectively.

Additional *in vitro* and *in vivo* studies on unscheduled DNA synthesis in rats were negative. Latanoprost has not been found to have any effect on male or female fertility in animal studies.

Pregnancy: Teratogenic Effects: Pregnancy Category C.

Reproduction studies have been performed in rats and rabbits. In rabbits an incidence of 4 of 16 dams had no viable fetuses at a dose that was approximately 80 times the maximum human dose, and the highest nonembryocidal dose in rabbits was approximately 15 times the maximum human dose. There are no adequate and well-controlled studies in pregnant women. XALATAN should be used during pregnancy only if the potential benefit justifies the potential risk to the fetus.

Nursing Mothers: It is not known whether this drug or its metabolites are excreted in human milk. Because many drugs are excreted in human milk, caution should be exercised when XALATAN is administered to a nursing woman.

Pediatric Use: Safety and effectiveness in pediatric patients have not been established.

Geriatric Use: No overall differences in safety or effectiveness have been observed between elderly and younger patients.

ADVERSE REACTIONS

Adverse events referred to in other sections of this insert:

Eyelash changes (increased length, thickness, pigmentation, and number of lashes); eyelid skin darkening; intraocular inflammation (iritis/uveitis); iris pigmentation changes; and macular edema, including cystoid macular edema (see **WARNINGS** and **PRECAUTIONS**).

Controlled Clinical Trials:

The ocular adverse events and ocular signs and symptoms reported in 5 to 15% of the patients on XALATAN Sterile Ophthalmic Solution in the three 6-month, multi-center, double-masked, active-controlled trials were blurred vision, burning and stinging, conjunctival hyperemia, foreign body sensation, itching, increased pigmentation of the iris, and punctate epithelial keratopathy.

Local conjunctival hyperemia was observed; however, less than 1% of the patients treated with XALATAN required discontinuation of therapy because of intolerance to conjunctival hyperemia.

In addition to the above listed ocular events/signs and symptoms, the following were reported in 1 to 4% of the patients: dry eye, excessive tearing, eye pain, lid crusting, lid discomfort/pain, lid edema, lid erythema, and photophobia.

The following events were reported in less than 1% of the patients: conjunctivitis, diplopia and discharge from the eye.

During clinical studies, there were extremely rare reports of the following: retinal artery embolus, retinal detachment, and vitreous hemorrhage from diabetic retinopathy.

The most common systemic adverse events seen with XALATAN were upper respiratory tract infection/cold/flu, which occurred at a rate of approximately 4%. Chest pain/angina pectoris, muscle/joint/back pain, and rash/allergic skin reaction each occurred at a rate of 1 to 2%.

Clinical Practice:

The following events have been identified during postmarketing use of XALATAN in clinical practice. Because they are reported voluntarily from a population of unknown size, estimates of frequency cannot be made. The events, which have been chosen for inclusion due to either their seriousness, frequency of reporting, possible causal connection to XALATAN, or a combination of these factors, include: asthma and exacerbation of asthma; corneal edema and erosions; dyspnea; eyelash and vellus hair changes (increased

Continued on next page

Xalatan—Cont.

length, thickness, pigmentation, and number); eyelid skin darkening; herpes keratitis; intraocular inflammation (iritis/uveitis); keratitis; macular edema, including cystoid macular edema; misdirected eyelashes sometimes resulting in eye irritation; and toxic epidermal necrolysis.

OVERDOSAGE

Apart from ocular irritation and conjunctival or episcleral hyperemia, the ocular effects of latanoprost administered at high doses are not known. Intravenous administration of large doses of latanoprost in monkeys has been associated with transient bronchoconstriction; however, in 11 patients with bronchial asthma treated with latanoprost, bronchoconstriction was not induced. Intravenous infusion of up to 3 µg/kg in healthy volunteers produced mean plasma concentrations 200 times higher than during clinical treatment and no adverse reactions were observed. Intravenous dosages of 5.5 to 10 µg/kg caused abdominal pain, dizziness, fatigue, hot flushes, nausea and sweating.

If overdosage with XALATAN Sterile Ophthalmic Solution occurs, treatment should be symptomatic.

DOSAGE AND ADMINISTRATION

The recommended dosage is one drop (1.5 µg) in the affected eye(s) once daily in the evening.

The dosage of XALATAN Sterile Ophthalmic Solution should not exceed once daily since it has been shown that more frequent administration may decrease the intraocular pressure lowering effect.

Reduction of the intraocular pressure starts approximately 3 to 4 hours after administration and the maximum effect is reached after 8 to 12 hours.

XALATAN may be used concomitantly with other topical ophthalmic drug products to lower intraocular pressure. If more than one topical ophthalmic drug is being used, the drugs should be administered at least five (5) minutes apart.

HOW SUPPLIED

XALATAN Sterile Ophthalmic Solution is a clear, isotonic, buffered, preserved colorless solution of latanoprost 0.005% (50 µg/mL). It is supplied as a 2.5 mL solution in a 5 mL clear low density polyethylene bottle with a clear low density polyethylene dropper tip, a turquoise high density polyethylene screw cap, and a tamper-evident clear low density polyethylene overcap.

2.5 mL fill, 0.005% (50 µg/mL)

Package of 1 bottle NDC 0013-8303-04

Storage: Protect from light. Store unopened bottle(s) under refrigeration at 2° to 8°C (36° to 46°F). During shipment to the patient, the bottle may be maintained at temperatures up to 40°C (104°F) for a period not exceeding 8 days. Once a bottle is opened for use, it may be stored at room temperature up to 25°C (77°F) for 6 weeks.

℞ only

U.S. Patent Nos. 4,599,353; 5,296,504 and 5,422,368.

Manufactured for:
Pharmacia & Upjohn Company
A subsidiary of Pharmacia Corporation
Kalamazoo, MI 49001, USA
By:
Cardinal Health
Woodstock, IL 60098, USA
Revised September 2003 818 057 207
691211

ZINECARD® ℞

[zī-nĕ-kard]
dexrazoxane for injection

Prescribing information for this product, which appears on pages 2806–2808 of the 2004 PDR, has been completely revised as follows. Please write "See Supplement A" next to the product heading.

DESCRIPTION

ZINECARD® (dexrazoxane for injection) is a sterile, pyrogen-free lyophilizate intended for intravenous administration. It is a cardioprotective agent for use in conjunction with doxorubicin.

Chemically, dexrazoxane is (S)-4,4′-(1-methyl-1,2-ethanediyl)bis-2,6-piperazinedione. The structural formula is as follows:

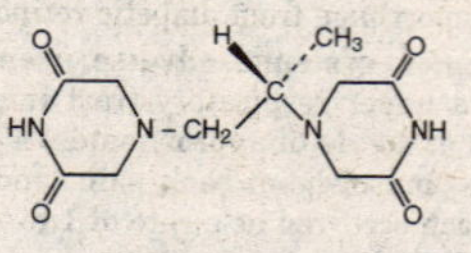

$C_{11}H_{16}N_4O_4$ M.W. 268.28

Dexrazoxane, a potent intracellular chelating agent is a derivative of EDTA. Dexrazoxane is a whitish crystalline powder which melts at 191° to 197°C. It is sparingly soluble in water and 0.1 N HCl, slightly soluble in ethanol and methanol and practically insoluble in nonpolar organic solvents. The pK_a is 2.1. Dexrazoxane has an octanol/water partition coefficient of 0.025 and degrades rapidly above a pH of 7.0. ZINECARD is available in 250 mg and 500 mg single use only vials.

Each **250 mg vial** contains dexrazoxane hydrochloride equivalent to 250 mg dexrazoxane. Hydrochloric Acid, NF is added for pH adjustment. When reconstituted as directed with the 25 mL vial of 0.167 Molar (M/6) Sodium Lactate Injection, USP diluent provided, each mL contains: 10 mg dexrazoxane. The pH of the resultant solution is 3.5 to 5.5. Each **500 mg vial** contains dexrazoxane hydrochloride equivalent to 500 mg dexrazoxane. Hydrochloric Acid, NF is added for pH adjustment. When reconstituted as directed with the 50 mL vial of 0.167 Molar (M/6) Sodium Lactate Injection, USP diluent provided, each mL contains: 10 mg dexrazoxane. The pH of the resultant solution is 3.5 to 5.5.

SUMMARY OF MEAN (%CV[a]) DEXRAZOXANE PHARMACOKINETIC PARAMETERS AT A DOSAGE RATIO OF 10:1 OF ZINECARD: DOXORUBICIN

Dose Doxorubicin (mg/m^2)	Dose Zinecard (mg/m^2)	Number of Subjects	Elimination Half-Life (h) *	Plasma Clearance ($L/h/m^2$)	Renal Clearance ($L/h/m^2$)	[b]Volume of Distribution (L/m^2)
50	500	10	2.5 (16)	7.88 (18)	3.35 (36)	22.4 (22)
60	600	5	2.1 (29)	6.25 (31)	—	22.0 (55)

[a] Coefficient of variation
[b] Steady-state volume of distribution

CLINICAL PHARMACOLOGY

Mechanism of Action: The mechanism by which ZINECARD exerts its cardioprotective activity is not fully understood. Dexrazoxane is a cyclic derivative of EDTA that readily penetrates cell membranes. Results of laboratory studies suggest that dexrazoxane is converted intracellularly to a ring-opened chelating agent that interferes with iron-mediated free radical generation thought to be responsible, in part, for anthracycline induced cardiomyopathy.

Pharmacokinetics: The pharmacokinetics of dexrazoxane have been studied in advanced cancer patients with normal renal and hepatic function. Generally, the pharmacokinetics of dexrazoxane can be adequately described by a two-compartment open model with first-order elimination. Dexrazoxane has been administered as a 15 minute infusion over a dose-range of 60 to 900 mg/m^2 with 60 mg/m^2 of doxorubicin, and at a fixed dose of 500 mg/m^2 with 50 mg/m^2 doxorubicin. The disposition kinetics of dexrazoxane are dose-independent, as shown by linear relationship between the area under plasma concentration-time curves and administered doses ranging from 60 to 900 mg/m^2. The mean peak plasma concentration of dexrazoxane was 36.5 µg/mL at the end of the 15 minute infusion of a 500 mg/m^2 dose of ZINECARD administered 15 to 30 minutes prior to the 50 mg/m^2 doxorubicin dose. The important pharmacokinetic parameters of dexrazoxane are summarized in the following table.

[See table above]

Following a rapid distributive phase (~0.2 to 0.3 hours), dexrazoxane reaches post-distributive equilibrium within two to four hours. The estimated steady-state volume of distribution of dexrazoxane suggests its distribution primarily in the total body water (25 L/m^2). The mean systemic clearance and steady-state volume of distribution of dexrazoxane in two Asian female patients at 500 mg/m^2 dexrazoxane along with 50 mg/m^2 doxorubicin were 15.15 $L/h/m^2$ and 36.27 L/m^2, respectively, but their elimination half-life and renal clearance of dexrazoxane were similar to those of the ten Caucasian patients from the same study. Qualitative metabolism studies with ZINECARD have confirmed the presence of unchanged drug, a diacid-diamide cleavage product, and two monoacid-monoamide ring products in the urine of animals and man. The metabolite levels were not measured in the pharmacokinetic studies.

Urinary excretion plays an important role in the elimination of dexrazoxane. Forty-two percent of the 500 mg/m^2 dose of ZINECARD was excreted in the urine.

Protein Binding: *In vitro* studies have shown that ZINECARD is not bound to plasma proteins.

Special Populations:

Pediatric: The pharmacokinetics of ZINECARD have not been evaluated in pediatric patients.

Gender: Analysis of pooled data from two pharmacokinetic studies indicate that male patients have a lower mean clearance value than female patients (110 $mL/min/m^2$ versus 133 $mL/min/m^2$). This gender effect is not clinically relevant.

Renal insufficiency: The pharmacokinetics of ZINECARD have not been evaluated in patients with renal impairment.

Hepatic insufficiency: The pharmacokinetics of ZINECARD have not been evaluated in patients with hepatic impairment. The ZINECARD dose is dependent upon the dose of doxorubicin (see **DOSAGE AND ADMINISTRATION**). Since a doxorubicin dose reduction is recommended in the presence of hyperbilirubinemia, the ZINECARD dosage is proportionately reduced in patients with hepatic impairment.

Drug Interactions: There was no significant change in the pharmacokinetics of doxorubicin (50 mg/m^2) and its predominant metabolite, doxorubicinol, in the presence of dexrazoxane (500 mg/m^2) in a crossover study in cancer patients.

Clinical Studies: The ability of ZINECARD to prevent/reduce the incidence and severity of doxorubicin-induced cardiomyopathy was demonstrated in three prospectively randomized placebo-controlled studies. In these studies, patients were treated with a doxorubicin-containing regimen and either ZINECARD or placebo starting with the first course of chemotherapy. There was no restriction on the cumulative dose of doxorubicin. Cardiac function was assessed by measurement of the left ventricular ejection fraction (LVEF), utilizing resting multigated nuclear medicine (MUGA) scans, and by clinical evaluations. Patients receiving ZINECARD had significantly smaller mean decreases from baseline in LVEF and lower incidences of congestive heart failure than the control group. The difference in decline from baseline in LVEF was evident beginning with a cumulative doxorubicin dose of 150 mg/m^2 and reached statistical significance in patients who received ≥400 mg/m^2 of doxorubicin. In addition to evaluating the effect of ZINECARD on cardiac function, the studies also assessed the effect of the addition of ZINECARD on the antitumor efficacy of the chemotherapy regimens. In one study (the largest of three breast cancer studies) patients with advanced breast cancer receiving fluorouracil, doxorubicin and cyclophosphamide (FAC) with ZINECARD had a lower response rate (48% vs 63%; p=0.007) and a shorter time to progression than patients who received FAC + placebo, although the survival of patients who did or did not receive ZINECARD with FAC was similar.

Two of the randomized breast cancer studies evaluating the efficacy and safety of FAC with either ZINECARD or placebo were amended to allow patients on the placebo arm who had attained a cumulative dose of doxorubicin of 300 mg/m^2 (six courses of FAC) to receive FAC with open-label ZINECARD for each subsequent course. This change in design allowed examination of whether there was a cardioprotective effect of ZINECARD even when it was started after substantial exposure to doxorubicin.

Retrospective historical analyses were then performed to compare the likelihood of heart failure in patients to whom ZINECARD was added to the FAC regimen after they had received six (6) courses of FAC (and who then continued treatment with FAC therapy) with the heart failure rate in patients who had received six (6) courses of FAC and continued to receive this regimen without added ZINECARD. These analyses showed that the risk of experiencing a cardiac event (see Table 1 for definition) at a given cumulative dose of doxorubicin above 300 mg/m^2 was substantially greater in the 99 patients who did *not* receive ZINECARD beginning with their seventh course of FAC than in the 102 patients who did receive ZINECARD (See Figure 1).

Table 1

The development of cardiac events is shown by:

1. Development of congestive heart failure, defined as having two or more of the following:
   a. Cardiomegaly by X-ray
   b. Basilar Rales
   c. S3 Gallop
   d. Paroxysmal nocturnal dyspnea and/or orthopnea and/or significant dyspnea on exertion.
2. Decline from baseline in LVEF by ≥10% and to below the lower limit of normal for the institution.
3. Decline in LVEF by ≥20% from baseline value.
4. Decline in LVEF to ≥5% below lower limit of normal for the institution.

Figure 1 displays the risk of developing congestive heart failure by cumulative dose of doxorubicin in patients who received ZINECARD starting with their seventh course of FAC compared to patients who did not. Patients unprotected by ZINECARD had a 13 times greater risk of developing congestive heart failure. Overall, 3% of patients treated with ZINECARD developed CHF compared with 22% of patients not receiving ZINECARD.

Figure 1
Doxorubicin Dose at Congestive Heart Failure (CHF)
FAC vs. FAC/ZINECARD Patients
Patients Receiving At Least Seven Courses of Treatment

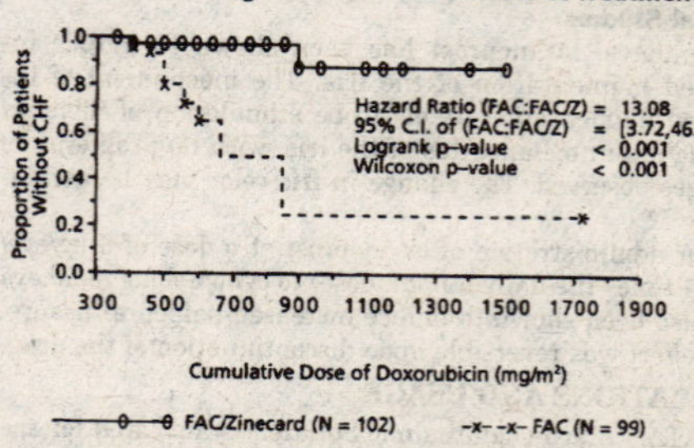

Because of its cardioprotective effect, ZINECARD permitted a greater percentage of patients to be treated with extended doxorubicin therapy. Figure 2 shows the number of patients still on treatment at increasing cumulative doses.

[See figure 2 at top of next column]

In addition to evaluating the cardioprotective efficacy of ZINECARD in this setting, the time to tumor progression and survival of these two groups of patients were also compared. There was a similar time to progression in the two groups and survival was at least as long for the group of

Figure 2
Cumulative Number of Patients On Treatment
FAC vs. FAC/ZINECARD Patients
Patients Receiving at Least Seven Courses of Treatment

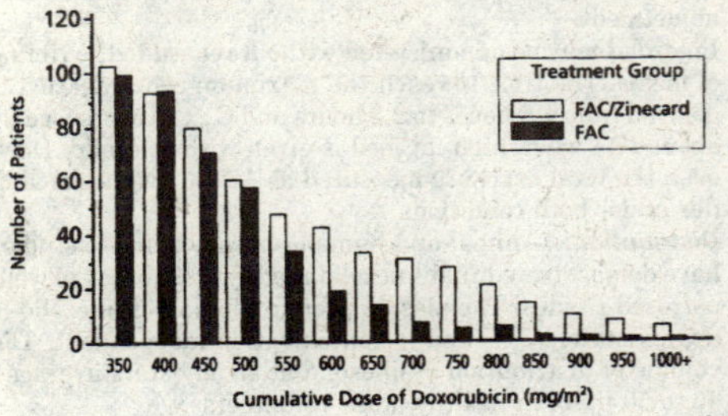

patients that received ZINECARD starting with their seventh course, i.e., starting after a cumulative dose of doxorubicin of 300 mg/m^2. These time to progression and survival data should be interpreted with caution, however, because they are based on comparisons of groups entered sequentially in the studies and are not comparisons of prospectively randomized patients.

INDICATIONS AND USAGE

ZINECARD is indicated for reducing the incidence and severity of cardiomyopathy associated with doxorubicin administration in women with metastatic breast cancer who have received a cumulative doxorubicin dose of 300 mg/m^2 and who will continue to receive doxorubicin therapy to maintain tumor control. It is not recommended for use with the initiation of doxorubicin therapy (see **WARNINGS**).

CONTRAINDICATIONS

ZINECARD should not be used with chemotherapy regimens that do not contain an anthracycline.

WARNINGS

ZINECARD may add to the myelosuppression caused by chemotherapeutic agents. There is some evidence that the use of dexrazoxane concurrently with the initiation of fluorouracil, doxorubicin and cyclophosphamide (FAC) therapy interferes with the antitumor efficacy of the regimen, and this use is not recommended. In the largest of three breast cancer trials, patients who received dexrazoxane starting with their first cycle of FAC therapy had a lower response rate (48% vs 63%; p=0.007) and shorter time to progression than patients who did not receive dexrazoxane (see **Clinical Studies** section of **CLINICAL PHARMACOLOGY**). Therefore, ZINECARD should only be used in those patients who have received a cumulative doxorubicin dose of 300 mg/m^2 and are continuing with doxorubicin therapy.

Although clinical studies have shown that patients receiving FAC with ZINECARD may receive a higher cumulative dose of doxorubicin before experiencing cardiac toxicity than patients receiving FAC without ZINECARD, the use of ZINECARD in patients who have already received a cumulative dose of doxorubicin of 300 mg/m^2 without ZINECARD, does not eliminate the potential for anthracycline induced cardiac toxicity. Therefore, cardiac function should be carefully monitored.

Secondary malignancies (primarily acute myeloid leukemia) have been reported in patients treated chronically with oral razoxane. Razoxane is the racemic mixture, of which dexrazoxane is the S(+)-enantiomer. In these patients, the total cumulative dose of razoxane ranged from 26 to 480 grams and the duration of treatment was from 42 to 319 weeks. One case of T-cell lymphoma, a case of B-cell lymphoma and six to eight cases of cutaneous basal cell or squamous cell carcinoma have also been reported in patients treated with razoxane.

PRECAUTIONS

General

Doxorubicin should not be given prior to the intravenous injection of ZINECARD. ZINECARD should be given by slow I.V. push or rapid drip intravenous infusion from a bag. Doxorubicin should be given within 30 minutes after beginning the infusion with ZINECARD. (See **DOSAGE AND ADMINISTRATION**).

As ZINECARD will always be used with cytotoxic drugs, patients should be monitored closely. While the myelosuppressive effects of ZINECARD at the recommended dose are mild, additive effects upon the myelosuppressive activity of chemotherapeutic agents may occur.

Laboratory tests

As ZINECARD may add to the myelosuppressive effects of cytotoxic drugs, frequent complete blood counts are recommended. (See **ADVERSE REACTIONS**).

Drug Interactions

ZINECARD does not influence the pharmacokinetics of doxorubicin. **Carcinogenesis, Mutagenesis, Impairment of Fertility** (see **WARNINGS** section for information on human carcinogenicity) - No long-term carcinogenicity studies have been carried out with dexrazoxane in animals. Dexrazoxane was not mutagenic in the Ames test but was found to be clastogenic to human lymphocytes *in vitro* and to mouse bone marrow erythrocytes *in vivo* (micronucleus test).

The possible adverse effects of ZINECARD on the fertility of humans and experimental animals, male or female, have not been adequately studied. Testicular atrophy was seen with dexrazoxane administration at doses as low as 30 mg/kg weekly for 6 weeks in rats (1/3 the human dose on a mg/m^2 basis) and as low as 20 mg/kg weekly for 13 weeks in dogs (approximately equal to the human dose on a mg/m^2 basis).

TABLE 2

ADVERSE EXPERIENCE	PERCENTAGE (%) OF BREAST CANCER PATIENTS WITH ADVERSE EXPERIENCE			
	FAC + ZINECARD		FAC + PLACEBO	
	Courses 1-6 N = 413	Courses ≥ 7 N = 102	Courses 1-6 N = 458	Course ≥ 7 N = 99
Alopecia	94	100	97	98
Nausea	77	51	84	60
Vomiting	59	42	72	49
Fatigue/Malaise	61	48	58	55
Anorexia	42	27	47	38
Stomatitis	34	26	41	28
Fever	34	22	29	18
Infection	23	19	18	21
Diarrhea	21	14	24	7
Pain on Injection	12	13	3	0
Sepsis	17	12	14	9
Neurotoxicity	17	10	13	5
Streaking/Erythema	5	4	4	2
Phlebitis	6	3	3	5
Esophagitis	6	3	7	4
Dysphagia	8	0	10	5
Hemorrhage	2	3	2	1
Extravasation	1	3	1	2
Urticaria	2	2	2	0
Recall Skin Reaction	1	1	2	0

Pregnancy - *Pregnancy Category C* - Dexrazoxane was maternotoxic at doses of 2 mg/kg (1/40 the human dose on a mg/m^2 basis) and embryotoxic and teratogenic at 8 mg/kg (approximately 1/10 the human dose on a mg/m^2 basis) when given daily to pregnant rats during the period of organogenesis. Teratogenic effects in the rat included imperforate anus, microphthalmia, and anophthalmia. In offspring allowed to develop to maturity, fertility was impaired in the male and female rats treated in utero during organogenesis at 8 mg/kg. In rabbits, doses of 5 mg/kg (approximately 1/10 the human dose on a mg/m^2 basis) daily during the period of organogenesis were maternotoxic and dosages of 20 mg/kg (1/2 the human dose on a mg/m^2 basis) were embryotoxic and teratogenic. Teratogenic effects in the rabbit included several skeletal malformations such as short tail, rib and thoracic malformations, and soft tissue variations including subcutaneous, eye and cardiac hemorrhagic areas, as well as agenesis of the gallbladder and of the intermediate lobe of the lung. There are no adequate and well-controlled studies in pregnant women. ZINECARD should be used during pregnancy only if the potential benefit justifies the potential risk to the fetus.

Nursing Mothers - It is not known whether dexrazoxane is excreted in human milk. Because many drugs are excreted in human milk and because of the potential for serious adverse reactions in nursing infants exposed to dexrazoxane, mothers should be advised to discontinue nursing during dexrazoxane therapy.

Pediatric Use - Safety and effectiveness of dexrazoxane in pediatric patients have not been established.

Geriatric Use - Clinical studies of ZINECARD did not include sufficient numbers of subjects aged 65 and over to determine whether they respond differently from younger subjects. Other reported clinical experience has not identified differences in responses between the elderly and younger patients. In general, elderly patients should be treated with caution due to the greater frequency of decreased hepatic, renal, or cardiac function, and concomitant disease or other drug therapy.

ADVERSE REACTIONS

ZINECARD at a dose of 500 mg/m^2 has been administered in combination with FAC in randomized, placebo-controlled, double-blind studies to patients with metastatic breast cancer. The dose of doxorubicin was 50 mg/m^2 in each of the trials. Courses were repeated every three weeks, provided recovery from toxicity had occurred. Table 2 below lists the incidence of adverse experiences for patients receiving FAC with either ZINECARD or placebo in the breast cancer studies. Adverse experiences occurring during courses 1 through 6 are displayed for patients receiving ZINECARD or placebo with FAC beginning with their first course of therapy (column 1 & 3, respectively). Adverse experiences occurring at course 7 and beyond for patients who received placebo with FAC during the first six courses and who then received either ZINECARD or placebo with FAC are also displayed (column 2 & 4, respectively).

[See table 2 above]

The adverse experiences listed above are likely attributable to the FAC regimen with the exception of pain on injection that was observed mainly on the ZINECARD arm.

Myelosuppression

Patients receiving FAC with ZINECARD experienced more severe leucopenia, granulocytopenia and thrombocytopenia at nadir than patients receiving FAC without ZINECARD, but recovery counts were similar for the two groups of patients.

Hepatic and Renal

Some patients receiving FAC + ZINECARD or FAC + placebo experienced marked abnormalities in hepatic or renal function tests, but the frequency and severity of abnormalities in bilirubin, alkaline phosphatase, BUN, and creatinine were similar for patients receiving FAC with or without ZINECARD.

OVERDOSAGE

There have been no instances of drug overdose in the clinical studies sponsored by either Pharmacia & Upjohn Company or the National Cancer Institute. The maximum dose administered during the cardioprotective trials was 1000 mg/m^2 every three weeks.

Disposition studies with ZINECARD have not been conducted in cancer patients undergoing dialysis, but retention of a significant dose fraction (>0.4) of the unchanged drug in the plasma pool, minimal tissue partitioning or binding, and availability of greater than 90% of the systemic drug levels in the unbound form suggest that it could be removed using conventional peritoneal or hemodialysis.

There is no known antidote for dexrazoxane. Instances of suspected overdose should be managed with good supportive care until resolution of myelosuppression and related conditions is complete. Management of overdose should include treatment of infections, fluid regulation, and maintenance of nutritional requirements.

DOSAGE AND ADMINISTRATION

The recommended dosage ratio of ZINECARD:doxorubicin is 10:1 (eg, 500 mg/m^2 ZINECARD:50 mg/m^2 doxorubicin). Since a doxorubicin dose reduction is recommended in the presence of hyperbilirubinemia, the ZINECARD dosage should be proportionately reduced (maintaining the 10:1 ratio) in patients with hepatic impairment. ZINECARD must be reconstituted with 0.167 Molar (M/6) Sodium Lactate Injection, USP, to give a concentration of 10 mg ZINECARD for each mL of sodium lactate. The reconstituted solution

Continued on next page

Zinecard—Cont.

should be given by slow I.V. push or rapid drip intravenous infusion from a bag. After completing the infusion of ZINECARD, and prior to a total elapsed time of 30 minutes (from the beginning of the ZINECARD infusion), the intravenous injection of doxorubicin should be given.

Reconstituted ZINECARD, when transferred to an empty infusion bag, is stable for 6 hours from the time of reconstitution when stored at controlled room temperature, 15° to 30°C (59° to 86°F) or under refrigeration, 2° to 8°C (36° to 46°F). DISCARD UNUSED SOLUTIONS.

The reconstituted ZINECARD solution may be diluted with either 0.9% Sodium Chloride Injection, USP or 5.0% Dextrose Injection, USP to a concentration range of 1.3 to 5.0 mg/mL in intravenous infusion bags. The resultant solutions are stable for 6 hours when stored at controlled room temperature, 15° to 30°C (59° to 86°F) or under refrigeration, 2° to 8°C (36° to 46°F). DISCARD UNUSED SOLUTIONS.

Incompatibility

ZINECARD should not be mixed with other drugs.

Parenteral drug products should be inspected visually for particulate matter and discoloration prior to administration, whenever solution and container permit.

Handling and Disposal: Caution in the handling and preparation of the reconstituted solution must be exercised and the use of gloves is recommended. If ZINECARD powder or solutions contact the skin or mucosae, immediately wash thoroughly with soap and water.

Procedures normally used for proper handling and disposal of anticancer drugs should be considered for use with ZINECARD. Several guidelines on this subject have been published.[1-8] There is no general agreement that all of the procedures recommended in the guidelines are necessary or appropriate.

HOW SUPPLIED

ZINECARD® (dexrazoxane for injection) is available in the following strengths as sterile, pyrogen-free lyophilizates.

NDC 0013-8715-62

250 mg single dose vial with a red flip-top seal, packaged in single vial packs. (This package also contains a 25 mL vial of 0.167 Molar (M/6) Sodium Lactate Injection, USP.)

NDC 0013-8725-89

500 mg single dose vial with a blue flip-top seal, packaged in single vial packs. (This package also contains a 50 mL vial of 0.167 Molar (M/6) Sodium Lactate Injection, USP.)

Store at 25°C (77°F); excursions permitted to 15° to 30°C (59° to 86°F) [see USP Controlled Room Temperature]. Reconstituted solutions of ZINECARD are stable for 6 hours at controlled room temperature or under refrigeration, 2° to 8°C (36° to 46°F). DISCARD UNUSED SOLUTIONS.

℞ only

REFERENCES:

1. ONS Clinical Practice Committee. Cancer Chemotherapy Guidelines and Recommendations for Practice. Pittsburgh, PA: Oncology Nursing Society. 1999; 32-41.
2. Recommendations for the Safe Handling of Parenteral Antineoplastic Drugs. Washington, DC: Division of Safety, Clinical Center Pharmacy Department and Cancer Nursing Services, National Institutes of Health; 1992. US Dept of Health and Human Services, Public Health Service Publication NIH 92-2621.
3. AMA Council on Scientific Affairs. Guidelines for Handling Parenteral Antineoplastics. *JAMA.* 1985; 253: 1590-1591.
4. National Study Commission on Cytotoxic Exposure-Recommendations for Handling Cytotoxic Agents. 1987. Available from Louis P. Jeffrey, Sc.D., Chairman, National Study Commission on Cytotoxic Exposure, Massachusetts College of Pharmacy and Allied Health Sciences, 179 Longwood Avenue, Boston, MA 02115.
5. Clinical Oncological Society of Australia. Guidelines and Recommendations for Safe Handling of Antineoplastic Agents. *Med J Australia.* 1983; 1:426-428.
6. Jones RB, Frank R, Mass T. Safe Handling of Chemotherapeutic Agents: A Report from the Mount Sinai Medical Center. CA - *A Cancer J for Clin.* 1983; 33: 258-263.
7. American Society of Hospital Pharmacists. ASHP Technical Assistance Bulletin on Handling Cytotoxic and Hazardous Drugs. *Am J Hosp Pharm.* 1990; 47:1033-1049.
8. Controlling Occupational Exposure to Hazardous Drugs. (OSHA Work Practice Guidelines.) *Am J Health-Syst Pharm.* 1996; 53: 1669-1685.

Manufactured for: Pharmacia & Upjohn Company
A subsidiary of Pharmacia Corporation
Kalamazoo, MI 49001, USA
By: Cardinal Health
Albuquerque, NM 87109, USA
Revised: September 2003 817 546 003

ZYVOX™ ℞

[*zī-vŏks*]

linezolid injection
linezolid tablets
linezolid for oral suspension

Prescribing information for this product, which appears on pages 2808–2815 of the 2004 PDR, has been completely revised as follows. Please write "See Supplement A" next to the product heading.

To reduce the development of drug-resistant bacteria and maintain the effectiveness of ZYVOX formulations and other antibacterial drugs, ZYVOX should be used only to treat or prevent infections that are proven or strongly suspected to be caused by bacteria.

DESCRIPTION

ZYVOX I.V. Injection, ZYVOX Tablets, and ZYVOX for Oral Suspension contain linezolid, which is a synthetic antibacterial agent of the oxazolidinone class. The chemical name for linezolid is (S)-N-[[3-[3-Fluoro-4-(4-morpholinyl)phenyl]-2-oxo-5-oxazolidinyl] methyl]-acetamide.

The empirical formula is $C_{16}H_{20}FN_3O_4$. Its molecular weight is 337.35, and its chemical structure is represented below:

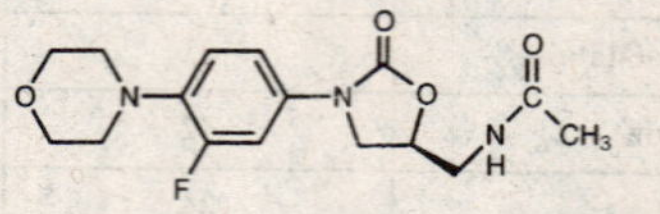

ZYVOX I.V. Injection is supplied as a ready-to-use sterile isotonic solution for intravenous infusion. Each mL contains 2 mg of linezolid. Inactive ingredients are sodium citrate, citric acid, and dextrose in an aqueous vehicle for intravenous administration. The sodium (Na^+) content is 0.38 mg/mL (5 mEq per 300-mL bag; 3.3 mEq per 200-mL bag; and 1.7 mEq per 100-mL bag).

ZYVOX Tablets for oral administration contain 400 mg or 600 mg linezolid as film-coated compressed tablets. Inactive ingredients are corn starch, microcrystalline cellulose, hydroxypropylcellulose, sodium starch glycolate, magnesium stearate, hypromellose, polyethylene glycol, titanium dioxide, and carnauba wax. The sodium (Na^+) content is 1.95 mg per 400-mg tablet and 2.92 mg per 600-mg tablet (0.1 mEq per tablet, regardless of strength).

ZYVOX for Oral Suspension is supplied as an orange-flavored granule/powder for constitution into a suspension for oral administration. Following constitution, each 5 mL contains 100 mg of linezolid. Inactive ingredients are sucrose, citric acid, sodium citrate, microcrystalline cellulose and carboxymethylcellulose sodium, aspartame, xanthan gum, mannitol, sodium benzoate, colloidal silicon dioxide, sodium chloride, and flavors (see **PRECAUTIONS, Information for Patients**). The sodium (Na^+) content is 8.52 mg per 5 mL (0.4 mEq per 5 mL).

CLINICAL PHARMACOLOGY

Pharmacokinetics

The mean pharmacokinetic parameters of linezolid in adults after single and multiple oral and intravenous (IV) doses are summarized in Table 1. Plasma concentrations of linezolid at steady-state after oral doses of 600 mg given every 12 hours (q12h) are shown in Figure 1.

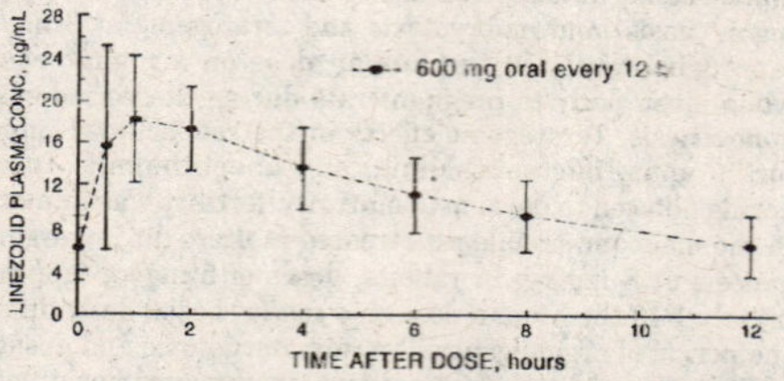

Figure 1. Plasma Concentrations of Linezolid in Adults at Steady-State Following Oral Dosing Every 12 Hours (Mean±Standard Deviation, n=16)

[See table 1 below]

Absorption: Linezolid is rapidly and extensively absorbed after oral dosing. Maximum plasma concentrations are reached approximately 1 to 2 hours after dosing, and the absolute bioavailability is approximately 100%. Therefore, linezolid may be given orally or intravenously without dose adjustment.

Linezolid may be administered without regard to the timing of meals. The time to reach the maximum concentration is delayed from 1.5 hours to 2.2 hours and C_{max} is decreased by about 17% when high fat food is given with linezolid. However, the total exposure measured as $AUC_{0-\infty}$ values is similar under both conditions.

Distribution: Animal and human pharmacokinetic studies have demonstrated that linezolid readily distributes to well-perfused tissues. The plasma protein binding of linezolid is approximately 31% and is concentration-independent. The volume of distribution of linezolid at steady-state averaged 40 to 50 liters in healthy adult volunteers.

Linezolid concentrations have been determined in various fluids from a limited number of subjects in Phase 1 volunteer studies following multiple dosing of linezolid. The ratio of linezolid in saliva relative to plasma was 1.2 to 1 and for sweat relative to plasma was 0.55 to 1.

Metabolism: Linezolid is primarily metabolized by oxidation of the morpholine ring, which results in two inactive ring-opened carboxylic acid metabolites: the aminoethoxyacetic acid metabolite (A), and the hydroxyethyl glycine metabolite (B). Formation of metabolite B is mediated by a non-enzymatic chemical oxidation mechanism in vitro. Linezolid is not an inducer of cytochrome P450 (CYP) in rats, and it has been demonstrated from in vitro studi that linezolid is not detectably metabolized by human cytochrome P450 and it does not inhibit the activities of clinically significant human CYP isoforms (1A2, 2C9, 2C19, 2D6, 2E1, 3A4).

Excretion: Nonrenal clearance accounts for approximately 65% of the total clearance of linezolid. Under steady-state conditions, approximately 30% of the dose appears in the urine as linezolid, 40% as metabolite B, and 10% as metabolite A. The renal clearance of linezolid is low (average 40 mL/min) and suggests net tubular reabsorption. Virtually no linezolid appears in the feces, while approximately 6% of the dose appears in the feces as metabolite B, and 3% as metabolite A.

A small degree of nonlinearity in clearance was observed with increasing doses of linezolid, which appears to be due to lower renal and nonrenal clearance of linezolid at higher concentrations. However, the difference in clearance was small and was not reflected in the apparent elimination half-life.

Special Populations

Geriatric: The pharmacokinetics of linezolid are not significantly altered in elderly patients (65 years or older). Therefore, dose adjustment for geriatric patients is not necessary.

Pediatric: The pharmacokinetics of linezolid following a single IV dose were investigated in pediatric patients ranging in age from birth through 17 years (including premature and full-term neonates), in healthy adolescent subjects ranging in age from 12 through 17 years, and in pediatric patients ranging in age from 1 week through 12 years. The pharmacokinetic parameters of linezolid are summarized in Table 2 for the pediatric populations studied and healthy adult subjects after administration of single IV doses.

The C_{max} and the volume of distribution (V_{ss}) of linezolid are similar regardless of age in pediatric patients. However, clearance of linezolid varies as a function of age. With the exclusion of pre-term neonates less than one week of age, clearance is most rapid in the youngest age groups ranging from >1 week old to 11 years, resulting in lower single-dose systemic exposure (AUC) and shorter half-life as compared with adults. As age of pediatric patients increases, the clearance of linezolid gradually decreases, and by adolescence

Table 1. Mean (Standard Deviation) Pharmacokinetic Parameters of Linezolid in Adults

Dose of Linezolid	C_{max} µg/mL	C_{min} µg/mL	T_{max} hrs	AUC* µg · h/mL	$t_{1/2}$ hrs	CL mL/min
400 mg tablet						
single dose†	8.10 (1.83)	—	1.52 (1.01)	55.10 (25.00)	5.20 (1.50)	146 (67)
every 12 hours	11.00 (4.37)	3.08 (2.25)	1.12 (0.47)	73.40 (33.50)	4.69 (1.70)	110 (49)
600 mg tablet						
single dose	12.70 (3.96)	—	1.28 (0.66)	91.40 (39.30)	4.26 (1.65)	127 (48)
every 12 hours	21.20 (5.78)	6.15 (2.94)	1.03 (0.62)	138.00 (42.10)	5.40 (2.06)	80 (29)
600 mg IV injection‡						
single dose	12.90 (1.60)	—	0.50 (0.10)	80.20 (33.30)	4.40 (2.40)	138 (39)
every 12 hours	15.10 (2.52)	3.68 (2.36)	0.51 (0.03)	89.70 (31.00)	4.80 (1.70)	123 (40)
600 mg oral suspension						
single dose	11.00 (2.76)	—	0.97 (0.88)	80.30 (35.10)	4.60 (1.71)	141 (45)

*AUC for single dose = $AUC_{0-\infty}$; for multiple-dose = $AUC_{0-\tau}$
† Data dose-normalized from 375 mg
‡ Data dose-normalized from 625 mg, IV dose was given as 0.5-hour infusion.
C_{max} = Maximum plasma concentration; C_{min} = Minimum plasma concentration; T_{max} = Time to C_{max};
AUC = Area under concentration-time curve; $t_{1/2}$ = Elimination half-life; CL = Systemic clearance

mean clearance values approach those observed for the adult population. There is wider inter-subject variability in linezolid clearance and systemic drug exposure (AUC) across all pediatric age groups as compared with adults. Similar mean daily AUC values were observed in pediatric patients from birth to 11 years of age dosed every 8 hours (q8h) relative to adolescents or adults dosed every 12 hours (q12h). Therefore, the dosage for pediatric patients up to 11 years of age should be 10 mg/kg q8h. Pediatric patients 12 years and older should receive 600 mg q12h (see **DOSAGE AND ADMINISTRATION**).

[See table 2 at right]

Gender: Females have a slightly lower volume of distribution of linezolid than males. Plasma concentrations are higher in females than in males, which is partly due to body weight differences. After a 600-mg dose, mean oral clearance is approximately 38% lower in females than in males. However, there are no significant gender differences in mean apparent elimination-rate constant or half-life. Thus, drug exposure in females is not expected to substantially increase beyond levels known to be well tolerated. Therefore, dose adjustment by gender does not appear to be necessary.

Renal Insufficiency: The pharmacokinetics of the parent drug, linezolid, are not altered in patients with any degree of renal insufficiency; however, the two primary metabolites of linezolid may accumulate in patients with renal insufficiency, with the amount of accumulation increasing with the severity of renal dysfunction (see Table 3). The clinical significance of accumulation of these two metabolites has not been determined in patients with severe renal insufficiency. Because similar plasma concentrations of linezolid are achieved regardless of renal function, no dose adjustment is recommended for patients with renal insufficiency. However, given the absence of information on the clinical significance of accumulation of the primary metabolites, use of linezolid in patients with renal insufficiency should be weighed against the potential risks of accumulation of these metabolites. Both linezolid and the two metabolites are eliminated by dialysis. No information is available on the effect of peritoneal dialysis on the pharmacokinetics of linezolid. Approximately 30% of a dose was eliminated in a 3-hour dialysis session beginning 3 hours after the dose of linezolid was administered; therefore, linezolid should be given after hemodialysis.

[See table 3 at right]

Hepatic Insufficiency: The pharmacokinetics of linezolid are not altered in patients (n=7) with mild-to-moderate hepatic insufficiency (Child-Pugh class A or B). On the basis of the available information, no dose adjustment is recommended for patients with mild-to-moderate hepatic insufficiency. The pharmacokinetics of linezolid in patients with severe hepatic insufficiency have not been evaluated.

Drug-Drug Interactions

Drugs Metabolized by Cytochrome P450: Linezolid is not an inducer of cytochrome P450 (CYP) in rats. It is not detectably metabolized by human cytochrome P450 and it does not inhibit the activities of clinically significant human CYP isoforms (1A2, 2C9, 2C19, 2D6, 2E1, 3A4). Therefore, no CYP450-induced drug interactions are expected with linezolid. Concurrent administration of linezolid does not substantially alter the pharmacokinetic characteristics of (S)-warfarin, which is extensively metabolized by CYP2C9. Drugs such as warfarin and phenytoin, which are CYP2C9 substrates, may be given with linezolid without changes in dosage regimen.

Antibiotics:

Aztreonam: The pharmacokinetics of linezolid or aztreonam are not altered when administered together.

Gentamicin: The pharmacokinetics of linezolid or gentamicin are not altered when administered together.

Monoamine Oxidase Inhibition: Linezolid is a reversible, nonselective inhibitor of monoamine oxidase. Therefore, linezolid has the potential for interaction with adrenergic and serotonergic agents.

Adrenergic Agents: A significant pressor response has been observed in normal adult subjects receiving linezolid and tyramine doses of more than 100 mg. Therefore, patients receiving linezolid need to avoid consuming large amounts of foods or beverages with high tyramine content (see **PRECAUTIONS, Information for Patients**).

A reversible enhancement of the pressor response of either pseudoephedrine HCl (PSE) or phenylpropanolamine HCl (PPA) is observed when linezolid is administered to healthy normotensive subjects (see **PRECAUTIONS, Drug Interactions**). A similar study has not been conducted in hypertensive patients. The interaction studies conducted in normotensive subjects evaluated the blood pressure and heart rate effects of placebo, PPA or PSE alone, linezolid alone, and the combination of steady-state linezolid (600 mg q12h for 3 days) with two doses of PPA (25 mg) or PSE (60 mg) given 4 hours apart. Heart rate was not affected by any of the treatments. Blood pressure was increased with both combination treatments. Maximum blood pressure levels were seen 2 to 3 hours after the second dose of PPA or PSE, and returned to baseline 2 to 3 hours after peak. The results of the PPA study follow, showing the mean (and range) maximum systolic blood pressure in mm Hg: placebo = 121 (103 to 158); linezolid alone = 120 (107 to 135); PPA alone = 125 (106 to 139); PPA with linezolid = 147 (129 to 176). The results from the PSE study were similar to those in the PPA study. The mean maximum increase in systolic blood pressure over baseline was 32 mm Hg (range: 20–52 mm Hg) and 38 mm Hg (range: 18–79 mm Hg) during co-administration of linezolid with pseudoephedrine or phenylpropanolamine, respectively.

Table 2. Pharmacokinetic Parameters of Linezolid in Pediatrics and Adults Following a Single Intravenous Infusion of 10 mg/kg or 600 mg Linezolid (Mean: (%CV); [Min, Max Values])

Age Group	C_{max} μg/mL	V_{ss} L/kg	AUC* μg•h/mL	$t_{1/2}$ hrs	CL mL/min/kg
Neonatal Patients					
Pre-term** <1 week (N = 9)†	12.7 (30%) [9.6, 22.2]	0.81 (24%) [0.43, 1.05]	108 (47%) [41, 191]	5.6 (46%) [2.4, 9.8]	2.0 (52%) [0.9, 4.0]
Full-term*** <1 week (N = 10)†	11.5 (24%) [8.0, 18.3]	0.78 (20%) [0.45, 0.96]	55 (47%) [19, 103]	3.0 (55%) [1.3, 6.1]	3.8 (55%) [1.5, 8.8]
Full-term*** ≥1 week to ≤28 days (N = 10)†	12.9 (28%) [7.7, 21.6]	0.66 (29%) [0.35, 1.06]	34 (21%) [23, 50]	1.5 (17%) [1.2, 1.9]	5.1 (22%) [3.3, 7.2]
Infant Patients > 28 days to < 3 Months (N = 12)†	11.0 (27%) [7.2, 18.0]	0.79 (26%) [0.42, 1.08]	33 (26%) [17, 48]	1.8 (28%) [1.2, 2.8]	5.4 (32%) [3.5, 9.9]
Pediatric Patients 3 months through 11 years† (N = 59)	15.1 (30%) [6.8, 36.7]	0.69 (28%) [0.31, 1.50]	58 (54%) [19, 153]	2.9 (53%) [0.9, 8.0]	3.8 (53%) [1.0, 8.5]
Adolescent Subjects and Patients 12 through 17 years‡ (N = 36)	16.7 (24%) [9.9, 28.9]	0.61 (15%) [0.44, 0.79]	95 (44%) [32, 178]	4.1 (46%) [1.3, 8.1]	2.1 (53%) [0.9, 5.2]
Adult Subjects§ (N = 29)	12.5 (21%) [8.2, 19.3]	0.65 (16%) [0.45, 0.84]	91 (33%) [53, 155]	4.9 (35%) [1.8, 8.3]	1.7 (34%) [0.9, 3.3]

* AUC = Single dose $AUC_{0-\infty}$
** In this data set, "pre-term" is defined as <34 weeks gestational age (Note: Only 1 patient enrolled was pre-term with a postnatal age between 1 week and 28 days)
*** In this data set, "full-term" is defined as ≥34 weeks gestational age
† Dose of 10 mg/kg
‡ Dose of 600 mg or 10 mg/kg up to a maximum of 600 mg
§ Dose normalized to 600 mg
C_{max} = Maximum plasma concentration; V_{ss}=Volume of distribution; AUC = Area under concentration-time curve;
$t_{1/2}$ = Apparent elimination half-life; CL = Systemic clearance normalized for body weight

Table 3. Mean (Standard Deviation) AUCs and Elimination Half-lives of Linezolid and Metabolites A and B in Patients with Varying Degrees of Renal Insufficiency After a Single 600-mg Oral Dose of Linezolid

Parameter	Healthy Subjects CL_{CR} > 80 mL/min	Moderate Renal Impairment 30 < CL_{CR} < 80 mL/min	Severe Renal Impairment 10 < CL_{CR} < 30 mL/min	Hemodialysis-Dependent	
				Off Dialysis*	On Dialysis
Linezolid					
$AUC_{0-\infty}$, μg h/mL	110 (22)	128 (53)	127 (66)	141 (45)	83 (23)
$t_{1/2}$, hours	6.4 (2.2)	6.1 (1.7)	7.1 (3.7)	8.4 (2.7)	7.0 (1.8)
Metabolite A					
AUC_{0-48}, μg h/mL	7.6 (1.9)	11.7 (4.3)	56.5 (30.6)	185 (124)	68.8 (23.9)
$t_{1/2}$, hours	6.3 (2.1)	6.6 (2.3)	9.0 (4.6)	NA	NA
Metabolite B					
AUC_{0-48}, μg h/mL	30.5 (6.2)	51.1 (38.5)	203 (92)	467 (102)	239 (44)
$t_{1/2}$, hours	6.6 (2.7)	9.9 (7.4)	11.0 (3.9)	NA	NA

* between hemodialysis sessions
NA = Not applicable

Serotonergic Agents: The potential drug-drug interaction with dextromethorphan was studied in healthy volunteers. Subjects were administered dextromethorphan (two 20-mg doses given 4 hours apart) with or without linezolid. No serotonin syndrome effects (confusion, delirium, restlessness, tremors, blushing, diphoresis, hyperpyrexia) have been observed in normal subjects receiving linezolid and dextromethorphan. The effects of other serotonin re-uptake inhibitors have not been studied.

MICROBIOLOGY

Linezolid is a synthetic antibacterial agent of a new class of antibiotics, the oxazolidinones, which has clinical utility in the treatment of infections caused by aerobic Gram-positive bacteria. The in vitro spectrum of activity of linezolid also includes certain Gram-negative bacteria and anaerobic bacteria. Linezolid inhibits bacterial protein synthesis through a mechanism of action different from that of other antibacterial agents; therefore, cross-resistance between linezolid and other classes of antibiotics is unlikely. Linezolid binds to a site on the bacterial 23S ribosomal RNA of the 50S subunit and prevents the formation of a functional 70S initiation complex, which is an essential component of the bacterial translation process. The results of time-kill studies have shown linezolid to be bacteriostatic against enterococci and staphylococci. For streptococci, linezolid was found to be bactericidal for the majority of strains.

In clinical trials, resistance to linezolid developed in 6 patients infected with *Enterococcus faecium* (4 patients received 200 mg q12h, lower than the recommended dose, and 2 patients received 600 mg q12h). In a compassionate use program, resistance to linezolid developed in 8 patients with *E. faecium* and in 1 patient with *Enterococcus faecalis*. All patients had either unremoved prosthetic devices or undrained abscesses. Resistance to linezolid occurs in vitro at a frequency of 1×10^{-9} to 1×10^{-11}. In vitro studies have shown that point mutations in the 23S rRNA are associated with linezolid resistance. Reports of vancomycin-resistant *E. faecium* becoming resistant to linezolid during its clinical use have been published.[1] In one report nosocomial spread of vancomycin- and linezolid-resistant *E. faecium* occurred[2]. There has been a report of *Staphylococcus aureus* (methicillin-resistant) developing resistance to linezolid during its clinical use.[3] The linezolid resistance in these organisms was associated with a point mutation in the 23S rRNA (substitution of thymine for guanine at position 2576) of the organism. When antibiotic-resistant organisms are encountered in the hospital, it is important to emphasize infection control policies.[4,5] Resistance to linezolid has not been reported in *Streptococcus* spp., including *Streptococcus pneumoniae*.

In vitro studies have demonstrated additivity or indifference between linezolid and vancomycin, gentamicin, rifampin, imipenemcilastatin, aztreonam, ampicillin, or streptomycin.

Linezolid has been shown to be active against most isolates of the following microorganisms, both in vitro and in clinical infections, as described in the **INDICATIONS AND USAGE** section.

Aerobic and facultative Gram-positive microorganisms

Enterococcus faecium (vancomycin-resistant strains only)
Staphylococcus aureus (including methicillin-resistant strains)
Streptococcus agalactiae
Streptococcus pneumoniae (penicillin-susceptible strains only)
Streptococcus pyogenes

The following in vitro data are available, but their clinical significance is unknown. At least 90% of the following microorganisms exhibit an in vitro minimum inhibitory concentration (MIC) less than or equal to the susceptible break-

Continued on next page

Zyvox—Cont.

point for linezolid. However, the safety and effectiveness of linezolid in treating clinical infections due to these microorganisms have not been established in adequate and well-controlled clinical trials.

Aerobic and facultative Gram-positive microorganisms

Enterococcus faecalis (including vancomycin-resistant strains)

Enterococcus faecium (vancomycin-susceptible strains)

Staphylococcus epidermidis (including methicillin-resistant strains)

Staphylococcus haemolyticus

Streptococcus pneumoniae (penicillin-resistant strains)

Viridans group streptococci

Aerobic and facultative Gram-negative microorganisms

Pasteurella multocida

Susceptibility Testing Methods

NOTE: Susceptibility testing by dilution methods requires the use of linezolid susceptibility powder.

When available, the results of in vitro susceptibility tests should be provided to the physician as periodic reports which describe the susceptibility profile of nosocomial and community-acquired pathogens. These reports should aid the physician in selecting the most effective antimicrobial.

Dilution Techniques: Quantitative methods are used to determine antimicrobial minimum inhibitory concentrations (MICs). These MICs provide estimates of the susceptibility of bacteria to antimicrobial compounds. The MICs should be determined using a standardized procedure. Standardized procedures are based on a dilution method[6,7] (broth or agar) or equivalent with standardized inoculum concentrations and standardized concentrations of linezolid powder. The MIC values should be interpreted according to criteria provided in Table 4.

Diffusion Techniques: Quantitative methods that require measurement of zone diameters also provide reproducible estimates of the susceptibility of bacteria to antimicrobial compounds. One such standardized procedure[7,8] requires the use of standardized inoculum concentrations. This procedure uses paper disks impregnated with 30 μg of linezolid to test the susceptibility of microorganisms to linezolid. The disk diffusion interpretive criteria are provided in Table 4.

Table 4. Susceptibility Interpretive Criteria for Linezolid

Pathogen	Susceptibility Interpretive Criteria: Minimal Inhibitory Concentrations (MIC in μg/mL)			Disk Diffusion (Zone Diameters in mm)		
	S	I	R	S	I	R
Enterococcus spp	≤2	4	≥8	≥23	21-22	≤20
Staphylococcus spp[a]	≤4	—	—	≥21	—	—
Streptococcus pneumoniae[a]	≤2[b]	—	—	≥21[c]	—	—
Streptococcus spp other than *S pneumoniae*[a]	≤2[b]	—	—	≥21[c]	—	—

[a] The current absence of data on resistant strains precludes defining any categories other than "Susceptible." Strains yielding test results suggestive of a "nonsusceptible" category should be retested, and if the result is confirmed, the isolate should be submitted to a reference laboratory for further testing.

[b] These interpretive standards for *S. pneumoniae* and *Streptococcus* spp. other than *S. pneumoniae* are applicable only to tests performed by broth microdilution using cation-adjusted Mueller-Hinton broth with 2 to 5% lysed horse blood inoculated with a direct colony suspension and incubated in ambient air at 35°C for 20 to 24 hours.

[c] These zone diameter interpretive standards are applicable only to tests performed using Mueller-Hinton agar supplemented with 5% defibrinated sheep blood inoculated with a direct colony suspension and incubated in 5% CO_2 at 35°C for 20 to 24 hours.

A report of "Susceptible" indicates that the pathogen is likely to be inhibited if the antimicrobial compound in the blood reaches the concentrations usually achievable. A report of "Intermediate" indicates that the result should be considered equivocal, and, if the microorganism is not fully susceptible to alternative, clinically feasible drugs, the test should be repeated. This category implies possible clinical applicability in body sites where the drug is physiologically concentrated or in situations where high dosage of drug can be used. This category also provides a buffer zone which prevents small uncontrolled technical factors from causing major discrepancies in interpretation. A report of "Resistant" indicates that the pathogen is not likely to be inhibited if the antimicrobial compound in the blood reaches the concentrations usually achievable; other therapy should be selected.

Quality Control

Standardized susceptibility test procedures require the use of quality control microorganisms to control the technical aspects of the test procedures. Standard linezolid powder should provide the following range of values noted in Table 5. **NOTE:** Quality control microorganisms are specific strains of organisms with intrinsic biological properties relating to resistance mechanisms and their genetic expression within bacteria; the specific strains used for microbiological quality control are not clinically significant.

Table 5. Acceptable Quality Control Ranges for Linezolid to be Used in Validation of Susceptibility Test Results

QC Strain	Acceptable Quality Control Ranges: Minimum Inhibitory Concentration (MIC in μg/mL)	Disk Diffusion (Zone Diameters in mm)
Enterococcus faecalis ATCC 29212	1–4	Not applicable
Staphylococcus aureus ATCC 29213	1–4	Not applicable
Staphylococcus aureus ATCC 25923	Not applicable	25–32
Streptococcus pneumoniae ATCC 49619[d]	0.50–2[e]	25–34[f]

[d] This organism may be used for validation of susceptibility test results when testing *Streptococcus* spp. other than *S. pneumoniae.*

[e] This quality control range for *S. pneumoniae* is applicable only to tests performed by broth microdilution using cation-adjusted Mueller-Hinton broth with 2 to 5% lysed horse blood inoculated with a direct colony suspension and incubated in ambient air at 35°C for 20 to 24 hours.

[f] This quality control zone diameter range is applicable only to tests performed using Mueller-Hinton agar supplemented with 5% defibrinated sheep blood inoculated with a direct colony suspension and incubated in 5% CO_2 at 35°C for 20 to 24 hours.

INDICATIONS AND USAGE

ZYVOX formulations are indicated in the treatment of the following infections caused by susceptible strains of the designated microorganisms (see **PRECAUTIONS, Pediatric Use** and **DOSAGE AND ADMINISTRATION**).

Vancomycin-Resistant *Enterococcus faecium* infections, including cases with concurrent bacteremia (see **CLINICAL STUDIES**).

Nosocomial pneumonia caused by *Staphylococcus aureus* (methicillin-susceptible and -resistant strains), or *Streptococcus pneumoniae* (penicillin-susceptible strains). Combination therapy may be clinically indicated if the documented or presumptive pathogens include Gram-negative organisms (see **CLINICAL STUDIES**).

Complicated skin and skin structure infections, including diabetic foot infections, without concomitant osteomyelitis, caused by *Staphylococcus aureus* (methicillin-susceptible and -resistant strains), *Streptococcus pyogenes,* or *Streptococcus agalactiae.* ZYVOX has not been studied in the treatment of decubitus ulcers. Combination therapy may be clinically indicated if the documented or presumptive pathogens include Gram-negative organisms (see **CLINICAL STUDIES**).

Uncomplicated skin and skin structure infections caused by *Staphylococcus aureus* (methicillin-susceptible only) or *Streptococcus pyogenes.*

Community-acquired pneumonia caused by *Streptococcus pneumoniae* (penicillin-susceptible strains only), including cases with concurrent bacteremia, or *Staphylococcus aureus* (methicillin-susceptible strains only).

To reduce the development of drug-resistant bacteria and maintain the effectiveness of ZYVOX and other antibacterial drugs, ZYVOX should be used only to treat or prevent infections that are proven or strongly suspected to be caused by susceptible bacteria. When culture and susceptibility information are available, they should be considered in selecting or modifying antibacterial therapy. In the absence of such data, local epidemiology and susceptibility patterns may contribute to the empiric selection of therapy.

CONTRAINDICATIONS

ZYVOX formulations are contraindicated for use in patients who have known hypersensitivity to linezolid or any of the other product components.

WARNINGS

Myelosuppression (including anemia, leukopenia, pancytopenia, and thrombocytopenia) has been reported in patients receiving linezolid. In cases where the outcome is known, when linezolid was discontinued, the affected hematologic parameters have risen toward pretreatment levels. Complete blood counts should be monitored weekly in patients who receive linezolid, particularly in those who receive linezolid for longer than two weeks, those with pre-existing myelosuppression, those receiving concomitant drugs that produce bone marrow suppression, or those with a chronic infection who have received previous or concomitant antibiotic therapy. Discontinuation of therapy with linezolid should be considered in patients who develop or have worsening myelosuppression.

In adult and juvenile dogs and rats, myelosuppression, reduced extramedullary hematopiesis in spleen and liver, and lymphoid depletion of thymus, lymph nodes, and spleen were observed (see **ANIMAL PHARMACOLOGY**).

Pseudomembranous colitis has been reported with nearly all antibacterial agents, including ZYVOX, and may range in severity from mild to life-threatening. Therefore, it is important to consider this diagnosis in patients who present with diarrhea subsequent to the administration of any antibacterial agent.

Treatment with antibacterial agents alters the normal flora of the colon and may permit overgrowth of clostridia. Studies indicated that a toxin produced by *Clostridium difficile* is a primary cause of "antibiotic-associated colitis."

After the diagnosis of pseudomembranous colitis has been established, appropriate therapeutic measures should be initiated. Mild cases of pseudomembranous colitis usually respond to drug discontinuation alone. In moderate to severe cases, consideration should be given to management with fluids and electrolytes, protein supplementation, and treatment with an antibacterial agent clinically effective against *Clostridium difficile.*

PRECAUTIONS

General

Lactic acidosis has been reported with the use of ZYVOX. In reported cases, patients experienced repeated episodes of nausea and vomiting. Patients who develop recurrent nausea or vomiting, unexplained acidosis, or a low bicarbonate level while receiving ZYVOX should receive immediate medical evaluation.

The use of antibiotics may promote the overgrowth of nonsusceptible organisms. Should superinfection occur during therapy, appropriate measures should be taken.

ZYVOX has not been studied in patients with uncontrolled hypertension, pheochromocytoma, carcinoid syndrome, or untreated hyperthyroidism.

The safety and efficacy of ZYVOX formulations given for longer than 28 days have not been evaluated in controlled clinical trials.

Prescribing ZYVOX in the absence of a proven or strongly suspected bacterial infection or a prophylactic indication is unlikely to provide benefit to the patient and increases the risk of the development of drug-resistant bacteria.

Information for Patients

Patients should be advised that:

- ZYVOX may be taken with or without food.
- They should inform their physician if they have a history of hypertension.
- Large quantities of foods or beverages with high tyramine content should be avoided while taking ZYVOX. Quantities of tyramine consumed should be less than 100 mg per meal. Foods high in tyramine content include those that may have undergone protein changes by aging, fermentation, pickling, or smoking to improve flavor, such as aged cheeses (0 to 15 mg tyramine per ounce); fermented or air-dried meats (0.1 to 8 mg tyramine per ounce); sauerkraut (8 mg tyramine per 8 ounces); soy sauce (5 mg tyramine per 1 teaspoon); tap beers (4 mg tyramine per 12 ounces); red wines (0 to 6 mg tyramine per 8 ounces). The tyramine content of any protein-rich food may be increased if stored for long periods or improperly refrigerated.[9,10]
- They should inform their physician if taking medications containing pseudoephedrine HCl or phenylpropanolamine HCl, such as cold remedies and decongestants.
- They should inform their physician if taking serotonin re-uptake inhibitors or other antidepressants.
- *Phenylketonurics:* Each 5 mL of the 100 mg/5 mL ZYVOX for Oral Suspension contains 20 mg phenylalanine. The other ZYVOX formulations do not contain phenylalanine. Contact your physician or pharmacist.

Patients should be counseled that antibacterial drugs including ZYVOX should only be used to treat bacterial infections. They do not treat viral infections (e.g., the common cold). When ZYVOX is prescribed to treat a bacterial infection, patients should be told that although it is common to feel better early in the course of therapy, the medication should be taken exactly as directed. Skipping doses or not completing the full course of therapy may (1) decrease the effectiveness of the immediate treatment and (2) increase the likelihood that bacteria will develop resistance and will not be treatable by ZYVOX or other antibacterial drugs in the future.

Drug Interactions (see also CLINICAL PHARMACOLOGY, Drug-Drug Interactions)

Monoamine Oxidase Inhibition: Linezolid is a reversible, nonselective inhibitor of monoamine oxidase. Therefore, linezolid has the potential for interaction with adrenergic and serotonergic agents.

Adrenergic Agents: Some individuals receiving ZYVOX may experience a reversible enhancement of the pressor response to indirect-acting sympathomimetic agents, vasopressor or dopaminergic agents. Commonly used drugs such as phenylpropanolamine and pseudoephedrine have been specifically studied. Initial doses of adrenergic agents, such as dopamine or epinephrine, should be reduced and titrated to achieve the desired response.

Serotonergic Agents: Co-administration of linezolid and serotonergic agents was not associated with serotonin syndrome in phase 1, 2 or 3 studies. Since there is limited experience with concomitant administration of linezolid and serotonergic agents, physicians should be alert to the possibility of signs and symptoms of serotonin syndrome (e.g., hyperpyrexia and cognitive dysfunction) in patients receiving such concomitant therapy.

Drug-Laboratory Test Interactions

There are no reported drug-laboratory test interactions.

Carcinogenesis, Mutagenesis, Impairment of Fertility

Lifetime studies in animals have not been conducted to evaluate the carcinogenic potential of linezolid. Neither mutagenic nor clastogenic potential was found in a battery of tests including: assays for mutagenicity (Ames bacterial reversion and CHO cell mutation), an in vitro unscheduled DNA synthesis (UDS) assay, an in vitro chromosome aberration assay in human lymphocytes, and an in vivo mouse micronucleus assay.

Linezolid did not affect the fertility or reproductive performance of adult female rats. It reversibly decreased fertility and reproductive performance in adult male rats when given at doses ≥50 mg/kg/day, with exposures approximately equal to or greater than the expected human exposure level (exposure comparisons are based on AUCs). The reversible fertility effects were mediated through altered spermatogenesis. Affected spermatids contained abnormally formed and oriented mitochondria and were non-viable. Epithelial cell hypertrophy and hyperplasia in the epididymis was observed in conjunction with decreased fertility. Similar epididymal changes were not seen in dogs.

In sexually mature male rats exposed to drug as juveniles, mildly decreased fertility was observed following treatment with linezolid through most of their period of sexual development (50 mg/kg/day from days 7 to 36 of age, and 100 mg/kg/day from days 37 to 55 of age), with exposures up to 1.7-fold greater than mean AUCs observed in pediatric patients aged 3 months to 11 years. Decreased fertility was not observed with shorter treatment periods, corresponding to exposure in utero through the early neonatal period (gestation day 6 through postnatal day 5), neonatal exposure (postnatal days 5 to 21), or to juvenile exposure (postnatal days 22 to 35). Reversible reductions in sperm motility and altered sperm morphology were observed in rats treated from postnatal day 22 to 35.

Pregnancy

Teratogenic Effects. Pregnancy Category C: Linezolid was not teratogenic in mice or rats at exposure levels 6.5-fold (in mice) or equivalent to (in rats) the expected human exposure level, based on AUCs. However, embryo and fetal toxicities were seen (see **Non-teratogenic Effects**). There are no adequate and well-controlled studies in pregnant women. ZYVOX should be used during pregnancy only if the potential benefit justifies the potential risk to the fetus.

Non-teratogenic Effects

In mice, embryo and fetal toxicities were seen only at doses that caused maternal toxicity (clinical signs and reduced body weight gain). A dose of 450 mg/kg/day (6.5-fold the estimated human exposure level based on AUCs) correlated with increased postimplantational embryo death, including total litter loss, decreased fetal body weights, and an increased incidence of costal cartilage fusion.

In rats, mild fetal toxicity was observed at 15 and 50 mg/kg/day (exposure levels 0.22-fold to approximately equivalent to the estimated human exposure, respectively based on AUCs). The effects consisted of decreased fetal body weights and reduced ossification of sternebrae, a finding often seen in association with decreased fetal body weights. Slight maternal toxicity, in the form of reduced body weight gain, was seen at 50 mg/kg/day.

When female rats were treated with 50 mg/kg/day (approximately equivalent to the estimated human exposure based on AUCs) of linezolid during pregnancy and lactation, survival of pups was decreased on postnatal days 1 to 4. Male and female pups permitted to mature to reproductive age, when mated, showed an increase in preimplantation loss.

Nursing Mothers

Linezolid and its metabolites are excreted in the milk of lactating rats. Concentrations in milk were similar to those in maternal plasma. It is not known whether linezolid is excreted in human milk. Because many drugs are excreted in human milk, caution should be exercised when ZYVOX is administered to a nursing woman.

Pediatric Use

The safety and effectiveness of ZYVOX for the treatment of pediatric patients with the following infections are supported by evidence from adequate and well-controlled studies in adults, pharmacokinetic data in pediatric patients, and additional data from a comparator-controlled study of Gram-positive infections in pediatric patients ranging in age from birth through 11 years (see **INDICATIONS AND USAGE** and **CLINICAL STUDIES**):

- nosocomial pneumonia
- complicated skin and skin structure infections
- community-acquired pneumonia (also supported by evidence from an uncontrolled study in patients ranging in age from 8 months through 12 years)
- vancomycin-resistant *Enterococcus faecium* infections

The safety and effectiveness of ZYVOX for the treatment of pediatric patients with the following infection have been established in a comparator-controlled study in pediatric patients ranging in age from 5 through 17 years (see **CLINICAL STUDIES**):

- uncomplicated skin and skin structure infections caused by *Staphylococcus aureus* (methicillin-susceptible strains only) or *Streptococcus pyogenes*

The C_{max} and the volume of distribution (V_{ss}) of linezolid are similar regardless of age in pediatric patients. However, linezolid clearance is a function of age. Excluding neonates less than a week of age, clearance is most rapid in the youngest age groups ranging from >1 week old to 11 years, resulting in lower single-dose systemic exposure (AUC) and shorter half-life as compared with adults. As age of pediatric patients increases, the clearance of linezolid gradually decreases, and by adolescence, mean clearance values approach those observed for the adult population. There is wider inter-subject variability in linezolid clearance and in systemic drug exposure (AUC) across all pediatric age groups as compared with adults.

Similar mean daily AUC values were observed in pediatric patients from birth to 11 years of age dosed q8h relative to adolescents or adults dosed q12h. Therefore, the dosage for pediatric patients up to 11 years of age should be 10 mg/kg q8h. Pediatric patients 12 years and older should receive 600 mg q12h.

Recommendations for the dosage regimen for pre-term neonates less than 7 days of age (gestational age less than 34 weeks) are based on pharmacokinetic data from 9 pre-term neonates. Most of these pre-term neonates have lower systemic linezolid clearance values and larger AUC values than many full-term neonates and older infants. Therefore, these pre-term neonates should be initiated with a dosing regimen of 10 mg/kg q12h. Consideration may be given to the use of a 10 mg/kg q8h regimen in neonates with a sub-optimal clinical response. All neonatal patients should receive 10 mg/kg q8h by 7 days of life (see **CLINICAL PHARMACOLOGY, Special Populations, Pediatric** and **DOSAGE AND ADMINISTRATION**).

In limited clinical experience, 5 out of 6 (83%) pediatric patients with infections due to Gram-positive pathogens with MICs of 4 μg/mL treated with ZYVOX had clinical cures. However, pediatric patients exhibit wider variability in linezolid clearance and systemic exposure (AUC) compared with adults. In pediatric patients with a sub-optimal clinical response, particularly those with pathogens with MIC of 4 μg/mL, lower systemic exposure, site and severity of infection, and the underlying medical condition should be considered when assessing clinical response (see **CLINICAL PHARMACOLOGY, Special Populations, Pediatric** and **DOSAGE AND ADMINISTRATION**).

Geriatric Use

Of the 2046 patients treated with ZYVOX in phase 3 comparator-controlled clinical trials, 589 (29%) were 65 years or older and 253 (12%) were 75 years or older. No overall differences in safety or effectiveness were observed between these patients and younger patients.

ANIMAL PHARMACOLOGY

Target organs of linezolid toxicity were similar in juvenile and adult rats and dogs. Dose- and time-dependent myelosuppression, as evidenced by bone marrow hypocellularity/decreased hematopoiesis, decreased extramedullary hematopoiesis in spleen and liver, and decreased levels of circulating erythrocytes, leukocytes, and platelets have been seen in animal studies. Lymphoid depletion occurred in thymus, lymph nodes, and spleen. Generally, the lymphoid findings were associated with anorexia, weight loss, and suppression of body weight gain, which may have contributed to the observed effects. These effects were observed at exposure levels that are comparable to those observed in some human subjects. The hematopoietic and lymphoid effects were reversible, although in some studies, reversal was incomplete within the duration of the recovery period.

ADVERSE REACTIONS

Adult Patients

The safety of ZYVOX formulations was evaluated in 2046 adult patients enrolled in seven phase 3 comparator-controlled clinical trials, who were treated for up to 28 days. In these studies, 85% of the adverse events reported with ZYVOX were described as mild to moderate in intensity. Table 6 shows the incidence of adverse events reported in at least 2% of patients in these trials. The most common adverse events in patients treated with ZYVOX were diarrhea (incidence across studies: 2.8% to 11.0%), headache (incidence across studies: 0.5% to 11.3%), and nausea (incidence across studies: 3.4% to 9.6%).

Table 6. Incidence (%) of Adverse Events Reported in ≥2% of Adult Patients in Comparator-Controlled Clinical Trials with ZYVOX

Event	ZYVOX (n=2046)	All Comparators* (n=2001)
Diarrhea	8.3	6.3
Headache	6.5	5.5
Nausea	6.2	4.6
Vomiting	3.7	2.0
Insomnia	2.5	1.7
Constipation	2.2	2.1
Rash	2.0	2.2
Dizziness	2.0	1.9
Fever	1.6	2.1

*Comparators included cefpodoxime proxetil 200 mg PO q12h; ceftriaxone 1 g IV q12h; clarithromycin 250 mg PO q12h; dicloxacillin 500 mg PO q6h; oxacillin 2 g IV q6h; vancomycin 1 g IV q12h.

Other adverse events reported in phase 2 and phase 3 studies included oral moniliasis, vaginal moniliasis, hypertension, dyspepsia, localized abdominal pain, pruritus, and tongue discoloration.

Table 7 shows the incidence of drug-related adverse events reported in at least 1% of adult patients in these trials by dose of ZYVOX.

[See table 7 above]

Table 7. Incidence (%) of Drug-Related Adverse Events Occurring in >1% of Adult Patients Treated with ZYVOX in Comparator-Controlled Clinical Trials

Adverse Events	Uncomplicated Skin and Skin Structure Infections		All Other Indications	
	ZYVOX 400 mg PO q12h (n=548)	Clarithromycin 250 mg PO q12h (n=537)	ZYVOX 600 mg q12h (n=1498)	All Other Comparators* (n=1464)
% of patients with 1 drug-related adverse event	25.4	19.6	20.4	14.3
% of patients discontinuing due to drug-related adverse events†	3.5	2.4	2.1	1.7
Diarrhea	5.3	4.8	4.0	2.7
Nausea	3.5	3.5	3.3	1.8
Headache	2.7	2.2	1.9	1.0
Taste alteration	1.8	2.0	0.9	0.2
Vaginal moniliasis	1.6	1.3	1.0	0.4
Fungal infection	1.5	0.2	0.1	<0.1
Abnormal liver function tests	0.4	0	1.3	0.5
Vomiting	0.9	0.4	1.2	0.4
Tongue discoloration	1.1	0	0.2	0
Dizziness	1.1	1.5	0.4	0.3
Oral moniliasis	0.4	0	1.1	0.4

*Comparators included cefpodoxime proxetil 200 mg PO q12h; ceftriaxone 1 g IV q12h; dicloxacillin 500 mg PO q6h; oxacillin 2 g IV q6h; vancomycin 1 g IV q12h.

†The most commonly reported drug-related adverse events leading to discontinuation in patients treated with ZYVOX were nausea, headache, diarrhea, and vomiting.

Pediatric Patients

The safety of ZYVOX formulations was evaluated in 215 pediatric patients ranging in age from birth through 11 years, and in 248 pediatric patients aged 5 through 17 years (146 of these 248 were age 5 through 11 and 102 were age 12 to 17). These patients were enrolled in two phase 3 comparator-controlled clinical trials and were treated for up to 28 days. In these studies, 83% and 99%, respectively, of the adverse events reported with ZYVOX were described as mild to moderate in intensity. In the study of hospitalized pedi-

Continued on next page

Zyvox—Cont.

atric patients (birth through 11 years) with Gram-positive infections, who were randomized 2 to 1 (linezolid:vancomycin), mortality was 6.0% (13/215) in the linezolid arm and 3.0% (3/101) in the vancomycin arm. However, given the severe underlying illness in the patient population, no causality could be established. Table 8 shows the incidence of adverse events reported in at least 2% of pediatric patients treated with ZYVOX in these trials.
[See table 8 below]
Table 9 shows the incidence of drug-related adverse events reported in more than 1% of pediatric patients (and more than 1 patient) in either treatment group in the comparator-controlled phase 3 trials.
[See table 9 at top of next page]

Laboratory Changes

ZYVOX has been associated with thrombocytopenia when used in doses up to and including 600 mg every 12 hours for up to 28 days. In phase 3 comparator-controlled trials, the percentage of adult patients who developed a substantially low platelet count (defined as less than 75% of lower limit of normal and/or baseline) was 2.4% (range among studies: 0.3 to 10.0%) with ZYVOX and 1.5% (range among studies: 0.4 to 7.0%) with a comparator. In a study of hospitalized pediatric patients ranging in age from birth through 11 years, the percentage of patients who developed a substantially low platelet count (defined as less than 75% of lower limit of normal and/or baseline) was 12.9% with ZYVOX and 13.4% with vancomycin. In an outpatient study of pediatric patients aged from 5 through 17 years, the percentage of patients who developed a substantially low platelet count was 0% with ZYVOX and 0.4% with cefadroxil. Thrombocytopenia associated with the use of ZYVOX appears to be dependent on duration of therapy, (generally greater than 2 weeks of treatment). The platelet counts for most patients returned to the normal range/baseline during the follow-up period. No related clinical adverse events were identified in phase 3 clinical trials in patients developing thrombocytopenia. Bleeding events were identified in thrombocytopenic patients in a compassionate use program for ZYVOX; the role of linezolid in these events cannot be determined (see **WARNINGS**).

Changes seen in other laboratory parameters, without regard to drug relationship, revealed no substantial differences between ZYVOX and the comparators. These changes were generally not clinically significant, did not lead to discontinuation of therapy, and were reversible. The incidence of adult and pediatric patients with at least one substantially abnormal hematologic or serum chemistry value is presented in Tables 10, 11, 12, and 13.
[See table 10 on next page]
[See table 11 on next page]
[See table 12 at top of page 396]
[See table 13 at top of page 396]

Postmarketing Experience

Myelosuppression (including anemia, leukopenia, pancytopenia, and thrombocytopenia) has been reported during postmarketing use of ZYVOX (see **WARNINGS**). Neuropathy (peripheral, optic) has been reported in patients treated with ZYVOX. Lactic acidosis has been reported with the use of ZYVOX (see **PRECAUTIONS**). Although these reports have primarily been in patients treated for longer than the maximum recommended duration of 28 days, these events have also been reported in patients receiving shorter courses of therapy. These events have been chosen for inclusion due to either their seriousness, frequency of reporting, possible causal connection to ZYVOX, or a combination of these factors. Because they are reported voluntarily from a population of unknown size, estimates of frequency cannot be made and causal relationship cannot be precisely established.

OVERDOSAGE

In the event of overdosage, supportive care is advised, with maintenance of glomerular filtration. Hemodialysis may facilitate more rapid elimination of linezolid. In a phase 1 clinical trial, approximately 30% of a dose of linezolid was removed during a 3-hour hemodialysis session beginning 3 hours after the dose of linezolid was administered. Data are not available for removal of linezolid with peritoneal dialysis or hemoperfusion. Clinical signs of acute toxicity in animals were decreased activity and ataxia in rats and vomiting and tremors in dogs treated with 3000 mg/kg/day and 2000 mg/kg/day, respectively.

Table 8. Incidence (%) of Adverse Events Reported in ≥2% of Pediatric Patients Treated with ZYVOX in Comparator-Controlled Clinical Trials

Event	Uncomplicated Skin and Skin Structure Infections*		All Other Indications†	
	ZYVOX (n=248)	Cefadroxil (n=251)	ZYVOX (n=215)	Vancomycin (n=101)
Fever	2.9	3.6	14.1	14.1
Diarrhea	7.8	8.0	10.8	12.1
Vomiting	2.9	6.4	9.4	9.1
Sepsis	0	0	8.0	7.1
Rash	1.6	1.2	7.0	15.2
Headache	6.5	4.0	0.9	0
Anemia	0	0	5.6	7.1
Thrombocytopenia	0	0	4.7	2.0
Upper respiratory infection	3.7	5.2	4.2	1.0
Nausea	3.7	3.2	1.9	0
Dyspnea	0	0	3.3	1.0
Reaction at site of injection or of vascular catheter	0	0	3.3	5.1
Trauma	3.3	4.8	2.8	2.0
Pharyngitis	2.9	1.6	0.5	1.0
Convulsion	0	0	2.8	2.0
Hypokalemia	0	0	2.8	3.0
Pneumonia	0	0	2.8	2.0
Thrombocythemia	0	0	2.8	2.0
Cough	2.4	4.0	0.9	0
Generalized abdominal pain	2.4	2.8	0.9	2.0
Localized abdominal pain	2.4	2.8	0.5	1.0
Apnea	0	0	2.3	2.0
Gastrointestinal bleeding	0	0	2.3	1.0
Generalized edema	0	0	2.3	1.0
Loose stools	1.6	0.8	2.3	3.0
Localized pain	2.0	1.6	0.9	0
Skin disorder	2.0	0	0.9	1.0

*Patients 5 through 11 years of age received ZYVOX 10 mg/kg PO q12h or cefadroxil 15 mg/kg PO q12h. Patients 12 years or older received ZYVOX 600 mg PO q12h or cefadroxil 500 mg PO q12h.
† Patients from birth through 11 years of age received ZYVOX 10 mg/kg IV/PO q8h or vancomycin 10 to 15 mg/kg IV q6-24h, depending on age and renal clearance.

DOSAGE AND ADMINISTRATION

The recommended dosage for ZYVOX formulations for the treatment of infections is described in Table 14.
[See table 14 on page 396]
Adult patients with infection due to MRSA should be treated with ZYVOX 600 mg q12h.
In limited clinical experience, 5 out of 6 (83%) pediatric patients with infections due to Gram-positive pathogens with MICs of 4 μg/mL treated with ZYVOX had clinical cures. However, pediatric patients exhibit wider variability in linezolid clearance and systemic exposure (AUC) compared with adults. In pediatric patients with a sub-optimal clinical response, particularly those with pathogens with MIC of 4 μg/mL, lower systemic exposure, site and severity of infection, and the underlying medical condition should be considered when assessing clinical response (see **CLINICAL PHARMACOLOGY, Special Populations, Pediatric** and **PRECAUTIONS, Pediatric Use**).
In controlled clinical trials, the protocol-defined duration of treatment for all infections ranged from 7 to 28 days. Total treatment duration was determined by the treating physician based on site and severity of the infection, and on the patient's clinical response.
No dose adjustment is necessary when switching from intravenous to oral administration. Patients whose therapy is started with ZYVOX I.V. Injection may be switched to either ZYVOX Tablets or Oral Suspension at the discretion of the physician, when clinically indicated.

Intravenous Administration

ZYVOX I.V. Injection is supplied in single-use, ready-to-use infusion bags (see **HOW SUPPLIED** for container sizes). Parenteral drug products should be inspected visually for particulate matter prior to administration. Check for minute leaks by firmly squeezing the bag. If leaks are detected, discard the solution, as sterility may be impaired.
ZYVOX I.V. Injection should be administered by intravenous infusion over a period of 30 to 120 minutes. **Do not use this intravenous infusion bag in series connections.** Additives should not be introduced into this solution. If ZYVOX I.V. Injection is to be given concomitantly with another drug, each drug should be given separately in accordance with the recommended dosage and route of administration for each product. In particular, physical incompatibilities resulted when ZYVOX I.V. Injection was combined with the following drugs during simulated Y-site administration: amphotericin B, chlorpromazine HCl, diazepam, pentamidine isothionate, erythromycin lactobionate, phenytoin sodium, and trimethoprimsulfamethoxazole. Additionally, chemical incompatibility resulted when ZYVOX I.V. Injection was combined with ceftriaxone sodium.
If the same intravenous line is used for sequential infusion of several drugs, the line should be flushed before and after infusion of ZYVOX I.V. Injection with an infusion solution compatible with ZYVOX I.V. Injection and with any other drug(s) administered via this common line (see **Compatible Intravenous Solutions**).

Compatible Intravenous Solutions

5% Dextrose Injection, USP
0.9% Sodium Chloride Injection, USP
Lactated Ringer's Injection, USP
Keep the infusion bags in the overwrap until ready to use. Store at room temperature. Protect from freezing. ZYVOX I.V. Injection may exhibit a yellow color that can intensify over time without adversely affecting potency.

Constitution of Oral Suspension

ZYVOX for Oral Suspension is supplied as a powder/granule for constitution. Gently tap bottle to loosen powder. Add a total of 123 mL distilled water in two portions. After adding the first half, shake vigorously to wet all of the powder. Then add the second half of the water and shake vigorously to obtain a uniform suspension. After constitution, each 5 mL of the suspension contains 100 mg of linezolid. Before using, gently mix by inverting the bottle 3 to 5 times. **DO NOT SHAKE.** Store constituted suspension at room temperature. Use within 21 days after constitution.

HOW SUPPLIED

Injection

ZYVOX I.V. Injection is available in single-use, ready-to-use flexible plastic infusion bags in a foil laminate overwrap. The infusion bags and ports are latex-free. The infusion bags are available in the following package sizes:

100 mL bag (200 mg linezolid)	NDC 0009-5137-01
200 mL bag (400 mg linezolid)	NDC 0009-5139-01
300 mL bag (600 mg linezolid)	NDC 0009-5140-01

Tablets

ZYVOX Tablets are available as follows:

Table 9. Incidence (%) of Drug-related Adverse Events Occurring in >1% of Pediatric Patients (and >1 Patient) in Either Treatment Group in Comparator-Controlled Clinical Trials

Event	Uncomplicated Skin and Skin Structure Infections*		All Other Indications†	
	ZYVOX (n=248)	Cefadroxil (n=251)	ZYVOX (n=215)	Vancomycin (n=101)
% of patients with ≥1 drug-related adverse event	19.2	14.1	18.8	34.3
% of patients discontinuing due to a drug-related adverse event	1.6	2.4	0.9	6.1
Diarrhea	5.7	5.2	3.8	6.1
Nausea	3.3	2.0	1.4	0
Headache	2.4	0.8	0	0
Loose stools	1.2	0.8	1.9	0
Thrombocytopenia	0	0	1.9	0
Vomiting	1.2	2.4	1.9	1.0
Generalized abdominal pain	1.6	1.2	0	0
Localized abdominal pain	1.6	1.2	0	0
Anemia	0	0	1.4	1.0
Eosinophilia	0.4	0.4	1.4	0
Rash	0.4	1.2	1.4	7.1
Vertigo	1.2	0.4	0	0
Oral moniliasis	0	0	0.9	4.0
Fever	0	0	0.5	3.0
Pruritus at non-application site	0.4	0	0	2.0
Anaphylaxis	0	0	0	10.1‡

*Patients 5 through 11 years of age received ZYVOX 10 mg/kg PO q12h or cefadroxil 15 mg/kg PO q12h. Patients 12 years or older received ZYVOX 600 mg PO q12h or cefadroxil 500 mg PO q12h.
† Patients from birth through 11 years of age received ZYVOX 10 mg/kg IV/PO q8h or vancomycin 10 to 15 mg/kg IV q6-24h, depending on age and renal clearance.
‡ These reports were of 'red-man syndrome', which were coded as anaphylaxis.

Table 10. Percent of Adult Patients who Experienced at Least One Substantially Abnormal* Hematology Laboratory Value in Comparator-Controlled Clinical Trials with ZYVOX

Laboratory Assay	Uncomplicated Skin and Skin Structure Infections		All Other Indications	
	ZYVOX 400 mg q12h	Clarithromycin 250 mg q12h	ZYVOX 600 mg q12h	All Other Comparators†
Hemoglobin (g/dL)	0.9	0.0	7.1	6.6
Platelet count (× 10^3/mm^3)	0.7	0.8	3.0	1.8
WBC (× 10^3/mm^3)	0.2	0.6	2.2	1.3
Neutrophils (× 10^3/mm^3)	0.0	0.2	1.1	1.2

* <75% (<50% for neutrophils) of Lower Limit of Normal (LLN) for values normal at baseline;
<75% (<50% for neutrophils) of LLN and of baseline for values abnormal at baseline.
† Comparators included cefpodoxime proxetil 200 mg PO q12h; ceftriaxone 1 g IV q12h; dicloxacillin 500 mg PO q6h; oxacillin 2 g IV q6h; vancomycin 1 g IV q12h.

Table 11. Percent of Adult Patients who Experienced at Least One Substantially Abnormal* Serum Chemistry Laboratory Value in Comparator-Controlled Clinical Trials with ZYVOX

Laboratory Assay	Uncomplicated Skin and Skin Structure Infections		All Other Indications	
	ZYVOX 400 mg q12h	Clarithromycin 250 mg q12h	ZYVOX 600 mg q12h	All Other Comparators†
AST (U/L)	1.7	1.3	5.0	6.8
ALT (U/L)	1.7	1.7	9.6	9.3
LDH (U/L)	0.2	0.2	1.8	1.5
Alkaline phosphatase (U/L)	0.2	0.2	3.5	3.1
Lipase (U/L)	2.8	2.6	4.3	4.2
Amylase (U/L)	0.2	0.2	2.4	2.0
Total bilirubin (mg/dL)	0.2	0.0	0.9	1.1
BUN (mg/dL)	0.2	0.0	2.1	1.5
Creatinine (mg/dL)	0.2	0.0	0.2	0.6

* >2 × Upper Limit of Normal (ULN) for values normal at baseline;
>2 × ULN and >2 × baseline for values abnormal at baseline.
† Comparators included cefpodoxime proxetil 200 mg PO q12h; ceftriaxone 1 g IV q12h; dicloxacillin 500 mg PO q6h; oxacillin 2 g IV q6h; vancomycin 1 g IV q12h.

400 mg (white, oblong, film-coated tablets printed with "ZYVOX 400mg")
100 tablets in HDPE bottle NDC 0009-5134-01
20 tablets in HDPE bottle NDC 0009-5134-02
Unit dose packages of 30 tablets NDC 0009-5134-03
600 mg (white, capsule-shaped, film-coated tablets printed with "ZYVOX 600 mg")
100 tablets in HDPE bottle NDC 0009-5135-01
20 tablets in HDPE bottle NDC 0009-5135-02
Unit dose packages of 30 tablets NDC 0009-5135-03

Oral Suspension

ZYVOX for Oral Suspension is available as a dry, white to off-white, orange-flavored granule/powder. When constituted as directed, each bottle will contain 150 mL of a suspension providing the equivalent of 100 mg of linezolid per each 5 mL. ZYVOX for Oral Suspension is supplied as follows:
100 mg/5 mL in 240-mL glass bottles NDC 0009-5136-01

Storage of ZYVOX Formulations

Store at 25°C (77°F); excursions permitted to 15-30°C (59-86°F) [see USP Controlled Room Temperature]. Protect from light. Keep bottles tightly closed to protect from moisture. It is recommended that the infusion bags be kept in the overwrap until ready to use. Protect infusion bags from freezing.

CLINICAL STUDIES

Adults

Vancomycin-Resistant Enterococcal Infections

Adult patients with documented or suspected vancomycin-resistant enterococcal infection were enrolled in a randomized, multi-center, double-blind trial comparing a high dose of ZYVOX (600 mg) with a low dose of ZYVOX (200 mg) given every 12 hours (q12h) either intravenously (IV) or orally for 7 to 28 days. Patients could receive concomitant aztreonam or aminoglycosides. There were 79 patients randomized to high-dose linezolid and 66 to low-dose linezolid. The intent-to-treat (ITT) population with documented vancomycin-resistant enterococcal infection at baseline consisted of 65 patients in the high-dose arm and 52 in the low-dose arm.

The cure rates for the ITT population with documented vancomycin-resistant enterococcal infection at baseline are presented in Table 15 by source of infection. These cure rates do not include patients with missing or indeterminate outcomes. The cure rate was higher in the high-dose arm than in the low-dose arm, although the difference was not statistically significant at the 0.05 level.

Table 15. Cure Rates at the Test-of-Cure Visit for ITT Adult Patients with Documented Vancomycin-Resistant Enterococcal Infections at Baseline

Source of Infection	Cured	
	ZYVOX 600 mg q12h n/N (%)	ZYVOX 200 mg q12h n/N (%)
Any site	39/58 (67)	24/46 (52)
Any site with associated bacteremia	10/17 (59)	4/14 (29)
Bacteremia of unknown origin	5/10 (50)	2/7 (29)
Skin and skin structure	9/13 (69)	5/5 (100)
Urinary tract	12/19 (63)	12/20 (60)
Pneumonia	2/3 (67)	0/1 (0)
Other*	11/13 (85)	5/13 (39)

*Includes sources of infection such as hepatic abscess, biliary sepsis, necrotic gall bladder, pericolonic abscess, pancreatitis, and catheter-related infection.

Nosocomial Pneumonia

Adult patients with clinically and radiologically documented nosocomial pneumonia were enrolled in a randomized, multi-center, double-blind trial. Patients were treated for 7 to 21 days. One group received ZYVOX I.V. Injection 600 mg q12h, and the other group received vancomycin 1 g q12h IV. Both groups received concomitant aztreonam (1 to 2 g every 8 hours IV), which could be continued if clinically indicated. There were 203 linezolid-treated and 193 vancomycin-treated patients enrolled in the study. One hundred twenty-two (60%) linezolid-treated patients and 103 (53%) vancomycin-treated patients were clinically evaluable. The cure rates in clinically evaluable patients were 57% for linezolid-treated patients and 60% for vancomycin-treated patients. The cure rates in clinically evaluable patients with ventilator-associated pneumonia were 47% for linezolid-treated patients and 40% for vancomycin-treated patients. A modified intent-to-treat (MITT) analysis of 94 linezolid-treated patients and 83 vancomycin-treated patients included subjects who had a pathogen isolated before treatment. The cure rates in the MITT analysis were 57% in linezolid-treated patients and 46% in vancomycin-treated patients. The cure rates by pathogen for microbiologically evaluable patients are presented in Table 16.

Continued on next page

Zyvox—Cont.

Table 16. Cure Rates at the Test-of-Cure Visit for Microbiologically Evaluable Adult Patients with Nosocomial Pneumonia

Pathogen	Cured	
	ZYVOX n/N (%)	Vancomycin n/N (%)
Staphylococcus aureus	23/38 (61)	14/23 (61)
Methicillin-resistant *S. aureus*	13/22 (59)	7/10 (70)
Streptococcus pneumoniae	9/9 (100)	9/10 (90)

Complicated Skin and Skin Structure Infections

Adult patients with clinically documented complicated skin and skin structure infections were enrolled in randomized, multi-center, double-blind, double-dummy trial comparing study medications administered IV followed by medications given orally for a total of 10 to 21 days of treatment. One group of patients received ZYVOX I.V. Injection 600 mg q12h followed by ZYVOX Tablets 600 mg q12h; the other group received oxacillin 2 g every 6 hours (q6h) IV followed by dicloxacillin 500 mg q6h orally. Patients could receive concomitant aztreonam if clinically indicated. There were 400 linezolid-treated and 419 oxacillin-treated patients enrolled in the study. Two hundred forty-five (61%) linezolid-treated patients and 242 (58%) oxacillin-treated patients were clinically evaluable. The cure rates in clinically evaluable patients were 90% in linezolid-treated patients and 85% in oxacillin-treated patients. A modified intent-to-treat (MITT) analysis of 316 linezolid-treated patients and 313 oxacillin-treated patients included subjects who met all criteria for study entry. The cure rates in the MITT analysis were 86% in linezolid-treated patients and 82% in oxacillin-treated patients. The cure rates by pathogen for microbiologically evaluable patients are presented in Table 17.

Table 17. Cure Rates at the Test-of-Cure Visit for Microbiologically Evaluable Adult Patients with Complicated Skin and Skin Structure Infections

Pathogen	Cured	
	ZYVOX n/N (%)	Oxacillin/ Dicloxacillin n/N (%)
Staphylococcus aureus	73/83 (88)	72/84 (86)
Methicillin-resistant *S. aureus*	2/3 (67)	0/0 (–)
Streptococcus agalactiae	6/6 (100)	3/6 (50)
Streptococcus pyogenes	18/26 (69)	21/28 (75)

A separate study provided additional experience with the use of ZYVOX in the treatment of methicillin-resistant *Staphylococcus aureus* (MRSA) infections. This was a randomized, open-label trial in hospitalized adult patients with documented or suspected MRSA infection.

One group of patients received ZYVOX I.V. Injection 600 mg q12h followed by ZYVOX Tablets 600 mg q12h. The other group of patients received vancomycin 1 g q12h IV. Both groups were treated for 7 to 28 days, and could receive concomitant aztreonam or gentamicin if clinically indicated. The cure rates in microbiologically evaluable patients with MRSA skin and skin structure infection were 26/33 (79%) for linezolid-treated patients and 24/33 (73%) for vancomycin-treated patients.

Diabetic Foot Infections

Adult diabetic patients with clinically documented complicated skin and skin structure infections ("diabetic foot infections") were enrolled in a randomized (2:1 ratio), multi-center, open-label trial comparing study medications administered IV or orally for a total of 14 to 28 days of treatment. One group of patients received ZYVOX 600 mg q12h IV or orally; the other group received ampicillin/sulbactam 1.5 to 3 g IV or amoxicillin/clavulanate 500 to 875 mg every 8 to 12 hours (q8–12h) orally. In countries where ampicillin/sulbactam is not marketed, amoxicillin/clavulanate 500 mg to 2 g every 6 hours (q6h) was used for the intravenous regimen. Patients in the comparator group could also be treated with vancomycin 1 g q12h IV if MRSA was isolated from the foot infection. Patients in either treatment group who had Gram-negative bacilli isolated from the infection site could also receive aztreonam 1 to 2 g q8–12h IV. All patients were eligible to receive appropriate adjunctive treatment methods, such as debridement and off-loading, as typically required in the treatment of diabetic foot infections, and most patients received these treatments. There were 241 linezolid-treated and 120 comparator-treated patients in the intent-to-treat (ITT) study population. Two hundred twelve (86%) linezolid-treated patients and 105 (85%) comparator-treated patients were clinically evaluable. In the ITT population, the cure rates were 68.5% (165/241) in linezolid-treated patients and 64% (77/120) in comparator-treated patients, where those with indeterminate and missing outcomes were considered failures. The cure rates in the clinically evaluable patients (excluding those with indeterminate and missing outcomes) were 83% (159/192) and 73% (74/101) in the linezolid- and comparator-treated patients, respectively. A critical post-hoc analysis focused on 121 linezolid-treated and 60 comparator-treated patients who had a Gram-positive pathogen isolated from the site of infection or from blood, who had less evidence of underlying osteomyelitis than the overall study population, and who did not receive prohibited antimicrobials. Based upon that analysis, the cure rates were 71% (86/121) in the linezolid-treated patients and 63% (38/60) in the comparator-treated patients. None of the above analyses were adjusted for the use of adjunctive therapies. The cure rates by pathogen for microbiologically evaluable patients are presented in Table 18.

Table 18. Cure Rates at the Test-of-Cure Visit for Microbiologically Evaluable Adult Patients with Diabetic Foot Infections

Pathogen	Cured	
	ZYVOX n/N (%)	Comparator n/N (%)
Staphylococcus aureus	49/63 (78)	20/29 (69)
Methicillin-resistant *S. aureus*	12/17 (71)	2/3 (67)
Streptococcus agalactiae	25/29 (86)	9/16 (56)

Pediatric Patients

Infections Due to Gram-positive Organisms

A safety and efficacy study provided experience on the use of ZYVOX in pediatric patients for the treatment of nosocomial pneumonia, complicated skin and skin structure infections, catheter-related bacteremia, bacteremia of unidentified source, and other infections due to Gram-positive bacterial pathogens, including methicillin-resistant and -susceptible *Staphylococcus aureus* and vancomycin-resistant *Enterococcus faecium*. Pediatric patients ranging in age from birth through 11 years with infections caused by the documented or suspected Gram-positive organisms were enrolled in a randomized, open-label, comparator-controlled trial. One group of patients received ZYVOX I.V. Injection 10 mg/kg every 8 hours (q8h) followed by ZYVOX for Oral Suspension 10 mg/kg q8h. A second group received vancomycin 10 to 15 mg/kg IV every 6 to 24 hours, depending on age and renal clearance. Patients who had confirmed VRE infections were placed in a third arm of the study and received ZYVOX 10 mg/kg q8h IV and/or orally. All patients were treated for a total of 10 to 28 days and could receive concomitant Gram-negative antibiotics if clinically indi-

Table 12. Percent of Pediatric Patients who Experienced at Least One Substantially Abnormal* Hematology Laboratory Value in Comparator-Controlled Clinical Trials with ZYVOX

Laboratory Assay	Uncomplicated Skin and Skin Structure Infections†		All Other Indications‡	
	ZYVOX	Cefadroxil	ZYVOX	Vancomycin
Hemoglobin (g/dL)	0.0	0.0	15.7	12.4
Platelet count (× 10³/mm³)	0.0	0.4	12.9	13.4
WBC (× 10³/mm³)	0.8	0.8	12.4	10.3
Neutrophils (× 10³/mm³)	1.2	0.8	5.9	4.3

* <75% (<50% for neutrophils) of Lower Limit of Normal (LLN) for values normal at baseline; <75% (<50% for neutrophils) of LLN and <75% (<50% for neutrophils, <90% for hemoglobin if baseline <LLN) of baseline for values abnormal at baseline.

† Patients 5 through 11 years of age received ZYVOX 10 mg/kg PO q12h or cefadroxil 15 mg/kg PO q12h. Patients 12 years or older received ZYVOX 600 mg PO q12h or cefadroxil 500 mg PO q12h.

‡ Patients from birth through 11 years of age received ZYVOX 10 mg/kg IV/PO q8h or vancomycin 10 to 15 mg/kg IV q6-24h, depending on age and renal clearance.

Table 13. Percent of Pediatric Patients who Experienced at Least One Substantially Abnormal* Serum Chemistry Laboratory Value in Comparator-Controlled Clinical Trials with ZYVOX

Laboratory Assay	Uncomplicated Skin and Skin Structure Infections†		All Other Indications‡	
	ZYVOX	Cefadroxil	ZYVOX	Vancomycin
ALT (U/L)	0.0	0.0	10.1	12.5
Lipase (U/L)	0.4	1.2	—	—
Amylase (U/L)	—	—	0.6	1.3
Total bilirubin (mg/dL)	—	—	6.3	5.2
Creatinine (mg/dL)	0.4	0.0	2.4	1.0

* >2 × Upper Limit of Normal (ULN) for values normal at baseline; >2 × ULN and >2 (>1.5 for total bilirubin) × baseline for values abnormal at baseline.

† Patients 5 through 11 years of age received ZYVOX 10 mg/kg PO q12h or cefadroxil 15 mg/kg PO q12h. Patients 12 years or older received ZYVOX 600 mg PO q12h or cefadroxil 500 mg PO q12h.

‡ Patients from birth through 11 years of age received ZYVOX 10 mg/kg IV/PO q8h or vancomycin 10 to 15 mg/kg IV q6-24h, depending on age and renal clearance.

Table 14. Dosage Guidelines for ZYVOX

Infection*	Dosage and Route of Administration		Recommended Duration of Treatment (consecutive days)
	Pediatric Patients† (Birth through 11 Years of Age)	Adults and Adolescents (12 Years and Older)	
Complicated skin and skin structure infections	10 mg/kg IV or oral‡ q8h	600 mg IV or oral‡ q12h	10 to 14
Community-acquired pneumonia, including concurrent bacteremia	10 mg/kg IV or oral‡ q8h	600 mg IV or oral‡ q12h	10 to 14
Nosocomial pneumonia	10 mg/kg IV or oral‡ q8h	600 mg IV or oral‡ q12h	10 to 14
Vancomycin-resistant *Enterococcus faecium* infections, including concurrent bacteremia	10 mg/kg IV or oral‡ q8h	600 mg IV or oral‡ q12h	14 to 28
Uncomplicated skin and skin structure infections	<5 yrs: 10 mg/kg oral‡ q8h 5-11 yrs: 10 mg/kg oral‡ q12h	Adults: 400 mg oral‡ q12h Adolescents: 600 mg oral‡ q12h	10 to 14

* Due to the designated pathogens (see **INDICATIONS AND USAGE**)

† **Neonates <7 days:** Most pre-term neonates <7 days of age (gestational age <34 weeks) have lower systemic linezolid clearance values and larger AUC values than many full-term neonates and older infants. These neonates should be initiated with a dosing regimen of 10 mg/kg q12h. Consideration may be given to the use of 10 mg/kg q8h regimen in neonates with a sub-optimal clinical response. All neonatal patients should receive 10 mg/kg q8h by 7 days of life (see **CLINICAL PHARMACOLOGY, Special Populations, Pediatric**).

‡ Oral dosing using either ZYVOX Tablets or ZYVOX for Oral Suspension

Table 19. Cure Rates at the Test-of-Cure Visit for Intent to Treat, Modified Intent to Treat, and Clinically Evaluable Pediatric Patients by Baseline Diagnosis

Population	ITT		MITT*		Clinically Evaluable	
	ZYVOX n/N (%)	Vancomycin n/N (%)	ZYVOX n/N (%)	Vancomycin n/N (%)	ZYVOX n/N (%)	Vancomycin n/N (%)
Any diagnosis	150/186 (81)	69/83 (83)	86/108 (80)	44/49 (90)	106/117 (91)	49/54 (91)
Bacteremia of unidentified source	22/29 (76)	11/16 (69)	8/12 (67)	7/8 (88)	14/17 (82)	7/9 (78)
Catheter-related bacteremia	30/41 (73)	8/12 (67)	25/35 (71)	7/10 (70)	21/25 (84)	7/9 (78)
Complicated skin and skin structure infections	61/72 (85)	31/34 (91)	37/43 (86)	22/23 (96)	46/49 (94)	26/27 (96)
Nosocomial pneumonia	13/18 (72)	11/12 (92)	5/6 (83)	4/4 (100)	7/7 (100)	5/5 (100)
Other infections	24/26 (92)	8/9 (89)	11/12 (92)	4/4 (100)	18/19 (95)	4/4 (100)

* MITT = ITT patients with an isolated Gram-positive pathogen at baseline

cated. In the intent-to-treat (ITT) population, there were 206 patients randomized to linezolid and 102 patients randomized to vancomycin. One hundred seventeen (57%) linezolid-treated patients and 55 (54%) vancomycin-treated patients were clinically evaluable. The cure rates in ITT patients were 81% in patients randomized to linezolid and 83% in patients randomized to vancomycin (95% Confidence Interval of the treatment difference; –13%, 8%). The cure rates in clinically evaluable patients were 91% in linezolid-treated patients and 91% in vancomycin-treated patients (95% CI; -11%, 11%). Modified intent-to-treat (MITT) patients included ITT patients who, at baseline, had a Gram-positive pathogen isolated from the site of infection or from blood. The cure rates in MITT patients were 80% in patients randomized to linezolid and 90% in patients randomized to vancomycin (95% CI; -23%, 3%). The cure rates for ITT, MITT, and clinically evaluable patients are presented in Table 19, and cure rates by pathogen for microbiologically evaluable patients are provided in Table 20.

[See table 19 above]

Table 20. Cure Rates at the Test-of-Cure Visit for Microbiologically Evaluable Pediatric Patients with Infections due to Gram-positive Pathogens

Pathogen	Microbiologically Evaluable	
	ZYVOX n/N (%)	Vancomycin n/N (%)
Vancomycin-resistant *Enterococcus faecium*	1/1 (100)	0/0 (–)
Staphylococcus aureus	36/38 (95)	23/24 (96)
Methicillin-resistant *S. aureus*	16/17 (94)	9/9 (100)
Streptococcus pyogenes	2/2 (100)	1/2 (50)

REFERENCES

1. Gonzales RD, PC Schreckenberger, MB Graham, et al. Infections due to vancomycin-resistant *Enterococcus faecium* resistant to linezolid. The Lancet 2001;357:1179.
2. Herrero IA, NC Issa, R Patel. Nosocomial spread of linezolid-resistant, vancomycin-resistant *Enterococcus faecium*. The New England Journal of Medicine 2002;346:867-869.
3. Tsiodras S, HS Gold, G Sakoulas, et al. Linezolid resistance in a clinical isolate of *Staphylococcus aureus.* The Lancet 2001;358:207-208.
4. Goldman DA, RA Weinstein, RP Wenzel, et al. Strategies to prevent and control the emergence and spread of antimicrobial-resistant microorganisms in hospitals. A challenge to hospital leadership. The Journal of the American Medical Association 1996;275:234-240.
5. Centers for Disease Control and Prevention. Guideline for hand hygiene in health-care settings: Recommendations of the Healthcare Infection Control Practices Advisory Committee and the HIPAC/SHEA/APIC/IDSA Hand Hygiene Task Force. Morbidity and Mortality Weekly Report 2002;51 (RR-16).
6. National Committee for Clinical Laboratory Standards. Methods for Dilution Antimicrobial Susceptibility Tests for Bacteria that Grow Aerobically. Fifth Edition. Approved Standard NCCLS Document M7-A5, Vol. 20, No. 2, NCCLS, Wayne, PA, January 2000.
7. National Committee for Clinical Laboratory Standards. Twelfth Informational Supplement. Approved NCCLS Document M100-S12, Vol. 21, No. 1, NCCLS, Wayne, PA, January 2002.
8. National Committee for Clinical Laboratory Standards. Performance Standards for Antimicrobial Disk Susceptibility Tests. Seventh Edition. Approved Standard NCCLS Document M2-A7, Vol. 20, No. 1, NCCLS, Wayne, PA, January 2000.
9. Walker SE et al. Tyramine content of previously restricted foods in monoamine oxidase inhibitor diets. Journal of Clinical Psychopharmacology 1996;16(5):383-388.
10. DaPrada M et al. On tyramine, food, beverages and the reversible MAO inhibitor moclobemide. Journal of Neural Transmission 1988; [Supplement] 26:31-56.

℞ only

US Patent Nos. 5,688,792; 6,559,305

Injection

Manufactured for: Pharmacia & Upjohn Company
A subsidiary of Pharmacia Corporation
Kalamazoo, Michigan 49001

By: Fresenius Kabi Norge AS
Halden, Norway

Tablets and Oral Suspension

Manufactured by: Pharmacia & Upjohn Company
A subsidiary of Pharmacia Corporation
Kalamazoo, Michigan 49001

Revised November 2003 818 073 306
693418

Roche Pharmaceuticals

Roche Laboratories Inc.
340 Kingsland Street
Nutley, NJ 07110-1199

For Medical Information:
(Including routine inquiries, adverse drug events and product complaints)
Call: (800) 526-6367
In Emergencies: 24-hour service
For the Medical Needs Program:
Call: (800) 285-4484
Write: Professional Product Information
Order Fulfillment
(800) 526-0625

FORTOVASE® ℞

[fŏr-tō-văs]
(saquinavir)
SOFT GELATIN CAPSULES
Rx only

Prescribing information for this product, which appears on pages 2905–2909 of the 2004 PDR, has been completely revised as follows. Please write "See Supplement A" next to the product heading.

Product identification in this document includes: INVIRASE® in reference to saquinavir mesylate; FORTOVASE in reference to saquinavir, and saquinavir in reference to the active base.

DESCRIPTION

FORTOVASE brand of saquinavir is an inhibitor of the human immunodeficiency virus (HIV) protease. FORTOVASE is available as beige, opaque, soft gelatin capsules for oral administration in a 200-mg strength (as saquinavir free base). Each capsule also contains the inactive ingredients medium chain mono- and diglycerides, povidone and dl-alpha tocopherol. Each capsule shell contains gelatin and glycerol 85% with the following colorants: red iron oxide, yellow iron oxide, and titanium dioxide. The chemical name for saquinavir is N-tert-butyl-decahydro-2-[2(R)-hydroxy-4-phenyl-3(S)-[[N-(2-quinolylcarbonyl)-L-asparaginyl]amino]butyl]-(4aS,8aS)-isoquinoline-3(S)-carboxamide which has a molecular formula $C_{38}H_{50}N_6O_5$ and a molecular weight of 670.86.

Saquinavir is a white to off-white powder and is insoluble in aqueous medium at 25°C.

MICROBIOLOGY

Mechanism of Action

Saquinavir is an inhibitor of HIV protease. HIV protease is an enzyme required for the proteolytic cleavage of viral polyprotein precursors into individual functional proteins found in infectious HIV. Saquinavir is a peptide-like substrate analogue that binds to the protease active site and inhibits the activity of the enzyme. Saquinavir inhibition prevents cleavage of the viral polyproteins resulting in the formation of immature noninfectious virus particles.

Antiviral Activity

In vitro antiviral activity of saquinavir was assessed in lymphoblastoid and monocytic cell lines and in peripheral blood lymphocytes. Saquinavir inhibited HIV activity in both acutely and chronically infected cells. IC_{50} and IC_{90} values (50% and 90% inhibitory concentrations) were in the range of 1 to 30 nM and 5 to 80 nM, respectively. In the presence of 40% human serum, the mean IC_{50} of saquinavir against laboratory strain HIV-1 RF in MT4 cells was 37.7 ± 5 nM, representing a 4-fold increase in IC_{50} value. In cell culture, saquinavir demonstrated additive to synergistic effects against HIV-1 in combination with reverse transcriptase inhibitors (didanosine, lamivudine, nevirapine, stavudine, zalcitabine and zidovudine) without enhanced cytotoxicity. Saquinavir in combination with the protease inhibitors amprenavir, atazanavir, or lopinavir resulted in synergistic antiviral activity.

Drug Resistance

HIV-1 mutants with reduced susceptibility to saquinavir have been selected during in vitro passage. Genotypic analyses of these isolates showed several substitutions in the HIV protease gene. Only the G48V and L90M substitutions were associated with reduced susceptibility to saquinavir, and conferred an increase in the IC_{50}value of 8- and 3-fold, respectively.

HIV-1 isolates with reduced susceptibility (≥4-fold increase in the IC_{50} value) to saquinavir emerged in some patients treated with INVIRASE. Genotypic analysis of these isolates identified resistance conferring primary mutations in the protease gene G48V and L90M, and secondary mutations L10I/R/V, I54V/L, A71V/T, G73S, V77I, V82A and I84V that contributed additional resistance to saquinavir. Forty-one isolates from 37 patients failing therapy with INVIRASE had a median decrease in susceptibility to saquinavir of 4.3 fold.

The degree of reduction in in vitro susceptibility to saquinavir of clinical isolates bearing substitutions G48V and L90M depends on the number of secondary mutations present. In general, higher levels of resistance are associated with greater number of mutations only in association with either or both of the primary mutations G48V and L90M. No data are currently available to address the development of resistance in patients receiving saquinavir/ritonavir.

Cross-resistance

Among protease inhibitors, variable cross-resistance has been observed. In one clinical study, 22 HIV-1 isolates with reduced susceptibility (>4-fold increase in the IC_{50} value) to saquinavir following therapy with INVIRASE were evaluated for cross-resistance to amprenavir, indinavir, nelfinavir and ritonavir. Six of the 22 isolates (27%) remained susceptible to all 4 protease inhibitors, 12 of the 22 isolates (55%) retained susceptibility to at least one of the PIs and 4 out of the 22 isolates (18%) displayed broad cross-resistance to all PIs.

Sixteen (73%) and 11 (50%) of the 22 isolates remained susceptible (<4-fold) to amprenavir and indinavir, respectively. Four of 16 (25%) and 9 of 21 (43%) with available data remained susceptible to nelfinavir and ritonavir, respectively.

After treatment failure with amprenavir, cross-resistance to saquinavir was evaluated. HIV-1 isolates from 22/22 patients failing treatment with amprenavir and containing one or more mutations M46L/I , I50V, I54L, V32I, I47V, and I84V were susceptible to saquinavir.

CLINICAL PHARMACOLOGY

Pharmacokinetics

The pharmacokinetic properties of saquinavir when administered as FORTOVASE have been evaluated in healthy volunteers (n=207) and HIV-infected patients (n=91) after single-oral doses (range: 300 mg to 1200 mg) and multiple-oral doses (range: 400 mg to 1200 mg tid). The disposition properties of saquinavir have been studied in healthy volunteers after intravenous doses of 6, 12, 36 or 72 mg (n=21).

HIV-infected patients administered FORTOVASE (1200 mg tid) had AUC and maximum plasma concentration (C_{max}) values approximately twice those observed in healthy volunteers receiving the same treatment regimen. The mean AUC values at week 1 were 4159 (CV 88%) and 8839 (CV 82%) ng•h/mL, and C_{max} values were 1420 (CV 81%) and 2477 (CV 76%) ng/mL for healthy volunteers and HIV-infected patients, respectively.

Absorption and Bioavailability in Adults

The absolute bioavailability of saquinavir administered as FORTOVASE has not been assessed. However, following single 600-mg doses, the relative bioavailability of saquinavir as FORTOVASE compared to saquinavir administered as INVIRASE was estimated as 331% (95% CI: 207% to 530%). The absolute bioavailability of saquinavir administered as INVIRASE averaged 4% (CV 73%, range: 1% to 9%) in 8 healthy volunteers who received a single 600-mg dose (3 x 200 mg) of INVIRASE following a high-fat breakfast (48 g protein, 60 g carbohydrate, 57 g fat; 1006 kcal). In healthy volunteers receiving single doses of FORTOVASE (300 mg to 1200 mg) and in HIV-infected patients receiving multiple doses of FORTOVASE (400 mg to 1200 mg tid), a greater than dose-proportional increase in saquinavir plasma concentrations has been observed.

Continued on next page

Fortovase—Cont.

Comparison of pharmacokinetic parameters between single- and multiple-dose studies shows that following multiple dosing of FORTOVASE (1200 mg tid) in healthy male volunteers (n=18), the steady-state AUC was 80% (95% CI: 22% to 176%) higher than that observed after a single 1200-mg dose (n=30).

Saquinavir plasma concentrations remained stable over a 60-week period of continued treatment in patients in a phase III substudy.

When administered as the sole protease inhibitor, it has been shown that FORTOVASE 1200 mg tid provides an 8-fold increase in AUC compared with INVIRASE 600 mg tid.

FORTOVASE in combination with ritonavir at doses of 400/400 mg bid, or 1000/100 mg bid provide saquinavir systemic exposures over a 24-hour period similar to or greater than those achieved with FORTOVASE 1200 mg tid.

[See table 1 above]

Food Effect

The mean 12-hour AUC after a single 800-mg oral dose of saquinavir in healthy volunteers (n=12) was increased from 167 ng•h/mL (CV 45%), under fasting conditions, to 1120 ng•h/mL (CV 54%) when FORTOVASE was given following a high-fat breakfast (45 g protein, 76 g carbohydrate, 55 g fat; 961 kcal). The effect of food with INVIRASE has been shown to persist for up to 2 hours. The mean 12-hour AUC after a single 1200-mg oral dose of FORTOVASE in healthy volunteers (n=12) was increased from 952 ng•h/mL, following a light meal (21 g protein, 50 g carbohydrate, 28 g fat; 524 kcal) to 1388 ng•h/mL when FORTOVASE was given following a high-fat breakfast (45 g protein, 76 g carbohydrate, 55 g fat; 961 kcal).

Saquinavir exposure was similar when FORTOVASE plus ritonavir (1000-mg/100-mg bid) was administered following a high-fat (45 g fat) or moderate-fat (20 g fat) breakfast.

Distribution in Adults

The mean steady-state volume of distribution following intravenous administration of a 12-mg dose of saquinavir (n=8) was 700 L (CV 39%), suggesting saquinavir partitions into tissues. It has been shown that saquinavir, up to 30 μg/mL, is approximately 97% bound to plasma proteins.

Metabolism and Elimination in Adults

In vitro studies using human liver microsomes have shown that the metabolism of saquinavir is cytochrome P450 mediated with the specific isoenzyme, CYP3A4, responsible for more than 90% of the hepatic metabolism. Based on in vitro studies, saquinavir is rapidly metabolized to a range of mono- and di-hydroxylated inactive compounds. In a mass balance study using 600 mg ^{14}C-saquinavir mesylate (n=8), 88% and 1% of the orally administered radioactivity was recovered in feces and urine, respectively, within 5 days of dosing. In an additional 4 subjects administered 10.5 mg ^{14}C-saquinavir intravenously, 81% and 3% of the intravenously administered radioactivity was recovered in feces and urine, respectively, within 5 days of dosing. In mass balance studies, 13% of circulating radioactivity in plasma was attributed to unchanged drug after oral administration and the remainder attributed to saquinavir metabolites. Following intravenous administration, 66% of circulating radioactivity was attributed to unchanged drug and the remainder attributed to saquinavir metabolites, suggesting that saquinavir undergoes extensive first-pass metabolism.

Systemic clearance of saquinavir was rapid, 1.14 L/h/kg (CV 12%) after intravenous doses of 6, 36, and 72 mg. The mean residence time of saquinavir was 7 hours (n=8).

Special Populations

Hepatic or Renal Impairment

Saquinavir pharmacokinetics in patients with hepatic or renal impairment has not been investigated (see PRECAUTIONS). Only 1% of saquinavir is excreted in the urine, so the impact of renal impairment on saquinavir elimination should be minimal.

Gender, Race and Age

The effect of gender was investigated in healthy volunteers receiving single 1200-mg doses of FORTOVASE (n=12 females, 18 males). No effect of gender was apparent on the pharmacokinetics of saquinavir in this study.

The effect of race on the pharmacokinetics of saquinavir has not been investigated.

Pediatric Patients

The pharmacokinetics of saquinavir in pediatric patients differs significantly from that in adults. Children have a markedly higher apparent clearance than adults and administration of saquinavir alone will not give consistently therapeutic plasma levels. The pharmacokinetics of saquinavir when coadministered with ritonavir to pediatric patients is under investigation.

Geriatric Patients

The pharmacokinetics of saquinavir when administered as FORTOVASE have not been sufficiently investigated in patients >65 years of age.

Drug Interactions (see PRECAUTIONS: Drug Interactions)

It is important to be aware that, when coadministered with ritonavir, the occurrence and magnitude of drug interactions may differ from those seen with FORTOVASE when administered as the sole protease inhibitor. When ritonavir is coadministered, prescribers should refer to the prescribing information for ritonavir regarding drug interactions associated with this drug.

Table 2 summarizes the effect of FORTOVASE on the geometric mean AUC and C_{max} of coadministered drugs. Table 3 summarizes the effect of coadministered drugs on the geometric mean AUC and C_{max} of saquinavir.

Table 1 Pharmacokinetic Parameters of Saquinavir at Steady-State After Administration of Different Regimens in HIV-Infected Patients

Dosing Regimen	n	$AUC_{0-\tau}$ (ng•h/mL)	AUC_{0-24h} (ng•h/mL)	C_{min} (ng/mL)
FORTOVASE 1200 mg tid (arithmetic mean)	31	7249	21747	216
INVIRASE 400 mg bid + ritonavir 400 mg bid (arithmetic mean± SD)	7	16000±8000	32000	480±360
INVIRASE 1000 mg bid + ritonavir 100 mg bid (geometric mean and 95% CI)	24	14607 (10218-20882)	29214	371 (245-561)
FORTOVASE 1000 mg bid + ritonavir 100 mg bid (geometric mean and 95% CI)	24	19085 (13943-26124)	38170	433 (301-622)

τ is the dosing interval (ie, 8h if tid and 12h if bid).

Table 2 Effect of FORTOVASE on the Pharmacokinetics of Coadministered Drugs

Coadministered Drug	FORTOVASE or FORTOVASE/ritonavir Dose	N	% Change for Coadministered Drug	
			AUC (95%CI)	C_{max} (95%CI)
Clarithromycin 500 mg bid × 7 days Clarithromycin 14-OH clarithromycin metabolite	1200 mg tid × 7 days	12V	 ↑45% (17-81%) ↓24% (5-40%)	 ↑39% (10-76%) ↓34% (14-50%)
Midazolam 7.5–mg oral single dose	1200 mg tid × 5 days	6V	↑514%	↑235%
Nelfinavir 750-mg single dose	1200 mg tid × 4 days	14P	↑18% (5-33%)	↔
Rifabutin 300 mg once daily	1200 mg tid	14P	↑44%	↑45%
Ritonavir 400 mg bid × 14 days	400 mg bid × 14 days	8V	↔	↔
Sildenafil 100-mg single dose	1200 mg tid × 8 days	27V	↑210% (150-300%)	↑140% (80-230%)
Terfenadine[ɸ] 60 mg bid × 11 days* Terfenadine Terfenadine acid metabolite	1200 mg tid × 4 days	12V	 ↑368% (257-514%) ↑120% (89-156%)	 ↑253% (164-373%) ↑93% (59-133%)
Efavirenz 600 mg	1200 mg tid	13V	↓12%	↓13%
Ketoconazole 400 mg once daily	1200 mg tid	12V	↔	↔
Enfuvirtide 90 mg SC q12h (bid) for 7 days	1000/100 mg bid	12 P	↔	↔

↑ Denotes an average increase in exposure by the percentage indicated.
↓ Denotes an average decrease in exposure by the percentage indicated.
↔Denotes no statistically significant change in exposure was observed.
* FORTOVASE should not be coadministered with terfenadine (see PRECAUTIONS: Drug Interactions).
P Patient
V Healthy Volunteers
ɸ No longer marketed in the US.

Table 3 Effect of Coadministered Drugs on FORTOVASE Pharmacokinetics

Coadministered Drug	FORTOVASE Dose	N	% Change for Saquinavir	
			AUC (95%CI)	C_{max} (95%CI)
Clarithromycin 500 mg bid × 7 days	1200 mg tid × 7 days	12V	↑177% (108-269%)	↑187% (105-300%)
Efavirenz 600 mg	1200 mg tid	13V	↓62%	↓50%
Indinavir 800 mg q8h × 2 days	1200-mg single dose	6V	↑364% (190-644%)	↑299% (138-568%)
Ketoconazole 400 mg once daily	1200 mg tid	12V	↑190%	↑171%
Nelfinavir 750 mg × 4 days	1200-mg single dose	14P	↑392% (271-553%)	↑179% (105-280%)
Rifabutin 300 mg once daily	1200 mg tid	14P	↓47%	↓31%
Rifampin 600 mg once daily	1200 mg tid × 14 days	14V	↓70%	↓65%
Ritonavir 100 mg bid	1000 mg bid†	24P	↑176%	↑153%
Ritonavir 400 mg bid × 14 days*	400 mg tid × 14 days†	8V	↑121% (7–359%)	↑64%§
Lopinavir/ritonavir 400/100 mg bid, 15 days	800 mg bid, 10 days combo vs. 1200 mg tid, 5 days alone	14V	↑9.62-fold (8.05, 11.49)^	↑6.34-fold (5.32, 7.55)^
400/100 mg bid, 20 days	1200 mg bid, 5 days combo vs. 1200 mg tid 5 days alone	10V	↑9.91-fold (8.28, 11.86)^	↑6.44-fold (5.59, 7.41)^

↑ Denotes an average increase in exposure by the percentage indicated.
↓ Denotes an average decrease in exposure by the percentage indicated.
* When ritonavir was combined with the same dose of either INVIRASE or FORTOVASE, actual mean plasma exposures (AUC_{0-12}, 18200 ng•h/mL, 20000 ng•h/mL, respectively) were not significantly different.
^ 90% CI reported
† Compared to standard FORTOVASE 1200 mg tid regimen (n=33).
P Patient
V Healthy Volunteers

[See table 2 above]
[See table 3 above]
For information regarding clinical recommendations, see PRECAUTIONS: Drug Interactions, Table 6.

INDICATIONS AND USAGE

FORTOVASE is indicated for use in combination with other antiretroviral agents for the treatment of HIV infection. This indication is based on studies that showed increased saquinavir concentrations and improved antiviral activity for FORTOVASE 1200 mg tid compared to INVIRASE 600 mg tid.

In treatment-naive and treatment-experienced patients, the efficacy of FORTOVASE (with or without ritonavir coadministration) has not been compared against the efficacy of antiretroviral regimens currently considered standard of care.

Description of Clinical Studies

When used in combination with other antiretroviral agents, FORTOVASE and INVIRASE have been shown to decrease plasma HIV RNA levels and increase CD4 cell counts in an open-label randomized study (NV15355) in treatment-naive, HIV-infected patients. In addition, in a randomized, double-blind study (NV14256) in ZDV-experienced, HIV-infected patients, a combination regimen of FORTOVASE and HIVID was shown to be superior to either INVIRASE or HIVID monotherapy in decreasing the cumulative incidence of clinical disease progression to AIDS-defining events or death. It should be noted that HIV treatment regimens that were used in the initial clinical studies of INVIRASE are no longer considered standard of care.

FORTOVASE 1000 mg bid coadministered with ritonavir 100 mg bid was studied in a heterogeneous population of 148 HIV infected patients (MaxCmin 1 study). At baseline 42 were treatment naive and 106 were treatment experienced (of which 52 had an HIV RNA level <400 copies/mL at baseline). Results showed that 91/148 (61%) subjects achieved and/or sustained and HIV RNA level <400 copies/mL at the completion of 48 weeks.

Study NV15182 was an open-label safety study of FORTOVASE in combination with other antiretroviral agents in HIV-infected patients. The 48-week safety results from this study are displayed in the ADVERSE REACTIONS section.

CONTRAINDICATIONS

FORTOVASE is contraindicated in patients with clinically significant hypersensitivity to saquinavir or to any of the components contained in the capsule.

FORTOVASE should not be administered concurrently with terfenadine, cisapride, astemizole, pimozide, triazolam, midazolam, or ergot derivatives, because competition for CYP3A4 by saquinavir could result in inhibition of the metabolism of these drugs and create the potential for serious and/or life-threatening reactions, such as cardiac arrhythmias or prolonged sedation (see PRECAUTIONS: Drug Interactions).

FORTOVASE is contraindicated in patients with severe hepatic impairment (see PRECAUTIONS: Hepatic Effects).

FORTOVASE should not be administered concurrently with drugs listed in Table 4 (also see PRECAUTIONS: Drug Interactions, Table 5).

Table 4 Drugs That Are Contraindicated With FORTOVASE

Drug Class	Drugs Within Class That Are Contraindicated With FORTOVASE
Antiarrhythmics	Amiodarone, bepridil, flecainide, propafenone, quinidine
Antihistamines	Astemizole*, terfenadine*
Ergot Derivatives	Dihydroergotamine, ergonovine, ergotamine, methylergonovine
Antimycobacterial Agents	Rifampin
GI Motility Agent	Cisapride*
Neuroleptics	Pimozide
Sedative/Hypnotics	Triazolam, midazolam

*No longer marketed in the US.

If FORTOVASE is coadministered with ritonavir, the ritonavir label should be reviewed for additional contraindicated drugs.

WARNINGS

ALERT: Find out about medicines that should not be taken with FORTOVASE. This statement is included on the product's bottle label.

Interaction with HMG-CoA Reductase Inhibitors

Concomitant use of FORTOVASE with lovastatin or simvastatin is not recommended. Caution should be exercised if HIV protease inhibitors, including FORTOVASE, are used concurrently with other HMG-CoA reductase inhibitors that are also metabolized by the CYP3A4 pathway (eg, atorvastatin). Since increased concentrations of statins can, in rare cases, cause severe adverse events such as myopathy including rhabdomyolysis, this risk may be increased when HIV protease inhibitors, including saquinavir, are used in combination with these drugs.

Interaction with St. John's Wort (hypericum perforatum)

Concomitant use of FORTOVASE and St. John's wort (hypericum perforatum) or products containing St. John's wort is not recommended. Coadministration of protease inhibitors, including FORTOVASE, with St. John's wort is expected to substantially decrease protease inhibitor concentrations and may result in sub-optimal levels of FORTOVASE and lead to loss of virologic response and possible resistance to FORTOVASE or to the class of protease inhibitors.

Interaction with Garlic Capsules

Garlic capsules should not be used while taking saquinavir as the sole protease inhibitor due to the risk of decreased saquinavir plasma concentrations. No data are available for the coadministration of FORTOVASE/ritonavir or INVIRASE/ritonavir and garlic capsules.

Diabetes Mellitus and Hyperglycemia

New onset diabetes mellitus, exacerbation of pre-existing diabetes mellitus and hyperglycemia have been reported during postmarketing surveillance in HIV-infected patients receiving protease-inhibitor therapy. Some patients required either initiation or dose adjustments of insulin or oral hypoglycemic agents for the treatment of these events. In some cases diabetic ketoacidosis has occurred. In those patients who discontinued protease-inhibitor therapy, hyperglycemia persisted in some cases. Because these events have been reported voluntarily during clinical practice, estimates of frequency cannot be made and a causal relationship between protease-inhibitor therapy and these events has not been established.

PRECAUTIONS

General

FORTOVASE (saquinavir) soft gelatin capsules and INVIRASE (saquinavir mesylate) capsules are not bioequivalent and cannot be used interchangeably when used as the sole protease inhibitor. Only FORTOVASE should be used for the initiation of therapy that includes saquinavir as a sole protease inhibitor (see DOSAGE AND ADMINISTRATION) since FORTOVASE soft gelatin capsules provide greater bioavailability and efficacy than INVIRASE capsules.

If a serious or severe toxicity occurs during treatment with FORTOVASE, FORTOVASE should be interrupted until the etiology of the event is identified or the toxicity resolves. At that time, resumption of treatment with full-dose FORTOVASE may be considered. For antiretroviral agents used in combination with FORTOVASE, physicians should refer to the complete product information for these drugs for dose adjustment recommendations and for information regarding drug-associated adverse reactions.

Hepatic Effects

The use of FORTOVASE by patients with hepatic impairment has not been studied. In the absence of such studies, caution should be exercised, as increases in saquinavir levels and/or increases in liver enzymes may occur. In patients with underlying hepatitis B or C, cirrhosis, chronic alcoholism and/or other underlying liver abnormalities there have been reports of worsening liver disease.

Renal Effects

Renal clearance is only a minor elimination pathway; the principal route of metabolism and excretion for saquinavir is by the liver. Therefore, no dose adjustment is necessary for patients with renal impairment. However, patients with severe renal impairment have not been studied and caution should be exercised when prescribing saquinavir in this population.

Hemophilia

There have been reports of spontaneous bleeding in patients with hemophilia A and B treated with protease inhibitors. In some patients additional factor VIII was required. In the majority of reported cases treatment with protease inhibitors was continued or restarted. A causal relationship between protease-inhibitor therapy and these episodes has not been established.

Hyperlipidemia

Elevated cholesterol and/or triglyceride levels have been observed in some patients taking saquinavir in combination with ritonavir. Marked elevation in triglyceride levels is a risk factor for development of pancreatitis. Cholesterol and triglyceride levels should be monitored prior to initiating combination dosing regimen of FORTOVASE or INVIRASE with ritonavir, and at periodic intervals while on such therapy. In these patients, lipid disorders should be managed as clinically appropriate.

Fat Redistribution

Redistribution/accumulation of body fat including central obesity, dorsocervical fat enlargement (buffalo hump), facial wasting, peripheral wasting, breast enlargement, and "cushingoid appearance" have been observed in patients receiving antiretroviral therapy. A causal relationship between protease inhibitor therapy and these events has not been established and the long-term consequences are currently unknown.

Resistance/Cross-resistance

Varying degrees of cross-resistance among protease inhibitors have been observed. Continued administration of FORTOVASE therapy following loss of viral suppression may increase the likelihood of cross-resistance to other protease inhibitors (see MICROBIOLOGY).

Information for Patients

A statement to patients and health care providers is included on the product's bottle label: **ALERT: Find out about medicines that should NOT be taken with FORTOVASE.** A Patient Package Insert (PPI) for FORTOVASE is available for patient information.

Patients should be informed that any change from INVIRASE to FORTOVASE or FORTOVASE to INVIRASE coadministered with ritonavir should be made only under the supervision of a physician.

FORTOVASE may interact with some drugs; therefore, patients should be advised to report to their doctor the use of any other prescription, nonprescription medication, or herbal products, particularly St. John's wort.

Patients should be informed that FORTOVASE is not a cure for HIV infection and that they may continue to acquire illnesses associated with advanced HIV infection, including opportunistic infections. Patients should be advised that FORTOVASE should be used only in combination with other active antiretroviral medications.

Patients should be informed that redistribution or accumulation of body fat may occur in patients receiving protease inhibitors and that the cause and long-term health effects of these conditions are not known at this time.

Patients should be told that the long-term effects of FORTOVASE are unknown at this time. They should be informed that FORTOVASE therapy has not been shown to reduce the risk of transmitting HIV to others through sexual contact or blood contamination.

Patients should be advised that FORTOVASE should be taken within 2 hours after a full meal. When FORTOVASE is coadministered with ritonavir a light meal is sufficient (see CLINICAL PHARMACOLOGY: Pharmacokinetics). Patients should be advised of the importance of taking their medication every day, as prescribed, to achieve maximum benefit. Patients should not alter the dose or discontinue therapy without consulting their physician. If a dose is missed, patients should take the next dose as soon as possible. However, the patient should not double the next dose.

Patients should be informed that refrigerated (36° to 46°F, 2° to 8°C) capsules of FORTOVASE remain stable until the expiration date printed on the label. Once brought to room temperature [at or below 77°F (25°C)], capsules should be used within 3 months.

Laboratory Tests

Clinical chemistry tests, viral load, and CD4 count should be performed prior to initiating FORTOVASE therapy and at appropriate intervals thereafter. Elevated nonfasting triglyceride levels have been observed in patients in saquinavir trials. Triglyceride levels should be periodically monitored during therapy. For comprehensive information concerning laboratory test alterations associated with use of other antiretroviral therapies, physicians should refer to the complete product information for these drugs.

Drug Interactions

Several drug interaction studies have been completed with both INVIRASE and FORTOVASE. Observations from drug interaction studies with FORTOVASE may not be predictive for INVIRASE. If ritonavir is coadministered, prescribers should also refer to the prescribing information for ritonavir regarding drug interactions associated with this agent.

The metabolism of saquinavir is mediated by cytochrome P450, with the specific isoenzyme CYP3A4 responsible for 90% of the hepatic metabolism. Additionally, saquinavir is a substrate for P-Glycoprotein (Pgp). Therefore, drugs that affect CYP3A4 and/or Pgp, may modify the pharmacokinetics of saquinavir. Similarly, saquinavir might also modify the pharmacokinetics of other drugs that are substrates for CYP3A4 or Pgp.

Drugs that are contraindicated specifically due to the expected magnitude of interaction and potential for serious adverse events are listed in Table 4 under CONTRAINDICATIONS. Additional drugs that are not recommended for coadministration with FORTOVASE are included in Table 5. These recommendations are based on either drug interaction studies or predicted interactions due to the expected magnitude of interaction and potential for serious events or loss of efficacy.

Drug interactions that have been established based on drug interaction studies are listed with the pharmacokinetic results in Table 2, which summarizes the effect of saquinavir, administered as FORTOVASE, on the geometric mean AUC and C_{max} of coadministered drugs and Table 3, which summarizes the effect of coadministered drugs on the geometric mean AUC and C_{max} of saquinavir. Clinical dose recommendations can be found in Table 6. The magnitude of interactions may be different when FORTOVASE is given with ritonavir.

[See table 5 at top of next page]

If FORTOVASE is coadministered with ritonavir, the ritonavir label should be reviewed for additional drugs that should not be coadministered.

[See table 6 on pages 400, 401 and 402]

Drugs That Are Mainly Metabolized by CYP3A4

Although specific studies have not been performed, coadministration with drugs that are mainly metabolized by CYP3A4 (eg, calcium channel blockers, dapsone, disopyramide, quinine, amiodarone, quinidine, warfarin, tacrolimus, cyclosporine, ergot derivatives, pimozide, carbamazepine, fentanyl, alfentanyl, alprazolam, nefazodone and triazolam) may have elevated plasma concentrations when coadministered with saquinavir; therefore, these combinations should be used with caution. If FORTOVASE is coadministered with ritonavir, the ritonavir label should be reviewed for additional drugs that should not be coadministered.

Inducers of CYP3A4

Coadministration with compounds that are potent inducers of CYP3A4 (eg, phenobarbital, phenytoin, dexamethasone, carbamazepine) may result in decreased plasma levels of saquinavir.

Carcinogenesis, Mutagenesis and Impairment of Fertility

Carcinogenesis

Carcinogenicity studies found no indication of carcinogenic activity in rats and mice administered saquinavir for approximately 2 years. The plasma exposures (AUC values) in the respective species were up to approximately 60% of (using rat) and equivalent to (using mouse) those obtained in humans at the recommended clinical dose (FORTOVASE 1200 mg tid).

Continued on next page

Fortovase—Cont.

Mutagenesis
Mutagenicity and genotoxicity studies, with and without metabolic activation where appropriate, have shown that saquinavir has no mutagenic activity in vitro in either bacterial (Ames test) or mammalian cells (Chinese hamster lung V79/HPRT test). Saquinavir does not induce chromosomal damage in vivo in the mouse micronucleus assay or in vitro in human peripheral blood lymphocytes and does not induce primary DNA damage in vitro in the unscheduled DNA synthesis test.
Impairment of Fertility
Fertility and reproductive performance were not affected in rats at plasma exposures (AUC values) approximately 50% of those achieved in humans at the recommended dose.
Pregnancy
Teratogenic Effects
Category B. Reproduction studies conducted with saquinavir in rats have shown no embryotoxicity or teratogenicity at plasma exposures (AUC values) approximately 50% of those achieved in humans at the recommended dose or in rabbits at plasma exposures approximately 40% of those achieved at the recommended clinical dose of FORTOVASE. Distribution studies in these species showed that placental transfer of saquinavir is low (less than 5% of maternal plasma concentrations).
Studies in rats indicated that exposure to saquinavir from late pregnancy through lactation at plasma concentrations (AUC values) approximately 50% of those achieved in humans at the recommended dose of FORTOVASE had no effect on the survival, growth and development of offspring to weaning. Clinical experience in pregnant women is limited. Saquinavir should be used during pregnancy only if the potential benefit justifies the potential risk to the fetus.
Antiretroviral Pregnancy Registry
To monitor maternal-fetal outcomes of pregnant women exposed to antiretroviral medications, including FORTOVASE, an Antiretroviral Pregnancy Registry has been established. Physicians are encouraged to register patients by calling 1-800-258-4263.
Nursing Mothers
The Centers for Disease Control and Prevention recommend that HIV-infected mothers not breast-feed their infants to avoid risking postnatal transmission of HIV. It is not known whether saquinavir is excreted in human milk. Because of both the potential for HIV transmission and the potential for serious adverse reactions in nursing infants, **mothers should be instructed not to breast-feed if they are receiving antiretroviral medications, including FORTOVASE.**
Pediatric Use
FORTOVASE should not be administered as a sole protease inhibitor to pediatric patients ≤16 years of age due to the risk of reduced saquinavir plasma concentrations compared to adults.
Safety and effectiveness of saquinavir when coadministered with ritonavir to pediatric patients is under investigation.
Geriatric Use
Clinical studies of FORTOVASE did not include sufficient numbers of subjects aged 65 and over to determine whether they respond differently from younger subjects. In general, caution should be taken when dosing FORTOVASE in elderly patients due to the greater frequency of decreased hepatic, renal, or cardiac function, and of concomitant disease or other drug therapy.

ADVERSE REACTIONS (see PRECAUTIONS)

The safety of FORTOVASE was studied in more than 500 patients who received the drug either alone or in combination with other antiretroviral agents. The majority of treatment-related adverse events were of mild intensity. The most frequently reported treatment-emergent adverse events among patients receiving FORTOVASE in combination with other antiretroviral agents were diarrhea, nausea, abdominal discomfort, and dyspepsia.
Clinical adverse events of at least moderate intensity, which occurred in ≥2% of patients in studies NV15182 (an open-label, single-arm safety study) and NV15355 (an open-label randomized study comparing FORTOVASE and INVIRASE) are summarized in Table 7. The median duration of treatment in studies NV15182 and NV15355 were 52 and 18 weeks, respectively. In NV15182, more than 300 patients were on treatment for approximately 1 year.
FORTOVASE did not appear to alter the pattern, frequency or severity of known major toxicities associated with the use of nucleoside analogues. Physicians should refer to the complete product information for other antiretroviral agents as appropriate for drug-associated adverse reactions to these other agents.
Rare occurrences of the following serious adverse experiences have been reported during clinical trials of FORTOVASE and/or INVIRASE and were considered at least possibly related to use of study drugs: confusion, ataxia and weakness; seizures; headache; acute myeloblastic leukemia; hemolytic anemia; thrombocytopenia; thrombocytopenia and intracranial hemorrhage leading to death; attempted suicide; Stevens-Johnson syndrome; bullous skin eruption and polyarthritis; severe cutaneous reaction associated with increased liver function tests; isolated elevation of transaminases; exacerbation of chronic liver disease with Grade 4 elevated liver function tests, jaundice, ascites, and right and left upper quadrant abdominal pain; pancreatitis leading to death; intestinal obstruction; portal hypertension; thrombophlebitis; peripheral vasoconstriction; drug fever; nephrolithiasis; and acute renal insufficiency.

Table 5 Drugs That Should Not Be Coadministered With FORTOVASE

Drug Class: Drug Name	Clinical Comment
Antiarrhythmics: Amiodarone, bepridil, flecainide, propafenone, quinidine	CONTRAINDICATED due to potential for serious and/or life-threatening reactions.
Antihistamines: astemizole*, terfenadine*	CONTRAINDICATED due to potential for serious and/or life-threatening cardiac arrhythmias.
Ergot Derivatives: Dihydroergotamine, ergonovine, ergotamine, methylergonovine	CONTRAINDICATED due to potential for serious and life-threatening reactions such as acute ergot toxicity characterized by peripheral vasospasm and ischemia of the extremities and other tissues.
Antimycobacterial Agents: rifampin	WARNING coadministration with rifampin is not recommended because rifampin markedly decreases the concentration of saquinavir. The safety and efficacy of this combination have not been established.
Garlic Capsules	Garlic capsules should not be used while taking saquinavir (FORTOVASE) as the sole protease inhibitor due to the risk of decreased saquinavir plasma concentrations. No data are available for the coadministration of INVIRASE/ritonavir or FORTOVASE/ritonavir and garlic capsules.
GI Motility Agent: cisapride*	CONTRAINDICATED due to potential for serious and/or life-threatening reactions such as cardiac arrhythmias.
Herbal Products: St. John's wort (hypericum perforatum)	WARNING coadministration may lead to loss of virologic response and possible resistance to FORTOVASE or to the class of protease inhibitors.
HMG-CoA Reductase Inhibitors: lovastatin, simvastatin	WARNING potential for serious reactions such as risk of myopathy including rhabdomyolysis.
Sedatives/Hypnotics: triazolam, midazolam	CONTRAINDICATED due to potential for serious and/or life-threatening reactions such as prolonged or increased sedation or respiratory depression.

* No longer marketed in the US.

Table 6 Established and Other Potentially Significant Drug Interactions: Alteration in Dose or Regimen May Be Recommended Based on Drug Interaction Studies or Predicted Interaction (Information in the table applies to FORTOVASE with or without ritonavir, unless otherwise indicated)

Concomitant Drug Class: Drug Name	Effect on Concentration of Saquinavir or Concomitant Drug	Clinical Comment
	HIV-Antiviral Agents	
Non-nucleoside reverse transcriptase inhibitor: Delavirdine	**FORTOVASE** ↑ Saquinavir Effect on delavirdine is not well established **FORTOVASE/ritonavir** Interaction has not been evaluated	Appropriate doses of the combination with respect to safety and efficacy have not been established.
Non-nucleoside reverse transcriptase inhibitor: Efavirenz*, nevirapine	**FORTOVASE** ↓ Saquinavir ↓ Efavirenz **FORTOVASE/ritonavir** Interaction has not been evaluated	FORTOVASE should not be given as the sole protease inhibitor to patients taking efavirenz or nevirapine. Appropriate doses of the combination of efavirenz or nevirapine and FORTOVASE/ritonavir with respect to safety and efficacy have not been established.
HIV protease inhibitor: Indinavir*	**FORTOVASE** ↑ Saquinavir Effect on indinavir is not well established **FORTOVASE/ritonavir** Interaction has not been evaluated	Appropriate doses of the combination with respect to safety and efficacy have not been established.
HIV protease inhibitor: Nelfinavir*	**FORTOVASE** ↑ Saquinavir ↑ Nelfinavir **FORTOVASE/ritonavir** Interaction has not been evaluated	Saquinavir 1200 mg bid with nelfinavir 1250 mg bid results in adequate plasma drug concentrations for both protease inhibitors.
HIV protease inhibitor: Ritonavir*	**FORTOVASE** ↑ Saquinavir ↔ Ritonavir	The recommended dose regimen when ritonavir is given to increase saquinavir concentrations is 1000 mg saquinavir plus ritonavir 100 mg twice daily.
HIV protease inhibitor: Lopinavir/ritonavir (coformulated capsule)*	**FORTOVASE** ↑ Saquinavir Effect on lopinavir is not well established	FORTOVASE (SQV) 800 mg bid + KALETRA produces ↑ AUC, ↑ C_{max}, and ↑ C_{min} relative to FORTOVASE 1200 mg tid (see CLINICAL PHARMACOLOGY: Table 3)
HIV fusion inhibitor: Enfuvirtide*	**FORTOVASE** Interaction has not been evaluated **FORTOVASE/ritonavir** ↔ Enfuvirtide	No clinically significant interaction was noted from a study in 12 HIV patients who received enfuvirtide concomitantly with FORTOVASE/ritonavir 1000/100 mg bid. No dose adjustments are required.
	Other Agents	
Antiarrhythmics: Lidocaine (systemic)	↑ Antiarrhythmics	Caution is warranted and therapeutic concentration monitoring, if available, is recommended for antiarrhythmics given with FORTOVASE or FORTOVASE/ritonavir
Anticoagulant: Warfarin		Concentrations of warfarin may be affected. It is recommended that INR (international normalized ratio) be monitored.

(Table continued on next page)

Table 6 *(cont.)* **Established and Other Potentially Significant Drug Interactions: Alteration in Dose or Regimen May Be Recommended Based on Drug Interaction Studies or Predicted Interaction (Information in the table applies to FORTOVASE with or without ritonavir, unless otherwise indicated)**

Concomitant Drug Class: Drug Name	Effect on Concentration of Saquinavir or Concomitant Drug	Clinical Comment
	Other	
Anticonvulsants: Carbamazepine, phenobarbital, phenytoin	**FORTOVASE** ↓ Saquinavir Effect on carbamazepine, phenobarbital, and phenytoin is not well established **FORTOVASE/ritonavir** Interaction has not been evaluated	Use with caution, FORTOVASE may be less effective due to decreased saquinavir plasma concentrations in patients taking these agents concomitantly.
Anti-infective: Clarithromycin*	**FORTOVASE** ↑ Saquinavir ↑ Clarithromycin **FORTOVASE/ritonavir** Interaction has not been evaluated	No dose adjustment is required when the two drugs are coadministered for a limited time at the doses studied (clarithromycin 500 mg bid and FORTOVASE 1200 mg tid for 7 days). For patients with renal impairment, the following dosage adjustments should be considered: • For patients with CL_{CR} 30 to 60 mL/min the dose of clarithromycin should be reduced by 50%. • For patients with CL_{CR} <30 mL/min the dose of clarithromycin should be decreased by 75%. No dose adjustment for patients with normal renal function is necessary.
Antifungal: Ketoconazole*, itraconazole	**FORTOVASE** ↑ Saquinavir ↔ Ketoconazole **FORTOVASE/ritonavir** Interaction has not been evaluated	No dose adjustment is required when the two drugs are coadministered for a limited time at the doses studied (ketoconazole 400 mg qd and FORTOVASE 1200 mg tid). A similar increase in plasma concentrations of saquinavir could occur with itraconazole.
Antimycobacterial Rifabutin*	↓ Saquinavir ↑ Rifabutin	FORTOVASE should not be given as the sole protease inhibitor to patients taking rifabutin. Appropriate doses of the combination of rifabutin and FORTOVASE/ritonavir with respect to safety and efficacy have not been established.
Antimycobacterial Rifampin*	**FORTOVASE** ↓ Saquinavir **FORTOVASE/ritonavir** Interaction has not been evaluated	FORTOVASE should not be given as the sole protease inhibitor to patients taking rifampin. Appropriate doses of the combination of rifampin and FORTOVASE/ritonavir with respect to safety and efficacy have not been established.
Benzodiazepines: Alprazolam, clorazepate, diazepam, flurazepam	↑ Benzodiazepines	Clinical significance is unknown; however, a decrease in benzodiazepine dose may be needed.
Calcium channel blockers: Diltiazem, felodipine, nifedipine, nicardipine, nimodipine, verapamil, amlodipine, nisoldipine, isradipine	↑ Calcium channel blockers	Caution is warranted and clinical monitoring of patients is recommended.
Corticosteroid: Dexamethasone	**FORTOVASE** ↓ Saquinavir **FORTOVASE/ritonavir** Interaction has not been evaluated	Use with caution, FORTOVASE may be less effective due to decreased saquinavir plasma concentrations in patients taking these agents concomitantly.
Histamine H_2-receptor antagonist: Ranitidine	**FORTOVASE** ↑ Saquinavir **FORTOVASE/ritonavir** Interaction has not been evaluated	The increase is not thought to be clinically relevant and no dose adjustment of FORTOVASE is recommended. Appropriate doses of the combination of ranitidine and FORTOVASE/ritonavir with respect to safety and efficacy have not been established.
HMG-CoA reductase inhibitors: Simvastatin, lovastatin, atorvastatin	↑ HMG-CoA reductase inhibitors	The combination of FORTOVASE with simvastatin and lovastatin should be avoided. Use lowest possible dose of atorvastatin and with careful monitoring or consider other HMG-CoA reductase inhibitors such as pravastatin, fluvastatin and rosuvastatin.
Immunosuppressants: Cyclosporine, tacrolimus, rapamycin	↑ Immunosuppressants	Therapeutic concentration monitoring is recommended for immunosuppressant agents when coadministered with FORTOVASE or FORTOVASE/ritonavir.
Narcotic analgesic: Methadone	**FORTOVASE/ritonavir** ↓ Methadone	Dosage of methadone may need to be increased when coadministered with FORTOVASE/ritonavir.
Oral contraceptives: Ethinyl estradiol	**FORTOVASE/ritonavir** ↓ Ethinyl estradiol	Alternative or additional contraceptive measures should be used when estrogen-based oral contraceptives and FORTOVASE/ritonavir are coadministered.
PDE5 inhibitor (phosphodiesterase type 5 inhibitors): Sildenafil*, vardenafil, tadalafil	↑ Sildenafil ↔ Saquinavir ↑ Vardenafil ↑ Tadalafil **FORTOVASE/ritonavir** Interaction has not been	Use sildenafil with caution at reduced doses of 25 mg every 48 hours with increased monitoring of adverse events when administered concomitantly with FORTOVASE or FORTOVASE/ritonavir. Use vardenafil with caution at reduced doses

(Table continued on next page)

Table 7 Percentage of Patients With Treatment-Emergent Adverse Events* of at Least Moderate Intensity, Occurring in ≥2% of Patients

	NV15182 (48 weeks)	NV15355 (48 weeks) Naive Patients
ADVERSE EVENT	**FORTOVASE + TOC† N=442**	**FORTOVASE + 2 RTIs‡ N=90**
Gastrointestinal		
Diarrhea	19.9	15.6
Nausea	10.6	13.3
Abdominal Discomfort	8.6	10.0
Dyspepsia	8.4	7.8
Flatulence	5.7	10.0
Vomiting	2.9	4.4
Abdominal Pain	2.3	4.4
Constipation	–	3.3
Body as a Whole		
Fatigue	4.8	8.9
Appetite Decreased	–	2.2
Chest Pain	–	2.2
Central and Peripheral Nervous System		
Headaches	5.0	5.6
Psychiatric Disorders		
Depression	2.7	–
Insomnia	–	5.6
Anxiety	–	2.2
Libido Disorder	–	3.3
Special Senses Disorders		
Taste Alteration	–	4.4
Musculoskeletal Disorders		
Pain	–	3.3
Dermatological Disorders		
Eczema	–	–
Rash	–	–
Verruca	–	2.2

*Includes adverse events at least possibly related to study drug or of unknown intensity and/or relationship to treatment (corresponding to ACTG Grade 2, 3 and 4).
†Antiretroviral Treatment of Choice.
‡Reverse Transcriptase Inhibitor.

Concomitant Therapy with Ritonavir

Table 8 Grade 2, 3 and 4 Adverse Events (All Causality) Reported in ≥2% of Adult Patients in the MaxCmin 1 Study of FORTOVASE in Combination with Ritonavir 1000/100 mg bid

	FORTOVASE 1000 mg plus Ritonavir 100 mg bid (48 weeks) N=148 n(%=n/N)
Endocrine Disorders	
Diabetes mellitus/ hyperglycemia	4 (2.7)
Lipodystrophy	8 (5.4)
Gastrointestinal Disorders	
Nausea	16 (10.8)
Vomiting	11 (7.4)
Diarrhea	12 (8.1)
Abdominal Pain	9 (6.1)
Constipation	3 (2.0)
General Disorders and Administration Site Conditions	
Fatigue	9 (6.1)
Fever	5 (3.4)
Musculoskeletal Disorders	
Back Pain	3 (2.0)
Respiratory Disorders	
Pneumonia	8 (5.4)
Bronchitis	4 (2.7)
Influenza	4 (2.7)
Sinusitis	4 (2.7)
Dermatological Disorders	
Rash	5 (3.4)
Pruritus	5 (3.4)
Dry lips/skin	3 (2.0)
Eczema	3 (2.0)

Includes events with unknown relationship to study drug.

Continued on next page

Fortovase—Cont.

Laboratory Abnormalities

In the MaxCmin 1 study, Grade 3 and 4 thrombocytopenia (2.0% of patients) and anemia (2.0%) were observed with FORTOVASE in combination with ritonavir. At 48 weeks, other lab abnormalities included increased ALT, increased AST, increased GGT, hyperglycemia, hypertriglyceridemia, increased TSH, neutropenia, raised amylase, and increased LDH.

Table 9 summarizes the percentage of patients with marked laboratory abnormalities in study NV15182 and NV15355 (median duration of treatment was 52 and 18 weeks, respectively). In study NV15182, by 48 weeks <1% of patients discontinued treatment due to laboratory abnormalities.

In the safety study (NV15182), 27% to 33% of subjects experienced 1 grade shifts in ALT and AST during the 48-week study period. In 46% of such events, there was a single abnormal transaminase level with no evidence of persistently elevated enzyme values during the course of study. Only 3% to 4% of patients had ≥3 grade shifts in transaminase levels and less than 0.5% of patients had to discontinue the study for increased liver function test values.

[See table 9 at right]

Additional marked lab abnormalities have been observed with INVIRASE. These include: calcium (low), phosphate (low), potassium (low), sodium (low).

Monotherapy and Combination Studies

Other clinical adverse experiences of any intensity, at least remotely related to FORTOVASE and INVIRASE, including those in <2% of patients, are listed below by body system.

Autonomic Nervous System

Mouth dry, night sweats, sweating increased

Body as a Whole

Allergic reaction, anorexia, appetite decreased, appetite disturbances, asthenia, chest pain, edema, fever, intoxication, malaise, olfactory disorder, pain body, pain pelvic, retrosternal pain, shivering, trauma, wasting syndrome, weakness generalized, weight decrease, redistribution/accumulation of body fat (see PRECAUTIONS: Fat Redistribution)

Cardiovascular/Cerebrovascular

Cyanosis, heart murmur, heart rate disorder, heart valve disorder, hypertension, hypotension, stroke, syncope, vein distended

Central and Peripheral Nervous System

Ataxia, cerebral hemorrhage, confusion, convulsions, dizziness, dysarthria, dysesthesia, hyperesthesia, hyperreflexia, hyporeflexia, light-headed feeling, myelopolyradiculoneuritis, neuropathy, numbness extremities, numbness face, paresis, paresthesis, peripheral neuropathy, poliomyelitis, prickly sensation, progressive multifocal leukoencephalopathy, spasms, tremor, unconsciousness

Dermatological

Acne, alopecia, chalazion, dermatitis, dermatitis seborrheic, erythema, folliculitis, furunculosis, hair changes, hot flushes, nail disorder, papillomatosis, papular rash, photosensitivity reaction, pigment changes skin, parasites external, pruritus, psoriasis, rash maculopapular, rash pruritic, red face, skin disorder, skin nodule, skin syndrome, skin ulceration, urticaria, verruca, xeroderma

Endocrine/Metabolic

Dehydration, diabetes mellitus, hyperglycemia, hypoglycemia, hypothyroidism, thirst, triglyceride increase, weight increase

Gastrointestinal

Abdominal distention, bowel movements frequent, buccal mucosa ulceration, canker sores oral, cheilitis, colic abdominal, dysphagia, esophageal ulceration, esophagitis, eructation, fecal incontinence, feces bloodstained, feces discolored, gastralgia, gastritis, gastroesophageal reflux, gastrointestinal inflammation, gingivitis, glossitis, hemorrhage rectum, hemorrhoids, infectious diarrhea, melena, painful defecation, parotid disorder, pruritus ani, pyrosis, salivary glands disorder, stomach upset, stomatitis, taste unpleasant, toothache, tooth disorder, ulcer gastrointestinal

Hematologic

Anemia, neutropenia, pancytopenia, splenomegaly

Liver and Biliary

Cholangitis sclerosing, cholelithiasis, hepatitis, hepatomegaly, hepatosplenomegaly, jaundice, liver enzyme disorder, pancreatitis

Musculoskeletal

Arthralgia, arthritis, back pain, cramps leg, cramps muscle, lumbago, musculoskeletal disorders, myalgia, myopathy, pain facial, pain jaw, pain leg, pain musculoskeletal, stiffness, tissue changes

Neoplasm

Kaposi's sarcoma, tumor

Platelet, Bleeding, Clotting

Bleeding dermal, hemorrhage, microhemorrhages, thrombocytopenia

Psychiatric

Agitation, amnesia, anxiety attack, behavior disturbances, dreaming excessive, euphoria, hallucination, intellectual ability reduced, irritability, lethargy, overdose effect, psychic disorder, psychosis, somnolence, speech disorder

Reproductive System

Epididymitis, erectile impotence, impotence, menstrual disorder, menstrual irregularity, penis disorder, prostate enlarged, vaginal discharge

Resistance Mechanism

Table 6 ***(cont.)*** **Established and Other Potentially Significant Drug Interactions: Alteration in Dose or Regimen May Be Recommended Based on Drug Interaction Studies or Predicted Interaction (Information in the table applies to FORTOVASE with or without ritonavir, unless otherwise indicated)**

Concomitant Drug Class: Drug Name	Effect on Concentration of Saquinavir or Concomitant Drug	Clinical Comment
Other Agents		
	evaluated, but expect increased concentrations of PDE5 inhibitors.	of no more than 2.5 mg every 72 hours with increased monitoring of adverse events when administered concomitantly with FORTOVASE or FORTOVASE/ritonavir. Use tadalafil with caution at reduced doses of no more than 10 mg every 72 hours with increased monitoring of adverse events when administered concomitantly with FORTOVASE or FORTOVASE/ritonavir.
Tricyclic antidepressants: Amitriptyline, imipramine	↑ Tricyclics	Therapeutic concentration monitoring is recommended for tricyclic antidepressants when coadministered with FORTOVASE/ritonavir.

*See CLINICAL PHARMACOLOGY: Pharmacokinetics, Tables 2 and 3 for magnitude of interactions

Table 9 Percentage of Patients with Marked Laboratory Abnormalities*

		NV15182 (48 weeks)	NV15355 (48 weeks) Naive Patients
BIOCHEMISTRY	**Limit**	**FORTOVASE + TOC†** **N=442**	**FORTOVASE + 2 RTIs‡** **N=90**
Alkaline Phosphatase (high)	>5 x ULN§	0.5	0.0
Calcium (high)	>12.5 mg/dL	0.2	0.0
Creatine Kinase (high)	>4 x ULN§	7.8	6.0
Gamma GT (high)	>5 x ULN§	5.7	5.0
Glucose (low)	<40 mg/dL	6.4	3.5
Glucose (high)	>250 mg/dL	1.4	0.0
Phosphate (low)	<1.5 mg/dL	0.5	1.0
Potassium (high)	>6.5 mEq/L	2.7	3.5
Serum Amylase (high)	>2 x ULN§	1.9	ND
SGOT (AST) (high)	>5 x ULN§	4.1	0.0
SGPT (ALT) (high)	>5 x ULN§	5.7	1.0
Sodium (high)	>157 mEq/L	0.7	0.0
Sodium (low)	<123 mEq/L	0.0	1.0
Total Bilirubin (high)	>2.5 x ULN§	1.6	0.0
Triglycerides (high)	>750 mg/dL	0.0	2.0
HEMATOLOGY			
Hemoglobin (low)	<7.0 gm/dL	0.7	1.0
Absolute Neutrophil Count (low)	<750 mm^3	2.9	1.0
Platelets (low)	<50,000 mm^3	0.9	0.0

* ACTG Grade 3 or above.
† Antiretroviral Treatment of Choice.
‡ Reverse Transcriptase Inhibitor.
§ ULN = Upper limit of normal range.
ND Not done.

Abscess, angina tonsillaris, candidiasis, cellulitis, herpes simplex, herpes zoster, infection bacterial, infection mycotic, infection staphylococcal, infestation parasitic, influenza, lymphadenopathy, molluscum contagiosum, moniliasis

Respiratory

Asthma bronchial, bronchitis, cough, dyspnea, epistaxis, hemoptysis, laryngitis, pharyngitis, pneumonia, pulmonary disease, respiratory disorder, rhinitis, rhinitis allergic atopic, sinusitis, upper respiratory tract infection

Special Senses

Blepharitis, conjunctivitis, cytomegalovirus retinitis, dry eye syndrome, earache, ear pressure, eye irritation, hearing decreased, otitis, taste unpleasant, tinnitus, visual disturbance, xerophthalmia

Urinary System

Micturition disorder, nocturia, renal calculus, renal colic, urinary tract bleeding, urinary tract infection

Postmarketing Experience with INVIRASE and FORTOVASE

Additional adverse events that have been observed during the postmarketing period are similar to those seen in clinical trials with INVIRASE and FORTOVASE and administration of INVIRASE and FORTOVASE in combination with ritonavir.

OVERDOSAGE

Two cases of FORTOVASE overdosage have been received (one case with unknown amount of FORTOVASE, the second case 3.6 to 4 grams at once). No adverse events have been reported in both cases. There were 2 patients who had overdoses with INVIRASE. No acute toxicities or sequelae were noted in the first patient after ingesting 8 grams of INVIRASE as a single dose. The patient was treated with induction of emesis within 2 to 4 hours after ingestion. The second patient ingested 2.4 grams of INVIRASE in combination with 600 mg of ritonavir and experienced pain in the throat that lasted for 6 hours and then resolved.

DOSAGE AND ADMINISTRATION

FORTOVASE (saquinavir) soft gelatin capsules and INVIRASE (saquinavir mesylate) capsules are not bioequivalent and cannot be used interchangeably When using saquinavir as the sole protease inhibitor in an antiviral regimen, FORTOVASE is the recommended formulation. INVIRASE may be considered only if it is combined with ritonavir, which significantly inhibits saquinavir's metabolism to provide plasma saquinavir levels at least equal to those achieved with FORTOVASE at the recommended dose of 1200 mg tid (see CLINICAL PHARMACOLOGY: Drug Interactions).

Adults (Over the Age of 16 Years)

FORTOVASE Administered Without Ritonavir:

- FORTOVASE 1200-mg tid (6 × 200-mg capsules)
- FORTOVASE should be taken with a meal or up to 2 hours after a meal

FORTOVASE Administered With Ritonavir:

- FORTOVASE 1000-mg bid (5 × 200-mg capsules) in combination with ritonavir 100-mg bid
- Ritonavir should be taken at the same time as FORTOVASE
- FORTOVASE and ritonavir should be taken within 2 hours after a meal

When used in combination with nucleoside analogues, the dosage of FORTOVASE should not be reduced as this will lead to greater than dose proportional decreases in saquinavir plasma levels.

Patients should be advised that FORTOVASE, like other protease inhibitors, is recommended for use in combination with active antiretroviral therapy. Greater activity has been observed when new antiretroviral therapies are begun at the same time as FORTOVASE. As with all protease inhibitors, adherence to the prescribed regimen is strongly recommended. Concomitant therapy should be based on a patient's prior drug exposure.

Monitoring of Patients

Clinical chemistry tests, viral load, and CD4 count should be performed prior to initiating FORTOVASE therapy and at appropriate intervals thereafter. For comprehensive patient monitoring recommendations for other antiretroviral therapies, physicians should refer to the complete product information for these drugs.

Dose Adjustment for Combination Therapy with FORTOVASE

For serious toxicities that may be associated with FORTOVASE, the drug should be interrupted. For recipients of combination therapy with FORTOVASE and other antiretroviral agents, dose adjustment of the other antiretroviral agents should be based on the known toxicity profile of the individual drug. FORTOVASE dose adjustments may be required with some other antiretroviral agents (see PRECAUTIONS: Drug Interactions). Physicians should refer to the complete product information for these drugs for comprehensive dose adjustment recommendations and drug-associated adverse reactions.

HOW SUPPLIED

FORTOVASE 200-mg capsules are beige, opaque, soft gelatin capsules with ROCHE and 0246 imprinted on the capsule shell — bottles of 180 (NDC 0004-0246-48).

The capsules should be refrigerated at 36° to 46°F (2° to 8°C) in tightly closed bottles until dispensed.

For patient use, refrigerated (36° to 46°F, 2° to 8°C) capsules of FORTOVASE remain stable until the expiration date printed on the label. Once brought to room temperature [at or below 77°F (25°C)], capsules should be used within 3 months.

HIVID and INVIRASE are registered trademarks of Hoffmann-La Roche Inc. KALETRA is a registered trademark of Abbott Laboratories.

Manufactured by:

F. Hoffmann-La Roche Ltd., Basel, Switzerland

Revised: December 2003

INVIRASE® ℞

[*In-vər-ās*]

(saquinavir mesylate)

CAPSULES

℞ only

Prescribing information for this product, which appears on pages 2917–2920 of the 2004 PDR, has been completely revised as follows. Please write "See Supplement A" next to the product heading.

WARNING

INVIRASE® (saquinavir mesylate) capsules and FORTOVASE® (saquinavir) soft gelatin capsules are not bioequivalent and cannot be used interchangeably. INVIRASE may be used only if it is combined with ritonavir, which significantly inhibits saquinavir's metabolism to provide plasma saquinavir levels at least equal to those achieved with FORTOVASE. When using saquinavir as the sole protease inhibitor in an antiviral regimen, FORTOVASE is the recommended formulation (see CLINICAL PHARMACOLOGY: Drug Interactions).

Product identification in this document includes: INVIRASE in reference to saquinavir mesylate; FORTOVASE in reference to saquinavir soft gel formulation, and saquinavir in reference to the active base.

DESCRIPTION

INVIRASE brand of saquinavir mesylate is an inhibitor of the human immunodeficiency virus (HIV) protease. INVIRASE is available as light brown and green, opaque hard gelatin capsules for oral administration in a 200-mg strength (as saquinavir free base). Each capsule also contains the inactive ingredients lactose, microcrystalline cellulose, povidone K30, sodium starch glycolate, talc, and magnesium stearate. Each capsule shell contains gelatin and water with the following dye systems: red iron oxide, yellow iron oxide, black iron oxide, FD&C Blue #2, and titanium dioxide. The chemical name for saquinavir mesylate is N-tert-butyl-decahydro-2-[2(R)-hydroxy-4-phenyl-3(S)-[[N-(2-quinolylcarbonyl)-L-asparaginyl]amino]butyl]-(4aS, 8aS)-isoquinoline-3(S)-carboxamide methanesulfonate with a molecular formula $C_{38}H_{50}N_6O_5 \bullet CH_4O_3S$ and a molecular weight of 766.96. The molecular weight of the free base is 670.86.

Saquinavir mesylate is a white to off-white, very fine powder with an aqueous solubility of 2.22 mg/mL at 25°C.

MICROBIOLOGY

Mechanism of Action

Saquinavir is an inhibitor of HIV protease. HIV protease is an enzyme required for the proteolytic cleavage of viral polyprotein precursors into individual functional proteins found in infectious HIV. Saquinavir is a peptide-like substrate analogue that binds to the protease active site and inhibits the activity of the enzyme. Saquinavir inhibition prevents cleavage of the viral polyproteins resulting in the formation of immature noninfectious virus particles.

Antiviral Activity

In vitro antiviral activity of saquinavir was assessed in lymphoblastoid and monocytic cell lines and in peripheral blood lymphocytes. Saquinavir inhibited HIV activity in both acutely and chronically infected cells. IC_{50} and IC_{90} values (50% and 90% inhibitory concentrations) were in the range of 1 to 30 nM and 5 to 80 nM, respectively. In the presence of 40% human serum, the mean IC_{50} of saquinavir against laboratory strain HIV-1 RF in MT4 cells was 37.7± 5nM representing a 4-fold increase in the IC_{50} value. In cell culture, saquinavir demonstrated additive to synergistic effects against HIV-1 in combination with reverse transcriptase inhibitors (didanosine, lamivudine, nevirapine, stavudine, zalcitabine and zidovudine) without enhanced cytotoxicity.

Table 1 Pharmacokinetic Parameters of Saquinavir at Steady-State After Administration of Different Regimens in HIV-Infected Patients

Dosing Regimen	N	AUC_τ (ng•h/mL)	AUC_{24h} (ng•h/mL)	C_{min} (ng/mL)
INVIRASE 600 mg tid (arithmetic mean, %CV)	10	866 (62)	2598	79
FORTOVASE 1200 mg tid (arithmetic mean)	31	7249	21747	216
INVIRASE 400 mg bid + ritonavir 400 mg bid (arithmetic mean ±SD)	7	16000±8000	32000	480±360
INVIRASE 1000 mg bid + ritonavir 100 mg bid (geometric mean and 95% CI)	24	14607 (10218-20882)	29214	371 (245-561)
FORTOVASE 1000 mg bid + ritonavir 100 mg bid (geometric mean and 95% CI)	24	19085 (13943-26124)	38170	433 (301-622)

τ is the dosing interval (ie, 8h if tid and 12h if bid)

Saquinavir in combination with the protease inhibitors amprenavir, atazanavir, or lopinavir resulted in synergistic antiviral activity.

Drug Resistance

HIV-1 mutants with reduced susceptibility to saquinavir have been selected during in vitro passage. Genotypic analyses of these isolates showed several substitutions in the HIV protease gene. Only the G48V and L90M substitutions were associated with reduced susceptibility to saquinavir, and conferred an increase in the IC_{50} value of 8- and 3-fold, respectively.

HIV-1 isolates with reduced susceptibility (≥4-fold increase in the IC_{50} value) to saquinavir emerged in some patients treated with INVIRASE. Genotypic analysis of these isolates identified resistance conferring primary mutations in the protease gene G48V and L90M, and secondary mutations L10I/R/V, I54V/L, A71V/T, G73S, V77I, V82A and I84V that contributed additional resistance to saquinavir. Forty-one isolates from 37 patients failing therapy with INVIRASE had a median decrease in susceptibility to saquinavir of 4.3 fold.

The degree of reduction in in vitro susceptibility to saquinavir of clinical isolates bearing substitutions G48V and L90M depends on the number of secondary mutations present. In general, higher levels of resistance are associated with greater number of mutations only in association with either or both of the primary mutations G48V and L90M. No data are currently available to address the development of resistance in patients receiving saquinavir/ritonavir.

Cross-resistance

Among protease inhibitors, variable crossresistance has been observed. In one clinical study, 22 HIV-1 isolates with reduced susceptibility (>4-fold increase in the IC_{50} value) to saquinavir following therapy with INVIRASE were evaluated for cross-resistance to amprenavir, indinavir, nelfinavir and ritonavir. Six of the 22 isolates (27%) remained susceptible to all 4 protease inhibitors, 12 of the 22 isolates (55%) retained susceptibility to at least one of the PIs and 4 out of the 22 isolates (18%) displayed broad cross- resistance to all PIs. Sixteen (73%) and 11 (50%) of the 22 isolates remained susceptible (<4-fold) to amprenavir and indinavir, respectively. Four of 16 (25%) and nine of 21 (43%) with available data remained susceptible to nelfinavir and ritonavir, respectively.

After treatment failure with amprenavir, cross-resistance to saquinavir was evaluated. HIV-1 isolates from 22/22 patients failing treatment with amprenavir and containing one or more mutations M46L/I, I50V, I54L, V32I, I47V, and I84V were susceptible to saquinavir.

CLINICAL PHARMACOLOGY

Pharmacokinetics

The pharmacokinetic properties of INVIRASE have been evaluated in healthy volunteers (n=351) and HIV-infected patients (n=270) after single- and multiple-oral doses of 25, 75, 200, and 600 mg tid and in healthy volunteers after intravenous doses of 6, 12, 36 or 72 mg (n=21). The pharmacokinetics of INVIRASE/ritonavir 400/400 mg bid and INVIRASE/ritonavir 1000/100 mg bid have also been evaluated in HIV-infected patients.

HIV-infected patients administered INVIRASE (600-mg TID) had AUC and maximum plasma concentration (C_{max}) values approximately 2–2.5 times those observed in healthy volunteers receiving the same treatment regimen.

Absorption and Bioavailability in Adults

Absolute bioavailability of saquinavir administered as INVIRASE averaged 4% (CV 73%, range: 1% to 9%) in 8 healthy volunteers who received a single 600-mg dose (3 × 200 mg) of saquinavir mesylate following a high-fat breakfast (48 g protein, 60 g carbohydrate, 57 g fat; 1006 kcal). The low bioavailability is thought to be due to a combination of incomplete absorption and extensive first-pass metabolism. Following single 600-mg doses, the relative bioavailability of saquinavir as FORTOVASE compared to saquinavir administered as INVIRASE was estimated at 331% (95% CI 207% to 530%).

When administered as the sole protease inhibitor, it has been shown that FORTOVASE 1200 mg tid provides an 8-fold increase in AUC compared with INVIRASE 600 mg tid (see Table 1).

INVIRASE in combination with ritonavir at doses of 1000/100 mg bid or 400/400 mg bid provides saquinavir systemic exposures over a 24-hour period similar to or greater than those achieved with FORTOVASE 1200 mg tid (see Table 1).

[See table 1 above]

Food Effect

No food effect data are available for INVIRASE in combination with ritonavir.

The mean 24-hour AUC after a single 600-mg oral dose (6 × 100 mg) in healthy volunteers (n=6) was increased from 24 ng•h/mL (CV 33%), under fasting conditions, to 161 ng•h/mL (CV 35%) when INVIRASE was given following a high-fat breakfast (48 g protein, 60 g carbohydrate, 57 g fat; 1006 kcal). Saquinavir 24-hour AUC and C_{max} (n=6) following the administration of a higher calorie meal (943 kcal, 54 g fat) were on average 2 times higher than after a lower calorie, lower fat meal (355 kcal, 8 g fat). The effect of food has been shown to persist for up to 2 hours.

Saquinavir exposure was similar when FORTOVASE plus ritonavir (1000-mg/100-mg bid) were administered following a high-fat (45 g fat) or moderate-fat (20 g fat) breakfast.

Distribution in Adults

The mean steady-state volume of distribution following intravenous administration of a 12-mg dose of saquinavir (n=8) was 700 L (CV 39%), suggesting saquinavir partitions into tissues. Saquinavir was approximately 98% bound to plasma proteins over a concentration range of 15 to 700 ng/mL. In 2 patients receiving saquinavir mesylate 600 mg tid, cerebrospinal fluid concentrations were negligible when compared to concentrations from matching plasma samples.

Metabolism and Elimination in Adults

In vitro studies using human liver microsomes have shown that the metabolism of saquinavir is cytochrome P450 mediated with the specific isoenzyme, CYP3A4, responsible for more than 90% of the hepatic metabolism. Based on in vitro studies, saquinavir is rapidly metabolized to a range of mono- and di-hydroxylated inactive compounds. In a mass balance study using 600 mg ^{14}C-saquinavir mesylate (n=8), 88% and 1% of the orally administered radioactivity was recovered in feces and urine, respectively, within 5 days of dosing. In an additional 4 subjects administered 10.5 mg ^{14}C-saquinavir intravenously, 81% and 3% of the intravenously administered radioactivity was recovered in feces and urine, respectively, within 5 days of dosing. In mass balance studies, 13% of circulating radioactivity in plasma was attributed to unchanged drug after oral administration and the remainder attributed to saquinavir metabolites. Following intravenous administration, 66% of circulating radioactivity was attributed to unchanged drug and the remainder attributed to saquinavir metabolites, suggesting that saquinavir undergoes extensive first-pass metabolism.

Systemic clearance of saquinavir was rapid, 1.14 L/h/kg (CV 12%) after intravenous doses of 6, 36, and 72 mg. The mean residence time of saquinavir was 7 hours (n=8).

Special Populations

Hepatic or Renal Impairment

Saquinavir pharmacokinetics in patients with hepatic or renal impairment has not been investigated (see PRECAUTIONS). Only 1% of saquinavir is excreted in the urine, so the impact of renal impairment on saquinavir elimination should be minimal.

Gender, Race, and Age

Pharmacokinetic data were available for 17 women in the Phase I/II studies. Pooled data did not reveal an apparent effect of gender on the pharmacokinetics of saquinavir.

The effect of race on the pharmacokinetics of saquinavir has not been investigated.

Pediatric Patients

The pharmacokinetics of saquinavir when administered as INVIRASE has not been sufficiently investigated in pediatric patients.

Geriatric Patients

The pharmacokinetics of saquinavir when administered as INVIRASE have not been sufficiently investigated in patients >65 years of age.

Drug Interactions (see PRECAUTIONS: Drug Interactions)

Several drug interaction studies have been completed with both INVIRASE and FORTOVASE. It is important to be aware that, when INVIRASE is coadministered with ritonavir, the occurrence and magnitude of drug interactions may differ from those seen with FORTOVASE when administered as the sole protease inhibitor. Because ritonavir is coadministered, prescribers should refer to the prescribing information for ritonavir regarding drug interactions associated with this drug.

Table 2 summarizes the effect of FORTOVASE on the geometric mean AUC and C_{max} of coadministered drugs. Table

Continued on next page

Invirase—Cont.

3 summarizes the effect of coadministered drugs on the geometric mean AUC and C_{max} of saquinavir.
[See table 2 at right]
[See table 3 at right]
For information regarding clinical recommendations, see PRECAUTIONS: Drug Interactions, Table 6.

INDICATIONS AND USAGE

INVIRASE in combination with ritonavir and other antiretroviral agents is indicated for the treatment of HIV infection. The twice daily administration of INVIRASE in combination with ritonavir is supported by safety data from the MaxCmin 1 study (see Table 7) and pharmacokinetic data (see Table 1). The efficacy of INVIRASE with ritonavir or FORTOVASE (with or without ritonavir coadministration) has not been compared against the efficacy of antiretroviral regimens currently considered standard of care.

Description of Clinical Studies

In a randomized, double-blind clinical study (NV14256) in ZDV-experienced, HIV-infected patients, INVIRASE in combination with HIVID was shown to be superior to either INVIRASE or HIVID monotherapy in decreasing the cumulative incidence of clinical disease progression to AIDS-defining events or death. Furthermore, in a randomized study (ACTG229/NV14255), patients with advanced HIV infection with history of prolonged ZDV treatment and who were given INVIRASE 600 mg tid + ZDV + HIVID experienced greater increases in CD4 cell counts as compared to those who received INVIRASE + ZDV or HIVID + ZDV. It should be noted that HIV treatment regimens that were used in these initial clinical studies of INVIRASE are no longer considered standard of care.

FORTOVASE 1000 mg bid coadministered with ritonavir 100 mg bid was studied in a heterogeneous population of 148 HIV-infected patients (MaxCmin 1 study). At baseline 42 were treatment naïve and 106 were treatment experienced (of which 52 had an HIV RNA level <400 copies/mL at baseline). Results showed that 91/148 (61%) subjects achieved and/or sustained an HIV RNA level <400 copies/mL at the completion of 48 weeks.

CONTRAINDICATIONS

INVIRASE may be used only if it is combined with ritonavir, which significantly inhibits saquinavir's metabolism and provides plasma saquinavir levels at least equal to those achieved with FORTOVASE.

INVIRASE is contraindicated in patients with clinically significant hypersensitivity to saquinavir or to any of the components contained in the capsule.

INVIRASE/ritonavir should not be administered concurrently with terfenadine, cisapride, astemizole, pimozide, triazolam, midazolam or ergot derivatives. Inhibition of CYP3A4 by saquinavir could result in elevated plasma concentrations of these drugs, potentially causing serious or life-threatening reactions, such as cardiac arrhythmias or prolonged sedation (see PRECAUTIONS: Drug Interactions).

INVIRASE when administered with ritonavir is contraindicated in patients with severe hepatic impairment.

INVIRASE should not be administered concurrently with drugs listed in Table 4 (also see PRECAUTIONS: Drug Interactions, Table 5).

Table 4 Drugs That Are Contraindicated With INVIRASE/Ritonavir

Drug Class	Drugs Within Class That Are Contraindicated With INVIRASE
Antiarrhythmics	Amiodarone, bepridil, flecainide, propafenone, quinidine
Antihistamines	Astemizole, terfenadine
Ergot Derivatives	Dihydroergotamine, ergonovine, ergotamine, methylergonovine
Antimycobacterial Agents	Rifampin*
GI Motility Agent	Cisapride
Neuroleptics	Pimozide
Sedative/Hypnotics	Triazolam, midazolam

*INVIRASE used as a sole protease inhibitor

WARNINGS

ALERT: Find out about medicines that should not be taken with INVIRASE. This statement is included on the product's bottle label.

Interaction with HMG-CoA Reductase Inhibitors

Concomitant use of INVIRASE with lovastatin or simvastatin is not recommended. Caution should be exercised if HIV protease inhibitors, including INVIRASE, are used concurrently with other HMG-CoA reductase inhibitors that are also metabolized by the CYP3A4 pathway (eg, atorvastatin). Since increased concentrations of statins can, in rare cases, cause severe adverse events such as myopathy including rhabdomyolysis, this risk may be increased when HIV protease inhibitors, including saquinavir, are used in combination with these drugs.

Table 2 Effect of FORTOVASE or INVIRASE on the Pharmacokinetics of Coadministered Drugs

Coadministered Drug	FORTOVASE or FORTOVASE/ ritonavir Dose	N	% Change for Coadministered Drug AUC (95%CI)	C_{max} (95%CI)
Clarithromycin 500 mg bid × 7 days	1200 mg tid × 7 days	12V		
Clarithromycin			↑45% (17-81%)	↑39% (10-76%)
14-OH clarithromycin metabolite			↓24% (5-40%)	↓34% (14-50%)
Midazolam 7.5-mg oral single dose	1200 mg tid ×5 days	6V	↑514%	↑235%
Ketoconazole 400 mg once daily	1200 mg tid	12V	↔	↔
Enfuvirtide 90 mg SCq 12h (bid) for 7 days	1000/100 mg bid	12P	↔	↔
Nelfinavir 750-mg single dose	1200 mg tid × 4 days	14P	↑18% (5-33%)	↔
Rifabutin 300 mg once daily	1200 mg tid	14P	↑44%	↑45%
Ritonavir 400 mg bid × 14 days	400 mg bid ×14 days	8V	↔	↔
Sildenafil 100-mg single dose	1200 mg tid ×8 days	27V	↑210% (150-300%)	↑140% (80-230%)
Terfenadine[ϕ] 60 mg bid × 11 days*	1200 mg tid × 4 days	12V		
Terfenadine			↑368% (257-514%)	↑253% (164-373%)
Terfendadine acid metabolite			↑120% (89-156%)	↑93% (59-133%)
Efavirenz 600 mg	1200 mg tid	13V	↓12%	↓13%

↑ Denotes an average increase in exposure by the percentage indicated.
↓ Denotes an average decrease in exposure by the percentage indicated.
↔ Denotes no statistically significant change in exposure was observed.
* FORTOVASE or INVIRASE/ritonavir should not be coadministered with terfenadine (see PRECAUTIONS: Drug Interactions).
P Patient
V Healthy Volunteers
ϕ No longer marketed in the US.

Table 3 Effect of Coadministered Drugs on FORTOVASE or INVIRASE Pharmacokinetics

Coadministered Drug	FORTOVASE Dose	N	% Change for Saquinavir AUC (95%CI)	C_{max} (95%CI)
Clarithromycin 500 mg bid × 7 days	1200 mg tid × 7 days	12V	↑177% (108-269%)	↑187% (105-300%)
Efavirenz 600 mg	1200 mg tid	13V	↓62%	↓50%
Indinavir 800 mg q8h × 2 days	1200-mg single dose	6V	↑364% (190-644%)	↑299% (138-568%)
Ketoconazole 400 mg once daily	1200 mg tid	12V	↑190%	↑171%
Nelfinavir 750 mg × 4 days	1200-mg single dose	14P	↑392% (271-553%)	↑179% (105-280%)
Rifabutin 300 mg once daily	1200 mg tid	14P	↓47%	↓39%
Rifampin 600 mg once daily	1200 mg tid × 14 days	14V	↓70%	↓65%
Ritonavir 100 mg bid	1000 mg bid†	24P	↑176%	↑153%
Ritonavir 400 mg bid × 14 days*	400 mg bid × 14 days†	8V	↑121% (7-359%)	↑64%§
Lopinavir/ritonavir 400/100 mg bid, 15 days	800 mg bid, 10 day combo vs. 1200 mg tid, 5 days alone	14V	↑9.62-fold (8.05, 11.49)^	↑6.34-fold (5.32, 7.55)^
400/100 mg bid, 20 days	1200 mg bid, 10 day combo vs. 1200 mg tid, 5 days alone	10V	↑9.91-fold (8.28, 11.86)^	↑6.44-fold (5.59, 7.41)^
Coadministered Drug	**INVIRASE Dose**	**N**	**% Change for Saquinavir AUC (95%CI)**	**C_{max} (95%CI)**
Rifabutin 150 mg every 3 days or 300 mg every 7 days	400 mg bid + 400 mg ritonavir bid	24P	↑19%	↑39%
Ritonavir 400 mg bid steady state*	400 mg bid steady state‡	7P	↑1587% (808-3034%)	↑1277% (577-2702%)
Ritonavir 100 mg bid	1000 mg bid‡	24P	↑1124%	↑1325%

↑ Denotes an average increase in exposure by the percentage indicated.
↓ Denotes an average decrease in exposure by the percentage indicated.
↔ Denotes no statistically significant change in exposure was observed.
* When ritonavir was combined with the same dose of either INVIRASE or FORTOVASE, actual mean plasma exposures (AUC_{12}, 18200 ng·h/mL, 20000 ng·h/mL, respectively) were not significantly different.
^ 90% CI reported
† Compared to standard FORTOVASE 1200 mg tid regimen (n=33).
‡ Compared to standard INVIRASE 600 mg tid regimen (n=114).
§ Did not reach statistical significance.
P Patient
V Healthy Volunteers

including rhabdomyolysis, this risk may be increased when HIV protease inhibitors, including saquinavir, are used in combination with these drugs.

Interaction with St. John's Wort (hypericum perforatum)
Concomitant use of INVIRASE and St. John's wort (hypericum perforatum) or products containing St. John's wort is not recommended. Coadministration of protease inhibitors, including INVIRASE, with St. John's wort is expected to substantially decrease protease-inhibitor concentrations and may result in sub-optimal levels of INVIRASE and lead to loss of virologic response and possible resistance to INVIRASE or to the class of protease inhibitors.

Interaction with Garlic Capsules
Garlic capsules should not be used while taking saquinavir as the sole protease inhibitor due to the risk of decreased saquinavir plasma concentrations. No data are available for the coadministration of INVIRASE/ritonavir or FORTOVASE/ritonavir and garlic capsules.

Diabetes Mellitus and Hyperglycemia
New onset diabetes mellitus, exacerbation of preexisting diabetes mellitus and hyperglycemia have been reported during postmarketing surveillance in HIV-infected patients receiving protease-inhibitor therapy. Some patients required either initiation or dose adjustments of insulin or oral hypoglycemic agents for the treatment of these events. In some cases diabetic ketoacidosis has occurred. In those patients who discontinued protease-inhibitor therapy, hyperglycemia persisted in some cases. Because these events have been reported voluntarily during clinical practice, estimates of frequency cannot be made and a causal relationship between protease-inhibitor therapy and these events has not been established.

PRECAUTIONS

General
INVIRASE (saquinavir mesylate) capsules and FORTOVASE (saquinavir) soft gelatin capsules are not bioequivalent and cannot be used interchangeably when used as the sole protease inhibitor. Only FORTOVASE should be used for the initiation of therapy that includes saquinavir as a sole protease inhibitor (see DOSAGE AND ADMINISTRATION) since FORTOVASE soft gelatin capsules provide greater bioavailability and efficacy than INVIRASE capsules.
If a serious or severe toxicity occurs during treatment with INVIRASE, INVIRASE should be interrupted until the etiology of the event is identified or the toxicity resolves. At that time, resumption of treatment with full-dose INVIRASE may be considered. For antiretroviral agents used in combination with INVIRASE, physicians should refer to the complete product information for these drugs for dose adjustment recommendations and for information regarding drug-associated adverse reactions.

Hepatic Effects
The use of INVIRASE (in combination with ritonavir) by patients with hepatic impairment has not been studied. In the absence of such studies, caution should be exercised, as increases in saquinavir levels and/or increases in liver enzymes may occur.
In patients with underlying hepatitis B or C, cirrhosis, chronic alcoholism and/or other underlying liver abnormalities there have been reports of worsening liver disease.

Renal Effects
Renal clearance is only a minor elimination pathway; the principal route of metabolism and excretion for saquinavir is by the liver. Therefore, no initial dose adjustment is necessary for patients with renal impairment. However, patients with severe renal impairment have not been studied, and caution should be exercised when prescribing saquinavir in this population.

Hemophilia
There have been reports of spontaneous bleeding in patients with hemophilia A and B treated with protease inhibitors. In some patients additional factor VIII was required. In the majority of reported cases treatment with protease inhibitors was continued or restarted. A causal relationship between protease inhibitor therapy and these episodes has not been established.

Hyperlipidemia
Elevated cholesterol and/or triglyceride levels have been observed in some patients taking saquinavir in combination with ritonavir. Marked elevation in triglyceride levels is a risk factor for development of pancreatitis. Cholesterol and triglyceride levels should be monitored prior to initiating combination dosing regimen of FORTOVASE or INVIRASE with ritonavir, and at periodic intervals while on such therapy. In these patients, lipid disorders should be managed as clinically appropriate.

Lactose Intolerance
Each capsule contains lactose (anhydrous) 63.3 mg. This quantity should not induce specific symptoms of intolerance.

Fat Redistribution
Redistribution/accumulation of body fat including central obesity, dorsocervical fat enlargement (buffalo hump), facial wasting, peripheral wasting, breast enlargement, and "cushingoid appearance" have been observed in patients receiving antiretroviral therapy. A causal relationship between protease-inhibitor therapy and these events has not been established and the long-term consequences are currently unknown.

Resistance/Cross-resistance
Varying degrees of cross-resistance among protease inhibitors have been observed. Continued administration of INVIRASE therapy following loss of viral suppression may increase the likelihood of cross-resistance to other protease inhibitors (see MICROBIOLOGY).

Information for Patients
A statement to patients and health care providers is included on the product's bottle label: **ALERT: Find out about medicines that should NOT be taken with INVIRASE.**
Patients should be informed that any change from INVIRASE to FORTOVASE or FORTOVASE to INVIRASE coadministered with a drug which inhibits its metabolism, such as ritonavir, should be made only under the supervision of a physician.
INVIRASE may interact with some drugs; therefore, patients should be advised to report to their doctor the use of any other prescription, nonprescription medication, or herbal products, particularly St. John's wort.

Patients should be informed that INVIRASE is not a cure for HIV infection and that they may continue to acquire illnesses associated with advanced HIV infection, including opportunistic infections. Patients should be advised that **INVIRASE may be used only if it is combined with ritonavir, which significantly inhibits saquinavir's metabolism to provide plasma saquinavir levels at least equal to those achieved with FORTOVASE.**
Patients should be informed that redistribution or accumulation of body fat may occur in patients receiving protease inhibitors and that the cause and long-term health effects of these conditions are not known at this time.
Patients should be told that the long-term effects of INVIRASE are unknown at this time. They should be informed that INVIRASE therapy has not been shown to reduce the risk of transmitting HIV to others through sexual contact or blood contamination.
Patients should be advised that INVIRASE administered with ritonavir should be taken within 2 hours after a full meal (see CLINICAL PHARMACOLOGY: Pharmacokinetics). When INVIRASE is taken without food, concentrations of saquinavir in the blood are substantially reduced and may result in no antiviral activity. Patients should be advised of the importance of taking their medication every day, as prescribed, to achieve maximum benefit. Patients should not alter the dose or discontinue therapy without consulting their physician. If a dose is missed, patients should take the next dose as soon as possible. However, the patient should not double the next dose.

Laboratory Tests
Clinical chemistry tests, viral load, and CD4 count should be performed prior to initiating INVIRASE therapy and at appropriate intervals thereafter. Elevated nonfasting triglyceride levels have been observed in patients in saquinavir trials. Triglyceride levels should be periodically monitored during therapy. For comprehensive information concerning laboratory test alterations associated with use of other antiretroviral therapies, physicians should refer to the complete product information for these drugs.

Drug Interactions
Several drug interaction studies have been completed with both INVIRASE and FORTOVASE. Observations from drug interaction studies with FORTOVASE may not be predictive for INVIRASE. Because ritonavir is coadministered, prescribers should also refer to the prescribing information for ritonavir regarding drug interactions associated with this agent.
The metabolism of saquinavir is mediated by cytochrome P450, with the specific isoenzyme CYP3A4 responsible for 90% of the hepatic metabolism. Additionally, saquinavir is a substrate for P-Glycoprotein (Pgp). Therefore, drugs that affect CYP3A4 and/or Pgp, may modify the pharmacokinetics of saquinavir. Similarly, saquinavir might also modify the pharmacokinetics of other drugs that are substrates for CYP3A4 or Pgp.
Drugs that are contraindicated specifically due to the expected magnitude of interaction and potential for serious adverse events are listed in Table 4 under CONTRAINDICATIONS. Additional drugs that are not recommended for coadministration with INVIRASE and ritonavir are included in Table 5. These recommendations are based on either drug interaction studies or predicted interactions due to the expected magnitude of interaction and potential for serious events or loss of efficacy.
Drug interactions that have been established based on drug interaction studies are listed with the pharmacokinetic results in Table 2, which summarizes the effect of saquinavir, administered as FORTOVASE or INVIRASE, on the geometric mean AUC and C_{max} of coadministered drugs and Table 3, which summarizes the effect of coadministered drugs on the geometric mean AUC and C_{max} of saquinavir. Clinical dose recommendations can be found in Table 6. The magnitude of the interactions may be different when INVIRASE or FORTOVASE are given with ritonavir.
When coadministering INVIRASE/ritonavir with any agent having a narrow therapeutic margin, such as anticoagulants, anticonvulsants, and antiarrhythmics, special attention is warranted. With some agents, the metabolism may be induced, resulting in decreased concentrations. Examples and clinical dose recommendations can be found in Table 6.

Table 5 Drugs That Should Not Be Coadministered With INVIRASE/Ritonavir

Drug Class: Drug Name	Clinical Comment
Antiarrhythmics: Amiodarone, bepridil, flecainide, propafenone, quinidine	CONTRAINDICATED due to potential for serious and/or life-threatening reactions.
Antihistamines: astemizole*, terfenadine*	CONTRAINDICATED due to potential for serious and/or life-threatening cardiac arrhythmias.
Ergot Derivatives: Dihydroergotamine, ergonovine, ergotamine, methylergonovine	CONTRAINDICATED due to potential for serious and life-threatening reactions such as acute ergot toxicity characterized by peripheral vasospasm and ischemia of the extremities and other tissues.
Antimycobacterial Agents: rifampin	CONTRAINDICATED since the coadministration of this product with saquinavir in an antiretroviral regimen reduces the plasma concentrations of saquinavir.
Garlic Capsules	Garlic capsules should not be used while taking saquinavir (FORTOVASE) as the sole protease inhibitor due to the risk of decreased saquinavir plasma concentrations. No data are available for the coadministration of INVIRASE/ritonavir or FORTOVASE/ritonavir and garlic capsules.
GI Motility Agent: cisapride*	CONTRAINDICATED due to potential for serious and/or life-threatening reactions such as cardiac arrhythmias.
Herbal Products: St. John's wort (hypericum perforatum)	WARNING coadministration may lead to loss of virologic response and possible resistance to INVIRASE or to the class of protease inhibitors.
HMG-CoA Reductase Inhibitors: lovastatin, simvastatin	WARNING potential for serious reactions such as risk of myopathy including rhabdomyolysis.
Sedatives/Hypnotics: triazolam, midazolam	CONTRAINDICATED due to potential for serious and/or life-threatening reactions such as prolonged or increased sedation or respiratory depression.

*No longer marketed in the US.

[See table 6 on pages 406, 407 and 408]

Drugs That Are Mainly Metabolized by CYP3A4
Although specific studies have not been performed, coadministration with drugs that are mainly metabolized by CYP3A4 (eg, calcium channel blockers, dapsone, disopyramide, quinine, amiodarone, quinidine, warfarin, tacrolimus, cyclosporine, ergot derivatives, pimozide, carbamazepine, fentanyl, alfentanyl, alprazolam, and triazolam) may have elevated plasma concentrations when coadministered with saquinavir; therefore, these combinations should be used with caution. Since INVIRASE is coadministered with ritonavir, the ritonavir label should be reviewed for additional drugs that should not be coadministered.

Inducers of CYP3A4
Coadministration with compounds that are potent inducers of CYP3A4 (eg, phenobarbital, phenytoin, dexamethasone, carbamazepine) may result in decreased plasma levels of saquinavir.

Carcinogenesis, Mutagenesis and Impairment of Fertility
Carcinogenesis
Carcinogenicity studies found no indication of carcinogenic activity in rats and mice administered saquinavir for approximately 2 years. The plasma exposures (AUC values) in the respective species were up to 6-fold (using rat) and 12-fold (using mouse) higher than those obtained in humans at the recommended clinical dose.

Mutagenesis
Mutagenicity and genotoxicity studies, with and without metabolic activation where appropriate, have shown that saquinavir has no mutagenic activity in vitro in either bacterial (Ames test) or mammalian cells (Chinese hamster

Continued on next page

Invirase—Cont.

lung V79/HPRT test). Saquinavir does not induce chromosomal damage in vivo in the mouse micronucleus assay or in vitro in human peripheral blood lymphocytes, and does not induce primary DNA damage in vitro in the unscheduled DNA synthesis test.

Impairment of Fertility

Fertility and reproductive performance were not affected in rats at plasma exposures (AUC values) up to 5 times those achieved in humans at the recommended dose.

Pregnancy

Teratogenic Effects: Category B

Reproduction studies conducted with saquinavir in rats have shown no embryotoxicity or teratogenicity at plasma exposures (AUC values) up to 5 times those achieved in humans at the recommended dose or in rabbits at plasma exposures 4 times those achieved at the recommended clinical dose. Studies in rats indicated that exposure to saquinavir from late pregnancy through lactation at plasma concentrations (AUC values) up to 5 times those achieved in humans at the recommended dose had no effect on the survival, growth, and development of offspring to weaning. Clinical experience in pregnant women is limited. Saquinavir should be used during pregnancy only if the potential benefit justifies the potential risk to the fetus.

Antiretroviral Pregnancy Registry

To monitor maternal-fetal outcomes of pregnant women exposed to antiretroviral medications, including INVIRASE, an Antiretroviral Pregnancy Registry has been established. Physicians are encouraged to register patients by calling 1-800-258-4263.

Nursing Mothers

The Centers for Disease Control and Prevention recommend that HIV-infected mothers not breast-feed their infants to avoid risking postnatal transmission of HIV. It is not known whether saquinavir is excreted in human milk. Because of both the potential for HIV transmission and the potential for serious adverse reactions in nursing infants, **mothers should be instructed not to breast-feed if they are receiving antiretroviral medications, including INVIRASE.**

Pediatric Use

Safety and effectiveness of INVIRASE in HIV-infected pediatric patients younger than 16 years of age have not been established.

Geriatric Use

Clinical studies of INVIRASE did not include sufficient numbers of subjects aged 65 and over to determine whether they respond differently from younger subjects. In general, caution should be taken when dosing INVIRASE in elderly patients due to the greater frequency of decreased hepatic, renal or cardiac function, and of concomitant disease or other drug therapy.

ADVERSE REACTIONS (see PRECAUTIONS)

INVIRASE may be used only if it is combined with ritonavir, which significantly inhibits saquinavir's metabolism to provide plasma saquinavir levels at least equal to those achieved with FORTOVASE. See Concomitant Therapy with Ritonavir Adverse Reactions for safety information with the recommended dosage regimen.

The safety of INVIRASE was studied in patients who received the drug either alone or in combination with zidovudine and/or HIVID (zalcitabine, ddC). The majority of adverse events were of mild intensity. The most frequently reported adverse events among patients receiving INVIRASE in clinical trials (excluding those toxicities known to be associated with zidovudine and HIVID when used in combinations) were diarrhea, abdominal discomfort, and nausea.

The following grade 2 to grade 4 adverse events, (considered at least possibly related to study drug or of unknown relationship) occurred in ≥2% of patients receiving INVIRASE 600 mg tid alone or in combination with zidovudine and/or HIVID: abdominal discomfort, abdominal pain, appetite disturbances, asthenia, buccal mucosa ulceration, diarrhea, dizziness, dyspepsia, extremity numbness, headache, mucosa damage, musculoskeletal pain, myalgia, nausea, paresthesia, peripheral neuropathy, pruritus, and rash.

Rare occurrences of the following serious adverse experiences have been reported during clinical trials of INVIRASE and were considered at least possibly related to use of study drugs: confusion, ataxia, and weakness; acute myeloblastic leukemia; hemolytic anemia; attempted suicide; Stevens-Johnson syndrome; seizures; severe cutaneous reaction associated with increased liver function tests; isolated elevation of transaminases; thrombophlebitis; headache; thrombocytopenia; exacerbation of chronic liver disease with Grade 4 elevated liver function tests, jaundice, ascites, and right and left upper quadrant abdominal pain; drug fever; bullous skin eruption and polyarthritis; pancreatitis leading to death; nephrolithiasis; thrombocytopenia and intracranial hemorrhage leading to death; peripheral vasoconstriction; portal hypertension; intestinal obstruction. These events were reported from a database of >6000 patients. Over 100 patients on INVIRASE therapy have been followed for >2 years.

Concomitant Therapy with Ritonavir Adverse Reactions

In combination with ritonavir the recommended dose of INVIRASE is 1000 mg two times daily with ritonavir 100 mg two times daily in combination with other antiretroviral agents. Table 7 lists grades 2, 3 and 4 related adverse events that occurred in ≥2% of patients receiving FORTOVASE with ritonavir (1000/100 mg bid).

Table 6 Established and Other Potentially Significant Drug Interactions: Alteration in Dose or Regimen May Be Recommended Based on Drug Interaction Studies or Predicted Interaction (Information in the table applies to INVIRASE/ritonavir)

Concomitant Drug Class: Drug Name	Effect on Concentration of Saquinavir or Concomitant Drug	Clinical Comment
HIV-Antiviral Agents		
Non-nucleoside reverse transcriptase inhibitor: Delavirdine	↑ Saquinavir Effect on delavirdine is not well established **INVIRASE/ritonavir** Interaction has not been evaluated	Appropriate doses of the combination with respect to safety and efficacy have not been established.
Non-nucleoside reverse transcriptase inhibitor: Efavirenz*, nevirapine	↓ Saquinavir ↓ Efavirenz **INVIRASE/ritonavir** Interaction has not been evaluated	INVIRASE should not be given as the sole protease inhibitor to patients. Appropriate doses of the combination of efavirenz or nevirapine and INVIRASE/ritonavir with respect to safety and efficacy have not been established.
HIV protease inhibitor: Indinavir*	↑ Saquinavir Effect on indinavir is not well established **INVIRASE/ritonavir** Interaction has not been evaluated	Appropriate doses of the combination of indinavir and INVIRASE/ritonavir with respect to safety and efficacy have not been established.
HIV protease inhibitor: Nelfinavir*	↑ Saquinavir ↑ Nelfinavir **INVIRASE/ritonavir** Interaction has not been evaluated	Saquinavir 1200 mg bid with nelfinavir 1250 mg bid results in adequate plasma drug concentrations for both protease inhibitors.
HIV protease inhibitor: Ritonavir*	↑ Saquinavir ↔Ritonavir	The recommended dose regimen when ritonavir is given to increase saquinavir concentrations is 1000 mg saquinavir plus ritonavir 100 mg twice daily.
HIV protease inhibitor: Lopinavir/ritonavir (coformulated capsule)*	↑ Saquinavir Effect on lopinavir is not well established	FORTOVASE (SQV) 800 mg bid + KALETRA produces ↑ AUC, ↑ C_{max}, and ↑ C_{min} relative to FORTOVASE 1200 mg tid (see CLINICAL PHARMACOLOGY: Table 3)
HIV fusion inhibitor: Enfuvirtide*	FORTOVASE Interaction has not been evaluated FORTOVASE/ritonavir ↔enfuvirtide	No clinically significant interaction was noted from a study in 12 HIV patients who received enfuvirtide concomitantly with FORTOVASE/ritonavir 1000/100 mg bid. No dose adjustments are required.

(Table continued on next page)

Table 7 Grade 2, 3 and 4 Related Adverse Events* (All Causality) Reported in ≥2% of Adult Patients in the MaxCmin 1 Study of FORTOVASE in Combination with Ritonavir 1000/100 mg bid

	FORTOVASE 1000 mg plus Ritonavir 100 mg bid (48 weeks) N=148 n(%=n/N)
Endocrine Disorders	
Diabetes mellitus/hyperglycemia	4 (2.7)
Lipodystrophy	8 (5.4)
Gastrointestinal Disorders	
Nausea	16 (10.8)
Vomiting	11 (7.4)
Diarrhea	12 (8.1)
Abdominal Pain	9 (6.1)
Constipation	3 (2.0)
General Disorders and Administration Site Conditions	
Fatigue	9 (6.1)
Fever	5 (3.4)
Musculoskeletal Disorders	
Back Pain	3 (2.0)
Respiratory Disorders	
Pneumonia	8 (5.4)
Bronchitis	4 (2.7)
Influenza	4 (2.7)
Sinusitis	4 (2.7)
Dermatological Disorders	
Rash	5 (3.4)
Pruritus	5 (3.4)
Dry lips/skin	3 (2.0)
Eczema	3 (2.0)

*Includes events with unknown relationship to study drug

Additionally, adverse events that occurred in clinical trials with FORTOVASE, which are not listed above, are listed for completeness. However, due to the higher bioavailability of FORTOVASE, these adverse events might not be predictive of the safety profile of INVIRASE.

Experience from Clinical Trials with FORTOVASE

The safety of FORTOVASE was studied in more than 500 patients who received the drug either alone or in combination with other antiretroviral agents. The most frequently reported adverse events among patients receiving FORTOVASE in combination with other antiretroviral agents were diarrhea, nausea, abdominal discomfort, and dyspepsia. Clinical adverse events of at least moderate intensity, which occurred in ≥2% of patients in 2 studies with FORTOVASE, which are not listed above, are listed below by body system.

Gastrointestinal Disorders: constipation, flatulence, vomiting

Body as a Whole: appetite decreased, chest pain, fatigue

Psychological: depression, insomnia, anxiety, libido disorder

Special Senses: taste alteration

Skin and Appendages: verruca, eczema

Laboratory Abnormalities with INVIRASE

Grade 3 and 4 lab abnormalities have been observed with FORTOVASE in combination with ritonavir. At 48 weeks, lab abnormalities included increased ALT, anemia, increased AST, increased GGT, hyperglycemia, hypertriglyceridemia, increased TSH, neutropenia, raised amylase, raised LDH, and thrombocytopenia.

INVIRASE may be used only if it is combined with ritonavir, which significantly inhibits saquinavir's metabolism to provide plasma saquinavir levels at least equal to those achieved with FORTOVASE.

In studies NV14255/ACTG 229 and NV14256, the following grade 3 or grade 4 abnormalities in laboratory tests were reported among patients receiving INVIRASE 600 mg tid alone or in combination with ZDV and/or HIVID:

Table 6 *(cont.)* **Established and Other Potentially Significant Drug Interactions: Alteration in Dose or Regimen May Be Recommended Based on Drug Interaction Studies or Predicted Interaction (Information in the table applies to INVIRASE/ritonavir)**

Concomitant Drug Class: Drug Name	Effect on Concentration of Saquinavir or Concomitant Drug	Clinical Comment
Other Agents		
Antiarrhythmics: Lidocaine (systemic)	↑ Antiarrhythmics	Caution is warranted and therapeutic concentration monitoring, if available, is recommended for antiarrhythmics given with INVIRASE/ritonavir
Anticoagulant: Warfarin		Concentrations of warfarin may be affected. It is recommended that INR (international normalized ratio) be monitored.
Anticonvulsants: Carbamazepine, phenobarbital, phenytoin	↓ Saquinavir Effect on carbamazepine, phenobarbital, and phenytoin is not well established **INVIRASE/ritonavir** Interaction has not been evaluated	Use with caution, saquinavir may be less effective due to decreased saquinavir plasma concentrations in patients taking these agents concomitantly.
Anti-infective: Clarithromycin*	↑ Saquinavir ↑ Clarithromycin **INVIRASE/ritonavir** Interaction has not been evaluated	No dose adjustment is required when the two drugs are coadministered for a limited time at the doses studied (clarithromycin 500 mg bid and FORTOVASE 1200 mg tid for 7 days). For patients with renal impairment, the following dosage adjustments should be considered: • For patients with CL_{CR} 30 to 60 mL/min the dose of clarithromycin should be reduced by 50%. • For patients with CL_{CR} <30 mL/min the dose of clarithromycin should be decreased by 75%. No dose adjustment for patients with normal renal function is necessary.
Antifungal: Ketoconazole*, itraconazole	↑ Saquinavir ↔Ketoconazole **INVIRASE/ritonavir** Interaction has not been evaluated	No dose adjustment is required when the two drugs are coadministered for a limited time at the doses studied (ketoconazole 400 mg qd and FORTOVASE 1200 mg tid). A similar increase in plasma concentrations of saquinavir could occur with itraconazole.
Antimycobacterial Rifabutin*	↓ Saquinavir ↑ Rifabutin	INVIRASE should not be given as the sole protease inhibitor to patients. Appropriate doses of the combination of rifabutin and INVIRASE/ritonavir with respect to safety and efficacy have not been established.
Antimycobacterial Rifampin*	↓ Saquinavir ↑ Rifabutin **INVIRASE/ritonavir** Interaction has not been evaluated	INVIRASE should not be given as the sole protease inhibitor to patients. Appropriate doses of the combination of rifampin and INVIRASE/ritonavir with respect to safety and efficacy have not been established.
Benzodiazepines: Alprazolam, clorazepate, diazepam, flurazepam	↑ Benzodiazepines	Clinical significance is unknown; however, a decrease in benzodiazepine dose may be needed.
Calcium channel blockers: Diltiazem, felodipine, nifedipine, nicardipine, nimodipine, verapamil, amlodipine, nisoldipine, isradipine	↑ Calcium channel blockers	Caution is warranted and clinical monitoring of patients is recommended.
Corticosteroid: Dexamethasone	↓ Saquinavir **INVIRASE/ritonavir** Interaction has not been evaluated	Use with caution, saquinavir may be less effective due to decreased saquinavir plasma concentrations in patients taking these agents concomitantly.
Histamine H_2-receptor antagonist: Ranitidine	↑ Saquinavir **INVIRASE/ritonavir** Interaction has not been evaluated	The increase is not thought to be clinically relevant and no dose adjustment of FORTOVASE is recommended. Appropriate doses of the combination of ranitidine and INVIRASE/ritonavir with respect to safety and efficacy have not been established.
HMG-CoA reductase inhibitors: Simvastatin, lovastatin, atorvastatin	↑ HMG-CoA reductase inhibitors	The combination of INVIRASE/ritonavir with simvastatin and lovastatin should be avoided. Use lowest possible dose of atorvastatin and with careful monitoring or consider other HMG-CoA reductase inhibitors such as pravastatin, fluvastatin and rosuvastatin.

(Table continued on next page)

Biochemistry
- Incidence between <1% and 4%-hypoglycemia, hyper- or hypocalcemia, hypophosphatemia, hyper- or hypokalemia, hyper- or hyponatremia, raised serum amylase grade 3 or 4 elevations in transaminases (SGOT [AST] SGPT [ALT]), hyperbilirubinemia
- Incidence of ≤5%: hyperglycemia. Incidence of between 7% and 12%: elevated creatine phosphokinase.

Hematology
- Incidence of ≤2%: thrombocytopenia and anemia. Incidence of between 1% and 8%: leucopenia.

Additional marked lab abnormalities have been observed with FORTOVASE. These include: alkaline phosphatase (high), gamma GT (high), and triglycerides (high).

Monotherapy and Combination Studies
Other clinical adverse experiences of any intensity, at least remotely related to INVIRASE, including those in <2% of patients on arms containing INVIRASE in studies NV14255/ACTG229 and NV14256, and those in smaller clinical trials, are listed below by body system.

Body as a Whole: allergic reaction, anorexia, chest pain, edema, fatigue, fever, intoxication, parasites external, retrosternal pain, shivering, wasting syndrome, weakness generalized, weight decrease, redistribution/accumulation of body fat (see PRECAUTIONS: Fat Redistribution)

Cardiovascular: cyanosis, heart murmur, heart valve disorder, hypertension, hypotension, syncope, vein distended

Endocrine/Metabolic: dehydration, diabetes mellitus, dry eye syndrome, hyperglycemia, weight increase, xerophthalmia

Gastrointestinal: cheilitis, colic abdominal, constipation, dyspepsia, dysphagia, esophagitis, eructation, feces bloodstained, feces discolored, flatulence, gastralgia, gastritis, gastrointestinal inflammation, gingivitis, glossitis, hemorrhage rectum, hemorrhoids, hepatitis, hepatomegaly, hepatosplenomegaly, infectious diarrhea, jaundice, liver enzyme disorder, melena, pain pelvic, painful defecation, pancreatitis, parotid disorder, salivary glands disorder, stomach upset, stomatitis, toothache, tooth disorder, vomiting

Hematologic: anemia, bleeding dermal, microhemorrhages, neutropenia, pancytopenia, splenomegaly, thrombocytopenia

Musculoskeletal: arthralgia, arthritis, back pain, cramps leg, cramps muscle, creatine phosphokinase increased, musculoskeletal disorders, stiffness, tissue changes, trauma

Neurological: ataxia, bowel movements frequent, confusion, convulsions, dysarthria, dysesthesia, heart rate disorder, hyperesthesia, hyperreflexia, hyporeflexia, light-headed feeling, mouth dry, myelopolyradiculoneuritis, numbness face, pain facial, paresis, poliomyelitis, prickly sensation, progressive multifocal leukoencephalopathy, spasms, tremor, unconsciousness

Psychological: agitation, amnesia, anxiety, anxiety attack, depression, dreaming excessive, euphoria, hallucination, insomnia, intellectual ability reduced, irritability, lethargy, libido disorder, overdose effect, psychic disorder, psychosis, somnolence, speech disorder, suicide attempt

Reproductive System: impotence, prostate enlarged, vaginal discharge

Resistance Mechanism: abscess, angina tonsillaris, candidiasis, cellulitis, herpes simplex, herpes zoster, infection bacterial, infection mycotic, infection staphylococcal, influenza, lymphadenopathy, moniliasis, tumor

Respiratory: bronchitis, cough, dyspnea, epistaxis, hemoptysis, laryngitis, pharyngitis, pneumonia, pulmonary disease, respiratory disorder, rhinitis, sinusitis, upper respiratory tract infection

Skin and Appendages: acne, alopecia, chalazion, dermatitis, dermatitis seborrheic, eczema, erythema, folliculitis, furunculosis, hair changes, hot flushes, nail disorder, night sweats, papillomatosis, photosensitivity reaction, pigment changes skin, rash maculopapular, skin disorder, skin nodule, skin ulceration, sweating increased, urticaria, verruca, xeroderma

Special Senses: blepharitis, earache, ear pressure, eye irritation, hearing decreased, otitis, taste alteration, tinnitus, visual disturbance

Urinary System: micturition disorder, renal calculus, urinary tract bleeding, urinary tract infection

Postmarketing Experience with INVIRASE and FORTOVASE
Additional adverse events that have been observed during the postmarketing period are similar to those seen in clinical trials with INVIRASE and FORTOVASE and administration of INVIRASE and FORTOVASE in combination with ritonavir.

OVERDOSAGE

No acute toxicities or sequelae were noted in 1 patient who ingested 8 grams of INVIRASE as a single dose. The patient was treated with induction of emesis within 2 to 4 hours after ingestion. A second patient ingested 2.4 grams of INVIRASE in combination with 600 mg of ritonavir and experienced pain in the throat that lasted for 6 hours and then resolved. In an exploratory Phase II study of oral dosing with INVIRASE at 7200 mg/day (1200 mg q4h), there were no serious toxicities reported through the first 25 weeks of treatment.

DOSAGE AND ADMINISTRATION

INVIRASE (saquinavir mesylate) capsules and FORTOVASE (saquinavir) soft gelatin capsules are not bioequivalent and cannot be used interchangeably. INVIRASE may be used only if it is combined with ritonavir, because it significantly inhibits saquinavir's metabolism to provide plasma saquinavir levels at least equal to those achieved with FOR-

Continued on next page

Invirase—Cont.

TOVASE at the recommended dose of 1200 mg tid. When using saquinavir as the sole protease inhibitor in an antiretroviral regimen, FORTOVASE is the recommended formulation (see CLINICAL PHARMACOLOGY: Drug Interactions).

Adults (Over the Age of 16 Years)

- INVIRASE 1000-mg bid (5 x 200-mg capsules) in combination with ritonavir 100-mg bid.
- Ritonavir should be taken at the same time as INVIRASE.
- INVIRASE and ritonavir should be taken within 2 hours after a meal.

Monitoring of Patients

Clinical chemistry tests, viral load, and CD4 count should be performed prior to initiating INVIRASE therapy and at appropriate intervals thereafter. For comprehensive patient monitoring recommendations for other nucleoside analogues, physicians should refer to the complete product information for these drugs.

Dose Adjustment for Combination Therapy with INVIRASE

For serious toxicities that may be associated with INVIRASE, the drug should be interrupted. INVIRASE at doses less than 1000 mg with 100 mg ritonavir bid are not recommended since lower doses have not shown antiviral activity. For recipients of combination therapy with INVIRASE and ritonavir, dose adjustments may be necessary. These adjustments should be based on the known toxicity profile of the individual agent and the pharmacokinetic interaction between saquinavir and the coadministered drug (see PRECAUTIONS: Drug Interactions). Physicians should refer to the complete product information for these drugs for comprehensive dose adjustment recommendations and drug-associated adverse reactions of nucleoside analogues.

HOW SUPPLIED

INVIRASE 200-mg capsules are light brown and green opaque capsules with ROCHE and 0245 imprinted on the capsule shell — bottles of 270 (NDC 0004-0245-15).

The capsules should be stored at 59° to 86°F (15° to 30°C) in tightly closed bottles.

HIVID, FORTOVASE and VERSED are registered trademarks of Hoffmann-La Roche Inc.

KALETRA is a registered trademark of Abbott Laboratories.

Manufactured by:
F. Hoffmann-La Roche Ltd., Basel, Switzerland
or Hoffmann-La Roche Inc., Nutley, New Jersey

Revised: December 2003

Table 6 *(cont.)* **Established and Other Potentially Significant Drug Interactions: Alteration in Dose or Regimen May Be Recommended Based on Drug Interaction Studies or Predicted Interaction (Information in the table applies to INVIRASE/ritonavir)**

Concomitant Drug Class: Drug Name	Effect on Concentration of Saquinavir or Concomitant Drug	Clinical Comment
	Other Agents	
Immunosuppressants: Cyclosporine, tacrolimus, rapamycin	↑ Immunosuppressants	Therapeutic concentration monitoring is recommended for immunosuppressant agents when coadministered with INVIRASE/ritonavir.
Narcotic analgesic: Methadone	↓ Methadone	Dosage of methadone may need to be increased when coadministered with INVIRASE/ritonavir.
Oral contraceptives: Ethinyl estradiol	↓ Ethinyl estradiol	Alternative or additional contraceptive measures should be used when estrogen-based oral contraceptives and INVIRASE/ritonavir are coadministered.
PDE5 inhibitors (phosphodiesterase type 5 inhibitors): Sildenafil*, vardenafil, tadalafil	↑ Sildenafil ↔Saquinavir ↑ Vardenafil ↑ Tadalafil	**Use sildenafil with caution at** reduced doses of 25 mg every 48 hours with increased monitoring of adverse events when administered concomitantly with INVIRASE/ritonavir. Use vardenafil with caution at reduced doses of no more than 2.5 mg every 72 hours with increased monitoring of adverse events when administered concomitantly with INVIRASE/ritonavir. Use tadalafil with caution at reduced doses of no more than 10 mg every 72 hours with increased monitoring of adverse events when administered concomitantly with INVIRASE/ritonavir.
Tricyclic antidepressants: Amitriptyline, imipramine	↑ Tricyclics	Therapeutic concentration monitoring is recommended for tricyclic antidepressants when coadministered with INVIRASE/ritonavir.

* See CLINICAL PHARMACOLOGY: Pharmacokinetics, Tables 2 and 3 for magnitude of interactions

PEGASYS®

(peginterferon alfa-2a) ℞

Prescribing information for this product, which appears on pages 2931–2935 of the 2004 PDR, has been revised as follows. Please write "See Supplement A" next to the product heading.

Alpha interferons, including PEGASYS (peginterferon alfa-2a), may cause or aggravate fatal or life-threatening neuropsychiatric, autoimmune, ischemic, and infectious disorders. Patients should be monitored closely with periodic clinical and laboratory evaluations. Therapy should be withdrawn in patients with persistently severe or worsening signs or symptoms of these conditions. In many, but not all cases, these disorders resolve after stopping PEGASYS therapy (see WARNINGS and ADVERSE REACTIONS).

Use with Ribavirin. Ribavirin, including COPEGUS®, may cause birth defects and/or death of the fetus. Extreme care must be taken to avoid pregnancy in female patients and in female partners of male patients. Ribavirin causes hemolytic anemia. The anemia associated with ribavirin therapy may result in a worsening of cardiac disease. Ribavirin is genotoxic and mutagenic and should be considered a potential carcinogen (see COPEGUS Package Insert for additional information and other WARNINGS).

DESCRIPTION

PEGASYS, peginterferon alfa-2a, is a covalent conjugate of recombinant alfa-2a interferon (approximate molecular weight [MW] 20,000 daltons) with a single branched bis-monomethoxy polyethylene glycol (PEG) chain (approximate MW 40,000 daltons). The PEG moiety is linked at a single site to the interferon alfa moiety via a stable amide bond to lysine. Peginterferon alfa-2a has an approximate molecular weight of 60,000 daltons. Interferon alfa-2a is produced using recombinant DNA technology in which a cloned human leukocyte interferon gene is inserted into and expressed in *Escherichia coli*.

PEGASYS is supplied as an injectable solution in vials and prefilled syringes.

180 µg/1.0 mL Vial: A vial contains approximately 1.2 mL of solution to deliver 1.0 mL of drug product. Subcutaneous (sc) administration of 1.0 mL delivers 180 µg of drug product (expressed as the amount of interferon alfa-2a), 8.0 mg sodium chloride, 0.05 mg polysorbate 80, 10.0 mg benzyl alcohol, 2.62 mg sodium acetate trihydrate, and 0.05 mg acetic acid. The solution is colorless to light yellow and the pH is 6.0 ± 0.5.

180 µg/0.5 mL Prefilled Syringe: Each syringe contains 0.6 mL of solution to deliver 0.5 mL of drug product. Subcutaneous (sc) administration of 0.5 mL delivers 180 µg of drug product (expressed as the amount of interferon alfa-2a), 4.0 mg sodium chloride, 0.025 mg polysorbate 80, 5.0 mg benzyl alcohol, 1.3085 mg sodium acetate trihydrate, and 0.0231 mg acetic acid. The solution is colorless to light yellow and the pH is 6.0 ± 0.5.

CLINICAL PHARMACOLOGY

Pharmacodynamics

Interferons bind to specific receptors on the cell surface initiating intracellular signaling via a complex cascade of protein-protein interactions leading to rapid activation of gene transcription. Interferon-stimulated genes modulate many biological effects including the inhibition of viral replication in infected cells, inhibition of cell proliferation and immunomodulation. The clinical relevance of these in vitro activities is not known.

PEGASYS stimulates the production of effector proteins such as serum neopterin and 2′, 5′-oligoadenylate synthetase.

Pharmacokinetics

Maximal serum concentrations (C_{max}) occur between 72 to 96 hours post-dose. The C_{max} and AUC measurements of PEGASYS increase in a dose-related manner. Week 48 mean trough concentrations (16 ng/mL; range 4 to 28) at 168 hours post-dose are approximately 2-fold higher than week 1 mean trough concentrations (8 ng/mL; range 0 to 15). Steady-state serum levels are reached within 5 to 8 weeks of once weekly dosing. The peak to trough ratio at week 48 is approximately 2.0.

The mean systemic clearance in healthy subjects given PEGASYS was 94 mL/h, which is approximately 100-fold lower than that for interferon alfa-2a (ROFERON®-A). The mean terminal half-life after sc dosing in patients with chronic hepatitis C was 80 hours (range 50 to 140 hours) compared to 5.1 hours (range 3.7 to 8.5 hours) for ROFERON®-A.

Special Populations

Gender and Age

PEGASYS administration yielded similar pharmacokinetics in male and female healthy subjects. The AUC was increased from 1295 to 1663 ng·h/mL in subjects older than 62 years taking 180 µg PEGASYS, but peak concentrations were similar (9 vs 10 ng/mL) in those older and younger than 62 years.

Pediatric Patients

The pharmacokinetics of PEGASYS have not been adequately studied in pediatric patients.

Renal Dysfunction

In patients with end stage renal disease undergoing hemodialysis, there is a 25% to 45% reduction in PEGASYS clearance (see **PRECAUTIONS: Renal Impairment**).

The pharmacokinetics of ribavirin following administration of COPEGUS have not been studied in patients with renal impairment and there are limited data from clinical trials on administration of COPEGUS in patients with creatinine clearance <50 mL/min. Therefore, patients with creatinine clearance <50 mL/min should not be treated with COPEGUS (see **WARNINGS** and **DOSAGE AND ADMINISTRATION**).

Effect of Food on Absorption of Ribavirin

Bioavailability of a single oral dose of ribavirin was increased by co-administration with a high-fat meal. The absorption was slowed (T_{max} was doubled) and the $AUC_{0\text{-}192h}$ and C_{max} increased by 42% and 66%, respectively, when COPEGUS was taken with a high-fat meal compared with fasting conditions (see **DOSAGE AND ADMINISTRATION**).

Drug Interactions

Nucleoside Analogues

Ribavirin has been shown in vitro to inhibit phosphorylation of zidovudine and stavudine, which could lead to decreased anti-retroviral activity. Exposure to didanosine or its active metabolite (dideoxyadenosine 5′-triphosphate) is increased when didanosine is co-administered with ribavirin (see **PRECAUTIONS: Drug Interactions**).

Methadone

The pharmacokinetics of concomitant administration of methadone and PEGASYS were evaluated in 24 PEGASYS naïve chronic hepatitis C patients (15 male, 9 female) who received 180 mg PEGASYS subcutaneously weekly. All patients were on stable methadone maintenance therapy (median dose 95 mg, range 30 mg to 150 mg) prior to receiving PEGASYS. Mean methadone PK parameters were 10% to 15% higher after 4 weeks of PEGASYS treatment as compared to baseline (see **PRECAUTIONS: Drug Interactions**). Methadone did not significantly alter the PK of PEGASYS as compared to a PK study of 6 chronic hepatitis C patients not receiving methadone.

CLINICAL STUDIES

PEGASYS Monotherapy (Studies 1, 2, and 3)

The safety and effectiveness of PEGASYS for the treatment of hepatitis C virus infection were assessed in three randomized, open-label, active-controlled clinical studies. All patients were adults, had compensated liver disease, detectable hepatitis C virus (HCV), liver biopsy diagnosis of chronic hepatitis, and were previously untreated with interferon. All patients received therapy by sc injection for 48 weeks, and were followed for an additional 24 weeks to assess the durability of response. In studies 1 and 2, approx-

Table 1 Sustained Response to Monotherapy Treatment

	Study 1			Study 2			Study 3		
	ROFERON-A 3 MIU (N=207)	PEGASYS 180 µg (N=208)	DIFF* (95% CI)	ROFERON-A 6/3 MIU (N=261)	PEGASYS 180 µg (N=265)	DIFF* (95% CI)	ROFERON-A 3 MIU (N=86)	PEGASYS 180 µg (N=87)	DIFF* (95% CI)
Combined Virologic and Biologic Sustained Response	11%	24%	13 (6, 20)	17%	35%	18 (11, 25)	7%	23%	16 (6, 26)
Sustained Virologic Response**	11%	26%	15 (8, 23)	19%	38%	19 (11, 26)	8%	30%	22 (11, 33)

* Percent difference between PEGASYS and Roferon-A treatment
** COBAS AMPLICOR® HCV Test, version 2.0

imately 20% of subjects had cirrhosis or bridging fibrosis. Study 3 enrolled patients with a histological diagnosis of cirrhosis (78%) or bridging fibrosis (22%).

In study 1 (n=630), patients received either ROFERON-A (interferon alfa-2a) 3 MIU three times/week (tiw), PEGASYS 135 µg once each week (qw) or PEGASYS 180 µg qw. In study 2 (n=526), patients received either ROFERON-A 6 MIU tiw for 12 weeks followed by 3 MIU tiw for 36 weeks or PEGASYS 180 µg qw. In study 3 (n=269), patients received ROFERON-A 3 MIU tiw, PEGASYS 90 µg qw or PEGASYS 180 µg once each week.

In all three studies, treatment with PEGASYS 180 µg resulted in significantly more patients who experienced a sustained response (defined as undetectable HCV RNA and normalization of ALT on or after study week 68) compared to treatment with ROFERON-A. In study 1, response to PEGASYS 135 µg was not different from response to 180 µg. In study 3, response to PEGASYS 90 µg was intermediate between PEGASYS 180 µg and ROFERON-A.

[See table 1 above]

Matched pre- and post-treatment liver biopsies were obtained in approximately 70% of patients. Similar modest reductions in inflammation compared to baseline were observed in all treatment groups.

Of the patients who did not demonstrate either undetectable HCV RNA or at least a $2\log^{10}$ drop in HCV RNA titer from baseline by 12 weeks of PEGASYS 180 µg therapy, 2% (3/156) achieved a sustained virologic response (see **DOSAGE AND ADMINISTRATION**).

Averaged over study 1, study 2, and study 3, response rates to PEGASYS were 23% among patients with viral genotype 1 and 48% in patients with other viral genotypes. The treatment response rates were similar in men and women.

PEGASYS/COPEGUS Combination Therapy (Studies 4 and 5)

The safety and effectiveness of PEGASYS in combination with COPEGUS for the treatment of hepatitis C virus infection were assessed in two randomized controlled clinical trials. All patients were adults, had compensated liver disease, detectable hepatitis C virus, liver biopsy diagnosis of chronic hepatitis, and were previously untreated with interferon. Approximately 20% of patients in both studies had compensated cirrhosis (Child-Pugh class A).

In study 4, patients were randomized to receive either PEGASYS 180 µg sc once weekly (qw) with an oral placebo, PEGASYS 180 µg qw with COPEGUS 1000 mg po (body weight <75 kg) or 1200 mg po (body weight ≥75 kg) or REBETRON™ (interferon alfa-2b 3 MIU sc tiw plus ribavirin 1000 mg or 1200 mg po). All patients received 48 weeks of therapy followed by 24 weeks of treatment-free follow-up. COPEGUS or placebo treatment assignment was blinded. PEGASYS in combination with COPEGUS resulted in a higher SVR (defined as undetectable HCV RNA at the end of the 24-week treatment-free follow-up period) compared to PEGASYS alone or interferon alfa-2b and ribavirin. In all treatment arms, patients with viral genotype 1, regardless of viral load, had a lower response rate.

[See table 2 at top of next page]

In study 5, all patients received PEGASYS 180 µg sc qw and were randomized to treatment for either 24 or 48 weeks and to a COPEGUS dose of either 800 mg or 1000 mg/1200 mg (for body weight <75 kg / ≥75 kg). Assignment to the four treatment arms was stratified by viral genotype and baseline HCV viral titer. Patients with genotype 1 and high viral titer (defined as $>2 \times 10^6$ HCV RNA copies/mL serum) were preferentially assigned to treatment for 48 weeks.

Genotype 1

Irrespective of baseline viral titer, treatment for 48 weeks with PEGASYS and 1000 mg or 1200 mg of COPEGUS resulted in higher SVR (defined as undetectable HCV RNA at the end of the 24-week treatment-free follow-up period) compared to shorter treatment (24 weeks) and/or 800 mg COPEGUS.

Genotype non-1

Irrespective of baseline viral titer, treatment for 24 weeks with PEGASYS and 800 mg of COPEGUS resulted in a similar SVR compared to longer treatment (48 weeks) and/or 1000 mg or 1200 mg of COPEGUS.

[See table 3 at top of next page]

Among the 36 patients with genotype 4, response rates were similar to those observed in patients with genotype 1 (data not shown). The numbers of patients with genotype 5 and 6 were too few to allow for meaningful assessment.

Treatment Response in Patient Subgroups

Treatment response rates are lower in patients with poor prognostic factors receiving pegylated interferon alpha therapy. In studies 4 and 5, treatment response rates were lower in patients older than 40 years (50% vs 66%), in patients with cirrhosis (47% vs 59%), in patients weighing over 85 kg (49% vs 60%), and in patients with genotype 1 with high vs low viral load (43% vs 56%). African American patients had lower response rates compared to Caucasians.

Paired liver biopsies were performed on approximately 20% of patients in studies 4 and 5. Modest reductions in inflammation compared to baseline were seen in all treatment groups.

In studies 4 and 5, lack of early virologic response at 12 weeks (defined as HCV RNA undetectable or $>2\log^{10}$ lower than baseline) was grounds for discontinuation of treatment. Of patients who lacked an early viral response at 12 weeks and completed a recommended course of therapy despite a protocol-defined option to discontinue therapy, 5/39 (13%) achieved an SVR. Of patients who lacked an early viral response at 24 weeks, nineteen completed a full course of therapy and none achieved an SVR.

INDICATIONS AND USAGE

PEGASYS, peginterferon alfa-2a, alone or in combination with COPEGUS, is indicated for the treatment of adults with chronic hepatitis C virus infection who have compensated liver disease and have not been previously treated with interferon alpha. Patients in whom efficacy was demonstrated included patients with compensated liver disease and histological evidence of cirrhosis (Child-Pugh class A).

CONTRAINDICATIONS

PEGASYS is contraindicated in patients with:

- Hypersensitivity to PEGASYS or any of its components
- Autoimmune hepatitis
- Hepatic decompensation (Child-Pugh class B and C) before or during treatment

PEGASYS is contraindicated in neonates and infants because it contains benzyl alcohol. Benzyl alcohol is associated with an increased incidence of neurologic and other complications in neonates and infants, which are sometimes fatal.

PEGASYS and COPEGUS combination therapy is additionally contraindicated in:

- Patients with known hypersensitivity to COPEGUS or to any component of the tablet
- Women who are pregnant
- Men whose female partners are pregnant
- Patients with hemoglobinopathies (eg, thalassemia major, sickle-cell anemia)

WARNINGS

General

Patients should be monitored for the following serious conditions, some of which may become life threatening. Patients with persistently severe or worsening signs or symptoms should have their therapy withdrawn (see **BOXED WARNING**).

Neuropsychiatric

Life-threatening or fatal neuropsychiatric reactions may manifest in patients receiving therapy with PEGASYS and include suicide, suicidal ideation, depression, relapse of drug addiction, and drug overdose. These reactions may occur in patients with and without previous psychiatric illness.

PEGASYS should be used with extreme caution in patients who report a history of depression. Neuropsychiatric adverse events observed with alpha interferon treatment include aggressive behavior, psychoses, hallucinations, bipolar disorders, and mania. Physicians should monitor all patients for evidence of depression and other psychiatric symptoms. Patients should be advised to report any sign or symptom of depression or suicidal ideation to their prescribing physicians. In severe cases, therapy should be stopped immediately and psychiatric intervention instituted (see **ADVERSE REACTIONS** and **DOSAGE AND ADMINISTRATION**).

Infections

Serious and severe bacterial infections, some fatal, have been observed in patients treated with alpha interferons including PEGASYS. Some of the infections have been associated with neutropenia. PEGASYS should be discontinued in patients who develop severe infections and appropriate antibiotic therapy instituted.

Bone Marrow Toxicity

PEGASYS suppresses bone marrow function and may result in severe cytopenias. Ribavirin may potentiate the neutropenia and lymphopenia induced by alpha interferons including PEGASYS. Very rarely alpha interferons may be associated with aplastic anemia. It is advised that complete blood counts (CBC) be obtained pre-treatment and monitored routinely during therapy (see **PRECAUTIONS: Laboratory Tests**).

PEGASYS and COPEGUS should be used with caution in patients with baseline neutrophil counts <1500 cells/mm³, with baseline platelet counts <90,000 cells/mm³ or baseline hemoglobin <10 g/dL. PEGASYS therapy should be discontinued, at least temporarily, in patients who develop severe decreases in neutrophil and/or platelet counts (see **DOSAGE AND ADMINISTRATION: Dose Modifications**).

Cardiovascular Disorders

Hypertension, supraventricular arrhythmias, chest pain, and myocardial infarction have been observed in patients treated with PEGASYS.

PEGASYS should be administered with caution to patients with pre-existing cardiac disease. Because cardiac disease may be worsened by ribavirin-induced anemia, patients with a history of significant or unstable cardiac disease should not use COPEGUS (see **WARNINGS: Anemia** and **COPEGUS Package Insert**).

Hypersensitivity

Severe acute hypersensitivity reactions (eg, urticaria, angioedema, bronchoconstriction, anaphylaxis) have been rarely observed during alpha interferon and ribavirin therapy. If such reaction occurs, therapy with PEGASYS and COPEGUS should be discontinued and appropriate medical therapy immediately instituted.

Endocrine Disorders

PEGASYS causes or aggravates hypothyroidism and hyperthyroidism. Hyperglycemia, hypoglycemia, and diabetes mellitus have been observed to develop in patients treated with PEGASYS. Patients with these conditions at baseline who cannot be effectively treated by medication should not begin PEGASYS therapy. Patients who develop these conditions during treatment and cannot be controlled with medication may require discontinuation of PEGASYS therapy.

Autoimmune Disorders

Development or exacerbation of autoimmune disorders including myositis, hepatitis, ITP, psoriasis, rheumatoid arthritis, interstitial nephritis, thyroiditis, and systemic lupus erythematosus have been reported in patients receiving alpha interferon. PEGASYS should be used with caution in patients with autoimmune disorders.

Pulmonary Disorders

Dyspnea, pulmonary infiltrates, pneumonia, bronchiolitis obliterans, interstitial pneumonitis and sarcoidosis, some resulting in respiratory failure and/or patient deaths, may be induced or aggravated by PEGASYS or alpha interferon therapy. Patients who develop persistent or unexplained pulmonary infiltrates or pulmonary function impairment should discontinue treatment with PEGASYS.

Colitis

Ulcerative, and hemorrhagic/ischemic colitis, sometimes fatal, have been observed within 12 weeks of starting alpha interferon treatment. Abdominal pain, bloody diarrhea, and fever are the typical manifestations of colitis. PEGASYS should be discontinued immediately if these symptoms develop. The colitis usually resolves within 1 to 3 weeks of discontinuation of alpha interferon.

Pancreatitis

Pancreatitis, sometimes fatal, has occurred during alpha interferon and ribavirin treatment. PEGASYS and COPEGUS should be suspended if symptoms or signs suggestive of pancreatitis are observed. PEGASYS and COPEGUS should be discontinued in patients diagnosed with pancreatitis.

Ophthalmologic Disorders

Decrease or loss of vision, retinopathy including macular edema, retinal artery or vein thrombosis, retinal hemorrhages and cotton wool spots, optic neuritis, and papilledema are induced or aggravated by treatment with PEGASYS or other alpha interferons. All patients should receive an eye examination at baseline. Patients with pre-existing ophthalmologic disorders (eg, diabetic or hypertensive retinopathy) should receive periodic ophthalmologic exams during interferon alpha treatment. Any patient who develops ocular symptoms should receive a prompt and complete eye examination. PEGASYS treatment should be discontinued in patients who develop new or worsening ophthalmologic disorders.

Pregnancy: Use with Ribavirin (also, see COPEGUS Package Insert.)

Ribavirin may cause birth defects and/or death of the exposed fetus. Extreme care must be taken to avoid pregnancy in female patients and in female partners of male patients taking PEGASYS and COPEGUS combination therapy. COPEGUS THERAPY SHOULD NOT BE STARTED UNLESS A REPORT OF A NEGATIVE PREGNANCY TEST HAS BEEN OBTAINED IMMEDIATELY PRIOR TO INITIATION OF THERAPY. Women of childbearing potential and men must use two forms of effective contraception during treatment and for at least six months after treatment has concluded. Routine monthly pregnancy tests must be performed during this time (see BOXED WARNING, CONTRAINDICATIONS, PRECAUTIONS: Information for Patients, and COPEGUS Package Insert).

Anemia

The primary toxicity of ribavirin is hemolytic anemia. Hemoglobin <10 g/dL was observed in approximately 13% of

Continued on next page

Pegasys—Cont.

Table 2 Sustained Virologic Response to Combination Therapy (Study 4)

	Interferon alfa-2b+ Ribavirin 1000 mg or 1200 mg	PEGASYS + Placebo	PEGASYS + COPEGUS 1000 mg or 1200 mg
All patients	197/444 (44%)	65/224 (29%)	241/453 (53%)
Genotype 1	103/285 (36%)	29/145 (20%)	132/298 (44%)
Genotypes 2-6	94/159 (59%)	36/79 (46%)	109/155 (70%)

Difference in overall treatment response (PEGASYS/COPEGUS – Interferon alfa-2b/ribavirin) was 9% (95% CI 2.3, 15.3).

Table 3 Sustained Virologic Response as a Function of Genotype (Study 5)

	24 Weeks Treatment		48 Weeks Treatment	
	PEGASYS + COPEGUS 800 mg (N=207)	PEGASYS + COPEGUS 1000 mg or 1200 mg* (N=280)	PEGASYS + COPEGUS 800 mg (N=361)	PEGASYS + COPEGUS 1000 mg or 1200 mg* (N=436)
Genotype 1	29/101 (29%)	48/118 (41%)	99/250 (40%)	138/271 (51%)
Genotype 2-3	79/96 (82%)	116/144 (81%)	75/99 (76%)	117/153 (76%)

*1000 mg for body weight <75 kg; 1200 mg for body weight ≥75 kg.

COPEGUS and PEGASYS treated patients in clinical trials (see PRECAUTIONS: Laboratory Tests). The anemia associated with COPEGUS occurs within 1 to 2 weeks of initiation of therapy with maximum drop in hemoglobin observed during the first eight weeks. BECAUSE THE INITIAL DROP IN HEMOGLOBIN MAY BE SIGNIFICANT, IT IS ADVISED THAT HEMOGLOBIN OR HEMATOCRIT BE OBTAINED PRE-TREATMENT AND AT WEEK 2 AND WEEK 4 OF THERAPY OR MORE FREQUENTLY IF CLINICALLY INDICATED. Patients should then be followed as clinically appropriate.

Fatal and nonfatal myocardial infarctions have been reported in patients with anemia caused by ribavirin. Patients should be assessed for underlying cardiac disease before initiation of ribavirin therapy. Patients with preexisting cardiac disease should have electrocardiograms administered before treatment, and should be appropriately monitored during therapy. If there is any deterioration of cardiovascular status, therapy should be suspended or discontinued (see **DOSAGE AND ADMINISTRATION: COPEGUS Dosage Modification Guidelines**). Because cardiac disease may be worsened by drug-induced anemia, patients with a history of significant or unstable cardiac disease should not use COPEGUS (see **COPEGUS Package Insert**).

Renal

It is recommended that renal function be evaluated in all patients started on COPEGUS. COPEGUS should not be administered to patients with creatinine clearance <50 mL/min (see **CLINICAL PHARMACOLOGY: Special Populations**).

PRECAUTIONS

General

The safety and efficacy of PEGASYS alone or in combination with COPEGUS for the treatment of hepatitis C have not been established in:

- Patients who have failed other alpha interferon treatments
- Liver or other organ transplant recipients
- Patients co-infected with human immunodeficiency virus (HIV) or hepatitis B virus (HBV)

Renal Impairment

A 25% to 45% higher exposure to PEGASYS is seen in subjects undergoing hemodialysis. In patients with impaired renal function, signs and symptoms of interferon toxicity should be closely monitored. Doses of PEGASYS should be adjusted accordingly. PEGASYS should be used with caution in patients with creatinine clearance <50 mL/min (see **DOSAGE AND ADMINISTRATION: Dose Modifications**).

Information for Patients

Patients receiving PEGASYS alone or in combination with COPEGUS should be directed in its appropriate use, informed of the benefits and risks associated with treatment, and referred to the PEGASYS and, if applicable, COPEGUS (ribavirin) MEDICATION GUIDES.

PEGASYS and COPEGUS combination therapy must not be used by women who are pregnant or by men whose female partners are pregnant. COPEGUS therapy should not be initiated until a report of a negative pregnancy test has been obtained immediately before starting therapy. Female patients of childbearing potential and male patients with female partners of childbearing potential must be advised of the teratogenic/embryocidal risks and must be instructed to practice effective contraception during COPEGUS therapy and for 6 months post-therapy. Patients should be advised to notify the physician immediately in the event of a pregnancy (see **CONTRAINDICATIONS** and **WARNINGS**).

Women of childbearing potential and men must use two forms of effective contraception during treatment and during the 6 months after treatment has concluded; routine monthly pregnancy tests must be performed during this time (see **CONTRAINDICATIONS** and **COPEGUS Package Insert**).

If pregnancy does occur during treatment or during 6 months post-therapy, the patient must be advised of the significant teratogenic risk of COPEGUS therapy to the fetus. To monitor maternal-fetal outcomes of pregnant women exposed to COPEGUS, the COPEGUS Pregnancy Registry has been established. Physicians and patients are strongly encouraged to register by calling 1-800-526-6367.

Patients should be advised that laboratory evaluations are required before starting therapy and periodically thereafter (see **Laboratory Tests**). Patients should be instructed to remain well hydrated, especially during the initial stages of treatment. Patients should be advised to take COPEGUS with food.

Patients should be informed that it is not known if therapy with PEGASYS alone or in combination with COPEGUS will prevent transmission of HCV infection to others or prevent cirrhosis, liver failure or liver cancer that might result from HCV infection. Patients who develop dizziness, confusion, somnolence, and fatigue should be cautioned to avoid driving or operating machinery.

If home use is prescribed, a puncture-resistant container for the disposal of used needles and syringes should be supplied to the patients. Patients should be thoroughly instructed in the importance of proper disposal and cautioned against any reuse of any needles and syringes. The full container should be disposed of according to the directions provided by the physician (see **MEDICATION GUIDE**).

Laboratory Tests

Before beginning PEGASYS or PEGASYS and COPEGUS combination therapy, standard hematological and biochemical laboratory tests are recommended for all patients. Pregnancy screening for women of childbearing potential must be performed.

After initiation of therapy, hematological tests should be performed at 2 weeks and 4 weeks and biochemical tests should be performed at 4 weeks. Additional testing should be performed periodically during therapy. In the clinical studies, the CBC (including hemoglobin level and white blood cell and platelet counts) and chemistries (including liver function tests and uric acid) were measured at 1, 2, 4, 6, and 8, and then every 4 weeks or more frequently if abnormalities were found. Thyroid stimulating hormone (TSH) was measured every 12 weeks. Monthly pregnancy testing should be performed during combination therapy and for 6 months after discontinuing therapy.

The entrance criteria used for the clinical studies of PEGASYS may be considered as a guideline to acceptable baseline values for initiation of treatment:

- Platelet count ≥90,000 cells/mm^3 (as low as 75,000 cells/mm^3 in patients with cirrhosis)
- Caution should be exercised in initiating treatment in any patient with baseline risk of severe anemia (eg, spherocytosis, history of GI bleeding).
- Absolute neutrophil count (ANC) ≥1500 cells/mm^3
- Serum creatinine concentration <1.5 × upper limit of normal
- TSH and T_4 within normal limits or adequately controlled thyroid function

PEGASYS treatment was associated with decreases in WBC, ANC, lymphocytes, and platelet counts often starting within the first 2 weeks of treatment (see **ADVERSE REACTIONS**). Dose reduction is recommended in patients with hematologic abnormalities (see **DOSAGE AND ADMINISTRATION: Dose Modifications**).

While fever is commonly caused by PEGASYS therapy, other causes of persistent fever must be ruled out, particularly in patients with neutropenia (see **WARNINGS: Infections**).

Transient elevations in ALT (2-fold to 5-fold above baseline) were observed in some patients receiving PEGASYS, and were not associated with deterioration of other liver function tests. When the increase in ALT levels is progressive despite dose reduction or is accompanied by increased bilirubin, PEGASYS therapy should be discontinued (see **DOSAGE AND ADMINISTRATION: Dose Modifications**).

Drug Interactions

Treatment with PEGASYS once weekly for 4 weeks in healthy subjects was associated with an inhibition of P450 1A2 and a 25% increase in theophylline AUC. Theophylline serum levels should be monitored and appropriate dose adjustments considered for patients given both theophylline and PEGASYS (see **PRECAUTIONS**). There was no effect on the pharmacokinetics of representative drugs metabolized by CYP 2C9, CYP 2C19, CYP 2D6 or CYP 3A4.

In a PK study of HCV patients concomitantly receiving methadone, treatment with PEGASYS once weekly for 4 weeks was associated with methadone levels that were 10% to 15% higher than at baseline (see **CLINICAL PHARMACOLOGY: Drug Interactions**). The clinical significance of this finding is unknown; however, patients should be monitored for the signs and symptoms of methadone toxicity.

In patients with chronic hepatitis C treated with PEGASYS in combination with COPEGUS, PEGASYS treatment did not affect ribavirin distribution or clearance.

Nucleoside Analogues

Didanosine

Co-administration of COPEGUS and didanosine is not recommended. Reports of fatal hepatic failure, as well as peripheral neuropathy, pancreatitis, and symptomatic hyperlactatemia/lactic acidosis have been reported in clinical trials (see **CLINICAL PHARMACOLOGY: Drug Interactions**).

Stavudine and Zidovudine

Ribavirin can antagonize the in vitro antiviral activity of stavudine and zidovudine against HIV. Therefore, concomitant use of ribavirin with either of these drugs should be avoided.

Carcinogenesis, Mutagenesis, Impairment of Fertility

Carcinogenesis

PEGASYS has not been tested for its carcinogenic potential.

Mutagenesis

PEGASYS did not cause DNA damage when tested in the Ames bacterial mutagenicity assay and in the in vitro chromosomal aberration assay in human lymphocytes, either in the presence or absence of metabolic activation.

Use With Ribavirin

Ribavirin is genotoxic and mutagenic. The carcinogenic potential of ribavirin has not been fully determined. In a p53 (+/-) mouse carcinogenicity study at doses up to the maximum tolerated dose of 100 mg/kg/day ribavirin was not oncogenic. However, on a body surface area basis, this dose was 0.5 times maximum recommended human 24-hour dose of ribavirin. A study in rats to assess the carcinogenic potential of ribavirin is ongoing (see COPEGUS Package Insert).

Impairment of Fertility

PEGASYS may impair fertility in women. Prolonged menstrual cycles and/or amenorrhea were observed in female cynomolgus monkeys given sc injections of 600 µg/kg/dose (7200 µg/m^2/dose) of PEGASYS every other day for one month, at approximately 180 times the recommended weekly human dose for a 60 kg person (based on body surface area). Menstrual cycle irregularities were accompanied by both a decrease and delay in the peak 17β-estradiol and progesterone levels following administration of PEGASYS to female monkeys. A return to normal menstrual rhythm followed cessation of treatment. Every other day dosing with 100 µg/kg (1200 µg/m^2) PEGASYS (equivalent to approximately 30 times the recommended human dose) had no effects on cycle duration or reproductive hormone status.

The effects of PEGASYS on male fertility have not been studied. However, no adverse effects on fertility were observed in male Rhesus monkeys treated with non-pegylated interferon alfa-2a for 5 months at doses up to 25 × 10^6 IU/kg/day.

Use With Ribavirin

Ribavirin has shown reversible toxicity in animal studies of male fertility (see **COPEGUS Package Insert**).

Pregnancy

Pregnancy: Category C

PEGASYS has not been studied for its teratogenic effect. Non-pegylated interferon alfa-2a treatment of pregnant Rhesus monkeys at approximately 20 to 500 times the human weekly dose resulted in a statistically significant increase in abortions. No teratogenic effects were seen in the offspring delivered at term. PEGASYS should be assumed to have abortifacient potential. There are no adequate and well-controlled studies of PEGASYS in pregnant women. PEGASYS is to be used during pregnancy only if the potential benefit justifies the potential risk to the fetus. PEGASYS is recommended for use in women of childbearing potential only when they are using effective contraception during therapy.

Pregnancy: Category X: Use With Ribavirin (see CONTRAINDICATIONS)

Significant teratogenic and/or embryocidal effects have been demonstrated in all animal species exposed to ribavirin. COPEGUS therapy is contraindicated in women who are pregnant and in the male partners of women who are pregnant (see CONTRAINDICATIONS, WARNINGS, and COPEGUS Package Insert).

If pregnancy occurs in a patient or partner of a patient during treatment or during the 6 months after treatment cessation, such cases should be reported to the COPEGUS Pregnancy Registry at 1-800-526-6367.

Nursing Mothers

It is not known whether peginterferon or ribavirin or its components are excreted in human milk. The effect of orally ingested peginterferon or ribavirin from breast milk on the nursing infant has not been evaluated. Because of the potential for adverse reactions from the drugs in nursing infants, a decision must be made whether to discontinue nursing or discontinue PEGASYS and COPEGUS treatment.

Pediatric Use

The safety and effectiveness of PEGASYS, alone or in combination with COPEGUS in patients below the age of 18 years have not been established.

PEGASYS contains benzyl alcohol. Benzyl alcohol has been

reported to be associated with an increased incidence of neurological and other complications in neonates and infants, which are sometimes fatal (see **CONTRAINDICATIONS**).

Geriatric Use

Younger patients have higher virologic response rates than older patients. Clinical studies of PEGASYS alone or in combination with COPEGUS did not include sufficient numbers of subjects aged 65 or over to determine whether they respond differently from younger subjects. Adverse reactions related to alpha interferons, such as CNS, cardiac, and systemic (eg, flu-like) effects may be more severe in the elderly and caution should be exercised in the use of PEGASYS in this population. PEGASYS and COPEGUS are excreted by the kidney, and the risk of toxic reactions to this therapy may be greater in patients with impaired renal function. Because elderly patients are more likely to have decreased renal function, care should be taken in dose selection and it may be useful to monitor renal function. PEGASYS should be used with caution in patients with creatinine clearance <50 mL/min and COPEGUS should not be administered to patients with creatinine clearance <50 mL/min.

ADVERSE REACTIONS

PEGASYS alone or in combination with COPEGUS causes a broad variety of serious adverse reactions (see **BOXED WARNING** and **WARNINGS**). In all studies, one or more serious adverse reactions occurred in 10% of patients receiving PEGASYS alone or in combination with COPEGUS.

The most common life-threatening or fatal events induced or aggravated by PEGASYS and COPEGUS were depression, suicide, relapse of drug abuse/overdose, and bacterial infections; each occurred at a frequency of <1%.

Nearly all patients in clinical trials experienced one or more adverse events. The most commonly reported adverse reactions were psychiatric reactions, including depression, irritability, anxiety, and flu-like symptoms such as fatigue, pyrexia, myalgia, headache, and rigors.

Overall 11% of patients receiving 48 weeks of therapy with PEGASYS either alone (7%) or in combination with COPEGUS (10%) discontinued therapy. The most common reasons for discontinuation of therapy were psychiatric, flu-like syndrome (eg, lethargy, fatigue, headache), dermatologic, and gastrointestinal disorders.

The most common reason for dose modification in patients receiving combination therapy was for laboratory abnormalities, neutropenia (20%) and thrombocytopenia (4%) for PEGASYS and anemia (22%) for COPEGUS.

PEGASYS dose was reduced in 12% of patients receiving 1000 mg to 1200 mg COPEGUS for 48 weeks and in 7% of patients receiving 800 mg COPEGUS for 24 weeks. COPEGUS dose was reduced in 21% of patients receiving 1000 mg to 1200 mg COPEGUS for 48 weeks and 12% in patients receiving 800 mg COPEGUS for 24 weeks.

Because clinical trials are conducted under widely varying and controlled conditions, adverse reaction rates observed in clinical trials of a drug cannot be directly compared to rates in the clinical trials of another drug. Also, the adverse event rates listed here may not predict the rates observed in a broader patient population in clinical practice.

[See table 4 at right]

Table 4 Adverse Reactions Occurring in ≥5% of Patients in Hepatitis C Clinical Trials (Pooled Studies 1, 2, 3, and Study 4)

Body System	PEGASYS 180 µg 48 week†	ROFERON-A*†	PEGASYS 180 µg + 1000 mg or 1200 mg COPEGUS 48 week**	Intron A + 1000 mg or 1200 mg REBETOL® 48 week**
	N=559	N=554	N=451	N=443
	%	%	%	%
Application Site Disorders				
Injection site reaction	22	18	23	16
Endocrine Disorders				
Hypothyroidism	3	2	4	5
Flu-like Symptoms and Signs				
Fatigue/Asthenia	56	57	65	68
Pyrexia	37	41	41	55
Rigors	35	44	25	37
Pain	11	12	10	9
Gastrointestinal				
Nausea/Vomiting	24	33	25	29
Diarrhea	16	16	11	10
Abdominal pain	15	15	8	9
Dry mouth	6	3	4	7
Dyspepsia	<1	1	6	5
Hematologic‡				
Lymphopenia	3	5	14	12
Anemia	2	1	11	11
Neutropenia	21	8	27	8
Thrombocytopenia	5	2	5	<1
Metabolic and Nutritional				
Anorexia	17	17	24	26
Weight decrease	4	3	10	10
Musculoskeletal, Connective Tissue and Bone				
Myalgia	37	38	40	49
Arthralgia	28	29	22	23
Back pain	9	10	5	5
Neurological				
Headache	54	58	43	49
Dizziness (excluding vertigo)	16	12	14	14
Memory impairment	5	4	6	5
Psychiatric				
Irritability/Anxiety/Nervousness	19	22	33	38
Insomnia	19	23	30	37
Depression	18	19	20	28
Concentration impairment	8	10	10	13
Mood alteration	3	2	5	6
Resistance Mechanism Disorders				
Overall	10	6	12	10
Respiratory, Thoracic and Mediastinal				
Dyspnea	4	2	13	14
Cough	4	3	10	7
Dyspnea exertional	<1	<1	4	7
Skin and Subcutaneous Tissue				
Alopecia	23	30	28	33
Pruritus	12	8	19	18
Dermatitis	8	3	16	13
Dry skin	4	3	10	13
Rash	5	4	8	5
Sweating increased	6	7	6	5
Eczema	1	1	5	4
Visual Disorders				
Vision blurred	4	2	5	2

† Pooled studies 1, 2, and 3
* Either 3 MIU or 6/3 MIU of ROFERON-A
** Study 4
‡ Severe hematologic abnormalities

Patients treated for 24 weeks with PEGASYS and 800 mg COPEGUS were observed to have lower incidence of serious adverse events (3% vs 10%), Hgb <10 g/dL (3% vs 15%), dose modification of PEGASYS (30% vs 36%) and COPEGUS (19% vs 38%) and of withdrawal from treatment (5% vs 15%) compared to patients treated for 48 weeks with PEGASYS and 1000 mg or 1200 mg COPEGUS. On the other hand the overall incidence of adverse events appeared to be similar in the two treatment groups.

The most common serious adverse event (3%) was bacterial infection (eg, sepsis, osteomyelitis, endocarditis, pyelonephritis, pneumonia). Other SAEs occurred at a frequency of <1% and included: suicide, suicidal ideation, psychosis, aggression, anxiety, drug abuse and drug overdose, angina, hepatic dysfunction, fatty liver, cholangitis, arrhythmia, diabetes mellitus, autoimmune phenomena (eg, hyperthyroidism, hypothyroidism, sarcoidosis, systemic lupus erythematosus, rheumatoid arthritis), peripheral neuropathy, aplastic anemia, peptic ulcer, gastrointestinal bleeding, pancreatitis, colitis, corneal ulcer, pulmonary embolism, coma, myositis, and cerebral hemorrhage.

Laboratory Test Values

Hemoglobin

The hemoglobin concentration decreased below 12 g/dL in 17% (median Hgb drop = 2.2 g/dL) of monotherapy and 52% (median Hgb drop = 3.7 g/dL) of combination therapy patients. Severe anemia (Hgb <10 g/dL) was encountered in 13% of patients receiving combination therapy and 2% of monotherapy recipients. Dose modification for anemia was required in 22% of ribavirin recipients treated for 48 weeks. Hemoglobin decreases in PEGASYS monotherapy were generally mild and did not require dose modification (see **DOSAGE AND ADMINISTRATION: Dose Modifications**).

Neutrophils

Decreases in neutrophil count below normal were observed in 95% of patients treated with PEGASYS either alone or in combination with COPEGUS. Severe potentially life-threatening neutropenia (ANC $<0.5 \times 10^9$/L) occurred in approximately 5% of patients receiving PEGASYS either alone or in combination with COPEGUS. Seventeen percent of patients receiving PEGASYS monotherapy and 20% to 24% of patients receiving PEGASYS/COPEGUS combination therapy required modification of interferon dosage for neutropenia. Two percent of patients required permanent reductions of PEGASYS dosage and <1% required permanent discontinuation. Median neutrophil counts return to pre-treatment levels 4 weeks after cessation of therapy (see **DOSAGE AND ADMINISTRATION: Dose Modifications**).

Lymphocytes

Decreases in lymphocyte count are induced by interferon alpha therapy. Lymphopenia was observed during both monotherapy (86%) and combination therapy with PEGASYS and COPEGUS (94%). Severe lymphopenia ($<0.5\times10^9$/L) occurred in approximately 5% of monotherapy patients and 14% of combination PEGASYS and COPEGUS therapy recipients. Dose adjustments were not required by protocol. Median lymphocyte counts return to pre-treatment levels after 4 to 12 weeks of the cessation of therapy. The clinical significance of the lymphopenia is not known.

Platelets

Platelet counts decreased in 52% of patients treated with PEGASYS alone (median drop 45% from baseline), 33% of patients receiving combination with COPEGUS (median drop 30% from baseline). Median platelet counts return to pre-treatment levels 4 weeks after the cessation of therapy.

Triglycerides

Triglyceride levels are elevated in patients receiving alfa interferon therapy and were elevated in the majority of patients participating in clinical studies receiving either PEGASYS alone or in combination with COPEGUS. Random levels higher ≥400 mg/dL were observed in about 20% of patients.

ALT Elevations

Less than 1% of patients experienced marked elevations (5- to 10-fold above baseline) in ALT levels during treatment. These transaminase elevations were on occasion associated with hyperbilirubinemia and were managed by dose reduction or discontinuation of study treatment. Liver function test abnormalities were generally transient. One case was attributed to autoimmune hepatitis, which persisted beyond study medication discontinuation (see **DOSAGE AND ADMINISTRATION: Dose Modifications**).

Continued on next page

Pegasys—Cont.

Thyroid Function
PEGASYS alone or in combination with COPEGUS was associated with the development of abnormalities in thyroid laboratory values, some with associated clinical manifestations. Hypothyroidism or hyperthyroidism requiring treatment, dose modification or discontinuation occurred in 4% and 1% of PEGASYS treated patients and 4% and 2% of PEGASYS and COPEGUS treated patients, respectively. Approximately half of the patients, who developed thyroid abnormalities during PEGASYS treatment, still had abnormalities during the follow-up period (see **PRECAUTIONS: Laboratory Tests**).

Immunogenicity
Nine percent (71/834) of patients treated with PEGASYS with or without COPEGUS developed binding antibodies to interferon alfa-2a, as assessed by an ELISA assay. Three percent of patients (25/835) receiving PEGASYS with or without COPEGUS, developed low-titer neutralizing antibodies (using an assay of a sensitivity of 100 INU/mL).

The clinical and pathological significance of the appearance of serum neutralizing antibodies is unknown. No apparent correlation of antibody development to clinical response or adverse events was observed. The percentage of patients whose test results were considered positive for antibodies is highly dependent on the sensitivity and specificity of the assays.

Additionally, the observed incidence of antibody positivity in these assays may be influenced by several factors including sample timing and handling, concomitant medications, and underlying disease. For these reasons, comparison of the incidence of antibodies to PEGASYS with the incidence of antibodies to these products may be misleading.

OVERDOSAGE

There is limited experience with overdosage. The maximum dose received by any patient was 7 times the intended dose of PEGASYS (180 μg/day for 7 days). There were no serious reactions attributed to overdosages. Weekly doses of up to 630 μg have been administered to patients with cancer. Dose-limiting toxicities were fatigue, elevated liver enzymes, neutropenia, and thrombocytopenia. There is no specific antidote for PEGASYS. Hemodialysis and peritoneal dialysis are not effective.

DOSAGE AND ADMINISTRATION

There are no safety and efficacy data on treatment for longer than 48 weeks. Consideration should be given to discontinuing therapy after 12 to 24 weeks of therapy if the patient has failed to demonstrate an early virologic response (see **CLINICAL STUDIES**).

PEGASYS

The recommended dose of PEGASYS monotherapy is 180 μg (1.0 mL vial or 0.5 mL prefilled syringe) once weekly for 48 weeks by subcutaneous administration in the abdomen or thigh.

PEGASYS and COPEGUS Combination

The recommended dose of PEGASYS when used in combination with ribavirin is 180 μg (1.0 mL vial or 0.5 mL prefilled syringe) once weekly. The recommended dose of COPEGUS and duration for PEGASYS/COPEGUS therapy is based on viral genotype (see Table 5).

The daily dose of COPEGUS is 800 mg to 1200 mg administered orally in two divided doses. The dose should be individualized to the patient depending on baseline disease characteristics (eg, genotype), response to therapy, and tolerability of the regimen.

Since COPEGUS absorption increases when administered with a meal, patients are advised to take COPEGUS with food.

[See table 5 below]

A patient should self-inject PEGASYS only if the physician determines that it is appropriate and the patient agrees to medical follow-up as necessary and training in proper injection technique has been provided to him/her (see illustrated PEGASYS **MEDICATION GUIDE** for directions on injection site preparation and injection instructions).

PEGASYS should be inspected visually for particulate matter and discoloration before administration, and not used if particulate matter is visible or product is discolored. Vials and prefilled syringes with particulate matter or discoloration should be returned to the pharmacist.

Dose Modifications

If severe adverse reactions or laboratory abnormalities develop during combination COPEGUS/PEGASYS therapy, the dose should be modified or discontinued, if appropriate, until the adverse reactions abate. If intolerance persists after dose adjustment, COPEGUS/PEGASYS therapy should be discontinued.

PEGASYS

General
When dose modification is required for moderate to severe adverse reactions (clinical and/or laboratory), initial dose reduction to 135 μg (which is 0.75 mL for the vials or adjustment to the corresponding graduation mark for the syringes) is generally adequate. However, in some cases, dose reduction to 90 μg (which is 0.5 mL for the vials or adjustment to the corresponding graduation mark for the syringes) may be needed. Following improvement of the adverse reaction, re-escalation of the dose may be considered (see **WARNINGS, PRECAUTIONS**, and **ADVERSE REACTIONS**).

Hematological
[See table 6 at bottom of next page]

Psychiatric: Depression
[See table 7 at bottom of next page]

Renal Function
In patients with end-stage renal disease requiring hemodialysis, dose reduction to 135 μg PEGASYS is recommended. Signs and symptoms of interferon toxicity should be closely monitored.

Liver Function
In patients with progressive ALT increases above baseline values, the dose of PEGASYS should be reduced to 135 μg. If ALT increases are progressive despite dose reduction or accompanied by increased bilirubin or evidence of hepatic decompensation, therapy should be immediately discontinued.

COPEGUS

[See table 8 at bottom of next page]

Once COPEGUS has been withheld due to a laboratory abnormality or clinical manifestation, an attempt may be made to restart COPEGUS at 600 mg daily and further increase the dose to 800 mg daily depending upon the physician's judgment. However, it is not recommended that COPEGUS be increased to the original dose (1000 mg or 1200 mg).

Renal Impairment
COPEGUS should not be used in patients with creatinine clearance <50 mL/min (see **WARNINGS** and **COPEGUS Package Insert**).

HOW SUPPLIED

Single Dose Vial

Each PEGASYS (peginterferon alfa-2a) 180 μg single use, clear glass vial provides 1.0 mL containing 180 μg peginterferon alfa-2a for sc injection. Each package contains 1 vial (NDC 0004-0350-09).

Vials Monthly Convenience Pack

Four vials of PEGASYS (peginterferon alfa-2a), 180 μg single use, clear glass vials, in a box with 4 syringes and 8 alcohol swabs (NDC 0004-0350-39). Each syringe is a 1 mL (1 cc) volume syringe supplied with a 27 gauge, 1/2 inch needle with needle-stick protection device.

Prefilled Syringes Monthly Convenience Pack

Four prefilled syringes of PEGASYS (peginterferon alfa-2a), 180 μg single use, graduated, clear glass prefilled syringes, in a box with 4 needles and 4 alcohol swabs (NDC 0004-0352-39). Each syringe is a 0.5 mL (1/2 cc) volume syringe supplied with a 27 gauge, 1/2 inch needle with needle-stick protection device.

Storage

Store in the refrigerator at 2° to 8°C (36° to 46°F). Do not freeze or shake. Protect from light. Vials and prefilled syringes are for single use only. Discard any unused portion.

REBETRON™ is a trademark of Schering Corporation.

Revised: December 2003

MEDICATION GUIDE
PEGASYS®
(peginterferon alfa-2a)

Before you start taking PEGASYS (PEG-ah-sis), alone or in combination with COPEGUS® (Co-PEG-UHS), please read this Medication Guide carefully. Read this Medication Guide each time you refill your prescription in case new information has been added and make sure the pharmacist has given you the medicine your healthcare provider prescribed for you. Reading the information in this Medication Guide does not take the place of talking with your healthcare provider.

If you are taking PEGASYS in combination with COPEGUS, you should also read the Medication Guide for COPEGUS (ribavirin, USP) Tablets.

What is the most important information I should know about PEGASYS therapy?

PEGASYS, taken alone or in combination with COPEGUS, is a treatment for some people who are infected with hepatitis C virus. However, PEGASYS and COPEGUS can have serious side effects that may cause death in rare cases. Before starting PEGASYS therapy, you should talk with your healthcare provider about the possible benefits and the possible side effects of treatment, to decide if either of these treatments is right for you. If you begin treatment you will need to see your healthcare provider regularly for examinations and blood tests to make sure your treatment is working and to check for side effects.

The most serious possible side effects of PEGASYS taken alone or in combination with COPEGUS include:

Risks to Pregnancy:

Taking PEGASYS in combination with COPEGUS tablets can cause death, serious birth defects or other harm to your unborn child. If you are a woman of childbearing age, you must have negative pregnancy tests just before beginning treatment, during treatment, and for 6 months after you have stopped treatment. You must not become pregnant while either you or your partner are being treated with the PEGASYS/COPEGUS combination therapy or for 6 months after stopping therapy. Men and women should use two forms of birth control while taking the combination therapy and for the 6 months after treatment is completed. If you are a man, one of the two forms of birth control should be a condom. You must use birth control even if you believe that you are not fertile or that your fertility is low. You should talk to your healthcare provider about birth control for you and your partner.

If you are pregnant, you or your male partner must not take PEGASYS/COPEGUS combination therapy. If you or your partner are being treated and you become pregnant either during treatment or within 6 months of stopping treatment, call your healthcare provider right away.

Mental health problems:

PEGASYS may cause some patients to develop mood or behavioral problems. Signs of these problems include irritability (getting easily upset), depression (feeling low, feeling bad about yourself or feeling hopeless), and anxiety. Some patients may have aggressive behavior. Some patients may develop thoughts about ending their lives (suicidal thoughts) and may attempt to do so. A few patients have even ended their lives. Former drug addicts may fall back into drug addiction or overdose. You must tell your healthcare provider if you are being treated for a mental illness or have a history of mental illness or if you are or have ever been addicted to drugs or alcohol. Call your healthcare provider immediately if you develop any of these problems while on PEGASYS treatment.

Blood problems:

Many patients taking PEGASYS have had a drop in the number of their white blood cells and their platelets. If the numbers of these blood cells are too low, you could be at risk for serious infections or bleeding.

COPEGUS causes a decrease in the number of your red blood cells (anemia). This can be dangerous, especially for patients who already have heart or circulatory (cardiovascular) problems. If you have or have ever had any cardiovascular problems, talk with your healthcare provider before taking the combination of PEGASYS and COPEGUS.

Infections:

Some patients taking interferon have had serious infections. Sometimes these infections have been fatal. If you develop a fever that does not go away or gets higher, call your healthcare provider right away. Your healthcare provider will need to examine you to rule out your having a serious infection.

Body organ problems:

Some patients may experience lung problems (such as difficulty breathing or pneumonia) and eye problems that can cause blurred vision or loss of your vision.

Call your healthcare provider immediately if you develop any of these conditions:

- **You become very depressed or think about suicide**
- **You have severe chest pain**
- **You have trouble breathing**
- **You have a change in your vision**
- **You become pregnant**
- **You notice unusual bleeding or bruising**
- **You have psoriasis (a skin disease) and it gets worse while taking PEGASYS**
- **High fever or a fever that does not go away**
- **You have severe stomach pain or lower back pain**
- **Bloody diarrhea**

*For more information on possible side effects with PEGASYS therapy, alone or in combination with COPEGUS, please read the section on **"What are the possible side effects of PEGASYS, and PEGASYS taken with COPEGUS?"** in this Medication Guide. You should also read the Medication Guide for COPEGUS tablets if you are taking that medicine with PEGASYS.*

What is PEGASYS?

PEGASYS is a drug used to treat adults who have a lasting (chronic) infection with hepatitis C virus and who show signs that the virus is damaging the liver. Patients with hepatitis C have the virus in their blood and in their liver. PEGASYS reduces the amount of virus in the body and helps the body's immune system fight the virus. The drug COPEGUS are tablets that may be taken with PEGASYS to help fight the virus infection. Do not take COPEGUS by itself.

In some patients that have received PEGASYS treatment for approximately one year, the amount of the hepatitis C virus in the body was decreased to a level so low that it could not be measured by blood tests. After 3 months of therapy, your healthcare provider may ask you to have a blood test to help determine how you are responding to your treatment.

Table 5 PEGASYS and COPEGUS Dosing Recommendations

Genotype	PEGASYS Dose	COPEGUS Dose	Duration
Genotype 1, 4	180 μg	<75 kg = 1000 mg ≥75 kg = 1200 mg	48 weeks 48 weeks
Genotype 2, 3	180 μg	800 mg	24 weeks

Genotypes 2 & 3 showed no increased response to treatment beyond 24 weeks (see Table 3). Data on genotypes 5 and 6 are insufficient for dosing recommendations.

It is not known if PEGASYS, used alone or in combination with COPEGUS, can cure hepatitis C (permanently eliminate the virus) or if it can prevent liver failure or liver cancer that is caused by hepatitis C infection.
It is also not known if PEGASYS, alone or in combination with COPEGUS, will prevent one infected person from infecting another person with hepatitis C.

Who should not take PEGASYS, or PEGASYS with COPEGUS?

Do not take PEGASYS or PEGASYS/COPEGUS therapy if you:

- are pregnant, planning to get pregnant during treatment or during the 6 months after treatment or breast-feeding
- are a male patient with a female sexual partner who is pregnant or plans to become pregnant at any time while you are being treated with COPEGUS or during the 6 months after your treatment has ended
- have hepatitis caused by your immune system attacking your liver (autoimmune hepatitis) or unstable liver disease
- had an allergic reaction to another alpha interferon or are allergic to any of the ingredients in PEGASYS or COPEGUS tablets
- Do not take PEGASYS, alone or in combination with COPEGUS, if you have abnormal red blood cells such as sickle-cell anemia or thalassemia major.

If you have ever had any of the following conditions or serious medical problems, tell your healthcare provider before you start taking PEGASYS:

- History of or current severe mental illness (such as depression or anxiety)
- History of drug or alcohol addiction or abuse
- History of heart disease or previous heart attack
- History of cancer
- Autoimmune disease (where the body's immune system attacks the body's own cells), such as psoriasis (a skin disease), systemic lupus erythematosus, rheumatoid arthritis
- Kidney problems
- Blood disorders
- You take a medicine called theophylline
- Diabetes (high blood sugar)
- Problems with the thyroid gland
- Liver problems, other than hepatitis C
- Hepatitis B infection
- HIV infection
- Colitis (an inflammation of the bowels)

You should tell your healthcare provider if you are taking or planning to take other prescription or nonprescription medicines or vitamin and mineral supplements or herbal medicines.

If you have any questions about your health condition or about taking PEGASYS alone or in combination with COPEGUS, you should talk to your healthcare provider.

How should I take PEGASYS, or PEGASYS with COPEGUS?

PEGASYS is given by injection under the skin (subcutaneous injection). PEGASYS comes in two different forms (a liquid in a single use vial and a liquid in a prefilled syringe). Your healthcare provider will determine which is best for you. Your healthcare provider will also decide whether you will take PEGASYS alone or with COPEGUS. Your dose of PEGASYS is given as a single injection once per week. At some point, your healthcare provider may change your dose of PEGASYS or COPEGUS. Do not change your dose unless your healthcare provider tells you to change it. It is important that you take PEGASYS and COPEGUS exactly as your healthcare provider tells you. Once you start treatment with PEGASYS, do not switch to another brand of interferon without talking to your healthcare provider. Other interferons may not have the same effect on the treatment of your disease. Switching brands will also require a change in your dose.

Take your prescribed dose of PEGASYS once a week, on the same day of each week and at approximately the same time. Your total dose of COPEGUS tablets should be divided so you take it twice a day with food (breakfast and dinner). Taking half your dose of COPEGUS in the morning and the other half at night will keep the medicine in your body at a steady level. Do not take more than your prescribed dose of PEGASYS or COPEGUS. **Be sure to read the Medication Guide for COPEGUS (ribavirin, USP) for complete instructions on how to take the COPEGUS tablets.**

Your healthcare provider will train you and/or the person that will be giving you the PEGASYS injections on the proper way to give injections. Whether you give yourself the injection or another person gives the injection to you, it is important that you are comfortable with preparing and injecting a dose of PEGASYS, and you understand the instructions in "How do I inject PEGASYS?" **At the end of this guide (see Appendix) there are detailed instructions on how to prepare and give yourself an injection of PEGASYS using the form your healthcare provider has prescribed for you.**

If you miss a dose and you remember **within 2 days** of when you should have taken PEGASYS, give yourself an injection of PEGASYS as soon as you remember. Take your next dose on the day you would usually take it. **If more than 2 days** have passed, ask your healthcare provider what you should do. If you miss a dose of COPEGUS, take the missed dose as soon as you remember during the same day. Do not take 2 doses too close together in time. If it is late in the day, wait until the next day and go back on schedule. **Do not double the next dose.**

If you take more than the prescribed amount of PEGASYS, call your healthcare provider right away. Your healthcare provider may want to examine you and take blood for testing.

You must get regular blood tests to help your healthcare provider check how the treatment is working and to check for side effects.

What should I avoid while taking PEGASYS, or PEGASYS with COPEGUS?

- If you are pregnant do not start taking or continue taking COPEGUS in combination with PEGASYS.
- Avoid becoming pregnant while taking PEGASYS, alone or in combination with COPEGUS. PEGASYS, alone or in combination with COPEGUS, may harm your unborn child (death or serious birth defects) or cause you to lose your baby (miscarry). **If you or your partner become pregnant during or within 6 months after treatment with COPEGUS, immediately report the pregnancy to your healthcare provider. You or your healthcare provider should call 1-800-526-6367.** When you call this number, you will be asked for information about you and/or your partner that will be added to a pregnancy registry. This information will be used to help you and your healthcare provider make decisions about your treatment for hepatitis in the future. You, your partner and/or your healthcare provider may also be asked follow-up information on the outcome of the pregnancy.
- Do not breast-feed your baby while on PEGASYS, alone or in combination with COPEGUS.

What are the possible side effects of PEGASYS, and PEGASYS taken with COPEGUS?

Possible, serious side effects include:

- **Risk to pregnancy, mental health problems including suicidal thoughts, blood problems, infections, and body organ problems:** *See "What is the most important information I should know about PEGASYS therapy?" in this Medication Guide.*
- **Autoimmune problems:** Some patients may develop a disease where the body's own immune system begins to attack itself (autoimmune disease) while on PEGASYS therapy. These diseases can include psoriasis or thyroid problems. In some patients who already have an autoimmune disease, the disease may worsen while on PEGASYS therapy.
- **Heart problems:** PEGASYS may cause some patients to experience chest pain, and very rarely a heart attack. Patients who already have heart disease could be at greatest risk. Tell your healthcare provider if you have or have had a heart problem in the past.

Common, but less serious, side effects include:

- **Flu-like symptoms:** Most patients who take PEGASYS have flu-like symptoms that usually lessen after the first few weeks of treatment. Flu-like symptoms may include fever, chills, muscle aches, joint pain, and headaches. Taking pain and fever reducers such as acetaminophen or ibuprofen before you take PEGASYS can help with these symptoms. You can also try taking PEGASYS at night. You may be able to sleep through the symptoms.
- **Extreme fatigue (tiredness):** Many patients may become extremely tired while on PEGASYS therapy.
- **Upset stomach:** Nausea, taste changes, diarrhea, and loss of appetite occur commonly.
- **Blood sugar problems:** Some patients may develop a problem with the way their body controls their blood sugar and may develop diabetes.
- **Skin reactions:** Some patients may develop rash, dry or itchy skin, and redness and swelling at the site of injection.
- **Hair thinning:** Temporary hair loss is not uncommon during treatment with PEGASYS.
- **Trouble sleeping**

These are not all of the side effects of PEGASYS, and PEGASYS taken with COPEGUS. Your healthcare provider or pharmacist can give you a more complete list.

Talk to your healthcare provider if you are worried about side effects or find them very bothersome.

General advice about prescription medicines

Medicines are sometimes prescribed for purposes other than those listed in a Medication Guide. If you have any concerns or questions about PEGASYS, contact your healthcare provider. Do not use PEGASYS for a condition or person other than that for which it is prescribed. If you want to know more about PEGASYS, your healthcare provider or pharmacist will be able to provide you with detailed information that is written for healthcare providers.

If you are taking COPEGUS (ribavirin, USP) in combination with PEGASYS, also read the Medication Guide supplied with that medicine.

Keep this and all drugs out of the reach of children.

This Medication Guide has been approved by the U.S. Food and Drug Administration.

Revised: December 2003

Medication Guide Appendix: Instructions for Preparing and Giving a Dose with a PEGASYS® Prefilled Syringe

How should I store PEGASYS Prefilled Syringes?

PEGASYS must be stored in the refrigerator at a temperature of 2°C to 8°C (36°F to 46°F). Do not leave PEGASYS outside of the refrigerator for more than 24 hours. Do not freeze PEGASYS. Keeping PEGASYS at temperatures outside the recommended range can destroy the medicine.

Each PEGASYS prefilled syringe can only be used once. Discard after use.

Continued on next page

Table 6 PEGASYS Hematological Dose Modification Guidelines

Laboratory Values	PEGASYS Dose Reduction	Discontinue PEGASYS if:
ANC <750/mm^3	135 μg	ANC <500/mm^3, treatment should be suspended until ANC values return to more than 1000/mm^3. Reinstitute at 90 μg and monitor ANC
Platelet <50,000/mm^3	90 μg	Platelet count <25,000/mm^3

Table 7 Guidelines for Modification or Discontinuation of PEGASYS and for Scheduling Visits for Patients with Depression

Depression Severity	Initial Management (4-8 weeks)		Depression		
	Dose modification	Visit schedule	Remains stable	Improves	Worsens
Mild	No change	Evaluate once weekly by visit and/or phone	Continue weekly visit schedule	Resume normal visit schedule	(See moderate or severe depression)
Moderate	Decrease PEGASYS dose to 135 μg (in some cases dose reduction to 90 μg may be needed)	Evaluate once weekly (office visit at least every other week)	Consider psychiatric consultation. Continue reduced dosing	If symptoms improve and are stable for 4 weeks, may resume normal visit schedule. Continue reduced dosing or return to normal dose	(See severe depression)
Severe	Discontinue PEGASYS permanently	Obtain immediate psychiatric consultation	Psychiatric therapy necessary		

Table 8 COPEGUS Dosage Modification Guidelines

Laboratory Values	Reduce Only COPEGUS Dose to 600 mg/day* if:	Discontinue COPEGUS if:
Hemoglobin in patients with no cardiac disease	<10 g/dL	<8.5 g/dL
Hemoglobin in patients with history of stable cardiac disease	≥2 g/dL decrease in hemoglobin during any 4 week period treatment	<12 g/dL despite 4 weeks at reduced dose

* One 200 mg tablet in the morning and two 200 mg tablets in the evening.

Pegasys—Cont.

Do not shake the prefilled syringe of PEGASYS. If PEGASYS is shaken too hard, it will not work properly. Protect PEGASYS from light during storage.

Keep this and all other medicines out of the reach of children.

How do I prepare and inject PEGASYS?

You should read through all of these directions and ask your healthcare provider for help if you have any questions before trying to give yourself an injection. It is important to follow these directions carefully. Talk to your healthcare provider if you have any questions about PEGASYS.

Your healthcare provider may not want you to take all the medicine that comes in the prefilled syringe. To appropriately administer the dose that your healthcare provider tells you to take, you may have to get rid of some of the medicine before injecting the medicine.

If you ever switch between using prefilled syringes and vials, talk to your healthcare provider about how much PEGASYS to use. Equal volumes of liquid from the prefilled syringes and the vials DO NOT contain the same amount of PEGASYS. If you switch between prefilled syringes and vials, you will have to adjust the volume of liquid that you use to give your injection. If you do not adjust this, you could accidentally take too much or too little of your medicine.

If you are giving this injection to someone else, a healthcare provider must teach you how to avoid needle sticks. Being stuck by a used needle can pass diseases on to you.

The prefilled syringes are used for injecting PEGASYS under the surface of the skin (subcutaneous).

1. Collect all the materials you will need before you start to give the injection:
   - One PEGASYS prefilled syringe Monthly Convenience Pack containing an inner carton holding the PEGASYS prefilled syringe
   - A puncture-resistant container for cleaning up when you are finished
2. Open the convenience pack and look at the contents.
   - Each convenience pack has everything you need for the PEGASYS injection.
     - 4 single use syringes filled with medicine (should be colorless to light yellow)
     - four 27 gauge, 1/2 inch needles with needle stick protection device
     - 4 alcohol swabs
   - Do not use PEGASYS if:
     - the medicine is cloudy
     - the medicine has particles floating in it
     - the medicine is any color besides colorless to light yellow
     - the expiration date has passed
3. Warm the refrigerated medicine by gently rolling it in the palms of your hands for about one minute. Do not shake.
4. Wash your hands with soap and warm water to prevent infection.
5. Attachment of the needle to the PEGASYS prefilled syringe:
   - Remove the needle from its package. Do not remove the needle shield yet. Keep the needle covered until just before you give the injection.

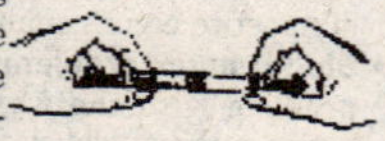

   - Remove and discard the rubber cap from the tip of the syringe barrel.
   - Put the needle onto the end of the syringe barrel so it fits tightly.
   - Here is a picture of the assembled syringe:

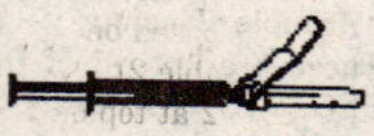

   - Keep the syringe in a horizontal position until ready for use.
   - If you need to set the syringe down, make sure the plastic shield covers the needle. Never let the needle touch any surface.
6. Decide where you will give the injection.
   - Pick a place on your stomach or thigh (see the picture at right). Avoid your navel and waistline. You should use a different place each time you give yourself an injection.

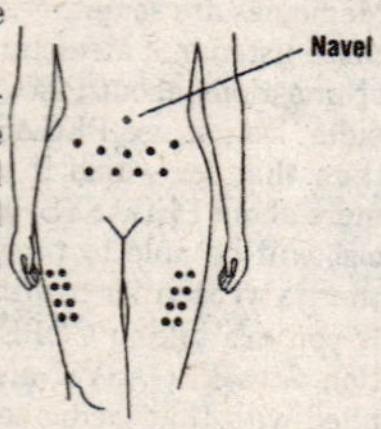

7. Prepare your skin for the injection.
   - To minimize the discomfort from injections, you may want to gently tap the area where you plan to give yourself an injection.
   - Clean the area using the alcohol pad. Let the skin dry for 10 seconds.
8. Uncover the needle.
   - Remove the plastic safety shield covering the needle. Do not remove the orange cap that is attached to the end of the syringe and above the needle that is the needle-stick protection device.

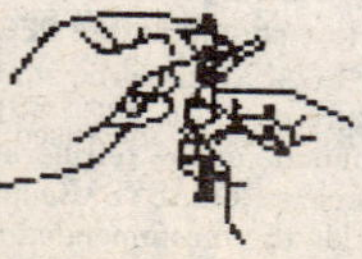

9. Remove air bubbles from the syringe.
   - Hold the syringe with the needle pointing up to the ceiling.
   - Using your thumb and finger, tap the syringe to bring air bubbles to the top.
   - Press the plunger in slightly to push air bubbles out of the syringe.
   - Your healthcare provider may not want you to take all the medicine that comes in the prefilled syringe.
   - To appropriately administer the dose that your healthcare provider tells you to take, you may have to get rid of some of the medicine before injecting the medicine.
   - The syringe has markings for 180 mcg, 135 mcg, and 90 mcg. Your healthcare provider will tell you which mark to use.

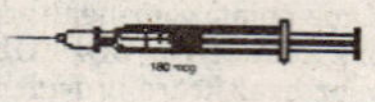

   - Once you know which mark to use, slowly and carefully press on the plunger rod of the syringe to push out medicine from the syringe. Keep pressing until the edge of the plunger stopper reaches the right mark on the side of the syringe.

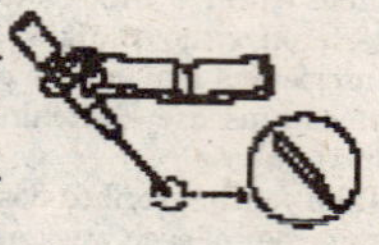

   - Do not decrease or increase your dose of PEGASYS unless your healthcare provider tells you to.
10. Give the injection of PEGASYS.
    - Position the point of the needle (the bevel) so it is facing up.
    - Pinch a fold of skin on your stomach or thigh firmly with your thumb and forefinger.

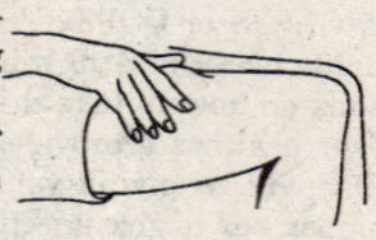

    - Hold the syringe like a pencil at a 45° to 90° angle to your skin. In one quick motion, insert the needle as far as it will go into the pinched area of skin. Pull the plunger of the syringe back very slightly. If blood comes into the syringe, the needle has entered a blood vessel. **Do not inject. Withdraw the needle and discard the syringe as outlined in step 11. Repeat the above steps with a new prefilled syringe and prepare a new site.**

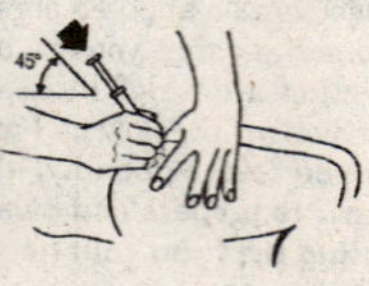

    - If no blood appears, release your skin and slowly push the plunger all the way down so that you get all of your medicine.
    - Pull out the needle at same angle you put it in.
    - Wipe the area with an alcohol swab.
11. For safety reasons, before you dispose of the syringe and needle, place the free end of the orange cap on a flat surface and push down on it until it clicks and covers over the needle. Always place used syringes and needles in a puncture-resistant container immediately after use and never reuse them. Keep your disposal container out of the reach of children.

How should I dispose of materials used to inject PEGASYS?

There may be special state and local laws for disposal of used needles and syringes. Your healthcare provider or pharmacist should provide you with instructions on how to properly dispose of your used syringes and needles. Always follow these instructions.

The instructions below should be used as a general guide for proper disposal:

- The needles and syringes should never be reused.
- Place all used needles and syringes in a puncture-proof disposable container that is available through your pharmacy or healthcare provider (Sharp's container).
- DO NOT use glass or clear plastic containers for disposal of needles and syringes.
- Dispose of the full container as instructed by your healthcare provider or pharmacist.

DO NOT throw the container in your household trash. DO NOT recycle. Keep the container out of the reach of children.

Appendix revision date: December 2003

Medication Guide Appendix: Instructions for Preparing and Giving a Dose with a PEGASYS® Vial

How should I store PEGASYS vials?

PEGASYS must be stored in the refrigerator at a temperature of 2°C to 8°C (36°F to 46°F). Do not leave PEGASYS outside of the refrigerator for more than 24 hours. Do not freeze PEGASYS. Keeping PEGASYS at temperatures outside the recommended range can destroy the medicine.

Each PEGASYS vial can only be used once. Discard after use.

Do not shake the vial of PEGASYS. If PEGASYS is shaken too hard, it will not work properly.

Protect PEGASYS from light during storage.

Keep this and all other medicines out of the reach of children.

How do I inject PEGASYS?

The following instructions will help you learn how to measure your dose and give yourself an injection of PEGASYS. You should read through all of these directions and ask your healthcare provider for help if you have any questions before trying to give yourself an injection. It is important to follow these directions carefully. Talk to your healthcare provider if you have any questions about PEGASYS.

If you are giving an injection to someone else, a healthcare provider must teach you how to avoid needle sticks. Being stuck by a used needle can pass diseases on to you.

1. Collect all the materials you will need before you start to give the injection:
   - One vial of PEGASYS
   - One syringe and needle
   - Several alcohol pads
   - A puncture-resistant container to dispose of the needle and syringe when you are finished

If you have received the PEGASYS Convenience Pack, it includes PEGASYS, safety syringes and needles with a needle-stick protection device attached, and alcohol swabs.

2. Check the date on the carton the PEGASYS comes in and make sure the expiration date has not passed, then remove a vial from the package and look at the medicine.
   - Do not use PEGASYS if:
     - the medicine is cloudy
     - the medicine has particles floating in it
     - the medicine is any color besides colorless to light yellow
     - the expiration date has passed
3. Warm the refrigerated medicine by gently rolling it in the palms of your hands for about one minute. Do not shake.
4. Wash your hands with soap and warm water to prevent infection.
5. Take the vial of PEGASYS and flip off the plastic top covering the vial opening, and clean the rubber stopper on the top of the vial with a different alcohol pad.

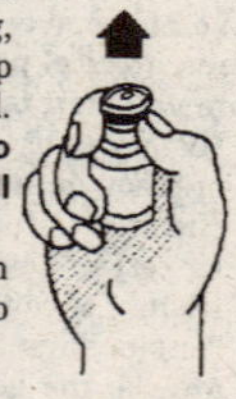

If you are not sure how much medicine to use or which mark to use, STOP and call your healthcare provider right away.

6. Remove the needle and syringe from their packaging and attach the needle to the end of the syringe.
   - If you are using a syringe and needle supplied with the PEGASYS Convenience Pack, the needle is already attached to the syringe and it will have a needle-stick protection device attached. Remove the clear protective cap from the end of the needle. Do not remove the orange cap that is attached to the end of the syringe and above the needle that is the needle-stick protection device.

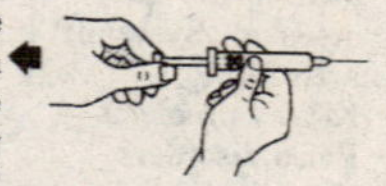

   - Pull the plunger back so the end of it is to the mark on the syringe barrel that matches the dose prescribed for you by your healthcare provider. This will pull air into the syringe barrel.
   - Push the needle through the center of the stopper on the vial.
   - Slowly inject all the air from the syringe into the air space above the solution. Do not inject air into the fluid.

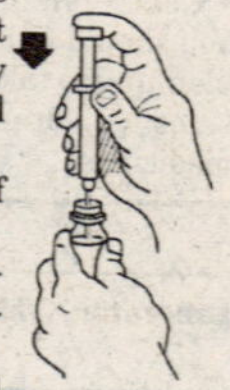

   - Keep the needle inside the vial and turn both upside down. Hold the vial and syringe straight up. Slowly pull back on the plunger until the medicine is in the syringe up to the mark that matches your dose. Make sure the needle tip always stays in the medicine (not in the air space above it).
   - When the medicine is up to the right mark on the syringe barrel, take the syringe and needle out of the rubber stopper on the vial.
   - Keep the syringe pointing up until you are ready to use it.
   - If you need to set the syringe down, make sure that you never let the needle touch any surface.

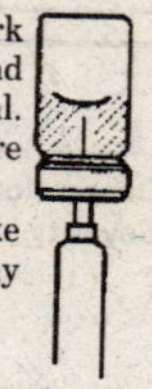

7. Remove air bubbles from the syringe.
   - Hold the syringe with the needle pointing up to the ceiling.
   - Using your thumb and finger, tap the syringe to bring air bubbles to top.
   - Press the plunger in slightly to push air bubbles out of the syringe.

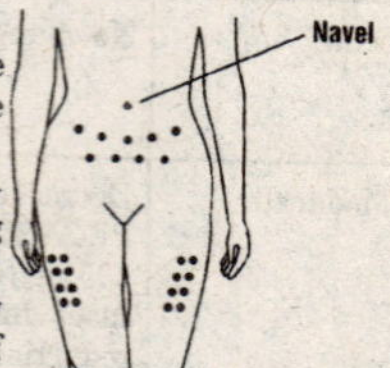

8. Decide where you will give the injection.
   - Pick a place on your stomach or thigh (see the picture below). Avoid your navel and waistline. You should use a different place each time you give yourself an injection.
9. Prepare your skin for the injection.
   - To minimize the discomfort from injections, you may want to gently tap the area where you plan to give yourself an injection.
   - Clean the area using an alcohol pad. Let the skin dry for 10 seconds.

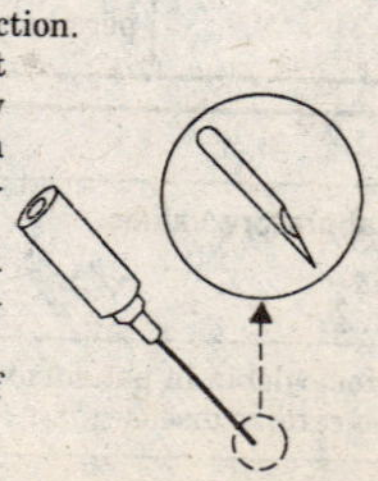

10. Give the injection of PEGASYS.
    - Position the point of the needle (the bevel) so it is facing up.
    - Pinch a fold of skin on your stomach or thigh firmly between your thumb and forefinger.

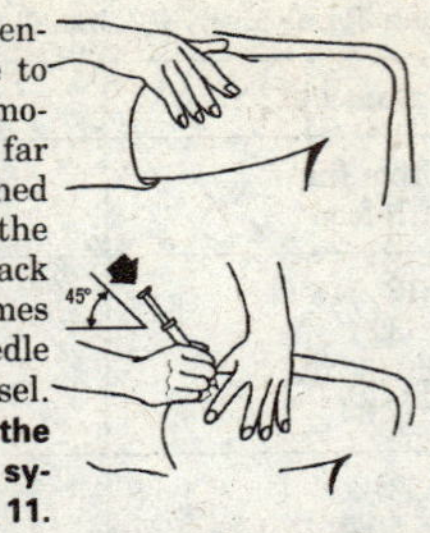

- Hold the syringe like a pencil at a 45° to 90° angle to your skin. In one quick motion, insert the needle as far as it will go into the pinched area of skin. Pull the plunger of the syringe back very slightly. If blood comes into the syringe, the needle has entered a blood vessel. **Do not inject. Withdraw the needle and discard the syringe as outlined in step 11. Repeat the above steps with a new vial and syringe and prepare a new site.**
- If no blood appears, release your skin and slowly push the plunger all the way down so that you get all of your medicine.
- Pull out the needle at same angle you put it in. Wipe the area with an alcohol pad.

11. For safety reasons, always place used syringes and needles in a puncture-resistant container immediately after use and never reuse them.
    - If you are using a syringe with a needle-stick protection device, before you dispose of the syringe and needle, place the free end of the orange cap on a flat surface and push down on it until it clicks and covers over the needle.

How should I dispose of materials used to inject PEGASYS?
There may be special state and local laws for disposal of used needles and syringes. Your healthcare provider or pharmacist should provide you with instructions on how to properly dispose of your used syringes and needles. Always follow these instructions.
The instructions below should be used as a general guide for proper disposal:
- The needles and syringes should never be reused.
- Place all used needles and syringes in a puncture-proof disposable container that is available through your pharmacy or healthcare provider (Sharp's container).
- DO NOT use glass or clear plastic containers for disposal of needles and syringes.
- Dispose of the full container as instructed by your healthcare provider or pharmacist.

DO NOT throw the container in your household trash. DO NOT recycle. Keep the container out of the reach of children.

Appendix revision date: December 2003

Hoffmann-La Roche Inc.
340 Kingsland Street
Nutley, New Jersey 07110-1199
U.S. Govt. Lic. No. 0136

VALCYTE®
(valganciclovir hydrochloride tablets)
Rx only ℞

Prescribing information for this product, which appears on pages 2970–2973 of the 2004 PDR, has been revised as follows. Please write "See Supplement A" next to the product heading.

> **WARNING**
> **THE CLINICAL TOXICITY OF VALCYTE, WHICH IS METABOLIZED TO GANCICLOVIR, INCLUDES GRANULOCYTOPENIA, ANEMIA AND THROMBOCYTOPENIA. IN ANIMAL STUDIES GANCICLOVIR WAS CARCINOGENIC, TERATOGENIC AND CAUSED ASPERMATOGENESIS.**

DESCRIPTION
Valcyte (valganciclovir HCl tablets) contains valganciclovir hydrochloride (valganciclovir HCl), a hydrochloride salt of the L-valyl ester of ganciclovir that exists as a mixture of two diastereomers. Ganciclovir is a synthetic guanine derivative active against cytomegalovirus (CMV).
Valcyte is available as a 450 mg tablet for oral administration. Each tablet contains 496.3 mg of valganciclovir HCl (corresponding to 450 mg of valganciclovir), and the inactive ingredients microcrystalline cellulose, povidone K-30, crospovidone and stearic acid. The film-coat applied to the tablets contains Opadry Pink®.
Valganciclovir HCl is a white to off-white crystalline powder with a molecular formula of $C_{14}H_{22}N_6O_5 \cdot HCl$ and a molecular weight of 390.83. The chemical name for valganciclovir HCl is L-Valine, 2-[(2-amino-1,6-dihydro-6-oxo-9H-purin-9-yl)methoxy]-3-hydroxypropyl ester, monohydrochloride. Valganciclovir HCl is a polar hydrophilic compound with a solubility of 70 mg/mL in water at 25°C at a pH of 7.0 and an n-octanol/water partition coefficient of 0.0095 at pH 7.0. The pKa for valganciclovir HCl is 7.6.
All doses in this insert are specified in terms of valganciclovir.

VIROLOGY
Mechanism of Action
Valganciclovir is an L-valyl ester (prodrug) of ganciclovir that exists as a mixture of two diastereomers. After oral administration, both diastereomers are rapidly converted to ganciclovir by intestinal and hepatic esterases. Ganciclovir is a synthetic analogue of 2′-deoxyguanosine, which inhibits replication of human cytomegalovirus in vitro and in vivo. In CMV-infected cells ganciclovir is initially phosphorylated to ganciclovir monophosphate by the viral protein kinase, pUL97. Further phosphorylation occurs by cellular kinases to produce ganciclovir triphosphate, which is then slowly metabolized intracellularly (half-life 18 hours). As the phosphorylation is largely dependent on the viral kinase, phosphorylation of ganciclovir occurs preferentially in virus-infected cells. The virustatic activity of ganciclovir is due to inhibition of viral DNA synthesis by ganciclovir triphosphate.

Antiviral Activity
The quantitative relationship between the in vitro susceptibility of human herpesviruses to antivirals and clinical response to antiviral therapy has not been established, and virus sensitivity testing has not been standardized. Sensitivity test results, expressed as the concentration of drug required to inhibit the growth of virus in cell culture by 50% (IC_{50}), vary greatly depending upon a number of factors. Thus the IC_{50} of ganciclovir that inhibits human CMV replication in vitro (laboratory and clinical isolates) has ranged from 0.02 to 5.75 µg/mL (0.08 to 22.94 µM). Ganciclovir inhibits mammalian cell proliferation (IC_{50}) in vitro at higher concentrations ranging from 10.21 to >250 µg/mL (40 to >1000 µM). Bone marrow-derived colony-forming cells are more sensitive (IC_{50} = 0.69 to 3.06 µg/mL; 2.7 to 12 µM).

Viral Resistance
Viruses resistant to ganciclovir can arise after prolonged treatment with valganciclovir by selection of mutations in either the viral protein kinase gene (UL97) responsible for ganciclovir monophosphorylation and/or in the viral DNA polymerase gene (UL54). Virus with mutations in the UL97 gene is resistant to ganciclovir alone, whereas virus with mutations in the UL54 gene may show cross-resistance to other antivirals that target the same sites on viral DNA polymerase.
The current working definition of CMV resistance to ganciclovir in in vitro assays is $IC_{50} \geq 1.5$ µg/mL (≥ 6.0 µM). CMV resistance to ganciclovir has been observed in individuals with AIDS and CMV retinitis who have never received ganciclovir therapy. Viral resistance has also been observed in patients receiving prolonged treatment for CMV retinitis with ganciclovir. The possibility of viral resistance should be considered in patients who show poor clinical response or experience persistent viral excretion during therapy.

CLINICAL PHARMACOLOGY
Pharmacokinetics
BECAUSE THE MAJOR ELIMINATION PATHWAY FOR GANCICLOVIR IS RENAL, DOSAGE REDUCTIONS ACCORDING TO CREATININE CLEARANCE ARE REQUIRED FOR VALCYTE TABLETS. FOR DOSING INSTRUCTIONS IN PATIENTS WITH RENAL IMPAIRMENT, REFER TO DOSAGE AND ADMINISTRATION.
The pharmacokinetic properties of valganciclovir have been evaluated in HIV- and CMV-seropositive patients, patients with AIDS and CMV retinitis and in solid organ transplant patients.
The ganciclovir pharmacokinetic measures following administration of 900 mg Valcyte and 5 mg/kg intravenous ganciclovir and 1000 mg three times daily oral ganciclovir in HIV-positive/CMV-positive patients are summarized in Table 1.
[See table 1 above]

Table 1 Mean Ganciclovir Pharmacokinetic* Measures in Healthy Volunteers and HIV-positive/CMV-positive Adults at Maintenance Dosage

Formulation	Valcyte Tablets	Cytovene®-IV	Cytovene®
Dosage	900 mg once daily with food	5 mg/kg once daily	1000 mg three times daily with food
$AUC_{0-24\ hr}$ (µg•h/mL)	29.1 ± 9.7 (3 studies, n=57)	26.5 ± 5.9 (4 studies, n=68)	Range of means 12.3 to 19.2 (6 studies, n=94)
C_{max} (µg/mL)	5.61 ± 1.52 (3 studies, n=58)	9.46 ± 2.02 (4 studies, n=68)	Range of means 0.955 to 1.40 (6 studies, n=94)
Absolute oral bioavailability (%)	59.4 ± 6.1 (2 studies, n=32)	Not Applicable	Range of means 6.22± 1.29 to 8.53 ± 1.53 (2 studies, n=32)
Elimination half-life (hr)	4.08 ± 0.76 (4 studies, n=73)	3.81 ± 0.71 (4 studies, n=69)	Range of means 3.86 to 5.03 (4 studies, n=61)
Renal clearance (mL/min/kg)	3.21 ± 0.75 (1 study, n=20)	2.99 ± 0.67 (1 study, n=16)	Range of means 2.67 to 3.98 (3 studies, n=30)

*Data were obtained from single and multiple dose studies in healthy volunteers, HIV-positive patients, and HIV-positive/CMV-positive patients with and without retinitis. Patients with CMV retinitis tended to have higher ganciclovir plasma concentrations than patients without CMV retinitis.

The area under the plasma concentration-time curve (AUC) for ganciclovir administered as Valcyte tablets is comparable to the ganciclovir AUC for intravenous ganciclovir. Ganciclovir C_{max} following Valcyte administration is 40% lower than following intravenous ganciclovir administration. During maintenance dosing, ganciclovir $AUC_{0-24\ hr}$ and C_{max} following oral ganciclovir administration (1000 mg three times daily) are lower relative to Valcyte and intravenous ganciclovir. The ganciclovir C_{min} following intravenous ganciclovir and Valcyte administration are less than the ganciclovir C_{min} following oral ganciclovir administration. The clinical significance of the differences in ganciclovir pharmacokinetics for these three ganciclovir delivery systems is unknown.
[See figure at top of next column]

Figure 1. Ganciclovir Plasma Concentration Time Profiles in HIV-positive/CMV-positive Patients*

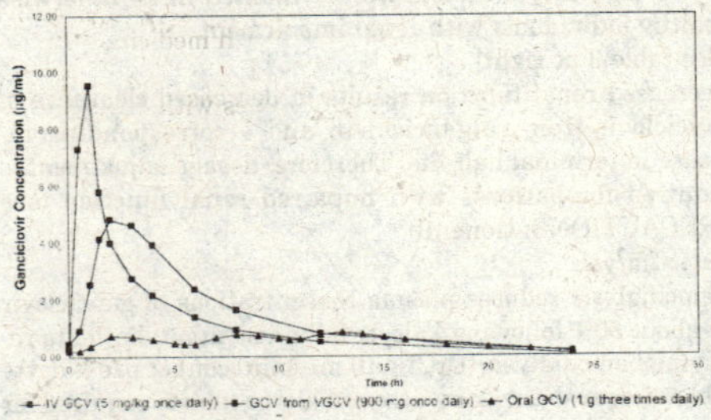

*Plasma concentration-time profiles for ganciclovir (GCV) from Valcyte (VGCV) and intravenous ganciclovir were obtained from a multiple dose study (study WV15376 n=21 and n=18, respectively) in HIV-positive/CMV-positive patients with CMV retinitis. The plasma concentration-time profile for oral ganciclovir was obtained from a multiple dose study (GAN2230 n=24) in HIV-positive/CMV-positive patients without CMV retinitis.

In solid organ transplant recipients, the mean systemic exposure to ganciclovir was 1.7 × higher following administration of 900 mg Valcyte tablets once daily versus 1000 mg ganciclovir capsules three times daily, when both drugs were administered according to their renal function dosing algorithms. The systemic ganciclovir exposures attained were comparable across kidney, heart and liver transplant recipients based on a population pharmacokinetics evaluation (see Table 2).
[See table 2 at top of next page]
In a pharmacokinetic study in liver transplant patients, the ganciclovir $AUC_{0-24\ hr}$ achieved with 900 mg valganciclovir was 41.7 ± 9.9 µg•h/mL (n=28) and the $AUC_{0-24\ hr}$ achieved with the approved dosage of 5 mg/kg intravenous ganciclovir was 48.2 ± 17.3 µg•h/mL (n=27).

Absorption
Valganciclovir, a prodrug of ganciclovir, is well absorbed from the gastrointestinal tract and rapidly metabolized in the intestinal wall and liver to ganciclovir. The absolute bioavailability of ganciclovir from Valcyte tablets following administration with food was approximately 60% (3 studies, n=18; n=16; n=28). Ganciclovir median T_{max} following administration of 450 mg to 2625 mg Valcyte tablets ranged from 1 to 3 hours. Dose proportionality with respect to ganciclovir AUC following administration of Valcyte tablets was demonstrated only under fed conditions. Systemic exposure to the prodrug, valganciclovir, is transient and low, and the AUC_{24} and C_{max} values are approximately 1% and 3% of those of ganciclovir, respectively.

Food Effects
When Valcyte tablets were administered with a high fat meal containing approximately 600 total calories (31.1 g fat, 51.6 g carbohydrates and 22.2 g protein) at a dose of 875 mg once daily to 16 HIV-positive subjects, the steady-state ganciclovir AUC increased by 30% (95% CI 12% to 51%), and the C_{max} increased by 14% (95% CI -5% to 36%), without any prolongation in time to peak plasma concentrations (T_{max}). Valcyte tablets should be administered with food (see DOSAGE AND ADMINISTRATION).

Continued on next page

Valcyte—Cont.

Distribution

Due to the rapid conversion of valganciclovir to ganciclovir, plasma protein binding of valganciclovir was not determined. Plasma protein binding of ganciclovir is 1% to 2% over concentrations of 0.5 and 51 μg/mL. When ganciclovir was administered intravenously, the steady-state volume of distribution of ganciclovir was 0.703 ± 0.134 L/kg (n=69).

After administration of Valcyte tablets, no correlation was observed between ganciclovir AUC and reciprocal weight; oral dosing of Valcyte tablets according to weight is not required.

Metabolism

Valganciclovir is rapidly hydrolyzed to ganciclovir; no other metabolites have been detected. No metabolite of orally administered radiolabeled ganciclovir (1000 mg single dose) accounted for more than 1% to 2% of the radioactivity recovered in the feces or urine.

Elimination

The major route of elimination of valganciclovir is by renal excretion as ganciclovir through glomerular filtration and active tubular secretion. Systemic clearance of intravenously administered ganciclovir was 3.07 ± 0.64 mL/min/kg (n=68) while renal clearance was 2.99 ± 0.67 mL/min/kg (n=16).

The terminal half-life ($t_{1/2}$) of ganciclovir following oral administration of Valcyte tablets to either healthy or HIV-positive/CMV-positive subjects was 4.08 ± 0.76 hours (n=73), and that following administration of intravenous ganciclovir was 3.81 ± 0.71 hours (n=69). In heart, kidney, kidney-pancreas, and liver transplant patients, the terminal elimination half-life of ganciclovir following oral administration of Valcyte was 6.48 ± 1.38 hours, and following oral administration of Cytovene was 8.56 ± 3.62.

Special Populations

Renal Impairment

The pharmacokinetics of ganciclovir from a single oral dose of 900 mg Valcyte tablets were evaluated in 24 otherwise healthy individuals with renal impairment.

[See table 3 at right]

Decreased renal function results in decreased clearance of ganciclovir from valganciclovir, and a corresponding increase in terminal half-life. Therefore, dosage adjustment is required for patients with impaired renal function (see PRECAUTIONS: General).

Hemodialysis

Hemodialysis reduces plasma concentrations of ganciclovir by about 50% following Valcyte administration. Patients receiving hemodialysis (CrCl <10 mL/min) cannot use Valcyte tablets because the daily dose of Valcyte tablets required for these patients is less than 450 mg (see PRECAUTIONS: General and DOSAGE AND ADMINISTRATION: Hemodialysis Patients).

Patients with Hepatic Impairment

The safety and efficacy of Valcyte tablets have not been studied in patients with hepatic impairment.

Race/Ethnicity and Gender

Insufficient data are available to demonstrate any effect of race or gender on the pharmacokinetics of valganciclovir.

Pediatrics

Valcyte tablets have not been studied in pediatric patients; the pharmacokinetic characteristics of Valcyte tablets in these patients have not been established (see PRECAUTIONS: Pediatric Use).

Geriatrics

No studies of Valcyte tablets have been conducted in adults older than 65 years of age (see PRECAUTIONS: Geriatric Use).

INDICATIONS AND USAGE

Valcyte tablets are indicated for the treatment of cytomegalovirus (CMV) retinitis in patients with acquired immunodeficiency syndrome (AIDS) (see CLINICAL TRIALS).

Valcyte is indicated for the prevention of cytomegalovirus (CMV) disease in kidney, heart, and kidney-pancreas transplant patients at high risk (Donor CMV seropositive/Recipient CMV seronegative [(D+/R-)]).

Valcyte is not indicated for use in liver transplant patients (see CLINICAL TRIALS and WARNINGS).

The safety and efficacy of Valcyte for the prevention of CMV disease in other solid organ transplant patients such as lung transplant patients have not been established.

CLINICAL TRIALS

Induction Therapy of CMV Retinitis

Study WV15376

In a randomized, open-label controlled study, 160 patients with AIDS and newly diagnosed CMV retinitis were randomized to receive treatment with either Valcyte tablets (900 mg twice daily for 21 days, then 900 mg once daily for 7 days) or with intravenous ganciclovir solution (5 mg/kg twice daily for 21 days, then 5 mg/kg once daily for 7 days). Study participants were: male (91%), White (53%), Hispanic (31%), and Black (11%). The median age was 39 years, the median baseline HIV-1 RNA was 4.9 $\log_{10}$, and the median CD_4 cell count was 23 cells/mm³. A determination of CMV retinitis progression by the masked review of retinal photographs taken at baseline and week 4 was the primary outcome measurement of the 3-week induction therapy. Table 4 provides the outcomes at 4 weeks.

Table 2 Mean Ganciclovir Pharmacokinetic Measures by Organ Type (Study PV 16000)

Parameter	Cytovene Capsules	Valcyte Tablets
Dosage	1000 mg three times daily with food	900 mg once daily with food
Heart Transplant Recipients	N=13	N=17
$AUC_{0-24\ hr}$ (μg•h/mL)	26.6 ± 11.6	40.2 ± 11.8
C_{max} (μg/ml)	1.4 ± 0.5	4.9 ± 1.1
Elimination half-life (hr)	8.47 ± 2.84	6.58 ± 1.50
Liver Transplant Recipients	N=33	N=75
$AUC_{0-24\ hr}$ (μg•h/mL)	24.9 ± 10.2	46.0 ± 16.1
C_{max} (μg/ml)	1.3 ± 0.4	5.4 ± 1.5
Elimination half-life (hr)	7.68 ± 2.74	6.18 ± 1.42
Kidney Transplant Recipients	N=36	N=68
$AUC_{0-24\ hr}$ (μg•h/mL)	31.3 ± 10.3	48.2 ± 14.6
C_{max} (μg/ml)	1.5 ± 0.5	5.3 ± 1.5
Elimination half-life (hr)	9.44 ± 4.37	6.77 ± 1.25

* Includes kidney-pancreas

Table 3 Pharmacokinetics of Ganciclovir From a Single Oral Dose of 900 mg Valcyte Tablets

Estimated Creatinine Clearance (mL/min)	N	Apparent Clearance (mL/min) Mean ± SD	AUC_{last} (μg•h/mL) Mean ± SD	Half-life (hours) Mean ± SD
51-70	6	249 ± 99	49.5 ± 22.4	4.85 ± 1.4
21-50	6	136 ± 64	91.9 ± 43.9	10.2 ± 4.4
11-20	6	45 ± 11	223 ± 46	21.8 ± 5.2
≤10	6	12.8 ± 8	366 ± 66	67.5 ± 34

Table 4 Week 4 Masked Review of Retinal Photographs in Study WV15376

	Cytovene-IV	Valcyte
Determination of CMV retinitis progression at Week 4	N=80	N=80
Progressor	7	7
Non-progressor	63	64
Death	2	1
Discontinuations due to Adverse Events	1	2
Failed to return	1	1
CMV not confirmed at baseline or no interpretable baseline photos	6	5

Maintenance Therapy of CMV Retinitis

No comparative clinical data are available on the efficacy of Valcyte for the maintenance therapy of CMV retinitis because all patients in study WV15376 received open-label Valcyte after week 4. However, the AUC for ganciclovir is similar following administration of 900 mg Valcyte tablets once daily and 5 mg/kg intravenous ganciclovir once daily. Although the ganciclovir C_{max} is lower following Valcyte administration compared to intravenous ganciclovir, it is higher than the C_{max} obtained following oral ganciclovir administration (see Figure 1 in CLINICAL PHARMACOLOGY). Therefore, use of Valcyte as maintenance therapy is supported by a plasma concentration-time profile similar to that of two approved products for maintenance therapy of CMV retinitis.

Prevention of CMV Disease in Heart, Kidney, Kidney-Pancreas, and Liver Transplantation

A double-blind, double-dummy active comparator study was conducted in 372 heart, liver, kidney, and kidney-pancreas transplant patients at high-risk for CMV disease (D+/R-). Patients were randomized (2 Valcyte: 1 oral ganciclovir) to receive either Valcyte (900 mg once daily) or oral ganciclovir (1000 mg three times a day) starting within 10 days of transplantation until Day 100 posttransplant. The proportion of patients who developed CMV disease, including CMV syndrome and/or tissue-invasive disease during the first 6 months posttransplant was similar between the Valcyte arm (12.1%, N=239) and the oral ganciclovir arm (15.2%, N=125). However, in liver transplant patients, the incidence of tissue-invasive CMV disease was significantly higher in the Valcyte group compared with the ganciclovir group. These results are summarized in Table 5.

Mortality at six months was 3.7% (9/244) in the Valcyte group and 1.6% (2/126) in the oral ganciclovir group.

[See table 5 below]

CONTRAINDICATIONS

Valcyte tablets are contraindicated in patients with hypersensitivity to valganciclovir or ganciclovir.

WARNINGS

THE CLINICAL TOXICITY OF VALCYTE, WHICH IS METABOLIZED TO GANCICLOVIR, INCLUDES GRANULOCYTOPENIA, ANEMIA AND THROMBOCYTOPENIA. IN ANIMAL STUDIES GANCICLOVIR WAS CARCINOGENIC, TERATOGENIC AND CAUSED ASPERMATOGENESIS.

Hematologic

Valcyte tablets should not be administered if the absolute neutrophil count is less than 500 cells/μL, the platelet count is less than 25,000/μL, or the hemoglobin is less than 8 g/dL. Severe leukopenia, neutropenia, anemia, thrombocytopenia, pancytopenia, bone marrow depression and aplastic anemia have been observed in patients treated with Valcyte tablets (and ganciclovir) (see PRECAUTIONS: Laboratory Testing and ADVERSE EVENTS).

Valcyte tablets should, therefore, be used with caution in patients with pre-existing cytopenias, or who have received or who are receiving myelosuppressive drugs or irradiation. Cytopenia may occur at any time during treatment and may increase with continued dosing. Cell counts usually begin to recover within 3 to 7 days of discontinuing drug.

Impairment of Fertility

Animal data indicate that administration of ganciclovir causes inhibition of spermatogenesis and subsequent infertility. These effects were reversible at lower doses and irreversible at higher doses (see PRECAUTIONS: Carcinogenesis, Mutagenesis and Impairment of Fertility). It is considered probable that in humans, Valcyte at the recommended doses may cause temporary or permanent inhibition of spermatogenesis. Animal data also indicate that suppression of fertility in females may occur.

Table 5 Percentage of Patients with CMV Disease and Tissue-Invasive CMV Disease by Organ Type: Endpoint Committee, 6 Month ITT Population

Organ	CMV Disease[1]		Tissue-Invasive CMV Disease		CMV Syndrome	
	VGCV (N=239)	GCV (N=125)	VGCV (N=239)	GCV (N=125)	VGCV (N=239)	GCV (N=125)
Liver (n=177)	19% (22/118)	12% (7/59)	14% (16/118)	3% (2/59)	5% (6/118)	9% (5/59)
Kidney (n=120)	6% (5/81)	23% (9/39)	1% (1/81)	5% (2/39)	5% (4/81)	18% (7/39)
Heart (n=56)	6% (2/35)	10% (2/21)	0% (0/35)	5% (1/21)	6% (2/35)	5% (1/21)
Kidney/Pancreas (n=11)	0% (0/5)	17% (1/6)	0% (0/5)	17% (1/6)	0% (0/5)	0% (0/6)

GCV = oral ganciclovir; VGCV = Valcyte

[1] Number of Patients with CMV Disease = Number of Patients with Tissue-Invasive CMV Disease + Number of Patients with CMV Syndrome.

Teratogenesis, Carcinogenesis and Mutagenesis

Because of the mutagenic and teratogenic potential of ganciclovir, women of childbearing potential should be advised to use effective contraception during treatment. Similarly, men should be advised to practice barrier contraception during, and for at least 90 days following, treatment with Valcyte tablets (see PRECAUTIONS: Carcinogenesis, Mutagenesis and Impairment of Fertility, and Pregnancy: Category C).

In animal studies, ganciclovir was found to be mutagenic and carcinogenic. Valcyte should, therefore, be considered a potential teratogen and carcinogen in humans with the potential to cause birth defects and cancers (see DOSAGE AND ADMINISTRATION: Handling and Disposal).

Tissue Invasive CMV Disease in Liver Transplant Patients

In liver transplant patients, there was a significantly higher incidence of tissue-invasive CMV disease in the Valcyte-treated group compared with the oral ganciclovir group (see CLINICAL TRIALS).

PRECAUTIONS

General

Strict adherence to dosage recommendations is essential to avoid overdose.

The bioavailability of ganciclovir from Valcyte tablets is significantly higher than from ganciclovir capsules. Patients switching from ganciclovir capsules should be advised of the risk of overdosage if they take more than the prescribed number of Valcyte tablets. Valcyte tablets cannot be substituted for Cytovene capsules on a one-to-one basis (see DOSAGE AND ADMINISTRATION).

Since ganciclovir is excreted by the kidneys, normal clearance depends on adequate renal function. IF RENAL FUNCTION IS IMPAIRED, DOSAGE ADJUSTMENTS ARE REQUIRED FOR VALCYTE TABLETS. Such adjustments should be based on measured or estimated creatinine clearance values (see DOSAGE AND ADMINISTRATION: Renal Impairment).

For patients on hemodialysis (CrCl <10 mL/min) it is recommended that ganciclovir be used (in accordance with the dose-reduction algorithm cited in the Cytovene®-IV and Cytovene® Capsules complete product information section on DOSAGE AND ADMINISTRATION: Renal Impairment) rather than Valcyte tablets (see DOSAGE AND ADMINISTRATION: Hemodialysis and CLINICAL PHARMACOLOGY: Special Populations: Hemodialysis).

Information for Patients (see Patient Information)

Valcyte tablets cannot be substituted for ganciclovir capsules on a one-to-one basis. Patients switching from ganciclovir capsules should be advised of the risk of overdosage if they take more than the prescribed number of Valcyte tablets (see OVERDOSAGE and DOSAGE AND ADMINISTRATION).

Valcyte is changed to ganciclovir once it is absorbed into the body. All patients should be informed that the major toxicities of ganciclovir include granulocytopenia (neutropenia), anemia and thrombocytopenia and that dose modifications may be required, including discontinuation. The importance of close monitoring of blood counts while on therapy should be emphasized. Patients should be informed that ganciclovir has been associated with elevations in serum creatinine. Patients should be instructed to take Valcyte tablets with food to maximize bioavailability.

Patients should be advised that ganciclovir has caused decreased sperm production in animals and may cause decreased fertility in humans. Women of childbearing potential should be advised that ganciclovir causes birth defects in animals and should not be used during pregnancy. Because of the potential for serious adverse events in nursing infants, mothers should be instructed not to breast-feed if they are receiving Valcyte tablets. Women of childbearing potential should be advised to use effective contraception during treatment with Valcyte tablets. Similarly, men should be advised to practice barrier contraception during and for at least 90 days following treatment with Valcyte tablets.

Although there is no information from human studies, patients should be advised that ganciclovir should be considered a potential carcinogen.

Convulsions, sedation, dizziness, ataxia and/or confusion have been reported with the use of Valcyte tablets and/or ganciclovir. If they occur, such effects may affect tasks requiring alertness including the patient's ability to drive and operate machinery.

Patients should be told that ganciclovir is not a cure for CMV retinitis, and that they may continue to experience progression of retinitis during or following treatment. Patients should be advised to have ophthalmologic follow-up examinations at a minimum of every 4 to 6 weeks while being treated with Valcyte tablets. Some patients will require more frequent follow-up.

Laboratory Testing

Due to the frequency of neutropenia, anemia and thrombocytopenia in patients receiving Valcyte tablets (see ADVERSE EVENTS), it is recommended that complete blood counts and platelet counts be performed frequently, especially in patients in whom ganciclovir or other nucleoside analogues have previously resulted in leukopenia, or in whom neutrophil counts are less than 1000 cells/μL at the beginning of treatment. Increased monitoring for cytopenias may be warranted if therapy with oral ganciclovir is changed to Valcyte, because of increased plasma concentrations of ganciclovir after Valcyte administration (see CLINICAL PHARMACOLOGY).

Table 6 Results of Drug Interaction Studies with Ganciclovir: Effects of Coadministered Drug on Ganciclovir Plasma AUC and C_{max} Values

Coadministered Drug	Ganciclovir Dosage	n	Ganciclovir Pharmacokinetic (PK) Parameter	Clinical Comment
Zidovudine 100 mg every 4 hours	1000 mg every 8 hours	12	AUC ↓ 17 ± 25% (range: -52% to 23%)	Zidovudine and Valcyte each have the potential to cause neutropenia and anemia. Some patients may not tolerate concomitant therapy at full dosage.
Didanosine 200 mg every 12 hours administered 2 hours before ganciclovir	1000 mg every 8 hours	12	AUC ↓ 21 ± 17% (range: -44% to 5%)	Effect not likely to be clinically significant.
Didanosine 200 mg every 12 hours stimultaneously administered with ganciclovir	1000 mg every 8 hours	12	No effect on ganciclovir PK parameters observed	No effect expected.
	IV ganciclovir 5 mg/kg twice daily	11	No effect on ganciclovir PK parameters observed	No effect expected.
	IV ganciclovir 5 mg/kg once daily	11	No effect on ganciclovir PK parameters observed	No effect expected.
Probenecid 500 mg every 6 hours	1000 mg every 8 hours	10	AUC ↑ 53 ± 91% (range: -14% to 299%) Ganciclovir renal clearance ↓ 22 ± 20% (Range: -54% to -4%)	Patients taking probenecid and Valcyte should be monitored for evidence of ganciclovir toxicity.
Zalcitabine 0.75 mg every 8 hours administered 2 hours before ganciclovir	1000 mg every 8 hours	10	AUC ↑ 13%	Effect not likely to be clinically significant.
Trimethoprim 200 mg once daily	1000 mg every 8 hours	12	Ganciclovir renal clearance ↓ 16.3% Half-life ↑ 15%	Effect not likely to be clinically significant.
Mycophenolate Mofetil 1.5 g single dose	IV ganciclovir 5 mg/kg single dose	12	No effect on ganciclovir PK parameters observed (patients with normal renal function)	Patients with renal impairment should be monitored carefully as levels of metabolites of both drugs may increase.

Table 7 Results of Drug Interaction Studies With Ganciclovir: Effects of Ganciclovir on Plasma AUC and C_{max} Values of Coadministered Drug

Coadministered Drug	Ganciclovir Dosage	N	Coadministered Drug Pharmacokinetic (PK) Parameter	Clinical Comment
Zidovudine 100 mg every 4 hours	1000 mg every 8 hours	12	AUC_{0-4} ↑ 19 ± 27% (range: -11% to 74%)	Zidovudine and Valcyte each have the potential to cause neutropenia and anemia. Some patients may not tolerate concomitant therapy at full dosage.
Didanosine 200 mg every 12 hours when administered 2 hours prior to or concurrent with ganciclovir	1000 mg every 8 hours	12	AUC_{0-12} ↑ 111 ± 114% (range: 10% to 493%)	Patients should be closely monitored for didanosine toxicity.
Didanosine 200 mg every 12 hours	IV ganciclovir 5 mg/kg twice daily	11	AUC_{0-12} ↑ 70 ± 40% (range: 3% to 121%) C_{max} ↑ 49 ± 48% (range: -28% to 125%)	Patients should be closely monitored for didanosine toxicity.
Didanosine 200 mg every 12 hours	IV ganciclovir 5 mg/kg once daily	11	AUC_{0-12} ↑ 50 ± 26% (range: 22% to 110%) C_{max} ↑ 36 ± 36% (range: -27% to 94%)	Patients should be closely monitored for didanosine toxicity.
Zalcitabine 0.75 mg every 8 hours administered 2 hours before ganciclovir	1000 mg every 8 hours	10	No clinically relevant PK parameter changes	No effect expected.
Trimethoprim 200 mg once daily	1000 mg every 8 hours	12	Increase (12%) in C_{min}	Effect not likely to be clinically significant.
Mycophenolate Mofetil (MMF) 1.5 g single dose	IV ganciclovir 5 mg/kg single dose	12	No PK interaction observed (patients with normal renal function)	Patients with renal impairment should be monitored carefully as levels of metabolites of both drugs may increase.

Increased serum creatinine levels have been observed in trials evaluating Valcyte tablets. Patients should have serum creatinine or creatinine clearance values monitored carefully to allow for dosage adjustments in renally impaired patients (see DOSAGE AND ADMINISTRATION: Renal Impairment). The mechanism of impairment of renal function is not known.

Drug Interactions

Drug Interaction Studies Conducted With Valcyte

No in vivo drug-drug interaction studies were conducted with valganciclovir. However, because valganciclovir is rapidly and extensively converted to ganciclovir, interactions associated with ganciclovir will be expected for Valcyte tablets.

Drug Interaction Studies Conducted With Ganciclovir

Binding of ganciclovir to plasma proteins is only about 1% to 2%, and drug interactions involving binding site displacement are not anticipated.

Drug-drug interaction studies were conducted in patients with normal renal function. Patients with impaired renal

Continued on next page

Valcyte—Cont.

function may have increased concentrations of ganciclovir and the coadministered drug following concomitant administration of Valcyte tablets and drugs excreted by the same pathway as ganciclovir. Therefore, these patients should be closely monitored for toxicity of ganciclovir and the coadministered drug.

[See table 6 at top of previous page]
[See table 7 on previous page]

Carcinogenesis, Mutagenesis and Impairment of Fertility‡
No long-term carcinogenicity studies have been conducted with Valcyte. However, upon oral administration, valganciclovir is rapidly and extensively converted to ganciclovir. Therefore, like ganciclovir, valganciclovir is a potential carcinogen.

Ganciclovir was carcinogenic in the mouse at oral doses that produced exposures approximately 0.1× and 1.4×, respectively, the mean drug exposure in humans following the recommended intravenous dose of 5 mg/kg, based on area under the plasma concentration curve (AUC) comparisons. At the higher dose there was a significant increase in the incidence of tumors of the preputial gland in males, forestomach (nonglandular mucosa) in males and females, and reproductive tissues (ovaries, uterus, mammary gland, clitoral gland and vagina) and liver in females. At the lower dose, a slightly increased incidence of tumors was noted in the preputial and harderian glands in males, forestomach in males and females, and liver in females. Ganciclovir should be considered a potential carcinogen in humans.

Valganciclovir increases mutations in mouse lymphoma cells. In the mouse micronucleus assay, valganciclovir was clastogenic. Valganciclovir was not mutagenic in the Ames Salmonella assay. Ganciclovir increased mutations in mouse lymphoma cells and DNA damage in human lymphocytes in vitro. In the mouse micronucleus assay, ganciclovir was clastogenic. Ganciclovir was not mutagenic in the Ames Salmonella assay.

Valganciclovir is converted to ganciclovir and therefore is expected to have similar reproductive toxicity effects as ganciclovir (see WARNINGS: Impairment of Fertility). Ganciclovir caused decreased mating behavior, decreased fertility, and an increased incidence of embryolethality in female mice following intravenous doses that produced an exposure approximately 1.7× the mean drug exposure in humans following the dose of 5 mg/kg, based on AUC comparisons. Ganciclovir caused decreased fertility in male mice and hypospermatogenesis in mice and dogs following daily oral or intravenous administration. Systemic drug exposure (AUC) at the lowest dose showing toxicity in each species ranged from 0.03 to 0.1× the AUC of the recommended human intravenous dose. Valganciclovir caused similar effects on spermatogenesis in mice, rats, and dogs. It is considered likely that ganciclovir (and valganciclovir) could cause inhibition of human spermatogenesis.

Pregnancy
Category C‡

Valganciclovir is converted to ganciclovir and therefore is expected to have reproductive toxicity effects similar to ganciclovir. Ganciclovir has been shown to be embryotoxic in rabbits and mice following intravenous administration, and teratogenic in rabbits. Fetal resorptions were present in at least 85% of rabbits and mice administered doses that produced 2× the human exposure based on AUC comparisons. Effects observed in rabbits included: fetal growth retardation, embryolethality, teratogenicity and/or maternal toxicity. Teratogenic changes included cleft palate, anophthalmia/microphthalmia, aplastic organs (kidney and pancreas), hydrocephaly and brachygnathia. In mice, effects observed were maternal/fetal toxicity and embryolethality.

Daily intravenous doses administered to female mice prior to mating, during gestation, and during lactation caused hypoplasia of the testes and seminal vesicles in the month-old male offspring, as well as pathologic changes in the nonglandular region of the stomach (see WARNINGS: Teratogenesis, Carcinogenesis and Mutagenesis). The drug exposure in mice as estimated by the AUC was approximately 1.7× the human AUC.

Data obtained using an ex vivo human placental model show that ganciclovir crosses the placenta and that simple diffusion is the most likely mechanism of transfer. The transfer was not saturable over a concentration range of 1 to 10 mg/mL and occurred by passive diffusion.

Valganciclovir may be teratogenic or embryotoxic at dose levels recommended for human use. There are no adequate and well-controlled studies in pregnant women. Valcyte tablets should be used during pregnancy only if the potential benefit justifies the potential risk to the fetus.

‡**Footnote:** All dose comparisons presented in the Carcinogenesis, Mutagenesis and Impairment of Fertility, and Pregnancy subsections are based on the human AUC following administration of a single 5 mg/kg infusion of intravenous ganciclovir.

Nursing Mothers
It is not known whether ganciclovir or valganciclovir is excreted in human milk. Because valganciclovir caused granulocytopenia, anemia and thrombocytopenia in clinical trials and ganciclovir was mutagenic and carcinogenic in animal studies, the possibility of serious adverse events from ganciclovir in nursing infants is possible (see WARNINGS). Because of potential for serious adverse events in nursing infants, **mothers should be instructed not to breast-feed if they are receiving Valcyte tablets.** In addition, the Centers for Disease Control and Prevention recommend that HIV-infected mothers not breast-feed their infants to avoid risking postnatal transmission of HIV.

Pediatric Use
Safety and effectiveness of Valcyte tablets in pediatric patients have not been established.

Geriatric Use
The pharmacokinetic characteristics of Valcyte in elderly patients have not been established. Since elderly individuals frequently have a reduced glomerular filtration rate, particular attention should be paid to assessing renal function before and during administration of Valcyte (see DOSAGE AND ADMINISTRATION).

Clinical studies of Valcyte did not include sufficient numbers of subjects aged 65 and over to determine whether they respond differently from younger subjects. In general, dose selection for an elderly patient should be cautious, reflecting the greater frequency of decreased hepatic, renal, or cardiac function, and of concomitant disease or other drug therapy. Valcyte is known to be substantially excreted by the kidney, and the risk of toxic reactions to this drug may be greater in patients with impaired renal function. Because elderly patients are more likely to have decreased renal function, care should be taken in dose selection. In addition, renal function should be monitored and dosage adjustments should be made accordingly (see PRECAUTIONS: General, CLINICAL PHARMACOLOGY: Special Populations: Renal Impairment, and DOSAGE AND ADMINISTRATION: Renal Impairment).

ADVERSE EVENTS

Experience With Valcyte Tablets
Valganciclovir, a prodrug of ganciclovir, is rapidly converted to ganciclovir after oral administration. Adverse events known to be associated with ganciclovir usage can therefore be expected to occur with Valcyte tablets.

Treatment of CMV Retinitis in AIDS Patients
As shown in Table 8, the safety profiles of Valcyte tablets and intravenous ganciclovir during 28 days of randomized therapy (21 days induction dose and 7 days maintenance dose) in 158 patients were comparable, with the exception of catheter-related infection, which occurred with greater frequency in patients randomized to receive IV ganciclovir.

Table 8 Percentage of Selected Adverse Events Occurring During the Randomized Phase of Study WV15376

Adverse Event	Valcyte Arm N=79	Intravenous Ganciclovir Arm N=79
Diarrhea	16%	10%
Neutropenia	11%	13%
Nausea	8%	14%
Headache	9%	5%
Anemia	8%	8%
Catheter-related infection	3%	11%

Tables 9 and 10 show the pooled adverse event data and abnormal laboratory values from two single arm, open-label clinical trials, study WV15376 and WV15705. A total of 370 patients received maintenance therapy with Valcyte tablets 900 mg once daily. Approximately 252 (68%) of these patients received Valcyte tablets for more than nine months (maximum duration was 36 months).

Table 9 Pooled Selected Adverse Events Reported in ≥5% of Patients in Two Clinical Studies in CMV Retinitis

	Patients with CMV Retinitis (Studies WV15376 and WV15705)
Adverse Events According to Body System	**Valcyte (N=370) (%)**
Gastrointestinal system	
Diarrhea	41
Nausea	30
Vomiting	21
Abdominal pain	15
Body as a whole	
Pyrexia	31
Headache	22
Hemic and lymphatic system	
Neutropenia	27
Anemia	26
Thrombocytopenia	6
Central and peripheral nervous system	
Insomnia	16
Peripheral neuropathy	9
Paresthesia	8
Special senses	
Retinal detachment	15

Table 10 Pooled Laboratory Abnormalities Reported in Two Clinical Studies in the Treatment of CMV Retinitis

	CMV Retinitis Patients (Studies WV15376 and WV15705)
Laboratory Abnormalities	**Valcyte (N=370) (%)**
Neutropenia: AUC /μL	
<500	19
500 – <750	17
750 – <1000	17
Anemia: Hemoglobin g/dL	
<6.5	7
6.5 – <8.0	13
8.0 – <9.5	16
Thrombocytopenia: Platelets/μL	
<25000	4
25000 – <50000	6
50000 – <100000	22
Serum Creatinine: mg/dL	
>2.5	3
>1.5 – 2.5	12

Prevention of CMV Disease in Selected Solid Organ Transplantation
Table 11 shows selected adverse events regardless of severity and drug relationship with an incidence of ≥5% from a clinical trial, PV16000 (up to 28 days after study treatment) where heart, kidney, kidney-pancreas and liver transplant patients received Valcyte (N=244) or oral ganciclovir (N=126). The majority of the adverse events were of mild or moderate intensity.

Table 11 Percentage of Selected Grades 1-4 Adverse Events Reported in ≥5% of Selected Solid Organ Transplant Patients in Study PV16000

Adverse Event	Valcyte (N=244) %	Oral Ganciclovir (N=126) %
Diarrhea	30	29
Tremors	28	25
Graft rejection	24	30
Nausea	23	23
Headache	22	27
Insomnia	20	16
Hypertension	18	15
Vomiting	16	14
Leukopenia	14	7
Pyrexia	13	14

Laboratory adverse events are those reported by investigators.

Adverse events not included in Table 11, which either occurred at a frequency of ≥5% in clinical study PV16000, or were selected serious adverse events reported in studies WV15376 , WV15705, or PV16000 with a frequency of <5% are listed below.

Allergic reactions: valganciclovir hypersensitivity
Bleeding complications: potentially life-threatening bleeding associated with thrombocytopenia
Central and peripheral nervous system: paresthesia, dizziness (excluding vertigo), convulsion
Gastrointestinal disorders: abdominal pain, constipation, dyspepsia, abdominal distention, ascites
General disorders and administration site disorders: fatigue, pain, edema, peripheral edema, weakness
Hemic system: anemia, neutropenia, thrombocytopenia, pancytopenia, bone marrow depression, aplastic anemia
Hepatobiliary disorders: abnormal hepatic function
Infections and infestations: pharyngitis/nasopharyngitis, upper respiratory tract infection, urinary tract infection, local and systemic infections and sepsis, postoperative wound infection
Injury, poisoning and procedural complications: postoperative complications, postoperative pain, increased wound drainage, wound dehiscence
Metabolism and nutrition disorders: hyperkalemia, hypokalemia, hypomagnesemia, hyperglycemia, appetite decreased, dehydration, hypophosphatemia, hypocalcemia

Musculoskeletal and connective tissue disorders: back pain, arthralgia, muscle cramps, limb pain
Psychiatric disorders: depression, psychosis, hallucinations, confusion, agitation
Renal and urinary disorders: renal impairment, dysuria, decreased creatinine clearance
Respiratory, thoracic and mediastinal disorders: cough, dyspnea, rhinorrhea, pleural effusion
Skin and subcutaneous tissue disorders: dermatitis, pruritus, acne
Vascular disorders: hypotension
Laboratory abnormalities reported with Valcyte tablets in one study in solid organ transplant patients are listed in Table 12.

Table 12 Laboratory Abnormalities Reported in Selected Solid Organ Transplant Patients in Study PV16000

Laboratory Abnormalities	Valcyte (N=244) %	Oral Cytovene (N=126) %
Neutropenia: ANC/µL		
<500	5	3
500 – <750	3	2
750 – <1000	5	2
Anemia: Hemoglobin g/dL		
<6.5	1	2
6.5 – <8.0	5	7
8.0 – <9.5	31	25
Thrombocytopenia: Platelets/µL		
<25000	0	2
25000 – <50000	1	3
50000 – <100000	18	21
Serum Creatinine: mg/dL		
>2.5	14	21
>1.5 – 2.5	45	47

Experience With Ganciclovir
Valganciclovir is rapidly converted to ganciclovir upon oral administration. Adverse events reported with Valcyte in general were similar to those reported with ganciclovir (Cytovene). Please refer to the Cytovene product information for more information on postmarketing adverse events associated with ganciclovir.

OVERDOSAGE

Overdose Experience With Valcyte Tablets
One adult developed fatal bone marrow depression (medullary aplasia) after several days of dosing that was at least 10-fold greater than recommended for the patient's estimated degree of renal impairment.
It is expected that an overdose of Valcyte tablets could also possibly result in increased renal toxicity (see PRECAUTIONS: General and DOSAGE AND ADMINISTRATION: Renal Impairment).
Since ganciclovir is dialyzable, dialysis may be useful in reducing serum concentrations in patients who have received an overdose of Valcyte tablets (see CLINICAL PHARMACOLOGY: Special Populations: *Hemodialysis*). Adequate hydration should be maintained. The use of hematopoietic growth factors should be considered (see CLINICAL PHARMACOLOGY: Special Populations: *Hemodialysis*).
Overdose Experience With Intravenous Ganciclovir
Reports of overdoses with intravenous ganciclovir have been received from clinical trials and during postmarketing experience. The majority of patients experienced one or more of the following adverse events:
Hematological toxicity: pancytopenia, bone marrow depression, medullary aplasia, leukopenia, neutropenia, granulocytopenia
Hepatotoxicity: hepatitis, liver function disorder
Renal toxicity: worsening of hematuria in a patient with pre-existing renal impairment, acute renal failure, elevated creatinine
Gastrointestinal toxicity: abdominal pain, diarrhea, vomiting
Neurotoxicity: generalized tremor, convulsion

DOSAGE AND ADMINISTRATION

Strict adherence to dosage recommendations is essential to avoid overdose. Valcyte tablets cannot be substituted for Cytovene capsules on a one-to-one basis.
Valcyte tablets are administered orally, and should be taken with food (see CLINICAL PHARMACOLOGY: Absorption). After oral administration, valganciclovir is rapidly and extensively converted into ganciclovir. The bioavailability of ganciclovir from Valcyte tablets is significantly higher than from ganciclovir capsules. Therefore the dosage and administration of Valcyte tablets as described below should be closely followed (see PRECAUTIONS: General and OVERDOSAGE).
For the Treatment of CMV Retinitis in Patients With Normal Renal Function

Induction:
For patients with active CMV retinitis, the recommended dosage is 900 mg (two 450 mg tablets) twice a day for 21 days with food.
Maintenance:
Following induction treatment, or in patients with inactive CMV retinitis, the recommended dosage is 900 mg (two 450 mg tablets) once daily with food.

Table 13 Dose Modifications for Patients With Impaired Renal Function

CrCl* (mL/min)	Induction Dose	Maintenance Prevention Dose
≥ 60	900 mg twice daily	900 mg once daily
40 – 59	450 mg twice daily	450 mg once daily
25 – 39	450 mg once daily	450 mg every 2 days
10 – 24	450 mg every 2 days	450 mg twice weekly

*An estimated creatinine clearance can be related to serum creatinine by the following formulas:

For males = $\frac{(140 - \text{age [years]}) \times (\text{body weight [kg]})}{(72) \times (\text{serum creatinine [mg/dL]})}$

For females = 0.85 × male value

For the Prevention of CMV Disease in Heart, Kidney, and Kidney-Pancreas Transplantation
For patients who have received a kidney, heart, or kidney-pancreas transplant, the recommended dose is 900 mg (two 450 mg tablets) once daily with food starting within 10 days of transplantation until 100 days posttransplantation.
Renal Impairment
Serum creatinine or creatinine clearance levels should be monitored carefully. Dosage adjustment is required according to creatinine clearance as shown in Table 13 (see PRECAUTIONS: General and CLINICAL PHARMACOLOGY: Special Populations: Renal Impairment). Increased monitoring for cytopenias may be warranted in patients with renal impairment (see PRECAUTIONS: Laboratory Testing). [See table 13 above]
Hemodialysis Patients
Valcyte should not be prescribed to patients receiving hemodialysis (see CLINICAL PHARMACOLOGY: Special Populations: Hemodialysis and PRECAUTIONS: General).
For patients on hemodialysis (CrCl <10 mL/min) a dose recommendation cannot be given (see CLINICAL PHARMACOLOGY: Special Populations: Hemodialysis).
Handling and Disposal
Caution should be exercised in the handling of Valcyte tablets. Tablets should not be broken or crushed. Since valganciclovir is considered a potential teratogen and carcinogen in humans, caution should be observed in handling broken tablets (see WARNINGS: Teratogenesis, Carcinogenesis and Mutagenesis). Avoid direct contact of broken or crushed tablets with skin or mucous membranes. If such contact occurs, wash thoroughly with soap and water, and rinse eyes thoroughly with plain water.
Because ganciclovir shares some of the properties of antitumor agents (ie, carcinogenicity and mutagenicity), consideration should be given to handling and disposal according to guidelines issued for antineoplastic drugs. Several guidelines on this subject have been published (see REFERENCES).
There is no general agreement that all of the procedures recommended in the guidelines are necessary or appropriate.

HOW SUPPLIED

Valcyte (valganciclovir HCl tablets) is available as 450 mg pink convex oval tablets with "VGC" on one side and "450" on the other side. Each tablet contains valganciclovir HCl equivalent to 450 mg valganciclovir. Valcyte is supplied in bottles of 60 tablets (NDC 0004-0038-22).
Storage
Store at 25°C (77°F); excursions permitted to 15°C to 30°C (59°F to 86°F) [See USP controlled room temperature].

REFERENCES

1. Recommendations for the Safe Handling of Cytotoxic Drugs. US Department of Health and Human Services, National Institutes of Health, Bethesda, MD, September 1992. NIH Publication No. 92-2621
2. American Society of Hospital Pharmacists technical assistance bulletin on handling cytotoxic and hazardous drugs. Am J Hosp Pharm. 1990; 47:1033-1049
3. Controlling Occupational Exposures to Hazardous Drugs. US Department of Labor. Occupational Health and Safety Administration. OSHA Technical Manual. Section VI - Chapter 2, January 20, 1999

PATIENT INFORMATION

Read the Patient Information that comes with Valcyte before you start using it and each time you get a refill. There may be new information. This information does not take the place of talking with your healthcare provider.
What is the most important information I should know about Valcyte?
- **Valcyte can affect your blood cells and bone marrow causing serious and life-threatening problems.** Valcyte can lower the amount of your white blood cells, red blood cells, and platelets. Your doctor may do regular blood tests to check your blood cells while you are taking Valcyte. Based on these tests, your doctor may change your dose or tell you to stop taking Valcyte.
- **Valcyte may cause cancer.** Valcyte causes cancer in animals. It is not known if Valcyte causes cancer in people.
- **Valcyte may cause birth defects.** Valcyte causes birth defects in animals. It is not known if Valcyte causes birth defects in people. Valcyte should not be used during pregnancy. **Tell your doctor right away if you get pregnant while taking Valcyte. If you can get pregnant, you should use effective birth control during treatment with Valcyte. Men should use a condom during treatment with Valcyte, and for 90 days after treatment, if their partner can get pregnant.** Talk to your doctor if you have questions about birth control. Valcyte may lower the amount of sperm in a man's body and cause fertility problems.
- **Valcyte changes into the medicine ganciclovir once it is in your body.** Ganciclovir is also the active ingredient in Cytovene® Capsules and Cytovene-IV®. Do not take Valcyte and Cytovene at the same time. The dose of medicine in Valcyte Tablets and Cytovene Capsules is different. **One tablet of Valcyte has more medicine than one capsule of Cytovene. This means that one Valcyte tablet cannot be substituted for one Cytovene Capsule. You could overdose and become very sick.** Talk to your doctor or pharmacist if you have questions about your medicine.

What is Valcyte?
Valcyte is an "antiviral" medicine used:
- to treat cytomegalovirus (CMV) retinitis in people who have acquired immunodeficiency syndrome (AIDS). When CMV virus infects the eyes, it is called CMV retinitis.
- to prevent cytomegalovirus (CMV) disease in people who have received a **heart, kidney, or kidney-pancreas** transplant and who have a chance for getting CMV disease.

Valcyte may:
- slow the growth of CMV virus in your body. CMV is an infection caused by a herpesvirus called cytomegalovirus. If CMV retinitis isn't treated, it can cause blindness. Valcyte may protect your eyesight from damage due to CMV disease. CMV can also infect other parts of the body.
- prevent CMV disease for up to 6 months after **heart, kidney, or kidney-pancreas** transplant. Valcyte may prevent CMV virus from spreading into healthy cells.

Valcyte does not cure CMV retinitis. You may still get retinitis or worsening of retinitis during or after treatment with Valcyte. Therefore, it is important to stay under a doctor's care and have your eyes checked regularly. Valcyte has not been studied in children or in adults older than age 65.
Who should not take Valcyte?
Do not take Valcyte if you:
- **are receiving hemodialysis.** The use of ganciclovir (Cytovene Capsules) rather than Valcyte tablets is recommended. Valcyte does not come in the right dose for people on hemodialysis.
- **are allergic to any of its ingredients or if you have ever had a serious reaction to ganciclovir (Cytovene Capsules or Cytovene-IV).** See the end of this leaflet for a list of the ingredients in Valcyte.

In addition, Valcyte is not for use in prevention of CMV disease in patients who have received a liver transplant. More research is needed before Valcyte can be recommended for use in the prevention of CMV disease in other organ transplant patients such as liver or lung transplant patients.
Before taking Valcyte, tell your doctor:
- **if you are pregnant or plan to become pregnant.** Valcyte may cause birth defects. (See "What is the most important information I should know about Valcyte?")
- **if you are breast-feeding.** It is not known if Valcyte passes into your milk and if it may harm your baby. You should not breast-feed if you are HIV-positive because of the chance of passing the HIV virus to your baby through your milk.
- **if you have kidney problems.** Your doctor may give you a lower dose of Valcyte, or check you more often if you are taking Valcyte.
- **if you have blood cell problems**
- **if you are having radiation treatment**
- **about all the medicines you take,** including prescription and non-prescription medicines, vitamins and herbal supplements. **Do not take Cytovene Capsules if you are taking Valcyte tablets.** Valcyte and other medicines may affect each other. These interactions may cause serious problems. The following medicines may need dose changes if you are also taking Valcyte:
  - Videx® (didanosine, ddI)
  - Retrovir® (zidovudine, ZDV, AZT)
  - Probenecid

  Tell your doctor if you take medicines such as chemotherapy medicines that can lower your bone marrow function.

How should I take Valcyte?
- Take Valcyte exactly as your doctor prescribes it. Your dose of Valcyte will depend on your medical condition. If you have kidney problems or are over age 65, your doctor may give you a lower dose of Valcyte.

Continued on next page

Valcyte—Cont.

- the usual dose for adults to get active CMV retinitis under control (induction therapy) is two 450 mg tablets twice a day for 21 days.
- the usual dose for adults to help keep CMV retinitis under control (maintenance therapy) is two 450 mg tablets once a day.
- the usual dose to prevent CMV in adults who have had a **heart, kidney, or kidney-pancreas** transplant is two 450 mg tablets once a day starting within 10 days of transplant and continuing until 100 days after the transplant.
- Take Valcyte with food.
- Do not break or crush Valcyte tablets.
- If you miss a dose of Valcyte, take the missed dose as soon as you remember. Then, take the next dose at the usual scheduled time. However, if it is almost time for your next dose, **do not take the missed dose.**
- Do not let your Valcyte run out. The amount of virus in your blood may increase if your medicine is stopped, even for a short time.
- If you take too much Valcyte, call your local poison control center or emergency room right away. You may need treatment in a hospital.
- Do not substitute Valcyte tablets for Cytovene capsules. Talk to your doctor, nurse or pharmacist if you have questions about your medicine.

What should I avoid while taking Valcyte?

- **Do not get pregnant.** Valcyte causes birth defects in animals. It is not known if Valcyte causes birth defects in people. Valcyte should not be used during pregnancy. **Tell your doctor right away if you get pregnant while taking Valcyte. If you can get pregnant, you should use effective birth control during treatment with Valcyte. Men should use a condom during treatment with Valcyte, and for 90 days after treatment, if their partner can get pregnant.** Talk to your doctor if you have questions about birth control. Valcyte may lower the amount of sperm in a man's body and cause fertility problems.
- **Do not breast-feed.** Valcyte may harm your baby. You should not breast-feed if you are HIV-positive because of the chance of passing the HIV virus to your baby through your milk.
- **Do not drive a car or operate other dangerous machinery until you know how Valcyte affects you.** Valcyte can cause seizures, sleepiness, dizziness, unsteady movements, and confusion.
- **Do not break or crush Valcyte tablets.** Avoid contact with broken Valcyte tablets on your skin, mucous membranes or eyes. If contact occurs, wash your skin well with soap and water or rinse your eyes well with plain water.

What are the possible side effects of Valcyte?

See "What is the most important information I should know about Valcyte?" for details on the most serious side effects.

Valcyte can also cause the following serious side effects:

- **kidney problems.** Valcyte may affect your kidney function. Your doctor may do regular blood tests called serum creatinine levels to check your kidney function while you are taking Valcyte.
- **brain and nerve problems.** Valcyte may cause seizures, sleepiness, dizziness, unsteady movements, and confusion.

Common side effects of Valcyte include diarrhea, nausea, vomiting, stomach pain, fever, headache, shaky movements (tremors), graft rejection, swelling of the legs, constipation, back pain, trouble sleeping, and high blood pressure.

Common changes in blood tests for people taking Valcyte include low white blood cells (neutropenia or leukopenia), low red blood cells (anemia), increased blood creatinine levels, increased calcium in the blood, and abnormal liver function.

Talk to your doctor about side effects that bother you or that won't go away.

These are not all the side effects of Valcyte. For more information, ask your doctor or pharmacist.

How do I store Valcyte?

- Store Valcyte at room temperature, 59° to 86° F (15° to 30° C.)
- **Keep Valcyte and all medicines out of the reach of children.**

General information about Valcyte.

Medicines are sometimes prescribed for conditions that are not mentioned in patient information leaflets. Do not use Valcyte for a condition for which it was not prescribed. Do not give Valcyte to other people, even if they have the same symptoms you have. It may harm them.

This leaflet summarizes the most important information about Valcyte. If you would like more information, talk with your doctor. You can ask your doctor or pharmacist for information about Valcyte that is written for health professionals. Information about Valcyte is also available at 1-800-526-6367 (toll-free).

What are the ingredients in Valcyte?

Active Ingredient: Valganciclovir HCl

Inactive Ingredients: microcrystalline cellulose, povidone K-30, crospovidone, and stearic acid. The film-coated applied to the tablets contains Opadry Pink®.

Cytovene is a registered trademark of Hoffmann-LaRoche Inc.

Videx is a registered trademark of Bristol-Myers Squibb Company.

Retrovir is a registered trademark of GlaxoSmithKline.

Valcyte tablets are manufactured by Patheon Inc., Mississauga, Ontario, Canada L5N 7K9

Revised: September 2003

XENICAL® ℞

[zen'i-cal]

(orlistat)

CAPSULES

℞ only

Prescribing information for this product, which appears on pages 2983–2986 of the 2004 PDR, has been completely revised as follows. Please write "See Supplement A" next to the product heading.

DESCRIPTION

XENICAL (orlistat) is a lipase inhibitor for obesity management that acts by inhibiting the absorption of dietary fats. Orlistat is (S)-2-formylamino-4-methyl-pentanoic acid (S)-1-[[(2S, 3S)-3-hexyl-4-oxo-2-oxetanyl] methyl]-dodecyl ester. Its empirical formula is $C_{29}H_{53}NO_5$, and its molecular weight is 495.7. It is a single diastereomeric molecule that contains four chiral centers, with a negative optical rotation in ethanol at 529 nm.

Orlistat is a white to off-white crystalline powder. Orlistat is practically insoluble in water, freely soluble in chloroform, and very soluble in methanol and ethanol. Orlistat has no pK_a within the physiological pH range.

XENICAL is available for oral administration in dark-blue, hard-gelatin capsules, with light-blue imprinting. Each capsule contains 120 mg of the active ingredient, orlistat. The capsules also contain the inactive ingredients microcrystalline cellulose, sodium starch glycolate, sodium lauryl sulfate, povidone, and talc. Each capsule shell contains gelatin, titanium dioxide, and FD&C Blue No.1, with printing of pharmaceutical glaze NF, titanium dioxide, and FD&C Blue No.1 aluminum lake.

CLINICAL PHARMACOLOGY

Mechanism of Action

Orlistat is a reversible inhibitor of lipases. It exerts its therapeutic activity in the lumen of the stomach and small intestine by forming a covalent bond with the active serine residue site of gastric and pancreatic lipases. The inactivated enzymes are thus unavailable to hydrolyze dietary fat in the form of triglycerides into absorbable free fatty acids and monoglycerides. As undigested triglycerides are not absorbed, the resulting caloric deficit may have a positive effect on weight control. Systemic absorption of the drug is therefore not needed for activity. At the recommended therapeutic dose of 120 mg three times a day, orlistat inhibits dietary fat absorption by approximately 30%.

Pharmacokinetics

Absorption

Systemic exposure to orlistat is minimal. Following oral dosing with 360 mg ^{14}C-orlistat, plasma radioactivity peaked at approximately 8 hours; plasma concentrations of intact orlistat were near the limits of detection (<5 ng/mL). In therapeutic studies involving monitoring of plasma samples, detection of intact orlistat in plasma was sporadic and concentrations were low (<10 ng/mL or 0.02 μM), without evidence of accumulation, and consistent with minimal absorption.

The average absolute bioavailability of intact orlistat was assessed in studies with male rats at oral doses of 150 and 1000 mg/kg/day and in male dogs at oral doses of 100 and 1000 mg/kg/day and found to be 0.12%, 0.59% in rats and 0.7%, 1.9% in dogs, respectively.

Distribution

In vitro orlistat was >99% bound to plasma proteins (lipoproteins and albumin were major binding proteins). Orlistat minimally partitioned into erythrocytes.

Metabolism

Based on animal data, it is likely that the metabolism of orlistat occurs mainly within the gastrointestinal wall. Based on an oral ^{14}C-orlistat mass balance study in obese patients, two metabolites, M1 (4-member lactone ring hydrolyzed) and M3 (M1 with N-formyl leucine moiety cleaved), accounted for approximately 42% of total radioactivity in plasma. M1 and M3 have an open β-lactone ring and extremely weak lipase inhibitory activity (1000- and 2500-fold less than orlistat, respectively). In view of this low inhibitory activity and the low plasma levels at the therapeutic dose (average of 26 ng/mL and 108 ng/mL for M1 and M3, respectively, 2 to 4 hours after a dose), these metabolites are considered pharmacologically inconsequential. The primary metabolite M1 had a short half-life (approximately 3 hours) whereas the secondary metabolite M3 disappeared at a slower rate (half-life approximately 13.5 hours). In obese patients, steady-state plasma levels of M1, but not M3, increased in proportion to orlistat doses.

Elimination

Following a single oral dose of 360 mg ^{14}C-orlistat in both normal weight and obese subjects, fecal excretion of the unabsorbed drug was found to be the major route of elimination. Orlistat and its M1 and M3 metabolites were also subject to biliary excretion. Approximately 97% of the administered radioactivity was excreted in feces; 83% of that was found to be unchanged orlistat. The cumulative renal excretion of total radioactivity was <2% of the given dose of 360 mg ^{14}C-orlistat. The time to reach complete excretion (fecal plus urinary) was 3 to 5 days. The disposition of orlistat appeared to be similar between normal weight and obese subjects. Based on limited data, the half-life of the absorbed orlistat is in the range of 1 to 2 hours.

Special Populations

Because the drug is minimally absorbed, studies in special populations (geriatric, different races, patients with renal and hepatic insufficiency) were not conducted.

Pediatrics

Plasma concentrations of orlistat and its metabolites M1 and M3 were similar to those found in adults at the same dose level. Daily fecal fat excretions were 27% and 7% of dietary intake in orlistat and placebo treatment groups, respectively.

Drug-Drug Interactions

Drug-drug interaction studies indicate that XENICAL had no effect on pharmacokinetics and/or pharmacodynamics of alcohol, digoxin, glyburide, nifedipine (extended-release tablets), oral contraceptives, phenytoin, pravastatin, or warfarin. Alcohol did not affect the pharmacodynamics of orlistat.

Other Short-term Studies

Adults

In several studies of up to 6-weeks duration, the effects of therapeutic doses of XENICAL on gastrointestinal and systemic physiological processes were assessed in normal-weight and obese subjects. Postprandial cholecystokinin plasma concentrations were lowered after multiple doses of XENICAL in two studies but not significantly different from placebo in two other experiments. There were no clinically significant changes observed in gallbladder motility, bile composition or lithogenicity, or colonic cell proliferation rate, and no clinically significant reduction of gastric emptying time or gastric acidity. In addition, no effects on plasma triglyceride levels or systemic lipases were observed with the administration of XENICAL in these studies. In a 3-week study of 28 healthy male volunteers, XENICAL (120 mg three times a day) did not significantly affect the balance of calcium, magnesium, phosphorus, zinc, copper, and iron.

Pediatrics

In a 3-week study of 32 obese adolescents aged 12 to 16 years, XENICAL (120 mg three times a day) did not significantly affect the balance of calcium, magnesium, phosphorus, zinc, or copper. The iron balance was decreased by 64.7 μmole/24 hours and 40.4 μmole/24 hours in orlistat and placebo treatment groups, respectively.

Dose-response Relationship

A simple maximum effect (E_{max}) model was used to define the dose-response curve of the relationship between XENICAL daily dose and fecal fat excretion as representative of gastrointestinal lipase inhibition. The dose-response curve demonstrated a steep portion for doses up to approximately 400 mg daily, followed by a plateau for higher doses. At doses greater than 120 mg three times a day, the percentage increase in effect was minimal.

CLINICAL STUDIES

Observational epidemiologic studies have established a relationship between obesity and visceral fat and the risks for cardiovascular disease, type 2 diabetes, certain forms of cancer, gallstones, certain respiratory disorders, and an increase in overall mortality. These studies suggest that weight loss, if maintained, may produce health benefits for obese patients who have or are at risk of developing weight-related comorbidities. The long-term effects of orlistat on morbidity and mortality associated with obesity have not been established.

The effects of XENICAL on weight loss, weight maintenance, and weight regain and on a number of comorbidities (eg, type 2 diabetes, lipids, blood pressure) were assessed in seven long-term (1- to 2-years duration) multicenter, double-blind, placebo-controlled clinical trials. During the first year of therapy, weight loss and weight maintenance were assessed. During the second year of therapy, some studies assessed continued weight loss and weight maintenance and others assessed the effect of orlistat on weight regain. These studies included over 2800 patients treated with XENICAL and 1400 patients treated with placebo. The majority of these patients had obesity-related risk factors and comorbidities. In these 7 studies, treatment with XENICAL and placebo designates treatment with XENICAL plus diet and placebo plus diet, respectively.

During the weight loss and weight maintenance period, a well-balanced, reduced-calorie diet that was intended to result in an approximate 20% decrease in caloric intake and provide 30% of calories from fat was recommended to all patients. In addition, all patients were offered nutritional counseling.

One-year Results: Weight Loss, Weight Maintenance, and Risk Factors

Weight loss was observed within 2 weeks of initiation of therapy and continued for 6 to 12 months.

Pooled data from five clinical trials indicated that the overall mean weight loss from randomization to the end of 6 months and 1 year of treatment in the intent-to-treat population were 12.4 lbs and 13.4 lbs in the patients treated with XENICAL and 6.2 lbs and 5.8 lbs in the placebo-treated patients, respectively. During the 4-week placebo lead-in period of the studies, an additional 5 to 6 lb weight loss was also observed in the same patients. Of the patients who completed 1 year of treatment, 57% of the patients treated with XENICAL (120 mg three times a day) and 31% of the placebo-treated patients lost at least 5% of their baseline body weight.

Table 1 Percentage of Patients Losing ≥5% and ≥10% of Body Weight From Randomization After 1-Year Treatment*

	Intent-to-Treat Population†									
	≥5% Weight Loss					≥10% Weight Loss				
Study No.	XENICAL	n	Placebo	n	p-value	XENICAL	n	Placebo	n	p-value
14119B	35.5%	110	21.3%	108	0.021	16.4%	110	6.5%	108	0.022
14119C	54.8%	343	27.4%	340	<0.001	24.8%	343	8.2%	340	<0.001
14149	50.6%	241	26.3%	236	<0.001	22.8%	241	11.9%	236	0.02
14161‡	37.1%	210	16.0%	212	<0.001	19.5%	210	3.8%	212	<0.001
14185	42.6%	657	22.4%	223	<0.001	17.7%	657	9.9%	223	0.006

The diet utilized during year 1 was a reduced-calorie diet.

* Treatment designates XENICAL 120 mg three times a day plus diet or placebo plus diet
† Last observation carried forward
‡ All studies, with the exception of 14161, were conducted at centers specialized in treating obesity and complications of obesity. Study 14161 was conducted with primary care physicians.

The percentages of patients achieving ≥5% and ≥10% weight loss after 1 year in five large multicenter studies for the intent-to-treat populations are presented in Table 1.
[See table 1 above]
The relative changes in risk factors associated with obesity following 1 year of therapy with XENICAL and placebo are presented for the population as a whole and for the population with abnormal values at randomization.

Population as a Whole

The changes in metabolic, cardiovascular and anthropometric risk factors associated with obesity based on pooled data for five clinical studies, regardless of the patient's risk factor status at randomization, are presented in Table 2. One year of therapy with XENICAL resulted in relative improvement in several risk factors.

Table 2 Mean Change in Risk Factors From Randomization Following 1-Year Treatment* Population as a Whole

Risk Factor	XENICAL 120 mg†	Placebo†
Metabolic:		
Total Cholesterol	-2.0%	+5.0%
LDL-Cholesterol	-4.0%	+5.0%
HDL-Cholesterol	+9.3%	+12.8%
LDL/HDL	-0.37	-0.20
Triglycerides	+1.34%	+2.9%
Fasting Glucose, mmol/L	-0.04	+0.0
Fasting Insulin, pmol/L	-6.7	+5.2
Cardiovascular:		
Systolic Blood Pressure, mm Hg	-1.01	+0.58
Diastolic Blood Pressure, mm Hg	-1.19	+0.46
Anthropometric:		
Waist Circumference, cm	-6.45	-4.04
Hip Circumference, cm	-5.31	-2.96

* Treatment designates XENICAL 120 mg three times a day plus diet or placebo plus diet
† Intent-to-treat population at week 52, observed data based on pooled data from 5 studies

Population With Abnormal Risk Factors at Randomization

The changes from randomization following 1-year treatment in the population with abnormal lipid levels (LDL ≥ 130 mg/dL, LDL/HDL ≥ 3.5, HDL <35 mg/dL) were greater for XENICAL compared to placebo with respect to LDL-cholesterol (-7.83% vs +1.14%) and the LDL/HDL ratio (-0.64 vs -0.46). HDL increased in the placebo group by 20.1% and in the XENICAL group by 18.8%. In the population with abnormal blood pressure at baseline (systolic BP ≥ 140 mm Hg), the change in SBP from randomization to 1 year was greater for XENICAL (-10.89 mm Hg) than placebo (-5.07 mm Hg). For patients with a diastolic blood pressure ≥90 mm Hg, XENICAL patients decreased by -7.9 mm Hg while the placebo patients decreased by -5.5 mm Hg. Fasting insulin decreased more for XENICAL than placebo (-39 vs -16 pmol/L) from randomization to 1 year in the population with abnormal baseline values (≥120 pmol/L). A greater reduction in waist circumference for XENICAL vs placebo (-7.29 vs -4.53 cm) was observed in the population with abnormal baseline values (≥100 cm).

Effect on Weight Regain

Three studies were designed to evaluate the effects of XENICAL compared to placebo in reducing weight regain after a previous weight loss achieved following either diet alone (one study, 14302) or prior treatment with XENICAL (two studies, 14119C and 14185). The diet utilized during the 1- year weight regain portion of the studies was a weight-maintenance diet, rather than a weight-loss diet, and patients received less nutritional counseling than patients in weight-loss studies. For studies 14119C and 14185, patients' previous weight loss was due to 1 year of treatment with XENICAL in conjunction with a mildly hypocaloric diet. Study 14302 was conducted to evaluate the effects of 1 year of treatment with XENICAL on weight regain in patients who had lost 8% or more of their body weight in the previous 6 months on diet alone.
In study 14119C, patients treated with placebo regained 52% of the weight they had previously lost while the patients treated with XENICAL regained 26% of the weight they had previously lost (p<0.001). In study 14185, patients treated with placebo regained 63% of the weight they had previously lost while the patients treated with XENICAL regained 35% of the weight they had lost (p<0.001). In study 14302, patients treated with placebo regained 53% of the weight they had previously lost while the patients treated with XENICAL regained 32% of the weight that they had lost (p<0.001).

Two-year Results: Long-term Weight Control and Risk Factors

The treatment effects of XENICAL were examined for 2 years in four of the five 1-year weight management clinical studies previously discussed (see Table 1). At the end of year 1, the patients' diets were reviewed and changed where necessary. The diet prescribed in the second year was designed to maintain patient's current weight. XENICAL was shown to be more effective than placebo in long-term weight control in four large, multicenter, 2-year double-blind, placebo-controlled studies.
Pooled data from four clinical studies indicate that 40% of all patients treated with 120 mg three times a day of XENICAL and 24% of patients treated with placebo who completed 2 years of the same therapy had ≥5% loss of body weight from randomization. Pooled data from four clinical studies indicate that the relative weight loss advantage between XENICAL 120 mg three times a day and placebo treatment groups was the same after 2 years as for 1 year, indicating that the pharmacologic advantage of XENICAL was maintained over 2 years. In the same studies cited in the **One-year Results** (see Table 1), the percentages of patients achieving a ≥5% and ≥10% weight loss after 2 years are shown in Table 3.
[See table 3 below]
The relative changes in risk factors associated with obesity following 2 years of therapy were also assessed in the population as a whole and the population with abnormal risk factors at randomization.

Population as a Whole

The relative differences in risk factors between treatment with XENICAL and placebo were similar to the results following 1 year of therapy for total cholesterol, LDL-cholesterol, LDL/HDL ratio, triglycerides, fasting glucose, fasting insulin, diastolic blood pressure, waist circumference, and hip circumference. The relative differences between treatment groups for HDL cholesterol and systolic blood pressure were less than that observed in the year one results.

Population With Abnormal Risk Factors at Randomization

The relative differences in risk factors between treatment with XENICAL and placebo were similar to the results following 1 year of therapy for LDL- and HDL-cholesterol, triglycerides, fasting insulin, diastolic blood pressure, and waist circumference. The relative differences between treatment groups for LDL/HDL ratio and isolated systolic blood pressure were less than that observed in the year one results.

Study of Patients With Type 2 Diabetes

A 1-year double-blind, placebo-controlled study in type 2 diabetics (N=321) stabilized on sulfonylureas was conducted. Thirty percent of patients treated with XENICAL achieved at least a 5% or greater reduction in body weight from randomization compared to 13% of the placebo-treated patients (p<0.001). Table 4 describes the changes over 1 year of treatment with XENICAL compared to placebo, in sulfonylurea usage and dose reduction as well as in hemoglobin HbA1c, fasting glucose, and insulin.

Table 4 Mean Changes in Body Weight and Glycemic Control From Randomization Following 1-Year Treatment in Patients With Type 2 Diabetes

	XENICAL 120 mg* (n=162)	Placebo* (n=159)	Statistical Significance
% patients who discontinued dose of oral sulfonylurea	11.7%	7.5%	†
% patients who decreased dose of oral sulfonylurea	31.5%	21.4%	
Average reduction in sulfonylurea medication dose	-22.8%	-9.1%	†
Body weight change (lbs)	-8.9	-4.2	†
HbA1c	-0.18%	+0.28%	†
Fasting glucose, mmol/L	-0.02	+0.54	†
Fasting insulin, pmol/L	-19.68	-18.02	ns

Statistical significance based on intent-to-treat population, last observation carried forward.
* Treatment designates XENICAL 120 mg three times a day plus diet or placebo plus diet
† Statistically significant (p ≤ 0.05) based on intent-to-treat, last observation carried forward
ns nonsignificant, p>0.05

In addition, XENICAL (n=162) compared to placebo (n=159) was associated with significant lowering for total cholesterol (-1.0% vs +9.0%, p≤0.05), LDL-cholesterol (-3.0% vs +10.0%, p≤0.05), LDL/HDL ratio (-0.26 vs -0.02, p≤0.05) and triglycerides (+2.54% vs +16.2%, p≤0.05), respectively. For HDL cholesterol, there was a +6.49% increase on XENICAL and +8.6% increase on placebo, p>0.05. Systolic blood pressure increased by +0.61 mm Hg on XENICAL and increased by +4.33 mm Hg on placebo, p>0.05. Diastolic blood pressure decreased by -0.47 mm Hg for XENICAL and by -0.5 mm Hg for placebo, p>0.05.

Glucose Tolerance in Obese Patients

Two-year studies that included oral glucose tolerance tests were conducted in obese patients not previously diagnosed or treated for type 2 diabetes and whose baseline oral glucose tolerance test (OGTT) status at randomization was either normal, impaired, or diabetic.
The progression from a normal OGTT at randomization to a diabetic or impaired OGTT following 2 years of treatment with XENICAL (n=251) or placebo (n=207) were compared. Following treatment with XENICAL, 0.0% and 7.2% of the

Table 3 Percentage of Patients Losing ≥5% and ≥10% of Body Weight From Randomization After 2-Year Treatment*

	Intent-to-Treat Population†									
	≥5% Weight Loss					≥10% Weight Loss				
Study No.	XENICAL	n	Placebo	n	p-value	XENICAL	n	Placebo	n	p-value
14119C	45.1%	133	23.6%	123	<0.001	24.8%	133	6.5%	123	<0.001
14149	43.3%	178	27.2%	158	0.002	18.0%	178	9.5%	158	0.025
14161‡	25.0%	148	15.0%	113	0.049	16.9%	148	3.5%	113	0.001
14185	34.0%	147	27.9%	122	0.279	17.7%	147	11.5%	122	0.154

The diet utilized during year 2 was designed for weight maintenance and not weight loss.

* Treatment designates XENICAL 120 mg three times a day plus diet or placebo plus diet
† Last observation carried forward
‡ All studies, with the exception of 14161 were conducted at centers specializing in treating obesity or complictions of obesity. Study 14161 was conducted with primary care physicians.

Continued on next page

Xenical—Cont.

patients progressed from normal to diabetic and normal to impaired, respectively, compared to 1.9% and 12.6% of the placebo treatment group, respectively.

In patients found to have an impaired OGTT at randomization, the percent of patients improving to normal or deteriorating to diabetic status following 1 and 2 years of treatment with XENICAL compared to placebo are presented. After 1 year of treatment, 45.8% of the placebo patients and 73% of the XENICAL patients had a normal oral glucose tolerance test while 10.4% of the placebo patients and 2.6% of the XENICAL patients became diabetic. After 2 years of treatment, 50% of the placebo patients and 71.7% of the XENICAL patients had a normal oral glucose tolerance test while 7.5% of placebo patients were found to be diabetic and 1.7% of XENICAL patients were found to be diabetic after treatment.

Pediatric Clinical Studies

The effects of XENICAL on body mass index (BMI) and weight loss were assessed in a 54-week multicenter, double-blind, placebo-controlled study in 539 obese adolescents (357 receiving XENICAL 120 mg three times a day, 182 receiving placebo), aged 12 to 16 years. All study participants had a baseline BMI that was 2 units greater than the US weighted mean for the 95th percentile based on age and gender. Body mass index was the primary efficacy parameter because it takes into account changes in height and body weight, which occur in growing children.

During the study, all patients were instructed to take a multivitamin containing fat-soluble vitamins at least 2 hours before or after ingestion of XENICAL. Patients were also maintained on a well-balanced, reduced-calorie diet that was intended to provide 30% of calories from fat. In addition, all patients were placed on a behavior modification program and offered exercise counseling.

Approximately 65% of patients in each treatment group completed the study.

Following one year of treatment, BMI decreased by an average of 0.55 kg/m^2 in the XENICAL-treated patients and increased by an average of 0.31 kg/m^2 in the placebo-treated patients (p=0.001).

The percentages of patients achieving ≥5% and ≥10% reduction in BMI and body weight after 52 weeks of treatment for the intent-to-treat population are presented in Table 5.

[See table 5 below]

INDICATIONS AND USAGE

XENICAL is indicated for obesity management including weight loss and weight maintenance when used in conjunction with a reduced-calorie diet. XENICAL is also indicated to reduce the risk for weight regain after prior weight loss. XENICAL is indicated for obese patients with an initial body mass index (BMI) ≥30 kg/m^2 or ≥27 kg/m^2 in the presence of other risk factors (eg, hypertension, diabetes, dyslipidemia).

Table 6 illustrates body mass index (BMI) according to a variety of weights and heights. The BMI is calculated by dividing weight in kilograms by height in meters squared. For example, a person who weighs 180 lbs and is 5′5″ would have a BMI of 30.

[See table 6 below]

CONTRAINDICATIONS

XENICAL is contraindicated in patients with chronic malabsorption syndrome or cholestasis, and in patients with known hypersensitivity to XENICAL or to any component of this product.

WARNINGS

Miscellaneous

Organic causes of obesity (eg, hypothyroidism) should be excluded before prescribing XENICAL.

Preliminary data from a XENICAL and cyclosporine drug interaction study indicate a reduction in cyclosporine plasma levels when XENICAL was coadministered with cyclosporine. Therefore, XENICAL and cyclosporine should not be coadministered. To reduce the chance of a drug-drug interaction, cyclosporine should be taken at least 2 hours before or after XENICAL in patients taking both drugs. In addition, in those patients whose cyclosporine levels are being measured, more frequent monitoring should be considered.

PRECAUTIONS

General

Patients should be advised to adhere to dietary guidelines (see DOSAGE AND ADMINISTRATION). Gastrointestinal events (see ADVERSE REACTIONS) may increase when XENICAL is taken with a diet high in fat (>30% total daily calories from fat). The daily intake of fat should be distributed over three main meals. If XENICAL is taken with any one meal very high in fat, the possibility of gastrointestinal effects increases.

Patients should be strongly encouraged to take a multivitamin supplement that contains fat-soluble vitamins to ensure adequate nutrition because XENICAL has been shown to reduce the absorption of some fat-soluble vitamins and beta-carotene (see DOSAGE AND ADMINISTRATION). In addition, the levels of vitamin D and beta-carotene may be low in obese patients compared with non-obese subjects. The supplement should be taken once a day at least 2 hours before or after the administration of XENICAL, such as at bedtime.

Table 7 illustrates the percentage of adult patients on XENICAL and placebo who developed a low vitamin level on two or more consecutive visits during 1 and 2 years of therapy in studies in which patients were not previously receiving vitamin supplementation.

Table 7 Incidence of Low Vitamin Values on Two or More Consecutive Visits (Nonsupplemented Adult Patients With Normal Baseline Values - First and Second Year)

	Placebo*	XENICAL*
Vitamin A	1.0%	2.2%
Vitamin D	6.6%	12.0%
Vitamin E	1.0%	5.8%
Beta-carotene	1.7%	6.1%

* Treatment designates placebo plus diet or XENICAL plus diet

Table 8 illustrates the percentage of adolescent patients on XENICAL and placebo who developed a low vitamin level on two or more consecutive visits during the 1-year study.

Table 8 Incidence of Low Vitamin Values on Two or More Consecutive Visits (Pediatric Patients With Normal Baseline Values*)

	Placebo**	XENICAL**
Vitamin A	0.0%	0.0%
Vitamin D	0.7%	1.4%
Vitamin E	0.0%	0.0%
Beta-carotene	0.8%	1.5%

*All patients were treated with vitamin supplementation throughout the course of the study

** Treatment designates placebo plus diet or XENICAL plus diet

Some patients may develop increased levels of urinary oxalate following treatment with XENICAL. Caution should be exercised when prescribing XENICAL to patients with a history of hyperoxaluria or calcium oxalate nephrolithiasis.

Weight-loss induction by XENICAL may be accompanied by improved metabolic control in diabetics, which might require a reduction in dose of oral hypoglycemic medication (eg, sulfonylureas, metformin) or insulin (see CLINICAL STUDIES).

Misuse Potential

As with any weight-loss agent, the potential exists for misuse of XENICAL in inappropriate patient populations (eg, patients with anorexia nervosa or bulimia). See INDICATIONS AND USAGE for recommended prescribing guidelines.

Information for Patients

Patients should read the Patient Information before starting treatment with XENICAL and each time their prescription is renewed.

Drug Interactions

Alcohol

In a multiple-dose study in 30 normal-weight subjects, coadministration of XENICAL and 40 grams of alcohol (eg, approximately 3 glasses of wine) did not result in alteration of alcohol pharmacokinetics, orlistat pharmacodynamics (fecal fat excretion), or systemic exposure to orlistat.

Cyclosporine

Preliminary data from a XENICAL and cyclosporine drug interaction study indicate a reduction in cyclosporine plasma levels when XENICAL was coadministered with cyclosporine (see WARNINGS).

Digoxin

In 12 normal-weight subjects receiving XENICAL 120 mg three times a day for 6 days, XENICAL did not alter the pharmacokinetics of a single dose of digoxin.

Fat-soluble Vitamin Supplements and Analogues

A pharmacokinetic interaction study showed a 30% reduction in beta-carotene supplement absorption when concomitantly administered with XENICAL. XENICAL inhibited absorption of a vitamin E acetate supplement by approximately 60%. The effect of orlistat on the absorption of supplemental vitamin D, vitamin A, and nutritionally-derived vitamin K is not known at this time.

Glyburide

In 12 normal-weight subjects receiving orlistat 80 mg three times a day for 5 days, orlistat did not alter the pharmacokinetics or pharmacodynamics (blood glucose-lowering) of glyburide.

Nifedipine (extended-release tablets)

In 17 normal-weight subjects receiving XENICAL 120 mg three times a day for 6 days, XENICAL did not alter the bioavailability of nifedipine (extended-release tablets).

Oral Contraceptives

In 20 normal-weight female subjects, the treatment of XENICAL 120 mg three times a day for 23 days resulted in no changes in the ovulation-suppressing action of oral contraceptives.

Phenytoin

In 12 normal-weight subjects receiving XENICAL 120 mg three times a day for 7 days, XENICAL did not alter the pharmacokinetics of a single 300-mg dose of phenytoin.

Pravastatin

In a 2-way crossover study of 24 normal-weight, mildly hypercholesterolemic patients receiving XENICAL 120 mg three times a day for 6 days, XENICAL did not affect the pharmacokinetics of pravastatin.

Warfarin

In 12 normal-weight subjects, administration of XENICAL 120 mg three times a day for 16 days did not result in any change in either warfarin pharmacokinetics (both R- and S-enantiomers) or pharmacodynamics (prothrombin time and serum Factor VII). Although undercarboxylated osteocalcin, a marker of vitamin K nutritional status, was unaltered with XENICAL administration, vitamin K levels tended to decline in subjects taking XENICAL. Therefore, as vitamin K absorption may be decreased with XENICAL, patients on chronic stable doses of warfarin who are prescribed XENICAL should be monitored closely for changes in coagulation parameters.

Carcinogenesis, Mutagenesis, Impairment of Fertility

Carcinogenicity studies in rats and mice did not show a carcinogenic potential for orlistat at doses up to 1000 mg/kg/day and 1500 mg/kg/day, respectively. For mice and rats, these doses are 38 and 46 times the daily human dose calculated on an area under concentration vs time curve basis of total drug-related material.

Orlistat had no detectable mutagenic or genotoxic activity as determined by the Ames test, a mammalian forward mutation assay (V79/HPRT), an in vitro clastogenesis assay in

Table 5 Percentages of Patients with ≥5% and ≥10% Decrease in Body Mass Index and Body Weight After 1-Year Treatment* (Protocol NM16189)

	Intent-to-Treat Population‡							
	≥5% Decrease				≥10% Decrease			
	XENICAL	n	Placebo	n	XENICAL	n	Placebo	n
BMI	26.5%	347	15.7%	178	13.3%	347	4.5%	178
Body Weight	19.0%	348	11.7%	180	9.5%	348	3.3%	180

* Treatment designates XENICAL 120 mg three times a day plus diet or placebo plus diet

‡ Last observation carried forward

Table 6 Body Mass Index (BMI), kg/m^{2*}

WEIGHT (lb)

HEIGHT (ft/in)	120	130	140	150	160	170	180	190	200	210	220	230	240	250	260	270	280	290	300	310	320
4'10"	25	27	29	31	34	36	38	40	42	44	46	48	50	52	54	57	59	61	63	65	67
4'11"	24	26	28	30	32	34	36	38	40	43	45	47	49	51	53	55	57	59	61	63	65
5'0"	23	25	27	29	31	33	35	37	39	41	43	45	47	49	51	53	55	57	59	61	63
5'1"	23	25	27	28	30	32	34	36	38	40	42	44	45	47	49	51	53	55	57	59	61
5'2"	22	24	26	27	29	31	33	35	37	38	40	42	44	46	48	49	51	53	55	57	59
5'3"	21	23	25	27	28	30	32	34	36	37	39	41	43	44	46	48	50	51	53	55	57
5'4"	21	22	24	26	28	29	31	33	34	36	38	40	41	43	45	46	48	50	52	53	55
5'5"	20	22	23	25	27	28	30	32	33	35	37	38	40	42	43	45	47	48	50	52	53
5'6"	19	21	23	24	26	27	29	31	32	34	36	37	39	40	42	44	45	47	49	50	52
5'7"	19	20	22	24	25	27	28	30	31	33	35	36	38	39	41	42	44	46	47	49	50
5'8"	18	20	21	23	24	26	27	29	30	32	34	35	37	38	40	41	43	44	46	47	49
5'9"	18	19	21	22	24	25	27	28	30	31	33	34	36	37	38	40	41	43	44	46	47
5'10"	17	19	20	22	23	24	26	27	29	30	32	33	35	36	37	39	40	42	43	45	46
5'11"	17	18	20	21	22	24	25	27	28	29	31	32	34	35	36	38	39	41	42	43	45
6'0"	16	18	19	20	22	23	24	26	27	29	30	31	33	34	35	37	38	39	41	42	43
6'1"	16	17	19	20	21	22	24	25	26	28	29	30	32	33	34	36	37	38	40	41	42
6'2"	15	17	18	19	21	22	23	24	26	27	28	30	31	32	33	35	36	37	39	40	41

* **Conversion Factors:**

Weight in lbs ÷ 2.2 = weight in kilograms (kg)

Height in inches x 0.0254 = height in meters (m)

1 foot = 12 inches

Table 9 Commonly Observed Adverse Events

	Year 1		Year 2	
Adverse Event	**XENICAL* % Patients (N=1913)**	**Placebo* % Patients (N=1466)**	**XENICAL* % Patients (N=613)**	**Placebo* % Patients (N=524)**
Oily Spotting	26.6	1.3	4.4	0.2
Flatus with Discharge	23.9	1.4	2.1	0.2
Fecal Urgency	22.1	6.7	2.8	1.7
Fatty/Oily Stool	20.0	2.9	5.5	0.6
Oily Evacuation	11.9	0.8	2.3	0.2
Increased Defecation	10.8	4.1	2.6	0.8
Fecal Incontinence	7.7	0.9	1.8	0.2

* Treatment designates XENICAL three times a day plus diet or placebo plus diet

Table 10 Other Treatment-Emergent Adverse Events From Seven Placebo-Controlled Clinical Trials

	Year 1		Year 2	
Body System/Adverse Event	**XENICAL* % Patients (N=1913)**	**Placebo* % Patients (N=1466)**	**XENICAL* % Patients (N=613)**	**Placebo* % Patients (N=524)**
Gastrointestinal System				
Abdominal Pain/Discomfort	25.5	21.4	–	–
Nausea	8.1	7.3	3.6	2.7
Infectious Diarrhea	5.3	4.4	–	–
Rectal Pain/Discomfort	5.2	4.0	3.3	1.9
Tooth Disorder	4.3	3.1	2.9	2.3
Gingival Disorder	4.1	2.9	2.0	1.5
Vomiting	3.8	3.5	–	–
Respiratory System				
Influenza	39.7	36.2	–	–
Upper Respiratory Infection	38.1	32.8	26.1	25.8
Lower Respiratory Infection	7.8	6.6	–	–
Ear, Nose & Throat Symptoms	2.0	1.6	–	–
Musculoskeletal System				
Back Pain	13.9	12.1	–	–
Pain Lower Extremities	–	–	10.8	10.3
Arthritis	5.4	4.8	–	–
Myalgia	4.2	3.3	–	–
Joint Disorder	2.3	2.2	–	–
Tendonitis	–	–	2.0	1.9
Central Nervous System				
Headache	30.6	27.6	–	–
Dizziness	5.2	5.0	–	–
Body as a Whole				
Fatigue	7.2	6.4	3.1	1.7
Sleep Disorder	3.9	3.3	–	–
Skin & Appendages				
Rash	4.3	4.0	–	–
Dry Skin	2.1	1.4	–	–
Reproductive, Female				
Menstrual Irregularity	9.8	7.5	–	–
Vaginitis	3.8	3.6	2.6	1.9
Urinary System				
Urinary Tract Infection	7.5	7.3	5.9	4.8
Psychiatric Disorder				
Psychiatric Anxiety	4.7	2.9	2.8	2.1
Depression	–	–	3.4	2.5
Hearing & Vestibular Disorders				
Otitis	4.3	3.4	2.9	2.5
Cardiovascular Disorders				
Pedal Edema	–	–	2.8	1.9

* Treatment designates XENICAL 120 mg three times a day plus diet or placebo plus diet
– None reported at a frequency ≥2% and greater than placebo

peripheral human lymphocytes, an unscheduled DNA synthesis assay (UDS) in rat hepatocytes in culture, and an in vivo mouse micronucleus test.

When given to rats at a dose of 400 mg/kg/day in a fertility and reproduction study, orlistat had no observable adverse effects. This dose is 12 times the daily human dose calculated on a body surface area (mg/m^2) basis.

Pregnancy

Teratogenic Effects: Pregnancy Category B.

Teratogenicity studies were conducted in rats and rabbits at doses up to 800 mg/kg/day. Neither study showed embryotoxicity or teratogenicity. This dose is 23 and 47 times the daily human dose calculated on a body surface area (mg/m^2) basis for rats and rabbits, respectively.

The incidence of dilated cerebral ventricles was increased in the mid- and high-dose groups of the rat teratology study. These doses were 6 and 23 times the daily human dose calculated on a body surface area (mg/m^2) basis for the mid- and high-dose levels, respectively. This finding was not reproduced in two additional rat teratology studies at similar doses.

There are no adequate and well-controlled studies of XENICAL in pregnant women. Because animal reproductive studies are not always predictive of human response, XENICAL is not recommended for use during pregnancy.

Nursing Mothers

It is not known if orlistat is secreted in human milk. Therefore, XENICAL should not be taken by nursing women.

Pediatric Use

The safety and efficacy of XENICAL have been evaluated in obese adolescent patients aged 12 to 16 years. Use of XENICAL in this age group is supported by evidence from adequate and well-controlled studies of XENICAL in adults with additional data from a 54-week efficacy and safety study and a 21-day mineral balance study in obese adolescent patients aged 12 to 16 years. Patients treated with XENICAL had a mean reduction in BMI of 0.55 kg/m^2 compared with an average increase of 0.31 kg/m^2 in placebo-treated patients (p=0.001). In both adolescent studies, adverse effects were generally similar to those described in adults and included fatty/oily stool, oily spotting, and oily evacuation. In a subgroup of 152 orlistat and 77 placebo patients from the 54-week study, changes in body composition measured by DEXA were similar in both treatment groups with the exception of fat mass, which was significantly reduced in patients treated with XENICAL compared to patients treated with placebo (-2.5 kg vs -0.6 kg, p=0.033). Because XENICAL can interfere with the absorption of fat-soluble vitamins, all patients should take a daily multivitamin that contains vitamins A, D, E, K, and beta-carotene. The supplement should be taken at least 2 hours before or after XENICAL (see CLINICAL PHARMACOLOGY: Other Short-term Studies; CLINICAL STUDIES: Pediatric Clinical Studies; ADVERSE REACTIONS: Pediatric Patients). XENICAL has not been studied in pediatric patients below the age of 12 years.

Geriatric Use

Clinical studies of XENICAL did not include sufficient numbers of patients aged 65 years and older to determine whether they respond differently from younger patients.

ADVERSE REACTIONS

Commonly Observed (based on first year and second year data - XENICAL 120 mg three times a day versus placebo): Gastrointestinal (GI) symptoms were the most commonly observed treatment-emergent adverse events associated with the use of XENICAL in double-blind, placebo-controlled clinical trials and are primarily a manifestation of the mechanism of action. (Commonly observed is defined as an incidence of ≥5% and an incidence in the XENICAL 120 mg group that is at least twice that of placebo.)

[See table 9 at left]

These and other commonly observed adverse reactions were generally mild and transient, and they decreased during the second year of treatment. In general, the first occurrence of these events was within 3 months of starting therapy. Overall, approximately 50% of all episodes of GI adverse events associated with orlistat treatment lasted for less than 1 week, and a majority lasted for no more than 4 weeks. However, GI adverse events may occur in some individuals over a period of 6 months or longer.

Discontinuation of Treatment

In controlled clinical trials, 8.8% of patients treated with XENICAL discontinued treatment due to adverse events, compared with 5.0% of placebo-treated patients. For XENICAL, the most common adverse events resulting in discontinuation of treatment were gastrointestinal.

Incidence in Controlled Clinical Trials

The following table lists other treatment-emergent adverse events from seven multicenter, double-blind, placebo-controlled clinical trials that occurred at a frequency of ≥2% among patients treated with XENICAL 120 mg three times a day and with an incidence that was greater than placebo during year 1 and year 2, regardless of relationship to study medication.

[See table 10 at left]

Other Clinical Studies or Postmarketing Surveillance

Rare cases of hypersensitivity have been reported with the use of XENICAL. Signs and symptoms have included pruritus, rash, urticaria, angioedema, and anaphylaxis.

Preliminary data from a XENICAL and cyclosporine drug interaction study indicate a reduction in cyclosporine plasma levels when XENICAL was coadministered with cyclosporine (see WARNINGS).

Pediatric Patients

In clinical trials with XENICAL in adolescent patients ages 12 to 16 years, the profile of adverse reactions was generally similar to that observed in adults.

OVERDOSAGE

Single doses of 800 mg XENICAL and multiple doses of up to 400 mg three times a day for 15 days have been studied in normal weight and obese subjects without significant adverse findings.

Should a significant overdose of XENICAL occur, it is recommended that the patient be observed for 24 hours. Based on human and animal studies, systemic effects attributable to the lipase-inhibiting properties of orlistat should be rapidly reversible.

DOSAGE AND ADMINISTRATION

The recommended dose of XENICAL is one 120-mg capsule three times a day with each main meal containing fat (during or up to 1 hour after the meal).

The patient should be on a nutritionally balanced, reduced-calorie diet that contains approximately 30% of calories from fat. The daily intake of fat, carbohydrate, and protein should be distributed over three main meals. If a meal is occasionally missed or contains no fat, the dose of XENICAL can be omitted.

Because XENICAL has been shown to reduce the absorption of some fat-soluble vitamins and beta-carotene, patients should be counseled to take a multivitamin containing fat-soluble vitamins to ensure adequate nutrition (see PRECAUTIONS: General). The supplement should be taken at least 2 hours before or after the administration of XENICAL, such as at bedtime.

Doses above 120 mg three times a day have not been shown to provide additional benefit.

Continued on next page

Xenical—Cont.

Based on fecal fat measurements, the effect of XENICAL is seen as soon as 24 to 48 hours after dosing. Upon discontinuation of therapy, fecal fat content usually returns to pretreatment levels within 48 to 72 hours.
The safety and effectiveness of XENICAL beyond 2 years have not been determined at this time.

HOW SUPPLIED

XENICAL is a dark-blue, hard-gelatin capsule containing pellets of powder.
XENICAL 120 mg Capsules: Dark-blue, two-piece, No. 1 opaque hard-gelatin capsule imprinted with Roche and XENICAL 120 in light-blue ink — bottle of 90 (NDC 0004-0256-52).

Storage Conditions

Store at 25°C (77°F); excursions permitted to 15° to 30°C (59° to 86°F) [see USP Controlled Room Temperature]. **Keep bottle tightly closed.**
XENICAL should not be used after the given expiration date.

Revised: December 2003

Sanofi-Synthelabo Inc.

90 PARK AVENUE
NEW YORK, NY 10016

Direct Inquiries to:
(212) 551-4000

For Medical Information Contact:
Product Information Services
(800) 446-6267

Sales and Ordering:
East Coast: (800) 223-1062
West Coast: (800) 223-5511

ELOXATIN™ ℞

[ē-lŏks-ă-tĭn]
(oxaliplatin for injection)

Prescribing information for this product, which appears on pages 3024–3028 of the 2004 PDR, has been completely revised as follows. Please write "See Supplement A" next to the product heading.

WARNING

ELOXATIN (oxaliplatin for injection) should be administered under the supervision of a qualified physician experienced in the use of cancer chemotherapeutic agents. Appropriate management of therapy and complications is possible only when adequate diagnostic and treatment facilities are readily available.
Anaphylactic-like reactions to ELOXATIN have been reported, and may occur within minutes of ELOXATIN administration. Epinephrine, corticosteroids, and antihistamines have been employed to alleviate symptoms (see WARNINGS and ADVERSE REACTIONS).

DESCRIPTION

ELOXATIN™ (oxaliplatin for injection) is an antineoplastic agent with the molecular formula $C_8H_{14}N_2O_4Pt$ and the chemical name of *cis*-[(1*R*,2*R*)-1,2-cyclohexanediamine-*N,N'*] [oxalato(2-)-*O,O'*] platinum. Oxaliplatin is an organoplatinum complex in which the platinum atom is complexed with 1,2-diaminocyclohexane (DACH) and with an oxalate ligand as a leaving group.

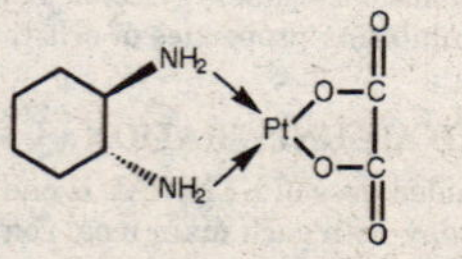

The molecular weight is 397.3. Oxaliplatin is slightly soluble in water at 6 mg/mL, very slightly soluble in methanol, and practically insoluble in ethanol and acetone.
ELOXATIN is supplied in vials containing 50 mg or 100 mg of oxaliplatin as a sterile, preservative-free lyophilized powder for reconstitution. Lactose monohydrate is present as an inactive ingredient at 450 mg and 900 mg in the 50 mg and 100 mg dosage strengths, respectively.

CLINICAL PHARMACOLOGY

Mechanism of Action

Oxaliplatin undergoes nonenzymatic conversion in physiologic solutions to active derivatives via displacement of the labile oxalate ligand. Several transient reactive species are formed, including monoaquo and diaquo DACH platinum, which covalently bind with macromolecules. Both inter- and intrastrand Pt-DNA crosslinks are formed. Crosslinks are formed between the *N*7 positions of two adjacent guanines (GG), adjacent adenine-guanines (AG), and guanines separated by an intervening nucleotide (GNG). These crosslinks inhibit DNA replication and transcription. Cytotoxicity is cell-cycle nonspecific.

Table 1 – Dosing Regimens in Patients Previously Untreated for Advanced Colorectal Cancer Clinical Trial

Treatment Arm	Dose	Regimen
ELOXATIN + 5-FU/LV FOLFOX4 (N=267)	**Day 1: ELOXATIN: 85 mg/m² (2-hour infusion) + LV 200 mg/m² (2-hour infusion), followed by 5-FU: 400 mg/m² (bolus), 600 mg/m² (22-hour infusion)** **Day 2: LV 200 mg/m² (2-hour infusion), followed by 5-FU: 400 mg/m² (bolus), 600 mg/m² (22-hour infusion)**	**q2w**
irinotecan + 5-FU/LV IFL (N=264)	Day 1: irinotecan 125 mg/m² as a 90-min infusion + LV 20 mg/m² as a 15-min infusion or IV push, followed by 5-FU 500 mg/m² IV bolus weekly × 4	q6w
ELOXATIN + irinotecan IROX (N=264)	Day 1: ELOXATIN: 85 mg/m² IV (2-hour infusion) + irinotecan 200 mg/m² IV over 30 minutes	q3w

Table 2 – Patient Demographics and Dosing in Patients Previously Untreated for Advanced Colorectal Cancer Clinical Trial

	ELOXATIN + 5-FU/LV N=267	irinotecan + 5-FU/LV N=264	ELOXATIN + irinotecan N=264
Sex: Male (%)	58.8	65.2	61.0
Female (%)	41.2	34.8	39.0
Median age (years)	61.0	61.0	61.0
<65 years of age (%)	61	62	63
≥65 years of age (%)	39	38	37
ECOG (%)			
0,1	94.4	95.5	94.7
2	5.6	4.5	5.3
Involved organs (%)			
Colon only	0.7	0.8	0.4
Liver only	39.3	44.3	39.0
Liver + other	41.2	38.6	40.9
Lung only	6.4	3.8	5.3
Other (including lymph nodes)	11.6	11.0	12.9
Not reported	0.7	1.5	1.5
Prior radiation (%)	3.0	1.5	3.0
Prior surgery (%)	74.5	79.2	81.8
Prior adjuvant (%)	15.7	14.8	15.2

Pharmacology

In vivo studies have shown antitumor activity of oxaliplatin against colon carcinoma. In combination with 5-fluorouracil (5-FU), oxaliplatin exhibits *in vitro* and *in vivo* antiproliferative activity greater than either compound alone in several tumor models [HT29 (colon), GR (mammary), and L1210 (leukemia)].

Human Pharmacokinetics

The reactive oxaliplatin derivatives are present as a fraction of the unbound platinum in plasma ultrafiltrate. The decline of ultrafilterable platinum levels following oxaliplatin administration is triphasic, characterized by two relatively short distribution phases ($t_{1/2\alpha}$; 0.43 hours and $t_{1/2\beta}$; 16.8 hours) and a long terminal elimination phase ($t_{1/2\gamma}$; 391 hours). Pharmacokinetic parameters obtained after a single 2-hour IV infusion of ELOXATIN at a dose of 85 mg/m² expressed as ultrafilterable platinum were C_{max} of 0.814 µg/mL and volume of distribution of 440 L.
Interpatient and intrapatient variability in ultrafilterable platinum exposure (AUC_{0-48}) assessed over 3 cycles was moderate to low (23% and 6%, respectively). A pharmacodynamic relationship between platinum ultrafiltrate levels and clinical safety and effectiveness has not been established.

Distribution

At the end of a 2-hour infusion of ELOXATIN, approximately 15% of the administered platinum is present in the systemic circulation. The remaining 85% is rapidly distributed into tissues or eliminated in the urine. In patients, plasma protein binding of platinum is irreversible and is greater than 90%. The main binding proteins are albumin and gammaglobulins. Platinum also binds irreversibly and accumulates (approximately 2-fold) in erythrocytes, where it appears to have no relevant activity. No platinum accumulation was observed in plasma ultrafiltrate following 85 mg/m² every two weeks.

Metabolism

Oxaliplatin undergoes rapid and extensive nonenzymatic biotransformation. There is no evidence of cytochrome P450-mediated metabolism *in vitro*.
Up to 17 platinum-containing derivatives have been observed in plasma ultrafiltrate samples from patients, including several cytotoxic species (monochloro DACH platinum, dichloro DACH platinum, and monoaquo and diaquo DACH platinum) and a number of noncytotoxic, conjugated species.

Elimination

The major route of platinum elimination is renal excretion. At five days after a single 2-hour infusion of ELOXATIN, urinary elimination accounted for about 54% of the platinum eliminated, with fecal excretion accounting for only about 2%. Platinum was cleared from plasma at a rate (10–17 L/h) that was similar to or exceeded the average human glomerular filtration rate (GFR; 7.5 L/h). There was no significant effect of gender on the clearance of ultrafilterable platinum. The renal clearance of ultrafilterable platinum is significantly correlated with GFR (see ADVERSE REACTIONS).

Pharmacokinetics in Special Populations

Renal Impairment

The AUC_{0-48hr} of platinum in the plasma ultrafiltrate increases as renal function decreases. The AUC_{0-48hr} of platinum in patients with mild (creatinine clearance, CL_{cr} 50 to 80 mL/min), moderate (CL_{cr} 30 to <50 mL/min) and severe renal (CL_{cr} <30 mL/min) impairment is increased by about 60, 140 and 190%, respectively, compared to patients with normal renal function (CL_{cr} >80 mL/min)] (see PRECAUTIONS and ADVERSE REACTIONS).

Drug - Drug Interactions

No pharmacokinetic interaction between 85 mg/m² of ELOXATIN and 5-FU has been observed in patients treated every 2 weeks, but increases of 5-FU plasma concentrations by approximately 20% have been observed with doses of 130 mg/m² of ELOXATIN administered every 3 weeks. *In vitro*, platinum was not displaced from plasma proteins by the fol-

lowing medications: erythromycin, salicylate, sodium valproate, granisetron, and paclitaxel. *In vitro*, oxaliplatin is not metabolized by, nor does it inhibit, human cytochrome P450 isoenzymes. No P450-mediated drug-drug interactions are therefore anticipated in patients.
Since platinum containing species are eliminated primarily through the kidney, clearance of these products may be decreased by co-administration of potentially nephrotoxic compounds, although this has not been specifically studied.

CLINICAL STUDIES

Combination Therapy with ELOXATIN and 5-FU/LV in Patients Previously Untreated for Advanced Colorectal Cancer

A North American, multicenter, open-label, randomized controlled study was sponsored by the National Cancer Institute (NCI) as an intergroup study led by the North Central Cancer Treatment Group (NCCTG). The study had 7 arms at different times during its conduct, four of which were closed due to either changes in the standard of care, toxicity, or simplification. During the study, the control arm was changed to irinotecan plus 5-FU/LV. The results reported below compared the efficacy and safety of two experimental regimens, ELOXATIN in combination with infusional 5-FU/LV and a combination of ELOXATIN plus irinotecan, to an approved control regimen of irinotecan plus 5-FU/LV in 795 concurrently randomized patients previously untreated for locally advanced or metastatic colorectal cancer. After completion of enrollment, the dose of irinotecan plus 5-FU/LV was decreased due to toxicity. Patients had to be at least 18 years of age, have known locally advanced, locally recurrent, or metastatic colorectal adenocarcinoma not curable by surgery or amenable to radiation therapy with curative intent, histologically proven colorectal adenocarcinoma, measurable or evaluable disease, with an ECOG performance status 0,1, or 2. Patients had to have granulocyte count $\geq 1.5 \times 10^9$/L, platelets $\geq 100 \times 10^9$/L, hemoglobin $\geq$9.0 gm/dL, creatinine $\leq$ 1.5 x ULN, total bilirubin $\leq$ 1.5 mg/dL, AST $\leq$ 5 x ULN, and alkaline phosphatase $\leq$ 5 x ULN. Patients may have received adjuvant therapy for resected Stage II or III disease without recurrence within 12 months. The patients were stratified for ECOG performance status (0, 1 vs. 2), prior adjuvant chemotherapy (yes vs. no), prior immunotherapy (yes vs. no), and age (<65 vs.$\geq$65 years). Although no post study treatment was specified in the protocol, 65 to 72% of patients received additional post study chemotherapy after study treatment discontinuation on all arms. Fifty eight percent of patients on the ELOXATIN plus 5-FU/LV arm received an irinotecan-containing regimen and 23% of patients on the irinotecan plus 5-FU/LV arm received oxaliplatin-containing regimens. Oxaliplatin was not commercially available during the trial.
The following table presents the dosing regimens of the three arms of the study.
[See table 1 at top of previous page]
The following table presents the demographics and dosing of the patient population entered into this study.
[See table 2 at top of previous page]
The length of a treatment cycle was 2 weeks for the ELOXATIN and 5-FU/LV regimen; 6 weeks for the irinotecan plus 5-FU/LV regimen; and 3 weeks for the ELOXATIN plus irinotecan regimen. The median number of cycles administered per patient was 10 (23.9 weeks) for the ELOXATIN and 5-FU/LV regimen, 4 (23.6 weeks) for the irinotecan plus 5-FU/LV regimen, and 7 (21.0 weeks) for the ELOXATIN plus irinotecan regimen.
Patients treated with the ELOXATIN and 5-FU/LV combination had a significantly longer time to tumor progression based on investigator assessment, longer overall survival, and a significantly higher confirmed response rate based on investigator assessment compared to patients given irinotecan plus 5-FU/LV. The following table summarizes the efficacy results.
[See table 3 above]

Table 3 – Summary of Efficacy

	ELOXATIN + 5-FU/LV N=267	irinotecan + 5-FU/LV N=264	ELOXATIN + irinotecan N=264
Survival (ITT)			
Number of deaths N (%)	155 (58.1)	192 (72.7)	175 (66.3)
Median survival (months)	19.4	14.6	17.6
Hazard Ratio and (95% confidence interval)	0.65 (0.53–0.80)*		
P-value	<0.0001*	–	–
TTP (ITT, investigator assessment)			
Percentage of progressors	82.8	81.8	89.4
Median TTP (months)	8.7	6.9	6.5
Hazard Ratio and (95% confidence interval)	0.74 (0.61–0.89)*		
P-value	0.0014*	–	–
Response Rate (investigator assessment)**			
Patients with measurable disease	210	212	215
Complete response N (%)	13 (6.2)	5 (2.4)	7 (3.3)
Partial response N (%)	82 (39.0)	64 (30.2)	67 (31.2)
Complete and partial response N (%)	95 (45.2)	69 (32.5)	74 (34.4)
95% confidence interval	(38.5–52.0)	(26.2–38.9)	(28.1–40.8)
P-value	0.0080*	–	–

*Compared to irinotecan plus 5-FU/LV (IFL) arm
**Based on all patients with measurable disease at baseline

The numbers in the response rate and TTP analysis are based on unblinded investigator assessment.
Figure 1 illustrates the Kaplan-Meier survival curves for the comparison of ELOXATIN and 5-FU/LV combination and ELOXATIN plus irinotecan to irinotecan plus 5-FU/LV.

Figure 1 illustrates the Kaplan-Meier survival curves for the comparison of ELOXATIN and 5-FU/LV combination and ELOXATIN plus irinotecan to irinotecan plus 5-FU/LV.

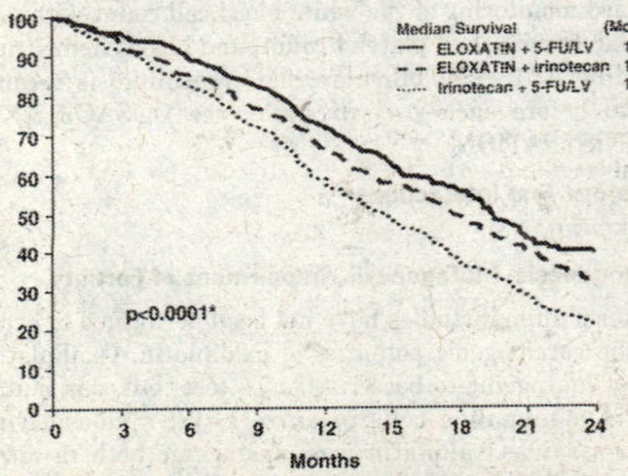

*Log rank test comparing Eloxatin plus 5-FU/LV to irinotecan plus 5-FU/LV.

A descriptive subgroup analysis demonstrated that the improvement in survival for ELOXATIN plus 5-FU/LV compared to irinotecan plus 5-FU/LV appeared to be maintained across age groups, prior adjuvant therapy, and number of organs involved. An estimated survival advantage in ELOXATIN plus 5-FU/LV versus irinotecan plus 5-FU/LV was seen in both genders; however it was greater among women than men. Insufficient subgroup sizes prevented analysis by race.

Table 4 – Dosing Regimens in Refractory and Relapsed Colorectal Cancer Clinical Trial

Treatment Arm	Dose	Regimen
ELOXATIN + 5-FU/LV (N=152)	**Day 1: ELOXATIN: 85 mg/m² (2-hour infusion) + LV 200 mg/m² (2-hour infusion), followed by 5-FU: 400 mg/m² (bolus), 600 mg/m² (22-hour infusion)** **Day 2: LV 200 mg/m² (2-hour infusion), followed by 5-FU: 400 mg/m² (bolus), 600 mg/m² (22-hour infusion)**	**q2w**
5-FU/LV (N=151)	Day 1: LV 200 mg/m² (2-hour infusion), followed by 5-FU: 400 mg/m² (bolus), 600 mg/m² (22-hour infusion) Day 2: LV 200 mg/m² (2-hour infusion), followed by 5-FU: 400 mg/m² (bolus), 600 mg/m² (22-hour infusion)	q2w
ELOXATIN (N=156)	Day 1: ELOXATIN 85 mg/m²(2-hour infusion)	q2w

Combination Therapy with ELOXATIN and 5-FU/LV in Previously Treated Patients with Advanced Colorectal Cancer

A multicenter, open-label, randomized, three arm controlled study was conducted in the US and Canada comparing the efficacy and safety of ELOXATIN in combination with an infusional schedule of 5-FU/LV to the same dose and schedule of 5-FU/LV alone and to single agent oxaliplatin in patients with advanced colorectal cancer who had relapsed/progressed during or within 6 months of first line therapy with bolus 5-FU/LV and irinotecan. The study was intended to be analyzed for response rate after 450 patients were enrolled. Survival will be subsequently assessed in all patients enrolled in the completed study. Accrual to this study is complete, with 821 patients enrolled. Patients in the study had to be at least 18 years of age, have unresectable, measurable, histologically proven colorectal adenocarcinoma, with a Karnofsky performance status >50%. Patients had to have SGOT(AST) and SGPT(ALT) $\leq$ 2x the institution's upper limit of normal (ULN), unless liver metastases were present and documented at baseline by CT or MRI scan, in which case $\leq$ 5x ULN was permitted. Patients had to have alkaline phosphatase $\leq$ 2x the institution's ULN, unless liver metastases were present and documented at baseline by CT or MRI scan, in which cases $\leq$ 5x ULN was permitted. Prior radiotherapy was permitted if it had been completed at least 3 weeks before randomization.
The dosing regimens of the three arms of the study are presented in the table below.
[See table 4 above]
Patients entered into the study for evaluation of response must have had at least one unidimensional lesion measuring $\geq$20mm using conventional CT or MRI scans, $\geq$10mm using a spiral CT scan. Tumor response and progression were assessed every 3 cycles (6 weeks) using the Response Evaluation Criteria in Solid Tumors (RECIST) until radiological documentation of progression or for 13 months following the first dose of study drug(s), whichever came first. Confirmed responses were based on two tumor assessments separated by at least 4 weeks.
The demographics of the patient population entered into this study are shown in the table below.
[See table 5 at top of next page]
The median number of cycles administered per patient was 6 for the ELOXATIN and 5-FU/LV combination and 3 each for 5-FU/LV alone and ELOXATIN alone.
Patients treated with the combination of ELOXATIN and 5-FU/LV had an increased response rate compared to patients given 5-FU/LV or oxaliplatin alone. The efficacy results are summarized in the tables below.
[See table 6 on next page]
[See table 7 on next page]
At the time of the interim analysis 49% of the radiographic progression events had occurred. In this interim analysis an estimated 2-month increase in median time to radiographic progression was observed compared to 5-FU/LV alone.
Of the 13 patients who had tumor response to the combination of ELOXATIN and 5-FU/LV, 5 were female and 8 were male, and responders included patients <65 years old and $\geq$65 years old. The small number of non-Caucasian participants made efficacy analyses in these populations uninterpretable.

INDICATIONS AND USAGE

ELOXATIN, used in combination with infusional 5-FU/LV, is indicated for the treatment of advanced carcinoma of the colon or rectum.

CONTRAINDICATIONS

ELOXATIN should not be administered to patients with a history of known allergy to ELOXATIN or other platinum compounds.

WARNINGS

As in the case for other platinum compounds, hypersensitivity and anaphylactic/anaphylactoid reactions to ELOXATIN have been reported (see ADVERSE REACTIONS). These allergic reactions were similar in nature and severity to those

Continued on next page

Eloxatin—Cont.

reported with other platinum-containing compounds, i.e., rash, urticaria, erythema, pruritus, and, rarely, bronchospasm and hypotension. These reactions occur within minutes of administration and should be managed with appropriate supportive therapy. Drug-related deaths associated with platinum compounds from this reaction have been reported.

Pregnancy Category D

ELOXATIN may cause fetal harm when administered to a pregnant woman. Pregnant rats were administered 1 mg/kg/day oxaliplatin (less than one-tenth the recommended human dose based on body surface area) during gestation days 1-5 (pre-implantation), 6-10, or 11-16 (during organogenesis). Oxaliplatin caused developmental mortality (increased early resorptions) when administered on days 6-10 and 11-16 and adversely affected fetal growth (decreased fetal weight, delayed ossification) when administered on days 6-10. If this drug is used during pregnancy or if the patient becomes pregnant while taking this drug, the patient should be apprised of the potential hazard to the fetus. Women of childbearing potential should be advised to avoid becoming pregnant while receiving treatment with ELOXATIN.

PRECAUTIONS

General

ELOXATIN should be administered under the supervision of a qualified physician experienced in the use of cancer chemotherapeutic agents. Appropriate management of therapy and complications is possible only when adequate diagnostic and treatment facilities are readily available.

Neuropathy

Neuropathy was graded using a study-specific neurotoxicity scale, which was different than the National Cancer Institute Common Toxicity Criteria, Version 2.0 (NCI CTC) (see below).

In the previously treated study, neuropathy information was collected to establish that ELOXATIN is associated with two types of neuropathy:

- **An acute, reversible, primarily peripheral, sensory neuropathy that is of early onset, occurring within hours or one to two days of dosing, that resolves within 14 days, and that frequently recurs with further dosing.** The symptoms may be precipitated or exacerbated by exposure to cold temperature or cold objects and they usually present as transient paresthesia, dysesthesia and hypoesthesia in the hands, feet, perioral area, or throat. Jaw spasm, abnormal tongue sensation, dysarthria, eye pain, and a feeling of chest pressure have also been observed. The acute, reversible pattern of sensory neuropathy was observed in about 56% of study patients who received ELOXATIN with 5-FU/LV. In any individual cycle acute neurotoxicity was observed in approximately 30% of patients. Ice (mucositis prophylaxis) should be avoided during the infusion of ELOXATIN because cold temperature can exacerbate acute neurological symptoms (see DOSAGE AND ADMINISTRATION: Dose Modifications).

  An acute syndrome of pharyngolaryngeal dysesthesia seen in 1-2% (grade 3/4) of patients previously untreated for advanced colorectal cancer, and the previously treated patients is characterized by subjective sensations of dysphagia or dyspnea, without any laryngospasm or bronchospasm (no stridor or wheezing).
- **A persistent (>14 days), primarily peripheral, sensory neuropathy that is usually characterized by paresthesias, dysesthesias, hypoesthesias, but may also include deficits in proprioception that can interfere with daily activities (e.g. writing, buttoning, swallowing, and difficulty walking from impaired proprioception).** These forms of neuropathy occurred in 48% of the study patients receiving ELOXATIN with 5-FU/LV. Persistent neuropathy can occur without any prior acute neuropathy event. The majority of the patients (80%) who developed grade 3 persistent neuropathy progressed from prior Grade 1 or 2 events. These symptoms may improve in some patients upon discontinuation of ELOXATIN.

Overall, neuropathy was reported in patients previously untreated for advanced colorectal cancer in 82% (all grades) and 19% (grade 3/4), and in the previously treated patients in 74% (all grades) and 7% (grade 3/4) events. Information regarding reversibility of neuropathy was not available from the trial for patients who had not been previously treated for colorectal cancer.

Neurotoxicity scale:

The grading scale for paresthesias/dysesthesias was: Grade 1, resolved and did not interfere with functioning; Grade 2, interfered with function but not daily activities; Grade 3, pain or functional impairment that interfered with daily activities; Grade 4, persistent impairment that is disabling or life-threatening.

Pulmonary Toxicity

ELOXATIN has been associated with pulmonary fibrosis (<1% of study patients), which may be fatal. The combined incidence of cough, dyspnea and hypoxia was 43% (any grade) and 7% (grade 3 and 4) in the ELOXATIN plus 5-FU/LV arm compared to 32% (any grade) and 5% (grade 3 and 4) in the irinotecan plus 5-FU/LV arm of unknown duration for patients with previously untreated colorectal cancer. In case of

Table 5 – Patient Demographics in Refractory and Relapsed Colorectal Cancer Clinical Trial

	5-FU/LV (N=151)	ELOXATIN (N=156)	ELOXATIN + 5-FU/LV (N=152)
Sex: Male (%)	54.3	60.9	57.2
Female (%)	45.7	39.1	42.8
Median age (years)	60.0	61.0	59.0
Range	21-80	27-79	22-88
Race (%)			
Caucasian	87.4	84.6	88.8
Black	7.9	7.1	5.9
Asian	1.3	2.6	2.6
Other	3.3	5.8	2.6
KPS (%)			
70–100	94.7	92.3	95.4
50–60	2.6	4.5	2.0
Not reported	2.6	3.2	2.6
Prior radiotherapy (%)	25.2	19.2	25.0
Prior pelvic radiation (%)	18.5	13.5	21.1
Number of metastatic sites (%)			
1	27.2	31.4	25.7
≥2	72.2	67.9	74.3
Liver involvement (%)			
Liver only	22.5	25.6	18.4
Liver + other	60.3	59.0	53.3

Table 6 - Response Rates (ITT Analysis)

Best Response	5-FU/LV (N=151)	ELOXATIN (N=156)	ELOXATIN + 5-FU/LV (N=152)
CR	0	0	0
PR	0	2 (1%)	13 (9%)
p-value	0.0002 for 5-FU/LV vs. ELOXATIN + 5-FU/LV		
95% CI	0-2.4%	0.2-4.6%	4.6-14.2%

Table 7 - Summary of Radiographic Time to Progression*

Arm	5-FU/LV (N=151)	ELOXATIN (N=156)	ELOXATIN + 5-FU/LV (N=152)
No. of Progressors	74	101	50
No. of patients with no radiological evaluation beyond baseline	22 (15%)	16 (10%)	17 (11%)
Median TTP (months)	2.7	1.6	4.6
95% CI	1.8-3.0	1.4-2.7	4.2-6.1

*This is not an ITT analysis. Events were limited to radiographic disease progression documented by independent review of radiographs. Clinical progression was not included in this analysis, and 18% of patients were excluded from the analysis based on unavailability of the radiographs for independent review.

unexplained respiratory symptoms such as non-productive cough, dyspnea, crackles, or radiological pulmonary infiltrates, ELOXATIN should be discontinued until further pulmonary investigation excludes interstitial lung disease or pulmonary fibrosis.

Information for Patients

Patients and patients' caregivers should be informed of the expected side effects of ELOXATIN, particularly its neurologic effects, both the acute, reversible effects, and the persistent neurosensory toxicity. Patients should be informed that the acute neurosensory toxicity may be precipitated or exacerbated by exposure to cold or cold objects. Patients should be instructed to avoid cold drinks, use of ice, and should cover exposed skin prior to exposure to cold temperature or cold objects.

Patients must be adequately informed of the risk of low blood cell counts and instructed to contact their physician immediately should fever, particularly if associated with persistent diarrhea, or evidence of infection develop.

Patients should be instructed to contact their physician if persistent vomiting, diarrhea, signs of dehydration, cough or breathing difficulties occur, or signs of allergic reaction appear.

Laboratory Tests

Standard monitoring of the white blood cell count with differential, hemoglobin, platelet count, and blood chemistries (including ALT, AST, bilirubin and creatinine) is recommended before each ELOXATIN cycle (see DOSAGE AND ADMINISTRATION).

Laboratory Test Interactions

None known.

Carcinogenesis, Mutagenesis, Impairment of Fertility

Long-term animal studies have not been performed to evaluate the carcinogenic potential of oxaliplatin. Oxaliplatin was not mutagenic to bacteria (Ames test) but was mutagenic to mammalian cells *in vitro* (L5178Y mouse lymphoma assay). Oxaliplatin was clastogenic both *in vitro* (chromosome aberration in human lymphocytes) and *in vivo* (mouse bone marrow micronucleus assay).

In a fertility study, male rats were given oxaliplatin at 0, 0.5, 1, or 2 mg/kg/day for five days every 21 days for a total of three cycles prior to mating with females that received two cycles of oxaliplatin on the same schedule. A dose of 2

Table 8 – Adverse Experience Reported in Patients Previously Untreated for Advanced Colorectal Cancer Clinical Trial (≥5% of all patients and with ≥1% NCI Grade 3/4 events)

	ELOXATIN + 5-FU/LV N=259		irinotecan + 5-FU/LV N=256		ELOXATIN + irinotecan N=258	
Adverse Event (WHO/Pref)	**All Grades (%)**	**Grade 3/4 (%)**	**All Grades (%)**	**Grade 3/4 (%)**	**All Grades (%)**	**Grade 3/4 (%)**
Any Event	99	82	98	70	99	76
Allergy/Immunology						
Hypersensitivity	12	2	5	0	6	1
Cardiovascular						
Thrombosis	6	5	6	6	3	3
Hypotension	5	3	6	3	4	3
Constitutional Symptoms/Pain/Ocular/Visual						
Fatigue	70	7	58	11	66	16
Abdominal Pain	29	8	31	7	39	10
Myalgia	14	2	6	0	9	2
Pain	7	1	5	1	6	1
Vision abnormal	5	0	2	1	6	1
Neuralgia	5	0	0	0	2	1
Dermatology/Skin						
Skin reaction–hand/foot	7	1	2	1	1	0
Injection site reaction	6	0	1	0	4	1
Gastrointestinal						
Nausea	71	6	67	15	83	19
Diarrhea	56	12	65	29	76	25
Vomiting	41	4	43	13	64	23
Stomatitis	38	0	25	1	19	1
Anorexia	35	2	25	4	27	5
Constipation	32	4	27	2	21	2
Diarrhea-colostomy	13	2	16	7	16	3
Gastrointestinal NOS	5	2	4	2	3	2
Hematology/Infection						
Infection no ANC	10	4	5	1	7	2
Infection—ANC	8	8	12	11	9	8
Lymphopenia	6	2	4	1	5	2
Febrile neutropenia	4	4	15	14	12	11
Hepatic/Metabolic/Laboratory/Renal						
Hyperglycemia	14	2	11	3	12	3
Hypokalemia	11	3	7	4	6	2
Dehydration	9	5	16	11	14	7
Hypoalbuminemia	8	0	5	2	9	1
Hyponatremia	8	2	7	4	4	1
Urinary frequency	5	1	2	1	3	1
Neurology						
Overall Neuropathy	82	19	18	2	69	7
Paresthesias	77	18	16	2	62	6
Pharyngo-laryngeal dysesthesias	38	2	1	0	28	1
Neuro-sensory	12	1	2	0	9	1
Neuro NOS	1	0	1	0	1	0
Pulmonary						
Cough	35	1	25	2	17	1
Dyspnea	18	7	14	3	11	2
Hiccups	5	1	2	0	3	2

mg/kg/day (less than one-seventh the recommended human dose on a body surface area basis) did not affect pregnancy rate, but caused developmental mortality (increased early resorptions, decreased live fetuses, decreased live births) and delayed growth (decreased fetal weight). Testicular damage, characterized by degeneration, hypoplasia, and atrophy, was observed in dogs administered oxaliplatin at 0.75 mg/kg/day x 5 days every 28 days for three cycles. A no effect level was not identified. This daily dose is approximately one-sixth of the recommended human dose on a body surface area basis.

Pregnancy Category D-See WARNINGS

Nursing Mothers - It is not known whether ELOXATIN or its derivatives are excreted in human milk. Because many drugs are excreted in human milk and because of the potential for serious adverse reactions in nursing infants from ELOXATIN, a decision should be made whether to discontinue nursing or delay the use of the drug, taking into account the importance of the drug to the mother.

Pediatric Use - The safety and effectiveness of ELOXATIN in pediatric patients have not been established.

Patients with Renal Impairment - The safety and effectiveness of the combination of ELOXATIN and 5-FU/LV in patients with renal impairment have not been evaluated. The combination of ELOXATIN and 5-FU/LV should be used with caution in patients with preexisting renal impairment since the primary route of platinum elimination is renal. Clearance of ultrafilterable platinum is decreased in patients with mild, moderate, and severe renal impairment. A pharmacodynamic relationship between platinum ultrafiltrate levels and clinical safety and effectiveness has not been established (see CLINICAL PHARMACOLOGY and ADVERSE REACTIONS).

Geriatric Use - No significant effect of age on the clearance of ultrafilterable platinum has been observed. In the previously untreated for advanced colorectal cancer randomized clinical trial (see CLINICAL STUDIES) of ELOXATIN, 160 patients treated with ELOXATIN and 5-FU/LV were < 65 years and 99 patients were ≥ 65 years. The same efficacy improvements in response rate, time to tumor progression, and overall survival were observed in the ≥ 65 year old patients as in the overall study population. In the previously treated randomized clinical trial (see CLINICAL STUDIES) of ELOXATIN, 95 patients treated with ELOXATIN and 5-FU/LV were < 65 years and 55 patients were ≥ 65 years. The rates of overall adverse events, including grade 3 and 4 events, were similar across and within arms in the different age groups in both studies. The incidence of diarrhea, dehydration, hypokalemia, leukopenia, fatigue and syncope were higher in patients ≥ 65 years old. No adjustment to starting dose was required in patients ≥ 65 years old.

Drug Interactions - No specific cytochrome P-450-based drug interaction studies have been conducted. No pharmacokinetic interaction between 85 mg/m^2 ELOXATIN and 5-FU/LV has been observed in patients treated every 2 weeks. Increases of 5-FU plasma concentrations by approximately 20% have been observed with doses of 130 mg/m^2 ELOXATIN dosed every 3 weeks. Since platinum containing species are eliminated primarily through the kidney, clearance of these products may be decreased by coadministration of potentially nephrotoxic compounds; although, this has not been specifically studied (see CLINICAL PHARMACOLOGY).

ADVERSE REACTIONS

More than 4,000 patients with advanced colorectal cancer have been treated in clinical studies with ELOXATIN either as a single agent or in combination with other medications. The most common adverse reactions were peripheral sensory neuropathies, fatigue, neutropenia, nausea, emesis, and diarrhea (see PRECAUTIONS).

Patients Previously Untreated for Advanced Colorectal Cancer

Two-hundred and fifty nine patients were treated in the ELOXATIN and 5-FU/LV combination arm of the randomized trial in patients previously untreated for advanced colorectal cancer (see CLINICAL STUDIES). The adverse event profile in this study was similar to that seen in other studies and the adverse reactions in this trial are shown in the tables below.

Both 5-FU and ELOXATIN are associated with gastrointestinal and hematologic adverse events. When ELOXATIN is administered in combination with 5-FU, the incidence of these events is increased.

The incidence of death within 30 days of treatment in the previously untreated for advanced colorectal cancer study, regardless of causality, was 3% with the ELOXATIN and 5-FU/LV combination, 5% with irinotecan plus 5-FU/LV, and 3% with ELOXATIN plus irinotecan. Deaths within 60 days from initiation of therapy were 2.3% with the ELOXATIN and 5-FU/LV combination, 5.1% with irinotecan plus 5-FU/LV, and 3.1% with ELOXATIN plus irinotecan.

The following table provides adverse events reported in the previously untreated for advanced colorectal cancer study (see CLINICAL STUDIES) by body system and decreasing order of frequency in the ELOXATIN and 5-FU/LV combination arm for events with overall incidences ≥5% and for grade 3/4 events with incidences ≥ 1%. This table does not include hematologic and blood chemistry abnormalities; these are shown separately below.

[See table 8 at left]

The following table provides adverse events reported in the previously untreated for advanced colorectal cancer study (see CLINICAL STUDIES) by body system and decreasing order of frequency in the ELOXATIN and 5-FU/LV combination arm for events with overall incidences ≥5% but with incidences < 1% NCI Grade 3/4 events.

Continued on next page

Eloxatin—Cont.

Table 9 - Adverse Experience Reported in Patients Previously Untreated for Advanced Colorectal Cancer Clinical Trial (≥5% of all patients but with < 1% NCI Grade 3/4 events)

	ELOXATIN + 5-FU/LV N=259	irinotecan + 5-FU/ LV N=256	ELOXATIN + irinotecan N=258
Adverse Event (WHO/Pref)	**All Grades (%)**	**All Grades (%)**	**All Grades (%)**
Allergy/Immunology			
Rash	11	4	7
Rhinitis allergic	10	6	6
Cardiovascular			
Edema	15	13	10
Constitutional Symptoms/Pain/Ocular/Visual			
Headache	13	6	9
Weight loss	11	9	11
Epistaxis	10	2	2
Tearing	9	1	2
Rigors	8	2	7
Dysphasia	5	3	3
Sweating	5	6	12
Arthralgia	5	5	8
Dermatology/Skin			
Alopecia	38	44	67
Flushing	7	2	5
Pruritus	6	4	2
Dry Skin	6	2	5
Gastrointestinal			
Taste perversion	14	6	8
Dyspepsia	12	7	5
Flatulence	9	6	5
Mouth Dryness	5	2	3
Hematology/Infection			
Fever no ANC	16	9	9
Hepatic/Metabolic/Laboratory/Renal			
Hypocalcemia	7	5	4
Elevated Creatinine	4	4	5
Neurology			
Insomnia	13	9	11
Depression	9	5	7
Dizziness	8	6	10
Anxiety	5	2	6

Adverse events were similar in men and women and in patients <65 and ≥65 years, but older patients may have been more susceptible to diarrhea, dehydration, hypokalemia, leukopenia, fatigue and syncope. The following additional adverse events, at least possibly related to treatment and potentially important, were reported in ≥2% and <5% of the patients in the ELOXATIN and 5-FU/LV combination arm (listed in decreasing order of frequency): metabolic, pneumonitis, catheter infection, vertigo, prothrombin time, pulmonary, rectal bleeding, dysuria, nail changes, chest pain, rectal pain, syncope, hypertension, hypoxia, unknown infection, bone pain, pigmentation changes, and urticaria.

Previously Treated Patients with Advanced Colorectal Cancer

Four hundred and fifty patients (about 150 receiving the combination of ELOXATIN and 5-FU/LV) were studied in a randomized trial in patients with refractory and relapsed colorectal cancer (see CLINICAL STUDIES). The adverse event profile in this study was similar to that seen in other studies and the adverse reactions in this trial are shown in the tables below.

Thirteen percent of patients in the ELOXATIN and 5-FU/LV combination arm and 18% in the 5-FU/LV arm of the previously treated study had to discontinue treatment because of adverse effects related to gastrointestinal, or hematologic adverse events, or neuropathies. Both 5-FU and ELOXATIN are associated with gastrointestinal and hematologic adverse events. When ELOXATIN is administered in combination with 5-FU, the incidence of these events is increased.

The incidence of death within 30 days of treatment in the previously treated study, regardless of causality, was 5% with the ELOXATIN and 5-FU/LV combination, 8% with ELOXATIN alone, and 7% with 5-FU/LV. Of the 7 deaths that occurred on the ELOXATIN and 5-FU/LV combination arm within 30 days of stopping treatment, 3 may have been treatment related, associated with gastrointestinal bleeding or dehydration.

The following table provides adverse events reported in the previously treated study (see CLINICAL STUDIES) by body system and in decreasing order of frequency in the ELOXATIN and 5-FU/LV combination arm for events with overall incidences ≥5% and for grade 3/4 events with incidences ≥ 1%. This table does not include hematologic and blood chemistry abnormalities; these are shown separately below.

[See table 10 on next page]

The following table provides adverse events reported in the previously treated study (see CLINICAL STUDIES) by body system and in decreasing order of frequency in the ELOXATIN and 5-FU/LV combination arm for events with overall incidences ≥5% but with incidences <1% NCI Grade 3/4 events.

Table 11 - Adverse Experience Reported in Previously Treated Colorectal Cancer Clinical Trial (≥5% of all patients but with < 1% NCI Grade 3/4 events)

	5-FU/LV (N = 142)	ELOXATIN (N = 153)	ELOXATIN +5-FU/LV (N = 150)
Adverse Event (WHO/Pref)	**All Grades (%)**	**All Grades (%)**	**All Grades (%)**
Allergy/Immunology			
Rhinitis	4	6	15
Allergic Reaction	1	3	10
Rash	5	5	9
Cardiovascular			
Peripheral Edema	11	5	10
Constitutional Symptoms/Pain/Ocular/Visual			
Headache	8	13	17
Arthralgia	10	7	10
Epistaxis	1	2	9
Abnormal Lacrimation	6	1	7
Rigors	6	9	7
Dermatology/Skin			
Hand-Foot Syndrome	13	1	11
Flushing	2	3	10
Alopecia	3	3	7
Gastrointestinal			
Constipation	23	31	32
Dyspepsia	10	7	14
Taste Perversion	1	5	13
Mucositis	10	2	7
Flatulence	6	3	5
Hepatic/Metabolic/Laboratory/Renal			
Hematuria	4	0	6
Dysuria	1	1	6
Neurology			
Dizziness	8	7	13
Insomnia	4	11	9
Pulmonary			
Upper Resp Tract Infection	4	7	10
Pharyngitis	10	2	9
Hiccup	0	2	5

Adverse events were similar in men and women and in patients <65 and ≥65 years, but older patients may have been more susceptible to dehydration, diarrhea, hypokalemia and fatigue. The following additional adverse events, at least possibly related to treatment and potentially important, were reported in ≥2% and <5% of the patients in the ELOXATIN and 5-FU/LV combination arm (listed in decreasing order of frequency): anxiety, myalgia, erythematous rash, increased sweating, conjunctivitis, weight decrease, dry mouth, rectal hemorrhage, depression, ataxia, ascites, hemorrhoids, muscle weakness, nervousness, tachycardia, abnormal micturition frequency, dry skin, pruritus, hemoptysis, purpura, vaginal hemorrhage, melena, somnolence, pneumonia, proctitis, involuntary muscle contractions, intestinal obstruction, gingivitis, tenesmus, hot flashes, enlarged abdomen, urinary incontinence.

Hematologic

The following tables list the hematologic changes occurring in ≥5% of patients, based on laboratory values and NCI grade, with the exception of anemia in the patients previously untreated for advanced colorectal cancer, which is based on AE reporting and NCI grade alone.

[See table 12 at bottom of next page]

[See table 13 at top of page 430]

Thrombocytopenia

Thrombocytopenia was frequently reported with the combination of ELOXATIN and 5-FU/LV. The incidence of Grade 3/4 thrombocytopenia in the patients previously untreated for advanced colorectal cancer and the previously treated patients was 3-5%. Grade 3/4 hemorrhagic events in both patient populations were reported at low frequency and the incidence of these events was greater for the combination of ELOXATIN and 5-FU/LV over the irinotecan plus 5-FU/LV or 5-FU/LV control groups. In the previously untreated patients, the incidence of epistaxis was 10% in the ELOXATIN and 5-FU/LV arm, and 2% and 1% respectively in the irinotecan plus 5-FU/LV or irinotecan plus ELOXATIN arms. The requirement for platelet transfusion was not increased in the ELOXATIN and 5-FU/LV arm. The incidence of all hemorrhagic events in the previously treated patients was also higher on the ELOXATIN combination arm compared to the 5-FU/LV arm. These events included gastrointestinal bleeding, hematuria and epistaxis.

Neutropenia

Neutropenia was frequently observed with the combination of ELOXATIN and 5-FU/LV, with Grade 3 and 4 events reported in 35% and 18% of the patients previously untreated for advanced colorectal cancer, respectively. Grade 3 and 4 events were reported in 27% and 17% of previously treated patients, respectively. The incidence of febrile neutropenia in the patients previously untreated for advanced colorectal cancer was 15% (3% of cycles) in the irinotecan plus 5-FU/LV arm and 4% (less than 1% of cycles) in the ELOXATIN and 5-FU/LV combination arm. Additionally, in this same population, infection with grade 3 or 4 neutropenia was 12% in the irinotecan plus 5-FU/LV, and 8% in the ELOXATIN and 5-FU/LV combination. The incidence of febrile neutropenia in the previously treated patients was 1% in the 5-FU/LV arm and 6% (less than 1% of cycles) in the ELOXATIN and 5-FU/LV combination arm.

Gastrointestinal

In patients previously untreated for advanced colorectal cancer receiving the combination of ELOXATIN and 5-FU/LV, the incidence of Grade 3 and 4 vomiting and diarrhea was less compared to irinotecan plus 5-FU/LV controls (see table). In previously treated patients receiving the combination of ELOXATIN and 5-FU/LV, the incidence of Grade 3 and 4 nausea, vomiting, diarrhea, and mucositis/stomatitis increased compared to 5-FU/LV controls (see table).

The incidence of gastrointestinal adverse events in the previously untreated and previously treated patients appears to be similar across cycles. Premedication with antiemetics, including 5-HT_3 blockers, is recommended. Diarrhea and mucositis may be exacerbated by the addition of ELOXATIN to 5-FU/LV, and should be managed with appropriate supportive care. Since cold temperature can exacerbate acute neurological symptoms, ice (mucositis prophylaxis) should be avoided during the infusion of ELOXATIN.

Dermatologic

ELOXATIN did not increase the incidence of alopecia compared to 5-FU/LV alone. No complete alopecia was reported. The incidence of hand-foot syndrome in patients previously untreated for advanced colorectal cancer was 2% in the irinotecan plus 5-FU/LV arm and 7% in the ELOXATIN and 5-FU/LV combination arm. The incidence of hand-foot syndrome in previously treated patients was 13% in the 5-FU/LV arm and 11% in the ELOXATIN and 5-FU/LV combination arm.

Care of Intravenous Site:

Extravasation may result in local pain and inflammation that may be severe and lead to complications, including necrosis. Injection site reaction, including redness, swelling, and pain, has been reported.

Neurologic

Overall, neuropathy was reported in patients previously untreated for advanced colorectal cancer in 82% (all grades) and 19% (grade 3/4), and in the previously treated patients in 74% (all grades) and 7% (grade 3/4) events. ELOXATIN is consistently associated with two types of peripheral neuropathy (see PRECAUTIONS, Neuropathy). In the previously treated patients, the incidence of overall and Grade 3/4 persistent peripheral neuropathy was 48% and 6%, respectively. The majority of the patients (80%) that developed grade 3 persistent neuropathy progressed from prior Grade 1 or 2 events. The median number of cycles administered on the ELOXATIN with 5-FU/LV combination arm in the previously treated patients was 6.

Pulmonary

ELOXATIN has been associated with pulmonary fibrosis (see PRECAUTIONS, Pulmonary Toxicity).

Allergic Reactions

Hypersensitivity to ELOXATIN has been observed (<2% Grade 3/4) in clinical studies. These allergic reactions which can be fatal, can occur at any cycle, and were similar in nature and severity to those reported with other platinum-containing compounds such as, rash, urticaria, erythema, pruritus, and, rarely, bronchospasm and hypotension. The symptoms associated with hypersensitivity reactions reported in the previously untreated patients were urticaria, pruritus, flushing of the face, diarrhea associated with oxaliplatin infusion, shortness of breath, bronchospasm, diaphoresis, chest pains, hypotension, disorientation and syncope. These reactions are usually managed with standard epinephrine, corticosteroid, antihistamine therapy, and may require discontinuation of therapy (see WARNINGS for anaphylactic/anaphylactoid reactions).

Anticoagulation and Hemorrhage

There have been reports while on study and from post-marketing surveillance of prolonged prothrombin time and INR occasionally associated with hemorrhage in patients who received ELOXATIN plus 5-FU/LV while on anticoagulants. Patients receiving ELOXATIN plus 5-FU/LV and requiring oral anticoagulants may require closer monitoring.

Renal

About 5-10% of patients in all groups had some degree of elevation of serum creatinine. The incidence of Grade 3/4 elevations in serum creatinine in the ELOXATIN and 5-FU/LV combination arm was 1% in the previously treated patients.

Table 10 – Adverse Experience Reported in Previously Treated Colorectal Cancer Clinical Trial (≥5% of all patients and with ≥1% NCI Grade 3/4 events)

Adverse Event (WHO/Pref)	5-FU/LV (N=142) All Grades (%)	5-FU/LV (N=142) Grade 3/4 (%)	ELOXATIN (N=153) All Grades (%)	ELOXATIN (N=153) Grade 3/4 (%)	ELOXATIN + 5-FU/LV (N=150) All Grades (%)	ELOXATIN + 5-FU/LV (N=150) Grade 3/4 (%)
Any Event	98	41	100	46	99	73
Cardiovascular						
Dyspnea	11	2	13	7	20	4
Coughing	9	0	11	0	19	1
Edema	13	1	10	1	15	1
Thromboembolism	4	2	2	1	9	8
Chest Pain	4	1	5	1	8	1
Constitutional Symptoms/Pain						
Fatigue	52	6	61	9	68	7
Back Pain	16	4	11	0	19	3
Pain	9	3	14	3	15	2
Dermatology/Skin						
Injection Site Reaction	5	1	9	0	10	3
Gastrointestinal						
Diarrhea	44	3	46	4	67	11
Nausea	59	4	64	4	65	11
Vomiting	27	4	37	4	40	9
Stomatitis	32	3	14	0	37	3
Abdominal Pain	31	5	31	7	33	4
Anorexia	20	1	20	2	29	3
Gastroesophageal Reflux	3	0	1	0	5	2
Hematology/Infection						
Fever	23	1	25	1	29	1
Febrile Neutropenia	1	1	0	0	6	6
Hepatic/Metabolic/Laboratory/Renal						
Hypokalemia	3	1	3	2	9	4
Dehydration	6	4	5	3	8	3
Neurology						
Neuropathy	17	0	76	7	74	7
Acute	10	0	65	5	56	2
Persistent	9	0	43	3	48	6

Table 12 – Adverse Hematologic Experiences in Patients Previously Untreated for Advanced Colorectal Cancer (≥5% of patients)

Hematology Parameter	ELOXATIN + 5-FU/LV N=259 All Grades (%)	ELOXATIN + 5-FU/LV N=259 Grade 3/4 (%)	irinotecan + 5-FU/LV N=256 All Grades (%)	irinotecan + 5-FU/LV N=256 Grade 3/4 (%)	ELOXATIN + irinotecan N=258 All Grades (%)	ELOXATIN + irinotecan N=258 Grade 3/4 (%)
Anemia	27	3	28	4	25	3
Leukopenia	85	20	84	23	76	24
Neutropenia	81	53	77	44	71	36
Thrombocytopenia	71	5	26	2	44	4

Hepatic

The following tables list the clinical chemistry changes associated with hepatic toxicity occurring in ≥5% of patients, based on adverse events reported and NCI CTC grade for patients previously untreated for advanced colorectal cancer, laboratory values and NCI CTC grade for previously treated patients.

[See table 14 at bottom of next page]
[See table 15 at bottom of next page]

Thromboembolism

The incidence of thromboembolic events was 6 and 9% of the patients previously untreated for advanced colorectal cancer and previously treated patients in the ELOXATIN and 5-FU/LV combination arm, respectively.

Postmarketing Experience

The following events have been reported from worldwide postmarketing experience.

Body as a whole:
-angioedema, anaphylactic shock

Central and peripheral nervous system disorders:
-loss of deep tendon reflexes, dysarthria, Lhermitte's sign, cranial nerve palsies, fasciculations

Gastrointestinal system disorders:
-severe diarrhea/vomiting resulting in hypokalemia, metabolic acidosis; ileus; intestinal obstruction, pancreatitis

Hearing and vestibular system disorders:
-deafness

Platelet, bleeding, and clotting disorders:
-immuno-allergic thrombocytopenia
-prolongation of prothrombin time and of INR in patients receiving anticoagulants

Red Blood Cell disorders:
-hemolytic uremic syndrome

Respiratory system disorders:
-pulmonary fibrosis, and other interstitial lung diseases

Vision disorders:
-decrease of visual acuity, visual field disturbance, optic neuritis

OVERDOSAGE

There have been five ELOXATIN overdoses reported. One patient received two 130 mg/m^2 doses of ELOXATIN (cumulative dose of 260 mg/m^2) within a 24 hour period. The patient experienced Grade 4 thrombocytopenia (<25,000/mm^3) without any bleeding, which resolved. Two other patients were mistakenly administered ELOXATIN instead of carboplatin. One patient received a total ELOXATIN dose of 500 mg and the other received 650 mg. The first patient experienced dyspnea, wheezing, paresthesia, profuse vomiting and chest pain on the day of administration. She developed respiratory failure and severe bradycardia, and subsequently did not respond to resuscitation efforts. The other patient also experienced dyspnea, wheezing, paresthesia, and vomiting. Her symptoms resolved with supportive care. Another patient who was mistakenly administered a 700 mg dose experienced rapid onset of dysesthesia. Inpatient supportive care was given, including hydration, electrolyte support, and platelet transfusion. Recovery occurred 15 days after the overdose. The last patient received an overdose of oxaliplatin at 360 mg instead of 120 mg over a 1-hour infusion by mistake. At the end of the infusion, the patient experienced 2 episodes of vomiting, laryngospasm, and paresthesia. The patient fully recovered from the laryngospasm within half an hour. At the time of reporting, 1 hour after onset of the event, the patient was recovering from paresthesia. There is no known antidote for ELOXATIN overdose. In addition to thrombocytopenia, the anticipated complications of an ELOXATIN overdose include myelosuppression, nausea and vomiting, diarrhea, and neurotoxicity. Patients suspected of receiving an overdose should be monitored, and supportive treatment should be administered.

DOSAGE AND ADMINISTRATION

The recommended dose schedule given every two weeks is as follows:

Day 1: ELOXATIN 85 mg/m^2 IV infusion in 250-500 mL D5W and leucovorin 200 mg/m^2 IV infusion in D5W both given over 120 minutes at the same time in separate bags using a Y-line, followed by 5-FU 400 mg/m^2 IV bolus given over 2-4 minutes, followed by 5-FU 600 mg/m^2 IV infusion in 500 mL D5W (recommended) as a 22-hour continuous infusion.

Day 2: Leucovorin 200 mg/m^2 IV infusion over 120 minutes, followed by 5-FU 400 mg/m^2 IV bolus given over 2-4 minutes, followed by 5-FU 600 mg/m^2 IV infusion in 500 mL D5W (recommended) as a 22-hour continuous infusion.

[See figure 2 on next page]

Repeat cycle every 2 weeks.

The administration of ELOXATIN does not require prehydration.

Premedication with antiemetics, including 5-HT$_3$ blockers with or without dexamethasone, is recommended.

For information on 5-fluorouracil and leucovorin, see the respective package inserts.

Dose Modification Recommendations

Prior to subsequent therapy cycles, patients should be evaluated for clinical toxicities and laboratory tests (see Laboratory Tests). Neuropathy was graded using a study-specific neurotoxicity scale (see PRECAUTIONS, Neuropathy). Other toxicities were graded by the NCI CTC, Version 2.0.

Continued on next page

Eloxatin—Cont.

Prolongation of infusion time for ELOXATIN from 2 hours to 6 hours decreases the C_{max} by an estimated 32% and may mitigate acute toxicities. The infusion times for 5-FU and leucovorin do not need to be changed.
For patients who experience persistent Grade 2 neurosensory events that do not resolve, a dose reduction of ELOXATIN to 65 mg/m^2 should be considered. For patients with persistent Grade 3 neurosensory events, discontinuing therapy should be considered. The 5-FU/LV regimen need not be altered.
A dose reduction of ELOXATIN to 65 mg/m^2 and 5-FU by 20% (300 mg/m^2 bolus and 500 mg/m^2 22 hour infusion) is recommended for patients after recovery from grade 3/4 gastrointestinal (despite prophylactic treatment) or grade 4 neutropenia or grade 3/4 thrombocytopenia. The next dose should be delayed until: neutrophils ≥1.5 x 10^9/L, and platelets ≥75 x 10^9/L.

Preparation of Infusion Solution

RECONSTITUTION OR FINAL DILUTION MUST NEVER BE PERFORMED WITH A SODIUM CHLORIDE SOLUTION OR OTHER CHLORIDE-CONTAINING SOLUTIONS.

The lyophilized powder is reconstituted by adding 10 mL (for the 50 mg vial) or 20 mL (for the 100 mg vial) of Water for Injection, USP or 5% Dextrose Injection, USP. **Do not administer the reconstituted solution without further dilution.** The reconstituted solution must be further diluted in an infusion solution of 250-500 mL of 5% Dextrose Injection, USP.
After reconstitution in the original vial, the solution may be stored up to 24 hours under refrigeration [2-8°C (36-46°F)]. After final dilution with 250-500 mL of 5% Dextrose Injection, USP, the shelf life is **6 hours at room temperature [20-25°C (68-77°F)] or up to 24 hours under refrigeration [2-8°C (36-46°F)].** ELOXATIN is not light sensitive.
ELOXATIN is incompatible in solution with alkaline medications or media (such as basic solutions of 5-FU) and must not be mixed with these or administered simultaneously through the same infusion line. **The infusion line should be flushed with D5W prior to administration of any concomitant medication.**
Parenteral drug products should be inspected visually for particulate matter and discoloration prior to administration and discarded if present.
Needles or intravenous administration sets containing aluminum parts that may come in contact with ELOXATIN should not be used for the preparation or mixing of the drug. Aluminum has been reported to cause degradation of platinum compounds.

HOW SUPPLIED

ELOXATIN is supplied in clear, glass, single-use vials with gray elastomeric stoppers and aluminum flip-off seals containing 50 mg or 100 mg of oxaliplatin as a sterile, preservative-free lyophilized powder for reconstitution. Lactose monohydrate is also present as an inactive ingredient.
NDC 0024-0596-02: 50 mg single-use vial with green flip-off seal individually packaged in a carton.
NDC 0024-0597-04: 100 mg single-use vial with dark blue flip-off seal individually packaged in a carton.

Storage

Store under normal lighting conditions at 25°C (77°F); excursions permitted to 15-30°C (59-86°F) [see USP controlled room temperature].

Handling and Disposal

As with other potentially toxic anticancer agents, care should be exercised in the handling and preparation of infusion solutions prepared from ELOXATIN. The use of gloves is recommended. If a solution of ELOXATIN contacts the skin, wash the skin immediately and thoroughly with soap and water. If ELOXATIN contacts the mucous membranes, flush thoroughly with water.
Procedures for the handling and disposal of anticancer drugs should be considered. Several guidelines on the subject have been published [1–8]. There is no general agreement that all of the procedures recommended in the guidelines are necessary or appropriate.

REFERENCES

1. ONS Clinical Practice Committee. Cancer Chemotherapy Guidelines and Recommendations for Practice. Pittsburgh, Pa: Oncology Nursing Society; 1999:32-41.
2. Recommendations for the safe handling of parenteral antineoplastic drugs. NIH Publication No. 83-2621. For sale by the Superintendent of Documents, U.S. Government Printing Office, Washington, D.C. 20402.
3. AMA Council Report. Guidelines for handling parenteral antineoplastics. *JAMA* 1985;253(11):1590-1592.
4. National Study Commission on Cytotoxic Exposure. Recommendations for handling cytotoxic agents. Available from Louis P. Jeffrey, Sc.D., Chairman, National Study Commission on Cytotoxic Exposure, Massachusetts College of Pharmacy and Allied Health Sciences, 179 Longwood Avenue, Boston, MA 02115.
5. Clinical Oncological Society of Australia. Guidelines and recommendations for safe handling of antineoplastic agents. *Med J Australia* 1983;1:426-428.
6. Jones RB, et al. Safe handling of chemotherapeutic agents: a report from the Mount Sinai Medical Center. *Ca - A Cancer Journal for Clinicians.* Sept./Oct. 1983:258-263.
7. American Society of Hospital Pharmacists. ASHP Technical Assistance Bulletin on handling cytotoxic and hazardous drugs. *Am J Hosp Pharm* 1990;47:1033-1049.
8. Controlling Occupational Exposure to Hazardous Drugs. (OSHA Work-Practice Guidelines). *Am J Hosp Pharm* 1996;53:1669-1685.

sanofi~synthelabo
Distributed by Sanofi-Synthelabo Inc.
New York, NY 10016
Manufactured for Sanofi-Synthelabo Inc. by Ben Venue Laboratories
Bedford, OH 44146-0568
ESS-5A Rev. 01/04

Figure 2

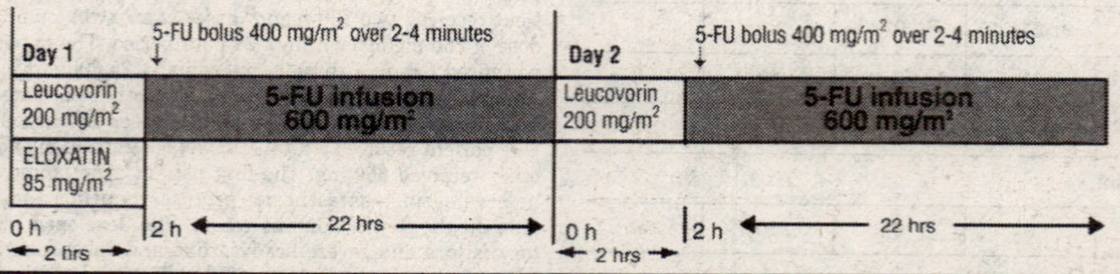

Table 13 – Adverse Hematologic Experiences in Previously Treated Patients (≥5% of patients)

Hematology Parameter	5-FU/LV (N=142)		ELOXATIN (N=153)		ELOXATIN + 5-FU/LV (N=150)	
	All Grades (%)	Grade 3/4 (%)	All Grades (%)	Grade 3/4 (%)	All Grades (%)	Grade 3/4 (%)
Anemia	68	2	64	1	81	2
Leukopenia	34	1	13	0	76	19
Neutropenia	25	5	7	0	73	44
Thrombocytopenia	20	0	30	3	64	4

Table 14 – Adverse Hepatic – Clinical Chemistry Experience in Patients Previously Untreated for Advanced Colorectal Cancer (≥5% of patients)

Clinical Chemistry	ELOXATIN + 5-FU/LV N=259		irinotecan + 5-FU/LV N=256		ELOXATIN + irinotecan N=258	
	All Grades (%)	Grade 3/4 (%)	All Grades (%)	Grade 3/4 (%)	All Grades (%)	Grade 3/4 (%)
ALT (SGPT-ALAT)	6	1	2	0	5	2
AST (SGOT-ASAT)	17	1	2	1	11	1
Alkaline Phosphatase	16	0	8	0	14	2
Total Bilirubin	6	1	3	1	3	2

Table 15 – Adverse Hepatic – Clinical Chemistry Experience in Previously Treated Patients (≥5% of patients)

Clinical Chemistry	5-FU/LV (N=142)		ELOXATIN (N=153)		ELOXATIN + 5-FU/LV (N=150)	
	All Grades (%)	Grade 3/4 (%)	All Grades (%)	Grade 3/4 (%)	All Grades (%)	Grade 3/4 (%)
ALT (SGPT-ALAT)	28	3	36	1	31	0
AST (SGOT-ASAT)	39	2	54	4	47	0
Total Bilirubin	22	6	13	5	13	1

PLAVIX® ℞

[*plă-vĭcks*]
(clopidogrel bisulfate tablets)

Prescribing information for this product, which appears on pages 3032–3036 of the 2004 PDR, has been completely revised as follows. Please write "See Supplement A" next to the product heading.

DESCRIPTION

PLAVIX (clopidogrel bisulfate) is an inhibitor of ADP-induced platelet aggregation acting by direct inhibition of adenosine diphosphate (ADP) binding to its receptor and of the subsequent ADP-mediated activation of the glycoprotein GPIIb/IIIa complex. Chemically it is methyl (+)-(*S*)-α-(2-chlorophenyl)-6,7-dihydrothieno[3,2-c]pyridine-5(4*H*)-acetate sulfate (1:1). The empirical formula of clopidogrel bisulfate is $C_{16}H_{16}ClNO_2S \bullet H_2SO_4$ and its molecular weight is 419.9.
The structural formula is as follows:

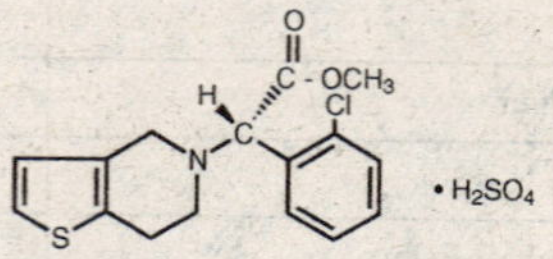

Clopidogrel bisulfate is a white to off-white powder. It is practically insoluble in water at neutral pH but freely soluble at pH 1. It also dissolves freely in methanol, dissolves sparingly in methylene chloride, and is practically insoluble in ethyl ether. It has a specific optical rotation of about +56°.
PLAVIX for oral administration is provided as pink, round, biconvex, debossed film-coated tablets containing 97.875 mg of clopidogrel bisulfate which is the molar equivalent of 75 mg of clopidogrel base.
Each tablet contains hydrogenated castor oil, hydroxypropylcellulose, mannitol, microcrystalline cellulose and polyethylene glycol 6000 as inactive ingredients. The pink film coating contains ferric oxide, hydroxypropyl methylcellulose 2910, lactose monohydrate, titanium dioxide and triacetin. The tablets are polished with Carnauba wax.

CLINICAL PHARMACOLOGY

Mechanism of Action

Clopidogrel is an inhibitor of platelet aggregation. A variety of drugs that inhibit platelet function have been shown to decrease morbid events in people with established cardiovascular atherosclerotic disease as evidenced by stroke or transient ischemic attacks, myocardial infarction, unstable angina or the need for vascular bypass or angioplasty. This indicates that platelets participate in the initiation and/or evolution of these events and that inhibiting them can reduce the event rate.

Pharmacodynamic Properties

Clopidogrel selectively inhibits the binding of adenosine diphosphate (ADP) to its platelet receptor and the subsequent ADP-mediated activation of the glycoprotein GPIIb/IIIa complex, thereby inhibiting platelet aggregation. Biotransformation of clopidogrel is necessary to produce inhibition of platelet aggregation, but an active metabolite responsible for the activity of the drug has not been isolated. Clopidogrel also inhibits platelet aggregation induced by agonists other than ADP by blocking the amplification of platelet activation by released ADP. Clopidogrel does not inhibit phosphodiesterase activity.

Clopidogrel acts by irreversibly modifying the platelet ADP receptor. Consequently, platelets exposed to clopidogrel are affected for the remainder of their lifespan.

Dose dependent inhibition of platelet aggregation can be seen 2 hours after single oral doses of PLAVIX. Repeated doses of 75 mg PLAVIX per day inhibit ADP-induced platelet aggregation on the first day, and inhibition reaches steady state between Day 3 and Day 7. At steady state, the average inhibition level observed with a dose of 75 mg PLAVIX per day was between 40% and 60%. Platelet aggregation and bleeding time gradually return to baseline values after treatment is discontinued, generally in about 5 days.

Pharmacokinetics and Metabolism

After repeated 75-mg oral doses of clopidogrel (base), plasma concentrations of the parent compound, which has no platelet inhibiting effect, are very low and are generally below the quantification limit (0.00025 mg/L) beyond 2 hours after dosing. Clopidogrel is extensively metabolized by the liver. The main circulating metabolite is the carboxylic acid derivative, and it too has no effect on platelet aggregation. It represents about 85% of the circulating drug-related compounds in plasma.

Following an oral dose of ^{14}C-labeled clopidogrel in humans, approximately 50% was excreted in the urine and approximately 46% in the feces in the 5 days after dosing. The elimination half-life of the main circulating metabolite was 8 hours after single and repeated administration. Covalent binding to platelets accounted for 2% of radiolabel with a half-life of 11 days.

Effect of Food: Administration of PLAVIX (clopidogrel bisulfate) with meals did not significantly modify the bioavailability of clopidogrel as assessed by the pharmacokinetics of the main circulating metabolite.

Absorption and Distribution: Clopidogrel is rapidly absorbed after oral administration of repeated doses of 75 mg clopidogrel (base), with peak plasma levels (≅3 mg/L) of the main circulating metabolite occurring approximately 1 hour after dosing. The pharmacokinetics of the main circulating metabolite are linear (plasma concentrations increased in proportion to dose) in the dose range of 50 to 150 mg of clopidogrel. Absorption is at least 50% based on urinary excretion of clopidogrel-related metabolites.

Clopidogrel and the main circulating metabolite bind reversibly *in vitro* to human plasma proteins (98% and 94%, respectively). The binding is nonsaturable *in vitro* up to a concentration of 100 μg/mL.

Metabolism and Elimination: *In vitro* and *in vivo*, clopidogrel undergoes rapid hydrolysis into its carboxylic acid derivative. In plasma and urine, the glucuronide of the carboxylic acid derivative is also observed.

Special Populations

Geriatric Patients: Plasma concentrations of the main circulating metabolite are significantly higher in elderly (≥75 years) compared to young healthy volunteers but these higher plasma levels were not associated with differences in platelet aggregation and bleeding time. No dosage adjustment is needed for the elderly.

Renally Impaired Patients: After repeated doses of 75 mg PLAVIX per day, plasma levels of the main circulating metabolite were lower in patients with severe renal impairment (creatinine clearance from 5 to 15 mL/min) compared to subjects with moderate renal impairment (creatinine clearance 30 to 60 mL/min) or healthy subjects. Although inhibition of ADP-induced platelet aggregation was lower (25%) than that observed in healthy volunteers, the prolongation of bleeding time was similar to healthy volunteers receiving 75 mg of PLAVIX per day.

Gender: No significant difference was observed in the plasma levels of the main circulating metabolite between males and females. In a small study comparing men and women, less inhibition of ADP-induced platelet aggregation was observed in women, but there was no difference in prolongation of bleeding time. In the large, controlled clinical study (Clopidogrel vs. Aspirin in Patients at Risk of Ischemic Events; CAPRIE), the incidence of clinical outcome events, other adverse clinical events, and abnormal clinical laboratory parameters was similar in men and women.

Race: Pharmacokinetic differences due to race have not been studied.

CLINICAL STUDIES

The clinical evidence for the efficacy of PLAVIX is derived from two double-blind trials: the CAPRIE study (Clopidogrel vs. Aspirin in Patients at Risk of Ischemic Events), a comparison of PLAVIX to aspirin, and the CURE study (Clopidogrel in Unstable Angina to Prevent Recurrent Ischemic Events), a comparison of PLAVIX to placebo, both given in combination with aspirin and other standard therapy.

The CAPRIE trial was a 19,185-patient, 304-center, international, randomized, double-blind, parallel-group study comparing PLAVIX (75 mg daily) to aspirin (325 mg daily). The patients randomized had: 1) recent histories of myocardial infarction (within 35 days); 2) recent histories of ischemic stroke (within 6 months) with at least a week of residual neurological signs; or 3) objectively established peripheral arterial disease. Patients received randomized treatment for an average of 1.6 years (maximum of 3 years). The trial's primary outcome was the time to first occurrence of new ischemic stroke (fatal or not), new myocardial infarction (fatal or not), or other vascular death. Deaths not easily attributable to nonvascular causes were all classified as vascular.

Table 1: Outcome Events in the CAPRIE Primary Analysis

Patients	PLAVIX 9599	aspirin 9586
IS (fatal or not)	438 (4.6%)	461 (4.8%)
MI (fatal or not)	275 (2.9%)	333 (3.5%)
Other vascular death	226 (2.4%)	226 (2.4%)
Total	939 (9.8%)	1020 (10.6%)

As shown in the table, PLAVIX (clopidogrel bisulfate) was associated with a lower incidence of outcome events of every kind. The overall risk reduction (9.8% vs. 10.6%) was 8.7%, P=0.045. Similar results were obtained when all-cause mortality and all-cause strokes were counted instead of vascular mortality and ischemic strokes (risk reduction 6.9%). In patients who survived an on-study stroke or myocardial infarction, the incidence of subsequent events was again lower in the PLAVIX group.

The curves showing the overall event rate are shown in Figure 1. The event curves separated early and continued to diverge over the 3-year follow-up period.

Figure 1: Fatal or Non-Fatal Vascular Events in the CAPRIE Study

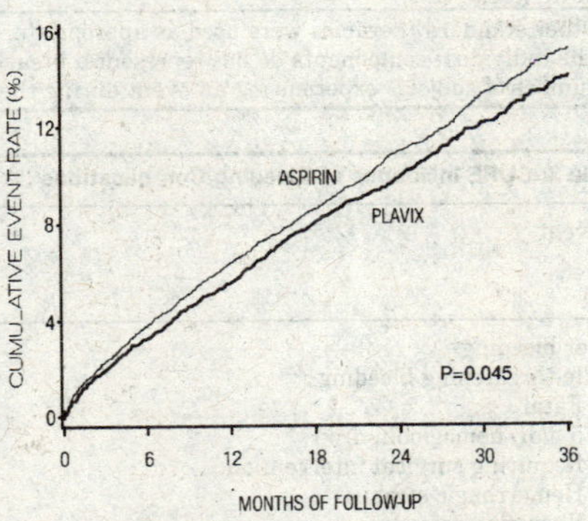

Although the statistical significance favoring PLAVIX over aspirin was marginal (P=0.045), and represents the result of a single trial that has not been replicated, the comparator drug, aspirin, is itself effective (vs. placebo) in reducing cardiovascular events in patients with recent myocardial infarction or stroke. Thus, the difference between PLAVIX and placebo, although not measured directly, is substantial. The CAPRIE trial included a population that was randomized on the basis of 3 entry criteria. The efficacy of PLAVIX relative to aspirin was heterogeneous across these randomized subgroups (P=0.043). It is not clear whether this difference is real or a chance occurrence. Although the CAPRIE trial was not designed to evaluate the relative benefit of PLAVIX over aspirin in the individual patient subgroups, the benefit appeared to be strongest in patients who were enrolled because of peripheral vascular disease (especially those who also had a history of myocardial infarction) and weaker in stroke patients. In patients who were enrolled in the trial on the sole basis of a recent myocardial infarction, PLAVIX was not numerically superior to aspirin.

In the meta-analyses of studies of aspirin vs. placebo in patients similar to those in CAPRIE, aspirin was associated with a reduced incidence of thrombotic events. There was a suggestion of heterogeneity in these studies too, with the effect strongest in patients with a history of myocardial infarction, weaker in patients with a history of stroke, and not discernible in patients with a history of peripheral vascular disease. With respect to the inferred comparison of PLAVIX to placebo, there is no indication of heterogeneity.

The CURE study included 12,562 patients with acute coronary syndrome without ST segment elevation (unstable angina or non-Q-wave myocardial infarction) and presenting within 24 hours of onset of the most recent episode of chest pain or symptoms consistent with ischemia. Patients were required to have either ECG changes compatible with new ischemia (without ST segment elevation) or elevated cardiac enzymes or troponin I or T to at least twice the upper limit of normal. The patient population was largely Caucasian (82%) and included 38% women, and 52% patients ≥65 years of age.

Patients were randomized to receive PLAVIX (300 mg loading dose followed by 75 mg/day) or placebo, and were treated for up to one year. Patients also received aspirin (75–325 mg once daily) and other standard therapies such as heparin. The use of GPIIb/IIIa inhibitors was not permitted for three days prior to randomization.

The number of patients experiencing the primary outcome (CV death, MI, or stroke) was 582 (9.30%) in the PLAVIX-treated group and 719 (11.41%) in the placebo-treated group, a 20% relative risk reduction (95% CI of 10%-28%; p=0.00009) for the PLAVIX-treated group (see Table 2).

At the end of 12 months, the number of patients experiencing the co-primary outcome (CV death, MI, stroke or refractory ischemia) was 1035 (16.54%) in the PLAVIX-treated group and 1187 (18.83%) in the placebo-treated group, a 14% relative risk reduction (95% CI of 6%-21%, p=0.0005) for the PLAVIX-treated group (see Table 2).

In the PLAVIX-treated group, each component of the two primary endpoints (CV death, MI, stroke, refractory ischemia) occurred less frequently than in the placebo-treated group.

[See table 2 at top of next page]

The benefits of PLAVIX were maintained throughout the course of the trial (up to 12 months).

Figure 2: Cardiovascular Death, Myocardial Infarction, and Stroke in the CURE Study

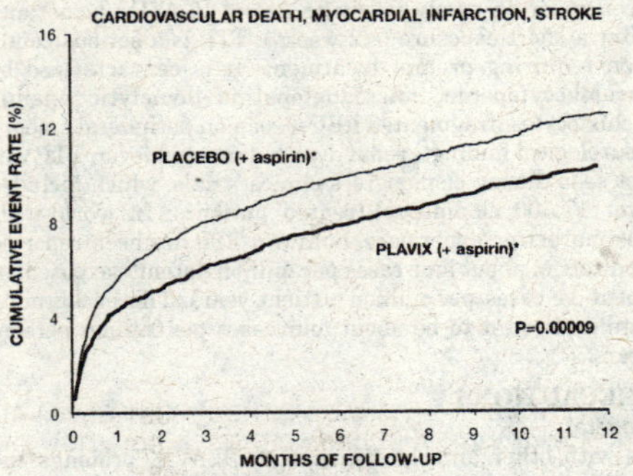

*Other standard therapies were used as appropriate

In CURE, the use of PLAVIX was associated with a lower incidence of CV death, MI or stroke in patient populations with different characteristics, as shown in Figure 3. The benefits associated with PLAVIX (clopidogrel bisulfate tablets) were independent of the use of other acute and long-term cardiovascular therapies, including heparin/LMWH (low molecular weight heparin), IV glycoprotein IIb/IIIa (GPIIb/IIIa) inhibitors, lipid-lowering drugs, beta-blockers, and ACE-inhibitors. The efficacy of PLAVIX was observed independently of the dose of aspirin (75-325 mg once daily). The use of oral anticoagulants, non-study anti-platelet drugs and chronic NSAIDs was not allowed in CURE.

Figure 3: Hazard Ratio for Patient Baseline Characteristics and On-Study Concomitant Medications/Interventions for the CURE Study

Baseline Characteristics		N	Percent Events PLAVIX (+aspirin)*	Percent Events Placebo (+aspirin)*
Overall		12562	9.3	11.4
Diagnosis	Non-Q-W	3295	12.7	15.5
	Unst Ang	8298	7.3	8.7
	Other	968	15.1	19.7
Elev Card Enzy	No	9381	8.8	10.9
	Yes	3176	10.7	13.0
ST Dcpr >1.0mm	No	7273	7.5	8.9
	Yes	5288	11.8	14.8
Diabetes	No	9721	7.9	9.9
	Yes	2840	14.2	16.7
Previous MI	No	8517	7.8	9.5
	Yes	4044	12.5	15.4
Previous Stroke	No	12055	8.9	11.0
	Yes	506	17.9	22.4
Concomitant Medication / Therapy				
Heparin/LMWH	No	951	4.9	7.7
	Yes	11611	9.7	11.7
Aspirin	<100mg	1927	8.5	9.7
	100-200mg	7428	9.2	10.9
	>200mg	3201	9.9	13.7
GPIIb/IIIa Antag	No	11739	8.9	10.8
	Yes	823	15.7	19.2
Beta-Blocker	No	2032	9.9	12.0
	Yes	10530	9.2	11.3
ACEI	No	4813	6.3	8.1
	Yes	7749	11.2	13.5
Lipid-Lowering	No	4461	10.9	13.1
	Yes	8101	8.4	10.5
PTCA/CABG	No	7977	8.1	10.0
	Yes	4585	11.4	13.8

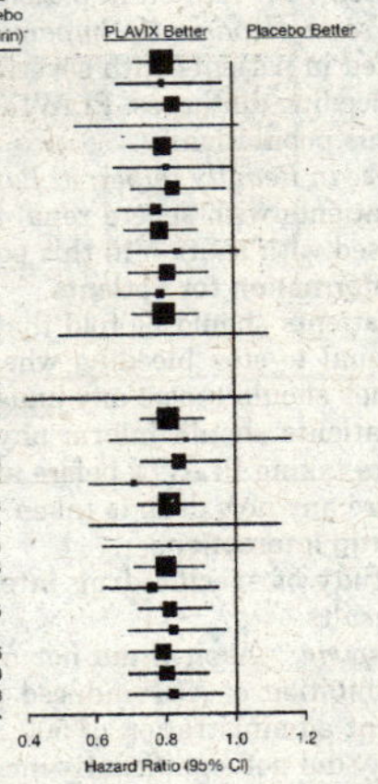

*Other standard therapies were used as appropriate

The use of PLAVIX in CURE was associated with a decrease in the use of thrombolytic therapy (71 patients [1.1%] in the PLAVIX group, 126 patients [2.0%] in the placebo group; relative risk reduction of 43%, P=0.0001), and GPIIb/IIIa inhibitors (369 patients [5.9%] in the PLAVIX group, 454 patients [7.2%] in the placebo group; relative risk reduction of 18%, P=0.003). The use of PLAVIX in CURE did not impact the number of patients treated with CABG or PCI (with or without stenting), (2253 patients [36.0%] in the PLAVIX group, 2324 patients [36.9%] in the placebo group; relative risk reduction of 4.0%, P=0.1658).

INDICATIONS AND USAGE

PLAVIX (clopidogrel bisulfate) is indicated for the reduction of thrombotic events as follows:

- **Recent MI, Recent Stroke or Established Peripheral Arterial Disease**
  For patients with a history of recent myocardial infarction (MI), recent stroke, or established peripheral arterial disease, PLAVIX has been shown to reduce the rate of a combined endpoint of new ischemic stroke (fatal or not), new MI (fatal or not), and other vascular death.
- **Acute Coronary Syndrome**
  For patients with acute coronary syndrome (unstable angina/non-Q-wave MI) including patients who are to be managed medically and those who are to be managed with percutaneous coronary intervention (with or without stent) or CABG, PLAVIX has been shown to decrease the rate of a combined endpoint of cardiovascular death, MI, or stroke as well as the rate of a combined endpoint of cardiovascular death, MI, stroke, or refractory ischemia.

CONTRAINDICATIONS

The use of PLAVIX is contraindicated in the following conditions:

- Hypersensitivity to the drug substance or any component of the product.

Continued on next page

Plavix—Cont.

- Active pathological bleeding such as peptic ulcer or intracranial hemorrhage.

WARNINGS

Thrombotic thrombocytopenic purpura (TTP): TTP has been reported rarely following use of PLAVIX, sometimes after a short exposure (<2 weeks). TTP is a serious condition requiring prompt treatment. It is characterized by thrombocytopenia, microangiopathic hemolytic anemia (schistocytes [fragmented RBCs] seen on peripheral smear), neurological findings, renal dysfunction, and fever. TTP was not seen during clopidogrel's clinical trials, which included over 17,500 clopidogrel-treated patients. In world-wide postmarketing experience, however, TTP has been reported at a rate of about four cases per million patients exposed, or about 11 cases per million patient-years. The background rate is thought to be about four cases per million person-years.

PRECAUTIONS

General

As with other antiplatelet agents, PLAVIX prolongs the bleeding time and therefore should be used with caution in patients who may be at risk of increased bleeding from trauma, surgery, or other pathological conditions (particularly gastrointestinal and intraocular). If a patient is to undergo elective surgery and an antiplatelet effect is not desired, PLAVIX should be discontinued 5 days prior to surgery.

Due to the risk of bleeding and undesirable hematological effects, blood cell count determination and/or other appropriate testing should be promptly considered, whenever such suspected clinical symptoms arise during the course of treatment (see **ADVERSE REACTIONS**).

GI Bleeding: In CAPRIE, PLAVIX was associated with a rate of gastrointestinal bleeding of 2.0%, vs. 2.7% on aspirin. In CURE, the incidence of major gastrointestinal bleeding was 1.3% vs. 0.7% (PLAVIX + aspirin vs. placebo + aspirin, respectively). PLAVIX should be used with caution in patients who have lesions with a propensity to bleed (such as ulcers). Drugs that might induce such lesions should be used with caution in patients taking PLAVIX.

Use in Hepatically Impaired Patients: Experience is limited in patients with severe hepatic disease, who may have bleeding diatheses. PLAVIX should be used with caution in this population.

Use in Renally-impaired Patients: Experience is limited in patients with severe renal impairment. PLAVIX should be used with caution in this population.

Information for Patients

Patients should be told that it may take them longer than usual to stop bleeding when they take PLAVIX, and that they should report any unusual bleeding to their physician. Patients should inform physicians and dentists that they are taking PLAVIX before any surgery is scheduled and before any new drug is taken.

Drug Interactions

Study of specific drug interactions yielded the following results:

Aspirin: Aspirin did not modify the clopidogrel-mediated inhibition of ADP-induced platelet aggregation. Concomitant administration of 500 mg of aspirin twice a day for 1 day did not significantly increase the prolongation of bleeding time induced by PLAVIX. PLAVIX potentiated the effect of aspirin on collagen-induced platelet aggregation. PLAVIX and aspirin have been administered together for up to one year.

Heparin: In a study in healthy volunteers, PLAVIX did not necessitate modification of the heparin dose or alter the effect of heparin on coagulation. Coadministration of heparin had no effect on inhibition of platelet aggregation induced by PLAVIX.

Nonsteroidal Anti-Inflammatory Drugs (NSAIDs): In healthy volunteers receiving naproxen, concomitant administration of PLAVIX was associated with increased occult gastrointestinal blood loss. NSAIDs and PLAVIX should be coadministered with caution.

Warfarin: Because of the increased risk of bleeding, the concomitant administration of warfarin with PLAVIX should be undertaken with caution. (See **Precautions–General**.)

Other Concomitant Therapy: No clinically significant pharmacodynamic interactions were observed when PLAVIX was coadministered with **atenolol**, **nifedipine**, or both atenolol and nifedipine. The pharmacodynamic activity of PLAVIX was also not significantly influenced by the coadministration of **phenobarbital**, **cimetidine** or **estrogen**.

The pharmacokinetics of **digoxin** or **theophylline** were not modified by the coadministration of PLAVIX (clopidogrel bisulfate).

At high concentrations *in vitro*, clopidogrel inhibits P_{450} (2C9). Accordingly, PLAVIX may interfere with the metabolism of **phenytoin**, **tamoxifen**, **tolbutamide**, **warfarin**, **torsemide**, **fluvastatin**, and many **non-steroidal anti-inflammatory agents**, but there are no data with which to predict the magnitude of these interactions. Caution should be used when any of these drugs is coadministered with PLAVIX.

In addition to the above specific interaction studies, patients entered into clinical trials with PLAVIX received a variety of concomitant medications including **diuretics**, **beta-blocking agents**, **angiotensin converting enzyme inhibitors**, **calcium antagonists**, **cholesterol lowering agents**, **coronary vasodilators**, **antidiabetic agents** (including **insulin**), **antiepileptic agents**, **hormone replacement therapy**, **heparins** (unfractionated and LMWH) and **GPIIb/IIIa antagonists** without evidence of clinically significant adverse interactions. The use of oral anticoagulants, non-study antiplatelet drug and chronic NSAIDs was not allowed in CURE and there are no data on their concomitant use with clopidogrel.

Table 2: Outcome Events in the CURE Primary Analysis

Outcome	PLAVIX (+ aspirin)* (n=6259)		Placebo (+ aspirin)* (n=6303)		Relative Risk Reduction (%) (95% CI)
Primary outcome (Cardiovascular death, MI, Stroke)	582	(9.3%)	719	(11.4%)	20% (10.3, 27.9) P=0.00009
Co-primary outcome (Cardiovascular death, MI, Stroke, Refractory Ischemia)	1035	(16.5%)	1187	(18.8%)	14% (6.2, 20.6) P=0.00052)
All Individual Outcome Events:†					
CV death	318	(5.1%)	345	(5.5%)	7% (-7.7, 20.6)
MI	324	(5.2%)	419	(6.6%)	23% (11.0, 33.4)
Stroke	75	(1.2%)	87	(1.4%)	14% (-17.7, 36.6)
Refractory ischemia	544	(8.7%)	587	(9.3%)	7% (-4.0, 18.0)

* Other standard therapies were used as appropriate.
† The individual components do not represent a breakdown of the primary and co-primary outcomes, but rather the total number of subjects experiencing an event during the course of the study.

Table 3: CURE Incidence of Bleeding Complications (% Patients)

Event	PLAVIX (+ aspirin)* (n=6259)	Placebo (+ aspirin)* (n=6303)	P-value
Major bleeding†	3.7‡	2.7§	0.001
Life-threatening bleeding	2.2	1.8	0.13
Fatal	0.2	0.2	
5 g/dL hemoglobin drop	0.9	0.9	
Requiring surgical intervention	0.7	0.7	
Hemorrhagic strokes	0.1	0.1	
Requiring inotropes	0.5	0.5	
Requiring transfusion (≥4 units)	1.2	1.0	
Other major bleeding	1.6	1.0	0.005
Significantly disabling	0.4	0.3	
Intraocular bleeding with significant loss of vision	0.05	0.03	
Requiring 2-3 units of blood	1.3	0.9	
Minor bleeding¶	5.1	2.4	<0.001

* Other standard therapies were used as appropriate.
† Life threatening and other major bleeding.
‡ Major bleeding event rate for PLAVIX + aspirin was dose-dependent on aspirin: <100 mg=2.6%; 100-200 mg=3.5%; >200 mg=4.9%
§ Major bleeding event rate for placebo + aspirin was dose-dependent on aspirin: <100 mg=2.0%; 100-200 mg=2.3%; >200 mg=4.0%
¶ Led to interruption of study medication.

Drug/Laboratory Test Interactions

None known.

Carcinogenesis, Mutagenesis, Impairment of Fertility

There was no evidence of tumorigenicity when clopidogrel was administered for 78 weeks to mice and 104 weeks to rats at dosages up to 77 mg/kg per day, which afforded plasma exposures >25 times that in humans at the recommended daily dose of 75 mg.

Clopidogrel was not genotoxic in four *in vitro* tests (Ames test, DNA-repair test in rat hepatocytes, gene mutation assay in Chinese hamster fibroblasts, and metaphase chromosome analysis of human lymphocytes) and in one *in vivo* test (micronucleus test by oral route in mice).

Clopidogrel was found to have no effect on fertility of male and female rats at oral doses up to 400 mg/kg per day (52 times the recommended human dose on a mg/m^2 basis).

Pregnancy

Pregnancy Category B. Reproduction studies performed in rats and rabbits at doses up to 500 and 300 mg/kg/day (respectively, 65 and 78 times the recommended daily human dose on a mg/m^2 basis), revealed no evidence of impaired fertility or fetotoxicity due to clopidogrel. There are, however, no adequate and well-controlled studies in pregnant women. Because animal reproduction studies are not always predictive of a human response, PLAVIX should be used during pregnancy only if clearly needed.

Nursing Mothers

Studies in rats have shown that clopidogrel and/or its metabolites are excreted in the milk. It is not known whether this drug is excreted in human milk. Because many drugs are excreted in human milk and because of the potential for serious adverse reactions in nursing infants, a decision should be made whether to discontinue nursing or to discontinue the drug, taking into account the importance of the drug to the nursing woman.

Pediatric Use

Safety and effectiveness in the pediatric population have not been established.

ADVERSE REACTIONS

PLAVIX has been evaluated for safety in more than 17,500 patients, including over 9,000 patients treated for 1 year or more. The overall tolerability of PLAVIX in CAPRIE was similar to that of aspirin regardless of age, gender and race, with an approximately equal incidence (13%) of patients withdrawing from treatment because of adverse reactions. The clinically important adverse events observed in CAPRIE and CURE are discussed below.

Hemorrhagic: In CAPRIE patients receiving PLAVIX, gastrointestinal hemorrhage occurred at a rate of 2.0%, and required hospitalization in 0.7%. In patients receiving aspirin, the corresponding rates were 2.7% and 1.1%, respectively. The incidence of intracranial hemorrhage was 0.4% for PLAVIX compared to 0.5% for aspirin.

In CURE, PLAVIX use with aspirin was associated with an increase in bleeding compared to placebo with aspirin (see Table 3). There was an excess in major bleeding in patients receiving PLAVIX plus aspirin compared with placebo plus aspirin, primarily gastrointestinal and at puncture sites. The incidence of intracranial hemorrhage (0.1%), and fatal bleeding (0.2%), was the same in both groups.

In patients receiving both PLAVIX and aspirin in CURE, the incidence of bleeding is described in Table 3.

[See table 3 above]

Ninety-two percent (92%) of the patients in the CURE study received heparin/LMWH, and the rate of bleeding in these patients was similar to the overall results.

There was no excess in major bleeds within seven days after coronary bypass graft surgery in patients who stopped therapy more than five days prior to surgery (event rate 4.4% PLAVIX + aspirin; 5.3% placebo + aspirin). In patients who remained on therapy within five days of bypass graft surgery, the event rate was 9.6% for PLAVIX + aspirin, and 6.3% for placebo + aspirin.

Neutropenia/agranulocytosis: Ticlopidine, a drug chemically similar to PLAVIX, is associated with a 0.8% rate of severe neutropenia (less than 450 neutrophils/μL). In CAPRIE severe neutropenia was observed in six patients, four on PLAVIX and two on aspirin. Two of the 9599 patients who received PLAVIX and none of the 9586 patients who received aspirin had neutrophil counts of zero. One of the four PLAVIX patients in CAPRIE was receiving cytotoxic chemotherapy, and another recovered and returned to the trial after only temporarily interrupting treatment with PLAVIX (clopidogrel bisulfate). In CURE, the numbers of patients with thrombocytopenia (19 PLAVIX + aspirin vs. 24 placebo + aspirin) or neutropenia (3 vs. 3) were similar. Although the risk of myelotoxicity with PLAVIX thus appears to be quite low, this possibility should be considered when a patient receiving PLAVIX demonstrates fever or other sign of infection.

Gastrointestinal: Overall, the incidence of gastrointestinal events (e.g. abdominal pain, dyspepsia, gastritis and constipation) in patients receiving PLAVIX (clopidogrel bisulfate) was 27.1%, compared to 29.8% in those receiving aspirin in the CAPRIE trial. In the CURE trial the incidence of these gastrointestinal events for patients receiving PLAVIX + aspirin was 11.7% compared to 12.5% for those receiving placebo + aspirin.

In the CAPRIE trial, the incidence of peptic, gastric or duodenal ulcers was 0.7% for PLAVIX and 1.2% for aspirin. In the CURE trial the incidence of peptic, gastric or duodenal ulcers was 0.4% for PLAVIX + aspirin and 0.3% for placebo + aspirin.

Cases of diarrhea were reported in the CAPRIE trial in 4.5% of patients in the PLAVIX group compared to 3.4% in the aspirin group. However, these were rarely severe (PLAVIX=0.2% and aspirin=0.1%). In the CURE trial, the incidence of diarrhea for patients receiving PLAVIX + aspirin was 2.1% compared to 2.2% for those receiving placebo + aspirin.

In the CAPRIE trial, the incidence of patients withdrawing from treatment because of gastrointestinal adverse reactions was 3.2% for PLAVIX and 4.0% for aspirin. In the CURE trial, the incidence of patients withdrawing from treatment because of gastrointestinal adverse reactions was 0.9% for PLAVIX + aspirin compared with 0.8% for placebo + aspirin.

Rash and Other Skin Disorders: In the CAPRIE trial, the incidence of skin and appendage disorders in patients receiving PLAVIX was 15.8% (0.7% serious); the corresponding rate in aspirin patients was 13.1% (0.5% serious). In the CURE trial the incidence of rash or other skin disorders in patients receiving PLAVIX + aspirin was 4.0% compared to 3.5% for those receiving placebo + aspirin.

In the CAPRIE trial, the overall incidence of patients withdrawing from treatment because of skin and appendage disorders adverse reactions was 1.5% for PLAVIX and 0.8% for aspirin. In the CURE trial, the incidence of patients withdrawing because of skin and appendage disorders adverse reactions was 0.7% for PLAVIX + aspirin compared with 0.3% for placebo + aspirin.

Adverse events occurring in ≥2.5% of patients on PLAVIX in the CAPRIE controlled clinical trial are shown below regardless of relationship to PLAVIX. The median duration of therapy was 20 months, with a maximum of 3 years.

Table 4: Adverse Events Occurring in ≥2.5% of PLAVIX Patients in CAPRIE

Body System / Event	% Incidence (% Discontinuation) PLAVIX [n=9599]	Aspirin [n=9586]
Body as a Whole-general disorders		
Chest Pain	8.3 (0.2)	8.3 (0.3)
Accidental/Inflicted Injury	7.9 (0.1)	7.3 (0.1)
Influenza-like symptoms	7.5 (<0.1)	7.0 (<0.1)
Pain	6.4 (0.1)	6.3 (0.1)
Fatigue	3.3 (0.1)	3.4 (0.1)
Cardiovascular disorders, general		
Edema	4.1 (<0.1)	4.5 (<0.1)
Hypertension	4.3 (<0.1)	5.1 (<0.1)
Central & peripheral nervous system disorders		
Headache	7.6 (0.3)	7.2 (0.2)
Dizziness	6.2 (0.2)	6.7 (0.3)
Gastrointestinal system disorders		
Abdominal pain	5.6 (0.7)	7.1 (1.0)
Dyspepsia	5.2 (0.6)	6.1 (0.7)
Diarrhea	4.5 (0.4)	3.4 (0.3)
Nausea	3.4 (0.5)	3.8 (0.4)
Metabolic & nutritional disorders		
Hypercholesterolemia	4.0 (0)	4.4 (<0.1)
Musculo-skeletal system disorders		
Arthralgia	6.3 (0.1)	6.2 (0.1)
Back Pain	5.8 (0.1)	5.3 (<0.1)
Platelet, bleeding, & clotting disorders		
Purpura/Bruise	5.3 (0.3)	3.7 (0.1)
Epistaxis	2.9 (0.2)	2.5 (0.1)
Psychiatric disorders		
Depression	3.6 (0.1)	3.9 (0.2)
Respiratory system disorders		
Upper resp tract infection	8.7 (<0.1)	8.3 (<0.1)
Dyspnea	4.5 (0.1)	4.7 (0.1)
Rhinitis	4.2 (0.1)	4.2 (<0.1)
Bronchitis	3.7 (0.1)	3.7 (0)
Coughing	3.1 (<0.1)	2.7 (<0.1)
Skin & appendage disorders		
Rash	4.2 (0.5)	3.5 (0.2)
Pruritus	3.3 (0.3)	1.6 (0.1)
Urinary system disorders		
Urinary tract infection	3.1 (0)	3.5 (0.1)

Incidence of discontinuation, regardless of relationship to therapy, is shown in parentheses.

Adverse events occurring in ≥2.0% of patients on PLAVIX in the CURE controlled clinical trial are shown below regardless of relationship to PLAVIX.

Table 5: Adverse Events Occurring in ≥2.0% of PLAVIX Patients in CURE

Body System / **Event**	% Incidence (% Discontinuation) PLAVIX (+ aspirin)* [n=6259]	Placebo (+ aspirin)* [n=6303]
Body as a Whole-general disorders		
Chest Pain	2.7 (<0.1)	2.8 (0.0)
Central & peripheral nervous system disorders		
Headache	3.1 (0.1)	3.2 (0.1)
Dizziness	2.4 (0.1)	2.0 (<0.1)
Gastrointestinal system disorders		
Abdominal pain	2.3 (0.3)	2.8 (0.3)
Dyspepsia	2.0 (0.1)	1.9 (<0.1)
Diarrhea	2.1 (0.1)	2.2 (0.1)

* Other standard therapies were used as appropriate.

Other adverse experiences of potential importance occurring in 1% to 2.5% of patients receiving PLAVIX (clopidogrel bisulfate) in the CAPRIE or CURE controlled clinical trials are listed below regardless of relationship to PLAVIX. In general, the incidence of these events was similar to that in patients receiving aspirin (in CAPRIE) or placebo + aspirin (in CURE).

Autonomic Nervous System Disorders: Syncope, Palpitation. *Body as a Whole-general disorders:* Asthenia, Fever, Hernia. *Cardiovascular disorders:* Cardiac failure. *Central and peripheral nervous system disorders:* Cramps legs, Hypoaesthesia, Neuralgia, Paraesthesia, Vertigo. *Gastrointestinal system disorders:* Constipation, Vomiting. *Heart rate and rhythm disorders:* Fibrillation atrial. *Liver and biliary system disorders:* Hepatic enzymes increased. *Metabolic and nutritional disorders:* Gout, hyperuricemia, non-protein nitrogen (NPN) increased. *Musculo-skeletal system disorders:* Arthritis, Arthrosis. *Platelet, bleeding & clotting disorders:* GI hemorrhage, hematoma, platelets decreased. *Psychiatric disorders:* Anxiety, Insomnia. *Red blood cell disorders:* Anemia. *Respiratory system disorders:* Pneumonia, Sinusitis. *Skin and appendage disorders:* Eczema, Skin ulceration. *Urinary system disorders:* Cystitis. *Vision disorders:* Cataract, Conjunctivitis.

Other potentially serious adverse events which may be of clinical interest but were rarely reported (<1%) in patients who received PLAVIX in the CAPRIE or CURE controlled clinical trials are listed below regardless of relationship to PLAVIX. In general, the incidence of these events was similar to that in patients receiving aspirin (in CAPRIE) or placebo + aspirin (in CURE).

Body as a whole: Allergic reaction, necrosis ischemic. *Cardiovascular disorders:* Edema generalized. *Gastrointestinal system disorders:* Gastric ulcer perforated, gastritis hemorrhagic, upper GI ulcer hemorrhagic. *Liver and Biliary system disorders:* Bilirubinemia, hepatitis infectious, liver fatty. *Platelet, bleeding and clotting disorders:* hemarthrosis, hematuria, hemoptysis, hemorrhage intracranial, hemorrhage retroperitoneal, hemorrhage of operative wound, ocular hemorrhage, pulmonary hemorrhage, purpura allergic, thrombocytopenia. *Red blood cell disorders:* Anemia aplastic, anemia hypochromic. *Reproductive disorders, female:* Menorrhagia. *Respiratory system disorders:* Hemothorax. *Skin and appendage disorders:* Bullous eruption, rash erythematous, rash maculopapular, urticaria. *Urinary system disorders:* Abnormal renal function, acute renal failure. *White cell and reticuloendothelial system disorders:* Agranulocytosis, granulocytopenia, leukemia, leukopenia, neutrophils decreased.

Postmarketing Experience

The following events have been reported spontaneously from worldwide postmarketing experience:

- *Body as a whole:*
  - hypersensitivity reactions, anaphylactoid reactions
- *Central and Peripheral Nervous System disorders:*
  - confusion, hallucinations, taste disorders
- *Liver and Biliary system disorders:*
  - abnormal liver function test, hepatitis (non-infectious)
- *Platelet, Bleeding and Clotting disorders:*
  - cases of bleeding with fatal outcome (especially intracranial, gastrointestinal and retroperitoneal hemorrhage)
  - agranulocytosis, aplastic anemia/pancytopenia, thrombotic thrombocytopenic purpura (TTP) — see **WARNINGS**.
  - conjunctival, ocular and retinal bleeding
- *Respiratory system disorders:*
  - bronchospasm
- *Skin and Appendage disorders:*
  - angioedema, erythema multiforme
- *Urinary system disorders:*
  - glomerulopathy, abnormal creatinine levels
- *Collagen disorders:*
  - vasculitis
- *Gastrointestinal disorders:*
  - colitis (including ulcerative or lymphocytic colitis)

OVERDOSAGE

One case of deliberate overdosage with PLAVIX was reported in the large, CAPRIE controlled clinical study. A 34-year-old woman took a single 1,050-mg dose of PLAVIX (equivalent to 14 standard 75-mg tablets). There were no associated adverse events. No special therapy was instituted, and she recovered without sequelae.

No adverse events were reported after single oral administration of 600 mg (equivalent to 8 standard 75-mg tablets) of PLAVIX in healthy volunteers. The bleeding time was prolonged by a factor of 1.7, which is similar to that typically observed with the therapeutic dose of 75 mg of PLAVIX per day.

A single oral dose of clopidogrel at 1500 or 2000 mg/kg was lethal to mice and to rats and at 3000 mg/kg to baboons. Symptoms of acute toxicity were vomiting (in baboons), prostration, difficult breathing, and gastrointestinal hemorrhage in all species.

Recommendations About Specific Treatment:

Based on biological plausibility, platelet transfusion may be appropriate to reverse the pharmacological effects of PLAVIX if quick reversal is required.

DOSAGE AND ADMINISTRATION

Recent MI, Recent Stroke, or Established Peripheral Arterial Disease

The recommended daily dose of PLAVIX is 75 mg once daily.

Acute Coronary Syndrome

For patients with acute coronary syndrome (unstable angina/non-Q-wave MI), PLAVIX should be initiated with a single 300 mg loading dose and then continued at 75 mg once daily. Aspirin (75 mg-325 mg once daily) should be initiated and continued in combination with PLAVIX. In CURE, most patients with Acute Coronary Syndrome also received heparin acutely (see **CLINICAL STUDIES**).

PLAVIX can be administered with or without food.

No dosage adjustment is necessary for elderly patients or patients with renal disease. (See **Clinical Pharmacology: Special Populations.**)

HOW SUPPLIED

PLAVIX (clopidogrel bisulfate) is available as a pink, round, biconvex, film-coated tablet debossed with "75" on one side and "1171" on the other. Tablets are provided as follows:

NDC 63653-1171-6 bottles of 30
NDC 63653-1171-1 bottles of 90
NDC 63653-1171-5 bottles of 500
NDC 63653-1171-3 blisters of 100

Storage

Store at 25° C (77° F); excursions permitted to 15°–30° C (59°–86° F) [See USP Controlled Room Temperature]

Distributed by:
Bristol-Myers Squibb/Sanofi Pharmaceuticals Partnership
New York, NY 10016
sanofi~synthelabo
Bristol-Myers Squibb Company

PLAVIX® is a registered trademark of Sanofi-Synthelabo.
51-021345-04

Revised July 2003

Schering Corporation

a wholly-owned subsidiary of Schering-Plough Corporation
GALLOPING HILL ROAD
KENILWORTH, NJ 07033

Direct Inquiries to:
(908) 298-4000
CUSTOMER SERVICE:
(800) 222-7579
FAX: (908) 595-3729

For Medical Information Contact:
Schering Laboratories
Drug Information Services
2000 Galloping Hill Road
Kenilworth, NJ 07033
(800) 526-4099
FAX: (973) 921-7228

CLARINEX® ℞

[*klă-rĭ-nĕks*]
(desloratadine)
TABLETS, REDITABS® TABLETS

Prescribing information for this product, which appears on pages 3044–3046 of the 2004 PDR, has been completely revised as follows. Please write "See Supplement A" next to the product heading.

DESCRIPTION

CLARINEX (desloratadine) Tablets are light blue, round, film coated tablets containing 5 mg desloratadine, an antihistamine, to be administered orally. It also contains the following excipients: dibasic calcium phosphate dihydrate USP, microcrystalline cellulose NF, corn starch NF, talc USP, carnauba wax NF, white wax NF, coating material consisting of lactose monohydrate, hydroxypropyl methylcellulose, titanium dioxide, polyethylene glycol, and FD&C Blue # 2 Aluminum Lake.

The CLARINEX RediTabs® brand of desloratadine orally-disintegrating tablets is a pink colored, round, tablet shaped unit with a "C" debossed on one side. Each RediTabs unit contains 5 mg of desloratadine. It also contains the following inactive ingredients: gelatin Type B NF, mannitol USP, aspartame NF, polarcrillin potassium NF, citric acid USP, red dye and tutti frutti flavoring.

Desloratadine is a white to off-white powder that is slightly soluble in water, but very soluble in ethanol and propylene glycol. It has an empirical formula: $C_{19}H_{19}ClN_2$ and a molecular weight of 310.8. The chemical name is 8-chloro-6,11-dihydro-11-(4-piperdinylidene)-5*H*-benzo[5,6]cyclohepta[1,2-*b*]pyridine and has the following structure:

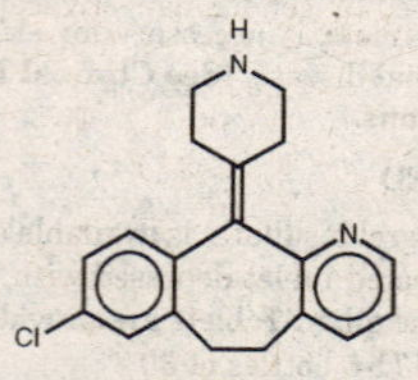

CLINICAL PHARMACOLOGY

Mechanism of Action: Desloratadine is a long-acting tricyclic histamine antagonist with selective H_1-receptor histamine antagonist activity. Receptor binding data indicates that at a concentration of 2-3 ng/mL (7 nanomolar), desloratadine shows significant interaction with the human histamine H_1-receptor. Desloratadine inhibited histamine release from human mast cells *in vitro*.

Results of a radiolabeled tissue distribution study in rats and a radioligand H_1-receptor binding study in guinea pigs showed that desloratadine did not readily cross the blood brain barrier.

Pharmacokinetics: Absorption: Following oral administration of desloratadine 5 mg once daily for 10 days to normal healthy volunteers, the mean time to maximum plasma concentrations (T_{max}) occurred at approximately 3 hours post dose and mean steady state peak plasma concentrations (C_{max}) and area under the concentration-time curve (AUC) of 4 ng/mL and 56.9 ng.hr/mL were observed, respectively. Neither food nor grapefruit juice had an effect on the bioavailability (C_{max} and AUC) of desloratadine.

The pharmacokinetic profile of CLARINEX RediTabs Tablets was evaluated in a three-way crossover study in 30 adult volunteers. A single CLARINEX RediTabs Tablet containing 5 mg of desloratadine was bioequivalent to a single 5 mg CLARINEX Tablet and was bioequivalent to 10 mL of CLARINEX Syrup containing 5 mg of desloratadine for both desloratadine and 3-hydroxydesloratadine. In a separate study with 30 adult volunteers, food or water had no effect on the bioavailability (AUC and C_{max}) of CLARINEX RediTabs Tablets, however, food shifted the desloratadine median T_{max} value from 2.5 to 4 hr.

Distribution: Desloratadine and 3-hydroxydesloratadine are approximately 82% to 87% and 85% to 89%, bound to plasma proteins, respectively. Protein binding of desloratadine and 3-hydroxydesloratadine was unaltered in subjects with impaired renal function.

Metabolism: Desloratadine (a major metabolite of loratadine) is extensively metabolized to 3-hydroxydesloratadine, an active metabolite, which is subsequently glucuronidated. The enzyme(s) responsible for the formation of 3-hydroxydesloratadine have not been identified. Data from clinical trials indicate that a subset of the general patient population has a decreased ability to form 3-hydroxydesloratadine, and are slow metabolizers of desloratadine. In pharmacokinetic studies (n=1087), approximately 7% of subjects were slow metabolizers of desloratadine (defined as a subject with an AUC ratio of 3-hydroxydesloratadine to desloratadine less than 0.1, or a subject with a desloratadine half-life exceeding 50 hours). The frequency of slow metabolizers is higher in Blacks (approximately 20% of Blacks were slow metabolizers in pharmacokinetic studies, n=276). The median exposure (AUC) to desloratadine in the slow metabolizers was approximately 6-fold greater than the subjects who are not slow metabolizers. Subjects who are slow metabolizers of desloratadine cannot be prospectively identified and will be exposed to higher levels of desloratadine following dosing with the recommended dose of desloratadine. Although not seen in these pharmacokinetic studies, patients who are slow metabolizers may be more susceptible to dose-related adverse events.

Elimination: The mean elimination half-life of desloratadine was 27 hours. C_{max} and AUC values increased in a dose proportional manner following single oral doses between 5 and 20 mg. The degree of accumulation after 14 days of dosing was consistent with the half-life and dosing frequency. A human mass balance study documented a recovery of approximately 87% of the ^{14}C-desloratadine dose, which was equally distributed in urine and feces as metabolic products. Analysis of plasma 3-hydroxydesloratadine showed similar T_{max} and half-life values compared to desloratadine.

Special Populations: Geriatric: In older subjects (≥ 65 years old; n=17) following multiple-dose administration of CLARINEX Tablets, the mean C_{max} and AUC values for desloratadine were 20% greater than in younger subjects (< 65 years old). The oral total body clearance (CL/F) when normalized for body weight was similar between the two age groups. The mean plasma elimination half-life of desloratadine was 33.7 hr in subjects ≥ 65 years old. The pharmacokinetics for 3-hydroxydesloratadine appeared unchanged in older versus younger subjects. These age-related differences are unlikely to be clinically relevant and no dosage adjustment is recommended in elderly subjects.

Renally Impaired: Desloratadine pharmacokinetics following a single dose of 7.5 mg were characterized in patients with mild (n=7; creatinine clearance 51–69 mL/min/1.73 m^2), moderate (n=6; creatinine clearance 34–43 mL/min/1.73 m^2), and severe (n=6; creatinine clearance 5–29 mL/min/1.73 m^2) renal impairment or hemodialysis dependent (n=6) patients. In patients with mild and moderate renal impairment, median C_{max} and AUC values increased by approximately 1.2- and 1.9-fold, respectively, relative to subjects with normal renal function. In patients with severe renal impairment or who were hemodialysis dependent, C_{max} and AUC values increased by approximately 1.7- and 2.5-fold, respectively. Minimal changes in 3-hydroxydesloratadine concentrations were observed. Desloratadine and 3-hydroxydesloratadine were poorly removed by hemodialysis. Plasma protein binding of desloratadine and 3-hydroxydesloratadine was unaltered by renal impairment. Dosage adjustment for patients with renal impairment is recommended (see **DOSAGE AND ADMINISTRATION** section).

Hepatically Impaired: Desloratadine pharmacokinetics were characterized following a single oral dose in patients with mild (n=4), moderate (n=4), and severe (n=4) hepatic impairment as defined by the Child-Pugh classification of hepatic function and 8 subjects with normal hepatic function. Patients with hepatic impairment, regardless of severity, had approximately a 2.4-fold increase in AUC as compared with normal subjects. The apparent oral clearance of desloratadine in patients with mild, moderate, and severe hepatic impairment was 37%, 36%, and 28% of that in normal subjects, respectively. An increase in the mean elimination half-life of desloratadine in patients with hepatic impairment was observed. For 3-hydroxydesloratadine, the mean C_{max} and AUC values for patients with hepatic impairment were not statistically significantly different from subjects with normal hepatic function. Dosage adjustment for patients with hepatic impairment is recommended (see **DOSAGE AND ADMINISTRATION** section).

Gender: Female subjects treated for 14 days with CLARINEX Tablets had 10% and 3% higher desloratadine C_{max} and AUC values, respectively, compared with male subjects. The 3-hydroxydesloratadine C_{max} and AUC values were also increased by 45% and 48%, respectively, in females compared with males. However, these apparent differences are not likely to be clinically relevant and therefore no dosage adjustment is recommended.

Race: Following 14 days of treatment with CLARINEX Tablets, the C_{max} and AUC values for desloratadine were 18% and 32% higher, respectively, in Blacks compared with Caucasians. For 3-hydroxydesloratadine there was a corresponding 10% reduction in C_{max} and AUC values in Blacks compared to Caucasians. These differences are not likely to be clinically relevant and therefore no dose adjustment is recommended.

Drug Interactions: In two controlled crossover clinical pharmacology studies in healthy male (n=12 in each study) and female (n=12 in each study) volunteers, desloratadine 7.5 mg (1.5 times the daily dose) once daily was coadministered with erythromycin 500 mg every 8 hours or ketoconazole 200 mg every 12 hours for 10 days. In 3 separate controlled, parallel group clinical pharmacology studies, desloratadine at the clinical dose of 5 mg has been coadministered with azithromycin 500 mg followed by 250 mg once daily for 4 days (n=18) or with fluoxetine 20 mg once daily for 7 days after a 23 day pretreatment period with fluoxetine (n=18) or with cimetidine 600 mg every 12 hours for 14 days (n=18) under steady state conditions to normal healthy male and female volunteers. Although increased plasma concentrations (C_{max} and AUC 0-24 hrs) of desloratadine and 3-hydroxydesloratadine were observed (see Table 1), there were no clinically relevant changes in the safety profile of desloratadine, as assessed by electrocardiographic parameters (including the corrected QT interval), clinical laboratory tests, vital signs, and adverse events.

[See table 1 above]

Table 1
Changes in Desloratadine and 3-Hydroxydesloratadine Pharmacokinetics in Healthy Male and Female Volunteers

	Desloratadine		3-Hydroxydesloratadine	
	C_{max}	AUC 0-24 hrs	C_{max}	AUC 0-24 hrs
Erythromycin (500 mg Q8h)	+24%	+14%	+43%	+40%
Ketoconazole (200 mg Q12h)	+45%	+39%	+43%	+72%
Azithromycin (500 mg day 1, 250 mg QD × 4 days)	+15%	+5%	+15%	+4%
Fluoxetine (20 mg QD)	+15%	+0%	+17%	+13%
Cimetidine (600 mg Q12h)	+12%	+19%	-11%	-3%

Pharmacodynamics: Wheal and Flare: Human histamine skin wheal studies following single and repeated 5 mg doses of desloratadine have shown that the drug exhibits an antihistaminic effect by 1 hour; this activity may persist for as long as 24 hours. There was no evidence of histamine-induced skin wheal tachyphylaxis within the desloratadine 5 mg group over the 28 day treatment period. The clinical relevance of histamine wheal skin testing is unknown.

Effects on QT_c: Single dose administration of desloratadine did not alter the corrected QT interval (QT_c) in rats (up to 12 mg/kg, oral), or guinea pigs (25 mg/kg, intravenous). Repeated oral administration at doses up to 24 mg/kg for durations up to 3 months in monkeys did not alter the QT_c at an estimated desloratadine exposure (AUC) that was approximately 955 times the mean AUC in humans at the recommended daily oral dose. See **OVERDOSAGE** section for information on human QT_c experience.

Table 2
TOTAL SYMPTOM SCORE (TSS)
Changes in a 2 Week Clinical Trial in Patients with Seasonal Allergic Rhinitis

Treatment Group (n)	Mean Baseline* (sem)	Change from Baseline** (sem)	Placebo Comparison (P-value)
CLARINEX 5.0 mg (171)	14.2 (0.3)	-4.3 (0.3)	P<0.01
Placebo (173)	13.7 (0.3)	-2.5 (0.3)	

* At baseline, a total nasal symptom score (sum of 4 individual symptoms) of at least 6 and a total non-nasal symptom score (sum of 4 individual symptoms) of at least 5 (each symptom scored 0 to 3 where 0=no symptom and 3=severe symptoms) was required for trial eligibility. TSS ranges from 0=no symptoms to 24=maximal symptoms.
**Mean reduction in TSS averaged over the 2-week treatment period.

Clinical Trials: Seasonal Allergic Rhinitis: The clinical efficacy and safety of CLARINEX Tablets were evaluated in over 2,300 patients 12 to 75 years of age with seasonal allergic rhinitis. A total of 1,838 patients received 2.5–20 mg/day of CLARINEX in 4 double-blind, randomized, placebo-controlled clinical trials of 2 to 4 weeks' duration conducted in the United States. The results of these studies demonstrated the efficacy and safety of CLARINEX 5 mg in the treatment of adult and adolescent patients with seasonal allergic rhinitis. In a dose ranging trial, CLARINEX 2.5-20 mg/day was studied. Doses of 5, 7.5, 10, and 20 mg/day were superior to placebo; and no additional benefit was seen at doses above 5.0 mg. In the same study, an increase in the incidence of somnolence was observed at doses of 10 mg/day and 20 mg/day (5.2% and 7.6%, respectively), compared to placebo (2.3%).

In 2 four-week studies of 924 patients (aged 15 to 75 years) with seasonal allergic rhinitis and concomitant asthma, CLARINEX Tablets 5 mg once daily improved rhinitis symptoms, with no decrease in pulmonary function. This supports the safety of administering CLARINEX Tablets to adult patients with seasonal allergic rhinitis with mild to moderate asthma.

CLARINEX Tablets 5 mg once daily significantly reduced the Total Symptom Scores (the sum of individual scores of nasal and non-nasal symptoms) in patients with seasonal allergic rhinitis. See Table 2.

[See table 2 at top of previous page]

There were no significant differences in the effectiveness of CLARINEX Tablets 5 mg across subgroups of patients defined by gender, age, or race.

Perennial Allergic Rhinitis: The clinical efficacy and safety of CLARINEX Tablets 5 mg were evaluated in over 1,300 patients 12 to 80 years of age with perennial allergic rhinitis. A total of 685 patients received 5 mg/day of CLARINEX in 2 double-blind, randomized, placebo-controlled clinical trials of 4 weeks' duration conducted in the United States and internationally. In one of these studies CLARINEX Tablets 5 mg once daily was shown to significantly reduce symptoms of perennial allergic rhinitis (Table 3).

[See table 3 at left]

Chronic Idiopathic Urticaria: The efficacy and safety of CLARINEX Tablets 5 mg once daily was studied in 416 chronic idiopathic urticaria patients 12 to 84 years of age, of whom 211 received CLARINEX. In two double-blind, placebo-controlled, randomized clinical trials of six weeks' duration, at the pre-specified one-week primary time point evaluation, CLARINEX Tablets significantly reduced the severity of pruritus when compared to placebo (Table 4). Secondary endpoints were also evaluated and during the first week of therapy CLARINEX Tablets 5 mg reduced the secondary endpoints, "Number of Hives" and the "Size of the Largest Hive," when compared to placebo.

[See table 4 at left]

Table 3
TOTAL SYMPTOM SCORE (TSS)
Changes in a 4 Week Clinical Trial in Patients with Perennial Allergic Rhinitis

Treatment Group (n)	Mean Baseline* (sem)	Change from Baseline** (sem)	Placebo Comparison (P-value)
CLARINEX 5.0 mg (337)	12.37 (0.18)	-4.06 (0.21)	P=0.01
Placebo (337)	12.30 (0.18)	-3.27 (0.21)	

* At baseline, average of total symptom score (sum of 5 individual nasal symptoms and 3 non-nasal symptoms, each symptom scored 0 to 3 where 0=no symptom and 3=severe symptoms) of at least 10 was required for trial eligibility. TSS ranges from 0=no symptoms to 24=maximal symptoms.
**Mean reduction in TSS averaged over the 4-week treatment period.

Table 4
PRURITUS SYMPTOM SCORE
Changes in the First Week of a Clinical Trial in Patients with Chronic Idiopathic Urticaria

Treatment Group (n)	Mean Baseline (sem)	Change from Baseline* (sem)	Placebo Comparison (P-value)
CLARINEX 5.0 mg (115)	2.19 (0.04)	-1.05 (0.07)	P<0.01
Placebo (110)	2.21 (0.04)	-0.52 (0.07)	

Pruritus scored 0 to 3 where 0=no symptom to 3=maximal symptom
*Mean reduction in pruritus averaged over the first week of treatment.

INDICATIONS AND USAGE

Allergic Rhinitis: CLARINEX Tablets 5 mg are indicated for the relief of the nasal and non-nasal symptoms of allergic rhinitis (seasonal and perennial) in patients 12 years of age and older.

Chronic Idiopathic Urticaria: CLARINEX Tablets are indicated for the symptomatic relief of pruritus, reduction in the number of hives, and size of hives, in patients with chronic idiopathic urticaria 12 years of age and older.

CONTRAINDICATIONS

CLARINEX Tablets 5 mg are contraindicated in patients who are hypersensitive to this medication or to any of its ingredients, or to loratadine.

PRECAUTIONS

Carcinogenesis, Mutagenesis, Impairment of Fertility: The carcinogenic potential of desloratadine was assessed using loratadine studies. In an 18-month study in mice and a 2-year study in rats, loratadine was administered in the diet at doses up to 40 mg/kg/day in mice (estimated desloratadine and desloratadine metabolite exposures were approximately 3 times the AUC in humans at the recommended daily oral dose) and 25 mg/kg/day in rats (estimated desloratadine and desloratadine metabolite exposures were approximately 30 times the AUC in humans at the recommended daily oral dose). Male mice given 40 mg/kg/day loratadine had a significantly higher incidence of hepatocellular tumors (combined adenomas and carcinomas) than concurrent controls. In rats, a significantly higher incidence of hepatocellular tumors (combined adenomas and carcinomas) was observed in males given 10 mg/kg/day and in males and females given 25 mg/kg/day. The estimated desloratadine and desloratadine metabolite exposures of rats given 10 mg/kg of loratadine were approximately 7 times the AUC in humans at the recommended daily oral dose. The clinical significance of these findings during long-term use of desloratadine is not known.

In genotoxicity studies with desloratadine, there was no evidence of genotoxic potential in a reverse mutation assay (*Salmonella*/*E. coli* mammalian microsome bacterial mutagenicity assay) or in two assays for chromosomal aberrations (human peripheral blood lymphocyte clastogenicity assay and mouse bone marrow micronucleus assay).

There was no effect on female fertility in rats at desloratadine doses up to 24 mg/kg/day (estimated desloratadine and desloratadine metabolite exposures were approximately 130 times the AUC in humans at the recommended daily oral dose). A male specific decrease in fertility, demonstrated by reduced female conception rates, decreased sperm numbers and motility, and histopathologic testicular changes, occurred at an oral desloratadine dose of 12 mg/kg in rats (estimated desloratadine exposures were approximately 45 times the AUC in humans at the recommended daily oral dose). Desloratadine had no effect on fertility in rats at an oral dose of 3 mg/kg/day (estimated desloratadine and desloratadine metabolite exposures were approximately 8 times the AUC in humans at the recommended daily oral dose).

Pregnancy Category C: Desloratadine was not teratogenic in rats at doses up to 48 mg/kg/day (estimated desloratadine and desloratadine metabolite exposures were approximately 210 times the AUC in humans at the recommended daily oral dose) or in rabbits at doses up to 60 mg/kg/day (estimated desloratadine exposures were approximately 230 times the AUC in humans at the recommended daily oral dose). In a separate study, an increase in pre-implantation loss and a decreased number of implantations and fetuses were noted in female rats at 24 mg/kg (estimated desloratadine and desloratadine metabolite exposures were approximately 120 times the AUC in humans at the recommended daily oral dose). Reduced body weight and slow righting reflex were reported in pups at doses of 9 mg/kg/day or greater (estimated desloratadine and desloratadine metabolite exposures were approximately 50 times or greater than the AUC in humans at the recommended daily oral dose). Desloratadine had no effect on pup development at an oral dose of 3 mg/kg/day (estimated desloratadine and desloratadine metabolite exposures were approximately 7 times the AUC in humans at the recommended daily oral dose). There are, however, no adequate and well-controlled studies in pregnant women. Because animal reproduction studies are not always predictive of human response, desloratadine should be used during pregnancy only if clearly needed.

Nursing Mothers: Desloratadine passes into breast milk, therefore a decision should be made whether to discontinue nursing or to discontinue desloratadine, taking into account the importance of the drug to the mother.

Pediatric Use: The safety and effectiveness of CLARINEX Tablets in pediatric patients under 12 years of age have not been established.

Geriatric Use: Clinical studies of desloratadine did not include sufficient numbers of subjects aged 65 and over to determine whether they respond differently from younger subjects. Other reported clinical experience has not identified differences between the elderly and younger patients. In general, dose selection for an elderly patient should be cautious, reflecting the greater frequency of decreased hepatic, renal, or cardiac function, and of concomitant disease or other drug therapy. (see **CLINICAL PHARMACOLOGY – Special Populations**).

Information for Patients: Patients should be instructed to use CLARINEX Tablets as directed. As there are no food effects on bioavailability, patients can be instructed that CLARINEX Tablets may be taken without regard to meals. Patients should be advised not to increase the dose or dosing frequency as studies have not demonstrated increased effectiveness at higher doses and somnolence may occur. Phenylketonurics: CLARINEX RediTabs Tablets contain phenylalanine 1.75 mg per tablet.

ADVERSE REACTIONS

Allergic Rhinitis: In multiple-dose placebo-controlled trials, 2,834 patients received CLARINEX Tablets at doses of 2.5 mg to 20 mg daily, of whom 1,655 patients received the recommended daily dose of 5 mg. In patients receiving 5 mg daily, the rate of adverse events was similar between CLARINEX and placebo-treated patients. The percent of patients who withdrew prematurely due to adverse events was 2.4% in the CLARINEX group and 2.6% in the placebo group. There were no serious adverse events in these trials in patients receiving desloratadine. All adverse events that were reported by greater than or equal to 2% of patients who received the recommended daily dose of CLARINEX Tablets (5.0 mg once-daily), and that were more common with CLARINEX Tablet than placebo, are listed in Table 5.

Table 5
Incidence of Adverse Events Reported by ≥ 2% of Allergic Rhinitis Patients in Placebo-Controlled, Multiple-Dose Clinical Trials

Adverse Experience	CLARINEX Tablets 5 mg (n=1,655)	Placebo (n=1,652)
Pharyngitis	4.1%	2.0%
Dry Mouth	3.0%	1.9%
Myalgia	2.1%	1.8%
Fatigue	2.1%	1.2%
Somnolence	2.1%	1.8%
Dysmenorrhea	2.1%	1.6%

The frequency and magnitude of laboratory and electrocardiographic abnormalities were similar in CLARINEX and placebo-treated patients.

There were no differences in adverse events for subgroups of patients as defined by gender, age, or race.

Chronic Idiopathic Urticaria: In multiple-dose, placebo-controlled trials of chronic idiopathic urticaria, 211 patients received CLARINEX Tablets and 205 received placebo. Adverse events that were reported by greater than or equal to 2% of patients who received CLARINEX Tablets and that were more common with CLARINEX than placebo were (rates for CLARINEX and placebo, respectively): headache (14%, 13%), nausea (5%, 2%), fatigue (5%, 1%), dizziness (4%, 3%), pharyngitis (3%, 2%), dyspepsia (3%, 1%), and myalgia (3%, 1%).

The following spontaneous adverse events have been reported during the marketing of desloratadine: tachycardia, palpitations and rarely hypersensitivity reactions (such as rash, pruritus, urticaria, edema, dyspnea, and anaphylaxis), and elevated liver enzymes including bilirubin.

DRUG ABUSE AND DEPENDENCE

There is no information to indicate that abuse or dependency occurs with CLARINEX Tablets.

OVERDOSAGE

Information regarding acute overdosage is limited to experience from clinical trials conducted during the development of the CLARINEX product. In a dose ranging trial, at doses of 10 mg and 20 mg/day somnolence was reported.

Single daily doses of 45 mg were given to normal male and female volunteers for 10 days. All ECGs obtained in this study were manually read in a blinded fashion by a cardiologist. In CLARINEX-treated subjects, there was an increase in mean heart rate of 9.2 bpm relative to placebo. The QT interval was corrected for heart rate (QT_c) by both the Bazett and Fridericia methods. Using the QT_c (Bazett) there was a mean increase of 8.1 msec in CLARINEX-treated subjects relative to placebo. Using QT_c (Fridericia) there was a mean increase of 0.4 msec in CLARINEX-treated subjects relative to placebo. No clinically relevant adverse events were reported.

In the event of overdose, consider standard measures to remove any unabsorbed drug. Symptomatic and supportive treatment is recommended. Desloratadine and 3-hydroxydesloratadine are not eliminated by hemodialysis.

Lethality occurred in rats at oral doses of 250 mg/kg or greater (estimated desloratadine and desloratadine metabolite exposures were approximately 120 times the AUC in humans at the recommended daily oral dose). The oral median lethal dose in mice was 353 mg/kg (estimated deslora-

Continued on next page

Clarinex—Cont.

tadine exposures were approximately 290 times the human daily oral dose on a mg/m[2] basis). No deaths occurred at oral doses up to 250 mg/kg in monkeys (estimated desloratadine exposures were approximately 810 times the human daily oral dose on a mg/m[2] basis).

DOSAGE AND ADMINISTRATION

In adults and children 12 years of age and over, the recommended dose of CLARINEX Tablets is 5 mg once daily. In patients with liver or renal impairment, a starting dose of one 5 mg tablet every other day is recommended based on pharmacokinetic data.

Administration of CLARINEX RediTabs Tablets: Place CLARINEX RediTabs Tablet on the tongue. Tablet disintegration occurs rapidly. Administer with or without water. Take tablet immediately after opening the blister.

HOW SUPPLIED

CLARINEX Tablets: Embossed "C5", light blue film coated tablets; that are packaged in high-density polyethylene plastic bottles of 100 (NDC 0085-1264-01) and 500 (NDC 0085-1264-02). Also available, CLARINEX Unit-of-Use package of 30 tablets (3 × 10; 10 blisters per card) (NDC 0085-1264-04); and Unit Dose-Hospital Pack of 100 Tablets (10 × 10; 10 blisters per card) (NDC 0085-1264-03).

Protect Unit-of-Use packaging and Unit Dose-Hospital Pack from excessive moisture.

Store at 25°C (77°F); excursions permitted to 15–30°C (59–86°F) [see USP Controlled Room Temperature]

Heat Sensitive. Avoid exposure at or above 30°C (86°F).

CLARINEX REDITABS (desloratadine orally-disintegrating tablets) 5 mg: "C" debossed, pink tablets in foil/foil blisters.

Packs of 30 tablets (containing 3 x 10's) NDC 0085-1280-01.

Store at 25°C (77°F); excursions permitted to 15–30°C (59–86°F) [see USP Controlled Room Temperature]

Schering®

Schering Corporation
Kenilworth, NJ 07033 USA
Rev. 7/03 **23882159T**

CLARINEX REDITABS brand of desloratadine orally-disintegrating tablets are manufactured for Schering Corporation by Cardinal Health UK. 416 Limited, England.

PEG-INTRON® ℞

[pĕg ĭn-trŏn]
(Peginterferon alfa-2b)
Powder for Injection

Prescribing information for this product, which appears on pages 3064–3069 of the 2004 PDR, has been completely revised as follows. Please write "See Supplement A" next to the product heading.

Alpha interferons, including PEG-Intron, may cause or aggravate fatal or life-threatening neuropsychiatric, autoimmune, ischemic, and infectious disorders. Patients should be monitored closely with periodic clinical and laboratory evaluations. Patients with persistently severe or worsening signs or symptoms of these conditions should be withdrawn from therapy. In many but not all cases these disorders resolve after stopping PEG-Intron therapy. See WARNINGS, ADVERSE REACTIONS.

Use with Ribavirin. Ribavirin may cause birth defects and/or death of the unborn child. Extreme care must be taken to avoid pregnancy in female patients and in female partners of male patients. Ribavirin causes hemolytic anemia. The anemia associated with REBETOL therapy may result in a worsening of cardiac disease. Ribavirin is genotoxic and mutagenic and should be considered a potential carcinogen. (See REBETOL package insert for additional information and other warnings).

DESCRIPTION

PEG-Intron®, peginterferon alfa-2b, Powder for Injection is a covalent conjugate of recombinant alfa-2b interferon with monomethoxypolyethylene glycol (PEG). The average molecular weight of the PEG portion of the molecule is 12,000 daltons. The average molecular weight of the PEG-Intron molecule is approximately 31,000 daltons. The specific activity of peginterferon alfa-2b is approximately 0.7×10^8 IU/mg protein.

Interferon alfa-2b, is a water-soluble protein with a molecular weight of 19,271 daltons produced by recombinant DNA techniques. It is obtained from the bacterial fermentation of a strain of *Escherichia coli* bearing a genetically engineered plasmid containing an interferon gene from human leukocytes.

PEG-Intron is supplied in both vials and the Redipen™ for subcutaneous use.

Vials

Each vial contains either 74 µg, 118.4 µg, 177.6 µg, or 222 µg of PEG-Intron as a white to off-white tablet-like solid, that is whole/in pieces or as a loose powder, and 1.11 mg dibasic sodium phosphate anhydrous, 1.11 mg monobasic sodium phosphate dihydrate, 59.2 mg sucrose and 0.074 mg polysorbate 80. Following reconstitution with 0.7 mL of the supplied Sterile Water for Injection, USP, each vial contains PEG-Intron at strengths of either 50 µg per 0.5 mL, 80 µg per 0.5 mL, 120 µg per 0.5 mL, or 150 µg per 0.5 mL.

Redipen™

Redipen™ is a dual-chamber glass cartridge containing lyophilized PEG-Intron as a white to off-white tablet or powder that is whole or in pieces in the sterile active chamber and a second chamber containing Sterile Water for Injection, USP. Each PEG-Intron Redipen™ contains either 67.5 µg, 108 µg, 162 µg, or 202.5 µg of PEG-Intron, and 1.013 mg dibasic sodium phosphate anhydrous, 1.013 mg monobasic sodium phosphate dihydrate, 54 mg sucrose and 0.0675 mg polysorbate 80. Each cartridge is reconstituted to allow for the administration of up to 0.5 mL of solution. Following reconstitution, each Redipen™ contains PEG-Intron at strengths of either 50 µg per 0.5 mL, 80 µg per 0.5 mL, 120 µg per 0.5 mL, or 150 µg per 0.5 mL for a single use. Because a small volume of reconstituted solution is lost during preparation of PEG-Intron, each Redipen™ contains an excess amount of PEG-Intron powder and diluent to ensure delivery of the labeled dose.

CLINICAL PHARMACOLOGY

General: The biological activity of PEG-Intron is derived from its interferon alfa-2b moiety. Interferons exert their cellular activities by binding to specific membrane receptors on the cell surface and initiate a complex sequence of intracellular events. These include the induction of certain enzymes, suppression of cell proliferation, immunomodulating activities such as enhancement of the phagocytic activity of macrophages and augmentation of the specific cytotoxicity of lymphocytes for target cells, and inhibition of virus replication in virus-infected cells. Interferon alfa upregulates the Th1 T-helper cell subset in *in vitro* studies. The clinical relevance of these findings is not known.

Pharmacodynamics: PEG-Intron raises concentrations of effector proteins such as serum neopterin and 2'5' oligoadenylate synthetase, raises body temperature, and causes reversible decreases in leukocyte and platelet counts. The correlation between the *in vitro* and *in vivo* pharmacologic and pharmacodynamic and clinical effects is unknown.

Pharmacokinetics: Following a single subcutaneous (SC) dose of PEG-Intron, the mean absorption half-life ($t_{½} k_a$) was 4.6 hours. Maximal serum concentrations (C_{max}) occur between 15–44 hours post-dose, and are sustained for up to 48–72 hours. The C_{max} and AUC measurements of PEG-Intron increase in a dose-related manner. After multiple dosing, there is an increase in bioavailability of PEG-Intron. Week 48 mean trough concentrations (320 pg/mL; range 0, 2960) are approximately 3-fold higher than Week 4 mean trough concentrations (94 pg/mL; range 0, 416). The mean PEG-Intron elimination half-life is approximately 40 hours (range 22 to 60 hours) in patients with HCV infection. The apparent clearance of PEG-Intron is estimated to be approximately 22.0 mL/hr•kg. Renal elimination accounts for 30% of the clearance. Single dose peginterferon alfa-2b pharmacokinetics following a subcutaneous 1.0 µg/kg dose suggest the clearance of peginterferon alfa-2b is reduced by approximately half in subjects with impaired renal function (creatinine clearance <50 mL/minute).

Pegylation of interferon alfa-2b produces a product (PEG-Intron) whose clearance is lower than that of non-pegylated interferon alfa-2b. When compared to INTRON A, PEG-Intron (1.0 µg/kg) has approximately a seven-fold lower mean apparent clearance and a five-fold greater mean half-life permitting a reduced dosing frequency. At effective therapeutic doses, PEG-Intron has approximately ten-fold greater C_{max} and 50-fold greater AUC than interferon alfa-2b.

The pharmacokinetics of geriatric subjects (>65 years of age) treated with a single subcutaneous dose of 1.0 µg/kg of PEG-Intron were similar in C_{max}, AUC, clearance, or elimination half-life as compared to younger subjects (28 to 44 years of age).

During the 48 week treatment period with PEG-Intron, no differences in the pharmacokinetic profiles were observed between male and female patients with chronic hepatitis C infection.

Effect of Food on Absorption of Ribavirin Both AUC_{tf} and C_{max} increased by 70% when REBETOL Capsules were administered with a high-fat meal (841 kcal, 53.8 g fat, 31.6 g protein, and 57.4 g carbohydrate) in a single-dose pharmacokinetic study. (See **DOSAGE AND ADMINISTRATION**).

Drug Interactions: It is not known if PEG-Intron therapy causes clinically significant drug-drug interactions with drugs metabolized by the liver in patients with hepatitis C. In 12 healthy subjects known to be CYP2D6 extensive metabolizers, a single subcutaneous dose of 1 µg/kg PEG-Intron did not inhibit CYP1A2, 2C8/9, 2D6, hepatic 3A4 or N-acetyltransferase; the effects of PEG-Intron on CYP2C19 were not assessed.

CLINICAL STUDIES

PEG-Intron Monotherapy-Study 1

A randomized study compared treatment with PEG-Intron (0.5, 1.0, or 1.5 µg/kg once weekly SC) to treatment with INTRON A, (3 million units three times weekly SC) in 1219 adults with chronic hepatitis from HCV infection. The patients were not previously treated with interferon alfa, had compensated liver disease, detectable HCV RNA, elevated ALT, and liver histopathology consistent with chronic hepatitis. Patients were treated for 48 weeks and were followed for 24 weeks post-treatment. Seventy percent of all patients were infected with HCV genotype 1, and 74 percent of all patients had high baseline levels of HCV RNA (more than 2 million copies per mL of serum), two factors known to predict poor response to treatment.

Response to treatment was defined as undetectable HCV RNA and normalization of ALT at 24 weeks posttreatment. The response rates to the 1.0 and 1.5 µg/kg PEG-Intron doses were similar (approximately 24%) to each other and were both higher than the response rate to INTRON A (12%). (See **Table 1**)

[See table 1 below]

TABLE 1. Rates of Response to Treatment-Study 1

	A PEG-Intron 0.5 µg/kg (N=315)	B PEG-Intron 1.0 µg/kg (N=298)	C INTRON A 3 MIU TIW (N=307)	B-C (95% CI) Difference between PEG-Intron 1.0 µg/kg and INTRON A
Treatment Response (Combined Virologic Response and ALT Normalization)	17%	24%	12%	11 (5, 18)
Virologic Response[a]	18%	25%	12%	12 (6, 19)
ALT Normalization	24%	29%	18%	11 (5, 18)

[a]Serum HCV is measured by a research-based quantitative polymerase chain reaction assay by a central laboratory.

Patients with both viral genotype 1 and high serum levels of HCV RNA at baseline were less likely to respond to treatment with PEG-Intron. Among patients with the two unfavorable prognostic variables, 8% (12/157) responded to PEG-Intron treatment and 2% (4/169) responded to INTRON A. Doses of PEG-Intron higher than the recommended dose did not result in higher response rates in these patients.

Patients receiving PEG-Intron with viral genotype 1 had a response rate of 14% (28/199) while patients with other viral genotypes had a 45% (43/96) response rate.

Ninety-six percent of the responders in the PEG-Intron groups and 100% of responders in the INTRON A group first cleared their viral RNA by week-24 of treatment. See **DOSAGE AND ADMINISTRATION**.

The treatment response rates were similar in men and women. Response rates were lower in African American and Hispanic patients and higher in Asians compared to Caucasians. Although African Americans had a higher proportion of poor prognostic factors compared to Caucasians the number of non-Caucasians studied (9% of the total) was insufficient to allow meaningful conclusions about differences in response rates after adjusting for prognostic factors.

Liver biopsies were obtained before and after treatment in 60% of patients. A modest reduction in inflammation compared to baseline that was similar in all four treatment groups was observed.

PEG-Intron/REBETOL Combination Therapy-Study 2

A randomized study compared treatment with two PEG-Intron/REBETOL regimens [PEG-Intron 1.5 µg/kg SC once weekly (QW)/REBETOL 800 mg PO daily (in divided doses); PEG-Intron 1.5 µg/kg SC QW for 4 weeks then 0.5 µg/kg SC QW for 44 weeks/REBETOL 1000/1200 mg PO daily (in divided doses)] with INTRON A [3 MIU SC thrice weekly (TIW)/REBETOL 1000/1200 mg PO daily (in divided doses)] in 1530 adults with chronic hepatitis C. Interferon naïve patients were treated for 48 weeks and followed for 24 weeks posttreatment. Eligible patients had compensated liver disease, detectable HCV RNA, elevated ALT, and liver histopathology consistent with chronic hepatitis.

Response to treatment was defined as undetectable HCV RNA at 24 weeks posttreatment. The response rate to the PEG-Intron 1.5 µg/kg plus ribavirin 800 mg dose was higher than the response rate to INTRON A/REBETOL (See **Table 2**). The response rate to PEG-Intron 1.5 → 0.5 µg/kg/REBETOL was essentially the same as the response to INTRON A/REBETOL (data not shown).

[See table 2 at top of next page]

Patients with viral genotype 1, regardless of viral load, had a lower response rate to PEG-Intron (1.5 µg/kg)/REBETOL compared to patients with other viral genotypes. Patients with both poor prognostic factors (genotype 1 and high viral load) had a response rate of 30% (78/256) compared to a response rate of 29% (71/247) with INTRON A/REBETOL.

Patients with lower body weight tended to have higher adverse event rates (see **ADVERSE REACTIONS**) and

TABLE 2. Rates of Response to Treatment-Study 2

	PEG-Intron 1.5 µg/kg QW REBETOL 800 mg QD	INTRON A 3 MIU TIW REBETOL 1000/1200 mg QD
Overall[1,2] response	52% (264/511)	46% (231/505)
Genotype 1	41% (141/348)	33% (112/343)
Genotype 2-6	75% (123/163)	73% (119/162)

[1]Serum HCV RNA is measured with a research-based quantitative polymerase chain reaction assay by a central laboratory.
[2]Difference in overall treatment response (PEG-Intron/REBETOL vs. INTRON A/REBETOL) is 6% with 95% confidence interval of (0.18, 11.63) adjusted for viral genotype and presence of cirrhosis at baseline.

higher response rates than patients with higher body weights. Differences in response rates between treatment arms did not substantially vary with body weight.

Treatment response rates with PEG-Intron/REBETOL were 49% in men and 56% in women. Response rates were lower in African American and Hispanic patients and higher in Asians compared to Caucasians. Although African Americans had a higher proportion of poor prognostic factors compared to Caucasians the number of non-Caucasians studied (11% of the total) was insufficient to allow meaningful conclusions about differences in response rates after adjusting for prognostic factors.

Liver biopsies were obtained before and after treatment in 68% of patients. Compared to baseline approximately 2/3 of patients in all treatment groups were observed to have a modest reduction in inflammation.

INDICATIONS AND USAGE

PEG-Intron, peginterferon alfa-2b, is indicated for use alone or in combination with REBETOL (ribavirin, USP) for the treatment of chronic hepatitis C in patients with compensated liver disease who have not been previously treated with interferon alpha and are at least 18 years of age.

CONTRAINDICATIONS

PEG-Intron is contraindicated in patients with:

- hypersensitivity to PEG-Intron or any other component of the product
- autoimmune hepatitis
- decompensated liver disease

PEG-Intron/REBETOL combination therapy is additionally contraindicated in:

- patients with hypersensitivity to ribavirin or any other component of the product
- women who are pregnant
- men whose female partners are pregnant
- patients with hemoglobinopathies (e.g., thalassemia major, sickle-cell anemia)

WARNINGS

Patients should be monitored for the following serious conditions, some of which may become life threatening. Patients with persistently severe or worsening signs or symptoms should be withdrawn from therapy.

Neuropsychiatric events

Life-threatening or fatal neuropsychiatric events, including suicide, suicidal and homicidal ideation, depression, relapse of drug addiction/overdose, and aggressive behavior have occurred in patients with and without a previous psychiatric disorder during PEG-Intron treatment and follow-up. Psychoses, hallucinations, bipolar disorders, and mania have been observed in patients treated with alpha interferons. PEG-Intron should be used with extreme caution in patients with a history of psychiatric disorders. Patients should be advised to report immediately any symptoms of depression and/or suicidal ideation to their prescribing physicians. Physicians should monitor all patients for evidence of depression and other psychiatric symptoms. In severe cases, PEG-Intron should be stopped immediately and psychiatric intervention instituted. (See **DOSAGE AND ADMINISTRATION: Dose Reduction.**)

Bone marrow toxicity

PEG-Intron suppresses bone marrow function, sometimes resulting in severe cytopenias. PEG-Intron should be discontinued in patients who develop severe decreases in neutrophil or platelet counts. (See **DOSAGE AND ADMINISTRATION: Dose Reduction**). Ribavirin may potentiate the neutropenia induced by interferon alpha. Very rarely alpha interferons may be associated with aplastic anemia.

Endocrine disorders

PEG-Intron causes or aggravates hypothyroidism and hyperthyroidism. Hyperglycemia has been observed in patients treated with PEG-Intron. Diabetes mellitus has been observed in patients treated with alpha interferons. Patients with these conditions who cannot be effectively treated by medication should not begin PEG-Intron therapy. Patients who develop these conditions during treatment and cannot be controlled with medication should not continue PEG-Intron therapy.

Cardiovascular events

Cardiovascular events, which include hypotension, arrhythmia, tachycardia, cardiomyopathy, angina pectoris, and myocardial infarction, have been observed in patients treated with PEG-Intron. PEG-Intron should be used cautiously in patients with cardiovascular disease. Patients with a history of myocardial infarction and arrhythmic disorder who require PEG-Intron therapy should be closely monitored (see **Laboratory Tests**). Patients with a history of significant or unstable cardiac disease should not be treated with PEG-Intron/REBETOL combination therapy. [See **REBETOL package insert.**]

Pulmonary disorders

Dyspnea, pulmonary infiltrates, pneumonia, bronchiolitis obliterans, interstitial pneumonitis and sarcoidosis some resulting in respiratory failure and/or patient deaths, may be induced or aggravated by PEG-Intron or alpha interferon therapy. Recurrence of respiratory failure has been observed with interferon rechallenge. PEG-Intron combination treatment should be suspended in patients who develop pulmonary infiltrates or pulmonary function impairment. Patients who resume interferon treatment should be closely monitored.

Colitis

Fatal and nonfatal ulcerative or hemorrhagic/ischemic colitis have been observed within 12 weeks of the start of alpha interferon treatment. Abdominal pain, bloody diarrhea, and fever are the typical manifestations. PEG-Intron treatment should be discontinued immediately in patients who develop these symptoms and signs. The colitis usually resolves within 1–3 weeks of discontinuation of alpha interferons.

Pancreatitis

Fatal and nonfatal pancreatitis have been observed in patients treated with alpha interferon. PEG-Intron therapy should be suspended in patients with signs and symptoms suggestive of pancreatitis and discontinued in patients diagnosed with pancreatitis.

Autoimmune disorders

Development or exacerbation of autoimmune disorders (e.g. thyroiditis, thrombocytopenia, rheumatoid arthritis, interstitial nephritis, systemic lupus erythematosus, psoriasis) have been observed in patients receiving PEG-Intron. PEG-Intron should be used with caution in patients with autoimmune disorders.

Ophthalmologic disorders

Decrease or loss of vision, retinopathy including macular edema, retinal artery or vein thrombosis, retinal hemorrhages and cotton wool spots, optic neuritis, and papilledema may be induced or aggravated by treatment with peginterferon alfa-2b or other alpha interferons. All patients should receive an eye examination at baseline. Patients with preexisting ophthalmologic disorders (e.g. diabetic or hypertensive retinopathy) should receive periodic ophthalmologic exams during interferon alpha treatment. Any patient who develops ocular symptoms should receive a prompt and complete eye examination. Peginterferon alfa-2b treatment should be discontinued in patients who develop new or worsening ophthalmologic disorders.

Hypersensitivity

Serious, acute hypersensitivity reactions (e.g., urticaria, angioedema, bronchoconstriction, anaphylaxis) have been rarely observed during alpha interferon therapy. If such a reaction develops during treatment with PEG-Intron, discontinue treatment and institute appropriate medical therapy immediately. Transient rashes do not necessitate interruption of treatment.

Use with Ribavirin-(See also REBETOL Package Insert)

REBETOL may cause birth defects and/or death of the unborn child. REBETOL therapy should not be started until a report of a negative pregnancy test has been obtained immediately prior to planned initiation of therapy. Patients should use at least two forms of contraception and have monthly pregnancy tests (See BOXED WARNING, CONTRAINDICATIONS and PRECAUTIONS: Information for Patients and REBETOL package insert).

Anemia

Ribavirin caused hemolytic anemia in 10% of PEG-Intron/REBETOL treated patients within 1–4 weeks of initiation of therapy. Complete blood counts should be obtained pretreatment and at week 2 and week 4 of therapy or more frequently if clinically indicated. Anemia associated with REBETOL therapy may result in a worsening of cardiac disease. Decrease in dosage or discontinuation of REBETOL may be necessary. (See **DOSAGE AND ADMINISTRATION: Dose Reduction.**)

PRECAUTIONS

- PEG-Intron alone or in combination with REBETOL has not been studied in patients who have failed other alpha interferon treatments.
- The safety and efficacy of PEG-Intron alone or in combination with REBETOL for the treatment of hepatitis C in liver or other organ transplant recipients have not been studied. Preliminary data indicates that interferon alpha therapy may be associated with an increased rate of kidney graft rejection. Liver graft rejection has also been reported but a causal association to interferon alpha therapy has not been established.
- The safety and efficacy of PEG-Intron/REBETOL for the treatment of patients with HCV co-infected with HIV or HBV have not been established.

Triglycerides: Elevated triglyceride levels have been observed in patients treated with interferons including PEG-Intron therapy. Elevated triglyceride levels should be managed as clinically appropriate. Hypertriglyceridemia may result in pancreatitis. Discontinuation of PEG-Intron therapy should be considered for patients with persistently elevated triglycerides (eg, triglycerides >1000 mg/dL) associated with symptoms of potential pancreatitis, such as abdominal pain, nausea, or vomiting.

Patients with renal failure: Increases in serum creatinine levels have been observed in patients with renal insufficiency treated with interferons, including PEG-Intron. Patients with impairment of renal function should be closely monitored for signs and symptoms of interferon toxicity, including increases in serum creatinine, and doses of PEG-Intron should be adjusted accordingly. PEG-Intron should be used with caution in patients with creatinine clearance <50 mL/min; in considering these patients for PEG-Intron therapy, the potential risks must be evaluated against the potential benefits of treatment. REBETOL must not be used in patients with creatinine clearance <50 mL/min. (See **DOSAGE AND ADMINISTRATION: Dose Reduction**).

Information for Patients: Patients receiving PEG-Intron alone or in combination with REBETOL should be directed in its appropriate use, informed of the benefits and risks associated with treatment, and referred to the **MEDICATION GUIDES for PEG-Intron and, if applicable, REBETOL (ribavirin, USP).**

Patients must be informed that REBETOL may cause birth defects and/or death of the unborn child. Extreme care must be taken to avoid pregnancy in female patients and in female partners of male patients during treatment with combination PEG-Intron/REBETOL therapy and for 6 months post-therapy. Combination PEG-Intron/REBETOL therapy should not be initiated until a report of a negative pregnancy test has been obtained immediately prior to initiation of therapy. It is recommended that patients undergo monthly pregnancy tests during therapy and for 6 months post-therapy. **(See CONTRAINDICATIONS and REBETOL package insert).**

Patients should be informed that there are no data regarding whether PEG-Intron therapy will prevent transmission of HCV infection to others. Also, it is not known if treatment with PEG-Intron will cure hepatitis C or prevent cirrhosis, liver failure, or liver cancer that may be the result of infection with the hepatitis C virus.

Patients should be advised that laboratory evaluations are required before starting therapy and periodically thereafter (see **Laboratory Tests**). It is advised that patients be well hydrated, especially during the initial stages of treatment. "Flu-like" symptoms associated with administration of PEG-Intron may be minimized by bedtime administration of PEG-Intron or by use of antipyretics.

Patients should be advised to use a puncture-resistant container for the disposal of used syringes, needles, and the Redipen™. The full container should be disposed of in accordance with state and local laws. Patients should be thoroughly instructed in the importance of proper disposal. Patients should also be cautioned against reusing or sharing needles, syringes, or the Redipen™.

Laboratory Tests: PEG-Intron alone or in combination with ribavirin may cause severe decreases in neutrophil and platelet counts, and hematologic, endocrine (e.g. TSH) and hepatic abnormalities. Transient elevations in ALT (2–5 fold above baseline) were observed in 10% of patients treated with PEG-Intron, and was not associated with deterioration of other liver functions.

Patients on PEG-Intron or PEG-Intron/REBETOL combination therapy should have hematology and blood chemistry testing before the start of treatment and then periodically thereafter. In the clinical trial CBC (including hemoglobin, neutrophil and platelet counts) and chemistries (including AST, ALT, bilirubin, and uric acid) were measured during the treatment period at weeks 2, 4, 8, 12, and then at 6-week intervals or more frequently if abnormalities developed. TSH levels were measured every 12 weeks during the treatment period.

HCV RNA should be measured at 6 months of treatment. PEG-Intron or PEG-Intron/REBETOL combination therapy should be discontinued in patients with persistent high viral levels.

Patients who have pre-existing cardiac abnormalities should have electrocardiograms administered before treatment with PEG-Intron/REBETOL.

Carcinogenesis, Mutagenesis, and Impairment of Fertility

Carcinogenesis and Mutagenesis: PEG-Intron has not been tested for its carcinogenic potential. Neither PEG-Intron, nor its components interferon or methoxypolyethylene glycol caused damage to DNA when tested in the standard battery of mutagenesis assays, in the presence and absence of metabolic activation.

Use with Ribavirin: Ribavirin is genotoxic and mutagenic and should be considered a potential carcinogen. See REBETOL package insert for additional warnings relevant to PEG-Intron therapy in combination with ribavirin.

Impairment of Fertility: PEG-Intron may impair human fertility. Irregular menstrual cycles were observed in female cynomolgus monkeys given subcutaneous injections of 4239 µg/m² PEG-Intron alone every other day for one month, (approximately 345 times the recommended weekly human dose based upon body surface area). These effects

Continued on next page

Peg-Intron—Cont.

included transiently decreased serum levels of estradiol and progesterone, suggestive of anovulation. Normal menstrual cycles and serum hormone levels resumed in these animals 2 to 3 months following cessation of PEG-Intron treatment. Every other day dosing with 262 µg/m^2 (approximately 21 times the weekly human dose) had no effects on cycle duration or reproductive hormone status. The effects of PEG-Intron on male fertility have not been studied.

Pregnancy Category C: PEG-Intron monotherapy: Non-pegylated Interferon alfa-2b, has been shown to have abortifacient effects in *Macaca mulatta* (rhesus monkeys) at 15 and 30 million IU/kg (estimated human equivalent of 5 and 10 million IU/kg, based on body surface area adjustment for a 60 kg adult). PEG-Intron should be assumed to also have abortifacient potential. There are no adequate and well-controlled studies in pregnant women. PEG-Intron therapy is to be used during pregnancy only if the potential benefit justifies the potential risk to the fetus. Therefore, PEG-Intron is recommended for use in fertile women only when they are using effective contraception during the treatment period.

Nursing Mothers: It is not known whether the components of PEG-Intron are excreted in human milk. Because of the potential for adverse reactions from the drug in nursing infants, a decision must be made whether to discontinue nursing or discontinue the treatment, taking into account the importance of the product to the mother.

Pregnancy Category X: Use with Ribavirin

Significant teratogenic and/or embryocidal effects have been demonstrated in all animal species exposed to ribavirin. REBETOL therapy is contraindicated in women who are pregnant and in the male partners of women who are pregnant. See CONTRAINDICATIONS and the REBETOL Package Insert.

If pregnancy occurs in a patient or partner of a patient during treatment with PEG-Intron and REBETOL during the 6 months after treatment cessation, physicians should report such cases by calling (800) 727-7064.

Pediatric. Safety and effectiveness in pediatric patients below the age of 18 years have not been established.

Geriatric. In general, younger patients tend to respond better than older patients to interferon-based therapies. Clinical studies of PEG-Intron alone or in combination with REBETOL did not include sufficient numbers of subjects aged 65 and over, however, to determine whether they respond differently than younger subjects. Treatment with alpha interferons, including PEG-Intron, is associated with neuropsychiatric, cardiac, pulmonary, GI and systemic (flu-like) adverse effects. Because these adverse reactions may be more severe in the elderly, caution should be exercised in use of PEG-Intron in this population. This drug is known to be substantially excreted by the kidney. Because elderly patients are more likely to have decreased renal function, the risk of toxic reactions to this drug may be greater in patients with impaired renal function. REBETOL should not be used in patients with creatinine clearance <50 mL/min. When using PEG-Intron/REBETOL therapy, refer also to the REBETOL Medication Guide.

ADVERSE REACTIONS

Nearly all study patients in clinical trials experienced one or more adverse events. In the PEG monotherapy trial the incidence of serious adverse events was similar (about 12%) in all treatment groups. In the PEG-Intron/REBETOL combination trial the incidence of serious adverse events was 17% in the PEG-Intron/REBETOL groups compared to 14% in the INTRON A/REBETOL group.

In many but not all cases, adverse events resolved after dose reduction or discontinuation of therapy. Some patients experienced ongoing or new serious adverse events during the 6-month follow-up period. In the PEG-Intron/REBETOL trial 13 patients experienced life-threatening psychiatric events (suicidal ideation or attempt) and one patient accomplished suicide.

There have been five patient deaths which occurred in clinical trials: one suicide in a patient receiving PEG-Intron monotherapy and one suicide in a patient receiving PEG-Intron/REBETOL combination therapy; two deaths among patients receiving INTRON A monotherapy (1 murder/suicide and 1 sudden death) and one patient death in the INTRON A/REBETOL group (motor vehicle accident).

Overall 10–14% of patients receiving PEG-Intron, alone or in combination with REBETOL, discontinued therapy compared with 6% treated with INTRON A alone and 13% treated with INTRON A in combination with REBETOL. The most common reasons for discontinuation of therapy were related to psychiatric, systemic (e.g. fatigue, headache), or gastrointestinal adverse events.

In the combination therapy trial, dose reductions due to adverse reactions occurred in 42% of patients receiving PEG-Intron (1.5 µg/kg)/REBETOL and in 34% of those receiving INTRON A/REBETOL. The majority of patients (57%) weighing 60 kg or less receiving PEG-Intron (1.5 µg/kg)/REBETOL required dose reduction. Reduction of interferon was dose related (PEG-Intron 1.5 µg/kg >PEG-Intron 0.5 µg/kg or INTRON A), 40%, 27%, 28%, respectively. Dose reduction for REBETOL was similar across all three groups, 33–35%. The most common reasons for dose modifications were neutropenia (18%), or anemia (9%). (see **Laboratory Values**). Other common reasons included depression, fatigue, nausea, and thrombocytopenia.

In the PEG-Intron/REBETOL combination trial the most common adverse events were psychiatric which occurred among 77% of patients and included most commonly depression, irritability, and insomnia, each reported by approximately 30-40% of subjects in all treatment groups. Suicidal behavior (ideation, attempts, and suicides) occurred in 2% of all patients during treatment or during follow-up after treatment cessation (see **WARNINGS**).

PEG-Intron induced fatigue or headache in approximately two-thirds of patients, and induced fever or rigors in approximately half of the patients. The severity of some of these systemic symptoms (e.g. fever and headache) tended to decrease as treatment continues. The incidence tends to be higher with PEG-Intron than with INTRON A therapy alone or in combination with REBETOL.

Application site inflammation and reaction (e.g. bruise, itchiness, irritation) occurred at approximately twice the incidence with PEG-Intron therapies (in up to 75% of patients) compared with INTRON A. However injection site pain was infrequent (2–3%) in all groups.

Other common adverse events in the PEG-Intron/REBETOL group included myalgia (56%), arthralgia (34%), nausea (43%), anorexia (32%), weight loss (29%), alopecia (36%), and pruritus (29%).

In the PEG-Intron monotherapy trial the incidence of severe adverse events was 13% in the INTRON A group and 17% in the PEG-Intron groups. In the PEG-Intron/REBETOL combination therapy trial the incidence of severe adverse events was 23% in the INTRON A/REBETOL group and 31–34% in the PEG-Intron/REBETOL groups. The incidence of life-threatening adverse events was ≤1% across all groups in the monotherapy and combination therapy trials.

Adverse events that occurred in the clinical trial at >5% incidence are provided in **Table 3** by treatment group. Due to potential differences in ascertainment procedures, adverse event rate comparisons across studies should not be made.

[See table 3 on next page]

Many patients continued to experience adverse events several months after discontinuation of therapy. By the end of the 6-month follow-up period the incidence of ongoing adverse events by body class in the PEG-Intron 1.5/REBETOL group was 33% (psychiatric), 20% (musculoskeletal), and 10% (for endocrine and for GI). In approximately 10–15% of patients weight loss, fatigue and headache had not resolved.

Individual serious adverse events occurred at a frequency ≤1% and included suicide attempt, suicidal ideation, severe depression; psychosis, aggressive reaction, relapse of drug addiction/overdose; nerve palsy (facial, oculomotor); cardiomyopathy, myocardial infarction, angina, pericardial effusion, retinal ischemia, retinal artery or vein thrombosis, blindness, decreased visual acuity, optic neuritis, transient ischemic attack, supraventricular arrhythmias, loss of consciousness; neutropenia, infection (sepsis, pneumonia, abscess, cellulitis); emphysema, bronchiolitis obliterans, pleural effusion, gastroenteritis, pancreatitis, gout, hyperglycemia, hyperthyroidism and hypothyroidism, autoimmune thrombocytopenia with or without purpura, rheumatoid arthritis, interstitial nephritis, lupus-like syndrome, sarcoidosis, aggravated psoriasis; urticaria, injection-site necrosis, vasculitis, phototoxicity.

Laboratory Values

Changes in selected laboratory values during treatment with PEG-Intron alone or in combination with REBETOL treatment are described below. **Decreases in hemoglobin, neutrophils, and platelets may require dose reduction or permanent discontinuation from therapy. (See DOSAGE AND ADMINISTRATION-Dose Reduction)**

Hemoglobin. REBETOL induced a decrease in hemoglobin levels in approximately two thirds of patients. Hemoglobin levels decreased to <11 g/dL in about 30% of patients. Severe anemia (<8 g/dL) occurred in <1% of patients. Dose modification was required in 9 and 13% of patients in the PEG-Intron/REBETOL and INTRON A/REBETOL groups. Hemoglobin levels become stable by treatment week 4–6 on average. Hemoglobin levels return to baseline between 4 and 12 weeks posttreatment. In the PEG-Intron monotherapy trial hemoglobin decreases were generally mild and dose modifications were rarely necessary. **(See DOSAGE AND ADMINISTRATION: Dose Reduction).**

Neutrophils. Decreases in neutrophil counts were observed in a majority of patients treated with PEG-Intron alone (70%) or as combination therapy with REBETOL (85%) and INTRON A/REBETOL (60%). Severe potentially life-threatening neutropenia (<0.5 × 10^9/L) occurred in 1% of patients treated with PEG-Intron monotherapy, 2% of patients treated with INTRON A/REBETOL and in 4% of patients treated with PEG-Intron/REBETOL. Two percent of patients receiving PEG-Intron monotherapy and 18% of patients receiving PEG-Intron/REBETOL required modification of interferon dosage. Few patients (≤1%) required permanent discontinuation of treatment. Neutrophil counts generally return to pre-treatment levels within 4 weeks of cessation of therapy. **(See DOSAGE AND ADMINISTRATION: Dose Reduction).**

Platelets. Platelet counts decrease in approximately 20% of patients treated with PEG-Intron alone or with REBETOL and in 6% of patients treated with INTRON A/REBETOL. Severe decreases in platelet counts (<50,000/mm^3) occur in <1% of patients. Patients may require discontinuation or dose modification as a result of platelet decreases. **(See DOSAGE AND ADMINISTRATION: Dose Reduction).** In the PEG-Intron/REBETOL combination therapy trial 1% or 3% of patients required dose modification of INTRON A or PEG-Intron respectively. Platelet counts generally returned to pretreatment levels within 4 weeks of the cessation of therapy.

Thyroid Function. Development of TSH abnormalities, with and without clinical manifestations, are associated with interferon therapies. Clinically apparent thyroid disorders occur among patients treated with either INTRON A or PEG-Intron (with or without REBETOL) at a similar incidence (5% for hypothyroidism and 3% for hyperthyroidism). Subjects developed new onset TSH abnormalities while on treatment and during the follow-up period. At the end of the follow-up period 7% of subjects still had abnormal TSH values.

Bilirubin and uric acid. In the PEG-Intron/REBETOL trial 10–14% of patients developed hyperbilirubinemia and 33–38% developed hyperuricemia in association with hemolysis. Six patients developed mild to moderate gout.

Postmarketing Experience

The following adverse reactions have been identified and reported during post-approval use of PEG-Intron therapy: seizures, hearing impairment, hearing loss, and peripheral neuropathy, cardiac ischemia, rhabdomyolysis, stomatitis, vertigo, renal insufficiency, renal failure, Stevens Johnson Syndrome, toxic epidermal necrolysis, and erythema multiforme. Because the reports of these reactions are voluntary and the population of uncertain size, it is not always possible to reliably estimate the frequency of the reaction or establish a causal relationship to drug exposure.

Immunogenicity: Approximately 2% of patients receiving PEG-Intron (32/1759) or INTRON A (11/728) with or without REBETOL developed low-titer (≤160) neutralizing antibodies to PEG-Intron or INTRON A. The clinical and pathological significance of the appearance of serum neutralizing antibodies is unknown. No apparent correlation of antibody development to clinical response or adverse events was observed. The incidence of post-treatment binding antibody ranged from 8 to 15 percent. The data reflect the percentage of patients whose test results were considered positive for antibodies to PEG-Intron in a Biacore assay that is used to measure binding antibodies, and in an antiviral neutralization assay, which measures serum-neutralizing antibodies. The percentage of patients whose test results were considered positive for antibodies is highly dependent on the sensitivity and specificity of the assays. Additionally the observed incidence of antibody positivity in these assays may be influenced by several factors including sample timing and handling, concomitant medications, and underlying disease. For these reasons, comparison of the incidence of antibodies to PEG-Intron with the incidence of antibodies to other products may be misleading.

OVERDOSAGE

There is limited experience with overdosage. In the clinical studies, a few patients accidentally received a dose greater than that prescribed. There were no instances in which a participant in the monotherapy or combination therapy trials received more than 10.5 times the intended dose of PEG-Intron. The maximum dose received by any patient was 3.45 µg/kg weekly over a period of approximately 12 weeks. The maximum known overdosage of REBETOL was an intentional ingestion of 10 g (fifty 200 mg capsules). There were no serious reactions attributed to these overdosages. In cases of overdosing, symptomatic treatment and close observation of the patient are recommended.

DOSAGE AND ADMINISTRATION

There are no safety and efficacy data on treatment for longer than one year. A patient should self-inject PEG-Intron only if the physician determines that it is appropriate and the patient agrees to medical follow-up as necessary and training in proper injection technique has been given to him/her. (See illustrated **MEDICATION GUIDE** for instructions.)

It is recommended that patients receiving PEG-Intron, alone or in combination with ribavirin, be discontinued from therapy if HCV viral levels remain high after 6 months of therapy.

PEG-Intron Monotherapy

The recommended dose of PEG-Intron regimen is 1.0 µg/kg/week subcutaneously for one year. The dose should be administered on the same day of the week.

The volume of PEG-Intron to be injected depends on the patient weight (see **Table 4** below).

[See table 4 at top of page 440]

PEG-Intron/REBETOL Combination Therapy

When administered in combination with REBETOL, the recommended dose of PEG-Intron is 1.5 micrograms/kg/week. The volume of PEG-Intron to be injected depends on the strength of PEG-Intron and patient's body weight. (See **Table 5** below).

[See table 5 at top of page 440]

The recommended dose of REBETOL is 800 mg/day in 2 divided doses: two capsules (400 mg) with breakfast and two capsules (400 mg) with dinner. REBETOL should not be used in patients with creatinine clearance <50 mL/min.

Dose Reduction

If a serious adverse reaction develops during the course of treatment (See **WARNINGS**) discontinue or modify the dosage of PEG-Intron and/or REBETOL until the adverse event abates or decreases in severity. If persistent or recurrent serious adverse events develop despite adequate dosage adjustment, discontinue treatment. For guidelines for dose modifications and discontinuation based on laboratory parameters, see **Tables 6 and 7**. In the combination therapy trial dose reductions occurred among 42% of patients receiving PEG-Intron 1.5 µg/kg/REBETOL 800 mg daily including 57% of those patients weighing 60 kg or less (see **ADVERSE REACTIONS**).

[See table 6 on next page]

[See table 7 on next page]

Preparation and Administration

PEG-Intron Redipen™

PEG-Intron Redipen™ consists of a dual-chamber glass cartridge with sterile, lyophilized peginterferon alfa-2b in the active chamber and Sterile Water for Injection, USP in the diluent chamber. The PEG-Intron in the glass cartridge should appear as a white to off-white tablet shaped solid that is whole or in pieces, or powder. To reconstitute the lyophilized peginterferon alfa-2b in the Redipen™, hold the Redipen™ upright (dose button down) and press the two halves of the pen together until there is an audible click. Gently invert the pen to mix the solution. DO NOT SHAKE. The reconstituted solution has a concentration of either 50 µg per 0.5 mL, 80 µg per 0.5 mL, 120 µg per 0.5 mL, or 150 µg per 0.5 mL for a single subcutaneous injection. Visually inspect the solution for particulate matter and discoloration prior to administration. The reconstituted solution should be clear and colorless. Do not use if the solution is discolored or cloudy, or if particulates are present.

Keeping the pen upright, attach the supplied needle and select the appropriate PEG-Intron dose by pulling back on the dosing button until the dark bands are visible and turning the button until the dark band is aligned with the correct dose. The prepared PEG-Intron solution is to be injected subcutaneously.

The PEG-Intron Redipen™ is a single use pen and does not contain a preservative. The reconstituted solution should be used immediately and cannot be stored for more than 24 hours at 2°–8°C (See **Storage**). **DO NOT REUSE THE REDIPEN™.** The sterility of any remaining product can no longer be guaranteed. **DISCARD THE UNUSED PORTION.** Pooling of unused portions of some medications has been linked to bacterial contamination and morbidity.

PEG-Intron Vials

Two B-D Safety-Lok™ syringes are provided in the package; one syringe is for the reconstitution steps and one for the patient injection. There is a plastic safety sleeve to be pulled over the needle after use. The syringe locks with an audible click when the green stripe on the safety sleeve covers the red stripe on the needle. Instructions for the preparation and administration of PEG-Intron Powder for Injection are provided below.

Reconstitute the PEG-Intron lyophilized product with only 0.7 mL of 1 mL of supplied diluent (Sterile Water for Injection, USP). **The diluent vial is for single use only. The remaining diluent should be discarded.** No other medications should be added to solutions containing PEG-Intron, and PEG-Intron should not be reconstituted with other diluents. Swirl gently to hasten complete dissolution of the powder. The reconstituted solution should be clear and colorless. Visually inspect the solution for particulate matter and discoloration prior to administration. The solution should not be used if discolored or cloudy, or if particulates are present.

The appropriate PEG-Intron dose should be withdrawn and injected subcutaneously. PEG-Intron vials are for single use only and do not contain a preservative. The reconstituted solution should be used immediately and cannot be stored for more than 24 hours at 2°–8°C (See **Storage**). **DO NOT REUSE THE VIAL.** The sterility of any remaining product can no longer be guaranteed. **DISCARD THE UNUSED PORTION.** Pooling of unused portions of some medications has been linked to bacterial contamination and morbidity.

After preparation and administration of the PEG-Intron for injection, it is essential to follow the state and or local procedures for proper disposal of syringes, needles, and the Redipen™. A puncture-resistant container should be used for disposal. Patients should be instructed in how to properly dispose of used syringes, needles, or the Redipen™ and be cautioned against the reuse of these items.

Storage

PEG-Intron Redipen™

PEG-Intron Redipen™ should be stored at 2° to 8°C (36° to 46°F). After reconstitution, the solution should be used immediately, but may be stored up to 24 hours at 2° to 8°C (36° to 46°F). The reconstituted solution contains no preservative, and is clear and colorless. **DO NOT FREEZE.**

PEG-Intron Vials

PEG-Intron should be stored at 25°C (77°F); excursions permitted to 15°–30°C (59°–86°F) [see USP Controlled Room Temperature]. After reconstitution with supplied Diluent the solution should be used immediately, but may be stored up to 24 hours at 2° to 8°C (36° to 46°F). The reconstituted solution contains no preservative, is clear and colorless. **DO NOT FREEZE.**

TABLE 3. Adverse Events Occurring in >5% of Patients

Adverse Events	*Percentage of Patients Reporting Adverse Events** Study 1: PEG-Intron 1.0 µg/kg (n=297)	Study 1: INTRON A 3 MIU (n=303)	Study 2: PEG-Intron 1.5 µg/kg/ REBETOL (n=511)	Study 2: INTRON A/ REBETOL (n=505)
Application Site				
Injection Site Inflammation/Reaction	47	20	75	49
Autonomic Nervous Sys.				
Mouth Dry	6	7	12	8
Sweating Increased	6	7	11	7
Flushing	6	3	4	3
Body as a Whole				
Fatigue/Asthenia	52	54	66	63
Headache	56	52	62	58
Rigors	23	19	48	41
Fever	22	12	46	33
Weight Decrease	11	13	29	20
RUQ Pain	8	8	12	6
Chest Pain	6	4	8	7
Malaise	7	6	4	6
Central/Periph. Nerv. Sys.				
Dizziness	12	10	21	17
Endocrine Disorders				
Hypothyroidism	5	3	5	4
Gastrointestinal				
Nausea	26	20	43	33
Anorexia	20	17	32	27
Diarrhea	18	16	22	17
Vomiting	7	6	14	12
Abdominal Pain	15	11	13	13
Dyspepsia	6	7	9	8
Constipation	1	3	5	5
Hematologic Disorders				
Neutropenia	6	2	26	14
Anemia	0	0	12	17
Leukopenia	<1	0	6	5
Thrombocytopenia	7	<1	5	2
Liver and Biliary System				
Hepatomegaly	6	5	4	4
Musculoskeletal				
Myalgia	54	53	56	50
Arthralgia	23	27	34	28
Musculoskeletal Pain	28	22	21	19
Psychiatric				
Insomnia	23	23	40	41
Depression	29	25	31	34
Anxiety/Emotional Lability/Irritability	28	34	47	47
Concentration Impaired	10	8	17	21
Agitation	2	2	8	5
Nervousness	4	3	6	6
Reproductive, Female				
Menstrual Disorder	4	3	7	6
Resistance Mechanism				
Infection Viral	11	10	12	12
Infection Fungal	<1	3	6	1
Respiratory System				
Dyspnea	4	2	26	24
Coughing	8	5	23	16
Pharyngitis	10	7	12	13
Rhinitis	2	2	8	6
Sinusitis	7	7	6	5
Skin and Appendages				
Alopecia	22	22	36	32
Pruritus	12	8	29	28
Rash	6	7	24	23
Skin Dry	11	9	24	23
Special Senses Other,				
Taste Perversion	<1	2	9	4
Vision Disorders				
Vision blurred	2	3	5	6
Conjunctivitis	4	2	4	5

* Patients reporting one or more adverse events. A patient may have reported more than one adverse event within a body system/organ class category.

HOW SUPPLIED

PEG-Intron Redipen™

PEG-Intron Redipen™ contains a dual-chamber glass cartridge with a white to off-white lyophilized powder active chamber and a sterile diluent chamber with Sterile Water for Injection, USP for subcutaneous use.

Each PEG-Intron Redipen™ Package Contains:	
A box containing one 50 µg per 0.5 mL PEG-Intron Redipen™ and 1 B-D needle and 2 alcohol swabs.	(NDC 0085-1323-01)
A box containing one 80 µg per 0.5 mL PEG-Intron Redipen™ and 1 B-D needle and 2 alcohol swabs.	(NDC 0085-1316-01)
A box containing one 120 µg per 0.5 mL PEG-Intron Redipen™ and 1 B-D needle and 2 alcohol swabs.	(NDC 0085-1297-01)
A box containing one 150 µg per 0.5 mL PEG-Intron Redipen™ and 1 B-D needle and 2 alcohol swabs.	(NDC 0085-1370-01)

PEG-Intron Vials

PEG-Intron is a white to off-white lyophilized powder supplied in 2-mL vials. The PEG-Intron Powder for Injection should be reconstituted with 0.7 mL of the supplied Diluent (Sterile Water for Injection, USP) prior to use.

Continued on next page

Peg-Intron—Cont.

Each PEG-Intron Package Contains:	
A box containing one 50 µg per 0.5 mL vial of PEG-Intron Powder for Injection and one 1 mL vial of Diluent (Sterile Water for Injection, USP), 2 B-D Safety-Lok™* syringes with a safety sleeve and 2 alcohol swabs.	(NDC 0085-1368-01)
A box containing one 80 µg per 0.5 mL vial of PEG-Intron Powder for Injection and one 1 mL vial of Diluent (Sterile Water for Injection, USP), 2 B-D Safety-Lok™* syringes with a safety sleeve and 2 alcohol swabs.	(NDC 0085-1291-01)
A box containing one 120 µg per 0.5 mL vial of PEG-Intron Powder for Injection and one 1 mL vial of Diluent (Sterile Water for Injection, USP), 2 B-D Safety-Lok™*syringes with a safety sleeve and 2 alcohol swabs.	(NDC 0085-1304-01)
A box containing one 150 µg per 0.5 mL vial of PEG-Intron Powder for Injection and one 1 mL vial of Diluent (Sterile Water for Injection, USP), 2 B-D Safety-Lok™*syringes with a safety sleeve and 2 alcohol swabs.	(NDC 0085-1279-01)

Schering Corporation
Kenilworth, NJ 07033 USA

Rev. 10/03 27664407T

*Safety-Lok is a trademark of Becton Dickinson and Company.

MEDICATION GUIDE
PEG-Intron® Redipen™
Single-dose
Delivery System
(Peginterferon alfa-2b)
Including appendix with instructions for using PEG-Intron® Redipen™ Single-dose Delivery System

Read this Medication Guide carefully before you start taking PEG-Intron (**Peg In-tron**) or PEG-Intron/REBETOL (**REB-eh-tole**) combination therapy. Read the Medication Guide each time you refill your prescription because there may be new information. The information in this Medication Guide does not take the place of talking with your doctor.

If you are taking PEG-Intron/REBETOL combination therapy, also read the Medication Guide for REBETOL (ribavirin, USP) Capsules.

What is the most important information I should know about PEG-Intron and PEG-Intron/REBETOL combination therapy?

PEG-Intron (peginterferon) is a treatment for some people who are infected with hepatitis C virus. However, PEG-Intron and PEG-Intron/ REBETOL combination therapy can have serious side effects that may cause death in rare cases. Before you decide to start treatment, you should talk to your doctor about the possible benefits and side effects of PEG-Intron or PEG-Intron/REBETOL combination therapy. If you begin treatment you will need to see your doctor regularly for medical examinations and lab tests to make sure your treatment is working and to check for side effects.

REBETOL capsules may cause birth defects and/or death of an unborn child. If you are pregnant, you or your male partner must not take PEG-Intron/ REBETOL combination therapy. You must not become pregnant while either you or your partner are being treated with the combination PEG-Intron/ REBETOL therapy, or for 6 months after stopping therapy. Men and women should use birth control while taking the combination therapy and for 6 months afterwards. If you or your partner are being treated and you become pregnant either during treatment or within 6 months of stopping treatment, call your doctor right away.

If you are taking PEG-Intron or PEG-Intron/REBETOL therapy you should call your doctor immediately if you develop any of these symptoms:

New or worsening mental health problems such as thoughts about killing or hurting yourself or others, trouble breathing, chest pain, severe stomach or lower back pain, bloody diarrhea or bloody bowel movements, high fever, bruising, bleeding, or decreased vision.

The most serious possible side effects of PEG-Intron and PEG-Intron/REBETOL therapy include:

Problems with Pregnancy. Combination PEG-Intron/ REBETOL therapy can cause death, serious birth defects, or other harm to your unborn child. If you are a woman of childbearing age you must not become pregnant during treatment and for 6 months after you have stopped therapy. You must have a negative pregnancy test immediately before beginning treatment, during treatment, and for 6 months after you have stopped therapy. Both male and female patients must use effective forms of birth control during treatment and for the 6 months after treatment is completed. Male patients should use a condom. If you are a female, you must use birth control even if you believe that you are not fertile or that your fertility is low. You should talk to your doctor about birth control for you and your partner.

Mental health problems and suicide. PEG-Intron and PEG-Intron/REBETOL therapies may cause patients to develop mood or behavioral problems. These can include irritability (getting easily upset) and depression (feeling low, feeling bad about yourself, or feeling hopeless). Some patients may have aggressive behavior. Former drug addicts may fall back into drug addiction or overdose. Some patients think about hurting or killing themselves or other people and some have killed (suicide) or hurt themselves or others. You must tell your doctor if you are being treated for a mental illness or had treatment in the past for any mental illness, including depression and suicidal behavior. You should tell your doctor if you have ever been addicted to drugs or alcohol.

Heart problems. Some patients taking PEG-Intron or PEG-Intron/REBETOL therapy may develop problems with their heart, including low blood pressure, fast heart rate, and very rarely, heart attacks. Tell your doctor if you have had any heart problems in the past.

Blood problems. PEG-Intron and PEG-Intron/REBETOL therapies commonly lower two types of blood cells (white blood cells and platelets). In some patients, these blood counts may fall to dangerously low levels. If your blood counts become very low, this could lead to infections or bleeding.

REBETOL therapy causes a decrease in the number of red blood cells you have (anemia). This can be dangerous, espe-

TABLE 4. Recommended PEG-Intron Monotherapy Dosing

Body weight (kg)	PEG-Intron Redipen™ or Vial Strength to Use	Amount of PEG-Intron (µg) to Administer	Volume (mL)* of PEG-Intron to Administer
≤45 46–56	50 µg per 0.5 mL	40 50	0.4 0.5
57–72 73–88	80 µg per 0.5 mL	64 80	0.4 0.5
89–106 107–136	120 µg per 0.5 mL	96 120	0.4 0.5
137–160	150 µg per 0.5 mL	150	0.5

* When reconstituted as directed

TABLE 5. Recommended PEG-Intron Combination Therapy Dosing

Body weight (kg)	PEG-Intron Redipen™ or Vial Strength to Use	Amount of PEG-Intron (µg) to Administer	Volume (mL)* of PEG-Intron to Administer
<40	50 µg per 0.5 mL	50	0.5
40–50 51–60	80 µg per 0.5 mL	64 80	0.4 0.5
61–75 76–85	120 µg per 0.5 mL	96 120	0.4 0.5
>85	150 µg per 0.5 mL	150	0.5

* When reconstituted as directed

TABLE 6. Guidelines for Modification or Discontinuation of PEG-Intron or PEG-Intron/REBETOL and for Scheduling Visits for Patients with Depression

Depression Severity[1]	Initial Management (4–8 wks)		Depression		
	Dose modification	Visit schedule	Remains stable	Improves	Worsens
Mild	No change	Evaluate once weekly by visit and/or phone.	Continue weekly visit schedule.	Resume normal visit schedule.	(See moderate or severe depression)
Moderate	Decrease IFN dose 50%	Evaluate once weekly (office visit at least every other week).	Consider psychiatric consultation. Continue reduced dosing.	If symptoms improve and are stable for 4 wks, may resume normal visit schedule. Continue reducing dosing or return to normal dose.	(See severe depression)
Severe	Discontinue IFN/R permanently.	Obtain immediate psychiatric consultation.	Psychiatric therapy necessary		

[1]See DSM-IV for definitions

TABLE 7. Guidelines for Dose Modification and Discontinuation of PEG-Intron or PEG-Intron/REBETOL for Hematologic Toxicity

Laboratory Values		PEG-Intron	REBETOL
Hgb*	<10.0 g/dL <8.5 g/dL	---------------------- Permanently discontinue	Decrease by 200 mg/day Permanently discontinue
WBC	$<1.5 \times 10^9$/L $<1.0 \times 10^9$/L	Reduce dose by 50% Permanently discontinue	---------------------- Permanently discontinue
Neutrophils	$<0.75 \times 10^9$/L $<0.5 \times 10^9$/L	Reduce dose by 50% Permanently discontinue	---------------------- Permanently discontinue
Platelets	$<80 \times 10^9$/L $<50 \times 10^9$/L	Reduce dose by 50% Permanently discontinue	---------------------- Permanently discontinue

* For patients with a history of stable cardiac disease receiving PEG-Intron in combination with ribavirin, the PEG-Intron dose should be reduced by half and the ribavirin dose by 200 mg/day if a >2g/dL decrease in hemoglobin is observed during any 4 week period. Both PEG-Intron and ribavirin should be permanently discontinued if patients have hemoglobin levels <12 g/dL after this ribavirin dose reduction.

cially for patients who already have heart or circulatory (cardiovascular) problems. Talk with your doctor before taking combination PEG-Intron/REBETOL therapy if you have or have ever had any cardiovascular problems.

Body organ problems. Certain symptoms like severe stomach pain may mean that your internal organs are being damaged.

For other possible side effects, see "What are the possible side effects of PEG-Intron and PEG-Intron/REBETOL" in this Medication Guide.

What is PEG-Intron and PEG-Intron/REBETOL combination therapy?

The PEG-Intron product is a drug used to treat adults who have a lasting (chronic) infection with hepatitis C virus and who show signs that the virus is damaging the liver.

PEG-Intron/REBETOL combination therapy consists of two medications also used to treat hepatitis C infection. Patients with hepatitis C have the virus in their blood and in their liver. PEG-Intron reduces the amount of virus in the body and helps the body's immune system fight the virus. REBETOL (ribavirin) is a drug that helps to fight the viral infection but does not work when used by itself to treat chronic hepatitis C.

It is not known if PEG-Intron or PEG-Intron/REBETOL therapies can cure hepatitis C (permanently eliminate the virus) or if it can prevent liver failure or liver cancer that is caused by hepatitis C infection.

It is also not known if PEG-Intron or PEG-Intron/REBETOL combination therapy will prevent one infected person from infecting another person with hepatitis C.

Who should not take PEG-Intron or PEG-Intron/REBETOL therapy?

Do not take PEG-Intron or PEG-Intron/REBETOL therapy if you:

- are pregnant, planning to get pregnant during treatment or during the 6 months after treatment, or breast-feeding.
- are a male patient with a female sexual partner who is pregnant or plans to become pregnant at any time while you are being treated with REBETOL or during the 6 months after your treatment has ended.
- have hepatitis caused by your immune system attacking your liver (autoimmune hepatitis) or unstable liver disease.
- had an allergic reaction to another alpha interferon or are allergic to any of the ingredients in PEG-Intron or REBETOL Capsules. If you have any doubts, ask your doctor.
- Do not take PEG-Intron/REBETOL combination therapy if you have abnormal red blood cells such as sickle-cell anemia or thalassemia major.

If you have any of the following conditions or serious medical problems, discuss them with your doctor before taking PEG-Intron or PEG-Intron/REBETOL therapy:

- depression or anxiety
- sleep problems
- high blood pressure
- previous heart attack, or other heart problems
- liver problems (other than hepatitis C infection)
- any kind of autoimmune disease (where the body's immune system attacks the body's own cells), such as psoriasis, systemic lupus erythematosus, rheumatoid arthritis
- thyroid problems
- diabetes
- colitis (inflammation of the bowels)
- cancer
- hepatitis B infection
- HIV infection
- kidney problems
- bleeding problems
- alcoholism
- drug abuse or addiction
- body organ transplant and are taking medicine that keeps your body from rejecting your transplant (suppresses your immune system).

How should I take PEG-Intron or PEG-Intron/REBETOL?

Your doctor will decide whether you will take PEG-Intron therapy alone or the combination of PEG-Intron/REBETOL, as well as the correct dose (based on your weight). PEG-Intron and PEG-Intron/REBETOL are given for one year. Take your prescribed dose of PEG-Intron once a week, on the same day of each week and at approximately the same time. Take the medicine for the full year and do not take more than the prescribed dose. REBETOL Capsules should be taken with food. When you take REBETOL with food, more of the medicine (70% more on average) is taken up by your body. You should take REBETOL the same way every day (twice a day with food) to keep the medicine in your body at a steady level. This will help your doctor to decide how your treatment is working and how to change the number of REBETOL capsules you take if you have side effects from REBETOL. **Be sure to read the Medication Guide for REBETOL (ribavirin, USP) for complete instructions on how to take the REBETOL capsules.**

You should be completely comfortable with how to prepare PEG-Intron; how to set the dose you take; and how to inject yourself before you use PEG-Intron for the first time. PEG-Intron comes in two different forms, a powder in a single-use vial and a Redipen™ single-use delivery system. See the attached appendix for detailed instructions for preparing and giving a dose of PEG-Intron.

If you miss a dose of the PEG-Intron product, take the missed dose as soon as possible during the same day or the next day, then continue on your regular dosing schedule. If several days go by after you miss a dose, check with your doctor about what to do. Do not double the next dose or take more than one dose a week without talking to your doctor. Call your doctor right away if you take more than your prescribed PEG-Intron dose. Your doctor may wish to examine you more closely, and take blood for testing.

If you miss a dose of REBETOL capsules, take the missed dose as soon as possible during the same day. If an entire day has gone by, check with your doctor about what to do. Do not double the next dose.

You must get regular blood tests to help your doctor check how the treatment is working and to check for side effects. Tell your doctor if you are taking or planning to take other prescription or non-prescription medicines, including vitamin and mineral supplements and herbal medicines.

What should I avoid while taking PEG-Intron or PEG-Intron/REBETOL therapies?

- If you are pregnant do not start taking PEG-Intron/REBETOL combination therapy.
- Avoid becoming pregnant while taking PEG-Intron or PEG-Intron/REBETOL.

PEG-Intron and PEG-Intron/REBETOL may harm your unborn child (death or serious birth defects) or cause you to lose your baby (miscarry). **If you or your partner become pregnant during treatment or during the 6 months after treatment with PEG-Intron/REBETOL combination therapy, immediately report the pregnancy to your doctor. You or your doctor should call (800) 727-7064.** By calling this number, information about you and/or your partner will be added to a pregnancy registry that will be used to help you and your doctor make decisions about your treatment for hepatitis in the future. You, your partner and/or your physician will be asked to provide follow-up information on the outcome of the pregnancy.

- Do not breast-feed your baby while taking PEG-Intron.

What are the possible side effects of PEG-Intron and PEG-Intron/REBETOL combination therapy?

Possible, serious side effects include:

Mental health problems including suicide, blood problems, heart problems, body organ problems. See "What is the most important information I should know about PEG-Intron and PEG-Intron/REBETOL combination therapy?"

Other body organ problems. A few patients have lung problems (such as pneumonia or inflammation of the lung tissue), inflammation of the kidney, and eye disorders.

New or worsening autoimmune disease. Some patients taking PEG-Intron or PEG-Intron/REBETOL develop autoimmune diseases (a condition where the body's immune cells attack other cells or organs in the body), including rheumatoid arthritis, systemic lupus erythematosus, and psoriasis. In some patients who already have an autoimmune disease, the disease worsens on PEG-Intron and PEG-Intron/REBETOL combination therapy.

Common but less serious side effects include:

Flu-like symptoms. Most patients who take PEG-Intron or PEG-Intron/REBETOL therapy have "flu-like" symptoms (headache, muscle aches, tiredness and fever). Some of these symptoms (fever, headache) usually lessen after the first few weeks of therapy. You can reduce some of these symptoms by injecting your PEG-Intron dose at bedtime. Over-the-counter pain and fever reducers, such as acetaminophen or ibuprofen, can be used to prevent or reduce the fever and headache.

Extreme fatigue (tiredness). Many patients become extremely tired while on PEG-Intron or PEG-Intron/REBETOL combination therapy.

Appetite problems. Nausea, loss of appetite, and weight loss, occur commonly.

Thyroid problems. Some patients develop changes in the function of their thyroid. Symptoms of thyroid changes include the inability to concentrate, feeling cold or hot all the time, a change in your weight and changes to your skin.

Blood sugar problems. Some patients develop problems with the way their body controls their blood sugar and may develop high blood sugar or diabetes.

Skin reactions. Redness, swelling, and itching are common at the site of injection. If after several days these symptoms do not disappear contact your doctor. You may get a rash during therapy. If this occurs, your doctor may recommend medicine to treat the rash.

Hair thinning. Hair thinning is common during PEG-Intron and PEG-Intron/ REBETOL treatment. Hair loss stops and hair growth returns after therapy is stopped.

These are not all of the side effects of PEG-Intron or PEG-Intron/REBETOL combination therapy. Your doctor or pharmacist can give you a more complete list.

General advice about prescription medicines:

Medicines are sometimes prescribed for purposes other than those listed in a Medication Guide. If you have any concerns about PEG-Intron, ask your doctor. Your doctor or pharmacist can give you information about PEG-Intron that was written for health care professionals. Do not use PEG-Intron for a condition for which it was not prescribed. Do not share this medication with other people.

If you are taking PEG-Intron/REBETOL combination therapy, also read the Medication Guide for REBETOL (ribavirin, USP) Capsules.

This Medication Guide has been approved by the U.S. Food and Drug Administration.

How do I prepare and inject the PEG-Intron Redipen™ Dose?

The PEG-Intron Redipen™ system is for a single use, by one person only. The Redipen™ must not be shared. Use only the injection needle provided in the packaging for the PEG-Intron Redipen™ system. If you have problems with the Redipen™ system or the PEG-Intron solution, you should contact your nurse, doctor, or pharmacist.

The following instructions explain how to prepare and inject yourself with the PEG-Intron Redipen™ system. Please read the instructions carefully and follow them step by step. Your health care provider will instruct you on how to self-inject with the PEG-Intron Redipen™. Do not attempt to inject yourself unless you are sure you understand the procedure and requirements for self-injection.

How to use the PEG-Intron Redipen™ single-dose delivery system.

Injection Needle

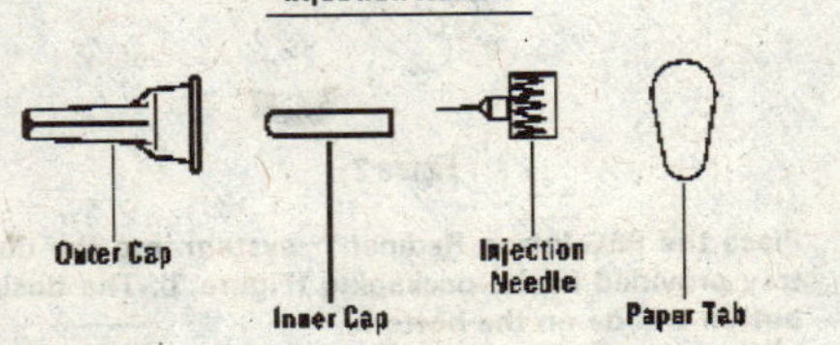

PEG-Intron Redipen™

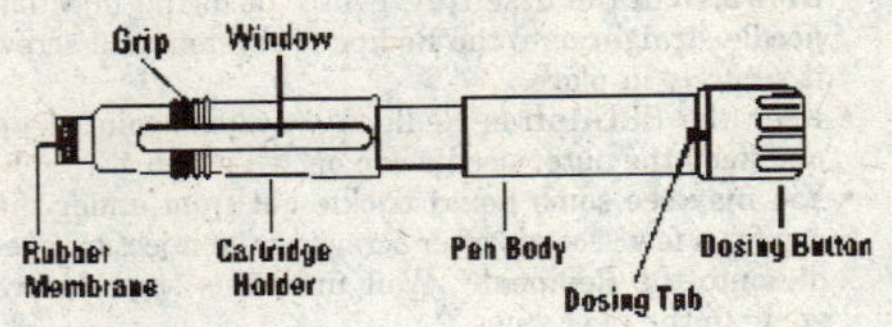

Storing PEG-Intron

PEG-Intron Redipen™ should be stored in the refrigerator at 2° to 8°C (36° to 46°F); avoid exposure to heat. After mixing, the PEG-Intron solution should be used immediately but may be stored in the refrigerator up to 24 hours at 2° to 8°C (36° to 46°F). The solution contains no preservatives. DO NOT FREEZE.

I: Preparation

1. Find a clean, well-lit, non-slip flat working surface and assemble all of the supplies you will need for an injection. All of the supplies you will need are in the PEG-Intron Redipen™ package. The package contains:
   - a PEG-Intron Redipen™ single-dose delivery system
   - one disposable needle
   - alcohol swabs, and
   - dose tray (the dose tray is the bottom half of the Redipen™ package)
2. Take the PEG-Intron Redipen™ system out of the refrigerator to allow the medicine to come to room temperature. Before removing the Redipen™ from the carton, check the expiration date printed on the PEG-Intron Redipen™ carton to make sure that the expiration date has not passed. Do not use if the expiration date has passed.
3. After taking the PEG-Intron Redipen™ system out of the carton, look in the window of the Redipen™ and make sure the PEG-Intron in the cartridge holder chamber is a white, to off-white tablet that is whole or in pieces or powder.
4. Wash your hands thoroughly with soap and water, rinse and towel dry. It is important to keep your work area, your hands, and injection site clean to minimize the risk of infection.

II: Mixing

Key points:

Before you mix the PEG-Intron, make sure it is at room temperature. It is important that you keep the PEG-Intron Redipen™ system UPRIGHT (dosing button down) as shown in Figure 1.

5. Hold the PEG-Intron Redipen™ system **UPRIGHT (Figure 1)** in the dose tray or on a flat non-slip surface with the dosing button down. You may want to hold the Redipen™ using the grip.
   - To mix the powder and the liquid, press the two halves of the pen together firmly until you hear the click.
   - Wait several seconds for the powder to completely dissolve.

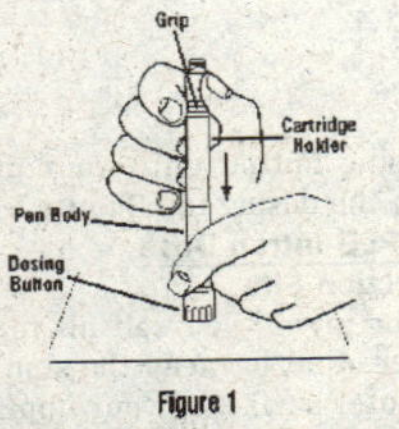

Figure 1

6. **Gently turn the PEG-Intron Redipen™ system upside down twice (Figure 2). To avoid excessive foaming, DO NOT SHAKE.**
   - Keeping the PEG-Intron Redipen™ system UPRIGHT, check through the Redipen™ window to see if the mixed PEG-Intron solution is completely dissolved. If there is still foam, wait until it settles. The solution should be clear, colorless, and without par-

Continued on next page

Peg-Intron—Cont.

ticles **before use**. It is normal to see some small bubbles near the top of the solution. Do not use if the solution is not clear, or if you see particles.

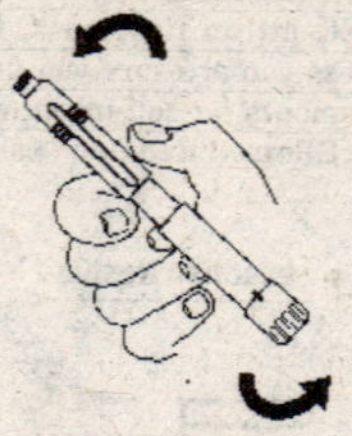

Figure 2

7. **Place the PEG-Intron Redipen™ system into the dose tray provided in the packaging (Figure 3). The dosing button will be on the bottom.**
   - Wipe the rubber membrane of the PEG-Intron Redipen™ system with one alcohol swab.
   - Remove the protective paper tab from the injection needle. Keeping the PEG-Intron Redipen™ system **UPRIGHT** in the dose tray, gently push the injection needle straight onto the Redipen™ system and screw it securely in place.
   - Keep the PEG-Intron Redipen™ system pointed up and keep the outer needle cap on.
   - You may see some liquid trickle out from under the cap for a few seconds after screwing the injection needle onto the Redipen™. Wait until this stops before going to the next step.

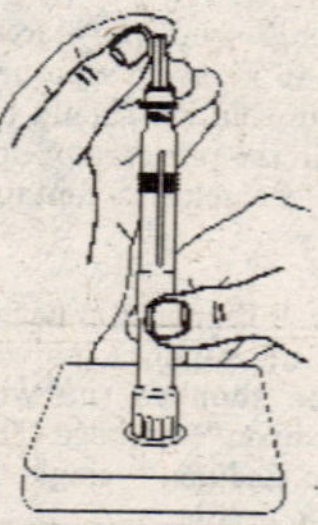

Figure 3

III: Setting the Dose

8. **Remove the PEG-Intron Redipen™ system from the dose tray (Figure 4).** Holding the PEG-Intron Redipen™ system firmly, pull the dosing button out as far as it will go, until you see the dark bands below the dosing button.

   Do not push the dosing button in until you are ready to self-inject the PEG-Intron dose.

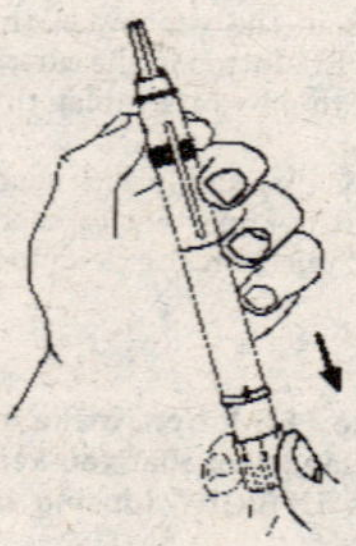

Figure 4

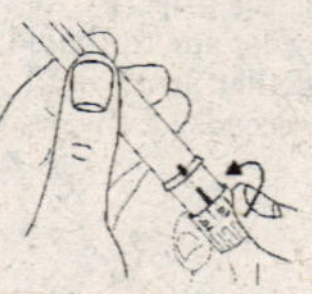

Figure 5

9. Turn the dosing button until your prescribed dose is lined up with the dosing tab (**Figure 5**).

IV: Injecting the PEG-Intron Dose

Choosing an Injection Site

The best sites for giving yourself an injection are those areas with a layer of fat between the skin and muscle, like your thigh, the outer surface of your upper arm, and abdomen. Do not inject yourself in the area near your navel or waistline. If you are very thin, you should only use the thigh or outer surface of the arm for injection.

You should use a different site each time you inject PEG-Intron to avoid soreness at any one site. Do not inject PEG-Intron into an area where the skin is irritated, red, bruised, infected, or has scars, stretch marks, or lumps.

10. Clean the skin where the injection is to be given with an alcohol swab, and wait for the area to dry.
11. Remove the outer cap from the needle (**Figure 6**). There may be some liquid around the inner needle cap. This is normal. Once the injection site is dry pull off the inner needle cap.

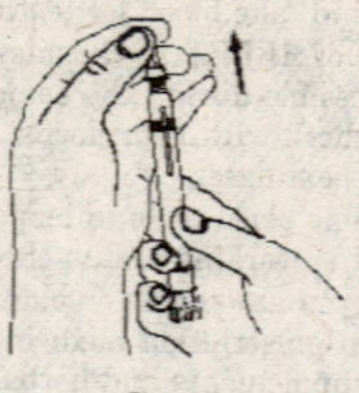

Figure 6

12. **Hold the PEG-Intron Redipen™ system with your fingers wrapped around the pen body barrel and your thumb on the dosing button (Figure 7).**
   - With your other hand, pinch the skin in the area you have cleaned for injection.
   - Insert the needle into the pinched skin at an angle of 45° to 90°.
   - Press the dosing button down slowly and firmly until you can't push it any further.
   - Keep your thumb pressed down on the dosing button for an additional 5 seconds to ensure that you get the complete dose.
   - Remove the needle from your skin.

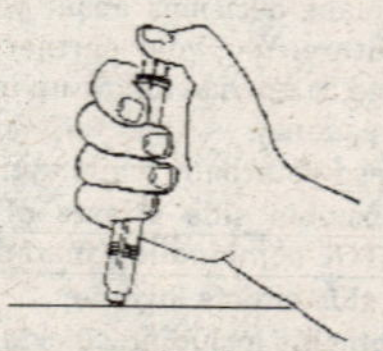

Figure 7

13. **Gently press the injection site with a small bandage or sterile gauze if necessary for a few seconds but** do not massage the injection site. If there is bleeding, cover with an adhesive bandage. Discard the PEG-Intron Redipen™ system with the needle still attached. DO NOT RECAP THE NEEDLE and DO NOT REUSE the Redipen™.
   - After 2 hours, check the injection site for redness, swelling, or tenderness. If you have a skin reaction and it doesn't clear up in a few days, contact your health care provider.

How do I dispose of the Redipen™?

Discard the Redipen™ system and needle and any solution remaining in the Redipen™ in a Sharps container or other puncture-proof container like a coffee can. DO NOT use glass or clear plastic containers. Your doctor or nurse will tell you how to dispose of a full container. Always keep the container out of reach of children.

Manufactured by:
Schering Corporation
Kenilworth, NJ 07033 USA
10/03 **27662404T**

REBETOL® ℞

[rĕ′bə-tōl]
(ribavirin, USP)
Capsules and Oral Solution

Prescribing information for this product, which appears on ages 3069–3073 of the 2004 PDR, has been completely revised as follows. Please write "See Supplement A" next to the product heading.

- **REBETOL monotherapy is not effective for the treatment of chronic hepatitis C virus infection and should not be used alone for this indication. (See WARNINGS).**
- **The primary toxicity of ribavirin is hemolytic anemia. The anemia associated with REBETOL therapy may result in worsening of cardiac disease that has led to fatal and nonfatal myocardial infarctions. Patients with a history of significant or unstable cardiac disease should not be treated with REBETOL. (See WARNINGS, ADVERSE REACTIONS and DOSAGE AND ADMINISTRATION).**
- **Significant teratogenic and/or embryocidal effects have been demonstrated in all animal species exposed to ribavirin. In addition, ribavirin has a multiple-dose half-life of 12 days, and so it may persist in nonplasma compartments for as long as 6 months. Therefore, REBETOL therapy is contraindicated in women who are pregnant and in the male partners of women who are pregnant. Extreme care must be taken to avoid pregnancy during therapy and for 6 months after completion of treatment in both female patients and in female partners of male patients who are taking REBETOL therapy. At least two reliable forms of effective contraception must be utilized during treatment and during the 6-month posttreatment follow-up-period. (See CONTRAINDICATIONS, WARNINGS, PRECAUTIONS—Information for Patients and Pregnancy Category X).**

DESCRIPTION

REBETOL®

REBETOL is Schering Corporation's brand name for ribavirin, a nucleoside analog. The chemical name of ribavirin is 1-β-D-ribofuranosyl-1*H*-1,2,4-triazole-3-carboxamide and has the following structural formula:

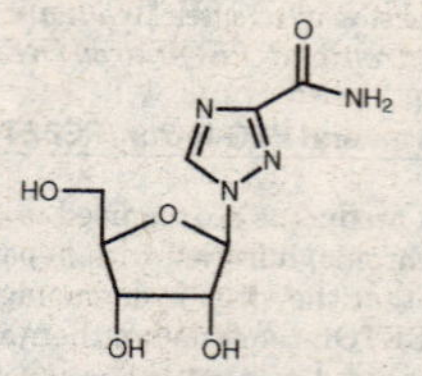

Ribavirin is a white, crystalline powder. It is freely soluble in water and slightly soluble in anhydrous alcohol. The empirical formula is $C_8H_{12}N_4O_5$ and the molecular weight is 244.21.

REBETOL Capsules consist of a white powder in a white, opaque, gelatin capsule. Each capsule contains 200 mg ribavirin and the inactive ingredients microcrystalline cellulose, lactose monohydrate, croscarmellose sodium, and magnesium stearate. The capsule shell consists of gelatin, sodium lauryl sulfate, silicon dioxide, and titanium dioxide. The capsule is printed with edible blue pharmaceutical ink which is made of shellac, anhydrous ethyl alcohol, isopropyl alcohol, n-butyl alcohol, propylene glycol, ammonium hydroxide, and FD&C Blue #2 aluminum lake.

REBETOL Oral Solution is a clear, colorless to pale or light yellow bubble gum-flavored liquid. Each milliliter of the solution contains 40 mg of ribavirin and the inactive ingredients sucrose, glycerin, sorbitol, propylene glycol, sodium citrate, citric acid, sodium benzoate, natural and artificial flavor for bubble gum #15864, and water.

Mechanism of Action

The mechanism of inhibition of hepatitis C virus (HCV) RNA by combination therapy with ribavirin and interferon products has not been established.

CLINICAL PHARMACOLOGY

Pharmacokinetics

Ribavirin Single- and multiple-dose pharmacokinetic properties in adults with chronic hepatitis C are summarized in **TABLE 1**. Ribavirin was rapidly and extensively absorbed following oral administration. However, due to first-pass metabolism, the absolute bioavailability averaged 64% (44%). There was a linear relationship between dose and AUC_{tf} (AUC from time zero to last measurable concentration) following single doses of 200–1200 mg ribavirin. The relationship between dose and C_{max} was curvilinear, tending to asymptote above single doses of 400–600 mg.

Upon multiple oral dosing, based on $AUC12_{hr}$, a sixfold accumulation of ribavirin was observed in plasma. Following oral dosing with 600 mg BID, steady-state was reached by approximately 4 weeks, with mean steady-state plasma concentrations of 2200 (37%) ng/mL. Upon discontinuation of dosing, the mean half-life was 298 (30%) hours, which probably reflects slow elimination from nonplasma compartments.

Effect of Food on Absorption of Ribavirin Both AUC_{tf} and C_{max} increased by 70% when REBETOL Capsules were administered with a high-fat meal (841 kcal, 53.8 g fat, 31.6 g protein, and 57.4 g carbohydrate) in a single-dose pharmacokinetic study. There are insufficient data to address the clinical relevance of these results. Clinical efficacy studies with REBETOL/INTRON A were conducted without instructions with respect to food consumption. During clinical studies with REBETOL/PEG-INTRON, all subjects were instructed to take REBETOL Capsules with food. (See **DOSAGE AND ADMINISTRATION**.)

Effect of Antacid on Absorption of Ribavirin Coadministration with an antacid containing magnesium, aluminum, and simethicone (Mylanta®[1]) resulted in a 14% decrease in mean ribavirin AUC_{tf}. The clinical relevance of results from this single-dose study is unknown.

TABLE 1. Mean (% CV) Pharmacokinetic Parameters for REBETOL When Administered Individually to Adults

Parameter	REBETOL		
	Single Dose 600 mg Oral Solution (N=14)	Single Dose 600 mg Capsules (N=12)	Multiple Dose 600 mg BID Capsules (N=12)
T_{max} (hr)	1.00(34)	1.7 (46)***	3 (60)
C_{max}*	872 (42)	782 (37)	3680 (85)
AUC_{tf}**	14098 (38)	13400 (48)	228000 (25)
$T_{½}$ (hr)		43.6 (47)	298 (30)
Apparent Volume of Distribution (L)		2825 (9)†	
Apparent Clearance (L/hr)		38.2 (40)	
Absolute Bioavailability		64% (44)††	

* ng/mL
** ng.hr/mL
*** N = 11
† data obtained from a single-dose pharmacokinetic study using ^{14}C labeled ribavirin; N = 5
†† N = 6

TABLE 3. Virologic and Histologic Responses: Previously Untreated Patients*

	US Study				International Study		
	24 weeks of treatment		48 weeks of treatment		24 weeks of treatment	48 weeks of treatment	
	INTRON A plus REBETOL (N=228)	INTRON A plus Placebo (N=231)	INTRON A plus REBETOL (N=228)	INTRON A plus Placebo (N=225)	INTRON A plus REBETOL (N=265)	INTRON A plus REBETOL (N=268)	INTRON A plus Placebo (N=266)
Virologic Response							
-Responder[1]	65 (29)	13 (6)	85 (37)	27 (12)	86 (32)	113 (42)	46 (17)
-Nonresponder	147 (64)	194 (84)	110 (48)	168 (75)	158 (60)	120 (45)	196 (74)
-Missing Data	16 (7)	24 (10)	33 (14)	30 (13)	21 (8)	35 (13)	24 (9)
Histologic Response							
-Improvement[1]	102 (45)	77 (33)	96 (42)	65 (29)	103 (39)	102 (38)	69 (26)
-No improvement	77 (34)	99 (43)	61 (27)	93 (41)	85 (32)	58 (22)	111 (41)
-Missing Data	49 (21)	55 (24)	71 (31)	67 (30)	77 (29)	108 (40)	86 (32)

*Number (%) of patients.
1. Defined as HCV RNA below limit of detection using a research-based RT-PCR assay at end of treatment and during follow-up period.
2. Defined as posttreatment (end of follow-up) minus pretreatment liver biopsy Knodell HAI score (I+II+III) improvement of ≥2 points.

TABLE 4. Virologic and Histologic Responses: Relapse Patients*

	US Study		International Study	
	INTRON A plus REBETOL (N=77)	INTRON A plus Placebo (N=76)	INTRON A plus REBETOL (N=96)	INTRON A plus Placebo (N=96)
Virologic Response				
-Responder[1]	33 (43)	3 (4)	46 (48)	5 (5)
-Nonresponder	36 (47)	66 (87)	45 (47)	91 (95)
-Missing Data	8 (10)	7 (9)	5 (5)	0 (0)
Histologic Response				
-Improvement[2]	38 (49)	27 (36)	49 (51)	30 (31)
-No improvement	23 (30)	37 (49)	29 (30)	44 (46)
-Missing Data	16 (21)	12 (16)	18 (19)	22 (23)

* Number (%) of patients.
1. Defined as HCV RNA below limit of detection using a research-based RT-PCR assay at end of treatment and during follow-up period.
2. Defined as posttreatment (end of follow-up) minus pretreatment liver biopsy Knodell HAI score (I+II+III) improvement of ≥2 points.

Ribavirin transport into nonplasma compartments has been most extensively studied in red blood cells, and has been identified to be primarily via an e_s-type equilibrative nucleoside transporter. This type of transporter is present on virtually all cell types and may account for the extensive volume of distribution. Ribavirin does not bind to plasma proteins.

Ribavirin has two pathways of metabolism: (i) a reversible phosphorylation pathway in nucleated cells; and (ii) a degradative pathway involving deribosylation and amide hydrolysis to yield a triazole carboxylic acid metabolite. Ribavirin and its triazole carboxamide and triazole carboxylic acid metabolites are excreted renally. After oral administration of 600 mg of ^{14}C-ribavirin, approximately 61% and 12% of the radioactivity was eliminated in the urine and feces, respectively, in 336 hours. Unchanged ribavirin accounted for 17% of the administered dose.

Results of *in vitro* studies using both human and rat liver microsome preparations indicated little or no cytochrome P450 enzyme-mediated metabolism of ribavirin, with minimal potential for P450 enzyme-based drug interactions.

No pharmacokinetic interactions were noted between INTRON A Injection and REBETOL Capsules in a multiple-dose pharmacokinetic study.

Drug Interactions Ribavirin has been shown *in vitro* to inhibit phosphorylation of zidovudine and stavudine which could lead to decreased antiretroviral activity. Exposure to didanosine or its active metabolite (dideoxyadenosine 5'-triphosphate) is increased when didanosine is co-administered with ribavirin, which could cause or worsen clinical toxicities (see **PRECAUTIONS: Drug Interactions**).

1. Trademark of Johnson & Johnson-Merck Consumer Pharmaceuticals Co.

Special Populations

Renal Dysfunction The pharmacokinetics of ribavirin were assessed after administration of a single oral dose (400 mg) of ribavirin to non HCV-infected subjects with varying degrees of renal dysfunction. The mean AUC_{tf} value was threefold greater in subjects with creatinine clearance values between 10 to 30 mL/min when compared to control subjects (creatinine clearance >90 mL/min). In subjects with creatinine clearance values between 30 to 60 mL/min, AUC_{tf} was twofold greater when compared to control subjects. The increased AUC_{tf} appears to be due to reduction of renal and non-renal clearance in these patients. Phase III efficacy trials included subjects with creatinine clearance values >50 mL/min. The multiple dose pharmacokinetics of ribavirin cannot be accurately predicted in patients with renal dysfunction. Ribavirin is not effectively removed by hemodialysis. Patients with creatinine clearance <50 mL/min should not be treated with REBETOL (See **WARNINGS**.)

Hepatic Dysfunction The effect of hepatic dysfunction was assessed after a single oral dose of ribavirin (600 mg). The mean AUC_{tf} values were not significantly different in subjects with mild, moderate, or severe hepatic dysfunction (Child-Pugh Classification A, B, or C) when compared to control subjects. However, the mean C_{max} values increased with severity of hepatic dysfunction and was twofold greater in subjects with severe hepatic dysfunction when compared to control subjects.

Elderly Patients Pharmacokinetic evaluations in elderly subjects have not been performed.

Gender There were no clinically significant pharmacokinetic differences noted in a single-dose study of eighteen male and eighteen female subjects.

Pediatric Patients Multiple-dose pharmacokinetic properties for REBETOL Capsules and INTRON A in pediatric patients with chronic hepatitis C between 5 and 16 years of age are summarized in **TABLE 2**. The pharmacokinetics of REBETOL and INTRON A (dose-normalized) are similar in adults and pediatric patients.

Complete pharmacokinetic characteristics of REBETOL Oral Solution have not been determined in pediatric patients. Ribavirin C_{min} values were similar following administration of REBETOL Oral Solution or REBETOL Capsules during 48 weeks of therapy in pediatric patients (3 to 16 years of age).

TABLE 2. Mean (% CV) Multiple-Dose Pharmacokinetic Parameters for INTRON A and REBETOL Capsules When Administered to Pediatric Patients With Chronic Hepatitis C

Parameter	REBETOL 15 mg/kg/day as 2 divided doses (n=17)	INTRON A 3 MIU/m² TIW (n=54)
T_{max} (hr)	1.9 (83)	5.9 (36)
C_{max} (ng/mL)	3275 (25)	51 (48)
AUC*	29774 (26)	622 (48)
Apparent clearance L/hr/kg	0.27 (27)	ND

*AUC_{12} (ng/hr/mL) for REBETOL; AUC_{0-24} (IU hr/mL) for INTRON A
ND=not done
In this section of the label, numbers in parenthesis indicate % coefficient of variation.

INDICATIONS AND USAGE

REBETOL (ribavirin, USP) Capsules and Oral Solution are indicated in combination with INTRON A (interferon alfa-2b, recombinant) Injection for the treatment of chronic hepatitis C in patients 3 years of age and older with compensated liver disease previously untreated with alpha interferon or in patients 18 years of age and older who have relapsed following alpha interferon therapy.

REBETOL Capsules are indicated in combination with PEG-INTRON (peginterferon alfa-2b, recombinant) Injection for the treatment of chronic hepatitis C in patients with compensated liver disease who have not been previously treated with interferon alpha and are at least 18 years of age.

The safety and efficacy of REBETOL Capsules or Oral Solution with interferons other than INTRON A or PEG-INTRON products have not been established.

<u>Pediatric Use</u>

Evidence of disease progression, such as hepatic inflammation and fibrosis, as well as prognostic factors for response, HCV genotype and viral load, should be considered when deciding to treat a pediatric patient. The benefits of treatment should be weighed against the safety findings observed (see **PRECAUTIONS Pediatric Use**) for pediatric subjects in the clinical trials.

Description of Clinical Studies

<u>REBETOL/INTRON A Combination Therapy</u>

Adult Patients

Previously Untreated Patients

Adults with compensated chronic hepatitis C and detectable HCV RNA (assessed by a central laboratory using a research-based RT-PCR assay) who were previously untreated with alpha interferon therapy were enrolled into two multicenter, double-blind trials (US and International) and randomized to receive REBETOL Capsules 1200 mg/day (1000 mg/day for patients weighing ≤75 kg) plus INTRON A Injection 3 MIU TIW or INTRON A Injection plus placebo for 24 or 48 weeks followed by 24 weeks of off-therapy follow-up. The International study did not contain a 24-week INTRON A plus placebo treatment arm. The US study enrolled 912 patients who, at baseline, were 67% male, 89% Caucasian with a mean Knodell HAI score (I+II+III) of 7.5, and 72% genotype 1. The International study, conducted in Europe, Israel, Canada, and Australia, enrolled 799 patients (65% male, 95% Caucasian, mean Knodell score 6.8, and 58% genotype 1).

Study results are summarized in **TABLE 3**.

[See table 3 above]

Of patients who had not achieved HCV RNA below the limit of detection of the research based assay by week 24 of REBETOL/INTRON A treatment, less than 5% responded to an additional 24 weeks of combination treatment.

Among patients with HCV Genotype 1 treated with REBETOL/INTRON A therapy who achieved HCV RNA below the detection limit of the research-based assay by 24 weeks, those randomized to 48 weeks of treatment had higher virologic responses compared to those in the 24 week treatment group. There was no observed increase in response rates for patients with HCV nongenotype 1 randomized to REBETOL/INTRON A therapy for 48 weeks compared to 24 weeks.

Relapse Patients

Patients with compensated chronic hepatitis C and detectable HCV RNA (assessed by a central laboratory using a research-based RT-PCR assay) who had relapsed following one or two courses of interferon therapy (defined as abnormal serum ALT levels) were enrolled into two multicenter, double-blind trials (US and International) and randomized to receive REBETOL 1200 mg/day (1000 mg/day for patients weighing ≤75 kg) plus INTRON A 3 MIU TIW or INTRON A plus placebo for 24 weeks followed by 24 weeks of off-therapy follow-up. The US study enrolled 153 patients who, at baseline, were 67% male, 92% Caucasian with a mean Knodell HAI score (I+II+III) of 6.8, and 58% genotype 1. The International study, conducted in Europe, Israel, Canada, and Australia, enrolled 192 patients (64% male, 95% Caucasian, mean Knodell score 6.6, and 56% genotype 1).

Study results are summarized in **TABLE 4**.

[See table 4 above]

Virologic and histologic responses were similar among male and female patients in both the previously untreated and relapse studies.

Pediatric Patients

Pediatric patients 3 to 16 years of age with compensated chronic hepatitis C and detectable HCV RNA (assessed by a central laboratory using a research-based RT-PCR assay) were treated with REBETOL 15 mg/kg per day plus INTRON A 3 MIU/m² TIW for 48 weeks followed by 24 weeks of off-therapy follow-up. A total of 118 patients received treatment who were 57% male, 80% Caucasian, and 78% genotype 1. Patients <5 years of age received REBETOL Oral Solution and those ≥5 years of age received either REBETOL Oral Solution or Capsules.

Study results are summarized in **TABLE 5**.

Continued on next page

Rebetol—Cont.

TABLE 5. Virologic Response: Previously Untreated Pediatric Patients*

	INTRON A 3 MIU/m² TIW Plus REBETOL 15 mg/kg/day
Overall Response[1] (n=118)	54 (46)
Genotype 1 (n=92)	33 (36)
Genotype non-1 (n=26)	21 (81)

*Number (%) of patients.

1. Defined as HCV RNA below limit of detection using a research-based RT-PCR assay at end of treatment and during follow-up.

Patients with viral genotype 1, regardless of viral load, had a lower response rate to INTRON A/REBETOL combination therapy compared to patients with genotype non-1, 36% versus 81%. Patients with both poor prognostic factors (genotype 1 and high viral load) had a response rate of 26% (13/50).

REBETOL/PEG-INTRON Combination Therapy

A randomized study compared treatment with two PEG-INTRON/ REBETOL regimens [PEG-INTRON 1.5 μg/kg SC once weekly (QW)/ REBETOL 800 mg PO daily (in divided doses); PEG-INTRON 1.5 μg/kg SC QW for 4 weeks then 0.5 μg/kg SC QW for 44 weeks/ REBETOL 1000/1200 mg PO daily (in divided doses)] with INTRON A [3 MIU SC thrice weekly (TIW)/REBETOL 1000/1200 mg PO daily (in divided doses)] in 1530 adults with chronic hepatitis C. Interferon naïve patients were treated for 48 weeks and followed for 24 weeks posttreatment. Eligible patients had compensated liver disease, detectable HCV RNA, elevated ALT, and liver histopathology consistent with chronic hepatitis.

Response to treatment was defined as undetectable HCV RNA at 24 weeks posttreatment (see **Table 6**).

TABLE 6. Rates of Response to Combination Treatment

	PEG-INTRON 1.5 μg/kg QW REBETOL 800 mg QD	INTRON A 3 MIU TIW REBETOL 1000/ 1200 mg QD
Overall[1,2] response	52% (264/511)	46% (231/505)
Genotype 1	41% (141/348)	33% (112/343)
Genotype 2-6	75% (123/163)	73% (119/162)

1. Serum HCV RNA was measured with a research-based quantitative polymerase chain reaction assay by a central laboratory.
2. Difference in overall treatment response (PEG-INTRON/ REBETOL vs. INTRON A/REBETOL) is 6% with 95% confidence interval of (0.18, 11.63) adjusted for viral genotype and presence of cirrhosis at baseline.

The response rate to PEG-INTRON 1.5→0.5μg/kg/ REBETOL was essentially the same as the response to INTRON A/REBETOL (data not shown).

Patients with viral genotype 1, regardless of viral load, had a lower response rate to PEG-INTRON (1.5 μg/kg)/ REBETOL combination therapy compared to patients with other viral genotypes. Patients with both poor prognostic factors (genotype 1 and high viral load) had a response rate of 30% (78/256) compared to a response rate of 29% (71/247) with INTRON A/ REBETOL combination therapy.

Patients with lower body weight tended to have higher adverse event rates (see **ADVERSE REACTIONS**) and higher response rates than patients with higher body weights. Differences in response rates between treatment arms did not substantially vary with body weight.

Treatment response rates with PEG-INTRON/REBETOL combination therapy were 49% in men and 56% in women. Response rates were lower in African American and Hispanic patients and higher in Asians compared to Caucasians. Although African Americans had a higher proportion of poor prognostic factors compared to Caucasians the number of non-Caucasians studied (11% of the total) was insufficient to allow meaningful conclusions about differences in response rates after adjusting for prognostic factors.

Liver biopsies were obtained before and after treatment in 68% of patients. Compared to baseline approximately $^2/_3$ of patients in all treatment groups were observed to have a modest reduction in inflammation.

CONTRAINDICATIONS

Pregnancy

REBETOL Capsules and Oral Solution may cause birth defects and/or death of the exposed fetus. REBETOL therapy is contraindicated for use in women who are pregnant or in men whose female partners are pregnant. (See **WARNINGS, PRECAUTIONS–Information for Patients and Pregnancy Category X**.)

REBETOL Capsules and Oral Solution are contraindicated in patients with a history of hypersensitivity to ribavirin or any component of the capsule.

Patients with autoimmune hepatitis must not be treated with combination REBETOL/INTRON A therapy because using these medicines can make the hepatitis worse.

Patients with hemoglobinopathies (eg, thalassemia major, sickle-cell anemia) should not be treated with REBETOL Capsules or Oral Solution.

WARNINGS

Based on results of clinical trials ribavirin monotherapy is not effective for the treatment of chronic hepatitis C virus infection; therefore, REBETOL Capsules or Oral Solution must not be used alone. The safety and efficacy of REBETOL Capsules and Oral Solution have only been established when used together with INTRON A (interferon alfa-2b, recombinant) as REBETRON Combination Therapy or with PEG-INTRON Injection.

There are significant adverse events caused by REBETOL/ INTRON A or PEG-INTRON therapy, including severe depression and suicidal ideation, hemolytic anemia, suppression of bone marrow function, autoimmune and infectious disorders, pulmonary dysfunction, pancreatitis, and diabetes. Suicidal ideation or attempts occurred more frequently among pediatric patients, primarily adolescents, compared to adult patients (2.4% versus 1%) during treatment and off-therapy follow-up. The REBETRON Combination Therapy and PEG-INTRON package inserts should be reviewed in their entirety prior to initiation of combination treatment for additional safety information.

Pregnancy

REBETOL Capsules and Oral Solution may cause birth defects and/or death of the exposed fetus. Extreme care must be taken to avoid pregnancy in female patients and in female partners of male patients. REBETOL has demonstrated significant teratogenic and/or embryocidal effects in all animal species in which adequate studies have been conducted. These effects occurred at doses as low as one twentieth of the recommended human dose of ribavirin. REBETOL THERAPY SHOULD NOT BE STARTED UNTIL A REPORT OF A NEGATIVE PREGNANCY TEST HAS BEEN OBTAINED IMMEDIATELY PRIOR TO PLANNED INITIATION OF THERAPY. Patients should be instructed to use at least two forms of effective contraception during treatment and during the six month period after treatment has been stopped based on multiple dose half-life of ribavirin of 12 days. Pregnancy testing should occur monthly during REBETOL therapy and for six months after therapy has stopped (see CONTRAINDICATIONS and PRECAUTIONS: Information for Patients and Pregnancy Category X).

Anemia

The primary toxicity of ribavirin is hemolytic anemia, which was observed in approximately 10% of REBETOL/ INTRON A-treated patients in clinical trials (see adverse reactions laboratory values—*hemoglobin*). The anemia associated with REBETOL capsules occurs within 1–2 weeks of initiation of therapy. BECAUSE THE INITIAL DROP IN HEMOGLOBIN MAY BE SIGNIFICANT, IT IS ADVISED THAT HEMOGLOBIN OR HEMATOCRIT BE OBTAINED PRETREATMENT AND AT WEEK 2 AND WEEK 4 OF THERAPY, OR MORE FREQUENTLY IF CLINICALLY INDICATED. Patients should then be followed as clinically appropriate.

Fatal and nonfatal myocardial infarctions have been reported in patients with anemia caused by REBETOL. Patients should be assessed for underlying cardiac disease before initiation of ribavirin therapy. Patients with preexisting cardiac disease should have electrocardiograms administered before treatment, and should be appropriately monitored during therapy. If there is any deterioration of cardiovascular status, therapy should be suspended or discontinued. (See DOSAGE AND ADMINISTRATION: Guidelines for Dose Modification.) Because cardiac disease may be worsened by drug induced anemia, patients with a history of significant or unstable cardiac disease should not use REBETOL. (See ADVERSE REACTIONS.)

REBETOL and INTRON A or PEG-INTRON therapy should be suspended in patients with signs and symptoms of pancreatitis and discontinued in patients with confirmed pancreatitis.

REBETOL should not be used in patients with creatinine clearance <50 mL/min. (See **Clinical Pharmacology, Special populations**.)

Pulmonary

Pulmonary symptoms, including dyspnea, pulmonary infiltrates, pneumonitis and pneumonia, have been reported during therapy with REBETOL/ INTRON A; occasional cases of fatal pneumonia have occurred. In addition, sarcoidosis or the exacerbation of sarcoidosis has been reported. If there is evidence of pulmonary infiltrates or pulmonary function impairment, the patient should be closely monitored, and if appropriate, combination REBETOL/ INTRON A treatment should be discontinued.

PRECAUTIONS

The safety and efficacy of REBETOL/INTRON A and PEG-INTRON therapy for the treatment of HIV infection, adenovirus, RSV, parainfluenza, or influenza infections have not been established. REBETOL Capsules should not be used for these indications. Ribavirin for inhalation has a separate package insert, which should be consulted if ribavirin inhalation therapy is being considered.

The safety and efficacy of REBETOL/INTRON A therapy has not been established in liver or other organ transplant patients, patients with decompensated liver disease due to hepatitis C infection, patients who are nonresponders to interferon therapy, or patients coinfected with HBV or HIV.

Information for Patients

Patients must be informed that REBETOL Capsules and Oral Solution may cause birth defects and/or death of the exposed fetus. REBETOL must not be used by women who are pregnant or by men whose female partners are pregnant. Extreme care must be taken to avoid pregnancy in female patients and in female partners of male patients taking REBETOL. REBETOL should not be initiated until a report of a negative pregnancy test has been obtained immediately prior to initiation of therapy. Patients must perform a pregnancy test monthly during therapy and for 6 months posttherapy. Women of childbearing potential must be counseled about use of effective contraception (two reliable forms) prior to initiating therapy. Patients (male and female) must be advised of the teratogenic/embryocidal risks and must be instructed to practice effective contraception during REBETOL and for 6 months posttherapy. Patients (male and female) should be advised to notify the physician immediately in the event of a pregnancy. (See **CONTRAINDICATIONS** and **WARNINGS**.)

If pregnancy does occur during treatment or during 6 months posttherapy, the patient must be advised of the teratogenic risk of REBETOL therapy to the fetus. Patients, or partners of patients, should immediately report any pregnancy that occurs during treatment or within 6 months after treatment cessation to their physician. Physicians should report such cases by calling 1-800-727-7064.

Patients receiving REBETOL Capsules should be informed of the benefits and risks associated with treatment, directed in its appropriate use, and referred to the patient **MEDICATION GUIDE**. Patients should be informed that the effect of treatment of hepatitis C infection on transmission is not known, and that appropriate precautions to prevent transmission of the hepatitis C virus should be taken.

The most common adverse experience occurring with REBETOL Capsules is anemia, which may be severe. (See **ADVERSE REACTIONS**.) Patients should be advised that laboratory evaluations are required prior to starting therapy and periodically thereafter. (See **Laboratory Tests**.) It is advised that patients be well hydrated, especially during the initial stages of treatment.

Laboratory Tests The following laboratory tests are recommended for all patients treated with REBETOL Capsules, prior to beginning treatment and then periodically thereafter.

- Standard hematologic tests—including hemoglobin (pretreatment, week 2 and week 4 of therapy, and as clinically appropriate [see **WARNINGS**]), complete and differential white blood cell counts, and platelet count.
- Blood chemistries—liver function tests and TSH.
- Pregnancy—including monthly monitoring for women of childbearing potential.
- ECG (See **WARNINGS**.)

Carcinogenesis and Mutagenesis Ribavirin did not cause an increase in any tumor type when administered for 6 months in the transgenic p53 deficient mouse model at doses up to 300 mg/kg (estimated human equivalent of 25 mg/kg based on body surface area adjustment for a 60 kg adult; approximately 1.9 times the maximum recommended human daily dose). Ribavirin was non-carcinogenic when administered for 2 years to rats at doses up to 40 mg/kg (estimated human equivalent of 5.71 mg/kg based on body surface area adjustment for a 60 kg adult). However, this dose was less than the maximum tolerated dose, and therefore the study was not adequate to fully characterize the carcinogenic potential of ribavirin.

Ribavirin demonstrated increased incidences of mutation and cell transformation in multiple genotoxicity assays. Ribavirin was active in the Balb/3T3 *In Vitro* Cell Transformation Assay. Mutagenic activity was observed in the mouse lymphoma assay, and at doses of 20–200 mg/kg (estimated human equivalent of 1.67–16.7 mg/kg, based on body surface area adjustment for a 60 kg adult; 0.1–1 X the maximum recommended human 24-hour dose of ribavirin) in a mouse micronucleus assay. A dominant lethal assay in rats was negative, indicating that if mutations occurred in rats they were not transmitted through male gametes.

Impairment of Fertility Ribavirin demonstrated significant embryocidal and/or teratogenic effects at doses well below the recommended human dose in all animal species in which adequate studies have been conducted.

Fertile women and partners of fertile women should not receive REBETOL unless the patient and his/her partner are using effective contraception (two reliable forms). Based on a multiple dose half-life ($t_{1/2}$) of ribavirin of 12 days, effective contraception must be utilized for 6 months posttherapy (eg, 15 half-lives of clearance for ribavirin).

REBETOL should be used with caution in fertile men. In studies in mice to evaluate the time course and reversibility of ribavirin-induced testicular degeneration at doses of 15 to 150 mg/kg/day (estimated human equivalent of 1.25–12.5 mg/kg/day, based on body surface area adjustment for a 60 kg adult; 0.1–0.8 X the maximum human 24-hour dose of ribavirin) administered for 3 or 6 months, abnormalities in sperm occurred. Upon cessation of treatment, essentially total recovery from ribavirin-induced testicular toxicity was apparent within 1 or 2 spermatogenesis cycles.

Animal Toxicology Long-term studies in the mouse and rat (18–24 months; doses of 20–75 and 10–40 mg/kg/day, respectively [estimated human equivalent doses of 1.67–6.25 and 1.43–5.71 mg/kg/day, respectively, based on body surface area adjustment for a 60 kg adult; approximately 0.1–0.4 X the maximum human 24-hour dose of ribavirin]) have demonstrated a relationship between chronic ribavirin exposure and increased incidences of vascular lesions (microscopic hemorrhages) in mice. In rats, retinal degeneration occurred in controls, but the incidence was increased in ribavirin-treated rats.

Pregnancy Category X (see **CONTRAINDICATIONS**)
Ribavirin produced significant embryocidal and/or teratogenic effects in all animal species in which adequate studies have been conducted. Malformations of the skull, palate, eye, jaw, limbs, skeleton, and gastrointestinal tract were noted. The incidence and severity of teratogenic effects increased with escalation of the drug dose. Survival of fetuses and offspring was reduced. In conventional embryotoxicity/teratogenicity studies in rats and rabbits, observed no effect dose levels were well below those for proposed clinical use (0.3 mg/kg/day for both the rat and rabbit; approximately 0.06 X the recommended human 24-hour dose of ribavirin). No maternal toxicity or effects on offspring were observed in a peri/postnatal toxicity study in rats dosed orally at up to 1 mg/kg/day (estimated human equivalent dose of 0.17 mg/kg based on body surface area adjustment for a 60 kg adult; approximately 0.01 X the maximum recommended human 24-hour dose of ribavirin).

Treatment and Posttreatment: Potential Risk to the Fetus
Ribavirin is known to accumulate in intracellular components from where it is cleared very slowly. It is not known whether ribavirin contained in sperm will exert a potential teratogenic effect upon fertilization of the ova. In a study in rats, it was concluded that dominant lethality was not induced by ribavirin at doses up to 200 mg/kg for 5 days (estimated human equivalent doses of 7.14–28.6 mg/kg, based on body surface area adjustment for a 60 kg adult; up to 1.7 X the maximum recommended human dose of ribavirin). However, because of the potential human teratogenic effects of ribavirin, male patients should be advised to take every precaution to avoid risk of pregnancy for their female partners.

Women of childbearing potential should not receive REBETOL unless they are using effective contraception (two reliable forms) during the therapy period. In addition, effective contraception should be utilized for 6 months post-therapy based on a multiple-dose half-life ($t_{1/2}$) of ribavirin of 12 days.

Male patients and their female partners must practice effective contraception (two reliable forms) during treatment with REBETOL and for the 6-month posttherapy period (eg, 15 half-lives for ribavirin clearance from the body).

If pregnancy occurs in a patient or partner of a patient during treatment or during the 6 months after treatment cessation, physicians should report such cases by calling 1-800-727-7064.

Nursing Mothers It is not known whether the REBETOL product is excreted in human milk. Because of the potential for serious adverse reactions from the drug in nursing infants, a decision should be made whether to discontinue nursing or to delay or discontinue REBETOL.

Geriatric Use Clinical studies of REBETOL/INTRON A or PEG-INTRON therapy did not include sufficient numbers of subjects aged 65 and over to determine if they respond differently from younger subjects.

REBETOL is known to be substantially excreted by the kidney, and the risk of toxic reactions to this drug may be greater in patients with impaired renal function. Because elderly patients often have decreased renal function, care should be taken in dose selection. Renal function should be monitored and dosage adjustments should be made accordingly. REBETOL should not be used in patients with creatinine clearance <50 mL/min. (See **WARNINGS.**)

In general, REBETOL Capsules should be administered to elderly patients cautiously, starting at the lower end of the dosing range, reflecting the greater frequency of decreased hepatic and/or cardiac function, and of concomitant disease or other drug therapy. In clinical trials, elderly subjects had a higher frequency of anemia (67%) than did younger patients (28%). (See **WARNINGS.**)

Pediatric Use **Suicidal ideation or attempts occurred more frequently among pediatric patients, primarily adolescents, compared to adult patients (2.4% versus 1%) during treatment and off-therapy follow-up (see WARNINGS).** As in adult patients, pediatric patients experienced other psychiatric adverse events (eg, depression, emotional lability, somnolence), anemia, and neutropenia (see **WARNINGS**). During a 48-week course of therapy there was a decrease in the rate of linear growth (mean percentile assignment decrease of 9%) and a decrease in the rate of weight gain (mean percentile assignment decrease of 13%). A general reversal of these trends was noted during the 24-week posttreatment period.

Drug Interactions

Didanosine: Co-administration of REBETOL Capsules or Oral Solution and didanosine is not recommended. Reports of fatal hepatic failure, as well as peripheral neuropathy, pancreatitis, and symptomatic hyperlactacemia/ lactic acidosis have been reported in clinical trials (see **CLINICAL PHARMACOLOGY: Drug Interactions**).

Stavudine and Zidovudine: Ribavirin may antagonize the in vitro antiviral activity of stavudine and zidovudine against HIV. Therefore, concomitant use of ribavirin with either of these drugs should be used with caution (see **CLINICAL PHARMACOLOGY: Drug Interactions**).

ADVERSE REACTIONS

The primary toxicity of ribavirin is hemolytic anemia. Reductions in hemoglobin levels occurred within the first 1–2 weeks of oral therapy. (See WARNINGS.) Cardiac and pulmonary events associated with anemia occurred in approximately 10% of patients. (See WARNINGS.)

TABLE 7. Selected Treatment-Emergent Adverse Events: Previously Untreated and Relapse Adult Patients and Previously Untreated Pediatric Patients

	Percentage of Patients						
	US Previously Untreated Study				US Relapse Study		Pediatric Patients
	24 weeks of treatment		48 weeks of treatment		24 weeks of treatment		48 weeks of treatment
Patients Reporting Adverse Events*	INTRON A plus REBETOL (N=228)	INTRON A plus Placebo (N=231)	INTRON A plus REBETOL (N=228)	INTRON A plus Placebo (N=225)	INTRON A plus REBETOL (N=77)	INTRON A plus Placebo (N=76)	INTRON A plus REBETOL (N=118)
Application Site Disorders							
Injection site inflammation	13	10	12	14	6	8	14
Injection site reaction	7	9	8	9	5	3	19
Body as a Whole - General Disorders							
Headache	63	63	66	67	66	68	69
Fatigue	68	62	70	72	60	53	58
Rigors	40	32	42	39	43	37	25
Fever	37	35	41	40	32	36	61
Influenza-like symptoms	14	18	18	20	13	13	31
Asthenia	9	4	9	9	10	4	5
Chest pain	5	4	9	8	6	7	5
Central & Peripheral Nervous System Disorders							
Dizziness	17	15	23	19	26	21	20
Gastrointestinal System Disorders							
Nausea	38	35	46	33	47	33	33
Anorexia	27	16	25	19	21	14	51
Dyspepsia	14	6	16	9	16	9	<1
Vomiting	11	10	9	13	12	8	42
Musculoskeletal System Disorders							
Myalgia	61	57	64	63	61	58	32
Arthralgia	30	27	33	36	29	29	15
Musculoskeletal pain	20	26	28	32	22	28	21
Psyciatric Disorders							
Insomnia	39	27	39	30	26	25	14
Irritability	23	19	32	27	25	20	10
Depression	32	25	36	37	23	14	13
Emotional lability	7	6	11	8	12	8	16
Concentration impaired	11	14	14	14	10	12	5
Nervousness	4	2	4	4	5	4	3
Respiratory System Disorders							
Dyspnea	19	9	18	10	17	12	5
Sinusitis	9	7	10	14	12	7	<1
Skin and Appendages Disorders							
Alopecia	28	27	32	28	27	26	23
Rash	20	9	28	8	21	5	17
Pruritus	21	9	19	8	13	4	12
Special Senses, Other Disorders							
Taste perversion	7	4	8	4	6	5	<1

*Patients reporting one or more adverse events. A patient may have reported more than one adverse event within a body system/organ class category.

REBETOL/INTRON A Combination Therapy
In clinical trials, 19% and 6% of previously untreated and relapse patients, respectively, discontinued therapy due to adverse events in the combination arms compared to 13% and 3% in the interferon arms. Selected treatment-emergent adverse events that occurred in the US studies with ≥5% incidence are provided in **TABLE 7** by treatment group. In general, the selected treatment-emergent adverse events were reported with lower incidence in the international studies as compared to the US studies with the exception of asthenia, influenza-like symptoms, nervousness, and pruritus.

Pediatric Patients
In clinical trials of 118 pediatric patients 3 to 16 years of age, 6% discontinued therapy due to adverse events. Dose modifications were required in 30% of patients, most commonly for anemia and neutropenia. In general, the adverse event profile in the pediatric population was similar to that observed in adults. Injection site disorders, fever, anorexia, vomiting, and emotional lability occurred more frequently in pediatric patients compared to adult patients. Conversely, pediatric patients experienced less fatigue, dyspepsia, arthralgia, insomnia, irritability, impaired concentration, dyspnea, and pruritus compared to adult patients. Selected treatment-emergent adverse events that occurred with ≥5% incidence among all pediatric patients who received the recommended dose of REBETOL/INTRON A combination therapy are provided in **Table 7**.
[See table 7 above]
In addition, the following spontaneous adverse events have been reported during the marketing surveillance of REBETOL/INTRON A therapy: hearing disorder and vertigo.

REBETOL/PEG-INTRON Combination Therapy
Overall, in clinical trials, 14% of patients receiving REBETOL in combination with PEG-INTRON, discontinued therapy compared with 13% treated with REBETOL in combination with INTRON A. The most common reasons for discontinuation of therapy were related to psychiatric, systemic (eg, fatigue, headache), or gastrointestinal adverse events. Adverse events that occurred in clinical trial at >5% incidence are provided in **Table 8** by treatment group. Safety and effectiveness of REBETOL in combination with PEG-INTRON has not been established in pediatric patients.

Continued on next page

Rebetol—Cont.

TABLE 8. Adverse Events Occurring in > 5% of Patients

Adverse Events	Percentage of Patients Reporting Adverse Events* PEG-INTRON 1.5 µg/kg/ REBETOL (N=511)	INTRON A/ REBETOL (N=505)
Application Site		
Injection Site Inflammation	25	18
Injection Site Reaction	58	36
Autonomic Nervous System		
Mouth Dry	12	8
Sweating Increased	11	7
Flushing	4	3
Body as a Whole		
Fatigue/Asthenia	66	63
Headache	62	58
Rigors	48	41
Fever	46	33
Weight Decrease	29	20
RUQ Pain	12	6
Chest Pain	8	7
Malaise	4	6
Central & Peripheral Nervous System		
Dizziness	21	17
Endocrine		
Hypothyroidism	5	4
Gastrointestinal		
Nausea	43	33
Anorexia	32	27
Diarrhea	22	17
Vomiting	14	12
Abdominal Pain	13	13
Dyspepsia	9	8
Constipation	5	5
Hematologic Disorders		
Neutropenia	26	14
Anemia	12	17
Leukopenia	6	5
Thrombocytopenia	5	2
Liver and Biliary System		
Hepatomegaly	4	4
Musculoskeletal		
Myalgia	56	50
Arthralgia	34	28
Musculoskeletal Pain	21	19
Psychiatric		
Insomnia	40	41
Depression	31	34
Anxiety/Emotional Lability/Irritability	47	47
Concentration Impaired	17	21
Agitation	8	5
Nervousness	6	6
Reproductive, Female		
Menstrual Disorder	7	6
Resistance Mechanism		
Infection Viral	12	12
Infection Fungal	6	1
Respiratory System		
Dyspnea	26	24
Coughing	23	16
Pharyngitis	12	13
Rhinitis	8	6
Sinusitis	6	5
Skin and Appendages		
Alopecia	36	32
Pruritus	29	28
Rash	24	23
Skin Dry	24	23
Special Senses, Other		
Taste Perversion	9	4
Vision Disorders		
Vision Blurred	5	6
Conjunctivitis	4	5

*Patients reporting one or more adverse events. A patient may have reported more than one adverse event within a body system/organ class category.

TABLE 9. Selected Hematologic Values During Treatment with REBETOL plus INTRON A: Previously Untreated and Relapse Adult Patients and Previously Untreated Pediatric Patients

	Percentage of Patients						
	US Previously Untreated Study				US Relapse Study		Pediatric Patients
	24 weeks of treatment		48 weeks of treatment		24 weeks of treatment		48 weeks of treatment
	INTRON A plus REBETOL (N=228)	INTRON A plus Placebo (N=231)	INTRON A plus REBETOL (N=228)	INTRON A plus Placebo (N=225)	INTRON A plus REBETOL (N=77)	INTRON A plus Placebo (N=76)	INTRON A plus REBETOL (N=118)
Hemoglobin (g/dL)							
9.5–10.9	24	1	32	1	21	3	24
8.0–9.4	5	0	4	0	4	0	3
6.5–7.9	0	0	0	0.4	0	0	0
<6.5	0	0	0	0	0	0	0
Leukocytes ($\times 10^9$/L)							
2.0–2.9	40	20	38	23	45	26	35
1.5–1.9	4	1	9	2	5	3	8
1.0–1.4	0.9	0	2	0	0	0	0
<1.0	0	0	0	0	0	0	0
Neutrophils ($\times 10^9$/L)							
1.0–1.49	30	32	31	44	42	34	37
0.75–0.99	14	15	14	11	16	18	15
0.5–0.74	9	9	14	7	8	4	16
<0.5	11	8	11	5	5	8	3
Platelets ($\times 10^9$/L)							
70–99	9	11	11	14	6	12	0.8
50–69	2	3	2	3	0	5	2
30–49	0	0.4	0	0.4	0	0	0
<30	0.9	0	1	0.9	0	0	0
Total Bilirubin (mg/dL)							
1.5–3.0	27	13	32	13	21	7	2
3.1–6.0	0.9	0.4	2	0	3	0	0
6.1–12.0	0	0	0.4	0	0	0	0
>12.0	0	0	0	0	0	0	0

Laboratory Values

REBETOL/INTRON A Combination Therapy

Changes in selected hematologic values (hemoglobin, white blood cells, neutrophils, and platelets) during therapy are described below. (See **TABLE 9**.)

Hemoglobin Hemoglobin decreases among patients receiving REBETOL therapy began at Week 1, with stabilization by Week 4. In previously untreated patients treated for 48 weeks the mean maximum decrease from baseline was 3.1 g/dL in the US study and 2.9 g/dL in the International study. In relapse patients the mean maximum decrease from baseline was 2.8 g/dL in the US study and 2.6 g/dL in the International study. Hemoglobin values returned to pretreatment levels within 4–8 weeks of cessation of therapy in most patients.

Bilirubin and Uric Acid Increases in both bilirubin and uric acid, associated with hemolysis, were noted in clinical trials. Most were moderate biochemical changes and were reversed within 4 weeks after treatment discontinuation. This observation occurs most frequently in patients with a previous diagnosis of Gilbert's syndrome. This has not been associated with hepatic dysfunction or clinical morbidity. [See table 9 above]

REBETOL/PEG-INTRON Combination Therapy

Changes in selected hematologic values (hemoglobin, white blood cells, neutrophils, and platelets) during therapy are described below. (See **TABLE 10**.)

Hemoglobin

REBETOL induced a decrease in hemoglobin levels in approximately two thirds of patients. Hemoglobin levels decreased to <11g/dL in about 30% of patients. Severe anemia (<8 g/dL) occurred in <1% of patients. Dose modification was required in 9 and 13% of patients in the PEG-INTRON/REBETOL and INTRON A/REBETOL groups.

Bilirubin and Uric Acid

In the REBETOL/PEG-INTRON combination trial 10–14% of patients developed hyperbilirubinemia and 33-38% developed hyperuricemia in association with hemolysis. Six patients developed mild to moderate gout.

TABLE 10. Selected Hematologic Values During Treatment with REBETOL plus PEG-INTRON

	Number (%) of Subjects	
	PEG-INTRON plus REBETOL (N=511)	INTRON A plus Placebo (N=505)
Hemoglobin (g/dL)		
9.5–10.9	26	27
8.0–9.4	3	3
6.5–7.9	0.2	0.2
<6.5	0	0
Leukocytes ($\times 10^9$/L)		
2.0–2.9	46	41
1.5–1.9	24	8
1.0–1.4	5	1
<1.0	0	0
Neutrophils ($\times 10^9$/L)		
1.0–1.49	33	37
0.75–0.99	25	13
0.5–0.74	18	7
<0.5	4	2
Platelets ($\times 10^9$/L)		
70–99	15	5
50–69	3	0.8
30–49	0.2	0.2
<30	0	0
Total Bilirubin (mg/dL)		
1.5–3.0	10	13
3.1–6.0	0.6	0.2
6.1–12.0	0	0.2
>12.0	0	0
ALT (SGPT)		
2 × Baseline	0.6	0.2
2.1–5 × Baseline	3	1
5.1–10 × Baseline	0	0
>10 × Baseline	0	0

OVERDOSAGE

There is limited experience with overdosage. Acute ingestion of up to 20 grams of REBETOL Capsules, INTRON A ingestion of up to 120 million units, and subcutaneous doses of INTRON A up to 10 times the recommended doses have been reported. Primary effects that have been observed are increased incidence and severity of the adverse events related to the therapeutic use of INTRON A and REBETOL. However, hepatic enzyme abnormalities, renal failure, hemorrhage, and myocardial infarction have been reported with administration of single subcutaneous doses of INTRON A that exceed dosing recommendations.

There is no specific antidote for INTRON A or REBETOL overdose, and hemodialysis and peritoneal dialysis are not effective for treatment of overdose of either agent.

DOSAGE AND ADMINISTRATION

(see **CLINICAL PHARMACOLOGY, Special Populations**; see **WARNINGS**)

REBETOL/INTRON A Combination Therapy

Adults The recommended dose of REBETOL Capsules depends on the patient's body weight. The recommended dose of REBETOL is provided in **TABLE 11**.

The recommended duration of treatment for patients previously untreated with interferon is 24 to 48 weeks. The duration of treatment should be individualized to the patient depending on baseline disease characteristics, response to therapy, and tolerability of the regimen. (See **Description of Clinical Studies** and **ADVERSE REACTIONS**.) After 24 weeks of treatment virologic response should be assessed. Treatment discontinuation should be considered in any patient who has not achieved an HCV RNA below the limit of detection of the assay by 24 weeks. There are no safety and efficacy data on treatment for longer than 48 weeks in the previously untreated patient population.

In patients who relapse following non-pegylated interferon monotherapy, the recommended duration of treatment is 24 weeks. There are no safety and efficacy data on treatment for longer than 24 weeks in the relapse patient population.

TABLE 11. Recommended Dosing

Body weight	REBETOL Capsules
≤ 75 kg	2 × 200-mg capsules AM, 3 × 200-mg capsules PM daily p.o.
> 75 kg	3 × 200 mg capsules AM, 3 × 200 mg capsules PM daily p.o.

Pediatrics The recommended dose of REBETOL is 15 mg/kg per day orally (divided dose AM and PM). For children weighing ≤25 kg or who cannot swallow capsules, REBETOL Oral Solution is supplied in a concentration of 40 mg/mL. For children weighing >25 kg, either the Oral Solution or 200-mg capsule may be administered. Refer to **TABLE 12** for dosing recommendations for the 200-mg capsule to achieve the recommended dose.

The recommended duration of treatment is 48 weeks for pediatric patients with genotype 1. After 24 weeks of treatment virologic response should be assessed. Treatment discontinuation should be considered in any patient who has not achieved an HCV RNA below the limit of detection of the assay by this time. The recommended duration of treatment for pediatric patients with genotype 2/3 is 24 weeks. There are no safety and efficacy data on treatment for longer than 48 weeks in pediatrics.

TABLE 12. Pediatric Dosing

Body weight	REBETOL Capsules	INTRON A Injection
25–36 kg	1 × 200-mg capsules AM, 1 × 200-mg capsules PM daily p.o.	3 million IU/m^2 3 times weekly s.c.
37–49 kg	1 × 200-mg capsules AM, 2 × 200-mg capsules PM daily p.o.	3 million IU/m^2 3 times weekly s.c.
50–61 kg	2 × 200-mg capsules AM, 2 × 200-mg capsules PM daily p.o.	3 million IU/m^2 3 times weekly s.c.
>61 kg	Refer to adult dosing table.	Refer to adult dosing table

REBETOL may be administered without regard to food, but should be administered in a consistent manner with respect to food intake. (See **CLINICAL PHARMACOLOGY**.)

REBETOL/PEG-INTRON Combination Therapy

The recommended dose of REBETOL Capsules is 800 mg/day in 2 divided doses: two capsules (400 mg) in the morning with food and two capsules (400 mg) in the evening with food.

***Dose Modifications* (TABLE 13)**

If severe adverse reactions or laboratory abnormalities develop during combination REBETOL/INTRON A therapy the dose should be modified, or discontinued if appropriate, until the adverse reactions abate. If intolerance persists after dose adjustment, REBETOL/INTRON A therapy should be discontinued.

REBETOL should not be used in patients with creatinine clearance <50 mL/min. (See **WARNINGS** and **CLINICAL PHARMACOLOGY, Special Populations**.)

REBETOL should be administered with caution to patients with preexisting cardiac disease. Patients should be assessed before commencement of therapy and should be appropriately monitored during therapy. If there is any deterioration of cardiovascular status, therapy should be stopped. (See **WARNINGS**.)

For patients with a history of stable cardiovascular disease, a permanent dose reduction is required if the hemoglobin decreases by ≥2 g/dL during any 4-week period. In addition, for these cardiac history patients, if the hemoglobin remains <12 g/dL after 4 weeks on a reduced dose, the patient should discontinue combination REBETOL/INTRON A therapy.

It is recommended that a patient whose hemoglobin level falls below 10 g/dL have his/her REBETOL dose reduced to 600 mg daily (1 × 200-mg capsule AM, 2 × 200-mg capsules PM) for adults and 7.5 mg/kg per day (divided dose AM and PM) for pediatric patients. A patient whose hemoglobin level falls below 8.5 g/dL should be permanently discontinued from REBETOL therapy. (See **WARNINGS**.)

TABLE 13. Guidelines for Dose Modifications and Discontinuation for Anemia

Hemoglobin	Dose Reduction* REBETOL- 600 mg daily adults 7.5 mg/kg daily for pediatrics	Permanent Discontinuation of REBETOL Treatment
No Cardiac History	**<10 g/dL**	**<8.5 g/dL**
Cardiac History Patients	**≥2 g/dL decrease during any 4-week period during treatment**	**<12 g/dL after 4 weeks of dose reduction**

HOW SUPPLIED

REBETOL 200-mg Capsules are white, opaque capsules with REBETOL, 200 mg, and the Schering Corporation logo imprinted on the capsule shell; the capsules are packaged in a bottle containing 42 capsules (NDC 0085-1327-04), 56 capsules (NDC 0085-1351-05), 70 capsules (NDC 0085-1385-07), and 84 capsules (NDC 0085-1194-03).

REBETOL Oral Solution 40 mg/mL is a clear, colorless to pale or light yellow bubble gum-flavored liquid and it is packaged in 4-oz. amber glass bottles (100 mL/bottle) with child-resistant closures (NDC 0085-1318-01).

Storage Conditions

The bottle of REBETOL Capsules should be stored at 25°C (77°F); excursions permitted to 15°–30°C (59°–86°F) [see USP Controlled Room Temperature].

REBETOL Oral Solution should be stored between 2° and 8°C (36° and 46°F) or at 25°C (77°F); excursions permitted to 15°–30°C (59°–86°F) [see USP Controlled Room Temperature].

Schering Corporation
Kenilworth, NJ 07033 USA
U.S. Patents 4,530,901 & 4,211,771

Rev. 3/03 **27002404T**

G.D. Searle & Co.

A Division of Pfizer
235 EAST 42ND ST
NEW YORK, NY 10017-5755

Direct Inquiries to:
212-733-2323

For Medical Information Contact:
800-323-4204

ARTHROTEC® ℞
[*är-thrō-tĕk*]
diclofenac sodium and misoprostol tablets

Prescribing information for this product, which appears on pages 3103–3107 of the 2004 PDR, has been completely revised as follows. Please write "See Supplement A" next to the product heading.

CONTRAINDICATIONS AND WARNINGS

ARTHROTEC (diclofenac sodium/misoprostol) ADMINISTRATION BY ANY ROUTE IS CONTRAINDICATED, BECAUSE ITS MISOPROSTOL COMPONENT CAN CAUSE ABORTION, IN WOMEN WHO ARE PREGNANT (See **WARNINGS** and **PRECAUTIONS**).

- Anecdotal reports have been received, primarily from Brazil, of congenital anomalies and reports of fetal death in pregnancies in which misoprostol has been used as an abortifacient.

PATIENTS MUST BE ADVISED OF THE ABORTIFACIENT PROPERTY AND WARNED NOT TO GIVE THE DRUG TO OTHERS.

UTERINE RUPTURE HAS BEEN REPORTED WHEN MISOPROSTOL WAS ADMINISTERED INTRAVAGINALLY IN PREGNANT WOMEN TO INDUCE LABOR OR TO INDUCE ABORTION BEYOND THE FIRST TRIMESTER OF PREGNANCY.

UTERINE PERFORATION HAS BEEN REPORTED FOLLOWING ADMINISTRATION OF COMBINED VAGINAL-AND-ORAL MISOPROSTOL IN PREGNANT WOMEN TO INDUCE ABORTION. IN EACH OF THESE REPORTED CASES, THE GESTATIONAL AGE OF THE PREGNANCIES WAS UNKNOWN.

ARTHROTEC should not be used in women of childbearing potential unless the patient requires nonsteroidal anti-inflammatory drug (NSAID) therapy and is at high risk of developing gastric or duodenal ulceration or for developing complications from gastric or duodenal ulcers associated with the use of the NSAID. (See *WARNINGS*). In such patients, ARTHROTEC may be prescribed if the patient:

- has had a negative serum pregnancy test within 2 weeks prior to beginning therapy.
- is capable of complying with effective contraceptive measures.
- has received both oral and written warnings of the hazards of misoprostol, the risk of possible contraception failure, and the danger to other women of childbearing potential should the drug be taken by mistake.
- will begin ARTHROTEC only on the second or third day of the next normal menstrual period.

DESCRIPTION

ARTHROTEC is a combination product containing diclofenac sodium, a nonsteroidal anti-inflammatory drug (NSAID) with analgesic properties, and misoprostol, a gastrointestinal (GI) mucosal protective prostaglandin E_1 analog. ARTHROTEC oral tablets are white to off-white, round, biconvex and approximately 11 mm in diameter. Each tablet consists of an enteric-coated core containing 50 mg (ARTHROTEC 50) or 75 mg (ARTHROTEC 75) diclofenac sodium surrounded by an outer mantle containing 200 mcg misoprostol.

Diclofenac sodium is a phenylacetic acid derivative that is a white to off-white, virtually odorless, crystalline powder. Diclofenac sodium is freely soluble in methanol, soluble in ethanol and practically insoluble in chloroform and in dilute acid. Diclofenac sodium is sparingly soluble in water. Its chemical formula and name are:

$C_{14}H_{10}Cl_2NO_2Na$ [M.W. = 318.14] 2-[(2,6-dichlorophenyl) amino] benzeneacetic acid, monosodium salt.

Misoprostol is a water-soluble, viscous liquid that contains approximately equal amounts of two diastereomers. Its chemical formula and name are:

$C_{22}H_{38}O_5$ [M.W. = 382.54] (±)methyl 11α, 16-dihydroxy-16-methyl-9-oxoprost-13E-en-1-oate.

Inactive ingredients in ARTHROTEC include: colloidal silicon dioxide; crospovidone; hydrogenated castor oil; hypromellose; lactose; magnesium stearate; methacrylic acid copolymer; microcrystalline cellulose; povidone (polyvidone) K-30; sodium hydroxide; starch (corn); talc; triethyl citrate.

CLINICAL PHARMACOLOGY

Pharmacodynamics and pharmacokinetics of diclofenac sodium

Diclofenac sodium is a nonsteroidal anti-inflammatory drug (NSAID). In pharmacologic studies, diclofenac sodium has shown anti-inflammatory, analgesic and antipyretic properties. The mechanism of action of diclofenac sodium, like other NSAIDs, is not completely understood but may be related to prostaglandin synthetase inhibition.

Diclofenac sodium is completely absorbed from the GI tract after fasting, oral administration. The diclofenac sodium in ARTHROTEC is in a pharmaceutical formulation that resists dissolution in the low pH of gastric fluid but allows a rapid release of drug in the higher pH environment of the duodenum. Only 50% of the absorbed dose is systemically available due to first pass metabolism. Peak plasma levels are achieved in 2 hours (range 1–4 hours), and the area under the plasma concentration curve (AUC) is dose proportional within the range of 25 mg to 150 mg. Peak plasma levels are less than dose proportional and are approximately 1.5 and 2.0 mcg/mL for 50 mg and 75 mg doses, respectively.

Plasma concentrations of diclofenac sodium decline from peak levels in a biexponential fashion, with the terminal phase having a half-life of approximately 2 hours. Clearance and volume of distribution are about 350 mL/min and 550 mL/kg, respectively. More than 99% of diclofenac sodium is reversibly bound to human plasma albumin.

Diclofenac sodium is eliminated through metabolism and subsequent urinary and biliary excretion of the glucuronide and the sulfate conjugates of the metabolites. Approximately 65% of the dose is excreted in the urine and 35% in the bile.

Conjugates of unchanged diclofenac account for 5–10% of the dose excreted in the urine and for less than 5% excreted in the bile. Little or no unchanged unconjugated drug is excreted. Conjugates of the principal metabolite account for 20–30% of the dose excreted in the urine and for 10–20% of the dose excreted in the bile.

Conjugates of three other metabolites together account for 10–20% of the dose excreted in the urine and for small amounts excreted in the bile. The elimination half-life values for these metabolites are shorter than those for the parent drug. Urinary excretion of an additional metabolite (half-life = 80 hours) accounts for only 1.4% of the oral dose. The degree of accumulation of diclofenac metabolites is unknown. Some of the metabolites may have activity.

Pharmacodynamics and pharmacokinetics of misoprostol

Misoprostol is a synthetic prostaglandin E_1 analog with gastric antisecretory and (in animals) mucosal protective properties. NSAIDs inhibit prostaglandin synthesis. A deficiency of prostaglandins within the gastric and duodenal mucosa may lead to diminishing bicarbonate and mucus secretion and may contribute to the mucosal damage caused by NSAIDs.

Continued on next page

Arthrotec—Cont.

Misoprostol can increase bicarbonate and mucus production, but in humans this has been shown at doses 200 mcg and above that are also antisecretory. It is therefore not possible to tell whether the ability of misoprostol to prevent gastric and duodenal ulcers is the result of its antisecretory effect, its mucosal protective effect, or both.

In vitro studies on canine parietal cells using tritiated misoprostol acid as the ligand have led to the identification and characterization of specific prostaglandin receptors. Receptor binding is saturable, reversible, and stereospecific. The sites have a high affinity for misoprostol, for its acid metabolite, and for other E type prostaglandins, but not for F or I prostaglandins and other unrelated compounds, such as histamine or cimetidine. Receptor-site affinity for misoprostol correlates well with an indirect index of antisecretory activity. It is likely that these specific receptors allow misoprostol taken with food to be effective topically, despite the lower serum concentrations attained.

Misoprostol produces a moderate decrease in pepsin concentration during basal conditions, but not during histamine stimulation. It has no significant effect on fasting or postprandial gastrin nor intrinsic factor output.

Effects on gastric acid secretion: Misoprostol, over the range of 50–200 mcg, inhibits basal and nocturnal gastric acid secretion, and acid secretion in response to a variety of stimuli, including meals, histamine, pentagastrin, and coffee. Activity is apparent 30 minutes after oral administration and persists for at least 3 hours. In general, the effects of 50 mcg were modest and shorter lived, and only the 200-mcg dose had substantial effects on nocturnal secretion or on histamine- and meal-stimulated secretion.

Orally administered misoprostol is rapidly and extensively absorbed, and it undergoes rapid metabolism to its biologically active metabolite, misoprostol acid. Misoprostol acid in ARTHROTEC reaches a maximum plasma concentration in about 20 minutes and is, thereafter, quickly eliminated with an elimination $t_{1/2}$ of about 30 minutes. There is high variability in plasma levels of misoprostol acid between and within studies, but mean values after single doses show a linear relationship with dose of misoprostol over the range of 200 to 400 mcg. No accumulation of misoprostol acid was found in multiple-dose studies, and plasma steady state was achieved within 2 days. The serum protein binding of misoprostol acid is less than 90% and is concentration-independent in the therapeutic range.

After oral administration of radiolabeled misoprostol, about 70% of detected radioactivity appears in the urine. Maximum plasma concentrations of misoprostol acid are diminished when the dose is taken with food, and total availability of misoprostol acid is reduced by use of concomitant antacid. Clinical trials were conducted with concomitant antacid; this effect does not appear to be clinically important.

Pharmacokinetic studies also showed a lack of drug interaction with antipyrine or propranolol given with misoprostol. Misoprostol given for 1 week had no effect on the steady state pharmacokinetics of diazepam when the two drugs were administered 2 hours apart.

Pharmacokinetics of ARTHROTEC

The pharmacokinetics following oral administration of a single dose (see Table 1) or multiple doses of ARTHROTEC (diclofenac sodium/misoprostol) to healthy subjects under fasted conditions are similar to the pharmacokinetics of the two individual components.

[See table 1 above]

Table 1.

MISOPROSTOL ACID Mean (SD)

Treatment (n=36)	C_{max} (pg/mL)	t_{max} (hr)	AUC (0–4 h) (pg•hr/mL)
ARTHROTEC 50	441 (137)	0.30 (0.13)	266 (95)
Cytotec®	478 (201)	0.30 (0.10)	295 (143)
ARTHROTEC 75	304 (110)	0.26 (0.09)	177 (49)
Cytotec	290 (130)	0.35 (0.12)	176 (58)

DICLOFENAC Mean (SD)

Treatment (n=36)	C_{max} (ng/mL)	t_{max} (hr)	AUC (0–12 h) (ng•hr/mL)
ARTHROTEC 50	1207 (364)	2.4 (1.0)	1380 (272)
Voltaren®	1298 (441)	2.4 (1.0)	1357 (290)
ARTHROTEC 75	2025 (2005)	2.0 (1.4)	2773 (1347)
Voltaren	2367 (1318)	1.9 (0.7)	2609 (1185)

SD: Standard deviation of the mean
AUC: Area under the curve
C_{max}: Peak concentration
t_{max}: Time to peak concentration

The rate and extent of absorption of both diclofenac sodium and misoprostol acid from ARTHROTEC 50 and ARTHROTEC 75 are similar to those from diclofenac sodium and misoprostol formulations each administered alone.

Neither diclofenac sodium nor misoprostol acid accumulated in plasma following repeated doses of ARTHROTEC given every 12 hours under fasted conditions. Food decreases the multiple-dose bioavailability profile of ARTHROTEC 50 and ARTHROTEC 75.

Special populations

A 4-week study, comparing plasma level profiles of diclofenac (50 mg bid) in younger (26–46 years) versus older (66–81 years) adults, did not show differences between age groups (10 patients per age group). In a multiple-dose (bid) cross-over study of 24 people aged 65 years or older, the misoprostol contained in ARTHROTEC did not affect the pharmacokinetics of diclofenac sodium.

Differences in the pharmacokinetics of diclofenac have not been detected in studies of patients with renal (50 mg intravenously) or hepatic impairment (100 mg oral solution). In patients with renal impairment (N=5, creatinine clearance 3 to 42 mL/min), AUC values and elimination rates were comparable to those in healthy people. In patients with biopsy-confirmed cirrhosis or chronic active hepatitis (variably elevated transaminases and mildly elevated bilirubins, N=10), diclofenac concentrations and urinary elimination values were comparable to those in healthy people.

Pharmacokinetic studies with misoprostol in patients with varying degrees of renal impairment showed an approximate doubling of $t_{1/2}$, C_{max} and AUC compared to healthy people. In people over 64 years of age, the AUC for misoprostol acid is increased.

Misoprostol does not affect the hepatic mixed function oxidase (cytochrome P-450) enzyme system in animals. In a study of people with mild to moderate hepatic impairment, mean misoprostol acid AUC and C_{max} showed approximately double the mean values obtained in healthy people. Three people who had the lowest antipyrine and lowest indocyanine green clearance values had the highest misoprostol acid AUC and C_{max} values.

CLINICAL STUDIES

Osteoarthritis

Diclofenac sodium, as a single ingredient or in combination with misoprostol, has been shown to be effective in the management of the signs and symptoms of osteoarthritis.

Rheumatoid arthritis

Diclofenac sodium, as a single ingredient or in combination with misoprostol, has been shown to be effective in the management of the signs and symptoms of rheumatoid arthritis.

Upper gastrointestinal safety

Diclofenac, and other NSAIDs, have caused serious gastrointestinal toxicity, such as bleeding, ulceration and perforation of the stomach, small intestine or large intestine. Misoprostol has been shown to reduce the incidence of endoscopically diagnosed NSAID-induced gastric and duodenal ulcers. In a 12-week, randomized, double-blind, dose response study, misoprostol 200 mcg administered qid, tid or bid, was significantly more effective than placebo in reducing the incidence of gastric ulcer in OA and RA patients using a variety of NSAIDs. The tid regimen was therapeutically equivalent to misoprostol 200 mcg qid with respect to the prevention of gastric ulcers. Misoprostol 200 mcg given bid was less effective than 200 mcg given tid or qid. The incidence of NSAID-induced duodenal ulcer was also significantly reduced with all three regimens of misoprostol compared to placebo (see Table 2).

Table 2.
Misoprostol 200 mcg Dosage Regimen

	Placebo	bid	tid	qid
Gastric ulcer	11%	6%*	3%*	3%*
Duodenal ulcer	6%	2%*	3%*	1%*

N=1623; 12 weeks.
*Misoprostol significantly different from placebo ($p<0.05$)

Results of a study in 572 patients with osteoarthritis demonstrate that patients receiving ARTHROTEC have a lower incidence of endoscopically defined gastric ulcers compared to patients receiving diclofenac sodium (see Table 3).

Table 3.

Osteoarthritis patients with history of ulcer or erosive disease (N=572), 6 weeks	Incidence of ulcers	
	Gastric	Duodenal
ARTHROTEC 50 tid	3%*	6%
ARTHROTEC 75 bid	4%*	3%
diclofenac sodium 75 mg bid	11%	7%
placebo	3%	1%

*Statistically significantly different from diclofenac ($p<0.05$)

INDICATIONS AND USAGE

ARTHROTEC is indicated for treatment of the signs and symptoms of osteoarthritis or rheumatoid arthritis in patients at high risk of developing NSAID-induced gastric and duodenal ulcers and their complications. See *WARNINGS—Gastrointestinal effects* for a list of factors that may increase the risk of NSAID-induced gastric and duodenal ulcers and their complications.

CONTRAINDICATIONS

See boxed ***CONTRAINDICATIONS AND WARNINGS*** related to misoprostol.

ARTHROTEC is contraindicated in patients with hypersensitivity to diclofenac or to misoprostol or other prostaglandins. ARTHROTEC should not be given to patients who have experienced asthma, urticaria, or other allergic-type reactions after taking aspirin or other NSAIDs. Severe, rarely fatal, anaphylactic-like reactions to diclofenac sodium have been reported.

WARNINGS

Regarding misoprostol:
See boxed ***CONTRAINDICATIONS AND WARNINGS***.
Regarding diclofenac:

Gastrointestinal (GI) effects—risk of GI ulceration, bleeding and perforation

Serious GI toxicity, such as inflammation, bleeding, ulceration and perforation of the stomach, small intestine or large intestine, can occur at any time, with or without warning symptoms, in patients treated with NSAIDs. Minor upper GI problems, such as dyspepsia, are common and may also occur at any time during NSAID therapy. Therefore, physicians and patients should remain alert for ulceration and bleeding, even in the absence of previous GI tract symptoms. Patients should be informed about the signs and/or symptoms and the steps to take if they occur. The utility of periodic laboratory monitoring has not been demonstrated, nor has it been adequately assessed. Only 1 in 5 patients who develop a serious upper GI adverse event on NSAID therapy is symptomatic. It has been demonstrated that upper GI ulcers, gross bleeding, or perforation, caused by NSAIDs, appear to occur in approximately 1% of patients treated for 3–6 months, and in 2–4% of patients treated for 1 year. These trends continue thus, increasing the likelihood of developing a serious GI event at some time during the course of therapy. However, even short-term therapy has risk.

NSAIDs should be prescribed with extreme caution in those with a prior history of ulcer disease or GI bleeding. Most spontaneous reports of fatal GI events are in elderly or debilitated patients and therefore special care should be taken in treating this population. **To minimize the potential risk for an adverse event, the lowest effective dose should be used for the shortest possible duration.** For very high-risk patients, alternate therapies that do not involve NSAIDs should be considered.

Studies have shown that patients with a history of peptic ulcer disease and/or GI bleeding, and who use NSAIDs, have a greater than 10-fold risk for developing a GI bleed than patients with neither of these risk factors. In addition to a past history of ulcer disease, pharmacoepidemiological studies have identified several other conditions or co-therapies that may increase the risk for GI bleeding, such as: treatment with oral corticosteroids, treatment with anticoagulants, longer duration of NSAID therapy, older age, smoking, alcoholism, poor general health and *Helicobacter pylori* positive status.

Hepatic effects

Elevations of one or more liver tests may occur during ARTHROTEC therapy. These laboratory abnormalities may progress, may remain unchanged, or may be transient with continued therapy. Borderline elevations (ie, less than 3 times the ULN [ULN = the upper limit of the normal range]), or greater elevations of transaminases occurred in about 15% of diclofenac-treated patients. Of the hepatic enzymes, ALT (SGPT) is the one recommended for the monitoring of liver injury.

In clinical trials, meaningful elevations (ie, more than 3 times the ULN) of AST (SGOT) (ALT was not measured in all studies) occurred in about 2% of approximately 5,700 patients at some time during diclofenac treatment. In a large, open, controlled trial, meaningful elevations of ALT and/or AST occurred in about 4% of 3,700 patients treated for 2–6 months, including marked elevations (ie, more than 8 times the ULN) in about 1% of the 3,700 patients. In that open-label study, a higher incidence of borderline (less than 3 times the ULN), moderate (3–8 times the ULN), and marked (>8 times the ULN) elevations of ALT or AST was observed in patients receiving diclofenac when compared to other NSAIDs. Transaminase elevations were seen more frequently in patients with osteoarthritis than in those with rheumatoid arthritis.

In addition to enzyme elevations seen in clinical trials, postmarketing surveillance has found rare cases of severe hepatic reactions, including liver necrosis, jaundice, and fulminant fatal hepatitis with and without jaundice. Some of these rare reported cases underwent liver transplantation. Physicians should measure transaminases periodically in patients receiving long-term therapy with diclofenac, because severe hepatotoxicity may develop without a prodrome of distinguishing symptoms. The optimum times for making the first and subsequent transaminase measurements are not known. In the largest U.S. trial (open-label) that involved 3,700 patients monitored first at 8 weeks and 1,200 patients monitored again at 24 weeks, almost all meaningful elevations in transaminases were detected before patients became symptomatic. In 42 of the 51 patients in all trials who developed marked transaminase elevations, abnormal tests occurred during the first 2 months of therapy with diclofenac. Postmarketing experience has shown severe hepatic reactions can occur at any time during treatment with diclofenac. Cases of drug-induced hepatotoxicity have been reported in the first month, and in some cases, the first 2 months of therapy. Based on these experiences, transaminases should be monitored within 4 to 8 weeks after initiating treatment with diclofenac (see *PRECAUTIONS—Laboratory tests*).

In clinical trials with ARTHROTEC, meaningful elevation of ALT (SGPT, more than 3 times the ULN) occurred in 1.6% of 2,184 patients treated with ARTHROTEC and in 1.4% of 1,691 patients treated with diclofenac sodium. These increases were generally transient, and enzyme levels returned to within the normal range upon discontinuation of ARTHROTEC therapy. The misoprostol component of ARTHROTEC does not appear to exacerbate the hepatic effects caused by the diclofenac sodium component. As with other NSAID containing products, if abnormal liver tests persist or worsen, if clinical signs and/or symptoms consistent with liver disease develop, or if systemic manifestations occur (eg, eosinophilia, rash, etc), ARTHROTEC should be discontinued immediately.

To minimize the possibility that hepatic injury will become severe between transaminase measurements, physicians should inform patients of the warning signs and symptoms of hepatotoxicity (eg, nausea, fatigue, lethargy, pruritus, jaundice, right upper quadrant tenderness, and "flu-like" symptoms), and the appropriate action patients should take if these signs and symptoms appear.

Anaphylactoid reactions

As with other NSAID containing products, anaphylactoid reactions may occur in patients without known prior exposure to ARTHROTEC or its components. ARTHROTEC should not be given to patients with the aspirin triad. The triad typically occurs in asthmatic patients who experience rhinitis with or without nasal polyps, or who exhibit severe, potentially fatal bronchospasm after taking aspirin or other NSAIDs (see *CONTRAINDICATIONS* and *PRECAUTIONS—Preexisting asthma*). Emergency help should be sought in cases where an anaphylactoid reaction occurs. Allergic reactions have been reported by less than 0.1% of patients who received ARTHROTEC in clinical trials, and there have been rare reports of anaphylaxis in the marketed use of ARTHROTEC outside of the United States.

Advanced renal disease

In patients with advanced kidney disease, treatment with ARTHROTEC is not recommended. If NSAID therapy must be initiated however, close monitoring of the patient's kidney function is advisable (see *PRECAUTIONS—Renal effects*).

PRECAUTIONS

Information for patients

Patients should be advised of the following:

SPECIAL NOTE FOR WOMEN: ARTHROTEC contains misoprostol. Because of its abortifacient property, misoprostol is contraindicated for use by pregnant women. Misoprostol may cause miscarriage if given to pregnant women at any time during pregnancy. Miscarriages caused by misoprostol may be incomplete, which could lead to dangerous bleeding, hospitalization, surgery, infertility, or maternal or fetal death.

See *PATIENT INFORMATION* at the end of this labeling for important information to discuss with the patient.

ARTHROTEC is available only as a unit-of-use package that includes a leaflet containing patient information. The patient should read the leaflet before taking ARTHROTEC and each time the prescription is renewed because the leaflet may have been revised. Keep ARTHROTEC out of the reach of children.

General

ARTHROTEC cannot be used to substitute for corticosteroids or to treat for corticosteroid insufficiency. Abrupt discontinuation of corticosteroids may lead to disease exacerbation. Patients on prolonged corticosteroid therapy should have their therapy tapered slowly if a decision is made to discontinue corticosteroids.

The pharmacological activity of ARTHROTEC in reducing inflammation may diminish the utility of this diagnostic sign in detecting complications of presumed noninfectious, painful conditions.

Renal effects

Caution should be used when initiating treatment with ARTHROTEC in patients with considerable dehydration. It is advisable to rehydrate patients first and then start therapy with ARTHROTEC. Caution is also recommended in patients with preexisting kidney disease (see *WARNINGS—Advanced renal disease*).

As with other NSAIDs, long-term administration of diclofenac has resulted in renal papillary necrosis and other renal medullary changes. Renal toxicity has also been seen in patients in which renal prostaglandins have a compensatory role in the maintenance of renal perfusion. In these patients, administration of an NSAID may cause a dose-dependent reduction in prostaglandin formation and, secondarily, in renal blood flow, which may precipitate overt renal decompensation. Patients at greatest risk of this reaction are those with impaired renal function, heart failure, or liver dysfunction, those taking diuretics and ACE inhibitors, and the elderly. Discontinuation of NSAID therapy is usually followed by recovery to the pretreatment state.

Diclofenac metabolites are eliminated primarily by the kidneys. The extent to which the metabolites may accumulate in patients with renal failure has not been studied. As with other NSAIDs, metabolites of which are excreted by the kidney, patients with significantly impaired renal function should be more closely monitored.

Hematologic effects

Anemia is sometimes seen in patients receiving diclofenac or other NSAIDs. This may be due to fluid retention, GI blood loss, or an incompletely described effect upon erythropoiesis. Patients on long-term treatment with NSAIDs, including ARTHROTEC, should have their hemoglobin or hematocrit checked if they exhibit any signs or symptoms of anemia.

All drugs that inhibit the biosynthesis of prostaglandins may interfere to some extent with platelet function and vascular responses to bleeding.

NSAIDs inhibit platelet aggregation and, unlike aspirin, their effect on platelet function is reversible, quantitatively less, and of shorter duration. ARTHROTEC does not generally affect platelet counts, prothrombin time (PT), or partial thromboplastin time (PTT). Patients receiving ARTHROTEC who may be adversely affected by alterations in platelet function, such as those with coagulation disorders or patients receiving anticoagulants, should be carefully monitored.

Aseptic meningitis

As with other NSAIDs, aseptic meningitis with fever and coma has been observed on rare occasions in patients on diclofenac therapy. Although it is probably more likely to occur in patients with systemic lupus and related connective tissue diseases, it has been reported in patients who do not have an underlying chronic disease. If signs or symptoms of meningitis develop in a patient on diclofenac, the possibility of its being related to diclofenac should be considered.

Fluid retention and edema

Fluid retention and edema have been observed in some patients taking NSAID containing products, including ARTHROTEC. Therefore, as with other NSAID containing products, ARTHROTEC should be used with caution in patients with a history of cardiac decompensation, hypertension, or other conditions predisposing to fluid retention.

Preexisting asthma

Patients with asthma may have aspirin-sensitive asthma. The use of aspirin in patients with aspirin-sensitive asthma has been associated with severe bronchospasm, which can be fatal. Since cross-reactivity, including bronchospasm, between aspirin and other NSAIDs has been reported in such aspirin-sensitive patients, ARTHROTEC should not be administered to patients with this form of aspirin sensitivity and should be used with caution in patients with preexisting asthma.

Porphyria

The use of ARTHROTEC in patients with hepatic porphyria should be avoided. To date, one patient has been described in whom diclofenac sodium probably triggered a clinical attack of porphyria. The postulated mechanism, demonstrated in rats, for causing such attacks by diclofenac sodium, as well as some other NSAIDs, is through stimulation of the porphyrin precursor delta-aminolevulinic acid (ALA).

Laboratory tests

Patients on long-term treatment with NSAIDs should have their CBC and a chemistry profile checked periodically. If clinical signs and symptoms consistent with liver or renal disease develop, systemic manifestations occur (eg, eosinophilia, rash, etc) or if abnormal liver tests persist or worsen, ARTHROTEC should be discontinued.

Effect on blood coagulation: Diclofenac sodium impairs platelet aggregation but does not affect bleeding time, plasma thrombin clotting time, plasma fibrinogen, or factors V and VII to XII. Statistically significant changes in prothrombin and partial thromboplastin times have been reported in normal volunteers. The mean changes were observed to be less than 1 second in both instances, however, and are unlikely to be clinically important. Diclofenac sodium is a prostaglandin synthetase inhibitor, however, and all drugs that inhibit prostaglandin synthesis interfere with platelet function to some degree; therefore, patients who may be adversely affected by such an action should be carefully observed. Misoprostol has not been shown to exacerbate the effects of diclofenac on platelet activity.

Drug interactions

Aspirin: Concomitant administration of ARTHROTEC and aspirin is not recommended because diclofenac sodium is displaced from its binding sites by aspirin, resulting in lower plasma concentrations, peak plasma levels and AUC values.

Digoxin: Elevated digoxin levels have been reported in patients receiving digoxin and diclofenac sodium. Patients receiving digoxin and ARTHROTEC should be monitored for possible digoxin toxicity.

Antihypertensive agents: NSAIDs can inhibit the activity of antihypertensives, including ACE inhibitors. Thus, caution should be taken when administering ARTHROTEC with such agents.

Warfarin: The effects of warfarin and NSAIDs on GI bleeding are synergistic, such that users of both drugs together have a risk of serious bleeding greater than users of either drug alone.

Oral hypoglycemics: Diclofenac sodium does not alter glucose metabolism in healthy people nor does it alter the effects of oral hypoglycemic agents. There are rare reports, however, from marketing experience, of changes in effects of insulin or oral hypoglycemic agents in the presence of diclofenac sodium that necessitated change in the doses of such agents. Both hypo- and hyperglycemic effects have been reported. A direct causal relationship has not been established, but physicians should consider the possibility that diclofenac sodium may alter a diabetic patient's response to insulin or oral hypoglycemic agents.

Methotrexate and cyclosporine: ARTHROTEC, like other NSAID containing products, may affect renal prostaglandins and increase the toxicity of certain drugs. Ingestion of ARTHROTEC may increase serum concentrations of methotrexate and increase cyclosporine nephrotoxicity. Patients who begin taking ARTHROTEC or who increase their dose of ARTHROTEC or any other NSAID containing product while taking methotrexate or cyclosporine may develop toxicity characteristic for these drugs. They should be observed closely, particularly if renal function is impaired.

Lithium: NSAIDs have produced an elevation of plasma lithium levels and a reduction in renal lithium clearance. The mean minimum lithium concentration increased 15% and the renal clearance was decreased by approximately 20%. These effects have been attributed to inhibition of renal prostaglandin synthesis by the NSAID. Thus, when NSAIDs and lithium are administered concurrently, subjects should be observed carefully for signs of lithium toxicity.

Antacids: Antacids reduce the bioavailability of misoprostol acid. Antacids may also delay absorption of diclofenac sodium. Magnesium-containing antacids exacerbate misoprostol-associated diarrhea. Thus, it is not recommended that ARTHROTEC be coadministered with magnesium-containing antacids.

Diuretics: The diclofenac sodium component of ARTHROTEC, like other NSAIDs, can inhibit the activity of diuretics. Concomitant therapy with potassium-sparing diuretics may be associated with increased serum potassium levels.

Other drugs: In small groups of patients (7–10 patients/interaction study), the concomitant administration of azathioprine, gold, chloroquine, D-penicillamine, prednisolone, doxycycline or digitoxin did not significantly affect the peak levels and AUC levels of diclofenac sodium. Phenobarbital toxicity has been reported to have occurred in a patient on chronic phenobarbital treatment following the initiation of diclofenac therapy. *In vitro*, diclofenac interferes minimally with the protein binding of prednisolone (10% decrease in binding). Benzylpenicillin, ampicillin, oxacillin, chlortetracycline, doxycycline, cephalothin, erythromycin, and sulfamethoxazole have no influence, *in vitro*, on the protein binding of diclofenac in human serum.

Animal toxicology

A reversible increase in the number of normal surface gastric epithelial cells occurred in the dog, rat, and mouse during long-term toxicology studies with misoprostol. No such increase has been observed in humans administered misoprostol for up to 1 year. An apparent response of the female mouse to misoprostol in long-term studies at 100 to 1000 times the human dose was hyperostosis, mainly of the medulla of sternebrae. Hyperostosis did not occur in long-term studies in the dog and rat and has not been seen in humans treated with misoprostol.

Carcinogenesis, mutagenesis, impairment of fertility

Long-term animal studies to evaluate the potential for carcinogenesis and animal studies to evaluate the effects on fertility have been performed with each component of ARTHROTEC given alone. ARTHROTEC itself (diclofenac sodium and misoprostol combinations in 250:1 ratio) was not genotoxic in the Ames test, the Chinese hamster ovary cell (CHO/HGPRT) forward mutation test, the rat lymphocyte chromosome aberration test or the mouse micronucleus test.

In a 24-month rat carcinogenicity study, oral misoprostol at doses up to 2.4 mg/kg/day (14.4 mg/m^2/day, 24 times the recommended maximum human dose of 0.6 mg/m^2/day) was not tumorigenic. In a 21-month mouse carcinogenicity study, oral misoprostol at doses up to 16 mg/kg/day (48 mg/m^2/day), 80 times the recommended maximum human dose based on body surface area, was not tumorigenic. Misoprostol, when administered to male and female breeding rats in an oral dose-range of 0.1 to 10 mg/kg/day (0.6 to 60 mg/m^2/day, 1 to 100 times the recommended maximum human dose based on body surface area) produced dose-related pre- and post-implantation losses and a significant decrease in the number of live pups born at the highest dose. These findings suggest the possibility of a general adverse effect on fertility in males and females.

In a 24-month rat carcinogenicity study, oral diclofenac sodium up to 2 mg/kg/day (12 mg/m^2/day) was not tumorigenic. For a 50-kg person of average height (1.46m^2 body surface area), this dose represents 0.08 times the recom-

Continued on next page

Arthrotec—Cont.

mended maximum human dose (148 mg/m^2) on a body surface area basis. In a 24-month mouse carcinogenicity study, oral diclofenac sodium at doses up to 0.3 mg/kg/day (0.9 mg/m^2/day, 0.006 times the recommended maximum human dose based on body surface area) in males and 1 mg/kg/day (3 mg/m^2/day, 0.02 times the recommended maximum human dose based on body surface area) in females was not tumorigenic. Diclofenac sodium at oral doses up to 4 mg/kg/day (24 mg/m^2/day, 0.16 times the recommended maximum human dose based on body surface area) was found to have no effect on fertility and reproductive performance of male and female rats.

Pregnancy

Pregnancy category X: See boxed ***CONTRAINDICATIONS AND WARNINGS*** regarding misoprostol. One case of amniotic fluid embolism, which resulted in maternal and fetal death, has been reported with use of misoprostol during pregnancy. Severe vaginal bleeding, retained placenta, shock, fetal bradycardia, and pelvic pain have also been reported. These women were administered misoprostol vaginally and/or orally over a range of doses.

Non-teratogenic effects

Misoprostol may endanger pregnancy (may cause miscarriage) and thereby cause harm to the fetus when administered to a pregnant woman. Misoprostol produces uterine contractions, uterine bleeding, and expulsion of the products of conception. Miscarriages caused by misoprostol may be incomplete. In studies in women undergoing elective termination of pregnancy during the first trimester, misoprostol caused partial or complete expulsion of the products of conception in 11% of the subjects and increased uterine bleeding in 41%.

Reports, primarily from Brazil, of congenital anomalies and reports of fetal death subsequent to use of misoprostol alone, as an abortifacient, have been received (see boxed ***CONTRAINDICATIONS AND WARNINGS***). If a woman is or becomes pregnant while taking this drug, the drug should be discontinued and the patient apprised of the potential hazard to the fetus.

The diclofenac sodium component of ARTHROTEC, like other NSAIDs which are prostaglandin-inhibiting drugs, may affect the fetal cardiovascular system causing premature closure of the ductus arteriosus. NSAIDs may also inhibit uterine contractions.

Teratogenic effects

An oral teratology study has been performed in pregnant rabbits at dose combinations (250:1 ratio) up to 10 mg/kg/day diclofenac sodium (120 mg/m^2/day, 0.8 times the recommended maximum human dose based on body surface area) and 0.04 mg/kg/day misoprostol (0.48 mg/m^2/day, 0.8 times the recommended maximum human dose based on body surface area) and has revealed no evidence of teratogenic potential for ARTHROTEC.

Oral teratology studies have been performed in pregnant rats at doses up to 1.6 mg/kg/day (9.6 mg/m^2/day, 16 times the recommended maximum human dose based on body surface area) and pregnant rabbits at doses up to 1.0 mg/kg/day (12 mg/m^2/day, 20 times the recommended maximum human dose based on body surface area) and have revealed no evidence of teratogenic potential for misoprostol.

Oral teratology studies have been performed in pregnant mice at doses up to 20 mg/kg/day (60 mg/m^2/day, 0.4 times the recommended maximum human dose based on body surface area), pregnant rats at doses up to 10 mg/kg/day (60 mg/m^2/day, 0.4 times the recommended maximum human dose based on body surface area) and pregnant rabbits at doses up to 10 mg/kg/day (120 mg/m^2/day, 0.8 times the recommended maximum human dose based on body surface area) and have revealed no evidence of teratogenic potential for diclofenac sodium.

Nursing mothers

Diclofenac sodium has been found in the milk of nursing mothers. It is unlikely that misoprostol is excreted into milk since the drug is rapidly metabolized throughout the body. Excretion of the active metabolite (misoprostol acid) into milk is possible, but has not been studied. Because of the potential for serious adverse reactions in nursing infants, ARTHROTEC is not recommended for use by nursing mothers.

Pediatric use

Safety and effectiveness of ARTHROTEC in pediatric patients have not been established.

Geriatric use

Of the more than 2,100 subjects in clinical studies with ARTHROTEC, 25% were 65 and over, while 6% were 75 and over. In studies with diclofenac, 31% of subjects were 65 and over. No overall differences in safety or effectiveness were observed between these subjects and younger subjects, and other reported clinical experience has not identified differences in responses between the elderly and younger patients, but greater sensitivity of some older individuals cannot be ruled out. As with any NSAID, the elderly are likely to tolerate adverse events less well than younger patients. Diclofenac is known to be substantially excreted by the kidney, and the risk of toxic reactions to ARTHROTEC may be greater in patients with impaired renal function. Because elderly patients are more likely to have decreased renal function, care should be taken in dose selection, and it may be useful to monitor renal function (see *PRECAUTIONS—Renal effects*).

Based on studies in the elderly, no adjustment of the dose of ARTHROTEC is necessary in the elderly for pharmacokinetic reasons (see *Pharmacokinetics of ARTHROTEC—Special populations*), although many elderly may need to receive a reduced dose because of low body weight or disorders associated with aging.

ADVERSE REACTIONS

Adverse reactions associated with ARTHROTEC

Adverse reaction information for ARTHROTEC is derived from Phase III multinational controlled clinical trials in over 2,000 patients, receiving ARTHROTEC 50 or ARTHROTEC 75, as well as from blinded, controlled trials of Voltaren® Delayed-Release Tablets (diclofenac) and Cytotec® Tablets (misoprostol).

Gastrointestinal

GI disorders had the highest reported incidence of adverse events for patients receiving ARTHROTEC. These events were generally minor, but led to discontinuation of therapy in 9% of patients on ARTHROTEC and 5% of patients on diclofenac. For GI ulcer rates, see *CLINICAL STUDIES—Upper gastrointestinal safety.*

GI disorder	ARTHROTEC	Diclofenac
Abdominal pain	21%	15%
Diarrhea	19%	11%
Dyspepsia	14%	11%
Nausea	11%	6%
Flatulence	9%	4%

ARTHROTEC can cause more abdominal pain, diarrhea and other GI symptoms than diclofenac alone.

Diarrhea and abdominal pain developed early in the course of therapy, and were usually self-limited (resolved after 2 to 7 days). Rare instances of profound diarrhea leading to severe dehydration have been reported in patients receiving misoprostol. Patients with an underlying condition such as inflammatory bowel disease, or those in whom dehydration, were it to occur, would be dangerous, should be monitored carefully if ARTHROTEC is prescribed. The incidence of diarrhea can be minimized by administering ARTHROTEC with food and by avoiding coadministration with magnesium-containing antacids.

Gynecological

Gynecological disorders previously reported with misoprostol use have also been reported for women receiving ARTHROTEC (see below). Postmenopausal vaginal bleeding may be related to ARTHROTEC administration. If it occurs, diagnostic workup should be undertaken to rule out gynecological pathology. There have been reports in which intravaginal administration of misoprostol in pregnant women resulted in rupture of the uterus and death of the infant. (See boxed ***CONTRAINDICATIONS AND WARNINGS***.)

Elderly

Overall, there were no significant differences in the safety profile of ARTHROTEC in over 500 patients 65 years of age or older compared with younger patients.

Other adverse experiences reported occasionally or rarely with ARTHROTEC, diclofenac or other NSAIDs, or misoprostol are:

Body as a whole: Asthenia, death, fatigue, fever, infection, malaise, sepsis.

Cardiovascular system: Arrhythmia, atrial fibrillation, congestive heart failure, hypertension, hypotension, increased CPK, increased LDH, myocardial infarction, palpitations, phlebitis, premature ventricular contractions, syncope, tachycardia, vasculitis.

Central and peripheral nervous system: Coma, convulsions, dizziness, drowsiness, headache, hyperesthesia, hypertonia, hypoesthesia, insomnia, meningitis, migraine, neuralgia, paresthesia, somnolence, tremor, vertigo.

Digestive: Anorexia, appetite changes, constipation, dry mouth, dysphagia, enteritis, esophageal ulceration, esophagitis, eructation, gastritis, gastroesophageal reflux, GI bleeding, GI neoplasm benign, glossitis, heartburn, hematemesis, hemorrhoids, intestinal perforation, peptic ulcer, stomatitis and ulcerative stomatitis, tenesmus, vomiting.

Female reproductive disorders: Breast pain, dysmenorrhea, intermenstrual bleeding, leukorrhea, menstrual disorder, menorrhagia, vaginal hemorrhage.

Hemic and lymphatic system: Agranulocytosis, anemia, aplastic anemia, coagulation time increased, ecchymosis, eosinophilia, epistaxis, hemolytic anemia, leukocytosis, leukopenia, lymphadenopathy, melena, pancytopenia, pulmonary embolism, purpura, rectal bleeding, thrombocythemia, thrombocytopenia.

Hypersensitivity: Angioedema, laryngeal/pharyngeal edema, urticaria.

Liver and biliary system: Abnormal hepatic function, bilirubinemia, hepatitis, jaundice, liver failure, pancreatitis.

Male reproductive disorders: Impotence, perineal pain.

Metabolic and nutritional: Alkaline phosphatase increased, BUN increased, dehydration, glycosuria, gout, hypercholesterolemia, hyperglycemia, hyperuricemia, hypoglycemia, hyponatremia, periorbital edema, porphyria, weight changes.

Musculoskeletal system: Arthralgia, myalgia.

Psychiatric: Anxiety, concentration impaired, confusion, depression, disorientation, dream abnormalities, hallucinations, irritability, nervousness, paranoia, psychotic reaction.

Respiratory system: Asthma, coughing, dyspnea, hyperventilation, pneumonia, respiratory depression.

Skin and appendages: Acne, alopecia, bruising, eczema, erythema multiforme, exfoliative dermatitis, pemphigoid reaction, photosensitivity, pruritus, pruritus ani, rash, skin ulceration, Stevens-Johnson syndrome, sweating increased, toxic epidermal necrolysis.

Special senses: Hearing impairment, taste loss, taste perversion, tinnitus.

Urinary system: Cystitis, dysuria, hematuria, interstitial nephritis, micturition frequency, nocturia, nephrotic syndrome, oliguria/polyuria, papillary necrosis, proteinuria, renal failure, urinary tract infection.

Vision: Amblyopia, blurred vision, conjunctivitis, diplopia, glaucoma, iritis, lacrimation abnormal, night blindness, vision abnormal.

OVERDOSAGE

The toxic dose of ARTHROTEC has not been determined. However, signs of overdosage from the components of the product have been described.

Diclofenac sodium

Clinical signs that may suggest diclofenac sodium overdose include GI complaints, confusion, drowsiness or general hypotonia. Reports of overdosage with diclofenac cover 66 cases. In approximately one-half of these reports of overdosage, concomitant medications were also taken. The highest dose of diclofenac was 5.0 g in a 17-year-old man who suffered loss of consciousness, increased intracranial pressure, and aspiration pneumonitis, and died 2 days after overdose. A 24-year-old woman who took 4.0 g and the 28- and 42-year-old women, each of whom took 3.75 g, did not develop any clinically significant signs or symptoms. However, there was a report of a 17-year-old female who experienced vomiting and drowsiness after an overdose of 2.37 g of diclofenac.

Animal studies show a wide range of susceptibilities to acute overdosage, with primates being more resistant to acute toxicity than rodents (LD_{50} in mg/kg: rats, 55; dogs, 500; monkeys, 3200).

Misoprostol

The toxic dose of misoprostol in humans has not been determined. Cumulative total daily doses of 1600 mcg have been tolerated, with only symptoms of GI discomfort being reported. In animals, the acute toxic effects are diarrhea, GI lesions, focal cardiac necrosis, hepatic necrosis, renal tubular necrosis, testicular atrophy, respiratory difficulties, and depression of the central nervous system. Clinical signs that may indicate an overdose are sedation, tremor, convulsions, dyspnea, abdominal pain, diarrhea, fever, palpitations, hypotension, or bradycardia.

ARTHROTEC

Symptoms of ARTHROTEC overdosage should be treated with supportive therapy. In case of acute overdosage, gastric lavage is recommended. Induced diuresis may be beneficial because diclofenac sodium and misoprostol metabolites are excreted in the urine. The effect of dialysis or hemoperfusion on the elimination of diclofenac sodium (99% protein bound) and misoprostol acid remains unproven. The use of oral activated charcoal may help to reduce the absorption of diclofenac sodium and misoprostol.

DOSAGE AND ADMINISTRATION

ARTHROTEC is administered as ARTHROTEC 50 (50 mg diclofenac sodium/200 mcg misoprostol) or as ARTHROTEC 75 (75 mg diclofenac sodium/200 mcg misoprostol).

Note: See *SPECIAL DOSING CONSIDERATIONS* section, below.

Osteoarthritis: The recommended dosage for maximal GI mucosal protection is ARTHROTEC 50 tid. For patients who experience intolerance, ARTHROTEC 75 bid or ARTHROTEC 50 bid can be used, but are less effective in preventing ulcers. This fixed combination product, ARTHROTEC, is not appropriate for patients who would not receive the appropriate dose of both ingredients. Doses of the components delivered with these regimens are as follows:

	OA regimen	Diclofenac sodium (mg/day)	Misoprostol (mcg/day)
ARTHROTEC 50	tid	150	600
	bid	100	400
ARTHROTEC 75	bid	150	400

Rheumatoid Arthritis: The recommended dosage is ARTHROTEC 50 tid or qid. For patients who experience intolerance, ARTHROTEC 75 bid or ARTHROTEC 50 bid can be used, but are less effective in preventing ulcers. This fixed combination product, ARTHROTEC, is not appropriate for patients who would not receive the appropriate dose of both ingredients. Doses of the components delivered with these regimens are as follows:

	RA regimen	Diclofenac sodium (mg/day)	Misoprostol (mcg/day)
ARTHROTEC 50	qid	200	800
	tid	150	600
	bid	100	400
ARTHROTEC 75	bid	150	400

SPECIAL DOSING CONSIDERATIONS: ARTHROTEC contains misoprostol, which provides protection against gastric and duodenal ulcers (see *CLINICAL STUDIES*). For gastric

ulcer prevention, the 200 mcg qid and tid regimens are therapeutically equivalent, but more protective than the bid regimen. For duodenal ulcer prevention, the qid regimen is more protective than the tid or bid regimens. However, the qid regimen is less well tolerated than the tid regimen because of usually self-limited diarrhea related to the misoprostol dose (see *ADVERSE REACTIONS—Gastrointestinal*), and the bid regimen may be better tolerated than tid in some patients.
Dosages may be individualized using the separate products (misoprostol and diclofenac), after which the patient may be changed to the appropriate ARTHROTEC dose. If clinically indicated, misoprostol co-therapy with ARTHROTEC, or use of the individual components to optimize the misoprostol dose and/or frequency of administration, may be appropriate. The total dose of misoprostol should not exceed 800 mcg/day, and no more than 200 mcg of misoprostol should be administered at any one time. Doses of diclofenac higher than 150 mg/day in osteoarthritis or higher than 225 mg/day in rheumatoid arthritis are not recommended. For additional information, it may be helpful to refer to the package inserts for Cytotec® tablets and Voltaren® tablets.

HOW SUPPLIED

ARTHROTEC (diclofenac sodium/misoprostol) is supplied as a film-coated tablet in dosage strengths of either 50 mg diclofenac sodium/200 mcg misoprostol or 75 mg diclofenac sodium/200 mcg misoprostol. The 50 mg/200 mcg dosage strength is a round, biconvex, white to off-white tablet imprinted with four "A's" encircling a "50" in the middle on one side and "SEARLE" and "1411" on the other. The 75 mg/200 mcg dosage strength is a round, biconvex, white to off-white tablet imprinted with four "A's" encircling a "75" in the middle on one side and "SEARLE" and "1421" on the other.
The dosage strengths are supplied in:

Strength	NDC Number	Size
50/200	0025–1411–60	bottle of 60
	0025–1411–90	bottle of 90
	0025–1411–34	carton of 100 unit dose
75/200	0025–1421–60	bottle of 60
	0025–1421–34	carton of 100 unit dose

Store at or below 25°C (77°F), in a dry area.

PATIENT INFORMATION

Read this leaflet before taking ARTHROTEC (diclofenac sodium 50 or 75 mg/misoprostol 200 mcg) and each time your prescription is renewed, because the leaflet may be changed.
ARTHROTEC is being prescribed by your doctor for treatment of your arthritis symptoms while at the same time providing protection from the development of stomach and intestinal ulcers due to the arthritis medication. ARTHROTEC contains diclofenac, an arthritis medication. ARTHROTEC also contains misoprostol to decrease the chance of getting stomach and intestinal ulcers that sometimes develop with NSAID medications. Serious side effects are still possible, however, and you should report to your physician any signs or symptoms of gastrointestinal ulceration or bleeding, skin rash, weight gain or swelling. If signs of liver toxicity occur (nausea, fatigue, lethargy, itching, jaundice, right upper quadrant tenderness, and "flu-like" symptoms) you should stop therapy and seek immediate medical attention.
Do not take ARTHROTEC if you are pregnant, because it contains misoprostol which can cause miscarriage if given at any stage of pregnancy. It is also important to avoid pregnancy while taking this medication and for at least one month or through one menstrual cycle after you stop taking it. Misoprostol may cause the uterus to rupture (tear) in pregnant women if it is used to bring on (induce) labor or to cause an abortion after the first trimester of pregnancy. Miscarriages or rupture of the uterus may result in severe bleeding, hospitalization, surgery, infertility or death.
If you become pregnant during ARTHROTEC therapy, stop taking ARTHROTEC and contact your doctor immediately. Remember that even if you are using a means of birth control, it is still possible to become pregnant. Should this occur, stop taking ARTHROTEC and consult your physician immediately.
ARTHROTEC may cause diarrhea, abdominal pain, upset stomach and/or nausea in some people. In most cases these problems develop during the first few weeks of therapy and stop after about a week with continued treatment. You can minimize possible diarrhea by making sure you take ARTHROTEC with meals and by avoiding the use of antacids containing magnesium (if needed, use one containing aluminum or calcium instead). ARTHROTEC tablets should be swallowed whole, and not chewed, crushed or dissolved. Because these side effects are usually mild to moderate and usually go away in a matter of days, most patients can continue to take ARTHROTEC. If you have prolonged difficulty (more than 7 days), or if you have severe diarrhea, cramping and/or nausea, call your doctor.
Take ARTHROTEC only according to the directions given by your doctor. Changes in dose should be made only with your doctor's approval.
Do not give ARTHROTEC to anyone else. It has been prescribed for your specific condition, may not be the correct treatment for another person, and could be dangerous for another person, especially a woman who may be, or could become, pregnant.
This information sheet does not cover all possible side effects of ARTHROTEC. See your doctor if you have questions.

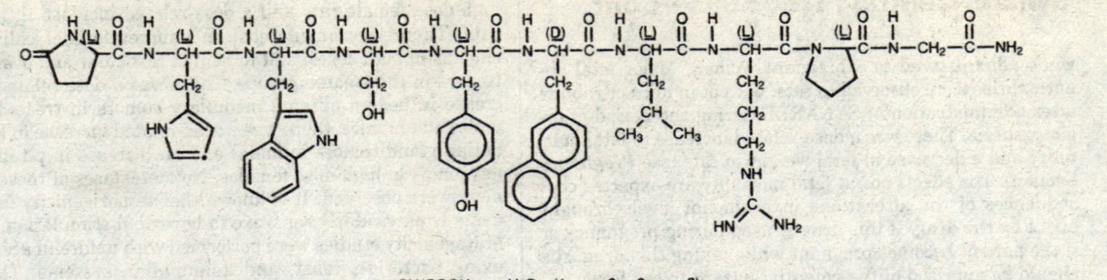

• x CH_3COOH • y H_2O (1 ≤ x ≤ 2; 2 ≤ y ≤ 8)

Keep out of reach of children.
℞ only Revised: July 2003
Manufactured for:
G.D. Searle LLC
A subsidiary of Pharmacia Corporation
Chicago, IL 60680, USA
by:
Pharmacia Limited
Morpeth, England
PHARMACIA
819 654 001 P04033-1

SYNAREL® ℞
[sĭn-ă-rĕl]
nafarelin acetate
nasal solution

Prescribing information for this product, which appears on pages 3111–3113 of the 2004 PDR, has been completely revised as follows. Please write "See Supplement A" next to the product heading.

CENTRAL PRECOCIOUS PUBERTY (FOR ENDOMETRIOSIS, SEE FOLLOWING SIDE)

PHYSICIAN LABELING

DESCRIPTION

SYNAREL (nafarelin acetate) Nasal Solution is intended for administration as a spray to the nasal mucosa. Nafarelin acetate, the active component of SYNAREL Nasal Solution, is a decapeptide with the chemical name: 5-oxo-L-prolyl-L-histidyl-L-tryptophyl-L-seryl-L-tyrosyl-3-(2-naphthyl)-D-alanyl-L-leucyl-L-arginyl-L-prolyl-glycinamide acetate. Nafarelin acetate is a synthetic analog of the naturally occurring gonadotropin-releasing hormone (GnRH).
Nafarelin acetate has the following chemical structure:
[See chemical structure above]
SYNAREL Nasal Solution contains nafarelin acetate (2 mg/mL, content expressed as nafarelin base) in a solution of benzalkonium chloride, glacial acetic acid, sodium hydroxide or hydrochloric acid (to adjust pH), sorbitol, and purified water.
After priming the pump unit for SYNAREL, each actuation of the unit delivers approximately 100 µL of the spray containing approximately 200 µg nafarelin base. The contents of one spray bottle are intended to deliver at least 60 sprays.

CLINICAL PHARMACOLOGY

Nafarelin acetate is a potent agonistic analog of gonadotropin-releasing hormone (GnRH). At the onset of administration, nafarelin stimulates the release of the pituitary gonadotropins, LH and FSH, resulting in a temporary increase of gonadal steroidogenesis. Repeated dosing abolishes the stimulatory effect on the pituitary gland. Twice daily administration leads to decreased secretion of gonadal steroids by about 4 weeks; consequently, tissues and functions that depend on gonadal steroids for their maintenance become quiescent.
In **children**, nafarelin acetate was rapidly absorbed into the systemic circulation after intranasal administration. Maximum serum concentrations (measured by RIA) were achieved between 10 and 45 minutes. Following a single dose of 400 µg base, the observed peak concentration was 2.2 ng/mL, whereas following a single dose of 600 µg base, the observed peak concentration was 6.6 ng/mL. The average serum half-life of nafarelin following intranasal administration of a 400 µg dose was approximately 2.5 hours. It is not known and cannot be predicted what the pharmacokinetics of nafarelin will be in children given a dose above 600 µg.
In **adult women**, nafarelin acetate was rapidly absorbed into the systemic circulation after intranasal administration. Maximum serum concentrations (measured by RIA) were achieved between 10 and 40 minutes. Following a single dose of 200 µg base, the observed average peak concentration was 0.6 ng/mL (range 0.2 to 1.4 ng/mL), whereas following a single dose of 400 µg base, the observed average peak concentration was 1.8 ng/mL (range 0.5 to 5.3 ng/mL). Bioavailability from a 400 µg dose averaged 2.8% (range 1.2 to 5.6%). The average serum half-life of nafarelin following intranasal administration was approximately 3 hours. About 80% of nafarelin acetate was bound to plasma proteins at 4°C. Twice daily intranasal administration of 200 or 400 µg of SYNAREL in 18 healthy women for 22 days did not lead to significant accumulation of the drug. Based on the mean C_{min} levels on Days 15 and 22, there appeared to be dose proportionality across the two dose levels.
After subcutaneous administration of ^{14}C-nafarelin acetate to men, 44–55% of the dose was recovered in urine and 18.5–44.2% was recovered in the feces. Approximately 3% of the administered dose appeared as unchanged nafarelin in urine. The ^{14}C serum half-life of the metabolites was about 85.5 hours. Six metabolites of nafarelin have been identified of which the major metabolite is Tyr-D(2)-Nal-Leu-Arg-Pro-Gly-NH_2(5–10). The activity of the metabolites, the metabolism of nafarelin by nasal mucosa, and the pharmacokinetics of the drug in hepatically- and renally-impaired patients have not been determined.
There appeared to be no significant effect of rhinitis, i.e., nasal congestion, on the systemic bioavailability of SYNAREL; however, if the use of a nasal decongestant for rhinitis is necessary during treatment with SYNAREL, the decongestant should not be used until at least 2 hours following dosing with SYNAREL.
When used regularly in girls and boys with **central precocious puberty (CPP)** at the recommended dose, SYNAREL suppresses LH and sex steroid hormone levels to prepubertal levels, affects a corresponding arrest of secondary sexual development, and slows linear growth and skeletal maturation. In some cases, initial estrogen withdrawal bleeding may occur, generally within 6 weeks after initiation of therapy. Thereafter, menstruation should cease.
In clinical studies the peak response of LH to GnRH stimulation was reduced from a pubertal response to a prepubertal response (< 15 mIU/mL) within one month of treatment.
Linear growth velocity, which is commonly pubertal in children with CPP, is reduced in most children within the first year of treatment to values of 5 to 6 cm/year or less. Children with CPP are frequently taller than their chronological age peers; height for chronological age approaches normal in most children during the second or third year of treatment with SYNAREL. Skeletal maturation rate (bone age velocity–change in bone age divided by change in chronological age) is usually abnormal (greater than 1) in children with CPP; in most children, bone age velocity approaches normal (1) during the first year of treatment. This results in a narrowing of the gap between bone age and chronological age, usually by the second or third year of treatment. The mean predicted adult height increases.
In clinical trials, breast development was arrested or regressed in 82% of girls, and genital development was arrested or regressed in 100% of boys. Because pubic hair growth is largely controlled by adrenal androgens, which are unaffected by nafarelin, pubic hair development was arrested or regressed only in 54% of girls and boys.
Reversal of the suppressive effects of SYNAREL has been demonstrated to occur in all children with CPP for whom one-year post-treatment follow-up is available (n=69). This demonstration consisted of the appearance or return of menses, the return of pubertal gonadotropin and gonadal sex steroid levels, and/or the advancement of secondary sexual development. Semen analysis was normal in the two ejaculated specimens obtained thus far from boys who have been taken off therapy to resume puberty. Fertility has not been documented by pregnancies and the effect of long-term use of the drug on fertility is not known.

INDICATIONS AND USAGE

FOR CENTRAL PRECOCIOUS PUBERTY

(For Endometriosis, *See Following Side*)
SYNAREL is indicated for treatment of **central precocious puberty (CPP)** (gonadotropin-dependent precocious puberty) in children of both sexes.
The diagnosis of **central precocious puberty (CPP)** is suspected when premature development of secondary sexual characteristics occurs at or before the age of 8 years in girls and 9 years in boys, and is accompanied by significant advancement of bone age and/or a poor adult height prediction. The diagnosis should be confirmed by pubertal gonadal sex steroid levels and a pubertal LH response to stimulation by native GnRH. Pelvic ultrasound assessment in girls usually reveals enlarged uterus and ovaries, the latter often with multiple cystic formations. Magnetic resonance imaging or CT-scanning of the brain is recommended to detect hypothalamic or pituitary tumors, or anatomical changes associated with increased intracranial pressure. Other causes of sexual precocity, such as congenital adrenal hyperplasia, testotoxicosis, testicular tumors and/or other autonomous feminizing or masculinizing disorders must be excluded by proper clinical hormonal and diagnostic imaging examinations.

CONTRAINDICATIONS

1. Hypersensitivity to GnRH, GnRH agonist analogs or any of the excipients in SYNAREL;
2. Undiagnosed abnormal vaginal bleeding;
3. Use in pregnancy or in women who may become pregnant while receiving the drug. SYNAREL may cause fetal harm

Continued on next page

Synarel-Central Precocious—Cont.

when administered to a pregnant woman. Major fetal abnormalities were observed in rats, but not in mice or rabbits after administration of SYNAREL during the period of organogenesis. There was a dose-related increase in fetal mortality and a decrease in fetal weight in rats (see ***Pregnancy*** Section). The effects on rat fetal mortality are expected consequences of the alterations in hormonal levels brought about by the drug. If this drug is used during pregnancy or if the patient becomes pregnant while taking this drug, she should be apprised of the potential hazard to the fetus;

4. Use in women who are breast-feeding (see ***Nursing Mothers*** Section).

WARNINGS

The diagnosis of central precocious puberty (CPP) must be established before treatment is initiated. Regular monitoring of CPP patients is needed to assess both patient response as well as compliance. This is particularly important during the first 6 to 8 weeks of treatment to assure that suppression of pituitary-gonadal function is rapid. Testing may include LH response to GnRH stimulation and circulating gonadal sex steroid levels. Assessment of growth velocity and bone age velocity should begin within 3 to 6 months of treatment initiation.

Some patients may not show suppression of the pituitary-gonadal axis by clinical and/or biochemical parameters. This may be due to lack of compliance with the recommended treatment regimen and may be rectified by recommending that the dosing be done by caregivers. If compliance problems are excluded, the possibility of gonadotropin independent sexual precocity should be reconsidered and appropriate examinations should be conducted. If compliance problems are excluded and if gonadotropin independent sexual precocity is not present, the dose of SYNAREL may be increased to 1800 µg administered as 600 µg tid.

PRECAUTIONS

General

As with other drugs that stimulate the release of gonadotropins or that induce ovulation, in adult women with endometriosis ovarian cysts have been reported to occur in the first two months of therapy with SYNAREL. Many, but not all, of these events occurred in women with polycystic ovarian disease. These cystic enlargements may resolve spontaneously, generally by about four to six weeks of therapy, but in some cases may require discontinuation of drug and/or surgical intervention. The relevance, if any, of such events in children is unknown.

Information for Patients, Patients' Parents or Guardians

An information pamphlet for patients is included with the product. Patients and their caregivers should be aware of the following information:

1. Reversibility of the suppressive effects of nafarelin has been demonstrated by the appearance or return of menses, by the return of pubertal gonadotropin and gonadal sex steroid levels, and/or by advancement of secondary sexual development. Semen analysis was normal in the two ejaculated specimens obtained thus far from boys who have been taken off therapy to resume puberty. Fertility has not been documented by pregnancies and the effect of long-term use of the drug on fertility is not known.

2. Patients and their caregivers should be adequately counseled to assure full compliance; irregular or incomplete daily doses may result in stimulation of the pituitary-gonadal axis.

3. During the first month of treatment with SYNAREL, some signs of puberty, e.g., vaginal bleeding or breast enlargement, may occur. This is the expected initial effect of the drug. Such changes should resolve soon after the first month. If such resolution does not occur within the first two months of treatment, this may be due to lack of compliance or the presence of gonadotropin independent sexual precocity. If both possibilities are definitively excluded, the dose of SYNAREL may be increased to 1800 µg/day administered as 600 µg tid.

4. Patients with intercurrent rhinitis should consult their physician for the use of a topical nasal decongestant. If the use of a topical nasal decongestant is required during treatment with SYNAREL, the decongestant should not be used until at least 2 hours following dosing with SYNAREL.

Sneezing during or immediately after dosing with SYNAREL should be avoided, if possible, since this may impair drug absorption.

Drug Interactions

No pharmacokinetic-based drug-drug interaction studies have been conducted with SYNAREL. However, because nafarelin acetate is a peptide that is primarily degraded by peptidase and not by cytochrome P-450 enzymes, and the drug is only about 80% bound to plasma proteins at 4°C, drug interactions would not be expected to occur.

Carcinogenesis, Mutagenesis, Impairment of Fertility

Carcinogenicity studies of nafarelin were conducted in rats (24 months) at doses up to 100 µg/kg/day and mice (18 months) at doses up to 500 µg/kg/day using intramuscular doses (up to 110 times and 560 times the maximum recommended human intranasal dose, respectively). These multiples of the human dose are based on the relative bioavailability of the drug by the two routes of administration. As seen with other GnRH agonists, nafarelin acetate given to laboratory rodents at high doses for prolonged periods induced proliferative responses (hyperplasia and/or neoplasia) of endocrine organs. At 24 months, there was an increase in the incidence of pituitary tumors (adenoma/carcinoma) in high-dose female rats and a dose-related increase in male rats. There was an increase in pancreatic islet cell adenomas in both sexes, and in benign testicular and ovarian tumors in the treated groups. There was a dose-related increase in benign adrenal medullary tumors in treated female rats. In mice, there was a dose-related increase in Harderian gland tumors in males and an increase in pituitary adenomas in high-dose females. No metastases of these tumors were observed. It is known that tumorigenicity in rodents is particularly sensitive to hormonal stimulation.

Mutagenicity studies were performed with nafarelin acetate using bacterial, yeast, and mammalian systems. These studies provided no evidence of mutagenic potential.

Reproduction studies in male and female rats have shown full reversibility of fertility suppression when drug treatment was discontinued after continuous administration for up to 6 months. The effect of treatment of prepubertal rats on the subsequent reproductive performance of mature animals has not been investigated.

Pregnancy, Teratogenic Effects

Pregnancy Category X. See ***'CONTRAINDICATIONS.'*** Intramuscular SYNAREL was administered to rats during the period of organogenesis at 0.4, 1.6, and 6.4 µg/kg/day (about 0.5, 2, and 7 times the maximum recommended human intranasal dose based on the relative bioavailability by the two routes of administration). An increase in major fetal abnormalities was observed in 4/80 fetuses at the highest dose. A similar, repeat study at the same doses in rats and studies in mice and rabbits at doses up to 600 µg/kg/day and 0.18 µg/kg/day, respectively, failed to demonstrate an increase in fetal abnormalities after administration during the period of organogenesis. In rats and rabbits, there was a dose-related increase in fetal mortality and a decrease in fetal weight with the highest dose.

Nursing Mothers

It is not known whether SYNAREL is excreted in human milk. Because many drugs are excreted in human milk, and because the effects of SYNAREL on lactation and/or the breastfed child have not been determined, SYNAREL should not be used by nursing mothers.

ADVERSE REACTIONS

In clinical trials of 155 pediatric patients, 2.6% reported symptoms suggestive of drug sensitivity, such as shortness of breath, chest pain, urticaria, rash, and pruritus.

In these 155 patients treated for an average of 41 months and as long as 80 months (6.7 years), adverse events most frequently reported (>3% of patients) consisted largely of episodes occurring during the first 6 weeks of treatment as a result of the transient stimulatory action of nafarelin upon the pituitary-gonadal axis:

- acne (10%)
- transient breast enlargement (8%)
- vaginal bleeding (8%)
- emotional lability (6%)
- transient increase in pubic hair (5%)
- body odor (4%)
- seborrhea (3%)

Hot flashes, common in adult women treated for endometriosis, occurred in only 3% of treated children and were transient. Other adverse events thought to be drug-related, and occurring in >3% of patients were rhinitis (5%) and white or brownish vaginal discharge (3%). Approximately 3% of patients withdrew from clinical trials due to adverse events.

In one male patient with concomitant congenital adrenal hyperplasia, and who had discontinued treatment 8 months previously to resume puberty, adrenal rest tumors were found in the left testis. Relationship to SYNAREL is unlikely.

Regular examinations of the pituitary gland by magnetic resonance imaging (MRI) or computer assisted tomography (CT) of children during long-term nafarelin therapy as well as during the post-treatment period has occasionally revealed changes in the shape and size of the pituitary gland. These changes include asymmetry and enlargement of the pituitary gland, and a pituitary microadenoma has been suspected in a few children. The relationship of these findings to SYNAREL is not known.

OVERDOSAGE

In experimental animals, a single subcutaneous administration of up to 60 times the recommended human dose (on a µg/kg basis, not adjusted for bioavailability) had no adverse effects. At present, there is no clinical evidence of adverse effects following overdosage of GnRH analogs.

Based on studies in monkeys, SYNAREL is not absorbed after oral administration.

DOSAGE AND ADMINISTRATION

For the treatment of central precocious puberty (CPP), the recommended daily dose of SYNAREL is 1600 µg. The dose can be increased to 1800 µg daily if adequate suppression cannot be achieved at 1600 µg/day.

The 1600 µg dose is achieved by two sprays (400 µg) into each nostril in the morning (4 sprays) and two sprays into each nostril in the evening (4 sprays), a total of 8 sprays per day. The 1800 µg dose is achieved by 3 sprays (600 µg) into alternating nostrils three times a day, a total of 9 sprays per day. The patient's head should be tilted back slightly, and 30 seconds should elapse between sprays.

If the prescribed therapy has been well tolerated by the patient, treatment of CPP with SYNAREL should continue until resumption of puberty is desired.

There appeared to be no significant effect of rhinitis, i.e., nasal congestion, on the systemic bioavailability of SYNAREL; however, if the use of a nasal decongestant for rhinitis is necessary during treatment with SYNAREL, the decongestant should not be used until at least 2 hours following dosing with SYNAREL.

Sneezing during or immediately after dosing with SYNAREL should be avoided, if possible, since this may impair drug absorption.

At 1600 µg/day, a bottle of SYNAREL provides about a 7-day supply (about 56 sprays). If the daily dose is increased, increase the supply to the patient to ensure uninterrupted treatment for the duration of therapy.

HOW SUPPLIED

Each 0.5 ounce bottle (NDC 0025-0166-08) contains 8 mL SYNAREL (nafarelin acetate) Nasal Solution 2 mg/mL (as nafarelin base), and is supplied with a metered spray pump that delivers 200 µg of nafarelin per spray. A dust cover and a leaflet of patient instructions are also included.

Store upright at 25°C (77°F); excursions permitted to 15–30°C (59–86°F) [see USP Controlled Room Temperature]. Protect from light.

℞ only Revised: November 2003

U.S. Patent No. 4,234,571.

PHARMACIA
G.D. Searle LLC
A subsidiary of Pharmacia Corporation
Chicago, IL 60680, USA

SYNAREL® ℞
nafarelin acetate
nasal solution

ENDOMETRIOSIS
(FOR CENTRAL PRECOCIOUS PUBERTY, SEE PREVIOUS SIDE)

Prescribing information for this product, which appears on pages 3113–3114 of the 2004 PDR, has been completely revised as follows. Please write "See Supplement A" next to the product heading.

PHYSICIAN LABELING

DESCRIPTION

SYNAREL (nafarelin acetate) Nasal Solution is intended for administration as a spray to the nasal mucosa. Nafarelin acetate, the active component of SYNAREL Nasal Solution, is a decapeptide with the chemical name: 5-oxo-L-prolyl-L-histidyl-L-tryptophyl-L-seryl-L-tyrosyl-3-(2-naphthyl)-D-alanyl-L-leucyl-L-arginyl-L-prolyl-glycinamide acetate. Nafarelin acetate is a synthetic analog of the naturally occurring gonadotropin-releasing hormone (GnRH).

Nafarelin acetate has the following chemical structure:

[See chemical structure at top of next column]

SYNAREL Nasal Solution contains nafarelin acetate (2 mg/mL, content expressed as nafarelin base) in a solution of benzalkonium chloride, glacial acetic acid, sodium hydroxide or hydrochloric acid (to adjust pH), sorbitol, and purified water.

After priming the pump unit for SYNAREL, each actuation of the unit delivers approximately 100 µL of the spray containing approximately 200 µg nafarelin base. The contents of one spray bottle are intended to deliver at least 60 sprays.

CLINICAL PHARMACOLOGY

Nafarelin acetate is a potent agonistic analog of gonadotropin-releasing hormone (GnRH). At the onset of administration, nafarelin stimulates the release of the pituitary gonadotropins, LH and FSH, resulting in a temporary increase of ovarian steroidogenesis. Repeated dosing abolishes the stimulatory effect on the pituitary gland. Twice daily administration leads to decreased secretion of gonadal steroids by about 4 weeks; consequently, tissues and functions that depend on gonadal steroids for their maintenance become quiescent.

Nafarelin acetate is rapidly absorbed into the systemic circulation after intranasal administration. Maximum serum concentrations (measured by RIA) were achieved between 10 and 40 minutes. Following a single dose of 200 µg base, the observed average peak concentration was 0.6 ng/mL (range 0.2 to 1.4 ng/mL), whereas following a single dose of 400 µg base, the observed average peak concentration was 1.8 ng/mL (range 0.5 to 5.3 ng/mL). Bioavailability from a 400 µg dose averaged 2.8% (range 1.2 to 5.6%). The average serum half-life of nafarelin following intranasal administration is approximately 3 hours. About 80% of nafarelin acetate is bound to plasma proteins at 4°C. Twice daily intranasal administration of 200 or 400 µg of SYNAREL in 18 healthy women for 22 days did not lead to significant accumulation of the drug. Based on the mean C_{min} levels on Days 15 and 22, there appeared to be dose proportionality across the two dose levels.

After subcutaneous administration of ^{14}C-nafarelin acetate to men, 44–55% of the dose was recovered in urine and 18.5–44.2% was recovered in feces. Approximately 3% of the administered dose appeared as unchanged nafarelin in urine. The ^{14}C serum half-life of the metabolites was about 85.5 hours. Six metabolites of nafarelin have been identified of which the major metabolite is Tyr-D(2)-Nal-Leu-Arg-Pro-Gly-NH_2(5-10). The activity of the metabolites, the metabolism of nafarelin by nasal mucosa, and the pharmacokinetics of the drug in hepatically- and renally-impaired patients have not been determined.

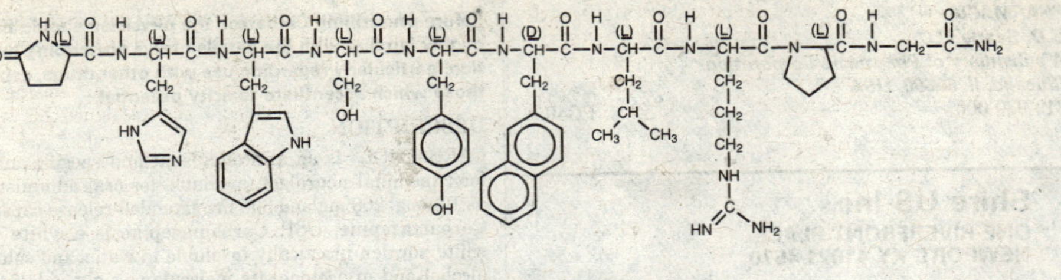

$\cdot x\, CH_3COOH \cdot y\, H_2O \quad (1 \le x \le 2;\ 2 \le y \le 8)$

There appeared to be no significant effect of rhinitis, i.e., nasal congestion, on the systemic bioavailability of SYNAREL; however, if the use of a nasal decongestant for rhinitis is necessary during treatment with SYNAREL, the decongestant should not be used until at least 2 hours following dosing of SYNAREL.
In controlled clinical studies, SYNAREL at doses of 400 and 800 µg/day for 6 months was shown to be comparable to danazol, 800 mg/day, in relieving the clinical symptoms of endometriosis (pelvic pain, dysmenorrhea, and dyspareunia) and in reducing the size of endometrial implants as determined by laparoscopy. The clinical significance of a decrease in endometriotic lesions is not known at this time and, in addition, laparoscopic staging of endometriosis does not necessarily correlate with severity of symptoms.
In a single controlled clinical trial, intranasal SYNAREL (nafarelin acetate) at a dose of 400 µg per day was shown to be clinically comparable to intramuscular leuprolide depot, 3.75 mg monthly, for the treatment of the symptoms (dysmenorrhea, dyspareunia and pelvic pain) associated with endometriosis.
SYNAREL 400 µg daily induced amenorrhea in approximately 65%, 80%, and 90% of the patients after 60, 90, and 120 days, respectively. In the first, second, and third post-treatment months, normal menstrual cycles resumed in 4%, 82%, and 100%, respectively, of those patients who did not become pregnant.
At the end of treatment, 60% of patients who received SYNAREL, 400 µg/day, were symptom free, 32% had mild symptoms, 7% had moderate symptoms, and 1% had severe symptoms. Of the 60% of patients who had complete relief of symptoms at the end of treatment, 17% had moderate symptoms 6 months after treatment was discontinued, 33% had mild symptoms, 50% remained symptom free, and no patient had severe symptoms.
During the first two months use of SYNAREL, some women experience vaginal bleeding of variable duration and intensity. In all likelihood, this bleeding represents estrogen withdrawal bleeding and is expected to stop spontaneously. If vaginal bleeding continues, the possibility of lack of compliance with the dosing regimen should be considered. If the patient is complying carefully with the regimen, an increase in dose to 400 µg twice a day should be considered.
There is no evidence that pregnancy rates are enhanced or adversely affected by the use of SYNAREL.

INDICATIONS AND USAGE FOR ENDOMETRIOSIS

(For Central Precocious Puberty, See *Previous Side*)
SYNAREL is indicated for management of endometriosis, including pain relief and reduction of endometriotic lesions. Experience with SYNAREL for the management of endometriosis has been limited to women 18 years of age and older treated for 6 months.

CONTRAINDICATIONS

1. Hypersensitivity to GnRH, GnRH agonist analogs or any of the excipients in SYNAREL;
2. Undiagnosed abnormal vaginal bleeding;
3. Use in pregnancy or in women who may become pregnant while receiving the drug. SYNAREL may cause fetal harm when administered to a pregnant woman. Major fetal abnormalities were observed in rats, but not in mice or rabbits after administration of SYNAREL during the period of organogenesis. There was a dose-related increase in fetal mortality and a decrease in fetal weight in rats (see ***Pregnancy*** Section). The effects on rat fetal mortality are expected consequences of the alterations in hormonal levels brought about by the drug. If this drug is used during pregnancy or if the patient becomes pregnant while taking this drug, she should be apprised of the potential hazard to the fetus;
4. Use in women who are breast-feeding (see ***Nursing Mothers*** Section).

WARNINGS

Safe use of nafarelin acetate in pregnancy has not been established clinically. Before starting treatment with SYNAREL, pregnancy must be excluded.
When used regularly at the recommended dose, SYNAREL usually inhibits ovulation and stops menstruation. Contraception is not insured, however, by taking SYNAREL, particularly if patients miss successive doses. Therefore, patients should use nonhormonal methods of contraception. Patients should be advised to see their physician if they believe they may be pregnant. If a patient becomes pregnant during treatment, the drug must be discontinued and the patient must be apprised of the potential risk to the fetus.

PRECAUTIONS

General
As with other drugs that stimulate the release of gonadotropins or that induce ovulation, ovarian cysts have been reported to occur in the first two months of therapy with SYNAREL. Many, but not all, of these events occurred in patients with polycystic ovarian disease. These cystic enlargements may resolve spontaneously, generally by about four to six weeks of therapy, but in some cases may require discontinuation of drug and/or surgical intervention.

Information for Patients
An information pamphlet for patients is included with the product. Patients should be aware of the following information:
1. Since menstruation should stop with effective doses of SYNAREL, the patient should notify her physician if regular menstruation persists. The cause of vaginal spotting, bleeding or menstruation could be noncompliance with the treatment regimen, or it could be that a higher dose of the drug is required to achieve amenorrhea. The patient should be questioned regarding her compliance. If she is careful and compliant, and menstruation persists to the second month, consideration should be given to doubling the dose of SYNAREL. If the patient has missed several doses, she should be counseled on the importance of taking SYNAREL regularly as prescribed.
2. Patients should not use SYNAREL if they are pregnant, breast-feeding, have undiagnosed abnormal vaginal bleeding, or are allergic to any of the ingredients in SYNAREL.
3. Safe use of the drug in pregnancy has not been established clinically. Therefore, a nonhormonal method of contraception should be used during treatment. Patients should be advised that if they miss successive doses of SYNAREL, breakthrough bleeding or ovulation may occur with the potential for conception. If a patient becomes pregnant during treatment, she should discontinue treatment and consult her physician.
4. Those adverse events occurring most frequently in clinical studies with SYNAREL are associated with hypoestrogenism; the most frequently reported are hot flashes, headaches, emotional lability, decreased libido, vaginal dryness, acne, myalgia, and reduction in breast size. Estrogen levels returned to normal after treatment was discontinued. Nasal irritation occurred in about 10% of all patients who used intranasal nafarelin.
5. The induced hypoestrogenic state results in a small loss in bone density over the course of treatment, some of which may not be reversible. During one six-month treatment period, this bone loss should not be important. In patients with major risk factors for decreased bone mineral content such as chronic alcohol and/or tobacco use, strong family history of osteoporosis, or chronic use of drugs that can reduce bone mass such as anticonvulsants or corticosteroids, therapy with SYNAREL may pose an additional risk. In these patients the risks and benefits must be weighed before therapy with SYNAREL is instituted. Repeated courses of treatment with gonadotropin-releasing hormone analogs are not advisable in patients with major risk factors for loss of bone mineral content.
6. Patients with intercurrent rhinitis should consult their physician for the use of a topical nasal decongestant. If the use of a topical nasal decongestant is required during treatment with SYNAREL, the decongestant should not be used until at least 2 hours following dosing with SYNAREL. Sneezing during or immediately after dosing with SYNAREL should be avoided, if possible, since this may impair drug absorption.
7. Retreatment cannot be recommended since safety data beyond 6 months are not available.

Drug Interactions
No pharmacokinetic-based drug-drug interaction studies have been conducted with SYNAREL. However, because nafarelin acetate is a peptide that is primarily degraded by peptidase and not by cytochrome P-450 enzymes, and the drug is only about 80% bound to plasma proteins at 4°C, drug interactions would not be expected to occur.

Drug/Laboratory Test Interactions
Administration of SYNAREL in therapeutic doses results in suppression of the pituitary-gonadal system. Normal function is usually restored within 4 to 8 weeks after treatment is discontinued. Therefore, diagnostic tests of pituitary gonadotropic and gonadal functions conducted during treatment and up to 4 to 8 weeks after discontinuation of therapy with SYNAREL may be misleading.

Carcinogenesis, Mutagenesis, Impairment of Fertility
Carcinogenicity studies of nafarelin were conducted in rats (24 months) at doses up to 100 µg/kg/day and mice (18 months) at doses up to 500 µg/kg/day using intramuscular doses (up to 110 times and 560 times the maximum recommended human intranasal dose, respectively). These multiples of the human dose are based on the relative bioavailability of the drug by the two routes of administration. As seen with other GnRH agonists, nafarelin acetate given to laboratory rodents at high doses for prolonged periods induced proliferative responses (hyperplasia and/or neoplasia) of endocrine organs. At 24 months, there was an increase in the incidence of pituitary tumors (adenoma/carcinoma) in high-dose female rats and a dose-related increase in male rats. There was an increase in pancreatic islet cell adenomas in both sexes, and in benign testicular and ovarian tumors in the treated groups. There was a dose-related increase in benign adrenal medullary tumors in treated female rats. In mice, there was a dose-related increase in Harderian gland tumors in males and an increase in pituitary adenomas in high-dose females. No metastases of these tumors were observed. It is known that tumorigenicity in rodents is particularly sensitive to hormonal stimulation.
Mutagenicity studies were performed with nafarelin acetate using bacterial, yeast, and mammalian systems. These studies provided no evidence of mutagenic potential.
Reproduction studies in male and female rats have shown full reversibility of fertility suppression when drug treatment was discontinued after continuous administration for up to 6 months. The effect of treatment of prepubertal rats on the subsequent reproductive performance of mature animals has not been investigated.

Pregnancy, Teratogenic Effects
Pregnancy Category X. See "***CONTRAINDICATIONS.***" Intramuscular SYNAREL was administered to rats during the period of organogenesis at 0.4, 1.6, and 6.4 µg/kg/day (about 0.5, 2, and 7 times the maximum recommended human intranasal dose based on the relative bioavailability by the two routes of administration). An increase in major fetal abnormalities was observed in 4/80 fetuses at the highest dose. A similar, repeat study at the same doses in rats and studies in mice and rabbits at doses up to 600 µg/kg/day and 0.18 µg/kg/day, respectively, failed to demonstrate an increase in fetal abnormalities after administration during the period of organogenesis. In rats and rabbits, there was a dose-related increase in fetal mortality and a decrease in fetal weight with the highest dose.

Nursing Mothers
It is not known whether SYNAREL is excreted in human milk. Because many drugs are excreted in human milk, and because the effects of SYNAREL on lactation and/or the breastfed child have not been determined, SYNAREL should not be used by nursing mothers.

Pediatric Use
Safety and effectiveness of SYNAREL for endometriosis in patients younger than 18 years have not been established.

ADVERSE REACTIONS

In formal clinical trials of 1509 healthy adult patients, symptoms suggestive of drug sensitivity, such as shortness of breath, chest pain, urticaria, rash and pruritus occurred in 3 patients (approximately 0.2%).
As would be expected with a drug which lowers serum estradiol levels, the most frequently reported adverse reactions were those related to hypoestrogenism.
In controlled studies comparing SYNAREL (400 µg/day) and danazol (600 or 800 mg/day), adverse reactions most frequently reported and thought to be drug-related are shown in the figure below:
[See figure at bottom of next page]
In addition, less than 1% of patients experienced paresthesia, palpitations, chloasma, maculopapular rash, eye pain, asthenia, lactation, breast engorgement, and arthralgia.

Changes in Bone Density
After six months of treatment with SYNAREL, vertebral trabecular bone density and total vertebral bone mass, measured by quantitative computed tomography (QCT), decreased by an average of 8.7% and 4.3%, respectively, compared to pretreatment levels. There was partial recovery of bone density in the post-treatment period; the average trabecular bone density and total bone mass were 4.9% and 3.3% less than the pretreatment levels, respectively. Total vertebral bone mass, measured by dual photon absorptiometry (DPA), decreased by a mean of 5.9% at the end of treatment.
After six months treatment with SYNAREL, bone mass as measured by dual x-ray bone densitometry (DEXA), decreased 3.2%. Mean total vertebral mass, re-examined by DEXA six months after completion of treatment, was 1.4% below pretreatment. There was little, if any, decrease in the mineral content in compact bone of the distal radius and second metacarpal. Use of SYNAREL for longer than the recommended six months or in the presence of other known risk factors for decreased bone mineral content may cause additional bone loss.

Changes in Laboratory Values During Treatment
Plasma enzymes. During clinical trials with SYNAREL, regular laboratory monitoring revealed that SGOT and SGPT levels were more than twice the upper limit of normal in only one patient each. There was no other clinical or laboratory evidence of abnormal liver function and levels returned to normal in both patients after treatment was stopped.
Lipids. At enrollment, 9% of the patients in the group taking SYNAREL 400 µg/day and 2% of the patients in the danazol group had total cholesterol values above 250 mg/dL. These patients also had cholesterol values above 250 mg/dL at the end of treatment.
Of those patients whose pretreatment cholesterol values were below 250 mg/dL, 6% in the group treated with SYNAREL and 18% in the danazol group, had post-treatment values above 250 mg/dL.
The mean (± SEM) pretreatment values for total cholesterol from all patients were 191.8 (4.3) mg/dL in the group treated with SYNAREL and 193.1 (4.6) mg/dL in the danazol group. At the end of treatment, the mean values for total cholesterol from all patients were 204.5 (4.8) mg/dL in the group treated with SYNAREL and 207.7 (5.1) mg/dL in the

Continued on next page

Synarel-Endometriosis—Cont.

danazol group. These increases from the pretreatment values were statistically significant ($p<0.05$) in both groups. Triglycerides were increased above the upper limit of 150 mg/dL in 12% of the patients who received SYNAREL and in 7% of the patients who received danazol.

At the end of treatment, no patients receiving SYNAREL had abnormally low HDL cholesterol fractions (less than 30 mg/dL) compared with 43% of patients receiving danazol. None of the patients receiving SYNAREL had abnormally high LDL cholesterol fractions (greater than 190 mg/dL) compared with 15% of those receiving danazol. There was no increase in the LDL/HDL ratio in patients receiving SYNAREL, but there was approximately a 2-fold increase in the LDL/HDL ratio in patients receiving danazol.

Other changes. In comparative studies, the following changes were seen in approximately 10% to 15% of patients. Treatment with SYNAREL was associated with elevations of plasma phosphorus and eosinophil counts, and decreases in serum calcium and WBC counts. Danazol therapy was associated with an increase of hematocrit and WBC.

OVERDOSAGE

In experimental animals, a single subcutaneous administration of up to 60 times the recommended human dose (on a µg/kg basis, not adjusted for bioavailability) had no adverse effects. At present, there is no clinical evidence of adverse effects following overdosage of GnRH analogs.

Based on studies in monkeys, SYNAREL is not absorbed after oral administration.

DOSAGE AND ADMINISTRATION

For the management of endometriosis, the recommended daily dose of SYNAREL is 400 µg. This is achieved by one spray (200 µg) into one nostril in the morning and one spray into the other nostril in the evening. Treatment should be started between days 2 and 4 of the menstrual cycle.

In an occasional patient, the 400 µg daily dose may not produce amenorrhea. For these patients with persistent regular menstruation after 2 months of treatment, the dose of SYNAREL may be increased to 800 µg daily. The 800 µg dose is administered as one spray into each nostril in the morning (a total of two sprays) and again in the evening.

The recommended duration of administration is six months. Retreatment cannot be recommended since safety data for retreatment are not available. If the symptoms of endometriosis recur after a course of therapy, and further treatment with SYNAREL is contemplated, it is recommended that bone density be assessed before retreatment begins to ensure that values are within normal limits.

There appeared to be no significant effect of rhinitis, i.e., nasal congestion, on the systemic bioavailability of SYNAREL; however, if the use of a nasal decongestant for rhinitis is necessary during treatment with SYNAREL, the decongestant should not be used until at least 2 hours following dosing with SYNAREL.

Sneezing during or immediately after dosing with SYNAREL should be avoided, if possible, since this may impair drug absorption.

At 400 µg/day, a bottle of SYNAREL provides a 30-day (about 60 sprays) supply. If the daily dose is increased, increase the supply to the patient to ensure uninterrupted treatment for the recommended duration of therapy.

HOW SUPPLIED

Each 0.5 ounce bottle (NDC 0025-0166-08) contains 8 mL SYNAREL (nafarelin acetate) Nasal Solution 2 mg/mL (as nafarelin base), and is supplied with a metered spray pump that delivers 200 µg of nafarelin per spray. A dust cover and a leaflet of patient instructions are also included.

Store upright at 25°C (77°F); excursions permitted to 15–30°C (59–86°F) [see USP Controlled Room Temperature]. Protect from light.

℞ only

U.S. Patent No. 4,234,571.

Revised: November 2003

ADVERSE EVENTS DURING 6 MONTHS TREATMENT WITH SYNAREL® 400 µg/day vs DANAZOL 600 OR 800 mg/day

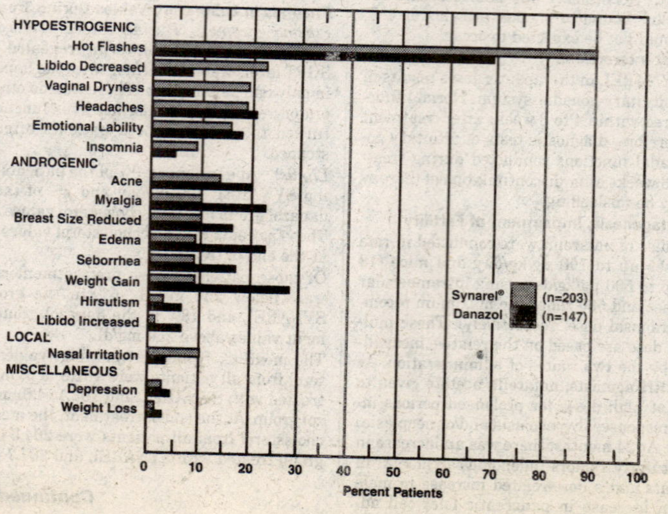

PHARMACIA
G.D. Searle LLC
A subsidiary of Pharmacia Corporation
Chicago, IL 60680, USA
819 930 000 PG4058

Shire US Inc.
ONE RIVERFRONT PLACE
NEWPORT, KY 41071-4570

Direct Inquiries to:
Customer Service
(800) 828-2088
(859) 669-8000
FAX: (859) 669-8420

For Medical Information Contact:
(800) 828-2088

CARBATROL® ℞

[căr-bō'trōl]

(carbamazepine extended-release capsules)

100 mg • 200 mg • 300 mg

Prescribing information for this product, which appears on pages 3148–3150 of the 2004 PDR, has been completely revised as follows. Please write "See Supplement A" next to the product heading.

Prescribing information

WARNING

APLASTIC ANEMIA AND AGRANULOCYTOSIS HAVE BEEN REPORTED IN ASSOCIATION WITH THE USE OF CARBAMAZEPINE. DATA FROM A POPULATION-BASED CASE-CONTROL STUDY DEMONSTRATE THAT THE RISK OF DEVELOPING THESE REACTIONS IS 5–8 TIMES GREATER THAN IN THE GENERAL POPULATION. HOWEVER, THE OVERALL RISK OF THESE REACTIONS IN THE UNTREATED GENERAL POPULATION IS LOW. APPROXIMATELY SIX PATIENTS PER ONE MILLION POPULATION PER YEAR FOR AGRANULOCYTOSIS AND TWO PATIENTS PER ONE MILLION POPULATION PER YEAR FOR APLASTIC ANEMIA.

ALTHOUGH REPORTS OF TRANSIENT OR PERSISTENT DECREASED PLATELET OR WHITE BLOOD CELL COUNTS ARE NOT UNCOMMON IN ASSOCIATION WITH THE USE OF CARBAMAZEPINE, DATA ARE NOT AVAILABLE TO ESTIMATE ACCURATELY THEIR INCIDENCE OR OUTCOME. HOWEVER, THE VAST MAJORITY OF THE CASES OF LEUKOPENIA HAVE NOT PROGRESSED TO THE MORE SERIOUS CONDITIONS OF APLASTIC ANEMIA OR AGRANULOCYTOSIS.

BECAUSE OF THE VERY LOW INCIDENCE OF AGRANULOCYTOSIS AND APLASTIC ANEMIA, THE VAST MAJORITY OF MINOR HEMATOLOGIC CHANGES OBSERVED IN MONITORING OF PATIENTS ON CARBAMAZEPINE ARE UNLIKELY TO SIGNAL THE OCCURRENCE OF EITHER ABNORMALITY. NONETHELESS, COMPLETE PRETREATMENT HEMATOLOGICAL TESTING SHOULD BE OBTAINED AS A BASELINE. IF A PATIENT IN THE COURSE OF TREATMENT EXHIBITS LOW OR DECREASED WHITE BLOOD CELL OR PLATELET COUNTS, THE PATIENT SHOULD BE MONITORED CLOSELY. DISCONTINUATION OF THE DRUG SHOULD BE CONSIDERED IF ANY EVIDENCE OF SIGNIFICANT BONE MARROW DEPRESSION DEVELOPS.

Before prescribing Carbatrol, the physician should be thoroughly familiar with the details of this prescribing information, particularly regarding use with other drugs, especially those which accentuate toxicity potential.

DESCRIPTION

CARBATROL® is an anticonvulsant and specific analgesic for trigeminal neuralgia, available for oral administration as 100 mg, 200 mg and 300 mg extended-release capsules of Carbamazepine, USP. Carbamazepine is a white to off-white powder, practically insoluble in water and soluble in alcohol and in acetone. Its molecular weight is 236.27. Its chemical name is 5H-dibenz[b,f]azepine-5-carboxamide, and its structural formula is:

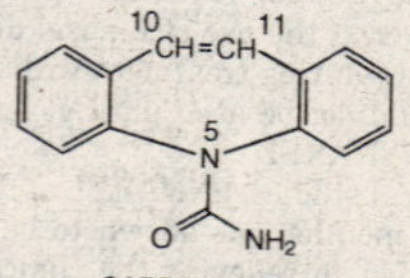

CARBAMAZEPINE

Carbatrol is a multi-component capsule formulation consisting of three different types of beads: immediate-release beads, extended-release beads, and enteric-release beads. The three bead types are combined in a specific ratio to provide twice daily dosing of Carbatrol.

Inactive ingredients: citric acid, colloidal silicon dioxide, lactose monohydrate, microcrystalline cellulose, polyethylene glycol, povidone, sodium lauryl sulfate, talc, triethyl citrate and other ingredients.

The 100 mg capsule shells contain gelatin-NF, FD&C Blue #2, Yellow Iron Oxide, and titanium dioxide and are imprinted with white ink; the 200 mg capsule shells contain gelatin-NF, FD&C Red #3, FD&C Yellow #6, Yellow Iron Oxide, FD&C Blue #2, and titanium dioxide, and are imprinted with white ink; and the 300 mg capsule shells contain gelatin-NF, FD&C Blue #2, FD&C Yellow #6, Red Iron Oxide, Yellow Iron Oxide, and titanium dioxide, and are imprinted with white ink.

CLINICAL PHARMACOLOGY

In controlled clinical trials, carbamazepine has been shown to be effective in the treatment of psychomotor and grand mal seizures, as well as trigeminal neuralgia.

Mechanism of Action

Carbamazepine has demonstrated anticonvulsant properties in rats and mice with electrically and chemically induced seizures. It appears to act by reducing polysynaptic responses and blocking the post-tetanic potentiation. Carbamazepine greatly reduces or abolishes pain induced by stimulation of the infraorbital nerve in cats and rats. It depresses thalamic potential and bulbar and polysynaptic reflexes, including the linguomandibular reflex in cats. Carbamazepine is chemically unrelated to other anticonvulsants or other drugs used to control the pain of trigeminal neuralgia. The mechanism of action remains unknown.

The principal metabolite of carbamazepine, carbamazepine-10,11-epoxide, has anticonvulsant activity as demonstrated in several *in vivo* animal models of seizures. Though clinical activity for the epoxide has been postulated, the significance of its activity with respect to the safety and efficacy of carbamazepine has not been established.

Pharmacokinetics

Carbamazepine (CBZ): Taken every 12 hours, carbamazepine extended-release capsules provide steady state plasma levels comparable to immediate-release carbamazepine tablets given every 6 hours, when administered at the same total mg daily dose. Following a single 200 mg oral extended-release dose of carbamazepine, peak plasma concentration was 1.9 ± 0.3 µg/mL and the time to reach the peak was 19 ± 7 hours. Following chronic administration (800 mg every 12 hours), the peak levels were 11.0 ± 2.5 µg/mL and the time to reach the peak was 5.9 ± 1.8 hours. The pharmacokinetics of extended-release carbamazepine is linear over the single dose range of 200–800 mg.

Carbamazepine is 76% bound to plasma proteins. Carbamazepine is primarily metabolized in the liver. Cytochrome P450 3A4 was identified as the major isoform responsible for the formation of carbamazepine-10,11-epoxide. Since carbamazepine induces its own metabolism, the half-life is also variable. Following a single extended-release dose of carbamazepine, the average half-life range from 35-40 hours and 12-17 hours on repeated dosing. The apparent oral clearance following a single dose was 25 ± 5 mL/min and following multiple dosing was 80 ± 30 mL/min.

After oral administration of ^{14}C-carbamazepine, 72% of the administered radioactivity was found in the urine and 28% in the feces. This urinary radioactivity was composed largely of hydroxylated and conjugated metabolites, with only 3% of unchanged carbamazepine.

Carbamazepine-10,11-epoxide (CBZ-E): Carbamazepine-10,11-epoxide is considered to be an active metabolite of carbamazepine. Following a single 200 mg oral extended-release dose of carbamazepine, the peak plasma concentration of carbamazepine-10,11-epoxide was 0.11 ± 0.012 µg/mL and the time to reach the peak was 36 ± 6 hours. Following chronic administration of a extended-release dose of carbamazepine (800 mg every 12 hours), the peak levels of carbamazepine-10,11-epoxide were 2.2 ± 0.9 µg/mL and the time to reach the peak was 14 ± 8 hours. The plasma half-life of carbamazepine-10,11-epoxide following administration of carbamazepine is 34 ± 9 hours. Following a single oral dose of extended-release carbamazepine (200-800 mg) the AUC and Cmax of carbamazepine-10,11-epoxide were less than 10% of carbamazepine. Following multiple dosing of extended-release carbamazepine (800-1600 mg daily for 14 days), the AUC and Cmax of carbamazepine-10,11-epoxide were dose related, ranging from 15.7 μg.hr/mL and 1.5 μg/mL at 800 mg/day to 32.6 μg.hr/mL and 3.2 μg/mL at 1600 mg/day, respectively, and were less than 30% of carbamazepine. Carbamazepine-10,11-epoxide is 50% bound to plasma proteins.

Food Effect: A high fat meal diet increased the rate of absorption of a single 400 mg dose (mean T_{max} was reduced from 24 hours, in the fasting state, to 14 hours and C_{max} increased from 3.2 to 4.3 μg/mL) but not the extent (AUC) of absorption. The elimination half-life remains unchanged between fed and fasting state. The multiple dose study conducted in the fed state showed that the steady-state C_{max} values were within the therapeutic concentration range. The pharmacokinetic profile of extended-release carbamazepine was similar when given by sprinkling the beads over applesauce compared to the intact capsule administered in the fasted state.

Special Populations

Hepatic Dysfunction: The effect of hepatic impairment on the pharmacokinetics of carbamazepine is not known. However, given that carbamazepine is primarily metabolized in the liver, it is prudent to proceed with caution in patients with hepatic dysfunction.

Renal Dysfunction: The effect of renal impairment on the pharmacokinetics of carbamazepine is not known.

Gender: No difference in the mean AUC and C_{max} of carbamazepine and carbamazepine-10,11-epoxide was found between males and females.

Age: Carbamazepine is more rapidly metabolized to carbamazepine-10,11-epoxide in young children than adults. In children below the age of 15, there is an inverse relationship between CBZ-E/CBZ ratio and increasing age.

Race: No information is available on the effect of race on the pharmacokinetics of carbamazepine.

INDICATIONS AND USAGE

Epilepsy

Carbatrol is indicated for use as an anticonvulsant drug. Evidence supporting efficacy of carbamazepine as an anticonvulsant was derived from active drug-controlled studies that enrolled patients with the following seizure types:

1. Partial seizures with complex symptomatology (psychomotor, temporal lobe). Patients with these seizures appear to show greater improvements than those with other types.
2. Generalized tonic-clonic seizures (grand mal).
3. Mixed seizure patterns which include the above, or other partial or generalized seizures. Absence seizures (petit mal) do not appear to be controlled by carbamazepine (see PRECAUTIONS, General).

Trigeminal Neuralgia

Carbatrol is indicated in the treatment of the pain associated with true trigeminal neuralgia. Beneficial results have also been reported in glossopharyngeal neuralgia. This drug is not a simple analgesic and should not be used for the relief of trivial aches or pains.

CONTRAINDICATIONS

Carbamazepine should not be used in patients with a history of previous bone marrow depression, hypersensitivity to the drug, or known sensitivity to any of the tricyclic compounds, such as amitriptyline, desipramine, imipramine, protriptyline and nortriptyline. Likewise, on theoretical grounds its use with monoamine oxidase inhibitors is not recommended. Before administration of carbamazepine, MAO inhibitors should be discontinued for a minimum of 14 days, or longer if the clinical situation permits.

WARNINGS

Usage in Pregnancy

Carbamazepine can cause fetal harm when administered to a pregnant woman.

Epidemiological data suggest that there may be an association between the use of carbamazepine during pregnancy and congenital malformations, including spina bifida. The prescribing physician will wish to weigh the benefits of therapy against the risks in treating or counseling women of childbearing potential. If this drug is used during pregnancy, or if the patient becomes pregnant while taking this drug, the patient should be apprised of the potential hazard to the fetus.

Retrospective case reviews suggest that, compared with monotherapy, there may be a higher prevalence of teratogenic effects associated with the use of anticonvulsants in combination therapy.

In humans, transplacental passage of carbamazepine is rapid (30–60 minutes), and the drug is accumulated in the fetal tissues, with higher levels found in liver and kidney than in brain and lung.

Carbamazepine has been shown to have adverse effects in reproduction studies in rats when given orally in dosages 10-25 times the maximum human daily dosage (MHDD) of 1200 mg on a mg/kg basis or 1.5-4 times the MHDD on a mg/m2 basis. In rat teratology studies, 2 of 135 offspring showed kinked ribs at 250 mg/kg and 4 of 119 offspring at 650 mg/kg showed other anomalies (cleft palate, 1; talipes, 1; anophthalmos, 2). In reproduction studies in rats, nursing offspring demonstrated a lack of weight gain and an unkempt appearance at a maternal dosage level of 200 mg/kg.

Antiepileptic drugs should not be discontinued abruptly in patients in whom the drug is administered to prevent major seizures because of the strong possibility of precipitating status epilepticus with attendant hypoxia and threat to life. In individual cases where the severity and frequency of the seizure disorder are such that removal of medication does not pose a serious threat to the patient, discontinuation of the drug may be considered prior to and during pregnancy, although it cannot be said with any confidence that even minor seizures do not pose some hazard to the developing embryo or fetus.

Tests to detect defects using current accepted procedures should be considered a part of routine prenatal care in childbearing women receiving carbamazepine.

General

Patients with a history of adverse hematologic reaction to any drug may be particularly at risk.

Severe dermatologic reactions, including toxic epidermal necrolysis (Lyell's syndrome) and Stevens-Johnson syndrome have been reported with carbamazepine. These reactions have been extremely rare. However, a few fatalities have been reported.

Carbamazepine has shown mild anticholinergic activity; therefore, patients with increased intraocular pressure should be closely observed during therapy.

Because of the relationship of the drug to other tricyclic compounds, the possibility of activation of a latent psychosis and, in elderly patients, of confusion or agitation should be considered.

PRECAUTIONS

General

Before initiating therapy, a detailed history and physical examination should be made.

Carbamazepine should be used with caution in patients with a mixed seizure disorder that includes atypical absence seizures, since in these patients carbamazepine has been associated with increased frequency of generalized convulsions (see INDICATIONS AND USAGE).

Therapy should be prescribed only after critical benefit-to-risk appraisal in patients with a history of cardiac, hepatic, or renal damage; adverse hematologic reaction to other drugs; or interrupted courses of therapy with carbamazepine.

Information for Patients

Patients should be made aware of the early toxic signs and symptoms of a potential hematologic problem, such as fever, sore throat, rash, ulcers in the mouth, easy bruising, petechial or purpuric hemorrhage, and should be advised to report to the physician immediately if any such signs or symptoms appear.

Since dizziness and drowsiness may occur, patients should be cautioned about the hazards of operating machinery or automobiles or engaging in other potentially dangerous tasks.

If necessary, the Carbatrol capsules can be opened and the contents sprinkled over food, such as a teaspoon of applesauce or other similar food products. Carbatrol capsules or their contents should not be crushed or chewed.

Laboratory Tests

Complete pretreatment blood counts, including platelets and possibly reticulocytes and serum iron, should be obtained as a baseline. If a patient in the course of treatment exhibits low or decreased white blood cell or platelet counts, the patient should be monitored closely. Discontinuation of the drug should be considered if any evidence of significant bone marrow depression develops.

Baseline and periodic evaluations of liver function, particularly in patients with a history of liver disease, must be performed during treatment with this drug since liver damage may occur. The drug should be discontinued immediately in cases of aggravated liver dysfunction or active liver disease.

Baseline and periodic eye examinations, including slit-lamp, funduscopy, and tonometry, are recommended since many phenothiazines and related drugs have been shown to cause eye changes.

Baseline and periodic complete urinalysis and BUN determinations are recommended for patients treated with this agent because of observed renal dysfunction.

Monitoring of blood levels (see CLINICAL PHARMACOLOGY) has increased the efficacy and safety of anticonvulsants. This monitoring may be particularly useful in cases of dramatic increase in seizure frequency and for verification of compliance. In addition, measurement of drug serum levels may aid in determining the cause of toxicity when more than one medication is being used.

Thyroid function tests have been reported to show decreased values with carbamazepine administered alone.

Hyponatremia has been reported in association with carbamazepine use, either alone or in combination with other drugs.

Interference with some pregnancy tests has been reported.

Drug Interactions

Clinically meaningful drug interactions have occurred with concomitant medications and include, but are not limited to the following:

Agents that may affect carbamazepine plasma levels:

CYP 3A4 inhibitors inhibit carbamazepine metabolism and can thus increase plasma carbamazepine levels.

Drugs that have been shown, or would be expected, to increase plasma carbamazepine levels include:

cimetidine, danazol, diltiazem, macrolides, erythromycin, troleandomycin, clarithromycin, fluoxetine, loratadine, terfenadine, isoniazid, niacinamide, nicotinamide, propoxyphene, ketoconazole, itraconazole, verapamil, valproate.*

CYP 3A4 inducers can increase the rate of carbamazepine metabolism and can thus decrease plasma carbamazepine levels. Drugs that have been shown, or would be expected, to decrease plasma carbamazepine levels include:

cisplatin, doxorubicin HCL, felbamate, rifampin*, phenobarbital, phenytoin, primidone, theophylline.

*increased levels of the active 10, 11-epoxide

Effect of carbamazepine on plasma levels of concomitant agents:

Carbatrol increases levels of clomipramine HCL, phenytoin and primidone.

Carbatrol induces hepatic CYP activity. Carbatrol causes, or would be expected to cause decreased levels of the following:

acetaminophen, alprazolam, clonazepam, clozapine, dicumarol, doxycycline, ethosuximide, haloperidol, methsuximide, oral contraceptives, phensuximide, phenytoin, theophylline, valproate, warfarin.

The doses of these drugs may therefore have to be increased when carbamazepine is added to the therapeutic regimen.

Concomitant administration of carbamazepine and lithium may increase the risk of neurotoxic side effects. Alterations of thyroid function have been reported in combination therapy with other anticonvulsant medications.

Breakthrough bleeding has been reported among patients receiving concomitant oral contraceptives and their reliability may be adversely affected.

Carcinogenesis, Mutagenesis, Impairment of Fertility

Administration of carbamazepine to Sprague-Dawley rats for two years in the diet at doses of 25, 75, and 250 mg/kg/day (low dose approximately 0.2 times the maximum human daily dose of 1200 mg on a mg/m^2 basis), resulted in a dose-related increase in the incidence of hepatocellular tumors in females and of benign interstitial cell adenomas in the testes of males.

Carbamazepine must, therefore, be considered to be carcinogenic in Sprague-Dawley rats. Bacterial and mammalian mutagenicity studies using carbamazepine produced negative results. The significance of these findings relative to the use of carbamazepine in humans is, at present, unknown.

Usage in Pregnancy

Pregnancy Category D (See WARNINGS)

Labor and Delivery

The effect of carbamazepine on human labor and delivery is unknown.

Nursing Mothers

Carbamazepine and its epoxide metabolite are transferred to breast milk and during lactation. The concentrations of carbamazepine and its epoxide metabolite are approximately 50% of the maternal plasma concentration. Because of the potential for serious adverse reactions in nursing infants from carbamazepine, a decision should be made whether to discontinue nursing or to discontinue the drug, taking into account the importance of the drug to the mother.

Pediatric Use

Substantial evidence of carbamazepine effectiveness for use in the management of children with epilepsy (see INDICATIONS for specific seizure types) is derived from clinical investigations performed in adults and from studies in several *in vitro* systems which support the conclusion that (1) the pathogenic mechanisms underlying seizure propagation are essentially identical in adults and children, and (2) the mechanism of action of carbamazepine in treating seizures is essentially identical in adults and children.

Taken as a whole, this information supports a conclusion that the generally acceptable therapeutic range of total carbamazepine in plasma (i.e., 4–12 μg/mL) is the same in children and adults.

The evidence assembled was primarily obtained from short-term use of carbamazepine. The safety of carbamazepine in children has been systematically studied up to 6 months. No longer term data from clinical trials is available.

Geriatric Use

No systematic studies in geriatric patients have been conducted.

ADVERSE REACTIONS

General: If adverse reactions are of such severity that the drug must be discontinued, the physician must be aware that abrupt discontinuation of any anticonvulsant drug in a responsive patient with epilepsy may lead to seizures or even status epilepticus with its life-threatening hazards.

The most severe adverse reactions previously observed with carbamazepine were reported in the hemopoietic system (see BOX WARNING), the skin, and the cardiovascular system.

The most frequently observed adverse reactions, particularly during the initial phases of therapy, are dizziness, drowsiness, unsteadiness, nausea, and vomiting. To minimize the possibility of such reactions, therapy should be initiated at the lowest dosage recommended.

The following additional adverse reactions were previously reported with carbamazepine:

Hemopoietic System: Aplastic anemia, agranulocytosis, pancytopenia, bone marrow depression, thrombocytopenia, leukopenia, leukocytosis, eosinophilia, acute intermittent porphyria.

Skin: Pruritic and erythematous rashes, urticaria, toxic epidermal necrolysis (Lyell's syndrome) (see WARNINGS),

Continued on next page

Carbatrol—Cont.

Stevens-Johnson syndrome (see WARNINGS), photosensitivity reactions, alterations in skin pigmentation, exfoliative dermatitis, erythema multiforme and nodosum, purpura, aggravation of disseminated lupus erythematosus, alopecia, and diaphoresis. In certain cases, discontinuation of therapy may be necessary. Isolated cases of hirsutism have been reported, but a causal relationship is not clear.
Cardiovascular System: Congestive heart failure, edema, aggravation of hypertension, hypotension, syncope and collapse, aggravation of coronary artery disease, arrhythmias and AV block, thrombophlebitis, thromboembolism, and adenopathy or lymphadenopathy. Some of these cardiovascular complications have resulted in fatalities. Myocardial infarction has been associated with other tricyclic compounds.
Liver: Abnormalities in liver function tests, cholestatic and hepatocellular jaundice, hepatitis.
Respiratory System: Pulmonary hypersensitivity characterized by fever, dyspnea, pneumonitis, or pneumonia.
Genitourinary System: Urinary frequency, acute urinary retention, oliguria with elevated blood pressure, azotemia, renal failure, and impotence. Albuminuria, glycosuria, elevated BUN, and microscopic deposits in the urine have also been reported.
Testicular atrophy occurred in rats receiving carbamazepine orally from 4-52 weeks at dosage levels of 50-400 mg/kg/day. Additionally, rats receiving carbamazepine in the diet for 2 years at dosage levels of 25, 75, and 250 mg/kg/day had a dose-related incidence of testicular atrophy and aspermatogenesis. In dogs, it produced a brownish discoloration, presumably a metabolite, in the urinary bladder at dosage levels of 50 mg/kg/day and higher. Relevance of these findings to humans is unknown.
Nervous System: Dizziness, drowsiness, disturbances of coordination, confusion, headache, fatigue, blurred vision, visual hallucinations, transient diplopia, oculomotor disturbances, nystagmus, speech disturbances, abnormal involuntary movements, peripheral neuritis and paresthesias, depression with agitation, talkativeness, tinnitus, and hyperacusis.
There have been reports of associated paralysis and other symptoms of cerebral arterial insufficiency, but the exact relationship of these reactions to the drug has not been established.
Isolated cases of neuroleptic malignant syndrome have been reported with concomitant use of psychotropic drugs.
Digestive System: Nausea, vomiting, gastric distress and abdominal pain, diarrhea, constipation, anorexia, and dryness of the mouth and pharynx, including glossitis and stomatitis.
Eyes: Scattered punctate cortical lens opacities, as well as conjunctivitis, have been reported. Although a direct causal relationship has not been established, many phenothiazines and related drugs have been shown to cause eye changes.
Musculoskeletal System: Aching joints and muscles, and leg cramps.
Metabolism: Fever and chills, inappropriate antidiuretic hormone (ADH) secretion syndrome has been reported. Cases of frank water intoxication, with decreased serum sodium (hyponatremia) and confusion have been reported in association with carbamazepine use (see PRECAUTIONS, Laboratory Tests). Decreased levels of plasma calcium have been reported.
Other: Isolated cases of a lupus erythematosus-like syndrome have been reported. There have been occasional reports of elevated levels of cholesterol, HDL cholesterol, and triglycerides in patients taking anticonvulsants.
A case of aseptic meningitis, accompanied by myoclonus and peripheral eosinophilia, has been reported in a patient taking carbamazepine in combination with other medications. The patient was successfully dechallenged, and the meningitis reappeared upon rechallenge with carbamazepine.

DRUG ABUSE AND DEPENDENCE

No evidence of abuse potential has been associated with carbamazepine, nor is there evidence of psychological or physical dependence in humans.

OVERDOSAGE

Acute Toxicity
Lowest known lethal dose: adults, >60 g (39-year-old man). Highest known doses survived: adults, 30 g (31-year-old woman); children, 10 g (6-year-old boy); small children, 5 g (3-year-old girl).
Oral LD_{50} in animals (mg/kg): mice, 1100-3750; rats, 3850-4025; rabbits, 1500–2680; guinea pigs, 920.
Signs and Symptoms
The first signs and symptoms appear after 1–3 hours. Neuromuscular disturbances are the most prominent. Cardiovascular disorders are generally milder, and severe cardiac complications occur only when very high doses (>60 g) have been ingested.
Respiration: Irregular breathing, respiratory depression.
Cardiovascular System: Tachycardia, hypotension or hypertension, shock, conduction disorders.
Nervous System and Muscles: Impairment of consciousness ranging in severity to deep coma. Convulsions, especially in small children. Motor restlessness, muscular twitching, tremor, athetoid movements, opisthotonos, ataxia, drowsiness, dizziness, mydriasis, nystagmus, adiadochokinesia, ballism, psychomotor disturbances, dysmetria. Initial hyperreflexia, followed by hyporeflexia.
Gastrointestinal Tract: Nausea, vomiting.
Kidneys and Bladder: Anuria or oliguria, urinary retention.
Laboratory Findings: Isolated instances of overdosage have included leukocytosis, reduced leukocyte count, glycosuria, and acetonuria. EEG may show dysrhythmias.
Combined Poisoning: When alcohol, tricyclic antidepressants, barbiturates, or hydantoins are taken at the same time, the signs and symptoms of acute poisoning with carbamazepine may be aggravated or modified.
Treatment
The prognosis in cases of severe poisoning is critically dependent upon prompt elimination of the drug, which may be achieved by inducing vomiting, irrigating the stomach, and by taking appropriate steps to diminish absorption. If these measures cannot be implemented without risk on the spot, the patient should be transferred at once to a hospital, while ensuring that vital functions are safeguarded. There is no specific antidote.
Elimination of the Drug: Induction of vomiting.
Gastric lavage. Even when more than 4 hours have elapsed following ingestion of the drug, the stomach should be repeatedly irrigated, especially if the patient has also consumed alcohol.
Measures to Reduce Absorption: Activated charcoal, laxatives.
Measures to Accelerate Elimination: Forced diuresis. Dialysis is indicated only in severe poisoning associated with renal failure. Replacement transfusion is indicated in severe poisoning in small children.
Respiratory Depression: Keep the airways free; resort, if necessary, to endotracheal intubation, artificial respiration, and administration of oxygen.
Hypotension, Shock: Keep the patient's legs raised and administer a plasma expander. If blood pressure fails to rise despite measures taken to increase plasma volume, use of vasoactive substances should be considered.
Convulsions: Diazepam or barbiturates.
Warning: Diazepam or barbiturates may aggravate respiratory depression (especially in children), hypotension, and coma. However, barbiturates should not be used if drugs that inhibit monoamine oxidase have also been taken by the patient either in overdosage or in recent therapy (within 1 week).
Surveillance: Respiration, cardiac function (ECG monitoring), blood pressure, body temperature, pupillary reflexes, and kidney and bladder function should be monitored for several days.
Treatment of Blood Count Abnormalities: If evidence of significant bone marrow depression develops, the following recommendations are suggested: (1) stop the drug, (2) perform daily CBC, platelet, and reticulocyte counts, (3) do a bone marrow aspiration and trephine biopsy immediately and repeat with sufficient frequency to monitor recovery.
Special periodic studies might be helpful as follows: (1) white cell and platelet antibodies, (2) ^{59}Fe-ferrokinetic studies, (3) peripheral blood cell typing, (4) cytogenetic studies on marrow and peripheral blood, (5) bone marrow culture studies for colony-forming units, (6) hemoglobin electrophoresis for A_2 and F hemoglobin, and (7) serum folic acid and B_{12} levels.
A fully developed aplastic anemia will require appropriate, intensive monitoring and therapy, for which specialized consultation should be sought.

DOSAGE AND ADMINISTRATION

Monitoring of blood levels has increased the efficacy and safety of anticonvulsants (see PRECAUTIONS, Laboratory Tests). Dosage should be adjusted to the needs of the individual patients. A low initial daily dosage with gradual increase is advised. As soon as adequate control is achieved, the dosage may be reduced very gradually to the minimum effective level. The Carbatrol capsules may be opened and the beads sprinkled over food, such as a teaspoon of applesauce or other similar food products if this method of administration is preferred. Carbatrol capsules or their contents should not be crushed or chewed. Carbatrol can be taken with or without meals.
Carbatrol is an extended-release formulation for twice a day administration. When converting patients from immediate release carbamazepine to Carbatrol extended-release capsules, the same total daily mg dose of carbamazepine should be administered.
Epilepsy (see INDICATIONS AND USAGE)
Adults and children over 12 years of age. Initial: 200 mg twice daily. Increase at weekly intervals by adding up to 200 mg/day until the optimal response is obtained. Dosage generally should not exceed 1000 mg per day in children 12-15 years of age, and 1200 mg daily in patients above 15 years of age. Doses up to 1600 mg daily have been used in adults. **Maintenance:** Adjust dosage to the minimum effective level, usually 800-1200 mg daily.
Children under 12 years of age: Children taking total daily dosages of immediate-release carbamazepine of 400 mg or greater may be converted to the same total daily dosage of Carbatrol extended-release capsules, using a twice daily regimen. Ordinarily, optimal clinical response is achieved at daily doses below 35 mg/kg. If satisfactory clinical response has not been achieved, plasma levels should be measured to determine whether or not they are in the therapeutic range. No recommendation regarding the safety of Carbatrol for use at doses above 35 mg/kg/24 hours can be made.
Combination Therapy: Carbatrol may be used alone or with other anticonvulsants. When added to existing anticonvulsant therapy, the drug should be added gradually while the other anticonvulsants are maintained or gradually decreased, except phenytoin, which may have to be increased (see PRECAUTIONS, Drug Interactions, and Pregnancy Category D).
Trigeminal Neuralgia (see INDICATIONS AND USAGE)
Initial: On the first day, start with one 200 mg capsule. This daily dose may be increased by up to 200 mg/day every 12 hours only as needed to achieve freedom from pain. Do not exceed 1200 mg daily. **Maintenance:** Control of pain can be maintained in most patients with 400-800 mg daily. However, some patients may be maintained on as little as 200 mg daily, while others may require as much as 1200 mg daily. At least once every 3 months throughout the treatment period, attempts should be made to reduce the dose to the minimum effective level or even to discontinue the drug.

HOW SUPPLIED

Carbatrol (carbamazepine extended-release capsules) is supplied in three dosage strengths.
100 mg-Two-piece hard gelatin capsule (bluish green opaque body and cap) printed with the Shire logo in white ink.
Supplied in bottles of 120 .... NDC 54092-171-12
Supplied in bottles of 14 .... NDC 54092-171-14
200 mg-Two-piece hard gelatin capsule (light gray opaque body with bluish green opaque cap) printed with the Shire logo in white ink.
Supplied in bottles of 120 .... NDC 54092-172-12
Supplied in bottles of 30 .... NDC 54092-172-30
300 mg-Two-piece hard gelatin capsule (black opaque body with bluish green opaque cap) printed with the Shire logo in white ink.
Supplied in bottles of 120 .... NDC 54092-173-12
Supplied in bottles of 30 .... NDC 54092-173-30
Store at 25°C (77°F). excursions 15-30°C (59-86°F).
Manufactured for:
Shire US Inc.
One River Front Place, Newport, KY 41071
1-800-828-2088, Made in U.S.A.

172 1207 002 (Rev 8/2003)

Takeda Pharmaceuticals America, Inc.

475 HALF DAY ROAD
LINCOLNSHIRE, IL 60069

Direct Inquiries to:
Sales and Ordering:
Customer Service
(877) 5 TAKEDA
(877) 582-5332

For Medical Information Contact:
General:
(877) TAKEDA 7
(877) 825-3327

Adverse Drug Experiences:
(877) TAKEDA 7
(877) 825-3327

ACTOS®

[*āk'tōs*] ℞
(pioglitazone hydrochloride) Tablets

Prescribing information for this product, which appears on pages 3186–3190 of the 2004 PDR, has been completely revised as follows. Please write "See Supplement A" next to the product heading.

DESCRIPTION

ACTOS (pioglitazone hydrochloride) is an oral antidiabetic agent that acts primarily by decreasing insulin resistance. ACTOS is used in the management of type 2 diabetes mellitus (also known as non-insulin-dependent diabetes mellitus [NIDDM] or adult-onset diabetes). Pharmacological studies indicate that ACTOS improves sensitivity to insulin in muscle and adipose tissue and inhibits hepatic gluconeogenesis. ACTOS improves glycemic control while reducing circulating insulin levels.
Pioglitazone [(±)-5-[[4-[2-(5-ethyl-2-pyridinyl)ethoxy]phenyl]methyl]-2,4-] thiazolidinedione monohydrochloride belongs to a different chemical class and has a different pharmacological action than the sulfonylureas, metformin, or the α-glucosidase inhibitors. The molecule contains one asymmetric carbon, and the compound is synthesized and used as the racemic mixture. The two enantiomers of pioglitazone interconvert in vivo. No differences were found in the pharmacologic activity between the two enantiomers. The structural formula is as shown:

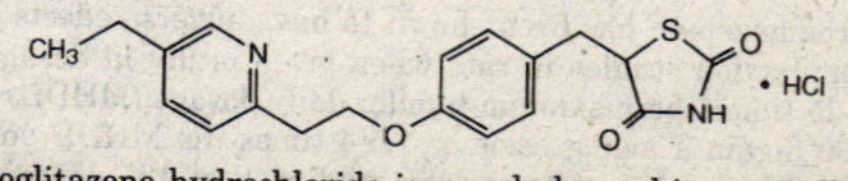

Pioglitazone hydrochloride is an odorless white crystalline powder that has a molecular formula of $C_{19}H_{20}N_2O_3S \bullet HCl$ and a molecular weight of 392.90 daltons. It is soluble in N,N-dimethylformamide, slightly soluble in anhydrous ethanol, very slightly soluble in acetone and acetonitrile, practically insoluble in water, and insoluble in ether.

ACTOS is available as a tablet for oral administration containing 15 mg, 30 mg, or 45 mg of pioglitazone (as the base) formulated with the following excipients: lactose monohydrate NF, hydroxypropylcellulose NF, carboxymethylcellulose calcium NF, and magnesium stearate NF.

CLINICAL PHARMACOLOGY

Mechanism of Action

ACTOS is a thiazolidinedione antidiabetic agent that depends on the presence of insulin for its mechanism of action. ACTOS decreases insulin resistance in the periphery and in the liver resulting in increased insulin-dependent glucose disposal and decreased hepatic glucose output. Unlike sulfonylureas, pioglitazone is not an insulin secretagogue. Pioglitazone is a potent and highly selective agonist for peroxisome proliferator-activated receptor-gamma (PPARγ). PPAR receptors are found in tissues important for insulin action such as adipose tissue, skeletal muscle, and liver. Activation of PPARγ nuclear receptors modulates the transcription of a number of insulin responsive genes involved in the control of glucose and lipid metabolism.

In animal models of diabetes, pioglitazone reduces the hyperglycemia, hyperinsulinemia, and hypertriglyceridemia characteristic of insulin-resistant states such as type 2 diabetes. The metabolic changes produced by pioglitazone result in increased responsiveness of insulin-dependent tissues and are observed in numerous animal models of insulin resistance.

Since pioglitazone enhances the effects of circulating insulin (by decreasing insulin resistance), it does not lower blood glucose in animal models that lack endogenous insulin.

Pharmacokinetics and Drug Metabolism

Serum concentrations of total pioglitazone (pioglitazone plus active metabolites) remain elevated 24 hours after once daily dosing. Steady-state serum concentrations of both pioglitazone and total pioglitazone are achieved within 7 days. At steady-state, two of the pharmacologically active metabolites of pioglitazone, Metabolites III (M-III) and IV (M-IV), reach serum concentrations equal to or greater than pioglitazone. In both healthy volunteers and in patients with type 2 diabetes, pioglitazone comprises approximately 30% to 50% of the peak total pioglitazone serum concentrations and 20% to 25% of the total area under the serum concentration-time curve (AUC).

Maximum serum concentration (C_{max}), AUC, and trough serum concentrations (C_{min}) for both pioglitazone and total pioglitazone increase proportionally at doses of 15 mg and 30 mg per day. There is a slightly less than proportional increase for pioglitazone and total pioglitazone at a dose of 60 mg per day.

Absorption: Following oral administration, in the fasting state, pioglitazone is first measurable in serum within 30 minutes, with peak concentrations observed within 2 hours. Food slightly delays the time to peak serum concentration to 3 to 4 hours, but does not alter the extent of absorption.

Distribution: The mean apparent volume of distribution (Vd/F) of pioglitazone following single-dose administration is 0.63 ± 0.41 (mean ± SD) L/kg of body weight. Pioglitazone is extensively protein bound (> 99%) in human serum, principally to serum albumin. Pioglitazone also binds to other serum proteins, but with lower affinity. Metabolites M-III and M-IV also are extensively bound (> 98%) to serum albumin.

Metabolism: Pioglitazone is extensively metabolized by hydroxylation and oxidation; the metabolites also partly convert to glucuronide or sulfate conjugates. Metabolites M-II and M-IV (hydroxy derivatives of pioglitazone) and M-III (keto derivative of pioglitazone) are pharmacologically active in animal models of type 2 diabetes. In addition to pioglitazone, M-III and M-IV are the principal drug-related species found in human serum following multiple dosing. At steady-state, in both healthy volunteers and in patients with type 2 diabetes, pioglitazone comprises approximately 30% to 50% of the total peak serum concentrations and 20% to 25% of the total AUC.

In vitro data demonstrate that multiple CYP isoforms are involved in the metabolism of pioglitazone. The cytochrome P450 isoforms involved are CYP2C8 and, to a lesser degree, CYP3A4 with additional contributions from a variety of other isoforms including the mainly extrahepatic CYP1A1. In vivo studies of pioglitazone in combination with P450 inhibitors and substrates have been performed (see Drug Interactions). Urinary 6β-hydroxycortisol/cortisol ratios measured in patients treated with ACTOS showed that pioglitazone is not a strong CYP3A4 enzyme inducer.

Excretion and Elimination: Following oral administration, approximately 15% to 30% of the pioglitazone dose is recovered in the urine. Renal elimination of pioglitazone is negligible, and the drug is excreted primarily as metabolites and their conjugates. It is presumed that most of the oral dose is excreted into the bile either unchanged or as metabolites and eliminated in the feces.

The mean serum half-life of pioglitazone and total pioglitazone ranges from 3 to 7 hours and 16 to 24 hours, respectively. Pioglitazone has an apparent clearance, CL/F, calculated to be 5 to 7 L/hr.

Special Populations

Renal Insufficiency: The serum elimination half-life of pioglitazone, M-III, and M-IV remains unchanged in patients with moderate (creatinine clearance 30 to 60 mL/min) to severe (creatinine clearance < 30 mL/min) renal impairment when compared to normal subjects. No dose adjustment in patients with renal dysfunction is recommended (see DOSAGE AND ADMINISTRATION).

Table 1 Lipids in a 26-Week Placebo-Controlled Monotherapy Dose-Ranging Study

	Placebo	ACTOS 15 mg Once Daily	ACTOS 30 mg Once Daily	ACTOS 45 mg Once Daily
Triglycerides (mg/dL)	N=79	N=79	N=84	N=77
Baseline (mean)	262.8	283.8	261.1	259.7
Percent change from baseline (mean)	4.8%	-9.0%	-9.6%	-9.3%
HDL Cholesterol (mg/dL)	N=79	N=79	N=83	N=77
Baseline (mean)	41.7	40.4	40.8	40.7
Percent change from baseline (mean)	8.1%	14.1%	12.2%	19.1%
LDL Cholesterol (mg/dL)	N=65	N=63	N=74	N=62
Baseline (mean)	138.8	131.9	135.6	126.8
Percent change from baseline (mean)	4.8%	7.2%	5.2%	6.0%
Total Cholesterol (mg/dL)	N=79	N=79	N=84	N=77
Baseline (mean)	224.6	220.0	222.7	213.7
Percent change from baseline (mean)	4.4%	4.6%	3.3%	6.4%

Hepatic Insufficiency: Compared with normal controls, subjects with impaired hepatic function (Child-Pugh Grade B/C) have an approximate 45% reduction in pioglitazone and total pioglitazone mean peak concentrations but no change in the mean AUC values.

ACTOS therapy should not be initiated if the patient exhibits clinical evidence of active liver disease or serum transaminase levels (ALT) exceed 2.5 times the upper limit of normal (see PRECAUTIONS, Hepatic Effects).

Elderly: In healthy elderly subjects, peak serum concentrations of pioglitazone and total pioglitazone are not significantly different, but AUC values are slightly higher and the terminal half-life values slightly longer than for younger subjects. These changes were not of a magnitude that would be considered clinically relevant.

Pediatrics: Pharmacokinetic data in the pediatric population are not available.

Gender: The mean C_{max} and AUC values were increased 20% to 60% in females. As monotherapy and in combination with sulfonylurea, metformin, or insulin, ACTOS improved glycemic control in both males and females. In controlled clinical trials, hemoglobin A_{1c} (HbA_{1c}) decreases from baseline were generally greater for females than for males (average mean difference in HbA_{1c} 0.5%). Since therapy should be individualized for each patient to achieve glycemic control, no dose adjustment is recommended based on gender alone.

Ethnicity: Pharmacokinetic data among various ethnic groups are not available.

Drug-Drug Interactions

The following drugs were studied in healthy volunteers with a co-administration of ACTOS 45 mg once daily. Listed below are the results:

Oral Contraceptives: Co-administration of ACTOS (45 mg once daily) and an oral contraceptive (1 mg norethindrone plus 0.035 mg ethinyl estradiol once daily) for 21 days, resulted in 11% and 11–14% decrease in ethinyl estradiol AUC (0–24h) and C_{max} respectively. There were no significant changes in norethindrone AUC (0–24h) and C_{max}. In view of the high variability of ethinyl estradiol pharmacokinetics, the clinical significance of this finding is unknown.

Fexofenadine HCl: Co-administration of ACTOS for 7 days with 60 mg fexofenadine administered orally twice daily resulted in no significant effect on pioglitazone pharmacokinetics. ACTOS had no significant effect on fexofenadine pharmacokinetics.

Glipizide: Co-administration of ACTOS and 5 mg glipizide administered orally once daily for 7 days did not alter the steady-state pharmacokinetics of glipizide.

Digoxin: Co-administration of ACTOS with 0.25 mg digoxin administered orally once daily for 7 days did not alter the steady-state pharmacokinetics of digoxin.

Warfarin: Co-administration of ACTOS for 7 days with warfarin did not alter the steady-state pharmacokinetics of warfarin. ACTOS has no clinically significant effect on prothrombin time when administered to patients receiving chronic warfarin therapy.

Metformin: Co-administration of a single dose of metformin (1000 mg) and ACTOS after 7 days of ACTOS did not alter the pharmacokinetics of the single dose of metformin.

Midazolam: Administration of ACTOS for 15 days followed by a single 7.5 mg dose of midazolam syrup resulted in a 26% reduction in midazolam C_{max} and AUC.

Ranitidine HCl: Co-administration of ACTOS for 7 days with ranitidine administered orally twice daily for either 4 or 7 days resulted in no significant effect on pioglitazone pharmacokinetics. ACTOS showed no significant effect on ranitidine pharmacokinetics.

Nifedipine ER: Co-administration of ACTOS for 7 days with 30 mg nifedipine ER administered orally once daily for 4 days to male and female volunteers resulted in least square mean (90% CI) values for unchanged nifedipine of 0.83 (0.73-0.95) for C_{max} and 0.88 (0.80-0.96) for AUC. In view of the high variability of nifedipine pharmacokinetics, the clinical significance of this finding is unknown.

Ketoconazole: Co-administration of ACTOS for 7 days with ketoconazole 200 mg administered twice daily resulted in least square mean (90% CI) values for unchanged pioglitazone of 1.14 (1.06-1.23) for C_{max}, 1.34 (1.26-1.41) for AUC and 1.87 (1.71-2.04) for C_{min}.

Atorvastatin Calcium: Co-administration of ACTOS for 7 days with atorvastatin calcium (LIPITOR®) 80 mg once daily resulted in least square mean (90% CI) values for unchanged pioglitazone of 0.69 (0.57-0.85) for C_{max}, 0.76 (0.65-0.88) for AUC and 0.96 (0.87-1.05) for C_{min}. For unchanged atorvastatin the least square mean (90% CI) values were 0.77 (0.66-0.90) for C_{max}, 0.86 (0.78-0.94) for AUC and 0.92 (0.82-1.02) for C_{min}.

Theophylline: Co-administration of ACTOS for 7 days with theophylline 400 mg administered twice daily resulted in no change in the pharmacokinetics of either drug.

Cytochrome P450: See **PRECAUTIONS**

Pharmacodynamics and Clinical Effects

Clinical studies demonstrate that ACTOS improves insulin sensitivity in insulin-resistant patients. ACTOS enhances cellular responsiveness to insulin, increases insulin-dependent glucose disposal, improves hepatic sensitivity to insulin, and improves dysfunctional glucose homeostasis. In patients with type 2 diabetes, the decreased insulin resistance produced by ACTOS results in lower plasma glucose concentrations, lower plasma insulin levels, and lower HbA_{1c} values. Based on results from an open-label extension study, the glucose lowering effects of ACTOS appear to persist for at least one year. In controlled clinical trials, ACTOS in combination with sulfonylurea, metformin, or insulin had an additive effect on glycemic control.

Patients with lipid abnormalities were included in clinical trials with ACTOS. Overall, patients treated with ACTOS had mean decreases in triglycerides, mean increases in HDL cholesterol, and no consistent mean changes in LDL and total cholesterol.

In a 26-week, placebo-controlled, dose-ranging study, mean triglyceride levels decreased in the 15 mg, 30 mg, and 45 mg ACTOS dose groups compared to a mean increase in the placebo group. Mean HDL levels increased to a greater extent in patients treated with ACTOS than in the placebo-treated patients. There were no consistent differences for LDL and total cholesterol in patients treated with ACTOS compared to placebo (Table 1).

[See table 1 above]

In the two other monotherapy studies (24 weeks and 16 weeks) and in combination therapy studies with sulfonylurea (24 weeks and 16 weeks) and metformin (24 weeks and 16 weeks), the results were generally consistent with the data above. In placebo-controlled trials, the placebo-corrected mean changes from baseline decreased 5% to 26% for triglycerides and increased 6% to 13% for HDL in patients treated with ACTOS. A similar pattern of results was seen in 24-week combination therapy studies of ACTOS with sulfonylurea or metformin.

In a combination therapy study with insulin (16 weeks), the placebo-corrected mean percent change from baseline in triglyceride values for patients treated with ACTOS was also decreased. A placebo-corrected mean change from baseline in LDL cholesterol of 7% was observed for the 15 mg dose group. Similar results to those noted above for HDL and total cholesterol were observed. A similar pattern of results was seen in a 24-week combination therapy study with ACTOS with insulin.

Clinical Studies

Monotherapy

In the U.S., three randomized, double-blind, placebo-controlled trials with durations from 16 to 26 weeks were conducted to evaluate the use of ACTOS as monotherapy in patients with type 2 diabetes. These studies examined ACTOS at doses up to 45 mg or placebo once daily in 865 patients.

In a 26-week dose-ranging study, 408 patients with type 2 diabetes were randomized to receive 7.5 mg, 15 mg, 30 mg, or 45 mg of ACTOS, or placebo once daily. Therapy with any previous antidiabetic agent was discontinued 8 weeks prior to the double-blind period. Treatment with 15 mg, 30 mg, and 45 mg of ACTOS produced statistically significant improvements in HbA_{1c} and fasting plasma glucose (FPG) at endpoint compared to placebo (see Figure 1, Table 2).

Figure 1 shows the time course for changes in FPG and HbA_{1c} for the entire study population in this 26-week study. Table 2 shows HbA_{1c} and FPG values for the entire study population.

[See figure 1 at top of next page]
[See table 2 at top of next page]

Continued on next page

Actos—Cont.

The study population included patients not previously treated with antidiabetic medication (naïve; 31%) and patients who were receiving antidiabetic medication at the time of study enrollment (previously treated; 69%). The data for the naïve and previously treated patient subsets are shown in Table 3. All patients entered an 8 week washout/run-in period prior to double-blind treatment. This run-in period was associated with little change in HbA_{1c} and FPG values from screening to baseline for the naïve patients; however, for the previously-treated group, washout from previous antidiabetic medication resulted in deterioration of glycemic control and increases in HbA_{1c} and FPG. Although most patients in the previously-treated group had a decrease from baseline in HbA_{1c} and FPG with ACTOS, in many cases the values did not return to screening levels by the end of the study. The study design did not permit the evaluation of patients who switched directly to ACTOS from another antidiabetic agent.

[See table 3 at right]

In a 24-week placebo-controlled study, 260 patients with type 2 diabetes were randomized to one of two forced-titration ACTOS treatment groups or a mock titration placebo group. Therapy with any previous antidiabetic agent was discontinued 6 weeks prior to the double-blind period. In one ACTOS treatment group, patients received an initial dose of 7.5 mg once daily. After four weeks, the dose was increased to 15 mg once daily and after another four weeks, the dose was increased to 30 mg once daily for the remainder of the study (16 weeks). In the second ACTOS treatment group, patients received an initial dose of 15 mg once daily and were titrated to 30 mg once daily and 45 mg once daily in a similar manner. Treatment with ACTOS, as described, produced statistically significant improvements in HbA_{1c} and FPG at endpoint compared to placebo (see Table 4).

[See table 4 at right]

For patients who had not been previously treated with antidiabetic medication (24%), mean values at screening were 10.1% for HbA_{1c} and 238 mg/dL for FPG. At baseline, mean HbA_{1c} was 10.2% and mean FPG was 243 mg/dL. Compared with placebo, treatment with ACTOS titrated to a final dose of 30 mg and 45 mg resulted in reductions from baseline in mean HbA_{1c} of 2.3% and 2.6% and mean FPG of 63 mg/dL and 95 mg/dL, respectively. For patients who had been previously treated with antidiabetic medication (76%), this medication was discontinued at screening. Mean values at screening were 9.4% for HbA_{1c} and 216 mg/dL for FPG. At baseline, mean HbA_{1c} was 10.7% and mean FPG was 290 mg/dL. Compared with placebo, treatment with ACTOS titrated to a final dose of 30 mg and 45 mg resulted in reductions from baseline in mean HbA_{1c} of 1.3% and 1.4% and mean FPG of 55 mg/dL and 60 mg/dL, respectively. For many previously-treated patients, HbA_{1c} and FPG had not returned to screening levels by the end of the study.

In a 16-week study, 197 patients with type 2 diabetes were randomized to treatment with 30 mg of ACTOS or placebo once daily. Therapy with any previous antidiabetic agent was discontinued 6 weeks prior to the double-blind period. Treatment with 30 mg of ACTOS produced statistically significant improvements in HbA_{1c} and FPG at endpoint compared to placebo (see Table 5).

[See table 5 at top of next page]

For patients who had not been previously treated with antidiabetic medication (40%), mean values at screening were 10.3% for HbA_{1c} and 240 mg/dL for FPG. At baseline, mean HbA_{1c} was 10.4% and mean FPG was 254 mg/dL. Compared with placebo, treatment with ACTOS 30 mg resulted in reductions from baseline in mean HbA_{1c} of 1.0% and mean FPG of 62 mg/dL. For patients who had been previously treated with antidiabetic medication (60%), this medication was discontinued at screening. Mean values at screening were 9.4% for HbA_{1c} and 216 mg/dL for FPG. At baseline, mean HbA_{1c} was 10.6% and mean FPG was 287 mg/dL. Compared with placebo, treatment with ACTOS 30 mg resulted in reductions from baseline in mean HbA_{1c} of 1.3% and mean FPG of 46 mg/dL. For many previously-treated patients, HbA_{1c} and FPG had not returned to screening levels by the end of the study.

Combination Therapy

Three 16-week, randomized, double-blind, placebo-controlled clinical studies and three 24-week randomized, double-blind, dose-controlled clinical studies were conducted to evaluate the effects of ACTOS on glycemic control in patients with type 2 diabetes who were inadequately controlled ($HbA_{1c} \geq 8\%$) despite current therapy with a sulfonylurea, metformin, or insulin. Previous diabetes treatment may have been monotherapy or combination therapy.

ACTOS Plus Sulfonylurea Studies

Two clinical studies were conducted with ACTOS in combination with a sulfonylurea. Both studies included patients with type 2 diabetes on sulfonylurea, either alone or in combination with another antidiabetic agent. All other antidiabetic agents were withdrawn prior to starting study treatment. In the first study, 560 patients were randomized to receive 15 mg or 30 mg of ACTOS or placebo once daily for 16 weeks in addition to their current sulfonylurea regimen. When compared to placebo at Week 16, the addition of ACTOS to the sulfonylurea significantly reduced the mean HbA_{1c} by 0.9% and 1.3% and mean FPG by 39 mg/dL and 58 mg/dL for the 15 mg and 30 mg doses, respectively.

In the second study, 702 patients were randomized to receive 30 mg or 45 mg of ACTOS once daily for 24 weeks in addition to their current sulfonylurea regimen. The mean reductions from baseline at Week 24 in HbA_{1c} were 1.55% and 1.67% for the 30 mg and 45 mg doses, respectively. Mean reductions from baseline in FPG were 51.5 mg/dL and 56.1 mg/dL.

The therapeutic effect of ACTOS in combination with sulfonylurea was observed in patients regardless of whether the patients were receiving low, medium, or high doses of sulfonylurea.

ACTOS Plus Metformin Studies

Two clinical studies were conducted with ACTOS in combination with metformin. Both studies included patients with type 2 diabetes on metformin, either alone or in combination with another diabetic agent. All other antidiabetic agents were withdrawn prior to starting study treatment. In the first study, 328 patients were randomized to receive either 30 mg of ACTOS or placebo once daily for 16 weeks in addition to their current metformin regimen. When compared to placebo at Week 16, the addition of ACTOS to metformin significantly reduced the mean HbA_{1c} by 0.8% and decreased the mean FPG by 38 mg/dL.

In the second study, 827 patients were randomized to receive either 30 mg or 45 mg of ACTOS once daily for 24 weeks in addition to their current metformin regimen. The

Figure 1 Mean Change from Baseline for FPG and HbA_{1c} in a 26-Week Placebo-Controlled Dose-Ranging Study

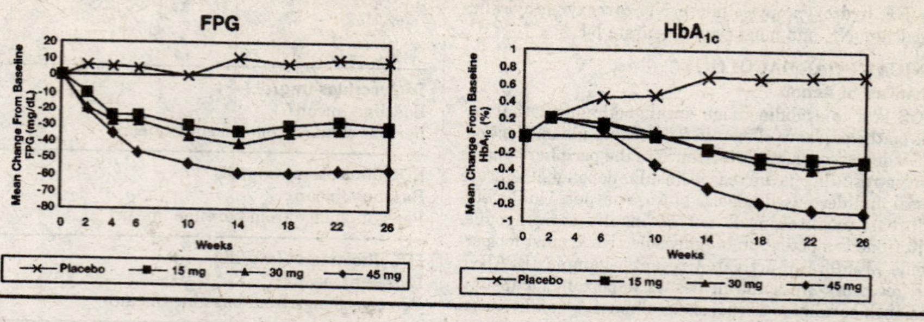

Table 2 Glycemic Parameters in a 26-Week Placebo-Controlled Dose-Ranging Study

	Placebo	ACTOS 15 mg Once Daily	ACTOS 30 mg Once Daily	ACTOS 45 mg Once Daily
Total Population				
HbA_{1c} (%)	N=79	N=79	N=85	N=76
Baseline (mean)	10.4	10.2	10.2	10.3
Change from baseline (adjusted mean⁺)	0.7	-0.3	-0.3	-0.9
Difference from placebo (adjusted mean⁺)		-1.0*	-1.0*	-1.6*
FPG (mg/dL)	N=79	N=79	N=84	N=77
Baseline (mean)	268	267	269	276
Change from baseline (adjusted mean⁺)	9	-30	-32	-56
Difference from placebo (adjusted mean⁺)		-39*	-41*	-65*

⁺ Adjusted for baseline, pooled center, and pooled center by treatment interaction
* $p \leq 0.050$ vs. placebo

Table 3 Glycemic Parameters in a 26-Week Placebo-Controlled Dose-Ranging Study

	Placebo	ACTOS 15 mg Once Daily	ACTOS 30 mg Once Daily	ACTOS 45 mg Once Daily
Naïve to Therapy				
HbA_{1c} (%)	N=25	N=26	N=26	N=21
Screening (mean)	9.3	10.0	9.5	9.8
Baseline (mean)	9.0	9.9	9.3	10.0
Change from baseline (adjusted mean*)	0.6	-0.8	-0.6	-1.9
Difference from placebo (adjusted mean*)		-1.4	-1.3	-2.6
FPG (mg/dL)	N=25	N=26	N=26	N=21
Screening (mean)	223	245	239	239
Baseline (mean)	229	251	225	235
Change from baseline (adjusted mean*)	16	-37	-41	-64
Difference from placebo (adjusted mean*)		-52	-56	-80
Previously Treated				
HbA_{1c} (%)	N=54	N=53	N=59	N=55
Screening (mean)	9.3	9.0	9.1	9.0
Baseline (mean)	10.9	10.4	10.4	10.6
Change from baseline (adjusted mean*)	0.8	-0.1	-0.0	-0.6
Difference from placebo (adjusted mean*)		-1.0	-0.9	-1.4
FPG (mg/dL)	N=54	N=53	N=58	N=56
Screening (mean)	222	209	230	215
Baseline (mean)	285	275	286	292
Change from baseline (adjusted mean*)	4	-32	-27	-55
Difference from placebo (adjusted mean*)		-36	-31	-59

* Adjusted for baseline and pooled center

Table 4 Glycemic Parameters in a 24-Week Placebo-Controlled Forced-Titration Study

	Placebo	ACTOS 30 mg⁺ Once Daily	ACTOS 45 mg⁺ Once Daily
Total Population			
HbA_{1c} (%)	N=83	N=85	N=85
Baseline (mean)	10.8	10.3	10.8
Change from baseline (adjusted mean⁺⁺)	0.9	-0.6	-0.6
Difference from placebo (adjusted mean⁺⁺)		-1.5*	-1.5*
FPG (mg/dL)	N=78	N=82	N=85
Baseline (mean)	279	268	281
Change from baseline (adjusted mean⁺⁺)	18	-44	-50
Difference from placebo (adjusted mean⁺⁺)		-62*	-68*

⁺ Final dose in forced titration
⁺⁺ Adjusted for baseline, pooled center, and pooled center by treatment interaction
* $p \leq 0.050$ vs. placebo

Table 5 Glycemic Parameters in a 16-Week Placebo-Controlled Study

	Placebo	ACTOS 30 mg Once Daily
Total Population		
HbA_{1c} (%)	N=93	N=100
Baseline (mean)	10.3	10.5
Change from baseline (adjusted mean+)	0.8	-0.6
Difference from placebo (adjusted mean+)		-1.4*
FPG (mg/dL)	N=91	N=99
Baseline (mean)	270	273
Change from baseline (adjusted mean+)	8	-50
Difference from placebo (adjusted mean+)		-58*

+ Adjusted for baseline, pooled center, and pooled center by treatment interaction

* $p \leq 0.050$ vs. placebo

Table 6 Weight Changes (kg) from Baseline during Double-Blind Clinical Trials with ACTOS

		Control Group (Placebo)	ACTOS 15 mg	ACTOS 30 mg	ACTOS 45 mg
		Median (25th / 75th percentile)	Median (25th / 75th percentile)	Median (25th / 75th percentile)	Median (25th / 75th percentile)
Monotherapy		-1.4 (-2.7/0.0) n=256	0.9 (-0.5/3.4) n=79	1.0 (-0.9/3.4) n=188	2.6 (0.2/5.4) n=79
Combination Therapy	Sulfonylurea	-0.5 (-1.8/0.7) n=187	2.0 (0.2/3.2) n=183	3.1 (1.1/5.4) n=528	4.1 (1.8/7.3) N=333
	Metformin	-1.4 (-3.2/0.3) n=160	N/A	0.9 (-0.3/3.2) n=567	1.8 (-0.9/5.0) N=407
	Insulin	0.2 (-1.4/1.4) n=182	2.3 (0.5/4.3) n=190	3.3 (0.9/6.3) n=522	4.1 (1.4/6.8) N=338

Note: Trial durations of 16 to 26 weeks

mean reductions from baseline at Week 24 in HbA_{1c} were 0.80% and 1.01% for the 30 mg and 45 mg doses, respectively. Mean reductions from baseline in FPG were 38.2 mg/dL and 50.7 mg/dL.

The therapeutic effect of ACTOS in combination with metformin was observed in patients regardless of whether the patients were receiving lower or higher doses of metformin.

ACTOS Plus Insulin Studies

Two clinical studies were conducted with ACTOS in combination with insulin. Both studies included patients with type 2 diabetes on insulin, either alone or in combination with another antidiabetic agent. All other antidiabetic agents were withdrawn prior to starting study treatment. In the first study, 566 patients receiving a median of 60.5 units per day of insulin were randomized to receive either 15 mg or 30 mg of ACTOS or placebo once daily for 16 weeks in addition to their insulin regimen. When compared to placebo at Week 16 the addition of ACTOS to insulin significantly reduced both HbA_{1c} by 0.7% and 1.0% and FPG by 35 mg/dL and 49 mg/dL for the 15 mg and 30 mg dose, respectively.

In the second study, 690 patients receiving a median of 60.0 units per day of insulin received either 30 mg or 45 mg of ACTOS once daily for 24 weeks in addition to their current insulin regimen. The mean reductions from baseline at Week 24 in HbA_{1c} were 1.17% and 1.46% for the 30 mg and 45 mg doses, respectively. Mean reductions from baseline in FPG were 31.9 mg/dL and 45.8 mg/dL. Improved glycemic control was accompanied by mean decreases from baseline in insulin dose requirements of 6.0% and 9.4% per day for the 30 mg and 45 mg dose, respectively.

The therapeutic effect of ACTOS in combination with insulin was observed in patients regardless of whether the patients were receiving lower or higher doses of insulin.

INDICATIONS AND USAGE

ACTOS is indicated as an adjunct to diet and exercise to improve glycemic control in patients with type 2 diabetes (non-insulin-dependent diabetes mellitus, NIDDM). ACTOS is indicated for monotherapy. ACTOS is also indicated for use in combination with a sulfonylurea, metformin, or insulin when diet and exercise plus the single agent does not result in adequate glycemic control.

Management of type 2 diabetes should also include nutritional counseling, weight reduction as needed, and exercise. These efforts are important not only in the primary treatment of type 2 diabetes, but also to maintain the efficacy of drug therapy.

CONTRAINDICATIONS

ACTOS is contraindicated in patients with known hypersensitivity to this product or any of its components.

WARNINGS

Cardiac Failure and Other Cardiac Effects

ACTOS, like other thiazolidinediones, can cause fluid retention when used alone or in combination with other antidiabetic agents, including insulin. Fluid retention may lead to or exacerbate heart failure. Patients should be observed for signs and symptoms of heart failure (see Information for Patients). ACTOS should be discontinued if any deterioration in cardiac status occurs. Patients with New York Heart Association (NYHA) Class III and IV cardiac status were not studied during these clinical trials; ACTOS is not recommended in these patients (see PRECAUTIONS, Cardiovascular).

In one 16-week U.S. double-blind, placebo-controlled clinical trial involving 566 patients with type 2 diabetes, ACTOS at doses of 15 mg and 30 mg in combination with insulin was compared to insulin therapy alone. This trial included patients with long-standing diabetes and a high prevalence of pre-existing medical conditions as follows: arterial hypertension (57.2%), peripheral neuropathy (22.6%), coronary heart disease (19.6%), retinopathy (13.1%), myocardial infarction (8.8%), vascular disease (6.4%), angina pectoris (4.4%), stroke and/or transient ischemic attack (4.1%), and congestive heart failure (2.3%).

In this study two of the 191 patients receiving 15 mg ACTOS plus insulin (1.1%) and two of the 188 patients receiving 30 mg ACTOS plus insulin (1.1%) developed congestive heart failure compared with none of the 187 patients on insulin therapy alone. All four of these patients had previous histories of cardiovascular conditions including coronary artery disease, previous CABG procedures, and myocardial infarction. In a 24-week dose-controlled study in which ACTOS was coadministered with insulin, 0.3% of patients (1/345) on 30 mg and 0.9% (3/345) of patients on 45 mg reported CHF as a serious adverse event.

Analysis of data from these studies did not identify specific factors that predict increased risk of congestive heart failure on combination therapy with insulin.

PRECAUTIONS

General

ACTOS exerts its antihyperglycemic effect only in the presence of insulin. Therefore, ACTOS should not be used in patients with type 1 diabetes or for the treatment of diabetic ketoacidosis.

Hypoglycemia: Patients receiving ACTOS in combination with insulin or oral hypoglycemic agents may be at risk for hypoglycemia, and a reduction in the dose of the concomitant agent may be necessary.

Cardiovascular: In U.S. placebo-controlled clinical trials that excluded patients with New York Heart Association (NYHA) Class III and IV cardiac status, the incidence of serious cardiac adverse events related to volume expansion was not increased in patients treated with ACTOS as monotherapy or in combination with sulfonylureas or metformin vs. placebo-treated patients. In insulin combination studies, a small number of patients with a history of previously existing cardiac disease developed congestive heart failure when treated with ACTOS in combination with insulin (see WARNINGS). Patients with NYHA Class III and IV cardiac status were not studied in these ACTOS clinical trials. ACTOS is not indicated in patients with NYHA Class III or IV cardiac status.

In postmarketing experience with ACTOS, cases of congestive heart failure have been reported in patients both with and without previously known heart disease.

Edema: ACTOS should be used with caution in patients with edema. In all U.S. clinical trials, edema was reported more frequently in patients treated with ACTOS than in placebo-treated patients and appears to be dose related (see ADVERSE REACTIONS). In postmarketing experience, reports of initiation or worsening of edema have been received.

Weight Gain: Dose related weight gain was seen with ACTOS alone and in combination with other hypoglycemic agents (Table 6). The mechanism of weight gain is unclear but probably involves a combination of fluid retention and fat accumulation.

[See table 6 at left]

Ovulation: Therapy with ACTOS, like other thiazolidinediones, may result in ovulation in some premenopausal anovulatory women. As a result, these patients may be at an increased risk for pregnancy while taking ACTOS. Thus, adequate contraception in premenopausal women should be recommended. This possible effect has not been investigated in clinical studies so the frequency of this occurrence is not known.

Hematologic: ACTOS may cause decreases in hemoglobin and hematocrit. Across all clinical studies, mean hemoglobin values declined by 2% to 4% in patients treated with ACTOS. These changes primarily occurred within the first 4 to 12 weeks of therapy and remained relatively constant thereafter. These changes may be related to increased plasma volume and have rarely been associated with any significant hematologic clinical effects (see ADVERSE REACTIONS, Laboratory Abnormalities).

Hepatic Effects: In pre-approval clinical studies worldwide, over 4500 subjects were treated with ACTOS. In U.S. clinical studies, over 4700 patients with type 2 diabetes received ACTOS. There was no evidence of drug-induced hepatotoxicity or elevation of ALT levels in the clinical studies. During pre-approval placebo-controlled clinical trials in the U.S., a total of 4 of 1526 (0.26%) patients treated with ACTOS and 2 of 793 (0.25%) placebo-treated patients had ALT values ≥ 3 times the upper limit of normal. The ALT elevations in patients treated with ACTOS were reversible and were not clearly related to therapy with ACTOS.

In postmarketing experience with ACTOS, reports of hepatitis and of hepatic enzyme elevations to 3 or more times the upper limit of normal have been received. Very rarely, these reports have involved hepatic failure with and without fatal outcome, although causality has not been established.

Pioglitazone is structurally related to troglitazone, a thiazolidinedione no longer marketed in the United States, which was associated with idiosyncratic hepatotoxicity and cases of liver failure, liver transplants and death during postmarketing clinical use. In pre-approval controlled clinical trials in patients with type 2 diabetes, troglitazone was more frequently associated with clinically significant elevations of hepatic enzymes (ALT > 3 times the upper limit of normal) compared to placebo, and cases of reversible jaundice were reported.

Pending the availability of the results of additional large, long-term controlled clinical trials and additional postmarketing safety data, it is recommended that patients treated with ACTOS undergo periodic monitoring of liver enzymes.

Serum ALT (alanine aminotransferase) levels should be evaluated prior to the initiation of therapy with ACTOS in all patients and periodically thereafter per the clinical judgment of the health care professional. Liver function tests should also be obtained for patients if symptoms suggestive of hepatic dysfunction occur, e.g., nausea, vomiting, abdominal pain, fatigue, anorexia, or dark urine. The decision whether to continue the patient on therapy with ACTOS should be guided by clinical judgment pending laboratory evaluations. If jaundice is observed, drug therapy should be discontinued.

Therapy with ACTOS should not be initiated if the patient exhibits clinical evidence of active liver disease or the ALT levels exceed 2.5 times the upper limit of normal. Patients with mildly elevated liver enzymes (ALT levels at 1 to 2.5 times the upper limit of normal) at baseline or any time during therapy with ACTOS should be evaluated to determine the cause of the liver enzyme elevation. Initiation or continuation of therapy with ACTOS in patients with mildly elevated liver enzymes should proceed with caution and include appropriate clinical follow-up which may include more frequent liver enzyme monitoring. If serum transaminase levels are increased (ALT > 2.5 times the upper limit of normal), liver function tests should be evaluated more frequently until the levels return to normal or pretreatment values. If ALT levels exceed 3 times the upper limit of normal, the test should be repeated as soon as possible. If ALT levels remain > 3 times the upper limit of normal or if the patient is jaundiced, ACTOS therapy should be discontinued.

There are no data available to evaluate the safety of ACTOS in patients who experienced liver abnormalities, hepatic dysfunction, or jaundice while on troglitazone. ACTOS should not be used in patients who experienced jaundice while taking troglitazone.

Laboratory Tests

FPG and HbA_{1c} measurements should be performed periodically to monitor glycemic control and the therapeutic response to ACTOS.

Liver enzyme monitoring is recommended prior to initiation of therapy with ACTOS in all patients and periodically thereafter per the clinical judgment of the health care professional (see PRECAUTIONS, General, Hepatic Effects and ADVERSE REACTIONS, Serum Transaminase Levels).

Information for Patients

It is important to instruct patients to adhere to dietary instructions and to have blood glucose and glycosylated hemoglobin tested regularly. During periods of stress such as fever, trauma, infection, or surgery, medication requirements may change and patients should be reminded to seek medical advice promptly.

Patients who experience an unusually rapid increase in weight or edema or who develop shortness of breath or other symptoms of heart failure while on ACTOS should immediately report these symptoms to their physician.

Continued on next page

Actos—Cont.

Patients should be told that blood tests for liver function will be performed prior to the start of therapy and periodically thereafter per the clinical judgment of the health care professional. Patients should be told to seek immediate medical advice for unexplained nausea, vomiting, abdominal pain, fatigue, anorexia, or dark urine.

Patients should be told to take ACTOS once daily. ACTOS can be taken with or without meals. If a dose is missed on one day, the dose should not be doubled the following day.

When using combination therapy with insulin or oral hypoglycemic agents, the risks of hypoglycemia, its symptoms and treatment, and conditions that predispose to its development should be explained to patients and their family members.

Therapy with ACTOS, like other thiazolidinediones, may result in ovulation in some premenopausal anovulatory women. As a result, these patients may be at an increased risk for pregnancy while taking ACTOS. Thus, adequate contraception in premenopausal women should be recommended. This possible effect has not been investigated in clinical studies so the frequency of this occurrence is not known.

Drug Interactions

In vivo drug-drug interaction studies have suggested that pioglitazone may be a weak inducer of CYP 450 isoform 3A4 substrate (see CLINICAL PHARMACOLOGY, Metabolism and Drug-Drug Interactions).

Carcinogenesis, Mutagenesis, Impairment of Fertility

A two-year carcinogenicity study was conducted in male and female rats at oral doses up to 63 mg/kg (approximately 14 times the maximum recommended human oral dose of 45 mg based on mg/m^2). Drug-induced tumors were not observed in any organ except for the urinary bladder. Benign and/or malignant transitional cell neoplasms were observed in male rats at 4 mg/kg/day and above (approximately equal to the maximum recommended human oral dose based on mg/m^2). A two-year carcinogenicity study was conducted in male and female mice at oral doses up to 100 mg/kg/day (approximately 11 times the maximum recommended human oral dose based on mg/m^2). No drug-induced tumors were observed in any organ.

During prospective evaluation of urinary cytology involving more than 1800 patients receiving ACTOS in clinical trials up to one year in duration, no new cases of bladder tumors were identified. Occasionally, abnormal urinary cytology results indicating possible malignancy were observed in both patients treated with ACTOS (0.72%) and patients treated with placebo (0.88%).

Pioglitazone HCl was not mutagenic in a battery of genetic toxicology studies, including the Ames bacterial assay, a mammalian cell forward gene mutation assay (CHO/HPRT and AS52/XPRT), an in vitro cytogenetics assay using CHL cells, an unscheduled DNA synthesis assay, and an in vivo micronucleus assay.

No adverse effects upon fertility were observed in male and female rats at oral doses up to 40 mg/kg pioglitazone HCl daily prior to and throughout mating and gestation (approximately 9 times the maximum recommended human oral dose based on mg/m^2).

Animal Toxicology

Heart enlargement has been observed in mice (100 mg/kg), rats (4 mg/kg and above) and dogs (3 mg/kg) treated orally with pioglitazone HCl (approximately 11, 1, and 2 times the maximum recommended human oral dose for mice, rats, and dogs, respectively, based on mg/m^2). In a one-year rat study, drug-related early death due to apparent heart dysfunction occurred at an oral dose of 160 mg/kg/day (approximately 35 times the maximum recommended human oral dose based on mg/m^2). Heart enlargement was seen in a 13-week study in monkeys at oral doses of 8.9 mg/kg and above (approximately 4 times the maximum recommended human oral dose based on mg/m^2), but not in a 52-week study at oral doses up to 32 mg/kg (approximately 13 times the maximum recommended human oral dose based on mg/m^2).

Pregnancy

Pregnancy Category C. Pioglitazone was not teratogenic in rats at oral doses up to 80 mg/kg or in rabbits given up to 160 mg/kg during organogenesis (approximately 17 and 40 times the maximum recommended human oral dose based on mg/m^2, respectively). Delayed parturition and embryotoxicity (as evidenced by increased postimplantation losses, delayed development and reduced fetal weights) were observed in rats at oral doses of 40 mg/kg/day and above (approximately 10 times the maximum recommended human oral dose based on mg/m^2). No functional or behavioral toxicity was observed in offspring of rats. In rabbits, embryotoxicity was observed at an oral dose of 160 mg/kg (approximately 40 times the maximum recommended human oral dose based on mg/m^2). Delayed postnatal development, attributed to decreased body weight, was observed in offspring of rats at oral doses of 10 mg/kg and above during late gestation and lactation periods (approximately 2 times the maximum recommended human oral dose based on mg/m^2).

There are no adequate and well-controlled studies in pregnant women. ACTOS should be used during pregnancy only if the potential benefit justifies the potential risk to the fetus.

Because current information strongly suggests that abnormal blood glucose levels during pregnancy are associated with a higher incidence of congenital anomalies, as well as increased neonatal morbidity and mortality, most experts recommend that insulin be used during pregnancy to maintain blood glucose levels as close to normal as possible.

Nursing Mothers

Pioglitazone is secreted in the milk of lactating rats. It is not known whether ACTOS is secreted in human milk. Because many drugs are excreted in human milk, ACTOS should not be administered to a breast-feeding woman.

Pediatric Use

Safety and effectiveness of ACTOS in pediatric patients have not been established.

Elderly Use

Approximately 500 patients in placebo-controlled clinical trials of ACTOS were 65 and over. No significant differences in effectiveness and safety were observed between these patients and younger patients.

ADVERSE REACTIONS

In worldwide clinical trials, over 5900 patients with type 2 diabetes have been treated with ACTOS. In U.S. clinical trials, over 4700 patients have received ACTOS, over 3300 patients have been treated for 6 months or longer, and over 450 patients for one year or longer.

The overall incidence and types of adverse events reported in placebo-controlled clinical trials of ACTOS monotherapy at doses of 7.5 mg, 15 mg, 30 mg, or 45 mg once daily are shown in Table 7.

Table 7 Placebo-Controlled Clinical Studies of ACTOS Monotherapy: Adverse Events Reported at a Frequency ≥ 5% of Patients Treated with ACTOS

(% of Patients)

	Placebo N=259	ACTOS N=606
Upper Respiratory Tract Infection	8.5	13.2
Headache	6.9	9.1
Sinusitis	4.6	6.3
Myalgia	2.7	5.4
Tooth Disorder	2.3	5.3
Diabetes Mellitus Aggravated	8.1	5.1
Pharyngitis	0.8	5.1

For most clinical adverse events the incidence was similar for groups treated with ACTOS monotherapy and those treated in combination with sulfonylureas, metformin, and insulin. There was an increase in the occurrence of edema in the patients treated with ACTOS and insulin compared to insulin alone.

In a 16-week, placebo-controlled ACTOS plus insulin trial (n=379), 10 patients treated with ACTOS plus insulin developed dyspnea and also, at some point during their therapy, developed either weight change or edema. Seven of these 10 patients received diuretics to treat these symptoms. This was not reported in the insulin plus placebo group.

The incidence of withdrawals from placebo-controlled clinical trials due to an adverse event other than hyperglycemia was similar for patients treated with placebo (2.8%) or ACTOS (3.3%).

In controlled combination therapy studies with either a sulfonylurea or insulin, mild to moderate hypoglycemia, which appears to be dose related, was reported (see PRECAUTIONS, General, Hypoglycemia and DOSAGE and ADMINISTRATION, Combination Therapy).

In U.S. double-blind studies, anemia was reported in ≤ 2% of patients treated with ACTOS plus sulfonylurea, metformin or insulin (see PRECAUTIONS, General, Hematologic).

In monotherapy studies, edema was reported for 4.8% of patients treated with ACTOS versus 1.2% of placebo-treated patients. In combination therapy studies, edema was reported for 7.2% of patients treated with ACTOS and sulfonylureas compared to 2.1% of patients on sulfonylureas alone. In combination therapy studies with metformin, edema was reported in 6.0% of patients on combination therapy compared to 2.5% of patients on metformin alone. In combination therapy studies with insulin, edema was reported in 15.3% of patients on combination therapy compared to 7.0% of patients on insulin alone. Most of these events were considered mild or moderate in intensity (see PRECAUTIONS, General, Edema).

In one 16-week clinical trial of insulin plus ACTOS combination therapy, more patients developed congestive heart failure on combination therapy (1.1%) compared to none on insulin alone (see WARNINGS, Cardiac Failure and Other Cardiac Effects).

Laboratory Abnormalities

Hematologic: ACTOS may cause decreases in hemoglobin and hematocrit. The fall in hemoglobin and hematocrit with ACTOS appears to be dose related. Across all clinical studies, mean hemoglobin values declined by 2% to 4% in patients treated with ACTOS. These changes generally occurred within the first 4 to 12 weeks of therapy and remained relatively stable thereafter. These changes may be related to increased plasma volume associated with ACTOS therapy and have rarely been associated with any significant hematologic clinical effects.

Serum Transaminase Levels: During all clinical studies in the U.S., 14 of 4780 (0.30%) patients treated with ACTOS had ALT values ≥ 3 times the upper limit of normal during treatment. All patients with follow-up values had reversible elevations in ALT. In the population of patients treated with ACTOS, mean values for bilirubin, AST, ALT, alkaline phosphatase, and GGT were decreased at the final visit compared with baseline. Fewer than 0.9% of patients treated with ACTOS were withdrawn from clinical trials in the U.S. due to abnormal liver function tests.

In pre-approval clinical trials, there were no cases of idiosyncratic drug reactions leading to hepatic failure (see PRECAUTIONS, Hepatic Effects).

CPK Levels: During required laboratory testing in clinical trials, sporadic, transient elevations in creatine phosphokinase levels (CPK) were observed. An isolated elevation to greater than 10 times the upper limit of normal was noted in 9 patients (values of 2150 to 11400 IU/L). Six of these patients continued to receive ACTOS, two patients had completed receiving study medication at the time of the elevated value and one patient discontinued study medication due to the elevation. These elevations resolved without any apparent clinical sequelae. The relationship of these events to ACTOS therapy is unknown.

OVERDOSAGE

During controlled clinical trials, one case of overdose with ACTOS was reported. A male patient took 120 mg per day for four days, then 180 mg per day for seven days. The patient denied any clinical symptoms during this period.

In the event of overdosage, appropriate supportive treatment should be initiated according to patient's clinical signs and symptoms.

DOSAGE AND ADMINISTRATION

ACTOS should be taken once daily without regard to meals. The management of antidiabetic therapy should be individualized. Ideally, the response to therapy should be evaluated using HbA_{1c} which is a better indicator of long-term glycemic control than FPG alone. HbA_{1c} reflects glycemia over the past two to three months. In clinical use, it is recommended that patients be treated with ACTOS for a period of time adequate to evaluate change in HbA_{1c} (three months) unless glycemic control deteriorates.

Monotherapy

ACTOS monotherapy in patients not adequately controlled with diet and exercise may be initiated at 15 mg or 30 mg once daily. For patients who respond inadequately to the initial dose of ACTOS, the dose can be increased in increments up to 45 mg once daily. For patients not responding adequately to monotherapy, combination therapy should be considered.

Combination Therapy

Sulfonylureas: ACTOS in combination with a sulfonylurea may be initiated at 15 mg or 30 mg once daily. The current sulfonylurea dose can be continued upon initiation of ACTOS therapy. If patients report hypoglycemia, the dose of the sulfonylurea should be decreased.

Metformin: ACTOS in combination with metformin may be initiated at 15 mg or 30 mg once daily. The current metformin dose can be continued upon initiation of ACTOS therapy. It is unlikely that the dose of metformin will require adjustment due to hypoglycemia during combination therapy with ACTOS.

Insulin: ACTOS in combination with insulin may be initiated at 15 mg or 30 mg once daily. The current insulin dose can be continued upon initiation of ACTOS therapy. In patients receiving ACTOS and insulin, the insulin dose can be decreased by 10% to 25% if the patient reports hypoglycemia or if plasma glucose concentrations decrease to less than 100 mg/dL. Further adjustments should be individualized based on glucose-lowering response.

Maximum Recommended Dose

The dose of ACTOS should not exceed 45 mg once daily in monotherapy or in combination with sulfonylurea, metformin or insulin.

Dose adjustment in patients with renal insufficiency is not recommended (see CLINICAL PHARMACOLOGY, Pharmacokinetics and Drug Metabolism).

Therapy with ACTOS should not be initiated if the patient exhibits clinical evidence of active liver disease or increased serum transaminase levels (ALT greater than 2.5 times the upper limit of normal) at start of therapy (see PRECAUTIONS, General, Hepatic Effects and CLINICAL PHARMACOLOGY Special Populations, Hepatic Insufficiency). Liver enzyme monitoring is recommended in all patients prior to initiation of therapy with ACTOS and periodically thereafter (see PRECAUTIONS, General, Hepatic Effects).

There are no data on the use of ACTOS in patients under 18 years of age; therefore, use of ACTOS in pediatric patients is not recommended.

No data are available on the use of ACTOS in combination with another thiazolidinedione.

HOW SUPPLIED

ACTOS is available in 15 mg, 30 mg, and 45 mg tablets as follows:

15 mg Tablet: white to off-white, round, convex, non-scored tablet with "ACTOS" on one side, and "15" on the other, available in:

NDC 64764-151-04 Bottle of 30
NDC 64764-151-05 Bottle of 90
NDC 64764-151-06 Bottle of 500

30 mg Tablet: white to off-white, round, flat, non-scored tablet with "ACTOS" on one side, and "30" on the other, available in:

NDC 64764-301-14 Bottle of 30
NDC 64764-301-15 Bottle of 90
NDC 64764-301-16 Bottle of 500
45 mg Tablet: white to off-white, round, flat, non-scored tablet with "ACTOS" on one side, and "45" on the other, available in:
NDC 64764-451-24 Bottle of 30
NDC 64764-451-25 Bottle of 90
NDC 64764-451-26 Bottle of 500

STORAGE

Store at 25°C (77°F); excursions permitted to 15-30°C (59-86°F) [see USP Controlled Room Temperature]. Keep container tightly closed, and protect from moisture and humidity.

Rx only

Manufactured by:
Takeda Chemical Industries, Ltd.
Osaka, Japan
Marketed by:
Takeda Pharmaceuticals America, Inc.
475 Half Day Road
Lincolnshire, IL 60069
and
Eli Lilly and Company
Lilly Corporate Center
Indianapolis, IN 46285

ACTOS® is a registered trademark of Takeda Chemical Industries, Ltd. and used under license by Takeda Pharmaceuticals America, Inc. and Eli Lilly and Co.
All other trademark names are the property of their respective owners.
5012100-07 Revised: December 2003

Wyeth Pharmaceuticals

Division of Wyeth
P.O. BOX 8299
PHILADELPHIA, PA 19101

For Product Information Contact:
(800) 934-5556
For Product Quality Contact:
(800) 999-9384
For Professional Services Contact:
(800) 395-9938
For Customer Service and Ordering Information Contact:
Pharmaceuticals: (800) 666-7248
Vaccines: (800) 572-8221
For Patient Assistance Program Contact:
(800) 568-9938
For All Other Inquiries:
(610) 688-4400
www.wyeth.com

Information on these Wyeth Pharmaceuticals products is based on labeling in effect as of April 2004. Since the publication of this reference book, there may have been revisions to the labeling of these products.
For further product information and current package inserts please visit www.wyeth.com or call our Global Medical Communications Department toll-free at 1-800-934-5556.

BENEFIX® ℞

[*bĕnĕ-fĭks*]
COAGULATION FACTOR IX (RECOMBINANT)

Prescribing information for this product, which appears on pages 3411–3413 of the 2004 PDR, has been revised as follows. Please write "See Supplement A" next to the product heading.
In the **WARNINGS** *section, the following statement has been added after the first paragraph:*
The diluent vial accompanying this product may contain dry natural rubber that may cause hypersensitivity reactions when handled by or administered to persons with known or possible latex sensitivity.
Manufactured by:
Wyeth Pharmaceuticals Inc.
Philadelphia, PA 19101
US Govt. License Number 3
Telephone: 1-800-934-5556
Imported and Distributed in Canada by:
Wyeth Canada
Montreal, Canada
W10483C002
ET02
Rev 12/03

EFFEXOR® ℞

[*ĕ-fĕks-ŏr*]
(venlafaxine hydrochloride)
Tablets
℞ only

Prescribing information for this product, which appears on pages 3413–3418 of the 2004 PDR, has been completely revised as follows. Please write "See Supplement A" next to the product heading.

DESCRIPTION

Effexor (venlafaxine hydrochloride) is a structurally novel antidepressant for oral administration. It is chemically unrelated to tricyclic, tetracyclic, or other available antidepressant agents. It is designated (R/S)-1-[2-(dimethylamino)-1-(4-methoxyphenyl)ethyl] cyclohexanol hydrochloride or (±)-1-[α-[(dimethyl-amino)methyl]-p-methoxybenzyl] cyclohexanol hydrochloride and has the empirical formula of $C_{17}H_{27}NO_2$ HCl. Its molecular weight is 313.87. The structural formula is shown below.

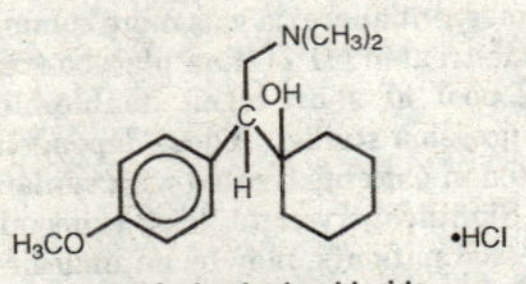

venlafaxine hydrochloride

Venlafaxine hydrochloride is a white to off-white crystalline solid with a solubility of 572 mg/mL in water (adjusted to ionic strength of 0.2 M with sodium chloride). Its octanol:water (0.2 M sodium chloride) partition coefficient is 0.43.
Compressed tablets contain venlafaxine hydrochloride equivalent to 25 mg, 37.5 mg, 50 mg, 75 mg, or 100 mg venlafaxine. Inactive ingredients consist of cellulose, iron oxides, lactose, magnesium stearate, and sodium starch glycolate.

CLINICAL PHARMACOLOGY

Pharmacodynamics
The mechanism of the antidepressant action of venlafaxine in humans is believed to be associated with its potentiation of neurotransmitter activity in the CNS. Preclinical studies have shown that venlafaxine and its active metabolite, O-desmethylvenlafaxine (ODV), are potent inhibitors of neuronal serotonin and norepinephrine reuptake and weak inhibitors of dopamine reuptake. Venlafaxine and ODV have no significant affinity for muscarinic, histaminergic, or α-1 adrenergic receptors in vitro. Pharmacologic activity at these receptors is hypothesized to be associated with the various anticholinergic, sedative, and cardiovascular effects seen with other psychotropic drugs. Venlafaxine and ODV do not possess monoamine oxidase (MAO) inhibitory activity.

Pharmacokinetics
Venlafaxine is well absorbed and extensively metabolized in the liver. O-desmethylvenlafaxine (ODV) is the only major active metabolite. On the basis of mass balance studies, at least 92% of a single dose of venlafaxine is absorbed. Approximately 87% of a venlafaxine dose is recovered in the urine within 48 hours as either unchanged venlafaxine (5%), unconjugated ODV (29%), conjugated ODV (26%), or other minor inactive metabolites (27%). Renal elimination of venlafaxine and its metabolites is the primary route of excretion. The relative bioavailability of venlafaxine from a tablet was 100% when compared to an oral solution. Food has no significant effect on the absorption of venlafaxine or on the formation of ODV.
The degree of binding of venlafaxine to human plasma is 27% ± 2% at concentrations ranging from 2.5 to 2215 ng/mL. The degree of ODV binding to human plasma is 30% ± 12% at concentrations ranging from 100 to 500 ng/mL. Protein-binding-induced drug interactions with venlafaxine are not expected.
Steady-state concentrations of both venlafaxine and ODV in plasma were attained within 3 days of multiple-dose therapy. Venlafaxine and ODV exhibited linear kinetics over the dose range of 75 to 450 mg total dose per day (administered on a q8h schedule). Plasma clearance, elimination half-life and steady-state volume of distribution were unaltered for both venlafaxine and ODV after multiple-dosing. Mean ± SD steady-state plasma clearance of venlafaxine and ODV is 1.3 ± 0.6 and 0.4 ± 0.2 L/h/kg, respectively; elimination half-life is 5 ± 2 and 11 ± 2 hours, respectively; and steady-state volume of distribution is 7.5 ± 3.7 L/kg and 5.7 ± 1.8 L/kg, respectively. When equal daily doses of venlafaxine were administered as either b.i.d. or t.i.d. regimens, the drug exposure (AUC) and fluctuation in plasma levels of venlafaxine and ODV were comparable following both regimens.

Age and Gender
A pharmacokinetic analysis of 404 venlafaxine-treated patients from two studies involving both b.i.d. and t.i.d. regimens showed that dose-normalized trough plasma levels of either venlafaxine or ODV were unaltered due to age or gender differences. Dosage adjustment based upon the age or gender of a patient is generally not necessary (see **DOSAGE AND ADMINISTRATION**).

Liver Disease
In 9 patients with hepatic cirrhosis, the pharmacokinetic disposition of both venlafaxine and ODV was significantly altered after oral administration of venlafaxine. Venlafaxine elimination half-life was prolonged by about 30%, and clearance decreased by about 50% in cirrhotic patients compared to normal subjects. ODV elimination half-life was prolonged by about 60% and clearance decreased by about 30% in cirrhotic patients compared to normal subjects. A large degree of intersubject variability was noted. Three patients with more severe cirrhosis had a more substantial decrease in venlafaxine clearance (about 90%) compared to normal subjects.
Dosage adjustment is necessary in these patients (see **DOSAGE AND ADMINISTRATION**).

Renal Disease
In a renal impairment study, venlafaxine elimination half-life after oral administration was prolonged by about 50% and clearance was reduced by about 24% in renally impaired patients (GFR = 10-70 mL/min), compared to normal subjects. In dialysis patients, venlafaxine elimination half-life was prolonged by about 180% and clearance was reduced by about 57% compared to normal subjects. Similarly, ODV elimination half-life was prolonged by about 40% although clearance was unchanged in patients with renal impairment (GFR = 10-70 mL/min) compared to normal subjects. In dialysis patients, ODV elimination half-life was prolonged by about 142% and clearance was reduced by about 56%, compared to normal subjects. A large degree of intersubject variability was noted.
Dosage adjustment is necessary in these patients (see **DOSAGE AND ADMINISTRATION**).

CLINICAL TRIALS

The efficacy of Effexor (venlafaxine hydrochloride) as a treatment for depression was established in 5 placebo-controlled, short-term trials. Four of these were 6-week trials in outpatients meeting DSM-III or DSM-III-R criteria for major depression: two involving dose titration with Effexor in a range of 75 to 225 mg/day (t.i.d. schedule), the third involving fixed Effexor doses of 75, 225, and 375 mg/day (t.i.d. schedule), and the fourth involving doses of 25, 75, and 200 mg/day (b.i.d. schedule). The fifth was a 4-week study of inpatients meeting DSM-III-R criteria for major depression with melancholia whose Effexor doses were titrated in a range of 150 to 375 mg/day (t.i.d. schedule). In these 5 studies, Effexor was shown to be significantly superior to placebo on at least 2 of the following 3 measures: Hamilton Depression Rating Scale (total score), Hamilton depressed mood item, and Clinical Global Impression-Severity of Illness rating. Doses from 75 to 225 mg/day were superior to placebo in outpatient studies and a mean dose of about 350 mg/day was effective in inpatients. Data from the 2 fixed-dose outpatient studies were suggestive of a dose-response relationship in the range of 75 to 225 mg/day. There was no suggestion of increased response with doses greater than 225 mg/day.
While there were no efficacy studies focusing specifically on an elderly population, elderly patients were included among the patients studied. Overall, approximately 2/3 of all patients in these trials were women. Exploratory analyses for age and gender effects on outcome did not suggest any differential responsiveness on the basis of age or sex.
In one longer-term study, outpatients meeting DSM-IV criteria for major depressive disorder who had responded during an 8-week open trial on Effexor XR (75, 150, or 225 mg, qAM) were randomized to continuation of their same Effexor XR dose or to placebo, for up to 26 weeks of observation for relapse. Response during the open phase was defined as a CGI Severity of Illness item score of ≤3 and a HAM-D-21 total score of ≤10 at the day 56 evaluation. Relapse during the double-blind phase was defined as follows: (1) a reappearance of major depressive disorder as defined by DSM-IV criteria and a CGI Severity of Illness item score of ≥4 (moderately ill), (2) 2 consecutive CGI Severity of Illness item scores of ≥4, or (3) a final CGI Severity of Illness item score of ≥4 for any patient who withdrew from the study for any reason. Patients receiving continued Effexor XR treatment experienced significantly lower relapse rates over the subsequent 26 weeks compared with those receiving placebo.
In a second longer-term trial, outpatients meeting DSM-III-R criteria for major depressive disorder, recurrent type, who had responded (HAM-D-21 total score ≤12 at the day 56 evaluation) and continued to be improved [defined as the following criteria being met for days 56 through 180: (1) no HAM-D-21 total score ≥20; (2) no more than 2 HAM-D-21 total scores >10; and (3) no single CGI Severity of Illness item score ≥4 (moderately ill)] during an initial 26 weeks of treatment on Effexor (100 to 200 mg/day, on a b.i.d. schedule) were randomized to continuation of their same Effexor dose or to placebo. The follow-up period to observe patients for relapse, defined as a CGI Severity of Illness item score ≥4, was for up to 52 weeks. Patients receiving continued Effexor treatment experienced significantly lower relapse rates over the subsequent 52 weeks compared with those receiving placebo.

INDICATIONS AND USAGE

Effexor (venlafaxine hydrochloride) is indicated for the treatment of depression.
The efficacy of Effexor in the treatment of depression was established in 6-week controlled trials of outpatients whose diagnoses corresponded most closely to the DSM-III or DSM-III-R category of major depressive disorder and in a 4-week controlled trial of inpatients meeting diagnostic criteria for major depressive disorder with melancholia (see **CLINICAL TRIALS**).
A major depressive episode implies a prominent and relatively persistent depressed or dysphoric mood that usually interferes with daily functioning (nearly every day for at least 2 weeks); it should include at least 4 of the following 8 symptoms: change in appetite, change in sleep, psychomotor agitation or retardation, loss of interest in usual activities or decrease in sexual drive, increased fatigue, feelings of guilt or worthlessness, slowed thinking or impaired concentration, and a suicide attempt or suicidal ideation.
The efficacy of Effexor XR in maintaining an antidepressant response for up to 26 weeks following 8 weeks of acute treat-

Continued on next page

Effexor—Cont.

ment was demonstrated in a placebo-controlled trial. The efficacy of Effexor in maintaining an antidepressant response in patients with recurrent depression who had responded and continued to be improved during an initial 26 weeks of treatment and were then followed for a period of up to 52 weeks was demonstrated in a second placebo-controlled trial (see **CLINICAL TRIALS**). Nevertheless, the physician who elects to use Effexor/Effexor XR for extended periods should periodically re-evaluate the long-term usefulness of the drug for the individual patient.

CONTRAINDICATIONS

Hypersensitivity to venlafaxine hydrochloride or to any excipients in the formulation.

Concomitant use in patients taking monoamine oxidase inhibitors (MAOIs) is contraindicated (see **WARNINGS**).

WARNINGS

Potential for Interaction with Monoamine Oxidase Inhibitors

Adverse reactions, some of which were serious, have been reported in patients who have recently been discontinued from a monoamine oxidase inhibitor (MAOI) and started on Effexor, or who have recently had Effexor therapy discontinued prior to initiation of an MAOI. These reactions have included tremor, myoclonus, diaphoresis, nausea, vomiting, flushing, dizziness, hyperthermia with features resembling neuroleptic malignant syndrome, seizures, and death. In patients receiving antidepressants with pharmacological properties similar to venlafaxine in combination with a monoamine oxidase inhibitor, there have also been reports of serious, sometimes fatal, reactions. For a selective serotonin reuptake inhibitor, these reactions have included hyperthermia, rigidity, myoclonus, autonomic instability with possible rapid fluctuations of vital signs, and mental status changes that include extreme agitation progressing to delirium and coma. Some cases presented with features resembling neuroleptic malignant syndrome. Severe hyperthermia and seizures, sometimes fatal, have been reported in association with the combined use of tricyclic antidepressants and MAOIs. These reactions have also been reported in patients who have recently discontinued these drugs and have been started on an MAOI. Therefore, it is recommended that Effexor not be used in combination with an MAOI, or within at least 14 days of discontinuing treatment with an MAOI. Based on the half-life of Effexor, at least 7 days should be allowed after stopping Effexor before starting an MAOI.

Sustained Hypertension

Venlafaxine treatment is associated with sustained increases in blood pressure in some patients. (1) In a premarketing study comparing three fixed doses of venlafaxine (75, 225, and 375 mg/day) and placebo, a mean increase in supine diastolic blood pressure (SDBP) of 7.2 mm Hg was seen in the 375 mg/day group at week 6 compared to essentially no changes in the 75 and 225 mg/day groups and a mean decrease in SDBP of 2.2 mm Hg in the placebo group. (2) An analysis for patients meeting criteria for sustained hypertension (defined as treatment-emergent SDBP ≥ 90 mm Hg *and* ≥ 10 mm Hg above baseline for 3 consecutive visits) revealed a dose-dependent increase in the incidence of sustained hypertension for venlafaxine:

Probability of Sustained Elevation in SDBP
(Pool of Premarketing Venlafaxine Studies)

Treatment Group	Incidence of Sustained Elevation in SDBP
Venlafaxine	
<100 mg/day	3%
101–200 mg/day	5%
201–300 mg/day	7%
>300 mg/day	13%
Placebo	2%

An analysis of the patients with sustained hypertension and the 19 venlafaxine patients who were discontinued from treatment because of hypertension (<1% of total venlafaxine-treated group) revealed that most of the blood pressure increases were in a modest range (10 to 15 mm Hg, SDBP). Nevertheless, sustained increases of this magnitude could have adverse consequences. Therefore, it is recommended that patients receiving venlafaxine have regular monitoring of blood pressure. For patients who experience a sustained increase in blood pressure while receiving venlafaxine, either dose reduction or discontinuation should be considered.

PRECAUTIONS

General

Anxiety and Insomnia

Treatment-emergent anxiety, nervousness, and insomnia were more commonly reported for venlafaxine-treated patients compared to placebo-treated patients in a pooled analysis of short-term, double-blind, placebo-controlled depression studies:

Symptom	Venlafaxine n = 1033	Placebo n = 609
Anxiety	6%	3%
Nervousness	13%	6%
Insomnia	18%	10%

Anxiety, nervousness, and insomnia led to drug discontinuation in 2%, 2%, and 3%, respectively, of the patients treated with venlafaxine in the Phase 2 and Phase 3 depression studies.

Changes in Appetite and Weight

Treatment-emergent anorexia was more commonly reported for venlafaxine-treated (11%) than placebo-treated patients (2%) in the pool of short-term, double-blind, placebo-controlled depression studies. A dose-dependent weight loss was often noted in patients treated with venlafaxine for several weeks. Significant weight loss, especially in underweight depressed patients, may be an undesirable result of venlafaxine treatment. A loss of 5% or more of body weight occurred in 6% of patients treated with venlafaxine compared with 1% of patients treated with placebo and 3% of patients treated with another antidepressant. However, discontinuation for weight loss associated with venlafaxine was uncommon (0.1% of venlafaxine-treated patients in the Phase 2 and Phase 3 depression trials).

The safety and efficacy of venlafaxine therapy in combination with weight loss agents, including phentermine, have not been established. Co-administration of Effexor and weight loss agents is not recommended. Effexor is not indicated for weight loss alone or in combination with other products.

Activation of Mania/Hypomania

During Phase 2 and Phase 3 trials, hypomania or mania occurred in 0.5% of patients treated with venlafaxine. Activation of mania/hypomania has also been reported in a small proportion of patients with major affective disorder who were treated with other marketed antidepressants. As with all antidepressants, Effexor (venlafaxine hydrochloride) should be used cautiously in patients with a history of mania.

Hyponatremia

Hyponatremia and/or the syndrome of inappropriate antidiuretic hormone secretion (SIADH) may occur with venlafaxine. This should be taken into consideration in patients who are, for example, volume-depleted, elderly, or taking diuretics.

Mydriasis

Mydriasis has been reported in association with venlafaxine; therefore patients with raised intraocular pressure or at risk of acute narrow angle glaucoma should be monitored.

Seizures

During premarketing testing, seizures were reported in 0.26% (8/3082) of venlafaxine-treated patients. Most seizures (5 of 8) occurred in patients receiving doses of 150 mg/day or less. Effexor should be used cautiously in patients with a history of seizures. It should be discontinued in any patient who develops seizures.

Abnormal Bleeding

There have been reports of abnormal bleeding (most commonly ecchymosis) associated with venlafaxine treatment. While a causal relationship to venlafaxine is unclear, impaired platelet aggregation may result from platelet serotonin depletion and contribute to such occurrences.

Serum Cholesterol Elevation

Clinically relevant increases in serum cholesterol were recorded in 5.3% of venlafaxine-treated patients and 0.0% of placebo-treated patients treated for at least 3 months in placebo-controlled trials (see **ADVERSE REACTIONS—Laboratory Changes**). Measurement of serum cholesterol levels should be considered during long-term treatment.

Suicide

The possibility of a suicide attempt is inherent in depression and may persist until significant remission occurs. Close supervision of high-risk patients should accompany initial drug therapy. Prescriptions for Effexor should be written for the smallest quantity of tablets consistent with good patient management in order to reduce the risk of overdose.

Use in Patients with Concomitant Illness

Clinical experience with Effexor in patients with concomitant systemic illness is limited. Caution is advised in administering Effexor to patients with diseases or conditions that could affect hemodynamic responses or metabolism.

Effexor has not been evaluated or used to any appreciable extent in patients with a recent history of myocardial infarction or unstable heart disease. Patients with these diagnoses were systematically excluded from many clinical studies during the product's premarketing testing. Evaluation of the electrocardiograms for 769 patients who received Effexor in 4- to 6-week double-blind placebo-controlled trials, however, showed that the incidence of trial-emergent conduction abnormalities did not differ from that with placebo. The mean heart rate in Effexor-treated patients was increased relative to baseline by about 4 beats per minute.

The electrocardiograms for 357 patients who received Effexor XR (the extended-release form of venlafaxine) and 285 patients who received placebo in 8- to 12-week double-blind, placebo-controlled trials were analyzed. The mean change from baseline in corrected QT interval (QTc) for Effexor XR-treated patients was increased relative to that for placebo-treated patients (increase of 4.7 msec for Effexor XR and decrease of 1.9 msec for placebo). In these same trials, the mean change from baseline in heart rate for Effexor XR-treated patients was significantly higher than that for placebo (a mean increase of 4 beats per minute for Effexor XR and 1 beat per minute for placebo). In a flexible-dose study, with Effexor doses in the range of 200 to 375 mg/day and mean dose greater than 300 mg/day, Effexor-treated patients had a mean increase in heart rate of 8.5 beats per minute compared with 1.7 beats per minute in the placebo group.

As increases in heart rate were observed, caution should be exercised in patients whose underlying medical conditions might be compromised by increases in heart rate (eg, patients with hyperthyroidism, heart failure, or recent myocardial infarction), particularly when using doses of Effexor above 200 mg/day.

In patients with renal impairment (GFR=10 to 70 mL/min) or cirrhosis of the liver, the clearances of venlafaxine and its active metabolite were decreased, thus prolonging the elimination half-lives of these substances. A lower dose may be necessary (see **DOSAGE AND ADMINISTRATION**). Effexor (venlafaxine hydrochloride), like all antidepressants, should be used with caution in such patients.

Information for Patients

Physicians are advised to discuss the following issues with patients for whom they prescribe Effexor:

Interference with Cognitive and Motor Performance

Clinical studies were performed to examine the effects of venlafaxine on behavioral performance of healthy individuals. The results revealed no clinically significant impairment of psychomotor, cognitive, or complex behavior performance. However, since any psychoactive drug may impair judgment, thinking, or motor skills, patients should be cautioned about operating hazardous machinery, including automobiles, until they are reasonably certain that Effexor therapy does not adversely affect their ability to engage in such activities.

Pregnancy

Patients should be advised to notify their physician if they become pregnant or intend to become pregnant during therapy.

Nursing

Patients should be advised to notify their physician if they are breast-feeding an infant.

Concomitant Medication

Patients should be advised to inform their physicians if they are taking, or plan to take, any prescription or over-the-counter drugs, including herbal preparations, since there is a potential for interactions.

Alcohol

Although Effexor has not been shown to increase the impairment of mental and motor skills caused by alcohol, patients should be advised to avoid alcohol while taking Effexor.

Allergic Reactions

Patients should be advised to notify their physician if they develop a rash, hives, or a related allergic phenomenon.

Laboratory Tests

There are no specific laboratory tests recommended.

Drug Interactions

As with all drugs, the potential for interaction by a variety of mechanisms is a possibility.

Alcohol

A single dose of ethanol (0.5 g/kg) had no effect on the pharmacokinetics of venlafaxine or ODV when venlafaxine was administered at 150 mg/day in 15 healthy male subjects. Additionally, administration of venlafaxine in a stable regimen did not exaggerate the psychomotor and psychometric effects induced by ethanol in these same subjects when they were not receiving venlafaxine.

Cimetidine

Concomitant administration of cimetidine and venlafaxine in a steady-state study for both drugs resulted in inhibition of first-pass metabolism of venlafaxine in 18 healthy subjects. The oral clearance of venlafaxine was reduced by about 43%, and the exposure (AUC) and maximum concentration (C_{max}) of the drug were increased by about 60%. However, co-administration of cimetidine had no apparent effect on the pharmacokinetics of ODV, which is present in much greater quantity in the circulation than is venlafaxine. The overall pharmacological activity of venlafaxine plus ODV is expected to increase only slightly, and no dosage adjustment should be necessary for most normal adults. However, for patients with pre-existing hypertension, and for elderly patients or patients with hepatic dysfunction, the interaction associated with the concomitant use of venlafaxine and cimetidine is not known and potentially could be more pronounced. Therefore, caution is advised with such patients.

Diazepam

Under steady-state conditions for venlafaxine administered at 150 mg/day, a single 10 mg dose of diazepam did not appear to affect the pharmacokinetics of either venlafaxine or ODV in 18 healthy male subjects. Venlafaxine also did not have any effect on the pharmacokinetics of diazepam or its active metabolite, desmethyldiazepam, or affect the psychomotor and psychometric effects induced by diazepam.

Haloperidol

Venlafaxine administered under steady-state conditions at 150 mg/day in 24 healthy subjects decreased total oral-dose clearance (Cl/F) of a single 2 mg dose of haloperidol by 42%, which resulted in a 70% increase in haloperidol AUC. In addition, the haloperidol C_{max} increased 88% when coadministered with venlafaxine, but the haloperidol elimination half-life ($t_{1/2}$) was unchanged. The mechanism explaining this finding is unknown.

Lithium
The steady-state pharmacokinetics of venlafaxine administered at 150 mg/day were not affected when a single 600 mg oral dose of lithium was administered to 12 healthy male subjects. O-desmethylvenlafaxine (ODV) also was unaffected. Venlafaxine had no effect on the pharmacokinetics of lithium (see also *CNS—Active Drugs*, below).
Drugs Highly Bound to Plasma Protein
Venlafaxine is not highly bound to plasma proteins; therefore, administration of Effexor to a patient taking another drug that is highly protein bound should not cause increased free concentrations of the other drug.
Drugs that Inhibit Cytochrome P450 Isoenzymes
CYP2D6 Inhibitors: In vitro and in vivo studies indicate that venlafaxine is metabolized to its active metabolite, ODV, by CYP2D6, the isoenzyme that is responsible for the genetic polymorphism seen in the metabolism of many antidepressants. Therefore, the potential exists for a drug interaction between drugs that inhibit CYP2D6-mediated metabolism and venlafaxine. However, although imipramine partially inhibited the CYP2D6-mediated metabolism of venlafaxine, resulting in higher plasma concentrations of venlafaxine and lower plasma concentrations of ODV, the total concentration of active compounds (venlafaxine plus ODV) was not affected. Additionally, in a clinical study involving CYP2D6-poor and -extensive metabolizers, the total concentration of active compounds (venlafaxine plus ODV), was similar in the two metabolizer groups. Therefore, no dosage adjustment is required when venlafaxine is coadministered with a CYP2D6 inhibitor.
CYP3A4 Inhibitors: In vitro studies indicate that venlafaxine is likely metabolized to a minor, less active metabolite, N-desmethylvenlafaxine, by CYP3A4. Because CYP3A4 is typically a minor pathway relative to CYP2D6 in the metabolism of venlafaxine, the potential for a clinically significant drug interaction between drugs that inhibit CYP3A4-mediated metabolism and venlafaxine is small.
The concomitant use of venlafaxine with a drug treatment(s) that potently inhibits both CYP2D6 and CYP3A4, the primary metabolizing enzymes for venlafaxine, has not been studied. Therefore, caution is advised should a patient's therapy include venlafaxine and any agent(s) that produce potent simultaneous inhibition of these two enzyme systems.
Drugs Metabolized by Cytochrome P450 Isoenzymes
CYP2D6: In vitro studies indicate that venlafaxine is a relatively weak inhibitor of CYP2D6. These findings have been confirmed in a clinical drug interaction study comparing the effect of venlafaxine to that of fluoxetine on the CYP2D6-mediated metabolism of dextromethorphan to dextrorphan.
Imipramine—Venlafaxine did not affect the pharmacokinetics of imipramine and 2-OH-imipramine. However, desipramine AUC, C_{max}, and C_{min} increased by about 35% in the presence of venlafaxine. The 2-OH-desipramine AUCs increased by at least 2.5 fold (with venlafaxine 37.5 mg q12h) and by 4.5 fold (with venlafaxine 75 mg q12h). Imipramine did not affect the pharmacokinetics of venlafaxine and ODV. The clinical significance of elevated 2-OH-desipramine levels is unknown.
Risperidone—Venlafaxine administered under steady-state conditions at 150 mg/day slightly inhibited the CYP2D6-mediated metabolism of risperidone (administered as a single 1 mg oral dose) to its active metabolite, 9-hydroxyrisperidone, resulting in an approximate 32% increase in risperidone AUC. However, venlafaxine coadministration did not significantly alter the pharmacokinetic profile of the total active moiety (risperidone plus 9-hydroxyrisperidone).
CYP3A4: Venlafaxine did not inhibit CYP3A4 in vitro. This finding was confirmed in vivo by clinical drug interaction studies in which venlafaxine did not inhibit the metabolism of several CYP3A4 substrates, including alprazolam, diazepam, and terfenadine.
Indinavir—In a study of 9 healthy volunteers, venlafaxine administered under steady-state conditions at 150 mg/day resulted in a 28% decrease in the AUC of a single 800 mg oral dose of indinavir and a 36% decrease in indinavir C_{max}. Indinavir did not affect the pharmacokinetics of venlafaxine and ODV. The clinical significance of this finding is unknown.
CYP1A2: Venlafaxine did not inhibit CYP1A2 in vitro. This finding was confirmed in vivo by a clinical drug interaction study in which venlafaxine did not inhibit the metabolism of caffeine, a CYP1A2 substrate.
CYP2C9: Venlafaxine did not inhibit CYP2C9 in vitro. The clinical significance of this finding is unknown.
CYP2C19: Venlafaxine did not inhibit the metabolism of diazepam which is partially metabolized by CYP2C19 (see *Diazepam* above).
Monoamine Oxidase Inhibitors
See **CONTRAINDICATIONS** and **WARNINGS**.
CNS-Active Drugs
The risk of using venlafaxine in combination with other CNS-active drugs has not been systematically evaluated (except in the case of those CNS-active drugs noted above). Consequently, caution is advised if the concomitant administration of venlafaxine and such drugs is required. Based on the mechanism of action of venlafaxine and the potential for serotonin syndrome, caution is advised when venlafaxine is co-administered with other drugs that may affect the serotonergic neurotransmitter systems, such as triptans, serotonin reuptake inhibitors (SRIs), or lithium.
Electroconvulsive Therapy
There are no clinical data establishing the benefit of electroconvulsive therapy combined with Effexor treatment.
Postmarketing Spontaneous Drug Interaction Reports
See **ADVERSE REACTIONS, Postmarketing Reports.**
Carcinogenesis, Mutagenesis, Impairment of Fertility
Carcinogenesis
Venlafaxine was given by oral gavage to mice for 18 months at doses up to 120 mg/kg per day, which was 16 times, on a mg/kg basis, and 1.7 times on a mg/m^2 basis, the maximum recommended human dose. Venlafaxine was also given to rats by oral gavage for 24 months at doses up to 120 mg/kg per day. In rats receiving the 120 mg/kg dose, plasma levels of venlafaxine were 1 times (male rats) and 6 times (female rats) the plasma levels of patients receiving the maximum recommended human dose. Plasma levels of the O-desmethyl metabolite were lower in rats than in patients receiving the maximum recommended dose. Tumors were not increased by venlafaxine treatment in mice or rats.
Mutagenicity
Venlafaxine and the major human metabolite, O-desmethylvenlafaxine (ODV), were not mutagenic in the Ames reverse mutation assay in Salmonella bacteria or the CHO/HGPRT mammalian cell forward gene mutation assay. Venlafaxine was also not mutagenic in the in vitro BALB/c-3T3 mouse cell transformation assay, the sister chromatid exchange assay in cultured CHO cells, or the in vivo chromosomal aberration assay in rat bone marrow. ODV was not mutagenic in the in vitro CHO cell chromosomal aberration assay. There was a clastogenic response in the in vivo chromosomal aberration assay in rat bone marrow in male rats receiving 200 times, on a mg/kg basis, or 50 times, on a mg/m^2 basis, the maximum human daily dose. The no effect dose was 67 times (mg/kg) or 17 times (mg/m^2) the human dose.
Impairment of Fertility
Reproduction and fertility studies in rats showed no effects on male or female fertility at oral doses of up to 8 times the maximum recommended human daily dose on a mg/kg basis, or up to 2 times on a mg/m^2 basis.
Pregnancy
Teratogenic Effects—Pregnancy Category C
Venlafaxine did not cause malformations in offspring of rats or rabbits given doses up to 11 times (rat) or 12 times (rabbit) the maximum recommended human daily dose on a mg/kg basis, or 2.5 times (rat) and 4 times (rabbit) the human daily dose on a mg/m^2 basis. However, in rats, there was a decrease in pup weight, an increase in stillborn pups, and an increase in pup deaths during the first 5 days of lactation, when dosing began during pregnancy and continued until weaning. The cause of these deaths is not known. These effects occurred at 10 times (mg/kg) or 2.5 times (mg/m^2) the maximum human daily dose. The no effect dose for rat pup mortality was 1.4 times the human dose on a mg/kg basis or 0.25 times the human dose on a mg/m^2 basis. There are no adequate and well-controlled studies in pregnant women. Because animal reproduction studies are not always predictive of human response, this drug should be used during pregnancy only if clearly needed.
Non-teratogenic Effects
If venlafaxine is used until or shortly before birth, discontinuation effects in the newborn should be considered.
Labor and Delivery
The effect of Effexor® (venlafaxine hydrochloride) on labor and delivery in humans is unknown.
Nursing Mothers
Venlafaxine and ODV have been reported to be excreted in human milk. Because of the potential for serious adverse reactions in nursing infants from Effexor, a decision should be made whether to discontinue nursing or to discontinue the drug, taking into account the importance of the drug to the mother.
Usage in Children
Safety and effectiveness in individuals below 18 years of age have not been established.
In pediatric clinical trials, there were increased reports of hostility and, especially in Major Depressive Disorder, suicide-related adverse events such as suicidal ideation and self-harm.
Geriatric Use
Of the 2,897 patients in Phase 2 and Phase 3 depression studies with Effexor, 12% (357) were 65 years of age or over. No overall differences in effectiveness or safety were observed between these patients and younger patients, and other reported clinical experience generally has not identified differences in response between the elderly and younger patients. However, greater sensitivity of some older individuals cannot be ruled out. As with other antidepressants, several cases of hyponatremia and syndrome of inappropriate antidiuretic hormone secretion (SIADH) have been reported, usually in the elderly.
The pharmacokinetics of venlafaxine and ODV are not substantially altered in the elderly (see **CLINICAL PHARMACOLOGY**). No dose adjustment is recommended for the elderly on the basis of age alone, although other clinical circumstances, some of which may be more common in the elderly, such as renal or hepatic impairment, may warrant a dose reduction (see **DOSAGE AND ADMINISTRATION**).

ADVERSE REACTIONS

Associated with Discontinuation of Treatment
Nineteen percent (537/2897) of venlafaxine patients in Phase 2 and Phase 3 depression studies discontinued treatment due to an adverse event. The more common events (≥ 1%) associated with discontinuation and considered to be drug-related (ie, those events associated with dropout at a rate approximately twice or greater for venlafaxine compared to placebo) included:

CNS	Venlafaxine	Placebo
Somnolence	3%	1%
Insomnia	3%	1%
Dizziness	3%	—
Nervousness	2%	—
Dry mouth	2%	—
Anxiety	2%	1%
Gastrointestinal		
Nausea	6%	1%
Urogenital		
Abnormal ejaculation*	3%	—
Other		
Headache	3%	1%
Asthenia	2%	—
Sweating	2%	—

* Percentages based on the number of males.
— Less than 1%

Incidence in Controlled Trials
Commonly Observed Adverse Events in Controlled Clinical Trials
The most commonly observed adverse events associated with the use of Effexor® (incidence of 5% or greater) and not seen at an equivalent incidence among placebo-treated patients (ie, incidence for Effexor at least twice that for placebo), derived from the 1% incidence table below, were asthenia, sweating, nausea, constipation, anorexia, vomiting, somnolence, dry mouth, dizziness, nervousness, anxiety, tremor, and blurred vision as well as abnormal ejaculation/orgasm and impotence in men.
Adverse Events Occurring at an Incidence of 1% or More Among Effexor-Treated Patients
The table that follows enumerates adverse events that occurred at an incidence of 1% or more, and were more frequent than in the placebo group, among Effexor-treated patients who participated in short-term (4- to 8-week) placebo-controlled trials in which patients were administered doses in a range of 75 to 375 mg/day. This table shows the percentage of patients in each group who had at least one episode of an event at some time during their treatment. Reported adverse events were classified using a standard COSTART-based Dictionary terminology.
The prescriber should be aware that these figures cannot be used to predict the incidence of side effects in the course of usual medical practice where patient characteristics and other factors differ from those which prevailed in the clinical trials. Similarly, the cited frequencies cannot be compared with figures obtained from other clinical investigations involving different treatments, uses and investigators. The cited figures, however, do provide the prescribing physician with some basis for estimating the relative contribution of drug and nondrug factors to the side effect incidence rate in the population studied.
[See table 1 at top of next page]
Dose Dependency of Adverse Events
A comparison of adverse event rates in a fixed-dose study comparing Effexor (venlafaxine hydrochloride) 75, 225, and 375 mg/day with placebo revealed a dose dependency for some of the more common adverse events associated with Effexor use, as shown in the table that follows. The rule for including events was to enumerate those that occurred at an incidence of 5% or more for at least one of the venlafaxine groups and for which the incidence was at least twice the placebo incidence for at least one Effexor group. Tests for potential dose relationships for these events (Cochran-Armitage Test, with a criterion of exact 2-sided p-value ≤ 0.05) suggested a dose-dependency for several adverse events in this list, including chills, hypertension, anorexia, nausea, agitation, dizziness, somnolence, tremor, yawning, sweating, and abnormal ejaculation.
[See table 2 at bottom of page 465]
Adaptation to Certain Adverse Events
Over a 6-week period, there was evidence of adaptation to some adverse events with continued therapy (eg, dizziness and nausea), but less to other effects (eg, abnormal ejaculation and dry mouth).
Vital Sign Changes
Effexor (venlafaxine hydrochloride) treatment (averaged over all dose groups) in clinical trials was associated with a mean increase in pulse rate of approximately 3 beats per minute, compared to no change for placebo. In a flexible-dose study, with doses in the range of 200 to 375 mg/day and mean dose greater than 300 mg/day, the mean pulse was increased by about 2 beats per minute compared with a decrease of about 1 beat per minute for placebo.
In controlled clinical trials, Effexor was associated with mean increases in diastolic blood pressure ranging from 0.7 to 2.5 mm Hg averaged over all dose groups, compared to mean decreases ranging from 0.9 to 3.8 mm Hg for placebo. However, there is a dose dependency for blood pressure increase (see **WARNINGS**).
Laboratory Changes
Of the serum chemistry and hematology parameters monitored during clinical trials with Effexor, a statistically significant difference with placebo was seen only for serum cholesterol. In premarketing trials, treatment with Effexor tablets was associated with a mean final on-therapy increase in total cholesterol of 3 mg/dL.
Patients treated with Effexor tablets for at least 3 months in placebo-controlled 12-month extension trials had a mean final on-therapy increase in total cholesterol of 9.1 mg/dL

Continued on next page

Effexor—Cont.

compared with a decrease of 7.1 mg/dL among placebo-treated patients. This increase was duration dependent over the study period and tended to be greater with higher doses. Clinically relevant increases in serum cholesterol, defined as 1) a final on-therapy increase in serum cholesterol ≥50 mg/dL from baseline and to a value ≥261 mg/dL or 2) an average on-therapy increase in serum cholesterol ≥50 mg/dL from baseline and to a value ≥261 mg/dL, were recorded in 5.3% of venlafaxine-treated patients and 0.0% of placebo-treated patients (see **PRECAUTIONS—General—** *Serum Cholesterol Elevation*).

ECG Changes

In an analysis of ECGs obtained in 769 patients treated with Effexor and 450 patients treated with placebo in controlled clinical trials, the only statistically significant difference observed was for heart rate, ie, a mean increase from baseline of 4 beats per minute for Effexor. In a flexible-dose study, with doses in the range of 200 to 375 mg/day and mean dose greater than 300 mg/day, the mean change in heart rate was 8.5 beats per minute compared with 1.7 beats per minute for placebo (see **PRECAUTIONS, General,** *Use in Patients with Concomitant Illness*).

Other Events Observed During the Premarketing Evaluation of Venlafaxine

During its premarketing assessment, multiple doses of Effexor were administered to 2897 patients in Phase 2 and Phase 3 studies. In addition, in premarketing assessment of Effexor XR (the extended release form of venlafaxine), multiple doses were administered to 705 patients in Phase 3 depression studies and Effexor was administered to 96 patients. During its premarketing assessment for Generalized Anxiety Disorder, multiple doses of Effexor XR were administered to 476 patients in Phase 3 studies. The conditions and duration of exposure to venlafaxine in both development programs varied greatly, and included (in overlapping categories) open and double-blind studies, uncontrolled and controlled studies, inpatient (Effexor only) and outpatient studies, fixed-dose and titration studies. Untoward events associated with this exposure were recorded by clinical investigators using terminology of their own choosing. Consequently, it is not possible to provide a meaningful estimate of the proportion of individuals experiencing adverse events without first grouping similar types of untoward events into a smaller number of standardized event categories.

In the tabulations that follow, reported adverse events were classified using a standard COSTART-based Dictionary terminology. The frequencies presented, therefore, represent the proportion of the 4174 patients exposed to multiple doses of either formulation of venlafaxine who experienced an event of the type cited on at least one occasion while receiving venlafaxine. All reported events are included except those already listed in Table 1 and those events for which a drug cause was remote. If the COSTART term for an event was so general as to be uninformative, it was replaced with a more informative term. It is important to emphasize that, although the events reported occurred during treatment with venlafaxine, they were not necessarily caused by it.

Events are further categorized by body system and listed in order of decreasing frequency using the following definitions: **frequent** adverse events are defined as those occurring on one or more occasions in at least 1/100 patients; **infrequent** adverse events are those occurring in 1/100 to 1/1000 patients; **rare** events are those occurring in fewer than 1/1000 patients.

TABLE 1
Treatment-Emergent Adverse Experience Incidence in 4- to 8-Week Placebo-Controlled Clinical Trials[1]

Body System	Preferred Term	Effexor (n=1033)	Placebo (n=609)
Body as a Whole	Headache	25%	24%
	Asthenia	12%	6%
	Infection	6%	5%
	Chills	3%	—
	Chest pain	2%	1%
	Trauma	2%	1%
Cardiovascular	Vasodilatation	4%	3%
	Increased blood pressure/hypertension	2%	—
	Tachycardia	2%	—
	Postural hypotension	1%	—
Dermatological	Sweating	12%	3%
	Rash	3%	2%
	Pruritus	1%	—
Gastrointestinal	Nausea	37%	11%
	Constipation	15%	7%
	Anorexia	11%	2%
	Diarrhea	8%	7%
	Vomiting	6%	2%
	Dyspepsia	5%	4%
	Flatulence	3%	2%
Metabolic	Weight loss	1%	—
Nervous System	Somnolence	23%	9%
	Dry mouth	22%	11%
	Dizziness	19%	7%
	Insomnia	18%	10%
	Nervousness	13%	6%
	Anxiety	6%	3%
	Tremor	5%	1%
	Abnormal dreams	4%	3%
	Hypertonia	3%	2%
	Paresthesia	3%	2%
	Libido decreased	2%	—
	Agitation	2%	—
	Confusion	2%	1%
	Thinking abnormal	2%	1%
	Depersonalization	1%	—
	Depression	1%	—
	Urinary retention	1%	—
	Twitching	1%	—
Respiration	Yawn	3%	—
Special Senses	Blurred vision	6%	2%
	Taste perversion	2%	—
	Tinnitus	2%	—
	Mydriasis	2%	—
Urogenital System	Abnormal ejaculation/orgasm	12%[2]	—[2]
	Impotence	6%[2]	—[2]
	Urinary frequency	3%	2%
	Urination impaired	2%	—
	Orgasm disturbance	2%[3]	—[3]

1 Events reported by at least 1% of patients treated with Effexor (venlafaxine hydrochloride) are included, and are rounded to the nearest %. Events for which the Effexor incidence was equal to or less than placebo are not listed in the table, but included the following: abdominal pain, pain, back pain, flu syndrome, fever, palpitation, increased appetite, myalgia, arthralgia, amnesia, hypesthesia, rhinitis, pharyngitis, sinusitis, cough increased, and dysmenorrhea[3].
—Incidence less than 1%.
2 Incidence based on number of male patients.
3 Incidence based on number of female patients.

Body as a whole—**Frequent:** chest pain substernal, neck pain; **Infrequent:** face edema, intentional injury, malaise, moniliasis, neck rigidity, pelvic pain, photosensitivity reaction, suicide attempt; **Rare:** appendicitis, bacteremia, carcinoma, cellulitis, withdrawal syndrome.

Cardiovascular system—**Frequent:** migraine; **Infrequent:** angina pectoris, arrhythmia, extrasystoles, hypotension, peripheral vascular disorder (mainly cold feet and/or cold hands), syncope, thrombophlebitis; **Rare:** aortic aneurysm, arteritis, first-degree atrioventricular block, bigeminy, bradycardia, bundle branch block, capillary fragility, cerebral ischemia, coronary artery disease, congestive heart failure, heart arrest, mitral valve disorder, mucocutaneous hemorrhage, myocardial infarct, pallor.

Digestive system—**Frequent:** eructation; **Infrequent:** bruxism, colitis, dysphagia, tongue edema, esophagitis, gastritis, gastroenteritis, gastrointestinal ulcer, gingivitis, glossitis, rectal hemorrhage, hemorrhoids, melena, stomatitis, mouth ulceration; **Rare:** cheilitis, cholecystitis, cholelithiasis, hematemesis, gastrointestinal hemorrhage, gum hemorrhage, hepatitis, ileitis, jaundice, intestinal obstruction, oral moniliasis, proctitis, increased salivation, soft stools, tongue discoloration.

Endocrine system—**Rare:** goiter, hyperthyroidism, hypothyroidism, thyroid nodule, thyroiditis.

Hemic and lymphatic system—**Frequent:** ecchymosis; **Infrequent:** anemia, leukocytosis, leukopenia, lymphadenopathy, thrombocythemia, thrombocytopenia; **Rare:** basophilia, bleeding time increased, cyanosis, eosinophilia, lymphocytosis, multiple myeloma, purpura.

Metabolic and nutritional—**Frequent:** edema, weight gain; **Infrequent:** alkaline phosphatase increased, glycosuria, hypercholesteremia, hyperglycemia, hyperuricemia, hypoglycemia, hypokalemia, SGOT increased, thirst; **Rare:** alcohol intolerance, bilirubinemia, BUN increased, creatinine increased, diabetes mellitus, dehydration, gout, healing abnormal, hemochromatosis, hypercalcinuria, hyperkalemia, hyperlipemia, hyperphosphatemia, hyponatremia, hypophosphatemia, hypoproteinemia, SGPT increased, uremia.

Musculoskeletal system—**Infrequent:** arthritis, arthrosis, bone pain, bone spurs, bursitis, leg cramps, myasthenia, tenosynovitis; **Rare:** pathological fracture, myopathy, osteoporosis, osteosclerosis, rheumatoid arthritis, tendon rupture.

Nervous system—**Frequent:** emotional lability, trismus, vertigo; **Infrequent:** apathy, ataxia, circumoral paresthesia, CNS stimulation, euphoria, hallucinations, hostility, hyperesthesia, hyperkinesia, hypotonia, incoordination, libido increased, manic reaction, myoclonus, neuralgia, neuropathy, paranoid reaction, psychosis, seizure, abnormal speech, stupor; **Rare:** akathisia, akinesia, alcohol abuse, aphasia, bradykinesia, buccoglossal syndrome, cerebrovascular accident, loss of consciousness, delusions, dementia, dystonia, facial paralysis, abnormal gait, Guillain-Barre Syndrome, hypokinesia, neuritis, nystagmus, paresis, psychotic depression, reflexes decreased, reflexes increased, suicidal ideation, torticollis.

Respiratory system—**Frequent:** bronchitis, dyspnea; **Infrequent:** asthma, chest congestion, epistaxis, hyperventilation, laryngismus, laryngitis, pneumonia, voice alteration; **Rare:** atelectasis, hemoptysis, hypoventilation, hypoxia, larynx edema, pleurisy, pulmonary embolus, sleep apnea.

Skin and appendages—**Infrequent:** acne, alopecia, brittle nails, contact dermatitis, dry skin, eczema, skin hypertrophy, maculopapular rash, psoriasis, urticaria; **Rare:** erythema nodosum, exfoliative dermatitis, lichenoid dermatitis, hair discoloration, skin discoloration, furunculosis, hirsutism, leukoderma, pustular rash, vesiculobullous rash, seborrhea, skin atrophy, skin striae.

Special senses—**Frequent:** abnormality of accommodation, abnormal vision; **Infrequent:** cataract, conjunctivitis, corneal lesion, diplopia, dry eyes, exophthalmos, eye pain, hyperacusis, otitis media, parosmia, photophobia, taste loss, visual field defect; **Rare:** blepharitis, chromatopsia, conjunctival edema, deafness, glaucoma, retinal hemorrhage, subconjunctival hemorrhage, keratitis, labyrinthitis, miosis, papilledema, decreased pupillary reflex, otitis externa, scleritis, uveitis.

Urogenital system—**Frequent:** metrorrhagia*, prostatitis*, vaginitis*; **Infrequent:** albuminuria, amenorrhea*, cystitis, dysuria, hematuria, female lactation*, leukorrhea*, menorrhagia*, nocturia, bladder pain, breast pain, polyuria, pyuria, urinary incontinence, urinary urgency, vaginal hemorrhage*; **Rare:** abortion*, anuria, breast discharge, breast engorgement, breast enlargement, endometriosis*, fibrocystic breast, calcium crystalluria, cervicitis*, ovarian cyst*, prolonged erection*, gynecomastia (male)*, hypomenorrhea*, kidney calculus, kidney pain, kidney function abnormal, mastitis, menopause*, pyelonephritis, oliguria, salpingitis*, urolithiasis, uterine hemorrhage*, uterine spasm.*

* Based on the number of men and women as appropriate.

Postmarketing Reports

Voluntary reports of other adverse events temporally associated with the use of venlafaxine that have been received since market introduction and that may have no causal relationship with the use of venlafaxine include the following: agranulocytosis, anaphylaxis, aplastic anemia, catatonia, congenital anomalies, CPK increased, deep vein thrombophlebitis, delirium, EKG abnormalities such as QT prolongation; cardiac arrhythmias including atrial fibrillation, supraventricular tachycardia, ventricular extrasystole, and rare reports of ventricular fibrillation and ventricular tachycardia, including torsade de pointes; epidermal necrosis/Stevens-Johnson Syndrome, erythema multiforme, extrapyramidal symptoms (including dyskinesia and tardive dyskinesia), hemorrhage (including eye and gastrointestinal bleeding), hepatic events (including GGT elevation; abnormalities of unspecified liver function tests; liver damage, necrosis, or failure; and fatty liver), involuntary movements, LDH increased, neuroleptic malignant syndrome-like events (including a case of a 10-year-old who may have been taking methylphenidate, was treated and recovered), neutropenia, night sweats, pancreatitis, pancytopenia, panic, prolactin increased, pulmonary eosinophilia, renal failure, rhabdomyolysis, serotonin syndrome, shock-like electrical sensations (in some cases, subsequent to the discontinuation of venlafaxine or tapering of dose), and syndrome of inappropriate antidiuretic hormone secretion (usually in the elderly).

There have been reports of elevated clozapine levels that were temporally associated with adverse events, including seizures, following the addition of venlafaxine. There have been reports of increases in prothrombin time, partial thromboplastin time, or INR when venlafaxine was given to patients receiving warfarin therapy.

DRUG ABUSE AND DEPENDENCE

Controlled Substance Class

Effexor (venlafaxine hydrochloride) is not a controlled substance.

Physical and Psychological Dependence

In vitro studies revealed that venlafaxine has virtually no affinity for opiate, benzodiazepine, phencyclidine (PCP), or N-methyl-D-aspartic acid (NMDA) receptors.

Venlafaxine was not found to have any significant CNS stimulant activity in rodents. In primate drug discrimination studies, venlafaxine showed no significant stimulant or depressant abuse liability.

Discontinuation effects have been reported in patients receiving venlafaxine (see **DOSAGE AND ADMINISTRATION**).

While Effexor has not been systematically studied in clinical trials for its potential for abuse, there was no indication of drug-seeking behavior in the clinical trials. However, it is not possible to predict on the basis of premarketing experience the extent to which a CNS active drug will be misused, diverted, and/or abused once marketed. Consequently, physicians should carefully evaluate patients for history of drug abuse and follow such patients closely, observing them for signs of misuse or abuse of Effexor (eg, development of tolerance, incrementation of dose, drug-seeking behavior).

OVERDOSAGE

Human Experience

There were 14 reports of acute overdose with Effexor (venlafaxine hydrochloride), either alone or in combination with other drugs and/or alcohol, among the patients included in the premarketing evaluation. The majority of the reports involved ingestions in which the total dose of Effexor taken was estimated to be no more than several-fold higher than the usual therapeutic dose. The 3 patients who took the highest doses were estimated to have ingested approximately 6.75 g, 2.75 g, and 2.5 g. The resultant peak plasma levels of venlafaxine for the latter 2 patients were 6.24 and 2.35 μg/mL, respectively, and the peak plasma levels of O-desmethylvenlafaxine were 3.37 and 1.30 μg/mL, respectively. Plasma venlafaxine levels were not obtained for the patient who ingested 6.75 g of venlafaxine. All 14 patients recovered without sequelae. Most patients reported no symptoms. Among the remaining patients, somnolence was the most commonly reported symptom. The patient who ingested 2.75 g of venlafaxine was observed to have 2 generalized convulsions and a prolongation of QTc to 500 msec, compared with 405 msec at baseline. Mild sinus tachycardia was reported in 2 of the other patients.

In postmarketing experience, overdose with venlafaxine has occurred predominantly in combination with alcohol and/or other drugs. Electrocardiogram changes (eg, prolongation of QT interval, bundle branch block, QRS prolongation), sinus and ventricular tachycardia, bradycardia, hypotension, altered level of consciousness (ranging from somnolence to coma), rhabdomyolysis, seizures, vertigo, and death have been reported.

Management of Overdosage

Treatment should consist of those general measures employed in the management of overdosage with any antidepressant.

Ensure an adequate airway, oxygenation, and ventilation. Monitor cardiac rhythm and vital signs. General supportive and symptomatic measures are also recommended. Induction of emesis is not recommended. Gastric lavage with a large-bore orogastric tube with appropriate airway protection, if needed, may be indicated if performed soon after ingestion or in symptomatic patients. Activated charcoal should be administered. Due to the large volume of distribution of this drug, forced diuresis, dialysis, hemoperfusion and exchange transfusion are unlikely to be of benefit. No specific antidotes for venlafaxine are known.

In managing overdosage, consider the possibility of multiple drug involvement. The physician should consider contacting a poison control center for additional information on the treatment of any overdose. Telephone numbers for certified poison control centers are listed in the *Physicians' Desk Reference (PDR)*.

DOSAGE AND ADMINISTRATION

Initial Treatment

The recommended starting dose for Effexor is 75 mg/day, administered in two or three divided doses, taken with food. Depending on tolerability and the need for further clinical effect, the dose may be increased to 150 mg/day. If needed, the dose should be further increased up to 225 mg/day. When increasing the dose, increments of up to 75 mg/day should be made at intervals of no less than 4 days. In outpatient settings there was no evidence of usefulness of doses greater than 225 mg/day for moderately depressed patients, but more severely depressed inpatients responded to a mean dose of 350 mg/day. Certain patients, including more severely depressed patients, may therefore respond more to higher doses, up to a maximum of 375 mg/day, generally in three divided doses (see **PRECAUTIONS, General,** *Use in Patients with Concomitant Illness*).

Dosage for Patients with Hepatic Impairment

Given the decrease in clearance and increase in elimination half-life for both venlafaxine and ODV that is observed in patients with hepatic cirrhosis compared to normal subjects (see **CLINICAL PHARMACOLOGY**), it is recommended that the total daily dose be reduced by 50% in patients with moderate hepatic impairment. Since there was much individual variability in clearance between patients with cirrhosis, it may be necessary to reduce the dose even more than 50%, and individualization of dosing may be desirable in some patients.

Dosage for Patients with Renal Impairment

Given the decrease in clearance for venlafaxine and the increase in elimination half-life for both venlafaxine and ODV that is observed in patients with renal impairment (GFR = 10 to 70 mL/min) compared to normals (see **CLINICAL PHARMACOLOGY**), it is recommended that the total daily dose be reduced by 25% in patients with mild to moderate renal impairment. It is recommended that the total daily dose be reduced by 50% and the dose be withheld until the dialysis treatment is completed (4 hrs) in patients undergoing hemodialysis. Since there was much individual variability in clearance between patients with renal impairment, individualization of dosing may be desirable in some patients.

Dosage for Elderly Patients

No dose adjustment is recommended for elderly patients on the basis of age. As with any antidepressant, however, caution should be exercised in treating the elderly. When individualizing the dosage, extra care should be taken when increasing the dose.

Maintenance Treatment

It is generally agreed that acute episodes of depression require several months or longer of sustained pharmacological therapy beyond response to the acute episode. In one study, in which patients responding during 8 weeks of acute treatment with Effexor XR were assigned randomly to placebo or to the same dose of Effexor XR (75, 150, or 225 mg/day, qAM) during 26 weeks of maintenance treatment as they had received during the acute stabilization phase, longer-term efficacy was demonstrated. A second longer-term study has demonstrated the efficacy of Effexor in maintaining an antidepressant response in patients with recurrent depression who had responded and continued to be improved during an initial 26 weeks of treatment and were then randomly assigned to placebo or Effexor for periods of up to 52 weeks on the same dose (100 to 200 mg/day, on a b.i.d. schedule) (see **CLINICAL TRIALS**). Based on these limited data, it is not known whether or not the dose of Effexor/Effexor XR needed for maintenance treatment is identical to the dose needed to achieve an initial response. Patients should be periodically reassessed to determine the need for maintenance treatment and the appropriate dose for such treatment.

Discontinuing Effexor (venlafaxine hydrochloride)

When discontinuing Effexor after more than 1 week of therapy, it is generally recommended that the dose be tapered to minimize the risk of discontinuation symptoms. Patients who have received Effexor for 6 weeks or more should have their dose tapered gradually over at least a 2-week period. Discontinuation symptoms have been systematically evaluated in patients taking venlafaxine, to include prospective analyses of clinical trials in Generalized Anxiety Disorder and retrospective surveys of trials in depression. Abrupt discontinuation or dose reduction of venlafaxine at various doses has been found to be associated with the appearance of new symptoms, the frequency of which increased with increased dose level and with longer duration of treatment. Reported symptoms include agitation, anorexia, anxiety, confusion, coordination impaired, diarrhea, dizziness, dry mouth, dysphoric mood, fasciculation, fatigue, headaches, hypomania, insomnia, nausea, nervousness, nightmares, seizures, sensory disturbances (including shock-like electrical sensations), somnolence, sweating, tinnitus, tremor, vertigo, and vomiting. It is therefore recommended that the dosage of Effexor be tapered gradually and the patient monitored. The period required for tapering may depend on the dose, duration of therapy and the individual patient. Discontinuation effects are well known to occur with antidepressants.

SWITCHING PATIENTS TO OR FROM A MONOAMINE OXIDASE INHIBITOR

At least 14 days should elapse between discontinuation of an MAOI and initiation of therapy with Effexor. In addition, at least 7 days should be allowed after stopping Effexor before starting an MAOI (see **CONTRAINDICATIONS** and **WARNINGS**).

HOW SUPPLIED

Effexor® (venlafaxine hydrochloride) Tablets are available as follows: 25 mg, peach, shield-shaped tablet with "25" and a "W" on one side and "701" on scored reverse side.

NDC 0008-0701-01, bottle of 100 tablets.

NDC 0008-0701-02, carton of 10 Redipak® blister strips of 10 tablets each.

37.5 mg, peach, shield-shaped tablet with "37.5" and a "W" on one side and "781" on scored reverse side.

NDC 0008-0781-01, bottle of 100 tablets.

NDC 0008-0781-02, carton of 10 Redipak® blister strips of 10 tablets each.

50 mg, peach, shield-shaped tablet with "50" and a "W" on one side and "703" on scored reverse side.

NDC 0008-0703-01, bottle of 100 tablets.

NDC 0008-0703-02, carton of 10 Redipak® blister strips of 10 tablets each.

75 mg, peach, shield-shaped tablet with "75" and a "W" on one side and "704" on scored reverse side.

NDC 0008-0704-01, bottle of 100 tablets.

NDC 0008-0704-02, carton of 10 Redipak® blister strips of 10 tablets each.

100 mg, peach, shield-shaped tablet with "100" and a "W" on one side and "705" on scored reverse side.

NDC 0008-0705-01, bottle of 100 tablets.

NDC 0008-0705-02, carton of 10 Redipak® blister strips of 10 tablets each.

The appearance of these tablets is a trademark of Wyeth Pharmaceuticals.

Store at controlled room temperature 20° to 25°C (68° to 77°F) in a dry place.

Dispense in a well-closed container as defined in the USP.

Wyeth®

Wyeth Pharmaceuticals Inc.

Continued on next page

TABLE 2
Treatment-Emergent Adverse Experience Incidence in a Dose Comparison Trial

Body System/ Preferred Term	Placebo (n=92)	Effexor (mg/day) 75 (n=89)	225 (n=89)	375 (n=88)
Body as a Whole				
Abdominal pain	3.3%	3.4%	2.2%	8.0%
Asthenia	3.3%	16.9%	14.6%	14.8%
Chills	1.1%	2.2%	5.6%	6.8%
Infection	2.2%	2.2%	5.6%	2.3%
Cardiovascular System				
Hypertension	1.1%	1.1%	2.2%	4.5%
Vasodilatation	0.0%	4.5%	5.6%	2.3%
Digestive System				
Anorexia	2.2%	14.6%	13.5%	17.0%
Dyspepsia	2.2%	6.7%	6.7%	4.5%
Nausea	14.1%	32.6%	38.2%	58.0%
Vomiting	1.1%	7.9%	3.4%	6.8%
Nervous System				
Agitation	0.0%	1.1%	2.2%	4.5%
Anxiety	4.3%	11.2%	4.5%	2.3%
Dizziness	4.3%	19.1%	22.5%	23.9%
Insomnia	9.8%	22.5%	20.2%	13.6%
Libido decreased	1.1%	2.2%	1.1%	5.7%
Nervousness	4.3%	21.3%	13.5%	12.5%
Somnolence	4.3%	16.9%	18.0%	26.1%
Tremor	0.0%	1.1%	2.2%	10.2%
Respiratory System				
Yawn	0.0%	4.5%	5.6%	8.0%
Skin and Appendages				
Sweating	5.4%	6.7%	12.4%	19.3%
Special Senses				
Abnormality of accommodation	0.0%	9.1%	7.9%	5.6%
Urogenital System				
Abnormal ejaculation/orgasm	0.0%	4.5%	2.2%	12.5%
Impotence	0.0%	5.8%	2.1%	3.6%
(Number of men)	(n=63)	(n=52)	(n=48)	(n=56)

Effexor—Cont.

Philadelphia, PA 19101

W10402C006
ET02
Rev 11/03

EFFEXOR® XR ℞

[ĕ-fĕks-ōr]

(venlafaxine hydrochloride)
Extended-Release Capsules
℞ only

Prescribing information for this product, which appears on pages 3418-3424 of the 2004 PDR, has been completely revised as follows. Please write "See Supplement A" next to the product heading.

DESCRIPTION

Effexor XR is an extended-release capsule for oral administration that contains venlafaxine hydrochloride, a structurally novel antidepressant. It is designated (R/S)-1-[2-(dimethylamino)-1-(4-methoxyphenyl)ethyl] cyclohexanol hydrochloride or (±)-1-[α-[(dimethylamino)methyl]-p-methoxybenzyl] cyclohexanol hydrochloride and has the empirical formula of $C_{17}H_{27}NO_2$ hydrochloride. Its molecular weight is 313.87. The structural formula is shown below.

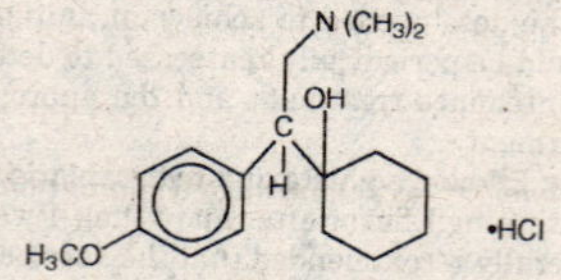

venlafaxine hydrochloride

Venlafaxine hydrochloride is a white to off-white crystalline solid with a solubility of 572 mg/mL in water (adjusted to ionic strength of 0.2 M with sodium chloride). Its octanol: water (0.2 M sodium chloride) partition coefficient is 0.43.

Effexor XR is formulated as an extended-release capsule for once-a-day oral administration. Drug release is controlled by diffusion through the coating membrane on the spheroids and is not pH dependent. Capsules contain venlafaxine hydrochloride equivalent to 37.5 mg, 75 mg, or 150 mg venlafaxine. Inactive ingredients consist of cellulose, ethylcellulose, gelatin, hypromellose, iron oxide, and titanium dioxide.

CLINICAL PHARMACOLOGY

Pharmacodynamics

The mechanism of the antidepressant action of venlafaxine in humans is believed to be associated with its potentiation of neurotransmitter activity in the CNS. Preclinical studies have shown that venlafaxine and its active metabolite, O-desmethylvenlafaxine (ODV), are potent inhibitors of neuronal serotonin and norepinephrine reuptake and weak inhibitors of dopamine reuptake. Venlafaxine and ODV have no significant affinity for muscarinic cholinergic, H_1-histaminergic, or α_1-adrenergic receptors in vitro. Pharmacologic activity at these receptors is hypothesized to be associated with the various anticholinergic, sedative, and cardiovascular effects seen with other psychotropic drugs. Venlafaxine and ODV do not possess monoamine oxidase (MAO) inhibitory activity.

Pharmacokinetics

Steady-state concentrations of venlafaxine and ODV in plasma are attained within 3 days of oral multiple dose therapy. Venlafaxine and ODV exhibited linear kinetics over the dose range of 75 to 450 mg/day. Mean±SD steady-state plasma clearance of venlafaxine and ODV is 1.3±0.6 and 0.4±0.2 L/h/kg, respectively; apparent elimination half-life is 5±2 and 11±2 hours, respectively; and apparent (steady-state) volume of distribution is 7.5±3.7 and 5.7±1.8 L/kg, respectively. Venlafaxine and ODV are minimally bound at therapeutic concentrations to plasma proteins (27% and 30%, respectively).

Absorption

Venlafaxine is well absorbed and extensively metabolized in the liver. O-desmethylvenlafaxine (ODV) is the only major active metabolite. On the basis of mass balance studies, at least 92% of a single oral dose of venlafaxine is absorbed. The absolute bioavailability of venlafaxine is about 45%.

Administration of Effexor XR (150 mg q24 hours) generally resulted in lower C_{max} (150 ng/mL for venlafaxine and 260 ng/mL for ODV) and later T_{max} (5.5 hours for venlafaxine and 9 hours for ODV) than for immediate release venlafaxine tablets (C_{max}'s for immediate release 75 mg q12 hours were 225 ng/mL for venlafaxine and 290 ng/mL for ODV; T_{max}'s were 2 hours for venlafaxine and 3 hours for ODV). When equal daily doses of venlafaxine were administered as either an immediate release tablet or the extended-release capsule, the exposure to both venlafaxine and ODV was similar for the two treatments, and the fluctuation in plasma concentrations was slightly lower with the Effexor XR capsule. Effexor XR, therefore, provides a slower rate of absorption, but the same extent of absorption compared with the immediate release tablet.

Food did not affect the bioavailability of venlafaxine or its active metabolite, ODV. Time of administration (AM vs PM) did not affect the pharmacokinetics of venlafaxine and ODV from the 75 mg Effexor XR capsule.

Metabolism and Excretion

Following absorption, venlafaxine undergoes extensive presystemic metabolism in the liver, primarily to ODV, but also to N-desmethylvenlafaxine, N,O-didesmethylvenlafaxine, and other minor metabolites. In vitro studies indicate that the formation of ODV is catalyzed by CYP2D6; this has been confirmed in a clinical study showing that patients with low CYP2D6 levels ("poor metabolizers") had increased levels of venlafaxine and reduced levels of ODV compared to people with normal CYP2D6 ("extensive metabolizers"). The differences between the CYP2D6 poor and extensive metabolizers, however, are not expected to be clinically important because the sum of venlafaxine and ODV is similar in the two groups and venlafaxine and ODV are pharmacologically approximately equiactive and equipotent.

Approximately 87% of a venlafaxine dose is recovered in the urine within 48 hours as unchanged venlafaxine (5%), unconjugated ODV (29%), conjugated ODV (26%), or other minor inactive metabolites (27%). Renal elimination of venlafaxine and its metabolites is thus the primary route of excretion.

Special Populations

Age and Gender: A population pharmacokinetic analysis of 404 venlafaxine-treated patients from two studies involving both b.i.d. and t.i.d. regimens showed that dose-normalized trough plasma levels of either venlafaxine or ODV were unaltered by age or gender differences. Dosage adjustment based on the age or gender of a patient is generally not necessary (see **DOSAGE AND ADMINISTRATION**).

Extensive/Poor Metabolizers: Plasma concentrations of venlafaxine were higher in CYP2D6 poor metabolizers than extensive metabolizers. Because the total exposure (AUC) of venlafaxine and ODV was similar in poor and extensive metabolizer groups, however, there is no need for different venlafaxine dosing regimens for these two groups.

Liver Disease: In 9 patients with hepatic cirrhosis, the pharmacokinetic disposition of both venlafaxine and ODV was significantly altered after oral administration of venlafaxine. Venlafaxine elimination half-life was prolonged by about 30%, and clearance decreased by about 50% in cirrhotic patients compared to normal subjects. ODV elimination half-life was prolonged by about 60%, and clearance decreased by about 30% in cirrhotic patients compared to normal subjects. A large degree of intersubject variability was noted. Three patients with more severe cirrhosis had a more substantial decrease in venlafaxine clearance (about 90%) compared to normal subjects. Dosage adjustment is necessary in these patients (see **DOSAGE AND ADMINISTRATION**).

Renal Disease: In a renal impairment study, venlafaxine elimination half-life after oral administration was prolonged by about 50% and clearance was reduced by about 24% in renally impaired patients (GFR=10 to 70 mL/min), compared to normal subjects. In dialysis patients, venlafaxine elimination half-life was prolonged by about 180% and clearance was reduced by about 57% compared to normal subjects. Similarly, ODV elimination half-life was prolonged by about 40% although clearance was unchanged in patients with renal impairment (GFR=10 to 70 mL/min) compared to normal subjects. In dialysis patients, ODV elimination half-life was prolonged by about 142% and clearance was reduced by about 56% compared to normal subjects. A large degree of intersubject variability was noted. Dosage adjustment is necessary in these patients (see **DOSAGE AND ADMINISTRATION**).

Clinical Trials

Major Depressive Disorder

The efficacy of Effexor XR (venlafaxine hydrochloride) extended-release capsules as a treatment for major depressive disorder was established in two placebo-controlled, short-term, flexible-dose studies in adult outpatients meeting DSM-III-R or DSM-IV criteria for major depressive disorder.

A 12-week study utilizing Effexor XR doses in a range 75 to 150 mg/day (mean dose for completers was 136 mg/day) and an 8-week study utilizing Effexor XR doses in a range 75 to 225 mg/day (mean dose for completers was 177 mg/day) both demonstrated superiority of Effexor XR over placebo on the HAM-D total score, HAM-D Depressed Mood Item, the MADRS total score, the Clinical Global Impressions (CGI) Severity of Illness item, and the CGI Global Improvement item. In both studies, Effexor XR was also significantly better than placebo for certain factors of the HAM-D, including the anxiety/somatization factor, the cognitive disturbance factor, and the retardation factor, as well as for the psychic anxiety score.

A 4-week study of inpatients meeting DSM-III-R criteria for major depressive disorder with melancholia utilizing Effexor (the immediate release form of venlafaxine) in a range of 150 to 375 mg/day (t.i.d. schedule) demonstrated superiority of Effexor over placebo. The mean dose in completers was 350 mg/day.

Examination of gender subsets of the population studied did not reveal any differential responsiveness on the basis of gender.

In one longer-term study, outpatients meeting DSM-IV criteria for major depressive disorder who had responded during an 8-week open trial on Effexor XR (75, 150, or 225 mg, qAM) were randomized to continuation of their same Effexor XR dose or to placebo, for up to 26 weeks of observation for relapse. Response during the open phase was defined as a CGI Severity of Illness item score of ≤3 and a HAM-D-21 total score of ≤10 at the day 56 evaluation. Relapse during the double-blind phase was defined as follows: (1) a reappearance of major depressive disorder as defined by DSM-IV criteria and a CGI Severity of Illness item score of ≥4 (moderately ill), (2) 2 consecutive CGI Severity of Illness item scores of ≥4, or (3) a final CGI Severity of Illness item score of ≥4 for any patient who withdrew from the study for any reason. Patients receiving continued Effexor XR treatment experienced significantly lower relapse rates over the subsequent 26 weeks compared with those receiving placebo.

In a second longer-term trial, outpatients meeting DSM-III-R criteria for major depressive disorder, recurrent type, who had responded (HAM-D-21 total score ≤12 at the day 56 evaluation) and continued to be improved [defined as the following criteria being met for days 56 through 180: (1) no HAM-D-21 total score ≥20; (2) no more than 2 HAM-D-21 total scores >10, and (3) no single CGI Severity of Illness item score ≥4(moderately ill)] during an initial 26 weeks of treatment on Effexor (100 to 200 mg/day, on a b.i.d. schedule) were randomized to continuation of their same Effexor dose or to placebo. The follow-up period to observe patients for relapse, defined as a CGI Severity of Illness item score ≥4, was for up to 52 weeks. Patients receiving continued Effexor treatment experienced significantly lower relapse rates over the subsequent 52 weeks compared with those receiving placebo.

Generalized Anxiety Disorder

The efficacy of Effexor XR capsules as a treatment for Generalized Anxiety Disorder (GAD) was established in two 8-week, placebo-controlled, fixed-dose studies, one 6-month, placebo-controlled, fixed-dose study, and one 6-month, placebo-controlled, flexible-dose study in outpatients meeting DSM-IV criteria for GAD.

One 8-week study evaluating Effexor XR doses of 75, 150, and 225 mg/day, and placebo showed that the 225 mg/day dose was more effective than placebo on the Hamilton Rating Scale for Anxiety (HAM-A) total score, both the HAM-A anxiety and tension items, and the Clinical Global Impressions (CGI) scale. While there was also evidence for superiority over placebo for the 75 and 150 mg/day doses, these doses were not as consistently effective as the highest dose.

A second 8-week study evaluating Effexor XR doses of 75 and 150 mg/day and placebo showed that both doses were more effective than placebo on some of these same outcomes; however, the 75 mg/day dose was more consistently effective than the 150 mg/day dose. A dose-response relationship for effectiveness in GAD was not clearly established in the 75 to 225 mg/day dose range utilized in these two studies.

Two 6-month studies, one evaluating Effexor XR doses of 37.5, 75, and 150 mg/day and the other evaluating Effexor XR doses of 75 to 225 mg/day, showed that daily doses of 75 mg or higher were more effective than placebo on the HAM-A total, both the HAM-A anxiety and tension items, and the CGI scale during 6 months of treatment. While there was also evidence for superiority over placebo for the 37.5 mg/day dose, this dose was not as consistently effective as the higher doses.

Examination of gender subsets of the population studied did not reveal any differential responsiveness on the basis of gender.

Social Anxiety Disorder (Social Phobia)

The efficacy of Effexor XR capsules as a treatment for Social Anxiety Disorder (also known as Social Phobia) was established in two double-blind, parallel group, 12-week, multicenter, placebo-controlled, flexible-dose studies in adult outpatients meeting DSM-IV criteria for Social Anxiety Disorder. Patients received doses in a range of 75 to 225 mg/day. Efficacy was assessed with the Liebowitz Social Anxiety Scale (LSAS). In these two trials, Effexor XR was significantly more effective than placebo on change from baseline to endpoint on the LSAS total score.

Examination of subsets of the population studied did not reveal any differential responsiveness on the basis of gender. There was insufficient information to determine the effect of age or race on outcome in these studies.

INDICATIONS AND USAGE

Major Depressive Disorder

Effexor XR (venlafaxine hydrochloride) extended-release capsules is indicated for the treatment of major depressive disorder.

The efficacy of Effexor XR in the treatment of major depressive disorder was established in 8- and 12-week controlled trials of outpatients whose diagnoses corresponded most closely to the DSM-III-R or DSM-IV category of major depressive disorder (see **Clinical Trials**).

A major depressive episode (DSM-IV) implies a prominent and relatively persistent (nearly every day for at least 2 weeks) depressed mood or the loss of interest or pleasure in nearly all activities, representing a change from previous functioning, and includes the presence of at least five of the following nine symptoms during the same two-week period: depressed mood, markedly diminished interest or pleasure in usual activities, significant change in weight and/or appetite, insomnia or hypersomnia, psychomotor agitation or retardation, increased fatigue, feelings of guilt or worthlessness, slowed thinking or impaired concentration, a suicide attempt or suicidal ideation.

The efficacy of Effexor (the immediate release form of venlafaxine) in the treatment of major depressive disorder in inpatients meeting diagnostic criteria for major depressive disorder with melancholia was established in a 4-week controlled trial (see **Clinical Trials**). The safety and efficacy of Effexor XR in hospitalized depressed patients have not been adequately studied.

The efficacy of Effexor XR in maintaining a response in major depressive disorder for up to 26 weeks following 8 weeks of acute treatment was demonstrated in a placebo-controlled trial. The efficacy of Effexor in maintaining a response in patients with recurrent major depressive disorder who had responded and continued to be improved during an initial 26 weeks of treatment and were then followed for a period of up to 52 weeks was demonstrated in a second placebo-controlled trial (see **Clinical Trials**). Nevertheless, the physician who elects to use Effexor/Effexor XR for extended periods should periodically re-evaluate the long-term usefulness of the drug for the individual patient (see **DOSAGE AND ADMINISTRATION**).

Generalized Anxiety Disorder

Effexor XR is indicated for the treatment of Generalized Anxiety Disorder (GAD) as defined in DSM-IV. Anxiety or tension associated with the stress of everyday life usually does not require treatment with an anxiolytic.

The efficacy of Effexor XR in the treatment of GAD was established in 8-week and 6-month placebo-controlled trials in outpatients diagnosed with GAD according to DSM-IV criteria (see **Clinical Trials**).

Generalized Anxiety Disorder (DSM-IV) is characterized by excessive anxiety and worry (apprehensive expectation) that is persistent for at least 6 months and which the person finds difficult to control. It must be associated with at least 3 of the following 6 symptoms: restlessness or feeling keyed up or on edge, being easily fatigued, difficulty concentrating or mind going blank, irritability, muscle tension, sleep disturbance.

Although the effectiveness of Effexor XR has been demonstrated in 6-month clinical trials in patients with GAD, the physician who elects to use Effexor XR for extended periods should periodically re-evaluate the long-term usefulness of the drug for the individual patient (see **DOSAGE AND ADMINISTRATION**).

Social Anxiety Disorder

Effexor XR is indicated for the treatment of Social Anxiety Disorder, also known as Social Phobia, as defined in DSM-IV (300.23).

Social Anxiety Disorder (DSM-IV) is characterized by a marked and persistent fear of 1 or more social or performance situations in which the person is exposed to unfamiliar people or to possible scrutiny by others. Exposure to the feared situation almost invariably provokes anxiety, which may approach the intensity of a panic attack. The feared situations are avoided or endured with intense anxiety or distress. The avoidance, anxious anticipation, or distress in the feared situation(s) interferes significantly with the person's normal routine, occupational or academic functioning, or social activities or relationships, or there is a marked distress about having the phobias. Lesser degrees of performance anxiety or shyness generally do not require psychopharmacological treatment.

The efficacy of Effexor XR in the treatment of Social Anxiety Disorder was established in two 12-week placebo-controlled trials in adult outpatients with Social Anxiety Disorder (DSM-IV). Effexor XR has not been studied in children or adolescents with Social Anxiety Disorder (see **Clinical Trials**).

The effectiveness of Effexor XR in the long-term treatment of Social Anxiety Disorder, ie, for more than 12 weeks, has not been systematically evaluated in adequate and well-controlled trials. Therefore, the physician who elects to use Effexor XR for extended periods should periodically re-evaluate the long-term usefulness of the drug for the individual patient (see **DOSAGE AND ADMINISTRATION**).

CONTRAINDICATIONS

Hypersensitivity to venlafaxine hydrochloride or to any excipients in the formulation.

Concomitant use in patients taking monoamine oxidase inhibitors (MAOIs) is contraindicated (see **WARNINGS**).

WARNINGS

Potential for Interaction with Monoamine Oxidase Inhibitors

Adverse reactions, some of which were serious, have been reported in patients who have recently been discontinued from a monoamine oxidase inhibitor (MAOI) and started on venlafaxine, or who have recently had venlafaxine therapy discontinued prior to initiation of an MAOI. These reactions have included tremor, myoclonus, diaphoresis, nausea, vomiting, flushing, dizziness, hyperthermia with features resembling neuroleptic malignant syndrome, seizures, and death. In patients receiving antidepressants with pharmacological properties similar to venlafaxine in combination with an MAOI, there have also been reports of serious, sometimes fatal, reactions. For a selective serotonin reuptake inhibitor, these reactions have included hyperthermia, rigidity, myoclonus, autonomic instability with possible rapid fluctuations of vital signs, and mental status changes that include extreme agitation progressing to delirium and coma. Some cases presented with features resembling neuroleptic malignant syndrome. Severe hyperthermia and seizures, sometimes fatal, have been reported in association with the combined use of tricyclic antidepressants and MAOIs. These reactions have also been reported in patients who have recently discontinued these drugs and have been started on an MAOI. The effects of combined use of venlafaxine and MAOIs have not been evaluated in humans or animals. Therefore, because venlafaxine is an inhibitor of both norepinephrine and serotonin reuptake, it is recommended that Effexor XR (venlafaxine hydrochloride) extended-release capsules not be used in combination with an MAOI, or within at least 14 days of discontinuing treatment with an MAOI. Based on the half-life of venlafaxine, at least 7 days should be allowed after stopping venlafaxine before starting an MAOI.

Sustained Hypertension

Venlafaxine treatment is associated with sustained increases in blood pressure in some patients. Among patients treated with 75 to 375 mg/day of Effexor XR in premarketing studies in patients with major depressive disorder, 3% (19/705) experienced sustained hypertension [defined as treatment-emergent supine diastolic blood pressure (SDBP) ≥ 90 mm Hg and ≥ 10 mm Hg above baseline for 3 consecutive on-therapy visits]. Among patients treated with 37.5 to 225 mg/day of Effexor XR in premarketing GAD studies, 0.5% (5/1011) experienced sustained hypertension. Among patients treated with 75 to 225 mg/day of Effexor XR in premarketing Social Anxiety Disorder studies, 1.4% (4/277) experienced sustained hypertension. Experience with the immediate-release venlafaxine showed that sustained hypertension was dose-related, increasing from 3% to 7% at 100 to 300 mg/day to 13% at doses above 300 mg/day. An insufficient number of patients received mean doses of Effexor XR over 300 mg/day to fully evaluate the incidence of sustained increases in blood pressure at these higher doses.

In placebo-controlled premarketing studies in patients with major depressive disorder with Effexor XR 75 to 225 mg/day, a final on-drug mean increase in supine diastolic blood pressure (SDBP) of 1.2 mm Hg was observed for Effexor XR-treated patients compared with a mean decrease of 0.2 mm Hg for placebo-treated patients. In placebo-controlled premarketing GAD studies with Effexor XR 37.5 to 225 mg/day, up to 8 weeks or up to 6 months, a final on-drug mean increase in SDBP of 0.3 mm Hg was observed for Effexor XR-treated patients compared with a mean decrease of 0.9 and 0.8 mm Hg, respectively, for placebo-treated patients. In placebo-controlled premarketing Social Anxiety Disorder studies with Effexor XR 75 to 225 mg/day up to 12 weeks, a final on-drug mean increase in SDBP of 1.6 mm Hg was observed for Effexor XR-treated patients compared with a mean decrease of 1.1 mm Hg for placebo-treated patients.

In premarketing major depressive disorder studies, 0.7% (5/705) of the Effexor XR-treated patients discontinued treatment because of elevated blood pressure. Among these patients, most of the blood pressure increases were in a modest range (12 to 16 mm Hg, SDBP). In premarketing GAD studies up to 8 weeks and up to 6 months, 0.7% (10/1381) and 1.3% (7/535) of the Effexor XR-treated patients, respectively, discontinued treatment because of elevated blood pressure. Among these patients, most of the blood pressure increases were in a modest range (12 to 25 mm Hg, SDBP up to 8 weeks; 8 to 28 mm Hg up to 6 months). In premarketing Social Anxiety Disorder studies up to 12 weeks, 0.4% (1/277) of the Effexor XR-treated patients discontinued treatment because of elevated blood pressure. In this patient, the blood pressure increase was modest (13 mm Hg, SDBP).

Sustained increases of SDBP could have adverse consequences. Therefore, it is recommended that patients receiving Effexor XR have regular monitoring of blood pressure. For patients who experience a sustained increase in blood pressure while receiving venlafaxine, either dose reduction or discontinuation should be considered.

PRECAUTIONS

General

Insomnia and Nervousness

Treatment-emergent insomnia and nervousness were more commonly reported for patients treated with Effexor XR (venlafaxine hydrochloride) extended-release capsules than with placebo in pooled analyses of short-term major depressive disorder, GAD, and Social Anxiety Disorder studies, as shown in Table 1.

Table 1
Incidence of Insomnia and Nervousness in Placebo-Controlled Major Depressive Disorder, GAD, and Social Anxiety Disorder Trials

	Major Depressive Disorder		GAD		Social Anxiety Disorder	
Symptom	Effexor XR n = 357	Placebo n = 285	Effexor XR n = 1381	Placebo n = 555	Effexor XR n = 277	Placebo n = 274
Insomnia	17%	11%	15%	10%	23%	7%
Nervousness	10%	5%	6%	4%	11%	3%

[See table 1 above]

Insomnia and nervousness each led to drug discontinuation in 0.9% of the patients treated with Effexor XR in major depressive disorder studies.

In GAD trials, insomnia and nervousness led to drug discontinuation in 3% and 2%, respectively, of the patients treated with Effexor XR up to 8 weeks and 2% and 0.7%, respectively, of the patients treated with Effexor XR up to 6 months.

In Social Anxiety Disorder trials, insomnia and nervousness led to drug discontinuation in 3% and 0%, respectively, of the patients treated with Effexor XR up to 12 weeks.

Changes in Appetite and Weight

Treatment-emergent anorexia was more commonly reported for Effexor XR-treated (8%) than placebo-treated patients (4%) in the pool of short-term studies in major depressive disorder. Significant weight loss, especially in underweight depressed patients, may be an undesirable result of Effexor XR treatment. A loss of 5% or more of body weight occurred in 7% of Effexor XR-treated and 2% of placebo-treated patients in placebo-controlled major depressive disorder trials. Discontinuation rates for anorexia and weight loss associated with Effexor XR were low (1.0% and 0.1%, respectively, of Effexor XR-treated patients in major depressive disorder studies).

In the pool of GAD studies, treatment-emergent anorexia was reported in 8% and 2% of patients receiving Effexor XR and placebo up to 8 weeks, respectively. A loss of 7% or more of body weight occurred in 3% of the Effexor XR-treated and 1% of the placebo-treated patients up to 6 months in these trials. Discontinuation rates for anorexia and weight loss were low for patients receiving Effexor XR up to 8 weeks (0.9% and 0.3%, respectively).

In the pool of Social Anxiety Disorder studies, treatment-emergent anorexia was reported in 20% and 2% of patients receiving Effexor XR and placebo up to 12 weeks, respectively. A loss of 7% or more of body weight occurred in none of the Effexor XR-treated or the placebo-treated patients up to 12 weeks in these trials. Discontinuation rates for anorexia and weight loss were low for patients receiving Effexor XR up to 12 weeks (0.4% and 0.0%, respectively).

The safety and efficacy of venlafaxine therapy in combination with weight loss agents, including phentermine, have not been established. Co-administration of Effexor XR and weight loss agents is not recommended. Effexor XR is not indicated for weight loss alone or in combination with other products.

Activation of Mania/Hypomania

During premarketing major depressive disorder studies, mania or hypomania occurred in 0.3% of Effexor XR-treated patients and 0.0% placebo patients. In premarketing GAD studies, 0.0% of Effexor XR-treated patients and 0.2% of placebo-treated patients experienced mania or hypomania. In premarketing Social Anxiety Disorder studies, no Effexor XR-treated patients and no placebo-treated patients experienced mania or hypomania. In all premarketing major depressive disorder trials with Effexor, mania or hypomania occurred in 0.5% of venlafaxine-treated patients compared with 0% of placebo patients. Mania/hypomania has also been reported in a small proportion of patients with mood disorders who were treated with other marketed drugs to treat major depressive disorder. As with all drugs effective in the treatment of major depressive disorder, Effexor XR should be used cautiously in patients with a history of mania.

Hyponatremia

Hyponatremia and/or the syndrome of inappropriate antidiuretic hormone secretion (SIADH) may occur with venlafaxine. This should be taken into consideration in patients who are, for example, volume-depleted, elderly, or taking diuretics.

Mydriasis

Mydriasis has been reported in association with venlafaxine; therefore patients with raised intraocular pressure or those at risk of acute narrow-angle glaucoma should be monitored.

Seizures

During premarketing experience, no seizures occurred among 705 Effexor XR-treated patients in the major depressive disorder studies, among 1381 Effexor XR-treated patients in GAD studies, or among 277 Effexor XR-treated patients in Social Anxiety Disorder studies. In all premarketing major depressive disorder trials with Effexor, seizures were reported at various doses in 0.3% (8/3082) of venlafaxine-treated patients. Effexor XR, like many antidepressants, should be used cautiously in patients with a history of seizures and should be discontinued in any patient who develops seizures.

Abnormal Bleeding

There have been reports of abnormal bleeding (most commonly ecchymosis) associated with venlafaxine treatment. While a causal relationship to venlafaxine is unclear, impaired platelet aggregation may result from platelet serotonin depletion and contribute to such occurrences.

Serum Cholesterol Elevation

Clinically relevant increases in serum cholesterol were recorded in 5.3% of venlafaxine-treated patients and 0.0% of placebo-treated patients treated for at least 3 months in placebo-controlled trials (see **ADVERSE REACTIONS-Laboratory Changes**). Measurement of serum cholesterol levels should be considered during long-term treatment.

Suicide

The possibility of a suicide attempt is inherent in major depressive disorder and may persist until significant remission occurs. Close supervision of high-risk patients should accompany initial drug therapy. Prescriptions for Effexor XR should be written for the smallest quantity of capsules consistent with good patient management in order to reduce the risk of overdose.

The same precautions observed when treating patients with major depressive disorder should be observed when treating patients with GAD or Social Anxiety Disorder.

Continued on next page

Effexor XR—Cont.

Use in Patients With Concomitant Illness

Premarketing experience with venlafaxine in patients with concomitant systemic illness is limited. Caution is advised in administering Effexor XR to patients with diseases or conditions that could affect hemodynamic responses or metabolism.

Venlafaxine has not been evaluated or used to any appreciable extent in patients with a recent history of myocardial infarction or unstable heart disease. Patients with these diagnoses were systematically excluded from many clinical studies during venlafaxine's premarketing testing. The electrocardiograms were analyzed for 275 patients who received Effexor XR and 220 patients who received placebo in 8- to 12-week double-blind, placebo-controlled trials in major depressive disorder, for 610 patients who received Effexor XR and 298 patients who received placebo in 8-week double-blind, placebo-controlled trials in GAD, and for 195 patients who received Effexor XR and 228 patients who received placebo in 12-week double-blind, placebo-controlled trials in Social Anxiety Disorder. The mean change from baseline in corrected QT interval (QTc) for Effexor XR-treated patients in major depressive disorder studies was increased relative to that for placebo-treated patients (increase of 4.7 msec for Effexor XR and decrease of 1.9 msec for placebo). The mean change from baseline in corrected QT interval (QTc) for Effexor XR-treated patients in the GAD studies did not differ significantly from that with placebo. The mean change from baseline in QTc for Effexor XR-treated patients in the Social Anxiety Disorder studies was increased relative to that for placebo-treated patients (increase of 2.8 msec for Effexor XR and decrease of 2.0 msec for placebo).

In these same trials, the mean change from baseline in heart rate for Effexor XR-treated patients in the major depressive disorder studies was significantly higher than that for placebo (a mean increase of 4 beats per minute for Effexor XR and 1 beat per minute for placebo). The mean change from baseline in heart rate for Effexor XR-treated patients in the GAD studies was significantly higher than that for placebo (a mean increase of 3 beats per minute for Effexor XR and no change for placebo). The mean change from baseline in heart rate for Effexor XR-treated patients in the Social Anxiety Disorder studies was significantly higher than that for placebo (a mean increase of 5 beats per minute for Effexor XR and no change for placebo).

In a flexible-dose study, with Effexor doses in the range of 200 to 375 mg/day and mean dose greater than 300 mg/day, Effexor-treated patients had a mean increase in heart rate of 8.5 beats per minute compared with 1.7 beats per minute in the placebo group.

As increases in heart rate were observed, caution should be exercised in patients whose underlying medical conditions might be compromised by increases in heart rate (eg, patients with hyperthyroidism, heart failure, or recent myocardial infarction), particularly when using doses of Effexor above 200 mg/day.

Evaluation of the electrocardiograms for 769 patients who received immediate release Effexor in 4- to 6-week double-blind, placebo-controlled trials showed that the incidence of trial-emergent conduction abnormalities did not differ from that with placebo.

In patients with renal impairment (GFR = 10 to 70 mL/min) or cirrhosis of the liver, the clearances of venlafaxine and its active metabolites were decreased, thus prolonging the elimination half-lives of these substances. A lower dose may be necessary (see **DOSAGE AND ADMINISTRATION**). Effexor XR, like all drugs effective in the treatment of major depressive disorder, should be used with caution in such patients.

Information for Patients

Physicians are advised to discuss the following issues with patients for whom they prescribe Effexor XR (venlafaxine hydrochloride) extended-release capsules:

Interference with Cognitive and Motor Performance

Clinical studies were performed to examine the effects of venlafaxine on behavioral performance of healthy individuals. The results revealed no clinically significant impairment of psychomotor, cognitive, or complex behavior performance. However, since any psychoactive drug may impair judgment, thinking, or motor skills, patients should be cautioned about operating hazardous machinery, including automobiles, until they are reasonably certain that venlafaxine therapy does not adversely affect their ability to engage in such activities.

Concomitant Medication

Patients should be advised to inform their physicians if they are taking, or plan to take, any prescription or over-the-counter drugs, including herbal preparations, since there is a potential for interactions.

Alcohol

Although venlafaxine has not been shown to increase the impairment of mental and motor skills caused by alcohol, patients should be advised to avoid alcohol while taking venlafaxine.

Allergic Reactions

Patients should be advised to notify their physician if they develop a rash, hives, or a related allergic phenomenon.

Pregnancy

Patients should be advised to notify their physician if they become pregnant or intend to become pregnant during therapy.

Nursing

Patients should be advised to notify their physician if they are breast-feeding an infant.

Laboratory Tests

There are no specific laboratory tests recommended.

Drug Interactions

As with all drugs, the potential for interaction by a variety of mechanisms is a possibility.

Alcohol

A single dose of ethanol (0.5 g/kg) had no effect on the pharmacokinetics of venlafaxine or O-desmethylvenlafaxine (ODV) when venlafaxine was administered at 150 mg/day in 15 healthy male subjects. Additionally, administration of venlafaxine in a stable regimen did not exaggerate the psychomotor and psychometric effects induced by ethanol in these same subjects when they were not receiving venlafaxine.

Cimetidine

Concomitant administration of cimetidine and venlafaxine in a steady-state study for both drugs resulted in inhibition of first-pass metabolism of venlafaxine in 18 healthy subjects. The oral clearance of venlafaxine was reduced by about 43%, and the exposure (AUC) and maximum concentration (C_{max}) of the drug were increased by about 60%. However, coadministration of cimetidine had no apparent effect on the pharmacokinetics of ODV, which is present in much greater quantity in the circulation than venlafaxine. The overall pharmacological activity of venlafaxine plus ODV is expected to increase only slightly, and no dosage adjustment should be necessary for most normal adults. However, for patients with pre-existing hypertension, and for elderly patients or patients with hepatic dysfunction, the interaction associated with the concomitant use of venlafaxine and cimetidine is not known and potentially could be more pronounced. Therefore, caution is advised with such patients.

Diazepam

Under steady-state conditions for venlafaxine administered at 150 mg/day, a single 10 mg dose of diazepam did not appear to affect the pharmacokinetics of either venlafaxine or ODV in 18 healthy male subjects. Venlafaxine also did not have any effect on the pharmacokinetics of diazepam or its active metabolite, desmethyldiazepam, or affect the psychomotor and psychometric effects induced by diazepam.

Haloperidol

Venlafaxine administered under steady-state conditions at 150 mg/day in 24 healthy subjects decreased total oral-dose clearance (Cl/F) of a single 2 mg dose of haloperidol by 42%, which resulted in a 70% increase in haloperidol AUC. In addition, the haloperidol C_{max} increased 88% when coadministered with venlafaxine, but the haloperidol elimination half-life ($t_{1/2}$) was unchanged. The mechanism explaining this finding is unknown.

Lithium

The steady-state pharmacokinetics of venlafaxine administered at 150 mg/day were not affected when a single 600 mg oral dose of lithium was administered to 12 healthy male subjects. ODV also was unaffected. Venlafaxine had no effect on the pharmacokinetics of lithium (see also *CNS-Active Drugs*, below).

Drugs Highly Bound to Plasma Proteins

Venlafaxine is not highly bound to plasma proteins; therefore, administration of Effexor XR to a patient taking another drug that is highly protein bound should not cause increased free concentrations of the other drug.

Drugs that Inhibit Cytochrome P450 Isoenzymes

CYP2D6 Inhibitors: In vitro and in vivo studies indicate that venlafaxine is metabolized to its active metabolite, ODV, by CYP2D6, the isoenzyme that is responsible for the genetic polymorphism seen in the metabolism of many antidepressants. Therefore, the potential exists for a drug interaction between drugs that inhibit CYP2D6-mediated metabolism of venlafaxine, reducing the metabolism of venlafaxine to ODV, resulting in increased plasma concentrations of venlafaxine and decreased concentrations of the active metabolite. CYP2D6 inhibitors such as quinidine would be expected to do this, but the effect would be similar to what is seen in patients who are genetically CYP2D6 poor metabolizers (see *Metabolism and Excretion* under **CLINICAL PHARMACOLOGY**). Therefore, no dosage adjustment is required when venlafaxine is coadministered with a CYP2D6 inhibitor.

The concomitant use of venlafaxine with drug treatment(s) that potentially inhibits both CYP2D6 and CYP3A4, the primary metabolizing enzymes for venlafaxine, has not been studied.

Therefore, caution is advised should a patient's therapy include venlafaxine and any agent(s) that produce simultaneous inhibition of these two enzyme systems.

Drugs Metabolized by Cytochrome P450 Isoenzymes

CYP2D6: In vitro studies indicate that venlafaxine is a relatively weak inhibitor of CYP2D6. These findings have been confirmed in a clinical drug interaction study comparing the effect of venlafaxine with that of fluoxetine on the CYP2D6-mediated metabolism of dextromethorphan to dextrorphan.

Imipramine—Venlafaxine did not affect the pharmacokinetics of imipramine and 2-OH-imipramine. However, desipramine AUC, C_{max}, and C_{min} increased by about 35% in the presence of venlafaxine. The 2-OH-desipramine AUC's increased by at least 2.5 fold (with venlafaxine 37.5 mg q12h) and by 4.5 fold (with venlafaxine 75 mg q12h). Imipramine did not affect the pharmacokinetics of venlafaxine and ODV. The clinical significance of elevated 2-OH-desipramine levels is unknown.

Risperidone—Venlafaxine administered under steady-state conditions at 150 mg/day slightly inhibited the CYP2D6-mediated metabolism of risperidone (administered as a single 1 mg oral dose) to its active metabolite, 9-hydroxyrisperidone, resulting in an approximate 32% increase in risperidone AUC. However, venlafaxine coadministration did not significantly alter the pharmacokinetic profile of the total active moiety (risperidone plus 9-hydroxyrisperidone).

CYP3A4: Venlafaxine did not inhibit CYP3A4 in vitro. This finding was confirmed in vivo by clinical drug interaction studies in which venlafaxine did not inhibit the metabolism of several CYP3A4 substrates, including alprazolam, diazepam, and terfenadine.

Indinavir—In a study of 9 healthy volunteers, venlafaxine administered under steady-state conditions at 150 mg/day resulted in a 28% decrease in the AUC of a single 800 mg oral dose of indinavir and a 36% decrease in indinavir C_{max}. Indinavir did not affect the pharmacokinetics of venlafaxine and ODV. The clinical significance of this finding is unknown.

CYP1A2: Venlafaxine did not inhibit CYP1A2 in vitro. This finding was confirmed in vivo by a clinical drug interaction study in which venlafaxine did not inhibit the metabolism of caffeine, a CYP1A2 substrate.

CYP2C9: Venlafaxine did not inhibit CYP2C9 in vitro. The clinical significance of this finding is unknown.

CYP2C19: Venlafaxine did not inhibit the metabolism of diazepam, which is partially metabolized by CYP2C19 (see *Diazepam* above).

Monoamine Oxidase Inhibitors

See **CONTRAINDICATIONS** and **WARNINGS**.

CNS-Active Drugs

The risk of using venlafaxine in combination with other CNS-active drugs has not been systematically evaluated (except in the case of those CNS-active drugs noted above). Consequently, caution is advised if the concomitant administration of venlafaxine and such drugs is required. Based on the mechanism of action of venlafaxine and the potential for serotonin syndrome, caution is advised when venlafaxine is co-administered with other drugs that may affect the serotonergic neurotransmitter systems, such as triptans, serotonin reuptake inhibitors (SRIs), or lithium.

Electroconvulsive Therapy

There are no clinical data establishing the benefit of electroconvulsive therapy combined with Effexor XR (venlafaxine hydrochloride) extended-release capsules treatment.

Postmarketing Spontaneous Drug Interaction Reports

See **ADVERSE REACTIONS**, **Postmarketing Reports**.

Carcinogenesis, Mutagenesis, Impairment of Fertility

Carcinogenesis

Venlafaxine was given by oral gavage to mice for 18 months at doses up to 120 mg/kg per day, which was 1.7 times the maximum recommended human dose on a mg/m^2 basis. Venlafaxine was also given to rats by oral gavage for 24 months at doses up to 120 mg/kg per day. In rats receiving the 120 mg/kg dose, plasma concentrations of venlafaxine at necropsy were 1 times (male rats) and 6 times (female rats) the plasma concentrations of patients receiving the maximum recommended human dose. Plasma levels of the O-desmethyl metabolite were lower in rats than in patients receiving the maximum recommended dose. Tumors were not increased by venlafaxine treatment in mice or rats.

Mutagenesis

Venlafaxine and the major human metabolite, O-desmethylvenlafaxine (ODV), were not mutagenic in the Ames reverse mutation assay in Salmonella bacteria or the Chinese hamster ovary/HGPRT mammalian cell forward gene mutation assay. Venlafaxine was also not mutagenic or clastogenic in the in vitro BALB/c-3T3 mouse cell transformation assay, the sister chromatid exchange assay in cultured Chinese hamster ovary cells, or in the in vivo chromosomal aberration assay in rat bone marrow. ODV was not clastogenic in the in vitro Chinese hamster ovary cell chromosomal aberration assay, but elicited a clastogenic response in the in vivo chromosomal aberration assay in rat bone marrow.

Impairment of Fertility

Reproduction and fertility studies in rats showed no effects on male or female fertility at oral doses of up to 2 times the maximum recommended human dose on a mg/m^2 basis.

Pregnancy

Teratogenic Effects - Pregnancy Category C

Venlafaxine did not cause malformations in offspring of rats or rabbits given doses up to 2.5 times (rat) or 4 times (rabbit) the maximum recommended human daily dose on a mg/m^2 basis. However, in rats, there was a decrease in pup weight, an increase in stillborn pups, and an increase in pup deaths during the first 5 days of lactation, when dosing began during pregnancy and continued until weaning. The cause of these deaths is not known. These effects occurred at 2.5 times (mg/m^2) the maximum human daily dose. The no effect dose for rat pup mortality was 0.25 times the human dose on a mg/m^2 basis. There are no adequate and well-controlled studies in pregnant women. Because animal reproduction studies are not always predictive of human response, this drug should be used during pregnancy only if clearly needed.

Table 2
Common Adverse Events Leading to Discontinuation of Treatment in Placebo-Controlled Trials[1]

Adverse Event	Percentage of Patients Discontinuing Due to Adverse Event: Major Depressive Disorder Indication[2]		GAD Indication[3,4]		Social Anxiety Disorder Indication	
	Effexor XR n=357	Placebo n=285	Effexor XR n=1381	Placebo n=555	Effexor XR n=277	Placebo n=274
Body as a Whole						
Asthenia	—	—	3%	<1%	1%	<1%
Headache	—	—	—	—	2%	<1%
Digestive System						
Nausea	4%	<1%	8%	<1%	4%	0%
Anorexia	1%	<1%	—	—	—	—
Dry Mouth	1%	0%	2%	<1%	—	—
Vomiting	—	—	1%	<1%	—	—
Nervous System						
Dizziness	2%	1%	—	—	2%	0%
Insomnia	1%	<1%	3%	<1%	3%	<1%
Somnolence	2%	<1%	3%	<1%	2%	<1%
Nervousness	—	—	2%	<1%	—	—
Tremor	—	—	1%	0%	—	—
Anxiety	—	—	—	—	1%	<1%
Skin						
Sweating	—	—	2%	<1%	1%	0%
Urogenital System						
Impotence[5]	—	—	—	—	3%	0%

[1]Two of the major depressive disorder studies were flexible dose and one was fixed dose. Four of the GAD studies were fixed dose and one was flexible dose. Both of the Social Anxiety Disorder studies were flexible dose.
[2]In U.S. placebo-controlled trials for major depressive disorder, the following were also common events leading to discontinuation and were considered to be drug-related for Effexor XR-treated patients (% Effexor XR [n = 192], % Placebo [n = 202]): hypertension (1%, <1%); diarrhea (1%, 0%); paresthesia (1%, 0%); tremor (1%, 0%); abnormal vision, mostly blurred vision (1%, 0%); and abnormal, mostly delayed, ejaculation (1%, 0%).
[3]In two short-term U.S. placebo-controlled trials for GAD, the following were also common events leading to discontinuation and were considered to be drug-related for Effexor XR-treated patients (% Effexor XR [n = 476]), % Placebo [n = 201]): headache (4%, <1%); vasodilatation (1%, 0%); anorexia (2%, <1%); dizziness (4%, 1%); thinking abnormal (1%, 0%); and abnormal vision (1%, 0%).
[4]In long-term placebo-controlled trials for GAD, the following was also a common event leading to discontinuation and was considered to be drug-related for Effexor XR-treated patients (% Effexor XR [n = 535], % Placebo [n = 257]): decreased libido (1%, 0%).
[5]Incidence is based on the number of men (Effexor XR = 158, placebo = 153).

Non-teratogenic Effects
If venlafaxine is used until or shortly before birth, discontinuation effects in the newborn should be considered.

Labor and Delivery
The effect of venlafaxine on labor and delivery in humans is unknown.

Nursing Mothers
Venlafaxine and ODV have been reported to be excreted in human milk. Because of the potential for serious adverse reactions in nursing infants from Effexor XR, a decision should be made whether to discontinue nursing or to discontinue the drug, taking into account the importance of the drug to the mother.

Pediatric Use
Safety and effectiveness in pediatric patients have not been established.
In pediatric clinical trials, there were increased reports of hostility and, especially in Major Depressive Disorder, suicide-related adverse events such as suicidal ideation and self-harm.

Geriatric Use
Approximately 4% (14/357), 6% (77/1381), and 2% (6/277) of Effexor XR-treated patients in placebo-controlled premarketing major depressive disorder, GAD, and Social Anxiety Disorder trials, respectively, were 65 years of age or over. Of 2,897 Effexor-treated patients in premarketing phase major depressive disorder studies, 12% (357) were 65 years of age or over. No overall differences in effectiveness or safety were observed between geriatric patients and younger patients, and other reported clinical experience generally has not identified differences in response between the elderly and younger patients. However, greater sensitivity of some older individuals cannot be ruled out. As with other antidepressants, several cases of hyponatremia and syndrome of inappropriate antidiuretic hormone secretion (SIADH) have been reported, usually in the elderly.
The pharmacokinetics of venlafaxine and ODV are not substantially altered in the elderly (see **CLINICAL PHARMACOLOGY**). No dose adjustment is recommended for the elderly on the basis of age alone, although other clinical circumstances, some of which may be more common in the elderly, such as renal or hepatic impairment, may warrant a dose reduction (see **DOSAGE AND ADMINISTRATION**).

ADVERSE REACTIONS
The information included in the **Adverse Findings Observed in Short-Term, Placebo-Controlled Studies with Effexor XR** subsection is based on data from a pool of three 8- and 12-week controlled clinical trials in major depressive disorder (includes two U.S. trials and one European trial), on data up to 8 weeks from a pool of five controlled clinical trials in GAD with Effexor XR®, and on data up to 12 weeks from a pool of two controlled clinical trials in Social Anxiety Disorder. Information on additional adverse events associated with Effexor XR in the entire development program for the formulation and with Effexor (the immediate release formulation of venlafaxine) is included in the **Other Adverse Events Observed During the Premarketing Evaluation of Effexor and Effexor XR** subsection (see also **WARNINGS** and **PRECAUTIONS**).

Adverse Findings Observed in Short-Term, Placebo-Controlled Studies with Effexor XR
Adverse Events Associated with Discontinuation of Treatment
Approximately 11% of the 357 patients who received Effexor® XR (venlafaxine hydrochloride) extended-release capsules in placebo-controlled clinical trials for major depressive disorder discontinued treatment due to an adverse experience, compared with 6% of the 285 placebo-treated patients in those studies. Approximately 18% of the 1381 patients who received Effexor XR capsules in placebo-controlled clinical trials for GAD discontinued treatment due to an adverse experience, compared with 12% of the 555 placebo-treated patients in those studies. Approximately 17% of the 277 patients who received Effexor XR capsules in placebo-controlled clinical trials for Social Anxiety Disorder discontinued treatment due to an adverse experience, compared with 5% of the 274 placebo-treated patients in those studies. The most common events leading to discontinuation and considered to be drug-related (ie, leading to discontinuation in at least 1% of the Effexor XR-treated patients at a rate at least twice that of placebo for either indication) are shown in Table 2.
[See table 2 above]
Adverse Events Occurring at an Incidence of 2% or More Among Effexor XR-Treated Patients
Tables 3, 4, and 5 enumerate the incidence, rounded to the nearest percent, of treatment-emergent adverse events that occurred during acute therapy of major depressive disorder (up to 12 weeks; dose range of 75 to 225 mg/day), of GAD (up to 8 weeks; dose range of 37.5 to 225 mg/day), and of Social Anxiety Disorder (up to 12 weeks; dose range of 75 to 225 mg/day), respectively, in 2% or more of patients treated with Effexor XR (venlafaxine hydrochloride) where the incidence in patients treated with Effexor XR was greater than the incidence for the respective placebo-treated patients. The table shows the percentage of patients in each group who had at least one episode of an event at some time during their treatment. Reported adverse events were classified using a standard COSTART-based Dictionary terminology. The prescriber should be aware that these figures cannot be used to predict the incidence of side effects in the course of usual medical practice where patient characteristics and other factors differ from those which prevailed in the clinical trials. Similarly, the cited frequencies cannot be compared with figures obtained from other clinical investigations involving different treatments, uses and investigators. The cited figures, however, do provide the prescribing physician with some basis for estimating the relative contribution of drug and nondrug factors to the side effect incidence rate in the population studied.
Commonly Observed Adverse Events from Tables 3, 4, and 5:
Major Depressive Disorder
Note in particular the following adverse events that occurred in at least 5% of the Effexor XR patients and at a rate at least twice that of the placebo group for all placebo-controlled trials for the major depressive disorder (Table 3): Abnormal ejaculation, gastrointestinal complaints (nausea, dry mouth, and anorexia), CNS complaints (dizziness, somnolence, and abnormal dreams), and sweating. In the two U.S. placebo-controlled trials, the following additional events occurred in at least 5% of Effexor XR-treated patients (n = 192) and at a rate at least twice that of the placebo group: Abnormalities of sexual function (impotence in men, anorgasmia in women, and libido decreased), gastrointestinal complaints (constipation and flatulence), CNS complaints (insomnia, nervousness, and tremor), problems of special senses (abnormal vision), cardiovascular effects (hypertension and vasodilatation), and yawning.

Generalized Anxiety Disorder
Note in particular the following adverse events that occurred in at least 5% of the Effexor XR patients and at a rate at least twice that of the placebo group for all placebo-controlled trials for the GAD indication (Table 4): Abnormalities of sexual function (abnormal ejaculation and impotence), gastrointestinal complaints (nausea, dry mouth, anorexia, and constipation), problems of special senses (abnormal vision), and sweating.
Social Anxiety Disorder
Note in particular the following adverse events that occurred in at least 5% of the Effexor XR patients and at a rate at least twice that of the placebo group for the 2 placebo-controlled trials for the Social Anxiety Disorder indication (Table 5): Asthenia, gastrointestinal complaints (anorexia, dry mouth, nausea), CNS complaints (anxiety, insomnia, libido decreased, nervousness, somnolence, dizziness), abnormalities of sexual function (abnormal ejaculation, orgasmic dysfunction, impotence), yawn, sweating, and abnormal vision.

Table 3
Treatment-Emergent Adverse Event Incidence in Short-Term Placebo-Controlled Effexor XR Clinical Trials in Patients with Major Depressive Disorder[1,2]

Body System Preferred Term	% Reporting Event: Effexor XR (n=357)	Placebo (n=285)
Body as a Whole		
Asthenia	8%	7%
Cardiovascular System		
Vasodilatation[3]	4%	2%
Hypertension	4%	1%
Digestive System		
Nausea	31%	12%
Constipation	8%	5%
Anorexia	8%	4%
Vomiting	4%	2%
Flatulence	4%	3%
Metabolic/Nutritional		
Weight Loss	3%	0%
Nervous System		
Dizziness	20%	9%
Somnolence	17%	8%
Insomnia	17%	11%
Dry Mouth	12%	6%
Nervousness	10%	5%
Abnormal Dreams[4]	7%	2%
Tremor	5%	2%
Depression	3%	<1%
Paresthesia	3%	1%
Libido Decreased	3%	<1%
Agitation	3%	1%
Respiratory System		
Pharyngitis	7%	6%
Yawn	3%	0%
Skin		
Sweating	14%	3%
Special Senses		
Abnormal Vision[5]	4%	<1%
Urogenital System		
Abnormal Ejaculation (male)[6,7]	16%	<1%
Impotence[7]	4%	<1%
Anorgasmia (female)[8,9]	3%	<1%

[1]Incidence, rounded to the nearest %, for events reported by at least 2% of patients treated with Effexor XR, except the following events which had an incidence equal to or less than placebo: abdominal pain, accidental injury, anxiety, back pain, bronchitis, diarrhea, dysmenorrhea, dyspepsia, flu syndrome, headache, infection, pain, palpitation, rhinitis, and sinusitis.
[2]<1% indicates an incidence greater than zero but less than 1%.
[3]Mostly "hot flashes."
[4]Mostly "vivid dreams," "nightmares," and "increased dreaming."
[5]Mostly "blurred vision" and "difficulty focusing eyes."
[6]Mostly "delayed ejaculation."
[7]Incidence is based on the number of male patients.
[8]Mostly "delayed orgasm" or "anorgasmia."
[9]Incidence is based on the number of female patients.

Continued on next page

Effexor XR—Cont.

Table 4
Treatment-Emergent Adverse Event Incidence in Short-Term Placebo-Controlled Effexor XR Clinical Trials in GAD Patients[1,2]

Body System	% Reporting Event	
Preferred Term	Effexor XR (n=1381)	Placebo (n=555)
Body as a Whole		
Asthenia	12%	8%
Cardiovascular System		
Vasodilatation[3]	4%	2%
Digestive System		
Nausea	35%	12%
Constipation	10%	4%
Anorexia	8%	2%
Vomiting	5%	3%
Nervous System		
Dizziness	16%	11%
Dry Mouth	16%	6%
Insomnia	15%	10%
Somnolence	14%	8%
Nervousness	6%	4%
Libido Decreased	4%	2%
Tremor	4%	<1%
Abnormal Dreams[4]	3%	2%
Hypertonia	3%	2%
Paresthesia	2%	1%
Respiratory System		
Yawn	3%	<1%
Skin		
Sweating	10%	3%
Special Senses		
Abnormal Vision[5]	5%	<1%
Urogenital System		
Abnormal Ejaculation[6,7]	11%	<1%
Impotence[7]	5%	<1%
Orgasmic Dysfunction (female)[8,9]	2%	0%

[1]Adverse events for which the Effexor XR reporting rate was less than or equal to the placebo rate are not included. These events are: abdominal pain, accidental injury, anxiety, back pain, diarrhea, dysmenorrhea, dyspepsia, flu syndrome, headache, infection, myalgia, pain, palpitation, pharyngitis, rhinitis, tinnitus, and urinary frequency.
[2]<1% means greater than zero but less than 1%.
[3]Mostly "hot flashes."
[4]Mostly "vivid dreams," "nightmares," and "increased dreaming."
[5]Mostly "blurred vision" and "difficulty focusing eyes."
[6]Includes "delayed ejaculation" and "anorgasmia."
[7]Percentage based on the number of males (Effexor XR = 525, placebo = 220).
[8]Includes "delayed orgasm," "abnormal orgasm," and "anorgasmia."
[9]Percentage based on the number of females (Effexor XR = 856, placebo = 335).

Table 5
Treatment-Emergent Adverse Event Incidence in Short-Term Placebo-Controlled Effexor XR Clinical Trials in Social Anxiety Disorder Patients[1,2]

Body System	% Reporting Event	
Preferred Term	Effexor XR (n=277)	Placebo (n=274)
Body as a Whole		
Headache	34%	33%
Asthenia	17%	8%
Flu Syndrome	6%	5%
Accidental Injury	5%	3%
Abdominal Pain	4%	3%
Cardiovascular System		
Hypertension	5%	4%
Vasodilatation[3]	3%	1%
Palpitation	3%	1%
Digestive System		
Nausea	29%	9%
Anorexia[4]	20%	1%
Constipation	8%	4%
Diarrhea	6%	5%
Vomiting	3%	2%
Eructation	2%	0%
Metabolic/Nutritional		
Weight Loss	4%	0%
Nervous System		
Insomnia	23%	7%
Dry Mouth	17%	4%
Dizziness	16%	8%
Somnolence	16%	8%
Nervousness	11%	3%
Libido Decreased	9%	<1%
Anxiety	5%	3%
Agitation	4%	1%
Tremor	4%	<1%
Abnormal Dreams[5]	4%	<1%
Paresthesia	3%	<1%
Twitching	2%	0%
Respiratory System		
Yawn	5%	<1%
Sinusitis	2%	1%
Skin		
Sweating	13%	2%
Special Senses		
Abnormal Vision[6]	6%	3%
Urogenital System		
Abnormal Ejaculation[7,8]	16%	1%
Impotence[8]	10%	1%
Orgasmic Dysfunction[9,10]	8%	0%

[1] Adverse events for which the Effexor XR reporting rate was less than or equal to the placebo rate are not included. These events are: back pain, depression, dysmenorrhea, dyspepsia, infection, myalgia, pain, pharyngitis, rash, rhinitis, and upper respiratory infection.
[2]<1% means greater than zero but less than 1%.
[3]Mostly "hot flashes."
[4]Mostly "decreased appetite" and "loss of appetite."
[5]Mostly "vivid dreams," "nightmares," and "increased dreaming."
[6]Mostly "blurred vision."
[7] Includes "delayed ejaculation" and "anorgasmia."
[8] Percentage based on the number of males (Effexor XR = 158, placebo = 153).
[9]Includes "abnormal orgasm" and "anorgasmia."
[10]Percentage based on the number of females (Effexor XR = 119, placebo = 121).

Vital Sign Changes
Effexor XR (venlafaxine hydrochloride) extended-release capsules treatment for up to 12 weeks in premarketing placebo-controlled major depressive disorder trials was associated with a mean final on-therapy increase in pulse rate of approximately 2 beats per minute, compared with 1 beat per minute for placebo. Effexor XR treatment for up to 8 weeks in premarketing placebo-controlled GAD trials was associated with a mean final on-therapy increase in pulse rate of approximately 2 beats per minute, compared with less than 1 beat per minute for placebo. Effexor XR treatment for up to 12 weeks in premarketing placebo-controlled Social Anxiety Disorder trials was associated with mean final on-therapy increase in pulse rate of approximately 4 beats per minute, compared with no change for placebo. (See the **Sustained Hypertension** section of **WARNINGS** for effects on blood pressure.)
In a flexible-dose study, with Effexor doses in the range of 200 to 375 mg/day and mean dose greater than 300 mg/day, the mean pulse was increased by about 2 beats per minute compared with a decrease of about 1 beat per minute for placebo.
Laboratory Changes
Effexor XR (venlafaxine hydrochloride) extended-release capsules treatment for up to 12 weeks in premarketing placebo-controlled trials for major depressive disorder was associated with a mean final on-therapy increase in serum cholesterol concentration of approximately 1.5 mg/dL compared with a mean final decrease of 7.4 mg/dL for placebo. Effexor XR treatment for up to 8 weeks and up to 6 months in premarketing placebo-controlled GAD trials was associated with mean final on-therapy increases in serum cholesterol concentration of approximately 1.0 mg/dL and 2.3 mg/dL, respectively while placebo subjects experienced mean final decreases of 4.9 mg/dL and 7.7 mg/dL, respectively. Effexor XR treatment for up to 12 weeks in premarketing placebo-controlled Social Anxiety Disorder trials was associated with mean final on-therapy increases in serum cholesterol concentration of approximately 11.4 mg/dL compared with a mean final decrease of 2.2 mg/dL for placebo. Patients treated with Effexor tablets (the immediate-release form of venlafaxine) for at least 3 months in placebo-controlled 12-month extension trials had a mean final on-therapy increase in total cholesterol of 9.1 mg/dL compared with a decrease of 7.1 mg/dL among placebo-treated patients. This increase was duration dependent over the study period and tended to be greater with higher doses. Clinically relevant increases in serum cholesterol, defined as 1) a final on-therapy increase in serum cholesterol ≥50 mg/dL from baseline and to a value ≥261 mg/dL, or 2) an average on-therapy increase in serum cholesterol ≥50 mg/dL from baseline and to a value ≥261 mg/dL, were recorded in 5.3% of venlafaxine-treated patients and 0.0% of placebo-treated patients (see **PRECAUTIONS-General**-*Serum Cholesterol Elevation*).
ECG Changes
In a flexible-dose study, with Effexor doses in the range of 200 to 375 mg/day and mean dose greater than 300 mg/day, the mean change in heart rate was 8.5 beats per minute compared with 1.7 beats per minute for placebo.
(See the *Use in Patients with Concomitant Illness* section of **PRECAUTIONS**).

Other Adverse Events Observed During the Premarketing Evaluation of Effexor and Effexor XR

During its premarketing assessment, multiple doses of Effexor XR were administered to 705 patients in Phase 3 major depressive disorder studies and Effexor was administered to 96 patients. During its premarketing assessment, multiple doses of Effexor XR were also administered to 1381 patients in Phase 3 GAD studies and 277 patients in Phase 3 Social Anxiety Disorder studies. In addition, in premarketing assessment of Effexor, multiple doses were administered to 2897 patients in Phase 2 to Phase 3 studies for major depressive disorder. The conditions and duration of exposure to venlafaxine in both development programs varied greatly, and included (in overlapping categories) open and double-blind studies, uncontrolled and controlled studies, inpatient (Effexor only) and outpatient studies, fixed-dose, and titration studies. Untoward events associated with this exposure were recorded by clinical investigators using terminology of their own choosing. Consequently, it is not possible to provide a meaningful estimate of the proportion of individuals experiencing adverse events without first grouping similar types of untoward events into a smaller number of standardized event categories.
In the tabulations that follow, reported adverse events were classified using a standard COSTART-based Dictionary terminology. The frequencies presented, therefore, represent the proportion of the 5356 patients exposed to multiple doses of either formulation of venlafaxine who experienced an event of the type cited on at least one occasion while receiving venlafaxine. All reported events are included except those already listed in Tables 3, 4, and 5 and those events for which a drug cause was remote. If the COSTART term for an event was so general as to be uninformative, it was replaced with a more informative term. It is important to emphasize that, although the events reported occurred during treatment with venlafaxine, they were not necessarily caused by it.
Events are further categorized by body system and listed in order of decreasing frequency using the following definitions: **frequent** adverse events are defined as those occurring on one or more occasions in at least 1/100 patients; **infrequent** adverse events are those occurring in 1/100 to 1/1000 patients; **rare** events are those occurring in fewer than 1/1000 patients.
Body as a whole—**Frequent:** chest pain substernal, chills, fever, neck pain; **Infrequent:** face edema, intentional injury, malaise, moniliasis, neck rigidity, pelvic pain, photosensitivity reaction, suicide attempt, withdrawal syndrome; **Rare:** appendicitis, bacteremia, carcinoma, cellulitis.
Cardiovascular system—**Frequent:** migraine, postural hypotension, tachycardia; **Infrequent:** angina pectoris, arrhythmia, extrasystoles, hypotension, peripheral vascular disorder (mainly cold feet and/or cold hands), syncope, thrombophlebitis; **Rare:** aortic aneurysm, arteritis, first-degree atrioventricular block, bigeminy, bradycardia, bundle branch block, capillary fragility, cerebral ischemia, coronary artery disease, congestive heart failure, heart arrest, cardiovascular disorder (mitral valve and circulatory disturbance), mucocutaneous hemorrhage, myocardial infarct, pallor.
Digestive system—**Frequent:** increased appetite; **Infrequent:** bruxism, colitis, dysphagia, tongue edema, esophagitis, gastritis, gastroenteritis, gastrointestinal ulcer, gingivitis, glossitis, rectal hemorrhage, hemorrhoids, melena, oral moniliasis, stomatitis, mouth ulceration; **Rare:** cheilitis, cholecystitis, cholelithiasis, esophageal spasms, duodenitis, hematemesis, gastrointestinal hemorrhage, gum hemorrhage, hepatitis, ileitis, jaundice, intestinal obstruction, parotitis, periodontitis, proctitis, increased salivation, soft stools, tongue discoloration.
Endocrine system—**Rare:** goiter, hyperthyroidism, hypothyroidism, thyroid nodule, thyroiditis.
Hemic and lymphatic system—**Frequent:** ecchymosis; **Infrequent:** anemia, leukocytosis, leukopenia, lymphadenopathy, thrombocythemia, thrombocytopenia; **Rare:** basophilia, bleeding time increased, cyanosis, eosinophilia, lymphocytosis, multiple myeloma, purpura.
Metabolic and nutritional—**Frequent:** edema, weight gain; **Infrequent:** alkaline phosphatase increased, dehydration, hypercholesteremia, hyperglycemia, hyperlipemia, hypokalemia, SGOT increased, SGPT increased, thirst; **Rare:** alcohol intolerance, bilirubinemia, BUN increased, creatinine increased, diabetes mellitus, glycosuria, gout, healing abnormal, hemochromatosis, hypercalcinuria, hyperkalemia, hyperphosphatemia, hyperuricemia, hypocholesteremia, hypoglycemia, hyponatremia, hypophosphatemia, hypoproteinemia, uremia.
Musculoskeletal system—**Frequent:** arthralgia; **Infrequent:** arthritis, arthrosis, bone pain, bone spurs, bursitis, leg cramps, myasthenia, tenosynovitis; **Rare:** pathological fracture, myopathy, osteoporosis, osteosclerosis, plantar fasciitis, rheumatoid arthritis, tendon rupture.
Nervous system—**Frequent:** amnesia, confusion, depersonalization, hypesthesia, thinking abnormal, trismus, vertigo; **Infrequent:** akathisia, apathy, ataxia, circumoral paresthesia, CNS stimulation, emotional lability, euphoria, hallucinations, hostility, hyperesthesia, hyperkinesia, hypotonia, incoordination, libido increased, manic reaction, myoclonus, neuralgia, neuropathy, psychosis, seizure, abnormal speech, stupor; **Rare:** akinesia, alcohol abuse, aphasia, bradykinesia, buccoglossal syndrome, cerebrovascular accident, feeling drunk, loss of consciousness, delusions, dementia, dystonia, facial paralysis, abnormal gait, Guillain-Barre Syndrome, hyperchlorhydria, hypokinesia, impulse control difficulties, neuritis, nystagmus, paranoid reaction, paresis, psychotic depression, reflexes decreased, reflexes increased, suicidal ideation, torticollis.
Respiratory system—**Frequent:** cough increased, dyspnea; **Infrequent:** asthma, chest congestion, epistaxis, hyperventilation, laryngismus, laryngitis, pneumonia, voice alteration; **Rare:** atelectasis, hemoptysis, hypoventilation, hypoxia, larynx edema, pleurisy, pulmonary embolus, sleep apnea.
Skin and appendages—**Frequent:** pruritus; **Infrequent:** acne, alopecia, brittle nails, contact dermatitis, dry skin, eczema, skin hypertrophy, maculopapular rash, psoriasis, urticaria; **Rare:** erythema nodosum, exfoliative dermatitis, lichenoid dermatitis, hair discoloration, skin discoloration,

furunculosis, hirsutism, leukoderma, petechial rash, pustular rash, vesiculobullous rash, seborrhea, skin atrophy, skin striae.

Special senses—**Frequent**: abnormality of accommodation, mydriasis, taste perversion; **Infrequent**: cataract, conjunctivitis, corneal lesion, diplopia, dry eyes, eye pain, hyperacusis, otitis media, parosmia, photophobia, taste loss, visual field defect; **Rare**: blepharitis, chromatopsia, conjunctival edema, deafness, exophthalmos, glaucoma, retinal hemorrhage, subconjunctival hemorrhage, keratitis, labyrinthitis, miosis, papilledema, decreased pupillary reflex, otitis externa, scleritis, uveitis.

Urogenital system—**Frequent**: metrorrhagia,* prostatic disorder (prostatitis and enlarged prostate),* urination impaired, vaginitis*; **Infrequent**: albuminuria, amenorrhea,* cystitis, dysuria, hematuria, leukorrhea,* menorrhagia,* nocturia, bladder pain, breast pain, polyuria, pyuria, urinary incontinence, urinary retention, urinary urgency, vaginal hemorrhage*; **Rare**: abortion,* anuria, breast discharge, breast engorgement, balanitis,* breast enlargement, endometriosis,* female lactation,* fibrocystic breast, calcium crystalluria, cervicitis,* orchitis,* ovarian cyst,* prolonged erection,* gynecomastia (male),* hypomenorrhea,* kidney calculus, kidney pain, kidney function abnormal, mastitis, menopause,* pyelonephritis, oliguria, salpingitis,* urolithiasis, uterine hemorrhage,* uterine spasm,* vaginal dryness.*

*Based on the number of men and women as appropriate.

Postmarketing Reports

Voluntary reports of other adverse events temporally associated with the use of venlafaxine that have been received since market introduction and that may have no causal relationship with the use of venlafaxine include the following: agranulocytosis, anaphylaxis, aplastic anemia, catatonia, congenital anomalies, CPK increased, deep vein thrombophlebitis, delirium, EKG abnormalities such as QT prolongation; cardiac arrhythmias including atrial fibrillation, supraventricular tachycardia, ventricular extrasystoles, and rare reports of ventricular fibrillation and ventricular tachycardia, including torsade de pointes; epidermal necrosis/Stevens-Johnson Syndrome, erythema multiforme, extrapyramidal symptoms (including dyskinesia and tardive dyskinesia), hemorrhage (including eye and gastrointestinal bleeding), hepatic events (including GGT elevation; abnormalities of unspecified liver function tests; liver damage, necrosis, or failure; and fatty liver), involuntary movements, LDH increased, neuroleptic malignant syndrome-like events (including a case of a 10-year-old who may have been taking methylphenidate, was treated and recovered), neutropenia, night sweats, pancreatitis, pancytopenia, panic, prolactin increased, pulmonary eosinophilia, renal failure, rhabdomyolysis, serotonin syndrome, shock-like electrical sensations (in some cases, subsequent to the discontinuation of venlafaxine or tapering of dose), and syndrome of inappropriate antidiuretic hormone secretion (usually in the elderly).

There have been reports of elevated clozapine levels that were temporally associated with adverse events, including seizures, following the addition of venlafaxine. There have been reports of increases in prothrombin time, partial thromboplastin time, or INR when venlafaxine was given to patients receiving warfarin therapy.

DRUG ABUSE AND DEPENDENCE

Controlled Substance Class

Effexor XR (venlafaxine hydrochloride) extended-release capsules is not a controlled substance.

Physical and Psychological Dependence

In vitro studies revealed that venlafaxine has virtually no affinity for opiate, benzodiazepine, phencyclidine (PCP), or N-methyl-D-aspartic acid (NMDA) receptors.

Venlafaxine was not found to have any significant CNS stimulant activity in rodents. In primate drug discrimination studies, venlafaxine showed no significant stimulant or depressant abuse liability.

Discontinuation effects have been reported in patients receiving venlafaxine (see **DOSAGE AND ADMINISTRATION**).

While venlafaxine has not been systematically studied in clinical trials for its potential for abuse, there was no indication of drug-seeking behavior in the clinical trials. However, it is not possible to predict on the basis of premarketing experience the extent to which a CNS active drug will be misused, diverted, and/or abused once marketed. Consequently, physicians should carefully evaluate patients for history of drug abuse and follow such patients closely, observing them for signs of misuse or abuse of venlafaxine (eg, development of tolerance, incrementation of dose, drug-seeking behavior).

OVERDOSAGE

Human Experience

Among the patients included in the premarketing evaluation of Effexor XR, there were 2 reports of acute overdosage with Effexor XR in major depressive disorder trials, either alone or in combination with other drugs. One patient took a combination of 6 g of Effexor XR and 2.5 mg of lorazepam. This patient was hospitalized, treated symptomatically, and recovered without any untoward effects. The other patient took 2.85 g of Effexor XR. This patient reported paresthesia of all four limbs but recovered without sequelae.

There were 2 reports of acute overdose with Effexor XR in GAD trials. One patient took a combination of 0.75 g of Effexor XR and 200 mg of paroxetine and 50 mg of zolpidem. This patient was described as being alert, able to communicate, and a little sleepy. This patient was hospitalized, treated with activated charcoal, and recovered without any untoward effects. The other patient took 1.2 g of Effexor XR. This patient recovered and no other specific problems were found. The patient had moderate dizziness, nausea, numb hands and feet, and hot-cold spells 5 days after the overdose. These symptoms resolved over the next week.

There were no reports of acute overdose with Effexor XR in Social Anxiety Disorder trials.

Among the patients included in the premarketing evaluation with Effexor, there were 14 reports of acute overdose with venlafaxine, either alone or in combination with other drugs and/or alcohol. The majority of the reports involved ingestion in which the total dose of venlafaxine taken was estimated to be no more than several-fold higher than the usual therapeutic dose. The 3 patients who took the highest doses were estimated to have ingested approximately 6.75 g, 2.75 g, and 2.5 g. The resultant peak plasma levels of venlafaxine for the latter 2 patients were 6.24 and 2.35 µg/mL, respectively, and the peak plasma levels of O-desmethylvenlafaxine were 3.37 and 1.30 µg/mL, respectively. Plasma venlafaxine levels were not obtained for the patient who ingested 6.75 g of venlafaxine. All 14 patients recovered without sequelae. Most patients reported no symptoms. Among the remaining patients, somnolence was the most commonly reported symptom. The patient who ingested 2.75 g of venlafaxine was observed to have 2 generalized convulsions and a prolongation of QTc to 500 msec, compared with 405 msec at baseline. Mild sinus tachycardia was reported in 2 of the other patients.

In postmarketing experience, overdose with venlafaxine has occurred predominantly in combination with alcohol and/or other drugs. Electrocardiogram changes (eg, prolongation of QT interval, bundle branch block, QRS prolongation), sinus and ventricular tachycardia, bradycardia, hypotension, altered level of consciousness (ranging from somnolence to coma), rhabdomyolysis, seizures, vertigo, and death have been reported.

Management of Overdosage

Treatment should consist of those general measures employed in the management of overdosage with any antidepressant.

Ensure an adequate airway, oxygenation, and ventilation. Monitor cardiac rhythm and vital signs. General supportive and symptomatic measures are also recommended. Induction of emesis is not recommended. Gastric lavage with a large bore orogastric tube with appropriate airway protection, if needed, may be indicated if performed soon after ingestion or in symptomatic patients.

Activated charcoal should be administered. Due to the large volume of distribution of this drug, forced diuresis, dialysis, hemoperfusion, and exchange transfusion are unlikely to be of benefit. No specific antidotes for venlafaxine are known.

In managing overdosage, consider the possibility of multiple drug involvement. The physician should consider contacting a poison control center for additional information on the treatment of any overdose. Telephone numbers for certified poison control centers are listed in the *Physicians' Desk Reference® (PDR).*

DOSAGE AND ADMINISTRATION

Effexor XR should be administered in a single dose with food either in the morning or in the evening at approximately the same time each day. Each capsule should be swallowed whole with fluid and not divided, crushed, chewed, or placed in water, or it may be administered by carefully opening the capsule and sprinkling the entire contents on a spoonful of applesauce. This drug/food mixture should be swallowed immediately without chewing and followed with a glass of water to ensure complete swallowing of the pellets.

Initial Treatment

Major Depressive Disorder

For most patients, the recommended starting dose for Effexor XR is 75 mg/day, administered in a single dose. In the clinical trials establishing the efficacy of Effexor XR in moderately depressed outpatients, the initial dose of venlafaxine was 75 mg/day. For some patients, it may be desirable to start at 37.5 mg/day for 4 to 7 days, to allow new patients to adjust to the medication before increasing to 75 mg/day. While the relationship between dose and antidepressant response for Effexor XR has not been adequately explored, patients not responding to the initial 75 mg/day dose may benefit from dose increases to a maximum of approximately 225 mg/day. Dose increases should be in increments of up to 75 mg/day, as needed, and should be made at intervals of not less than 4 days, since steady state plasma levels of venlafaxine and its major metabolites are achieved in most patients by day 4. In the clinical trials establishing efficacy, upward titration was permitted at intervals of 2 weeks or more; the average doses were about 140 to 180 mg/day (see **Clinical Trials** under **CLINICAL PHARMACOLOGY**).

It should be noted that, while the maximum recommended dose for moderately depressed outpatients is also 225 mg/day for Effexor (the immediate release form of venlafaxine), more severely depressed inpatients in one study of the development program for that product responded to a mean dose of 350 mg/day (range of 150 to 375 mg/day). Whether or not higher doses of Effexor XR are needed for more severely depressed patients is unknown; however, the experience with Effexor XR doses higher than 225 mg/day is very limited. (See **PRECAUTIONS-General**-*Use in Patients with Concomitant Illness.*)

Generalized Anxiety Disorder

For most patients, the recommended starting dose for Effexor XR is 75 mg/day, administered in a single dose. In clinical trials establishing the efficacy of Effexor XR in outpatients with Generalized Anxiety Disorder (GAD), the initial dose of venlafaxine was 75 mg/day. For some patients, it may be desirable to start at 37.5 mg/day for 4 to 7 days, to allow new patients to adjust to the medication before increasing to 75 mg/day. Although a dose-response relationship for effectiveness in GAD was not clearly established in fixed-dose studies, certain patients not responding to the initial 75 mg/day dose may benefit from dose increases to a maximum of approximately 225 mg/day. Dose increases should be in increments of up to 75 mg/day, as needed, and should be made at intervals of not less than 4 days. (See the *Use in Patients with Concomitant Illness* section of **PRECAUTIONS**.)

Social Anxiety Disorder (Social Phobia)

For most patients, the recommended starting dose for Effexor XR is 75 mg/day, administered in a single dose. In clinical trials establishing the efficacy of Effexor XR in outpatients with Social Anxiety Disorder, the initial dose of Effexor XR was 75 mg/day and the maximum dose was 225 mg/day. For some patients, it may be desirable to start at 37.5 mg/day for 4 to 7 days, to allow new patients to adjust to the medication before increasing to 75 mg/day. Although a dose-response relationship for effectiveness in patients with Social Anxiety Disorder was not clearly established in fixed-dose studies, certain patients not responding to the initial 75 mg/day dose may benefit from dose increases to a maximum of approximately 225 mg/day. Dose increases should be in increments of up to 75 mg/day, as needed, and should be made at intervals of not less than 4 days. (See the *Use in Patients with Concomitant Illness* section of **PRECAUTIONS**).

Switching Patients from Effexor Tablets

Depressed patients who are currently being treated at a therapeutic dose with Effexor may be switched to Effexor XR at the nearest equivalent dose (mg/day), eg, 37.5 mg venlafaxine two-times-a-day to 75 mg Effexor XR once daily. However, individual dosage adjustments may be necessary.

Patients with Hepatic Impairment

Given the decrease in clearance and increase in elimination half-life for both venlafaxine and ODV that is observed in patients with hepatic cirrhosis compared with normal subjects (see **CLINICAL PHARMACOLOGY**), it is recommended that the starting dose be reduced by 50% in patients with moderate hepatic impairment. Because there was much individual variability in clearance between patients with cirrhosis, individualization of dosage may be desirable in some patients.

Patients with Renal Impairment

Given the decrease in clearance for venlafaxine and the increase in elimination half-life for both venlafaxine and ODV that is observed in patients with renal impairment (GFR = 10 to 70 mL/min) compared with normal subjects (see **CLINICAL PHARMACOLOGY**), it is recommended that the total daily dose be reduced by 25% to 50%. In patients undergoing hemodialysis, it is recommended that the total daily dose be reduced by 50% and that the dose be withheld until the dialysis treatment is completed (4 hrs). Because there was much individual variability in clearance between patients with renal impairment, individualization of dosage may be desirable in some patients.

Elderly Patients

No dose adjustment is recommended for elderly patients solely on the basis of age. As with any drug for the treatment of major depressive disorder, Generalized Anxiety Disorder, or Social Anxiety Disorder, however, caution should be exercised in treating the elderly. When individualizing the dosage, extra care should be taken when increasing the dose.

Maintenance Treatment

There is no body of evidence available from controlled trials to indicate how long patients with major depressive disorder, Generalized Anxiety Disorder, or Social Anxiety Disorder should be treated with Effexor XR.

It is generally agreed that acute episodes of major depressive disorder require several months or longer of sustained pharmacological therapy beyond response to the acute episode. In one study, in which patients responding during 8 weeks of acute treatment with Effexor XR were assigned randomly to placebo or to the same dose of Effexor XR (75, 150, or 225 mg/day, qAM) during 26 weeks of maintenance treatment as they had received during the acute stabilization phase, longer-term efficacy was demonstrated. A second longer-term study has demonstrated the efficacy of Effexor in maintaining a response in patients with recurrent major depressive disorder who had responded and continued to be improved during an initial 26 weeks of treatment and were then randomly assigned to placebo or Effexor for periods of up to 52 weeks on the same dose (100 to 200 mg/day, on a b.i.d. schedule) (see **Clinical Trials** under **CLINICAL PHARMACOLOGY**). Based on these limited data, it is not known whether or not the dose of Effexor/Effexor XR needed for maintenance treatment is identical to the dose needed to achieve an initial response. Patients should be periodically reassessed to determine the need for maintenance treatment and the appropriate dose for such treatment.

In patients with Generalized Anxiety Disorder, Effexor XR has been shown to be effective in 6-month clinical trials. The

Continued on next page

Effexor XR—Cont.

need for continuing medication in patients with GAD who improve with Effexor XR treatment should be periodically reassessed.

In patients with Social Anxiety Disorder, there are no efficacy data beyond 12 weeks of treatment with Effexor XR. The need for continuing medication in patients with Social Anxiety Disorder who improve with Effexor XR treatment should be periodically reassessed.

Discontinuing Effexor XR

When discontinuing Effexor XR after more than 1 week of therapy, it is generally recommended that the dose be tapered to minimize the risk of discontinuation symptoms. Patients who have received Effexor XR for 6 weeks or more should have their dose tapered over at least a 2-week period. In clinical trials with Effexor XR, tapering was achieved by reducing the daily dose by 75 mg at 1 week intervals. Individualization of tapering may be necessary.

Discontinuation symptoms have been systematically evaluated in patients taking venlafaxine, to include prospective analyses of clinical trials in Generalized Anxiety Disorder and retrospective surveys of trials of major depressive disorder. Abrupt discontinuation or dose reduction of venlafaxine at various doses has been found to be associated with the appearance of new symptoms, the frequency of which increased with increased dose level and with longer duration of treatment. Reported symptoms include agitation, anorexia, anxiety, confusion, coordination impaired, diarrhea, dizziness, dry mouth, dysphoric mood, fasciculation, fatigue, headaches, hypomania, insomnia, nausea, nervousness, nightmares, seizures, sensory disturbances (including shock-like electrical sensations), somnolence, sweating, tinnitus, tremor, vertigo, and vomiting. It is therefore recommended that the dosage of Effexor XR be tapered gradually and the patient monitored. The period required for tapering may depend on the dose, duration of therapy and the individual patient. Discontinuation effects are well known to occur with antidepressants.

Switching Patients To or From a Monoamine Oxidase Inhibitor

At least 14 days should elapse between discontinuation of an MAOI and initiation of therapy with Effexor XR. In addition, at least 7 days should be allowed after stopping Effexor XR before starting an MAOI (see **CONTRAINDICATIONS** and **WARNINGS**).

HOW SUPPLIED

Effexor® XR (venlafaxine hydrochloride) extended-release capsules are available as follows:

37.5 mg, grey cap/peach body with W and "Effexor XR" on the cap and "37.5" on the body.

NDC 0008-0837-01, bottle of 100 capsules.

NDC 0008-0837-03, carton of 10 Redipak® blister strips of 10 capsules each.

Store at controlled room temperature, 20°C to 25°C (68°F to 77°F).

75 mg, peach cap and body with W and "Effexor XR" on the cap and "75" on the body.

NDC 0008-0833-01, bottle of 100 capsules.

NDC 0008-0833-03, carton of 10 Redipak® blister strips of 10 capsules each.

Store at controlled room temperature, 20°C to 25°C (68°F to 77°F).

150 mg, dark orange cap and body with W and "Effexor XR" on the cap and "150" on the body.

NDC 0008-0836-01, bottle of 100 capsules.

NDC 0008-0836-03, carton of 10 Redipak® blister strips of 10 capsules each.

Store at controlled room temperature, 20°C to 25°C (68°F to 77°F).

The appearance of these capsules is a trademark of Wyeth Pharmaceuticals.

Wyeth®

Wyeth Pharmaceuticals Inc. W10404C008
Philadelphia, PA 19101 ET02
Rev 12/03

HibTITER® ℞

[*hĭb-tī-tər*]

HAEMOPHILUS b CONJUGATE VACCINE
(Diphtheria CRM_{197} Protein Conjugate)
℞ only

Prescribing information for this product, which appears on page(s) 3427–3430 of the 2004 PDR, has been completely revised as follows. Please write "See Supplement A" next to the product heading.

This product's label may have been revised after this insert was used in production. For further product information and current package insert, please visit www.wyeth.com or call our medical communications department toll-free at 1-800-934-5556.

DESCRIPTION

Haemophilus b Conjugate Vaccine (Diphtheria CRM_{197} Protein Conjugate) HibTITER is a sterile solution of a conjugate of oligosaccharides of the capsular antigen of *Haemophilus influenzae* type b (Haemophilus b) and diphtheria CRM_{197} protein (CRM_{197}) dissolved in 0.9% sodium chloride. The oligosaccharides are derived from highly purified capsular polysaccharide, polyribosylribitol phosphate, isolated from Haemophilus b strain Eagan grown in a chemically defined medium (a mixture of mineral salts, amino acids, and cofactors). The oligosaccharides are purified and sized by diafiltrations through a series of ultrafiltration membranes, and coupled by reductive amination directly to highly purified CRM_{197}.[1,2] CRM_{197} is a nontoxic variant of diphtheria toxin isolated from cultures of *Corynebacterium diphtheriae* C7 (β197) grown in a casamino acids and yeast extract-based medium that is ultrafiltered before use. CRM_{197} is purified through ultrafiltration, ammonium sulfate precipitation, and ion-exchange chromatography to high purity. The conjugate is purified to remove unreacted protein, oligosaccharides, and reagents; sterilized by filtration; and filled into vials. HibTITER is intended for intramuscular use.

The vaccine is a clear, colorless solution. Each single dose of 0.5 mL is formulated to contain 10 µg of purified Haemophilus b saccharide and approximately 25 µg of CRM_{197} protein. The potency of HibTITER is determined by chemical assay for polyribosylribitol.

CLINICAL PHARMACOLOGY

For several decades *Haemophilus influenzae* type b (Haemophilus b) was the most common cause of invasive bacterial disease, including meningitis, in young children in the United States. Although nonencapsulated *H. influenzae* are common and six capsular polysaccharide types are known, strains with the type b capsule caused most of the invasive Haemophilus diseases.[3]

Haemophilus b diseases occurred primarily in children under 5 years of age prior to immunization with *Haemophilus influenzae* type b vaccines. In the US, the cumulative risk of developing invasive Haemophilus b disease during the first 5 years of life was estimated to be about 1 in 200. Approximately 60% of cases were meningitis. Cellulitis, epiglottitis, pericarditis, pneumonia, sepsis, or septic arthritis made up the remaining 40%. An estimated 12,000 cases of Haemophilus b meningitis occurred annually prior to the routine use of conjugate vaccines in toddlers.[3,4] The mortality rate can be 5%, and neurologic sequelae have been observed in up to 38% of survivors.[5]

The incidence of invasive Haemophilus b disease peaks between 6 months and 1 year of age, and approximately 55% of disease occurs between 6 and 18 months of age.[3] Interpersonal transmission of Haemophilus b occurs and risk of invasive disease is increased in children younger than 4 years of age who are exposed in the household to a primary case of disease. Clusters of cases in children in day care have been reported and recent studies suggest that the rate of secondary cases may also be increased among children exposed to a primary case in the daycare setting.[3,6]

The incidence of invasive Haemophilus b disease is increased in certain children, such as those who are native Americans, black, or from lower socioeconomic status, and those with medical conditions such as asplenia, sickle cell disease, malignancies associated with immunosuppression, and antibody deficiency syndromes.[3,4,6]

The protective activity of antibody to Haemophilus b polysaccharide was demonstrated by passive antibody studies in animals and in children with agammaglobulinemia or with Haemophilus b disease[7] and confirmed with the efficacy study of Haemophilus b polysaccharide (HbPs) vaccine.[8] Data from passive antibody studies indicate that a preexisting titer of antibody to HbPs of 0.15 µg/mL correlates with protection.[9] Data from a Finnish field trial in children 18 to 71 months of age indicate that a titer of > 1.0 µg/mL 3 weeks after vaccination is associated with long-term protection.[10,11]

Linkage of Haemophilus b saccharides to a protein such as CRM_{197} converts the saccharide (HbO) to a T-dependent (HbOC) antigen, and results in an enhanced antibody response to the saccharide in young infants that primes for an anamnestic response and is predominantly of the IgG class.[12] Laboratory evidence indicates that the native state of the CRM_{197} protein and the use of oligosaccharides in the formulation of HibTITER enhances its immunogenicity.[13–15]

Prior to licensure, the immunogenicity of HibTITER was evaluated in US infants and children.[15] Infants 1 to 6 months of age at first immunization received three doses at approximately 2-month intervals.[16] Children 7 to 11 and 12 to 14 months of age received 2 doses at the same interval.[15] Children 15 to 23 months of age received a single dose.[17] HibTITER was highly immunogenic in all age groups studied, with 97% to 100% of 1,232 infants attaining titers of ≥ 1 µg/mL and 92% to 100% for bactericidal activity.[15–17]

Long-term persistence of the antibody response was observed. More than 80% of 235 infants who received three doses of vaccine had an anti-HbPs antibody level ≥ 1 µg/mL at 2 years of age.[18]

The vaccine generated an immune response characteristic of a protein antigen. IgG anti-HbPs antibodies of IgG_1 subclass predominated and the immune system was primed for a booster response to HibTITER. There is some evidence suggesting natural increases in antibody levels over time after vaccination, most probably the result of contact with Haemophilus type b organisms or cross-reactive antigens.[18] These studies were carried out at a time when significant levels of Haemophilus b disease were still present in the community.

Antibody generated by HibTITER has been found to have high avidity, a measure of the functional affinity of antibody to bind to antigen. High-avidity antibody is more potent than low-avidity antibody in serum bactericidal assays.[19] The contribution to clinical protection is unknown.

Immunogenicity of HibTITER was evaluated in 26 children 22 months to 5 years of age who had not responded to earlier vaccination with Haemophilus b polysaccharide vaccine. One dose of HibTITER was immunogenic in all 26 children and generated titers of ≥ 1 µg/mL in 25 of the 26 infants.[20] HibTITER has been found to be immunogenic in children with sickle cell disease, a condition that may cause increased susceptibility to Haemophilus b disease.[21] HibTITER has also been shown to be immunogenic in native American infants, such as the group of 50 studied in Alaska who received three doses at 2, 4, and 6 months of age.[20] Antibody levels achieved were comparable to those seen in healthy US infants who received their first dose at 1 to 2 months of age and subsequent doses at 4 to 6 months of age.[15,16,20]

Postlicensure surveillance of immunogenicity was conducted during the distribution of the first 30 million doses of HibTITER and during the time period over which Haemophilus b disease in children has been decreasing significantly in areas of extensive vaccine usage.[20,22–29] After three doses, titers ranged from 2.37 to 8.45 µg/mL with 67% to 94% attaining ≥ 1 µg/mL.[20,24,25]

Persistence of antibody was examined in several cohorts of subjects that received either a selected commercial lot or that were part of the initial efficacy trial in northern California. Geometric mean titers for these cohorts were between 0.51 and 1.96 just prior to boosting at 15 to 18 months. These lots not only induced persistent antibody but also provided effective priming for a booster dose with commercial lots, with postboosting titers greater than 1.0 µg/mL in 80% to 97% of subjects.[20]

HibTITER (HbOC) was shown to be effective in a large-scale controlled clinical trial in a multiethnic population in northern California carried out between February 1988 and June 1990.[30,31] There were no (0) vaccine failures in infants who received three doses of HibTITER and 12 cases of Haemophilus b disease (6 cases of meningitis) in the control group. The estimate of efficacy is 100% (P = .0002) with 95% confidence intervals of 68% to 100%. Through the end of 1991, with an additional 49,000 person-years of follow-up, there were still no cases of Haemophilus b disease in fully vaccinated infants less than 2 years of age.[22,23] One case of disease has been reported in a 3 1/2-year-old child who did not receive a booster dose as recommended.

A comparative clinical trial was performed in Finland where approximately 53,000 infants received HibTITER at 4 and 6 months of age and a booster dose at 14 months in a trial conducted from January 1988 through December 1990. Only two children developed Haemophilus b disease after receiving the two-dose primary immunization schedule. One child became ill at 15 months of age and the other at 18 months of age; neither child received the scheduled booster at 14 months of age. No vaccine failure has been reported in children who received the two-dose primary series and the booster dose at 14 months of age. Based on more than 32,000 person-years of follow-up time, the estimate of efficacy is about 95% when compared to historical control groups followed between 1985 and 1988.[20] Historical controls were used since all infants received one of two Haemophilus b conjugate vaccines during the period of the trial.

Evidence of efficacy postlicensure includes significant reductions in Haemophilus b disease that are closely associated with increases in the net doses of Haemophilus b Conjugate Vaccine distributed in the US.[20,22–29] In the northern California Kaiser Permanente there has been a 94% decrease in Haemophilus disease incidence in 1991 for children younger than 18 months of age, compared to 1984-1988, when HibTITER was not available for this age group.[22,23] Furthermore, active surveillance by the Centers for Disease Control and Prevention (CDC) has shown a 71% decrease in Haemophilus b disease in children less than 15 months old, between 1989 and 1991, which corresponds temporally and geographically with increases in net doses of Haemophilus b conjugate vaccine distributed in the US.[26] As with all vaccines, this conjugate vaccine cannot be expected to be 100% effective. There have been rare reports to the Vaccine Adverse Event Reporting System (VAERS) of Haemophilus b disease following full primary immunization.

INDICATIONS AND USAGE

Haemophilus b Conjugate Vaccine (Diphtheria CRM_{197} Protein Conjugate) HibTITER is indicated for the immunization of children 2 months to 71 months of age against invasive diseases caused by *H. influenza* type b.

As with any vaccine, HibTITER may not protect 100% of individuals receiving the vaccine.

The American Academy of Pediatrics (AAP), the Advisory Committee on Immunization Practices (ACIP) and the American Academy of Family Physicians (AAFP) encourage the routine simultaneous administration of *Haemophilus influenzae* type b vaccines with other currently recommended vaccines, but at different sites (see **DRUG INTERACTIONS**).[32,33,34,35]

CONTRAINDICATIONS

Hypersensitivity to any component of the vaccine, including diphtheria toxoid, is a contraindication to the use of HibTITER.

The occurrence of an allergic or anaphylactic reaction following a prior dose of HibTITER is a contraindication to the use of HibTITER.

The decision to administer or delay vaccination because of a current or recent febrile illness depends largely on the severity of the symptoms and their etiology. Although a severe or even moderate febrile illness is sufficient reason to postpone vaccinations, minor illnesses, such as a mild respiratory infection with or without low-grade fever, are not generally contraindications.

WARNINGS

HibTITER WILL NOT PROTECT AGAINST *H. INFLUENZA* OTHER THAN TYPE b STRAINS, NOR WILL HibTITER PROTECT AGAINST OTHER MICROORGANISMS THAT CAUSE MENINGITIS OR SEPTIC DISEASE.

AS WITH ANY INTRAMUSCULAR INJECTION, HibTITER SHOULD BE GIVEN WITH CAUTION TO INFANTS OR CHILDREN WITH THROMBOCYTOPENIA OR ANY COAGULATION DISORDER, OR TO THOSE RECEIVING ANTICOAGULANT THERAPY (SEE **DRUG INTERACTIONS**).

ANTIGENURIA HAS BEEN DETECTED FOLLOWING RECEIPT OF HAEMOPHILUS b CONJUGATE VACCINE[36] AND THEREFORE ANTIGEN DETECTION IN URINE MAY NOT HAVE DIAGNOSTIC VALUE IN SUSPECTED HAEMOPHILUS b DISEASE WITHIN 2 WEEKS OF IMMUNIZATION.

The vial stopper contains dry natural rubber that may cause hypersensitivity reactions when handled by or when the product is injected in persons with known or possible latex sensitivity.

PRECAUTIONS

GENERAL

1. CARE IS TO BE TAKEN BY THE HEALTH CARE PROVIDER FOR SAFE AND EFFECTIVE USE OF THIS PRODUCT.
2. PRIOR TO ADMINISTRATION OF ANY DOSE OF HibTITER, THE PARENT OR GUARDIAN SHOULD BE ASKED ABOUT THE PERSONAL HISTORY, FAMILY HISTORY, AND RECENT HEALTH STATUS OF THE VACCINE RECIPIENT. THE HEALTH CARE PROVIDER SHOULD ASCERTAIN PREVIOUS IMMUNIZATION HISTORY, CURRENT HEALTH STATUS, AND OCCURRENCE OF ANY SYMPTOMS AND/OR SIGNS OF AN ADVERSE EVENT AFTER PREVIOUS IMMUNIZATION IN THE CHILD TO BE IMMUNIZED, IN ORDER TO DETERMINE THE EXISTENCE OF ANY CONTRAINDICATION TO IMMUNIZATION WITH HibTITER AND TO ALLOW AN ASSESSMENT OF BENEFITS AND RISKS.
3. BEFORE THE INJECTION OF ANY BIOLOGICAL, THE HEALTH CARE PROVIDER SHOULD TAKE ALL PRECAUTIONS KNOWN FOR THE PREVENTION OF ALLERGIC OR ANY OTHER SIDE REACTIONS. This should include: a review of the patient's history regarding possible sensitivity; the ready availability of epinephrine 1:1,000 and other appropriate agents used for control of immediate allergic reactions; and a knowledge of the recent literature pertaining to use of the biological concerned, including the nature of side effects and adverse reactions that may follow its use.
4. Children with impaired immune responsiveness, whether due to the use of immunosuppressive therapy (including irradiation, corticosteroids, antimetabolites, alkylating agents, and cytotoxic agents), a genetic defect, human immunodeficiency virus (HIV) infection, or other causes, may have reduced antibody response to active immunization procedures.[37,38] Deferral of administration of vaccine may be considered in individuals receiving immunosuppressive therapy.[37] Other groups should receive this vaccine according to the usual recommended schedule.[37–39] (See **DRUG INTERACTIONS**.)
5. This product is not contraindicated based on the presence of human immunodeficiency virus infection.[40]
6. As reported with Haemophilus b polysaccharide vaccine, cases of Haemophilus b disease may occur prior to the onset of the protective effects of the vaccine.[3,41]
7. The vaccine should not be injected intradermally, subcutaneously, or intravenously since the safety and immunogenicity of these routes have not been evaluated. The vaccine should be given intramuscularly.
8. A separate sterile syringe and needle or a sterile disposable unit should be used for each individual patient to prevent transmission of infectious agents from one person to another. Needles should be disposed of properly and should not be recapped.
9. Special care should be taken to prevent injection into a blood vessel.
10. The vaccine is to be administered immediately after being drawn up into a syringe. Single dose 0.5 mL vial contains no preservative. Use one dose per vial; do not reenter vial. Discard unused portions.

ALTHOUGH SOME ANTIBODY RESPONSE TO DIPHTHERIA TOXIN OCCURS, IMMUNIZATION WITH HibTITER DOES NOT SUBSTITUTE FOR ROUTINE DIPHTHERIA IMMUNIZATION.

The vial stopper contains dry natural rubber that may cause hypersensitivity reactions when handled by or when the product is injected in persons with known or possible latex sensitivity.

INFORMATION FOR PATIENT

PRIOR TO ADMINISTRATION OF HibTITER, HEALTH CARE PERSONNEL SHOULD INFORM THE PARENT, GUARDIAN OR OTHER RESPONSIBLE ADULT, OF THE RECOMMENDED IMMUNIZATION SCHEDULE FOR PROTECTION AGAINST HAEMOPHILUS b DISEASE AND THE BENEFITS AND RISKS TO THE CHILD RECEIVING THIS VACCINE. GUIDANCE SHOULD BE PROVIDED ON MEASURES TO BE TAKEN SHOULD ADVERSE EVENTS OCCUR, SUCH AS, ANTIPYRETIC MEASURES FOR ELEVATED TEMPERATURES AND THE NEED TO REPORT ADVERSE EVENTS TO THE HEALTH CARE PROVIDER. Parents should be provided with vaccine information pamphlets at the time of each vaccination, as stated in the National Childhood Vaccine Injury Act.[42]

PATIENTS, PARENTS, OR GUARDIANS SHOULD BE INSTRUCTED TO REPORT ANY SERIOUS ADVERSE REACTIONS TO THEIR HEALTH CARE PROVIDER.

DRUG INTERACTIONS

Children receiving therapy with immunosuppressive agents (large amounts of corticosteroids, antimetabolites, alkylating agents, cytotoxic agents) may not respond optimally to active immunization.[37,38,39] (See **PRECAUTIONS, GENERAL.**)

As with other intramuscular injections, HibTITER should be given with caution to children on anticoagulant therapy.

No impairment of the antibody response to the individual antigens was demonstrated when HibTITER was given at the same time but at separate sites as DTP plus OPV to children 2 to 20 months of age or MMR to children 15 ± 1 month of age.[20,43,44]

There are no clinical studies where a direct comparison of the immune responses to HibTITER was compared with the concurrent administration of diphtheria and tetanus toxoids and acellular pertussis vaccine (DTaP), hepatitis B vaccine (Hep B), inactivated poliovirus vaccine (IPV), 7-valent Conjugate Vaccine-Diphtheria CRM_{197} Protein (Prevnar), or Varicella vaccine. However, in clinical trials where HibTITER and DTaP or HibTITER, DTaP, IPV, and Hep B vaccines were administered concurrently with or without Prevnar in children at 2, 4, and 6 months of age, the percentage of children achieving Hib antibody levels of ≥0.15 or ≥1.0 μg/mL were similar.[45,46] In one study where children 12-15 months of age were administered a booster dose of HibTITER concurrently with DTaP and Prevnar, some suppression of the Hib antibody response was observed, but over 97% of children achieved titers of ≥1.0 μg/mL.[47,48] However, in another study where a booster dose of HibTITER was administered to children at 12-15 months of age concurrently with or without Prevnar the percentage of children achieving Hib antibody levels of ≥0.15 or ≥1.0 μg/mL was found to be similar.[49,50]

HibTITER and DTaP administered concurrently with and without Prevnar at 2, 4, and 6, and 12–15 months of age did not impair immune responses to the seven Pneumococcal vaccine serotypes in Prevnar.[47,48,51,52]

There are no clinical trials where the local and systemic reactogenicity of HibTITER was directly compared with the concurrent administration of DTaP, Hep B, IPV, Prevnar, or Varicella vaccines.

The American Academy of Pediatrics (AAP), the Advisory Committee on Immunization Practices (ACIP) and the American Academy of Family Physicians (AAFP) encourage routine simultaneous administration of DTaP, IPV, *Haemophilus influenzae* type b vaccine, pneumococcal conjugate vaccine, measles-mumps-rubella (MMR), varicella vaccine and hepatitis B vaccine for children who are the recommended age to receive these vaccines and for whom no specific contraindications exist at the time of the visit, unless, in the judgment of the provider, complete vaccination of the child will not be compromised by administering different vaccines at different visits. Simultaneous administration is particularly important if the child might not return for subsequent vaccinations.[32,33,34,35]

CARCINOGENESIS, MUTAGENESIS, IMPAIRMENT OF FERTILITY

HibTITER has not been evaluated for its carcinogenic, mutagenic potential, or impairment of fertility.

PREGNANCY

REPRODUCTIVE STUDIES— PREGNANCY CATEGORY C

Animal reproduction studies have not been conducted with HibTITER. It is also not known whether HibTITER can cause fetal harm when administered to a pregnant woman or can affect reproduction capability. HibTITER is NOT recommended for use in a pregnant woman.

GERIATRIC USE

This vaccine is NOT recommended for use in adult populations.

PEDIATRIC USE

The safety and effectiveness of HibTITER in children below the age of 6 weeks have not been established.

ADVERSE REACTIONS

Adverse reactions associated with HibTITER have been evaluated in 401 infants who were vaccinated initially at 1 to 6 months of age and were given 1,118 doses independent of DTP vaccine. Observations were made during the day of vaccination and days 1 and 2 postvaccination. A temperature > 38.3°C was recorded at least once during the observation period following 2% of the vaccinations. Local erythema, warmth, or swelling (≥ 2 cm) was observed following 3.3% of vaccinations. The incidence of temperature > 38.3°C was greater during the first postvaccination day than during the day of vaccination or the second postvaccination day. The incidence of local erythema, warmth, or swelling was similar during the day of vaccination and the first postvaccination day; it was lower during the second postvaccination day. All side effects have been infrequent, mild, and transient with no serious sequelae (Table 1). No difference in the rates of these complaints was reported after dose 1, 2, or 3.

[See table 1 above]

TABLE 1

Number of Subjects (Percent) Manifesting Side Effects Associated with HibTITER Administered Independently from DTP* (Infants Vaccinated Initially at 1–6 Months of Age)

	Dose 1 n = 401			Dose 2 n = 383			Dose 3 n = 334		
Symptoms	Same Day As Vacc.	+1 Day	+2 Days	Same Day As Vacc.	+1 Day	+2 Days	Same Day As Vacc.	+1 Day	+2 Days
Temp > 38.3°C	0	2	2	2	3	2	2	6	5
	-	< 1%	< 1%	< 1%	< 1%	< 1%	< 1%	1.8%	1.5%
Redness ≥ 2 cm	1	0	0	1	6	0	5	4	0
	< 1%	-	-	< 1%	1.6%	-	1.5%	1.2%	-
Warmth ≥ 2 cm	1	1	0	2	1	0	1	6	0
	< 1%	< 1%	-	< 1%	< 1%	-	< 1%	1.8%	-
Swelling ≥ 2 cm	5	1	0	2	2	0	1	0	0
	1.2%	< 1%	-	< 1%	< 1%	-	< 1%	-	-

*DTP and HibTITER given 2 weeks apart with DTP having been given first.

The following complaints were also observed after 1,118 vaccinations with HibTITER: irritability (133), sleepiness (91), prolonged crying [≥4 hours] (38), appetite loss (23), vomiting (9), diarrhea (2), and rash (1).

Additional safety data with HibTITER are available from the efficacy studies conducted in young infants.[30] There were 79,483 doses given to 30,844 infants at approximately 2, 4, and 6 months of age in California, usually at the same time as DTP (but at a separate injection site) and OPV; approximately 100,000 doses have been given to 53,000 infants at 4 and 6 months in Finland at the same time as a combined DTP and inactivated polio (IPV) vaccine (but at a separate injection site). The rate and type of reactions associated with the vaccinations were no different from those seen when DTP or DTP-IPV was administered alone. These included fever, local reactions, rash, and one hyporesponsive episode with a single seizure. The safety of HibTITER was also evaluated in the California study by direct phone questioning of the parents or guardians of 6,887 vaccine recipients. The incidence and type of side effects reported within 24 hours of vaccination were similar to those cited in Table 1. In addition, analysis of emergency room (ER) visits within 30 days and hospitalization within 60 days after receipt of 23,800 doses of HibTITER showed no increase in the rates of any type of ER visit or hospitalization.

Table 2 details the side effects associated with a single vaccination of HibTITER given (without DTP) to infants of 15 to 23 months of age.

TABLE 2

Selected Adverse Reactions* in Children of 15–23 Months of Age Following Vaccination with HibTITER

Adverse Reaction	No. of Subjects	Reaction Within 24 h	% Postvaccination At 48 h
Fever >38.3°C	354	1.4	0.6
Erythema	354	2.0	—
Swelling	354	1.7	—
Tenderness	354	3.7	0.3

*The following complaints were reported after vaccination of these 354 children in the indicated number of children: diarrhea (9), vomiting (5), prolonged crying [>4 hours] (4), and rashes (2).

Similar results have been observed in the analysis of 2,285 subjects of 18 to 60 months of age, vaccinated as part of a postmarketing safety study of HibTITER.[20] These data were collected by telephone survey 24 to 48 hours postvaccination. Additional observations included irritability, restless sleep, and GI symptoms (diarrhea, vomiting, and loss of appetite) in the group that received HibTITER alone. A cause and effect relationship between these observations and the vaccinations has not been established.

Post Approval Experience

The following adverse reactions have been identified during post approval use of HibTITER. Because these reactions are reported voluntarily from a population of uncertain size, it is not always possible to reliably estimate their frequency or establish a causal relationship to drug exposure. Decisions to include these reactions in labeling are typically based on one or more of the following factors: (1) seriousness of the reaction, (2) frequency of reporting, or (3) strength of causal connection to the vaccine for post marketing surveillance information.

Continued on next page

Hibtiter—Cont.

Injection Site Reactions
Injection site reactions including hypersensitivity (including urticaria), induration, inflammation, mass, and skin discoloration.
Systemic Events
Anaphylactoid/anaphylactic reactions (including shock), angioneurotic edema, convulsions,[53] erythema multiforme, facial edema, febrile seizures, Guillain-Barré syndrome,[54] headache, hives (urticaria), hypersensitivity reaction, lethargy, and malaise. Also reported, hypotonia or hyporesponsive-hypotonic-episodes (in many instances pertussis-containing vaccine was coadministered).

Reporting of Adverse Reactions

Any suspected adverse events following immunization should be reported by the healthcare professional to the US Department of Health and Human Services (DHHS). The National Vaccine Injury Compensation Program requires that the manufacturer and lot number of the vaccine administered be recorded by the healthcare professional in the vaccine recipient's permanent medical record (or in a permanent office log or file), along with the date of administration of the vaccine and the name, address, and title of the person administering the vaccine. The DHHS has established the Vaccine Adverse Event Reporting System (VAERS) to accept all reports of suspected adverse events after the administration of any vaccine, including but not limited to the reporting of events required by the National Childhood Vaccine Injury Act of 1986.[42] The VAERS FDA web site is:
http://www.fda.gov/cber/vaers/vaers.htm
The VAERS toll-free number for VAERS forms and information is 800-822-7967.
There have been spontaneous reports of apnea in temporal association with the administration of HibTITER. In most cases HibTITER was administered concomitantly with other vaccines including diphtheria tetanus pertussis vaccine (DTP), diphtheria tetanus acellular pertussis vaccine (DTaP), hepatitis B vaccine, inactivated polio vaccine (IPV), oral polio vaccine (OPV), pneumococcal 7-valent conjugate vaccine, measles-mumps-rubella (MMR), and/or meningococcal group C conjugate vaccine (not licensed in the US). In addition, in some of the reports existing medical conditions such as prematurity and/or history of apnea were present.

OVERDOSAGE

There have been reports of overdose with HibTITER. Many cases were due to inadvertent coadministration with another Haemophilus b conjugate-containing vaccine. Most individuals were asymptomatic. In general, adverse events reported with overdosage have also been reported with recommended single doses of HibTITER.

DOSAGE AND ADMINISTRATION

HibTITER is for intramuscular use only.

Any parenteral drug product should be inspected visually for particulate matter and/or discoloration prior to administration whenever solution and container permit. If these conditions exist, or if cloudy, HibTITER should not be administered.
Before injection, the skin over the site to be injected should be cleansed with a suitable germicide. After insertion of the needle, aspirate to help avoid inadvertent injection into a blood vessel.
The vaccine should be injected intramuscularly, preferably into the midlateral muscles of the thigh or deltoid, with care to avoid major peripheral nerve trunks. Do not inject in the gluteal area.
The vaccine is to be administered immediately after being drawn up into a syringe. Single dose 0.5 mL vial contains no preservative. Use one dose per vial; do not re-enter vial. Discard unused portions.
HibTITER is indicated for children 2 months to 71 months of age for the prevention of invasive Haemophilus b disease. For infants 2 to 6 months of age, the immunizing dose is three separate injections of 0.5 mL given at approximately 2-month intervals. Previously unvaccinated infants from 7 through 11 months of age should receive two separate injections approximately 2 months apart. Children from 12 through 14 months of age who have not been vaccinated previously receive one injection. All vaccinated children receive a single booster dose at 15 months of age or older, but not less than 2 months after the previous dose. Previously unvaccinated children 15 to 71 months of age receive a single injection of HibTITER.[32,33] Preterm infants should be vaccinated with HibTITER according to their chronological age, from birth.[32]

Recommended Immunization Schedule

Age at First Immunization (Mo)	No. of Doses	Booster
2–6	3	Yes
7–11	2	Yes
12–14	1	Yes
15 and over	1	No

Interruption of the recommended schedules with a delay between doses does not interfere with the final immunity achieved nor does it necessitate starting the series over again, regardless of the length of time elapsed between doses.[32,33]

Data support that HibTITER may be interchanged with other *Haemophilus influenzae* type b conjugate vaccines for the primary immunization series[55,56]
Each dose of 0.5 mL is formulated to contain 10 µg of purified Haemophilus b saccharide and approximately 25 µg of CRM_{197} protein.

STORAGE

DO NOT FREEZE. Store refrigerated away from freezer compartments at 2°C-8°C (36°F-46°F). Discard if the vaccine has been frozen.

HOW SUPPLIED

Vial, 1 Dose (5 per package) – Product No. 0005-0104-32

REFERENCES

1. United States Patent Number 4,902,506 by Anderson PW, Eby filed May 5, 1986 issued February 20, 1990.
2. Seid RC Jr, Boykins RA, Liu DF, et al. Chemical evidence for covalent linkage of a semi-synthetic glycoconjugate vaccine for *Haemophilus influenzae* type b disease. *Glycoconjugate J.* 1989;6:489-498.
3. Wenger JD, Ward JL, Broome CV. Prevention of *Haemophilus influenzae* type b disease: vaccines and passive prophylaxis. In: Remington JS, Swartz MS, eds. *Current Clinical Topics in Infectious Diseases.* New York, NY: McGraw-Hill Inc; 1989;10: 306-339.
4. Recommendation of the Immunization Practices Advisory Committee (ACIP) – polysaccharide vaccine for prevention of *Haemophilus influenzae* type b disease. *MMWR.* 1985;34:201-205.
5. Sell SH. Long term sequelae of bacterial meningitis in children. *Pediatr Infect Dis J.* 1983;2:90-93.
6. Broome CV. Epidemiology of *Haemophilus influenzae* type b infections in the United States. *Pediatr Infect Dis J.* 1987;6:779-782.
7. Alexander HE. The productive or curative element in type b *Haemophilus influenzae* rabbit serum. *Yale J Biol Med.* 1944;16:425-434.
8. Peltola H, Kayhty H, Sivonen A. *Haemophilus influenzae* type b capsular polysaccharide vaccine in children: a double-blind field study of 100,000 vaccinees 3 months to 5 years of age in Finland. *Pediatrics.* 1977;60:730-737.
9. Robbins JB, Parke JC Jr, Schneerson R. Quantitative measurement of "natural" and immunization-induced *Haemophilus influenzae* type b capsular polysaccharide antibodies. *Pediatr Res.* 1973;7:103-110.
10. Kayhty H, Peltola H, Karanko V, et al. The protective level of serum antibodies to the capsular polysaccharide of *Haemophilus influenzae* type b. *J Infect Dis.* 1983;147:1100.
11. Kayhty H, Karanko V, Peltola H, et al. Serum antibodies after vaccination with *Haemophilus influenzae* type b capsular polysaccharide and responses to reimmunization: no evidence immunologic tolerance or memory. *Pediatrics.* 1984;74:857-865.
12. Weinberg GA, Granoff DM. Polysaccharide-protein conjugate vaccines for the prevention of *Haemophilus influenzae* type b disease. *J Pediatr.* 1988;113:621-631.
13. Makela O, Péterfy F, Outshoorn IG, et al. Immunogenic properties of a (1–6) dextran, its protein conjugates, and conjugates of its breakdown products in mice. *Scand J Immunol.* 1984;19:541-550.
14. Anderson P, Pichichero ME, Insel RA. Immunogens consisting of oligosaccharides from *Haemophilus influenzae* type b coupled to diphtheria toxoid or the toxin protein CRM197. *J Clin Invest.* 1985;76:52-59.
15. Madore DV, Phipps DC, Eby R, et al. Immune response of young children vaccinated with *Haemophilus influenzae* type b conjugate vaccines. In: Cruse JM, Lewis RE, eds. *Contributions to Microbiology and Immunology: Conjugate Vaccines.* New York, NY: Karger Medical and Scientific Publishers; 1989;10:125-150.
16. Madore DV, Phipps DC, Eby R, et al. Safety and immunologic response to *Haemophilus influenzae* type b oligosaccharide-CRM197 conjugate vaccine in 1- to 6-month-old infants. *Pediatrics.* 1990;85:331-337.
17. Madore DV, Johnson CL, Phipps DC, et al. Safety and immunogenicity of *Haemophilus influenzae* type b oligosaccharide-CRM197 conjugate vaccine in infants aged 15–23 months. *Pediatrics.* 1990;86:527-534.
18. Rothstein EP, Madore DV, Long S. Antibody persistence four years after primary immunization of infants and toddlers with *Haemophilus influenzae* type b CRM197 conjugate vaccine. *J Pediatr.* 1991; 119:655-657.
19. Schlesinger Y, Granoff DM. Avidity and bactericidal activity of antibodies elicited by different *Haemophilus influenzae* type b conjugate vaccines. *JAMA.* 1992;267:1489-1494.
20. Unpublished data available from Lederle Laboratories.
21. Gigliotti F, Feldman S, Wang WC, et al. Immunization of young infants with sickle cell disease with a *Haemophilus influenzae* type b saccharide-diphtheria CRM197 protein conjugate vaccine. *J Pediatr.* 1989;114:1006-1010.
22. Black SB, Shinefield HR, The Kaiser Permanente Pediatric Vaccine Study Group. Immunization with oligosaccharide conjugate *Haemophilus influenzae* type b (HbOC) vaccine on a large health maintenance organization population: extended follow-up and impact on *Haemophilus influenzae* disease epidemiology. *Pediatric Infect Dis J.* 1992;11:610-613.
23. Black SB, Shinefield HR, Fireman B, et al. Safety, immunogenicity, and efficacy in infancy of oligosaccharide conjugate *Haemophilus influenzae* type b vaccine in a United States Population: possible implications for optimal use. *J Infect Dis.* 1992;165 (suppl 1):S139-S143.
24. Granoff DM, Anderson EL, Osterholm MT, et al. Differences in the immunogenicity of three *Haemophilus influenzae* type b conjugate vaccines in infants. *J Pediatr.* 1992;121:187-194.
25. Decker MD, Edwards KM, Bradley R, et al. Comparative trial in infants of four conjugate *Haemophilus influenzae* type b vaccines. *J Pediatr.* 1992;120:184-189.
26. Adams WG, Deaver KA, Cochi SL, et al. Decline of childhood *Haemophilus influenzae* type b (Hib) disease in the Hib vaccine era. *JAMA.* 1993;269:221-226.
27. Murphy TV, White KE, Pastor P, et al. Declining incidence of *Haemophilus influenzae* type b disease since introduction of vaccination. *JAMA.* 1993;269:246-248.
28. Broadhurst LE, Erickson RL, Kelley PW. Decreases in invasive *Haemophilus influenzae* diseases in US Army children, 1984 through 1991. *JAMA.* 1993;269:227-231.
29. Shapiro ED. Infections caused by *Haemophilus influenzae* type b: the beginning of the end? *JAMA.* 1993;269:264-266.
30. Black SB, Shinefield HR, Lampert D, et al. Safety and immunogenicity of oligosaccharide conjugate *Haemophilus influenzae* type b (HbOC) vaccine in infancy. *Pediatr Infect Dis J.* 1991;10:92-96.
31. Black SB, Shinefield HR, Fireman B, et al. Efficacy in infancy of oligosaccharide conjugate *Haemophilus influenzae* type b (HbOC) vaccine in a United States Population of 61,080 children. *Pediatr Infect Dis J.* 1991;10:97-104.
32. Recommendations of the AAP: *Haemophilus influenzae* type b conjugate vaccines: recommendations for immunization of infants and children 2 months of age and older: update. *Pediatrics.* 1991;88:169-172.
33. Recommendation of the ACIP: Haemophilus b conjugate vaccines for prevention of *Haemophilus influenzae* type b disease among infants and children two months of age and older. *MMWR.* 1991;40:1-7.
34. Centers for Disease Control and Prevention. General recommendations on immunization: Recommendations of the Advisory Committee on Immunization Practices (ACIP) and the American Academy of Family Physicians (AAFP). *MMWR.* 2002;51(No. RR-2):1-36.
35. 2000 Red Book: Report of the Committee on Infectious Diseases. 25th ed. Elk Grove Village, IL: American Academy of Pediatrics; 2000: 26, 266-72.
36. Jones RG, Bass JW, Weisse ME, et al. Antigenuria after immunization with *Haemophilus influenzae* oligosaccharide CRM197 conjugate (HbOC) vaccine. *Pediatr Infect Dis J.* 1991;10:557-559.
37. American Academy of Pediatrics: Report of the Committee on Infectious Diseases. 22nd ed. Elk Grove Village, Ill: American Academy of Pediatrics; 1991.
38. Recommendation of the ACIP: Immunization of children infected with human T-lymphotrophic virus type III/lymphadenopathy-associated virus. *MMWR.* 1986; 35(38):595-606.
39. Immunization of children infected with human immunodeficiency virus – supplementary ACIP statement. *MMWR.* 1988;37(12):181-183.
40. General Recommendations on Immunization: Recommendations of the Immunization Practices Advisory Committee (ACIP). *MMWR.* 1989;38(13):221.
41. Spinola SM, Sheaffer CI, Philbrick KB, et al. Antigenuria after *Haemophilus influenzae* type b polysaccharide immunization: a prospective study. *J Pediatr.* 1986;109:835-837.
42. CDC. Vaccine Adverse Event Reporting System – United States. *MMWR.* 1990;39:730-733.
43. Paradiso PR. Combined childhood immunizations. *JAMA.* 1992;268:1685.
44. Paradiso PR, Hogerman DA, Madore DV, et al. Safety and immunogenicity of a combined diphtheria, tetanus, pertussis and *Haemophilus influenzae* type b vaccine in young infants. *Pediatrics.* 1993;92(6):827-32.
45. Wyeth Pharmaceuticals, Data on File: Prevnar Study D118-P12.
46. Wyeth Pharmaceuticals, Data on File: Prevnar Study D118-P16.
47. Wyeth Pharmaceuticals, Data on File: Prevnar Study D118-P7.
48. Shinefield H, Black S, Ray P, et al. Safety and immunogenicity of heptavalent pneumococcal CRM_{197} conjugate vaccine in infants and toddlers. *Pediatr Infect Dis J.* 1999;18:757-63.
49. Wyeth Pharmaceuticals, Data on File: Prevnar Study D118-P3.
50. Rennels MB, Edwards KM, Keyserling HL, et al. Safety and immunogenicity of heptavalent pneumococcal vaccine conjugated to CRM_{197} in United States infants. *Pediatrics.* 1998;101(4):604-11.
51. Wyeth Pharmaceuticals, Data on File: Prevnar Study D118-P8.
52. Black S, Shinefield H, Fireman B, et al. Efficacy, safety and immunogenicity of heptavalent pneumococcal conjugate vaccine in children. *Pediatr Infect Dis J.* 2000;19:187-95.
53. Milstein JB, Gross TP, Kuritsky JN. Adverse reactions reported following receipt of *Haemophilus influenzae* type b vaccine: an analysis after one year of marketing. *Pediatrics.* 1987;80:270-274.
54. D'Cruz DF, Shapiro ED, Spiegelman KN, et al. Acute inflammatory demyelinating polyradiculoneuropathy

(Guillain-Barré syndrome) after immunization with *Haemophilus influenzae* type b conjugate vaccine. *J Pediatr*. 1989;115:743-746.
55. Greenberg DP, Lieberman JM, Marcy SM, et al. Enhanced antibody responses in infants given different sequences of heterogeneous *Haemophilus influenzae* type b conjugate vaccines. *J Pediatr*. 1995;126:206-11.
56. Anderson EL, Decker MD, Englund JA, et al. Interchangeability of conjugated *Haemophilus influenzae* type b vaccines in infants. *JAMA*. 1995;273:849-53.

Wyeth®
Manufactured by: W10461C003
Wyeth Pharmaceuticals Inc. ET01
Philadelphia, PA 19101 Rev 01/04
US Govt. License No. 3

INDERAL® LA ℞
[*In' der-āl*]
(propranolol hydrochloride)
Long-Acting Capsules
℞ only

Prescribing information for this product, which appears on pages 3430–3431 of the 2004 PDR, has been revised as follows. Please write "See Supplement A" next to the product heading.

In the **WARNINGS** *section, the following has been added to the beginning of the section:*
Hypersensitivity reactions, including anaphylactic/anaphylactoid reactions, have been associated with the administration of propranolol (see "**ADVERSE REACTIONS**").

In the **WARNINGS** *section, the following has been added to the end of the section:*
Skin Reactions: Cutaneous reactions, including Stevens-Johnson Syndrome, toxic epidermal necrolysis, exfoliative dermatitis, erythema multiforme, and urticaria, have been reported with use of propranolol (see "**ADVERSE REACTIONS**").

In the **ADVERSE REACTIONS** *section, the "Allergic" subsection has been revised as follows:*
Allergic: Hypersensitivity reactions, including anaphylactic/anaphylactoid reactions, pharyngitis and agranulocytosis, erythematous rash, fever combined with aching and sore throat, laryngospasm, and respiratory distress.

In the **ADVERSE REACTIONS** *section, the following subsection has been added to the end of the section:*
Skin: Stevens-Johnson Syndrome, toxic epidermal necrolysis, exfoliative dermatitis, erythema multiforme, and urticaria.

Wyeth Pharmaceuticals Inc.
Philadelphia, PA 19101
W10478C002 ET01
Rev 11/03

LO/OVRAL®-28 ℞
[*lō' ōvrăl*]
Tablets
(NORGESTREL AND ETHINYL ESTRADIOL TABLETS)

℞ only

Prescribing information for this product, which appears on pages 3431–3437 of the 2004 PDR, has been completely revised as follows. Please write "See Supplement A" next to the product heading.

Patients should be counseled that oral contraceptives do not protect against transmission of HIV (AIDS) and other sexually transmitted diseases (STDs) such as chlamydia, genital herpes, genital warts, gonorrhea, hepatitis B, and syphilis.

DESCRIPTION

21 white LO/OVRAL tablets, each containing 0.3 mg of norgestrel (*dl*-13-beta-ethyl-17-alpha-ethinyl-17-beta-hydroxygon-4-en-3-one), a totally synthetic progestogen, and 0.03 mg of ethinyl estradiol (19-nor-17α-pregna-1,3,5 (10)-trien-20-yne-3,17-diol), and 7 pink inert tablets. The inactive ingredients present are cellulose, D&C Red 30, lactose, magnesium stearate, and polacrilin potassium.

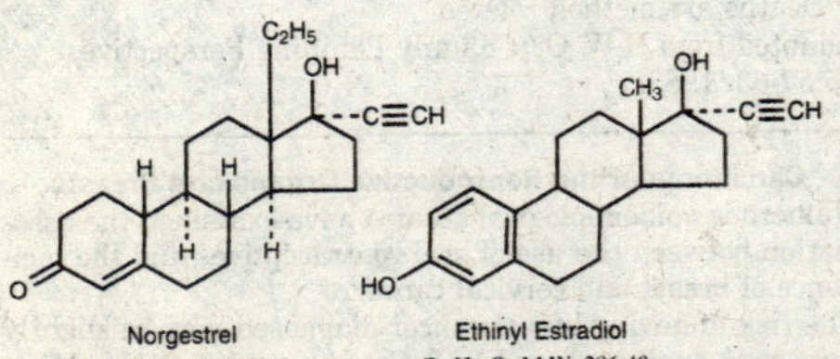

Norgestrel — $C_{21}H_{28}O_2$ M.W. 312.45
Ethinyl Estradiol — $C_{20}H_{24}O_2$ M.W. 296.40

CLINICAL PHARMACOLOGY

Mode of Action

Combination oral contraceptives act by suppression of gonadotropins. Although the primary mechanism of this action is inhibition of ovulation, other alterations include changes in the cervical mucus (which increase the difficulty of sperm entry into the uterus) and the endometrium (which reduce the likelihood of implantation).

Table I: Percentage Of Women Experiencing An Unintended Pregnancy During The First Year Of Typical Use And The First Year Of Perfect Use Of Contraception And The Percentage Continuing Use At The End Of The First Year. United States.

Method (1)	% of Women Experiencing an Unintended Pregnancy within the First Year of Use — Typical Use[1] (2)	Perfect Use[2] (3)	% of Women Continuing Use at One Year[3] (4)
Chance[4]	85	85	
Spermicides[5]	26	6	40
Periodic abstinence	25		63
Calendar		9	
Ovulation Method		3	
Sympto-Thermal[6]		2	
Post-Ovulation		1	
Cap[7]			
Parous Women	40	26	42
Nulliparous Women	20	9	56
Sponge			
Parous Women	40	20	42
Nulliparous Women	20	9	56
Diaphragm[7]	20	6	56
Withdrawal	19	4	
Condom[8]			
Female (Reality)	21	5	56
Male	14	3	61
Pill	5		71
Progestin only		0.5	
Combined		0.1	
IUD			
Progesterone T	2.0	1.5	81
Copper T380A	0.8	0.6	78
LNg 20	0.1	0.1	81
Depo-Provera®	0.3	0.3	70
Levonorgestrel Implants (Norplant®)	0.05	0.05	88
Female Sterilization	0.5	0.5	100
Male Sterilization	0.15	0.10	100

Lactation Amenorrhea Method: LAM is a highly effective, temporary method of contraception.[9]

Source: Trussell J. Contraceptive efficacy. In: Hatcher RA, Trussell J, Stewart F, Cates W, Stewart GK, Kowel D, Guest F. Contraceptive Technology: Seventeenth Revised Edition. New York NY: Irvington Publishers; 1998.

1. Among *typical* couples who initiate use of a method (not necessarily for the first time), the percentage who experience an accidental pregnancy during the first year if they do not stop use for any other reason.
2. Among couples who initiate use of a method (not necessarily for the first time) and who use it *perfectly* (both consistently and correctly), the percentage who experience an accidental pregnancy during the first year if they do not stop use for any other reason.
3. Among couples attempting to avoid pregnancy, the percentage who continue to use a method for one year.
4. The percents becoming pregnant in columns (2) and (3) are based on data from populations where contraception is not used and from women who cease using contraception in order to become pregnant. Among such populations, about 89% become pregnant within one year. This estimate was lowered slightly (to 85%) to represent the percent who would become pregnant within one year among women now relying on reversible methods of contraception if they abandoned contraception altogether.
5. Foams, creams, gels, vaginal suppositories, and vaginal film.
6. Cervical mucus (ovulation) method supplemented by calendar in the pre-ovulatory and basal body temperature in the post-ovulatory phases.
7. With spermicidal cream or jelly.
8. Without spermicides.
9. However, to maintain effective protection against pregnancy, another method of contraception must be used as soon as menstruation resumes, the frequency or duration of breastfeeds is reduced, bottle feeds are introduced, or the baby reaches 6 months of age.

INDICATIONS AND USAGE

Oral contraceptives are indicated for the prevention of pregnancy in women who elect to use this product as a method of contraception.

Oral contraceptives are highly effective. Table I lists the typical accidental pregnancy rates for users of combination oral contraceptives and other methods of contraception. The efficacy of these contraceptive methods, except sterilization, the IUD, and implants depends upon the reliability with which they are used. Correct and consistent use of methods can result in lower failure rates.

[See table I above]

CONTRAINDICATIONS

Combination oral contraceptives should not be used in women with any of the following conditions:

Thrombophlebitis or thromboembolic disorders
A past history of deep-vein thrombophlebitis or thromboembolic disorders
Cerebral-vascular or coronary-artery disease (current or history)
Thrombogenic valvulopathies
Thrombogenic rhythm disorders
Major surgery with prolonged immobilization
Diabetes with vascular involvement
Headaches with focal neurological symptoms
Uncontrolled hypertension
Known or suspected carcinoma of the breast or personal history of breast cancer

Continued on next page

Lo/Ovral-28—Cont.

Carcinoma of the endometrium or other known or suspected estrogen-dependent neoplasia
Undiagnosed abnormal genital bleeding
Cholestatic jaundice of pregnancy or jaundice with prior pill use
Hepatic adenomas or carcinomas, or active liver disease, as long as liver function has not returned to normal
Known or suspected pregnancy
Hypersensitivity to any of the components of Lo/Ovral-28

WARNINGS

Cigarette smoking increases the risk of serious cardiovascular side effects from oral-contraceptive use. This risk increases with age and with the extent of smoking (in epidemiologic studies, 15 or more cigarettes per day was associated with a significantly increased risk) and is quite marked in women over 35 years of age. Women who use oral contraceptives should be strongly advised not to smoke.

The use of oral contraceptives is associated with increased risks of several serious conditions including venous and arterial thrombotic and thromboembolic events (such as myocardial infarction, thromboembolism, and stroke), hepatic neoplasia, gallbladder disease, and hypertension, although the risk of serious morbidity or mortality is very small in healthy women without underlying risk factors. The risk of morbidity and mortality increases significantly in the presence of other underlying risk factors such as certain inherited or acquired thrombophilias, hypertension, hyperlipidemias, obesity, diabetes, and surgery or trauma with increased risk of thrombosis.

Practitioners prescribing oral contraceptives should be familiar with the following information relating to these risks.

The information contained in this package insert is based principally on studies carried out in patients who used oral contraceptives with higher doses of estrogens and progestogens than those in common use today. The effect of long-term use of the oral contraceptives with lower doses of both estrogens and progestogens remains to be determined.

Throughout this labeling, epidemiological studies reported are of two types: retrospective or case control studies and prospective or cohort studies. Case control studies provide a measure of the relative risk of disease, namely, a ratio of the incidence of a disease among oral-contraceptive users to that among nonusers. The relative risk does not provide information on the actual clinical occurrence of a disease. Cohort studies provide a measure of attributable risk, which is the difference in the incidence of disease between oral-contraceptive users and nonusers. The attributable risk does provide information about the actual occurrence of a disease in the population. For further information, the reader is referred to a text on epidemiological methods.

1. **Thromboembolic Disorders And Other Vascular Problems**

a. *Myocardial infarction*

An increased risk of myocardial infarction has been attributed to oral-contraceptive use. This risk is primarily in smokers or women with other underlying risk factors for coronary-artery disease such as hypertension, hypercholesterolemia, morbid obesity, and diabetes. The relative risk of heart attack for current oral-contraceptive users has been estimated to be two to six. The risk is very low under the age of 30.

Smoking in combination with oral-contraceptive use has been shown to contribute substantially to the incidence of myocardial infarctions in women in their mid-thirties or older with smoking accounting for the majority of excess cases. Mortality rates associated with circulatory disease have been shown to increase substantially in smokers over the age of 35 and nonsmokers over the age of 40 (Table II) among women who use oral contraceptives.

[See table II at top of next column]

CIRCULATORY DISEASE MORTALITY RATES PER 100,000 WOMAN YEARS BY AGE, SMOKING STATUS AND ORAL-CONTRACEPTIVE USE

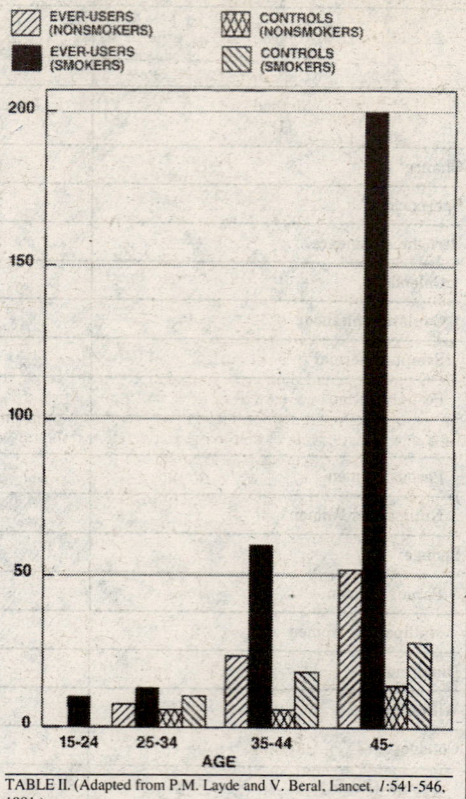

TABLE II. (Adapted from P.M. Layde and V. Beral, Lancet, *1*:541-546, 1981.)

Oral contraceptives may compound the effects of well-known risk factors, such as hypertension, diabetes, hyperlipidemias, age, and obesity. In particular, some progestogens are known to decrease HDL cholesterol and cause glucose intolerance, while estrogens may create a state of hyperinsulinism. Oral contraceptives have been shown to increase blood pressure among users (see section 9 in **WARNINGS**). Similar effects on risk factors have been associated with an increased risk of heart disease. Oral contraceptives must be used with caution in women with cardiovascular disease risk factors.

b. *Venous thrombosis and thromboembolism*

An increased risk of venous thromboembolic and thrombotic disease associated with the use of oral contraceptives is well established. Case control studies have found the relative risk of users compared to nonusers to be 3 for the first episode of superficial venous thrombosis, 4 to 11 for deep-vein thrombosis or pulmonary embolism, and 1.5 to 6 for women with predisposing conditions for venous thromboembolic disease. Cohort studies have shown the relative risk to be somewhat lower, about 3 for new cases and about 4.5 for new cases requiring hospitalization. The approximate incidence of deep-vein thrombosis and pulmonary embolism in users of low dose (<50 mcg ethinyl estradiol) combination oral contraceptives is up to 4 per 10,000 woman-years compared to 0.5-3 per 10,000 woman-years for non-users. However, the incidence is substantially less than that associated with pregnancy (6 per 10,000 woman-years). The excess risk is highest during the first year a woman ever uses a combined oral contraceptive. Venous thromboembolism may be fatal. The risk of venous thrombotic and thromboembolic events is further increased in women with conditions predisposing for venous thrombosis and thromboembolism. The risk of thromboembolic disease due to oral contraceptives is not related to length of use and gradually disappears after pill use is stopped.

A two- to four-fold increase in relative risk of postoperative thromboembolic complications has been reported with the use of oral contraceptives. The relative risk of venous thrombosis in women who have predisposing conditions is twice that of women without such medical conditions. If feasible, oral contraceptives should be discontinued at least four weeks prior to and for two weeks after elective surgery of a type associated with an increase in risk of thromboembolism and during and following prolonged immobilization. Since the immediate postpartum period is also associated with an increased risk of thromboembolism, oral contraceptives should be started no earlier than four weeks after delivery in women who elect not to breast-feed, or a midtrimester pregnancy termination.

c. *Cerebrovascular diseases*

Oral contraceptives have been shown to increase both the relative and attributable risks of cerebrovascular events (thrombotic and hemorrhagic strokes), although, in general, the risk is greatest among older (>35 years), hypertensive women who also smoke. Hypertension was found to be a risk factor for both users and nonusers, for both types of strokes, while smoking interacted to increase the risk for hemorrhagic strokes.

In a large study, the relative risk of thrombotic strokes has been shown to range from 3 for normotensive users to 14 for users with severe hypertension. The relative risk of hemorrhagic stroke is reported to be 1.2 for nonsmokers who used oral contraceptives, 2.6 for smokers who did not use oral contraceptives, 7.6 for smokers who used oral contraceptives, 1.8 for normotensive users, and 25.7 for users with severe hypertension. The attributable risk is also greater in older women. Oral contraceptives also increase the risk for stroke in women with other underlying risk factors such as certain inherited or acquired thrombophilias, hyperlipidemias, and obesity.

Women with migraine (particularly migraine/headaches with focal neurological symptoms, see **CONTRAINDICATIONS**) who take combination oral contraceptives may be at an increased risk of stroke.

d. *Dose-related risk of vascular disease from oral contraceptives*

A positive association has been observed between the amount of estrogen and progestogen in oral contraceptives and the risk of vascular disease. A decline in serum high-density lipoproteins (HDL) has been reported with many progestational agents. A decline in serum high-density lipoproteins has been associated with an increased incidence of ischemic heart disease. Because estrogens increase HDL cholesterol, the net effect of an oral contraceptive depends on a balance achieved between doses of estrogen and progestogen and the nature and absolute amount of progestogen used in the contraceptive. The amount of both hormones should be considered in the choice of an oral contraceptive.

Minimizing exposure to estrogen and progestogen is in keeping with good principles of therapeutics. For any particular estrogen/progestogen combination, the dosage regimen prescribed should be one which contains the least amount of estrogen and progestogen that is compatible with a low failure rate and the needs of the individual patient. New acceptors of oral-contraceptive agents should be started on preparations containing the lowest estrogen content which is judged appropriate for the individual patient.

e. *Persistence of risk of vascular disease*

There are two studies which have shown persistence of risk of vascular disease for ever-users of oral contraceptives. In a study in the United States, the risk of developing myocardial infarction after discontinuing oral contraceptives persists for at least 9 years for women 40 to 49 years who had used oral contraceptives for five or more years, but this increased risk was not demonstrated in other age groups. In another study in Great Britain, the risk of developing cerebrovascular disease persisted for at least 6 years after discontinuation of oral contraceptives, although excess risk was very small. However, both studies were performed with oral-contraceptive formulations containing 50 mcg or higher of estrogen.

2. **Estimates of Mortality from Contraceptive Use**

One study gathered data from a variety of sources which have estimated the mortality rate associated with different methods of contraception at different ages (Table III). These estimates include the combined risk of death associated with contraceptive methods plus the risk attributable to pregnancy in the event of method failure. Each method of contraception has its specific benefits and risks. The study concluded that with the exception of oral-contraceptive users 35 and older who smoke and 40 and older who do not smoke, mortality associated with all methods of birth control is less than that associated with childbirth. The observation of a possible increase in risk of mortality with age for oral-contraceptive users is based on data gathered in the 1970's—but not reported until 1983. However, current clinical practice involves the use of lower estrogen dose formulations combined with careful restriction of oral-contraceptive use to women who do not have the various risk factors listed in this labeling.

Because of these changes in practice and, also, because of some limited new data which suggest that the risk of cardiovascular disease with the use of oral contraceptives may now be less than previously observed, the Fertility and Maternal Health Drugs Advisory Committee was asked to review the topic in 1989. The Committee concluded that although cardiovascular-disease risks may be increased with oral-contraceptive use after age 40 in healthy nonsmoking women (even with the newer low-dose formulations), there are greater potential health risks associated with pregnancy in older women and with the alternative surgical and medical procedures which may be necessary if such women do not have access to effective and acceptable means of contraception.

Therefore, the Committee recommended that the benefits of oral-contraceptive use by healthy nonsmoking women over 40 may outweigh the possible risks. Of course, older women, as all women who take oral contraceptives, should take the lowest possible dose formulation that is effective.

TABLE III–ANNUAL NUMBER OF BIRTH-RELATED OR METHOD-RELATED DEATHS ASSOCIATED WITH CONTROL OF FERTILITY PER 100,000 NONSTERILE WOMEN, BY FERTILITY-CONTROL METHOD AND ACCORDING TO AGE

Method of control and outcome	15-19	20-24	25-29	30-34	35-39	40-44
No fertility-control methods*	7.0	7.4	9.1	14.8	25.7	28.2
Oral contraceptives nonsmoker**	0.3	0.5	0.9	1.9	13.8	31.6
Oral contraceptives smoker**	2.2	3.4	6.6	13.5	51.1	117.2
IUD**	0.8	0.8	1.0	1.0	1.4	1.4
Condom*	1.1	1.6	0.7	0.2	0.3	0.4
Diaphragm/ spermicide*	1.9	1.2	1.2	1.3	2.2	2.8
Periodic abstinence*	2.5	1.6	1.6	1.7	2.9	3.6

*Deaths are birth related
**Deaths are method related
Adapted from H.W. Ory, Family Planning Perspectives, *15*:57-63, 1983.

3. **Carcinoma of the Reproductive Organs and Breasts**

Numerous epidemiological studies have examined the association between the use of oral contraceptives and the incidence of breast and cervical cancer.

The risk of having breast cancer diagnosed may be slightly increased among current and recent users of COCs. However, this excess risk appears to decrease over time after COC discontinuation and by 10 years after cessation the increased risk disappears. Some studies report an increased risk with duration of use while other studies do not and no consistent relationships have been found with dose or type of steroid. Some studies have reported a small increase in risk for women who first use COCs at a younger age. Most studies show a similar pattern of risk with COC use regardless of a woman's reproductive history or her family breast cancer history.

Breast cancers diagnosed in current or previous OC users tend to be less clinically advanced than in nonusers.
Women with known or suspected carcinoma of the breast or personal history of breast cancer should not use oral contraceptives because breast cancer is usually a hormonally-sensitive tumor.
Some studies suggest that oral-contraceptive use has been associated with an increase in the risk of cervical intraepithelial neoplasia or invasive cervical cancer in some populations of women. However, there continues to be controversy about the extent to which such findings may be due to differences in sexual behavior and other factors.
In spite of many studies of the relationship between combination oral-contraceptive use and breast and cervical cancers, a cause-and-effect relationship has not been established.

4. **Hepatic Neoplasia**
Benign hepatic adenomas are associated with oral-contraceptive use, although the incidence of benign tumors is rare in the United States. Indirect calculations have estimated the attributable risk to be in the range of 3.3 cases/100,000 for users, a risk that increases after four or more years of use. Rupture of rare, benign, hepatic adenomas may cause death through intra-abdominal hemorrhage.
Studies from Britain have shown an increased risk of developing hepatocellular carcinoma in long-term (>8 years) oral-contraceptive users.
However, these cancers are extremely rare in the U.S., and the attributable risk (the excess incidence) of liver cancers in oral-contraceptive users approaches less than one per million users.

5. **Ocular Lesions**
There have been clinical case reports of retinal thrombosis associated with the use of oral contraceptives that may lead to partial or complete loss of vision. Oral contraceptives should be discontinued if there is unexplained partial or complete loss of vision; onset of proptosis or diplopia; papilledema; or retinal vascular lesions. Appropriate diagnostic and therapeutic measures should be undertaken immediately.

6. **Oral-Contraceptive Use Before or During Early Pregnancy**
Extensive epidemiological studies have revealed no increased risk of birth defects in infants born to women who have used oral contraceptives prior to pregnancy. Studies also do not suggest a teratogenic effect, particularly insofar as cardiac anomalies and limb-reduction defects are concerned, when taken inadvertently during early pregnancy (see **CONTRAINDICATIONS** section).
The administration of oral contraceptives to induce withdrawal bleeding should not be used as a test for pregnancy. Oral contraceptives should not be used during pregnancy to treat threatened or habitual abortion.
It is recommended that for any patient who has missed two consecutive periods, pregnancy should be ruled out before continuing oral-contraceptive use. If the patient has not adhered to the prescribed schedule, the possibility of pregnancy should be considered at the time of the first missed period. Oral-contraceptive use should be discontinued if pregnancy is confirmed.

7. **Gallbladder Disease**
Combination oral contraceptives may worsen existing gallbladder disease and may accelerate the development of this disease in previously asymptomatic women. Earlier studies have reported an increased lifetime relative risk of gallbladder surgery in users of oral contraceptives and estrogens. More recent studies, however, have shown that the relative risk of developing gallbladder disease among oral-contraceptive users may be minimal. The recent findings of minimal risk may be related to the use of oral-contraceptive formulations containing lower hormonal doses of estrogens and progestogens.

8. **Carbohydrate and Lipid Metabolic Effects**
Oral contraceptives have been shown to cause glucose intolerance in a significant percentage of users. Oral contraceptives containing greater than 75 mcg of estrogens cause hyperinsulinism, while lower doses of estrogen cause less glucose intolerance. Progestogens increase insulin secretion and create insulin resistance, this effect varying with different progestational agents. However, in the nondiabetic woman, oral contraceptives appear to have no effect on fasting blood glucose. Because of these demonstrated effects, prediabetic and diabetic women should be carefully observed while taking oral contraceptives.
A small proportion of women will have persistent hypertriglyceridemia while on the pill. As discussed earlier (see **WARNINGS**, 1a. and 1d.; **PRECAUTIONS**, 3.), changes in serum triglycerides and lipoprotein levels have been reported in oral-contraceptive users.

9. **Elevated Blood Pressure**
Women with uncontrolled hypertension should not be started on hormonal contraception. An increase in blood pressure has been reported in women taking oral contraceptives, and this increase is more likely in older oral-contraceptive users and with continued use. Data from the Royal College of General Practitioners and subsequent randomized trials have shown that the incidence of hypertension increases with increasing quantities of progestogens.
Women with a history of hypertension or hypertension-related diseases, or renal disease, should be encouraged to use another method of contraception. If women with hypertension elect to use oral contraceptives, they should be monitored closely, and if significant elevation of blood pressure occurs, oral contraceptives should be discontinued (see **CONTRAINDICATIONS** section). For most women, elevated blood pressure will return to normal after stopping oral contraceptives, and there is no difference in the occurrence of hypertension among ever- and never-users.

10. **Headache**
The onset or exacerbation of migraine or development of headache with a new pattern that is recurrent, persistent, or severe requires discontinuation of oral contraceptives and evaluation of the cause. (See **WARNINGS**, 1c. and **CONTRAINDICATIONS**.)

11. **Bleeding Irregularities**
Breakthrough bleeding and spotting are sometimes encountered in patients on oral contraceptives, especially during the first three months of use. The type and dose of progestogen may be important. If bleeding persists or recurs, nonhormonal causes should be considered and adequate diagnostic measures taken to rule out malignancy or pregnancy in the event of breakthrough bleeding, as in the case of any abnormal vaginal bleeding. If pathology has been excluded, time or a change to another formulation may solve the problem. In some women withdrawal bleeding may not occur during the "tablet-free" or "inactive-tablet" interval. If the COC has not been taken according to directions prior to the first missed withdrawal bleed, or if two consecutive withdrawal bleeds are missed, tablet-taking should be discontinued and a nonhormonal method of contraception should be used until the possibility of pregnancy is excluded.
Some women may encounter post-pill amenorrhea or oligomenorrhea (possibly with anovulation), especially when such a condition was pre-existent.

12. **Ectopic Pregnancy**
Ectopic as well as intrauterine pregnancy may occur in contraceptive failures.

PRECAUTIONS

1. **General**
Patients should be counseled that oral contraceptives do not protect against transmission of HIV (AIDS) and other sexually transmitted diseases (STDs) such as chlamydia, genital herpes, genital warts, gonorrhea, hepatitis B, and syphilis.

2. **Physical Examination and Follow-Up**
A periodic personal and family medical history and complete physical examination are appropriate for all women, including women using oral contraceptives. The physical examination, however, may be deferred until after initiation of oral contraceptives if requested by the woman and judged appropriate by the clinician. The physical examination should include special reference to blood pressure, breasts, abdomen and pelvic organs, including cervical cytology, and relevant laboratory tests. In case of undiagnosed, persistent or recurrent abnormal vaginal bleeding, appropriate diagnostic measures should be conducted to rule out malignancy. Women with a strong family history of breast cancer or who have breast nodules should be monitored with particular care.

3. **Lipid Disorders**
Women who are being treated for hyperlipidemias should be followed closely if they elect to use oral contraceptives. Some progestogens may elevate LDL levels and may render the control of hyperlipidemias more difficult. (See **WARNINGS**, 1a., 1d., and 8.)
In patients with defects of lipoprotein metabolism, estrogen-containing preparations may be associated with rare but significant elevations of plasma triglycerides which may lead to pancreatitis.

4. **Liver Function**
If jaundice develops in any woman receiving hormonal contraceptives, the medication should be discontinued. Steroid hormones may be poorly metabolized in patients with impaired liver function.

5. **Fluid Retention**
Oral contraceptives may cause some degree of fluid retention. They should be prescribed with caution, and only with careful monitoring, in patients with conditions which might be aggravated by fluid retention.

6. **Emotional Disorders**
Patients becoming significantly depressed while taking oral contraceptives should stop the medication and use an alternate method of contraception in an attempt to determine whether the symptom is drug-related. Women with a history of depression should be carefully observed and the drug discontinued if significant depression occurs.

7. **Contact Lenses**
Contact-lens wearers who develop visual changes or changes in lens tolerance should be assessed by an ophthalmologist.

8. **Gastrointestinal**
Diarrhea and/or vomiting may reduce hormone absorption resulting in decreased serum concentrations.

9. **Drug Interactions**
Changes in contraceptive effectiveness associated with coadministration of other products:
Contraceptive effectiveness may be reduced when hormonal contraceptives are coadministered with antibiotics, anticonvulsants, and other drugs that increase the metabolism of contraceptive steroids. This could result in unintended pregnancy or breakthrough bleeding. Examples include rifampin, rifabutin, barbiturates, primidone, phenylbutazone, phenytoin, dexamethasone, carbamazepine, felbamate, oxcarbazepine, topiramate, griseofulvin, and modafinil.
Several cases of contraceptive failure and breakthrough bleeding have been reported in the literature with concomitant administration of antibiotics such as ampicillin and other penicillins, and tetracyclines, possibly due to a decrease of enterohepatic recirculation of estrogens. However, clinical pharmacology studies investigating drug interactions between combined oral contraceptives and these antibiotics have reported inconsistent results. Enterohepatic recirculation of estrogens may also be decreased by substances that reduce gut transit time.
Several of the anti-HIV protease inhibitors have been studied with coadministration of oral combination hormonal contraceptives; significant changes (increase and decrease) in the plasma levels of the estrogen and progestin have been noted in some cases. The safety and efficacy of oral contraceptive products may be affected with coadministration of anti-HIV protease inhibitors. Health-care professionals should refer to the label of the individual anti-HIV protease inhibitors for further drug-drug interaction information.
Herbal products containing St. John's Wort (Hypericum perforatum) may induce hepatic enzymes (cytochrome P 450) and p-glycoprotein transporter and may reduce the effectiveness of contraceptive steroids. This may also result in breakthrough bleeding.
During concomitant use of ethinyl estradiol containing products and substances that may lead to decreased plasma steroid hormone concentrations, it is recommended that a nonhormonal back-up method of birth control be used in addition to the regular intake of Lo/Ovral-28. If the use of a substance which leads to decreased ethinyl estradiol plasma concentrations is required for a prolonged period of time, combination oral contraceptives should not be considered the primary contraceptive.
After discontinuation of substances that may lead to decreased ethinyl estradiol plasma concentrations, use of a nonhormonal back-up method of birth control is recommended for 7 days. Longer use of a back-up method is advisable after discontinuation of substances that have led to induction of hepatic microsomal enzymes, resulting in decreased ethinyl estradiol concentrations. It may take several weeks until enzyme induction has completely subsided, depending on dosage, duration of use, and rate of elimination of the inducing substance.
Increase in plasma levels associated with coadministered drugs:
Coadministration of atorvastatin and certain oral contraceptives containing ethinyl estradiol increase AUC values for ethinyl estradiol by approximately 20%. The mechanism of this interaction is unknown. Ascorbic acid and acetaminophen increase the bioavailability of ethinyl estradiol since these drugs act as competitive inhibitors for sulfation of ethinyl estradiol in the gastrointestinal wall, a known pathway of elimination for ethinyl estradiol. CYP 3A4 inhibitors such as indinavir, itraconazole, ketoconazole, fluconazole, and troleandomycin may increase plasma hormone levels. Troleandomycin may also increase the risk of intrahepatic cholestasis during coadministration with combination oral contraceptives.
Changes in plasma levels of coadministered drugs:
Combination hormonal contraceptives containing some synthetic estrogens (eg, ethinyl estradiol) may inhibit the metabolism of other compounds. Increased plasma concentrations of cyclosporin, prednisolone and other corticosteroids, and theophylline have been reported with concomitant administration of oral contraceptives. Decreased plasma concentrations of acetaminophen and increased clearance of temazepam, salicylic acid, morphine, and clofibric acid, due to induction of conjugation (particularly glucuronidation), have been noted when these drugs were administered with oral contraceptives.
The prescribing information of concomitant medications should be consulted to identify potential interactions.

10. **Interactions With Laboratory Tests**
Certain endocrine- and liver-function tests and blood components may be affected by oral contraceptives:
a. Increased prothrombin and factors VII, VIII, IX, and X; decreased antithrombin 3; increased norepinephrine-induced platelet aggregability.
b. Increased thyroid-binding globulin (TBG) leading to increased circulating total thyroid hormone, as measured by protein-bound iodine (PBI), T_4 by column or by radioimmunoassay. Free T_3 resin uptake is decreased, reflecting the elevated TBG; free T_4 concentration is unaltered.
c. Other binding proteins may be elevated in serum ie, corticosteroid binding globulin (CBG), sex hormone-binding globulins (SHBG) leading to increased levels of total circulating corticosteroids and sex steroids respectively. Free or biologically active hormone concentrations are unchanged.
d. Triglycerides may be increased and levels of various other lipids and lipoproteins may be affected.
e. Glucose tolerance may be decreased.
f. Serum folate levels may be depressed by oral-contraceptive therapy.
This may be of clinical significance if a woman becomes pregnant shortly after discontinuing oral contraceptives.

11. **Carcinogenesis**
See **WARNINGS** section.

12. **Pregnancy**
Pregnancy Category X. See **CONTRAINDICATIONS** and **WARNINGS** sections.

13. **Nursing Mothers**
Small amounts of oral-contraceptive steroids and/or metabolites have been identified in the milk of nursing mothers, and a few adverse effects on the child have been reported, including jaundice and breast enlargement. In addition, combination oral contraceptives given in the postpartum period may interfere with lactation by decreasing the quantity

Continued on next page

Lo/Ovral-28—Cont.

and quality of breast milk. If possible, the nursing mother should be advised not to use combination oral contraceptives but to use other forms of contraception until she has completely weaned her child.

14. **Fertility Following Discontinuation**
Users of combination oral contraceptives may experience some delay in becoming pregnant after discontinuation of COCs, especially those women who had irregular menstrual cycles prior to use. Conception may be delayed an average of 1–2 months among women stopping COCs compared to women stopping nonhormonal contraceptive methods.
Women who do not wish to become pregnant after discontinuation of COCs should be advised to use another method of birth control.

15. **Pediatric Use**
Safety and efficacy of Lo/Ovral-28 tablets have been established in women of reproductive age. Safety and efficacy are expected to be the same for postpubertal adolescents under the age of 16 and for users 16 years and older. Use of this product before menarche is not indicated.

16. **Geriatric Use**
This product has not been studied in women over 65 years of age and is not indicated in this population.

Information for the Patient
See Patient Labeling Printed Below.

ADVERSE REACTIONS

An increased risk of the following serious adverse reactions (see **WARNINGS** section for additional information) has been associated with the use of oral contraceptives:
Thromboembolic and thrombotic disorders and other vascular problems (including thrombophlebitis and venous thrombosis with or without pulmonary embolism, mesenteric thrombosis, arterial thromboembolism, myocardial infarction, cerebral hemorrhage, cerebral thrombosis), carcinoma of the reproductive organs and breasts, hepatic neoplasia (including hepatic adenomas or benign liver tumors), ocular lesions (including retinal vascular thrombosis), gallbladder disease, carbohydrate and lipid effects, elevated blood pressure, and headache including migraine.
The following adverse reactions have been reported in patients receiving oral contraceptives and are believed to be drug-related (alphabetically listed):

Acne
Amenorrhea
Anaphylactic/anaphylactoid reactions, including urticaria, angioedema, and severe reactions with respiratory and circulatory symptoms
Breakthrough bleeding
Breast changes: tenderness, pain, enlargement, secretion
Budd-Chiari syndrome
Cervical erosion and secretion, change in
Cholestatic jaundice
Chorea, exacerbation of
Colitis
Corneal curvature (steepening), change in
Diminution in lactation when given immediately postpartum
Dizziness
Edema/fluid retention
Erythema multiforme
Erythema nodosum
Gastrointestinal symptoms (such as abdominal pain, cramps, and bloating)
Hirsutism
Intolerance to contact lenses
Libido, changes in
Loss of scalp hair
Melasma/chloasma which may persist
Menstrual flow, change in
Mood changes, including depression
Nausea
Nervousness
Pancreatitis
Porphyria, exacerbation of
Rash (allergic)
Serum folate levels, decrease in
Spotting
Systemic lupus erythematosus, exacerbation of
Temporary infertility after discontinuation of treatment
Vaginitis, including candidiasis
Varicose veins, aggravation of
Vomiting
Weight or appetite (increase or decrease), change in

The following adverse reactions have been reported in users of oral contraceptives:
Cataracts
Cystitis-like syndrome
Dysmenorrhea
Hemolytic uremic syndrome
Hemorrhagic eruption
Optic neuritis, which may lead to partial or complete loss of vision
Porphyria
Premenstrual syndrome
Renal function, impaired

OVERDOSAGE

Symptoms of oral contraceptive overdosage in adults and children may include nausea, vomiting, and drowsiness/fatigue; withdrawal bleeding may occur in females. There is no specific antidote and further treatment of overdose, if necessary, is directed to the symptoms.

NONCONTRACEPTIVE HEALTH BENEFITS
The following noncontraceptive health benefits related to the use of oral contraceptives are supported by epidemiological studies which largely utilized oral-contraceptive formulations containing doses exceeding 0.035 mg of ethinyl estradiol or 0.05 mg of mestranol.

Effects on menses:
Increased menstrual cycle regularity
Decreased blood loss and decreased incidence of iron-deficiency anemia
Decreased incidence of dysmenorrhea

Effects related to inhibition of ovulation:
Decreased incidence of functional ovarian cysts
Decreased incidence of ectopic pregnancies

Effects from long-term use:
Decreased incidence of fibroadenomas and fibrocystic disease of the breast
Decreased incidence of acute pelvic inflammatory disease
Decreased incidence of endometrial cancer
Decreased incidence of ovarian cancer

DOSAGE AND ADMINISTRATION

To achieve maximum contraceptive effectiveness, Lo/Ovral-28 must be taken exactly as directed and at intervals not exceeding 24 hours. The possibility of ovulation and conception prior to initiation of medication should be considered.
The dosage of Lo/Ovral-28 is one white tablet daily for 21 consecutive days, followed by one pink inert tablet daily for 7 consecutive days, according to prescribed schedule. It is recommended that tablets be taken at the same time each day.
During the first cycle of medication, the patient is instructed to begin taking Lo/Ovral-28 on the first Sunday after the onset of menstruation. If menstruation begins on a Sunday, the first tablet (white) is taken that day. One white tablet should be taken daily for 21 consecutive days followed by one pink inert tablet daily for 7 consecutive days. Withdrawal bleeding should usually occur within three days following discontinuation of white tablets and may not have finished before the next pack is started. During the first cycle, contraceptive reliance should not be placed on Lo/Ovral-28 until a white tablet has been taken daily for 7 consecutive days and a nonhormonal back-up method of birth control should be used during those 7 days. The possibility of ovulation and conception prior to initiation of medication should be considered.
The patient begins her next and all subsequent 28-day courses of tablets on the same day of the week (Sunday) on which she began her first course, following the same schedule: 21 days on white tablets—7 days on pink inert tablets. If in any cycle the patient starts tablets later than the proper day, she should protect herself against pregnancy by using a nonhormonal back-up method of birth control until she has taken a white tablet daily for 7 consecutive days.
When the patient is switching from a 21-day regimen of tablets, she should wait 7 days after her last tablet before she starts Lo/Ovral-28. She will probably experience withdrawal bleeding during that week. She should be sure that no more than 7 days pass after her previous 21-day regimen. When the patient is switching from a 28-day regimen of tablets, she should start her first pack of Lo/Ovral-28 on the day after her last tablet. She should not wait any days between packs. The patient may switch any day from a progestin-only pill and should begin Lo/Ovral-28 the next day. If switching from an implant or injection, the patient should start Lo/Ovral-28 on the day of implant removal or the day the next injection would be due. In switching from a progestin-only pill, injection, or implant, the patient should be advised to use a nonhormonal back-up method of birth control for the first 7 days of tablet-taking.
If spotting or breakthrough bleeding occurs, the patient is instructed to continue on the same regimen. This type of bleeding is usually transient and without significance; however, if the bleeding is persistent or prolonged, the patient is advised to consult her health-care professional. Although pregnancy is unlikely if Lo/Ovral-28 is taken according to directions, if withdrawal bleeding does not occur, the possibility of pregnancy must be considered. If the patient has not adhered to the prescribed schedule (missed one or more tablets or started taking them on a day later than she should have), the probability of pregnancy should be considered at the time of the first missed period and appropriate diagnostic measures taken. If the patient has adhered to the prescribed regimen and misses two consecutive periods, pregnancy should be ruled out. Hormone contraception should be discontinued if pregnancy is confirmed.
For additional patient instructions regarding missed tablets, see the **WHAT TO DO IF YOU MISS PILLS** section in the **DETAILED PATIENT LABELING** below.
Any time the patient misses two or more white tablets, she should also use another method of contraception until she has taken a white tablet daily for seven consecutive days. If the patient misses one or more pink tablets, she is still protected against pregnancy **provided** she begins taking white tablets again on the proper day.
If breakthrough bleeding occurs following missed white tablets, it will usually be transient and of no consequence. The possibility of ovulation increases with each successive day that scheduled white tablets are missed.
Lo/Ovral-28 may be initiated no earlier than day 28 postpartum in the nonlactating mother or after a second-trimester abortion due to the increased risk for thromboembolism (see **CONTRAINDICATIONS**, **WARNINGS**, and **PRECAUTIONS** concerning thromboembolic disease). The patient should be advised to use a nonhormonal back-up method for the first 7 days of tablet-taking. However, if intercourse has already occurred, pregnancy should be excluded before the start of combined oral contraceptive use or the patient must wait for her first menstrual period. In the case of first-trimester abortion, if the patient starts Lo/Ovral-28 immediately, additional contraceptive measures are not needed.

HOW SUPPLIED

Lo/Ovral®-28 Tablets (0.3 mg norgestrel and 0.03 mg ethinyl estradiol) are available in packages of 6 PILPAK® dispensers, each containing 28 tablets as follows:
21 active tablets, NDC 0008-0078, white, round tablet marked "WYETH" and "78".
7 inert tablets, NDC 0008-0486, pink, round tablet marked "WYETH" and "486".
Store at controlled room temperature 20°C to 25°C (68°F to 77°F).
References available upon request.

Brief Summary Patient Package Insert

This product (like all oral contraceptives) is intended to prevent pregnancy. Oral contraceptives do not protect against transmission of HIV (AIDS) and other sexually transmitted diseases (STDs) such as chlamydia, genital herpes, genital warts, gonorrhea, hepatitis B, and syphilis.
Oral contraceptives, also known as "birth-control pills" or "the pill," are taken to prevent pregnancy, and when taken correctly, have a failure rate of approximately 1% per year when taken without missing any pills. The average failure rate is approximately 5% per year when women who miss pills are included. For most women oral contraceptives are also free of serious or unpleasant side effects. However, forgetting to take pills considerably increases the chances of pregnancy.
For the majority of women, oral contraceptives can be taken safely. But there are some women who are at high risk of developing certain serious diseases that can be life-threatening or may cause temporary or permanent disability or death. The risks associated with taking oral contraceptives increase significantly if you:

- smoke
- have high blood pressure, diabetes, high cholesterol, or a tendency to form blood clots, or are obese
- have or have had clotting disorders, heart attack, stroke, angina pectoris, cancer of the breast or sex organs, jaundice, malignant or benign liver tumors, or major surgery with prolonged immobilization
- have headaches with neurological symptoms

You should not take the pill if you suspect you are pregnant or have unexplained vaginal bleeding.

> **Cigarette smoking increases the risk of serious adverse effects on the heart and blood vessels from oral-contraceptive use. This risk increases with age and with the amount of smoking (15 or more cigarettes per day has been associated with a significantly increased risk) and is quite marked in women over 35 years of age. Women who use oral contraceptives should not smoke.**

Most side effects of the pill are not serious. The most common such effects are nausea, vomiting, bleeding between menstrual periods, weight gain, breast tenderness, and difficulty wearing contact lenses. These side effects, especially nausea and vomiting, may subside within the first three months of use.
The serious side effects of the pill occur very infrequently, especially if you are in good health and do not smoke. However, you should know that the following medical conditions have been associated with or made worse by the pill:
1. Blood clots in the legs (thrombophlebitis), lungs (pulmonary embolism), stoppage or rupture of a blood vessel in the brain (stroke), blockage of blood vessels in the heart (heart attack and angina pectoris) or other organs of the body. As mentioned above, smoking increases the risk of heart attacks and strokes and subsequent serious medical consequences. Women with migraine also may be at increased risk of stroke with pill use.
2. Liver tumors, which may rupture and cause severe bleeding. A possible but not definite association has been found with the pill and liver cancer. However, liver cancers are extremely rare. The chance of developing liver cancer from using the pill is thus even rarer.
3. High blood pressure, although blood pressure usually returns to normal when the pill is stopped.
The symptoms associated with these serious side effects are discussed in the detailed leaflet given to you with your supply of pills. Notify your health-care professional if you notice any unusual physical disturbances while taking the pill. In addition, drugs such as rifampin, as well as some anticonvulsants and some antibiotics, herbal preparations containing St. John's Wort (Hypericum perforatum), and HIV/AIDS drugs may decrease oral-contraceptive effectiveness.
Various studies give conflicting reports on the relationship between breast cancer and oral-contraceptive use.
Oral-contraceptive use may slightly increase your chance of having breast cancer diagnosed, particularly if you started using hormonal contraceptives at a younger age.
After you stop using hormonal contraceptives, the chances of having breast cancer diagnosed begin to go down and disappear 10 years after stopping use of the pill. It is not known whether this slightly increased risk of having breast

cancer diagnosed is caused by the pill. It may be that women taking the pill were examined more often, so that breast cancer was more likely to be detected.

You should have regular breast examinations by a health-care professional and examine your own breasts monthly. Tell your health-care professional if you have a family history of breast cancer or if you have had breast nodules or an abnormal mammogram. Women who currently have or have had breast cancer should not use oral contraceptives because breast cancer is usually a hormone-sensitive tumor.

Some studies have found an increase in the incidence of cancer of the cervix in women who use oral contraceptives. However, this finding may be related to factors other than the use of oral contraceptives. There is insufficient evidence to rule out the possibility that the pill may cause such cancers.

Taking the combination pill provides some important non-contraceptive health benefits. These include less painful menstruation, less menstrual blood loss and anemia, fewer pelvic infections, and fewer cancers of the ovary and the lining of the uterus.

Be sure to discuss any medical condition you may have with your health-care professional. Your health-care professional will take a medical and family history before prescribing oral contraceptives and will examine you. The physical examination may be delayed to another time if you request it and the health-care professional believes that it is appropriate to postpone it. You should be reexamined at least once a year while taking oral contraceptives. The detailed patient information leaflet gives you further information which you should read and discuss with your health-care professional.

This product (like all oral contraceptives) is intended to prevent pregnancy. It does not protect against transmission of HIV (AIDS) and other sexually transmitted diseases such as chlamydia, genital herpes, genital warts, gonorrhea, hepatitis B, and syphilis.

DETAILED PATIENT LABELING

This product (like all oral contraceptives) is intended to prevent pregnancy. Oral contraceptives do not protect against transmission of HIV (AIDS) and other sexually transmitted diseases (STDs) such as chlamydia, genital herpes, genital warts, gonorrhea, hepatitis B, and syphilis.

INTRODUCTION

Any woman who considers using oral contraceptives (the "birth-control pill" or "the pill") should understand the benefits and risks of using this form of birth control. This leaflet will give you much of the information you will need to make this decision and will also help you determine if you are at risk of developing any of the serious side effects of the pill. It will tell you how to take the pill properly so that it will be as effective as possible. However, this leaflet is not a replacement for a careful discussion between you and your health-care professional. You should discuss the information provided in this leaflet with him or her, both when you first start taking the pill and during your revisits. You should also follow your health-care professional's advice with regard to regular check-ups while you are on the pill.

EFFECTIVENESS OF ORAL CONTRACEPTIVES

Oral contraceptives or "birth-control pills" or "the pill" are used to prevent pregnancy and are more effective than most other nonsurgical methods of birth control. When they are taken correctly without missing any pills, the chance of becoming pregnant is approximately 1% per year. Average failure rates are approximately 5% per year when women who miss pills are included. The chance of becoming pregnant increases with each missed pill during the menstrual cycle.

In comparison, average failure rates for other methods of birth control during the first year of use are as follows:

IUD: 0.1-2%	Female condom alone: 21%
Depo-Provera® (injectable progestogen): 0.3%	Cervical cap
Norplant® System (levonorgestrel implants): 0.05%	Never given birth: 20%
Diaphragm with spermicides: 20%	Given birth: 40%
Spermidices alone: 26%	Periodic abstinence: 25%
Male condom alone: 14%	No methods: 85%

WHO SHOULD NOT TAKE ORAL CONTRACEPTIVES

Cigarette smoking increases the risk of serious adverse effects on the heart and blood vessels from oral-contraceptive use. This risk increases with age and with the amount of smoking (15 or more cigarettes per day has been associated with a significantly increased risk) and is quite marked in women over 35 years of age. Women who use oral contraceptives should not smoke.

Some women should not take the pill. You should not take the pill if you have any of the following conditions:

- History of heart attack or stroke
- History of blood clots in the legs (thrombophlebitis), lungs (pulmonary embolism), or eyes
- History of blood clots in the deep veins of your legs
- Known or suspected breast cancer or cancer of the lining of the uterus, cervix, or vagina or certain hormonally-sensitive cancers
- Liver tumor (benign or cancerous)
- Chest pain (angina pectoris)
- Unexplained vaginal bleeding (until a diagnosis is reached by your health-care professional)
- Yellowing of the whites of the eyes or of the skin (jaundice) during pregnancy or during previous use of the pill
- Known or suspected pregnancy
- Heart valve or heart rhythm disorders that may be associated with formation of blood clots
- Diabetes affecting your circulation
- Headaches with neurological symptoms
- Uncontrolled high blood pressure
- Active liver disease with abnormal liver function tests
- Allergy or hypersensitivity to any of the components of Lo/Ovral-28
- A need for surgery with prolonged bedrest

Tell your health-care professional if you have any of these conditions. Your health-care professional can recommend another method of birth control.

OTHER CONSIDERATIONS BEFORE TAKING ORAL CONTRACEPTIVES

Tell your health-care professional if you or any family member has ever had:

- Breast nodules, fibrocystic disease of the breast, an abnormal breast X-ray or mammogram
- Diabetes
- Elevated cholesterol or triglycerides
- High blood pressure
- A tendency to form blood clots
- Migraine or other headaches or epilepsy
- Depression
- Gallbladder, liver, heart, or kidney disease
- History of scanty or irregular menstrual periods

Women with any of these conditions should be checked often by their health-care professional if they choose to use oral contraceptives. Also, be sure to inform your health-care professional if you smoke or are on any medications.

RISKS OF TAKING ORAL CONTRACEPTIVES

1. *Risk of developing blood clots*

Blood clots and blockage of blood vessels are the most serious side effects of taking oral contraceptives and can cause death or serious disability. In particular, a clot in the legs can cause thrombophlebitis and a clot that travels to the lungs can cause a sudden blocking of the vessel carrying blood to the lungs. Rarely, clots occur in the blood vessels of the eye and may cause blindness, double vision, or impaired vision.

Users of COCs have a higher risk of developing blood clots compared to nonusers. This risk is highest during the first year of COC use.

If you take oral contraceptives and need elective surgery, need to stay in bed for a prolonged illness or injury, or have recently delivered a baby, you may be at risk of developing blood clots. You should consult your health-care professional about stopping oral contraceptives three to four weeks before surgery and not taking oral contraceptives for two weeks after surgery or during bed rest. You should also not take oral contraceptives soon after delivery of a baby or a midtrimester pregnancy termination. It is advisable to wait for at least four weeks after delivery if you are not breast-feeding. If you are breast-feeding, you should wait until you have weaned your child before using the pill. (See also the section on breast-feeding in GENERAL PRECAUTIONS.)

2. *Heart attacks and strokes*

Oral contraceptives may increase the tendency to develop strokes (stoppage or rupture of blood vessels in the brain) and angina pectoris and heart attacks (blockage of blood vessels in the heart). Any of these conditions can cause death or serious disability.

Smoking greatly increases the possibility of suffering heart attacks and strokes. Furthermore, smoking and the use of oral contraceptives greatly increase the chances of developing and dying of heart disease.

Women with migraine (especially migraine/headache with neurological symptoms) who take oral contraceptives also may be at higher risk of stroke.

3. *Gallbladder disease*

Oral-contraceptive users probably have a greater risk than nonusers of having gallbladder disease. This risk may be related to pills containing high doses of estrogens. Oral contraceptives may worsen existing gallbladder disease or accelerate the development of gallbladder disease in women previously without symptoms.

4. *Liver tumors*

In rare cases, oral contraceptives can cause benign but dangerous liver tumors. These benign liver tumors can rupture and cause fatal internal bleeding. In addition, a possible but not definite association has been found with the pill and liver cancers in two studies in which a few women who developed these very rare cancers were found to have used oral contraceptives for long periods. However, liver cancers are extremely rare. The chance of developing liver cancer from using the pill is thus even rarer.

5. *Cancer of the reproductive organs and breasts*

Various studies give conflicting reports on the relationship between breast cancer and oral-contraceptive use.

Oral-contraceptive use may slightly increase your chance of having breast cancer diagnosed, particularly if you started using hormonal contraceptives at a younger age.

After you stop using hormonal contraceptives, the chances of having breast cancer diagnosed begin to go down and disappear 10 years after stopping use of the pill. It is not known whether this slightly increased risk of having breast cancer diagnosed is caused by the pill. It may be that women taking the pill were examined more often, so that breast cancer was more likely to be detected.

You should have regular breast examinations by a health-care professional and examine your own breasts monthly. Tell your health-care professional if you have a family history of breast cancer or if you have had breast nodules or an abnormal mammogram. Women who currently have or have had breast cancer should not use oral contraceptives because breast cancer is usually a hormone-sensitive tumor.

Some studies have found an increase in the incidence of cancer of the cervix in women who use oral contraceptives. However, this finding may be related to factors other than the use of oral contraceptives. There is insufficient evidence to rule out the possibility that the pill may cause such cancers.

6. *Lipid metabolism and inflammation of the pancreas*

In patients with abnormal lipid levels, there have been reports of significant increases in plasma triglycerides during estrogen therapy. This has led to inflammation of the pancreas in some cases.

ESTIMATED RISK OF DEATH FROM A BIRTH-CONTROL METHOD OR PREGNANCY

All methods of birth control and pregnancy are associated with a risk of developing certain diseases which may lead to disability or death. An estimate of the number of deaths associated with different methods of birth control and pregnancy has been calculated and is shown in the following table.

ANNUAL NUMBER OF BIRTH-RELATED OR METHOD-RELATED DEATHS ASSOCIATED WITH CONTROL OF FERTILITY PER 100,000 NONSTERILE WOMEN, BY FERTILITY-CONTROL METHOD AND ACCORDING TO AGE

Method of control and outcome	15-19	20-24	25-29	30-34	35-39	40-44
No fertility-control methods*	7.0	7.4	9.1	14.8	25.7	28.2
Oral contraceptives nonsmoker**	0.3	0.5	0.9	1.9	13.8	31.6
Oral contraceptives smoker**	2.2	3.4	6.6	13.5	51.1	117.2
IUD**	0.8	0.8	1.0	1.0	1.4	1.4
Condom*	1.1	1.6	0.7	0.2	0.3	0.4
Diaphragm/ spermicide*	1.9	1.2	1.2	1.3	2.2	2.8
Periodic abstinence*	2.5	1.6	1.6	1.7	2.9	3.6

*Deaths are birth related

**Deaths are method related

In the above table, the risk of death from any birth-control method is less than the risk of childbirth, except for oral-contraceptive users over the age of 35 who smoke and pill users over the age of 40 even if they do not smoke. It can be seen in the table that for women aged 15 to 39, the risk of death was highest with pregnancy (7 to 26 deaths per 100,000 women, depending on age). Among pill users who do not smoke, the risk of death was always lower than that associated with pregnancy for any age group, except for those women over the age of 40, when the risk increases to 32 deaths per 100,000 women, compared to 28 associated with pregnancy at that age. However, for pill users who smoke and are over the age of 35, the estimated number of deaths exceeds those for other methods of birth control. If a woman is over the age of 40 and smokes, her estimated risk of death is four times higher (117/100,000 women) than the estimated risk associated with pregnancy (28/100,000 women) in that age group.

The suggestion that women over 40 who do not smoke should not take oral contraceptives is based on information from older high-dose pills. An Advisory Committee of the FDA discussed this issue in 1989 and recommended that the benefits of oral-contraceptive use by healthy, nonsmoking women over 40 years of age may outweigh the possible risks. Older women, as all women who take oral contraceptives, should take an oral contraceptive which contains the least amount of estrogen and progestogen that is compatible with the individual patient needs.

WARNING SIGNALS

If any of these adverse effects occur while you are taking oral contraceptives, call your health-care professional immediately:

- Sharp chest pain, coughing of blood, or sudden shortness of breath (indicating a possible clot in the lung)
- Pain in the calf (indicating a possible clot in the leg)
- Crushing chest pain or heaviness in the chest (indicating a possible heart attack)
- Sudden severe headache or vomiting, dizziness or fainting, disturbances of vision or speech, weakness, or numbness in an arm or leg (indicating a possible stroke)
- Sudden partial or complete loss of vision (indicating a possible clot in the eye)
- Breast lumps (indicating possible breast cancer or fibrocystic disease of the breast; ask your health-care professional to show you how to examine your breasts)

Continued on next page

Lo/Ovral-28—Cont.

- Severe pain or tenderness in the stomach area (indicating a possibly ruptured liver tumor)
- Difficulty in sleeping, weakness, lack of energy, fatigue, or change in mood (possibly indicating severe depression)
- Jaundice or a yellowing of the skin or eyeballs, accompanied frequently by fever, fatigue, loss of appetite, dark-colored urine, or light-colored bowel movements (indicating possible liver problems)

SIDE EFFECTS OF ORAL CONTRACEPTIVES

1. *Irregular vaginal bleeding*
Irregular vaginal bleeding or spotting may occur while you are taking the pills. Irregular bleeding may vary from slight staining between menstrual periods to breakthrough bleeding which is a flow much like a regular period. Irregular bleeding occurs most often during the first few months of oral-contraceptive use, but may also occur after you have been taking the pill for some time. Such bleeding may be temporary and usually does not indicate any serious problems. It is important to continue taking your pills on schedule. If the bleeding occurs in more than one cycle or lasts for more than a few days, talk to your health-care professional.
2. *Contact lenses*
If you wear contact lenses and notice a change in vision or an inability to wear your lenses, contact your health-care professional.
3. *Fluid retention*
Oral contraceptives may cause edema (fluid retention) with swelling of the fingers or ankles and may raise your blood pressure. If you experience fluid retention, contact your health-care professional.
4. *Melasma*
A spotty darkening of the skin is possible, particularly of the face.
5. *Other side effects*
Other side effects may include nausea, breast tenderness, change in appetite, headache, nervousness, depression, dizziness, loss of scalp hair, rash, vaginal infections, inflammation of the pancreas, and allergic reactions.
If any of these side effects bother you, call your health-care professional.

GENERAL PRECAUTIONS

1. *Missed periods and use of oral contraceptives before or during early pregnancy*
There may be times when you may not menstruate regularly after you have completed taking a cycle of pills. If you have taken your pills regularly and miss one menstrual period, continue taking your pills for the next cycle but be sure to inform your health-care professional. If you have not taken the pills daily as instructed and missed a menstrual period, or if you missed two consecutive menstrual periods, you may be pregnant. Check with your health-care professional immediately to determine whether you are pregnant. Stop taking oral contraceptives if pregnancy is confirmed.
There is no conclusive evidence that oral-contraceptive use is associated with an increase in birth defects when taken inadvertently during early pregnancy. Previously, a few studies had reported that oral contraceptives might be associated with birth defects, but these findings have not been confirmed in more recent studies. Nevertheless, oral contraceptives should not be used during pregnancy. You should check with your health-care professional about risks to your unborn child of any medication taken during pregnancy.
2. *While breast-feeding*
If you are breast-feeding, consult your health-care professional before starting oral contraceptives. Some of the drug will be passed on to the child in the milk. A few adverse effects on the child have been reported, including yellowing of the skin (jaundice) and breast enlargement. In addition, oral contraceptives may decrease the amount and quality of your milk. If possible, do not use oral contraceptives while breast-feeding. You should use another method of contraception since breast-feeding provides only partial protection from becoming pregnant, and this partial protection decreases significantly as you breast-feed for longer periods of time. You should consider starting oral contraceptives only after you have weaned your child completely.
3. *Laboratory tests*
If you are scheduled for any laboratory tests, tell your health-care professional you are taking birth-control pills. Certain blood tests may be affected by birth-control pills.
4. *Drug interactions*
Certain drugs may interact with birth-control pills to make them less effective in preventing pregnancy or cause an increase in breakthrough bleeding. Such drugs include rifampin, drugs used for epilepsy such as barbiturates (for example, phenobarbital) and phenytoin (Dilantin® is one brand of this drug), primidone (Mysoline®), topiramate (Topamax®), carbamazepine (Tegretol® is one brand of this drug), phenylbutazone (Butazolidin® is one brand of this drug), some drugs used for HIV or AIDS such as ritonavir (Norvir®), modafinil (Provigil®), possibly certain antibiotics (such as ampicillin and other penicillins, and tetracyclines), and herbal products containing St. John's Wort (Hypericum perforatum). You may also need to use a nonhormonal method of contraception (such as condoms and/or spermicide) during any cycle in which you take drugs that can make oral contraceptives less effective.
You may be at a higher risk of a specific type of liver dysfunction if you take troleandomycin and oral contraceptives at the same time.
Be sure to tell your health-care professional if you are taking or start taking any other medications, including nonprescription products or herbal products while taking birth control pills.
5. *Sexually transmitted diseases*
This product (like all oral contraceptives) is intended to prevent pregnancy. It does not protect against transmission of HIV (AIDS) and other sexually transmitted diseases such as chlamydia, genital herpes, genital warts, gonorrhea, hepatitis B, and syphilis.

HOW TO TAKE THE PILL

IMPORTANT POINTS TO REMEMBER

BEFORE YOU START TAKING YOUR PILLS:
1. BE SURE TO READ THESE DIRECTIONS:
Before you start taking your pills.
And
Anytime you are not sure what to do.
2. THE RIGHT WAY TO TAKE THE PILL IS TO TAKE ONE PILL EVERY DAY AT THE SAME TIME.
If you miss pills you could get pregnant. This includes starting the pack late. The more pills you miss, the more likely you are to get pregnant.
3. MANY WOMEN HAVE SPOTTING OR LIGHT BLEEDING, OR MAY FEEL SICK TO THEIR STOMACH DURING THE FIRST 1-3 PACKS OF PILLS.
If you feel sick to your stomach, do not stop taking the pill. The problem will usually go away. If it doesn't go away, check with your health-care professional.
4. MISSING PILLS CAN ALSO CAUSE SPOTTING OR LIGHT BLEEDING, even when you make up these missed pills.
On the days you take 2 pills to make up for missed pills, you could also feel a little sick to your stomach.
5. IF YOU HAVE VOMITING (within 4 hours after you take your pill), you should follow the instructions for WHAT TO DO IF YOU MISS PILLS. IF YOU HAVE DIARRHEA, or IF YOU TAKE SOME MEDICINES, including some antibiotics, your pills may not work as well. Use a back-up nonhormonal method (such as condoms and/or spermicide) until you check with your health-care professional.
6. IF YOU HAVE TROUBLE REMEMBERING TO TAKE THE PILL, talk to your health-care professional about how to make pill-taking easier or about using another method of birth control.
7. IF YOU HAVE ANY QUESTIONS OR ARE UNSURE ABOUT THE INFORMATION IN THIS LEAFLET, call your health-care professional.

LO/OVRAL® & LO/OVRAL®-28 TABLETS (norgestrel and ethinyl estradiol tablets).

***BEFORE* YOU START TAKING YOUR PILLS**

1. DECIDE WHAT TIME OF DAY YOU WANT TO TAKE YOUR PILL.
It is important to take it at about the same time every day.
2. LOOK AT YOUR PILL PACK TO SEE IF IT HAS 21 OR 28 PILLS:
The *21-pill pack* has 21 "active" white pills (with hormones) to take for 3 weeks, followed by 1 week without pills.
The *28-pill pack* has 21 "active" white pills (with hormones) to take for 3 weeks, followed by 1 week of reminder pink pills (without hormones).
3. ALSO FIND:
1) where on the pack to start taking pills, and
2) in what order to take the pills (follow the arrows).

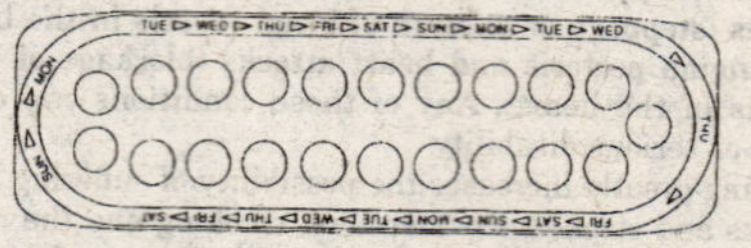

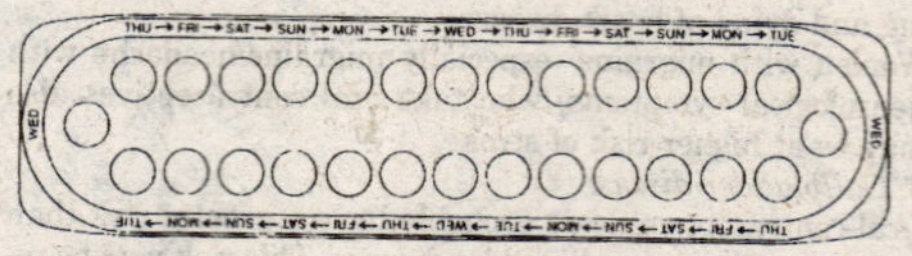

4. BE SURE YOU HAVE READY AT ALL TIMES:
ANOTHER KIND OF BIRTH CONTROL (such as condoms and/or spermicide) to use as a back-up in case you miss pills.
AN EXTRA, FULL PILL PACK.

WHEN TO START THE *FIRST* PACK OF PILLS

For the 21-day pill pack you have two choices of which day to start taking your first pack of pills. (See **DAY 1 START** or **SUNDAY START** directions below.) Decide with your health-care professional which is the best day for you. The 28-day pill pack accommodates a **SUNDAY START** only. For either pill pack pick a time of day which will be easy to remember.

DAY 1 START:
These instructions are for the 21-day pill pack only. The 28-day pill pack does not accommodate a **DAY 1 START** dosage regimen.
1. Take the first "active" white pill of the first pack during the *first 24 hours of your period.*
2. You will not need to use a back-up nonhormonal method of birth control, since you are starting the pill at the beginning of your period.

SUNDAY START:
These instructions are for either the 21-day or the 28-day pill pack.
1. Take the first "active" white pill of the first pack on the *Sunday after your period starts,* even if you are still bleeding. If your period begins on Sunday, start the pack that same day.
2. *Use a nonhormonal method of birth control* (such as condoms and/or spermicide) as a back-up method if you have sex anytime from the Sunday you start your first pack until the next Sunday (7 days).

WHAT TO DO DURING THE MONTH

1. **TAKE ONE PILL AT THE SAME TIME EVERY DAY UNTIL THE PACK IS EMPTY.**
Do not skip pills even if you are spotting or bleeding between monthly periods or feel sick to your stomach (nausea).
Do not skip pills even if you do not have sex very often.
2. **WHEN YOU FINISH A PACK OR SWITCH YOUR BRAND OF PILLS:**
21 pills: Wait 7 days to start the next pack. You will probably have your period during that week. Be sure that no more than 7 days pass between 21-day packs.
28 pills: Start the next pack on the day after your last "reminder" pill. Do not wait any days between packs.

WHAT TO DO IF YOU MISS PILLS

The pill may not be as effective if you miss white "active" pills, and particularly if you miss the first few or the last few white "active" pills in a pack.
If you **MISS 1** white "active" pill:
1. Take it as soon as you remember. Take the next pill at your regular time. This means you may take 2 pills in 1 day.
2. You COULD BECOME PREGNANT if you have sex in the *7 days* after you miss pills. You MUST use a nonhormonal birth-control method (such as condoms and/or spermicide) as a back-up for those 7 days.
If you **MISS 2** white "active" pills in a row in **WEEK 1 OR WEEK 2** of your pack:
1. Take 2 pills on the day you remember and 2 pills the next day.
2. Then take 1 pill a day until you finish the pack.
3. You COULD BECOME PREGNANT if you have sex in the *7 days* after you miss pills. You MUST use a nonhormonal birth-control method (such as condoms and/or spermicide) as a back-up for those 7 days.
If you **MISS 2** white "active" pills in a row in **THE 3rd WEEK:**
The ***Day 1 Starter*** instructions are for the 21-day pill pack only. The 28-day pill pack does not accommodate a **DAY 1 START** dosage regimen. The ***Sunday Starter*** instructions are for either the 21-day or 28-day pill pack.
1. ***If you are a Day 1 Starter:***
THROW OUT the rest of the pill pack and start a new pack that same day.
If you are a Sunday Starter:
Keep taking 1 pill every day until Sunday.
On Sunday, THROW OUT the rest of the pack and start a new pack of pills that same day.
2. You may not have your period this month but this is expected. However, if you miss your period 2 months in a row, call your health-care professional because you might be pregnant.
3. You COULD BECOME PREGNANT if you have sex in the *7 days* after you miss pills. You MUST use a nonhormonal birth-control method (such as condoms and/or spermicide) as a back-up for those 7 days.
If you **MISS 3 OR MORE** white "active" pills in a row (during the first 3 weeks):
The ***Day 1 Starter*** instructions are for the 21-day pill pack only. The 28-day pill pack does not accommodate a **DAY 1 START** dosage regimen. The ***Sunday Starter*** instructions are for either the 21-day or 28-day pill pack.
1. ***If you are a Day 1 Starter:***
THROW OUT the rest of the pill pack and start a new pack that same day.
If you are a Sunday Starter:
Keep taking 1 pill every day until Sunday.
On Sunday, THROW OUT the rest of the pack and start a new pack of pills that same day.
2. You may not have your period this month but this is expected. However, if you miss your period 2 months in a row, call your health-care professional because you might be pregnant.
3. You COULD BECOME PREGNANT if you have sex in the *7 days* after you miss pills. You MUST use a nonhormonal birth-control method (such as condoms and/or spermicide) as a back-up for those 7 days.

A REMINDER FOR THOSE ON 28-DAY PACKS
If you forget any of the 7 pink "reminder" pills in Week 4:
THROW AWAY the pills you missed.
Keep taking 1 pill each day until the pack is empty.
You do not need a back-up nonhormonal birth-control method if you start your next pack on time.

FINALLY, IF YOU ARE STILL NOT SURE WHAT TO DO ABOUT THE PILLS YOU HAVE MISSED
Use a BACK-UP NONHORMONAL BIRTH-CONTROL METHOD anytime you have sex.
KEEP TAKING ONE PILL EACH DAY until you can reach your health-care professional.

PREGNANCY DUE TO PILL FAILURE
The incidence of pill failure resulting in pregnancy is approximately 1% if taken every day as directed, but the average failure rate is approximately 5% including women who do not always take the pill exactly as directed without missing any pills. If you do become pregnant, the risk to the fetus is minimal, but you should stop taking your pills and discuss the pregnancy with your health-care professional.
PREGNANCY AFTER STOPPING THE PILL
There may be some delay in becoming pregnant after you stop using oral contraceptives, especially if you had irregular menstrual cycles before you used oral contraceptives. It may be advisable to postpone conception until you begin menstruating regularly once you have stopped taking the pill and desire pregnancy.
There does not appear to be any increase in birth defects in newborn babies when pregnancy occurs soon after stopping the pill.
If you do not desire pregnancy, you should use another method of birth control immediately after stopping the oral contraceptive pill.
OVERDOSAGE
Overdosage may cause nausea, vomiting, and fatigue/drowsiness. Withdrawal bleeding may occur in females. In case of overdosage, contact your health-care professional or pharmacist.
OTHER INFORMATION
Your health-care professional will take a medical and family history before prescribing oral contraceptives and will examine you. The physical examination may be delayed to another time if you request it and the health-care professional believes that it is appropriate to postpone it. You should be reexamined at least once a year. Be sure to inform your health-care professional if there is a family history of any of the conditions listed previously in this leaflet. Be sure to keep all appointments with your health-care professional, because this is a time to determine if there are early signs of side effects of oral-contraceptive use.
Do not use the drug for any condition other than the one for which it was prescribed. This drug has been prescribed specifically for you; do not give it to others who may want birth-control pills.
HEALTH BENEFITS FROM ORAL CONTRACEPTIVES
In addition to preventing pregnancy, use of oral contraceptives may provide certain benefits. They are:
- Menstrual cycles may become more regular.
- Blood flow during menstruation may be lighter, and less iron may be lost. Therefore, anemia due to iron deficiency is less likely to occur.
- Pain or other symptoms during menstruation may be encountered less frequently.
- Ovarian cysts may occur less frequently.
- Ectopic (tubal) pregnancy may occur less frequently.
- Noncancerous cysts or lumps in the breast may occur less frequently.
- Acute pelvic inflammatory disease may occur less frequently.
- Oral-contraceptive use may provide some protection against developing two forms of cancer: cancer of the ovaries and cancer of the lining of the uterus.

If you want more information about birth-control pills, ask your health-care professional or pharmacist. They have a more technical leaflet called the Professional Labeling which you may wish to read.
Wyeth Laboratories
A Wyeth-Ayerst Company
Philadelphia, PA 19101

W10468C001
ET02
Rev 07/03

MYLOTARG® ℞
[*mī'lō-tärg*]
(gemtuzumab ozogamicin for Injection)
FOR INTRAVENOUS USE ONLY

Prescribing information for this product, which appears on pages 3437–3440 of the 2004 PDR, has been revised as follows. Please write "See Supplement A" next to the product heading.
In the **ADVERSE REACTIONS** *section, the "Other Clinical Experience" subsection was revised as follows:*
Other Clinical Experience:
In postmarketing experience and other clinical trials, additional cases of VOD have been reported, some in association with the use of other chemotherapeutic agents, underlying hepatic disease/abnormal liver function, or a history of prior or subsequent HSCT. Renal failure secondary to TLS, hypersensitivity reactions, anaphylaxis, pulmonary events, and gastrointestinal hemorrhage have also been reported in association with the use of Mylotarg (gemtuzumab ozogamicin for Injection). (See **WARNINGS** section).
Wyeth Laboratories
Division of Wyeth-Ayerst Pharmaceuticals Inc.
Philadelphia, PA 19101
W10477C001 ET01
Rev 07/03

OVRAL®-28 ℞
[*ō'vrăl*]
Tablets
(NORGESTREL AND ETHINYL ESTRADIOL TABLETS)
℞ only

Prescribing information for this product, which appears on pages 3443–3449 of the 2004 PDR, has been completely revised as follows. Please write "See Supplement A" next to the product heading.

Patients should be counseled that oral contraceptives do not protect against transmission of HIV (AIDS) and other sexually transmitted diseases (STDs) such as chlamydia, genital herpes, genital warts, gonorrhea, hepatitis B, and syphilis.

DESCRIPTION
21 white Ovral tablets, each containing 0.5 mg of norgestrel, (*dl*-13-beta-ethyl-17-alpha-ethinyl-17-beta-hydroxygon-4-en-3-one), a totally synthetic progestogen, and 0.05 mg of ethinyl estradiol, (19-nor-17α-pregna-1,3,5 (10)-trien-20-yne-3,17-diol), and 7 pink inert tablets. The inactive ingredients present are cellulose, D&C Red 30, lactose, magnesium stearate, and polacrilin potassium.

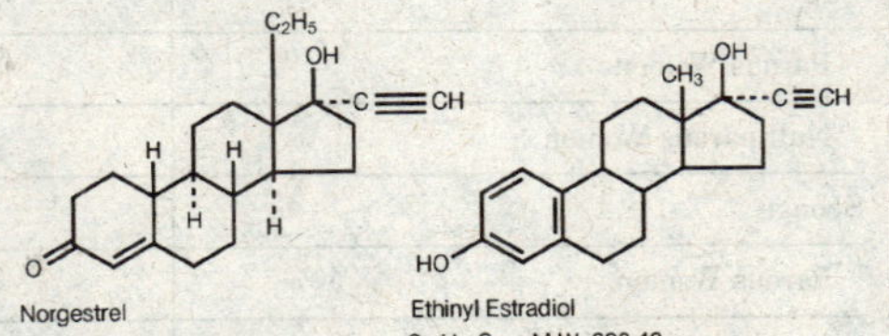

Norgestrel $C_{21}H_{28}O_2$ M.W. 312.45   Ethinyl Estradiol $C_{20}H_{24}O_2$ M.W. 296.40

CLINICAL PHARMACOLOGY
Mode of Action
Combination oral contraceptives act by suppression of gonadotropins. Although the primary mechanism of this action is inhibition of ovulation, other alterations include changes in the cervical mucus (which increase the difficulty of sperm entry into the uterus) and the endometrium (which reduce the likelihood of implantation).
INDICATIONS AND USAGE
Oral contraceptives are indicated for the prevention of pregnancy in women who elect to use this product as a method of contraception. Oral contraceptive products such as Ovral® or Ovral®-28 (norgestrel and ethinyl estradiol tablets), which contain 50 mcg of estrogen, should not be used unless medically indicated.
Oral contraceptives are highly effective. Table I lists the typical accidental pregnancy rates for users of combination oral contraceptives and other methods of contraception. The efficacy of these contraceptive methods, except sterilization, the IUD, and implants depends upon the reliability with which they are used. Correct and consistent use of methods can result in lower failure rates.
[See table I at top of next page]
CONTRAINDICATIONS
Combination oral contraceptives should not be used in women with any of the following conditions:
Thrombophlebitis or thromboembolic disorders
A past history of deep-vein thrombophlebitis or thromboembolic disorders
Cerebral-vascular or coronary-artery disease (current or history)
Thrombogenic valvulopathies
Thrombogenic rhythm disorders
Major surgery with prolonged immobilization
Diabetes with vascular involvement
Headaches with focal neurological symptoms
Uncontrolled hypertension
Known or suspected carcinoma of the breast or personal history of breast cancer
Carcinoma of the endometrium or other known or suspected estrogen-dependent neoplasia
Undiagnosed abnormal genital bleeding
Cholestatic jaundice of pregnancy or jaundice with prior pill use
Hepatic adenomas or carcinomas, or active liver disease, as long as liver function has not returned to normal
Known or suspected pregnancy
Hypersensitivity to any of the components of Ovral-28
WARNINGS

Cigarette smoking increases the risk of serious cardiovascular side effects from oral-contraceptive use. This risk increases with age and with the extent of smoking (in epidemiologic studies, 15 or more cigarettes per day was associated with a significantly increased risk) and is quite marked in women over 35 years of age. Women who use oral contraceptives should be strongly advised not to smoke.

The use of oral contraceptives is associated with increased risks of several serious conditions including venous and arterial thrombotic and thromboembolic events (such as myocardial infarction, thromboembolism, and stroke), hepatic neoplasia, gallbladder disease, and hypertension, although the risk of serious morbidity or mortality is very small in healthy women without underlying risk factors. The risk of morbidity and mortality increases significantly in the presence of other underlying risk factors such as certain inherited or acquired thrombophilias, hypertension, hyperlipidemias, obesity, diabetes, and surgery or trauma with increased risk of thrombosis.
Practitioners prescribing oral contraceptives should be familiar with the following information relating to these risks.
The information contained in this package insert is based principally on studies carried out in patients who used oral contraceptives with higher doses of estrogens and progestogens than those in common use today. The effect of long-term use of the oral contraceptives with lower doses of both estrogens and progestogens remains to be determined.
Throughout this labeling, epidemiological studies reported are of two types: retrospective or case control studies and prospective or cohort studies. Case control studies provide a measure of the relative risk of disease, namely, a ratio of the incidence of a disease among oral-contraceptive users to that among nonusers. The relative risk does not provide information on the actual clinical occurrence of a disease. Cohort studies provide a measure of attributable risk, which is the difference in the incidence of disease between oral-contraceptive users and nonusers. The attributable risk does provide information about the actual occurrence of a disease in the population. For further information, the reader is referred to a text on epidemiological methods.
1. **Thromboembolic Disorders and Other Vascular Problems**
a. Myocardial infarction
An increased risk of myocardial infarction has been attributed to oral-contraceptive use. This risk is primarily in smokers or women with other underlying risk factors for coronary-artery disease such as hypertension, hypercholesterolemia, morbid obesity, and diabetes. The relative risk of heart attack for current oral-contraceptive users has been estimated to be two to six. The risk is very low under the age of 30.
Smoking in combination with oral-contraceptive use has been shown to contribute substantially to the incidence of myocardial infarction in women in their mid-thirties or older with smoking accounting for the majority of excess cases. Mortality rates associated with circulatory disease have been shown to increase substantially in smokers over the age of 35 and nonsmokers over the age of 40 (Table II) among women who use oral contraceptives.

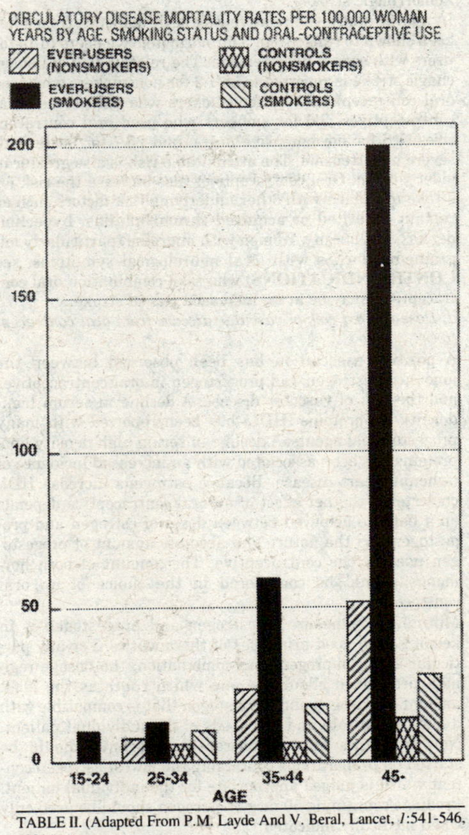

TABLE II. (Adapted From P.M. Layde And V. Beral, Lancet, *1*:541-546, 1981.)

Oral contraceptives may compound the effects of well-known risk factors, such as hypertension, diabetes, hyperlipidemias, age, and obesity. In particular, some progestogens are known to decrease HDL cholesterol and cause glucose intolerance, while estrogens may create a state of hyperinsulinism. Oral contraceptives have been shown to increase blood pressure among users (see section 9 in **WARNINGS**). Similar effects on risk factors have been associated with an increased risk of heart disease. Oral contraceptives must be used with caution in women with cardiovascular disease risk factors.
b. Venous thrombosis and thromboembolism
An increased risk of venous thromboembolic and thrombotic disease associated with the use of oral contraceptives is well established. Case control studies have found the relative risk of users compared to nonusers to be 3 for the first episode of superficial venous thrombosis, 4 to 11 for deep-vein thrombosis or pulmonary embolism, and 1.5 to 6 for women

Continued on next page

Ovral-28—Cont.

with predisposing conditions for venous thromboembolic disease. Cohort studies have shown the relative risk to be somewhat lower, about 3 for new cases and about 4.5 for new cases requiring hospitalization. Some epidemiological studies suggest that COCs with 50 mcg or more of ethinyl estradiol may be associated with a higher risk of such events than COCs with a lower dose of ethinyl estradiol. However, the incidence is substantially less than that associated with pregnancy (6 per 10,000 woman-years). The excess risk is highest during the first year a woman ever uses a combined oral contraceptive. Venous thromboembolism may be fatal. The risk of venous thrombotic and thromboembolic events is further increased in women with conditions predisposing for venous thrombosis and thromboembolism. The risk of thromboembolic disease due to oral contraceptives is not related to length of use and gradually disappears after pill use is stopped.

A two- to four-fold increase in relative risk of postoperative thromboembolic complications has been reported with the use of oral contraceptives. The relative risk of venous thrombosis in women who have predisposing conditions is twice that of women without such medical conditions. If feasible, oral contraceptives should be discontinued at least four weeks prior to and for two weeks after elective surgery of a type associated with an increase in risk of thromboembolism and during and following prolonged immobilization. Since the immediate postpartum period is also associated with an increased risk of thromboembolism, oral contraceptives should be started no earlier than four weeks after delivery in women who elect not to breast-feed, or a midtrimester pregnancy termination.

c. Cerebrovascular diseases

Oral contraceptives have been shown to increase both the relative and attributable risks of cerebrovascular events (thrombotic and hemorrhagic strokes), although, in general, the risk is greatest among older (>35 years), hypertensive women who also smoke. Hypertension was found to be a risk factor for both users and nonusers, for both types of strokes, while smoking interacted to increase the risk for hemorrhagic strokes.

In a large study, the relative risk of thrombotic strokes has been shown to range from 3 for normotensive users to 14 for users with severe hypertension. The relative risk of hemorrhagic stroke is reported to be 1.2 for nonsmokers who used oral contraceptives, 2.6 for smokers who did not use oral contraceptives, 7.6 for smokers who used oral contraceptives, 1.8 for normotensive users, and 25.7 for users with severe hypertension. The attributable risk is also greater in older women. Oral contraceptives also increase the risk for stroke in women with other underlying risk factors such as certain inherited or acquired thrombophilias, hyperlipidemias, and obesity. Women with migraine (particularly migraine/headaches with focal neurological symptoms, see **CONTRAINDICATIONS**) who take combination oral contraceptives may be at an increased risk of stroke.

d. Dose-related risk of vascular disease from oral contraceptives

A positive association has been observed between the amount of estrogen and progestogen in oral contraceptives and the risk of vascular disease. A decline in serum high-density lipoproteins (HDL) has been reported with many progestational agents. A decline in serum high-density lipoproteins has been associated with an increased incidence of ischemic heart disease. Because estrogens increase HDL cholesterol, the net effect of an oral contraceptive depends on a balance achieved between doses of estrogen and progestogen and the nature and absolute amount of progestogen used in the contraceptive. The amount of both hormones should be considered in the choice of an oral contraceptive.

Minimizing exposure to estrogen and progestogen is in keeping with good principles of therapeutics. For any particular estrogen/progestogen combination, the dosage regimen prescribed should be one which contains the least amount of estrogen and progestogen that is compatible with a low failure rate and the needs of the individual patient. New acceptors of oral-contraceptive agents should be started on preparations containing the lowest estrogen content which is judged appropriate for the individual patient. Products containing 50 mcg of estrogen should be used only when medically indicated.

e. Persistence of risk of vascular disease

There are two studies which have shown persistence of risk of vascular disease for ever-users of oral contraceptives. In a study in the United States, the risk of developing myocardial infarction after discontinuing oral contraceptives persists for at least 9 years for women 40 to 49 years who had used oral contraceptives for five or more years, but this increased risk was not demonstrated in other age groups. In another study in Great Britain, the risk of developing cerebrovascular disease persisted for at least 6 years after discontinuation of oral contraceptives, although excess risk was very small. Both studies were performed with oral-contraceptive formulations containing 50 mcg or higher of estrogen.

2. Estimates of Mortality from Contraceptive Use

One study gathered data from a variety of sources which have estimated the mortality rate associated with different methods of contraception at different ages (Table III). These estimates include the combined risk of death associated with contraceptive methods plus the risk attributable to pregnancy in the event of method failure. Each method of contraception has its specific benefits and risks. The study concluded that with the exception of oral-contraceptive users 35 and older who smoke and 40 and older who do not smoke, mortality associated with all methods of birth control is less than that associated with childbirth. The observation of a possible increase in risk of mortality with age for oral-contraceptive users is based on data gathered in the 1970's—but not reported until 1983. However, current clinical practice involves the use of lower estrogen dose formulations combined with careful restriction of oral-contraceptive use to women who do not have the various risk factors listed in this labeling.

Because of these changes in practice and, also, because of some limited new data which suggest that the risk of cardiovascular disease with the use of oral contraceptives may now be less than previously observed, the Fertility and Maternal Health Drugs Advisory Committee was asked to review the topic in 1989. The Committee concluded that although cardiovascular-disease risks may be increased with oral-contraceptive use after age 40 in healthy nonsmoking women (even with the newer low-dose formulations), there are greater potential health risks associated with pregnancy in older women and with the alternative surgical and medical procedures which may be necessary if such women do not have access to effective and acceptable means of contraception.

Therefore, the Committee recommended that the benefits of oral-contraceptive use by healthy nonsmoking women over 40 may outweigh the possible risks. Of course, older women, as all women who take oral contraceptives, should take the lowest possible dose formulation that is effective.

Table I: Percentage Of Women Experiencing An Unintended Pregnancy During The First Year Of Typical Use And The First Year Of Perfect Use Of Contraception And The Percentage Continuing Use At The End Of The First Year. United States.

	% of Women Experiencing an Unintended Pregnancy within the First Year of Use		% of Women Continuing Use at One Year[3]
Method (1)	Typical Use[1] (2)	Perfect Use[2] (3)	(4)
Chance[4]	85	85	
Spermicides[5]	26	6	40
Periodic abstinence	25		63
Calendar		9	
Ovulation Method		3	
Sympto-Thermal[6]		2	
Post-Ovulation		1	
Cap[7]			
Parous Women	40	26	42
Nulliparous Women	20	9	56
Sponge			
Parous Women	40	20	42
Nulliparous Women	20	9	56
Diaphragm[7]	20	6	56
Withdrawal	19	4	
Condom[8]			
Female (Reality)	21	5	56
Male	14	3	61
Pill	5		71
Progestin only		0.5	
Combined		0.1	
IUD			
Progesterone T	2.0	1.5	81
Copper T380A	0.8	0.6	78
LNg 20	0.1	0.1	81
Depo-Provera®	0.3	0.3	70
Levonorgestrel Implants (Norplant®)	0.05	0.05	88
Female Sterilization	0.5	0.5	100
Male Sterilization	0.15	0.10	100

Lactation Amenorrhea Method: LAM is a highly effective, temporary method of contraception.[9]

Source: Trussell J. Contraceptive efficacy. In: Hatcher RA, Trussell J, Stewart F, Cates W, Stewart GK, Kowel D, Guest F. Contraceptive Technology: Seventeenth Revised Edition. New York NY: Irvington Publishers; 1998.

1. Among *typical* couples who initiate use of a method (not necessarily for the first time), the percentage who experience an accidental pregnancy during the first year if they do not stop use for any other reason.
2. Among couples who initiate use of a method (not necessarily for the first time) and who use it *perfectly* (both consistently and correctly), the percentage who experience an accidental pregnancy during the first year if they do not stop use for any other reason.
3. Among couples attempting to avoid pregnancy, the percentage who continue to use a method for one year.
4. The percents becoming pregnant in columns (2) and (3) are based on data from populations where contraception is not used and from women who cease using contraception in order to become pregnant. Among such populations, about 89% become pregnant within one year. This estimate was lowered slightly (to 85%) to represent the percent who would become pregnant within one year among women now relying on reversible methods of contraception if they abandoned contraception altogether.
5. Foams, creams, gels, vaginal suppositories, and vaginal film.
6. Cervical mucus (ovulation) method supplemented by calendar in the pre-ovulatory and basal body temperature in the post-ovulatory phases.
7. With spermicidal cream or jelly.
8. Without spermicides.
9. However, to maintain effective protection against pregnancy, another method of contraception must be used as soon as menstruation resumes, the frequency or duration of breastfeeds is reduced, bottle feeds are introduced, or the baby reaches 6 months of age.

TABLE III–ANNUAL NUMBER OF BIRTH-RELATED OR METHOD-RELATED DEATHS ASSOCIATED WITH CONTROL OF FERTILITY PER 100,000 NONSTERILE WOMEN, BY FERTILITY-CONTROL METHOD AND ACCORDING TO AGE

Method of control and outcome	15-19	20-24	25-29	30-34	35-39	40-44
No fertility-control methods*	7.0	7.4	9.1	14.8	25.7	28.2
Oral contraceptives nonsmoker**	0.3	0.5	0.9	1.9	13.8	31.6
Oral contraceptives smoker**	2.2	3.4	6.6	13.5	51.1	117.2
IUD**	0.8	0.8	1.0	1.0	1.4	1.4
Condom*	1.1	1.6	0.7	0.2	0.3	0.4
Diaphragm/ spermicide*	1.9	1.2	1.2	1.3	2.2	2.8
Periodic abstinence*	2.5	1.6	1.6	1.7	2.9	3.6

*Deaths are birth related
**Deaths are method related
Adapted from H.W. Ory, Family Planning Perspectives, *15*:57-63, 1983.

3. Carcinoma of the Reproductive Organs and Breasts
Numerous epidemiological studies have examined the association between the use of oral contraceptives and the incidence of breast and cervical cancer.
The risk of having breast cancer diagnosed may be slightly increased among current and recent users of COCs. However, this excess risk appears to decrease over time after COC discontinuation and by 10 years after cessation the increased risk disappears. Some studies report an increased risk with duration of use while other studies do not and no consistent relationships have been found with dose or type of steroid. Some studies have reported a small increase in risk for women who first use COCs at a younger age. Most studies show a similar pattern of risk with COC use regardless of a woman's reproductive history or her family breast cancer history.
Breast cancers diagnosed in current or previous OC users tend to be less clinically advanced than in nonusers.
Women with known or suspected carcinoma of the breast or personal history of breast cancer should not use oral contraceptives because breast cancer is usually a hormonally-sensitive tumor.
Some studies suggest that oral-contraceptive use has been associated with an increase in the risk of cervical intraepithelial neoplasia or invasive cervical cancer in some populations of women. However, there continues to be controversy about the extent to which such findings may be due to differences in sexual behavior and other factors.
In spite of many studies of the relationship between combination oral-contraceptive use and breast and cervical cancers, a cause-and-effect relationship has not been established.

4. Hepatic Neoplasia
Benign hepatic adenomas are associated with oral-contraceptive use, although the incidence of benign tumors is rare in the United States. Indirect calculations have estimated the attributable risk to be in the range of 3.3 cases/100,000 for users, a risk that increases after four or more years of use. Rupture of rare, benign, hepatic adenomas may cause death through intra-abdominal hemorrhage.
Studies from Britain have shown an increased risk of developing hepatocellular carcinoma in long-term (>8 years) oral-contraceptive users.
However, these cancers are extremely rare in the U.S., and the attributable risk (the excess incidence) of liver cancers in oral-contraceptive users approaches less than one per million users.

5. Ocular Lesions
There have been clinical case reports of retinal thrombosis associated with the use of oral contraceptives that may lead to partial or complete loss of vision. Oral contraceptives should be discontinued if there is unexplained partial or complete loss of vision; onset of proptosis or diplopia; papilledema; or retinal vascular lesions. Appropriate diagnostic and therapeutic measures should be undertaken immediately.

6. Oral-Contraceptive Use Before or During Early Pregnancy
Extensive epidemiological studies have revealed no increased risk of birth defects in infants born to women who have used oral contraceptives prior to pregnancy. Studies also do not suggest a teratogenic effect, particularly insofar as cardiac anomalies and limb-reduction defects are concerned, when taken inadvertently during early pregnancy (see **CONTRAINDICATIONS** section).
The administration of oral contraceptives to induce withdrawal bleeding should not be used as a test for pregnancy. Oral contraceptives should not be used during pregnancy to treat threatened or habitual abortion.
It is recommended that for any patient who has missed two consecutive periods, pregnancy should be ruled out before continuing oral-contraceptive use. If the patient has not adhered to the prescribed schedule, the possibility of pregnancy should be considered at the time of the first missed period. Oral-contraceptive use should be discontinued if pregnancy is confirmed.

7. Gallbladder Disease
Combination oral contraceptives may worsen existing gallbladder disease and may accelerate the development of this disease in previously asymptomatic women. Earlier studies have reported an increased lifetime relative risk of gallbladder surgery in users of oral contraceptives and estrogens. More recent studies, however, have shown that the relative risk of developing gallbladder disease among oral-contraceptive users may be minimal. The recent findings of minimal risk may be related to the use of oral-contraceptive formulations containing lower hormonal doses of estrogens and progestogens.

8. Carbohydrate and Lipid Metabolic Effects
Oral contraceptives have been shown to cause glucose intolerance in a significant percentage of users. Oral contraceptives containing greater than 75 mcg of estrogens cause hyperinsulinism, while lower doses of estrogen cause less glucose intolerance. Progestogens increase insulin secretion and create insulin resistance, this effect varying with different progestational agents. However, in the nondiabetic woman, oral contraceptives appear to have no effect on fasting blood glucose. Because of these demonstrated effects, prediabetic and diabetic women should be carefully observed while taking oral contraceptives.
A small proportion of women will have persistent hypertriglyceridemia while on the pill. As discussed earlier (see **WARNINGS** 1a and 1d; **PRECAUTIONS** 3), changes in serum triglycerides and lipoprotein levels have been reported in oral-contraceptive users.

9. Elevated Blood Pressure
Women with uncontrolled hypertension should not be started on hormonal contraception. An increase in blood pressure has been reported in women taking oral contraceptives, and this increase is more likely in older oral-contraceptive users and with continued use. Data from the Royal College of General Practitioners and subsequent randomized trials have shown that the incidence of hypertension increases with increasing quantities of progestogens.
Women with a history of hypertension or hypertension-related diseases, or renal disease, should be encouraged to use another method of contraception. If women with hypertension elect to use oral contraceptives, they should be monitored closely, and if significant elevation of blood pressure occurs, oral contraceptives should be discontinued (see **CONTRAINDICATIONS** section). For most women, elevated blood pressure will return to normal after stopping oral contraceptives, and there is no difference in the occurrence of hypertension among ever- and never-users.

10. Headache
The onset or exacerbation of migraine or development of headache with a new pattern that is recurrent, persistent, or severe requires discontinuation of oral contraceptives and evaluation of the cause. (See **WARNINGS** 1c and **CONTRAINDICATIONS**.)

11. Bleeding Irregularities
Breakthrough bleeding and spotting are sometimes encountered in patients on oral contraceptives, especially during the first three months of use. The type and dose of progestogen may be important. If bleeding persists or recurs, nonhormonal causes should be considered and adequate diagnostic measures taken to rule out malignancy or pregnancy in the event of breakthrough bleeding, as in the case of any abnormal vaginal bleeding. If pathology has been excluded, time or a change to another formulation may solve the problem. In some women withdrawal bleeding may not occur during the "tablet-free" or "inactive-tablet" interval. If the COC has not been taken according to directions prior to the first missed withdrawal bleed, or if two consecutive withdrawal bleeds are missed, tablet-taking should be discontinued and a nonhormonal method of contraception should be used until the possibility of pregnancy is excluded.
Some women may encounter post-pill amenorrhea or oligomenorrhea (possibly with anovulation), especially when such a condition was preexistent.

12. Ectopic Pregnancy
Ectopic as well as intrauterine pregnancy may occur in contraceptive failures.

PRECAUTIONS

1. General
Patients should be counseled that oral contraceptives do not protect against transmission of HIV (AIDS) and other sexually transmitted diseases (STDs) such as chlamydia, genital herpes, genital warts, gonorrhea, hepatitis B, and syphilis.

2. Physical Examination and Follow-Up
A periodic personal and family medical history and complete physical examination are appropriate for all women, including women using oral contraceptives. The physical examination, however, may be deferred until after initiation of oral contraceptives if requested by the woman and judged appropriate by the clinician. The physical examination should include special reference to blood pressure, breasts, abdomen and pelvic organs, including cervical cytology, and relevant laboratory tests. In case of undiagnosed, persistent or recurrent abnormal vaginal bleeding, appropriate diagnostic measures should be conducted to rule out malignancy. Women with a strong family history of breast cancer or who have breast nodules should be monitored with particular care.

3. Lipid Disorders
Women who are being treated for hyperlipidemias should be followed closely if they elect to use oral contraceptives. Some progestogens may elevate LDL levels and may render the control of hyperlipidemias more difficult. (See **WARNINGS** 1a, 1d, and 8.)
In patients with defects of lipoprotein metabolism, estrogen-containing preparations may be associated with rare but significant elevations of plasma triglycerides which may lead to pancreatitis.

4. Liver Function
If jaundice develops in any woman receiving such drugs, the medication should be discontinued. Steroid hormones may be poorly metabolized in patients with impaired liver function.

5. Fluid Retention
Oral contraceptives may cause some degree of fluid retention. They should be prescribed with caution, and only with careful monitoring, in patients with conditions which might be aggravated by fluid retention.

6. Emotional Disorders
Patients becoming significantly depressed while taking oral contraceptives should stop the medication and use an alternate method of contraception in an attempt to determine whether the symptom is drug related. Women with a history of depression should be carefully observed and the drug discontinued if significant depression occurs.

7. Contact Lenses
Contact-lens wearers who develop visual changes or changes in lens tolerance should be assessed by an ophthalmologist.

8. Gastrointestinal
Diarrhea and/or vomiting may reduce hormone absorption resulting in decreased serum concentrations.

9. Drug Interactions
Changes in contraceptive effectiveness associated with coadministration of other products:
Contraceptive effectiveness may be reduced when hormonal contraceptives are coadministered with antibiotics, anticonvulsants, and other drugs that increase the metabolism of contraceptive steroids. This could result in unintended pregnancy or breakthrough bleeding. Examples include rifampin, rifabutin, barbiturates, primidone, phenylbutazone, phenytoin, dexamethasone, carbamazepine, felbamate, oxcarbazepine, topiramate, griseofulvin, and modafinil.
Several cases of contraceptive failure and breakthrough bleeding have been reported in the literature with concomitant administration of antibiotics such as ampicillin and other penicillins, and tetracyclines, possibly due to a decrease of enterohepatic recirculation of estrogens. However, clinical pharmacology studies investigating drug interactions between combined oral contraceptives and these antibiotics have reported inconsistent results. Enterohepatic recirculation of estrogens may also be decreased by substances that reduce gut transit time.
Several of the anti-HIV protease inhibitors have been studied with coadministration of oral combination hormonal contraceptives; significant changes (increase and decrease) in the plasma levels of the estrogen and progestin have been noted in some cases. The safety and efficacy of oral contraceptive products may be affected with coadministration of anti-HIV protease inhibitors. Health-care professionals should refer to the label of the individual anti-HIV protease inhibitors for further drug-drug interaction information.
Herbal products containing St. John's Wort (Hypericum perforatum) may induce hepatic enzymes (cytochrome P 450) and p-glycoprotein transporter and may reduce the effectiveness of contraceptive steroids. This may also result in breakthrough bleeding.
During concomitant use of ethinyl estradiol containing products and substances that may lead to decreased plasma steroid hormone concentrations, it is recommended that a nonhormonal back-up method of birth control be used in addition to the regular intake of Ovral. If the use of a substance which leads to decreased ethinyl estradiol plasma concentrations is required for a prolonged period of time, combination oral contraceptives should not be considered the primary contraceptive.
After discontinuation of substances that may lead to decreased ethinyl estradiol plasma concentrations, use of a nonhormonal back-up method of birth control is recommended for 7 days. Longer use of a back-up method is advisable after discontinuation of substances that have led to induction of hepatic microsomal enzymes, resulting in decreased ethinyl estradiol concentrations. It may take several weeks until enzyme induction has completely subsided, depending on dosage, duration of use, and rate of elimination of the inducing substance.
Increase in plasma levels associated with coadministered drugs:
Coadministration of atorvastatin and certain oral contraceptives containing ethinyl estradiol increase AUC values for ethinyl estradiol by approximately 20%. The mechanism of this interaction is unknown. Ascorbic acid and acetaminophen increase the bioavailability of ethinyl estradiol since these drugs act as competitive inhibitors for sulfation of ethinyl estradiol in the gastrointestinal wall, a known pathway of elimination for ethinyl estradiol. CYP 3A4 inhibitors such as indinavir, itraconazole, ketoconazole, fluconazole, and troleandomycin may increase plasma hormone levels. Troleandomycin may also increase the risk of intrahepatic cholestasis during coadministration with combination oral contraceptives.
Changes in plasma levels of coadministered drugs:
Combination hormonal contraceptives containing some synthetic estrogens (eg, ethinyl estradiol) may inhibit the me-

Continued on next page

Ovral-28—Cont.

tabolism of other compounds. Increased plasma concentrations of cyclosporin, prednisolone and other corticosteroids, and theophylline have been reported with concomitant administration of oral contraceptives. Decreased plasma concentrations of acetaminophen and increased clearance of temazepam, salicylic acid, morphine, and clofibric acid, due to induction of conjugation (particularly glucuronidation), have been noted when these drugs were administered with oral contraceptives.
The prescribing information of concomitant medications should be consulted to identify potential interactions.

10. **Interactions with Laboratory Tests**
Certain endocrine- and liver-function tests and blood components may be affected by oral contraceptives:
a. Increased prothrombin and factors VII, VIII, IX, and X; decreased antithrombin 3; increased norepinephrine-induced platelet aggregability.
b. Increased thyroid-binding globulin (TBG) leading to increased circulating total thyroid hormone, as measured by protein-bound iodine (PBI), T_4 by column or by radioimmunoassay. Free T_3 resin uptake is decreased, reflecting the elevated TBG; free T_4 concentration is unaltered.
c. Other binding proteins may be elevated in serum ie, corticosteroid binding globulin (CBG), sex hormone-binding globulins (SHBG) leading to increased levels of total circulating corticosteroids and sex steroids, respectively. Free or biologically active hormone concentrations are unchanged.
d. Triglycerides may be increased and levels of various other lipids and lipoproteins may be affected.
e. Glucose tolerance may be decreased.
f. Serum folate levels may be depressed by oral-contraceptive therapy. This may be of clinical significance if a woman becomes pregnant shortly after discontinuing oral contraceptives.

11. **Carcinogenesis**
See **WARNINGS** section.

12. **Pregnancy**
Pregnancy Category X. See **CONTRAINDICATIONS** and **WARNINGS** sections.

13. **Nursing Mothers**
Small amounts of oral-contraceptive steroids and/or metabolites have been identified in the milk of nursing mothers, and a few adverse effects on the child have been reported, including jaundice and breast enlargement. In addition, combination oral contraceptives given in the postpartum period may interfere with lactation by decreasing the quantity and quality of breast milk. If possible, the nursing mother should be advised not to use combination oral contraceptives but to use other forms of contraception until she has completely weaned her child.

14. **Fertility Following Discontinuation**
Users of combination oral contraceptives may experience some delay in becoming pregnant after discontinuation of COCs, especially those women who had irregular menstrual cycles prior to use. Conception may be delayed an average of 1–2 months among women stopping COCs compared to women stopping nonhormonal contraceptive methods.
Women who do not wish to become pregnant after discontinuation of COCs should be advised to use another method of birth control.

15. **Pediatric Use**
Safety and efficacy of Ovral-28 tablets have been established in women of reproductive age. Safety and efficacy are expected to be the same for postpubertal adolescents under the age of 16 and for users 16 years and older. Use of this product before menarche is not indicated.

16. **Geriatric Use**
This product has not been studied in women over 65 years of age and is not indicated in this population.

Information for the Patient
See Patient Labeling Printed Below.

ADVERSE REACTIONS

An increased risk of the following serious adverse reactions (see **WARNINGS** section for additional information) has been associated with the use of oral contraceptives:
Thromboembolic and thrombotic disorders and other vascular problems (including thrombophlebitis and venous thrombosis with or without pulmonary embolism, mesenteric thrombosis, arterial thromboembolism, myocardial infarction, cerebral hemorrhage, cerebral thrombosis), carcinoma of the reproductive organs and breasts, hepatic neoplasia (including hepatic adenomas or benign liver tumors), ocular lesions (including retinal vascular thrombosis), gallbladder disease, carbohydrate and lipid effects, elevated blood pressure, and headache including migraine.
The following adverse reactions have been reported in patients receiving oral contraceptives and are believed to be drug related (alphabetically listed):
Acne
Amenorrhea
Anaphylactic/anaphylactoid reactions, including urticaria, angioedema, and severe reactions with respiratory and circulatory symptoms
Breakthrough bleeding
Breast changes: tenderness, pain, enlargement, secretion
Budd-Chiari syndrome
Cervical erosion and secretion, change in
Cholestatic jaundice
Chorea, exacerbation of
Colitis
Corneal curvature (steepening), change in
Diminution in lactation when given immediately postpartum
Dizziness
Edema/fluid retention
Erythema multiforme
Erythema nodosum
Gastrointestinal symptoms (such as abdominal pain, cramps, and bloating)
Hirsutism
Intolerance to contact lenses
Libido, changes in
Loss of scalp hair
Melasma/chloasma which may persist
Menstrual flow, change in
Mood changes, including depression
Nausea
Nervousness
Pancreatitis
Porphyria, exacerbation of
Rash (allergic)
Serum folate levels, decrease in
Spotting
Systemic lupus erythematosus, exacerbation of
Temporary infertility after discontinuation of treatment
Vaginitis, including candidiasis
Varicose veins, aggravation of
Vomiting
Weight or appetite (increase or decrease), change in

The following adverse reactions have been reported in users of oral contraceptives:
Cataracts
Cystitis-like syndrome
Dysmenorrhea
Hemolytic uremic syndrome
Hemorrhagic eruption
Optic neuritis, which may lead to partial or complete loss of vision
Porphyria
Premenstrual syndrome
Renal function, impaired

OVERDOSAGE

Symptoms of oral contraceptive overdosage in adults and children may include nausea, vomiting, and drowsiness/fatigue; withdrawal bleeding may occur in females. There is no specific antidote and further treatment of overdose, if necessary, is directed to the symptoms.

NONCONTRACEPTIVE HEALTH BENEFITS

The following noncontraceptive health benefits related to the use of oral contraceptives are supported by epidemiological studies which largely utilized oral-contraceptive formulations containing doses exceeding 0.035 mg of ethinyl estradiol or 0.05 mg of mestranol.

Effects on menses:
Increased menstrual cycle regularity
Decreased blood loss and decreased incidence of iron-deficiency anemia
Decreased incidence of dysmenorrhea

Effects related to inhibition of ovulation:
Decreased incidence of functional ovarian cysts
Decreased incidence of ectopic pregnancies

Effects from long-term use:
Decreased incidence of fibroadenomas and fibrocystic disease of the breast
Decreased incidence of acute pelvic inflammatory disease
Decreased incidence of endometrial cancer
Decreased incidence of ovarian cancer

DOSAGE AND ADMINISTRATION

To achieve maximum contraceptive effectiveness, Ovral-28 must be taken exactly as directed and at intervals not exceeding 24 hours. The possibility of ovulation and conception prior to initiation of medication should be considered.
The dosage of Ovral-28 is one white tablet daily for 21 consecutive days, followed by one pink inert tablet daily for 7 consecutive days, according to prescribed schedule.
It is recommended that Ovral-28 tablets be taken at the same time each day.
During the first cycle of medication, the patient is instructed to begin taking Ovral-28 on the first Sunday after the onset of menstruation. If menstruation begins on a Sunday, the first tablet (white) is taken that day. One white tablet should be taken daily for 21 consecutive days followed by one pink inert tablet daily for 7 consecutive days. Withdrawal bleeding should usually occur within three days following discontinuation of white tablets and may not have finished before the next pack is started. During the first cycle, contraceptive reliance should not be placed on Ovral-28 until a white tablet has been taken daily for 7 consecutive days and a nonhormonal back-up method of birth control should be used during those 7 days. The possibility of ovulation and conception prior to initiation of medication should be considered.
The patient begins her next and all subsequent 28-day courses of tablets on the same day of the week (Sunday) on which she began her first course, following the same schedule: 21 days on white tablets—7 days on pink inert tablets. If in any cycle the patient starts tablets later than the proper day, she should protect herself against pregnancy by using a nonhormonal back-up method of birth control until she has taken a white tablet daily for 7 consecutive days.
When the patient is switching from a 21-day regimen of tablets, she should wait 7 days after her last tablet before she starts Ovral-28. She will probably experience withdrawal bleeding during that week. She should be sure that no more than 7 days pass after her previous 21-day regimen. When the patient is switching from a 28-day regimen of tablets, she should start her first pack of Ovral-28 on the day after her last tablet. She should not wait any days between packs. The patient may switch any day from a progestin-only pill and should begin Ovral-28 the next day. If switching from an implant or injection, the patient should start Ovral-28 on the day of implant removal or the day the next injection would be due. In switching from a progestin-only pill, injection, or implant, the patient should be advised to use a nonhormonal back-up method of birth control for the first 7 days of tablet-taking.
If spotting or breakthrough bleeding occurs, the patient is instructed to continue on the same regimen. This type of bleeding is usually transient and without significance; however, if the bleeding is persistent or prolonged, the patient is advised to consult her health-care professional. Although pregnancy is unlikely if Ovral-28 is taken according to directions, if withdrawal bleeding does not occur, the possibility of pregnancy must be considered. If the patient has not adhered to the prescribed schedule (missed one or more tablets or started taking them on a day later than she should have), the probability of pregnancy should be considered at the time of the first missed period and appropriate diagnostic measures taken. If the patient has adhered to the prescribed regimen and misses two consecutive periods, pregnancy should be ruled out. Hormone contraception should be discontinued if pregnancy is confirmed.
For additional patient instructions regarding missed tablets, see the **"WHAT TO DO IF YOU MISS PILLS"** section in the **DETAILED PATIENT LABELING** below.
Any time the patient misses two or more white tablets, she should also use another method of contraception until she has taken a white tablet daily for seven consecutive days. If the patient misses one or more pink tablets, she is still protected against pregnancy **provided** she begins taking white tablets again on the proper day.
If breakthrough bleeding occurs following missed white tablets, it will usually be transient and of no consequence. The possibility of ovulation increases with each successive day that scheduled white tablets are missed.
Ovral-28 may be initiated no earlier than day 28 postpartum in the nonlactating mother or after a second-trimester abortion due to the increased risk for thromboembolism (see **CONTRAINDICATIONS**, **WARNINGS**, and **PRECAUTIONS** concerning thromboembolic disease). The patient should be advised to use a nonhormonal back-up method for the first 7 days of tablet-taking. However, if intercourse has already occurred, pregnancy should be excluded before the start of combined oral contraceptive use or the patient must wait for her first menstrual period.
In the case of first-trimester abortion, if the patient starts Ovral-28 immediately, additional contraceptive measures are not needed.

HOW SUPPLIED

Ovral®-28 Tablets (0.5 mg norgestrel and 0.05 mg ethinyl estradiol) are available in packages of 6 PILPAK® dispensers, each containing 28 tablets as follows:
21 active tablets, NDC 0008-0056, white, round tablet marked "WYETH" and "56".
7 inert tablets, NDC 0008-0445, pink, round tablet marked "WYETH" and "445".
Store at controlled room temperature 20°C to 25°C (68°F to 77°F).
References available upon request.

Brief Summary Patient Package Insert

This product (like all oral contraceptives) is intended to prevent pregnancy. Oral contraceptives do not protect against transmission of HIV (AIDS) and other sexually transmitted diseases (STDs) such as chlamydia, genital herpes, genital warts, gonorrhea, hepatitis B, and syphilis.

Oral contraceptives, also known as "birth-control pills" or "the pill," are taken to prevent pregnancy, and when taken correctly, have a failure rate of approximately 1% per year when taken without missing any pills. The average failure rate of large numbers of pill users is approximately 5% per year when women who miss pills are included. For most women oral contraceptives are also free of serious or unpleasant side effects. However, forgetting to take pills considerably increases the chances of pregnancy.
For the majority of women, oral contraceptives can be taken safely. But there are some women who are at high risk of developing certain serious diseases that can be life-threatening or may cause temporary or permanent disability or death. The risks associated with taking oral contraceptives increase significantly if you:
- smoke
- have high blood pressure, diabetes, high cholesterol, or a tendency to form blood clots, or are obese
- have or have had clotting disorders, heart attack, stroke, angina pectoris, cancer of the breast or sex organs, jaundice, malignant or benign liver tumors, or major surgery with prolonged immobilization
- have headaches with neurological symptoms

You should not take the pill if you suspect you are pregnant or have unexplained vaginal bleeding.

Cigarette smoking increases the risk of serious adverse effects on the heart and blood vessels from oral-contraceptive use. This risk increases with age and with the amount of smoking (15 or more cigarettes per day

has been associated with a significantly increased risk) and is quite marked in women over 35 years of age. Women who use oral contraceptives should not smoke.

Most side effects of the pill are not serious. The most common such effects are nausea, vomiting, bleeding between menstrual periods, weight gain, breast tenderness, and difficulty wearing contact lenses. These side effects, especially nausea and vomiting, may subside within the first three months of use.

The serious side effects of the pill occur very infrequently, especially if you are in good health and do not smoke. However, you should know that the following medical conditions have been associated with or made worse by the pill:

1. Blood clots in the legs (thrombophlebitis), lungs (pulmonary embolism), stoppage or rupture of a blood vessel in the brain (stroke), blockage of blood vessels in the heart (heart attack and angina pectoris) or other organs of the body. As mentioned above, smoking increases the risk of heart attacks and strokes and subsequent serious medical consequences. Women with migraine also may be at increased risk of stroke with pill use.

2. Liver tumors, which may rupture and cause severe bleeding. A possible but not definite association has been found with the pill and liver cancer. However, liver cancers are extremely rare. The chance of developing liver cancer from using the pill is thus even rarer.

3. High blood pressure, although blood pressure usually returns to normal when the pill is stopped.

The symptoms associated with these serious side effects are discussed in the detailed leaflet given to you with your supply of pills. Notify your health-care professional if you notice any unusual physical disturbances while taking the pill. In addition, drugs such as rifampin, as well as some anticonvulsants and some antibiotics, herbal preparations containing St. John's Wort (Hypericum perforatum), and HIV/AIDS drugs may decrease oral-contraceptive effectiveness.

Various studies give conflicting reports on the relationship between breast cancer and oral-contraceptive use.

Oral-contraceptive use may slightly increase your chance of having breast cancer diagnosed, particularly if you started using hormonal contraceptives at a younger age.

After you stop using hormonal contraceptives, the chances of having breast cancer diagnosed begin to go down and disappear 10 years after stopping use of the pill. It is not known whether this slightly increased risk of having breast cancer diagnosed is caused by the pill. It may be that women taking the pill were examined more often, so that breast cancer was more likely to be detected.

You should have regular breast examinations by a health-care professional and examine your own breasts monthly. Tell your health-care professional if you have a family history of breast cancer or if you have had breast nodules or an abnormal mammogram. Women who currently have or have had breast cancer should not use oral contraceptives because breast cancer is usually a hormone-sensitive tumor.

Some studies have found an increase in the incidence of cancer of the cervix in women who use oral contraceptives. However, this finding may be related to factors other than the use of oral contraceptives. There is insufficient evidence to rule out the possibility that the pill may cause such cancers.

Taking the combination pill provides some important noncontraceptive health benefits. These include less painful menstruation, less menstrual blood loss and anemia, fewer pelvic infections, and fewer cancers of the ovary and the lining of the uterus.

Be sure to discuss any medical condition you may have with your health-care professional. Your health-care professional will take a medical and family history before prescribing oral contraceptives and will examine you. The physical examination may be delayed to another time if you request it and the health-care professional believes that it is appropriate to postpone it. You should be reexamined at least once a year while taking oral contraceptives. The detailed patient information leaflet gives you further information which you should read and discuss with your health-care professional.

This product (like all oral contraceptives) is intended to prevent pregnancy. It does not protect against transmission of HIV (AIDS) and other sexually transmitted diseases such as chlamydia, genital herpes, genital warts, gonorrhea, hepatitis B, and syphilis.

DETAILED PATIENT LABELING

This product (like all oral contraceptives) is intended to prevent pregnancy. Oral contraceptives do not protect against transmission of HIV (AIDS) and other sexually transmitted diseases (STDs) such as chlamydia, genital herpes, genital warts, gonorrhea, hepatitis B, and syphilis.

INTRODUCTION

You should not use Ovral or Ovral-28, which contain higher doses of estrogen than other oral contraceptives, unless specifically recommended by your health-care professional. Any woman who considers using oral contraceptives (the "birth-control pill" or "the pill") should understand the benefits and risks of using this form of birth control. This leaflet will give you much of the information you will need to make this decision and will also help you determine if you are at risk of developing any of the serious side effects of the pill. It will tell you how to take the pill properly so that it will be as effective as possible. However, this leaflet is not a replacement for a careful discussion between you and your health-care professional. You should discuss the information provided in this leaflet with him or her, both when you first start taking the pill and during your revisits. You should also follow your health-care professional's advice with regard to regular check-ups while you are on the pill.

EFFECTIVENESS OF ORAL CONTRACEPTIVES

Oral contraceptives or "birth-control pills" or "the pill" are used to prevent pregnancy and are more effective than most other nonsurgical methods of birth control. When they are taken correctly, without missing any pills the chance of becoming pregnant is approximately 1% per year. Average failure rates are approximately 5% per year when women who miss pills are included. The chance of becoming pregnant increases with each missed pill during the menstrual cycle. In comparison, average failure rates for other methods of birth control during the first year of use are as follows:

IUD: 0.1-2%	Female condom alone: 21%
Depo-Provera® (injectable progestogen): 0.3%	Cervical cap
Norplant® System (levonorgestrel implants): 0.05%	Never given birth: 20%
Diaphragm with spermicides: 20%	Given birth: 40%
Spermidices alone: 26%	Periodic abstinence: 25%
Male condom alone: 14%	No methods: 85%

WHO SHOULD NOT TAKE ORAL CONTRACEPTIVES

Cigarette smoking increases the risk of serious adverse effects on the heart and blood vessels from oral-contraceptive use. This risk increases with age and with the amount of smoking (15 or more cigarettes per day has been associated with a significantly increased risk) and is quite marked in women over 35 years of age. Women who use oral contraceptives should not smoke.

Some women should not take the pill. You should not take the pill if you have any of the following conditions:

- History of heart attack or stroke
- History of blood clots in the legs (thrombophlebitis), lungs (pulmonary embolism), or eyes
- History of blood clots in the deep veins of your legs
- Chest pain (angina pectoris)
- Known or suspected breast cancer or cancer of the lining of the uterus, cervix, or vagina or certain hormonally-sensitive cancers
- Unexplained vaginal bleeding (until a diagnosis is reached by your health-care professional)
- Liver tumor (benign or cancerous)
- Yellowing of the whites of the eyes or of the skin (jaundice) during pregnancy or during previous use of the pill
- Known or suspected pregnancy
- A need for surgery with prolonged bedrest
- Heart valve or heart rhythm disorders that may be associated with formation of blood clots
- Diabetes affecting your circulation
- Headaches with neurological symptoms
- Uncontrolled high blood pressure
- Active liver disease with abnormal liver function tests
- Allergy or hypersensitivity to any of the components of Ovral-28

Tell your health-care professional if you have any of these conditions. Your health-care professional can recommend another method of birth control.

OTHER CONSIDERATIONS BEFORE TAKING ORAL CONTRACEPTIVES

Tell your health-care professional if you or any family member has ever had:

- Breast nodules, fibrocystic disease of the breast, an abnormal breast X-ray or mammogram
- Diabetes
- Elevated cholesterol or triglycerides
- High blood pressure
- A tendency to form blood clots
- Migraine or other headaches or epilepsy
- Depression
- Gallbladder, liver, heart, or kidney disease
- History of scanty or irregular menstrual periods

Women with any of these conditions should be checked often by their health-care professional if they choose to use oral contraceptives. Also, be sure to inform your health-care professional if you smoke or are on any medications.

RISKS OF TAKING ORAL CONTRACEPTIVES

1. Risk of developing blood clots

Blood clots and blockage of blood vessels are the most serious side effects of taking oral contraceptives and can cause death or serious disability. In particular, a clot in the legs can cause thrombophlebitis and a clot that travels to the lungs can cause a sudden blocking of the vessel carrying blood to the lungs. Rarely, clots occur in the blood vessels of the eye and may cause blindness, double vision, or impaired vision.

Users of COCs have a higher risk of developing blood clots compared to nonusers. This risk is highest during the first year of COC use.

If you take oral contraceptives and need elective surgery, need to stay in bed for a prolonged illness or injury, or have recently delivered a baby, you may be at risk of developing blood clots. You should consult your health-care professional about stopping oral contraceptives three to four weeks before surgery and not taking oral contraceptives for two weeks after surgery or during bed rest. You should also not take oral contraceptives soon after delivery of a baby or a midtrimester pregnancy termination. It is advisable to wait for at least four weeks after delivery if you are not breast-feeding. If you are breast-feeding, you should wait until you have weaned your child before using the pill. (See also the section on breast-feeding in GENERAL PRECAUTIONS.)

2. Heart attacks and strokes

Oral contraceptives may increase the tendency to develop strokes (stoppage or rupture of blood vessels in the brain) and angina pectoris and heart attacks (blockage of blood vessels in the heart). Any of these conditions can cause death or serious disability.

Smoking greatly increases the possibility of suffering heart attacks and strokes. Furthermore, smoking and the use of oral contraceptives greatly increase the chances of developing and dying of heart disease.

Women with migraine (especially migraine/headache with neurological symptoms) who take oral contraceptives also may be at higher risk of stroke.

3. Gallbladder disease

Oral-contraceptive users probably have a greater risk than nonusers of having gallbladder disease. This risk may be related to pills containing high doses of estrogens. Oral contraceptives may worsen existing gallbladder disease or accelerate the development of gallbladder disease in women previously without symptoms.

4. Liver tumors

In rare cases, oral contraceptives can cause benign but dangerous liver tumors. These benign liver tumors can rupture and cause fatal internal bleeding. In addition, a possible but not definite association has been found with the pill and liver cancers in two studies in which a few women who developed these very rare cancers were found to have used oral contraceptives for long periods. However, liver cancers are extremely rare. The chance of developing liver cancer from using the pill is thus even rarer.

5. Cancer of the reproductive organs and breasts

Various studies give conflicting reports on the relationship between breast cancer and oral-contraceptive use.

Oral-contraceptive use may slightly increase your chance of having breast cancer diagnosed, particularly if you started using hormonal contraceptives at a younger age.

After you stop using hormonal contraceptives, the chances of having breast cancer diagnosed begin to go down and disappear 10 years after stopping use of the pill. It is not known whether this slightly increased risk of having breast cancer diagnosed is caused by the pill. It may be that women taking the pill were examined more often, so that breast cancer was more likely to be detected.

You should have regular breast examinations by a health-care professional and examine your own breasts monthly. Tell your health-care professional if you have a family history of breast cancer or if you have had breast nodules or an abnormal mammogram. Women who currently have or have had breast cancer should not use oral contraceptives because breast cancer is usually a hormone-sensitive tumor.

Some studies have found an increase in the incidence of cancer of the cervix in women who use oral contraceptives. However, this finding may be related to factors other than the use of oral contraceptives. There is insufficient evidence to rule out the possibility that the pill may cause such cancers.

6. Lipid metabolism and inflammation of the pancreas

In patients with abnormal lipid levels, there have been reports of significant increases in plasma triglycerides during estrogen therapy. This has led to inflammation of the pancreas in some cases.

ESTIMATED RISK OF DEATH FROM A BIRTH-CONTROL METHOD OR PREGNANCY

All methods of birth control and pregnancy are associated with a risk of developing certain diseases which may lead to disability or death. An estimate of the number of deaths associated with different methods of birth control and pregnancy has been calculated and is shown in the following table.

ANNUAL NUMBER OF BIRTH-RELATED OR METHOD-RELATED DEATHS ASSOCIATED WITH CONTROL OF FERTILITY PER 100,000 NONSTERILE WOMEN, BY FERTILITY-CONTROL METHOD AND ACCORDING TO AGE

Method of control and outcome	15-19	20-24	25-29	30-34	35-39	40-44
No fertility-control methods*	7.0	7.4	9.1	14.8	25.7	28.2
Oral contraceptives nonsmoker**	0.3	0.5	0.9	1.9	13.8	31.6
Oral contraceptives smoker**	2.2	3.4	6.6	13.5	51.1	117.2
IUD**	0.8	0.8	1.0	1.0	1.4	1.4
Condom*	1.1	1.6	0.7	0.2	0.3	0.4
Diaphragm/ spermicide*	1.9	1.2	1.2	1.3	2.2	2.8
Periodic abstinence*	2.5	1.6	1.6	1.7	2.9	3.6

Continued on next page

Ovral-28—Cont.

*Deaths are birth related
**Deaths are method related

In the above table, the risk of death from any birth-control method is less than the risk of childbirth, except for oral-contraceptive users over the age of 35 who smoke and pill users over the age of 40 even if they do not smoke. It can be seen in the table that for women aged 15 to 39, the risk of death was highest with pregnancy (7 to 26 deaths per 100,000 women, depending on age). Among pill users who do not smoke, the risk of death was always lower than that associated with pregnancy for any age group, except for those women over the age of 40, when the risk increases to 32 deaths per 100,000 women, compared to 28 associated with pregnancy at that age. However, for pill users who smoke and are over the age of 35, the estimated number of deaths exceeds those for other methods of birth control. If a woman is over the age of 40 and smokes, her estimated risk of death is four times higher (117/100,000 women) than the estimated risk associated with pregnancy (28/100,000 women) in that age group.

The suggestion that women over 40 who do not smoke should not take oral contraceptives is based on information from older high-dose pills. An Advisory Committee of the FDA discussed this issue in 1989 and recommended that the benefits of oral-contraceptive use by healthy, nonsmoking women over 40 years of age may outweigh the possible risks. Older women, as all women who take oral contraceptives, should take an oral contraceptive which contains the least amount of estrogen and progestogen that is compatible with the individual patient needs.

WARNING SIGNALS

If any of these adverse effects occur while you are taking oral contraceptives, call your health-care professional immediately:

- Sharp chest pain, coughing of blood, or sudden shortness of breath (indicating a possible clot in the lung)
- Pain in the calf (indicating a possible clot in the leg)
- Crushing chest pain or heaviness in the chest (indicating a possible heart attack)
- Sudden severe headache or vomiting, dizziness or fainting, disturbances of vision or speech, weakness, or numbness in an arm or leg (indicating a possible stroke)
- Sudden partial or complete loss of vision (indicating a possible clot in the eye)
- Breast lumps (indicating possible breast cancer or fibrocystic disease of the breast; ask your health-care professional to show you how to examine your breasts)
- Severe pain or tenderness in the stomach area (indicating a possibly ruptured liver tumor)
- Difficulty in sleeping, weakness, lack of energy, fatigue, or change in mood (possibly indicating severe depression)
- Jaundice or a yellowing of the skin or eyeballs, accompanied frequently by fever, fatigue, loss of appetite, dark-colored urine, or light-colored bowel movements (indicating possible liver problems)

SIDE EFFECTS OF ORAL CONTRACEPTIVES

1. *Irregular vaginal bleeding*

Irregular vaginal bleeding or spotting may occur while you are taking the pills. Irregular bleeding may vary from slight staining between menstrual periods to breakthrough bleeding which is a flow much like a regular period. Irregular bleeding occurs most often during the first few months of oral-contraceptive use, but may also occur after you have been taking the pill for some time. Such bleeding may be temporary and usually does not indicate any serious problems. It is important to continue taking your pills on schedule. If the bleeding occurs in more than one cycle or lasts for more than a few days, talk to your health-care professional.

2. *Contact lenses*

If you wear contact lenses and notice a change in vision or an inability to wear your lenses, contact your health-care professional.

3. *Fluid retention*

Oral contraceptives may cause edema (fluid retention) with swelling of the fingers or ankles and may raise your blood pressure. If you experience fluid retention, contact your health-care professional.

4. *Melasma*

A spotty darkening of the skin is possible, particularly of the face.

5. *Other side effects*

Other side effects may include nausea, breast tenderness, change in appetite, headache, nervousness, depression, dizziness, loss of scalp hair, rash, vaginal infections, inflammation of the pancreas, and allergic reactions.

If any of these side effects bother you, call your health-care professional.

GENERAL PRECAUTIONS

1. *Missed periods and use of oral contraceptives before or during early pregnancy*

There may be times when you may not menstruate regularly after you have completed taking a cycle of pills. If you have taken your pills regularly and miss one menstrual period, continue taking your pills for the next cycle but be sure to inform your health-care professional. If you have not taken the pills daily as instructed and missed a menstrual period, or if you missed two consecutive menstrual periods, you may be pregnant. Check with your health-care professional immediately to determine whether you are pregnant. Stop taking oral contraceptives if pregnancy is confirmed.

There is no conclusive evidence that oral-contraceptive use is associated with an increase in birth defects when taken inadvertently during early pregnancy. Previously, a few studies had reported that oral contraceptives might be associated with birth defects, but these findings have not been confirmed in more recent studies. Nevertheless, oral contraceptives should not be used during pregnancy. You should check with your health-care professional about risks to your unborn child of any medication taken during pregnancy.

2. *While breast-feeding*

If you are breast-feeding, consult your health-care professional before starting oral contraceptives. Some of the drug will be passed on to the child in the milk. A few adverse effects on the child have been reported, including yellowing of the skin (jaundice) and breast enlargement. In addition, oral contraceptives may decrease the amount and quality of your milk. If possible, do not use oral contraceptives while breast-feeding. You should use another method of contraception since breast-feeding provides only partial protection from becoming pregnant, and this partial protection decreases significantly as you breast-feed for longer periods of time. You should consider starting oral contraceptives only after you have weaned your child completely.

3. *Laboratory tests*

If you are scheduled for any laboratory tests, tell your health-care professional you are taking birth-control pills. Certain blood tests may be affected by birth-control pills.

4. *Drug interactions*

Certain drugs may interact with birth-control pills to make them less effective in preventing pregnancy or cause an increase in breakthrough bleeding. Such drugs include rifampin, drugs used for epilepsy such as barbiturates (for example, phenobarbital) and phenytoin (Dilantin® is one brand of this drug), primidone (Mysoline®), topiramate (Topamax®), carbamazepine (Tegretol® is one brand of this drug), phenylbutazone (Butazolidin® is one brand of this drug), some drugs used for HIV or AIDS such as ritonavir (Norvir®), modafinil (Provigil®) and possibly certain antibiotics (such as ampicillin and other penicillins, and tetracyclines), and herbal products containing St. John's Wort (Hypericum perforatum). You may also need to use a nonhormonal method of contraception (such as condoms and/or spermicide) during any cycle in which you take drugs that can make oral contraceptives less effective.

You may be at higher risk of a specific type of liver dysfunction if you take troleandomycin and oral contraceptives at the same time.

Be sure to tell your health-care professional if you are taking or start taking any other medications, including nonprescription products or herbal products while taking birth control pills.

5. *Sexually transmitted diseases*

This product (like all oral contraceptives) is intended to prevent pregnancy. It does not protect against transmission of HIV (AIDS) and other sexually transmitted diseases such as chlamydia, genital herpes, genital warts, gonorrhea, hepatitis B, and syphilis.

HOW TO TAKE THE PILL

IMPORTANT POINTS TO REMEMBER

BEFORE YOU START TAKING YOUR PILLS:

1. BE SURE TO READ THESE DIRECTIONS:

Before you start taking your pills.

And

Anytime you are not sure what to do.

2. THE RIGHT WAY TO TAKE THE PILL IS TO TAKE ONE PILL EVERY DAY AT THE SAME TIME.

If you miss pills you could get pregnant. This includes starting the pack late. The more pills you miss, the more likely you are to get pregnant.

3. MANY WOMEN HAVE SPOTTING OR LIGHT BLEEDING, OR MAY FEEL SICK TO THEIR STOMACH DURING THE FIRST 1–3 PACKS OF PILLS.

If you feel sick to your stomach, do not stop taking the pill. The problem will usually go away. If it doesn't go away, check with your health-care professional.

4. MISSING PILLS CAN ALSO CAUSE SPOTTING OR LIGHT BLEEDING, even when you make up these missed pills.

On the days you take 2 pills to make up for missed pills, you could also feel a little sick to your stomach.

5. IF YOU HAVE VOMITING (within 4 hours after you take your pill), you should follow the instructions for WHAT TO DO IF YOU MISS PILLS. IF YOU HAVE DIARRHEA or IF YOU TAKE SOME MEDICINES, including some antibiotics, your pills may not work as well. Use a back-up nonhormonal method (such as condoms and/or spermicide) until you check with your health-care professional.

6. IF YOU HAVE TROUBLE REMEMBERING TO TAKE THE PILL, talk to your health-care professional about how to make pill-taking easier or about using another method of birth control.

7. IF YOU HAVE ANY QUESTIONS OR ARE UNSURE ABOUT THE INFORMATION IN THIS LEAFLET, call your health-care professional.

OVRAL® AND OVRAL®-28 (norgestrel and ethinyl estradiol tablets)

BEFORE YOU START TAKING YOUR PILLS

1. DECIDE WHAT TIME OF DAY YOU WANT TO TAKE YOUR PILL.

It is important to take it at about the same time every day.

2. LOOK AT YOUR PILL PACK TO SEE IF IT HAS 21 OR 28 PILLS:

The *21-pill* pack has 21 "active" white pills (with hormones) to take for 3 weeks, followed by 1 week without pills.

The *28-pill* pack has 21 "active" white pills (with hormones) to take for 3 weeks, followed by 1 week of reminder pink pills (without hormones).

3. ALSO FIND:

1) where on the pack to start taking pills, and

2) in what order to take the pills (follow the arrows).

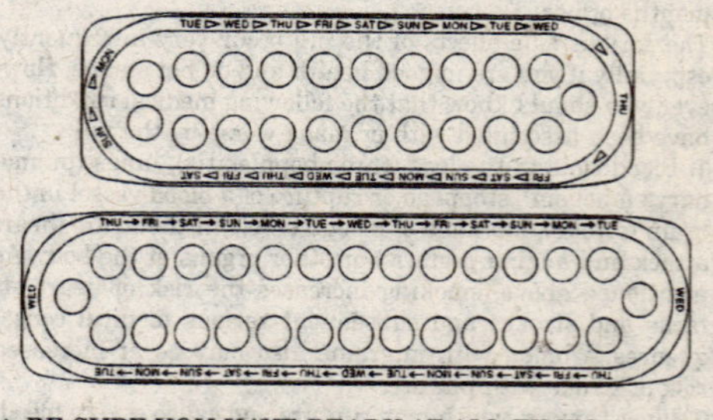

4. BE SURE YOU HAVE READY AT ALL TIMES:

ANOTHER KIND OF BIRTH CONTROL (such as condoms and/or spermicide) to use as a back-up in case you miss pills.

AN EXTRA, FULL PILL PACK.

WHEN TO START THE _FIRST_ PACK OF PILLS

For the 21-day pill pack you have two choices of which day to start taking your first pack of pills. (See DAY 1 START or SUNDAY START directions below.) Decide with your health-care professional which is the best day for you. The 28-day pill pack accommodates a SUNDAY START only. For either pill pack pick a time of day which will be easy to remember.

DAY 1 START:

These instructions are for the 21-day pill pack only. The 28-day pill pack does not accommodate a **DAY 1 START** dosage regimen.

1. Take the first "active" white pill of the first pack during the *first 24 hours of your period.*

2. You will not need to use a back-up nonhormonal method of birth control, since you are starting the pill at the beginning of your period.

SUNDAY START:

These instructions are for either the 21-day or the 28-day pill pack.

1. Take the first "active" white pill of the first pack on the *Sunday after your period starts,* even if you are still bleeding. If your period begins on Sunday, start the pack that same day.

2. *Use a nonhormonal method of birth control* (such as condoms and/or spermicide) as a back-up method if you have sex anytime from the Sunday you start your first pack until the next Sunday (7 days).

WHAT TO DO DURING THE MONTH

1. TAKE ONE PILL AT THE SAME TIME EVERY DAY UNTIL THE PACK IS EMPTY.

Do not skip pills even if you are spotting or bleeding between monthly periods or feel sick to your stomach (nausea).

Do not skip pills even if you do not have sex very often.

2. WHEN YOU FINISH A PACK OR SWITCH YOUR BRAND OF PILLS:

21 pills: Wait 7 days to start the next pack. You will probably have your period during that week. Be sure that no more than 7 days pass between 21-day packs.

28 pills: Start the next pack on the day after your last "reminder" pill. Do not wait any days between packs.

WHAT TO DO IF YOU MISS PILLS

The pill may not be as effective if you miss white "active" pills, and particularly if you miss the first few or the last few white "active" pills in a pack.

If you **MISS 1** white "active" pill:

1. Take it as soon as you remember. Take the next pill at your regular time. This means you may take 2 pills in 1 day.

2. You COULD BECOME PREGNANT if you have sex in the *7 days* after you miss pills. You MUST use a nonhormonal birth-control method (such as condoms and/or spermicide) as a back-up for those 7 days.

If you **MISS 2** white "active" pills in a row in **WEEK 1 OR WEEK 2** of your pack:

1. Take 2 pills on the day you remember and 2 pills the next day.

2. Then take 1 pill a day until you finish the pack.

3. You COULD BECOME PREGNANT if you have sex in the *7 days* after you miss pills. You MUST use a nonhormonal birth-control method (such as condoms and/or spermicide) as a back-up for those 7 days.

If you **MISS 2** white "active" pills in a row in **THE 3rd WEEK**:

The ***Day 1 Starter*** instructions are for the 21-day pill pack only. The 28-day pill pack does not accommodate a **DAY 1 START** dosage regimen. The ***Sunday Starter*** instructions are for either the 21-day or 28-day pill pack.

1. ***If you are a Day 1 Starter:***

THROW OUT the rest of the pill pack and start a new pack that same day.

If you are a Sunday Starter:

Keep taking 1 pill every day until Sunday.
On Sunday, THROW OUT the rest of the pack and start a new pack of pills that same day.
2. You may not have your period this month but this is expected. However, if you miss your period 2 months in a row, call your health-care professional because you might be pregnant.
3. You COULD BECOME PREGNANT if you have sex in the *7 days* after you miss pills. You MUST use a nonhormonal birth-control method (such as condoms and/or spermicide) as a back-up for those 7 days.
If you **MISS 3 OR MORE** white "active" pills in a row (during the first 3 weeks):
The ***Day 1 Starter*** instructions are for the 21-day pill pack only. The 28-day pill pack does not accommodate a **DAY 1 START** dosage regimen. The ***Sunday Starter*** instructions are for either the 21-day or 28-day pill pack.
1. ***If you are a Day 1 Starter:***
THROW OUT the rest of the pill pack and start a new pack that same day.
If you are a Sunday Starter:
Keep taking 1 pill every day until Sunday.
On Sunday, THROW OUT the rest of the pack and start a new pack of pills that same day.
2. You may not have your period this month but this is expected. However, if you miss your period 2 months in a row, call your health-care professional because you might be pregnant.
3. You COULD BECOME PREGNANT if you have sex in the 7 days after you miss pills. You MUST use a nonhormonal birth-control method (such as condoms and/or spermicide) as a back-up for those 7 days.

A REMINDER FOR THOSE ON 28-DAY PACKS
If you forget any of the 7 pink "reminder" pills in Week 4:
THROW AWAY the pills you missed.
Keep taking 1 pill each day until the pack is empty.
You do not need a back-up nonhormonal birth-control method if you start your next pack on time.

FINALLY, IF YOU ARE STILL NOT SURE WHAT TO DO ABOUT THE PILLS YOU HAVE MISSED
Use a BACK-UP NONHORMONAL BIRTH-CONTROL METHOD anytime you have sex.
KEEP TAKING ONE PILL EACH DAY until you can reach your health-care professional.

PREGNANCY DUE TO PILL FAILURE
The incidence of pill failure resulting in pregnancy is approximately 1% if taken every day as directed, but the average failure rate is approximately 5% including women who do not always take the pill exactly as directed without missing any pills. If you do become pregnant, the risk to the fetus is minimal, but you should stop taking your pills and discuss the pregnancy with your health-care professional.
PREGNANCY AFTER STOPPING THE PILL
There may be some delay in becoming pregnant after you stop using oral contraceptives, especially if you had irregular menstrual cycles before you used oral contraceptives. It may be advisable to postpone conception until you begin menstruating regularly once you have stopped taking the pill and desire pregnancy.
There does not appear to be any increase in birth defects in newborn babies when pregnancy occurs soon after stopping the pill.
If you do not desire pregnancy, you should use another method of birth control immediately after stopping the oral contraceptive pill.
OVERDOSAGE
Overdosage may cause nausea, vomiting, and fatigue/drowsiness. Withdrawal bleeding may occur in females. In case of overdosage, contact your health-care professional or pharmacist.
OTHER INFORMATION
Your health-care professional will take a medical and family history before prescribing oral contraceptives and will examine you. The physical examination may be delayed to another time if you request it and the health-care professional believes that it is appropriate to postpone it. You should be reexamined at least once a year. Be sure to inform your health-care professional if there is a family history of any of the conditions listed previously in this leaflet. Be sure to keep all appointments with your health-care professional, because this is a time to determine if there are early signs of side effects of oral-contraceptive use.
Do not use the drug for any condition other than the one for which it was prescribed. This drug has been prescribed specifically for you; do not give it to others who may want birth-control pills.
HEALTH BENEFITS FROM ORAL CONTRACEPTIVES
In addition to preventing pregnancy, use of oral contraceptives may provide certain benefits. They are:
- Menstrual cycles may become more regular.
- Blood flow during menstruation may be lighter, and less iron may be lost. Therefore, anemia due to iron deficiency is less likely to occur.
- Pain or other symptoms during menstruation may be encountered less frequently.
- Ovarian cysts may occur less frequently.
- Ectopic (tubal) pregnancy may occur less frequently.
- Noncancerous cysts or lumps in the breast may occur less frequently.
- Acute pelvic inflammatory disease may occur less frequently.
- Oral-contraceptive use may provide some protection against developing two forms of cancer: cancer of the ovaries and cancer of the lining of the uterus.

If you want more information about birth-control pills, ask your health-care professional or pharmacist. They have a more technical leaflet called the Professional Labeling which you may wish to read.

Wyeth®
Wyeth Pharmaceuticals Inc.
Philadelphia, PA 19101

W10442C003
ET02
Rev 08/03

OVRETTE® Tablets ℞
[*ō'vrĕt*]
(norgestrel tablets)
℞ only

Prescribing information for this product, which appears on pages 3449–3452 of the 2004 PDR, has been completely revised as follows. Please write "See Supplement A" next to the product heading.

Patients should be counseled that oral contraceptives do not protect against transmission of HIV (AIDS) and other sexually transmitted diseases (STDs) such as chlamydia, genital herpes, genital warts, gonorrhea, hepatitis B, and syphilis.

DESCRIPTION
Each OVRETTE tablet contains 0.075 mg of norgestrel (*dl*-13-beta-ethyl-17-alpha-ethinyl-17-beta-hydroxygon-4-en-3-one). The inactive ingredients present are cellulose, FD&C Yellow 5, lactose, magnesium stearate, and polacrilin potassium.
Each OVRETTE tablet contains 0.075 mg of a single active steroid ingredient, norgestrel, a totally synthetic progestogen. The available data suggest that the d (-) enantiomeric form of norgestrel is the biologically active portion. This form amounts to 0.0375 mg per OVRETTE tablet.

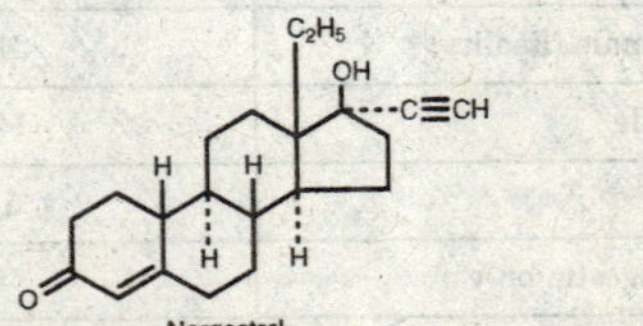

Norgestrel

$C_{21}H_{28}O_2$ M.W. 312.45

CLINICAL PHARMACOLOGY
1. Mode of Action
Progestin-only oral contraceptives such as OVRETTE prevent conception by suppressing ovulation in approximately half of users, thickening the cervical mucus to inhibit sperm penetration, lowering the midcycle LH and FSH peaks, slowing the movement of the ovum through the fallopian tubes, and altering the endometrium.
2. Pharmacokinetics
Serum progestin levels peak about two hours after oral administration, followed by rapid distribution and elimination. By 24 hours after drug ingestion, serum levels are near baseline, making efficacy dependent upon rigid adherence to the dosing schedule. There are large variations in serum levels among individual users. Progestin-only administration results in lower steady-state progestin levels and a shorter elimination half-life than concomitant administration with estrogens.

INDICATIONS AND USAGE
1. Indications
Progestin-only oral contraceptives are indicated for the prevention of pregnancy.
2. Efficacy
Oral contraceptives are highly effective. Table 1 lists the typical accidental pregnancy rates for users of oral contraceptives and other methods of contraception. The efficacy of these contraceptive methods except sterilization, the IUD, and the NORPLANT System, depends upon the reliability with which they are used correctly. Consistent use of these methods can result in lower failure rates.
[See table 1 at top of next page]

CONTRAINDICATIONS
Progestin-only oral contraceptives should not be used by women who currently have the following conditions:
- Known or suspected pregnancy
- Known or suspected carcinoma of the breast
- Undiagnosed abnormal genital bleeding
- Hypersensitivity to any component of this product
- Benign or malignant liver tumors
- Acute liver disease

WARNINGS
Cigarette smoking increases the risk of serious cardiovascular disease. Women who use oral contraceptives should be strongly advised not to smoke.
OVRETTE does not contain estrogen and, therefore, this insert does not discuss the serious health risks that have been associated with the estrogen component of combination oral contraceptives (COCs). The health-care professional is referred to the prescribing information of COCs for a discussion of those risks. The relationship between progestin-only oral contraceptives and these risks is not fully defined. The physician should remain alert to the earliest manifestation of symptoms of any serious disease and discontinue oral contraceptive therapy when appropriate.
1. Ectopic Pregnancy
The incidence of ectopic pregnancies for progestin-only oral contraceptive users is 5 per 1000 woman-years. Up to 10% of pregnancies reported in clinical studies of progestin-only oral contraceptive users are extrauterine. Although symptoms of ectopic pregnancy should be watched for, a history of ectopic pregnancy need not be considered a contraindication to use of this contraceptive method. Health-care professionals should be alert to the possibility of an ectopic pregnancy in women who become pregnant or complain of lower abdominal pain while on progestin-only oral contraceptives.
2. Delayed Follicular Atresia/Ovarian Cysts
If follicular development occurs, atresia of the follicle is sometimes delayed, and the follicle may continue to grow beyond the size it would attain in a normal cycle. Generally these enlarged follicles disappear spontaneously. Often they are asymptomatic; in some cases they are associated with mild abdominal pain. Rarely they may twist or rupture, requiring surgical intervention.
3. Irregular Genital Bleeding
Irregular menstrual patterns are common among women using progestin-only oral contraceptives. If genital bleeding is suggestive of infection, malignancy, pregnancy, or other conditions, such nonpharmacologic causes should be ruled out. If prolonged amenorrhea occurs, the possibility of pregnancy should be evaluated. If one menstrual period is missed and the progestin-only oral contraceptive has not been taken according to directions, or if two consecutive periods are missed, tablet-taking should be discontinued and a nonhormonal back-up method of contraception should be used until the possibility of pregnancy is excluded.
4. Carcinoma of the Breast and Reproductive Organs
Some epidemiological studies of oral contraceptive users have reported a slightly increased risk of having breast cancer diagnosed in women who were currently using combination oral contraceptives (COCs). The increased risk gradually disappeared within 10 years after stopping use of combination oral contraceptives. Breast cancers diagnosed in ever-users tend to be less clinically advanced than the cancers diagnosed in never-users. These studies have predominantly involved COCs and there are insufficient data to determine whether the use of progestin-only oral contraceptives similarly increases the risk. However, women with breast cancer should not use oral contraceptives because the role of female hormones in breast cancer has not been fully determined.
Some studies suggest that oral contraceptive use has been associated with an increase in the risk of cervical intraepithelial neoplasia or invasive cervical cancer in some populations of women. However, there continues to be controversy about the extent to which such findings may be due to differences in sexual behavior and other factors.
There are insufficient data to determine whether the use of progestin-only oral contraceptives increases the risk of developing cervical intraepithelial neoplasia.
5. Hepatic Neoplasia/Liver Disease
Benign hepatic adenomas are associated with COC use, although the incidence of benign tumors is rare in the United States. Rupture of benign, hepatic adenomas may cause death through intra-abdominal hemorrhage.
Studies from Britain and the US have shown an increased risk of developing hepatocellular carcinoma in COC-users. However, these cancers are rare. There are insufficient data to determine whether progestin-only oral contraceptives increase the risk of developing hepatic neoplasia.
Women with a history of oral contraceptive related cholestasis or women with cholestasis during pregnancy are more likely to have this condition with oral contraceptive use. If these women receive a progestin-only oral contraceptive they should be carefully monitored and, if the condition recurs, progestin-only oral contraceptive use should be discontinued.
6. Thromboembolic Disorders and Other Vascular Problems
An increased risk of venous and arterial thrombotic and thromboembolic events have been found to be associated with the use of COCs. These events include superficial venous thrombosis, deep-vein thrombosis, pulmonary embolism, retinal vascular thrombosis, myocardial infarction, and cerebrovascular events (thrombotic and hemorrhagic strokes). There are insufficient data to determine whether the use of progestin-only contraceptives increases the risk of developing thrombotic disease and/or other vascular problems. However, there have been reports of some of these conditions coincident with the use of progestin-only oral contraceptives; therefore, the possibility of thrombosis should be considered.
Care should be used when prescribing progestin-only oral contraceptives to women predisposed to thromboembolic disorders (eg, a history of thromboembolic events, thrombophilia, cardiovascular disease; women who are obese or experience prolonged immobilization).

PRECAUTIONS
1. General
Patients should be counseled that oral contraceptives do not protect against transmission of HIV (AIDS) and other

Continued on next page

Ovrette—Cont.

sexually transmitted diseases (STDs) such as chlamydia, genital herpes, genital warts, gonorrhea, hepatitis B, and syphilis.

2. Physical Examination and Follow Up

A complete personal and family medical history and physical examination is appropriate for all women, including women using oral contraceptives. The physical examination may be deferred until after initiation of oral contraceptives if requested by the woman and judged appropriate by the clinician. Such examinations should be repeated periodically during the use of progestin-only oral contraceptives.

3. Carbohydrate and Lipid Effects

Some progestin-only oral contraceptive users may experience slight deterioration in glucose tolerance with increases in plasma insulin, but women with diabetes mellitus who use progestin-only oral contraceptives do not generally experience changes in their insulin requirements. Nonetheless, diabetic women should be carefully observed while taking progestin-only oral contraceptives.

Lipid metabolism is occasionally affected in that HDL, HDL_2, and apolipoprotein A-I and A-II may be decreased; hepatic lipase may be increased. There is usually no effect on total cholesterol, HDL_3, LDL, or VLDL.

4. Drug Interactions

The effectiveness of progestin-only pills is reduced by hepatic enzyme-inducing drugs such as the anticonvulsants, phenytoin, carbamazepine; barbiturates; the antituberculosis drug rifampin; protease inhibitors; and herbal preparations containing St. John's Wort (hypericum perforatum). This could result in unintended pregnancy or breakthrough bleeding. There are anecdotal reports of reduced efficacy of combination oral contraceptives when used concomitantly with broad-spectrum antibiotics. No significant interaction has been found with progestin-only oral contraceptives and broad-spectrum antibiotics.

During concomitant use of OVRETTE and substances that may affect its efficacy, it is recommended that a nonhormonal back-up method of contraception be used in addition to the regular intake of OVRETTE. Use of a nonhormonal back-up method is advisable after discontinuation of substances that have led to induction of hepatic microsomal enzymes. It may take several weeks until enzyme induction has subsided, depending on dosage, duration of use, and rate of elimination of the inducing substance. For women receiving long-term therapy with hepatic enzyme inducers, another method of contraception should be considered.

Substances that reduce gastrointestinal transit time may affect contraceptive efficacy.

The product information of concomitant medications/substances should be consulted to identify potential interactions.

5. Interactions with Laboratory Tests

The following endocrine tests may be affected by progestin-only oral contraceptive use:

- Sex hormone-binding globulin (SHBG) concentrations may be decreased.
- Total thyroxine concentrations may be decreased, due to a decrease in thyroid binding globulin (TBG). However, free thyroxine level should remain unchanged.

6. Carcinogenesis

See **WARNINGS** section.

7. Pregnancy

Many epidemiological studies have found no effects on fetal development associated with long-term use of contraceptive doses of oral progestins. The few studies of infant growth and development that have been conducted have not demonstrated significant adverse effects. It is nonetheless prudent to rule out suspected pregnancy before initiating any hormonal contraceptive use. Epidemiological studies also do not suggest a teratogenic effect of oral contraceptives when taken inadvertently during early pregnancy. (See **CONTRAINDICATIONS**.)

8. Nursing Mothers

Small amounts of progestin pass into the breast milk, resulting in steroid levels in infant plasma. No adverse effects have been found on breastfeeding performance. Very rarely, adverse effects in the infant/child have been reported, including jaundice.

9. Fertility Following Discontinuation

The limited available data do not indicate a significant delay in the return of normal ovulation and fertility following discontinuation of progestin-only oral contraceptives.

10. Migraine/Headache

The onset or exacerbation of migraine, or development of headache with a new pattern that is recurrent, persistent, or severe requires discontinuation of oral contraceptives and evaluation of the cause.

Women with migraine (particularly migraine with aura) who take progestin-only oral contraceptives may be at increased risk of stroke.

11. Gastrointestinal

Diarrhea and/or vomiting may reduce hormone absorption.

12. Pediatric Use

Safety and efficacy of OVRETTE has been established in women of reproductive age. Safety and efficacy are expected to be the same for postpubertal adolescents under the age of 16 and users 16 and older. Use of this product before menarche is not indicated.

13. FD&C Yellow No. 5

This product contains FD&C Yellow No. 5 (tartrazine) which may cause allergic-type reactions (including bronchial asthma) in certain susceptible persons. Although the overall incidence of FD&C Yellow No. 5 (tartrazine) sensitivity in the general population is low, it is frequently seen in patients who also have aspirin hypersensitivity. (See **CONTRAINDICATIONS**.)

14. Geriatric Use

This product has not been studied in women over 65 years of age and is not indicated in this population.

INFORMATION FOR THE PATIENT

1. See **PATIENT LABELING** for detailed information.
2. Counseling issues

The following points should be discussed with prospective users before prescribing progestin-only oral contraceptives:

- The necessity of taking pills at the same time every day, including throughout all bleeding episodes.
- The need to use a nonhormonal back-up method of contraception (such as condoms and/or spermicides) for the next 48 hours whenever a progestin-only oral contraceptive is taken 3 or more hours late.
- The potential side effects of progestin-only oral contraceptives, particularly menstrual irregularities.

Table 1: Percentage Of Women Experiencing An Unintended Pregnancy During The First Year Of Typical Use And The First Year Of Perfect Use Of Contraception And The Percentage Continuing Use At The End Of The First Year
United States

	% of Women Experiencing an Unintended Pregnancy within the First Year of Use		% of Women Continuing Use at One Year[3]
Method (1)	Typical Use[1] (2)	Perfect Use[2] (3)	(4)
Chance[4]	85	85	
Spermicides[5]	26	6	40
Periodic abstinence	25		63
Calendar		9	
Ovulation Method		3	
Sympto-Thermal[6]		2	
Post-Ovulation		1	
Cap[7]			
Parous Women	40	26	42
Nulliparous Women	20	9	56
Sponge			
Parous Women	40	20	42
Nulliparous Women	20	9	56
Diaphragm[7]	20	6	56
Withdrawal	19	4	
Condom[8]			
Female (Reality)	21	5	56
Male	14	3	61
Pill	5		71
Progestin only		0.5	
Combined		0.1	
IUD			
Progesterone T	2.0	1.5	81
Copper T380A	0.8	0.6	78
LNg 20	0.1	0.1	81
Depo-Provera®	0.3	0.3	70
Levonorgestrel Implants (Norplant®)	0.05	0.05	88
Female Sterilization	0.5	0.5	100
Male Sterilization	0.15	0.10	100

Lactation Amenorrhea Method: LAM is a highly effective, temporary method of contraception.[9]

Source: Trussell J, Contraceptive efficacy. In: Hatcher RA, Trussell J, Stewart F, Cates W, Stewart GK, Kowel D, Guest F. Contraceptive Technology: Seventeenth Revised Edition. New York NY: Irvington Publishers; 1998.

[1]Among *typical* couples who initiate use of a method (not necessarily for the first time), the percentage who experience an accidental pregnancy during the first year if they do not stop use for any other reason.

[2]Among couples who initiate use of a method (not necessarily for the first time) and who use it *perfectly* (both consistently and correctly), the percentage who experience an accidental pregnancy during the first year if they do not stop use for any other reason.

[3]Among couples attempting to avoid pregnancy, the percentage who continue to use a method for one year.

[4]The percents becoming pregnant in columns (2) and (3) are based on data from populations where contraception is not used and from women who cease using contraception in order to become pregnant. Among such populations, about 89% become pregnant within one year. This estimate was lowered slightly (to 85%) to represent the percent who would become pregnant within one year among women now relying on reversible methods of contraception if they abandoned contraception altogether.

[5]Foams, creams, gels, vaginal suppositories, and vaginal film.

[6]Cervical mucus (ovulation) method supplemented by calendar in the pre-ovulatory and basal body temperature in the post-ovulatory phases.

[7]With spermicidal cream or jelly.

[8]Without spermicides.

[9]However, to maintain effective protection against pregnancy, another method of contraception must be used as soon as menstruation resumes, the frequency or duration of breastfeeds is reduced, bottle feeds are introduced, or the baby reaches 6 months of age.

- The need to inform the clinician of prolonged episodes of bleeding, amenorrhea or severe abdominal pain.
- The importance of using a barrier method in addition to progestin-only oral contraceptives if a woman is at risk of contracting or transmitting STDs/HIV.

ADVERSE REACTIONS

An increased risk of the following adverse reactions has been reported with the use of progestin-only oral contraceptives (see **WARNINGS** section for additional information):
Ectopic pregnancy
Delayed follicular atresia/ovarian cysts
Menstrual irregularity, changes in menstrual flow; breakthrough bleeding/spotting; amenorrhea, prolonged bleeding

The following adverse reactions also have been reported with the use of progestin-only oral contraceptives:
Abdominal pain, cramps, distention
Acne
Alopecia
Anaphylactic/anaphylactoid reactions, including urticaria, throat tightness, and facial edema
Appetite increase or decrease
AST, ALT, bilirubin increase
Blood pressure increase
Breast pain, enlargement, secretion, and tenderness
Chloasma/melasma that may persist
Cholestasis
Dizziness
Edema
Fatigue
Galactorrhea
Glucose intolerance
HDL decrease
Hirsutism
Leg cramps/pain
Libido decrease
Migraine/headache
Mood disturbances, including depression
Myocardial infarction
Nausea
Nervousness
Rash
Stroke
Vaginal discharge
Vomiting
Weight change (increase or decrease)
See **WARNINGS** section for discussion of:
Carcinoma of the breast and reproductive organs
Hepatic neoplasia
Arterial and venous thromboembolic events

OVERDOSAGE

Symptoms of oral contraceptive overdosage may include nausea, vomiting, breast tenderness, dizziness, somnolence (drowsiness/fatigue), and withdrawal bleeding in females. There is no specific antidote and further treatment of overdose, if necessary, is directed to the symptoms.

DOSAGE AND ADMINISTRATION

To achieve maximum contraceptive effectiveness, OVRETTE must be taken exactly as directed. One tablet is taken every day, at the same time. Administration is continuous, with no interruption between pill packs. See **PATIENT LABELING** for detailed instructions.

If one menstrual period is missed and the progestin-only oral contraceptive has not been taken according to directions, or if two consecutive periods are missed, tablet-taking should be discontinued and a nonhormonal back-up method of contraception should be used until the possibility of pregnancy is excluded.

HOW SUPPLIED

OVRETTE® tablets (0.075 mg norgestrel) are available in packages of 6 PILPAK® dispensers with 28 tablets each as follows: NDC 0008-0062-01, yellow, round tablet marked "WYETH" on one side and "62" on reverse side.

STORAGE

Store at controlled room temperature 20° to 25°C (68° to 77°F).

References available upon request.

DETAILED PATIENT LABELING

OVRETTE® (norgestrel) TABLETS

This product (like all oral contraceptives) is used to prevent pregnancy. It does not protect against HIV infection (AIDS) or other sexually transmitted diseases (STDs) such as chlamydia, genital herpes, genital warts, gonorrhea, hepatitis B, and syphilis.

DESCRIPTION

Each OVRETTE® tablet contains 0.075 mg of norgestrel. The inactive ingredients present are cellulose, FD&C Yellow 5, lactose, magnesium stearate, and polacrilin potassium.

INTRODUCTION

This leaflet is about birth control pills that contain one hormone, a progestin. Please read this leaflet before you begin to take your pills. It is meant to be used along with talking with your health-care professional.

Progestin-only pills are often called "POPs" or "the mini-pill." POPs have less progestin than the combined birth control pill (or "the pill") which contains both an estrogen and a progestin.

HOW EFFECTIVE ARE POPs?

POPs or "birth-control pills" or "the pill" are used to prevent pregnancy and are more effective than other nonsurgical methods of birth control. When they are taken correctly, without missing any pills the chance of becoming pregnant is approximately 1.0% per year. Average failure rates are approximately 5% per year when women who miss pills are included. The chance of becoming pregnant increases with each missed pill during the menstrual cycle.

In comparison, average failure rates for other methods of birth control during the first year of use are as follows:

IUD: 0.1-2%	Female condom alone: 21%
Depo-Provera® (injectable progestogen): 0.3%	Cervical cap
Norplant® System (levonorgestrel implants): 0.05%	Never given birth: 20%
Diaphragm with spermicides: 20%	Given birth: 40%
Spermicides alone: 26%	Periodic abstinence: 25%
Male condom alone: 14%	No methods: 85%

HOW DO POPs WORK?

POPs can prevent pregnancy in different ways including:
- They make the cervical mucus at the entrance to the womb (the uterus) too thick for the sperm to get through to the egg.
- They prevent ovulation (release of the egg from the ovary) in about half of the cycles.
- They also affect other hormones, the fallopian tubes, and the lining of the uterus.

YOU SHOULD NOT TAKE POPs
- If there is any chance you may be pregnant.
- If you have breast cancer.
- If you have bleeding between your periods which has not been diagnosed.
- If you are hypersensitive or allergic to any component of this product.
- If you have liver tumors, either non-cancerous or cancerous.
- If you have acute liver disease.

RISKS OF TAKING POPs

Cigarette smoking greatly increases the possibility of suffering heart attacks and strokes. Women who use oral contraceptives are strongly advised not to smoke.

Warning: If you have sudden or severe pain in your lower abdomen or stomach area, you may have an ectopic pregnancy or an ovarian cyst. If this happens, you should contact your health-care professional immediately.

Ectopic Pregnancy

An ectopic pregnancy is a pregnancy outside the womb. Because POPs protect against pregnancy, the chance of having a pregnancy outside the womb is very low. If you do get pregnant while taking POPs, you have a slightly higher chance that the pregnancy will be ectopic than do users of some other birth control methods.

Ovarian Cysts

These cysts are small sacs of fluid in the ovary. They are more common among POP-users than among users of most other birth control methods. They usually disappear without treatment and rarely cause problems.

Cancer of the Reproductive Organs and Breasts

Some studies reported a slightly increased risk of the diagnosis of breast cancer in women who were currently using oral contraceptives, which contained both estrogen and progestin. The risk gradually disappeared within 10 years after stopping use of the combination oral contraceptive. There is not enough information to determine whether the use of POPs increases this risk in a similar way.

Some studies have found an increase in the incidence of cancer or precancerous lesions of the cervix in women who use combination oral contraceptives (COCs). However, this finding may be related to factors other than the use of oral contraceptives and there is not enough information to determine whether the use of POPs increases the risk of developing cancer of the cervix.

Liver Tumors or Diseases

In rare cases, use of COCs has been associated with non-cancerous but dangerous liver tumors. These non-cancerous liver tumors can rupture and cause fatal internal bleeding. In addition, a possible association has been found with COCs and liver cancer in studies in which a few women who developed these very rare cancers were found to have used COCs for long periods of time. There is not enough information to determine if POPs increase the risk of liver tumors. Talk with your health-care professional if you have or have had liver problems.

Headache/Migraine

If you develop or have worsening of migraine or develop headache with a new pattern that is recurrent, persistent, or severe, you should discontinue taking oral contraceptives and see your health-care professional for an evaluation of the cause.

Women with migraine (particularly migraine with aura) who take POPs may be at increased risk of stroke.

Abnormal Blood Clotting

Changes in the blood clotting system have been reported in users of COCs. These changes allow the blood to clot more easily, possibly allowing clots to form in the bloodstream. If blood clots do form in the bloodstream, they can cause serious problems by cutting off the blood supply to vital organs. These problems may include a stroke (if the clot is in a blood vessel of the brain), a heart attack (if the clot is in a blood vessel of the heart), a pulmonary embolus (if the clot forms in the legs or pelvis, then breaks off and travels to the lungs), retinal thrombosis (if the clot is in a blood vessel of the eye) or other problems. Any of these conditions may cause death or serious long term disability.

There is not enough information to determine whether the use of POPs is associated with the development of blood clots, blockage of blood vessels, heart attack, and stroke. However, there have been reports of some of these conditions with the use of POPs. Therefore, the possibility of blood clots should be considered.

Diabetic Women

Diabetic women taking POPs do not generally require changes in the amount of insulin they are taking. However, your health-care professional may monitor you more closely under these conditions.

FD&C Yellow No. 5 (tartrazine)

Ovrette contains FD&C Yellow No. 5 (tartrazine) which may cause allergic-type reactions (including bronchial asthma) in certain susceptible persons. Although the overall incidence of FD&C Yellow No. 5 (tartrazine) sensitivity in the general population is low, it is frequently seen in patients who also have aspirin sensitivity.

SEXUALLY TRANSMITTED DISEASES (STDs)

Warning: POPs DO NOT PROTECT AGAINST GETTING OR GIVING SOMEONE HIV (AIDS) OR ANY OTHER STD SUCH AS CHLAMYDIA, GONORRHEA, GENITAL WARTS, HERPES, HEPATITIS B, AND SYPHILIS.

SIDE EFFECTS

An increased risk of the following side effects (see **RISKS OF TAKING POPs** for additional information) has been associated with the use of POPs:

Irregular bleeding - The most common side effect of POPs is a change in menstrual bleeding. Your periods may be either early or late, shorter or longer, heavier or lighter and/or you may have some spotting between periods. Taking pills late or missing pills can also result in some spotting or bleeding.
Ectopic pregnancy (pregnancy outside of the uterus)
Ovarian cysts

Other Side Effects:
Abdominal pain, cramps, bloating
Acne
Allergic/hypersensitivity reactions, including hives, rash, throat tightness, and facial swelling
Appetite increase or decrease
Blood pressure increase
Blood sugar increase
Breast pain, enlargement, secretion, and tenderness
Changes in liver function tests (AST, ALT, bilirubin increase)
Darkening areas of skin, especially on the face that may persist
Dizziness
Excessive hair growth on the face and body
Fatigue
Fluid retention
Hair loss
HDL decrease
Headache/migraine
Heart attack
Jaundice
Leg cramps/pain
Milky breast discharge
Mood disturbances, including depression
Nausea
Nervousness
Rash
Sex drive decrease
Stroke
Vaginal discharge
Vomiting
Weight changes (increase or decrease)
See also **RISKS OF TAKING POPs** for information on:
Abnormal blood clotting
Cancer of the reproductive organs and breast
Liver tumors
If you are concerned about any of these side effects, check with your health-care professional.

USING POPs WITH OTHER MEDICINES

Before taking a POP, inform your health-care professional if you are taking medicines for seizures (epilepsy), tuberculosis (TB), HIV/AIDS, or any other medication, including over-the-counter medicine and herbal products.

These medicines can make POPs less effective:

Medicines for seizures such as:
- Phenytoin (Dilantin®)
- Carbamazepine (Tegretol®)
- Phenobarbital

Medicine for TB:
- Rifampin (Rifadin®, Rimactane®)

Herbal Preparations such as:
- St. John's Wort (hypericum perforatum)

HIV/AIDS drugs such as:
- Zidovudine (Retrovir®)
- Indinavir (Crixivan®)

Before you begin taking any new medicines, be sure your health-care professional knows you are taking a progestin-only birth control pill.

Continued on next page

Ovrette—Cont.

HOW TO TAKE POPs

Important Points to Remember

- POPs must be taken at the same time every day, so choose a time and then take the pill at that same time every day. Every time you take a pill late, and especially if you miss a pill, you are more likely to get pregnant.
- Start the next pack the day after the last pack is finished. There is no break between packs. Always have your next pack of pills ready.
- You may have some bleeding between periods. Do not stop taking your pills if this happens. This is usually temporary and without significance; however, if bleeding is prolonged (more than 8 days) or unusually heavy, consult your health-care professional.
- If 1 menstrual period is missed and Ovrette has not been taken according to directions or if 2 consecutive periods are missed, tablet-taking should be discontinued and a nonhormonal back-up method of birth control (such as a condom and/or a spermicide) should be used until the possibility of pregnancy is excluded.
- If you vomit within 4 hours after taking a pill, or have diarrhea, absorption may not be complete; therefore, use a nonhormonal back-up method of birth control every time you have sex during the next 48 hours. (See **If You Are Late or Miss Taking Your POPs**.)
- If you want to stop taking POPs, you can do so at any time, but, if you remain sexually active and don't wish to become pregnant, be certain to use another birth control method.
- If you are not sure about how to take POPs, ask your health-care professional.

Starting POPs

- It's best to take your first POP on the first day of your menstrual period.
- If you decide to take your first POP on another day, use a nonhormonal back-up method of birth control (such as a condom and/or a spermicide) every time you have sex during the first 48 hours.
- If you have had a miscarriage, an abortion, or gave birth and are NOT breastfeeding, you can start POPs the next day. In addition, a nonhormonal back-up method of birth control should be used for the first 48 hours.

If You Are Late or Miss Taking Your POPs

- If one tablet is missed, but is less than three hours late, it should be taken as soon as it is remembered. Further tablets should be taken at the usual time.
- If one tablet is missed and is more than three hours late or if more than one consecutive tablet is missed, the last missed tablet should be taken as soon as it is remembered, even if this means taking two tablets in one day. Further tablets should be taken at the usual time, and a nonhormonal back-up method of birth control (such as a condom and/or a spermicide) should be used for the next 48 hours.
- In addition, if three or more tablets have been missed, the possibility of pregnancy should be considered before tablet-taking is resumed.
- If you are not sure what to do about the pills you have missed, keep taking POPs and use a nonhormonal back-up method of birth control until you can talk to your health-care professional.

If You Are Breastfeeding

- If you are breastfeeding (not giving your baby any food or formula), you may start your pills 6 weeks after delivery.
- When you begin taking your pills, a nonhormonal back-up method of birth control (such as a condom and/or a spermicide) should be used for the first 48 hours.

If You Are Switching Pills

- If you are switching from the combined pills to POPs, take the first POP the day after you finish the last active combined pill. Do not take any of the 7 inactive pills from the combined pill pack. You should know that many women have irregular periods after switching to POPs, but this is normal and to be expected.
- If you are switching from POPs to the combined pills, take the first active combined pill on the first day of your period, even if your POPs pack is not finished.
- If you switch to another brand of POPs, start the new brand anytime.
- If you are breastfeeding, you can switch to another method of birth control (such as a condom and/or a spermicide) at any time, except do not switch to the combined pills until you stop breastfeeding.

CHANGING FROM ANOTHER TYPE OF PROGESTIN-ONLY METHOD (IMPLANT, INJECTION)

Tablet-taking should start on the day of an implant removal or, if using an injection, the day the next injection would be due. In addition, a nonhormonal back-up method of birth control should be used for the first 48 hours.

PREGNANCY WHILE ON THE PILL

If you become pregnant or think you might be pregnant contact your health-care professional. You should stop taking POPs if pregnancy is confirmed. Even though POPs have not been shown to cause harm to the unborn baby, it is always best to avoid taking any drugs or medicines that you do not need when you are pregnant.

You should get a pregnancy test:

- If your period is late and you took one or more pills late or missed taking them and had sex without a nonhormonal back-up method of birth control.
- Anytime you miss 2 periods in a row.

WILL POPs AFFECT YOUR ABILITY TO GET PREGNANT LATER?

If you want to become pregnant, simply stop taking POPs. POPs will not delay your ability to get pregnant.

BREASTFEEDING

POPs have not been shown to affect breastfeeding performance. As with other medications taken while breastfeeding, small amounts of Ovrette can pass into the breast milk. Very rarely, adverse effects in the infant/child have been reported, including jaundice.

OVERDOSE

Overdosage may cause nausea, vomiting, breast tenderness, dizziness, somnolence (fatigue/drowsiness), and withdrawal bleeding in females. In case of overdosage, contact your health-care professional or pharmacist.

OTHER QUESTIONS OR CONCERNS

If you have any questions or concerns, check with your health-care professional. You can also ask for the more detailed "Professional Labeling" written for health-care professionals.

HOW TO STORE OVRETTE®

Store at controlled room temperature, 20° to 25°C (68° to 77°F).

Wyeth®
Wyeth Pharmaceuticals Inc.
Philadelphia, PA 19101

W10454C003
ET02
Rev 10/03

PREMARIN® ℞

[*prĕm'ă-rĭn*]
(conjugated estrogens tablets, USP)
℞ only

Prescribing information for this product, which appears on pages 3456–3462 of the 2004 PDR, has been completely revised as follows. Please write "See Supplement A" next to the product heading.

ESTROGENS INCREASE THE RISK OF ENDOMETRIAL CANCER

Close clinical surveillance of all women taking estrogens is important. Adequate diagnostic measures, including endometrial sampling when indicated, should be undertaken to rule out malignancy in all cases of undiagnosed persistent or recurring abnormal vaginal bleeding. There is no evidence that the use of "natural" estrogens results in a different endometrial risk profile than synthetic estrogens of equivalent estrogen dose.

CARDIOVASCULAR AND OTHER RISKS

Estrogens with or without progestins should not be used for the prevention of cardiovascular disease.

The Women's Health Initiative (WHI) study reported increased risks of myocardial infarction, stroke, invasive breast cancer, pulmonary emboli, and deep vein thrombosis in postmenopausal women during 5 years of treatment with conjugated equine estrogens (0.625 mg) combined with medroxyprogesterone acetate (2.5 mg) relative to placebo (see **CLINICAL PHARMACOLOGY, Clinical Studies**). Other doses of conjugated estrogens and medroxyprogesterone acetate, and other combinations of estrogens and progestins were not studied in the WHI and, in the absence of comparable data, these risks should be assumed to be similar. Because of these risks, estrogens with or without progestins should be prescribed at the lowest effective doses and for the shortest duration consistent with treatment goals and risks for the individual woman.

DESCRIPTION

Premarin® (conjugated estrogens tablets, USP) for oral administration contains a mixture of conjugated equine estrogens obtained exclusively from natural sources, occurring as the sodium salts of water-soluble estrogen sulfates blended to represent the average composition of material derived from pregnant mares' urine. It is a mixture of sodium estrone sulfate and sodium equilin sulfate. It contains as concomitant components, as sodium sulfate conjugates, 17α-dihydroequilin, 17α-estradiol, and 17β-dihydroequilin. Tablets for oral administration are available in 0.3 mg, 0.45 mg, 0.625 mg, 0.9 mg, 1.25 mg, and 2.5 mg strengths of conjugated estrogens.

Premarin tablets contain the following inactive ingredients: calcium phosphate tribasic, calcium sulfate, carnauba wax, cellulose, glyceryl monooleate, lactose, magnesium stearate, methylcellulose, pharmaceutical glaze, polyethylene glycol, stearic acid (not present in 0.45 mg tablet), sucrose, and titanium dioxide.

— 0.3 mg tablets also contain: D&C Yellow No. 10, FD&C Blue No. 1, FD&C Blue No. 2, FD&C Yellow No. 6; these tablets comply with USP Drug Release Test 1.
— 0.45 mg tablets also contain: FD&C Blue No. 2; these tablets comply with USP Drug Release Test 1.
— 0.625 mg tablets also contain: FD&C Blue No. 2, D&C Red No. 27, FD&C Red No. 40; these tablets comply with USP Drug Release Test 1.
— 0.9 mg tablets also contain: D&C Red No. 6, D&C Red No. 7; these tablets comply with USP Drug Release Test 2.
— 1.25 mg tablets also contain: black iron oxide, D&C Yellow No. 10, FD&C Yellow No. 6; these tablets comply with USP Drug Release Test 3.
— 2.5 mg tablets also contain: FD&C Blue No. 2, D&C Red No. 7; these tablets comply with USP Drug Release Test 3.

CLINICAL PHARMACOLOGY

Endogenous estrogens are largely responsible for the development and maintenance of the female reproductive system and secondary sexual characteristics. Although circulating estrogens exist in a dynamic equilibrium of metabolic interconversions, estradiol is the principal intracellular human estrogen and is substantially more potent than its metabolites, estrone and estriol, at the receptor level.

The primary source of estrogen in normally cycling adult women is the ovarian follicle, which secretes 70 to 500 mcg of estradiol daily, depending on the phase of the menstrual cycle. After menopause, most endogenous estrogen is produced by conversion of androstenedione, secreted by the adrenal cortex, to estrone by peripheral tissues. Thus, estrone and the sulfate-conjugated form, estrone sulfate, are the most abundant circulating estrogens in postmenopausal women.

Estrogens act through binding to nuclear receptors in estrogen-responsive tissues. To date, two estrogen receptors have been identified. These vary in proportion from tissue to tissue.

Circulating estrogens modulate the pituitary secretion of the gonadotropins, luteinizing hormone (LH) and follicle stimulating hormone (FSH) through a negative feedback mechanism. Estrogens act to reduce the elevated levels of these gonadotropins seen in postmenopausal women.

Pharmacokinetics

Absorption

Conjugated estrogens are soluble in water and are well absorbed from the gastrointestinal tract after release from the drug formulation. The Premarin tablet releases conjugated estrogens slowly over several hours. Table 1 summarizes the mean pharmacokinetic parameters for unconjugated and conjugated estrogens following administration of 2 × 0.3 mg, 2 × 0.45 mg, and 2 × 0.625 mg tablets to healthy postmenopausal women.

[See table 1 at top of next page]

Distribution

The distribution of exogenous estrogens is similar to that of endogenous estrogens. Estrogens are widely distributed in the body and are generally found in higher concentration in the sex hormone target organs. Estrogens circulate in the blood largely bound to sex hormone binding globulin (SHBG) and albumin.

Metabolism

Exogenous estrogens are metabolized in the same manner as endogenous estrogens. Circulating estrogens exist in a dynamic equilibrium of metabolic interconversions. These transformations take place mainly in the liver. Estradiol is converted reversibly to estrone, and both can be converted to estriol, which is the major urinary metabolite. Estrogens also undergo enterohepatic recirculation via sulfate and glucuronide conjugation in the liver, biliary secretion of conjugates into the intestine, and hydrolysis in the gut followed by reabsorption. In postmenopausal women a significant proportion of the circulating estrogens exists as sulfate conjugates, especially estrone sulfate, which serves as a circulating reservoir for the formation of more active estrogens.

Excretion

Estradiol, estrone, and estriol are excreted in the urine along with glucuronide and sulfate conjugates.

Special Populations

No pharmacokinetic studies were conducted in special populations, including patients with renal or hepatic impairment.

Drug Interactions

Data from a single-dose drug-drug interaction study involving conjugated estrogens and medroxyprogesterone acetate indicate that the pharmacokinetic dispositions of both drugs are not significantly altered. No other clinical drug-drug interaction studies have been conducted with conjugated estrogens.

In vitro and in vivo studies have shown that estrogens are metabolized partially by cytochrome P450 3A4 (CYP3A4). Therefore, inducers or inhibitors of CYP3A4 may affect estrogen drug metabolism. Inducers of CYP3A4 such as St. John's Wort preparations (Hypericum perforatum), phenobarbital, carbamazepine, and rifampin may reduce plasma concentrations of estrogens, possibly resulting in a decrease in therapeutic effects and/or changes in the uterine bleeding profile. Inhibitors of CYP3A4 such as erythromycin, clarithromycin, ketoconazole, itraconazole, ritonavir and grapefruit juice may increase plasma concentrations of estrogens and may result in side effects.

TABLE 1. PHARMACOKINETIC PARAMETERS FOR PREMARIN

PK Parameter Arithmetic Mean (%CV)	C_{max}	t_{max} (h)	$t_{1/2}$ (h)	AUC
Pharmacokinetic Profile of Unconjugated Estrogens Following a Dose of 2 × 0.3 mg				
PK Parameter Arithmetic Mean (%CV)	C_{max} (pg/mL)	t_{max} (h)	$t_{1/2}$ (h)	AUC (pg•h/mL)
Estrone	82 (33)	7.8 (27)	54.7 (42)	5390 (50)
Baseline-adjusted estrone	58 (42)	7.8 (27)	21.1 (45)	1467 (41)
Equilin	31 (47)	7.2 (28)	18.3 (110)	652 (68)
Pharmacokinetic Profile of Conjugated Estrogens Following a Dose of 2 × 0.3 mg				
PK Parameter Arithmetic Mean (%CV)	C_{max} (ng/mL)	t_{max} (h)	$t_{1/2}$ (h)	AUC (ng•h/mL)
Estrone	2.5 (32)	6.5 (29)	25.4 (22)	61.0 (43)
Baseline-adjusted total estrone	2.4 (32)	6.5 (29)	16.2 (34)	40.8 (36)
Equilin	1.6 (40)	5.9 (27)	11.8 (21)	22.4 (42)
Pharmacokinetic Profile of Unconjugated Estrogens Following a Dose of 2 × 0.45 mg				
PK Parameter Arithmetic Mean (%CV)	C_{max} (pg/mL)	t_{max} (h)	$t_{1/2}$ (h)	AUC (pg•h/mL)
Estrone	92 (32)	8.7 (28)	56.4 (68)	6344 (56)
Baseline-adjusted estrone	65 (40)	8.7 (28)	20.3 (38)	1940 (40)
Equilin	35 (49)	7.6 (33)	21.9 (113)	849 (60)
Pharmacokinetic Profile of Conjugated Estrogens Following a Dose of 2 × 0.45 mg				
PK Parameter Arithmetic Mean (%CV)	C_{max} (ng/mL)	t_{max} (h)	$t_{1/2}$ (h)	AUC (ng•h/mL)
Total estrone	2.8 (46)	7.1 (27)	27.6 (35)	77 (34)
Baseline-adjusted total estrone	2.6 (46)	7.1 (27)	14.7 (42)	48 (38)
Total equilin	1.9 (53)	5.9 (32)	11.8 (32)	29 (55)
Pharmacokinetic Profile of Unconjugated Estrogens Following a Dose of 2 × 0.625 mg				
PK Parameter Arithmetic Mean (%CV)	C_{max} (pg/mL)	t_{max} (h)	$t_{1/2}$ (h)	AUC (pg•h/mL)
Estrone	139 (37)	8.8 (20)	28.0 (30)	5016 (34)
Baseline-adjusted estrone	120 (41)	8.8 (20)	17.4 (37)	2956 (39)
Equilin	66 (42)	7.9 (19)	13.6 (52)	1210 (37)
Pharmacokinetic Profile of Conjugated Estrogens Following a Dose of 2 × 0.625 mg				
PK Parameter Arithmetic Mean (%CV)	C_{max} (ng/mL)	t_{max} (h)	$t_{1/2}$ (h)	AUC (ng•h/mL)
Total estrone	7.3 (41)	7.3 (24)	15.0 (25)	134 (42)
Baseline-adjusted total estrone	7.1 (41)	7.3 (24)	13.6 (23)	122 (38)
Total equilin	5.0 (42)	6.2 (26)	10.1 (26)	65 (44)

TABLE 2. SUMMARY TABULATION OF THE NUMBER OF HOT FLUSHES PER DAY–MEAN VALUES AND COMPARISONS BETWEEN THE ACTIVE TREATMENT GROUPS AND THE PLACEBO GROUP: PATIENTS WITH AT LEAST 7 MODERATE TO SEVERE FLUSHES PER DAY OR AT LEAST 50 PER WEEK AT BASELINE, LOCF

Treatment (No. of Patients) Time Period (week)	No. of Hot Flushes/Day: Baseline Mean ± SD	Observed Mean ± SD	Mean Change ± SD	p-Values vs. Placebo[a]
0.625 mg CE (n = 27)				
4	12.29 ± 3.89	1.95 ± 2.77	-10.34 ± 4.73	<0.001
12	12.29 ± 3.89	0.75 ± 1.82	-11.54 ± 4.62	<0.001
0.45 mg CE (n = 32)				
4	12.25 ± 5.04	5.04 ± 5.31	-7.21 ± 4.75	<0.001
12	12.25 ± 5.04	2.32 ± 3.32	-9.93 ± 4.64	<0.001
0.3 mg CE (n = 30)				
4	13.77 ± 4.78	4.65 ± 3.71	-9.12 ± 4.71	<0.001
12	13.77 ± 4.78	2.52 ± 3.23	-11.25 ± 4.60	<0.001
Placebo (n = 28)				
4	11.69 ± 3.87	7.89 ± 5.28	-3.80 ± 4.71	—
12	11.69 ± 3.87	5.71 ± 5.22	-5.98 ± 4.60	—

a: Based on analysis of covariance with treatment as factor and baseline as covariate.

Clinical Studies

Effects on Vasomotor Symptoms

In the first year of the Health and Osteoporosis, Progestin and Estrogen (HOPE) Study, a total of 2805 postmenopausal women (average age 53.3 ± 4.9 years) were randomly assigned to one of eight treatment groups, receiving either placebo or conjugated estrogens with or without medroxyprogesterone acetate. Efficacy for vasomotor symptoms was assessed during the first 12 weeks of treatment in a subset of symptomatic women (n = 241) who had at least 7 moderate to severe hot flushes daily or at least 50 moderate to severe hot flushes during the week before randomization. Premarin (0.3 mg, 0.45 mg, and 0.625 mg tablets) was shown to be statistically better than placebo at weeks 4 and 12 for relief of both the frequency and severity of moderate to severe vasomotor symptoms. Table 2 shows the adjusted mean number of hot flushes in the Premarin 0.3 mg, 0.45 mg, and 0.625 mg and placebo treatment groups over the initial 12-week period.

[See table 2 above]

Effects on Vulvar and Vaginal Atrophy

Results of vaginal maturation indexes at cycles 6 and 13 showed that the differences from placebo were statistically significant (p<0.001) for all treatment groups (conjugated estrogens alone and conjugated estrogens/medroxyprogesterone acetate treatment groups).

Effects on Bone Mineral Density

Health and Osteoporosis, Progestin and Estrogen (HOPE) Study

The HOPE study was a double-blind, randomized, placebo/active-drug-controlled, multicenter study of healthy postmenopausal women with an intact uterus. Subjects (mean age 53.3 ± 4.9 years) were 2.3 ± 0.9 years, on average, since menopause, and took one 600-mg tablet of elemental calcium (Caltrate) daily. Subjects were not given vitamin D supplements. They were treated with Premarin 0.625 mg, 0.45 mg, 0.3 mg, or placebo. Prevention of bone loss was assessed by measurement of bone mineral density (BMD), primarily at the anteroposterior lumbar spine (L_2 to L_4). Secondarily, BMD measurements of the total body, femoral neck, and trochanter were also analyzed. Serum osteocalcin, urinary calcium, and N-telopeptide were used as bone turnover markers (BTM) at cycles 6, 13, 19, and 26.

Intent-to-treat subjects

All active treatment groups showed significant differences from placebo in each of the 4 BMD endpoints at cycles 6, 13, 19, and 26. The mean percent increases in the primary efficacy measure (L_2 to L_4 BMD) at the final on-therapy evaluation (cycle 26 for those who completed and the last available evaluation for those who discontinued early) were 2.46% with 0.625 mg, 2.26% with 0.45 mg, and 1.13% with 0.3 mg. The placebo group showed a mean percent decrease from baseline at the final evaluation of 2.45%. These results show that the lower dosages of Premarin were effective in increasing L_2 to L_4 BMD compared with placebo and, therefore, support the efficacy of the lower doses.

The analysis for the other 3 BMD endpoints yielded mean percent changes from baseline in femoral trochanter that were generally larger than those seen for L_2 to L_4 and changes in femoral neck and total body that were generally smaller than those seen for L_2 to L_4. Significant differences between groups indicated that each of the Premarin treatments was more effective than placebo for all 3 of these additional BMD endpoints. With regard to femoral neck and total body, the active treatment groups all showed mean percent increases in BMD while placebo treatment was accompanied by mean percent decreases. For femoral trochanter, each of the Premarin dose groups showed a mean percent increase that was significantly greater than the small increase seen in the placebo group. The percent changes from baseline to final evaluation are shown in Table 3.

[See table 3 at top of next page]

Figure 1 shows the cumulative percentage of subjects with changes from baseline equal to or greater than the value shown on the x-axis.

Figure 1: CUMULATIVE PERCENT OF SUBJECTS WITH CHANGES FROM BASELINE IN SPINE BMD OF GIVEN MAGNITUDE OR GREATER IN PREMARIN AND PLACEBO GROUPS

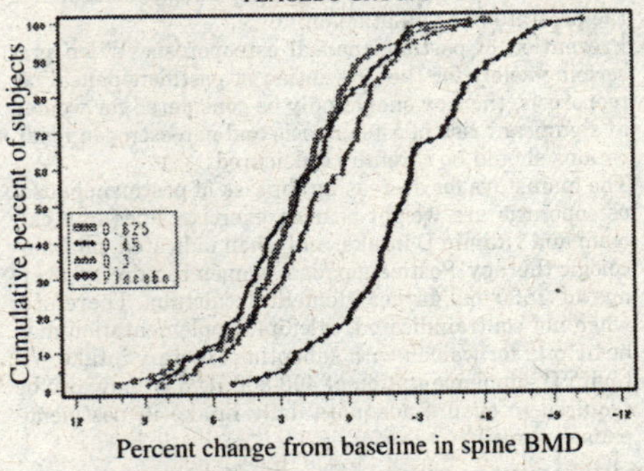

The mean percent changes from baseline in L_2 to L_4 BMD for women who completed the bone density study are shown with standard error bars by treatment group in Figure 2. Significant differences between each of the Premarin dosage groups and placebo were found at cycles 6, 13, 19, and 26.

Figure 2. ADJUSTED MEAN (SE) PERCENT CHANGE FROM BASELINE AT EACH CYCLE IN SPINE BMD: SUBJECTS COMPLETING IN PREMARIN GROUPS AND PLACEBO

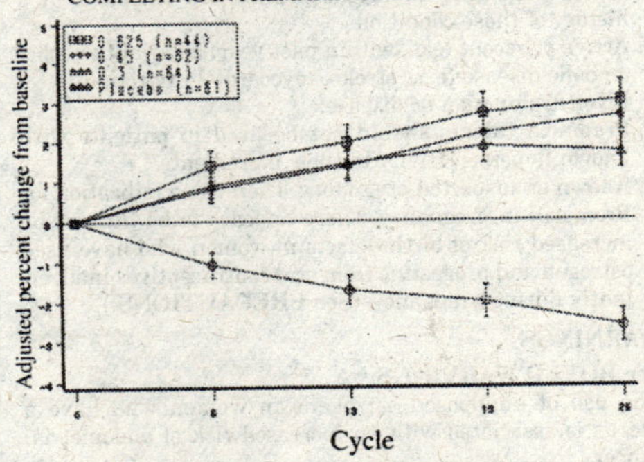

The bone turnover markers serum osteocalcin and urinary N-telopeptide significantly decreased (p<0.001) in all active-treatment groups at cycles 6, 13, 19, and 26 compared with the placebo group. Larger mean decreases from baseline were seen with the active groups than with the placebo group. Significant differences from placebo were seen less frequently in urine calcium.

Women's Health Initiative Studies

The Women's Health Initiative (WHI) enrolled a total of 27,000 predominantly healthy postmenopausal women to assess the risks and benefits of either the use of Premarin (0.625 mg conjugated equine estrogens per day) alone or the use of Prempro (0.625 mg conjugated equine estrogens plus 2.5 mg medroxyprogesterone acetate per day) compared to placebo in the prevention of certain chronic diseases. The primary endpoint was the incidence of coronary heart disease (CHD) (nonfatal myocardial infarction and CHD death), with invasive breast cancer as the primary adverse outcome studied. A "global index" included the earliest occurrence of CHD, invasive breast cancer, stroke, pulmonary embolism (PE), endometrial cancer, colorectal cancer, hip fracture, or death due to other cause. The study did not evaluate the effects of Premarin or Prempro on menopausal symptoms.

The Premarin-only substudy is continuing and results have not been reported. The Prempro substudy was stopped early because, according to the predefined stopping rule, the in-

Continued on next page

Premarin—Cont.

creased risk of breast cancer and cardiovascular events exceeded the specified benefits included in the "global index." Results of the Prempro substudy, which included 16,608 women (average age of 63 years, range 50 to 79; 83.9% White, 6.5% Black, 5.5% Hispanic), after an average follow-up of 5.2 years are presented in Table 4 below.

[See table 4 at right]

For those outcomes included in the "global index," absolute excess risks per 10,000 person-years in the group treated with Prempro were 7 more CHD events, 8 more strokes, 8 more PEs, and 8 more invasive breast cancers, while absolute risk reductions per 10,000 person-years were 6 fewer colorectal cancers and 5 fewer hip fractures. The absolute excess risk of events included in the "global index" was 19 per 10,000 person-years. There was no difference between the groups in terms of all-cause mortality. (See **BOXED WARNINGS, WARNINGS**, and **PRECAUTIONS**.)

INDICATIONS AND USAGE

Premarin therapy is indicated in the:

1. Treatment of moderate to severe vasomotor symptoms associated with the menopause.
2. Treatment of moderate to severe symptoms of vulvar and vaginal atrophy associated with the menopause. When prescribing solely for the treatment of symptoms of vulvar and vaginal atrophy, topical vaginal products should be considered.
3. Treatment of hypoestrogenism due to hypogonadism, castration or primary ovarian failure.
4. Treatment of breast cancer (for palliation only) in appropriately selected women and men with metastatic disease.
5. Treatment of advanced androgen-dependent carcinoma of the prostate (for palliation only).
6. Prevention of postmenopausal osteoporosis. When prescribing solely for the prevention of postmenopausal osteoporosis, therapy should only be considered for women at significant risk of osteoporosis and non-estrogen medications should be carefully considered.

   The mainstays for decreasing the risk of postmenopausal osteoporosis are weight-bearing exercise, adequate calcium and vitamin D intake, and when indicated, pharmacologic therapy. Postmenopausal women require an average of 1500 mg/day of elemental calcium. Therefore, when not contraindicated, calcium supplementation may be helpful for women with suboptimal dietary intake. Vitamin D supplementation of 400-800 IU/day may also be required to ensure adequate daily intake in postmenopausal women.

CONTRAINDICATIONS

Estrogens should not be used in individuals with any of the following conditions:

1. Undiagnosed abnormal genital bleeding.
2. Known, suspected, or history of cancer of the breast except in appropriately selected patients being treated for metastatic disease.
3. Known or suspected estrogen-dependent neoplasia.
4. Active deep vein thrombosis, pulmonary embolism or a history of these conditions.
5. Active or recent (e.g., within past year) arterial thromboembolic disease (e.g., stroke, myocardial infarction).
6. Liver dysfunction or disease.
7. Premarin tablets should not be used in patients with known hypersensitivity to their ingredients.
8. Known or suspected pregnancy. There is no indication for Premarin in pregnancy. There appears to be little or no increased risk of birth defects in women who have used estrogen and progestins from oral contraceptives inadvertently during pregnancy. (See **PRECAUTIONS**.)

WARNINGS

See **BOXED WARNINGS**.

The use of unopposed estrogens in women who have a uterus is associated with an increased risk of endometrial cancer.

1. **Cardiovascular Disorders.** Estrogen and estrogen/progestin therapy have been associated with an increased risk of cardiovascular events such as myocardial infarction and stroke, as well as venous thrombosis and pulmonary embolism (venous thromboembolism or VTE). Should any of these occur or be suspected, estrogens should be discontinued immediately.

   Risk factors for arterial vascular disease (e.g., hypertension, diabetes mellitus, tobacco use, hypercholesterolemia, and obesity) and/or venous thromboembolism (e.g., personal history or family history of VTE, obesity, and systemic lupus erythematosus) should be managed appropriately.

a. ***Coronary heart disease and stroke.*** In the Premarin substudy of the Women's Health Initiative study (WHI), an increase in the number of myocardial infarctions and strokes has been observed in women receiving Premarin compared to placebo. These observations are preliminary, and the study is continuing. (See **CLINICAL PHARMACOLOGY, Clinical Studies.**)

In the Prempro substudy of WHI, an increased risk of coronary heart disease (CHD) events (defined as non-fatal myocardial infarction and CHD death) was observed in women receiving Prempro compared to women receiving placebo (37 vs 30 per 10,000 person-years). The increase in risk was observed in year one and persisted.

In the same substudy of WHI, an increased risk of stroke was observed in women receiving Prempro compared to women receiving placebo (29 vs 21 per 10,000 person-years). The increase in risk was observed after the first year and persisted.

In postmenopausal women with documented heart disease (n = 2,763, average age 66.7 years) a controlled clinical trial of secondary prevention of cardiovascular disease (Heart and Estrogen/progestin Replacement Study; HERS) treatment with Prempro (0.625 mg conjugated equine estrogen plus 2.5 mg medroxyprogesterone acetate per day) demonstrated no cardiovascular benefit. During an average follow-up of 4.1 years, treatment with Prempro did not reduce the overall rate of CHD events in postmenopausal women with established coronary heart disease. There were more CHD events in the Prempro-treated group than in the placebo group in year 1, but not during the subsequent years. Two thousand three hundred and twenty one women from the original HERS trial agreed to participate in an open label extension of HERS, HERS II. Average follow-up in HERS II was an additional 2.7 years, for a total of 6.8 years overall. Rates of CHD events were comparable among women in the Prempro group and the placebo group in HERS, HERS II, and overall.

Large doses of estrogen (5 mg conjugated estrogens per day), comparable to those used to treat cancer of the prostate and breast, have been shown in a large prospective clinical trial in men to increase the risk of nonfatal myocardial infarction, pulmonary embolism, and thrombophlebitis.

b. ***Venous thromboembolism (VTE).*** In the Premarin substudy of the Women's Health Initiative (WHI), an increase in VTE has been observed in women receiving Premarin compared to placebo. These observations are preliminary, and the study is continuing. (See **CLINICAL PHARMACOLOGY, Clinical Studies.**)

In the Prempro substudy of WHI, a 2-fold greater rate of VTE, including deep venous thrombosis and pulmonary embolism, was observed in women receiving Prempro compared to women receiving placebo. The rate of VTE was 34 per 10,000 woman-years in the Prempro group compared to 16 per 10,000 woman-years in the placebo group. The increase in VTE risk was observed during the first year and persisted.

If feasible, estrogens should be discontinued at least 4 to 6 weeks before surgery of the type associated with an increased risk of thromboembolism, or during periods of prolonged immobilization.

2. **Malignant neoplasms.**

a. ***Endometrial cancer.*** The use of unopposed estrogens in women with intact uteri has been associated with an increased risk of endometrial cancer. The reported endometrial cancer risk among unopposed estrogen users with an intact uterus is about 2- to 12-fold greater than in non-users, and appears dependent on duration of treatment and on estrogen dose. Most studies show no significant increased risk associated with the use of estrogens for less than one year. The greatest risk appears associated with prolonged use, with increased risks of 15- to 24-fold for five to ten years or more, and this risk has been shown to persist for at least 8 to 15 years after estrogen therapy is discontinued.

Clinical surveillance of all women taking estrogen/progestin combinations is important. Adequate diagnostic measures, including endometrial sampling when indicated, should be undertaken to rule out malignancy in all cases of undiagnosed persistent or recurring abnormal vaginal bleeding. There is no evidence that the use of natural estrogens results in a different endometrial risk profile than synthetic estrogens of equivalent estrogen dose.

TABLE 3. PERCENT CHANGE IN BONE MINERAL DENSITY: COMPARISON BETWEEN ACTIVE AND PLACEBO GROUPS IN THE INTENT-TO-TREAT POPULATION, LAST OBSERVATION CARRIED FORWARD

Region Evaluated Treatment Group[a]	No. of Subjects	Baseline (g/cm^2) Mean ± SD	Change from Baseline (%) Adjusted Mean ± SE	p-Value vs Placebo
L_2 to L_4 BMD				
0.625	83	1.17 ± 0.15	2.46 ± 0.37	<0.001
0.45	91	1.13 ± 0.15	2.26 ± 0.35	<0.001
0.3	87	1.14 ± 0.15	1.13 ± 0.36	<0.001
Placebo	85	1.14 ± 0.14	-2.45 ± 0.36	
Total Body BMD				
0.625	84	1.15 ± 0.08	0.68 ± 0.17	<0.001
0.45	91	1.14 ± 0.08	0.74 ± 0.16	<0.001
0.3	87	1.14 ± 0.07	0.40 ± 0.17	<0.001
Placebo	85	1.13 ± 0.08	-1.50 ± 0.17	
Femoral Neck BMD				
0.625	84	0.91 ± 0.14	1.82 ± 0.45	<0.001
0.45	91	0.89 ± 0.13	1.84 ± 0.44	<0.001
0.3	87	0.86 ± 0.11	0.62 ± 0.45	<0.001
Placebo	85	0.88 ± 0.14	-1.72 ± 0.45	
Femoral Trochanter BMD				
0.625	84	0.78 ± 0.13	3.82 ± 0.58	<0.001
0.45	91	0.76 ± 0.12	3.16 ± 0.56	0.003
0.3	87	0.75 ± 0.10	3.05 ± 0.57	0.005
Placebo	85	0.75 ± 0.12	0.81 ± 0.58	

a: Identified by dosage (mg) of Premarin or placebo.

TABLE 4. RELATIVE AND ABSOLUTE RISK SEEN IN THE PREMPRO SUBSTUDY OF WHI[a]

Event[c]	Relative Risk Prempro vs Placebo at 5.2 Years (95% CI*)	Placebo n = 8102	Prempro n = 8506
		Absolute Risk per 10,000 Person-years	
CHD events	1.29 (1.02-1.63)	30	37
Non-fatal MI	*1.32 (1.02-1.72)*	*23*	*30*
CHD death	*1.18 (0.70-1.97)*	*6*	*7*
Invasive breast cancer[b]	1.26 (1.00-1.59)	30	38
Stroke	1.41 (1.07-1.85)	21	29
Pulmonary embolism	2.13 (1.39-3.25)	8	16
Colorectal cancer	0.63 (0.43-0.92)	16	10
Endometrial cancer	0.83 (0.47-1.47)	6	5
Hip fracture	0.66 (0.45-0.98)	15	10
Death due to causes other than the events above	0.92 (0.74-1.14)	40	37
Global Index[c]	1.15 (1.03-1.28)	151	170
Deep vein thrombosis[d]	2.07 (1.49-2.87)	13	26
Vertebral fractures[d]	0.66 (0.44-0.98)	15	9
Other osteoporotic fractures[d]	0.77 (0.69-0.86)	170	131

a: Adapted from JAMA, 2002; 288:321-333
b: Includes metastatic and non-metastatic breast cancer with the exception of in situ breast cancer
c: A subset of the events was combined in a "global index," defined as the earliest occurrence of CHD events, invasive breast cancer, stroke, pulmonary embolism, endometrial cancer, colorectal cancer, hip fracture, or death due to other causes
d: Not included in Global Index
* Nominal confidence intervals unadjusted for multiple looks and multiple comparisons

Adding a progestin to postmenopausal estrogen therapy has been shown to reduce the risk of endometrial hyperplasia, which may be a precursor to endometrial cancer.

b. ***Breast cancer.*** Estrogen and estrogen/progestin therapy in postmenopausal women has been associated with an increased risk of breast cancer. In the Prempro substudy of the Women's Health Initiative study (WHI), a 26% increase of invasive breast cancer (38 vs 30 per 10,000 woman-years) after an average of 5.2 years of treatment was observed in women receiving Prempro compared to women receiving placebo. The increased risk of breast cancer became apparent after 4 years on Prempro. The women reporting prior postmenopausal use of estrogen and/or estrogen with progestin had a higher relative risk for breast cancer associated with Prempro than those who had never used these hormones. (See **CLINICAL PHARMACOLOGY, Clinical Studies.**)

In the Premarin substudy of the WHI study, no increased risk of breast cancer in estrogen-treated women compared to placebo was reported after an average of 5.2 years of therapy. These data are preliminary and that substudy of WHI is continuing.

Epidemiologic studies have reported an increased risk of breast cancer in association with increasing duration of postmenopausal treatment with estrogens, with or without progestin. This association was reanalyzed in original data from 51 studies that involved treatment with various doses and types of estrogens, with and without progestin. In the reanalysis, an increased risk of having breast cancer diagnosed became apparent after about 5 years of continued treatment, and subsided after treatment had been discontinued for about 5 years. Some later studies have suggested that treatment with estrogen and progestin increases the risk of breast cancer more than treatment with estrogen alone.

A postmenopausal woman without a uterus who requires estrogen should receive estrogen-alone therapy and should not be exposed unnecessarily to progestins. All postmenopausal women should receive yearly breast exams by a healthcare provider and perform monthly breast self-examinations. In addition, mammography examinations should be scheduled based on patient age and risk factors.

3. **Dementia.** In a study of women 65 years of age and older (a randomized controlled sub-study of the Women's Health Initiative, the Women's Health Initiative Memory Study; n=4,532, 54% older than 70), those treated with PREMPRO (0.625 mg, conjugated equine estrogen, plus 2.5 mg medroxyprogesterone acetate) were reported to have a two-fold increase in the risk of developing probable dementia. After an average follow-up of 4 years, the absolute risk of probable dementia was 45 per 10,000 woman-years in the PREMPRO group and 22 per 10,000 woman-years in the placebo group. It is unknown whether these findings apply to younger postmenopausal women.

   The estrogen-alone sub-study of the Women's Health Initiative Memory Study is currently ongoing. No data are available. It is unknown whether these findings apply to estrogen alone therapy.

4. **Gallbladder Disease.** A 2- to 4-fold increase in the risk of gallbladder disease requiring surgery in postmenopausal women receiving estrogens has been reported.
5. **Hypercalcemia.** Estrogen administration may lead to severe hypercalcemia in patients with breast cancer and bone metastases. If hypercalcemia occurs, use of the drug should be stopped and appropriate measures taken to reduce the serum calcium level.
6. **Visual abnormalities.** Retinal vascular thrombosis has been reported in patients receiving estrogens. Discontinue medication pending examination if there is sudden partial or complete loss of vision, or a sudden onset of proptosis, diplopia, or migraine. If examination reveals papilledema or retinal vascular lesions, estrogens should be discontinued.

PRECAUTIONS

A. General

1. ***Addition of a progestin when a woman has not had a hysterectomy.***
   Studies of the addition of a progestin for 10 or more days of a cycle of estrogen administration, or daily with estrogen in a continuous regimen, have reported a lowered incidence of endometrial hyperplasia than would be induced by estrogen treatment alone. Endometrial hyperplasia may be a precursor to endometrial cancer.
   There are, however, possible risks that may be associated with the use of progestins with estrogens compared to estrogen-alone regimens. These include: a possible increased risk of breast cancer, adverse effects on lipoprotein metabolism (e.g., lowering HDL, raising LDL) and impairment of glucose tolerance.
2. ***Elevated blood pressure.***
   In a small number of case reports, substantial increases in blood pressure have been attributed to idiosyncratic reactions to estrogens. In a large, randomized, placebo-controlled clinical trial, a generalized effect of estrogen therapy on blood pressure was not seen. Blood pressure should be monitored at regular intervals during estrogen use.
3. ***Hypertriglyceridemia.***
   In patients with pre-existing hypertriglyceridemia, estrogen therapy may be associated with elevations of plasma triglycerides leading to pancreatitis and other complications. In the HOPE study, the mean percent increase from baseline in serum triglycerides after one year of treatment with Premarin 0.625 mg, 0.45 mg, and 0.3 mg compared with placebo were 34.3, 30.2, 25.1, and 10.7, respectively. After two years of treatment, the mean percent changes were 47.6, 32.5, 19.0, and 5.5, respectively.
4. ***Impaired liver function and past history of cholestatic jaundice.***
   Estrogens may be poorly metabolized in patients with impaired liver function. For patients with a history of cholestatic jaundice associated with past estrogen use or with pregnancy, caution should be exercised and in the case of recurrence, medication should be discontinued.
5. ***Hypothyroidism.***
   Estrogen administration leads to increased thyroid-binding globulin (TBG) levels. Patients with normal thyroid function can compensate for the increased TBG by making more thyroid hormone, thus maintaining free T_4 and T_3 serum concentrations in the normal range. Patients dependent on thyroid hormone replacement therapy who are also receiving estrogens may require increased doses of their thyroid replacement therapy. These patients should have their thyroid function monitored in order to maintain their free thyroid hormone levels in an acceptable range.
6. ***Fluid retention.***
   Because estrogens may cause some degree of fluid retention, patients with conditions that might be influenced by this factor, such as cardiac or renal dysfunction, warrant careful observation when estrogens are prescribed.
7. ***Hypocalcemia.***
   Estrogens should be used with caution in individuals with severe hypocalcemia.
8. ***Ovarian cancer.***
   Use of estrogen-only products, in particular for ten or more years, has been associated with an increased risk of ovarian cancer in some epidemiological studies. Other studies did not show a significant association. Data are insufficient to determine whether there is an increased risk with combined estrogen/progestin therapy in postmenopausal women.
9. ***Exacerbation of endometriosis.***
   Endometriosis may be exacerbated with administration of estrogens.
   A few cases of malignant transformation of residual endometrial implants have been reported in women treated post-hysterectomy with estrogen-only therapy. For patients known to have residual endometriosis post-hysterectomy, the addition of progestin should be considered.
10. ***Exacerbation of other conditions.***
    Estrogen therapy may cause an exacerbation of asthma, diabetes mellitus, epilepsy, migraine, porphyria, systemic lupus erythematosus, and hepatic hemangiomas and should be used with caution in patients with these conditions.

B. Patient Information

Physicians are advised to discuss the contents of the PATIENT INFORMATION leaflet with patients for whom they prescribe Premarin.

C. Laboratory Tests

Estrogen administration should be initiated at the lowest dose for the treatment of postmenopausal moderate to severe vasomotor symptoms and moderate to severe symptoms of postmenopausal vulvar and vaginal atrophy and then guided by clinical response rather than by serum hormone levels (e.g., estradiol, FSH). Laboratory parameters may be useful in guiding dosage for the treatment of hypoestrogenism due to hypogonadism, castration and primary ovarian failure.

D. Drug/Laboratory Test Interactions

1. Accelerated prothrombin time, partial thromboplastin time, and platelet aggregation time; increased platelet count; increased factors II, VII antigen, VIII antigen, VIII coagulant activity, IX, X, XII, VII-X complex, II-VII-X complex, and beta-thromboglobulin; decreased levels of anti-factor Xa and antithrombin III, decreased antithrombin III activity; increased levels of fibrinogen and fibrinogen activity; increased plasminogen antigen and activity.
2. Increased thyroid binding globulin (TBG) levels leading to increased circulating total thyroid hormone levels as measured by protein-bound iodine (PBI), T_4 levels (by column or by radioimmunoassay) or T_3 levels by radioimmunoassay. T_3 resin uptake is decreased, reflecting the elevated TBG. Free T_4 and free T_3 concentrations are unaltered. Patients on thyroid replacement therapy may require higher doses of thyroid hormone.
3. Other binding proteins may be elevated in serum, i.e., corticosteroid binding globulin (CBG), sex hormone binding globulin (SHBG), leading to increased circulating corticosteroids and sex steroids, respectively. Free or biologically active hormone concentrations are unchanged. Other plasma proteins may be increased (angiotensinogen/renin substrate, alpha-1-antitrypsin, ceruloplasmin).
4. Increased plasma HDL and HDL_2 cholesterol subfraction concentrations, reduced LDL cholesterol concentrations, increased triglyceride levels.
5. Impaired glucose tolerance.
6. Reduced response to metyrapone test.

E. Carcinogenesis, Mutagenesis, Impairment of Fertility

Long term continuous administration of natural and synthetic estrogens in certain animal species increases the frequency of carcinomas of the breast, uterus, cervix, vagina, testis, and liver. (See **BOXED WARNINGS, CONTRAINDICATIONS,** and **WARNINGS**).

F. Pregnancy

Premarin should not be used during pregnancy. (See **CONTRAINDICATIONS**).

G. Nursing Mothers

Estrogen administration to nursing mothers has been shown to decrease the quantity and quality of the milk. Detectable amounts of estrogens have been identified in the milk of mothers receiving this drug. Caution should be exercised when Premarin is administered to a nursing woman.

H. Pediatric Use

Estrogen therapy has been used for the induction of puberty in adolescents with some forms of pubertal delay. Safety and effectiveness in pediatric patients have not otherwise been established.

Large and repeated doses of estrogen over an extended time period have been shown to accelerate epiphyseal closure, which could result in short stature if treatment is initiated before the completion of physiologic puberty in normally developing children. If estrogen is administered to patients whose bone growth is not complete, periodic monitoring of bone maturation and effects on epiphyseal centers is recommended during estrogen administration.

Estrogen treatment of prepubertal girls also induces premature breast development and vaginal cornification, and may induce vaginal bleeding. In boys, estrogen treatment may modify the normal pubertal process and induce gynecomastia. See **INDICATIONS** and **DOSAGE AND ADMINISTRATION** sections.

I. Geriatric Use

Of the total number of subjects in the Prempro substudy of the Women's Health Initiative study, 44% (n=7,320) were 65 years and over, while 6.6% (n=1,095) were 75 and over (see **CLINICAL PHARMACOLOGY, Clinical Studies**). No significant differences in safety were observed between subjects 65 years and over compared to younger subjects. There was a higher incidence of stroke and invasive breast cancer in women 75 and over compared to younger subjects.

With respect to efficacy in the approved indications, there have not been sufficient numbers of geriatric patients involved in studies utilizing Premarin to determine whether those over 65 years of age differ from younger subjects in their response to Premarin.

ADVERSE REACTIONS

See **BOXED WARNINGS, WARNINGS,** and **PRECAUTIONS.**

Because clinical trials are conducted under widely varying conditions, adverse reaction rates observed in the clinical trials of a drug cannot be directly compared to rates in the clinical trials of another drug and may not reflect the rates observed in practice. The adverse reaction information from clinical trials does, however, provide a basis for identifying the adverse events that appear to be related to drug use and for approximating rates.

During the first year of a 2-year clinical trial with 2333 postmenopausal women between 40 and 65 years of age (88% Caucasian), 1012 women were treated with conjugated estrogens and 332 were treated with placebo. Table 5 summarizes adverse events that occurred at a rate of ≥ 5%.

[See table 5 at top of next page]

The following additional adverse reactions have been reported with estrogen and/or progestin therapy:

1. *Genitourinary system*
Changes in vaginal bleeding pattern and abnormal withdrawal bleeding or flow; breakthrough bleeding, spotting, dysmenorrhea
Increase in size of uterine leiomyomata
Vaginitis, including vaginal candidiasis
Change in amount of cervical secretion
Change in cervical ectropion
Ovarian cancer
Endometrial hyperplasia
Endometrial cancer

2. *Breasts*
Tenderness, enlargement, pain, discharge, galactorrhea
Fibrocystic breast changes
Breast cancer

3. *Cardiovascular*
Deep and superficial venous thrombosis
Pulmonary embolism
Thrombophlebitis
Myocardial infarction
Stroke
Increase in blood pressure

4. *Gastrointestinal*
Nausea, vomiting
Abdominal cramps, bloating
Cholestatic jaundice
Increased incidence of gallbladder disease
Pancreatitis
Enlargement of hepatic hemangiomas

5. *Skin*
Chloasma or melasma that may persist when drug is discontinued
Erythema multiforme
Erythema nodosum
Hemorrhagic eruption
Loss of scalp hair
Hirsutism

Continued on next page

Premarin—Cont.

Pruritus, rash
6. *Eyes*
Retinal vascular thrombosis
Steepening of corneal curvature
Intolerance to contact lenses
7. *Central Nervous System*
Headache
Migraine
Dizziness
Mental depression
Chorea
Nervousness
Mood disturbances
Irritability
Exacerbation of epilepsy
Dementia
8. *Miscellaneous*
Increase or decrease in weight
Reduced carbohydrate tolerance
Aggravation of porphyria
Edema
Arthralgias
Leg cramps
Changes in libido
Urticaria, angioedema, anaphylactoid/anaphylactic reactions
Hypocalcemia
Exacerbation of asthma
Increased triglycerides

OVERDOSAGE

Serious ill effects have not been reported following acute ingestion of large doses of estrogen-containing oral contraceptives by young children. Overdosage of estrogen may cause nausea and vomiting, and withdrawal bleeding may occur in females.

DOSAGE AND ADMINISTRATION

When estrogen is prescribed for a postmenopausal woman with a uterus, progestin should also be initiated to reduce the risk of endometrial cancer. A woman without a uterus does not need progestin. Use of estrogen, alone or in combination with a progestin, should be limited to the shortest duration consistent with treatment goals and risks for the individual woman. Patients should be re-evaluated periodically as clinically appropriate (e.g., at 3-month to 6-month intervals) to determine if treatment is still necessary (see **BOXED WARNINGS** and **WARNINGS**). For women with a uterus, adequate diagnostic measures, such as endometrial sampling, when indicated, should be undertaken to rule out malignancy in cases of undiagnosed persistent or recurring abnormal vaginal bleeding.

1. For treatment of moderate to severe vasomotor symptoms and/or moderate to severe symptoms of vulvar and vaginal atrophy associated with the menopause. When prescribing solely for the treatment of moderate to severe symptoms of vulvar and vaginal atrophy, topical vaginal products should be considered.
   Patients should be treated with the lowest effective dose. Generally women should be started at 0.3 mg Premarin daily. Subsequent dosage adjustment may be made based upon the individual patient response. This dose should be periodically reassessed by the healthcare provider.
   Premarin therapy may be given continuously with no interruption in therapy, or in cyclical regimens (regimens such as 25 days on drug followed by five days off drug) as is medically appropriate on an individualized basis.
2. For prevention of postmenopausal osteoporosis:
   When prescribing solely for the prevention of postmenopausal osteoporosis, therapy should be considered only for women at significant risk of osteoporosis and non-estrogen medications should be carefully considered. Patients should be treated with the lowest effective dose. Generally women should be started at 0.3 mg Premarin daily. Subsequent dosage adjustment may be made based upon the individual clinical and bone mineral density responses. This dose should be periodically reassessed by the healthcare provider.
   Premarin therapy may be given continuously with no interruption in therapy, or in cyclical regimens (regimens such as 25 days on drug followed by five days off drug) as is medically appropriate on an individualized basis.
3. For treatment of female hypoestrogenism due to hypogonadism, castration, or primary ovarian failure:
   Female hypogonadism—0.3 mg or 0.625 mg daily, administered cyclically (e.g., three weeks on and one week off). Doses are adjusted depending on the severity of symptoms and responsiveness of the endometrium.
   In clinical studies of delayed puberty due to female hypogonadism, breast development was induced by doses as low as 0.15 mg. The dosage may be gradually titrated upward at 6 to 12 month intervals as needed to achieve appropriate bone age advancement and eventual epiphyseal closure. Clinical studies suggest that doses of 0.15 mg, 0.3 mg, and 0.6 mg are associated with mean ratios of bone age advancement to chronological age progression ($\Delta BA/\Delta CA$) of 1.1, 1.5, and 2.1, respectively. (Premarin in the dose strength of 0.15 mg is not available commercially). Available data suggest that chronic dosing with 0.625 mg is sufficient to induce artificial cyclic menses with sequential progestin treatment and to maintain bone mineral density after skeletal maturity is achieved.
   Female castration or primary ovarian failure—1.25 mg daily, cyclically. Adjust dosage, upward or downward, according to severity of symptoms and response of the patient. For maintenance, adjust dosage to lowest level that will provide effective control.
4. For treatment of breast cancer, for palliation only, in appropriately selected women and men with metastatic disease:
   Suggested dosage is 10 mg three times daily for a period of at least three months.
5. For treatment of advanced androgen-dependent carcinoma of the prostate, for palliation only:
   1.25 mg to 2.5 mg three times daily. The effectiveness of therapy can be judged by phosphatase determinations as well as by symptomatic improvement of the patient.

TABLE 5. NUMBER (%) OF PATIENTS REPORTING ≥ 5% TREATMENT EMERGENT ADVERSE EVENTS

Body System Adverse event	--Conjugated Estrogens Treatment Group-- 0.625 mg (n = 348)	0.45 mg (n = 338)	0.3 mg (n = 326)	Placebo (n = 332)
Any adverse event	323 (93%)	305 (90%)	292 (90%)	281 (85%)
Body as a Whole				
Abdominal pain	56 (16%)	50 (15%)	54 (17%)	37 (11%)
Accidental injury	21 (6%)	41 (12%)	20 (6%)	29 (9%)
Asthenia	25 (7%)	23 (7%)	25 (8%)	16 (5%)
Back pain	49 (14%)	43 (13%)	43 (13%)	39 (12%)
Flu syndrome	37 (11%)	38 (11%)	33 (10%)	35 (11%)
Headache	90 (26%)	109 (32%)	96 (29%)	93 (28%)
Infection	61 (18%)	75 (22%)	74 (23%)	74 (22%)
Pain	58 (17%)	61 (18%)	66 (20%)	61 (18%)
Digestive System				
Diarrhea	21 (6%)	25 (7%)	19 (6%)	21 (6%)
Dyspepsia	33 (9%)	32 (9%)	36 (11%)	46 (14%)
Flatulence	24 (7%)	23 (7%)	18 (6%)	9 (3%)
Nausea	32 (9%)	21 (6%)	21 (6%)	30 (9%)
Musculoskeletal System				
Arthralgia	47 (14%)	42 (12%)	22 (7%)	39 (12%)
Leg cramps	19 (5%)	23 (7%)	11 (3%)	7 (2%)
Myalgia	18 (5%)	18 (5%)	29 (9%)	25 (8%)
Nervous System				
Depression	25 (7%)	27 (8%)	17 (5%)	22 (7%)
Dizziness	19 (5%)	20 (6%)	12 (4%)	17 (5%)
Insomnia	21 (6%)	25 (7%)	24 (7%)	33 (10%)
Nervousness	12 (3%)	17 (5%)	6 (2%)	7 (2%)
Respiratory System				
Cough increased	13 (4%)	22 (7%)	14 (4%)	14 (4%)
Pharyngitis	35 (10%)	35 (10%)	40 (12%)	38 (11%)
Rhinitis	21 (6%)	30 (9%)	31 (10%)	42 (13%)
Sinusitis	22 (6%)	36 (11%)	24 (7%)	24 (7%)
Upper respiratory infection	42 (12%)	34 (10%)	28 (9%)	35 (11%)
Skin and Appendages				
Pruritus	14 (4%)	17 (5%)	16 (5%)	7 (2%)
Urogenital System				
Breast pain	38 (11%)	41 (12%)	24 (7%)	29 (9%)
Leukorrhea	18 (5%)	22 (7%)	13 (4%)	9 (3%)
Vaginal hemorrhage	47 (14%)	14 (4%)	7 (2%)	0
Vaginal moniliasis	20 (6%)	18 (5%)	17 (5%)	6 (2%)
Vaginitis	24 (7%)	20 (6%)	16 (5%)	4 (1%)

HOW SUPPLIED

Premarin (conjugated estrogens tablets, USP)
— Each oval purple tablet contains 2.5 mg, in bottles of 100 (NDC 0046-0865-81) and 1,000 (NDC 0046-0865-91).
— Each oval yellow tablet contains 1.25 mg, in bottles of 100 (NDC 0046-0866-81); 1,000 (NDC 0046-0866-91); and Unit-Dose packages of 100 (NDC 0046-0866-99).
— Each oval white tablet contains 0.9 mg, in bottles of 100 (NDC 0046-0864-81).
— Each oval maroon tablet contains 0.625 mg, in bottles of 100 (NDC 0046-0867-81); 1,000 (NDC 0046-0867-91); and Unit-Dose Packages of 100 (NDC 0046-0867-99).
— Each oval blue tablet contains 0.45 mg, in bottles of 100 (NDC 0046-0936-81).
— Each oval green tablet contains 0.3 mg, in bottles of 100 (NDC 0046-0868-81) and 1,000 (NDC 0046-0868-91).

The appearance of these tablets is a trademark of Wyeth Pharmaceuticals.

Store at 20-25° C (68-77° F); excursions permitted to 15-30° C (59-86° F) [see USP Controlled Room Temperature].
Dispense in a well-closed container as defined in the USP.

PATIENT INFORMATION

(Updated July 16, 2003)
Premarin®
(conjugated estrogens tablets, USP)

Read this PATIENT INFORMATION before you start taking Premarin and read what you get each time you refill Premarin. There may be new information. This information does not take the place of talking to your healthcare provider about your medical condition or your treatment.

What is the most important information I should know about Premarin (an estrogen mixture)?

- Estrogens increase the chances of getting cancer of the uterus.
  Report any unusual vaginal bleeding right away while you are taking Premarin. Vaginal bleeding after menopause may be a warning sign of cancer of the uterus (womb). Your healthcare provider should check any unusual vaginal bleeding to find out the cause.
- Do not use estrogens with or without progestins to prevent heart disease, heart attacks, or strokes.
  Using estrogens with or without progestins may increase your chances of getting heart attacks, strokes, breast cancer, and blood clots. You and your healthcare provider should talk regularly about whether you still need treatment with estrogens.

What is Premarin?

Premarin is a medicine that contains a mixture of estrogen hormones.

Premarin is used after menopause to:

- **reduce moderate to severe hot flashes.** Estrogens are hormones made by a woman's ovaries. The ovaries normally stop making estrogens when a woman is between 45 and 55 years old. This drop in body estrogen levels causes the "change of life" or menopause (the end of monthly menstrual periods). Sometimes both ovaries are removed during an operation before natural menopause takes place. The sudden drop in estrogen levels causes "surgical menopause."
  When the estrogen levels begin dropping, some women get very uncomfortable symptoms, such as feelings of warmth in the face, neck, and chest, or sudden strong feelings of heat and sweating ("hot flashes" or "hot flushes"). In some women the symptoms are mild, and they will not need to take estrogens. In other women, symptoms can be more severe. You and your healthcare provider should talk regularly about whether you still need treatment with Premarin.
- **treat moderate to severe dryness, itching, and burning, in and around the vagina.** You and your healthcare provider should talk regularly about whether you still need treatment with Premarin to control these problems.
- **help reduce your chances of getting osteoporosis (thin weak bones).** Osteoporosis from menopause is a thinning of the bones that makes them weaker and easier to break. If you use Premarin only to prevent osteoporosis from menopause, talk with your healthcare provider about whether a different treatment or medicine without estrogens might be better for you. You and your healthcare provider should talk regularly about whether you should continue with Premarin.
  Weight-bearing exercise, like walking or running, and taking calcium and vitamin D supplements may also lower your chances for getting postmenopausal osteoporosis. It is important to talk about exercise and supplements with your healthcare provider before starting them.

Premarin is also used to:

- **treat certain conditions in women before menopause if their ovaries do not make enough estrogen naturally.**
- **ease symptoms of certain cancers that have spread through the body, in men and women.**

Who should not take Premarin?

Do not start taking Premarin if you:

- **have unusual vaginal bleeding.**
- **currently have or have had certain cancers.** Estrogens may increase the chances of getting certain types of cancers, including cancer of the breast or uterus. If you have or have had cancer, talk with your healthcare provider about whether you should take Premarin.
- **had a stroke or heart attack in the past year.**
- **currently have or have had blood clots.**

- **are allergic to Premarin tablets or any of its ingredients.** See the end of this leaflet for a list of all the ingredients in Premarin.
- **think you may be pregnant.**

Tell your healthcare provider:

- **if you are breast feeding.** The hormones in Premarin can pass into your milk.
- **about all of your medical problems.** Your healthcare provider may need to check you more carefully if you have certain conditions, such as asthma (wheezing), epilepsy (seizures), migraine, endometriosis, lupus, problems with your heart, liver, thyroid, kidneys, or have high calcium levels in your blood.
- **about all the medicines you take,** including prescription and nonprescription medicines, vitamins, and herbal supplements. Some medicines may affect how Premarin works. Premarin may also affect how your other medicines work.
- **if you are going to have surgery or will be on bedrest.** You may need to stop taking estrogens.

How should I take Premarin?

- Take one Premarin tablet at the same time each day.
- If you miss a dose, take it as soon as possible. If it is almost time for your next dose, skip the missed dose and go back to your normal schedule. Do not take 2 doses at the same time.
- Estrogens should be used only as long as needed. You and your healthcare provider should talk regularly (for example, every 3 to 6 months) about whether you still need treatment with Premarin.

What are the possible side effects of Premarin?

Less common but serious side effects include:

- Breast cancer
- Cancer of the uterus
- Stroke
- Heart attack
- Blood clots
- Dementia
- Gallbladder disease
- Ovarian cancer

These are some of the warning signs of serious side effects:

- Breast lumps
- Unusual vaginal bleeding
- Dizziness and faintness
- Changes in speech
- Severe headaches
- Chest pain
- Shortness of breath
- Pains in your legs
- Changes in vision
- Vomiting

Call your healthcare provider right away if you get any of these warning signs, or any other unusual symptom that concerns you.

Common side effects include:

- Headache
- Breast pain
- Irregular vaginal bleeding or spotting
- Stomach/abdominal cramps, bloating
- Nausea and vomiting
- Hair loss

Other side effects include:

- High blood pressure
- Liver problems
- High blood sugar
- Fluid retention
- Enlargement of benign tumors of the uterus ("fibroids")
- Vaginal yeast infections

These are not all the possible side effects of Premarin. For more information, ask your healthcare provider or pharmacist.

What can I do to lower my chances of getting a serious side effect with Premarin?

- Talk with your healthcare provider regularly about whether you should continue taking Premarin.
- If you have a uterus, talk to your healthcare provider about whether the addition of a progestin is right for you.
- See your healthcare provider right away if you get vaginal bleeding while taking Premarin.
- Have a breast exam and mammogram (breast X-ray) every year unless your healthcare provider tells you something else. If members of your family have had breast cancer or if you have ever had breast lumps or an abnormal mammogram, you may need to have breast exams more often.
- If you have high blood pressure, high cholesterol (fat in the blood), diabetes, are overweight, or if you use tobacco, you may have higher chances for getting heart disease. Ask your healthcare provider for ways to lower your chances for getting heart disease.

General information about the safe and effective use of Premarin

Medicines are sometimes prescribed for conditions that are not mentioned in patient information leaflets. Do not take Premarin for conditions for which it was not prescribed. Do not give Premarin to other people, even if they have the same symptoms you have. It may harm them.

Keep Premarin out of the reach of children.

This leaflet provides a summary of the most important information about Premarin. If you would like more information, talk with your healthcare provider or pharmacist. You can ask for information about Premarin that is written for health professionals. You can get more information by calling the toll free number 800-934-5556.

What are the ingredients in Premarin?

Premarin contains a mixture of conjugated equine estrogens, which are a mixture of sodium estrone sulfate and sodium equilin sulfate and other components including sodium sulfate conjugates, 17 α-dihydroequilin, 17 α-estradiol, and 17 β-dihydroequilin. Premarin also contains calcium phosphate tribasic, calcium sulfate, carnauba wax, cellulose, glyceryl monooleate, lactose, magnesium stearate, methylcellulose, pharmaceutical glaze, polyethylene glycol, stearic acid, sucrose, and titanium dioxide. The tablets come in different strengths and each strength tablet is a different color. The color ingredients are:

- 0.3 mg tablet (green color): D&C Yellow No. 10, FD&C Blue No. 1, FD&C Blue No. 2, and FD&C Yellow No. 6.
- 0.45 mg tablet (blue color): FD&C Blue No. 2.
- 0.625 mg tablet (maroon color): FD&C Blue No. 2, D&C Red No. 27, and FD&C Red No. 40.
- 0.9 mg tablet (white color): D&C Red No. 6 and D&C Red No. 7.
- 1.25 mg tablet (yellow color): black iron oxide, D&C Yellow No. 10, and FD&C Yellow No. 6.
- 2.5 mg tablet (purple color): FD&C Blue No. 2 and D&C Red No. 7.

The appearance of these tablets is a trademark of Wyeth Pharmaceuticals.

Wyeth®

Wyeth Pharmaceuticals Inc.
Philadelphia, PA 19101 W10405C008
ET05
Revised July 16, 2003

PREVNAR® ℞

[*prĕv′năr*]

Pneumococcal 7-valent Conjugate Vaccine (Diphtheria CRM_{197} Protein)

Prescribing information for this product, which appears on pages 3471–3478 of the 2004 PDR, has been revised as follows. Please write "See Supplement A" next to the product heading.

The copy preceding the **DESCRIPTION SECTION** *was revised as follows:*

Pneumococcal 7-valent Conjugate Vaccine (Diphtheria CRM_{197} Protein)
FOR PEDIATRIC USE ONLY
℞ only
For Intramuscular Injection Only

This product's label may have been revised after this insert was used in production. For further product information and current package insert, please visit www.wyeth.com or call our medical communications department toll-free at 1-800-934-5556.

Manufactured by:
Wyeth Pharmaceuticals Inc.
Philadelphia, PA 19101
US Govt. License No. 3
W10430C003
ET01
Rev 01/04

PROTONIX® ℞

[*prŏ′tō-nĭks*]

(pantoprazole sodium)
Delayed-Release Tablets
℞ only

Prescribing information for this product, which appears on pages 3478–3480 of the 2004 PDR, has been completely revised as follows. Please write "See Supplement A" next to the product heading.

DESCRIPTION

The active ingredient in PROTONIX® (pantoprazole sodium) Delayed-Release Tablets is a substituted benzimidazole, sodium 5-(difluoromethoxy)-2-[[(3,4-dimethoxy-2-pyridinyl)methyl] sulfinyl]-1*H*-benzimidazole sesquihydrate, a compound that inhibits gastric acid secretion. Its empirical formula is $C_{16}H_{14}F_2N_3NaO_4S \times 1.5\ H_2O$, with a molecular weight of 432.4. The structural formula is:

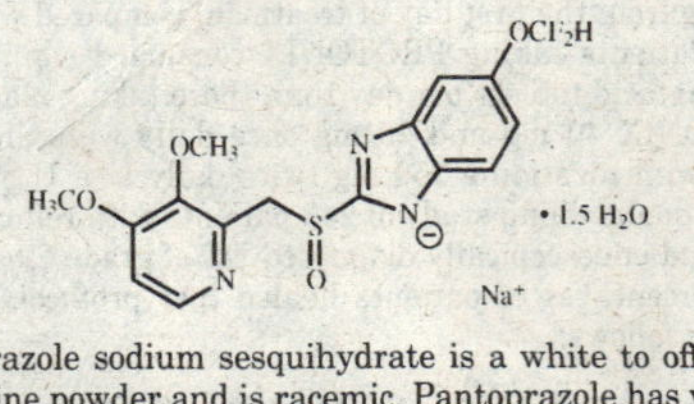

Pantoprazole sodium sesquihydrate is a white to off-white crystalline powder and is racemic. Pantoprazole has weakly basic and acidic properties. Pantoprazole sodium sesquihydrate is freely soluble in water, very slightly soluble in phosphate buffer at pH 7.4, and practically insoluble in n-hexane.

The stability of the compound in aqueous solution is pH-dependent. The rate of degradation increases with decreasing pH. At ambient temperature, the degradation half-life is approximately 2.8 hours at pH 5.0 and approximately 220 hours at pH 7.8.

PROTONIX is supplied as a delayed-release tablet for oral administration, available in 2 strengths. Each delayed-release tablet contains 45.1 mg or 22.6 mg of pantoprazole sodium sesquihydrate (equivalent to 40 mg or 20 mg pantoprazole, respectively) with the following inactive ingredients: calcium stearate, crospovidone, hypromellose, iron oxide, mannitol, methacrylic acid copolymer, polysorbate 80, povidone, propylene glycol, sodium carbonate, sodium lauryl sulfate, titanium dioxide, and triethyl citrate.

CLINICAL PHARMACOLOGY

Pharmacokinetics

PROTONIX is prepared as an enteric-coated tablet so that absorption of pantoprazole begins only after the tablet leaves the stomach. Peak serum concentration (C_{max}) and area under the serum concentration time curve (AUC) increase in a manner proportional to oral and intravenous doses from 10 mg to 80 mg. Pantoprazole does not accumulate and its pharmacokinetics are unaltered with multiple daily dosing. Following oral or intravenous administration, the serum concentration of pantoprazole declines biexponentially with a terminal elimination half-life of approximately one hour. In extensive metabolizers (see Metabolism section) with normal liver function receiving an oral dose of the enteric-coated 40 mg pantoprazole tablet, the peak concentration (C_{max}) is 2.5 μg/mL, the time to reach the peak concentration (t_{max}) is 2.5 h and the total area under the plasma concentration versus time curve (AUC) is 4.8 μg•hr/mL. When pantoprazole is given with food, its t_{max} is highly variable and may increase significantly. Following intravenous administration of pantoprazole to extensive metabolizers, its total clearance is 7.6-14.0 L/h and its apparent volume of distribution is 11.0-23.6L.

Absorption

The absorption of pantoprazole is rapid, with a C_{max} of 2.5 μg/mL that occurs approximately 2.5 hours after single or multiple oral 40-mg doses. Pantoprazole is well absorbed; it undergoes little first-pass metabolism resulting in an absolute bioavailability of approximately 77%. Pantoprazole absorption is not affected by concomitant administration of antacids. Administration of pantoprazole with food may delay its absorption up to 2 hours or longer; however, the C_{max} and the extent of pantoprazole absorption (AUC) are not altered. Thus, pantoprazole may be taken without regard to timing of meals.

Distribution

The apparent volume of distribution of pantoprazole is approximately 11.0-23.6L, distributing mainly in extracellular fluid. The serum protein binding of pantoprazole is about 98%, primarily to albumin.

Metabolism

Pantoprazole is extensively metabolized in the liver through the cytochrome P450 (CYP) system. Pantoprazole metabolism is independent of the route of administration (intravenous or oral). The main metabolic pathway is demethylation, by CYP2C19, with subsequent sulfation; other metabolic pathways include oxidation by CYP3A4. There is no evidence that any of the pantoprazole metabolites have significant pharmacologic activity. CYP2C19 displays a known genetic polymorphism due to its deficiency in some sub-populations (e.g. 3% of Caucasians and African-Americans and 17-23% of Asians). Although these sub-populations of slow pantoprazole metabolizers have elimination half-life values of 3.5 to 10.0 hours, they still have minimal accumulation (≤ 23%) with once daily dosing.

Elimination

After a single oral or intravenous dose of ^{14}C-labeled pantoprazole to healthy, normal metabolizer volunteers, approximately 71% of the dose was excreted in the urine with 18% excreted in the feces through biliary excretion. There was no renal excretion of unchanged pantoprazole.

Special Populations

Geriatric

Only slight to moderate increases in pantoprazole AUC (43%) and C_{max} (26%) were found in elderly volunteers (64 to 76 years of age) after repeated oral administration, compared with younger subjects. No dosage adjustment is recommended based on age.

Pediatric

The pharmacokinetics of pantoprazole have not been investigated in patients <18 years of age.

Gender

There is a modest increase in pantoprazole AUC and C_{max} in women compared to men. However, weight-normalized clearance values are similar in women and men. No dosage adjustment is needed based on gender (Also see **Use in Women**).

Renal Impairment

In patients with severe renal impairment, pharmacokinetic parameters for pantoprazole were similar to those of healthy subjects. No dosage adjustment is necessary in patients with renal impairment or in patients undergoing hemodialysis.

Hepatic Impairment

In patients with mild to severe hepatic impairment, maximum pantoprazole concentrations increased only slightly (1.5-fold) relative to healthy subjects. Although serum half-life values increased to 7-9 hours and AUC values increased by 5- to 7-fold in hepatic-impaired patients, these increases were no greater than those observed in slow CYP2C19 metabolizers, where no dosage frequency adjustment is warranted. These pharmacokinetic changes in hepatic-impaired patients result in minimal drug accumulation following once daily multiple-dose administration. No dosage adjust-

Continued on next page

Protonix Tablets—Cont.

ment is needed in patients with mild to severe hepatic impairment. Doses higher than 40 mg/day have not been studied in hepatically-impaired patients.

Drug-Drug Interactions

Pantoprazole is metabolized mainly by CYP2C19 and to minor extents by CYPs 3A4, 2D6 and 2C9. In *in vivo* drug-drug interaction studies with CYP2C19 substrates (diazepam [also a CYP3A4 substrate] and phenytoin [also a CYP3A4 inducer]), nifedipine, midazolam, and clarithromycin (CYP3A4 substrates), metoprolol (a CYP2D6 substrate), diclofenac, naproxen and piroxicam (CYP2C9 substrates) and theophylline (a CYP1A2 substrate) in healthy subjects, the pharmacokinetics of pantoprazole were not significantly altered. It is, therefore, expected that other drugs metabolized by CYPs 2C19, 3A4, 2D6, 2C9 and 1A2 would not significantly affect the pharmacokinetics of pantoprazole. *In vivo* studies also suggest that pantoprazole does not significantly affect the kinetics of other drugs (cisapride, theophylline, diazepam [and its active metabolite, desmethyldiazepam], phenytoin, warfarin, metoprolol, nifedipine, carbamazepine, midazolam, clarithromycin, naproxen, piroxicam and oral contraceptives [levonorgestrel/ethinyl estradiol]) metabolized by CYPs 2C19, 3A4, 2C9, 2D6 and 1A2. Therefore, it is expected that pantoprazole would not significantly affect the pharmacokinetics of other drugs metabolized by these isozymes. Dosage adjustment of such drugs is not necessary when they are co-administered with pantoprazole. In other *in vivo* studies, digoxin, ethanol, glyburide, antipyrine, caffeine, metronidazole, and amoxicillin had no clinically relevant interactions with pantoprazole. Although no significant drug-drug interactions have been observed in clinical studies, the potential for significant drug-drug interactions with more than once daily dosing with high doses of pantoprazole has not been studied in poor metabolizers or individuals who are hepatically impaired.

Pharmacodynamics

Mechanism of Action

Pantoprazole is a proton pump inhibitor (PPI) that suppresses the final step in gastric acid production by covalently binding to the (H^+,K^+)-ATPase enzyme system at the secretory surface of the gastric parietal cell. This effect leads to inhibition of both basal and stimulated gastric acid secretion irrespective of the stimulus. The binding to the (H^+,K^+)-ATPase results in a duration of antisecretory effect that persists longer than 24 hours for all doses tested.

Antisecretory Activity

Under maximal acid stimulatory conditions using pentagastrin, a dose-dependent decrease in gastric acid output occurs after a single dose of oral (20-80 mg) or a single dose of intravenous (20-120 mg) pantoprazole in healthy volunteers. Pantoprazole given once daily results in increasing inhibition of gastric acid secretion. Following the initial oral dose of 40 mg pantoprazole, a 51% mean inhibition was achieved by 2.5 hours. With once a day dosing for 7 days the mean inhibition was increased to 85%. Pantoprazole suppressed acid secretion in excess of 95% in half of the subjects. Acid secretion had returned to normal within a week after the last dose of pantoprazole; there was no evidence of rebound hypersecretion.

In a series of dose-response studies pantoprazole, at oral doses ranging from 20 to 120 mg, caused dose-related increases in median basal gastric pH and in the percent of time gastric pH was > 3 and > 4. Treatment with 40 mg of pantoprazole produced optimal increases in gastric pH which were significantly greater than the 20-mg dose. Doses higher than 40 mg (60, 80, 120 mg) did not result in further significant increases in median gastric pH. The effects of pantoprazole on median pH from one double-blind crossover study are shown below.

Effect of Single Daily Doses of Oral Pantoprazole on Intragastric pH

	Median pH on day 7			
Time	Placebo	20 mg	40 mg	80 mg
8 a.m. - 8 a.m. (24 hours)	1.3	2.9*	3.8*#	3.9*#
8 a.m. - 10 p.m. (Daytime)	1.6	3.2*	4.4*#	4.8*#
10 p.m. - 8 a.m. (Nighttime)	1.2	2.1*	3.0*	2.6*

* Significantly different from placebo
\# Significantly different from 20 mg

Serum Gastrin Effects

Fasting serum gastrin levels were assessed in two double-blind studies of the acute healing of erosive esophagitis (EE) in which 682 patients with gastroesophageal reflux disease (GERD) received 10, 20, or 40 mg of PROTONIX for up to 8 weeks. At 4 weeks of treatment there was an increase in mean gastrin levels of 7%, 35%, and 72% over pretreatment values in the 10, 20, and 40 mg treatment groups, respectively. A similar increase in serum gastrin levels was noted at the 8 week visit with mean increases of 3%, 26%, and 84% for the three pantoprazole dose groups. Median serum gastrin levels remained within normal limits during maintenance therapy with PROTONIX (pantoprazole sodium) Delayed-Release Tablets.

In long-term international studies involving over 800 patients, a 2- to 3-fold mean increase from the pretreatment fasting serum gastrin level was observed in the initial months of treatment with pantoprazole at doses of 40 mg per day during GERD maintenance studies and 40 mg or higher per day in patients with refractory GERD. Fasting serum gastrin levels generally remained at approximately 2 to 3 times baseline for up to 4 years of periodic follow-up in clinical trials.

Following healing of gastric or duodenal ulcers with pantoprazole treatment, elevated gastrin levels return to normal by at least 3 months.

Enterochromaffin-Like (ECL) Cell Effects

In 39 patients treated with oral pantoprazole 40 mg to 240 mg daily (majority receiving 40 mg to 80 mg) for up to 5 years, there was a moderate increase in ECL-cell density starting after the first year of use which appeared to plateau after 4 years.

In a nonclinical study in Sprague-Dawley rats, lifetime exposure (24 months) to pantoprazole at doses of 0.5 to 200 mg/kg/day resulted in dose-related increases in gastric ECL-cell proliferation and gastric neuroendocrine (NE)-cell tumors. Gastric NE-cell tumors in rats may result from chronic elevation of serum gastrin concentrations. The high density of ECL cells in the rat stomach makes this species highly susceptible to the proliferative effects of elevated gastrin concentrations produced by proton pump inhibitors. However, there were no observed elevations in serum gastrin following the administration of pantoprazole at a dose of 0.5 mg/kg/day. In a separate study, a gastric NE-cell tumor without concomitant ECL-cell proliferative changes was observed in 1 female rat following 12 months of dosing with pantoprazole at 5 mg/kg/day and a 9 month off-dose recovery. (See **PRECAUTIONS, Carcinogenesis, Mutagenesis, Impairment of Fertility**).

Other Effects

No clinically relevant effects of pantoprazole on cardiovascular, respiratory, ophthalmic, or central nervous system function have been detected. In a clinical pharmacology study, pantoprazole 40 mg given once daily for 2 weeks had no effect on the levels of the following hormones: cortisol, testosterone, triiodothyronine (T3), thyroxine (T4), thyroid-stimulating hormone (TSH), thyronine-binding protein, parathyroid hormone, insulin, glucagon, renin, aldosterone, follicle-stimulating hormone, luteinizing hormone, prolactin and growth hormone.

In a 1-year study of GERD patients treated with pantoprazole 40 mg or 20 mg, there were no changes from baseline in overall levels of T3, T4, and TSH.

Clinical Studies

PROTONIX Delayed-Release Tablets were used in all clinical trials.

Erosive Esophagitis (EE) Associated with Gastroesophageal Reflux Disease (GERD)

A U.S. multicenter double-blind, placebo-controlled study of PROTONIX 10 mg, 20 mg, or 40 mg once daily was conducted in 603 patients with reflux symptoms and endoscopically diagnosed EE of grade 2 or above (Hetzel-Dent scale). In this study, approximately 25% of enrolled patients had severe EE of grade 3 and 10% had grade 4. The percentages of patients healed (per protocol, n=541) in this study were as follows:

Erosive Esophagitis Healing Rates (per protocol)

	PROTONIX			Placebo
Week	10 mg QD (n = 153)	20 mg QD (n = 158)	40 mg QD (n = 162)	(n = 68)
4	45.6%+	58.4%+#	75.0%+*	14.3%
8	66.0%+	83.5%+#	92.6%+*	39.7%

\+ ($p < 0.001$) PROTONIX versus placebo.
* ($p < 0.05$) versus 10 mg, or 20 mg PROTONIX
\# ($p < 0.05$) versus 10 mg PROTONIX

In this study, all PROTONIX treatment groups had significantly greater healing rates than the placebo group. This was true regardless of *H. pylori* status for the 40-mg and 20-mg PROTONIX treatment groups. The 40-mg dose of PROTONIX resulted in healing rates significantly greater than those found with either the 20- or 10-mg dose.

A significantly greater proportion of patients taking PROTONIX 40 mg experienced complete relief of daytime and nighttime heartburn and the absence of regurgitation starting from the first day of treatment compared with placebo. Patients taking PROTONIX consumed significantly fewer antacid tablets per day than those taking placebo.

PROTONIX 40 mg and 20 mg once daily were also compared with nizatidine 150 mg twice daily in a U.S. multicenter, double-blind study of 243 patients with reflux symptoms and endoscopically diagnosed EE of grade 2 or above. The percentages of patients healed (per protocol, n=212) were as follows:

Erosive Esophagitis Healing Rates (per protocol)

	PROTONIX		Nizatidine
Week	20 mg QD (n = 72)	40 mg QD (n = 70)	150 mg BID (n = 70)
4	61.4%+	64.0%+	22.2%
8	79.2%+	82.9%+	41.4%

\+ ($p < 0.001$) PROTONIX versus nizatidine.

Once daily treatment with PROTONIX 40 or 20 mg resulted in significantly superior rates of healing at both 4 and 8 weeks compared with twice daily treatment with 150 mg of nizatidine. For the 40 mg treatment group, significantly greater healing rates compared to nizatidine were achieved regardless of the *H. pylori* status.

A significantly greater proportion of the patients in the PROTONIX treatment groups experienced complete relief of nighttime heartburn and regurgitation starting on the first day and of daytime heartburn on the second day compared with those taking nizatidine 150 mg twice daily. Patients taking PROTONIX consumed significantly fewer antacid tablets per day than those taking nizatidine.

Long-Term Maintenance of Healing of Erosive Esophagitis

Two independent, multicenter, randomized, double-blind, comparator-controlled trials of identical design were conducted in GERD patients with endoscopically-confirmed healed erosive esophagitis to demonstrate efficacy of PROTONIX in long-term maintenance of healing. The two U.S. studies enrolled 386 and 404 patients, respectively, to receive either 10 mg, 20 mg, or 40 mg of PROTONIX (pantoprazole sodium) Delayed-Release Tablets once daily or 150 mg of ranitidine twice daily. As demonstrated in the table below, PROTONIX 40 mg and 20 mg were significantly superior to ranitidine at every time point with respect to the maintenance of healing. In addition, PROTONIX 40 mg was superior to all other treatments studied.

Long-Term Maintenance of Healing of Erosive Gastroesophageal Reflux Disease (GERD Maintenance): Percentage of Patients Who Remained Healed

	PROTONIX 20 mg QD	PROTONIX 40 mg QD	Ranitidine 150 mg BID
Study 1	n = 75	n = 74	n = 75
Month 1	91*	99*	68
Month 3	82*	93*#	54
Month 6	76*	90*#	44
Month 12	70*	86*#	35
Study 2	n = 74	n = 88	n = 84
Month 1	89*	92*#	62
Month 3	78*	91*#	47
Month 6	72*	88*#	39
Month 12	72*	83*	37

* ($p < 0.05$ vs ranitidine)
\# ($p < 0.05$ vs PROTONIX 20 mg)
Note: PROTONIX 10 mg was superior ($p < 0.05$) to ranitidine in study 2 but not study 1.

PROTONIX 40 mg was superior to ranitidine in reducing the number of daytime and nighttime heartburn episodes from the first through the twelfth month of treatment. PROTONIX 20 mg, administered once daily, was also effective in reducing episodes of daytime and nighttime heartburn in one trial.

Number of Episodes of Heartburn (mean ± SD)

		PROTONIX 40 mg QD	Ranitidine 150 mg BID
Month 1	Daytime	5.1 ± 1.6*	18.3 ± 1.6
	Nighttime	3.9 ± 1.1*	11.9 ± 1.1
Month 12	Daytime	2.9 ± 1.5*	17.5 ± 1.5
	Nighttime	2.5 ± 1.2*	13.8 ± 1.3

* ($p < 0.001$ vs ranitidine, combined data from the 2 U.S. studies)

Pathological Hypersecretory Conditions Including Zollinger-Ellison Syndrome

In a multicenter, open-label trial of 35 patients with pathological hypersecretory conditions, such as Zollinger-Ellison syndrome with or without multiple endocrine neoplasia-type I, PROTONIX successfully controlled gastric acid secretion. Doses ranging from 80 mg daily to 240 mg daily maintained gastric acid output below 10mEq/h in patients without prior acid-reducing surgery and below 5 mEq/h in patients with prior acid-reducing surgery.

Doses were initially titrated to the individual patient needs, and adjusted in some patients based on the clinical response with time. (See DOSAGE AND ADMINISTRATION.) PROTONIX was well tolerated at these dose levels for prolonged periods (greater than 2 years in some patients).

INDICATIONS AND USAGE

Short-Term Treatment of Erosive Esophagitis Associated With Gastroesophageal Reflux Disease (GERD)

PROTONIX® (pantoprazole sodium) Delayed-Release Tablets are indicated for the short-term treatment (up to 8 weeks) in the healing and symptomatic relief of erosive esophagitis. For those patients who have not healed after 8 weeks of treatment, an additional 8 week course of PROTONIX may be considered.

Maintenance of Healing of Erosive Esophagitis

PROTONIX Delayed-Release Tablets are indicated for maintenance of healing of erosive esophagitis and reduction in relapse rates of daytime and nighttime heartburn symptoms in patients with gastroesophageal reflux disease (GERD). Controlled studies did not extend beyond 12 months.

Pathological Hypersecretory Conditions Including Zollinger-Ellison Syndrome

PROTONIX Delayed-Release Tablets are indicated for the long-term treatment of pathological hypersecretory conditions, including Zollinger-Ellison syndrome.

CONTRAINDICATIONS

PROTONIX Delayed-Release Tablets are contraindicated in patients with known hypersensitivity to any component of the formulation.

PRECAUTIONS

General

Symptomatic response to therapy with pantoprazole does not preclude the presence of gastric malignancy.

Owing to the chronic nature of erosive esophagitis, there may be a potential for prolonged administration of pantoprazole. In long-term rodent studies, pantoprazole was carcinogenic and caused rare types of gastrointestinal tumors. The relevance of these findings to tumor development in humans is unknown.

Generally, daily treatment with any acid-suppressing medications over a long period of time (e.g. longer than 3 years) may lead to malabsorption of cyanocobalamin (Vitamin B-12) caused by hypo- or achlorhydria. Rare reports of cyanocobalamin deficiency occurring with acid-suppressing therapy have been reported in the literature. This possibility should be considered if clinical symptoms consistent with cyanocobalamin deficiency are observed.

Information for Patients

Patients should be cautioned that PROTONIX Delayed-Release Tablets should not be split, crushed or chewed. The tablets should be swallowed whole, with or without food in the stomach. Concomitant administration of antacids does not affect the absorption of pantoprazole.

Drug Interactions

Pantoprazole is metabolized through the cytochrome P450 system, primarily the CYP2C19 and CYP3A4 isozymes, and subsequently undergoes Phase II conjugation. Based on studies evaluating possible interactions of pantoprazole with other drugs, no dosage adjustment is needed with concomitant use of the following: theophylline, cisapride, antipyrine, caffeine, carbamazepine, diazepam (and its active metabolite, desmethyldiazepam), diclofenac, naproxen, piroxicam, digoxin, ethanol, glyburide, an oral contraceptive (levonorgestrel/ethinyl estradiol), metoprolol, nifedipine, phenytoin, warfarin, midazolam, clarithromycin, metronidazole, or amoxicillin. Clinically relevant interactions of pantoprazole with other drugs with the same metabolic pathways are not expected. Therefore, when co-administered with pantoprazole, adjustment of the dosage of pantoprazole or of such drugs may not be necessary. There was also no interaction with concomitantly administered antacids.

Because of profound and long lasting inhibition of gastric acid secretion, pantoprazole may interfere with absorption of drugs where gastric pH is an important determinant of their bioavailability (e.g., ketoconazole, ampicillin esters, and iron salts).

Carcinogenesis, Mutagenesis, Impairment of Fertility

In a 24-month carcinogenicity study, Sprague-Dawley rats were treated orally with doses of 0.5 to 200 mg/kg/day, about 0.1 to 40 times the exposure on a body surface area basis, of a 50-kg person dosed at 40 mg/day. In the gastric fundus, treatment at 0.5 to 200 mg/kg/day produced enterochromaffin-like (ECL) cell hyperplasia and benign and malignant neuroendocrine cell tumors in a dose-related manner. In the forestomach, treatment at 50 and 200 mg/kg/day (about 10 and 40 times the recommended human dose on a body surface area basis) produced benign squamous cell papillomas and malignant squamous cell carcinomas. Rare gastrointestinal tumors associated with pantoprazole treatment included an adenocarcinoma of the duodenum at 50 mg/kg/day, and benign polyps and adenocarcinomas of the gastric fundus at 200 mg/kg/day.

In the liver, treatment at 0.5 to 200 mg/kg/day produced dose-related increases in the incidences of hepatocellular adenomas and carcinomas. In the thyroid gland, treatment at 200 mg/kg/day produced increased incidences of follicular cell adenomas and carcinomas for both male and female rats.

Sporadic occurrences of hepatocellular adenomas and a hepatocellular carcinoma were observed in Sprague-Dawley rats exposed to pantoprazole in 6-month and 12-month toxicity studies.

In a 24-month carcinogenicity study, Fischer 344 rats were treated orally with doses of 5 to 50 mg/kg/day, approximately 1 to 10 times the recommended human dose based on body surface area. In the gastric fundus, treatment at 5 to 50 mg/kg/day produced enterochromaffin-like (ECL) cell hyperplasia and benign and malignant neuroendocrine cell tumors. Dose selection for this study may not have been adequate to comprehensively evaluate the carcinogenic potential of pantoprazole.

In a 24-month carcinogenicity study, B6C3F1 mice were treated orally with doses of 5 to 150 mg/kg/day, 0.5 to 15 times the recommended human dose based on body surface area. In the liver, treatment at 150 mg/kg/day produced increased incidences of hepatocellular adenomas and carcinomas in female mice. Treatment at 5 to 150 mg/kg/day also produced gastric fundic ECL cell hyperplasia.

A 26-week p53 +/- transgenic mouse carcinogenicity study was not positive.

Pantoprazole was positive in the *in vitro* human lymphocyte chromosomal aberration assays, in one of two mouse micronucleus tests for clastogenic effects, and in the *in vitro* Chinese hamster ovarian cell/HGPRT forward mutation assay for mutagenic effects. Equivocal results were observed in the *in vivo* rat liver DNA covalent binding assay. Pantoprazole was negative in the *in vitro* Ames mutation assay, the *in vitro* unscheduled DNA synthesis (UDS) assay with rat hepatocytes, the *in vitro* AS52/GPT mammalian cell-forward gene mutation assay, the *in vitro* thymidine kinase mutation test with mouse lymphoma L5178Y cells, and the *in vivo* rat bone marrow cell chromosomal aberration assay.

Pantoprazole at oral doses up to 500 mg/kg/day in male rats (98 times the recommended human dose based on body surface area) and 450 mg/kg/day in female rats (88 times the recommended human dose based on body surface area) was found to have no effect on fertility and reproductive performance.

Pregnancy

Teratogenic Effects

Pregnancy Category B

Teratology studies have been performed in rats at oral doses up to 450 mg/kg/day (88 times the recommended human dose based on body surface area) and rabbits at oral doses up to 40 mg/kg/day (16 times the recommended human dose based on body surface area) and have revealed no evidence of impaired fertility or harm to the fetus due to pantoprazole. There are, however, no adequate and well-controlled studies in pregnant women. Because animal reproduction studies are not always predictive of human response, this drug should be used during pregnancy only if clearly needed.

Nursing Mothers

Pantoprazole and its metabolites are excreted in the milk of rats. Pantoprazole excretion in human milk has been detected in a study of a single nursing mother after a single 40 mg oral dose. The clinical relevance of this finding is not known. Many drugs which are excreted in human milk have a potential for serious adverse reactions in nursing infants. Based on the potential for tumorigenicity shown for pantoprazole in rodent carcinogenicity studies, a decision should be made whether to discontinue nursing or to discontinue the drug, taking into account the benefit of the drug to the mother.

Pediatric Use

Safety and effectiveness in pediatric patients have not been established.

Use in Women

Erosive esophagitis healing rates in the 221 women treated with PROTONIX (pantoprazole sodium) Delayed-Release Tablets in U.S. clinical trials were similar to those found in men. In the 122 women treated long-term with PROTONIX 40 mg or 20 mg, healing was maintained at a rate similar to that in men. The incidence rates of adverse events were also similar for men and women.

Use in Elderly

In short-term U.S. clinical trials, erosive esophagitis healing rates in the 107 elderly patients (≥ 65 years old) treated with PROTONIX were similar to those found in patients under the age of 65. The incidence rates of adverse events and laboratory abnormalities in patients aged 65 years and older were similar to those associated with patients younger than 65 years of age.

Laboratory Tests

There have been reports of false-positive urine screening tests for tetrahydrocannabinol (THC) in patients receiving most proton pump inhibitors, including pantoprazole. An alternative confirmatory method should be considered to verify positive results.

ADVERSE REACTIONS

Worldwide, more than 11,100 patients have been treated with pantoprazole in clinical trials involving various dosages and duration of treatment. In general, pantoprazole has been well tolerated in both short-term and long-term trials.

In two U.S. controlled clinical trials involving PROTONIX 10-, 20-, or 40-mg doses for up to 8 weeks, there were no dose-related effects on the incidence of adverse events. The following adverse events considered by investigators to be possibly, probably or definitely related to drug occurred in 1% or more in the individual studies of GERD patients on therapy with PROTONIX.

Most Frequent Adverse Events Reported as Drug Related in Short-term Domestic Trials

	% Incidence			
	Study 300-US		Study 301-US	
Study Event	PROTONIX (n = 521)	Placebo (n = 82)	PROTONIX (n = 161)	Nizatidine (n = 82)
Headache	6	6	9	13
Diarrhea	4	1	6	6
Flatulence	2	2	4	0
Abdominal pain	1	2	4	4
Rash	<1	0	2	0
Eructation	1	1	0	0
Insomnia	<1	2	1	1
Hyperglycemia	1	0	<1	0

Note: Only adverse events with an incidence greater than or equal to the comparators are shown.

In international short-term double-blind or open-label, clinical trials involving 20 to 80 mg per day, the following adverse events were reported to occur in 1% or more of 2805 GERD patients receiving pantoprazole for up to 8 weeks.

Adverse Events in GERD Patients in Short-term International Trials

	% Incidence			
Study Event	Pantoprazole Total (n=2805)	Ranitidine 300 mg (n=594)	Omeprazole 20 mg (n=474)	Famotidine 40 mg (n=239)
Headache	2	3	2	1
Diarrhea	2	2	2	<1
Abdominal Pain	1	1	<1	<1

In two U.S. controlled clinical trials involving PROTONIX 10-, 20-, or 40-mg doses for up to 12 months, the following adverse events considered by investigators to be possibly, probably or definitely related to drug occurred in 1% or more of GERD patients on long-term therapy.

Most Frequent Adverse Events Reported as Drug Related in Long-term Domestic Trials

	% Incidence	
Study Event	PROTONIX (n = 536)	Ranitidine (n = 185)
Headache	5	2
Abdominal pain	3	1
Liver function tests abnormal	2	<1
Nausea	2	2
Vomiting	2	2

Note: Only adverse events with an incidence greater than or equal to the comparators are shown.

In addition, in these short- and long-term domestic and international trials, the following treatment-emergent events, regardless of causality, occurred at a rate of ≥ 1% in pantoprazole-treated patients: anxiety, arthralgia, asthenia, back pain, bronchitis, chest pain, constipation, cough increased, dizziness, dyspepsia, dyspnea, flu syndrome, gastroenteritis, gastrointestinal disorder, hyperlipemia, hypertonia, infection, liver function tests abnormal, migraine, nausea, neck pain, pain, pharyngitis, rectal disorder, rhinitis, SGPT increased, sinusitis, upper respiratory tract infection, urinary frequency, urinary tract infection, and vomiting.

Additional treatment-emergent adverse experiences occurring in <1% of pantoprazole-treated patients from these trials are listed below by body system. In most instances the relationship to pantoprazole was unclear.

BODY AS A WHOLE: abscess, allergic reaction, chills, cyst, face edema, fever, generalized edema, heat stroke, hernia, laboratory test abnormal, malaise, moniliasis, neoplasm, non-specified drug reaction, photosensitivity reaction.

CARDIOVASCULAR SYSTEM: abnormal electrocardiogram, angina pectoris, arrhythmia, atrial fibrillation/flutter, cardiovascular disorder, chest pain substernal, congestive heart failure, hemorrhage, hypertension, hypotension, myocardial infarction, myocardial ischemia, palpitation, retinal vascular disorder, syncope, tachycardia, thrombophlebitis, thrombosis, vasodilatation.

DIGESTIVE SYSTEM: anorexia, aphthous stomatitis, cardiospasm, colitis, dry mouth, duodenitis, dysphagia, enteritis, esophageal hemorrhage, esophagitis, gastrointestinal carcinoma, gastrointestinal hemorrhage, gastrointestinal moniliasis, gingivitis, glossitis, halitosis, hematemesis, increased appetite, melena, mouth ulceration, oral moniliasis, periodontal abscess, periodontitis, rectal hemorrhage, stomach ulcer, stomatitis, stools abnormal, tongue discoloration, ulcerative colitis.

ENDOCRINE SYSTEM: diabetes mellitus, glycosuria, goiter.

HEPATO-BILIARY SYSTEM: biliary pain, hyperbilirubinemia, cholecystitis, cholelithiasis, cholestatic jaundice, hepatitis, alkaline phosphatase increased, gamma glutamyl transpeptidase increased, SGOT increased.

HEMIC AND LYMPHATIC SYSTEM: anemia, ecchymosis, eosinophilia, hypochromic anemia, iron deficiency anemia, leukocytosis, leukopenia, thrombocytopenia.

METABOLIC AND NUTRITIONAL: dehydration, edema, gout, peripheral edema, thirst, weight gain, weight loss.

MUSCULOSKELETAL SYSTEM: arthritis, arthrosis, bone disorder, bone pain, bursitis, joint disorder, leg cramps, neck rigidity, myalgia, tenosynovitis.

NERVOUS SYSTEM: abnormal dreams, confusion, convulsion, depression, dry mouth, dysarthria, emotional lability, hallucinations, hyperkinesia, hypesthesia, libido decreased, nervousness, neuralgia, neuritis, neuropathy, paresthesia, reflexes decreased, sleep disorder, somnolence, thinking abnormal, tremor, vertigo.

RESPIRATORY SYSTEM: asthma, epistaxis, hiccup, laryngitis, lung disorder, pneumonia, voice alteration.

SKIN AND APPENDAGES: acne, alopecia, contact dermatitis, dry skin, eczema, fungal dermatitis, hemorrhage, herpes simplex, herpes zoster, lichenoid dermatitis, maculopapular rash, pruritus, skin disorder, skin ulcer, sweating, urticaria.

SPECIAL SENSES: abnormal vision, amblyopia, cataract specified, deafness, diplopia, ear pain, extraocular palsy, glaucoma, otitis externa, taste perversion, tinnitus.

UROGENITAL SYSTEM: albuminuria, balanitis, breast pain, cystitis, dysmenorrhea, dysuria, epididymitis, hema-

Continued on next page

Protonix Tablets—Cont.

turia, impotence, kidney calculus, kidney pain, nocturia, prostatic disorder, pyelonephritis, scrotal edema, urethral pain, urethritis, urinary tract disorder, urination impaired, vaginitis.

In an open-label US clinical trial conducted in 35 patients with pathological hypersecretory conditions treated with PROTONIX for up to 27 months, the adverse events reported were consistent with the safety profile of the drug in other populations.

Postmarketing Reports

There have been spontaneous reports of adverse events with the postmarketing use of pantoprazole. These reports include anaphylaxis (including anaphylactic shock); angioedema (Quincke's edema); anterior ischemic optic neuropathy; elevated CPK (creatine phosphokinase); severe dermatologic reactions, including erythema multiforme, Stevens-Johnson syndrome, and toxic epidermal necrolysis (TEN, some fatal); hepatocellular damage leading to jaundice and hepatic failure; interstitial nephritis; pancreatitis; pancytopenia; and rhabdomyolysis. In addition, also observed have been confusion, hypokinesia, speech disorder, increased salivation, vertigo, nausea, tinnitus, and blurred vision.

Laboratory Values

In two U.S. controlled, short-term trials in patients with erosive esophagitis associated with GERD, 0.4% of the patients on PROTONIX 40 mg experienced SGPT elevations of greater than three times the upper limit of normal at the final treatment visit. In two U.S. controlled, long-term trials in patients with erosive esophagitis associated with GERD, none of 178 patients (0%) on PROTONIX 40 mg and two of 181 patients (1.1%) on PROTONIX 20 mg, experienced significant transaminase elevations at 12 months (or earlier if a patient discontinued prematurely). Significant elevations of SGOT or SGPT were defined as values at least three times the upper limit of normal that were non-sporadic and had no clear alternative explanation. The following changes in laboratory parameters were reported as adverse events: creatinine increased, hypercholesterolemia, and hyperuricemia.

OVERDOSAGE

Experience in patients taking very high doses of pantoprazole is limited. There have been spontaneous reports of overdosage with pantoprazole, including a suicide in which pantoprazole 560 mg and undetermined amounts of chloroquine and zopiclone were also ingested. There have also been spontaneous reports of patients taking similar amounts of pantoprazole (400 and 600 mg) with no adverse effects.

Pantoprazole is not removed by hemodialysis. In case of overdosage, treatment should be symptomatic and supportive.

Single oral doses of pantoprazole at 709 mg/kg, 798 mg/kg and 887 mg/kg were lethal to mice, rats and dogs, respectively. The symptoms of acute toxicity were hypoactivity, ataxia, hunched sitting, limb-splay, lateral position, segregation, absence of ear reflex, and tremor.

DOSAGE AND ADMINISTRATION

Treatment of Erosive Esophagitis

The recommended adult oral dose is 40 mg given once daily for up to 8 weeks. For those patients who have not healed after 8 weeks of treatment, an additional 8-week course of PROTONIX may be considered. (See **INDICATIONS AND USAGE**.)

Maintenance of Healing of Erosive Esophagitis

The recommended adult oral dose is one PROTONIX 40 mg Delayed-Release Tablet, taken daily. (See **Clinical Studies**.)

Pathological Hypersecretory Conditions Including Zollinger-Ellison Syndrome

The dosage of PROTONIX in patients with pathological hypersecretory conditions varies with the individual patient. The recommended adult starting dose is 40 mg twice daily. Dosage regimens should be adjusted to individual patient needs and should continue for as long as clinically indicated. Doses up to 240 mg daily have been administered. Some patients have been treated continuously with PROTONIX for more than 2 years.

No dosage adjustment is necessary in patients with renal impairment, hepatic impairment, or for elderly patients. Doses higher than 40 mg/day have not been studied in hepatically-impaired patients. No dosage adjustment is necessary in patients undergoing hemodialysis.

PROTONIX delayed-release Tablets should be swallowed whole, with or without food in the stomach. If patients are unable to swallow a 40 mg tablet, two 20 mg tablets may be taken. Concomitant administration of antacids does not affect the absorption of PROTONIX.

Patients should be cautioned that PROTONIX delayed-release Tablets should not be split, chewed or crushed.

HOW SUPPLIED

PROTONIX® (pantoprazole sodium) Delayed-Release Tablets are supplied as 40 mg yellow oval biconvex delayed-release tablets imprinted with PROTONIX (brown ink) on one side.

They are available as follows:

NDC 0008-0841-10 bottles of 100
NDC 0008-0841-81 bottles of 90
NDC 0008-0841-91 bottles of 1000
NDC 0008-0841-99 carton of 10 Redipak® blister strips of 10 tablets each

PROTONIX is supplied as 20 mg yellow oval biconvex delayed-release tablets imprinted with P20 (brown ink) on one side.

They are available as follows:

NDC 0008-0843-81 bottles of 90

Storage

Store PROTONIX® delayed-release Tablets at 20°–25°C (68°–77°F); excursions permitted to 15°-30°C (59°-86°F). [See USP Controlled Room Temperature].

U.S. Patent No. 4,758,579

Packaged by Wyeth Laboratories
A Wyeth-Ayerst Company
Philadelphia, PA 19101
under license from
ALTANA Pharma
D78467 Konstanz, Germany

W10438C007
ET01
Rev 03/04

PROTONIX® I.V. ℞

[*prō'tō-nĭks*]
(pantoprazole sodium)
for Injection
℞ only

Prescribing information for this product, which appears on pages 3480–3483 of the 2004 PDR, has been completely revised as follows. Please write "See Supplement A" next to the product heading.

DESCRIPTION

The active ingredient in PROTONIX® I.V. (pantoprazole sodium) for Injection is a substituted benzimidazole, sodium 5-(difluoromethoxy)-2-[[(3,4-dimethoxy-2-pyridinyl)methyl] sulfinyl]-1H-benzimidazole, a compound that inhibits gastric acid secretion. Its empirical formula is $C_{16}H_{14}F_2N_3NaO_4S$, with a molecular weight of 405.4. The structural formula is:

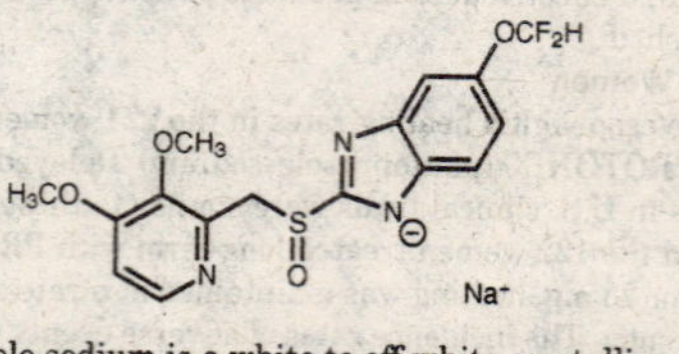

Pantoprazole sodium is a white to off-white crystalline powder and is racemic. Pantoprazole has weakly basic and acidic properties. Pantoprazole sodium is freely soluble in water, very slightly soluble in phosphate buffer at pH 7.4, and practically insoluble in n-hexane. The stability of the compound in aqueous solution is pH-dependent. The rate of degradation increases with decreasing pH. The reconstituted solution of PROTONIX I.V. for Injection is in the pH range 9.0 to 10.5.

PROTONIX I.V. for Injection is supplied as a freeze-dried powder in a clear glass vial fitted with a rubber stopper and crimp seal containing pantoprazole sodium, equivalent to 40 mg of pantoprazole, edetate disodium (1 mg), and hydroxide to adjust pH.

CLINICAL PHARMACOLOGY

Pharmacokinetics

Pantoprazole peak serum concentration (C_{max}) and area under the serum concentration-time curve (AUC) increase in a manner proportional to intravenous doses from 10 mg to 80 mg. Pantoprazole does not accumulate and its pharmacokinetics are unaltered with multiple daily dosing. Following the administration of PROTONIX I.V. for Injection, the serum concentration of pantoprazole declines biexponentially with a terminal elimination half-life of approximately one hour. In extensive metabolizers (see **CLINICAL PHARMACOLOGY, Metabolism**) with normal liver function receiving a 40 mg dose of PROTONIX I.V. for Injection by constant rate over 15 minutes, the peak concentration (C_{max}) is 5.52 μg/mL and the total area under the plasma concentration versus time curve (AUC) is 5.4 μg · hr/mL. The total clearance is 7.6-14.0 L/h and the apparent volume of distribution is 11.0-23.6 L.

Distribution

The apparent volume of distribution of pantoprazole is approximately 11.0-23.6 L, distributing mainly in extracellular fluid. The serum protein binding of pantoprazole is about 98%, primarily to albumin.

Metabolism

Pantoprazole is extensively metabolized in the liver through the cytochrome P450 (CYP) system. Pantoprazole metabolism is independent of the route of administration (intravenous or oral). The main metabolic pathway is demethylation, by CYP2C19, with subsequent sulfation; other metabolic pathways include oxidation by CYP3A4. There is no evidence that any of the pantoprazole metabolites have significant pharmacologic activity. CYP2C19 displays a known genetic polymorphism due to its deficiency in some sub-populations (e.g., 3% of Caucasians and African-Americans and 17-23% of Asians). Although these sub-populations of slow pantoprazole metabolizers have elimination half-life values from 3.5 to 10.0 hours, they still have minimal accumulation (≤23%) with once daily dosing.

Elimination

After administration of a single intravenous dose of ^{14}C-labeled pantoprazole to healthy, normal metabolizer subjects, approximately 71% of the dose was excreted in the urine with 18% excreted in the feces through biliary excretion. There was no renal excretion of unchanged pantoprazole.

Special Populations

Geriatric

After repeated I.V. administration in elderly subjects (65 to 76 years of age), pantoprazole AUC and elimination half-life values were similar to those observed in younger subjects. No dosage adjustment is recommended based on age.

Pediatric

The pharmacokinetics of pantoprazole have not been investigated in patients <18 years of age.

Gender

After oral administration there is a modest increase in pantoprazole AUC and C_{max} in women compared to men. However, weight-normalized clearance values are similar in women and men. No dosage adjustment is warranted based on gender (also see **Use in Women**).

Renal Impairment

In patients with severe renal impairment, pharmacokinetic parameters for pantoprazole were similar to those of healthy subjects. No dosage adjustment is necessary in patients with renal impairment or in patients undergoing hemodialysis.

Hepatic Impairment

Oral administration studies (absolute bioavailability is approximately 70%) were performed in patients with mild to severe hepatic impairment. Maximum pantoprazole concentrations increased only slightly (1.5-fold) relative to healthy subjects. Although serum elimination half-life values increased to 7-9 hours and AUC values increased by 5- to 7-fold in hepatic-impaired patients, these increases were no greater than those observed in slow CYP2C19 metabolizers, where no dosage adjustment is warranted. These pharmacokinetic changes in hepatic-impaired patients result in minimal drug accumulation following once daily multiple-dose administration equal to or less than 21%. No dosage adjustment is needed in patients with mild to severe hepatic impairment. Doses higher than 40 mg/day have not been studied in hepatically-impaired patients.

Drug-Drug Interactions

Pantoprazole is metabolized mainly by CYP2C19 and to minor extents by CYPs 3A4, 2D6 and 2C9. In *in vivo* drug-drug interaction studies with CYP2C19 substrates (diazepam [also a CYP3A4 substrate] and phenytoin [also a CYP3A4 inducer]), nifedipine, midazolam, and clarithromycin (CYP3A4 substrates), metoprolol (a CYP2D6 substrate), diclofenac, naproxen and piroxicam (CYP2C9 substrates) and theophylline (a CYP1A2 substrate) in healthy subjects, the pharmacokinetics of pantoprazole were not significantly altered. It is, therefore, expected that other drugs metabolized by CYPs 2C19, 3A4, 2D6, 2C9 and 1A2 would not significantly affect the pharmacokinetics of pantoprazole. *In vivo* studies also suggest that pantoprazole does not significantly affect the kinetics of other drugs (cisapride, theophylline, diazepam [and its active metabolite, desmethyldiazepam], phenytoin, warfarin, metoprolol, nifedipine, carbamazepine, midazolam, clarithromycin, naproxen, piroxicam and oral contraceptives [levonorgestrel/ethinyl estradiol]) metabolized by CYPs 2C19, 3A4, 2D6, 2C9 and 1A2. Therefore, it is expected that pantoprazole would not significantly affect the pharmacokinetics of other drugs metabolized by these isozymes. Dosage adjustment of such drugs is not necessary when they are co-administered with pantoprazole. In other *in vivo* studies, digoxin, ethanol, glyburide, antipyrine, caffeine, metronidazole, and amoxicillin had no clinically relevant interactions with pantoprazole. Although no significant drug-drug interactions have been observed in clinical studies, the potential for significant drug-drug interactions with more than once daily dosing with high doses of pantoprazole has not been studied in poor metabolizers or individuals who are hepatically impaired.

Because of profound and long lasting inhibition of gastric acid secretion, pantoprazole may interfere with absorption of drugs where gastric pH is an important determinant of their bioavailability (e.g., ketoconazole, ampicillin esters, and iron salts).

Pharmacodynamics

Mechanism of Action

Pantoprazole is a proton pump inhibitor (PPI) that suppresses the final step in gastric acid production by covalently binding to the (H^+, K^+)-ATPase enzyme system at the secretory surface of the gastric parietal cell. This effect leads to inhibition of both basal and stimulated gastric acid secretion irrespective of the stimulus. The binding to the (H^+, K^+)-ATPase results in a duration of antisecretory effect that persists longer than 24 hours for all doses tested.

Antisecretory Activity

The magnitude and time course for inhibition of pentagastrin-stimulated acid output (PSAO) by single doses (20 to 120 mg) of PROTONIX I.V. for Injection were assessed in a single-dose, open-label, placebo-controlled, dose-response study. The results of this study are shown in the table below. Healthy subjects received a continuous infusion for 25 hours of pentagastrin (PG) at 1 μg/kg/h, a dose known to produce submaximal gastric acid secretion. The placebo group showed a sustained, continuous acid output for 25 hours, validating the reliability of the testing model. PROTONIX I.V. for Injection had an onset of antisecretory activity within 15 to 30 minutes of administration. Doses of 20 to 80 mg of PROTONIX I.V. for Injection substantially reduced the 24-hour cumulative PSAO in a dose-dependent manner, despite a short plasma elimination half-life. Complete suppression of PSAO was achieved with 80 mg within approximately 2 hours and no further significant suppression was seen with 120 mg. The duration of action of PROTONIX I.V. for Injection was 24 hours.

[See first table at right]

In one study of gastric pH in healthy subjects, pantoprazole was administered orally (40 mg enteric coated tablets) or intravenously (40 mg) once daily for 5 days and pH was measured for 24 hours following the fifth dose. The outcome measure was median percent of time that pH was ≥ 4 and the results were similar for intravenous and oral medications; however, the clinical significance of this parameter is unknown.

Serum Gastrin Effects

Serum gastrin concentrations were assessed in a placebo-controlled five-day study of oral pantoprazole with 40 and 60 mg doses in healthy subjects. Following the last dose on day 5, the median 24-hour serum gastrin concentrations were elevated by 3-4 fold compared to placebo in both 40 and 60 mg dose groups. However, by 24 hours following the last dose median serum gastrin concentrations for both groups returned to normal levels.

During 6 days of repeated administration of PROTONIX I.V. for Injection in patients with Zollinger-Ellison Syndrome, consistent changes of serum gastrin concentrations from baseline were not observed.

Enterochromaffin-Like (ECL) Cell Effects

There are no data available on the effects of intravenous pantoprazole on ECL cells.

In a nonclinical study in Sprague-Dawley rats, lifetime exposure (24 months) to pantoprazole at doses of 0.5 to 200 mg/kg/day resulted in dose-related increases in gastric ECL-cell proliferation and gastric neuroendocrine (NE)-cell tumors. Gastric NE-cell tumors in rats may result from chronic elevation of serum gastrin concentrations. The high density of ECL cells in the rat stomach makes this species highly susceptible to the proliferative effects of elevated gastrin concentrations produced by proton pump inhibitors. However, there were no observed elevations in serum gastrin following the administration of pantoprazole at a dose of 0.5 mg/kg/day. In a separate study, a gastric NE-cell tumor without concomitant ECL-cell proliferative changes was observed in 1 female rat following 12 months of dosing with pantoprazole at 5 mg/kg/day and a 9 month off-dose recovery (see **PRECAUTIONS, Carcinogenesis, Mutagenesis, Impairment of Fertility**).

Other Effects

No clinically relevant effects of pantoprazole on cardiovascular, respiratory, ophthalmic, or central nervous system function have been detected. In a clinical pharmacology study, pantoprazole 40 mg given orally once daily for 2 weeks had no effect on the levels of the following hormones: cortisol, testosterone, triiodothyronine (T3), thyroxine (T4), thyroid-stimulating hormone, thyronine-binding protein, parathyroid hormone, insulin, glucagon, renin, aldosterone, follicle-stimulating hormone, luteinizing hormone, prolactin and growth hormone.

Clinical Studies

Gastroesophageal Reflux Disease (GERD) Associated With a History of Erosive Esophagitis

A multicenter, double-blind, two-period placebo-controlled study was conducted to assess the ability of PROTONIX® I.V. (pantoprazole sodium) for Injection to maintain gastric acid suppression in patients switched from the oral dosage form of pantoprazole to the intravenous dosage form. Gastroesophageal reflux disease (GERD) patients (n=65, 26 to 64 years; 35 female; 9 black, 11 Hispanic, 44 white, 1 other) with a history of erosive esophagitis were randomized to receive either 20 or 40 mg of oral pantoprazole once per day for 10 days (period 1) and, then were switched in period 2 to either daily intravenous pantoprazole or placebo for 7 days, matching their respective dose level from period 1. Patients were administered all test medication with a light meal. Maximum acid output (MAO) and basal acid output (BAO) were determined 24 hours following the last day of oral medication (day 10), the first day (day 1) of intravenous administration and the last day of intravenous administration (day 7). MAO was estimated from a 1 hour continuous collection of gastric contents following subcutaneous injection of 6.0 μg/kg of pentagastrin.

This study demonstrated that, after 10 days of repeated oral administration followed by 7 days of intravenous administration, the oral and intravenous dosage forms of PROTONIX 40 mg are similar in their ability to suppress MAO and BAO in patients having GERD with a history of erosive esophagitis (see table below). Also, patients on oral PROTONIX who were switched to intravenous placebo experienced a significant increase in acid output within 48 hours of their last oral dose. However, at 48 hours after their last oral dose, patients treated with PROTONIX I.V. for Injection had a significantly lower mean basal acid output than those treated with placebo.

[See second table above]

Data comparing PROTONIX I.V. for Injection to other proton pump inhibitors (oral or I.V.) or H2 receptor antagonists (oral or I.V.) are limited, and therefore, are inadequate to support any conclusions regarding comparative efficacy.

Pathological Hypersecretion Associated with Zollinger-Ellison Syndrome

Two studies measured the pharmacodynamic effects of 6 day treatment with PROTONIX I.V. for Injection in patients with Zollinger-Ellison Syndrome (with and without multiple endocrine neoplasia type I). In one of these studies, an initial treatment with PROTONIX I.V. for Injection in 21 patients (29 to 75 years; 8 female; 4 black, 1 Hispanic, 16

Gastric Acid Output (mEq/hr, Mean ± SD) and Percent Inhibition[a] (Mean ± SD) of Pentagastrin-Stimulated Acid Output Over 24 Hours Following a Single Dose of PROTONIX I.V. for Injection[b] in Healthy Subjects

Treatment Dose	—2 hours— Acid Output	—2 hours— % Inhibition	—4 hours— Acid Output	—4 hours— % Inhibition	—12 hours— Acid Output	—12 hours— % Inhibition	—24 hours— Acid Output	—24 hours— % Inhibition
0 mg (Placebo, n=4)	39 ± 21	NA	26 ± 14	NA	32 ± 20	NA	38 ± 24	NA
20 mg (n=4–6)	13 ± 18	47 ± 27	6 ± 8	83 ± 21	20 ± 20	54 ± 44	30 ± 23	45 ± 43
40 mg (n=8)	5 ± 5	82 ± 11	4 ± 4	90 ± 11	11 ± 10	81 ± 13	16 ± 12	52 ± 36
80 mg (n=8)	0.1 ± 0.2	96 ± 6	0.3 ± 0.4	99 ± 1	2 ± 2	90 ± 7	7 ± 4	63 ± 18

a: Compared to individual subject baseline prior to treatment with PROTONIX I.V. for Injection.
NA = not applicable.
b: Inhibition of gastric acid output and the percent inhibition of stimulated acid output in response to PROTONIX I.V. for Injection may be higher after repeated doses.

ANTISECRETORY EFFECTS (mEq/h) OF 40 mg PROTONIX I.V. for INJECTION AND 40 mg ORAL PROTONIX IN GERD PATIENTS WITH A HISTORY OF EROSIVE ESOPHAGITIS

Parameter	PROTONIX Delayed-Release Tablets DAY 10	PROTONIX I.V. for Injection DAY 7	Placebo I.V. DAY 7
Mean maximum acid output	6.49 n=30	6.62 n=23	29.19* n=7
Mean basal acid output	0.80 n=30	0.53 n=23	4.14* n=7

*P<0.0001 Significantly different from PROTONIX I.V. for Injection.

white) reduced acid output to the target level (≤ 10 mEq/h) and significantly reduced H+ concentration and the volume of gastric secretions; target levels were achieved within 45 minutes of drug administration.

In the other study of 14 patients (38 to 67 years; 5 female; 2 black, 12 white) with Zollinger-Ellison Syndrome, treatment was switched from an oral proton pump inhibitor to PROTONIX I.V. for Injection. PROTONIX I.V. for Injection maintained or improved control of gastric acid secretion.

In both studies, PROTONIX I.V. for Injection 160 or 240 mg per day in divided doses maintained basal acid secretion below target levels in all patients. Target levels were 10 mEq/h in patients without prior gastric surgery, and 5 mEq/h in all patients with prior gastric acid-reducing surgery. Once gastric acid secretion was controlled, there was no evidence of tolerance during this 7 day study. Basal acid secretion was maintained below target levels for at least 24 hours in all patients and through the end of treatment in these studies (3 to 7 days) in all but 1 patient who required a dose adjustment guided by acid output measurements until acid control was achieved. In both studies, doses were adjusted to the individual patient need, but gastric acid secretion was controlled in greater than 80% of patients by a starting regimen of 80 mg q12h.

INDICATIONS AND USAGE

Treatment of Gastroesophageal Reflux Disease Associated With a History of Erosive Esophagitis

PROTONIX I.V. for Injection is indicated for short-term treatment (7 to 10 days) of patients having gastroesophageal reflux disease (GERD) with a history of erosive esophagitis, **as an alternative to oral therapy in patients who are unable to continue taking PROTONIX (pantoprazole sodium) Delayed-Release Tablets.** Safety and efficacy of PROTONIX I.V. for Injection as an initial treatment of patients having GERD with a history of erosive esophagitis have not been demonstrated.

Pathological Hypersecretion Associated with Zollinger-Ellison Syndrome

PROTONIX I.V. for Injection is indicated for the treatment of pathological hypersecretory conditions associated with Zollinger-Ellison Syndrome or other neoplastic conditions.

CONTRAINDICATIONS

PROTONIX I.V. for Injection is contraindicated in patients with known hypersensitivity to the formulation.

PRECAUTIONS

General

Immediate hypersensitivity reactions: Anaphylaxis has been reported with use of intravenous pantoprazole. This may require emergency medical treatment.

Injection site reactions: Thrombophlebitis was associated with the administration of intravenous pantoprazole.

Hepatic effects: Mild, transient transaminase elevations have been observed in clinical studies. The clinical significance of this finding in a large population of subjects administered intravenous pantoprazole is unknown. (See **ADVERSE REACTIONS** section).

Symptomatic response to therapy with pantoprazole does not preclude the presence of gastric malignancy.

As with any other intravenous product containing edetate disodium (the salt form of EDTA) which is a potent chelator of metal ions including zinc, zinc supplementation should be considered in patients treated with PROTONIX I.V. for Injection who are prone to zinc deficiency. Caution should be used when other EDTA containing products are also co-administered intravenously.

Treatment with PROTONIX® I.V. (pantoprazole sodium) for Injection should be discontinued as soon as the patient is able to resume treatment with PROTONIX Delayed-Release Tablets.

Drug Interactions (see **CLINICAL PHARMACOLOGY, Drug-Drug Interactions**)

Carcinogenesis, Mutagenesis, Impairment of Fertility

In a 24-month carcinogenicity study, Sprague-Dawley rats were treated orally with doses of 0.5 to 200 mg/kg/day, about 0.1 to 40 times the exposure on a body surface area basis, of a 50-kg person dosed at 40 mg/day. In the gastric fundus, treatment at 0.5 to 200 mg/kg/day produced enterochromaffin-like (ECL) cell hyperplasia and benign and malignant neuroendocrine cell tumors in a dose-related manner. In the forestomach, treatment at 50 and 200 mg/kg/day (about 10 and 40 times the recommended human dose on a body surface area basis) produced benign squamous cell papillomas and malignant squamous cell carcinomas. Rare gastrointestinal tumors associated with pantoprazole treatment included an adenocarcinoma of the duodenum at 50 mg/kg/day, and benign polyps and adenocarcinomas of the gastric fundus at 200 mg/kg/day. In the liver, treatment at 0.5 to 200 mg/kg/day produced dose-related increases in the incidences of hepatocellular adenomas and carcinomas. In the thyroid gland, treatment at 200 mg/kg/day produced increased incidences of follicular cell adenomas and carcinomas for both male and female rats.

Sporadic occurrences of hepatocellular adenomas and a hepatocellular carcinoma were observed in Sprague-Dawley rats exposed to pantoprazole in 6-month and 12-month oral toxicity studies.

In a 24-month carcinogenicity study, Fischer 344 rats were treated orally with doses of 5 to 50 mg/kg/day, approximately 1 to 10 times the recommended human dose based on body surface area. In the gastric fundus, treatment at 5 to 50 mg/kg/day produced enterochromaffin-like (ECL) cell hyperplasia and benign and malignant neuroendocrine cell tumors. Dose selection for this study may not have been adequate to comprehensively evaluate the carcinogenic potential of pantoprazole.

In a 24-month carcinogenicity study, B6C3F1 mice were treated orally with doses of 5 to 150 mg/kg/day, 0.5 to 15 times the recommended human dose based on body surface area. In the liver, treatment at 150 mg/kg/day produced increased incidences of hepatocellular adenomas and carcinomas in female mice. Treatment at 5 to 150 mg/kg/day also produced gastric fundic ECL cell hyperplasia.

Pantoprazole was positive in the *in vitro* human lymphocyte chromosomal aberration assays, in one of two mouse micronucleus tests for clastogenic effects, and in the *in vitro* Chinese hamster ovarian cell/HGPRT forward mutation assay for mutagenic effects. Equivocal results were observed in the *in vivo* rat liver DNA covalent binding assay. Pantoprazole was negative in the *in vitro* Ames mutation assay, the *in vitro* unscheduled DNA synthesis (UDS) assay with rat hepatocytes, the *in vitro* AS52/GPT mammalian cell-forward gene mutation assay, the *in vitro* thymidine kinase mutation test with mouse lymphoma L5178Y cells, and the *in vivo* rat bone marrow cell chromosomal aberration assay. A 26-week p53 +/- transgenic mouse carcinogenicity study was not positive.

Pantoprazole at oral doses up to 500 mg/kg/day in male rats (98 times the recommended human dose based on body surface area) and 450 mg/kg/day in female rats (88 times the recommended human dose based on body surface area) was found to have no effect on fertility and reproductive performance.

Pregnancy

Teratogenic Effects

Pregnancy Category B

Teratology studies have been performed in rats at intravenous doses up to 20 mg/kg/day (4 times the recommended

Continued on next page

Protonix I.V.—Cont.

human dose based on body surface area) and rabbits at intravenous doses up to 15 mg/kg/day (6 times the recommended human dose based on body surface area) and have revealed no evidence of impaired fertility or harm to the fetus due to pantoprazole. There are, however, no adequate and well-controlled studies in pregnant women. Because animal reproduction studies are not always predictive of human response, this drug should be used during pregnancy only if clearly needed.

Nursing Mothers

Pantoprazole and its metabolites are excreted in the milk of rats. Pantoprazole excretion in human milk has been detected in a study of a single nursing mother after a single 40 mg oral dose. The clinical relevance of this finding is not known. Many drugs which are excreted in human milk have a potential for serious adverse reactions in nursing infants. Based on the potential for tumorigenicity shown for pantoprazole in rodent carcinogenicity studies, a decision should be made whether to discontinue nursing or to discontinue the drug, taking into account the benefit of the drug to the mother.

Pediatric Use

Safety and effectiveness in pediatric patients have not been established.

Use in Women

No gender-related differences in the safety profile of intravenous pantoprazole were seen in international trials involving 166 men and 120 women with erosive esophagitis associated with GERD. Erosive esophagitis healing rates in the 221 women treated with oral pantoprazole in U.S. clinical trials were similar to those found in men. The incidence rates of adverse events were also similar between men and women.

Use in Elderly

No age-related differences in the safety profile of intravenous pantoprazole were seen in international trials involving 86 elderly (≥ 65 years old) and 200 younger (< 65 years old) patients with erosive esophagitis associated with GERD. Erosive esophagitis healing rates in the 107 elderly patients (≥ 65 years old) treated with oral pantoprazole in U.S. clinical trials were similar to those found in patients under the age of 65. The incidence rates of adverse events and laboratory abnormalities in patients aged 65 years and older were similar to those associated with patients younger than 65 years of age.

Laboratory Tests

There have been reports of false-positive urine screening tests for tetrahydrocannabinol (THC) in patients receiving most proton pump inhibitors, including pantoprazole. An alternative confirmatory method should be considered to verify positive results.

ADVERSE REACTIONS

Safety Experience with Intravenous Pantoprazole

Intravenous pantoprazole has been studied in clinical trials in several populations including patients having GERD with a history of erosive esophagitis, patients with Zollinger-Ellison Syndrome and healthy subjects. Adverse experiences occurring in >1% of patients treated with intravenous pantoprazole (n=714) in domestic or international clinical trials are shown below by body system. In most instances, the relationship to pantoprazole was unclear.

BODY AS A WHOLE: abdominal pain, headache, injection site reaction (including thrombophlebitis and abscess).
DIGESTIVE SYSTEM: constipation, dyspepsia, nausea, diarrhea.
NERVOUS SYSTEM: insomnia.
RESPIRATORY SYSTEM: rhinitis.

Head-to-head comparative studies between PROTONIX I.V. for Injection and oral PROTONIX, other proton pump inhibitors (oral or I.V.), or H2 receptor antagonists (oral or I.V.) have been limited. The available information does not provide sufficient evidence to distinguish the safety profile of these regimens.

Safety Experience with Oral Pantoprazole

In short-term clinical trials in patients with erosive esophagitis associated with GERD treated with oral pantoprazole, the following adverse events, regardless of causality, occurred at a rate of ≥1%.

BODY AS A WHOLE: headache, asthenia, back pain, chest pain, neck pain, flu syndrome, infection, pain.
CARDIOVASCULAR SYSTEM: migraine.
DIGESTIVE SYSTEM: diarrhea, flatulence, abdominal pain, eructation, constipation, dyspepsia, gastroenteritis, gastrointestinal disorder, nausea, rectal disorder, vomiting.
HEPATO-BILIARY SYSTEM: liver function tests abnormal, SGPT increased.
METABOLIC AND NUTRITIONAL: hyperglycemia, hyperlipemia.
MUSCULOSKELETAL SYSTEM: arthralgia.
NERVOUS SYSTEM: insomnia, anxiety, dizziness, hypertonia.
RESPIRATORY SYSTEM: bronchitis, cough increased, dyspnea, pharyngitis, rhinitis, sinusitis, upper respiratory tract infection.
SKIN AND APPENDAGES: rash.
UROGENITAL SYSTEM: urinary frequency, and urinary tract infection.

Additional adverse experiences occurring in <1% of patients with erosive esophagitis associated with GERD receiving oral pantoprazole based on pooled results from either short-term domestic or international trials are shown below within each body system. In most instances, the relationship to pantoprazole was unclear.

BODY AS A WHOLE: abscess, allergic reaction, chills, cyst, face edema, fever, generalized edema, heat stroke, hernia, laboratory test abnormal, malaise, moniliasis, neoplasm, non-specified drug reaction.
CARDIOVASCULAR SYSTEM: abnormal electrocardiogram, angina pectoris, arrhythmia, cardiovascular disorder, chest pain substernal, congestive heart failure, hemorrhage, hypertension, hypotension, myocardial ischemia, palpitation, retinal vascular disorder, syncope, tachycardia, thrombophlebitis, thrombosis, vasodilatation.
DIGESTIVE SYSTEM: anorexia, aphthous stomatitis, cardiospasm, colitis, dry mouth, duodenitis, dysphagia, enteritis, esophageal hemorrhage, esophagitis, gastrointestinal carcinoma, gastrointestinal hemorrhage, gastrointestinal moniliasis, gingivitis, glossitis, halitosis, hematemesis, increased appetite, melena, mouth ulceration, oral moniliasis, periodontal abscess, periodontitis, rectal hemorrhage, stomach ulcer, stomatitis, stools abnormal, tongue discoloration, ulcerative colitis.
ENDOCRINE SYSTEM: diabetes mellitus, glycosuria, goiter.
HEPATO-BILIARY SYSTEM: biliary pain, hyperbilirubinemia, cholecystitis, cholelithiasis, cholestatic jaundice, hepatitis, alkaline phosphatase increased, gamma glutamyl transpeptidase increased, SGOT increased.
HEMIC AND LYMPHATIC SYSTEM: anemia, ecchymosis, eosinophilia, hypochromic anemia, iron deficiency anemia, leukocytosis, leukopenia, thrombocytopenia.
METABOLIC AND NUTRITIONAL: dehydration, edema, gout, peripheral edema, thirst, weight gain, weight loss.
MUSCULOSKELETAL SYSTEM: arthritis, arthrosis, bone disorder, bone pain, bursitis, joint disorder, leg cramps, neck rigidity, myalgia, tenosynovitis.
NERVOUS SYSTEM: abnormal dreams, confusion, convulsion, depression, dry mouth, dysarthria, emotional lability, hallucinations, hyperkinesia, hypesthesia, libido decreased, nervousness, neuralgia, neuritis, paresthesia, reflexes decreased, sleep disorder, somnolence, thinking abnormal, tremor, vertigo.
RESPIRATORY SYSTEM: asthma, epistaxis, hiccup, laryngitis, lung disorder, pneumonia, voice alteration.
SKIN AND APPENDAGES: acne, alopecia, contact dermatitis, dry skin, eczema, fungal dermatitis, hemorrhage, herpes simplex, herpes zoster, lichenoid dermatitis, maculopapular rash, pain, pruritus, skin disorder, skin ulcer, sweating, urticaria.
SPECIAL SENSES: abnormal vision, amblyopia, cataract specified, deafness, diplopia, ear pain, extraocular palsy, glaucoma, otitis externa, taste perversion, tinnitus.
UROGENITAL SYSTEM: albuminuria, balanitis, breast pain, cystitis, dysmenorrhea, dysuria, epididymitis, hematuria, impotence, kidney calculus, kidney pain, nocturia, prostatic disorder, pyelonephritis, scrotal edema, urethral pain, urethritis, urinary tract disorder, urination impaired, vaginitis.

Postmarketing Reports

The postmarketing safety profile of intravenous pantoprazole is not substantially different from that of oral pantoprazole (described below).

There have been spontaneous reports of adverse events with postmarketing use of intravenous or oral pantoprazole. These reports include anaphylaxis (including anaphylactic shock); angioedema (Quincke's edema); anterior ischemic optic neuropathy; elevated CPK (creatine phosphokinase); severe dermatologic reactions, including erythema multiforme, Stevens-Johnson syndrome, and toxic epidermal necrolysis (TEN, some fatal); hepatocellular damage leading to jaundice and hepatic failure; interstitial nephritis; pancreatitis; pancytopenia; and rhabdomyolysis. In addition, also observed have been confusion, hypokinesia, speech disorder, increased salivation, vertigo, nausea, tinnitus, and blurred vision.

Laboratory Values

In U.S. clinical trials of patients having GERD with a history of erosive esophagitis and international clinical trials of patients with erosive esophagitis associated with GERD, the overall percentages of transaminase elevations did not increase during treatment with intravenous pantoprazole. For other laboratory parameters, there were no clinically important changes identified.

In two U.S. controlled trials of oral pantoprazole in patients with erosive esophagitis associated with GERD, 0.4% of the patients on 40 mg oral pantoprazole experienced SGPT elevations of greater than three times the upper limit of normal at the final treatment visit. Except in those patients where there was a clear alternative explanation for a laboratory value change, such as intercurrent illness, the elevations tended to be mild and sporadic. The following changes in laboratory parameters were reported as adverse events: creatinine increased, hypercholesterolemia, and hyperuricemia.

OVERDOSAGE

Experience in patients taking very high doses of pantoprazole is limited. There have been spontaneous reports of overdosage with pantoprazole, including a suicide in which pantoprazole 560 mg and undetermined amounts of chloroquine and zopiclone were also ingested. There have also been spontaneous reports of patients taking similar amounts of pantoprazole (400 and 600 mg) with no adverse effects.

Pantoprazole is not removed by hemodialysis. In case of overdose, treatment should be symptomatic and supportive. Single intravenous doses of pantoprazole at 378, 230, and 266 mg/kg (38, 46, and 177 times the recommended human dose based on body surface area) were lethal to mice, rats and dogs, respectively. The symptoms of acute toxicity were hypoactivity, ataxia, hunched sitting, limb-splay, lateral position, segregation, absence of ear reflex, and tremor.

DOSAGE AND ADMINISTRATION

PROTONIX I.V. for Injection may be administered intravenously through a dedicated line or through a Y-site. The intravenous line should be flushed before and after administration of PROTONIX I.V. for Injection with either 5% Dextrose Injection, USP, 0.9% Sodium Chloride Injection, USP, or Lactated Ringer's Injection, USP. When administered through a Y-site, PROTONIX I.V. for Injection is compatible with the following solutions: 5% Dextrose Injection, USP, 0.9% Sodium Chloride Injection, USP, or Lactated Ringer's Injection, USP.

Midazolam HCl has been shown to be incompatible with Y-site administration of PROTONIX I.V. for Injection. PROTONIX I.V. for Injection may not be compatible with products containing zinc. When PROTONIX I.V. for Injection is administered through a Y-site, immediately stop use if precipitation or discoloration occurs.

Parenteral drug products should be inspected visually for particulate matter and discoloration prior to and during administration whenever solution and container permit.

Treatment with PROTONIX I.V. for Injection should be discontinued as soon as the patient is able to resume treatment with PROTONIX Delayed-Release Tablets. Also, data on the safe and effective dosing for conditions other than those described in **INDICATIONS AND USAGE**, such as life-threatening upper gastrointestinal bleeds, are not available. PROTONIX I.V. 40 mg once daily does not raise gastric pH to levels sufficient to contribute to the treatment of such life-threatening conditions.

Parenteral routes of administration other than intravenous are not recommended.

No dosage adjustment is necessary in patients with renal impairment, hepatic impairment, or for elderly patients. Doses higher than 40 mg/day have not been studied in hepatically-impaired patients. No dosage adjustment is necessary in patients undergoing hemodialysis.

Treatment of Gastroesophageal Reflux Disease Associated With a History of Erosive Esophagitis

The recommended adult dose, **as an alternative to continued oral therapy**, is 40-mg pantoprazole given once daily by intravenous infusion for 7 to 10 days. Safety and efficacy of PROTONIX I.V. for Injection as a treatment of patients having GERD with a history of erosive esophagitis for more than 10 days have not been demonstrated (see **INDICATIONS AND USAGE**).

Fifteen Minute Infusion

PROTONIX I.V. for Injection should be reconstituted with 10 mL of 0.9% Sodium Chloride Injection, USP, and further diluted (admixed) with 100 mL of 5% Dextrose Injection, USP, 0.9% Sodium Chloride Injection, USP, or Lactated Ringer's Injection, USP, to a final concentration of approximately 0.4 mg/mL. The reconstituted solution may be stored for up to 2 hours at room temperature prior to further dilution; the admixed solution may be stored for up to 22 hours at room temperature prior to intravenous infusion. Both the reconstituted solution and the admixed solution do not need to be protected from light.

PROTONIX I.V. for Injection admixtures should be administered intravenously over a period of approximately 15 minutes at a rate of approximately 7 mL/min.

Two Minute Infusion

PROTONIX I.V. for Injection should be reconstituted with 10 mL of 0.9% Sodium Chloride Injection, USP, to a final concentration of approximately 4 mg/mL. The reconstituted solution may be stored for up to 2 hours at room temperature prior to intravenous infusion and does not need to be protected from light. PROTONIX I.V. for Injection should be administered intravenously over a period of at least 2 minutes.

Pathological Hypersecretion Associated with Zollinger-Ellison Syndrome

The dosage of PROTONIX I.V. for Injection in patients with pathological hypersecretory conditions associated with Zollinger-Ellison Syndrome or other neoplastic conditions varies with individual patients. The recommended adult dosage is 80 mg q12h. The frequency of dosing can be adjusted to individual patient needs based on acid output measurements. In those patients who need a higher dosage, 80 mg q8h is expected to maintain acid output below 10 mEq/h. Daily doses higher than 240 mg or administered for more than 6 days have not been studied. (See **Clinical Studies** section.) Transition from oral to I.V. and from I.V. to oral formulations of gastric acid inhibitors should be performed in such a manner to ensure continuity of effect of suppression of acid secretion. Patients with Zollinger-Ellison Syndrome may be vulnerable to serious clinical complications of increased acid production even after a short period of loss of effective inhibition.

Fifteen Minute Infusion

Each vial of PROTONIX I.V. for Injection should be reconstituted with 10 mL of 0.9% Sodium Chloride Injection, USP. The contents of the two vials should be combined and further diluted (admixed) with 80 mL of 5% Dextrose Injection, USP, 0.9% Sodium Chloride Injection, USP, or Lactated Ringer's Injection, USP, to a total volume of 100 mL with a final concentration of approximately 0.8 mg/mL. The reconstituted solution may be stored for up to 2 hours at room temperature prior to further dilution; the admixed solution may be stored for up to 22 hours at room temperature prior to intravenous infusion. Both the reconstituted solution and the admixed solution do not need to be protected from light.

PROTONIX I.V. for Injection should be administered intravenously over a period of approximately 15 minutes at a rate of approximately 7 mL/min.

Two Minute Infusion

PROTONIX I.V. for Injection should be reconstituted with 10 mL of 0.9% Sodium Chloride Injection, USP, per vial to a final concentration of approximately 4 mg/mL. The reconstituted solution may be stored for up to 2 hours at room temperature prior to intravenous infusion and does not need to be protected from light. The total volume from both vials should be administered intravenously over a period of at least 2 minutes.

HOW SUPPLIED

PROTONIX® I.V. (pantoprazole sodium) for Injection is supplied as a freeze-dried powder containing 40 mg of pantoprazole per vial.

PROTONIX I.V. for Injection is available as follows:

NDC 0008-0923-51 One carton containing 1 vial of PROTONIX I.V. for Injection (each vial containing 40-mg pantoprazole).

Storage

Store PROTONIX I.V. for Injection at 2°C - 8°C (36°F - 46°F) and protect from light.

Caution: the reconstituted product should not be frozen.

U.S. Patent No. 4,758,579

Marketed by Wyeth Pharmaceuticals Inc.
Philadelphia, PA 19101
under license from
ALTANA Pharma
D78467 Konstanz, Germany

W10447C008
ET01
Rev 04/04

RAPAMUNE® ℞

[*rāp-ā-mūn*]
(sirolimus)
Oral Solution and Tablets
℞ only

Prescribing information for this product, which appears on pages 3483–3490 of the 2004 PDR, has been completely revised as follows. Please write "See Supplement A" next to the product heading.

> WARNING:
> Increased susceptibility to infection and the possible development of lymphoma may result from immunosuppression. Only physicians experienced in immunosuppressive therapy and management of renal transplant patients should use Rapamune®. Patients receiving the drug should be managed in facilities equipped and staffed with adequate laboratory and supportive medical resources. The physician responsible for maintenance therapy should have complete information requisite for the follow-up of the patient.

DESCRIPTION

Rapamune® (sirolimus) is an immunosuppressive agent. Sirolimus is a macrocyclic lactone produced by *Streptomyces hygroscopicus*. The chemical name of sirolimus (also known as rapamycin) is (3*S*,6*R*,7*E*,9*R*,10*R*,12*R*,14*S*,15*E*,17*E*,19*E*,21*S*,23*S*,26*R*,27*R*,34a*S*)-9,10,12,13,14,21,22,23,24,25,26,27,32,33,34,34a-hexadecahydro-9,27-dihydroxy-3-[(1*R*)-2-[(1*S*,3*R*,4*R*)-4-hydroxy-3-methoxycyclohexyl]-1-methylethyl]-10,21-dimethoxy-6,8,12,14,20,26-hexamethyl-23,27-epoxy-3*H*-pyrido[2,1-c][1,4] oxaazacyclohentriacontine-1,5,11,28,29 (4*H*,6*H*,31*H*)-pentone. Its molecular formula is $C_{51}H_{79}NO_{13}$ and its molecular weight is 914.2. The structural formula of sirolimus is shown below.

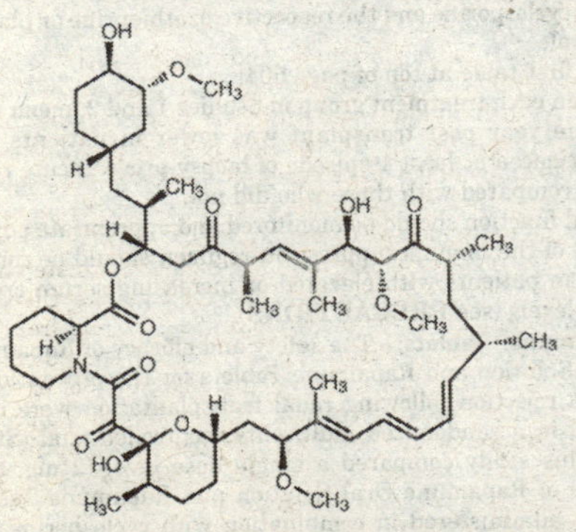

Sirolimus is a white to off-white powder and is insoluble in water, but freely soluble in benzyl alcohol, chloroform, acetone, and acetonitrile.

Rapamune® is available for administration as an oral solution containing 1 mg/mL sirolimus. Rapamune is also available as a white, triangular-shaped tablet containing 1-mg sirolimus, and as a yellow to beige triangular-shaped tablet containing 2-mg sirolimus.

SIROLIMUS PHARMACOKINETIC PARAMETERS (MEAN ± SD) IN RENAL TRANSPLANT PATIENTS (MULTIPLE DOSE ORAL SOLUTION)[a,b]

N	Dose	$C_{max,ss}$[c] (ng/mL)	$t_{max,ss}$ (h)	$AUC_{\tau,ss}$[c] (ng•h/mL)	CL/F/WT[d] (mL/h/kg)
19	2 mg	12.2 ± 6.2	3.01 ± 2.40	158 ± 70	182 ± 72
23	5 mg	37.4 ± 21	1.84 ± 1.30	396 ± 193	221 ± 143

a: Sirolimus administered four hours after cyclosporine oral solution (MODIFIED) (e.g., Neoral® Oral Solution) and/or cyclosporine capsules (MODIFIED) (e.g., Neoral® Soft Gelatin Capsules).
b: As measured by the Liquid Chromatographic/Tandem Mass Spectrometric Method (LC/MS/MS).
c: These parameters were dose normalized prior to the statistical comparison.
d: CL/F/WT = oral dose clearance.

The inactive ingredients in Rapamune® Oral Solution are Phosal 50 PG® (phosphatidylcholine, propylene glycol, mono- and di-glycerides, ethanol, soy fatty acids, and ascorbyl palmitate) and polysorbate 80. Rapamune Oral Solution contains 1.5% - 2.5% ethanol.

The inactive ingredients in Rapamune® Tablets include sucrose, lactose, polyethylene glycol 8000, calcium sulfate, microcrystalline cellulose, pharmaceutical glaze, talc, titanium dioxide, magnesium stearate, povidone, poloxamer 188, polyethylene glycol 20,000, glyceryl monooleate, carnauba wax, and other ingredients. The 2 mg dosage strength also contains iron oxide yellow 10 and iron oxide brown 70.

CLINICAL PHARMACOLOGY

Mechanism of Action

Sirolimus inhibits T lymphocyte activation and proliferation that occurs in response to antigenic and cytokine (Interleukin [IL]-2, IL-4, and IL-15) stimulation by a mechanism that is distinct from that of other immunosuppressants. Sirolimus also inhibits antibody production. In cells, sirolimus binds to the immunophilin, FK Binding Protein-12 (FKBP-12), to generate an immunosuppressive complex. The sirolimus:FKBP-12 complex has no effect on calcineurin activity. This complex binds to and inhibits the activation of the mammalian Target Of Rapamycin (mTOR), a key regulatory kinase. This inhibition suppresses cytokine-driven T-cell proliferation, inhibiting the progression from the G_1 to the S phase of the cell cycle.

Studies in experimental models show that sirolimus prolongs allograft (kidney, heart, skin, islet, small bowel, pancreatico-duodenal, and bone marrow) survival in mice, rats, pigs, and/or primates. Sirolimus reverses acute rejection of heart and kidney allografts in rats and prolongs the graft survival in presensitized rats. In some studies, the immunosuppressive effect of sirolimus lasts up to 6 months after discontinuation of therapy. This tolerization effect is alloantigen specific.

In rodent models of autoimmune disease, sirolimus suppresses immune-mediated events associated with systemic lupus erythematosus, collagen-induced arthritis, autoimmune type I diabetes, autoimmune myocarditis, experimental allergic encephalomyelitis, graft-versus-host disease, and autoimmune uveoretinitis.

Pharmacokinetics

Sirolimus pharmacokinetic activity has been determined following oral administration in healthy subjects, pediatric dialysis patients, hepatically-impaired patients, and renal transplant patients.

Absorption

Following administration of Rapamune® Oral Solution, sirolimus is rapidly absorbed, with a mean time-to-peak concentration (t_{max}) of approximately 1 hour after a single dose in healthy subjects and approximately 2 hours after multiple oral doses in renal transplant recipients. The systemic availability of sirolimus was estimated to be approximately 14% after the administration of Rapamune Oral Solution. The mean bioavailability of sirolimus after administration of the tablet is about 27% higher relative to the oral solution. Sirolimus oral tablets are not bioequivalent to the oral solution; however, clinical equivalence has been demonstrated at the 2-mg dose level. (See **Clinical Studies** and **DOSAGE AND ADMINISTRATION**). Sirolimus concentrations, following the administration of Rapamune Oral Solution to stable renal transplant patients, are dose proportional between 3 and 12 mg/m².

Food effects: In 22 healthy volunteers receiving Rapamune Oral Solution, a high-fat meal (861.8 kcal, 54.9% kcal from fat) altered the bioavailability characteristics of sirolimus. Compared with fasting, a 34% decrease in the peak blood sirolimus concentration (C_{max}), a 3.5-fold increase in the time-to-peak concentration (t_{max}), and a 35% increase in total exposure (AUC) was observed. After administration of Rapamune Tablets and a high-fat meal in 24 healthy volunteers, C_{max}, t_{max}, and AUC showed increases of 65%, 32%, and 23%, respectively. To minimize variability, both Rapamune Oral Solution and Tablets should be taken consistently with or without food (See **DOSAGE AND ADMINISTRATION**).

Distribution

The mean (± SD) blood-to-plasma ratio of sirolimus was 36 ± 18 in stable renal allograft recipients after administration of oral solution, indicating that sirolimus is extensively partitioned into formed blood elements. The mean volume of distribution (V_{ss}/F) of sirolimus is 12 ± 8 L/kg. Sirolimus is extensively bound (approximately 92%) to human plasma proteins. In man, the binding of sirolimus was shown mainly to be associated with serum albumin (97%), α_1-acid glycoprotein, and lipoproteins.

Metabolism

Sirolimus is a substrate for both cytochrome P450 IIIA4 (CYP3A4) and P-glycoprotein (P-gp). Sirolimus is extensively metabolized by the CYP3A4 isozyme in the intestinal wall and liver and undergoes counter-transport from enterocytes of the small intestine into the gut lumen by the P-gp drug efflux pump. Sirolimus is potentially recycled between enterocytes and the gut lumen to allow continued metabolism by CYP3A4. Therefore, absorption and subsequent elimination of systemically absorbed sirolimus may be influenced by drugs that affect these proteins. Inhibitors of CYP3A4 and P-gp increase sirolimus levels. Inducers of CYP3A4 and P-gp decrease sirolimus levels. (See **WARNINGS** and **PRECAUTIONS, Drug Interactions** and **Other drug interactions**). Sirolimus is extensively metabolized by O-demethylation and/or hydroxylation. Seven (7) major metabolites, including hydroxy, demethyl, and hydroxydemethyl, are identifiable in whole blood. Some of these metabolites are also detectable in plasma, fecal, and urine samples. Glucuronide and sulfate conjugates are not present in any of the biologic matrices. Sirolimus is the major component in human whole blood and contributes to more than 90% of the immunosuppressive activity.

Excretion

After a single dose of [^{14}C]sirolimus oral solution in healthy volunteers, the majority (91%) of radioactivity was recovered from the feces, and only a minor amount (2.2%) was excreted in urine.

Pharmacokinetics in renal transplant patients

Rapamune Oral Solution: Pharmacokinetic parameters for sirolimus oral solution given daily in combination with cyclosporine and corticosteroids in renal transplant patients are summarized below based on data collected at months 1, 3, and 6 after transplantation (Studies 1 and 2; see **CLINICAL STUDIES**). There were no significant differences in any of these parameters with respect to treatment group or month.

[See table above]

Whole blood sirolimus trough concentrations (mean ± SD), as measured by immunoassay, for the 2 mg/day and 5 mg/day dose groups were 8.6 ± 4.0 ng/mL (n = 226) and 17.3 ± 7.4 ng/mL (n = 219), respectively. Whole blood trough sirolimus concentrations, as measured by LC/MS/MS, were significantly correlated (r^2 = 0.96) with $AUC_{\tau,ss}$. Upon repeated twice daily administration without an initial loading dose in a multiple-dose study, the average trough concentration of sirolimus increases approximately 2 to 3-fold over the initial 6 days of therapy at which time steady state is reached. A loading dose of 3 times the maintenance dose will provide near steady-state concentrations within 1 day in most patients. The mean ± SD terminal elimination half life ($t_{½}$) of sirolimus after multiple dosing in stable renal transplant patients was estimated to be about 62 ± 16 hours.

Rapamune Tablets: Pharmacokinetic parameters for sirolimus tablets administered daily in combination with cyclosporine and corticosteroids in renal transplant patients are summarized below based on data collected at months 1 and 3 after transplantation (Study 3; see **CLINICAL STUDIES**).

[See first table at top of next page]

Whole blood sirolimus trough concentrations (mean ± SD), as measured by immunoassay, for 2 mg of oral solution and 2 mg of tablets over 6 months, were 8.9 ± 4.4 ng/mL (n = 172) and 9.5 ± 3.9 ng/mL (n = 179), respectively. Whole blood trough sirolimus concentrations, as measured by LC/MS/MS, were significantly correlated (r^2 = 0.85) with $AUC_{\tau,ss}$. Mean whole blood sirolimus trough concentrations in patients receiving either Rapamune Oral Solution or Rapamune Tablets with a loading dose of three times the maintenance dose achieved steady-state concentrations within 24 hours after the start of dose administration.

Average Rapamune doses and sirolimus whole blood trough concentrations for tablets administered daily in combination with cyclosporine and following cyclosporine withdrawal, in combination with corticosteroids in renal transplant patients (Study 4; see **CLINICAL STUDIES**) are summarized in the table below.

[See second table at top of next page]

The withdrawal of cyclosporine and concurrent increases in sirolimus trough concentrations to steady-state required approximately 6 weeks. Larger Rapamune® doses were required due to the absence of the inhibition of sirolimus metabolism and transport by cyclosporine and to achieve higher target concentrations during concentration-controlled administration following cyclosporine withdrawal.

Continued on next page

Rapamune—Cont.

Special Populations

Hepatic impairment: Sirolimus oral solution (15 mg) was administered as a single oral dose to 18 subjects with normal hepatic function and to 18 patients with Child-Pugh classification A or B hepatic impairment, in which hepatic impairment was primary and not related to an underlying systemic disease. Shown below are the mean ± SD pharmacokinetic parameters following the administration of sirolimus oral solution.

[See third table at right]

Compared with the values in the normal hepatic group, the hepatic impairment group had higher mean values for sirolimus AUC (61%) and $t_{1/2}$ (43%) and had lower mean values for sirolimus CL/F/WT (33%). The mean $t_{1/2}$ increased from 79 ± 12 hours in subjects with normal hepatic function to 113 ± 41 hours in patients with impaired hepatic function. The rate of absorption of sirolimus was not altered by hepatic disease, as evidenced by C_{max} and t_{max} values. However, hepatic diseases with varying etiologies may show different effects and the pharmacokinetics of sirolimus in patients with severe hepatic dysfunction is unknown. Dosage adjustment is recommended for patients with mild to moderate hepatic impairment (see **DOSAGE AND ADMINISTRATION**).

Renal impairment: The effect of renal impairment on the pharmacokinetics of sirolimus is not known. However, there is minimal (2.2%) renal excretion of the drug or its metabolites.

Pediatric: Limited pharmacokinetic data are available in pediatric patients. The table below summarizes pharmacokinetic data obtained in pediatric dialysis patients with chronically impaired renal function.

[See fourth table at right]

Geriatric: Clinical studies of Rapamune did not include a sufficient number of patients >65 years of age to determine whether they will respond differently than younger patients. After the administration of Rapamune Oral Solution, sirolimus trough concentration data in 35 renal transplant patients >65 years of age were similar to those in the adult population (n = 822) 18 to 65 years of age. Similar results were obtained after the administration of Rapamune Tablets to 12 renal transplant patients >65 years of age compared with adults (n = 167) 18 to 65 years of age.

Gender: After the administration of Rapamune Oral Solution, sirolimus oral dose clearance in males was 12% lower than that in females; male subjects had a significantly longer $t_{1/2}$ than did female subjects (72.3 hours versus 61.3 hours). A similar trend in the effect of gender on sirolimus oral dose clearance and $t_{1/2}$ was observed after the administration of Rapamune Tablets. Dose adjustments based on gender are not recommended.

Race: In large phase 3 trials (Studies 1 and 2) using Rapamune Oral Solution and cyclosporine oral solution (MODIFIED) (e.g., Neoral® Oral Solution) and/or cyclosporine capsules (MODIFIED) (e.g., Neoral® Soft Gelatin Capsules), there were no significant differences in mean trough sirolimus concentrations over time between black (n = 139) and non-black (n = 724) patients during the first 6 months after transplantation at sirolimus doses of 2 mg/day and 5 mg/day. Similarly, after administration of Rapamune Tablets (2 mg/day) in a phase III trial, mean sirolimus trough concentrations over 6 months were not significantly different among black (n = 51) and non-black (n = 128) patients.

CLINICAL STUDIES

Rapamune® Oral Solution: The safety and efficacy of Rapamune® Oral Solution for the prevention of organ rejection following renal transplantation were assessed in two randomized, double-blind, multicenter, controlled trials. These studies compared two dose levels of Rapamune Oral Solution (2 mg and 5 mg, once daily) with azathioprine (Study 1) or placebo (Study 2) when administered in combination with cyclosporine and corticosteroids. Study 1 was conducted in the United States at 38 sites. Seven hundred nineteen (719) patients were enrolled in this trial and randomized following transplantation; 284 were randomized to receive Rapamune Oral Solution 2 mg/day, 274 were randomized to receive Rapamune Oral Solution 5 mg/day, and 161 to receive azathioprine 2-3 mg/kg/day. Study 2 was conducted in Australia, Canada, Europe, and the United States, at a total of 34 sites. Five hundred seventy-six (576) patients were enrolled in this trial and randomized before transplantation; 227 were randomized to receive Rapamune Oral Solution 2 mg/day, 219 were randomized to receive Rapamune Oral Solution 5 mg/day, and 130 to receive placebo. In both studies, the use of antilymphocyte antibody induction therapy was prohibited. In both studies, the primary efficacy endpoint was the rate of efficacy failure in the first 6 months after transplantation. Efficacy failure was defined as the first occurrence of an acute rejection episode (confirmed by biopsy), graft loss, or death.

The tables below summarize the results of the primary efficacy analyses from these trials. Rapamune Oral Solution, at doses of 2 mg/day and 5 mg/day, significantly reduced the incidence of efficacy failure (statistically significant at the <0.025 level; nominal significance level adjusted for multiple [2] dose comparisons) at 6 months following transplantation compared with both azathioprine and placebo.

[See fifth table at right]
[See first table at top of next page]

SIROLIMUS PHARMACOKINETIC PARAMETERS (MEAN ± SD) IN RENAL TRANSPLANT PATIENTS (MULTIPLE DOSE TABLETS)[a,b]

n	Dose (2 mg/day)	$C_{max,ss}$[c] (ng/mL)	$t_{max,ss}$ (h)	$AUC_{\tau,ss}$[c] (ng•h/mL)	CL/F/WT[d] (mL/h/kg)
17	Oral solution	14.4 ± 5.3	2.12 ± 0.84	194 ± 78	173 ± 50
13	Tablets	15.0 ± 4.9	3.46 ± 2.40	230 ± 67	139 ± 63

a: Sirolimus administered four hours after cyclosporine oral solution (MODIFIED) (e.g., Neoral® Oral Solution) and/or cyclosporine capsules (MODIFIED) (e.g., Neoral® Soft Gelatin Capsules).
b: As measured by the Liquid Chromatographic/Tandem Mass Spectrometric Method (LC/MS/MS).
c: These parameters were dose normalized prior to the statistical comparison.
d: CL/F/WT = oral dose clearance.

AVERAGE RAPAMUNE DOSES AND SIROLIMUS TROUGH CONCENTRATIONS (MEAN ± SD) IN RENAL TRANSPLANT PATIENTS AFTER MULTIPLE DOSE TABLET ADMINISTRATION

	Rapamune with Cyclosporine Therapy[a]	Rapamune Following Cyclosporine Withdrawal[a]
Rapamune Dose (mg/day)		
Months 4 to 12	2.1 ± 0.7	8.2 ± 4.2
Months 12 to 24	2.0 ± 0.8	6.4 ± 3.0
Sirolimus C_{min} (ng/mL)[b]		
Months 4 to 12	10.7 ± 3.8	23.3 ± 5.0
Months 12 to 24	11.2 ± 4.1	22.5 ± 4.8

a: 215 patients were randomized to each group.
b: Expressed by immunoassay and equivalence.

SIROLIMUS PHARMACOKINETIC PARAMETERS (MEAN ± SD) IN 18 HEALTHY SUBJECTS AND 18 PATIENTS WITH HEPATIC IMPAIRMENT (15 MG SINGLE DOSE – ORAL SOLUTION)

Population	$C_{max,ss}$[a] (ng/mL)	t_{max} (h)	$AUC_{0-\infty}$ (ng•h/mL)	CL/F/WT (mL/h/kg)
Healthy subjects	78.2 ± 18.3	0.82 ± 0.17	970 ± 272	215 ± 76
Hepatic impairment	77.9 ± 23.1	0.84 ± 0.17	1567 ± 616	144 ± 62

a: As measured by (LC/MS/MS).

SIROLIMUS PHARMACOKINETIC PARAMETERS (MEAN ± SD) IN PEDIATRIC PATIENTS WITH STABLE CHRONIC RENAL FAILURE MAINTAINED ON HEMODIALYSIS OR PERITONEAL DIALYSIS (1, 3, 9, 15 MG/M² SINGLE DOSE)

Age Group (y)	n	t_{max} (h)	$t_{1/2}$ (h)	CL/F/WT (mL/h/kg)
5-11	9	1.1 ± 0.5	71 ± 40	580 ± 450
12-18	11	0.79 ± 0.17	55 ± 18	450 ± 232

INCIDENCE (%) OF EFFICACY FAILURE AT 6 AND 24 MONTHS FOR STUDY 1[a,b]

Parameter	Rapamune® Oral Solution 2 mg/day (n = 284)	Rapamune® Oral Solution 5 mg/day (n = 274)	Azathioprine 2-3 mg/kg/day (n = 161)
Efficacy failure at 6 months[c]	18.7	16.8	32.3
Components of efficacy failure			
Biopsy-proven acute rejection	16.5	11.3	29.2
Graft loss	1.1	2.9	2.5
Death	0.7	1.8	0
Lost to follow-up	0.4	0.7	0.6
Efficacy failure at 24 months	32.8	25.9	36.0
Components of efficacy failure			
Biopsy-proven acute rejection	23.6	17.5	32.3
Graft loss	3.9	4.7	3.1
Death	4.2	3.3	0
Lost to follow-up	1.1	0.4	0.6

a: Patients received cyclosporine and corticosteroids.
b: Includes patients who prematurely discontinued treatment.
c: Primary endpoint.

Patient and graft survival at 1 year were co-primary endpoints. The table below shows graft and patient survival at 1 and 2 years in Study 1 and 1 and 3 years in Study 2. The graft and patient survival rates were similar in patients treated with Rapamune and comparator-treated patients.

[See second table at top of next page]

The reduction in the incidence of first biopsy-confirmed acute rejection episodes in patients treated with Rapamune compared with the control groups included a reduction in all grades of rejection.

In Study 1, which was prospectively stratified by race within center, efficacy failure was similar for Rapamune Oral Solution 2 mg/day and lower for Rapamune Oral Solution 5 mg/day compared with azathioprine in black patients. In Study 2, which was not prospectively stratified by race, efficacy failure was similar for both Rapamune Oral Solution doses compared with placebo in black patients. The decision to use the higher dose of Rapamune Oral Solution in black patients must be weighed against the increased risk of dose-dependent adverse events that were observed with the Rapamune Oral Solution 5-mg dose (see **ADVERSE REACTIONS**).

[See third table on next page]

Mean glomerular filtration rates (GFR) post transplant were calculated by using the Nankivell equation at 12 and 24 months for Study 1, and 12 and 36 months for Study 2. Mean GFR was lower in patients treated with cyclosporine and Rapamune Oral Solution compared with those treated with cyclosporine and the respective azathioprine or placebo control.

[See first table at top of page 504]

Within each treatment group in Studies 1 and 2, mean GFR at one year post transplant was lower in patients who experienced at least 1 episode of biopsy-proven acute rejection, compared with those who did not.

Renal function should be monitored and appropriate adjustment of the immunosuppression regimen should be considered in patients with elevated or increasing serum creatinine levels (see **PRECAUTIONS**).

Rapamune® Tablets: The safety and efficacy of Rapamune Oral Solution and Rapamune Tablets for the prevention of organ rejection following renal transplantation were compared in a randomized multicenter controlled trial (Study 3). This study compared a single dose level (2 mg, once daily) of Rapamune Oral Solution and Rapamune Tablets when administered in combination with cyclosporine and corticosteroids. The study was conducted at 30 centers in Australia, Canada, and the United States. Four hundred seventy-seven (477) patients were enrolled in this study and randomized before transplantation; 238 patients were randomized to receive Rapamune Oral Solution 2 mg/day and 239 patients were randomized to receive Rapamune Tablets 2 mg/day. In this study, the use of antilymphocyte antibody induction therapy was prohibited. The primary efficacy end-

INCIDENCE (%) OF EFFICACY FAILURE AT 6 AND 36 MONTHS FOR STUDY 2[a,b]

Parameter	Rapamune® Oral Solution 2 mg/day (n = 227)	Rapamune® Oral Solution 5 mg/day (n = 219)	Placebo (n = 130)
Efficacy failure at 6 months[c]	30.0	25.6	47.7
Components of efficacy failure			
Biopsy-proven acute rejection	24.7	19.2	41.5
Graft loss	3.1	3.7	3.9
Death	2.2	2.7	2.3
Lost to follow-up	0	0	0
Efficacy failure at 36 months	44.1	41.6	54.6
Components of efficacy failure			
Biopsy-proven acute rejection	32.2	27.4	43.9
Graft loss	6.2	7.3	4.6
Death	5.7	5.9	5.4
Lost to follow-up	0	0.9	0.8

a: Patients received cyclosporine and corticosteroids.
b: Includes patients who prematurely discontinued treatment.
c: Primary endpoint.

GRAFT AND PATIENT SURVIVAL (%) FOR STUDY 1 (12 AND 24 MONTHS) AND STUDY 2 (12 AND 36 MONTHS)[a,b]

Parameter	Rapamune® Oral Solution 2 mg/day	Rapamune® Oral Solution 5 mg/day	Azathioprine 2-3 mg/kg/day	Placebo
Study 1	(n = 284)	(n = 274)	(n = 161)	
Graft survival				
• Month 12	94.7	92.7	93.8	
Month 24	85.2	89.1	90.1	
Patient survival				
Month 12	97.2	96.0	98.1	
Month 24	92.6	94.9	96.3	
Study 2	(n = 227)	(n = 219)		(n = 130)
Graft survival				
Month 12	89.9	90.9		87.7
Month 36	81.1	79.9		80.8
Patient survival				
Month 12	96.5	95.0		94.6
Month 36	90.3	89.5		90.8

a: Patients received cyclosporine and corticosteroids.
b: Includes patients who prematurely discontinued treatment.

PERCENTAGE OF EFFICACY FAILURE BY RACE AT 6 MONTHS[a,b]

Parameter	Rapamune® Oral Solution 2 mg/day	Rapamune® Oral Solution 5 mg/day	Azathioprine 2-3 mg/kg/day	Placebo
Study 1				
Black (n = 166)	34.9 (n = 63)	18.0 (n = 61)	33.3 (n = 42)	
Non-black (n = 553)	14.0 (n = 221)	16.4 (n = 213)	31.9 (n = 119)	
Study 2				
Black (n = 66)	30.8 (n = 26)	33.7 (n = 27)		38.5 (n = 13)
Non-black (n = 510)	29.9 (n = 201)	24.5 (n = 192)		48.7 (n = 117)

a: Patients received cyclosporine and corticosteroids.
b: Includes patients who prematurely discontinued treatment.

point was the rate of efficacy failure in the first 3 months after transplantation. Efficacy failure was defined as the first occurrence of an acute rejection episode (confirmed by biopsy), graft loss, or death.

The table below summarizes the result of the efficacy failure analysis at 3 and 6 months from this trial. The overall rate of efficacy failure at 3 months, the primary endpoint, in the tablet treatment group was equivalent to the rate in the oral solution treatment group.

[See second table at top of next page]

Graft and patient survival at 12 months were co-primary endpoints. There was no significant difference between the oral solution and tablet formulations for both graft and patient survival. Graft survival was 92.0% and 88.7% for the oral solution and tablet treatment groups, respectively. The patient survival rates in the oral solution and tablet treatment groups were 95.8% and 96.2%, respectively.

The mean GFR at 12 months, calculated by the Nankivell equation, were not significantly different for the oral solution group and for the tablet group.

The table below summarizes the mean GFR at one-year post-transplantation for all patients in Study 3 who had serum creatinine measured at 12 months.

OVERALL CALCULATED GLOMERULAR FILTRATION RATES (CC/MIN) BY NANKIVELL EQUATION AT 12 MONTHS POST TRANSPLANT: STUDY 3[a,b]

	Rapamune® Oral Solution	Rapamune® Tablets
Mean ± SEM	53.1 ± 1.7 (n = 229)	51.7 ± 1.7 (n = 225)

a: Includes patients who prematurely discontinued treatment.
b: Patients who had a graft loss were included in the analysis with GFR set to 0.0.

In Study 4, the safety and efficacy of Rapamune as a maintenance regimen were assessed following cyclosporine withdrawal at 3 to 4 months post renal transplantation. Study 4 was a randomized, multicenter, controlled trial conducted at 57 centers in Australia, Canada, and Europe. Five hundred twenty-five (525) patients were enrolled. All patients in this study received the tablet formulation. This study compared patients who were administered Rapamune, cyclosporine, and corticosteroids continuously with patients who received the same standardized therapy for the first 3 months after transplantation (prerandomization period) followed by the withdrawal of cyclosporine. During cyclosporine withdrawal the Rapamune dosages were adjusted to achieve targeted sirolimus whole blood trough concentration ranges (20 to 30 ng/mL, experimental immunoassay). At 3 months, 430 patients were equally randomized to either Rapamune with cyclosporine therapy or Rapamune as a maintenance regimen following cyclosporine withdrawal. Eligibility for randomization included no Banff Grade 3 acute rejection episode or vascular rejection in the 4 weeks before random assignment; serum creatinine ≤ 4.5 mg/dL; and adequate renal function to support cyclosporine withdrawal (in the opinion of the investigator). The primary efficacy endpoint was graft survival at 12 months after transplantation. Secondary efficacy endpoints were the rate of biopsy-confirmed acute rejection, patient survival, incidence of efficacy failure (defined as the first occurrence of either biopsy-proven acute rejection, graft loss, or death), and treatment failure (defined as the first occurrence of either discontinuation, acute rejection, graft loss, or death).

The safety and efficacy of cyclosporine withdrawal in high-risk patients have not been adequately studied and it is therefore not recommended. This includes patients with Banff grade III acute rejection or vascular rejection prior to cyclosporine withdrawal, those who are dialysis-dependent, serum creatinine > 4.5 mg/dL, black patients, re-transplants, multi-organ transplants, or patients with high panel of reactive antibodies (See **INDICATIONS AND USAGE**).

The table below summarizes the resulting graft and patient survival at 12, 24, and 36 months for this trial. At 12, 24, and 36 months, graft and patient survival were similar for both groups.

GRAFT AND PATIENT SURVIVAL (%): STUDY 4[a]

Parameter	Rapamune with Cyclosporine Therapy (n = 215)	Rapamune Following Cyclosporine Withdrawal (n = 215)
Graft Survival		
Month 12[b]	95.8	97.2
Month 24	91.2	93.5
Month 36	85.1	91.2
Patient Survival		
Month 12	97.2	98.1
Month 24	94.0	95.3
Month 36	88.4	93.5

a: Includes patients who prematurely discontinued treatment.
b: Primary efficacy endpoint.

The table below summarizes the results of first biopsy-proven acute rejection at 12 and 36 months. There was a significant difference in first biopsy-proven rejection between the two groups during post-randomization through 12 months. Most of the post-randomization acute rejections occurred in the first 3 months following randomization.

INCIDENCE OF FIRST BIOPSY-PROVEN ACUTE REJECTION (%) BY TREATMENT GROUP AT 36 MONTHS: STUDY 4[a]

Period	Rapamune with Cyclosporine Therapy (n = 215)	Rapamune Following Cyclosporine withdrawal (n = 215)
Prerandomization[b]	9.3	10.2
Postrandomization through 12 months[b]	4.2	9.8
Postrandomization from 12 to 36 months	1.4	0.5
Postrandomization through 36 months	5.6	10.2
Total at 36 months	14.9	20.5

a: Includes patients who prematurely discontinued treatment.
b: Randomization occurred at 3 months ± 2 weeks.

Patients receiving renal allografts with ≥ 4 HLA mismatches experienced significantly higher rates of acute rejection following randomization to the cyclosporine withdrawal group compared with patients who continued cyclosporine (15.3% vs 3.0%). Patients receiving renal allografts with ≤ 3 HLA mismatches, demonstrated similar rates of acute rejection between treatment groups (6.8% vs 7.7%) following randomization.

The table below summarizes the mean calculated GFR in Study 4.

CALCULATED GLOMERULAR FILTRATION RATES (mL/min) BY NANKIVELL EQUATION AT 12, 24, AND 36 MONTHS POST TRANSPLANT: STUDY 4[a,b]

Parameter	Rapamune with Cyclosporine Therapy	Rapamune Following Cyclosporine Withdrawal
Month 12		
Mean ± SEM	53.2 ± 1.5 n = 208	59.3 ± 1.5 n = 203
Month 24		
Mean ± SEM	48.4 ± 1.7 n = 203	58.4 ± 1.6 n = 201
Month 36		
Mean ± SEM	47.3 ± 1.8 (n = 194)	59.4 ± 1.8 (n = 194)

a: Includes patients who prematurely discontinued treatment.
b: Patients who had a graft loss were included in the analysis and had their GFR set to 0.0.

The mean GFR at 12, 24, and 36 months, calculated by the Nankivell equation, was significantly higher for patients receiving Rapamune as a maintenance regimen following cyclosporine withdrawal than for those in the Rapamune with cyclosporine therapy group. Patients who had an acute rejection prior to randomization had a significantly higher GFR following cyclosporine withdrawal compared to those in the Rapamune with cyclosporine group. There was no significant difference in GFR between groups for patients who experienced acute rejection postrandomization.

INDICATIONS AND USAGE

Rapamune® (sirolimus) is indicated for the prophylaxis of organ rejection in patients receiving renal transplants. It is

Continued on next page

Rapamune—Cont.

recommended that Rapamune be used initially in a regimen with cyclosporine and corticosteroids. In patients at low to moderate immunologic risk cyclosporine should be withdrawn 2 to 4 months after transplantation and Rapamune® dose should be increased to reach recommended blood concentrations (See **DOSAGE AND ADMINISTRATION**).

The safety and efficacy of cyclosporine withdrawal in high-risk patients have not been adequately studied and it is therefore not recommended. This includes patients with Banff grade III acute rejection or vascular rejection prior to cyclosporine withdrawal, those who are dialysis-dependent, or with serum creatinine > 4.5 mg/dL, black patients, retransplants, multi-organ transplants, patients with high panel of reactive antibodies (See **CLINICAL STUDIES**).

CONTRAINDICATIONS

Rapamune is contraindicated in patients with a hypersensitivity to sirolimus or its derivatives or any component of the drug product.

WARNINGS

Increased susceptibility to infection and the possible development of lymphoma and other malignancies, particularly of the skin, may result from immunosuppression (see **ADVERSE REACTIONS**). Oversuppression of the immune system can also increase susceptibility to infection including opportunistic infections, fatal infections, and sepsis. Only physicians experienced in immunosuppressive therapy and management of organ transplant patients should use Rapamune. Patients receiving the drug should be managed in facilities equipped and staffed with adequate laboratory and supportive medical resources. The physician responsible for maintenance therapy should have complete information requisite for the follow-up of the patient.

Hypersensitivity reactions, including anaphylactic/anaphylactoid reactions, have been associated with the administration of sirolimus (see **ADVERSE REACTIONS**).

As usual for patients with increased risk for skin cancer, exposure to sunlight and UV light should be limited by wearing protective clothing and using a sunscreen with a high protection factor.

Increased serum cholesterol and triglycerides, that may require treatment, occurred more frequently in patients treated with Rapamune compared with azathioprine or placebo controls (see **PRECAUTIONS**).

In Studies 1 and 2, from month 6 through months 24 and 36, respectively, mean serum creatinine was increased and mean glomerular filtration rate was decreased in patients treated with Rapamune and cyclosporine compared with those treated with cyclosporine and placebo or azathioprine controls. The rate of decline in renal function was greater in patients receiving Rapamune and cyclosporine compared with control therapies (see **CLINICAL STUDIES**).

Renal function should be closely monitored during the administration of Rapamune® in combination with cyclosporine since long-term administration can be associated with deterioration of renal function. Appropriate adjustment of the immunosuppression regimen, including discontinuation of Rapamune and/or cyclosporine, should be considered in patients with elevated or increasing serum creatinine levels. Caution should be exercised when using other drugs which are known to impair renal function. In patients at low to moderate immunologic risk continuation of combination therapy with cyclosporine beyond 4 months following transplantation should only be considered when the benefits outweigh the risks of this combination for the individual patients (see **PRECAUTIONS**).

In clinical trials, Rapamune has been administered concurrently with corticosteroids and with the following formulations of cyclosporine:

- Sandimmune® Injection (cyclosporine injection)
- Sandimmune® Oral Solution (cyclosporine oral solution)
- Sandimmune® Soft Gelatin Capsules (cyclosporine capsules)
- Neoral® Soft Gelatin Capsules (cyclosporine capsules [MODIFIED])
- Neoral® Oral Solution (cyclosporine oral solution [MODIFIED])

The efficacy and safety of the use of Rapamune in combination with other immunosuppressive agents has not been determined.

Liver Transplantation – Excess Mortality, Graft Loss, and Hepatic Artery Thrombosis (HAT):

The use of sirolimus in combination with tacrolimus was associated with excess mortality and graft loss in a study in de novo liver transplant recipients. Many of these patients had evidence of infection at or near the time of death.

In this and another study in de novo liver transplant recipients, the use of sirolimus in combination with cyclosporine or tacrolimus was associated with an increase in HAT; most cases of HAT occurred within 30 days post-transplantation and most led to graft loss or death.

Lung Transplantation – Bronchial Anastomotic Dehiscence:

Cases of bronchial anastomotic dehiscence, most fatal, have been reported in de novo lung transplant patients when sirolimus has been used as part of an immunosuppressive regimen.

The safety and efficacy of Rapamune® (sirolimus) as immunosuppressive therapy have not been established in liver or lung transplant patients, and therefore, such use is not recommended.

OVERALL CALCULATED GLOMERULAR FILTRATION RATES (Mean ± SEM, cc/min) BY NANKIVELL EQUATION POST TRANSPLANT[a,b]

Parameter	Rapamune® Oral Solution 2 mg/day	Rapamune® Oral Solution 5 mg/day	Azathioprine 2-3 mg/kg/day	Placebo
Study 1				
Month 12	57.4 ± 1.3 (n = 269)	54.6 ± 1.3 (n = 248)	64.1 ± 1.6 (n = 149)	
Month 24	58.4 ± 1.5 (n = 221)	52.6 ± 1.5 (n = 222)	62.4 ± 1.9 (n = 132)	
Study 2				
Month 12	52.4 ± 1.5 (n = 211)	51.5 ± 1.5 (n = 199)		58.0 ± 2.1 (n = 117)
Month 36	48.1 ± 1.8 (n = 183)	46.1 ± 2.0 (n = 177)		53.4 ± 2.7 (n = 102)

a: Includes patients who prematurely discontinued treatment.
b: Patients who had a graft loss were included in the analysis with GFR set to 0.0.

INCIDENCE (%) OF EFFICACY FAILURE AT 3 AND 6 MONTHS: STUDY 3[a,b]

	Rapamune® Oral Solution (n = 238)	Rapamune® Tablets (n = 239)
Efficacy Failure at 3 months[c]	23.5	24.7
Components of efficacy failure		
Biopsy-proven acute rejection	18.9	17.6
Graft loss	3.4	6.3
Death	1.3	0.8
Efficacy Failure at 6 months	26.1	27.2
Components of efficacy failure		
Biopsy-proven acute rejection	21.0	19.2
Graft loss	3.4	6.3
Death	1.7	1.7

a: Patients received cyclosporine and corticosteroids.
b: Includes patients who prematurely discontinued treatment.
c: Efficacy failure at 3 months was the primary endpoint.

Co-administration of sirolimus with strong inhibitors of CYP3A4 and/or P-gp (such as ketoconazole, voriconazole, itraconazole, telithromycin, or clarithromycin) or strong inducers of CYP3A4 and/or P-gp (such as rifampin or rifabutin) is not recommended (see **CLINICAL PHARMACOLOGY, Metabolism,** and **PRECAUTIONS, Drug Interactions** and **Other drug interactions**).

PRECAUTIONS

General

Rapamune is intended for oral administration only.

Lymphocele, a known surgical complication of renal transplantation, occurred significantly more often in a dose-related fashion in patients treated with Rapamune. Appropriate operative measures should be considered to minimize this complication.

Lipids

The use of Rapamune® in renal transplant patients was associated with increased serum cholesterol and triglycerides that may require treatment.

In Studies 1 and 2, in *de novo* renal transplant recipients who began the study with normal, fasting, total serum cholesterol (<200 mg/dL) or normal, fasting, total serum triglycerides (<200 mg/dL), there was an increased incidence of hypercholesterolemia (fasting serum cholesterol >240 mg/dL) or hypertriglyceridemia (fasting serum triglycerides >500 mg/dL), respectively, in patients receiving both Rapamune® 2 mg and Rapamune® 5 mg compared with azathioprine and placebo controls.

Treatment of new-onset hypercholesterolemia with lipid-lowering agents was required in 42–52% of patients enrolled in the Rapamune arms of Studies 1 and 2 compared with 16% of patients in the placebo arm and 22% of patients in the azathioprine arm.

In Study 4 during the prerandomization period, mean fasting serum cholesterol and triglyceride values rapidly increased, and peaked at 2 months with mean cholesterol values > 240 mg/dL and triglycerides > 250 mg/dL. After randomization mean cholesterol and triglyceride values remained higher in the cyclosporine withdrawal arm compared to the Rapamune® and cyclosporine combination.

Renal transplant patients have a higher prevalence of clinically significant hyperlipidemia. Accordingly, the risk/benefit should be carefully considered in patients with established hyperlipidemia before initiating an immunosuppressive regimen including Rapamune.

Any patient who is administered Rapamune should be monitored for hyperlipidemia using laboratory tests and if hyperlipidemia is detected, subsequent interventions such as diet, exercise, and lipid-lowering agents, as outlined by the National Cholesterol Education Program guidelines, should be initiated.

In clinical trials, the concomitant administration of Rapamune and HMG-CoA reductase inhibitors and/or fibrates appeared to be well tolerated.

During Rapamune therapy with cyclosporine, patients administered an HMG-CoA reductase inhibitor and/or fibrate should be monitored for the possible development of rhabdomyolysis and other adverse effects as described in the respective labeling for these agents.

Renal Function

Patients treated with cyclosporine and Rapamune were noted to have higher serum creatinine levels and lower glomerular filtration rates compared with patients treated with cyclosporine and placebo or azathioprine controls (Studies 1 and 2). The rate of decline in renal function in these studies was greater in patients receiving Rapamune and cyclosporine compared with control therapies. In patients at low to moderate immunologic risk (See **CLINICAL STUDIES**) continuation of combination therapy with cyclosporine beyond 4 months following transplantation should only be considered when the benefits outweigh the risks of this combination for the individual patients. (see **WARNINGS**).

Renal function should be monitored during the administration of Rapamune® in combination with cyclosporine. Appropriate adjustment of the immunosuppression regimen, including discontinuation of Rapamune and/or cyclosporine, should be considered in patients with elevated or increasing serum creatinine levels. Caution should be exercised when using agents (e.g., aminoglycosides, and amphotericin B) that are known to have a deleterious effect on renal function.

Antimicrobial Prophylaxis

Cases of *Pneumocystis carinii* pneumonia have been reported in patients not receiving antimicrobial prophylaxis. Therefore, antimicrobial prophylaxis for *Pneumocystis carinii* pneumonia should be administered for 1 year following transplantation.

Cytomegalovirus (CMV) prophylaxis is recommended for 3 months after transplantation, particularly for patients at increased risk for CMV disease.

Interstitial Lung Disease

Cases of interstitial lung disease (including pneumonitis, and infrequently bronchiolitis obliterans organizing pneumonia [BOOP] and pulmonary fibrosis), some fatal, with no identified infectious etiology have occurred in patients receiving immunosuppressive regimens including Rapamune. In some cases, the interstitial lung disease has resolved upon discontinuation or dose reduction of Rapamune. The risk may be increased as the trough Rapamune concentration increases (see **ADVERSE REACTIONS, Other clinical experience**).

Information for Patients

Patients should be given complete dosage instructions (see **Patient Instructions**). Women of childbearing potential should be informed of the potential risks during pregnancy and that they should use effective contraception prior to initiation of Rapamune therapy, during Rapamune therapy and for 12 weeks after Rapamune therapy has been stopped (see **PRECAUTIONS: Pregnancy**).

Patients should be told that exposure to sunlight and UV light should be limited by wearing protective clothing and using a sunscreen with a high protection factor because of the increased risk for skin cancer (see **WARNINGS**).

Laboratory Tests

Whole blood sirolimus concentrations should be monitored in patients receiving concentration-controlled Rapamune.

Monitoring is also necessary in patients likely to have altered drug metabolism, in patients ≥13 years who weigh less than 40 kg, in patients with hepatic impairment, and during concurrent administration of potent CYP3A4 inducers and inhibitors (see **PRECAUTIONS: Drug Interactions**).

Drug Interactions

Sirolimus is known to be a substrate for both cytochrome CYP3A4 and P-gp. The pharmacokinetic interaction between sirolimus and concomitantly administered drugs is discussed below. Drug interaction studies have not been conducted with drugs other than those described below.

Cyclosporine capsules MODIFIED:

Cyclosporine is a substrate and inhibitor of CYP3A4 and P-gp.

Because of the effect of cyclosporine capsules (MODIFIED), it is recommended that sirolimus should be taken 4 hours after administration of cyclosporine oral solution (MODIFIED) and/or cyclosporine capsules (MODIFIED) (see DOSAGE AND ADMINISTRATION).

Studies assessing the effect of concomitant administration of cyclosporine capsules (MODIFIED) with sirolimus oral solution and with sirolimus tablets are summarized below.

Rapamune Oral Solution: In a single dose drug-drug interaction study, 24 healthy volunteers were administered 10 mg sirolimus either simultaneously or 4 hours after a 300 mg dose of Neoral® Soft Gelatin Capsules (cyclosporine capsules [MODIFIED]). For simultaneous administration, the mean C_{max} and AUC of sirolimus were increased by 116% and 230%, respectively, relative to administration of sirolimus alone. However, when given 4 hours after Neoral® Soft Gelatin Capsules (cyclosporine capsules [MODIFIED]) administration, sirolimus C_{max} and AUC were increased by 37% and 80%, respectively, compared with administration of sirolimus alone.

Mean cyclosporine C_{max} and AUC were not significantly affected when sirolimus was given simultaneously or when administered 4 hours after Neoral® Soft Gelatin Capsules (cyclosporine capsules [MODIFIED]). However, after multiple-dose administration of sirolimus given 4 hours after Neoral® in renal post-transplant patients over 6 months, cyclosporine oral-dose clearance was reduced, and lower doses of Neoral® Soft Gelatin Capsules (cyclosporine capsules [MODIFIED]) were needed to maintain target cyclosporine concentration.

Rapamune Tablets: In a single-dose drug-drug interaction study, 24 healthy volunteers were administered 10 mg sirolimus (Rapamune Tablets) either simultaneously or 4 hours after a 300-mg dose of Neoral® Soft Gelatin Capsules (cyclosporine capsules [MODIFIED]). For simultaneous administration, mean C_{max} and AUC were increased by 512% and 148%, respectively, relative to administration of sirolimus alone. However, when given 4 hours after cyclosporine administration, sirolimus C_{max} and AUC were both increased by only 33% compared with administration of sirolimus alone.

Cyclosporine oral solution: In a multiple-dose study in 150 psoriasis patients, sirolimus 0.5, 1.5, and 3 mg/m²/day was administered simultaneously with Sandimmune® Oral Solution (cyclosporine Oral Solution) 1.25 mg/kg/day. The increase in average sirolimus trough concentrations ranged between 67% to 86% relative to when sirolimus was administered without cyclosporine. The intersubject variability (%CV) for sirolimus trough concentrations ranged from 39.7% to 68.7%. There was no significant effect of multiple-dose sirolimus on cyclosporine trough concentrations following Sandimmune® Oral Solution (cyclosporine oral solution) administration. However, the %CV was higher (range 85.9%–165%) than those from previous studies.

Sandimmune® Oral Solution (cyclosporine oral solution) is not bioequivalent to Neoral® Oral Solution (cyclosporine oral solution MODIFIED), and should not be used interchangeably. Although there is no published data comparing Sandimmune® Oral Solution (cyclosporine oral solution) to SangCya® Oral Solution (cyclosporine oral solution [MODIFIED]), they should not be used interchangeably. Likewise, Sandimmune® Soft Gelatin Capsules (cyclosporine capsules) are not bioequivalent to Neoral® Soft Gelatin Capsules (cyclosporine capsules [MODIFIED]) and should not be used interchangeably.

Diltiazem: Diltiazem is a substrate and inhibitor of CYP3A4 and P-gp; sirolimus levels should be monitored and a dose adjustment may be necessary. The simultaneous oral administration of 10 mg of sirolimus oral solution and 120 mg of diltiazem to 18 healthy volunteers significantly affected the bioavailability of sirolimus. Sirolimus C_{max}, t_{max}, and AUC were increased 1.4-, 1.3-, and 1.6-fold, respectively. Sirolimus did not affect the pharmacokinetics of either diltiazem or its metabolites desacetyldiltiazem and desmethyldiltiazem.

Ketoconazole: Ketoconazole is a strong inhibitor of CYP3A4 and P-gp; co-administration of sirolimus oral solution or tablets and ketoconazole is not recommended (see **WARNINGS**). Multiple-dose ketoconazole administration significantly affected the rate and extent of absorption and sirolimus exposure after administration of Rapamune® Oral Solution, as reflected by increases in sirolimus C_{max}, t_{max}, and AUC of 4.3-fold, 38%, and 10.9-fold, respectively. However, the terminal $t_{1/2}$ of sirolimus was not changed. Single-dose sirolimus did not affect steady-state 12-hour plasma ketoconazole concentrations.

Rifampin: Rifampin is a strong inducer of CYP3A4 and P-gp; co-administration of sirolimus oral solution or tablets and rifampin is not recommended (see **WARNINGS**). Pretreatment of 14 healthy volunteers with multiple doses of rifampin, 600 mg daily for 14 days, followed by a single 20-mg dose of sirolimus oral solution, greatly increased sirolimus oral-dose clearance by 5.5-fold (range = 2.8 to 10), which represents mean decreases in AUC and C_{max} of about 82% and 71%, respectively. In patients where rifampin is indicated, alternative therapeutic agents with less enzyme induction potential should be considered.

Drugs which may be coadministered without dose adjustment

Clinically significant pharmacokinetic drug-drug interactions were not observed in studies of drugs listed below. A synopsis of the type of study performed for each drug is provided. Sirolimus and these drugs may be coadministered without dose adjustments.

Acyclovir: Acyclovir, 200 mg, was administered once daily for 3 days followed by a single 10-mg dose of sirolimus oral solution on day 3 in 20 adult healthy volunteers.

Digoxin: Digoxin, 0.25 mg, was administered daily for 8 days and a single 10-mg dose of sirolimus oral solution was given on day 8 to 24 healthy volunteers.

Glyburide: A single 5-mg dose of glyburide and a single 10-mg dose of sirolimus oral solution were administered to 24 healthy volunteers. Sirolimus did not affect the hypoglycemic action of glyburide.

Nifedipine: A single 60-mg dose of nifedipine and a single 10-mg dose of sirolimus oral solution were administered to 24 healthy volunteers.

Norgestrel/ethinyl estradiol (Lo/Ovral®): Sirolimus oral solution, 2 mg, was given daily for 7 days to 21 healthy female volunteers on norgestrel/ethinyl estradiol.

Prednisolone: Pharmacokinetic information was obtained from 42 stable renal transplant patients receiving daily doses of prednisone (5-20 mg/day) and either single or multiple doses of sirolimus oral solution (0.5-5 mg/m² q 12h).

Sulfamethoxazole/trimethoprim (Bactrim®): A single oral dose of sulfamethoxazole (400 mg)/trimethoprim (80 mg) was given to 15 renal transplant patients receiving daily oral doses of sirolimus (8 to 25 mg/m²).

Other drug interactions

Co-administration of sirolimus with strong inhibitors of CYP3A4 and/or P-gp (such as ketoconazole, voriconazole, itraconazole, telithromycin, or clarithromycin) or strong inducers of CYP3A4 and/or P-gp (such as rifampin or rifabutin) is not recommended (see **WARNINGS**). Sirolimus is extensively metabolized by the CYP3A4 isoenzyme in the intestinal wall and liver and undergoes counter-transport from enterocytes of the small intestine into the gut lumen by the P-gp drug efflux pump. Sirolimus is potentially recycled between enterocytes and the gut lumen to allow continued metabolism by CYP3A4. Therefore, absorption and the subsequent elimination of systemically absorbed sirolimus may be influenced by drugs that affect these proteins. Strong inhibitors of CYP3A4 and P-gp significantly decrease the metabolism of sirolimus and increase sirolimus concentrations, while strong inducers of CYP3A4 and P-gp significantly increase the metabolism of sirolimus and decrease sirolimus concentrations.

In patients in whom strong inhibitors or inducers of CYP3A4 are indicated, alternative therapeutic agents with less potential for inhibition or induction of CYP3A4 should be considered.

Sirolimus is a substrate for the multidrug efflux pump, P-gp in the small intestine. Therefore, absorption of sirolimus may be influenced by drugs that affect P-gp.

Aside from those mentioned above, other drugs that increase sirolimus blood concentrations include (but are not limited to):

Calcium channel blockers: nicardipine, verapamil.
Antifungal agents: clotrimazole, fluconazole.
Antibiotics: erythromycin, troleandomycin.
Gastrointestinal prokinetic agents: cisapride, metoclopramide.
Other drugs: bromocriptine, cimetidine, danazol, HIV-protease inhibitors (e.g., ritonavir, indinavir).

Aside from those mentioned above, other drugs that decrease sirolimus concentrations include (but are not limited to):

Anticonvulsants: carbamazepine, phenobarbital, phenytoin.
Antibiotics: rifapentine.

Care should be exercised when drugs or other substances that are metabolized by CYP3A4 are administered concomitantly with Rapamune. Grapefruit juice reduces CYP3A4-mediated metabolism of Rapamune and must not be used for dilution (see **DOSAGE AND ADMINISTRATION**).

Herbal Preparations

St. John's Wort (*hypericum perforatum*) induces CYP3A4 and P-gp. Since sirolimus is a substrate for both cytochrome CYP3A4 and P-gp, there is the potential that the use of St. John's Wort in patients receiving Rapamune could result in reduced sirolimus concentrations.

Vaccination

Immunosuppressants may affect response to vaccination. Therefore, during treatment with Rapamune, vaccination may be less effective. The use of live vaccines should be avoided; live vaccines may include, but are not limited to measles, mumps, rubella, oral polio, BCG, yellow fever, varicella, and TY21a typhoid.

Drug-Laboratory Test Interactions

There are no studies on the interactions of sirolimus in commonly employed clinical laboratory tests.

Carcinogenesis, Mutagenesis, and Impairment of Fertility

Sirolimus was not genotoxic in the in vitro bacterial reverse mutation assay, the Chinese hamster ovary cell chromosomal aberration assay, the mouse lymphoma cell forward mutation assay, or the in vivo mouse micronucleus assay.

Carcinogenicity studies were conducted in mice and rats. In an 86-week female mouse study at dosages of 0, 12.5, 25 and 50/6 (dosage lowered from 50 to 6 mg/kg/day at week 31 due to infection secondary to immunosuppression) there was a statistically significant increase in malignant lymphoma at all dose levels (approximately 16 to 135 times the clinical doses adjusted for body surface area) compared with controls. In a second mouse study at dosages of 0, 1, 3 and 6 mg/kg (approximately 3 to 16 times the clinical dose adjusted for body surface area), hepatocellular adenoma and carcinoma (males), were considered Rapamune related. In the 104-week rat study at dosages of 0, 0.05, 0.1, and 0.2 mg/kg/day (approximately 0.4 to 1 times the clinical dose adjusted for body surface area), there was a statistically significant increased incidence of testicular adenoma in the 0.2 mg/kg/day group.

There was no effect on fertility in female rats following the administration of sirolimus at dosages up to 0.5 mg/kg (approximately 1 to 3 times the clinical doses adjusted for body surface area). In male rats, there was no significant difference in fertility rate compared to controls at a dosage of 2 mg/kg (approximately 4 to 11 times the clinical doses adjusted for body surface area). Reductions in testicular weights and/or histological lesions (e.g., tubular atrophy and tubular giant cells) were observed in rats following dosages of 0.65 mg/kg (approximately 1 to 3 times the clinical doses adjusted for body surface area) and above and in a monkey study at 0.1 mg/kg (approximately 0.4 to 1 times the clinical doses adjusted for body surface area) and above. Sperm counts were reduced in male rats following the administration of sirolimus for 13 weeks at a dosage of 6 mg/kg (approximately 12 to 32 times the clinical doses adjusted for body surface area), but showed improvement by 3 months after dosing was stopped.

Pregnancy

Pregnancy Category C: Sirolimus was embryo/feto toxic in rats at dosages of 0.1 mg/kg and above (approximately 0.2 to 0.5 the clinical doses adjusted for body surface area). Embryo/feto toxicity was manifested as mortality and reduced fetal weights (with associated delays in skeletal ossification). However, no teratogenesis was evident. In combination with cyclosporine, rats had increased embryo/feto mortality compared with Rapamune alone. There were no effects on rabbit development at the maternally toxic dosage of 0.05 mg/kg (approximately 0.3 to 0.8 times the clinical doses adjusted for body surface area). There are no adequate and well controlled studies in pregnant women. Effective contraception must be initiated before Rapamune therapy, during Rapamune therapy, and for 12 weeks after Rapamune therapy has been stopped. Rapamune should be used during pregnancy only if the potential benefit outweighs the potential risk to the embryo/fetus.

Use during lactation

Sirolimus is excreted in trace amounts in milk of lactating rats. It is not known whether sirolimus is excreted in human milk. The pharmacokinetic and safety profiles of sirolimus in infants are not known. Because many drugs are excreted in human milk and because of the potential for adverse reactions in nursing infants from sirolimus, a decision should be made whether to discontinue nursing or to discontinue the drug, taking into account the importance of the drug to the mother.

Pediatric use

The safety and efficacy of Rapamune in pediatric patients below the age of 13 years have not been established.

Geriatric use

Clinical studies of Rapamune Oral Solution or Tablets did not include sufficient numbers of patients aged 65 years and over to determine whether safety and efficacy differ in this population from younger patients. Data pertaining to sirolimus trough concentrations suggest that dose adjustments based upon age in geriatric renal patients are not necessary.

ADVERSE REACTIONS

Rapamune® Oral Solution: The incidence of adverse reactions was determined in two randomized, double-blind, multicenter controlled trials in which 499 renal transplant patients received Rapamune Oral Solution 2 mg/day, 477 received Rapamune Oral Solution 5 mg/day, 160 received azathioprine, and 124 received placebo. All patients were treated with cyclosporine and corticosteroids. Data (≥ 12 months post-transplant) presented in the table below show the adverse reactions that occurred in any treatment group with an incidence of ≥ 20%.

Specific adverse reactions associated with the administration of Rapamune (sirolimus) Oral Solution occurred at a significantly higher frequency than in the respective control group. For both Rapamune Oral Solution 2 mg/day and 5 mg/day these include hypercholesterolemia, hyperlipemia, hypertension, and rash; for Rapamune Oral Solution 2 mg/day acne; and for Rapamune Oral Solution 5 mg/day anemia, arthralgia, diarrhea, hypokalemia, and thrombocytopenia. The elevations of triglycerides and cholesterol and decreases in platelets and hemoglobin occurred in a dose-related manner in patients receiving Rapamune.

Patients maintained on Rapamune Oral Solution 5 mg/day, when compared with patients on Rapamune Oral Solution

Continued on next page

Rapamune—Cont.

2 mg/day, demonstrated an increased incidence of the following adverse events: anemia, leukopenia, thrombocytopenia, hypokalemia, hyperlipemia, fever, and diarrhea.
In general, adverse events related to the administration of Rapamune were dependent on dose/concentration.
[See table below]
With longer term follow-up, the adverse event profile remained similar. Some new events became significantly different among the treatment groups. For events which occurred at a frequency of ≥ 20% by 24 months for Study 1 and 36 months for Study 2, only the incidence of edema became significantly higher in both Rapamune groups as compared with the control group. The incidence of headache became significantly more common in the Rapamune 5mg/day group as compared with control therapy.
At 24 months for Study 1, the following treatment-emergent infections were significantly different among the treatment groups: bronchitis, Herpes simplex, pneumonia, pyelonephritis, and upper respiratory infections. In each instance, the incidence was highest in the Rapamune 5 mg/day group, lower in the Rapamune 2 mg/day group and lowest in the azathioprine group. Except for upper respiratory infections in the Rapamune 5 mg/day group, the remainder of events occurred with a frequency of < 20%.
At 36 months in Study 2 only the incidence of treatment-emergent Herpes simplex was significantly different among the treatment groups, being higher in the Rapamune 5 mg/day group than either of the other groups.
The table below summarizes the incidence of malignancies in the two controlled trials for the prevention of acute rejection. At 24 (Study 1) and 36 months (Study 2) there were no significant differences among treatment groups.
[See first table at bottom of next page]
Among the adverse events that were reported at a rate of ≥3% and <20% at 12 months, the following were more prominent in patients maintained on Rapamune 5 mg/day, when compared with patients on Rapamune 2 mg/day: epistaxis, lymphocele, insomnia, thrombotic thrombocytopenic purpura (hemolytic-uremic syndrome), skin ulcer, increased LDH, hypotension, facial edema.
The following adverse events were reported with ≥3% and <20% incidence in patients in any Rapamune treatment group in the two controlled clinical trials for the prevention of acute rejection, BODY AS A WHOLE: abdomen enlarged, abscess, ascites, cellulitis, chills, face edema, flu syndrome, generalized edema, hernia, *Herpes zoster* infection, lymphocele, malaise, pelvic pain, peritonitis, sepsis; CARDIOVASCULAR SYSTEM: atrial fibrillation, congestive heart failure, hemorrhage, hypervolemia, hypotension, palpitation, peripheral vascular disorder, postural hypotension, syncope, tachycardia, thrombophlebitis, thrombosis, vasodilatation, venous thromboembolism; DIGESTIVE SYSTEM: anorexia, dysphagia, eructation, esophagitis, flatulence, gastritis, gastroenteritis, gingivitis, gum hyperplasia, ileus, liver function tests abnormal, mouth ulceration, oral moniliasis, stomatitis; ENDOCRINE SYSTEM: Cushing's syndrome, diabetes mellitus, glycosuria; HEMIC AND LYMPHATIC SYSTEM: ecchymosis, leukocytosis, lymphadenopathy, polycythemia, thrombotic thrombocytopenic purpura (hemolytic-uremic syndrome); METABOLIC AND NUTRITIONAL: acidosis, alkaline phosphatase increased, BUN increased, creatine phosphokinase increased, dehydration, healing abnormal, hypercalcemia, hyperglycemia, hyperphosphatemia, hypocalcemia, hypoglycemia, hypomagnesemia, hyponatremia, lactic dehydrogenase increased, AST/SGOT increased, ALT/SGPT increased, weight loss; MUSCULOSKELETAL SYSTEM: arthrosis, bone necrosis, leg cramps, myalgia, osteoporosis, tetany; NERVOUS SYSTEM: anxiety, confusion, depression, dizziness, emotional lability, hypertonia, hypesthesia, hypotonia, insomnia, neuropathy, paresthesia, somnolence; RESPIRATORY SYSTEM: asthma, atelectasis, bronchitis, cough increased, epistaxis, hypoxia, lung edema, pleural effusion, pneumonia, rhinitis, sinusitis; SKIN AND APPENDAGES: fungal dermatitis, hirsutism, pruritus, skin hypertrophy, skin ulcer, sweating; SPECIAL SENSES: abnormal vision, cataract, conjunctivitis, deafness, ear pain, otitis media, tinnitus; UROGENITAL SYSTEM: albuminuria, bladder pain, dysuria, hematuria, hydronephrosis, impotence, kidney pain, kidney tubular necrosis, nocturia, oliguria, pyelonephritis, pyuria, scrotal edema, testis disorder, toxic nephropathy, urinary frequency, urinary incontinence, urinary retention.
Less frequently occurring adverse events included: mycobacterial infections, Epstein-Barr virus infections, and pancreatitis.
Among the events which were reported at an incidence of ≥ 3% and < 20% by 24 months for Study 1 and 36 months for Study 2, tachycardia and Cushing's syndrome were reported significantly more commonly in both Rapamune groups as compared with the control therapy. Events that were reported more commonly in the Rapamune 5 mg/day group than either the Rapamune 2 mg/day group and/or control group were: abnormal healing, bone necrosis, chills, congestive heart failure, dysuria, hernia, hirsutism, urinary frequency, and lymphadenopathy.
Rapamune® Tablets: The safety profile of the tablet did not differ from that of the oral solution formulation. The incidence of adverse reactions up to 12 months was determined in a randomized, multicenter controlled trial (Study 3) in which 229 renal transplant patients received Rapamune Oral Solution 2 mg once daily and 228 patients received Rapamune Tablets 2 mg once daily. All patients were treated with cyclosporine and corticosteroids. The adverse reactions that occurred in either treatment group with an incidence of ≥ 20% in Study 3 are similar to those reported for Studies 1 and 2. There was no notable difference in the incidence of these adverse events between treatment groups (oral solution versus tablets) in Study 3, with the exception of acne, which occurred more frequently in the oral solution group, and tremor which occurred more frequently in the tablet group, particularly in Black patients.
The adverse events that occurred in patients with an incidence of ≥3% and <20% in either treatment group in Study 3 were similar to those reported in Studies 1 and 2. There was no notable difference in the incidence of these adverse events between treatment groups (oral solution versus tablets) in Study 3, with the exception of hypertonia, which occurred more frequently in the oral solution group and diabetes mellitus which occurred more frequently in the tablet group. Hispanic patients in the tablet group experienced hyperglycemia more frequently than Hispanic patients in the oral solution group. In Study 3 alone, menorrhagia, metrorrhagia, and polyuria occurred with an incidence of ≥3% and <20%.
The clinically important opportunistic or common transplant-related infections were identical in all three studies and the incidences of these infections were similar in Study 3 compared with Studies 1 and 2. The incidence rates of these infections were not significantly different between the oral solution and tablet treatment groups in Study 3.
In Study 3 (at 12 months), there were two cases of lymphoma/lymphoproliferative disorder in the oral solution treatment group (0.8%) and two reported cases of lymphoma/lymphoproliferative disorder in the tablet treatment group (0.8%). These differences were not statistically significant and were similar to the incidences observed in Studies 1 and 2.
Rapamune following cyclosporine withdrawal: The incidence of adverse reactions was determined through 36 months in a randomized, multicenter controlled trial (Study 4) in which 215 renal transplant patients received Rapamune as a maintenance regimen following cyclosporine withdrawal and 215 patients received Rapamune with cyclosporine therapy. All patients were treated with corticosteroids. The safety profile prior to randomization (start of cyclosporine withdrawal) was similar to that of the 2-mg Rapamune groups in Studies 1, 2, and 3. Following randomization (at 3 months) patients who had cyclosporine eliminated from their therapy experienced significantly higher incidences of abnormal liver function tests (including increased AST/SGOT and increased ALT/SGPT), hypokalemia, thrombocytopenia, abnormal healing, ileus, and rectal disorder. Conversely, the incidence of hypertension, cyclosporine toxicity, increased creatinine, abnormal kidney function, toxic nephropathy, edema, hyperkalemia, hyperuricemia, and gum hyperplasia was significantly higher in patients who remained on cyclosporine than those who had cyclosporine withdrawn from therapy. Mean systolic and diastolic blood pressure improved significantly following cyclosporine withdrawal.
In Study 4, at 36 months, the incidence of Herpes zoster infection was significantly lower in patients receiving Rapamune following cyclosporine withdrawal compared with patients who continued to receive Rapamune and cyclosporine.
The incidence of malignancies in Study 4 is presented in the table below. In Study 4, the incidence of lymphoma/lymphoproliferative disease was similar in all treatment groups. The overall incidence of malignancy was higher in patients receiving Rapamune plus cyclosporine compared with patients who had cyclosporine withdrawn.
[See second table at bottom of next page]
Other clinical experience: Cases of interstitial lung disease (including pneumonitis, and infrequently bronchiolitis obliterans organizing pneumonia [BOOP] and pulmonary fibrosis), some fatal, with no identified infectious etiology have occurred in patients receiving immunosuppressive regimens including Rapamune. In some cases, the interstitial lung disease has resolved upon discontinuation or dose reduction of Rapamune. The risk may be increased as the sirolimus trough concentration increases (see **PRECAUTIONS, General, *Interstitial Lung Disease***). There have been reports of neutropenia and rare reports of pancytopenia. Hypersensitivity reactions, including anaphylactic/anaphylactoid reactions, have been associated with the administration of sirolimus (see **WARNINGS**). Hepatotoxicity has been reported, including fatal hepatic necrosis with elevated sirolimus trough concentrations. Abnormal healing

ADVERSE EVENTS OCCURRING AT A FREQUENCY OF ≥ 20% IN ANY TREATMENT GROUP IN PREVENTION OF ACUTE RENAL REJECTION TRIALS (%) AT ≥ 12 MONTHS POST-TRANSPLANTATION FOR STUDIES 1 AND 2[a]

Body System	Rapamune® Oral Solution -------2 mg/day-------		Rapamune® Oral Solution -------5 mg/day-------		Azathioprine 2-3 mg/kg/day	Placebo
Adverse Event	Study 1 (n = 281)	Study 2 (n = 218)	Study 1 (n = 269)	Study 2 (n = 208)	Study 1 (n = 160)	Study 2 (n = 124)
Body As A Whole						
Abdominal pain	28	29	30	36	29	30
Asthenia	38	22	40	28	37	28
Back pain	16	23	26	22	23	20
Chest pain	16	18	19	24	16	19
Fever	27	23	33	34	33	35
Headache	23	34	27	34	21	31
Pain	24	33	29	29	30	25
Cardiovascular System						
Hypertension	43	45	39	49	29	48
Digestive System						
Constipation	28	36	34	38	37	31
Diarrhea	32	25	42	35	28	27
Dyspepsia	17	23	23	25	24	34
Nausea	31	25	36	31	39	29
Vomiting	21	19	25	25	31	21
Hemic And Lymphatic System						
Anemia	27	23	37	33	29	21
Leukopenia	9	9	15	13	20	8
Thrombocytopenia	13	14	20	30	9	9
Metabolic And Nutritional						
Creatinine increased	35	39	37	40	28	38
Edema	24	20	16	18	23	15
Hypercholesteremia (See **WARNINGS** and **PRECAUTIONS**)	38	43	42	46	33	23
Hyperkalemia	15	17	12	14	24	27
Hyperlipemia (See **WARNINGS** and **PRECAUTIONS**)	38	45	44	57	28	23
Hypokalemia	17	11	21	17	11	9
Hypophosphatemia	20	15	23	19	20	19
Peripheral edema	60	54	64	58	58	48
Weight gain	21	11	15	8	19	15
Musculoskeletal System						
Arthralgia	25	25	27	31	21	18
Nervous System						
Insomnia	14	13	22	14	18	8
Tremor	31	21	30	22	28	19
Respiratory System						
Dyspnea	22	24	28	30	23	30
Pharyngitis	17	16	16	21	17	22
Upper respiratory infection	20	26	24	23	13	23
Skin And Appendages						
Acne	31	22	20	22	17	19
Rash	12	10	13	20	6	6
Urogenital System						
Urinary tract infection	20	26	23	33	31	26

a: Patients received cyclosporine and corticosteroids.

following transplant surgery has been reported, including fascial dehiscence and anastomotic disruption (e.g., wound, vascular, airway, ureteral, biliary).

The safety and efficacy of conversion from calcineurin inhibitors to sirolimus in maintenance renal transplant population has not been established. In an ongoing study evaluating the safety and efficacy of conversion from calcineurin inhibitors to sirolimus (target levels of 12–20 ng/mL) in maintenance renal transplant patients; enrollment was stopped in the subset of patients (n=90) with a baseline glomerular filtration rate of less than 40 mL/min. There was a higher rate of serious adverse events including pneumonia, acute rejection, graft loss and death in this sirolimus treatment arm.

OVERDOSAGE

Reports of overdose with Rapamune have been received; however, experience has been limited. In general, the adverse effects of overdose are consistent with those listed in the **ADVERSE REACTIONS** section (see **ADVERSE REACTIONS**).

General supportive measures should be followed in all cases of overdose. Based on the poor aqueous solubility and high erythrocyte and plasma protein binding of sirolimus, it is anticipated that sirolimus is not dialyzable to any significant extent. In mice and rats, the acute oral lethal dose was greater than 800 mg/kg.

DOSAGE AND ADMINISTRATION

It is recommended that Rapamune Oral Solution and Tablets be used initially in a regimen with cyclosporine and corticosteroids. Cyclosporine withdrawal is recommended 2 to 4 months after transplantation in patients at low to moderate immunologic risk.

The safety and efficacy of cyclosporine withdrawal in high-risk patients have not been adequately studied and it is therefore not recommended. This includes patients with Banff grade III acute rejection or vascular rejection prior to cyclosporine withdrawal, those who are dialysis-dependent, or with serum creatinine > 4.5 mg/dL, black patients, re-transplants, multi-organ transplants, patients with high panel of reactive antibodies (See **INDICATIONS AND USAGE** and **CLINICAL STUDIES**).

Two-mg of Rapamune oral solution has been demonstrated to be clinically equivalent to 2-mg Rapamune oral tablets and hence, are interchangeable on a mg to mg basis. However, it is not known if higher doses of Rapamune oral solution are clinically equivalent to higher doses of tablets on a mg to mg basis. (See **CLINICAL PHARMACOLOGY: Absorption**). Rapamune is to be administered orally once daily.

Rapamune and cyclosporine combination therapy: The initial dose of Rapamune should be administered as soon as possible after transplantation. For *de novo* transplant recipients, a loading dose of Rapamune of 3 times the maintenance dose should be given. A daily maintenance dose of 2-mg is recommended for use in renal transplant patients, with a loading dose of 6 mg. Although a daily maintenance dose of 5 mg, with a loading dose of 15 mg was used in clinical trials of the oral solution and was shown to be safe and effective, no efficacy advantage over the 2-mg dose could be established for renal transplant patients. Patients receiving 2 mg of Rapamune Oral Solution per day demonstrated an overall better safety profile than did patients receiving 5 mg of Rapamune Oral Solution per day.

Rapamune following cyclosporine withdrawal: Initially, patients considered for cyclosporine withdrawal should be receiving Rapamune and cyclosporine combination therapy. At 2 to 4 months following transplantation, cyclosporine should be progressively discontinued over 4 to 8 weeks and the Rapamune® dose should be adjusted to obtain whole blood trough concentrations within the range of 12 to 24 ng/mL (chromatographic method). Therapeutic drug monitoring should not be the sole basis for adjusting Rapamune therapy. Careful attention should be made to clinical signs/symptoms, tissue biopsy, and laboratory parameters. Cyclosporine inhibits the metabolism and transport of sirolimus, and consequently, sirolimus concentrations will decrease when cyclosporine is discontinued unless the Rapamune dose is increased. The Rapamune® dose will need to be approximately 4-fold higher to account for both the absence of the pharmacokinetic interaction (approximately 2-fold increase) and the augmented immunosuppressive requirement in the absence of cyclosporine (approximately 2-fold increase).

Frequent Rapamune® dose adjustments based on non-steady-state sirolimus concentrations can lead to overdosing or underdosing because sirolimus has a long half-life. Once Rapamune® maintenance dose is adjusted, patients should be retained on the new maintenance dose at least for 7 to 14 days before further dosage adjustment with concentration monitoring. In most patients dose adjustments can be based on simple proportion: new Rapamune® dose = current dose x (target concentration / current concentration). A loading dose should be considered in addition to a new maintenance dose when it is necessary to considerably increase sirolimus trough concentrations: Rapamune® loading dose = 3 x (new maintenance dose - current maintenance dose). The maximum Rapamune® dose administered on any day should not exceed 40 mg. If an estimated daily dose exceeds 40 mg due to the addition of a loading dose, the loading dose should be administered over 2 days. Sirolimus trough concentrations should be monitored at least 3 to 4 days after a loading dose(s).

To minimize the variability of exposure to Rapamune, this drug should be taken consistently with or without food. Grapefruit juice reduces CYP3A4-mediated drug metabolism and potentially enhances P-gp mediated drug counter-transport from enterocytes of the small intestine. This juice must not be administered with Rapamune or used for dilution.

It is recommended that sirolimus be taken 4 hours after administration of cyclosporine oral solution (MODIFIED) and/or cyclosporine capsules (MODIFIED).

Dosage Adjustments

The initial dosage in patients ≥13 years who weigh less than 40 kg should be adjusted, based on body surface area, to 1 mg/m²/day. The loading dose should be 3 mg/m².

It is recommended that the maintenance dose of Rapamune be reduced by approximately one third in patients with hepatic impairment. It is not necessary to modify the Rapamune loading dose. Dosage need not be adjusted because of impaired renal function.

Blood Concentration Monitoring

Whole blood trough concentrations of sirolimus should be monitored in patients receiving concentration-controlled Rapamune®. Monitoring is also necessary in pediatric patients, in patients with hepatic impairment, during concurrent administration of CYP3A4 and/or P-gp inducers and inhibitors, and/or if cyclosporine dosage is markedly changed or discontinued (see **DOSAGE AND ADMINISTRATION**).

In controlled clinical trials with concomitant cyclosporine (Studies 1 and 2), mean sirolimus whole blood trough concentrations through month 12 following transplantation, as measured by immunoassay, were 9 ng/mL (range 4.5–14 ng/mL [10th to 90th percentile]) for the 2 mg/day treatment group, and 17 ng/mL (range 10–28 ng/mL [10th to 90th percentile]) for the 5 mg/day dose.

In a controlled clinical trial with cyclosporine withdrawal (Study 4), the mean sirolimus whole blood trough concentrations during months 4 through 12 following transplantation, as measured by immunoassay, were 10.7 ng/mL (range 6.3–16.0 ng/mL [10th to 90th percentile]) in the concomitant Rapamune and cyclosporine treatment group (n = 205) and were 23.3 ng/mL (range 17.0–29.0 ng/mL [10th to 90th percentile]) in the cyclosporine withdrawal treatment group (n = 200).

Results from other assays may differ from those with an immunoassay. On average, chromatographic methods (HPLC UV or LC/MS/MS) yield results that are approximately 20% lower than the immunoassay for whole blood concentration determinations. Adjustments to the targeted range should be made according to the assay utilized to determine sirolimus trough concentrations. Therefore, comparison between concentrations in the published literature and an individual patient concentration using current assays must be made with detailed knowledge of the assay methods employed. A discussion of the different assay methods is contained in *Clinical Therapeutics*, Volume 22, Supplement B, April 2000.

Instructions for Dilution and Administration of Rapamune® Oral Solution Bottles

The amber oral dose syringe should be used to withdraw the prescribed amount of Rapamune® Oral Solution from the bottle. Empty the correct amount of Rapamune from the syringe into only a glass or plastic container holding at least two (2) ounces (1/4 cup, 60 mL) of water or orange juice. No other liquids, including grapefruit juice, should be used for dilution. Stir vigorously and drink at once. Refill the container with an additional volume (minimum of four [4] ounces [1/2 cup, 120 mL]) of water or orange juice, stir vigorously, and drink at once.

Handling and Disposal

Since Rapamune is not absorbed through the skin, there are no special precautions. However, if direct contact with the skin or mucous membranes occurs, wash thoroughly with soap and water; rinse eyes with plain water.

HOW SUPPLIED

Rapamune® Oral Solution is supplied at a concentration of 1 mg/mL in:

Cartons:

NDC # 0008-1030-06, containing a 2 oz (60 mL fill) amber glass bottle.

In addition to the bottles, each carton is supplied with an oral syringe adapter for fitting into the neck of the bottle, sufficient disposable amber oral syringes and caps for daily dosing, and a carrying case.

Rapamune® Tablets are available as follows:

1 mg, white, triangular-shaped tablets marked "RAPAMUNE 1 mg" on one side.

NDC # 0008-1031-05, bottle of 100 tablets.

NDC # 0008-1031-10, Redipak® cartons of 100 tablets (10 blister cards of 10 tablets each).

2 mg, yellow to beige triangular-shaped tablets marked "RAPAMUNE 2 mg" on one side.

NDC # 0008-1032-05, bottle of 100 tablets.

NDC # 0008-1032-10, Redipak® cartons of 100 tablets (10 blister cards of 10 tablets each [2 x 5]).

Storage

Rapamune® Oral Solution bottles should be stored protected from light and refrigerated at 2°C to 8°C (36°F to 46°F). Once the bottle is opened, the contents should be used within one month. If necessary, the patient may store the bottles at room temperatures up to 25°C (77°F) for a short period of time (e.g., not more than 15 days for the bottles).

An amber syringe and cap are provided for dosing and the product may be kept in the syringe for a maximum of 24 hours at room temperatures up to 25°C (77°F) or refrigerated at 2°C to 8°C (36°F to 46°F). The syringe should be discarded after one use. After dilution, the preparation should be used immediately.

Rapamune Oral Solution provided in bottles may develop a slight haze when refrigerated. If such a haze occurs allow the product to stand at room temperature and shake gently until the haze disappears. The presence of this haze does not affect the quality of the product.

Rapamune® Tablets should be stored at 20° to 25°C (USP Controlled Room Temperature) (68° to 77°F). Use cartons to protect blister cards and strips from light. Dispense in a tight, light-resistant container as defined in the USP.

US Pat. Nos.: 5,100,899; 5,212,155; 5,308,847; 5,403,833; 5,536,729.

INCIDENCE (%) OF MALIGNANCIES IN STUDY 1 (24 MONTHS) AND STUDY 2 (36 MONTHS) POST-TRANSPLANT[a,b]

Malignancy	Rapamune® Oral Solution 2 mg/day Study 1 (n = 284)	Rapamune® Oral Solution 2 mg/day Study 2 (n = 227)	Rapamune® Oral Solution 5 mg/day Study 1 (n = 274)	Rapamune® Oral Solution 5 mg/day Study 2 (n = 219)	Azathioprine 2-3 mg/kg/day Study 1 (n = 161)	Placebo Study 2 (n = 130)
Lymphoma/ lymphoproliferative disease	**0.7**	**1.8**	**1.1**	**3.2**	**0.6**	**0.8**
Skin Carcinoma						
Any Squamous Cell[c]	0.4	2.7	2.2	0.9	3.8	3.0
Any Basal Cell[c]	0.7	2.2	1.5	1.8	2.5	5.3
Melanoma	0.0	0.4	0.0	1.4	0.0	0.0
Miscellaneous/Not Specified	0.0	0.0	0.0	0.0	0.0	0.8
Total	**1.1**	**4.4**	**3.3**	**4.1**	**4.3**	**7.7**
Other Malignancy	**1.1**	**2.2**	**1.5**	**1.4**	**0.6**	**2.3**

a: Patients received cyclosporine and corticosteroids.
b: Includes patients who prematurely discontinued treatment.
c: Patients may be counted in more than one category.

INCIDENCE (%) OF MALIGNANCIES IN STUDY 4 AT 36 MONTHS POST-TRANSPLANT[a,b]

Malignancy	Nonrandomized (n = 95)	Rapamune with Cyclosporine Therapy (n = 215)	Rapamune Following Cyclosporine Withdrawal (n = 215)
Lymphoma/lymphoproliferative disease	**1.1**	**1.4**	**0.5**
Skin Carcinoma			
Any Squamous Cell[c]	1.1	1.9	2.3
Any Basal Cell[c]	3.2	4.7	2.3
Melanoma	0.0	0.5	0.0
Miscellaneous/Not Specified	1.1	0.9	0.0
Total	**4.2**	**6.5**	**3.7**
Other Malignancy	**1.1**	**3.3**	**1.4**

a: Patients received cyclosporine and corticosteroids.
b: Includes patients who prematurely discontinued treatment.
c: Patients may be counted in more than one category.

Continued on next page

Rapamune—Cont.

PATIENT INSTRUCTIONS FOR RAPAMUNE® (SIROLIMUS) ORAL SOLUTION ADMINISTRATION

Bottles

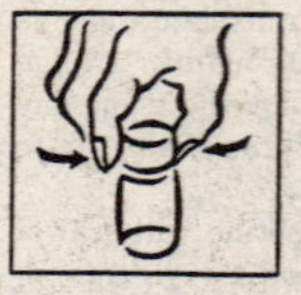

1. Open the solution bottle. Remove the safety cap by squeezing the tabs on the cap and twisting counter-clockwise.

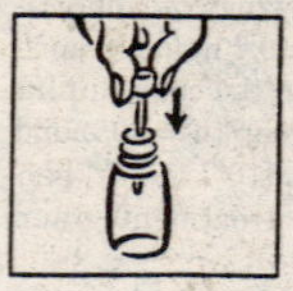

2. On first use, insert the adapter assembly (plastic tube with stopper) tightly into the bottle until it is even with the top of the bottle. Do not remove the adapter assembly from the bottle once inserted.

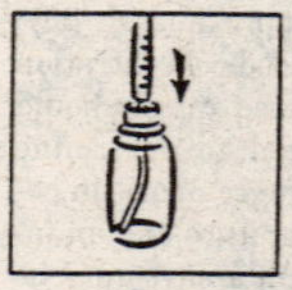

3. For each use, tightly insert one of the amber syringes with the plunger fully depressed into the opening in the adapter.

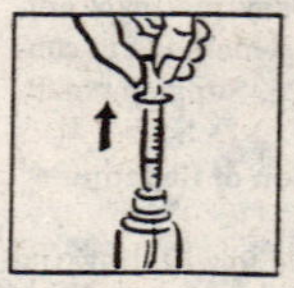

4. Withdraw the prescribed amount of Rapamune® Oral Solution by gently pulling out the plunger of the syringe until the bottom of the black line of the plunger is even with the appropriate mark on the syringe. Always keep the bottle in an upright position. If bubbles form in the syringe, empty the syringe into the bottle and repeat the procedure.

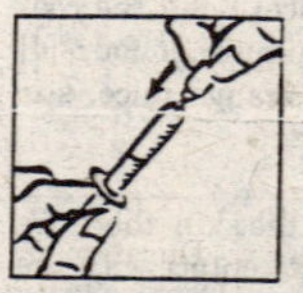

5. You may have been instructed to carry your medication with you. If it is necessary to carry the filled syringe, place a cap securely on the syringe – the cap should snap into place.

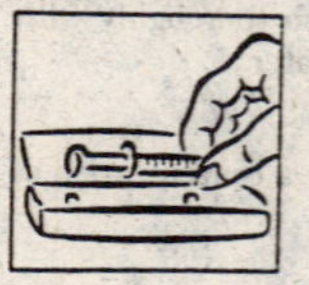

6. Then place the capped syringe in the enclosed carrying case. Once in the syringe, the medication may be kept at room temperature or refrigerated and should be used within 24 hours. Extreme temperatures (below 36°F and above 86°F) should be avoided. Remember to keep this medication out of the reach of children.

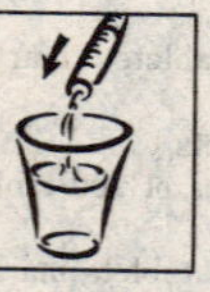

7. Empty the syringe into a glass or plastic cup containing at least 2 ounces (1/4 cup, 60 mL) of water or orange juice, stir vigorously for one (1) minute and drink immediately. Refill the container with at least 4 ounces (1/2 cup, 120 mL) of water or orange juice, stir vigorously again and drink the rinse solution. Apple juice, grapefruit juice, or other liquids are NOT to be used. Only glass or plastic cups should be used to dilute Rapamune® Oral Solution. The syringe and cap should be used once and then discarded.

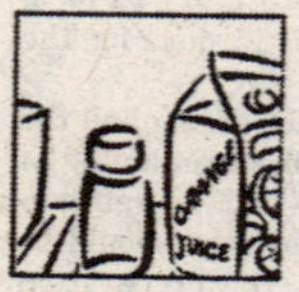

8. Always store the bottles of medication in the refrigerator. When refrigerated, a slight haze may develop in the solution. The presence of a haze does not affect the quality of the product. If this happens, bring the Rapamune® Oral Solution to room temperature and shake until the haze disappears. If it is necessary to wipe clean the mouth of the bottle before returning the product to the refrigerator, wipe with a dry cloth to avoid introducing water, or any other liquid, into the bottle.

Wyeth Laboratories
A Wyeth-Ayerst Company
Philadelphia, PA 19101

W10431C004
ET01
Rev 1/04

REFACTO® ℞

[*rē-făk'tō*]
Antihemophilic Factor, Recombinant
℞ only

Prescribing information for this product, which appears on pages 3490–3492 of the 2004 PDR, has been revised as follows. Please write "See Supplement A" next to the product heading.

The **DESCRIPTION** *section has been revised as follows:*

ReFacto® Antihemophilic Factor (Recombinant) is a purified protein produced by recombinant DNA technology for use in therapy of factor VIII deficiency. ReFacto is a glycoprotein with an approximate molecular mass of 170 kDa consisting of 1438 amino acids. It has an amino acid sequence that is comparable to the 90 + 80 kDa form of factor VIII, and post-translational modifications that are similar to those of the plasma-derived molecule. ReFacto has *in vitro* functional characteristics comparable to those of endogenous factor VIII.

ReFacto is produced by a genetically engineered Chinese hamster ovary (CHO) cell line. The CHO cell line secretes B-domain deleted recombinant factor VIII into a defined cell culture medium that contains human serum albumin and recombinant insulin, but does not contain any proteins derived from animal sources. The protein is purified by a chromatography purification process that yields a high-purity, active product. The potency expressed in international units (IU) is determined using the European Pharmacopoeial chromogenic assay against the WHO standard. The specific activity of ReFacto is 9110-13700 IU per milligram of protein. ReFacto is not purified from human blood and contains no preservatives or added human components in the final formulation. ReFacto is formulated as a sterile, nonpyrogenic, lyophilized powder preparation for intravenous (IV) injection. It is available in single-use vials containing the labeled amount of factor VIII activity (IU). Each vial contains nominally 250, 500, 1000 or 2000 IU of ReFacto per vial. The formulated product is a clear colorless solution upon reconstitution and contains sodium chloride, sucrose, L-histidine, calcium chloride, and polysorbate 80.

Genetics Institute, Inc.
Cambridge MA 02140-2387, USA
US License Number 1163
Telephone: 1-800-934-5556
W10403C003
ET01
Rev 06/03

SYNVISC® ℞

[*sĭn'vĭsk*]
HYLAN G-F 20

Prescribing information for this product, which appears on pages 3492–3494 of the 2004 PDR, has been completely revised as follows. Please write "See Supplement A" next to the product heading.

Caution: Federal law restricts this device to sale by or on the order of a physician (or properly licensed practitioner).

DESCRIPTION

Synvisc® (hylan G-F 20) is an elastoviscous fluid containing hylan polymers produced from chicken combs. Hylans are derivatives of hyaluronan (sodium hyaluronate), a natural complex sugar of the glycosaminoglycan family. Hyaluronan is a long-chain polymer containing repeating disaccharide units of Na-glucuronate-N-acetylglucosamine.

INDICATIONS

Synvisc is indicated for the treatment of pain in osteoarthritis (OA) of the knee in patients who have failed to respond adequately to conservative nonpharmacologic therapy and simple analgesics, e.g., acetaminophen.

CONTRAINDICATIONS

- Do not administer to patients with known hypersensitivity (allergy) to hyaluronan (sodium hyaluronate) preparations.
- Do not inject Synvisc in the knees of patients having knee joint infections or skin diseases or infections in the area of the injection site.

WARNINGS

- Do not concomitantly use disinfectants containing quaternary ammonium salts for skin preparation because hyaluronan can precipitate in their presence.
- Do not inject Synvisc extra-articularly or into the synovial tissues and capsule. Local and systemic adverse events, generally in the area of the injection, have occurred following extra-articular injection of Synvisc.
- Intravascular injections of Synvisc may cause systemic adverse events.

PRECAUTIONS

General

- The effectiveness of a single treatment cycle of less than three injections of Synvisc has not been established.
- The safety and effectiveness of Synvisc in locations other than the knee and for conditions other than osteoarthritis have not been established.
- Do not inject anesthetics or other medications into the knee joint during Synvisc therapy. Such medications may dilute Synvisc and affect its safety and effectiveness.
- Use caution when injecting Synvisc into patients who are allergic to avian proteins, feathers and egg products.
- The safety and effectiveness of Synvisc in severely inflamed knee joints have not been established.
- Strict aseptic administration technique must be followed.
- STERILE CONTENTS. The syringe is intended for single use. The contents of the syringe must be used immediately after its packaging is opened. Discard any unused Synvisc.
- Do not use Synvisc if package is opened or damaged. Store in original packaging (protected from light) at room temperature below 86°F (30°C). DO NOT FREEZE.
- Remove synovial fluid or effusion before each Synvisc injection.
- Synvisc should be used with caution when there is evidence of lymphatic or venous stasis in that leg.

Information for Patients

- Provide patients with a copy of the Patient Labeling prior to use.
- Transient pain, swelling and/or effusion of the injected joint may occur after intra-articular injection of Synvisc. In some cases the effusion may be considerable and can cause pronounced pain; cases where swelling is extensive should be discussed with the physician.
- As with any invasive joint procedure, it is recommended that the patient avoid any strenuous activities or prolonged weight-bearing activities such as jogging or tennis following the intra-articular injection.
- The packaging of this product contains dry natural rubber latex.

Use in Specific Populations

- **Pregnancy:** The safety and effectiveness of Synvisc have not been established in pregnant women.
- **Nursing mothers:** It is not known if Synvisc is excreted in human milk. The safety and effectiveness of Synvisc have not been established in lactating women.
- The safety and effectiveness of Synvisc have not been established in children.

ADVERSE EVENTS

Adverse Events Involving the Injected Joint

Clinical Trials: A total of 511 patients (559 knees) received 1771 injections in seven clinical trials of Synvisc. There were 39 reports in 37 patients (2.2% of injections, 7.2% of patients) of knee pain and/or swelling after these injections. Ten patients (10 knees) were treated with arthrocentesis and removal of joint effusion. Two additional patients (two knees) received treatment with intra-articular steroids. Two patients (two knees) received NSAIDs. One of these patients also received arthrocentesis. One patient was treated with arthroscopy. The remaining patients with adverse events localized to the knee received no treatment or only analgesics.

Postmarket Experience: The most common adverse events reported have been pain, swelling and/or effusion in the injected knee. In some cases the effusion was considerable and caused pronounced pain. In some instances, patients have presented with knees that were tender, warm and red. It is important to rule out infection or crystalline arthropathies in such cases. Synovial fluid aspirates of varying volumes have revealed a range of cell counts, from very few to over 50,000 cells/mm^3. Reported treatments included symptomatic therapy (e.g., rest, ice, heat, elevation, simple analgesics and NSAIDs) and/or arthrocentesis. Intra-articular corticosteroids have been used when infection was excluded. Rarely, arthroscopy has been performed. The occurrence of post-injection effusion may be associated with patient history of effusion, advanced stage of disease and/or the number of injections or treatment courses a patient receives. Reactions generally abate within a few days. Clinical benefit from the treatment may still occur after such reactions.

The clinical trials described above included 38 patients who received a second course of Synvisc injections (132 injections). There were twelve reports in nine patients (9.1% of injections, 23.7% of patients) of knee pain and/or swelling after these injections. Reports of two additional clinical trials in which patients received repeated courses of Synvisc treatment have appeared during the post-marketing period. One of these trials included 48 patients who received 210 injections during a second course of Synvisc treatment[1]; the other contained 71 patients who received 211 injections during a second course of Synvisc treatment.

A total of 157 patients have received 553 injections in the three clinical trials of repeated courses of Synvisc treatment. The reports in these trials describe a total of 48 reports of adverse events localized to the injected knee in 35 patients that occurred after injections that patients had received during their second course of treatment. These adverse events accounted for 6.3% of injections in 22.3% of patients as compared to 2.2% of injections in 7.2% of patients in a single course of Synvisc injections. In addition, reports of two retrospective studies during the post-marketing period have described adverse events localized to the injected knee that have occurred after 4.4% and 8.5% of injections that patients had received during one or more repeated courses of Synvisc treatment.[2,3]

Intra-articular infections did not occur in any of the clinical trials and have been reported only rarely during clinical use of Synvisc.

Other Adverse Events

Clinical Trials: In three concurrently controlled clinical trials with a total of 112 patients who received Synvisc and 110 patients who received either saline or arthrocentesis, there were no statistically significant differences in the numbers or types of adverse events between the group of patients that received Synvisc and the group that received control treatments.

TABLE 2
CONCURRENT OSTEOARTHRITIS THERAPIES[1]

CONCURRENT MEDICATIONS[2]	TREATED KNEES TOTAL	Synvisc	Control	P Synvisc/ Control
German Multicenter	N[3]=109	N=52	N=57	
Medications [N (%)][4]	27 (25%)	5 (10%)	22 (39%)	0.001
NSAIDS	17 (16%)	4 (8%)	13 (23%)	0.03
Acetaminophen	7 (6%)	1 (2%)	6 (11%)	0.07
Other medications[5]	3 (3%)	3 (5%)	0 (0%)	0.09
German Single Center[6]	N=29	N=14	N=15	
Any concurrent medication [N (%)]	NA[7]	NA	NA	NA
U.S. Multicenter[8]	N=103	N=51	N=52	
Acetaminophen [N (%)]	100 (97%)	50 (98%)	50 (96%)	0.6

Footnotes:
[1] Patients ≥ 40 years old and received the complete treatment course
[2] Individual patients may be represented by more than one therapy
[3] N = number of knees
[4] Number and percentage of subjects
[5] Medications not approved in the U.S.
[6] No concurrent therapies were recorded
[7] Data not collected
[8] Only acetaminophen was allowed

TABLE 3A
EFFECTIVENESS OF WEIGHT-BEARING PAIN[1]
EVALUATED BY PATIENTS

	Baseline	Improvement (Change from Baseline)						
Week	0	1	2	3	4	8	12	26[6]
German Multicenter								
Synvisc-treated								
Mean[2]	69.7	12.0	26.5	37.9	NA[5]	45.9	46.5	34.0
P[3]		0.0001	0.0001	0.0001		0.0001	0.0001	0.0001
Saline-treated								
Mean	75.1	9.0	17.0	23.0	NA	16.8	16.4	19.1
P[3]		0.0001	0.0001	0.0001		0.0001	0.0002	0.0001
P[4]	0.1	0.3	0.01	0.0008	NA	<0.0001	<0.0001	0.005
German Single Center								
Synvisc-treated								
Mean	65.2	10.6	31.8	43.9	NA	51.7	53.5	44.5
P[3]		0.02	0.0001	0.0001		0.0001	0.0001	0.0001
Saline-treated								
Mean	69.8	5.4	19.3	25.4	NA	24.4	26.8	21.2
P[3]		0.01	0.0001	0.0001		0.0001	0.0001	0.002
P[4]	0.4	0.2	0.03	0.01	NA	0.0001	0.0001	0.001
U.S. Multicenter								
Synvisc-treated								
Mean	67.3	12.9	18.9	NA	21.3	NA	NA	NA
P[3]		0.0002	0.0001		0.0001			
Arthrocenteses								
Mean	69.4	9.4	21.2	NA	19.1	NA	NA	NA
P[3]		0.01	0.0001		0.0002			
P[4]	0.6	0.5	0.7	NA	0.7	NA	NA	NA

Footnotes:
[1] Patients ≥ 40 years old and received the complete treatment course
[2] Mean of assessments on VAS of 0 to 100 mm
[3] Significance from baseline
[4] Significance between Synvisc and control
[5] NA = no measurement taken
[6] Week 26 data based on patient telephone interviews rather than patient office visit

Systemic adverse events each occurred in 10 (2.0%) of the Synvisc-treated patients. There was one case each of rash (thorax and back) and itching of the skin following Synvisc injections in these studies. These symptoms did not recur when these patients received additional Synvisc injections. The remaining generalized adverse events reported were calf cramps, hemorrhoid problems, ankle edema, muscle pain, tonsillitis with nausea, tachyarrythmia, phlebitis with varicosities and low back sprain.

Postmarket Experience: Other adverse events reported include: rash, *hives*, itching, *fever*, nausea, *headache*, *dizziness*, *chills*, muscle cramps, *paresthesia*, peripheral edema, *malaise*, *respiratory difficulties*, *flushing* and *facial swelling*. There have been rare reports of *thrombocytopenia* coincident with Synvisc injection. These medical events occurred under circumstances where causal relationship to Synvisc is uncertain. (Adverse events reported *only* in worldwide postmarketing experience, not seen in clinical trials, are considered more rare and are *italicized*.)

CLINICAL STUDIES

The safety and effectiveness of Synvisc were studied in patients ≥40 years old in the three concurrently controlled clinical trials. The three studies investigated a total of 136 women and 81 men. The demographics of trial participants were comparable across treatment groups with regard to age, gender and duration of osteoarthritis, except that there was a significantly greater ($p = 0.04$) number of men in the Synvisc group and women in the control group in one study (see Table 1).

One study was a multicenter study conducted at four sites in Germany. This was a randomized, double-blind prospective clinical trial with two treatment groups. The study compared the safety and effectiveness of three weekly intra-articular injections of Synvisc and of physiological saline in 103 subjects (109 knees) with osteoarthritis of the knee over a 26-week period.

A significantly greater number of saline-treated patients took concurrent osteoarthritis medications than did patients treated with Synvisc (see Table 2). While both the Synvisc and the saline-treated groups improved significantly as compared to baseline in all effectiveness measures, the Synvisc group showed a significantly greater improvement in all outcome measures than did the saline-treated patients over a 26-week period (see Tables 3A and 3B).

A second study conducted at a single center in Germany[4] was a concurrently controlled, randomized, double-blind prospective clinical trial with two treatment groups. This study compared the safety and effectiveness over a 26-week period of three weekly intra-articular injections of Synvisc and of physiological saline in 29 subjects (29 knees) with osteoarthritis of the knee. The results of the study were similar to those in the German multicenter study, except that the significance levels in most comparisons were smaller (see Tables 3A and 3B). In both of these studies the most pain relief and the greatest amount of treatment success occurred 8 to 12 weeks after Synvisc treatment began. Investigators obtained data at 26 weeks by telephone interviews. A validation study suggested that the results obtained in telephone interviews are equivalent to those obtained in office visits. Since investigators did not follow patients beyond week 26, the duration of pain relief beyond 26 weeks is not known.

A third study was a prospective, concurrently controlled, randomized, double-blind multicenter study conducted in 90 subjects (103 knees) at five U.S. sites. The study compared the safety and effectiveness of three weekly intra-articular injections of Synvisc and of three weekly arthrocenteses in subjects with osteoarthritis of the knee over a four-week period after the first injection or arthrocentesis.

Both the Synvisc-treated and the arthrocentesis-treated groups improved significantly as compared to baseline in all effectiveness measures. However, there were no significant differences between the Synvisc-treated and arthrocentesis-treated patients at any time during the four-week evaluation period (see Tables 3A and 3B).

Covariate analyses with the covariates of center, presence or absence of previous treatments, baseline levels of outcome measures, age, gender, body mass, effusion, baseline X-ray score, duration of osteoarthritis, treatment of contralateral knee, and presence or absence of concurrent therapies, did not reveal any factors that significantly affected the results of any of the three studies.

The German studies and the U.S. study differed in several respects, including inclusion of patients with effusions, length of no treatment period prior to Synvisc injection, nature of control treatment, final evaluation time, mean duration of disease, mean weight, prior treatments for OA, pain and X-ray inclusion criteria. Thus, the German and the U.S. studies, which gave different results, investigated different patient populations and compared Synvisc with different control treatments.

Although success criteria for safety were not specified in any of the three studies, adverse events were enumerated in each study. These events are included in the "Adverse Events" section.

TABLE 1
DEMOGRAPHIC DATA[1]

	DEMOGRAPHIC VARIABLE Age	Gender [N[2] (%)] M	F	Duration of Osteoarthritis (years)
German Multicenter[3]				
Synvisc	62.3	21 (45%)	26 (55%)	5.4
Saline	64.7	13 (25%)	39 (75%)	5.6
P (Synvisc/Saline)	0.3	0.04		0.9
German Single Center				
Synvisc	59.8	10 (71%)	4 (29%)	2.4
Saline	59.5	8 (53%)	7 (47%)	2.5
P (Synvisc/Saline)	0.9	0.3		1.0
U.S. Multicenter[4]				
Synvisc	62.9	17 (39%)	27 (61%)	8.9
Arthrocenteses	67.1	12 (29%)	30 (71%)	7.9
P (Synvisc/ Arthrocenteses)	0.06	0.3		0.5

Footnotes:
[1] Patients ≥ 40 years old and received the complete treatment course
[2] N = number of patients
[3] In addition, 1 male and 3 females were treated with Synvisc in one knee and saline in the other
[4] In addition, 4 females were treated with Synvisc in one knee and arthrocenteses in the other

[See table 2 above]
[See table 3A above]
[See table 3B at top of next page]

DETAILED DEVICE DESCRIPTION

Synvisc contains hylan A (average molecular weight 6,000,000) and hylan B hydrated gel in a buffered physiological sodium chloride solution, pH 7.2. Synvisc has an elasticity (storage modulus G') at 2.5 Hz of 111 ± 13 Pascals (Pa) and a viscosity (loss modulus G") of 25 ± 2 Pa (elasticity and viscosity of knee synovial fluid of 18 to 27-year-old humans measured with a comparable method at 2.5 Hz: G' = 117 ± 13 Pa; G" = 45 ± 8 Pa.)

Each syringe of Synvisc contains:

Hylan polymers (hylan A + hylan B)	16 mg
Sodium chloride	17 mg

Continued on next page

Synvisc—Cont.

Disodium hydrogen phosphate	0.32 mg
Sodium dihydrogen phosphate monohydrate	0.08 mg
Water for injection	q.s. to 2.0 mL

HOW SUPPLIED

Synvisc is supplied in a 2.25 mL glass syringe containing 2 mL Synvisc.

Product Number: 0008-9149-02 3 disposable syringes

The contents of the syringe are sterile and nonpyrogenic.

DIRECTIONS FOR USE

Synvisc is administered by intra-articular injection once a week (one week apart) for a total of three injections.

Precaution: Do not use Synvisc if the package has been opened or damaged. Store in original packaging (protected from light) at room temperature below 86°F (30°C). DO NOT FREEZE.

Precaution: Strict aseptic administration technique must be followed.

Precaution: Do not concomitantly use disinfectants containing quaternary ammonium salts for skin preparation because hyaluronan can precipitate in their presence.

Precaution: Remove synovial fluid or effusion before each Synvisc injection.

Do not use the same syringe for removing synovial fluid and for injecting Synvisc, but the same needle should be used.

Take particular care to remove the tip cap of the syringe and needle aseptically.

Twist the gray tip cap before pulling it off, as this will minimize product leakage.

Inject Synvisc into the knee joint through an 18 to 22 gauge needle.

To ensure a tight seal and prevent leakage during administration, secure the needle tightly while firmly holding the luer hub.

Precaution: Do not over tighten or apply excessive leverage when attaching the needle or removing the needle guard, as this may break the tip of the syringe.

Do not inject anesthetics or any other medications intra-articularly into the knee while administering Synvisc therapy. This may dilute Synvisc and affect its safety and effectiveness.

Precaution: The syringe containing Synvisc is intended for single use. The contents of the syringe must be used immediately after the syringe has been removed from its packaging. Inject the full 2 mL in one knee only. If treatment is bilateral, a separate syringe must be used for each knee. Discard any unused Synvisc.

DISTRIBUTED BY:
Wyeth-Ayerst Pharmaceuticals
Philadelphia, Pennsylvania 19101
Telephone: 1-800-99-WYETH

DEVELOPED AND MANUFACTURED BY:
Genzyme Biosurgery
a division of Genzyme Corporation
1125 Pleasant View Terrace
Ridgefield, New Jersey 07657

Covered by U.S. patents #4,636,524, #4,713,448, #5,099,013, #5,143,724.

REFERENCES

1. Raynauld, J.P., Bellamy, N., Goldsmith, C.H., Tugwell, P., Torrance, G.W., Pericak, D., et al. (2002). An evaluation of the safety and effectiveness of repeat courses of hylan G-F 20 for treating patients with knee osteoarthritis. Osteoarthritis Research Society International, 2002 OARSI World Congress on Osteoarthritis, Sydney, Australia [Paper reference # PS128]. Presentation on File.
2. Leopold, S.S., Warme, W.J., Pettis, P.D. and Shott, S. (2002). Increased frequency of acute local reaction to intra-articular Hylan GF-20 (Synvisc) in patients receiving more than one course of treatment. J. Bone Joint Surg. 84-A (9): 1619–1623.

TABLE 3B
EFFECTIVENESS OF NIGHT PAIN[1]
EVALUATED BY PATIENTS

	Baseline	Improvement (Change from Baseline)						
Week	0	1	2	3	4	8	12	26[6]
German Multicenter								
Synvisc-treated								
Mean[2]	41.6	9.2	20.0	26.4	NA[5]	28.3	29.8	24.3
P[3]		0.0001	0.0001	0.0001		0.0001	0.0001	0.0001
Saline-treated								
Mean	45.7	9.5	15.2	21.2	NA	18.4	17.3	12.8
P[3]		0.0001	0.0001	0.0001		0.0001	0.0001	0.002
P[4]	0.5	0.9	0.2	0.3	NA	0.05	0.02	0.03
German Single Center								
Synvisc-treated								
Mean	31.8	8.4	17.7	24.8	NA	28.9	29.5	25.4
P[3]		0.04	0.005	0.004		0.005	0.005	0.004
Saline-treated								
Mean	33.3	4.5	13.1	16.1	NA	16.1	17.9	14.9
P[3]		0.1	0.001	0.0007		0.0001	0.0001	0.01
P[4]	0.9	0.4	0.4	0.3	NA	0.1	0.2	0.2
U.S. Multicenter								
Synvisc-treated								
Mean	61.0	19.0	17.9	NA	22.8	NA	NA	NA
P[3]		0.0001	0.0001		0.0001			
Arthrocenteses								
Mean	76.0	23.3	36.3	NA	29.8	NA	NA	NA
P[3]		0.0001	0.0001		0.0001			
P[4]	0.002	0.5	0.004	NA	0.3	NA	NA	NA

Footnotes:
[1] Patients ≥ 40 years old and received the complete treatment course
[2] Mean of assessments on VAS of 0 to 100 mm
[3] Significance from baseline
[4] Significance between Synvisc and control
[5] NA = no measurement taken
[6] Week 26 data based on patient telephone interviews rather than patient office visit

3. Waddell, D.D., Estey, D.J. and Bricker, D. (2001). Retrospective tolerance of Hylan G-F 20 using fluoroscopically-confirmed injection and effectiveness of retreatment in knee osteoarthritis. Proceedings of the American College of Rheumatology Annual Meeting 2001. Presentation on File.
4. Scale, D., Wobig, and Wolpert, W. (1994). Viscosupplementation of osteoarthritic knees with hylan: a treatment schedule study. Curr. Ther. Res. 55: 220–232.

CI 6082-5 Revised October 7, 2003

ZOSYN® ℞

[zō′sĭn]

(Piperacillin and Tazobactam for Injection)

℞ only

Prescribing information for this product, which appears on pages 3501–3505 of the 2004 PDR, has been revised as follows. Please write "See Supplement A" next to the product heading.

The following has been added above the **DESCRIPTION** *section:*

To reduce the development of drug-resistant bacteria and maintain the effectiveness of Zosyn (piperacillin and tazobactam) injection and other antibacterial drugs, Zosyn (piperacillin and tazobactam) should be used only to treat or prevent infections that are proven or strongly suspected to be caused by bacteria.

In the **INDICATIONS AND USAGE** *section, the following has been added to the end of the section:*

To reduce the development of drug-resistant bacteria and maintain the effectiveness of Zosyn (piperacillin and tazobactam) injection and other antibacterial drugs, Zosyn (piperacillin and tazobactam) should be used only to treat or prevent infections that are proven or strongly suspected to be caused by susceptible bacteria. When culture and susceptibility information are available, they should be considered in selecting or modifying antibacterial therapy. In the absence of such data, local epidemiology and susceptibility patterns may contribute to the empiric selection of therapy.

In the **PRECAUTIONS** *section, the following has been added to the end of the "General" subsection:*

Prescribing Zosyn (piperacillin and tazobactam) in the absence of a proven or strongly suspected bacterial infection or a prophylactic indication is unlikely to provide benefit to the patient and increases the risk of development of drug-resistant bacteria.

In the **PRECAUTIONS** *section, the following has been added to the end of the "Drug/Laboratory Test Interactions" subsection:*

There have been reports of positive test results using the Bio-Rad Laboratories Platelia *Aspergillus* EIA test in patients receiving piperacillin/tazobactam injection who were subsequently found to be free of *Aspergillus* infection. Cross-reactions with non-*Aspergillus* polysaccharides and polyfuranoses with the Bio-Rad Laboratories Platelia *Aspergillus* EIA test have been reported. Therefore, positive test results in patients receiving piperacillin/tazobactam should be interpreted cautiously and confirmed by other diagnostic methods.

Wyeth Pharmaceuticals Inc.
Philadelphia, PA 19101
W10414C004 ET02
Rev 10/03

U.S. FOOD AND DRUG ADMINISTRATION

Medical Product Reporting Programs

MedWatch (24-hour service) **800-332-1088**
Reporting of problems with drugs, devices, biologics (except vaccines), medical foods, and dietary supplements.

Vaccine Adverse Event Reporting System (24-hour service) **800-822-7967**
Reporting of vaccine-related problems.

Mandatory Medical Device Reporting **301-827-0360**
Reporting required from user facilities regarding device-related deaths and serious injuries.

Veterinary Adverse Drug Reaction Program **888-332-8387**
Reporting of adverse drug events in animals.

Division of Drug Marketing, Advertising, and Communication (DDMAC) **301-827-2828**
Inquiries from health professionals regarding product promotion.

USP Medication Errors **800-233-7767**
Reporting of medication errors or near-errors to help avoid future problems through improvement in product names and packaging.

Information for Health Professionals

Center for Drug Evaluation and Research Drug Information Hotline **301-827-4573**
Information on human drugs including hormones.

Center for Biologics Office of Communications **301-827-2000**
Information on biological products including vaccines and blood.

Emergency Operations **301-443-1240**
Emergencies involving FDA-regulated products, tampering reports, and emergency Investigational New Drug requests.

Office of Orphan Products Development **301-827-3666**
Information on products for rare diseases.

General Information

General Consumer Inquiries **888-463-6332**
Consumer information on regulated products/issues.

Freedom of Information **301-827-6500**
Requests for publicly available FDA documents.

Office of Public Affairs **301-827-6250**
Interviews/press inquiries on FDA activities.

Center for Food Safety and Applied Nutrition **888-723-3366**
Information on food safety, seafood, dietary supplements, women's nutrition, and cosmetics.

Consumer Information Service, Center for Devices and Radiological Health **301-443-4190**
Information on medical devices, mammography facilities, and radiation-emitting products.

Key to Controlled Substances Categories

Products listed with the symbols shown below are subject to the Controlled Substances Act of 1970. These drugs are categorized according to their potential for abuse. The greater the potential, the more severe the limitations on their prescription.

CATEGORY	INTERPRETATION
C-II	**HIGH POTENTIAL FOR ABUSE.** Use may lead to severe physical or psychological dependence. Prescriptions must be written in ink, or typewritten and signed by the practitioner. Verbal prescriptions must be confirmed in writing within 72 hours, and may be given only in a genuine emergency. No renewals are permitted.
C-III	**SOME POTENTIAL FOR ABUSE.** Use may lead to low-to-moderate physical dependence or high psychological dependence. Prescriptions may be oral or written. Up to five renewals are permitted within six months.
C-IV	**LOW POTENTIAL FOR ABUSE.** Use may lead to limited physical or psychological dependence. Prescriptions may be oral or written. Up to five renewals are permitted within six months.
C-V	**SUBJECT TO STATE AND LOCAL REGULATION.** Abuse potential is low; a prescription may not be required.

Key to FDA Use-in-Pregnancy Ratings

The U.S. Food and Drug Administration's use-in-pregnancy rating system weighs the degree to which available information has ruled out risk to the fetus against the drug's potential benefit to the patient. The ratings, and their interpretation, are as follows:

CATEGORY	INTERPRETATION
A	**CONTROLLED STUDIES SHOW NO RISK.** Adequate, well-controlled studies in pregnant women have failed to demonstrate a risk to the fetus in any trimester of pregnancy.
B	**NO EVIDENCE OF RISK IN HUMANS.** Adequate, well-controlled studies in pregnant women have not shown increased risk of fetal abnormalities despite adverse findings in animals, or, in the absence of adequate human studies, animal studies show no fetal risk. The chance of fetal harm is remote, but remains a possibility.
C	**RISK CANNOT BE RULED OUT.** Adequate, well-controlled human studies are lacking, and animal studies have shown a risk to the fetus or are lacking as well. There is a chance of fetal harm if the drug is administered during pregnancy; but the potential benefits may outweigh the potential risk.
D	**POSITIVE EVIDENCE OF RISK.** Studies in humans, or investigational or post-marketing data, have demonstrated fetal risk. Nevertheless, potential benefits from the use of the drug may outweigh the potential risk. For example, the drug may be acceptable if needed in a life-threatening situation or serious disease for which safer drugs cannot be used or are ineffective.
X	**CONTRAINDICATED IN PREGNANCY.** Studies in animals or humans, or investigational or post-marketing reports, have demonstrated positive evidence of fetal abnormalities or risk which clearly outweighs any possible benefit to the patient.

WEBSITE: www.vaers.org   E-MAIL: info@vaers.org   FAX: 1-877-721-0366

VAERS

VACCINE ADVERSE EVENT REPORTING SYSTEM

24 Hour Toll-Free Information 1-800-822-7967
P.O. Box 1100, Rockville, MD 20849-1100
PATIENT IDENTITY KEPT CONFIDENTIAL

For CDC/FDA Use Only
VAERS Number ______
Date Received ______

Patient Name: ______ Last First M.I.	Vaccine administered by (Name): ______	Form completed by (Name): ______
Address ______	Responsible Physician ______ Facility Name/Address ______	Relation to Patient ☐ Vaccine Provider ☐ Patient/Parent ☐ Manufacturer ☐ Other Address *(if different from patient or provider)* ______
City State Zip Telephone no. (____) ______	City State Zip Telephone no. (____) ______	City State Zip Telephone no. (____) ______

1. State
2. County where administered
3. Date of birth __/__/__ mm dd yy
4. Patient age
5. Sex ☐ M ☐ F
6. Date form completed __/__/__ mm dd yy

7. Describe adverse events(s) (symptoms, signs, time course) and treatment, if any

8. Check all appropriate:
- ☐ Patient died (date __/__/__ mm dd yy)
- ☐ Life threatening illness
- ☐ Required emergency room/doctor visit
- ☐ Required hospitalization (______days)
- ☐ Resulted in prolongation of hospitalization
- ☐ Resulted in permanent disability
- ☐ None of the above

9. Patient recovered ☐ YES ☐ NO ☐ UNKNOWN

10. Date of vaccination __/__/__ mm dd yy Time ______ AM PM

11. Adverse event onset __/__/__ mm dd yy Time ______ AM PM

12. Relevant diagnostic tests/laboratory data

13. Enter all vaccines given on date listed in no. 10

	Vaccine (type)	Manufacturer	Lot number	Route/Site	No. Previous Doses
a.					
b.					
c.					
d.					

14. Any other vaccinations within 4 weeks prior to the date listed in no. 10

	Vaccine (type)	Manufacturer	Lot number	Route/Site	No. Previous doses	Date given
a.						
b.						

15. Vaccinated at:
- ☐ Private doctor's office/hospital
- ☐ Public health clinic/hospital
- ☐ Military clinic/hospital
- ☐ Other/unknown

16. Vaccine purchased with:
- ☐ Private funds
- ☐ Public funds
- ☐ Military funds
- ☐ Other/unknown

17. Other medications

18. Illness at time of vaccination (specify)

19. Pre-existing physician-diagnosed allergies, birth defects, medical conditions (specify)

20. Have you reported this adverse event previously? ☐ No ☐ To doctor ☐ To health department ☐ To manufacturer

21. Adverse event following prior vaccination (check all applicable, specify)

	Adverse Event	Onset Age	Type Vaccine	Dose no. in series
☐ In patient				
☐ In brother or sister				

Only for children 5 and under

22. Birth weight ______ lb. ______ oz.

23. No. of brothers and sisters

Only for reports submitted by manufacturer/immunization project

24. Mfr./imm. proj. report no.

25. Date received by mfr./imm.proj.

26. 15 day report? ☐ Yes ☐ No

27. Report type ☐ Initial ☐ Follow-Up

Health care providers and manufacturers are required by law (42 USC 300aa-25) to report reactions to vaccines listed in the Table of Reportable Events Following Immunization. Reports for reactions to other vaccines are voluntary except when required as a condition of immunization grant awards.

Form VAERS-1(FDA)

VACCINE ADVERSE EVENT REPORTS

DIRECTIONS FOR COMPLETING FORM

(Additional pages may be attached if more space is needed)

GENERAL

Use a separate form for each patient. Complete the form to the best of your abilities. Items 3, 4, 7, 8, 10, 11, and 13 are considered essential and should be completed whenever possible. Parents/Guardians may need to consult the facility where the vaccine was administered for some of the information (such as manufacturer, lot number or laboratory data.)
Refer to the Reportable Events Table (RET) for events mandated for reporting by law. Reporting for other serious events felt to be related but not on the RET is encouraged.
Health care providers other than the vaccine administrator (VA) treating a patient for a suspected adverse event should notify the VA and provide the information about the adverse event to allow the VA to complete the form to meet the VA's legal responsibility.
These data will be used to increase understanding of adverse events following vaccination and will become part of CDC Privacy Act System 09-20-0136, "Epidemiologic Studies and Surveillance of Disease Problems". Information identifying the person who received the vaccine orthat person's legal representativewill not be made available tothe public, but may be available to the vaccinee or legal representative.

SPECIFIC INSTRUCTIONS

Form Completed By: To be used by parents/guardians, vaccine manufacturers/distributors, vaccine administrators, and/or the person completing the form on behalf of the patient or the health professional who administered the vaccine.

Item 7: Describe the suspected adverse event. Such things as temperature, local and general signs and symptoms, time course, duration of symptoms diagnosis, treatment and recovery should be noted.

Item 9: Check "YES" if the patient's health condition is the same as it was prior to the vaccine, "NO" if the patient has not returned to the pre-vaccination state of health, or "UNKNOWN" if the patient's condition is not known.

Item 10: Give dates and times as specifically as you can remember. If you do not know the exact time, please

Item 11: indicate "AM" or "PM" when possible if this information is known. If more than one adverse event, give the onset date and time for the most serious event.

Item 12: Include "negative" or "normal" results of any relevant tests performed as well as abnormal findings.

Item 13: List ONLY those vaccines given on the day listed in Item 10.

Item 14: List any other vaccines that the patient received within 4 weeks prior to the date listed in Item 10.

Item 16: This section refers to how the person who gave the vaccine purchased it, not to the patient's insurance.

Item 17: List any prescription or non-prescription medications the patient was taking when the vaccine(s) was given.

Item 18: List any short term illnesses the patient had on the date the vaccine(s) was given (i.e., cold, flu, ear infection).

Item 19: List any pre-existing physician-diagnosed allergies, birth defects, medical conditions (including developmental and/or neurologic disorders) for the patient.

Item 21: List any suspected adverse events the patient, or the patient's brothers or sisters, may have had to previous vaccinations. If more than one brother or sister, or if the patient has reacted to more than one priorvaccine, use additional pages to explain completely. For the onset age of a patient, provide the age in months if less than two years old.

Item 26: This space is for manufacturers' use only.